This text belongs to Richard Sullivan

cursèd be he who steals this book

D0217921

# THROMBOSIS
# AND
# HEMORRHAGE

*Second Edition*

# THROMBOSIS AND HEMORRHAGE

## Second Edition

### Editors

**JOSEPH LOSCALZO, M.D., Ph.D.**

Wade Professor and Chairman
Department of Medicine
Director, Whitaker Cardiovascular Institute
Boston University School of Medicine
Physician-in-Chief
Boston Medical Center
Boston, Massachusetts

**ANDREW I. SCHAFER, M.D.**

The Bob and Vivian Smith Professor and Chairman
Department of Medicine
Baylor College of Medicine
Chief
Internal Medicine Service
The Methodist Hospital
Houston, Texas

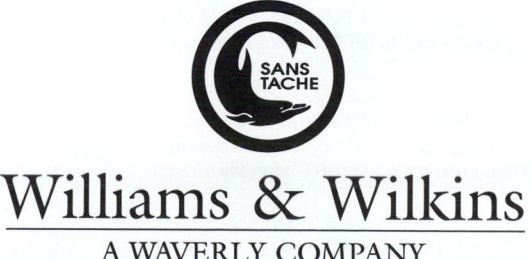

## Williams & Wilkins

### A WAVERLY COMPANY

BALTIMORE • PHILADELPHIA • LONDON • PARIS • BANGKOK
BUENOS AIRES • HONG KONG • MUNICH • SYDNEY • TOKYO • WROCLAW

*Editor:* Jonathan W. Pine, Jr.
*Managing Editor:* Leah Ann Kiehne Hayes
*Marketing Manager:* Daniell T. Griffin
*Production Coordinator:* Danielle Hagan
*Project Editor:* Ulita Lushnycky
*Text/Cover Designer:* Shepherd, Inc.
*Illustration Planner:* Ray Lowman
*Typesetter:* Maryland Composition, Inc.
*Printer/Binder:* RR Donnelley & Sons Company

Copyright © 1998 Williams & Wilkins

351 West Camden Street
Baltimore, Maryland 21201-2436 USA

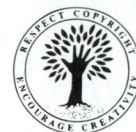

Rose Tree Corporate Center
1400 North Providence Road
Building II, Suite 5025
Media, Pennsylvania 19063-2043 USA

Accurate indications, adverse reactions and dosage schedules for drugs are provided in this book, but it is possible that they may change. The reader is urged to review the package information data of the manufacturers of the medications mentioned.

*Printed in the United States of America*

First Edition, 1994

**Library of Congress Cataloging-in-Publication Data**

Thrombosis and hemorrhage / editors, Joseph Loscalzo, Andrew
  I. Schafer. — 2nd ed.
     p.     cm.
   Includes bibliographical references and index.
   ISBN 0-683-30114-4
    1. Blood—Coagulation—Disorders.   2. Thrombosis.     I. Loscalzo,
Joseph.     II. Schafer, Andrew I.
   [DNLM: 1. Hemorrhagic Diathesis.   2. Thrombosis.   3. Hemostasis.
WH 322 T5312 1998]
RC647.C55T47   1998
616.1'57—dc21
DNLM/DLC
for Library of Congress                                             97-48547
                                                                       CIP

*The publishers have made every effort to trace the copyright holders for borrowed material. If they have inadvertently overlooked any, they will be pleased to make the necessary arrangements at the first opportunity.*

To purchase additional copies of this book, call our customer service department at **(800) 638-0672** or fax orders to **(800) 447-8438.** For other book services, including chapter reprints and large quantity sales, ask for the Special Sales department.

Canadian customers should call **(800) 665-1148,** or fax **(800) 665-0103.** For all other calls originating outside of the United States, please call **(410) 528-4223** or fax us at **(410) 528-8550.**

**Visit Williams & Wilkins on the Internet:** **http://www.wwilkins.com** or contact our customer service department at **custserv©wwilkins.com.** Williams & Wilkins customer service representatives are available from 8:30 am to 6:00 pm, EST, Monday through Friday, for telephone access.

                                98  99  00  01  02
                  1   2   3   4   5   6   7   8   9   10

*To our wives, Anita and Pauline,*
*and to our children, Julia and Alex Loscalzo,*
*and Kate, Pamela, and Eric Schafer*

# PREFACE

Exquisitely regulated hemostatic mechanisms have evolved within the animal kingdom to protect against the ever-present danger of fatal hemorrhage. Platelets and clotting factors interact to generate the protective hemostatic plug, which staunches the flow of blood at sites of vascular injury. The fibrinolytic system has evolved to recanalize occluded vessels as healing occurs to restore perfusion through an injured vessel in which a protective clot has formed. In conjunction with physiologic antithrombotic systems, the fibrinolytic system is also responsible for the maintenance of blood fluidity under normal conditions.

Despite the many fail-safe mechanisms designed to regulate hemostasis (or, perhaps, because of them), a variety of disorders exist that are associated either with an hemorrhagic or a prothrombotic diathesis; in some cases, both abnormalities are present as part of a complex set of pathophysiologic responses (such as disseminated intravascular coagulopathy). These disorders have served as the basis for the development of the clinical hematologic field of coagulation.

In this book, we have endeavored to provide a comprehensive and systematic review of the biology, pathobiology, and clinical disorders of the hemostatic system. The first three parts of the book review the basic elements of hemostasis and include chapters on the fundamental determinants of fibrin formation and stabilization, the normal function and response of platelets, and the components of the vessel wall that interact with and regulate hemostatic responses. The specific clinical disorders are then introduced by chapters in which the clinical and laboratory approaches to the diagnosis of bleeding and thrombosis are outlined. This is followed by a detailed review of specific bleeding disorders, which includes abnormalities of platelets, coagulation factors, and fibrinolysis; specific thrombotic disorders; and complex hemostatic abnormalities. The last two parts of the book present practical information on the management of patients with hemorrhagic and thrombotic disorders. New chapters in this edition of the book include a discussion of the genetics of coagulation proteins, genetic models of hemostatic disorders, maternal hemostasis, and gene therapy of thrombotic and hemorrhagic disorders.

We believe that a book of this nature will provide information that is timely, comprehensive, and logically organized in the rapidly expanding and increasingly complex field of hemostasis. The text should prove useful both to basic investigators in the fields of coagulation and vascular biology as well as to clinicians who manage patients with hemorrhagic and thrombotic disorders. In contemporary medicine, a variety of subspecialists are increasingly confronted with a need to understand the hemostatic system. Not only do the subspecialists include hematologist-"clotters," but they also include cardiologists, neurologists, transplant surgeons, cardiothoracic and general surgeons, clinical pathologists, blood bankers, and vascular medicine specialists. We hope that this text will meet the needs of these diverse investigators and clinicians and provide the basis for a continuing appreciation of the magnificent complexities inherent in this rapidly growing field of medicine.

J.L.
A.I.S.

# ACKNOWLEDGMENT

We wish to express our heartfelt thanks to Ms. Stephanie Tribuna, Ms. Denise Lewis, Ms. Suzanne Clive, Dr. Germaine Welch, Ms. Emily Zermeño, and Ms. Patty Ryan for their assistance throughout the many phases of the development of this text. We would also like to express our gratitude to Ms. Leah Hayes of Williams & Wilkins for her expert editorial assistance. Without their help, the final product would not have been possible. We also wish to thank Ms. Anita B. Loscalzo for her assistance in the preparation of reference citations.

# CONTRIBUTORS

**M. Nadir Ali, M.D.**
Assistant Professor of Medicine
Division of Cardiology
Baylor College of Medicine
Director, Cardiac Catheterization Laboratory
Veterans Affairs Medical Center
Houston, Texas

**Barbara Rita Alevriadou, Ph.D.**
Assistant Professor of Biomedical Engineering
Johns Hopkins University School of Medicine
Baltimore, Maryland

**Barbara M. Alving, M.D.**
Professor of Medicine
The Uniformed Services University
    of the Health Sciences
Bethesda, Maryland
Director, Hematology and Medical Oncology Section
Washington Cancer Institute at the Washington
    Hospital Center
Washington, D.C.

**H. Vernon Anderson, M.D.**
Associate Professor of Medicine
Division of Cardiology
University of Texas Health Science Center at Houston
Houston, Texas

**Maureen Andrew, Ph.D.**
Professor of Pediatrics and Pathology
Hamilton Civic Hospitals Research Centre
Hamilton, Ontario, Canada

**Robert K. Andrews, M.D.**
Senior Research Officer
Hazel and Pip Appel Vascular Biology Laboratory
Baker Medical Research Institute
Prahran, Australia

**Richard H. Aster, M.D.**
Clinical Professor of Medicine and Pathology
Medical College of Wisconsin
Senior Investigator
Blood Research Institute
Blood Center of Southeastern Wisconsin
Milwaukee, Wisconsin

**Kenneth A. Ault, M.D.**
Associate Professor of Medicine
Research Director
Maine Medical Center Research Institute
Maine Medical Center
Portland, Maine

**Tiziano Barbui, Ph.D.**
Professor of Hematology
Ospedali Riuniti
Bergamo, Italy

**Carl Barsigian, M.D., Ph.D.**
Resident in Internal Medicine
Cardeza Foundation for Hematologic Research
Jefferson Medical College of Thomas Jefferson
    University
Philadelphia, Pennsylvania

**Kenneth A. Bauer, M.D.**
Associate Professor in Medicine
Harvard Medical School
Beth Israel Deaconess Medical Center
Boston, Massachusetts
Chief, Section of Hematology and Oncology
Brockton-West Roxbury Department of Veterans
    Affairs Medical Center
West Roxbury, Massachusetts

**Joshua A. Beckman, M.D.**
Fellow in Cardiovascular Medicine
Brigham and Women's Hospital
Boston, Massachusetts

**Michael C. Berndt, Ph.D.**
Associate Director, Department of Vascular Biology
Baker Medical Research Institute
Melbourne, Australia

**M. Daniel Bingham, M.D.**
Fellow in Hematology and Oncology
University of North Carolina, Chapel Hill
Chapel Hill, North Carolina

**Paula L. Bockenstedt, M.D.**
Assistant Professor of Internal Medicine
Director, Adult Coagulation Disorder Program
Division of Hematology and Oncology
University of Michigan Medical Center
Ann Arbor, Michigan

**D. Ware Branch, M.D.**
Professor of Maternal and Fetal Medicine
Department of Obstetrics and Gynecology
University of Utah School of Medicine
Salt Lake City, Utah

**George J. Broze, Jr., M.D.**
Professor of Medicine, Cell Biology, and Physiology
Division of Hematology
Washington University Medical Center
St. Louis, Missouri

**Carlo Brugnara, M.D.**
Associate Professor of Laboratory Medicine
  and Pathology
Harvard Medical School
The Children's Hospital
Department of Medicine
Brigham and Women's Hospital
Boston, Massachusetts

**Peter Carmeliet, M.D., Ph.D.**
Associate Professor and Adjunct Director
Center for Transgene Technology and Gene Therapy
Flanders Interuniversity Institute for Biotechnology
Campus Gasthuisberg
Leuven, Belgium

**W. Hallowell Churchill, M.D.**
Associate Professor of Medicine
Division of Hematology and Oncology
Harvard Medical School
Brigham and Women's Hospital
Departments of Pathology and Laboratory Medicine
The Children's Hospital
Boston, Massachusetts

**Douglas B. Cines, M.D.**
Professor of Pathology and Laboratory Medicine and
  Medicine
Director, Hematology and Coagulation Laboratories
University of Pennsylvania School of Medicine
Hospital of the University Pennsylvania
Philadelphia, Pennsylvania

**Ira S. Cohen, M.D.**
Associate Professor of Medicine
Division of Cardiovascular Disease
Yale University School of Medicine
New Haven, Connecticut
Chief, Non-invasive Cardiology
West Haven Veterans Affairs Medical Center
West Haven, Connecticut

**Richard A. Cohen, M.D.**
Professor of Medicine and Physiology
Vascular Medicine and Biology
Robert Dawson Evans Department of Clinical
  Research
Department of Medicine
Boston University Medical Center
Boston, Massachusetts

**Désiré Collen, M.D., Ph.D.**
Center for Transgene Technology and Gene Therapy
Flanders Interuniversity Institute for Biotechnology
Campus Gasthuisberg
Leuven, Belgium

**Kathleen A. Cooney, M.D.**
Assistant Professor of Internal Medicine and Surgery
University of Michigan School of Medicine
Department of Veterans Affairs Medical Center
Ann Arbor, Michigan

**Mark A. Creager, M.D.**
Associate Professor of Medicine
Harvard Medical School
Director, Vascular Center
Director, Noninvasive Vascular Laboratory
Division of Cardiovascular Medicine
Brigham and Women's Hospital
Boston, Massachusetts

**George L. Dale, Ph.D.**
Associate Professor of Medicine
University of Oklahoma Health Science Center
Oklahoma City, Oklahoma

**Paul J. Declerck, Ph.D.**
Professor
Laboratory of Pharmaceutical Biology
Katholieke Universiteit Leuven
Leuven, Belgium

**Gregory J. del Zoppo, M.D.**
Associate Professor of Molecular
  and Experimental Medicine
The Scripps Research Institute
Division of Hematology and Medical Oncology
Scripps Clinic and Research Foundation
La Jolla, California

**Donna M. DiMichele, M.D.**
Assistant Professor of Pediatrics
Director, Regional Comprehensive Hemophilia
  Diagnostic and Treatment Center
The New York Hospital—Cornell Medical Center
New York, New York

**David R. Dobroski, M.D.**
Fellow in Cardiology
Department of Medicine
Boston University School of Medicine
Boston, Massachusetts

**Lindsay C. Dunlop, M.D., Ph.D., F.R.A.C.P.,
F.R.C.P.A.**
Conjoint Senior Lecturer in Pathology and Medicine
University of New South Wales
Consultant Haematologist
Department of Haematology
Liverpool Hospital
Liverpool, New South Wales, Australia

**Mary E. Eberst, M.D.**
Assistant Professor of Emergency Medicine
  and Medicine
University of North Carolina at Chapel Hill
Chapel Hill, North Carolina

**Michael D. Ezekowitz, M.D., Ph.D.**
Professor of Medicine
Department of Cardiology
Yale University School of Medicine
New Haven, Connecticut

**Jawed Fareed, Ph.D.**
Professor of Pathology and Pharmacology
Director, Hemostasis Research Laboratories
Loyola University Medical Center
Maywood, Illinois

**Guido Finazzi, M.D.**
Senior Consultant in Hematology
Ospedali Riuniti
Bergamo, Italy

**Charles W. Francis, M.D.**
Professor of Medicine and Pathology
  and Laboratory Medicine
Acting Chief, Vascular Medicine Unit
University of Rochester School of Medicine
  and Dentistry
Rochester, New York

**Jane E. Freedman, M.D.**
Assistant Professor of Medicine
Divisions of Clinical Pharmacology and Cardiology
Georgetown University School of Medicine
Washington, DC

**Gary H. Gibbons, M.D.**
Department of Medicine
Brigham and Women's Hospital
Boston, Massachusetts

**David Ginsburg, M.D.**
Professor of Internal Medicine and Human Genetics
Investigator, Howard Hughes Medical Institute
University of Michigan Medical School
Ann Arbor, Michigan

**Noyan Gokce, M.D.**
Fellow in Cardiology
Department of Medicine
Boston University School of Medicine
Boston, Massachusetts

**Herman K. Gold, M.D.**
Associate Professor of Medicine
Harvard Medical School
Massachusetts General Hospital
Boston, Massachusetts

**Charles S. Gornick, M.D.**
Associate Professor of Medicine
Director, Cardiac Arrhythmia Unit
University of Minnesota Medical School
Veterans Affairs Medical Center
Minneapolis, Minnesota

**David Green, M.D., Ph.D.**
Professor of Medicine
Director, Hemophilia Program
Northwestern University Medical School
Chicago, Illinois

**Charles S. Greenberg, M.D.**
Associate Professor of Medicine and Pathology
Division of Hematology
Duke University Medical Center
Durham, North Carolina

**Jerome E. Groopman, M.D.**
Professor of Medicine
Chief, Division of Experimental Medicine
Harvard Medical School
Beth Israel Deaconess Medical Center
Boston, Massachusetts

**John H. Hartwig, Ph.D.**
Associate Professor of Medicine
Experimental Medical Division
Brigham and Women's Hospital
Boston, Massachusetts

**Joann M. Hettasch, Ph.D.**
Research Associate in Medicine
Division of Hematology
Duke University Medical Center
Durham, North Carolina

**Katherine A. High, M.D.**
William H. Bennett Associate Professor of Pediatrics
    and Pathology
Research Director, Hematology Division
University of Pennsylvania School of Medicine
Director, Hematology and Coagulation Laboratories
The Children's Hospital of Philadelphia
Philadelphia, Pennsylvania

**Paul Imbach, M.D.**
Professor of Pediatrics
Division of Hematology and Oncology
University Children's Hospital
Basel, Switzerland

**Nancy Swords Jenny, Ph.D.**
Postdoctoral Associate
Department of Biochemistry
University of Vermont College of Medicine
Burlington, Vermont

**Walter Jeske, Ph.D.**
Research Fellow in Pathology
Cardiovascular Institute
Loyola University Medical Center
Maywood, Illinois

**Kenneth Kaushansky, M.D.**
Professor of Medicine
Division of Hematology
University of Washington
Seattle, Washington

**John F. Keaney, Jr., M.D.**
Assistant Professor of Medicine
Boston University School of Medicine
Boston, Massachusetts

**Shukri F. Khuri, M.D.**
Professor of Surgery
Harvard Medical School
Boston, Massachusetts
Chief, Surgical Service
Brockton and West Roxbury Veterans Affairs
    Medical Center
West Roxbury, Massachusetts

**Michael H. Kroll, M.D.**
Associate Professor of Medicine
Section of Hematology and Oncology
Baylor College of Medicine
Veterans Administration Medical Center
Houston, Texas

**David A. Lane, M.D.**
Professor of Molecular Haematology
Imperial College School of Medicine
Charing Cross and Westminister Hospital
University of London
Hammersmith, London, United Kingdom

**Peter J. Larson, M.D.**
Associate Professor of Pediatrics
Department of Pediatrics
University of Pennsylvania School of Medicine
The Children's Hospital of Philadelphia
Philadelphia, Pennsylvania

**Charles A. Lawson, M.D.**
Assistant Professor of Anesthesiology
Columbia University College of Physicians
    and Surgeons
New York, New York

**Jane A. Leopold, M.D.**
Fellow in Interventional Cardiology
Department of Medicine
Boston University School of Medicine
Boston, Massachusetts

**James D. Levine, M.D.**
Assistant Professor of Medicine
Beth Israel Deaconess Medical Center
Harvard Medical School
Boston, Massachusetts

**Glenn N. Levine, M.D.**
Assistant Professor of Medicine
Division of Cardiology
Baylor College of Medicine
Co-Director, Cardiac Catheterization Laboratory
Houston Veterans Affairs Medical Center
Houston, Texas

**Moise L. Levy, M.D.**
Associate Professor of Dermatology and Pediatrics
Baylor College of Medicine
Chief, Dermatology Service
Texas Children's Hospital
Houston, Texas

**José A. López, M.D.**
Associate Professor
Departments of Internal Medicine
    and Molecular and Human Genetics
Baylor College of Medicine
Houston, Texas

**Joseph Loscalzo, M.D., Ph.D.**
Wade Professor and Chairman
Department of Medicine
Director, Whitaker Cardiovascular Institute
Boston University School of Medicine
Physician-in-Chief
Boston Medical Center
Boston, Massachusetts

**Savvas C. Makrides, Ph.D.**
Director, Cell Biology
Praecis Pharmaceuticals, Inc.
Cambridge, Massachusetts

**Kenneth G. Mann, Ph.D.**
Professor and Chairman
Department of Biochemistry
University of Vermont College of Medicine
Burlington, Vermont

**Pier Mannuccio Mannucci, M.D.**
Professor of Medicine
Angelo Bianchi Bonomi Hemophilia
    and Thrombosis Center
Institute of Internal Medicine
IRCCS Maggiore Hospital
University of Milan
Milan, Italy

**Jose Martinez, M.D.**
Professor of Medicine
Associate Director
Cardeza Foundation for Hematologic Research
Jefferson Medical College of Thomas Jefferson
    University
Philadelphia, Pennsylvania

**Philip L. McCarthy, Jr., M.D.**
Assistant Professor of Medicine
Section of Malignant Hematology and Bone Marrow
    Transplantation
Roswell Park Cancer Institute
Buffalo, New York

**Keith R. McCrae, M.D.**
Associate Professor of Medicine
Section of Hematology
Sol Sherry Thrombosis Research Center
Temple University School of Medicine
Philadelphia, Pennsylvania

**Rodger P. McEver, M.D.**
Professor of Medicine and Biochemistry
    and Molecular Biology
University of Oklahoma Health Sciences Center
Investigator, W.P. Warren Medical Research Institute
Cardiovascular Biology Research Program
Oklahoma Medical Research Foundation
Oklahoma City, Oklahoma

**Janice G. McFarland, M.D.**
Clinical Associate Professor of Medicine
Medical College of Wisconsin
Vice President of Medical Affairs
Director, Platelet Antibody Laboratory
The Blood Center of Southwestern Wisconsin
Milwaukee, Wisconsin

**Larry Vern McIntire, Ph.D.**
E.D. Butcher Professor and Chair
Institute of Biosciences and Bioengineering
Rice University
Houston, Texas

**Robert McMillan, M.D.**
Division of Hematology and Oncology
The Scripps Research Institute
La Jolla, California

**Harry L. Messmore, Jr., M.D.**
Attending Physician
Departments of Medicine and Pathology
Hines Veterans Administration Hospital
Maywood, Illinois

**Alan D. Michelson, M.D.**
Professor of Pediatrics and Pathology
Director, Center for Platelet Function Studies
University of Massachusetts Medical Center
Worcester, Massachusetts

**Lindsey A. Miles, Ph.D.**
Associate Professor of Vascular Biology
The Scripps Research Institute
La Jolla, California

**Joel L. Moake, M.D.**
Professor of Medicine
Baylor College of Medicine
Associate Director, Biomedical Engineering
    Laboratory
Rice University
Houston, Texas

**Scott Murphy, M.D.**
Professor of Medicine
Jefferson Medical College
Thomas Jefferson University
Chief Medical Officer
American Red Cross Blood Services
Penn-Jersey Region
Philadelphia, Pennsylvania

**Elizabeth G. Nabel, M.D.**
Professor of Internal Medicine and Physiology
Chief, Division of Cardiology
Cardiovascular Research Center
University of Michigan Medical Center
Ann Arbor, Michigan

**Peter J. Newman, Ph.D.**
Senior Investigator
Blood Research Institute
The Blood Center of Southeastern Wisconsin
Milwaukee, Wisconsin

**William C. Nichols, Ph.D.**
Research Investigator
Department of Internal Medicine
University of Michigan Medical School
Ann Arbor, Michigan

**Bryan T. Oshiro, M.D.**
Assistant Professor of Obstetrics and Gynecology
University of Utah School of Medicine
Salt Lake City, Utah
Director of Perinatology
McKay-Dee Hospital
Ogden, Utah

**Carlo Patrono, M.D.**
Professor of Pharmacology
Cattedra di Farmacologia I
Universita' degli Studi ''G. D'Annunzio''
Chieti, Italy

**Ellinor I. B. Peerschke, Ph.D.**
Professor of Pathology
Cornell Medical College
Director, Laboratories for Clinical Hematology
The New York Hospital
New York, New York

**Martin D. Phillips, M.D.**
Director, Medical Affairs
Centeon
King of Prussia, Pennsylvania

**David J. Pinsky, M.D.**
Assistant Professor of Medicine
Columbia University College of Physicians
   and Surgeons
New York, New York

**Edward F. Plow, Ph.D.**
Head of Research
Joseph J. Jacobs Center for Thrombosis
   and Vascular Biology
Chairman, Department of Molecular Cardiology
Cleveland Clinic Foundation
Cleveland, Ohio

**LeRoy E. Rabbani, M.D.**
Assistant Professor of Medicine
Columbia University College of Physicians
   and Surgeons
Assistant Attending Physician
Columbia-Presbyterian Medical Center
New York, New York

**Harold R. Roberts, M.D.**
Sarah Graham Keasan Professor of Medicine
University of North Carolina
Division of Hematology and Oncology
University of North Carolina Hospitals
Chapel Hill, North Carolina

**Michael J. Rohrer, M.D.**
Associate Professor of Surgery
Division of Vascular Surgery
University of Massachusetts Medical School
Worcester, Massachusetts

**Julia Myers Ross, Ph.D.**
Assistant Professor of Chemical and Biochemical
   Engineering
University of Maryland
Baltimore, Maryland

**Zaverio M. Ruggeri, M.D.**
Professor of Molecular and Experimental Medicine
   and Vascular Biology
Division of Experimental Thrombosis and Hemostasis
Roon Research Laboratory for Arteriosclerosis
   and Thrombosis
The Scripps Research Institute
La Jolla, California

**Una S. Ryan, Ph.D.**
President, Chief Executive Officer, and Chief Scientific
   Officer
T Cell Sciences, Inc.
Needham, Massachusetts

**Andrew I. Schafer, M.D.**
The Bob and Vivian Smith Professor and Chairman
Department of Medicine
Baylor College of Medicine
Chief
Internal Medicine Service
The Methodist Hospital
Houston, TX

**Jonathan S. Scharfstein, M.D.**
Assistant Professor of Medicine
Division of Cardiology
Case Western Reserve School of Medicine
Cleveland, Ohio

**Alvin H. Schmaier, M.D.**
Professor of Internal Medicine and Pathology
Division of Hematology and Oncology
University of Michigan
Ann Arbor, Michigan

**Ann Marie Schmidt, M.D.**
Assistant Professor of Medicine
Columbia University College of Physicians
    and Surgeons
New York, New York

**Rachel E. Simmonds**
Candidate for Doctoral Degree
Department of Haematology
Imperial College School of Medicine
Charing Cross Hospital
Hammersmith, London, United Kingdom

**Brian Richard Smith, M.D.**
Professor of Medicine, Laboratory Medicine
    and Pediatrics
Yale University School of Medicine
New Haven, Connecticut

**Bernardo Stein, M.D.**
Clearwater Cardiovascular Consultants, M.D., P.A.
Clearwater, Florida

**David M. Stern, M.D.**
Professor of Physiology and Cellular Biophysics
    in Surgery
Columbia University College of Physicians
    and Surgeons
New York, New York

**Richard Sullivan, M.D.**
Associate Professor of Medicine, Molecular
    Physiology, and Biophysics
Baylor College of Medicine
Veterans Affairs Medical Center
Houston, Texas

**Tatiana Ugarova, Ph.D.**
Project Scientist
Department of Molecular Cardiology
Cleveland Clinic Foundation
Cleveland, Ohio

**C. Robert Valeri, M.D., F.A.C.P.**
Professor of Medicine and Research Professor
    of Surgery
Director, Naval Blood Research Laboratory
Boston University School of Medicine
Boston, Massachusetts

**Douglas E. Vaughan, M.D.**
Professor of Medicine and Pharmacology
Vanderbilt University Medical Center
Nashville Veterans Affairs Medical Center
Nashville, Tennessee

**Joseph A. Vita, M.D.**
Associate Professor of Medicine
Whitaker Cardiovascular Institute
Boston University School of Medicine
Boston, Massachusetts

**Jerry Ware, Ph.D.**
Associate Professor of Molecular
    and Experimental Medicine
The Scripps Research Institute
La Jolla, California

**James T. Willerson, M.D.**
Edward Randall III Professor and Chairman
Department of Internal Medicine
University of Texas-Houston Medical School
Hermann Hospital
Medical Director and Chief of Cardiology
Texas Heart Institute
St. Johns Episcopal Hospital
Houston, Texas

**Eliot Williams, M.D., Ph.D.**
Associate Professor of Medicine
Section of Hematology
University of Wisconsin
Madison, Wisconsin

# CONTENTS

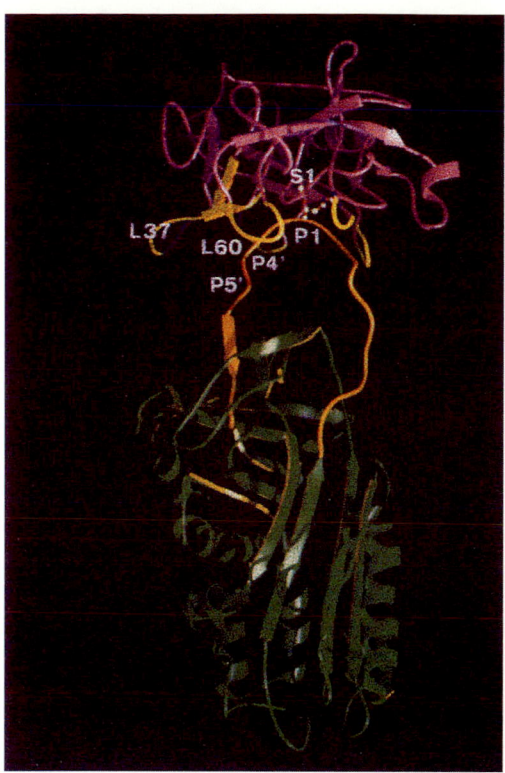

**FIGURE 7.5.** Model depicting proposed structure of active PAI-1 in contact with a molecule of low molecular weight urokinase.

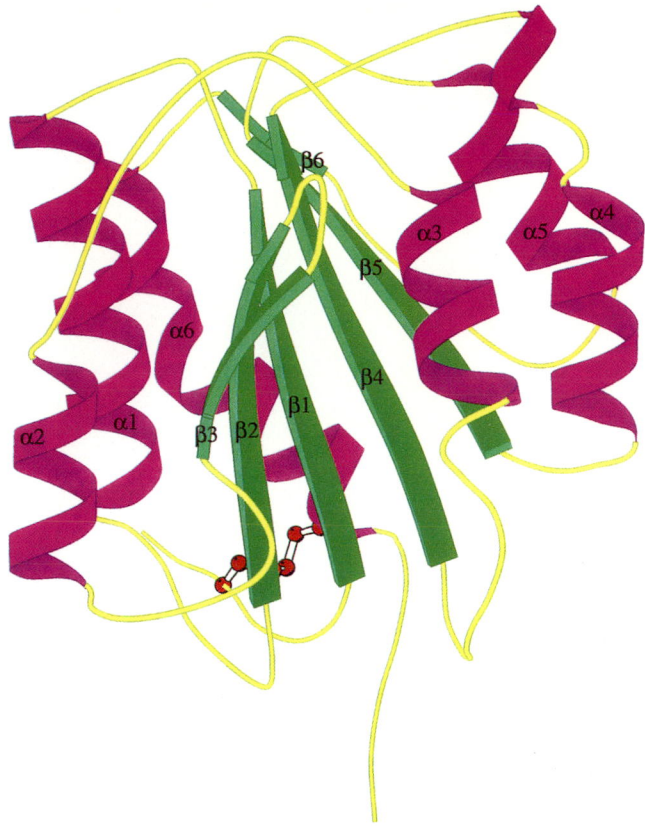

**FIGURE 16.13.** Ribbon representation of the three-dimensional structure of the von Willebrand factor (vWf) A1 domain. α-Helices are shown in purple, β-strands in green, and loops in yellow. The side chains of Cys[509] and Cys[695], linked in an intrachain disulfide bond, appear in dark red near the bottom of the molecule. (This figure was prepared with the help of Reha Celikel and Kottayil I. Varughese.)

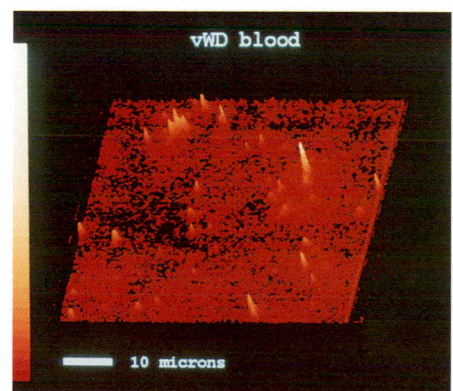
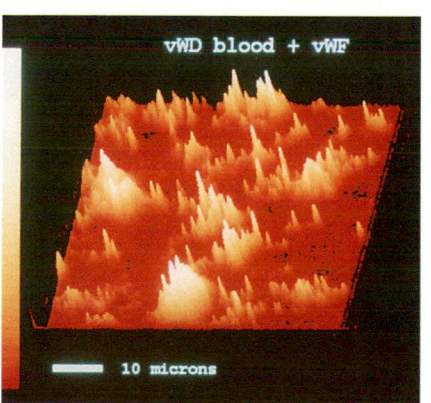

A                                                                      B

**FIGURE 20.6.** Three-dimensional reconstructions of platelets deposited from flowing whole blood onto collagen type I-coated surfaces. Citrated whole blood from a patient with severe von Willebrand disease was incubated for 5 minutes (**A**) in the absence and (**B**) in the presence of von Willebrand factor and perfused at 37°C for 1 minute at a wall shear rate of 1500/s (approximately 57 dyn/cm²). Digital analysis was performed on video images taken at 0.38 mm downstream from the beginning of the collagen coating at the end of the 1 minute perfusion. Blood flow was from left to right and magnification ×290.

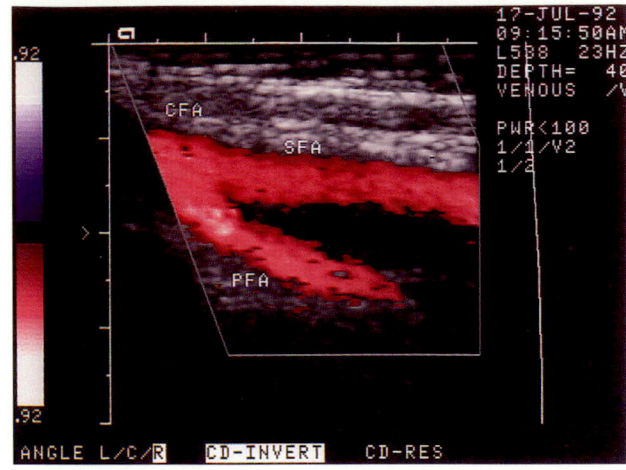
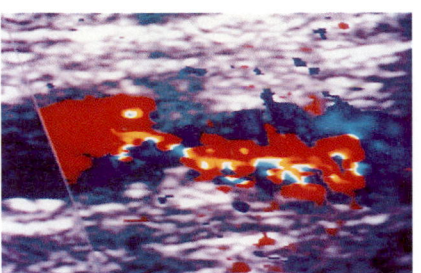

**FIGURE 25.6.** **A.,** Color-assisted duplex ultrasound examination of a normal common femoral artery bifurcation. The consistency of color and hue reflect the laminar flow through a normal artery. **B.,** Color-assisted duplex ultrasound examination of a common femoral artery stenosis. Color desaturation reflects accelerated flow through a stenosis. The multiple colors are indicative of the turbulence at the site of the stenosis.

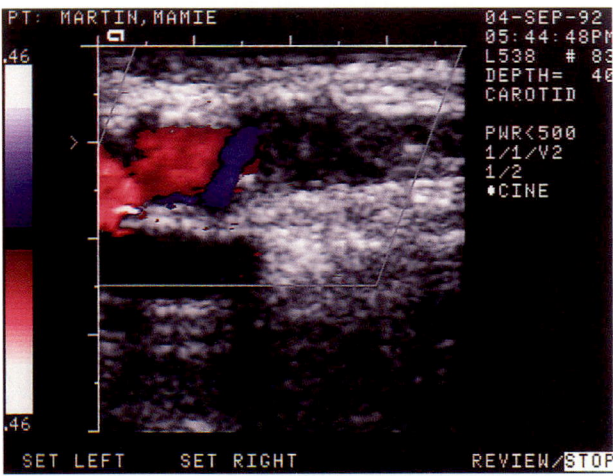

**FIGURE 25.7.** Acute arterial occlusion detected by color Doppler. The color display within the artery is abruptly terminated by thrombotic occlusion.

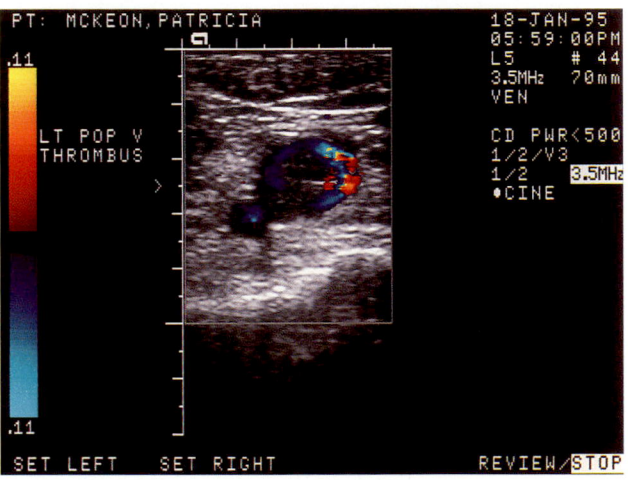

**FIGURE 25.18.** Transverse color Doppler display of partially obstructing venous thrombus within the common femoral vein (CFV). Note that blood cells, depicted by color Doppler (*blue*), course around an intraluminal filling defect. The contiguous common femoral artery (CFA) is also detected by color Doppler (*red*).

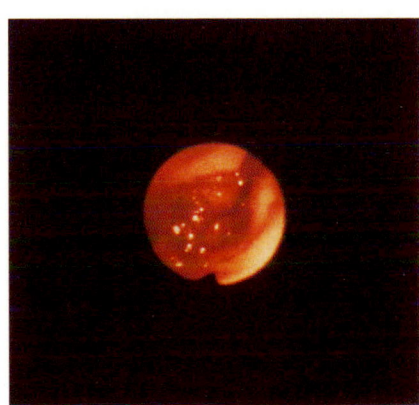

**FIGURE 25.13.** Demonstration of a femoral artery thrombus by intravascular angioscopy. (Courtesy of Dr. George Abela and reproduced with permission [Seeger JM, Abela GS. J Vasc Surg 1986;4:315–320]).

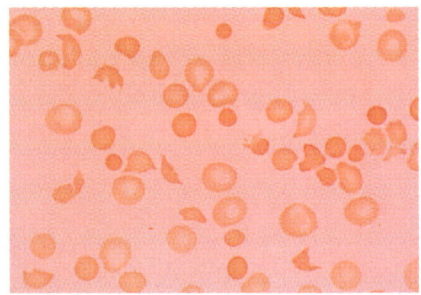

**FIGURE 27.1.** Peripheral blood smear from a patient with an acute episode of thrombotic thrombocytopenic purpura. Schistocytes of different forms, as well as spherocytes and microspherocytes, are present.

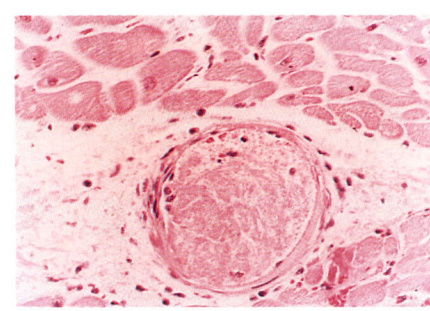
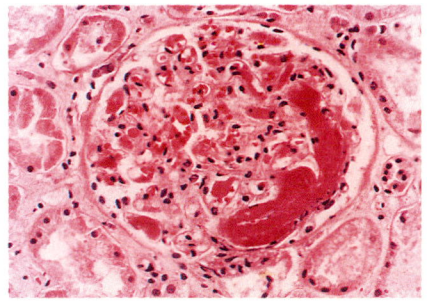

A                                                                                        B

**FIGURE 27.3.**    **A.,** Myocardial arteriole containing one hyaline thrombus, composed predominantly of platelets and platelet-derived material, from a patient who died during an episode of thrombotic thrombocytopenic pupura. **B.,** Glomerular arterioles with clots composed predominantly of fibrin and red cells from a patient who died with disseminated intravascular coagulation. (Courtesy of Dr. A. Saleem.)

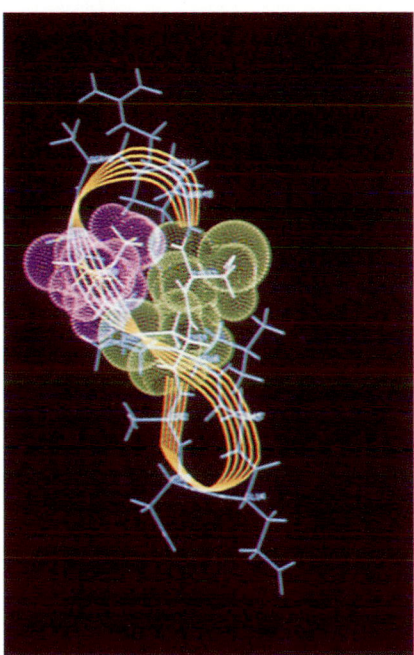
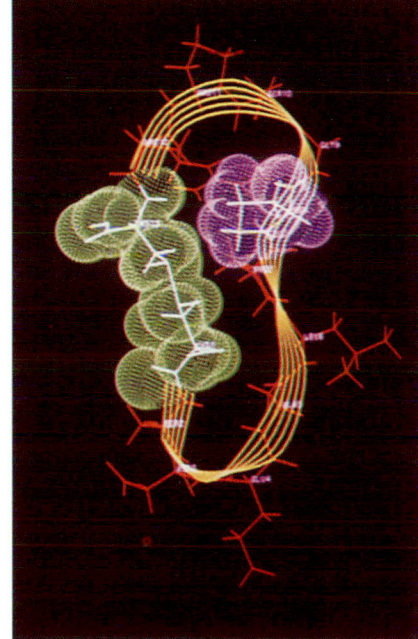

**FIGURE 28.2.**    Three-dimensional conformation of GP IIIa residues 26–38. Molecular modeling of the loop formed by $Cys_{26}$-$Cys_{38}$ (green space–filling amino acids), performed on an Evans and Sutherland minicomputer using Sybyl energy minimalization software, shows that simple substitution of a proline for a leucine at residue 33 (purple) imparts significant local conformational changes in this region. The loop on the left represents the $Leu_{33}$ allele, while the loop on the right represents the $Pro_{33}$ form. Note that the single amino acid substitution causes this small loop to shift from a "Figure 8" shape to that of an oblong circle. This difference in conformation is likely responsible for eliciting the alloimmune response in both PTP and NATP. (Figure provided by Drs. Jack Gorski and Peter J. Newman, Blood Research Institute, The Blood Center of Southeastern Wisconsin.)

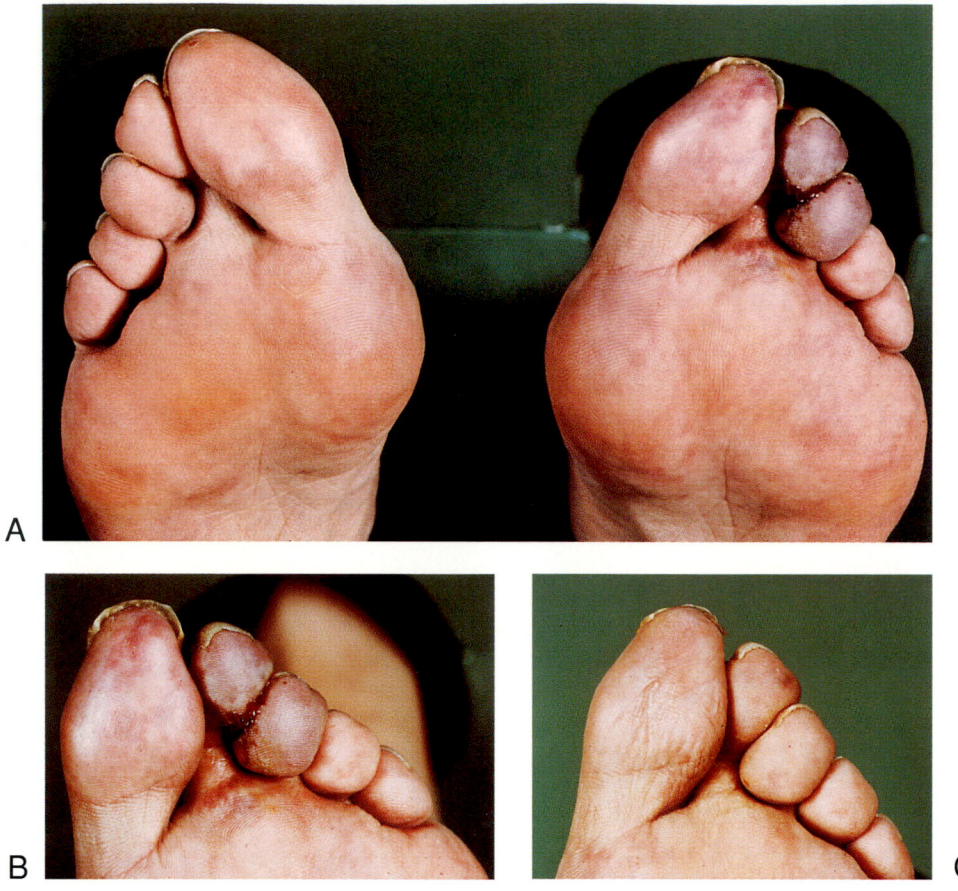

**FIGURE 31.2.** **A.,** Severe and disabling burning pain, warmth and red congestion of the sole of the forefoot and big toe, and bluish discoloration of very painful $2^{nd}$ and $3^{rd}$ toes of the left foot in a patient with essential thrombocythemia (platelet count $767 \times 10^9/L$). **B** and **C.,** Details of the involved big, $2^{nd}$, and $3^{rd}$ toes with erythromelalgia, which completely disappeared after treatment with low-dose aspirin. (Courtesy of Dr. J.J. Michiels.)

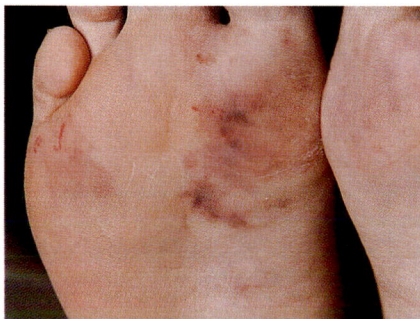

**FIGURE 31.3.** Erythromelalgia in its most typical appearance with severe burning and aching pain, congestion, and mottled red-blue discoloration of the sole of the right forefoot in a patient with essential thrombocythemia (platelet count $576 \times 10^9/L$). (Courtesy of Dr. J.J. Michiels.)

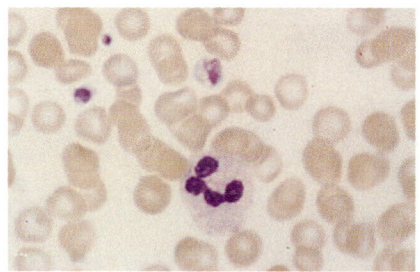

**FIGURE 32.1.** Wright-stained peripheral blood smear from a patient with Bernard-Soulier syndrome showing large platelets.

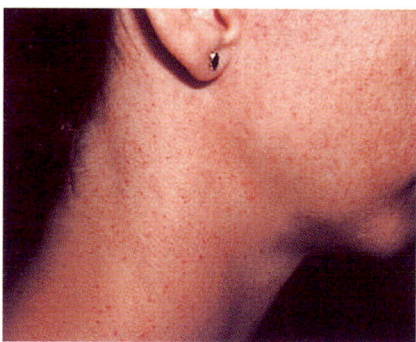

**FIGURE 43.1.**    Mechanical petechiae caused by vomiting.

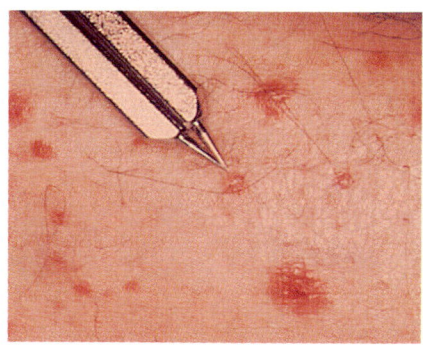

**FIGURE    43.5.**    Perifollicular hemorrhage and corkscrew hairs (tip of pointer) in scurvy. (Courtesy of Dr. Andrew I. Schafer.)

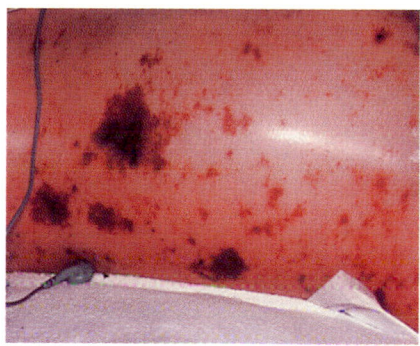

**FIGURE 43.2.**    Purpura in a patient with meningiococcemia.

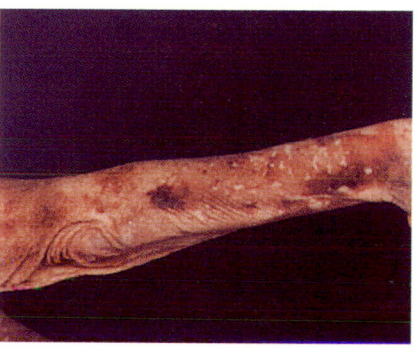

**FIGURE 43.6.**    Ecchymoses on the arm of a patient with Cushing's disease. (Courtesy of Dr. Robert F. Gagel.)

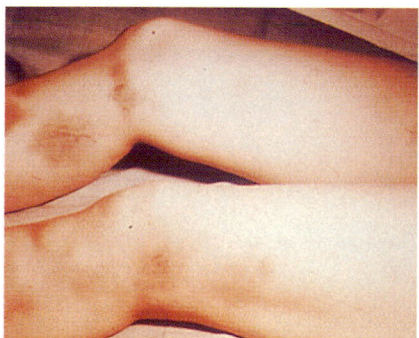

**FIGURE 43.3.**    Self-inflicted ecchymoses (i.e., bruises) on a patient's lower extremities. (Courtesy of Dr. Andrew I. Schafer.)

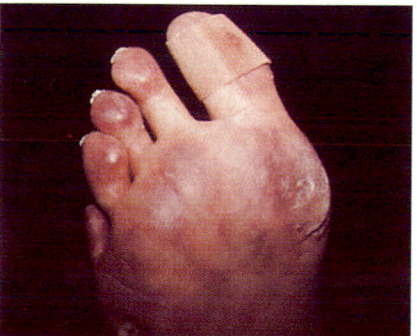

**Figure 43.7.**    Ecchymoses on the third and fourth toes and livedo reticularis on the sole of the foot of a patient with cholesterol emboli.

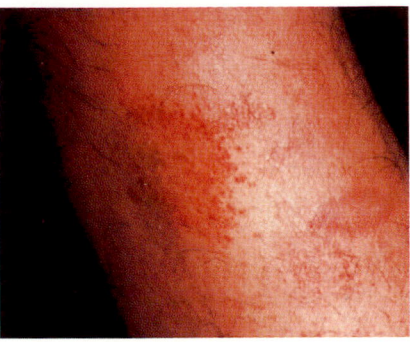

**FIGURE 43.8.**    Pigmented purpura on the distal lower extremity.

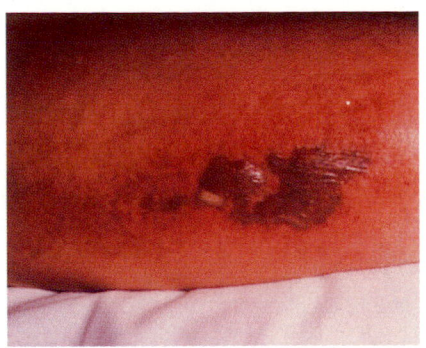

**FIGURE 43.9.**    Warfarin-induced skin necrosis on the distal lower extremity.

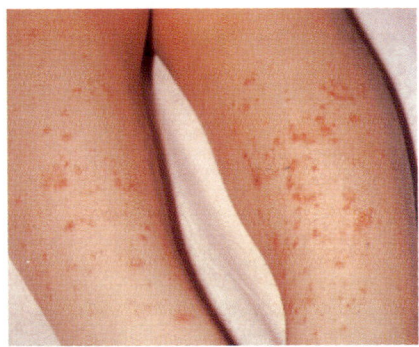

**FIGURE 43.10.**    Palpable purpura of Henoch-Schoenlein purpura on the legs of a child.

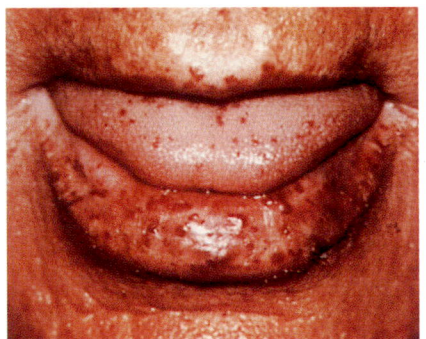

**FIGURE 43.11.**    Telangiectasia on the lips and face of a patient with hereditary hemorrhagic telangiectasia. (Courtesy of Dr. Andrew I. Schafer.)

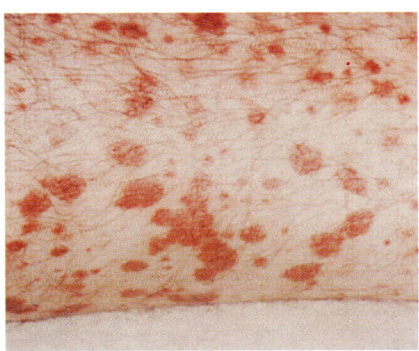

**FIGURE 43.12.**    Classic Kaposi's sarcoma on the lower extremity of an elderly man.

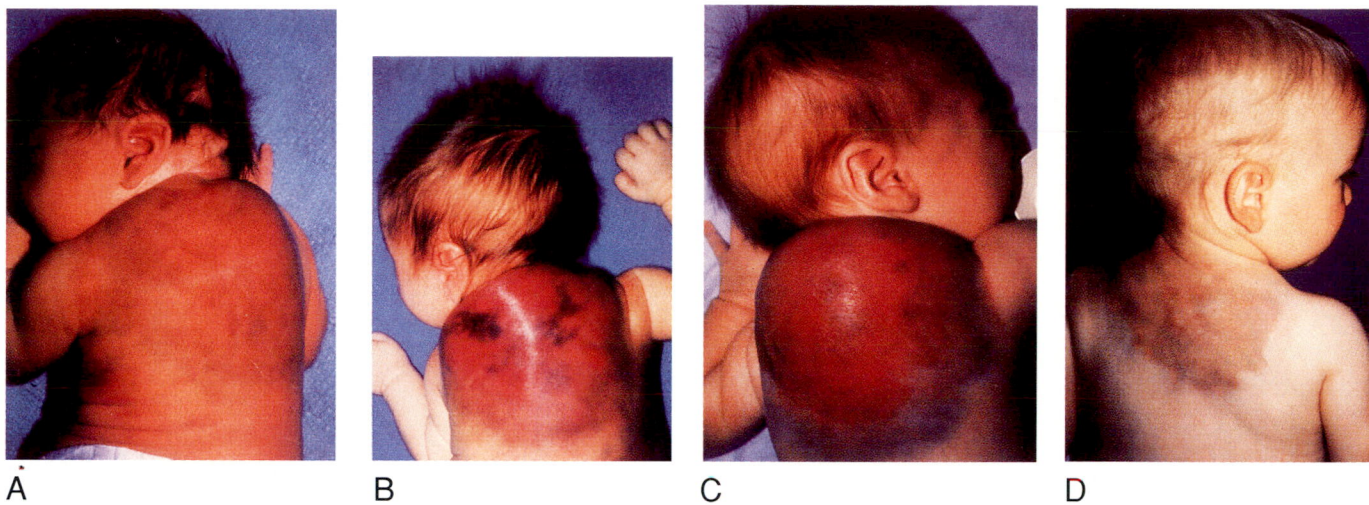

A          B          C          D

**FIGURE 44.5.** Kasabach-Merritt syndrome. Hemangioma of the posterior thorax at birth **(A);** at 2 weeks of age, showing rapid enlargement associated with DIC **(B);** after 1 month of interferon-α treatment, showing early regression **(C);** at 1 year of age, after 11 months of interferon-α treatment, showing nearly complete involution and disappearance of DIC **(D).** (Reprinted with permission from Ezekowitz RA, Mulliken JB, Folkman J. Interferon alfa-2a therapy for life-threatening hemangiomas of infancy. N Engl J Med 1992;326:1456–1463.)

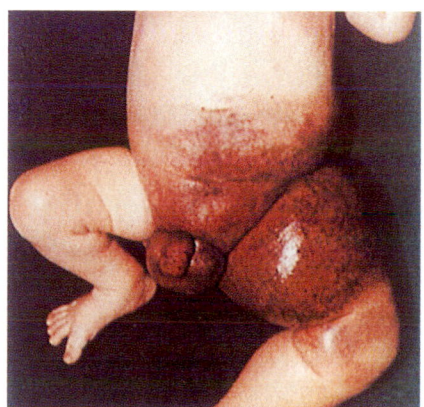

**FIGURE 47.4.** Kasabach-Merritt syndrome. (Reproduced with permission from Simon C, Janner M. Color atlas of pediatric diseases. Toronto: Marcel Dekker, 1987.)

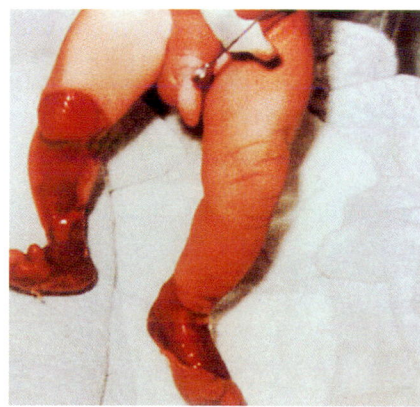

**FIGURE 47.7.** Purpura fulminans. (Reproduced with permission from Weinberg S, Prose NS. Color atlas of dermatology. 2nd ed. New York: McGraw-Hill, 1990.)

# SECTION 1

# COAGULATION AND FIBRINOLYSIS

# CHAPTER 1

# COAGULATION CASCADE: AN OVERVIEW

Nancy Swords Jenny and Kenneth G. Mann

Hemostasis is maintained by the processes involved in blood coagulation and consists of interactions ranging from clot formation to tissue regeneration. In response to vascular damage, clotting reactions are initiated that create an insoluble fibrin/platelet plug, arrest blood loss, and eventually result in the restoration of vascular integrity. These processes occur on a continuous basis and are governed by a series of subprocesses that define the outcome. The subprocesses of a coagulation response include initiation of the event through vascular injury, propagation of the procoagulant response, termination of the response subsequent to clot formation, elimination of the clot, and repair and regeneration of the damaged tissue (1). Due to the manner in which these subprocesses occur, the coagulation response is localized to the area of injury, molamplified to the appropriate degree according to the severity of the injury, attenuated to systemic activation, and modulated to allow for subsequent repair mechanisms.

The coagulation cascade was initially described as a series of sequential proteolytic actions (2, 3). The emerging picture of coagulation, however, defines a complex, threshold-limited, highly interwoven array of physical, cellular, and biochemical processes that contribute to hemostasis. The subprocesses of the coagulation cascade (i.e., initiation, propagation, termination, elimination, and repair) illustrate the intricate choreography involved in maintenance of vascular integrity (1).

## COAGULATION CASCADE

### INITIATION

Initiation of the procoagulant response occurs when the vascular endothelium and circulating blood cells are perturbed and the normally antithrombogenic nature of the vascular system is altered due to mechanical injury or inflammatory stimulus. In the case of a perforating injury, prothrombotic subendothelial tissue elements are exposed and peripheral blood cells such as platelets accumulate at the site of injury. This exposure and accumulation provides receptors and membrane surfaces that promote the binding of circulating procoagulant proteins. The initiation phase provides a tableau for the subsequent stages of coagulation.

### PROPAGATION

Propagation of coagulation results from the activities of the procoagulant enzymatic complexes that assemble on the sites provided by the subendothelial matrix and peripheral blood cells. These surface-associated multicomponent complexes are composed of serine proteases, nonenzymatic cofactor proteins, calcium ions ($Ca^{2+}$), and cellular membrane components. Two distinct pathways of blood clotting that proceed from either the intrinsic or extrinsic initiating complexes have been identified (Fig. 1.1) (4–7). Both pathways converge to form a common pathway leading to $\alpha$-thrombin generation (Fig. 1.1). The intrinsic, or contact activation pathway,

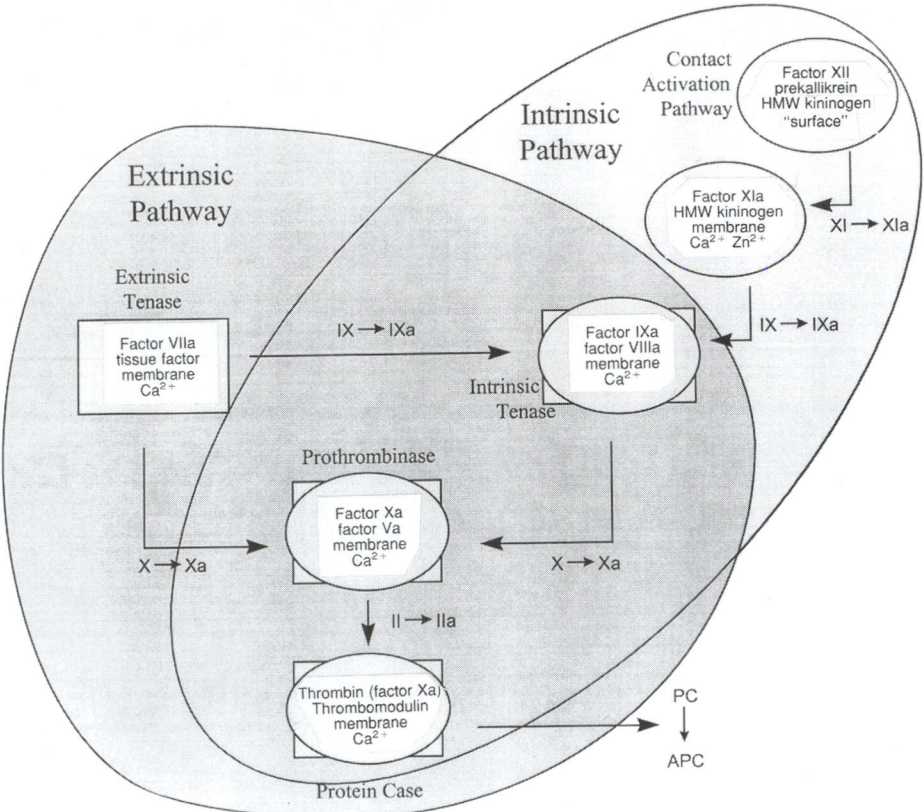

**FIGURE 1.1.** The enzymatic complexes of the coagulation cascade. The multi-protein complexes required for hemostasis each involve a serine protease, one or more cofactor proteins, divalent cations ($Ca^{2+}$ and/or $Zn^{2+}$), and a surface. Factor XII of the contact activation pathway is activated subsequent to exposure of a negatively charged surface. The other serine protease components, factors XIa, VIIa, IXa, and Xa, and α-thrombin (IIa), are generated from their respective zymogen forms (factors XI, VII, IX, and X and prothrombin [II]) as part of the cascade. The cofactor proteins, most notably tissue factor and factors VIIIa and Va, mediate the binding of their respective protease components to phospholipid membranes and significantly enhance the efficiency of protease function. The protein Case complex is responsible for activating protein C (PC) to form activated protein C (APC).

consists of several plasma proteins activated by contact with negatively charged surfaces (6, 7) (Fig. 1.1). Deficiencies in proteins associated with initiation of the intrinsic pathway (prekallikrein, high-molecular-weight kininogen, and factor XII) are known to exist but are not associated with bleeding tendencies (8–10). However, individuals with protein deficiencies in the extrinsic and common pathways (prothrombin and factors V, VIII, VII, IX, and X) can present with severe bleeding diatheses (11–15). Individuals with factor XI deficiency have also had bleeding episodes associated with surgical challenge (16, 17). The physiologic relevance of the initial complex of the contact activation system in hemorrhage control is therefore unknown (18), although factor XI appears to play an important role in the hemostatic response (19). Factor XI's role in hemostasis probably does not result from its activation by factor XIIa in the intrinsic pathway. Instead, factor XI may be activated by α-thrombin as part of a positive feedback loop stemming from α-thrombin generation. Factor XIa would then

function in the (auto)propagation of α-thrombin formation (20).

The extrinsic (or tissue factor) pathway of coagulation (Fig. 1.1) is initiated or triggered by the interaction of plasma-derived factor VIIa with tissue factor (4, 21, 22) (see Chapter 4). Tissue factor is an integral membrane protein that can present mechanically with acute vascular damage (23). The tissue factor protein is not normally expressed on vascular cell surfaces; however, it is constitutively expressed on extravascular cell surfaces (23–28) and exposed to blood flow as a result of endothelial cell damage. Tissue factor can also be presented by peripheral blood cells and endothelial cells influenced by inflammatory cytokines (29, 30). Low levels of factor VIIa circulate in blood (31). This factor VIIa can bind to tissue factor and initiate the coagulation process upon injury and exposure or expression of tissue factor. Free factor VIIa displays remarkably poor enzymatic activity and is not inhibited by circulating inhibitors in the absence of complex formation with tissue

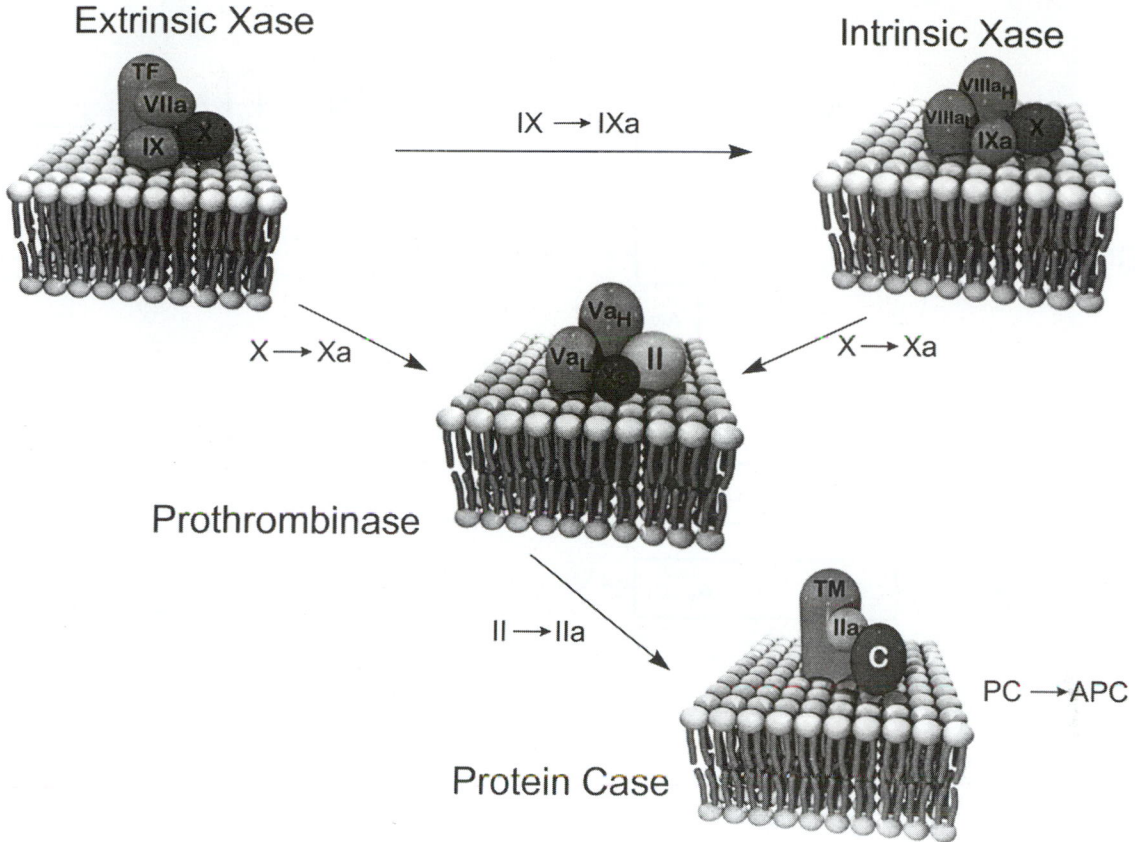

**FIGURE 1.2.**   Schematic representation of the phospholipid membrane-associated enzyme complexes of coagulation. Each vitamin K-dependent serine protease (factors VIIa, IXa, and Xa and $\alpha$-thrombin [IIa]) is shown in association with its cofactor protein (tissue factor [TF], factors VIIIa and Va, and thrombomodulin [TM]) and zymogen substrate(s) (factors IX and X, prothrombin [II] and protein C [C]) on the membrane surface. The cofactor proteins, factor VIIIa and factor Va, are characterized by a two domain structure and consist of heavy (H) and light (L) chains that are bridged together by $Ca^{2+}$ ions. Both domains are required for cofactor-membrane association and cofactor-protease binding. Tissue factor, thrombomodulin, and cell-membrane associated cofactors assist protease binding to the membrane and cofactor through their extracellular domains.

factor (32, 33). The tissue factor-factor VIIa complex may activate additional low levels of factor VII, but the most probable promoter of factor VII activation is $\alpha$-thrombin or the factor Xa-phospholipid complex. Factor Xa associated with phospholipid (without factor Va, its cofactor in the prothrombinase complex) activates factor VII at a 24-fold higher rate than tissue factor-factor VIIa (34). $\alpha$-thrombin is a less active but more abundant activator. Enhancement of the initial stage of blood coagulation via formation of higher levels of tissue factor-factor VIIa complexes is, therefore, most likely dependent on factor Xa and $\alpha$-thrombin (34).

The proteases required for normal blood coagulation through the extrinsic pathway express their functions as components of membrane-dependent enzyme complexes (Fig. 1.2). There are three procoagulant complexes (prothrombinase, intrinsic tenase, and extrinsic tenase) and one anticoagulant complex (protein Case) (Fig. 1.2). Prothrombinase and the intrinsic tenase contain homologous plasma-derived cofactors while the ex-

trinsic tenase and protein Case contain cofactor proteins that are tissue- or cell-derived (Fig. 1.3)(35, 36).

The vitamin K-dependent zymogens (prothrombin, protein C, and factors VII, IX, and X) are characterized by an $NH_2$-terminal Gla-domain that contains 10 to 12 $\gamma$-carboxyglutamate residues (35) (Fig. 1.4). The $\gamma$-carboxylation of glutamate residues is a post-translational modification of these proteins that requires a vitamin K-dependent carboxylase (37). The $\gamma$-carboxyglutamate or Gla residues play an essential role in modulating the three-dimensional structures of these proteins and in the binding of the serine proteases and zymogens to the membrane surface (38–41).

The plasma-derived procofactors, factor V and factor VIII, are synthesized as single-chain molecules and are highly homologous, sharing many structural and functional similarities (42, 43) (Fig. 1.3). Upon activation, the central B domains of these proteins are excised by proteolysis. The heavy chain regions (A1 and A2 domains) and light chain regions (A3, C1, and C2 domains)

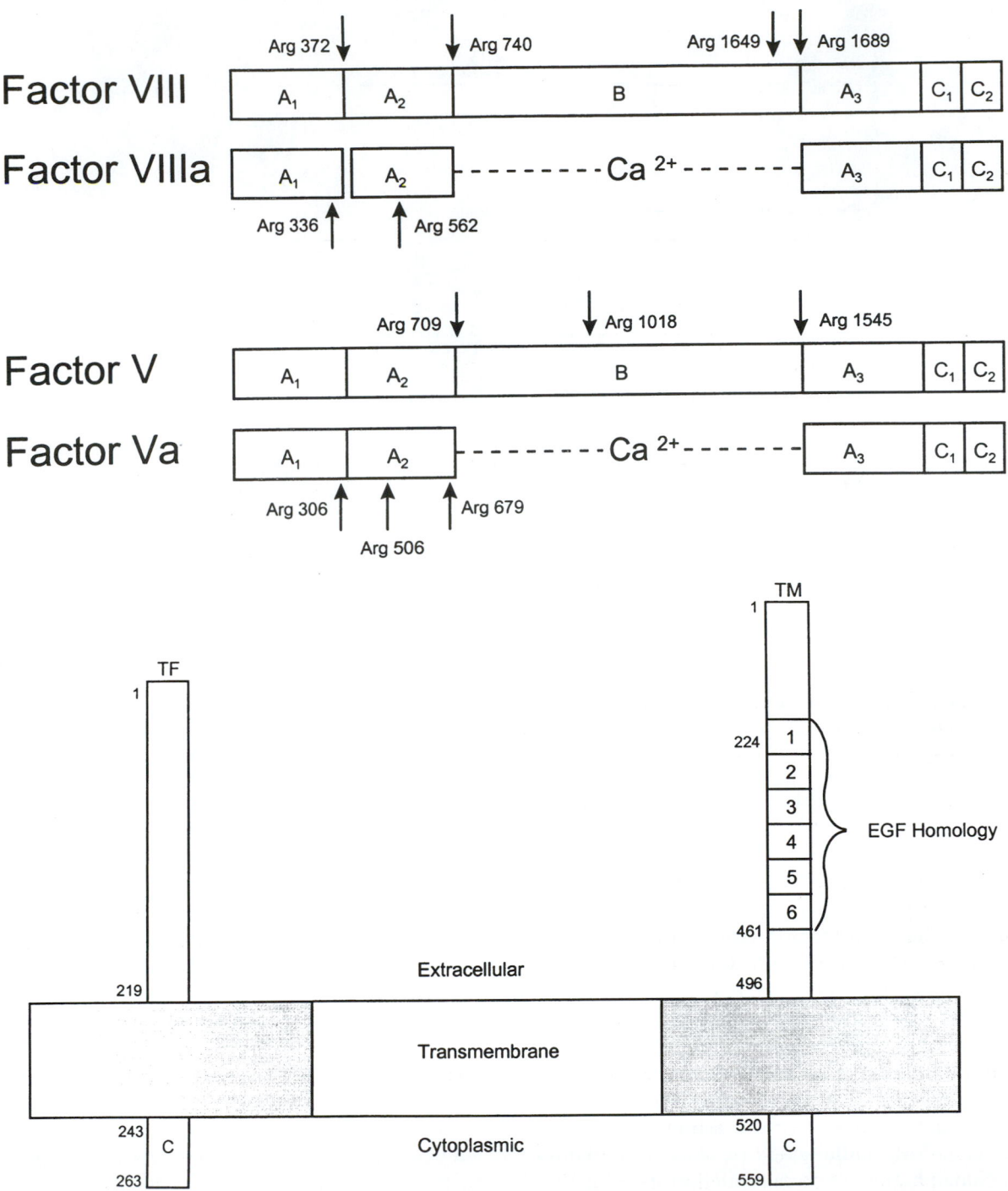

**FIGURE 1.3.**   Structural organization of the plasma-derived and cell membrane-associated cofactors. A, The circulating procofactors, factor V and factor VIII, are activated by α-thrombin. Both cofactor proteins are composed of internally triplicated A domains (A1, A2, and A3) and internally duplicated C domains (C1 and C2). The B domains in the procofactor molecules are not homologous. Factor Va is composed of two domains, the A1-A2 and A3-C1-C2 regions, while factor VIIIa is composed of three domains, the A1, A2, and A3-C1-C2 regions. Noncovalent Ca$^{2+}$ interactions are responsible for the association of the heavy (A1 and A2) and light (A3, C1, and C2) chains of the cofactors. B, Tissue factor (TF) and thrombomodulin (TM) are composed of extracellular domains, transmembrane domains, and cytoplasmic regions. Tissue factor is expressed by a variety of vascular and circulating cells while thrombomodulin is predominantly an endothelial cell associated protein.

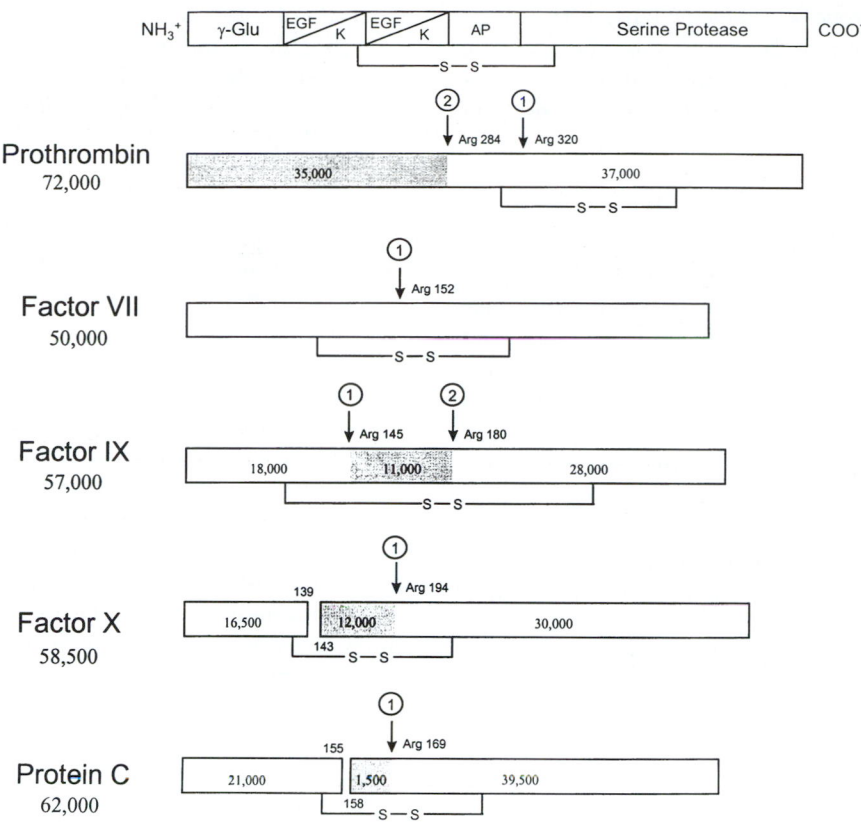

**FIGURE 1.4.**   Schematic representation of the structures of the vitamin K-dependent proteins. The $NH_2$-terminal portion of the vitamin K-dependent serine protease contain the $\gamma$-carboxyglutamate $\gamma$-Glu residues and the domain comprised of epidermal growth factor-like (EGF) structures (factors VII, IX, and X and protein C) or kringle (K) structures (prothrombin). The activation peptide (AP), which is cleaved subsequent to zymogen activation, and the serine protease domain, which contains the active site, are indicated. The structural organization of the individual vitamin K-dependent zymogens are also illustrated. The cleavage sites that result in zymogen activation are indicated.

of the cofactor molecules remain associated through a $Ca^{2+}$-dependent mechanism (Fig. 1.3). The A1 and A2 domains remain covalently connected in factor Va. In contrast, factor VIIIa has an additional cleavage site required for its activation between the A1 and A2 domains at $Arg_{372}$ (42, 43). While the two-chain factor Va is reasonably stable, the three-chain factor VIIIa spontaneously decomposes with release of the A2 domain. The cofactors provided by cellular membranes (Fig. 1.3) are composed of extracellular and cytoplasmic domains and transmembrane regions.

The principal result of coagulation propagation through the activities of membrane-dependent enzyme complexes is prothrombin activation to provide $\alpha$-thrombin activity. $\alpha$-thrombin, in turn, activates circulating platelets to add to the cellular accumulation at the site of vascular injury or activation and converts soluble fibrinogen into an insoluble fibrin matrix. $\alpha$-thrombin also participates in positive feedback by activating a number of protein components of the coagulation cascade. $\alpha$-thrombin activates the procofactors, factors V and VIII, and the zymogens, factors VII and XI (20,

44–52). $\alpha$-thrombin also activates factor XIII (fibrin-stabilizing factor) to factor XIIIa (53), a transglutaminase enzyme that stabilizes the fibrin clot with cross-links, thus strengthening the fibrin clot matrix (54–57) (see Chapter 6). Fibrin, the substrate of factor XIIIa, acts to accelerate the formation of factor XIIIa by $\alpha$-thrombin (58, 59). This feedback loop ensures factor XIIIa is not produced until its substrate is available (58, 59). The thrombin-activatable fibrinolysis inhibitor (TAFI), also known as carboxypeptidase U (60) or procarboxypeptidase B (61), is a procarboxypeptidase B activated in an $\alpha$-thrombin-dependent manner (62). The active form, TAFIa, protects the fibrin clot from degradation during the termination phase of coagulation. The propagation phase of blood coagulation thus results in generation of a stable plug at the site of injury and cessation of blood loss.

## TERMINATION

Termination of clot formation involves at least two constitutive inhibitory processes and a dynamic, clotting-initiated, inhibitory process (35) (see Chapter 3). Termination leads to inhibition of the procoagulant enzymatic complexes either by direct inhibition of protease components or by inactivation of the cofactor proteins. The constitutive inhibitory system consists mainly of circulating protease inhibitors antithrombin III (AT-III) and tissue factor pathway inhibitor (TFPI) (35). AT-III, a member of the serpin family of protease inhibitors (63), circulates at a relatively high plasma concentration (2 to 3 μM [64, 65]) and inhibits most enzymes in the procoagulant system; the inhibition of α-thrombin and factor Xa is probably AT-III's most significant role (66, 67). Complex formation between AT-III and its target enzymes is enhanced up to 2000-fold by heparin and is a major contributor to the clinical heparin anticoagulation process (68, 69). *In vivo*, endothelial cells are althought to provide surface-bound heparin sulfate proteoglycan biopolymers that function as the natural agonist for which clinically administered heparin is a surrogate (70, 71).

TFPI, which circulates at a relatively low plasma concentration (2.4 nM [72]), is a member of the Kunitz family of enzyme inhibitors (73) and reversibly inhibits free factor Xa but does not appear to have a significant inhibitory effect toward other serine proteases when present at normal plasma concentrations (74). TFPI's major function is the elimination of the extrinsic tenase trigger of coagulation through a factor Xa-dependent mechanism (75, 76). TFPI binds noncovalently at or near the active site of factor Xa and inhibits factor Xa. The TFPI-factor Xa complex then reversibly inhibits the tissue factor-factor VIIa complex through quaternary complex formation. The quaternary complex may also be formed by TFPI binding directly to the tissue factor-factor VIIa-factor Xa tertiary complex (75, 76). In either instance, TFPI utilizes an enzymatic product of the extrinsic tenase (Fig. 1.2) to inhibit the complex and shut off the procoagulant triggering mechanism.

The protein C pathway regulates procoagulant events through a dynamic inhibitory system (35). Activated protein C (APC), the product of the thrombomodulin-α-thrombin complex (protein Case) (77, 78) (Fig. 1.2), inactivates prothrombinase and intrinsic tenase by cleaving and inactivating their respective cofactors, factor Va and factor VIIIa (Fig. 1.3) (47, 79–82). Under physiological conditions, the inactivation of factor VIIIa also occurs rapidly by an APC-independent mechanism through dissociation of the A2 domain (83–85). APC's primary role is the inactivation of factor Va and the arrest of prothrombinase activity (86, 87). The extent of expression of protein Case and APC is directly and paradoxically related to the generation of the procoagulant end product α-thrombin and prothrombinase activity (35). Complex formation between α-thrombin and its anticoagulant cofactor, thrombomodulin, changes the

reactivity of α-thrombin so the enzyme no longer serves a procoagulant role in activating platelets and cofactor proteins or in cleaving fibrinogen: the thrombomodulin-α-thrombin complex functions mainly to produce APC (88, 89). Protein S, a vitamin K-dependent protein, is also involved in the APC inhibitory pathway and appears to serve as a cofactor for APC in a limited capacity (90). Protein S contains a Gla domain (91), associates with phospholipid membranes (92), and is cleaved by α-thrombin (93). However, while the physiologic importance of protein S is secure, its precise biological function has not yet been clarified.

Individuals deficient in protein C or protein S are known to have thrombotic tendencies (see Chapter 40). Failure of the clot termination process in these individuals leads to clinically relevant pathology. Deficiencies in either of these proteins may occur congenitally or during the initiation of warfarin therapy (91, 94–100). Likewise, individuals with diminished levels of AT-III have thrombotic tendencies (101–103). Although TFPI deficiency does not have an established clinical syndrome, models of hemostasis indicate TFPI is an important regulator of coagulation (104–106).

A mutation in factor V caused by an $Arg_{506}$ to Gln substitution (factor $V^{Leiden}$) is also associated with thrombotic tendencies (107–111) (see Chapter 40). The point mutation which leads to factor $V^{Leiden}$ is associated with a condition termed "APC resistance" (107–111). Inactivation of factor Va by APC occurs in a membrane-dependent sequential fashion (87). Initial cleavage of factor Va by APC at $Arg_{506}$ gives rise to an intermediate, partially active species. Subsequent cleavages at $Arg_{306}$ and $Arg_{679}$ are required for complete loss of cofactor activity (87). Individuals with the factor $V^{Leiden}$ defect display normal factor Va cofactor activity with respect to prothrombinase function but lack the crucial site at $Arg_{506}$ that enhances cofactor inactivation by APC. Factor $Va^{Leiden}$ is therefore inactivated at a markedly slower rate than normal factor Va (112). Prolongation of factor Va cofactor activity and α-thrombin generation by the prothrombinase complex increases the extent of clot formation, resulting in an increased risk of venous thrombosis, which is manifest in individuals with the factor $V^{Leiden}$ defect (112).

The termination phase of the blood clotting event is critical in mediating the extent of clot formation. Termination of clot generation after the appropriate plug has formed is necessary to prevent unwanted thrombotic events that result from systemic and/or excessive clot formation. This is demonstrated by the clinical thrombotic disorders in individuals with deficiencies in inhibitory pathways.

## ELIMINATION

Elimination of the clot is an essential step in the tissue repair process and requires the enzyme plasmin (see

Chapter 7). The fibrin-based clot is "dissolved" by plasmin cleavage of the fibrin matrix to produce soluble fibrin peptides (113, 114). Plasmin is generated from the circulating zymogen plasminogen through the action of urokinase (u-PA) or tissue-type plasminogen activator (t-PA) (113, 114). Plasmin activity is required for fibrin matrix proteolysis and activation of various metalloproteinases (115), which degrade the damaged tissue components to allow for cell migration and the final stages of vascular repair.

The plasminogen/plasminogen-activator system (see Chapter 7) is as complex as the procoagulant cascade. Plasmin activity is regulated by vascular cells that secrete the plasminogen activators and plasminogen activator inhibitor 1 (PAI-1) (116–118). Plasmin functions in a positive feedback loop to cleave full length plasminogen (glu-plasminogen) to generate an intermediate species (des 1–76 or lys-plasminogen) that is more readily activated by t-PA and u-PA (116–118). Complex formation between plasminogen and various receptors on cell surfaces and extracellular matrices also enhances plasminogen activation and protects plasmin from inactivation by the circulating inhibitor $\alpha_2$-antiplasmin (119–124).

Additionally, factors Va and Xa have been reported to enhance plasmin generation (125). Plasmin cleaves both factors V and Va, resulting in transient activation of factor V to factor Va and subsequent inactivation to factor Va$_{iPM}$ (126). The inactivation process exposes a plasminogen binding site on the inactive factor Va molecule (125). This process is phospholipid- and Ca$^{2+}$-dependent. Factor Va$_{iPM}$ may function as a cofactor for t-PA in plasminogen activation (125). Factor Xa also accelerates the rate of t-PA activation of plasminogen, with both factor Va$_{iPM}$ and factor Xa accelerating plasmin generation approximately 150-fold (125). Interactions among factor Va$_{iPM}$, factor Xa, and plasmin generation may provide a direct link between procoagulant events and fibrinolysis and ensure both events are localized to the membrane area exposed or provided at the site of vessel injury (125).

TAFIa, produced by the thrombomodulin-$\alpha$-thrombin complex (62), decreases the rate at which glu-plasminogen is activated by t-PA, most likely by modifying fibrin (62). TAFIa excises COOH-terminal lysine residues from the fibrin/fibrin fragment molecules, thus interfering with plasminogen association with the fibrin matrix and reducing the rate of plasmin generation (62).

TAFIa is althought to be responsible for a profibrinolytic effect of APC (127, 128). In the absence of APC, prothrombin conversion to $\alpha$-thrombin continues without any significant inhibition of explosive $\alpha$-thrombin generation. The continuous generation of $\alpha$-thrombin results in higher levels of TAFIa, which in turn reduces the rate of fibrinolysis. The generation of $\alpha$-thrombin is significantly reduced in the presence of APC, thus reducing the activation of TAFI. APC indirectly attenuates fibrinolysis through inhibition of TAFI activation (127). The interplay among $\alpha$-thrombin, APC, and TAFI directly link the processes of propagation, termination, and elimination of the fibrin clot (127). Although the processes of coagulation are broken down into individual components, none of these processes functions independently.

## REPAIR

Repair and regeneration of the damaged tissue constitute the final steps in the coagulation process. These processes require plasmin activity to activate the metalloproteinases that degrade the damaged extracellular matrix to allow for cell migration into the damaged area (115). $\alpha$-thrombin, which plays multiple procoagulant and anticoagulant roles, also potentially performs key functions in the repair mechanism. $\alpha$-thrombin is a potent growth factor and chemo-attractant with noted active site-dependent and -independent effects on fibroblasts, macrophages, and smooth muscle cells (129, 130). $\alpha$-thrombin activation of platelets results in the release of vasoactive compounds and growth factors, such as transforming growth factor-$\beta$ (TGF-$\beta$), platelet-derived growth factor (PDGF), and epidermal growth factor (131–136). These growth factors stimulate proliferation of a number of cell types (137, 138). $\alpha$-thrombin also mediates growth factor production by the endothelium (139). The action of the primary procoagulant protein is a principal component of the process that allows cells to repopulate the damaged area, which recreates the endothelial and subendothelial elements required to form the antithrombogenic vascular-blood interface. Although the cycle of coagulation is presented here as a linear sequence of reactions, the overall process occurs in a highly interwoven, non-sequential fashion that results in the prevention of blood loss from injury and regeneration and maintenance of vascular integrity.

# MODEL SYSTEMS
## SYNTHETIC MEMBRANE SYSTEMS

The propagation phase of blood coagulation consists of the membrane-dependent events of coagulation and illustrates the complex sequence of the blood coagulation event. The "activated cell" membrane is a key element in complex formation and function. Although the true nature of the cellular elements is not currently understood, the cellular membrane system can be imitated by synthetic phospholipid membranes. The membrane functions as a surface for condensing the procoagulant protein molecules and as a vital component in the assembly and expression of the procoagulant and anticoagulant complexes (140). *In vivo*, the procoagulant membrane surface is althought to be primarily contributed by platelets which circulate as quiescent discoid cell particles. However, when platelets are stimulated as a result of vascular injury, they undergo a shape change, reveal anionic phospholipids on their surfaces, release numerous proteins from storage granules, and aggregate to participate in clot formation (141, 142). Other circulating blood cells (monocytes and lymphocytes) and vascular lining cells may also contribute to this membrane requirement. *In vitro* studies frequently take advantage of a far less complex, but unregulated, membrane system composed of synthetic phospholipid mixtures. The most commonly used synthetic phospholipid surfaces are small (350 Å diameter) unilamellar vesicles composed of 70 to 80% phosphatidylcholine (PC), a neutral phospholipid, and 20 to 30% phosphatidylserine (PS), an anionic lipid moiety. The phosphatidylcholine/phosphatidylserine (PCPS) mixture has been found to function in a manner kinetically similar to membrane surfaces provided by cellular components. Five to 15 mole percent anionic phospholipid is required for optimum membrane-dependent complex activity (143). Vitamin K-dependent enzymes and zymogens associate with the phospholipid membrane via $Ca^{2+}$-bridging between the Gla residues on the $NH_2$-terminal domains of the molecules and the negatively charged phospholipid surface (38–41). The anionic lipid is also required for plasma derived-cofactor binding interactions (143).

Studies of the properties, assembly, and kinetics of membrane-dependent procoagulant and anticoagulant complexes have focused on the prothrombinase complex and have been extrapolated to the other complexes. The prothrombinase complex consists of the serine protease factor Xa; its protein cofactor, factor Va; $Ca^{2+}$; and an anionic phospholipid-containing membrane (Fig. 1.2). Initial studies of the prothrombinase system showed that both factor Va and factor Xa interact with the membrane surface and with each other (144). The dissociation constant for the factor Va-lipid interaction, $K_d = 2.9$ nM (145) (Table 1.1), suggests a high-affinity interaction. The factor Va-lipid association occurs by hydrophobic and electrostatic interactions and involves two regions (the A3 and C2 domains) of the light chain of the factor Va molecule (87, 146, 147) (Fig. 1.3). The factor Va-membrane interaction also may involve penetration of the factor Va molecule into the membrane bilayer (148). This interaction is reported to be dependent on the A3 domain of the factor Va molecule, which is althought to penetrate the bilayer subsequent to the association of factor Va on the bilayer surface, leading to the tight protein-membrane complex (149). The dissociation constant for the factor Xa-lipid complex, $K_d = 110$ nM (150) (Table 1.1), is more than two orders of magnitude higher than that for the factor Va-lipid complex

**TABLE 1.1.** Dissociation Constants for the Protein-Protein and Protein-Membrane Interactions Involved in Prothrombinase Complex Assembly

| Interaction | $K_d$ (nM) | References |
|---|---|---|
| Factor Va-PCPS | 3 | 145 |
| Factor Xa-PCPS | 110 | 150 |
| Prothrombin-PCPS | 1000 | 152 |
| Factor Va-factor Xa | 800 | 153–155 |
| Factor Va-PCPS-factor Xa | 1 | 38 |
| Factor Va-prothrombin | 10,000 | 82 |

*PCPS, phosphatidylcholine/phosphatidylserine synthetic membrane.*

and far higher than the estimated concentration of factor Xa produced in plasma during blood clotting. Zymogen factor X circulates at a plasma concentration of 170 nM (151), and a maximum concentration of 2 nM factor Xa would be available during the propagation phase if the coagulation reaction were to proceed with approximately 1% zymogen to enzyme conversion. This level of factor Xa, which is probably an overestimation, would not be sufficient to enable factor Xa-phospholipid complexes to exist without other stabilizing interactions. In the solution phase, the factor Va-factor Xa protein-protein interaction is also a low affinity event, which is characterized by a dissociation constant of 800 nM (152) (Table 1.1). Thus, protein-protein interaction alone does not provide the stabilizing energy required for prothrombinase complex assembly. The fully assembled complex on a phospholipid surface, however, has an effective dissociation constant of approximately 1 nM (153–155) (Table 1.1), which indicates membrane-protein-protein-membrane interactions stabilize the complex and lead to functional complex assembly at biologically relevant concentrations of protein reactants. The membrane-dependent protein-protein interactions also ensure the procoagulant reaction is localized to the specific area of vascular damage on the membrane sites provided by the cellular response to injury.

The substrate of the prothrombinase complex, prothrombin, also interacts with the phospholipid membrane and factor Va. The prothrombin-phospholipid interaction, $K_d = 1000$ nM (38) (Table 1.1), is of lower affinity than the factor Va-factor Xa interaction in solution. However, since prothrombin circulates at a plasma concentration of approximately 1400 nM (156), the low affinity prothrombin-membrane interaction is sufficient to ensure that prothrombin can associate with the membrane surface at the relevant *in vivo* concentration and would be available to interact with membrane-bound factor Va-factor Xa complex. The factor Va-prothrombin interaction, $K_d = 10$ μM (82) (Table 1.1), is mediated through the A1-A2 domains of factor Va. This interaction is unlikely to serve a biological function without the other protein-protein and protein-phospholipid interactions.

The factor Va-factor Xa-phospholipid interaction that stabilizes prothrombinase is mediated by the A1 and A3 domains of factor Va (157) (Fig. 1.3) and the Gla and serine protease domains of factor Xa (158, 159) (Fig. 1.4). Kinetic measurements using small synthetic substrates for factor Xa indicate the short range catalytic efficiency of the active site of factor Xa is not altered by cofactor-enzyme-phospholipid binding interactions. However, the active site region appears to undergo a conformational change that alters the accessibility and orientation of the region to its macromolecular substrate, prothrombin (158). The stabilization of the factor Xa-membrane interaction by factor Va and the alteration in the active site and potentially exosite regions of factor Xa lead to enhanced prothrombin activation. The fully assembled prothrombinase complex catalyzes α-thrombin generation at a rate that is at least 300,000 times more efficient than factor Xa acting alone (153) (Table 1.2). For comparison, the amount of α-thrombin produced by the prothrombinase complex in one minute would require six months if produced by an equivalent concentration of factor Xa alone acting on 1.4 μM prothrombin in solution (35).

The association of factor Va with factor Xa and the lipid membrane may result in conformational changes in factor Va and factor Xa. These changes may be the primary contribution to the enhanced affinity of the factor Va-factor Xa-lipid interaction as compared to the individual protein-phospholipid and protein-protein in-

teractions (143). The approximate 1000-fold increase in affinity of the factor Va-factor Xa interaction in the presence of a phospholipid surface may also be explained by the loss in degrees of freedom for protein motion and orientation when factor Va and factor Xa are membrane-bound, creating an oriented, two-dimensional system rather than the three-dimensional, random process found in solution (143, 150).

Multiple factors are operable in the development of a model of prothrombinase complex assembly. The assembly process depends on the initial formation of factor Va-lipid and factor Xa-lipid complexes. These protein-lipid products subsequently associate, resulting in prothrombinase complex formation. The formation of the individual protein-lipid complexes on separate sites of the membrane surface constitute the rate-limiting steps of prothrombinase assembly (143, 150) (Fig. 1.5). The factor Va-factor Xa interaction, which completes complex assembly, results from extremely rapid translational and/or rotational diffusion of the proteins on the membrane surface (143, 150) (Fig. 1.5).

The lipid-dependent membrane exchange model of prothrombinase complex assembly via factor Va-lipid and factor Xa-lipid interactions on separate vesicles has been examined. A 500-fold decrease in the rate of prothrombinase complex assembly is observed when factor Va is provided bound to one pool of phospholipid vesicles and factor Xa is contributed bound to a second pool of lipids versus adding both proteins from solution to the same membrane surface (150). Factor Va-factor Xa interactions under the former condition depend on dissociation of the proteins from one surface and reassociation on a second surface to complete prothrombinase complex assembly. A similar decrease in the rate of complex assembly is observed with excess phospholipid,

**TABLE 1.2.** Relative Efficiencies of the Procoagulant Vitamin K-Dependent Enzymes and Co-factor-Enzyme Complexes. The turnover number ($k_{cat}$) and Michaelis constant ($K_m$) for the free vitamin K-dependent enzymes and the fully assembled procoagulant complexes are compared to estimate the efficiencies ($k_{cat}/K_m$) of zymogen activation by free enzymes versus complexes.

| Enzyme | Substrate | $K_m$ (μM) | $k_{cat}$ (min$^{-1}$) | $k_{cat}/K_m$ (M·min$^{-1}$) | Efficiency Ratio |
|---|---|---|---|---|---|
| VIIa | IX | NA | NA | | |
| VIIa/TF/PCPS/Ca$^{2+}$ | IX | 0.243 | 15.6 | $6.42 \times 10^7$ | — |
| VIIa | X | 4.87 | 0.024 | $4.93 \times 10^3$ | |
| VIIa/TF/PCPS/Ca$^{2+}$ | X | 0.45 | 69.0 | $1.53 \times 10^8$ | $3.10 \times 10^4$ |
| IXa | X | 299.0 | 0.002 | 6.69 | |
| IXa/VIIIa/PCPS/Ca$^{2+}$ | X | 0.063 | 500.0 | $7.94 \times 10^9$ | $1.19 \times 10^9$ |
| Xa | II | 131.0 | 0.6 | $4.58 \times 10^3$ | |
| Xa/Va/PCPS/Ca$^{2+}$ | II | 1.0 | 1800.0 | $1.80 \times 10^9$ | $3.93 \times 10^5$ |

TF, tissue factor: PCPS, phosphatidylcholine/phosphotidylserine synthetic membrane.

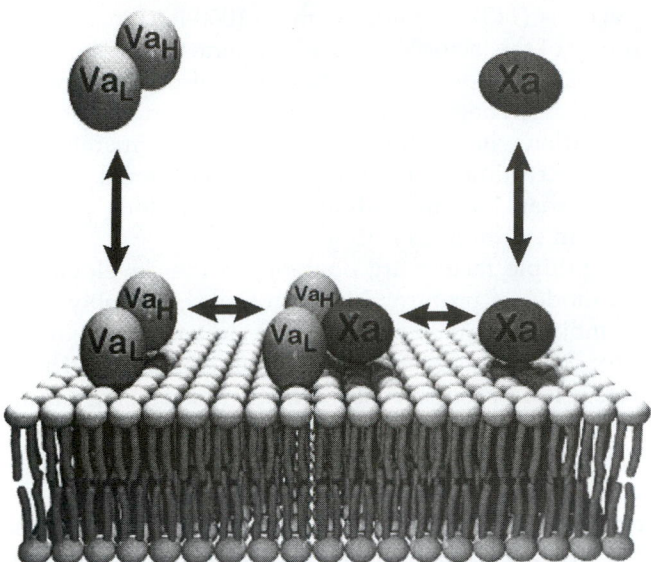

**FIGURE 1.5.** Membrane-associated assembly of the prothrombinase complex. Prothrombinase complex assembly proceeds through initial formation of factor Va-lipid and factor Xa-lipid complexes. The individual binary protein-lipid complexes then combine on the membrane surface through translational or rotational diffusion to form the prothrombinase complex. The light chain of factor Va ($Va_L$) mediates factor Va-lipid interaction while both the heavy ($Va_H$) and light chains are involved in factor Va-factor Xa-lipid interaction.

which results in separation and dilution of the cofactor and enzyme proteins (150). The dissociation rate constants of factor Va and factor Xa are 10 to 100 million times slower than their respective association rate constants (143, 150), creating a significant kinetic advantage for α-thrombin generation in the presence of the geographically located membrane surface.

Studies of the assembly of membrane-bound factor Xa and factor Va into the prothrombinase complex have used non-fluid phospholipid vesicles composed of saturated fatty acids or frozen lipids (140, 160). The fluidities of the vesicle preparations were altered by changing the temperature or varying the fatty acyl side chains of the lipids incorporated into the vesicles. Unsaturated phospholipids promote procoagulant activity (150, 160–162) while saturated phospholipids are associated with a decrease in prothrombinase activity (162). The fluidities of the vesicle preparations in the studies of prothrombinase complex assembly and function do not significantly influence the steady-state rate of α-thrombin generation; however, the time required to reach the maximum rate of α-thrombin production increased as the fluidity of the vesicles decreased. This lag probably corresponds to a decrease in the diffusion rates of factor Va and factor Xa on non-fluid membranes and a decrease in the rate of prothrombin delivery to the complex (140, 160). These assembly experiments establish the importance of the

qualities of protein-lipid interactions and the nature of the membrane surface in prothrombinase complex formation.

The influence of the membrane fatty acid composition is also shown in mechanistic alteration in the activation of prothrombin (162). Prothrombinase activates prothrombin by two sequential cleavages in the presence of a fluid, unsaturated membrane surface (163–165) (Fig. 1.6). The first cleavage produces the intermediate product meizothrombin and the second cleavage generates α-thrombin and prothrombin fragment 1.2. Without a phospholipid membrane, factor Xa activates prothrombin at a slow rate, the prothrombin cleavage pattern is reversed, and meizothrombin is not formed (Fig. 1.6) (163–165). Although the importance of meizothrombin in plasma during blood coagulation has been debated (166–168), meizothrombin is a membrane binding enzyme (163) and may contribute specialized functions during the blood clotting event.

In the presence of nonfluid phospholipids with saturated fatty acid chains, the proteolysis of prethrombin-1, a cleavage product of prothrombin that lacks the Gla domain and kringle 1 region of the parent molecule, is also altered versus the proteolytic pattern observed on fluid vesicle preparations (140). The prethrombin-1 substrate is not delivered to the prothrombinase complex via the lipid surface since it lacks the Gla-domain required for lipid interaction. Hence, the differences in the cleavage patterns of prethrombin-1 are not solely the result of altered reactivity of the substrate with the membrane but are the result of a fundamental alteration in prothrombinase assembly on the non-fluid membrane surface (140). Prethrombin-1 is cleaved to generate meizothrombin des fragment 1 in the presence of prothrombinase assembled on an unsaturated fluid membrane surface. A second cleavage step yields α-thrombin and fragment 2. The cleavage pattern occurs in the opposite direction and no meizothrombin-des-fragment 1 intermediate is formed when the prothrombinase complex is formed on saturated phospholipid vesicles (140). The membrane surface contributes elements beyond mere binding sites that provide for functional complex assembly.

The assembly and function of the intrinsic tenase complex, factor VIIIa-factor IXa (Fig. 1.2), which activates factor X to factor Xa, is also a membrane-dependent phenomenon and shows remarkable homology to the prothrombinase complex. The serine proteases, factor IXa and factor Xa, and the cofactor proteins, factor VIIIa and factor Va, of the two complexes share numerous similarities (42, 43). Although the factor VIIIa-factor IXa complex has not been as thoroughly characterized as the prothrombinase complex, the assembly of the complex on a membrane surface increases the rate of factor Xa generation approximately

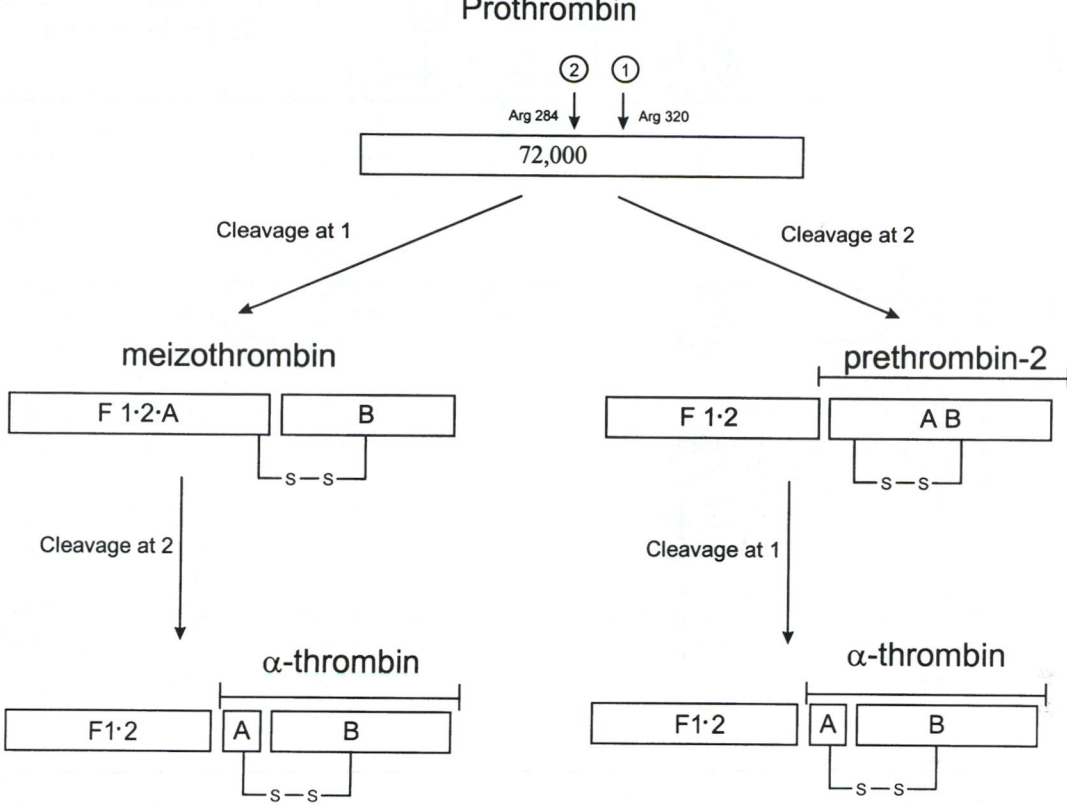

**FIGURE 1.6.** Schematic diagram of membrane-dependent prothrombin activation. Prothrombin activation by prothrombinase on a membrane surface proceeds through two sequential cleavages of the zymogen. Meizothrombin, the active intermediate formed only with the full complex and a membrane surface, is generated by peptide bond cleavage at $Arg_{320}$. A second bond cleavage at $Arg_{284}$ generates α-thrombin (domains A and B bridged by a disulfide bond) and releases prothrombin fragment 1.2 (F1·2). Without an appropriate membrane surface, prothrombin cleavage occurs in the opposite direction with generation of prethrombin-2 and fragment 1.2 as the first step and subsequent cleavage to generate α-thrombin. No meizothrombin intermediate is formed without a membrane surface.

$10^9$-fold more than that of factor IXa alone (169, 170) (Table 1.2). Additionally, association of factor VIIIa with factor IXa on the membrane surface stabilizes the cofactor and prolongs the functional lifetime of the intrinsic tenase (171, 172). Factor VIII is stabilized by forming a complex with the large, multimeric protein, von Willebrand factor (vWf) in the blood circulation prior to activation (11) (see Chapter 16). However, when factor VIIIa is released from this complex upon activation, the newly formed factor VIIIa undergoes spontaneous dissociation to generate an inactive cofactor (83, 84, 173). Complex formation between factor VIIIa and factor IXa on a membrane bilayer stabilizes the activity of factor VIIIa (171, 172). The protein-protein interaction between factor VIIIa and factor IXa is also enhanced 10-fold in the presence of a phospholipid membrane. The $K_d$ for the factor VIIIa-factor IXa interaction in solution, 46 nM, is reduced to 4.3 nM in the presence of a phospholipid bilayer, which indicates a significantly higher affinity interaction as a consequence of complex assembly on a surface (174).

Complex formation and an anionic membrane surface contribute to an increase in enzyme efficiency and protein stabilization for both the intrinsic tenase and prothrombinase complexes.

The cofactor-enzyme combination of the extrinsic tenase, tissue factor-factor VIIa, dramatically alters the active site of the protease (175) and enhances the efficiency of activation of its substrates, factors IX and X, approximately $10^4$-fold versus factor VIIa alone (176). However, assembly of the extrinsic tenase does not display the same essential requirements for an anionic phospholipid-equivalent membrane surface as the other procoagulant complexes (4). Factor VIIa interaction with tissue factor without membrane-governed interactions is sufficient to elevate the catalytic efficiency of the enzyme toward small synthetic substrates (175). Furthermore, although this protein-protein interaction is enhanced by $Ca^{2+}$, the divalent cation is not an essential requirement. The membrane-dependent nature of the extrinsic tenase arises from requirements for substrate delivery via two-dimensional transfer on

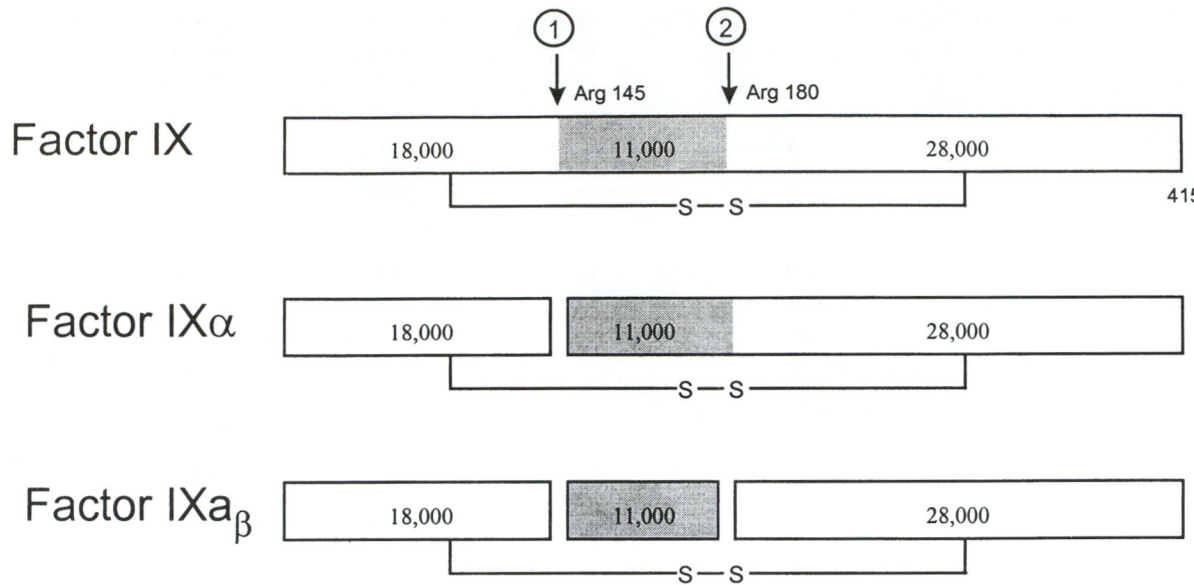

**FIGURE 1.7.** Schematic diagram of factor IX activation. Peptide bond cleavage by the tissue factor-factor VIIa or factor Xa-lipid complex at $Arg_{145}$ yields factor IXα, an inactive intermediate in the pathway. A second cleavage at $Arg_{180}$, which is mediated by the extrinsic tenase, generates the active enzyme factor IXa.

the phospholipid surface (177–180). Factors IX and X initially form zymogen-lipid complexes mediated by the Gla domains of proteins and are then transferred to the catalytic complex along the membrane surface (177–180). The Gla domain of factor VIIa may also associate with anionic phospholipid to generate effective tissue factor-factor VIIa activity toward the natural substrates, factors IX and X (181). This membrane-dependent mechanism of substrate-complex interaction supports the enhanced efficiency of zymogen activation by the extrinsic tenase assembled on a lipid bilayer versus the slow rate of zymogen cleavage without a membrane (31, 177, 178). Without a surface, the tenase complex and zymogen substrates would depend on diffusion with random orientations in three dimensions to allow the zymogen to interact with the catalytic site.

The extrinsic tenase also displays different requirements than the other procoagulant complexes in terms of generation of its serine protease component. Factor VII may be activated by factors IXa, Xa, or XIIa or α-thrombin (182–184). The zymogen may also undergo a lipid-dependent autoactivation process when associated with its cofactor, tissue factor (185). Additionally, tissue factor-factor VIIa complexes formed from the low level of circulating factor VIIa may be responsible for activating factor VII bound to tissue factor and enhancing extrinsic tenase activity. Although the pathway of physiologic factor VIIa generation is unknown, the importance of the extrinsic tenase trigger of coagulation is well documented.

The extrinsic tenase complex, tissue factor-factor VIIa (Fig. 1.2), provides factor IXa and factor Xa during the propagation stage of blood coagulation (177, 186–188). Evaluation of the activation of factor IX and factor X individually by the tissue factor-factor VIIa complex showed factor X is the preferred substrate (177, 186–188). However, if the extrinsic tenase could provide significant amounts of factor Xa in vivo, the severe bleeding disorders associated with deficiencies in the factor VIIIa-factor IXa complex (hemophilia A and hemophilia B) would not exist. Activation of factor X by the extrinsic tenase might in theory, offset the lack of factor X activation by the intrinsic tenase in hemophilias A and B and thus provide factor Xa to form the prothrombinase complex. The extrinsic tenase is, in fact, able to provide sufficient factor Xa to allow for coagulation at high concentrations achieved by clinical administration of recombinant factor VIIa. However, normal physiological levels are inadequate to reverse the documented pathology of hemophilias A and B.

When factors IX and X are simultaneously presented to the extrinsic tenase complex, factor IXa generation is increased while factor Xa generation is suppressed by almost 50% compared to the activation of factor X alone (169, 176). This suggests factor IX, not factor X, is an equivalent or preferred substrate for the extrinsic tenase in the complex plasma milieu (169, 176). Additionally, the intermediate species in factor IX activation, factor IXα (Fig. 1.7), is generated more rapidly in the presence of factor X. The intermediate factor IXα is activated by the extrinsic tenase at a higher rate than factor IX. These data implicate the low level of factor Xa generated by tissue factor-factor VIIa in the activation of factor IX. A model for the role of the extrinsic tenase suggests the conversion of factor IX to the intermediate factor IXα (Fig. 1.7) occurs by the tissue factor-factor VIIa complex or by a factor Xa-phospholipid complex. In a second step, factor IXα is converted to the active enzyme factor IXa (Fig. 1.7) by the extrinsic tenase (169, 176). Additional support for extrinsic tenase as a provider of factor IXa, not factor Xa, is shown by measurements of second order rate constants of factor X activation by the extrinsic and intrinsic tenase complexes. Factor Xa generation by tissue factor-factor VIIa occurs at only 1/50th the rate of factor X activation by the factor VIIIa-factor IXa complex (169, 170, 176). Thus, both complexes have specific and noninterchangeable roles in the procoagulant response.

The interaction between factor Xa and the tissue factor-factor VIIa complex is proposed to play an important role in triggering the procoagulant response and generation of α-thrombin (169, 176). The extrinsic tenase generates low levels of factors IXa and Xa in the initial stages of the hemostatic event (Fig. 1.8). Factor Xa-membrane complexes assist extrinsic tenase in activating higher levels of factor IXa. Factor IXa forms complexes with factor VIIIa on the phospholipid surface, and the fully assembled intrinsic tenase accelerates the formation of factor Xa by more than 50-fold (Fig. 1.8). The burst of factor Xa overcomes the levels of factor Xa inhibitors such as TFPI and achieves maximal levels of prothrombinase activity leading to a propagation of the procoagulant event (Fig. 1.8). Formation of prothrombinase leads to fibrin/platelet clot formation and eventually termination of the procoagulant response (169, 176).

The membrane-dependent mechanism of complex

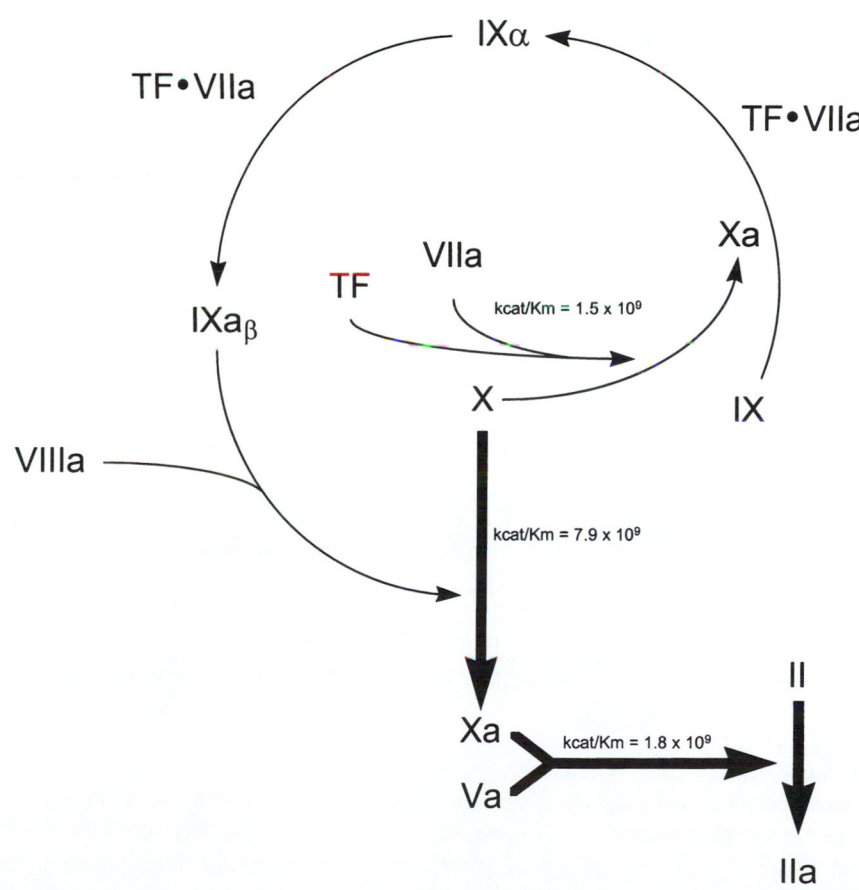

**FIGURE 1.8.**   Schematic model of the activation of factors IX and X by the extrinsic tenase. The tissue factor (TF)-factor VIIa complex triggers the procoagulant response by activation of small amounts of factors IX and X. The factor Xa that is generated assists in converting factor IX to factor IXα, which is the intermediate species in factor IX activation. Fully active factor IXaβ can then be rapidly generated by the extrinsic tenase. Complex formation between factor IXa and factor VIIIa significantly accelerates factor X activation and leads to a burst of factor Xa that exceeds levels of circulating factor Xa inhibitors and allows for formation of the prothrombinase complex. The prothrombinase complex (factor Va:factor Xa) activates prothrombin (II) to α-thrombin (IIa). The relative efficiencies, turnover number/Michaelis constant (kcal/Km), of the complexes are indicated. (With permission from Lawson JH, Mann KG. Cooperative activation of human factor IX by the human extrinsic pathway of blood coagulation. J Biol Chem 1991;266:11317–11327.)

assembly can be expanded to encompass the myriad of interactions observed under various experimental conditions. Upon exposure of tissue factor that results from vascular injury, the circulating factor VIIa forms the extrinsic tenase and activates circulating factors VII and IX and low levels of factor X (169, 176). Factors IXa and Xa would activate their respective procofactors, factor VIII and factor V, to generate the intrinsic tenase and prothrombinase complexes. The low levels of α-thrombin produced would activate more factor VIII and factor V in a positive feedback loop, which leads to a sustained and elevated level of factor Xa generation by the intrinsic tenase, maximal prothrombinase complex assembly, and an explosive burst of α-thrombin formation. α-thrombin activation of factor XI also promotes further α-thrombin generation (20). Factor XIa is able to activate factor IX and sustains factor Xa generation by the intrinsic tenase complex subsequent to inhibition of the tissue factor-factor VIIa complex through the action of TFPI (20). The constitutive protein Case anticoagulant pathway would also be initiated to regulate the extent of clot formation, hence mediating clot dissolution and subsequent repair of injured tissue (35, 189).

Analysis of the assembly of prothrombinase and intrinsic tenase complexes on phospholipid membranes and membrane-dependent substrate delivery to these complexes as well as the extrinsic tenase suggests the entire array of hemostatic enzyme complex reactions may interact on the same membrane (35, 143) (Fig. 1.9). The procoagulant vitamin K-dependent enzyme complexes are stabilized and exhibit large increases in cata-

lytic efficiency when interacting with the lipid surface (Table 1.2). In addition to more efficient generation of enzyme products, the intermediate products of the intrinsic and extrinsic tenase complexes would be transferred more rapidly in two dimensions on the membrane surface. Surface-dependent two-dimensional transfer of factor IXa and factor Xa between complexes would sufficiently increase the rate of intrinsic tenase and prothrombinase assembly and function to create the burst of α-thrombin required for clot formation (Fig. 1.9). Dissociation and reassociation of the enzyme constituents, factors IXa and Xa, would not only increase the time required for complex formation, but would expose free enzymes to inhibitors and dilution in circulation. Complex formation between enzyme and cofactor has also been shown to protect enzymes and cofactors from inactivation by circulating inhibitory proteins (64, 190–193) (see Chapter 3). The surface association of the blood coagulation process decreases the risk of enzyme product inhibition and loss of the products in the blood flow past the injured area. Channeled surface-dependent interactions increase catalytic efficiency, sequester enzyme products at the site of injury, and protect enzyme products from inhibition (35, 143).

The concept of membrane-dependent, interwoven reactions developed from synthetic phospholipid systems is supported, to a limited extent, by *in vitro* studies utilizing platelets as the membrane source and plasma concentrations of the participating protein components (194). The results of these studies indicate the tissue factor-factor VIIa complex activates minute quantities of

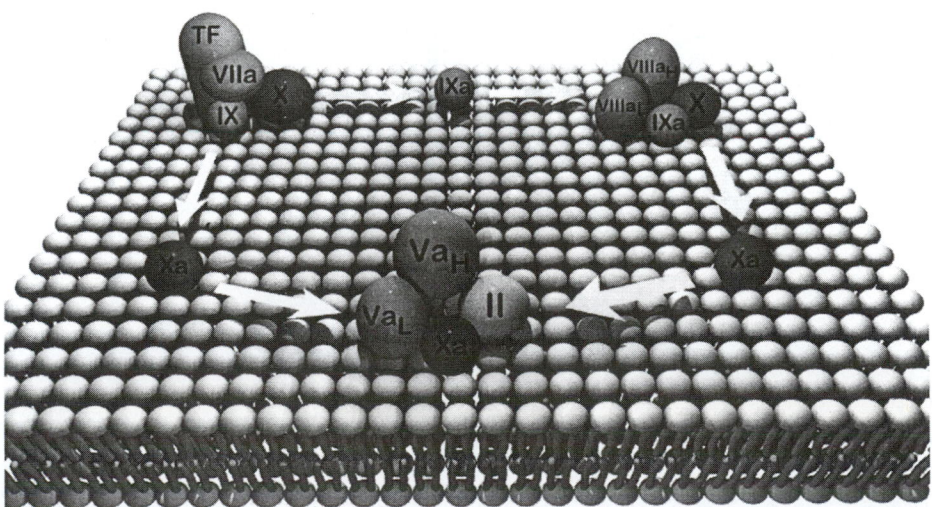

**FIGURE 1.9.** Illustration of the proposed mechanism of two-dimensional transfer of enzyme intermediates between membrane-dependent complexes. Factor IXa is transferred via membrane surface from the extrinsic tenase (tissue factor [TF]: factor VIIa) to factor VIIIa bound at a separate site on the membrane. The extrinsic tenase and intrinsic tenase complexes participate in activation of factor X and transfer of factor Xa to factor Va in the same lipid-dependent manner. Prothrombin (II)-membrane interactions are also important in efficient generation of α-thrombin. Diffusion of factor IXa and factor Xa enzymes along the lipid surface serves to accelerate the rate of complex assembly and protect the free enzymes from inactivation by circulating inhibitors.

factors IX and X. Factor Xa generates low levels of α-thrombin, which leads to platelet activation and presentation of the surface required for membrane-dependent complex assembly. Factor IXa, in complex with its cofactor, factor VIIIa, propagates α-thrombin production by activating higher levels of factor X and promoting prothrombinase complex formation (194). In this system, explosive α-thrombin generation is only observed when factor X and prothrombin are activated by the intrinsic tenase and prothrombinase complexes functioning in tandem on the same membrane surface (194).

## CELLULAR MEMBRANE SYSTEMS

The phospholipid-dependent model systems developed from experiments with synthetic vesicles have also been extended to other studies of cellular systems. Cellular systems provide levels of complexity not encountered with the synthetic model system because the cellular membranes not only express an equivalent to an anionic phospholipid surface, but also express one that is physiologically regulated to ensure appropriate and adequate expression of the hemostatic response. Regulation occurs before injury and during response to a challenge. The endothelium actively maintains a selective barrier between blood components and the subendothelium (195). However, numerous interactions between endothelial and subendothelial elements, platelets and other peripheral blood cells, and circulating procoagulant proteins must be choreographed to initiate the necessary hemostatic event when the endothelial barrier is breached.

Platelet membranes provide the most quantitatively abundant cellular surface for expression of the hemostatic response. Platelets are activated as part of the procoagulant response and a number of platelet agonists (e.g., ADP, serotonin, α-thrombin, and collagen) are present or generated at the site of vascular damage. Platelet adhesion and/or aggregation at the injury site minimally requires receptors for the adhesive molecules vWf, fibrinogen, and collagen (196) (see Chapter 11).

The semi-discoid platelets (197) undergo a dramatic morphological change in which the cells become spherical and extend numerous pseudopods when exposed to an agonist (198, 199). The morphological change is accompanied by a redistribution of the phospholipids in the platelet membrane (142). In the unstimulated state, the negatively charged phospholipids (phosphatidylserine and phosphatidylinositol) are almost exclusively located in the inner platelet membrane and not exposed to blood components. Upon activation, a transbilayer movement of anionic phospholipids is hypothesized to occur, which allows presentation of the requisite membrane surface for promotion of the procoagulant response (142). Platelet activation is also reported to involve shedding of small membranous particles, or mi-crovesicles, from the platelet surface (200, 201). The formation and function of these particles is not yet understood. Microvesicle shedding may be the result of the natural aging process of circulating platelets (202, 203) or the result of an underlying pathophysiology such as thrombocytopenia or cardiopulmonary bypass surgery (204–207). The platelet microvesicles support procoagulant activity (200, 201, 207–209) and may have a role in disseminated intravascular coagulation (204–207).

Scott syndrome (a defect in the platelet membrane that may cause hemorrhagic complications) is associated with lack of procoagulant sites on the activated platelet membrane (207, 210, 211). Platelets from an individual with Scott syndrome have a normal platelet phospholipid content but do not express sites for prothrombinase and intrinsic tenase complex assembly (210–212) or shed microvesicles upon stimulation (213). The individual with Scott syndrome demonstrated normal platelet secretion and aggregation, which indicates the bleeding disorder associated with the syndrome may result from abnormalities in the putative $Ca^{2+}$-mediated transbilayer movement of anionic phospholipids upon platelet stimulation (210–212). This platelet defect would decrease the anionic phospholipid components available for procoagulant complex assembly. Microvesicle formation may be linked to the transbilayer movement of phospholipids, and both processes may be directly associated with the support of coagulation events by the activated platelet membrane (213). Regardless of the mechanism, the normal platelet activation process provides a membrane surface functionally similar to synthetic PCPS vesicles.

Studies of the kinetics of prothrombinase complex assembly and function on platelet membranes have shown a more intricate mechanism than that reported for synthetic phospholipid vesicles. Not only do human platelets provide binding sites for factors V and Va, but they also possess an internal store that comprises 18 to 25% of the total available factor V pool (214). This platelet factor V pool is a key element of prothrombinase function *in vivo*. Factor V Quebec is a bleeding disorder characterized by normal levels of functional plasma factor V but reduced platelet factor V activity (215). The factor V Quebec defect results from proteolytic degradation of platelet factor V before release upon platelet activation (216). Although affected individuals have sufficient plasma factor V (66 to 75% of total available factor V) to saturate platelet binding sites, the lack of platelet factor V results in severe bleeding episodes (215). Release of platelet factor V directly to binding sites on the platelet membrane is an essential step in promoting coagulation.

In contrast, normal levels of platelet factor V without plasma factor V activity appear sufficient to ensure coagulation (217). An individual with an acquired immune inhibitor to factor V did not demonstrate bleeding abnormalities, even upon surgical challenge, despite a plasma factor V activity level of less than 1% of normal. The factor V pool in this individual's platelets was apparently inaccessible to the inhibitory antibody and was able to promote normal hemostasis (217).

Many studies have used bovine platelets that contain only 2 to 5% of the total bovine factor V pool to avoid complications presented by the large platelet reserve of factor V in human platelets (218). Direct binding measurements of bovine factors V and Va to activated bovine platelets indicate factor Va interacts with higher affinity than the procofactor, factor V (218). Bovine factor Va binds to approximately 900 high affinity sites ($K_d$ = 0.3 nM) and up to 3500 lower affinity sites ($K_d$ = 3.0 nM). The procofactor, however, only interacts with 800 to 900 lower affinity sites ($K_d$ = 3.0 nM). Factor Va can displace bound factor V completely, but factor V can displace only a small amount of factor Va from the lower affinity sites (218). The plasma concentration of factor V is close to 100 nM in the bovine system. This concentration is sufficient to suggest factor V may be associated with the bovine platelet membrane at all times *in vivo*. Procofactor activation would result in the higher affinity interaction demonstrated for factor Va (218). Bovine platelet activation does not appear to effect the binding interactions of the procofactor or cofactor (218). Factor Va also appears to form at least part of the receptor for factor Xa on the surface of bovine platelets (155). Although bovine platelets express an average of 2200 factor Va binding sites (high and low affinity sites), only 900 of these sites appear to be actively involved in functional complex assembly and α-thrombin production (155).

The general characteristics of prothrombinase complex assembly and function on platelet membranes and phospholipid vesicles appear to be similar. Factor Va forms at least part of the receptor for factor Xa on platelet membranes (219). The light chain of factor Va mediates the binding of the cofactor to platelets and mediates the factor Va-factor Xa interaction (220–223). However, evidence indicates specific receptors are expressed by cellular membranes that distinguish these cell membranes from those of synthetic model systems (224). First, factor Va interaction with the platelet membrane is of higher affinity than factor Va association with phospholipid vesicles. The latter factor Va-vesicle interaction ($K_d$ = 2.9 nM) (145), is equivalent to the lower affinity factor Va-bovine platelet interaction, but significantly higher affinity sites exist on bovine ($K_d$ = 0.3 nM) (218) and human ($K_d$ = 0.1 nM) (225) platelets. A separate and more complex class of binding sites may exist on the platelet membrane (224). This class of high-affinity receptors on bovine platelets is also specific for factor Va,

and factor V does not interact with these sites (218). Second, factors V and VIII do not compete for binding sites on the human platelet membrane (226). The procofactors are highly homologous and share the same requirements for phospholipid interaction. If these molecules bound solely to phospholipids present on the platelet surface, both proteins would bind indiscriminately and competitively. Separate binding sites for factors V and VIII may likewise exist on platelet membranes (226). Third, a monoclonal antibody has been identified that blocks factor Va interaction with the platelet membrane but has no effect on factor Va binding to phospholipid vesicles (227). Fourth, the binding of factor IXa is mediated by a specific receptor on the membranes of α-thrombin-activated human platelets (228, 229). Although these data may have alternative explanations, they do suggest the platelet membrane is a more complex system than a simple mixture of phospholipids (224).

Recent findings support theories on the complex nature of platelet membranes and the importance of the platelet activation event in hemostasis (230). Little factor Va binding is detected on the unactived human platelet surface. However, only trace levels (0.5 nM) of α-thrombin (insufficient for "conventional" platelet activation and release) are required for maximal factor Va binding. Approximately 6000 factor Va binding sites exist on the activated human platelet surface, and saturation of these sites requires platelet-released and plasma factor Va pools (230). Although factor Xa binding depends on factor Va binding, factor Va binding alone is not sufficient to promote factor Xa association with the human platelet membrane. A 20-fold higher concentration of α-thrombin (10 nM) is required for optimal factor Xa binding (approximately 2800 sites per platelet) with saturating concentrations of factor Va (230). Human platelets express effector cell protease receptor-1 (EPR-1) or an EPR-1-like molecule subsequent to activation with higher levels of α-thrombin (230). EPR-1 is reported to be a membrane-imbedded receptor for factor Xa (231–234). The platelet-expressed EPR-1 molecule and factor Va are proposed to form a heterodimer that functions as a membrane receptor for factor Xa (224, 230). A model of prothrombinase complex assembly on the human platelet membrane has been developed based on these observations. No association of factor Va or factor Xa with the platelet membrane occurs before platelet activation in this model. The binding of the cofactor and enzyme proteins each occur as distinct interactions dependent on the level of platelet activation subsequent to platelet stimulation. Factor Xa binding and prothrombinase function are only possible when EPR-1 has been expressed, and EPR-1 and factor Va interact to create the factor Xa receptor (230). Platelet activation and EPR-1 expression are key elements in establishing prothrombinase function on the human platelet membrane.

*In vivo*, platelets can adhere to extracellular matrix components exposed by damage to the endothelial cell layer without other stimulatory events (196). At least one of these molecules, vWf, promotes platelet adhesion without promoting the release of platelet protein stores (235). Under static conditions, platelets adhere to a vWf matrix and undergo a morphologic change, which includes extension of pseudopods, but do not release internal platelet protein stores (235). These vWf-adherent platelets support the same level of prothrombinase activity with and without α-thrombin stimulation (236). The morphologic changes that accompany adhesion may promote the expression of the procoagulant membrane surface and any other receptors required for prothrombinase complex assembly and function. Platelet adherence at sites of vascular damage may therefore play a key role by providing for prothrombinase activity before the generation of high levels of α-thrombin. The α-thrombin thus produced could then activate additional circulating platelets, adding to the platelet plug and increasing the number of potential prothrombinase sites (235, 236).

The intrinsic tenase complex also interacts with platelet membranes. Factor VIII binding is directly influenced by platelet activation (226), and the number of sites occupied by factor VIII increases 23-fold subsequent to platelet activation (226). Assays of intrinsic tenase activity indicate approximately 1000 functional sites on membranes of α-thrombin–activated human platelets (237).

Although factors V and VIII do not compete for binding sites on the platelet membrane (226), a reciprocal competition has been reported for factor Va and factor VIII (238). Low concentrations of factor Va (1–30 nM) enhance the binding of factor VIII and enhance the activity of the intrinsic tenase complex (238). Higher concentrations of factor Va have an inhibitory effect on factor VIII binding and intrinsic tenase activity. Factor VIII appears to have the same effects on factor Va binding and prothrombinase complex function (238). Interactions between factor Va and factor VIII may be important in modulating the procoagulant activity on platelet membranes (238). Platelet participation in the hemostatic response highlights the key features of the lipid-dependent mechanism: localization of the response to injured area, amplification of procoagulant activity, and interplay between the lipid-dependent complexes.

In contrast to the prothrombinase and intrinsic tenase complexes, which require plasma-derived cofactors to interact with cellular membranes and membrane receptor molecules, the cofactor protein of the extrinsic tenase, tissue factor, is expressed on cellular membranes in response to vascular injury (4, 21, 22). Tissue factor is constitutively expressed by cellular components of the subendothelium and exposed to factors VII and VIIa in the blood flow upon damage to the endothelium (23–25, 239). Endothelial cells and circulating monocytes may also express tissue factor in response to stimulation by inflammatory agents such as cytokines and immune complexes (29, 30). However, these cells require 4 to 8 hours *in vitro* to express maximal levels of tissue factor and return to a basal level of cofactor expression after 24 to 40 hours (29, 30). The tissue factor associated with the subendothelium most likely forms the procoagulant triggering complex with factor VIIa in response to vascular damage, while the tissue factor expressed on monocytes and endothelial cells may have a role in inflammatory reactions. The functional properties of the extrinsic tenase complex on stimulated, cultured umbilical vein endothelial cells appear to be identical to the properties of the complex assembled on synthetic phospholipid vesicles (240–246). *In vivo*, however, the activity of the complex is regulated.

## RECONSTITUTED "PLASMA" MODEL SYSTEMS

A reconstituted empirical model has been used for analyses of the procoagulant and anticoagulant activities in the hemostatic mechanism (19, 247, 248). The model consists of a mixture of procoagulant enzymes and cofactor precursors at average physiologic plasma concentrations in the presence of phospholipid vesicles and $Ca^{2+}$. The addition of the tissue factor-factor VIIa complex at preselected concentrations initiates the procoagulant process. This model illustrates the threshold-limited concept of blood coagulation: the levels of procoagulant reactants must reach a certain level, which is determined by the concentration of the extrinsic tenase trigger, before achieving the phase of explosive α-thrombin generation (19).

The extrinsic tenase role in factor Xa generation may also supersede the intrinsic tenase role under some conditions (19). At high concentrations of tissue factor-factor VIIa, production of factor Xa by the extrinsic route dominates production by the intrinsic complex (19). These data are in accord with the demonstration that high levels of recombinant factor VIIa will alleviate bleeding complications in individuals with hemophilia A (249, 250). Evidence that elevated levels of extrinsic tenase components are capable of superseding the intrinsic tenase role is also observed in the prothrombin time (PT) assay, which is a clinical clotting assay that measures the function of the extrinsic and common pathways. The assay is initiated by the addition of tissue factor (thromboplastin) and is insensitive to deficiencies in the intrinsic tenase components, factor VIII and factor IX. Overall, however, the reconstituted empirical model leads to the hypothesis that the expression or exposure of tissue factor *in vivo* with normal physiologic levels of procoagulant proteins is

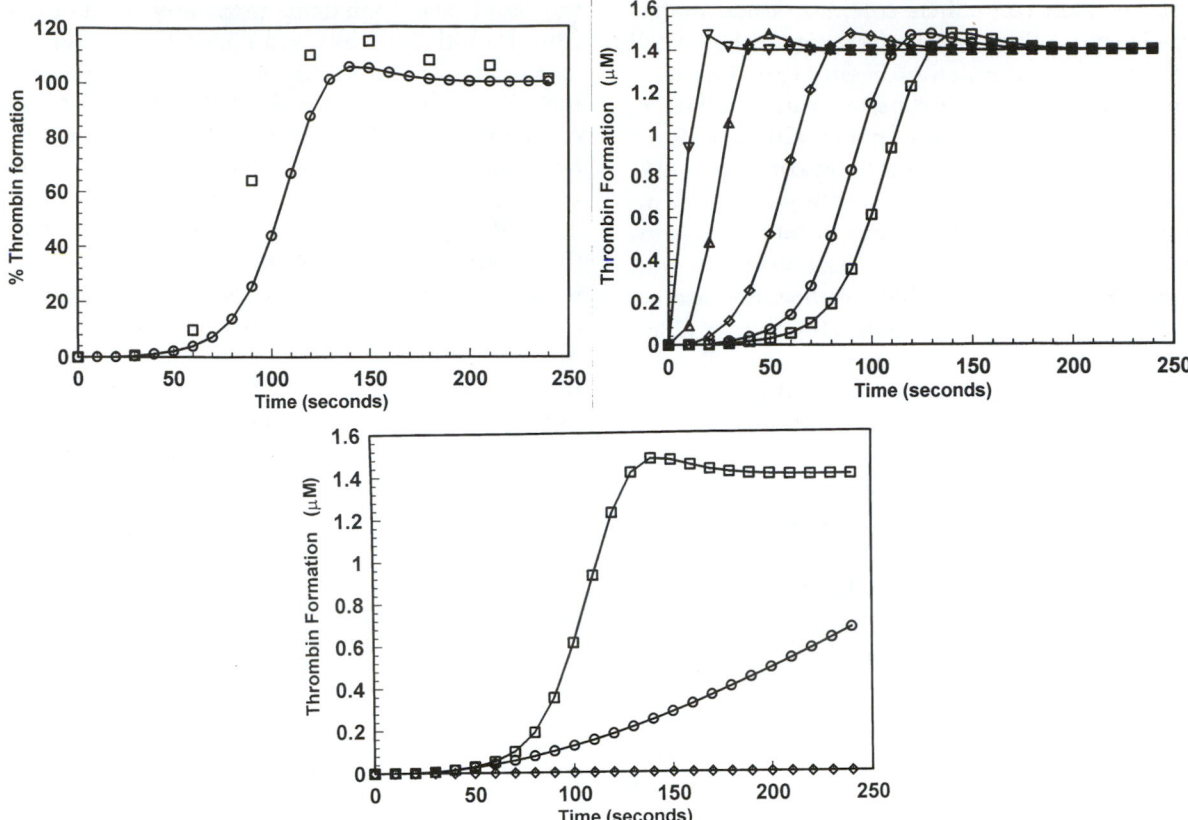

**FIGURE 1.10.** α-thrombin generation triggered by extrinsic tenase function as predicted by a theoretical model of the procoagulant event. A, A comparison of α-thrombin generation using the reconstituted empirical experimental system (□) and theoretical model (○). 5 pM Tissue factor-factor VIIa was used as the triggering catalyst for both model systems. B, Effect of varying tissue factor-factor VIIa concentration in the theoretical model. The concentration range included 5 pM (□), 10 pM (○), 50 pM (◇), 500 pM (△), and 5 nM (▽) tissue factor-factor VIIa. C, Theoretical simulation of factor V and factor VIII deficiencies. α-thrombin generation without factor VIII (○) and factor V (◇) was compared to α-thrombin generation with all protein components (□). (With permission from Jones KC, Mann KG. A model for the tissue factor pathway to thrombin. II. A mathematical simulation [published erratum appears in J Biol Chem 1995 Apr 14;270 (15):9026]. J Biol Chem 1994;269:23367–23373.)

the initiating step in the procoagulant reaction to injury and serves to launch activation of factors IX and X, factors V and VIII, and prothrombin (19).

Mathematical simulations of the procoagulant events in the clotting cascade have been developed from estimated and measured rate constants for the individual procoagulant reactions (251). These models provide reasonable approximations of procoagulant events initiated by a range of tissue factor-factor VIIa concentrations (5 pM to 5 nM) (Fig. 1.10).

The initial reconstituted plasma empirical system has been expanded to include the termination reactions of blood coagulation (252, 253). APC reduces the rate of α-thrombin generation without influencing the lag or initial phase of α-thrombin generation. Initial α-thrombin formation occurs within the same time frame regardless of the presence of elements of the protein C system. In contrast, TFPI, which shuts down the extrinsic tenase trigger of the coagulation response, is the major inhibitor

of the initiation phase of α-thrombin generation (247, 248). TFPI extends the lag phase leading to α-thrombin production and slightly reduces the rate of α-thrombin generation during the propagation phase. AT-III, the major serpin inhibitor, exerts its major influence in slowing thrombin generation and arresting the procoagulant event (247).

The protein C system TFPI and AT-III act synergistically in mediating α-thrombin generation (248). TFPI inactivates the tissue factor-factor VIIa-factor Xa trigger of coagulation limiting intrinsic tenase and prothrombinase activities. The APC subsequently formed and circulating AT-III inactivate factor Va, thrombin, factor Xa, and factor IXa. The complementary nature of these inhibitory processes effectively terminates α-thrombin production (247, 248).

Overall, the models suggest the following sequence of events in the procoagulant pathway initiated by the tissue factor-factor VIIa complex:

1. The tissue factor-factor VIIa complex activates factors IX and X. The steady state rate of factor IX activation is approximately 0.5 pM factor IXa/second. The rate of factor Xa generation, 1.0 pM factor Xa/second, is slightly higher. Changes in the level of procoagulant triggering complex reduces the lag phase of α-thrombin generation but does not influence the maximal rate of α-thrombin formation.

2. The factor Xa activated by the extrinsic tenase trigger of coagulation activates factor V to generate factor Va.

3. Factor Va complexes with factor Xa and generates traces of α-thrombin via the meizothrombin intermediate.

4. The initial formation of α-thrombin accelerates the activation of factor V and generates factor VIIIa.

5. Formation of the intrinsic tenase, factor VIIIa-factor IXa complex, enhances the rate of factor Xa generation. Acceleration of factor Xa generation sets the stage for the explosive formation of α-thrombin.

# WHOLE BLOOD CLOTTING

Most studies of clot formation in a blood or plasma milieu make use of chelators, which sequesters $Ca^{2+}$. However, since many of the molecular and cellular events in blood clotting are $Ca^{2+}$-dependent, the recalcification process influences the rates of cellular and enzymatic processes. We have developed a whole blood system in which the contact activation pathway is blocked, which permits studies of whole blood clotting initiated by exogenous tissue factor. The clot time is the endpoint of analyses for most clinical clot-based assays. However, most α-thrombin generation occurs subsequent to clot formation during whole blood coagulation induced by tissue factor. Significant levels of prothrombin remain uncleaved, which indicates the procoagulant event is terminated before a large fraction of the available zymogen is converted to α-thrombin. The initial fibrin-based clot is formed with incorporation of uncleaved fibrinogen and results with little α-thrombin (approximately 5 to 10 nM). Indeed, the concentration of prothrombinase

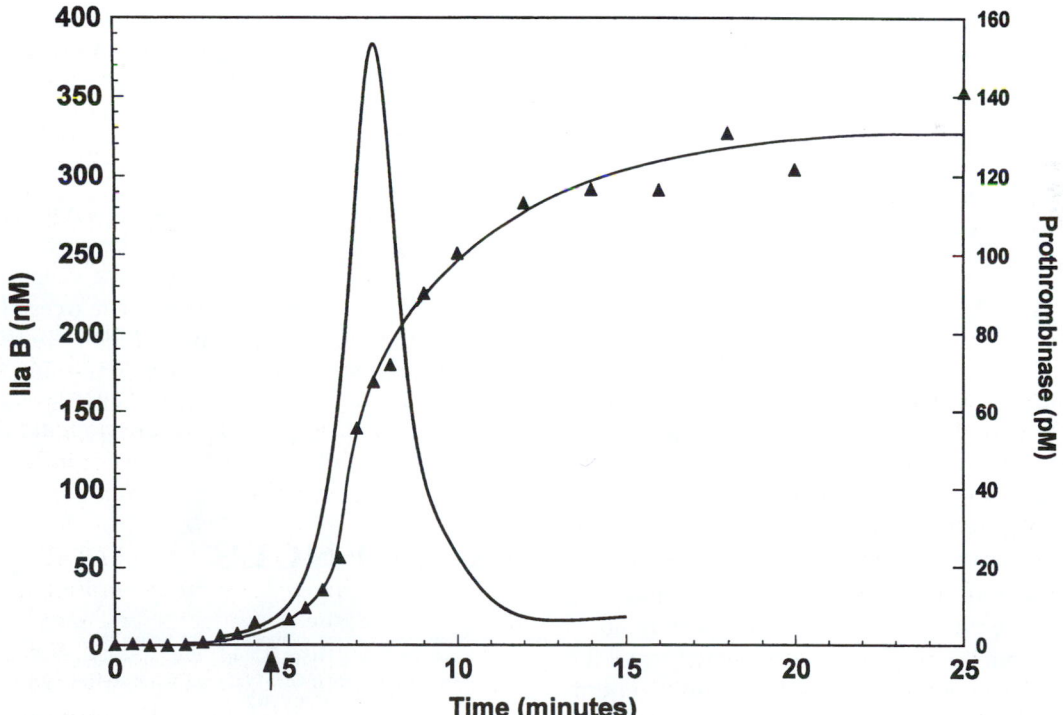

**FIGURE 1.11.** α-thrombin concentration and prothrombinase complex generation in the fluid phase of minimally altered clotting blood. The B-chain of α-thrombin, which contains the active site, was quantitated at time points throughout the blood clotting process (▲). The clot time (4.5 minutes) is indicated by the bold arrow. Maximum α-thrombin concentration (360 nM) is not reached until 60 minutes. The molar concentration of prothrombinase (solid line) is inferred from the generation of α-thrombin. (With permission from Rand MD, Lock JB, van't Veer C, et al. Blood clotting in minimally altered whole blood. Blood 1996;88:3432–3445.)

**TABLE 1.3.** Maximum Potential Enzyme Complex Concentrations and Observed Enzyme Complex Concentrations. The plasma protein concentrations of protein components of the vitamin K-dependent enzyme complexes were used to calculate the maximum possible catalyst concentration. The actual enzyme concentrations observed in the whole blood clotting system are listed for comparison.

| Catalyst | Protein | Plasma Concentrations (nM)[a] | Maximum Catalyst Concentrations (nM) | Observed Catalyst Concentrations (nM)[b] |
|---|---|---|---|---|
| Prothrombinase | Prothrombin | 1400 | 20 | 0.16 |
|  | Factor X | 170 |  |  |
|  | Factor V | 20 |  |  |
| Extrinsic tenase | Factor IX | 90 | 10 |  |
|  | Factor X | 170 |  |  |
|  | Factor VII | 10 |  |  |
|  | Tissue factor | — |  |  |
| Intrinsic tenase | Factor X | 170 | 0.7 | ≤0.001 |
|  | Factor IX | 90 |  |  |
|  | Factor VIII | 0.7 |  |  |

[a] *References for plasma concentrations of protein components: 11, 28, 40, 156, 254–256.*
[b] *Catalyst concentration observed at clot time in whole blood as recorded in Rand MD, Lock JB, van't Veer C, et al. Blood clotting in minimally altered whole blood. Blood 1996;88.*

complex formed at clot time is only 0.007 nM (Fig. 1.11) (253), and prothrombinase complex reaches a maximum of only 0.16 nM, a value achieved well after clot time (253) (Fig. 1.11). The maximal prothrombinase level appears to be only 1% of the potential concentration (20 nM) (Table 1.3). Approximately 50% of the platelet protein stores are released before clot formation.

The whole blood system, in combination with the other model systems, permits detailed relevant biological analyses of blood coagulation pathways.

# SUMMARY

Examination of the model systems and known clinical manifestations of protein deficiencies and defects shows hemostasis is achieved through complex interwoven interactions between cellular elements of the vascular system and the circulating procoagulant and anticoagulant components. Stimulation of the procoagulant response is a threshold-limited event in which the level of the response is triggered at limiting levels of the initiating components. Once the procoagulant initiator is sufficient, the membrane-dependent enzyme reactions of the propagation phase lead to explosive α-thrombin generation and clot formation. The membrane surface acts as a component of the multiprotein complexes and sequesters and protects the procoagulant enzymes from dilution and inhibition.

Initiation and propagation of coagulation also result in simultaneous activation and participation of its terminators. The constitutive inhibitory processes act syner-

gistically with the protein C pathway to limit α-thrombin activity. The elimination phase may also begin during termination to initiate breakdown of the clot and start the subsequent repair processes, which likewise may be dependent on α-thrombin activity.

The highly interactive subprocesses of the coagulation cascade function to ensure the procoagulant response is appropriate to the extent of vascular injury, localized only to the specific site of damage, and controlled to prevent systemic thrombus formation. Coincidental repair mechanisms return the vascular system to its actively antithrombotic state. The overall hemostatic cycle is thus able to maintain blood fluidity, prevent blood loss, and repair vascular damage effectively under all but the most extreme conditions involving absence of vital components of the procoagulant and anticoagulant complexes.

# REFERENCES

1. Mann KG. Normal hemostasis. In: Kelley WN, ed. Textbook of internal medicine. 2nd ed. Philadelphia: JB Lippincott, Co. 1992:1240–1245.
2. Davie EW, Ratnoff OD. Waterfall sequence for intrinsic blood clotting. Science 1964;145:1310–1312.
3. MacFarlane RG. An enzyme cascade in the blood clotting mechanism and its function as a biochemical amplifier. Nature 1964;202:498–499.
4. Nemerson Y. Tissue factor and hemostasis. Blood 1988;71:1–8.
5. Forman SD, Nemerson Y. Membrane-dependent coagulation reaction is independent of the concentration of phospholipid-bound substrate: fluid phase factor X regulates the extrinsic system. Proc Natl Acad Sci U S A 1986;83:4675–4679.
6. Bouma BN, Griffin JH. Human blood coagulation Factor XI. Purification, properties, and mechanism of activation by activated Factor XII. J Biol Chem 1977;252:6432–6437.

7. Fujikawa K, Heimark RL, Kurachi K et al. Activation of bovine factor XII (Hageman factor) by plasma kallikrein. Biochemistry 1980;19:1322–1330.

8. Hathaway WE, Belhasen LP, Hathaway HS. Evidence for a new plasma thromboplastin factor. I. Case report, coagulation studies and physiochemical properties. Blood 1965;26:521–532.

9. Colman RW, Bagdasarian A, Talamo RC et al. Williams Trait. Human kininogen deficiency with diminished levels of plasminogen proactivator and prekallikrein associated with abnormalities of the Hageman factor-dependent pathways. J Clin Invest 1975;56:1650–1662.

10. Hoak JC, Swanson LW, Warner ED et al. Myocardial infarction associated with severe factor XII deficiency. Lancet 1966;2:884–886.

11. Hoyer LW. Factor VIII. In: Colman RW, Hirsh J, Marder VJ et al, eds. Hemostasis and thrombosis: basic principles and clinical practice. Philadelphia: JB Lippincott, 1987:48–59.

12. Biggs R, Douglas AS, MacFarlane RG. Christmas disease: a condition previously mistaken for hemophilia. BMJ 1952;2:1378–1384.

13. Telfer TP, Denson KW, Wright DR. A "new" coagulation defect. Br J Haematol 1956;2:308–312.

14. Owren PA Jr, Cooper T. Parahemophilia. Arch Intern Med 1955;95:194–201.

15. Roberts HR, Foster PA. Inherited disorders of prothrombin conversion. In: Colman RW, Hirsh J, Marder VJ et al, eds. Hemostasis and thrombosis: basic principles and clinical practice. Philadelphia: JB Lippincott, 1987:162–181.

16. Rapaport SI, Proctor RR, Patch MJ et al. The mode of inheritance of PTA deficiency: evidence for the existence of major PTA deficiency and minor PTA deficiency. Blood 1961;18:149–155.

17. Sidi A, Seligsohn U, Jonas P et al. Factor XI deficiency: detection and management during urological surgery. J Urol 1978;119:528–530.

18. Schmaier AH, Silverberg M, Kaplan AP et al. Contact activation and its abnormalities. In: Colman RW, Hirsh J, Marder VJ et al, eds. Hemostasis and thrombosis: basic principles and clinical practice. Philadelphia: JB Lippincott, 1987:18–33.

19. Lawson JH, Kalafatis M, Stram S et al. A model for the tissue factor pathway to thrombin. J Biol Chem 1994;269:23357–23366.

20. Gailani D, Broze GJ Jr. Factor XI activation in a revised model of blood coagulation. Science 1991;253:909–912.

21. Edgington TS, Mackman N, Brand K et al. The structural biology of expression and function of tissue factor. Thromb Haemost 1991;66:67–79.

22. Nakagaki T, Foster DC, Berkner KL et al. Initiation of the extrinsic pathway of blood coagulation: evidence for the tissue factor-dependent autoactivation of human coagulation factor VII. Biochemistry 1991;30:10819–10824.

23. Drake TA, Morrissey JH, Edgington TS. Selective cellular expression of tissue factor in human tissues. Implications for disorders of hemostasis and thrombosis. Am J Pathol 1989;134:1087–1097.

24. Rodgers GM, Greenberg CS, Shuman MA. Characterization of the effects of cultured vascular cells on the activation of blood coagulation. Blood 1983;61:1155–1162.

25. Maynard JR, Dreyer BE, Stemerman MB et al. Tissue-factor coagulant activity of cultured human endothelial and smooth muscle cells and fibroblasts. Blood 1977;50:387–396.

26. Wilcox JN, Smith KM, Schwartz SM et al. Localization of tissue factor in the normal vessel wall and in the atherosclerotic plaque. Proc Natl Acad Sci U S A 1989;86:2839–2843.

27. Callander NS, Varki N, Rao LV. Immunohistochemical identification of tissue factor in solid tumors. Cancer 1992;70:1194–1201.

28. Fleck RA, Rao LV, Rapaport SI et al. Localization of human tissue factor antigen by immunostaining with monospecific, polyclonal anti-human tissue factor antibody. Thromb Res 1990;57:765–781.

29. Rodgers GM. Hemostatic properties of normal and perturbed vascular cells. FASEB J 1988;2:116–123.

30. Conkling PR, Greenberg CS, Weinberg JB. Tumor necrosis factor induces tissue factor-like activity in human leukemia cell line U937 and peripheral blood monocytes. Blood 1988;72:128–133.

31. Morrissey JH, Macik BG, Neuenschwander PF et al. Quantitation of activated factor VII levels in plasma using a tissue factor mutant selectively deficient in promoting factor VII activation. Blood 1993;81:734–744.

32. Kondo S, Kisiel W. Regulation of factor VIIa activity in plasma: evidence that antithrombin III is the sole plasma protease inhibitor of human factor VIIa. Thromb Res 1987;436:325–335.

33. Broze GJ Jr, Majerus PW. Purification and properties of human coagulation factor VII. J Biol Chem 1980;255:1242–1247.

34. Butenas S, Mann KG. Kinetics of human factor VII activation. Biochemistry 1996;35:1904–1910.

35. Kalafatis M, Swords NA, Rand MD et al. Membrane dependent reactions in blood coagulation: role of the vitamin K-dependent enzyme complexes. Biochem Biophys Acta 1994;1227:113–129.

36. Colman R, Marder VJ, Salzman EW et al. Plasma coagulation factors. In: Colman RW, Hirsh J, Marder VJ et al, eds. Hemostasis and thrombosis: basic principles and clinical practice. 3rd ed. Philadelphia: JB Lippincott, 1994:3–18.

37. Esmon CT, Sadowski JA, Suttie JW. A new carboxylation reaction. The vitamin K-dependent incorporation of $H^{14}CO_3^-$ into prothrombin. J Biol Chem 1975;250:4744–4748.

38. Mann KG. Prothrombin. Methods Enzymol 1976;45:123–156.

39. Nesheim ME, Abbott T, Jenny R et al. Evidence that the thrombin-catalyzed feedback cleavage of fragment 1.2 at Arg[154]-Ser[155] promotes the release of thrombin from the catalytic surface during the activation of bovine prothrombin. J Biol Chem 1988;263:1037–1044.

40. Thompson AR. Structure, function, and molecular defects of factor IX. Blood 1986;67:565–572.

41. Nelsestuen GL, Kisiel W, Di Scipio RG. Interaction of vitamin K-dependent proteins with membranes. Biochemistry 1978;17:2134–2138.

42. Mann KG, Jenny RJ, Krishnaswamy S. Cofactor proteins in the assembly and expression of blood clotting enzyme complexes. Annu Rev Biochem 1988;57:915–956.

43. Kane WH, Davie EW. Blood coagulation factors V and VIII: structural and functional similarities and their relationship to hemorrhagic and thrombotic disorders [Review]. Blood 1988;71:539–555.

44. Radcliffe R, Nemerson Y. Activation and control of factor VII by activated factor X and thrombin. J Biol Chem 1975;250:388–395.

45. Toole JJ, Knopf JL, Wozney JM et al. Molecular cloning of a cDNA encoding human antihaemophilic factor. Nature 1984;312:342–347.

46. Hill-Eubanks DC, Parker CG, Lollar P. Differential proteolytic activation of factor VIII-von Willebrand factor complex by thrombin. Proc Natl Acad Sci U S A 1989;86:6508–6512.

47. Eaton D, Rodriguez H, Vehar GA. Proteolytic processing of human factor VIII. Correlation of specific cleavages by thrombin, factor Xa and activated protein C with activation and inactivation of factor VIII coagulant activity. Biochemistry 1986;25:505–512.

48. Lollar P, Hill-Eubanks DC, Parker CG. Association of the factor VIII light chain with von Willebrand factor. J Biol Chem 1988;263:10451–10455.

49. Nesheim ME, Mann KG. Thrombin-catalyzed activation of single chain bovine factor V. J Biol Chem 1979;254:1326–1334.

50. Nesheim ME, Foster WB, Hewick R et al. Characterization of factor V activation intermediates. J Biol Chem 1984;259:3187–3196.

51. Suzuki K, Dahlback B, Stenflo J. Thrombin-catalyzed activation of human coagulation factor V. J Biol Chem 1982;257:6556–6564.

52. Naito K, Fujikawa K. Activation of human blood coagulation factor XI independent of factor XII. Factor XI is activated by thrombin and factor XIa in the presence of negatively charged surfaces. J Biol Chem 1991;266:7353–7358.

53. Lorand L, Konishi K. Activation of the fibrin stabilizing factor of plasma by thrombin. Arch Biochem Biophys 1964;105:58–67.

54. Roberts WW, Lorand L, Mockros LF. Viscoelastic properties of fibrin clots. Biorheology 1973;10:29–42.

55. Mockros LF, Roberts WW, Lorand L. Viscoelastic properties of ligation-inhibited fibrin clots. Biophys Chem 1974;2:164–169.

56. Shen LL, McDonagh RP, McDonagh J et al. Fibrin gel structure: influence of calcium and covalent crosslinking on the elasticity. Biochem Biophys Res Commun 1974;56:793–798.

57. Shen L, Lorand L. Contribution of fibrin stabilization to clot strength. Supplementation of factor XIII-deficient plasma with the purified zymogen. J Clin Invest 1983;71:1336–1341.

58. Lewis SD, Janus TJ, Lorand L et al. Regulation of formation of factor XIIIa by its fibrin substrates. Biochemistry 1985;24:6772–6777.

59. Naski MC, Lorand L, Shafer JA. Characterization of the kinetic pathway for fibrin promotion of α-thrombin-catalyzed activation of plasma factor XIII. Biochemistry 1991;30:934–941.

60. Hendriks D, Wang W, Scharpe S et al. Purification and characterization of a new arginine carboxypeptidase in human serum. Biochim Biophys Acta 1990;1034:86–92.

61. Eaton DL, Malloy BE, Tsai SP et al. Isolation, molecular cloning and partial characterization of a novel carboxypeptidase B from human plasma. J Biol Chem 1991;266:21833–21838.

62. Bajzar L, Manuel R, Nesheim ME. Purification and characterization of TAFI, a thrombin-activatable fibrinolysis inhibitor. J Biol Chem 1995;270:14477–14484.

63. Harper PL, Carrell RW. The Serpins. In: Bloom AL, Forbes CD, Thomas DP et al, eds. Haemostasis and thrombosis. New York: Churchill Livingston, 1997:641–653.

64. Rosenberg RD, Rosenberg JS. Natural anticoagulant mechanisms [Review]. J Clin Invest 1984;74:1–6.

65. Petersen TE, Dudek-Wojciechowska G, Sottrup-Jensen L et al. Primary structure of antithrombin-III (heparin cofactor). In: Collen D, Wiman B, Verstrate M, eds. The physiological inhibitors of coagulation and fibrinolysis. Amsterdam: Elsevier, 1979:43–54.

66. Lane DA, Olds RJ, Thein SL. Antithrombin and its deficiency. In: Bloom AL, Forbes CD, Thomas DP et al, eds. Haemostasis and thrombosis. 3rd ed. New York: Churchill Livingstone, 1994:655–670.

67. Olson ST, Bjork I, Shore JD. Kinetic characterization of heparin-catalyzed and uncatalyzed inhibition of blood coagulation proteinases by antithrombin. Methods Enzymol 1997;222:525–559.

68. Lindahl U, Backstrom G, Thunberg L et al. Evidence for a 3-0-sulfated D-glucosamine residue in the antithrombin-binding sequence of heparin. Proc Natl Acad Sci U S A 1980;77:6551–6555.

69. Casu B, Oreste P, Torri G et al. The structure of heparin oligosaccharide

fragments with high anti-(factor Xa) activity containing the minimal anti-thrombin III-binding sequence. Chemical and 13C nuclear-magnetic-resonance studies. Biochem J 1981;197:599–609.

70. Marcum JA, Rosenberg RD. Anticoagulantly active heparin-like molecules from vascular tissue. Biochemistry 1984;23:1730–1737.

71. Marcum JA, Rosenberg RD. Heparinlike molecules with anticoagulant activity are synthesized by cultured endothelial cells. Biochem Biophys Res Commun 1985;126:365–372.

72. Novotny WF, Brown SG, Miletich JP et al. Plasma antigen levels of the lipoprotein-associated coagulation inhibitor in individual samples. Blood 1991;78:387–393.

73. Wun TC, Kretzmer KK, Girard TJ et al. Cloning and characterization of cDNA coding for the lipoprotein-associated coagulation inhibitor shows that it consists of three tandem Kunitz-type inhibitory domains. J Biol Chem 1988;263:6001–6004.

74. Broze GJ Jr. Tissue-factor inhibitior is also a factor Xa inhibitor [Abstract]. Clin Res 1987;35:597.

75. Rapaport SI. The extrinsic pathway inhibitor: a regulator of tissue factor-dependent blood coagulation. Thromb Haemost 1991;66:6–15.

76. Broze GJ Jr, Warren LA, Novotny WF et al. The lipoprotein-associated coagulation inhibitor that inhibits the factor VII-tissue factor complex also inhibits factor Xa: insight into its possible mechanism of action. Blood 1988;71:335–343.

77. Dahlbäck B, Stenflo J. A natural anticoagulant pathway: Proteins C, S, C4b-binding protein and thrombomodulin. In: Bloom AL, Forbes CD, Thomas DP et al, eds. Haemostasis and thrombosis. 3rd ed. New York: Churchill Livingstone, 1994:671–698.

78. Esmon CT, Esmon NL, Le Bonniec BF et al. Protein C activation. Methods Enzymol 1993;222:359–385.

79. Canfield W, Nesheim ME, Kisiel W et al. Proteolytic inactivation of bovine factor Va by bovine activated protein C [Abstract]. Circulation 1978;210.

80. Walker FJ, Sexton PW, Esmon CT. The inhibition of blood coagulation by activated protein C through the selective inactivation of activated factor V. Biochim Biophys Acta 1979;571:333–342.

81. Suzuki K, Stenflo J, Dahlback B et al. Inactivation of human coagulation factor V by activated protein C. J Biol Chem 1983;258:1914–1920.

82. Guinto ER, Esmon CT. Loss of prothrombin and of factor Xa-factor Va interactions upon inactivation of factor Va by activated protein C. J Biol Chem 1984;259:13986–13992.

83. Fay PJ, Haidaris PJ, Smudzin TM. Human factor VIIIa subunit structure. Reconstitution of factor VIIIa from the isolated A1/A3-C1-C2 dimer and A2 subunit. J Biol Chem 1991;266:8957–8962.

84. Lollar P, Parker CG. pH-dependent denaturation of thrombin-activated porcine factor VIII. J Biol Chem 1990;265:1688–1692.

85. Lu D, Kalafatis M, Mann KG et al. Comparison of activated protein C/protein S-mediated inactivation of human factor VIII and factor V. Blood 1997;87:4708–4717.

86. Kalafatis M, Mann KG. Role of the membrane in the inactivation of factor Va by activated protein C. J Biol Chem 1993;268:27246–27257.

87. Kalafatis M, Rand MD, Mann KG. The mechanism of inactivation of human factor V and human factor Va by activated protein C. J Biol Chem 1994;269:31869–31880.

88. Esmon CT. The roles of protein C and thrombomodulin in the regulation of blood coagulation. J Biol Chem 1989;264:4743–4746.

89. Walker FJ, Fay PJ. Regulation of blood coagulation by the protein C system. FASEB J 1992;6:2561–2567.

90. Esmon CT. The regulation of natural anticoagulant pathways. Science 1987;235:1348–1352.

91. Di Scipio RG, Davie EW. Characterization of protein S, a ã-carboxy-glutamic acid containing protein from bovine and human plasma. Biochemistry 1979;18:899–904.

92. Walker FJ. Regulation of activated protein C by protein S. The role of phospholipid in factor Va inactivation. J Biol Chem 1981;256:11128–11131.

93. Dahlback B, Lundwall A, Stenflo J. Localization of thrombin cleavage sites in the aminoterminal region of bovine protein S. J Biol Chem 1986;261:5111–5115.

94. Schwarz HP, Fischer M, Hopmeier P et al. Plasma protein S deficiency in familial thrombotic disease. Blood 1984;64:1297–1300.

95. Comp PC, Esmon CT. Recurrent venous thromboembolism in individuals with a partial deficiency of protein S. N Engl J Med 1984;311:1525–1528.

96. Craig A, Taberner DA, Fisher AH et al. Type 1 protein S deficiency and skin necrosis. Postgrad Med J 1990;66:389–391.

97. Grimaudo V, Gueissaz F, Hauert J et al. Necrosis of skin induced by coumarin in an individual deficient in protein S. BMJ 1989;298:233–234.

98. Griffin JH, Evatt B, Zimmerman TS et al. Deficiency of protein C in congenital thrombotic disease. J Clin Invest 1981;68:1370–1373.

99. Bertina RM, Broekmans AW, van der Linden IK et al. Protein C deficiency in a Dutch family with thrombotic disease. Thromb Haemost 1982;48:1–5.

100. Bovill EG, Bauer KA, Dickerman JD et al. The clinical spectrum of heterozygous protein C deficiency in a large New England kindred. Blood 1989;73:712–717.

101. Thaler E, Lechner K. Antithrombin III deficiency and thromboembolism. Bailliere's Clinical Haematology 1981;10:369–390.

102. Demers C, Ginsberg JS, Hirsh J et al. Thrombosis in antithrombin-III-deficient persons. Report of a large kindred and literature Review. Ann Intern Med 1992;116:754–761.

103. Hathaway WE. Clinical aspects of antithrombin III deficiency. Semin Hematol 1991;28:19–23.

104. Sandset PM, Sirnes PA, Abildgaard U. Factor VII and extrinsic pathway inhibitor in acute coronary disease. Br J Haematol 1989;72:391–396.

105. Sandset PM, Warn-Cramer BJ, Rao LV et al. Depletion of extrinsic pathway inhibitor (EPI) sensitizes rabbits to disseminated intravascular coagulation induced with tissue factor: evidence supporting a physiologic role for EPI as a natural anticoagulant. Proc Natl Acad Sci U S A 1991;88:708–712.

106. Day KC, Hoffman LC, Palmier MO et al. Recombinant lipoprotein-associated coagulation inhibitor inhibits tissue thromboplastin-induced intravascular coagulation in the rabbit. Blood 1990;76:1538–1545.

107. Dahlback B, Carlsson M, Svensson PJ. Familial thrombophilia due to a previously unrecognized mechanism characterized by poor anticoagulant response to activated protein C: See attached. Proc Natl Acad Sci U S A 1993;90:1004–1008.

108. Bertina RM, Koeleman BP, Koster T et al. Mutation in blood coagulation factor V associated with resistance to activated protein C. Nature 1994;369:64–67.

109. Sun X, Evatt B, Griffin JH. Blood coagulation factor Va abnormality associated with resistance to activated protein C in venous thrombophilia. Blood 1994;83:3120–3125.

110. Koeleman BP, Reitsma PH, Allaart CF et al. Activated protein C resistance as an additional risk factor for thrombosis in protein C-deficient families. Blood 1994;84:1031–1035.

111. Rosendaal FR, Koster T, Vandenbroucke JP et al. High risk of thrombosis in individuals homozygous for factor V Leiden (activated protein C resistance). Blood 1995;85:1504–1508.

112. Kalafatis M, Bertina RM, Rand MD et al. Characterization of the molecular defect in factor V$^{R506Q}$. J Biol Chem 1995;270:4053–4057.

113. Collen D, Lijnen HR. Molecular basis of fibrinolysis, as relevant for thrombolytic therapy. Thromb Haemost 1995;74:167–171.

114. Henkin J, Marcotte P, Yang HC. The plasminogen-plasmin system. Prog Cardiovasc Dis 1991;34:135–164.

115. Ellis V, Pyke C, Eriksen J et al. The urokinase receptor: involvement in cell surface proteolysis and cancer invasion. Ann N Y Acad Sci 1992;667:13–31.

116. Hoylaerts M, Rijken DC, Lijnen HR et al. Kinetics of the activation of plasminogen by human tissue plasminogen activator. Role of fibrin. J Biol Chem 1982;257:2912–2919.

117. Markus G, Evers JL, Hobika GH. Comparison of some properties of native (Glu) and modified (Lys) human plasminogen. J Biol Chem 1978;253:733–739.

118. Markus G, Priore RL, Wissler FC. The binding of tranexamic acid to native (Glu) and modified (Lys) human plasminogen and its effect on conformation. J Biol Chem 1979;254:1211–1216.

119. Hajjar KA, Nachman RL. Endothelial cell-mediated conversion of Glu-plasminogen to Lys-plasminogen. Further evidence for assembly of the fibrinolytic system on the endothelial cell surface. J Clin Invest 1988;82:1769–1778.

120. Ellis V, Behrendt N, Dano K. Plasminogen activation by receptor-bound urokinase. A kinetic study with both cell-associated and isolated receptor. J Biol Chem 1991;266:12752–12758.

121. Miles LA, Plow EF. Binding and activation of plasminogen on the platelet surface. J Biol Chem 1985;260:4303–4311.

122. Blasi F, Behrendt N, Cubellis MV et al. The urokinase receptor and regulation of cell surface plasminogen activation. Cell Differentiation Development 1990;32:247–253.

123. Vaheri A, Stephens RW, Salonen EM et al. Plasminogen activation at the cell surface-matrix interface. Cell Differ Dev 1990;32:255–262.

124. Knudsen BS, Silverstein RL, Leung LL et al. Binding of plasminogen to extracellular matrix. J Biol Chem 1986;261:10765–10771.

125. Pryzdial EL, Bajzar L, Nesheim ME. Prothrombinase components can accelerate tissue plasminogen activator-catalyzed plasminogen activation. J Biol Chem 1995;270:17871–17877.

126. Lee CD, Mann KG. Activation/inactivation of human factor V by plasmin. Blood 1989;73:185–190.

127. Bajzar L, Nesheim ME, Tracy PB. The profibrinolytic effect of activated protein C in clots formed from plasma is TAFI-dependent. Blood 1996;88:2093–2100.

128. Bajzar L, Nesheim M. The effect of activated protein C on fibrinolysis in cell-free plasma can be attributed specifically to attenuation of prothrombin activation. J Biol Chem 1993;268:8608–8616.

129. Bar-Shavit R, Benezra M, Eldor A et al. Thrombin immobilized to extracellular matrix is a potent mitogen for vascular smooth muscle cells: nonenzymatic mode of action. Cell Regulation 1990;1:453–463.

130. Bar-Shavit R, Kahn AJ, Mann KG et al. Identification of a thrombin sequence with growth factor activity on macrophages. Proc Natl Acad Sci U S A 1986;83:976–980.

131. Singh JP, Chaikin MA, Stiles CD. Phylogenetic analysis of platelet-derived growth factor by radio-receptor assay. J Cell Biol 1982;95:667–671.

132. Huang JS, Huang SS, Deuel TF. Human platelet-derived growth factor: radioimmunoassay and discovery of specific plasma-binding protein. J Cell Biol 1983;97:383–388.

133. Antoniades HN, Scher CD, Stiles CD. Purification of human platelet-derived growth factor. Proc Natl Acad Sci U S A 1979;76:1809–1813.

134. Assoian RK, Komoriya A, Meyers CA et al. Transforming growth factor-beta in human platelets. Identifcation of a major storage site, purification, and characterization. J Biol Chem 1983;258:7155–7160.

135. Hsuan JJ. Transforming growth factors β. Br Med Bull 1989;45:425–437.

136. Oka Y, Orth DN. Human plasma epidermal growth factor/β-urogastrone is associated with blood platelets. J Clin Invest 1983;72:249–259.

137. Berk BC, Alexander RW. Vasoactive effects of growth factors. Biochem Pharmacol 1989;38:219–225.

138. Niewiarowski S, Holt JC, Cook JJ. Biochemistry and physiology of secreted platelet proteins. In: Colman RW, Hirsh J, Marder VJ et al, eds. Hemostasis and thrombosis: basic principles and clinical practice. Philadelphia: JB Lippincott, 1994:546–556.

139. Daniel TO, Gibbs VC, Milfay DF et al. Thrombin stimulates c-sis gene expression in microvascular endothelial cells. J Biol Chem 1986;261:9579–9582.

140. Kung C, Hayes E, Mann KG. A membrane-mediated catalytic event in prothrombin activation. J Biol Chem 1994;269:25838–25848.

141. Walsh PN. Platelet coagulant activities and hemostasis: a hypothesis. Blood 1974;43:597–605.

142. Bevers EM, Comfurius P, Zwaal RF. Changes in membrane phospholipid distribution during platelet activation. Biochim Biophys Acta 1983;736:57–66.

143. Mann KG, Nesheim ME, Church WR et al. Surface-dependent reactions of the vitamin K-dependent enzyme complexes. Blood 1990;76:1–16.

144. Papahadjopoulos D, Hanahan DJ. Observations on the interaction of phospholipids and certain clotting factors in prothrombin activator formation. Biochim Biophys Acta 1964;90:436–439.

145. Krishnaswamy S, Mann KG. The binding of factor Va to phospholipid vesicles. J Biol Chem 1988;263:5714–5723.

146. Ortel TL, Devore-Carter D, Quinn-Allen M et al. Deletion analysis of recombinant human factor V. J Biol Chem 1992;267:4189–4198.

147. Kalafatis M, Jenny RJ, Mann KG. Identification and characterization of a phospholipid-binding site of bovine factor Va. J Biol Chem 1990;265:21580–21589.

148. Lecompte MF, Krishnaswamy S, Mann KG et al. Membrane penetration of bovine factor V and Va detected by labeling with 5-iodonaphthalene-1-azide. J Biol Chem 1987;262:1935–1937.

149. Lecompte MF, Bouix G, Mann KG. Electrostatic and hydrophobic interactions are involved in factor Va binding to membranes containing acidic phospholipids. J Biol Chem 1994;269:1905–1910.

150. Krishnaswamy S, Jones KC, Mann KG. Prothrombinase complex assembly: Kinetic mechanism of enzyme assembly on phospholipid vesicles. J Biol Chem 1988;263:3823–3834.

151. Di Scipio RG, Hermodson MA, Yates SG et al. A comparison of human prothrombin, factor IX (Christmas factor), factor X (Stuart factor), and protein S. Biochemistry 1977;16:698–706.

152. Pryzdial EL, Mann KG. The association of coagulation factor Xa and factor Va. J Biol Chem 1991;266:8969–8977.

153. Nesheim ME, Taswell JB, Mann KG. The contribution of bovine factor V and factor Va to the activity of prothrombinase. J Biol Chem 1979;254:10952–10962.

154. Krishnaswamy S. Prothrombinase complex assembly. Contributions of protein-protein and protein-membrane interactions toward complex formation. J Biol Chem 1990;265:3708–3718.

155. Tracy PB, Nesheim ME, Mann KG. Coordinate binding of factor Va and factor Xa to the unstimulated platelet. J Biol Chem 1981;256:743–751.

156. Lundblad RL, Kingdon HS, Mann KG. Thrombin. Methods Enzymol 1976;45:156–176.

157. Kalafatis M, Xue J, Lawler CM et al. Contribution of the heavy and light chains of factor Va to the interaction with factor Xa. Biochemistry 1994;33:6538–6545.

158. Walker RK, Krishnaswamy S. The influence of factor Va on the active site of factor Xa. J Biol Chem 1993;268:13920–13929.

159. Nesheim ME, Tracy RP, Mann KG. "Clotspeed," a mathematical simulation of the functional properties of prothrombinase. J Biol Chem 1984;259:1447–1453.

160. Higgins DL, Callahan PJ, Prendergast FG et al. Lipid mobility in the assembly and expression of the activity of the prothrombinase complex. J Biol Chem 1985;260:3604–3612.

161. Jones ME, Lentz BR, Dombrose FA et al. Comparison of the abilities of synthetic and platelet-derived membranes to enhance thrombin formation. Thromb Res 1985;39:711–724.

162. Govers-Reimslag JW, Janssen MP, Zwall RF et al. Effect of membrane fluidity and fatty acid composition on the prothrombin-converting activity of phospholipid vesicles. Biochemistry 1992;31:10000–10008.

163. Krishnaswamy S, Mann KG, Nesheim ME. The prothrombinase-catalyzed activation of prothrombin proceeds through the intermediate meizithrombin in an ordered, sequential reaction. J Biol Chem 1986;261:8977–8984.

164. Heldebrant CM, Butkowski RJ, Bajaj SP et al. The activation of prothrombin. II. Partial reactions, physical and chemical characterization of the intermediates of activation. J Biol Chem 1973;248:7149–7163.

165. Malhotra OP, Nesheim ME, Mann KG. The kinetics of activation of normal and gamma-carboxyglutamic acid-deficient prothrombins. J Biol Chem 1985;260:279–287.

166. Giesen PLA, Willems GM, Hemker HC et al. Membrane-mediated assembly of the prothrombinase complex. J Biol Chem 1991;266:18720–18725.

167. Tans G, Janssen-Claessen T, Hemker HC et al. Meizothrombin formation during factor Xa-catalyzed prothrombin activation. J Biol Chem 1991;266:21864–21873.

168. Tans G, Nicolaes GA, Thomassen MC et al. Activation of human factor V by meizothrombin. J Biol Chem 1994;269:15969–15972.

169. Mann KG, Krishnaswamy S, Lawson JH. Surface-dependent hemostasis. Semin Hematol 1992;29:213–226.

170. Ahmad SS, Rawala-Sheikh R, Walsh PN. Components and assembly of the factor X activating complex. Semin Thromb Hemost 1992;18:311–323.

171. Lamphear BJ, Fay PJ. Factor IXa enhances reconstitution of factor VIIIa from isolated A2 subunit and A1/A3-C1-C2 dimer. J Biol Chem 1992;267:3725–3730.

172. Curtis JE, Helgerson SL, Parker ET et al. Isolation and characterization of thrombin-activated human factor VIII. J Biol Chem 1994;269:6246–6251.

173. Lollar P, Parker CG. Subunit structure of thrombin-activated porcine factor VIII. Biochemistry 1989;28:666–674.

174. Gilbert GE, Arena AA. Activation of the factor VIIIa-factor IXa enzyme complex of blood coagulation by membranes containing phosphatidyl-L-serine. J Biol Chem 1996;271:11120–11125.

175. Lawson JH, Butenas S, Mann KG. The evaluation of complex-dependent alterations in human factor VIIa. J Biol Chem 1992;267:4834–4843.

176. Lawson JH, Mann KG. Cooperative activation of human factor IX by the human extrinsic pathway of blood coagulation. J Biol Chem 1991;266:11317–11327.

177. Krishnaswamy S, Field KA, Edgington TS et al. Role of the membrane surface in the activation of human coagulation factor X. J Biol Chem 1992;267:26110–26120.

178. Ruf W, Rehemtulla A, Morrissey JH et al. Phospholipid-independent and -dependent interactions required for tissue factor receptor and cofactor function. J Biol Chem 1991;266:16256.

179. Fiore MM, Neuenschwander PF, Morrissey JH. The biochemical basis for the apparent defect of soluble mutant tissue factor in enhancing the proteolytic activities of factor VIIa. J Biol Chem 1994;269:143–149.

180. Rezaie AR, Neuenschwander PF, Morrissey JH et al. Analysis of the functions of the first epidermal growth factor-like domain of factor X. J Biol Chem 1993;268:8176–8180.

181. Neuenschwander PF, Morrissey JH. Roles of the membrane-interactive regions of factor VIIa and tissue factor. J Biol Chem 1994;269:8007–8013.

182. Nemerson Y, Repke D. Tissue factor accelerates the activation of coagulation factor VII: the role of a bifunctional coagulation cofactor. Thromb Res 1985;40:351–358.

183. Nemerson Y, Esnouf MP. Activation of a proteolytic system by a membrane lipoprotein: mechanism of action of tissue factor. Proc Natl Acad Sci U S A 1973;70:310–314.

184. Seligsohn U, Osterud B, Brown SF et al. Activation of human factor VII in plasma and in purified systems: roles of activated factor IX, kallikrein, and activated factor XII. J Clin Invest 1979;64:1056–1065.

185. Neuenschwander PF, Fiore MM, Morrissey JH. Factor VII autoactivation proceeds via interaction of distinct protease-cofactor and zymogen-cofactor complexes. Implications of a two-dimensional enzyme kinetic mechanism. J Biol Chem 1993;268:21489–21492.

186. Jesty J, Silverberg SA. Kinetics of the tissue factor-dependent activation of coagulation Factors IX and X in a bovine plasma system. J Biol Chem 1979;254:12337–12345.

187. Morrison SA, Jesty J. Tissue factor-dependent activation of tritium-labeled factor IX and factor X in human plasma. Blood 1984;63:1338–1347.

188. Osterud B, Rapaport SI. Activation of factor IX by the reaction product of tissue factor and factor VII: additional pathway for initiating blood coagulation. Proc Natl Acad Sci U S A 1977;74:5260–5264.

189. Kalafatis M, Mann KG. The coagulation explosion. Cerebrovascular Diseas 1995;5:93–97.

190. Lawson JH, Butenas S, Ribarik N et al. Complex-dependent inhibition of factor VIIa by antithrombin III and heparin. J Biol Chem 1993;268:767–770.

191. Shigematsu Y, Miyata T, Higashi S et al. Expression of human soluble tissue factor in yeast and enzymatic properties of its complex with factor VIIa. J Biol Chem 1992;267:21329–21337.

192. Rao LV, Rapaport SI, Hoang AD. Binding of factor VIIa to tissue factor permits rapid antithrombin III/heparin inhibition of factor VIIa. Blood 1993;81:2600–2607.

193. Hamamoto T, Yamamoto M, Nordfang O et al. Inhibitory properties of full-length and truncated recombinant tissue factor pathway inhibitor (TFPI). J Biol Chem 1993;268:8704–8710.

194. Hoffman M, Monroe DM, Oliver JA et al. Factors IXa and Xa play distinct roles in tissue factor-dependent initiation of coagulation. Blood 1995;86:1794–1801.

195. Stern D, Nawroth P, Handley D et al. An endothelial cell-dependent pathway of coagulation. Proc Natl Acad Sci U S A 1985;82:2523–2527.

196. Hawiger J, Steer ML, Salzman EW. Intracellular regulatory processes in platelets. In: Colman RW, Hirsh J, Marder VJ et al, eds. Hemostasis and thrombosis: basic principles and clinical practice. Philadelphia: JB Lippincott, 1987:710–725.

197. White JG. Platelet ultrastructure. In: Bloom AL, Forbes CD, Duncan PT et al, eds. Hemostasis and thrombosis. Churchill Livingstone, 1994:49–88.

198. White JG. Anatomy and structural organization of the platelet. In: Colman RW, Hirsh J, Marder VJ et al, eds. Hemostasis and thrombosis: basic principles and clinical practice. Philadelphia: JB Lippincott, 1994:397–413.

199. Nachmias VT. Platelet and megakaryocyte shape change: triggered alterations in the cytoskeleton [Review]. Semin Hematol 1983;20:261–281.

200. Bode AP, Sandberg H, Dombrose FA et al. Association of factor V activity with membranous vesicles released from human platelets: requirement for platelet stimulation. Thromb Res 1985;39:49–61.

201. Sandberg H, Bode AP, Dombrose FA et al. Expression of coagulant activity in human platelets: release of membranous vesicles providing platelet factor 1 and platelet factor 3. Thromb Res 1985;39:63–79.

202. George JN, Lewis PC. Studies on platelet plasma membranes. III. Membrane glycoprotein loss from circulating platelets in rabbits: inhibition of aspirin-dipyridamole and acceleration by thrombin. J Lab Clin Med 1978; 91:301–306.

203. Blajchman MA, Senyi AF, Hirsh J et al. Hemostatic function, survival, and membrane glycoprotein changes in young versus old rabbit platelets. J Clin Invest 1981;68:1289–1294.

204. Khan I, Zucker-Franklin D, Karpatkin S. Microthrombocytosis and platelet fragmentation associated with idiopathic/autoimmune thrombocytopenic purpura. Br J Haematol 1975;31:449–460.

205. Zucker-Franklin D, Karpatkin S. Red cell and platelet fragmentation in idiopathic autoimmune thrombocytopenic purpura. N Engl J Med 1977; 297:517–523.

206. George JN, Pickett EB, Saucerman S et al. Platelet surface glycoproteins. J Clin Invest 1986;78:340–348.

207. Warkentin TE, Hayward CP, Boshkov LK et al. Sera from individuals with heparin-induced thrombocytopenia generate platelet-derived microparticles with procoagulant activity: an explanation for the thrombotic complications of heparin-induced thrombocytopenia. Blood 1994;84:3691–3699.

208. Fox JE, Austin CD, Reynolds CC et al. Evidence that agonist-induced activation of calpain causes the shedding of procoagulant-containing microvesicles from the membrane of aggregating platelets. J Biol Chem 1991; 266:13289–13295.

209. Wiedmer T, Shattil SJ, Cunningham M et al. Role of calcium and calpain in complement-induced vesiculation of the platelet plasma membrane and in the exposure of the platelet factor Va receptor. Biochemistry 1990;29: 623–632.

210. Miletich JP, Kane WH, Hofmann SL et al. Deficiency of factor Xa-factor Va binding sites on the platelets of a individual with a bleeding disorder. Blood 1979;54:1015–1022.

211. Rosing J, Bevers EM, Comfurius P et al. Impaired factor X and prothrombin activation associated with decreased phospholipid exposure in platelets from a individual with a bleeding disorder. Blood 1985;65:1557–1561.

212. Weiss HJ, Vicic WJ, Lages BA et al. Isolated deficiency of platelet procoagulant activity. Am J Med 1979;67:206–213.

213. Sims PJ, Wiedmer T, Esmon CT et al. Assembly of the platelet prothrombinase complex is linked to vesiculation of the platelet plasma membrane. Studies in Scott syndrome: an isolated defect in platelet procoagulant activity. J Biol Chem 1989;264:17049–17057.

214. Tracy PB, Eide LL, Bowie EJ et al. Radioimmunoassay of factor V in human plasma and platelets. Blood 1982;60:59–63.

215. Tracy PB, Giles AR, Mann KG et al. Factor V (Quebec): a bleeding diathesis associated with a qualitative platelet Factor V deficiency. J Clin Invest 1984;74:1221–1228.

216. Janeway CM, Rivard GE, Tracy PB et al. Factor V Quebec revisited. Blood 1996;87:3571–3578.

217. Nesheim ME, Nichols WL, Cole TL et al. Isolation and study of an acquired inhibitor of human coagulation factor V. J Clin Invest 1986;77:405–415.

218. Tracy PB, Peterson JM, Nesheim ME et al. Interaction of coagulation factor V and factor Va with platelets. J Biol Chem 1979;254:10354–10361.

219. Saitoh M, Ishikawa T, Matsushima S et al. Selective inhibition of catalytic activity of smooth muscle myosin light chain kinase. J Biol Chem 1987; 262:7796–7801.

220. Higgins DL, Mann KG. The interaction of bovine factor V and factor V-derived peptides with phospholipid vesicles. J Biol Chem 1983;258: 6503–6508.

221. van de Waart P, Bruls H, Hemker HC et al. Interaction of bovine blood clotting factor Va and its subunits with phospholipid vesicles. Biochemistry 1983;22:2427–2432.

222. Tracy PB, Mann KG. Prothrombinase complex assembly on the platelet surface is mediated through the 74,000-dalton component of factor Va. Proc Natl Acad Sci U S A 1983;80:2380–2384.

223. Tucker MM, Foster WB, Katzmann JA et al. A monoclonal antibody which inhibits the factor Va:factor Xa interaction. J Biol Chem 1983;258: 1210–1214.

224. Nesheim ME, Furmaniak-Kazmierczak E, Henin C et al. On the existence of platelet receptors for factor V(a) and factor VIII (a) [Review]. Thromb Haemost 1993;70:80–86.

225. Tracy PB, Eide LL, Mann KG. Human prothrombinase complex assembly and function on isolated peripheral blood cell populations. J Biol Chem 1985;260:2119–2124.

226. Nesheim ME, Pittman DD, Wang JH et al. The binding of 35S-labeled recombinant factor VIII to activated and unactivated human platelets. J Biol Chem 1988;263:16467–16470.

227. Mann KG, Tracy PB. Platelet involvement in coagulation. In: Holmsen H, ed. Platelet responses and metabolism. Boca Raton: CRC Press, 1986: 297–324.

228. Ahmad SS, Rawala-Sheikh R, Walsh PN. Comparative interactions of factor IX and factor IXa with human platelets. J Biol Chem 1989;264: 3244–3251.

229. Ahmad SS, Rawala-Sheikh R, Walsh PN. Platelet receptor occupancy with factor IXa promotes factor X activation. J Biol Chem 1989;264:20012–20016.

230. Bouchard BA, Catcher CS, Thrash B et al. Effector cell protease receptor-1, a platelet activation-dependent membrane protein, regulates prothrombinase-catalyzed thrombin generation. J Biol Chem 1997;272:9244–9251.

231. Altieri DC, Edgington TS. Sequential receptor cascade for coagulation proteins on monocytes. Constitutive biosynthesis and functional prothrombinase acitivty of a membrane form of factor V/Va. J Biol Chem 1989;264: 2969–2972.

232. Altieri DC, Edgington TS. Identification of effector cell protease receptor-1. A leukocyte-distributed receptor for the serine protease factor Xa. J Immunol 1990;145:246–253.

233. Altieri DC, Stamnes SJ. Protease-dependent T cell activation: ligation of effector cell protease receptor-1 (EPR-1) stimulates lymphocyte proliferation. Cell Immunol 1994;155:372–383.

234. Bouchard BA, Shatos MA, Tracy PB. Human brain pericytes differentially regulate expression of procoagulant enzyme complexes comprising the extrinsic pathway of blood coagulation. Arterioscler Thromb Vasc Biol 1997;17:1–9.

235. Swords NA, Mann KG. The assembly of prothrombinase complex on adherent platelets. Arterioscler Thromb 1993;13:1602–1612.

236. Swords NA, Tracy PB, Mann KG. Intact platelet membranes, not platelet-released microvesicles, support the procoagulant activity of adherent platelets. Arterioscler Thromb 1993;13:1613–1622.

237. Rosing J, van Rijn JL, Bevers EM et al. The role of activated human platelets in prothrombin and factor X activation. Blood 1985;65:319–332.

238. Gilbert GE, Sims PJ, Wiedmer T et al. Platelet derived microparticles express high affinity receptors for factor VIII. J Biol Chem 1991;266: 17261–17268.

239. Nemerson Y, Bach R. Tissue factor revisited [Review]. Prog Hemost Thromb 1982;6:237–261.

240. Almdahl SM, Brox JH, Osterud B. Mononuclear phagocyte thromboplastin and endotoxin in individuals with secondary bacterial periotonitis. Scand J Gastroenterol 1987;22:914–918.

241. Morgan D, Edwards RL, Rickles FR. Monocyte procoagulant activity as a peripheral marker of clotting activation in cancer individuals [Review]. Haemostasis 1998;18:55–65.

242. Idell S, James KK, Levin EG et al. Local abnormalities in coagulation and fibrinolytic pathways predispose to alveolar fibrin deposition in the adult respiratory distress syndrome. J Clin Invest 1989;84:695–705.

243. Nygaard OP, Unneberg K, Reikeras O et al. Thromboplastin activity of blood monocytes after total hip replacement. Scand J Clin Lab Invest 1990; 50:183–186.

244. Rivers RP, Hathaway WE, Weston WL. The endotoxin-induced coagulant activity of human monocytes. Br J Haematol 1975;30:311–316.

245. Osterud B, Flaegstad T. Increased tissue thromboplastin activity in monocytes of individuals with meningococcal infection: related to an unfavorable prognosis. Thromb Haemost 1983;49:5–7.

246. Goodnight SH, Kenoyer G, Rapaport SI et al. Defibrination after brain-tissue destruction: a serious complication of head injury. N Engl J Med 1974;290:1043–1047.

247. van't Veer C, Mann KG. Regulation of tissue factor initiated thrombin generation by the stoichiometric inhibitors tissue factor pathway inhibitor, antithrombin-III, and heparin cofactor II. J Biol Chem 1997;272:4367–4377.

248. van't Veer C, Golden NJ, Kalafatis M et al. Inhibitory mechanism of the protein C pathway on tissue factor-induced thrombin generation: synergistic effect in combination with tissue factor pathway inhibitor. J Biol Chem 1997;272:In press.

249. Hedner U, Kisiel W. Use of human factor VIIa in the treatment of two hemophilia A individuals with high-titer inhibitors. J Clin Invest 1983;71: 1836–1841.

250. Hedner U, Glazer S, Pingel K et al. Successful use of recombinant factor VIIa in individual with severe haemophilia A during synovectomy [Letter]. Lancet 1988;2:1193.

251. Mann KG, Golden NJ, van't Veer C. Tissue factor pathway to thrombin: analyses of normal concentration variations in procoagulant and anticoagulant factors [Abstract]. Thromb Haemost 1997

252. Jones KC, Mann KG. A model for the tissue factor pathway to thrombin.

II. A mathematical simulation [published erratum appears in J Biol Chem 1995 Apr 14;270 (15):9026]. J Biol Chem 1994;269:23367–23373.

253. Rand MD, Lock JB, van't Veer C et al. Blood clotting in minimally altered whole blood. Blood 1996;88:3432–3445.

254. Nesheim ME, Katzmann JA, Tracy PB et al. Factor V [Review]. Methods Enzymol 1981;80:249–274.

255. Bajaj SP, Rapaport SI, Brown SF. Isolation and characterization of human factor VII. Activation of factor VII by factor Xa. J Biol Chem 1981;256:253–259.

256. Kisiel W, Davie EW. Isolation and characterization of bovine factor VII. Biochemistry 1975;14:4928–4934.

# CHAPTER 2

# MOLECULAR GENETICS OF BLOOD COAGULATION

Peter J. Larson and Katherine A. High

## INTRODUCTION

The determination of the amino acid sequences of the major procoagulant proteins was hampered for years by the fact that many of these proteins are present in plasma in very low concentrations. They are extremely labile, so that purification of amounts sufficient for protein sequencing proved a formidable task. Thus, the introduction of straightforward and universally applicable techniques for gene cloning represented a major advance in that it allowed the isolation of the genes encoding the blood coagulation factors. This task, begun in the early 1980s and essentially completed by the end of the decade, has allowed deduction of amino acid sequences from the cloned cDNAs, characterization of mutations responsible for inherited abnormalities, production of large quantities of recombinant protein for research and for therapeutic purposes, and the development of animal models of disease through transgenic and gene knockout technologies. It has also made possible the contemplation of a novel approach to the treatment of bleeding diatheses—that of gene transfer.

For all of the human coagulation factors, cDNA sequence and chromosomal localization are available (Table 2.1), and for most, complete genomic sequence as well. The study of the genes encoding the coagulation factors has shed light on the evolution of the clotting system; these data will be reviewed, as will the gene organization and the regulation of expression of these genes. Mechanisms by which mutations arise in the nucleotide sequence will also be discussed, and available databases of mutations reviewed.

## EVOLUTION OF COAGULATION

All organisms with a closed vascular system face the challenge of ensuring that any breach in the vascular tree does not result in exsanguination, and that the response to such a break does not result in thrombosis through the entire system. Thus, the human coagulation system has evolved, in part, to prevent the loss of intravascular fluid and formed elements of the blood after vascular injury while maintaining the fluid state of the blood. In more primitive organisms without closed circulatory systems, coagulation provides a defense against invading microorganisms. Analysis of the molecular evolution of blood coagulation and the complement system suggests that they arose from a single ancestral system that provided a dual defense against invading microorganisms and loss of body fluids. Without the complete characterization of the coagulation systems of lower animals, much of the current model of evolution of the coagulation system is speculative; however, determination of the coding sequences of the coagulation proteins and their alignment and codon usage has allowed an estimation of the order of appearance and age of divergence of some of these proteins.

Doolittle has proposed that the coagulation system of humans and higher mammals represents a progressive development and refinement of a primitive system in which disruption of the circulatory system resulted in the exposure of a "tissue factor" (1). This factor likely

**TABLE 2.1.** Chromosome Mapping of Human Coagulation Factor Genes

| Factor | Chromosomal Location | Reference |
|---|---|---|
| Fibrinogen γ-α-β | 4q23-q32 | Kant, et al, 1985 (19) |
| Prothrombin | 11p11-q12 | Royle, et al, 1987 (136) |
| Factor V | 1q21-q25 | Wang, et al, 1988 (137) |
| Factor VIII | Xq28 | Tantravahi, et al, 1986 (138) |
| | | Purello, et al, 1985 (139) |
| Factor IX | Xq27.1 | Camerino, et al, 1984 (140) |
| | | Purello, et al, 1985 (139) |
| Tissue Factor | 1p21-p22 | Kao, et al, 1988 (141) |
| Factor VII | 13q34-qter | DeGrouchy, et al, 1984 (142) |
| | | Cox and Gedde-Dahl, 1985 (143) |
| Factor X | 13q34-qter | DeGrouchy, et al, 1984 (142) |
| | | Scambler and Williamson, 1985 (144) |
| | | Royle, et al, 1986 (145) |
| Factor XI | 4q32-q35 | Kato, et al, 1989 (107) |
| Prekallikrein | 4q35 | Beaubien, et al, 1991 (106) |
| Factor XII | 5q33-qter | Royle, et al, 1988 (146) |
| Factor XIII | A: 6p24-p25 | A: Board, et al, 1988 (147) |
| | | A: Weisberg, et al, 1987 (148) |
| | B: 1q31-q32 | B: Webb, et al, 1989 (149) |
| High-molecular-weight kininogen | 3q26-qter | Cheung, et al, 1992 (150) |

evolved from a cytokine receptor based on the homology of human tissue factor to the interferon receptors (2), and was able to activate a circulating protein (a primitive prothrombin). Upon activation, the prothrombin-like protein formed the ligand for a receptor (like the thrombin receptor) on an effector cell in the circulation. Occupation of this receptor conferred on the effector cell the ability to clump with other "sticky white cells." This simple system blocked the loss of body fluid and attracted effector cells to sites of microbial invasion. Effector cell-mediated hemostasis is extant in modern coelomate animals such as the hydra (1). The addition of steps and modifications to this basic reaction has resulted in a hemostatic system that includes the formation of a protein gel, localization of reactions to an activated membrane surface, and increased regulation of coagulation both by additional activations of procoagulant and anticoagulant proteases, and by protein cofactors. The complement system diverged to provide a defense against cellular pathogens. The fibrinolytic system likely developed separately and early, as evidenced by its responsiveness to bacterial proteases.

The formation of a protein gel to effect hemostasis is a common feature of coagulation in vertebrates and some invertebrates. In crustaceans and arachnids, hemostatic systems have evolved in which a protein gel is formed as a vascular plug. Proteolysis is not involved in the crustacean system; rather the formation of cross-linked "fibrinogen" is the result of a transglutaminase

reaction. An unrelated system has evolved in arachnids in which a cascade of serine protease zymogen activations results in the cleavage of a target protein, coagulogen, which then forms a polymer, coagulin (3). This system, studied most extensively in the horseshoe crab, has other similarities to the coagulation cascade of vertebrates, such as the presence of mosaic proteases with modules related to those in the coagulation proteases of higher vertebrates, the cleavage of an arginyl-glycine bond in coagulogen by the final enzyme in the cascade (thrombin catalyzes the cleavage of arginyl-glycine bonds in the α and β chains of fibrinogen), and crosslinking of the resultant coagulin by a transglutaminase related to factor XIIIa. However, the arachnid system differs markedly from the vertebral coagulation system in that it is activated in response to bacterial endotoxins (4); the noncatalytic domains of the serine proteases are not related to vertebral coagulation serine proteases; and coagulogen is not homologous to vertebrate fibrinogen (3).

A zymogen present in the horseshoe crab clotting system provides evidence for the development of coagulation from an ancestral system with components of both the complement and coagulation systems (5). The endotoxin-sensitive horseshoe crab factor C has a noncatalytic portion that contains five complement B-type units, a growth factor domain, and a lectin domain (6). The catalytic domain is similar to that of prothrombin. It is likely that the complement system developed from a lectin-based recognition system, and, before the appearance of immunoglobulins, lectins fulfilled the role of recognition of invading microorganisms by binding to the polysaccharide components of their cell walls (7). Evidence for lectin-based recognition of foreign targets in humans includes the observations that lectins are capable of activating the complement system (7–9), and that lectins on the surface of cells in the reticuloendothelial system are important for the recognition of senescent desialated red cells (7). Sequence similarities between human complement serine proteases C1r and C1s and the closely related haptoglobin, a noncatalytic scavenger of free hemoglobin, suggest that the primitive complement system was composed of three components that recognized, lysed, and scavenged the toxic residua of target cells (5).

Based on evidence obtained during the past 40 years from experiments in comparative enzymology, protein purification and sequencing, the isolation of the genes for coagulation proteins and the computer-assisted alignment of their nucleotide sequences, it is likely that the coagulation proteases in vertebrates have evolved from a trypsin-like digestive enzyme by a series of gene duplications (10, 11). The genealogy of these events has been partially ordered through the analysis of acquisition of similar functional domains (1), by the codon usage for the active site serine (12), and through the determination of intron location in homologous genes, such as the three chains of fibrinogen and the vitamin K-dependent proteases (13–15) (Fig. 2.1). The promiscuous activity of the parent digestive protease became restricted in the coagulation enzymes by subsequent point mutations and the acquisition, through exon shuffling, of modules (or domains) from other proteins (1, 11). This specialization resulted in enzymes that effect limited proteolysis in which the protein substrates are not destroyed, but instead are modified to perform the more complex functions of physiologic regulation.

The importance of domain acquisition as an evolutionary mechanism is appreciated when one considers that most regulatory proteases have been constructed from modules common to other proteins (5). For example, a distinguishing feature of vertebrate coagulation is the localization of reactions to anionic membrane surfaces. This localization is the result of the acquisition of a calcium binding domain (Gla domain) in the vitamin K-dependent proteases and lipid binding of their cofactors (Fig. 2.2). These proteases have also acquired one or more epidermal growth factor (EGF)-like modules; EGF domains are althought to be involved in binding to other macromolecules such as cofactors, activators, or substrates. As compared to evolution by point mutation,

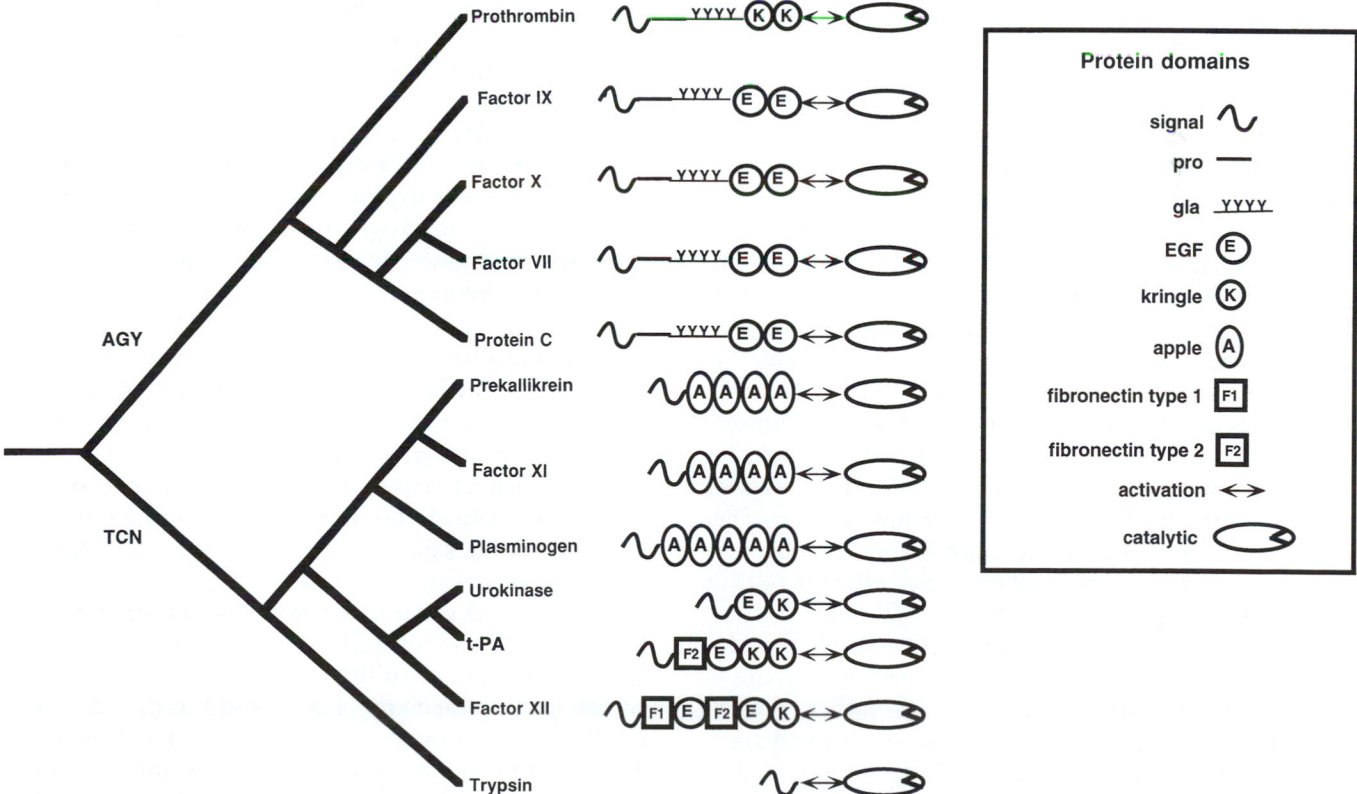

**FIGURE 2.1.** Proposed evolutionary divergence from an ancestral serine protease leading to the proteases of coagulation. (1, 5). AGY (AGY = AG[C or T]), TCN (TCN = TC [any nucleotide]) denote codon usage for the active site serine (5).

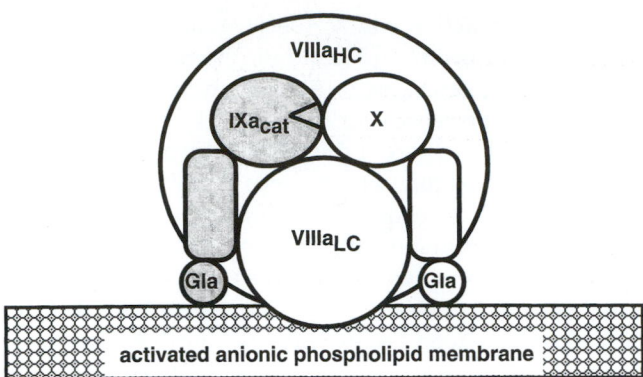

**FIGURE 2.2.** The activation of factor X by factor IXa (in the intrinsic tenase complex) is localized to activated anionic membrane surfaces by the calcium binding domains (Gla domains) of these vitamin K-dependent coagulation factors. The cofactor (factor VIIIa) is localized to the membrane surface through lipid binding by its light chain Gla domain. VIIIa$_{HC}$, factor VIIIa heavy chain; VIIIa$_{LC}$, factor VIIIa light chain, IXa$_{cat}$, catalytic domain of factor IXa. (Modified from Brandstetter H, Bauer M, Huber R, et al X-ray structure of clotting factor IXa: Active site and module structure related to Xase activity and hemophilia B. Proc Natl Acad Sci U S A 1995;92:9796–9800.)

the acquisition of additional protein modules immediately affords new specificity to the protein without abrogation of the original specificity or function. As a consequence of module acquisition, the noncatalytic domains of the coagulation proteases now comprise the larger portions of these proteins, rendering them more specific with respect to their activation and activity (5). In the cases of factors IX and X, further specificity and catalytic efficiency have been gained by interaction with the noncatalytic mosaic protein cofactors (factors V and VIII) (see Fig. 2.2).

The primitive fibrinogen was likely derived from an adhesive molecule (5). Cytotactin, an extracellular adhesion molecule (16, 17), and a second protein that is specific to cytotoxic T-lymphocytes (althought to serve as a cellular adhesive for target cells [18]) both share sequence homology with fibrinogen. An adhesive molecule that forms a hemostatic plug is also in keeping with the development of coagulation from a primitive system of defense against microbial invasion in which the adhesive protein would serve to immobilize bacteria and parasites and to enhance adherence of effector cells at sites of injury (5).

Human fibrinogen is composed of three homologous chains: Aα, Bβ, and γ. The genes encoding the α, β, and γ chains are closely linked to each other on chromosome 4, and they are likely to have resulted from duplication of a primitive adhesive protein gene (19). Three-chain fibrinogen is present in the most primitive extant vertebrates, such as the lamprey, but a molecule that is homologous to fibrinogen has not been identified

in invertebrates. Comparison of the amino acid structure of the three chains, however, suggests that the gene triplication occurred at a time corresponding to the divergence of plants and animals (5).

Without better characterization of lower vertebrate and invertebrate hemostatic and complement systems, the time scale of evolution of the human coagulation system remains uncertain (1, 5). Estimates for the appearance of proteins in human coagulation have been made based on analysis of sequence homology (20). The earliest proteins, including fibrinogen, prothrombin, and tissue factor were likely present 600 million years ago. Acquisition of the Gla and EGF-like domains and gene duplications resulted in the vitamin K-dependent factors VII and X approximately 500 million years ago. Factors V and XII appeared at the same time. Factor VIII, factor IX, and factor XI appeared about 450 million years ago, and the most recent divergence was prekallikrein from factor XI, 124 million years ago.

# GENE ORGANIZATION AND REGULATION OF EXPRESSION

## FIBRINOGEN

The regulatory mechanisms governing the expression of the closely linked genes encoding the three chains of fibrinogen are some of the best characterized of all human genes. The coordinate regulation of the expression of fibrinogen in the liver is of interest for two reasons. First, an increased risk of ischemic heart disease has been associated with high levels of circulating fibrinogen (21–24). Second, expression of fibrinogen, along with other hepatically synthesized proteins, such as haptoglobin, α-2 macroglobulin, and α-1 antitrypsin, is increased during infection and inflammatory processes; these proteins together are known as acute phase reactants.

The genes for each of the three chains of human fibrinogen are located within a 50-kb region on chromosome 4 (q23–q32). The degree of homology between, and the intronic organization of, the α, β, and γ genes suggest that they arose by successive duplication of a single ancestral gene more than 1 billion years ago (19, 25). A candidate ancestor gene has not been identified. The genes are organized in the order β-α-γ, centromere →telomere, with the α and γ genes transcribed toward the β gene.

Fibrinogen is a multimeric protein; each monomer consists of a single chain of α, β, and γ fibrinogen. Mature fibrinogen consists of two monomers that dimerize by association of all six chains at their amino termini (Fig. 2.3). Histologic evidence derived from transfected cell lines and from individuals with mutations affecting transcription of one of the fibrinogen genes demon-

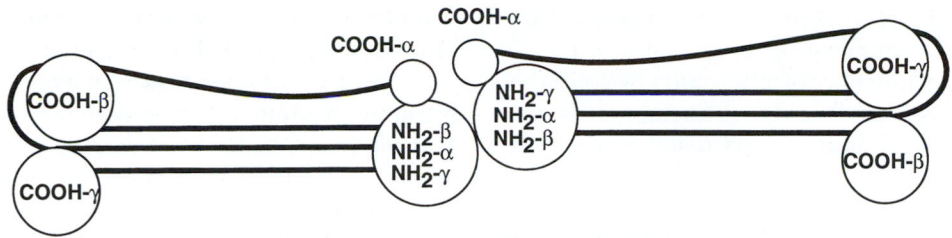

**FIGURE 2.3.** The structure of fibrinogen derived from electron microscopy and x-ray diffraction studies shows a central dimerization of two monomers each composed of heterotrimers formed from the association of single α, β, and γ chains. The aminotermini of the six polypeptides are represented by adjacent globular regions and are stabilized by three intermonomer disulfide bonds (one between the N-termini of the two β chains and two between the N-termini of the γ chains). The three chains of each monomer extend out from the central N-termini in a helical arrangement (denoted by parallel lines). The β and γ chains fold into globular domains at the distal ends of the molecule, whereas the hydrophilic C-terminus of each α chain folds centrally and together form a domain located above the N-termini. (Modified from Hoyer LW, Whyshock EG, Colman RW. Coagulation cofactors: Factors V and VIII. In: Colman RW, Hirsh J, Marder VJ, et al., eds. Hemostasis and thrombosis: Basic principles and clinical practice. 3d ed. Philadelphia: JB Lippincott, 1994;109–133.)

strates that the hepatocyte does not secrete improperly assembled fibrinogen (26–29). Overexpression of any of the three chains in a human hepatoma cell line increased transcription of the genes for the other two chains (30); the mechanism by which this up-regulation occurs is unknown. Studies of untransfected Hep G2 cells suggest that synthesis of β-fibrinogen is rate limiting for assembly of 6-chain mature fibrinogen (31, 32). *In vivo*, coordinate regulation of the three fibrinogen genes has been documented in studies of rats in which a 12.5-fold increase in hepatic mRNA of all three chains was observed to peak at 12 to 16 hours after defibrination with snake venom. This response depended partially on corticosteroid, as adrenalectomized rats had threefold to fourfold lower mRNA levels after defibrination (33).

There appears to be no region similar to the locus control region of the hemoglobin genes governing the expression of fibrinogen. The coordinate regulation of expression of the three genes is instead due to similar *cis*-acting transcription control elements in their respective promoters (34, 35). Each of the three genes possesses a TATA sequence (35–37), a conserved element that allows accurate and efficient transcription by RNA polymerase II.

Hepatic specific expression depends on the presence, in the α and β genes, of *cis* sequences that bind HNF-1, a hepatic-specific transcription factor first identified by Courtois et al in a study of the rat β-fibrinogen gene (38). Because HNF-1 expression is not restricted to the liver, the HNF-1 binding site is insufficient to limit the synthesis of the α and β chains to the liver. Indeed, HNF-1 is also expressed in the kidney, and α and β transcripts have been identified in renal tissue (39). A recently described HNF-1 cofactor (DCoH) may be required to confer liver specificity to the α and β genes (40). The γ transcript has been found in liver, brain, lung, and marrow by Northern analysis (41, 42). Although

γ chain expression is not limited to the liver, hepatic synthesis in the human gene is supported by an upstream stimulatory factor (USF) binding site approximately 70 bases 5′ to the transcription start site (35). As with the observed transcription of α and β genes in the kidney, the significance of extrahepatic transcription of the γ gene is not known. A recent study of cultured lung epithelial cells in the presence of interleukin (IL)-6 and dexamethasone demonstrated up-regulation of transcription of Aα and Bβ genes and the secretion of intact three-chain fibrinogen. This work suggests that local inflammatory processes can induce the production of fibrinogen that may in turn play a role in wound repair (43).

Each of the three fibrinogen genes possesses a single type II IL-6 responsive sequence that mediates the increase in fibrinogen expression observed with infection or inflammation (acute phase response) (35–37, 44). In the promoters of the α and β genes, the IL-6 site is adjacent to a C/EBP site (36, 37, 44), and in the case of the α gene, IL-6 response requires that both sites be intact (37). A C/EBP consensus binding site has not been identified in the promoter of the γ chain gene.

Other elements have been identified in the three promoters (35). A glucocorticoid response element has been localized between 1 and 3 kb from the start site of transcription in the β gene. Both positive and negative regulatory *cis* elements are present in the α and β genes. There is an AGGA motif 50 bases 5′ to the IL-6 site in the γ gene that exerts a negative influence on transcription (35). Sequences in the γ promoter adjacent to the CAAT site bind to the adenovirus major late transcriptional protein (45).

The γ transcript undergoes alternative processing that results in two species—the predominant shorter species and a second species elongated by 16 amino acids. This longer species arises from an alternative polyadenylation signal present in intron 8 (46, 47). Plasma fibrinogen contains $\gamma:\gamma'$ chains at a 9:1 ratio ($\gamma:\gamma'$) (47–49). The function of alternatively spliced $\gamma$ chain and fibrinogen containing $\gamma'$-fibrinogen is unknown. The additional amino acids result in a highly charged carboxylterminus with 7 acidic and 1 basic amino acids (overall charge = −6) (46, 49). It has been hypothesized that this highly charged terminus may prevent uptake of $\gamma'$-containing fibrinogen into platelets, thus accounting for the absence of this fibrinogen species in platelets (50).

## VITAMIN K-DEPENDENT PROCOAGULANT PROTEINS AND OTHER SERINE PROTEASES

The liver is the major site of synthesis of the vitamin K-dependent procoagulant proteins, but recent experimental data have disproven the longstanding assumption that they are expressed exclusively in the liver. Northern analysis demonstrates that both prothrombin (51) and factor X (52) are expressed at low levels in other tissues, including uterus, placenta, kidney, spleen, and small intestine for prothrombin, and lung, heart, ovary, and small intestine for factor X. Factor VII (53) and factor IX (54), however, are expressed exclusively in the liver. The significance of extrahepatic expression of prothrombin and factor X is unclear, but the recent discovery of widely distributed specific cell surface receptors that activate intracellular signaling cascades (G protein-coupled receptors for thrombin [55], EPR-1 for factor Xa [56]) after occupation of the receptors by these proteins suggests that they may have physiologic roles beyond those already delineated in coagulation.

For both prothrombin and factor X, levels of mRNA expression in liver are tenfold to twentyfold higher than in other tissues, and, as noted above, factors VII and IX are expressed exclusively in the liver. Thus expression of the first two is liver-predominant, and that of the latter two is liver-restricted. Most often, tissue specific expression is controlled at the level of transcription (57), although alternative mechanisms exist (for example, transcript stability, translational efficiency). As noted earlier, control at the level of transcription results from the interaction of specific nuclear proteins (transcription factors and coactivators, collectively referred to as trans-acting factors) and elements in the DNA sequence to which they bind (cis elements). For all four of the vitamin K-dependent procoagulant proteins, expression in liver depends on the binding of both liver-enriched and ubiquitous transcription factors to specific sequences in the 5' flanking regions of the genes (Fig. 2.4). In the case of prothrombin, an HNF-1 binding site is present at $-887 \rightarrow -875$, and additional protein binding sites are found in the region between $-919 \rightarrow -790$, although the cognate binding proteins are not yet identified (58, 59). The promoters of factors VII, IX, and X have

been more extensively characterized; they all contain a binding site for HNF-4, a member of the nuclear receptor superfamily that is expressed in liver, kidney, and small intestine. An intact HNF-4 site is critical for expression of these genes, as demonstrated by in vitro reporter gene assays, and in the case of factors VII and IX, by the occurrence of severe clotting factor deficiencies in individuals with mutations at these sites (60–62). Except for the HNF-4 binding site, these promoters have little in common. The factor VII and factor X promoters both have binding sites for the ubiquitous transcription factor Sp1, and the promoters of factor IX and factor X contain the cis element 5'-CCAAT-3', although this cis element binds NF-IL in the factor IX promoter (63) and the unrelated transcription factor NF-Y in the factor X promoter (52).

Many examples exist of disease due to mutations in the promoter regions of genes; indeed, mutations in the globin gene promoter that give rise to thalassemia were instrumental in defining the critical elements of Pol II promoters (64). The field of blood coagulation can lay claim to what is arguably the most fascinating of all promoter mutations, the hemophilia B Leyden variants. The unique feature of these variants is that individuals exhibit "recovery" from severe hemophilia with the onset of puberty. Thus the disease is characterized by the absence of factor IX expression in childhood (factor IX levels less than 2%), and a gradual rise in factor IX levels after the onset of puberty (~4 to 5% per year until the age of 20 or so, reaching a stable maximum of 30 to 60%). The hemophilia B Leyden variants were first described in 1970 (65); the same group published a more extensive longitudinal study of eight related individuals in 1982 (66) (Fig. 2.5). Affected individuals demonstrate concordance of factor IX antigen and activity levels throughout the course of the disease. The relationship of the recovery phenomenon to androgens was explored in a clinical study carried out by Bri't et al (67), who documented that short-term treatment with testosterone elevated the factor IX level to 5% in a child with hemophilia B Leyden, as did treatment with anabolic steroids (levels rose to 10 to 15%). Mutation detection in individuals with hemophilia B Leyden has revealed a heterogeneous group of mutations, all clustered at the 5' end of the gene. Defects at −21 (61), −20 (62, 68), −6 (69, 70), −5 (71), +6 (72), +8 (73), and +13 (74–76) have been reported (77). These mutations fall into three different protein-binding domains (see Fig. 2.4), but all display a similar phenotype.

The absence of factor IX expression during childhood in these individuals is theoretically straightforward to explain, inasmuch as all the mutations disrupt protein binding sites in the 5' flanking sequence, but the pathophysiologic basis for the gradual recovery after the onset of puberty has been more difficult to establish. An early hypothesis proposed by Crossley et al (78) was

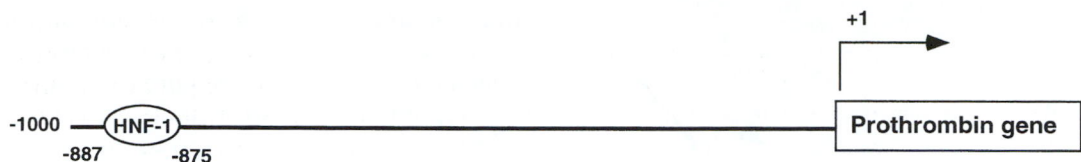

**A. Prothrombin promoter**

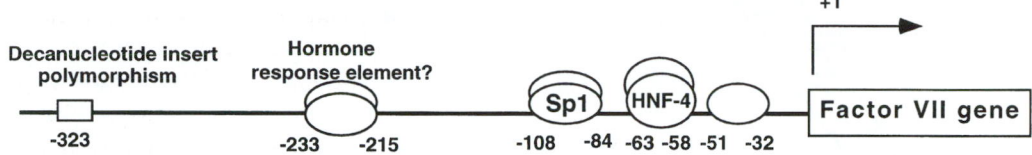

**B. Factor VII promoter**

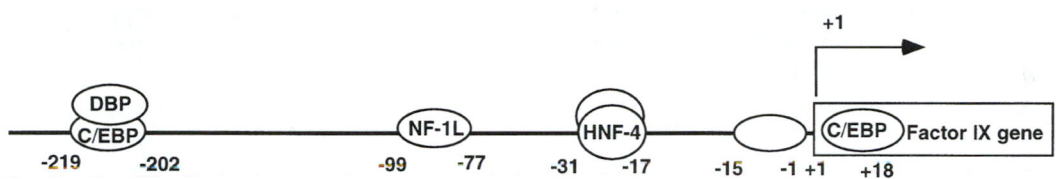

**C. Factor IX promoter**

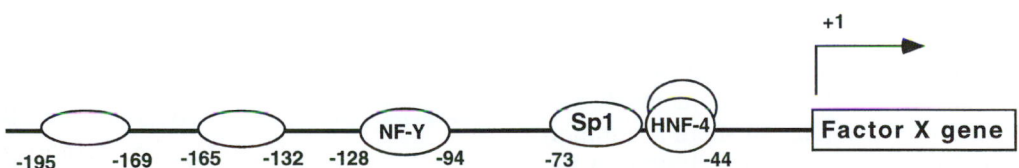

**D. Factor X promoter**

**FIGURE 2.4.**   Identified regulatory elements in the promoters of prothrombin, factor VII, factor IX, and factor X. Lines represent 5′ flanking sequences, ellipses denote protein-binding sites in the DNA sequence, and labels within ellipses denote the proteins that bind at these sites. Unlabeled ellipses denote sites that bind as yet unidentified proteins. HNF-1, hepatocyte nuclear factor 1: *DBP,* D site binding protein; *C/EBP,* CCAAT/enhancer binding protein; *NF-1L,* nuclear factor-1, liver; *HNF-4,* hepatocyte nuclear factor 4; *NF-Y,* nuclear factor Y. **A,** Prothrombin promoter. The cognate proteins that bind at the more proximal site (see text) have not been identified. **B,** Factor VII promoter. The presence of the decanucleotide insert is associated with reduced promoter activity (53); the protein binding sequence at −233 to −215 has homology to nuclear hormone receptor response element; the protein binding at −51 to −32 has not been identified. **C,** Factor IX promoter: D-site binding protein is although to enhance binding of C/EBP at the distal site. The protein that binds at the −15 to −1 site has not been identified. Note the presence of a C/EBP binding site within the 5′ untranslated region. **D,** Factor X promoter: methylation interference data suggest that HNF-4 and Sp1 bind at overlapping sites and compete for the binding site. NF-Y is a ubiquitous transcription factor. The proteins that bind at the two upstream sites have not yet been identified.

that the effects of a weak androgen-response element located at −36 to −22 become apparent when a mutation within this region abolishes binding of HNF-4 (see Fig. 2.4). Such a hypothesis does not account for the recovery seen in Leyden mutations that fall outside the HNF-4 binding site. An alternate hypothesis proposed by Lillicrap et al (71) is that the D-site binding protein, which is developmentally regulated in the rat, with expression commencing at puberty, enhances the binding of C/EBP to its cognate site at −219 to −202, result-

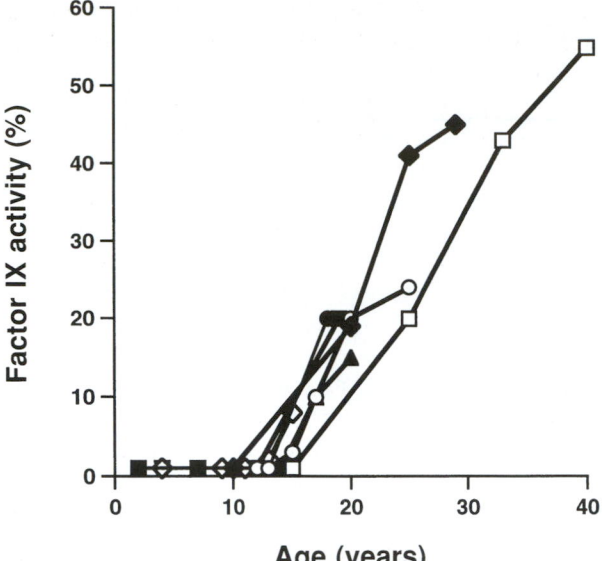

**FIGURE 2.5.** Factor IX levels measured over time in eight individuals with Leyden variant hemophilia B. These mutations in the promoter result in severe factor IX deficiency until puberty when factor IX levels rise gradually to approximately 30%. (Adapted from Bri't E, Bertina RM, Van Tilburg NH, et al Haemophilia B Leyden: A sex-linked hereditary disorder that improves after puberty. N Engl J Med 1982;306:788–790.)

ing in improved factor IX expression postpuberty. This hypothesis has the advantage of accounting for all genotypes so far encountered. Whether either, or both, of these is correct remains to be established.

The proteolytic enzymes of the clotting cascade, including prekallikrein, factor XII, factor XI, factor IX, factor VII, factor X, and prothrombin, all share a common structure (see Fig. 2.1), with a catalytic domain at the carboxyterminus of the protein. This catalytic domain is a serine protease, homologous to the digestive enzyme trypsin. Like trypsin, the active site of these enzymes is composed of a catalytic triad containing histidine, aspartate, and serine in a precise spatial arrangement; the coagulation enzymes cleave peptide bonds by a mechanism similar to that of trypsin (79). In contrast to trypsin, however, which cleaves peptide bonds indiscriminately, the clotting enzymes display a remarkable substrate specificity. The enzymes are secreted into the plasma as zymogens or inactive precursors; exposure of the active site requires proteolysis of a specific peptide bond within the activation peptide, a short sequence located between the aminoterminus and the catalytic domain (see Fig. 2.1).

A subset of the serine proteases, factors II, VII, IX, and X, are distinguished by the presence of an unusual posttranslational modification, the addition of a carboxyl group to the γ-carbon of glutamic acid residues in the aminoterminus of the protein. This reaction is catalyzed by the enzyme γ-glutamylcarboxylase and re-

quires vitamin K as a cofactor (80). These γ-carboxyglutamic acid residues, known as Gla residues, generate a negative charge that is required for calcium binding; calcium binding in turn induces a conformational change in the protein that exposes phospholipid binding sites, thus allowing localization of reactions onto a membrane surface. The exon-intron organization of these four proteins is similar, especially for factors VII, IX, and X. Indeed, the genes for factor VII and X are located directly adjacent to one another on chromosome 13 and appear to have arisen by gene duplication. The exons of factors VII, IX, and X correlate in an approximate way with the domains of the protein; thus exon 1 encodes the signal sequence, exon 2 the propeptide and the Gla domain, exon 3 an aromatic acid-rich connecting sequence, exons 4 and 5 the two epidermal growth factor-like domains, exon 6 the activation peptide, and exon 7 and 8 the catalytic domain (and in the case of factor IX, the long 3' untranslated region). The gene organization for prothrombin, including the placement of intervening sequences, is similar for the first three exons, but then diverges, with exon 4 encoding a cysteine loop, exons 5 and 6 the first kringle domain, exon 7 the second kringle, exons 8 to 10 the activation peptide, and exons 11 to 14 the catalytic domain. For the genes encoding factors VII, IX, and X, the placement of the intervening sequences is remarkably similar, and the splice junction types are identical (Table 2.2). The lengths of the introns vary considerably, and this variation in intron size accounts to a great extent for the differences in the overall size of

**TABLE 2.2.** Intron Lengths and Splice Junction Types for Human Coagulation Factors IX, VII, and X

| Intron | IX | VII | X[1] | Splice Junction Type |
|---|---|---|---|---|
| A | 6206 | 1067[2] 2574 | Unknown | 1 |
| B | 188 | 1919 | 8000 | 0 |
| C | 3689 | 68 | 920 | 1 |
| D | 7163 | 1908 | 1400 | 1 |
| E | 2565 | 971 | 3000 | 1 |
| F | 9473 | 595 | 3300 | 0 |
| G | 668 | 816 | 1400 | 1 |

[1] Intron lengths for factor X are approximate. The length of intron A has not been determined.

[2] The two intron lengths are for the introns following exons 1a and 1b in factor VII.

Modified from High KA and Roberts HR. Factor IX. In: High KA and Roberts HR, eds. Molecular basis of hemostasis and thrombosis. New York: Marcel Dekker, Inc., 1995.

the genes (34 kb for factor IX, 20 kb for factor X, and 12.3 kb for factor VII), because the sizes of the coding regions are similar.

## FACTOR V AND FACTOR VIII

Factor V and factor VIII are homologous lipid-binding proteins that function in coagulation as cofactors for the serine proteases factor Xa and factor IXa, respectively. As homologous complexes, the intrinsic tenase (factor IXa–factor VIIIa) and prothrombinase (factor Xa–factor Va) assemble on the phospholipid membrane surfaces of activated platelets (see Chapter 1). The two complexes differ in their abilities to effect limited proteolysis of their specific macromolecular substrates, factor X and prothrombin, respectively. Factor V and factor VIII circulate as inactive forms in trace amounts in plasma and are converted to the biologically active form by thrombin cleavage. Activation of factor V and factor VIII results in the formation of a heavy and a light chain; these two chains form a heterodimer that is held together by a single calcium ion. In both cases, the large (~40% of the inactive cofactor), heavily glycosylated intervening B domain is cleaved out by thrombin activation. A function for the B domain has not been identified. Both cofactors are inactivated at the membrane surface by several proteolytic cleavages by activated protein C.

The protein structures and gene organizations of factor V and factor VIII are similar, suggesting that they arose from duplication of a common primordial precursor gene. Each contains a triplicated A domain with sequence homology to the triplicated A domains of plasma ceruloplasmin (Fig. 2.6). Factor V and factor VIII also contain duplicated C domains; these are homologous to duplicated domains present in human and murine breast epithelial cell protein (81, 82) and may function in interactions with phospholipid surfaces (83). The domain organization of the factor V and factor VIII proteins are identical; A1-A2-B-A3-C1-C2. Interestingly, the intervening B domains share no homology between the two proteins (84, 85). The presence of the B domain is likely to have occurred by insertion of a large exon into the ancestor gene with subsequent divergence of sequence (83). Evidence of divergence of B domain sequence between factor V and factor VIII and between the sequences of these cofactors from different species suggests little selective pressure to conserve the amino acid sequence of the B domain. The exon-intron organization of both cofactor genes correlates with the protein domains and is nearly identical for factor V and factor VIII (86, 87). The gene for factor V is ~80 kb and is located on chromosome 1 (q21–25), whereas the gene for factor VIII is present on the X chromosome and is much larger (~180 kb), the difference being accounted for by six intronic sequences that are significantly larger in the factor VIII gene (86).

The A domains of factor VIII and factor V are ~30% identical to each other and to ceruloplasmin, a copper oxidase that binds 5 to 6 copper atoms (88). Although a single copper ion has been identified in bovine factor V (89), the copper binding ligands present in ceruloplasmin are not conserved in factor V or factor VIII (90–92). Thus, based on overall sequence homology, these three proteins constitute a family of related proteins that is

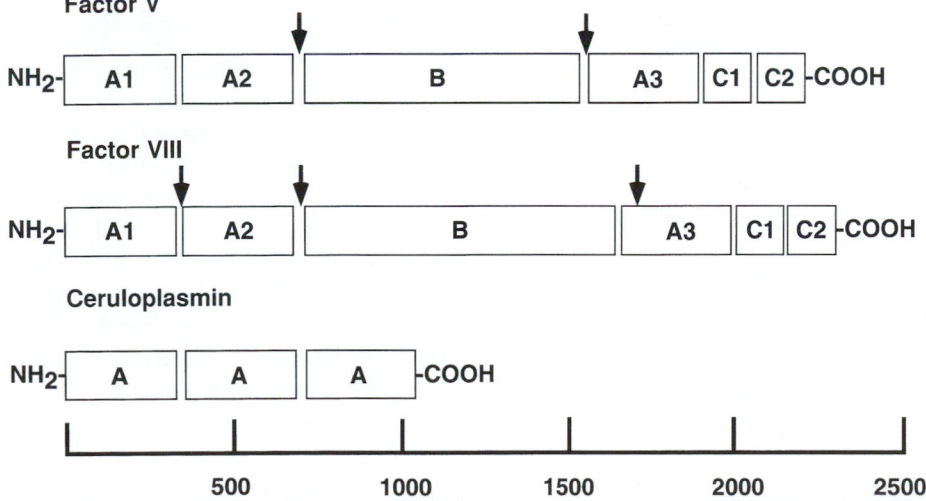

**FIGURE 2.6.**  The protein domains (and gene organization) of human factor V and human factor VIII are homologous and contain triplicated A domains similar to the gene for human ceruloplasmin. Factor V and factor VIII also contain duplicated C domains, which are homologous to domains present in breast epithelial cell protein and are althought to function in phospholipid binding. The intervening B domains share little homology. The arrows denote thrombin cleavage sites. The scale below represents size of the proteins in amino acid residues.

undergoing evolutionary divergence (93). The crystal structure for ceruloplasmin has recently been solved and, in the absence of nuclear magnetic resonance (NMR) or crystal structure for factor VIII, the coordinates for ceruloplasmin have been used to model the A domains of factor VIII (94). This model has been used to predict the binding sites on the A domains of factor VIII for factor IXa, BiP, a chaperone protein present in the lumen of the endoplasmic reticulum, and activated protein C, as well as the single copper ion binding site in the molecule.

Factor VIII is expressed primarily but not exclusively in the liver, factor VIII mRNA having been found in spleen, kidney, lymph nodes, placenta, pancreas, and muscle. As is the case for other coagulation factors, this liver-predominant expression appears to be controlled by a combination of ubiquitous and liver-enriched transcription factors. Using RNase protection, Gitschier et al (87) mapped the transcription start site for factor VIII to a site 170 bp upstream from the translation start site. Figueiredo and Brownlee (95), using DNase footprinting, identified 19 protein binding sites within the first 1175 bp upstream from the translation start site. Reporter gene assays document that the sequence from $-279$ to $-64$ directs maximal promoter expression in liver cell lines, and gel shift and supershift experiments have been used to define the cognate binding proteins for the three protein binding sites within this region, two of which bind the liver-specific factor C/EBP and one the ubiquitous factor NFκB. The role of binding sites for HNF-4 and HNF-1, which lie just outside the defined maximal promoter sequence at the 5' and 3' boundaries, respectively, is unclear. The factor V promoter has not been studied in detail.

A syndrome of combined deficiency of factors V and VIII has been described in more than 58 kindreds (96–100). The syndrome has been estimated to occur with a frequency of up to 1:100,000 in some populations and is inherited in an autosomal recessive fashion. Typical individuals have a moderate bleeding tendency and have factor V and factor VIII levels in the range of 5 to 30%. In recent work using homozygosity mapping, Nichols et al have identified a 2.5 cM candidate locus responsible for this combined deficiency syndrome on the long arm of chromosome 18 (101A). The gene product is likely to play a role in a biosynthetic pathway common to both factor V and factor VIII. It should be noted that this syndrome is distinct from a coinheritance of both factor V and factor VIII deficiencies reported in four families (101B–104).

## PREKALLIKREIN AND FACTOR XI

The genes for human factor XI and prekallikrein are closely linked on the long arm of chromosome 4 (4q35) (105–107). Comparison of the two cDNA sequences, po-

sitions of the introns, and linkage of the two genes are all consistent with a recent gene duplication event. This divergence is estimated to have occurred around the time of the appearance of mammals, approximately 124 million years ago (108).

As noted earlier, catalytic domains of these two proteins (the light chains of the activated zymogens) share sequence homology with other coagulation serine proteases. The heavy chains contain four tandem repeat "apple" domains that confer on these proteins the ability to bind high molecular weight kininogen (HK) (109–111). The apple domains are each 90 to 91 amino acids long and are characterized by three intradomain disulfide bonds. In factor XI, the first and fourth apple domains each contain single cysteine residues; these two single cysteines form a disulfide bond. The fourth apple domain in prekallikrein contains a fourth intradomain disulfide bond. Binding of these proteins in complex with HK to negatively charged surfaces such as dextran sulfate, heparin, or kaolin enhances their activation by factor XIIa (112).

Because HK and factor XII deficiencies do not lead to bleeding diatheses, the contact activation of prekallikrein and factor XI likely does not play a significant role in normal hemostasis (113, 114). Contact activation of these factors may function instead to enhance hemostasis in pathologic conditions such as infection, myocardial infarction, and contact with foreign materials (115–117). Thrombin activation of factor XI has recently been described, and it has been hypothesized that factor XI has importance in a feedback enhancement of further thrombin generation once coagulation is initiated through the extrinsic (tissue factor) pathway (118–120).

## Mutations: Mechanisms and Databases (See Chapters 35 and 36)

The types of mutations found in genes encoding coagulation factors are, for the most part, the same as those involved in other genetic disorders, such as small insertions and deletions, missense mutations, and nonsense mutations. At least two genetic mechanisms of disease were first described in coagulation factors: insertion of a transposable element into the factor VIII gene (121) and an intrachromosomal recombination event that is responsible for approximately 40% of cases of severe hemophilia A (122). Because mutations at CpG dinucleotides are heavily represented in coagulation factor mutation databases, this mechanism will also be briefly reviewed.

### CpG Dinucleotides

A common cause of spontaneous mutation in vertebrate genomes involves the methylation of cytosine residues. Methylation of DNA is althought to suppress transcription in some genes, although this is not a universal find-

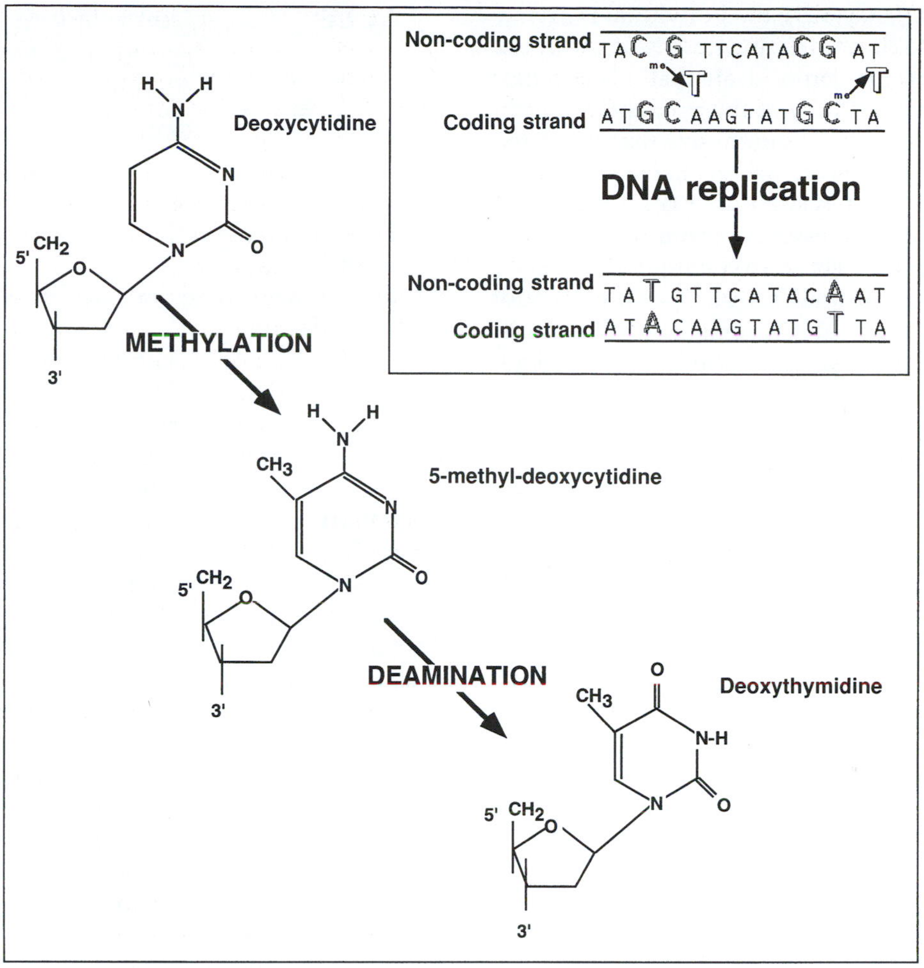

**FIGURE 2.7.** Deamination of methylated cytosines is responsible for some point mutations. Inset: when deamination of methylcytosine occurs in one strand, it results in a C→T transition in that strand and a G→A transition in the opposite strand.

ing (123). Of methylated cytosine residues in eukaryotic genomes, 90% occur within CG dinucleotides (124, 125). Spontaneous deamination of methylated cytosine residues (which occurs with a slow but detectable frequency) results in the formation of thymidine; subsequent daughter strands then maintain the C→T change (Fig. 2.7), as thymidine, so generated, is not repaired. When the change occurs in the coding strand, it causes a C→T transition in the coding strand. If the deamination of methylcytosine occurs in the noncoding strand, a G→A transition occurs in the coding strand (inset to Fig. 2.7). Up to 35% of mutations in the human genome have been found to occur within CG dinucleotides representing a 42-fold increase above that predicted from random mutation (125). Thus, CG dinucleotides are "hot spots" for mutation because of the high frequency of methylated cytosines in these dinucleotides and the propensity of these methylated cytosine residues to undergo deamination (126).

Koeberl et al have characterized mutations in the human factor IX gene due to spontaneous deamination of methylated cytosines. They found up to a 77-fold enhancement at CG dinucleotides without a measurable effect of flanking nucleotides (75). In a study of 38 families with hemophilia B, and from information available in the hemophilia B database, mutations at CG dinucleotides causing disease were found at all evolutionarily conserved sites where the transition would cause a nonconservative substitution except A-10→T, and R338→Q (127, 128). Two other conserved sites (R29→Q and R116→TGA[STOP]) were found at frequencies much lower than predicted. The authors speculated that these CG dinucleotides may undergo methylation at a lower rate or be unmethylated. As an alternative explanation, they postulated that the A-10 and R338 mutations may cause diseases other than hemophilia B or may be gestational lethals, and they predicted that as more mutations are defined, transitions at these two residues would be observed. Of interest in this regard is the recent report by Chu et al describing an individual with warfarin sensitivity resulting in unmeasureable factor IX levels on therapeutic doses of warfarin, due to an A-10→T mutation in the factor IX gene (129); the individual is asymptomatic when not taking warfarin and has factor IX levels of 100%. The authors demonstrate that this mutation results in a decreased affinity of the propeptide for the γ-glutamylcarboxylase and hypothesize that the defect becomes clinically significant when there is increased competition for the carboxylase under conditions, such as warfarin therapy, that result in accumulation of substrates for the enzyme. These two studies underscore the predictive value of analysis of CpG dinucleotide transitions resulting in substitutions at evolutionarily conserved amino acid residues in the human genome.

## Inversion Mutation Caused by Intrachromosomal Recombination within Exon 22 of the Factor VIII Gene

Genetic analysis of the coding sequences and exon-intron junctions in individuals with mild or moderate hemophilia A has allowed the identification of causative mutations in almost all cases. However, before 1993, such analysis failed to explain the etiology of the genetic defect in approximately half the cases of severe hemophilia A. Naylor et al used polymerase chain reaction (PCR) amplification of reverse transcribed mRNA and found that amplification across the boundary of exons 22 and 23 was not possible in 10 of 24 severely affected hemophilia A individuals (130). Levinson et al identified two ubiquitously expressed genes within this region (intron 22); one of these, factor VIII-associated-gene A is transcribed in the opposite direction to the factor VIII gene (131, 132). Two other copies of gene A are located ~500 kb upstream of the factor VIII gene. It has been shown subsequently that the majority of severely affected individuals with defects unexplained by coding sequence mutations have an inversion of exons 1–22 of the factor VIII gene caused by an intrachromosomal homologous recombination of the intron 22 gene A with one of the two upstream gene A copies (122). Family studies have documented that this mutation most commonly arises in the germline cells; it is then transmitted silently through a carrier daughter and is first manifested in her male offspring.

## Databases of Mutations in the Genes of Coagulation Proteins

Over the past decade, several groups have undertaken the compilation of described mutations in the genes for coagulation factors that result in a measurable change in phenotype. These databases are useful to clinicians (for example, the relationship of specific factor VIII and IX mutations to inhibitor formation) and investigators interested in both regulation of expression and structure-function analyses of these proteins. Some of these databases have been published within broader reviews or chapters on the individual coagulation proteins. Oth-

**TABLE 2.3.** Compilations of Naturally Occurring Mutations in the Genes of Human Coagulation Factors

| Factor | Reference |
|---|---|
| Fibrinogen (factor I) | Lord, 1995 (151) |
| Prothrombin (factor II) | Friezner Degen, 1995 (152) |
| Factor V | Girolami, et al, 1985 (153) |
| | Seeler, 1972 (154) |
| | Melliger and Duckert, 1971 (155) |
| | Tracy and Mann, 1987 (156) |
| Factor VII | Cooper, et al, 1994 (157) |
| Factor VIII | Tuddenham, et al, 1994 (158) |
| | Kemball-Cook and Tuddenham, 1997 (159) |
| Factor IX | Giannelli, et al, 1997 (133) |
| Factor X | Cooper, et al, 1997 (160) |
| Factor XI | Asakai, et al, 1989 (161) |
| | Fujikawa, et al, 1995 (117) |
| Factor XII | Saito and Kojima, 1995 (162) |
| Factor XIII | Anwar, et al, 1995 (163) |
| | Lai and Greenburg, 1995 (164) |
| Prekallikrein | Saito, 1987 (113) |
| | Saito and Kojima, 1995 (162) |
| High-molecular-weight kininogen | Saito and Kojima, 1995 (162) |

ers have been specifically published and updated periodically as catalogues of mutations affecting the protein. References that catalogue described mutations for a given coagulation protein are listed in Table 2.3.

The first such database, published in 1991 by Giannelli, compiled the known mutations of factor IX resulting in hemophilia B (128). Currently this is one of the largest such databases of naturally occurring mutations assembled for any human gene (133). Its size is accounted for by the location of the gene on the X chromosome and the severe phenotype associated with factor IX deficiency, as well as the relatively small size of the coding region, which makes the gene amenable to direct sequence analysis. The database includes mutations in all exons, intron-exon junctions, and the 5' flanking region of the gene, and has been useful to basic scientists, making readily available the functional effects of specific amino acid substitutions within the factor IX molecule (c.f. Brandstetter et al [134]). The availability of similar databases for other coagulation proteins will be useful in the more complete definition of structure-function relationships.

# REFERENCES

1. Doolittle RF. The evolution of vertebrate blood coagulation: a case of Yin and Yang [review]. Thromb Haemost 1993;70:24–28.
2. Bazan JF. Structural design and molecular evolution of a cytokine receptor superfamily. Proc Natl Acad Sci U S A 1990;87:6934–6938.
3. Iwanaga S. Primitive coagulation systems and their message to modern biology. Thromb Haemost 1993;70:48–55.
4. Tokunaga F, Miyata T, Nakamura T et al. Lipopolysaccharide-sensitive serine-protease zymogen (factor C) of horseshoe crab hemocytes. Identification and alignment of proteolytic fragments produced during the activation show that it is a novel type of serine protease. Eur J Biochem 1987;167:405–416.
5. Patthy L. Evolution of blood coagulation and fibrinolysis. Blood Coagul Fibrinolysis 1990;1:153–166.
6. Muta T, Miyata T, Misumi Y et al. Limulus factor C. An endotoxin-sensitive serine protease zymogen with a mosaic structure of complement-like, epidermal growth factor-like, and lectin-like domains. J Biol Chem 1991;266:6554–6561.
7. Sharon N, Lis H. Lectins as cell recognition molecules. Science 1989;246:227–234.
8. Sharon N. Carbohydrates as recognition determinants in phagocytosis and in lectin-mediated killing of target cells [review]. Biol Cell 1984;51:239–245.
9. Patthy L. Homology of cytotoxic protein of eosinophilic leukocytes with IgE receptor Fc RII: Implications for its structure and function. Mol Immunol 1989;26:1151–1154.
10. Krawczak M, Wacey A, Cooper DN. Molecular reconstruction and homology modelling of the catalytic domain of the common ancestor of the haemostatic vitamin K-dependent serine proteinases. Hum Genet 1996;98:351–370.
11. Neurath H. Evolution of proteolytic enzymes [review]. Science 1984;224:350–357.
12. Brenner S. The molecular evolution of genes and proteins: A tale of two serines. Nature 1988;334:528–530.
13. Crabtree GR, Comeau CM, Fowlkes DM et al. Evolution and structure of the fibrinogen genes. Random insertion of introns or selective loss? J Mol Biol 1985;185:1–19.
14. Long GL. Structure and evolution of the human genes encoding protein C and coagulation factors VII, IX, and X. Cold Spring Harb Symp Quant Biol 1986;51:525–529.
15. Rogers J. Exon shuffling and intron insertion in serine protease genes [news]. Nature 1985;315:458–459.
16. Jones FS, Burgoon MP, Hoffman S et al. A cDNA clone for cytotactin contains sequences similar to epidermal growth factor-like repeats and segments of fibronectin and fibrinogen. Proc Natl Acad Sci U S A 1988;85:2186–2190.
17. Jones FS, Hoffman S, Cunningham BA et al. A detailed structural model of cytotactin: protein homologies, alternative RNA splicing, and binding regions. Proc Natl Acad Sci U S A 1989;86:1905–1909.
18. Koyama T, Hall LR, Haser WG et al. Structure of a cytotoxic T-lymphocyte-specific gene shows a strong homology to fibrinogen and chains. Proc Natl Acad Sci U S A 1987;84:1609–1613.
19. Kant JA, Fornace AJ Jr, Saxe D et al. Evolution and organization of the fibrinogen locus on chromosome 4: Gene duplication accompanied by transposition and inversion. Proc Natl Acad Sci U S A 1985;82:2344–2348.
20. Doolittle RF, Feng DF. Reconstructing the evolution of vertebrate blood coagulation from a consideration of the amino acid sequences of clotting proteins. Cold Spring Harb Symp Quant Biol 1987;52:869–874.
21. Meade TW, Mellows S, Brozovic M et al. Haemostatic function and ischaemic heart disease: Principal results of the Northwick Park Heart Study. Lancet 1986;2:533–537.
22. Wilhelmsen L, Svardsudd K, Korsan-Bengtsen K et al. Fibrinogen as a risk factor for stroke and myocardial infarction. N Engl J Med 1984;311:501–505.
23. Stone MC, Thorp JM. Plasma fibrinogen—A major coronary risk factor. J R Coll Gen Pract 1985;35:565–569.
24. Kannel WB, Wolf PA, Castelli WP et al. Fibrinogen and risk of cardiovascular disease. The Framingham Study. JAMA 1987;258:1183–1186.
25. Doolittle RF, Watt KW, Cottrell BA et al. The amino acid sequence of the alpha-chain of human fibrinogen. Nature 1979;280:464–468.
26. Binnie CG, Hettasch JM, Strickland E et al. Characterization of purified recombinant fibrinogen: Partial phosphorylation of fibrinopeptide A. Biochemistry 1993;32:107–113.
27. Pfeifer U, Ormanns W, Klinge O. Hepatocellular fibrinogen storage in familial hypofibrinogenemia. Virchows Arch B Cell Pathol Incl Mol Pathol 1981;36:247–255.
28. Roy SN, Procyk R, Kudryk BJ et al. Assembly and secretion of recombinant human fibrinogen. J Biol Chem 1991;266:4758–4763.
29. Hartwig R, Danishefsky KJ. Studies on the assembly and secretion of fibrinogen. J Biol Chem 1991;266:6578–6585.
30. Roy SN, Overton O, Redman CM. Overexpression of any fibrinogen chain by Hep G2 cells specifically elevates the expression of the other two chains. J Biol Chem 1994;269:691–695.
31. Roy SN, Mukhopadhyay G, Redman CM. Regulation of fibrinogen assembly. Transfection of Hep G2 cells with B cDNA specifically enhances synthesis of the three component chains of fibrinogen. J Biol Chem 1990;265:6389–6393.
32. Yu S, Sher B, Kudryk B et al. Intracellular assembly of human fibrinogen. J Biol Chem 1983;258:13407–13410.
33. Crabtree GR, Kant JA. Coordinate accumulation of the mRNAs for the alpha, beta, and gamma chains of rat fibrinogen following defibrination. J Biol Chem 1982;257:7277–7279.
34. Fowlkes DM, Mullis NT, Comeau CM et al. Potential basis for regulation of the coordinately expressed fibrinogen genes: Homology in the 5′ flanking regions. Proc Natl Acad Sci U S A 1984;81:2313–2316.
35. Mizuguchi J, Hu CH, Cao Z et al. Characterization of the 5′-flanking region of the gene for the gamma chain of human fibrinogen. J Biol Chem 1995;270:28350–28356.
36. Anderson GM, Shaw AR, Shafer JA. Functional characterization of promoter elements involved in regulation of human B beta-fibrinogen expression. Evidence for binding of novel activator and repressor proteins. J Biol Chem 1993;268:22650–22655.
37. Hu CH, Harris JE, Davie EW et al. Characterization of the 5′-flanking region of the gene for the alpha chain of human fibrinogen. J Biol Chem 1995;270:28342–28349.
38. Courtois G, Morgan JG, Campbell LA et al. Interaction of a liver-specific nuclear factor with the fibrinogen and alpha 1-antitrypsin promoters. Science 1987;238:688–692.
39. Baumhueter S, Mendel DB, Conley PB et al. HNF-1 shares three sequence motifs with the POU domain proteins and is identical to LF-B1 and APF. Genes Dev 1990;4:372–379.
40. Hansen LP, Crabtree GR. Regulation of the HNF-1 homeodomain proteins by DcoH [review]. Curr Opin Genet Dev 1993;3:246–253.
41. Haidaris PJ, Courtney MA. Tissue-specific and ubiquitous expression of fibrinogen gamma-chain mRNA. Blood Coagul Fibrinolysis 1990;1:433–437.
42. Courtney MA, Stoler MH, Marder VJ et al. Developmental expression of mRNAs encoding platelet proteins in rat megakaryocytes. Blood 1991;77:560–568.
43. Haidaris PJ. Induction of fibrinogen biosynthesis and secretion from cultured pulmonary epithelial cells. Blood 1997;89:873–882.
44. Dalmon J, Laurent M, Courtois G. The human beta fibrinogen promoter contains a hepatocyte nuclear factor 1-dependent interleukin-6-responsive element. Mol Cell Biol 1993;13:1183–1193.
45. Morgan JG, Courtois G, Fourel G et al. Sp1, a CAAT-binding factor, and the adenovirus major late promoter transcription factor interact with functional regions of the gamma-fibrinogen promoter. Mol Cell Biol 1988;8:2628–2637.
46. Crabtree GR, Kant JA. Organization of the rat gamma-fibrinogen gene: alternative mRNA splice patterns produce the gamma A and gamma B (gamma ′) chains of fibrinogen. Cell 1982;31:159–166.
47. Fornace AJ Jr, Cummings DE, Comeau CM et al. Structure of the human gamma-fibrinogen gene. Alternate mRNA splicing near the 3′ end of the gene produces gamma A and gamma B forms of gamma-fibrinogen. J Biol Chem 1984;259:12826–12830.
48. Chung DW, Davie EW. Gamma and gamma′ chains of human fibrinogen are produced by alternative mRNA processing. Biochemistry 1984;23:4232–4236.
49. Wolfenstein-Todel C, Mosesson MW. Carboxyterminal amino acid sequence of a human fibrinogen gamma-chain variant (g′). Biochemistry 1981;20:6146–6149.
50. Handagama PJ, Amrani DL, Shuman MA. Endocytosis of fibrinogen into hamster megakaryocyte alpha granules is dependent on a dimeric gamma A configuration. Blood 1995;85:1790–1795.
51. Jamison CS, Degen SJ. Prenatal and postnatal expression of mRNA coding for rat prothrombin. Biochem Biophys Acta 1991;1088:208–216.
52. Hung HL, High KA. Liver-enriched transcription factor HNF-4 and ubiquitous factor NF-Y are critical for expression of blood coagulation factor X. J Biol Chem 1996;271:2323–2331.
53. Pollak ES, Hung HL, Godin W et al. Functional characterization of the human factor VII 5′-flanking region. J Biol Chem 1996;271:1738–1747.
54. Salier JP, Hirosawa S, Kurachi K. Functional characterization of the 5′-regulatory region of human factor IX gene. J Biol Chem 1990;265:7062–7068.
55. Coughlin SR, Vu TK, Hung DT et al. Characterization of a functional thrombin receptor. Issues and opportunities. J Clin Invest 1992;89:351–355.
56. Altieri DC. Xa receptor EPR-1 [review]. FASEB J 1995;9:860–865.
57. Darnell JE Jr. Variety in the level of gene control in eukaryotic cells. Nature 1982;297:365–371.
58. Chow BK, Ting V, Tufaro F et al. Characterization of a novel liver-specific enhancer in the human prothrombin gene. J Biol Chem 1991;266:18927–18933.
59. Bancroft JD, McDowell SA, Degen SJ. The human prothrombin gene: transcriptional regulation in HepG2 cells. Biochemistry 1992;31:12469–12476.

60. Arbini AA, Pollak ES, Bayleran JK et al. Severe factor VII deficiency due to a mutation disrupting a hepatocyte nuclear factor 4 binding site in the factor VII promoter. Blood 1997;89:176–182.

61. Reijnen MJ, Peerlinck K, Maasdam D et al. Hemophilia B Leyden: Substitution of thymine for guanine at position −21 results in a disruption of a hepatocyte nuclear factor 4 binding site in the factor IX promoter. Blood 1993;82:151–158.

62. Reitsma PH, Bertina RM, Ploos van Amstel JK et al. The putative factor IX gene promoter in hemophilia B Leyden. Blood 1988;72:1074–1076.

63. Crossley M, Brownlee GG. Disruption of a C/EBP binding site in the factor IX promoter is associated with haemophilia B. Nature 1990;345:444–446.

64. Weatherall DJ. The thalassemias. In: Stamatoyannopoulos G, Nienhuis AW, Majerus PW, Varmus H, eds. The molecular basis of blood diseases. 2nd ed. Philadelphia: WB Saunders Co., 1994;157–205.

65. Veltkamp JJ, Meilof J, Remmelts HG et al. Another genetic variant of haemophilia B: Haemophilia B Leyden. Scand J Haematol 1970;7:82–90.

66. Bri't E, Bertina RM, Van Tilburg NH et al. Haemophilia B Leyden: A sex-linked hereditary disorder that improves after puberty. N Engl J Med 1982;306:788–790.

67. Bri't E, Wijnands MC, Veltkamp JJ. The prophylactic treatment of haemophilia B Leyden with anabolic steroids. Ann Intern Med 1986;103:225–226.

68. Ghanem N, Costes B, Martin J et al. Twenty-four novel hemophilia B mutations revealed by rapid scanning of the whole factor IX gene in a French population sample. Eur J Hum Genet 1993;1:144–155.

69. Crossley M, Winship PR, Austen DE et al. A less severe form of haemophilia B Leyden. Nucleic Acids Res 1990;18:4633.

70. Hirosawa S, Fahner JB, Salier JP et al. Structural and functional basis of the developmental regulation of human coagulation factor IX gene: Factor IX Leyden. Proc Natl Acad Sci U S A 1990;87:4421–4425.

71. Picketts DJ, Lillicrap DP, Mueller CR. Synergy between transcription factors DBP and C/EBP compensates for a haemophilia B Leyden factor IX mutation. Nat Genet 1993;3:175–179.

72. Freedenberg DL, Black B. Altered developmental control of the factor IX gene: A new T to A mutation at position +6 of the F-IX gene resulting in hemophilia B Leyden [abstract]. Thromb Haemost 1991;65:964.

73. Royle G, Van De Water NS, Berry E et al. Haemophilia B Leyden arising de novo by point mutation in the putative factor IX promoter region. Br J Haematol 1991;77:191–194.

74. Reitsma PH, Mandalaki T, Kasper CK et al. Two novel point mutations correlate with an altered developmental expression of blood coagulation factor IX (hemophilia B Leyden phenotype). Blood 1989;73:743–746.

75. Koeberl DD, Bottema CD, Buerstedde JM et al. Functionally important regions of the factor IX gene have a low rate of polymorphism and a high rate of mutation in the dinucleotide CpG. Am J Hum Genet 1989;45:448–457.

76. Crossley PM, Winship PR, Black A et al. Unusual case of haemophilia B [letter]. Lancet 1989;1:960.

77. Anson DS, Choo KH, Rees DJ et al. The gene structure of human antihaemophilic factor IX. EMBO J 1984;3:1053–1060.

78. Crossley M, Ludwig M, Stowell KM et al. Recovery from hemophilia B Leyden: An androgen-responsive element in the factor IX promoter. Science 1992;257:377–379.

79. Sprang S, Standing T, Fletterick RJ et al. The three-dimensional structure of Asn 102 mutant of trypsin: role of Asp 102 in serine protease catalyst. Science 1987;237:905–909.

80. Wu SM, Cheung WF, Frazier D et al. Cloning and expression of the cDNA for human gamma-glutamyl carboxylase. Science 1991;254:1634–1636.

81. Larocca D, Peterson JA, Urrea R et al. A Mr 46,000 human milk fat globule protein that is highly expressed in human breast tumors contains factor VIII-like domains. Cancer Res 1991;51:4994–4998.

82. Stubbs JD, Lekutis C, Singer KL et al. cDNA cloning of a mouse mammary epithelial cell surface protein reveals the existence of epidermal growth factor-like domains linked to factor VIII-like sequences. Proc Natl Acad Sci U S A 1990;87:8417–8421.

83. Ortel T, Keller F, Kane W. Factor V. In: High K, Roberts H, eds. Molecular basis of hemostasis and thrombosis. New York: Marcel Dekker, 1995:119–146.

84. Toole JJ, Knopf JL, Wozney JM et al. Molecular cloning of a cDNA encoding human antihaemophilic factor. Nature 1984;312:342–347.

85. Vehar GA, Keyt B, Eaton DL et al. Structure of human factor VIII. Nature 1984;312:337–342.

86. Cripe LD, Moore KD, Kane WH. Structure of the gene for human coagulation factor V. Biochemistry 1992;31:3777–3785.

87. Gitschier J, Wood WI, Goralka TM et al. Characterization of the human factor VIII gene. Nature 1984;312:326–330.

88. Ryden L. Copper proteins and copper enzymes. 3rd ed. Boca Raton: CRC Press, 1984;37–100.

89. Mann KG, Lawler CM, Vehar GA et al. Coagulation factor V contains copper ion. J Biol Chem 1984;259:12949–12951.

90. Kane WH, Davie EW. Cloning of a cDNA coding for human factor V, a blood coagulation factor homologous to factor VIII and ceruloplasmin. Proc Natl Acad Sci U S A 1986;83:6800–6804.

91. Kane WH, Ichinose A, Hagen FS et al. Cloning of cDNAs coding for the heavy chain region and connecting region of human factor V, a blood coagulation factor with four types of internal repeats. Biochemistry 1987;26:6508–6514.

92. Jenny RJ, Pittman DD, Toole JJ et al. Complete cDNA and derived amino acid sequence of human factor V. Proc Natl Acad Sci U S A 1987;84:4846–4850.

93. Church WR, Jernigan RL, Toole J et al. Coagulation factors V and VIII and ceruloplasmin constitute a family of structurally related proteins. Proc Natl Acad Sci U S A 1984;81:6934–6937.

94. Pemberton S, Lindley P, Zaitsev V et al. A molecular model for the triplicated A domains of human factor VIII based on the crystal structure of human ceruloplasmin. Blood 1997;89:2413–2421.

95. Figueiredo MS, Brownlee GG. cis-acting elements and transcription factors involved in the promoter activity of the human factor VIII gene. J Biol Chem 1995;270:11828–11838.

96. Oeri J, Matter M, Isenschmid H et al. Angeborener mangel an faktor V (parahaemophilie) verbunden mit echter haemophilie A bein zwei bruden. Med Probl Pediatr 1954;1:575–588.

97. Seligsohn U, Zivelin A, Zwang E. Combined factor V and factor VIII deficiency among non-Ashkenazi Jews. N Engl J Med 1982;307:1191–1195.

98. Seligsohn U. Combined factor V and factor VIII deficiency. In: Seghatchian MJ, Savidge GT, eds. Factor VIII-von Willebrand Factor. Boca Raton, FL: CRC Press, 1989.

99. Seligsohn U, Ramot B. Combined factor V and factor VIII deficiency: Report of four cases. Br J Haematol 1969;16:475–486.

100. Seligsohn UA, Zivelin A, Zwang E. Decreased factor VIII clotting antigen levels in the combined factor V and VIII deficiency. Thromb Res 1984;33:95–98.

101A. Nichols WC, Seligsohn U, Zirelin A et al. Linkage of combined Factors V and VIII deficiencies to chromosome 18q by homozygosity mapping. J Clin Invest 1997;99:596–601.

101B. Ozsoylu S. Combined congenital deficiency of factor V and factor VIII [letter]. Acta Haematol 1983;70:207–208.

102. Mazzone D, Fichera A, Pratico G et al. Combined congenital deficiency of factor V and factor VIII. Acta Haematol 1982;68:337–338.

103. Girolami A, Gastaldi G, Patrassi G et al. Combined congenital deficiency of factor V and factor VIII. Report of a further case with some considerations on the hereditary transmission of this disorder. Acta Haematol 1976;55:234–243.

104. Bartlett JA, Sweeney JD, Sadowsky D. Exodontia in combined factor V and factor VIII deficiency. J Oral Maxillofac Surg 1985;43:537–539.

105. Chung DW, Fujikawa K, McMullen BA et al. Human plasma prekallikrein, a zymogen to a serine protease that contains four tandem repeats. Biochemistry 1986;25:2410–2417.

106. Beaubien G, Rosinski-Chupin I, Mattei MG et al. Gene structure and chromosomal localization of plasma kallikrein. Biochemistry 1991;30:1628–1635.

107. Kato A, Asakai R, Davie EW et al. Factor XI gene (F11) is located on the distal end of the long arm of human chromosome 4. Cytogenet Cell Genet 1989;52:77–78.

108. Veloso D, Shilling J, Shine J et al. Recent evolutionary divergence of plasma prekallikrein and factor XI. Thromb Res 1986;43:153–160.

109. Page JD, Colman RW. Localization of distinct functional domains on prekallikrein for interaction with both high molecular weight kininogen and activated factor XII in a 28-kDa fragment (amino acids 141–371). J Biol Chem 1991;266:8143–8148.

110. Baglia FA, Jameson BA, Walsh PN. Fine mapping of the high molecular weight kininogen binding site on blood coagulation factor XI through the use of rationally designed synthetic analogs. J Biol Chem 1992;267:4247–4252.

111. Baglia FA, Jameson BA, Walsh PN. Localization of the high molecular weight kininogen binding site in the heavy chain of human factor XI to amino acids phenylalanine 56 through serine 86. J Biol Chem 1990;265:4149–4154.

112. Wiggins RC, Bouma BN, Cochrane CG et al. Role of high-molecular-weight kininogen in surface-binding and activation of coagulation factor XI and prekallikrein. Proc Natl Acad Sci U S A 1977;74:4636–4640.

113. Saito H. Contact factors in health and disease. Semin Thromb Hemost 1987;13:36–49.

114. Kaplan AP, Silverberg M. The coagulation-kinin pathway of human plasma [review]. Blood 1987;70:1–15.

115. Kelleher CC, Mitropoulos KA, Imeson J et al. Hageman factor and risk of myocardial infarction in middle-aged men. Atherosclerosis 1992;97:67–73.

116. Colman RW. Contact systems in infectious disease [review]. Rev Infect Dis 1989;11(Suppl 4):S689–S699.

117. Fujikawa K, Chung D. Factor XI. In: High K, Roberts H, eds. Molecular basis of hemostasis and thrombosis. New York: Marcel Dekker, 1995;257–268.

118. Davie EW, Fujikawa K, Kisiel W. The coagulation cascade: Initiation, maintenance, and regulation [review]. Biochemistry 1991;30:10363–10370.

119. Gailani D, Broze GJ Jr. Factor XI activation in a revised model of blood coagulation. Science 1991;253:909–912.

120. Naito K, Fujikawa K. Activation of human blood coagulation factor XI

independent of factor XII. Factor XI is activated by thrombin and factor XIa in the presence of negatively charged surfaces. J Biol Chem 1991;266: 7353–7358.

121. Kazazian HH Jr, Wong C, Youssoufian H et al. Haemophilia A resulting from *de novo* insertion of L1 sequences represents a novel mechanism for mutation in man. Nature 1988;332:164–166.

122. Lakich D, Kazazian HH Jr, Antonarkis SE et al. Inversions disrupting the factor VIII gene are a common cause of severe haemophilia A. Nat Genet 1993;5:236–241.

123. van der Ploeg LH, Flavell RA. DNA methylation in the human gamma delta beta-globin locus in erythroid and nonerythroid tissues. Cell 1980; 19:947–958.

124. Grippo P, Iaccarino M, Parisi E et al. Methylation of DNA in developing sea urchin embryos. J Mol Biol 1968;36:195–208.

125. Cooper DN, Youssoufian H. The CpG dinucleotide and human genetic disease. Hum Genet 1988;78:151–155.

126. Barker D, Schafer M, White R. Restriction sites containing CpG show a higher frequency of polymorphism in human DNA. Cell 1984;36:131–138.

127. Bottema CD, Ketterling RP, Vielhaber E et al. The pattern of spontaneous germ-line mutation: Relative rates of mutation at or near CpG dinucleotides in the factor IX gene. Hum Genet 1993;91:496–503.

128. Giannelli F, Green PM, High KA et al. Haemophilia B: Database of point mutations and short additions and deletions. Nucleic Acids Res 1990;18: 4053–4059.

129. Chu K, Wu SM, Stanley T et al. A mutation in the propeptide of factor IX leads to warfarin sensitivity by a novel mechanism. J Clin Invest 1996;98: 1619–1625.

130. Naylor JA, Green PM, Rizza CR et al. Analysis of factor VIII mRNA reveals defects in everyone of 28 haemophilia A individuals. Hum Mol Genet 1993;2:11–17.

131. Levinson B, Kenwrick S, Gamel P et al. Evidence for a third transcript from the human factor VIII gene. Genomics 1992;14:585–589.

132. Levinson B, Kenwrick S, Lakich D et al. A transcribed gene in an intron of the human factor VIII gene. Genomics 1990;7:1–11.

133. Giannelli F, Green PM, Sommer SS et al. Haemophilia B: Database of point mutations and short additions and deletions, 7th edition. Nucleic Acids Res 1997;25:133–135.

134. Brandstetter H, Bauer M, Huber R et al. X-ray structure of clotting factor IXa: Active site and module structure related to Xase activity and hemophilia B. Proc Natl Acad Sci U S A 1995;92:9796–9800.

135. Hoyer LW, Whyshock EG, Colman RW. Coagulation cofactors: Factors V and VIII. In: Colman RW, Hirsh J, Marder VJ et al, eds. Hemostasis and thrombosis: Basic principles and clinical practice. 3d ed. Philadelphia: JB Lippincott, 1994;109–133.

136. Royle NJ, Irwin DM, Koschinsky ML et al. Human genes encoding prothrombin and ceruloplasmin map to 11p11-q12 and 3q21-24, respectively. Somat Cell Mol Genet 1987;13:285–292.

137. Wang H, Riddell DC, Guinto ER et al. Localization of the gene encoding human factor V to chromosome 1q21-25. Genomics 1988;2:324–328.

138. Tantravahi U, Murty VV, Jhanwar SC et al. Physical mapping of the factor VIII gene proximal to two polymorphic DNA probes in human chromosome band Xq28: Implications for factor VIII gene segregation analysis. Cytogenet Cell Genet 1986;42:75–79.

139. Purello M, Alhadeff B, Esposito D et al. The human genes for hemophilia A and hemophilia B flank the X chromosome fragile site at Xq27.3. EMBO J 1985;4:725–729.

140. Camerino G, Grzeschik KH, Jaye M et al. Regional localization on the human X chromosome and polymorphism of the coagulation factor IX gene (hemophilia B locus). Proc Natl Acad Sci U S A 1984;81:498–502.

141. Kao FT, Hartz J, Horton R et al. Regional assignment of human tissue factor gene (F3) to chromosome 1p21-p22. Somat Cell Mol Genet 1988;14: 407–410.

142. de Grouchy J, Dautzenberg MD, Turleau C et al. Regional mapping of clotting factors VII and X to 13q34. Expression of factor VII through chromosome 8. Hum Genet 1984;66:230–233.

143. Cox DR, Gedde-Dahl T Jr. Report of the Committee on the Genetic Constitution of Chromosomes 13, 14, 15 and 16. Cytogenet Cell Genet 1985;40: 206–241.

144. Scambler PJ, Williamson R. The structural gene for human coagulation factor X is located on chromosome 13q34. Cytogenet Cell Genet 1985;39: 231–233.

145. Royle NJ, Fung MR, MacGillivray RT et al. The gene for clotting factor 10 is mapped to 13q32–qter. Cytogenet Cell Genet 1986;41:185–188.

146. Royle NJ, Nigli M, Cool D et al. Structural gene encoding human factor XII is located at 5q33–qter. Somat Cell Mol Genet 1988;14:217–221.

147. Board PG, Chapple R, Coggan M. Haplotypes of the coagulation factor XIII A subunit locus in normal and deficient subjects. Am J Hum Genet 1988;42:712–717.

148. Weisberg LJ, Shiu DT, Greenberg CS et al. Localization of the gene for coagulation factor XIII a-chain to chromosome 6 and identification of sites of synthesis. J Clin Invest 1987;79:649–652.

149. Webb GC, Coggan M, Ichinose A et al. Localization of the coagulation factor XIII B subunit gene (F13B) to chromosome bands 1q31-32.1 and restriction fragment length polymorphism at the locus. Hum Genet 1989; 81:157–160.

150. Cheung PP, Cannizzaro LA, Colman RW. Chromosomal mapping of human kininogen gene (KNG) to 3q26—qter. Cytogenet Cell Genet 1992; 59:24–26.

151. Lord S. Fibrinogen. In: High K, Roberts H, eds. Molecular basis of hemostasis and thrombosis. New York: Marcel Dekker, 1995;51–74.

152. Friezner Degen S. Prothrombin. In: High K, Roberts H, eds. Molecular basis of hemostasis and thrombosis. New York: Marcel Dekker, 1995; 75–100.

153. Girolami A, De Marco L, Dal Bo Zanon R et al. Rarer quantitative and qualitative abnormalities of coagulation [review]. Clin Haematol 1985;14: 385–411.

154. Seeler RA. Parahemophilia. Factor V deficiency [review]. Med Clin North Am 1972;56:119–125.

155. Melliger EJ, Duckert F. Major surgery in a subject with factor V deficiency. Cholecystectomy in a parahaemophilic woman and Review of the literature. Thromb Diath Haemorrh 1971;25:438–446.

156. Tracy PB, Mann KG. Abnormal formation of the prothrombinase complex: Factor V deficiency and related disorders. Hum Pathol 1987;18:162–169.

157. Cooper DN, Millar DS, Wacey A et al. Inherited factor VII deficiency: Molecular genetics and pathophysiology. Thromb Haemost 1997;78: 151–160.

158. Tuddenham EG, Schwaab R, Seehafer J et al. Haemophilia A: Database of nucleotide substitutions, deletions, insertions and rearrangements of the factor VIII gene, 2nd edition [corrected and republished article originally printed in Nucleic Acids Res 1994;17:3511–3533]. Nucleic Acids Res 1994; 22:4851–4868.

159. Kemball-Cook G, Tuddenham EG. The factor VIII mutation database on the world wide web: The haemophilia A mutation, search, test and resource site. HAMSTeRS update (version 3.0). Nucleic Acids Res 1997;25: 128–132.

160. Cooper DN, Millar DS, Wacey A et al. Inherited factor X deficiency: Molecular genetics and pathophysiology. Thromb Haemost 1997;78:161–172.

161. Asakai R, Chung DW, Ratnoff OD et al. Factor XI (plasma thromboplastin antecedent) deficiency in Ashkenazi Jews is a bleeding disorder that can result from three types of point mutations. Proc Natl Acad Sci U S A 1989; 86:7667–7671.

162. Saito H, Kojima T. Factor XII, prekallikrein, and high-molecular-weight kininogen. In: High K, Roberts H, eds. Molecular basis of hemostasis and thrombosis. New York: Marcel Dekker, 1995;269–286.

163. Anwar R, Stewart AD, Miloszewski KJ et al. Molecular basis of inherited factor XIII deficiency: Identification of multiple mutations provides insights into protein function. Br J Haematol 1995;91:728–735.

164. Lai TS, Greenberg CS. Factor XIII. In: High K, Roberts H, eds. Molecular basis of hemostasis and thrombosis. New York: Marcel Dekker, 1995; 287–308.

# CHAPTER 3

# REGULATION OF COAGULATION

Rachel E. Simmonds and David A. Lane

## INTRODUCTION

The coagulation cascade is essential for repairing damage to the vasculature and preventing blood loss. It consists of a series of protein activation steps that produce proteinases or cofactors, which sequentially activate additional zymogens and procofactors. The endpoint of the cascade is the generation of thrombin, which transforms fibrinogen to a fibrin clot. Initiation of the cascade occurs potentially via two pathways. One of these, the extrinsic (or tissue factor) pathway, is triggered by tissue factor exposure in the damaged vasculature. This forms a complex with factor VII which is activated by activated factor X (factor Xa), thrombin, activated factor VII (factor VIIa), or activated factor IX (factor IXa). The tissue factor/factor VIIa complex can then activate factor IX or factor X. Initiation of coagulation can also occur via the intrinsic (or contact activation) pathway. Factors XI and XII are activated on a negatively charged surface and activated factor XI then activates factor IX.

As described in Chapter 1, the initiation pathways converge at the point of factor IX activation. Factor IXa activates factor X, which in turn activates prothrombin (generating thrombin). Both reactions are greatly augmented by the presence of a cofactor, activated factor VIII (factor VIIIa) or activated factor V (factor Va), respectively, which are activated from their precursors by thrombin or factor Xa (in the case of factor V). The complex of factor IXa and factor VIIIa is known as the 'factor X activating' (or 'tenase') complex, whereas the complex of factor Xa and factor Va is known as the 'prothrombinase' complex; in this latter case, the presence of factor Va increases the rate of thrombin generation 100,000

fold. This is achieved by increasing the affinity of the proteinase for phospholipid membranes.

The circulating levels of prothrombin are at least 100 times that required for complete clot formation. Therefore, it is essential for the coagulation cascade to be carefully regulated to maintain intravascular fluidity. Many inhibitory proteins are involved in regulation, at least one for each proteinase. Inhibitory proteins belong to inhibitor families that have specialized regulatory functions. While inhibitory proteins have been well characterized in inhibitory function *in vitro*, their biological roles have not always been demonstrated through the association of their deficiencies with clinical thrombotic events. This chapter will focus primarily on the two known principle anticoagulant pathways—the protein C and the heparan sulfate/antithrombin III pathways (antithrombin III is now more usually termed antithrombin). The roles of these pathways in pathology are established. The inhibitory roles of heparin cofactor II and the tissue factor pathway inhibitor (TFPI), components of two other pathways, will be mentioned briefly. The pathophysiological role of the former inhibitor is uncertain and TFPI is described in detail in Chapter 4.

The pathways described herein do not operate in isolation; recent reports suggest a synergistic suppression of thrombin generation between TFPI and either antithrombin or the protein C anticoagulant pathways (1, 2). In normal healthy individuals, the balance of procoagulant and anticoagulant forces is towards the latter in the absence of tissue damage. The two principle regulatory pathways discussed are summarized in Fig. 3.1. The importance of these regulatory mechanisms is illustrated frequently by the thrombotic manifestations in

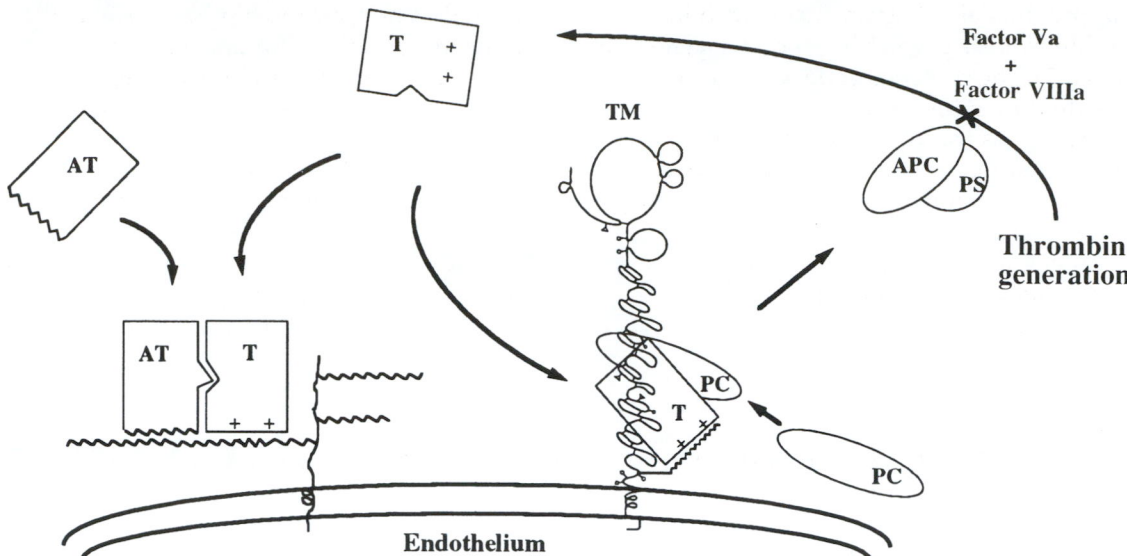

**FIGURE 3.1.**   Simplified view of the two principle regulatory mechanisms controlling coagulation proteinase activity in the blood. To the left is a heparan sulfate proteoglycan, which is an integral cell membrane protein of which the glycosaminoglycan side chains can contain essential elements of the pentasaccharide binding fragment of heparin (drawn as a sawtooth). This negatively charged glycosaminoglycan forms a template upon which thrombin (T) and antithrombin (AT) can bind and be approximated, thereby accelerating the rate of thrombin inhibition. To the right is thrombomodulin (TM), which is another membrane intercalated proteoglycan that can contain a glucosaminoglycan side chain (chondroitin sulfate, drawn as a sawtooth). Thrombomodulin acts as a receptor for thrombin, which is prevented from acting on fibrinogen once bound and instead activates protein C (PC). Activated protein C (APC), with protein S (PS) as a cofactor, inactivates factor Va and factor VIIIa, which in turn down-regulates thrombin generation. Protein S normally forms an equilibrium complex with C4b binding protein in plasma (not shown), and it is only the fraction of free (unbound) protein S that is able to act in this way. Fig. adapted from Bourin MC, Lindahl U. Glycosaminoglycans in the regulation of blood coagulation. Biochem J 1993;289:313–330 and Dahlback B, Stenflo J. The protein C anticoagulant system. In: Stamatoyannopoulos G, Nienhuis AW, Majerus PW, Varmus H, eds. The molecular basis of blood diseases. 2nd ed: Philadelphia: WB Saunders, 1994:599–627.

heterozygous and homozygous carriers of defects in the genes coding for the proteins that constitute these pathways (3, 4) (see Chapter 40).

## THE PROTEIN C ANTICOAGULANT SYSTEM

The protein C anticoagulant system regulates coagulation by inactivating factors VIIIa and Va, the cofactors to factors IXa and Xa (5, 6) (Fig. 3.1), in reactions that are strongly influenced by calcium ions ($Ca^{2+}$). In the first step, thrombin binds to thrombomodulin (TM), a transmembrane protein that alters the substrate specificity of the proteinase (7). Protein C is then activated by thrombin/TM complex via the cleavage of an internal peptide bond and release of an activation peptide. $Ca^{2+}$ ions play an important role in the activation of protein C and are a requirement for activation by the thrombin/TM complex (8). Activation of protein C by free thrombin has been demonstrated in purified systems; however, $Ca^{2+}$ strongly inhibits this reaction (9). Protein C activation by free thrombin is not expected to occur *in*

*vivo* because the physiologic concentration of $Ca^{2+}$ ions is between 1 and 2 mM. Once released from the thrombin/TM complex, activated protein C (APC) inactivates factors VIIIa and Va by sequential cleavage of specific peptide bonds (10–12). These reactions are augmented by a nonenzymic cofactor, protein S (13), that does not require activation. The anticoagulant functions of APC and protein S also require the presence of $Ca^{2+}$ ions and a negatively charged phospholipid membrane (10, 13). A second endothelial cell transmembrane protein, the endothelial cell protein C/APC receptor (EPCR), that may influence the rate of protein C activation has recently been identified (14).

The synthesis of protein C and protein S depends on post-translational γ-carboxylation of aminoterminal Glu residues to produce functionally active molecules (15). This modification is carried out by vitamin K-dependent γ-carboxylase (16), which also modifies other procoagulant factors (factors VII, IX, and X and prothrombin). These proteins are collectively known as the vitamin K-dependent proteins. Examination of the modular structure of the mature proteins of this group shows that all proteins contain a homologous aminoterminal portion of approximately 37 amino acids with between nine and 11 Glu residues, which are γ-carboxylated before secretion (15). The presence of these γ-carboxylated Glu (Gla) residues identifies a structural and functional domain referred to as the Gla domain. Factors IX and X each contain an additional Gla residue within the adjacent domain, which is known as the aromatic stack; the aromatic stack is another module found in all vitamin K-dependent coagulation factors (15). This small domain contains residues with aromatic side chains and is predicted to form an α-helix.

Studies of prothrombin have provided much information on the structure and function of Gla domains and can be used as a model for other vitamin K-dependent proteins because of the high sequence similarity. An alignment of the amino acid sequences of the Gla and aromatic stack domains of bovine and human prothrombin, human protein C, and human protein S is shown in Fig. 3.2A. The presence of Gla residues confers Ca$^{2+}$ binding properties that are essential for binding to negatively charged phospholipids; once bound, Ca$^{2+}$ ions are generally althought to mediate the interaction

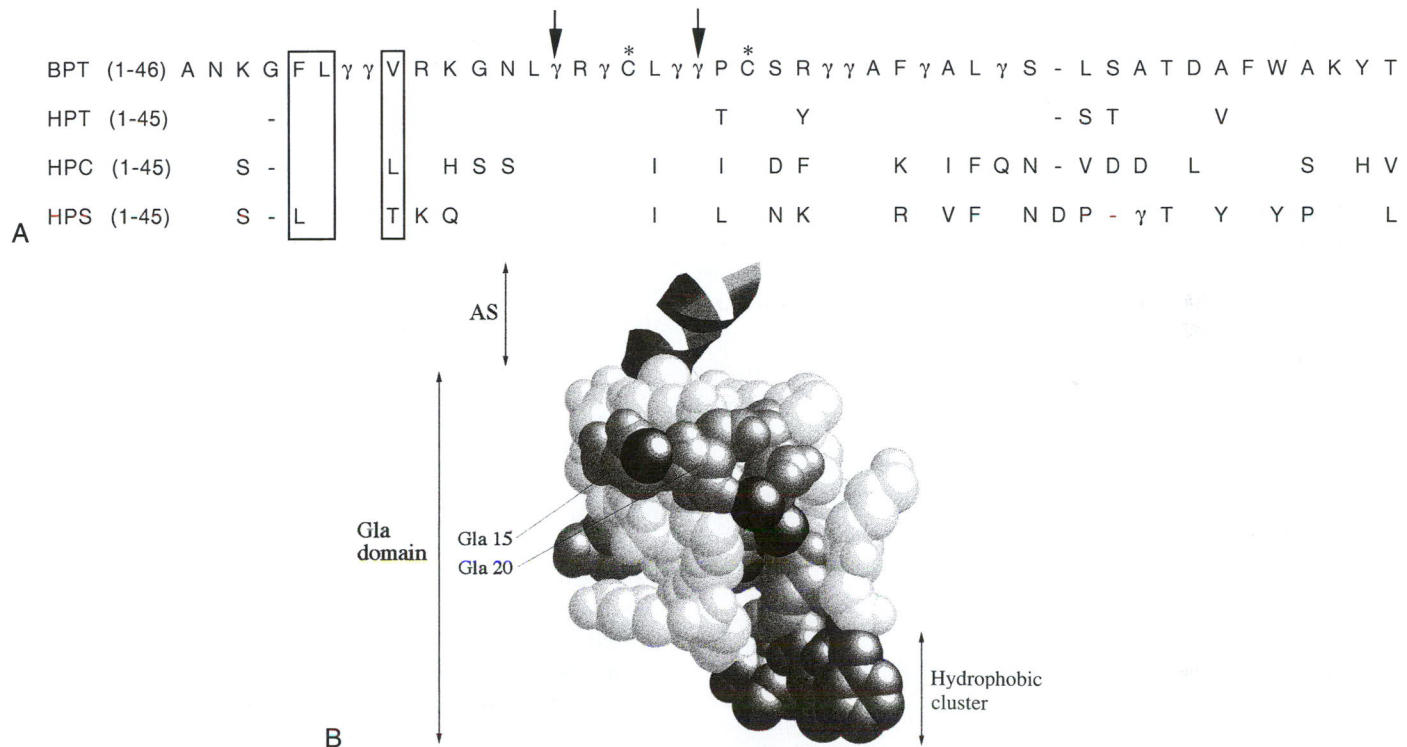

**FIGURE 3.2.** The crystal structure of the Gla and aromatic stack (AS) domains of bovine prothrombin fragment 1 and their similarity to the components of the protein C anticoagulant pathway, protein C and protein S. Several coagulation factors, including the components of the protein C anticoagulant pathway, protein S, and protein C, have a homologous aminoterminal portion termed the Gla domain. It is so called because of the presence of several γ-carboxylated Glu residues (Gla, γ), which require vitamin K for synthesis. Much knowledge has come from studies of bovine prothrombin fragment 1 (in particular the Ca$^{2+}$-dependent crystal structure of this region) that can be applied to other vitamin K-dependent proteins because of the high sequence similarity. A; An alignment of amino acid residues constituting the Gla and aromatic stack domains of bovine and human prothrombin (BPT and HPT, respectively), human protein C (HPC), and human protein S (HPS), using the single letter code. Asterisks (*) indicate the two Cys residues that form a disulfide bond. Identical residues in human prothrombin, protein C and protein S are indicated by a blank space, and gaps are indicated by a hyphen (-). Hydrophobic residues corresponding to residues 5, 6, and 9 of bovine prothrombin are boxed. In the crystal structure, these residues form an unusual solvent-exposed cluster that plays a role in phospholipid binding (panel B, hydrophobic cluster). The Gla residues corresponding to residues 14 and 19 of protein C are indicated with an arrow. These have been found to be unimportant for Ca$^{2+}$ and phospholipid binding and biological activity, and coordinate the binding of a single Ca$^{2+}$ ion (panel B). The sequences are bovine prothrombin (331), human prothrombin (332), human protein C (117), and human protein S (160). B; Representation of the Ca$^{2+}$ dependent crystal structure of bovine prothrombin fragment 1 (Gla and aromatic stack domains only), using coordinates provided by Soriano-Garcia et al (25). All residues of the Gla domain are represented by space filling, whereas the helical arrangement of the aromatic stack (AS) is shown with a ribbon. Gla residues are shaded light gray, and the hydrophobic residues corresponding to Phe 4, Leu 5, and Leu 8 of protein C (see text) are shaded dark gray. All other residues of the Gla domain are in pale gray. Also visible as black spheres are four of the seven Ca$^{2+}$ ions bound to this region. Binding of Ca$^{2+}$ ions brings together residues that are remote with respect to linear sequence, for example Gla 15 and 20 (corresponding to Gla 14 and 19 of protein C).

between the Gla domain and phospholipid. When synthesized in the presence of vitamin K-antagonist drugs such as warfarin, the Glu residues are not γ-carboxylated and the resulting molecule has reduced affinity for $Ca^{2+}$ ions and phospholipids (15, 17). Phospholipid binding of prothrombin in the presence of $Ca^{2+}$ ions reduces the $K_m$ for factor Xa-mediated prothrombin activation by greater than two orders of magnitude (15). Much of the $Ca^{2+}$ dependence of this and additional interactions of prothrombin and other coagulation factors is due to the Gla domain. Binding of vitamin K-dependent proteins to phospholipid in the presence of $Ca^{2+}$ provides a mechanism by which functionally important domains are oriented correctly (18).

There appear to be at least two stages involved in $Ca^{2+}$ binding. First, two or three cation binding sites are occupied, which induces a conformation change and brings together amino acids that are remote with respect to primary amino acid sequence. This change can be detected by changes in intrinsic fluorescence (19, 20) and in the specificity of conformation-specific antibodies (21–23). Various multivalent cations can substitute for $Ca^{2+}$ in this step (21–24). Second, another group of four or five cation binding sites that are required for the interaction with phospholipid vesicles and have more specificity for $Ca^{2+}$ ions are occupied (20, 23). The X-ray crystal structure of the $Ca^{2+}$-dependent conformation of bovine prothrombin fragment 1 that includes the Gla domain and the aromatic stack shows three $Ca^{2+}$ binding sites buried within the peptide and four solvent-exposed $Ca^{2+}$ ions within the Gla domain. As predicted, the aromatic stack has an α-helical conformation. A representation of the crystal structure of the Gla and aromatic stack domains of bovine prothrombin fragment 1 is shown in Fig. 3.2B.

All vitamin K-dependent precursor proteins also have a prepropeptide that is removed by two proteolytic cleavages prior to secretion. The first cleavage removes the prepeptide (or signal peptide), which is a stretch of hydrophobic residues essential for transport of protein through the endoplasmic reticulum and for secretion. The regions in this group of proteins are structurally unremarkable compared to the signal peptides of other secreted proteins. The second cleavage removes the propeptide, which contains elements that are recognized by vitamin K-dependent γ-carboxylase (26, 27). Recombinant vitamin K-dependent proteins lacking the propeptide are not γ-carboxylated before secretion. Although the precise mechanism by which γ-carboxylase recognizes the individual Glu residues that need to be modified remains uncertain, human γ-carboxylase and a γ-carboxylase-associated protein have recently been purified from mammalian cells expressing factor IX (28). *In vitro* carboxylase activity towards a synthetic substrate is stimulated by the addition of isolated propeptide, which suggests that the propeptide binding to γ-carboxylase activates the enzyme. Recent progress in understanding the mechanism of action of the vitamin K-dependent γ-carboxylase is outlined elsewhere (29, 30).

A second structural module homologous to the epidermal growth factor (EGF) precursor, known as the EGF-like domain, has been identified in many proteins including the coagulation factors VII, IX, X, and XII and three components of the protein C anticoagulant pathway, protein C, protein S, and TM (31, 32). The EGF precursor is a small protein consisting of 53 amino acids including six Cys residues that form three internal disulfide bonds in the pattern 1 to 3, 2 to 4, and 5 to 6. Many EGF-like domains of coagulation factors contain a high affinity $Ca^{2+}$ binding site, and a five-amino acid $Ca^{2+}$ binding consensus has been described (Asp/Asn, Asp/Asn, Gln/Glu, Asp/Asn, Tyr/Phe; the fourth residue in this sequence may be β-hydroxylated) (33).

The low resolution solution structures of EGF (34) and a $Ca^{2+}$ free form of the first EGF-like domain of factor X (35) have been resolved. Recently, the high resolution $Ca^{2+}$-dependent crystal structure of the first EGF-like domain isolated from factor IX (residues 46 to 84) has also been determined (36). These studies show that the main structural feature of the EGF-like domain is two antiparallel β-sheets. In the $Ca^{2+}$-dependent crystal structure, each domain occupies an elongated area (35 Å × 15 Å × 15 Å), and the overall arrangement of molecules in the crystal is helical (36). The structure of each domain is somewhat strained, with more residues than expected lying in unfavored positions, but these regions of strain are in the loops between the Cys residues, which suggests an important role for the disulfide bonds in maintaining the correct conformation. Binding of $Ca^{2+}$ ions induces a conformational change in the aminoterminus of this domain, and two molecules bind a total of three $Ca^{2+}$ ions (36). Two of these are rigidly defined and involve seven ligand interactions, six of which are contributed by one domain and the seventh contributed by a second domain, which forms a pentagonal bipyramid. The $Ca^{2+}$-binding site that involves two EGF-like domains provides a model for the role of these domains in stabilizing the structure of proteins that contain multiple copies (such as protein S) just like binding of $Ca^{2+}$ to one domain would promote binding of $Ca^{2+}$ to the others. In proteins with few EGF-like domains (such as factors IX and X and protein C), the seventh $Ca^{2+}$ ligand could conceivably be donated by the Gla domain with the same effect (36).

## THROMBOMODULIN

TM is a transmembrane proteoglycan with a molecular size of approximately 105 Kda expressed primarily in endothelial cells; TM has also been detected in the brain of rabbits (37) and in platelets (38). TM has been found on the vascular surface of endothelial cells of arteries, veins, capillaries, and lymphatic vessels, with more than 30,000 molecules per cell, but not in central nervous system vessels (39, 40). A soluble form also circulates in plasma at a concentration of approximately 20 μg/L (41). TM is expressed in the developing fetus, and its absence causes embryonic lethality in transgenic mice before the development of a cardiovascular system (42). Cell surface TM was identified when it was shown that protein C was rapidly activated by thrombin reversibly bound to an endothelial cell receptor (7) in a $Ca^{2+}$-dependent manner. The thrombin receptor was named TM because of its ability to alter the substrate specificity of thrombin by reversing its procoagulant role to that of an anticoagulant. Inhibition of the procoagulant functions of thrombin also proceeds by following two events: stearic hindrance as TM, fibrinogen, and factor V compete for binding to thrombin (43) and the stimulation of thrombin inhibition by antithrombin (44).

Although meizothrombin, an intermediate in prothrombin activation, is a poor procoagulant protein (45), it has been reported to be approximately sixfold more efficient in the activation of protein C (46). This effect was seen in a purified system when meizothrombin was complexed with soluble TM, in the presence of saturating levels of phospholipid vesicles. Although another report was unable to demonstrate an interaction between cell surface TM and meizothrombin (47), a possible specific role for meizothrombin in anticoagulation is suggested by these findings.

An additional role for the thrombin/TM complex has recently been elucidated (48). The complex acts as part of the fibrinolytic system because it is able to increase the activation of thrombin activatable fibrinolysis inhibitor (TAFI) approximately 1000-fold more than the activation rate by free thrombin (49). Activated TAFI (TAFIa) is a carboxypeptidase B-like enzyme with substrate specificity directed towards terminal arginine and lysine residues of proteins and polypeptides; TAFIa is a potent inhibitor of fibrinolysis (50, 51). At 10 mM TAFIa, the clot lysis time is increased approximately fourfold (49, 52), and induced activation of this zymogen could disrupt the fibrinolytic processes as the circulating concentration of TAFI is approximately 50 nM (53).

## The TM Molecule

The mature human protein consists of 557 amino acid residues following cleavage of an 18-amino acid signal peptide (54–56). The signal peptide seems unessential for the localization of TM within the cell membrane (57). Mature TM has a modular structure containing an aminoterminal lectin-like domain (residues 1 to 154) followed by a hydrophobic region (residues 155 to 222), six EGF-like domains (residues 223 to 462), a Ser/Thr rich region (residues 463 to 497), a transmembrane re-

gion (residues 498 to 521), and a short cytoplasmic tail at the carboxyterminus (residues 522 to 557). A schematic representation of the domain structure of TM is shown in Fig. 3.3. In human TM, there are five potential N-linked glycosylation and seven potential O-linked glycosylation sites located in the Ser/Thr rich, hydrophobic, and EGF-like domains (54). The third to the sixth EGF-like domains contain the consensus for β-hydroxylation of Asn residues, which are partially hydroxylated and could play a role in $Ca^{2+}$ binding (58). The shape of a soluble form of TM has been determined by electron microscopy (59). This investigation showed that TM is an elongated molecule, which is approximately 20 nm in length, and has a bulge at either terminus.

The lectin-like domain of TM displays approximately 20% homology to proteins of the selectin family, although it is unknown whether TM has lectin-like properties (60, 61). An important role for this region in regulating cell surface expression of TM has been identified (57). The EGF-like domains are critical for TM function because they contain enough structural information for acceleration of protein C activation (62) and include the binding sites for thrombin and protein C; these domains also include the putative $Ca^{2+}$-dependent binding site within the fifth EGF-like domain (63) and the regions responsible for TAFI activation (48). Removal of the first and second or first to third EGF-like domains does not significantly impair the ability to either bind thrombin or increase the rate of protein C activation (64–66). The predominant thrombin binding site is located in the fifth and sixth EGF-like domains (67), while the fourth EGF-like domain interacts with protein C (65, 66, 68). Two synthetic peptides derived from the latter half of the fifth EGF-like domain inhibited thrombin binding to TM, which suggests that this region contains residues important for this interaction (43, 66). A unique disulfide bonding pattern in the fifth EGF-like domain of TM has recently been determined. In this domain, disulfide bonds occur in the pattern 1 to 2, 3 to 4, and 5 to 6, which could result in greater flexibility (69). In a purified system, the fifth EGF-like domain with this unusual binding pattern has a greater affinity for thrombin than a form with the consensus 1 to 3, 2 to 4, 5 to 6 bonding pattern (70). The crystal structure of a peptide consisting of Glu 408 to Glu 426 (the third loop of the fifth EGF-like domain of TM) has been resolved, and here, two molecules of thrombin bind to the nonadecapeptide (71). The fifth and sixth EGF-like domains interact with anion binding exosite 1 of thrombin (72, 73), which is an extended groove structure that also constitutes the binding site for hirudin (74), the leech anticoagulant. Once bound to TM, the active site of thrombin is located approximately 66 Å above the membrane surface, as determined by fluorescence energy transfer (75). Consequently, the thrombin molecule may not be in contact with the membrane surface.

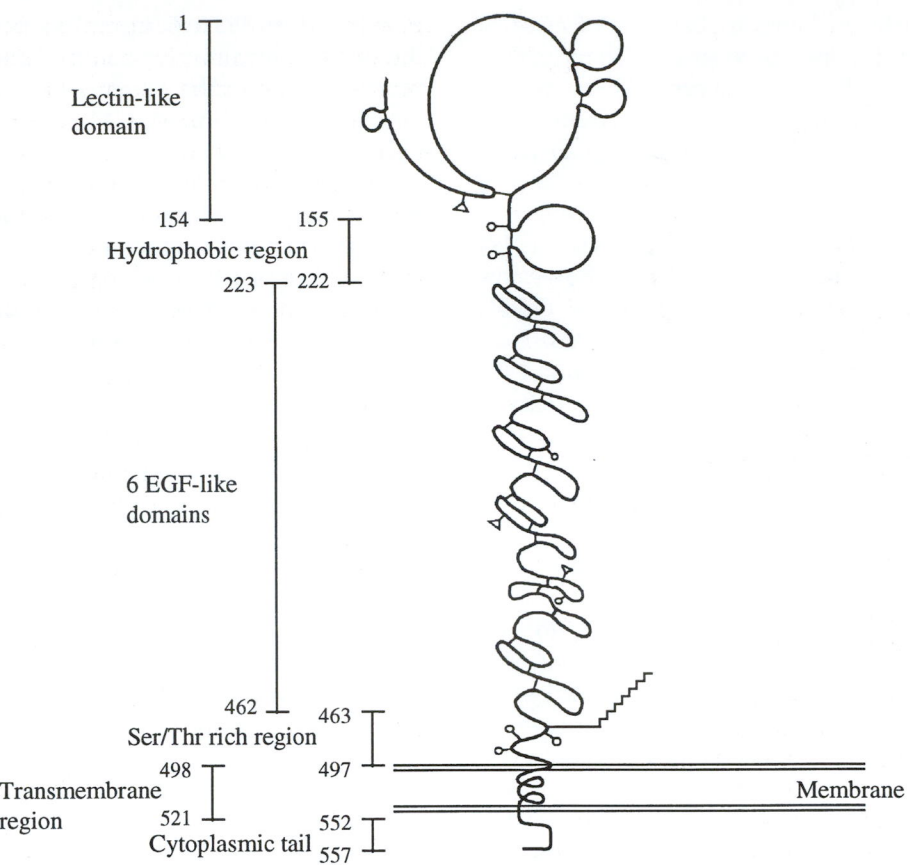

**FIGURE 3.3.** Schematic representation of the domain structure of thrombomodulin (TM). TM is a multimodular transmembrane proteoglycan and is shown imbedded in a cell membrane with its domains and amino acid residue numbers that constitute those domains indicated. Potential N- and O-linked glycosylation sites are indicated with a triangle and circle, respectively. An important moiety of TM, chondroitin sulfate, is shown as a sawtooth. The disulfide bonding pattern shown is largely based on homology with the appropriate domains of related proteins. Six regions homologous to epidermal growth factor (EGF-like domains) are shown. The bonding patterns of the fourth and fifth EGF-like domains have been determined experimentally. Whereas the fourth EGF-like domain has the normal bonding pattern, the fifth EGF-like domain is bonded in the pattern 1 to 2, 3 to 4, and 5 to 6, which confers a high thrombin affinity on this region (see text). Adapted, with permission, from Dahlback B, Stenflo J. The protein C anticoagulant system. In: Stamatoyannopoulos G, Nienhuis AW, Majerus PW, Varmus H, eds. The molecular basis of blood diseases. 2nd ed: Philadelphia: WB Saunders, 1994:599–627.

Alanine scanning mutagenesis of individual residues between Cys 333 and Cys 462 (i.e., the third to sixth EGF-like domains of TM [all residues except Ala, Cys, Gly, and Pro]) has identified important residues for protein C activation by the thrombin/TM complex (63). These include Asp 349, Glu 357, Tyr 358, and Phe 376 (within the fourth EGF-like domain), Asp 398, Asp 400, Asn 402, Glu 408, Tyr 413 to Asp 417, Asp 423 to Glu 426, Asn 429, Asn 439, Leu 440, and Phe 444 (within the fifth and the sixth EGF-like (Fig. 3.4). Eleven of these 22 residues are negative in charge, and none have a positive charge, suggesting that ionic interactions between TM and thrombin are important for binding. However, mutation of Asp 398, Glu 408, Asp 417, and Asn 439 did not alter the apparent $K_d$ for thrombin of such mutants, suggesting an alternative mechanism for the reduced

activity. The importance of the $Ca^{2+}$ binding site within the fifth EGF-like domain is highlighted by the observation that mutation of all residues of the consensus sequence (76) results in less activation of the protein C variants (63). The Asp 349 residue, which is located in the loop between the third and fourth EGF-like domain, has been shown independently to be important for the $Ca^{2+}$-dependence of the protein C/TM interaction (77).

The short loop between the fourth and fifth EGF-like domains (Gln 387, Met 388, and Phe 389) plays a critical role in TM function. If Met 388 is oxidized, the molecule loses biological activity (78), whereas replacement with a Leu residue is associated with increased activity by increasing the catalytic activity of thrombin. Furthermore, deletion of any one of these three residues or the insertion of a fourth amino acid into this region

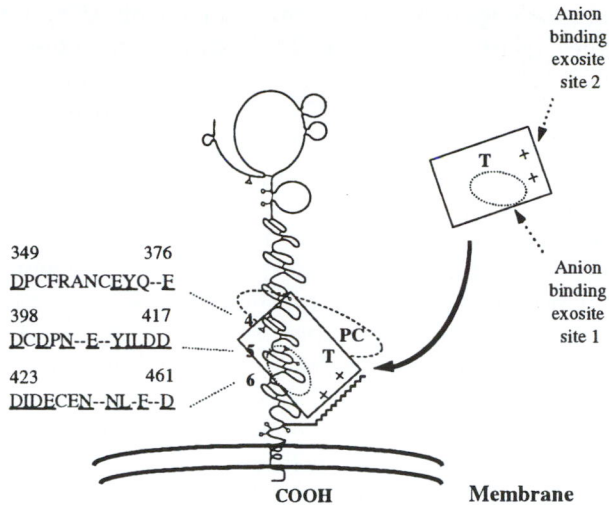

349          376
DPCFRANCEYQ--E

398          417
DCDPN--E--YILDD

423          461
DIDECEN--NL-E-D

COOH          **Membrane**

Anion binding exosite site 2

Anion binding exosite site 1

**FIGURE 3.4.** Residues of thrombomodulin involved in thrombin binding and protein C activation. Thrombin (T), which contains two anion binding exosites (1 and 2, labeled), binds to thrombomodulin (TM) by interacting with the chondroitin sulfate side chain and specific residues contained in the fifth and sixth EGF-like domains (numbered vertically). Additional residues in the fourth EGF-like domain are involved in protein C (PC) activation. The residues identified by alanine scanning mutagenesis in the fourth to sixth EGF-like domains are shown to the left with single letter codes with particularly important residues underlined. Adapted with permission from Dahlback B, Stenflo J. The protein C anticoagulant system. In: Stamatoyannopoulos G, Nienhuis AW, Majerus PW, Varmus H, eds. The molecular basis of blood diseases. 2nd ed: Philadelphia: WB Saunders, 1994:599–627.

results in almost complete loss of activity (79). This suggests an essential role for this spacer region in maintaining optimal alignment of the fourth EGF-like domain (protein C binding) with respect to the fifth and sixth EGF-like domains (thrombin binding). Substitution of any of these three residues (apart from Met 388 to Leu) results in a variant TM molecule with reduced activity, although Phe 389 is the least sensitive to substitution.

An important element identified in rabbit TM, chondroitin sulfate (44, 80–82), enhances the binding of thrombin to TM approximately 13-fold. Chondroitin sulfate consists of approximately 20 disaccharide repeats (glucuronic acid-N-acetylgalactosamine-4/6-monosulfate) with a trisaccharide at its terminus (N-acetylgalactosamine-4,6-disulfate-glucuronic acid-N-acetylgalactosamine-4,6-disulfate) (82, 83). It is strongly negative in charge and has a molecular mass of 10 to 12 Kda. For a period, it remained uncertain whether *in vivo* human TM contains this glucosaminoglycan because it could not be identified in TM purified from human endothelial cells. However, inhibition of glucosaminoglycan addition by β-D-xyloside in cultured endothelial

cells results in reduced thrombin receptor activity (84). Certain cell types display a larger amount of TM-associated chondroitin sulfate than others. Therefore, it seems human TM can be present in either form. Chondroitin sulfate is attached to TM in the Ser/Thr rich domain where there are four potential sites for addition; these sites for addition are based on the homology to the proposed xylosyltransferase acceptor consensus of which Ser 472 and Ser 474 are of particular interest. Mutation of Ser 474 to Gly in recombinant soluble TM reduces chondroitin sulfate attachment to below detectable levels, which suggests that this is the primary site of addition (85). The Ser 472 residue appears to represent a secondary attachment site (85). The point of attachment does not seem critical because no apparent difference in cofactor activity exists between TM that has chondroitin sulfate added to one of the two sites. TM containing a chondroitin sulfate moiety is referred to here as intact TM.

The mechanism by which the chondroitin sulfate modulates TM activity involves alteration of the $Ca^{2+}$-dependence of thrombin binding, which reduces the $K_d$ for this interaction and thus alters the $Ca^{2+}$-dependence of protein C activation (86). A direct binding has been demonstrated between purified chondroitin sulfate and thrombin ($K_d$ approximately 20 nM) (87). TM lacking chondroitin sulfate displays unusual $Ca^{2+}$-dependent binding characteristics with maximal binding at 200 to 500 μM $Ca^{2+}$, which is below physiologic concentration (86). Thrombin binding to intact TM is maximal at the normal $Ca^{2+}$ concentration in plasma, and at least two thrombin molecules appear to bind to one molecule of intact TM, each with different affinities (59, 87). The higher affinity site involves the interaction of thrombin, the fifth and sixth EGF-like domains of TM, and chondroitin sulfate (87). The lower affinity binding site may only involve chondroitin sulfate, possibly via the repeating disaccharide units that make up this moiety. The expected binding site for chondroitin sulfate on thrombin is anion binding exosite 2 (which contains basic amino acid residues) because the fifth and sixth EGF-like domains of TM (which bind exosite 1) do not inhibit this interaction (87). Chondroitin sulfate appears to affect the $Ca^{2+}$-dependence of protein C activation by neutralizing the charge within this exosite. Removal of the positive charge within anion binding exosite 2 by mutation of Arg 93, 97, and 101 to Ala results in a thrombin molecule with normal procoagulant activity and normal protein C activation by TM-lacking chondroitin sulfate. However, the presence of this proteoglycan no longer enhances protein C activation (88). Once bound to anion binding exosite 2 of thrombin, chondroitin sulfate induces a conformation change in thrombin, as detected by probes for its active center. In addition to promoting the binding of thrombin to TM, chondroitin sulfate also stimulates inhibition of thrombin by antithrombin (89).

Several cationic proteins, which circulate at high concentrations in the blood, are potent inhibitors of both soluble and membrane-bound TM. These include the eosinophil specific granule proteins: major basic protein, eosinophil peroxidase, and eosinophil cationic protein (90). Platelet factor 4, which is a component of platelet granules, inhibits TM because of its interaction with the chondroitin sulfate side chain (80). A contradictory report suggests that platelet factor 4 acts as a potent stimulator of TM cofactor activity (91).

Regulation of TM proceeds partly by internalization that is induced by thrombin binding (92) followed by degradation of thrombin; however, TM appears to be recycled and returned to the membrane surface. Internalization is blocked when protein C but not APC is bound to TM. Initially it was althought that the cytoplasmic tail was important in this process; however, deletion of this region did not have significant effect (93). More recently, the aminoterminal lectin-like domain has been implicated in the signaling mechanism for internalization (57). Recombinant TM molecules with deletions of either the entire aminoterminal portion (signal peptide, lectin-like domain, hydrophobic region, and 12 residues of the first EGF-like domain) or only the lectin-like domain are transported to the cell membrane normally and exhibit equivalent protein C activation characteristics as compared to wild type TM. However, constitutive endocytosis of TM following thrombin binding (as observed using electron microscopy and immunofluorescence) no longer occurs. Deletion of the hydrophobic region did not affect any of these functions.

## The Molecular Genetics of TM

The full length cDNA transcript of TM is 3.7 kbp and was first isolated using an expression library with selection for clones expressing a protein recognized by antibodies against TM (54, 55). The transcript includes between 123 and 168 bp of 5' untranslated sequence, 1725 bp of coding sequence, 1779 bp of 3' untranslated sequence, and a poly-A tail of 40 bp. The TM gene has been cloned and exists as a single copy on chromosome 20 at position p12 to cen (55, 94, 95). An unusual feature of this gene is the absence of introns; thus, the cDNA sequence corresponds precisely to that of the genomic sequence (56). The reason for the lack of introns is unknown. A single polymorphic site has been identified in the TM gene that results in the substitution of Ala 455 for Val (96). The allele frequency of Val 455 is 0.18 in a European population. Several transcription start sites have been identified and are located 123, 163, and 168 bp upstream of the translation start (AUG) codon (97–99). Several numbering systems have been used to describe the TM promoter region, which has been extensively studied. Here, we adhere to the designation +1 for the transcription start site 168 bp upstream of the AUG translation initiation codon.

Potentially important sequences for gene regulation were identified when the human TM gene was cloned (56). These included a TATA box-like sequence (TATAA) in position -21 to -26; a CAAT box at -106 to -109; and four potential Sp1 binding sites at -123 to -128, -135 to -140, -201 to -206, and -264 to -269. A separate study using reporter gene analysis and mutation of residues representing putative Sp1 binding sequences showed that only those at -135 to -140 and -201 to -206 were important for expression (Fig. 3.5) (100). Although mutation of residues within the potential Sp1 site located at -264 to -269 did not reduce reporter gene activity, deletion of sequence between -233 and -290 reduced the level of expression, which suggests that a positive-

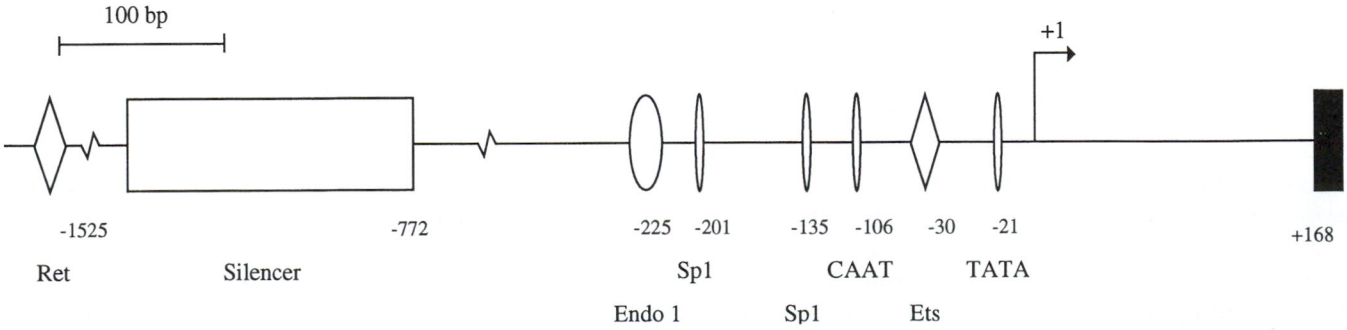

**FIGURE 3.5.** Transcriptional regulation of the gene for thrombomodulin (TM). The gene encoding TM is regulated by multiple cis-acting elements which interact with trans-acting factors, the best defined of which are shown here. The predominant transcription start site is indicated (+1), which is 168 bp upstream of the Met initiation codon. The coding region is shown as the black boxed area. Positive-acting elements are shown as ovals, negative-acting elements as a rectangle, and cellular response elements as diamonds. The numbering corresponds to the 3' base of each element on the coding strand, relative to +1. Abbreviations; Endo 1, region homologous to the endothelin 1 gene involved in endothelial cell specific expression; Ets, motif which responds to Ets, the likely downstream target for tumor necrosis factor a; Ret, retinoic acid response element.

acting element other than Sp1 is located in this region (100). Mutation of the CAAT box reduced expression; although in this case, deletion of residues -100 to -130 increased reporter gene activity. This region is therefore likely to contain both positive and negative transcriptional regulating elements.

Several regions containing positive enhancer elements (-29 to -72, -225 to -245, and -314 to -337) have been identified using a combination of deletion mutants and DNase footprinting analysis (97). Two regions within the sequence of -29 to -72 are protected from cleavage by DNase I, which are -65 to -43 on the coding strand (corresponding to -58 to -46 on the non-coding strand) and -58 to -30 on both strands (Fig. 3.5). The components interacting with these two regions are essential for transcription of the TM gene. The region -245 to -225 has homology to an area of the endothelin I gene, which is involved in endothelial cell-specific expression (101). Elimination of this sequence resulted in a 40-fold reduction of transcriptional activity, which indicates the presence of an essential positive-acting element (Fig. 3.5). A silencer localized at -772 to -947 that reduces reporter gene activity regardless of localization and orientation is also apparent (Fig. 3.5) (100).

Cellular regulation of TM has been observed by various compounds. Inflammatory mediators such as endotoxin, interleukin 1, and tumor necrosis factor (TNF) down-regulate TM expression (102–105) and may therefore play a role in the increased tendency towards thrombosis in such conditions as gram-negative septicemia. This expression reduction may be neutralized by interleukin 4. An atherogenic lipoprotein, which is an oxidized low density lipoprotein, also down-regulates TM expression. The down-regulation occurs because of inhibition of transcription by an unspecified lysosomal degradation product of the oxidized low density lipoprotein (106). Up-regulation of TM expression can be stimulated by tumor-promoting phorbol esters (105, 107), histamine, retinoic acid (99), or by agents that increase the intracellular concentration of cyclic adenosine monophosphate (cyclic AMP) (108–111).

The mechanisms by which three of the above regulators affect TM expression have been investigated. A TNFα-response element is located in the region -56 to -74, which, in isolation, stimulates the heterologous herpes simplex virus thymidine kinase promoter approximately fivefold regardless of orientation, and confers sensitivity to TNFα (98). Nuclear proteins bind to this region of DNA, and deletion of this sequence from the TM promoter results in a 90% reduction in reporter gene activity, although the remaining activity can no longer be repressed by TNFα. The loss of repression can be explained by the presence of Ets motifs (GGAA) in this region because mutation of these elements also eliminates TNFα repression. An Ets-like transcription factor

is the downstream target for TNFα in endothelial cells. A closely spaced direct repeat of the retinoic acid response element (*TGGTCACTGCAGGTCA*) has been identified at position -1525 to -1539 and this is sufficient to confer responsiveness in U937 cells (99). Mutation within the repeats destroys the ability to respond, whereas mutation outside the repeats does not. The retinoic acid response differs between cell lines, and cells with normally high levels of TM expression undergo less changes following culture with retinoic acid. The role of cyclic AMP has only been studied for mouse TM and indicates multiple promoter/enhancer elements in the -50 to -237 region (112).

## PROTEIN C

Protein C was first isolated from plasma as a vitamin K-dependent protein with unknown function (113). Subsequently it was found to be the zymogen of a serine proteinase possessing potent anticoagulant properties (10) with substrate specificity directed towards factor V, factor Va, and factor VIIIa, which it inactivates. Protein C is synthesized primarily in the liver (114) as a single chain plasma glycoprotein of approximately 62 Kda. Protein C is also synthesized in human male reproductive organs (115). Protein C circulates in plasma at an approximate concentration of 4 mg/L.

### The Protein C Molecule

The complete amino acid sequence of human and bovine protein C was derived from cDNA sequence (116, 117); as a vitamin K-dependent protein and the zymogen of a serine proteinase, it has homology with other vitamin K-dependent serine proteinases of the coagulation cascade (factors VII, IX, X, and prothrombin). The prepropeptide of 42 amino acids is removed by two proteolytic cleavages prior to secretion of the mature 419 residue protein. The hydrophobic prepeptide is removed by cleavage at Gly -25 and the propeptide necessary for γ-carboxylation of the Gla domain (26) is removed by cleavage at Arg -1. A dipeptide, Lys 156-Arg 157, is removed from approximately 85% of protein C before secretion (118). The resulting molecule consists of two polypeptide chains that remain linked by a disulfide bond between Cys 141 and Cys 277. The single chain protein C appears to have equivalent biological activity to the two-chain form once they are activated. The light chain of two-chain protein C consists of the vitamin K-dependent Gla domain (residues 1 to 37), an aromatic stack (residues 38 to 45), and two EGF-like domains (residues 46 to 137). The heavy chain consists of the catalytic domain (residues 170 to 419) and the 12 residue activation peptide, which is released following cleavage of the Arg 169-Leu 170 peptide bond by the thrombin/TM complex (Fig. 3.6).

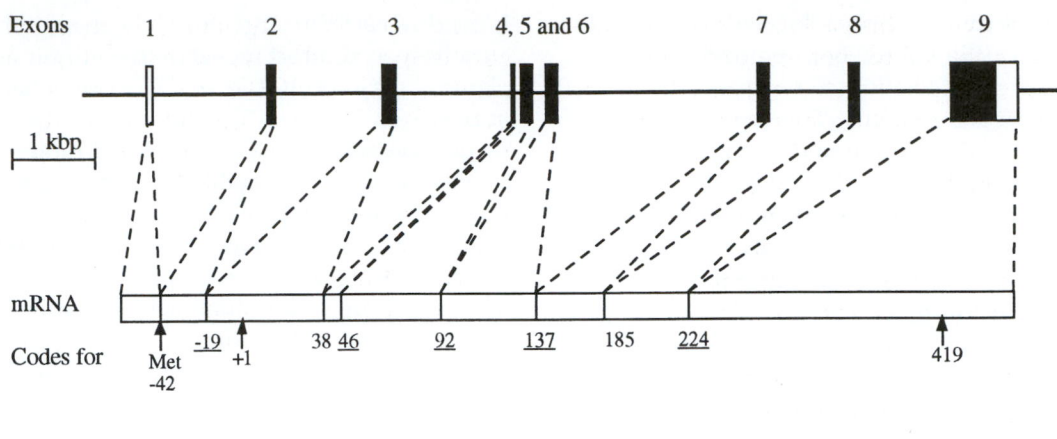

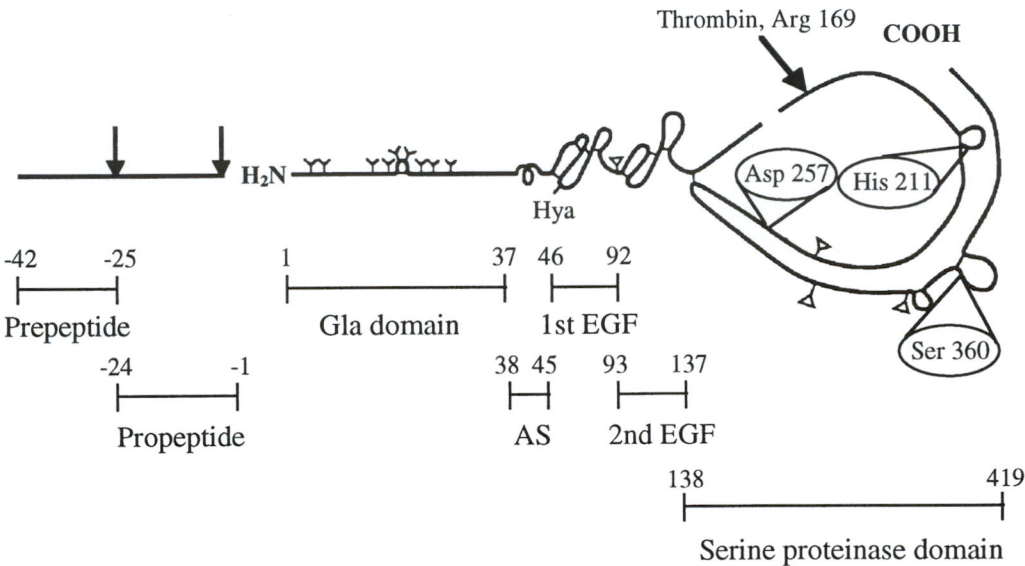

**FIGURE 3.6.** Organization of the gene encoding human protein C and the modular structure of the gene product. The exons of the gene encoding human protein C (upper panel) spanning 11 kbp are numbered 1 to 9 and code for a 42 residue prepropeptide and 419 residue mature protein (lower panel). The 5' and 3' untranslated regions of the gene are indicated by open boxes, and the mRNA shows the codons at which splice junctions in the gene occur. Exon 1 codes for 5' untranslated sequence only, and the Met initiation codon is the first 3 bases of exon 2. An underlined number indicates that the codon, coding for the residue shown, is interrupted by an intron. If not underlined, the codon is the first of that exon. The initiation codon, the first residue of the mature protein (+1), and the final coding residue are indicated (419). Comparison of the numbering for the amino acids encoded by separate exons and the modular structure of protein C shows that each exon (or group of exons) encodes a discrete structural domain. The prepropeptide is shown with the position of the proteolytic cleavages that occur prior to secretion indicated with arrows. Another arrow at Arg 169 indicates the thrombin cleavage site. The catalytic triad of the activated protein, His 211, Asp 257, and Ser 360, is also shown. Human protein C undergoes extensive post-translational modification, including γ-carboxylation (Y), β-hydroxylation of an Asp residue (Hya), and N-linked glycosylation (four potential sites, triangle). Abbreviations: AS, aromatic stack; EGF, epidermal growth factor-like domain. Adapted with permission from Dahlback B, Stenflo J. The protein C anticoagulant system. In: Stamatoyannopoulos G, Nienhuis AW, Majerus PW, Varmus H, eds. The molecular basis of blood diseases. 2nd ed: Philadelphia: WB Saunders, 1994:599–627.

The Gla domain of human protein C contains nine γ-carboxylated glutamic acid residues (Gla 6, 7, 14, 16, 19, 20, 25, 26, and 29) and an internal disulfide loop between Cys 17 and Cys 22 (Figs. 3.2 and 3.6). Several naturally occurring mutations have been identified in this region that result in a variant protein C molecule with reduced biological activity, which includes the substitution of Gla 20, 25, and 26 (119). However, not all the Gla residues are essential for the Gla domain to achieve the correct $Ca^{2+}$-dependent conformation and bind phospholipid. Neither conservative nor nonconservative mutation of Gla 14 or 19 alter the above properties or the biological activity of the variants (120–123). These two residues are expected to coordinate the binding of one solvent-exposed $Ca^{2+}$ ion by analogy to the resolved 3-dimensional structure of prothrombin fragment 1 (Fig. 3.2B), which suggests $Ca^{2+}$ binding in this position is not required for full activity (120, 122). Gla 6 plays a more complex role because nonconservative mutation to Val totally destroys activity, although conservative mutation to Asp does not alter it (122). In this case, a single carboxyl group of this Gla residue may be involved in binding one internal and one solvent-exposed $Ca^{2+}$ ion, which explains the near full biological activity of the Gla 6 to Asp mutation. The Gla 6 to Val mutation did not alter phospholipid binding of the variant protein, possibly because of the hydrophobic effect described below, which is surprising in view of the loss of activity. This suggests that not only is phospholipid binding of the Gla domain of protein C important but this must also result in the proper orientation on the membrane surface to maintain activity.

The presence of hydrophobic components in the Gla domain also contribute a significant portion of the binding energy of protein C to phospholipids (124–126). The $Ca^{2+}$-dependent X-ray crystal structure of bovine prothrombin fragment 1 shows an unusual cluster of solvent-exposed hydrophobic residues (Phe 4, Leu 5, and Leu 8) that are highly conserved amongst all the vitamin K-dependent proteins (Fig. 3.2) (25). Mutation of human protein C, with replacement of each of these hydrophobic residues by a hydrophilic one, does not alter overall $Ca^{2+}$ binding but does reduce the activity of the variants by 70 to 98% (125). The affinity for phospholipid was reduced by the presence of hydrophilic residues at positions 5 and 8, and the substitution of Leu 5 for a hydrophobic Trp slightly increases phospholipid binding (126). The presence of a hydrophilic residue at position 4 does not greatly alter phospholipid binding, but the loss of activity in such a variant APC molecule suggests it plays a role in the orientation with respect to its substrates (125).

Isolated Gla domain binds directly to the soluble thrombin/TM complex, as demonstrated by ultracentrifugation experiments (127), and also competes with protein C or APC for binding to soluble TM and thrombin even in the absence of $Ca^{2+}$. This suggests a role for the Gla domain in the interaction of protein C with thrombin and TM. However, it is unlikely that the Gla domain accounts for all the binding between protein C and thrombin because excess Gla peptide was unable to inhibit binding fully. The aromatic stack region has been reported both to aid formation of the correct $Ca^{2+}$-dependent conformation of the Gla domain and not to be required for macroscopic phospholipid binding, $Ca^{2+}$-dependent conformation, or activation by the thrombin/TM complex (128).

The first EGF-like domain of protein C is unusual because it is predicted to contain four internal disulfide bonds. The additional bond (between Cys 59 and Cys 64) is not expected to greatly affect the conformation of this region. However, the recently determined crystal structure of APC indicates some differences in conformation between the second EGF-like domain of APC and the first EGF-like domain of factor IX (129). This domain also contains a β-hydroxylated Asp residue (Hya), located at position 71 (130), that has been implicated in the $Ca^{2+}$ binding properties of this domain (131). $Ca^{2+}$ binding to a high affinity binding site induces a conformational change in the heavy chain of protein C. The second EGF-like domain contains a N-linked carbohydrate side chain at Asn 97. Glycosylation at this site is critical for efficient secretion of protein C (132).

The catalytic domain of protein C has approximately 70% sequence homology to the other serine proteinases, prothrombin, factor IX, and factor X and contains seven Cys residues, one of which is involved in the disulfide bond linking the heavy chain to the light chain. All remaining Cys residues are involved in internal disulfide bonds in positions conserved between the serine proteinases, between Cys 196 and Cys 212, Cys 331 and Cys 345, and Cys 356 and Cys 384. There are three potential N-linked glycosylation sites within the catalytic domain at positions Asn 248, Asn 313, and Asn 329. The latter of these is situated in the sequence Asn-X-Cys, which is unusual compared to the consensus Asn-X-Ser/Thr sequence (117). Glycosylation of Asn 97 (within the second EGF-like domain) affects glycosylation at this position (132), and approximately 30% of circulating protein C remains unmodified at Asn 329, although this appears not to greatly affect biological activity. The catalytic triad consists of His 211, Asp 257, and Ser 360, and mutations of His 211 and Arg 352 and Asp 359 (in the vicinity of Ser 360) have been identified as causes of reduced protein C activity in individuals with thrombosis (119). An additional $Ca^{2+}$ binding site is present in the proteinase domain involving the region between Glu 225 and Glu 235 (known as the $Ca^{2+}$ binding loop) (133). The intrinsic fluorescence of Trp 231 and Trp 234 within this loop is quenched upon $Ca^{2+}$ binding because of conformational changes (134). It has been suggested that acidic residues near the thrombin cleavage site of protein C move adjacent to Trp 231 upon $Ca^{2+}$ binding and form part of the $Ca^{2+}$ binding pocket. Mutation of Asp 167 and Asp 172 (at the P3 and P3′ positions) reduces the $Ca^{2+}$-dependent fluorescence quenching twofold and the $Ca^{2+}$ affinity of the variants (135).

The crystal structure of D-Phe-Pro-Arg chlormethyl ketone-inhibited Gla-domainless APC has recently been resolved to 2.8 Å (129). The catalytic domain is approximately spherical (45 Å × 45 Å × 50 Å) and has several points of contact with the second EGF-like domain. One of the features of this domain is a positively charged groove, similar to anion binding exosite 1 of thrombin, including eight clustered basic residues: Lys 191, Lys 192, Lys 193, Arg 222, Arg 229, Arg 230, Lys 233, and Arg 314. The exosite may also include Lys 308, Lys 311, and Arg 314, although the orientation of these side chains has not been defined. No region similar to anion binding exosite 2 of thrombin is present, which is a possible explanation of the resistance of APC to serpins. In general, most of the loops surrounding the active site are analogous to those of the other serine proteinases.

## Activation of Protein C

The activation of protein C by the thrombin/TM complex is dependent on $Ca^{2+}$ whether or not the activation complex is membrane-associated or in solution. The Gla domain of protein C was a contender for providing this $Ca^{2+}$-dependence because of its well-characterized $Ca^{2+}$ binding properties described above. However, a variant protein C molecule lacking the Gla domain still requires $Ca^{2+}$ ions for activation by the thrombin/TM complex (136). Wild type and Gla-domainless protein C are activated at the same rate in solution with saturating levels of $Ca^{2+}$. However, activation by membrane-associated thrombin/TM complex is much less rapid, and the $Ca^{2+}$-dependence of activation is altered (half maximal activation at 50 $\mu$M $Ca^{2+}$ for Gla-domainless protein C and 250 $\mu$M $Ca^{2+}$ for intact protein C). Activation of Gla-domainless protein C by free thrombin is still inhibited by $Ca^{2+}$, which suggests the conformation of this variant is shifted towards the $Ca^{2+}$-dependent form (136). Such studies indicate the $Ca^{2+}$-dependence of protein C activation depends on residues outside the Gla domain. The high affinity $Ca^{2+}$ binding site located within the first EGF-like domain also does not appear to be important because a variant lacking both the Gla domain and the first EGF-like domain has similar $Ca^{2+}$-dependent activation characteristics to that of Gla-domainless protein C (137). As mentioned above, $Ca^{2+}$ binding appears to result in a conformation change in the region around the scissile bond of protein C. Taken together, this implicates the $Ca^{2+}$ binding loop within the serine proteinase domain in providing the $Ca^{2+}$-dependence of protein C activation. In thrombin, which does not have these $Ca^{2+}$-dependent properties, a homologous loop is maintained by a salt bridge between Lys 225 and Glu 235 (protein C numbering). The $Ca^{2+}$-dependence of Gla domainless protein C activation can be removed by introducing a Glu 235 to Lys mutation (i.e., introducing a salt bridge at an analogous position to that of thrombin) (133), which suggests this variant is similar to the $Ca^{2+}$-stabilized conformation of the wild type protein and it does not have this $Ca^{2+}$ binding site.

Several residues surrounding the thrombin cleavage site of protein C are also involved in $Ca^{2+}$-dependent activation. Disruption of the $Ca^{2+}$ binding pocket by mutation of the acidic residues at the P3 and P3′ positions alters the $Ca^{2+}$-dependent activation by the thrombin/TM complex (135). Mutation of Pro, which is situated at the P2 position of protein C (Pro 168 to Val), has a similar effect and also influences activation by free thrombin (138). This variant requires 100 times more $Ca^{2+}$ for equivalent activation by the thrombin/TM complex (saturating levels), but $Ca^{2+}$ no longer inhibits activation by free thrombin. A cluster of basic residues, at the P5′ (Lys 174), P8′ (Arg 177), and P9′ (Arg 178) positions, suggests a mechanism by which protein C activation by free thrombin remains low. Conversion of these residues to Glu does not alter the catalytic ability of the variant APC but increases the rate of protein C activation by free thrombin 12-fold in the presence of $Ca^{2+}$ (139). No effect was observed in the absence of $Ca^{2+}$, and activation by the thrombin/TM complex was diminished. This can be explained by electrostatic repulsion between this basic cluster in wild type protein C and the anion binding exosite 1 of thrombin. Altering the charge eliminates repulsion and promotes activation by free thrombin. Upon binding of thrombin to TM, this anion binding exosite is masked (72); therefore, the basic cluster of protein C also appears to play a role in the protein C/TM interaction.

## The Inactivation of Factors V, Va, and VIIIa by APC

Factor V and factor VIII are highly homologous proteins, neither of which has procoagulant function until activated by either thrombin or factor Xa (140). Both factor V and factor VIII contain two types of internal repeats (termed A and C modules). The aminoterminal region of the single chain procofactors consist of two A modules (A1 and A2) and the carboxyterminus consists of another A module and two C modules (A3, C1, and C2), which are separated from the aminoterminus by an additional domain (the B module). Activation occurs by the cleavage of at least three peptide bonds. Both proteins are then composed of a heavy and a light chain, following the release of activation peptides derived from the B module. The heavy chain of factor V, consisting of A1 and A2, is noncovalently attached to the light chain, consisting of A3, C1, and C2, via $Ca^{2+}$-dependent interactions. A phospholipid binding site is located in the A3 domain.

The anticoagulant function of APC appears to be species specific because the bovine protein does not prolong the clotting time of human plasma. In contrast, human APC can function in both human and bovine plasma. The mechanism of *in vitro* inactivation of bovine and human factor V and factor Va have been well studied. Inactivation of human factor Va on membrane surfaces is an ordered event and progresses by sequential cleavage of peptide bonds at Arg 506 (within the A2 domain) followed by cleavage at Arg 306 and Arg 679 (1, 141). The fragments produced by cleavage at Arg 506 are intermediate, which suggests it is a requirement for complete exposure of the other scissile bonds. Only cleavage at Arg 306 (between the A1 and A2 domains) is associated with immediate and complete loss of cofactor activity towards factor Xa. Conversely, the first cleavage by APC in membrane-bound factor V is Arg 306, followed by those at Arg 506, Arg 679, and Lys 994, which suggests the functionally important cleavage site is already available in this case (141). All these cleavage sites are in the heavy chain of the factor V/Va molecule, and no cleavage occurs in the light chain (1). Bovine factor V/Va differs from the human form because cleavages within the light chain also occur. The phospholipid-dependent inactivation of factor V by APC has recently been reported to be enhanced by heparin (142).

The inactivation of human factor VIIIa by APC proceeds similarly to that of factor Va. Arg 336 of factor VIIIa corresponds to Arg 306 of factor Va, and cleavage in this position also results in immediate and complete loss of cofactor activity. A cleavage within the A2 domain of factor VIIIa is required to expose this cleavage site.

A recent study using a reconstituted model of tissue factor-induced thrombin generation suggests APC exerts its effect solely by the proteolytic inactivation of factor Va (1). In this study, the suppression of thrombin formation correlated with degradation of the factor Va heavy chain and slowed generation of the factor Va light chain. The cleavage of factor VIIIa did not alter the generation of thrombin or activation of factor X.

A variant protein C molecule with the substitution Glu 357 to Gln (close to Ser 360 of the catalytic triad) was produced in a recombinant system in an attempt to increase the activity of APC towards factor Va (143). This was based on a similar mutation at the homologous position in thrombin that increased its activity to substrates containing an Asp residue at the P3 and P3′ sites. Factor Va also has an Asp residue at the P3 site. *In vitro*, the variant inactivated factor Va two- to threefold more rapidly than the wild type. The anticoagulant activity was slightly reduced in plasma; this finding is explained by the increased susceptibility of the variant to proteinase inhibitors. Therefore, it would appear the evolution of protein C has been such that protease activity is submaximal whilst maintaining resistance to the wide range of circulating inhibitors.

The helical conformation of the aromatic stack is important in presenting the active site of APC in the correct alignment to its substrates, although the precise amino acid content is not vital. The Gla domain dependent $Ca^{2+}$ binding, macroscopic phospholipid binding, or rate of activation by the thrombin/TM complex is not significantly altered if the aromatic stack domain of protein C is replaced with the equivalent found in factor IX or the helical formation is disrupted by single residue substitutions (128). However, disruption of the helical stack results in an approximate 60 to 70% loss in APC activity towards natural substrates as measured by the aPTT and factor VIIIa inactivation; replacement does not significantly alter these functions (128).

## The Molecular Genetics of Protein C

Several cDNAs encoding human protein C spanning the entire coding region have been isolated (117, 144). Two different mRNA species, which are 1650 and 1850 bp in length, are present, as visualized by Northern blot. These represent the use of alternate polyadenylation sites 68 and 294 bp downstream of the translation termination codon. The full-length cDNA therefore includes approximately 75 bp of 5′ untranslated region, 68 or 294 bp 3′ untranslated region, in addition to 1383 bp coding for the 461 residue precursor protein.

The gene for protein C has been fully sequenced and is located on chromosome 2 (145, 146), position q13-q14 (147, 148), which spans approximately 11 kbp of genomic DNA (149, 150). Initially, Foster et al detected only eight exons; however, a ninth exon was subsequently identified that codes for the 5′ untranslated sequence. Intron/exon boundaries obey the GT-AG rule and are of a similar type to those found in related proteins. The intron/exon structure of the gene also provides insights into the domain structure of the mature protein because in many cases each exon encodes a discrete domain (Fig. 3.6). Thus, exon 1 encodes 5′ untranslated sequence, exon 2 encodes the signal peptide, exon 3 encodes the propeptide and the Gla domain, exon 4 encodes the aromatic stack, and exons 5 and 6 encode each of the two EGF-like domains. The final three exons code for the serine proteinase domain, which has exons and splice junctions in similar positions and of the same phase class to those of factors VII, IX, and X. In contrast, protein C and prothrombin are dissimilar with respect to location of exons in other regions and only have exons 2, 3, and 4 in homologous positions. This supports a model for the evolution of these proteins from a common ancestral gene.

The 5′ sequence of the protein C gene has recently been characterized, approximately 800 bp of additional sequence obtained, and the transcription initiation site further characterized (Fig. 3.7) (151). Nearly 80% of transcripts start 65 bp upstream of the first intron/exon boundary (denoted here as +1), another 18% start at -7, and 2% start at +13 (previously assigned as +1). It would therefore appear exon 1 can be of variable length, although it is uncertain if this heterogeneity occurs during *in vivo* protein C expression. About 66 bp of exon 1

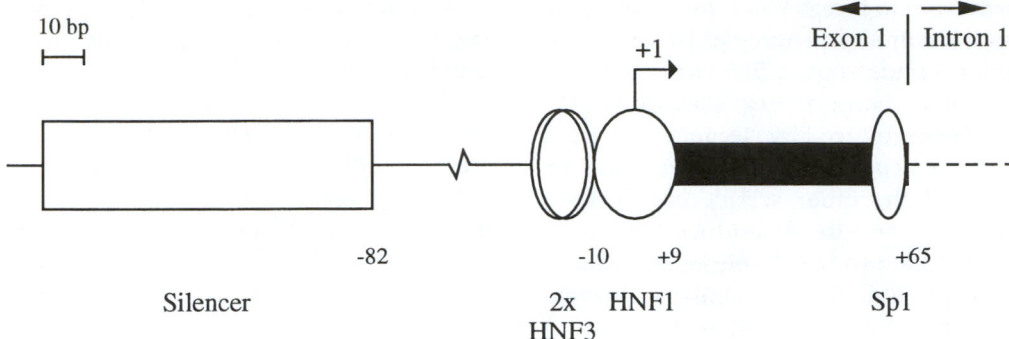

**FIGURE 3.7.** Transcriptional regulation of the gene for human protein C. The 5' area gene encoding protein C does not contain any region with TATA box similarity and must therefore be regulated by TATA-less promoters, which are commonly characterized by a clustering of transcription initiation sites surrounding +1 in the absence of alternative initiator sequences. The predominant transcription start site is indicated (+1), which is 65 bp upstream of the first intron/exon boundary, and exon 1 is shown as the black boxed area. Positive-acting elements are shown as ovals, and negative-acting elements as a rectangle. The numbering corresponds to the 3' base of each element on the coding strand, relative to +1. Abbreviation: HNF, hepatic nuclear factor.

and 1.5 kbp of upstream sequence are sufficient to promote high level expression of a reporter gene in cultured liver cells. However, the protein C gene belongs to a class of genes that lacks a TATA box element and must be regulated by TATA-less promoters, which are commonly characterized by a clustering of transcription initiation start sites surrounding +1.

The region from -42 to +66 contains strong liver specific elements because it drives reporter gene expression in HepG2 but not HeLa cells. DNA footprint analysis shows two areas protected by HepG2 cell nuclear proteins. Although there is no homology between one of these (+20 to +30) and known recognition sequences for transcription factors, the other contains one region homologous to the hepatic nuclear factor (HNF) 1 recognition sequence (-10 to +9) and two overlapping, oppositely oriented, HNF 3 binding sites (-25 to -11). Four naturally occurring point mutations identified in individuals with reduced protein C levels occur within these enhancer sequences at positions -20, -15, -2, and +3 (119). *In vitro* mutagenesis confirmed these mutations reduce reporter gene expression between 75 and 90% (151, 152). Double stranded sequences, which are derived from the three potential binding sites, bind nuclear proteins derived from liver cells alone. Introducing mutations at -20, -2, and +3 abolished the binding of these liver-specific proteins (151). The importance of the overlapping HNF 3 binding sites has been further emphasized as mutation at -20 was found to completely abolish binding of HNF 3, whereas mutation at -15 reduced the binding of this transcription factor (152). Two molecules of HNF 3 bind to this region, probably on opposite faces of the DNA helix. Exon 1 also contains a potential Sp1 binding site (+58 to +65), and this sequence binds HepG2 nuclear proteins that are displaced by the Sp1 binding consensus oligonucleotide.

Several promoters, which may lack the TATA box, have an initiator element that can replace or assist in directing transcription initiation. However, sequences surrounding the three possible initiation sites of protein C have no similarity to any known initiator elements (151). An unknown initiator element may be responsible for assembling the transcription apparatus. Alternatively, this function may be carried out by the cluster of regulatory elements described above. Silencer elements may also exist in the region -82 to -162, although this has not been examined in detail (151).

## PROTEIN S

Protein S circulates as an approximately 64 Kda single chain glycoprotein with a plasma concentration of 20-25 mg/L. It is expressed in many tissues including the liver (114), endothelial cells (153, 154), Leydig cells of the testis (155), brain, and megakaryocytes (156, 157). The anticoagulant function of protein S was originally althought to be solely as a nonenzymic cofactor for APC in the degradation of factors Va and VIIIa (13). However, APC-independent functions have also been proposed, although their physiologic relevance remains to be determined. Protein S may also play a role in the complement pathway because a proportion is noncovalently bound to C4b-binding protein (C4bBP) (158), which is a component of this pathway; however, any such role remains to be defined. The protein S/C4bBP complex affects certain functions of protein S; most importantly protein S can no longer act as a cofactor to APC.

### The Protein S Molecule

The primary structure of human and bovine protein S was derived from cDNA sequence (159-162), which revealed a domain structure regionally homologous to other vitamin K-dependent proteins. The mature molecule is 635 amino acids in length and results from two proteolytic cleavages prior to secretion. Cleavage at Ala - 18 removes the 22 residue hydrophobic signal (pre-) peptide, and a further 17 residues representing the propeptide are removed by cleavage at Arg -1. The mature protein consists of a Gla domain (residues 1 to 37), an aromatic stack (residues 38 to 46), a thrombin sensitive region (TSR, residues 47 to 75), four EGF-like domains (residues 76 to 242), and a region homologous to sex hormone binding globulin (SHBG-like domain, residues 243 to 63) (Fig. 3.8).

The Gla domain contains 11 γ-carboxylated glutamic acid residues (6, 7, 14, 16, 19, 20, 25, 26, 29, 32, and 36) and a small disulfide loop between Cys 17 and Cys 22 (Fig. 3.2). As in other vitamin K-dependent proteins, the $Ca^{2+}$-dependent conformation of the Gla domain is essential for protein S to bind to negatively charged phospholipid and for its biological functions. Immediately adjacent to the aromatic stack is the TSR, which is formed by a disulfide bond between Cys 47 and Cys 72. The term 'TSR' reflects an important feature of this loop because it is sensitive to cleavage by thrombin (163, 164). Two Arg residues, 52 and 70, are responsible for the thrombin sensitivity in bovine protein S. There are three thrombin cleavage sites in human protein S: Arg 49, Arg 60, and Arg 70 (165). Following thrombin cleavage, the Gla domain of protein S is no longer capable of binding $Ca^{2+}$ ions (166) or assuming the $Ca^{2+}$-dependent conformation required for binding to phospholipids. This change suggests the TSR is intimately involved in the folding of the Gla domain in protein S. Thrombin cleaved protein S has no APC cofactor activity (167, 168). However, protein S is protected from this cleavage at physiologic concentrations of $Ca^{2+}$ and high concentrations of phospholipid (166, 169). The TSR, together with the first EGF-like domain, is likely to be involved in the interaction with APC (170, 171).

The first EGF-like domain contains a β-hydroxyaspartic acid residue (Hya 95), and each of the second to the fourth EGF-like domains contains a β-hydroxyasparagine residue (Hyn 136, 178 and 217) (76). Each of the Hyn containing EGF-like domains contain a very high affinity $Ca^{2+}$ binding site ($K_d$ in the nanomolar range), which is important for protein S/C4bBP interaction and achieving native conformation and protease resistance (172). This binding site explains the $Ca^{2+}$ binding properties retained by Gla-domainless protein S (166). However, presence of the Hya and Hyn residues does not appear to be required for protein S to demonstrate APC cofactor function or to bind C4bBP (173). Although the crystal structure of protein S remains to be determined, conformation of the aminoterminal domains of the molecule can be inferred by analogy to prothrombin fragment 1 (Gla domain and aromatic stack) (25) and the EGF-like domains of other proteins (such as factor IX) (36).

The carboxyterminal region of protein S is unlike the other vitamin K-dependent proteins and is homologous to SHBG and androgen binding protein (174–176). Little is known of the conformation of this region, which contains only three disulfide bonds. One of these (between Cys 245 and Cys 527) forms a large loop, with another internal loop between Cys 408 and Cys 434. The third disulfide loop (between Cys 598 and Cys 625) is situated at the extreme carboxyterminus of protein S. There are three potential N-glycosylation sites within the SHBG-like domain at Asn 458, 468, and 489, which should account for the 7 to 8% carbohydrate found in protein S purified from plasma. Although the SHBG-like domain does not appear to confer the ability to bind steroids on protein S (155), this domain does contain the binding site for C4bBP. The binding site has been partly localized to residues 605 to 614 (within the carboxyterminal disulfide loop) (177) and may also include amino acids 413 to 433 (the internal disulfide loop) (178). A more recent investigation has identified another region of the SHBG-like domain that is important for binding of protein S to C4bBP. Using a bacteriophage display library, which expresses random six and 15-mer peptides on the surface of bacteriophages, peptides with high homology to residues surrounding position 450 were found to bind to the C4bBP β-chain. A synthetic peptide corresponding to residues 447 to 468 was subsequently found to inhibit the binding of protein S to C4bBP and to bind directly to C4bBP.

## Protein S and C4b Binding Protein

In normal individuals, approximately 60% of circulating protein S is in complex with C4bBP, which is a multimeric protein consisting of six or seven α-chains and either one or no β-chain (180–182). C4bBP has several functions, including cofactor activity in the degradation of C4b by serine protease factor I (180). The α-chains contain the binding site for C4b, whereas the β-chain contains the binding site for protein S (183, 184). The protein S/C4bBP complex does not appear to interfere with the functions of C4bBP in the complement pathway. The amount of unbound (or free) protein S is equal to the molar excess of total protein S over β-chain containing C4bBP (185, 186) because of the low dissociation constant for this reaction (0.5 to 1 nM in the presence of $Ca^{2+}$). The levels of C4bBP may increase by as much as 400% during the acute phase reaction. However, near constant levels of free protein S are maintained by differential regulation of the α- and β-chains of C4bBP, and the majority of C4bBP does not contain the β-chain in this circumstance (186).

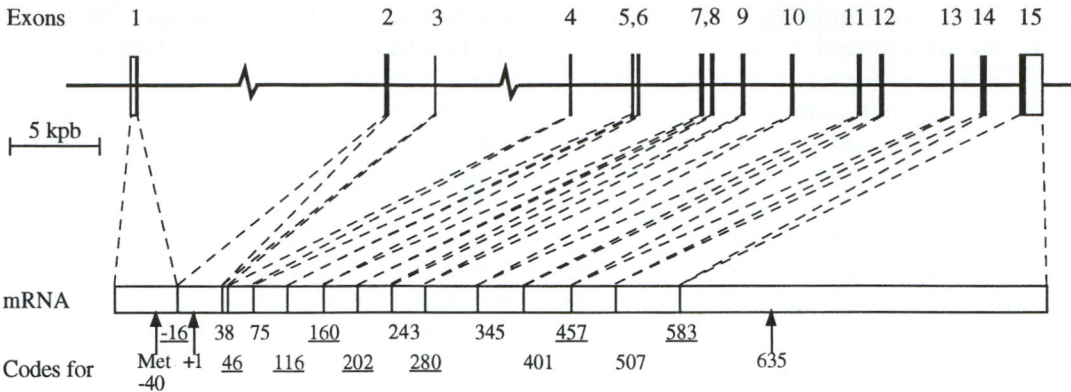

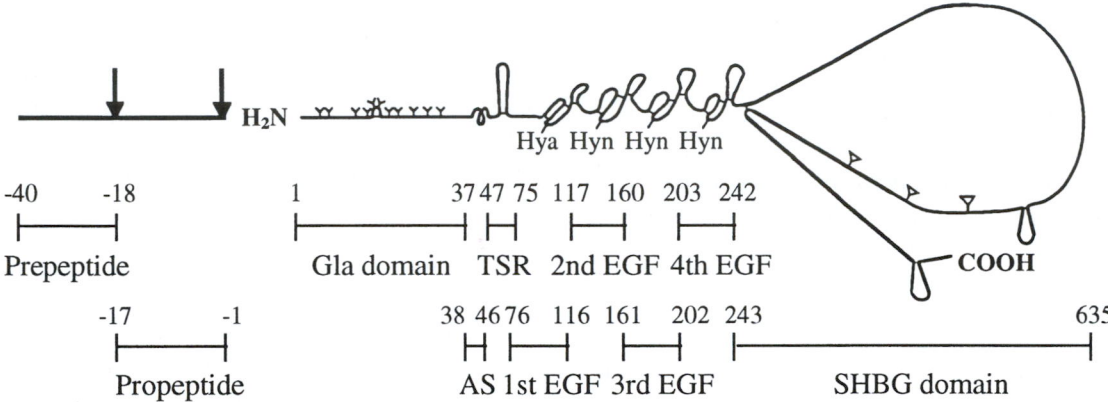

**FIGURE 3.8.** Organization of the gene encoding human protein S and the modular structure of the gene product. The exons of the gene encoding human protein S (upper panel) spanning more than 80 kbp are numbered 1 to 15 and code for a 40 residue prepropeptide and a 635 residue mature protein (lower panel). The 5′ and 3′ untranslated regions of the gene are indicated by open boxes, and the mRNA shows the codons at which splice junctions in the gene occur. An underlined number indicates that the codon (coding for the residue shown) is interrupted by an intron. If not underlined, the codon is the first of that exon. The initiation codon, the first residue of the mature protein ($+1$), and the final coding residue are indicated (635). Comparison of the numbering for the amino acids encoded by separate exons and the modular structure of protein S shows that each exon (or group of exons) encodes a discrete structural domain. Here, the prepropeptide is shown with the position of the proteolytic cleavages that occur prior to secretion indicated with arrows. Human protein S undergoes extensive post-translational modification, including γ-carboxylation (Y), β-hydroxylation of an Asp residue (Hya) and three Asn (Hyn) residues, and N-linked glycosylation (three potential sites, triangle). Other abbreviations: AS, aromatic stack; EGF, epidermal growth factor-like domain; SHBG, sex hormone binding globulin-like domain; TSR, thrombin sensitive region. Adapted with permission from Dahlback B, Stenflo J. The protein C anticoagulant system. In: Stamatoyannopoulos G, Nienhuis AW, Majerus PW, Varmus H, eds. The molecular basis of blood diseases. 2nd ed: Philadelphia: WB Saunders, 1994:599–627.

A naturally occurring mutation causing a Ser 460 to Pro substitution (187) results in a variant protein S molecule with abnormal C4bBP binding characteristics (188). The variant (named protein S Heerlen) displays a biphasic binding to C4bBP, which is immobilized on microtitre plates instead of the monophasic binding observed with native protein S. These results suggest two molecules of the variant can bind to one molecule of C4bBP, a potential explanation for the normal total levels of protein S antigen, but reduced levels of free protein S antigen, observed in most individuals who carry this mutation.

## The Anticoagulant Activity of Protein S

The principle anticoagulant activity of protein S is to function as a cofactor to APC in the inactivation of factors Va and VIIIa (13). This activity is blocked when protein S is in complex with C4bBP (189); thus, only free protein S has APC cofactor activity *in vivo*. While it has not been possible to demonstrate an interaction between protein S and APC in the fluid phase, on a lipid surface they form a 1:1 stoichiometric complex. In purified systems, the rate of inactivation of factors Va and VIIIa by APC is increased approximately twofold by the presence of protein S. The increase primarily occurs because of an increase in the affinity of APC for phospholipid vesicles (190), which results in a complex on the surface of endothelial cells (191, 192) and platelets (193, 194). This weak cofactor activity was surprising, given the severe clinical consequences of homozygous protein S deficiency and the risk for thrombosis associated with heterozygous protein S deficiency in clinically affected families (3). However, three observations have recently been made that are more in keeping with these clinical observations: 1) protein S stimulates APC cleavage of Arg 306 in factor Va 20-fold; 2) protein S competes with factor Xa for a binding site on factor Va; this removes the protective effect of factor Xa in APC proteolysis of factor Va that has been observed in the absence of protein S (195, 196). A similar reaction takes place between factor IXa and factor VIIIa, and in this case, protein S removes the protective effect of factor IXa; 3) intact factor V and protein S appear to act as synergistic cofactors for APC in the inactivation of factor VIIIa (197). Factor V alone confers no additional increase in the rate of inactivation in the presence of APC, but the inactivation rate is increased approximately 10-fold in the presence of factor V and protein S. This represents a fivefold increase compared to the effect of protein S alone. However, the significance of this role is disputed because protein S did not greatly increase the proteolytic cleavage of factor VIIIa in a reconstituted system (1). Intact factor V and factor Va may increase the affinity of APC for the phospholipid membrane.

Functionally important domains of protein S have been identified using monoclonal antibodies mapped to its aminoterminal epitopes (170). Monoclonal antibodies against the Gla domain inhibit APC cofactor function by blocking phospholipid binding to protein S. Monoclonal antibodies against the TSR and the first EGF-like domain inhibit the APC cofactor activity of protein S without affecting phospholipid binding, which suggests these two regions constitute the point of interaction between protein S and APC. Chimeric human/bovine protein S molecules have been used to confirm the roles of these two domains (171). The species specificity of the anticoagulant function of APC in human plasma is restored if both bovine APC and bovine protein S are present. Thus, human protein S can display cofactor activity to human but not bovine APC, and bovine protein S can display cofactor activity to both (189). This suggests human protein S and bovine APC are unable to form a complex on the phospholipid surface. The cofactor activity of human protein S to bovine APC is restored if the TSR and the first EGF-like bovine protein S are used to replace the homologous regions in the human protein. Replacement of the TSR alone is not sufficient to restore cofactor activity.

A natural point mutation in the gene for protein S,

$+5$ G to A in intron 5, has recently been described in an individual with normal levels of protein S antigen and 30% levels of protein S activity with respect to APC cofactor function (198). This mutation results in the deletion of the first EGF-like domain of the protein S molecule, and the truncated form was present in the individual's plasma. This supports the conclusion of the *in vitro* studies discussed above that concluded the first EGF-domain is critical for protein S to act as a cofactor to APC.

Rhesus monkey and porcine protein S are able to act as cofactors to only human or bovine APC, respectively (199), and rabbit protein S has a higher activity in bovine compared to human APC (200). The amino acid sequence of protein S from these species has been predicted from cDNA clones (199, 201), and their comparison have implicated amino acids Arg 49, Gln 52, Gln 61, Ser 81, Ser 92, Lys 97, Thr 103, and Pro 106 in the interaction between human protein S and APC (199). The third EGF-like domain does not appear to be important for APC cofactor function because this region can be removed from recombinant human protein S without effect on activity in a plasma system (202).

Protein S also has *in vitro* anticoagulant properties that are independent of APC by directly inhibiting both the prothrombinase complex and the factor X activating complex. Initially a direct binding between factor Va and protein S was demonstrated that was $Ca^{2+}$-dependent, saturable, reversible, and blocked the binding of prothrombin to factor Va (203). Protein S also binds to factor Xa and inhibits the amidolytic activities of this serine proteinase. Efficiency is increased in the presence of $Ca^{2+}$ and factor Va, but phospholipids have no effect in the absence of factor Va (204). Inhibition of the prothrombinase complex is achieved to the same extent by thrombin-cleaved and C4bBP-associated protein S. Half maximal inhibition is observed around the physiologic concentration of free protein S and appears to be dependent on $Ca^{2+}$ and phospholipid binding. Intact and thrombin-cleaved protein S bind directly to factor V and factor Va. However, the protein S/C4bBP complex can no longer bind factor V or factor Va, which suggests this complex formation blocks the factor V/Va binding site. Factor Xa activity is reduced by free protein S and the protein S/C4bBP complex through noncompetitive inhibition. Thrombin-cleaved protein S loses its inhibitory activity, which suggests the conformational change induced by this cleavage results in loss of the factor Xa binding site (205). A more recent report suggests the inhibitory effect of protein S on the prothrombinase complex is through competition for phospholipid binding sites (206).

Protein S inhibition of the factor X activating complex requires the presence of phospholipid, is unaltered by thrombin cleavage and is increased when protein S is in complex with C4bBP (207). Protein S binds directly to factor VIII, in a reversible, specific, and saturable manner, and the affinity of the protein S/C4bBP complex for factor VIII is fivefold greater than that of protein S alone. C4bBP also binds factor VIII (208). The presence of the carrier protein of factor VIII, von Willebrand factor, decreases its ability to bind protein S by approximately 40%.

In addition to the functions mentioned above, protein S may also play a role in vascular injury repair because it acts as a mitogen towards smooth muscle cells (209, 210). Although a receptor for protein S has not been identified to date, it may be similar to a tyrosine kinase receptor of the Axl family. This is because bovine protein S activates human Sky; a member of this group of transmembrane proteins and a homologue of protein S (human Gas6) stimulates human Sky (211, 212). Furthermore, protein S stimulates osteoblasts and may have a role in bone development (213).

## The Molecular Genetics of Protein S

The full length cDNA encoding human protein S has been cloned by several groups (160–162), and reports on its length range from 2.6 to 4 kbp, of which 2028 bp represents the coding region. The remainder is between 108 and 120 bp of 5' untranslated sequence and approximately 1140 bp of 3' untranslated region, including a poly-A tail. The 3' untranslated region contains two putative polyadenylation signal sequences (AATAAA) 1096 and 1131 bp downstream of the translation stop codon (161). The site of polyadenylation is 20 bp downstream of this latter site. The human protein S cDNA has 87.5% nucleotide identity to bovine protein S (159).

Two genes for human protein S have been mapped near the centromere of chromosome 3 (146, 214) in position p11.1 to 11.2 (215) situated within 4 cM of each other. One is the active gene (PROS1 or PSα), which is comprised of 15 exons and 14 introns (216–218). The other (PROS2 or PSβ) shares approximately 97% nucleic acid identity within the coding regions with the active gene but lacks exon 1. The 3% difference in sequence within PROS2 gives rise to multiple frameshifts and stop codons. PROS2 has no open reading frame and is considered to be an inactive pseudogene. The chimpanzee and gorilla also have two protein S genes, whereas the rhesus monkey, orangutan, and African green monkey have only one, which suggests a gene duplication event in the evolution of the orangutan from African apes (217). The active gene spans approximately 80 kbp, of which only a small percentage is coding sequence. In most cases, the complete sequence of these regions has not been determined because of the size of the introns of PROS1 (ranging from 0.8 to more than 20 kbp). However, all obey the GT-AT rule and are of identical phase class to other vitamin K-dependent proteins and SHBG when they are optimally aligned. Six repetitive Alu elements have been identified, which have 82% homology to each other.

Each exon (or group of exons) of PROS1 encodes a discrete structural domain (Fig. 3.8) (216). Exon 1 codes for the 5' untranslated region and prepeptide. Similar to protein C, a single exon codes for both the propeptide and the Gla domain (exon 2). Exon 3 encodes the aromatic stack, and the unique TSR is encoded by exon 4. Each of the EGF-like domains are encoded by exons 5 through 8 and the SHBG-like domain by exons 9 to 15, with introns positioned similarly to those of the SHBG gene. This is compatible with the suggestion the coagulation factors evolved from a common ancestral gene through exon shuffling.

Primer extension experiments suggest the presence of two major transcription start sites, which are 174 and 286 bp upstream of the translation initiation codon (217). Both of these sites represent a longer 5' untranslated region than the longest protein S cDNA isolated. Although approximately 700 bp of 5' untranscribed sequence has been published, the PROS1 regulatory elements remain poorly characterized and no region with TATA box-like similarity has been identified. However, several clustered GC-rich sequences exist in the region 30 to 80 bp upstream of the translation start codon (*AUG*) that resemble the consensus for Sp1 binding sites (216). It remains possible that similar to protein C, an additional exon may be present upstream of that containing the translation start site. This is supported by the presence of two potential splice acceptor sites, 138 and 251 bp upstream of the translation start site, which could give rise to the two different transcription start sites by alternative splicing (217).

## THE ENDOTHELIAL CELL PROTEIN C/APC RECEPTOR

The recent identification of a second endothelial cell receptor involved in protein C activation, which is the endothelial cell protein C/APC receptor (EPCR), suggests the model of protein C activation by thrombin and TM alone is a simplification. The presence of an additional component on the surface of endothelial cells was originally postulated by Esmon et al in their description of Gla-domainless protein C (136). In the presence of components at their physiologic concentrations, they observed intact protein C was activated 50 times more rapidly than Gla-domainless protein C over the cell surface, in contrast with the identical activation rates by the soluble thrombin/TM complex. A 1.3 kbp cDNA was isolated using an expression library with selection for clones expressing a cell surface protein that could bind protein C (14). This codes for a 238 residue precursor protein that binds both protein C and APC. The Gla domain of protein C is a requirement for this interaction. The EPCR has a mass of approximately 46 Kda, which is larger than predicted based on amino acid sequence (25 Kda) and is probably due to the presence of carbohydrate located at four potential N-glycosylation sites within the coding region. The EPCR is expressed primarily on the surface of the endothelial cells of the large-vessels of the vasculature and is only present at low levels in the capillaries (219).

The EPCR itself does not have any direct anticoagulant effect; its addition to plasma does not increase the clotting time, and APC bound to the EPCR loses its ability to inactivate its natural substrate, factor Va (220). However, the use of monoclonal antibodies that inhibit the binding of protein C to the EPCR has shown the EPCR influences the rate of activation of protein C by the thrombin/TM complex on endothelium (221). If access to EPCR is blocked, then the rate to protein C activation is reduced approximately 80%. This suggests protein C activation on endothelial cells requires both the thrombin/TM complex and the interaction of the Gla domain of protein C with the EPCR. Crucially, it provides a potentially important mechanism of enhancing the initiation of the protein C anticoagulant system in the large-vessels, especially the arteries (219). It has also been proposed that binding of APC to the EPCR modulates the activity of this serine proteinase similarly to that of the effect of TM on thrombin (219). This suggestion arose primarily from the crystal structure of Gla-domainless APC (129), which showed this protein had a groove similar in structure and location to anion binding exosite 1 of thrombin. However, alternative substrates for the EPCR/APC complex have yet to be identified.

The amino acid sequence of the EPCR predicted from cDNA sequence and homology searches suggests similarities to the CD1/MHC class I superfamily (approximately 60% homology at the amino acid level) (14). The extracellular region of the EPCR may have two distinct domains based on this homology. It was initially predicted 15 residues of the 238 amino acids represented the signal sequence for receptor transport to the cell surface (14). This was consistent with a two-domain structure because there would be four Cys residues available to form two disulfide bonds in the extracellular region. However, sequencing of the aminoterminal amino acids of a soluble form of the EPCR indicated 17 residues are removed and, as such, the mature molecule consists of 221 residues, including only three Cys residues available to form disulfide bonds (222). This undermines the proposed two domain.main structure, and the native conformation of the molecule remains uncertain.

The contribution of the EPCR in coagulation regulation and prevention of thrombus formation is unknown. These preliminary studies suggest an important physiologic role will be defined in the future.

# THE HEPARAN SULFATE/ ANTITHROMBIN PATHWAY

Antithrombin is the most important direct inhibitor of coagulation proteinases and circulates at an approximate concentration in plasma of 150 mg/L. It inhibits the activity of thrombin, factor Xa, factor IXa, factor XIa, and factor XIIa by forming equimolar tight complexes that block the accessibility of respective substrates to the proteinase active sites (223). The inhibition of thrombin by antithrombin may be most effective at suppressing coagulation because of the key role of thrombin in accelerating its own generation by participating in factor V and factor VIII activation. Antithrombin also plays a role in the inhibition of factor VIIa by complementing the action of TFPI. In its free state, factor VIIa is not inhibited by antithrombin probably because its active site is not fully exposed. However, inhibition by antithrombin occurs once factor VIIa is in complex with its obligatory cell surface cofactor, tissue factor, which further exposes the active center of the proteinase (2).

The inhibitory action of antithrombin can be greatly accelerated by heparin (223–225), a highly charged linear polysaccharide, structurally related to heparan sulfate, the latter being found as a proteoglycan on the endothelial cell surface. Subpopulations of vascular heparan sulfate can accelerate the inhibitory action of antithrombin against coagulation proteinases and this mechanism of accelerated proteinase inhibition is a natural anticoagulant pathway (226–228). Amino acid sequence composition determination of antithrombin identifies its membership of a superfamily of related inhibitors, which are the serpins (serine proteinase inhibitors) (229, 230), that regulate proteinase activities in several processes. These processes include coagulation, the complement pathway, matrix remodeling, cell differentiation, and inflammation. The importance of the superfamily has been highlighted by a common mechanism of pathologies arising from natural mutations of the various inhibitors. Images of the surface topography of the protein family derived from crystal structures suggest the detailed mechanisms of the inhibitory action of the serpins (231–233). The importance of antithrombin as an inhibitor of coagulation is highlighted by the thrombotic problems of individuals with inherited disorders or deficiency of this serpin (234, 235) (see Chapter 40).

## THE ANTITHROMBIN MOLECULE

The antithrombin gene codes for a nascent protein containing a signal peptide of 32 amino acids cleaved prior to secretion, which results in a mature polypeptide of 432 amino acids (236). Post-translational modifications include disulfide bond formation at Cys 8 to Cys 128,

Cys 21 to Cys 95, and Cys 247 to Cys 430 and also glycosylation at Asn 96, Asn 135, Asn 155, and Asn 192 (Fig. 3.9). Glycosylation at Asn 135 is incomplete because of the presence of a Ser residue at the third position of the N-glycosylation consensus sequence (237). Variable glycosylation accounts for much of the heterogeneity of the plasma protein visible on isoelectric focusing. Proximity of Asn 135 to elements comprising the heparin interaction site (see below) gives a potential functional importance to heterogeneity at this site. The β isoform, which is the small fraction (approximately 5%) of antithrombin lacking an oligosaccharide side chain, is able to bind heparin with higher affinity with an approximate 10-fold decrease in the $K_d$ for this interaction (the major fraction with the side chain at Asn 135 is known as the α isoform) (238).

The structure of the 432 residue protein has been elucidated by several analyses of crystal structure. Antithrombin has a highly ordered tertiary structure that is folded as three β-sheets (A to C) and nine α-helices (A to I). The inhibitory action of antithrombin against proteinases, as is 50 the case for all serpins, involves recognition of the reactive site bond (Arg 393 to Ser 394 for antithrombin, also known as the P1-P1' bond) by the active site of the proteinase (Fig. 3.10). In antithrombin, the reactive site is located in a reactive loop which protrudes above the main body of the inhibitor (the reactive loop may adopt a helical conformation in other serpins). The first step in the interaction between antithrombin and proteinase is the formation of a Michaelis complex between reactive loop and proteinase. A substrate reaction then begins in which the proteinase attempts to cleave the P1-P1' bond of antithrombin.

In the crystal structure of cleaved antithrombin (and other cleaved serpins) the reactive bond is separated to opposite ends of the molecule, with the polypeptide aminoterminal to Arg 393 inserting into the sheet A structure (Fig. 3.10). A similar complete loop insertion is observed in denatured or 'latent' antithrombin, which is not cleaved but is functionally inactive. However, during normal inhibitory function, the substrate reaction proceeds next to an acyl intermediate stage. Then a conformational change is induced in antithrombin that stabilizes the complex with thrombin. The conformational change in the reactive loop necessary for stabilization of the complex involves partial insertion of the reactive loop into sheet A (Fig. 3.10) (239). It appears there is competition between partial loop insertion and the substrate reaction, the outcome of which determines the ultimate fate of the antithrombin-proteinase interaction (cleaved, inactive free antithrombin and proteinase on the one hand, or stabilized antithrombin-proteinase complex on the other hand).

This model of complex stabilization is supported by studies of natural variants of antithrombin found in individuals with a predisposition to thrombotic disease (see Chapter 40). The variant antithrombins with substitutions 10 to 12 residues aminoterminal to the reactive site bond (denoted P10-P12 residues), such as Ala 384 to Pro and Ala 382 to Thr, are unable to form stabilized complexes with proteinases (240). Instead, a substrate reaction with cleavage at the reactive site bond takes place, which releases thrombin (241, 242). In this circumstance, it appears the rate of reactive loop insertion into the sheet A structure may be delayed by the substitution, which enables the substrate reaction to go to completion.

The model is also supported by investigations of another group of natural variants that have substitution mutations carboxyterminal to the reactive site bond: the variants designated as having pleiotropic effects. These

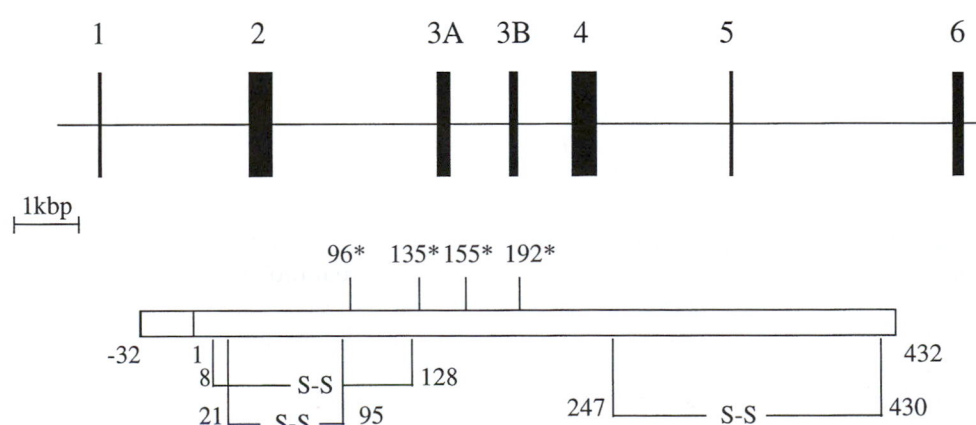

**FIGURE 3.9.** Organization of the gene coding for antithrombin (also referred to as antithrombin III) and its polypeptide. The exons of the gene encoding antithrombin (upper panel), which span 13.4 kbp of genomic DNA, are numbered 1, 2, 3A, 3B, 4, 5, and 6 and code for a nascent polypeptide (lower panel) with a signal peptide of 32 amino acids that is cleaved prior to secretion of the mature 432 residue protein. Post-translational modifications include glycosylation at positions indicated with an asterisk (*) and disulfide bond formation indicated below the polypeptide. Note that residue 135 is variably glycosylated.

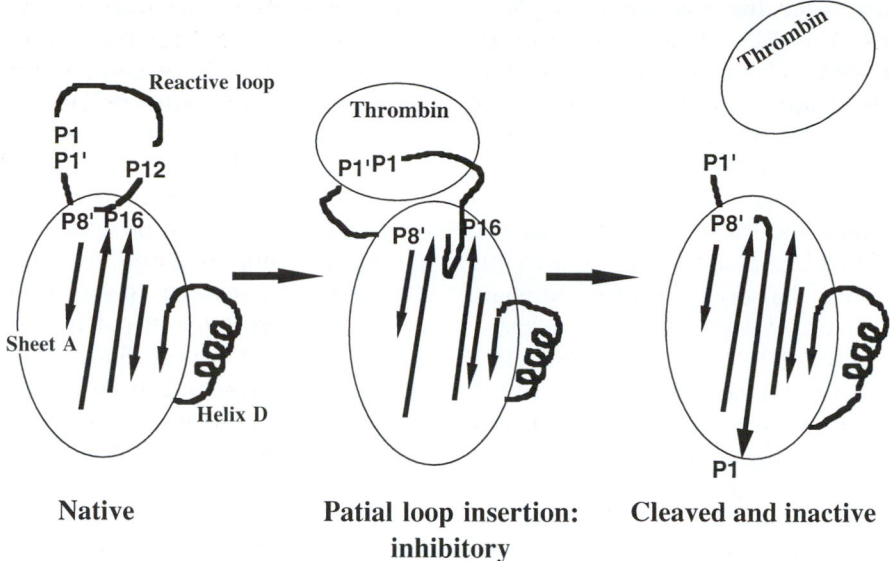

**Native**          **Patial loop insertion:**          **Cleaved and inactive**
                    **inhibitory**

**FIGURE 3.10.** Representation of antithrombin structural changes based upon serpin crystal structure images. Antithrombin has several structural elements, three of which are illustrated ("Native"): a mobile protruding reactive loop containing the reactive site bond (P1-P1'), helix D around which the heparin binding site is centered, and a sheet A structure with five (arrowed) strands. During the inhibition of proteinases such as thrombin, the proteinase attempts to cleave the reactive site bond in a substrate reaction, but a conformational change in the reactive loop, which results in partial loop insertion into sheet A, traps the thrombin in a stabilized complex ("Partial loop insertion"). Under certain circumstances, for example mutation of the P12 residue, the rate of partial loop insertion is delayed, which enables the substrate reaction to be completed. Then, thrombin is released and the reactive loop fully inserts into sheet A ("Cleaved and inactive").

variants, with substitutions largely affecting or adjacent to strand 1C (Phe 402, Ala 404, Asn 405, Arg 406, Pro 407, and, perhaps, Pro 429) (243, 244) are unable to inactivate proteinases, probably because their substitutions are adjacent to the reactive center, or they are in extremely mobile elements that must undergo large structural transitions during complex stabilization.

Inhibition of proteinases by antithrombin is slow in relation to other serpin-proteinase reactions. Heparin, although, has an appreciable accelerating effect upon the formation of antithrombin-proteinase complexes. The formation of the antithrombin-thrombin complex is accelerated at least 2000-fold under optimum conditions (rate constant of inhibition of $1.5 \times 10^7$ to $3 \times 10^8$ $M^{-1}s^{-1}$), and this reduces the half-time of inhibition of thrombin in plasma to about 10 ms (245). Similar rate enhancements have been observed for the inactivation of factors Xa and IXa by antithrombin. The accelerating effect of heparin occurs in concentrations much below those of antithrombin and the proteinases with each molecule accelerating the formation of many antithrombin-proteinase complexes.

Heparin promotes the formation of a ternary complex of antithrombin and proteinase (246–248) in which the active site of the proteinase is brought into contact with the reactive site of antithrombin (see Chapter 55). Assembly of the ternary complex proceeds preferen-

tially through formation of a heparin-antithrombin complex because of antithrombin's high affinity for heparin. The binding of heparin to antithrombin induces a conformational change in the protein that further enhances heparin binding. Thrombin and other proteinases that bind with quite high affinity to heparin will bind to the heparin chain adjacent to antithrombin on the relatively non-specific regions of the polysaccharide chain that adjoin the antithrombin binding pentasaccharide sequence (249). In this circumstance, a crucial role of heparin seems to be the bringing together of inhibitor and proteinase (termed "approximation"), rather than just the induction of a conformational change (250). Binding to the heparin chain and approximation are essential for thrombin's accelerated inhibition (251). In contrast, factor Xa and other proteinases that bind only weakly to heparin are inhibited directly by the heparin-antithrombin complex, and approximation of antithrombin and proteinase on heparin does not need to take place. Rather, the conformational change induced in the inhibitor by heparin appears to enable the inhibition reaction to proceed more rapidly. Recent work (using a reactive site labeled variant and a monoclonal antibody that recognizes the strand 1C/4B region) has confirmed that binding of heparin or its essential pentasaccharide to antithrombin results directly in perturbation of the reactive center environment (252, 253). Once an acyl intermediate has formed between the reactive site of antithrombin and the active site of the proteinase (factor Xa or thrombin), the change in conformation in antithrombin results in a reduced binding affinity of the complex for heparin, which enables its release and participation in additional antithrombin-proteinase reactions.

Early attempts at characterization of the interaction between heparin and antithrombin used heparin heterogeneous with respect to size and ability to interact with antithrombin. The finding that only a fraction of commercial heparin binds with high affinity to the protein was a major advance (254, 255) (see Chapter 55). The minimal binding sequence of heparin has been localized to a unique pentasaccharide sequence by a series of subsequent studies (256–260). This essential pentasaccharide of heparin is comprised of three glucosamine and two hexuronic acid (one glucuronic and one iduronic acid) residues. Two of the glucosamine units are N-sulfated, and the third may be either N-acetylated or N-sulfated. O-sulfate groups occur on the iduronic acid unit and two, but possibly all, of the glucosamine units (256). At least four sulfate groups are essential for antithrombin binding, including a unique 3-O-sulfate residue located on the internal glucosamine unit. This latter sulfate is a critical determinant of the specificity of the glycosaminoglycan-antithrombin interaction.

While heparin is exposed to blood only following its administration during clinical use, the vasculature is surrounded by large quantities of heparan sulfate, which is part of proteoglycans with core proteins intercalated into cell membranes. Heparan sulfate itself is greatly heterogeneous but is structurally and biosynthetically related to heparin (261). It has been proposed these two glycosaminoglycans can be distinguished on the basis of their sulfate content and distribution, with heparin having more than 80% of its glucosamine residues N-sulfated and the concentration of O-sulfate groups exceeding that of the N-sulfate groups (262). The core proteins define families of heparan sulfate proteoglycans, with the major ones in the cardiovascular system being syndecan, glypican, and perlecan. These heparan sulfate proteoglycans mediate several biological processes, including mesodermal cell fate, positioning of the heart, vasculogenesis and angiogenesis after vascular injury, interaction with adhesive proteins on cells, and anticoagulation. These complex processes have recently been comprehensively reviewed (263). Isolated organ perfusion studies revealed antithrombin-thrombin complex formation could be significantly accelerated in anticoagulation (226, 227). Cultured endothelial cells synthesize small amounts of anticoagulantly active proteoglycan (264). Histologic investigations demonstrated while the luminal surface of the endothelium contains a small amount of the active heparan sulfate, most of the active heparan sulfate is present in the subendothelial

space. This observation and results of inhibitory experiments conducted with damaged vessel sections obtained following balloon injury (265) suggest a role for such species in regulating thrombin at sites of damaged vessels, perhaps acting with the $\beta$ isoform of antithrombin (described above).

The biosynthesis of heparin and heparan sulfate is an ordered sequential process, involving formation of the glycosaminoglycan-protein linkage region, formation of the glycosaminoglycan chains, and modification of these chains (261). The last process alone requires deacetylation of N-acetylglucosamine residues, N-sulfation of glucosamine residues, formation of iduronic acid units, and incorporation of O-sulfate groups. It is only recently that the nature of the many biosynthetic enzymes involved is being fully defined. A critical but late step of biosynthesis endows the heparan sulfate chain with anticoagulant activity (266–268). This step adds the 3-O sulfate mentioned above to the chain, is rate limiting, and depends on the presence of the responsible glucosaminyl 3-O sulfotransferase, which is an enzyme that is not abundant in the endothelial cell. This explains the very low fractional concentration of active proteoglycans in the vasculature. Nevertheless, independent support for this small fraction's important role is supported by the observation that individuals experience early onset and severe thromboembolic disease when they are homozygous for genetic defects solely altering the heparin binding properties of antithrombin (see Chapter 40).

Heparin binds through the essential pentasaccharide with a $K_d$ of approximately 20 nM (249, 269). Binding strongly depends on ionic strength and pH. It appears a maximum of five to six charged groups on each molecule is involved, with the negatively charged sulfates of the glycosaminoglycan interacting with positively charged residues (Lys and Arg) on antithrombin. Heparin binding alters the overall fluorescence spectrum of antithrombin, which suggests the interaction has resulted in a conformational change (270, 271).

The heparin binding domain of antithrombin appears to consist principally of three regions encompassing the aminoterminal polypeptide, amino acids 41 to 49, and amino acids 107 to 156. Within these regions are clusters of basic amino acids that may be spatially coordinated to provide the heparin binding site. The delineation of these regions was based on biochemical experiments and characterization of natural mutants affecting these sites. Little information exists on the precise role of the aminoterminal polypeptide, other than the identification of Arg 24 as a probable pentasaccharide contact residue from a study of a natural variant (272). The second region has been investigated with several techniques. Chemical or genetic modification of Trp 49 results in impaired binding of heparin to antithrombin (271, 273). Using a combination of limited digestion with the enzyme proteinase V8 and quantitative aminoterminal sequence analysis, Liu and Chang suggest cleavage of Glu 34 to Gly 35, Glu 42 to Ala 43, and Glu 50 to Leu 51 was drastically inhibited by preincubation of antithrombin with heparin (274). The results suggest Glu 34 to Leu 51 may be involved in heparin binding. Further, studies of natural variants found in affected individuals with antithrombin deficiency have demonstrated that substitutions at Arg 24 (272), Pro 41 (275), and Arg 47 (276) interfere with heparin binding.

The third region involved in heparin binding consists of positively charged amino acids which form helix D; Lys 107, Lys 114, Lys 125, Arg 129, Arg 132, and Lys 133, at the surface of the antithrombin molecule (277). Chemical modification studies of antithrombin with water soluble reagents that are specific for lysine residues suggest Lys 107, Lys 114, Lys 125, and Lys 136 are involved in heparin binding (278, 279). Chemical modification is extremely difficult to control at the individual residue level, and the suggestion of a role for each of these residues should be viewed cautiously. Further evidence that the region encompassing residues 124 to 145 may be important in heparin binding comes from studies by Smith et al (280). Smith et al showed polyclonal antibodies with specificity against a synthetic peptide comprising residues 124 to 145 block the binding of heparin to antithrombin. Recombinant antithrombin with Lys 125 replaced by Met has approximately a 170-fold reduction in heparin affinity and approximately a 30-fold reduction in pentasaccharide affinity compared to wild type antithrombin. Remarkably, these reductions in affinity do not seem to alter the maximal accelerating effect of these polysaccharides on antithrombin-proteinase reactions (281). A naturally occurring variant with a substitution at Arg 129 greatly reduced binding to heparin, which establishes an important role for this residue and helix D in the binding interaction (282). As mentioned above, the β form of antithrombin has no carbohydrate at Asn 135. Recombinant carbohydrate isoforms of antithrombin with substituted Asn 135 have higher heparin affinity than wild type antithrombin (238, 283).

A serpin tertiary structure model, based on the crystal structure of cleaved $\alpha_1$-antitrypsin, was used initially as a template to visualize the heparin binding domains of antithrombin. Borg et al (277) proposed seven basic residues are aligned to form a positive site stretching across the molecule from the A helix (Arg 47) to the D helix (Lys 125, Arg 129, Arg 132) and the adjacent Lys 133. Thus, two of the putative heparin binding regions are adjacent to each other in this 3-dimensional structure (the aminoterminal polypeptide is not clearly identified in any structures described to date). This model appears to provide a partial explanation for many of the features of the heparin binding site of antithrombin. In this con-

text, integrity of the disulfide bond between Cys 8 and Cys 128 (Cys 128 is located within the second heparin binding region) is important for binding heparin to antithrombin. The crystal structures of both cleaved and intact antithrombin provided further support for a surface orientated primary contact site comprised of elements of helices D, A, and perhaps C (231, 233). From a consideration of the cleaved bovine antithrombin structure, it has been proposed Arg 13, Lys 39, Arg 46, Arg 47, Arg 129, and Arg 132 comprise the primary pentasaccharide contact surface (232).

Specific basic residues are important in the heparin binding site because they provide the points of contact with negatively charged groups of the pentasaccharide. The overall conformation of the heparin binding domain must also be incorporated into a binding model, along with any structural changes that may occur as part of the heparin-induced conformational change. This consideration arose when results of variants having pleiotropic effects were reported. In addition to the properties noted above, variants with pleiotropic effects have impaired interaction with heparin and its pentasaccharide (243, 284, 285). It appears the hydrophobic region at the carboxyterminus is essential either for the maintenance of the 3-dimensional structure of the molecule or for propagation of the heparin-induced conformation change.

Residues adjacent to the proposed heparin interaction site can undermine its integrity by distorting the positive contact site or by preventing the induced conformational change that occurs on binding. Thus, Pro 41 (275), Leu 99 (286, 287), Ser 116 (288), and Gln 118 (287), substituted in natural variants with abnormal heparin binding, may alter heparin binding in this way (285).

The nature of the conformational change in antithrombin induced by heparin binding is still under investigation; some suggest partial insertion of the reactive loop is required for heparin activation (233) and others favor expulsion of a previously inserted loop (289, 290).

## THE ANTITHROMBIN GENE

A cDNA encoding human antithrombin has been isolated by several groups (291–293). A single copy of the gene for human antithrombin is located on chromosome 1q23-25 (294) and spans approximately 14 kbp of genomic DNA. There are seven exons numbered 1, 2, 3A, 3B, 4, 5, and 6 (Fig. 3.9) and all splice junctions obey the GT-AG rule (236). Initially, it was althought there were only six exons; however, an additional 1 kbp intron was subsequently identified within exon 3 (295), and these two exons are referred to as 3A and 3B. There are 10 Alu repeat elements within the gene, which is higher than average for the human genome; two of these (within intron 4) have polymorphic trinucleotide (ATT) repeats. Other identified polymorphic sites include a 76 bp length polymorphism located in the 5' region (296), a Pst I site in codon 305 (297), a Nhe I site in intron 4 (298), and a Dde I site in intron 5 (299). Antithrombin is synthesized primarily in the liver, but messenger RNA can also be detected in the kidney and brain. A single transcription start site has been identified 72 bp upstream of the *A*UG initiation codon (denoted +1) using primer extension studies (300). The polyadenylation signal (AATAAA) is located 49 bp downstream of the termination codon, and poly-A tail addition usually begins 24 bp 3' of this site (291, 292, 301).

Similar to protein C, the antithrombin gene belongs to a class of genes regulated by TATA-less promoters; the closest TATA box consensus sequence is distant (155 bp upstream) from the transcription start site and no CAAT box-like element has been identified. However, the consensus sequence for an alternative initiator element (CCACCC) is present in close proximity (-43 to -38). There is also a potential GAGA box (-14 to +1), which is a growth hormone controlled regulatory element that partly determines basal promoter activity in the rat serine protease inhibitor 2.1 gene (Fig. 3.11).

An 800 bp fragment of the 5' region of the antithrombin gene is sufficient to enhance expression of a reporter gene in both liver and kidney cells, regardless of orientation (302). Within this fragment, regions homologous to an enhancer core element of immunoglobulin, chymotrypsin, and insulin genes (-41 to -51) and sequences found in eukaryotic viral enhancers and the human insulin gene (-2 to -10) are present. Furthermore, a region of the antithrombin gene (-84 to -73) was found to interact with a specific trans-acting factor, Tf-LF1, while investigating gene regulation in the liver (303).

Another study noted maximal reporter gene activity in a fragment containing the sequence -1100 to +68 by deletion analysis of a construct containing 6 kbp of antithrombin gene sequence (304). Further 5' deletion did not significantly reduce expression until sequences 3' of nucleotide -150 were removed. This indicated the presence of enhancer elements in the region -150 to +68. DNA footprint analysis showed three regions within this sequence protected from digestion by DNase I; A, -65 to -89 on the coding strand (corresponding to -68 to -92 on the noncoding strand); B, -14 to +37 (corresponding to -8 to +30 on the noncoding strand); and C, -101 to -124 on the noncoding strand only. The liver specific transcription factor HNF 4 binds to two of these, A and C; the sequences -74 to -86, -104 to -116, and -111 to -123 match the HNF 4 binding consensus sequence in 10, nine and 11 out of 13 nucleotides, respectively (Fig. 3.11). CAAT-enhancer binding protein A binds to region B, and the binding site was further localized to the region +4 to +11 by mutational analysis (Fig. 3.11). Nuclear extracts of non-liver cells also bind to these regions, such as chicken ovalbumin upstream promoter transcription factor 1 and thyroid hormone receptor α (both of which repress the activity of HNF 4), retinoid X receptor α, peroxisome proliferator-activated receptor α, and the single stranded DNA binding proteins PYBP and pTB.

A second enhancer-like element was identified within intron 1 of the antithrombin gene (+300 to +700), although only when orientation was reversed. Reporter gene activity is reduced but not completely abolished when this element is present in its normal orientation together with the upstream sequences mentioned above (304). Thus, this second region appears to act in opposition to the first. The sequence -97 to -49,

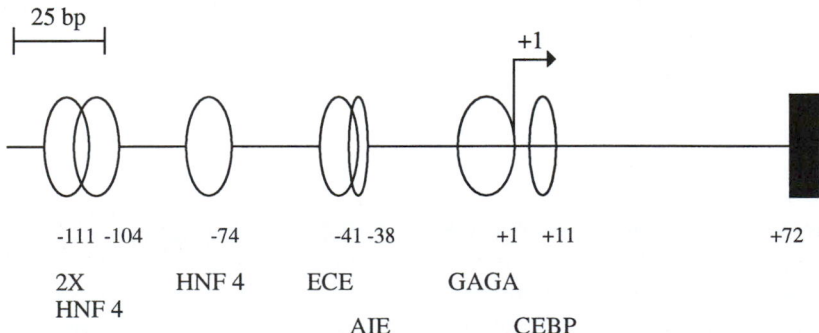

**FIGURE 3.11.** Transcriptional regulation of the gene for human antithrombin. Similar to protein C, the area of the gene encoding antithrombin, which is in close proximity to the transcription start site, does not contain any region with TATA box similarity. However, in this case there is a potential alternative initiator element (AIE) and a GAGA box which could substitute the role of the TATA box. The single transcription start site is indicated (+1) and is 72 bp upstream of the initiator (Met) codon. The coding region is shown as the black boxed area. Some of the positive-acting elements controlling expression of the gene are shown (ovals). The numbering corresponds to the 3' base of each element relative to +1 on the coding strand. A potential silencer region, which acts as an enhancer if the orientation is reversed, is present in intron 1, but is not illustrated. Other abbreviations: CEBP, CAAT-enhancer binding protein; ECE, enhancer core element; HNF, hepatic nuclear factor.

which contains three consensus AGGTCA hormone response element halfsites, has also been defined in the noncoding strand (305). The site responds to all-trans retinoic acid (ATRA) and L-3,5,3'-tri-iodothyronine (T3). ATRA acts in the presence of the nuclear receptor RXRα and T3 in the presence of its receptor TRβ.

# HEPARIN COFACTOR II

The suppression of thrombin activity in blood by direct inhibition (as opposed to inhibition of thrombin generation) is primarily mediated by antithrombin. However, a second serpin, heparin cofactor II, also inhibits thrombin; its action is greatly accelerated by heparin, heparan sulfate, and, uniquely, dermatan sulfate (306–310). Endothelial cells do not accelerate inhibition of thrombin by heparin cofactor II. However, certain vascular cells that synthesize dermatan sulfate can function in this way (309). The proteoglycans biglycan and decorin, which contain dermatan sulfate, both accelerate heparin cofactor II activity; this activity suggests a vascular or extravascular cell/site-specific role for this inhibitor in regions in which such proteoglycans dominate. Interest in the role of heparin cofactor II was excited by early reports showing partial deficiency of the protein in individuals with thromboembolic disease. However, a causal relationship between deficiency and disease has been opposed by the finding of similar prevalences of deficiency in normal subjects and individuals with thrombosis (311). While the physiologic role of this inhibitor remains to be clarified, the detailed mechanism of its action has been elucidated by kinetic studies utilizing recombinant wild type and mutant proteins (310).

The gene for heparin cofactor II is distributed over 16 kbp of genomic DNA and is located on chromosome 22q11 (312). Synthesis of the protein is in the liver (plasma concentration approximately 70 μg/L) and results in secretion of a mature polypeptide of 480 amino acids (approximately 66 Kda) once the signal peptide of 19 amino acids has been cleaved. Heparin cofactor II has approximately 30% sequence identity with antithrombin, which reflects its common serpin ancestral origin. However, it differs in several important respects. First, while it undergoes post-translational modifications, including N-linked glycosylation, and it contains three cysteine residues, its folding is not stabilized by disulfide bond formation since these bonds are absent. Second, the aminoterminal region contains two highly acidic regions each containing an O-sulfated tyrosine residue (313). Third, the reactive site residues (P1-P1' bond) is Leu 444-Ser 445. The primary determinant of specificity is provided by the nature of the P1-P1' bond. Leucine at position 444 is an unusual target residue for thrombin, and its presence accounts for the low inhibition rate of thrombin, with its mutation to arginine in-

creasing the inhibition rate approximately 100-fold (314). Inhibition of thrombin involves similar structural changes in the reactive loop of heparin cofactor II to those indicated above for antithrombin. Partial reactive loop insertion will probably stabilize the inhibitor-proteinase complex. However, such a prediction is currently unsupported by crystallographic images of different conformations of this particular serpin.

The second determinant of specificity of heparin cofactor II is the aminoterminal (acidic) regions. These regions resemble the carboxyterminal acidic sequence of hirudin that confer to it very high thrombin specificity because of the ability of the acidic region to bind to the anion-binding exosite of the proteinase. However, deletion of the acidic regions of heparin cofactor II does not dramatically impair thrombin inhibition when conducted in the absence of a rate enhancing glycosaminoglycan. In contrast, in the presence of heparin or dermatan sulfate, aminoterminal deletion of the inhibitor has a large effect on function (315). These observations have been rationalized into a model of accelerated inhibition of thrombin by heparin cofactor II (310). In its unstimulated state, heparin cofactor II folds such that the aminoterminal acidic regions are associated with a basic cluster of residues that form the interaction site on the protein for glycosaminoglycans when the residues are unmasked. This latter interaction site has been defined by investigation of natural and recombinant mutants (316–318). Optimum heparin binding requires Lys 173, Arg 184, and Arg 185, while optimum dermatan sulfate binding requires Arg 184, Arg 185, Arg 189, Arg 192, and Arg 193. This differential requirement for binding points to overlapping binding sites for these two glycosaminoglycans. Unmasking of this domain occurs upon contact with either heparin or dermatan sulfate, and, unlike antithrombin, a highly specific polysaccharide sequence is not required. Once the glycosaminoglycan has bound the inhibitor, the displaced aminoterminal acidic regions are available for interaction with thrombin, are able to bind to the anion binding exosite of that proteinase, and thereby direct the proteinase to the reactive site bond.

# TISSUE FACTOR PATHWAY INHIBITOR (SEE CHAPTER 4)

TFPI was first identified in the 1950s, but it was not until the last decade that it has been fully characterized (319, 320). TFPI regulatory activity is directed towards the extrinsic initiation pathway of the coagulation cascade involving binding and direct inhibition of factor Xa. It also inhibits the tissue factor/factor VIIa complex in a factor Xa dependent fashion. Although the role of TFPI in preventing thrombus formation *in vivo* has not yet been defined, in animal models, immunodepletion of

TFPI results in a reduction of the threshold at which tissue factor induces disseminated intravascular coagulation (321).

Full length TFPI contains 276 amino acids, including a negatively charged aminoterminus, three Kunitz domains, and a positively charged carboxyterminus (322). The second Kunitz domain contains the binding site for factor Xa, whereas the factor VIIa binding site is located in the first Kunitz domain (323). However, endogenous TFPI is heterogeneous with regard to localization and content. The majority (50 to 80%) is attached to the surface of endothelial cells and is released following infusion of heparin (324), perhaps suggesting the binding site for TFPI is heparan sulfate, although it is possible other receptor sites are involved. Between 10 and 50% of total TFPI circulates in complex with lipoproteins at an approximate concentration of 50 to 150 mg/L (325). Small amounts have also been detected in platelets. Compared to TFPI released by heparin, TFPI in complex with lipoproteins has low anticoagulant properties measured by prolongation of clotting time (326). TFPI is truncated at the carboxyterminus and lacks a portion of the third Kunitz domain and the positively charged carboxyterminal domain when in complex with low density lipoprotein (327). Furthermore, TFPI can be covalently bound to apolipoprotein AII via a disulfide bond when in complex with high density lipoprotein.

Antithrombin and TFPI cooperate in the regulation of factor X activation (2, 328). Antithrombin, but not TFPI, inhibits factor Xa-mediated activation of factor VII in the factor VII/tissue factor complex. TFPI, but not antithrombin, inhibits excess factor X activation by the factor VII/tissue factor complex. TFPI in conjunction with APC strongly suppresses thrombin generation caused by tissue factor/factor VIIa (1). Together, these regulatory pathways play a key role in modulating extrinsic (tissue factor) activation of the coagulation cascade. Although mutations in the gene for TFPI have not been identified in individuals with thrombosis, this is most likely because of the problems of selecting suitable probands for genetic analysis due to the heterogeneity mentioned above, rather than because of the absence of a inherited TFPI deficiency. TFPI is reviewed in detail in Chapter 4.

# ACKNOWLEDGMENT

The work of the authors is supported by grants from the British Heart Foundation and the Special Trustees of Charing Cross Hospital.

# REFERENCES

1. van't Veer C, Golden NJ, Kalafatis M et al. Inhibitory mechanism of the protein C pathway on tissue factor-induced thrombin generation. Synergistic effect in combination with tissue factor pathway inhibitor. J Biol Chem 1997;272:7983–7994.
2. van't Veer C, Mann KG. Regulation of tissue factor initiated thrombin generation by the stoichiometric inhibitors tissue factor pathway inhibitor, antithrombin-III and heparin cofactor II. J Biol Chem 1997;272:4367–4377.
3. Lane DA, Mannucci PM, Bauer KA et al. Inherited thrombophilia: part 1. Thromb Haemost 1996;76:651–662.
4. Lane DA, Mannucci PM, Bauer KA et al. Inherited thrombophilia: part 2. Thromb Haemost 1996;76:824–834.
5. Esmon CT. The protein C anticoagulant pathway. Arterioscler Thromb 1992;12:135–145.
6. Dahlback B. The protein C anticoagulant system: inherited defects as basis for venous thrombosis. Thromb Res 1995;77:1–43.
7. Esmon CT, Owen WG. Identification of an endothelial cell cofactor for thrombin-catalyzed activation of protein C. Proc Natl Acad Sci U S A 1981; 78:2249–2252.
8. Esmon NL, Owen WG, Esmon CT. Isolation of a membrane-bound cofactor for thrombin-catalyzed activation of protein C. J Biol Chem 1982;257: 859–864.
9. Amphlett GW, Kisiel W, Castellino FJ. Interaction of calcium with bovine plasma protein C. Biochemistry 1981;20:2156–2161.
10. Kisiel W, Canfield WM, Ericsson LH et al. Anticoagulant properties of bovine plasma protein C following activation by thrombin. Biochemistry 1977;16:5824–5831.
11. Walker FJ, Sexton PW, Esmon CT. The inhibition of blood coagulation by activated protein C through the selective inactivation of activated factor V. Biochim Biophys Acta 1979;571:333–342.
12. Marlar RA, Kleiss AJ, Griffin JH. Mechanism of action of human activated protein C, a thrombin-dependent anticoagulant enzyme. Blood 1982;59: 1067–1072.
13. Walker FJ. Regulation of activated protein C by a new protein. A possible function for bovine protein S. J Biol Chem 1980;255:5521–5524.
14. Fukudome K, Esmon CT. Identification, cloning and regulation of a novel endothelial protein C/activated protein C receptor. J Biol Chem 1994;269: 26486–26491.
15. Stenflo J, Dahlback B. Vitamin K-dependent proteins. In: Stamatoyannopoulos G, Nienhuis AW, Majerus PW, Varmus H, eds. The molecular basis of blood diseases. 2nd ed. Philadelphia: WB Saunders, 1994:565–598.
16. Suttie JW. Vitamin K-dependent carboxylase [Review]. Annu Rev Biochem 1985;54:459–477.
17. Nelsestuen GL, Suttie JW. Mode of action of vitamin K. Calcium binding properties of bovine prothrombin. Biochemistry 1972;11:4961–4964.
18. Mann KG, Nesheim ME, Church WR et al. Surface dependent reactions of the vitamin K-dependent enzyme complexes [Review]. Blood 1990;76: 1–16.
19. Astermark J, Bjork I, Ohlin AK et al. Structural requirements for $Ca^{2+}$ binding to the gamma-carboxyglutamic acid and epidermal growth factor-like regions of factor IX. Studies using intact domains isolated from controlled proteolytic digests of bovine factor IX. J Biol Chem 1991;266: 2430–2437.
20. Nelsestuen GL. Role of gamma-carboxyglutamic acid. An unusual protein transition required for the calcium-dependent binding of prothrombin to phospholipid. J Biol Chem 1976;251:5648–5656.
21. Liebman HA, Furie BC, Furie R. The factor IX phospholipid binding site is required for calcium dependent activation of factor IX by factor XIa. J Biol Chem 1987;262:7605–7612.
22. Church WR, Boulanger LL, Messier TL et al. Evidence for a common metal ion-dependent transition in the 4-carboxyglutamic acid domains of several vitamin K-dependent proteins. J Biol Chem 1989;264:17882–17887.
23. Borowski M, Furie B, Bauminger S et al. Prothrombin requires two sequential metal-dependent conformational transitions to bind phospholipid. Conformation-specific antibodies directed against the phospholipid-binding site on prothrombin. J Biol Chem 1986;261:14969–14975.
24. Prendergast FG, Mann KG. Differentiation of metal ion-induced transitions of prothrombin fragment 1. J Biol Chem 1977;252:840–850.
25. Soriano-Garcia M, Park CH, Tulinsky A et al. Structure of $Ca^{2+}$ prothrombin fragment 1 including the conformation of the Gla domain. Biochemistry 1989;28:6805–6810.
26. Foster DC, Rudinski MS, Schach BG et al. Propeptide of human protein C is necessary for gamma-carboxylation. Biochemistry 1987;26:7003–7011.
27. Jorgensen MJ, Cantor AB, Furie BC et al. Recognition site directing vitamin K-dependent gamma-carboxylation resides on the propeptide of factor IX. Cell 1987;48:185–191.
28. Lingenfelter SE, Berkner KL. Isolation of the human γ-carboxylase and a γ-carboxylase-associated protein from factor IX-expressing mammalian cells. Biochemistry 1996;35:8234–8243.
29. Furie BC, Furie B. Structure and mechanism of action of the vitamin K-dependent γ-glutamyl carboxylase: recent advances from mutagenesis studies. Thromb Haemost 1997;78:595–598.
30. Wu SM, Stanley TB, Mutucumarana VP et al. Characterization of the γ-glutamyl carboxylase. Thromb Haemost 1997;78:599–604.
31. Appella E, Weber IT, Blasi F. Structure and function of epidermal growth factor-like regions in proteins [Review]. FEBS Lett 1988;231:1–4.

32. Stenflo J. Structure-function relationships of epidermal growth factor modules in vitamin K-dependent clotting factors [Review]. Blood 1991;78:1637–1651.

33. Handford PA, Mayhew M, Baron M et al. Key residues involved in calcium-binding motifs in EGF-like domains. Nature 1991;351:164–167.

34. Cooke RM, Wilkinson AJ, Baron M et al. The solution structure of human epidermal growth factor. Nature 1987;327:339–341.

35. Selander M, Persson E, Stenflo J et al. 1H NMR assignment and secondary structure of the $Ca^{2+}$-free form of the aminoterminal epidermal growth factor like domain in coagulation factor X. Biochemistry 1990;29:8111–8118.

36. Rao Z, Handford P, Mayhew M et al. The structure of a $Ca^{2+}$-binding epidermal growth factor-like domain: its role in protein-protein interactions. Cell 1995;82:131–141.

37. DeBault LE, Esmon NL, Olson JR et al. Distribution of the thrombomodulin antigen in the rabbit vasculature. Lab Invest 1986;54:172–178.

38. Suzuki K, Nishioka J, Hayashi T et al. Functionally active thrombomodulin is present in human platelets. J Biochem (Tokyo) 1988;104:628–632.

39. Maruyama I, Bell CE, Majerus PW. Thrombomodulin is found on endothelium of arteries, veins, capillaries, and lymphatics, and on syncytiotrophoblast of human placenta. J Cell Biol 1985;101:363–371.

40. Ishii H, Salem HH, Bell CE et al. Thrombomodulin, an endothelial anticoagulant protein, is absent from the human brain. Blood 1986;67:362–365.

41. Ishii H, Majerus PW. Thrombomodulin is present in human plasma and urine. J Clin Invest 1985;76:2178–2181.

42. Rosenberg RD. Thrombomodulin gene disruption and mutation in mice. Thromb Haemost 1997;78:705–709.

43. Tsiang M, Lentz SR, Dittman WA et al. Equilibrium binding of thrombin to recombinant human thrombomodulin: effect of hirudin, fibrinogen, factor Va, and peptide analogues. Biochemistry 1990;29:10602–10612.

44. Bourin MC, Boffa MC, Bjork I et al. Functional domains of rabbit thrombomodulin. Proc Natl Acad Sci U S A 1986;83:5924–5928.

45. Stevens WK, Côté HCF, MacGillivray RT et al. Calcium ion modulation of meizothrombin autolysis at Arg55 to Asp56 and catalytic activity. J Biol Chem 1996;271:8062–8067.

46. Côté HC, Bajzar L, Stevens WK et al. Functional characterization of recombinant human meizothrombin and Meizothrombin(desF1). Thrombomodulin-dependent activation of protein C and thrombin-activatable fibrinolysis inhibitor (TAFI), platelet aggregation, antithrombin-III inhibition. J Biol Chem 1997;272:6194–6200.

47. Wu Q, Picard V, Aiach M et al. Activation-induced exposure of the thrombin anion-binding exosite. Interactions of recombinant mutant prothrombins with thrombomodulin and a thrombin exosite-specific antibody. J Biol Chem 1994;269:3725–3730.

48. Nesheim M, Wang W, Boffa M et al. Thrombin, thrombomodulin and TAFI in the molecular link between coagulation and fibrinolysis. Thromb Haemost 1997;78:386–391.

49. Bajzar L, Morser J, Nesheim M. TAFI, or plasma procarboxypeptidase B, couples the coagulation and fibrinolytic cascades through the thrombin-thrombomodulin complex. J Biol Chem 1996;271:16603–16608.

50. Eaton DL, Malloy BE, Tsai SP et al. Isolation, molecular cloning, and partial characterization of a novel carboxypeptidase B from human plasma. J Biol Chem 1991;266:21833–21838.

51. Tan AK, Eaton DL. Activation and characterization of procarboxypeptidase B from human plasma. Biochemistry 1995;34:5811–5816.

52. Sakharov DV, Plow EF, Rijken DC. On the mechanism of the antifibrinolytic activity of plasma carboxypeptidase B. J Biol Chem 1997;272:14477–14482.

53. Bajzar L, Manuel R, Nesheim ME. Purification and characterization of TAFI, a thrombin-activable fibrinolysis inhibitor. J Biol Chem 1995;270:14477–14484.

54. Suzuki K, Kusumoto H, Deyashiki Y et al. Structure and expression of human thrombomodulin, a thrombin receptor on endothelium acting as a cofactor for protein C activation. EMBO J 1987;6:1891–1897.

55. Wen DZ, Dittman WA, Ye RD et al. Human thrombomodulin: complete cDNA sequence and chromosome localization of the gene. Biochemistry 1987;26:4350–4357.

56. Jackman RW, Beeler DL, Fritze L et al. Human thrombomodulin gene is intron depleted: nucleic acid sequences of the cDNA and gene predict protein structure and suggest sites of regulatory control. Proc Natl Acad Sci U S A 1987;84:6425–6429.

57. Conway EM, Pollefeyt S, Collen D et al. The aminoterminal lectin-like domain of thrombomodulin is required for constitutive endocytosis. Blood 1997;89:652–661.

58. Stenflo J, Ohlin AK, Owen WG et al. beta-Hydroxyaspartic acid or beta-hydroxyasparagine in bovine low density lipoprotein receptor and in bovine thrombomodulin. J Biol Chem 1988;263:21–24.

59. Weisel JW, Nagaswami C, Young TA et al. The shape of thrombomodulin and interactions with thrombin as determined by electron microscopy. J Biol Chem 1996;271:31485–31490.

60. Patthy L. Detecting distant homologies of mosaic proteins. Analysis of the sequences of thrombomodulin, thrombospondin complement components C9, C8 alpha and C8 beta, vitronectin and plasma cell membrane glycoprotein PC-1. J Mol Biol 1988;202:689–696.

61. Petersen TE. The aminoterminal domain of thrombomodulin and pancreatic stone protein are homologous with lectins. FEBS Lett 1988;231:51–53.

62. Kurosawa S, Galvin JB, Esmon NL et al. Proteolytic formation and properties of functional domains of thrombomodulin. J Biol Chem 1987;262:2206–2212.

63. Nagashima M, Lundh E, Leonard JC et al. Alanine-scanning mutagenesis of the epidermal growth factor-like domains of human thrombomodulin identifies critical residues for its cofactor activity. J Biol Chem 1993;268:2888–2892.

64. Stearns DJ, Kurosawa S, Esmon CT. Microthrombomodulin. Residues 310–486 from the epidermal growth factor precursor homology domain of thrombomodulin will accelerate protein C activation. J Biol Chem 1989;264:3352–3356.

65. Zushi M, Gomi K, Yamamoto S et al. The last three consecutive epidermal growth factor-like structures of human thrombomodulin comprise the minimum functional domain for protein C-activating cofactor activity and anticoagulant activity. J Biol Chem 1989;264:10351–10353.

66. Hayashi T, Zushi M, Yamamoto S et al. Further localization of binding sites for thrombin and protein C in human thrombomodulin. J Biol Chem 1990;265:20156–20159.

67. Kurosawa S, Stearns DJ, Jackson KW et al. A 10-kDa cyanogen bromide fragment from the epidermal growth factor homology domain of rabbit thrombomodulin contains the primary thrombin binding site. J Biol Chem 1988;263:5993–5996.

68. Suzuki K, Hayashi T, Nishioka J et al. A domain composed of epidermal growth factor-like structures of human thrombomodulin is essential for thrombin binding and for protein C activation. J Biol Chem 1989;264:4872–4876.

69. White CE, Hunter MJ, Meininger DP et al. The fifth epidermal growth factor-like domain of thrombomodulin does not have an epidermal growth factor-like disulfide bonding pattern. Proc Natl Acad Sci U S A 1996;93:10177–10182.

70. Hunter MJ, Komives EA. Thrombin-binding affinities of different disulfide-bonded isomers of the fifth EGF-like domain of thrombomodulin. Protein Sci 1995;4:2129–2137.

71. Mathews II, Padmanabhan KP, Tulinksy A et al. Structure of a nonadecapeptide of the fifth EGF domain of thrombomodulin complexed with thrombin. Biochemistry 1994;33:13547–13552.

72. Ye J, Liu LW, Esmon CT et al. The fifth and sixth growth factor-like domains of thrombomodulin bind to the anion-binding exosite of thrombin and alter its specificity. J Biol Chem 1992;267:11023–11028.

73. Hofsteenge J, Taguchi H, Stone SR. Effect of thrombomodulin on the kinetics of the interaction of thrombin with substrates and inhibitors. Biochem J 1986;237:243–251.

74. Rydel TJ, Ravichandran KG, Tulinsky A et al. The structure of a complex of recombinant hirudin and human alpha-thrombin. Science 1990;249:277–280.

75. Lu RL, Esmon NL, Esmon CT et al. The active site of the thrombin-thrombomodulin complex. A fluorescence energy transfer measurement of its distance above the membrane surface. J Biol Chem 1989;264:12956–12962.

76. Stenflo J, Lundwall A, Dahlback B. beta-Hydroxyasparagine in domains homologous to the epidermal growth factor precursor in vitamin K-dependent protein S. Proc Natl Acad Sci U S A 1987;84:368–372.

77. Zushi M, Gomi K, Honda G et al. Aspartic acid 349 in the fourth epidermal growth factor-like structure of human thrombomodulin plays a role in its $Ca(2+)$-mediated binding to protein C. J Biol Chem 1991;266:19886–19889.

78. Glaser CB, Morser J, Clarke JH et al. Oxidation of a specific methionine in thrombomodulin by activated neutrophil products blocks cofactor activity. A potential rapid mechanism for modulation of coagulation. J Clin Invest 1992;90:2565–2573.

79. Clarke JH, Light DR, Blasko E et al. The short loop between epidermal growth factor-like domains 4 and 5 is critical for human thrombomodulin function. J Biol Chem 1993;268:6309–6315.

80. Bourin MC, Ohlin AK, Lane DA et al. Relationship between anticoagulant activities and polyanionic properties of rabbit thrombomodulin. J Biol Chem 1988;263:8044–8052.

81. Bourin MC, Lindahl U. Functional role of the polysaccharide component of rabbit thrombomodulin proteoglycan. Effects on inactivation of thrombin by antithrombin, cleavage of fibrinogen by thrombin and thrombin-catalyzed activation of factor V. Biochem J 1990;270:419–425.

82. Bourin MC, Lundgren Akerlund E, Lindahl U. Isolation and characterization of the glycosaminoglycan component of rabbit thrombomodulin proteoglycan. J Biol Chem 1990;265:15424–15431.

83. Nawa K, Sakano K, Fujiwara H et al. Presence and function of chondroitin-4-sulfate on recombinant human soluble thrombomodulin. Biochem Biophys Res Commun 1990;171:729–737.

84. Parkinson JF, Garcia JG, Bang NU. Decreased thrombin affinity of cell-surface thrombomodulin following treatment of cultured endothelial cells with beta-D-xyloside. Biochem Biophys Res Commun 1990;169:177–183.

85. Gerlitz B, Hassell T, Vlahos CJ et al. Identification of the predominant glycosaminoglycan-attachment site in soluble recombinant human thrombomodulin: potential regulation of functionality by glycosyltransferase competition for serine 474. Biochem J 1993;295:131–140.

86. Parkinson JF, Grinnell BW, Moore RE et al. Stable expression of a secretable deletion mutant of recombinant human thrombomodulin in mammalian cells. J Biol Chem 1990;265:12602–12610.

87. Ye J, Esmon CT, Johnson AE. The chondroitin sulfate moiety of thrombomodulin binds a second molecule of thrombin. J Biol Chem 1993;268:2373–2379.

88. Ye J, Rezaie AR, Esmon CT. Glycosaminoglycan contributions to both protein C activation and thrombin inhibition involve a common arginine-rich site in thrombin that includes residues arginine 93, 97, and 101. J Biol Chem 1994;269:17965–17970.

89. Koyama T, Parkinson JF, Sie P et al. Different glycoforms of human thrombomodulin. Their glycosaminoglycan-dependent modulatory effects on thrombin inactivation by heparin cofactor II and antithrombin III. Eur J Biochem 1991;198:563–570.

90. Slungaard A, Vercellotti GM, Tran T et al. Eosinophil cationic granule proteins impair thrombomodulin function. A potential mechanism for thromboembolism in hypereosinophilic heart disease. J Clin Invest 1993;91:1721–1730.

91. Slungaard A, Key NS. Platelet factor 4 stimulates thrombomodulin protein C-activating cofactor activity. A structure-function analysis. J Biol Chem 1994;269:25549–25556.

92. Conway EM, Boffa MC, Nowakowski B et al. An ultrastructural study of thrombomodulin endocytosis: internalization occurs via clathrin-coated and non-coated pits. J Cell Physiol 1992;151:604–612.

93. Conway EM, Nowakowski B, Steiner-Mosonyi M. Thrombomodulin lacking the cytoplasmic domain efficiently internalizes thrombin via non-clathrin-coated, pit-mediated endocytosis. J Cell Physiol 1994;158:285–298.

94. Espinosa R 3d, Sadler JE, Le Beau MM. Regional localization of the human thrombomodulin gene to 20p12-cen. Genomics 1989;5:649–650.

95. Shirai T, Shiojiri S, Ito H et al. Gene structure of human thrombomodulin, a cofactor for thrombin-catalyzed activation of protein C. J Biochem (Tokyo) 1988;103:281–285.

96. van der Velden PA, Krommenhoek-Van Es T, Allaart CF et al. A frequent thrombomodulin amino acid dimorphism is not associated with thrombophilia. Thromb Haemost 1991;65:511–513.

97. Yu K, Morioka H, Fritze LM et al. Transcriptional regulation of the thrombomodulin gene. J Biol Chem 1992;267:23237–23247.

98. von der Ahe D, Nischan C, Kunz C et al. Ets transcription factor binding site is required for positive and TNF alpha-induced negative promoter regulation. Nucleic Acids Res 1993;21:5636–5643.

99. Dittman WA, Nelson SC, Greer PK et al. Characterization of thrombomodulin expression in response to retinoic acid and identification of a retinoic acid response element in the human thrombomodulin gene. J Biol Chem 1994;269:16925–16932.

100. Tazawa R, Hirosawa S, Suzuki K et al. Functional characterization of the 5'-regulatory region of the human thrombomodulin gene. J Biochem (Tokyo) 1993;113:600–606.

101. Lee ME, Bloch KD, Clifford JA et al. Functional analysis of the endothelin-1 gene promoter. Evidence for an endothelial cell-specific cis-acting sequence. J Biol Chem 1990;265:10446–10450.

102. Moore KL, Andreoli SP, Esmon NL et al. Endotoxin enhances tissue factor and suppresses thrombomodulin expression of human vascular endothelium in vitro. J Clin Invest 1987;79:124–130.

103. Conway EM, Rosenberg RD. Tumor necrosis factor suppresses transcription of the thrombomodulin gene in endothelial cells. Mol Cell Biol 1988;8:5588–5592.

104. Moore KL, Esmon CT, Esmon NL. Tumor necrosis factor leads to the internalization and degradation of thrombomodulin from the surface of bovine aortic endothelial cells in culture. Blood 1989;73:159–165.

105. Archipoff G, Beretz A, Freyssinet JM et al. Heterogeneous regulation of constitutive thrombomodulin or inducible tissue-factor activities on the surface of human saphenous-vein endothelial cells in culture following stimulation by interleukin-1, tumour necrosis factor, thrombin or phorbol ester. Biochem J 1991;273:679–684.

106. Ishii H, Kizaki K, Horie S et al. Oxidized low density lipoprotein reduces thrombomodulin transcription in cultured human endothelial cells through degradation of the lipoprotein in lysosomes. J Biol Chem 1996;271:8458–8465.

107. Dittman WA, Kumada T, Sadler JE et al. The structure and function of mouse thrombomodulin. Phorbol myristate acetate stimulates degradation and synthesis of thrombomodulin without affecting mRNA levels in hemangioma cells. J Biol Chem 1988;263:15815–15822.

108. Imada S, Imada M. Increase of a surface glycoprotein by cyclic AMP in Chinese hamster ovary cells. Dependence on cell-cell interaction. J Biol Chem 1982;257:9108–9113.

109. Ito T, Ogura M, Morishita Y et al. Enhanced expression of thrombomodulin by intracellular cyclic AMP-increasing agents in two human megakaryoblastic leukemia cell lines. Thromb Res 1990;58:615–624.

110. Ishii H, Kizaki K, Uchiyama H et al. Cyclic AMP increases thrombomodulin expression on membrane surface of cultured human umbilical vein endothelial cells. Thromb Res 1990;59:841–850.

111. Maruyama I, Soejima Y, Osame M et al. Increased expression of thrombomodulin on the cultured human umbilical vein endothelial cells and mouse hemangioma cells by cyclic AMP. Thromb Res 1991;61:301–310.

112. Shirayoshi Y, Imada S, Katayanagi S et al. Cyclic AMP-mediated augmentation of thrombomodulin gene expression: cell type-dependent usage of control regions. Exp Cell Res 1993;208:75–83.

113. Stenflo J. A new vitamin K-dependent protein. Purification from bovine plasma and preliminary characterization. J Biol Chem 1976;251:355–363.

114. Fair DS, Marlar RA. Biosynthesis and secretion of factor VII, protein C, protein S, and the protein C inhibitor from a human hepatoma cell line. Blood 1986;67:64–70.

115. He X, Shen L, Bjartell A et al. The gene encoding vitamin K-dependent anticoagulant protein C is expressed in human male reproductive tissues. J Histochem Cytochem 1995;43:563–570.

116. Long GL, Belagaje RM, MacGillivray RT. Cloning and sequencing of liver cDNA coding for bovine protein C. Proc Natl Acad Sci U S A 1984;81:5653–5656.

117. Foster D, Davie EW. Characterization of a cDNA coding for human protein C. Proc Natl Acad Sci U S A 1984;81:4766–4770.

118. Miletich JP, Leykam JF, Broze GJ Jr. Detection of single chain protein C in human plasma [Abstract]. Blood (Suppl I) 1983;62:306a.

119. Reitsma PH, Bernardi F, Doig RG et al. Protein C deficiency: a database of mutations, 1995 update. On behalf of the Subcommittee on Plasma Coagulation Inhibitors of the Scientific and Standardization Committee of the ISTH. Thromb Haemost 1995;73:876–889.

120. Zhang L, Castellino FJ. Influence of specific gamma-carboxyglutamic acid residues on the integrity of the calcium-dependent conformation of human protein C. J Biol Chem 1992;267:26078–26084.

121. Zhang L, Jhingan A, Castellino FJ. Role of individual gamma-carboxyglutamic acid residues of activated human protein C in defining its in vitro anticoagulant activity. Blood 1992;80:942–952.

122. Christiansen WT, Tulinsky A, Castellino FJ. Functions of individual γ-carboxyglutamic acid (Gla) residues of human protein C. Determination of functionally nonessential Gla residues and correlations with their mode of binding to calcium. Biochemistry 1994;33:14993–15000.

123. Jhingan A, Zhang L, Christiansen WT et al. The activities of recombinant gamma-carboxyglutamic-acid-deficient mutants of activated human protein C toward human coagulation factor Va and factor VIII in purified systems and in plasma. Biochemistry 1994;33:1869–1875.

124. Zhang L, Castellino FJ. The binding energy of human coagulation protein C to acidic phospholipid vesicles contains a major contribution from leucine 5 in the gamma-carboxyglutamic acid domain. J Biol Chem 1994;269:3590–3595.

125. Christiansen WT, Jalbert LR, Robertson RM et al. Hydrophobic amino acid residues of human anticoagulation protein C that contribute to its functional binding to phospholipid vesicles. Biochemistry 1995;34:10376–10382.

126. Jalbert LR, Chan JC, Christiansen WT et al. The hydrophobic nature of residue-5 of human protein C is a major determinant of its functional interactions with acidic phospholipid vesicles. Biochemistry 1996;35:7093–7099.

127. Olsen PH, Esmon NL, Esmon CT et al. Ca²⁺ dependence of the interactions between protein C, thrombin, and the elastase fragment of thrombomodulin. Analysis by ultracentrifugation. Biochemistry 1992;31:746–754.

128. Christiansen WT, Geng JP, Castellino FJ. Structure-function assessment of the role of the helical stack domain in the properties of human recombinant protein C and activated protein C. Biochemistry 1995;34:8082–8090.

129. Mather T, Oganessyan V, Hof P et al. The 2.8 Å crystal structure of Gla-domainless activated protein C. EMBO J 1996;15:6822–6831.

130. Drakenberg T, Fernlund P, Roepstorff P et al. beta-Hydroxyaspartic acid in vitamin K-dependent protein C. Proc Natl Acad Sci U S A 1983;80:1802–1806.

131. Ohlin AK, Landes G, Bourdon P et al. Beta-hydroxyaspartic acid in the first epidermal growth factor-like domain of protein C. Its role in Ca²⁺ binding and biological activity. J Biol Chem 1988;263:19240–19248.

132. Grinnell BW, Walls JD, Gerlitz B. Glycosylation of human protein C affects its secretion, processing, functional activities and activation by thrombin. J Biol Chem 1991;266:9778–9785.

133. Rezaie AR, Mather T, Sussman F et al. Mutation of Glu-80 to Lys results in a protein C mutant that no longer requires Ca²⁺ for rapid activation by the thrombin-thrombomodulin complex. J Biol Chem 1994;269:3151–3154.

134. Rezaie AR, Esmon CT. Tryptophans 231 and 234 in protein C report the Ca²⁺-dependent conformational change required for activation by the thrombin-thrombomodulin complex. Biochemistry 1995;34:12221–12226.

135. Rezaie AR, Esmon CT. The function of calcium in protein C activation by thrombin and the thrombin-thrombomodulin complex can be distinguished by mutational analysis of protein C derivatives. J Biol Chem 1992;267:26104–26109.

136. Esmon NL, DeBault LE, Esmon CT. Proteolytic formation and properties of γ-carboxyglutamic acid-domainless protein C. J Biol Chem 1983;258:5548–5553.

137. Rezaie AR, Esmon NL, Esmon CT. The high affinity calcium-binding site involved in protein C activation is outside the first epidermal growth factor homology domain. J Biol Chem 1992;267:11701–11704.

138. Rezaie AR, Esmon CT. Proline at the P2 position in protein C is important for calcium-mediated regulation of protein C activation and secretion. Blood 1994;83:2526–2531.

139. Grinnell BW, Gerlitz B, Berg DT. Identification of a region in protein C involved in thrombomodulin-stimulated activation by thrombin: potential repulsion at anion-binding site I in thrombin. Biochem J 1994;303:929–933.

140. Kane WH, Davie EW. Blood coagulation factors V and VIII: structural and functional similarities and their relationship to hemorrhagic and thrombotic disorders. Blood 1988;71:539–555.

141. Kalafatis M, Rand MD, Mann KG. The mechanism of inactivation of human factor V and human factor Va by activated protein C. J Biol Chem 1994;269:31869–31880.

142. Petäjä J, Fernández JA, Gruber A et al. Anticoagulant synergism of heparin and activated protein C in vitro. J Clin Invest 1997;99:2655–2663.

143. Rezaie AR, Esmon CT. Conversion of glutamic acid 192 to glutamine in activated protein C changes the substrate specificity and increases reactivity toward macromolecular inhibitors. J Biol Chem 1993;268:19943–19948.

144. Beckmann RJ, Schmidt RJ, Santerre RF et al. The structure and evolution of a 461 amino acid human protein C precursor and its messenger RNA, based upon the DNA sequence of cloned human liver cDNAs. Nucleic Acids Res 1985;13:5233–5247.

145. Rocchi M, Roncuzzi L, Santamaria R et al. Mapping through somatic cell hybrids and cDNA probes of protein C to chromosome 2, factor X to chromosome 13, and alpha 1-acid glycoprotein to chromosome 9. Hum Genet 1986;74:30–33.

146. Long GL, Marshall A, Gardner JC et al. Genes for human vitamin K-dependent plasma proteins C and S are located on chromosomes 2 and 3, respectively. Somat Cell Mol Genet 1988;14:93–98.

147. Kato A, Miura O, Sumi Y et al. Assignment of the human protein C gene (PROC) to chromosome region 2q14-q21 by in situ hybridisation. Cytogenet Cell Genet 1988;47:46–47.

148. Patracchini P, Aiello V, Palazzi P et al. Sublocalisation of the human protein C gene on chromosome 2q13-q14. Hum Genet 1989;81:191–192.

149. Foster DC, Yoshitake S, Davie EW. The nucleotide sequence of the gene for human protein C. Proc Natl Acad Sci U S A 1985;82:4673–4677.

150. Plutzky J, Hoskins JA, Long GL et al. Evolution and organization of the human protein C gene. Proc Natl Acad Sci U S A 1986;83:546–550.

151. Miao CH, Ho WT, Greenberg DL et al. Transcriptional regulation of the gene coding for human protein C. J Biol Chem 1996;271:9587–9594.

152. Spek CA, Greengard JS, Griffin JH et al. Two mutations in the promoter region of the human protein C gene both cause type I protein C deficiency by disruption of two HNF-3 binding sites. J Biol Chem 1995;270: 24216–24221.

153. Fair DS, Marlar RA, Levin EG. Human endothelial cells synthesize protein S. Blood 1986;67:1168–1171.

154. Stern D, Brett J, Harris K et al. Participation of endothelial cells in the protein C-protein S anticoagulant pathway: the synthesis and release of protein S. J Cell Biol 1986;102:1971–1978.

155. Malm J, He XH, Bjartell A et al. Vitamin K-dependent protein S in Leydig cells of human testis. Biochem J 1994;302:845–850.

156. Schwarz HP, Heeb MJ, Wencel-Drake JD et al. Identification and quantitation of protein S in human platelets. Blood 1985;66:1452–1455.

157. Ogura M, Tanabe N, Nishioka J et al. Biosynthesis and secretion of functional protein S by a human megakaryoblastic cell line (MEG-01). Blood 1987;70:301–306.

158. Dahlback B, Stenflo J. High molecular weight complex in human plasma between vitamin K-dependent protein S and complement component C4b-binding protein. Proc Natl Acad Sci U S A 1981;78:2512–2516.

159. Dahlback B, Lundwall A, Stenflo J. Primary structure of bovine vitamin K-dependent protein S. Proc Natl Acad Sci U S A 1986;83:4199–4203.

160. Lundwall A, Dackowski W, Cohen E et al. Isolation and sequence of the cDNA for human protein S, a regulator of blood coagulation. Proc Natl Acad Sci U S A 1986;83:6716–6720.

161. Hoskins J, Norman DK, Beckmann RJ et al. Cloning and characterisation of human liver cDNA encoding a protein S precursor. Proc Natl Acad Sci U S A 1987;84:349–353.

162. Ploos van Amstel HK, van der Zanden AL, Reitsma PH et al. Human protein S cDNA encodes Phe-16 and Tyr-222 in consensus sequences for the post-translational processing. FEBS Lett 1987;222:186–190.

163. Dahlback B. Purification of human vitamin K-dependent protein S and its limited proteolysis by thrombin. Biochem J 1983;209:837–846.

164. Dahlback B, Lundwall A, Stenflo J. Localization of thrombin cleavage sites in the aminoterminal region of bovine protein S. J Biol Chem 1986;261: 5111–5115.

165. Chang GT, Aaldering L, Hackeng TM et al. Construction and characterization of thrombin-resistant variants of recombinant human protein S. Thromb Haemost 1994;72:693–697.

166. Sugo T, Dahlback B, Holmgren A et al. Calcium binding of bovine protein S. Effect of thrombin cleavage and removal of the gamma-carboxyglutamic acid-containing region. J Biol Chem 1986;261:5116–5120.

167. Suzuki K, Nishioka J, Hashimoto S. Regulation of activated protein C by thrombin-modified protein S. J Biochem (Tokyo) 1983;94:699–705.

168. Walker FJ. Regulation of vitamin K-dependent protein S. Inactivation by thrombin. J Biol Chem 1984;259:10335–10339.

169. Mitchell CA, Hau L, Salem HH. Control of thrombin mediated cleavage of protein S. Thromb Haemost 1986;56:151–154.

170. Dahlback B, Hildebrand B, Malm J. Characterization of functionally important domains in human vitamin K-dependent protein S using monoclonal antibodies. J Biol Chem 1990;265:8127–8135.

171. He X, Shen L, Dahlback B. Expression and functional characterization of chimeras between human and bovine vitamin K-dependent protein-S-defining modules important for the species specificity of the activated protein C cofactor activity. Eur J Biochem 1995;227:433–440.

172. Dahlback B, Hildebrand B, Linse S. Novel type of very high affinity calcium-binding sites in beta-hydroxyasparagine-containing epidermal growth factor-like domains in vitamin K-dependent protein S. J Biol Chem 1990;265:18481–18489.

173. Nelson RM, VanDusen WJ, Friedman PA et al. β-Hydroxyaspartic acid and β-hydroxyasparagine residues in recombinant human protein S are not required for anticoagulant cofactor activity or for binding to C4b-binding protein. J Biol Chem 1991;266:20586–20589.

174. Gershagen S, Fernlund P, Lundwall A. A cDNA coding for human sex hormone binding globulin. Homology to vitamin K-dependent protein S. FEBS Lett 1987;220:129–135.

175. Baker ME, French FS, Joseph DR. Vitamin K-dependent protein S is similar to rat androgen-binding protein. Biochem J 1987;243:293–296.

176. Gershagen S, Fernlund P, Edenbrandt CM. The genes for SHBG/ABP and the SHBG-like region of vitamin K-dependent protein S have evolved from a common ancestral gene. J Steroid Biochem Mol Biol 1991;40:763–769.

177. Walker FJ. Characterization of a synthetic peptide that inhibits the interaction between protein S and C4b-binding protein. J Biol Chem 1989;264: 17645–17648.

178. Fernandez JA, Heeb MJ, Griffin JH. Identification of residues 413–433 of plasma protein S as essential for binding to C4b-binding protein. J Biol Chem 1993;268:16788–16794.

179. Linse S, Härdig Y, Schultz DA et al. A region of vitamin K-dependent protein S that binds to C4b binding protein (C4BP) identified using bacteriophage peptide display libraries. J Biol Chem 1997;272:14658–14665.

180. Dahlback B. Protein S and C4b-binding protein: components involved in the regulation of the protein C anticoagulant system [Review]. Thromb Haemost 1991;66:49–61.

181. Hillarp A, Dahlback B. Cloning of cDNA coding for the β-chain of human complement component C4b-binding protein: sequence homology with the α-chain. Proc Natl Acad Sci U S A 1990;87:1183–1187.

182. Hillarp A, Dahlback B. Novel subunit in C4b-binding protein required for protein S binding. J Biol Chem 1988;263:12759–12764.

183. Hardig Y, Rezaie A, Dahlback B. High affinity binding of human vitamin K-dependent protein S to a truncated recombinant beta-chain of C4b-binding protein expressed in Escherichia coli. J Biol Chem 1993;268:3033–3036.

184. Fernandez JA, Griffin JH. A protein S binding site on C4b-binding protein involves beta chain residues 31–45. J Biol Chem 1994;269:2535–2540.

185. Griffin JH, Gruber A, Fernandez JA. Reevaluation of total, free, and bound protein S and C4b-binding protein levels in plasma anticoagulated with citrate or hirudin. Blood 1992;79:3203–3211.

186. Garcia de Frutos P, Alim RI, Hardig Y et al. Differential regulation of alpha and beta chains of C4b-binding protein during acute-phase response resulting in stable plasma levels of free anticoagulant protein S. Blood 1994;84:815–822.

187. Bertina RM, Ploos van Amstel HK, van Wijngaarden A et al. Heerlen polymorphism of protein S, an immunologic polymorphism due to dimorphism of residue 460. Blood 1990;76:538–548.

188. Duchemin J, Gandrille S, Borgel D et al. The Ser 460 to Pro substitution of the protein S α (PROS1) gene is a frequent mutation associated with free protein S (type IIa) deficiency. Blood 1995;86:3436–3443.

189. Dahlback B. Inhibition of protein Ca cofactor function of human and bovine protein S by C4b-binding protein. J Biol Chem 1986;261:12022–12027.

190. Walker FJ. Regulation of activated protein C by protein S. The role of phospholipid in factor Va inactivation. J Biol Chem 1981;256:11128–11131.

191. Hackeng TM, Hessing M, van 't Veer C et al. Protein S binding to human endothelial cells is required for expression of cofactor activity for activated protein C. J Biol Chem 1993;268:3993–4000.

192. Stern DM, Nawroth PP, Harris K et al. Cultured bovine aortic endothelial cells promote activated protein C-protein S-mediated inactivation of factor Va. J Biol Chem 1986;261:713–718.

193. Suzuki K, Nishioka J, Matsuda M et al. Protein S is essential for the activated protein C-catalyzed inactivation of platelet-associated factor Va. J Biochem (Tokyo) 1984;96:455–460.

194. Harris KW, Esmon CT. Protein S is required for bovine platelets to support activated protein C binding and activity. J Biol Chem 1985;260:2007–2010.

195. Rosing J, Hoekema L, Nicolaes GA et al. Effects of protein S and factor Xa on peptide bond cleavages during inactivation of factor Va and factor Va(R506Q) by activated protein C. J Biol Chem 1995;270:27852–27858.

196. Solymoss S, Tucker MM, Tracy PB. Kinetics of inactivation of membrane-bound factor Va by activated protein C. Protein S modulates factor Xa protection. J Biol Chem 1988;263:14884–14890.

197. Shen L, Dahlback B. Factor V and protein S as synergistic cofactors to activated protein C in degradation of factor VIIIa. J Biol Chem 1994;269: 18735–18738.

198. Leroy-Matheron C, Gouault-Heilmann M, Borgel D et al. Aberrant spliced

transcripts generated during PROS1 gene expression in a family with type II protein S (PS) deficiency [Abstract]. Thromb Haemost 1997;Suppl:187.

199. Greengard JS, Fernandez JA, Radtke KP et al. Identification of candidate residues for interaction of protein S with C4b binding protein and activated protein C. Biochem J 1995;305:397–403.

200. He X, Dahlback B. Rabbit plasma, unlike its human counterpart, contains no complex between protein S and C4b-binding protein. Thromb Haemost 1994;71:446–451.

201. He X, Dahlback B. Molecular cloning, expression and functional characterization of rabbit anticoagulant vitamin K-dependent protein S. Eur J Biochem 1993;217:857–865.

202. Chang GT, Maas BH, Ploos van Amstel HK et al. Studies of the interaction between human protein S and human C4b-binding protein using deletion variants of recombinant human protein S. Thromb Haemost 1994;71:461–467.

203. Heeb MJ, Mesters RM, Tans G et al. Binding of protein S to factor Va associated with inhibition of prothrombinase that is independent of activated protein C. J Biol Chem 1993;268:2872–2877.

204. Heeb MJ, Rosing J, Bakker HM et al. Protein S binds to and inhibits factor Xa. Proc Natl Acad Sci U S A 1994;91:2728–2732.

205. Hackeng TM, van 't Veer C, Meijers JC et al. Human protein S inhibits prothrombinase complex activity on endothelial cells and platelets via direct interactions with factors Va and Xa. J Biol Chem 1994;269:21051–21058.

206. van't Veer C, Golden NJ, Mann KG. Regulation of prothrombinase activity by protein S [Abstract]. Thromb Haemost 1997;Suppl:186.

207. Koppelman SJ, Hackeng TM, Sixma JJ et al. Inhibition of the intrinsic factor X activating complex by protein S: evidence for specific binding of protein S to Factor VIII. Blood 1995;86:1062–1071.

208. Koppelman SJ, Hackeng TM, Sixma JJ et al. Inhibition of the intrinsic factor X activating reaction by complement C4b-binding protein, evidence for a specific binding between factor VIII and C4b-binding protein [Abstract]. Br J Haematol 1994;87:52.

209. Gasic GP, Arenas CP, Gasic TB et al. Coagulation factors X, Xa, and protein S as potent mitogens of cultured aortic smooth muscle cells. Proc Natl Acad Sci U S A 1992;89:2317–2320.

210. Benzakour O, Formstone C, Rahman S et al. Evidence for a protein S receptor(s) on human vascular smooth muscle cells. Analysis of the binding characteristics and mitogenic properties of protein S on human vascular smooth muscle cells. Biochem J 1995;308:481–485.

211. Stitt TN, Conn G, Gore M et al. The anticoagulation factor protein S and its relative, Gas6, are ligands for the Tyro 3/Axl family of receptor tyrosine kinases. Cell 1995;80:661–670.

212. Godowski PJ, Mark MR, Chen J et al. Reevaluation of the roles of protein S and Gas6 as ligands for the receptor tyrosine kinase Rse/Tyro 3. Cell 1995;82:355–358.

213. Maillard C, Berruyer M, Serre CM et al. Protein-S, a vitamin K-dependent protein, is a bone matrix component synthesized and secreted by osteoblasts. Endocrinology 1992;130:1599–1604.

214. Ploos van Amstel JK, van der Zanden AL, Bakker E et al. Two genes homologous with human protein S cDNA are located on chromosome 3. Thromb Haemost 1987;58:982–987.

215. Watkins PC, Eddy R, Fukushima Y et al. The gene for protein S maps near the centromere of human chromosome 3. Blood 1988;71:238–241.

216. Schmidel DK, Tatro AV, Phelps LG et al. Organization of the human protein S genes. Biochemistry 1990;29:7845–7852.

217. Ploos van Amstel HK, Reitsma PH, van der Logt CP et al. Intron-exon organization of the active human protein S gene PS alpha and its pseudogene PS beta: duplication and silencing during primate evolution. Biochemistry 1990;29:7853–7861.

218. Edenbrandt CM, Lundwall A, Wydro R et al. Molecular analysis of the gene for vitamin K-dependent protein S and its pseudogene. Cloning and partial gene organization. Biochemistry 1990;29:7861–7868.

219. Esmon CT, Ding W, Yasuhiro K et al. The protein C pathway: new insights. Thromb Haemost 1997;78:70–74.

220. Regan LM, Stearns-Kurosawa DJ, Kurosawa S et al. The endothelial cell protein C receptor. Inhibition of activated protein C anticoagulant function without modulation of reaction with proteinase inhibitors. J Biol Chem 1996;271:17499–17503.

221. Stearns-Kurosawa DJ, Kurosawa S, Mollica JS et al. The endothelial cell protein C receptor augments protein C activation by the thrombin-thrombomodulin complex. Proc Natl Acad Sci U S A 1996;93:10212–10216.

222. Fukudome K, Kurosawa S, Stearns-Kurosawa DJ et al. The endothelial cell protein C receptor. Cell surface expression and direct ligand binding by the soluble receptor. J Biol Chem 1996;271:17491–17498.

223. Olson ST, Bjork I, Shore JD. Kinetic characterization of heparin-catalyzed and uncatalyzed inhibition of blood coagulation proteinases by antithrombin. Methods Enzymol 1993;222:525–559.

224. Abildgaard U. Binding of thrombin to antithrombin III. Scand J Clin Lab Invest 1969;24:23–27.

225. Rosenberg RD, Damus PS. The purification and mechanism of action of human antithrombin-heparin cofactor. J Biol Chem 1973;248:6490–6505.

226. Marcum JA, Rosenberg RD. Anticoagulantly active heparin-like molecules from vascular tissue. Biochemistry 1984;23:1730–1737.

227. Marcum JA, Rosenberg RD. Heparin-like molecules with anticoagulant activity are synthesized by cultured endothelial cells. Biochem Biophys Res Commun 1985;126:365–372.

228. Felsch JS, Owen WG. Endogenous antithrombin associated with microvascular endothelium. Quantitative analysis in perfused rat hearts. Biochemistry 1994;33:818–822.

229. Huber R, Carrell RW. Implications of the three-dimensional structure of α1-antitrypsin for structure and function of serpins [Review]. Biochemistry 1989;28:8951–8966.

230. Hunt LT, Dayhoff MO. A surprising new protein superfamily containing ovalbumin, antithrombin III, and α1-proteinase inhibitor. Biochem Biophys Res Commun 1980;95:864–871.

231. Schreuder HA, de Boer B, Dijkema R et al. The intact and cleaved human antithrombin III complex as a model for serpin-proteinase interactions. Nat Struct Biol 1994;1:48–54.

232. Mourey L, Samama JP, Delarue M et al. Crystal structure of cleaved bovine antithrombin III at 3.2 Å resolution. J Mol Biol 1993;232:223–241.

233. Carrell RW, Stein PE, Fermi G et al. Biological implications of a 3 Å structure of dimeric antithrombin. Structure 1994;2:257–270.

234. Thaler E, Lechner K. Antithrombin III deficiency and thromboembolism [Review]. Clin Haematol 1981;10:369–390.

235. Lane DA, Kunz G, Olds RJ et al. Molecular genetics of antithrombin deficiency [Review]. Blood Rev 1996;10:59–74.

236. Olds RJ, Lane DA, Chowdhury V et al. Complete nucleotide sequence of the antithrombin gene: evidence for homologous recombination causing thrombophilia. Biochemistry 1993;32:4216–4224.

237. Picard V, Ersdal-Badju E, Bock SC. Partial glycosylation of antithrombin III asparagine 135 is caused by the serine in the third position of its N-glycosylation consensus sequence and is responsible for production of the β-antithrombin III isoform with enhanced heparin affinity. Biochemistry 1995;34:8433–8440.

238. Turko IV, Fan B, Gettins PG. Carbohydrate isoforms of antithrombin variant N135Q with different heparin affinities. FEBS Lett 1993;335:9–12.

239. Skriver K, Wikoff WR, Patston PA et al. Substrate properties of C1 inhibitor Ma (alanine 434–glutamic acid). Genetic and structural evidence suggesting that the P12-region contains critical determinants of serine protease inhibitor/substrate status. J Biol Chem 1991;266:9216–9221.

240. Devraj-Kizuk R, Chui DH, Prochownik EV et al. Antithrombin-III-Hamilton: a gene with a point mutation (guanine to adenine) in codon 382 causing impaired serine protease reactivity. Blood 1988;72:1518–1523.

241. Caso R, Lane DA, Olds RJ et al. Antithrombin Vicenza, Ala 384 to Pro (GCA to CCA) mutation, transforming the inhibitor into a substrate. Br J Haematol 1991;77:87–92.

242. Ireland H, Lane DA, Thompson E et al. Antithrombin Glasgow II: alanine 382 to threonine mutation in the serpin P12 position, resulting in a substrate reaction with thrombin. Br J Haematol 1991;79:70–74.

243. Lane DA, Olds RJ, Conard J et al. Pleiotropic effects of antithrombin strand 1C substitution mutations. J Clin Invest 1992;90:2422–2433.

244. Olds RJ, Lane DA, Caso R et al. Antithrombin III Budapest: a single amino acid substitution (429Pro to Leu) in a region highly conserved in the serpin family. Blood 1992;79:1206–1212.

245. Bjork I, Olson ST, Shore JD. Molecular mechanisms of the accelerating effect of heparin on the reactions between antithrombin and the clotting proteinases. In: Lane DA, Lindahl U, eds. Heparin: chemical and biological properties, clinical applications. London: Edward Arnold, 1989:229–255.

246. Pomerantz MW, Owen WG. A catalytic role for heparin. Evidence for a ternary complex of heparin cofactor thrombin and heparin. Biochim Biophys Acta 1978;535:66–77.

247. Griffith MJ. Kinetics of the heparin-enhanced antithrombin III/thrombin reaction. Evidence for a template model for the mechanism of action of heparin. J Biol Chem 1982;257:7360–7365.

248. Griffith MJ. The heparin enhanced antithrombin III/thrombin reaction is saturable with respect to both thrombin and antithrombin III. J Biol Chem 1982;257:13899–13902.

249. Olson ST, Halvorson HR, Bjork I. Quantitative characterisation of the thrombin-heparin interaction. Discrimination between specific and nonspecific binding models. J Biol Chem 1991;266:6342–6352.

250. Olson ST, Bjork I. Predominant contribution of surface approximation to the mechanism of heparin acceleration of the antithrombin-thrombin reaction. Elucidation from salt concentration effects. J Biol Chem 1991;266:6353–6364.

251. Lane DA, Denton J, Flynn AM et al. Anticoagulant activities of heparin oligosaccharides and their neutralization by platelet factor 4. Biochem J 1984;218:725–732.

252. Gettins PG, Fan BC, Crews BC et al. Transmission of conformational change from the heparin binding site to the reactive center of antithrombin. Biochemistry 1993;32:8385–8389.

253. Dawes J, James K, Lane DA. The conformational change in antithrombin induced by heparin, probed with a monoclonal antibody against the 1C/4B region. Biochemistry 1994;33:4375–4383.

254. Hook M, Bjork I, Hopwood J et al. Anticoagulant activity of heparin: separation of high activity and low activity heparin species by affinity chromatography on immobilized antithrombin. FEBS Lett 1976;66:90–93.

255. Lam LH, Silbert JE, Rosenberg RD. The separation of active and inactive forms of heparin. Biochem Biophys Res Commun 1976;69:570–577.

256. Lindahl U, Backstrom G, Thunberg L et al. Evidence for a 3-O-sulfated D-glucosamine residue in the antithrombin-binding sequence of heparin. Proc Natl Acad Sci U S A 1980;77:6551–6555.

257. Casu B, Oreste P, Torri G et al. The structure of heparin oligosaccharide fragments with high anti-(factor Xa) activity containing the minimal antithrombin III binding sequence. Chemical and 13C nuclear-magnetic-resonance studies. Biochem J 1981;197:599–609.

258. Thunberg L, Backstrom G, Lindahl U. Further characterisation of the antithrombin-binding sequence in heparin. Carbohydr Res 1982;100: 393–410.

259. Choay J, Petitou M, Lormeau JC et al. Structure-activity relationship in heparin: a synthetic pentasaccharide with high affinity for antithrombin III and eliciting high anti-factor Xa activity. Biochem Biophys Res Commun 1983;116:492–499.

260. Atha DH, Stephens AW, Rosenberg RD. Evaluation of critical groups required for the binding of heparin to antithrombin. Proc Natl Acad Sci U S A 1984;81:1030–1034.

261. Lindahl U. Biosynthesis of heparin and related polysaccharides. In: Lane DA, Lindahl U, eds. Heparin: chemical and biological properties, clinical applications. London: Edward Arnold, 1989:159–189.

262. Lane DA, Lindahl U, eds. Heparin: chemical and biological properties, clinical applications. London: Edward Arnold, 1989.

263. Rosenberg RD, Shworak NW, Liu J et al. Heparan sulfate proteoglycans of the cardiovascular system. Specific structures emerge but how is synthesis regulated? J Clin Invest 1997;99:2062–2070.

264. Marcum JA, Rosenberg RD. The biochemistry, cell biology, and pathophysiology of anticoagulantly active heparin-like molecules of the vessel wall. In: Lane DA, Lindahl U, eds. Heparin: chemical and biological properties, clinical applications. London: Edward Arnold, 1989:275–294.

265. Frebelius S, Isaksson S, Swedenborg J. Thrombin inhibition by antithrombin III on the subendothelium is explained by the isoform ATβ. Arterioscler Thromb Vasc Biol 1996;16:1292–1297.

266. Colliec-Jouault S, Shworak NW, Liu J et al. Characterization of a cell mutant specifically defective in the synthesis of anticoagulantly active heparan sulfate. J Biol Chem 1994;269:24953–24958.

267. Shworak NW, Shirakawa M, Colliec-Jouault S et al. Pathway-specific regulation of the synthesis of anticoagulantly active heparan sulfate. J Biol Chem 1994;269:24941–24952.

268. Shworak NW, Fritze LMS, Liu J et al. Cell-free synthesis of anticoagulant heparan sulfate reveals a limiting converting activity modifies an excess precursor pool. J Biol Chem 1996;271:27063–27071.

269. Jordan R, Beeler D, Rosenberg R. Fractionation of low-molecular-weight heparin species and their interaction with antithrombin. J Biol Chem 1979; 254:2902–2913.

270. Nordenman B, Danielsson A, Bjork I. The binding of low-affinity and high-affinity heparin to antithrombin. Fluorescence studies. Eur J Biochem 1978; 90:1–6.

271. Blackburn MN, Sibley CC. The heparin binding site of antithrombin III. Evidence for a critical tryptophan residue. J Biol Chem 1980;255:824–826.

272. Borg JY, Brennan SO, Carrell RW et al. Antithrombin Rouen-IV 24 Arg to Cys. The aminoterminal contribution to heparin binding. FEBS Lett 1990; 266:163–166.

273. Gettins P, Choay J, Crews BC et al. Role of tryptophan 49 in the heparin cofactor activity of human antithrombin III. J Biol Chem 1992;267: 21946–21953.

274. Liu CS, Chang JY. Probing the heparin-binding domain of human antithrombin III with V8 protease. Eur J Biochem 1987;167:247–252.

275. Chang JY, Tran TH. Antithrombin III Basel. Identification of a Pro-Leu substitution in a hereditary abnormal antithrombin with impaired heparin cofactor activity. J Biol Chem 1986;261:1174–1176.

276. Koide T, Odani S, Takahashi K et al. Antithrombin III Toyama: replacement of arginine 47 by cysteine in hereditary abnormal antithrombin III that lacks heparin-binding ability. Proc Natl Acad Sci U S A 1984;81:289–293.

277. Borg JY, Owen MC, Soria C et al. Proposed heparin binding site in antithrombin based on arginine 47. A new variant Rouen-II, 47 Arg to Ser. J Clin Invest 1988;81:1292–1296.

278. Liu CS, Chang JY. The heparin binding site of human antithrombin III. Selective chemical modification at Lys114, Lys 125 and Lys 287 impairs its heparin cofactor activity. J Biol Chem 1987;262:17356–17361.

279. Chang JY. Binding of heparin to human antithrombin III activates selective chemical modification at lysine 236. Lys107, Lys125 and Lys136 are situated within the heparin-binding site of antithrombin III. J Biol Chem 1989; 264:3111–3115.

280. Smith JW, Dey N, Knauer DJ. Heparin binding domain of antithrombin III: characterization using a synthetic peptide directed polyclonal antibody. Biochemistry 1990;29:8950–8957.

281. Fan B, Turko IV, Gettins PG. Lysine-heparin interactions in antithrombin. Properties of K125M and K290M, K294M, K297M variants. Biochemistry 1994;33:14156–14161.

282. Gandrille S, Aiach M, Lane DA et al. Important role of arginine 129 in heparin-binding site of antithrombin III. Identification of a novel mutation arginine 129 to glutamine. J Biol Chem 1990;265:18997–19001.

283. Ersdal-Badju E, Lu A, Peng X et al. Elimination of glycosylation heterogeneity affecting heparin affinity of recombinant human antithrombin III

by expression of a beta-like variant in baculovirus-infected insect cells. Biochem J 1995;310:323–330.

284. Watton J, Longstaff C, Lane DA et al. Heparin binding affinity of normal and genetically modified antithrombin III measured using a monoclonal antibody to the heparin binding site of antithrombin III. Biochemistry 1993; 32:7286–7293.

285. Mille B, Watton J, Barrowcliffe TW et al. Role of N and C terminal amino acids in antithrombin binding to pentasaccharide. J Biol Chem 1994;269: 29435–29443.

286. Olds RJ, Lane DA, Boisclair M et al. Antithrombin Budapest 3. An antithrombin variant with reduced heparin affinity resulting from the substitution L99F. FEBS Lett 1992;300:241–246.

287. Chowdhury V, Mille B, Olds RJ et al. Antithrombin Southport (Leu99 to Val) and Vienna (Gln118 to Pro): two novel antithrombin variants with abnormal heparin binding. Br J Haematol 1995;89:602–609.

288. Okajima K, Abe H, Maeda S et al. Antithrombin III Nagasaki (Ser116-Pro): a heterozygous variant with defective heparin binding associated with thrombosis. Blood 1993;81:1300–1305.

289. van Boeckel CA, Grootenhuis D, Visser A. A mechanism for heparin-induced potentiation of antithrombin III [Letter]. Nat Struct Biol 1994;1: 423–425.

290. Huntington JA, Olson ST, Fan B et al. Mechanisms of heparin activation of antithrombin. Evidence for reactive centre loop preinsertion with expulsion upon heparin binding. Biochemistry 1996;35:8495–8503.

291. Bock SC, Wion KL, Vehar GA et al. Cloning and expression of the cDNA for human antithrombin III [Letter]. Nucleic Acids Res 1982;10:8113–8125.

292. Prochownik EV, Markham AF, Orkin SH. Isolation of a cDNA clone for human antithrombin III. J Biol Chem 1983;258:8389–8394.

293. Chandra T, Stackhouse R, Kidd VJ et al. Isolation and sequence characterisation of a cDNA clone of human antithrombin III. Proc Natl Acad Sci U S A 1983;80:1845–1848.

294. Bock SC, Harris JF, Balazs I et al. Assignment of the human antithrombin III structural gene to chromosome 1q23-25. Cytogenet Cell Genet 1985;39: 67–69.

295. Bock SC, Marrinan JA, Radziejewska E. Antithrombin III Utah: proline-407 to leucine mutation in a highly conserved region near the inhibitor reactive site [published erratum appears in Biochemistry 1989;28:3628]. Biochemistry 1988;27:6171–6178.

296. Bock SC, Levitan DJ. Characterisation of an unusual DNA length polymorphism 5′ to the human antithrombin III gene. Nucleic Acids Res 1983;11: 8569–8582.

297. Prochownik EV, Antonarakis S, Bauer KA et al. Molecular heterogeneity of inherited antithrombin III deficiency. N Engl J Med 1983;308:1549–1552.

298. Bock SC, Radziejewska E. A Nhe I RFLP in the human antithrombin III gene (1q23-25) (AT3). Nucleic Acids Res 1991;19:2519.

299. Daly ME, Perry DJ. DdeI polymorphism in intron 5 of the ATIII gene. Nucleic Acids Res 1990;18:5583.

300. Prochownik EV, Orkin SH. In vivo transcription of a human antithrombin III "minigene." J Biol Chem 1984;259:15386–15392.

301. Prochownik EV, Smith MJ, Markham A. Two regions downstream of AA-TAAA in the human antithrombin III gene are important for cleavage-polyadenylation. J Biol Chem 1987;262:9004–9010.

302. Prochownik EV. Relationship between an enhancer element in the human antithrombin III gene and an immunoglobulin light-chain gene enhancer. Nature 1985;316:845–848.

303. Ochoa A, Brunel F, Mendelzon D et al. Different liver nuclear proteins binds to similar DNA sequences in the 5′ flanking regions of three hepatic genes. Nucleic Acids Res 1989;17:119–133.

304. Fernandez-Rachubinski FA, Weiner JH, Blajchman MA. Regions flanking exon 1 regulate constitutive expression of the human antithrombin gene. J Biol Chem 1996;271:29502–29512.

305. Niessen RW, Rezaee F, de Vijlder JJ et al. Human antithrombin III gene expression is probably regulated by a hormone receptor response element. Thromb Haemost 1995;73:1251.

306. Tollefsen DM, Majerus DW, Blank MK. Heparin cofactor II. Purification and properties of a heparin-dependent inhibitor of thrombin in human plasma. J Biol Chem 1982;257:2162–2169.

307. Tollefsen DM, Pestka CA, Monafo WJ. Activation of heparin cofactor II by dermatan sulfate. J Biol Chem 1983;258:6713–6716.

308. Ragg H. A new member of the plasma protease inhibitor gene family. Nucleic Acids Res 1986;14:1073–1088.

309. McGuire EA, Tollefsen DM. Activation of heparin cofactor II by fibroblasts and vascular smooth muscle cells. J Biol Chem 1987;262:169–175.

310. Tollefsen DM. Insight into the mechanisms of action of heparin cofactor II [Review]. Thromb Haemost 1995;74:1209–1214.

311. Bertina RM, van der Linden IK, Engesser L et al. Hereditary heparin cofactor II deficiency and the risk of development of thrombosis. Thromb Haemost 1987;57:196–200.

312. Herzog R, Lutz S, Blin N et al. Complete nucleotide sequence of the gene for human heparin cofactor II and mapping to chromosomal band 22q11.Biochemistry 1991;30:1350–1357.

313. Hortin G, Tollefsen DM, Strauss AW. Identification of two sites of sulfation of human heparin cofactor II. J Biol Chem 1986;261:15827–15830.

314. Derechin VM, Blinder MA, Tollefsen DM. Substitution of arginine for Leu444 in the reactive site of heparin cofactor II enhances the rate of thrombin inhibition. J Biol Chem 1990;265:5623–5628.

315. Van Deerlin VM, Tollefsen DM. The N-terminal acidic domain of heparin cofactor II mediates the inhibition of α-thrombin in the presence of glycosaminoglycans. J Biol Chem 1991;266:20223–20231.

316. Blinder MA, Andersson TR, Abildgaard U et al. Heparin cofactor II Oslo. Mutation of Arg-189 to His decreases the affinity for dermatansulfate. J Biol Chem 1989;264:5128–5133.

317. Ragg H, Ulshofer T, Gerewitz J. On the activation of human leuserpin-2, a thrombin inhibitor, by glycosaminoglycans. J Biol Chem 1990;265:5211–5218.

318. Blinder MA, Tollefsen DM. Site-directed mutagenesis of arginine 103 and lysine 185 in the proposed glycosaminoglycan-binding site of heparin cofactor II. J Biol Chem 1990;265:286–291.

319. Sanders NL, Bajaj SP, Zivelin A et al. Inhibition of tissue factor/factor VIIa activity in plasma requires factor X and an additional plasma component. Blood 1985;66:204–212.

320. Broze GJ Jr, Miletich JP. Characterisation of the inhibition of tissue factor in serum. Blood 1987;69:150–155.

321. Sandset PM, Warn-Cramer BJ, Maki SL et al. Depletion of extrinsic pathway inhibitor (EPI) sensitizes rabbits to disseminated intravascular coagulation induced with tissue factor: evidence supporting a physiologic role for EPI as a natural anticoagulant. Proc Natl Acad Sci U S A 1991;88:708–712.

322. Wun TC, Kretzmer KK, Girard TJ et al. Cloning and characterisation of a cDNA coding for the lipoprotein-associated coagulation inhibitor shows that it consists of three tandem Kunitz-type inhibitory domains. J Biol Chem 1988;13:6001–6004.

323. Girard TJ, Warren LA, Novotny WF et al. Functional significance of the Kunitz type inhibitor domains of lipoprotein-associated coagulation inhibitor. Nature 1989;338:518–520.

324. Hubbard AR, Weller LJ, Gray E. Measurement of tissue factor pathway inhibitor in normal and post-heparin plasma. Blood Coagul Fibrinolysis 1994;5:819–823.

325. Novotny WF, Girard JP, Miletich JP et al. Purification and characterisation of the lipoprotein-associated coagulation inhibitor from human plasma. J Biol Chem 1989;264:18832–18837.

326. Lindahl AK, Jacobsen PB, Sandset PM et al. Tissue factor pathway inhibitor with high anticoagulant activity is increased in post-heparin plasma and in plasma from cancer individuals. Blood Coagul Fibrinolysis 1991;2:713–721.

327. Broze GJ Jr, Lange GW, Duffin KL et al. Heterogeneity of plasma tissue factor pathway inhibitor. Blood Coagul Fibrinolysis 1994;5:551–559.

328. Jesty J, Lorenz A, Rodriguez J et al. Initiation of the tissue factor pathway of coagulation in the presence of heparin: control by antithrombin III and tissue factor pathway inhibitor. Blood 1996;87:2301–2307.

329. Bourin MC, Lindahl U. Glycosaminoglycans in the regulation of blood coagulation. Biochem J 1993;289:313–330.

330. Dahlback B, Stenflo J. The protein C anticoagulant system. In: Stamatoyannopoulos G, Nienhuis AW, Majerus PW, Varmus H, eds. The molecular basis of blood diseases. 2nd ed: Philadelphia: WB Saunders, 1994:599–627.

331. MacGilivray RT, Davie EW. Characterisation of bovine prothrombin mRNA and its translation product. Biochemistry 1984;23:1626–1634.

332. Degen SJ, MacGillivray RT, Davie EW. Characterization of the complementary deoxyribonucleic acid and gene coding for human prothrombin. Biochemistry 1983;22:2087–2097.

# CHAPTER 4

# THE TISSUE FACTOR PATHWAY OF COAGULATION

George J. Broze Jr.

Investigators noted in the early 19th century that damaged tissues induced the clotting of blood. In 1892, Schmidt (1) suggested that tissues contained a substance, which was later termed thromboplastin or tissue factor (factor III), that directly converted prothrombin to thrombin. Morawitz (2) subsequently proposed a two-step theory of coagulation in which thromboplastin acted on prothrombin to produce thrombin and thrombin converted fibrinogen to fibrin. The simplified theory of Morawitz required modification with the development of improved assays for thrombin generation and identification of specific hereditary coagulation deficiencies of factor V, factor VII (3), and factor X (4, 5). Nevertheless, throughout the first half of this century, it was widely accepted that the exposure of blood to tissue factor was responsible for triggering hemostasis.

Studies suggesting an alternative coagulation pathway that did not require tissue factor were initially ignored. Although Manteuffel (6) had shown in 1893 that hemophiliac blood normally clotted following the addition of tissue factor, it was 50 years later that mounting evidence, including the further definition of hemophilia A (factor VIII deficiency) and hemophilia B (factor IX deficiency), forced a reassessment of the hemostatic mechanism. Morawitz's theory did not explain the bleeding patterns of hemophiliacs since their blood appeared to clot normally after the addition of tissue factor.

In 1964, the "cascade" (7) and "waterfall" (8) theories proposed an intrinsic pathway of coagulation. An integral part of these theories was the amplification of coagulation that could be achieved through the sequential activation of protease zymogens to active enzymes. Coagulation was initiated in the intrinsic pathway through exposure of the contact factors (factor XII, high-molecular-weight kininogen, and prekallikrein) in plasma to a surface, which lead to the activation of factor XI. Factor XIa, in turn, activated factor IX and factor IXa, along with factor VIII, then activated factor X. The alternative extrinsic pathway, in which the exposure of factor VII in plasma to tissue factor produced direct activation of factor X, was relegated to a minor, ancillary role in hemostasis since the intrinsic pathway required factors VIII and IX, which are the factors missing in hemophiliacs.

The cascade and waterfall hypotheses of blood coagulation, which segregated the known coagulation factors into intrinsic, extrinsic, and common pathways, and the availability of *in vitro* tests for coagulation initiated by contact (partial thromboplastin time [PTT]) and tissue factor (prothrombin time [PT]) proved invaluable in the laboratory diagnosis of clinical bleeding disorders. These theories that emphasized intrinsic coagulation however, did not accurately reflect *in vivo* hemostasis. Individuals deficient in one of the contact factors are asymptomatic (9), whereas people deficient in factor VII bleed abnormally (10, 11). These clinical observations and the *in vitro* demonstration by Osterud and Rapaport (12) that factor VIIa-tissue factor can activate factor IX of the intrinsic pathway as well as factor X have led to a renewed appreciation of the role of tissue factor in the initiation of coagulation.

The severe hemorrhage that is seen in hemophiliacs despite an intact extrinsic coagulation pathway appears partially due to an endogenous inhibitor of tissue factor-induced coagulation. The properties of this tissue factor pathway inhibitor (TFPI) have led to a reformulation of the coagulation cascade (13, 14). Tissue factor is responsible for the initiation of coagulation, but subsequent amplification of the clotting process through the action of factors VIII and IX is required for hemostasis.

This chapter reviews the biochemistry, molecular biology and physiology of factor VII, tissue factor, and TFPI; and role of these proteins in hemostasis. The contribution of tissue factor-induced coagulation to specific pathologic conditions is discussed in Chapters 36, 44, and 45.

# FACTOR VII

In Morawitz's (2) original two-step theory of coagulation, thromboplastin directly converted prothrombin to thrombin in the presence of calcium ions. With improved one-stage and two-stage assay techniques for prothrombin activation, it became apparent that additional factors were required for thromboplastin-induced thrombin generation. Factor V was the first such factor to be identified and was initially called proaccelerin or labile factor (the latter term referring to its instability during the storage of plasma and its absence in human serum). A second factor, which remained stable in plasma during storage and was present at high levels in serum, was also required for thromboplastin-induced prothrombin activation. This activity was termed stable factor by Quick, proconvertin by Owren, serum prothrombin conversion accelerator (SPCA) by Alexander, and factor VII by Koller (15). A individual who was congenitally deficient in this factor was initially identified by Alexander and et al (3); a separation between the activities of factor VII and a third factor required for thromboplastin-induced coagulation was accomplished with the subsequent description of individuals with factor X deficiency (4, 5).

The isolation of factor VII was hampered by its trace concentration in plasma and its sensitivity to proteolytic activation and degradation. Bovine factor VII was eventually purified using benzamidine-agarose chromatography (16, 17), and the subsequent isolation of human factor VII relied on the difference in its affinity for an ion-exchange matrix in the presence and absence of calcium ions (18, 19). Factor VII complementary DNA (cDNA) has been isolated and cloned (20), and the entire nucleotide sequence of the factor VII gene has been reported (21). The cDNA for rabbit and mouse factor VII has been isolated (22, 23), and the nucleotide sequence of exon 8, which encodes the catalytic domain, has also been reported for the factor VII genes of the rhesus monkey and dog (24).

## MOLECULAR BIOLOGY

The factor VII gene is 12.8 kb long and contains nine exons and eight introns; it is located adjacent to the gene for factor X on the long arm of chromosome 13 (q34) (21, 25). Expression of the factor VII gene may be regulated by a separate gene on chromosome 8 (25, 26). The organization of the factor VII gene is strikingly similar to that of the genes for the vitamin K-dependent proteins, factor IX, factor X, and protein C (27); the conservation of discrete protein domains, intron positions, and phases of intron splice sites supports the theory that the members of this protein family arose through a process of gene duplication, gene modification, and exon shuffling.

The 5' flanking region of the factor VII gene lacks typical TATA and CAAT sequences, and the major transcription start site is located approximately 50 bp upstream of the codon for the initiation methionine (+1) (28–30). The liver-enriched transcription factor hepatocyte nuclear factor-4 (HNF-4) and the ubiquitous transcription factor Sp1 bind the factor VII promoter and are required for optimal *in vitro* transcription. HNF-4 produces a similar positive regulatory effect on the transcription of the genes for factor IX, factor X, and several apolipoproteins (31). Severe factor VII deficiency due to a mutation within the HNF-4 binding site in the factor VII promoter has been reported (32).

The signal peptide (residues -60 to -18) that is removed during the intracellular processing of factor VII is encoded by exons 1a and 1b (21). Alternative splicing of exon 1b leads to messenger RNAs (mRNAs) that code for leader sequences of either 38 or 60 amino acids; both messages direct the expression of active factor VII, but the mRNA lacking exon 1b is more abundant in normal liver (33). The propeptide (-17 to -1), which is also excised during protein processing, and the γ-carboxyglutamic acid (Gla)-rich domain (residues 1–37) are encoded by exon 2. Exon 3 encodes the short aromatic amino acid stack domain (residues 38–45), and exons 4 (residues 46–83) and 5 (residues 84–130) each code for an epidermal growth factor (EGF)-like domain. Exons 6, 7, and 8 code for the catalytic domain of factor VII (residues 131–406) and a 1.17 kb untranslated region that contains a poly (A) signal and three alternative sites for polyadenylation.

Three genetic polymorphisms that affect the plasma antigenic level of factor VII have been identified. An insertion of a decanucleotide at position -323 in the factor VII gene reduces promoter activity *in vitro* (29) and is associated with lower plasma levels of factor VII *in vivo* (34). A DNA base change from G to A in exon 8 results in the loss of an Msp I restriction endonuclease site and the substitution of a glutamine for an arginine at residue 353 in the catalytic domain of factor VII. The lower frequency allele, termed M2, is associated with a decrease in plasma factor VII (35). Finally, the number of tandem repeats within minisatellite DNA in the intron between exons 7 and 8 is also related to the level of factor VII (31).

## BIOCHEMISTRY

Ten glutamic acid residues near the aminoterminus of the factor VII molecule are post-translationally modified to Glas by a carboxylase enzyme, which requires reduced vitamin K as an obligate cofactor (Fig. 4.1). The carboxylation of the glutamic acid residues in the Gla domains of the vitamin K-dependent proteins is directed by polypeptides located between the signal pep-

tide and the aminotermini of the mature proteins (36). The propeptides of these proteins are homologous and contain a binding site for the vitamin K-dependent carboxylase. The propeptide is subsequently removed from the mature protein through the action of a basic dipeptidase in the subtilisin family of enzymes (37).

Calcium ion binding mediated by the Gla residues in vitamin K-dependent proteins, including factor VII, induces a conformational change that leads to the expression of membrane and cofactor binding properties. In the crystal structure of recombinant factor VIIa where Glu35 is apparently not γ-carboxylated (38), seven bound calcium ions are observed in the Gla do-

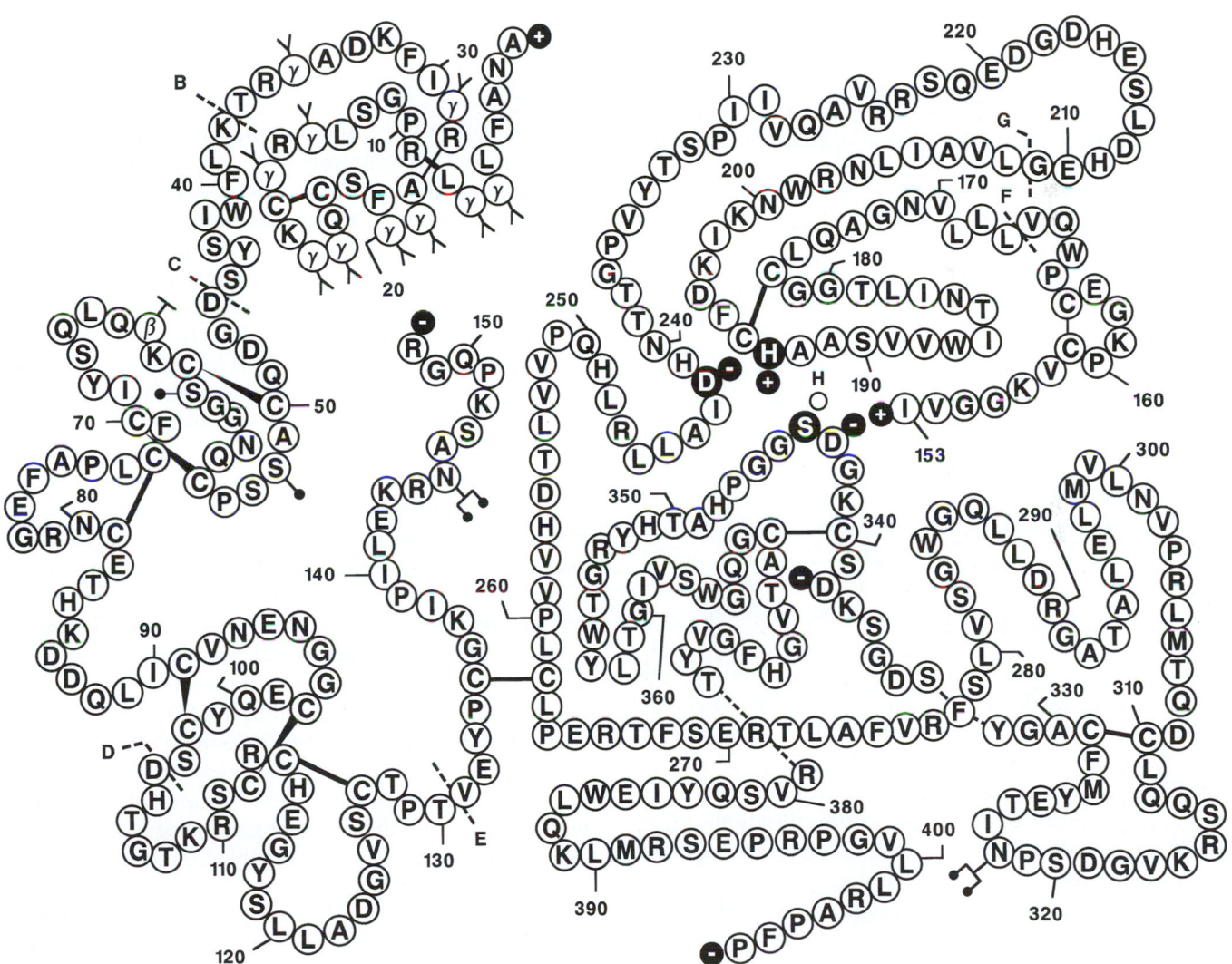

**FIGURE 4.1.**   Structure of activated factor VII. The amino-terminal light chain (left) and carboxy-terminal heavy chain (right) of factor VIIa are depicted in the figure linked by a disulfide bond between Cys135 and Cys262. Amino acids are identified by the single letter code: ⅄ and γ denote γ-carboxyglutamic acid; ⅄ and β denote β-hydroxyaspartic acid; ⅄ denotes site of N-linked glycosylation; and ⅄ denotes sites of O-linked glycosylation. The catalytic triad of residues His193, Asp242, and Ser344 is shown in bold, and the charged side chains of other residues believed to be involved in the cleavage of substrates by the enzyme are depicted (see text). Sites of introns in the factor VII gene are labeled with capital letters. The structure of the Gla domain, epidermal growth factor domains, and catalytic domain of factor VII are patterned after Thompson [619].

main, six of which are arranged in a linear fashion. In the calcium-bound configuration, residues Phe4, Leu5, and Leu8 within the Gla domain form a hydrophobic epitope that may mediate phospholipid binding (39–40).

A short, helical, hydrophobic segment that contains the sequence Phe-Trp-Ile-Ser-Tyr follows the Gla domain of factor VII (see Fig. 4.1). A similar segment, termed the aromatic amino acid stack, is present in the other vitamin K-dependent coagulation factors and is a target for chymotrypsin cleavage.

The regions of factor VII encompassing residues 46–83 (exon 4) and 84–130 (exon 5) are called EGF domains because of their homology with a module in the EGF precursor. A single calcium ion is bound by EGF-1 with high affinity ($K_D \sim 200$ μM) (41). Its coordination sphere is octahedral and involves residues Gln49, Gln64, Gly47, Asp46, and Asp63 (38). Although Asp67 in EGF-1 resides within a consensus sequence for the action of the enzyme β-aspartyl hydroxylase, it apparently is not hydroxylated (42).

The $Arg_{152}$-$Ile_{153}$ site that is proteolytically cleaved during the activation of factor VII lies within the domain encoded by exon 6 (residues 131–167). Following proteolysis, the aminoterminal light chain and carboxyterminal heavy chain of factor VIIa are connected by a disulfide bond between $Cys_{135}$ in this domain and $Cys_{262}$ in the catalytic domain. The structure of the catalytic domain of factor VII is similar to those of the serine proteases trypsin and chymotrypsin and contains the typical active site triad of $Ser_{344}$, $Asp_{242}$, and $His_{193}$ (see Fig. 4.1). Studies suggest that $Asp_{343}$ and the free amino group of $Ile_{153}$, which is generated following the proteolytic formation of factor VIIa, are involved in the activation of $Ser_{344}$ (43). $Asp_{338}$ is in the substrate-binding pocket of the enzyme and serves to tether the arginine at the $P_1$ site in the substrates cleaved by factor VIIa. Similar to trypsin and factors IX and X, the catalytic domain of factor VII contains a high-affinity ($K_D \sim 200$ μM) divalent cation binding site involving residues between Glu210 and Glu220 of a surface loop (38, 41).

The predicted protein mass of factor VII is 45.5 Kda (20), and it migrates on sodium dodecyl sulfate (SDS) polyacrylamide gel electrophoresis with an apparent molecular mass of 50 Kda. N-linked glycosylation occurs at $Asn_{145}$ and $Asn_{322}$; and glucose-, xylose-glucose-, or (xylose)2-glucose- is linked to $Ser_{52}$ while fucose- is linked to $Ser_{60}$ by O-glycosylation (44, 45). The role of these oligosaccharides in the function or physiology of factor VII is unknown.

Zymogen factor VII lacks intrinsic catalytic activity (46). Factor VII is proteolytically activated *in vitro* by thrombin and factor XIIa in the absence of cofactors and by factor Xa and factor IXa in the presence of calcium ions and procoagulant phospholipids. *In vitro*, factor Xa

is the most potent activator of factor VII (47), and the actions of factor Xa and factor IXa are accelerated when factor VII is bound to tissue factor (48–50). Factor VIIa-mediated activation of factor VII bound to tissue factor has also been demonstrated *in vitro* (49, 51–54). The autoactivation of factor VII in the absence of tissue factor has been reported in the presence of poly-D-lysine and sphingosine-containing phospholipid vesicles (52, 55). A soluble, truncated form of tissue factor lacking the transmembrane and cytoplasmic domains of the molecule fails to promote the activation of factor VII under appropriate conditions and has been used to construct a specific assay for factor VIIa in plasma (49, 53, 56). Hepsin and the prothrombin activator from Taipan snake venom are additional nonphysiologic activators of factor VII (57, 58).

## PHYSIOLOGY

Human factor VII circulates in plasma at a concentration of 10 nmol/l (500 ng/ml). It is synthesized predominantly by the liver, but stimulated monocytes/macrophages may provide an important source of factor VII at local sites in tissues (59). A second form of factor VII, which appears to lack the aminoterminal Gla domain, is secreted by cultured hepatoma cells (HepG2) and constitutes approximately 5 to 8% of the total plasma factor VII (60). The half-life of factor VII in plasma is approximately 4 to 5 hours (61), which is the shortest half-life of the vitamin K-dependent coagulation factors. The half-life of factor VIIa in plasma is 2.5 hours, which is much longer than that of other activated coagulation factors (62). Following infusion in the rat, radio-labeled factor VII and VIIa accumulate predominantly in the liver, and receptor-mediated internalization and degradation of factor VIIa has been described in a human hepatoma cell line (63–65). A potent inhibitor of factor VIIa has not been described, and antithrombin III slowly inhibits factor VIIa even in the presence of heparin (18, 66).

The low level of coagulation activation found in healthy individuals is predominantly due to factor VII(a) and is tissue factor–dependent (67–69). Factor VIIa circulates in plasma at a concentration approximately 0.5 to 1.0% that of zymogen factor VII, and factor IX(a) appears primarily responsible for these basal levels of factor VIIa (56, 70, 71).

Plasma factor VII antigen (factor VIIag), total procoagulant activity (factor VIIc), and factor VIIa increase with age; this trend is most striking in women (56, 72, 73). Hormone replacement therapy reduces the increase in factor VII parameters that is seen following menopause (72). Warfarin therapy produces reduced levels of factor VIIag (~50%), factor VIIc (~35%), and factor VIIa (~40%). An accentuated rebound in factor VIIa may occur after warfarin is discontinued (74, 75). Factor VIIc is positively correlated with dietary fat intake and the level of serum lipid, particularly triglycerides (76). The association between factor VIIc and hyperlipidemia in the fasting state may be related to an increase in factor VII mass, which is due to increased synthesis or decreased catabolism of the molecule (77–79). The increase in factor VIIc that occurs during postprandial lipemia is due to factor VII activation and depends on factor IX (80).

In the prospective Northwick Park Heart Study, factor VIIc was a dramatic independent predictor of subsequent fatal ischemic events (see Chapter 39) (81, 82). The Prospective Cardiovascular Munster (PROCAM) study reported a trend toward higher factor VIIc values and fatal events at six-year follow-up (p = 0.06) (83), and a significant (although apparently not independent) association between factor VIIc and total ischemic events at eight-year follow-up (p < 0.05) (84). Several large cross-sectional studies have failed to detect a relationship between factor VIIc levels and the prevalence of vascular disease (85–89). Differences in technique, including the use of non-fasting blood samples and a factor VIIc assay more sensitive to factor VIIa, could contribute to the stronger relationship between factor VIIc and vascular complications that was reported in the Northwick Park study (90). Nevertheless, the extent of the association between increased factor VII and arterial disease is unknown, and whether the risk is due to an increase in factor VII mass or factor VIIa is controversial (91–94). Plasma levels of factor VII do not appear to be related to venous thrombotic disease (95).

Acquired factor VII deficiency is usually due to liver disease, oral anticoagulant therapy, or vitamin K deficiency (see Chapters 45 and 55). Reduced levels of factor VII, however, have been reported in association with the following: hepatic syndromes of Dubin-Johnson, Rotor, and Gilbert (96–98); retroperitoneal fibrosis (99); homocystinuria (100); Hodgkin's disease (101); aplastic anemia (102); antithymocyte globulin and methylprednisolone treatment (103); high-dose chemotherapy; bone marrow transplantation (104); liposarcoma (105); and a familial syndrome of carotid body tumors in which factor X is reduced (106). Congenital factor VII deficiency is discussed in Chapter 36.

# TISSUE FACTOR

Tissue factor functions as a lipoprotein cofactor to enhance the proteolytic activity of factor VIIa toward its substrates, factor IX and factor X. Its lipoprotein nature was initially suggested by Howell (107) and confirmed by Chargaff (108). Early recombination experiments showed that both the lipid and protein components of tissue factor are required for optimal coagulant activity (109).

The tissue factor apoprotein is an integral membrane protein. Early attempts to isolate the apoprotein were hampered by the following factors: the need to use detergents to extract it from tissues, the need to relipidate it into phospholipid vesicles before functional assay, and its trace concentration in tissues. Early work, however, suggested the molecular mass of the tissue factor apoprotein is approximately 50 Kda (110) and the apoprotein contains carbohydrate that is bound by concanavalin A (111). In 1981, the tissue factor apoprotein from bovine brain was isolated by Bach et al (112) using immunoaffinity chromatography. The human tissue factor apoprotein was purified from brain (113) and placenta (114) using factor VII-affinity chromatography 4 years later. Soon thereafter, human tissue factor cDNA was isolated and cloned (115, 116) and the complete sequence of the human tissue factor gene was determined (117). Mouse tissue factor cDNA (118) and genomic DNA (119) and rabbit (120, 121), bovine (122), and rat (123) tissue factor cDNA have also been isolated.

## MOLECULAR BIOLOGY

The human tissue factor gene resides on the short arm of chromosome 1 (p21–22) (124, 125). It is 12.4 kb in length and contains six exons and five introns. Exon 1 (amino acids -32 to +1) encodes the aminoterminal signal peptide, which is removed during post-translational processing of the protein. Exon 2 (residues 2–39), exon 3 (residues 40–105), exon 4 (residues 106–165), and exon 5 (residues 166–218) encode the extracellular portion of the tissue factor molecule; exon 6 (residues 219–263) codes for the transmembrane and cytoplasmic domains of the tissue factor apoprotein and 1.14 kb of 3' untranslated sequence (117).

The tissue factor transcript contains 123 bp of 5' untranslated sequence with the transcription start site located 26 bp downstream from a TATA promoter element. The transcriptional regulation of the human tissue factor gene is complex and has been examined in a limited number of cell types. Sp1 sites within a minimal promoter (−111 to +14 bp) are required for basal expression, and overlapping Sp1/Egr-1 sites within this region are important for phorbol myristate acetate (PMA) and serum induction of tissue factor expression in epithelial cells (126–128). A distal enhancer (−227 to −172 bp) contains two AP-1 sites and an overlapping imperfect kB/Ets site that are important for lipopolysaccharide (LPS) and cytokine induction of the tissue factor gene in monocytes and endothelial cells (127, 129–131). LPS-stimulated tissue factor expression is associated with the following: the concerted binding of c-Jun/Fos heterodimers at the AP-1 sites and transcription factor occupation of the kB/Ets site in the distal enhancer, and Egr-1 binding in the proximal enhancer. Conflicting reports have identified c-Rel/p65 heterodimers (132) and Ets-1/2 (131) as transcription factors responsible for binding the kB/Ets site in the tissue factor promoter. An additional kB site (−441 bp) may be involved in the tissue factor induction mediated by advanced glycosylation end products (133). Treatment of monocytes and endothelial cells with the protein synthesis inhibitor cycloheximide produces superinduction of tissue factor mRNA. This phenomenon may result from both the release of transcription from the control of a short-lived repressor protein and increased stability of the tissue factor mRNA (134–138).

A CpG island (139) encompasses the promoter and exon 1 of the tissue factor gene. This region is highly enriched in C + G nucleotides (70%) and contains a high proportion of CpG dinucleotides (117). CpG islands have been noted in the 5′ region of several "housekeeping" genes, but their function is unknown. There are one partial and three full-length Alu repeats in the tissue factor gene. One of these Alu repeats is in the 3′ untranslated region of exon 6 and is flanked by 11-nucleotide palindromic direct repeats that contain Hind III sites (117, 140). The significance of this common repetitive sequence in the mRNA coding for human tissue factor is unknown.

The size of the predominant tissue factor mRNA species in cells and tissues is 2.3 kb (116, 140). Less abundant tissue factor transcripts of higher molecular weight have occasionally been noted and appear to arise through incomplete or alternative splicing (141). An AU-rich domain occurs near the end of the 3′ untranslated sequence of the tissue factor message. Similar AU-rich regions in the messages coding for inflammatory mediators have been shown to direct their rapid degradation. This AU-rich sequence in tissue factor mRNA may be related (142) to the short half-lives reported for tissue factor messages in endothelial cells treated with phorbol myristate acetate (~50 minutes) (135) and monocytes stimulated by LPS (90 minutes) (134).

An apparent genetic polymorphism occurs in exon 6 of the tissue factor gene (140). A T or C at nucleotide 11,184 in the gene results in either a valine or alanine being encoded at residue 228 within the membrane spanning domain of the tissue factor molecule. Two additional polymorphisms have been described in intron E of the tissue factor gene that produce Msp I and Pst I restriction fragment length polymorphisms (RFLPs) (117, 124).

## BIOCHEMISTRY

Based on its predicted primary amino acid sequence (Fig. 4.2), the tissue factor apoprotein contains three domains: 1) an aminoterminal extracellular domain, residues 1–219; 2) a transmembrane domain, residues 220–242; and 3) a carboxyterminal cytoplasmic domain, residues 243–263. It is a member of the Class II cytokine receptor superfamily that also contains the interferon-α, -β, and -γ, and interleukin-10 receptors. Crystallographic analysis of the extracellular domain shows two fibronectin III domains linked end-to-end with an extensive hydrophobic interface that creates a rigid structure with a 120° elbow (143).

The calculated molecular mass of the apoprotein is 29.6 Kda, whereas estimates of the molecular mass of the apoprotein determined by SDS polyacrylamide gel electrophoresis range from 42 to 47 Kda. This difference in molecular mass is explained in part by N-linked glycosylation of $Asn_{11}$, $Asn_{124}$, and $Asn_{137}$ in the extracellular domain (144). A fourth potential site for N-linked glycosylation in the cytoplasmic domain is not used, and the apoprotein does not appear to contain O-linked carbohydrate (144, 145). Glycosylation does not affect the procoagulant activity of tissue factor. The amino acid sequences of bovine (122), rabbit (120, 121), rat (123), and mouse (118, 138) tissue factor are 72%, 72%, 54%, and 54%, respectively, homologous with that of human tissue factor.

The aminoterminal sequence of human tissue factor apoprotein is heterogeneous; 60% of the apoprotein molecules isolated from human brain begin with $Ser_1$ and 40% begin with $Thr_3$ (140). This heterogeneity likely results from alternative sites of signal peptidase cleavage during intracellular processing of the apoprotein, but a later proteolytic event has not been excluded.

Two disulfide bonds are formed by the four cysteines in the extracellular domain of the apoprotein (Fig. 4.2) (146), and the disulfide bond between $Cys_{186}$ and $Cys_{209}$ is required for tissue factor functional activity (147). A fifth cysteine in the cytoplasmic tail of tissue factor ($Cys_{245}$) is coupled through a thioester bond to either palmitate or stearate (146). A similar linkage between an intracellular cysteine and a fatty acid has been reported in other integral membrane proteins, but its physiologic significance is unknown, and deacylation of tissue factor does not affect its biologic activity (146). $Cys_{245}$ also mediates the formation of the disulfide-bonded tissue factor homodimers and the tissue factor α-globin heterodimers that are present in some preparations of purified tissue factor (113, 114, 116, 148–150). These disulfide-linked conjugates likely represent artifacts that are introduced during the purification of the apoprotein, since the reducing environment within the cytoplasm would not favor the formation of a disulfide bond.

A cluster of four basic amino acids exists at the boundary between the transmembrane domain and the cytoplasmic tail of the tissue factor apoprotein (see Fig. 4.2). This motif is typical for integral membrane proteins that are inserted in the aminoterminus—extracellular orientation (151). Ionic interactions between the charged side chains of these amino acids with acidic phospholipid head groups and an interaction between membrane phospholipids and the fatty acid linked to

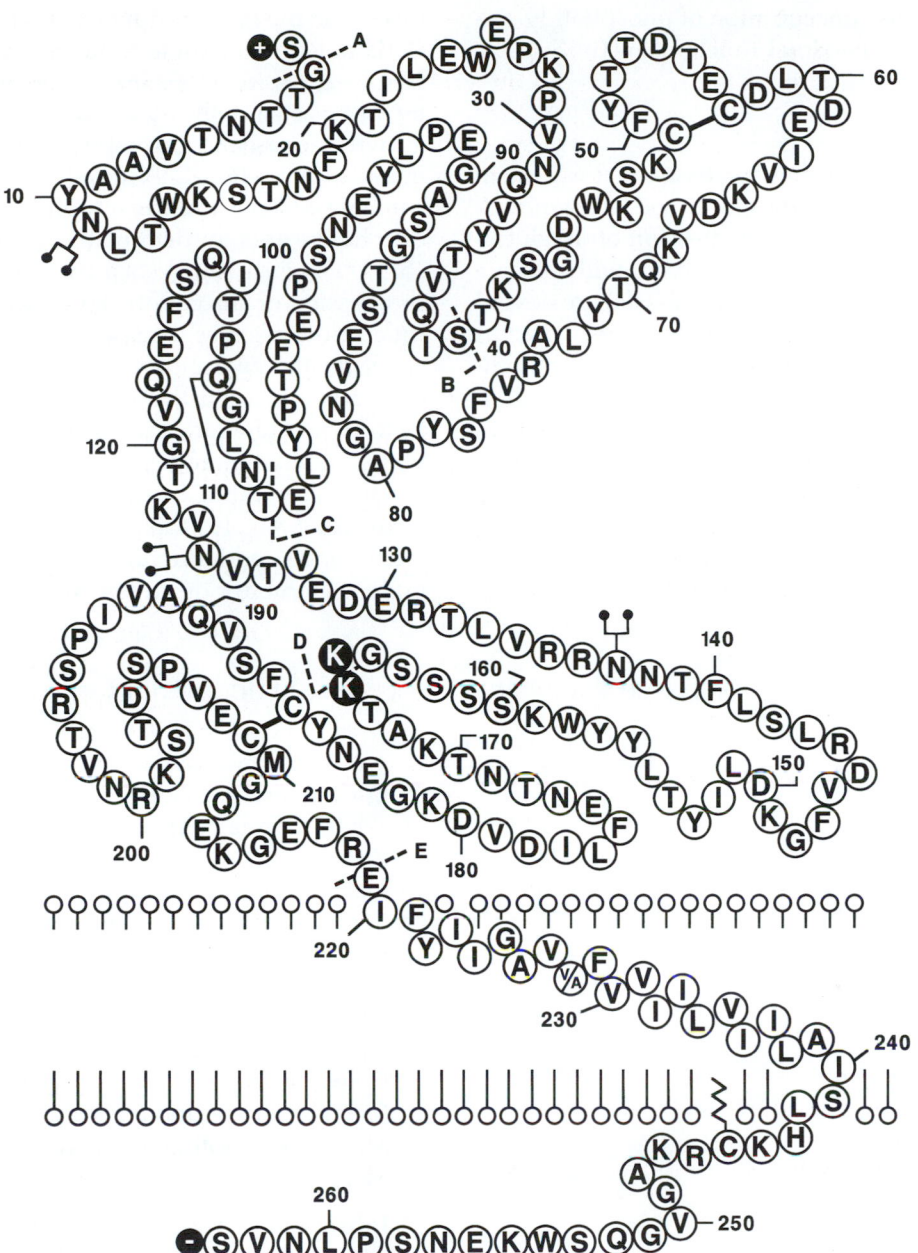

**FIGURE 4.2.** Structure of tissue factor. The predicted transmembrane domain traverses the plasma membrane of a cell and is followed by a short cytoplasmic tail. The single-letter amino acid code is used to identify amino acids; ⌇ denotes sites of carbohydrate attachment; and ⌇ represents palmitate or stearate. Shown in bold are $Lys_{165}$ and $Lys_{166}$, which are important for substrate and factor Xa-TFPI binding. Sites of introns in the tissue factor gene are labeled with capital letters.

$Cys_{245}$ that is at the center of this basic cluster may serve to tether the cytoplasmic tail to the inner leaflet of the cell membrane (146). The role of protein kinase C–dependent phosphorylation of serine residue(s) in the cytoplasmic domain of tissue factor is unknown (152).

To express optimal coagulant activity, the tissue factor apoprotein must be anchored on a phospholipid membrane. The mechanism for this apoprotein-phospholipid interaction, however, does not appear to be critical; chimeric proteins produced by linking the extracellular domain of tissue factor with a glycosyl-phosphatidyl-inositol (GPI) anchor or the transmembrane domain of a heterologous protein possess procoagulant activity (153, 154). A combination of neutral and acidic phospholipids (e.g., 70% phosphatidylcholine and 30% phosphatidylserine) is required when purified phospholipids are used for relipidation of the apoprotein (109). The inclusion of phosphatidylethanolamine dramatically reduces the concentration of phosphatidylserine needed to restore maximal functional activity (155).

## CELL BIOLOGY

Immunohistochemical studies for tissue factor protein and *in situ* hybridization studies for tissue factor mRNA have demonstrated the cellular expression of tissue factor is selective. Cells typically in contact with plasma (e.g., blood cells and endothelium of vessels) are devoid of tissue factor under normal circumstances, whereas prominent tissue factor expression is found in the vascular adventitia, astroglia, organ capsules, and epithelium of the skin, mucosa, bronchus, and glomeruli (156–161). Tissue factor expression by endometrial stromal cells is hormonally regulated (162, 163). The central nervous system, lungs, and placenta contain relatively large amounts of tissue factor. Certain neoplasms directly express tissue factor; others induce tissue factor expression

by cells in the surrounding tissues (164, 165). The metastatic potential of some tumor cells is related to tissue factor expression (166, 167). Expression of tissue factor by vascular smooth muscle cells is rapidly induced by growth factors and thrombin *in vitro* and by vascular injury *in vivo* (168–170). In addition, tissue factor presumably derived from macrophages or smooth muscle cells has been identified in atherosclerotic plaques (156, 157, 171), which suggests a role for tissue factor in the progression or thrombotic complications of atherosclerotic cardiovascular disease.

With the exception of blood cells and endothelial cells, most cells constitutively produce detectable tissue factor when they are grown in tissue culture. In fibroblasts, stimulation by serum, TGFβ$_1$ EGF, FGF, or PDGF produces the rapid but transient appearance of tissue factor mRNA (118, 138, 172). Its activation by growth factors and superinduction in the presence of cycloheximide, an inhibitor of protein synthesis, led to the inclu-

**TABLE 4.1.** Expression of Tissue Factor in Monocytes or Endothelial Cells *in vitro*

| | References | | References |
|---|---|---|---|
| **Induction** | | **Enhancement** | |
| Endotoxin | 422, 423 | T-lymphocyte collaboration | 471–474 |
| Interleukin-1 | 424, 425 | Platelets | 475 |
| Interleukin-2 | 425 | Platelet-activating factor | 476 |
| Tumor necrosis factor | 426, 427 | CD11/CD18 receptor occupancy | 477 |
| Interferon-γ | 428 | Inhibitors of calmodulin/protein | |
| Thrombin | 429 | kinase C | 478 |
| Phorbol ester | 430, 431 | High glucose concentrations | 479 |
| Adherence | 432 | Apoptosis | 212 |
| Infections and phagocytes | 433–441 | Hemoglobin | 480 |
| Activated complement | 442, 443 | Mercury compounds | 481 |
| Immune complexes | 444, 445 | Monocyte/endothelial cell coculture | 482 |
| Anti-cardiolipin antibodies, | 446, 447 | Mechanical strain | 483 |
| anti-phospholipid sera | | | |
| Allogeneic stimulation | 448, 449 | **Inhibition** | |
| C-reactive protein | 450 | Glucocorticoids | 484 |
| Cholesterol | 451 | Dipyridamole | 203, 204 |
| Native and modified lipoproteins | 452–454 | Iloprost/prostaglandin E$_1$ | 205, 206 |
| Oxidizing conditions | 455 | Pentoxifyllin | 207 |
| Oxygen free radicals | 456 | Retinoic acid | 201, 202 |
| Modified albumin | 457 | Polyunsaturated fatty acids | 485 |
| Advanced glycosylation end products | 458 | K+ channel blockers | 486 |
| Monocyte chemoattractant protein 1 | 459 | Interleukin-4 | 487 |
| Platelet-derived growth factor | 459 | Interleukin-10 | 199, 487 |
| Vascular endothelial cell growth factor | 460, 461 | Interleukin-13 | 487 |
| P-Selectin | 462 | | |
| Engagement of β1 or α4 integrin chains | 463 | | |
| Cytotoxic agents | 464–466 | | |
| Tumor cell exposure | 467–468 | | |
| Humic acid | 469 | | |
| Tuftsin | 470 | | |

sion of the tissue factor gene in a family of "immediate-early" genes, the products of which are althought to mediate the growth response (173). That tissue factor expression has been detected in a variety of developing tissues during early embryogenesis is perhaps consistent with this notion (174). Recent studies suggest a role for tissue factor in processes unrelated to coagulation, such as transmembrane signaling (175–177), tumor growth and angiogenesis (178), embryonic vasculogenesis (179), and cancer metastasis (166).

Monocytes and endothelial cells express tissue factor *in vitro* by physiologically relevant agents, many of which are associated with the inflammatory response (Table 4.1). Thus, it is tempting to speculate that the local coagulation and propensity for systemic thrombosis that accompany many diseases are due to the aberrant production of tissue factor by these cells, which are normally not thrombogenic. Indirect evidence supports such a role for monocyte-generated tissue factor. Increased levels of tissue factor have been detected *ex vivo* in peripheral blood monocytes (at the time of their isolation or following *in vitro* incubation) in a variety of pathologic states. Enhanced tissue factor generation has been described in tissue macrophages isolated from diseased organs (Table 4.2). The demonstration of tissue factor expression by endothelial cells *in vivo* has been more difficult (159, 180), but endothelial tissue factor expression has been detected in splenic capillaries in a baboon model of septic shock, in the microvasculature of tumors, in the placenta, and at inflammatory sites (181–187). Perhaps the best evidence for a direct link between the induction of tissue factor expression and pathologic coagulation *in vivo* is the ability of anti-tissue factor antibodies to ameliorate the disseminated intravascular coagulation that develops following Escherichia coli infusion in baboons and endotoxin infusion in rabbits and chimpanzees (188–190).

The expression of tissue factor by stimulated monocytes and endothelial cells requires mRNA and protein synthesis. Following induction, tissue factor mRNA appears early, peaks at 1 to 2 hours, and returns to baseline by 6 hours. Tissue factor activity is detectable in 1 to 2 hours, peaks at 4 to 10 hours, and returns to baseline by 20 to 30 hours. Protein kinase C and perhaps protein tyrosine kinase are involved in the response of monocytes and endothelial cells to LPS, PMA, and cytokines (191–194). In the activation process, pre-existing cytoplasmic NFκB-Rel complexes dissociate from the inhibitor protein IκBα, the IκBα is proteolytically degraded, and the transcription factors translocate to the nucleus and initiate the expression of target genes. Proteinase inhibitors, pyrrolidine dithiocarbamate, and salicylates (including aspirin), which block the proteolysis of IκBα, inhibit LPS and cytokine induction of tissue factor expression (195–197). Interleukin-4 (IL-4), IL-10,

**TABLE 4.2.** Monocyte/Macrophage Generation of Tissue Factor *in vivo* and *ex vivo*

| | References |
|---|---|
| **Peripheral blood monocytes** | |
| Inflammatory diseases | 488, 489 |
|    Inflammatory bowel disease | 490, 491 |
|    Systemic lupus erythematosus | 492, 493 |
| Infections | 494, 495 |
| Shwartzman reaction | 496 |
| Trauma and surgery | 497–500 |
| Coronary artery disease | 501 |
| Diabetes mellitus | 502 |
| Cancer | 503–506 |
| Renal transplant rejection | 507–509 |
| Parenteral nutrition solutions | 510, 511 |
| OKT3 monoclonal antibody | 512 |
| **Tissue macrophages** | |
| Spleen | |
|    Systemic lupus erythematosus | 513 |
|    Atherogenic diet | 514 |
| Kidney | |
|    Transplant rejection | 515, 516 |
|    Glomerulonephritis | 517–519 |
| Neoplastic tissue | 520 |
| Endocarditis | 521 |
| Atheromatous plaques | 522, 523 |
| Bronchoalveolar lavage fluid | |
|    Sarcoidosis | 524 |
|    Granulomatous pneumonitis | 525 |
|    Respiratory distress syndrome | 526, 527 |
|    Cancer | 528 |
|    Asbestos exposure | 529 |
|    Ozone | 530 |

IL-13, retinoic acid, and agents that increase intracellular cyclic adenosine monophosphate (cAMP) levels (e.g., dipyridamole, Iloprost, pentoxifylline) also suppress the cellular expression of tissue factor (189, 198–208).

Tissue factor activity measured after the lysis of cells is consistently more than the activity detectable on the surface of the cells when they are intact. Agents that perturb the cell membrane or induce the shedding of membrane vesicles also increase tissue factor activity (209–215). Although intracellular stores of tissue factor have been detected in certain cells (216, 217), in most cells this process represents the activation of previously surface exposed, encrypted tissue factor. Studies using cultured fibroblasts or carcinoma cells and stimulated monocytes or endothelial cells have shown more than 90% of the total tissue factor antigen in these cells is present at their surface and binds factor VIIa. However, the measurable tissue factor activity does not reflect the extent of factor VIIa/tissue factor binding and is increased more than fivefold when the cells are lysed or further stimulated with a calcium ionophore (218–220). The mechanism(s) by which these manipulations enhance factor VIIa/tissue factor catalytic activity is not certain but may involve the redistribution of acidic phospholipids from the inner leaflet of the plasma membrane to the surface with a change in the phospholipid milieu surrounding the tissue factor apoprotein (221). Alternative explanations and a combination of effects are certainly possible (222–224).

The surface distribution of tissue factor differs between cells, and this apical versus basal-lateral sorting of the tissue factor molecule does not require the presence of its cytoplasmic domain (225). Downregulation of endothelial cell surface factor VIIa/tissue factor activity occurs through the formation of a factor Xa-TFPI-factor VIIa/tissue factor complex (see below) and the translocation of the complex into caveolae (226). An additional, GP I-anchored moiety that may represent the surface binding site for TFPI is also involved in the process.

That human tissue factor deficiency has not been reported is consistent with the observation that tissue factor gene deletion in mice produces intrauterine lethality with more than 85% of the TF($-$/$-$) mice dying during mid-gestation (embryonic day E9.5–11.5) (181, 227, 228). A loss of vascular integrity within the extraembryonic vasculature precipitates the lethal outcome, but whether the defect is due to the lack of tissue factor's procoagulant function or some other function of tissue factor is uncertain.

# FACTOR VIIa-TISSUE FACTOR COMPLEX

Factor VII and factor VIIa bind to tissue factor with 1:1 stoichiometry. This binding is dependent on calcium ions and is mediated predominantly through an interaction between factor VII(a) and the apoprotein portion of tissue factor. Although a wide range of dissociation constants has been reported for the factor VIIa-tissue factor interaction, there is general agreement that the binding is of very high affinity ($K_d < 1$ nM). The binding of zymogen factor VII may be modestly less avid than that of factor VIIa (approximately fivefold) (43, 49, 229). The affinity of factor VIIa for tissue factor is enhanced by its macromolecular substrate, factor X, (230) or the covalent attachment of a small molecular weight peptidyl substrate (e.g., dansyl-glu-gly-arg chloromethyl ketone treatment) (43). Positive cooperation has been described in some (48, 229, 231, 232) studies investigating the binding of factor VIIa to tissue factor. Thus, the binding process may involve the association of factor VIIa with dimeric or multimeric complexes of tissue factor apoprotein. Crosslinking studies of cell surface tissue factor are consistent with this notion and suggest the transmembrane portion of tissue factor is necessary for interaction between tissue factor molecules (156, 223).

Crystallographic analysis of factor VIIa bound to the extracellular domain of tissue factor shows an elongated shape of the complex and intertwining of the molecules in an anti-parallel orientation (38). An extensive area of contact between factor VIIa and tissue factor can be divided into three major regions: 1) interaction between the hydrophobic stack of factor VIIa and the carboxyterminal fibronectin III domain of tissue factor near the presumed membrane surface; 2) interaction between the EGF-1 domain of factor VII and portions of fibronectin III domains at the "elbow" region of tissue factor; and 3) interaction between the EGF-2 and catalytic domains of factor VIIa and the top of the aminoterminal fibronectin III domain of tissue factor. The residues in factor VIIa and tissue factor found in these regions of contact correlate well with previous studies that used mutational analysis and other methods to investigate the factor VIIa-tissue factor interaction (38, 222, 233). The active site of factor VIIa in the complex has been estimated to be approximately 80 Ångstroms above the membrane surface (38, 234).

The binding of factor VIIa to tissue factor enhances its proteolytic activity toward the physiologic substrates, factors IX and X, several thousandfold (235). This dramatic effect is mediated by two mechanisms: 1) tissue factor binding allosterically alters the active site of factor VIIa thereby increasing its intrinsic catalytic activity 20- to 100-fold (as measured by small molecular weight substrates) (43, 236–238); and 2) factor VIIa/tissue factor complexation enhances the assembly of macromolecular substrate. The phospholipid membrane (232, 239, 240), an epitope on tissue factor that involves Lys165 and Lys166 (241, 242), and the Gla domain of factor VIIa contribute to this effect on substrate recognition (243).

Factor IX and factor X compete for the factor VIIa/tissue factor catalytic complex (244). Most investigators have found that factor X is the preferred substrate *in vitro*, but whether the same is true *in vivo* is unknown. The catalytic efficiency of factor X activation by factor VIIa in the presence of tissue factor and calcium ions is more than 1000-fold greater than that by factor VIIa in the presence of procoagulant phospholipids and calcium ions (235). The inefficient activation of factor X by factor VIIa with phospholipids and calcium ions alone, however, appears to account for the shortening in the plasma-activated PTT (aPTT) seen following the infusion of high doses of factor VIIa (245, 246). The *in vivo* procoagulant effect of factor VIIa treatment is tissue factor-dependent and thus may involve the exchange of factor VIIa for factor VII at tissue factor binding sites (69, 247–249). Although the factor VIIa/tissue factor complex is a potent activator of factor X, it is kinetically much less efficient than the alternative pathway for factor X activation that involves factor VIIIa and factor IXa (250).

The interaction between factor VII and tissue factor demonstrates considerable species specificity. Whereas human tissue factor induces coagulation in rodent plasmas, the tissue factors from mice, guinea pigs, rats, and hamsters possess little procoagulant activity in human plasma (251, 252). Further, human tissue factor interacts poorly with bovine factor VII, and the coagulation of human plasma induced by bovine tissue factor (as opposed to human tissue factor) is more sensitive to the level of factor VIIa (253, 254). Certain abnormal forms of factor VII interact with the tissue factor from different species in a distinctive fashion (255–257). The activities of factor VII$_{Padua}$(Arg$_{304}$→Gln) and factor VII$_{Nagoya}$ (Arg$_{304}$→Trp) are least with rabbit tissue factor (<10%), intermediate with human tissue factor, and near normal with bovine tissue factor (50, 255).

In contrast to its marginal inhibition of free factor VIIa, antithrombin III inactivates factor VIIa bound to tissue factor in the presence of heparin (258, 259). This inhibitory effect is most apparent when factor VIIa is limiting in the reaction (i.e., all VIIa bound to tissue factor). The decrease in factor VIIa/tissue factor-mediated activation of factor X produced by antithrombin/heparin is modest under presumably more physiologic conditions in which factor VII(a) is in excess and tissue factor limiting (260, 261). The modest decrease is due to the exchange of free factor VII(a) with factor VIIa-antithrombin III complexes at tissue factor binding sites (262). A potentially more important effect of antithrombin III/heparin on tissue factor initiated coagulation is the suppression of feedback activation of factor VII by factors Xa, IXa, and thrombin (260, 261, 263). The procoagulant activity of factor VIIa and tissue factor is also inhibited *in vitro* by sphingosine, apolipoprotein AII, and C-reactive protein, which interfere with the binding of factor VIIa to tissue factor (264–266), and by members of the annexin family of proteins, which bind in a calcium-dependent manner to acidic phospholipids in the lipid portion of the tissue factor lipoprotein (267, 268). It has not been proven, however, that any of these agents serve to modulate the induction of coagulation by tissue factor *in vivo*.

# TISSUE FACTOR PATHWAY INHIBITOR

The work of Loeb et al (269, 270) first suggested serum contained a moiety that inhibits the procoagulant activity of tissue extracts in 1922. Later, Thomas (271) and Schneider (272) independently demonstrated the *in vivo* correlate of this observation by showing that the preincubation of tissue thromboplastin with serum prevented its lethal effect when infused into animals. Thomas (271) also noted the following: the inhibitory effect of serum required calcium ions, the inhibitor appeared to bind to thromboplastin, and the effect could be reversed by calcium ion chelators.

Hjort (273) reported in 1957 that the previously described serum inhibitor of thromboplastin recognized the factor VIIa-Ca$^{2+}$-tissue factor complex, which he termed convertin, rather than factor VII (proconvertin) or thromboplastin alone. He ascribed the calcium dependence and reversibility of the inhibition by calcium chelation to the requirement for convertin formation and suggested through indirect means that the binding of the inhibitor to convertin was also calcium ion-dependent. Approximately at the same time, Biggs et al (274, 275) reported that coagulation was delayed and incomplete following the addition of low concentrations of tissue factor to hemophiliac plasma. The possible connection between this observation and the previously described thromboplastin inhibitor was not explored further because of the advent of the intrinsic pathway of coagulation (7, 8).

Nearly 25 years later, Carson (276) reported that plasma lipoproteins inhibited the catalytic activity of the factor VIIa-tissue factor complex. Carson showed this inhibitory activity was contained in the protein component of the lipoprotein, particularly in high-density lipoproteins (HDL). Near the same time, Dahl et al (277) demonstrated that the anticonvertin activity of Hjort eluted as two high-molecular-weight peaks following the gel filtration of plasma. Marlar et al (278), extending the work of Biggs (274, 275), showed that much less factor X was activated in hemophiliac plasma than in normal plasma when coagulation was induced by small amounts of tissue factor. Subsequently, Morrison and Jesty (279) reported the activation of factor IX and factor X in normal plasma was also incomplete following the addition of tissue factor and this apparent inhibition of factor VIIa-tissue factor enzymatic activity was directly related to factor X or brief pretreatment of plasma with factor Xa. Finally, Sanders et al (280) documented factor X and an inhibitor present in the total lipoprotein fraction of plasma following density centrifugation was required for this apparent inhibition of tissue factor-mediated coagulation.

Additional studies confirmed the work of Sanders et al (280) and showed the inhibition of factor VIIa-tissue factor is reversed by chelation of calcium ions, which releases functionally active factor VIIa and tissue factor (281–283). Thus, the rediscovered inhibitor appears to be identical to the one originally characterized by Thomas (271) and Hjort (273).

Factor Xa was shown to be the specific cofactor required for the optimal effect of the inhibitor on the factor VIIa-tissue factor complex; active site-inhibited factor Xa was without effect (282–284). With the subsequent isolation of TFPI, it was discovered that TFPI inhibited factor VIIa-tissue factor complex in a factor Xa-dependent fashion and directly inactivated factor Xa (13). Thus, in retrospect, the same inhibitor may have been the subject of previous studies describing a fast-acting factor Xa inhibitor that is carried by the plasma lipoproteins (285) and the plasma concentration of which increases following the *in vivo* administration of a heparin analog (286).

The inhibitor was initially purified from the conditioned media of HepG2 (human hepatoma) cells (287, 288) using factor Xa affinity chromatography, and later TFPI from human plasma (289, 290) was also isolated. cDNAs for human (291, 292), rhesus monkey (293), canine (294), rabbit (295, 296), and rat (297) TFPI have been isolated and cloned, and the organization of the human TFPI gene has been determined (298, 299).

This inhibitor has been called antithromboplastin (272), anticonvertin (273), the factor Xa-dependent factor VIIa-tissue factor inhibitor, tissue factor inhibitor (287), extrinsic pathway inhibitor (283), and lipoprotein-associated coagulation inhibitor (288) because of its many attributes. In 1991, a subcommittee of the Scientific and Standardization Committee of the International Society on Thrombosis and Haemostasis proposed the currently used name, which is TFPI.

## MOLECULAR BIOLOGY

The TFPI gene spans approximately 70 kb on the long arm of chromosome 2 (q32) and contains nine exons and eight introns (298–300). Exons 1 and 2 encode a 5' untranslated region, and exon 3 encodes the signal peptide, which is removed during processing of the protein, and the aminoterminus of the mature TFPI. The TFPI molecule contains three tandem Kunitz-type proteinase inhibitor domains that are encoded by separate exons (4, 6, and 8). The intervening peptides between Kunitz domains are encoded by exons 5 and 7 (Fig. 4.3). The carboxyterminus of the TFPI protein and an extensive 3' untranslated region are encoded by exon 9. All the splice junctions between exons are of the same type (type 1), which suggests that the TFPI gene was assembled during evolution through a process of gene duplication and exon shuffling. A Pst I RFLP has been described in the TFPI gene (301).

The putative promoter region of the TFPI gene contains one NF1 sequence and two imperfect AP1 sequences. AP1 binding sites have been shown to act as phorbol ester-responsive elements in several other genes (302), and the induction of TFPI expression in cultured monocytic cells (U937) following phorbol myristate acetate treatment has been reported (303). A GATA consensus element lies approximately 400 bp upstream of the transcription initiation sites (304). This DNA motif appears essential for the expression of certain genes by erythroid, megakaryocytic, and endothelial cells. The 5' flanking region of the gene, however, does not contain a TATA box or CAAT sequence, which may account for the use of multiple, alternative transcriptional start sites (298, 299). Alternative splicing of the short exon 2 in the 5' untranslated region of the TFPI message occurs, but its significance is uncertain. Cells that constitutively express TFPI produce TFPI mRNA of two sizes, which are 1.4 and 4.0 kb, that arise through the use of alternative polyadenylation signals (292). The 3' untranslated region of the 4.0 kb message contains many AUUU motifs and two UAAUUUAU sequences, which have been associated with mRNA instability in other messages. Preliminary evidence, however, suggests that both the 1.4 and 4.0 kb TFPI mRNAs are relatively stable (292).

## BIOCHEMISTRY

The primary structure of TFPI, as predicted by cDNA sequencing, is unique (291, 292). After a 24 or 28 amino acid signal peptide, the mature protein has 276 residues (32 Kda) and contains an acidic aminoterminal region followed by three tandem Kunitz-type protease inhibitory domains and a basic carboxyterminal region (see Fig. 4.3). The molecule contains N-linked carbohydrate at $Asn_{117}$ and $Asn_{167}$ and O-linked carbohydrate at $Ser_{174}$ and $Thr_{175}$ (305). The oligosaccharides in TFPI expressed by certain cells *in vitro* (e.g., endothelial and kidney cells) are sulfated (306–308). $Ser_2$ is partially phosphorylated in the TFPI expressed by some cells in tissue culture, but similar phosphorylation has not been detected in TFPI circulating in plasma (309). These post-translational modifications do not appear to affect the known functional properties of TFPI (309–311).

Kunitz-type inhibitors appear to act by the standard mechanism (312) in which the inhibitor feigns to be a good substrate, but, after the enzyme binds, the subsequent cleavage between the $P_1$ and $P_1'$ amino acid residues at the active site cleft of the inhibitor occurs slowly or not at all. The $P_1$ residue is an important determinant of the specificity of these inhibitors, and alterations of the residue in the $P_1$ position can profoundly affect their inhibitory activity. In kinetic terms, Kunitz-type inhibitors typically produce slow, tight-binding, competitive, and reversible enzyme inhibition. "Slow" implies that the final degree of inhibition does not occur immediately, and "tight-binding" refers to the inhibition produced at concentrations near that of the enzyme being inhibited. The known structure of the prototype Kunitz-type inhibitor, bovine basic pancreatic trypsin inhibitor (i.e., aprotinin, Trasylol), and its interaction with trypsin, disulfide bonds, active site cleft, and residues, which are predicted to be in close contact with the catalytic domain in a target

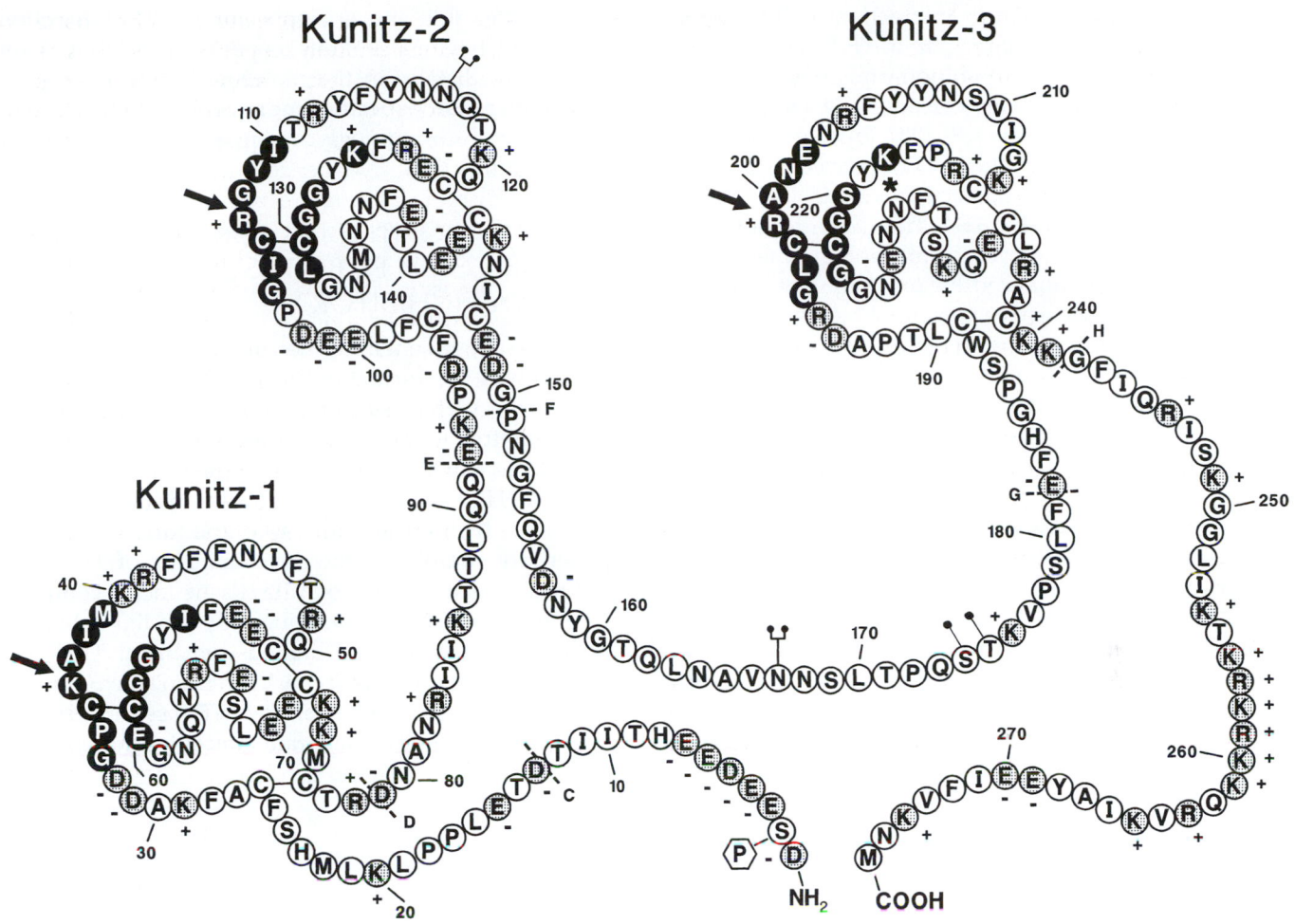

**FIGURE 4.3.**    Structures of tissue factor pathway inhibitor (TFPI). The three Kunitz-type inhibitory domains of TFPI are labeled, and arrows indicate the location of the respective active-site inhibitory clefts ($P_1$-$P_1'$). Based on the structure of the bovine pancreatic trypsin inhibitor-trypsin complex, the residues in each TFPI Kunitz-type domain, which are predicted to be in close contact with the catalytic domains of target proteinases, are shown in bold. Charged residues are stippled. N-linked glycosylation is denoted as ⚡; O-linked glycosylation as ❯; a site for potential N-linked glycosylation in the Kunitz 3 that is apparently not used is labeled with an *. Potential phosphorylation at $Ser_2$ is also shown. Sites of introns in the TFPI gene are labeled with capital letters.

protease, is depicted in Fig. 4.3 for each of the three Kunitz modules of the TFPI molecule (313).

Experiments in which the $P_1$ residue of each Kunitz domain in TFPI was individually altered have shown that the second Kunitz domain of TFPI mediates factor Xa binding and inhibition, whereas the first Kunitz domain is necessary for the inhibition of the factor VIIa-tissue factor complex (314). Alteration of the $P_1$ residue in the third Kunitz domain does not affect either of these functions of TFPI. Studies examining the inhibitory properties of the isolated Kunitz domains of TFPI have reached the same conclusions (315). The Kunitz-3 domain appears to lack proteinase inhibitory activity (315), and the physiologic role of this domain is unknown. TFPI also inhibits trypsin and chymotrypsin reasonably well and inhibits cathepsin G, plasmin, and activated

protein C poorly (315–317); the physiologic significance of these inhibitory reactions is doubtful.

## INHIBITION OF FACTOR Xa BY TISSUE FACTOR PATHWAY INHIBITOR

TFPI inhibits the factor VIIa-tissue factor enzymatic complex in a factor Xa-dependent manner, and it produces direct inhibition of factor Xa by binding at or near its serine active site (13). The factor Xa-TFPI complex demonstrates 1:1 stoichiometry, and its formation does not require calcium ions. The factor Xa-TFPI interaction is reversed by treatment with SDS or high concentrations of the serine protease inhibitor benzamidine, which binds to the active site of factor Xa (13, 288).

Other parts of the TFPI molecule besides the Kunitz-

2 domain are involved in its interaction with factor Xa. The basic carboxyterminal region of TFPI is required for rapid, efficient factor Xa inhibition, and carboxyterminal truncated forms of TFPI are considerably less potent inhibitors of factor Xa (315, 318–320). Further, neutrophil elastase–mediated cleavage of TFPI between Kunitz domains 1 and 2 dramatically reduces the ability of TFPI to inhibit factor Xa (317, 321). The inhibition of factor Xa by TFPI in the presence of physiologic calcium ion concentrations is enhanced by procoagulant phospholipids (322), and the carboxyterminal region of the TFPI molecule is important for this effect (319, 320). Physiologic concentrations of TFPI, however, do not effectively inhibit prothrombin activation by factor Xa in a preformed prothrombinase complex (323, 324).

Heparin and other polyanions accelerate TFPI-mediated inhibition of factor Xa (319). The heparin dose–response for this effect exhibits an optima, which suggests that the polyanion forms a template to which factor Xa and TFPI simultaneously bind (319, 322). Basic residues within the carboxyterminal region of TFPI are required for optimal heparin binding, and progressive carboxyterminal truncation of the TFPI molecule produces proteins with decreasing affinity for heparin (319). The Kunitz-3 domain contains a heparin binding site(s),

but whether this site is important for TFPI function above and beyond separate heparin binding sites located more distally in the molecule is uncertain (319, 325). Rather than a specific binding epitope, charge density on the glycosaminoglycan appears to be crucial for TFPI binding (326).

## INHIBITION OF THE FACTOR VIIa-TISSUE FACTOR COMPLEX BY TISSUE FACTOR PATHWAY INHIBITOR

Factor Xa-dependent inhibition of factor VIIa/tissue factor involves the formation of a quaternary factor Xa-TFPI-factor VIIa/tissue factor complex (Fig. 4.4) (13). This inhibitory complex can result from the initial binding of factor Xa to TFPI with subsequent binding of the factor Xa-TFPI complex to factor VIIa/tissue factor. An alternative theoretical pathway to the formation of the quaternary complex is the direct binding of TFPI to a preformed factor Xa-factor VIIa/tissue factor complex. A chimeric molecule containing only the light chain of factor Xa linked to the Kunitz-1 domain of TFPI is a potent direct inhibitor of factor VIIa/tissue factor, which suggests the binding of factor Xa to TFPI serves to juxtapose these domains on separate molecules thereby pro-

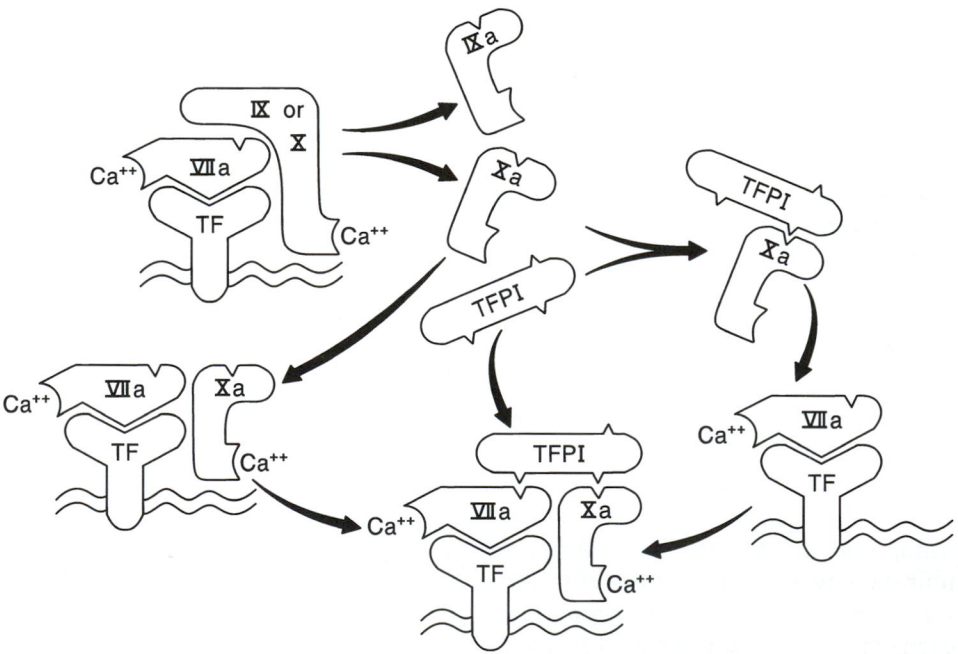

**FIGURE 4.4.** Proposed mechanism for the inhibition of factor Xa and the factor VIIa-tissue factor (TF) complex by tissue factor pathway inhibitor (TFPI). The indentations represent the active sites of factor VIIa and factor Xa; the protrusions represent the three Kunitz-type domains of TFPI. In the factor Xa-TFPI complex, the active site of factor Xa is bound to the second Kunitz domain of TFPI. In the final quaternary factor Xa-TFPI-factor VIIa-tissue factor complex, factor Xa is bound at its active site to the second Kunitz domain of TFPI and factor VIIa is bound at its active site to the first Kunitz domain of TFPI. Two potential pathways for the formation of the final quaternary inhibitory complex are depicted: on the left, TFPI binds to a preformed factor Xa-factor VIIa-tissue factor complex; on the right, TFPI binds to factor Xa and the factor Xa-TFPI complex then binds to factor VIIa-tissue factor.

ducing a complex that binds the factor VIIa/tissue factor complex with high affinity (327). The Gla domain of factor Xa and $Lys_{165}$-$Lys_{166}$ of tissue factor, which are structures required for the optimal recognition of factor X by factor VIIa/tissue factor, are also important for the inhibition of factor VIIa/tissue factor by factor Xa-TFPI (13, 328, 329). Studies of the effects of heparin on factor Xa-dependent factor VIIa/tissue factor inhibition by TFPI have produced conflicting results (330, 331).

Some researchers report the inhibition of factor X activation by factor VIIa/tissue factor is more rapid (10-fold) with full-length TFPI than carboxyterminal truncated forms of TFPI and relate this difference to the relative rates at which the TFPI forms bind factor Xa (320). Other researchers have found full-length and carboxy-truncated TFPI to produce comparable rates of factor VIIa/tissue factor inhibition (331, 332). The ultimate affinity of the quaternary inhibitory complex formed with full-length TFPI, however, is greater than that of complexes formed with truncated TFPI; the latter inhibitory complexes dissociate more rapidly (332, 333). The anticoagulant effect of exogenously added full-length TFPI is considerably more than that of carboxy-truncated TFPI in one stage plasma coagulation assays (318, 319, 334). The disparity in anticoagulant effect between the TFPI forms reflects their ability to inhibit factor Xa when plasma coagulation is induced by factor Xa or the factor X-coagulant protein (XCP) from Russels Viper venom. The difference seen when tissue factor is used to induce coagulation (PT) presumably represents the combination of anti-factor Xa and anti-factor VIIa/tissue factor activities.

The requirement of factor Xa for the inhibition of factor VIIa/tissue factor by TFPI is not absolute, and high concentrations of TFPI will inhibit factor VIIa/tissue factor without factor Xa (315, 335–337). This factor Xa-independent inhibition of factor VIIa/tissue factor by TFPI is of uncertain physiologic relevance but could be important when TFPI is used as a therapeutic agent and plasma levels of TFPI are more than 50-fold that of normal plasma (338–340).

## CELL BIOLOGY AND CATABOLISM

The endothelium is presumed to be the major source of TFPI *in vivo*. Immunohistochemic studies of normal tissues have detected TFPI in the endothelium of the microvasculature, megakaryocytes, macrophages, and the microglia of the brain (341, 342). A range of TFPI mRNA levels are detected through Northern analysis of tissues; mRNA levels are highest in the placenta and lung and lowest in the brain (343). Cell lines derived from a wide variety of tissues synthesize TFPI in tissue culture. The production of TFPI by these cells in tissue culture, however, may not reflect sites of TFPI expression *in vivo*. For example, several hepatoma cell lines

express TFPI in culture, yet TFPI is not detected in hepatocytes in primary culture or by immunohistochemic staining of liver sections (341, 344).

Cultured endothelial cells and adherent monocytes and macrophages express TFPI. A significant fraction of TFPI in cultured endothelial cells and adherent monocytes appears to remain membrane-associated (303, 344–346). A recent report suggests TFPI is stored in granules distinct from Weibel-Palade bodies in cultured endothelial cells, is redistributed to the cell surface, and is released into the media following thrombin treatment (347). Other researchers report that more than 90% of the cell-associated TFPI in an endothelial cell line stimulated with tissue necrosis factor is on the cell surface (226). Heparin and thrombin treatment increases the release of TFPI from cells in culture (347, 348). Whereas the stimulation of endothelial cells and adherent monocytes with inflammatory mediators induces a dramatic induction of tissue factor synthesis, such treatment produces minimal changes in TFPI expression (304, 349). Megakaryocytes synthesize TFPI and the TFPI carried by circulating blood platelets is released following their stimulation with thrombin or other agonists (350).

Following its infusion in animals, full-length TFPI is cleared rapidly from plasma ($\alpha$-phase $t\frac{1}{2}$ ~ 2 minutes; $\beta$-phase $t\frac{1}{2}$ ~ 80 minutes) and predominantly taken up by the liver and kidney (351, 352). At least two separate processes contribute to this phenomenon: 1) reversible binding of TFPI at cell surfaces (presumably the endothelium *in vivo*); and 2) cellular endocytosis and degradation of TFPI mediated by the low-density lipoproteins (LDL) receptor-related protein/$a_2$-macroglobulin receptor (LRP).

TFPI binds to a wide variety of cells *in vitro*. Most of this binding is mediated by low affinity sites that require the basic carboxyterminus of TFPI for binding and whose interaction with TFPI is inhibited by heparin or protamine (336, 353–355). Whether these TFPI binding sites involve phospholipids (356), heparan sulfate glycosaminoglycans (357), specific cell surface proteins, or a combination of these elements has not been established. Nevertheless, the characteristics of the cell surface TFPI binding *in vitro* may explain the following: the markedly lower recovery of full-length versus carboxyterminal truncated forms of TFPI following their infusion in animals and the inhibition of full-length TFPI clearance produced by concomitant heparin or protamine infusion (352, 358, 359).

LRP functions as an endocytosis receptor for TFPI and several other proteins, including $\alpha_2$-macroglolin-protease complexes, free plasminogen activators and plasminogen activators complexed with their inhibitors, lipoprotein lipase, and $\beta$-migrating very low density lipoproteins enriched with apolipoprotein-E (353–355, 360). A 39 Kda protein that copurifies with LRP (i.e., receptor-associated protein [RAP]) competes with all known LRP ligands for binding. LRP is particularly abundant in the liver, brain, and placenta. A closely related receptor, glycoprotein 330, that binds many of the same ligands is produced predominantly in the kidney (360, 361). In mice, the combination of high levels of protamine to prevent presumed cell surface binding at the endothelium and high levels of the 39 Kda protein to inhibit LRP-mediated endocytosis dramatically slows the clearance of infused TFPI from plasma (359).

An additional pathway for the endocytosis and degradation of TFPI has been recently identified (362). *In vitro* studies show that the uptake and degradation of factor Xa by hepatoma cells and embryonic fibroblasts requires cell surface TFPI, and, further, the uptake and degradation of surface bound TFPI is also markedly stimulated in response to factor Xa binding. The cellular kinetics of factor Xa and TFPI internalization and degradation are similar, which suggests factor Xa and surface bound TFPI are taken up as a bimolecular complex. This TFPI-factor Xa endocytic pathway is independent of LRP and does not require tissue factor. Indirect studies in rabbits suggest a similar process is operational *in vivo* because the clearance of heparin releasable, presumably endothelial cell–surface bound, TFPI-factor Xa complexes is faster than that of TFPI alone (363).

TFPI also appears to participate in the down-regulation of factor VIIa/tissue factor complexes at the surface of stimulated endothelial cells (226). This process requires the formation of the quaternary factor Xa-TFPI-factor VIIa/tissue factor inhibitory complex and involves translocation of the complex into caveolae. Differential detergent solubility and the effect of phosphotidylinositol-specific phospholipase C suggest that a GP I-anchored membrane protein, which may represent a cell surface TFPI binding site, is involved in the internalization mechanism. The effect of staurosporine, which inhibits the phosphorylation of the cytoplasmic domain of tissue factor and blocks down-regulation of tissue factor in stimulated monocytes, on this translocation process in endothelial cells has not been tested (364). The relationship between this pathway and the factor Xa-TFPI degradation pathway described above is not certain.

## PHYSIOLOGY

There is a broad range of plasma TFPI concentrations in normal individuals (mean ~ 2.5 nM or ~100 ng/ml) (365–367). Much of the circulating TFPI is bound to lipoproteins (284, 289, 368). Plasma concentrations of TFPI correlate with LDL levels because LDL is a major carrier; plasma concentrations increase with diet-induced hypercholesterolemia in animals and decrease in response to drug therapy in individuals with familial hypercholesterolemia (369–373). Individuals with abetalipopro-

teinemia who lack LDL have low levels of TFPI in plasma (366).

Predominant forms of TFPI in plasma have molecular weights of 34 and 41 Kda, and less abundant forms of higher molecular mass are also present (289, 374, 375). The size heterogeneity of plasma TFPI reflects, in part, the carboxyterminal truncation of the molecule and the formation of mixed disulfide complexes with apolipoprotein-AII and potentially other proteins (374, 375). The major form of TFPI bound to LDL has a molecular weight of 34 Kda and lacks the distal portion of full-length TFPI, including at least a large portion of the Kunitz-3 domain. The 41 Kda form of TFPI that circulates with HDL is a similar carboxy-truncated form of TFPI that is disulfide-linked to monomeric apolipoprotein-AII. Additional forms with less extensive carboxyterminal truncation and full-length TFPI (43 Kda) also circulate in plasma. The mechanism underlying the association of the 34 Kda carboxy-truncated form of TFPI with LDL has not been determined. Proteolytic processing by as yet unidentified proteinases is likely responsible for the circulating forms of TFPI with modest truncation of the carboxyterminal tail (334). Additional or alternative modifications may be involved in the production of the 34 Kda form of TFPI that is bound tightly in LDL. Oxidation of LDL *in vitro* reduces its associated TFPI activity (376).

Estimates of the proportion of total plasma TFPI that circulates "free" of lipoproteins range from 10 to 60% (290, 377, 378). The *in vitro* manipulations required to separate lipoprotein-bound TFPI from "free" TFPI (e.g., gel filtration, density gradient lipoprotein isolation) result in reduced recovery of "free" TFPI (358, 381) and, conversely, may separate loosely bound TFPI from the lipoproteins. A TFPI immunoassay based on an antibody against the Kunitz-3 domain, which does not recognize lipoprotein-bound TFPI (378), detected $19.2 \pm 4.0$ ng/ml of "free" TFPI in nine normal individuals (379). The concentration of full-length TFPI normally circulating in plasma has not been established.

The parenteral administration of heparin, low-molecular-weight heparin and other polyanions increases the circulating levels of TFPI in plasma (365, 366, 380). The source of this additional TFPI is presumed to be the endothelium. The mechanism(s) underlying the heparin-induced release phenomenon is unknown but may involve the displacement of TFPI from binding sites (perhaps glycosaminoglycans) at the endothelial cell surface. Following the intravenous infusion of a heparin bolus, the plasma TFPI level peaks at 3 to 5 minutes and then returns to the pretreatment level with a half-life that mirrors that of the administered heparin. Protamine treatment during this time causes the TFPI level to immediately return to the baseline level (380, 381). Heparin-releasable TFPI is not associated with lipoproteins.

Based on its molecular weight, tight-binding to heparin-agarose, and potent anticoagulant activity, heparin-releasable TFPI *is* althought to represent full-length or a near full-length form of TFPI (290). The extent of TFPI release decreases with repeated (every 4 hours) and continuous heparin infusion (379).

Quantitative assessment of the heparin-induced increase in plasma TFPI levels is hampered by discrepancies between the results of functional and antigenic assays (382). Two-stage (end-point) functional assays based on factor VIIa/tissue factor inhibition show a post-heparin increase in plasma TFPI levels of approximately two- to threefold, whereas antigen based assays typically suggest a considerably greater increase. This discrepancy may be because lipoprotein-bound and carboxyterminal truncated forms of TFPI are under-represented in antigen assays, whereas their contribution to factor VIIa/tissue factor inhibition is detected by functional assay. The substantial extra-plasma reservoir of TFPI defined by heparin-releasability is probably physiologically significant. Although individuals with abetalipoproteinemia have low baseline plasma levels of TFPI (<25% of normal), they have normal levels of heparin-releasable TFPI and do not have an increased risk of thrombosis (366). It is not known whether TFPI contributes to the antithrombotic effect of heparin therapy.

Plasma TFPI concentrations in normal individuals are stable, with little variation during the day, following meals, and over many months' time (367). TFPI levels slightly increase with age in adults, which likely reflects plasma lipoprotein levels (73, 367, 383); low levels are present in mid-gestation fetuses (~30%) and newborn infants (~55%) (384). Unlike levels of tissue plasminogen activator and von Willebrand factor, which are also synthesized by endothelial cells, TFPI levels in plasma are not increased by infusion of desmopressin (DDAVP) or venous occlusion (365–367). TFPI is not elevated in individuals with pneumonia and does not increase postoperatively, which suggests TFPI does not behave as an acute-phase reactant (367, 385–387). Increased levels of TFPI have been noted with advanced cancer (388), uremia, and regular hemodialysis (389) and in late pregnancy (366, 367, 390); decreased levels have been reported in thrombotic thrombocytopenic purpura (391). Levels of TFPI are normal in individuals with the lupus anticoagulant and those treated with warfarin (365–367). Although low levels of plasma TFPI are occasionally seen in septicemia and disseminated intravascular coagulation, more often the TFPI concentrations are normal or elevated (366, 387, 392–394). Clinical studies have failed to demonstrate a clear relationship between TFPI levels and arterial or venous thrombotic disease (366, 395–398).

Animal studies have shown the depletion of endogenous TFPI sensitizes rabbits to the disseminated intravascular coagulation induced by tissue factor or endotoxin infusion (399, 400). Similar depletion of endogenous TFPI does not effect the coagulopathy produced by the infusion of a complex of factor Xa and phospholipids, which suggests the major physiologic role of TFPI is the regulation of factor VIIa/tissue factor activity (401). TFPI gene-disruption in mice is associated with embryonic hemorrhage and intrauterine lethality presumably related to a consumptive coagulopathy (402). The absence of TFPI may produce a similar fate in humans because an individual with TFPI deficiency has not been identified.

# PLACENTAL PROTEIN 5/TISSUE FACTOR PATHWAY INHIBITOR-2

The cDNA for placental protein 5/TFPI-2 (PP5/TFPI-2) was isolated in 1994 by screening a placental cDNA library with an oligonucleotide probe designed to detect Kunitz domain-related DNA sequences (403). The encoded protein was named TFPI-2 due to its ability to inhibit factor VIIa/tissue factor and overall structural resemblance to TFPI. Subsequent studies have shown TFPI-2 is identical to a previously studied heparin binding protein called PP5 (404, 405). The PP5/TFPI-2 cDNA has a 705 bp open reading frame and encodes a 235 amino acid protein. After a classic signal peptide, PP5/TFPI-2 has a short aminoterminal peptide followed by three tandem Kunitz-like domains and a basic carboxy-terminal tail. The structure of domain 2 is atypical for a Kunitz-type inhibitor because it contains an additional amino acid inserted between the first and second cysteines and two additional amino acids inserted between the fourth and fifth cysteines of the domain loops. The residues at the presumed $P_1$ reactive sites of Kunitz domains 1, 2, and 3 are Arg, Glu, and Ser, respectively.

PP5/TFPI-2 mRNA (~1.4 kb) has been detected in placenta, liver, and endothelial cells through Northern analysis (403). Cultured umbilical vein endothelial cells, dermal microvascular endothelial cells, keratinocytes, foreskin fibroblasts, and certain cancer cells express PP5/TFPI-2 (406, 407). Under tissue culture conditions, approximately 70% of the expressed protein is deposited in the extracellular matrix and the remainder, approximately 30%, remains cell-associated with little PP5/TFPI-2 found in conditioned media (406). Variable glycosylation leads to three isoforms (27, 31, and 33 Kda) of PP5/TFPI-2 (406).

In contrast to TFPI, factor X(a) appears to have a minimal effect on the inhibition of factor VIIa/tissue factor produced by PP5/TFPI-2 (403). Heparin enhances PP5/TFPI-2 mediated factor VIIa/tissue factor inhibition 20-fold, but the affinity of the inhibitory complex is modest (Ki = 10 nM) (408). PP5/TFPI-2 also inhibits trypsin, plasmin, factor XIa, chymotrypsin, and plasma kallikrein (408).

The level of PP5/TFPI-2 circulating in plasma is normally low (~15 pM), but it increases 40- to 70-fold during pregnancy (409). The elevated levels of PP5/TFPI-2 in the plasma of pregnant women are further increased by the infusion of heparin (410). Similar to TFPI, the source of this heparin-releasable PP5/TFPI-2 is althought to be the endothelium. The physiologic role of PP5/TFPI-2 is unknown.

## THE TISSUE FACTOR PATHWAY AND THE COAGULATION CASCADE

In the current scheme (411), the critical role of the tissue factor pathway is to initiate the coagulation process (Fig. 4.5). Plasma gains access to tissue factor exposed at subendothelial locations at the site of a wound. Factors VII and VIIa in plasma bind this tissue factor, and the factor VIIa/tissue factor catalytic complex activates limited quantities of factor X and factor IX. Additional local activation of factor VII may be produced by factor VIIa (autoactivation) or through feedback activation by other proteinases (e.g., factor Xa, factor IXa). Some factor Xa generates thrombin that produces the local activation of platelets and the critical cofactors V and VIII (412–414). TFPI dampens the clotting process by producing factor

Xa-dependent feedback inhibition of the factor VIIa/tissue factor complex. Persistent and amplified production of factor Xa and thrombin then proceeds through the actions of factor IXa with its cofactor VIIIa. Factor XIa, possibly activated by thrombin (415, 416) or through other means, produces additional factor IXa to supplement that initially generated by the factor VIIa/tissue factor complex before its inactivation by TFPI.

Based on the clinical phenotype of individuals with severe factor VII deficiency, it is clear factor VIIa/tissue factor-mediated initiation of coagulation is important for normal hemostatic function. Individuals lacking factors of the "contact" system, including factor XII, high-molecular-weight kininogen, and prekallikrein, do not bleed. Thus, contact activation is not required for hemostasis but may contribute to coagulation in certain pathologic conditions. The severe hemorrhagic diathesis seen in hemophilia demonstrates that the amplified and perhaps sustained generation of thrombin by factor Xa, which is produced by factor IXa/VIIIa, is critical for ultimate hemostasis. This augmentation phase of coagulation is required to: 1) overcome the effects of plasma proteinase inhibitors of coagulation enzymes and 2) prevent premature lysis of the clot through thrombin-mediated activation of carboxypeptidase-U (plasma pro-carboxypeptidase-B, thrombin-activatable fibrinolysis inhibitor) (417, 418). The factor VIIa/tissue factor-mediated "initiation phase" of coagulation contributes to this secondary phase by priming the system through the

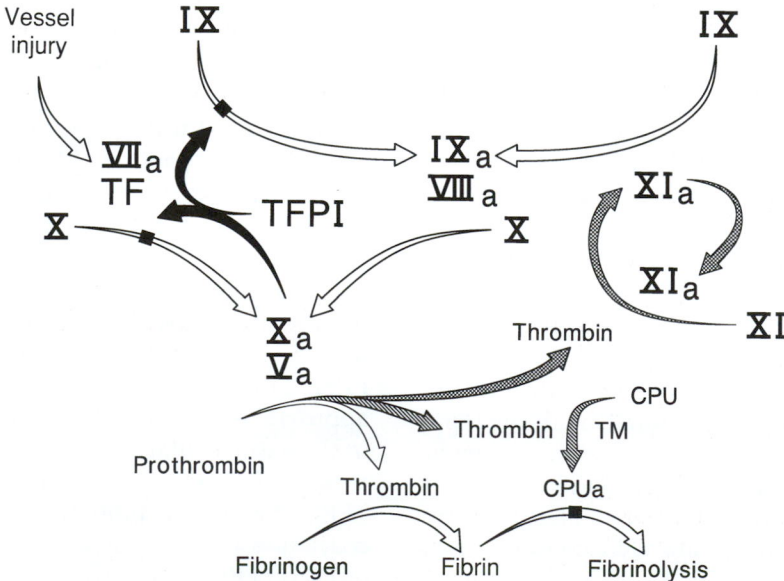

**FIGURE 4.5.** Tissue factor pathway of coagulation. Hemostasis is initiated when factor VII and factor VIIa in plasma gain access to tissue factor at a site of blood vessel injury. Limited quantities of factor IXa and factor Xa are generated before feedback inhibition of the factor VIIa/tissue factor complex mediated by TFPI and factor Xa. The generation of factor Xa and thrombin is then amplified through the action of factor VIIIa and factor IXa, the latter produced initially by factor VIIa/tissue factor and supplemented by factor XIa that is generated through the action of thrombin or by other means. Thrombin activation of carboxypeptidase-U (CPU), which is enhanced by the cofactor thrombomodulin (TM), inhibits subsequent fibrinolysis of the clot.

activation of platelets and the production of factors Va and VIIIa, and by producing the initial factor IXa. Under certain conditions and particularly in locations with high endogenous fibrinolytic activity, additional factor IXa generated by factor XIa is required for hemostasis (419–421).

# REFERENCES

1. Schmidt A. Zur Blutlehre. Leipzig: Vogel, 1892.
2. Morawitz P. The chemistry of blood coagulation. Ergeb Physiol 1905;4:307–422.
3. Alexander B, Goldstein, R, Landwehr G et al. Congenital SPCA deficiency: a hitherto unrecognized coagulation defect with hemorrhage rectified by serum and serum fractions. J Clin Invest 1951;30:596–608.
4. Telfer TP, Denson KW, Wright DR. A "new" coagulation defect. Br J Haematol 1956;2:308–316.
5. Hougie E, Barrow EM, Graham JB. Stuart clotting defect. I. Segregation of an hereditary hemorrhagic state from the heterogeneous group heretofore called "stable factor" (SPCA, proavertin, factor VII) deficiency. J Clin Invest 1957;36:485–496.
6. Manteuffel ZV. Bemerkungen zur Blustillung bein Haemophilie. Dtsch Med Wochenschr 1893;19:665–667.
7. MacFarlane RG. An enzyme cascade in the blood clotting mechanism, and its function as a biochemical amplifier. Nature 1964;202:498–499.
8. Davie EW, Ratnoff OD. Waterfall sequence for intrinsic blood clotting. Science 1964;145:1310–1312.
9. Kaplan AP, Silverberg M. The coagulation-kinin pathway of human plasma. Blood 1987;70:1–15.
10. Ragni MV, Lewis JH, Spero JA et al. Factor VII deficiency. Am J Hematol 1981;10:79–88.
11. Triplett DA, Brandt JT, Batard MA et al. Hereditary factor VII deficiency: heterogeneity defined by combined functional and immunochemical analysis. Blood 1985;66:1284–1287.
12. Osterud B, Rapaport SI. Activation of factor IX by the reaction product of tissue factor and factor VII: additional pathway for initiating blood coagulation. Proc Natl Acad Sci U S A 1977;74:5260–5264.
13. Broze GJ Jr, Warren LA, Novotny WF et al. The lipoprotein-associated coagulation inhibitor that inhibits the factor VII-tissue factor complex also inhibits factor Xa: insight into its possible mechanism of action. Blood 1988;71:335–343.
14. Broze GJ Jr, Girard TJ, Novotny WF. Regulation of coagulation by a multivalent Kunitz-type inhibitor. Biochemistry 1990;29:7539–7546.
15. Owren PA. Prothrombin and accessory factors: clinical significance. Am J Med 1953;14:201–215.
16. Radcliffe R, Nemerson Y. Activation and control of factor VII by activated factor X and thrombin. Isolation and characterization of a single chain form of factor VII. J Biol Chem 1975;250:388–395.
17. Kisiel W, Davie EW. Isolation and characterization of bovine factor VII. Biochemistry 1975;14:4928–4934.
18. Broze GJ Jr, Majerus PW. Purification and properties of human coagulation factor VII. J Biol Chem 1980;255:1242–1247.
19. Bajaj SP, Rapaport SI, Brown SF. Isolation and characterization of human factor VII. Activation of factor VII by factor Xa. J Biol Chem 1981;256:253–259.
20. Hagen FS, Gray CL, O'Hara P et al. Characterization of a cDNA coding for human factor VII. Proc Natl Acad Sci U S A 1986;83:2412–2416.
21. O'Hara PJ, Grant FJ, Haldeman BA et al. Nucleotide sequence of the gene coding for human factor VII, a vitamin K-dependent protein participating in blood coagulation. Proc Natl Acad Sci U S A 1987;84:5158–5162.
22. Brothers AB, Clarke BJ, Sheffield WP et al. Complete nucleotide sequence of the cDNA encoding rabbit coagulation factor VII. Thromb Res 1993;69:231–238.
23. Idusogie E, Rosen E, Geng JP et al. Characterization of a cDNA encoding murine coagulation factor VII. Thromb Haemost 1996;75:481–487.
24. Murakawa M, Okamura T, Kamura T et al. Analysis of the partial nucleotide sequences and deduced primary structures of the protease domains of mammalian blood coagulation factors VII and X. Eur J Haematol 1994;52:162–168.
25. deGrouchy J, Dauitzenberg MD, Turleau C et al. Regional mapping of clotting factors VII and X to 13q34. Expression of factor VII through chromosome 8. Hum Genet 1984;66:230–233.
26. Fagan K, Wilkinson I, Allen M et al. The coagulation factor VII regulator is located on 8p23.1. Hum Genet 1988;79:365–367.
27. Furie B, Furie BC. The molecular basis of blood coagulation. Cell 1988;53:505–518.
28. Erdmann D, Heim J. Orphan nuclear receptor HNF-4 binds to the human coagulation factor VII promoter. J Biol Chem 1995;270:22988–22996.
29. Pollak ES, Hung HL, Godin W et al. Functional characterization of the human factor VII 5-lanking region. J Biol Chem 1996;271:1738–1747.
30. Greenberg D, Miao CH, Ho WT et al. Liver-specific expression of the human factor VII gene. Proc Natl Acad Sci U S A 1995;92:12347–12351.
31. Reijnen MJ, Sladek FM, Bertina RM et al. Disruption of a binding site for hepatocyte nuclear factor 4 results in hemophilia B Leyden. Proc Natl Acad Sci U S A 1992;89:6300–6303.
32. Arbini AA, Pollak ES, Bayleran JK et al. Severe factor VII deficiency due to a mutation disrupting a hepatocyte nuclear factor 4 binding site in the factor VII promoter. Blood 1996;89:176–182.
33. Berkner K, Busby S, Davie E et al. Isolation and expression of cDNAs encoding human factor VII. Cold Spring Harb Symp Quant Biol 1986;51:531–541.
34. Bernardi F, Marchetti G, Pinotti M et al. Factor VII gene polymorphisms contribute about one third of the factor VII level variation in plasma. Arterioscler Thromb Vasc Biol 1996;16:72–76.
35. Green F, Kelleher C, Wilkes H et al. A common genetic polymorphism associated with lower coagulation factor VII levels in healthy individuals. Arterioscler Thromb 1991;11:540–546.
36. Furie B, Furie BC. Molecular basis of vitamin K-dependent gamma-carboxylation. [Review]. Blood 1990;75:1753–1762.
37. Barr PJ. Mammalian subtilisins: the long-sought dibasic processing endoproteases. Cell 1991;66:1–3.
38. Banner DW, D-Arcy A, Chene C et al. The crystal structure of the complex of blood coagulation factor VIIa with soluble tissue factor. Nature 1996;380:41–46.
39. Freedman SJ, Furie BC, Furie B et al. Structure of the calcium ion-bound gamma carboxyglutamic acid-rich domain of factor IX. Biochemistry 1995;34:12126–12137.
40. Sunnerhagen M, Forsen S, Hoffren AM et al. Structure of the Ca(2+)-free Gla domain sheds light on membrane binding of blood coagulation proteins. Nat Struct Biol 1995;2:504–509.
41. Sabharwal AK, Birktoft JJ, Gorka J et al. High affinity Ca2+-binding site in the serine protease domain of human factor VIIa and its role in tissue factor binding and development of catalytic activity. J Biol Chem 1995;270:15523–15530.
42. Thim L, Bjoern S, Christensen M et al. Amino acid sequence and posttranslational modifications of human factor VIIa from plasma and transfected baby hamster kidney cells. Biochemistry 1988;27:7785–7793.
43. Higashi S, Matsumoto N, Iwanga S. Molecular mechanism of tissue factor-mediated acceleration of factor VIIa activity. J Biol Chem 1996;271:26569–26574.
44. Nishimura H, Kawabata S, Kisiel W et al. Identification of a disaccharide (Xyl-Glc) and a trisaccharide (Xyl2-Glc) O-glycosidically linked to a serine residue in the first epidermal growth factor-like domain of human factors VII and IX and protein Z and bovine protein Z. J Biol Chem 1989;264:20320–20325.
45. Bjoern S, Foster DC, Thim L et al. Human plasma and recombinant factor VII. Characterization of O-glycosylations at serine residues 52 and 60 and effects of site-directed mutagenesis of serine 52 to alanine. J Biol Chem 1991;266:11051–11057.
46. Chaing S, Clarke B, Sridhara S et al. Severe factor VII deficiency caused by mutations abolishing the cleavage site for activation and altering binding to tissue factor. Blood 1994;83:3524–3535.
47. Butenas S, Mann KG. Kinetics of human factor VII activation. Biochemistry 1996;35:1904–1910.
48. Wildgoose P, Kisiel W. Activation of human factor VII by factors IXa and Xa on human bladder carcinoma cells. Blood 1989;73:1888–1895.
49. Neuenschwander PF, Morrissey JH. Deletion of the membrane anchoring region of tissue factor abolishes autoactivation of factor VII but not cofactor function. Analysis of a mutant with a selective deficiency in activity. J Biol Chem 1992;267:14477–14482.
50. Matsushita T, Kojima T, Emi N et al. impaired human tissue factor-mediated activity in blood clotting factor VII$_{Nagoya}$ (Arg$^{304}$-Trp). J Biol Chem 1994;269:7355–7363.
51. Nakagaki T, Foster DC, Berkner KL et al. Initiation of the extrinsic pathway of blood coagulation: evidence for the tissue factor dependent autoactivation of human coagulation factor VII. Biochemistry 1991;30:10819–10824.
52. Pedersen AH, Lund-Hansen T, Bisgaard FH et al. Autoactivation of human recombinant coagulation factor VII. Biochemistry 1989;28:9331–9336.
53. Fiore MM, Neuenschwander PF, Morrissey JH. The biochemical basis for the apparent defect of soluble mutant tissue factor in enhancing the proteolytic activities of factor VIIa. J Biol Chem 1994;269:143–149.
54. Sakai T, Lund-Hansen T, Paborsky L et al. Binding of human factors VII and VIIa to a human bladder carcinoma cell line (J82). Implications for the initiation of the extrinsic pathway of blood coagulation. J Biol Chem 1989;264:9980–9988.
55. Iino M, Kisiel W. Sphingosine-containing phospholipid vesicles support human factor VII autoactivation in the absence of tissue factor. Thromb Res 1996;82:119–127.
56. Morrissey JH, Macik BG, Neuenschwander PF et al. Quantitation of activated factor VII levels in plasma using a tissue factor mutant selectively deficient in promoting factor VII activation. Blood 1993;81:734–744.

57. Kazama Y, Hamamoto T, Foster DC et al. Hepsin, a putative membrane-associated serin protease, activates human factor VII and initiates a pathway of blood coagulation on the cell surface leading to thrombin formation. J Biol Chem 1995;270:66–72.

58. Nakagaki T, Lin P, Kisiel W. Activation of human factor VII by the prothrombin activator from the venom of Oxyuranus scutellatus (Taipan snake). Thromb Res 1992;65:105–116.

59. Tsao BP, Fair DS, Curtiss LK et al. Monocytes can be induced by lipopolysaccharide-triggered lymphocytes to express functional factor VII/VIIa protease activity. J Exp Med 1984;159:1042–1057.

60. Broze GJ Jr, Hickman S, Miletich JP. Monoclonal anti-human factor VII antibodies. Detection in plasma of a second protein antigenically and genetically related to factor VII. J Clin Invest 1985;76:937–946.

61. Dike DW, Griffiths D, Bidwell E et al. A factor VII concentrate for therapeutic use. Br J Haematol 1980;45:107–118.

62. Seligsohn U, Kasper CK, Osterud B et al. Activated factor VII: presence in factor IX concentrates and persistence in the circulation after infusion. Blood 1979;53:828–837.

63. Thomsen MK, Diness V, Nilsson P et al. Pharmacokinetics of recombinant factor VIIa in the rat; a comparison of bio-, immuno- and isotope assays. Thromb Haemost 1993;70:458–464.

64. Beeby TL, Chasseaud LF, Taylor T et al. Distribution of the recombinant coagulation factor $^{125}$I-rFVIIa in rats. Thromb Haemost 1993;70:465–468.

65. Chang GT, Kisiel W. Internalization and degradation of recombinant human coagulation factor VIIa by the human hepatoma cell line HuH7. Thromb Haemost 1995;73:231–238.

66. Kondo S, Kisiel W. Regulation of factor VIIa activity in plasma: evidence that antithrombin III is the sole plasma protease inhibitor of human factor VIIa. Thromb Res 1987;46:325–335.

67. Bauer KA, Kass BL, ten Cate H et al. Factor IX is activated in vivo by the tissue factor mechanism. Blood 1990;76:731–736.

68. Bauer KA, Mannucci PM, Gringeri A et al. Factor IXa-factor VIIIa-cell surface complex does not contribute to the basal activation of the coagulation mechanism in vivo. Blood 1992;79:2039–2047.

69. ten Cate H, Bauer KA, Levi M et al. The activation of factor X and prothrombin by recombinant factor VIIa in vivo is mediated by tissue factor. J Clin Invest 1993;92:1207–1212.

70. Wildgoose P, Nemerson Y, Hansen LL et al. Measurement of basal levels of factor VIIa in hemophilia A and B individuals. Blood 1992;80:25–28.

71. Eichinger S, Mannucci PM, Tradati F et al. Determinants of plasma factor VIIa levels in humans. Blood 1995;86:3021–3025.

72. Scarabin PY, Vissac AM, Kirzin JM et al. Population correlates of coagulation factor VII: importance of age, sex, and menopausal status as determinants of activated factor VII. Arterioscler Thromb Vasc Biol 1996;16:1170–1176.

73. Ariens RA, Coppola R, Mannucci PM. The increase with age of the components of the tissue factor coagulation pathway is gender-dependent. Blood Coagul Fibrinolysis 1995;6d:433–437.

74. Sakata T, Kario K, Matsuo T et al. Suppression of plasma-activated factor VII levels by warfarin therapy. Arterioscler Thromb Vasc Biol 1995;15:241–246.

75. Raskob GE, Durica SS, Morrissey JH et al. Effect of treatment with low-dose warfarin-aspirin on activated factor VII. Blood 1995;85:3034–3039.

76. Mennen LI, Schouten EG, Grobbee DE et al. Coagulation factor VII, dietary fat, and blood lipids: a Review. Thromb Haemost 1966;76:492–499.

77. Hoffman CJ, Lawson WE, Miller RH et al. Correlation of vitamin K-dependent clotting factors with cholesterol and triglycerides in healthy young adults. Arterioscler Thromb 1994;14:1737–1740.

78. Miller GH, Stirling Y, Howard DJ et al. Dietary fat intake and plasma factor VII antigen concentration. Thromb Haemost 1995;73:893.

79. Zitoun D, Bara L, Basdevant A et al. Levels of factor VIIc associated with decreased tissue factor pathway inhibitor and increased plasminogen activator inhibitor-1 in dyslipidemias. Arterioscler Thromb Vasc Biol 1996;16:77–81.

80. Miller GJ, Martin JC, Mitropoulos KA et al. Activation of factor VII during alimentary lipemia occurs in healthy adults and individuals with congenital factor XII or factor XI deficiency, but not in individuals with factor IX deficiency. Blood 1996;87:4187–4196.

81. Meade TW, Mellows S, Brozovic M et al. Haemostatic function and ischaemic heart disease: principal results of the Northwick Park Heart Study. Lancet 1986;2:533–537.

82. Ruddock V, Meade TW. Factor VII activity and ischaemic heart disease: fatal and non-fatal events. QJM 1994;87:403–406.

83. Heinrich J, Balleisen L, Schulte H et al. Fibrinogen and factor VII in the prediction of coronary risk. Arterioscler Thromb 1994;12:54–59.

84. Assmann G, Cullen P, Heinrich J et al. Hemostatic variables in the prediction of coronary risk: results of the 8 year follow-up of healthy men in the Munster Heart Study (PROCAM). Isr J Med Sci 1996;32:364–370.

85. Folsom AR, Wu KK, Shahar E et al. Association of hemostatic variables with prevalent cardiovascular disease and asymptomatic carotid artery atherosclerosis. The Atherosclerosis Risk in Communities (ARIC) study. Arterioscler Thromb 1993;13:1829–1836.

86. Salomaa V, Rasi V, Pekkanen J et al. Haemostatic factors and prevalent coronary heart disease; the FINRISK haemostasis study. Eur Heart J 1994;15:1293–1299.

87. Cushman M, Yanez D, Psaty BM et al. Association of fibrinogen and coagulation factors VII and VIII with cardiovascular risk factors in the elderly. Am J Epidemiol 1996;143:665–676.

88. Lee AJ, Fowkes G, Lowe GDO et al. Fibrin D-dimer, haemostatic factors and peripheral arterial disease. Thromb Haemost 1995;74:828–832.

89. Tracy RP, Bovill EG, Yanez D et al. Fibrinogen and factor VIII, but not factor VII, are associated with measures of subclinical cardiovascular disease in the elderly. Results from the Cardiovascular Health Study. Arterioscler Thromb Vasc Biol 1995;15:1269–1279.

90. Miller GJ, Stirling Y, Esnouf MP et al. Factor VII-deficient substrate plasmas depleted of protein C raise the sensitivity of the factor VII bioassay to activated factor VII: an international study. Thromb Haemost 1994;71:38–48.

91. Hoffman C, Shah A, Sodums M et al. Factor VII activity state in coronary artery disease. J Lab Clin Med 1988;111:475–481.

92. Moor E, Silveira A, van't Hooft F et al. Coagulation factor VII mass and activity in young men with myocardial infarction at a young age: role of plasma lipoproteins and factor VII genotype. Arterioscler Thromb 1995;15:655–665.

93. Merlini PA, Ardissino D, Oltrona L et al. Heightened thrombin formation but normal plasma levels of activated factor VII in individuals with acute coronary syndromes. Arterioscler Thromb Vasc Biol 1995;15:1675–1679.

94. Kario K, Miyata T, Sakata T et al. Fluorigenic assay of activated factor VII. Plasma factor VIIa levels in relation to arterial diseases in Japanese. Arterioscler Thromb 1994;14:265–274.

95. Koster T, Rosendaal FR, Reitsma PH et al. Factor VII and fibrinogen levels as risk factors for venous thrombosis. Thromb Haemost 1994;71:719–722.

96. Seligsohn U, Shani M, Ramot B et al. Hereditary deficiency of blood clotting factor VII and Dubin-Johnson syndrome in an Israeli family. Isr J Med Sci 1959;5:1060–1065.

97. Seligsohn U, Shani M, Ramot B. Gilbert syndrome and factor VII deficiency. Lancet 1970;1:1398.

98. Levanon M, Rimon S, Shani M et al. Active and inactive factor VII in Dubin-Johnson syndrome with factor VII deficiency, hereditary factor VII deficiency and on coumadin treatment. Br J Haemat 1972;23:669–677.

99. Popham BI, Stevenson TD. Idiopathic retroperitoneal fibrosis associated with a coagulation defect (factor VII deficiency): report of a case and Review of the literature. Ann Intern Med 1960;52:894–906.

100. Munnich A, Saudubray JM, Dautzenberg MD et al. Diet-responsive proconvertin (factor VII) deficiency in homocystinuria. J Pediatr 1983;102:730–734.

101. Slease RB, Schumacher HR. Deficiency of coagulation factors VII and XII in an individual with Hodgkin's disease. Arch Int Med 1977;1633–1635.

102. Weisdorf D, Hasegawa D, Fair DS. Acquired factor VII deficiency associated with aplastic anaemia: correction with bone marrow transplantation. Br J Haemat 1989;71:409–413.

103. Fischer M, Lechner K, Hinterberger W et al. Deficiency of fibrinogen and factor VII following treatment of severe aplastic anaemia with anti-thymocyte globulin and high-dose methylprednisolone. Scand J Haemat 1985;34:312–316.

104. Kaufman PA, Jones RB, Greenberg CS et al. Autologous bone marrow transplantation and factor XII, factor VII, and protein C deficiencies. Report of a new association and its possible relationship to endothelial cell injury. Cancer 1990;66:515–521.

105. de Raucourt E, Dumont MD, Tourani JM et al. Acquired factor VII deficiency associated with pleural liposarcoma. Blood Coagul Fibrinolysis 1994;5:833–836.

106. Kroll AJ, Alexander B, Cochizo F et al. Hereditary deficiencies of clotting VII and X associated with carotid body tumors. N Engl J Med 1964;279:6–13.

107. Howell WH. The nature and action of the thromboplastic (zymoplastic) substance of the tissues. Am J Physiol 1912;31:1–21.

108. Chargaff E, Bendich A, Cohen S. The thromboplastic protein: structure, properties, disintegration. J Biol Chem 1944;156:161–178.

109. Bjorklid E, Storm E, Osterud B et al. The interaction of the protein and phospholipid components of tissue thromboplastin (factor III) with the factors VII and X. Scand J Haemat 1975;14:65–70.

110. Bjorklid E, Storm E. Purification and some properties of the protein component of tissue thromboplastin from human brain. Biochem J 1977;165:89–96.

111. Pitlick FA. Binding of bovine brain tissue factor to concanavalin A-Sepharose. Partial purification of coagulant, arylamidase, and alkaline phosphatase activities. Biochim Biophys Acta 1976;428:27–34.

112. Bach R, Nemerson Y, Konigsberg W. Purification and characterization of bovine tissue factor. J Biol Chem 1981;256:8324–8331.

113. Broze GJ Jr, Leykam JE, Schwartz BD et al. Purification of human brain tissue factor. J Biol Chem 1985;260:10917–10920.

114. Guha A, Bach R, Konigsberg W et al. Affinity purification of human tissue factor: interaction of factor VII and tissue factor in detergent micelles. Proc Natl Acad Sci U S A 1986;83:299–302.

115. Spicer EK, Horton R, Bloem L et al. Isolation of cDNA clones coding for

human tissue factor: primary structure of the protein and cDNA. Proc Natl Acad Sci U S A 1987;84:5148–5152.

116. Morrissey JH, Fakhrai H, Edgington TS. Molecular cloning of the cDNA for tissue factor, the cellular receptor for the initiation of the coagulation protease cascade. Cell 1987;50:129–135.

117. Mackman N, Morrissey JH, Fowler B et al. Complete sequence of the human tissue factor gene, a highly regulated cellular receptor that initiates the coagulation protease cascade. Biochemistry 1989;28:1755–1762.

118. Hartzell S, Ryder K, Lanahan A et al. A growth factor-responsive gene of murine BALB/c 3T3 cells encodes a protein homologous to human tissue factor. Mol Cell Biol 1989;9:2567–2573.

119. Mackman N, Imes S, Maske WH et al. Structure of the murine tissue factor gene. Chromosome location and conservation of regulatory elements in the promoter. Arterioscler Thromb 1992;12:474–483.

120. Pawashe A, Ezekowitz M, Lin TC et al. Molecular cloning, characterization and expression of cDNA for rabbit brain tissue factor. Thromb Haemost 1991;66:315–320.

121. Andrews BS, Rehemtulla A, Fowler BJ et al. Conservation of tissue factor primary sequence among three mammalian species. Gene 1991;98:265–269.

122. Takayenoki Y, Muta T, Miyata T et al. cDNA and amino acid sequences of bovine tissue factor. Biochem Biophys Res Comm 1991;181:1145–1150.

123. Taby O, Rosenfield CL, Bogdanov V et al. Cloning of the rat tissue factor cDNA and promoter: identification of a serum-response region. Thromb Haemost 1996;76:697–702.

124. Scarpati EM, Sadler JE, O'Connell P et al. Identification and mapping of RFLPs for human tissue factor (HTF) to chromosome 1p. Nucleic Acids Res 1987:15.

125. Kao FT, Hartz J, Horton R et al. Regional assignment of human tissue factor gene (F3) to chromosome 1p21-p22. Somat Cell Mol Genet 1988;14:407–410.

126. Cui MZ, Parry GC, Edgington TS et al. Regulation of tissue factor gene expression in epithelial cells. Induction by serum and phorbol 12-myristate 13-acetate. Arterioscler Thromb 1994;14:807–814.

127. Mackman N. Regulation of the tissue factor gene. FASEB J 1995;9:883–889.

128. Cui MZ, Parry GC, Oeth P et al. Transcriptional regulation of the tissue factor gene in human epithelial cells is mediated by SP1 and EGR-1. J Biol Chem 1996;271:2731–2739.

129. Parry GC, Mackman N. Transcriptional regulation of tissue factor expression in human endothelial cells. Arterioscler Thromb 1995;15:612–621.

130. Bierhaus A, Zhang Y, Deng Y et al. Mechanism of the tumor necrosis factor alpha-mediated induction of endothelial tissue factor. J Biol Chem 1995;270:26419–26432.

131. Groupp ER, Donovan-Peluso M. Lipopolysaccharide induction of the THP-1 cells activates binding of c-Jun, Ets, and Egr-1 to the tissue factor promoter. J Biol Chem 1996;271:12423–12430.

132. Oeth PA, Parry GCN, Kunsch C et al. Lipopolysaccharide induction of tissue factor gene expression in monocytic cells is mediated by binding of c-Rel/p65 heterodimers to a kB-like site. Mol Cell Biol 1994;14:3772–3781.

133. Bierhaus A, Sernau T, Quehenberger P et al. A newly identified NFkB-like site in the tissue factor promoter is involved in advanced glycosylation end products (AGEs) mediated induction of tissue factor [Abstract]. Thromb Haemost 1995;73:1185.

134. Gregory SA, Morrissey JH, Edgington TS. Regulation of tissue factor gene expression in the monocyte procoagulant response to endotoxin. Mol Cell Biol 1989;9:2752–2755.

135. Scarpati EM, Sadler JE. Regulation of endothelial cell coagulant properties. Modulation of tissue factor, plasminogen activator inhibitors, and thrombomodulin by phorbol 12-myristate 13-acetate and tumor necrosis factor [published erratum appears in J Biol Chem 1990 Aug 25;265:14696]. J Biol Chem 1989;264:20705–20713.

136. Conway EM, Bach R, Rosenberg RD et al. Tumor necrosis factor enhances expression of tissue factor mRNA in endothelial cells. Thromb Res 1989;53:231–241.

137. Crossman DC, Carr DP, Tuddenham EG et al. The regulation of tissue factor mRNA in human endothelial cells in response to endotoxin or phorbol ester. J Biol Chem 1990;.265:9782–9787.

138. Ranganathan G, Blatti SP, Subramaniam M et al. Cloning of murine tissue factor and regulation of gene expression by transforming growth factor type beta 1. J Biol Chem 1991;266:496–501.

139. Bird AP. CpG-rich islands and the function of DNA methylation. Nature 1986;321:209–213.

140. Scarpati EM, Wen D, Broze GJ et al. Human tissue factor: cDNA sequence and chromosome localization of the gene. Biochemistry 1987;26:5234–5238.

141. van der Logt CP, Reitsma PH, Bertina RM. Alternative splicing is responsible for the presence of two tissue factor mRNA species in LPS stimulated human monocytes. Thromb Haemost 1992;67:272–276.

142. Ahern SM, Miyata T, Sadler JE. Regulation of human tissue factor expression by mRNA turnover. J Biol Chem 1993;268:2154–2159.

143. Muller YA, Ultsch MN, de Vos AM. The crystal structure of the extracellular domain of human tissue factor refined to 1.7 A resolution. J Mol Biol 1996;256:144–159.

144. Paborsky LR, Harris RJ. Post-translational modifications of recombinant human tissue factor. Thromb Res 1990;60:367–376.

145. Bach RR. Initiation of coagulation by tissue factor. CRC Crit Rev Biochem 1988;23:339–368.

146. Bach R, Konigsberg WH, Nemerson Y. Human tissue factor contains thio-ester-linked palmitate and stearate on the cytoplasmic half-cystine. Biochemistry 1988;27:4227–4231.

147. Rehemtulla A, Ruf W, Edgington TS. The integrity of the cysteine 186-cysteine 209 bond of the second disulfide loop of tissue factor is required for binding of factor VII. J Biol Chem 1991;266:10294–10299.

148. Carson SD, Ross SE, Gramzinski RA. Protein co-isolated with human tissue factor impairs recovery of activity. Blood 1988;71:520–523.

149. Morrissey JH, Revak D, Tejada P et al. Resolution of monomeric and heterodimeric forms of tissue factor, the high-affinity cellular receptor for factor VII. Thromb Res 1988;50:481–493.

150. Paborsky LR, Tate KM, Harris RJ et al. Purification of recombinant human tissue factor. Biochemistry 1989;28:8072–8077.

151. Beltzer JP, Fiedler K, Fuhrer C et al. Charged residues are major determinants of the transmembrane orientation of a signal-anchor sequence. J Biol Chem 1991;266:973–978.

152. Zioncheck TF, Roy S, Vehar GA. The cytoplasmic domain of tissue factor is phosphorylated by a protein kinase C-dependent mechanism. J Biol Chem 1992;267:3561–3564.

153. Paborsky LR, Caras IW, Fisher KL et al. Lipid association, but not the transmembrane domain, is required for tissue factor activity: substitution of the transmembrane domain with a phosphatidyl inositol anchor. J Biol Chem 1991;266:21911–21916.

154. Roy S, Paborsky LR, Vehar GA. Self-association of tissue factor is revealed by chemical crosslinking. J Biol Chem 1991;266:4665–4668.

155. Neuenschwander PF, Bianco-Fisher E, Rezaie AR et al. Phosphatidylethanolamine augments factor VIIa-tissue factor activity: enhancement of sensitivity to phosphatidyl serine. Biochemistry 1995;34:13988–13993.

156. Wilcox JN, Smith KM, Schwartz SM et al. Localization of tissue factor in the normal vessel wall and in the atherosclerotic plaque. Proc Natl Acad Sci U S A 1989;86:2839–2843.

157. Drake TA, Morrissey JH, Edgington TS. Selective cellular expression of tissue factor in human tissues. Implications for disorders of hemostasis and thrombosis. Am J Pathol 1989;134:1087–1097.

158. Fleck RA, Rao LV, Rapaport SI et al. Localization of human tissue factor antigen by immunostaining with monospecific, polyclonal anti-human tissue factor antibody [corrected and republished article originally printed in Thromb Res 1990 Mar 1;57:765–781]. Thromb Res 1990;59:421–437.

159. Mackman N, Sawdey MS, Keeton MR et al. Murine tissue factor gene expression in vivo: tissue and cell specificity and regulation by lipopolysaccharide. Am J Pathol 1993;143:76–84.

160. Eddleston M, de la Torre J, Oldstone MBA et al. Astrocytes are the primary source of tissue factor in the murine central nervous system—a role for astrocytes in cerebral hemostasis. J Clin Invest 1993;92:349–358.

161. Faulk WP, Labarrere CA, Carson SD. Tissue factor: identification and characterization of cell types in human placentae. Blood 1990;76:86–96.

162. Henrikson KP, Greenwood JA, Pentecost BT et al. Estrogen control of uterine tissue factor messenger ribonucleic acid levels. Endocrinology 1992;130:2669–2674.

163. Lockwood CJ, Krikun G, Papp C et al. Biological mechanisms underlying RU 486 clinical effects: inhibition of endometrial stromal cell tissue factor content. J Clin Endocrinol Metab 1994;79:786–790.

164. Callander NS, Varki N, Rao LV. Immunohistochemical identification of tissue factor in solid tumors. Cancer 1992;70:1194–1201.

165. Rao LV. Tissue factor as a tumor procoagulant. Cancer Metastasis Rev 1992;89:11832–11836.

166. Bromberg ME, Konigsberg WH, Madison JF et al. Tissue factor promotes melanoma metastasis by a pathway independent of blood coagulation. Proc Natl Acad Sci U S A 1995;92:8205–8209.

167. Meuller BM, Reisfeld RA, Edgington TS et al. Expression of tissue factor by melanoma cells promotes efficient hematogenous metastasis. Proc Natl Acad Sci U S A 1992;89:11832–11836.

168. Taubman MB, Marmur JD, Rosenfield CL et al. Agonist-mediated tissue factor expression in cultured vascular smooth muscle cells. Role of Ca2+ mobilization and protein kinase C activation. J Clin Invest 1993;91:547–552.

169. Marmur JD, Rossikhina M, Guha A et al. Tissue factor is rapidly induced in arterial smooth muscle after balloon injury. J Clin Invest 1993;91:2253–2259.

170. Speidel C, Eisenberg PR, Ruf W et al. Tissue factor mediates prolonged procoagulant activity on the luminal surface of balloon-injured aortas in rabbits. Circulation 1995;92:3323–3330.

171. Thiruvikraman SV, Guha A, Roboz J et al. In situ localization of tissue factor in human atherosclerotic plaques by binding of digoxigenin-labeled factors VIIa and X. Lab Invest 1996;75:451–461.

172. Bloem LJ, Chen L, Konigsberg WH et al. Serum stimulation of quiescent human fibroblasts induces the synthesis of tissue factor mRNA followed by the appearance of tissue factor antigen and procoagulant activity. J Cell Physiol 1989;139:418–423.

173. Lau LF, Nathans D. Expression of a set growth-related immediate early genes in BALB/c 3T3 cells: coordinate regulation with c-fos or c-myc. Proc Natl Acad Sci U S A 1987;84:1182–1186.

174. Luther T, Flossel C, Mackman N et al. Tissue factor expression during human and mouse development. Am J Pathol 1996;149:101–112.

175. Rottingen JA, Enden T, Camerer E et al. Binding of human factor VIIa to tissue factor induces cytosolic Ca2+-signals J82 cells, transfected COS-1 cells, Madin-Darby canine kidney cells and in human endothelial cells induced to synthesize tissue factor. J Biol Chem 1995;270:4650–4660.

176. Masuda M, Nakamura S, Murakami T et al. Association of tissue factor with a gamma chain homodimer of the IgE receptor type I in cultured human monocytes. Eur J Immunol 1996;26:2529–2532.

177. Camerer E, Rottingen JA, Iversen JG et al. Coagulation factors VII and X induce Ca2+ oscillations in Madin-Darby canine kidney cells only when proteolytically active. J Biol Chem 1996;271:29034–29042.

178. Zhang YM, Deng YH, Luther T et al. Tissue factor controls the balance of angiogenic and antiangiogenic properties of tumor cells in mice. J Clin Invest 1994;94:1320–1327.

179. Carmeliet P, Mackman N, Moons L et al. Role of tissue factor in embryonic blood vessel development. Nature 1996;383:73–75.

180. Solberg S, Osterud B, Larsen T et al. Lack of ability to synthesize tissue factor by endothelial cells in intact human saphenous veins. Blood Coagul Fibrinolysis 1990;1:595–600.

181. Drake TA, Cheng J, Chang A et al. Expression of tissue factor thrombomodulin, and E-selectin in baboons with lethal Escherichia coli sepsis. Am J Pathol 1993;142:1–13.

182. Contrino J, Hair G, Kreutzer DL et al. In situ detection of tissue factor in vascular endothelial cells: correlation with the malignant phenotype of human breast disease. Nature Med 1996;2:209–215.

183. Zhang Y, Deng Y, Wendt T et al. Intravenous somatic gene transfer with antisense tissue factor restores blood flow by reducing tumor necrosis factor-induced tissue factor expression and fibrin deposition in mouse meth-A sarcomas. J Clin Invest 1996;97:2213–2224.

184. More L, Sim R, Hudson M et al. Immunohistochemical study of tissue factor expression in normal intestine and idiopathic inflammatory bowel disease. J Clin Pathol 1993;46:703–708.

185. Weinberg JB, Pippen AM, Greenberg CS. Extravascular fibrin formation and dissolution in synovial tissue of individuals with osteoarthritis and rheumatoid arthritis. Arthritis Rheum 1991;34:996–1005.

186. Labarrere CA, Esmon CT, Carson SD et al. Concordant expression of tissue factor and class II MHC antigens in human placental endothelium. Placenta 1990;11:309–318.

187. Lang IM, Mackman N, Kriett JM et al. Prothrombotic activation of pulmonary arterial endothelial cells in an individual with tuberculosis. Hum Pathol 1996;27:423–427.

188. Taylor FB Jr, Chang A, Ruf W et al. Lethal E. coli septic shock is prevented by blocking tissue factor with monoclonal antibody. Circ Shock 1991;33:127–134.

189. Warr TA, Rao LV, Rapaport SI. Disseminated intravascular coagulation in rabbits induced by administration of endotoxin or tissue factor: effect of anti-tissue factor antibodies and measurement of plasma extrinsic pathway inhibitor activity. Blood 1990;75:1481–1489.

190. Marcel L, ten Cate H, Bauer KA et al. Inhibition of endotoxin-induced activation of coagulation and fibrinolysis by pentoxifyllin or by a monoclonal anti-tissue factor antibody in chimpanzees. J Clin Invest 1994;93:114–120.

191. Pettersen KS, Wiiger MT, Narahara N et al. Induction of tissue factor synthesis in human umbilical vein endothelial cells involves protein kinase C. Thromb Haemost 1992;67:472–477.

192. Ternisien C, Ramani M, Ollivier V et al. Endotoxin-induced tissue factor in human monocytes is dependent upon protein kinase C activation. Thromb Haemost 1993;70:800–806.

193. Terry CM, Callahan KS. Protein kinase C regulates cytokine-induced tissue factor transcription and procoagulant activity in human endothelial cells. J Lab Clin Med 1996;127:81–93.

194. Ternisien C, Ollivier V, Khechai F et al. Protein tyrosine kinase activation is required for LPS and PMA induction of tissue factor mRNA in human blood monocytes. Thromb Haemost 1995;73:413–420.

195. Mackman N. Protease inhibitors block lipopolysaccharide induction of tissue factor gene expression in human monocytic cells by preventing activation of c-Rel/p65 heterodimers. J Biol Chem 1994;269:26363–26367.

196. Orthner CL, Rodgers GM, Fitzgerald LA. Pyrrolidine dithiocarbamate abrogates tissue factor (TF) expression by endothelial cells: evidence implicating nuclear factor-B in TF induction by diverse agonists. Blood 1995;86:436–443.

197. Oeth P, Mackman N. Salicylates inhibit lipopolysaccharide-induced transcriptional activation of the tissue factor gene in human monocytic cells. Blood 1995;86:4144–4152.

198. Herbert JM, Savi P, Laplace MC et al. IL-4 inhibits LPS-, IL-1β- and TNF alpha-induced expression of tissue factor in endothelial cells and monocytes. FEBS Lett 1992;310:31–33.

199. Ramani M, Khechai F, Ollivier V et al. Interleukin-10 and pentoxifyllin inhibit C-reactive protein-induced tissue factor gene expression in peripheral human blood monocytes. FEBS Lett 1994;356:86–88.

200. Herbert JM, Savi P, Laplace MC et al. IL-4 and IL-3 exhibit comparable abilities to reduce pyrogen-induced expression of procoagulant activity in endothelial cells and monocytes. FEBS Lett 1993;328:268–270.

201. Ishii H, Horie S, Kizaki K et al. Retinoic acid counteracts both the down-regulation of thrombomodulin and the induction of tissue factor in cultured human endothelial cells exposed to tumor necrosis factor. Blood 1992;80:2556–2562.

202. Barstad RM, Hamers MJ, Stephens RW et al. Retinoic acid reduces induction of monocyte tissue factor and tissue factor/factor VIIa-dependent arterial thrombus formation. Blood 1995;86:212–218.

203. Hasday JD, Sitrin RG. Dipyridamole stimulates urokinase production and suppresses procoagulant activity of rabbit alveolar macrophages: a possible mechanism of antithrombotic action. Blood 1987;69:660–667.

204. Brozna JP, Horan M, Carson SD. Dipyridamole inhibits O2-release and expression of tissue factor activity by peripheral blood monocytes stimulated with lipopolysaccharide. Thromb Res 1990;60:141–156.

205. Crutchley DJ, Hirsh MJ. The stable prostacyclin analog, iloprost, and prostaglandin E1 inhibit monocyte procoagulant activity in vitro. Blood 1991;78:382–386.

206. Crutchley DJ, Solomon DE, Conanan LB. Prostacyclin analogues inhibit tissue factor expression in the human monocytic cell line THP-1 via a cyclic AMP-dependent mechanism. Arterioscler Thromb 1992;12:664–670.

207. de Prost D, Ollivier V, Hakim J. Pentoxifyllin inhibition of procoagulant activity generated by activated mononuclear phagocytes. Mol Pharmacol 1990;38:562–566.

208. Ollivier V, Parry GCN, Cobb RR et al. Elevated cyclic AMP inhibits NF-(B-mediated transcription in human monocytic cells and endothelial cells. J Biol Chem 1996;271:20828–20835.

209. Carson SD, Perry GA, Pirruccello SJ. Fibroblast tissue factor: Calcium and ionophore induce shape changes, release of membrane vesicles, and redistribution of tissue factor antigen in addition to increased procoagulant activity. Blood 1994;84:526–534.

210. Dvorak HF, Van DeWater L, Bitzer AM et al. Procoagulant activity associated with plasma membrane vesicles shed by cultured tumor cells. Cancer Res 1983;43:4434–4442.

211. Satta N, Toti F, Feugeas O et al. Monocyte vesiculation is a possible mechanism for dissemination of membrane-associated procoagulant activities and adhesion molecules after stimulation by lipopolysaccharide. J Immunol 1994;153:3245–3255.

212. Greeno EW, Bach RR, Moldow CF. Apoptosis is associated with increased cell surface tissue factor procoagulant activity. Lab Invest 1996;75:281–289.

213. Bona R, Lee E, Rickles F. Tissue factor apoprotein: intracellular transport and expression in shed membrane vesicles. Thromb Res 1987;48:487–500.

214. Schorer AE, Rick PD, Swaim WR et al. Structural features of endotoxin required for stimulation of endothelial cell tissue factor production; exposure of preformed tissue factor after oxidant-mediated endothelial cell injury. J Lab Clin Med 1985;106:38–42.

215. Carson SD, Johnson DR. Consecutive enzyme cascades: complement activation at the cell surface triggers increased tissue factor activity. Blood 1990;76:361–367.

216. Carson SD, Pirruccello SJ, Haire WD. Tissue factor antigen and activity are not expressed on the surface of intact cells isolated from an acute promyelocytic leukemia individual. Thromb Res 1990;59:159–170.

217. Leoni P, Dean RT. An intracellular pool of the procoagulant thromboplastin in human monocytes. Thromb Res 1985;40:199–205.

218. Drake TA, Ruf W, Morrissey JH et al. Functional tissue factor is entirely cell surface expressed on lipopolysaccharide-stimulated human blood monocytes and a constitutively tissue factor-producing neoplastic cell line. J Cell Biol 1989;109:389–395.

219. Bach R, Rifkin DB. Expression of tissue factor procoagulant activity: regulation by cytosolic calcium. Proc Natl Acad Sci U S A 1990;87:6995–6999.

220. Le DT, Rapaport SI, Rao LV. Relations between factor VIIa binding and expression of factor VIIa/tissue factor catalytic activity on cell surfaces. J Biol Chem 1992;267:15447–15454.

221. Le DT, Rapaport SI, Rao LV. Studies of the mechanism for enhanced cell surface factor VIIa/tissue factor activation on fibroblast monolayers after their exposure to N-ethylmaleimide. Thromb Haemost 1994;72:848–855.

222. Martin DM, Boys CW, Ruf W. Tissue factor: molecular recognition and cofactor function. FASEB J 1995;9:852–859.

223. Bach RR, Moldow CF. Activation of tissue factor procoagulant activity on HL-60 cells [Abstract]. Blood 1996;88:282a.

224. Mulder AB, Smit JW, Bom VJ et al. Association of smooth muscle cell tissue factor with caveolae. Blood 1996;88:1306–1313.

225. Camerer E, Pringle S, Skartlien AH et al. Opposite sorting of tissue factor in human umbilical vein endothelial cells and Madin-Darby canine kidney epithelial cells. Blood 1996;88:1339–1349.

226. Sevinsky JR, Rao LV, Ruf W. Ligand induced protease receptor translocation into caveolae: a mechanism for regulating cell surface proteolysis of the tissue factor-dependent coagulation pathway. J Cell Biol 1996;133:293–304.

227. Bugge TH, Xiao Q, Kombrinck KW et al. Fatal embryonic bleeding events in mice lacking tissue factor, the cell-associated initiator of blood coagulation. Proc Natl Acad Sci U S A 1996;93:6258–6263.

228. Toomey JR, Kratzer KE, Lasky NM et al. Targeted disruption of the murine tissue factor gene results in embryonic lethality. Blood 1996;88:1583–1587.

229. Bach R, Gentry R, Nemerson Y. Factor VII binding to tissue factor in reconstituted phospholipid vesicles: induction of cooperativity by phosphatidylserine. Biochemistry 1986;25:4007–4020.

230. Nemerson Y, Gentry R. An ordered addition, essential activation model of the tissue factor pathway of coagulation: evidence for a conformational cage [published erratum appears in Biochemistry 1987 Feb 10;26:974]. Biochemistry 1986;25:4020–4033.

231. Fair DS, MacDonald MJ. Cooperative interaction between factor VII and cell surface-expressed tissue factor. J Biol Chem 1987;262:11692–11698.

232. Krishnaswamy S. The interaction of human factor VIIa with tissue factor. J Biol Chem 1992;267:23696–23706.

233. Tuddenham EG, Pemberton S, Cooper DN. Inherited factor VII deficiency: genetics and molecular pathology. Thromb Haemost 1995;74:313–321.

234. McCallum CD, Hapak RC, Neuenschwander PF et al. The location of the active site of blood coagulation factor VIIa above the membrane surface and its reorientation upon association with tissue factor. J Biol Chem 1996;271:28168–28175.

235. Bom VJ, Bertina RM. The contributions of Ca2+, phospholipids and tissue-factor apoprotein to the activation of human blood-coagulation factor X by activated factor VII. Biochem J 1990;265:327–336.

236. Higashi S, Nishimura H, Fujii S et al. Tissue factor potentiates the factor VIIa-catalyzed hydrolysis of an ester substrate. J Biol Chem 1992;267:17990–17996.

237. Freskgard PO, Olsen OH, Persson E. Structural changes in factor VIIa induced by Ca2+ and tissue factor studied using circular dichroism spectroscopy. Protein Sci 1996;5:1531–1540.

238. Lawson JH, Butenas S, Mann KG. The evaluation of complex-dependent alterations in human factor VIIa. J Biol Chem 1992;267:4834–4843.

239. Ruf W, Rehemtulla A, Morrissey JH et al. Phospholipid-independent and -dependent interactions required for tissue factor receptor and cofactor function. J Biol Chem 1991;266:2158–2166.

240. Krishnaswamy S, Field KA, Edgington TS et al. Role of the membrane surface in the activation of human coagulation factor X. J Biol Chem 1992;267:26110–26120.

241. Ruf W, Miles DJ, Rehemtulla A et al. Tissue factor residues 157-167 are required for efficient proteolytic activation of factor X and factor VII. J Biol Chem 1992;267:22206–22210.

242. Huang Q, Neuenschwander PF, Rezaie et al. Substrate recognition by tissue factor-factor VIIa. Evidence for interaction of residues Lys165 and Lys166 of tissue factor with the 4-carboxyglutamate-rich domain of factor X. J Biol Chem 1996;271:21752–21757.

243. Neuenschwander PF, Morrissey JH. Roles of the membrane-interactive regions of factor VIIa and tissue factor. The factor VIIa Gla domain is dispensable for binding to tissue factor but important for activation of factor X. J Biol Chem 1994;269:8007–8013.

244. Jesty J, Silverberg SA. Kinetics of the tissue factor-dependent activation of coagulation Factors IX and X in a bovine plasma system. J Biol Chem 1979;254:12337–12345.

245. Telgt DS, Macik BG, McCord DM et al. Mechanism by which recombinant factor VIIa shortens the aPTT: activation of factor X in the absence of tissue factor. Thromb Res 1989;56:603–609.

246. Rao LV, Rapaport SI. Factor VIIa-catalyzed activation of factor X independent of tissue factor: its possible significance for control of hemophilic bleeding by infused factor VIIa. Blood 1990;75:1069–1073.

247. Hedner U, Kisiel W. Use of human factor VIIa in the treatment of two hemophilia A individuals with high-titer inhibitors. J Clin Invest 1983;71:1836–1841.

248. Brinkhous KM, Hedner U, Garris JB et al. Effect of recombinant factor VIIa on the hemostatic defect in dogs with hemophilia A, hemophilia B, and von Willebrand disease. Proc Natl Acad Sci U S A 1989;86:1382–1386.

249. Rao LV, Williams T, Rapaport SI. Studies of the activation of factor VII bound to tissue factor. Blood 1996;87:3738–3748.

250. McGee MP, Li LC. Functional difference between intrinsic and extrinsic coagulation pathways. Kinetics of factor X activation on human monocytes and alveolar macrophages. J Biol Chem 1991;266:8079–8085.

251. Kadish JL, Wenc KM, Dvorak HF. Tissue factor activity of normal and neoplastic cells: quantitation and species specificity. J Natl Cancer Inst 1983;70:551–557.

252. Janson TL, Stormorken H, Prydz H. Species specificity of tissue thromboplastin. Haemostasis 1984;14:440–444.

253. Hemker HC, Muller AD, Gonggrijp R. The estimation of activated human blood coagulation factor VII. J Mol Med 1976;1:127–134.

254. van Deijk WA, van Dam-Mieras MC, Muller AD et al. Evaluation of a coagulation assay determining the activity state of factor VII in plasma. Haemostasis 1983;13:192–197.

255. Girolami A, Fabris F, Dal Bo Zanon R et al. Factor VII Padua: a congenital coagulation disorder due to an abnormal factor VII with a peculiar activation pattern. J Lab Clin Med 1978;91:387–395.

256. Girolami A, Falezza G, Patrassi G et al. Factor VII Verona coagulation disorder: double heterozygosis with an abnormal factor VII and heterozygous factor VII deficiency. Blood 1977;50:603–610.

257. Girolami A, Cattarozzi G, Dal Bo Zanon R et al. Factor VII Padua 2: another factor VII abnormality with defective ox brain thromboplastin activation and a complex hereditary pattern. Blood 1979;54:46–53.

258. Lawson JH, Butenas S, Ribarik N et al. Complex-dependent inhibition of factor VIIa by antithrombin III and heparin. J Biol Chem 1993;268:767–770.

259. Rao LV, Rapaport SI, Hoang AD. Binding of factor VIIa to tissue factor permits rapid antithrombin III/heparin inhibition of factor VIIa. Blood 1993;81:2600–2607.

260. Broze GJ Jr. Inhibition of Factor VIIa/tissue factor by antithrombin III and tissue factor pathway inhibitor. Blood 1993;82:1679–1680.

261. Jesty J, Lorenz A, Rodriguez J et al. Initiation of the tissue factor pathway of coagulation in the presence of heparin: Control by antithrombin III and tissue factor pathway inhibitor. Blood 1996;87:2301–2307.

262. Rao LV, Nordfang O, Hoang AD et al. Mechanism of antithrombin III inhibition of factor VIIa/tissue factor activity on cell surfaces. Comparison with tissue factor pathway inhibitor/factor Xa-induced inhibition of factor VIIa/tissue factor activity. Blood 1995;85:121–129.

263. Rao LV, Rapaport SI. Activation of factor VII bound to tissue factor: a key early step in the tissue factor pathway of blood coagulation. Proc Natl Acad Sci U S A 1988;85:6687–6691.

264. Conkling PR, Patton KL, Hannun YA et al. Sphingosine inhibits monocyte tissue factor-initiated coagulation by altering factor VII binding. J Biol Chem 1989;264:18440–18444.

265. Carson SD. Tissue factor (coagulation factor III) inhibition by apolipoprotein A-II. J Biol Chem 1987;262:718–721.

266. Carson SD, Ross SE. Effects of lipid-binding proteins apo A-I, apo A-II, beta 2-glycoprotein I, and C-reactive protein in activation of factor X by tissue factor-factor VIIa. Thromb Res 1988;50:669–678.

267. Kondo S, Noguchi M, Funakoshi T et al. Inhibition of human factor VIIa-tissue factor activity by placental anticoagulant protein. Thromb Res 1987;48:449–459.

268. Gramzinski RA, Broze GJ Jr, Carson SD. Human fibroblast tissue factor is inhibited by lipoprotein-associated coagulation inhibitor and placental anticoagulant protein but not by apolipoprotein A-II. Blood 1989;73:983–989.

269. Loeb L, Fleisher MS, Tuttle L. The interaction between blood serum and tissue extract in the coagulation of the blood: I. The combined action of serum and tissue extract on fluoride, hirudin, and peptone plasma; the effect of heating on the serum. J Biol Chem 1922;51:461–483.

270. Loeb L, Fleisher MS, Tuttle L. The interaction between blood serum and tissue extract in the coagulation of blood: II. A comparison between the effects of the stroma of erythrocytes and of tissue extracts, unheated and heated, on the coagulation of the blood, and on the mechanism of the interaction of these substances with blood serum. J Biol Chem 1922;51:485–506.

271. Thomas L. Studies on the intravascular thromboplastin effect of tissue suspensions in mice: II. A factor in normal rabbit serum which inhibits the thromboplastin effect of the sedimentable tissue component. Bull Johns Hopkins Hosp 1947;81:26–42.

272. Schneider CL. The active principle of placental toxin: thromboplastin; its inactivator in blood: antithromboplastin. Am J Physiol 1947;149:123–129.

273. Hjort PF. Intermediate reactions in the coagulation of blood with tissue thromboplastin. Scand J Clin Lab Invest 1957;9:1–182.

274. Biggs R, MacFarlane RG. The reaction of hemophiliac plasma to thromboplastin. J Clin Invest 1951;4:445–459.

275. Biggs R, Nossel HL. Tissue extract and the contact reaction in blood coagulation. Thromb Diath Haemorrh 1961;6:1–14.

276. Carson SD. Plasma high density lipoproteins inhibit the activation of coagulation factor X by factor VIIa and tissue factor. FEBS Lett 1981;132:37–40.

277. Dahl PE, Abildgaard U, Larsen ML et al. Inhibition of activated coagulation factor VII by normal human plasma. Thromb Haemost 1982;48:253–256.

278. Marlar RA, Kleiss AJ, Griffin JH. An alternative extrinsic pathway of human blood coagulation. Blood 1982;60:1353–1358.

279. Morrison SA, Jesty J. Tissue factor-dependent activation of tritium-labeled factor IX and factor X in human plasma. Blood 1984;63:1338–1347.

280. Sanders NL, Bajaj SP, Zivelin A et al. Inhibition of tissue factor/factor VIIa activity in plasma requires factor X and an additional plasma component. Blood 1985;66:204–212.

281. Hubbard AR, Jennings CA. Inhibition of tissue thromboplastin-mediated blood coagulation. Thromb Res 1986;42:489–498.

282. Broze GJ Jr, Miletich JP. Characterization of the inhibition of tissue factor in serum. Blood 1987;69:150–155.

283. Rao LV, Rapaport SI. Studies of a mechanism inhibiting the initiation of the extrinsic pathway of coagulation. Blood 1987;69:645–651.

284. Hubbard AR, Jennings CA. Inhibition of the tissue factor-factor VII complex: involvement of factor Xa and lipoproteins. Thromb Res 1987;46:527–537.

285. Barrowcliffe TW, Eggleton CA, Stocks J. Studies of anti-Xa activity in human plasma. II: The role of lipoproteins. Thromb Res 1982;27:185–195.

286. Thomas DP, Barrowcliffe TW, Merton RE et al. In vivo release of anti-Xa clotting activity by a heparin analogue. Thromb Res 1980;17:831–840.

287. Broze GJ Jr, Miletich JP. Isolation of the tissue factor inhibitor produced by HepG2 hepatoma cells. Proc Natl Acad Sci U S A 1987;84:1886–1890.

288. Broze GJ Jr, Warren LA, Girard TJ et al. Isolation of the lipoprotein associated coagulation inhibitor produced by HepG2 (human hepatoma) cells using bovine factor Xa affinity chromatography. Thromb Res 1987;48:253–259.

289. Novotny WF, Girard TJ, Miletich JP et al. Purification and characterization of the lipoprotein-associated coagulation inhibitor from human plasma. J Biol Chem 1989;264:18832–18837.

290. Novotny WF, Palmier M, Wun TC et al. Purification and properties of heparin-releasable lipoprotein-associated coagulation inhibitor. Blood 1991;78:394–400.

291. Wun TC, Kretzmer KK, Girard TJ et al. Cloning and characterization of a cDNA coding for the lipoprotein-associated coagulation inhibitor shows that it consists of three tandem Kunitz-type inhibitory domains. J Biol Chem 1988;263:6001–6004.

292. Girard TJ, Warren LA, Novotny WF et al. Identification of the 1.4 kb and 4.0 kb messages for the lipoprotein associated coagulation inhibitor and expression of the encoded protein. Thromb Res 1989;55:37–50.

293. Kamei S, Kamikubo Y, Hamuro T et al. Amino acid sequence and inhibitory activity of rhesus monkey tissue factor pathway inhibitor (TFPI): Comparison with human TFPI. J Biochem 1994;115:708–714.

294. Girard TJ, Gailani D, Broze GJ Jr. Complementary DNA sequencing of canine tissue factor pathway inhibitor reveals a unique nanomeric repetitive sequence between the second and third Kunitz domains. J Biochem 1994;303:923–928.

295. Wesselschmidt RL, Girard TJ, Broze GJ Jr. cDNA sequence of rabbit LACI. Nucleic Acids Res 1990;18:6440.

296. Belaaouaj A, Kuppuswamy MN, Birktoft JJ et al. Revised cDNA sequence of rabbit tissue factor pathway inhibitor. Thromb Res 1993;69:547–553.

297. Enjyoji K, Emi M, Mukai T et al. cDNA cloning and expression of rat tissue factor pathway inhibitor (TFPI). J Biochem 1992;111:681–687.

298. van der Logt CP, Reitsma PH, Bertina RM. Intron-exon organization of the human gene coding for the lipoprotein-associated coagulation inhibitor: the factor Xa dependent inhibitor of the extrinsic pathway of coagulation. Biochemistry 1991;30:1571–1577.

299. Girard TJ, Eddy R, Wesselschmidt RL et al. Structure of the human lipoprotein-associated coagulation inhibitor gene. Intron/exon gene organization and localization of the gene to chromosome 2. J Biol Chem 1991;266:5036–5041.

300. van der Logt CP, Kluck PM, Wiegant J et al. Refined regional assignment of the human tissue factor pathway inhibitor (TFPI) gene to chromosome band 2q32 by non-isotopic in situ hybridization. Hum Genet 1992;89:577–578.

301. van der Logt CP, Reitsma PH, Bertina RM. A PstI RFLP of the LACI gene. Nucleic Acids Res 1990;18:5920.

302. Angel P, Baumann I, Stein B, Delius H et al. 12-O-tetradecanoyl-phorbol-13-acetate induction of the human collagenase gene is mediated by an inducible enhancer element located in the 5'-flanking region. Mol Cell Biol 1987;7:2256–2266.

303. Rana SV, Reimers HJ, Pathikonda MS et al. Expression of tissue factor and factor VIIa/tissue factor inhibitor activity in endotoxin or phorbol ester stimulated U937 monocyte-like cells. Blood 1988;71:259–262.

304. Ameri A, Kuppuswamy MN, Basu S et al. Expression of tissue factor and tissue factor pathway inhibitor by cultured endothelial cells in response to inflammatory mediators. Blood 1992;79:3219–3226.

305. Nakahara Y, Miyata T, Hamuro T et al. Amino acid sequence and carbohydrate structure of a recombinant human tissue factor pathway inhibitor expressed in Chinese hamster ovary cells: One N- and two O-linked carbohydrate chains are located between Kunitz domains 2 and 3 and one N-linked carbohydrate is in Kunitz domain 2. Biochemistry 1996;35:233–241.

306. Colburn P, Buonassisi V. Identification of an endothelial cell product as an inhibitor of tissue factor activity. In Vitro Cell & Dev Biol 1988;24:1133–1136.

307. Warn-Cramer BJ, Maki SL, Rapaport SI. A sulfated rabbit endothelial cell glycoprotein that inhibits factor VIIa/tissue factor is functionally and immunologically identical to rabbit extrinsic pathway inhibitor (EPI). Thromb Res 1991;61:515–527.

308. Smith PL, Skelton TP, Fiete D et al. The asparagine-linked oligosaccharides on tissue factor pathway inhibitor terminate with SO4-4GalNAc beta 1,4GlcNAc beta 1,2 Mana alpha.1 J Biol Chem 1992;267:19140–19146.

309. Girard TJ, McCourt D, Novotny WF et al. Endogenous phosphorylation of the lipoprotein-associated coagulation inhibitor at serine-2. J Biochem 1990;270:621–625.

310. Gustafson ME, Junger KD, Wun TC et al. Renaturation and purification of human tissue factor pathway inhibitor expressed in recombinant E. coli. Protein Expr Purif 1994;5:233–241.

311. Holst J, Lindblad B, Nordfang O et al. Does glycosylation influence the experimental antithrombotic effect of a two-domain tissue factor pathway inhibitor? Haemostasis 1996;26:23–30.

312. Laskowski MJ, Kato I. Protein inhibitors of proteinases. Annu Rev Biochem 1980;49:593–626.

313. Gebhard W, Tschesche H, Fritz H. Biochemistry of aprotinin and aprotinin-like inhibitors. In: Barrett AJ, Salvese G, eds. Protease Inhibitors. Amsterdam: Elsevier Science, 1986:375.

314. Girard TJ, Warren LA, Novotny WF et al. Functional significance of the Kunitz-type inhibitory domains of lipoprotein-associated coagulation inhibitor. Nature 1989;338:518–520.

315. Petersen LC, Bjorn SE, Olsen OH et al. Inhibitory properties of separate recombinant Kunitz-type inhibitor domains from tissue factor pathway inhibitor. Eur J Biochem 1996;235:310–316.

316. Hamamoto T, Kisiel W. Full-length human tissue factor pathway inhibitor inhibits human activated protein C in the presence of heparin. Thromb Res 1995;80:291–297.

317. Petersen LC, Bjorn SE, Nordfang O. Effect of leukocyte proteinases on tissue factor pathway inhibitor. Thromb Haemost 1992;67:537–541.

318. Wesselschmidt R, Likert K, Girard T et al. Tissue factor pathway inhibitor: the carboxyterminus is required for optimal inhibition of factor Xa. Blood 1992;79:2004–2010.

319. Wesselschmidt RI, Likert KM, Huang ZF et al. Structural requirements for tissue factor pathway inhibitor interactions with factor Xa and heparin. Blood Coagul Fibrinolysis 1993;4:661–669.

320. Lindhout T, Franssen J, Willems G. Kinetics of the inhibition of tissue factor-factor VIIa by tissue factor pathway inhibitor. Thromb Haemost 1995;74:910–915.

321. Higuchi DA, Wun TC, Likert KM et al. The effect of leukocyte elastase on tissue factor pathway inhibitor. Blood 1992;79:1712–1719.

322. Huang ZF, Wun TC, Broze GJ Jr. et al. Kinetics of factor Xa inhibition by tissue factor pathway inhibitor. J Biol Chem 1993;268:26950–26955.

323. van't Veer C, Hackeng TM, Delahaye C et al. Activated factor X and thrombin formation triggered by tissue factor on endothelial cell matrix in a flow model: effect of the tissue factor pathway inhibitor. Blood 1994;84:1132–1142.

324. Mast AE, Broze GJ Jr. Physiological concentrations of tissue factor pathway inhibitor do not inhibit prothrombinase. Blood 1996;87:1845–1850.

325. Enjyoji K, Miyata T, Kamikubo Y et al. Effect of heparin on the inhibition of factor Xa by tissue factor pathway inhibitor. A segment, Gly212-Phe243, in the third Kunitz domain is a heparin binding site. Biochemistry 1995;34:5725–5735.

326. Valentin S, Larnkjer A, Ostergaard P et al. Characterization of the binding between tissue factor pathway inhibitor and glycosaminoglycans. Thromb Res 1994;75:173–183.

327. Girard TJ, MacPhail LA, Likert KM et al. Inhibition of factor VIIa-tissue factor coagulation activity by a hybrid protein. Science 1990;248:1421–1424.

328. Warn-Cramer BJ, Rao LV, Maki SL et al. Rapaport SI. Modifications of extrinsic pathway inhibitor (EPI) and factor Xa that affect their ability to interact and to inhibit factor VIIa/tissue factor: evidence for a two-step model of inhibition. Thromb Haemost 1988;60:453–456.

329. Rao LVM, Ruf W. Tissue factor residues Lys165 and Lys166 are essential for rapid formation of the quaternary complex of tissue factor VIIa with Xa-tissue factor pathway inhibitor. Biochemistry 1995;34:10867–10871.

330. Jesty J, Wun TC, Lorenz A. Kinetics of the inhibition of factor Xa and the tissue factor-factor VIIa complex by the tissue factor pathway inhibitor in the presence and absence of heparin. Biochemistry 1994;33:12686–12694.

331. Hamamoto T, Kisiel W. The effect of heparin on the regulation of factor VIIa-tissue factor activity by tissue factor pathway inhibitor. Blood Coagul Fibrinolysis 1996;7:470–476.

332. Valentin S, Reutlingsperger CP, Nordfang O et al. Inhibition of factor X activation at extracellular matrix of fibroblasts during flow conditions: A comparison between tissue factor pathway inhibitor and inactive factor VIIa. Thromb Haemost 1995;74:1478–1485.

333. Petersen LC, Valentin S, Hedner U. Regulation of the extrinsic pathway system of health and disease: The role of factor VIIa and tissue factor pathway inhibitor. Thromb Res 1995;79:1–47.

334. Nordfang O, Bjorn SE, Valentin S et al. The C-terminus of tissue factor pathway inhibitor is essential to its anticoagulant activity. Biochemistry 1991;30:10371–10376.

335. Pedersen AH, Nordfang O, Norris F et al. Recombinant human extrinsic pathway inhibitor. Production, isolation, and characterization of its inhibitory activity on tissue factor-initiated coagulation reactions. J Biol Chem 1990;265:16786–16793.

336. Callander NS, Rao LV, Nordfang O et al. Mechanisms of binding of recombinant extrinsic pathway inhibitor (rEPI) to cultured cell surfaces. Evidence that rEPI can bind to and inhibit factor VIIa-tissue factor complexes in the absence of factor Xa. J Biol Chem 1992;267:876–882.

337. Girard TJ, Broze GJ Jr. Tissue factor pathway inhibitor. In: Lorand L, Mann KG eds. Methods in enzymology. Orlando: Academic Press, 1993:196–209.

338. Day KC, Hoffman LC, Palmier MO et al. Recombinant lipoprotein-associated coagulation inhibitor inhibits tissue thromboplastin-induced intravascular coagulation in the rabbit. Blood 1990;76:1538–1545.

339. Haskel EJ, Torr SR, Day KC et al. Prevention of arterial reocclusion after thrombolysis with recombinant lipoprotein-associated coagulation inhibitor. Circulation 1991;84:821–827.

340. Creasey AA, Chang AC, Feigen L et al. Tissue factor pathway inhibitor reduces mortality from Escherichia coli septic shock. J Clin Invest 1993;91:2850–2856.

341. Werling RW, Zacharski LR, Kisiel W et al. Distribution of tissue factor

pathway inhibitor in normal and malignant human tissues. Thromb Haemost 1993;69:366–369.

342. Hollister RD, Kisiel W, Hyman BT. Immunohistochemical localization of tissue factor pathway inhibitor-1 (TFPI-1), a Kunitz proteinase inhibitor, in Alzheimer's disease. Brain Res 1996;728:13–19.

343. Bajaj MS, Kuppuswamy MN, Leingang K et al. Transcriptional expression of tissue factor pathway inhibitor in normal human tissues. Blood 1993; 82:271a (abstract 1071).

344. Bajaj MS, Kuppuswamy MN, Saito H et al. Cultured normal human hepatocytes do not synthesize lipoprotein-associated coagulation inhibitor: evidence that endothelium is the principal site of its synthesis. Proc Natl Acad Sci U S A 1990;87:8869–8873.

345. McGee MP, Foster S, Wang X. Simultaneous expression of tissue factor and tissue factor pathway inhibitor by human monocytes. J Exp Med 1994; 179:1847–1854.

346. Bajaj MS, Ameri A, Kuppuswamy MN et al. Expression of tissue factor pathway inhibitor (TFPI) and GATA-2 transcription factor by activated human monocytes. Blood 1993;8:343a.

347. Lupu C, Lupu F, Dennehy U et al. Thrombin induces the redistribution and acute release of tissue factor pathway inhibitor from specific granules within human endothelial cells in culture. Arterioscler Thromb 1995;15: 2055–2062.

348. Yamabe H, Osawa H, Inuma H et al. Tissue factor pathway inhibitor production by human mesangial cells in culture. Thromb Haemost 1996;76: 215–219.

349. van der Logt CP, Dirven RJ, Reitsma PH et al. Expression of tissue factor and tissue factor pathway inhibitor in response to bacterial lipopolysaccharide and phorbol ester. Blood Coagul Fibrinolysis 1994;5:211–220.

350. Novotny WF, Girard TJ, Miletich JP et al. Platelets secrete a coagulation inhibitor functionally and antigenically similar to the lipoprotein associated coagulation inhibitor. Blood 1988;72:2020–2025.

351. Palmier MO, Hall LJ, Reisch CM et al. Clearance of recombinant tissue factor pathway inhibitor (TFPI) in rabbits. Thromb Haemost 1992;68: 33–36.

352. Bregengaard C, Nordfang O, Ostergaard P et al. Pharmacokinetics of full-length and two-domain tissue factor pathway inhibitor in combination with heparin in rabbits. Thromb Haemost 1993;70:454–457.

353. Warshawsky I, Broze GJ Jr, Schwartz AL. The low density lipoprotein receptor-related protein mediates the cellular degradation of tissue factor pathway inhibitor. Proc Natl Acad Sci U S A 1994;91:6664–6668.

354. Warshawsky I, Bu G, Mast A et al. The carboxyterminus of tissue factor pathway inhibitor is required for interacting with hepatoma cells *in vitro* and *in vivo*. J Clin Invest 1995;95:1773–1781.

355. Warshawsky I, Herz J, Broze GJ Jr et al. The low density lipoprotein receptor-related protein can function independently from heparan sulfate proteoglycans in tissue factor pathway inhibitor endocytosis. J Biol Chem 1996;271:25873–25879.

356. Valentin S, Schousboe I. Factor Xa enhances the binding of tissue factor pathway inhibitor to acidic phospholipids. Thromb Haemost 1996;75: 796–800.

357. Kojima T, Ksumi A, Yamazaki T et al. Human ryudocan from endothelium-like cells binds basic fibroblast growth factor, midkine, and tissue factor pathway inhibitor. J Biol Chem 1996;271:5914–5920.

358. Valentin S, Nordfang O, Bregengard C et al. Evidence that the C-terminus of tissue factor pathway inhibitor (TFPI) is essential for its *in vitro* and *in vivo* interaction with lipoproteins. Blood Coagul Fibrinolysis 1993;4: 713–720.

359. Narita M, Bu G, Olins GM et al. Two receptor systems are involved in the plasma clearance of tissue factor pathway inhibitor *in vivo*. J Biol Chem 1995;270:24800–24804.

360. Krieger M, Herz J. Structures and functions of multiligand lipoprotein receptors: Macrophage scavenger receptors and LDL receptor-related protein (LRP). Annu Rev Biochem 1994;63:601–637.

361. Willnow TE, Goldstein JL, Orth K et al. Low density in lipoprotein receptor-related protein and gp330 bind similar ligands, including plasminogen activator-inhibitor complexes and lactoferrin, an inhibitor of chylomicron remnant clearance. J Biol Chem 1992;267:26172–26180.

362. Ho G, Toomey JR, Broze GJ Jr et al. Receptor-mediated endocytosis of coagulation factor Xa requires cell surface-bound tissue factor pathway inhibitor. J Biol Chem 1996;271:9497–9502.

363. Kamikubo Y, Hamuro T, Matsuda J et al. The clearance of proteoglycan-associated human recombinant tissue factor pathway inhibitor (h-rTFPI) in rabbits: A complex formation of h-rTFPI with factor Xa promotes a clearance rate of h-rTFPI. Thromb Res 1996;83:161–175.

364. Brozna JP, Forman M, Carson SD. Staurosporine blocks down-regulation of monocyte-associated tissue factor. Blood Coagul Fibrinolysis 1994;5: 929–938.

365. Sandset PM, Abildgaard U, Larsen ML. Heparin induces release of extrinsic coagulation pathway inhibitor (EPI). Thromb Res 1988;50:803–813.

366. Novotny WF, Brown SG, Miletich JP et al. Plasma antigen levels of the lipoprotein-associated coagulation inhibitor in individual samples. Blood 1991;78:387–393.

367. Warr TA, Warn-Cramer BJ, Rao LV et al. Human plasma extrinsic pathway inhibitor activity: I. Standardization of assay and evaluation of physiologic variables. Blood 1989;74:201–206.

368. Lesnik P, Vonica A, Guerin M et al. Anticoagulant activity of tissue factor pathway inhibitor in human plasma is preferentially associated with dense subspecies of LDL and HDL and with Lp(a). Arterioscler Thromb 1993; 13:1066–1075.

369. Sandset PM, Lund H, Norseth J et al. Treatment with hydroxymethylglutaryl-coenzyme A reductase inhibitors in hypercholesterolemia induces changes in the components of the extrinsic coagulation system. Arterioscler Thromb 1991;11:138–145.

370. Hansen JB, Huseby NE, Sandset PM et al. Tissue factor pathway inhibitor and lipoproteins. Evidence for association with and regulation by LDL in human plasma. Arterioscler Thromb 1994;14:223–229.

371. Abumiya T, Nakamura S, Takenaka A et al. Response of plasma tissue factor pathway inhibitor to diet-induced hypercholesterolemia in crab-eating monkeys. Arterioscler Thromb 1994;14:483–488.

372. Hansen JB, Huseby KR, Huseby NE et al. Effect of cholesterol lowering on intravascular pools of TFPI and its anticoagulant potential in type II hyperlipoproteinemia. Arterioscler Thromb Vasc Biol 1995; 15:879–885.

373. Moor E, Hamsten A, Karpe F et al. Relationship of tissue factor pathway inhibitor activity to plasma lipoproteins and myocardial infarction at a young age. Thromb Haemost 1994;71:707–712.

374. Warn-Cramer BJ, Maki SL, Zivelin A et al. Partial purification and characterization of extrinsic pathway inhibitor (the factor Xa-dependent plasma inhibitor of factor VIIa/tissue factor). Thromb Res 1987;48:11–22.

375. Broze GJ Jr, Lange GW, Duffin KL et al. Heterogeneity of plasma tissue factor pathway inhibitor. Blood Coagul Fibrinolysis 1994;5:551–559.

376. Lesnik P, Dentan C, Vonica A et al. Tissue factor pathway inhibitor activity associated with LDL is inactivated by cell- and copper-mediated oxidation. Arterioscler Thromb Vasc Biol 1995;15:1121–1130.

377. Kokawa T, Abumiya T, Kimura T et al. Tissue factor pathway inhibitor activity in human plasma. Measurement of lipoprotein-associated and free forms in hyperlipidemia. Arterioscler Thromb 1995;15:504–510.

378. Abumiya T, Enjyoji K, Kokawa T et al. An anti-tissue factor pathway inhibitor (TFPI) monoclonal antibody recognizes the third Kunitz domain (K3) of free-form TFPI but not lipoprotein-associated forms in plasma. J Biochem 1995;118:178–182.

379. Hansen JB, Sandset PM, Huseby KR et al. Depletion of intravascular pools of tissue factor pathway inhibitor (TFPI) during repeated or continuous intravenous infusion of heparin in man. Thromb Haemost 1996;76: 703–709.

380. Holst J, Lindblad B, Bergqvist D et al. Effect of protamine sulfate on tissue factor pathway inhibitor released by iv or sc standard or low-molecular-weight heparin [Abstract]. Thromb Haemost 1993;69:1114.

381. Harenberg J, Siegele M, Dempfle CE et al. Protamine neutralization of the release of tissue factor pathway inhibitor activity by heparins. Thromb Haemost 1993;70:942–945.

382. Hubbard AR, Weller IJ, Gray E. Measurement of tissue factor pathway inhibitor in normal and post-heparin plasma. Blood Coagul Fibrinolysis 1994;5:819–823.

383. Sandset PM, Larsen ML, Abildgaard U et al. Chromogenic substrate assay of extrinsic pathway inhibitor (EPI): levels in the normal population and relation to cholesterol. Blood Coagul Fibrinolysis 1991; 2:425–433.

384. Reverdiau-Moalic P, Delahousse B, Body G et al. Evolution of blood coagulation activators and inhibitors in the healthy human fetus. Blood 1996; 88:900–906.

385. Sandset PM, Andersson TR. Coagulation inhibitor levels in pneumonia and stroke: changes due to consumption and acute phase reaction. J Intern Med 1989;225:311–316.

386. Sandset PM, Hogevold HE, Lyberg T et al. Extrinsic pathway inhibitor in elective surgery: a comparison with other coagulation inhibitors. Thromb Haemost 1989;62:856–860.

387. Abildgaard U, Sandset PM, Andersson TR et al. The inhibitor of F VIIa in plasma measured with a sensitive chromogenic substrate assay: comparison with antithrombin, protein C and heparin cofactor II in a clinical material. Folia Haematol 1988;115:274–277.

388. Lindahl AK, Sandset PM, Abildgaard U et al. High plasma levels of extrinsic pathway inhibitor and low levels of other coagulation inhibitors in advanced cancer. Acta Chir Scand 1989;155:389–393.

389. Kario K, Matsuo T, Yamada T et al. Increased tissue factor pathway inhibitor levels in uremic individuals on regular hemodialysis. Thromb Haemost 1994;71:275–279.

390. Sandset PM, Hellgren U, Uvebrandt M et al. Extrinsic pathway inhibitor and heparin cofactor II during normal and hypertension pregnancy. Thromb Res 1989;55:6645–6670.

391. Kobayashi M, Wada H, Wakita Y et al. Decreased plasma tissue factor pathway inhibitor levels in individuals with thrombotic thrombocytopenic purpura. Thromb Haemost 1995;73:10–14.

392. Warr TA, Rao LV, Rapaport SI. Human plasma extrinsic pathway inhibitor activity: II. Plasma levels in disseminated intravascular coagulation and hepatocellular disease. Blood 1989;74:994–998.

393. Takahashi H, Sato N, Shibata A. Plasma tissue factor pathway inhibitor in disseminated intravascular coagulation: Comparison of its behavior with plasma tissue factor. Thromb Res 1995;80:339–348.

394. Sandset PM, Roise O, Aasen AO et al. Extrinsic pathway inhibitor in postoperative/posttraumatic septicemia: increased levels in fatal cases. Haemostasis 1989;19:189–195.

395. Sandset PM, Sirnes PA, Abildgaard U. Factor VII and extrinsic pathway inhibitor in acute coronary disease. Br J Haematol 1989;72:391–396.

396. Abumiya T, Yamaguchi T, Terasaki T et al. Decreased plasma tissue factor pathway inhibitor activity in ischemic stroke individuals. Thromb Haemost 1995;74:1050–1054.

397. Holst J, Lindblad B, Wedeberg E et al. Tissue factor pathway inhibitor (TFPI) and its response to heparin in individuals with spontaneous deep vein thrombosis. Thromb Res 1993;72:467–470.

398. Llobet D, Falkon L, Mateo J et al. Low levels of tissue factor pathway inhibitor (TFPI) in two out of three members of a family with thrombophilia. Thromb Res 1995;80:413–418.

399. Sandset PM, Warn-Cramer BJ, Rao LV et al. Depletion of extrinsic pathway inhibitor (EPI) sensitizes rabbits to disseminated intravascular coagulation induced with tissue factor: evidence supporting a physiologic role for EPI as a natural anticoagulant. Proc Natl Acad Sci U S A 1991;88:708–712.

400. Sandset PM, Warn-Cramer BJ, Maki SL et al. Immunodepletion of extrinsic pathway inhibitor sensitizes rabbits to endotoxin-induced intravascular coagulation and the generalized Shwartzman reaction. Blood 1991;78:1496–1502.

401. Warn-Cramer BJ, Rapaport SI. Studies of factor Xa/phospholipid induced intravascular coagulation in rabbits. Effects of immunodepletion of tissue factor pathway inhibitor. Arterioscler Thromb 1993;13:1551–1557.

402. Huang ZF, Higuchi DA, Lasky N et al. Tissue-factor pathway inhibitor (TFPI) gene-deletion in mice produces intrauterine lethality. Blood 1996;88:470a.

403. Sprecher CA, Kisiel W, Amathewes S et al. Molecular cloning, expression, and partial characterization of a second human tissue-factor-pathway inhibitor. Proc Natl Acad Sci U S A 1994;91:3353–3357.

404. Bohn H, Winckler W. Isolierung und charakterisierung des plazenta-proteins PP5. (Isolation and characterization of the placental protein pp5 [author's transl]) Arch Gyneco 1977;223:179–186.

405. Rice A, Chard T. A method for the purification of placental protein 5 (PP5) from placental extracts. Clin Chim Acta 1983;131:289–294.

406. Rao CN, Reddy P, Liu Y et al. Extracellular matrix-associated serine protease inhibitors (Mr 33,000, 31,000, and 27,000) are single-gene products with differential glycosylation: cDNA cloning of the 33-kDa inhibitor reveals its identity to tissue factor pathway inhibitor-2. Arch Biochem Biophys 1996;335:82–92.

407. Miyagi Y, Koshikawa N, Yasumitsu H et al. cDNA cloning and mRNA expression of a serine proteinase secreted by cancer cells: identification as placental protein 5 and tissue factor pathway inhibitor. J Biochem 1994;116:939–942.

408. Petersen LC, Sprecher CA, Foster DC et al. Inhibitory properties of a novel human Kunitz-type protease inhibitor homologous to tissue factor pathway inhibitor. Biochemistry 1996;35:266–272.

409. Butzow R, Alfthan H, Stenman UH et al. Immunofluorometric demonstration and quantification of placental protein 5 in the absence of pregnancy. Clin Chem 1988;34:1591–1593.

410. Menabawey M, Silman R, Rice A et al. Dramatic increase in placental protein 5 levels following injection of small doses of heparin. Br J Obstet Gynaecol 1985;92:207–210.

411. Broze GJ Jr. Tissue factor pathway inhibitor and the revised theory of coagulation. Annu Rev Med 1995;46:103–112.

412. Monroe DM, Roberts HM, Hoffman M. Platelet procoagulant complex assembly in a tissue factor-initiated system. Br J Haematol 1994;88:364–371.

413. Hoffman M, Monroe DM, Oliver JA et al. Factors IXa and Xa play distinct roles in tissue factor-dependent initiation of coagulation. Blood 1995;86:1794–1801.

414. Rand MD, Lock JB, van't Veer C et al. Blood clotting in minimally altered whole blood. Blood 1996;88:3432–3445.

415. Naito K, Fujikawa K. Activation of human blood coagulation factor XI independent of factor XII. Factor XI is activated by thrombin and factor XI a in the presence of negatively charged surfaces. J Biol Chem 1991;266:7353–7358.

416. Gailani D, Broze GJ Jr. Factor XI activation in a revised model of blood coagulation. Science 1991;253:909–912.

417. Bajzar L, Manuel R, Nesheim ME. Purification and characterization of TAFI, a thrombin-activatable fibrinolysis inhibitor. J Biol Chem 1995;270:14477–14484.

418. Broze GJ Jr, Higuchi DA. Coagulation-dependent inhibition of fibrinolysis: Role of carboxypeptidase-U and the premature lysis of clots from hemophilic plasma. Blood 1996;88:3815–3823.

419. von dem Borne PA, Meijers JC, Bouma BN. Feedback activation of factor XI by thrombin in plasma results in additional formation of thrombin that protects fibrin clots from fibrinolysis. Blood 1995;86:3035–3042.

420. Asakai R, Chung DW, Davie EW et al. Factor XI deficiency in Ashkenazi Jews in Israel. N Engl J Med 1991;325:153–158.

421. Berliner S, Horowitz I, Martinowitz U et al. Dental surgery in individuals with severe factor XI deficiency without plasma replacement. Blood Coagul Fibrinolysis 1992;3:465–468.

422. Colucci M, Balconi G, Lorenzet R et al. Cultured human endothelial cells generate tissue factor in response to endotoxin. J Clin Invest 1983;71:1893–1896.

423. Rivers RP, Hathaway WE, Weston WL. The endotoxin-induced coagulant activity of human monocytes. Br J Haematol 1975;30:311–316.

424. Bevilacqua MP, Pober JS, Majeau GR et al. Interleukin 1 (IL-1) induces biosynthesis and cell surface expression of procoagulant activity in human vascular endothelial cells. J Exp Med 1984;160:618–623.

425. Carlsen E, Flatmark A, Prydz H. Cytokine-induced procoagulant activity in monocytes and endothelial cells. Further enhancement by cyclosporine. Transplantation 1988;46:575–580.

426. Conkling PR, Greenberg CS, Weinberg JB. Tumor necrosis factor induces tissue factor-like activity in human leukemia cell line U937 and peripheral blood monocytes. Blood 1988;72:128–133.

427. Bevilacqua MP, Pober JS, Majeau GR et al. Recombinant tumor necrosis factor induces procoagulant activity in cultured human vascular endothelium: characterization and comparison with the actions of interleukin 1. Proc Natl Acad Sci U S A 1986;83:4533–4537.

428. Scheibenbogen C, Moser H, Krause S et al. Interferon-gamma-induced expression of tissue factor activity during human monocyte to macrophage maturation. Haemostasis 1992;22:173–178.

429. Brox JH, Osterud B, Bjorklid E et al. Production and availability of thromboplastin in endothelial cells: the effects of thrombin, endotoxin and platelets. Br J Haematol 1984;57:239–246.

430. Lyberg T, Galdal KS, Evensen SA et al. Cellular cooperation in endothelial cell thromboplastin synthesis. Br J Haematol 1983;53:85–95.

431. Lyberg T, Prydz H. Phorbol esters induce synthesis of thromboplastin activity in human monocytes. Biochem J. 1981;194:699–706.

432. van Ginkel CJ, van Akin WG, Oh JI et al. Stimulation of monocyte procoagulant activity by adherence to different surfaces. Br J Haematol 1977;37:35–45.

433. Key NS, Vercellotti GM, Winkelmann JC et al. Infection of vascular endothelial cells with herpes simplex virus enhances tissue factor activity and reduces thrombomodulin expression. Proc Natl Acad Sci U S A 1990;87:7095–7099.

434. van Ginkel CJ, Thorig L, Thompson J et al. Enhancement of generation of monocyte tissue thromboplastin by bacterial phagocytosis: possible pathway for fibrin formation on infected vegetations in bacterial endocarditis. Infect Immun 1979;25:388–395.

435. Levy GA, Leibowitz JL, Edgington TS. Induction of monocyte procoagulant activity by murine hepatitis virus type 3 parallels disease susceptibility in mice. J Exp Med 1981;154:1150–1163.

436. Drake TA, Pang M. Staphylococcus aureus induces tissue factor expression in cultured human cardiac valve endothelium. J Infect Dis 1988;157:749–756.

437. Teysseire N, Arnoux D, George F et al. von Willebrand factor release and thrombomodulin and tissue factor expression in Rickettsia conorii-infected endothelial cells. Infect Immun 1992;60:4388–4393.

438. Penrod G, Polack B, Peyron F et al. Monocyte tissue factor expression induced by Plasmodium falciparum-infected erythrocytes. Thromb Haemost 1992;68:111–114.

439. Sporn LA, Haidaris PJ, Shi RJ et al. Rickettsia rickettsii infection of cultured human endothelial cells induces tissue factor expression. Blood 1994;83:1527–1534.

440. Mazure G, Grundy JE, Nygard G et al. Measles virus induction of human endothelial cell tissue factor procoagulant activity *in vivo*. J Gen Virol 1994;75:2863–2871.

441. Bancsi MJ, Thompson J, Bertina RM. Stimulation of monocyte tissue factor expression in an *in vitro* model of bacterial endocarditis. Infect Immun 1994;62:5669–5672.

442. Prydz H, Allison AC, Schorlemmer HU. Further link between complement activation and blood coagulation. Nature 1977;270:173–174.

443. Galdal KS. Thromboplastin synthesis in endothelial cells. Haemostasis 1984;14:378–385.

444. Tannenbaum SH, Finko R, Cines DB. Antibody and immune complexes induce tissue factor production by human endothelial cells. J Immunol 1986;137:1532–1537.

445. Prydz H, Lyberg T, Deteix P et al. *In vitro* stimulation of tissue thromboplastin (factor III) activity in human monocytes by immune complexes and lectins. Thromb Res 1979;15:465–474.

446. Kornberg A, Blank M, Kaufman S et al. Induction of tissue factor-like activity in monocytes by anti-cardiolipin antibodies. J Immunol 1994;153:1328–1332.

447. Branch DW, Rodgers GM. Induction of endothelial cell tissue factor activity by sera from individuals with antiphospholipid syndrome: a possible mechanism of thrombosis. Am J Obstet Gynecol 1993;168:206–210.

448. Rothberger H, Zimmerman TS, Vaughan JH. Increased production and

expression of tissue thromboplastin-like procoagulant activity *in vitro* by allogeneically stimulated human leukocytes. J Clin Invest 1978;62:649–655.

449. van Ginkel CJ, Zeijlemaker WP, Stricker LA et al. Enhancement of monocyte thromboplastin activity by antigenically stimulated lymphocytes: a link between immune reactivity and blood coagulation. Eur J Immunol 1981;11:579–583.

450. Cermak J, Key NS, Bach RR et al. C-reactive protein induces human peripheral blood monocytes to synthesize tissue factor. Blood 1993;82: 513–520.

451. Lesnik P, Rouis M, Skarlatos S et al. Uptake of exogenous free cholesterol induces up-regulation of tissue factor expression in human monocyte-derived macrophages. Proc Natl Acad Sci U S A 1992;89:10370–10374.

452. Levy GA, Schwartz BS, Curtiss LK et al. Plasma lipoprotein induction and suppression of the generation of cellular procoagulant activity *in vitro*. J Clin Invest 1981;67:1614–1622.

453. Schuff-Werner P, Claus G, Armstrong VW et al. Enhanced procoagulatory activity (PCA) of human monocytes/macrophages after *in vitro* stimulation with chemically modified LDL. Atherosclerosis 1989;78:109–112.

454. Drake TA, Hannani K, Fei HH et al. Minimally oxidized low-density lipoprotein induces tissue factor expression in cultured human endothelial cells. Am J Pathol 1991;138:601–607.

455. Crutchley DJ, Que BG. Copper-induced tissue factor expression in human monocytic THP-1 cells and its inhibition by antioxidants. Circulation 1995; 92:238–243.

456. Golino P, Ragni M, Cirillo P et al. Effects of tissue factor induced by oxygen free radicals on coronary flow during reperfusion. Nat Med 1996;2:35–40.

457. Faucette KJ, Parker CJ, McCluskey T et al. Induction of tissue factor activity in endothelial cells and monocytes by a modified form of albumin present in normal human plasma. Blood 1992;79:2888–2895.

458. Esposito C, Gerlach H, Brett J et al. Endothelial receptor-mediated binding of glycose-modified albumin is associated with increased monolayer permeability and modulation of cell surface coagulant properties. J Exp Med 1989;170:1387–1407.

459. Ernofsson M, Siegbahn A. Platelet-derived growth factor-BB and monocyte chemotactic protein-1 induce human peripheral blood monocytes to express tissue factor. Thromb Res 1996;83:307–320.

460. Clauss M, Murray JC, Vianna M et al. A polypeptide factor produced by fibrosarcoma cells that induces endothelial tissue factor and enhances the procoagulant response to tumor necrosis factor/cachectin. J Biol Chem 1990;265:7078–7083.

461. Clauss M, Gerlach M, Gerlach H et al. Vascular permeability factor: a tumor-derived polypeptide that induces endothelial cell and monocyte procoagulant activity, and promotes monocyte migration. J Exp Med 1990; 172:1535–1545.

462. Celi A, Pellegrini G, Lorenzet R et al. P-selectin induces the expression of tissue factor on monocytes. Proc Natl Acad Sci U S A 1994;91:8767–8771.

463. Fan ST, Mackman N, Cui MZ et al. Integrin regulation of an inflammatory effector gene. Direct induction of the tissue factor promoter by engagement of beta 1 or alpha 4 integrin chains. J Immunol 1995;154:3266–3274.

464. Fibach E, Treves A, Korenberg A et al. *In vitro* generation of procoagulant activity by leukemic promyelocytes in response to cytotoxic drugs. Am J Hematol 1985;20:257–265.

465. Wheeler HR, Geczy CL. Induction of macrophage procoagulant expression by cisplatin, daunorubicin and doxorubicin. Int J Cancer 1990;46:626–632.

466. Walsh J, Wheeler HR, Geczy CL. Modulation of tissue factor on human monocytes by cisplatin and adriamycin. Br J Haematol 1992;81:480–488.

467. Rambaldi A, Alessio G, Casali B et al. Induction of monocyte-macrophage procoagulant activity by transformed cell lines. J Immunol 1986:136: 3848–3855.

468. Murray JC, Clauss M, Denekamp J et al. Selective induction of endothelial cell tissue factor in the presence of a tumour-derived mediator: a potential mechanism of flavone acetic acid action in tumour vasculature. Int J Cancer 1991;49:254–259.

469. Yang HL, Lu FJ, Wung SL et al. Humic acid induces expression of tissue factor by cultured endothelial cells: regulation by cytosolic calcium and protein kinase C. Thromb Haemost 1994;71:325–330.

470. Kornberg A, Catane R, Peller S et al. Tuftsin induces tissue factor-like activity in human mononuclear cells and in monocytic cell lines. Blood 1990;76:814–819.

471. Levy GA, Schwartz BS, Edgington TS. The kinetics and metabolic requirements for direct lymphocyte induction of human procoagulant monokines by bacterial lipopolysaccharide. J Immunol 1981;127:357–363.

472. Edwards RL, Rickles FR, Bobrove AM. Mononuclear cell tissue factor: cell of origin and requirements for activation. Blood 1979;54:359–370.

473. Gregory SA, Kornbluth RS, Helin H et al. Monocyte procoagulant inducing factor: a lymphokine involved in the T cell-instructed monocyte procoagulant response to antigen. J Immunol 1986;137:3231–3239.

474. Del Prete G, De Carli M, Lammel RM et al. Th1 and T-helper cells exert opposite regulatory effects on procoagulant activity and tissue factor production by human monocytes. Blood 1995;86:250–257.

475. Johnsen UL, Lyberg T, Galdal KS et al. Platelets stimulate thromboplastin synthesis in human endothelial cells. Thromb Haemost 1983;49:69–72.

476. Kucey DS, Kubicki EI, Rotstein OD. Platelet-activating factor primes endotoxin-stimulated macrophage procoagulant activity. J Surg Res 1991;50: 436–441.

477. Fan ST, Edgington TS. Coupling of the adhesive receptor CD11b/CD18 to functional enhancement of effector macrophage tissue factor response. J Clin Invest 1991;87:50–57.

478. Zuckerman SH, Suprenant YM. Augmentation of procoagulant activity in monokine stimulated human endothelial cells by calmodulin/protein kinase C inhibitors. Thromb Res 1988;49:205–214.

479. Boeri D, Almus FE, Maiello M et al. Modification of tissue-factor mRNA and protein response to thrombin and interleukin 1 by high glucose in cultured human endothelial cells. Diabetes 1989;38:212–218.

480. Roth RI. Hemoglobin enhances the production of tissue factor by endothelial cells in response to bacterial endotoxin. Blood 1994;83:2860–2865.

481. Kaneko H, Kakkar VV, Scully MF. Mercury compounds induce a rapid increase in procoagulant activity of monocyte-like U937 cells. Br J Haematol 1994;87:87–93.

482. Collins PW, Noble KE, Reittie JR et al. Induction of tissue factor expression in human monocyte/endothelium cocultures. Br J Haematol 1995;91: 963–970.

483. Silverman MD, Manalopoulos VG, Unsworth BR et al. Tissue factor expression is differentially modulated by cyclic mechanical strain in various human endothelial cells. Blood Coagul Fibrinolysis 1996;7:281–288.

484. Muhlfelder TW, Khan I, Niemetz J. Factors influencing the release of procoagulant-tissue factor activity from leukocytes. J Lab Clin Med 1978;92: 65–72.

485. Lale A, Herbert JM. Polyunsaturated fatty acids reduce pyrogen-induced tissue factor expression in human monocytes. Biochem Pharmacol 1994; 48:429–431.

486. Crutchley DJ, Conanan LB, Que BG. K+ channel blockers inhibit tissue factor expression by human monocytic cells. Circ Res 1995;76:16–20.

487. Ernofsson M, Tenno T, Siegbahn A. Inhibition of tissue factor surface expression in human peripheral blood monocytes exposed to cytokines. Br J Haematol 1996;95:249–257.

488. van Ginkel CW, Oh JI, Vreeken J et al. Monocyte production of thromboplastin activity in inflammatory and malignant disease. Leukocytes and Blood Coagulation. Amsterdam. Chapter Vi, Thesis.

489. Thiagarajan P, Niemetz J. Procoagulant-tissue factor activity of circulating peripheral blood leukocytes. Results of *in vivo* studies. Thromb Res 1980; 17:891–896.

490. Shelly WB, Juhlin L. Fibrin star. JAMA 1982;247:3066.

491. Edwards RL, Levine JB, Green R et al. Activation of blood coagulation in Crohn's disease. Increased plasma fibrinopeptide A levels and enhanced generation of monocyte tissue factor activity. Gastroenterology 1987;92: 329–337.

492. Cole EH, Schulman J, Urowitz M et al. Monocyte procoagulant activity in glomerulonephritis associated with systemic lupus erythematosus. J Clin Invest 1985;75:861–868.

493. de Prost D, Ollivier V, Ternisien C et al. Increased monocyte procoagulant activity independent of the lupus anticoagulant in individuals with systemic lupus erythematosus. Thromb Haemost 1990;64:216–221.

494. Osterud B, Flaegstad T. Increased tissue thromboplastin activity in monocytes of individuals with meningococcal infection: related to an unfavourable prognosis. Thromb Haemost 1983;49:5–7.

495. Rivers RP, Cattermole HE, Wright I. The expression of surface tissue factor apoprotein by blood monocytes in the course of infections in early infancy. Pediatr Res 1992;31:567–573.

496. Rothberger H, Dove FB, Lee TK et al. Procoagulant activity of lymphocyte-macrophage populations in rabbits: selective increases in marrow, blood, and spleen cells during Shwartzman reactions. Blood 1983;61:712–717.

497. Miller CL, Graziano C, Lim RC et al. Generation of tissue factor by individual monocytes: correlation to thromboembolic complications. Thromb Haemost 1981;46:489–495.

498. Osterud B, Due J Jr. Blood coagulation in individuals with benign and malignant tumours before and after surgery. Special reference to thromboplastin generation in monocytes. Scand J Haematol 1984;32:258–264.

499. Blakowski SA, Zacharski LR, Beck JR. Postoperative elevation of human peripheral blood monocyte tissue factor coagulant activity. J Lab Clin Med 1986;108:117–120.

500. Ollivier V, Sheibani A, Chollet MS et al. Monocyte procoagulant activity and membrane-associated D dimer after knee replacement surgery. Thromb Res 1989;55:179–185.

501. Leatham EW, Bath PM, Tooze JA et al. Increased monocyte tissue factor expression in coronary disease. Br Heart J 1995;73:10–13.

502. Jude B, Watel A, Fontaine O et al. Distinctive features of procoagulant response of monocytes from diabetic individuals. Haemostasis 1989; 19:65–73.

503. Edwards RL, Rickles FR, Cronlund M. Abnormalities of blood coagulation in individuals with cancer. Mononuclear cell tissue factor generation. J Lab Clin Med 1981;98:917–928.

504. Gonmori H, Maekawa T, Kobayashi N et al. The role of tissue thromboplastin in the development of DIC accompanying neoplastic diseases. Bibl Haematol 1983;49:23–39.

505. Lando PA, Edgington TS. An innate host response to the neoplastic cell:

syngeneic rat tumor cells can elicit a rapid *de novo* lymphoid procoagulant response. J Immunol 1985;135:3587–3595.

506. Morgan D, Edwards RL, Rickles FR. Monocyte procoagulant activity as a peripheral marker of clotting activation in cancer individuals. Haemostasis 1988;18:55–65.

507. Halloran P, Aprile M, Haddad G et al. The significance of elevated procoagulant activity in the monocytes of renal transplant recipients. Transplant Proc 1982;14:669–672.

508. Cole EH, Cardella CJ, Schulman J et al. Monocyte procoagulant activity and plasminogen activator. Role in human renal allograft rejection. Transplantation 1985;40:363–371.

509. Rothberger H, Meredith J, Mutton T et al. Increased tissue factor activity generation *in vitro* by canine blood leukocytes associated with allogeneic kidney transplantation and rejection. Thromb Haemost 1985;53:1–4.

510. Montemurro P, Lattanzio A, Chetta G et al. Increased *in vitro* and *in vivo* generation of procoagulant activity (tissue factor) by mononuclear phagocytes after intralipid infusion in rabbits. Blood 1985;65:1391–1395.

511. Wakefield A, Cohen Z, Rosenthal A et al. Thrombogenicity of total parenteral nutrition solutions: II. Effect on induction of endothelial cell procoagulant activity. Gastroenterology 1989;97:1220–1228.

512. Pradier O, Surquin M, Stordeur P et al. Monocyte procoagulant activity induced by *in vivo* administration of the OKT3 monoclonal antibody. Blood 1996;87:3768–3774.

513. Cole EH, Sweet J, Levy GA. Expression of macrophage procoagulant activity in murine systemic lupus erythematosus. J Clin Invest 1986;78:8879–893.

514. Semeraro N, Montemurro P, Giordano D et al. Increased macrophage procoagulant activity but normal endothelial thrombomodulin in rabbits fed an atherogenic diet. Haemostasis 1990;20:54–61.

515. Hattler BJ, Rocklin RE, Ward PA et al. Functional features of lymphocytes recovered from a human renal allograft. Cell Immunol 1973;9:289–296.

516. Rothberger H, Barringer M, Meredith J. Increased tissue factor activity of monocytes/macrophages isolated from canine renal allografts. Blood 1984;63:623–628.

517. Holdsworth SR, Tipping PG. Macrophage-induced glomerular fibrin deposition in experimental glomerulonephritis in the rabbit. J Clin Invest 1985;76:1367–1374.

518. Tipping PG, Holdsworth SR. The participation of macrophages, glomerular procoagulant activity, and factor VIII in glomerular fibrin deposition. Studies on anti-GBM antibody-induced glomerulonephritis in rabbits. Am J Pathol 1986;124:10–17.

519. Tipping PG, Lowe MG, Holdsworth SR. Glomerular macrophages express augmented procoagulant activity in experimental fibrin-related glomerulonephritis in rabbits. J Clin Invest 1988;82:1253–1259.

520. Lorenzet R, Peri G, Locati D et al. Generation of procoagulant activity by mononuclear phagocytes: a possible mechanism contributing to blood clotting activation within malignant tissues. Blood 1983;62:271–273.

521. Drake TA, Rogers GM, Sande MA. Tissue factor is a major stimulus for vegetation formation in enterococcal endocarditis in rabbits. J Clin Invest 1984;73:1750–1753.

522. Tipping PG, Malliaros J, Holdsworth SR. Procoagulant activity expression by macrophages from atheromatous vascular plaques. Atherosclerosis 1989;79:237–243.

523. Kato K, Elsayed YA, Namoto M et al. Enhanced expression of tissue factor activity in the atherosclerotic aortas of cholesterol-fed rabbits. Thromb Res 1996;82:334–347.

524. Chapman HAJ, Allen CL, Stone OL et al. Human alveolar macrophages synthesize factor VII *in vitro*. Possible role in interstitial lung disease. J Clin Invest 1985;75:2030–2037.

525. Rothberger H, McGee MP, Lee TK. Tissue factor activity. A marker of alveolar macrophage maturation in rabbits. Effects of granulomatous pneumonitis. J Clin Invest 1984;73:1524–1531.

526. Idell S, Gonzalez K, Bradford H et al. Procoagulant activity in bronchoalveolar lavage in the adult respiratory distress syndrome. Contribution of tissue factor associated with factor VII. Am Rev Respir Dis 1987;136:1466–1474.

527. Seeger W, Hubel J, Klapettek K et al. Procoagulant activity in bronchoalveolar lavage of severely traumatized individuals-relation to the development of acute respiratory distress. Thromb Res 1991;61:53–64.

528. Semeraro N, De Lucia O, Lattanzio A et al. Procoagulant activity of human alveolar macrophages: different expression in individuals with lung cancer. Int J Cancer 1986;37:525–529.

529. Callahan KS, Griffith DE, Garcia JG. Asbestos exposure results in increased lung procoagulant activity *in vivo* and *in vitro*. Chest 1990;98:112–119.

530. McGee MP, Devlin R, Saluta G et al. Tissue factor and factor VII messenger RNAs in human alveolar macrophages: effects of breathing ozone. Blood 1990;75:122–127.

# CHAPTER 5

# CONTACT ACTIVATION

Alvin H. Schmaier

## INTRODUCTION

The kallikrein-kinin system was first recognized as a plasma and tissue proteolytic system responsible for the liberation of the vasoactive proinflammatory mediator, bradykinin (BK) (1). BK, a nonapeptide released from kininogens by kallikrein, can reproduce many of the characteristics of an inflammatory state such as changes in local blood pressure, edema, and pain resulting in vasodilation and increased microvessel permeability. In 1975, three individuals were described with a deficiency of high-molecular-weight kininogen (HK), which is the precursor of BK; these three individuals also had a prolonged activated partial thromboplastin time (aPTT) (2–4). Even although none of these individuals had a hemorrhagic state, the focus of studies in the plasma kallikrein-kinin system was altered to define the procoagulant property of HK Deficiency of factor XII and prekallikrein, which are two related zymogens required for the enzymatic cleavage of HK to yield BK, does not lead to bleeding. These plasma proteins were grouped as the "contact system" because they required contact with artificial negatively-charged surfaces for zymogen activation *in vitro*. Many investigators in hemostasis have considered this proteolytic system unimportant because the deficiencies of these proteins does not lead to a bleeding state and *in vitro* activation of this system requires artificial negatively-charged surfaces. However, recent evidence indicates the elusive physiologic, negatively-charged surface for contact system activation is the assembly of these proteins on endothelial cell membranes and activation of prekallikrein by an endothelial cell membrane protease, which is independent of factor XII. Thus, contact activation and the

contact system are really misnamed descriptions of this group of proteins, and the erroneous description arises from an incomplete understanding of how these constituents assemble to be activated and regulated *in vivo*. Furthermore, by ignoring that deficiencies of these proteins prolong the aPTT without being associated with bleeding and by observing the activities of the contact proteins, the reader will realize these proteins alone and when assembled are anti-thrombotic and profibrinolytic agents that contribute to the constitutive anticoagulant environment of the intravascular compartment.

## STRUCTURE-FUNCTION CHARACTERISTICS OF THE CONTACT SYSTEM

The structure and function of the three proteins, HK, prekallikrein (PK), and factor XII (FXII) will be considered. Other proteins will be referred to only as they interact with these three constituents.

### HIGH-MOLECULAR-WEIGHT KININOGEN (WILLIAMS, FITZGERALD TRAIT)

#### Gene Expression and Regulation

The two forms of plasma kininogen, HK and low-molecular-weight kininogen (LK), are the products of a single gene (5, 6). This gene maps to 3q26-qter, which is the location of the homologous $\alpha_2$HS-glycoprotein and histidine-rich glycoprotein (7–9). The single kininogen gene of 11 exons consisting of 27 kb produces a unique mRNA

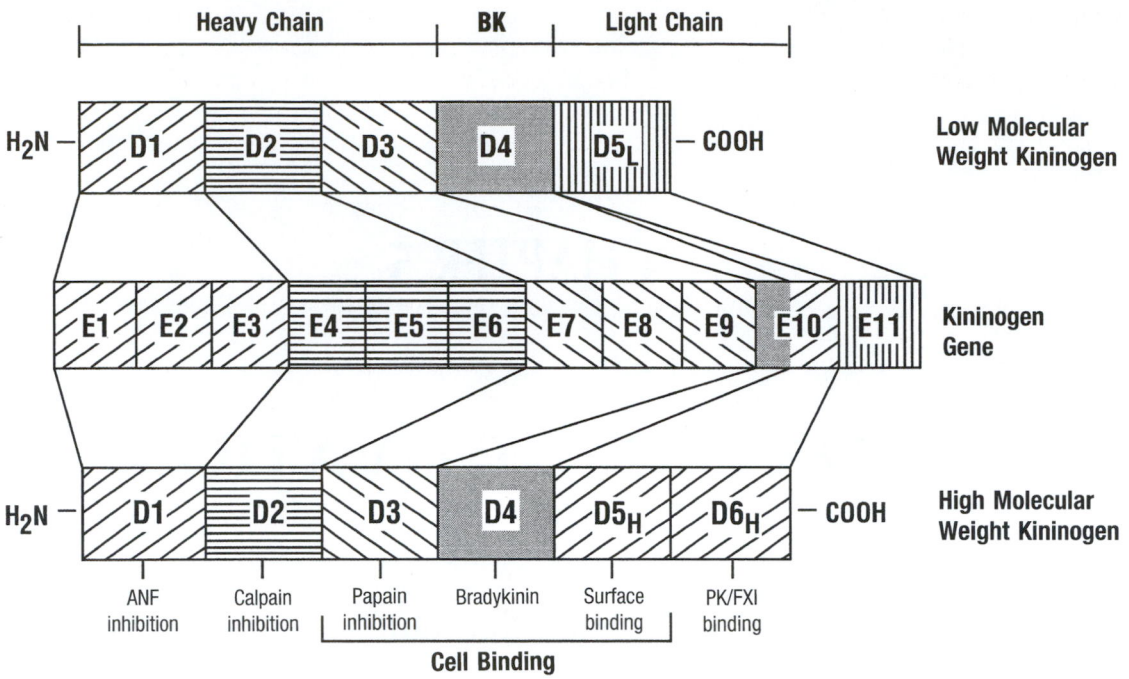

**FIGURE 5.1.** The domain structure of the kininogens. The kininogens are produced by one gene with 11 exons (E1–E11). E1–E3 codes for domain 1 (D1) on both HK (high-molecular-weight kininogen) and LK (low-molecular-weight kininogen). Parts of domain 1 inhibit atrial naturetic factor. E4–E6 codes for domain 2 (D2), which has papain and unique calpain inhibitory sequences. E7–E9 codes for domain 3 (D3), which has papain inihibitory sequences. Domain 4 (D4) is coded by part of E10; it is the bradykinin sequence on kininogens and the first 12 amino acids of the light chains of HK and LK. The remainder of E10 codes for HK's light chain, which consists of domain 5 (D5$_H$) and domain 6 (D6$_H$). D5$_H$ is an artificial surface binding region; D6$_H$ has the prekallikrein and factor XI binding regions. Domains 3, 4, and 5 on HK also participate in cell binding. E11 codes for the remainder of the unique light chain of LK (D5$_L$).

for HK and LK by alternative splicing (Fig. 5.1) (6). HK and LK share the coding region of the first nine exons, a part of exon 10 containing the BK sequence, and the first 12 amino acids after the carboxyterminal sequence of BK. Exon 11 codes for a unique 4 Kda light chain of LK. Complete exon 10 contains the full coding sequence for the unique 56 Kda light chain of HK. HK is produced from exon 10 through a process of alternative RNA processing events. A novel mechanism occurs for alternative RNA processing in the rat kininogen gene (10). Splicing efficiency is controlled by the interaction of U1 small nuclear ribonucleoprotein and the U1 small nuclear RNA (snRNA)-complementary repetitive sequences of the kininogen pre-mRNA. The mRNA for LK and HK are 1.7 and 3.5 kb, respectively.

The molecular basis for homozygous total kininogen deficiency, Williams trait, has been determined (11). Finding no gross DNA deletion or insertion by Southern blot, a C to T transition at nucleotide 587 occurred, which changed a CGA (Arg) codon to TGA (Stop) mutation in exon 5 and resulted in the prevention of HK and LK synthesis (11). The phenotype of this defect is similar to that seen in Brown-Norway Katholiek rats that have absent plasma kininogen;

however, the defect in the rats is the result of a single point mutation, Ala$_{163}$Thr, which results in defective secretion from the liver (12). Little is known about what regulates gene expression of kininogen. In the rat, ovariectomy results in a reduction of kininogen transcripts in the liver, while estrogens increase kininogen mRNA levels (13). This result is consistent with the clinical observation that HK concentrations increase during pregnancy (14). In contrast, progesterone treatment reduces kininogen gene expression, which results in a slight reduction of plasma kininogen levels (15). Murine fibroblasts synthesize and secrete kininogen in response to cyclic AMP, forskolin, prostaglandin E$_2$, and tumor necrosis factor α (15). Similarly, tumor necrosis factor α has been recognized to increase kininogen expression in Hep G2 cells (16). Little else is known to influence kininogen levels because this aspect of kininogen metabolism has not been studied extensively.

## Protein Chemistry and Structure of Kininogen

The two mRNAs of the kininogen code for two separate proteins (Fig. 5.1). LK is a 66 Kda β-globulin with a plasma concentration of 160 μg/ml (2.4 μM) and an isoelectric point of 4.7 (17, 18). HK is a 120 Kda α-globulin with a plasma concentration of 80 μg/ml (0.67 μM) and an isoelectric point of 4.3 (18, 19). Human liver is a source for cDNA for both kininogens (5, 6), but human umbilical vein endothelial cells have been shown to contain HK mRNA and synthesize the protein (20). Kininogen antigen also has been found in platelets, granulocytes, renal tubular cells, and skin (19–24). LK was also known as $\alpha_1$-cysteine protease inhibitor until its cloning (25). HK and LK are globular proteins. LK gel filters at 66 Kda and behaves as a true globular protein; HK, although 120 Kda, gel filters at 220 Kda, which indicates a high axial ratio (Fig. 5.1). Physical evidence for HK being a complex of globular units was obtained through electron microscopy studies (26). On electron microscopy, HK appeared to be a linear array of three linked centralized globular regions with the two ends thinly connected (26). Cleavage of HK through plasma kallikrein leads to a striking change in conformation in HK The central globular region is separated after bradykinin liberation and rearranged with the cysteine protease inhibitory region opposite the prekallikrein binding region (26). The regions of kininogen are divided into domains (Fig. 5.1). Serine protease sensitive regions separate these domains (27–29). Contiguity of these domains is important for several biologic functions of kininogen such as calpain inhibition and HK and LK binding to endothelial cells (30–32). Alternatively, disruption of the contiguity of HK develops a new function, i.e., its cell antiadhesive activity (33). The major activity of kininogen, which is to deliver bradykinin, is the programmed disruption of protein since bradykinin is not active as a biologic peptide unless liberated from its precursor.

## Domain Structure of Kininogen

The kininogens are proteins composed of multiple domains, each with associated specific activities (Fig. 5.1). Although each domain of the protein has specific activity(ies), the protein as a whole participates in biologic processes. One function of the kininogen that is facilitated by binding to cell receptors is that bradykinin can be liberated in a defined environment where the peptide can bind to bradykinin receptors and influence local cellular responses. Thus, one can view each function of the domains of the kininogen as participating in the whole protein's kinin delivery activity. The kininogen can be divided into three portions: the heavy chain, which is common to HK and LK; the bradykinin moiety; and the light chains, which are unique to HK and LK (Fig. 5.1). Domains 1–3 consists of kininogen's heavy chain. Little is known about the function of domain 1 except it has a low-affinity calcium binding site (34), and the role of this calcium binding site is

unknown. Although calcium ion is important for phorbol 12-myristate 13-acetate up-regulation of LK and heavy chain binding to endothelial cells (35), no reliable evidence exists that calcium ion participates in HK binding to cells (31, 36) (contrary to the work of other laboratories [37, 38]). Recent evidence also indicates domain 1 may have some inhibitory activity against atrial naturetic peptide (39).

Domains 2 and 3 contain the highly conserved amino acid sequence, QVVAG, found in cysteine protease inhibitors (27). LK and HK are potent, tight-binding, reversible cysteine protease inhibitors with $K_i$s of 2 and 0.5 nM, respectively, for platelet calpain (18, 40). Domain 2 is the calpain inhibitory region on kininogen (28, 30, 40). Calpain is inhibited by domain 2, whereas papain and cathepsin L are effectively inhibited by domains 2 and 3 (27, 30). A peptide containing $Q_{170}VVAG_{174}$ blocks HK inhibition of calpain, and thus functions as a binding site (Fig. 5.2). A peptide C-terminal, C211-C227, is a direct inhibitor of calpain (IC$_{50}$ = 35 μM). The two probably form a continuous binding site. A third peptide (V128-L138) N-terminal to the QVVAG region inhibited papain, but not calpain, which indicates the inhibitory sites of domain 2 for the two cysteine protease are overlapping but not identical. In contrast, the optimal inhibition of cathepsin B and H requires three loops of domain 3 (41, 42). Although inhibitors of cysteine protease, kininogen are also substrates of this class of enzyme when a molar excess of enzyme to inhibitor is present (44, 45). Since kininogen are extracellular or contained within granules in platelets and granulocytes, it is unclear how kininogen interact with cellular cysteine protease, which are mostly bound to internal membrane or cytosolic in location (19, 21, 44). However, when platelets are activated, calpain translocates to the external membrane where it could be inhibited by HK in plasma or in externalized platelet α-granule HK (44, 46, 47).

Domain 3 has other functions (Fig. 5.2). The finding that LK and its isolated heavy chain bind to platelets and endothelial cells indicates a cell binding region exists on the kininogen heavy chain (35, 48, 49). This is confirmed by direct studies using isolated and recombinant domain 3, which contain the heavy chain cell–binding region on platelets (50) and neutrophils (51). Using a computerized model of domain 3 based upon the crystalline structure of cystatin (52), the sequential amino acid structure of domain 3 was drawn to show three surface-exposed regions: a disulfide loop connecting it to domain 2 and two hairpin loops. The cysteine protease inhibitory region of domain 3 consists of these three loops. We sought to determine which of these three surface-exposed loops was the domain 3 cell binding site(s) for endothelial cells (43). Synthetic peptides of these surface-exposed regions, $K_{244}ICVGCPRDIP_{254}$

# High Molecular Weight Kininogen

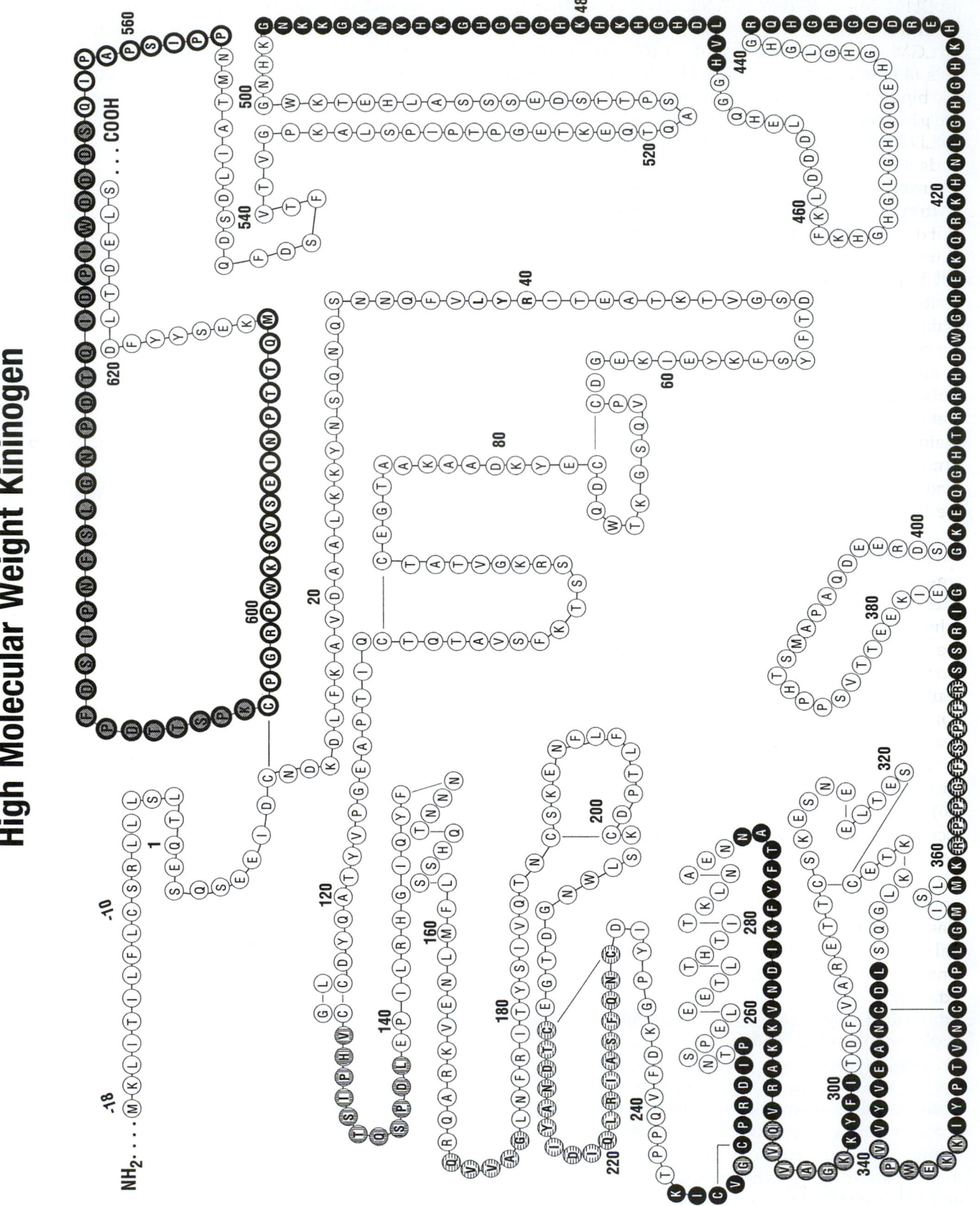

(KIC11), $N_{276}$ATFYFKIDNVKKARVQVVAGKKYFI$_{301}$ (NAT26), and $L_{331}$DCNAEVYVVPWEKKIY-PTVNC-QPLGM$_{357}$ (LDC27) inhibit HK binding to endothelial cells (43). KIC11, NAT26, and LDC27 inhibited biotin-HK binding to endothelial cells with IC$_{50}$'s of 1000 $\mu$M, 258 $\mu$M, and 60 $\mu$M, respectively. The minimal sequence in LDC27 required to inhibit binding was 13 amino acids, $C_{333}$NAEVYVVPWEKK$_{345}$ (IC$_{50}$ = 113 $\mu$M) (53). A similar peptide also blocked binding of [$^{125}$I]-HK to neutrophils. In addition, preliminary evidence indicates that domain 3 may contain an additional site for binding to neutrophils, Leu$_{271}$-Ala$_{277}$ (54). Since papain blocked HK binding to endothelial cells, the cysteine protease inhibitory site overlaps with the cell binding site on domain 3. Thus, the last 27 amino acids of domain 3, which are contiguous to domain 4, the bradykinin region, are an endothelial cell binding site. Thrombospondin (TSP), a platelet $\alpha$-granule protein secreted upon platelet stimulation, also binds to HK both to a site on the heavy chain requiring calcium ions and to the light chain independent of calcium ions (53). TSP's interaction with kininogen heavy chain may be on domain 3 overlapping the KIC11 sequence (53).

The last function ascribed to domain 3 was $\alpha$-thrombin inhibitory activity (48, 50, 55). Inhibition of $\alpha$-thrombin–induced platelet activation was shown using isolated domain 3 prepared by tryptic digestion of LK in solution (50). The thrombin inhibitory region was not the same as the platelet binding region because one monoclonal antibody, which did not block cell binding, neutralized HK's ability to inhibit $\alpha$-thrombin's activation of platelets (50). Further investigations have revealed, however, that the $\alpha$-thrombin inhibitory region on kininogens is not one of the cell binding regions described in the previous paragraph (43, 56). Hasan et al (56) suggest the thrombin inhibitory activity previously ascribed to domain 3, which is prepared by proteolytic cleavage, is really domain 4 or the kinin moiety remaining attached to domain 3 (56). Bradykinin is liberated from its parent protein in three ways when pure or plasma HK is cleaved by plasma kallikrein on an artificial surface (57, 58). The first cleavage yields a "nicked" kininogen composed of two disulfide-linked 64 and 56 Kda chains. The second cleavage yields bradykinin (0.9 Kda) and an intermediate kinin-free protein of approximately similar molecular weight to "nicked" HK. The third cleavage results in a stable kinin-free protein composed of two disulfide-linked 64 and 46 Kda chains.

However, this sequence does not necessarily occur when kininogens are cleaved in solution without a surface, and bradykinin can remain attached to heavy or light chain kininogen (59). Trypsin-cleaved LK and domain 3 prepared by tryptic digestion have the bradykinin moiety attached to LK's heavy chain and isolated domain 3 (32). Bradykinin and its analogs have been shown to be inhibitors of $\alpha$-thrombin–induced platelet aggregation by preventing $\alpha$-thrombin from cleaving its cloned receptor (i.e., PAR1) (56).

Domain 4, which is the bradykinin region, has many functions assigned to this nanopeptide in addition to its newest function, which is $\alpha$-thrombin inhibition (56). It is beyond the scope of this review to discuss the many functions of bradykinin except to say that its activity is supportive of the antithrombin-profibrinolytic activity of its parent proteins, the kininogens. In the liberation of bradykinin, HK is a better substrate of plasma kallikrein and LK is a better substrate of tissue kallikrein. However, both kininogens are substrates for both forms of kallikrein. Factor XIIa cleaves HK similarly to plasma kallikrein (60). Factor XIa initially cleaves HK into 76 and 46 Kda bands. The 46 Kda light chain of HK is proteolyzed into smaller inactive fragments upon prolonged exposure to factor XIa (61). Elastase treatment of LK renders the protein a better substrate of plasma kallikrein to liberate bradykinin and Met-Lys-bradykinin (62), but it destroys HK's procoagulant activity. Cathepsin D inactivates kininogen's cysteine protease inhibitory activity (63). Domain 4 also serves as a cell binding region (65). The carboxyterminal portion of bradykinin and the aminoterminal portion of kininogen's common light chain participate by providing a low-affinity ($K_d$ = 1 mM) binding site for endothelial cells. The importance of the domain 4 cell binding region is not its isolated affinity to the cell surface, but its ability to hold kininogen's in the proper conformation for optimal cell binding (26). For example, intact HK binds to endothelial cells with a $K_d$ of 7 nM and $1 \times 10^7$ molecules/cell versus kinin-free kininogen, which binds to endothelial cells with a $K_d$ of 30 nM and $1–2.6 \times 10^6$ molecules/cell (31, 65). These different data for intact or kinin-free HK's interaction with biologic surfaces are not surprising considering the major change in the shape of HK that occurs when it is cleaved on an artificial surface (26).

LK's light chain is 4 Kda and consists of one domain (D5$_L$) whose function is unknown. HK's light chain is

**FIGURE 5.2.**   The structure of high-molecular-weight kininogen. An amino acid sequence diagram of high-molecular-weight kininogen. ◍ represents a papain inhibitory domain. ⊜ represents a calpain inhibitory domain. ● represents a cell surface binding domain. ◓ represents overlapping papain inhibitory activity and cell surface binding activity. ◒ represents bradykinin. ○ represents the factor XI binding domain. ● represents overlapping prekallikrein and factor XI binding domain.

56 Kda and consists of two domains, which are domains 5 ($D5_H$) and 6 (Figs. 5.1 and 5.2). HK's domain 5 has also been shown to have another cell binding site. Initial investigations showed that $D5_H$ serves as an additional cell binding site on platelets, granulocytes, and endothelial cells (35, 49, 51, 66). Two areas of $D5_H$ were found to participate in cell binding (67). One is on the aminoterminal end of the domain and consists of sequences $G_{402}$KEQGHTRRHDWGHEKQRK$_{420}$ (GKE19) and $H_{421}$NLGHGHKHERDQGH-GHQRGH$_{441}$ (HNL21). These peptides inhibit biotin-HK binding with $IC_{50}$'s of 792 μM and 215 μM, respectively. The other region is on the carboxyterminal region of $D5_H$. It consists of two overlapping peptides $H_{479}$KHGHGHGKHKNKGKKNGKH$_{498}$ (HKH20) and $H_{471}$VLDHGHKHKHGHGHGKHKNKGKK$_{494}$ (HVL-24), which inhibit HK binding with $IC_{50}$'s of 0.23 μM and 0.8 μM, respectively (67). Independent of its cell binding region, $D5_H$ has been recognized as HK's artificial surface binding region (28, 64, 68). $D5_H$'s histidine- and glycine-rich regions have the ability to bind to anionic surfaces, zinc, and heparin (68–70). A 7.3 Kda peptide (57 amino acids), which was isolated on an immunoaffinity column with an antibody that neutralized HK coagulant activity, was identified as $H_{441}$-$K_{497}$ (28, 68). This peptide inhibits coagulant activity and can bind to anionic surfaces with an $IC_{50}$ = 30 μM. $D5_H$ contains two histidine- and glycine-rich regions, one on its carboxyterminal side, which is also rich in lysine ($H_{457}$-$K_{502}$) similar to HKH20, and the other on its aminoterminal side ($K_{420}$-$H_{458}$), which is similar to HNL21. Using a deletion mutagenesis strategy on $D5_H$, the anionic surface–binding region was found to be associated with both histidine-glycine-rich regions of $D5_H$ (64). Either region can support coagulant activity when it is associated with D6 (64). Synthetic peptides HKH20 and HVL24, which comprise its high-affinity cell–binding regions on the carboxyterminal region of $D5_H$, also inhibit the procoagulant activity of HK (Fig. 5.2) (67). No other peptides from $D5_H$ inhibit procoagulant activity and endothelial cell membrane–binding. Further, a polyclonal antibody raised to HKH20 prolongs the procoagulant activity of HK in plasma (67). These data indicate the endothelial cell and the artificial surface binding region on HK are overlapping within the same highly conserved domain (67). Peptide HKH20 and its parent HK have the additional ability to interact with M protein on *Staphylococcus pyogenes* (71). The highest affinity

cell–binding site for $D5_H$ is the artificial surface binding site. Efforts by many researchers during the last two decades to characterize HK binding to artificial surfaces indicate the location of HK's cell binding site. This fact is important because HK binding modulates prekallikrein activation. Lastly, when HK is bradykinin free, the residual kinin-free kininogen has the ability to prevent vitronectin's adhesive interaction with tumor cells, endothelial cells, platelets, and monocytes (33). This property is much weaker in intact non-proteolyzed HK This result was anticipated by the finding that the resulting kinin-free kininogen binds much more tightly to anionic surfaces than the uncleaved HK following the cleavage of bradykinin from HK (72).

HK's domain 6 has prekallikrein (residues 556–595) and factor XI binding sites (residues 556–613) (73–75). Prekallikrein's affinity for its binding site on the light chain of HK is approximately 17 nM (76, 77). The prekallikrein and factor XI binding sites consist of a 31-residue sequence that contains predominantly β-turn elements (78). An N-terminally and C-terminally truncated 27-mer (residue 569–95) has the essential structural elements for prekallikrein binding (79, 80). HK's procoagulant activity depends on two activities: the ability to bind to anionic surfaces via $D5_H$ and the ability to bind prekallikrein and factor XI to domain 6. Inhibition of either interaction with monoclonal antibodies directed to these regions will inhibit HK's procoagulant activity (28, 81, 82). HK's domain 6 also serves as the acceptor protein for factor XI and prekallikrein binding to platelets, neutrophils, and endothelial cells (37, 83, 84).

## PREKALLIKREIN (FLETCHER FACTOR)

Prekallikrein (PK) is produced by a single gene that maps to chromosome 4 (85). PK's gene structure is similar to that of factor XI (86). Its mRNA codes for a 371 amino acid heavy chain and a 248 amino acid light chain, which are held together by a disulfide bond (86). The amino acid sequence of PK has 58% homology to factor XI (86). The protein has four tandem repeats in the aminoterminal portion of the molecule due to the linking of the first and sixth, second and fifth, and third and fourth half cysteine residues present in each repeat (Fig. 5.3). This arrangement results in four groups of 90 or 91 amino acids that are arranged in "apple domains" (87, 88). These same structures have been de-

**FIGURE 5.3.** The structure of prekallikrein. The letters $A_1$ to $A_4$ represent the apple domains of prekallikrein's heavy chain. The notation "Factor XIIa" and arrow at arginine$_{371}$ represents the factor XIIa activation site on prekallikrein. Histidine$_{415}$, aspartic acid$_{464}$, and serine$_{559}$ represent kallikrein's catalytic active site. ● represents the regions involved in binding to high molecular weight kininogen. This figure is adapted from McMullen and associates (Ref #88).

# Prekallikrein

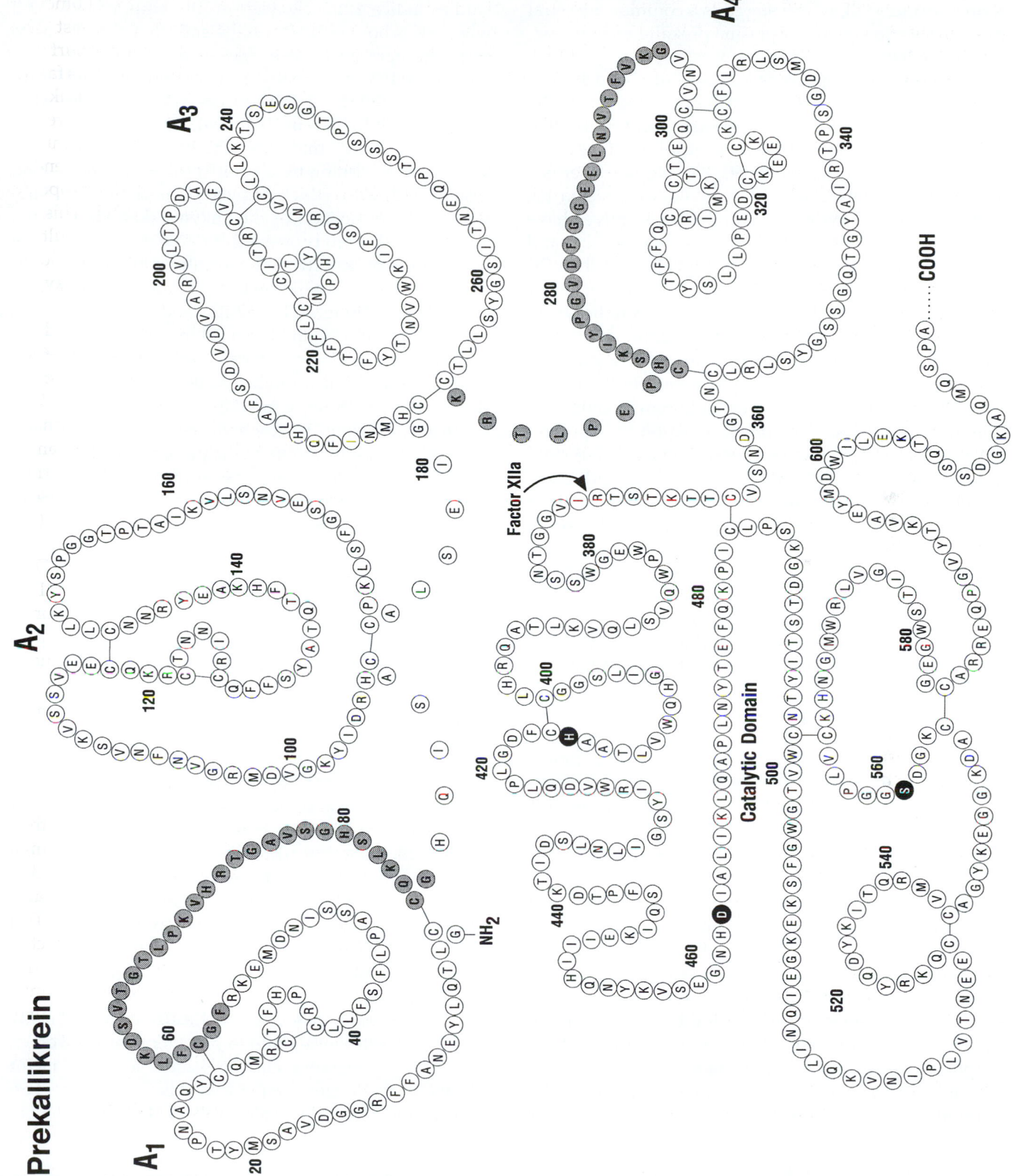

scribed in factor XI, which suggests a common ancestral gene duplication event for plasma prekallikrein and factor XI (85, 89).

In plasma, PK appears as a doublet of 85 and 88 Kda, whether or not the protein has undergone reduction (90, 91). PK is a fast γ-globulin (isoelectric point = 8.5–9.0) in plasma, with a circulating concentration estimated at 35–50 μg/ml (0.41–0.56 μM) (92, 93). Human liver is a source for PK cDNA (87). In liver disease, plasma PK is decreased (92). Women on oral contraceptives have increased PK levels, but women in their second and third trimesters of pregnancy do not (14, 92). When PK is activated to kallikrein (α-kallikrein) by either factor XIIa or factor XII fragments, the protein on reduced sodium dodecyl sulfate (SDS) gel electrophoresis has two subunits: a heavy chain of approximately 52 Kda and two light chains variants of approximately 36 and 33 Kda (90, 91). The active site of kallikrein is contained within its light chain because this region incorporates tritiated diisopropyl fluorophosphate in a covalent linkage with serine$_{559}$ (Fig. 5.3) (94). Histidine$_{415}$ and aspartic acid$_{464}$ comprise the other two amino acids involved in catalytic activity (Fig. 5.3). Prolonged incubation of kallikrein with itself results in autodigestion of its heavy chain into 33 and 20 Kda bands, as seen on reduced SDS gel electrophoresis, to yield β-kallikrein (95). These cleavages occur through the tandem repeats in the heavy chain and result in a protein that cleaves HK more slowly and fails to activate neutrophils or induce the secretion of elastase (87, 96). Immunoblot assay of artificial surface–activated plasma shows kallikrein in complex with α$_2$-macroglobulin (α$_2$M) and C1 inhibitor and the appearance of a 50 Kda prekallikrein/kallikrein fragment containing a portion of the native protein's heavy chain (14). At least 75% of PK circulates bound, noncovalently, to HK (97). The binding regions on PK for HK are on apple domains 1 (F56-G86) and 4 (K266-G295) (Fig. 5.3) (98–102).

The *in vitro* conversion of human plasma PK to activated kallikrein is catalyzed by activated factor XII on a surface augmented by HK or by Hageman factor fragment (βFXIIa) in the fluid phase (94). Prekallikrein will not become activated on an artificial surface without factor XII. It is because of this finding that this system is called the contact system. A single bond (Arg$_{371}$-Ile$_{372}$) is split and generates a heavy chain of 371 amino acids still linked to a light chain by a single disulfide bridge without a change in molecular weight. However, recent

studies indicate this cleavage occurs without factor XII when PK is bound to HK on the endothelial cell surface (84). The light chain of kallikrein reacts with protease inhibitors (103), principally α$_2$-macroglobulin and C1 inhibitor (C1-INH). C1-INH forms a 1:1 stoichiometric complex with kallikrein (104–108), which results in loss of proteolytic and amidolytic activity. HK protects kallikrein from inhibition by C1-INH and α$_2$M in a purified system (103, 108), which suggests a mechanism of substrate (HK) protection of the enzyme (kallikrein) from active site–directed protease inhibitors. α$_2$M inhibits the kinin-forming activity and partially inhibits the amidolytic activity of kallikrein by forming a covalent complex (106). Although C1 inhibitor and α$_2$M account for an equal amount of kallikrein inhibition in plasma, C1 inhibitor in plasma acts more rapidly than α$_2$M (109). Antithrombin III also inhibits kallikrein, but it does so slowly, even with heparin (110). Heparin, which binds to HK (68, 70), significantly accelerates the inhibition of kallikrein by antithrombin in the presence of HK Protein C inhibitor is also a potent inhibitor of kallikrein (111, 112). The major protein substrates of plasma kallikrein are factor XII, HK, and prourokinase (113, 114).

## FACTOR XII (HAGEMAN FACTOR)

Factor XII is produced by a single gene that maps to chromosome 5 (115, 116). The gene for factor XII is 12 kb comprised of 13 introns and 14 exons (117). Factor XII has multiple domains with extensive sequence homology to regions of tissue-type plasminogen activator (t-PA) (the epidermal growth factor [EGF]-like region and the kringle region) and fibronectin (Fig. 5.4) (117–119). The factor XII intron/exon gene structure is similar in organization to the serine protease family of t-PA and urokinase-type plasminogen activator (u-PA) genes, which are different from most other coagulation protein genes (117). Its 2.4 kb messenger RNA (mRNA) codes for a 596 amino acid, single chain β-globulin with a molecular mass of 80–90 Kda and an isoelectric point of 6.1–6.5 (120). Its concentration in plasma is estimated to be 30 μg/ml (0.375 μM) (range 15–47 μg/ml) (121, 122). Human liver is a source for factor XII DNA (118), and cultured rat hepatocytes synthesize factor XII (123). In humans, estrogens given to postmenopausal women and during pregnancy elevate plasma levels of factor XII, and its expression is enhanced in isolated livers of estrogen- and prolactin-treated rats (124–126). Rat liver

**FIGURE 5.4.** The structure of factor XII. Proteolysis at arginines 334, 343, and 353 (See arrows) result in activated factor XII (β-factor XIIa). The catalytic triad of factor XIIa consists of histidine$_{393}$, aspartic acid$_{442}$, and serine$_{544}$. ⬤ represents the artificial surface binding domains on factor XII's heavy chain. ◉ represent two of factor XII's zinc binding domains. This figure is adapted from Cool and MacGillivray (Ref# 117).

# FACTOR XII

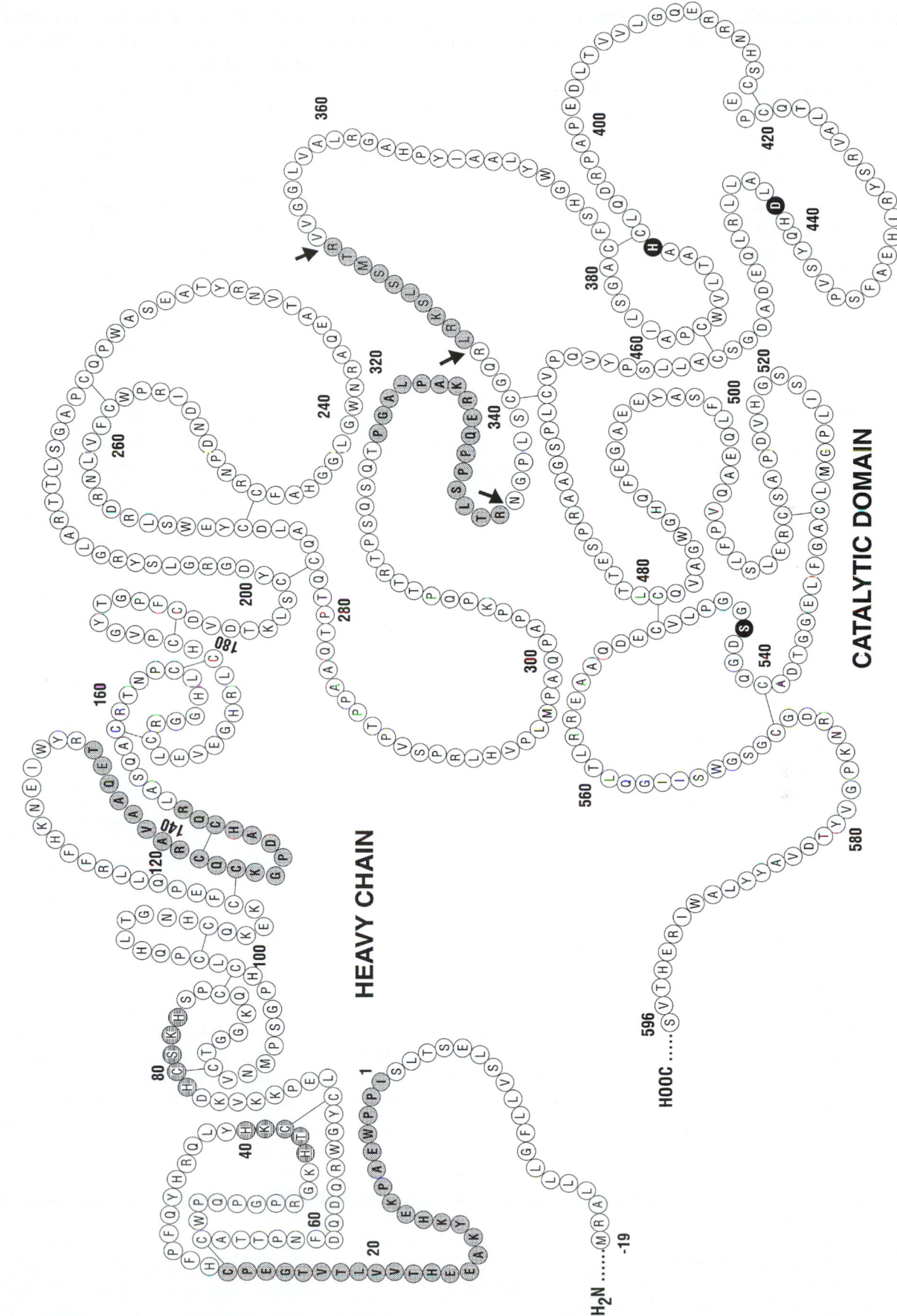

**HEAVY CHAIN**

**CATALYTIC DOMAIN**

DNA has been shown to have a functional estrogen regulatory element contained in its 5′ untranslated region, which is modulated by 17β-estradiol (127). Factor XII, which contains an EGF domain, enhances HepG2 cell proliferation and thymidine and leucine incorporation, which suggests that it is a mitogen for these cells (128). Factor XII functions through its EGF domain as a mitogen and stimulates a signal transduction pathway by a mitogen-induced protein kinase (129). This activity is independent of activated factor XII's proteolytic activities.

Factor XII can be divided into two regions, a heavy chain and a light chain (Fig. 5.4). The heavy chain contains two artificial surface binding regions, one at its aminoterminus (I1-C28) and another on its fibronectin type I region (T134-R153) (130, 131). Recent studies using recombinant deletion mutants of factor XII confirm these findings and also indicate that another region on factor XII's heavy chain, on the second EGF-like or kringle domain (P313-R334, L344-R353), also participates in artificial surface binding (132). Factor XII is autoactivated (solid phase activation) upon contact with negatively-charged surfaces (133). Binding to the surface and the cleavage during autoactivation results in distinct, defined conformational changes (134). Plasma proteases, including plasma kallikrein and plasmin, activate factor XII (FXII) to factor XIIa (αFXIIa), which cleaves the bond connecting $Arg_{353}$-$Val_{354}$, and generates a two-chain molecule composed of a heavy chain (353 residues) and a light chain (243 residues) held together by a disulfide bond (118). The light chain of factor XIIa is a typical serine protease containing the canonical $Asp_{412}$, $His_{393}$, $Ser_{554}$ and is the site for inhibition by its major plasma inhibitor, C1-inhibitor (135). Hageman factor fragments or factor XII fragments (FXIIf, bFXIIa) (Mr = 30 Kda) are produced by further proteolytic cleavage, which results in a chain of 243 residues expressing catalytic activity attached to a fragment of the former heavy chain by a single disulfide bond. Defects in the light chain of factor XII result in disorders of the enzymatic activity of the protein. Coagulation factor XII Washington DC has a $Cys_{571}Ser$ substitution, which results in complete loss of procoagulant activity (136). Coagulation factor XII Bern is a protein, which is unable to activate factor XI or prekallikrein when it is kallikrein-cleaved (137). Contact activation arises from the activation of factor XII on negatively-charged surfaces or by addition of a protease that produced enzymatic cleavage. These two mechanisms have been referred to as solid- and fluid-phase activation, respectively (138).

The activation of factor XII that arises from binding with negatively-charged surfaces (138, 139–141) is termed autoactivation (142–147). The autoactivation phenomena of factor XII is probably an *in vitro* event arising from working with this protein on artificial surfaces. No evidence exists that it occurs *in vivo*. Nonphysi-

ologic substances with a negative surface charge that activate factor XII include glass, kaolin, celite, dextran sulfate, ellagic acid, and bismuth subgallate (148–150). Furthermore, factor XII, like other plasma proteins, is adsorbed onto biomedical polymers such as Dacron, polyethylene, silicone rubber, polytetrafluoroethylene, and polydimethylsiloxane (151). Biologic components that are exposed in pathophysiologic situations that can induce factor XII activation include articular cartilage (149), skin (152), fatty acids (153, 154), endotoxin (155), sodium urate crystals (156), calcium pyrophosphate, L-homocysteine (157), hematin (158), and protoporphyrin (159). Physiologic, negatively-charged surfaces of cell membranes include sulfatides (cerebroside sulfates), heparins, chondroitin sulfate E, and other glycosaminoglycans (159–165). It is also possible that a wide range of substances, including phosphatidylserine, phosphatidylglycerol, phosphatidic acid, and phosphatidylinositol under certain conditions, can promote factor XII activation (166). Although many physiologic, negatively-charged surfaces can be associated *in vitro* with factor XII autoactivation, the concept of autoactivation has never been a sufficiently convincing mechanism to explain activation of factor XII and associated contact system activation. It is unclear whether the activity of factor XII arises from a conformational change in the protein when it binds to a negatively-charged surface or if autoactivation is simply an *in vitro* event resulting from autocatalysis of small quantities of activated factor XII contaminating zymogen factor XII used in the experiments. Some evidence suggests that $Zn^{2+}$ binding to factor XII induces a conformational change that makes the protein more susceptible for development of enzymatic activity when associated with negatively-charged surfaces (167–169). Four zinc binding sites exist, two of which have been identified (H40-H44, H78-H82) (Fig. 5.4) (170). Alternative mechanisms have been sought for factor XII activation *in vivo*. A rabbit endothelial cell activator of factor XII has been described, but no corresponding example in humans have been found (171). Other studies indicate that incubation of zymogen factor XII with human umbilical vein endothelial cells does not result in human factor XII activation (unpublished). However, assembly of PK bound to HK on human umbilical vein endothelial cells results in PK activation independent of factor XII by a cell-associated membrane proteinase (84). Furthermore, factor XII activation by this pathway can occur secondary to PK activation.

Enzymatic activation of factor XII gives rise to successively smaller proteins, each with the same active site serine. Activation of zymogen factor XII by plasma kallikrein, trypsin, or plasmin results in a smaller-sized enzyme, a decrease in its surface-binding properties, and a decrease in its coagulant activity. Two major forms of activated Hageman factor: factor XIIa (α-HFa, HFa, or α XIIa) exist, an 80 Kda protein that consists of two disulfide-linked polypeptide chains and factor XIIf (Hageman factor fragments, HFf, β-HFa, β XIIa), which is a 28-30 Kda fragment derived from factor XIIa (172–176). The 80 Kda form of activated factor XII has the ability to bind to negatively-charged surfaces and to activate factor XI (131, 132). The 28–30 Kda enzymatic form of factor XII has no surface-binding properties but retains its ability to activate prekallikrein and C1 (138, 177, 178).

The major plasma protease inhibitor of activated factor XIIa and XIIf is C1 inhibitor, which accounts for more than 90% of the inhibition of these proteases in plasma (179–182). C1 inhibitor will bind both proteins and irreversibly inactivate them. Factor XIIa is protected from C1 inhibitor inactivation when associated with a kaolin surface (183). Antithrombin III has some inhibitory activity on factor XIIa (184, 185). Plasminogen activator inhibitor-1 (PAI-1) also inhibits factor XIIa (186). Endothelial cells may also produce a protein that impairs factor XII activation but not its coagulant or amidolytic activity once formed (187).

# EXPRESSION OF KININOGENS ON BIOLOGIC MEMBRANES

The major impediment in understanding the contact system is the pervasive notion that the system has no biologic relevance because it is entirely activated on artificial surfaces. Although much work has been performed to describe physiologic, negatively-charged surfaces (e.g., acidic phospholipids, cholesterol sulfate, sulfatides, gout crystals, etc.), none have been convincing as a single unifying activator of this system. It may be that the physiologic, negatively-charged surface for contact system activation is the assembly of these proteins on biologic surfaces, i.e., on cell membranes. In the protected milieu of the cell membrane, the assembly of contact proteins on endothelial cell membranes leads to a multiprotein complex that results in prekallikrein activation independent of activated factor XII (84). This mechanism will be discussed in a later section. Many detailed investigations of the proteins of the contact system interacting with cells have led to the current hypothesis of the way in which the system is physiologically activated. Although some individual cell differences exist, the common features of contact protein expression and interaction with cells in the intravascular compartment will be discussed first.

The pivotal protein for contact system assembly on cell membranes is HK. Unoccupied binding sites for HK exists on each of these cells and are also contained within platelets, granulocytes, and endothelial cells (19–21, 36–38, 46, 188, 189). Why each of these cells contain ki-

ninogens and also have unoccupied binding sites for them is unknown. In platelets, less than 8% of total platelet HK is tightly bound to the platelet membrane (19, 46). Upon platelet activation, 40% of total platelet HK is secreted and another 40% of the total becomes expressed upon the activated platelet membrane (46). The total platelet contribution to plasma HK is 0.23% (19, 190). The local concentration of HK on or around the activated platelet membrane may exceed 10 times the plasma concentration of this protein since platelets excrete their granule contents by exocytosis (19, 46).

The majority of granulocyte-associated HK appears to be exogenous HK, which is tightly bound and nonexchangeable with the granulocyte surface (191). Granulocytes have the ability to assemble all proteins of the contact system (191). Elastase liberated from granulocytes proteolyses cell-bound HK (192). Initial investigations suggested that human umbilical vein endothelial cells were able to internalize HK (20, 189). However, more recent investigations indicate no mechanism exists for HK internalization by endothelial cells (31). The difference in the amount of HK associated with the endothelial cell membrane when cells are maintained at 4°C versus 37°C is that at the higher temperature there is increased expression of kininogen-binding sites (20, 31, 35, 189, 193).

There are characteristic features of kininogen binding to all cells. First, kininogen binding to cells has an absolute requirement for $Zn^{2+}$ (20, 21, 36, 38, 188, 189). The requirement for $Zn^{2+}$ is probably not limited to mediate HK binding to cells by its zinc binding region of domain 5 (68, 69). LK binding to platelets and endothelial cells also has an absolute requirement for $Zn^{2+}$. These data indicate that $Zn^{2+}$ is necessary for membrane expression of the kininogen-binding site (35, 48). Although some authors suggest that calcium is a cofactor for binding to endothelial cells and platelets, our investigations reveal that it does not influence HK binding to unstimulated platelets, endothelial cells, or granulocytes (21, 31, 36). However, calcium was a requirement for maximal up-regulation of LK or isolated heavy chain binding to endothelial cells after stimulation with phorbol esters (35). When HK or LK binds to platelets, granulocytes, or endothelial cells, the binding affinities are similar (Table 5.1). Since the affinity of HK binding to cells in the intravascular compartment is between 7 and 52 nM and the plasma concentration of HK is 670 nM, we postulate that all kininogen-binding sites in the intravascular compartment are saturated *in vivo*. The number of binding sites for the kininogens on cells in the intravascular compartment varies with the cell type. Platelets have ~1000 binding sites/cell; granulocytes, 50,000 sites/cell; and endothelial cells, ~1,000,000 sites/cell when chilled to 4°C and ~10,000,000 sites/cell when maintained at 37°C (Table 5.1) (20, 21, 31, 35, 36, 50).

**TABLE 5.1.**   Kininogen Expression on Cells in the Intravascular Compartment

| Cell Type | $K_d$ (nM)† | No. of Sites |
|---|---|---|
| Platelets | | |
| [125]I-HK | 15 ± 4§ | 911 ± 239 |
| [125]I-LK | 27 ± 2 | 647 ± 147 |
| [125]I-D3 | 39 ± 8 | 1227 ± 404 |
| Granulocytes | | |
| [125]I-HK | 10 ± 1.3 | $4.8 \times 10^4$ |
| Endothelial Cells | | |
| [125]I-HK @ 4°C | 52 ± 13 | $9.3 \times 10^5$ |
| [125]I-LK @ 4°C | 43 ± 8 | $9.7 \times 10^5$ |
| biotin-HK @ 4°C | 46 ± 8 | $2.6 \times 10^6$ |
| biotin-HK @ 37°C | 7 ± 3 | $1.0 \times 10^7$ |

† Values presented were determined by direct binding studies.

§ Values presented represent the mean ± SD.

The expression of kininogens on cell membranes is a complex process. Multiple regions on kininogen allow it to interact with its various cellular receptors. The first indication of this was the finding that HK binds to platelets, endothelial cells, and granulocytes by regions on their heavy and light chains (35, 51, 49, 66). HK has three domains that fit into the putative kininogen receptor(s) on endothelial cells (65). The interaction sites between HK and its putative receptor may be multiple locations, such as 3 in domain 3, 1 in domain 4, and 2 in domain 5 (43, 54, 65, 67). The sequence of peptide LDC27 from domain 3 and HKH20 from domain 5 are at present the known highest affinity binding regions on HK for endothelial cells (43, 67). It is important to appreciate that the binding of even a low-affinity sequence from domain 4 will block whole HK from binding to endothelial cells (65). This information suggests that HK and, presumably, LK have a tight fit in its binding site(s). Since the $K_i$ and $K_d$ calculated from binding studies for HK, LK, and all of their subunits are the same, the two chains of kininogens do not bind to cells in an optimal manner (49, 194). This kind of noncooperative interaction is characterized by a loss of entropy on binding and suggests whole HK bends to fit into its binding site (194). In support of this theory, when bradykinin is liberated from HK, kinin-free HK binds to endothelial cells with lower affinity and number of binding sites (31, 65). Likewise, when LK is cleaved between domains 1 and 2 so a change in the conformation of the LK occurs, a decrease in LK binding to endothelial cells occurs compared with intact LK (37). These changes in the biology of HK expression on cell membranes when

bradykinin is removed from the protein are, in retrospect, predictable from the major conformational changes that take place between HK and kinin-free kininogen as shown in functional characteristics (32, 72), in electron microscopy (26), and documented by circular dichroism (32, 195).

The putative kininogen receptor(s) and binding site(s) on endothelial cells are a structure that may be regulated. First, treatment of endothelial cells with metabolic inhibitors of anaerobic and aerobic metabolism and the hexose monophosphate shunt abolish HK binding to the cells (31). Cycloheximide has no effect on HK binding to endothelial cells. Second, temperature or the bradykinin sequence in kininogens contributes to the level of kininogen binding to endothelial cells (31, 32). Third, bradykinin treatment of endothelial cells results in increased HK and LK binding, and this pathway is mediated by protein kinase C and the endothelial cell B1 bradykinin receptor (35). Fourth, heavy chain and LK have a $Ca^{2+}$ requirement for the phorbol 12-myristate 13-acetate 4-0-methyl ether–induced up-regulation of endothelial cell binding sites, whereas HK does not (35). Fifth, angiotensin converting enzyme inhibitors potentiate the effect of bradykinin on up-regulating the HK binding site on endothelial cells (35). Last, when HK binds to endothelial cells, it initiates a series of events that allow for a membrane-associated enzyme to activate prekallikrein bound to HK (84). Thus, bradykinin up regulates kininogen binding on endothelial cells, and kininogens can influence bradykinin formation through prekallikrein localization and activation. These data indicate this system is tightly controlled in an autocrine-like manner.

The combined data presented above indicate there should be a physiochemical receptor(s) for kininogens on blood and endothelial cells. Recent evidence proposes several candidate proteins as the kininogen receptor(s). The putative kininogen receptor binding site may be a multiprotein complex. Antibody inhibition studies suggest that Mac-1 (CD11b/CD18) may be a HK binding site on granulocytes (51). Fibrinogen is a noncompetitive inhibitor of HK binding to granulocytes and ADP-stimulated platelets (192). HK could bind directly to CD11b/CD18 on granulocytes or could interact with a receptor complexed to that integrin (see below). Herwald et al (196, 197) have isolated a 33 Kda protein, which was identified as gC1qR, on a HK affinity column from EA.hy926 cells, which is a human umbilical vein endothelial cell line. gC1qR is a known C1 receptor protein (198), which binds HK and peptides from domain 5 but not LK or binding peptides from domain 3. Further, its ability to bind HK does not require $Zn^{2+}$, although other researchers claim $Zn^{2+}$ is required for ligand blots (199). Moreover, a small portion of total endothelial cell gC1qR is found on the external membrane of endothelial cells. These data indicate that gC1qR cannot explain all characteristics of the kininogen receptor. Factor XII blocks HK binding to gC1qR (197). These data support the previous finding that factor XII partially blocks HK binding to endothelial cells (200). The kininogen-binding protein just described may form part of a multiprotein receptor complex in order to explain the features of HK and LK binding to cells. Recently, evidence has been presented indicating cleaved HK also binds to the urokinase receptor on endothelial cells (201). An antibody to domain 2/3 of the urokinase receptor completely inhibits cleaved HK binding to endothelial cells, as does vitronectin, which is a ligand for this receptor domain. Soluble urokinase receptor markedly inhibits the binding of cleaved HK and forms a complex in a cell-free system. The finding that integrins are tightly associated with the urokinase receptor (202) and can enhance the binding of ligands to domain 2/3 of the urokinase receptor could be relevant to the interaction of kininogens with neutrophils, which display both integrins and the urokinase receptor. This interaction could explain why antibodies to CD11b/CD18 (MAC1) influence HK binding to granulocytes (51). However, since platelets do not express the urokinase receptor, this candidate binding site cannot be the major kininogen receptor.

Most recently, a third kininogen-binding protein has been recognized (203). Human cytokeratin 1 was affinity purified on a HK column from endothelial cell lysates. Cytokeratin 1 is found on endothelial cell, plalelet, and granulocyte membranes. HK specifically binds to cytokeratin 1 when zinc ion is present. Further, HK, LK, and their domain 3 and 5 peptides block HK binding to cytokeratin. gC1qR and su-PAR also block HK binding to cytokeratin. These data along with the recent finding that cytokeratin 8 is a cellular plasminogen receptor suggest that these proteins may represent a new class of presentation receptors on cells (204, 205).

# HK AND CELLULAR ACTIVATION

Kininogen binding modulates activation of the contact system on endothelial cells and platelets. Platelet and endothelial cell-bound HK is protected from activation by exogenous plasma kallikrein (49, 206). Moreover, HK serves as the binding site or receptor for factor XI and prekallikrein on platelets and endothelial cells (37, 83, 84, 207). No evidence indicates platelet-associated factor XI is activated to factor XIa in any favorable fashion (208). However, prekallikrein bound to HK on platelets or endothelial cells can result in its activation to kallikrein by factor XIIa-dependent (84, 209) or -independent

(84) mechanisms. Both situations result in bradykinin generation (84). Thus, cell membrane assembly of contact proteins through binding can result in a complex that can be activated through physiologic mechanisms to result in bradykinin liberation and kininogen-dependent activities.

In addition to the general characteristics of contact proteins interacting with cells of the intravascular compartment, some unique protein-cell interactions exist as well. Kallikrein, but not PK, is chemotactic for neutrophils (210). Exposure of neutrophils to concentrations of kallikrein capable of eliciting chemotaxis increased aerobic glycolysis and activity of the hexose-monophosphate shunt (211). Neutrophils aggregate in response to kallikrein in the presence of calcium (212). This interaction is associated with stimulation of the respiratory burst in neutrophils, as indicated by an increase in oxygen uptake (212). Kallikrein also induces neutrophils to release human neutrophil elastase from their azurophilic granules (213) and primes neutrophils for superoxide production (214).

Human neutrophils in plasma release elastase during blood coagulation (213, 214), but neutrophils resuspended in either PK- or factor XII-deficient plasma release less than 33% of the amount of elastase released in normal human plasma (213). A skin window technique assessing the *in vivo* chemotaxis of leukocytes in response to tissue or microvascular injury shows a significant impairment in chemotaxis in factor XII- and PK-deficient individuals (215). This suggests that kallikrein and factor XIIa are important in the release of elastase from neutrophils in plasma. In addition, kallikrein induces *in vitro* release of elastase from neutrophils, which requires the presence of both the active site of kallikrein (on its light chain) and an intact heavy chain (216). The requirement for an uncleaved heavy chain can be explained by the requirement for apple 1 and apple 4 sequences for binding of kallikrein to HK on neutrophils (102). Factor XIIa has also been shown to cause neutrophil aggregation (217) and degranulation (release of elastase). Factor XIIf does not stimulate neutrophils, and, thus, a domain on the heavy chain is required. However, the catalytic activity of factor XIIa is required because the active site inhibitors, which are D-Pro-Phe-Arg-CH$_2$Cl and corn trypsin inhibitor, abolish the reaction.

Factor XIIa can decrease the number of FcγR1 (immunoglobulin) receptors on monocytes without affecting the affinity of this receptor for immunoglobulin. This interaction requires the heavy chain, but, in contrast to the effect of factor XIIa on neutrophils, does not require the catalytic apparatus of the light chain (218). The site on factor XII responsible for the down-regulation of FcγR1 may be within the N-terminal 18 amino acids (219), and this decrease could impair the clearance of immune complexes. Toossi et al (220) have found factor

XII induces monocyte synthesis and secretion of interleukins 1 and 6, and they found that LPS-stimulated secretion of these interleukins is also potentiated by factor XII.

# PHYSIOLOGIC INTERACTIONS OF CONTACT SYSTEM PROTEINS

The simple fact that HK, prekallikrein, and factor XII prolong artificial surface–activated clotting assays without being associated with bleeding has been confounding. The absence of any hemostatic defect suggests no direct role exists for these proteins in hemostasis. However, three individuals have been reported to have naturally occurring antibodies to the HK binding site on the heavy chain of factor XI and have clinical bleeding states (221, 222). How these antibodies influenced factor XI's procoagulant activity is unknown. Independent of these proteins' general lack of effect on hemostasis, contact system activation influences several aspects related to vascular biology. The kininogens have several activities either within the intact protein or manifest when the intact protein is proteolyzed by plasma, tissue kallikreins, or activated forms of factor XII. This system is a potent regulator of local blood pressure because of its ability to deliver bradykinin. It also has selective antithrombin and profibrinolytic activities. Cleaved kininogen also has unmasked antiadhesive activity.

## BLOOD PRESSURE REGULATION

The first and most enduring function of the plasma kininogens is the generation of bradykinin, a potent biologically active peptide (1). In many ways, kininogens and bradykinin, which is a domain 4 activation peptide, contribute to vessel patency, increased blood flow, and anti-thrombotic/profibrinolytic activities (Table 5.2). Bradykinin itself is a potent stimulator of endothelial cell prostacyclin synthesis, which inhibits platelet function (223, 224), superoxide formation (225), tissue-type plasminogen activator release (226, 227), nitric oxide formation (228), and endothelial cell-dependent smooth muscle hyperpolarization factor formation (229). Further, bradykinin provides a major stimulus to prevent subendothelial smooth muscle proliferation through its ability to stimulate NO and cGMP formation in endothelial cells (230, 231). Kinins appear to prevent vascular smooth muscle growth and proliferation in the presence of an intact endothelium (232, 233). Alternatively, when vessels are injured, bradykinin stimulates protein kinase C and subsequently MAP kinases, which can result in vascular smooth muscle growth and proliferation (234,

**TABLE 5.2.** Kininogens' Antithrombin, Antiadhesive and Profibrinolytic Activities

| Domain | Activity |
|---|---|
| Bradykinin | Stimulates Prostacyclin Formation |
| Bradykinin | Stimulates NO Formation |
| Bradykinin | Stimulates Superoxide Formation |
| Bradykinin | Stimulates Tissue Plasminogen Activator Secretion |
| RPPGF | Prevents α-Thrombin from Cleaving Its Receptor |
| Domain 2 | Prevents Calpain-Related Platelet Aggregation |
| Domain 5 | Prevents Cells from Sticking to Artificial Surfaces |
| Domain 5 | Displaces Fibrinogen from Surfaces and Cells |
| Domain 6 | Prekallikrein Receptor on Endothelial Cells and Neutrophils |

235). Thus the sum of bradykinin activities in an intact vessel is to maintain blood flow and vessels patency. Bradykinin without endothelium stimulates repair of vessels, which could lead to smooth muscle proliferation and intimal hypertrophy. The ability of kininogens to bind to cells orders the assembly and activation of PK and factor XII, which are the first critical steps for kinin liberation. The ability of kininogens to localize to cell membranes and liberate bradykinin makes them important blood pressure regulators. The major bradykinin degrading enzyme in the intravascular compartment is kininase II, which is identical to angiotensin-converting enzyme (ACE) (236). The net effect of this enzyme is to raise blood pressure by destroying bradykinin, which is a vasodilator, and producing angiotensin II, which is a vasoconstrictor (237).

Modulation of bradykinin liberation also has a direct effect on blood pressure *in vivo*. Transgenic mice overexpressing tissue kallikrein are hypotensive (238). Intramuscular delivery of rat kallikrein-binding protein, which is a tissue kallikrein inhibitor, reverses hypotension in transgenic mice overexpressing human tissue kallikrein (239). Rat kallikrein-binding protein or kallistatin is the cognate serine protease inhibitor of tissue kallikrein (240–242). Gene delivery of tissue kallikrein reduces mean blood pressure of spontaneous hypertensive rats, and this inhibition is blocked by kallistatin (243, 244). These molecular genetic studies indicate presumed tissue kallikrein–induced bradykinin liberation directly modifies local and, if sufficiently diffuse, systemic blood pressure regulation. The latter situation may occur in such conditions as systemic inflammatory response syndromes.

# THROMBIN INHIBITION

In addition to the salutary effects of kinins to maintain vessel patency, bradykinin's precursor proteins, which are the kininogens, have been shown to inhibit selective α-thrombin induced platelet activation. Kininogens influence α-thrombin induced platelet and endothelial cell activation by way of at least two mechanisms (31, 48, 50) (Table 5.2). The first mechanism is an indirect one and is probably mediated by kininogen's ability to inhibit platelet calpain. When α-thrombin activates platelets, cytosolic or internal membrane–associated platelet calpain translocates to be externalized on the activated platelet surface (44, 47). Externalized platelet calpain is able to proteolyze platelet surface membrane glycoproteins like glycoprotein Ibα (245). Platelet calpain also proteolyses a putative platelet ADP receptor, which exposes the platelet fibrinogen receptor and thus allows for platelet aggregation (246, 247). Thus, inhibition of externalized platelet calpain by leupeptin or HK (i.e., inhibitors of calpains) results in inhibition of α-thrombin–mediated platelet aggregation by preventing fibrinogen binding (58, 247). These data have been used to develop a group of compounds modeled after kininogen domain 2, which prevent α- and γ-thrombin induced platelet aggregation without interfering with other platelet agonists and thrombin-induced intracellular platelet activation (56, 248). Selective thrombin induced platelet aggregation inhibitors can be developed by designing peptides modeled after kininogen domain 2.

Although the above information on HK's inhibition of α-thrombin induced platelet aggregation is an indirect pathway, additional studies suggest more than one mechanism by which kininogens inhibit α-thrombin induced platelet activation. HK and LK were found to inhibit α-thrombin induced platelet aggregation and secretion (48, 55). Since α-thrombin induced platelet secretion is independent of and occurs before platelet aggregation, there must be another mechanism(s) by which the kininogens interfere with α-thrombin induced platelet activation and the inhibition of calpain-related platelet aggregation (249). HK and LK inhibit α-thrombin noncompetitively, but not Phe-Pro-Arg-chloromethylketone-treated thrombin, from binding to the platelet high-affinity site and endothelial cells (31, 48, 55, 250). This result offered one explanation for the blockade of platelet activation by α-thrombin by large molecular mass proteins like HK and LK. The ability to inhibit α-thrombin binding to platelets was initially localized to the kininogen domain 3 (50). However, one monoclonal antibody to domain 3, which did not block binding, neutralized HK's ability to inhibit α-thrombin induced platelet activation; this suggests that the cell binding site and α-thrombin inhibitory regions are different (50). In support of this assessment, peptides of each of the surface-exposed segments of kininogen domain 3, all of which inhibited HK binding to endothelial cells, did not block α-thrombin induced activation of platelets (56). These results prompted additional studies to find the α-thrombin inhibitory domain on kininogens, which was found to be domain 4 attached to the carboxyterminus of domain 3 prepared by proteolytic cleavage.

The second mechanism by which fragments from kininogens inhibit α-thrombin induced platelet activation has been described by Hasan et al (56). Peptides derived from kininogen domain 4 inhibit α-thrombin induced platelet activation by blocking the enzyme's ability to proteolyze the cloned thrombin receptor, $PAR_1$. Although large molecular mass HK, LK, and domain 3 inhibit α-thrombin binding to platelets, isolated domain 4, i.e., bradykinin (RPPGFSPFR) and MKRPPGFSPFRSSRIG, do not inhibit binding (48, 50, 56). These data indicate another mechanism is operative for these peptides to block α-thrombin induced platelet activation. Like the parent proteins HK and LK, domain 4 peptides also do not inhibit α-thrombin's ability to cleave a tripeptide substrate or clot fibrinogen, which suggests that these peptides do not interact with α-thrombin's active site or anion binding exosite (31, 48, 50, 56). Moreover, like HK and LK, these peptides are not substrates of α-thrombin, and they do not form complexes with α-thrombin (31, 48, 56). Domain 4 peptides do not block ADP-, collagen-, or U46619-induced platelet aggregation in vitro (56). They block α-thrombin induced calcium mobilization and γ-thrombin induced platelet aggregation in plasma in vitro (56). The minimal form of domain 4 that inhibits α-thrombin induced platelet activation is the peptide RPPGF (56). RPPGF is the angiotensin-converting enzyme–breakdown product of bradykinin and the major plasma breakdown product of bradykinin with a metabolic degradation rate in plasma of 4.2 h (251, 252). It is of interest to speculate that the known cardioprotective effects of ACE inhibitors may be contributed to in part by their ability to elevate bradykinin and inhibit intracoronary activation of platelets by thrombin. Knowing this peptide possesses the α-thrombin inhibitory activity indicates the α-thrombin inhibitory activity persists when this sequence is in kininogens, free as bradykinin, or degraded into a bradykinin metabolite. Additional studies were performed to ascertain the mechanism by which RPPGF and related domain 4 peptides inhibit α-thrombin induced platelet activation. RPPGF does not block the thrombin receptor activation peptide, SFLLRN, from inducing platelet activation (56). Domain 4 peptides prevented α-thrombin from eliminating an epitope on the cloned thrombin receptor (PAR1) where α-thrombin cleaves this receptor during the activation process. This result indicates domain 4 peptides prevent α-thrombin from cleaving the cloned thrombin receptor after arginine[41], which is a critical step in α-thrombin activation of cells through this receptor (56). When a peptide was prepared that spanned the α-thrombin cleavage site on the cloned thrombin receptor (NATLDPRSFLLR), RPPGF and HK prevented α-thrombin from cleaving this peptide between the arginine and the serine (56). RPPGF specifically interferes with thrombin's ability to cleave the cloned thrombin receptor to activate platelets without interfering with its procoagulant activity.

## PARTICIPATION IN FIBRINOLYSIS

HK also participates in cellular fibrinolysis in addition to these unique mechanisms of α-thrombin inhibition. From the time of recognition of HK deficiency, this protein has been ascribed to have a role in the fibrinolytic process, although the specific, physiologic mechanism has been unknown (2, 4). It has been known for more than 35 years that contact activation can increase total plasma fibrinolysis (253). Kallikrein, factor XIIa, and factor XIa cleave plasminogen directly, albeit much less efficiently than tissue-type plasminogen activator or urokinase plasminogen activator (254–257). However, plasma kallikrein has been characterized to be a kinetically favorable activator of single chain urokinase *in vitro* (114). More recent studies suggest single chain urokinase activation by kallikrein can best occur on the platelet and endothelial cell surface (83, 209, 258).

These studies prompted us to examine the relationship of prekallikrein assembly on endothelial cells and how it may participate in single-chain urokinase activation (Table 5.2) (84). When prekallikrein binds to HK on endothelial cells, the zymogen becomes activated to kallikrein as indicated by elaboration of amidolytic activity, changes in the structure of prekallikrein to kallikrein on gel electrophoresis, and cleavage of HK (84). Prekallikrein activation occurs independent of any activated forms of factor XII. The prekallikrein activating enzyme(s) is not a serine protease, but a calcium-requiring sulfhydryl(thiol) membrane proteinase (84). Prekallikrein activation over endothelial cells is kinetically similar to prekallikrein activation by factor XII on an artificial surface. Thus contact protein assembly on endothelial cells results in prekallikrein activation without factor XII and an artificial surface (84). This assembly of contact proteins allows for a physiologic pathway for this system to be activated. The degree of prekallikrein activation is regulated by HK. Increasing HK concentrations up regulates the enzyme that activates cell-bound prekallikrein. Thus HK regulates prekallikrein activation which, in turn, liberates more bradykinin from cell-bound HK and removes HK from the surface to slow prekallikrein activation (84). In support of this mechanism, peptides derived from D6 of HK down-regulate plasmin formation by interfering with prekallikrein binding to HK on the endothelial cell surface (259).

The prekallikrein activation pathway on endothelial cells results in the kinetically favorable conversion of single chain urokinase into two chain urokinase in an environment that has a constitutive molar excess secretion of endothelial cell plasminogen activator inhibitor-1 (84, 259). Formation of two chain urokinase results in a 4.3-fold increase in plasminogen activation. This system for plasminogen activation occurs in an environment that contains no tissue plasminogen activator and fibrin and contains an excess of the factor XIIa inhibitor, which is corn trypsin inhibitor. This mechanism for single chain urokinase activation is another pathway for cellular fibrinolysis that is either independent of or conjoined with single chain urokinase activation associated with its binding to its receptor (260). The binding of HK (and, thus, kallikrein) to domain 2/3 of the urokinase receptor (201) on the same molecule as prourokinase, which binds to domain 1 of the receptor, allows an efficient cleavage of the latter by kallikrein. In addition, HK can compete with vitronectin, which also binds to domain 2/3 of the urokinase receptor, and displace vitronectin and its associated molecule, which is plasminogen activator inhibitor-1, thereby enhancing fibrinolysis. This pathway is an explanation of how two-chain urokinase can be formed in plasminogen knockout mice (261).

## ANTIADHESIVE PROPERTIES

HK has been postulated to be an antiadhesive protein. This property has been observed under three different situations. First, cleaved, kinin-free kininogen (HKa) can compete for deposition with adhesive proteins on negatively-charged surfaces such as those that occur on biomaterials. Second, HKa can compete with adhesive proteins for binding to cells. Third, HK on surfaces or in solution can prevent cells from attaching to protein-covered surfaces.

Vroman and Adams (262) found fibrinogen can be immunochemically detected on a negatively-charged surface within seconds, but not within minutes, of normal human plasma contact of the surface. This phenomenon is the result of the displacement of fibrinogen by HK after surface-dependent autoactivation of factor XII (263, 264). Factor XIIa directly and indirectly (through the formation of kallikrein) generates HKa from HK. HKa (but not HK or LK) displaces fibrinogen from the surface (61). Therefore, the "Vroman effect" is the result of the time- and surface-dependent generation of HKa via contact activation of plasma, which results in the physical displacement of adherent fibrinogen from the surface (264). Extensive proteolysis results in HKi (61), which does not displace fibrinogen (264).

As previously mentioned, HK is a non-competitive inhibitor of fibrinogen binding to granulocytes and activated platelets (192). Asakura et al (33) also have shown that HKa, but not HK, HKi, or LK, inhibits the adhesion and spreading of human osteosarcoma cells to vitronectin-coated polystyrene plates. HKa was also demonstrated to inhibit the attachment of platelets and monocytes to extracellular matrix proteins and the spread of bovine aortic endothelial cells on fibrinogen and vitronectin (33). The inhibition by HK of cell attachment to vitronectin can be explained by the cells competition for occupancy of domain 2/3 on the urokinase receptor (201). Additional studies also indicate that HKa and kallikrein inhibit u-PA-induced monocyte adhesion, although factor XII and plasminogen up regulate it (265).

# DISEASE STATE INTERACTIONS

## HEREDITARY ANGIOEDEMA

Hereditary angioedema (HAE) is a congenital condition associated with a deficiency or defect in the C1 inhibitor. Acute attacks of HAE are associated with contact system activation (14, 266–268). Characteristically, in acute attacks of HAE, plasma prekallikrein activity is reduced while plasma prekallikrein antigen levels are normal and HK activity and antigen levels are reduced (14, 267, 269). Contact activation arises from the absence of protease inhibition as a result of lowered C1 inhibitor levels. Bradykinin liberation may be a major mediator of the edema seen in that condition (270). The phenomena of cold activation of factor VII is the result of cold inactivation of C1 inhibitor and factor XII activation in a tube with resultant factor VII activation (271–273). Lowering temperatures below 37°C decreases the reactivity of C1 inhibitor for its enzymes (274).

## SYSTEMIC INFLAMMATORY RESPONSE SYNDROME AND SEPSIS

Activation of the contact system occurs in individuals with systemic inflammatory response syndrome (SIRS) and sepsis. Although contact activation is not the only system that gets activated in individuals with sepsis, its activation contributes to the vascular instability associated with these illnesses. Older investigations of individuals with gram negative sepsis showed that functional factor XII, prekallikrein, and C1-INH decreased in individuals with hypotensive septicemia (275). Individuals with clinical and laboratory criteria for disseminated intravascular coagulation (DIC), which is associated with septicemia or viremia, experience a decrease of functional factor XII, prekallikrein, and C1-INH. In contrast, no significant changes occur in the kallikrein-kinin system in individuals with neoplasia (275). Decreased prekallikrein activity and elevated bradykinin were associated with positive blood cultures and hypotension in a group of individuals with postoperative

septicemia (276). During a vaccine trial of human individuals who were experimentally infected with typhoid fever, all individuals with typhoid fever showed a decrease in functional prekallikrein and C1-INH, but the corresponding antigens remained unaffected (277). Individuals with adult respiratory distress syndrome (ARDS) have significantly reduced plasma levels of factor XII, PK, and HK with increased levels of C1-INH antigen with decreased levels of C1-INH activity (278, 279). Decreased levels of PK have been documented in bacteremia and septicemia as a result of viruses, fungi, and *Rickettsia*. Individuals with Rocky Mountain spotted fever have decreased PK levels with increased kallikrein-C1-inhibitor complexes (280). In most cases of septic shock, kallikrein-C1-inhibitor complexes are rapidly cleared and thus cannot be measured (281). However, $\alpha_2$M-Kal complexes are slowly cleared from plasma and are readily measured as a marker for sepsis (282).

Healthy human volunteers who receive a low dose of *Escherichia coli* endotoxin (0.4 ng/kg body weight) develop a flu-like illness associated with a hyperdynamic cardiovascular state lasting 24 hours (283). Functional prekallikrein levels are lower in the endotoxin group compared with controls at 2 hours after infusion and remain low throughout the rest of the experimental protocol at 5 and 24 hours. The concentration of $\alpha_2$M-Kal complexes was elevated fourfold in the endotoxin-treated group by 3 hours and fivefold by 5 hours; a decrease to normal occurred in the circulating levels of complexes by 24 hours (284). In a baboon animal model where two concentrations of *E. coli* were used to produce lethal and non-lethal hypotension, the lethal group developed irreversible hypotension, which correlated with the decline in functional levels of HK and an increase in $\alpha_2$M-Kal complexes (285). The non-lethal group experienced reversible hypotension, a less striking decline in HK, and a slight elevation in $\alpha_2$M-Kal. This study suggests that irreversible hypotension correlates with activation of the contact system. Using a concentration of monoclonal antibody to human factor XII that was able to inhibit *in vitro* factor XII coagulant activity in baboon plasma by 60%, plasma HK levels remained stable or rose in the group treated with the monoclonal antibody to factor XII whereas a 40% decline from baseline levels occurred in the untreated group. Further, in the untreated group, there was a rise of $\alpha_2$M-Kal complexes, which was completely blocked by the monoclonal antibody in the treated group. Comparison of group survival rates using a Kaplan-Meier plot showed that treated animals survived significantly longer than untreated animals. This study indicates that inhibition of contact system activation with a monoclonal antibody to factor XII modulates blood pressure in primates treated with lethal quantities of *E. coli*. It also indicates that this system is one of the important regulators of blood pressure during infection.

## THROMBOSIS RISK FACTOR

Independent of the multiple mechanisms by which kininogens are selective antithrombins that modulate α-thrombin's activation of platelets and endothelial cells *in vitro* and the proposed physiologic mechanism for cellular fibrinolysis resulting from assembly of HK and PK on endothelium, clinical observation suggests total deficiencies of these proteins may be additional risk factors for thrombosis. John Hageman (Hageman factor) and Mayme Williams (Williams trait) died of pulmonary emboli (286, 287). However, extenuating circumstances existed in both individuals. Mr. Hageman had a fractured pelvis, and Ms. Williams had lung cancer. Some clinical studies suggest that contact protein deficiencies may be associated with impaired contact factor–dependent fibrinolysis. This finding may contribute to an increased incidence of thrombosis in individuals with congenital factor XII deficiency (288–292) and in acquired thrombotic disorders such as myocardial infarction (293) and rethrombosis of coronary arteries after thrombolytic therapy (294). However, careful investigation in 350 Dutch individuals with idiopathic deep venous thrombosis did not result in an increase in heterozygous factor XII deficiency over controls (295). These studies suggest that complete contact protein deficiencies may be the only risk factor for thrombosis, if it is a risk factor at all.

## ACKNOWLEDGMENTS

This research was supported in part by HL35553, HL52799, and HL56415.

## REFERENCES

1. Roche e Silva M, Beraldo WT, Rosenfeld G. Bradykinin, a hypotensive and smooth muscle stimulating factor released from plasma globulin by snake venoms and by trypsin. Am J Physiol 1949;156:261–273.
2. Colman RW, Bagdasarian A, Talamo RC et al. Williams trait. Human kininogen deficiency with diminished levels of plasminogen proactivator and prekallikrein associated with abnormalities of the Hageman factor-dependent pathways. J Clin Invest 1975;56:1650–1662.
3. Wuepper KD, Miller DR, Lacombe MJ. Flaujeac trait. Deficiency of human plasma kininogen. J Clin Invest 1975;56:1663–1672.
4. Saito H, Ratnoff OD, Waldmann R et al. Fitzgerald trait. Deficiency of a hitherto unrecognized agent, Fitzgerald factor, participating in surface mediated reactions of clotting, fibrinolysis, generation of kinins, and the property of diluted plasma enhancing vascular permeability (PF/DIL). J Clin Invest 1975;55:1082–1089.
5. Takagaki Y, Kitamura N, Nakanishi S. Cloning and sequence analysis of cDNAs for human high molecular weight and low-molecular-weight prekininogens. Primary structures of two human prekininogens. J Biol Chem 1985;260:8601–8609.
6. Kitamura N, Kitagawa H, Fukushima D et al. Structural organization of the human kininogen gene and a model for its evolution. J Biol Chem 1985;260:8610–8617.
7. Fong D, Smith DI, Hsieh WT. The human kininogen gene (KNG) mapped to chromosome 3q26-qter by analysis of somatic cell hybrids using the polymerase chain reaction. Hum Genet 1991;87:189–192.
8. Cheung PP, Cannizzaro LA, Colman RW. Chromosomal mapping of human kininogen gene (KNG) to 3q26–qter. Cytogenet Cell Genet 1992;59:24–26.
9. Rizzu P, Baldini A. Three members of the human cystatin gene superfamily, AHSG, HRG, and KNG, map within one megabase of genomic DNA at 3q27. Cytogenet Cell Genet 1995;70:26–28.
10. Kakizuka A, Ingi T, Murai T et al. A set of U1 snRNA-complementary sequences involved in governing alternative RNA splicing of the kininogen genes. J Biol Chem 1990;265:10102–10108.
11. Cheung PP, Kunapuli SP, Scott CF et al. Genetic basis of total kininogen deficiency in Williams' trait. J Biol Chem 1993;268:23361–23365.
12. Hayashi I, Hoshiko S, Makabe O et al. A point mutation of alanine 163 to threonine is responsible for the defective secretion of high molecular weight kininogen by the liver of brown Norway Katholiek rats. J Biol Chem 1993;268:17219–17224.
13. Chen LM, Chung P, Chao S et al. Differential regulation of kininogen gene expression by estrogen and progesterone *in vivo*. Biochim Biophys Acta 1992;1131:145–151.
14. Chhibber G, Cohen A, Lane S et al. Immunoblotting of plasma in a pregnant individual with hereditary angioedema. J Lab Clin Med 1990;115:112–121.
15. Takano M, Yokoyama K, Yayama K et al. Murine fibroblasts synthesize and secrete kininogen in response to cyclic-AMP, prostaglandin E2 and tumor necrosis factor. Biochim Biophys Acta 1995;1265:189–195.
16. Scott CF, Colman RW. Sensitive antigenic determinations of high molecular weight kininogen performed by covalent coupling of capture antibody. J Lab Clin Med 1992;119:77–86.
17. Jacobsen S, Kriz M. Some data on two purified kininogens from human plasma. Br J Pharmacol 1967;29:25–36.
18. Schmaier AH, Bradford H, Silver LD et al. High molecular weight kininogen is an inhibitor of platelet calpain. J Clin Invest 1986;77:1565–1573.
19. Schmaier AH, Zuckerberg A, Silverman C et al. High-molecular weight kininogen. A secreted platelet protein. J Clin Invest 1983;71:1477–1489.
20. Schmaier AH, Kuo A, Lundberg D et al. The expression of high molecular weight kininogen on human umbilical vein endothelial cells. J Biol Chem 1988;263:16327–16333.
21. Gustafson EJ, Schmaier AH, Wachtfogel YT et al. Human neutrophils contain and bind high molecular weight kininogen. J Clin Invest 1989;84:28–35.
22. Proud D, Perkins M, Pierce JV et al. Characterization and localization of human renal kininogen. J Biol Chem 1981;256:10634–10639.
23. Hallbach J, Adams G, Wirthensohn G et al. Quantification of kininogen in human renal medulla. Biol Chem Hoppe Seyler 1987;368:1151–1155.
24. Yamamoto T, Tsuruta J, Kambara T. Interstitial-tissue localization of high-molecular-weight kininogen in guinea-pig skin. Biochim Biophys Acta 1987;916:332–342.
25. Ohkubo I, Kurachi K, Takasawa T et al. Isolation of a human cDNA for alpha 2-thiol proteinase inhibitor and its identity with low-molecular-weight kininogen. Biochemistry 1984;23:5691–5697.
26. Weisel JW, Nagaswami C, Woodhead JL et al. The shape of high molecular weight kininogen: organization into structural domains, changes with activation, and interactions with prekallikrein, as determined by electron microscopy. J Biol Chem 1994;269:10100–10106.
27. Salvesen G, Parkes C, Abrahamson M et al. Human low-Mr kininogen contains three copies of a cystatin sequence that are divergent in structure and in inhibitory activity for cysteine proteinases. Biochem J 1986;234:429–434.
28. Schmaier AH, Schutsky D, Farber A et al. Determination of the bifunctional properties of high molecular weight kininogen by studies with monoclonal antibodies directed to each of its chains. J Biol Chem 1987;262:1405–1411.
29. Vogel R, Assfalg-Machleidt I, Esterl A et al. Proteinase-sensitive regions in the heavy chain of low-molecular-weight kininogen map to the interdomain junctions. J Biol Chem 1988;263:12661–12668.
30. Bradford HN, Jameson BA, Adam AA et al. Contiguous binding and inhibitory sites on kininogens required for the inhibition of platelet calpain. J Biol Chem 1993;268:26546–26551.
31. Hasan AA, Cines DB, Ngaiza JR et al. High-molecular-weight kininogen is exclusively membrane bound on endothelial cells to influence activation of vascular endothelium. Blood 1995;85:3134–3143.
32. Hasan AA, Zhang J, Samuel M et al. Conformational changes in low-molecular-weight kininogen alters its ability to bind to endothelial cells. Thromb Haemost 1995;74:1088–1095.
33. Asakura S, Hurley RW, Skorstengaard K et al. Inhibition of cell adhesion by high molecular weight kininogen. J Cell Biol 1992;116:465–476.
34. Ishiguro H, Higashiyama S, Ohkubo I et al. Heavy chain of human high molecular weight and low-molecular-weight kininogen binds calcium ion. Biochemistry 1987;26:7450–7458.
35. Zini JM, Schmaier AH, Cines DB. Bradykinin regulates the expression of kininogen binding sites on endothelial cells. Blood 1993;81:2936–2946.
36. Gustafson EJ, Schutsky D, Knight L et al. High molecular weight kininogen binds to unstimulated platelets. J Clin Invest 1986;78:310–318.
37. Greengard JS, Heeb MJ, Ersdal E et al. Binding of coagulation factor XI to washed human platelets. Biochemistry 1986;25:3884–3890.
38. van Iwaarden F, de Groot PG, Bouma BN. The binding of high molecular weight kininogen to cultured human endothelial cells. J Biol Chem 1988;263:4698–4703.

39. Croxatto HR, Boric MP, Roblero J et al. Digestive process and regulation of renal excretory function. Pepsanurin and prokinins inhibitors of diuresis mediated by atrial natriuretic peptide. Rev Med Chil 1995;122:1162–1172.
40. Bradford HN, Schmaier AH, Colman RW. Kinetics of inhibition of platelet calpain II by human kininogens. Biochem J 1990;270:83–90.
41. Auerswald EA, Rossler D, Mentele R et al. Cloning, expression and characterization of human kininogen domain 3. FEBS Lett 1993;321:93–97.
42. Ylinenjarvi K, Prasthofer TW, Martin NC et al. Interaction of cysteine proteinases with recombinant kininogen domain 2, expressed in Escherichia coli. FEBS Lett 1995;357:309–311.
43. Herwald H, Hasan AA, Godovac-Zimmermann J et al. Identification of an endothelial cell binding site on kininogen domain D3. J Biol Chem 1995;270:14634–14642.
44. Schmaier AH, Bradford HN, Lundberg D et al. Membrane expression of platelet calpain. Blood 1990;75:1273–1281.
45. Scott CF, Whitaker EJ, Hammond BF et al. Purification and characterization of a potent 70-kDa thiol lysyl-proteinase (Lys-gingivain) from Porphyromonas gingivalis that cleaves kininogens and fibrinogen. J Biol Chem 1993;268:7935–7942.
46. Schmaier AH, Smith PM, Purdon AD et al. High molecular weight kininogen: localization in the unstimulated and activated platelet and activation by a platelet calpain(s). Blood 1986;67:119–130.
47. Saido TC, Suzuki H, Yamazaki H et al. In situ capture of m-calpain activation of platelets. J Biol Chem 1993;268:7422–7426.
48. Meloni FJ, Schmaier AH. Low-molecular-weight kininogen binds to platelets to modulate thrombin-induced platelet activation. J Biol Chem 1991;266:6786–6794.
49. Meloni FJ, Gustafson EJ, Schmaier AH. High molecular weight kininogen binds to platelets by its heavy and light chains and when bound has altered susceptibility to kallikrein cleavage. Blood 1992;79:1233–1244.
50. Jiang YP, Muller-Esterl W, Schmaier AH. Domain 3 of kininogens contains a cell-binding site and a site that modifies thrombin activation of platelets. J Biol Chem 1992;267:3712–3717.
51. Wachtfogel YT, DeLa Cadena RA, Kunapuli SP et al. High molecular weight kininogen binds to Mac-1 on neutrophils by its heavy chain (domain 3) and its light chain (domain 5). J Biol Chem 1994;269:19307–19312.
52. Bode W, Engh R, Musil D et al. The 2.0 Å X-ray crystal structure of chicken egg white cystatin and its possible mode of interaction with cysteine proteinases. EMBO J 1988;7:2593–2599.
53. DeLa Cadena RA, Wyshock EG, Kunapuli SP et al. Platelet thrombospondin interactions with human high and low-molecular-weight kininogens. Thromb Haemost 1994;72:125–131.
54. Khan M, Punia N, Majluf-Cruz A et al. The binding sites on high molecular weight kininogen (HK) to activated human neutrophils are localized to K263-Q292, Q329-M357, and H493-K520 [Abstract]. Blood 1995;86:33a.
55. Puri RN, Zhou F, Hu CJ et al. High molecular weight kininogen inhibits thrombin-induced platelet aggregation and cleavage of aggregin by inhibiting binding of thrombin to platelets. Blood 1991;77:500–507.
56. Hasan AA, Amenta S, Schmaier AH. Bradykinin and its metabolite, Arg-Pro-Pro-Gly-Phe, are selective inhibitors of a-thrombin-induced platelet activation. Circulation 1996;94:517–528.
57. Mori K, Nagasawa S. Studies on human high molecular weight (HMW) kininogen. II. Structural change of HMW kininogen by the action of human plasma kallikrein. J Biochem 1981;89:1465–1473.
58. Schmaier AH, Farber A, Schein R et al. Structural changes of plasma high molecular weight kininogen after in vitro activation and in sepsis. J Lab Clin Med 1988;112:182–192.
59. Tayeh MA, Olson ST, Shore JD. Surface-induced alterations in the kinetic pathway for cleavage of human high molecular weight kininogen by plasma kallikrein. J Biol Chem 1994;269:16318–16325.
60. Wiggins RC. Kinin release from high molecular weight kininogen by the action of Hageman factor in the absence of kallikrein. J Biol Chem 1983;258:8963–8970.
61. Scott CF, Silver LD, Purdon AD et al. Cleavage of human high molecular weight kininogen by factor XIa in vitro. Effect on structure and function. J Biol Chem 1985;260:10856–10863.
62. Sato F, Nagasawa S. Mechanism of kinin release from human low-molecular-mass-kininogen by the synergistic action of human plasma kallikrein and leukocyte elastase. Biol Chem Hoppe Seyler 1988;369:1009–1017.
63. Kleniewski J, Donaldson V. Granulocyte elastase cleaves human high molecular weight kininogen and destroys its clot-promoting activity. J Exp Med 1988;167:1895–1907.
64. Kunapuli SP, DeLa Cadena RA, Colman RW. Deletion mutagenesis of high molecular weight kininogen light chain. Identification of two anionic surface binding subdomains. J Biol Chem 1993;268:2486–2492.
65. Hasan AA, Cines DB, Zhang J et al. The carboxyterminus of bradykinin and aminoterminus of the light chain of kininogens comprise an endothelial cell binding domain. J Biol Chem 1994;269:31822–31830.
66. Reddigari SR, Kuna P, Miragliotta G et al. Human high molecular weight kininogen binds to human umbilical vein endothelial cells via its heavy and light chains. Blood 1993;81:1306–1311.
67. Hasan AA, Cines DB, Herwald H et al. Mapping the cell binding site on high molecular weight kininogen domain 5. J Biol Chem 1995;270:19256–19261.
68. DeLa Cadena RA, Colman RW. The sequence HGLGHGHEQQHGLGHGH in the light chain of high molecular weight kininogen serves as a primary structural feature for zinc-dependent binding to an anionic surface. Protein Sci 1992;1:151–160.
69. Retzios AD, Rosenfeld R, Schiffman S. Effects of chemical modifications on the surface- and protein-binding properties of the light chain of human high molecular weight kininogen. J Biol Chem 1987;262:3074–3081.
70. Bjork I, Olson ST, Sheffer RG et al. Binding of heparin to human high molecular weight kininogen. Biochemistry 1989;28:1213–1221.
71. Ben Nasr AB, Herwald H, Muller-Esterl W et al. Human kininogens interact with M protein, a bacterial surface protein and virulence determinant. Biochem J 1995;305:173–180.
72. Scott CF, Silver LD, Schapira M et al. Cleavage of human high molecular weight kininogen markedly enhances its coagulant activity. Evidence that this molecule exists as a procofactor. J Clin Invest 1984;73:954–962.
73. Tait JF, Fujikawa K. Identification of the binding site for plasma prekallikrein in human high molecular weight kininogen. A region from residues 185 to 224 of the kininogen light chain retains full binding activity. J Biol Chem 1986;261:15396–15401.
74. Tait JF, Fujikawa K. Primary structure requirements for the binding of human high molecular weight kininogen to plasma prekallikrein and factor XI. J Biol Chem 1987;262:11651–11656.
75. Vogel R, Kaufmann J, Chung DW et al. Mapping of the prekallikrein binding site of human H-kininogen by ligand screening of lambda gt11 expression libraries: mimicking of the predicted binding site by anti-idiotypic antibodies. J Biol Chem 1990;265:12494–12502.
76. Bock PE, Shore JD. Protein-protein interactions in contact activation of blood coagulation. Characterization of fluorescein-labeled human high molecular weight kininogen-light chain as a probe. J Biol Chem 1983;258:15079–15086.
77. Bock PE, Shore JD, Tans G et al. Protein-protein interactions in contact activation of blood coagulation. Binding of high molecular weight kininogen and the 5-(iodo-acetamido) fluorescein-labeled kininogen light chain to prekallikrein, kallikrein, and the separated kallikrein heavy and light chains. J Biol Chem 1985;260:12434–12443.
78. Scarsdale JN, Harris RB. Solution phase conformation studies of the prekallikrein binding domain of high molecular weight kininogen. J Protein Chem 1990;9:647–659.
79. You JL, Scarsdale JN, Harris RB. Calorimetric and spectroscopic examination of the solution phase structures of prekallikrein binding domain peptides of high molecular weight kininogen. J Protein Chem 1991;10:301–311.
80. You JL, Page JD, Scarsdale JN et al. Conformational analysis of synthetic peptides encompassing the factor XI and prekallikrein overlapping binding domains of high molecular weight kininogen. Peptides 1993;14:867–876.
81. Reddigari S, Kaplan AP. Monoclonal antibody to human high molecular weight kininogen recognizes its prekallikrein binding site and inhibits coagulant activity. Blood 1989;74:695–702.
82. Kaufmann J, Haasemann M, Modrow S et al. Structural dissection of the multidomain kininogens. Fine mapping of the target epitopes of antibodies interfering with their functional properties. J Biol Chem 1993;268:9079–9091.
83. Lenich C, Pannell R, Gurewich V. Assembly and activation of the intrinsic fibrinolytic pathway on the surface of human endothelial cells in culture. Thromb Haemost 1995;74:698–703.
84. Motta G, Rojkjaee R, Hasan AAK et al. High molecular weight kininogen regulates prekallikrein assembly and activation on endothelial cells: A novel mechanism for contact activation. Blood. In press, 1998.
85. Beaubien G, Rosinski-Chupin I, Mattei MG et al. Gene structure and chromosomal localization of plasma kallikrein. Biochemistry 1991;30:1628–1635.
86. Asakai R, Davie EW, Chung DW. Organization of the gene for human factor XI. Biochemistry 1987;26:7221–7228.
87. Chung DW, Fujikawa K, McMullen BA et al. Human plasma prekallikrein, a zymogen to a serine protease that contains four tandem repeats. Biochemistry 1986;25:2410–2417.
88. McMullen BA, Fujikawa K, Davie EW. Location of the disulfide bonds in human plasma prekallikrein: the presence of four novel apple domains in the aminoterminal portion of the molecule. Biochemistry 1991;30:2050–2056.
89. McMullen BA, Fugikawa K, Davie EW. Location of the disulfide bonds in human coagulation factor XI: the presence of Tandem apple domains. Biochemistry 1991;30:2056–2060.
90. Mandle R Jr, Kaplan AP. Hageman factor substrates. Human plasma prekallikrein: mechanism of activation by Hageman factor and participation in Hageman factor-dependent fibrinolysis. J Biol Chem 1977;252:6097–6104.
91. Scott CF, Liu CY, Colman RW. Human plasma prekallikrein: a rapid high yield method for purification. Eur J Biochem 1979;100:77–83.
92. Fisher CA, Schmaier AH, Addonizio VP et al. Assay of prekallikrein in human plasma: comparison of amidolytic, esterolytic, coagulation, and immunochemical assays. Blood 1982;59:963–970.
93. McConnell DJ, Mason B. The isolation of human plasma prekallikrein. Br J Pharmacol 1970;38:490–502.

94. Wuepper KD, Cochrane CG. Plasma prekallikrein: isolation, characterization, and mechanism of action. J Exp Med 1972;135:1–20.
95. Burger D, Schleuning WD, Schapira M. Human plasma prekallikrein: immunoaffinity purification and activation to α and β kallikrein. J Biol Chem 1986;261:324–327.
96. Colman RW, Wachtfogel YT, Kucich U et al. Effect of cleavage of the heavy chain of human plasma kallikrein on its functional properties. Blood 1985;65:311–318.
97. Mandle RJ, Colman RW, Kaplan AP. Identification of prekallikrein and high molecular weight kininogen as a complex in human plasma. Proc Natl Acad Sci U S A 1976;73:4179–4183.
98. Page JD, Colman RW. Localization of distinct functional domains on prekallikrein for interaction with both high molecular weight kininogen and activated factor XII in a 28-kDa fragment (amino acids 141–371). J Biol Chem 1991;266:8143–8148.
99. Page JD, You JL, Harris RB et al. Localization of the binding site on plasma kallikrein for high molecular weight kininogen to both apple 1 and apple 4 domains of the heavy chain. Arch Biochem Biophys 1994;314:159–164.
100. Hock J, Vogel R, Linke RP et al. High molecular weight kininogen-binding site of prekallikrein probed by monoclonal antibodies. J Biol Chem 1990;265:12005–12011.
101. Lin Y, Shenoy SS Harris RB et al. Direct evidence for multi-facial contacts between high molecular weight kininogen and plasma prekallikrein. Biochemistry 1996;35:12945–12949.
102. Herwald H, Renne T, Meijers JCM et al. Mapping of the discontinuous kininogen binding site of prekallikrein. A distal binding segment is located in the heavy chain domain A4. J Biol Chem 1996;271:13061–13067.
103. Schapira M, Scott CF, Colman RW. Protection of human plasma kallikrein from inactivation by C1 inhibitor and other protease inhibitors. The role of high molecular weight kininogen. Biochemistry 1981;20:2738–2743.
104. Gigli I, Mason JW, Colman RW et al. Interaction of plasma kallikrein with the C1 inhibitor. J Immunol 1970;104:574–581.
105. Van der Graff F, Koedam JA, Bouma BA. Inactivation of Kallikrein in plasma. J Clin Invest 1983;71:149–158.
106. Schapira M, Scott CF, Colman RW. Contribution of plasma protease inhibitors to the inactivation of kallikrein in plasma. J Clin Invest 1982;69:462–468.
107. Van der Graff F, Koedam JA, Griffin JH et al. Interaction of human plasma kallikrein and its light chain with C1 inhibitor. Biochemistry 1983;22:4860–4866.
108. Schapira M, Scott CF, James A et al. High molecular weight kininogen or its light chain protects human plasma kallikrein from inactivation by plasma protease inhibitors. Biochemistry 1982;21:567–572.
109. Schmaier AH, Gustafson E, Idell S et al. Plasma prekallikrein assay: reversible inhibition of C1 inhibitor by chloroform and its use in measuring prekallikrein in different mammalian species. J Lab Clin Med 1984;104:882–892.
110. Lahiri B, Bagdasarian A, Mitchell B et al. Antithrombin-heparin cofactor: an inhibitor of plasma Kallikrein. Arch Biochem Biophys 1976;175:737–747.
111. Meijers JC, Kanters DH, Vlooswijk RA et al. Inactivation of human plasma kallikrein and factor XIa by protein C inhibitor. Biochemistry 1988;27:4231–4237.
112. Espana F, Estelles A, Griffin JH et al. Interaction of plasma kallikrein with protein C inhibitor in purified mixtures and in plasma. Thromb Haemost 1991;65:46–51.
113. Hauert J, Nicoloso G, Schleuning WD et al. Plasminogen activators in dextran sulfate-activated euglobulin fractions: a molecular analysis of factor XII and prekallikrein-dependent fibrinolysis. Blood 1989;73:994–999.
114. Ichinose A, Fujikawa K, Suyama T. The activation of prourokinase by plasma kallikrein and its inactivation by thrombin. J Biol Chem 1986;261:3486–3489.
115. Citarella F, Tripodi M, Fantoni A et al. Assignment of human coagulation factor XII (fXII) to chromosome 5 by cDNA hybridization to DNA from somatic cell hybrids. Hum Genet 1988;80:397–398.
116. Royle NJ, Nigli M, Cool D et al. Structural gene encoding human factor XII is located at 5q33-qter. Somat Cell Mol Genet 1988;14:217–221.
117. Cool DE, MacGillivray RT. Characterization of the human blood coagulation factor XII gene. J Biol Chem 1987;262:13662–13673.
118. Cool DE, Edgell CJS, Louie GV et al. Characterization of human blood coagulation factor XII cDNA. J Biol Chem 1985;260:13666–13676.
119. Que BG, Davie EW. Characterization of a cDNA coding for human factor XII (Hageman factor). Biochemistry 1986;25:1525–1528.
120. Griffin JH, Cochrane CG. Human factor XII (Hageman factor). Methods Enzymol 1976;45:56–65.
121. Revak SD, Cochrane CC, Johnston A et al. Structural changes accompanying enzymatic activation of Hageman factor. J Clin Invest 1974;54:619–627.
122. Saito H, Ratnoff OD, Pensky J. Radioimmunoassay of human Hageman factor (factor XII). J Lab Clin Med 1976;88:506–514.
123. Gordon EM, Gallagher CA, Johnson TR et al. Hepatocytes express blood coagulation factor XII (Hageman factor). J Lab Clin Med 1990;115:463–469.
124. Gordon EM, Williams SR, Frenchek B et al. Dose-dependent effects of postmenopausal estrogen and progestin on antithrombin III and factor XII. J Lab Clin Med 1988;111:52–56.
125. Mitropoulos KA, Martin JC, Burgess A et al. The increased rate of activation of factor XII in late pregnancy can contribute to the increased reactivity of factor VII. Thromb Haemost 1990;63:349–355.
126. Gordon EM, Johnson TR, Ramos LP et al. Enhanced expression of factor XII (Hageman factor) in isolated livers of estrogen- and prolactin-treated rats. J Lab Clin Med 1991;117:353–358.
127. Farsetti A, Misiti S, Citarella F et al. Molecular basis of estrogen regulation of Hageman factor XII gene expression. Endocrinology 1995;136:5076–5083.
128. Schmeidler-Sapiro KT, Ratnoff OD, Gordon EM. Mitogenic effects of coagulation factor XII and factor XIIa on HepG2 cells. Proc Natl Acad Sci U S A 1991;88:4382–4385.
129. Gordon EM, Venkatesan N, Salazar R et al. Factor XII-induced mitogenesis is mediated via a distinct signal transduction pathway that activates a mitogen-activated protein kinase. Proc Natl Acad Sci U S A. 1996;93:2174–2179.
130. Pixley RA, Stumpo LG, Birkmeyer K et al. A monoclonal antibody recognizing an icosapeptide sequence in the heavy chain of human factor XII inhibits surface-catalyzed activation. J Biol Chem 1987;262:10140–10145.
131. Clarke BJ, Cote HC, Cool DE et al. Mapping of a putative surface-binding site of human coagulation factor XII. J Biol Chem 1989;264:11497–11502.
132. Citarella F, Ravon DM, Pascucci B et al. Structure/function analysis of human factor XII using recombinant deletion mutants. Evidence for an additional region involved in the binding to negatively charged surfaces. Eur J Biochem 1996;238:240–249.
133. Cochrane CG, Revak SD, Wuepper KD. Activation of Hageman factor in solid and fluid phases. A critical role of kallikrein. J Exp Med 1973;138:1564–1583.
134. Samuel M, Pixley RA, Villanueva MA et al. Human factor XII (Hageman factor) autoactivation by dextran sulfate: circular dichroism, fluorescence, and ultraviolet difference spectroscopic studies. J Biol Chem 1992;267:19691–19697.
135. Pixley RA, Schapira M, Colman RW. Effect of heparin on the inactivation rate of human activated factor XII by antithrombin III. Blood 1985;66:198–203.
136. Miyata T, Kawabata S, Iwanaga S et al. Coagulation factor XII (Hageman factor) Washington DC: inactive factor XIIa results from $Cys_{571}$–Ser substitution. Proc Natl Acad Sci U S A 1989;86:8319–8322.
137. Wuillemin WA, Huber I, Furlan M et al. Functional characterization of an abnormal factor XII molecule (F XII Bern). Blood 1991;78:997–1004.
138. Cochrane CG, Revak SD, Wuepper KD. Activation of Hageman factor in solid and fluid phases: a critical role of kallikrein. J Exp Med 1973;138:1564–1583.
139. Revak SD, Cochrane CG, Griffin JH. The binding and cleavage characteristics of human Hageman factor during contact activation. A comparison of normal plasma with plasma deficient in factor XI, prekallikrein or high molecular weight kininogen. J Clin Invest 1977;59:1167–1175.
140. Griffin JH. Role of surface in the surface-dependent activation of Hageman factor (blood coagulation factor XII). Proc Natl Acad Sci U S A 1978;75:1998–2002.
141. Kirby EP, McDevitt PJ. The binding of bovine factor XII to kaolin. Blood 1983;61:652–659.
142. Wiggins RC, Cochrane CC. The autoactivation of rabbit Hageman factor. J Exp Med 1979;150:1122–1133.
143. Miller G, Silverberg M, Kaplan AP. Autoactivability of human Hageman factor. Biochem Biophys Res Commun 1980;92:803–810.
144. Silverberg M, Dunn JT, Garen L et al. Autoactivation of human Hageman factor: demonstration utilizing a synthetic substrate. J Biol Chem 1980;255:7281–7286.
145. Dunn JT, Silverberg M, Kaplan AP. The cleavage and formation of activated human Hageman factor by autodigestion and by kallikrein. J Biol Chem 1982;257:1779–1784.
146. Espana F, Ratnoff OD. Activation of Hageman factor (factor XII) by sulfatides and other agents in the absence of plasma proteases. J Lab Clin Med 1983;102:31–45.
147. Tankersley DL, Finlayson JS. Kinetics of activation and autoactivation of human factor XII. Biochemistry 1984;23:273–279.
148. Margolis J. The interrelationship of coagulation of plasma and release of peptides. Ann N Y Acad Sci 1963;104:133–145.
149. Ratnoff OD. The biology and pathology of the initiation of coagulation. In: Brown EB, Moore CV, eds. Progress in hematology. New York: Grune & Stratton, 1966;V:204.
150. Thorisdottir H. Ratnoff OD, Maniglia AJ. Activation of Hageman factor (factor XII) by bismuth subgallate, a hemostatic agent. J Lab Clin Med 1988;112:481–486.
151. Ziats NP, Pankowsky DA, Tierney BP et al. Adsorption of Hageman factor (factor XII) and other human plasma proteins to biomedical polymers. J Lab Clin Med 1990;116:687–696.
152. Margolis J. Activation of Hageman factor by saturated fatty acids. Aust J Exp Biol Med Sci 1962;40:505–514.
153. Didisheim P, Mibasham RS. Activation of Hageman factor (factor XII) by long chain saturated fatty acids. Thromb Diath Haemorrh 1963;9:346–353.
154. Nossel HL. Activation of factors XII (Hageman) and XI (PTA) by skin contact. Proc Soc Exp Biol Med 1966;122:16–17.

155. Botti RE, Ratnoff OD. Studies on the pathogenesis of thrombosis: an experimental "hypercoagulable" state induced by the intravenous injection of ellagic acid. J Lab Clin Med 1964;64:385–398.
156. Kellermeyer RW, Breckenridge RT. The inflammatory process in acute gouty arthritis. I. Activation of Hageman factor by sodium urate crystals. J Lab Clin Med 1965;65:307–315.
157. Ratnoff OD. Activation of Hageman factor by L-homocysteine. Science 1968;162:1007–1009.
158. Becker CG, Wagner M, Kaplan AP et al. Activation of factor XII-dependent pathways in human plasma by hematin and protoporphyrin. J Clin Invest 1985;76:413–419.
159. Kurachi K, Fujikawa K, Davie EW. Mechanism of activation of bovine factor XI by factor XII and XIIa. Biochemistry 1980;19:1330–1338.
160. Fujikawa K, Heimark RL, Kurachi K et al. Activation of bovine factor XII (Hageman factor) by plasma kallikrein. Biochemistry 1980;19:1322–1330.
161. Tans G, Rosing J, Griffin JH. Sulfatide-dependent autoactivation of human blood coagulation factor XII (Hageman factor). J Biol Chem 1983;258:8215–8222.
162. Hojima Y, Cochrane CG, Wiggins RC et al. In vitro activation of the contact (Hageman factor) system of plasma by heparin and chondroitin sulfate E. Blood 1984;63:1453–1459.
163. Koenig JM, Chahine A, Ratnoff OD. Inhibition of the activation of Hageman factor (factor XII) by soluble human placental collagens types III, IV, and V. J Lab Clin Med 1991;117:523–527.
164. Silverberg M, Diehl SV. The autoactivation of factor XII (Hageman factor) induced by low-Mr heparin and dextran sulfate. Biochem J 1987;248:715–720.
165. Tans G, Verklei AJ, Yu J et al. Sulfatide bilayers as a surface for contact activation in human plasma. Biochem Biophys Res Commun 1987;149:1002–1007.
166. Griep MA, Fujikawa K, Nelsestuen GL. Possible basis for the apparent surface selectivity of the contact activation of human blood coagulation factor XII. Biochemistry 1986;25:6688–6694.
167. Schousboe I. Contact activation in human plasma is triggered by zinc ion modulation of factor XII (Hageman Factor). Blood Coagul Fibrinolysis 1993;4:671–678.
168. Bernardo MM, Day DE, Olson ST et al. Surface-independent acceleration of factor XII activation by zinc ions. I. Kinetic characterization of the metal ion rate enhancement. J Biol Chem 1993;268:12468–12476.
169. Bernardo MM, Day DE, Halvorson HR et al. Surface-independent acceleration of factor XII activation by zinc ions. II. Direct binding and fluorescence studies. J Biol Chem 1993;268:12477–12483.
170. Rojkjaer R, Schousboe I. Identification of the $Zn^{2+}$ binding sites in factor XII and its activation derivatives. Eur J Biochem 1997;247:491–496.
171. Wiggins RC, Loskutoff DJ, Cochrane CG et al. Activation of rabbit Hageman factor by homogenates of cultured rabbit endothelial cells. J Clin Invest 1980;65:197–206.
172. Bagdasarian A, Talamo RC, Colman RW. Isolation of the high molecular weight activators of human plasma prekallikrein. J Biol Chem 1973;248:3456-3463.
173. Kaplan AP, Austen KF. A prealbumin activator of prekallikrein. J Immunol 1970;105:802–811.
174. Wuepper KD, Tucker ES III, Cochrane CG. Plasma kinin system: proenzyme components. J Immunol 1970;105:1307–1311.
175. Cochrane CG, Griffin JH. Molecular assembly in the contact phase of the Hageman factor system. Am J Med 1979;67:657–664.
176. Kaplan AP, Austen KF. A prealbumin activator of prekallikrein. II. Derivation of activators of prekallikrein from active Hageman factor by digestion with plasmin. J Exp Med 1971;133:696–712.
177. Revak SD, Cochrane CG, Bouma BN et al. Surface and fluid phase activities of two forms of activated Hageman factor produced during contact activation of plasma. J Exp Med 1978;147:719–729.
178. Revak SD, Cochrane CG. The relationship of structure and function in human Hageman factor. The association of enzymatic and binding activities with separate regions of the molecule. J Clin Invest 1976;57:852–860.
179. Forbes CD, Pensky J, Ratnoff OD. Inhibition of activated Hageman factor and activated plasma thromboplastin antecedent by purified C1-inactivator. J Lab Clin Med 1970;76:809–815.
180. Schreiber AD, Kaplan AP, Austen KF. Inhibition by C1-INH of Hageman factor fragment activation of coagulation, fibrinolysis and kinin-generation. J Clin Invest 1973;52:1402–1409.
181. de Agostini A, Lijnen HR, Pixley RA et al. Inactivation of factor XII active fragment in normal plasma. Predominant role of C1-inhibitor. J Clin Invest 1984;73:1542–1549.
182. Pixley RA, Schapira M, Colman RW. The regulation of human factor XIIa by plasma proteinase inhibitors. J Biol Chem 1985;260:1723–1729.
183. Pixley RA, Schmaier A, Colman RW. Effect of negatively charged activating compounds on inactivation of factor XIIa by C1 inhibitor. Arch Biochem Biophys 1987;256:490–498.
184. Stead N, Kaplan AP, Rosenberg RD. Inhibition of activated factor XII by antithrombin-heparin cofactor. J Biol Chem 1976;251:6481–6488.
185. Pixley RA, Colman RW. Effect of heparin on the inactivation rate of human activated factor XII by antithrombin III. Blood 1985;66:198–203.
186. Berrettini M, Schleef RR, Espana F et al. Interaction of type 1 plasminogen activator inhibitor with the enzymes of the contact activation system. J Biol Chem 1989;264:11738–11743.
187. Kleniewski J, Donaldson VH. Endothelial cells produce a substance that inhibits contact activation of coagulation by blocking the activation of Hageman factor. Proc Natl Acad Sci U S A 1993;90:198–202.
188. Greengard JS, Griffin JH. Receptors for high molecular weight kininogen on stimulated washed human platelets. Biochemistry 1984;23:6863–6869.
189. van Iwaarden F, de Groot PG, Sixma JJ et al. High-molecular weight kininogen is present in cultured human endothelial cells: localization, isolation, and characterization. Blood 1988;71:1268–1276.
190. Kerbiriou-Nabias DM, Garcia FO, Larrieu MJ. Radioimmunoassays of human high and low-molecular-weight kininogens in plasmas and platelets. Br J Haematol 1984;56:273–286.
191. Figueroa CD, Henderson LM, Kaufmann J et al. Immunovisualization of high (HK) and low (LK) molecular weight kininogens on isolated human neutrophils. Blood 1992;79:754–759.
192. Gustafson EJ, Lukasiewicz H, Wachtfogel YT et al. High molecular weight kininogen inhibits fibrinogen binding to cytoadhesins of neutrophils and platelets. J Cell Biol 1989;109:377–387.
193. Berrettini M, Schleef RR, Heeb MJ et al. Assembly and expression of an intrinsic factor IX activator complex on the surface of cultured human endothelial cells. J Biol Chem 1992;267:19833–19839.
194. Jencks WP. On the attribution and additivity of binding energies. Proc Natl Acad Sci U S A 1981;78:4046–4050.
195. Villanueva GB, Leung L, Bradford H et al. Conformation of high molecular weight kininogen: effects of kallikrein and factor XIa cleavage. Biochem Biophys Res Commun 1989;158:72–79.
196. Edgell CJ, McDonald CC, Graham JB. Permanent cell lines expressing human factor VIII-related antigen established by hybridization. Proc Natl Acad Sci U S A 1983;80:3734–3737.
197. Herwald H, Dedio J, Kellner R et al. Isolation and characterization of the kininogen-binding protein p33 from endothelial cells. Identity with the gC1q receptor. J Biol Chem 1996;271:13040–13047.
198. Ghebrehiwet B, Lim BL, Peerschke EI et al. Isolation, cDNA cloning, and overexpression of a 33-kD cell surface glycoprotein that binds to the globular "heads" of C1q. J Exp Med 1994;179:1809–1821.
199. Joseph K, Ghebrehiwet B, Peerschke EI et al. Identification of the zinc-dependent endothelial cell binding protein for high molecular weight kininogen and factor XII: identity with the receptor that binds to the globular "heads" of C1q (gC1q-R). Proc Natl Acad Sci U S A 1996;93:8552–8557.
200. Reddigari SR, Shibayama Y, Brunnee T et al. Human Hageman factor (factor XII) and high molecular weight kininogen compete for the same binding site on human umbilical vein endothelial cells. J Biol Chem 1993;268:11982–11987.
201. Colman RW, Pixley RA, Najamunnisa S et al. Binding of high molecular weight kininogen to human endothelial cells is mediated via a site within Domains 2 and 3 of the urokinase receptor. J Clin Invest 1997;100:1481–1487.
202. Wei Y, Lukashev M, Simon DI et al. Regulation of integrin function by the urokinase receptor. Science 1996;273:1551–1555.
203. Hasan AAK, Zisman T, Schmaier AH. Cytokeratin 1 is the major endothelial cell receptor for kininogens [Abstract]. Thromb Haemost 1997;77(Suppl 1):141.
204. Hembrough TA, Vasudevan J, Allietta MM et al. A cytokeratin 8-like protein with plasminogen-binding activity is present on the external surface of hepatocytes, HepG2 cells, and breast carcinoma cell line. J Cell Sci 1995;108:1071–1082.
205. Hembrough TA, Li L, Gonias SL. Cell-surface cytokeratin 8 is the major plasminogen receptor on breast cancer cells and is required for the accelerated activation of cell-associated plasminogen by tissue-type plasminogen activator. J Biol Chem 1996;271:25684–25691.
206. Nishikawa K, Shibayama Y, Kuna P et al. Generation of vasoactive peptide bradykinin from human umbilical vein endothelium-bound high molecular weight kininogen by plasma kallikrein. Blood 1992;80:1980–1988.
207. Sinha D, Seaman FS, Koshy A et al. Blood coagulation factor XIa binds specifically to a site on activated human platelets distinct from that for factor XI. J Clin Invest 1984;73:1550–1556.
208. Walsh PN, Sinha D, Koshy A et al. Functional characterization of platelet-bound factor XIa: retention of factor XIa activity on the platelet surface. Blood 1986;68:225–230.
209. Loza JP, Gurewich V, Johnstone M et al. Platelet-bound prekallikrein promotes pro-urokinase-induced clot lysis: a mechanism for targeting the factor XII dependent intrinsic pathway of fibrinolysis. Thromb Haemost 1994;71:347–352.
210. Kaplan AP, Kay AB, Austen KF. A prealbumen activator of prekallikrein II. Appearance of chemotactic activity for human neutrophils by the conversion of prekallikrein to kallikrein. J Exp Med 1972;135:81–97.
211. Schapira M, Despland E, Scott CF et al. Purified human plasma kallikrein aggregates human blood neutrophils. J Clin Invest 1982;69:1199–1202.
212. Wachtfogel YT, Kucich U, James HL et al. Human plasma kallikrein releases neutrophil elastase during blood coagulation. J Clin Invest 1983;72:1672–1677.

213. Zimmerli W, Huber I, Bouma BN et al. Purified human plasma kallikrein does not stimulate but primes neutrophils for superoxide production. Thromb Haemost 1989;62:1121–1125.

214. Plow EF. Leukocyte elastase release during blood coagulation: a potential mechanism for activation of the alternative fibrinolytic pathway. J Clin Invest 1982;69:564–572.

215. Rebuck JW. The skin window as a monitor of leukocytic functions in contact activation factor deficiencies in man. Am J Clin Pathol 1983;79:405–413.

216. Colman RW, Wachtfogel YT, Kucich U et al. Effect of cleavage of the heavy chain of human plasma kallikrein on its functional properties. Blood 1985;65:311–318.

217. Wachtfogel YT, Pixley RA, Kucich U et al. Purified plasma factor XIIa aggregates human neutrophils and causes degranulation. Blood 1986;67:1731–1737.

218. Chien P, Pixley RA, Stumpo LG et al. Modulation of the human monocyte binding site for monomeric immunoglobulin G by activated Hageman factor. J Clin Invest 1988;82:1554–1559.

219. Chien P, Pixley RA, Ruiz P et al. Modulation of monocyte FcgR1 by activated Hageman factor: mapping the functional XIIa site [Abstract]. Blood 1990;76:178a.

220. Toossi Z, Sedor JR, Mettler MA et al. Induction of expression of monocyte interleukin 1 by Hageman factor (factor XII). Proc Natl Acad Sci U S A 1992;89:11969–11972.

221. Stern DM, Nossel HL, Owen J. Acquired antibody to factor XI in a individual with congenital factor XI deficiency. J Clin Invest 1982;69:1270–1276.

222. DeLa Cadena R, Baglia FA, Johnson CA et al. Naturally occurring human antibodies against two distinct functional domains in the heavy chain of FXI/FXIa. Blood 1988;72:1748–1754.

223. Crutchley DJ, Ryan JW, Ryan US et al. Bradykinin-induced release of prostacyclin and thromboxanes from bovine pulmonary artery endothelial cells. Studies with lower homologs and calcium antagonists. Biochim Biophys Acta 1983;751:99–107.

224. Hong SL. Effect of bradykinin and thrombin on prostacyclin synthesis in endothelial cells from calf and pig aorta and human umbilical cord vein. Thromb Res 1980;18:787–795.

225. Holland JA, Pritchard KA, Pappolla MA et al. Bradykinin induces superoxide anion release from human endothelial cells. J Cell Physiol 1990;143:21–25.

226. Smith D, Gilbert M, Owen WG. Tissue plasminogen activator release *in vivo* in response to vasoactive agents. Blood 1985;66:835–839.

227. Brown NJ, Nadeau JH, Vaughan DE. Selective stimulation of tissue-type plasminogen activator (t-PA) *in vivo* by infusion of bradykinin. Thromb Haemost 1997;77:522–525.

228. Palmer RM, Ferrige AG, Moncada S. Nitric oxide release accounts for the biologic activity of endothelium-derived relaxing factor. Nature 1987;327:524–526.

229. Nakashima M, Mombouli JV, Taylor AA et al. Endothelium-dependent hyperpolarization caused by bradykinin in human coronary arteries. J Clin Invest 1993;92:2867–2871.

230. Boulanger C, Schini VB, Moncada S et al. Stimulation of cyclic GMP production in cultured endothelial cells of the pig by bradykinin, adenosine diphosphate, calcium ionophore A23187 and nitric oxide. Br J Pharmacol 1990;101:152–156.

231. Schini VB, Boulanger C, Regoli D et al. Bradykinin stimulates the production of cyclic GMP via activation of B2 kinin receptors in cultured porcine aortic endothelial cells. J Pharmacol Exp Ther 1990;252:581–585.

232. Busse R, Mulsch A. Induction of nitric oxide synthase by cytokines in vascular smooth muscle cells. FEBS Lett 1990;275:87–90.

233. Imai T, Hirata Y, Kanno K et al. Induction of nitric oxide synthase by cyclic AMP in rat vascular smooth muscle cells. J Clin Invest 1994;93:543–549.

234. Dixon BS, Breckon R, Fortune J et al. Effects of kinins on cultured arterial smooth muscle. Am J Physiol 1990;258:C299–308.

235. Dixon BS, Sharma RV, Dickerson T et al. Bradykinin and angiotensin II: activation of protein kinase C in arterial smooth muscle. Am J Physiol 1994;266:C1406–1420.

236. Yang HY, Erdos EG. Second kininase in human blood plasma. Nature 1967;215:1402–1403.

237. Sofer RL. Angiotensin-converting enzyme and the regulation of vasoactive peptides. Annu Rev Biochem 1976;45:73–94.

238. Wang J, Xiong W, Yang Z et al. Human tissue kallikrein induces hypotension in transgenic mice. Hypertension 1994;23:236–243.

239. Ma JX, Yang Z, Chao J et al. Intramuscular delivery of rat kallikrein-binding protein gene reverses hypotension in transgenic mice expressing human tissue kallikrein. J Biol Chem 1995;270:451–455.

240. Chao J, Tillman DM, Wang MY et al. Identification of a new tissue-kallikrein-binding protein. Biochem J 1986;239:325–331.

241. Chao J, Chai KX, Chen LM et al. Tissue kallikrein-binding protein is a serpin. I. Purification, characterization, and distribution in normotensive and spontaneously hypertensive rats. J Biol Chem 1990;265:16394–16401.

242. Zhou GX, Chao L, Chao J. Kallistatin: a novel human tissue kallikrein inhibitor. Purification, characterization, and reactive center sequence. J Biol Chem 1992;267:25873–25880.

243. Wang C, Chao L, Chao J. Direct gene delivery of human tissue kallikrein reduces blood pressure in spontaneously hypertensive rats. J Clin Invest 1995;95:1710–1716.

244. Xiong W, Chao J, Chao L. Muscle delivery of human kallikrein gene reduces blood pressure in hypertensive rats. Hypertension 1995;25:715–719.

245. Coller BS. Effects of tertiary amine local anesthetics on von Willebrand factor-dependent platelet function: alteration of membrane reactivity and degradation of GP Ib by a calcium-dependent protease(s). Blood 1982;60:731–743.

246. Puri RN, Gustafson EJ, Zhou F et al. Inhibition of thrombin-induced platelet aggregation by high molecular weight kininogen. Trans Assoc Am Physicians 1987;100:232–240.

247. Puri RN, Matsueda R, Umeyama H et al. Modulation of thrombin-induced platelet aggregation by inhibition of calpain by a synthetic peptide derived from the thiol-protease inhibitory sequence of kininogens and S-(3-nitro-2-pyridinesulfenyl)-cysteine. Eur J Biochem 1993;214:233–241.

248. Matsueda R, Umeyama H, Puri RN et al. Design and synthesis of a kininogen-based selective inhibitor of thrombin-induced platelet aggregation. Pept Res 1994;7:32–35.

249. Charo IF, Feinman RD, Detwiler TC. Interrelations of platelet aggregation and secretion. J Clin Invest 1977;60:866–873.

250. Schmaier AH, Meloni FJ, Nawarawong W et al. PPACK-thrombin is a noncompetitive inhibitor of alpha-thrombin binding to human platelets. Thromb Res 1992;67:479–489.

251. Majima M, Sunahara N, Harada Y et al. Detection of the degradation products of bradykinin by enzyme immunoassays as markers for the release of kinin *in vivo*. Biochem Pharmacol 1993;45:559–567.

252. Shima C, Majima M, Katori M. A stable metabolite, Arg-Pro-Pro-Gly-Phe, of bradykinin in the degradation pathway in human plasma. Jpn J Pharmacol 1992;60:111–119.

253. Niewiarowski S, Prou-Wartelle O. Role of the contact factor (Hageman factor) in fibrinolysis. Thromb Diath Haemorrh 1959;3:593–603.

254. Colman RW. Activation of plasminogen by human plasma kallikrein. Biochem Biophys Res Commun 1969;35:273–279.

255. Mandle R Jr, Kaplan AP. Hageman factor substrates. Human plasma prekallikrein: mechanism of activation by Hageman factor and participation in Hageman factor-dependent fibrinolysis. J Biol Chem 1977;252:6097–6104.

256. Goldsmith GH Jr, Saito H, Ratnoff OD. The activation of plasminogen by Hageman factor (factor XII) and Hageman factor fragments. J Clin Invest 1978;62:54–60.

257. Mandle RJ Jr, Kaplan AP. Hageman-factor-dependent fibrinolysis. Generation of fibrinolytic activity by the interaction of human activated factor XI and plasminogen. Blood 1979;54:850–862.

258. Gurewich V, Johnstone M, Loza JP et al. Pro-urokinase and prekallikrein are both associated with platelets. Implications for the intrinsic pathway of fibrinolysis and for therapeutic thrombolysis. FEBS Lett 1993;318:317–321.

259. Lin Y, Harris RB, Yan W et al. High molecular weight kininogen peptides inhibit the formation of kallikrein on endothelial cell surfaces and subsequent urokinase-dependent plasmin formation. Blood, 1997;90:690–697.

260. Higazi A, Cohen RL, Henkin J et al. Enhancement of the enzymatic activity of single-chain urokinase plasminogen activator by soluble urokinase receptor. J Biol Chem 1995;270:17375–17380.

261. Carmeliet P, Collen D. Gene targeting and gene transfer studies of the plasminogen/plasmin system: implications in thrombosis, hemostasis, neointima formation, and atherosclerosis. FASEB J 1995;9:934–938.

262. Vroman L, Adams A. Possible involvement of fibrinogen and proteolysis in surface activation. A study with the recording ellipsometer. Thromb Diath Haemorrh 1967;18:510–524.

263. Schmaier AH, Silver L, Adams AL et al. The effect of high molecular weight kininogen on surface-adsorbed fibrinogen. Thromb Res 1984;33:51–67.

264. Brash JL, Scott CF, ten Hove P et al. Mechanism of transient adsorption of fibrinogen from plasma to solid surfaces: role of the contact and fibrinolytic systems. Blood 1988;71:932–939.

265. Li C, Gurewich V, Liu JN. Urokinase-type plasminogen activator-induced monocyte adhesion is modulated by kininogen, kallikrein, factor XII, and plasminogen. Exp Cell Res 1996;226:239–242.

266. Landerman NS. Hereditary angioneurotic edema. I. Case reports and review of the literature. J Allergy Clin Immunol 1962;33:316–329.

267. Schapira M, Sliver LD, Scott CF et al. Prekallikrein activation and high molecular weight kininogen consumption in hereditary angioedema. N Engl J Med 1983;308:1050–1053.

268. Cugno M, Hack CE, de Boer JP et al. Generation of plasmin during acute attacks of hereditary angioedema. J Lab Clin Med 1993;121:38–43.

269. Berrettini M, Lammle B, White T et al. Detection of *in vitro* and *in vivo* cleavage of high molecular weight kininogen in human plasma by immunblotting with monoclonal antibodies. Blood 1986;68:455–462.

270. Fields T, Ghebrehiwet B, Kaplan AP. Kinin formation in hereditary angioedema plasma: evidence against kinin derivation from C2 and in support of "spontaneous" formation of bradykinin. J Allergy Clin Immunol 1983;72:54–60.

271. Rapaport SI, Aas K, Owren PA. The effect of glass upon the activity of the various plasma clotting factors. J Clin Invest 1955;34:9–19.

272. Gjonnaess H. Cold-promoted activation of factor VII. III. Relation to the kallikrein system. Thromb Diath Haemorrh 1972;28:182–193.
273. Seligsohn U, Osterud B, Brown SF et al. Activation of human factor VII in plasma and in purified systems. J Clin Invest 1979;64:239–243.
274. Weiss R, Kaplan AP. The effect of C1 inhibitor upon Hageman factor autoactivation. Blood 1986;68:239–243.
275. Mason JW, Colman RW. The role of Hageman factor in disseminated intravascular coagulation induced by septicemia, neoplasia, or liver disease. Thromb Diath Haemorrh 1971;26:325–331.
276. O'Donnell TF Jr, Clowes GH Jr, Talamo RC et al. Kinin activation in the blood of individuals with sepsis. Surg Gynecol Obstet 1976;143:539–545.
277. Colman RW, Edelman R, Scott CF et al. Plasma kallikrein activation and inhibition during typhoid fever. J Clin Invest 1978;61:287–296.
278. Schapira M, Gardaz JP, Py P et al. Prekallikrein activation in the adult respiratory distress syndrome. Bull Eur Physiopathol Respir 1985;21:237–241.
279. Carvalho AC, DeMarinis S, Scott CF et al. Activation of the contact system of plasma proteolysis in the adult respiratory distress syndrome. J Lab Clin Med 1988;112:270–277.
280. Rao AK, Schapira M, Clements ML et al. A prospective study of platelets and plasma proteolytic systems during the early stages of Rocky Mountain spotted fever. N Engl J Med 1988;318:1021–1028.
281. Nuijens JH, Huijbregts CC, Eerenberg Belmer AJ et al. Quantification of plasma factor XIIa-Cl(-)-inhibitor and kallikrein-Cl(-)-inhibitor complexes in sepsis. Blood 1988;72:1841–1848.
282. Kaufman N, Page JD, Pixley RA et al. Alpha 2-macroglobulin-kallikrein complexes detect contact system activation in hereditary angioedema and human sepsis. Blood 1991;77:2660–2667.
283. DeLa Cadena RA, Suffredini AF, Page JD et al. Activation of the kallikrein-kinin system after endotoxin administration to normal human volunteers. Blood 1993;81:3313–3317.
284. Pixley RA, DeLa Cadena RA, Page JD et al. Activation of the contact system in lethal hypotensive bacteremia in a baboon model. Am J Pathol 1992;140:897–906.
285. Pixley RA, DeLa Cadena RA, Page JD et al. The contact system contributes to hypotension but not disseminated intravascular coagulation in lethal bacteremia: *In vivo* use of a monoclonal anti-factor XII antibody to block contact activation in baboons. J Clin Invest 1993;91:61–68.
286. Ratnoff OD, Busse RJ Jr, Sheon RP. The demise of John Hageman. N Engl J Med 1968;279:760–761.
287. Colman RW. Contributions of Mayme Williams to the elucidation of the multiple functions of the plasma kininogens. Thromb Haemost 1992;68:99–101.
288. Goodnough LT, Saito H, Ratnoff OD. Thrombosis or myocardial infarction in congenital clotting factor abnormalities and chronic thrombocytopenias: a report of 21 individuals and a review of 50 previously reported cases. Medicine 1983;62:248–255.
289. Mannhalter C, Fisher M, Hopmeier P et al. Factor XII activity and antigen concentrations in individuals suffering from recurrent thrombosis. Fibrinolysis 1987;1:259.
290. Lammle B, Wuillemin WA, Huber I et al. Thromboembolism and bleeding tendency in congenital factor XII deficiency: a study on 74 subjects from 14 Swiss families. Thromb Haemost 1991;65:117–121.
291. Halbmayer WM, Mannhalter C, Feichtinger C et al. The prevalence of factor XII deficiency in 103 orally anticoagulated outpatients suffering from recurrent venous and/or arterial thromboembolism. Thromb Haemost 1992;68:285–290.
292. von Kanel R, Wuillemin WA, Furlan M et al. Factor XII clotting activity and antigen levels in individuals with thromboembolic disease. Blood Coagul Fibrinolysis 1992;3:555–561.
293. Jespersen J, Munkvad S, Pedersen OD et al. Evidence for a role of factor XII-dependent fibrinolysis in cardiovascular diseases. Ann N Y Acad Sci 1992;667:454–456.
294. Munkvad S, Jespersen J, Gram J et al. Long-lasting depression of the factor XII-dependent fibrinolytic system in individuals with myocardial infarction undergoing thrombolytic therapy with recombinant tissue-type plasminogen activator: a randomized placebo-controlled study. J Am Coll Cardiol 1991;17:957–962.
295. Koster T, Rosendaal FR, Bri't E et al. John Hageman's factor and deep-vein thrombosis: Leiden Thrombophilia Study. Br J Haematol 1994;87:422–424.

# CHAPTER 6

# FIBRIN FORMATION AND STABILIZATION

## Joann M. Hettasch and Charles S. Greenberg

## FIBRIN FORMATION AND STABILIZATION

Fibrin formation and stabilization are the processes by which soluble fibrinogen is converted into an insoluble fibrin clot by the action of thrombin and factor XIIIa. Fibrinogen conversion to an insoluble fibrin matrix occurs in three major phases: 1) fibrinopeptide cleavage by thrombin; 2) fibrin polymerization; and 3) covalent stabilization by factor XIIIa. Congenital or acquired abnormalities in the blood coagulation proteins involved in fibrin stabilization can lead to serious hemorrhagic and thrombotic disorders, demonstrating the importance of these proteins in regulating hemostasis. Fibrin formed in the absence of factor XIIIa fails to provide an adequate matrix for wound healing or a permanent barrier to blood loss. In this chapter, an overview of the structure of the fibrinogen molecule and fibrin formation will be presented. In addition, the plasma and cellular factors involved in the covalent modification of fibrin by factor XIIIa will be discussed.

## FORMATION OF FIBRIN

### THE FIBRINOGEN MOLECULE

The fibrinogen molecule is a large, trinodular, disulfide-bonded glycoprotein that is composed of two symmetrical half-molecules each containing three distinct polypeptide chains designated A$\alpha$, B$\beta$, and $\gamma$ (Fig. 6.1) (1–3). The human fibrinogen molecule is 340 Kda and can be described by the formula A$\alpha_2$B$\beta_2\gamma_2$. The A$\alpha$, B$\beta$, and $\gamma$ chain are 63.5, 56.0, and 47.0 Kda, respectively (4, 5).

The earliest studies of fibrinogen demonstrated that the fibrinogen molecule had the properties of a fibrous protein. X-ray diffraction studies of fibrinogen and fibrin depicted a pattern characteristic of other fibrous proteins, including keratin and myosin (6). The diffraction pattern was derived from the triple stranded $\alpha$-helices known as coiled-coil regions (Fig 6.1) (6, 7). Electron microscopy was the first technique used to demonstrate that the fibrinogen molecule folded into a trinodular structure (8–11).

The fibrinogen molecule is 45 nm long and 9 nm in diameter. The central nodule called the E-domain is 5 nm in diameter and the aminoterminal ends of all six polypeptide chains form the N-terminal disulfide knot (Fig. 6.1) (8–10). The two D-domains form the outer two nodules and are made up of the carboxyterminal two-thirds of the B$\beta$ and $\gamma$ chains (11). The D-domain can be further defined by x-ray diffraction studies into two subdomains that are formed by the independent folding of the B$\beta$ and $\gamma$ chains. These subdomains appear to be located diagonally from the long axis of the molecule (Fig. 6.1) (7).

The E- and D-domains are separated from each other by a stretch of 111 to 112 amino acids from each polypeptide chain, which forms the triple-stranded $\alpha$-helical structure called the coiled-coil domain (12). The coiled-coil region is supported on either side by a set of disulfide bonds called disulfide rings (Fig. 6.1) (13–18). The disulfide rings and the coiled-coil region impart mechanical stability to the molecule.

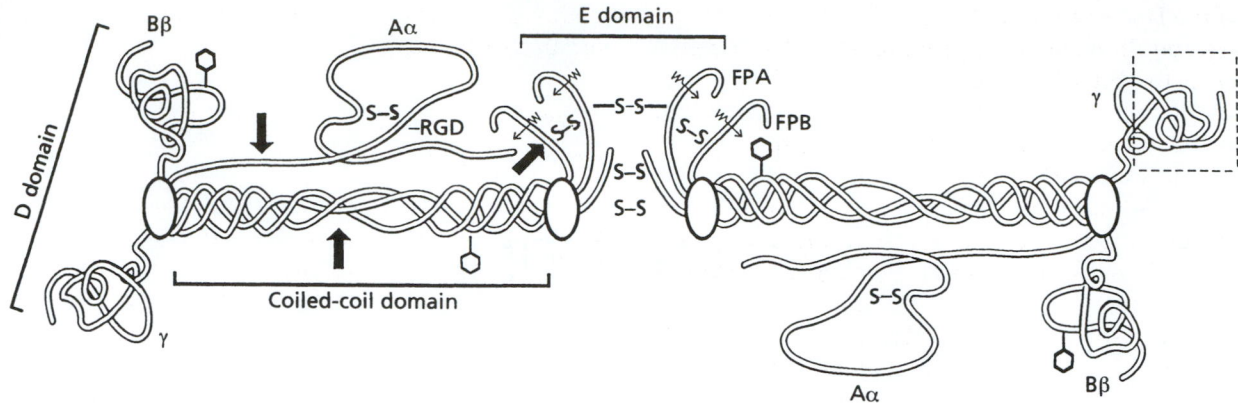

**FIGURE 6.1.** Model structure of fibrinogen. The fibrinogen model is a large glycoprotein that forms a trinodular structure. Three distinct polypeptide chains designated Aα, Bβ, and γ are disulfide bonded to produce two symmetrical half molecules. The entire molecule is 45 nm long and 9 nm in diameter. The two D-domains form the outer nodules and are made up of the carboxyterminal two thirds of the Bβ and γ chains. X-ray diffraction studies suggest that the D-domain has two subdomains formed by the independent folding of the Bβ and γ chains. These subdomains are located diagonally from the long axis. Within the carboxyterminal γ chain domain (*dashed box*) there exists the glutamine and lysine crosslinking sites, calmodulin-like, calcium binding site, and a platelet binding domain. The central E domain nodule is 5 nm in diameter and is formed by disulfide bonding the six aminotermini of each polypeptide chain. The D and E domains are separated from each other by a set of disulfide bonds called disulfide rings and a stretch of amino acids called the coiled-coil domain. Plasmin sequentially degrades the molecule by cleaving the Bβ chain, then the Aα and four sites in the coiled-coil region (marked in *dark arrows*). Thrombin cleaves fibrinopeptides A and B from the aminotermini from the Aα and Bβ-chains. A platelet-binding RGD sequence is also present in the Aα-chain. FPA, fibrinopeptide A; FPB, fibrinopeptide B; RGD, Arginine, Glycine, Aspartic Acid. (Modified from Mosesson MW. Fibrin polymerization and its regulatory role in hemostasis. J Lab Clin Med 1990;116:8.)

The tertiary structure of fibrinogen makes the molecule susceptible to a selective pattern of proteolytic cleavage. Plasmin initially removes the carboxyterminal hydrophilic third of the Aα-chain (dark arrow, Fig. 6.1) and the first 42 amino acids of the Bβ chain, producing the clottable fragment X (molecular weight 240 to 260 Kda) (Fig. 6.1) (19, 20). Fragment X is then cleaved at one of the two coiled-coil regions, producing fragment D (approximately 100 Kda) and fragment Y molecules (approximately 150 Kda). Fragment Y is subsequently cleaved at the remaining coiled-coil region to produce a second fragment D and fragment E (approximately 45 Kda). These fragments are immunologically distinct and readily separated by ion-exchange chromatography (19, 20).

The complete primary structure for each of the human polypeptide chains has been established by amino acid and nucleic acid sequencing (21–28). The primary structures of the individual polypeptide chains of fibrinogen demonstrate significant homology and suggest a common ancestral gene (29). The homology between the chains is most readily defined by the conservation in the placement of the disulfide rings in each of the chains (15–18).

The Aα chain, 610 amino acids in length, is divided into three sections of equivalent size (24). The aminoterminal section from amino acids 1 to 194 is linked by disulfide bonds to both the Bβ and the γ chains. The section from amino acid 195 to 239 is a protease-sensitive domain containing a high content of prolines and four plasmin cleavage sites (dark arrow, Fig. 6.1) (30, 31). The middle third of the Aα chain (amino acid 240 to 424) is very rich in apolar amino acids and contains ten tandem repeats, each 13 amino acids long (24). Two glutamine residues at amino acid 328 and 366 serve as Aα-chain crosslinking acceptor sites (24). The fibronectin (32) and α2-antiplasmin (33) crosslinking sites are present in the carboxyterminus of the Aα-chain (24).

The Bβ chain, 461 amino acids in length, may also be subdivided into thirds. The first 80 amino acids are about 15% identical to the Aα-chain and are held together with the N-terminals of the other chains to form the central E-domain, or N-terminal disulfide knot (Fig. 6.1). The middle section (amino acids 81 to 192) contains the two sets of disulfide rings that delineate the coiled-coil region (Fig. 6.1). The third section, amino acids 193 to 461, folds to form a subsection of the D-domain (Fig. 6.1) (1, 2).

The γ chain, which is only 411 amino acids long, is also readily subdivided into three sections. The first section of only 18 amino acids is formed due to gene deletion, removing the cleavable fibrinopeptide domains which are present in the Aα and Bβ genes (29). The middle segment, amino acids 19 to 129, contains the disulfide rings and the coiled-coil region (12). The final section, amino acids 130 to 411, forms the globular segment of the D-domain (Fig. 6.1) (34, 35). The γ- and Bβ-chains can be aligned with approximately 35% sequence identity in the final third of the molecules. The alignment of the Bβ and γ chains demonstrates that the γ chain has gained a carboxyterminal extension of 18 amino acids that participate in factor XIIIa mediated crosslinking (36). The carboxyterminus of the γ chain also contains the sequences known to promote staphylococcal clumping, cell adhesion, and platelet aggregation (Fig. 6.1) (37–39).

Calcium ions modulate the structure and function of fibrinogen (40). There are three calcium binding sites identified within the fibrinogen molecule (40–42). Two of the sites are located within the amino acid sequence defined by residues 311 to 336 of the γ chains in the D-domain. The amino acid sequence in this region of the molecule is homologous to the calcium binding domain of calmodulin. When calcium ions occupy this site, the γ chain is protected from plasmin degradation. The third site for calcium binding is located in the E-domain (41).

The three binding sites have sufficient affinity for calcium ($Kd \sim \times 10^{-5}$ M) such that at physiologic plasma conditions (1.5 mM free calcium), all sites are occupied. Calcium ions also regulate fibrin polymerization by enhancing the rate and the extent of lateral association of protofibrils to form fibrin strands (40).

Carbohydrates attached to both the β- and γ chains play a role in fibrin polymerization (43–45). The carbohydrates are linked to fibrinogen by N-glycosidic bonds to asparagines with the sequence Asn-X-Thr (45). Defective fibrin polymerization occurs when abnormal carbohydrates, especially sialic acid residues, are added to the fibrinogen, as occurs in cirrhosis (46).

Two distinct molecular forms of the γ chain are detectable in the human plasma fibrinogen molecule. These forms are distinguishable by both size and charge. The γ chain, present in approximately 85% of the fibrinogen molecules, is shorter and more positively charged than the longer, more negatively charged γ' chain (approximately 15% of the molecules). These two forms of the γ chain are always present in human fibrinogen, although their relative proportions are not under any known physiologic control mechanism (47–51). The human γ chain is formed by alternative polyadenylation of the last intron (52). A polyadenylation signal in the middle of the last intron produces the γ' mRNA, which causes the last intron to remain unspliced in approximately 15% of the transcripts producing a new C-terminus. The C-terminal extension does not modify fibrin crosslinking but does interfere with the ability of fibrinogen containing these γ'-chains to support platelet aggregation (53, 54). Platelets contain exclusively γ chains in their alpha-granules which could be selectively imported into the platelet. Recent studies indicate that the γ'-chain is a carrier for the zymogen of factor XIII in circulating blood (55).

## X-RAY CRYSTALLOGRAPHY OF FIBRINOGEN

Most of the current information regarding the structure of fibrinogen comes from biochemical and biophysical studies on the molecule, but the x-ray crystal structure of this 340 Kda glycoprotein has not been determined. However, there is new information available on the structure of various domains of fibrinogen. Preliminary diffraction studies on fragment D have been reported (56, 57). The x-ray crystal structure of this fragment will provide detailed information on the extent of the coiled-coil region, and the orientation of the β and γ domains at the atomic level. Fragment D was also co-crystallized with the Gly-Pro-Arg-Pro-amide peptide, and the diffraction studies on this structure should indicate the nature of the interactions leading to polymerization (56).

There has been a great deal of interest in the structure of the carboxyterminal domain of the γ chain of fibrinogen because this domain binds to platelets, certain bacteria, and contains the reciprocal γ chain crosslinking site for factor XIIIa. Elucidation of the structure of this region of the γ chain should give a clearer picture of how the fibrin clot is stabilized at the molecular level. Nuclear magnetic resonance (NMR) studies on a synthetic peptide (residues 392 to 411) of the carboxyterminus of the γ chain revealed the presence of a type II β turn in this region (58). In other studies, a 14 amino acid segment (397 to 411) of the carboxyterminus of the γ chain was added as an extension to lysozyme (59). This hybrid protein was expressed, crystallized, and its structure was determined. This peptide also had a turn but it was not located in the same position as in the NMR studies. More recently, a preliminary study on the crystal structure of a 30 Kda γ chain domain corresponding to residues 147 to 411 was reported in abstract form (60). This structure may resolve the discrepancy between the data obtained by NMR on the synthetic peptide and the x-ray crystal structure of the lysozyme extension peptide. However, until the 340 Kda protein is crystallized, there will also be some concern over whether the fragments are folded in the native conformation in the absence of the rest of the molecule.

## RELEASE OF FIBRINOPEPTIDES A AND B

In the first phase of fibrin formation thrombin cleaves two specific Arg-Gly bonds in the Aα- and Bβ-chains of fibrinogen, releasing fibrinopeptides A and B from the aminoterminus (Fig. 6.1 ) (61). Release of fibrinopeptide A (Aα 1 to 16) initiates the process by which fibrin assembles into a gel composed of interconnecting fibrin strands (Fig. 6.2) (62).

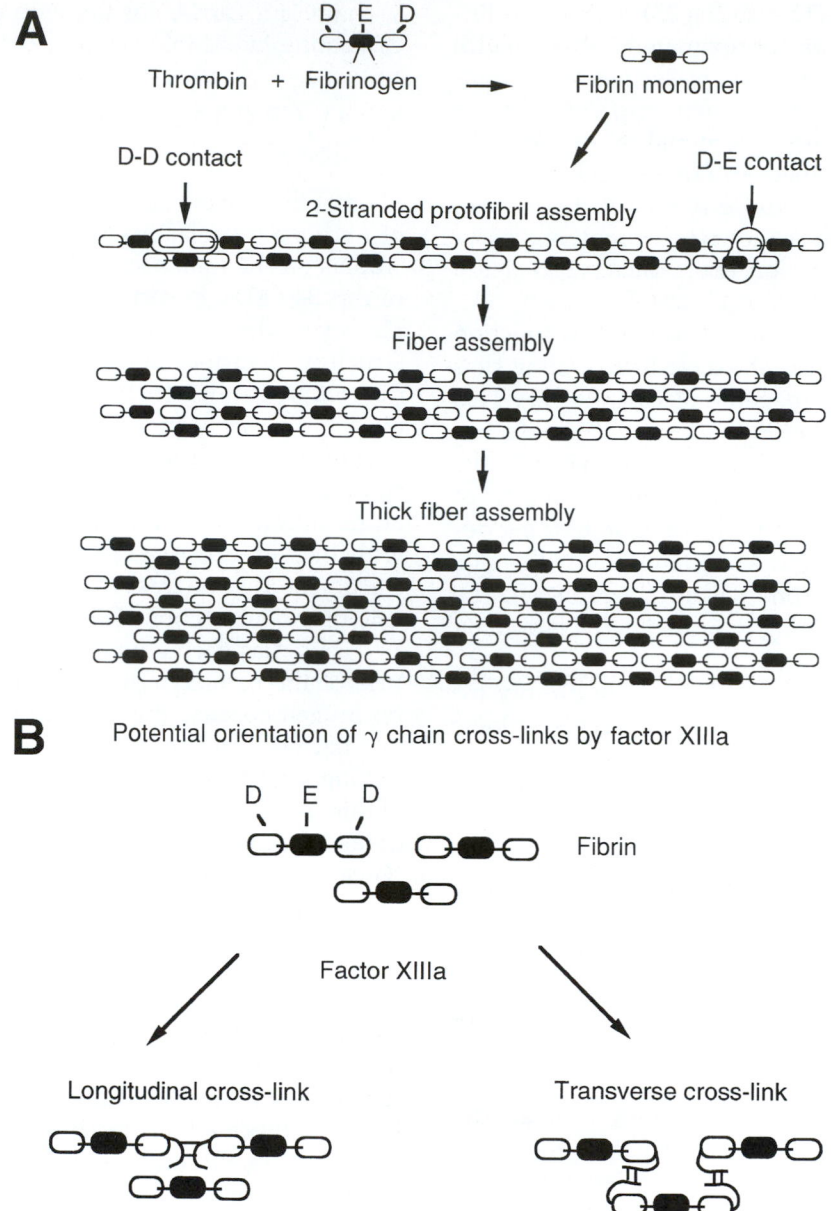

**FIGURE 6.2.**   Model of fibrin polymerization and crosslinking. **A,** Fibrinogen and fibrin molecules are shown as trinodular structures. The central E domain is shown as a closed oval and the outer D-domains are shown as open ovals. Thrombin catalyzes the release of the fibrinopeptides A and B from the central E domain. Then fibrin monomer molecules align in a staggered half overlapping orientation. The molecule is held together by the D–E contacts to form a two-stranded protofibril. The protofibrils will also polymerize laterally to form thicker fibers that will branch to form a three-dimensional gel. **B,** In the presence of $Ca^{2+}$, plasma factor XIII and thrombin, the fibrin polymers are crosslinked initially by isopeptide bonds between the $\gamma$ chains in the D-domain. The orientation of the isopeptide bond formed between the $\gamma$-chains in the D-domains of assembled fibrin fibers remains unresolved. One possibility is that these bonds are oriented parallel to the direction of fiber growth in a longitudinal (end-to-end) manner. The other possibility is that the isopeptide bonds occur in a transverse (or half-staggered) manner between two strands of the protofibril. The longitudinal and transverse crosslink patterns are illustrated in Fig. 6.2B. Both types of crosslinking could occur during clot formation *in vivo.*

Initial studies of thrombin cleavage suggested that fibrinopeptide A release occurred more rapidly than fibrinopeptide B release (61, 63). However, fibrinopeptide B cleavage occurs at a slower rate, making it appear that fibrinopeptide A release occurs first (64, 65). During the assembly of fibrin fibers, the rate of fibrinopeptide B cleavage increases significantly. Fibrinopeptide B cleavage by thrombin could be promoted by either a conformational change induced by fibrin polymerization or by the preferential release of fibrinopeptide B from soluble fibrin polymers (66–68).

## ASSEMBLY OF FIBRIN POLYMERS

In the second phase of fibrin formation, thrombin-catalyzed release of fibrinopeptides A and B exposes two types of binding sites in the central E-domain and produces fibrin monomer molecules that cooperate in the assembly of fibrin polymers (Fig. 6.2) (69). Binding sites on the central E-domain of fibrin monomers will interact with complementary sites on the $\gamma$ chain of the D-domain of adjacent fibrin monomers (69). The noncovalent interaction between the half-overlapped monomers is called the D-E contact site (Fig. 6.2) (70). The D-E contacts provide stability to the elongating intermediate fibrin polymers composed of overlapping fibrin molecules described as protofibrils (Fig. 6.2) (71).

The localization of the $\gamma$ chain sequence involved in the D-E contact site has been studied extensively by several investigators. The $\gamma$ chain site is reportedly located between either $\gamma$ 373–410 (72), $\gamma$ 374–396 (73), $\gamma$ 356–411 (74), $\gamma$ 303–405 (75), or $\gamma$ 337–379 (76, 77). These studies demonstrate that the carboxyterminus of the $\gamma$ chain plays an important role in fibrin polymerization.

Complementary binding sites involved in D-E contacts of the central E-domain are located at the aminoterminus of the $A\alpha$-chain in the region that is exposed after thrombin releases fibrinopeptide A (78). Synthetic peptides mimicking the new aminoterminus sequence GPR bind to fibrinogen and inhibit fibrin polymerization (78). This is in distinct contrast to the peptide sequence GHRP identical to the aminoterminus of the $\beta$-chain which binds to a separate site on fibrinogen but fails to block fibrin polymerization (79).

The process by which the half-staggered overlapping molecules elongate involves formation of a trimeric structure by the addition of fibrin monomers to a dimer held together by D-E contacts. The additional monomer forms a D-D contact as well as another D-E contact (Fig. 6.2) (70). A two-stranded protofibril is formed as this elongation process continues (70, 80–82). After long protofibrils form they assemble into thicker fibers of fibrin (70, 71, 81). The protofibrils associate with other protofibrils through lateral associations which are held together by a set of weak interactions. These noncovalent interactions are distinct from the D-E contacts and are sensitive to changes in pH, ionic strength, and temperature (80, 83–85). The sites on the fibrin molecules responsible for the lateral association of fibrin protofibrils are not well established. Release of the negatively charged fibrinopeptide B enhances the rate and extent of fibrin fiber formation (80, 83, 84).

Fibrin polymerization is a reversible and exothermic reaction (86, 87). The exothermic nature of the process is althought to derive from hydrogen bonding between fibrin molecules. The hydrogen-bonded molecules are in a reversible equilibrium that can be influenced by changes in pH (88). Histidine residues are postulated to be the acceptor molecules and tyrosine residues the donors based upon the pH dependence of polymerization and the uptake of protons occurring with polymerization (88). Studies of photo-oxidation to modify histidine residues have demonstrated that histidine 16 of the $B\beta$-chain is essential for fibrin polymerization (89). Protofibrils and their fibers ultimately interconnect and form a network of fibrin fibers. Only 20% of the fibrin gel's volume is composed of protein, with 80% being solvent (90).

## RECOMBINANT HUMAN FIBRINOGEN

The expression of recombinant human fibrinogen from mammalian cells has been described by several laboratories (91–94). The ability to produce recombinant fibrinogen in mammalian cells has provided a means to understand the structure and function of this important plasma glycoprotein. Site-directed mutagenesis of the cysteine residues involved in the disulfide linkages between the three chains of fibrinogen has been used to understand the interaction of the subunits and the intermediates formed during the assembly of the intact molecule (95, 96). Based on these studies, the steps in fibrinogen assembly appear to be a progression from single chains, to 2-chain complexes, to half-molecules. The $A\alpha\beta\gamma$ half-molecule then dimerizes to form intact fibrinogen.

Recombinant human fibrinogen isolated from mammalian cells has also been used to determine which domains are involved in cell adhesion events. Fibrinogen binds to both platelets and endothelial cells and can mediate cell adhesion, spreading, and angiogenesis. The $A\alpha$ chain of fibrinogen contains the RGD cellular adhesion sequence (97) at residues $A\alpha95-97$ and $A\alpha572-574$. The $\gamma$ chain of fibrinogen contains another potential cellular adhesion site, the dodecapeptide sequence at the carboxyterminus of the $\gamma$ chain, $\gamma$ 400-411 (98–100). Studies using recombinant fibrinogen molecules with mutations at these sites provide evidence that platelet aggregation is supported by the $\gamma$ chain site (39, 101), and that endothelial cell adhesion relies on the RGD-domain at $A\alpha572-574$ (102) in human fibrinogen. Another study using mutant recombinant fibrinogen demonstrated that the $\gamma$ chain domain involved in platelet aggregation (AGDV) (54) is not required for clot retraction (103); this finding implies that other domains are important for this process.

# FIBRIN COFACTOR FUNCTION AND FIBRIN STABILIZATION

Fibrin plays an important cofactor function by modulating the action of thrombin, plasmin(ogen), tissue-type plasminogen activator (t-PA), and factor XIIIa within the clot.

## REGULATION OF THROMBIN

The binding of thrombin to fibrin protects thrombin from inactivation by antithrombin III and the heparin-antithrombin III complex (104). Thrombin bound to fibrin remains active and can play a role in the propagation of fibrin and activation of factor XIII.

Thrombin utilizes a site distinct from its active site, called the exosite, to bind fibrin (105, 106). The thrombin binding and anticoagulant nature of fibrin was first reported by Seegers' group (107), and thrombin binding to fibrin has been studied in detail by several laboratories (108–111). The congenital dysfibrinogen New York I, is missing Bβ 9-72, producing a defect in thrombin binding associated with a thrombotic disorder (112, 113). The congenital dysfibrinogen Naples also has a defect in thrombin binding that correlates with a thrombotic tendency (114). The fibrinogen Naples molecule has a Ala 68 to Thr mutation in the Bβ chain. The rapid lysis of fibrin by fibrinolytic agents releases thrombin activity which can cleave fibrinogen and may promote rethrombosis *in vivo* (115, 116).

## MODULATION OF FIBRINOLYTIC PATHWAYS

Fibrin modulates fibrinolysis by regulating factor XIIIa, t-PA, plasminogen, and $\alpha_2$-antiplasmin binding to the clot. Lysine residue 303 on the Aα chain is covalently crosslinked to $\alpha_2$-antiplasmin by factor XIIIa (38). This reaction is important in making fibrin resistant to plasmin degradation (117–120). Individuals deficient in $\alpha_2$-antiplasmin experience a serious lifelong bleeding disorder clinically similar to factor XIII deficiency (121).

Plasminogen molecules bind noncovalently to fibrin (122), and the number of plasminogen molecules that bind increases as plasmin cleaves fibrin and exposes new lysine residues with affinity for the lysine binding sites on plasminogen (123–128). The increased binding of plasminogen to partially degraded fibrin increases the amount of plasmin generated on the fibrin surface and enhances fibrinolysis; however, plasminogen binding to fibrin is not necessary for fibrin to enhance plasmin formation, because t-PA-fibrin complexes can efficiently bind plasminogen and convert it to plasmin (129). Factor XIIIa crosslinking of fibrin will make exposure of these lysine binding sites more difficult.

Binding of t-PA to fibrin enhances the rate of plasminogen cleavage and the formation of plasmin (129). Occupancy of the fibrin binding site on t-PA increases activity several-hundred-fold. This acceleration of t-PA's activity by fibrin is present in the fibrinogen molecule in a latent form (130–134). It appears to be localized within the lysine containing region of the Aα-chains (residues 148 to 161). Chemical modification of lysine 157 of the Aα-chain in fibrin results in a loss of t-PA binding activity (134). The Gly-Pro-Arg-Pro binding site on the fibrin(ogen) molecule is important for t-PA activation and is a binding site for t-PA in the initial interaction between t-PA and fibrin (135). Crosslinking of fibrin by factor XIIIa masks the high affinity binding sites for t-PA, resulting in an additional mechanism for the regulation of fibrinolysis (136).

## ROLE OF FIBRIN(OGEN) IN TISSUE INJURY AND ANGIOGENESIS

Wound healing, tumor stroma generation, and inflammation are processes in which fibrin and fibrin degradation products are generated. The formation of fibrin and fibrin degradation products stimulate a variety of responses in vascular cells designed to restore the tissue to its normal physiologic state. The fibrin network provides the initial provisional matrix that supports revascularization of injured tissue (137–140). Fibrin is formed after activation of blood coagulation pathways during thrombosis, tumor growth, and inflammation and plays an important role in the pathologic response of the tissue (141). After tissue injury, fibrinogen extravasates from blood vessels into the extravascular space and forms a provisional fibrin matrix by activation of the coagulation cascade (139). Inflammatory cells and endothelial cells migrate into this matrix and stimulate the repair process. Tissue remodeling involves a series of events that includes detachment of endothelial cells from the established matrix, migration and attachment to the provisional matrix composed of fibrin and other plasma-derived components.

The role of fibrin in these processes is to stimulate specific responses in a number of different cell types including fibroblasts, blood cells, and endothelial cells. In vascular injury, the accumulation of fibrin, fibrinogen, and fibrin(ogen) degradation products influence endothelial cell function. Fibrinogen influences the adhesion, motility, and cytoskeletal organization of endothelial cells (142–145) and fibroblasts (146). Exposure of endothelial cells to fibrin *in vitro* can elicit a number of responses such as secretion of von Willebrand factor (147), loss of monolayer organization, disruption of cell-cell contacts, and migration (148, 149). Cleavage of fibrinopeptide B from fibrinogen by thrombin results in the exposure of β15-42 on the fibrin β-chain, and this domain has been shown to enhance cellular proliferation (150) and modulate cytoskeletal organization (151). Fibrin matrices also induce endothelial cell migration and capillary tube formation (152, 153). Fibrin(ogen) degradation products can stimulate the release of endothelial-derived growth factors (154), promote endothelial cell detachment (155) and retraction (156), and increase vascular permeability (157). In addition, fragment D has been shown to increase the secretion of plasminogen activator and enhance the generation of plasmin (155). This may ultimately lead to the proteolysis of extracellular matrix and cellular detachment.

At early phases of wound healing, the fibrin clot is the primary extracellular matrix in which endothelial cells and fibroblasts migrate and proliferate with the development of new blood vessels. The importance of fibrin as the provisional matrix that regulates wound healing was recently demonstrated in fibrinogen-deficient transgenic mice. Histologic evaluation of hepatic and renal hematomas in these transgenic mice revealed an unusual organization of cells around the injured area (158). Thick bands of fibroblasts encapsulated pools of blood, but there was no evidence of cells infiltrating the injured site. These observations strongly support the hypothesis that fibrin is the provisional matrix necessary for the movement of cells into wound sites and this in turn results in tissue repair. Fibronectin crosslinked to the provisional fibrin network can enhance endothelial cell growth by modulating cell adhesion and cell spreading (159–161). The three-dimensional matrix of the fibrin clot induces endothelial cells to round up and form tube-like structures (152, 153, 155, 156). The deposited fibrin network influences the cytoskeletal organization of endothelial cells and therefore plays a role in cellular adhesion, migration, and the maintenance of cell shape (144, 145, 151, 162). Recent studies have also found that the integrin receptor $\alpha_v\beta_3$ is transiently expressed during cutaneous wound healing (163). This integrin receptor mediates the attachment of endothelial cells to fibrinogen, fibronectin, and vitronectin, three adhesive glycoproteins that are present in the provisional fibrin matrix (162). The $\alpha_v\beta_3$ receptor has been implicated in endothelial cell migration (164), and there is evidence that this receptor modulates angiogenesis in the chick chorioallantoic membrane assay (165, 166). Although changes in integrin expression are important to blood vessel development, another critical component in this process is proteolytic degradation of the provisional matrix. Urokinase activity coupled with the presence of angiogenic factors has recently been shown to be required for the formation of capillary tubes by microvascular endothelial cells in a three-dimensional fibrin matrix (155, 156, 167). The presence of fibrin(ogen) receptors coupled with the cellular effects of fibrin(ogen) on endothelium suggest that fibrin(ogen) modulates events essential to the development of the neovasculature during tissue repair.

The generation of stroma surrounding the tumor is a key factor in the development of the tumor vascular supply (137, 168–170). The extravasation of fibrinogen from leaky or damaged blood vessels also occurs during tumor development (168, 169). Extravascular plasma fibrinogen and plasma fibronectin through coagulation events initiated by tumor cell tissue factor form a fibrin network. This provisional matrix stimulates the migration of inflammatory cells, platelets, and endothelial cells into an environment that supports vascularization. Angiogenic factors, such as vascular endothelial cell growth factor, are expressed in injured tissues and in tumor cells (171). The development of a vascular supply that nourishes the tumor requires communication between endothelial cells, inflammatory cells, fibroblasts, proteases, angiogenic factors, and the provisional fibrin matrix. Thus, the environment of wounded tissue and that of developing tumors are similar in nature and both are supportive of the angiogenic process.

The production of fibrin and fibrin degradation products is also associated with tissue inflammation (172) (see Chapter 15). Recent studies suggest that fibrin deposition modulates leukocyte accumulation at sites of inflammation by increasing ICAM-1 on the endothelial surface (173, 174). Qi and Kreutzer (173) demonstrated that fibrin could induce leukocyte chemotaxis by stimulating the production of interleukin-8 (IL-8) in vascular endothelium. In addition, other investigators found that the adhesion of leukocytes to cytokine-stimulated endothelium is modulated by fibrinogen (175). Residues 117 to 133 of the fibrinogen γ chain were identified as the domain that binds to ICAM-1 on endothelium (176). Integrin-dependent adhesion to fibrin under flow conditions has also been demonstrated (177, 178). Thus, fibrinogen acts as a bridging molecule between endothelium activated by inflammatory cytokines and monocytes. In addition, it was recently shown that cultured pulmonary epithelial cells secrete fibrinogen in response to proinflammatory mediators, such as IL-6 (179). These results suggest that extrahepatic epithelial cells may promote wound healing by up-regulating fibrinogen synthesis and secretion in response to local inflammation. Other studies have examined the molecular basis of fibrinogen-mediated acute inflammatory responses to implanted biomaterials, such as artificial joints and prosthetic devices (180). In these situations, the proinflammatory activity of adsorbed fibrinogen appears to reside in the γ chain sequence 190 to 202 (181). This domain on the fibrinogen molecule has also been shown to bind the integrin, CD11b/CD18 (Mac-1), on leukocytes (181). Further studies are needed to define both the direct and indirect effects of fibrin(ogen) and fibrin degradation products on cellular adhesion, chemotaxis, and signal transduction in the inflammatory process.

# FIBRIN STABILIZATION

The final phase of fibrin formation involves the covalent modification of fibrin molecules by factor XIIIa. The for-

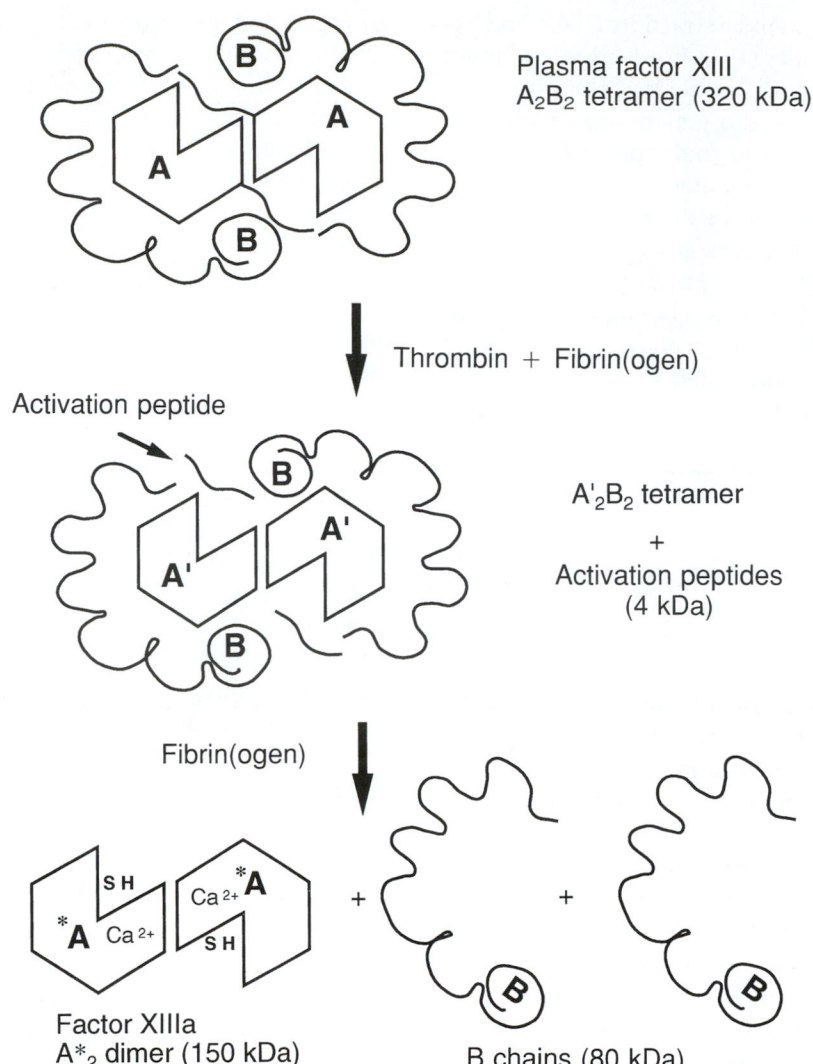

Plasma factor XIII
$A_2B_2$ tetramer (320 kDa)

Thrombin + Fibrin(ogen)

Activation peptide

$A'_2B_2$ tetramer
+
Activation peptides
(4 kDa)

Fibrin(ogen)

Factor XIIIa
$A*_2$ dimer (150 kDa)

B chains (80 kDa)

**FIGURE 6.3.** Plasma factor XIII activation pathway. The thrombin-catalyzed activation of the plasma factor XIII ($A_2B_2$) tetramer occurs in two steps. In the first step, thrombin releases the activation peptides from the A-chains producing the inactive intermediate $A'_2B_2$. Fibrinogen, factor XIII, and thrombin interactions promote this event. In the second step, calcium ions cause the B-chains to dissociate, exposing the active site Cysteine 314. The enzyme $A_2$ is now capable of crosslinking fibrin and other molecules. In this model, the A-chains are packed such that they are oriented to promote crosslinking of fibrin molecules polymerized in an antiparallel configuration. The B-chains are depicted as flexible rod shaped molecules made up of several disulfide loops which apparently can wrap around the A-chains. A-chains are shown as a tightly packed dimeric molecule.

mation of fibrin and factor XIIIa are closely related events involving interactions between factor XIII, fibrin, and thrombin (Fig. 6.3) (182, 183). The biochemistry of these interactions will be reviewed.

# FACTOR XIII: STRUCTURE AND SYNTHESIS

## PLASMA FACTOR XIII

The plasma factor XIII molecule is composed of two nonidentical protein subunits that form a tetrameric molecule containing two A-chains and two B-chains, as indicated in Table 6.1 and Fig. 6.3 (182, 183). The tetra-

mer is held together by high affinity noncovalent forces and has a molecular weight of 320 Kda (182, 183). The A-subunit contains the catalytic domain (184) and has sequence homology with other enzymes called transglutaminases that are involved in tissue stabilization by covalently crosslinking proteins with isopeptide bonds (185–187). The B-chain has sequence homology to the family of complement regulatory proteins (188, 189) that exist on chromosome 1 (190) and plays an important role in the regulation of plasma factor XIII activation (191). Unlike the A-chain, the B-chain (79.7 Kda) has a large number of intrachain disulfide bonds and does not contain any free sulfhydryl groups (188).

**TABLE 6.1.**   Properties of the A- and B-chains of Plasma Factor XIII

| | A-chain Properties | B-chain Properties |
|---|---|---|
| Molecular mass (kDa) | 83.15 | 79.7 |
| Chromosome | 6p24-25[a] | 1q31-q32.1[b] |
| Binding Properties | Fibrin | A-chains |
| Carbohydrate | None | 8.5% |
| Homology | Keratinocyte, tissue, and prostate transglutaminases, erythrocyte band 4.2 | β2-glycoprotein I, decay-accelerating factor, complement receptor type I, haptoglobin, complement regulatory proteins C1r, C1s, C2, factor B, C4b-binding protein, factor H, and C7 |

[a] *Board PG, Webb GC, McKee J et al. Localization of the coagulation factor XIII A subunit gene (F13A) to chromosome bands 6p24 — p25. Cytogenet Cell Genet 1988;48:25–27.*
[b] *Webb GC, Coggan M, Ichinose A et al. Localization of the coagulation factor XIII B subunit gene (F13B) to chromosome bands 1q31-32.1 and restriction fragment length polymorphism at the locus. Hum Genet 1989;81:157–160.*

Approximately 15 µg/mL of the A-subunit (192) and 14 µg/mL of the B-subunit circulate in human plasma (193). Therefore, all the plasma A-chains and B-chains circulate in tetrameric form, yielding a plasma factor XIII concentration of 0.90 µmol/L. Plasma factor XIII is activated during blood coagulation through the action of thrombin (182, 194). Thrombin-activated factor XIIIa is the only enzyme of the blood coagulation cascade with an active site cysteine. After fibrin formation, the noncatalytic B-chains remain in serum, whereas the A-chains are firmly attached to the fibrin clot (194, 195).

## FACTOR XIII A-CHAINS

Megakaryocytes in the bone marrow synthesize factor XIII A-chains, as do the mononuclear progenitor cells that lead to the development of monocytes and macrophages (196, 197). Placental factor XIII A-chain is directly derived from tissue macrophages existing in the placenta (198). Platelet factor XIII is composed solely of two A-subunits and has a molecular weight of approximately 160 Kda (182, 183, 194). Platelets contain an estimated 50% of the total potential factor XIIIa activity in blood (199). Within the platelets, most of the factor XIII is localized to the cytoplasm (199). However, during fibrin formation, platelet factor XIII contributes to the cross-linking of extracellular fibrin (199, 200). Plasma factor XIII A-chains also bind to thrombin-activated platelets after the A-chains are cleaved by thrombin (201). Platelet factor XIII A-chains may be released and then bound to the platelet surface during platelet activation (202). The association of the factor XIIIa molecule with the activated platelet surface allows it to participate at the platelet-fibrin interface, thereby stabilizing hemostatic plugs.

The factor XIIIa binding site on platelets is degraded by plasmin (202).

The platelet factor XIII A-chain molecule is immunologically similar to the plasma factor XIII A-chain molecule; they share similar amino acid compositions and electrophoretic mobilities (194, 203). Furthermore, the properties of the factor XIIIa enzymes generated by thrombin from either plasma or platelet factor XIII are similar (182, 183, 194). Plasma factor XIII B-chains assemble with the platelet A-chains to form a tetrameric complex that is virtually indistinguishable from native plasma factor XIII (182, 194, 204).

The factor XIII A-chain sequence was derived from both direct protein sequence analysis of purified placental factor XIII A-chains (185) and complementary DNA (cDNA) sequence analysis (Fig. 6.4A) (186, 187). Amino acid sequence analysis of factor XIII A-chains reveals 45% identity to the human keratinocyte transglutaminase (type I) and 39% identity to human tissue transglutaminase (type II) (205). Furthermore, the factor XIII A-chain is highly homologous to the human erythrocyte membrane protein, band 4.2 (205). The factor XIII A-chain gene has been localized to bands p24-25 on chromosome 6 (206). Polymorphisms have been detected in the A-subunit by both protein sequencing, cDNA sequencing, and isoelectric focusing (185–187).

When comparing the factor XIII A-chain gene structure with the keratinocyte transglutaminase gene, the activation peptide in the aminoterminus is encoded by a unique and separate exon (205). In contrast, the intron-exon boundaries of the remainder of the molecule are similar. The amino acid sequences surrounding the active site cysteine of the keratinocyte, tissue transglutaminase, and factor XIII are virtually identical (205). The

**A**

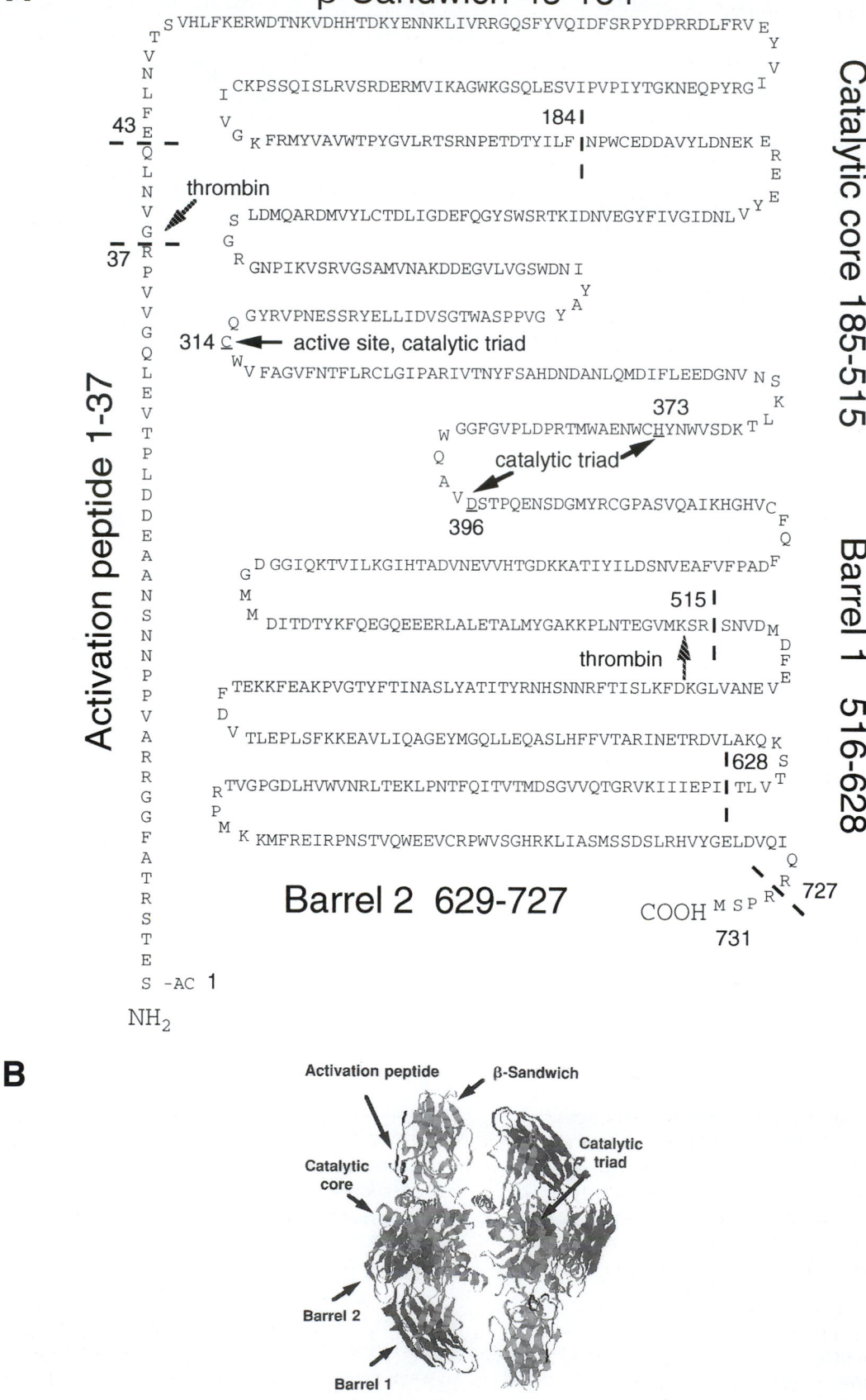

β-Sandwich 43-184

Catalytic core 185-515

Barrel 1    516-628

Activation peptide 1-37

thrombin

active site, catalytic triad

catalytic triad

Barrel 2    629-727

COOH

**B**

Activation peptide    β-Sandwich

Catalytic triad

Catalytic core

Barrel 2

Barrel 1

putative calcium binding domains are similar to those in the keratinocyte and tissue transglutaminases (type I and type II) and share sequence homology to calmodulin (185, 205).

The active site cysteine in the A-chain is located at amino acid residue 314, and it is found in a cryptic form in both platelet and plasma factor XIII (194). After thrombin cleaves the activation peptide between Arg$_{37}$ and Gly$_{38}$ (207), calcium ions promote a conformational change in the A-chain that allows the Cys$_{314}$ to be exposed (Fig. 6.3) (208–210). Unlike plasma factor XIII, in which there is a significant lag phase between thrombin cleavage and expression of the active site, platelet factor XIII is rapidly activated by thrombin (211). The lag phase in plasma factor XIIIa formation is due to the B-chain, because they must dissociate before factor XIIIa activity is fully expressed (210).

Electron microscopy has revealed that the A-chains exist as globular particles, 6 × 9 nm (212). Based on x-ray crystallography data, partial specific volume, molecular mass, and sedimentation coefficient, the dimensions of the dimer were calculated to be 6.4 × 9.4 nm (213). The three-dimensional structure of the zymogen of human recombinant factor XIII A-chain has been solved at 2.8 angstroms resolution by x-ray crystallography (214). This structure revealed that the A-chain is folded into four sequential domains (Fig. 6.4B). These four distinct domains are the β-sandwich, the catalytic core, barrel 1, and barrel 2. The structure of the β-sandwich, barrel 1, and barrel 2 domains is predominantly β-sheet. The largest domain, the catalytic core, is composed of both α-helix and β-sheet and contains the active site cysteine. The activation peptide is a small domain (residues 1 to 37) located at the aminoterminus of the molecule and cleavage at Arg 37 by thrombin results in activation of factor XIII. The x-ray diffraction studies of the factor XIII A-chain revealed a catalytic triad similar in structure to that observed in cysteine proteases in the core domain. The residues that compose this catalytic triad are Cys 314, His 373, and Asp 396 (214). Site-directed mutagenesis performed on recombinant factor XIII supports the structural evidence (215) that these residues are indeed essential for catalytic activity (216, 217).

The A-chains have nine cysteine residues but no intrasulfide or interdisulfide bonds (185). The aminoterminal residue of the A-chain is N-acetyl serine, and the function of this acetylation reaction is not well established (185). Furthermore, the process by which the factor XIII A-chain is secreted into plasma remains unexplained. Bone marrow transplantation studies suggest that the plasma factor XIII A-chains are derived from bone marrow cells that are either megakaryocytic or monocytic in origin (197, 218). In other studies, hepatocytes were shown to synthesize A-chains *in vitro* (219). Release of the A-chains from platelets or monocytes upon cell death could play a role in regulating plasma factor XIII concentrations. Additional studies need to be performed to explain the mechanism(s) regulating plasma factor XIII levels.

## FACTOR XIII B-CHAINS

The complete primary sequence of factor XIII B-chain has been deduced from the cDNA sequence (188). Twenty potential glycosylation sites have been identified (188). This protein is composed of 641 amino acids with a molecular weight of 80,000 after the addition of carbohydrate (8.5%) (188). Ten tandem repeats, each containing about sixty amino acids with two disulfide bonds, represent almost 95% of the amino acid sequence (Fig. 6.5). These 10 tandem repeats are similar in structure to the repeats in at least 15 other proteins, including β$_2$ glycoprotein I, decay accelerating factor, complement receptor type I, haptoglobin, IL-2 receptor, and complement regulating proteins (C1r, C1s, C2, factor B, C4b-binding protein, factor H, and C7) (188, 220). The cell

**FIGURE 6.4.** Factor XIII. A-chain structure. **A,** illustrates the amino acid sequence of factor XIII A-chain. This enzyme is composed of 731 amino acids. The aminoterminal serine residue is acetylated. The activation peptide is cleaved by thrombin at the R$_{37}$ bond. Four distinct domains make up the factor XIII monomer: the β-sandwich, residues 43–184; the catalytic core, residues 185–515; barrel 1, residues 516–628; and barrel 2, residues 629–727. The secondary structure of the β-sandwich, barrel 1 and barrel 2 domains, is predominantly β-sheet, whereas the catalytic core is a mixture of β-sheet and α-helix. Thrombin-cleaved factor XIII A-chains acquire catalytic activity after calcium ions induce exposure of the active site C$_{314}$. The catalytic triad is composed of residues C314, H373, and D396. A second thrombin cleavage site exits at K$_{513}$-S$_{514}$ and the action of thrombin at this bond releases a 50 Kda fibrin binding fragment and a carboxyterminal domain. The 50 Kda fragment binds fibrin and is catalytically active, suggesting that it contains the substrate recognition sites. The A subunit of human factor XIII exhibits genetic polymorphism. (From Suzuki K, Henke J, Iwata M et al Novel polymorphisms and haplotypes in the human coagulation factor XIII A-subunit gene. Hum Genet 1996;98:393–395.) The polymorphic sites have been described. (From Suzuki K, Iwata M, Ito S et al Molecular basis for subtypic differences of the "a" subunit of coagulation factor XIII with description of the genesis of the subtypes. Hum Genet 1994;94:129–135.) **B,** A model of factor XIII, highlights the domains characterized from the resolved crystal structure. This image was created using the atomic coordinates of the x-ray crystal structure of factor XIII deposited in the Protein Data Bank at Brookhaven National Laboratory and the graphics program, RASMOL.

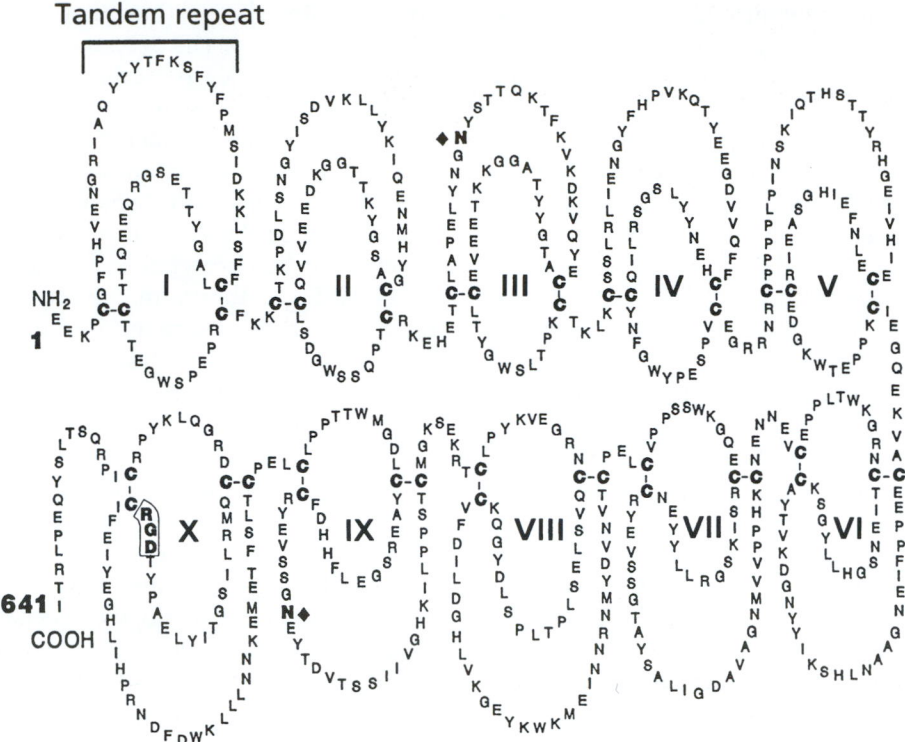

**FIGURE 6.5.** Factor XIII. B-chain structure. The B-chain contains a total 641 amino acids and a series of ten homologous tandem repeats composed of two disulfide bonds. The disulfide bridges between the first and the third cysteine residue and the second and fourth cysteines are diagrammed based on the sequence homology to β2-glycoprotein I in which the disulfide pairing is established. There are two potential glycosylation sites diagrammed as closed diamonds (♦). In addition, the cell adhesion peptide RGD is located in the tenth tandem repeat. The B-chain forms a flexible rod-shaped molecule. (From Chung D, Ichinose A. Hereditary disorders related to fibrinogen and factor XIII. In: Scriver CR, Beaudet AL, Sly WS, Valle D, eds. The metabolic basis of inherited disease. New York: McGraw-Hill, 1989;2:2135–2153.)

attachment sequence RGD (Arg-Gly-Asp) is located near the carboxyterminus of the B-chain and could possibly contribute to an adhesive function of this molecule. In preliminary studies, the B-chains were found to enhance the binding of the A-chains to fibrinogen and fibrin (221).

The B-chains stabilize the structure of the A-chains and limit the susceptibility of A-chains to proteolysis (191). The B-chains also interfere with the contact activation pathway of blood coagulation (222); the physiologic significance of this effect *in vivo* remains to be determined.

## CELL-ASSOCIATED FACTOR XIII

Factor XIII A-chains have been detected by immunologic techniques in monocytes and macrophages (223–225) and a wide variety of tissues including lymph nodes (226), uterus (227), and the skin (228). The factor XIII A-chain in the uterus is associated with monocyte-derived tissue macrophages (227). Factor XIII A-chains have been used by several investigators as a reliable

marker of the normal proliferation of monocytic cell lines in leukemias and lymphomas (223, 229). Monocyte factor XIII is expressed on the surface of these cells and can regulate the crosslinking of extracellular fibrin (224, 225). The factors regulating the surface expression of monocyte factor XIII are not well established.

## MECHANISMS OF ACTION OF FACTOR XIII

### THROMBIN PROTEOLYSIS

Thrombin plays a dual role in fibrin stabilization by catalyzing the conversion of fibrinogen to fibrin and the proteolytic activation of factor XIII to factor XIIIa (Fig. 6.6) These reactions are very carefully regulated to generate factor XIIIa during fibrin formation. Thrombin initially releases fibrinopeptide A from fibrinogen and then hydrolyzes the $Arg_{37}$-$Gly_{38}$ bond at the aminoterminus of the A-chain of factor XIII to release the activation peptide (207). The rate of thrombin cleavage of plasma factor XIII is greatly accelerated by the presence of fibrin polymers (230–233). The ability of fibrin polymers to

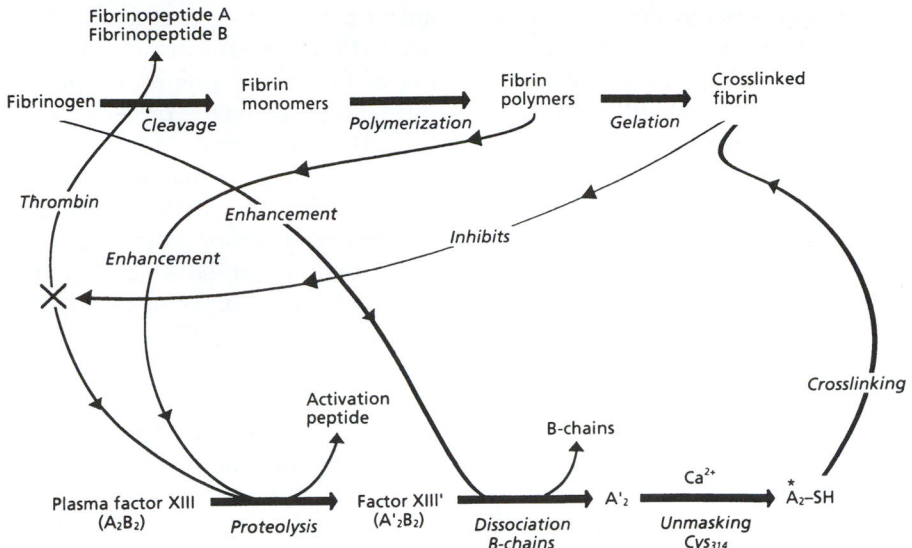

**FIGURE 6.6.** Regulation of fibrin crosslinking by factor XIII-fibrin(ogen) interactions: The complex interactions between thrombin, factor XIII, and different molecular forms of fibrin crosslinking are diagrammed. The activation of plasma factor XIII and the formation of crosslinked fibrin are processes that are very closely related to each other. Thrombin cleavage of plasma factor XIII is enhanced by fibrin polymers. Fibrinogen and fibrin promote the calcium dependent dissociation of thrombin-cleaved factor XIII $A'_2B_2$ to yield the active enzyme, factor XIIIa (A-SH), which has the active site $Cys_{314}$ residues exposed for catalytic crosslinking of fibrin polymers. Once factor XIIIa crosslinks fibrin, thrombin cleavage of factor XIII is inhibited (x). All molecular forms of factor XIII will interact and bind to fibrinogen and fibrin.

promote factor XIIIa formation helps to ensure that factor XIIIa is generated as the fibrin network assembles during the hemostatic response. Thrombin cleavage of the activation peptide of plasma factor XIII A-chains is 80-fold faster when plasma factor XIII forms a complex with fibrin (230). In addition, fibrin provides binding sites for α-thrombin. In contrast, γ-thrombin, which does not readily associate with fibrin, fails to increase the rate of proteolysis of plasma factor XIII in the presence of fibrin polymers (234–236). Therefore, thrombin proteolysis of plasma factor XIII requires a complex set of interactions occurring between thrombin and factor XIII on the fibrin polymer surface.

Thrombin proteolysis of platelet factor XIII appears to be less complex. The release of only one activation peptide from the platelet dimer is required for optimum expression of factor XIIIa activity (237). Furthermore, fibrin does not promote the α-thrombin cleavage of the activation peptide of platelet factor XIII (234). When the B-chains of factor XIII are added to platelet factor XIII A-chains, the A-chains are protected from proteolysis (191, 234).

## ROLE OF CALCIUM IONS IN UNMASKING THE ACTIVE SITE OF FACTOR XIII

The proteolysis of factor XIII to the thrombin-cleaved intermediate is an essential step in the formation of factor XIIIa, but this reaction alone is insufficient to gener-

ate fibrin stabilizing activity (Fig. 6.3). Thrombin-cleaved plasma factor XIII retains its tetrameric structure by noncovalent interactions, and the active site of the A-chains cannot be readily labeled with radioactive iodoacetamide (210, 211, 238). Once calcium ions are added to the thrombin activated form of plasma factor XIII, the B-chains dissociate, the active site cysteine ($Cys_{314}$) is exposed, and factor XIIIa activity is generated (210, 211, 238). Furthermore, this appears to be a reversible set of interactions since chelating the calcium ions reverses these events.

Detailed studies of the effect of calcium ions on the dissociation of the B-chain and expression of the active site have demonstrated that this is the slow, rate-limiting step in plasma factor XIIIa formation. Calcium ion concentrations greater than 10 mM are required for full expression of plasma factor XIIIa activity (210, 239). This concentration of calcium ions is significantly higher than that which exists in human plasma, which suggests that there must be another plasma cofactor to regulate the rapid activation of plasma factor XIII in the presence of physiologic calcium concentrations (239). Fibrinogen is the plasma cofactor that promotes the dissociation of the B-chains from thrombin-cleaved plasma factor XIII in the presence of calcium ions (239). In the presence of normal plasma concentrations of fibrinogen, thrombin-cleaved factor XIII is fully activated at plasma calcium ion concentrations of 1.5 mmol/L (239). In contrast, thrombin-cleaved platelet factor XIII A-chains are rapidly activated at plasma calcium ion concentrations. Therefore, the B-chains limit the expression of the active site in the plasma factor XIII molecule (239). The ability of fibrinogen to promote the dissociation of the B-chain from thrombin-cleaved plasma factor XIII is mediated by a specific interaction with the central region in the Aα-chain of fibrinogen defined by amino acid residues 242 to 424 (238).

The portion of the factor XIII A-chain that modulates thrombin recognition of the activation peptide of factor XIII A-chains is not well defined. Although thrombin is presumed to be the major plasma protease required for factor XIII activation, the activation of factor XIII by factor Xa (240), calpain (241), and a platelet protease (242) have been reported. Plasmin, the major fibrin degrading enzyme formed during fibrinolysis, is unable to activate factor XIII and does not degrade the purified factor XIII molecule (243). However, plasmin releases factor XIIIa from the fibrin clot where it retains enzymatic activity (244). This action has at least two consequences: the release of factor XIIIa could a) contribute to the local stabilization of fibrin at the site of vascular occlusion, and b) produce an adverse effect on thrombolysis by promoting the rapid stabilization of newly formed fibrin.

## ROLE OF FIBRINOGEN AND FIBRIN IN THE ACTIVATION OF FACTOR XIII

It was noted for many years that fibrinogen preparations were contaminated by plasma factor XIII, suggesting a strong interaction between the two proteins (245). The association constant for the binding of plasma factor XIII and platelet factor XIII to fibrinogen has been reported between 10 nmol/L (246) and 14 μmol/L (247). Therefore, at normal plasma concentrations of fibrinogen (8 μmol/L), plasma factor XIII could be expected to associate reversibly with fibrinogen (246). The interactions between factor XIII, fibrinogen, and its intermediates have been studied by several investigators (195, 245–247). The B-chains of factor XIII do not prevent the A-chains from interacting with the fibrinogen molecule (195, 246). Platelet factor XIII, plasma factor XIII, and thrombin-cleaved plasma factor XIII bind in a calcium-independent manner to fibrin (195). These studies demonstrate that localization of plasma factor XIII A-chains to the fibrin clot does not require proteolysis of fibrin by thrombin. Furthermore, factor XIII could bind to fibrinogen molecules polymerized by protamine sulfate (195). Therefore, release of fibrinopeptides A and B from the fibrin molecule is not necessary for plasma factor XIII binding to the fibrin clot.

Factor XIIIa formation regulates its own production by a negative feedback pathway (Fig. 6.6). Once fibrin is covalently crosslinked by factor XIIIa, it no longer serves as a cofactor to promote thrombin cleavage of plasma factor XIII (232). This provides an efficient mech-

anism for ensuring that factor XIIIa is formed only as needed during hemostasis. Once factor XIIIa crosslinking of fibrin γ chains is complete, new sites of fibrin formation become the preferred location for further factor XIIIa formation.

Hornyack and Shafer studied the interaction of factor XIII and factor XIIIa with fibrin and demonstrated that the zymogen of plasma factor XIII and factor XIIIa bind to different sites on the fibrin molecule (247). Thrombin-cleaved A-chains bind with approximately sevenfold higher affinity to fibrin than the native A-chains (247). Saturation of fibrin with the zymogen of plasma factor XIII did not influence binding of thrombin-cleaved factor XIII, strongly suggesting that the zymogen and thrombin-cleaved forms of factor XIII bind to distinct and noninteracting sites on fibrin (247). Further support for separate binding sites comes from experiments demonstrating that the zymogen of plasma factor XIII does not interfere with the ability of fibrinogen to promote B-chain dissociation from thrombin-cleaved plasma factor XIII (247).

Activation of platelet factor XIII under conditions in which all the platelet factor XIII molecules were associated with fibrin was not promoted by the presence of fibrin polymers (247). This finding is in contrast with the ability of fibrin to accelerate plasma factor XIII activation and demonstrates that the B-chains play an important role in regulating the three-dimensional organization of the tetrameric factor XIII molecule within the thrombin-fibrin complex. In summary, factor XIIIa formation in plasma is regulated by a complex set of interactions between fibrinogen and fibrin, ensuring that factor XIIIa is formed during fibrin network assembly.

# MECHANISMS OF ACTION OF FACTOR XIII

## TRANSGLUTAMINASE REACTION

Factor XIIIa catalyzes the covalent modification of fibrin by a transglutaminase reaction. This reaction involves the formation of an amide bond between the carbonyl group of a glutamine residue in one fibrin molecule and the ε-amino group of a lysine residue in another fibrin molecule (Fig. 6.7) (235). The active site cysteine in factor XIIIa reacts with the γ-carbonyl group of a glutamine residue in the protein substrate forming a γ-glutamyl ester intermediate which undergoes aminolysis (Fig. 6.7) (235). Calcium ions are required for the formation of the active site thioester intermediate (235, 248). During this reaction, the ε-amino group of lysine reacts and the γ-glutamyl ε-lysyl bond is formed. Ammonia is then released from the glutamine residue of the protein substrate (235, 248). A wide variety of synthetic compounds containing primary amino groups can replace lysine in

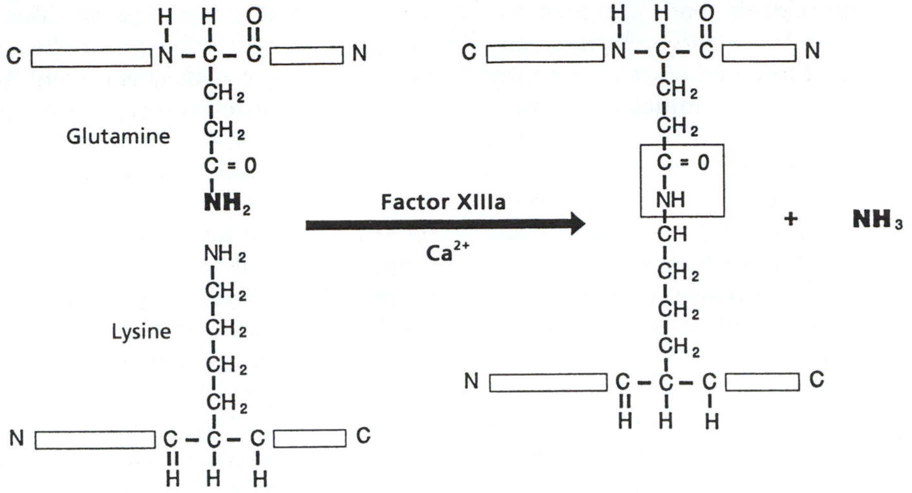

**FIGURE 6.7.** Formation of factor XIIIa-catalyzed isopeptide bond. Factor XIIIa recognizes glutamine containing side chains in several different plasma proteins. In this diagram, two separate fibrin molecules are aligned in an anti-parallel configuration. (Note opposite orientation of amino- and carboxytermini of the individual proteins.) Factor XIIIa's active site cysteine (Cys$_{314}$) will form a calcium dependent thioester complex with the glutamine residue. Then a neighboring lysine residue aligned by fibrin polymerization will serve as an electron acceptor and an isopeptide γ-glutaminyl ε-lysyl bond will form between the proteins. Ammonia is released during the catalytic process from the glutamine residue. Intermolecular covalent bonds provide structural stability and prevent fibrin proteolysis and the chemical and physical disruption of hemostatic plugs.

this reaction and are used in quantitative factor XIIIa activity assays (249–251).

The x-ray crystal structure of the zymogen of factor XIII A-chain has revealed a similarity in structure between the active site of factor XIII and the cysteine proteases (214, 215). This similarity implies that the catalytic mechanism of transglutaminases is similar to the reverse hydrolysis reaction of the proteinases. The isopeptide crosslink between two proteins that results from the catalytic action of factor XIII is diagrammed in Fig. 6.7. The reaction is extremely specific since only a select group of protein-bound glutamine residues can form this bond with factor XIIIa. The determinants for substrate specificity reside both in the enzyme and in the conformation of the protein substrates (248, 252). The glutamine residue must be accessible to factor XIIIa and cannot be buried inside the protein structure. Furthermore, charged amino acids within 5 amino acids of the glutamine interfere with an exposed glutamine serving as a substrate (253). In the absence of a reactive lysine residue, the primary reaction product from the transglutaminase reaction is the release of ammonia from the glutamine and the formation of glutamic acid (235). There is also evidence that the amino acid residue preceding the peptide-bound lysine modulates the recognition of this lysine as a crosslink site (254, 255).

Most of the crosslinking reactions of factor XIIIa proceed with little reversibility. However, α$_2$-antiplasmin crosslinking to fibrinogen and fibrin by factor XIIIa is reversible, with approximately 30% of the plasma α$_2$-antiplasmin molecules covalently attached to fibrin (118,

256). Studies by Mosesson et al, suggest that γ-γ crosslinking may also be reversible, because D-dimer formation can proceed to the formation of D-trimers and D-tetramers after all the D-dimers are formed (257).

Factor XIII zymogens may undergo conformational changes in the presence of high salt concentrations (258), chaotropic agents (258), and high calcium ion concentrations (210) allowing the expression of catalytic activity. This noncatalytic activation pathway is proposed to be an alternate mechanism for the activation of intracellular factor XIII A-chains (258).

The factor XIIIa molecule consists of a dimer with two potential active site residues available for catalysis. There has been controversy regarding the ability of factor XIIIa to express both active sites. There appears to be a set of noncooperative interactions that allow only one set of active site-cysteine residues to be expressed at a time (237). This would allow one of the A-chains to crosslink a pair of fibrin γ chains, followed by the other A-chain crosslinking the other set of γ chains oriented in the antiparallel configuration. Steric hindrance or conformational changes in the A-chains could control this catalytic mechanism. Additional studies are needed to delineate the mechanism by which factor XIIIa produces the antiparallel γ chain crosslinks as well as the other protein crosslinking reactions described below.

## PROTEINS CROSSLINKED BY FACTOR XIIIA

### Fibrin γ Chain  Crosslinking

As many as six isopeptide bonds can be formed between one fibrin molecule and its neighbor (235, 259), a process ensuring that the fibrin clot is both mechanically strengthened and relatively resistant to chemical and enzymatic degradation compared with the un-crosslinked polymer (260–264). The initial fibrin cross-linking reaction involves the γ chains. The pair of donor lysine (K406) and acceptor glutamine (Q398, or Q399) molecules, which are only a short distance apart on the γ chain, are covalently held together by an isopeptide bond (36, 265). The crosslinking reaction occurs via molecules that are closely aligned with the proper geometry to allow the isopeptide bond to be placed in an antiparallel orientation (Fig. 6.7) (266).

There has been some controversy regarding the spatial orientation of crosslinking between fibrin molecules (267–269). Studies performed with factor XIIIa crosslinking of fibrinogen suggested that the isopeptide bond was formed between two fibrin molecules aligned end-to-end in the same strand of the protofibril (267, 270). However, other studies using fibrin crosslinked by factor XIIIa suggest that the γ-γ crosslink is oriented between two fibrin molecules aligned across the fibrin protofibril in a transorientation, as diagrammed in Fig. 6.3 (268, 269, 271). The transorientation of the covalent bond is likely to be a direct result of the conformational constraints imposed by the noncovalent association between the D- and E-domains of fibrin molecules that regulate fibrin polymerization (268, 269). There is evidence that the γ chain crosslink may be reversible and result in the production of higher-ordered crosslinked γ chain products; namely D-trimers and D-tetramers (257). Although direct protein sequencing and analysis of crosslinked products in these D-trimeric and D-tetrameric structures have not been reported, it is assumed that these structures use K406 and the glutamine residues that exist in D-dimer formation. The formation of the D-trimers and D-tetramers is promoted by the formation of fibrin in the presence of high salt and high calcium ion concentrations (272). Mosesson proposed that D-trimers originate at interfibrillar junctions or tri-molecular branch points in the fibrin strands (Fig. 6.3) (273). In contrast, the D-tetramers are althought to arise at either interfibrillar junctions or tetramolecular branch points in the fibrin network (Fig. 6.3) (273). The formation of D-trimers and D-tetramers strongly supports the concept that intermolecular crosslinking of fibrin occurs across the γ chains in the so called transorientation. However, it does not exclude the possibility that both the *cis-* and *trans-*modes of crosslinking could be involved *in vivo*.

## Fibrin Aα-Chain Crosslinking

The crosslinking of the Aα-chains of fibrin to form Aα-polymers is an extremely complex process and occurs much more slowly than the crosslinking of the γ chains (274). Each Aα-chain has at least two glutamine acceptor sites located at amino acid residues 328 and 366 (275) and five potential lysine sites between residues 518 and 584 (275). This provides the possibility for a highly complex and intricate crosslinking network to be formed in the portion of Aα-chain that is highly flexible and protrudes from the surface of the molecule. The extent of Aα-chain crosslinking plays a very important role in the regulation of fibrinolysis (276–279). Most investigators agree that the Aα-chain appears to stabilize and promote the association of fibrin protofibrils into thick bundles of opaque fibers with higher tensile strength (280). The exact orientation of the Aα-chain crosslinks in relationship to the fibrin network is not thoroughly established. The Aα-chain crosslinked network appears to form a protective barrier that impedes the ability of plasmin to degrade the coiled coil regions of the fibrin molecule maintaining the structure of the fibrin network. Plasmin must degrade fibrin between the D- and E-domains in the coiled coil regions to allow fibrin to release soluble fragments and lose its structure (281–284). When crosslinked fibrin is degraded by plasmin, a dimeric form of the fragment D-domain (called D-dimer) containing the intermolecular γ chain crosslink is released in association with fragment E (281–284).

## Fibrin α-γ Chain Crosslinking

The covalent crosslinking by factor XIIIa between the Aα and γ chains of fibrin has recently been described (285). The Aα-γ crosslink is promoted by the formation of the γ-γ crosslinking. The function of the Aα-γ crosslink is still unknown; however, it could play an important role in the stabilization of clot structure. Direct sequence analysis of the amino acids participating in the crosslinking remains to be established.

## Fibrinogen Crosslinking

Factor XIIIa will crosslink fibrinogen in the same pattern as fibrin, with γ chain dimers occurring first, followed by Aα-chain polymer formation (286). However, the crosslinking reaction of fibrinogen occurs at a much slower rate. This is apparently due to the difference in protein conformation and alignment of the γ chains in the fibrin polymer, rather than the exposure of crosslink sites after the fibrinopeptides are removed from the fibrinogen molecules. Kinetic analysis of fibrinogen and fibrin crosslinking reactions has demonstrated zero order kinetics for fibrin and first order kinetics for fibrinogen (286). Therefore, under conditions of high fibrinogen concentrations, the crosslinking of γ chains can occur at a rate that is actually more rapid than that of fibrin (286). Factor XIIIa crosslinks fibrinogen to form a gel *in vitro* (286–289), but the physiologic role of fibrinogen crosslinking has not been defined. Factor XIIIa can also crosslink soluble fibrinogen to fibrin before it has formed an insoluble fibrin clot. Soluble fibrinogen-fibrin crosslinked complexes have been demonstrated to be present *in vivo* (290–292). Furthermore, high concentrations of fibrinogen inhibit fibrin crosslinking and may prevent fibrin stabilization (276).

## $\alpha_2$-Plasmin Inhibitor ($\alpha_2$-Antiplasmin)

$\alpha_2$-Antiplasmin is the major physiologic inhibitor of plasmin *in vivo* (293, 294). Factor XIIIa rapidly crosslinks $\alpha_2$-antiplasmin to the A$\alpha$-chain of fibrinogen (33, 117). This crosslinking reaction occurs at the glutamine residue in the second position from the aminoterminus of $\alpha_2$-antiplasmin (295) and the lysine residue at position 313 in the A$\alpha$-chain of fibrin (33). The rates of crosslinking of $\alpha_2$-antiplasmin to fibrinogen and fibrin are very similar (32). The $\alpha_2$-antiplasmin, when covalently crosslinked to fibrin, is an efficient plasmin inhibitor and plays a major role in the regulation of fibrinolysis (118, 119). Individuals congenitally deficient in $\alpha_2$-antiplasmin experience a serious bleeding disorder, with major hemorrhage occurring after trauma. The clinical presentation is similar to that of individuals with congenital factor XIII deficiency (121).

Synthetic peptides containing the amino acid sequences surrounding the glutamine crosslinking site in the $\alpha_2$-antiplasmin are crosslinked by factor XIIIa to fibrin. This reaction inhibits $\alpha_2$-antiplasmin crosslinking to fibrin and promotes fibrinolysis (295). Monoclonal antibodies to $\alpha_2$-antiplasmin also block $\alpha_2$-antiplasmin crosslinking to fibrin and promote fibrinolysis (296).

The initial $\alpha_2$-antiplasmin complex occurring during early fibrin clot formation exists in a heterodimeric form containing monomeric A$\alpha$-chains (117). The $\alpha_2$-antiplasmin molecule bound to the A$\alpha$-chain undergoes further crosslinking to form high molecular weight complexes containing A$\alpha$-chain polymers. Thus, $\alpha_2$-antiplasmin is localized to the A$\alpha$-chain crosslinked network surrounding fibrin and protects the inner protofibrils from plasmin degradation. It is surprising that only 30% of the $\alpha_2$-antiplasmin inhibitor is covalently crosslinked to the plasma clot (118, 297). This finding is apparently due to the reversible nature of the bond (32). The $\alpha_2$-antiplasmin may be in a reversible equilibrium reaction with the fibrin surface and may play an important role in the modulation of early fibrinolytic events. However, the amount of $\alpha_2$-antiplasmin in the clot is extremely low relative to the amount of plasmin that can be generated during fibrinolysis (124–126). Therefore, under conditions in which plasmin is being generated at high rates, the crosslinked $\alpha_2$-antiplasmin offers fibrin limited protection from degradation.

## Fibronectin

Fibronectin is one of the major plasma protein substrates for factor XIIIa (298, 299). Fibronectin circulates in plasma and is also associated with the extracellular matrix surrounding fibroblasts, endothelial cells, and a wide variety of other cells (300). Cells synthesize fibronectin (300, 301), and both the cellular and plasma forms of fibronectin are factor XIIIa substrates (300). The major glutamine residue involved in the covalent crosslinking of fibronectin appears to be located at the aminoterminal end of the molecule at amino acid 3 (300, 301). Fibronectin can be crosslinked to both itself (300) and collagen (302, 303). However, when fibrin is present, fibronectin-fibrin complexes are the preferred crosslinked products (304). Fibronectin crosslinking to fibrin occurs through the A$\alpha$-chain of the fibrin molecule (299). Fibronectin can actually inhibit fibrin crosslinking and lead to the formation of soluble fibrin (289, 304, 305). Fibronectin crosslinking to fibrin does not modify $\alpha_2$-antiplasmin crosslinking (306). Fibroblasts can bind factor XIIIa and crosslink fibronectin on the surface where it is assembled into the extracellular matrix (307). *In vitro* studies suggest that fibronectin alters the mechanical properties of fibrin (305, 307–309). However, in plasma fibronectin crosslinking does not appear to alter the properties of fibrin (310).

## Collagen

The concept that factor XIIIa plays an essential role in forming the provisional matrix necessary for tissue repair developed from early clinical observations on defective wound healing in factor XIII-deficient individuals (311, 312). The covalent attachment of fibrin to collagen at the site of vascular injury could play a very important role in preventing fibrin from being dislodged from the vessel wall. Factor XIIIa crosslinks fibronectin to fibrin *in vitro*, and this reaction could occur *in vivo* at the site of vascular injury. Furthermore, crosslinking of fibronectin to collagen molecules has been demonstrated. Collagen types I, II, III, and V can be crosslinked to fibronectin by factor XIIIa, whereas collagen type IV is not a suitable substrate (303). In these crosslinking reactions, collagen provides the lysine residues necessary to form an isopeptide bond with a glutamine residue in fibronectin.

## Platelet Cytoskeleton Proteins

Several platelet cytoskeletal proteins, including actin and myosin (see Chapter 10), reportedly serve as factor XIIIa substrates. The physiologic significance of these reactions is not established. In purified systems, actin can be crosslinked to fibrin, forming crosslinked A$\alpha$-chain polymers (313). The crosslinking of actin is inhibited by several nucleotide triphosphate molecules (adenosine, guanosine, and cytosine triphosphate) but is not inhibited by cyclic adenosine monophosphate or adenosine monophosphate. The nucleotide effect is a direct effect on the actin and not on factor XIIIa (314).

Therefore, once platelets have undergone dense body degranulation to deplete their stores of nucleotide triphosphates, crosslinking of actin would no longer be inhibited. Myosin isolated from platelets and skeletal muscle tissue can also incorporate primary amines and form high molecular weight crosslinked products when incubated with factor XIIIa (315). The crosslinking reaction occurs predominantly through the heavy chains of myosin (315).

Factor XIIIa incorporates lysine analogs into specific glutamine sites in the fibrinogen receptor (glycoprotein IIb-IIIa) on platelet membranes, demonstrating that the receptor is a substrate for factor XIIIa (316). The physiologic significance of this reaction remains unclear; however, it is possible that covalent crosslinks between fibrinogen, the platelet fibrinogen receptor, and cytoskeletal proteins could provide a stable attachment site increasing platelet-fibrin plug structural integrity during hemostasis.

Factor XIIIa crosslinking appears to play an important role in clot retraction and the attachment of platelets to fibrin during the retraction process (317). The platelet protein, vinculin (318), is a factor XIIIa substrate. Factor V, a molecule essential for the generation of thrombin, is also reported to be a factor XIIIa substrate (319, 320) and may be crosslinked to platelet actin (321). Localization of factor V to sites at which factor XIIIa is formed could provide fibrin, platelets, and extracellular matrices with a source of factor V, thereby accelerating thrombin formation and hemostasis.

## Other Factor XIIIa Substrates

von Willebrand factor (Chapter 16) is crosslinked to fibrin when blood clots slowly (322). *In vitro*, von Willebrand factor is reported to be a factor XIIIa substrate and can be crosslinked to fibrin or other extracellular matrix molecules, including collagen (323). These reactions could promote platelet adhesion and facilitate the hemostatic response. The high molecular weight forms of von Willebrand factor have likewise been reported to bind noncovalently to the crosslinked forms of fibrin (324). Vitronectin, another extracellular matrix molecule present in platelet α-granules, is also crosslinked by factor XIIIa (325). The major glutamine crosslinking site *in vitro*nectin has been localized to glutamine 93 (326), with minor sites at glutamine 73, 84, and 86. Thrombospondin is another factor XIIIa substrate that undergoes covalent incorporation into fibrin during fibrin polymerization (327).

## ROLE OF FACTOR XIII IN PREGNANCY

Factor XIII-deficient women experience spontaneous abortions unless they receive regular supplementation of factor XIII by the intravenous infusion of pasteurized placental factor XIII (328). This suggests that the plasma-derived factor XIII is absolutely necessary for successful pregnancy. Maternal plasma factor XIII may be essential for the control of placental or uterine hemorrhage at the maternal-fetal interface. Alternatively, maternal plasma factor XIII may be needed to provide the proper matrix to promote the growth and proliferation of the placenta. There is a large amount of tissue invasion and remodeling that occurs during pregnancy, and it is possible that both the hemostatic properties of factor XIII and its effects on fibrin and extracellular matrices are essential for the normal growth and development of the fetus. The use of a short tandem repeat polymorphism, (AAAG)n, upstream of the coding region of the factor XIII A-subunit gene has recently been described as a gene marker for factor XIII A-subunit deficiency carrier detection, and this gene marker is the first to be used as a prenatal diagnosis for this disorder (329).

## ROLE OF FACTOR XIII IN WOUND HEALING

Fibrin provides the provisional extracellular matrix during wound healing. The association of factor XIII with fibrin places it in a pivotal position to modify cellular migration, cell attachment, and cellular lysis of fibrin during tissue regeneration (Fig. 6.8A, B). It is estimated that approximately 25% of factor XIII-deficient individuals experience abnormal wound healing (194).

Additional clinical and experimental observations demonstrate that factor XIII activity is involved in tissue repair mechanisms. Crosslinking of fibrin is essential for the provision of an optimal environment for fibroblast growth (330–332). During major surgery, plasma factor XIII concentrations decrease to levels that are suboptimal for fibroblast proliferation (333). When factor XIII concentration is increased in animal studies, there are reports of improved healing of experimental wounds (334). The association of factor XIII with the fibroblast surface and the crosslinking of fibronectin and collagen could explain the beneficial effects of factor XIII on wound healing. Monocyte migration into fibrin gels is greatly influenced by factor XIIIa crosslinking of fibronectin (335, 336). Because monocytes are involved in orchestrating tissue remodeling, failure to crosslink fibronectin to the gel may reduce cell proliferation and monocyte migration essential for wound healing. Monocyte factor XIII concentrations are reduced in factor XIII-deficient individuals which could also contribute to wound healing defects (337). The migration of human fibroblasts into fibrin is enhanced by factor XIIIa crosslinking the Aα-chains in the absence of fibronectin. In contrast, γ chain crosslinking does not promote fibroblast migration into fibrin gels. Therefore, Aα-chain crosslinking by factor XIIIa is an important factor in modulating fibroblast migration during wound healing processes (338).

**A**

**Clot forms in response to injury:
provisional fibrin matrix crosslinked by FXIIIa**

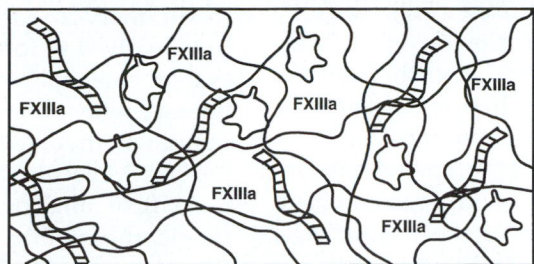

- Plasma fibrinogen, fibrin, fibronectin and platelets form
  the provisional matrix

- Platelets secrete growth factors such as PDGF, TGFβ and TGFα

- Platelets release extracellular matrix components :
  fibrinogen, fibronectin, thrombospondin and von Willebrand factor

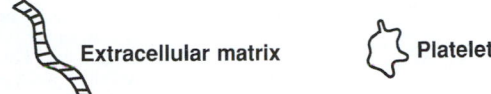

Extracellular matrix            Platelet

**B**   **Influx of inflammatory cells to promote tissue repair**

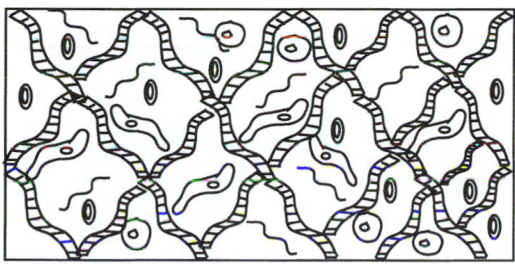

- Migration of fibroblasts, monocytes and endothelial cells

- Secretion of growth factors and proliferation of cells

- Production, deposition and assembly of extracellular matrix

- Blood vessel development

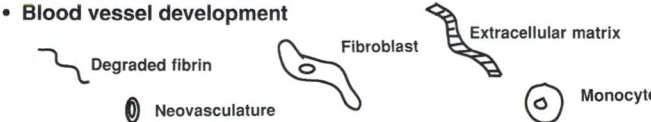

Degraded fibrin        Fibroblast        Extracellular matrix

Neovasculature                    Monocyte

**FIGURE 6.8.** Fibrin and factor XIII in wound healing. **A** and **B** illustrate different stages of tissue remodeling that occur in response to vascular injury. A clot forms at the site of vascular damage and is initially composed mainly of crosslinked fibrin and fibronectin as well as platelets. Activation of platelets at the site of injury leads to the secretion of growth factors and extracellular matrix molecules. This provisional crosslinked matrix enhances the influx of inflammatory cells to promote the production of early granulation tissue. As the migration of fibroblasts, monocytes, and endothelial cells occurs, growth factor production is enhanced, leading to cellular proliferation and extracellular matrix production. The fibrin matrix is gradually degraded and replaced by extracellular matrix molecules such as fibronectin, hyaluronan, SPARC, tenascin, proteoglycans, and collagen. The interactions of the inflammatory cells, cytokines, and matrix ultimately leads to remodeled tissue containing new blood vessels.

## ROLE OF FACTOR XIII IN OTHER DISEASE STATES

Remarkable clinical responses to factor XIII infusion therapy have been reported (339). First, factor XIII con-

centrations are diminished during the acute phase of ulcerative colitis and replacement of factor XIII diminishes the duration of gastrointestinal bleeding (340, 341). Second, plasma factor XIII levels are also decreased in Crohn's disease (342). In these individuals, factor XIII

A-chains were localized to capillary thrombi in the bowel wall, suggesting a role for factor XIIIa formation in the pathogenesis of Crohn's disease (342). Third, a beneficial effect of factor XIII transfusion therapy in scleroderma (343) has also been reported. Fourth, Henoch-Schonlein purpura, a disease of children associated with renal failure and low factor XIII concentrations, has been reported to respond to replacement therapy with factor XIII (344). Finally, the topical application of recombinant factor XIII A-chains prevented intracerebral hemorrhage in rats that were anticoagulated (345). Therefore, recombinant factor XIII A-chains could have a beneficial effect in some individuals at a high risk of postoperative intracranial hemorrhage. Clinical studies using recombinant factor XIII A-chains are needed to establish the clinical utility of this protein in man.

## CLINICAL USE OF FIBRIN SEALANTS (SEE CHAPTER 53)

Initially, fibrin sealants were used to reduce blood loss under clinical circumstances such as thoracic and cardiovascular, neurosurgical, plastic surgical, and general trauma applications (346). Examples of specific applications include using the fibrin sealants at suture lines or at sites of vascular anastomoses to reduce and control perioperative bleeding during cardiac surgery (347). Fibrin sealants have also been successfully used to reduce postoperative cerebral spinal fluid leakage following dural closures (348). This adhesive sealant has also been effective in reducing bleeding and promoting skin graft adherence following burn debridement (349). The versatility of fibrin sealants is becoming more apparent as it is used in various circumstances (350). Other applications that have been reported include its use in controlling hemostasis in individuals with coagulation disorders (351); repairing dural defects in craniofacial resections (352); achieving hemostasis after tooth extraction in anticoagulated individuals (353); closing rectovaginal (354) and bronchopleural fistulas (355); closing ventricular septal defects (356); and treatment of pneumothoraces in premature infants (357). In the United States, fibrin sealants are prepared from single-donor plasma (358) or autologous cryoprecipitate (359, 360). In Europe, multidonor fibrinogen concentrates are used to prepare sealants. These preparations must be virally inactivated by either pasteurization (361), steam heat (362), or solvent-detergent (363). Combinations of these methods including UV-irradiation are also being used to ensure viral safety. The compositions of commercially available fibrin sealants differ greatly. The use of recombinant proteins may provide a means to determine the exact composition of sealant necessary for different applications and ensure the safe commercial use of this product.

## SUMMARY

In summary, the fibrinogen and factor XIII molecules have evolved to form a well-regulated fibrin stabilizing system essential for normal hemostasis. Both proteins interact with proteases, cells, and extracellular matrix molecules involved in tissue remodeling and wound healing. Molecular defects or acquired antibodies to factor XIII or fibrinogen can manifest as serious hemorrhagic, thrombotic, or wound healing defects. Clinical disorders of factor XIII and fibrinogen are discussed further in Chapters 36 and 47.

## REFERENCES

1. Hermans J, McDonagh J. Fibrin: structure and interactions [Review]. Semin Thromb Hemost 1982;8:11–24.
2. Doolittle RF. The structure and evolution of vertebrate fibrinogen. Ann N Y Acad Sci 1983;408:13–27.
3. Henschen A, Lottspeich F, Kehl M et al. Covalent structure of fibrinogen. Ann N Y Acad Sci 1983;408:28–43.
4. McKee PA, Rogers LA, Marler E et al. The subunit polypeptides of human fibrinogen. Arch Biochem Biophys 1966;116:271–279.
5. McKee PA, Mattock P, Hill RL. Subunit structure of human fibrinogen, soluble fibrin, and crosslinked insoluble fibrin. Proc Natl Acad Sci U S A 1970;66:738–744.
6. Bailey K, Astbury WT, Rudall KM. Fibrinogen and fibrin as members of the keratin-myosin group. Nature 1943;151:716–717.
7. Weisel JW, Stauffacher CV, Bullitt E et al. A model for fibrinogen: domains and sequence. Science 1985;230:1388–1391.
8. Hall CE, Slayter HS. The fibrinogen molecule: its size, shape and mode of polymerization. J Biophys Biochem Cytol 1959;5:11–15.
9. Weisel JW, Phillips GN Jr, Cohen C. A model from electron microscopy for the molecular structure of fibrinogen and fibrin. Nature 1981;289:263–267.
10. Fowler WE, Erickson HP. Trinodular structure of fibrinogen. Confirmation by both shadowing and negative stain electron microscopy. J Mol Biol 1979;134:241–249.
11. Mosesson MW, Hainfeld J, Wall J et al. Identification and mass analysis of human fibrinogen molecules and their domains by scanning transmission electron microscopy. J Mol Biol 1981;153:695–718.
12. Doolittle RF, Goldbaum DM, Doolittle LR. Designation of sequences involved in the "coiled-coil" interdomainal connections in fibrinogen: constructions of an atomic scale model. J Mol Biol 1978;120:311–325.
13. Henschen A. Number and reactivity of disulfide bonds in fibrinogen and fibrin. Arkiv Kemi 1964;22:355–359.
14. Gardlund B, Hessel B, Marguerie G et al. Primary structure of human fibrinogen. Characterization of disulfide-containing cyanogen-bromide fragments. Eur J Biochem 1977;77:595–610.
15. Blomback B, Blomback M, Henschen A et al. N-terminal disulphide knot of human fibrinogen. Nature 1968;218:130–134.
16. Blomback B, Hessel B, Hogg D. Disulfide bridges in nh2-terminal part of human fibrinogen. Thromb Res 1976;8:639–658.
17. Bouma H, Takagi T, Doolittle RF. The arrangement of disulfide bonds in fragment D from human fibrinogen. Thromb Res 1978;13:557–562.
18. Henschen A. Disulfide bridges in the middle part of human fibrinogen. Hoppe Seylers Z Physiol Chem 1978;359:1757–1770.
19. Marder VJ, Budzynski AZ. The structure of the fibrinogen degradation products [Review]. Prog Hemost Thromb 1974;2:141–174.
20. Gaffney PJ. The biochemistry of fibrinogen and fibrin degradation products. In: Ogston D, Bennett B, eds. Haemostasis: biochemistry, physiology and pathology. London: John Wiley, 1977;105–168.
21. Lottspeich F, Henschen A. Amino acid sequence of human fibrin. Preliminary note on the completion of the gamma-chain sequence. Hoppe Seylers Z Physiol Chem 1977;358:935–938.
22. Henschen A, Lottspeich F. Amino acid sequence of human fibrin. Preliminary note on the completion of the beta-chain sequence. Hoppe Seylers Z Physiol Chem 1977;358:1643–1646.
23. Watt KW, Takagi T, Doolittle RF. Amino acid sequence of the beta chain of human fibrinogen: homology with the gamma chain. Proc Natl Acad Sci U S A 1978;75:1731–1735.
24. Doolittle RF, Watt KW, Cottrell BA et al. The amino acid sequence of the alpha-chain of human fibrinogen. Nature 1979;280:464–468.
25. Chung DW, Chan WY, Davie EW. Characterization of a complementary deoxyribonucleic acid coding for the gamma chain of human fibrinogen. Biochemistry 1983;22:3250–3256.

26. Chung DW, Que BG, Rixon MW et al. Characterization of complementary deoxyribonucleic acid and genomic deoxyribonucleic acid for the beta chain of human fibrinogen. Biochemistry 1983;22:3244–3250.

27. Rixon MW, Chan WY, Davie EW et al. Characterization of a complementary deoxyribonucleic acid coding for the alpha chain of human fibrinogen. Biochemistry 1983;22:3237–3244.

28. Chung DW, Rixon MW, MacGillivray RT et al. Characterization of a cDNA clone coding for the beta chain of bovine fibrinogen. Proc Natl Acad Sci U S A 1981;78:1466–1470.

29. Crabtree GR, Comeau CM, Fowlkes DM et al. Evolution and structure of the fibrinogen genes. Random insertion of introns or selective loss? J Mol Biol 1985;185:1–19.

30. Takagi T, Doolittle RF. Amino acid sequence studies on the alpha chain of human fibrinogen. Location of four plasmin attack points and a covalent crosslinking site. Biochemistry 1975;14:5149–5156.

31. Takagi T, Doolittle RF. The amino acid sequences of those portions of human fibrinogen fragment E which are not included in the aminoterminal disulfide knot. Thromb Res 1975;7:813–818.

32. Mosher DF. Crosslinking of cold-insoluble globulin by fibrin-stabilizing factor. J Biol Chem 1975;250:6614–6621.

33. Kimura S, Aoki N. Crosslinking site in fibrinogen for alpha 2-plasmin inhibitor. J Biol Chem 1986;261:15591–15595.

34. Telford JN, Nagy JA, Hatcher PA et al. Location of peptide fragments in the fibrinogen molecule by immunoelectron microscopy. Proc Natl Acad Sci U S A 1980;77:2372–2376.

35. Norton PA, Slayter HS. Immune labeling of the D and E regions of human fibrinogen by electron microscopy. Proc Natl Acad Sci U S A 1981;78:1661–1665.

36. Chen R, Doolittle RF. γ-γ crosslinking sites in human and bovine fibrin. Biochemistry 1971;10:4487–4491.

37. Hawiger J, Timmons S, Kloczewiak M et al. Gamma and alpha chains of human fibrinogen possess sites reactive with human platelet receptors. Proc Natl Acad Sci U S A 1982;79:2068–2071.

38. Strong DD, Laudano AP, Hawiger J et al. Isolation, characterization, and synthesis of peptides from human fibrinogen that block the staphylococcal clumping reaction and construction of a synthetic clumping particle. Biochemistry 1982;21:1414–1420.

39. Farrell DH, Thiagarajan P, Chung DW et al. Role of fibrinogen alpha and gamma chain sites in platelet aggregation. Proc Natl Acad Sci U S A 1992; 89:10729–10732.

40. Hardy JJ, Carrell NA, McDonagh J. Calcium ion functions in fibrinogen conversion to fibrin. Ann N Y Acad Sci 1983;408:279–287.

41. Nieuwenhuizen W, Haverkate F. Calcium-binding regions in fibrinogen. Ann N Y Acad Sci 1983;408:92–96.

42. Dang CV, Ebert RF, Bell WR. Localization of a fibrinogen calcium binding site between gamma-subunit positions 311 and 336 by terbium fluorescence. J Biol Chem 1985;260:9713–9719.

43. Topfer-Peterson E, Lottspeich F, Henschen A. Carbohydrate linkage site in the beta-chain of human fibrin. Hoppe Seylers Z Physiol Chem 1976; 357:1509–1513.

44. Nickerson JM, Fuller GM. Modification of fibrinogen chains during synthesis: glycosylation of B beta and gamma chains. Biochemistry 1981;20:2818–2821.

45. Townsend RR, Hilliker E, Li YT et al. Carbohydrate structure of human fibrinogen. Use of 300-MHz 1H-NMR to characterize glycosidase-treated glycopeptides. J Biol Chem 1982;257:9704–9710.

46. Martinez J, Palascak JE, Kwasniak D. Abnormal sialic acid content of the dysfibrinogenemia associated with liver disease. J Clin Invest 1978;61:535–538.

47. Mosesson MW, Finlayson JS, Umfleet RA. Human fibrinogen heterogeneities. 3. Identification of chain variants. J Biol Chem 1972;247:5223–5227.

48. Mosesson MW. Fibrinogen heterogeneity. Ann N Y Acad Sci 1983;408:97–113.

49. Wolfenstein-Todel C, Mosesson MW. Human plasma fibrinogen heterogeneity: evidence for an extended carboxyl terminal sequence in a normal gamma chain variant (gamma'). Proc Natl Acad Sci U S A 1980;77:5069–5073.

50. Wolfenstein-Todel C, Mosesson MW. Carboxyterminal amino acid sequence of a human fibrinogen gamma-chain variant (gamma'). Biochemistry 1981;20:6146–6149.

51. Francis CW, Kraus DH, Marder VJ. Structural and chromatographic heterogeneity of normal plasma fibrinogen associated with the presence of three gamma-chain types with distinct molecular weights. Biochim Biophys Acta 1983;744:155–164.

52. Fornace AJ Jr, Cummings DE, Comeau CM et al. Structure of the human gamma-fibrinogen gene. Alternate mRNA splicing near the 3' end of the gene produces gamma A and gamma B forms of gamma-fibrinogen. J Biol Chem 1984;259:12826–12830.

53. Mosesson MW, Homandberg GA, Amrani DL. Human platelet fibrinogen gamma chain structure. Blood 1984;63:990–995.

54. Hettasch JM, Bolyard MG, Lord ST. The residues AGDV of recombinant gamma chains of human fibrinogen must be carboxyterminal to support human platelet aggregation. Thromb Haemost 1992;68:701–706.

55. Siebenlist KR, Meh DA, Mosesson MW. Plasma factor XIII binds specifically to fibrinogen molecules containing gamma chains. Biochemistry 1996;35:10448–10453.

56. Everse SJ, Pelletier H, Doolittle RF. Crystallization of fragment D from human fibrinogen. Protein Sci 1995;4:1013–1016.

57. Doolittle RF, Everse SJ, Spraggon G. Human Fibrinogen: anticipating a 3-dimensional structure [Review]. FASEB J 1996;10:1464–1470.

58. Blumenstein M, Matsueda GR, Timmons S et al. A beta-turn is present in the 392-411 segment of the human fibrinogen gamma-chain. Effects of structural changes in this segment on affinity to antibody 4A5. Biochemistry 1992;31:10692–10698.

59. Donahue JP, Patel H, Anderson WF et al. Three-dimensional structure of the platelet integrin recognition segment of the fibrinogen gamma chain obtained by carrier protein-driven crystallization. Proc Natl Acad Sci U S A 1994;91:12178–12182.

60. Yee VC, Pratt KP, Cote HC et al. Gamma-fibrinogen: crystal structure of a 30kDa C-terminus fragment at 2.1 resolution [Abstract]. Int Union Crystal XVII Congr Gen Assembly 1996.

61. Blomback B, Vestermark A. Isolation of fibrinopeptides by chromatography. Arkiv Kemi 1958;12:173.

62. Blomback B, Hessel B, Hogg D et al. A two-step fibrinogen-fibrin transition in blood coagulation. Nature 1978;275:501–505.

63. Bailey K, Bettelheim FR, Lorand L et al. Action of thrombin in the clotting of fibrinogen. Nature 1951;167:233–234.

64. Martinelli RA, Scheraga HA. Steady-state kinetic study of the bovine thrombin-fibrinogen interaction. Biochemistry 1980;19:2343–2350.

65. Higgins DL, Lewis SD, Shafer JA. Steady state kinetic parameters for the thrombin-catalyzed conversion of human fibrinogen to fibrin. J Biol Chem 1983;258:9276–9282.

66. Hurlet-Jensen A, Cummins HZ, Nossel HL et al. Fibrin polymerization and release of fibrinopeptide B by thrombin. Thromb Res 1982;27:419–427.

67. Hanna LS, Scheraga HA, Francis CW et al. Comparison of structures of various human fibrinogens and a derivative thereof by a study of the kinetics of release of fibrinopeptides. Biochemistry 1984;23:4681–4687.

68. Lewis SD, Shields PP, Shafer JA. Characterization of the kinetic pathway for liberation of fibrinopeptides during assembly of fibrin. J Biol Chem 1985;260:10192–10199.

69. Olexa SA, Budzynski AZ. Evidence for four different polymerization sites involved in human fibrin formation. Proc Natl Acad Sci U S A 1980;77:1374–1378.

70. Fowler WE, Hantgan RR, Hermans J et al. Structure of the fibrin protofibril. Proc Natl Acad Sci U S A 1981;78:4872–4876.

71. Ferry JD. The mechanism of polymerization of fibrinogen. Proc Natl Acad Sci U S A 1952;38:566–569.

72. Olexa SA, Budzynski AZ. Localization of a fibrin polymerization site. J Biol Chem 1981;256:3544–3549.

73. Horwitz BH, Varadi A, Scheraga HA. Localization of a fibrin gamma-chain polymerization site within segment Thr-374 to Glu-396 of human fibrinogen. Proc Natl Acad Sci U S A 1984;81:5980–5984.

74. Varadi A, Scheraga HA. Localization of segments essential for polymerization and for calcium binding in the gamma-chain of human fibrinogen. Biochemistry 1986;25:519–528.

75. Southan C, Thompson E, Panico M et al. Characterization of peptides cleaved by plasmin from the C-terminal polymerization domain of human fibrinogen. J Biol Chem 1985;260:13095–13101.

76. Shimizu A, Nagel GM, Doolittle RF. Photoaffinity labeling of the primary fibrin polymerization site: isolation and characterization of a labeled cyanogen bromide fragment corresponding to gamma-chain residues 337-379. Proc Natl Acad Sci U S A 1992;89:2888–2892.

77. Yamazumi K, Doolittle RF. Photoaffinity labeling of the primary fibrin polymerization site: localization of the label to gamma-chain Tyr-363. Proc Natl Acad Sci U S A 1992;89:2893–2896.

78. Laudano AP, Doolittle RF. Synthetic peptide derivatives that bind to fibrinogen and prevent the polymerization of fibrin monomers. Proc Natl Acad Sci U S A 1978;75:3085–3089.

79. Laudano AP, Doolittle RF. Studies on synthetic peptides that bind to fibrinogen and prevent fibrin polymerization. Structural requirements, number of binding sites, and species differences. Biochemistry 1980;19:1013–1019.

80. Hantgan R, Fowler W, Erickson H et al. Fibrin assembly: a comparison of electron microscopic and light scattering results. Thromb Haemost 1980;44:119–124.

81. Krakow W, Endres GF, Siegel BM et al. An electron microscopic investigation of the polymerization of bovine fibrin monomer. J Mol Biol 1972;71:95–103.

82. Siegel BM, Mernan JP, Scheraga HA. The configuration of native and partially polymerized fibrinogen. Biochem Biophys Acta 1953;11:329–336.

83. Shen LL, Hermans J, McDonagh J et al. Role of fibrinopeptide B release: comparison of fibrins produced by thrombin and Ancrod. Am J Physiol 1977;232:H629–H633.

84. Wiltzius P, Dietler G, Kanzig W et al. Fibrin aggregation before sol-gel transition. Biophys J 1982;38:123–132.

85. Shainoff JR, Dardik BN. Fibrinopeptide B and aggregation of fibrinogen. Science 1979;204:200–202.

86. Sturtevant JM, Laskowski M Jr, Donnelly TH et al. Equilibria in the fibrinogen-fibrin conversion. III. Heats of polymerization and clotting of fibrin monomer. J Am Chem Soc 1955;77:6168–6172.

87. Blomback B, Hessel B, Okada M et al. Mechanism of fibrin formation and its regulation. Ann N Y Acad Sci 1981;370:536–544.

88. Scheraga HA. Interaction of thrombin and fibrinogen and the polymerization of fibrin monomer. Ann N Y Acad Sci 1983;408:330–343.

89. Shimizu A, Saito Y, Matsushima A et al. Identification of an essential histidine residue for fibrin polymerization. Essential role of histidine 16 of the B beta-chain. J Biol Chem 1983;258:7915–7917.

90. Carr ME Jr, Hermans J. Size and density of fibrin fibers from turbidity. Macromolecules 1978;11:46–50.

91. Roy SN, Procyk R, Kudryk BJ et al. Assembly and secretion of recombinant human fibrinogen. J Biol Chem 1991;266:4758–4763.

92. Hartwig R, Danishefsky KJ. Studies on the assembly and secretion of fibrinogen. J Biol Chem 1991;266:6578–6585.

93. Farrell DH, Mulvihill ER, Huang SM et al. Recombinant human fibrinogen and sulfation of the gamma' chain. Biochemistry 1991;30:9414–9420.

94. Binnie CG, Hettasch JM, Strickland E et al. Characterization of purified recombinant fibrinogen: partial phosphorylation of fibrinopeptide A. Biochemistry 1993;32:107–113.

95. Zhang JZ, Kudryk B, Redman CM. Symmetrical disulfide bonds are not necessary for assembly and secretion of human fibrinogen. J Biol Chem 1993;268:11278–11282.

96. Huang S, Mulvihill ER, Farrell DH et al. Biosynthesis of human fibrinogen. Subunit interactions and potential intermediates in the assembly. J Biol Chem 1993;268:8919–8926.

97. Ruoslahti E, Pierschbacher MD. New perspectives in cell adhesion: rGD and integrins [Review]. Science 1987;238:491–497.

98. Kloczewiak M, Timmons S, Hawiger J. Localization of a site interacting with human platelet receptor on carboxyterminal segment of human fibrinogen gamma chain. Biochem Biophys Res Commun 1982;107:181–187.

99. Kloczewiak M, Timmons S, Hawiger J. Recognition site for the platelet receptor is present on the 15-residue carboxyterminal fragment of the gamma chain of human fibrinogen and is not involved in the fibrin polymerization reaction. Thromb Res 1983;29:249–255.

100. Kloczewiak M, Timmons S, Lukas TJ et al. Platelet receptor recognition site on human fibrinogen. Synthesis and structure-function relationship of peptides corresponding to the carboxyterminal segment of the gamma chain. Biochemistry 1984;23:1767–1774.

101. Farrell DH, Thiagarajan P. Binding of recombinant fibrinogen mutants to platelets. J Biol Chem 1994;269:226–231.

102. Thiagarajan P, Rippon AJ, Farrell DH. Alternative adhesion sites in human fibrinogen for vascular endothelial cells. Biochemistry 1996;35:4169–4175.

103. Rooney MM, Parise LV, Lord ST. Dissecting clot retraction and platelet aggregation. Clot retraction does not require an intact fibrinogen gamma chain C terminus. J Biol Chem 1996;271:8553–8555.

104. Hogg PJ, Jackson CM. Fibrin monomer protects thrombin from inactivation by heparin-antithrombin III: implications for heparin efficacy. Proc Natl Acad Sci U S A 1989;86:3619–3623.

105. Liu CY, Nossel HL, Kaplan KL. The binding of thrombin by fibrin. J Biol Chem 1979;254:10421–10425.

106. Wilner GD, Danitz MP, Mudd MS et al. Selective immobilization of alpha-thrombin by surface-bound fibrin. J Lab Clin Med 1981;97:403–411.

107. Seegers WH, Nieft M, Loomis EC. Note on the adsorption of thrombin on fibrin. Science 1945;101:520–521.

108. Kaminski M, McDonagh J. Studies on the mechanism of thrombin. Interaction with fibrin. J Biol Chem 1983;258:10530–10535.

109. Francis CW, Markham RE Jr, Barlow GH et al. Thrombin activity of fibrin thrombi and soluble plasmic derivatives. J Lab Clin Med 1983;102:220–230.

110. Berliner LJ, Sugawara Y, Fenton JW 2d. Human alpha-thrombin binding to nonpolymerized fibrin-Sepharose: evidence for an anionic binding region. Biochemistry 1985;24:7005–7009.

111. Fenton JW 2d, Olson TA, Zabinski MP et al. Anion-binding exosite of human alpha-thrombin and fibrin(ogen) recognition. Biochemistry 1988;27:7106–7112.

112. Liu CY, Koehn JA, Morgan FJ. Characterization of fibrinogen New York 1. A dysfunctional fibrinogen with a deletion of B beta(9–72) corresponding exactly to exon 2 of the gene. J Biol Chem 1985;260:4390–4396.

113. Al-Mondhiry H, Bilezikian SB, Nossel HL. Fibrinogen "New York"—an abnormal fibrinogen associated with thromboembolism: functional evaluation. Blood 1975;45:607–619.

114. Koopman J, Haverkate F, Lord ST et al. Molecular basis of fibrinogen Naples associated with defective thrombin binding and thrombophilia. Homozygous substitution of B beta 68 Ala——Thr. J Clin Invest 1992;90:238–244.

115. Mirshahi M, Soria J, Soria C et al. Evaluation of the inhibition by heparin and hirudin of coagulation activation during r-tPA-induced thrombolysis. Blood 1989;74:1025–1030.

116. Owen J, Friedman KD, Grossman BA et al. Thrombolytic therapy with tissue plasminogen activator or streptokinase induces transient thrombin activity. Blood 1988;72:616–620.

117. Sakata Y, Aoki N. Crosslinking of alpha 2-plasmin inhibitor to fibrin by fibrin-stabilizing factor. J Clin Invest 1980;65:290–297.

118. Sakata Y, Aoki N. Significance of crosslinking of alpha 2-plasmin inhibitor to fibrin in inhibition of fibrinolysis and in hemostasis. J Clin Invest 1982;69:536–542.

119. Mimuro J, Kimura S, Aoki N. Release of alpha 2-plasmin inhibitor from plasma fibrin clots by activated coagulation factor XIII. Its effect on fibrinolysis. J Clin Invest 1986;77:1006–1013.

120. Tamaki T, Aoki N. Crosslinking of alpha 2-plasmin inhibitor to fibrin catalyzed by activated fibrin-stabilizing factor. J Biol Chem 1982;257:14767–14772.

121. Aoki N, Saito H, Kamiya T et al. Congenital deficiency of alpha 2-plasmin inhibitor associated with severe hemorrhagic tendency. J Clin Invest 1979;63:877–884.

122. Bok RA, Mangel WF. Quantitative characterization of the binding of plasminogen to intact fibrin clots, lysine-sepharose, and fibrin cleaved by plasmin. Biochemistry 1985;24:3279–3236.

123. Tran-Thang C, Kruithof EK, Bachmann F. Tissue-type plasminogen activator increases the binding of glu-plasminogen to clots. J Clin Invest 1984;74:2009–2016.

124. Suenson E, Lutzen O, Thorsen S. Initial plasmin-degradation of fibrin as the basis of a positive feed-back mechanism in fibrinolysis. Eur J Biochem 1984;140:513–522.

125. Harpel PC, Chang TS, Verderber E. Tissue plasminogen activator and urokinase mediate the binding of Glu-plasminogen to plasma fibrin I. Evidence for new binding sites in plasmin-degraded fibrin I. J Biol Chem 1985;260:4432–4440.

126. Tran-Thang C, Kruithof EK, Atkinson J et al. High-affinity binding sites for human Glu-plasminogen unveiled by limited plasmic degradation of human fibrin. Eur J Biochem 1986;160:599–604.

127. Suenson E, Petersen LC. Fibrin and plasminogen structures essential to stimulation of plasmin formation by tissue-type plasminogen activator. Biochim Biophys Acta 1986;870:510–519.

128. Varadi A, Patthy L. Beta(Leu121-Lys122) segment of fibrinogen is in a region essential for plasminogen binding by fibrin fragment E. Biochemistry 1984;23:2108–2112.

129. Hoylaerts M, Rijken DC, Lijnen HR et al. Kinetics of the activation of plasminogen by human tissue plasminogen activator. Role of fibrin. J Biol Chem 1982;257:2912–2919.

130. Varadi A, Patthy L. Location of plasminogen-binding sites in human fibrin(ogen). Biochemistry 1983;22:2440–2446.

131. Verheijen JH, Nieuwenhuizen W, Wijngaards G. Activation of plasminogen by tissue activator is increased specifically in the presence of certain soluble fibrin(ogen) fragments. Thromb Res 1982;27:377–385.

132. Nieuwenhuizen W, Vermond A, Voskuilen M et al. Identification of a site in fibrin(ogen) which is involved in the acceleration of plasminogen activation by tissue-type plasminogen activator. Biochim Biophys Acta 1983;748:86–92.

133. Nieuwenhuizen W, Verheijen JH, Vermond A et al. Plasminogen activation by tissue activator is accelerated in the presence of fibrin(ogen) cyanogen bromide fragment FCB-2. Biochim Biophys Acta 1983;755:531–533.

134. Voskuilen M, Vermond A, Veeneman GH et al. Fibrinogen lysine residue A alpha 157 plays a crucial role in the fibrin-induced acceleration of plasminogen activation, catalyzed by tissue-type plasminogen activator. J Biol Chem 1987;262:5944–5946.

135. Kaczmarek E, Lee MH, McDonagh J. Initial interaction between fibrin and tissue plasminogen activator (t-PA). The Gly-Pro-Arg-Pro binding site on fibrin(ogen) is important for t-PA activity. J Biol Chem 1993;268:2474–2479.

136. Husain SS, Hasan AA, Budzynski AZ. Differences between binding of one-chain and two-chain tissue plasminogen activators to non-crosslinked and crosslinked fibrin clots. Blood 1989;74:999–1006.

137. Dvorak HF. Tumors: Wounds that do not heal. Similarities between tumor stroma generation and wound healing [Review]. N Engl J Med 1986;315:1650–1659.

138. Brown LF, Dvorak AM, Dvorak HF. Leaky vessels, fibrin deposition, and fibrosis: a sequence of events common to solid tumors and to many other types of disease [Review]. Am Rev Respir Dis 1989;140:1104–1107.

139. Brown LF, Van de Water L, Harvey VS et al. Fibrinogen influx and accumulation of crosslinked fibrin in healing wounds and in tumor stroma. Am J Pathol 1988;130:455–465.

140. Gailit J, Clark RA. Wound repair in the context of extracellular matrix [Review]. Curr Opin Cell Biol 1994;6:717–725.

141. Dvorak HF, Nagy JA, Berse B et al. Vascular permeability factor, fibrin, and the pathogenesis of tumor stroma formation [Review] Ann N Y Acad Sci 1992;667:101–111.

142. Albelda SM, Daise M, Levine EM et al. Identification and characterization of cell-substratum adhesion receptors on cultured human endothelial cells. J Clin Invest 1989;83:1992–2002.

143. Cheresh DA. Human endothelial cells synthesize and express an Arg-Gly-Asp-directed adhesion receptor involved in attachment to fibrinogen and von Willebrand factor. Proc Natl Acad Sci U S A 1987;84:6471–6475.

144. Dejana E, Languino LR, Polentarutti N et al. Interaction between fibrinogen and cultured endothelial cells. Induction of migration and specific binding. J Clin Invest 1985;75:11–18.

145. Dejana E, Lampugnani MG, Giorgi M et al. Fibrinogen induces endothelial cell adhesion and spreading via the release of endogenous matrix proteins and the recruitment of more than one integrin receptor. Blood 1990;75:1509–1517.

146. Farrell DH, al-Mondhiry HA. Human fibroblast adhesion to fibrinogen. Biochemistry 1997;36:1123–1128.

147. Ribes JA, Francis CW, Wagner DD. Fibrin induces release of von Willebrand factor from endothelial cells. J Clin Invest 1987;79:117–123.

148. Weimar B, Delvos U. The mechanism of fibrin-induced disorganization of cultured human endothelial cell monolayers. Arteriosclerosis 1986;6:139–145.

149. Kadish JL, Butterfield CE, Folkman J. The effect of fibrin on cultured vascular endothelial cells. Tissue Cell 1979;11:99–108.

150. Sporn LA, Bunce LA, Francis CW. Cell proliferation on fibrin: modulation by fibrinopeptide cleavage. Blood 1995;86:1802–1810.

151. Bunce LA, Sporn LA, Francis CW. Endothelial cell spreading on fibrin requires fibrinopeptide B cleavage and amino acid residues 15-42 of the beta chain. J Clin Invest 1992;89:842–850.

152. Chalupowicz DG, Chowdhury ZA, Bach TL et al. Fibrin II induces endothelial cell capillary tube formation. J Cell Biol 1995;130:207–215.

153. Dvorak HF, Harvey VS, Estrella P et al. Fibrin containing gels induce angiogenesis. Implications for tumor stroma generation and wound healing. Lab Invest 1987;57:673–686.

154. Lorenzet R, Sobel JH, Bini A et al. Low-molecular-weight fibrinogen degradation products stimulate the release of growth factors from endothelial cells. Thromb Haemost 1992;68:357–363.

155. Ge M, Tang G, Ryan TJ et al. Fibrinogen degradation product fragment D induces endothelial cell detachment by activation of cell-mediated fibrinolysis. J Clin Invest 1992;90:2508–2516.

156. Conforti G, Dominguez-Jimenez C, Ronne E. Cell-surface plasminogen activation causes a retraction of in vitro cultured human umbilical vein endothelial cell monolayer. Blood 1994;83:994–1005.

157. Ge M, Ryan TJ, Lum H et al. Fibrinogen degradation product fragment D increases endothelial monolayer permeability. Am J Physiol 1991;261:L283–L289.

158. Suh TT, Holmback K, Jensen NJ et al. Resolution of spontaneous bleeding events but failure of pregnancy in fibrinogen-deficient mice. Genes Dev 1995;9:2020–2033.

159. Clark RA, Quinn JH, Winn HJ et al. Fibronectin is produced by blood vessels in response to injury. J Exp Med 1982;156:646–651.

160. Clark RA, Lanigan JM, DellaPelle P et al. Fibronectin and fibrin provide a provisional matrix for epidermal cell migration during wound reepithelialization. J Invest Dermatol 1982;79:264–269.

161. Clark RA, DellaPelle P, Manseau E et al. Blood vessel fibronectin increases in conjunction with endothelial cell proliferation and capillary ingrowth during wound healing. J Invest Dermatol 1982;79:269–276.

162. Cheresh DA, Berliner SA, Vicente V et al. Recognition of distinct adhesive sites on fibrinogen by related integrins on platelets and endothelial cells. Cell 1989;58:945–953.

163. Clark RA, Tonnesen MG, Gailit J et al. Transient functional expression of alphaVbeta 3 on vascular cells during wound repair. Am J Pathol 1996;148:1407–1421.

164. Leavesley DI, Schwartz MA, Rosenfeld M et al. Integrin beta 1- and beta 3-mediated endothelial cell migration is triggered through distinct signaling mechanisms. J Cell Biol 1993;121:163–170.

165. Brooks PC, Clark RA, Cheresh DA. Requirement of vascular integrin alpha v beta 3 for angiogenesis. Science 1994;264:569–571.

166. Friedlander M, Brooks PC, Shaffer RW et al. Definition of two angiogenic pathways by distinct alpha v integrins. Science 1995;270:1500–1502.

167. Koolwijk P, van Erck MG, de Vree WJ et al. Cooperative effect of TNFalpha, bFGF, and VEGF on the formation of tubular structures of human microvascular endothelial cells in a fibrin matrix. Role of urokinase activity. J Cell Biol 1996;132:1177–1188.

168. Dvorak HF. Leaky tumor vessels: consequences for tumor stroma generation and for solid tumor therapy [Review]. Prog Clin Biol Res 1990;354A:317–330.

169. Nagy JA, Brown LF, Senger DR et al. Pathogenesis of tumor stroma generation: a critical role for leaky blood vessels and fibrin deposition [Review]. Biochim Biophys Acta 1989;948:305–326.

170. Senger DR, Brown LF, Claffey KP et al. Vascular permeability factor, tumor angiogenesis and stroma generation [Review]. Invasion Metastasis 1994;14:385–394.

171. Dvorak HF, Brown LF, Detmar M et al. Vascular permeability factor/vascular endothelial growth factor microvascular hyperpermeability and angiogenesis [Review]. Am J Pathol 1995;146:1029–1039.

172. Altieri DC. Inflammatory cell participation in coagulation [Review]. Semin Cell Biol 1995;6:269–274.

173. Qi J, Kreutzer DL. Fibrin activation of vascular endothelial cells. Induction of IL-8 expression. J Immunol 1995;155:867–876.

174. Qi J, Kreutzer DL, Piela-Smith TH. Fibrin induction of ICAM-1 expression in human vascular endothelial cells. J Immunol 1997;158:1880–1886.

175. Languino LR, Plescia J, Duperray A et al. Fibrinogen mediates leukocyte adhesion to vascular endothelium through an ICAM-1-dependent pathway. Cell 1993;73:1423–1434.

176. Altieri DC, Duperray A, Plescia J et al. Structural recognition of a novel fibrinogen gamma chain sequence (117-133) by intercellular adhesion molecule-1 mediates leukocyte-endothelium interaction. J Biol Chem 1995;270:696–699.

177. Kuijper PH, Gallardo Torres HI, Lammers JW et al. Platelet and fibrin deposition at the damaged vessel wall: cooperative substrates for neutrophil adhesion under flow conditions. Blood 1997;89:166–175.

178. Kuijper PH, Gallardo Torres HI, van der Linden JA et al. Neutrophil adhesion to fibrinogen and fibrin under flow conditions is diminished by activation and L-selectin shedding. Blood 1997;89:2131–2138.

179. Haidaris PJ. Induction of fibrinogen biosynthesis and secretion from cultured pulmonary epithelial cells. Blood 1997;89:873–882.

180. Tang L, Ugarova TP, Plow EF et al. Molecular determinants of acute inflammatory responses to biomaterials. J Clin Invest 1996;97:1329–1334.

181. Altieri DC, Plescia J, Plow EF. The structural motif glycine 190-valine 202 of the fibrinogen gamma chain interacts with CD11b/CD18 integrin (alpha M beta 2, Mac-1) and promotes leukocyte adhesion. J Biol Chem 1993;268:1847–1853.

182. Schwartz ML, Pizzo SV, Hill RL et al. Human Factor XIII from plasma and platelets. Molecular weights, subunit structures, proteolytic activation, and crosslinking of fibrinogen and fibrin. J Biol Chem 1973;248:1395–1407.

183. Chung SI, Lewis MS, Folk JE. Relationships of the catalytic properties of human plasma and platelet transglutaminases (activated blood coagulation factor XIII) to their subunit structures. J Biol Chem 1974;249:940–950.

184. Folk JE, Chung SI. Blood coagulation factor XIII: relationship of some biological properties to subunit structure. In: reich E, Rifkin DB, Shaw E, eds. Proteases and biological control. Cold Spring Harbor, NY: cold Spring Harbor Laboratory 1975;157–170.

185. Takahashi N, Takahashi Y, Putnam FW. Primary structure of blood coagulation factor XIIIa (fibrinoligase, transglutaminase) from human placenta. Proc Natl Acad Sci U S A 1986;83:8019–8023.

186. Grundmann U, Amann E, Zettlmeissl G et al. Characterization of cDNA coding for human factor XIIIa. Proc Natl Acad Sci U S A 1986;83:8024–8028.

187. Ichinose A, Hendrickson LE, Fujikawa K et al. Amino acid sequence of the a subunit of human factor XIII. Biochemistry 1986;25:6900–6906.

188. Ichinose A, McMullen BA, Fujikawa K et al. Amino acid sequence of the b subunit of human factor XIII, a protein composed of ten repetitive segments. Biochemistry 1986;25:4633–4638.

189. Kristensen T, D'Eustachio P, Ogata RT et al. The superfamily of C3b/C4b-binding proteins [Review]. Fed Proc 1987;46:2463–2469.

190. Webb GC, Coggan M, Ichinose A et al. Localization of the coagulation factor XIII B subunit gene (F13B) to chromosome bands 1q31-32.1 and restriction fragment length polymorphism at the locus. Hum Genet 1989;81:157–160.

191. Mary A, Achyuthan KE, Greenberg CS. B-chains prevent the proteolytic inactivation of the A-chains of plasma factor XIII. Biochim Biophys Acta 1988;966:328–335.

192. Skrzynia C, Reisner HM, McDonagh J. Characterization of the catalytic subunit of factor XIII by radioimmunoassay. Blood 1982;60:1089–1095.

193. Yorifuji H, Anderson K, Lynch GW et al. B protein of factor XIII: differentiation between free B and complexed B. Blood 1988;72:1645–1650.

194. Lorand L, Losowsky MS, Miloszewski KJ. Human factor XIII: fibrin-stabilizing factor. Prog Hemost Thromb 1980;5:245–290.

195. Greenberg CS, Dobson JV, Miraglia CC. Regulation of plasma factor XIII binding to fibrin in vitro. Blood 1985;66:1028–1034.

196. Weisberg LJ, Shiu DT, Conkling PR et al. Identification of normal human peripheral blood monocytes and liver as sites of synthesis of coagulation factor XIII a-chain. Blood 1987;70:579–582.

197. Wolpl A, Lattke H, Board PG et al. Coagulation factor XIII A and B subunits in bone marrow and liver transplantation. Transplantation 1987;43:151–153.

198. Adany R, Muszbek L. Immunohistochemical detection of factor XIII subunit a in histiocytes of human uterus. Histochemistry 1989;91:169–174.

199. McDonagh J, McDonagh RP Jr, Delage JM et al. Factor XIII in human plasma and platelets. J Clin Invest 1969;48:940–946.

200. Francis CW, Marder VJ. Rapid formation of large molecular weight alphapolymers in crosslinked fibrin induced by high factor XIII concentrations. Role of platelet factor XIII. J Clin Invest 1987;80:1459–1465.

201. Greenberg CS, Shuman MA. Specific binding of blood coagulation factor XIIIa to thrombin-stimulated platelets. J Biol Chem 1984;259:14721–14727.

202. Kreager JA, Devine DV, Greenberg CS. Cytofluorometric identification of plasmin-sensitive factor XIIIa binding to platelets. Thromb Haemost 1988;60:88–93.

203. McDonagh J, Waggoner WG, Hamilton EG et al. Affinity chromatography of human plasma and platelet factor XIII on organomercurial agarose. Biochim Biophys Acta 1976;446:345–357.

204. Radek JT, Jeong JM, Wilson J et al. Association of the A subunits of recombinant placental factor XIII with the native carrier B subunits from human plasma. Biochemistry 1993;32:3527–3534.

205. Greenberg CS, Birckbichler PJ, Rice RH. Transglutaminases: multifunctional crosslinking enzymes that stabilize tissues [Review]. FASEB J 1991; 5:3071–3077.

206. Board PG, Webb GC, McKee J et al. Localization of the coagulation factor XIII A subunit gene (F13A) to chromosome bands 6p24—p25. Cytogenet Cell Genet 1988;48:25–27.

207. Takagi T, Doolittle RF. Amino acid sequence studies on factor XIII and the peptide released during its activation by thrombin. Biochemistry 1974; 13:750–756.

208. Cooke RD, Holbrook JJ. The calcium-induced dissociation of human plasma clotting factor XIII. Biochem J 1974;141:79–84.

209. Cooke RD, Pestell TC, Holbrook JJ. Calcium and thiol reactivity of human plasma clotting factor XIII. Biochem J 1974;141:675–682.

210. Curtis CG, Brown KL, Credo RB et al. Calcium-dependent unmasking of active center cysteine during activation of fibrin stabilizing factor. Biochemistry 1974;13:3774–3780.

211. Hornyak TJ, Shafer JA. Role of calcium ion in the generation of factor XIII activity. Biochemistry 1991;30:6175–6182.

212. Carrell NA, Erickson HP, McDonagh J. Electron microscopy and hydrodynamic properties of factor XIII subunits. J Biol Chem 1989;264:551–556.

213. Bishop PD, Lasser GW, Le Trong I et al. Human recombinant factor XIII from Saccharomyces cerevisiae. Crystallization and preliminary x-ray data. J Biol Chem 1990;265:13888–13889.

214. Yee VC, Pedersen LC, Le Trong I et al. Three-dimensional structure of a transglutaminase: human blood coagulation factor XIII. Proc Natl Acad Sci U S A 1994;91:7296–7300.

215. Pedersen LC, Yee VC, Bishop PD et al. Transglutaminase factor XIII uses proteinase-like catalytic triad to crosslink macromolecules. Protein Sci 1994;3:1131–1135.

216. Hettasch JM, Greenberg CS. Analysis of the catalytic activity of human factor XIIIa by site-directed mutagenesis. J Biol Chem 1994;269: 28309–28313.

217. Micanovic R, Procyk R, Lin W et al. Role of histidine 373 in the catalytic activity of coagulation factor XIII. J Biol Chem 1994;269:9190–9194.

218. Poon MC, Russell JA, Low S et al. Hemopoietic origin of factor XIII A subunits in platelets, monocytes, and plasma. Evidence from bone marrow transplantation studies. J Clin Invest 1989;84:787–792.

219. Nagy JA, Kradin RL, McDonagh J. Biosynthesis of factor XIII A B subunits. Adv Exp Med Biol 1988;231:29–49.

220. Bottenus RE, Ichinose A, Davie EW. Nucleotide sequence of the gene for the b subunit of human factor XIII. Biochemistry 1990;29:11195–11209.

221. Santiago MA, Santiago RJ, Achyuthan KE et al. Factor XIII b-chains enhance the binding of a-chains to fibrin(ogen): role of the c-terminus of the a-chains [Abstract]. Blood 1994;84(Suppl):391a.

222. Halkier T, Magnusson S. Contact activation of blood coagulation is inhibited by plasma factor XIII b-chain. Thromb Res 1988;51:313–324.

223. Adany R, Kiss A, Muszbek L. Factor XIII: a marker of mono- and megakaryocytopoiesis. Br J Haematol 1987;67:167–172.

224. Henriksson P, Becker S, Lynch G et al. Identification of intracellular factor XIII in human monocytes and macrophages. J Clin Invest 1985;76:528–534.

225. Conkling PR, Achyuthan KE, Greenberg CS et al. Human mononuclear phagocyte transglutaminase activity crosslinks fibrin. Thromb Res 1989; 55:57–68.

226. Adany R, Nemes Z, Muszbek L. Characterization of factor XIII containing-macrophages in lymph nodes with Hodgkin's disease. Br J Cancer 1987; 55:421–426.

227. Adany R, Fodor F, Molnar P et al. Increased density of histiocytes in uterine leiomyomas. Int J Gynecol Pathol 1990;9:137–144.

228. Cerio R, Griffiths CE, Cooper KD et al. Characterization of factor XIIIa positive dermal dendritic cells in normal and inflamed skin. Br J Dermatol 1989;121:421–431.

229. Nemes Z, Thomazy V. Diagnostic significance of histiocyte-related markers in malignant histiocytosis and true histiocytic lymphoma. Cancer 1988; 62:1970–1980.

230. Naski MC, Lorand L, Shafer JA. Characterization of the kinetic pathway for fibrin promotion of alpha-thrombin-catalyzed activation of plasma factor XIII. Biochemistry 1991;30:934–941.

231. Janus TJ, Lewis SD, Lorand L et al. Promotion of thrombin-catalyzed activation of factor XIII by fibrinogen. Biochemistry 1983;22:6269–6272.

232. Lewis SD, Janus TJ, Lorand L et al. Regulation of formation of factor XIIIa by its fibrin substrates. Biochemistry 1985;24:6772–6777.

233. Greenberg CS, Miraglia CC, Rickles FR et al. Cleavage of blood coagulation factor XIII and fibrinogen by thrombin during in vitro clotting. J Clin Invest 1985;75:1463–1470.

234. Greenberg CS, Achyuthan KE, Fenton JW 2d. Factor XIIIa formation promoted by complexing of alpha-thrombin, fibrin, and plasma factor XIII. Blood 1987;69:867–871.

235. Folk JE, Finlayson JS. The epsilon-(gamma-glutamyl)lysine crosslink and the catalytic role of transglutaminases [Review]. Adv Protein Chem 1977; 31:1–133.

236. Lewis SD, Lorand L, Fenton JW 2d et al. Catalytic competence of human alpha- and gamma-thrombin in the activation of fibrinogen and factor XIII. Biochemistry 1987;26:7597–7603.

237. Hornyak TJ, Bishop PD, Shafer JA. Alpha-thrombin-catalyzed activation of human platelet factor XIII: relationship between proteolysis and factor XIIIa activity. Biochemistry 1989;28:7326–7332.

238. Credo RB, Curtis CG, Lorand L. Alpha-chain domain of fibrinogen controls generation of fibrinoligase (coagulation factor XIIIa). Calcium ion regulatory aspects. Biochemistry 1981;20:3770–3778.

239. Credo RB, Curtis CG, Lorand L. Ca2+-related regulatory function of fibrinogen. Proc Natl Acad Sci U S A 1978;75:4234–4237.

240. McDonagh J, McDonagh RP. Alternative pathways for the activation of factor XIII. Br J Haematol 1975;30:465–477.

241. Ando Y, Imamura S, Yamagata Y et al. Platelet factor XIII is activated by calpain. Biochem Biophys Res Commun 1987;144:484–490.

242. Lynch GW, Pfueller SL. Thrombin-independent activation of platelet factor XIII by endogenous platelet acid protease. Thromb Haemost 1988;59: 372–377.

243. Rider DM, McDonagh J. Resistance of factor XIII to degradation or activation by plasmin. Biochim Biophys Acta 1981;675:171–177.

244. Miloszewski K, Sheltawy MJ, Losowsky MS. Fibrinolysis and factor XIII. Acta Haematol 1974;52:40–46.

245. Becker CM. Separation of human plasma fibrin stabilizing factor (factor XIII) from fibrinogen by fibrinogen polymer formation. Biochem Biophys Res Commun 1986;134:678–684.

246. Greenberg CS, Shuman MA. The zymogen forms of blood coagulation factor XIII bind specifically to fibrinogen. J Biol Chem 1982;257:6096–6101.

247. Hornyak TJ, Shafer JA. Interactions of factor XIII with fibrin as substrate and cofactor. Biochemistry 1992;31:423–429.

248. Chung SI, Folk JE. Kinetic studies with transglutaminases. The human blood enzymes (activated coagulation factor 13) and the guinea pig hair follicle enzyme. J Biol Chem 1972;247:2798–2807.

249. Parameswaran KN, Lorand L. New thioester substrates for fibrinoligase (coagulation factor XIIIa) and for transglutaminase. Transfer of the fluorescently labeled acyl group to amines and alcohols. Biochemistry 1981;20: 3703–3711.

250. Lorand L, Parameswaran KN, Velasco PT et al. New colored and fluorescent amine substrates for activated fibrin stabilizing factor (Factor XIIIa) and for transglutaminase. Anal Biochem 1983;131:419–425.

251. Gross M, Whetzel NK, Folk JE. Amine binding sites in acyl intermediates of transglutaminases. Human blood plasma enzyme (activated coagulation factor XIII) and guinea pig liver enzyme. J Biol Chem 1977;252: 3752–3759.

252. Gorman JJ, Folk JE. Structural features of glutamine substrates for human plasma factor XIIIa (activated blood coagulation factor XIII). J Biol Chem 1980;255:419–427.

253. Coussons PJ, Price NC, Kelly SM et al. Factors that govern the specificity of transglutaminase-catalysed modification of proteins and peptides [Letter]. Biochem J 1992;282:929–930.

254. Groenen PJ, Smulders RH, Peters RF et al. The amine-donor substrate specificity of tissue-type transglutaminase. Influence of amino acid residues flanking the amine-donor lysine residue. Eur J Biochem 1994;220: 795–799.

255. Grootjans JJ, Groenen PJ, de Jong WW. Substrate requirements for transglutaminases. Influence of the amino acid residue preceding the amine donor lysine in a native protein. J Biol Chem 1995;270:22855–22858.

256. Ichinose A, Aoki N. Reversible crosslinking of alpha 2-plasmin inhibitor to fibrinogen by fibrin-stabilizing factor. Biochim Biophys Acta 1982;706: 158–164.

257. Mosesson MW, Siebenlist KR, Amrani DL et al. Identification of covalently linked trimeric and tetrameric D domains in crosslinked fibrin. Proc Natl Acad Sci U S A 1989;86:1113–1117.

258. Polgar J, Hidasi V, Muszbek L. Non-proteolytic activation of cellular protransglutaminase (placenta macrophage factor XIII). Biochem J 1990;267: 557–560.

259. Pisano JJ, Finlayson JS, Peyton MP. Crosslink in fibrin polymerized by factor 13:epsilon-(gamma-glutamyl)lysine. Science 1968;160:892–893.

260. Shen LL, Hermans J, McDonagh J et al. Effects of calcium ion and covalent crosslinking on formation and elasticity of fibrin cells. Thromb Res 1975; 6:255–265.

261. Gerth C, Roberts WW, Ferry JD. Rheology of fibrin clots. II. Linear viscoelastic behavior in shear creep. Biophys Chem 1974;2:208–217.

262. Robbins KC. A study on the conversion of fibrinogen to fibrin. Am J Physiol 1944;142:581–588.

263. Cottrell BA, Strong DD, Watt KW et al. Amino acid sequence studies on the alpha chain of human fibrinogen. Exact location of crosslinking acceptor sites. Biochemistry 1979;18:5405–5410.

264. Laki K, Lorand L. On the solubility of fibrin clots. Science 1948;108:280.

265. Purves L, Purves M, Brandt W. Cleavage of fibrin-derived D-dimer into monomers by endopeptidase from puff adder venom (Bitis arietans) acting at crosslinked sites of the gamma-chain. Sequence of carboxyterminal cyanogen bromide gamma-chain fragments. Biochemistry 1987;26: 4640–4646.

266. Hoeprich PD Jr, Doolittle RF. Dimeric half-molecules of human fibrinogen are joined through disulfide bonds in an antiparallel orientation. Biochemistry 1983;22:2049–2055.

267. Fowler WE, Erickson HP, Hantgan RR et al. Crosslinked fibrinogen dimers demonstrate a feature of the molecular packing in fibrin fibers. Science 1981;211:287–289.

268. Selmayr E, Mahn I, Muller-Berghaus G. Crosslinking of soluble fibrin and fibrinogen. Thromb Res 1985;39:467–474.

269. Selmayr E, Deffner M, Bachmann L et al. Chromatography and electron microscopy of crosslinked fibrin polymers—a new model describing the crosslinking at the DD-trans contact of the fibrin molecules. Biopolymers 1988;27:1733–1748.

270. Weisel JW, Francis CW, Nagaswami C et al. Determination of the topology of factor XIIIa-induced fibrin gamma-chain crosslinks by electron microscopy of ligated fragments. J Biol Chem 1993;268:26618–26624.

271. Siebenlist KR, Meh DA, Wall JS et al. Orientation of the carboxyterminal regions of fibrin gamma chain dimers determined from the crosslinked products formed in mixtures of fibrin fragment D, and factor XIIIa. Thromb Haemost 1995;74:1113–1119.

272. Siebenlist KR, Mosesson MW. Factors affecting gamma-chain multimer formation in crosslinked fibrin. Biochemistry 1992;31:936–941.

273. Mosesson MW. Fibrin polymerization and its regulatory role in hemostasis. J Lab Clin Med 1990;116:8–17.

274. Schwartz ML, Pizzo SV, Hill RL et al. The effect of fibrin-stabilizing factor on the subunit structure of human fibrin. J Clin Invest 1971;50:1506–1513.

275. Fretto LJ, Ferguson EW, Steinman HM et al. Localization of the alpha-chain crosslink acceptor sites of human fibrin. J Biol Chem 1978;253:2184–2195.

276. Shen LL, McDonagh RP, McDonagh J et al. Early events in the plasmin digestion of fibrinogen and fibrin. Effects of plasmin on fibrin polymerization. J Biol Chem 1977;252:6184–6189.

277. Gaffney PJ, Whitaker AN. Fibrin crosslinks and lysis rates. Thromb Res 1979;14:85–94.

278. Rampling MW. Factor XIII crosslinking and the rate of fibrinolysis induced by streptokinase and urokinase. Thromb Res 1978;12:287–295.

279. McDonagh RP Jr, McDonagh J, Duckert F. The influence of fibrin crosslinking on the kinetics of urokinase-induced clot lysis. Br J Haematol 1971;21:323–332.

280. Gaffney PJ, Lane DA, Kakkar VV et al. Characterisation of a soluble D dimer-E complex in crosslinked fibrin digests. Thromb Res 1975;7:89–99.

281. Muller MF, Ris H, Ferry JD. Electron microscopy of fine fibrin clots and fine and coarse fibrin films. Observations of fibers in cross-section and in deformed states. J Mol Biol 1984;174:369–384.

282. Francis CW, Marder VJ, Barlow GH. Plasmic degradation of crosslinked fibrin. Characterization of new macromolecular soluble complexes and a model of their structure. J Clin Invest 1980;66:1033–1043.

283. Pizzo SV, Taylor LM Jr, Schwartz ML et al. Subunit structure of fragment D from fibrinogen and crosslinked fibrin. J Biol Chem 1973;248:4584–4590.

284. Gaffney PJ, Brasher M. Subunit structure of the plasmin-induced degradation products of crosslinked fibrin. Biochim Biophys Acta 1973;295:308–313.

285. Shainoff JR, Urbanic DA, DiBello PM. Immunoelectrophoretic characterizations of the crosslinking of fibrinogen and fibrin by factor XIIIa and tissue transglutaminase. Identification of a rapid mode of hybrid alpha-/gamma-chain crosslinking that is promoted by the gamma-chain crosslinking. J Biol Chem 1991;266:6429–6437.

286. Dardik BN, Shainoff JR. Crosslinking of monomeric fibrin by factor XIIIa. Thromb Haemost 1979;42:864–872.

287. Seelich T, Furlan M, Beck EA. Reactivity of fibrinogen crosslinking sites in the absence of thrombin. Thromb Haemost 1976;35:620–627.

288. Shimizu A, Ferry JD. Ligation of fibrinogen by factor XIIIa with dithiothreitol: mechanical properties of ligated fibrinogen gels. Biopolymers 1988;27:703–713.

289. Procyk R, Blomback B. Factor XIII-induced crosslinking in solutions of fibrinogen and fibronectin. Biochim Biophys Acta 1988;967:304–313.

290. von Hugo R, Hafter R, Stemberger A et al. Complex formation of crosslinked fibrin oligomers with agarose-coupled fibrinogen and fibrin. Hoppe Seylers Z Physiol Chem 1977;358:1359–1363.

291. Shainoff JR, Page IH. Cofibrins and fibrin-intermediates as indicators of thrombin activation *in vivo*. Circ Res 1960;8:1013–1022.

292. Kierulf P. Studies on soluble fibrin in plasma. V. Isolation and characterization of the clottable proteins obtained from individual plasmas upon gelation with ethanol. Thromb Res 1974;4:183–187.

293. Collen D. Identification and some properties of a new fast-reacting plasmin inhibitor in human plasma. Eur J Biochem 1976;69:209–216.

294. Moroi M, Aoki N. Isolation and characterization of alpha2-plasmin inhibitor from human plasma. A novel proteinase inhibitor which inhibits activator-induced clot lysis. J Biol Chem 1976;251:5956–5965.

295. Kimura S, Tamaki T, Aoki N. Acceleration of fibrinolysis by the N-terminal peptide of alpha 2-plasmin inhibitor. Blood 1985;66:157–160.

296. Reed GL 3d, Matsueda GR, Haber E. Inhibition of clot-bound alpha 2-antiplasmin enhances *in vivo* thrombolysis. Circulation 1990;82:164–168.

297. Sakata Y, Eguchi Y, Mimuro J et al. Clot lysis induced by a monoclonal antibody against alpha 2-plasmin inhibitor. Blood 1989;74:2692–2697.

298. Mosher DF. Action of fibrin-stabilizing factor on cold-insoluble globulin and alpha2-macroglobulin in clotting plasma. J Biol Chem 1976;251:1639–1645.

299. Mosher DF. Fibronectin. Prog Hemost Thromb 1980;5:111–151.

300. Mosher DF, Fogerty FJ, Chernousov MA et al. Assembly of fibronectin into extracellular matrix [Review] Ann N Y Acad Sci 1991;614:167–180.

301. Mosher DF, Schad PE, Vann JM. Crosslinking of collagen and fibronectin by factor XIIIa. Localization of participating glutaminyl residues to a tryptic fragment of fibronectin. J Biol Chem 1980;255:1181–1188.

302. Mosher DF, Schad PE, Kleinman HK. Inhibition of blood coagulation factor XIIIa-mediated crosslinking between fibronectin and collagen by polyamines. J Supramol Struct 1979;11:227–235.

303. Mosher DF, Schad PE. Crosslinking of fibronectin to collagen by blood coagulation Factor XIIIa. J Clin Invest 1979;64:781–787.

304. Procyk R, Adamson L, Block M et al. Factor XIII catalyzed formation of fibrinogen-fibronectin oligomers—a thiol enhanced process. Thromb Res 1985;40:833–852.

305. Niewiarowska J, Cierniewski CS. Inhibitory effect of fibronectin on the fibrin formation. Thromb Res 1982;27:611–618.

306. Tamaki T, Aoki N. Crosslinking of alpha 2-plasmin inhibitor and fibronectin to fibrin by fibrin-stabilizing factor. Biochim Biophys Acta 1981;661:280–286.

307. Barry EL, Mosher DF. Factor XIIIa-mediated crosslinking of fibronectin in fibroblast cell layers. Crosslinking of cellular and plasma fibronectin and of aminoterminal fibronectin fragments. J Biol Chem 1989;264:4179–4185.

308. Okada M, Blomback B, Chang MD et al. Fibronectin and fibrin gel structure. J Biol Chem 1985;260:1811–1820.

309. Kamykowski GW, Mosher DF, Lorand L et al. Modification of shear modulus and creep compliance of fibrin clots by fibronectin. Biophys Chem 1981;13:25–28.

310. Chow TW, McIntire LV, Peterson DM. Importance of plasma fibronectin in determining PFP and PRP clot mechanical properties. Thromb Res 1983;29:243–248.

311. Duckert F, Jung E, Shmerling DH. A hitherto undescribed congenital haemorrhagic diathesis probably due to fibrin stabilizing factor deficiency. Thromb Diath Haemorrh 1960;5:179–186.

312. Duckert F. Documentation of the plasma factor XIII deficiency in man. Ann N Y Acad Sci 1972;202:190–199.

313. Mui PT, Ganguly P. Crosslinking of actin and fibrin by fibrin-stabilizing factor. Am J Physiol 1977;233:H346–H349.

314. Cohen I, Blankenberg TA, Borden D et al. Factor XIIIa-catalyzed crosslinking of platelet and muscle actin. Regulation by nucleotides. Biochim Biophys Acta 1980;628:365–375.

315. Cohen I, Young-Bandala L, Blankenberg TA et al. Fibrinoligase-catalyzed crosslinking of myosin from platelet and skeletal muscle. Arch Biochem Biophys 1979;192:100–111.

316. Cohen I, Lim CT, Kahn DR et al. Disulfide-linked and transglutaminase-catalyzed protein assemblies in platelets. Blood 1985;66:143–151.

317. Cohen I, Gerrard JM, White JG. Ultrastructure of clots during isometric contraction. J Cell Biol 1982;93:775–787.

318. Asijee GM, Muszbek L, Kappelmayer J et al. Platelet vinculin: a substrate of activated factor XIII. Biochim Biophys Acta 1988;954:303–308.

319. Francis RT, McDonagh J, Mann KG. Factor V is a substrate for the transamidase factor XIIIa. J Biol Chem 1986;261:9787–9792.

320. Huh MM, Schick BP, Schick PK et al. Covalent crosslinking of human coagulation factor V by activated factor XIII from guinea pig megakaryocytes and human plasma. Blood 1988;71:1693–1702.

321. Wang DL, Annamalai AE, Ghosh S et al. Human platelet factor V is crosslinked to actin by FXIIIa during platelet activation by thrombin. Thromb Res 1990;57:39–57.

322. Hada M, Kaminski M, Bockenstedt P et al. Covalent crosslinking of von Willebrand factor to fibrin. Blood 1986;68:95–101.

323. Bockenstedt P, McDonagh J, Handin RI. Binding and covalent crosslinking of purified von Willebrand factor to native monomeric collagen. J Clin Invest 1986;78:551–556.

324. Ribes JA, Francis CW. Multimer size dependence of von Willebrand factor binding to crosslinked or noncrosslinked fibrin. Blood 1990;75:1460–1465.

325. Sane DC, Moser TL, Greenberg CS. Vitronectin in the substratum of endothelial cells is crosslinked and phosphorylated. Biochem Biophys Res Commun 1991;174:465–469.

326. Skorstengaard K, Halkier T, Hojrup P et al. Sequence location of a putative transglutaminase crosslinking site in human vitronectin. FEBS Lett 1990;262:269–274.

327. Bale MD, Westrick LG, Mosher DF. Incorporation of thrombospondin into fibrin clots. J Biol Chem 1985;260:7502–7508.

328. Rodeghiero F, Castaman GC, Di Bona E et al. Successful pregnancy in a woman with congenital factor XIII deficiency treated with substitutive therapy. Report of a second case. Blut 1987;55:45–48.

329. Kangsadalampai S, Coggan M, Caglayan SH et al. Application of HUMF13A01 (AAAG) (n) STR polymorphism to the genetic diagnosis of coagulation factor XIII deficiency. Thromb Haemost 1996;76:879–882.

330. Bruhn HD, Zurborn KH. Influences of clotting factors (thrombin, factor

XIII) and of fibronectin on the growth of tumor cells and leukemic cells *in vitro.* Blut 1983;46:85–88.

331. Beck E, Duckert F, Ernst M. The influence of fibrin stabilizing factor on the growth of fibroblasts *in vitro* and wound healing. Thromb Diath Haemorrh 1961;6:485–491.

332. Ueyama M, Urayama T. The role of factor XIII in fibroblast proliferation. Jpn J Exp Med 1978;48:135–142.

333. Letheby BA, Davis RB, Larsen AE. The effect of major surgical procedures on plasma and platelet levels of Factor VIII. Thromb Diath Haemorrh 1974;31:20–29.

334. Powanda MC, Moyer ED. Plasma proteins and wound healing. Surg Gynecol Obstet 1981;153:749–755.

335. Knox P, Crooks S, Rimmer CS. Role of fibronectin in the migration of fibroblasts into plasma clots. J Cell Biol 1986;102:2318–2323.

336. Lanir N, Ciano PS, Van de Water L et al. Macrophage migration in fibrin gel matrices. II. Effects of clotting factor XIII, fibronectin, and glycosaminoglycan content on cell migration. J Immunol 1988;140:2340–2349.

337. Muszbek L, Adany R, Kavai M et al. Monocytes of individuals congenitally deficient in plasma factor XIII lack factor XIII subunit a antigen and transglutaminase activity. Thromb Haemost 1988;59:231–235.

338. Brown LF, Lanir N, McDonagh J et al. Fibroblast migration in fibrin gel matrices. Am J Pathol 1993;142:273–283.

339. Suzuki R, Toda H, Takamura Y. Dynamics of blood coagulation factor XIII in ulcerative colitis and preliminary study of the factor XIII concentrate. Blut 1989;59:162–164.

340. Lorenz R, Heinmuller M, Classen M et al. Substitution of factor XIII: a therapeutic approach to ulcerative colitis. Haemostasis 1991;21:5–9.

341. Stadnicki A, Kloczko J, Nowak A et al. Factor XIII subunits in relation to some other hemostatic parameters in ulcerative colitis. Am J Gastroenterol 1991;86:690–693.

342. Hudson M, Wakefield AJ, Hutton RA et al. Factor XIIIA subunit and Crohn's disease. Gut 1993;34:75–79.

343. Guillevin L, Euller-Ziegler L, Chouvet B et al. Traitement de la sclerodermie systemique par le facteur XIII chez 86 malades suivis a long terme. Presse Med 1985;14:2327–2329.

344. Kamitsuji H, Tani K, Yasui M et al. Activity of blood coagulation factor XIII as a prognostic indicator in individuals with Henoch-Schonlein purpura. Efficacy of factor XIII substitution. Eur J Pediatr 1987;146:519–523.

345. Laohaprasit V, Edwards MW, Mayberg MR. Prevention of postoperative intracerebral hemorrhage with topical recombinant factor XIII in the rat. Neurosurgery 1993;32:630–634.

346. Spotnitz WD. Fibrin sealant in the United States: clinical use at the University of Virginia [Review]. Thromb Haemost 1995;74:482–485.

347. Spotnitz WD, Dalton MS, Baker JW et al. Reduction of perioperative hemorrhage by anterior mediastinal spray application of fibrin glue during cardiac operations. Ann Thorac Surg 1987;44:529–531.

348. Shaffrey CI, Spotnitz WD, Shaffrey ME et al. Neurosurgical applications of fibrin glue: augmentation of dural closure in 134 individuals. Neurosurgery 1990;26:207–210.

349. Stuart JD, Kenney JG, Lettieri J et al. Application of single-donor fibrin glue to burns. J Burn Care Rehabil 1988;9:619–622.

350. Featherstone C. Fibrin sealants for haemostasis and drug delivery [News]. Lancet 1997;349:334.

351. Kram HB, Nathan RC, Stafford FJ et al. Fibrin glue achieves hemostasis in individuals with coagulation disorders. Arch Surg 1989;124:385–387.

352. Toma AG, Fisher EW, Cheesman AD. Autologous fibrin glue in the repair of dural defects in craniofacial resections. J Laryngol Otol 1992;106:356–357.

353. Zusman SP, Lustig JP, Bin Nun G. Cost evaluation of two methods of post tooth extraction hemostasis in individuals on anticoagulant therapy. Community Dent Health 1993;10:167–173.

354. Abel ME, Chiu YS, Russell TR et al. Autologous fibrin glue in the treatment of rectovaginal and complex fistulas. Dis Colon Rectum 1993;36:447–449.

355. Glover W, Chavis TV, Daniel TM et al. Fibrin glue application through the flexible fiberoptic bronchoscope: closure of bronchopleural fistulas. J Thorac Cardiovasc Surg 1987;93:470–472.

356. Leca F, Karam J, Vouhe PR et al. Surgical treatment of multiple ventricular septal defects using a biologic glue. J Thorac Cardiovasc Surg 1994;107:96–102.

357. Berger JT, Gilhooly J. Fibrin glue treatment of persistent pneumothorax in a premature infant. J Pediatr 1993;122:958–960.

358. DePalma L, Criss VR, Luban NL. The preparation of fibrinogen concentrate for use as fibrin glue by four different methods. Transfusion 1993;33:717–720.

359. Saltz R, Dimick A, Harris C et al. Application of autologous fibrin glue in burn wounds. J Burn Care Rehabil 1989;10:504–507.

360. Casali B, Rodeghiero F, Tosetto A et al. Fibrin glue from single-donation autologous plasmapheresis. Transfusion 1992;32:641–643.

361. Hilfenhaus J, Weidmann E. Fibrin glue safety: inactivation of potential viral contaminants by pasteurization of the human plasma components. Arzneimittelforschung 1985;35:1617–1619.

362. Cuthbertson B, Reid KG, Foster PR. Viral contamination of human plasma products and procedures for preventing virus transmission by plasma products. Blood separation and plasma fractionation. Wiley-Liss, 1991:385–435.

363. Burnouf-Radosevich M, Burnouf T, Huart JJ. Biochemical and physical properties of a solvent-detergent-treated fibrin glue. Vox Sang 1990;58:77–84.

364. Suzuki K, Henke J, Iwata M et al. Novel polymorphisms and haplotypes in the human coagulation factor XIII A-subunit gene. Hum Genet 1996;98:393–395.

365. Suzuki K, Iwata M, Ito S et al. Molecular basis for subtypic differences of the "a" subunit of coagulation factor XIII with description of the genesis of the subtypes. Hum Genet 1994;94:129–135.

366. Chung D, Ichinose A. Hereditary disorders related to fibrinogen and factor XIII. In: scriver CR, Beaudet AL, Sly WS, Valle D, eds. The metabolic basis of inherited disease. New York: mcGraw-Hill, 1989;2:2135–2153.

# CHAPTER 7

# FIBRINOLYSIS AND ITS REGULATION

## Douglas E. Vaughan and Paul J. Declerck

## FIBRINOLYTIC COMPONENTS: REGULATION OF SYNTHESIS AND SECRETION

Fibrinolysis is defined narrowly as the plasmin-mediated degradation of fibrin. The fibrinolytic system is composed of several proteins (serine proteinases and inhibitors) that interact to regulate the generation of plasmin (Fig.7.1). Control of the fibrinolytic process occurs at many levels, including protein-protein interactions, but also at the cellular level where the synthesis and secretion of proteins involved in fibrinolysis is highly regulated. This system serves as one of the endogenous defense mechanisms in the prevention of intravascular thrombosis. As such, it complements the endogenous anticoagulants (see Chapter 3) and endothelial-derived platelet inhibitors (see Chapter 13) in retarding clot formation. During the past several years, there has been a growing appreciation for the role plasminogen activators (PA) play in tissue remodeling as well.

## PLASMINOGEN

### SOURCES AND CHARACTERIZATION

Plasminogen circulates in abundant ($\mu$M) concentrations in plasma and is synthesized primarily in the liver (1). The zymogen plasminogen is a single-chain glycoprotein of 92 Kd, containing approximately 2% carbohydrate. Complete amino acid sequencing revealed that human plasminogen comprises 790 amino acids (2), including a preactivation peptide that is 77 amino acids in length, five homologous triple-loop structures called "kringle" domains, an activation cleavage site ($Arg^{560}$-$Val^{561}$), and the catalytic domain comprising the three amino acids of the active site ($His^{602}$, $Asp^{645}$, and $Ser^{740}$) (Fig. 7.2).

Cleavage of the $Arg^{560}$-$Val^{561}$ bond by a PA yields the active enzyme plasmin (3). This two-chain molecule consists of a heavy chain (or A-chain) originating from the amino$_2$-terminal part of plasminogen and a light chain (or B-chain) originating from the carboxyterminal part. The active site is located in the B-chain. The plasmin A-chain contains "lysine binding sites" that are also available in the plasminogen molecule. These domains mediate its interaction with fibrin and with $\alpha_2$-antiplasmin ($\alpha_2$-AP) and contribute to the "fibrin-specificity" of the endogenous fibrinolytic system.

## STRUCTURE OF THE GENE; REGULATION OF SYNTHESIS

The full length cDNA for plasminogen has been cloned and characterized (4). The gene for human plasminogen is localized on the long arm of chromosome 6 at band q26-27 (5) and has also been cloned (6). The gene consists of 19 exons spanning 52.5 kb of DNA. Nucleotide sequence analysis revealed a striking similarity with other serine proteases and with apolipoprotein(a) (7). The close relationship between the gene encoding for plasminogen and that for apolipoprotein(a) (8) suggests that

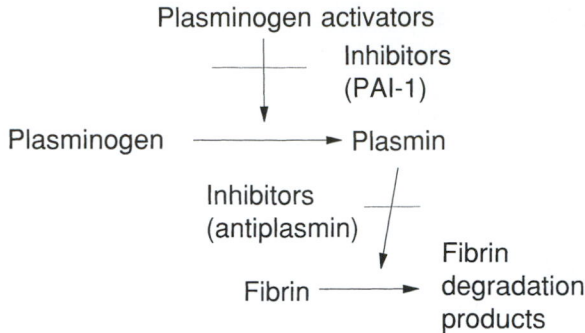

**FIGURE 7.1.** Schematic representation of the mammalian fibrinolytic system.

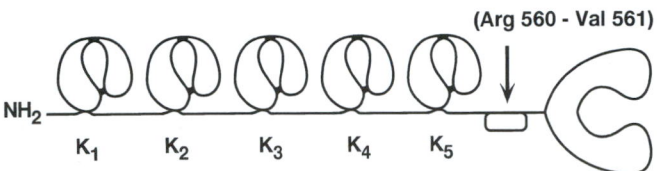

**FIGURE 7.2.** Schematic representation of the structure of plasminogen. Cleavage of the indicated peptide bond converts plasminogen to plasmin. Adapted from Handin R, Loscalzo J. In: Braunwald E, ed. Heart disease—A textbook of cardiovascular medicine. 4th ed. Philadelphia: WB Saunders, 1992; 1767–1789.

the latter may have evolved through exon shuffling. Analysis of DNA sequence also revealed that the 5'-upstream region of the plasminogen gene contains two clusters of regulatory elements for transcription, that is, CCAAT boxes and TATAA sequences (6). Sequence elements (CTGGGA), common to genes for acute-phase reactants, are also present in the 5'-upstream region. Although extensive data have been generated with respect to the organization of the gene for plasminogen, further detailed studies will be needed to gain insight into the regulation of its expression.

# TISSUE-TYPE PLASMINOGEN ACTIVATOR

## SOURCES AND CHARACTERIZATION OF PROTEIN

Plasma tissue-type plasminogen activator (t-PA) is derived primarily from vascular endothelial cells. It circulates in low (pM) concentrations in plasma and has a half-life of 5 to 7 minutes. Free t-PA is cleared via mannose receptors in the liver, whereas t-PA/plasminogen activator inhibitor (PAI)-1 complexes are cleared via the low density lipoprotein receptor-related protein (LRP)

(9) and by the urokinase-type plasminogen activator receptor (u-PAR) (10). Tissue-type plasminogen activator is a serine protease of 68 Kd synthesized as a single-chain molecule consisting of 527 amino acids (Fig. 7.3). Direct determination of the amino acid sequence of the entire protein confirmed the primary structure of the protein as predicted from the nucleotide sequence (11). Tissue-type plasminogen activator is synthesized as a precursor protein that undergoes posttranslational modifications (12). The 20 to 23 residues at the aminoterminal end of the protein constitute a typical hydrophobic signal peptide required for secretion of t-PA. A presequence of 12 to 15 hydrophilic residues precedes the aminoterminus of mature t-PA. Based on the striking homology between distinct portions of the amino acid sequence of t-PA with corresponding domains of other proteins, the following subdomains can be distinguished in the mature protein: a finger domain (residues 4 to 50), which is homologous to the type I fingers (F) of fibronectin; residues 51 to 87, which form a domain that is homologous to epidermal growth factor (EGF); and residues 88 to 176 ($K_1$) and 177 to 262 ($K_2$), two triple disulfide loop structures homologous to the kringles found in plasminogen. The F, EGF, $K_1$, and $K_2$ domains comprise the heavy or A chain of t-PA. The carboxyter-

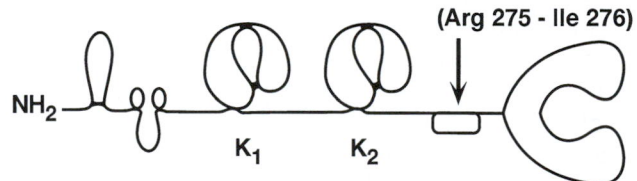

**FIGURE 7.3.** Schematic representation of the structure of t-PA. Cleavage of the indicated peptide bond converts single-chain t-PA to two-chain t-PA. Adapted from Handin R, Loscalzo J. In: Braunwald E, ed. Heart disease—A textbook of cardiovascular medicine. 4th ed. Philadelphia: WB Saunders, 1992;1767–1789.

**TABLE 7.1.** Agents That Regulate Vascular Tissue-Type Plasminogen Activator Production

| Agent | Effect |
| --- | --- |
| Butyrate | ⇈ |
| Phorbol esters | ↑ |
| Histamine | ↑ |
| Retinoids | ↑ |
| Shear stress | ↑ |
| Forskolin | ↓ |
| Ethanol | ↑ |
| Bradykinin | ↑ |

minal region, comprising amino acids 276 to 527, constitutes the light or B chain and is homologous to that of other serine proteinases (13). The catalytic site of t-PA is located in the B-chain, and is composed of $His^{322}$, $Asp^{371}$, and $Ser^{478}$. Hydrolysis of the $Arg^{275}$-$Ile^{276}$ bond by plasmin converts t-PA to a two-chain molecule in which the heavy and light chain are connected by a disulfide bond. Although t-PA undergoes a conformational change during the conversion from the single-chain to two-chain form, both forms are catalytically active.

## STRUCTURE OF THE TISSUE-TYPE PLASMINOGEN ACTIVATOR GENE; REGULATION OF SYNTHESIS

The cDNA of t-PA has been cloned and the complete amino acid sequence has been determined (12, 14, 15). The human t-PA gene is localized on chromosome 8 (16, 17) and nearly 36 kb of the human t-PA genomic sequence have been determined (18, 19, 20). The t-PA gene consists of 14 exons, and the intron-exon organization suggests that the assembly is an example of the "exon shuffling" principle (21), which proposes that the distinct structural domains are encoded by a single exon or by adjacent exons. The proximal promoter sequences in the human gene contain typical TATA and CAAT boxes, and potential recognition sequences for transcription factors (for example, AP1, NF1, SP1, AP2) have been identified that may have a functional role in the regulation of t-PA expression (20). A sequence very similar to the consensus sequences of the cyclic adenosine monophosphate (cAMP)-responsive element (CRE) and a sequence exhibiting homology with the consensus sequence of the AP2 binding site have been identified between position −102 and −115 and between +60 and +74, respectively (22). Both elements were suggested to have a cooperative effect on constitutive t-PA gene expression. A typical retinoid-response element has been described far upstream from the transcription start site of t-PA (23). Studies on t-PA gene expression at the mRNA level using endothelial cells have revealed relatively small changes induced by a variety of agonists. Conflicting results were obtained with agents modulating cAMP levels. Inhibition of secreted t-PA (24) or a small increase in t-PA expression was observed using butyrate (25). Tissue-type plasminogen activator gene expression in endothelial cells and in HeLa cells increases after treatment with the tumor-promoting phorbol ester, PMA (26–28). Only a few compounds have thus far been identified that primarily or exclusively stimulate t-PA synthesis without affecting PAI-1 synthesis. These include histamine (29), butyrate (25), or a combination of cAMP with protein kinase agonists (27). Retinoids have been shown to induce an increase of t-PA

mRNA *in vitro* as well as *in vivo* (30, 31). Another study reported twofold to threefold selective stimulation of t-PA secretion rate by endothelial cells subjected to arterial levels of shear stress, whereas no changes were observed in PAI-1 secretion (32). The synthetic glucocorticoid, dexamethasone, has also been reported to induce a moderate increase in t-PA gene expression by HT-1080 cells (33).

## UROKINASE-TYPE PLASMINOGEN ACTIVATOR

### SOURCES AND CHARACTERISTICS OF THE PROTEIN

Similar to t-PA, urokinase-type plasminogen activator (u-PA) circulates in trace concentrations in plasma and is an endothelial product. Mature u-PA is a single-chain glycoprotein with $M_r$ 54,000 and consists of 411 amino acids (34) (Fig. 7.4). Single-chain u-PA (scu-PA) has minimal activity. Hydrolysis of $Lys^{158}$-$Ile^{159}$ peptide bond by plasmin or kallikrein converts the molecule to its two-chain active form (35, 36). The aminoterminal chain consists of 158 amino acids and contains one region homologous to human epidermal growth factor (residues 5 to 49) and one region homologous to the plasminogen kringles. The carboxyterminal chain consists of 253 amino

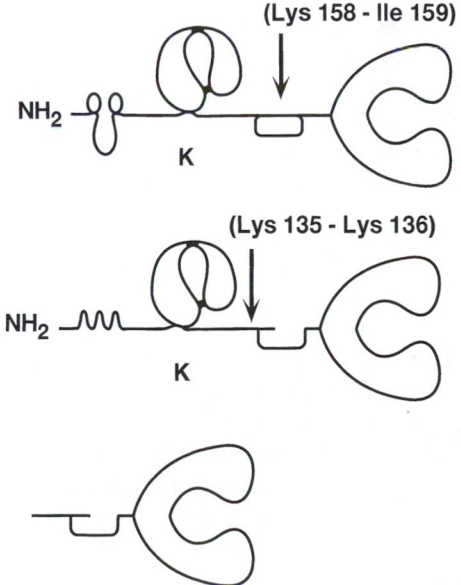

**FIGURE 7.4.** Schematic representation of the various structures of u-PA. (**Upper**) Single-chain u-PA; (**middle**) Two-chain u-PA; (**bottom**) Low-molecular-weight urokinase. Adapted from Handin R, Loscalzo J, In: Braunwald E, ed. Heart disease—A textbook of cardiovascular medicine. 4th ed. Philadelphia: WB Saunders, 1992;1767–1789.

**TABLE 7.2.**   Agents that Regulate Plasminogen Activator Inhibitor Synthesis in Cultured Endothelium

| Agent | Effect |
|---|---|
| Lipopolysaccharide | ↑ |
| Interleukin 1 | ↑ |
| TNF-α | ↑ |
| TGF-β | ↑ |
| bFGF | ↑ |
| Phorbol esters | ↑ |
| Thrombin | ↑ |
| HTG-VLDL | ↑ |
| Lp(a) | ↑ |
| Angiotensin II | ↑ |
| Glucose | ↑ |
| Forskolin | ↓ |
| ECG + heparin | ↓ |
| Ethanol | ↓ |

acids and contains the catalytic center composed of His[204], Arg[255], and Ser[256]. A single carbohydrate moiety is attached to Asn[302]. The two chains are connected by a Cys[148]–Cys[279] interchain disulfide bond. A low $M_r$ derivative ($M_r$ 33,000) of two-chain urokinase can be generated through hydrolysis of the Lys[135]–Lys[136] peptide bond subsequent to cleavage of the Lys[158]–Ile[159] bond (37, 38). Cleavage of the Arg[156]–Phe[157] peptide bond in scu-PA by thrombin results in an inactive two-chain urokinase derivative (36).

## STRUCTURE OF THE GENE; REGULATION OF SYNTHESIS

The cDNA of human u-PA has been isolated and the nucleotide sequence has been determined (39). The human gene for u-PA has been localized on chromosome 10 and spans 6.4 kb (40). It contains 11 exons and the intron-exon organization closely resembles that of the t-PA gene (39), with several important exceptions. Exon III of t-PA is totally absent and exon IV is partially missing in the u-PA gene, which accounts for the absence of the finger domain in u-PA; exons VIII and IX, which together code for the second kringle in t-PA, are totally missing as well. Exon II of the u-PA gene codes for a signal peptide composed of 20 amino acids; exons III and IV code for the growth factor domain and exon V and VI for the kringle region. The 5′-region of exon VII, which codes for the peptide connecting the light and heavy chain, is 39 bp longer than the corresponding exon of the t-PA gene. The 3′-region of exon VII and exons VIII to XI code for the heavy chain.

Urokinase-type plasminogen activator expression is induced during neoplastic transformation as well as by exposure to a wide variety of agents including hormonal factors, growth factors, phorbol esters, and cAMP. Several of these effects have been shown to occur at the mRNA level. It has been proposed that the transcription factors AP1 and AP2 may be involved in tumor promoter modulation of u-PA expression (40). Although this rather complex regulatory system may play an important role in cellular migration, invasion, and tumor metastasis, its influence on fibrinolysis is less well understood. Functional analysis of the human u-PA promoter has revealed the presence of a potential enhancer element approximately 2 kb upstream of the transcription start site and potential negative regulatory elements approximately 1.5 kb. Interleukin-1 and lipopolysaccharide induce small increases in u-PA expression by endothelial cells, whereas tumor necrosis factor (TNF), which has negligible effect on t-PA, has been shown to increase u-PA mRNA levels in endothelial cells by a factor of fivefold to thirtyfold (41, 42). The cytokine transforming growth factor-β1 (TGF-β1) has been reported to induce an approximately fivefold increase of u-PA gene expression in human epithelial cells (43). Urokinase-plasminogen activator gene expression in HT-1080 cells is strongly downregulated by dexamethasone (33).

## α₂-ANTIPLASMIN

### SOURCES AND CHARACTERISTICS

α₂-Antiplasmin is a single-chain glycoprotein of approximately 70 Kd consisting of 452 amino acids and containing two disulfide bridges (44, 45). α₂-antiplasmin shows a significant homology with other members of the serine proteinase inhibitor family (46). α₂-antiplasmin was identified in plasma (47, 48) from which it was purified and characterized (49). It is produced and secreted by liver cells (50). In normal plasma, α₂-AP is heterogeneous and consists of functionally active and inactive forms. Approximately 30% of the α₂-AP antigen appears to be functionally inactive (51). The apparently inactive form still has the intact reactive site but lacks 26 residues from the carboxyterminus presumably containing the plasminogen binding site (52). Therefore, this truncated form does not bind to plasminogen (53) and reacts much more slowly with plasmin. It has been suggested that α₂-AP is synthesized as the plasminogen binding form and that it is partly converted to the nonbinding form in the circulation (54, 55).

### STRUCTURE OF THE GENE

The cDNA encoding for α₂-AP has been isolated and characterized. The predicted amino acid sequence confirms its homology with other serpins to a degree of 23 to 28% (46). The human α₂-AP gene has been characterized

(56). The gene spans 16,000 base pairs and consists of 10 exons. The promoter region contains typical elements, including a TATA box, a CCAAT box, and several GC-rich sequences. Sequences in the 5'-flanking region closely resembling a hepatitis B enhancer element have been suggested to be involved in tissue specific expression of $\alpha_2$-AP (56). The functional role of these sequences has not been elucidated.

# PLASMINOGEN ACTIVATOR INHIBITOR-1

## SOURCES AND CHARACTERIZATION OF THE PROTEIN

Plasminogen activator inhibitor-1 (PAT-1) was first identified in conditioned media of [human] endothelial cells (57, 58) and rat hepatoma cells (59). It has subsequently been identified in plasma (60–63), platelets (64), and a variety of other tissues and conditioned media (65–67). In plasma, PAI-1 concentrations vary widely (68). The PAI-1 that is present in plasma is likely derived from multiple sources, including endothelial cells, adipose tissue, the liver, and platelets (69).

Plasminogen activator inhibitor-1 is a single-chain glycoprotein with an apparent $M_r$ of 50,000 consisting of 379 amino acids, and lacking any cysteine residues or disulfide bonds to stabilize its structure (69) (Fig. 7.4). It is synthesized in an active form, but exhibits marked functional instability and has a functional half-life of approximately 2 hours at 37°C (70) (Fig. 7.5; see color plate 7.5). At least four different conformations of PAI-1 have been described (71, 73): 1) the active form that reacts with, and is cleaved by, plasminogen activator (74); 2) the latent form, which is nonreactive and noncleavable (75); 3) a substrate form, which can be cleaved by plasminogen activators, but is noninhibitory in nature (76); and 4) the inert form of PAI-1 generated by the cleavage of the reactive site of active PAI-1 by plasminogen activators (77). The structural basis of latency was elucidated when the structure of intact latent PAI-1 was determined by single-crystal x-ray diffraction (75). In latent PAI-1, the intact reactive site loop inserts as a fourth strand into the major $\beta$-sheet of the molecule, which reduces its ability to be cleaved by, and complex with, a PA (78).

Although active PAI-1 has not been crystallized, its structure has been deduced based on alignment studies using the structure of latent PAI-1 and other intact serpins (74) (Fig. 7.5; see color plate 7.5). Active PAI-1 in plasma is stabilized by a noncovalent association with vitronectin (79, 80), which is also the major component responsible for binding of active PAI-1 to the extracellular matrix of cultured human endothelial cells (81). Binding to vitronectin also broadens the reactivity of PAI-1 and converts it into a moderately active inhibitor of thrombin (82). Latent PAI-1 can be reactivated by pro-

tein denaturants, such as sodium dodecylsulfate (SDS), guanidinium HCl, or urea (83) by heat, or by negatively charged phospholipids (84). There is limited evidence indicating that latent PAI-1 can be reactivated *in vivo* by a fast-acting mechanism likely localized to vascular surfaces (85).

The full length cDNA encoding human PAI-1 has been cloned and sequenced (86, 87). The predicted amino acid sequences show a significant homology between PAI-1 and members of the serpin family (88). In the amino acid (AA) region ($AA^{328}$–$AA^{359}$), including the reactive site, it has 55% homology with antithrombin (AT)-III, 41% with PAI-2, 39% with $\alpha_2$-AP, 32% with $C_1$ inhibitor, and 21% with $\alpha_1$-protease inhibitor.

## STRUCTURE OF THE GENE; REGULATION OF SYNTHESIS

The human and rat PAI-1 genes have been characterized (89–91). The human PAI-1 gene has been mapped on chromosome 7 (q21.3–q22) close to the locus for cystic fibrosis (92). The gene spans approximately 12,200 base pairs and consists of 9 exons and 8 introns. The gene organization of the PAI-1 gene is distinct from that of other serpins (89). However, comparison of the intron positions in the PAI-1 gene with the typical subdomain structure of serpins revealed a nonrandom distribution for 7 of the 8 introns; that is, the introns are positioned close to the boundary of individual structural subdomains or in the random coil regions of the protein (89). This similarity has led to the suggestion of an evolutionary process called "intron-sliding" (93) within the genes of the serpin family, allowing variation in the amino acid sequence without affecting the overall folding structure of these proteins.

The promoter contains a typical TATA box but no CAAT sequence (91, 94, 95) (Fig. 7.6). Promoter deletion mapping has revealed the presence of a strong and tissue-specific promoter within the first 187 base pairs of the 5'-flanking region of the PAI-1 gene. Two regions in this promoter have been identified to be inducible by the synthetic glucocorticoid, dexamethasone, with one element localized between nucleotides $-90$ and $+75$ and a second region located between $-800$ and $-549$ (96). The proximal element appears to contain the glucocorticoid responsive enhancer element (96). Transforming growth factor-$\beta$ (TFG-$\beta$) responsive elements have also been identified in the PAI-1 5'-flanking DNA region between the nucleotides $-791$ and $-546$, and $-328$ and $-186$ upstream of the transcription start site (97, 98). It has also been suggested that in HepG2 cells, PAI-1 gene regulation by TGF-$\beta$ is also mediated by posttranscriptional mechanisms (98). The regulatory region localized between bases $-791$ and $-546$ appears to be 74% homologous to the equivalent region in the murine PAI-1 gene sequence (99) and 80% identical to the region in the rat PAI-1 gene sequence (91), suggesting that con-

**FIGURE 7.6.** Location of promoter elements in the upstream regulatory region of the PAI-1 gene. Potential carbohydrate response elements labeled Cho RE.

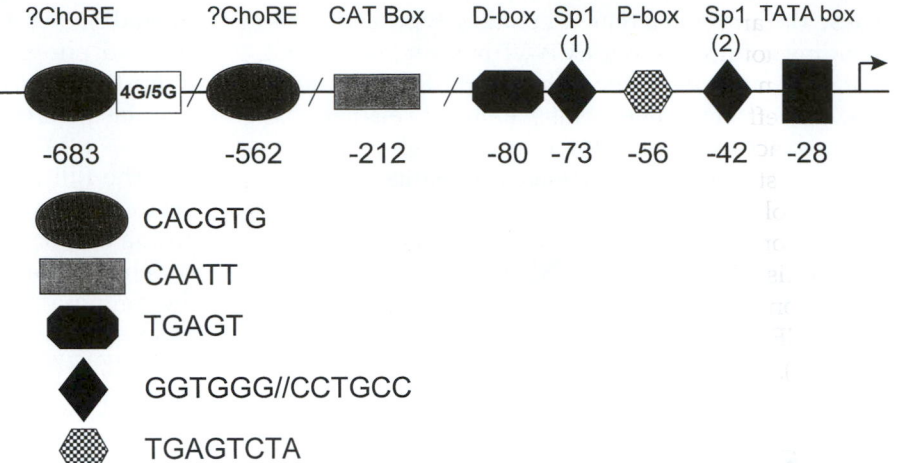

**FIGURE 7.7.** Representation of the 4G/5G polymorphism at −675 of the PAI-1 gene as it appears on a sequencing gel.

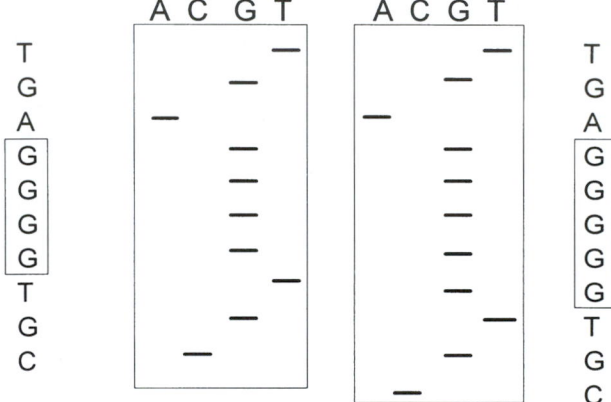

served *cis*-acting sequences are involved in the TGF-β inducibility. TGF-β is known to stimulate the expression of *c-fos* and *c-jun,* two components of the AP-1 complex. The human PAI-1 gene has an AP-1-like binding site (GGAGTCA) at position −672 to −666 base pairs upstream of the transcription start site. This sequence is 100% identical in both the murine and the rat 5′ flanking DNA (98). A common dialleleic polymorphism has been identified in a guanosine tract at −675 from the transcription start site (100). The two alleles differ by only a single guanosine in a run of four or five bases (Fig. 7.7). Individuals that are homozygous for the 4G allele have relatively high plasma levels of PAI-1, whereas homozygotes for the 5G allele tend to have lower levels. These observations have been explained mechanistically by the binding of a transcriptional activator to the 4G allele, whereas a repressor and an activator bind to the 5G allele. Recent studies have also linked the 4G allele with increased risk of myocardial infarction (101).

Two PAI-1 mRNA species have been observed with lengths of 2.3 and 3.4 kb, respectively (86, 87). The occurrence of two distinct PAI-1 mRNA forms is due to alternative polyadenylation with an additional 3′ untranslated region (approximately 1 kb) in the larger mRNA species containing a 75 base pair AT-rich sequence that has been proposed to play a role in PAI-1 gene regulation by a posttranslational mechanism (102). A 120 base pair sequence in the 3′ untranslated region preceding the AT-rich sequence is highly conserved between the human, bovine, mouse, and rat genes (87, 99, 103, 104). This fragment has no similarity to other sequences, but the high degree of homology has been suggested to be consistent with a putative regulatory role.

Although the existence of posttranscriptional regulation of PAI-I mRNA levels has been suggested, the majority of studies examining regulation of PAI-1 mRNA expression have demonstrated an effect at the transcriptional level. Plasminogen activator inhibitor-1 is synthesized by a wide variety of established cell lines and primary cell cultures in which its expression can be modulated by various agonists such as hormones, growth factors, endotoxin, cytokines, and phorbol esters. Regulation of PAI-1 expression is cell specific. In endothelial cells, PAI-1 gene expression is stimulated by lipopolysaccharide (LPS) (105–107), IL-1 (108), TNF-α (107), TGF-β (107), basic fibroblast growth factor (bFGF) (109), phorbol esters (110), thrombin (111, 112), very low density lipoprotein (VLDL) (113), lipoprotein(a) (114), and angiotensin II (115). The stimulatory effect of platelet releasates on PAI-1 synthesis by endothelial cells was suggested to be mediated mainly by TGF-β (116). Only a few agents have been reported to down-regulate PAI-1 expression in endothelial cells, including forskolin (27, 31, 117), endothelial cell growth factor supplement combined with heparin (118), and ethanol (119).

In contrast to endothelial cells, PAI-1 expression in

human hepatocytes is not modulated by TNF-α (120), nor by dexamethasone (67). On the other hand, insulin has a pronounced effect on PAI-1 synthesis in Hep G2 cells and in isolated human hepatocytes (121, 122), but has little effect on endothelial PAI-1 expression. Plasminogen activator inhibitor-1 synthesis in Hep G2 cells is further stimulated by TGF-β (123), by EGF (124), and by phorbol esters. Treatment of HTC rat hepatoma cells with 8-bromo-cAMP results in a strong decrease of PAI-1 synthesis (125). Plasminogen activator inhibitor-1 gene expression in HT-1080 cells is stimulated by TNF-α (126), TGF-β (127), dexamethasone (33), and phorbol esters (128).

# PLASMINOGEN ACTIVATOR INHIBITOR-2

## SOURCES AND CHARACTERIZATION OF THE PROTEIN

Plasminogen activator inhibitor-2 (PAI-2) or placental-type PAI was first demonstrated in extracts of human placenta (129–133) and is localized in the trophoblastic epithelium (134). Very high PAI-2 frequently can be identified in plasma during pregnancy (135, 136), but can also be identified in men and nonpregnant women (137). Plasminogen activator inhibitor-2 has been identified in human leukocytes (138), and is also secreted by monocytes, macrophages, and fibrosarcoma cells (139–142).

Plasminogen activator inhibitor-2 was purified to homogeneity from placenta (134, 143), from leukocytes (138), and from the conditioned medium of phorbol ester-stimulated U-937 cells (139). It can occur in two different forms: an intracellular nonglycosylated form with $M_r$ 47,000 and pI 5.0 and a secreted glycosylated form with $M_r$ 60,000 and pI 4.4 (144). Plasminogen activator inhibitor-2 also belongs to the serpin superfamily and contains 393 amino acids, with the reactive site constituted by the peptide bond $Arg^{358}$-$Thr^{359}$. In contrast to PAI-1, no latent form of PAI-2 has been identified (144).

## STRUCTURE OF THE GENE; REGULATION OF SYNTHESIS

The cDNA encoding PAI-2 has been isolated and sequenced (145–147). The gene for PAI-2 has been localized on chromosome 18 q21-23 (146). The PAI-2 gene spans 16.5 kb and contains 8 exons. A consensus sequence TATAAAA is found 22 bp 5′ (upstream) of the proposed transcription initiation site. The structure of the gene is quite different from that of the PAI-1 gene, but is similar to that of the chicken ovalbumin gene (148, 149). No shared regulatory sequences are evident between PAI-1

and PAI-2 and, although both are induced transcriptionally by TNF in HT-1080 cells (33), they do not appear to be coordinately expressed. Downstream from the 3′-end, a poly(A) addition signal AATAAA is found and a 14 A residue stretch was observed 16 bp further downstream (147). The 3′-untranslated region also contains the TTATTTAT motif, which has been identified in the cDNAs of inflammatory mediators (147, 150).

Secretion of PAI-2 can be increased in macrophages by endotoxin (140) and in lymphoid cells by phorbol esters (139, 151), which was demonstrated to stimulate the gene transcription of PAI-2 more than 50-fold (147). A 60-fold increase in PAI-2 mRNA was observed in U-937 cells treated with PMA and was shown to be mainly transcriptionally mediated (147). Dexamethasone induces a moderate decrease of PAI-2 gene expression by HT-1080 cells (33). Angiotensin II induces endothelial expression of PAI-1 and PAI-2 (152).

# FUNCTIONAL REGULATION OF PHYSIOLOGICAL FIBRINOLYSIS

## INTRODUCTION

Fibrinolysis depends on the conversion of the inactive proenzyme, plasminogen, into the active serine protease, plasmin, via the hydrolysis of a single arginyl-valyl-peptide bond ($Arg^{560}$-$Val^{561}$). This activation can be induced by PAs, which have a high specificity toward their natural substrate, plasminogen. Plasminogen, which is the central component responsible for the degradation of fibrin, has limited substrate specificity and may also degrade several other plasma proteins, including fibrinogen, factor V, and factor VIII. Extensive activation of the fibrinolytic system, such as during infusion of non–fibrin-specific thrombolytic agents (such as streptokinase and urokinase), is, therefore, usually associated with a "systemic fibrinolytic state," characterized by plasminogen activation, depletion of $α_2$-AP, and fibrinogen breakdown. Physiologic fibrinolysis, which is responsible for the removal of excess fibrin from the vascular bed, is, however, highly fibrin specific and not associated with a systemic fibrinolytic state. This fibrin-specificity results from specific molecular interactions between the reactants: PA, plasminogen, fibrin, $α_2$-AP, and PAIs.

Because of its central role in the regulation of fibrinolytic activity, fibrin deserves particular attention for its contribution to the mechanism of fibrin-specific plasminogen activation by t-PA and scu-PA. Other proteins localize and catalyze PAs, including specific cell surface receptors. The role of physiologic serine protease inhibitors will be discussed in terms of their contribution to the regulation of fibrinolysis.

# CATALYTIC PROTEINS

## FIBRIN

Plasminogen has specific affinity for fibrin, a property that is derived from "lysine-binding" sites localized to kringles 1 and 4 of the plasminogen molecule (153). The presence of t-PA increases the binding of plasminogen to a fibrin clot (154). Tissue-plasminogen activator has a specific affinity for fibrin, with a dissociation constant of the t-PA fibrin complex of 0.14 µM. Urokinase-plasminogen activator, single-chain, as well as two-chain, does not bind specifically to fibrin (155).

Plasminogen activation by t-PA occurs at a slow rate in the absence of fibrin, whereas addition of fibrin strikingly enhances the rate of plasminogen activation (154, 156, 157). The kinetic data support a mechanism in which fibrin provides a surface to which t-PA and plasminogen adsorb in a sequential and ordered way, yielding a cyclic ternary complex. Fibrin essentially increases the local plasminogen concentration by creating an additional interaction between t-PA and its substrate. The high affinity of t-PA for plasminogen (low $K_m$) in the presence of fibrin thus allows efficient activation on the fibrin clot, whereas plasminogen activation by t-PA in plasma is a comparatively inefficient process. However, other evidence has been presented that fibrin influences both the $K_m$ and $k_{cat}$ of the activation of plasminogen by t-PA (158).

Both the finger domain and kringle 2 mediate binding of t-PA to fibrin (156, 159). Initial binding of t-PA to fibrin is governed by the finger domain and, after partial degradation of fibrin, newly exposed carboxylterminal lysine residues result in enhanced binding of t-PA via kringle 2 (160). Indeed, during plasmin degradation of fibrin (157), new t-PA binding sites with much lower (2 to 4 orders of magnitude) dissociation constants are formed. Thus, early fibrin digestion by plasmin may accelerate fibrinolysis by increasing the binding of both t-PA (159) and plasminogen (158). Conversely, the removal of these carboxyterminal lysines in fibrin by the action of plasma carboxypeptidases (161) may impair the efficiency of fibrinolysis (162, 163).

The interaction between fibrin and the finger domain of t-PA probably plays only a minor role in the observed stimulation of PA activity of t-PA in the presence of fibrin. In contrast, kringle 2 likely plays an important role in this respect (164). In addition, it has been reported that t-PA mutants lacking either kringle 1 or kringle 2 are indistinguishable from wild-type t-PA, and that mutants lacking both kringles are not stimulated by t-PA (164). The activity of t-PA can also be stimulated by β-amyloid (165) and by cell surface receptors that colocalize t-PA and plasminogen. Annexin II has been reported to enhance plasminogen activation and to serve as a specific binding site for t-PA in vascular endothelium (166).

Urokinase-type plasminogen activator can be obtained as single-chain (scu-PA) or as a two-chain molecule (tcu-PA). Neither form has any affinity for fibrin. Two-chain molecule u-PA activates fibrin-bound and circulating plasminogen relatively indiscriminately (167). Extensive plasminogen activation and depletion of $\alpha_2$-AP may occur after thrombolytic treatment with tcu-PA, leading to systemic fibrinogenolysis.

Single-chain form u-PA, in contrast to tcu-PA, exhibits a significant fibrin-specific activity in human plasma. Because scu-PA does not bind to fibrin, its mechanism of fibrin specificity is entirely different than that of t-PA. Several hypotheses for the mechanism of plasminogen activation and the fibrin-specificity of clot lysis with scu-PA in plasma have been proposed. One hypothesis states that scu-PA has intrinsic plasminogen activating potential that is counteracted by a competitive inhibitory mechanism in plasma, which is reversed by fibrin (155). Alternatively, it has been proposed that u-PA is inactive toward circulating plasminogen but active toward conformationally altered plasminogen bound to partially digested fibrin (168). Thirdly, scu-PA has been proposed to be a genuine proenzyme with negligible activity toward plasminogen (167), and fibrinolysis with scu-PA would thus entirely depend on generation on tcu-PA. The original hypothesis that scu-PA exerts its fibrin-specific fibrinolytic action via binding to fibrin has been abandoned.

Several methodologic difficulties have hampered the quantitative investigation of these alternative hypotheses and the interpretation of results. These include: a) variability in kinetic properties of scu-PA obtained from different sources (169, 170); b) different sensitivity to activation of alternative molecular or conformational forms of plasminogen (glu-plasminogen-like or lys-plasminogen-like); c) efficient conversion of scu-PA to tcu-PA by generated plasmin, which is associated with a marked increase in catalytic efficiency towards plasminogen (170); and d) positive feedback of partial degradation of fibrin on the activation of plasminogen (155, 171, 172). In addition, dose-response curves of clot lysis with scu-PA in a plasma milieu are strongly nonlinear (169), which invalidates linear extrapolation of potencies derived from clot lysis versus time curves (173).

In a study using a cleavage-resistant mutant, scu-PA-Glu[158], it was suggested that conversion of scu-PA to tcu-PA during clot lysis constitutes a primary feedback system (174). Binding of plasminogen to fibrin or predigestion of fibrin was found to result in relatively minor additional acceleration of fibrinolysis. Using a monoclonal antibody (MA-12E6A8)-based enzyme-linked immunosorbent assay (ELISA) reacting specifically with two-chain forms of u-PA, it was demonstrated that the levels of tcu-PA generated in plasma do not contribute significantly to clot lysis with scu-PA, and that clot lysis with scu-PA does not require extensive systemic conversion of scu-PA to tcu-PA (173). In this study, it was also observed that systemic fibrinogen breakdown during thrombolysis with scu-PA occurs only as a consequence of extensive systemic conversion of scu-PA to the relatively non–fibrin-specific form, tcu-PA. Taken together, these data add evidence to the hypothesis that the mechanism of clot selectivity of scu-PA involves the conversion of tcu-PA at the fibrin surface, which in plasma may be prevented by a mechanism of competitive inhibition that is reversed by fibrin. Recently, it has also been demonstrated that circulating $\alpha_2$-AP may play an important role in the fibrin-specific activity of scu-PA by preventing the conversion of scu-PA to tcu-PA in plasma (175). It cannot be excluded, however, that other plasma components may also contribute to the fibrin-specificity of plasminogen activator in plasma.

## RECEPTORS

The presence of u-PAR, a specific cellular receptor for u-PA, was first demonstrated by Vassalli et al, who reported the specific and saturable binding of u-PA to monocytes (176). Subsequently, the presence of u-PA receptors has been identified on a variety of cell types, including endothelial cells (177, 178).

The purified human receptor for u-PA is a single-chain, heavily glycosylated protein with an apparent molecular weight of approximately 55 Kd (179). The cDNA-derived amino acid sequence corresponds with a polypeptide consisting of 313 residues (180). The u-PAR is inserted into the cell membrane through a glycosylphosphatidylinositol (GP I) anchor and lacks a cytoplasmic domain (181). The u-PAR is composed of three repeating sequences comprising approximately 90 amino acids each, which constitute the entire molecule (182). It has been suggested that each of these three units constitutes autonomous structural entities. The amino-terminal unit (amino acids 1–87) can be released by limited proteolytic cleavage and retains full u-PA binding capacity (182, 183).

The u-PAR plays an important role in localizing u-PA-catalyzed plasminogen activation by confining u-PA activity to the cell surface (184, 185). The u-PAR also enhances the catalytic efficiency of u-PA by up to twentyfold compared with u-PA in solution (186). The biological significance of the u-PAR in terms of intravascular fibrinolysis is debatable (187), whereas u-PA-catalyzed plasminogen activation does appear to play a crucial role in the degradation of extracellular matrix during cell migration and invasion (184, 188).

Recent studies have identified additional functional roles for the u-PAR in clearing u-PA/PAI complexes (10, 189, 190), in intracellular signaling (191), which may occur via an interaction with integrin receptors on the cell surface (192, 193), and in gene expression (191, 194). In some systems, there is evidence that u-PAR occupancy promotes cellular differentiation and proliferation (195). The u-PAR also appears to function as a receptor for vitronectin (196–198). Dewerchin et al have recently shown that u-PAR-deficient mice display normal lysis of a murine plasma clot injected via the jugular vein with reduced rates of u-PA-mediated plasminogen activation *in vitro* (199). In addition, macrophage function is apparently preserved in u-PAR deficient mice.

There is evidence of specific binding sites for plasminogen and t-PA on cell surfaces. These binding sites catalyze plasminogen activation and are clearly distinct from the u-PAR. Hajjar et al have defined a role for annexin II as a receptor for t-PA and plasminogen on the surface of endothelial cells (166). Cell-surface proteins with carboxyterminal lysyl residues also appear to function as plasminogen binding sites, and $\alpha$-enolase has been identified as a prominent representative of this class of receptors (200). Conversely, plasma carboxypeptidase B can reduce the binding of plasminogen to cell surfaces, thereby reducing fibrinolytic activity (162, 201).

## PHYSIOLOGIC INHIBITORS

Inhibition of the fibrinolytic system may occur at the level of plasmin or at the level of PAs. More than a decade ago, $\alpha_2$-AP was identified as the main plasmin inhibitor in human plasma. $\alpha_2$-Macroglobulin acts as a slower reacting inhibitor of plasmin than $\alpha_2$-AP. Because it acts as a second line inhibitor and is only of limited importance in the regulation of fibrinolysis, $\alpha_2$-macroglobulin will not be discussed. Inhibition of the physiologic plasminogen activators t-PA and u-PA in human plasma occurs primarily by PAI-1 and PAI-2.

### $\alpha_2$-ANTIPLASMIN

### Physiochemical Properties

$\alpha_2$-Antiplasmin belongs to the serine protease inhibitor family (44, 46), and forms a 1:1 stoichiometric complex with plasmin that is devoid of protease or esterase activity (47, 48, 51, 202). $\alpha_2$-Antiplasmin, like many other plasma protease inhibitors, has a broad *in vitro* inhibitory spectrum, but its physiologic role as an inhibitor of proteinases other than plasmin seems negligible. $\alpha_2$-Antiplasmin reacts very rapidly with plasmin in solution, with a second-order rate constant of $2–4 \times 10^7$ $M^{-1}s^{-1}$. The presence of free lysine binding sites and a free active center in the plasmin molecule are prerequisites for this rapid inhibition to occur (203). Crosslinking of $\alpha_2$-AP to fibrin, when blood is clotted in the presence of $Ca^{2+}$-ions and activated factor XIII, contributes to inhibition of endogenous fibrinolysis (204, 205).

## Kinetics of the Reaction

The kinetics of the inhibition of human plasmin by $\alpha_2$-AP have been studied in detail (54, 203). This model can be presented by:

$$P + A \underset{k_{-1}}{\overset{k_1}{\rightleftharpoons}} PA \overset{k_2}{\rightarrow} PA'$$

in which P is plasmin, A is $\alpha_2$-AP, PA is reversible inactive complex, and PA' is irreversible, inactive complex. The second order rate constant $(K_1) \approx 3 \times 10^7\,M^{-1}s^{-1}$ (203).

The inhibition rate relies strongly on the availability of both free lysine binding site(s) and the free active site of plasmin (54, 203, 206). Competition for the lysine-binding sites also explains why the reaction rate between plasmin and $\alpha_2$-AP in plasma may be reduced by the presence of plasmin proteins, such as histidine-rich glycoprotein (207) or fibrinogen (208). Owing to interferences with the lysine-binding site and the active site, the half-life of plasmin molecules on the fibrin surface is estimated to be two to three orders of magnitude longer than that of free plasmin (203). Therefore, the preferential inhibition of plasmin in the circulation, in contrast to the plasmin at the fibrin surface, constitutes the contribution of $\alpha_2$-AP to the fibrin specificity. Although circulating $\alpha_2$-AP makes an important contribution to the fibrin specificity of clot lysis by preferentially neutralizing plasmin activity in the circulation, its presence at the fibrin surface probably has but a limited effect on the initial phase of the lysis.

## PLASMINOGEN ACTIVATOR INHIBITOR-1

Plasminogen activator inhibitor-1 is the primary inhibitor of t-PA and u-PA in human plasma (61). It reacts with single-chain and two-chain t-PA and with tcu-PA, but not with scu-PA or streptokinase (61, 63, 209). The second order rate constant for the inhibition of single-chain t-PA by PAI-1 is on the order of $10^7\,M^{-1}s^{-1}$ (60, 67, 210), whereas inhibition of two-chain t-PA and tcu-PA is even more rapid. Platelets contain a significant amount of PAI-1 (64, 211, 212), which is released during platelet aggregation, resulting in a twofold to fivefold increased PAI-1 activity level and a sixfold to tenfold increase in PAI-1 antigen levels (48, 213–215). These high local concentrations may thus contribute to the resistance of a platelet-rich clot to lysis.

Plasminogen activator inhibitor-1 influences fibrinolysis via a direct interaction with PAs. The result is a net decrease of the fibrinolytic activity. Plasminogen activator inhibitor-1 or PAI-2 most likely does not influence the fibrin-specificity of fibrinolysis. In plasma, PAI-1 circulates in excess over t-PA, thereby severely limiting fibrinolytic activity in the circulation. Plasminogen activator inhibitor-1 also has the ability to bind to and inhibit fibrin-bound t-PA (216) and receptor-bound urokinase (217). Some evidence also exists that receptor-bound t-PA may be protected from inactivation by PAI-1 (218).

The formation of a covalent complex between t-PA and PAI-1 involves an interaction between the active site of t-PA and the "bait" residues ($Arg^{346}$-$Met^{347}$) of PAI-1. These two proteins interact via a noncovalent, electrostatic interaction, in which positively charged residues located in a surface loop near the active site of t-PA (residues 296-302) interact with negatively charged residues (350-355) near the reactive center of PAI-1 (219, 220). The importance of this "second-site" interaction has been demonstrated by the design and expression of site-specific mutants of t-PA with negatively charged residues in this loop, yielding mutant molecules with significant resistance to inactivation by PAI-1 (219, 221).

Although PAI-1 is a relatively specific inhibitor of PAs, it has recently been shown that binding to vitronectin endows PAI-1 with thrombin-inhibitory properties (82). This observation has additional significance when one considers that the PAI-1-vitronectin complex may be the physiologically relevant form of PAI-1 (222), because active PAI-1 binds to, and is stabilized by, this interaction in plasma and in the subendothelial matrix.

Recent evidence suggests that the interaction between PAI-1 and vitronectin may have other consequences on cell function. Stefansson et al reported that vitronectin enhances the migration of smooth muscle cells (SMCs), and that the specific integrin receptor for vitronectin ($\alpha_v\beta_3$) is required for cell motility (223). They also reported that the integrin attachment site on vitronectin overlaps with the binding site for PAI-1, and that the active conformation of PAI-1 blocks SMC migration. This effect requires high affinity binding to vitronectin and does not depend on the ability of PAI-1 to inhibit PAs. Thus, it appears that PAI-1 can reduce cellular migration by inhibiting plasmin generation and matrix degradation and by blocking the interaction between vitronectin and the integrin receptor $\alpha_v\beta_3$ (223).

## PLASMINOGEN ACTIVATOR INHIBITOR-2

Plasminogen activator inhibitor-2 inhibits tcu-PA with a second-order rate constant $(k_1) \approx 9 \times 10^5\,M^{-1}s^{-1}$ (139), which is about tenfold slower than PAI-1. Plasminogen activator inhibitor-2 also efficiently inhibits two-chain t-PA ($k_1 = 2 \times 10^5 \, M^{-1}s^{-1}$), less efficiently single-chain t-PA ($k_1 = 9 \times 10^3 \, M^{-1}s^{-1}$), and it does not inhibit scu-PA (139). Plasminogen activator inhibitor-2 does not occur in a latent form (70). Although PAI-2 in plasma occurs most frequently in association with pregnancy, it has occasionally been identified in men and nonpregnant women (135). Given its comparatively slow rate of interaction with t-PA, it is unlikely that PAI-2 plays a major role in the regulation of vascular fibrinolysis. Its major function is likely to be related to the maintenance of hemostasis during pregnancy and delivery.

# PHYSIOLOGIC REGULATION OF VASCULAR FIBRINOLYTIC BALANCE

During the past several years, there has been a growing appreciation for the role the PA system plays in fibrinolysis and in extracellular proteolysis. Plasmin generation is important in cell migration, angiogenesis (188), tissue remodeling (including wound healing), and other processes (224, 225). Thus, although very little plasminogen activation occurs in plasma in the absence of fibrin, it appears that plasmin generation in tissues occurs in a variety of physiologic processes.

Under normal circumstances, there is an abundance of plasminogen present in blood that is potentially available for activation. Plasminogen deficiency is associated with some increased risk of clotting (226–229). Mice that have been genetically engineered to lack plasminogen develop spontaneous fibrin deposits and a markedly reduced capacity for wound healing (230). Plasminogen-deficient mice survive embryonic development but develop spontaneous fibrin deposition due to impaired thrombolysis and suffer retarded growth and reduced fertility and survival. The Plg-/- phenotype is quite similar to that of the combined t-PA-/-:u-PA-/- phenotype described by Carmeliet et al (231).

Relative excess of PA is rare in humans under normal circumstances, except in the setting of acute administration of thrombolytic agents. Several individuals have been described with hereditary deficiencies of PAI-1. This disorder is typically manifested by posttraumatic or postsurgical bleeding (232–236).

The most common acquired abnormality of fibrinolysis is an excess of PAI-1. Increased plasma PAI-1 levels have been associated with venous thromboembolic disease and recurrent myocardial infarction (237–239). Several groups have recently demonstrated that PAI-1 is increased in the vicinity of atherosclerotic lesions (240–242). This may retard the local generation of plasmin that is needed for normal tissue and vascular

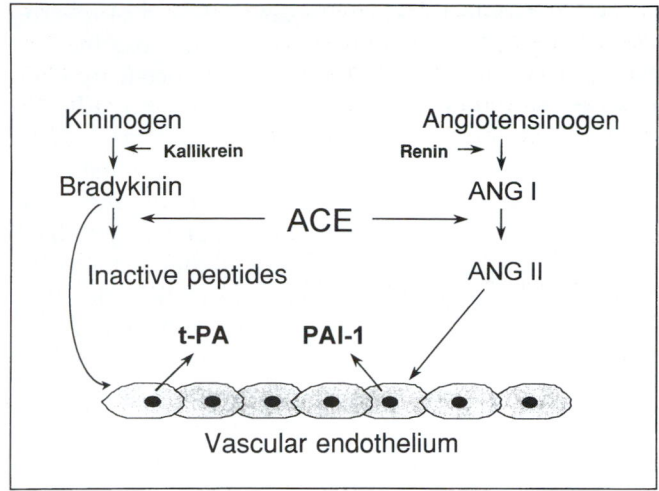

**FIGURE 7.8.** Strategic location of ACE in regulating vascular fibrinolytic balance. ANG II, angiotensin II; PAI-1, plasminogen activator inhibitor-1; t-PA, tissue-type plasminogen activator.

"housekeeping." In recent years, angiotensin II and glucose have emerged as physiologic regulators of PAI-1 production and present a shared mechanism for development of vascular disease in common disorders such as hypertension and diabetes mellitus.

There is a compelling body of evidence that the renin-angiotensin system plays an important role in the regulation of fibrinolytic balance (115, 152, 243–247). Angiotensin-converting enzyme (ACE) is strategically positioned to regulate vascular fibrinolytic balance (Fig. 7.8) by virtue of its endothelial localization and bifunctional role in degrading bradykinin and activating angiotensin (248). Bradykinin is one of the most potent stimuli regulating the production and secretion of t-PA (249–251), whereas angiotensin appears to be an important regulator of PAI-1 production and secretion in vascular tissue (115, 245, 246). Angiotensin II has been shown to stimulate PAI-1 mRNA expression in cultured endothelial and vascular smooth muscle cells (115, 247). There is a significant correlation between plasma PAI-1 levels and plasma renin activity and aldosterone (252).

Increased PAI-1 production has also been identified in diabetes, and probably contributes to the development of vascular complications in this disorder (253–258). Two mechanisms are implicated at present. First, plasma PAI-1 levels correlate significantly with insulin levels (259, 260), and insulin directly stimulates PAI-1 expression in cultured hepatocytes (121). Second, glucose also stimulates PAI-1 expression, but in a tissue-specific manner. In contrast with insulin, glucose increases PAI-1 expression in cultured endothelial cells (261). This latter effect may be particularly important in view of increasing evidence that PAI-1 is overexpressed in atherosclerotic lesions (240, 242) and that PAI-1 deficiency may protect against the development of atherosclerosis (187, 262). Insulin resistance, glucose intolerance, and elevated PAI-1 levels frequently occur together in obese individuals. Recent data indicate that adipose tissue is an important source of circulating PAI-1 (263). Thus, hypertension and diabetes, two of the most common disorders leading to the development of premature cardiovascular disease in humans, can be characterized as hormonal/metabolic disturbances that lead to increased PAI-1 production. Therapeutic strategies that alter vascular fibrinolytic balance by reducing PAI-1 expression merit investigation for potential use in reducing the vascular complications of diabetes and hypertension.

# REFERENCES

1. Raum D, Marcus D, Alper CA et al. Synthesis of human plasminogen by the liver. Science 1980;208:1036–1037.
2. Wiman B. Primary structure of the B-chain of human plasmin. Eur J Biochem 1977;76:129–137.
3. Robbins KC, Summaria L, Hsieh B et al. The peptide chains of human plasmin. Mechanism of activation of human plasminogen to plasmin. J Biol Chem 1967;242:2333–2342.
4. Forsgren M, Raden B, Israelsson M et al. Molecular cloning and characterization of a full-length cDNA clone for human plasminogen. FEBS Lett 1987;213:254–260.
5. Murray JC, Buetow KH, Donovan M et al. Linkage disequilibrium of plasminogen polymorphisms and assignment of the gene to human chromosome 6q26-6q27. Am J Hum Genet 1987;40:338–350.
6. Petersen TE, Martzen MR, Ichinose A et al. Characterization of the gene for human plasminogen, a key proenzyme in the fibrinolytic system. J Biol Chem 1990;265:6104–6111.
7. McLean JW, Tomlinson JE, Kuang WJ et al. cDNA sequence of human apolipoprotein(a) is homologous to plasminogen. Nature 1987;330:132–137.
8. Tomlinson JE, McLean JW, Lawn RM. Rhesus monkey apolipoprotein(a). Sequence, evolution, and sites of synthesis. J Biol Chem 1989;264:5957–5965.
9. Narita M, Bu G, Herz J et al. Two receptor systems are involved in the plasma clearance of tissue-type plasminogen activator (t-PA) *in vivo*. J Clin Invest 1995;96:1164–1168.
10. Andreasen PA, Sottrup-Jensen L, Kjoller L et al. Receptor-mediated endocytosis of plasminogen activators and activator/inhibitor complexes [Review]. FEBS Lett 1994;338:239–245.
11. Pohl G, Kallstrom M, Bergsdorf N et al. Tissue plasminogen activator: Peptide analyses confirm an indirectly derived amino acid sequence, identify the active site serine residue, establish glycosylation sites, and localize variant differences. Biochemistry 1984;23:3701–3707.
12. Pennica D, Holmes WE, Kohr WJ et al. Cloning and expression of human tissue-type plasminogen activator cDNA in *E coli*. Nature 1983;301:214–221.
13. Davie EW, Ichinose A, Leytus SP. Structural features of the proteins participating in blood coagulation and fibrinolysis. Cold Spring Harb Symp Quant Biol 1986;51:509–514.
14. Edlund T, Ny T, Ranby M et al. Isolation of cDNA sequences coding for apart of human tissue plasminogen activator. Proc Natl Acad Sci U S A 1983;80:349–352.
15. Fisher R, Waller EK, Grossi G et al. Isolation and characterization of the human tissue-type plasminogen activator structural gene including its 5′ flanking region. J Biol Chem 1985;260:11223–11230.
16. Verheijen JH, Visse R, Wijnen JT et al. Assignment of the human tissue-type plasminogen activator gene (PLAT) to chromosome 8. Hum Genet 1986;72:153–156.
17. Rajput B, Degen SF, Reich E et al. Chromosomal locations of human tissue plasminogen activator and urokinase genes. Science 1985;230:672–674.
18. Browne MJ, Tyrrell AW, Chapman CG et al. Isolation of a human tissue-type plasminogen-activator genomic DNA clone and its expression in mouse L cells. Gene 1985;33:279–284.
19. Degen SJ, Rajput B, Reich E. The human tissue plasminogen activator gene. J Biol Chem 1986;261:6972–6985.
20. Feng P, Ohlsson M, Ny T. The structure of the TATA-less rat tissue-type plasminogen activator gene. Species-specific sequence divergences in the promoter predict differences in regulation of gene expression. J Biol Chem1990;265:2022–2027.
21. Patthy L. Evolution of the proteases of blood coagulation and fibrinolysis by assembly from modules. Cell 1985;41:657–663.
22. Medcalf RL, Ruegg M, Schleuning WD. A DNA motif related to the cAMP-responsive element and an exon-located activator protein-2 binding site in the human tissue-type plasminogen activator gene promoter cooperate in basal expression and convey activation by phorbol ester and cAMP. J Biol Chem 1990;265:14618–14626.
23. Bulens F, Ibanez-Tallon I, Van Acker P et al. Retinoic acid inductionof human tissue-type plasminogen activator gene expression via a directrepeat element (DR5) located at −7 kilobases. J Biol Chem 1995;270:7167–7175.
24. Francis RB Jr, Neely S. Inhibition of endothelial secretion oftissue-type plasminogen activator and its rapid inhibitor by agents which increase intracellular cyclic AMP. Biochim Biophys Acta 1989;1012:207–213.
25. Kooistra T, van den Berg J, Tons A et al. Butyrate stimulates tissue-type plasminogen-activator synthesis in cultured human endothelial cells. Biochem J 1987;247:605–612.
26. Waller EK, Schleuning WD. Induction of fibrinolytic activity in HeLa cells by phorbol myristate acetate. Tissue-type plasminogen activator antigen and mRNA augmentation require intermediate protein biosynthesis. J Biol Chem 1985;260:6354–6360.
27. Santell L, Levin EG. Cyclic AMP potentiates phorbol ester stimulation of tissue plasminogen activator release and inhibits secretion of plasminogen activator inhibitor-1 from human endothelial cells. J Biol Chem 1988;263:16802–16808.
28. Levin EG, Marotti KR, Santell L. Protein kinase C and the stimulation of tissue plasminogen activator release from human endothelial cells. Dependence on the elevation of messenger RNA. J Biol Chem 1989;264:16030–16036.
29. Hanss M, Collen D. Secretion of tissue-type plasminogen activator and plasminogen activator inhibitor by cultured human endothelial cells: Modulation by thrombin, endotoxin, and histamine. J Lab Clin Med 1987;109:97–104.
30. Thompson EA, Nelles L, Collen D. Effect of retinoic acid on the synthesis of tissue-type plasminogen activator and plasminogen activator inhibitor-1 in human endothelial cells. Eur J Biochem 1991;201:627–632.
31. Kooistra T, Bosma PJ, Toet K et al. Role of protein kinase C and cyclicadenosine monophosphate in the regulation of tissue-type plasminogen activator, plasminogen activator inhibitor-1, and platelet-derived growth factor mRNA levels in human endothelial cells. Possible involvement of protooncogenes *c-jun* and *c-fos*. Arterioscler Thromb 1991;11:1042–1052.
32. Diamond SL, Eskin SG, McIntire LV. Fluid flow stimulates tissue plasminogen activator secretion by cultured human endothelial cells. Science 1989;243:1483–1485.
33. Medcalf RL, Van den Berg E, Schleuning WD. Glucocorticoid-modulated gene expression of tissue- and urinary-type plasminogen activator and plasminogen activator inhibitor 1 and 2. J Cell Biol 1988;106:971–978.
34. Wun TC, Schleuning WD, Reich E. Isolation and characterization of urokinase from human plasma. J Biol Chem 1982;257:3276–3283.
35. Kasai S, Arimura H, Nishida M et al. Proteolytic cleavage of single-chain pro-urokinase induces conformational change which follows activation of the zymogen and reduction of its high affinity for fibrin. J Biol Chem 1985;260:12377–12381.
36. Ichinose A, Fujikawa K, Suyama T. The activation of pro-urokinase by plasma kallikrein and its inactivation by thrombin. J Biol Chem 1986;261:3486–3489.
37. Steffens GJ, Gunzler WA, Otting F et al. The complete amino acid sequence of low molecular mass urokinase from human urine. Hoppe Seylers Z Physiol Chem 1982;363:1043–1058.
38. Stump DC, Thienpont M, Collen D. Urokinase-related proteins in human urine. Isolation and characterization of single-chain urokinase (pro-urokinase) and urokinase-inhibitor complex. J Biol Chem 1986;261:1267–1273.
39. Riccio A, Grimaldi G, Verde P et al. The human urokinase-plasminogen activator gene and its promoter. Nucleic Acids Res 1985;13:2759–2771.
40. Blasi F, Riccio A, Sebastio G. Human plasminogen activators. Genes and proteins structure [Review]. Horiz Biochem Biophys 1986;8:377–414.
41. Medina R, Socher SH, Han JH et al. Interleukin-1, endotoxin or tumor necrosis factor/cachectin enhance the level of plasminogen activator inhibitor messenger RNA in bovine aortic endothelial cells. Thromb Res 1989;54:41–52.
42. van Hinsbergh VW, van den Berg EA, Fiers W et al. Tumor necrosis factor induces the production of urokinase-type plasminogen activator by human endothelial cells. Blood 1990;75:1991–1998.
43. Gerwin BI, Keski-Oja J, Seddon M et al. TGF-beta 1 modulation of urokinase and PAI-1 expression in human bronchial epithelial cells. Am J Physiol 1990;259:L262–L269.
44. Lijnen HR, Wiman B, Collen D. Partial primary structure of human alpha 2-antiplasmin-homology with other plasma protease inhibitors. Thromb Haemost 1982;48:311–314.
45. Lijnen HR, Holmes WE, van Hoef B et al. Amino acid sequence of human alpha 2-antiplasmin. Eur J Biochem 1987;166:565–574.

46. Holmes WE, Nelles L, Lijnen HR et al. Primary structure of human alpha 2-antiplasmin, a serine protease inhibitor (serpin). J Biol Chem 1987;262: 1659–1664.

47. Collen D. Identification and some properties of a new fast-reacting plasmin inhibitor in human plasma. Eur J Biochem 1976;69:209–216.

48. Moroi M, Aoki N. Isolation and characterization of alpha2-plasmin inhibitor from human plasma. A novel proteinase inhibitor which inhibits activator-induced clot lysis. J Biol Chem 1976;251:5956–5965.

49. Wiman B. Affinity-chromatographic purification of human alpha 2-antiplasmin. Biochem J 1980;191:229–232.

50. Hogstorp H, Saldeen T. Synthesis of alpha 2-antiplasmin by rat liver cells. Thromb Res 1982;28:19–25.

51. Mullertz S, Clemmensen I. The primary inhibitor of plasmin in human plasma. Biochem J 1976;159:545–553.

52. Kluft C, Los N. Demonstration of two forms of alpha 2-antiplasmin in plasma by modified crossed immunoelectrophoresis. Thromb Res 1981; 21:65–71.

53. Sugiyama N, Sasaki T, Iwamoto M et al. Binding site of alpha 2-plasmin inhibitor to plasminogen. Biochim Biophys Acta 1988;952:1–7.

54. Christensen U, Clemmensen I. Purification and reaction mechanisms of the primary inhibitor of plasmin from human plasma. Biochem J 1978; 175:635–641.

55. Wiman B, Nilsson T, Cedergren B. Studies on a form of alpha 2-antiplasmin in plasma which does not interact with the lysine-binding sites in plasminogen. Thromb Res 1982;28:193–199.

56. Hirosawa S, Nakamura Y, Miura O et al. Organization of the human alpha 2-plasmin inhibitor gene. Proc Natl Acad Sci U S A 1988;85:6836–6840.

57. Loskutoff DJ, Edgington TS. An inhibitor of plasminogen activator in rabbit endothelial cells. J Biol Chem 1981;256:4142–4145.

58. Loskutoff DJ, van Mourik JA, Erickson LA et al. Detection of an unusually stable fibrinolytic inhibitor produced by bovine endothelial cells. Proc Natl Acad Sci U S A 1983;80:2956–2960.

59. Coleman PL, Barouski PA, Gelehrter TD. The dexamethasone-induced inhibitor of fibrinolytic activity in hepatoma cells. A cellular product which specifically inhibits plasminogen activation. J Biol Chem 1982;257: 4260–4264.

60. Kruithof EK, Tran-Thang C, Ransijn A et al. Demonstration of a fast-acting inhibitor of plasminogen activators in human plasma. Blood 1984;64: 907–913.

61. Wiman B, Chmielewska J, Ranby M. Inactivation of tissue plasminogen activator in plasma. Demonstration of a complex with a new rapid inhibitor. J Biol Chem 1984;259:3644–3647.

62. Juhan-Vague I, Moerman B, De Cock F et al. Plasma levels of a specific inhibitor of tissue-type plasminogen activator (and urokinase) in normal and pathological conditions. Thromb Res 1984;33:523–530.

63. Verheijen JH, Chang GT, Kluft C. Evidence for the occurrence of a fast-acting inhibitor for tissue-type plasminogen activator in human plasma. Thromb Haemost 1984;51:392–395.

64. Erickson LA, Ginsberg MH, Loskutoff DJ. Detection and partial characterization of an inhibitor of plasminogen activator in human platelets. J Clin Invest 1984;74:1465–1472.

65. Andreasen PA, Nielsen LS, Kristensen P et al. Plasminogen activator inhibitor from human fibrosarcoma cells binds urokinase-type plasminogen activator, but not its proenzyme. J Biol Chem 1986;261:7644–7651.

66. Sprengers ED, Princen HM, Kooistra T et al. Inhibition of plasminogen activators by conditioned medium of human hepatocytes and hepatoma cell line Hep G2. J Lab Clin Med 1985;105:751–758.

67. Coleman PL, Patel PD, Cwikel BJ et al. Characterization of the dexamethasone-induced inhibitor of plasminogen activator in HTC hepatoma cells. J Biol Chem 1986;261:4352–4357.

68. Nicoloso G, Hauert J, Kruithof EK et al. Fibrinolysis in normal subjects—Comparison between plasminogen activator inhibitor and other components of the fibrinolytic system. Thromb Haemost 1988;59:299–303.

69. Sprengers ED, Kluft C. Plasminogen activator inhibitors [Review]. Blood 1987;69:381–387.

70. Hekman CM, Loskutoff DJ. Endothelial cells produce a latent inhibitor of plasminogen activators that can be activated by denaturants. J Biol Chem 1985;260:11581–11587.

71. Vaughan DE, Declerck PJ, Reilly TM et al. Dynamic structural and functional relationships in recombinant plasminogen activator inhibitor-1(rPAI-1). Biochim Biophys Acta 1993;1202:221–229.

72. Lawrence DA, Olson ST, Palaniappan S et al. Engineering plasminogen activator inhibitor 1 mutants with increased functional stability. Biochemistry 1994;33:3643–3648.

73. Lawrence DA, Palaniappan S, Stefansson S et al. Characterization of the binding of different conformational forms of plasminogen activator inhibitor-1 to vitronectin. Implications for the regulation of pericellular proteolysis. J Biol Chem 1997;272:7676–7680.

74. Aertgeerts K, De Rantner CJ, Booth NA et al. Rational design of complex formation between plasminogen activator inhibitor-1 and target proteinases. J Struct Biol 1997;118:236–242.

75. Mottonen J, Strand A, Symersky J et al. Structural basis of latency in plasminogen activator inhibitor-1. Nature 1992;355:270–273.

76. Declerck PJ, De Mol M, Vaughan DE et al. Identification of a conformationally distinct form of plasminogen activator inhibitor-1, acting as a noninhibitory substrate for tissue-type plasminogen activator. J Biol Chem 1992; 267:11693–11696.

77. Aertgeerts K, De Bondt HL, De Ranter C et al. Crystallization and x-ray diffraction data of the cleaved form of plasminogen activator inhibitor-1. Proteins 1995;23:118–121.

78. Goldsmith EJ, Mottonen J. Serpins: The uncut version [Review]. Structure 1994;2:241–244.

79. Declerck PJ, De Mol M, Alessi MC et al. Purification and characterization of a plasminogen activator inhibitor 1 binding protein from human plasma. Identification as a multimeric form of S protein (vitronectin). J Biol Chem 1988;263:15454–15461.

80. Wiman B, Almquist A, Sigurdardottir O et al. Plasminogen activator inhibitor 1 (PAI) is bound to vitronectin in plasma. FEBS Lett 1988;242:125–128.

81. Mimuro J, Loskutoff DJ. Purification of a protein from bovine plasma that binds to type 1 plasminogen activator inhibitor and prevents its interaction with extracellular matrix. Evidence that the protein is vitronectin. J Biol Chem 1989;264:936–939.

82. Ehrlich HJ, Gebbink RK, Keijer J et al. Alteration of serpin specificity by a protein cofactor. Vitronectin endows plasminogen activator inhibitor 1 with thrombin inhibitory properties. J Biol Chem 1990;265:13029–13035.

83. Hekman CM, Loskutoff DJ. Fibrinolytic pathways and the endothelium [Review]. Semin Thromb Hemost 1987;13:514–527.

84. Lambers JW, Cammenga M, Konig BW et al. Activation of human endothelial cell-type plasminogen activator inhibitor (PAI-1) by negatively charged phospholipids. J Biol Chem 1987;262:17492–17496.

85. Vaughan DE, Declerck PJ, Van Houtte E et al. Studies of recombinant plasminogen activator inhibitor-1 in rabbits. Pharmacokinetics and evidence for reactivation of latent plasminogen activator inhibitor-1 in vivo. Circ Res 1990;67:1281–1286.

86. Ny T, Sawdey M, Lawrence D et al. Cloning and sequence of a cDNA coding for the human beta-migrating endothelial cell-type plasminogen activator inhibitor. Proc Natl Acad Sci U S A 1986;83:6776–6780.

87. Ginsburg D, Zeheb R, Yang AY et al. cDNA cloning of human plasminogen activator-inhibitor from endothelial cells. J Clin Invest 1986;78:1673–1680.

88. Pannekoek H, Veerman H, Lambers H et al. Endothelial plasminogen activator inhibitor (PAI): A new member of the Serpin gene family. EMBO J 1986;5:2539–2544.

89. Loskutoff DJ, Linders M, Keijer J et al. Structure of the human plasminogen activator inhibitor 1 gene: Nonrandom distribution of introns. Biochemistry 1987;26:3763–3768.

90. Strandberg L, Lawrence D, Ny T. The organization of the human-plasminogen-activator-inhibitor-1 gene. Implications on the evolution of the serine-protease inhibitor family. Eur J Biochem 1988;176:609–616.

91. Bruzdzinski CJ, Riordan-Johnson M, Nordby EC et al. Isolation and characterization of the rat plasminogen activator inhibitor-1 gene. J Biol Chem 1990;265:2078–2085.

92. Klinger KW, Winqvist R, Riccio A et al. Plasminogen activator inhibitor type 1 gene is located at region q21.3-q22 of chromosome 7 and genetically linked with cystic fibrosis. Proc Natl Acad Sci U S A 1987;84:8548–8552.

93. Craik CS, Rutter WJ, Fletterick R. Splice junctions: Association with variation in protein structure. Science 1983;220:1125–1129.

94. Bruzdzinski CJ, Johnson MR, Goble CA et al. Mechanism of glucocorticoid induction of the rat plasminogen activator inhibitor-1 gene in HTC rat hepatoma cells: Identification of cis-acting regulatory elements. Mol Endocrinol 1993;7:1169–1177.

95. Bosma PJ, van den Berg EA, Kooistra T et al. Human plasminogen activator-1 gene. Promoter and structural gene nucleotide sequences. J Biol Chem 1988;263:9129–9141.

96. van Zonneveld AJ, Curriden SA, Loskutoff DJ. Type 1 plasminogen activator inhibitor gene: Functional analysis and glucocorticoid regulation of its promoter. Proc Natl Acad Sci U S A 1988;85:5525–5529.

97. Keeton MR, Curriden SA, van Zonneveld AJ et al. Identification of regulatory sequences in the type 1 plasminogen activator inhibitor gene responsive to transforming growth factor beta. J Biol Chem 1991;266:23048–23052.

98. Westerhausen DR Jr, Hopkins WE, Billadello JJ. Multiple transforming growth factor-beta-inducible elements regulate expression of the plasminogen activator inhibitor type-1 gene in Hep G2 cells. J Biol Chem 1991; 266:1092–1100.

99. Prendergast GC, Diamond LE, Dahl D et al. The c-myc-regulated gene mrl encodes plasminogen activator inhibitor 1. Mol Cell Biol 1990;10: 1265–1269.

100. Dawson SJ, Wiman B, Hamsten A et al. The two allele sequences of a common polymorphism in the promoter of the plasminogen activator inhibitor-1 (PAI-1) gene respond differently to interleukin-1 in HepG2 cells. J Biol Chem 1993;268:10739–10745.

101. Eriksson P, Kallin B, van 't Hooft FM et al. Allele-specific increase in basal transcription of the plasminogen-activator-inhibitor 1 gene is associated with myocardial infarction. Proc Natl Acad Sci U S A 1995;92:1851–1855.

102. van den Berg EA, Sprengers ED, Jaye M et al. Regulation of plasminogen activator inhibitor-1 mRNA in human endothelial cells. Thromb Haemost 1988;60:63–67.

103. Zeheb R, Gelehrter TD. Cloning and sequencing of cDNA for the rat plasminogen activator inhibitor-1. Gene 1988;73:459–468.

104. Mimuro J, Sawdey M, Hattori M et al. cDna for bovine type 1 plasminogen activator inhibitor (Pai-1). Nucleic Acid Res 1989;17:8872.

105. Colucci M, Paramo JA, Collen D. Generation in plasma of a fast-acting inhibitor of plasminogen activator in response to endotoxin stimulation. J Clin Invest 1985;75:818–824.

106. Crutchley DJ, Conanan LB. Endotoxin induction of an inhibitor of plasminogen activator in bovine pulmonary artery endothelial cells. J Biol Chem 1986;261:154–159.

107. Sawdey M, Podor TJ, Loskutoff DJ. Regulation of type 1 plasminogen activator inhibitor gene expression in cultured bovine aortic endothelial cells. Induction by transforming growth factor-beta, lipopolysaccharide, and tumor necrosis factor-alpha. J Biol Chem 1989;264:10396–10401.

108. Schleef RR, Bevilacqua MP, Sawdey M et al. Cytokine activation of vascular endothelium. Effects on tissue-type plasminogen activator and type 1 plasminogen activator inhibitor. J Biol Chem 1988;263:5797–5803.

109. Saksela O, Moscatelli D, Rifkin DB. The opposing effects of basic fibroblast growth factor and transforming growth factor beta on the regulation of plasminogen activator activity in capillary endothelial cells. J Cell Biol 1987;105:957–963.

110. Scarpati EM, Sadler JE. Regulation of endothelial cell coagulant properties. Modulation of tissue factor, plasminogen activator inhibitors, and thrombomodulin by phorbol 12-myristate 13-acetate and tumor necrosis factor. J Biol Chem 1989;264:20705–20713.

111. Gelehrter TD, Sznycer-Laszuk R. Thrombin induction of plasminogen activator-inhibitor in cultured human endothelial cells. J Clin Invest 1986;77:165–169.

112. Dichek D, Quertermous T. Thrombin regulation of mRNA levels of tissue plasminogen activator and plasminogen activator inhibitor-1 in cultured human umbilical vein endothelial cells. Blood 1989;74:222–228.

113. Stiko-Rahm A, Wiman B, Hamsten A et al. Secretion of plasminogen activator inhibitor-1 from cultured human umbilical vein endothelial cells is induced by very low density lipoprotein. Arteriosclerosis 1990;10:1067–1073.

114. Etingin OR, Hajjar DP, Hajjar KA et al. Lipoprotein (a) regulates plasminogen activator inhibitor-1 expression in endothelial cells. A potential mechanism in thrombogenesis. J Biol Chem 1991;266:2459–2465.

115. Vaughan DE, Lazos SA, Tong K. Angiotensin II regulates the expression of plasminogen activator inhibitor-1 in cultured endothelial cells. A potential link between the renin-angiotensin system and thrombosis. J Clin Invest 1995;95:995–1001.

116. Fujii S, Hopkins WE, Sobel BE. Mechanisms contributing to increased synthesis of plasminogen activator inhibitor type 1 in endothelial cells by constituents of platelets and their implications for thrombolysis. Circulation 1991;83:645–651.

117. Georg B, Riccio A, Andreasen P. Forskolin down-regulates type-1 plasminogen activator inhibitor and tissue-type plasminogen activator and their mRNAs in human fibrosarcoma cells. Mol Cell Endocrinol 1990;72:103–110.

118. Konkle BA, Ginsburg D. The addition of endothelial cell growth factor and heparin to human umbilical vein endothelial cell cultures decreases plasminogen activator inhibitor-1 expression. J Clin Invest 1988;82:579–585.

119. Venkov CD, Su M, Shyr Y et al. Ethanol-induced alterations in the expression of endothelial-derived fibrinolytic components. Fibrinolysis Proteolysis 1997;11:115–118.

120. van Hinsbergh VW, Kooistra T, van den Berg EA et al. Tumor necrosis factor increases the production of plasminogen activator inhibitor in human endothelial cells *in vitro* and in rats *in vivo*. Blood 1988;72:1467–1473.

121. Alessi MC, Juhan-Vague I, Kooistra T et al. Insulin stimulates the synthesis of plasminogen activator inhibitor 1 by the human hepatocellular cell line Hep G2. Thromb Haemost 1988;60:491–494.

122. Kooistra T, Bosma PJ, Tons HA et al. Plasminogen activator inhibitor 1: Biosynthesis and mRNA level are increased by insulin in cultured human hepatocytes. Thromb Haemost 1989;62:723–728.

123. Fujii S, Lucore CL, Hopkins WE et al. Potential attenuation of fibrinolysis by growth factors released from platelets and their pharmacologic implications. Am J Cardiol 1989;63:1505–1511.

124. Hopkins WE, Westerhausen DR Jr, Sobel BE et al. Transcriptional regulation of plasminogen activator inhibitor type-1 mRNA in Hep G2 cells by epidermal growth factor. Nucleic Acid Res 1991;19:163–168.

125. Heaton JH, Gelehrter TD. Cyclic nucleotide regulation of plasminogen activator and plasminogen activator-inhibitor messenger RNAs in rat hepatoma cells. Mol Endocrinol 1990;4:171–178.

126. Georg B, Helseth E, Lund LR et al. Tumor necrosis factor-alpha regulates mRNA for urokinase-type plasminogen activator and type-1 plasminogen activator inhibitor in human neoplastic cell lines. Mol Cell Endocrinol 1989;61:87–96.

127. Laiho M, Weis FM, Boyd FT et al. Responsiveness to transforming growth factor-beta (TGF-beta) restored by genetic complementation between cells defective in TGF-beta receptors I and II. J Biol Chem 1991;266:9108–9112.

128. Mayer M, Lund LR, Riccio A et al. Plasminogen activator inhibitor type-1 protein, mRNA and gene transcription are increased by phorbol esters in human rhabdomyosarcoma cells. J Biol Chem 1988;263:15688–15693.

129. Kawano T, Morimoto K, Uemura Y. Urokinase inhibitor in human placenta. Nature 1968;217:253–254.

130. Kawano T, Morimoto K, Uemura Y. Partial purification and properties of urokinase inhibitor from human placenta. J Biochem 1970;67:333–342.

131. Kawano T, Uemura Y. Inhibition of tissue activator by urokinase inhibitor. Thromb Diath Haemorrh 1971;25:129–133.

132. Astedt B, Lecander I, Brodin T et al. Purification of a specific placental plasminogen activator inhibitor by monoclonal antibody and its complex formation with plasminogen activator. Thromb Haemost 1985;53:122–125.

133. Holmberg L, Lecander I, Persson B et al. An inhibitor from placenta specifically binds urokinase and inhibits plasminogen activator released from ovarian carcinoma in tissue culture. Biochim Biophys Acta 1978;544:128–137.

134. Astedt B, Hagerstrand I, Lecander I. Cellular localisation in placenta of placental type plasminogen activator inhibitor. Thromb Haemost 1986;56:63–65.

135. Lecander I, Astedt B. Isolation of a new specific plasminogen activator inhibitor from pregnancy plasma. Br J Haematol 1986;62:221–228.

136. Kruithof EK, Tran-Thang C, Gudinchet A et al. Fibrinolysis in pregnancy: A study of plasminogen activator inhibitors. Blood 1987;69:460–466.

137. Lecander I, Astedt B. Occurrence of a specific plasminogen activator inhibitor of placental type, PAI-2, in men and non-pregnant women. Fibrinolysis 1989;3:27–30.

138. Kopitar M, Rozman B, Babnik J et al. Human leucocyte urokinase inhibitor-purification, characterization and comparative studies against different plasminogen activators. Thromb Haemost 1985;54:750–755.

139. Kruithof EK, Vassalli JD, Schleuning WD et al. Purification and characterization of a plasminogen activator inhibitor from the histiocytic lymphoma cell line U-937. J Biol Chem 1986;261:11207–11213.

140. Chapman HA Jr, Stone OL. A fibrinolytic inhibitor of human alveolar macrophages. Induction with endotoxin. Am Rev Respir Dis 1985;132:569–575.

141. Saksela O, Hovi T, Vaheri A. Urokinase-type plasminogen activator and its inhibitor secreted by cultured human monocyte-macrophages. J Cell Physiol 1985;122:125–132.

142. Wohlwend A, Belin D, Vassalli JD. Plasminogen activator-specific inhibitors produced by human monocytes/macrophages. J Exp Med 1987;165:320–339.

143. Wun TC, Reich E. An inhibitor of plasminogen activation from human placenta. Purification and characterization. J Biol Chem 1987;262:3646–3653.

144. Kruithof EK, Baker MS, Bunn CL. Biological and clinical aspects of plasminogen activator inhibitor type 2 [Review]. Blood 1995;86:4007–4024.

145. Ye RD, Wun TC, Sadler JE. cDNA cloning and expression in *Escherichia coli* of a plasminogen activator inhibitor from human placenta. J Biol Chem 1987;262:3718–3725.

146. Webb AC, Collins KL, Snyder SE et al. Human monocyte Arg-Serpin cDNA. Sequence, chromosomal assignment, and homology to plasminogen activator-inhibitor. J Exp Med 1987;166:77–94.

147. Schleuning WD, Medcalf RL, Hession C et al. Plasminogen activator inhibitor 2: Regulation of gene transcription during phorbol ester-mediated differentiation of U-937 human histiocytic lymphoma cells. Mol Cell Biol 1987;7:4564–4567.

148. Ye RD, Ahern SM, Le Beau MM et al. Structure of the gene for human plasminogen activator inhibitor-2. The nearest mammalian homologue of chicken ovalbumin. J Biol Chem 1989;264:5495–5502.

149. Samia JA, Alexander SJ, Horton KW et al. Chromosomal organization and localization of the human urokinase inhibitor gene: Perfect structural conservation with ovalbumin. Genomics 1990;6:159–167.

150. Antalis TM, Clark MA, Barnes T et al. Cloning and expression of a cDNA coding for a human monocyte-derived plasminogen activator inhibitor. Proc Natl Acad Sci U S A 1988;85:985–989.

151. Genton C, Kruithof EK, Schleuning WD. Phorbol ester induces the biosynthesis of glycosylated and nonglycosylated plasminogen activator inhibitor 2 in high excess over urokinase-type plasminogen activator in human U-937 lymphoma cells. J Cell Biol 1987;104:705–712.

152. Feener EP, Northrup JM, Aiello LP et al. Angiotensin II induces plasminogen activator inhibitor-1 and -2 expression in vascular endothelial and smooth muscle cells. J Clin Invest 1995;95:1353–1362.

153. Lijnen HR, Collen D. Molecular mechanism of fibrinolysis. Adv Exp Med Biol 1984;164:217–228.

154. Hoylaerts M, Rijken DC, Lijnen HR et al. Kinetics of the activation of plasminogen by human tissue plasminogen activator. Role of fibrin. J Biol Chem 1982;257:2912–2919.

155. Lijnen HR, Zamarron C, Blaber M et al. Activation of plasminogen by pro-urokinase. I. Mechanism. J Biol Chem 1986;261:1253–1258.

156. Verheijen JH, Caspers MP, Chang GT et al. Involvement of finger domain and kringle 2 domain of tissue-type plasminogen activator in fibrin binding and stimulation of activity by fibrin. EMBO J 1986;5:3525–3530.

157. Higgins DL, Vehar GA. Interaction of one-chain and two-chain tissue plas-

minogen activator with intact and plasmin-degraded fibrin. Biochemistry 1987;26:7786–7791.

158. Nieuwenhuizen W, Voskuilen M, Vermond A et al. The influence of fibrin-(ogen) fragments on the kinetic parameters of the tissue-type plasminogen-activator-mediated activation of different forms of plasminogen. Eur J Biochem 1988;174:163–169.

159. van Zonneveld AJ, Veerman H, Pannekoek H. On the interaction of the finger and the kringle-2 domain of tissue-type plasminogen activator with fibrin. Inhibition of kringle-2 binding to fibrin by epsilon-amino caproic acid. J Biol Chem 1986;261:14214–14218.

160. van Zonneveld AJ, Veerman H, Pannekoek H. Autonomous functions of structural domains on human tissue-type plasminogen activator. Proc Natl Acad Sci U S A 1986;83:4670–4674.

161. Sakharov DV, Plow EF, Rijken DC. On the mechanism of the antifibrinolytic activity of plasma carboxypeptidase B. J Biol Chem 1997;272:14477–14482.

162. Redlitz A, Tan AK, Eaton DL et al. Plasma carboxypeptidases as regulators of the plasminogen system. J Clin Invest 1995;96:2534–2538.

163. Redlitz A, Nicolini FA, Malycky JL et al. Inducible carboxypeptidase activity. A role in clot lysis in vivo. Circulation 1996;93:1328–1330.

164. Gething MJ, Adler B, Boose JA et al. Variants of human tissue-type plasminogen activator that lack specific structural domains of the heavy chain. EMBO J 1988;7:2731–2740.

165. Kingston IB, Castro MT, Anderson S. In vitro stimulation of tissue-type plasminogen activator by Alzheimer amyloid beta-peptide analogues. Nat Med 1995;1:138–142.

166. Hajjar KA, Jacovina AT, Chacko J. An endothelial cell receptor for plasminogen/tissue plasminogen activator. I. Identity with annexin II. J Biol Chem 1994;269:21191–21197.

167. Lijnen HR, Van Hoef B, De Cock F et al. The mechanism of plasminogen activation and fibrin dissolution by single chain urokinase-type plasminogen activator in a plasma milieu in vitro. Blood 1989;73:1864–1872.

168. Pannell R, Gurewich V. Activation of plasminogen by single-chain urokinase or by two-chain urokinase-a demonstration that single-chain urokinase has a low catalytic activity (pro-urokinase). Blood 1987;69:22–26.

169. Collen D, Zamarron C, Lijnen HR et al. Activation of plasminogen by pro-urokinase. II. Kinetics. J Biol Chem 1986;261:1259–1266.

170. Lijnen HR, Van Hoef B, Collen D. Comparative kinetic analysis of the activation of human plasminogen by natural and recombinant single-chain urokinase-type plasminogen activator. Biochim Biophys Acta 1986;884:402–408.

171. Lijnen HR, Collen D. Molecular mechanisms of thrombolytic therapy. Haemostasis 1986;16:3–15.

172. Lijnen HR, Collen D. Mechanisms of plasminogen activation by mammalian plasminogen activators [Review]. Enzyme 1988;40:90–96.

173. Declerck PJ, Lijnen HR, Verstreken M et al. A monoclonal antibody specific for two-chain urokinase-type plasminogen activator. Application to the study of the mechanism of clot lysis with single-chain urokinase-type plasminogen activator in plasma. Blood 1990;75:1794–1800.

174. Lijnen HR, Van Hoef B, Nelles L et al. Plasminogen activation with single-chain urokinase-type plasminogen activator (scu-PA). Studies with active site mutagenized plasminogen (Ser740——Ala) and plasmin-resistant scu-PA (Lys158——Glu). J Biol Chem 1990;265:5232–5236.

175. Declerck PJ, Lijnen HR, Verstreken M et al. Role of alpha 2-antiplasmin in fibrin-specific clot lysis with single-chain urokinase-type plasminogen activator in human plasma. Thromb Haemost 1991;65:394–398.

176. Vassalli JD, Baccino D, Belin D. A cellular binding site for the Mr 55,000 form of the human plasminogen activator, urokinase. J Cell Biol 1985;100:86–92.

177. Miles LA, Levin EG, Plescia J et al. Plasminogen receptors, urokinase receptors, and their modulation on human endothelial cells. Blood 1988;72:628–635.

178. Barnathan ES, Kuo A, Kariko K et al. Characterization of human endothelial cell urokinase-type plasminogen activator receptor protein and messenger RNA. Blood 1990;76:1795–1806.

179. Estreicher A, Wohlwend A, Belin D et al. Characterization of the cellular binding site for the urokinase-type plasminogen activator. J Biol Chem 1989;264:1180–1189.

180. Roldan AL, Cubellis MV, Masucci MT et al. Cloning and expression of the receptor for human urokinase plasminogen activator, a central molecule in cell surface, plasmin dependent proteolysis. EMBO J 1990;9:467–474.

181. Ploug M, Ronne E, Behrendt N et al. Cellular receptor for urokinase plasminogen activator. Carboxylterminal processing and membrane anchoring by glycosyl-phosphatidylinositol. J Biol Chem 1991;266:1926–1933.

182. Behrendt N, Ronne E, Ploug M et al. The human receptor for urokinase plasminogen activator. NH2-terminal amino acid sequence and glycosylation variants. J Biol Chem 1990;265:6453–6460.

183. Hoyer-Hansen G, Ronne E, Solberg H et al. Urokinase plasminogen activator cleaves its cell surface receptor releasing the ligand-binding domain. J Biol Chem 1992;267:18224–18229.

184. Blasi F. Urokinase and urokinase receptor: A paracrine/autocrine system regulating cell migration and invasiveness [Review]. Bioessays 1993;15:105–111.

185. Ellis V, Behrendt N, Dano K. Cellular receptor for urokinase-type plasminogen activator: Function in cell-surface proteolysis. Methods Enzymol 1993;223:223–233.

186. Ellis V, Behrendt N, Dano K. Plasminogen activation by receptor-bound urokinase. A kinetic study with both cell-associated and isolated receptor. J Biol Chem 1991;266:12752–12758.

187. Carmeliet P, Moons L, Dewerchin M et al. Insights in vessel development and vascular disorders using targeted inactivation and transfer of vascular endothelial growth factor, the tissue factor receptor, and the plasminogen system [Review]. Ann N Y Acad Sci 1997;811:191–206.

188. Pepper MS, Vassalli JD, Montesano R et al. Urokinase-type plasminogen activator is induced in migrating capillary endothelial cells. J Cell Biol 1987;105:2535–2541.

189. Nykjaer A, Conese M, Christensen EI et al. Recycling of the urokinase receptor upon internalization of the u-PA:serpin complexes. EMBO J 1997;16:2610–2620.

190. Estreicher A, Muhlhauser J, Carpentier JL et al. The receptor for urokinase type plasminogen activator polarizes expression of the protease to the leading edge of migrating monocytes and promotes degradation of enzyme inhibitor complexes. J Cell Biol 1990;111:783–792.

191. Del Rosso M, Anichini E, Pedersen N et al. Urokinase-urokinase receptor interaction: Non-mitogenic signal transduction in human epidermal cells. Biochem Biophys Res Commun 1993;190:347–352.

192. Bianchi E, Ferrero E, Fazioli F et al. Integrin-dependent induction of functional urokinase receptors in primary T lymphocytes. J Clin Invest 1996;98:1133–1141.

193. Wei Y, Lukashev M, Simon DI et al. Regulation of integrin function by the urokinase receptor. Science 1996;273:1551–1555.

194. Rao NK, Shi GP, Chapman HA. Urokinase receptor is a multifunctional protein: Influence of receptor occupancy on macrophage gene expression. J Clin Invest 1995;96:465–474.

195. Wells JM, Strickland S. Regulated localization confers multiple functions on the protease urokinase plasminogen activator. J Cell Physiol 1997;171:217–225.

196. Deng G, Curriden SA, Wang S et al. Is plasminogen activator inhibitor-1 the molecular switch that governs urokinase receptor-mediated cell adhesion and release? J Cell Biol 1996;134:1563–1571.

197. Kanse SM, Kost C, Wilhelm OG et al. The urokinase receptor is a major vitronectin-binding protein on endothelial cells. Exp Cell Res 1996;224:344–353.

198. Wei Y, Waltz DA, Rao N et al. Identification of the urokinase receptor as an adhesion receptor for vitronectin. J Biol Chem 1994;269:32380–32388.

199. Dewerchin M, Nuffelen AV, Wallays G et al. Generation and characterization of urokinase receptor-deficient mice. J Clin Invest 1996;97:870–878.

200. Miles LA, Dahlberg CM, Plescia J et al. Role of cell-surface lysines in plasminogen binding to cells: Identification of alpha-enolase as a candidate plasminogen receptor. Biochemistry 1991;30:1682–1691.

201. Loskutoff DJ. Carboxypeptidases: New regulators of plasminogen activation in vivo? [Editorial]. J Clin Invest 1995;96:2104–2105.

202. Wiman B, Collen D. Purification and characterization of human antiplasmin, the fast-acting plasmin inhibitor in plasma. Eur J Biochem 1977;78:19–26.

203. Wiman B, Collen D. On the kinetics of the reaction between human antiplasmin and plasmin. Eur J Biochem 1978;84:573–578.

204. Tamaki T, Aoki N. Crosslinking of alpha 2-plasmin inhibitor and fibronectin to fibrin by fibrin-stabilizing factor. Biochim Biophys Acta 1981;661:280–286.

205. Sakata Y, Aoki N. Crosslinking of alpha 2-plasmin inhibitor to fibrin by fibrin-stabilizing factor. J Clin Invest 1980;65:290–297.

206. Wiman B, Boman L, Collen D. On the kinetics of the reaction between human antiplasmin and a low-molecular weight form of plasmin. Eur J Biochem 1978;87:143–146.

207. Lijnen HR, Hoylaerts M, Collen D. Isolation and characterization of a human plasma protein with affinity for the lysine binding sites in plasminogen. Role in the regulation of fibrinolysis and identification as histidine-rich glycoprotein. J Biol Chem 1980;255:10214–10222.

208. Wiman B, Lijnen HR, Collen D. On the specific interaction between the lysine-binding sites in plasmin and complementary sites in alpha2-antiplasmin and in fibrinogen. Biochim Biophys Acta 1979;579:142–154.

209. Thorsen S, Philips M. Isolation of tissue-type plasminogen activator-inhibitor complexes from human plasma. Evidence for a rapid plasminogen activator inhibitor. Biochim Biophys Acta 1984;802:111–118.

210. Chmielewska J, Ranby M, Wiman B. Evidence for a rapid inhibitor to tissue plasminogen activator in plasma. Thromb Res 1983;31:427–436.

211. Booth NA, Anderson JA, Bennett B. Platelet release protein which inhibits plasminogen activators. J Clin Pathol 1985;38:825–830.

212. Sprengers ED, Akkerman JW, Jansen BG. Blood platelet plasminogen activator inhibitor: Two different pools of endothelial cell type plasminogen activator in human blood. Thromb Haemost 1986;55:325–329.

213. Erickson LA, Hekman CM, Loskutoff DJ. The primary plasminogen-activator inhibitors in endothelial cells, platelets, serum, and plasma are immunologically related. Proc Natl Acad Sci U S A 1985;82:8710–8714.

214. Kruithof EK, Tran-Thang C, Bachmann F. Studies on the release of a plas-

minogen activator inhibitor by human platelets. Thromb Haemost 1986; 55:201–205.

215. Declerck PJ, Alessi MC, Verstreken M et al. Measurement of plasminogen activator inhibitor 1 in biologic fluids with a murine monoclonal antibody-based enzyme-linked immunosorbent assay. Blood 1988;71:220–225.

216. Wagner OF, de Vries C, Hohmann C et al. Interaction between plasminogen activator inhibitor type 1 (PAI-1) bound to fibrin and either tissue-type plasminogen activator (t-PA) or urokinase-type plasminogen activator (u-PA). Binding of t-PA/PAI-1 complexes to fibrin mediated by both the finger and the kringle-2 domain of t-PA. J Clin Invest 1989;84:647–655.

217. Cubellis MV, Andreasen P, Ragno P et al. Accessibility of receptor-bound urokinase to type-1 plasminogen activator inhibitor. Proc Natl Acad Sci U S A 1989;86:4828–4832.

218. Hajjar KA, Hamel NM, Harpel PC et al. Binding of tissue plasminogen activator to cultured human endothelial cells. J Clin Invest 1987;80: 1712–1719.

219. Madison EL, Goldsmith EJ, Gerard RD et al. Serpin-resistant mutants of human tissue-type plasminogen activator. Nature 1989;339:721–724.

220. Madison EL, Goldsmith EJ, Gerard RD et al. Amino acid residues that affect interaction of tissue-type plasminogen activator with plasminogen activator inhibitor 1. Proc Natl Acad Sci U S A 1990;87:3530–3533.

221. Keyt BA, Paoni NF, Refino CJ et al. A faster-acting and more potent form of tissue plasminogen activator. Proc Natl Acad Sci U S A 1994;91:3670–3674.

222. Keijer J, Ehrlich HJ, Linders M et al. Vitronectin governs the interaction between plasminogen activator inhibitor 1 and tissue-type plasminogen activator. J Biol Chem 1991;266:10700–10707.

223. Stefansson S, Lawrence DA. The serpin PAI-1 inhibits cell migration by blocking integrin alpha V beta3 binding to vitronectin. Nature 1996;383: 441–443.

224. Mignatti P, Rifkin DB. Plasminogen activators and matrix metalloproteinases in angiogenesis [Review]. Enzyme Protein 1996;49:117–137.

225. Vassalli JD, Sappino AP, Belin D. The plasminogen activator/plasmin system. J Clin Invest 1991;88:1067–1072.

226. Ichinose A, Espling ES, Takamatsu J et al. Two types of abnormal genes for plasminogen in families with a predisposition for thrombosis. Proc Natl Acad Sci U S A 1991;88:115–119.

227. Robbins KC. Dysplasminogenemias [Review]. Prog Cardiovasc Dis 1992; 34:295–308.

228. Sartori MT, Patrassi GM, Theodoridis P et al. Heterozygous type I plasminogen deficiency is associated with an increased risk for thrombosis: A statistical analysis in 20 kindreds. Blood Coagul Fibrinolysis 1994;5: 889–893.

229. Azuma H, Uno Y, Shigekiyo T et al. Congenital plasminogen deficiency caused by a Ser572 to Pro mutation. Blood 1993;82:475–480.

230. Bugge TH, Flick MJ, Daugherty CC et al. Plasminogen deficiency causes severe thrombosis but is compatible with development and reproduction. Genes Dev 1995;9:794–807.

231. Carmeliet P, Schoonjans L, Kieckens L et al. Physiological consequences of loss of plasminogen activator gene function in mice. Nature 1994;368: 419–424.

232. Fay WP, Shapiro AD, Shih JL et al. Brief report: Complete deficiency of plasminogen-activator inhibitor type 1 due to a frame-shift mutation. N Engl J Med 1992;327:1729–1733.

233. Takahashi Y, Tanaka T, Minowa H et al. Hereditary partial deficiency of plasminogen activator inhibitor-1 associated with a lifelong bleeding tendency. Int J Hematol 1996;64:61–68.

234. Tanimura LK, Weddell JA, McKown CG et al. Oral management of a individual with a plasminogen activator inhibitor (PAI-1) deficiency: Case report. Pediatr Dent 1994;16:133–135.

235. Lee MH, Vosburgh E, Anderson K et al. Deficiency of plasma plasminogen activator inhibitor 1 results in hyperfibrinolytic bleeding. Blood 1993;81: 2357–2362.

236. Fay WP, Parker AC, Condrey LR et al. Human plasminogen activator inhibitor-1 (PAI-1) deficiency: Characterization of a large kindred with a null mutation in the PAI-1 gene. Blood 1997;90:204–208.

237. Hamsten A, Wiman B, de Faire U et al. Increased plasma levels of a rapid inhibitor of tissue plasminogen activator in young survivors of myocardial infarction. N Engl J Med 1985;313:1557–1563.

238. Hamsten A, de Faire U, Walldius G et al. Plasminogen activator inhibitor in plasma: Risk factor for recurrent myocardial infarction. Lancet 1987;2: 3–9.

239. Meade TW, Ruddock V, Stirling Y et al. Fibrinolytic activity, clotting factors, and long-term incidence of ischaemic heart disease in the Northwick Park Heart Study. Lancet 1993;342:1076–1079.

240. Schneiderman J, Sawdey MS, Keeton MR et al. Increased type 1 plasminogen activator inhibitor gene expression in atherosclerotic human arteries. Proc Natl Acad Sci U S A 1992;89:6998–7002.

241. Lupu F, Bergonzelli GE, Heim DA et al. Localization and production of plasminogen activator inhibitor-1 in human healthy and atherosclerotic arteries. Arterioscler Thromb 1993;13:1090–1100.

242. Robbie LA, Booth NA, Brown AJ et al. Inhibitors of fibrinolysis are elevated in atherosclerotic plaque. Arterioscler Thromb Vasc Biol 1996;16: 539–545.

243. Ridker PM, Gaboury CL, Conlin PR et al. Stimulation of plasminogen activator inhibitor in vivo by infusion of angiotensin II. Evidence of a potential interaction between the renin-angiotensin system and fibrinolytic function. Circulation 1993;87:1969–1973.

244. Olson JA Jr, Shiverick KT, Ogilvie S et al. Angiotensin II induces secretion of plasminogen activator inhibitor 1 and a tissue metalloprotease inhibitor-related protein from rat brain astrocytes. Proc Natl Acad Sci U S A 1991; 88:1928–1932.

245. Hamdan AD, Quist WC, Gagne JB et al. Angiotensin-converting enzyme inhibition suppresses plasminogen activator inhibitor-1 expression in the neointima of balloon-injured rat aorta. Circulation 1996;93:1073–1078.

246. Kerins DM, Hao Q, Vaughan DE. Angiotensin induction of PAI-1 expression in endothelial cells is mediated by the hexapeptide angiotensin IV. J Clin Invest 1995;96:2515–2520.

247. van Leeuwen RT, Kol A, Andreotti F et al. Angiotensin II increases plasminogen activator inhibitor type 1 and tissue-type plasminogen activator messenger RNA in cultured rat aortic smooth muscle cells. Circulation 1994;90:362–368.

248. Erdos E, Skidgel RA. The angiotensin 1-converting enzyme. Lab Invest 1987;56:345–348.

249. Smith D, Gilbert M, Owen WG. Tissue plasminogen activator release in vivo in response to vasoactive agents. Blood 1985;66:835–839.

250. Emeis JJ, Tranquille N. On the role of bradykinin in secretion from vascular endothelium. Agents Actions 1992;38:285–291.

251. Brown NJ, Nadeau JH, Vaughan DE. Selective stimulation of tissue-type plasminogen activator (t-PA) in vivo by infusion of bradykinin. Thromb Haemost 1997;77:522–525.

252. Vaughan DE, Rouleau JL, Pfeffer MA. Role of the fibrinolytic system in preventing myocardial infarction. Eur Heart J 1995;16:31–36.

253. Gough SC, Rice PJ, McCormack L et al. The relationship between plasminogen activator inhibitor-1 and insulin resistance in newly diagnosed type 2 diabetes mellitus. Diabet Med 1993;10:638–642.

254. Ito Y, Okeda T, Sato Y et al. Plasminogen activator inhibitor-1 in nonobese subjects with non-insulin-dependent diabetes mellitus. Proc Soc Exp Biol Med 1996;211:287–291.

255. Mansfield MW, Stickland MH, Grant PJ. Environmental and genetic factors in relation to elevated circulating levels of plasminogen activator inhibitor-1 in Caucasian individuals with non-insulin-dependent diabetes mellitus. Thromb Haemost 1995;74:842–847.

256. Schneider DJ, Nordt TK, Sobel BE. Attenuated fibrinolysis and accelerated atherogenesis in type II diabetic individuals [review]. Diabetes 1993;42: 1–7.

257. Juhan-Vague I, Roul C, Alessi MC et al. Increased plasminogen activator inhibitor activity in non insulin dependent diabetic individuals-relationship with plasma insulin. Thromb Haemost 1989;61:370–373.

258. Juhan-Vague I, Alessi MC, Vague P. Increased plasma plasminogen activator inhibitor 1 levels. A possible link between insulin resistance and atherothrombosis. Diabetologia 1991;34:457–462.

259. Vague P, Juhan-Vague I, Aillaud MF et al. Correlation between blood fibrinolytic activity, plasminogen activator inhibitor level, plasma insulin level, and relative body weight in normal and obese subjects. Metabolism 1986;35:250–253.

260. Nordt TK, Sawa H, Fujii S et al. Induction of plasminogen activator inhibitor type-1 (PAI-1) by proinsulin and insulin in vivo. Circulation 1995;91: 764–770.

261. Nordt TK, Klassen KJ, Schneider DJ et al. Augmentation of synthesis of plasminogen activator inhibitor type-1 in arterial endothelial cells by glucose and its implications for local fibrinolysis. Arterioscler Thromb 1993; 13:1822–1828.

262. Eitzman DT, Nabel EG, Gordon D et al. Atherosclerosis in transgenic mice that either overexpress or lack the murine plasminogen activator inhibitor-1 gene [Abstract]. Circulation 1996;94:I-460.

263. Samad F, Yamamoto K, Loskutoff DJ. Distribution and regulation of plasminogen activator inhibitor-1 in murine adipose tissue in vivo. Induction by tumor necrosis factor-alpha and lipopolysaccharide. J Clin Invest 1996; 97:37–46.

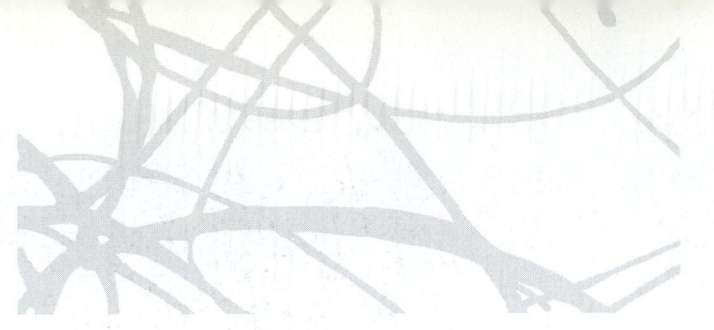

# SECTION 2

# PLATELETS

# CHAPTER 8

# REGULATION OF MEGAKARYOPOIESIS

## Kenneth Kaushansky

## INTRODUCTION

Platelet production is an enormous task. Each day the adult human produces approximately $1 \times 10^{11}$ platelets, a level of production that can increase tenfold in times of increased demand. Production of each of the blood cell lineages depends on hematopoietic stem and progenitor cells, a supportive marrow stroma consisting of cells and matrix glycosaminoglycans, and a growing family of protein hormones and cytokines. In contrast to erythropoiesis or myelopoiesis, some of the cellular and humoral components necessary for platelet production have only recently been identified. Nevertheless, in the past few years our understanding of this previously enigmatic process has rapidly expanded. This chapter will focus on the development of megakaryocytes, their precursors and their progeny, and on the hematopoietic growth factors that support the survival, proliferation, and differentiation of these cells. However, it will not deal with the therapeutic use of the proteins; instead the reader is referred to recently published reviews on this subject (1, 2).

## A MODEL OF HEMATOPOIESIS

The basic concepts leading to our present understanding of blood cell production were formulated by Till and McCulloch in the early 1960s (3). The capacity to transplant marrow cells and reconstitute all of hematopoiesis in lethally irradiated recipients provided an *in vivo* assay for the hematopoietic stem cell, but it was not until the development of clonal *in vitro* assays of hematopoietic progenitors that a coherent model of blood cell production emerged. The pioneering work of Pluznik and Sachs (4) and of Bradley and Metcalf (5) provided a convenient method to enumerate and characterize marrow cells committed to various hematopoietic lineages.

The assays for hematopoietic progenitor cells consist of marrow cells, either unfractionated or purified to varying degrees; a semisolid support (either methylcellulose or agar, which prevent cellular migration); and a source of hematopoietic growth factors. This latter requirement was initially fulfilled by using cellular underlayers containing fibroblasts, lymphocytes, or monocytes, but was soon replaced by tissue culture medium conditioned by a variety of normal and neoplastic cellular sources. Such colony-stimulating activity rich media rapidly became the starting material of choice to biochemically purify a number of hematopoiesis restricted polypeptide growth factors (see below). However, the assays themselves served a greater purpose. By using various sources of colony-stimulating activity, a number of investigators identified colonies containing cells of single hematopoietic lineages or those composed of multiple combinations of specific cell types. As the marrow cells in these culture systems were immobilized by the semisolid supporting matrix, all of the cells in such colonies were derived from a single progenitor, allowing one to retrospectively determine the developmental capacity of individual, marrow-derived progenitor cells, termed colony-forming units (CFU). Present concepts of hematopoiesis emerged from the range of cellular compositions of colony types identified in such assays (6) (Fig. 8.1). In this model, mature blood cells are derived

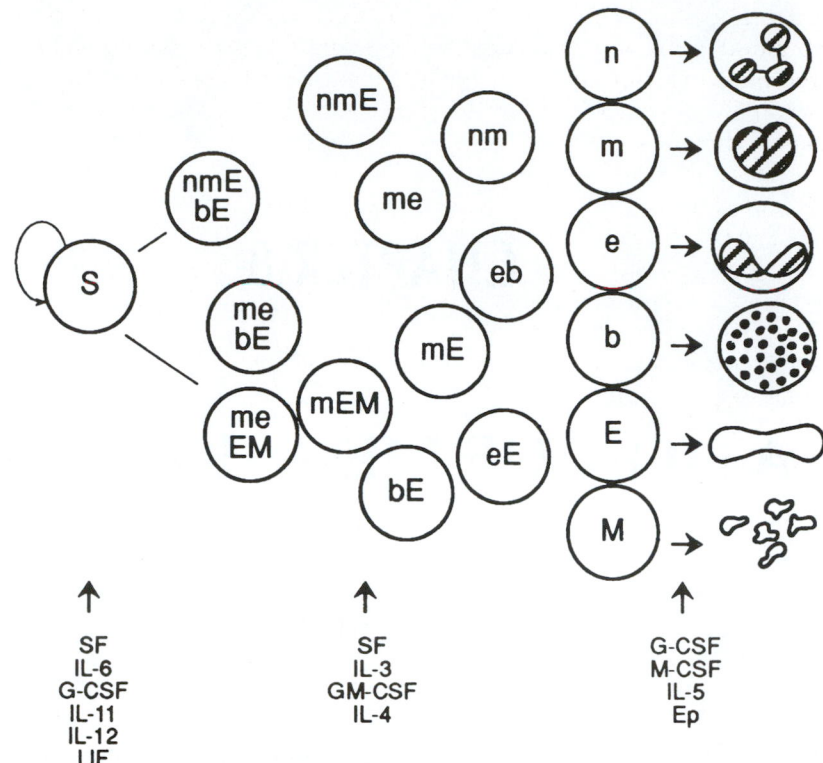

**FIGURE 8.1.**   A model of hematopoiesis. The model is based on results derived from *in vitro* semi-solid cultures of marrow cells. As such cultures are clonal (i.e., all of the cells in a colony are derived from a single hematopoietic progenitor cell), the presence of a colony containing a mixture of neutrophils (n), erythrocytes (E), and monocytes (m) implies the presence of a progenitor cell (in this case termed a colony-forming unit [CFU]-nmE) in the initial marrow innoculum, which has the developmental capacity for these three lineages. By using different combinations of purified hematopoietic growth factors, the cytokines necessary for each of these progenitors have been determined. Other progenitor cell types include those for basophils (b), megakaryocytes (M), and eosinophils (e). The hematopoietic proteins can be classified as acting on stem cells (KL [here termed SF], IL-6, G-CSF, IL-11, IL-12, LIF), on immature, multipotent progenitors (e.g., IL-3, KL, GM-CSF, IL-4), or on lineage committed cells (e.g., Epo, G-CSF, IL-5, M-CSF). For the most part, the conclusions obtained from analysis of such culture systems have been substantiated *in vivo*. Reprinted with permission from Ogawa M. Differentiation and proliferation of hematopoietic stem cells. Blood 1993;81:2844–2853.

from lineage-committed and pluripotent progenitors, each derived ultimately from the hematopoietic stem cell.

Using the colony-forming assay to evaluate the cell types supported by various conditioned, tissue culture media, a number of colony-stimulating activities were defined. For example, granulocyte-macrophage colony-stimulating factor (GM-CSF) was defined as the substance that supports the formation of colonies containing granulocytes and macrophages from a bipotential hematopoietic progenitor (CFU-GM). In a similar way M-CSF was defined as supporting monocyte proliferation from CFU-M, G-CSF as supporting granulocyte (actually only neutrophil) growth from CFU-G, and Multi-CSF as supporting the development of several hematopoietic colony types (including mixed erythroid and nonerythroid) from a multipotential progenitor (CFU-GEMM or CFU-Mix). More recent efforts involving pro-

tein purification and cloning by functional expression have yielded at least 13 distinct proteins that influence the proliferation of hematopoietic progenitor cells (Fig. 8.1). However, rather than each of these cytokines supporting cellular development from the earliest stem cell to the mature blood cell, they appear to support primarily particular aspects of the development of each lineage.

Hematopoietic development can be conveniently divided into early and late phases. Hematopoietic stem cells first undergo a progressive loss of developmental potential and commit to a specific cellular lineage, a maturational stage represented by unipotent progenitors (CFU-M, CFU-Eo, CFU-G, CFU-MK, etc.). Subsequent development of each of these lineage committed cells into their mature counterparts comprise the later aspects of hematopoiesis. This model of blood cell development is best illustrated by considering erythropoiesis. Erythropoietin (EPO) is necessary and sufficient for the maturation of late erythroid progenitors (CFU-E) into reticulocytes and mature red blood cells *in vitro*. Genetic elimination of EPO or the EPO receptor supports this conclusion; either EPO or EPO receptor deficiency are lethal embryonic events, occurring at the earliest stages of fetal liver erythrocyte production. However, the livers of such nullizygous mice contain BFU-E (burst-forming unit-erythroid) and CFU-E (colony-forming unit-erythroid), indicating that hematopoietic stem cells can develop into erythroid progenitors in the absence of erythropoietin function (7). The growth factors responsible for this early aspect of erythropoiesis were revealed by *in vitro* studies. Collectively termed ''burst promoting activities,'' interleukin (IL)-3, GM-CSF, and the *c-kit* ligand (KL; also termed steel factor [SF], stem cell factor [SCF], or mast cell growth factor [MGF]) were found to act on primitive hematopoietic cells to induce erythroid colony formation from cells with extensive developmental potential (i.e., BFU-E) (8, 9). Of the three proteins, KL is the most important *in vivo*, as alteration of either KL or its receptor results in a severe macrocytic anemia (10). Thus erythropoiesis depends on at least two distinct growth factors, one supporting the proliferation of primitive progenitors and their development into cells capable of responding to erythropoietin and the other allowing their differentiation into mature erythrocytes.

## MEGAKARYOCYTIC PROGENITOR CELLS

Culture conditions that support the proliferation of megakaryocytic progenitors have been established in the past 10 years (11, 12). Using either methylcellulose, agar, or a plasma clot, multiple investigators have demonstrated two colony morphologies that contain megakaryocytes exclusively. The colony-forming unit megakaryocyte (CFU-MK) is a cell that develops into a simple colony containing from 3 to 50 mature MKs. Larger, more complex colonies that include satellite collections of MKs and contain up to several hundred cells are derived from the burst-forming unit-megakaryocyte (BFU-MK). Such lineage restricted colonies have been described using marrow cells from both human and murine sources. Because of the difference in their proliferative potential and by analogy to erythroid progenitors, BFU-MK and CFU-MK are althought to represent primitive and mature progenitors restricted to the MK lineage.

Megakaryocytes have also been noted mixed into colonies containing cells of one or more additional hematopoietic lineages. The most primitive colony-forming cell is termed a CFU-GEMM, or CFU-Mix, and often contains several megakaryocytes. However, more recently, particular attention has been paid to the mixed erythroid/MK progenitor cell. The colonies derived from these bipotent cells usually contain large numbers of both erythroid and megakaryocytic cells. The existence of such a cell is felt by many to provide additional evidence for the commonality of the two lineages (13–16). This close relationship of erythropoiesis and megakaryopoiesis correlates with the common effects of the hormones althought to be restricted to each single lineage (erythropoietin and thrombopoietin, respectively; see below).

## MEGAKARYOCYTIC CYTOKINES AND THEIR ACTIVITIES

Initial studies yielding colonies containing MKs were nearly always conducted using plasma. The application of various conditioned culture media and then purified cytokines revealed that IL-3, GM-CSF, and KL support the proliferation of MK progenitors in plasma containing cultures (17–19). IL-3 is a monomeric, 25- to 30-kDa polypeptide produced by T-lymphocytes and mast cells (20). The mature human polypeptide contains 133 amino acids, but significant amounts of carbohydrate modification account for its larger than expected molecular weight. GM-CSF, an 18- to 30-kDa monomeric protein, is produced by T lymphocytes, endothelial cells, monocytes, and fibroblasts, and like IL-3, is highly modified with both N-linked and O-linked carbohydrate (21). Although the two proteins display limited primary sequence homology, their tertiary structures are highly related (22, 23). In contrast to the hematopoietic cytokine family, KL is more closely related to other hematopoietic proteins that utilize protein tyrosine kinase receptors, such as M-CSF (24) and the flt-3 ligand (FL) (25). KL was first cloned in 1990 and reported under a variety of names (in addition to kit ligand, stem cell factor, mast cell growth factor, and steel factor were used), reflecting the diverse nature of the assays utilized to identify the protein (26–29).

The soluble form of KL is a dimeric protein composed of two identical noncovalently linked polypeptides of 165 residues (30). Soluble KL is released from a membrane-bound form of the molecule (31) by a membrane-associated protease, which cleaves the protein a fixed distance from the cell surface (32). The dimeric membrane-bound form is also active (29) and is the critical physiologic form, as its signal persists in receptor bearing cells much longer than that of soluble KL (33). Also, a naturally occurring mutation of the KL gene (Sl$^d$), which allows production of the soluble but not the membrane-bound form of KL, results in a phenotype nearly identical to deletion of the entire locus (31). More recently, effects of FL on megakaryocyte formation have been investigated. This growth factor was initially identified as the ligand for a novel member of the protein tyrosine kinase family of receptors most closely related to *c-kit*, the receptor for KL (25). Like the latter, FL appears in both soluble and membrane-bound forms, is a noncovalently linked dimer, and affects primarily primitive hematopoietic cells (25, 34–37). Although several studies have shown that when used alone FL does not support megakaryocyte colony formation, some but not all studies suggest that it works in synergy with other MK-CSFs to augment the growth of CFU-MK in semisolid media (38, 39). However, FL administration to animals clearly expands the number of marrow and splenic progenitor cells that can give rise to megakaryocytes in culture (40).

Like their effects on erythropoiesis, IL-3, KL, GM-CSF, and FL are althought to act early in megakaryopoiesis, expanding the number and/or proliferative state of megakaryocytic progenitors, but not supporting their terminal differentiation. Most investigators believed that the plasma in such megakaryocyte colony-containing cultures contributed a critical megakaryocyte differentiation activity. A likely candidate was thrombopoietin, the agent in thrombocytopenic plasma posited nearly 40 years ago to be responsible for the thrombocytosis that follows thrombocytopenia (41). However, such a protein proved difficult to purify or to clone, and the active component of plasma remained enigmatic.

In the late 1980s and early 1990s three molecules were obtained that display effects on megakaryocyte production. Interleukin (IL)-6, cloned by several groups using a number of different assays (hepatocyte growth, myeloma cell growth, immunoglobulin secretion, antiviral activity), was later found to display megakaryocytic effects as well. IL-6 is a 26-kDa polypeptide produced in almost all tissues from T cells, fibroblasts, macrophages, and stromal cells (42). The mature protein is composed of 184 amino acids, contains two disulfide bonds, and displays both N-linked and O-linked carbohydrate modification. Although not an MK-CSF when used alone, IL-6 augments the number of colonies obtained in the presence of IL-3 or KL (43–46). In such culture systems IL-6 was althought to exert primarily a differentiating effect, as its levels correlate with megakaryocyte size and ploidy in long-term marrow cultures and its neutralization reduces these parameters (47, 48). Similar effects on megakaryocyte maturation were noted in suspension culture of murine and human marrow cells (47, 49, 50). The administration of IL-6 to mice, dogs, or humans results in a modest thrombocytosis (43, 51–56). These findings suggested that IL-6 might be responsible for megakaryocyte formation *in vivo*, a conclusion supported by its production by tumor cells in selected cases of paraneoplastic thrombocytosis (see below). It should also be noted that the effects of IL-1 on megakaryopoiesis are indirect, acting to increase megakaryocyte formation through its induction of IL-6 production (56, 57).

When IL-11 and leukemia inhibitory factor (LIF) were cloned a short time later, both cytokines were shown to act in synergy with IL-3 or KL to augment mega-

karyocyte formation. Interleukin-11 was initially cloned from a gibbon marrow stromal cell line as an activity that supported the proliferation of an IL-6-responsive, myeloma cell line (58). It is a 23-kDa polypeptide that contains 199 amino acids but, unlike the other hematopoietic growth factors, is devoid of cysteine residues and does not contain sites of N-linked carbohydrate modification (59). LIF was initially cloned as a human interleukin that induced DA-1 cells to proliferate or leukemic M1 cells to differentiate (60). The protein is composed of 180 amino acids, contains three disulfide bonds, and seven sites of N-linked carbohydrate modification (61). The latter feature is responsible for its highly heterogeneous molecular mass of 38 to 67 Kda. LIF displays a wide range of activities (62), including effects on the liver (acute phase response), neurons (adrenergic to cholinergic switch), adipocytes (inhibition of lipoprotein lipase), and embryonic cells (to maintain pluripotentiality).

Like IL-6, IL-11 and LIF display multiple effects on hematopoiesis, including megakaryocytic activities. IL-11 and LIF act to enhance MK maturation *in vitro* (50, 63). Moreover, IL-6 and IL-11 were also found to augment the effects of IL-3 and KL on the proliferation of primitive hematopoietic cells, suggesting that these cytokines augment MK development at multiple levels. Consistent with these *in vitro* findings, the administration of either recombinant IL-11 or LIF to rodents, nonhuman primates, or humans produces a modest thrombocytosis (60, 64–69). Together, such findings suggested to many that these pleiotropic cytokines might provide the equivalent of the postulated hormone, thrombopoietin. However, several investigators argued that neither IL-6 nor IL-11 were thrombopoietin (70–73), the primary regulator of platelet formation.

## THE CLONING AND CHARACTERIZATION OF THROMBOPOIETIN

One of the key observations leading to the cloning and characterization of thrombopoietin was identification of the myeloproliferative leukemia virus (mplV). An acute murine transforming retrovirus, mplV induces a pan-myeloid transformation in infected animals characterized by erythroid, myeloid, and megakaryocytic expansion and eventual hematopoietic failure (74). The transforming oncogene (*v-mpl*) was reported on in 1990 (75), and the corresponding cellular proto-oncogene (*c-mpl*) cloned from the human erythroleukemia cell line HEL in 1992 (76). Based on the predicted primary sequence of the two genes, it became clear that the *c-mpl* locus encodes a hematopoietic growth factor receptor. This conclusion was based on recognition of the cytokine receptor motif in the predicted polypeptide sequence, a 200 amino acid region that contains four spatially conserved cysteine residues and a Trp-Ser-Xaa-Trp-Ser (where Xaa is any amino acid) pentapeptide closely adjacent to a single transmembrane domain (77). As the predicted *c-mpl* protein contained two such motifs, it was almost certain to represent an orphan hematopoietic cytokine receptor.

As noted, *c-mpl* was first cloned from HEL cells. Although primarily erythroid in nature, these cells can also be induced to display megakaryocytic features (78). Additional findings suggested that the mpl ligand might function in megakaryopoiesis. Messenger RNA for *c-mpl* was found restricted to megakaryocytes, their precursors or progeny, or to leukemic cell lines which can be induced to display features of megakaryocytic differentiation (76, 79). Also, antisense oligodeoxynucleotide-mediated elimination of *c-mpl* expression was reported to substantially reduce the capacity of CD-34-selected marrow cells to develop into megakaryocytic, but not erythroid or myeloid colonies (80). Based on these findings, a number of investigators began efforts to purify and clone the mpl ligand.

Using three distinct strategies, five separate groups have reported the purification or cloning of thrombopoietin, the mpl ligand (81–85). Using thrombocytopenic plasma, two groups used conventional protein purification techniques to obtain the rat and ovine homologues (84, 85). Porcine or canine thrombocytopenic plasma was the starting material for two additional purification efforts, making use of mpl-receptor affinity chromatography (81, 83). Finally, functional expression cloning methods were used to obtain a murine thrombopoietin cDNA from an mpl receptor-bearing cell line growing autonomously because of mutagenesis-induced mpl ligand expression (82). Despite these differences in the approaches taken, all five groups reported on the identical molecule (except for species-specific differences) within several months of one another.

The cloned human thrombopoietin cDNA predicts a polypeptide of 353 amino acids and includes a 21 amino acid secretory leader sequence. It can be conveniently divided into two domains: the aminoterminal 154 residues of the mature polypeptide bear striking sequence homology with erythropoietin and bind to the mpl receptor; the carboxyterminal domain bears no resemblance to any known proteins, but contains multiple sites of both N- and O-linked carbohydrate. This latter feature accounts for the large discrepancy between the predicted and actual molecular weight of the protein; nearly 50% of the 70-kDa thrombopoietin molecule is carbohydrate.

Two forms of the hormone have been tested for *in vitro* and *in vivo* effects: the full-length polypeptide produced in mammalian cell culture (Genentech, Kirin, and ZymoGenetics) and a polyethylene glycol-modified, truncated form (which includes only the mpl-binding domain) produced in *Escherichia coli* (Amgen). At present there are no definitive data to suggest that the two forms of the hormone differ in any biologic assay. Therefore, for the remainder of this discussion, both molecules will be referred to as thrombopoietin.

Recombinant thrombopoietin exerts profound effects on megakaryocyte differentiation. When used in suspension cultures containing unfractionated or purified marrow cells, thrombopoietin induces the expression of platelet-specific glycoproteins, high levels of polyploidy, and all of the ultrastructural features of highly developed marrow megakaryocytes (45, 86, 87). Moreover, such cultures produce platelets, which function normally in assays of agonist-induced expression of activation markers (88). Thrombopoietin is also a potent MK-CSF. When used alone, the hormone induces whole marrow cells or purified hematopoietic progenitors to develop into small to medium sized, megakaryocyte-containing colonies in semisolid medium (86, 87, 89–92). It also acts in synergy with IL-3, KL, FL, IL-11, or erythropoietin to augment MK colony formation above that found when each of these cytokines are used alone (93, 94). In addition, at least for IL-3 plus thrombopoietin or KL plus thrombopoietin, the resultant colonies are larger, with more cells per colony than when grown in the presence of IL-3, KL, or thrombopoietin alone. Taken together, these *in vitro* effects of thrombopoietin correlate well with the profound expansion and maturation of marrow megakaryocytes and the peripheral blood thrombocytosis that follows administration of the protein to rodents, dogs, monkeys, or humans (81, 86, 95–99). The use of modest doses of the hormone are associated with up to tenfold increases in marrow megakaryocyte numbers and blood steady-state platelet levels.

## A UNIFIED MODEL OF MEGAKARYOPOIESIS

Accumulating evidence supports the conclusion that the full maturation of platelets from the hematopoietic stem cell requires at least two cytokines: an early acting agent, such as IL-3, and a hormone capable of supporting the differentiation of megakaryocytic progenitors, such as thrombopoietin (Fig. 8.2). Other cytokines such as KL, FL, IL-6, IL-11, or LIF, agents shown to influence megakaryocyte production, may play an accessory role in megakaryopoiesis, acting in concert with IL-3 or thrombopoietin. Both *in vitro* and *in vivo* findings support this model: (a) the addition of a soluble form of the mpl receptor, which neutralizes the effects of thrombopoietin on megakaryocytic progenitor cells, eliminates KL-, IL-6-, or IL-11-induced MK colony formation, but not that which results from IL-3 stimulation (45); (b) the lack of a significant megakaryocytic phenotype in IL-6 or IL-11 receptor knock-out mice (100; Begley, personal communication); and (c) genetic elimination of thrombopoietin or its receptor results in profound thrombocytopenia (101, 102).

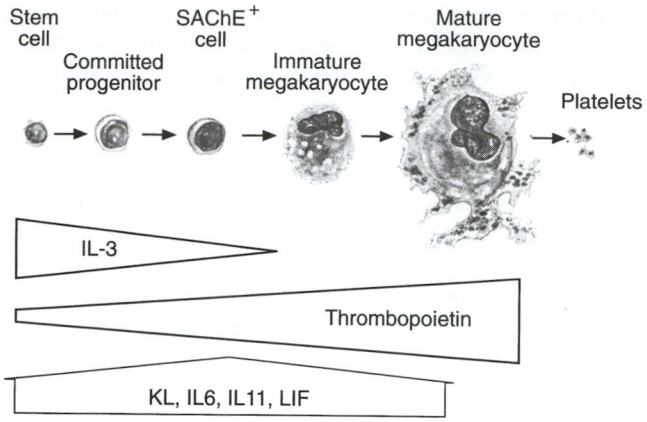

**FIGURE 8.2.** The roles of specific cytokines in megakaryopoiesis. From a number of studies a model of megakaryopoiesis has emerged. IL-3 can independently support the formation of megakaryocytes; however, such cells do not develop beyond the immature stage and do not become polyploid. In contrast, thrombopoietin alone supports all aspects of this process, from the earliest stem cell through the mature, highly polyploid megakaryocyte. Other cytokines such as KL, IL-6, IL-11, and LIF act at multiple stages of the process, but act only in synergy with either IL-3 or thrombopoietin. Note that none of these cytokines appear necessary for the final stages of platelet formation. SAChE$^+$ refers to the small, acetylcholinesterase positive cell, which represents the earliest histochemically identified megakaryocytic precursor described.

Although the model presented in Fig. 8.2 is consistent with much of the available data, there are some aspects of megakaryopoiesis that are not absolutely certain. For example, elimination of T cells, the primary source of IL-3, or genetic elimination of IL-3 has no megakaryocytic phenotype (103, 104). In contrast, naturally occurring mutations of KL (Sl/Sl$^d$ mice) display effects on megakaryocyte physiology, albeit of limited impact (105). Unfortunately, the double KL/mpl knockout has not yet been reported. Also, although genetic elimination of thrombopoietin results in profound thrombocytopenia, a modicum of platelet production (about 10% of normal) is still possible (101, 102), levels that are partially responsive to the administration of IL-6 or IL-11 (Frederic deSauvage, personal communication). Whether the residual platelet production in the mpl or thrombopoietin knockout mice is due to some combination of KL, IL-3, IL-6, or IL-11 awaits combining these genetic defects, studies that are currently underway.

## MEGAKARYOCYTE DIFFERENTIATION

### Endomitosis

One of the most characteristic features of megakaryocyte development is polyploidy, brought about by continued DNA replication in the absence of nuclear or cyto-

plasmic division. This process occurs following standard cell divisions necessary to expand the number of immediate megakaryocytic precursor cells, but prior to megakaryocyte cytoplasmic expansion and maturation (106). Although poorly understood for many years, the recent ability to produce large numbers of normal megakaryocytes in culture has begun to shed some light on this previously enigmatic process. Endomitosis is not simply the absence of mitosis but rather an abbreviated mitosis. Following typical, mitotic cell cycles, megakaryocytic progenitor cells enter the endo cycle, characterized by a short $G_1$ phase, a normal-length DNA-synthesis phase, a short $G_2$ phase, and an endomitosis phase (107). During the latter phase, megakaryocytic chromosomes condense, the nuclear membrane breaks down, and centrioles form mitotic spindles on which the replicated chromosomes assemble. However, following chromosomal separation, individual chromatids fail to migrate to opposite poles of the cell, the spindle dissociates, and the cell once again enters $G_1$ phase (108, 109). Attempts at biochemical analysis of this process have come from leukemic cell lines and normal cultured megakaryocytes.

An attractive hypothesis to explain endomitosis is a failure to form a normal mitosis promoting factor, recently identified as the cyclin B/cdc2 complex (110). This M phase kinase participates in several aspects of mitosis, including chromosomal condensation, nuclear membrane breakdown, and inhibition of previous phases of the cell cycle. It is of some interest that yeast strains, carrying temperature-sensitive mutations of either cyclin B or cdc2 homologues, undergo an extra round of DNA synthesis when grown at the nonpermissive temperature and then returned to the permissive temperature (111, 112). Working with the bipotential erythro/megakaryocytic cell line HEL, Long et al have found endomitotic cells to contain high levels of cyclin B, but to lack cdc2 (113). In contrast, Meg T cells, derived from transformation of murine marrow with a temperature-sensitive SV40 large T antigen, driven by a megakaryocyte-specific promoter, fail to produce cyclin B during their endomitotic phase (114). Thus both cell lines fail to express a functional mitotic kinase during endomitotic development, but by very different mechanisms.

In contrast to these findings, results from normal murine megakaryocytes argue for normal mitotic kinase activity during endomitosis. Using thrombopoietin to expand marrow cell cultures *in vitro*, two groups have provided evidence for the presence of both cyclin B and cdc2 in endomitotic megakaryocytes and for their associated kinase activity (109, 115). Although such studies are only in their infancy, it appears that other mechanisms are required to explain the absence of nuclear and cytoplasmic separation characteristic of megakaryocyte development.

## Cytoplasmic Maturation

Several investigators have identified both *cis*-acting genetic elements and *trans*-acting factors essential for the expression of MK-specific genes, providing beginning insights into the molecular mechanisms of lineage-specific differentiation. The promoters for the glycoprotein (GP) IIb, GP Ib, platelet factor 4 (PF 4), and mpl genes have been the focus of several recent studies. Most investigators have identified consensus sequences for both GATA-1 and members of the Ets family of transcription factors in the 5′ flanking regions of these genes, deletion of which reduces or eliminates reporter gene expression (116–120). However, in addition to their role in driving expression of some of the genes that underlie mature megakaryocyte and platelet function, GATA proteins appear to be an integral part of triggering the entire megakaryocytic developmental program.

The GATA family of transcription factors were first identified in erythroid cells and were initially althought to be specific for that lineage (121). However, further study revealed that megakaryocytes and mast cells also express the protein (122, 123). The first convincing evidence that GATA proteins may be essential for initiating megakaryocyte development came from studies of the myeloid leukemia cell line 416B. Forced expression of GATA1, but not the usually coexpressed protein SCL, lead to the megakaryocytic differentiation of these cells (124). More recently, a unique, GATA-1-altered mouse was reported in which *cis*-acting elements required for full GATA expression were modified, resulting in reduced but not absent expression of the protein (125). Unlike GATA-1 knockout mice, which die of erythroid failure (126), such "knockdown" animals are anemic, but survive, allowing analysis of the effects of GATA-1 deficiency on other lineages. In addition to the anemia, the mice are severely thrombocytopenic, and display normal to increased numbers of underdeveloped megakaryocytes (125). The cells undergo endomitosis, resulting in polyploid megakaryocytes, but cytoplasmic development is severely altered; the scant cytoplasm is deficient in demarcation membranes and platelet-specific granules and contains excess, rough endoplasmic reticulum and peripheral clear zones. Thus GATA-1 appears essential for postendomitotic MK cytoplasmic maturation.

A second transcription factor also appears to play an important role in the final stages of MK maturation. NF-E2 was initially described as a heterodimeric protein belonging to the basic leucine zipper family of transcription factors, which binds to tandem AP-1-like motifs in the second DNAse hypersensitive site of the β-globin locus control region (LCR) (127). Although the p18 subunit of NF-E2 is ubiquitously expressed, the p45 subunit is present exclusively in cells of the erythroid and megakaryocytic lineages. Due to its binding to elements of the β-globin LCR and the necessity of these elements

for expression of β-globin in transgenic mice and reporter gene analyses, an important erythroid role for NF-E2 was inferred. However, genetic elimination of p45 failed to affect erythropoiesis (128). Rather, p45 nullizygous mice display prominent alterations in megakaryocyte development. Although interbreeding of heterozygous p45 mice results in live births with the expected Mendelian ratios, nullizygous mice die soon after birth of widespread hemorrhage. The reason is absolute thrombocytopenia. Examination of the animals reveals a modest expansion of marrow megakaryocytes but a failure of the cells to produce platelets. Additional studies localize the NF-E2 defect to cytoplasmic maturation. Megakaryocytes from knockout mice proliferate normally in response to thrombopoietin; they become polyploid and express mpl, acetylcholinesterase, the megakaryocyte-specific marker 4A5 (althought to be GP V), platelet factor 4, and GP IIb. However, megakaryocytes from the knockout mice are deficient in platelet granules and platelet fields, the regions of megakaryocyte cytoplasm destined to become mature platelets. Thus the loss of either GATA-1 or NF-E2 results in a failure of late aspects of cellular maturation. The target genes on which these two transcription factors exert their effects on cellular maturation are not known; however, the availability of the GATA-1 knockdown and NF-E2 knockout mice should provide an opportunity to study this aspect of megakaryocyte development more fully.

## Platelet Formation

Platelets form by fragmentation of megakaryocyte cytoplasm. Following the completion of endomitosis, megakaryocyte cytoplasm expands and develops demarcation membranes and specific granules. Electron microscopic study of marrow megakaryocytes reveals this developmental process to occur in juxtaposition to sinusoidal endothelial cells. Fully mature megakaryocytes develop cytoplasmic extensions through the endothelial barrier into the sinusoidal lumen, where platelet-sized particles are released (129). It is also possible that the final stages of megakaryocyte fragmentation occur in the lung, at least for some megakaryocytes. Howell and Donahue reported many years ago that platelet levels in pulmonary venous blood exceed those found in the pulmonary artery, suggesting platelet production in the lung (130). Whether this represents the migration and fragmentation of intact megakaryocytes in the lung or merely the final size reduction of large fragments of megakaryocyte cytoplasm is not clear. Lung megakaryocytes have been characterized by Slater et al, who believe they contribute much to blood platelet production (131). However, in our recent preclinical studies of thrombopoietin in mice, we failed to detect any denuded megakaryocyte nuclei in the lungs of mice sacrificed with platelet counts as high as 4 million/mm³. Moreover, cultured megakaryocytes can form functional platelets *in vitro* in the absence of endothelial surfaces or the pulmonary circulation (see below). Thus the role of pulmonary bed platelet production remains controversial.

Although much is known of the morphologic basis of cytoplasmic fragmentation of megakaryocytic cytoplasm, little is understood of the molecular basis for the final stages of platelet release. These features are described more completely in Chapter 10, but the role of thrombopoietin in one aspect of this process has been explored and will be reviewed here.

The *in vitro* counterpart of platelet formation may be the development of proplatelet processes, long cytoplasmic exvaginations that occur toward the terminal phases of megakaryocyte cultures (88). These processes are believed to represent platelet formation as similar exvaginations of megakaryocyte cytoplasm are frequently observed *in vivo*, insinuating between marrow sinusoidal endothelial cells (129). Moreover, proplatelets break up into platelet-sized fragments, which both morphologically and functionally resemble normal blood platelets (88, 132). However, despite its importance in the growth and development of megakaryocytes and their progenitors, thrombopoietin does not appear to be essential for the final stages of megakaryocyte proplatelet formation and fragmentation (88) and has been reported to inhibit the process (133).

## THE EFFECTS OF MEGAKARYOCYTIC GROWTH FACTORS ON PLATELET FUNCTION

In addition to affecting the proliferation and differentiation of stem and progenitor cells, hematopoietic growth factors often affect the function of the mature cells they help to produce. This was first realized for GM-CSF; in addition to inducing the production of monocytes and neutrophils, the cytokine also primes these mature cell types to respond to previously sub-threshold levels of their normal activators. For example, GM-CSF enhances the neutrophil response to calcium ionophore, leukotrienes, or bacterial products. In a similar way, GM-CSF primes eosinophils and monocytes; IL-3 affects monocytes, basophils, and eosinophils; and M-CSF activates monocytes (134–140). It is believed that these effects may be responsible for the toxicity of these myelopoietic agents found in recent clinical trials. Comparable with these effects, proteins that stimulate thrombopoiesis may display the capacity to activate or prime platelet function. Many such studies have begun to appear on the effects of thrombopoietin on platelet activation.

Although little evidence suggests that thrombopoietin can act as a direct and independent platelet agonist,

several *ex vivo* studies have found synergistic effects of thrombopoietin on platelet aggregation or activation in response to ADP, other platelet agonists, or shear stress (141–145). Many of these studies measure the expression of P-selectin, an α-granule membrane protein that is expressed on the surface of activated platelets (99). Most but not all studies indicate that these effects to "prime" platelets to respond to subthreshold levels of other platelet agonists can be blocked with prostaglandin inhibitors. However, the physiologic relevance of these findings are not revealed by *in vitro* studies. Thus preclinical and clinical trials of the effects of thrombopoietic cytokines on platelet activation have attempted to address this potentially important issue.

Interleukin-6 has been evaluated for its effects on platelet activation *in vivo*. In both preclinical models and clinical trials, the cytokine was found to activate platelets directly and to heighten the sensitivity of platelets to physiologic agonists. Peng et al (146) administered 40 μg/kg/day human IL-6 to dogs and found that the dose of thrombin required to externalize P-selectin fell by more than 70%. Oleksowicz et al (147) have monitored the effects of IL-6 on platelet function in individuals who received the cytokine as treatment for cancer. They found evidence for platelet activation; maximal aggregatory response, platelet thromboxane production, and PF 4 release were all increased in response to standard platelet agonists, and glycoprotein (GP) IIb-IIIa internalization was also noted. Like the *in vitro* effects of thrombopoietin on platelet priming, these IL-6 effects were inhibitable with prostaglandin blockade (148). In contrast to the reported platelet activation with IL-6, a preclinical trial published in abstract form reports no effects of IL-11 on platelet morphology or activation *in vivo* (149). Using doses of the recombinant protein sufficient to increase the platelet count 150%, these investigators found no evidence of "platelet priming"; exteriorization of P-selectin in response to thrombin stimulation was identical in platelets derived from vehicle-treated and IL-11–treated animals. As IL-6 and IL-11 are althought to signal in precisely the same ways (see below), differences between IL-6 and IL-11 on platelet function might be related to differential receptor display on platelets, differences in the methodologies employed by these investigators, or differences in the dosing applied in the studies.

Peng et al (146) also reported on the platelet effects of thrombopoietin administration to dogs. In contrast to the proaggregatory effects of IL-6, thrombopoietin administration failed to alter platelet function, assessed by comparing thrombin dose-response curves for P-selectin exteriorization. In a more extensive study Harker et al (97) found that, although the use of thrombopoietin in dogs was associated with *in vitro* evidence of primed platelets, their deposition on an exteriorized vascular shunt was in proportion to the animals' platelet count. The authors concluded that, as long as the platelet count does not become excessively increased, the administration of thrombopoietin is unlikely to trigger pathologic thrombosis in individuals who receive it. However, given this growing body of preclinical data, clinical trials of the agent should pay particular attention to this aspect of its safety. In this regard the initial clinical experience has been favorable.

The expression of several platelet surface markers was examined during the administration of thrombopoietin to individuals in the initial clinical trials of the hormone (99, 150). GP Ib, the von Willebrand factor receptor, mediates the initial wave of platelet adhesion at sites of vascular injury (Chapter 11). Upon platelet activation the majority of GP Ib becomes inaccessible due to internalization. However, platelet GP Ib expression remained unchanged following the administration of 0.3 or 1.0 $\mu$g/kg/day of MGDF to seven individuals. Platelet aggregation is mediated by binding of fibrinogen to the $\beta_3$-integrin complex, GP IIb-IIIa (Chapter 11). The level of surface GP IIb-IIIa expression approximately doubles on platelet activation (151). In addition, platelet activation results in changes in the structure of the complex, mediated by cytoplasmic binding of $\beta 3$ endonexin (152), a conformational change that can be detected by the monoclonal antibody D3GP3 (153, 154). There were no changes in the surface expression of the GP IIb-IIIa complex, expression of its active conformation, or surface expression of P-selectin following administration of thrombopoietin. Thus there was no evidence for platelet activation occurring in response to thrombopoietin treatment.

Using *in vitro* assays, the platelets circulating in subjects treated with thrombopoietin also display normal function. Platelet aggregation and ATP release in response to ristocetin, thrombin-receptor agonist peptide, collagen, and ADP were virtually identical to that measured in the placebo controls either 24 hours after administration of thrombopoietin or on the final day of the study (99). The lack of change in both platelet function and platelet surface activation establishes that thrombopoietin induces the production of normal platelets.

## THE MOLECULAR MECHANISMS OF MEGAKARYOPOIETIC CYTOKINE ACTION

It is clear that a number of hematopoietic growth factors exert physiologic effects on hematopoietic stem and progenitor cells, allowing their development into platelet-producing megakaryocytes. Several important paradigms for hematopoietic-growth-factor action have emerged in recent years. First, as best exemplified by the work of Koury and Bondurant (155) with erythropoietin, is the capacity of growth factors to prevent developing cells from undergoing programmed cell death, or apoptosis. The withdrawal of erythropoietin from purified erythroid progenitor cells leads to DNA fragmentation; the presence of the hormone greatly reduces apoptosis (155), mediated in erythroid cells by *bcl-2* and *bcl-$x_L$* (156). A second important insight into the molecular mechanisms of growth factor action was gleaned from studies of M-CSF (or CSF-1) and IL-2. Initiation of DNA synthesis depends on activation of $G_1$ phase, cyclin-dependent kinases (cdks). The catalytic subunit of the cdks are present throughout the cell cycle in an inactive form. Kinase activity depends on the presence of a specific activator, members of the cyclin D family during $G_1$ phase (157), and elimination of inhibitors of the cyclin/kinase complex (158), small proteins termed p16Ink, p21 and p27. Hematopoietic growth factors affect both aspects of $G_1$ cdk activation. Transcription of the cyclin D gene is one of the earliest events that follows M-CSF binding to its receptor (159), and culture with IL-2 reduces levels of p27 (160). A complete description of the action of hematopoietic growth factors on megakaryocytic expansion will require a thorough understanding of how IL-3, KL, IL-6, IL-11, and thrombopoietin binding lead to suppression of apoptosis and initiation of the cell cycle.

The first step in hematopoietic growth factor action is binding to specific, cell-surface receptors. Recent study of many of these receptors has begun to provide initial molecular insights into cytokine-induced signaling. It is clear that protein tyrosine phosphorylation is an integral part of the cellular response to hematopoietic growth factor stimulation. For example, protein tyrosine kinase inhibitors block growth induced by many hematopoietic cytokines, and phosphatase inhibitors have the opposite effect (161, 162). However, neither the IL-3, IL-6, IL-11, nor thrombopoietin receptors contain any enzymatic activity. Rather, these receptors recruit cytoplasmic kinases to activate signaling molecules. The erythropoietin receptor was the first member of the hematopoietic cytokine receptor family shown to enlist and activate a member of the Janus family of cytoplasmic tyrosine kinases (JAKs). Subsequent work has shown that JAK kinases mediate much of the secondary protein tyrosine phosphorylation triggered by the binding of hematopoietic growth factors to their cognate receptors (163, 164). The role of other cytoplasmic kinases in growth factor-induced signaling such as the *src*-related kinases is also under active investigation (165, 166). Although many of the signals involved in thrombopoietic cytokine action are rapidly being identified, major challenges lie ahead in deciphering the molecular basis of signal specificity. For example, the cellular response generated on thrombopoietin binding is distinct from that originating at the IL-3 receptor, but many of the same molecules are activated on binding of both cytokines (see below). The answer may lie in the identification of molecules that lend specificity to the particular combination of JAKs and STATs (signal transduction and activators of transcription), activated by each receptor (167). A thorough analysis of the specific patterns of signaling intermediates orchestrated by each of the cytokines, which act directly on megakaryocytes, will be required to more fully understand the role played by each during thrombopoiesis.

The IL-3 receptor is composed of two distinct subunits, a polypeptide specific for IL-3 (IL-3R$\alpha$) and a molecule common to the IL-3, GM-CSF, and IL-5 receptors (termed $\beta_C$). IL-3R$\alpha$ binds IL-3 with low affinity; recruitment of $\beta_C$ enhances ligand affinity and leads to signaling. The stoichiometry of this process for GM-CSF binding has recently been discerned. On ligand binding to GM-CSFR$\alpha$, a preformed $\beta_C$ homodimer is recruited to the complex resulting in $\beta_C$-induced signal transduction (168). It is thus very likely that similar events occur on IL-3 binding to IL-3R$\alpha$. In addition, once the IL-3R$\alpha$ chain interacts with $\beta_C$, a disulfide bond stabilizes the complex and induces signaling (169).

Like the IL-3 receptor, the IL-6, IL-11, and LIF receptors are each composed of two subunits. The IL-6R$\alpha$, IL-11R$\alpha$, and LIFR bind their respective ligands with low affinity, but these events alone are not sufficient to transduce a proliferative or differentiative signal. All three receptors utilize the gp130 polypeptide as an affinity conversion and signaling subunit. Ligand binding leads to dimerization of the signaling subunits; either homodimerization of gp130 by IL-6 or IL-11, or heterodimerization of gp130 with the LIFR for LIF (170, 171). It is likely that the signals induced by these cytokines are identical, at least for IL-6 and IL-11. In addition to their use of a common signaling subunit, the soluble forms of their receptors, which lack cytoplasmic domains, signal as well as the corresponding full-length receptors do (at least as far as has been tested) (172, 173), thus eliminating a role for the distinct cytoplasmic domains of the receptor $\alpha$ chains. Thus, since megakaryocytes display gp130, IL-6R$\alpha$, and IL-11R$\alpha$ (149, 174), it is likely that IL-6 induces an identical response in megakaryocytes as IL-11. Experimental evidence for this view is accumulating in both hepatic and nonhepatic cells (175).

In contrast to these heterodimeric receptors, the mplreceptor polypeptide alone appears sufficient for thrombopoietin signaling; the receptor does not utilize the gp130, $\beta_C$, or IL-2R$\gamma$ polypeptides as a coreceptor (176, 177), and mplreceptor homodimerization leads to proliferative signaling (178, 179).

Many studies of IL-3 receptor signaling have been completed. As noted above, IL-3 receptor engagement by its ligand leads to the dimerization of the signaling subunit, $\beta_C$, on the membrane of the cell. The hematopoietic cytokine receptors do not possess any enzymatic activities. Nevertheless, within seconds of binding ligand these receptors and a number of other cytoplasmic proteins become tyrosine phosphorylated. Multiple studies have indicated this to be accomplished by members of the JAK family of cytoplasmic tyrosine kinases, which bind constitutively to the cytoplasmic domain of the receptor through the box1 and box2 motifs (164, 180). Once two molecules of JAK kinase are brought together by ligand-induced receptor dimerization, the JAKs are cross-phosphorylated, thereby increasing kinase activity and leading to the phosphorylation of a number of tethered substrates, and the receptor itself. Of the Janus kinases, most studies have identified JAK2 as interacting with the membrane proximal region of the $\beta_C$ subunit of the IL-3 receptor (181–183). Once activated, JAK2 phosphorylates a number of other substrates. Among the best studied are the STAT family of proteins. There are presently at least seven distinct STAT family members, STAT1 through STAT4, STAT5a, STAT5b, and STAT6, most of which do not appear to be receptor-specific. For example, although STAT 5 was initially recognized as a response element of the prolactin receptor, it has now been shown to associate with and contribute to *in vitro* signaling from the erythropoietin, IL-3, thrombopoietin, and many other receptors (164, 184–188). However, these conclusions are based primarily on results from *in vitro* experiments using transformed cell lines. A more rigorous test of these conclusions should be based on studies of normal cell populations (189) and the phenotypes of individual STAT knockout mice, experiments that are currently under way.

Signal specificity is althought to depend on the entire spectrum of membrane-bound and cytoplasmic intermediates modified by ligand binding, rather than on activation of a single signaling molecule. As their name implies, STATs are transcription factors. However, in the dephosphorylated form they are latent; only on JAK-mediated phosphorylation do STAT proteins dimerize by virtue of their SH2 domains (which are also responsible for their recruitment to the receptor) and then translocate to the nucleus where they bind to the promoters of cytokine responsive genes (163). The STAT proteins also appear to require phosphorylation on serine or threonine for activation (185, 190, 191), possibly mediated by MAP kinases (192) (see below). Nearly every study of IL-3 signaling implicates STAT5 as the primary if not exclusive STAT family member activated (184, 186, 187). Unfortunately, the targets of IL-3 activated STAT5 are not yet known, and much work remains to determine the molecular mechanisms of IL-3–induced proliferation. It should also be noted that an *in vivo* role for STAT5 in hematopoiesis has not yet been established.

Additional substrates that are phosphorylated and activated on IL-3 binding include Raf-1, a serine/threonine kinase that initiates the MAP kinase cascade (193), MAP kinases (194, 195), Shc (196–199), Grb2 (196, 200),

**TABLE 8.1.**   Signaling Intermediates Identified for the Megakaryopoietic Cytokines

| | JAKs | STATs | Adaptors | PI3K | MAPK | Others |
|---|---|---|---|---|---|---|
| IL-3 | JAK2[181–183] | STATS[184, 186, 187, 239] | Grb2[196] | p85[183, 200, 202] | Raf-1[193] MAPK[194,195] | bcl-2[205] fes[183] vav[201] fyn, hck[203] lyn[183, 203, 204] |
| SF | JAK2[211] | STAT3[215] | Grb2[196] | p85[202, 208, 212, 213] | Raf-1[212] MAPK[194, 195] | FAK[214] vav[201, 216] cbl[217] PLCγ[212] |
| IL-6/IL-11 | JAK1[206, 218] JAK2[206, 218, 220] JYK2[206, 218] | STAT1[224, 225] STAT3[219, 226] | Grb2[228, 230] Shc[228] | p85[227] | MAPK[229, 230] | vav[230] NF-IL-6[231] yes[254] hck[255] btk, tek[256] |
| TPO | JAK[185, 189, 235–237, 239–241] TYK[189, 236, 241] | STAT3[185, 189, 239, 241] STAT5[185, 188, 189, 239, 241, 242] | Grb2[239] Shc[239–241, 244, 246, 252] | p85[141] | Raf-1[243] MAPK[239, 243, 245] | sos[240] vav[239–241] cbl[240, 241] |

Vav (201), and PI 3 kinase (183, 200, 202). In addition, a number of other kinases are activated in response to IL-3 binding, including fes (183), fyn (203), hck (203), and lyn (183, 203, 204). Finally, JAK-independent transcriptional up-regulation and activation of the proto-oncogenes *c-myc* and *bcl-2* occurs following IL-3 signaling (197, 205). However, none of these signaling molecules appear to be specific to IL-3-induced stimulation, and the role of each of these proteins in megakaryocytic cell survival and proliferation cannot be discerned at this time; only by gain of function and loss-of-function strategies can the importance of individual molecules be assessed. A summary of the signaling molecules activated by IL-3 and other megakaryopoietic cytokines is presented in Table 8.1. These results must be viewed in their proper context, the use of purified cytokines to induce proliferation of a large number of very different leukemic cell lines. The heterogeneity of conclusions that derive from such an approach is apparent in the report of Stahl et al (206). Studying the response to IL-6, these authors report three different patterns of activation of JAK kinase family members in three different cell lines. Unfortunately, very few studies report on the signaling molecules activated in primary cells, the most relevant source for study, and in contrast to multiple studies of cytokine-induced proliferation, investigators are only now beginning to address the pathways involved in megakaryocytic differentiation.

The signaling cascades initiated by IL-3 binding are of limited duration. Multiple mechanisms to govern this process must exist. One such mechanism depends on dephosphorylation of the IL-3 receptor. Following JAK2-mediated receptor activation, the hematopoietic cell phosphatase (HCP, also termed SHPTP1) binds to the $\beta_C$ subunit and dephosphorylates the IL-3 receptor. Overexpression of the phosphatase is associated with diminished, IL-3-induced proliferation (207), strongly suggesting that this mechanism serves to limit ligand-induced signaling. A similar mechanism has been shown to limit erythropoietin-induced signaling; genetic elimination of the site of phosphatase binding leads to congenital erythrocytosis.

Although the SF receptor, c-kit, contains an intrinsic tyrosine kinase activity and bears no homology to any of the other hematopoietic receptors under discussion, its signaling pathway is very similar to that induced by the IL-3 receptor. On binding of SF, the c-kit receptor dimerizes, cross-phosphorylating its cytoplasmic domains on tyrosine (208–210). However, additional kinases are also activated on c-kit binding of SF, including JAK2 (211), PI-3 kinase (202, 212, 213), and focal adhesion kinase (FAK) (214). The role of the STATs in c-kit signaling is somewhat different from that found with IL-3 or the other hematopoietic receptor family members. Whereas IL-3, IL-6, IL-11, and TPO all induce tyrosine phosphorylation of various STATs, engagement of the c-kit receptor leads to serine phosphorylation only (215). Activation of c-kit leads to recruitment of a number of adapter molecules to the signaling complex, including Shc and Grb2 (196, 199), Vav (216) and Cbl (217), and to activation of the Raf/MAP kinase pathway (194, 195, 212) and PL-Cγ (212). Unfortunately, little is known of the downstream targets activated or suppressed by engagement of these signaling pathways.

Like other members of the hematopoietic cytokine receptor family, gp130, the signaling component of the IL-6 and IL-11 receptors, does not possess any obvious enzymatic activities. Nevertheless, within seconds of binding of IL-6 or IL-11 to its receptor complex gp130 becomes phosphorylated on specific tyrosine residues. The gp130 subunit has been shown to bind JAK1, JAK2, and TYK2, depending on the cell line utilized (206). Once two of these kinases are brought together by ligand-induced gp130 dimerization, JAK1 becomes cross-phosphorylated by either JAK2 or TYK2 (218–220), increasing its activity and leading to the phosphorylation of multiple cytoplasmic substrates, including several tyrosine residues of gp130 itself. The gp130 molecule then acts, like the $\beta_C$ of the IL-3 receptor, as a scaffold on which a complex of signaling molecules assemble. For the gp130-related cytokines, the concept has emerged that distinct signaling intermediates subserve specific cellular processes. For example, by generating truncation mutants of the receptor, Murakami et al (221) demonstrated that only the membrane-proximal 61 residues (which includes the box1 and box2 motifs) are required for gp130-induced proliferation in leukemic cell lines. However, additional regions (box3) are required for gp 130-induced differentiation. The middle third of the gp130 cytoplasmic domain contains YXXQ (where Y = tyrosine, X = any amino acid, and Q = glutamine) and NXXY (where N = asparagine) motifs. When phosphorylated, these sequences serve as docking sites for molecules containing SH2 domains (222, 223). Among the important substrates that interact with these more distal cytoplasmic regions of the receptor are STAT1 and STAT3 (219, 224–226) and the adapter proteins Grb2 and Shc, which are then phosphorylated by the JAK kinases bound to gp130 (224, 227, 228).

On phosphorylation, STAT1 and STAT3 both homodimerize and heterodimerize via their phosphotyrosine residues, bind to each others' SH2 domains to form three distinct complexes (164), and acquire the capacity to translocate to the nucleus and bind to a specific DNA sequence (for STAT3 dimers, a type 2 IL-6 response element, CTGGGA). Among the hepatic genes althought to be activated by STAT3 are fibrinogen, α1-acid glycoprotein, T-kininogen, α2-macroglobulin, C-reactive protein, and haptoglobin (224). Much less is known about megakaryocytic genes that might possess binding sites for STAT3 dimers, or the role of STAT1 in gp130-mediated processes.

The second pathway by which gp130 signaling affects gene transcription is initiated by the phosphorylation of Grb2 and Shc. These proteins contain multiple docking motifs, allowing them to serve as bridging molecules, thereby bringing together and activating arrays of proteins. One such target of gp130-activated Grb2 and Shc is the Ras/MAPK signaling pathway (228–230). Although the complete details have not yet been elucidated, it is presently althought that recruitment of membrane-bound Ras alters the ratio of bound GTP to GDP, activating a cascade of signaling intermediates, including Raf-1, MAP kinase kinase, and MAP kinase. When activated, MAP kinase phosphorylates NF-IL-6 on serine/threonine residues (231), a nuclear transcription factor that then becomes competent to bind and activate type 1 IL-6 response elements (T[T/G]NNGNAA[T/G]), which are present in several hepatic (α1-acid glycoprotein, hemopexin, C-reactive protein, and haptoglobin) (227) and macrophage (G-CSF, tumor necrosis factor, IL-1, IL-6, IL-8, lysozyme, and nitric oxide synthetase) (232–234) gp130-responsive genes. As for the STAT pathway, less is known of megakaryocytic targets of gp130-induced NF-IL-6 activation. However, even at this elementary stage of understanding of IL-3 and IL-6/IL-11/LIF signaling, it is tempting to speculate that distinct pathways are utilized by cytokines that support primarily a proliferative response (e.g., IL-3) and those that induce predominantly differentiative events (e.g., IL-6/IL-11) in megakaryocytes.

Although only recently cloned, progress has been rapid in deciphering the pathways by which thrombopoietin signals. Because of the homology between erythropoietin and thrombopoietin, and between mpl and the rest of the cytokine receptor family, initial studies of how mpl signals concentrated on the JAK and STAT families of proteins. The first reports focused on leukemic cell lines that naturally express the mpl receptor, or ones engineered to do so. These studies identified JAK2 and TYK2 as the immediate kinases which bind to mpl and become activated on exposure to thrombopoietin (185, 189, 235–241). Whether both of these kinases are essential for signaling is not yet clear. Other proteins reported in various megakaryocytic cell lines to be phosphorylated in response to thrombopoietin include STAT3 and STAT5 (185, 188, 189, 239, 241, 242); the adapter proteins Grb2 (239), Vav (239–241), Cbl (240, 241), and SOS (240); Shc and its related phosphatase SHIP (189, 239–241, 244); the Raf-1/MAP kinase (239, 243, 245); and hematopoietic cytokine receptor-related phosphatases such as SHPTP-2 (239).

Several lines of evidence are consistent with the hypothesis that cytokine-induced megakaryocyte differentiation is supported by activation of STAT3 and Shc. First, the sites at which these signaling intermediates bind to mpl colocalize, but are distinct from the predominant STAT5 binding site. STAT5 activation persists if the membrane proximal 69 residues of mpl are intact, even when both of the endogenous tyrosine residues in this region are mutated to phenylalanine (242). In contrast, STAT3 and Shc dock to one of the two terminal tyrosine residues at positions 112 or 117 of the murine mpl receptor cytoplasmic domain (242, 246). These results are consistent with previous findings indicating that recognition elements for STAT3 and STAT5 are distinct (247). Second, a dominant negative form of STAT5 blocks IL-3-induced proliferation (184, 248), but a dominant negative form of Shc inhibits mpl-induced differentiation, albeit in 32DM.2 cells, which can only differentiate along a granulocytic pathway (244). A recent study also supports the role of Shc in mpl-induced differentiation of WEHI3B-D cells (246), and deletion of the region of the mpl receptor that binds STAT3 and Shc (residues 101-116) eliminated thrombopoietin-induced differentiation of UT-7/Epo cells in which the mpl receptor was expressed (249). Third, deletion of residues 71–94 eliminates the capacity of the mpl receptor to induce differentiation toward the megakaryocyte lineage (induction of GP Ib and IIb-IIIa) in UT-7 cells, but not their proliferation in response to thrombopoietin (250). This same region also inhibits thrombopoietin-induced proliferation of BaF3 cells (242), consistent with the common observation that differentiation requires the cessation of proliferation. Fourth, although cell lines that proliferate in response to thrombopoietin display prominent phosphorylation of both STAT3 and STAT5, highly polyploid normal megakaryocytes have lost most of their capacity to activate STAT5 (189). Fifth, gp130-related cytokines, which promote differentiation rather than proliferation of megakaryocytes, activate STAT3 rather than STAT5 (219, 224, 247). In contrast, IL-3, which only supports the proliferation of megakaryocytes, predominantly activates STAT5 (186, 187). Finally, 32D cells, which proliferate in response to IL-3 and partially differentiate in response to thrombopoietin, display a predominance of STAT5 activation over STAT3 in IL-3 but a predominance of STAT3 phosphorylation over STAT5 in thrombopoietin (239). Although consistent with the hypothesis that STAT3 and Shc are responsible for megakaryocytic differentiation, it must be remembered that different cell lines possess varying capacities for thrombopoietin-induced proliferation and differentiation. Thus, as with signaling studies done with other hematopoietic cytokines in transformed cells, the properties of each cell line should be carefully considered when interpreting these results (e.g., all of the "thrombopoietin-induced differentiation" in the above studies was actually myeloid differentiation in myeloid leukemic cell lines expressing c-mpl). Ideally, the profile of signaling molecules displayed by normal cells during various stages of megakaryocytic development should be sought.

The nature of thrombopoietin signaling in mature platelets has also been explored (144, 251–253) and reveals that the hormone stimulates the phosphorylation

and activation of JAK2, STAT3, and STAT5. As the hormone has been shown to prime platelets for an enhanced response to classical platelet agonists, future studies are concentrating on how these signaling intermediates might participate in the pathways of platelet activation. An obvious target for such studies is the recently cloned β3 endonexin molecule, a cytoplasmic protein that enhances the affinity of the GP IIb-IIIa complex for fibrinogen in activated platelets (152).

Finally, although most recent studies of the molecular mechanisms of signaling by the hematopoietic cytokines have focused on the JAK family of protein tyrosine kinases, it should be emphasized that several other src-related kinases have been shown to associate with hematopoietic receptors, including the btk, tec, yes, and hck kinases with the gp130 family of cytokine receptors (254–256) and the fyn, lyn, fes, and hck kinases with the IL-3 receptor (166, 183, 257). Although these molecules do not appear to be required for mitogenesis in response to cytokine stimulation, the role that these molecules play in transducing other critical signals initiated by cytokine binding will only come from continued study.

## THE THROMBOPOIETIC RESPONSE TO THROMBOCYTOPENIA

The induction of acute immune-mediated thrombocytopenia results in a relatively rapid restoration of platelet levels followed by a brief period of rebound thrombocytosis (258–263). As discussed previously, the plasma substance posited to be responsible for recovery was termed thrombopoietin 40 years ago (41). With the recent cloning of the mpl ligand investigators sought to test this tenet. In both acute, antibody-mediated and myelosuppressive therapy-induced thrombocytopenia, plasma concentrations of mpl ligand vary inversely with platelet counts, rising to maximal levels within 24 hours of the onset of profound thrombocytopenia (87, 264–266). Two models have been advanced to explain the inverse relationship between platelet count and thrombopoietin levels. In the first, thrombopoietin production is constitutive, but its consumption, and hence the level remaining in the blood to affect megakaryopoiesis, is determined by the mass of mpl receptors (i.e., platelets and megakaryocytes) accessible to the plasma (267, 268). In this way, states of thrombocytosis result in increased thrombopoietin consumption (by the expanded platelet mass of mpl receptors), reducing megakaryopoiesis. Conversely, thrombocytopenia reduces peripheral blood thrombopoietin destruction, resulting in elevated blood levels of the hormone, which drive megakaryopoiesis and platelet recovery. This model is based on one advanced for the regulation of M-CSF levels by monocyte uptake and destruction (269). The weight of current evidence supports an important role for this mechanism in the regulation of thrombopoietin production. First, platelets bear mpl receptors (76), which can deplete plasma of thrombopoietin (267). Second, thrombopoietin mRNA levels in the liver and kidney, the two most prominent tissue sources of specific transcripts, do not vary in states of profound thrombocytopenia or thrombocytosis (268, 270, 271). Third, transfusion of normal platelets into thrombocytopenic mpl receptor-deficient mice, which display high thrombopoietin levels, temporarily depresses these levels until thrombocytopenia returns (267). Finally, thrombopoietin knockout mice display a gene dosage effect (272); platelet levels in heterozygous mice are intermediate between the wild type and nullizygous animals, suggesting that active regulation of the remaining thrombopoietin locus cannot compensate for the reduced level of mRNA derived from the remaining normal allele.

An alternative model suggests that thrombopoietin expression is a regulated event; low platelet levels can induce enhanced mRNA production. Evidence for this model of thrombopoietin regulation has been slower to develop. However, two studies argue that mRNA levels are modulated in response to thrombocytopenia, at least in the marrow. By using a semiquantitative assay of thrombopoietin transcripts, McCarty et al found increased thrombopoietin-specific mRNA in the marrow of mice made thrombocytopenic by both immune and myelosuppressive methods (270). As noted above, mRNA levels in the liver and kidney in these experiments were unaffected by severe thrombocytopenia in both sets of animals. These findings were confirmed in a more recent study utilizing *in situ* hybridization; marrow but not liver or kidney mRNA signals were increased in individuals with thrombocytopenia (273). However, the relative importance of thrombopoietin gene regulation in the marrow is presently uncertain.

In addition to the modulation of thrombopoietin concentration in response to alterations in platelet count, levels of many of the other cytokines found to affect megakaryocyte production have been investigated in conditions of altered platelet production. IL-3 has not been detected in any states other than severe immunologic reactions, appearing to minimize its role in the modulation of platelet homeostasis. IL-6 levels rise in states of inflammation, but do not vary with immune-mediated thrombocytopenia (72). However, in some individuals, its levels have been shown to correlate with tumor-induced thrombocytosis (274–276). KL levels are detectable in the plasma of normal persons (~ 3 ng/ml) (30), but are not modulated in states of pancytopenia (277). In contrast, both FL and IL-11 levels have been reported to vary inversely with platelet counts (265, 278), although FL levels have only been reported in states of pancytopenia, not isolated thrombocytopenia. However, these results argue that mechanisms in addition to variation in thrombopoietin levels may contribute to the regulation of thrombopoiesis.

## mpl AND PATHOLOGIC ASPECTS OF HEMATOPOIESIS

Two general categories of pathologic thrombocytosis can be identified: those cases with normal megakaryocytes, including both reactive and tumor-associated thrombocytosis, and those in which platelet production is likely independent of humoral influences, the myeloproliferative stem cell disorders. Although the cause of both classes of thrombocytosis are only poorly understood, some correlative data are available for the former group. Most of the published cases of reactive thrombocytosis are reported to involve IL-6. Individuals with thrombocytosis and rheumatoid arthritis, psoriasis, and many solid tumors (mesothelioma, lung and ovarian carcinoma) often display elevated levels of IL-6 (274, 275, 279–282). However, thrombocytosis in these individuals may be more complex; the degree of thrombocytosis does not correlate with the IL-6 level, and the concentrations found in such individuals are rarely as high as those found necessary to produce thrombocytosis when the exogenous cytokine is administered to individuals (283, 284).

Although surprisingly little data are available on the levels of thrombopoietin in individuals with inflammatory conditions, an initial report suggests that elevated levels of the hormone are an infrequent cause of reactive thrombocytosis (285). However, this report covered only six individuals; many more cases need to be reported before this conclusion can be considered rigorous.

Multiple lines of evidence indicate that megakaryocytes are part of the neoplastic clone in individuals with myeloproliferative and myelodysplastic syndromes. Therefore, should thrombocytosis arise in these individuals, it is likely that the loss of thrombopoietic control would reside within the abnormal megakaryocyte itself. However, it is distinctly possible that the mpl receptor is directly or indirectly involved in the pathophysiology of these disorders. Several lines of evidence support this concept. First, the thrombopoietin receptor was first identified as a viral oncogene, *v-mpl*, the cause of an acute myeloproliferative syndrome in mice (75). In addition, factor-independent growth of cells expressing single amino acid substitutions of *c-mpl* have been described (179, 286), raising the possibility that naturally occurring mutations of the gene might be identified as part of a neoplastic process. Second, the chronic expression of thrombopoietin in murine marrow cells *in vivo* leads to a chronic hematologic disease reminiscent of essential thrombocythemia, with extramedullary hematopoiesis and myelofibrosis (287). Third, fresh marrow cells from a substantial proportion of individuals with chronic myelodysplastic, myeloproliferative syndromes or acute leukemia display mpl receptors on their surface, and many of these cells proliferate in response to exogenous thrombopoietin (Table 8.2) (79, 288–293). Fourth, marrow and peripheral blood hematopoietic progeni-

**TABLE 8.2.**   The Role of mpl in Myeloproliferative Disorders

| Reference | n | % mpl⁺ | | | % Tpo-Induced Growth | % Tpo⁺ | Comments |
|-----------|---|-----|-----|-----|------------------|--------|----------|
| | | AML | MDS | MPS | | | |
| 79 | 67 | 51 | 31 | | | | M1–M7 |
| 288[a] | 50 | 52 | | | 85 | | Short-term culture |
| 289[a] | 15 | | | | 27 | | Long-term culture |
| 290 | 20 | 75 | | | 55 | | M1–M5, M7 |
| 291 | 21 | 60 | | | 23 | | M2, M7 |
| 292[a] | 50 | 54 | | | | 36 | RT-PCR [CM⁻] |
| 293 | 15 | | | 100 | | 0 | spont col forming AS reduced col |

*n, number of individuals with myeloid phenotype; M1–M7, FAB classification of acute leukemia; rt-PCR [CM⁻], indicates that although these cases were positive by the reverse-transcriptase polymerase chain reaction method, the conditioned culture medium did not contain detectable thrombopoietin by biological assay; spont col forming AS reduced col, indicates that antisense oligodeoxynucleotides to c-mpl eliminated spontaneous colony formation in this study.*

[a] *It is unclear if these three reports represent overlapping individual samples.*

tors from individuals with myeloproliferative disorders often grow in culture in the absence of exogenous growth factors. Such "spontaneous colony growth" is a useful diagnostic marker for many of these disorders. Of considerable interest, antisense inhibition of *c-mpl* eliminated spontaneous colony formation in all nine individuals studied with mpl⁺ myeloproliferative disorders in one recent report (293). Additional studies in which gain-of-function or loss-of-function intervention strategies are employed will be required to firmly establish a role for the mpl receptor in neoplastic hematopoiesis.

In addition to these instances of mpl involvement in multiple myeloproliferative disorders, a special case for a role for thrombopoietin in essential thrombocythemia can be made. It is presently felt that a majority of the regulation of thrombopoietin levels can be accounted for by platelet and megakaryocyte uptake and destruction of the hormone (267, 268, 271, 272). If so, then a defect in that process could account for a resetting of the steady-state platelet level seen in essential thrombocythemia. The somewhat higher levels of thrombopoietin responsible for this process would not have to be large; as the platelet count climbs, a new rate of thrombopoietin destruction is achieved, bringing about a new steady-state level of the hormone. In support of this hypothesis is the finding that thrombopoietin levels in individuals with essential thrombocythemia are somewhat higher than normal (285), especially when viewed in the context of the extremely high platelet counts present in these individuals. However, other than the thrombocytosis, this hypothesis does not account for the other manifestations of essential thrombocythemia, the thrombotic tendency or impaired platelet function of many of these individuals, the spontaneous colony formation, or the multilineage nature of the disease. Clearly, additional work in this interesting field

will be necessary to more clearly define the role of thrombopoietin and its receptor in essential thrombocythemia.

## FUTURE DIRECTIONS

Thrombopoietin has moved from theory to reality and from cloning to the clinic in just 3 short years. With it has come a new era in our understanding of thrombopoiesis. Although much has now been learned about the production, cellular effects, and *in vivo* biology of many of the cytokines and hormones that affect this process, many important physiologic questions remain. For example, what is the relative importance of local marrow thrombopoietin production compared with that derived from the circulating pool, what property of thrombocytopenia is responsible for the marrow regulation of IL-11 and thrombopoietin, what molecular intermediates are unique to mpl receptor signaling and are they permissive or directive for cellular differentiation, and what is the molecular basis for the synergy shown between thrombopoietin and the other cytokines that affect megakaryocyte proliferation and differentiation? The availability of these hormones and cytokines has also opened new windows into the physiology of the megakaryocyte, allowing investigators to study what distinguishes the erythroid from the megakaryocytic program of differentiation and to determine the molecular mechanisms that underlie endomitosis and cytoplasmic fragmentation. We can now reexamine the pathophysiology of both benign and malignant myeloproliferation, hopefully providing new diagnostic insights and therapeutic opportunities. The answers to these and other previously unapproachable physiologic and pathologic questions of megakaryocyte and platelet biology and the results from clinical trials of these agents in individuals with iatrogenic or natural states of marrow failure are eagerly awaited. The cloning of thrombopoietin was an important step in our understanding of megakaryopoiesis, but many more important questions remain.

# REFERENCES

1. Gordon MS, Hoffman R. Growth factors affecting human thrombocytopoiesis: potential agents for the treatment of thrombocytopenia [Editorial]. Blood 1992;80:302–307.
2. Kaushansky K. The thrombocytopenia of cancer. Prospects for effective cytokine therapy. Hematol Oncol Clin North Am 1996;10:431–455.
3. Till JE, McCulloch EA. A direct measurement of the radiation sensitivity of normal mouse bone marrow cells. Radiat Res 1961;14:213–222.
4. Pluznik DH, Sachs L. The cloning of normal "mast" cells in tissue culture. J Cell Physiol 1965;66:319–324.
5. Bradley TR, Metcalf D. The growth of mouse bone marrow cells *in vitro*. Aust J Exp Biol Med Sci 1966;44:287–299.
6. Ogawa M. Differentiation and proliferation of hematopoietic stem cells. Blood 1993;81:2844–2853.
7. Kieran MW, Perkins AC, Orkin SH et al. Thrombopoietin rescues *in vitro* erythroid colony formation from mouse embryos lacking erythropoietin receptor. Proc Natl Acad Sci U S A 1996;93:9126–9131.
8. Emerson SG, Thomas S, Ferrara JL et al. Developmental regulation of erythropoiesis by hematopoietic growth factors: analysis on populations of BFU-E from bone marrow, peripheral blood, and fetal liver. Blood 1989; 74:49–55.
9. Dai CH, Krantz SB, Zsebo KM. Human burst-forming units-erythroid need direct interaction with stem cell factor for further development. Blood 1991;78:2493–2497.
10. Witte ON. Steel locus defines new multipotent growth factor. Cell 1990; 63:5–6.
11. Williams N, Eger RR, Jackson HM et al. Two-factor requirement for murine megakaryocyte colony formation. J Cell Physiol 1982;110:101–104.
12. Long MW, Gragowski LL, Heffner CH et al. Phorbol diesters stimulate the development of an early murine progenitor cell. The burst-forming unit-megakaryocyte. J Clin Invest 1985;76:431–438.
13. McDonald TP, Sullivan PS. Megakaryocytic and erythrocytic cell lines share a common precursor cell. Exp Hematol 1993;21:1316–1320.
14. Hunt P. A bipotential megakaryocyte/erythrocyte progenitor cell: the link between erythropoiesis and megakaryopoiesis becomes stronger [Editorial]. J Lab Clin Med 1995;125:303–304.
15. Papayannopoulou T, Brice M, Farrer D et al. Insights into the cellular mechanisms of erythropoietin-thrombopoietin synergy. Exp Hematol 1996;24:660–669.
16. Debili N, Coulombel L, Croisille L et al. Characterization of a bipotent erythro-megakaryocytic progenitor in human bone marrow. Blood 1996; 88:1284–1296.
17. Kaushansky K, O'Hara PJ, Berkner K et al. Genomic cloning, characterization, and multilineage growth-promoting activity of human granulocyte-macrophage colony-stimulating factor. Proc Natl Acad Sci U S A 1986;83: 3101–3105.
18. Segal GM, Stueve T, Adamson JW. Analysis of murine megakaryocyte colony size and ploidy: effects of interleukin-3. J Cell Physiol 1988;137: 537–544.
19. Briddell RA, Bruno E, Cooper RJ et al. Effect of c-kit ligand on *in vitro* human megakaryocytopoiesis. Blood 1991;78:2854–2859.
20. Yang YC, Ciarletta AB, Temple PA et al. Human IL-3 (multi-CSF): identification by expression cloning of a novel hematopoietic growth factor related to murine IL-3. Cell 1986;47:3–10.
21. Wong GG, Witek JS, Temple PA et al. Human GM-CSF: molecular cloning of the complementary DNA and purification of the natural and recombinant proteins. Science 1985;228:810–815.
22. Diederichs K, Boone T, Karplus PA. Novel fold and putative receptor binding site of granulocyte-macrophage colony-stimulating factor. Science 1991;254:1779–1782.
23. Feng Y, Klein BK, Vu L et al. $^1$H, $^{13}$C, and $^{15}$N NMR resonance assignments, secondary structure, and backbone topology of a variant of human interleukin-3. Biochemistry 1995;34:6540–6551.
24. Bazan JF. Genetic and structural homology of stem cell factor and macrophage colony–stimulating factor [Letter]. Cell 1991;65:9–10.
25. Lyman SD, James L, Vanden Bos T et al. Molecular cloning of a ligand for the flt3/flk-2 tyrosine kinase receptor: a proliferative factor for primitive hematopoietic cells. Cell 1993;75:1157–1167.
26. Flanagan JG, Leder P. The kit ligand: a cell surface molecule altered in steel mutant fibroblasts. Cell 1990;63:185–194.
27. Martin FH, Suggs SV, Langley KE et al. Primary structure and functional expression of rat and human stem cell factor. Cell 1990;63:203–210.
28. Huang E, Nocka K, Beier DR et al. The hematopoietic growth factor KL is encoded by the Sl locus and is the ligand of the c-kit receptor, the gene product of the W locus. Cell 1990;63:225–233.
29. Anderson DM, Lyman SD, Baird A et al. Molecular cloning of mast cell growth factor, a hemopoietin that is active in both membrane bound and soluble forms. Cell 1990;63:235–243.
30. Langley KE, Bennett LG, Wypych J et al. Soluble stem cell factor in human serum. Blood 1993;81:656–660.
31. Flanagan JG, Chan DC, Leder P. Transmembrane form of the kit ligand growth factor is determined by alternative splicing and is missing in the Sl$^d$ mutant. Cell 1991;64:1025–1035.
32. Cheng HJ, Flanagan JG. Transmembrane kit ligand cleavage does not require a signal in the cytoplasmic domain and occurs at a site dependent on spacing from the membrane. Mol Biol Cell 1994;5:943–953.
33. Miyazawa K, Williams DA, Gotoh A et al. Membrane bound steel factor induces more persistent tyrosine kinase activation and longer life span of c-kit gene–encoded protein than its soluble form. Blood 1995;85:641–649.
34. Lyman SD, James L, Johnson L et al. Cloning of the human homologue of the murine flt3 ligand: a growth factor for early hematopoietic progenitor cells. Blood 1994;83:2795–2801.
35. Hudak S, Hunte B, Culpepper J et al. Flt3/flk2 ligand promotes the growth of murine stem cells and the expansion of colony-forming cells and spleen colony-forming units. Blood 1995;85:2747–2755.
36. Hirayama F, Lyman SD, Clark SC et al. The flt3 ligand supports proliferation of lymphohematopoietic progenitors and early B-lymphoid progenitors. Blood 1995;85:1762–1768.
37. Rusten LS, Lyman SD, Veiby OP et al. The flt3 ligand is a direct and potent stimulator of the growth of primitive and committed human CD34 + bone marrow progenitor cells *in vitro*. Blood 1996;87:1317–1325.
38. Piacibello W, Garetto L, Sanavio F et al. The effects of human flt3 ligand on *in vitro* human megakaryocytopoiesis. Exp Hematol 1996;24:340–346.
39. Ratajczak MZ, Ratajczak J, Ford J et al. FLT3/FLK-2 (STK-1) ligand does not stimulate human megakaryopoiesis *in vitro*. Stem Cells 1996;14: 146–150.
40. Brasel K, McKenna HJ, Morrissey PJ et al. Hematologic effects of flt3 ligand *in vivo* in mice. Blood 1996;88:2004–2012.
41. Kelemen E, Cserhati I, Tanos B. Demonstration and some properties of human thrombopoietin in thrombocythemic sera. Acta Haematol 1958;20: 350–355.
42. Kishimoto T. The biology of interleukin-6. Blood 1989;74:1–10.
43. Ishibashi T, Kimura H, Shikama Y et al. Interleukin-6 is a potent thrombopoietic factor *in vivo* in mice. Blood 1989;74:1241–1244.
44. Quesenberry PJ, McGrath HE, Williams ME et al. Multifactor stimulation of megakaryocytopoiesis: effects of interleukin 6. Exp Hematol 1991;19: 35–41.
45. Kaushansky K, Broudy VC, Lin N et al. Thrombopoietin, the mpl-ligand, is essential for full megakaryocyte development. Proc Natl Acad Sci U S A 1995;92:3234–3238.
46. Ayala IA, Tomer A, Kellar KL. Flow cytometric analysis of megakaryocyte-associated antigens on CD34 cells and their progeny in liquid culture. Stem Cells 1996;14:320–329.
47. Kimura H, Ishibashi T, Uchida T et al. Interleukin 6 is a differentiation factor for human megakaryocytes *in vitro*. Eur J Immunol 1990;20: 1927–1931.
48. Mei RL, Burstein SA. Megakaryocytic maturation in murine long-term bone marrow culture: role of interleukin-6. Blood 1991;78:1438–1447.
49. Williams N, De Giorgio T, Banu N et al. Recombinant interleukin 6 stimulates immature murine megakaryocytes. Exp Hematol 1990;18:69–72.
50. Debili N, Massé JM, Katz A et al. Effects of the recombinant hematopoietic growth factors interleukin-3, interleukin-6, stem cell factor, and leukemia inhibitory factor on the megakaryocytic differentiation of CD34 + cells. Blood 1993;82:84–95.
51. Asano S, Okano A, Ozawa K et al. *In vivo* effects of recombinant human interleukin-6 in primates: stimulated production of platelets. Blood 1990; 75:1602–1605.
52. Hill RJ, Warren MK, Levin J. Stimulation of thrombopoiesis in mice by human recombinant interleukin 6. J Clin Invest 1990;85:1242–1247.
53. Carrington PA, Hill RJ, Stenberg PE et al. Multiple *in vivo* effects of interleukin-3 and interleukin-6 on murine megakaryocytopoiesis. Blood 1991;77:34–41.
54. Burstein SA, Downs T, Friese P et al. Thrombocytopoiesis in normal and sublethally irradiated dogs: response to human interleukin-6. Blood 1992; 80:420–428.
55. Zeidler C, Kanz L, Hurkuck F et al. *In vivo* effects of interleukin-6 on thrombopoiesis in healthy and irradiated primates. Blood 1992;80: 2740–2745.
56. Warren MK, Conroy LB, Rose JS. The role of interleukin 6 and interleukin 1 in megakaryocyte development. Exp Hematol 1989;17:1095–1099.
57. Dan K, Gomi S, Inokuchi K et al. Effects of interleukin-1 and tumor necrosis factor on megakaryocytopoiesis: mechanism of reactive thrombocytosis. Acta Haematol 1995;93:67–72.
58. Paul SR, Bennett F, Calvetti JA et al. Molecular cloning of a cDNA encoding interleukin 11, a stromal cell-derived lymphopoietic and hematopoietic cytokine. Proc Natl Acad Sci U S A 1990;87:7512–7516.
59. Du XX, Williams DA. Interleukin-11: a multifunctional growth factor de-

rived from the hematopoietic microenvironment. Blood 1994;83: 2023–2030.

60. Metcalf D, Nicola NA, Gearing DP. Effects of injected leukemia inhibitory factor on hematopoietic and other tissues in mice. Blood 1990;76:50–56.

61. Gough NM. Molecular genetics of leukemia inhibitory factor (LIF) and its receptor. Growth Factors 1992;7:175–179.

62. Hilton DJ. LIF: lots of interesting functions. Trends Biochem Sci 1992;17: 72–76.

63. Teramura M, Kobayashi S, Hoshino S et al. Interleukin-11 enhances human megakaryocytopoiesis *in vitro*. Blood 1992;79:327–331.

64. Neben TY, Loebelenz J, Hayes L et al. Recombinant human interleukin-11 stimulates megakaryocytopoiesis and increases peripheral platelets in normal and splenectomized mice. Blood 1993;81:901–908.

65. Yonemura Y, Kawakita M, Masuda T et al. Effect of recombinant human interleukin 11 on rat megakaryopoiesis and thrombopoiesis *in vivo*: comparative study with interleukin 6. Br J Haematol 1993;84:16–23.

66. Hangoc G, Yin T, Cooper S et al. *In vivo* effects of recombinant interleukin-11 on myelopoiesis in mice. Blood 1993;81:965–972.

67. Farese AM, Myers LA, MacVittie TJ. Therapeutic efficacy of recombinant human leukemia inhibitory factor in a primate model of radiation-induced marrow aplasia. Blood 1994;84:3675–3678.

68. Goldman SJ. Preclinical biology of interleukin 11: a multifunctional hematopoietic cytokine with potent thrombopoietic activity. Stem Cells 1995; 13:462–471.

69. Gordon MS, McCaskill-Stevens WJ, Battiato LA et al. A phase I trial of recombinant interleukin-11 (neumega rhIL-11 growth factor) in women with breast cancer receiving chemotherapy. Blood 1996;87:3615–3624.

70. Williams N. Is thrombopoietin interleukin 6? Exp Hematol 1991;19: 714–718.

71. Straneva JE, van Besien KW, Derigs G et al. Is interleukin 6 the physiological regulator of thrombopoiesis? Exp Hematol 1992;20:47–50.

72. Hill RJ, Warren MK, Levin J et al. Evidence that interleukin-6 does not play a role in the stimulation of platelet production after induction of acute thrombocytopenia. Blood 1992;80:346–351.

73. Tsukada J, Misago M, Ogawa R et al. Synergism between serum factor(s) and erythropoietin in inducing murine megakaryocyte colony formation: the synergistic factor in serum is distinct from interleukin-11 and stem cell factor (c-kit ligand) [Letter]. Blood 1993;81:866–867.

74. Wendling F, Varlet P, Charon M et al. A retrovirus complex inducing an acute myeloproliferative leukemia disorder in mice. Virology 1986;149: 242–246.

75. Souyri M, Vigon I, Penciolelli JF et al. A putative truncated cytokine receptor gene transduced by the myeloproliferative leukemia virus immortalizes hematopoietic progenitors. Cell 1990;63:1137–1147.

76. Vigon I, Mornon JP, Cocault L et al. Molecular cloning and characterization of mpl, the human homolog of the *v-mpl* oncogene: identification of a member of the hematopoietic growth factor receptor superfamily. Proc Natl Acad Sci U S A 1992;89:5640–5644.

77. Cosman D. The hematopoietin receptor superfamily. Cytokine 1993;5: 95–106.

78. Long MW, Heffner CH, Williams JL et al. Regulation of megakaryocyte phenotype in human erythroleukemia cells. J Clin Invest 1990;85: 1072–1084.

79. Vigon I, Dreyfus F, Melle J et al. Expression of the *c-mpl* proto-oncogene in human hematologic malignancies. Blood 1993;82:877–883.

80. Methia N, Louache F, Vainchenker W et al. Oligodeoxynucleotides antisense to the proto-oncogene *c-mpl* specifically inhibit *in vitro* megakaryocytopoiesis. Blood 1993;82:1395–1401.

81. de Sauvage FJ, Hass PE, Spencer SD et al. Stimulation of megakaryocytopoiesis and thrombopoiesis by the *c-mpl* ligand. Nature 1994;369:533–538.

82. Lok S, Kaushansky K, Holly RD et al. Cloning and expression of murine thrombopoietin cDNA and stimulation of platelet production *in vivo*. Nature 1994;369:565–568.

83. Bartley TD, Bogenberger J, Hunt P et al. Identification and cloning of a megakaryocyte growth and development factor that is a ligand for the cytokine receptor mpl. Cell 1994;77:1117–1124.

84. Kuter DJ, Beeler DL, Rosenberg RD. The purification of megapoietin: a physiological regulator of megakaryocyte growth and platelet production. Proc Natl Acad Sci U S A 1994;91:11104–11108.

85. Sohma Y, Akahori H, Seki N et al. Molecular cloning and chromosomal localization of the human thrombopoietin gene. FEBS Lett 1994;353:57–61.

86. Kaushansky K, Lok S, Holly RD et al. Promotion of megakaryocyte progenitor expansion and differentiation by the *c-mpl* ligand thrombopoietin. Nature 1994;369:568–571.

87. Wendling F, Maraskovsky E, Debili N et al. *c-mpl* ligand is a humoral regulator of megakaryocytopoiesis. Nature 1994;369:571–574.

88. Choi ES, Nichol JL, Hokom MM et al. Platelets generated *in vitro* from proplatelet-displaying human megakaryocytes are functional. Blood 1995; 85:402–413.

89. Debili N, Wendling F, Katz A et al. The mpl-ligand or thrombopoietin or megakaryocyte growth and differentiative factor has both direct proliferative and differentiative activities on human megakaryocyte progenitors. Blood 1995;86:2516–2525.

90. Nichol JL, Hokom MM, Hornkohl A et al. Megakaryocyte growth and development factor. Analyses of *in vitro* effects on human megakaryopoiesis and endogenous serum levels during chemotherapy-induced thrombocytopenia. J Clin Invest 1995;95:2973–2978.

91. Kato T, Horie K, Hagiwara T et al. GP IIb-IIIa+ subpopulation of rat megakaryocyte progenitor cells exhibits high responsiveness to human thrombopoietin. Exp Hematol 1996;24:1209–1214.

92. Angchaisuksiri P, Carlson PL, Dessypris EN. Effects of recombinant human thrombopoietin on megakaryocyte colony formation and megakaryocyte ploidy by human CD34 + cells in a serum-free system. Br J Haematol 1996;93:13–17.

93. Broudy VC, Lin NL, Kaushansky K. Thrombopoietin (*c-mpl* ligand) acts synergistically with erythropoietin, stem cell factor, and interleukin-11 to enhance murine megakaryocyte colony growth and increases megakaryocyte ploidy *in vitro*. Blood 1995;85:1719–1726.

94. Petzer AL, Zandstra PW, Piret JM et al. Differential cytokine effects on primitive (CD34+ CD38-) human hematopoietic cells: novel responses to Flt-3 ligand and thrombopoietin. J Exp Med 1996;183:2551–2558.

95. Farese AM, Hunt P, Boone T et al. Recombinant human megakaryocyte growth and development factor stimulates thrombocytosis in normal nonhuman primates. Blood 1995;86:54–59.

96. Akahori H, Shibuya K, Obuchi M et al. Effect of recombinant human thrombopoietin in nonhuman primates with chemotherapy-induced thrombocytopenia. Br J Haematol 1996;94:722–728.

97. Harker LA, Hunt P, Marzek UM et al. Regulation of platelet production and function by megakaryocyte growth and development factor in nonhuman primates. Blood 1996;87:1833–1844.

98. Ulich TR, del Castillo J, Senaldi G et al. Systemic hematologic effects of PEG-rHuMGDF-induced megakaryocyte hyperplasia in mice. Blood 1996; 87:5006–5015.

99. O'Malley CJ, Rasko JE, Basser RL et al. Administration of pegylated human megakaryocyte growth and development factor to humans stimulates the production of functional platelets that show no evidence of *in vivo* activation. Blood 1996;88:3288–3298.

100. Bernad A, Kopf M, Kulbacki R et al. Interleukin-6 is required *in vivo* for the regulation of stem cells and committed progenitors of the hematopoietic system. Immunity 1994;1:725–731.

101. Gurney AL, Carver-Moore K, de Sauvage FJ et al. Thrombocytopenia in c-mpl-deficient mice. Science 1994;265:1445–1447.

102. Alexander WS, Roberts AW, Nicola NA et al. Deficiencies in progenitor cells of multiple hematopoietic lineages and defective megakaryocytopoiesis in mice lacking the thrombopoietin receptor *c-mpl*. Blood 1996;87: 2162–2170.

103. Ebbe S, Levin J, Miller K et al. Thrombocytopoietic response to immunothrombocytopenia in nude mice. Blood 1987;69:192–198.

104. Nishinakamura R, Miyajima A, Mee PJ et al. Hematopoiesis in mice lacking the entire granulocyte-macrophage colony-stimulating factor/interleukin-3/interleukin-5 functions. Blood 1996;88:2458–2464.

105. Ebbe S, Phalen E, Stohlman F Jr. Abnormalities of megakaryocytes in S1/S1^d mice. Blood 1973;42:865–871.

106. Long MW, Hoffman R. Thrombocytopoiesis. In: Hoffman R, Benz EJ Jr, Shattil SJ et al., eds. Hematology: basic principles and practice. 2nd ed. New York: Churchill Livingstone, 1995; p. 274.

107. Odell TT Jr, Jackson CW, Reiter RS. Generation cycle of rat megakaryocytes. Exp Cell Res 1968;53:321.

108. Rolovic Z. Ploidy value of endoreduplicating human megakaryocytes in immune and hypersplenic thrombocytopenia. In: Bardini MG, Ebbe S, eds. Platelets: production, function, transfusion and storage. New York: Grune & Stratton, 1974; pp. 143–155.

109. Vitrat N, Le Couedic JP, Pique C et al. Megakaryocyte endomitosis are really abortive mitosis [Abstract]. Blood 1996;88(Suppl 1):287a.

110. King RW, Jackson PK, Kirschner MW. Mitosis in transition. Cell 1994;79: 563–568.

111. Broek D, Bartlett R, Crawford K et al. Involvement of p34cdc2 in establishing the dependency of S phase on mitosis. Nature 1991;349:388–393.

112. Hayles J, Fisher D, Woollard A et al. Temporal order of S phase and mitosis in fission yeast is determined by the state of the p34$^{cdc2}$-mitotic B cyclin complex. Cell 1994;78:813–822.

113. Datta NS, Williams JL, Caldwell J et al. Novel alterations in cdk 1/cyclin B1 kinase complex formation occur during the acquistion of a polyploid DNA content. Mol Biol Cell 1996;7:209–223.

114. Zhang Y, Wang Z, Ravid K. The cell cycle in polyploid megakaryocytes is associated with reduced activity of cyclin B1-dependent cdc2 kinase. J Biol Chem 1996;271:4266–4272.

115. Carow CE, Fox NE, Kaushansky K. Purified endomitotic megakaryocytes display a funcitonal cyclin B1-associated mitotic kinase [Abstract]. Blood 1996;88(Suppl 1):287a.

116. Ravid K, Doi T, Beeler DL et al. Transcriptional regulation of the rat platelet factor 4 gene:interaction between an enhancer/silencer domain and the GATA site. Mol Cell Biol 1992;11:6116–6127.

117. Lemarchandel V, Ghysdael J, Mignotte V et al. GATA and Ets *cis*-acting sequences mediate megakaryocyte-specific expression. Mol Cell Biol 1993; 13:668–676.

118. Block KL, Ravid K, Phung QH et al. Characterization of regulatory elements in the 5′ flanking region of the rat GP IIb gene by studies in primary rat marrow culture system. Blood 1994;84:3385–3393.

119. Ramachandran B, Surrey S, Schwartz E. Megakaryocyte-specific positive regulatory sequence 5′ to the human PF4 gene. Exp Hematol 1995;23: 49–57.

120. Deveaux S, Filipe A, Lemarchandel V et al. Analysis of the thrombopoietin receptor (mpl) promoter implicates GATA and Ets proteins in the coregulation of megakaryocyte-specific genes. Blood 1996;87:4678–4685.

121. Martin DI, Tsai SF, Orkin SH. Increased gamma-globin expression in a nondeletion HPFH mediated by an erythroid-specific DNA-binding factor. Nature 1989;338:435–438.

122. Martin DI, Zon LI, Mutter G et al. Expression of an erythroid transcription factor in megakaryocytic and mast cell lineages. Nature 1990;344:444–447.

123. Romeo PH, Prandini MH, Joulin V et al. Megakaryocytic and erythrocytic lineages share specific transcription factors. Nature 1990;344:447–449.

124. Visvader JE, Elefanty AG, Strasser A et al. GATA-1 but not SCL induces megakaryocytic differentiation in an early myeloid cell line. EMBO J 1992; 11:4557–4564.

125. Shivdasani RA, McDevitt M, Fujiwara Y et al. A lineage restricted gene knockout reveals the critical role of erythroid transcription factor GATA-1 in regulating megakaryocyte growth and platelet formation in vivo [Abstract]. Blood 1996;88(Suppl 1):472a.

126. Pevny L, Simon MC, Robertson E et al. Erythroid differentiation in chimaeric mice blocked by a targeted mutation in the gene for transcription factor GATA-1. Nature 1991;349:257–260.

127. Andrews NC, Erdjument-Bromage H, Davidson MB et al. Erythroid transcription factor NF-E2 is a haematopoietic-specific basic-leucine zipper protein. Nature 1993;362:722–728.

128. Shivdasani RA, Rosenblatt MF, Zucker-Franklin D et al. Transcription factor NF-E2 is required for platelet formation independent of the actions of thrombopoietin/MGDF in megakaryocyte development. Cell 1995;81: 695–704.

129. Tavassoli M, Aoki M. Localization of megakaryocytes in the bone marrow. Blood Cells 1989;15:3–14.

130. Howell WH, Donahue DP. The production of blood platelets in the lungs. J Exp Med 1939;65:177–204.

131. Slater DN, Trowbridge EA, Martin JF. The megakaryocyte in thrombocytopenia: a microscopic study which supports the theory that platelets are produced in the pulmonary circulation. Thromb Res 1983;31:163–176.

132. Zeigler FC, de Sauvage F, Widmer HR et al. In vitro megakaryocytopoietic and thrombopoietic activity of c-mpl ligand (TPO) on purified murine hematopoietic stem cells. Blood 1994;84:4045–4052.

133. Ito T, Ishida Y, Kashiwagi R et al. Recombinant human c-mpl ligand is not a direct stimulator of proplatelet formation immature human megakaryocytes. Br J Haematol 1996;94:387–390.

134. Wing EJ, Waheed A, Shadduck RK et al. Effect of colony-stimulating factor on murine macrophages. J Clin Invest 1982;69:270–276.

135. Metcalf D, Begley CG, Johnson GR et al. Biological properties in vitro of a recombinant human granulocyte-macrophage colony-stimulating factor. Blood 1986;67:37–45.

136. Weisbart RH, Kwan L, Golde DW et al. Human GM-CSF primes neutrophils for enhanced oxidative metabolism in response to the major physiological chemoattractants. Blood 1987;69:18–21.

137. DiPersio JF, Billing P, Williams R et al. Human granulocyte-macrophage colony-stimulating factor and other cytokines prime human neutrophils for enhanced arachidonic acid release and leukotriene B$_4$ synthesis. J Immunol 1988;140:4315–4322.

138. Fabian I, Kletter Y, Mor S et al. Activation of human eosinophil and neutrophil functions by haematopoietic growth factors: comparisons of IL-1, IL-3, IL-5 and GM-CSF. Br J Haematol 1992;80:137–143.

139. Rothenberg ME, Owen WF Jr, Silberstein DS et al. Human eosinophils have prolonged survival, enhanced functional properties, and become hypodense when exposed to human interleukin 3. J Clin Invest 1988;81: 1986–1992.

140. Valent P, Besemer J, Muhm M et al. Interleukin 3 activates human blood basophils via high-affinity binding sites. Proc Natl Acad Sci U S A 1989; 86:5542–5546.

141. Chen J, Herceg-Harjacek L, Groopman JE et al. Regulation of platelet activation in vitro by the c-mpl ligand, thrombopoietin. Blood 1995;86: 4054–4062.

142. Kojima H, Hamazaki Y, Nagata Y et al. Modulation of platelet activation in vitro by thrombopoietin. Thromb Haemost 1995;74:1541–1545.

143. Montrucchio G, Brizzi MF, Calosso G et al. Effects of recombinant megakaryocyte growth and development factor on platelet activation. Blood 1996;87:2762–2768.

144. Oda A, Miyakawa Y, Druker B et al. Thrombopoietin primes human platelet aggregation induced by shear stress and multiple agonists. Blood 1996; 87:4664–4670.

145. Wun T, Paglieroni T, Hammond WP et al. Thrombopoietin is synergistic with other hematopoietic growth factors and physiologic platelet agonists for platelet activation in vitro. Am J Hematol 1997;54:225–232.

146. Peng J, Friese P, Wolf RF et al. Relative reactivity of platelets from thrombopoietin and interleukin-6 treated dogs. Blood 1996;87:4158–4163.

147. Oleksowicz L, Puszkin E, Mrowiec Z et al. Alterations in platelet function in individuals receiving interleukin-6 as cytokine therapy. Cancer Invest 1996;14:307–316.

148. Oleksowicz L, Mrowiec Z, Zuckerman D et al. Platelet activation induced by interleukin-6: evidence for a mechanism involving arachadonic acid metabolism. Thromb Haemost 1994;72:302–308.

149. Kaviani MD, Mason LE, Bree AG et al. Effects of recombinant human interleukin 11 on the activation and morphology of peripheral blood platelets and megakaryocytes in nonhuman primates [Abstract]. Blood 1996; 88(Suppl 1):26a.

150. Basser RL, Rasko JE, Clarke K et al. Thrombopoietic effects of pegylated recombinant human megakaryocyte growth and development factor (PEG-rHuMGDF) in individuals with advanced cancer. Lancet 1996;348: 1279–1281.

151. Abrams C, Shattil SJ. Immunological detection of activated platelets in clinical disorders. Thromb Haemost 1991;65:467–473.

152. Kashiwagi H, Eigenthaler M, Ginsberg MH et al. Affinity modulation of the platelet fibrinogen receptor by β3 endonexin, a selective binding partner of the β3 integrin cytoplasmic tail [Abstract]. Blood 1996;88(Suppl 1): 140a.

153. Kouns WC, Wall CD, White MM et al. A conformation-dependent epitope of human platelet glycoprotein IIIa. J Biol Chem 1990;265:20594–20601.

154. Honda S, Tomiyama Y, Pelletier AJ et al. Topography of ligand-induced binding sites, including a novel cation-sensitive epitope (Albert Park 5) at the aminoterminus, of the human integrin beta 3 subunit. J Biol Chem 1995;270:11947–11954.

155. Koury MJ, Bondurant MC. Erythropoietin retards DNA breakdown and prevents programmed death in erythroid progenitor cells. Science 1990; 248:378–381.

156. Silva M, Grillot D, Benito A et al. Erythropoietin can promote erythroid progenitor survival by repressing apoptosis through Bcl-x$_L$ and Bcl-2. Blood 1996;88:1576–1582.

157. Sherr CJ. G1 phase progression: cycling on cue. Cell 1994;79:551–555.

158. Peter M, Herskowitz I. Joining the complex: cyclin-dependent kinase inhibitory proteins and the cell cycle. Cell 1994;79:181–184.

159. Matsushime H, Roussel MF, Ashmun RA et al. Colony-stimulating factor 1 regulates novel cyclins during the G1 phase of the cell cycle. Cell 1991; 65:701–713.

160. Firpo EJ, Koff A, Solomon MJ et al. Inactivation of Cdk2 inhibitor during interleukin 2-induced proliferation of human T lymphocytes. Mol Cell Biol 1994;14:4889–4901.

161. Tojo A, Kasuga M, Urabe A et al. Vanadate can replace interleukin 3 for transient growth of factor-dependent cells. Exp Cell Res 1987;171:16–23.

162. Satoh T, Uehara Y, Kaziro Y. Inhibition of interleukin 3 and granulocyte-macrophage colony-stimulating factor stimulated increase of active ras.GTP by herbimycin A, a specific inhibitor of tyrosine kinases. J Biol Chem 1992;267:2537–2541.

163. Darnell JE, Kerr IM, Stark GR. Jak-STAT pathways and transcriptional activation in response to IFNs and other extracellular signaling proteins. Science 1994;264:1415–1420.

164. Ihle JN, Kerr IM. Jaks and Stats in signaling by the cytokine receptor superfamily. Trends Genet 1995;11:69–74.

165. Corey SJ, Burkhardt AL, Bolen JB et al. Granulocyte colony-stimulating factor receptor signaling involves the formation of a three-component complex with Lyn and Syk protein-tyrosine kinases. Proc Natl Acad Sci U S A 1994;91:4683–4687.

166. Anderson SM, Jorgensen B. Activation of src-related tyrosine kinases by IL-3. J Immunol 1995;155:1660–1670.

167. Bluyssen AR, Durbin JE, Levy DE. ISGF3γp48, a specificity switch for interferon-activated transcription factors. Cytokine Growth Factor Rev 1996;7:11–17.

168. Muto A, Watanabe S, Miyajima A et al. The β subunit of human granulocyte-macrophage colony-stimulating factor receptor forms a homodimer and is activated via association with the α subunit. J Exp Med 1996;183: 1911–1916.

169. Stomski FC, Sun Q, Bagley CJ et al. Human interleukin-3 (IL-3) induces disulfide-linked IL-3 receptor α- and β-chain heterodimerization, which is required for receptor activation but not high-affinity binding. Mol Cell Biol 1996;16:3035–3046.

170. Kishimoto T, Taga T, Akira S. Cytokine signal transduction. Cell 1994;6: 253–262.

171. Hilton DJ, Hilton AA, Raicevic A et al. Cloning of a murine IL-11 receptor alpha-chain; requirement for gp130 for high affinity binding and signal transduction. EMBO J 1994;13:4765–4775.

172. Taga T, Hibi M, Hirata Y et al. Interleukin-6 triggers the association of its receptor with a possible signal transducer, gp130. Cell 1989;58:573–581.

173. Karow J, Hudson KR, Hall MA et al. Mediation of interleukin-11–dependent biological responses by a soluble form of the interleukin-11 receptor. Biochem J 1996;318:489–495.

174. Navarro S, Debili N, LeCouedic JP et al. Interleukin-6 and its receptor are

expressed by human megakaryocytes: *in vitro* effects on proliferation and endoreduplication. Blood 1991;77:461–471.

175. Baumann H, Wang Y, Morella KK et al. Complex of the soluble IL-11 receptor and IL-11 acts as IL-6-type cytokine in hepatic and nonhepatic cells. J Immunol 1996;157:284–290.

176. Broudy VC, Lin NL, Fox N et al. Thrombopoietin stimulates colony-forming unit-megakaryocyte proliferation and megakaryocyte maturation independently of cytokines that signal through the gp130 receptor subunit. Blood 1996;88:2026–2032.

177. Kaushansky K, Broudy VC, Drachman JG. The TPO receptor and signal transduction. In: Kuter D, Hunt P, Sheridan WP, Zucker-Franklin D, eds. Thrombopoiesis and the mpl ligand: molecular, cellular, preclinical and clinical biology. Totawa, NJ: Humana Press, 1996.

178. Vigon I, Florindo C, Fichelson S et al. Characterization of the murine mpl proto-oncogene, a member of the hematopoietic cytokine receptor family: molecular cloning, chromosomal location and evidence for a function in cell growth. Oncogene 1993;8:2607–2615.

179. Alexander WS, Metcalf D, Dunn AR. Point mutations within a dimer interface homology domain of c-mpl induce constitutive receptor activity and tumorigenicity. EMBO J 1995;14:5569–5578.

180. Tanner JW, Chen W, Young RL et al. The conserved box 1 motif of cytokine receptors is required for association with JAK kinases. J Biol Chem 1995; 270:6523–6530.

181. Silvennoinen O, Witthuhn BA, Quelle FW et al. Structure of the murine Jak2 protein-tyrosine kinase and its role in interleukin 3 signal transduction. Proc Natl Acad Sci U S A 1993;90:8429–8433.

182. Quelle F, Sato N, Witthuhn BA et al. JAK2 associates with the $\beta_C$ chain of the receptor for granulocyte-macrophage colony-stimulating factor, and its activation requires the membrane-proximal region. Mol Cell Biol 1994; 14:4335–4341.

183. Rao P, Mufson RA. A membrane proximal domain of the human interleukin-3 receptor $\beta_C$ subunit that signals DNA synthesis in NIH 3T3 cells specifically binds a complex of Src and Janus family tyrosine kinases and phosphatidylinositol 3-kinase. J Biol Chem 1995;270:6886–6893.

184. Azam M, Erdjument-Bromage H, Kreider BL et al. Interleukin-3 signals through multiple isoforms of Stat5. EMBO J 1995;14:1402–1411.

185. Bacon CM, Tortolani PJ, Shimosaka A et al. Thrombopoietin (TPO) induces tyrosine phosphorylation and activation of STAT5 and STAT3. FEBS Lett 1995;370:63–68.

186. Mui AL, Wakao H, O'Farrell AM et al. Interleukin-3, granulocyte-macrophage colony-stimulating factor and interleukin-5 transduce signals through two STAT5 homologs. EMBO J 1995;14:1166–1175.

187. Chin H, Nakamura N, Kamiyama R et al. Physical and functional interactions between stat5 and tyrosine phosphorylated receptors for erythropoietin and interleukin-3. Blood 1996;88:4415–4425.

188. Pallard C, Gouilleux F, Benit L et al. Thrombopoietin activates a STAT5-like factor in hematopoietic cells. EMBO J 1995;14:2847–2856.

189. Drachman JG, Sabath DF, Fox NE et al. Thrombopoietin signal transduction in purified murine megakaryocytes. Blood 1997;89:483–492.

190. Zhang X, Blenis J, Li HC et al. Requirement of serine phosphorylation for formation of STAT-promoter complexes. Science 1995;267:1990–1994.

191. Wen Z, Zhong Z, Darnell JE Jr. Maximal activation of transcription by Stat1 and Stat3 requires both tyrosine and serine phosphorylation. Cell 1995;82:241–250.

192. David M, Petricoin E, Benjamin C et al. Requirement for MAP kinase (ERK2) activity in interferon α– and interferon β–stimulated gene expression through STAT proteins. Science 1995;269:1721–1723.

193. Kanakura Y, Druker B, Wood KW et al. Granulocyte-macrophage colony-stimulating factor and interleukin-3 induce rapid phosphorylation and activation of the proto-oncogene Raf-1 in a human factor-dependent myeloid cell line. Blood 1991;77:243–248.

194. Welham MJ, Duronio V, Sanghera JS et al. Multiple hemopoietic growth factors stimulate activation of mitogen-activated protein kinase family members. J Immunol 1992;149:1683–1693.

195. Okuda K, Sanghera JS, Pelech SL et al. Granulocyte-macrophage colony-stimulating factor, interleukin-3, and steel factor induce rapid tyrosine phosphorylation of p42 and p44 MAP kinase. Blood 1992;79:2880–2887.

196. Cutler RL, Liu L, Damen JE et al. Multiple cytokines induce the tyrosine phosphorylation of Shc and its association with Grb2 in hemopoietic cells. J Biol Chem 1993;268:21463–21465.

197. Sato N, Sakamaki K, Terada N et al. Signal transduction by the high affinity GM-CSF receptor: two distinct cytoplasmic regions of the common b subunit responsible for different signaling. EMBO J 1993;12:4181–4189.

198. Dorsch M, Hock H, Diamantstein T. Tyrosine phosphorylation of Shc is induced by IL-3, IL-5 and GM-CSF. Biochem Biophys Res Commun 1994; 200:562–568.

199. Matsuguchi T, Salgia R, Hallek M et al. Shc phosphorylation in myeloid cells is regulated by granulocyte macrophage colony-stimulating factor, interleukin 3 and steel factor and is constitutively increased by p210BCR/ABL. J Biol Chem 1994;269:5016–5021.

200. Welham MJ, Dechert U, Leslie KB et al. Interleukin-3 and granulocyte/macrophage colony-stimulating factor, but not IL-4, induce tyrosine phos-

201. Matsuguchi T, Inhorn RC, Carlesso N et al. Tyrosine phosphorylation of p95Vav in myeloid cells is regulated by GM-CSF, IL-3 and steel factor and is constitutively increased by p210BCR/ABL. EMBO J 1995;14:257–265.

phorylation, activation and association of SHPTP-2 with Grb2 and phosphatidylinositol 3'-kinase. J Biol Chem 1994;269:23764–23768.

202. Gold MR, Duronio V, Saxena SP et al. Multiple cytokines activate phosphatidylinositol 3-kinase in hemopoietic cells. J Biol Chem 1994;269: 5403–5412.

203. Anderson SM, Jorgensen B. Activation of src-related tyrosine kinases by IL-3. J Immunol 1995;155:1660–1670.

204. Torigoe T, O'Conner R, Santoli D et al. Interleukin-3 regulates the activity of the LYN protein-tyrosine kinase in myeloid-committed leukemic cell lines. Blood 1992;80:617–624.

205. Rinaudo MS, Su K, Falk LA et al. Human interleukin-3 receptor modulates bcl-2 mRNA and protein levels through protein kinase C in TF-1 cells. Blood 1995;86:80–88.

206. Stahl N, Boulton TG, Farruggella T et al. Association and activation of Jak-Tyk kinases by CNTF-LIF-OSM-IL-6 β-receptor components. Science 1994;263:92–95.

207. Yi T, Mui ALF, Krystal G et al. Hematopoietic cell phosphatase associates with the interleukin-3 (IL-3) receptor β chain and down-regulates IL-3-induced tyrosine phosphorylation and mitogenesis. Mol Cell Biol 1993; 13:7577–7586.

208. Lev S, Yarden Y, Givol D. Dimerization and activation of the kit receptor by monovalent and bivalent binding of the stem cell factor. J Biol Chem 1992;267:15970–15977.

209. Philo JS, Wen J, Wypych J et al. Human stem cell factor dimer forms a complex with two molecules of the extracellular domain of its receptor, kit. J Biol Chem 1996;271:6895–6902.

210. Broudy VC. Stem cell factor and hematopoiesis. [Review] Blood 1997;90: 1345–1364.

211. Weiler SR, Mou S, DeBerry CS et al. JAK2 is associated with the c-kit proto-oncogene product and is phosphorylated in response to stem cell factor. Blood 1996;87:3688–3693.

212. Lev S, Givol D, Yarden Y. A specific combination of substrates is involved in signal transduction by the kit-encoded receptor. EMBO J 1991;10: 647–654.

213. Serve H, Hsu YC, Besmer P. Tyrosine residue 719 of the c-kit receptor is essential for binding of the p85 subunit of phosphotidyl (PI) 3-kinase and for c-kit associated PI 3-kinase activity on COS-1 cells. J Biol Chem 1994; 269:6026–6030.

214. Takahira H, Gotoh A, Ritchie A et al. Steel factor enhances integrin-mediated tyrosine phosphorylation of focal adhesion kinase (pp125FAK) and paxillin. Blood 1997;89:1574–1584.

215. Gotoh A, Takahira H, Mantel C et al. Steel factor induces serine phosphorylation of Stat3 in human growth factor–dependent myeloid cell lines. Blood 1996;88:138–145.

216. Alai M, Mui ALF, Cutler RL et al. Steel factor stimulates the tyrosine phosphorylation of the proto-oncogene product p95vav, in human hemopoietic cells. J Biol Chem 1992;267:18021–18025.

217. Wisniewski D, Strife A, Clarkson B. c-kit ligand stimulates tyrosine phosphorylation of the c-Cbl protein in human hematopoietic cells. Leukemia 1996;10:1436–1442.

218. Guschin D, Rogers N, Briscoe J et al. A major role for the protein tyrosine kinase JAK1 in the JAK/STAT signal transduction pathway in response to interleukin-6. EMBO J 1995;14:1421–1431.

219. Zhong Z, Wen Z, Darnell JE Jr. Stat3: a STAT family member activated by tyrosine phosphorylation in response to epidermal growth factor and interleukin-6. Science 1994;264:95–98.

220. Yin T, Yasukawa K, Taga T et al. Identification of a 130 kilodalton tyrosine-phosphorylated protein induced by interleukin-11 as JAK2 tyrosine kinase, which associates with gp130 signal transducer. Exp Hematol 1994; 22:467–472.

221. Murakami M, Narazaki M, Hibi M et al. Critical cytoplasmic region of the interleukin 6 signal transducer gp130 is conserved in the cytokine receptor family. Proc Natl Acad Sci U S A 1991;88:11349–11353.

222. Stahl N, Farruggella TJ, Boulton TG et al. Choice of STATs and other substrates specified by modular tyrosine-based motifs in cytokine receptors. Science 1995;267:1349–1353.

223. Laminet AA, Apell G, Conroy L et al. Affinity, specificity, and kinetics of the interaction of the SHC phosphotyrosine binding domain with asparagine-X-X-phosphotyrosine motifs of growth factor receptors. J Biol Chem 1996;271:264–269.

224. Akiro S, Nishio Y, Inoue M et al. Molecular cloning of APRF, a novel IFN-stimulated gene factor 3 p91-related transcription factor involved in the gp130-mediated signaling pathway. Cell 1994;77:63–71.

225. Sadowski HB, Shuai K, Darnell JE Jr et al. A common nuclear signal transduction pathway activated by growth factor and cytokine receptors. Science 1993;261:1739–1744.

226. Baumann H, Wang Y, Morella KK et al. Complex of the soluble IL-11 receptor and IL-11 acts as IL-6-type cytokine in hepatic and nonhepatic cells. J Immunol 1996;157:284–290.

227. Boulton TG, Stahl N, Yancopoulos GD. Ciliary neurotrophic factor/leuke-

mia inhibitory factor/interleukin 6/oncostatin M family of cytokines induces tyrosine phosphorylation of a common set of proteins overlapping those induced by other cytokines and growth factors. J Biol Chem 1994; 269:11648–11655.

228. Neumann C, Zehentmaier G, Danhauser-Riedl S et al. Interleukin-6 induces tyrosine phosphorylation of the Ras activating protein Shc, and its complex formation with Grb2 in the human multiple myeloma cell line LP-1. Eur J Immunol 1996;26:379–384.

229. Yin T, Yang YC. Mitogen activated protein kinases and ribosomal S6 protein kinases are involved in signaling pathways shared by interleukin-11, interleukin-6, leukemia inhibitory factor, and oncostatin M in mouse 3T3-L1 cells. J Biol Chem 1994;269:3731–3738.

230. Lee IS, Liu Y, Narazaki M et al. Vav is associated with signal transducing molecules gp130, Grb2 and Erk2, and is tyrosine phosphorylated in response to interleukin-6. FEBS Lett 1997;401:133–137.

231. Nakajima T, Kinoshita S, Sasagawa T et al. Phosphorylation at threonine-235 by a ras-dependent mitogen-activated protein kinase cascade is essential for transcription factor NF-IL6. Proc Natl Acad Sci U S A 1993;90: 2207–2211.

232. Nishizawa M, Nagata S. Regulatory elements responsible for inducible expression of the granulocyte colony-stimulating factor gene in macrophages. Mol Cell Biol 1990;10:2002–2011.

233. Mukaida N, Mahe Y, Matsushima K. Cooperative interaction of nuclear factor-κB- and cis-regulatory enhancer binding protein-like factor binding elements in activating the interleukin-8 gene by pro-inflammatory cytokines. J Biol Chem 1990;265:21128–21133.

234. Natsuka S, Akira S, Nishio Y et al. Macrophage differentiation-specific expression of NF-IL6, a transcription factor for interleukin-6. Blood 1992; 79:460–466.

235. Drachman J, Griffin JD, Kaushansky K. The c-mpl ligand (thrombopoietin) stimulates tyrosine phosphorylation of Jak2, Shc, and c-mpl. J Biol Chem 1995;270:4979–4982.

236. Sattler M, Durstin MA, Frank DA et al. The thrombopoietin receptor c-mpl activates JAK2 and TYK2 tyrosine kinases. Exp Hematol 1995;23: 1040–1048.

237. Tortolani PJ, Johnston JA, Bacon CM et al. Thrombopoietin induces tyrosine phosphorylation and activation of the Janus kinase, JAK2. Blood 1995; 85:3444–3451.

238. Morella KK, Bruno E, Kumaki S et al. Signal transduction by the receptors for thrombopoietin (c-mpl) and interleukin-3 in hematopoietic and nonhematopoietic cells. Blood 1995;86:557–571.

239. Mu SX, Xia M, Elliott G et al. Megakaryocyte growth and development factor and interleukin-3 induce patterns of protein-tyrosine phosphorylation that correlate with dominant differentiation over proliferation of mpl-transfected 32D cells. Blood 1995;86:4532–4543.

240. Sasaki K, Odai H, Hanazono Y et al. TPO/c-mpl ligand induces tyrosine phosphorylation of multiple cellular proteins including proto-oncogene products, Vav and c-Cbl, and Ras signaling molecules. Biochem Biophys Res Commun 1995;216:338–347.

241. Morita H, Tahara T, Matsumoto A et al. Functional analysis of the cytoplasmic domain of the human mpl receptor for tyrosine-phosphorylation of the signaling molecules, proliferation and differentiation. FEBS Lett 1996;395:228–234.

242. Drachman JG, Kaushansky K. Dissecting the thrombopoietin receptor: functional elements of the mpl cytoplasmic domain. Proc Natl Acad Sci U S A 1997;94:2350–2355.

243. Nagata Y, Todokoro K. Thrombopoietin induces activation of at least two distinct signaling pathways. FEBS Lett 1995;377:497–501.

244. Hill RJ, Zozulya S, Lu YL et al. Differentiation induced by the c-mpl cytokine receptor is blocked by mutant Shc adaptor protein. Cell Growth Differ 1996;7:1125–1134.

245. Yamada M, Komatsu N, Okada K et al. Thrombopoietin induces tyrosine phosphorylation and activation of mitogen-activated protein kinases in a human thrombopoietin-dependent cell line. Biochem Biophys Res Commun 1995;217:230–237.

246. Alexander WS, Maurer AB, Novak U et al. Tyrosine-599 of the c-mpl receptor is required for Shc phosphorylation and the induction of cellular differentiation. EMBO J 1996;15:6531–6540.

247. Lai CF, Ripperger J, Morella KK et al. STAT3 and STAT5B are targets of two different signal pathways activated by hematopoietin receptors and control transcription via separate cytokine response elements. J Biol Chem 1995;270:23254–23257.

248. Mui AL, Wakao H, Kinoshita T et al. Suppression of interleukin-3 induced gene expression by a C-terminal truncated Stat5: role of Stat5 in proliferation. EMBO J 1996;15:2425–2433.

249. Takatoku M, Kametaka M, Shimizu R et al. Identification of functional domains of the human thrombopoietin receptor required for growth and differentiation of megakaryocytic cells. J Biol Chem 1997;272:7259–7263.

250. Porteu F, Rouyez MC, Cocault L et al. Functional regions of the mouse thrombopoietin receptor cytoplasmic domain: evidence for a critical region which is involved in differentiation and can be complemented by erythropoietin. Mol Cell Biol 1996;16:2473–2482.

251. Ezumi Y, Takayama H, Okuma M. Thrombopoietin, c-mpl ligand, induces

252. Miyakawa Y, Oda A, Druker BJ et al. Recombinant thrombopoietin induces rapid protein tyrosine phosphorylation of Janus kinase 2 and Shc in human blood platelets. Blood 1995;86:23–27.

253. Rodriguez-Linares B, Watson SP. Thrombopoietin potentiates activation of human platelets in association with JAK2 and TYK2 phosphorylation. Biochem J 1996;316:93–98.

254. Schieven GL, Kallestad JC, Brown TJ et al. Oncostatin M induces tyrosine phosphorylation in endothelial cells and activation of p62yes tyrosine kinase. J Immunol 1992;149:1676–1682.

255. Ernst M, Gearing DP. Functional and biochemical association of Hck with the LIF/IL-6 receptor signal transducing subunit gp130 in embryonic stem cells. EMBO J 1994;13:1574–1584.

256. Matsuda T, Takahashi-Tezuka M, Fukada T et al. Association and activation of btk and tec tyrosine kinases by gp130, a signal transducer of the interleukin-6 family of cytokines. Blood 1995;85:627–633.

257. Torigoe T, O'Connor R, Santoli D et al. Interleukin-3 regulates the activity of the LYN protein-tyrosine kinase in myeloid-committed leukemic cell lines. Blood 1992;80:617–624.

258. Kelemen E, Lehoczky D, Perkedy J et al. Serum thrombopoietic activity in idiopathic thrombocytopenic purpura. Lancet 1960;1:1134.

259. Odell TT, McDonald TP, Detwiler TC. Stimulation of platelet production by serum of platelet-depleted rats. Proc Soc Exp Biol Med 1961;108:428.

260. De Gabriele G, Penington DG. Regulation of platelet production: "thrombopoietin." Br J Haematol 1967;13:210–215.

261. McDonald TP. Bioassay for thrombopoietin utilizing mice in rebound thrombocytosis. Proc Soc Exp Biol Med 1973;144:1006–1012.

262. Hill RJ, Levin J. Regulators of thrombopoiesis: their biochemistry and physiology. Blood Cells 1989;15:141–166.

263. McDonald TP. Thrombopoietin: its biology, purification, and characterization. Exp Hematol 1988;16:201–205.

264. Nichol JL, Hokom MM, Hornkohl A et al. Megakaryocyte growth and development factor: analyses of in vitro effects on human megakaryopoiesis and endogenous serum levels during chemotherapy-induced thrombocytopenia. J Clin Invest 1995;95:2973–2978.

265. Chang M, Suen Y, Meng G et al. Differential mechanisms in the regulation of endogenous levels of thrombopoietin and interleukin-11 during thrombocytopenia: insight into the regulation of platelet production. Blood 1996; 88:3354–3362.

266. Emmons RV, Reid DM, Cohen RL et al. Human thrombopoietin levels are high when thrombocytopenia is due to megakaryocyte deficiency and low when due to increased platelet destruction. Blood 1996;87:4068–4071.

267. Kuter DJ, Rosenberg RD. The reciprocal relationship of thrombopoietin (c-mpl ligand) to changes in the platelet mass during busulfan-induced thrombocytopenia in the rabbit. Blood 1995;85:2720–2730.

268. Stoffel R, Wiestner A, Skoda RC. Thrombopoietin in thrombocytopenic mice: evidence against regulation at the mRNA level and for a direct regulatory role of platelets. Blood 1996;87:567–573.

269. Bartocci A, Mastrogiannis DS, Migliorati G et al. Macrophages specifically regulate the concentration of their own growth factor in the circulation. Proc Natl Acad Sci U S A 1987;84:6179–6183.

270. McCarty JM, Sprugel KH, Fox NE et al. Murine thrombopoietin mRNA levels are modulated by platelet count. Blood 1995;86:3668–3675.

271. Cohen-Solal K, Villeval JL, Titeux M et al. Constitutive expression of mpl ligand transcripts during thrombocytopenia or thrombocytosis. Blood 1996;88:2578–2584.

272. de Sauvage FJ, Carver-Moore K, Luoh SM et al. Physiological regulation of early and late stages of megakaryocytopoiesis by thrombopoietin. J Exp Med 1996;183:651–656.

273. Sungaran R, Markovic B, Chong BH. Localization and regulation of thrombopoietin mRNA expression in human kidney, liver, bone marrow and spleen using in situ hybridization. Blood 1997;89:101–107.

274. Gastl G, Plante M, Finstad CL et al. High IL-6 levels in ascitic fluid correlate with reactive thrombocytosis in individuals with epithelial ovarian cancer. Br J Haematol 1993;83:433–441.

275. Blay JY, Favrot M, Rossi JF et al. Role of interleukin-6 in paraneoplastic thrombocytosis [Letter]. Blood 1993;82:2261–2262.

276. Tefferi A, Ho TC, Ahmann GJ et al. Plasma interleukin-6 and C-reactive protein levels in reactive versus clonal thrombocytosis. Am J Med 1994; 97:374–378.

277. Nimer SD, Leung DH, Wolin MJ et al. Serum stem cell factor levels in individuals with aplastic anemia. Int J Hematol 1994;60:185–189.

278. Lyman SD, Seaberg M, Hanna R et al. Plasma/serum levels of flt3 ligand are low in normal individuals and highly elevated in individuals with Fanconi anemia and acquired aplastic anemia. Blood 1995;86:4091–4096.

279. Tange T, Hasegawa Y, Oka T et al. Establishment and characterization of a new human mesothelioma cell line (T-85) from malignant peritoneal mesothelioma with remarkable thrombocytosis. Pathol Int 1995;45: 791–800.

280. Yasumoto S, Imayama S, Hori Y. Increased serum level of interleukin-6 in individuals with psoriatic arthritis and thrombocytosis. J Dermatol 1995; 22:718–722.

281. Takeuchi E, Ito M, Mori M et al. Lung cancer producing interleukin-6. Intern Med 1996;35:212–214.
282. Haznedaroglu IC, Ertenli I, Ozcebe OI et al. Megakaryocyte-related interleukins in reactive thrombocytosis versus autonomous thrombocythemia. Acta Haematol 1996;95:107–111.
283. Hollen CW, Henthorn J, Koziol JA et al. Serum interleukin-6 levels in individuals with thrombocytosis. Leuk Lymphoma 1992;8:235–241.
284. Estrov Z, Talpaz M, Mavligit G et al. Elevated plasma thrombopoietic activity in individuals with metastatic cancer-related thrombocytosis. Am J Med 1995;98:551–558.
285. Nichol J. Serum levels of thrombopoietin in health and disease. In: Kuter DJ, Hunt P, Sheridan W, Zucker-Franklin D, eds. Thrombopoiesis and thrombopoietins: molecular, cellular, preclinical and clinical biology. Totowa, NJ: Humana Press, 1997; pp. 359–376.
286. Onishi M, Mui AL, Morikawa Y et al. Identification of an oncogenic form of the thrombopoietin receptor mpl using retrovirus-mediated gene transfer. Blood 1996;88:1399–1406.
287. Yan XQ, Lacey D, Fletcher F et al. Chronic exposure to retroviral vector encoded MGDF (mpl-ligand) induces lineage-specific growth and differentiation of megakaryocytes in mice. Blood 1995;86:4025–4033.

288. Matsumura I, Kanakura Y, Kato T et al. Growth response of acute myeloblastic leukemia cells to recombinant human thrombopoietin. Blood 1995;86:703–709.
289. Matsumura I, Kanakura Y, Kato T et al. The biological properties of recombinant human thrombopoietin in the proliferation and megakaryocytic differentiation of acute myeloblastic leukemia cells. Blood 1996;88:3074–3082.
290. Motoji T, Takanashi M, Motomura S et al. Growth stimulatory effect of thrombopoietin on the blast cells of acute myelogenous leukaemia. Br J Haematol 1996;94:513–516.
291. Quentmeier H, Zaborski M, Graf G et al. Expression of the receptor mpl and proliferative effects of its ligand thrombopoietin on human leukemia cells. Leukemia 1996;10:297–310.
292. Matsumura I, Kanakura Y, Ikeda H et al. Coexpression of thrombopoietin and c-mpl genes in human acute myeloblastic leukemia cells. Leukemia 1996;10:91–94.
293. Li Y, Hetet G, Kiladjian JJ et al. Proto-oncogene c-mpl is involved in spontaneous megakaryocytopoiesis in myeloproliferative disorders. Br J Haematol 1996;92:60–66.

# CHAPTER 9

# PLATELET TURNOVER

## George L. Dale

Platelets in man have a maximum circulating life span of approximately 10 days. In normal individuals the majority of platelets survive to this endpoint to then be removed by senescence mechanisms; however, a small but significant proportion are consumed by hemostatic processes associated with maintenance of vascular integrity. During this 10 day circulating life span a decline in platelet functional capabilities is assumed but unproven. This brief summary of the platelet life cycle is based on 4 decades of experimentation, although for many years investigation in this area was hindered by numerous technical obstacles. Included among these were difficulties with precise cell enumeration, anticoagulants unsuitable for maintaining platelet viability, and suboptimal labeling reagents. As each of these hurdles was overcome, a clearer picture of platelet kinetics emerged, and this chapter will focus on the empirical understanding of platelet turnover currently available. In addition, hypotheses and supporting data concerning age-dependent changes and senescence mechanisms in platelets will be presented, although further understanding of the molecular events controlling the platelet life span will depend on additional technical advances.

## RADIOISOTOPIC MEASUREMENT OF PLATELET LIFE SPAN

Platelet labeling with [51Cr]-chromate gave the first reliable estimates of platelet survival (1); however, [51Cr] labeling suffered from serious shortcomings, including poor incorporation efficiencies, an unacceptable isotope-leakage rate, and a decay energy too low for facile external monitoring of isotopic decay (2). [111In]-indium-oxine was first proposed as a substitute for [51Cr] in 1976 by Thakur et al (3); [111In] exhibited an excellent incorporation efficiency, enhanced label stability, and improved capabilities for external monitoring. [111In] (2.81-day half-life) remains the standard today for isotopic quantitation of platelet survival (2), even although numerous other labels have been described (4). However, it should be appreciated that technical obstacles associated with isotopic labeling still hinder the routine determination of platelet survival in individuals.

## STANDARD LABELING PROCEDURE

In 1988 the International Committee for Standardization in Hematology published detailed protocols for the use of [111In]-oxine in determining platelet survival (2). These recommendations, which were an extension of an earlier protocol for [51Cr]-chromate-labeling (5), describe exact conditions for drawing blood, isolating platelets, and isotopic labeling in normal and thrombocytopenic individuals. A brief outline of the protocol will be provided here to serve as a focal point for subsequent discussions; the reader is referred to the original protocol (2) for detailed methods. For a normal individual ~50 mL of blood is drawn sterilely into acid-citrate-dextrose. Platelet-rich plasma (PRP) is prepared by low-speed centrifugation of the whole blood; platelets are pelleted from the PRP with high-speed centrifugation and then gently resuspended in a protein-free medium for labeling with [111In]-oxine. After labeling, a final centrifugation is used to remove unincorporated label. The

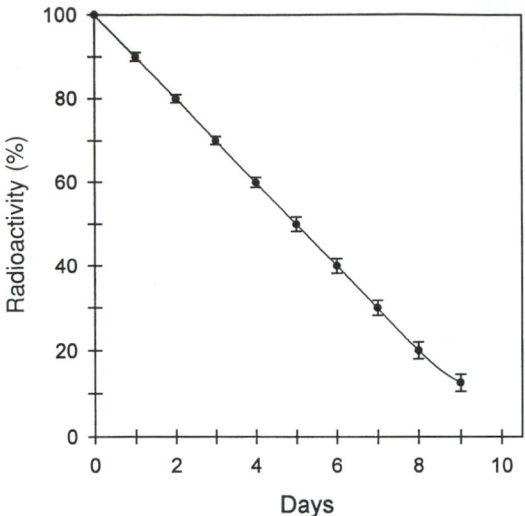

**FIGURE 9.1.** Platelet survival in 28 normal humans. Platelets were labeled with [$^{111}$In]-oxine and reinfused into the donor, and plasma radioactivity was monitored over 10 days (abscissa). Data are expressed as the percent of radioactivity in the first sample from each subject (ordinate); values represent mean ± 1SE (n = 28). Mean platelet survival was 9.3 ± 1.0 days. (Adapted from Wessels P, Heyns AD, Pieters H et al. An improved method for the quantification of the *in vivo* kinetics of a representative population of $^{111}$-In-labeled human platelets. Eur J Nucl Med 1985;10:522–527.)

labeled platelets are reinfused, and periodic blood samples are obtained for calculating the rate of disappearance of [$^{111}$In] from the circulation (2). A typical survival curve utilizing [$^{111}$In]-labeled platelets is shown in Fig. 9.1 (analysis of this curve will be discussed below). Subsequent enhancements in this methodology have been published (6–8); of particular importance are procedures for utilizing as little as 15 mL of blood from normals and <100 mL from thrombocytopenic individuals (6). With these modifications, individuals with platelet counts as low as 10,000/μl can be studied.

As mentioned, the strengths of [$^{111}$In] as a label for platelets include high labeling efficiency, minimal leakage of the label, a superior decay energy for [$^{111}$In], and a short isotopic half-life which allows repeat analyses (3). However, the weaknesses of this labeling technique include the necessity of isolating platelets free of plasma proteins and other cellular elements, the potential that the subfraction of platelets present in the PRP is not representative of the total population, and the general problem of radioisotope utilization in vulnerable populations such as pediatric or obstetric individuals. The negative consequences associated with labeling isolated platelets are discussed below in the section on Collection Injury. The representative nature of platelets in PRP has been addressed (9) with little difference observed between the PRP and total platelet population. However,

this potential caveat must be considered when assaying individual samples with abnormal platelet density distributions and therefore with the potential for an unusual allocation of platelets into a PRP preparation.

## CHEMISTRY OF INDIUM LABELING

Indium (In$^{+3}$) is available commercially as a complex with oxine (8-hydroxy quinoline). Oxine acts as a low-affinity chelator for the indium ion (3), but, more importantly, the indium-oxine complex is lipophilic and thereby passes through cell membranes to allow intracellular labeling (4). Presumably various cellular proteins, with higher affinity for indium than that exhibited by oxine, bind the In$^{+3}$ ion since free oxine is lost from the cell during labeling (10). Analysis of intracellular binding indicates that [$^{111}$In$^{+3}$] is bound to cytoplasmic proteins and cellular membranes (10). Two important consequences ensue from these observations. First, the binding of indium to platelet proteins is neither irreversible nor specific. Therefore labeling of platelets needs to be done in plasma-free media (transferrin strongly binds indium), as well as in the absence of other cellular components (leukocytes, erythrocytes) that also label with indium (3). These restrictions necessitate isolation of pure platelets and thereby create the most significant problem associated with this technique as discussed in the next section. Other chelators (4) of indium have been described (tropolone, mercaptopyridine-*N*-oxide, and acetylacetone); all serve the same purpose of providing a lipophilic, low affinity binding reservoir able to transfer [$^{111}$In$^{+3}$] to more stable binding sites within the cell.

## COLLECTION INJURY

Harker in 1978 (11) used the term "collection injury" to describe the damage resulting from *in vitro* processing and labeling of platelets. This vague but useful term covers all the negative consequences of isolating platelets and incubating them in protein-free, nonphysiologic media. While platelets are sensitive to a number of *in vitro* insults (e.g., small gauge needles and basic pH), the most damaging aspect of radioisotopic labeling is the need to centrifugally pellet the cells. A number of studies have discussed the collection injury associated with pelleting and resuspension of the platelets (11, 12). Presumably, the combination of centrifugal force, a plastic surface, and the extremely high concentration of platelets achieved in the cell pellet produces conditions where even a small number of activated platelets can affect the total population. Utilization of low pH buffers for pelleting of platelets (2) minimizes activation, and various other inhibitors of platelet activation have been suggested, although none has gained acceptance (13, 14). A significant improvement in [$^{111}$In]-labeling technology was the introduction of incubation conditions that allow essentially quantitative uptake of the [$^{111}$In], thereby eliminating the need for a final platelet wash after labeling (6).

However, even with the optimization of labeling conditions that has occurred over the last several years, the collection injury is still considered a significant problem and the main cause for failure of this technique in the hands of inexperienced users. The subtle nature of the collection injury, even in expert laboratories, was shown in a report by Badenhorst et al (12). Dog platelets were labeled with [$^{111}$In] by standard techniques and reinfused into the original donor. Twenty-four hours later blood from this donor dog was drawn and infused into a matched, recipient animal, and the fate of the [$^{111}$In] platelets in both dogs was monitored. While there was a modest, but insignificant, change in the calculated life spans in the two groups of animals, the shape of the platelet survival curves was different. The initial recipients of labeled platelets gave typical curves with modest curvilinear characteristics. However, the secondary recipients gave more linear survival curves. The authors' interpretation was that the first set of dogs served as a "filter" to remove or sequester platelets damaged during *in vitro* handling, that is, those representing the collection injury, and that without this damaged population the survival of the platelets in the secondary recipient dogs was more linear.

## ALTERNATIVE ISOTOPIC LABELING TECHNIQUES

Other isotopic labels previously utilized for determination of platelet survival in humans and primates include [$^{99m}$Tc] (15), meta-[$^{123}$I]-iodobenzylguanidine (4), [$^{32}$P]-diisopropyl fluorophosphate (DFP) (16), [$^{14}$C]-serotonin (17), diazotized-[$^{125}$I]-iodosulfanilic acid (18), and [$^{51}$Cr]-chromate (8). Of these alternative labels, only [$^{51}$Cr] is used to any extent currently, and its frequency is small compared with that for [$^{111}$In]. Additionally, cohort labeling studies with biosynthetic labels such as [$^{75}$Se]-selenomethionine (19) have been reported; however, these labels produce parabolic survival curves and are complicated by high reutilization rates for the isotopic labels.

## PLATELET DISTRIBUTION

Initial experiments with isotopically labeled platelets indicated that a significant proportion of the platelets (25 to 35%) were lost from the peripheral circulation immediately after infusion (20). External imaging demonstrated that the majority of these platelets were pooled in the spleen (20). In agreement with these observations, essentially 100% of infused radioactivity remains in the

peripheral circulation in splenectomized individuals (21). While splenic pooling is compatible with a closed, two-compartment model (22, 23), the mechanism responsible for splenic pooling is not clear. The extent of the splenic pool is known to be a function of splenic blood flow and platelet transit time, which is approximately 10 minutes (24). There are at least two possible explanations for this prolonged residence time. The most likely explanation is that the small size of platelets facilitates passage into the sluggish sinusoidal circulation where particles less than 2 μm tend to accumulate (25); however, selective, cell-cell, adhesive interactions concentrating platelets in the spleen cannot be excluded (26).

While splenic pooling in normals generally represents less than 35% of all platelets (24), the proportion can rise as high as 90% in severe splenomegaly (20, 27). In addition, it is clear that splenic pooling is subject to pharmacologic and physiologic manipulation. As demonstrated in Fig. 9.2, platelets present in the spleen can be mobilized with intravenous epinephrine (20). In this example, epinephrine, administered several hours after infusion of radiolabeled platelets, resulted in an increase in peripheral platelet count and a decrease in radioactiv-

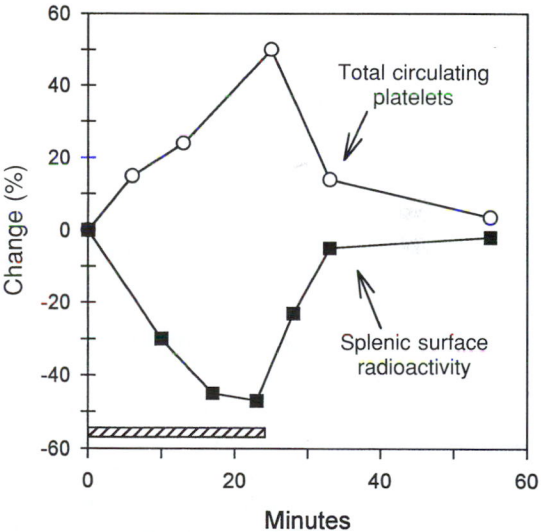

**FIGURE 9.2.** Effect of epinephrine on splenic pooling of radiolabeled platelets in normals. Intravenous epinephrine was administered to an individual 4 hours after infusion of autologous [$^{51}$Cr]-labeled platelets. Circulating platelet counts were monitored (open circles); radioactivity concentrated in the spleen was quantitated with a radiation spectrometer (solid squares). Both measurements were normalized to pretreatment values. The epinephrine infusion continued for 25 minutes (hatched bar). Epinephrine induced an increase in peripheral platelet count and a decrease in splenic sequestration of radiolabeled platelets; both changes reversed on cessation of epinephrine. (Adapted from Aster RH. Pooling of platelets in the spleen: role in the pathogenesis of hypersplenic thrombocytopenia. J Clin Invest 1966;45:645–657.)

ity monitored over the spleen (20). No effect of epineph-rine is observed in asplenic individuals. Epinephrine presumably functions by attenuation of splenic blood flow since the percentage of blood diverted to the spleen decreases from the normal 5% of total blood flow to approximately 1.5% (28). In addition, exercise (23, 29) and apheresis (30) can mobilize platelets sequestered in the spleen.

Platelets sequestered in the spleen are larger than those in the general circulation. With exercise-induced release of platelets (23, 31), mean platelet volume (MPV) for the total population increased 1.5 to 3.7%. Since the net increase in platelet count was 11 to 24%, the MPV of the released platelets was approximately 20% larger than that of platelets in the peripheral circulation. How-ever, some investigators have also suggested that only the youngest, most hemostatically active platelets are sequestered in the spleen (32); this is not supported by studies utilizing valid monitors of platelet age (23, 29). The increased platelet size after splenic clearance may explain reported increases in reactivity and the false con-clusion that younger cells are sequestered; as discussed below, platelet size, which does affect reactivity, does not change with cell age (33, 34).

# MATHEMATICAL ANALYSIS OF PLATELET SURVIVAL CURVES

The analysis of survival data assumes that blood vol-ume, platelet production, and platelet destruction re-main constant throughout the experiment. With these constraints numerous mathematical models have been utilized for analysis of platelet survival curves (35). These models were developed primarily to allow an ob-jective evaluation of survivals for comparisons between individuals and laboratories; however, there has also been an expectation by some investigators that the sur-vival patterns may offer clues as to the mechanisms in-volved in platelet loss. While there are over a dozen analysis methods available in the literature (35), the most frequently utilized is the multiple-hit model of Murphy and Francis (36), also referred to as the gamma-fit analysis. The multiple-hit model is based on the premise that platelets accumulate "hits" as they circu-late and that a threshold level of these hits must be achieved before the platelet is recognized as damaged and removed from the circulation. No assumption is made as to the nature of these hits other than the likeli-hood that they will be damaging to platelet function (36). However, a mechanism that tracks the platelet cir-culating life span without impairing or damaging the cell (the so-called odometer model) fits equally well with this mathematical analysis. It should be appreciated that

the gamma-fit analysis gives increased weight to early time points in the survival curve (36) and that a mean survival is estimated rather than a maximum life span. While the multiple-hit analysis remains the most fre-quently utilized method and the one recommended by the International Committee for Standardization in He-matology (2), many investigators recommend at least two types of analyses for most survival curves (35).

The nearly linear survival curve in Fig. 9.1 indi-cates that the majority of platelets synthesized in normal individuals survive to a defined life span to be removed from the circulation by senescence mechanisms; how-ever, some platelets are clearly utilized daily for mainte-nance of vascular integrity. To quantitate this consump-tion, Hanson and Slichter (37) examined platelet survival curves in normals and in individuals with vary-ing degrees of thrombocytopenia due to bone marrow hypoplasia. Normal individuals had survival patterns similar to that in Fig. 9.1, while individuals with low platelet counts (<50,000/μl) had shortened mean life spans with more curvilinear survival curves, suggesting a higher proportion of random disappearance (Fig. 9.3). The data are compatible with a model where approxi-mately 7000 platelets/μl/day are consumed for hemo-static purposes. In normal individuals, when the splenic pool is taken into account, this represents 15 to 20% of

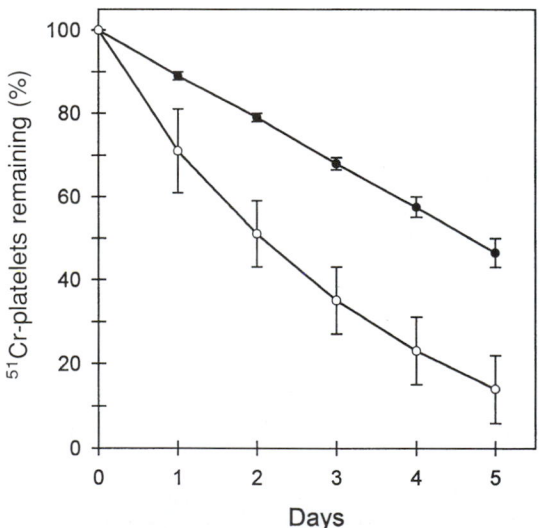

**FIGURE 9.3.** Effect of platelet count on survival of autol-ogous platelets. Survival of [$^{51}$Cr]-labeled platelets in 16 nor-mals (solid circles) and 6 individuals with severe thrombocyto-penia due to bone marrow hypoplasia (platelet counts 19,000 ± 6,000/μl; open circles). Note the curvilinear nature of the survival curve in individuals with low platelet numbers, indi-cating that random clearance of platelets in thrombocytopenic individuals represents a significant proportion of total platelet turnover. (Adapted from Hanson SR, Slichter SJ. Platelet kinet-ics in individuals with bone marrow hypoplasia: evidence for a fixed platelet requirement. Blood 1985;66:1105–1109.)

the daily turnover of all platelets. However, in individuals with low platelet production and presumably normal hemostatic requirements, this level of random destruction can represent a significant proportion of total platelet turnover, resulting in a curvilinear survival curve (37). While the term random destruction suggests all platelets may participate, it should be emphasized that the characteristics of those platelets lost for maintenance of hemostatic integrity is not known. They may represent predominantly young, hyperreactive platelets or the total population.

In summary, accurate evaluation of platelet survival remains a technically demanding procedure and one fraught with pitfalls for the experimentally naive. These technical obstacles are the primary reason that this assay is not routinely available in most medical centers.

# NONISOTOPIC ANALYSIS OF PLATELET SURVIVAL

Two techniques have been reported for nonisotopic analysis of platelet survival in humans. The first example was described by Schwartz (38) and refined by Stuart et al (39). Specifically, aspirin was used to irreversibly inactivate platelet cyclooxygenase, a key enzyme in the synthesis of thromboxanes and prostaglandins. Since mature platelets have essentially no protein synthesis, the aspirin-treated cell remains cyclooxygenase-deficient for the remainder of its life span. However, platelets synthesized after aspirin exposure have a normal level of cyclooxygenase, resulting in a progressive return to initial enzyme levels for the total population as aspirin-treated cells age. Estimation of platelet survival relies on quantitation of cyclooxygenase enzymatic activity (39), which is frequently measured indirectly as agonist-induced generation of malondialdehyde, a side product of thromboxane synthesis. Survival curves obtained after aspirin treatment often have a delay period before recovery of cyclooxygenase activity occurs (40, 41); this lag may be due to aspirin inactivation of megakaryocyte cyclooxygenase resulting in the release of newly synthesized, but cyclooxygenase-deficient, platelets. Additionally, the overall shape of the survival curves depends on the analytical technique utilized (41). The technical obstacles associated with this assay do not necessarily negate its utility, but they do present problems when comparisons with data obtained with traditional methodologies are attempted.

Another nonisotopic assay for platelet survival utilizes tranylcypromine or phenelzine, irreversible inhibitors of monoamine oxidase. Chamberlain et al (42, 43) demonstrated that a single dose of tranylcypromine will inactivate >80% of platelet monoamine oxidase; and similar to aspirin treatment, enzyme activity only recovers with new platelet synthesis (43). However, survival curves have a lag phase (43) analogous to that observed with aspirin-recovery curves, and investigators have utilized these antidepressants for examining platelet survival. It is noteworthy that both the aspirin and monoamine oxidase techniques have two advantages over isotopic labeling: they allow *in vivo* tagging of platelets, which avoids any collection injury, and all platelets are labeled instead of a subpopulation. Other nonisotopic procedures for determining platelet life span in animals are detailed below.

# INDIRECT MEASURES OF PLATELET SURVIVAL

Identification of age-dependent markers in platelets would allow one to estimate the mean age of a platelet population and thereby the mean survival if certain conditions are met (i.e., steady state of platelet production and degradation). In practice, the most frequently utilized markers determine the percentage of newly synthesized platelets, a parameter that offers additional information on the platelet production rate. A number of reports detailed below have proposed the use of these measurements for discriminating between synthetic and destructive mechanisms in thrombocytopenic individuals.

## THIAZOLE ORANGE STAINING

Staining platelets with methylene blue demonstrates a small fraction with reticulated bodies (44), analogous to those observed in reticulocytes. These ''reticulated platelets'' can also be stained with RNA/DNA fluorochromes such as thiazole orange (45) and auramine O (46), which allow quantitation by flow cytometry. The assumption has been that reticulated platelets contain vestigial mRNA from their megakaryocyte precursors and represent the very youngest platelets in the circulation. Recently, studies in dogs (47) and mice (48) used biotinylation (see below) to verify that thiazole orange-positive ($TO^+$) platelets in these experimental animals are less than 24 hours old. If the data on $TO^+$ platelet age in experimental animals are applicable to humans, it may be possible to infer the mean age of the total platelet population from the percentage represented by these youngest cells.

Numerous reports have demonstrated that the percentage of reticulated platelets is elevated in clinical settings where platelet production would be expected to be increased. Kienast and Schmitz (49) examined thrombocytopenic individuals whose marrow contained normal or increased numbers of megakaryocytes and found the percentage of $TO^+$ platelets elevated on average threefold above control, an observation consistent with potentiated production and decreased life span. In contrast, thrombocytopenic individuals with reduced numbers of megakaryocytes had normal percentages of TO[+] platelets, a finding compatible with attenuated platelet synthesis and relatively normal life span. Subsequent studies (50–52) have reiterated the finding that the percentage of TO[+] platelets is elevated in thrombocytopenia associated with premature platelet destruction and normal when associated with marrow suppression. Additional insight can be gained by considering the absolute numbers of TO[+] platelets (i.e., TO[+] cells/μl blood). In thrombocytopenic individuals, the absolute number of TO[+] platelets can be either normal or low with premature platelet destruction, but it is always low with impaired synthesis (49).

Even although an assay for TO[+] platelets probably represents the best opportunity to estimate platelet survival without invasive testing, several technical hurdles keep this assay out of routine use. The primary obstacle is the difficulty of standardizing TO[+] measurements; values from different laboratories for the percentage of TO[+] platelets in normals range from 0.9% (53) to 11.6% (51) with others in between (49, 50, 54). As a result, assays for TO[+] platelets are still primarily the province of research laboratories.

## PLATELET SEROTONIN CONTENT

Another surrogate marker of mean platelet age is serotonin content. Studies in dogs have documented that platelets accumulate serotonin as they age (55, 56), presumably as a result of active incorporation of plasma serotonin into platelet dense granules. Recently, Aranda et al (57) extended these studies into humans and demonstrated a correlation between serotonin levels and experimentally determined platelet life spans in 25 normals and 11 individuals with immune thrombocytopenic purpura (ITP). While there is a reasonable correlation between serotonin content and platelet life span, the data show sufficient variability to suggest that individual determinations will have rather large confidence limits. Two caveats with serotonin as a surrogate marker of platelet age are the role of dense granule secretion during platelet activation (57) and the unavailability of routine serotonin analysis.

# MEASUREMENT OF PLATELET TURNOVER IN ANIMALS

Historically, all of the methodologies detailed above have been either developed or utilized in experimental animals. In addition, nonisotopic approaches for quantitating platelet life span have been developed in experimental animals, but have not yet been used in humans. These methods are described below.

## PLATELET BIOTINYLATION

Heilmann et al (58) demonstrated that dog platelets incubated *in vitro* with N-hydroxy succinimido biotin (NHS-biotin) were covalently labeled with biotin. Biotinylated platelets, which can be enumerated by flow cytometry after labeling with fluorochrome-labeled streptavidin (58), have an *in vivo* life span indistinguishable from isotopically labeled platelets. Franco et al (59) have verified that rabbit platelets can also be biotinylated without affecting *in vivo* survival and have further extended this technique by demonstrating that two populations of platelets can be simultaneously monitored by labeling with different levels of biotin (Fig. 9.4). Recently, dual-level biotinylation was utilized in dogs to examine the survival of autologous and homologous platelets in splenectomized dogs (60). Platelets can also be biotinylated *in vivo* in dogs and mice by intravenous infusion of activated-biotin derivatives; these *in vivo* derivatized platelets survive normally (61, 62).

The potential utility of biotinylation in humans has been questioned by recent studies demonstrating naturally occurring antibiotin antibodies in normal humans (63); interestingly, high-affinity titers of antibiotin antibodies were observed in several laboratory workers routinely exposed to biotinylation reagents. Additionally, Cordle et al (64) have shown that infusion of biotinyl-

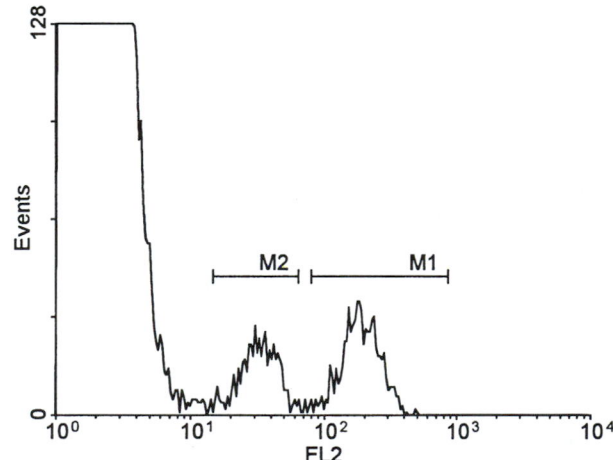

**FIGURE 9.4.** Flow cytometric analysis of dual-level biotinylation of dog platelets. Two samples of whole blood from a dog were labeled *in vitro* with different concentrations of NHS-biotin as described (60). Three hours after reinfusion of the two samples blood was drawn and analyzed for biotinylated platelets by their ability to bind phycoerythrin-streptavidin (FL2) and a platelet-specific monoclonal antibody. The histogram demonstrates the number of events (ordinate) versus phycoerythrin fluorescence (abscissa). Regions M1 (high-level biotinylation) and M2 (low-level biotinylation) represent 5.1 and 3.8%, respectively, of the total platelet population. Each biotinylated platelet population can be monitored independently.

ated red cells into humans results in generation of a weak immune response, one not capable of affecting the survival of the biotinylated erythrocytes but sufficient to cause concern over the feasibility of using biotinylated cells in man. On the other hand, considerable experience with biotinylated red cells and biotinylated platelets in experimental animals has not demonstrated any significant problem with immunization against biotinylated cells (61).

## FLUORESCENT LABELING OF PLATELETS

Cat platelets have been fluorescently labeled by incubation with fluorescein isothiocyanate (FITC) and found to have a normal life span (65). However, repeat experiments indicated a strong immunologic response was elicited against FITC-labeled platelets. Recent work in dogs has substantiated that FITC is sufficiently antigenic that an animal can only be used once for infusion of FITC-platelets (GL Dale, unpublished observation).

Platelets can also be labeled with a fluorescent probe, PKH2, which intercalates into the lipid bilayer and serves as a stable marker for cells. Recently, PKH2 has been used for short-term, *in vivo* monitoring of baboon platelets (66). While a similar fluorescent dye has been utilized successfully in erythrocytes (67), no report of a rigorous examination of platelet life span after PKH2 labeling has been published.

# FACTORS AFFECTING PLATELET SURVIVAL

Platelet survival is shortened in numerous pathologic conditions, including ITP (6), drug-induced thrombocytopenia (68), diabetes (69), coronary atherosclerosis (70), and AIDS (71). Each of these is discussed in separate chapters of this volume. Below are additional circumstances affecting platelet life span.

## SPLENECTOMY

The impact of splenectomy on platelet life span in humans has been a contentious issue. Some studies have reported normal life spans in asplenic individuals (20, 72) while other reports indicate platelet life spans are prolonged as much as 33% after splenectomy (21, 73). The anecdotal nature of trauma-induced splenectomy does not lend itself to systematic studies on the effect of this surgery; furthermore, splenectomies performed in response to systemic causes (e.g., ITP) also do not offer an opportunity to examine this question. To address this problem, controlled experiments in dogs were performed to determine platelet life span presplenectomy and postsplenectomy (60). These data in dogs demonstrated a 47% increase in platelet life span post-

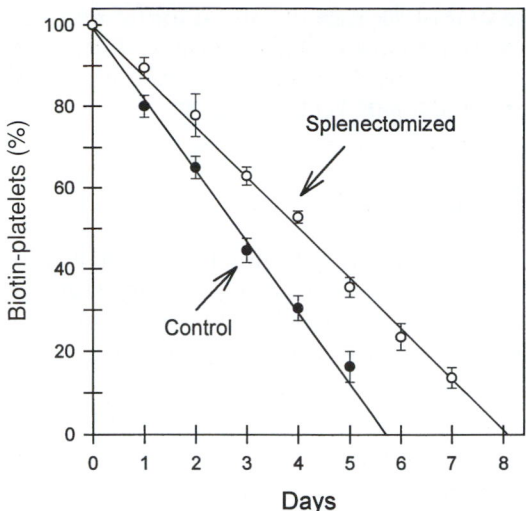

**FIGURE 9.5.** Effect of splenectomy on platelet survival in the dog. Survival of biotinylated platelets was quantitated presplenectomy and postsplenectomy. Control survival (solid circles) was 131 ± 15 hours, while postsplenectomy survival (open circles) increased to 193 ± 7 hours representing a 47% increase in platelet survival. (Adapted from Dale GL, Wolf RF, Hynes LA et al. Quantitation of platelet life span in splenectomized dogs. Exp Hematol 1996;24:518–523.)

splenectomy (Fig. 9.5). Interestingly, the curvilinear nature of the platelet survival curve was modestly attenuated after splenectomy, an observation reported earlier in asplenic humans (21).

## CYTOKINE INFLUENCES ON PLATELET LIFE SPAN

Cytokines modulate platelet synthesis and reactivity (74); however, cytokines can also affect platelet survival. Granulocyte-macrophage colony-stimulating factor (GM-CSF) has been shown to induce a significant, dose-dependent thrombocytopenia in dogs concomitant with a profound decrease in platelet life span (75). Platelet survival in GM-CSF treated animals is shortened up to 75%; however, platelets from cytokine-treated animals transfused into control dogs have a normal life span, indicating no endogenous defect in the platelets (75). The mechanism responsible for this change is not clear, although activation of monocytes or macrophages of the reticuloendothelial system (76) with a resultant lowering of the threshold for recognition and removal of damaged cells is one possible explanation. In support of this hypothesis, increased hepatic uptake of [$^{111}$In]-labeled platelets in GM-CSF treated dogs was observed (75). However, similar studies in rhesus monkeys demonstrated no thrombocytopenia and a small, but not statistically significant, decrease in platelet survival (77), even although GM-CSF significantly impacts megakaryocytopoiesis in humans (78) and primates (79).

# AGE-DEPENDENT ALTERATIONS IN PLATELETS

There has been a long-standing interest in alterations in platelets during their *in vivo* life span. However, the reader is cautioned that the validity of reports in this field is often compromised by the techniques used to identify or isolate platelets of different ages as discussed in the following sections. The best data are available in experimental animals; however, credible information on human platelets has been published, especially regarding density and volume changes associated with cellular age.

## PLATELET SIZE AND DENSITY WITH AGE

Several investigators have utilized radioisotopic labeling of human and baboon platelets to follow *in vivo* aging changes (34, 80–82). These studies, in general, have agreed that platelet density increases with age for these two species (80, 82); however, the magnitude of the age-dependent change may not be sufficient to explain the entire density spectrum present in a normal platelet population (81). Similar results were obtained with tranylcypromine-treated platelets (42). In contrast, platelet volume normally does not change appreciably with cell age (34, 82), but reflects heterogeneity generated at the time of fragmentation of the megakaryocyte. Caution is required, however, in extrapolating this observation to all circumstances since it is not known if the larger platelets produced under the influence of extreme thrombopoiesis (83) or cytokine treatment (84) also maintain a stable volume during aging.

Demonstration that young and old platelets have different densities has led some investigators to assume that pure populations of young and old platelets can be obtained by density fractionation. This misconception hindered the study of red cell aging for several decades (85) and led to the generalization that old red cells may be dense but not all dense red cells are old (86). Similar skepticism is warranted in the study of platelet aging.

One final caveat is the problematic role of animal models in examining platelet aging. Rabbit platelets decrease in density with cell age (87, 88), the exact opposite of that observed with human and baboon platelets, providing a good example of the caution necessary in this field.

## AGE-DEPENDENT CHANGES IN PLATELET COMPOSITION

Dense granule serotonin content increases with platelet age in both dogs (55, 56) and humans (57), data obtained

with multiple experimental approaches. Numerous other changes reported for aged platelets are based only on observations made with density fractionated platelets, including alterations in class I HLA antigens (89), changes in glycolytic enzymes (90), and alteration of total sialic acid content (91). These findings await verification with additional experimental approaches.

Biotinylation, described above for determination of platelet life span, can also be used in experimental animals for delineating age-dependent changes in platelet content or platelet function. Examination of the survival curves in Fig. 9.5 demonstrates that biotinylated platelets in a dog 5 days after biotinylation are by definition greater than or equal to 5 days old. Isolation or identification of these biotinylated platelets allows one to quantitate age-dependent changes. Heilmann et al (92) utilized biotinylation in the dog to determine that α-granule fibrinogen content of platelets increases with *in vivo* age, presumably due to continuous receptor-mediated uptake of plasma fibrinogen during the cellular life span.

## AGE-DEPENDENT CHANGES IN PLATELET REACTIVITY

It has been assumed that aged platelets are functionally less competent than are young platelets, although there are relatively few unassailable data on this point. Observations in ITP individuals with very low platelet counts but few bleeding problems support the premise that young platelets are hemostatically more competent (93, 94). Furthermore, transfusions of normal platelets into thrombocytopenic individuals have suggested that old platelets are less proficient at correcting bleeding times even although they are indistinguishable from young platelets when assayed *in vitro* for aggregation with ADP or collagen (95). Biosynthetic labeling experiments in baboons indicate that young (2 days old) platelets are more reactive than are 9 day old platelets (33); however, the impact of heterogeneity needs to be considered since large platelets at every age are more reactive than age-matched smaller platelets (33). Additional, qualitative data on the reactivity of aged platelets in various species are available from a number of studies (96–98); however, direct identification of aged platelets has been problematic and most studies have exploited experimental manipulation of animals (e.g., recovery from experimentally induced thrombocytopenia) or clinical conditions where a majority of platelets fall within certain age limits, but the populations are not pure (95, 96).

Quantitative data on reactivity of aged platelets are primarily limited to animal models. Peng et al (61) used biotinylation in dogs to demonstrate that old platelets are less easily activated by thrombin than are young platelets (Fig. 9.6), a result consistent with the observation that TO$^+$ platelets (i.e., less than 24 hours old) are

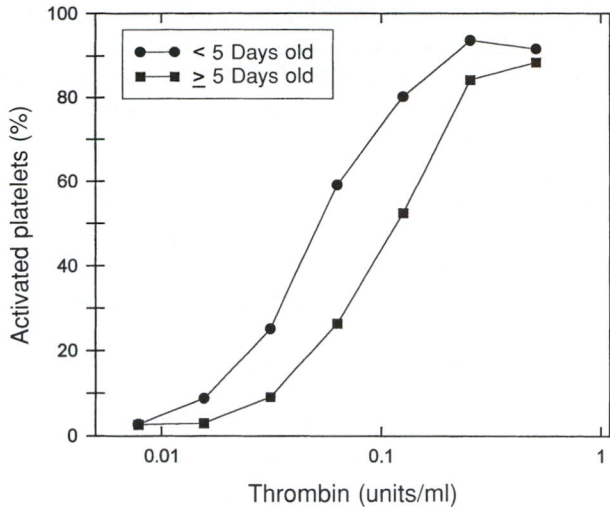

**FIGURE 9.6.** Thrombin reactivity of aged platelets from dogs. Aged, biotinylated platelets were identified 5 days after *in vivo* biotinylation in dogs. Platelet reactivity (ordinate) was quantitated as the percentage of platelets demonstrating cell surface P-selectin (an α-granule membrane protein) after stimulation with increasing concentrations of thrombin (abscissa). Aged (≥5 days old), biotinylated platelets (squares) are less easily activated by thrombin than are younger (<5 days old), nonbiotinylated platelets (circles). (Adapted from Peng J, Friese P, Heilmann E et al. Aged platelets have an impaired response to thrombin as quantitated by P-selectin expression. Blood 1994;83:161–166.)

more reactive toward thrombin than are TO-negative platelets (99). However, a surprising observation was that treatment of experimental animals with some cytokines results in increased reactivity for not only the total platelet population but also for the TO⁺ platelets. For example, interleukin-6 administration to dogs increases the percentage of TO⁺ platelets as well as the thrombin reactivity of these TO⁺ platelets; however, thrombopoietin administration results in increased synthesis of TO⁺ platelets with normal reactivity (99). These data indicate that platelet synthesis and reactivity are under separate control and that cytokine-induced platelets may be hyperreactive when compared to age-matched, normal platelets. These observations demonstrate the peril of generalizations concerning cell age and platelet reactivity.

## PLATELET SENESCENCE

While the above section lists numerous changes associated with platelet aging, there is no indication as to the mechanism of platelet senescence. If the multiple hit theory of platelet aging is correct, the biologic clock determining the life span of platelets is simply one of accumulated insults, which are presumably recognized by tissue

macrophages responsible for phagocytosis of senescent platelets. Senescent platelets are removed primarily by macrophages in the spleen, although the larger blood flow of the liver allows severely damaged platelets to be removed more quickly by hepatic macrophages (22, 100). Proposals for senescence changes in aging platelets include decreased levels of sialic acid (91), accumulation of surface IgG (101), or generation of a senescence antigen associated with glycoprotein IIIa (102). None of these proposals have yet been verified in valid model systems.

## REFERENCES

1. Aster RH, Jandl JH. Platelet sequestration in man. I. Methods. J Clin Invest 1964;43:843–855.
2. Anonymous. Recommended method for indium-111 platelet survival studies. International Committee for Standardization in Hematology. Panel on Diagnostic Applications of Radionuclides. J Nucl Med 1988;29:564–566.
3. Thakur ML, Welch MJ, Joist JH, Coleman RE. Indium-111–labeled platelets: studies on preparation and evaluation of *in vitro* and *in vivo* functions. Thromb Res 1976;9:345–357.
4. Rodrigues M, Sinzinger H. Platelet labeling-methodology and clinical applications [Review]. Thromb Res 1994;76:399–432.
5. Anonymous. Recommended methods for radioisotope platelet survival studies: by the panel on Diagnostic Application of Radioisotopes in Hematology, International Committee for Standardization in Hematology. Blood 1977;50:1137–1144.
6. Tomer A, Hanson SR, Harker LA. Autologous platelet kinetics in individuals with severe thrombocytopenia: discrimination between disorders of production and destruction. J Lab Clin Med 1991;118:546–554.
7. De Vries RA, De Bruin M, Oldenburg SJ et al. A new dual-label technique for platelet survival studies with the use of ¹¹¹indium and ¹¹⁴ᵐindium tropolonate. Br J Haematol 1991;78:236–241.
8. Wadenvik H, Kutti J. The *in vivo* kinetics of ¹¹¹In- and ⁵¹Cr-labelled platelets: a comparative study using both stored and fresh platelets. Br J Haematol 1991;78:523–528.
9. Wessels P, Heyns AD, Pieters H et al. An improved method for the quantification of the *in vivo* kinetics of a representative population of 111-In-labeled human platelets. Eur J Nucl Med 1985;10:522–527.
10. Mathias CJ, Welch MJ. Labeling mechanism and localization of indium-111 in human platelets. J Nucl Med 1979;20:659.
11. Harker LA. Platelet survival time: its measurement and use. Prog Hemost Thromb 1978;4:321–347.
12. Badenhorst PN, Lotter MG, Heyns AD et al. The influence of the collection injury on the survival and distribution of Indium-111 canine platelets. Br J Haematol 1982;52:233–240.
13. Radomski MW, Palmer RM, Read NG et al. Isolation and washing of human platelets with nitric oxide. Thromb Res 1988;50:537–546.
14. Bode AP, Holme S, Heaton WA et al. Sustained elevation of intracellular cyclic 3′-5′ adenosine monophosphate is necessary for preservation of platelet integrity during long-term storage at 22 degrees C. Blood 1994;83:1235–1243.
15. Becker W, Borner W, Borst U. 99m-Tc hexamethylpropyleneamineoxine as a platelet label: evaluation of labeling parameters and first *in vivo* result. Nucl Med Commun 1988;9:831–842.
16. Bithell TC, Athens JW, Cartwright GE et al. Radioactive diisopropyl fluorophosphate as a platelet label: an evaluation of *in vitro* and *in vivo* technics. Blood 1967;29:354–372.
17. Heyssel RM. Determination of human platelet survival utilizing C14-labeled serotonin. J Clin Invest 1961;40:2134.
18. Hanson SR, Harker LA. Survival of baboon platelets labeled with diazotized I-125-iodosulfanilic acid: no effect of drugs that modify platelet behavior. Thromb Res 1981;23:133–143.
19. Amorosi E, Garg SK, Karpatkin S. Heterogeneity of human platelets. Identification of a young platelet population with 75-Se-selenomethionine. Br J Haematol 1971;21:227–232.
20. Aster RH. Pooling of platelets in the spleen: role in the pathogenesis of hypersplenic thrombocytopenia. J Clin Invest 1966;45:645–657.
21. Heyns AD, Lotter MG, Badenhorst PN et al. Kinetics and fate of In-111-oxine-labelled blood platelets in asplenic subjects. Thromb Haemost 1980;44:100–104.
22. Heyns AD, Lotter MG, Badenhorst PN et al. Kinetics of distribution and sites of destruction of 111-Indium-labeled human platelets. Br J Haematol 1980;44:269–280.

23. Chamberlain KG, Tong M, Penington DG. Properties of the exchangeable splenic platelets released into the circulation during exercise-induced thrombocytosis. Am J Hematol 1990;34:161–168.
24. Wadenvik H, Kutti J. The spleen and pooling of blood cells. Eur J Haematol 1988; 41:1–5.
25. Bjorkman SE. The splenic circulation. Acta Med Scand 1947;191(Suppl): 7–89.
26. Weiss LA. A scanning electron micrographic study of the spleen. Blood 1974;43:665–691.
27. Heyns AD, Badenhorst PN, Lotter MG et al. Platelet turnover and kinetics in immune thrombocytopenia purpura: results with autologous In-111-labeled platelets and homologous Cr-51-labeled platelets differ. Blood 1986;67:86–92.
28. Wadenvik H, Kutti J. The effect of an adrenaline infusion on the splenic blood flow and intrasplenic platelet kinetics. Br J Haematol 1987;67: 187–192.
29. Schmidt KG, Rasmussen JW. Are young platelets released in excess from the spleen in response to short-term physical exercise? Scand J Haematol 1984;32:207–214.
30. Heyns AD, Badenhorst PN, Lotter MG et al. Kinetics and mobilization from the spleen of 111-Indium-labeled platelets during apheresis. Transfusion 1985;25:215–218.
31. Jensen PN, Glud TK, Arnfred T. Platelet number and platelet volume in healthy young men during exercise and changes in posture. Scand J Clin Lab Invest 1984;44:735–738.
32. Shulman NR, Watkins SP, Itscoitz SB et al. Evidence that the spleen retains the youngest and hemostatically most effective platelets. Trans Assoc Am Phys 1968;81:302–313.
33. Thompson CB, Jakubowski JA, Quinn PG et al. Platelet size and age determine platelet function independently. Blood 1984;63:1372–1375.
34. Thompson CB, Love DG, Quinn PG et al. Platelet size does not correlate with platelet age. Blood 1983;62:487–494.
35. Lotter MG, Heyns AD, Badenhorst PN et al. Evaluation of mathematic models to assess platelet kinetics. J Nucl Med 1986;27:1192–1201.
36. Murphy EA, Francis ME. The estimation of blood platelet survival. II. The multiple hit model. Thromb Diath Haemorrh 1971;25:53–80.
37. Hanson SR, Slichter SJ. Platelet kinetics in individuals with bone marrow hypoplasia: evidence for a fixed platelet requirement. Blood 1985;66: 1105–1109.
38. Schwartz AD. A method for demonstrating shortened platelet survival utilizing recovery from aspirin effect. J Pediatr 1974;84:350–354.
39. Stuart MJ, Murphy S, Oski FA. A simple nonradioisotope technic for the determination of platelet life span. N Engl J Med 1975;292:1310–1313.
40. De Haas HA, Clark SE, Zahavi J et al. A modified non-radioisotopic method for measurement of platelet production time. Br J Haematol 1979; 43:137–141.
41. Catalano PM, Smith JB, Murphy S. Platelet recovery from aspirin inhibition in vivo: differing patterns under various assay conditions. Blood 1981; 57:99–105.
42. Chamberlain KG, Tong M, Chiu E et al. The relationship of human platelet density to platelet age: platelet population labeling by monoamine oxidase inhibition. Blood 1989;73:1218–1225.
43. Chamberlain KG, Tong M, Chiu E et al. The use of monoamine oxidase inhibition to estimate megakaryocyte-platelet regeneration time. Thromb Res 1988;49:425–435.
44. Ingram M, Coopersmith A. Reticulated platelets following acute blood loss. Br J Haematol 1969;17:225–229.
45. Lee LG, Chen CH, Chiu LA. Thiazole orange: a new dye for reticulocyte analysis. Cytometry 1986;7:508–517.
46. Watanabe K, Takeuchi K, Kawai Y et al. Automated measurement of reticulated platelets in estimating thrombopoiesis. Eur J Haematol 1995;54: 163–171.
47. Dale GL, Friese P, Hynes LA et al. Demonstration that thiazole orange-positive platelets in the dog are less than twenty-four hours old. Blood 1995;85:1822–1825.
48. Ault KA, Knowles C. In vivo biotinylation demonstrates that reticulated platelets are the youngest platelets in circulation. Exp Hematol 1995;23: 996–1001.
49. Kienast J, Schmitz G. Flow cytometric analysis of thiazole orange uptake by platelets: a diagnostic aid in the evaluation of thrombocytopenic disorders. Blood 1990;75:116–121.
50. Richards EM, Baglin TP. Quantitation of reticulated platelets: methodology and clinical application. Br J Haematol 1995;91:445–451.
51. Chavda N, Mackie IJ, Porter JB et al. Rapid flow cytometric quantitation of reticulated platelets in whole blood. Platelets 1996;7:189–194.
52. Rinder HM, Bonan JL, Anandan S et al. Noninvasive measurement of platelet kinetics in normal and hypertensive pregnancies. Am J Obstet Gynecol 1994;170:117–122.
53. Ault KA, Rinder HM, Mitchell J et al. The significance of platelets with increased RNA content (reticulated platelets). Am J Clin Pathol 1992;98: 637–646.
54. Bonan JL, Rinder HM, Smith BR. Determination of the percentage of thiazole orange (TO)-positive, "reticulated" platelets using autologous erythrocyte TO fluorescence as an internal standard. Cytometry 1993;14: 690–694.
55. Mezzano D, Del Pino GE, Montesinos M et al. Platelet 5-hydroxytryptamine increases with platelet age in dogs. Thromb Haemost 1991;66: 254–258.
56. Aranda E, Pizarro M, Pereira J et al. Accumulation of 5-hydroxytryptamine by aging platelets: studies in a model of suppressed thrombopoiesis in dogs. Thromb Haemost 1994;71:488–492.
57. Aranda E, Pereira J, Ajenjo C et al. Human intraplatelet 5-hydroxytryptamine is correlated with mean platelet survival time. Thromb Res 1996;84: 67–72.
58. Heilmann E, Friese P, Anderson S et al. Biotinylated platelets: a new approach to the measurement of platelet life span. Br J Haematol 1993;85: 729–735.
59. Franco RS, Lee KN, Barker-Gear R et al. Use of bi-level biotinylation for concurrent measurement of in vivo recovery and survival in two rabbit platelet populations. Transfusion 1994;34:784–789.
60. Dale GL, Wolf RF, Hynes LA et al. Quantitation of platelet life span in splenectomized dogs. Exp Hematol 1996;24:518–523.
61. Peng J, Friese P, Heilmann E et al. Aged platelets have an impaired response to thrombin as quantitated by P-selectin expression. Blood 1994; 83:161–166.
62. Manning KL, Novinger S, Sullivan PS et al. Successful determination of platelet life span in C3H mice by in vivo biotinylation. Lab Anim Sci 1996; 46:545–548.
63. Dale GL, Gaddy P, Pikul FJ. Antibodies against biotinylated proteins are present in normal human sera. J Lab Clin Med 1994;123:365–371.
64. Cordle DG, Strauss RG, Lankford G et al. Antibodies provoked by transfusion of biotin-labeled red blood cells [Abstract]. Transfusion 1996; 36(Suppl):46S.
65. Jacobs RM, Boyce JT, Kociba GJ. Flow cytometric and radioisotopic determinations of platelet survival time in normal cats and feline leukemia virus-infected cats. Cytometry 1986;7:64–69.
66. Michelson AD, Barnard MR, Hechtman HB et al. In vivo tracking of platelets: circulating degranulated platelets rapidly lose surface P-selectin but continue to circulate and function. Proc Natl Acad Sci U S A 1996;93: 11877–11882.
67. Slezak SE, Horan PK. Fluorescent in vivo tracking of hematopoietic cells. I. Technical considerations. Blood 1989;74:2172–2177.
68. Harker LA. The kinetics of platelet production and destruction in man. Clin Haematol 1977;6:671–693.
69. Winocour PD. Platelet turnover in advanced diabetes. Eur J Clin Invest 1994;24(Suppl 1):34–37.
70. Ritchie JL, Harker LA. Platelet and fibrinogen survival in coronary atherosclerosis. Am J Cardiol 1977;39:595–598.
71. Najean Y, Rain JD. The mechanism of thrombocytopenia in individuals with HIV infection. J Lab Clin Med 1994;123:415–420.
72. Kutti J, Safai-Kutti S. In vitro labeling of platelets: an experimental study on healthy asplenic subjects using two different incubation media. Br J Haematol 1975;31:57–64.
73. Hill-Zobek RL, McCandless B, Kang SA et al. Organ distribution and fate of human platelets: studies of asplenic and splenomegalic individuals. Am J Hematol 1986;23:231–238.
74. Burstein SA, Peng J, Friese P et al. Cytokine-induced alteration of platelet and hemostatic function. Stem Cells 1996;14(Suppl 1):154–162.
75. Nash RA, Burstein SA, Storb R et al. Thrombocytopenia in dogs induced by granulocyte-macrophage colony-stimulating factor: increased destruction of circulating platelets. Blood 1995;86:1765–1775.
76. Hallett MB, Lloyds D. Neutrophil priming: the cellular signals that say "amber" but not "green." Immunol Today 1995;16:264–268.
77. Tomer A, Stahl CP, McClure HM et al. Effects of recombinant human granulocyte-macrophage colony-stimulating factor on platelet survival and activation using a nonhuman primate model. Exp Hematol 1993;21: 1577–1582.
78. Aglietta M, Monzeglio C, Sanavio F et al. In vivo effect of granulocyte-macrophage colony-stimulating factor on megakaryocytopoiesis. Blood 1991;77:1191–1194.
79. Stahl CP, Winton EF, Monroe MC et al. Recombinant human granulocyte-macrophage colony-stimulating factor promotes megakaryocyte maturation in nonhuman primates. Exp Hematol 1991;19:810–816.
80. Mezzano D, Aranda E, Rodriguez S et al. Increase in density and accumulation of serotonin by human aging platelets. Am J Hematol 1984;17:11–21.
81. Savage B, McFadden PR, Hanson SR et al. The relation of platelet density to platelet age: survival of low- and high-density Indium-111-labeled platelets in baboons. Blood 1986;68:386–393.
82. Mezzano D, Hwang KI, Catalano P et al. Evidence that platelet buoyant density, but not size, correlates with platelet age in man. Am J Hematol 1981;11:61–76.
83. Corash L, Chen HY, Levin J et al. Regulation of thrombopoiesis: effects of the degree of thrombocytopenia on megakaryocyte ploidy and platelet volume. Blood 1987;70:177–185.
84. Burstein SA. Effects of interleukin-6 on megakaryocytes and on canine platelet function. Stem Cells 1994;12:386–393.

85. Beutler E. Isolation of the aged. Blood Cells 1988;14:1–5.
86. Dale GL, Norenberg SL. Density fractionation of erythrocytes by Percoll/hypaque results in only a slight enrichment for aged cells. Biochim Biophys Acta 1990;1036:183–187.
87. Corash L, Shafer B. Use of asplenic rabbits to demonstrate that platelet age and density are related. Blood 1982;60:166–172.
88. Rand ML, Packham MA, Mustard JF. Survival of density subpopulations of rabbit platelets: use of Cr-51- or In-111-labeled platelets to measure survival of least-dense and most-dense platelets concurrently. Blood 1983;61:362–367.
89. Cretney PC, Aster RH. Variation of class I HLA antigen expression among platelet density cohorts: a possible index of platelet age? Blood 1988;71:516–519.
90. Karpatkin S, Strick N. Heterogeneity of human platelets. V. Differences in glycolytic and related enzymes with possible relation to platelet age. J Clin Invest 1972;51:1235–1243.
91. Rand ML, Greenberg JP, Packham MA et al. Density subpopulations of rabbit platelets: size, protein, and sialic acid content, and specific radioactivity changes following labeling with S35-sulfate *in vivo*. Blood 1981;57:741–746.
92. Heilmann E, Hynes LA, Friese P et al. Dog platelets accumulate intracellular fibrinogen as they age. J Cell Physiol 1994;161:23–30.
93. Harker LA, Slichter SJ. The bleeding time as a screening test for evaluation of platelet function. N Engl J Med 1972;287:155–159.
94. Harker LA, Hanson SR. Platelet factors predisposing to arterial thrombosis. Baillieres Clin Haematol 1994;7:499–522.
95. Johnson CA, Abildgaard CF, Schulman I. Functional studies of young versus old platelets in a individual with chronic thrombocytopenia. Blood 1971;37:163–171.
96. Ginsburg AD, Aster RH. Changes associated with platelet aging. Thromb Diath Haemorrh 1972;27:406–415.
97. Hirsh J. Platelet age: its relationship to platelet size, function and metabolism. Br J Haematol 1972;23:209–215.
98. Hirsh J, Glynn MF, Mustard JF. The effect of platelet age on platelet adherence to collagen. J Clin Invest 1968;47:466–473.
99. Peng J, Friese P, Wolf RF et al. Relative reactivity of platelets from thrombopoietin- and interleukin-6-treated dogs. Blood 1996;87:4158–4163.
100. Kaplan JE, Saba TM. Platelet removal from the circulation by the liver and spleen. Am J Physiol 1978;235:H314–H320.
101. Kotzé HF, van Wyk V, Badenhorst PN et al. Influence of platelet membrane sialic acid and platelet-associated IgG on ageing and sequestration of blood platelets in baboons. Thromb Haemost 1993;70:676–680.
102. Nugent DJ, Kunicki TJ, Berglund C et al. A human monoclonal autoantibody recognizes a neoantigen on glycoprotein IIIa expressed on stored and activated platelets. Blood 1987;70:16–22.

# CHAPTER 10

# PLATELET MORPHOLOGY

John H. Hartwig

## INTRODUCTION

Platelets, subcellular fragments derived from megakaryocytes, circulate in blood as small discs having a precise and reproducible structure. During normal circulation these small discs are frequently pushed into the surface of endothelial cells by the flow of the larger blood-borne elements, yet they circulate without damage and without interacting with the surface of the vascular lining. However, when challenged by localized vascular damage or by activating agents released by damaged endothelial cells, platelets are rapidly activated to prevent vascular leakage. Platelet activation requires rapid structural and chemical changes that (a) activate platelet adhesion receptors, (b) remodel the cell cytoskeleton to allow cell spreading and aggregation, (c) change the composition of the plasma membrane, and (d) lead to secretion and synthesis of platelet activating factors. This chapter focuses on the structure of the resting blood platelet and on the changes in this structure that accompany cell activation.

Studies over the past 30 years have clearly shown that the discoid shape of the platelet as it circulates in the vascular system is maintained by a unique, actin-based cytoskeleton. This cytoskeleton is constructed as the platelet forms within the cortex of the megakaryocyte. It has, at its core, a three-dimensional scaffolding of actin and tubulin polymers. This cytoplasmic framework connects to a specialized membrane-adherent, two-dimensional network whose main component is spectrin. Once assembly of the cytoskeleton is complete in the megakaryocyte, the mature platelet is shed from its surface. In the circulatory system the cytoskeleton provides the mechanical basis by which the cell resists deformation by fluid shear forces. The cytoskeleton in discoid platelets also has been designed with a second purpose in mind. It has been constructed in a special way that facilitates the rapid and extensive changes in cell shape required for these cells to act as vascular plugs. On demand, the actin filaments of the cytoplasmic framework are fragmented. Fragmentation leads to a new cell shape. First, it releases the constraints imposed on the plasma membrane by the membrane skeleton. This event allows the membrane to flow outward. Second, it creates a template onto which actin assembles. Elongation of actin filaments is the driving force for the formation of surface projections.

## STRUCTURE OF THE PLATELET AT REST

Resting human platelets circulate in blood as anucleated discs (Figs. 10.1 through 10.4). Discs are heterogeneous in size, having average dimensions of ~3.0 × 0.5 μm (Figs. 10.1 and 10.3) and have a small cytoplasmic volume of 7 fL (1). Viewed from the outside, discs are flat and have featureless surfaces except for periodic invaginations or pits that demarcate the entrances into the open canalicular system (OCS) of the platelet (arrows in Figs. 10.3 and 10.4). Freeze fracture studies have shown the OCS to be an intricate membrane system of interconnected and anastomosing conduits within the cell (2).

Although the membrane surface appears featureless in micrographs, the lipid bilayer of resting cells is a transmembrane receptor concentrate (Table 10.1). Receptors expressed on the cell surface (see Chapter 11) include (a) the major serpentine receptors of the cell, that is, receptors for thrombin, ADP, thromboxane $A_2$ and epinephrine; (b) the glycoprotein receptor for von Willebrand factor; (c) $\beta_3$ and $\beta_1$ integrin receptors for fibrinogen and collagen; (d) and the Fc receptor, Fc$\gamma$RIIA. The most abundant receptors on the cell surface are highly glycosylated proteins. The major surface glycoprotein receptor is an integrin, GP IIb-IIIa, which can bind both fibrinogen and von Willebrand factor (vWf). GP IIb-IIIa is a complex of the platelet unique $\alpha$ (GP IIb, $M_r$ 145,000, 1008 amino acids) and one $\beta$ (GP IIIa, $M_r$ 95,000, 762 amino acids) integrin subunit ($\alpha_{IIb}\beta_3$). Both the $\alpha$ and $\beta$ subunits have short cytoplasmic tails of 20 and 41 residues at their carboxyltermi-

nals, respectively. The $\alpha$ subunit is composed of a heavy and light chain covalently linked by a single disulfide bond. Both chains derive from a pro-IIb molecule that is enzymatically cleaved and processed in the megakaryocyte. GP IIb-IIIa lies dormant on the surface of the resting cell. Its ligand binding activity is initiated by intracellular signals generated by other receptor-agonist interactions (see Chapters 11 and 12). These intracellular signals have the capacity to induce a conformational change in the molecule that opens its ligand binding site (3–7). The ligand binding site recognizes all proteins having an Arg-Gly-Asp (RGD) sequence which is present in the two major platelet ligands, fibrinogen and vWf (8). There are 50,000 molecules of GP IIb-IIIa in a platelet, 80 to 90% of which are exposed on the resting cell sur-

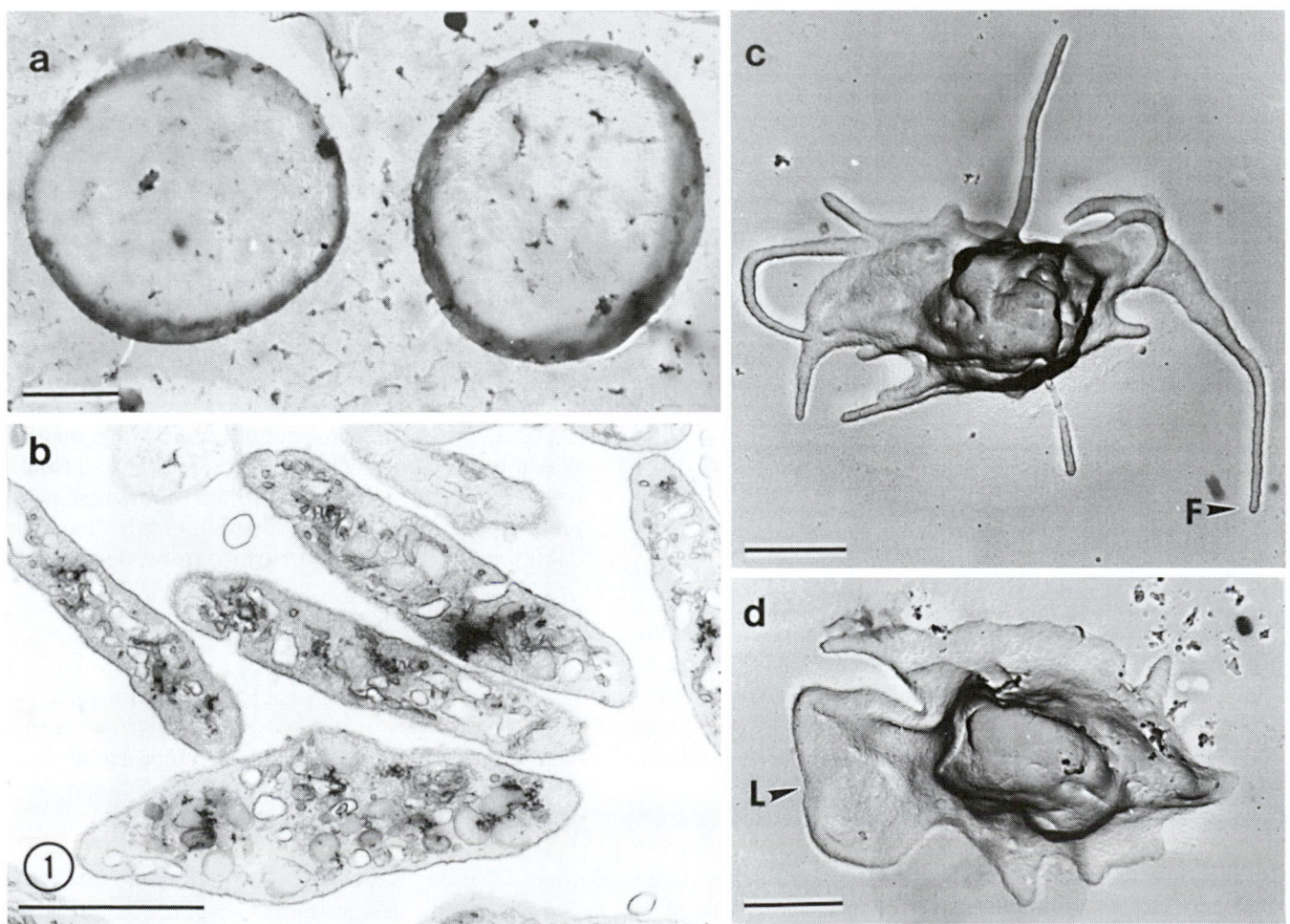

**FIGURE 10.1.**   The resting and active forms of the human blood platelet. **a** and **b,** Morphology of resting cells. **a,** Metal replica of rapidly frozen and freeze-dried specimens showing the surface of two resting cells. In this view only the thick axis of the cell (the plate-like surface) is visible. **b,** Transverse sections through the thin axis of resting cells. **c** and **d,** Metal replicas showing the surface topology of activated cells. Platelets convert from discs into two general morphologies. Platelets spread circumferentially by extension of 1 to 5 μm long filopods and broad sheets of thin lamellae. **c,** Filopodial form. Some cells extend only filopodia when activated. Filopodia (F) grow from the surface of the cell. **d,** Spread or lamellipodial form. Inspection of the surface of cells after spreading reveals that many of the openings of the OCS have been lost (compare with Fig. 10.4B). This cell has spread on the surface using a number of large, flat lamellipodia (L). The bars are 1 μm.

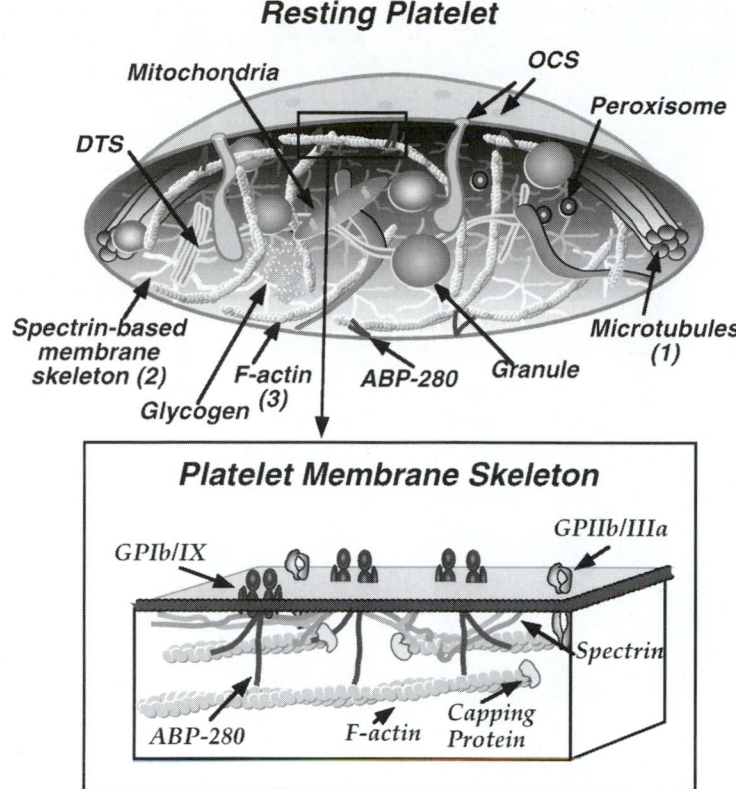

**FIGURE 10.2.**   Schematic showing the structural features of the resting blood platelet and its membrane skeleton. Resting cells have discoid shapes. Structural elements that support this shape are **(1)** a marginal microtubule coil; **(2)** a spectrin-based membrane skeleton; and **(3)** a rigid network of crosslinked cytoplasmic actin filaments (only a small number of the actin filaments have been added to this illustration because they would obscure the rest of the structures in the cell). The microtubule coil is formed from a single microtubule that has rolled up on itself. Resting cells have also been reported to have some intermediate filaments but of unknown function. The rest of the cytoplasmic space is filled with soluble proteins, glycogen particles, and intracellular granules and organelles. Granules that can be identified in electron micrographs are the dense granules, which have electron dense cores after heavy metal staining, and $\alpha$-granules, which stain less well. Components contained within these granules are listed in Table 10.2. Organelles found in the cell are mitochondria, lysosomes, and peroxisomes. Two important membrane systems are also present: the dense tubular system (DTS) and the open canalicular system (OCS). The DTS is an internal system of membrane throughout the cell that is analogous to the smooth endoplasmic reticular system of nucleated cells. The DTS has two primary functions: calcium storage and release and steroid lipid synthesis. The OCS is a second membrane-bounded system of tunnels woven throughout the cytoplasm of the cell. It, however, is in direct communication with the extracellular space. **Inset.** Platelets have a specialized membrane skeleton. This membrane skeleton is composed of spectrin, actin, and many associated proteins. Spectrin dimers (100 nm in length and 5 nm in width), each with a single, actin-filament binding site, self-associate into stable tetramers under physiologic conditions. Tetramers are 200 nm long, bipolar molecules that have an actin filament binding site at each molecular end. The membrane skeleton is held in compression between the plasma membrane and the cytoplasmic actin by ABP-280 connections from the sides of actin filaments to the membrane glycoprotein GP $Ib_{\alpha\beta}$-IX-V. Greater than 98% of all of the barbed ends of actin filaments are capped in the resting cell.

face. A small amount of the receptor, 10 to 15%, shuttles to the surface on cell activation, in the membranes of the storage granules.

The other protein present in copious amounts on the surface of the resting cell is the receptor for vWf (see Chapter 11). This highly glycosylated receptor, a member of the leucine-rich family, is a complex of four subunits: GP $Ib_{\alpha}$ ($M_r$ 143,000, 610 amino acids, 96 C-T cytoplasmic residues), GP $Ib_{\beta}$ ($M_r$ 22,000, 181 amino acids, 34 cytoplasmic residues), GP IX ($M_r$ 20,000, 160

amino acids, 6-8 cytoplasmic residue), and GPV ($M_r$ 82,000, 544 amino acids, 16 cytoplasmic residues [9]). GP $Ib_{\alpha}$, GP $Ib_{\beta}$, and GP IX assemble into a GP $Ib_{\alpha\beta}$-IX complex with equal stoichiometry (1 GP $Ib_{\alpha}$:1 GP $Ib_{\beta}$:1 GP IX). There are 25,000 GP $Ib_{\alpha\beta}$-IX complexes on the resting cell surface. Two of each complex are further linked together by a single GPV (9), a linkage mediated between GPV and GP $Ib_{\alpha}$ (10). Each vWf receptor complex (GP $Ib_{\alpha\beta}$-IX)$_2$-V is coupled to the underlying actin filaments through one molecule of ABP-280, which binds to both

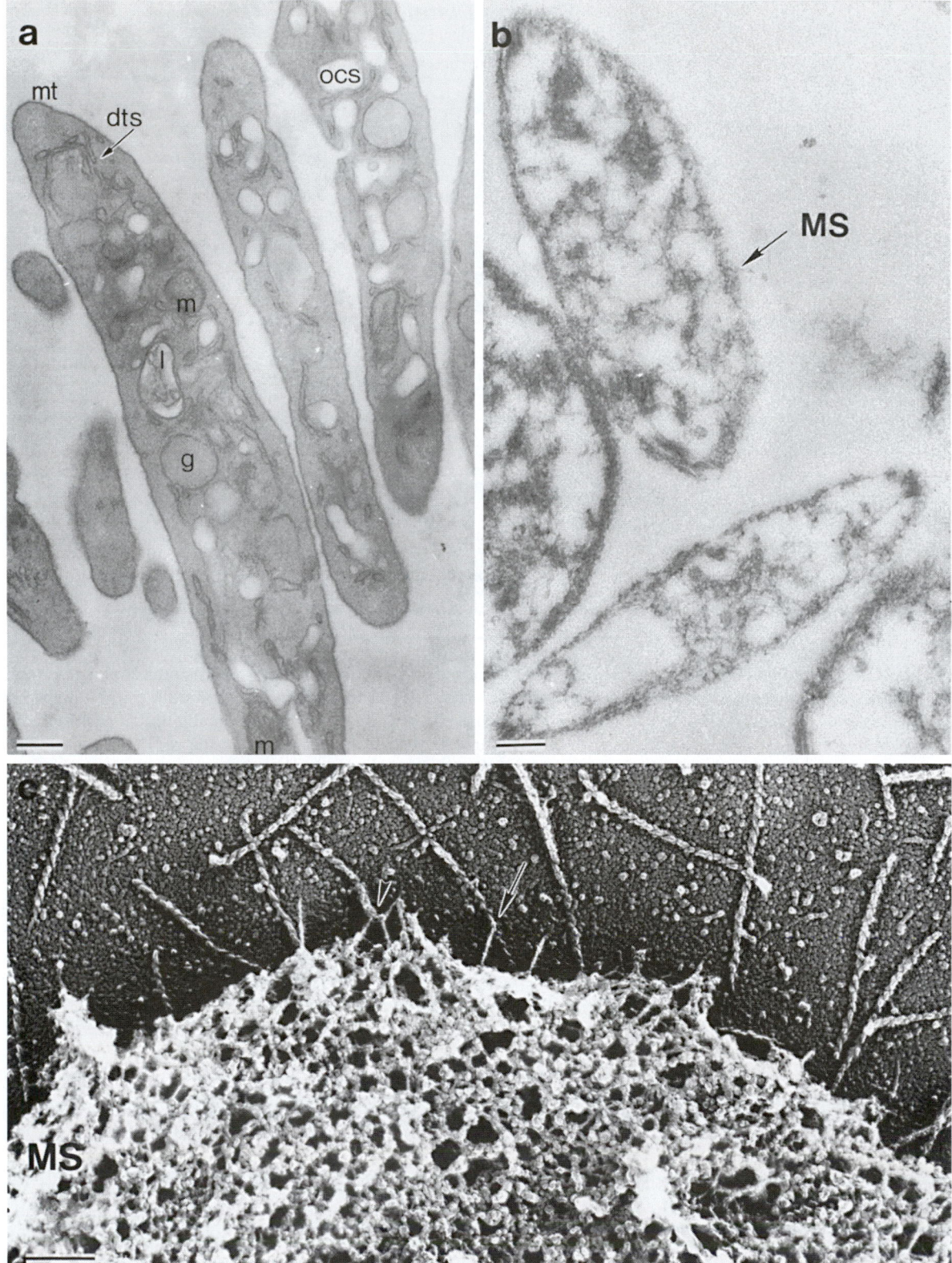

**FIGURE 10.3.** Electron micrographs showing the structural features of the resting platelet illustrated in Fig. 10.2. **a,** Transverse section through resting cells. At higher magnification, other structural components of the cell are visible. Resting cells are densely filled with granules (g), mitochondria (m), and the internal membranes of the dense tubular system (dts) and the open canalicular system (OCS). The dts is a system of smooth endoplasmic membranes responsible for calcium storage and release. The open canalicular system opens to the cell surface at a number of points (arrowheads), as well as branching internally

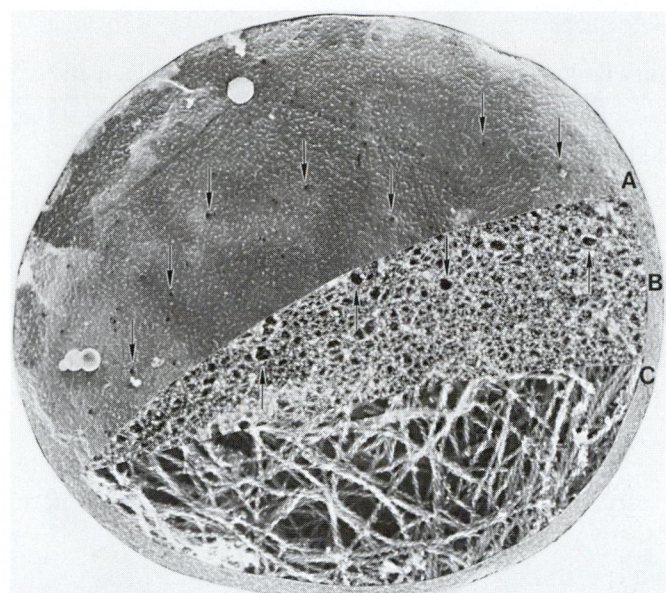

**FIGURE 10.4.** Composite illustrating the two major structural layers of the resting cytoskeleton. **A,** The plasma membrane of the resting cell is decorated with invaginations into the open canalicular system (OCS) of tunnels (arrows). **B,** The membrane of the cell is supported by an underlying spectrin network. This network tightly laminates the plasma membrane. The openings to the OCS are preserved in the membrane skeleton. As discussed in Fig. 10.3, this network is both directly and indirectly attached to the underlying actin filaments. Filament ends are bound by spectrin molecules. Filament sides are linked to the plasma membrane receptor, GP Ib$_{\alpha\beta}$-IX-V, by molecules of ABP-280. **C,** The cytoplasmic space has a dense filling of actin filaments. Actin filaments from the cell center radiate outward. As the filaments approach the plasma membrane, they turn and run in parallel with it. The actin filaments have been labeled with myosin S1 fragment.

of the GP Ib$_\alpha$ chains in the complex. This transmembrane receptor-ABP-280-actin filament complex is important for the mechanical resilience of the resting platelet. Forced expression studies in cultured cells have demonstrated all subunit components of this complex with the exception of GPV to be necessary for stable expression at the surface of cells (11, 12). Unlike GP IIb-IIIa, the vWf receptor is ligand competent on the surface of the resting cell. Binding to vWf in plasma does not occur under normal homeostatic conditions because vWf must first bind to the exposed basement membrane and be linearized by fluid flow before it can interact with the platelet receptor (13). The first interaction between platelets and the damaged vascular surface is mediated by this receptor-ligand complex. However, the binding of GP Ib$_{\alpha\beta}$-IX-V to vWf is transient under blood flow because GP Ib$_{\alpha\beta}$-IX-V has a high off-rate constant. Hence, under flow, the interaction of platelets with activated vWf initiates the rolling of platelets over the vascular surface but not tight adherence. To establish a firm contact with the damaged vascular endothelium, GP IIb-IIIa on the platelet surface must also activate and engage the tethered vWf (14, 15).

Other integrin receptors are also found in platelets. The next most abundant integrin is the collagen receptor, GP Ia-IIa. GP Ia-IIa is found at considerably lower density on the surface than the fibrinogen or von Willebrand receptors. GP Ia-IIa is probably not the only receptor on the platelet surface that can bind collagen.

## INTRACELLULAR COMPONENTS OF RESTING PLATELETS

The plasma membrane of the cell is separated from all cytoplasmic inclusions by a small thin zone of peripheral cytoplasm (Fig. 10.3*A*). This peripheral zone appears

---

**FIGURE 10.3.** *(Continued)*

(arrows). The dense tubular system is distributed throughout the cytoplasm of the cell except for the most peripheral band (50 to 100 nm thick) of featureless cytoplasm. This band is occupied by the membrane skeleton (ms) of the cell. The peripheral microtubule ring is cut in cross-section at the two ends of the cell (mt). **b,** The cytoskeleton of the resting cell in transverse section. The cytoskeleton remains after removal of lipids and soluble proteins using detergents (Triton X-100). Note that the cytoskeleton retains the discoid shape of the cell and is covered by a dense matte of material, 50 to 100 nm in thickness. This proteinaceous matte corresponds to the membrane skeleton (MS) of the cell (see panel c). The cytoplasmic space has a lacy filling of filaments revealed by other techniques to be actin (Fig. 10.4, zone C). **c,** The membrane skeleton (MS) of the resting cell and its attachments to actin filaments. In metal replicas of rapidly frozen and freeze-dried cells, both the structure of the membrane skeleton and its actin filament attachments are clarified. The MS is a two-dimensional network composed of spectrin tetramers that are coated with globular material such as residual membrane proteins and cytoplasmic proteins associated with this network. Two types of actin filament connections are made with this network. The actin filaments have been decorated using myosin subfragment 1 (S1), which gives them a twisted cable–like appearance in frozen samples. Myosin S1 labeling reveals the polarity of the actin filament and "pointed" (p) and "barbed (b)" ends are definable. The ends of actin filament are bound by the ends of spectrin molecules on the edges of the membrane network (arrowhead). Multiple spectrin molecules can be observed to be bound at the "pointed" end of one actin filament. Elongated strands also link the membrane skeleton to the sides of actin filaments. The strands are molecules of ABP-280. The bars are 0.5 μm.

**TABLE 10.1.**   Receivers of the Platelet Plasma Membrane

| Receptor | # Exposed on Platelet Surface vs Total | Membrane Density/$\mu^2$ |
|---|---|---|
| vWf (GP Ib$_{\alpha\beta}$-IX-V) | 25,000/28,000 | 2000 |
| Fibrinogen (GP IIb-IIIa or $\alpha_{IIb}\beta_3$) | 50,000/55,000 | 4000 |
| Collagen (GP Ia-IIa or $\alpha_2\beta_1$) | Minor | |
| Laminin ($\alpha_6\beta_1$ or VLA-6) | Minor | |
| Fibronectin ($\alpha_5\beta_1$ or VLA-2) | Minor | |
| Vitronectin ($\alpha_5\beta_3$) | Minor | |
| Fc$_\gamma$RIIA | 1000–2000 | 80 |
| Thrombin | 1500–2000/3000 (130) | 80 |
| ADP | ND | |
| Thromboxane A$_2$ | ND | |
| P-selectin (CD 62) | None on resting cell | |
| Collagen, thrombospondin (GP IV, CD 36) | Minor | |

**TABLE 10.2.**   Contents of Platelet Granules

| α-Granules | Dense Granules |
|---|---|
| **Soluble adhesive proteins:** fibrinogen, fibronectin, thrombospondin, von Willebrand factor | **Activating agents:** ADP, ATP, serotonin, guanine nucleotides |
| **Enzymes and inhibitors:** plasminogen, $\alpha_2$ antiplasmin | **Other:** Ca$^{2+}$, pyrophosphate |
| **Procoagulants:** factor V, PF4 | **Membrane bounded adhesion proteins:** P-selectin, granulophysin (132) |
| **Growth factors:** PDGF, TGF-$\alpha$, TGF-$\beta$, GGF, ECGF | |
| **Membrane bounded adhesion proteins:** P-selectin (131) | |
| **Bactericidal:** $\beta$-lysin | |
| **Other:** Mg$^{2+}$, guanine nucleotide | |

featureless in cell sections, but is occupied by the membrane skeleton of the cell which will be discussed below. Underneath this zone is the cytoplasmic space that is filled with granules, organelles, and the specialized membrane systems of the cell.

## Granules

Activated platelets recruit blood-borne cells to areas of vascular damage. Release of preformed mediators, packaged in intracellular granules, initiates the secondary homeostatic interaction. In the resting cell many granules are present, and in many cases they sit juxtaposed to the membranes of the OCS. The release reaction of platelets differs from that of other cells in that the granules fuse with the membranes of the OCS and release their contents into this system of internal tubes (see below). Granules are unable to approach the plasma membrane of the activated cell because actin filament assembly densely fills the cortical cytoplasm and compresses the cellular granules and organelles into the cell center where they can release only by fusing with the OCS. Actin filaments thus form an extensive barrier that prevents granule movements to, and fusion with, the plasma membrane.

Platelets have two recognized storage granules, α- and dense granules (Fig. 10.3) (Table 10.2). The α-granules are the most abundant and contain proteins that function to enhance the adhesive process, promote cell-cell interactions, and stimulate vascular repair. These granules also carry the bulk of the cellular P-selectin molecules in their membrane. Once inserted into the plasma membrane, P-selectin recruits neutrophils through the neutrophil counter-receptor, the P-selectin glycoprotein ligand (PSGL1), to sites where platelets have adhered (16). Dense granules (or dense bodies), identified in electron micrographs by virtue of their electron dense cores, function primarily to recruit additional platelets to sites of injury. Critical, platelet activating components released from the dense granules on cell activation include serotonin and ADP. ADP is a potent platelet agonist, activating platelet shape change, the granule release reaction, and aggregation.

## Organelles

Platelets contain at least three different types of intracellular organelles. Each cell contains a small number of mitochondria that are easily identified under the electron microscope by their internal system of membrane cistrae. Less obvious in sections, but identifiable after specific cytologic staining procedures, are lysosomes and peroxisomes. Platelet peroxisomes are small organelles that contain the enzyme catalase. Lysosomes are also small in size when compared with those in other cells. They contain, however, the usual battery of degradative enzymes, including acid phosphatases, aryl sulfatase, β-glucuronidase, cathepsin, and β-galactosidase. These organelles function in the degradation of materials ingested by pinocytosis or phagocytosis.

## Membrane Compartments

### Open Canalicular System

The open canalicular system (OCS) is an extensive system of internal membrane tunnels that serves as a conduit system for the cell. One function noted previously is as a passage into which granular contents are released. A second function is a storage site for membrane receptors and proteins. For example, about 30% of the thrombin receptors are localized in the OCS of the resting cell awaiting movement to the surface of the activated cells. Membrane receptors are also removed from the cell surface into this membrane reservoir, a process termed down-regulation, following cell activation. The best understood surface protein in this regard is the vWf receptor. After activation of platelets in suspension, a centrifugal flow of surface GP $Ib_{\alpha\beta}$-IX-V into the cell center and OCS ensues. Although contiguous with the plasma membrane, not all proteins on the cell surface can enter the OCS. Factors controlling the movement into the OCS remain to be defined. Entry restriction, however, occurs at the necks of the OCS infoldings; for example, IgG molecules fail to penetrate into the OCS. The third function of the OCS is to serve as a source of redundant plasma membrane for cell spreading. OCS membrane is disgorged to the surface following cell activation. When cells are activated in solution, much of this membrane is subsequently reabsorbed into the remnants of the OCS.

### Dense Tubular System

The dense tubular system (DTS) is a membranous compartment that is randomly woven through the cytoplasmic volume. It is believed to be analogous in function to the smooth, endoplasmic, reticular system and serves as the major, calcium-storage system in the platelet. The membranes forming the DTS have inwardly directed $Ca^{2+}$-pumps ($Ca^{2+}/Mg^{2+}$ ATPase). Their pumps maintain cytosolic calcium concentrations in the nanomolar range in a cell at rest. Calcium pumped from the cytoplasm is bound in the cavity of the DTS by the calcium binding protein, calreticulin. The DTS also contains ligand-responsive calcium gates. Calcium is released by the soluble messenger inositol 1,4,5 trisphosphate ($IP_3$), which binds to a special receptor in the membrane of the DTS. The DTS is also the major site of prostaglandin and thromboxane synthesis in the platelet.

### Cytoplasmic Inclusions

The only major cytoplasmic inclusions observed in platelets are glycogen particles.

## THE CYTOSKELETON OF THE RESTING PLATELET

The discoid shape of the resting platelet is maintained by a specialized membrane skeleton that is buttressed by underlying actin filaments and by a peripheral microtubule coil. Important structural and signaling components of the cytoskeleton are listed in Tables 10.3 and 10.4.

## The Marginal Microtubule Coil

The resting platelets have a prominent peripheral microtubule coil (17, 18) composed of a single microtubule that has rolled up on itself (Fig. 10.5). The microtubule coil positions at the periphery of the cell, along the thin axis of the resting discoid shape (see Figs. 10.1 and 10.3). Microtubules are hollow polymers, 25 nm in diameter, composed of 13 protofilaments. Each protofilament is a linear array of end-to-end stacked αβ tubulin subunits. In cells, microtubules are coated with many associated proteins that regulate polymer stability. In nucleated cells, αβ tubulin subunits are in dynamic equilibrium with microtubules such that reversible cycles of assembly-disassembly of microtubules are frequently observed. The critical concentration for tubulin assembly *in vitro* is 5 μM. Platelets have a high tubulin concentration, ~70 μM, 60% of which is assembled into polymer (19). The polymerized tubulin fraction assembles into a single microtubule ~ 100 μm in length which is coiled 8 to 12 times within the platelet. Activation leads to fragmentation of the single microtubule forming this coil, and many individual microtubules are subsequently found in the cell. Cooling platelets to 4°C also leads to the loss of the peripheral microtubule coil (20), causing it to either dissolve or the microtubule to become dispersed throughout the cell.

Microtubules have associated motor proteins that can move over their surface. Microtubule motor proteins are dynein and the kinesin family of proteins (21). The kinesin family encompasses proteins that share a conserved motor domain but diverge with respect to other portions of the protein. *In vitro* studies have defined the different directions microtubule motor proteins move over the surface of microtubules. With one exception, the family of kinesin proteins move on the surface of the microtubule toward its positive end; dynein moves toward the negative end of microtubule.

The function of the peripheral microtubule coil re-

**TABLE 10.3.** Platelet Cytoskeletal Proteins

| Protein | Function | References |
|---|---|---|
| Actin | 42 Kda protein that reversibly assembles into filaments. Present in platelet cytoplasm at a concentration of 0.55 mM. | |
| ABP-280 | 560 Kda homodimeric actin crosslinking protein. Subunits self-associate tail-to-tail to form a 160-nm molecule with actin binding sites on each end. Crosslinks actin filaments within platelet cytoplasm; attaches GP Ib-IX to underlying actin filaments. Molar ratio of ABP-280 to F-actin is 6:1. | (46, 47, 50, 55) |
| α-Actinin | 200-kda homodimeric protein that crosslinks actin filaments into loose bundles. Subunits assemble into antiparallel rods, 35 nm in length. | (50) |
| β4-Thymosin | 5 Kda (44 amino acids) constitutive actin monomer binding protein present at an equal molar ratio to actin. Binding affinity ($k_d$) for ATP-actin monomer of 2 μM. | (30, 31, 133) |
| CapZ | Heterodimer composed of 36 and 32 Kda subunits. Constitutively binds to the barbed ends of actin filaments. In the resting platelet, capZ sequesters the bulk of the barbed filament ends. | (41) |
| Cofilin | Small actin binding protein (20 kda) that accelerates the depolymerization of actin filaments. Preferentially binds to ADP-actin. Inactivated by phosphorylation and ppIs. | (86, 88) |
| Dystrophin | Large, elongated protein believed to crosslink actin filaments and link them to membranes. It has been identified by immunohistochemistry as a component of the testing membrane skeleton. Its function is unknown. Present in very low amounts. | (134) |
| Fightless 1 | 130 Kda barbed end capping protein. Participates in capping the filaments of the resting cell and helps cap filaments assembled following cell stimulation. | (42) |
| Fimbrin (L-plastin) | 68 Kda actin filament bundling protein found in microvilli. | |
| Gelsolin | 80 Kda calcium-activated actin filament severing protein. The activation of gelsolin is required for conversion of resting discoid cells into their normal activated forms. Is inactivated by ppIs. | (37, 79, 135, 136) |
| GP Ib-IX | Multicomponent membrane receptor of vWf that is also a critical structural component of the resting cytoskeleton. The link between actin and GP Ib-IX stabilizes the resting membrane skeleton. | (65–67) |
| GP IIb-IIIa | The major platelet integrin receptor. This receptor links to the cytoskeleton of the activated cell and is used to mechanically connect the actin cytoskeleton to matrix components. | (120) |
| Moesin | Protein of the erzin family that is involved in the connection of actin filaments to membranes, primarily at the tips of filopodia. | (137) |
| Myosin II | 500 Kda hexameric contractile protein (2 × 200 Kda heavy chain, 2 × 20 and 2 × 15 Kda light chains). Reversibly assembles into bipolar filaments, 300 nm in length containing 28 myosin molecules. Component of the membrane skeleton of the resting cell. Centralizes GP Ib-IX on the surface of the activated cell. Moves actin filaments in the pointed direction. | (113) |
| Spectrin | Large, elongated, tetrameric protein ($\alpha_2\beta_2$). α and β chains assemble into antiparallel dimers. One end of the dimer strand has an actin binding site, the other a self-association site. Dimers self-associate to form the 200 nm long strands that compose the membrane skeleton of platelets and erythrocytes. | (44, 69) |
| Talin | 200 Kda adhesion site protein involved in attaching integrin receptors to the cytoskeleton. Has been reported to directly bind actin. | (138, 139) |
| Tensin | 210 Kda actin capping protein of adhesion sites. Expressed in low abundance in platelets. Function ill-defined. | (140–142) |
| Tropomyosin | Rod shaped, 30 nm long protein that binds along the actin filament groves. Each molecular binds to six actin subunits in filaments. Amplifies myosin II actin-activated ATPase activity. Other functions unclear in nonmuscle cells. | |
| VASP | 50 Kda protein component of the spatial actin monomer delivery system. Self-associates into tetramers. Each subunit has four profilin binding sites. VASP binds to vinculin and zyxin. VASP is related in structure to a *Drosophila* protein called Ena. The mammalian homolog of ENA is called MENA. | (106) |
| Vinculin | 130 Kda protein of adhesion sites. Although its precise function is unclear, vinculin is involved in attaching actin filaments to adhesion sites. Vinculin contains a cryptic actin binding site in its N-terminal head domain. It also has ppI and VASP binding sites. | (111) |
| WASP | Protein mutated, or lacking, in myeloid cells from individuals having Wiskott-Aldrich syndrome. Binds the small GTPase Cdc42. WASP contains pH, GBD, polyproline, cofilin, and verprolin domains. N-WASP is the ubiguious isoform of WASP, first identified in neuronal cells. | (94–97) |
| WIP | Recently identified protein that binds WASP. Highly enriched in proline residues. Contains a verprolin-like domain. | |
| Zyxin | Protein of adhesion sites that binds VASP. | (109) |

| Protein | Function | References |
|---|---|---|
| cdc42 | Small GTPase that regulates the growth of filopodia in fibroblasts. Binds to the WASP protein. | (93) |
| 14-3-3 | Small adaptor protein associated with the cytoplasmic tails of the vWf receptor. | |
| PI-3 kinase | Family of enzymes that phosphorylate phosphoinositides in the D3 position. Platelets have at least two forms of this enzyme. One is regulated by trimeric G proteins (βγ-p110). The other is activated through tyrosine kinase receptors (p85/p110). Rho has been reported to also activate the latter form of the kinase in platelets. | (143, 144) |
| PI$_4$P-5 kinase | Kinase that phosphorylates PI$_4$P in the D3 position. This enzyme has been shown to bind to both the rac and rho GTPases, although its activity state is affected by GTPase binding. Also activated by phosphatidic acid. | (145–147) |
| Pleckstrin | Adaptor protein involved in the coupling of different signaling cascades in the platelet. Contains two pH domains. These domains bind either PIP$_2$ or βγ-G-protein subunits. On platelet activation, pleckstrin is phosphorylated in three positions by PKCs. | (148–150) |
| PLC | Enzymes that hydrolyze PI$_{45}$, P$_2$ into IP$_3$ and DAG. | |
| PKC | A family of kinases activated by D3 containing ppIs and DAG. | (104, 151, 152) |
| pp60$^{src}$ | Kinases involved in signal transduction. | |
| pp125$^{Fak}$ | Tyrosine kinase associated with adhesion sites. | (153) |
| Rac | Small GTPase that directs the assembly of lamellipods and ruffles. In platelets, rac is involved in the activation of PI$_4$P-5 kinase. | (91, 154, 155) |
| rap1b | Small GTPase involved in either the regulation of GP IIb-IIIa activity or downstream signaling from this receptor to other signaling cascades. | (156) |
| RATFK | A FAK related tyrosine kinase enriched in platelets and megakaryocytes. | (157) |
| Rho | Small GTPase that initiates stress-fiber and adhesion site formation. | (91, 154) |
| Trimeric G proteins | Critical signaling proteins that couple serpentine receptors to cellular functions. | |

mains ambiguous to this day. One role hypothesized for the microtubule ring is the maintenance of discoid shape. While this notion is attractive, experimental evidence exists both for and against this idea. Destabilizers such as colchicine, vincristine, or nocodazole have been used to depolymerize the platelet microtubule ring. Human platelets are reported to round (lose discoid shape) after extensive colchicine treatment (17) . However, in bovine platelets, microtubule disassembly has no detrimental effect on the cells and they remain discoid in shape (22). The microtubule ring has also been suggested to be of importance in thrombopoiesis. Thrombopoietin (see Chapter 8) induces the shedding of platelet-like particles from megakaryocytes *in vitro*. Platelets are first observed at the cell margins in defined "proplatelet" territories. Next, the proplatelet territories at the periphery of the megakaryocyte elongate in a process that correlates with the formation of a central longitudinal microtubule bundle (23). The proplatelets are then shed from the cell surface. In this process the microtubule bundle could participate in defining the boundaries of individual platelets within the megakaryocyte

and act as a ruler to size the platelets to be shed. Microtubules could also serve as tracks in the translocation of components into the proplatelet bodies. Microtubules also may be involved in the transport of material when the cells are activated. The microtubule coil reorganizes in activated cells, forming a radial array from which individual microtubules exit and run to the cell surface, particularly into filopods and pseudopods (Fig. 10.6). Microtubules are therefore in the correct position to serve as tracks in the delivery of material across the cell.

## Organization of Actin in the Resting Cell

Platelets contain high concentrations of actin, 0.5 mM, which, like tubulin, is in a dynamic, monomer-polymer equilibrium (24). In the resting platelet only a portion of the cytoplasmic actin is polymerized into filaments. Forty percent of the total actin is polymerized into ~ 2000 filaments within the platelet cytoplasm. The average length of each filament is ~ 1.1 μm. Actin polymers are double helical polarized structures. Because of this inherent polarity, the kinetics of monomer addition and subtraction from the two filament ends are different in

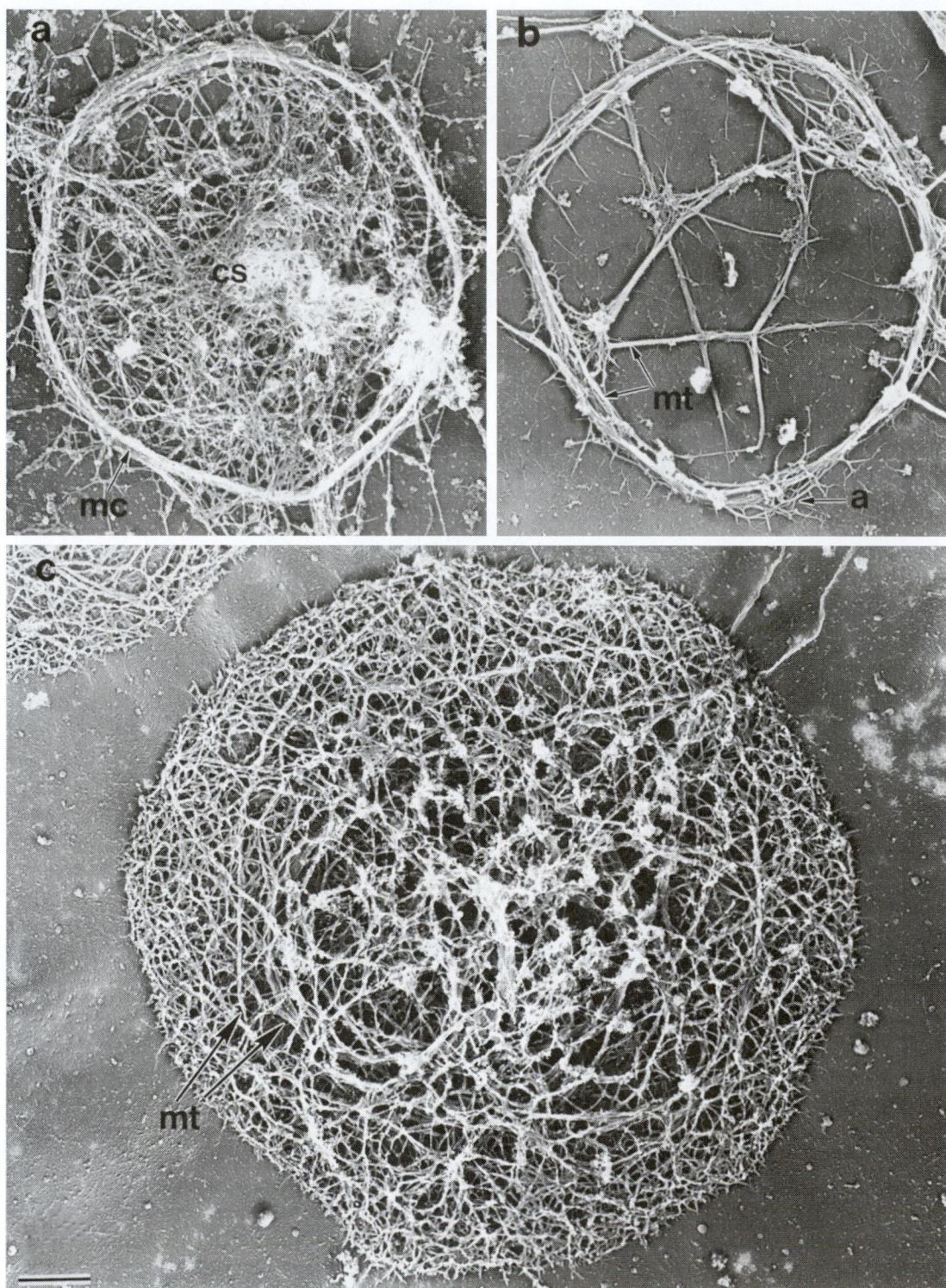

**FIGURE 10.5.** **a** and **b,** The microtubule ring of the resting platelet. **a,** Removal of the membrane skeleton unveils the structure of the underlying microtubule coil (mc) and the actin cytoskeleton (cs). The microtubule ring retains the dimensions of the resting cell; for example, the diameter of the cytoskeleton and coil is 9 μm. **b,** Structure of an isolated microtubule ring. Isolated specimens retain the size and shape of the ring in cytoskeletal preparations (compare with panel A). In addition to microtubules, isolated rings also have many intermingled actin fibers. **c,** Calcium mediated fragmentation of the resting cytoskeleton converts discs into spheres. Organization of a representative cytoskeleton from an activated cell using cytochalasin to trap cytoskeletal changes independent of those mediated by actin assembly. There is an increase in the cytoskeletal surface area relative to a cytoskeleton from a resting cell (compare with panel A). The cortex of the cytoskeleton is replete with short actin filaments arranged in a three-dimensional network. Microtubules (mt) are indicated by the arrows. The bars are 0.5 μm.

the presence of ATP (25). The affinity of monomer is highest for the end of the filament defined as "barbed" by decoration of filaments with myosin subfragment 1. During filament assembly (26), monomers add most rapidly to this filament end. This end of the actin filament is also the site to which the fungal metabolites, the cytochalasins, bind (27). Since actin filament assembly is completely inhibited by cytochalasin in agonist-treated cells, filament growth is restricted to the barbed filament end (28, 29). Growth at the opposing, or "pointed" end can also occur *in vitro* but at a rate tenfold slower than at the barbed end. Growth from the pointed end does not, however, occur in activated cells. Growth at the pointed end is prevented by the proteins that bind to and sequester actin into a nonpolymerizable or monomeric pool. In the resting platelet 60% of the total actin is stored in such a pool, primarily in a 1:1 complex with β4-thymosin, a small protein present at equal molar concentration to actin in platelet cytoplasm (30–32). The affinity of β4-thymosin for actin monomer is greater than that of the pointed filament end for monomer but less than that of the barbed end for monomer. Hence, to maintain a stable population of filaments in the resting cell, all the barbed ends of the filaments must be sequestered. Barbed end sequestration is mediated by another group of proteins, including gelsolin (33–37), capZ, or capping protein (38–41), and flightless1 (42). CapZ is responsible for protecting filament ends in the resting cell. CapZ binds constitutively to actin filament ends with high affinity (43). In the resting cell, 30 to 35% of capZ is bound to actin, an amount sufficient to cap all of the barbed filament ends.

Cytoplasmic actin filaments fill ~10% of the cytoplasmic space of the resting cell. These filaments arise in the center of the cell where they are joined together into a three-dimensional network (44). In general, the filaments then radiate outward from the cell center, and as the ends approach the plasma membrane, they turn to run in parallel with the membrane (see Fig. 10.4). Within cytoplasm, the architecture of actin filaments is determined by filament crosslinking proteins. These proteins bind along the sides of actin filaments and organize actin into higher order ultrastuctures. The most abundant proteins having this function in platelets are ABP-280 (45, 46), a large ($M_r$ 561,000) elongated dimeric molecule (47–49), and α-actinin, a smaller ($M_r$ 200,000) homodimer with its subunits arranged side-by-side in an antiparallel configuration (50–54). ABP-280 and α-actinin are present at 5- to 10-μM concentrations in platelets. This corresponds to a molar ratio of crosslinking protein to actin of 1:50 to 100.

ABP-280 subunits self-associate end-to-end, forming bipolar molecules. Molecules have their actin binding sites on their free ends. The orientation of these ends in solution provides the protein with the capacity to crosslink actin filaments into orthogonal networks. ABP-280 also constitutively adheres actin fibers to the plasma membrane through binding to the vWf receptor (55, 56). Each ABP-280 subunit has an extended rod domain that is formed from 24 repetitive elements, each composed of ~100 amino acids and that fold into an Ig-like barrel structure (57). The actin binding domain is localized at the N-terminus of each subunit. Proteolytic experiments first indicated that the binding site for GP $Ib_\alpha$ is in the carboxyl portion of ABP-280 subunits (55, 56, 58–60). Truncation experiments next revealed that the GP $Ib_\alpha$ binding site lies between residues 2099 and 2136 of the ABP-280 subunit or repeats 17-19, which is near to the self-association site on the molecule. Since each ABP-280 subunit strand is 80 nm long, the GP $Ib_\alpha$ binding site is ~60 nm in distance from the actin binding domain. Subunits dimerize at the C-T using the last repetitive element, repeat 24, forming a molecule having two binding sites for GP $Ib_\alpha$. Andrews and Fox have restricted the site of ABP-280 attachment to the vWf receptor to the α-chain of GP Ib. The α-chain extends a cytoplasmic tail of 96 amino acids (residues 515-610 of GP $Ib_\alpha$). Synthetic peptides spanning from residues 536-568 compete efficiently with GP $Ib_\alpha$ for ABP-280 binding *in vitro*.

The stoichiometry of ABP-280 to GP $Ib_{\alpha\beta}$-IX-V in the platelet is 1:2. Experiments have shown that each ABP-280 molecule is bound to the cytoplasmic domain of two GP Iα chains; >90% of the GP $Ib_{\alpha\beta}$-IX-V is irreversibly complexed to ABP-280. The binding of ABP to GP $Ib_\alpha$ is not affected by the activation state of the platelet. Linkage of actin filaments to the vWf receptor is essential for the assembly and maintenance of the discoid cell morphology. The most damaging of platelet structure defects in humans is found when platelets lack this connection. This disease in humans is Bernard-Soulier syndrome (BSS) (see Chapter 32). Platelets from individuals with BBS have <10% of the normal surface compliment of GP $Ib_{\alpha\beta}$-IX. Failure to express surface GP $Ib_{\alpha\beta}$-IX results from destabilizing mutations in any one of the three component receptor subunits, GP $Ib_\alpha$, GP $Ib_\beta$, or GP IX (61–66). The hallmarks of this platelet specific disease are enlarged and fragile platelets (67). As discussed below, these defects result from loss of the ABP-280-actin filament linkage that normally stabilizes the interaction of actin with the platelet plasma membrane.

## THE MEMBRANE SKELETON OF THE RESTING PLATELET

The most remarkable ultrastructure found in the resting platelet lies just beneath its plasma membrane where an elaborate membrane skeleton is found (Fig. 10.3). This skeleton is a planar network of elongated spectrin molecules that laminates the underside of and provides support for the plasma membrane (Figs. 10.3 and 10.4). This

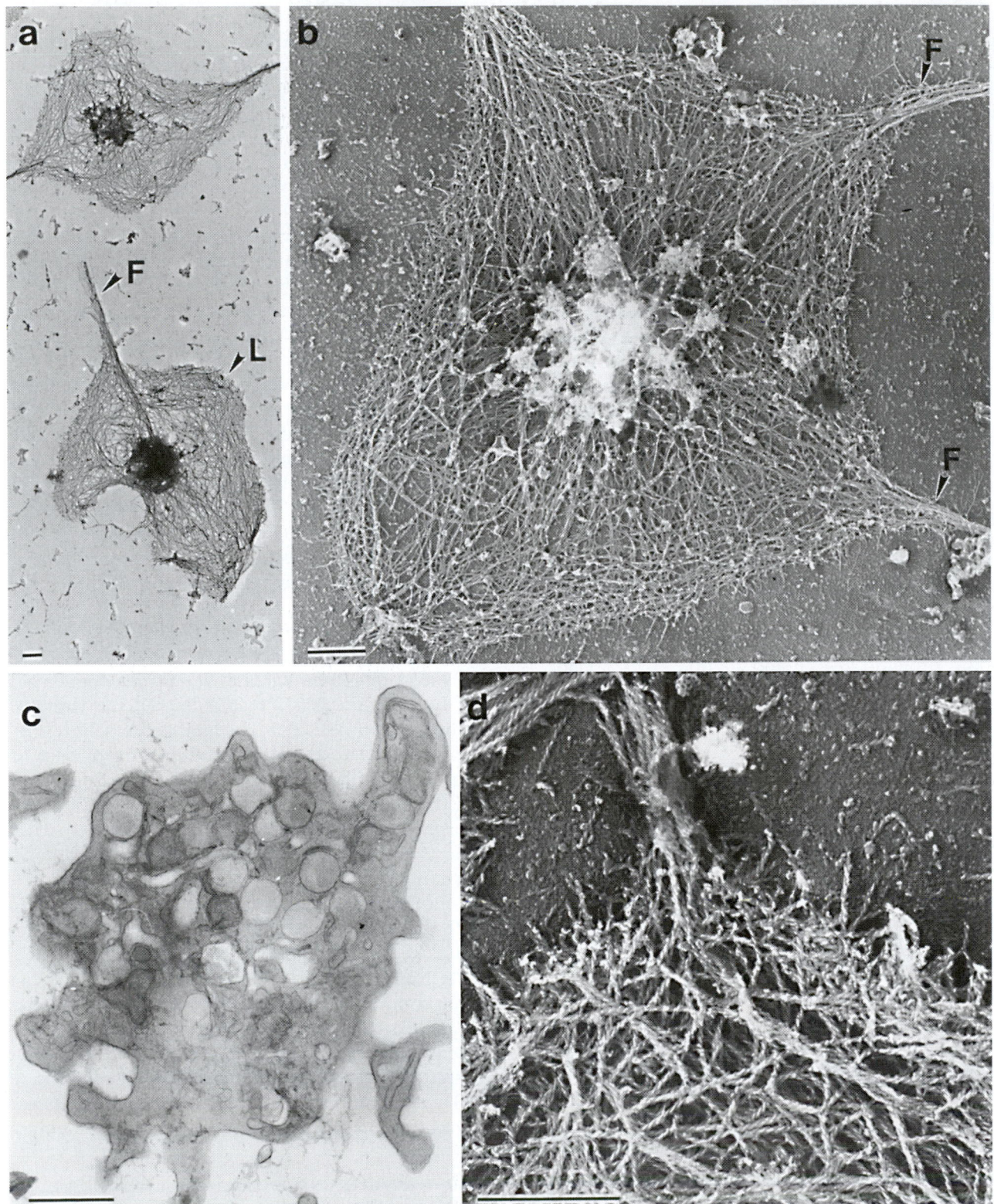

**FIGURE 10.6.** Structure of the activated platelet and its cytoskeleton. In accordance with the work of many laboratories (73, 158, 159, 160), a dramatic remodeling of the cytoskeleton accompanies the extension of cellular processes. **a,** Low magnification micrograph of the cytoskeleton of two platelets activated by adherence to a glass surface. In rapidly frozen and freeze-dried specimens, a reproducible reordering of cytoskeletal actin is found as they spread on the glass surface. **a and b,** Two distinct zones of new actin filament assembly are observed. Filopods (F) contain bundles of long actin fibers that radiate in parallel out from the center of the cytoskeleton. The bundle fibers originate from diverse points within the internal actin filament core and

membrane skeleton, first appreciated in biochemical studies (68–70), has striking ultrastructural resemblance to its erythrocyte counterpart (44). This two-dimensional network is composed of thin, elongated spectrin tetramers that are interconnected by actin. The actin junctions between the spectrin molecules in the platelet, however, differ from those of the erythrocyte. Spectrin molecules connect on short actin filaments: 14-mers of actin (37 nm long filaments) in the erythrocyte, while in the platelet spectrin joins into a network by binding to the ends of actin filaments in close apposition to the plasma membrane (Fig. 10.3).

The platelet spectrin-actin filament membrane network is fortified by a second major actin filament membrane connection: ABP-280 molecules that fasten GP Ib$_{\alpha\beta}$-IX-V to the sides of cytoplasmic actin filaments. To complete this connection, ABP-280 molecules link GP Ib$_{\alpha\beta}$-IX-V to the sides of actin filaments using the pores of the spectrin network. This feat is possible because ABP-280 molecules are long strands that are able to both crosslink actin filaments in the peripheral cytoplasm and to reach the cytoplasmic tail of GP Ib$_\alpha$ at the plasma membrane. Each actin filament in the resting cell is bound to an average of six (GP Ib$_{\alpha\beta}$-IX)$_2$-V complexes; for example, the stoichiometry of ABP-280 molecules to (GP Ib$_{\alpha\beta}$-IX)$_2$-V complexes is 1:1 in the platelet, and >90% of the (GP Ib$_{\alpha\beta}$-IX)$_2$-V complexes are always bound to ABP-280. The underlying actin filament system, therefore, through the ABP-280-GP Ib-IX linkage, is tightly laminated to the spectrin-membrane network. In the resting cell, the connection of GP Ib-IX to underlying actin filament rails restricts the mobility of the spectrin network, holding it in a state of compression. In the activated cell, fragmentation of the underlying actin filaments is used to rapidly alter the mechanical properties of the membrane skeleton.

The importance of this second actin filament membrane linkage to cell stability is established by the fragility of BSS platelets. Although these cells have a normal spectrin based network, the loss of the ABP-280-GP Ib$_{\alpha\beta}$-IX-V linkage causes the membrane skeleton to be loosely attached to actin filaments, only through the actin binding domains of the spectrin molecules. Absence of this linkage results in platelets of aberrant morphology and large size. The increase in size occurs because the spectrin network is free to expand in the absence of the constraints imposed by the ABP-280-GP Ib$_{\alpha\beta}$-IX-V system.

## Intermediate Filaments

Platelets contain the intermediate filament protein, vimentin, as a minor cellular component (71). In the resting cell, vimentin filaments have been reported to distribute throughout the cytoplasm and to be concentrated in the peripheral microtubule ring, suggesting a role in stabilizing this structure.

# STRUCTURE OF THE ACTIVATED PLATELET

Platelets, when exposed to a variety of agonists, undergo rapid and dramatic changes in cell shape (72, 73) and can convert from discs into spiny forms within seconds. Shape change follows a reproducible temporal sequence of events during which the resting platelet actin-cytoskeleton is disassembled and replaced. The first observable change following activation is the conversion of discs into spherical or rounded shapes. Filopodia and lamellipodia then extend from the surfaces of the spherical forms (Fig. 10.7). Protrusion of membrane-bounded cytoplasmic extensions depends on new actin filament assembly. As protrusions form, intracellular granules, organelles, and the microtubule coil are compressed into the cell center, forming an electron dense mass. Consolidation of material in the cell center is mediated by two factors. First, the cortical actin filament assembly restricts the entry of large cellular inclusions into the cor-

**FIGURE 10.6.** *(Continued)* converge at the base of the filopodia. These are referred to as filopodial bundles. A second type of filament organization is found within the lamellae (L). Filaments within lamellae are short and ordered into space-filling orthogonal networks. These are referred to as lamellipodial or orthogonal networks. Microtubules also reorder on cell activation. The microtubule ring can either become compressed in the cell center or fragmented; for example, multiple single microtubules are now found. In cells where fragmentation has occurred, one or more of the microtubules generally run into filopodia along with the actin bundles. One important change in the cytoskeleton on activation is the apparent loss of the membrane skeleton. The membrane skeleton has been rearranged such that it is no longer readily visible in the activated cytoskeleton. Immunogold studies have revealed that this is not due to the removal of the spectrin molecules from near the cell surface but to a dilution of spectrin molecules over the enlarged cell surface. **c,** Thin sections reveal the generalized remodeling of the cell on activation, but fail to delineate the dramatic nature of the changes in the membrane skeleton or actin skeleton. **d,** Labeling of cytoskeletons from activated cells with skeletal myosin S1 demonstrates that almost every 10 nm diameter filament in the cytoskeleton of an activated platelet is actin and that the short filaments near the cytoskeletal margin and the long filaments that are bundled within the filopods have their barbed filament ends pointing out. The bars are 0.5 μm.

## Actin Changes During Platelet Activation

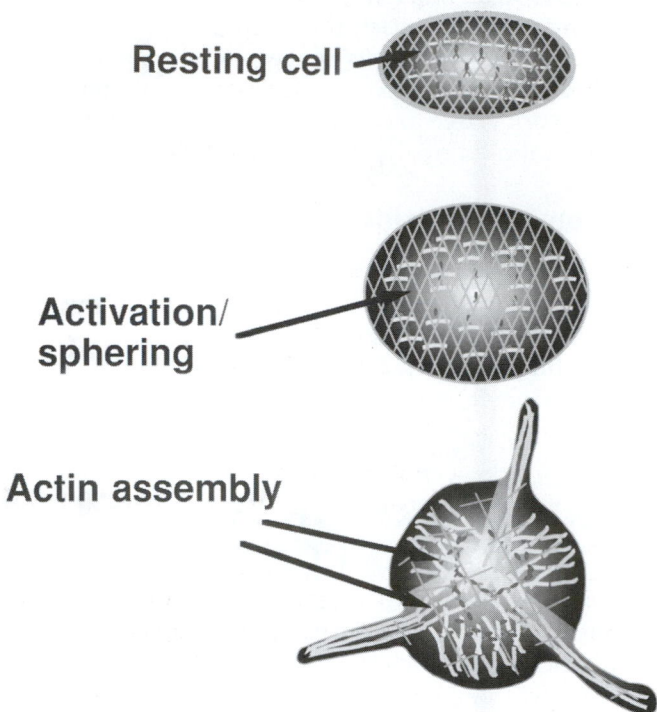

Resting cell

Activation/
sphering

Actin assembly

**FIGURE 10.7.** Sequence of changes in the actin cytoskeleton during platelet activation. **The Resting Cell.** The plasma membrane of the resting human platelet is invested with a dense coat composed of three primary elements: spectrin, ABP-280, and the attached ends and sides of actin filaments. Actin filaments also form a three-dimensional actin filament core stabilized by ABP-280 molecules. Actin filaments from the core run to the membrane skeleton and end. Barbed actin-filament ends are capped in the resting cell by capZ. The sides of these filaments are fastened to the membrane by GP $Ib_{\alpha\beta}$-IX-V-ABP-280 complexes. **Activation/Sphering.** Shape change during activation requires the severing of portions of the radial actin filaments that are in the proximity of cellular membranes. This unlocks the membrane skeleton and frees it to expand. This step requires an increase in cytosolic calcium concentrations into the μM level. The calcium-dependent fragmentation of cortical filaments can be observed by trapping the short filaments in cells activated in the presence of cytochalasin B. Cytochalasin B treated and activated cells enlarge and have cytoskeletons replete with marginal, short, actin filaments. **Actin Assembly.** Severing is followed by the uncapping of filaments and elongation of these fragments by addition of actin monomers previously in storage. Two zones of assembly are found: filopodia elongating from core actin fibers and lamellipodia growing from the short, actin filament templates.

tex. Second, the activation of platelet myosin II provides inward contractile forces (1, 74). Once shape change is complete, the actin filament cytoskeleton is used as a platform for contraction, and contractile tension is ex-

erted between cells. This process causes the syneresis of clots.

## CONVERSION OF DISCS INTO SPHERICAL SHAPES

Transformation of the disc into a spherical shape occurs if cytoplasmic calcium concentrations are allowed to rise into the micromolar range (75). Resting cells maintain cytosolic calcium at 10 to 20 nM (76). Ligand binding to serpentine receptors activates, in a trimeric G protein dependent manner, phospholipase $C_\beta$ (77, 78) (see Chapter 12). Phospholipase $C_\beta$ hydrolyzes membrane bound phosphatidylinositol-4,5-bisphosphate to inositol 1,4,5 trisphosphate ($IP_3$) and diacylglycerol (Fig. 10.8). Formation of the soluble inositol trisphosphate messenger is maximal within seconds following receptor ligation. $IP_3$ diffuses to and binds receptors on the dense tubular system, effecting the release of calcium. Release of calcium from this system alone is capable of generating a rise in cytosolic calcium concentrations to 3 to 5 μM. Calcium can also be imported through the plasma membrane from the extracellular fluid. The combined effort of these two systems can raise cytoplasmic calcium to 10 μM.

While calcium can alter the activity of many actin-

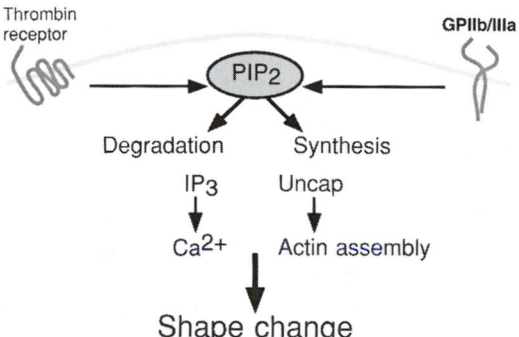

**FIGURE 10.8.** Central role of polyphosphoinositides in the control of platelet shape change. Shape change is regulated by both the degradation of phosphatidylinositol 4,5-bisphosphate ($PI_{4,5}P_2$) by phospholipase C into diacylglycerol (DAG) and inositol 1,4,5 trisphosphate ($IP_3$) and by the synthesis of $PI_{4,5}P_2$ and $PI_{3,4}P_2$ in the plasma membrane. Synthesis of the $PI_{4,5}P_2$ is also initiated by receptor ligation. The thrombin receptor is an example of a receptor that activates both pathways. Thrombin leads to phospholipase $C_\beta$ activation through trimeric G proteins to degrade $PI_{4,5}P_2$ into $IP_3$ and DAG. $IP_3$ binds to a receptor in the DTS to effect the release of calcium. Thrombin also activates, through unknown signals, the cytoplasmic GTPase rac to activate phosphatidylinositol kinases. $PI_{4,5}P_2$ starts actin assembly and lamellipodial growth by binding to and inactivating barbed end capping proteins. The active form of GP IIb-IIIa activates the synthesis of polyphosphoinositides, particularly $PI_{3,4}P_2$.

associated proteins, one particularly important platelet protein that becomes active is gelsolin (34, 37, 79). Gelsolin, an 80,000 dalton protein, is present in platelets at a concentration of 5 μM (41). It is a calcium-binding protein that, when bound to calcium, binds actin filaments. Once bound, gelsolin intercalates into the filament, severs it, and then remains bound to the newly formed barbed filament end. Since the molar ratio of gelsolin to actin filaments is 1:55 in the platelet, activation of gelsolin can convert the 2000 filaments of 1.1-μm lengths in the resting cell into 15,000 filaments of 135-nm lengths (Fig. 10.9). Critically, the filament severing process releases the constraints imposed by the underlying actin filament/ABP-280/GP $Ib_{\alpha\beta}$-IX-V connections on the membrane skeleton in the resting cell, allowing the spectrin-based membrane skeleton to expand, the plasma membrane to flow outward, and the cell to round. The importance of gelsolin in this function has been established using platelets from mice genetically engineered to lack gelsolin. These cells fail to sever filaments on activation and have altered kinetics of GP $Ib_{\alpha\beta}$-IX-V down-regulation.

## RELATIONSHIP OF PLATELET ROUNDING TO GRANULE SECRETION

Platelet activation is accompanied not only by actin reordering but by the exocytosis of platelet storage granules. Mediators released from platelet granules enhance platelet plug formation by attracting additional platelets into the surface of the wound and initiating cellular-repair reactions. The platelet release reaction is unique. The majority of platelet intracellular granules release their contents into the OCS from whence they diffuse into the surrounding fluids. Because of the complex enfolding of the OCS of membrane, granules, even in the resting cells, are always in close apposition to the OCS, explaining, in part, this mechanism of granule secretion. Another factor driving this unique release mechanism is the dramatic cortical actin assembly reaction. Actin assembly begins immediately following activation of cells and results in the formation of an enhanced cortical filament network. The cortical actin network represents a formidable barrier to the exocytosis of granules.

The fusion and release of granule contents following platelet activation depends on a rise of cytosolic calcium concentrations into the micromolar range and is diminished greatly by activities that blunt this transient calcium increase. In many secretory cells it has been proposed that actin filaments form a barrier to exocytosis and must be removed to allow granules to approach the plasma membrane. One proposed role for calcium is to activate protein(s) that function in this capacity. In the platelet it is the gelsolin-mediated filament fragmentation, which also causes the cells to round, that disrupts actin filaments whose cytoplasmic orientation hinders

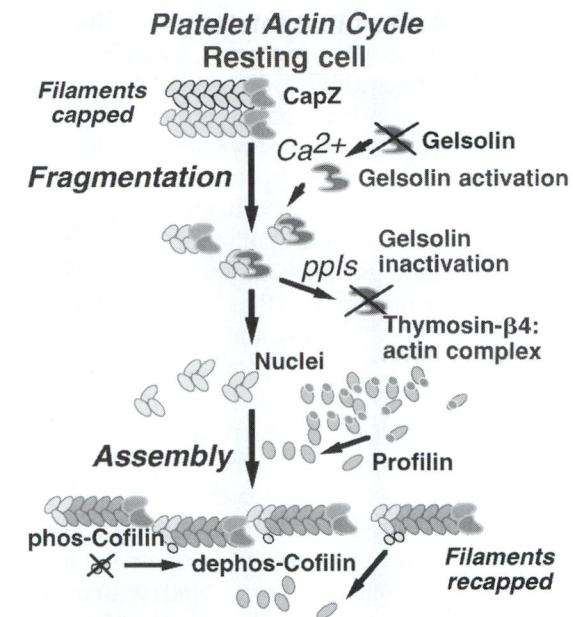

**FIGURE 10.9.** Protein interactions that control actin assembly in the platelet. The 2000 actin filaments in the resting cell are maintained in a stable pool because actin disassembly is prevented by capZ binding to the barbed ends of filaments and because cofilin is maintained in an inactive state by phosphorylation. A large pool of soluble inactive gelsolin is present in the cytoplasm. Agonist binding induces a cytosolic calcium transient. This activates soluble gelsolin to bind and sever the preexisting actin fibers, increasing dramatically the filament number, while decreasing the lengths to 0.2 to 0.3 μm. Filament pieces initially remain capped by gelsolin and capZ. The actin-assembly phase of activation begins when signals are generated that dissociate capping proteins from filament ends. These signals are limited to the plasma membrane and, for activation of actin assembly through the thrombin receptor, are the new synthesis of polyphosphoinositides in the plasma membrane. Polyphosphoinositides bind to and inactivate capping proteins. Filament ends, freed of their caps, act as templates for actin assembly. Profilin now functions to transfer actin monomers stored in complex with β4-thymosin to the barbed filament ends. The assembly reaction ends when filaments become recapped by capZ. Dephosphorylation of cofilin can also lead to reversal of a portion of the new actin assembly by increasing the off rate of monomers from the pointed filament ends, returning the monomers to the storage pool.

the approach of granules to the cytoplasmic membrane surface. Calcium-calmodulin also activates myosin light chain kinase to phosphorylate myosin II (74, 80). Activation of the contractile activity of myosin II generates a centrifugal collapse of granules into the cell center. This promotes fusion of granules by bringing them into intimate contact with the OCS.

## PROTRUSIVE ACTIN ASSEMBLY

Rounding of the cell is followed by a massive assembly of actin filaments. As a result, the filament content of cells doubles. Assembly is initiated from the barbed ends of preexisting actin filaments (28, 29, 81) when barbed end capping proteins dissociate (Fig. 10.9). Uncapping of barbed ends occurs at the cytoplasmic face of the plasma membrane where phospholipids that bind to and inactivate the capping proteins are generated in sufficient concentrations to be effective (Figs. 10.8 and 10.9). Potent phospholipids that inhibit the activity of capping proteins both *in vitro* and *in vivo* are phosphatidylinositol 4,5 bisphosphate ($PI_{4,5}P_2$), phosphatidylinositol 3,4 bisphosphate ($PI_{3,4}P_2$), and phosphatidylinositol 3,4,5 trisphosphate ($PI_{3,4,5}P_3$) (82, 83). Once barbed ends are exposed, the equilibrium between actin monomer and sequestration proteins is altered because, as noted above, the barbed end of the filament has a higher affinity for actin monomer than does the monomer storage protein β4-thymosin. Transfer of monomers from β4-thymosin to the barbed ends of filaments is facilitated by profilin, a small, actin binding protein with the capacity to accelerate filament growth at the barbed filament end from actin-β4-thymosin complexes (84, 85). Filament ends remain open for net assembly for a short time because of the ~3 $\mu M^{-1} s^{-1}$ on-rate constant for capZ (43). Once filaments have elongated, the assembly reaction is terminated by three factors: (a) the diminished size of the actin monomer pool; (b) recapping of the filaments by capZ, a protein with 0.1 nM affinity for the barbed ends of actin filaments; and (c) the dephosphorylation of cofilin (86), a process that activates this protein, accelerating the rate of actin filament depolymerization (87, 88).

Although bulk actin filament assembly is initiated by agonists, the question remains as to how different actin filament ultrastructures are built within the cytoplasm, that is, lamellipods or filopods.

## LAMELLIPODIAL ACTIN ASSEMBLY

Lamellipodial growth is driven by a robust, cortical actin assembly process. Structural examination of lamellipods reveals them to be replete with actin filaments that are organized into orthogonal networks. Such a network is biologically efficient because it uses a minimal amount of polymer to fill a maximal cytoplasmic volume. The structural constraints for this reaction are established by actin filament crosslinking proteins, of which ABP-280 plays the crucial role. ABP-280 binds actin filaments into orthogonal networks *in vitro* and organizes the actin filaments of the resting cell into such a network, as well as laminating these filaments to the plasma membrane. Actin filaments are attached at multiple points to GP $Ib_{\alpha\beta}$-IX-V in the plasma membrane by ABP-280 (Fig. 10.7). Activation leads to the fragmentation of the orthogonal network into short pieces by gelsolin. Despite the short lengths of the filament fragments, however, they remain linked into a contiguous network in perme-abilized cells, connected into a network by the crosslinking activities of ABP-280, α-actinin, and spectrin molecules (Fig. 10.5C). Expansion of the orthogonal network forms lamellipodia during platelet activation. Actin assembly is induced, and filaments elongate off the barbed ends of the filament fragments. It is the spatial orientation of ends of the actin fragments, as defined by ABP-280 crosslinking, that serves as the template for the ensuing growth of the orthogonal network. The ABP-280/GP $Ib_{\alpha\beta}$-IX-V connection further confines the filament pieces to the membrane where second messenger phosphoinositides are synthesized.

Recent work has elucidated how different stimuli can promote particular types of actin assembly within cells (89, 90). In addition, the signaling system for lamellipodial growth from the thrombin receptor has been partially defined. The key ingredients for the specification of different forms of actin architecture are the species of small GTPase recruited by the stimulus. For example, the GTPase Rac, through growth factor receptors in fibroblasts, directs actin remodeling into pleatlike protrusions or ruffles (91). In permeabilized platelets that retain sufficient signaling components to uncap actin filaments in response to thrombin receptor ligation, the addition of physiologic concentrations of Rac quickly stimulates actin filament uncapping. This small GTPase completes signaling to actin in platelets by initiating the net synthesis of polyphosphoinositides, in particular the synthesis of phosphatidylinositol-4 monophosphate ($PI_4P$) and $PI_{4,5}P_2$. These polyphosphoinositides as a family represent only a small amount (~2%) of the total platelet lipids. They are the only phospholipids that have been found to rapidly change in concentration following cell activation. In the resting cell, $PI_4P$ and $PI_{4,5}P_2$ are present in the plasma membrane at concentrations of 150 to 200 μM. Following cell activation, these two phospholipids are made in large quantities, increasing their concentration in the platelet plasma membrane to 250 to 280 μM. $PI_4P$ and $PI_{4,5}P_2$ bind to, inactivate, and dissociate capping proteins from the actin cytoskeleton of the platelet to start the actin assembly reaction (41, 82). Similarly, microinjection of $PI_4P$-5 kinase induces a massive actin polymerization reaction in cultured cells (92). Upstream signaling events that couple the receptor to the GTPase are less clear, although inhibitory experiments have shown that the thrombin receptor couples initially to actin assembly through trimeric G proteins; that is, actin assembly and cell shape change are inhibited by pertussis toxin (77).

## FILOPODIAL ACTIN ASSEMBLY

Filopodial growth is a very different process from lamellipodial assembly. To protrude a filopod, only a small cluster of nucleation sites is necessary. Filopods can be seen to grow from the surface of the cell. Under the electron microscope, they are cored by long actin filaments that originate in the cell center (Fig. 10.6). These filaments begin as loose collections in the cell center. By the time they enter the filopodia, however, they collect into tight bundles. As mentioned above, microtubules can also, along with actin, enter filopodia.

The cytoplasmic signaling system for assembling filopodia is less well defined than that producing lamellipodia. Microinjection and forced expression experiments with cells other than platelets have shown that another GTPase, Cdc42hs, appears to program the actin-based assembly that results in protrusion of hair-like filopodia from the cell surface (93). Signaling to Cdc42hs is known to be initiated by bradykinin, whose receptor is a member of the seven membrane spanning, serpentine receptor family. The signaling molecules that connect this receptor to Cdc42hs are undefined. One platelet protein that has been found to interact with Cdc42hs is the Wiskott-Aldrich syndrome protein (WASP) (94). WASP has a GBD (GTPase binding domain) and 2 PH (pleckstrin homology) domains, a polyproline domain, and cofilin and verprolin related sequence domains (95–97). Pleckstrin homology domains bind specifically to $PI_{4,5}P_2$ (98–100) and to the $\beta\gamma$ subunits of the trimeric G proteins (101, 102). As discussed above, cofilin is a protein that binds to the actin subunits in filaments promoting filament disassembly from the pointed end and N-WASP, a protein related to WASP in structure that has been shown recently to interact with actin (103).

In platelets the following information on filopodial formation exists. First, certain agonists are capable of inducing predominant filopodia growth. Platelets lack the receptor for bradykinin, but treatment of cells with the tumorgenic agent phorbol myristate acetate generates a filopodial transformation. Key in this process is that this agent converts GP IIb-IIIa to its active form. Once activated, GP IIb-IIIa, through outside-in signaling

(see Chapters 11 and 12), causes actin assembly and filopodia growth. The actin assembly reaction differs from that induced by thrombin. The kinetics of filament assembly are slow and the extent of assembly small. Actin assembly is driven by exposing a small number of barbed, equivalent, nucleation sites (83). Once again, polyphosphoinositides are important messengers in this signaling cascade. In particular, a D3 containing polyphosphoinositide, phosphatidylinositol 3,4-bisphosphate ($PI_{3,4}P_2$), and a D4 containing polyphosphoinositide, $PI_4P$, are synthesized in response to activation and ligation of GP IIb-IIIa. Inhibitory experiments have revealed the actin response to be greatly blunted if GP IIb-IIIa is crippled or if D3 phospholipid production is inhibited (104).

Experiments in cells other than platelets have implicated other components to be of importance for filopodial assembly. One multiprotein system implicated in filopodial actin assembly is a specialized, spatial actin-monomer delivery system (Fig. 10.10). This system functions by attracting large concentrations of actin monomers to focal points in the cytoplasm. Actin monomers concentrate on the abundant (20 to 30 $\mu$M in platelets) cytoplasmic actin monomer binding protein, profilin. This protein binds monomers and facilitates the transfer of monomers to the barbed ends of actin filaments. Profilin, in turn, is bound by proteins that carry a small, profilin binding domain composed of 6 amino acids having the sequence XPPPPP, defined recently as ABM-2 (actin binding motif 2) where X is generally A or G (105). This motif binds profilin and is found repeated multiple times in the proteins VASP and Mena. VASP is an abundant platelet protein (106) with four ABM-2 motifs. Tetramers of VASP, believed to be the native species, can therefore bind up to 16 profilin molecules (107). Mena, a protein related in sequence to VASP, is present in mammalian cells (108) and has three ABM-2 motifs.

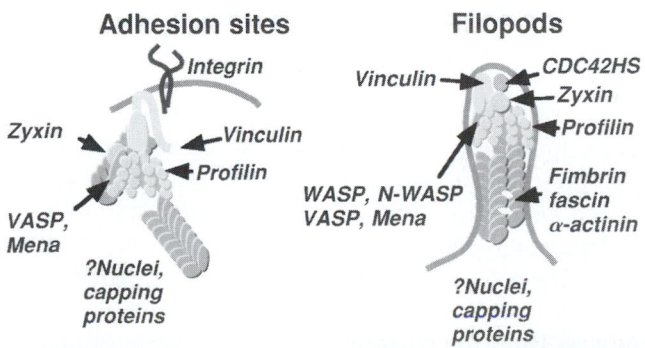

**FIGURE 10.10.**   Proteins implicated in filopodial assembly—spatial actin monomer delivery. Actin monomers are transferred to sites of filopodial assembly by profilin. High concentrations of profilin result from the expression of multiple profilin binding sites on VASP (Table 10.3), WASP, N-WASP (neuronal WASP), and/or Mena (Mammalian Enabled) (108). Spatial targeting is directed by vinculin and zyxin, which bind VASP and/or Mena. Vinculin (161–163) and zyxin (109) are also components of adhesion sites and may promote filament growth at these focal sites in a similar fashion to filopodial growth.

Whether Mena is found in platelets has not been determined. WASP is another protein implicated in microspike formation. WASP shares homology with VASP and possesses three ABM-2 motifs (97). The ability of WASP to bind Cdc42hs indicates a central role in this process in platelets (95–97).

ABM-2 carrying proteins that bind profilin are in turn bound to another group of proteins found at focal adhesions through a second site called ABM-1. The ABM-1 motif is also a polyproline-based sequence of five amino acids that begins with a conserved phenylalanine residue followed by a minimum of four proline residues. Adhesion site proteins containing these sites are vinculin and zyxin. Binding of vinculin and zyxin to VASP has been demonstrated *in vitro* (109–111). This system therefore provides the targeting information necessary to deliver actin monomers to sites of filopodial growth and the capacity to concentrate profilin molecules and facilitate actin delivery to filament ends. The origin of filament nucleation sites in this system has not been defined. Filament ends could be recruited for those present in platelets, or, in addition to supplying monomer, this system might also nucleate filament assembly.

Control of this system is considerably less well defined. As noted above, Cdc42hs is implicated in signals that turn on filopodia growth. VASP is also a phosphoprotein that is, like cofilin, dephosphorylated on cell activation (112). Dephosphorylation may therefore potentiate VASP's function in this system or regulate its oligomeric state. Similarly, vinculin is a molecule that exists in open and closed conformations. In the closed conformation both the actin and VASP binding sites are sequestered.

## MOVEMENTS OF SURFACE RECEPTORS IN ACTIVATED PLATELETS

Membrane proteins rearrange following platelet activation. The most widely studied movements are made by the major surface glycoproteins GP Ib$_{\alpha\beta}$-IX-V and GP IIb-IIIa (see Chapter 11).

## GP Ib$_{\alpha\beta}$-IX-V

GP Ib$_{\alpha\beta}$-IX-V molecules are at their highest density on the surface of resting cells. GP Ib$_{\alpha\beta}$-IX-V complexes decorate the surface in linear rows that correspond to the location of the underlying actin filaments to which they are linked (113). On activation of cells in solution, GP Ib$_{\alpha\beta}$-IX-V molecules of the cell surface become drawn into the cell center and are removed from the surface into remnants of the OCS (114–118). The inward collapse of the receptor begins rapidly (within a minute) following cell activation at a time after which all the actin cytoskeleton assembly has been completed. Centralization becomes maximal after 5 to 10 minutes, and

>80% of the receptor may be removed from the cell surface. Aggregation into the cell center occurs in a process that is analogous to receptor capping in lymphocytes except that the inward movement of GP Ib$_{\alpha\beta}$-IX-V is constitutive, without the necessity of receptor cross-linking. Removal of receptors into the OCS is maximal when cells are in suspension and in buffers lacking calcium. When cells are adherent, the centralization process is greatly slowed, most likely because the actin filaments composing the cytoskeleton become tethered to the substratum, inhibiting their inward collapse. The mechanism of centralization is poorly defined except that it is known to be a contractile process requiring the activation and participation of myosin II (113). Myosin II is a prominent component in the membrane skeleton of the resting cell and is quickly activated following treatment of cells with agonists (74, 80).

## GP IIb-IIIa

GP IIb-IIIa also redistributes on the surface of activated platelets. The surface movements made by this receptor are, however, more complex than those of GP Ib$_{\alpha\beta}$-IX-V. Activation first leads to an initial increase in the amount of total GP IIb-IIIa on the cell surface. A small amount of the total GP IIb-IIIa, stored in α-granular membranes, is carried to the plasma membranes by exocytosis (119). Once at the surface, GP IIb-IIIa can exist in both active and inactive forms. Only the active form binds ligand. Activation requires intracellular signals that mediate a conformational change in the receptor and mediate the interaction of GP IIb-IIIa with the cytoskeleton (120). Linkage to the cytoskeleton stabilizes the ligand-receptor complex. Molecules involved in the linkage of GP IIb-IIIa to the cytoskeleton have not been clearly defined. Talin, a platelet protein of abundance, has been reported to bind directly to the cytoplasmic tails of both the α and β chains (121). Two other adhesion site related proteins, tensin and ppFAK[125], arrive early after integrin receptor activation (122, 123). Inactive receptor distributes over the entire surface of the cell. Active receptor-ligand complexes redistribute from the cell periphery into the central cell mass. Hence, after cell activation, receptor-ligand complexes accumulate over the dense central mass of the cell and into the OCS of cells in movements that are temporally and spatially similar to those of GP Ib$_{\alpha\beta}$-IX-V. Centralization occurs along linear tracks from the cell periphery to the cell center (124). Since centralization is inhibited by cytochalasin B, it is likely that these tracks are actin filaments (125, 126).

## THE AGGREGATION REACTION

After platelets convert into their activated forms, they bind to one another (aggregate) and contract. Aggregation of platelets begins after the actin assembly and cytoskeletal reorganization processes are complete and is mediated by fibrinogen bridging of GP IIb-IIIa receptors. Crosslinking of GP IIb-IIIa receptors induces outside-in signaling by this receptor that recruits additional proteins to the cytoskeleton, particularly to the sites of receptor clusters (127). Proteins procured by signals generated by clustered GP IIb-IIIa include myosin II, tyrosine kinases, adhesion site-related proteins, polyphosphoinositide kinases, and small GTPases. In many cases the functions of these proteins are not known, but many must function to enhance the connection between the membrane and the cytoskeleton or to generate subsequent signals to initiate the contractile process.

The anatomy of platelets in clots has been widely characterized at the level of the electron microscope. Contracting cells within clots have elongated morphologies and much of the cytoplasmic actin is reorganized into retractile fibers that are cored by actin filament bundles. Bundles are pulled into the cell center by a myosin II mediated mechanical process, the same process that moves surface receptors into the OCS of membranes following cell activation. The cell center becomes an electron dense mass composed of entangled cytoskeletal proteins and vesicular concentrates. The retraction of cytoplasmic extensions, as noted previously, recovers plasma membrane that was disgorged during lamellipodial spreading and filopodial formation. The contractile forces applied to the cells in many cases exceed the strength of the cell. Aggregation is associated with the mechanical rupture of cells and the release of microvesicles from cells (128, 129).

Fragmented platelets must be removed from clotted blood. Clarification of clots requires the participation of an enzymatic blood system for removing fibrin (see Chapter 7) and plasmaborne proteins that depolymerize actin polymer released from dying cells. Surprisingly, some of the same proteins that are used inside cells to regulate actin structure are also present in plasma. Most important in this regard are plasma gelsolin and vitamin D-binding protein. Under the divalent cation concentrations of plasma, the calcium binding site in gelsolin is saturated, allowing plasma gelsolin to fragment actin polymers. Vitamin D-binding protein binds actin monomers with high affinity, preventing reassembly, a process strongly promoted by ionic conditions in plasma.

# REFERENCES

1. Nachmias VT, Yoshida K. The cytoskeleton of the blood platelet: a dynamic structure. Adv Mol Cell Biol 1988;2:181–211.
2. Zucker-Franklin D. The ultrastructure of megakaryocytes and platelets. In: Gordon AS, ed. Regulation of hematopoiesis. New York: Appleton-Century-Crofts. 1970;55:1553–1586.
3. Shattil SJ, Hoxie JA, Cunningham M et al. Changes in platelet membrane glycoprotein IIb-IIIa complex during platelet activation. J Biol Chem 1985;260:11107–11114.
4. Shattil SJ, Brass LF. Induction of the fibrinogen receptor on human platelets by intracellular mediators. J Biol Chem 1987;262:992–1000.
5. Shattil SJ, Cunningham M, Hoxie JA. Detection of activated platelets in whole blood using activation-dependent monoclonal antibodies and flow cytometry. Blood 1987;70:307–315.
6. Du X, Plow EF, Frelinger AL et al. Ligands "activate" integrin αIIbβ3 (platelet GP IIb-IIIa). Cell 1991;65:409–416.
7. Ginsberg MH, Du X, Plow EF. Inside-out integrin signaling. Curr Opin Cell Biol 1992;4:766–771.
8. Savage B, Shattil SJ, Ruggeri ZM. Modulation of platelet function through adhesion receptors. A dual role for glycoprotein IIb-IIIa (integrin αIIbβ3) mediated by fibrinogen and glycoprotein Ib-von Willebrand factor. J Biol Chem 1992;267:11300–11306.
9. Lanza F, Morales M, de la Salle C et al. Cloning and characterization of the gene encoding the human platelet glycoprotein V. A member of the leucine-rich glycoprotein family cleaved during thrombin-induced platelet activation. J Biol Chem 1993;268:20801–20807.
10. Li CQ, Dong JF, Lanza F et al. Expression of platelet glycoprotein (GP) V in heterologous cells and evidence for its association with GP Ib-IX-V complex on the cell surface. J Biol Chem 1995;270:16302–16307.
11. López JA, Weisman S, Sanan DA et al. Glycoprotein (GP) Ibβ is the critical subunit linking GP Ibα and GP IX in the GP Ib-IX complex. J Biol Chem 1994;269:23716–23721.
12. López JA, Leung B, Reynolds CC et al. Efficient plasma membrane expression of a functional platelet glycoprotein Ib-IX complex requires the presence of its three subunits. J Biol Chem 1992;267:12851–12859.
13. Siediecki CA, Lestini BJ, Kottke-Marchant KK et al. Shear-dependent changes in the three-dimensional structure of human von Willebrand factor. Blood 1996;88:2939–2950.
14. Savage B, Shattil SJ, Ruggeri ZM. Modulation of platelet function through adhesion receptors. A dual role for glycoprotein IIb-IIIa (integrin αIIbβ3) mediated by fibrinogen and glycoprotein Ib-von Willebrand factor. J Biol Chem 1992;267:11300–11306.
15. Ruggeri ZM. von Willebrand factor and fibrinogen. Curr Opin Cell Biol 1993;5:898–906.
16. Diacovo TG, Roth SJ, Buccola JM et al. Neutrophil rolling, arrest, and transmigration across activated, surface-adherent platelets via sequential action of P-selectin and the β2-integrin CD11b/CD18. Blood 1996;88:146–157.
17. White JG. Effects of colchicine and vinca alkaloids on human platelets. Am J Pathol 1968;53:281–291.
18. White JG, Krivit W. An ultrastructural basis for the shape changes induced in platelets by chilling. Blood 1967;30:625–635.
19. Kenney DM, Linck RW. The cytoskeleton of unstimulated blood platelets: structure and composition of the isolated marginal microtubular band. J Cell Sci 1985;78:1–22.
20. White JG, Krivit W. An ultrastructural basis for the shape changes induced in platelets by chilling. Blood 1967;30:625–635.
21. Sheetz MP. Microtubule motor complexes moving membranous organelles. Cell Struct Funct 1996;21:369–373.
22. Takeuchi K, Kuroda K, Ishigami M et al. Actin cytoskeleton of resting bovine platelets. Exp Cell Res 1990;186:374–380.
23. Cramer EM, Norol F, Guichard J et al. Ultrastructure of platelet formation by human megakaryocytes cultured with the mpl ligand. Blood 1997;89:2336–2346.
24. Markey F, Persson T, Lindberg U. Characterization of platelet extracts before and after stimulation with respect to the possible role of profilactin as microfilament precursor. Cell 1981;23:145–153.
25. Pollard TD, Mooseker MS. Direct measurement of actin polymerization rate constants by electron microscopy of actin filaments nucleated by isolated microvillus cores. J Cell Biol 1981;88:654–659.
26. Huxley H. Electron microscopic studies on the structure of natural and synthetic protein filaments from striated muscle. J Mol Biol 1963;3:281–308.
27. Cooper JA. Effects of cytochalasin and phalloidin on actin. J Cell Biol 1987;105:1473–1478.
28. Fox JE, Phillips DR. Inhibition of actin polymerization in blood platelets by cytochalasins. Nature 1981;292:650–652.
29. Flanagan MD, Lin S. Cytochalasins block actin filament elongation by binding to high-affinity sites associated with f-actin. J Biol Chem 1980;255:835–838.
30. Safer D, Golla R, Nachmias VT. Isolation of a 5-kilodalton actin-sequestering peptide from human blood platelets. Proc Natl Acad Sci U S A 1990;87:2536–2539.
31. Safer D, Elzinga M, Nachmias VT. Thymosin B4 and Fx, an actin-sequestering peptide, are indistinguishable. J Biol Chem 1991;266:4029–4032.
32. Safer D, Nachmais VT. Beta thymosins as actin-binding peptides. Bioessays 1994;16:590.
33. Yin HL, Stossel TP. Control of cytoplasmic actin gel-sol transformation by gelsolin, a calcium-dependent regulatory protein. Nature 1979;281:583–586.
34. Yin HL, Zaner KS, Stossel TP. Ca$^{2+}$ control of actin gelation. Interaction of gelsolin with actin filaments and regulation of actin gelation. J Biol Chem 1980;255:9494–9500.

35. Yin HL, Kwiatkowski DJ, Mole JE et al. Structure and biosynthesis of cytoplasmic and secreted variants of gelsolin. J Biol Chem 1984;259: 5271–5276.

36. Yin HL. Gelsolin: calcium- and polyphosphoinositide-regulated actin-modulating protein. Bioessays 1987;7:176–179.

37. Lind SE, Janmey PA, Chaponnier C et al. Reversible binding of actin to gelsolin and profilin in human platelet extracts. J Cell Biol 1987;105: 833–842.

38. Isenberg G, Aebi U, Pollard TD. An actin-binding protein from Acanthamoeba regulater actin filament polymeriztion and interactions. Nature 1980;288:455–459.

39. Cooper JA, Pollard TD. Effect of capping protein on the kinetics of actin polymerization. Biochemistry 1985;24:793–799.

40. Cooper JA, Blum J, Williams RC Jr et al. Purification and characterization of actophorin, a new 15,000-dalton actin-binding protein from acanthamoeba castellanii. J Biol Chem 1986;261:477–485.

41. Barkalow K, Witke W, Kwiatkowski DJ et al. Coordinated regulation of platelet actin filament barbed ends by gelsolin and capping protein. J Cell Biol 1996;134:389–399.

42. Claudianos C, Campbell HD. The novel flightless-I gene brings together two gene families, actin-binding proteins related to gelsolin and leucine-rich-repeat proteins involved in Ras signal transduction. Mol Biol Evol 1995;12:405–414.

43. Schafer D, Jennings P, Cooper JA. Dynamics of capping protein and actin assembly in vitro: uncapping barbed ends by polyphosphoinositides. J Cell Biol 1996;135:169–179.

44. Hartwig JH, DeSisto M. The cytoskeleton of the resting human blood platelet: structure of the membrane skeleton and its attachment to actin filaments. J Cell Biol 1991;112:407–425.

45. Rosenberg S, Stracher A, Lucas RC. Isolation and characterization of actin and actin-binding protein from human platelets. J Cell Biol 1981;91: 201–211.

46. Rosenberg S, Stracher A. Effect of actin-binding protein on the sedimentation properties of actin. J Cell Biol 1982;94:51–55.

47. Gorlin JB, Yamin R, Egan S et al. Human endothelial actin-binding protein (ABP-280, non-muscle filamin): a molecular leaf spring. J Cell Biol 1990; 111:1089–1105.

48. Gorlin JB, Henske E, Warren ST et al. Actin-binding protein (ABP-280) filamin gene (FLN) maps telomeric to the color vision locus (R/GCP) and centromeric to G6PD in Xq28. Genomics 1993;17:496–498.

49. Hartwig JH, Stossel TP. Structure of macrophage actin-binding protein molecules in solution and interacting with actin filaments. J Mol Biol 1981; 145:563–581.

50. Rosenberg S, Stracher A, Burridge K. Isolation and characterization of a calcium-sensitive α-actinin-like protein from human platelet cytoskeletons. J Biol Chem 1981;256:12986–12991.

51. Sixma JJ, van den Berg A, Jockusch BM et al. Immunoelectron microscopic localization of actin, α-actinin, actin-binding protein and myosin in resting and activated human blood platelets. Eur J Cell Biol 1989;48:271–281.

52. Imamura M, Endo T, Kuroda M et al. Substructure and higher structure of chicken smooth muscle α-actinin molecule. J Biol Chem 1988;263: 7800–7805.

53. Landon F, Olomucki A. Isolation and physio-chemical properties of blood platelet α-actinin. Biochim Biophys Acta 1983;742:129–134.

54. Langer BG, Gonnella PA, Nachmias VT. α-Actinin and vinculin in normal and thrombasthenic platelets. Blood 1984;63:606–614.

55. Fox JE. Identification of actin-binding protein as the protein linking the membrane skeleton to glycoproteins on platelet plasma membrane. J Biol Chem 1985;260:11970–11977.

56. Okita JR, Pidard D, Newman PJ et al. On the association of glycoprotein Ib and actin-binding protein in human platelets. J Cell Biol 1985;100:317–321.

57. Fucini P, Renner C, Herberhold C et al. The repeating segments of the F-actin crosslinking gelation factor (ABP-120) have an immunoglobulin-like fold. Nature Struct Biol 1997;4:223–230.

58. Aakhus AM, Wilkinson JM, Solum NO. Glycoprotein Ib- and actin-binding regions in human platelet actin-binding protein. Biochem Soc Trans 1991; 19:1133–1134.

59. Aakhus AM, Wilkinson J, Solum NO. Binding of human platelet glycoprotein Ib and actin to fragments of actin-binding protein. Thromb Haemost 1992;67:252–257.

60. Ezzell RM, Kenney DM, Egan S et al. Localization of the domain of actin-binding protein that binds to membrane glycoprotein Ib and actin in human platelets. J Biol Chem 1988;263:13303–13309.

61. Ludlow LB, Schick BP, Budarf ML et al. Identification of a mutation in the GATA binding site of the platelet glycoprotein Ibβ promoter resulting in the Bernard-Soulier syndrome. J Biol Chem 1996;271:22076–22080.

62. Ware J, Russell SR, Vicente V et al. Nonsense mutation in the glycoprotein Ibα coding sequence associated with Bernard-Soulier syndrome. Proc Natl Acad Sci U S A 1990;87:2026–2030.

63. Marco L, Mazzucato M, Fabris F et al. Variant Bernard-Soulier syndrome type bolzano. A congenital bleeding disorder due to a structural and functional abnormality of the platelet glycoprotein Ib-IX complex. J Clin Invest 1990;86:25–31.

64. Drouin J, McGregor JL, Parmentier S et al. Residual amounts of glycoprotein Ib concomitant with near-absence of glycoprotein IX in platelets of Bernard-Soulier individuals. Blood 1988;72:1086–1088.

65. Berndt MC, Gregory C, Chong BH et al. Additional glycoprotein defects in Bernard-Soulier's syndrome: confirmation of genetic basis by parental analysis. Blood 1983;62:800–807.

66. Clemetson KJ, McGregor JL, James E et al. Characterization of the platelet membrane glycoprotein abnormalities in Bernard-Soulier syndrome and comparison with normal by surface-labeling techniques and high-resolution two-dimensional gel electrophoresis. J Clin Invest 1982;70:304–311.

67. McGill M, Jamieson GA, Drouin J et al. Morphometric analysis of platelets in Bernard-Soulier syndrome: size and configuration in individuals and carriers. Thromb Haemost 1984;52:37–41.

68. Fox JE, Goll DE, Reynolds CC et al. Identification of two proteins (actin-binding protein and p235) that are hydrolyzed by endogenous Ca$^{2+}$-dependent protease during platelet aggregation. J Biol Chem 1985;260: 1060–1066.

69. Fox JE, Reynolds CC, Morrow JS et al. Spectrin is associated with membrane-bound actin filaments in platelets and is hydrolyzed by the Ca$^{2+}$-dependent protease during platelet activation. Blood 1987;69:537–545.

70. Fox JE, Boyles JK, Berndt MC et al. Identification of a membrane skeleton in platelets. J Cell Biol 1988;107:1525–1538.

71. Tablin F, Taube D. Platelet intermediate filaments detection of a vimentin-like protein in human and bovine platelets. Cell Motil Cytoskeleton 1987; 8:61–67.

72. Carlsson L, Markey F, Blikstad I et al. Reorganization of actin in platelets stimulated by thrombin as measured by the DNase I inhibition assay. Proc Natl Acad Sci U S A 1979;76:6376–6380.

73. Karlsson R, Lassing I, Hoglund AS et al. The organization of microfilaments in spreading platelets: a comparison with fibroblasts and glial cells. J Cell Physiol 1984;121:96–113.

74. Nachmias VT, Kavaler J, Jacubowitz S. Reversible association of myosin with the platelet cytoskeleton. Nature 1985;313:70–72.

75. Davies T, Drotts D, Weil GJ et al. Cytoplasmic Ca$^{2+}$ is necessary for thrombin-induced platelet activation. J Biol Chem 1989;264:19600–19606.

76. Brass LF. Ca$^{2+}$ hemostasis in unstimulated platelets. J Biol Chem 1984; 259:12563–12570.

77. Brass LF, Laposata M, Banga HS et al. Regulation of the phosphoinositide hydrolysis pathway in thrombin-stimulated platelets by a pertussis toxin–sensitive guanine nucleotide–binding protein. Evaluation of its contribution to platelet activation and comparisons with protein Gi. J Biol Chem 1986;261:16838–16847.

78. Brass LF, Joseph SA. A role for inositol triphosphate in intracellular Ca$^{2+}$ mobilization and granule secretion in platelets. J Biol Chem 1985;260: 15172–15179.

79. Witke W, Sharpe AH, Hartwig JH et al. Hemostatic, inflammatory, and fibroblast responses are blunted in mice lacking gelsolin. Cell 1995;81: 41–51.

80. Adelstein RS, Conti MA. Phosphorylation of platelet myosin increases actin-activated myosin ATPase activity. Nature 1975;256:597–598.

81. Casella JF, Flanagan MD, Lin S. Cytochalasin D inhibits actin polymerization and induces depolymerization of actin filaments formed during platelet shape change. Nature 1981;293:302–305.

82. Hartwig JH, Bokoch GM, Carpenter CL et al. Thrombin receptor ligation and activated Rac uncap actin filament barbed ends through phosphoinositide synthesis in permeabilized human platelets. Cell 1995;82:643–653.

83. Hartwig JH, Kung S, Kovacsovics TJ et al. D3 Phosphoinositides and outside-in integrin signaling by GP IIb-IIIa mediate platelet actin assembly and filopodial extension induced by phorbol 12-myristate 13-acetate. J Biol Chem 1996;271:32986–32993.

84. Goldschmidt-Clermont PJ, Furman MI, Safer D et al. The control of actin nucleotide exchange by thymosin β4 and profilin. A potential regulatory mechanism for actin polymerization in cells. Mol Biol Cell 1992;3: 1015–1024.

85. Pantaloni D, Carlier MF. How profilin promotes actin filament assembly in the presence of thymosin beta 4. Cell 1993;75:1007–1014.

86. Davidson MM, Haslam RJ. Dephosphorylation of cofilin in stimulated platelets: roles for GTP-binding protein and Ca$^{2+}$. Biochem J 1994;301: 41–47.

87. Rosenblatt J, Agnew B, Abe H et al. Xenopus actin depolymerizing factor/cofilin (XAC) is responsible for the turnover of actin filaments in Listeria monocytogenes tails. J Cell Biol 1997;136:1323–1332.

88. Carlier MF, Laurent V, Santolini J et al. Actin depolymerizing factor (ADF/cofilin) enhances the rate of filament turnover: implication in actin-based motility. J Cell Biol 1997;136:1307–1322.

89. Hall A. Ras-related proteins. Curr Opin Cell Biol 1993;5:265–268.

90. Hall A. Small GTP-binding proteins and the regulation of the actin cytoskeleton. Annu Rev Cell Biol 1994;10:31–54.

91. Ridley AJ, Paterson HF, Johnston C et al. The small GTP-binding protein rac regulates growth factor–induced membrane ruffling. Cell 1992;70: 401–410.

92. Shibasaki Y, Ishihara H, Kizuki N et al. Massive actin polymerization

induced by phosphatidylinositol-4-phosphate 5-kinase *in vivo*. J Biol Chem 1997;272:7578–7581.

93. Nobes CD, Hall A. Rac, rho, and cdc42 GTPase regulate the assembly of multi-molecular focal complexes associated with actin stress fibers, lamellipodia, and filopodia. Cell 1995;81:53–62.

94. Derry JM, Ochs HD, Francke U. Identification of a novel gene mutated in Wiskott-Aldrich syndrome. Cell 1994;78:635–644.

95. Aspenstrom P, Lindberg U, Hall A. Two GTPases, Cdc42 and Rac, bind directly to a protein implicated in the immunodeficiency disorder Wiskott-Aldrich syndrome. Curr Biol 1996;6:70–75.

96. Kolluri R, Tolias KF, Carpenter C et al. Direct interaction of the Wiskott-Aldrich syndrome protein with the GTPase, Cdc42. Proc Natl Acad Sci U S A 1996;93:5615–5618.

97. Symons M, Derry JM, Karlak B et al. Wiskott-Aldrich syndrome protein, a novel effector for the GTPase CDC42Hs, is implicated in actin polymerization. Cell 1996;84:723–734.

98. Harlan JE, Yoon HS, Hajduk PJ et al. Structural characterization of the interaction between a pleckstrin homology domain and phosphatidylinositol 4,5-bisphosphate. Biochemistry 1995;34:9859–9864.

99. Harlan JE, Hajduk PJ, Yoon HS et al. Pleckstrin homology domains bind to phosphatidylinositol-4,5-bisphosphate. Nature 1994;371:168–170.

100. Lemmon MA, Ferguson KM, Obrien R et al. Specific and high-affinity binding of inositol phosphates to an isolated pleckstrin homology domain. Proc Natl Acad Sci U S A 1995;92:10472–10476.

101. Touhara K, Inglese J, Pitcher JA et al. Binding of G protein beta-gamma-subunits to pleckstrin homology domains. J Biol Chem 1994;269:10217–10220.

102. Touhara K, Koch WJ, Hawes BE et al. Mutational analysis of the pleckstrin homology domain of the beta-adrenergic receptor kinase—differential effects on G(beta-gamma) and phosphatidylinositol 4,5-bisphosphate binding. J Biol Chem 1995;270:17000–17005.

103. Miki H, Miura K, Takenawa T. N-WASP, a novel actin-depolymerizing protein, regulates the cortical cytoskeletal rearrangement in a PIP2-dependent manner downstream of tyrosine kinases. EMBO J 1996;15:5326–5335.

104. Kovacsovics TJ, Bachelot C, Toker A et al. Phosphoinositide 3-kinase inhibition spares actin assembly in activating platelets but reverses platelet aggregation. J Biol Chem 1995;270:11358–11366.

105. Purich DL, Southwick FS. ABM-1 and ABM-2 homology sequences: consensus docking sites for actin-based motility defined by oligoproline regions in Listeria Acta surface protein and human VASP. Biochem Biophys Res Comm 1997;231:686–691.

106. Reinhard M, Halbrügge M, Scheer U et al. The 46/50 Kda phosphoprotein VASP purified from human platelets is a novel protein associated with actin filaments and focal contacts. EMBO J 1992;11:2063–2070.

107. Reinhard M, Giehl K, Abel K et al. The proline-rich focal adhesion and microfilament protein VASP is a ligand for profilins. EMBO J 1995;14:1583–1589.

108. Gertler FB, Niebuhr K, Reinhard M et al. Mena, a relative of VASP and drosophila enabled, is implicated in the control of microfilament dynamics. Cell 1996;87:227–239.

109. Reinhard M, Jouvenal K, Tripier D et al. Identification, purification and characterization of a zyxin-related protein that binds the focal adhesion and microfilament protein VASP (vasodilator-stimulated phosphoprotein). Proc Natl Acad Sci U S A 1995;92:7956–7960.

110. Reinhard M, Rudiger M, Jockusch BM et al. VASP interaction with vinculin: a recurring theme of interactions with proline-rich motifs. FEBS Lett 1996;399:103–107.

111. Brindle NP, Holt MR, Davies JE et al. The focal-adhesion vasodilator-stimulated phosphoprotein (VASP) binds to the proline-rich domain in vinculin. Biochem J 1996;318:753–757.

112. Abel K, Mieskes G, Walter U. Dephosphorylation of the focal adhesion protein VASP *in vitro* and in intact human platelets. FEBS Lett 1995;370:184–188.

113. Kovacsovics TJ, Hartwig JH. Thrombin-induced GP Ib-IX centralization on the platelet surface requires actin assembly and myosin II activation. Blood 1996;87:618–629.

114. Michelson AD, Benoit SE, Kroll MH et al. The activation-induced decrease in the platelet surface expression of the glycoprotein Ib-IX complex is reversible. Blood 1994;83:3562–3573.

115. Michelson AD. Thrombin-induced down-regulation of the platelet membrane glycoprotein Ib-IX complex. Semin Thromb Hemost 1992;18:18–27.

116. Michelson AD, Elis PA, Barnard MR et al. Downregulation of the platelet surface glycoprotein Ib-IX complex in whole blood stimulated by thrombin, adenosine diphosphate, or an *in vivo* wound. Blood 1991;77:770–779.

117. Michelson A, Barnard MR. Thrombin-induced changes in platelet membrane glycoproteins Ib, IX, and IIb-IIIa complex. Blood 1987;70:1673–1678.

118. Hourdille P, Heilmann E, Combrie R et al. Thrombin induces a rapid redistribution of glycoprotein Ib-IX complexes within the membrane systems of activated human platelets. Blood 1990;76:1503–1513.

119. Nurden P, Humbert M, Piotrowicz RS et al. Distribution of ligand-occupied αIIbβ3 in resting and activated platelets determined by expression of a novel class of ligand-induced binding site recognized by monoclonal antibody AP6. Blood 1996;88:887–899.

120. Fox JE, Shattil SJ, Kinlough-Rathbone RL et al. The platelet cytoskeleton stabilizes the interaction between αIIbβ3 and its ligand and induces selective movement of ligand-occupied integrin. J Biol Chem 1996;271:7004–7011.

121. Knezevic I, Leisner T, Lam SC. Direct binding of the platelet integrin αIIbβ3 (GP IIb-IIIa) to talin. Evidence that interaction is mediated through the cycoplasmic domains of both alpha IIb and beta 3. J Biol Chem 1996;271:16416–16421.

122. Miyamoto S, Teramoto H, Coso O et al. Integrin function: molecular hierarchies of cytoskeletal and signaling molecules. J Cell Biol 1995;131:791–805.

123. Miyamoto S, Akiyama S, Yamada KM. Synergistic roles for receptor occupancy and aggregation in integrin transmembrane function. Science 1995;267:883–885.

124. Albrecht RM, Goodman SL, Simmons SR. Distribution and movement of membrane-associated platelet glycoproteins: use of colloidal gold with correlative video-enhanced light microscopy, low-voltage high-resolution scanning microscopy, and high-voltage transmission electron microscopy. Am J Anat 1989;185:149–164.

125. Olorundare OE, Simmons SR, Albrecht RM. Evidence for two mechanisms of ligand-receptor movement on surface-activated platelets. Eur J Cell Biol 1993;60:131–145.

126. Olorundare OE, Simmons SR, Albrecht RM. Cytochalasin D and E: effects on fibrinogen receptor movement and cytoskeletal reorganization in fully spread, surface-activated platelets: a correlative light and electron microscopic investigation. Blood 1992;79:99–109.

127. Fox JE. The platelet cytoskeleton. Thromb Haemost 1993;70:884–893.

128. Wencel-Drake JD, Dieter MG, Lam SC. Immunolocalization of β1 integrins in platelets and platelet-derived microvesicles. Blood 1993;82:1197–1203.

129. Fox JE, Austin CD, Boyles JK et al. Role of the membrane skeleton in preventing the shedding of procoagulant-rich microvesicles from the platelet plasma membrane. J Cell Biol 1990;111:483–493.

130. Molino M, Bainton DF, Hoxie JA et al. Thrombin receptors on human platelets. Initial localization and subsequent redistribution during platelet activation. J Biol Chem 1997;272:6011–6017.

131. Stenberg PE, McEver RP, Shuman MA et al. A platelet α-granule membrane protein (GMP-140) is expressed on the plasma membrane after activation. J Cell Biol 1985;101:880.

132. Israels SJ, Gerrard JM, Jacques YU et al. Platelet dense granule membranes contain both granulophysin and P-selectin (GMP-140). Blood 1992;80:143–152.

133. Carlier MF, Jean C, Rieger KJ et al. Modulation of the interaction between G-actin and thymosin β4 by the ATP/ADP ratio: possible implication in the regulation of actin dynamics. Proc Natl Acad Sci U S A 1993;90:5034–5038.

134. Earnest JP, Santos GF, Zuerbig S et al. Dystrophin-related protein in platelet membrane skeleton. J Biol Chem 1995;270:27259–27265.

135. Lind SE, Yin HL, Stossel TP. Human platelets contain gelsolin, a regulator of actin filament length. J Clin Invest 1982;69:1384–1387.

136. Hartwig JH. Mechanism of actin rearrangements mediating platelet activation. J Cell Biol 1992;118:1421–1442.

137. Hirao M, Sato N, Kondo T et al. Regulation mechanism of ERM (ezrin/radixin/moesin) protein/plasma membrane association: possible involvement of phosphatidylinositol turnover and rho-dependent signaling pathway. J Cell Biol 1996;135:37–51.

138. Beckerle MC, Miller DE, Bertagnolli ME et al. Activation-dependent redistribution of the adhesion plaque protein, talin, in intact human platelets. J Cell Biol 1989;109:3333–3346.

139. Burridge K, Nuckolls G, Otey C et al. Actin-membrane interaction in focal adhesions. Cell Differ Dev 1990;32:337–342.

140. Auger KR, Songyang Z, Lo SH et al. Platelet-derived growth factor-induced formation of tensin and phosphoinositide 3-kinase complexes. J Biol Chem 1996;271:23452–23457.

141. Lo SH, Janmey PA, Hartwig JH et al. Interaction of tensin with actin and identification of its three distinct actin-binding domains. J Cell Biol 1994;125:1067–1075.

142. Lo SH, An Q, Bao S et al. Molecular cloning of chick cardiac muscle tensin: full-length cDNA sequence, expression and characterization. J Biol Chem 1994;269:22310–22319.

143. Zhang J, Zhang J, Shattil SJ et al. Phosphoinositide 3-kinase γ and p85/phosphoinositide 3-kinase in platelets: relative activation by thrombin receptor or β-phorbol myristate acetate and roles in promoting the ligand-binding function of αIIbβ3 integrin. J Biol Chem 1996;271:6265–6272.

144. Zhang J, King WG, Dillon S et al. Activation of platelet phosphatidylinositide 3-kinase requires the small GTP-binding protein rho. J Biol Chem 1993;268:22251–22254.

145. Chong LD, Traynor-Kaplan A, Bokoch GM et al. The small GTP-binding protein rho regulates a phosphatidylinositol 4-phosphate 5-kinase in mammalian cells. Cell 1994;79:507–513.

146. Tolias KF, Cantley LC, Carpenter CL. Rho family GTPases bind to phosphoinositide kinases. J Biol Chem 1995;270:17656–17659.

147. Hinchliffe KA, Irvine RF, Divecha N. Aggregation-dependent, integrin-mediated increases in cytoskeletally associated PtdInsP$_2$ (4, 5) levels in

human platelets are controlled by translocation of PtdIns 4-P 5-kinase C to the cytoskeleton. EMBO J 1996;15:6516–6524.

148. Abrams CS, Zhao W, Belmonte E et al. Protein kinase C regulates pleckstrin by phosphorylation of sites adjacent to the N-terminal pleckstrin homology domain. J Biol Chem 1995;270:23317–23321.

149. Abrams CS, Zhao W, Brass LF. A site of interaction between pleckstrins pH domains and G$\beta\gamma$. Biochim Biophys Acta 1996;1314:233–238.

150. Ma AD, Brass LF, Abrams CS. Pleckstrin associates with plasma membrane and induces the formation of membrane projections: requirements for phosphorylation and the NH2-terminal PH domain. J Cell Biol 1997; 136:1071–1079.

151. Toker A, Meyer M, Kishta Reddy KK et al. Activation of protein kinase C family members by the novel polyphosphoinositides PtdIns-3,4-P2 and PtdIns-3,4,5-P3. J Biol Chem 1994;269:32358–32367.

152. Toker A, Bachelot C, Chen CS et al. Phosphorylation of the platelet p47 phosphoprotein is mediated by the lipid products of phosphoinositide 3-kinase. J Biol Chem 1995;270:29525–29531.

153. Schaller MD, Borgman CA, Cobb BS et al. pp125FAK, a structurally distinctive protein-tyrosine kinase associated with focal adhesions. Proc Natl Acad Sci U S A 1992;89:5192–5196.

154. Ridley AJ, Hall A. The small GTP-binding protein rho regulates the assembly of focal adhesions and actin stress fibers in response to growth factors. Cell 1992;70:389–399.

155. Hartwig JH, De Groot NJ, Jugloff LS et al. The ligand-induced membrane IgM association with the cytoskeletal matrix of B-cells is not mediated through the Ig$\alpha$/$\beta$ heterodimer. J Immunol 1995;155:3769–3779.

156. Franke B, Akkerman JW, Bos JL. Rapid Ca$^{2+}$-mediated activation of Rap1 in human platelets. EMBO J 1997;16:252–259.

157. Avraham S, London R, Fu Y et al. Identification and characterization of a novel related adhesion focal tyrosine kinase (RAFTK) from megakaryocytes and brain. J Biol Chem 1995;270:27742–27751.

158. Nachmias VT, Sullender J, Fallon J et al. Observations on the "cytoskeleton" of human platelets. Thromb Haemost 1979;42:1661–1666.

159. Nachmias VT. Cytoskeleton of human platelets at rest and after spreading. J Cell Biol 1980;86:795–802.

160. White JG. Arrangements of actin filaments in the cytoskeleton of human platelets. Am J Pathol 1984;117:207–217.

161. Asijee GM, Sturk A, Bruin T et al. Vinculin is a permanent component of the membrane skeleton and is incorporated into the (re)organising cytoskeleton upon platelet activation. Eur J Biochem 1990;189:131–136.

162. Horvath AR, Asijee GM, Muszbek L. Cytoskeletal assembly and vinculin-cytoskeleton interaction in different phases of the activation of bovine platelets. Cell Motil Cytoskeleton 1992;21:123–131.

163. Nachmias VT, Golla R. Vinculin in relation to stress fibers in spread platelets. Cell Motil Cytoskeleton 1991;20:190–202.

# CHAPTER 11

# PLATELET MEMBRANES AND RECEPTORS

Ellinor I. B. Peerschke and José A. López

Platelets participate in hemostasis and thrombosis by adhering to injured blood vessel walls and accumulating at sites of injury (1). Although platelet deposition at these sites is responsible for the primary arrest of bleeding under physiologic conditions, it can also lead to vascular occlusion with ensuing ischemic tissue damage and thrombus embolization under pathologic conditions. Interactions of platelets with their environment and with each other represent complex processes that are initiated at the cell surface. The surface membrane, therefore, provides a reactive interface between the external medium, including components of the blood vessel wall and plasma, and the platelet interior.

## MEMBRANE STRUCTURE: GENERAL PROPERTIES

Like all cell membranes, the platelet surface membrane consists of a bilayer of amphipathic lipids made up of glycolipids and phospholipids (2, 3). Glycolipids reside exclusively in the outer leaflet of the membrane, whereas phospholipids are asymmetrically distributed between the two halves of the bilayer. Sphingomyelin and phosphatidyl choline are predominantly found in the outer half of the bilayer. Phosphatidyl inositol and phosphatidyl serine, involved in intracellular signaling (see Chapter 12) and the enhancement of fluid phase coagulation (see Platelet Membrane Receptors for Coagulant and Fibrinolytic Proteins), are located primarily in the inner half of the bilayer.

Cholesterol is a major structural component of plasma membranes. Like phospholipids, cholesterol is asymmetrically distributed between the inner and outer membrane phospholipid bilayer, with the outer leaflet containing twice as much cholesterol as the inner leaflet. Cholesterol functions to maintain membrane fluidity and influences membrane transport and permeability (4). Perturbations in the phospholipid:cholesterol ratio result in changes in membrane microviscosity, which can influence membrane protein expression by altering the lateral mobility of proteins in the membrane and affecting the degree of protein exposure relative to the plane of the membrane. Indeed, changes in platelet function have been ascribed to modifications in membrane cholesterol content *in vitro* and *in vivo* (5, 6).

In addition to lipids, all biologic membranes, including the platelet surface membrane, contain proteins, many of which are endowed with carbohydrate side chains (3). Carbohydrate side chains are commonly attached to the protein backbone via the amide group of asparagine, and consist of core and terminal sugars. The core sugars often contain the sequence *N*-acetylglucosamine-*N*-acetylglucosamine-mannose-mannose, whereas terminal sugars include galactose, *N*-acetyl derivatives of glucosamine and galactosamine, and sialic acid (*N*-acetylneuraminic acid). Sialic acid usually represents the terminal residue and contributes significantly to the overall platelet membrane negative charge.

Receptors constitute one of the most important categories of cell membrane proteins. They usually represent glycoproteins present at the cell surface, but receptor pools may also be held in reserve in intracellular membranes. Receptors are crucial for transducing a wide range of external stimuli and signals into intracellular events (see Chapter 12). Thus most receptors traverse the membrane and consist of external, transmembrane, and cytoplasmic domains.

Membrane proteins and receptors diffuse laterally in the plane of the phospholipid bilayer (3). This diffusion tends to be slow in resting cells, but can be influenced by interactions with the membrane glycocalyx and the intracellular cytoskeleton (see Chapter 10). The glycocalyx is a predominantly carbohydrate containing region external to the lipid bilayer (3). It is made up of the extracellular domains of integral membrane glycoproteins, glycosylated molecules bound ionically to these domains, and proteoglycans.

Platelet membrane receptors can be classified operationally according to protein structure, function, nature of bound ligand, and expression requirements. Based on recent cDNA sequence analysis, many platelet membrane glycoproteins have been shown to share structural features with receptors from other cells also involved in adhesive interactions with their environment. This has allowed the classification of certain platelet membrane glycoproteins within a number of large gene families. Receptors supporting hemostasis and thrombosis include members of the integrin gene family, the leucine-rich glycoprotein gene family, the selectin gene family, and the immunoglobulin gene superfamily. In addition, several glycoproteins have been identified that, thus far, appear unrelated to any known gene family or have not as yet been cloned and sequenced.

# PLATELET ACTIVATION RECEPTORS

Platelets can be activated by a variety of substances, including small molecules, enzymes, and macromolecular protein complexes. Platelets generally respond to stimulation by changing shape, interacting with each other in a process called aggregation, and releasing their granule contents (7). Chapter 12 includes a more detailed discussion of the platelet activation receptors described below as they relate to cell activation.

## ADENOSINE DIPHOSPHATE (ADP) RECEPTORS

The demonstration of specific ADP receptors has been fraught with technical difficulty, and to date no receptor has been identified. The importance of such receptors for normal hemostasis, however, is demonstrated by an inherited bleeding disorder linked to defective platelet interactions with ADP (8). Studies using a synthetic

ADP analog, 2-methylthioadenosine ($\beta$-$^{32}$P) diphosphate, suggest the presence of a single class of 765 binding sites whose occupancy prevents the accumulation of intracellular cAMP by agents such as prostaglandin, but fails to inhibit ADP-induced platelet shape change (9). This receptor has been identified as a 43 Kd–molecular-weight (mol wt) protein by photoaffinity labeling studies and appears to be a member of the $P_{2y}$ nucleotide receptor family of G protein–coupled, seven transmembrane domain receptors (10). In addition, a 100,000-mol-wt platelet surface membrane protein, designated aggregin, has been identified by affinity labeling with the synthetic ADP analog, 5'-$p$-fluorosulfonyl benzoyl adenosine (FSBA) (11, 12). Although FSBA inhibits ADP-induced shaped change, it fails to prevent ADP-induced increases in platelet cytosolic calcium or ADP's action on adenylate cyclase.

Other studies have identified a 43 Kda protein as a potential ADP receptor (13), and an adenine nucleotide binding site has been identified on GP IIb alpha (14). Thus, platelets may contain several classes of ADP binding sites on the same or different proteins capable of interaction with ADP with varying affinity. The relevance of each of these for platelet activation and signal transduction requires further study.

## EPINEPHRINE RECEPTORS

Platelet stimulation by epinephrine occurs without a change in platelet shape (15) and is mediated by $\alpha_2$-adrenergic receptors coupled to the $G_i$ type of G protein (16). The platelet epinephrine receptor has been purified to homogeneity and migrates as a single protein band with a mol wt of 64,000 on SDS-polyacrylamide gels (17). Approximately 300 $\alpha_2$-adrenergic receptors have been demonstrated per platelet (18). Although epinephrine binding to platelets is decreased in several disease states, including essential thrombocythemia (19), and after antidepressant drug therapy (20), it is unclear whether these decreases reflect the down-regulation of epinephrine receptor numbers or the presence of occupied or blocked receptors. A reduction in the number of platelet $\alpha_2$-adrenergic receptors, however, has been described in family members whose platelets demonstrate impaired platelet aggregation and secretion in response to epinephrine (21).

The gene for the platelet $\alpha_2$-adrenergic receptor has been cloned and sequenced (22). This gene contains no introns and codes for a 450 amino acid protein containing seven hydrophobic membrane spanning domains, similar to those found in several other G protein–linked receptors. The externally oriented regions of the amino-terminal transmembrane domains are predicted to form an agonist binding pocket, whereas the cytoplasmic domain and associated membrane spanning loops are thought to interact with G proteins. In addition, a consensus sequence potentially involved in signal transduction via phosphorylation of serine and threonine has been identified in one of the cytoplasmic loops.

## SEROTONIN RECEPTORS

Serotonin is another small molecule capable of stimulating platelets. Platelet activation occurs at $10^{-6}$ M concentrations via receptors of the $S_2$ subtype (23, 24) that have been cloned and sequenced (25). Receptor occupancy leads to platelet aggregation and secretion via G protein–coupled mechanisms (26). Recent evidence suggests that the same receptor is present on megakaryocytes and stimulates megakaryopoiesis (27).

Platelets also possess a transport system for the uptake of serotonin into dense granules (28). Serotonin transport is $Na^+$ dependent and is stimulated by $K^+$ or a pH gradient across the plasma membrane. Platelet serotonin uptake is similar to the uptake of biogenic amines by presynaptic nerve endings, making platelets a useful model for the study of neuronal serotonin transport.

## THROMBOXANE A₂ RECEPTORS

Arachidonic acid metabolites, including thromboxane $A_2$ and its precursor $PGH_2$, stimulate platelet shape change, aggregation, and secretion (29). Both compounds bind to the same cell-surface receptor, and direct binding studies with radiolabeled endoperoxide analogs have demonstrated approximately 2000 binding sites per platelet with a Kd of 100 nM (30, 31). Platelet activation by another prostaglandin analog, 8-epi-prostaglandin $F_{2a}$, however, appears to be mediated by separate binding sites, unrelated to thromboxane $A_2$ receptor isoforms (32).

The human platelet thromboxane $A_2$ receptor has been cloned (33). Its cDNA sequence encodes a protein of 343 amino acids and contains seven putative transmembrane domains and one extramembrane loop althought to contain the ligand binding site. Five histidine residues have been identified in the deduced amino acid sequence, two of which are located in the putative extramembranous loop. These histidine residues may modulate ligand binding by influencing both receptor number and affinity, particularly at low pH (31).

Interestingly, platelet thromboxane receptors are acutely and reversibly up-regulated following acute myocardial infarction (34). Gene expression can be regulated by activation of protein kinase C via induction of an AP-2-like nuclear factor binding to upstream promotor elements. Up-regulation of thromboxane receptors following myocardial infarction is consistent with increased gene transcription in platelet progenitor cells (34).

## VASOPRESSIN RECEPTORS

Photoaffinity labeling techniques have been used to identify a 125 Kda platelet membrane protein serving as a receptor for vasopressin (35). Radioligand binding studies using arginine vasopressin have demonstrated the presence of approximately 95 binding sites per platelet with a Kd of 1 nM (35, 36).

## PLATELET ACTIVATING FACTOR RECEPTORS

Platelets are also stimulated by acetyl glycerol ether phosphoryl choline or platelet activating factor (PAF). This agonist is synthesized by a variety of inflammatory cells and platelets and induces platelet shape change, aggregation, and secretion (7). Platelets possess approximately 300 PAF receptors (Kd = 0.2 nM), which are under close intracellular control, possibly via a calcium-calmodulin dependent phosphorylation/dephosphorylation process (37). Studies using rabbit platelets suggest that PAF binding is enhanced by $Mg^{+2}$ and inhibited by guanosine triphosphate (GTP), characteristic of ligand interactions with receptors coupled to G proteins (38). The receptor has been cloned and found to be a member of a family of proteins consisting of single polypeptide chains expressing seven transmembrane domains (39).

## THROMBIN RECEPTORS

Thrombin activates platelets by multiple pathways, depending on its concentration (16). A high-affinity human platelet thrombin receptor (1700 to 1800 copies/cell) has been identified by expression cloning and belongs to a family of peptide receptors (40). The deduced receptor amino acid sequence reveals a putative thrombin cleavage site and a sequence resembling an acidic region in the carboxyterminus of hirudin, a potent thrombin inhibitor. Signal transduction by this thrombin receptor occurs via a novel activation pathway that involves the thrombin-induced cleavage of the receptor's large aminoterminal extracellular extension, creating a new receptor aminoterminus and a tethered ligand that serves to activate the receptor (see Chapter 12). A synthetic peptide mimicking this ligand possesses full agonist activity (41). Whereas the synthetic peptide is fully capable of activating platelets, its activity is quite different from that of native thrombin (42).

In addition, GP Ib has been shown to contain both high-affinity and moderate-affinity thrombin binding sites (43), and GPV cleavage accompanies thrombin stimulation of human platelets (44). Current evidence suggests that both GP Ib and the seven-transmembrane-domain thrombin receptor contribute to platelet stimulation by thrombin (45).

## COLLAGEN RECEPTORS

Several different platelet membrane components may participate in collagen-induced platelet adhesion and activation. The platelet GP Ia-IIa complex (VLA-2) (see Platelet Adhesion Receptors) serves as a major, magnesium-dependent binding site for monomeric collagen (46, 47) and participates in platelet secretion and aggregation in response to fibrillar collagen. GP IV (CD36), an 88 Kda major platelet membrane glycoprotein, also participates in collagen-induced platelet adhesion and aggregation (48). GP IV (see Platelet Adhesion Receptors) recognizes Type I collagen fibrils with a Kd of 0.34 $\mu$M. Other collagen binding proteins include a 65 Kda protein, purified from detergent extracts of platelets by affinity chromatography on Type I collagen (49), and a platelet membrane receptor for the complement component C1q (50) (see Platelet Membrane Proteins Involved in Immunoregulatory Functions). C1q possesses a collagen-like aminoterminus and modulates collagen-induced platelet aggregation at low collagen concentrations ($<$5 $\mu$g/ml). The C1q receptor, which recognizes both collagen and the collagen-like domain of C1q, migrates with an apparent mol wt of 67 Kda on SDS-polyacrylamide gels, but appears to be distinct from the 65 Kda, collagen binding protein isolated by Chiang et al (51, 52). Additional platelet collagen binding sites may include GP IIb (53) and GP VI (54) (see Platelet Adhesion Receptors).

## RECEPTORS FOR AGGREGATED IgG, IMMUNE COMPLEXES, AND SELECTED MONOCLONAL ANTIBODIES

Platelets can be activated by aggregated IgG or immune complexes. This requires the occupancy of platelet Fc receptors (55) (see Platelet Membrane Receptors Involved in Immunoregulatory Functions) by macromolecular, multivalent ligand complexes, which crosslink these receptors in the platelet membrane (56). In addition, a variety of monoclonal antibodies have been reported to induce platelet aggregation (57). Some of these recognize epitopes either in GP IIb-IIIa (see Platelet Adhesion Receptors), the platelet CD9 antigen (see Platelet Antigens Shared With Leukocytes), or GP IV (see Platelet Adhesion Receptors). Platelet activation by these antibodies is dependent on Fc receptor occupancy, as well as the interaction of antibodies with their antigen-combining site on the same or adjacent platelets. Platelet stimulation occurs primarily through the activation of phospholipase C (58, 59), although a thromboxane $A_2$–dependent pathway may also play a role (58).

## THROMBOPOIETIN RECEPTORS (mpl-R)

The thrombopoietin receptor is a cytokine receptor belonging to the hematopoietin receptor superfamily. Both the receptor and its ligand, thrombopoietin, have been cloned and sequenced and are discussed in detail in Chapter 8. Briefly, the thrombopoietin receptor is expressed on megakaryocytes and platelets (60) and, when occupied on platelets, leads to tyrosine phosphorylation of several intracellular proteins (61–63) and enhances aggregation induced by epinephrine, ADP, or shear stress (64).

## PLATELET INHIBITOR RECEPTORS

Agents that stimulate adenylate cyclase and increase intracellular levels of cyclic AMP inhibit platelet function (30). Some of the most potent inhibitors of platelet activation and aggregation in this category are $PGE_1$ and $PGD_2$ (65). These inhibitors interact with platelets via distinct receptors, both coupled to G proteins. $PGI_2$ is the major metabolite of arachidonic acid in vascular tissue and is althought to play an important role in maintaining a nonthrombogenic barrier between circulating platelets and the blood vessel wall. Approximately 2700 high-affinity receptors, which bind prostacyclin with a Kd of 6 to 12 nM, have been identified per platelet (66, 67). This receptor has been purified to homogeneity (68) and migrates with an apparent mol wt of 190,000 on SDS-polyacrylamide gels. It is composed of two nonidentical subunits with molecular weights of 85,000 and 95,000. $PGD_2$ binding sites (Kd = 10 nM, B max 200 to 800 sites/platelet) have as yet not been identified (69).

Adenosine also inhibits platelet function. Evidence for the presence of high-affinity binding sites (Kd = 0.16 $\mu$M, Bmax 5500 sites per platelet) and low-affinity binding sites (Kd = 2.9 $\mu$M, 22,000 sites per platelet) has been presented (70).

## PLATELET ADHESION RECEPTORS

Surface membrane glycoproteins (GP) are critical for normal platelet adhesion to components of the blood vessel wall and platelet interactions with each other. Initial studies made use of SDS-polyacrylamide gel electrophoresis to examine surface-membrane glycoproteins (71) and revealed the absence of key receptors involved in inherited bleeding disorders (14) (see Chapter 32). The separation of major platelet membrane glycoproteins by two-dimensional, nonreduced-reduced SDS-polyacrylamide gel electrophoresis is depicted in Fig. 11.1.

### ADHESION RECEPTORS OF THE INTEGRIN FAMILY

Integrins are $\alpha/\beta$ heterodimer protein complexes involved in cell-matrix and cell-cell interactions (72, 73).

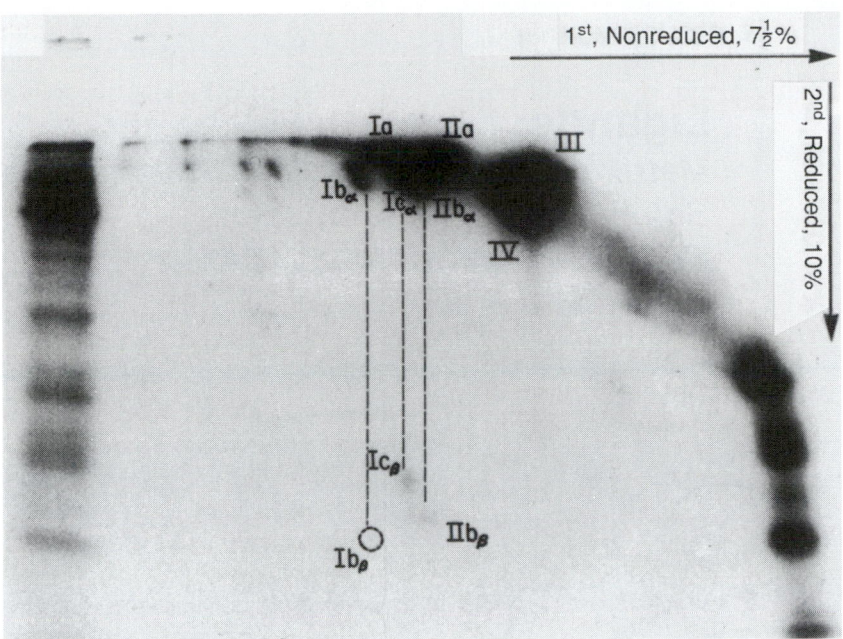

**FIGURE 11.1.**   Analysis of [$^{125}$I]–surface-labeled platelets by one-dimensional, reduced (1) and two-dimensional, nonreduced-reduced (2) SDS-polyacrylamide gel electrophoresis. (Reprinted by permission of the Amer Soc of Biochem and Molec Biol from Phillips DR, Agin PP. Platelet plasma membrane glycoproteins. Evidence for the presence of nonequivalent disulfide bonds using nonreduced-reduced two-dimensional gel electrophoresis. J Biol Chem 1977;252:2121–2126.

The general structure of these receptors is presented in Fig. 11.2. Integrins are widely distributed on the surface of nearly all eukaryotic adherent cells. Each receptor in the superfamily contains an alpha and a β subunit. Individual integrins can often bind to more than one ligand, and individual ligands may be recognized by more than one integrin. The majority of integrin receptor ligands are extracellular matrix proteins involved in cell-substratum adhesion. Some integrins, but not all, mediate cell adhesion by interacting with a variety of extracellular glycoprotein ligands sharing the amino acid recognition sequence ARG-GLY-ASP (RGD), first identified in fibronectin (74).

### The Fibrinogen Receptor: GP IIb-IIIa

The glycoprotein IIb-IIIa complex is probably the most abundant receptor on the platelet membrane (75). Its α subunit, GP IIb, is expressed exclusively on platelets and cells of megakaryocyte lineage, whereas its β$_3$ subunit, GP IIIa, is shared by other integrins in the cytoadhesion subfamily (72, 73).

Normal platelets contain approximately 80,000 molecules of GP IIb-IIIa (76). Additional GP IIb-IIIa complexes are present in membranes of the platelet surface–connected canalicular system (77) and α granules (78). These intracellular receptor pools can be expressed at the cell surface following platelet activation.

### GP IIb-IIIa Structure

GP IIb has a molecular weight of 136,000 and is composed of a larger α (125, 000) and a smaller β (23, 000) subunit, linked by a single disulfide bridge (75) (Fig. 11.3). The β subunit serves to anchor GP IIb in the platelet membrane. The disulfide-linked α subunit is entirely extracellular.

GP IIIa is also an integral membrane protein. It is a disulfide bond-rich, single-chain protein with an apparent mol wt of 90,000 on nonreduced, SDS-polyacrylamide gels and an apparent mol wt of 110,000 following disulfide-bond reduction (75). GP IIIa contains 56 cysteine residues, each involved in an intrachain disulfide bond (79). A large, disulfide-bonded loop, consisting of at least 325 to 384 amino acids (80, 81), is susceptible to proteolytic cleavage by chymotrypsin, trypsin, and plasmin. Because the residual membrane-bound GP IIIa no longer interacts with adhesive proteins, it is likely that a portion of the receptor's ligand binding site resides in the proteolytic fragment (82–84).

Glycoproteins IIb and IIIa form a calcium-dependent heterodimer complex (85, 86) that can be dissociated by divalent cation chelators. Although mM concentrations of either calcium or magnesium prevent complex dissociation, only calcium supports GP IIb-IIIa reassociation (87). The precise relationship between the role of calcium in maintaining subunit association and its role in mediating ligand binding is as yet unclear.

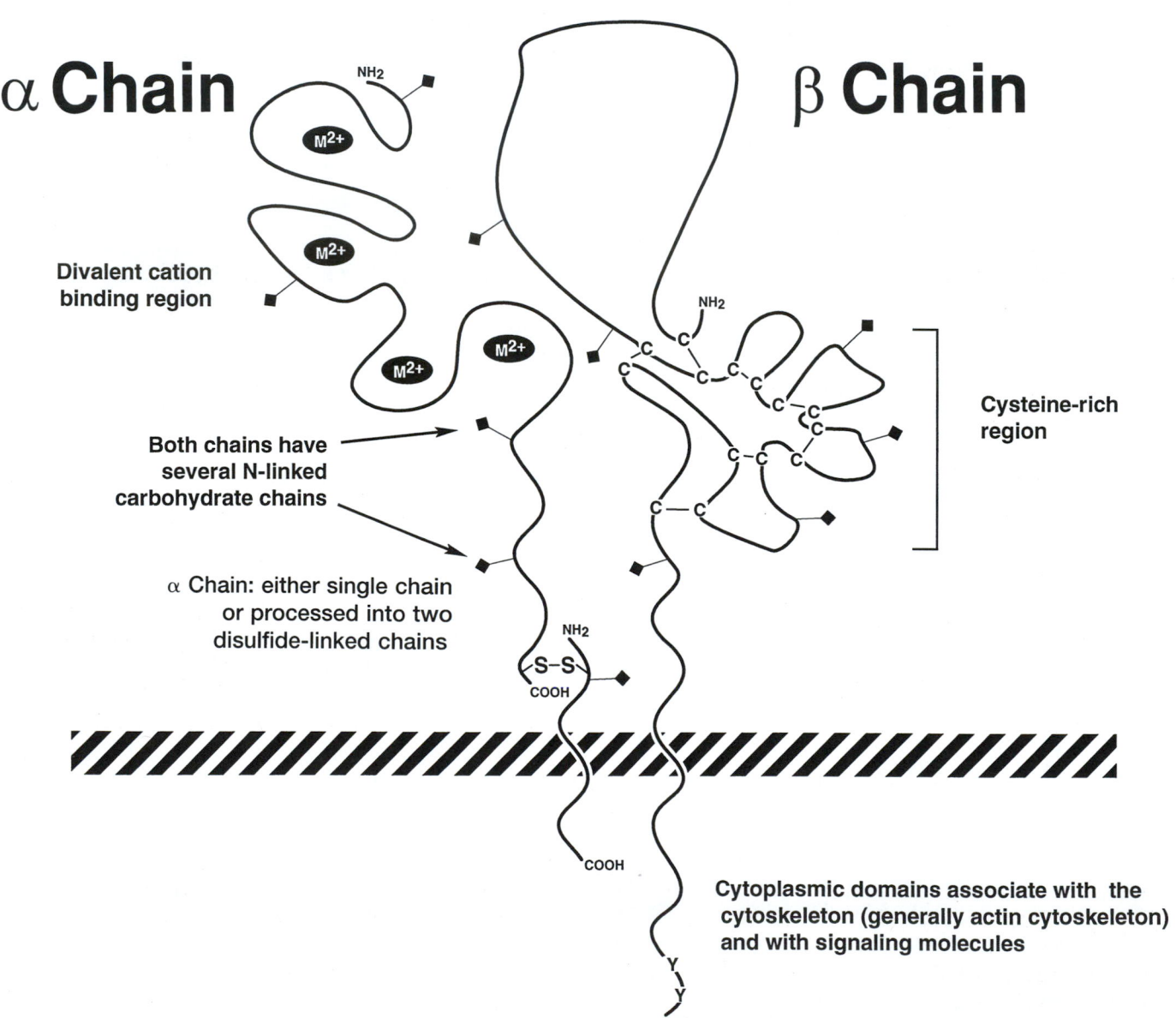

**Ligands:**
*Matrix proteins: generally RGD mediated*
*Soluble proteins: fibrinogen*
*Counter-receptors: e.g., ICAM-1*

α **Chain**

NH₂

M²⁺

M²⁺

**Divalent cation binding region**

M²⁺    M²⁺

**Both chains have several N-linked carbohydrate chains**

α Chain: either single chain or processed into two disulfide-linked chains

NH₂

S–S

COOH

COOH

β **Chain**

NH₂

C  C
C  C  C  C
C  C  C  C
C  C  C

C  C

**Cysteine-rich region**

NH₂

Y
Y
COOH

**Cytoplasmic domains associate with the cytoskeleton (generally actin cytoskeleton) and with signaling molecules**

**FIGURE 11.2.**   Generic structural features of integrin receptors. (M⁺²) metal ion binding regions; (◆) *N*-linked carbohydrate side chains; (Y) tyrosine phosphorylation sites; (S-S) disulfide bonds; (C) cysteine; (NH₂) aminoterminus; (COOH) carboxyterminus.

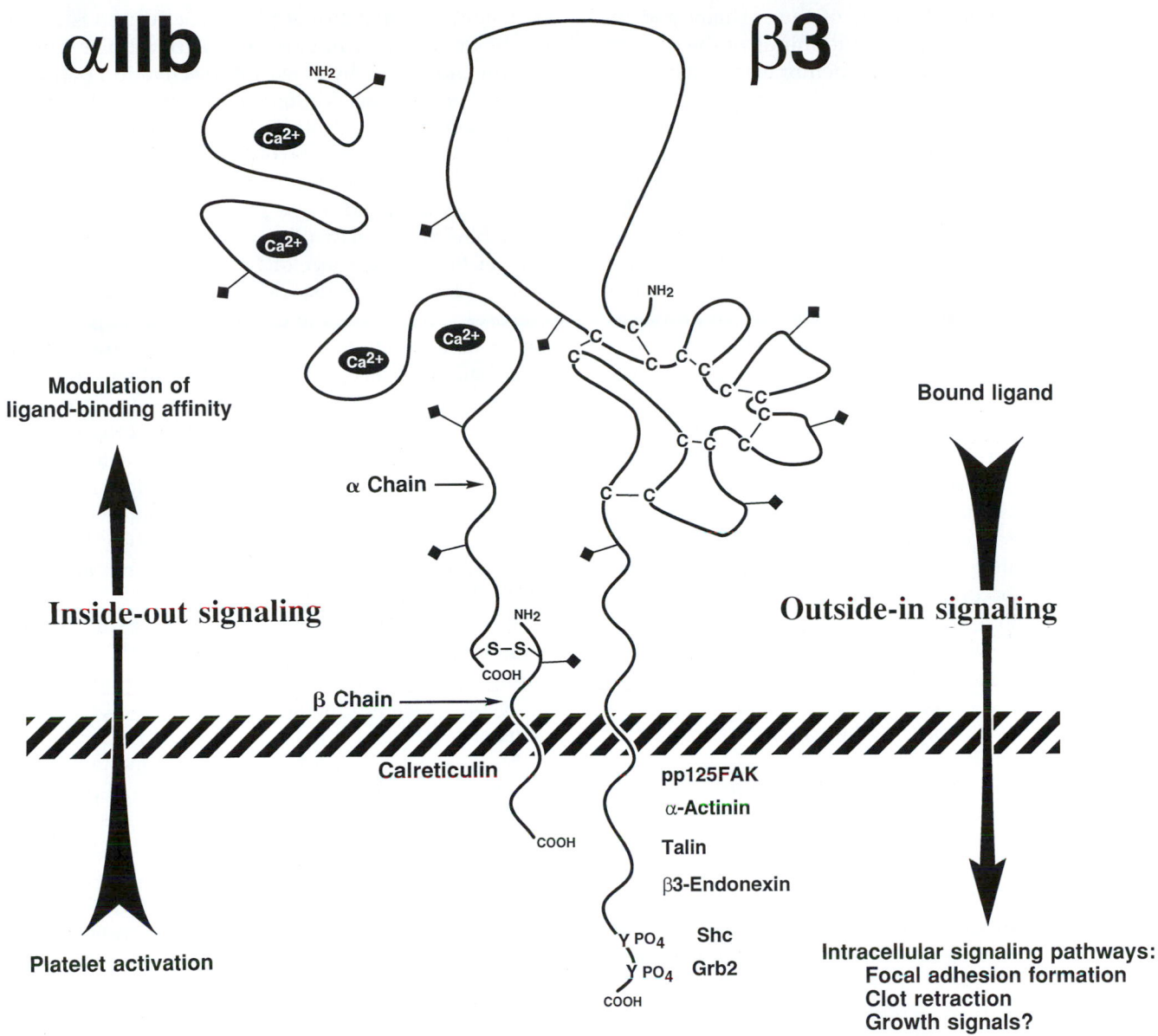

**FIGURE 11.3.** Summary of GP IIb ($\alpha_{IIb}$) and GP IIIa ($\beta_3$) structure deduced from molecular, biochemical, and functional studies. (◆) N-linked carbohydrate side chains; (Y) tyrosine phosphorylation sites; (S-S) disulfide bonds; (C) cysteine; (NH$_2$) aminoterminus; (COOH) carboxyterminus; (PO$_4$) phosphorylation sites.

Two high-affinity (Kd = 9 nM) and approximately six intermediate-affinity (Kd 400 nM) calcium binding sites have been identified within the GP IIb-IIIa complex (88, 89). In addition, GP IIb-IIIa contains a class of low-affinity binding sites for divalent cations, which support adhesive protein binding (90, 91).

Although dissociation of the GP IIb-IIIa complex by divalent cation chelators is reversible initially, progressive monomer self-association occurs at 37°C, producing nonfunctional, high-mol-wt, irreversible, glycoprotein aggregates (87). The inability to reform heterodimer complexes is primarily associated with a calcium-dependent transition in GP IIIa, which results in subunit

unfolding and subsequent GP IIIa aggregation (87). A similar structural transition is observed in GP IIb, but at tenfold-lower calcium concentrations.

## Molecular Biology

The genes for GP IIb and GP IIIa are each located in the proximal portion of the long arm of chromosome 17 at q21–23 (92) and are in linkage disequilibrium. A diagram summarizing the salient structural features of GP IIb and GP IIIa deduced from cDNA sequencing (92) is presented in Fig. 11. 3. GP IIb contains two strongly hydrophobic regions, one representing a typical signal peptide at the aminoterminus of the α chain, and the other, located near the carboxyterminus of the β chain, representing a putative transmembrane domain. The latter is followed by 20 hydrophilic amino acids constituting the cytoplasmic tail. The extracellular domain of GP IIb β contains a single potential *N*-linked glycosylation site, whereas GP IIb α contains four possible *N*-linked glycosylation sites, and four stretches of 12 amino acids, each resembling calcium binding regions.

The cDNA sequence of GP IIIa reveals the presence of an aminoterminal hydrophobic region representing a signal peptide, and a carboxyterminal hydrophobic sequence representing the transmembrane domain. The latter is followed by a 41 amino acid cytoplasmic tail, which contains a tyrosine residue in a region similar to the major autophosphorylation site of the epidermal-growth factor receptor (92). Although there is no evidence that this tyrosine is phosphorylated, there is evidence that phosphorylation of serine and threonine does occur as a consequence of both "outside-in" and "inside-out" signaling events involving GP IIb-IIIa activation, receptor occupancy, and receptor clustering, respectively (93). GP IIIa also contains four cysteine-rich tandem repeats, which are reminiscent of cysteine-rich repeats containing the ligand-binding sites of LDL and insulin receptors. There is no evidence, however, supporting a similar function for these structures in GP IIIa.

The intracellular assembly and membrane expression of the GP IIb-IIIa complex has been followed in cultured megakaryocytes, HEL cells, and heterologous cells transfected with GP IIb and GP IIIa cDNA (92). These studies indicate that GP IIb is synthesized as an approximately 130,000-mol-wt, single-chain precursor that undergoes core glycosylation, disulfide bond formation, and folding in the endoplasmic reticulum (ER). Calcium binding domains of GP IIb play an important role in maintaining the overall conformation of GP IIb-IIIa, allowing further intracellular processing or transport to the cell surface (94). Posttranslational processing, consisting of cleavage into two subunits and final carbohydrate modification, does not go to completion, however, unless the GP IIb-IIIa heterodimer has been assembled in the ER. In contrast, GP IIIa precursors are fully processed even without GP IIb. Like GP IIb, GP IIIa does not insert into the cell membrane without first engaging in complex formation.

## GP IIb-IIIa Activation

Although unstimulated platelets express surface membrane GP IIb-IIIa, these complexes do not interact with adhesive macromolecules unless platelets are stimulated (95) (Fig. 11.4). Interestingly, GP IIb-IIIa-ligand complexes have been identified in the α granule membranes of unstimulated platelets (96). The process by which surface membrane GP IIb-IIIa is converted into a competent receptor during platelet activation is incompletely understood, but requires extracellular ionized calcium and occurs by at least two activation pathways (93, 97), one of which is initiated by G protein dependent phosphoinositide hydrolysis leading to a rise in cytosolic calcium and activation of protein kinase C. Interestingly, receptors rendered competent by ADP or epinephrine without adhesive proteins rapidly lose their ligand binding capacity (98), whereas thrombin triggers a longer lasting exposure of GP IIb-IIIa (99).

In addition to agonists described previously, certain proteases can activate the GP IIb-IIIa complex (95). Exposure of platelets to chymotrypsin, for example, induces ligand binding sites and also results in digestion of GP IIIa, leaving a 66 KdA, membrane-associated fragment that does not recognize RGD-containing peptides (82, 83). Although attempts have been made to correlate GP IIb or GP IIIa proteolysis with activation, the "gain-of-function" cleavage has not been identified (82, 83, 100). Recent evidence suggests that $Na^+/Ca^{2+}$ exchanger operating in the reverse mode is a critical step in GP IIb-IIIa activation (101).

Exposure of platelets to plasmin also results in activation of GP IIb-IIIa ligand binding sites (102, 103). This finding may be of clinical relevance in individuals undergoing plasmin-mediated fibrinolysis for vascular occlusions (103).

Studies using monoclonal or polyclonal antibodies to probe GP IIb-IIIa structural and functional properties have suggested that conformational changes in the receptor and/or its microenvironment are associated with GP IIb-IIIa activation (104). Direct evidence that agonist-induced activation of GP IIb-IIIa in intact platelets indeed involves conformational changes in the receptor has been obtained using fluorescence resonance energy transfer techniques (105).

Although the precise mechanism of receptor activation is still uncertain, considerable attention has been focused on the cytoplasmic tails of GP IIb and GP IIIa. Evidence suggests that the cytoplasmic domains of both integrin α and β subunits control ligand binding affinity. Deletion of $\beta_3$ Leu$^{717}$–Asp$^{723}$, as well as disruption of the α 991–995 GFFKP sequence, leads to energy independent, constitutive GP IIb-IIIa activation (106, 107). The ability of integrin cytoplasmic domains to regulate integrin affinity may be due to their interaction with cytosolic constituents. Isolated β cytoplasmic domains for example associate with focal adhesions and initiate phosphorylation of pp125$^{FAK}$ (108), as does deletion of the α cytoplasmic domain of intact integrins (109). Thus, interaction between the conserved regions of integrin cytosolic domains may constrain these receptors into a low-affinity conformation. Although agonist induced phosphorylation of GP IIIa has been described, the extent of phosphorylation is extremely limited and unlikely to participate in receptor activation (110).

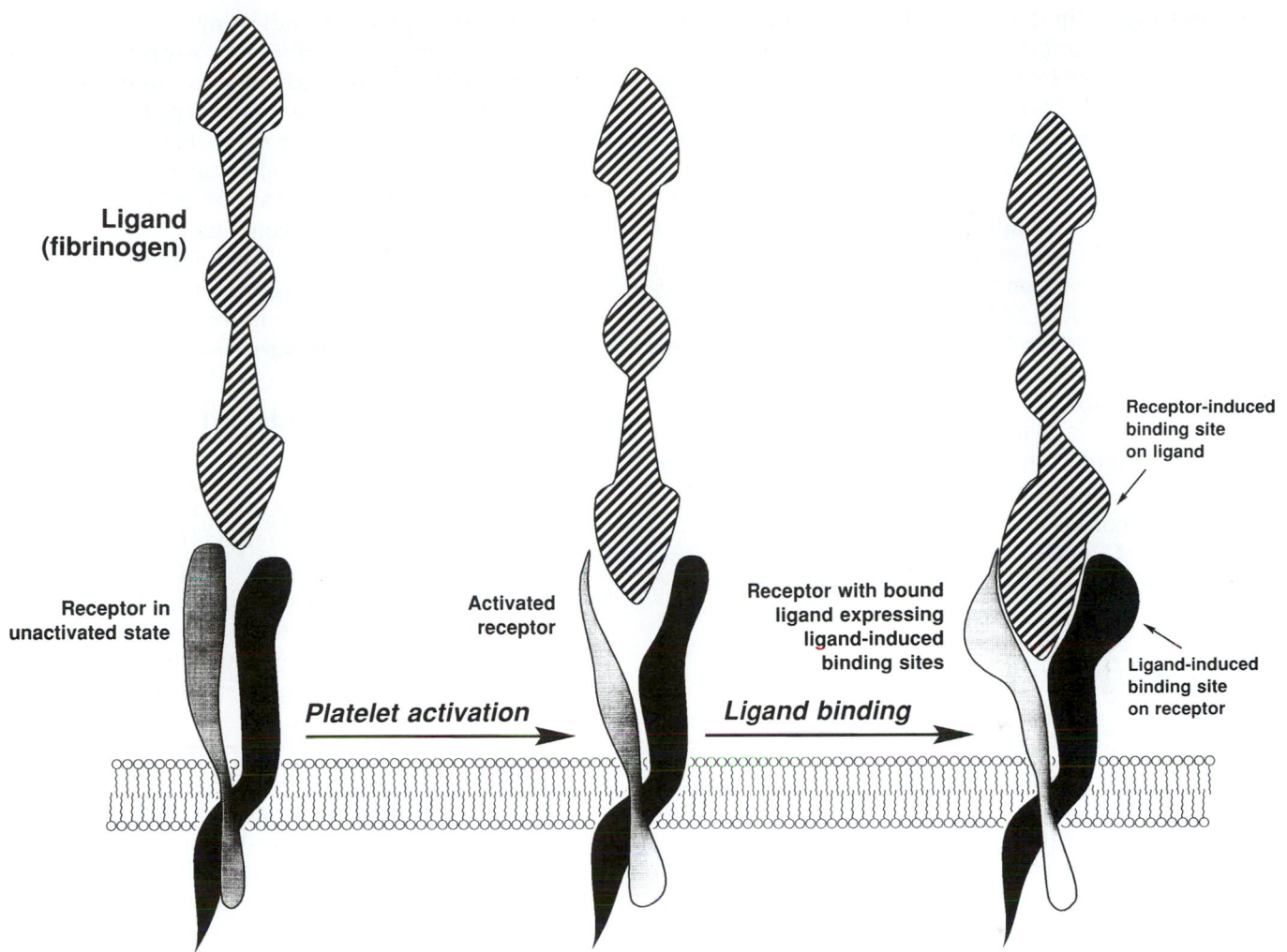

**FIGURE 11.4.** A model of GP IIb-IIIa activation and fibrinogen binding, depicting the exposure of ligand binding sites in the receptor following platelet activation, and the expression of ligand induced binding sites (LIBS) in GP IIb-IIIa, as well as receptor-induced binding sites (RIBS), in the fibrinogen ligand following GP IIb-IIIa occupancy.

In addition to conventional agonists and proteases, RGD peptides reversibly activate GP IIb-IIIa in intact cells and cell membranes (111, 112). Nuclear magnetic-resonance studies indicate that RGD peptides induce conformational transitions in purified GP IIb-IIIa SDS systems, yielding multiple binding states for fibrinogen γ chain peptides, and modify peptide-binding affinity (113). Further, GP IIb-IIIa function also may be influenced by lipids, particularly lysophosphatidic acid generated during platelet activation by agonists (114).

## Adhesive Protein Binding

Competent GP IIb-IIIa complexes can bind a variety of soluble adhesive proteins: fibrinogen, von Willebrand Factor (vWf), fibronectin, thrombospondin, and vitronectin (73, 115). Studies using inhibitory, anti–GP IIb-IIIa, monoclonal antibodies suggest a related binding mechanism for these adhesive proteins (115, 116). These ligand-receptor interactions are important for normal hemostasis and pathologic thrombus formation and have been implicated in tumor metastasis and propagation (117).

Recognition of ligands by the GP IIb-IIIa hetero-dimer complex, in part, involves the RGD tripeptide sequence (72, 73). In the case of fibrinogen, RGD sequences are located at positions 95–97 and 572–574 of each of two Aα chains. In addition to RGD sequences, fibrinogen contains GP IIb-IIIa recognition domains encompassing residues 400–411 in the C-terminal of each of two λ chains (118). Synthetic peptides, representing both α-chain RGD and γ chain platelet-recognition sequences, completely inhibit not only fibrinogen binding but also vWf and fibronectin binding, despite the absence of γ chain–like receptor recognition sequences in the latter ligands (72, 73). Studies with natural variants of fibrinogen, mutant forms of recombinant fibrinogen, and proteolytically derived fibrinogen fragments have emphasized the importance of the carboxyterminus of the fibrinogen γ chain in fibrinogen binding and platelet aggregation (119, 120).

Using a variety of biochemical and genetic approaches, the fibrinogen-binding site in GP IIb-IIIa has been mapped to the aminoterminal portion of GP IIb and GP IIIa (121). A highly conserved region in GP IIIa ($D^{109}$–$E^{171}$) is likely to be involved in ligand recognition because point mutations in this region abrogate ligand binding (122, 123). In addition, the N-terminal region of GP IIb, particularly a 21 amino acid stretch bounded by $A^{294}$–$M^{314}$ (123), appears to be involved in ligand binding, and a peptide from GP IIb, corresponding to amino acids 300–312, inhibits clot retraction, platelet aggregation, and binds fibrinogen (124). Although the fine structure of the binding site for fibrinogen or other RGD ligands has not been established, current evidence favors a model in which several discontinuous regions of both glycoproteins form a three dimensional, ligand binding pocket (121).

### Calcium Transport

In addition to serving as a receptor for fibrinogen and other adhesive proteins, the GP IIb-IIIa complex is involved in calcium homeostasis (125). Indeed, GP IIb-IIIa can function as a calcium channel in liposomes (126). Calcium movement into phospholipid vesicles is dependent on GP IIb-IIIa complex formation and is inhibited by some but not all monoclonal antibodies directed against the receptor complex and by some calcium channel blockers. Interestingly, overall calcium exchange in thrombasthenic platelets, lacking GP IIb-IIIa, is half that observed in normal platelets (127), and dissociation of the GP IIb-IIIa complex in normal platelets is associated with a decrease in basal calcium influx (125). In contrast, dissociation of GP IIb-IIIa in human erythroleukemia (HEL) cell membranes apparently has no effect on calcium transport (128), and calcium influx into either HEL cells or activated platelets appears only partially dependent, if at all, on the presence of functional GP IIb-IIIa complexes (128, 129). These observations suggest that GP IIb-IIIa may exert an indirect rather than a direct effect on calcium transport.

### Binding of Snake Venom Proteins

A variety of snake venom proteins, particularly from pit vipers, have been shown to interact with GP IIb-IIIa. A group of venom proteins termed disintegrins constitute a family of low-molecular-weight, cysteine-rich, RGD-containing peptides. These are potent inhibitors of platelet aggregation and fibrinogen binding and may be useful clinically as antithrombotic agents (130).

Unlike physiologic adhesive proteins, however, these venom-derived proteins bind to both stimulated and unstimulated platelets, indicating that a competent, RGD binding site is constitutively expressed on the platelet membrane and is accessible to small molecules. Indeed, synthetic, RGD-containing peptides and peptides resembling the fibrinogen γ chain 400–411 sequence also do not require platelet activation for interaction with GP IIb-IIIa (131). Studies using a series of immobilized RGD peptides containing variable numbers of glycine residues on polyacrylonitrile beads revealed that the majority of RGD binding sites on GP IIb-IIIa can be reached by peptides that extend out approximately 11–32 A from the surface of the bead (132).

### Binding of Other Ligands: IgE and *Borrelia burgdorferi*

A relationship between binding sites for IgE on human platelets and GP IIb-IIIa has emerged (133). IgE binding is althought to mediate IgE-dependent cytotoxic functions of platelets against helminth parasites. Platelets from individuals with thrombasthenia lacking GP IIb-IIIa fail to bind IgE. Moreover, a variety of polyclonal and monoclonal antibodies against GP IIb-IIIa inhibit IgE binding.

In addition, the tickborne spirochete *Borrelia burgdorferi*, which causes Lyme disease, interacts with platelets via GP IIb-IIIa. Interactions of the spirochete requires GP IIb-IIIa activation; thus binding is seen only to activated platelets. Binding is independent of fibrinogen binding, but is inhibited by a synthetic-RGD peptide and a synthetic peptide based on the γ chain of fibrinogen that blocks binding to GP IIb-IIIa (134).

### GP IIb-IIIa Mediated Platelet Aggregation and Adhesion

Fibrinogen is althought to aggregate platelets directly by forming bridges between GP IIb-IIIa receptors on adjacent platelets (Fig. 11.5) (118). This model of platelet-platelet interactions is supported by experimental evidence demonstrating not only a direct relationship between platelet aggregation and fibrinogen binding, but also decreased platelet aggregation at high fibrinogen concentrations, when platelet receptors become saturated with fibrinogen and insufficient free receptors remain to link platelets into aggregates (95, 135). These platelet-platelet interactions may be reinforced by the release of α-granule thrombospondin (136). Thrombospondin has been shown to bind to both platelet-associated fibrinogen and GP IV (see Other Platelet Membrane Proteins Involved in Hemostasis and Thrombosis) on the platelet surface. This interaction appears to stabilize fibrinogen binding to GP IIb-IIIa and is essential for the secondary wave of "irreversible" platelet aggregation. In addition, agonist-induced actin polymerization is re-

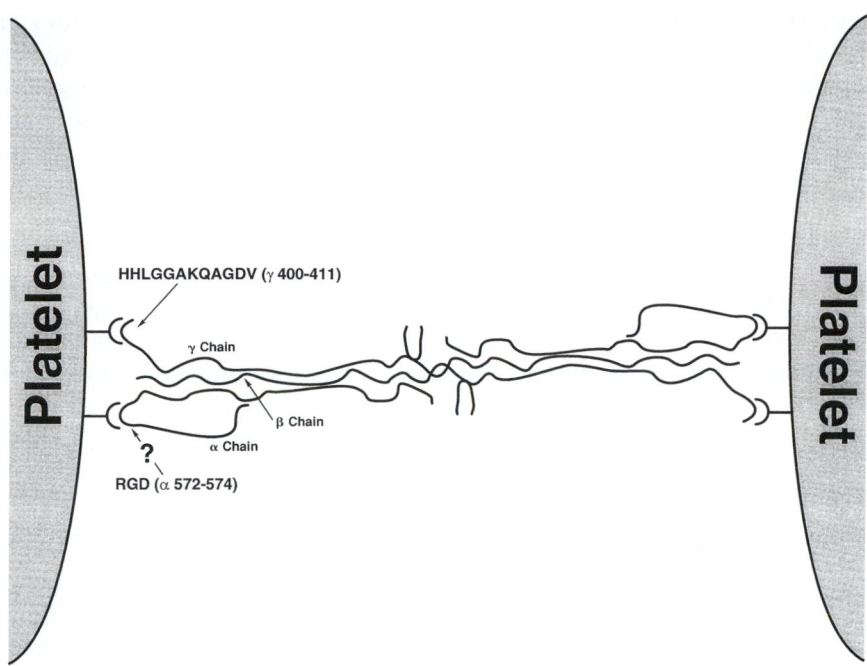

**FIGURE 11.5.**  A model of platelet aggregation mediated by fibrinogen bridging between adjacent platelets. The involvement of the fibrinogen carboxyterminal $\gamma^{400-411}$ dodecapeptide is shown, as well as potential contributions from the carboxyterminal fibrinogen $\alpha^{572-574}$ RGD sequence.

quired for irreversible platelet aggregation (137) and irreversible fibrinogen binding (138).

The first indication that GP IIb-IIIa was directly involved in fibrinogen binding and platelet aggregation came from studies of individuals with Glanzmann's thrombasthenia (see Chapter 32), a bleeding disorder characterized by GP IIb-IIIa deficient platelets that fail to aggregate following agonist-induced stimulation (14, 95). In addition, human recombinant GP IIb-IIIa complexes, expressed on the surface of Chinese hamster ovary cells, have been shown to support cell-cell interactions (139, 140) at low shear rates by mechanisms requiring that the glycoprotein complex be in an activated state. Recombinant GP IIb-IIIa, however, fail to support cell aggregation at high shear rates, suggesting that fibrinogen binding to GP IIb-IIIa *per se* may not be sufficient for platelet aggregation under high-shear conditions, such as in the microvasculature or in an aggregometer. Post–fibrinogen binding events (see Changes in Ligand-Receptor Interactions and Membrane Expression), including receptor reorganization and stabilization of fibrinogen binding, may strengthen platelet-platelet interactions.

In addition to platelet aggregation, fibrinogen plays an important role in platelet adhesion to artificial surfaces (141) and the extracellular matrix via interaction with fibulin-1, an intercellular component of a wide range of connective tissues (142). It has been suggested that presentation of platelets with multivalent ligands,

such as fibrinogen on a surface, contributes to platelet activation and accumulation. Recent studies have compared the recognition of fibrinogen by GP IIb-IIIa on unstimulated and stimulated platelets (143). The adhesion of unstimulated platelets was supported exclusively by residues in the carboxyterminal of the A$\alpha$ chain (RGD 572–574), whereas stimulated platelets recognized a variety of proteolytic-fibrinogen digests lacking A$\alpha$ RGD 572–574 but retaining the $\gamma$ chain 400–411 sequence. Furthermore, adhesion of stimulated platelets under static conditions is supported by plasmic fibrinogen digests that contain no known platelet recognition sequence (144). Thus, it is possible that distinct fibrinogen domains participate in the interaction with platelets and become engaged as a function of platelet activation. Platelets in whole blood perfused at a wall shear rate of 50 sec$^{-1}$ adhere to fibrinogen, fragment X, but not to fragments D or E (143). At wall shear rates of 200 sec$^{-1}$, only intact fibrinogen supports platelet adhesion.

## Changes in Ligand-Receptor Interactions and Membrane Expression

The interaction of fibrinogen with GP IIb-IIIa is a multiphasic process (138). The initial interaction occurs rapidly and is readily reversible, either by removing divalent cations with chelating agents or by adding excess unlabeled fibrinogen as competitor. After stimulation and ligand binding, this interaction becomes increasingly less reversible with time. Additional studies indicate that irreversible binding is an intrinsic property of GP IIb-IIIa (145). In addition, conformational changes in both receptor and ligand have been reported as a direct consequence of ligand binding (146–148) (Fig. 11.4). These sites may play important roles in post–receptor occupancy events such as second wave platelet aggregation, adhesion to collagen, and clot retraction. Moreover, GP IIb-IIIa clustering and sequestration in areas of the open canalicular system (149) and transport to α granules (150) have been noted following receptor occupancy with either fibrinogen or specific monoclonal antibodies. Furthermore, studies using confocal microscopy have demonstrated the selective GP IIb-IIIa mediated, actin-dependent clearance of bound fibrinogen from the activated platelet surface, suggesting a mechanism for preventing and limiting thrombus development (151). However, some controversy exists with regard to ligand-induced GP IIb-IIIa clustering and internalization as detected by electron microscopy, since recent studies suggest that the observed reorganization of membrane GP IIb-IIIa is more a function of the binding of large, electron dense gold or ferritin labeled probes to the receptor rather than specific, adhesive protein binding (152). Studies of platelets from individuals with Glanzmann's thrombasthenia, however, provide evidence that GP IIb-IIIa is indeed likely to be involved in fibrinogen trafficking between the surface membrane and α granules (153).

## GP IIb-IIIa Interactions with the Platelet Cytoskeleton

Following platelet activation and aggregation, the GP IIb-IIIa complex becomes associated with actin filaments in the platelet cytoskeleton (154). The association of GP IIb-IIIa with submembranous actin filaments is likely mediated by an intermediary protein such as talin (P235). Other potential protein intermediates forming the link between the actin cytoskeleton and ligand bound integrins are vinculin, fibrin, α actinin, or tensin (155). These interactions may be controlled by small, GTP binding proteins such as Rho. Presumably, the association of GP IIb-IIIa with the platelet cytoskeleton facilitates the contractile response, particularly clot retraction, which requires the interaction of fibrin with GP IIb-IIIa, the GP IIb-IIIa association with actin, and the interaction of actin with myosin (156). Activation of the platelet cytoskeleton has also been implicated in the exposure of fibrinogen receptors and the stabilization of platelet-fibrinogen interactions (138).

## GP IIb-IIIa Dependent Protein Signaling

The binding of fibrinogen to GP IIb-IIIa initiates intracellular signaling events distinct from initial signals required for GP IIb-IIIa activation (157). These outside-in signaling events are manifested by GP IIb-IIIa clustering within the plane of the membrane; sequential activation of protein tyrosine kinases such as $pp72^{syk}$, $pp60^{src}$, and $pp125^{FAK}$; and tyrosine phosphorylation of multiple platelet proteins (157, 158). Recently, GP IIIa phosphorylation on $Tyr^{747}$ and $Tyr^{759}$ was described following fibrinogen binding and platelet aggregation, as well as the interaction of the cytoplasmic tail of GP IIIa residues 740-762 with signaling proteins SHC and GRB2 (159), which belong to the Ras signaling pathway (160). These reactions are accompanied by a dramatic reorganization of the actin cytoskeleton and redistribution of the tyrosine kinases and other signaling elements to detergent-insoluble cytoskeletal fractions of the cell.

## GP IIb-IIIa Antigenic Determinants

Both GP IIb and IIIa are known to bear a number of clinically important alloantigenic determinants that are responsible for eliciting the immune response in post-transfusion purpura and neonatal alloimmune thrombocytopenic purpura (161, 162), disorders that are discussed in greater detail in Chapter 28. The alloantigen system most frequently implicated in these disorders is $PL^A$, expressed on GP IIIa. GP IIIa also contains the Pen(Yuk) antigens and the $Zw^a$ antigen (161), as well as the $Sr^a$ antigen system (161). Moreover, autoantibodies against GP IIb or GP IIIa in thrombocytopenia associated with HIV infection have been described (163).

GP IIb also expresses alloantigens. The Bak(lek) alloantigen system is found on GP IIb (161). In addition, GP IIb exhibits IgM binding associated with EDTA and temperature-dependent pseudothrombocytopenia (164) (see Chapter 23).

## THE VITRONECTIN RECEPTOR

The vitronectin receptor ($\alpha_v\beta_3$) has been described on platelets, endothelial cells, smooth muscle cells (92), and melanoma cells (165). It represents a relatively minor platelet integrin with copy numbers ranging from 100 to 1400 per platelet. The vitronectin receptor consists of an α subunit ($\alpha_v$), which is composed of a larger subunit (mol wt 135,000) that is disulfide bonded to a smaller subunit (mol wt 25,000) and expresses 35% sequence identity with GP IIb. Its β subunit ($\beta_3$) (mol wt 110,000) is identical to GP IIIa.

Platelet vitronectin receptors from a group of individuals expressing the thrombasthenic phenotype have been characterized (166). Whereas platelets from these individuals lack GP IIb-IIIa fibrinogen receptors, they express normal quantities of vitronectin receptors.

Like GP IIb-IIIa, the vitronectin receptor binds a variety of RGD-containing adhesive proteins such as vitronectin, fibronectin, vWf, and thrombospondin. Although other thrombospondin binding sites have been described, most notably GP IV, $\alpha_v\beta_3$ binds thrombospondin in an RGD dependent manner (167). RGD binding domains have been localized to residues 139–349 of the vitronectin-receptor $\alpha$ subunit (168), and residues 61–203 of the $\beta$ subunit using photoaffinity labeling techniques. Unlike the GP IIb-IIIa fibrinogen receptor, however, the vitronectin receptor function is constitutive and is inhibited only by RGD containing peptides and not the $\gamma$ chain dodecapeptide sequence (169). Although the vitronectin receptor may mediate platelet interactions with vitronectin and thrombospondin, its precise biologic role has not been established.

## THE FIBRONECTIN RECEPTOR: GPIc-IIa

The fibronectin receptor ($\alpha_5$, $\beta_1$) is another minor integrin on platelet membranes (92). It constitutes one of three platelet $\beta_1$ integrins thus far identified. The receptor $\alpha$ subunit, GP Ic, consists of a 135,000-mol-wt larger subunit, identical to VLA$\alpha_5$ (170), disulfide bonded to a 27 Kda smaller subunit. The $\beta$ subunit, GP IIa ($\beta_1$), migrates with an apparent mol wt of 130 Kda on SDS-polyacrylamide gels.

The fibronectin receptor interacts with fibronectin and laminin (92). Like the vitronectin receptor, it does not require platelet activation to support RGD dependent ligand binding. The fibronectin receptor participates in the adhesion of platelets from healthy individuals and individuals with Glanzmann's thrombasthenia, lacking GP IIb-IIIa, to fibronectin-coated surfaces under both static and flow conditions.

## THE LAMININ RECEPTOR

The platelet laminin receptor consists of a 125,000-mol-wt $\alpha$ subunit and a 130,000-mol-wt $\beta_1$ subunit (92). This receptor mediates platelet adhesion to laminin-coated surfaces, particularly under flow conditions (171). Platelet interaction with laminin is divalent cation dependent and specifically inhibited by monoclonal antibodies directed against VLA-6. Platelets adhere to laminin and spread on laminin-coated surfaces, but do not aggregate (172). The $\alpha$ subunit of VLA-6 ($\alpha_6$) is difficult to distinguish from GP Ic of the fibronectin receptor by one-dimensional SDS-polyacrylamide gel electrophoresis. However, the two proteins are readily distinguished by peptide mapping and two dimensional gel electrophoresis using isoelectric focusing in the first dimension and SDS-polyacrylamide gel electrophoresis in the second dimension (71).

## THE COLLAGEN RECEPTOR: GP Ia-IIa

Platelets adhere to and aggregate in response to collagen types I, II, III, and IV (172). In contrast to platelet adhesion

which can be supported by collagen monomers, platelet aggregation requires the native, triple-helix, collagen structure. Although several platelet proteins have been suggested as possible binding sites for collagen (see Platelet Activation Receptors), the GP Ia-IIa complex is likely to play a major role (46, 47). The platelets of individuals lacking GP Ia, for example, fail to adhere to and/or aggregate in response to collagen and present with a mild bleeding diathesis (173), as described in Chapter 32. In addition, recent evidence from studies with monoclonal antibodies directed against GP IIa suggest a potential role for this glycoprotein in signal transduction. The antibody inhibits platelet adhesion to type III collagen, as well as aggregation and secretion in response to collagen, thrombin, and arachidonic acid (174).

The interaction of GP Ia-IIa with collagen is magnesium dependent and inhibited by calcium. Distinct binding sites for both calcium and magnesium have been identified (175). It appears that these divalent cations stabilize different conformations of the complex. Experiments with both intact platelets and liposomes containing the purified GP Ia-IIa complex indicate that the receptor specifically recognizes a cyanogen bromide fragment of the $\alpha$ 1(I) chain of collagen, designated $\alpha$ 1(I)CB3 (176).

GP Ia-IIa is present at about 2000 copies per platelet (92). The complex is identical to VLA-2 ($\alpha_{IIb}/\beta_3$) and consists of a 167 Kda $\alpha$ subunit and a 130 Kda–mol-wt $\beta$ subunit. Although only 2000 copies of GP Ia have been detected on the platelet surface, approximately 5000 copies of GP IIa have been reported. This excess likely reflects GP IIa complexed with $\alpha_6$ and GP Ic to form the laminin and fibronectin receptors, respectively. Considerable variability in GP Ia-IIa activity has been described among normal individuals, and this correlates well with the ability of platelets to adhere to collagen types I and III under static conditions (177).

The complete amino acid sequence of VLA 2$\alpha$ has been deduced by molecular cloning and cDNA sequencing (178). The sequence reflects an overall 18 to 25% similarity with known amino acid sequences of other integrin $\alpha$ subunits and includes a signal peptide (29 amino acids) followed by an extracellular domain (1103 amino acids), a transmembrane domain (27 amino acids), and a short (22 amino acid) cytoplasmic tail. Interestingly, the deduced $\alpha_2$ sequence matches that of other integrin $\alpha$ chains in the position of 17 of 20 cysteine residues, the presence of three metal binding domains, and the transmembrane domain sequence. In addition, the $\alpha_2$ sequence contains a 191 amino acid insert (I domain) previously found only in leukocyte integrins of the $\beta_2$ family. This $\alpha_2$ I domain expresses 23 to 41% sequence similarity with domains in cartilage matrix proteins and vWf, which are also associated with collagen binding. There is recent evidence that this I-domain is functional in the interaction of GP Ia with collagen (179).

Platelet adhesion to collagen under flow conditions differs from adhesion under static conditions in that it has an absolute requirement for vWf (180). vWf has two collagen binding sites, one located in the A1 repeat and one in the A3 repeat. The latter is essential for collagen binding. vWf mediated platelet-collagen interactions require the platelet GP Ib-IX complex (see below).

The VLA-2 antigen carries the HPA-5 (BR) alloantigen system. The $Br^a/Br^b$ system is one of the most commonly encountered and is often associated with neonatal alloimmune thrombocytopenia. This system has been ascribed to a $Glu^{515}$ ($Br^b$) to Leu ($Br^a$) polymorphism in GP Ia (181).

# ADHESION RECEPTORS OF THE LEUCINE-RICH GLYCOPROTEIN GENE FAMILY

## THE VON WILLEBRAND FACTOR RECEPTOR: THE GP Ib-IX-V COMPLEX

The GP Ib-IX-V complex is a unique adhesion receptor, which, unlike members of the integrin family or other adhesion receptors on platelets, is not a member of an adhesion receptor family from which clues can be drawn as to its function. Nevertheless, each of its individual polypeptide components are members of the leucine rich glycoprotein family, whose common feature is the presence of a motif with one or several tandemly repeated copies of a leucine-rich sequence of 23 to 27 amino acids (182, 183). Within the leucine-rich family is a subfamily of proteins that do function as adhesion receptors, but their overall structures and modes of operation have little in common except their involvement in protein-protein interactions (182).

## GP Ib-IX-V Structure

The GP Ib-IX-V complex comprises four polypeptides, GP Ibα, GP Ibβ, GP IX, and GP V, present in a stoichiometry of 2:2:2:1, respectively (Fig. 11.6). The complex is the second most abundant receptor on the platelet surface (after GP IIb-IIIa), with 25,000 copies of GP Ibα, GP Ibβ, and GP IX and half as many copies of GP V (184). It represents the major sialoglycoprotein on the platelet surface and thus the major contributor to the dense negative charge of the platelet (185). GP Ib consists of two disulfide-linked subunits, GP Ibα (mol wt 145,000) and GP Ibβ (mol wt 24,000), and is tightly but noncovalently complexed with GP IX (mol wt 17,000). GP V is also noncovalently associated with the complex, but more loosely (Fig. 11.6), and associates directly with GP Ibα (186). All of the polypeptides span the platelet plasma membrane once and are typical type I transmembrane

proteins, with their aminotermini oriented to the outside of the platelet and their carboxytermini in the cytoplasm. All contain leucine-rich repeats (fifteen in GP V, seven in GP Ibα, and one each in GP IX and GP Ibβ) and conserved sequences that flank these repeats (182). Glycoprotein Ibβ and GP IX are the most similar to each other, with 60% sequence similarity in their extracellular domains (182). GP Ibα and GP V are similar to GP Ibβ and GP IX, but contain more leucine-rich repeats and additional sequences not present in the smaller polypeptides (Fig. 11.6).

Four molecular weight variants of GP Ib have been identified by SDS-PAGE (187). These arise from a genetic polymorphism and are designated A (mol wt 168,000), B (mol wt 162,000), C (mol wt 159,000), and D (mol wt 153,000). The polymorphism has been localized to the rod-shaped macroglycopeptide portion of GP Ibα (188), and results from duplication of a 13-amino acid sequence present in the smallest form that is duplicated once, twice, or thrice to yield the larger forms (189, 190). The macroglycopeptide region lies between the plasma membrane and the aminoterminal ligand-binding region of GP Ibα and, because of its elongated conformation, may act as a spacer, keeping the ligand-binding region high above the platelet surface. Added repeats are predicted to increase the distance of this region from the cell membrane and possibly to affect the susceptibility of the molecule to shear-induced changes in conformation (189). In all populations examined, the C isoform is the most common (182). The D variant is much more frequent in Asian populations than in Caucasians, and the A isoform appears to be found almost exclusively in Asians, in whom the frequency of this allele is close to 10% (187–190). The length polymorphism is linked to the $Sib^a$ and HPA-2 (Ko) alloantigen systems (190), which are based on dimorphism at residue 145 (90% of alleles have threonine in this position; 10% have methionine) (191). Methionine at position 145 is only seen in the two larger isoforms of GP Ibα (190).

The extracellular domain of GP Ibα is susceptible to proteolysis by a number of enzymes (192). Trypsin and chymotrypsin release this domain (the soluble fragment is called glycocalicin), leaving a GP Ibα remnant of approximately 25,0000 mol wt that is disulfide linked to GP Ibβ. GP Ibα is also susceptible to cleavage by platelet calcium-dependent proteases that may become expressed on the platelet surface, a mechanism that has been postulated to contribute to the thrombopathy of the Wiskott-Aldrich syndrome. Loss of membrane glycocalicin significantly reduces the platelet net negative charge (193).

## Molecular Biology

The complete amino acid sequences of GP Ibα, GP Ibβ, and GP IX have been deduced from analysis of the nu-

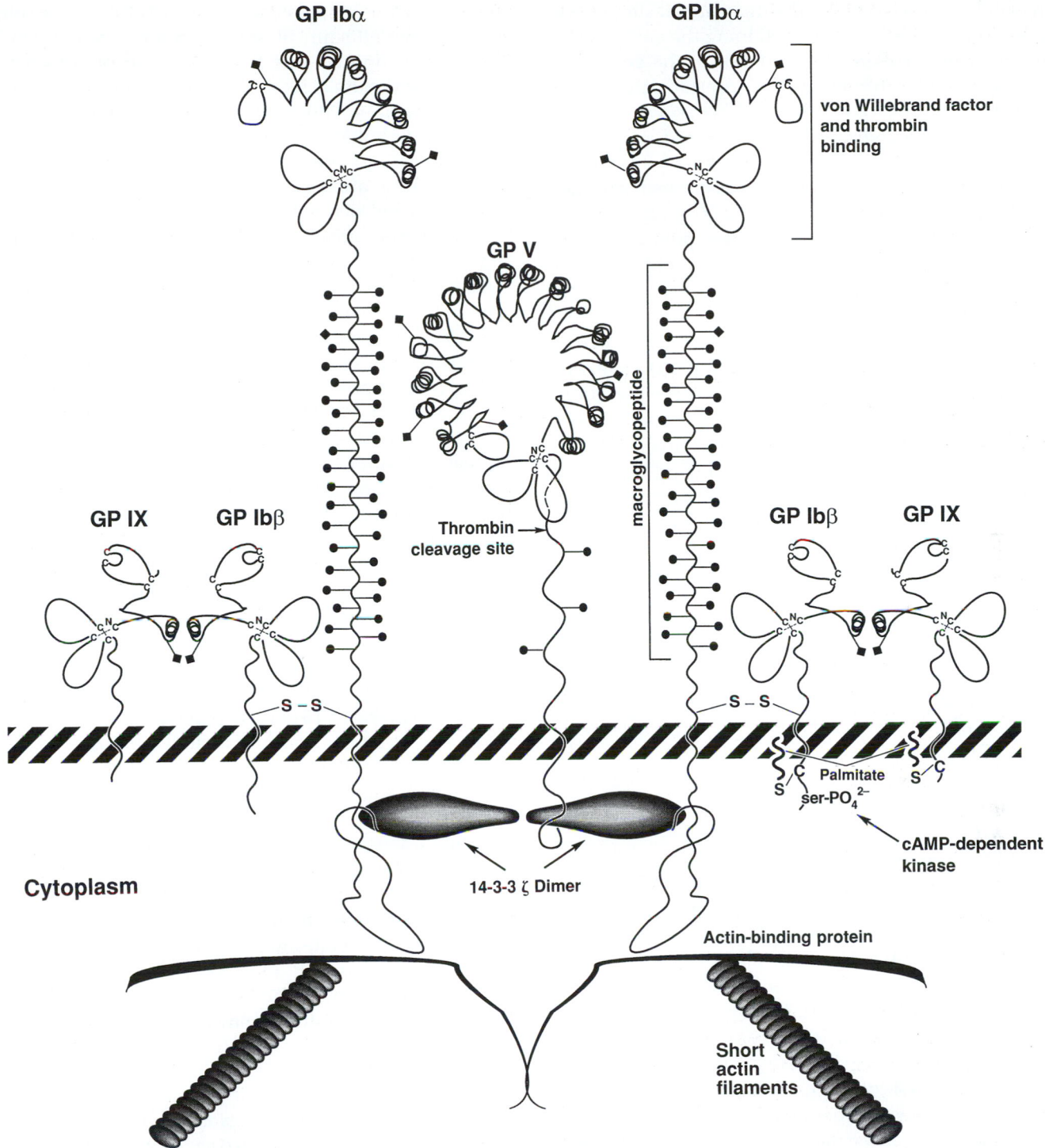

**FIGURE 11.6.** Structural characteristics of the GP Ib-IX-V complex deduced from molecular, biochemical, and functional studies. (⬳) leucine-rich glycoprotein domain; (S-S) disulfide bonds; (◆) N-linked carbohydrate side chain; (●) O-linked carbohydrate side chain; (serPO₄) serine phosphorylation site; (C) cysteine; (S) serine.

cleotide sequences of the respective HEL cell cDNA clones (194–196), and the sequence of GP V was determined by directly sequencing its gene (197, 198). All of the polypeptides are encoded by distinct genes, which themselves are in different regions of the human genome. The genes are located on 17p12-pter for GP Ibα (199), 22q11.2 for GP Ibβ (200), 3q21 for GP IX (201), and 3q29 for GP V (201). The genes, like the polypeptides, are similar to each other in that they are all simple, with all but the gene for GP Ibβ containing the entire protein coding region within one exon. All of the genes have only one or two introns in the 5' untranslated region, with the exception of GP Ibβ, which has a small intron interrupting the coding sequence six codons from the initiation codon (202). These simple structures have facilitated the search for mutations associated with deficiency disorders of the complex (see Chapter 32).

The cDNA sequence for GP Ibα predicts a short, hydrophobic, aminoterminal signal peptide that precedes the known aminoterminal sequence histidine, proline, isoleucine (HIS, PRO, ILE) (194). A second stretch of hydrophobic amino acids begins at residue 486 and probably represents the transmembrane domain. The cDNA sequence of GP Ibα also predicts the presence of nine cysteine residues, all located on the aminoterminal side of this putative transmembrane domain. Seven of these lie within the aminoterminal ligand-binding region, where they have been shown to form three disulfide loops (203) (Fig. 11.6), with one free cysteine residue remaining unpaired in this region. The two remaining cysteine residues lie immediately aminoterminal to the putative transmembrane domain and at least one is involved in the disulfide bond with GP Ibβ. Following the transmembrane domain is a 96-amino acid carboxyterminal cytoplasmic domain that contains regions that interact with actin-binding protein (204) and the ζ isoform of the signaling molecule 14.3.3 (205, 206), a known activator of the MAP kinase, Raf-1 (207–209).

GP Ibα is heavily glycosylated, containing four potential sites for N-linked glycosylation and a large cluster of serine and threonine residues in the macroglycopeptide region that are likely O-glycosylated. The latter region contains five tandem repeats with the consensus sequence threonine-threonine-X-glutamic acid-proline-threonine-proline-X-proline (THR-THR-X-GLU-PRO-THR-PRO-X-PRO) (194) and is also the region affected by the tandem duplication associated with size polymorphism of GP Ibα. Thus, the larger GP Ibα variants are expected to contain a larger complement of O-linked sugars and also a higher charge density secondary to the sialic-acid residues on each carbohydrate chain. The disparity between the predicted molecular mass based on the cDNA sequence (67, 192 daltons) and the molecular mass of 135,000 daltons deduced from SDS-polyacrylamide gels is consistent with extensive GP Ibα glycosylation.

The full-length cDNA for GP Ibβ encodes a 181-amino acid polypeptide with a calculated mol wt of 19,319. The sequence contains two hydrophobic stretches, one at the aminoterminus, representing the signal peptide, and the other near the carboxyterminus representing a likely transmembrane domain. The presence of 10 cysteine residues is predicted (195), one expressed in the cytoplasmic domain (210), which may serve as the attachment site for palmitic acid (211). It has been proposed that the interaction of membrane proteins with fatty acids may serve to stabilize glycoprotein interactions either with the plasma membrane or with hydrophobic portions of other membrane proteins. The cDNA sequence also predicts a single potential site for N-glycosylation in the extracellular domain and a single, leucine-rich repeat. In addition, GP Ibβ contains two potential sites for cyclic AMP–dependent phosphorylation in its cytoplasmic domain (195), one of which has been demonstrated to become phosphorylated (212).

GP IX is composed of 160 amino acids, and has a calculated mol wt of 17,259, excluding carbohydrate (196). This polypeptide is similar to GP Ibβ except in its cytoplasmic domain, which diverges greatly from the GP Ibβ sequence. It also contains only one leucine-rich repeat and contains nine cysteine residues, all in similar positions to those of GP Ibβ (182). The extra cysteine of GP Ibβ is presumably the one involved in the disulfide link with GP Ibα (see Fig. 11.6). The cytoplasmic cysteine of GP IX, like that of GP Ibβ, is also posttranslationally modified by fatty acylation (211). In addition, this polypeptide also appears to undergo myristoylation, in a process involving an amide linkage (213).

GP V is also similar to the other polypeptides of the complex. It is predicted to contain 560 amino acids, of which 360 make up 15 leucine-rich repeats. The distribution of extracellular cysteines is similar to that of GP Ibβ and GP IX, predicting a similar disulfide bond pattern (Fig. 11.6). This polypeptide is unique in that it is the only one of the four that contains a cleavage site for thrombin, within a sequence Gly-Pro-Arg-Gly-Pro-Pro, with the cleavage splitting the Arg-Gly peptide bond. Unlike other known thrombin substrates, GP V does not contain an anionic region for docking to thrombin's anion-binding exosite. Such a sequence is present in the aminoterminus of GP Ibα, which is not cleaved by thrombin, suggesting that the two polypeptides may cooperate in allowing thrombin cleavage of GP V.

## vWf Binding

GP Ib functions primarily in platelet adhesion to vascular subendothelium, recognizing immobilized vWf in the vessel wall (214). This was established initially by studying platelets from individuals with the Bernard-Soulier syndrome (215) (see Chapter 32). Platelets from these individuals do not bind vWf and lack the GP Ib-IX-V complex. Monoclonal antibodies directed against GP Ibα can mimic the platelet dysfunction associated with the Bernard-Soulier syndrome. The function of GP IX is unknown, but it does appear to be a target for many quinine/quinidine-dependent antibodies (216).

Although platelets are exposed to plasma vWf in

the circulation, GP Ib preferentially recognizes vWf present in the subendothelium (217). Adhesion to subendothelium increases as shear rates increase, a mechanism that underlies the importance of platelet adhesion in arresting blood loss in high-flow regions of the vasculature, such as small arteries and capillaries. If fluid shear stresses reach pathologic levels not normally found in the circulation (such as in regions of arterial stenosis), vWf and GP Ib can interact in the fluid phase, a process that activates platelets and leads to their aggregation (218). This phenomenon may underlie such clinical syndromes as unstable angina and transient ischemic attacks of the brain.

*In vitro*, the interaction between GP Ib and vWf can be induced by modulators, such as the peptide antibiotic ristocetin or the snake venom protein botrocetin (219). The interaction can also be induced by removal of the terminal sialic acid residues from vWf carbohydrate side chains (220), or with fibrin monomer (221–223). Platelet adhesion to fibrin in whole blood at high shear rates is dependent on both GP IIb-IIIa and secondary interactions between GP Ib and vWf. vWf must first bind to platelets before it can interact with fibrin and promote platelet adhesion. Thus, platelet interactions with vWf may be the result of specific functional conformation(s) assumed by vWf when associated with components of the vessel wall or developing fibrin thrombi and/or may reflect changes in the GP Ib receptor induced by agonists or rheologic conditions. Indeed, point mutations have been identified in both GP Ibα (224, 225) and vWf (226) that lead to spontaneous interaction between the ligand and the receptor, indicating that either is subject to activation. These mutations lead to platelet-type von Willebrand disease and type 2b von Willebrand disease, respectively.

The intrachain disulfide loop between $Cys^{509}$ and $Cys^{695}$ and flanking residues in the A1 domain of vWf are associated with GP Ib binding functions (219). Based on the functional consequences of single point mutations observed in individuals with type 2b von Willebrand disease, conformational changes within the A1 domain are likely responsible for regulation of vWf affinity for GP Ib. The observation that recombinant vWf molecules carrying two type-2b mutations do not bind platelets with higher affinity than those with only one mutation suggests that vWf can only adopt either "on" or "off" conformations, with no states of intermediate affinity (226).

The binding site(s) for vWf within the GP Ib-IX-V complex has been localized to a 45 Kda fragment at the aminoterminus of GP Ibα (227). Several different sequences within this region are involved in the binding. Studies with synthetic peptides have identified two sequences, $Ser^{251}–Tyr^{279}$ and $Gly^{271}–Gly^{285}$, that inhibit vWf binding (228). The inhibition appears to be modula-

tor-specific in that the latter peptide was more potent in inhibiting the interaction induced by botrocetin and the former had a more pronounced effect on ristocetin-induced binding. The latter sequence is rich in anionic amino acid residues and contains three tyrosines that become posttranslationally sulfated, a modification that is required for optimal binding of the complex to vWf, whether induced by ristocetin or botrocetin (229, 230). The modification is also required for the shear-dependent agglutination of mammalian cells expressing recombinant GP Ib-IX complexes (231). These sequences are located on the carboxyterminal side of the leucine-rich repeats. The leucine-rich repeats themselves also have an important role in vWf binding, as demonstrated by the fact that several Bernard-Soulier syndrome mutations produce normal surface levels of dysfunctional polypeptides that fail to interact with vWf (232, 233). Also important for modulating the interaction between the complex and vWf is a disulfide loop between $Cys^{211}$ and $Cys^{248}$, which is the region affected by the mutations associated with platelet-type vWf (for a review, see reference 182). This region can apparently exist in two possible conformations, with the higher-energy conformation promoting the interaction with vWf (234). The gain-of-function mutations of platelet-type von Willebrand disease apparently favor the active conformation.

vWf in its native form consists of 230 Kda monomers disulfide linked into large multimers of $10^3$ to $>10^4$ Kda (see Chapter 16). Each monomer of 250 amino acids has several modular functional domains, termed A, B, C, and D, arranged in the order D'-D3-A1-A2-A3-D4-B1-B2-B3-C1-C2. An Arg-Gly-Asp (RGD) sequence within the C1 domain mediates binding of vWf to integrins, including the GP IIb-IIIa complex. The binding site for the GP Ib-IX-V complex has been localized to the A1 domain by selective proteolysis of native vWf and functional analysis of the resultant fragments. Two fragments, a reduced and alkylated 52/48 Kda tryptic fragment (spanning residues $Val^{449}–Lys^{728}$) (235) and a monomeric 39/34 Kda dispase fragment ($Leu^{480}–Gly^{718}$) (236), were both shown to inhibit vWf binding to platelets. Furthermore, the 39/34 Kda dispase fragment could be directly cross-linked to the GP Ib-IX-V complex on platelets (236). The region encompassed by these fragments in native vWf contains a disulfide bond between $Cys^{509}$ and $Cys^{695}$ and encloses a sequence that is predominantly positively charged. Flanking the two cysteines is a region rich in proline and sialylated *O*-linked carbohydrate, which probably contains the region through which vWf interacts with ristocetin (237). Studies with synthetic peptides have identified the region spanning Asp514–Glu542 within the disulfide loop as a potential GP Ib-IX-V–binding site (237).

The binding of vWf to GP Ib-IX-V on the platelet surface transduces transmembrane signals that result in phospholipid metabolism, activation of protein kinase C and other protein kinases, elevation of cytosolic-calcium concentration, thromboxane $A_2$ synthesis, cytoskeletal reorganization, and changes in the ligand-binding function of other adhesion receptors (238–241). Although the mechanism of signal transduction by GP Ib to cytoplasmic constituents to initiate the above response is unclear, it has been reported recently that a 29 Kda protein corresponding to the $\zeta$ isoform of 14-3-3 proteins associates with GP Ib-IX-V (205). A number of functions have been attributed to 14-3-3 $\zeta$, including phospholipase $A_2$ activity, activation of the MAP kinase pathway via Raf protein kinase, and regulation of protein kinase C (242).

## Thrombin Binding

In addition to its well known role as a receptor for vWf, GP Ib is one of the major thrombin binding proteins on the platelet (243). Previous studies localized the thrombin binding site on GP Ibα to within the sequence $Phe^{216}$–$Ala^{274}$ (244), which appears to overlap with the binding domain described for vWf (228). This region has been further dissected, with one study demonstrating that several synthetic peptides derived from the sequence $Trp^{219}$–$Val^{227}$ are capable of inhibiting thrombin-induced platelet aggregation, with a requirement for the presence of $Ala^{224}$–$Asn^{226}$ (Ala-Glu-Asn) (245). The anionic region identified as important for vWf binding has also been shown to be an important determinant of thrombin binding and also requires posttranslational sulfation of tyrosines (246). Thus, as is the case for vWf binding, the sequence requirements for thrombin binding are complex. Further complexity is indicated by the polypeptide requirements for high-affinity thrombin binding. Studies of the recombinant complex expressed in mouse L cells indicate that on the cell surface, high-affinity binding to the complex only occurs with GP V (247). The high-affinity site does not itself reside on GP V, as it can be removed by a protease that cleaves off the N-terminus of GP Ibα but not GP V.

Binding of thrombin to the GP Ib-IX-V complex is important in mediating the responses to this agonist, as evidenced by the attenuated response to thrombin of Bernard-Soulier syndrome platelets and the recent demonstration that both GP Ib and the seven-transmembrane domain thrombin receptor contribute to increases in cytosolic calcium following platelet exposure to thrombin (248). Alternatively or in addition, two forms of GP Ib, one acting as a high-affinity, α-thrombin receptor and the other a vWf receptor, exhibit different sensitivities to digestion with Serratia protease (249).

## Interactions with the Cytoskeleton

The GP Ib-IX-V complex constitutes the major attachment site between the platelet membrane skeleton and the plasma membrane (Fig. 11.6). This interaction is mediated by actin-binding protein and may play a role in organizing actin polymerization, perhaps by regulating the addition of actin monomers onto short actin filaments in the membrane skeleton. This interaction is specific, with a Kd of $10^{-7}$ M (250). Approximately 20% of total actin-binding protein in platelets is associated with the GP Ib-IX-V complex (251).

Linkage of the membrane skeleton to GP Ib-IX-V also appears to regulate the ability of GP Ib to bind ligand (252). For example, the ability of platelets to agglutinate with vWf is decreased immediately following thrombin stimulation of platelets (see Activation Dependent Receptor Redistribution), an effect that is abolished by cytochalasins (253). Similarly, the ability of GP Ib to bind vWf is inhibited by agents that elevate cAMP concentrations in platelets, and the effect of these agents is inhibited by cytochalasins (254). Moreover, GP Ib becomes phosphorylated when platelets are treated with agents such as prostaglandin $E_1$ that elevate intracellular cAMP concentrations, and phosphorylation is associated with inhibition of actin polymerization when platelets are activated by collagen (255). Thus it has been postulated that inhibition of actin polymerization may prevent collagen-induced release of a capping protein from actin filaments, resulting in the observed functional inhibition.

## Activation-Dependent Receptor Redistribution

GP Ib undergoes marked redistribution following *in vitro* platelet stimulation with thrombin, ADP, A23187, and PAF (253, 256). Thrombin reduces binding of anti-GP Ib-IX-V monoclonal antibodies to platelets by 60 to 90% (253). This phenomenon is not due to proteolytic removal of GP Ib from the platelet membrane, however, but rather to receptor sequestration in the open canalicular system (257). Receptor redistribution requires actin polymerization and activation of myosin, as indicated by its inhibition by both cytochalasins and inhibitors of myosin light-chain kinase (258). A similar mechanism has been proposed for the observed inhibition of ristocetin-induced platelet agglutination following platelet exposure to plasmin (259).

It is not universally agreed that receptor redistribution occurs on thrombin activation of platelets, as other investigators, using methods different from those that have demonstrated redistribution, have failed to detect redistribution of the complex (260). Interestingly, results obtained on platelets in an experimental thrombosis system *in vivo* indicate that GP Ib remains on the surface of activated platelets (261).

# ADHESION RECEPTORS OF THE SELECTIN GENE FAMILY

## P-SELECTIN

The selectins are a family of vascular cell surface receptors that are characterized by lectin-like domains at their aminotermini, an adjacent, epidermal growth factor–like domain, followed by multiple, short consensus repeat units homologous to those of the complement regulatory proteins (262). Blood cells possess three members of the selectin family: L-selectin, expressed on leukocytes (lymphoid and myeloid cells); E-selectin, expressed on the endothelium; and P-selectin, expressed on platelets and on endothelium (262). P-selectin (CD62, older designations GMP-140 and PADGEM) is a 140 Kda integral membrane protein that is stored in both the Weibel-Palade bodies of endothelium and the α-granules of platelets. On activation of these cells, their granules fuse with the plasma membrane, and P-selectin is detectable on the cell surface within minutes. Approximately 13,000 molecules can be detected with monoclonal antibodies on the surfaces of activated platelets. In addition to this rapid expression on the surfaces of platelets and endothelial cells, transcription of the P-selectin gene increases with activation of endothelium by lipopolysaccharide, tumor necrosis factor–α, or interleukin-1 (263–265).

P-selectin on activated platelets mediates platelet attachment to neutrophils and monocytes, and P-selectin on endothelium mediates the rolling of these leukocytes on endothelium during an inflammatory response, especially early in response to inflammatory stimuli (262). Consistent with this role in early inflammation, P-selectin knockout mice demonstrated delayed entry of leukocytes into the peritoneum in response to an inflammatory stimulus (266). Leukocyte rolling is also supported at sites of vessel damage by adherent platelets, which express P-selectin on their surfaces (267).

A number of other roles have been postulated for P-selectin in the inflammatory response, including participation in late monocyte egress from the vasculature and in T cell–dependent hypersensitivity reactions (262). In addition, adhesion of activated platelets to monocytes through P-selectin induces tissue factor expression, which initiates blood coagulation and fibrin deposition at sites of vascular injury or inflammation (268).

P-selectin is a cysteine rich, highly glycosylated, integral membrane protein with a nonreduced mol wt of 140,000 (269). Its gene spans more than 50 kilobases and contains 17 exons, almost all of which encode distinct structural domains (269).

The P-selectin protein sequence deduced from the cDNA (270) reveals a typical type I transmembrane protein, with an aminoterminal hydrophobic signal peptide that transports the N-terminus into the endoplasmic reticulum, and a second hydrophobic sequence that anchors the protein in the membrane. The N-terminus of the mature protein is a region homologous to C-type lectins and is followed by a domain similar to repeated motifs of epidermal growth factor (EGF) (Fig. 11.7). This is then followed by nine short consensus repeats, or sushi domains, similar to those of complement regulatory proteins (262) and the factor XIII b subunit (271), each containing approximately 60 amino acids. After the sushi domains is a hydrophobic transmembrane domain, followed by a cytoplasmic domain of 35 amino acids. This cytoplasmic domain specifies P-selectin sorting to granules (272), internalization from the cell surface (273), and targeting for lysosomal degradation (274). These processes are likely regulated by phosphorylation of cytoplasmic residues; phosphorylation has been demonstrated of serine (275), threonine (275), tyrosine (276), and histidine (277) residues. A cysteine that becomes acylated by palmitic acid or stearic acid is also found in the P-selectin cytoplasmic domain (278).

Examination of deglycosylated P-selectin reveals four distinct polypeptides ranging in mol wt from 80,000 to 92,000 (92, 269). The smaller mol wt forms may arise from alternative splicing during the processing of P-selectin mRNA, as indicated by isolation of individual cDNA clones that lack either the seventh sushi domain or the transmembrane domain (270).

Studies of the molecular basis of selectin adhesion have focused on carbohydrate recognition by lectin domains (279). Ligand recognition by P-selectin requires both carbohydrate and polypeptide motifs. The carbohydrate specificity is rather narrow, with the prototype carbohydrates being of the O-linked type, with fucose and sialic acid important components of the recognition motif. Specific α1,3 fucosyl transferases are necessary for synthesis of the selectin carbohydrate ligands, with the transferase FucT-VII being the enzyme expressed on cells that express the P-selectin ligand (280). The recent finding that mice with targeted deletions of their FucT-VII gene are virtually devoid of E- and P-selectin ligands on their leukocytes supports the important role for this enzyme in synthesizing the ligand for P-selectin (281) and suggests as well that tissue-specificity of ligand expression can be determined by the appropriate expression of fucosyl transferases.

In addition to the carbohydrate determinant, P-selectin binding to leukocytes requires peptide determinants from the glycoprotein termed P-selectin glycoprotein ligand-1 (PSGL-1). PSGL-1 is expressed on blood neutrophils, monocytes, and lymphocytes and contains an anionic sulfated region near its N-terminus similar to the sulfated region of GP Ibα. Sulfation of tyrosines in this region is required for the P-selectin–PSGL-1 interaction (282–285).

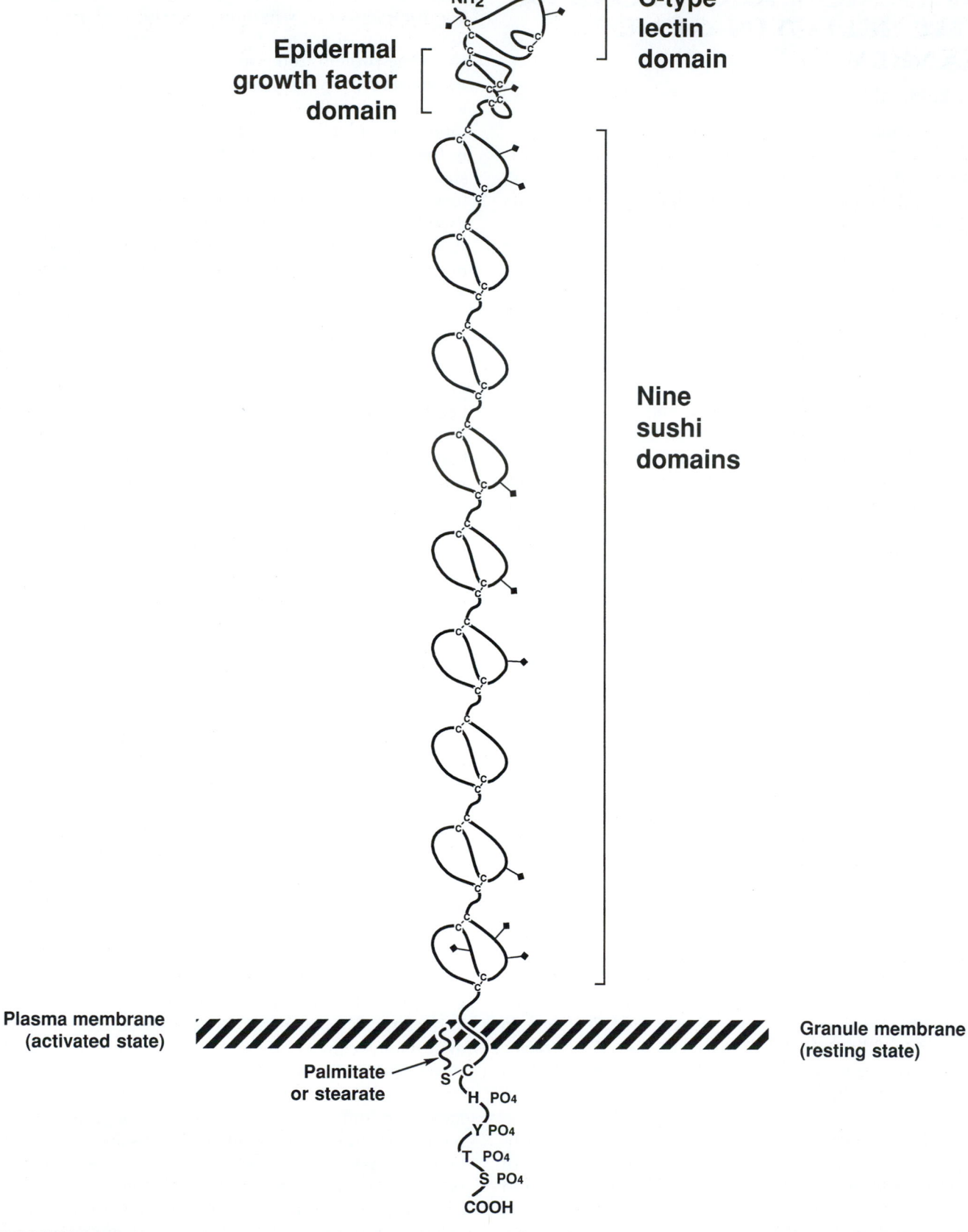

**FIGURE 11.7.**   Summary of structural features of P-selectin. (◆) *N*-linked carbohydrate side chains; (PO₄) phosphorylation sites; (H) histidine; (Y) tyrosine; (T) threonine; (S) serine; (C) cysteine; (NH₂) aminoterminus; (COOH) carboxyterminus.

# ADHESION RECEPTORS OF THE IMMUNOGLOBULIN GENE SUPERFAMILY

## PECAM-1 AND ICAM-2

The platelet endothelial cell adhesion molecule-1 (PECAM-1) is a 130 Kd glycoprotein identical to the CD31 differentiation antigen described on blood monocytes, neutrophils, and mitogen induced lymphoblasts (92, 286). The primary structure deduced from cDNA sequencing (287) reveals the presence of six immunoglobulin-like homology units, shared by other members of this gene superfamily. These domains are located extracellularly and are of the $C_2$ subgroup, predominantly found in the cell adhesion molecules (CAM) subfamily of immunoglobulin-like proteins. The cDNA-deduced primary structure further predicts an N-terminal extracellular domain of 574 amino acids with nine potential asparagine linked glycosylation sites and 12 cysteine residues spaced approximately 50 amino acids apart. A 19 residue transmembrane domain is deduced, followed by a 188 residue cytoplasmic domain, which contains a tyrosine that may serve as a phosphorylation site for tyrosine kinase. PECAM-1 is also present on endothelial cell membranes, particularly at intercellular junctions.

The cell surface distribution of PECAM-1 suggests a potential role in cell recognition events. The presence of a cytoplasmic tyrosine residue that may serve as a phosphorylation site by tyrosine kinases may also suggest participation in signal transduction. In addition, it has been hypothesized that the presence of PECAM-1 in a thrombus provides a surface for monocyte and granulocyte adhesion. This "homing activity" could initiate cellular events involved in inflammation and wound healing. Moreover, as several closely related members of the immunoglobulin gene superfamily have been shown to serve as receptors for viruses, including rhinovirus, human immunodeficiency virus, and poliovirus, it has been speculated that PECAM-1 may likewise participate in the entry of viruses into platelets and endothelial cells (287).

In addition to PECAM-1, platelets constitutively express approximately 3000 copies of ICAM-2 (intracellular adhesion molecule-2) on their surface (288). This number remains unchanged after platelet activation. To date, ICAM-2 is the only known $\beta_2$-integrin ligand present on platelets. It has a molecular weight of 59,000 daltons as determined by gel electrophoresis. ICAM-2 facilitates resting and activated platelet interactions with purified leukocyte function associated antigen-1 (LFA-1) and may therefore play an important role in leukocyte-platelet interactions in inflammation and thrombosis.

# OTHER PLATELET MEMBRANE PROTEINS INVOLVED IN HEMOSTASIS AND THROMBOSIS

## GLYCOPROTEIN IV

A major platelet membrane glycoprotein that appears unrelated to any presently known gene family is GP IV, also designated GP IIIb (289, 290). It appears later in megakaryocyte development than GP IIb-IIIa or GP Ib and is related to the leukocyte differentiation antigen CD36. GP IV also expresses the OKM-5 antigen.

Approximately 12,000 copies of GP IV are present per platelet. GP IV is not unique to cells of megakaryocyte lineage (92), however, and has been identified on endothelial cells, on melanoma cells where it functions in cell attachment and spreading, and on monocytes where it participates in signal transduction and platelet rosetting. GP IV is composed of 26% carbohydrate and exhibits an apparent molecular weight of 85 to 95 Kd on SDS-polyacrylamide gels and an isoelectric point between 4.4 and 6.3. The isoelectric heterogeneity probably reflects a variable GP IV sialic-acid content. Indeed, GP IV is highly glycosylated and is distinguished by its high resistance to proteolytic digestion in intact platelets.

GP IV is detected in widely varying amounts on platelets from normal donors (291), and its expression is increased in myeloproliferative syndromes (292). This glycoprotein is lacking in individuals that are negative for the NAK$^a$ isoantigen (293), but this has not been associated with any recognized hemostatic problem.

cDNA clones for GP IV have been isolated from a placental cDNA library (92). The GP IV cDNA sequence codes for a protein consisting of 471 amino acids with a calculated mol wt of 53,000. The sequence also indicates the presence of 10 potential sites for asparagine-linked glycosylation and a potential signal peptide at the aminoterminus. Interestingly, the aminoterminal sequence of the isolated protein is identical to the aminoterminal sequence deduced from cDNA sequences, suggesting that it is not cleaved from the body of the protein during translocation to the endoplasmic reticulum.

GP IV functions as a receptor for the α-granule protein thrombospondin on activated platelets (294). GP IV activation occurs through a process that appears to be dependent on the dephosphorylation of Thr$^{92}$ in the extracellular domain (295). GP IV binds type I collagen fibrils, and antibodies raised against GP IV inhibit collagen-induced platelet aggregation (48). Recent evidence suggests that GP IV plays a role in the early stages of platelet adhesion to physiologically relevant subendothelial surfaces at a shear rate of 800 sec$^{-1}$ (296).

Endothelial cell GP IV mediates the binding of *Plasmodium falciparum*–infected erythrocytes (297). This activity may be separate from the receptor's capacity to bind either thrombospondin or collagen, as expression of c-DNA encoding placental GP IV in Cos-7 cells supports cytoadherence of *Plasmodium falciparum*–infected red cells but not thrombospondin binding (298). Expression of CD 36 in Jurkat cells, however, did result in demonstrable thrombospondin binding (294).

Despite uncertainty as to the identity of the ligand for GP IV, a role for this glycoprotein in platelet signaling is suggested by recent findings that GP IV is physically associated with at least three Src-related protein tyrosine kinases in platelets: pp60$^{fyn}$, pp62$^{yes}$, and pp54/58$^{lyn}$ (157). A similar association was found in GP IV-containing cell lines. Further support for the possibility that GP IV functions in signal transduction comes from evidence that monoclonal antibodies to GP IV can induce platelet aggregation and secretion (299).

## GLYCOPROTEIN VI

GPVI represents a 61 Kda platelet membrane glycoprotein. It is either absent or reduced in some individuals suffering from mild bleeding disorders (54). Platelets from these individuals fail to adhere to or aggregate in response to collagen. The mechanism by which GP VI contributes to collagen-platelet interactions is ill defined. Recent studies suggest that under conditions of high shear (800 sec$^{-1}$), GP VI is involved in platelet-platelet interactions (300) and may play a role in regulating protein-tyrosine phosphorylation induced by collagen via cyclic AMP-insensitive activation of c-Src and Syk tyrosine kinases (301).

## THE PLATELET TETRASPAN ANTIGEN, PETA-3

Monoclonal antibodies directed against the PETA-3 antigen (platelet endothelial cell tetraspan antigen -3), recognizing a 27 Kda glycoprotein on human platelets and endothelial cells have been characterized (302). These antibodies induce platelet aggregation by mechanisms dependent on binding both Fc and Fab regions on the antibody (302). GP27 has been cloned (303) and shown to be a novel member of the transmembrane 4 superfamily also known as Tetraspans. This family includes other platelet proteins, namely CD9 and CD63 (304). While their precise function is unknown, these molecules appear to be part of multicomponent signaling complexes that affect a variety of cell adhesion, proliferation, and migration functions.

## ACTIVATION DEPENDENT EXPRESSION OF GLYCOPROTEINS FROM INTRACELLULAR STORES

A number of granule membrane proteins become expressed on the surface membrane of platelets following stimulation with strong agonists. In addition to α granule membrane proteins, the exposure of dense body and lysosomal granule membrane constituents has been described. P-selectin (see Adhesion Receptors of the Selectin Gene Family) is probably the best known platelet granule membrane protein to be expressed on the platelet surface membrane. Recently, another α granule membrane protein, mol wt 33 KdA, designated GMP33, was recognized on the surface of platelets following thrombin-induced secretion (305). Its function is presently unknown. In addition to these α granule membrane proteins, a 40 Kda dense granule membrane protein becomes accessible on the platelet surface following secretion (306).

Expression of a 53,000-mol-wt lysosomal membrane protein has been described also following platelet activation and secretion (307). Monoclonal antibodies directed against this protein recognize 650 binding sites on unstimulated platelets compared with 12,600 binding sites on thrombin-activated platelets, assuming a 1:1 relationship between antibody binding and antigen. Interestingly, surface expression of the 53,000-mol-wt lysosomal membrane protein increased during coronary artery bypass surgery. This protein was recently cloned and found to represent the CD63 antigen (308).

Two other glycoproteins of lysosomal membrane origin are surface expressed following the release of platelet granule contents. These are heavily glycosylated 110 Kda proteins, designated LAMP-1 (309) and LAMP-2 (310). LAMP-1 and LAMP-2 are homologous proteins belonging to a family of lysosomal membrane proteins that have been characterized in several species. Their surface expression is seen only following lysosomal granule release, effected by platelet stimulation with thrombin or collagen, but not ADP or epinephrine. Thrombin activation can induce the exposure of approximately 1000 LAMP-1 or LAMP-2 molecules per platelet, compared with the presence of less than 50 to 100 molecules per platelet in the resting state.

Another granule protein, multimerin (P-155) is released from activated platelets and binds to the platelet surface (311). Multimerin is a secreted protein, composed of variously sized, large multimers held together by disulfide bonds. Factor V is complexed with multimerin in resting platelet lysates and colocalizes with multimerin in platelet α granules (312). The cDNA sequence of human endothelial cell multimerin suggests a unique protein with RGDS, coiled-coil, and epidermal growth factor–like domains and a carboxylterminus similar to the globular domain of complement C1q and collagens type VIII and X (313).

# PLATELET MEMBRANE PROTEINS INVOLVED IN IMMUNOREGULATORY FUNCTIONS

## PLATELET Fc RECEPTORS

Platelets possess type II Fc receptors, mol wt 40,000, which recognize the Fc domain of IgG (55). These receptors play a significant role in transmembrane signaling and have been shown to mediate platelet activation by a variety of monoclonal antibodies (see Platelet Activation Receptors). Fc receptors are expressed on both megakaryocytes and platelets. Site-directed mutagenesis and epitope mapping experiments suggest that the extracellular domain closest to the membrane is responsible for ligand binding, especially amino acids 141–169. Additional platelet activation by thrombin or PMA results in a substantial increase in surface receptors, suggesting that receptors are translocated to the surface on activation (314). In megakaryocytes, interferon γ has been shown to increase Fc receptor transcription and expression (315). In addition, a soluble isoform of the Fc γ RII receptor, which lacks the transmembrane domain, has been characterized (316). A candidate for the soluble form of Fc γ RII has been found in platelet and megakaryocytic culture supernatants by immunochemical techniques.

Two allelic polymorphisms for the Fc γ RII receptor have been described (317). One consists of a glutamine (Q) to tryptophan (W) substitution at amino acid 27 in the extracellular domain without known structural or functional consequences. The second involves an arginine (R) to histidine (H) substitution at amino acid 131. This substitution appears to dictate ligand specificity (318).

Considerable individual variation in the number of Fc receptors has been reported on human platelets. Using monoclonal antibodies specific for the Fcγ RII receptor, between 575 and 1534 antibody binding sites have been detected per platelet, assuming a 1:1 interaction between antibody and the membrane receptor. Interestingly, a novel, 40 KdA protein, distinct from the Fcγ RII receptor based on amino acid sequence analysis, appears to be associated with the Fcγ RII receptor (319). Unlike the Fc receptor, however, the associated moiety is detected on thrombin activated platelets but not resting platelets, suggesting that it may represent a granule protein, which binds to the platelet membrane following platelet activation and secretion.

A larger mol wt, IgG-binding protein has also been identified on platelets. This molecule has been designated GP210, based on its migration as a 210 Kda protein on SDS-polyacrylamide gels (320). Since antibodies to GP210 crossreact with the 40 Kda Fcγ RII receptor (320), it has been suggested that GP210 represents a complex between a larger membrane protein and the 40 Kda Fcγ RII receptor. This larger mol wt protein may be GP Ib, as the GP210 antigen appears to be lacking on platelets from individuals with the Bernard Soulier syndrome, and is altered following ristocetin-induced vWf binding to GP Ib. The GP210 antigen remains unchanged, however, following platelet exposure to chymotrypsin which cleaves the amino-terminal, glycocalicin moiety from GP Ib.

# PLATELET RECEPTORS FOR COMPLEMENT COMPONENTS AND REGULATORY PROTEINS

Platelets possess receptors for select complement components and complement regulatory proteins (321). Specific receptors for both the collagen-like and globular domains of C1q, a subcomponent of the first component of complement (C1), have been described (322, 323). These have been designated cC1qR and gC1qR, respectively.

The cC1qR appears to function in the modulation of platelet interactions with collagen at low collagen concentrations, but is distinct from other platelet collagen receptors, as platelet interactions with collagen and C1q can be modulated separately using distinct monoclonal antibodies (322). The purified C1q receptor has a mol wt of 60 to 67 Kda by SDS-polyacrylamide gel electrophoresis and contains intrachain disulfide bonds, whose reduction results in an increase in the receptor's apparent mol wt to 72 to 75 Kda. It shares sequence homology with calreticulin (324). The cC1qR participates in immune complex localization to platelets, and when crosslinked by aggregated C1q, induces platelet activation, aggregation, secretion, and expression of procoagulant activity (325) via phosphatidyl inositol mediated signaling pathways.

The gC1qR is a 28 to 33 Kda protein that has been cloned and sequenced (326). Chromosomal mapping has located the gC1qR gene to Chromosome 17. The gC1qR is present on platelets and a variety of other cells. It is identical to the high molecular weight kininogen receptor purified from human endothelial cells (327) and may thus participate in modulation of contact activation and kinin generation at sites of blood vessel or tissue injury.

Platelets also express a C3 specific binding protein (328). Isolation of this moiety by affinity chromatography reveals the presence of two entities migrating with mol wts of 64 Kda and 53 Kda on SDS-polyacrylamide gels. This material is similar to the human leukocyte iC3 and C3b binding glycoprotein termed GP45-70. This glycoprotein also migrates as a doublet on SDS-polyacrylamide gel electrophoresis, and the amount of high- and low-mol-wt forms differs among individuals. It has been suggested that the difference in apparent mol wt is due to the differences in the sialic acid content of the two species.

Although platelets do not possess CR1 or CR2, they do possess the immunoregulatory protein DAF (decay accelerating factor) (321). DAF is a 70,000-mol-wt membrane constituent that facilitates the decay of both classical and alternative pathway-generated C3 convertase. These collective observations have led to the hypothesis that DAF and GP45-70 function to prevent autologous complement activation on human platelets, as well as on leukocytes.

# PLATELET ANTIGENS SHARED WITH LEUKOCYTES

Platelets express a variety of leukocyte surface antigens, designated CD, which are defined by clusters of monoclonal antibodies (329). In addition to CD31 (see PECAM-1), CD36 (see GP IV), and CD62 (see GMP140), platelet CD9 and CD69 have been described.

CD9 is a nontransmembrane, 24 Kda, surface glycoprotein that is involved in platelet activation (see also Platelet Activation Receptors) (58, 59), when combined with specific monoclonal antibodies that also interact with platelet Fc receptors (57). Although the function of CD9 is not understood, particularly as its physiologic ligand is unknown, it may associate with GP IIb-IIIa in the platelet membrane (330).

CD69 consists of a homodimer complex composed of two chains, mol wts 28 and 32 Kda (331). Both chains have the same 24 Kda protein backbone but are differently glycosylated by *N*-linked sugars. Both chains are constitutively phosphorylated and are likely to be integral membrane proteins. Although a physiologic ligand for CD69 has not been identified, experimental evidence suggests that, like CD9, it also may be capable of signal transduction.

In addition to numerous CD antigens, platelets share the PTA1 antigen with T lymphocytes (332). Platelets constitutively express approximately 1200 PTA1 antigens per cell. PTA1 represents a 67 Kda membrane protein, which is extensively glycosylated. Removal of *N*-linked carbohydrate reveals a 35 Kda protein core. The interaction of monoclonal antibodies with PTA1 induces platelet activation and aggregation and is accompanied by PTA1 phosphorylation. The PTA1 antigen is also phosphorylated during collagen-induced and thrombin-induced platelet aggregation.

# PLATELET MEMBRANE RECEPTORS FOR COAGULANT AND FIBRINOLYTIC PROTEINS

One of the earliest recognized effects of platelets on blood coagulation is the shortening of the plasma clotting time by stimulated platelets. The relevant platelet activity is termed platelet factor 3 or PF3 (333, 334) and results from the combined effects of the surface expression of procoagulant phospholipids (phosphatidyl serine, phosphatidyl inositol) and the receptor mediated interaction between coagulation proteins. In addition to its role in coagulation, the platelet membrane provides receptors for proteins involved in anticoagulation and fibrinolysis (335).

Although phospholipid movement in the cell membrane was originally althought to be limited to the lateral plane of the membrane, it is now appreciated that movement from one leaflet to the other also occurs in a process called flip-flop (336). Transbilayer movement of membrane phospholipids may be facilitated by physical properties between phospholipid monolayers, the presence of membrane spanning proteins, and/or irregularities of normal bilayer structure. In addition, modification of the cell cytoskeleton has been shown to enhance transbilayer movement of phospholipids (252). Moreover, membrane glycoproteins, particularly platelet GP Ib, play a role in mediating the interaction between the cytoskeleton and the cell membrane. Interestingly, platelets from individuals with Bernard Soulier syndrome, lacking GP Ib, exhibit enhanced procoagulant activity and increased phosphatidylserine exposure on nonactivated platelets (337, 338).

In some studies the number of binding sites for factor Va on activated platelets has been estimated at 2000 to 3000 per cell (339, 340). Binding of factor Va does not require but is enhanced by factor Xa and prothrombin. Only 200 to 300 high-affinity binding sites for factor Xa (Kd 30–70 pM) have been detected (339, 340). The presence of saturable, reversible, and calcium dependent binding sites for factor X on human platelets (Kd 320 $\pm$ 40 nM, Bmax 16,000 $\pm$ 2000 sites/platelet) has been reported on platelets activated with either thrombin or the thrombin receptor agonist peptide SFLLRN-amide, but not with ADP (341). Platelet bound factor X represents a kinetically important pool of substrate that is preferentially activated on the surface of activated platelets (342). Prothrombin is an effective competitor for Factor X binding. The gla-domains of factors X and II appear to contain regions necessary for platelet binding.

Specific binding sites have also been reported for factors VIII (343), IX (344), and XI (345), as well as high molecular weight kininogen (HK) (346). Interestingly, platelet-bound HK is proteolyzed at a slower rate by kallikrein and plasmin than its fluid phase counterpart, suggesting that cell binding may modify the rate of bradykinin liberation from HK.

In addition to serving in a procoagulant capacity, the platelet membrane functions in anticoagulation. Platelets interact with activated protein C, which inactivates factors Va and VIIIa. There are approximately 200 specific binding sites for activated protein C per platelet (Kd $10^{-8}$ M) (347). Once bound, activated protein C is approximately 8000 fold more active than its free counterpart.

Platelets also participate in the regulation of fibrinolysis by presenting binding sites for plasminogen, t-PA, and plasmin (348, 349). The zymogen, glu-plasminogen, binds to isolated human platelets in a time dependent, specific, and saturable manner with a Kd of 1.9 $\mu$M and a Bmax of 37,000 sites per platelet. Following platelet stimulation with thrombin, the number of plasminogen binding sites increases to 190,000 with a Kd of 2.6 $\mu$M. Plasminogen binds to the GP IIb-IIIa complex, either alone or in association with proteins antigenically related to $\alpha_2$ macroglobulin receptor associated protein (350). Plasminogen binding is inhibited by lysine or lysine analogs, particularly peptides with carboxyterminal, but not internal or aminoterminal lysyl residues. Peptides corresponding to the carboxyterminal 19 amino acids of $\alpha_2$ antiplasmin represent the most potent inhibitors of plasminogen binding.

# PLATELET MICROPARTICLES/ MICROVESICLES

Platelet stimulation by strong agonists such as thrombin or collagen or both can lead to the shedding of small membrane vesicles from the surface. These microparticles were first described by Wolf (351) and were noted to contain most of the platelet-related coagulant activity in whole blood and serum. Small quantities of platelet microparticles are detected in normal plasma, and increased concentrations are observed in response to shear stress, in stored platelet concentrates, and in the cryoprecipitate fraction of plasma, normal serum, and plasma from individuals having undergone cardiopulmonary bypass or individuals suffering from disorders associated with complement activation (352–354). Platelets from a indi-

**TABLE 11.1.** Adhesive Platelet Membrane Glycoproteins

| | | Mol Wt (Reduced)[a] | | | | | |
|---|---|---|---|---|---|---|---|
| | Alternate Designation | Alpha Subunit | Beta Subunit | Gene Family | Ligand[b] | Function | Glycoprotein Expression[c] |
| GP IIb-IIIa | $\alpha_{IIb}/\beta_3$ | 125 Kda, 23 Kda | 110 Kda | Integrin | Fibr, vWf, FN, VN | Aggregation Adhesion | C, S |
| Vitronectin receptor | $\alpha_v\beta_3$ | 135 Kda, 25 Kda | 110 Kda | Integrin | VN, ?vWf, Fibr | Adhesion | C |
| GP Ic-IIa | VLA-5 | 135 Kda, 27 Kda | 130 Kda | Integrin | FN, ?Laminin | Adhesion | C |
| Alpha$_6$/IIa | VLA-6 | 125 Kda | 130 Kda | Integrin | Laminin | Adhesion | C |
| GP Ia/IIa | VLA-2 | 167 Kda | 130 Kda | Integrin | Collagen | Adhesion | C |
| GP Ib-IX | | 145 Kda, 24 Kda | 17 Kda | Leucine-rich glycoprotein | VWF, THR | Adhesion | C |
| P-Selectin | GMP 140 PADGEM CD-62 | 140 Kda | | Selectin | PSGL-1[d], O-linked carbohydrate | Platelet-leukocyte interactions | S |
| PECAM-1 | CD31 | 130 Kda | | Immunoglobulin | ? | Platelet-endothelial cell interactions | C |
| GP IV | GP IIIb, CD36 | 88 Kda | ? | | TSP, Collagen | Adhesion | C |
| GP VI | | 61 Kda | ? | | Collagen | Aggregation | C |
| PETA-3[e] | | 27 Kda | | Tetraspan | ? | ?Aggregation | C |

[a] Numbers separated by commas represent the molecular weight of disulfide-linked alpha and beta chains of the respective receptor alpha or beta subunit.

[b] vWf, von Willebrand Factor; Fibr, fibrinogen; FN, fibronectin; VN, vitronectin; TSP, thrombospondin; THR, thrombin.

[c] C, constitutive expression; S, membrane expression requires platelet stimulation.

[d] P-selectin–glycoprotein ligand-1.

[e] Platelet–endothelial cell tetraspan antigen-3.

vidual with Scott syndrome express markedly reduced procoagulant activity linked to a defect in calcium mediated vesiculation of the plasma membrane and decreased membrane exposure of phosphatidyl serine (355).

Evidence suggests that the shedding of membrane microparticles correlates with the disruption of the platelet membrane cytoskeleton, specifically, calpain-mediated hydrolysis of actin-binding protein and the disruption of actin filament association with the surface membrane (356). Additional evidence indicates that the shedding of microvesicles from the platelet surface may be metabolically regulated by the activity of one or more calcium-dependent protein kinases (354).

Ultrastructurally, platelet microvesicles resemble membrane enclosed, amorphous cytoplasm or small, empty vesicles. They contain GP IIb-IIIa and express glycoproteins associated with platelet activation and secretion, such as GMP140 (P-Selectin) and thrombospondin (357). In addition, microvesicles derived from activated platelets exhibit factor VIII and factor Va binding sites (358). Thus increases in circulating platelet microvesicles is likely to reflect *in vivo* platelet activation or destruction and may be associated with a hypercoagulable state. Indeed, recent observations demonstrate microparticle association with fibrin strands (359), suggesting that microparticles modulate thrombus formation by providing sustained catalytic surfaces for coagulation factors and their regulators.

## SUMMARY

The platelet membrane and its receptors serve to organize the hemostatic response and recognize inflammatory and thrombotic stimuli. The large number of platelet membrane receptors can be classified into various structural and/or functional subgroups as summarized in Table 11.1. These receptors mediate the interactions of platelets with their microenvironment leading to homotypic and heterotypic cell-cell interactions, interactions with the subendothelial matrix, and the transduction of signals from the outside to the inside of the platelet to elicit or enhance various adhesive responses. Through a variety of technical advances in the areas of cell and molecular biology, many of the platelet membrane receptors have been cloned and sequenced. This has led to a better understanding of platelet physiology in health and disease and has contributed to the development of new therapeutic modalities to inhibit platelet function (360, 361), particularly in the treatment of cardiovascular occlusions. In addition, the role of membrane proteins in platelet tumor-cell interactions and tumor metastasis is emerging (117), and antiplatelet agents based on an enhanced understanding of platelet membrane biology may provide new, targeted therapy in this setting.

# REFERENCES

1. Weiss HJ. Platelet pathophysiology and antiplatelet drug therapy. New York: Liss, 1982.
2. Chap H, Perret B, Plantavid M et al. Topography of platelet membrane phospholipids. In: MacIntyre DE, Gordon JI, eds. Platelets in biology and pathology III. Amsterdam: Elsevier Science, 1987; pp. 191–204.
3. Evans WH, Graham JM. Membrane structure and function. Oxford, England: Oxford IRL Press, Oxford University Press, 1988.
4. Le AV, Doyle O. General theory of membrane structure and function. In: Venters JC, Harrison LC, eds. Membranes, detergents, and receptor solubilization. New York: AR Liss, 1984; pp. 1–25.
5. Shattil SJ, Copper RA. Role of membrane lipid composition, organization, and fluidity in human platelet function. In: Spaet TH, ed. Progress in hemostasis and thrombosis. Vol. 4. New York: Grune & Stratton, 1978; pp. 59–86.
6. Tandon N, Harmon JT, Rodbard D et al. Thrombin receptors define responsiveness of cholesterol modified platelets. J Biol Chem 1983;258:11840–11845.
7. Zucker MB, Nachmias VT. Platelet activation. Arteriosclerosis 1985;5:2–18.
8. Nurden P, Savi P, Heilmann E et al. An inherited bleeding disorder linked to a defective interaction between ADP and its receptor on platelets. Its influence on glycoprotein IIb-IIIa complex function. J Clin Invest 1995;95:1612–1622.
9. MacFarlane DE. 2-methylthioadenosine [beta-32P] diphosphate: synthesis and use as probe of platelet ADP receptors. Methods Enzymol 1992;215:137–142.
10. Mills DC. ADP-receptors on platelets. Thromb Haemost 1996;76:835–856.
11. Colman RW. Aggregin: a platelet ADP receptor that mediates activation. FASEB J 1990;4:1425–1435.
12. Puri RN, Kumar A, Chen H et al. Inhibition of ADP-induced platelet responses by covalent modification of aggregin, a putative ADP receptor, by 8-(4-bromo-2, 3-dioxybutylthio)ADP. J Biol Chem 1995;270:24482–24488.
13. Cristalli G, Mills DC. Identification of a receptor for ADP on blood platelets by photoaffinity labeling. Biochem J 1993;291:875–881.
14. Greco NJ, Yamamoto N, Jackson BW et al. Identification of a nucleotide-binding site on glycoprotein IIb. Relationship to ADP-induced platelet activation. J Biol Chem 1991;266:13627–13633.
15. Shattil SJ. Activation of human platelets by epinephrine. In: Insel PA, ed. Adrenergic receptors in man. New York: Marcel Dekker, 1987; pp. 303–353.
16. Brass LF, Manning DR, Shattil SJ. GTP-binding proteins and platelet activation. In: Coller BS, ed. Progress in hemostasis and thrombosis. Vol. 10. Philadelphia: WB Saunders, 1991; pp. 127–174.
17. Regan JW, Nakata H, DeMarinis RM et al. Purification and characterization of the human platelet alpha2-adrenergic receptor. J Biol Chem 1986;261:3894–3900.
18. McFarlane DE, Wright BL, Stump DC. Use of (methyl-3H)yohimbine as a radioligand for alpha2 adrenoreceptors on intact platelets. Comparison with dihydroergocryptine. Thromb Res 1981;23:31–43.
19. Kaywin P, McDonough M, Insel PA et al. Platelet function in essential thrombocythemia. Decreased epinephrine response associated with a defect of platelet alpha2-adrenergic receptors. N Engl J Med 1978;299:505–509.
20. Smith CB, Hollingsworth PJ, Garcia-Sevilla JA et al. Platelet alpha2-adrenoreceptors are decreased in number after anti-depressant therapy. Prog Neuropsychopharmacol Biol Psychiatry 1983;7:241–247.
21. Rao K, Willis J, Kowalska MA et al. Differential requirements for platelet aggregation and inhibition of adenylate cyclase by epinephrine. Studies of a familial platelet alpha2-adrenergic receptor defect. Blood 1988;71:494–501.
22. Kobilka BK, Matsui H, Kobilka TS et al. Cloning, sequencing, and expression of the gene coding for the human platelet alpha2 adrenergic receptor. Science 1987;238:650–656.
23. De Chaffoy de Courcelles D, Leysen JE, De Clerck F et al. Evidence that phospholipid turnover in the signal transducing system is coupled to serotonin S2 receptor sites. J Biol Chem 1985;260:7603–7608.
24. Scrutton MC, Thompson NT. Agonists and receptors: serotonin. In: Holmsen H, ed. Platelet responses and metabolism II. Receptors and metabolism. Boca Raton, FL: CRC Press, 1986; pp. 57–72.
25. Saltzman AG, Morse B, Whitman MM et al. Cloning of the human serotonin 5-HT2 and 5HT1C receptor subtypes. Biochem Biophys Res Commun 1991;181:1469–1478.
26. Peroutka SJ. Phylogenotic tree analysis of G protein–coupled 5HT receptors: implications for receptor nomenclature. Neuropharmacology 1992;31:609–613.
27. Yang H, Srikiatkhachorn A, Anthony M et al. Serotonin stimulates megakaryocytopoiesis via the 5HT2 receptor. Blood Coagul Fibrinolysis 1996;7:127–133.
28. Rudnick G, Humphreys CJ. Platelet serotonin transporter. Methods Enzymol 1992;215:213–224.
29. Hamberg M, Svensson J, Samuelsson B. Thromboxanes: a new group of

biologically active compounds derived from prostaglandin endoperoxides. Proc Natl Acad Sci U S A 1975;72:2994–2998.

30. Armstrong RA, Jones RL, Wilson NH. Ligand binding to thromboxane receptors on human platelets. Correlation with biological activity. Br J Pharmacol 1983;79:953–964.

31. Mayeux PR, Morinelli TA, Williams TC et al. Differential effect of pH on thromboxane $A_2$/prostaglandin $H_2$ receptor agonist and antagonist binding to human platelets. J Biol Chem 1991;266:13752–13758.

32. Pratico D, Smyth EM, Violi F et al. Local amplification of platelet function by 8-epi prostaglandin $F_{2\alpha}$ is not mediated by thromboxane receptor isoforms. J Biol Chem 1996;271:14916–14924.

33. Hirata M, Hayashi Y, Ushikubi F et al. Cloning and expression of cDNA from a human thromboxane $A_2$ receptor. Nature 1991;49:617–620.

34. D'Angelo DD, Davis MG, Houser WA et al. Characterization of 5' end of human thromboxane receptor gene. Organizational analysis and mapping of protein kinase C-responsive elements regulating expression in platelets. Circ Res 1995;77:466–474.

35. Thibonnier M. The human platelet vasopressin receptor. Identification by direct photoaffinity labeling. J Biol Chem 1987;262:10960–10964.

36. Vittet D, Rondot A, Cantan B et al. Nature and properties of human platelet vasopressin receptor. Biochem J 1986;233:631–636.

37. Burgers JA, Akkerman JWN. Regulation of the receptor for platelet-activating factor on human platelets. Biochem J 1993;291:157–161.

38. Hwang SB, Lam MH, Pong SS. Ionic and GTP regulation of binding of platelet activating factor to receptors and platelet activating factor induced activation of GTPase in rabbit platelet membranes. J Biol Chem 1986;261:532–537.

39. Honda Z, Nakamura M, Miki I et al. Cloning by functional expression of platelet-activating factor receptor from guinea pig lung. Nature 1991;349:342–346.

40. Vu TK, Hung DT, Wheaton VI et al. Molecular cloning of a functional thrombin receptor reveals a novel proteolytic mechanism of receptor activation. Cell 1991;64:1057–1068.

41. Coughlin SR. Molecular mechanisms of thrombin signaling. Semin Hematol 1994;31:270–277.

42. Kinlough-Rathbone RL, Perry DW, Packham MA. Contrasting effects of thrombin and the thrombin receptor peptide, SFLLRN, on aggregation and release of $^{14}$C-serotonin by human platelets pretreated with chymotrypsin or serratia marcescens protease. Thromb Haemost 1995;73:122–125.

43. Harmon JT, Jamieson GA. The glycocalicin portion of platelet glycoprotein Ib expresses both high and moderate affinity receptor sites for thrombin. A soluble radio-receptor assay for the interaction of thrombin with platelets. J Biol Chem 1986;261:13224–13229.

44. Phillips DR. Receptors for platelet agonists. In: George JN, Nurden AT, Phillips DR., eds. Platelet membrane glycoproteins. New York: Plenum Press, 1985; pp. 145–169.

45. Greco NJ, Tandon NN, Jones GD et al. Contributions of glycoprotein IB and the seven transmembrane domain receptor to increases in platelet cytoplasmic [$Ca^{2+}$] induced by alpha thrombin. Biochemistry 1996;35:906–911.

46. Kunicki TJ, Nugent DJ, Staats SJ et al. The human fibroblast class II extracellular matrix receptor mediates platelet adhesion to collagen and is identical to the platelet glycoprotein Ia-IIa complex. J Biol Chem 1988;263:4516–4519.

47. Coller BS, Beer JH, Scudder LE et al. Collagen-platelet interactions: evidence for a direct interaction of collagen with platelet GP Ia-IIa and an indirect interaction with platelet GP IIb-IIIa mediated by adhesive proteins. Blood 1989;74:182–192.

48. Tandon NN, Kralisz U, Jamieson GA. Identification of glycoprotein IV (CD36) as a primary receptor for platelet collagen adhesion. J Biol Chem 1989;264:7576–7583.

49. Chiang TM, Kang AH. Isolation and purification of collagen alpha 1(I)receptor from human platelet membranes. J Biol Chem 1982;257:7581–7586.

50. Peerschke EIB, Ghebrehiwet B. Human blood platelets possess specific binding sites for C1q. J Immunol 1987;138:1537–1541.

51. Chiang TM, Kang AH, Dale JB et al. Immunochemical studies of the purified human platelet receptor for the alpha 1(I)chain of chick skin collagen. J Immunol 1984;133:872–876.

52. Chiang TM, Jin A, Hasty KA et al. Collagen-platelet interaction: inhibition by a monoclonal antibody which binds a 90,000 dalton platelet glycoprotein. Thromb Res 1989;53:129–142.

53. Santoro SA. Identification of a 160,000 dalton platelet membrane protein that mediates the initial divalent cation-dependent adhesion of platelets to collagen. Cell 1986;46:913–920.

54. Moroi M, Jung SM, Okuma M et al. A individual with platelets deficient in GP VI that lack both collagen induced aggregation and adhesion. J Clin Invest 1989;84:1440–1445.

55. Anderson CL, Chacko GW, Osborne JM et al. The Fc receptor for immunoglobulin G (Fc$_{gamma}$RII) on human platelets. Semin Thromb Hemost 1995;21:1–9.

56. Hensen PM, Ginsberg MH. Immunologic reactions of platelets. In: Gordon JI, ed. Platelets in biology and pathology 2. Amsterdam: Elsevier/N. Holland, 1981; pp. 265–308.

57. Horsewood P, Hayward CP, Warkentin TE et al. Investigation of the mechanism of monoclonal antibody induced platelet activation. Blood 1991;78:1019–1026.

58. Carroll RC, Worthington RE, Boucheix C. Stimulus-response coupling in human platelet activation by monoclonal antibodies to the CD9 antigen, a 24 Kda surface-membrane glycoprotein. Biochem J 1990;266:527–535.

59. Jennings LK, Fox CF, Kouns WC et al. The activation of human platelets mediated by anti human platelet p24/CD9 monoclonal antibodies. J Biol Chem 1990;265:3815–3822.

60. DeBili N, Wendling F, Cosman D et al. The mpl receptor is expressed in the megakaryocytic lineage from late progenitors to platelets. Blood 1995;85:391–401.

61. Miyakawa Y, Oda A, Druker BJ et al. Recombinant thrombopoietin induces rapid protein tyrosine phosphorylation of Janus kinase 2 and shc in human blood platelets. Blood 1995;86:23–27.

62. Miyakawa Y, Oda A, Druker BJ et al. Thrombopoietin induces tyrosine phosphorylation of Stat 3 and Stat 5 in human blood platelets. Blood 1996;87:439–446.

63. Oda A, Ozaki K, Druker BJ et al. p120$^{c\text{-}cbl}$ is present in human blood platelets and is differentially involved in signaling by thrombopoietin and thrombin. Blood 1996;88:1330–1338.

64. Oda A, Miyakawa Y, Druker BJ et al. Thrombopoietin primes human platelet aggregation induced by shear stress and by multiple agonists. Blood 1996;87:4664–4670.

65. Miller OV, Gorman RR. Evidence for distinct prostaglandin $I_2$ and $D_2$ receptors in human platelets. J Pharmacol Exp Ther 1979;210:134–140.

66. Schafer AI, Cooper B, O'Hara D et al. Identification of platelet receptors for prostaglandin $I_2$ and $D_2$. J Biol Chem 1979;254:2914–2917.

67. Siegl AM, Smith JB, Silver MJ et al. Selective binding site for ($^3$H) prostacyclin on platelets. J Clin Invest 1979;63:215–220.

68. Dutta-Roy AK, Sinha AK. Purification and properties of prostaglandin $E_1$/prostacyclin receptor of human blood platelets. J Biol Chem 1987;262:12685–12691.

69. Siegl AM, Smith JB, Silver MJ. Specific binding sites for prostaglandin $D_2$ on human platelets. Biochim Biophys Res Comm 1979;90:291–296.

70. Blockmans D, Deckmyn H, Vermylen J. Platelet activation. Blood Rev 1995;9:143–156.

71. Phillips DR, Agin PP. Platelet plasma membrane glycoproteins. Evidence for the presence of nonequivalent disulfide bonds using nonreduced-reduced, two dimensional gel electrophoresis. J Biol Chem 1977;252:2121–2126.

72. Ginsberg MH, Du X, O'Toole TE et al. Platelet integrins. Thromb Haemost 1995;74:352–359.

73. Hynes RO. The complexity of platelet adhesion to extracellular matrixes. Thromb Haemost 1991;66:40–43

74. Mohri H. Fibronectin and integrins interactions. J Invest Med 1996;44:429–441.

75. Phillips DR, Charo IF, Parise LV et al. The platelet membrane glycoprotein IIb-IIIa complex. Blood 1988;71:831–843.

76. Wagner CL, Mascelli MA, Neblock DS et al. Analysis of GP IIb-IIIa receptor number by quantification of 7E3 binding to human platelets. Blood 1996;88:907–914.

77. Woods VL Jr, Wolff LE, Keller DM. Resting platelets contain a substantial centrally located pool of glycoprotein IIb-IIIa complexes which may be accessible to some but not other extracellular proteins. J Biol Chem 1986;261:15242–15251.

78. Cramer EM, Savidge GF, Vainchenker W et al. Alpha-granule pool of glycoprotein IIb-IIIa in normal and pathologic platelets and megakaryocytes. Blood 1990;75:1220–1227.

79. Calvete JJ, Henschen A, Gonzalez-Rodriguez J. Assignment of disulfide bonds in human platelet GP IIIa. A disulfide pattern for the beta-subunits of the integrin family. Biochem J 1991;274:63–71.

80. Kouns WC, Newman PJ, Puckett KJ et al. Further characterization of the loop structure of platelet glycoprotein IIIa: partial mapping of functionally significant glycoprotein IIIa epitopes. Blood 1991;78:3215–3233.

81. Calvete JJ, Mann K, Schafer W et al. Proteolytic degradation of the RGD-binding and non-RGD-binding conformers of human platelet integrin glycoprotein IIb-IIIa: clues for identification of regions involved in the receptor's activation. Biochem J 1994;298:1–7.

82. Peerschke EIB, Coller BS. A murine monoclonal antibody that blocks fibrinogen binding to normal platelets also inhibits fibrinogen interactions with chymotrypsin-treated platelets. Blood 1984;64:59–63.

83. Niewiarowski S, Norton KJ, Eckardt A et al. Structural and functional characterization of major platelet membrane components derived by limited proteolysis of glycoprotein IIIa. Biochim Biophys Acta 1989;983:91–99.

84. Calvete JJ, Arias J, Alvarez MV et al. Further studies on the topography of the N-terminal region of human platelet glycoprotein IIIa. Biochem J 1991;274:457–463.

85. Kunicki TJ, Pidard D, Rosa JP, Nurden AT. The formation of $Ca^{++}$-dependent complexes of platelet membrane glycoproteins IIb and IIIa in solution as determined by crossed immunoelectrophoresis. Blood 1981;58:268–278.

86. Jennings LK, Phillips DR. Purification of glycoproteins IIb and III from human platelet plasma membranes and characterization of a calcium dependent glycoprotein IIb-III complex. J Biol Chem 1982;257:10458–10463.

87. Steiner B, Parise LV, Leung B, Phillips DR. $Ca^{+2}$ dependent structural transitions of the platelet glycoprotein IIb-IIIa complex. Preparation of stable glycoprotein IIb and IIIa monomers. J Biol Chem 1991;266:14986–14991.

88. Brass LF, Shattil SJ. Identification and function of the high-affinity binding sites for $Ca^{2+}$ on the surface of platelets. J Clin Invest 1984;73:626–632.

89. Brass LF, Shattil SJ. Changes in surface bound and exchangeable calcium during platelet activation. J Biol Chem 1982;257:14000–14005.

90. D'Souza SE, Haas TA, Piotrowicz RS et al. Ligand and cation binding are dual functions of a discrete segment of the integrin $beta_3$ subunit: cation displacement is involved in ligand binding. Cell 1994;79:659–667.

91. Gulino D, Boudignon C, Zhang L et al. Ca(2+)-binding properties of the platelet glycoprotein IIb ligand interaction domain. J Biol Chem 1992;267:1001–1007.

92. Bennett JS. The molecular biology of platelet membrane proteins. Semin Hematol 1990;27:186–204.

93. Shattil SJ. Function and regulation of the $beta_3$ integrins in hemostasis and vascular biology. Thromb Haemost 1995;74:149–155.

94. Basani RB, Vilaire G, Shattil SJ et al. Glanzmann thrombasthenia due to a two amino acid deletion in the fourth calcium binding domain of $alpha_{IIb}$: demonstration of the importance of calcium binding domains in the conformation of $alpha_{IIb}beta_3$. Blood 1996;88:167–173.

95. Peerschke EIB. The platelet fibrinogen receptor. Semin Hematol 1985;22:241–259.

96. Nurden P, Humbert M, Piotrowicz RS et al. Distribution of ligand-occupied $alpha_{IIb}beta_3$ in resting and activated human platelets determined by expression of a novel class of ligand-induced binding sites recognized by monoclonal antibody AP6. Blood 1996;88:887–899.

97. Blockman D, Deckmyn H, Vermylen J. Platelet activation. Blood Reviews 1995;9:143–156.

98. van Willigen G, Akkerman JWN. Protein kinase C and cyclic AMP regulate reversible exposure of binding sites for fibrinogen on the glycoprotein IIB-IIIA complex of human platelets. Biochem J 1991;273:115–120.

99. van Willigen G, Akkerman JWN. Regulation of glycoprotein IIB/IIIA exposure on platelets stimulated with alpha-thrombin. Blood 1992;79:82–90.

100. Pidard D, Frelinger AL, Bouillot C et al. Activation of the fibrinogen receptor on human platelets exposed to alpha chymotrypsin. Relationship with a major proteolytic cleavage at the carboxyterminus of the membrane glycoprotein IIb heavy chain. Eur J Biochem 1991;200:437–447.

101. Shiraga M, Tomiyama Y, Honda S et al. Affinity modulation of the platelet integrin $alpha_{IIb}beta_3$ by alpha chymotrypsin: a possible role for $Na^+$/$Ca^{2+}$ exchanger. Blood 1996;88:2594–2602.

102. Cramer EM, Lu H, Caen JP et al. Differential redistribution of platelet glycoprotein Ib and IIb-IIIa after plasmin stimulation. Blood 1991;77:694–699.

103. Rao GHR, Wilson RF, White CW et al. Influence of thrombolytic agents on human platelet function. Thromb Res 1991;62:319–334.

104. Coller BS. Activation-specific platelet antigens. In: Kunicki TJ, George JN, eds. Platelet immunobiology: molecular and clinical aspects. New York: JB Lippincott, 1989; pp. 166–192.

105. Sims PJ, Ginsberg MH, Plow EF et al. Effect of platelet activation on the conformation of the plasma membrane glycoprotein IIb-IIIa complex. J Biol Chem 1991;266:7345–7352.

106. Hughes PE, O'Toole TE, Ylanne J et al. The conserved membrane-proximal region of an integrin cytoplasmic domain specifies ligand binding affinity. J Biol Chem 1995;270:12411–12417.

107. Peter K, Bode C. A deletion in the alpha subunit locks platelet integrin $alpha_{IIb}beta_3$ into a high affinity state. Blood Coagul Fibrinolysis 1996;7:233–236.

108. Akiyama SK, Yamada SS, Yamada KM et al. Transmembrane signal transduction by integrin cytoplasmic domains expressed in single-subunit chimeras. J Biol Chem 1994;269:15961–15964.

109. Ylanne J, Chen Y, O'Toole TE et al. Distinct functions of integrin alpha and beta subunit cytoplasmic domains in cell spreading and formation of focal adhesions. J Cell Biol 1993;122:223–233.

110. Hillery CA, Smyth SS, Parise LV. Phosphorylation of human platelet glycoprotein IIIa (GP IIIa). Dissociation from fibrinogen receptor activation and phosphorylation of GP IIIa in vitro. J Biol Chem 1991;266:14663–14669.

111. Du X, Plow EF, Frelinger AL et al. Ligands "activate" integrin $alpha_{IIb}beta_3$ (platelet GP IIb-IIIa). Cell 1991;65:408–416.

112. Smyth SS, Parise LV. Regulation of ligand binding to glycoprotein IIb-IIIa (integrin alpha IIb beta 3) in isolated platelet membranes. Biochem J 1993;292:749–758.

113. Mayo KH, Fan F, Beavers MP et al. RGD induces conformational transitions in purified platelet integrin GP IIb-IIIa-SDS system yielding multiple binding states for fibrinogen gamma chain C-terminal peptide. FEBS Lett 1996;378:79–82.

114. Smyth SS, Hillery CA, Parise LV. Fibrinogen binding to purified platelet glycoproteins IIb-IIIa (integrin $alpha_{IIb}beta_3$) is modulated by lipids. J Biol Chem 1992;267:15568–15577.

115. Asch E, Podack E. Vitronectin binds to activated human platelets and plays a role in platelet aggregation. J Clin Invest 1990;85:1372–1378.

116. Plow EF, McEver RP, Coller BS et al. Related binding mechanisms for fibrinogen, fibronectin, von Willebrand Factor, and thrombospondin on thrombin-stimulated human platelets. Blood 1985;66:724–727.

117. Nierodzik ML, Klepfish A, Karpatkin S. Role of platelet integrin GP IIb-GP IIIa, fibronectin, von Willebrand Factor, and thrombin in platelet-tumor interaction in vitro and metastasis in vivo. Semin Hematol 1994;31:278–288.

118. Hawiger J. Adhesive interactions of platelets and their blockade. Ann N Y Acad Sci 1991;614:270–278.

119. Kirschbaum NE, Mosesson MW, Amrani DL. Characterization of the gamma chain platelet binding site on fibrinogen fragment D. Blood 1992;79:2643–2648.

120. Farrell DH, Thiagarajan P, Chung DW et al. Role of fibrinogen alpha and gamma chain sites in platelet aggregation. Proc Natl Acad Sci U S A 1992;89:10729–10732.

121. Plow EF, D'Souza SE, Ginsberg MH. Ligand binding to GP IIb-IIIa. A status report. Semin Thromb Hemost 1992;18:324–332.

122. Loftus JC, O'Toole TE, Plow EF et al. A $beta_3$ integrin mutation abolishes ligand binding and alters divalent cation-dependent conformation. Science 1990;249:915–918.

123. D'Souza SE, Ginsberg MH, Matsueda GR et al. A discrete sequence in a platelet integrin is involved in ligand recognition. Nature 1991;350:66–68.

124. Taylor DB, Gartner T. A peptide corresponding to GP $IIb_{alpha}$ 300-312, a presumptive fibrinogen gamma-chain binding site on the platelet integrin GP IIb-IIIa, inhibits the adhesion of platelets to at least four adhesive ligands. J Biol Chem 1992;267:11729–11733.

125. Brass LF. $Ca^{+2}$ transport across the platelet membrane: a role for glycoproteins IIb and IIIa. J Biol Chem 1985;260:2231–2236.

126. Rybak ME, Renzulli LA. Ligand inhibition of the platelet GP IIb-IIIa complex function as a calcium channel in liposomes. J Biol Chem 1989;264:14617–14620.

127. Peerschke EI, Grant RA, Zucker MB. Decreased association of $^{45}$calcium with platelets unable to aggregate due to thrombasthenia or prolonged calcium deprivation. Br J Haematol 1980;46:247–256.

128. Suldan Z, Brass LF. Role of the glycoprotein IIb-IIIa complex in plasma membrane $Ca^{+2}$ transport: a comparison of results obtained with platelets from human erythroleukemia cells. Blood 1991;78:2887–2893.

129. Powling MJ, Hardisty RM. Glycoprotein IIb-IIIa complex and $Ca^{++}$ influx into stimulated platelets. Blood 1985;66:731–734.

130. Niewiarowski S, McLane MA, Kloczewiak M et al. Disintegrins and other naturally occurring antagonists of platelet fibrinogen receptors. Semin Hematol 1994;31:289–300.

131. Ginsberg MH, Frelinger AL, Lam SCT et al. Analysis of platelet aggregation disorders based on flow cytometric analysis of membrane glycoprotein IIb-IIIa with conformation-specific monoclonal antibodies. Blood 1990;76:2017–2023.

132. Beer JH, Springer KT, Coller BS. Immobilized Arg-Gly-Asp (RGD) peptides of varying lengths as structural probes of the platelet glycoprotein IIb-IIIa receptor. Blood 1992;79:117–128.

133. Ameisen JC, Joseph M, Caen JP et al. A role for glycoprotein IIb-IIIa complexes in the binding of IgE to human platelets and platelet IgE-dependent cytolytic function. Br J Haematol 1986;64:21–32.

134. Coburn J, Leong JM, Ergan JK. Integrin $alpha_{IIb}beta_3$ mediates binding of the Lyme disease agent Borrelia burgdorferi to human platelets. Proc Natl Acad Sci U S A 1993;90:7059–7063.

135. Hawiger J, Kloczewiak M, Bednarek MA et al. Platelet receptor recognition domains of the alpha chain of human fibrinogen: structure-functions analysis. Biochemistry 1989;28:2909–2914.

136. Asch AS, Nachman RL. Thrombospondin: phenomenology to function. In: Coller BS, ed. Progress in hemostasis and thrombosis. Vol 9. Philadelphia: WB Saunders, 1989; pp. 157–175.

137. Torti M, Festetics ET, Bertoni A et al. Agonist-induced actin polymerization is required for the irreversibility of platelet aggregation. Thromb Haemost 1996;76:444–449.

138. Peerschke EIB. Events occurring after thrombin-induced fibrinogen binding to platelets. Semin Thromb Hemost 1992;18:34–43.

139. Frojmovic MM, O'Toole TE, Plow EF et al. Platelet glycoprotein IIb-IIIa ($alpha_{IIb}$, $beta_3$ integrin) confers fibrinogen- and activation-dependent aggregation on heterologous cells. Blood 1991;78:369–376.

140. Sung KLP, Frojmovic MM, O'Toole TE et al. Determination of adhesion force between single cell pairs generated by activated GP IIb-IIIa receptors. Blood 1993;81:419–423.

141. Lindon JN, McManama GP, Kushner L et al. Does the conformation of adsorbed fibrinogen dictate platelet interaction with artificial surfaces? Blood 1986;68:355–362.

142. Godyna S, Diaz-Ricart M, Argraves WS. Fibulin-1 mediates platelet adhesion via a bridge of fibrinogen. Blood 1996;88:2569–2577.

143. Ruggeri ZM. The role of von Willebrand Factor and fibrinogen in the initiation of platelet adhesion to thrombogenic surfaces. Thromb Haemost 1995;74:460–463.

144. Peerschke EIB, Galanakis DK. Platelet adhesion to late fibrinogen degradation products. Blood Coag Fibrinolysis 1996;7:353–360.

145. Muller V, Zerwes HG, Tangemann K et al. Two step binding mechanism of fibrinogen to alphaIIB/beta 3 integrin reconstituted into planar lipid bilayers. J Biol Chem 1993;268:6800–6808.

146. Frelinger AL III, Cohen I, Plow EF et al. Selective inhibition of integrin function by antibodies specific for ligand-occupied receptor conformers. J Biol Chem 1990;265:6346–6352.

147. Mondoro TH, Wall CD, White MM et al. Selective induction of a glycoprotein IIIa ligand-induced binding site by fibrinogen and von Willebrand Factor. Blood 1996;88:3824–3830.

148. Ugarova T, Agbanyo F, Plow EF. Conformational changes in adhesive proteins modulate their adhesive function. Thromb Haemost 1995;74: 253–358.

149. Leistikow EA, Barnhart MI, Albrecht RM et al. Redistribution of fibrinogen receptors on surface activated platelets. In: Mosesson MW, ed. Fibrinogen 3. Biochemistry, biological functions, gene regulation, and expression. New York: Elsevier Science, 1988; pp. 215–220.

150. Morgenstern E, Ruf A, Patscheke H. Transport of anti-glycoprotein IIb-IIIa-antibodies into the alpha-granules of unstimulated human blood platelets. Thromb Haemost 1992;67:121–125.

151. Peerschke EIB. Bound fibrinogen distribution on stimulated platelets. Examination by confocal scanning laser microscopy. Am J Pathol 1995;147: 678–687.

152. White JG, Escolar G. Fibrinogen receptors do not undergo spontaneous redistribution on surface-activated platelets. Arteriosclerosis 1990;10: 738–744.

153. Coller BS, Seligsohn U, West SM et al. Platelet fibrinogen and vitronectin in Glanzmann thrombasthenia: evidence consistent with specific roles for glycoprotein IIb-IIIa and alpha_v/beta_3 integrins in platelet protein trafficking. Blood 1991;78:2603–2610.

154. Carroll RC, Butler RG, Morris PA et al. Separable assembly of platelet pseudopodal and contractile cytoskeletons. Cells 1982;30:385–393.

155. Furman MI, Gardner TM, Goldschmidt-Clermont PJ. Mechanisms of cytoskeletal reorganization during platelet activation. Thromb Haemost 1993; 70:229–232.

156. Cohen I. The mechanism of clot retraction. In: George JN, Nurden AT, Phillips DR, eds. Platelet membrane glycoproteins. New York: Plenum Press, 1985; pp. 299–323.

157. Shattil SJ, Brugge JS. Protein tyrosine phosphorylation and the adhesive functions of platelets. Curr Opin Cell Biol 1991;3:869–879.

158. Clark EA, Brugge JS. Integrins and signal transduction pathways: the road taken. Science 1995;268:233–239.

159. Law DA, Nannizzi-Alaimo L, Phillips DR. Outside-in integrin signal transduction. J Biol Chem 1996;271:10811–10815.45

160. Egan SE, Giddings BW, Brooks MW et al. Association of Sos Ras exchange protein with Grb2 is implicated in tyrosine kinase signal transduction and transformation. Nature 1993;363:45–51.

161. Newman PJ. Platelet GP IIb-IIIa: molecular variations and alloantigens. Thromb Haemost 1991;66:111–118.

162. Santoso S, Kalb R, Kroll H et al. A point mutation leads to an unpaired cysteine residue and a molecular weight polymorphism of a functional platelet beta_3 integrin subunit. J Biol Chem 1994;269:8439–8444.

163. Gonzalez-Canejero R, Rivera J, Rosillo MC et al. Association of autoantibodies against platelet glycoprotein Ib-IX and IIb-IIIa, and platelet reactive anti-HIV antibodies in thrombocytopenic narcotic addicts. Br J Haematol 1996;93:464–471.

164. van Vliet HHDM, Kappers-Klumm MC, Abel J. Pseudothrombocytopenia: a cold autoantibody against platelet glycoprotein IIb. Br J Haematol 1986; 62:505–511.

165. McGregor BC, McGregor JL, Weiss LM. Presence of cytoadhesins (IIb-IIIa–like glycoproteins) on human metastatic melanoma but not on benign melanocytes. Am J Clin Pathol 1989;92:495–499.

166. Coller BS, Cheresh DA, Asch E et al. Platelet vitronectin receptor expression differentiates Iraqi-Jewish from Arab individuals with Glanzmann thrombasthenia in Israel. Blood 1991;77:75–83.

167. Lawler J, Hynes RO. An integrin receptor on normal and thrombasthenic platelets that binds thrombospondin. Blood 1989;74:2022–2027.

168. Smith JW, Cheresh DA. Integrin (alpha_v, beta_3) ligand interactions. Identification of a heterodimeric RGD binding site on the vitronectin receptor. J Biol Chem 1990;265:2168–2172.

169. Smith JW, Ruggeri ZM, Kunicki TJ et al. Interaction of integrins alpha_v beta_3 and glycoprotein IIb-IIIa with fibrinogen. Differential peptide recognition accounts for distinct binding sites. J Biol Chem 1990;265: 12267–12271.

170. Pischel KD, Bluestein HG, Woods VL Jr. Platelet glycoprotein Ia, Ic and IIa are physicochemically indistinguishable from the very late activation antigens adhesion-related proteins of lymphocytes and other cell types. J Clin Invest 1988;81:505–513.

171. Hindriks G, Ijsseldijk MJW, Sonnenberg A et al. Platelet adhesion to laminin: role of Ca^{2+} and Mg^{2+} ions, shear rate, and platelet membrane glycoproteins. Blood 1992;79:928–935.

172. Sixma JJ, van Zanten GH, Banga JD et al. Platelet adhesion. Semin Hematol 1995;32:89–98.

173. Nieuwenhuis HK, Akkerman JWN, Houdijk WPM et al. Human blood

174. Parmentier S, Catimel B, McGregor L et al. Role of glycoprotein IIa (beta_1 subunit of very late activation antigens) in platelet functions. Blood 1991; 78:2021–2026.

175. Staatz WD, Peter KJ, Santoro SA. Divalent cation-dependent structures in the platelet membrane GP Ia-IIa (VLA_2) complex. Biochem Biophys Res Commun 1990;168:107–114.

176. Staatz WD, Walsh JJ, Pexton T et al. The alpha_2beta_1 integrin cell surface collagen receptor binds to the alpha 1(I)-CB3 peptide of collagen. J Biol Chem 1990;265:4778–4781.

177. Kunicki TJ, Orchekowski R, Annis D et al. Variability of integrin alph_2 beta_1 activity on human platelets. Blood 1993;82:2693–2703.

178. Takada Y, Hemler ME. The primary structure of the VLA-2/collagen receptor alpha_2 subunit (platelet GP Ia): homology to other integrins and the presence of a possible collagen-binding domain. J Cell Biol 1987;109: 397–407.

179. Kamata T, Puzon W, Takada Y. Identification of putative ligand binding sites within the I domain of integrin alpha_2beta_1 (VLA-2, CD49b/CD29). J Biol Chem 1994;269:9659–9663.

180. Sixma JJ, van Zanten GH, Saelman EUM et al. Platelet adhesion to collagen. Thromb Haemost 1995;74:454–459.

181. Santoso S, Kalb R, Kiefel V et al. The human platelet alloantigen, Br^a and Br^b, are associated with a single amino acid polymorphism on glycoprotein Ia (integrin alpha_2 subunit). J Clin Invest 1993;92:2427–2432.

182. López JA. The platelet glycoprotein Ib-IX complex. Blood Coagul Fibrinolysis 1994;5:97–119.

183. Kobe B, Deisenhofer J. The leucine-rich repeat: a versatile binding motif. Trends Biochem Sci 1994;19:415–421.

184. Modderman PW, Admiraal LG, Sonnenberg A et al. Glycoproteins V and Ib-IX form a noncovalent complex in the platelet membrane. J Biol Chem 1992;267:364–369.

185. Madoff MA, Ebbe S, Baldini M. Sialic acid of human blood platelets. J Clin Invest 1964;43:870–877.

186. Li CQ, Dong J, Lanza F et al. Expression of platelet glycoprotein (GP) V in heterologous cells and evidence for its association with GP Ibá in forming a GP Ib-IX-V complex on the cell surface. J Biol Chem 1995;270:16302–16307.

187. Moroi M, Jung SM, Yoshida N. Genetic polymorphism of platelet glycoprotein Ib. Blood 1984;64:622–629.

188. Meyer M, Schellenberg I. Platelet membrane glycoprotein Ib: genetic polymorphism detected in the intact molecule and in proteolytic fragments. Thromb Res 1990;58:233–242.

189. López JA, Ludwig EH, McCarthy BJ. Polymorphism of human glycoprotein Ibá results from a variable number of tandem repeats of a 13-amino acid sequence in the mucin-like macroglycopeptide region. Structure/function implications. J Biol Chem 1992;267:10055–10061.

190. Ishida F, Furihata K, Ishida K et al. The largest variant of platelet glycoprotein Ibá has four tandem repeats of 13 amino acids in the macroglycopeptide region and a genetic linkage with methionine 145. Blood 1995;86: 1357–1360.

191. Kuijpers RW, Faber NM, Cuypers HT et al. NH2-terminal globular domain of human platelet glycoprotein Ibá has a methionine145/threonine145 amino acid polymorphism, which is associated with the HPA-2 (Ko) alloantigens. J Clin Invest 1992;89:381–384.

192. Solum NO, Hagen I, Filion-Myklebust C et al. Platelet glycocalicin: its membrane association and solubilization in aqueous media. Biochim Biophys Acta 1980;597:235–246.

193. Clemetson KJ. Glycoproteins of the platelet plasma membrane. In: George JN, Nurden AT, Phillips DR, eds. Platelet membrane glycoproteins. New York: Plenum Press, 1985; pp. 51–85.

194. Lopez JA, Chung DW, Fujikawa K et al. Cloning of the á chain of human platelet glycoprotein Ib: a transmembrane protein with homology to leucine-rich á2-glycoprotein. Proc Natl Acad Sci U S A 1987;84:5615–5619.

195. Lopez JA, Chung DW, Fujikawa K et al. The á and â chains of human platelet glycoprotein Ib are both transmembrane proteins containing a leucine-rich amino acid sequence. Proc Natl Acad Sci U S A 1988;85: 2135–2139.

196. Hickey MJ, Williams SA, Roth GJ. Human platelet glycoprotein IX: an adhesive prototype of leucine-rich glycoproteins with flank-center-flank structures. Proc Natl Acad Sci U S A 1989;86:6773–6777.

197. Hickey MJ, Hagen FS, Yagi M et al. Human platelet glycoprotein V: characterization of the polypeptide and the related Ib-V-IX receptor system of adhesive, leucine-rich glycoproteins. Proc Natl Acad Sci U S A 1993;90: 8327–8331.

198. Lanza F, Morales M, de La Salle C et al. Cloning and characterization of the gene encoding the human platelet glycoprotein V. A member of the leucine-rich glycoprotein family cleaved during thrombin-induced platelet activation. J Biol Chem 1993;268:20801–20807.

199. Wenger RH, Wicki AN, Kieffer N et al. The 5' flanking region and chromosomal localization of the gene encoding human platelet membrane glycoprotein Ibá. Gene 1989;85:517–524.

200. Budarf ML, Konkle BA, Ludlow LB et al. Identification of a individual with Bernard-Soulier syndrome and a deletion in the DiGeorge/Velo-

platelets showing no response to collagen fail to express surface glycoprotein IA. Nature 1985;318:470–472.

cardio-facial chromosomal region in 22q11.2. Hum Mol Genet 1995;4: 763–766.

201. Yagi M, Edelhoff S, Disteche CM et al. Human platelet glycoprotein V and IX: mapping of two leucine-rich glycoprotein genes to chromosome 3 and analysis of structures. Biochemistry 1995;34:16132–16137.

202. Yagi M, Edelhoff S, Disteche CM et al. Structural characterization and chromosomal location of the gene encoding human platelet glycoprotein Ibb. J Biol Chem 1994;269:17424–17427.

203. Hess D, Schaller J, Rickli EE et al. Identification of the disulphide bonds in human platelet glycocalicin. Eur J Biochem 1991;199:389–393.

204. Andrews RK, Fox JE. Identification of a region in the cytoplasmic domain of the platelet membrane glycoprotein Ib-IX complex that binds to purified actin-binding protein. J Biol Chem 1992;267:18605–18611.

205. Du X, Harris SJ, Tetaz TJ et al. Association of a phospholipase A₂ (14-3-3 protein) with the platelet glycoprotein Ib-IX complex. J Biol Chem 1994;269:18287–18290.

206. Du X, Fox JE, Pei S. Identification of a binding sequence for the 14-3-3 protein within the cytoplasmic domain of the adhesion receptor, platelet glycoprotein Ibâ. J Biol Chem 1996;271:7362–7367.

207. Fantl WJ, Muslin AJ, Kikuchi A et al. Activation of Raf-1 by 14-3-3 proteins. Nature 1994;371:612–614.

208. Freed E, Symons M, Macdonald SG et al. Binding of 14-3-3 proteins to the protein kinase Raf and effects on its activation. Science 1994;265:1713-1716.

209. Fu H, Xia K, Pallas DC et al. Interaction of the protein kinase Raf-1 with 14-3-3 proteins. Science 1994;266:126–129.

210. Kalomiris EL, Coller BS. Thiol-specific probes indicate that the â-chain of platelet glycoprotein Ib is a transmembrane protein with a reactive endofacial sulfhydryl group. Biochemistry 1985;24:5430–5436.

211. Muzbarek L, Laposata M. Glycoprotein Ib and glycoprotein IX in human platelets are acylated with palmitic acid through thioester linkages. J Biol Chem 1989;264:9716–9719.

212. Wardell MR, Reynolds CC, Berndt MC et al. Platelet glycoprotein Ibâ is phosphorylated on serine 166 by cyclic AMP-dependent protein kinase. J Biol Chem 1989;264:15656–15661.

213. Schick PK, Walker J. The acylation of megakaryocyte proteins-glycoprotein IX is primarily myristoylated while glycoprotein IB is palmitoylated. Blood 1996;87:1377–1384.

214. George JN, Nurden AT, Phillips DR. Molecular defects in interactions of platelets with the vessel wall. N Engl J Med 1984;311:1084–1098.

215. Weiss HJ, Tschopp TB, Baumgartner HR et al. Decreased adhesion of giant (Bernard-Soulier) platelets to subendothelium. Further implications on the role of the von Willebrand factor in hemostasis. Am J Med 1974;57:920–925.

216. Berndt MC, Chong BH, Bull HA et al. Molecular characterization of quinine/quinidine drug-dependent antibody platelet interaction using monoclonal antibodies. Blood 1985;66:1292–1301.

217. Turitto VT, Weiss HJ, Zimmerman TS et al. Factor VIII/von Willebrand factor in subendothelium mediates platelet adhesion. Blood 1985;65:823–831.

218. Kroll MH, Hellums JD, McIntire LV et al. Platelets and shear stress. Blood 1996;88:1525–1541.

219. Andrews RK, López JA, Berndt MC. Molecular mechanisms of platelet adhesion and activation. Int J Biochem Cell Biol 1997;29:91–105.

220. De Marco L, Shapiro SS. Properties of human asialo-Factor VIII. A ristocetin-independent platelet-aggregating agent. J Clin Invest 1981;68:321–328.

221. Loscalzo J, Inbal A, Handin RI. von Willebrand protein facilitates platelet incorporation into polymerizing fibrin. J Clin Invest 1986;78:1112–1119.

222. Parker RI, Gralnick HR. Fibrin monomer induces binding of endogenous platelet von Willebrand factor to the glycocalicin portion of platelet glycoprotein IB. Blood 1987;70:1589–1594.

223. Endenburg SC, Hantgan RR, Lindeboom-Blokzijl L et al. On the role of von Willebrand factor in promoting platelet adhesion to fibrin in flowing blood. Blood 1995;86:4158–4165.

224. Miller JL, Cunningham D, Lyle VA et al. Mutation in the gene encoding the á chain of platelet glycoprotein Ib in platelet-type von Willebrand disease. Proc Natl Acad Sci U S A 1991;88:4761–4765.

225. Russell SD, Roth GJ. Pseudo–von Willebrand disease: a mutation in the platelet glycoprotein Ibâ gene associated with a hyperactive surface receptor. Blood 1993;81:1787–1791.

226. Cooney KA, Ginsburg D. Comparative analysis of type 2b von Willebrand disease mutations: implications for the mechanism of von Willebrand factor binding to platelets. Blood 1996;87:2322–2328.

227. Wicki AN, Clemetson KJ. Structure and function of platelet membrane glycoproteins Ib and V. Effects of leukocyte elastase and other proteases on platelets response to von Willebrand factor and thrombin. Eur J Biochem 1985;153:1–11.

228. Vicente V, Houghten RA, Ruggeri ZM. Identification of a site in the á chain of platelet glycoprotein Ib that participates in von Willebrand factor binding. J Biol Chem 1990;265:274–280.

229. Dong JF, Li CQ, López JA. Tyrosine sulfation of the GP Ib-IX complex: identification of sulfated residues and effect on ligand binding. Biochemistry 1994;33:13946–13953.

230. Ward CM, Andrews RK, Smith AI et al. Mocarhagin, a novel cobra venom metalloproteinase, cleaves the platelet von Willebrand factor receptor glycoprotein Ibá. Identification of the sulfated tryosine/anionic sequence Tyr-276-Glu-282 of glycoprotein Ibá as a binding site for von Willebrand factor and á-thrombin. Biochemistry 1996;35:4929–4938.

231. Dong J, Hyun W, López JA. Aggregation of mammalian cells expressing the platelet glycoprotein (GP) Ib-IX complex and the requirement for tyrosine sulfation of GP Ibá. Blood 1995;86:4175–4183.

232. Miller JL, Lyle VA, Cunningham D. Mutation of leucine-57 to phenylalanine in a platelet glycoprotein Ibá leucine tandem repeat occurring in individuals with an autosomal dominant variant of Bernard-Soulier disease. Blood 1992;79:439–446.

233. Ware J, Russell SR, Marchese P et al. Point mutation in a leucine-rich repeat of platelet glycoprotein Ibá resulting in the Bernard-Soulier syndrome. J Clin Invest 1993;92:1213–1220.

234. Pincus MR, Dykes DC, Carty RP et al. Conformational energy analysis of the substitution of Val for Gly 233 in a functional region of platelet GP Ibá in platelet-type von Willebrand disease. Biochim Biophys Acta 1991;1097:133–139.

235. Fujimura Y, Titani K, Holland LZ et al. A heparin-binding domain of human von Willebrand factor. Characterization and localization to a tryptic fragment extending from amino acid residue Val-449 to Lys-728. J Biol Chem 1987;262:1734–1739.

236. Andrews RK, Gorman JJ, Booth WJ et al. Crosslinking of a monomeric 39/34-kDa dispase fragment of von Willebrand factor (Leu-480/Val-481-Gly-718) to the N-terminal region of the á-chain of membrane glycoprotein Ib on intact platelets with bis(sulfosuccinimidyl) suberate. Biochemistry 1989;28:8326–8336.

237. Berndt MC, Ward CM, Booth WJ et al. Identification of aspartic acid 514 through glutamic acid 542 as a glycoprotein Ib-IX complex receptor recognition sequence in von Willebrand factor. Mechanism of modulation of von Willebrand factor by ristocetin and botrocetin. Biochemistry 1992;31:11144–11151.

238. Kroll MH, Harris TS, Moake JL et al. von Willebrand factor binding to platelet GP Ib initiates signals for platelet activation. J Clin Invest 1991;88:1568–1573.

239. Chow TW, Hellums JD, Moake JL et al. Shear stress-induced von Willebrand factor binding to platelet glycoprotein Ib initiates calcium influx associated with aggregation. Blood 1992;80:113–120.

240. Ikeda Y, Handa M, Kamata T et al. Transmembrane calcium influx associated with von Willebrand factor binding to GP Ib in the initiation of shear-induced platelet aggregation. Thromb Haemost 1993;69:496–502.

241. Jackson SP, Schoenwaelder SM, Yuan Y et al. Adhesion receptor activation of phosphatidylinositol 3-kinase. von Willebrand factor stimulates the cytoskeletal association and activation of phosphatidylinositol 3-kinase and pp⁶⁰ᶜ⁻ˢʳᶜ in human platelets. J Biol Chem 1994;269:27093–27099.

242. Aitken A. 14-3-3 proteins on the MAP. Trends Biochem Sci 1995;20:95–97.

243. Harmon JT, Jamieson GA. The glycocalicin portion of platelet glycoprotein Ib expresses both high and moderate affinity receptor sites for thrombin. A soluble radioreceptor assay for the interaction of thrombin with platelets. J Biol Chem 1986;261:13224–13229.

244. Katagiri Y, Hayashi Y, Yamamoto K et al. Localization of von Willebrand factor and thrombin-interactive domains on human platelet glycoprotein Ib. Thromb Haemost 1990;63:122–126.

245. McKeown LP, Williams SB, Hansmann KE et al. Glycoprotein Ibá peptides inhibit thrombin and SFLLRN-induced platelet aggregation. J Lab Clin Med 1996;128:492–494.

246. Marchese P, Murata M, Mazzucato M et al. Identification of three-tyrosine residues of glycoprotein Ibá with distinct roles in von Willebrand factor and á-thrombin binding. J Biol Chem 1995;270:9571–9578.

247. Dong JF, Sae-Tung G, López JA. Role of glycoprotein V in the formation of the platelet high affinity thrombin-binding site. Blood 1997;89:4355–4363.

248. Greco NJ, Tandon NN, Jones GD et al. Contribution of glycoprotein Ib and the seven transmembrane domain receptor to increases in platelet cytoplasmic [Ca²⁺] induced by á-thrombin. Biochemistry 1996;35:906–914.

249. Greco NJ, Jones GD, Tandon NN et al. Differentiation of the two forms of GP Ib functioning as receptors for á-thrombin and von Willebrand factor: Ca²⁺ responses of protease-treated human platelets activated with á-thrombin and the tethered ligand peptide. Biochemistry 1996;35:915–921.

250. Andrews RK, Fox JE. Interaction of purified actin-binding protein with the platelet membrane glycoprotein Ib-IX complex. J Biol Chem 1991;266:7144–7147.

251. Ezzell RM, Kenney DM, Egan S et al. Localization of the domain of actin-binding protein that binds to membrane glycoprotein Ib and actin in human platelets. J Biol Chem 1988;263:13303–13309.

252. Fox JEB. The platelet cytoskeleton. In: Verstraete M, Vermylen J, Lijnen HR, Arnout J, eds. Thrombosis and haemostasis. Leuven, Belgium: Leuven University Press, 1987; pp. 175–225.

253. George JN, Torres MM. Thrombin decreases von Willebrand factor binding to platelet glycoprotein Ib. Blood 1988;71:1253–1259.

254. Coller BS. Inhibition of von Willebrand factor–dependent platelet function

by increased platelet cyclic AMP and its prevention by cytoskeleton-disrupting agents. Blood 1981;57:846-855.

255. Fox JE, Berndt MC. Cyclic AMP–dependent phosphorylation of glycoprotein Ib inhibits collagen-induced polymerization of actin in platelets. J Biol Chem 1989;264:9520–9526.

256. McPherson J, Zucker MB, Mauss EA et al. The effect of agonists and antagonists of platelet aggregation on von Willebrand factor–mediated platelet agglutination. Thromb Haemost 1991;65:573–577.

257. Michelson AD, Ellis PA, Barnard MR et al. Downregulation of the platelet surface glycoprotein Ib-IX complex in whole blood stimulated by thrombin, adenosine diphosphate, or an *in vivo* wound. Blood 1991;77:770–779.

258. Kovacsovics TJ, Hartwig JH. Thrombin-induced GP Ib-IX centralization on the platelet surface requires actin assembly and myosin II activation. Blood 1996;87:618–629.

259. Cramer EM, Lu H, Caen JP et al. Differential redistribution of platelet glycoproteins Ib and IIb-IIIa after plasmin stimulation. Blood 1991;77:694–699.

260. White JG, Krumwiede MD, Cocking-Johnson D et al. Retention of glycoprotein Ib-IX receptors on external surfaces of thrombin-activated platelets in suspension. Blood 1995;86:3468–3478.

261. Lozano M, Escolar G, White JG et al. Redistribution of membrane glycoproteins in platelet activation under flow conditions. Blood Coagul Fibrinolysis 1996;7:214–217.

262. Kansas GS. Selectins and their ligands: current concepts and controversies. Blood 1996;88:3259–3287.

263. Gotsch U, Jager U, Dominis M et al. Expression of P-selectin on endothelial cells is upregulated by LPS and TNF-á *in vivo*. Cell Adhes Commun 1994;2:7–14.

264. Bischoff J, Brasel C. Regulation of P-selectin by tumor necrosis factor-á. Biochem Biophys Res Commun 1995;210:174–180.

265. Weller A, Isenmann S, Vestweber D. Cloning of the mouse endothelial selectins. Expression of both E- and P-selectin is inducible by tumor necrosis factor á. J Biol Chem 1992;267:15176–15183.

266. Mayadas TN, Johnson RC, Rayburn H et al. Leukocyte rolling and extravasation are severely compromised in P selectin–deficient mice. Cell 1993;74:541–554.

267. Diacovo TG, Roth SJ, Buccola JM et al. Neutrophil rolling, arrest, and transmigration across activated, surface-adherent platelets via sequential action of P-selection and the beta 2-integrin CD11b/CD18. Blood 1996;88:146–157.

268. Celi A, Pellegrini G, Lorenzet R et al. P-selectin induces the expression of tissue factor on monocytes. Proc Natl Acad Sci U S A 1994;91:8767–8771.

269. Johnston GI, Bliss GA, Newman PJ et al. Structure of the human gene encoding granule membrane protein-140, a member of the selectin family of adhesion receptors for leukocytes. J Biol Chem 1990;265:21381–21385.

270. Johnston GI, Cook RG, McEver RP. Cloning of GMP-140, a granule membrane protein of platelets and endothelium: sequence similarity to proteins involved in cell adhesion and inflammation. Cell 1989;56:1033–1044.

271. Bottenus RE, Ichinose A, Davie EW. Nucleotide sequence of the gene for the â subunit of human factor VIII. Biochemistry 1990;29:11195–11209.

272. Disdier M, Morrissey JH, Fugate RD et al. Cytoplasmic domain of P-selectin (CD62) contains the signal for sorting into the regulated secretory pathway. Molec Biol Cell 1992;3:309–321.

273. Setiadi H, Disdier M, Green SA et al. Residues throughout the cytoplasmic domain affect the internalization efficiency of P-selectin. J Biol Chem 1995;270:26818–26826.

274. Green SA, Setiadi H, McEver RP et al. The cytoplasmic domain of P-selectin contains a sorting determinant that mediates rapid degradation in lysosomes. J Cell Biol 1994;124:435–448.

275. Fujimoto T, McEver RP. The cytoplasmic domain of P-selectin is phosphorylated on serine and threonine residues. Blood 1993;82:1758–1766.

276. Modderman PW, von dem Borne AE, Sonnenberg A. Tyrosine phosphorylation of P-selectin in intact platelets and in a disulphide-linked complex with immunoprecipitated pp60c-src. Biochem J 1994;299:613-621.

277. Crovello CS, Furie BC, Furie B. Histidine phosphorylation of P-selectin upon stimulation of human platelets: a novel pathway for activation-dependent signal transduction. Cell 1995;82:279–286.

278. Fujimoto T, Stroud E, Whatley RE et al. P-selectin is acylated with palmitic acid and stearic acid at cysteine 766 through a thioester linkage. J Biol Chem 1993;268:11394–11400.

279. Rosen SD, Bertozzi CR. The selectins and their ligands. Curr Opin Cell Biol 1994;6:663–673.

280. Natsuka S, Gersten KM, Zenita K et al. Molecular cloning of a cDNA encoding a novel human leukocyte á-1,3,-fucosyltransferase capable of synthesizing the sialy Lewis x determinant. J Biol Chem 1994;269:16789–16794.

281. Maly P, Thall AD, Petryniak B et al. The á(1, 3) fucosyltrasnferase Fuc-TVII controls leukocyte trafficking through an essential role in L-, E-, and P-selectin ligand biosynthesis. Cell 1996;86:643–653.

282. Pouyani T, Seed B. PSGL-1 recognition of P-selectin is controlled by a tyrosine sulfation consensus at the PSGL-1 aminoterminus. Cell 1995;83:333–343.

283. Sako D, Comess KM, Barone KM et al. A sulfated peptide segment at the aminoterminus of PSGL-1 is critical for P-selectin binding. Cell 1995;83:323–331.

284. Wilkins PP, Moore KL, McEver RP, Cummings RD. Tyrosine sulfation of P-selectin glycoprotein ligand-1 is required for high affinity binding to P-selectin. J Biol Chem 1995;270:22677–22680.

285. De Luca M, Dunlop LC, Andrews RK et al. A novel cobra venom metalloproteinase, mocarhagin, cleaves a 10-amino acid peptide from the mature N terminus of P-selectin glycoprotein ligand receptor, PSGL-1, and abolishes P-selectin binding. J Biol Chem 1995;270:26734–26737.

286. Newman PJ. The biology of PECAM. J Clin Invest 1997;99:3–8.

287. Newman PJ, Berndt NC, Gorski J et al. PECAM-1 (CD-31) cloning and relation to adhesion molecules of the immunoglobulin gene superfamily. Science 1990;247:1219–1222.

288. Diavco TG, deFougerolles AR, Bainton DF et al. A functional integrin ligand on the surface of platelets: intercellular adhesion molecule-2. J Clin Invest 1994;94:1242–1251.

289. McGregor JL, Catimel B, Parmentier S et al. Rapid purification and partial characterization of human platelet glycoprotein IIIb. Interaction with thrombospondin and its role in platelet aggregation. J Biol Chem 1989;264:501–506.

290. Tandon NN, Lipski RH, Burgess WH et al. Isolation and characterization of platelet glycoprotein IV (CD36). J Biol Chem 1989;264:7570–7575.

291. Jamieson GA, Okumura T, Fishback B et al. Platelet membrane glycoproteins in thrombasthenia, Bernard Soulier syndrome, and storage pool disease. J Lab Clin Med 1979;93:652–660.

292. Eche N, Sie P, Caranobe C et al. Platelets in myeloproliferative disorders. III. Glycoprotein profile in relation to platelet function and platelet density. Scand J Haematol 1981;26:123–129.

293. Yamamoto N, Ikeda H, Tandon NN et al. A platelet membrane glycoprotein (GP) deficiency in healthy blood donors: Naka- platelets lack detectable GP IV (CD36). Blood 1990;76:1698–1703.

294. Frazier WA. Thrombospondins. Curr Opin Cell Biol 1991;3:792–799.

295. Asch AS, Liu I, Briccetti FM et al. Analysis of CD36 binding domains: ligand specificity controlled by dephosphorylation of an ectodomain. Science 1993;262:1436–1440.

296. Diaz-Ricart M, Tandon NN, Gomez-Ortiz G et al. Antibodies to CD36 (GP IV) inhibit platelet adhesion to subendothelial surfaces under flow conditions. Arterioscler Thromb Vasc Biol 1996;16:883–888.

297. Howard RJ, Gilladoga AD. Molecular studies related to the pathogenesis of cerebral malaria. Blood 1989;74:2603–2618.

298. Oquendo P, Hundt E, Lawler J et al. CD36 directly mediates cytoadherence of *Plasmodium falciparum*–parasitized erythrocytes. Cell 1989;58:95–101.

299. Aiken ML, Ginsberg MH, Byers-Ward V et al. Effect of OKM5, a monoclonal antibody to GP IV, on platelet aggregation and thrombospondin surface expression. Blood 1990;76:2501–2509.

300. Moroi M, Jung SM, Shinmyozu K et al. Analysis of platelet adhesion to a collagen-coated surface under flow conditions: the involvement of GP VI in platelet adhesion. Blood 1996;88:2081–2092.

301. Ichinohe T, Takayama H, Ezumi Y et al. Collagen-stimulated activation of Syk but not c-Src is severely compromised in human platelets lacking membrane glycoprotein VI. J Biol Chem 1997;272:63–68.

302. Roberts JP, Rogers S, Drury J et al. Platelet activation induced by a murine monoclonal antibody directed against a novel tetraspan antigen. Br J Haematol 1995;89:853–860.

303. Fitter S, Tetaz TJ, Berndt MC et al. Molecular cloning of cDNA encoding a novel platelet-endothelial cell tetra-span antigen, PETA-3. Blood 1995;86:1348–1355.

304. Wright MD, Tomlinson MG. The ins and outs of the transmembrane 4 superfamily. Immunol Today 1994;15:588–594.

305. Metzelaar MJ, Heijnen HFG, Sixma JJ et al. Identification of a 33-Kd protein associated with the alpha-granule membrane (GMP-33) that is expressed on the surface of activated platelets. Blood 1992;79:372–379.

306. Gerrard JM, Lint D, Sims PJ et al. Identification of a platelet dense granule membrane protein that is deficient in a individual with the Hermansky-Pudlak syndrome. Blood 1991;77:101–102.

307. Nieuwenhuis KH, van Oosterhout JJP, Rozemuller EIF et al. Studies with a monoclonal antibody against activated platelets: evidence that a secreted 53,000–molecular weight lysosome-like granule protein is exposed on the surface of activated platelets in the circulation. Blood 1987;70:838–845.

308. Metzelaar MJ, Wijngaard PJ, Peters PJ et al. CD63 Antigen. A novel lysosomal membrane glycoprotein cloned by a screening procedure for intracellular antigens in eukaryotic cells. J Biol Chem 1991;266:3239–3245.

309. Febbraio M, Silverstein RL. Identification and characterization of LAMP-1 as an activation dependent platelet surface glycoprotein. J Biol Chem 1990;265:18531–18537.

310. Silverstein RL, Febbraio M. Identification of lysosome-associated protein-2 as an activation dependent platelet surface glycoprotein. Blood 1992;80:1470–1475.

311. Hayward CPM, Smith JW, Horsewood P et al. P155, a multimeric platelet protein that is expressed on activated platelets. J Biol Chem 1991;266:7114–7120.

312. Hayward CP, Furmaniak-Kazmierczak E, Cieutat AM et al. Factor V is

complexed with multimerin in resting platelet lysates and colocalizes with multimerin in platelet alpha granules. J Biol Chem 1995;270:19217–19224.

313. Hayward CP, Hassell JA, Denomme GA et al. The cDNA sequence of human endothelial cell multimerin. A unique protein with RGDS, coiled-coil, and epidermal growth factor–like domains and a carboxylterminus similar to the globular domain of complement C1q and collagens type VIII and X. J Biol Chem 1995;270:18246–18251.

314. McCrae KR, Shattil SJ, Cines DB. Platelet activation induces increased Fc gamma receptor expression. J Immunol 1990;144:3920–3927.

315. Petroni KL, Shen L, Guyre PM. Modulation of human polymorphonuclear leukocyte IgG Fc receptor and receptor mediated function by interferon gamma and glucocorticoids. J Immunol 1988;140:3467–3472.

316. Rappaport EF, Cassel DL, Walterhouse DO et al. A soluble form of the human Fc receptor Fc gamma RIIA: cloning, transcript analysis and detection. Exp Hematol 1993;21:689–696.

317. Tate BJ, Witort E, McKenzie IFC et al. Expression of the high responder/nonresponder human Fc gamma RII: analysis by PCR and transfection into FcR-COS cells. Immunol Cell Biol 1992;70:79–87.

318. Bachelot R, Saffroy R, Gandrille S et al. Role of Fc$_{gamma}$RIIA gene polymorphism in human platelet activation by monoclonal antibodies. Thromb Haemost 1995;74:1557–1563.

319. Hildreth JE, Derr D, Azorsa DO. Characterization of a novel self-associating Mr40,000 platelet glycoprotein. Blood 1991;77:121–132.

320. Stricker RB, Reyes PT, Corash L et al. Evidence that a 210,000 molecular weight glycoprotein (GP210) serves as a platelet Fc receptor. J Clin Invest 1987;79:1589–1594.

321. Sims PJ, Wiedmer T. The response of human platelets to activated components of the complement system. Immunol Today 1991;12:338–342.

322. Peerschke EIB, Ghebrehiwet B. Platelet membrane receptors for the complement component C1q. Semin Hematol 1994;31:320–328.

323. Peerschke EIB, Reid KBM, Ghebrehiwet B. Identification of a novel 33kDa C1q binding site on human platelets. J Immunol 1994;152:5896–5901.

324. Eggleton P, Lieu TS, Zappi EG et al. Calreticulin is released from activated neutrophils and binds to C1q and mannan binding protein. Clin Immunol Immunopathol 1994;72:405–409.

325. Peerschke EIB, Reid KBM, Ghebrehiwet B. Platelet activation by C1q results in the induction of alpha$_{IIB}$/beta$_3$ integrins (GP IIb-IIIa) and the expression of P-selectin and procoagulant activity. J Exp Med 1993;178:579–587.

326. Ghebrehiwet B, Lim BL, Peerschke EIB et al. Isolation, cDNA cloning, and overexpression of a 33-kD cell surface glycoprotein that binds to the globular "heads" of C1q. J Exp Med 1994;179:1809–1821.

327. Joseph K, Ghebrehiwet B, Peerschke EIB et al. Identification of the zinc-dependent endothelial cell binding protein for high molecular weight kininogen and factor XII: identification with the receptor that binds to the globular "heads" of C1q (gC1qR). Proc Natl Acad Sci U S A 1996;93:8552–8557.

328. Yu GH, Holers VM, Seya T et al. Identification of a third component of complement-binding glycoprotein of human platelets. J Clin Invest 1986;78:494–501.

329. Roitt I. Essential immunology. 7th ed. Oxford: Blackwell Scientific, 1991; pp. 115–116.

330. Slupsky JR, Seehafer JG, Tang S et al. Evidence that monoclonal antibodies against CD9 antigen induce specific association between CD9 and the platelet glycoprotein IIb-IIIa complex. J Biol Chem 1989;264:12289–12293.

331. Testi R, Pucinelli F, Frati L et al. CD69 is expressed on platelets and mediates platelet activation and aggregation. J Exp Med 1990;172:701–707.

332. Scott JL, Dunn SM, Jin B et al. Characterization of a novel membrane glycoprotein involved in platelet activation. J Biol Chem 1989;264:13475–13482.

333. Zwaal RFA. Membrane and lipid involvement in blood coagulation. Biochim Biophys Acta 1978;515:163–205.

334. Mann KG, Nesheim ME, Church WR et al. Surface-dependent reactions of the vitamin K-dependent enzyme complexes. Blood 1990;76:1–16.

335. Bevers EM, Rosing J, Zwaal RFA. Platelets and coagulation. In: MacIntyre DE, Gordon JI, eds. Platelets in biology and pathology III. Amsterdam: Elsevier Science, 1987; pp. 127–160.

336. Van Deenen LLM. Topology and dynamics of phospholipids in membranes. FEBS Lett 1981;123:3–15.

337. Solum NO, Olsen TM, Gogstad GO et al. Demonstration of a new glycoprotein Ib-related component in platelet extracts prepared in the presence of leupeptin. Biochim Biophys Acta 1983;729:53–61.

338. Okita JR, Pidard D, Newman PJ et al. On the association of glycoprotein Ib and actin-binding protein in human platelets. J Cell Biol 1985;100:317–321.

339. Kane WH, Linhout MJ, Jackson CM et al. Factor Va-dependent binding of Factor Xa to human platelets. J Biol Chem 1980;255:1170–1174.

340. Tracy PB, Nesheim ME, Mann KG. Coordinate binding of factor Va and factor Xa to the unstimulated platelet. J Biol Chem 1981;256:743–751.

341. Scandura JM, Ahmad SS, Walsh PN. A binding site expressed on the surface of activated human platelets is shared by Factor X and prothrombin. Biochemistry 1996;35:8890–8902.

342. Scandura JM, Walsh PN. Factor X bound to the surface of activated human platelets is preferentially activated by platelet bound Factor IX a. Biochemistry 1996;35:8903–8913.

343. Nesheim ME, Pittman DD, Wang JH et al. The binding of $^{35}$S-labeled recombinant factor VIII to activated and unactivated human platelets. J Biol Chem 1988;263:16467–16470.

344. Ahmad SS, Rawala–Sheikh R, Walsh PN. Comparative interactions of factor IX and factor IXa with human platelets. J Biol Chem 1989;264:3244–3251.

345. Walsh PN, Baglia FA, Jameson BA. Factor XI and platelets. Activation and regulation. Thromb Haemost 1993;70:75–79.

346. Meloni FJ, Gustafson EJ, Schmaier AH. High molecular weight kininogen binds to platelets by its heavy and light chains and when bound has altered susceptibility to kallikrein cleavage. Blood 1992;79:1233–1244.

347. Harris KW, Esmon CT. Protein S is required for bovine platelets to support activated protein C binding and activity. J Biol Chem 1985;260:2007–2010.

348. Ouimet H, Freedman JE, Loscalzo J. Kinetics and mechanism of platelet-surface plasminogen activity by tissue-type plasminogen activator. Biochem 1994;33:2970–2976.

349. Hajjar KA. Cellular receptors in the regulation of plasmin generation. Thromb Haemost 1995;74:294–301.

350. Mills LA, Ginsberg MH, Plow EF. Plasminogen interacts with human platelets through two distinct mechanisms. J Clin Invest 1986;77:2001–2009.

351. Wolf P. The nature and significance of platelet products in human plasma. Br J Haematol 1967;13:269–288.

352. Miyazaki Y, Nomura S, Miyake T et al. High shear-stress can initiate both platelet aggregation and shedding of procoagulant containing microparticles. Blood 1996;88:3456–3464.

353. George JN, Thoi LL, McManus LM et al. Isolation of human platelet membrane microparticles from plasma and serum. Blood 1982;60:834–840.

354. Wiedmer T, Sims PJ. Participation of protein kinase in complement C5b-9-induced shedding of platelet plasma membrane vesicles. Blood 1991;78:2880–2886.

355. Weiss HJ. Scott syndrome; a disorder of platelet coagulant activity. Semin Hematol 1994;31:312–319.

356. Fox JEB, Boyles JK. The membrane skeleton. A distinct structure that regulates the function of cells. Bioessays 1988;8:14–18.

357. George JN, Pickett EB, Saucerman S et al. Platelet surface glycoproteins. Studies on resting and activated platelets and platelet membrane microparticles in normal subjects, and observations in individuals during adult respiratory distress syndrome and cardiac surgery. J Clin Invest 1986;78:340–348.

358. Gilbert GE, Sims PJ, Wiedmer T et al. Platelet-derived microparticles express high affinity receptors for Factor VIII. J Biol Chem 1991;266:17261–17268.

359. Siljander P, Carpen O, Lassila R. Platelet derived microparticles associate with fibrin during thrombosis. Blood 1996;87:4651–4663.

360. Peerschke EIB. Platelet membrane glycoproteins: functional characterization and clinical applications. Am J Clin Pathol 1992;98:455–463.

361. Coller BS, Anderson K, Weisman HF. New antiplatelet agents: platelet GP IIb-IIIa antagonists. Thromb Haemost 1995;74:302–308.

# CHAPTER 12

# MECHANISMS OF PLATELET ACTIVATION

## Michael H. Kroll and Richard Sullivan

## INTRODUCTION

Platelets are necessary for normal hemostasis and are vital participants in the development of pathologic thromboses, particularly in the arterial circulation where flow-associated, elevated wall shear stresses prevent early fibrin deposition. "Primary hemostasis" is defined as the platelet/blood vessel interactions that initiate physiologic thrombus formation. When primary hemostasis is triggered by a pathologic stimulus (such as a ruptured atherosclerotic plaque) platelet adhesion coupled to platelet activation leads to the development of a self-amplifying series of cellular responses that result in the formation of a platelet plug (the so-called "white thrombus"), vasoocclusion, and ischemia or infarction (1). This pathogenetic schema is clearly established for coronary, cerebral, and peripheral arterial diseases (2).

Individual platelets circulate in an inactivated state through a complex vascular system lined by a monolayer of endothelial cells. In response to vessel wall injury, alterations in blood flow, or chemical stimuli, platelets manifest a triad of linked functional responses: adhesion, secretion, and aggregation (Fig. 12.1). These functional responses occur via a series of carefully coordinated signals that convert extracellular stimuli into intracellular chemical messengers that direct specific enzymatic reactions.

The state of platelet activation is regulated dynamically by the actions of a diverse array of excitatory and inhibitory extracellular stimuli. Platelets are equipped with specific plasma membrane receptors (see Chapter 11) that organize these various stimuli and transform them into biologic responses (3). This transformation occurs to a large extent through classical mechanisms of transmembranous, stimulus-response coupling that results in the generation of specific, intracellular, second messengers. The primary activation pathway of platelets employs two second messengers derived from enzymatic hydrolysis of inositol phospholipids: inositol 1,4,5-trisphosphate ($IP_3$) and $sn$-1,2-diacylglycerol (DG). The major inhibitory signaling pathways in platelets employ the cyclic nucleotides, adenosine 3'5'-cyclic monophosphate (cAMP) and guanosine 3'5'-cyclic monophosphate (cGMP), as the second messenger. The generation of $IP_3$, DG, and cAMP is triggered by specific extracellular molecules occupying cell surface receptors, and these second messengers are generated intracellularly by the activation of membrane-associated enzymes through receptor-linked changes of membrane-associated, heterotrimeric, guanosine triphosphate (GTP)–binding regulatory proteins (G proteins). In each case, the activated signal-generating enzyme converts highly phosphorylated precursors into intracellular second messengers: phospholipase C (PLC) cleaves membrane phosphatidylinositol 4,5-bisphosphate ($PIP_2$) into $IP_3$ and DG, and adenylyl or guanylyl cyclase converts adenosine or guanosine triphosphate (ATP or GTP) into cAMP or cGMP. The second messengers formed by these reactions cause important intracellular responses by inducing conformational changes in target proteins either directly or indirectly by the activation of protein

## Platelet Responses

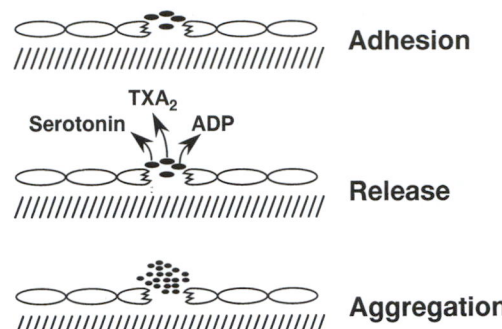

**FIGURE 12.1.** Platelet function comprises a triad of responses: adhesion, release (or secretion), and aggregation. These responses arise from the activation of carefully regulated transmembranous signal pathways that ultimately result in the generation of a platelet thrombus. EC, endothelial cell; SE, subendothelium; TXA$_2$, thromboxane A$_2$; ADP, adenosine diphosphate.

kinases: IP$_3$ releases calcium (Ca$^{2+}$), which causes activation of various Ca$^{2+}$-dependent enzymes, DG causes activation of protein kinase C; and cAMP and cGMP cause activation of cAMP- and cGMP-dependent protein kinases.

In addition to these second messenger–mediated signal pathways, tertiary biochemical responses branching from the major activation pathways are initiated intracellularly, and these responses fine-tune, dampen, or amplify the signals caused by classical second messengers. Thus, a network of carefully regulated reactions governs physiologic and pathophysiologic platelet function. Elucidation of these complex reactions is not yet complete. Nonetheless, knowledge about the fundamental mechanisms of platelet activation has contributed substantially to an understanding of human biology, both because the platelet has often served as the cell-type from which basic and general principles of cell signaling have been developed and because advances in understanding basic mechanisms of platelet activation have often led to clinical advances in the prevention and treatment of atherothrombotic diseases. Despite being "terminally" differentiated, platelets have taught us much about the molecular basis of highly conserved and ubiquitous systems for signaling, as well as their functional significance in adhesion, cohesion (aggregation), secretion, and even cell growth. Furthermore, recent characterizations of unique aspects of platelet activation hold out the promise of novel means by which the prevention and treatment of platelet-dependent thrombosis can be accomplished without imposing major defects in the hemostatic system (4).

# LIGAND-RECEPTOR INTERACTIONS

Physiologic platelet activation or inhibition is initiated when an extracellular stimulus interacts with the platelet surface. This interaction often involves a ligand-receptor coupling wherein extracellular molecules bind to one or more specific membrane receptors. There is great diversity in the structure and sites of production of the different extracellular stimuli that regulate platelet function. Included are plasma constituents such as proteases (thrombin, plasmin) and catecholamines; vascular wall products such as prostacyclin (PGI$_2$) and collagen; platelet products, including adenosine diphosphate (ADP) and serotonin; molecules potentially derived from multiple blood cell and vascular sources such as ADP, platelet activating factor (PAF), von Willebrand factor (vWf), the prostaglandin endoperoxides PGG$_2$/PGH$_2$, and thromboxane A$_2$ (TXA$_2$); and components of the extracellular matrix such as collagen.

Soluble extracellular signals that elicit platelet responses through receptor-mediated events are grouped as follows: (a) "strong agonists" (thrombin, prostaglandin endoperoxides, TXA$_2$, collagen, platelet activating factor, and vasopressin) that cause platelet aggregation that does not depend on secretion and that is not inhibited by blocking platelet PGG$_2$/PGH$_2$ synthase ("cyclooxygenase"); (b) "weak agonists" (ADP, epinephrine, and serotonin) that depend on secretion to effect a full aggregation response; and (c) antagonists (PGI$_2$ and PGD$_2$) that inhibit platelet responses to many different stimuli by causing elevations of platelet cytosolic cAMP. "Weak agonists" cause aggregation that may demonstrate a "second wave" blocked by inhibitors of cyclooxygenase (e.g., aspirin).

The structures of the platelet receptors for many of these ligands have been identified, but there are large gaps in current knowledge about the molecular mechanisms by which ligand binding initiates receptor signaling across the plasma membrane (Table 12.1) (4–14). Analyses of receptor structure demonstrate that a ligand may have more than one receptor and that receptor heterogeneity may be an important mechanism by which an extracellular stimulus is directed to the appropriate physiologic response. Receptor heterogeneity also occurs between cell-types, for example, the platelet and the vascular smooth muscle cell TXA$_2$ receptors (5), thus providing additional regulation of the organization of an extracellular stimulus into an appropriate multicellular response.

## THROMBIN

The "strong agonist" thrombin is an important extracellular stimulus for platelet activation *in vivo* (15). There

**TABLE 12.1.**  Activating Ligand-Receptor Interactions

| Receptor | Structure | Binding | G Protein | Effector | Other |
|---|---|---|---|---|---|
| Thrombin 1. High affinity | ?GP Ib-IX-V | $K_d \approx 300$ pM $B_{max} \approx 50$–$100$ (sites/platelet) | ? | $Ca^{2+}$ influx pathway? | May cooperate with moderate affinity receptor |
| 2. Moderate affinity | 425 aa 7 transmembrane domains | $K_d \approx 11$ nM $B_{max} \approx 1700$ | $G_p$, $G_Q$: $G_i$ | PLC Down-regulate AC | Unique proteolytic mechanism creates "tethered ligand peptide" |
| 3. Low affinity | ? | $K_d \approx 2.9$ µM $B_{max} \approx 590,000$ | ? | ? | Probably not a functional receptor |
| $TXA_2$/$PGG_i$/ $PGH_i$ 1. High affinity | ? | $K_d \approx 234$ pM $B_{max} \approx 670$ | ? | direct ↑ $[Ca^{2+}]i$ | May "prime" platelets |
| 2. Moderate affinity | 343 aa 7 transmembrane domains | $K_d \approx 2$ nM $B_{max} \approx 670$ | $G_q$: pertusis toxin–insensitive | PLC | Primary functional receptor |
| PAF | 342 aa $M_r$ 39,000 7 transmembrane domains | $K_d \approx 100$–$500$ pM $B_{max} \approx 1400$ | $G_p$: pertusis toxin–sensitive | PLC | Wide range of published $K_d$ and $B_{max}$ data |
| Collagen 1. GP Ia-IIa (Integrin $\alpha_2\beta_1$) | $\alpha_2$ $M_r$ 167,000 $\beta_2$ $M_r$ 130,000 | $K_d \approx 500$ pM $B_{max} \approx 1400$ | ? | Uncertain: with $\geq 10$ µg/ml type I collage, PLC is directly activated; at lower concentrations, $PLA_2$ is first activated | $Mg^{2+}$-dependent binding that is inhibited by $Ca^{2+}$ |
| 2. GP IV (CD36) | $M_r$ 85,000–95,000 (highly glycosylated) | $K_d \approx 340$ pM $B_{max} \approx 12,000$ ? | ? | | Platelet thrombospondin receptor |
| 3. GP VI | $M_r$ 62,000 | | ? | | Based on clinical evidence |
| Vasopressin $V_1$ | $M_r$ 125,000 7 transmembrane domains | $K_d \approx 1$ nM $B_{max} \approx 95$ | $G_p$: pertussis toxin–sensitive | PLC | Physiologic relevance is questionable |
| Epinephrine | 450 AA $M_r$ 64,000 7 transmembrane domains | $K_d \approx 2.5$ nM $B_{max} \approx 300$ | $G_i$-pertussis toxin–sensitive | Down-regulate AC | May be coupled to $PLA_2$ through an $Na^+$/$H^+$ exchange and GP IIb-IIIa dependent mechanism |
| ADP 1. "Aggregin" | $M_r$ 100,000 | ? | No | ? | ADP binding induces a $Ca^{2+}$-dependent cleavage that causes shape change and activates GP IIb-IIIa |
| 2. GP IIIbα | $M_r$ 125,000 | $K_d \approx 30$ nM $B_{max} \approx 280,000$ | ? | ? | May be directly coupled to $PLA_2$ |
| 3. $P_{2t}$ | 7 transmembrane domains | $K_d \approx 5$ nM $B_{max} \approx 600$ | G protein (?$G_i$) | PLC Down-regulate AC | |
| Serotonin ($S_2$) | 475 aa | $K_d \approx 2$ nM $B_{max}$ 6–60 fmol per mg membrane protein | $G_p$, $G_i$: pertussin toxin–sensitive | PLC Down-regulate AC | $K_d$ determined by binding to COS cells expressing cloned human $S_2$ receptor; $B_{max}$ measurements in intact platelets complicated by active uptake of ligand |

PLC, phospholipase C; PLA$_2$, phospholipase A$_2$; AC, adenylyl cyclase; aa, amino acid.

are three classes of binding sites having affinities designated as low (590,000 sites/platelet; $K_d \sim 2900$ nM), moderate (1700 sites/platelet; $K_d \sim 11$ nM), and high (50 sites/platelet; $K_d \sim 0.3$ nM). The relationship between thrombin's binding and proteolytic activities was clarified by the cDNA cloning and expression of a functional human platelet thrombin receptor (16). The binding characteristics of this receptor correspond with the pre-

# Thrombin Receptor Schematic

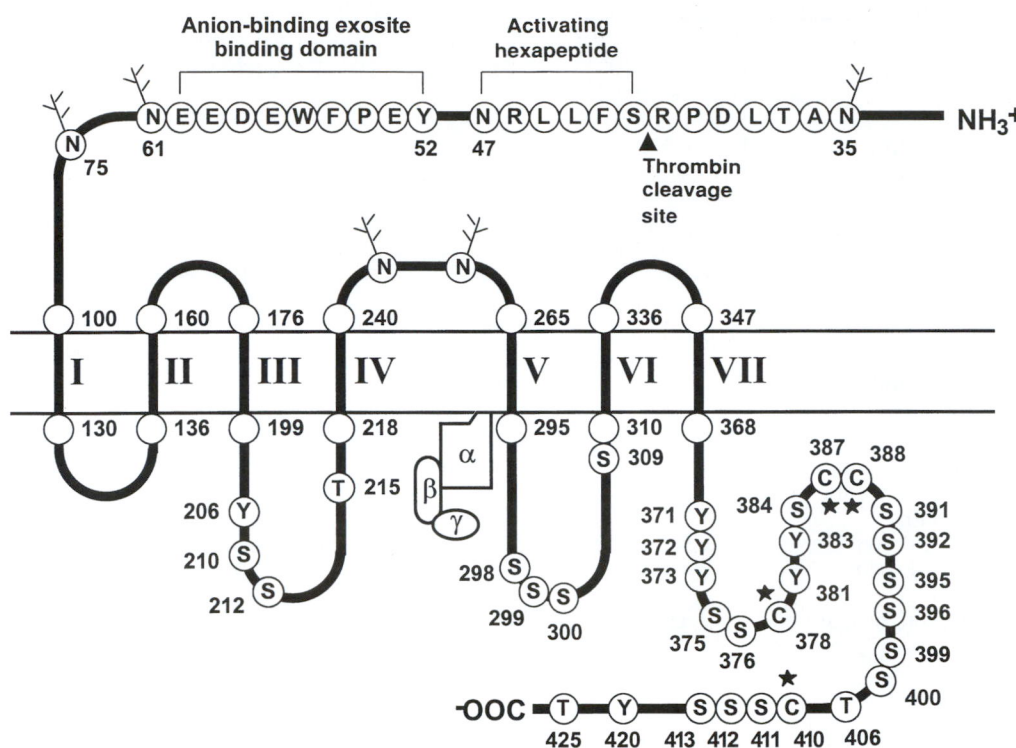

**FIGURE 12.2.** Schematic representation of the moderate affinity thrombin receptor. It is a member of the family of receptors with seven transmembranous domains (heptahelical). Thrombin binds to the anionic domain (amino acids 52–61) and cleaves at the arginine 41/serine 42. This exposes a tethered ligand domain (SFLLRN) that interacts elsewhere with the receptor to activate it. Extracellular *N*-glycosylation sites are marked and potential intracellular phosphorylation sites are designated (S, T, or Y). Sites of potential cysteine-linked lipid anchors are asterisked.

viously described platelet moderate affinity thrombin binding site (17–19). This structure reveals a 425 amino acid protein that belongs to the family of receptor proteins that have seven transmembranous domains (heptahelical) (20). The extracellular *N*-terminal domain possesses a thrombin cleavage site adjacent to a stretch of negatively charged amino acids that interact with the anion-binding exosite of thrombin (Fig. 12.2). Thrombin binding to and cleavage of this receptor results in cellular activation through a mechanism that begins with the exposure of a new "tethered-ligand peptide" that binds to some (as yet unspecified) receptor domain probably nearer to the carboxyterminus of the receptor. The soluble ligand peptide is, itself, a potent stimulus for platelet activation. The thrombin receptor has homology with adrenergic receptors, and both thrombin and adrenergic receptors are coupled to effector (or signal-generating) enzymes by heterotrimeric G proteins (see below). Thrombin activates PLC through two heterotrimeric G proteins—a pertussis toxin–sensitive homologue designated $G_P$ and the pertussis toxin–insensitive protein $G_q$—and inhibits adenylyl cyclase through a (probably different) pertussis toxin-sensitive G protein designated $G_i$ (21, 22).

Based on the interaction of α thrombin with the glycocalicin component of glycoprotein (GP) Ib (see Chapter 11) and on observations that platelets from individuals with Bernard-Soulier syndrome bind less thrombin and demonstrate decreased thrombin-induced aggregation, it has been proposed that the extracellular domain of GP Ibα is a functionally significant high-affinity thrombin receptor that couples thrombin binding to platelet activation (23). Evidence indicates that both GP Ibα and the heptahelical receptor work in concert to effect thrombin-induced platelet activation (24). It appears that GP Ibα is not involved in the trigger reaction, but could modulate additional signaling after thrombin binds to its receptor, particularly transmembranous calcium influx (25). The mechanism by which ligand engagement by the GP Ib-IX-V complex signals platelet activation is incompletely understood (4). It is interesting to note that GPV may be the critical component of the GP Ib-IX-V complex involved in thrombin binding (26). The importance of the GP Ib-IX-V complex in platelet responses to α thrombin *in vivo* has attracted increasing recent attention, in part because of observations that adult mice completely deficient in the moderate affinity seven transmembrane domain thrombin receptor have no bleeding diathesis and that their platelets respond completely normally to α thrombin (27).

## $TXA_2/PGG_2/PGH_2$

The arachidonic-acid metabolites that stimulate platelets are the prostaglandin endoperoxides ($PGG_2/PGH_2$) and $TXA_2$ (28). These are considered "strong agonists" because they directly activate PLC. A moderate affinity ($K_d \sim 2$ nM), endoperoxide/$TXA_2$-receptor is coupled to PLC by a pertussis toxin-insensitive, heterotrimeric, GTP-binding protein designated $G_q$ that is distinct from that which couples thrombin to PLC (29). There is a second, high affinity, endoperoxide/$TXA_2$ receptor isomer ($K_d \sim 234$ pM) that directly mediates changes in platelet cytosolic ionized calcium ($[Ca^{2+}]_i$) and shape change independent of PLC activity and may "prime" the platelet for activation by other agonists (30). Cloning and expression of a 343 amino acid platelet endoperoxide/$TXA_2$ receptor indicates that it, like thrombin, is a member of the family of receptor proteins that have seven transmembranous domains. Recent molecular analyses point to two isoforms of the human platelet $TXA_2$ receptor that differ only in the functional importance of a single arginine residue in the first cytoplasmic loop (31). Neither platelet endoperoxide/$TXA_2$ receptor is coupled to inhibition of adenylyl cyclase. It appears that an identical species of endoperoxide/$TXA_2$ receptor is present on platelets and vascular cells.

## PLATELET ACTIVATING FACTOR

Platelet-activating factor (PAF) is a complex lipid molecule (1-O-alkyl-2-O-acetyl-*sn*-glycerol-3-phosphorylcholine) derived from various inflammatory cells (neutrophils, macrophages, and eosinophils) as well as from the vascular endothelium and platelets. This molecule is a particularly potent activator of neutrophils and is a "strong agonist" for platelet activation *in vitro* (32), although its role in platelet-mediated thrombus formation *in vivo* is probably small. PAF has a specific receptor that has been cloned from guinea pig lung (33) and human leukocytes (34) and that has been shown to be another member of the family of receptor proteins that have seven transmembranous domains. As would be predicted by its primary amino acid sequence, the PAF receptor (like the thrombin and $TXA_2$ receptors) is coupled to the activation of PLC by a pertussis toxin-sensitive, heterotrimeric G protein (35); like the $TXA_2$ receptor, the platelet PAF receptor is not coupled to the inhibition of adenylyl cyclase (21).

## COLLAGEN

Platelets are activated by collagen types I, III, IV, V, and VI (types I, III, and VI are found in the vessel wall) (36, 37). Collagen must be in a native, triple-helix conformation for binding to occur, and platelets are capable of binding both soluble and insoluble collagen. At higher concentrations ($> \sim 10$ mg/ml), collagen functions as a "strong agonist" to activate platelet PLC independent of functional cyclooxygenase activity. At lower concentrations, collagen-induced aggregation of platelets involves a long lag phase during which the release of arachidonic acid and ADP contribute to the rate and magnitude of aggregation (i.e., collagen functions as a "weak agonist"). Several potential integrin and nonintegrin platelet receptors for collagen have been identified, which include GP Ia-IIa (integrin $\alpha_2\beta_1$) (36), GP IV (CD 36) (38), and GP VI (39). Each of these receptors mediates platelet adhesion, secretion, and aggregation, suggesting that collagen induces direct adhesion-activation coupling. The relative physiologic importance of the different collagen receptors is presently unknown. A single report suggests that an $M_r$ 85,000- to 90,000-membrane protein may participate in collagen binding to human platelets (40).

GP Ia/IIa is a heterodimeric member of the integrin superfamily ($\alpha_2\beta_1$). Molecular cloning reveals that the larger $\alpha_2$ subunit (GP Ia) contains a single transmembrane domain (41). Individuals congenitally deficient in this platelet protein have been noted to have a mild bleeding diathesis (42). Collagen binding to GP Ia-IIa is dependent on $Mg^{2+}$ and inhibited by $Ca^{2+}$. GP Ia-IIa may become activated in response to ADP and may mediate subsequent platelet adhesion to collagen (43).

GP IV is a highly glycosylated protein having $M_r$ 85,000 to 95,000. It has at least one, but no more than two, transmembrane domains. GP IV also functions as the platelet thrombospondin receptor. *In vitro*, a monoclonal antibody (mAB) to GP IV activates platelets (44). This may involve protein tyrosine kinases related to the c-*src* proto oncogene, since many *src*-related proteins are associated with GP IV in the resting platelet membrane (45). The importance of GP IV *in vivo* is, however, uncertain; up to 11% of healthy Japanese blood donors lack this platelet protein without any detectable clinical effect (46). Similarly, there is no evidence that thrombospondin binding to platelet GP IV is a signal transducing event, although in other cell types this has been associated with tyrosine kinase signaling activity (47).

The role of GP VI in physiologic platelet function is unknown. Its possible importance is based on two clinical observations: one individual with a mild bleeding problem associated with a deficiency of the 62,000 dalton membrane GP VI and absent platelet adhesion and aggregation in response to collagen (39), and another individual with immune thrombocytopenia associated with defective collagen-induced platelet aggregation and serum antibodies to GP VI (48).

The activation pathways initiated by platelet binding to collagen have not been rigorously defined, but include PLC-mediated production of phosphatidic acid (PA) and elevations of cytosolic ionized calcium ($[Ca^{2+}]_i$) (49) and involves the expression of a functional GP IIb-IIIa complex (50). Of note, collagen activates the $\gamma$ isoform of PLC, probably through the activation of nonreceptor SH2 containing tyrosine kinases that assemble on a tyrosine phosphorylated $\gamma$ chain of the platelet Fc receptor (51, 52) (see below). The initiating receptor for this may be GP Ia-IIa (integrin $\alpha_2\beta_1$).

## VASOPRESSIN

Vasopressin is an extracellular mediator of platelet activation that functions *in vitro* like other "strong agonists," although its physiologic and pathologic importance *in vivo* is probably minimal. This may be because platelets have only a small number of $M_r$ 124,000 specific $V_1$ receptors (approximately 90 binding sites per platelet) (53). The occupancy of $V_1$ receptors is associated with pertussis toxin sensitive, G protein mediated activation of PLC, but, like the $TXA_2$ and PAF receptors, the platelet $V_1$ receptor is not coupled to the inhibition of adenylyl cyclase. Molecular cloning of the rat liver $V_{1a}$ receptor demonstrates that this protein is a member of the family of receptor molecules containing seven transmembranous domains (54).

## EPINEPHRINE

The only adrenergic receptors that human platelets possess are $\alpha_2$ adrenergic receptors. The structure of the platelet $\alpha_2$ adrenergic receptor has been determined (55). The membrane topology of the platelet $\alpha_2$ adrenergic receptor provides the structural paradigm (seven transmembranous domains) for the functions of a number of platelet receptors for important extracellular stimulatory ligands, including thrombin, eicosanoids, and PAF. Each of these ligands stimulates intracellular activation pathways through a transmembranous signal involving a heterotrimeric G protein that interacts with a specific domain (comprised, in part, of the third intracellular loop) of the receptor protein. Epinephrine binding to platelets is associated with an aspirin-sensitive activation of PLC; therefore the $\alpha_2$ receptor is not directly coupled to PLC. There is evidence that the $\alpha_2$ receptor is coupled by a G protein to phospholipase $A_2$ ($PLA_2$) through a mechanism that depends on $Na^+/H^+$ exchange and fibrinogen binding to GP IIb-IIIa (as will be discussed further below). Activation of $PLA_2$ causes the release and metabolism of arachidonic acid, which then leads to the activation of PLC. The $\alpha_2$ receptor is also

coupled by a different heterotrimeric G protein to the inhibition of adenylyl cyclase (like thrombin), and this may account in part for the mechanism by which epinephrine "primes" the platelet for activation by other agonists.

## ADENOSINE DIPHOSPHATE

Platelets are unique in that the adenine nucleotide ADP, rather than ATP, is preferred by the platelet purinergic receptor. ADP functions as an important physiologic "weak agonist," while ATP antagonizes ADP-induced platelet responses. Quantitative analyses of ADP binding to platelets have been, until recently, complicated by the rapid hydrolysis of bound ADP by platelet surface ADPases. Using an affinity reagent, one platelet ADP receptor has been partially characterized as an $M_r$ 100,000 protein called "aggregin" (56). More recently, the binding sites for ADP have been studied using formalin-fixed platelets and radiolabeled adenine nucleotides (57). These studies indicate that there are two ADP receptors ($K_{d1} \sim 30$ nM, 25,600 sites/platelets; $K_{d2} \sim 3$ mM, 383,000 sites/platelet), with the high affinity receptor identical to the 125,000-dalton subunit of GP IIb.

There is evidence that ADP binding to aggregin induces a $Ca^{2+}$-dependent cleavage of this receptor that signals a conformational change in platelet GP IIb-IIIa to permit fibrinogen binding (56). This may be associated with $PLA_2$ activation (as with epinephrine), since ADP-induced platelet PLC activation is blocked by inhibiting cyclooxygenase. The ADP/aggregin interaction is essential for epinephrine-induced platelet activation and may contribute to the amplification of platelet responses to many physiologic stimuli.

The presence and function of the $P_{2t}$ purinergic receptor in human platelets is established, although the molecular structure of this novel purinergic receptor is not yet elucidated. There are $\sim 600$ $P_{2t}$ receptors per platelet with a $K_d$ of $\sim 5$ nM (58). These are presumed heptahelical structures that trigger both G protein mediated PLC activation and the inhibition of adenylyl cyclase. Platelets also express $P_{2tu}$ purinergic receptors that bind ATP and activate adenylyl cyclase (59).

## SEROTONIN

Serotonin (5-hydroxytryptamine) is a "weak" platelet agonist that has received recent attention concerning its potential role in acute coronary artery thrombosis (60) and as a biologic marker for many psychiatric disorders (61). Platelets have specific $S_2$ receptors. The human $S_2$ receptor has been cloned and is another member of the seven transmembrane domain receptor family (62). Occupation of this receptor is associated with PLC activation (63) that is generally dependent on intact arachidonic acid metabolism (9). The role of G proteins in serotonin-induced platelet activation is poorly understood. Quantitative binding studies of intact platelets are difficult because platelets have an active transporter of extracellular serotonin (with a $K_m$ similar to that of neuronal tissue).

## PLATELET ADHESION RECEPTORS THAT MEDIATE ACTIVATION (SEE CHAPTER 11)

### GP Ib-IX-V

Soluble or solid-phase von Willebrand factor (vWf) does not bind to resting platelets in static or stirring systems. Under the influence of chemical modulators or mechanical shearing forces, vWf binds to platelet GP Ib$\alpha$ and stimulates platelet signaling pathways leading to important functional consequences (see below) (4, 64).

### GP IIb-IIIa

GP IIb-IIIa ($\alpha_{IIb}/\beta_3$) is a member of the integrin family of proteins (65) found only on platelets and megakaryocytes (discussed in Chapter 11). It is the single most abundant species of glycoprotein on the platelet surface (~50,000 copies), and its functions are to effect platelet adhesion under static or low-shear conditions and to mediate platelet cohesion (aggregation) in response to chemical agonists or high-shear dependent vWf binding to GP Ib$\alpha$. Its primary ligands are fibrinogen and vWf, but it also binds to fibrin, fibronectin, vitronectin and thrombospondin. Ligand binding requires the "activation" of the GP IIb-IIIa complex (see below). This activation occurs in response to all chemical agonists, as well as vWf binding to GP Ib$\alpha$, and involves receptor clustering into a new conformer receptive for ligand binding through an RGD motif (e.g., fibrinogen). Activation also upregulates the number of surface complexes by ~50%, as they translocate from the surface-connected open canalicular system and the $\alpha$ granules.

GP IIb ($M_r$ 136,000) is a heterodimer of an extracellular heavy chain ($M_r$ 125,000) linked by a single disulfide bridge to a smaller subunit ($M_r$ 23,000) containing one transmembranous domain and a short (20 amino acids), cytoplasmic tail; GP IIb forms a $Ca^{2+}$-dependent complex with GP IIIa ($M_r$ 110,000 unreduced), which has a large, disulfide bound loop that forms a globular structure with an RGD-recognition site (characteristic of the integrins) near its aminoterminus and a 47 amino acid, C-terminal cytoplasmic tail.

Ligand binding to GP IIb-IIIa initiates submembranous biochemical responses ("outside-in signaling"), although their functional importance in platelets (and megakaryocytes) is uncertain. GP IIb-IIIa undergoes an additional conformational change following ligand binding, suggesting one potential role for GP IIb-IIIa-mediated "outside-in" signaling; it participates as part of a bidirectional signaling loop that regulates GP IIb-IIIa avidity and "locks" fibrinogen to its receptor (66). This process involves ligand-induced, GP IIb-IIIa-mediated alterations in GP IIb-IIIa anchorage to the cytoskeleton. This altered association actually stabilizes the ligand-receptor interaction, perhaps tightening the bonds formed extracellularly (67).

GP IIb-IIIa of resting platelets binds to immobilized fibrinogen, which causes GP IIb-IIIa activation, tyrosine phosphorylation, cytoskeletal reorganization, and platelet spreading (68, 69). This demonstrates that GP IIb-IIIa-mediated signaling is involved in functionally important responses *in vitro*, although the physiologic relevance of static platelet adhesion to insoluble fibrinogen is unproved (70). This signaling does, however, involve protein tyrosine phosphorylation, as sequential activation of the tyrosine kinases pp72$^{syc}$, pp60$^{c\text{-}src}$, and pp125$^{FAK}$ is associated with fibrinogen binding to GP IIb-IIIa, and these tyrosine kinases catalyze the phosphorylation of numerous platelet proteins, most of which are not identified (71). The phosphorylation of these nonreceptor tyrosine kinases could be initiated by *src*-mediated tyrosine phosphorylation of the cytoplasmic tail of GP IIIa, triggering a docking with the adaptor proteins growth factor receptor binding protein 2 (Grb2) and Shc, both of which have been implicated in integrin-mediated signaling in other cell types (see below) (72, 73).

GP IIb-IIIa may also be involved in regulating the direct activation of phospholipase $A_2$ by epinephrine or ADP and in regulating of tyrosine kinase activity following platelet stimulation by chemical agonists. Both will be discussed in more details below.

### Other Platelet Integrins

The integrin $\alpha_2\beta_1$ (GP Ia-IIa) is a collagen receptor that induces functionally important platelet signals, possibly through the activation of phospholipase C$\gamma$2 (74). Phospholipase C$\gamma$2, as well as pp60$^{c\text{-}src}$ and pp125$^{FAK}$, are tyrosine phosphorylated in an $\alpha_2\beta_1$-specific manner (70). As described above, there are additional putative platelet collagen receptors, and ranking their relative significance *in vivo* has, to date, been impossible.

Another platelet integrin is the $\alpha_v\beta_3$ complex that binds to vitronectin (fibronectin, vWf, and thrombospondin); there is no evidence that this receptor transduces signals for platelet activation. Platelets also have the fibronectin receptor (GP Ic-IIa [$\alpha_5/\beta_1$]) and the laminin receptor ($\alpha_6/\beta_1$); no signaling functions have been ascribed to these receptor molecules.

## OTHER ACTIVATION-INITIATING RECEPTORS

The platelet contains $F_c$ receptors designated as the $M_r$ 40,000 $F_c\gamma$RII. These $F_c\gamma$RII molecules transduce activation signals following antibody binding. This signal pathway involves phospholipase Cγ activation following receptor crosslinking (75). $F_c\gamma RII$ crosslinking may also be coupled to the *ras* → mitogen activated protein (MAP) kinase → phospholipase $A_2$ pathway (see below) (76). Platelet $F_c\gamma RII$-mediated signaling is a nonspecific response to intact immunoglobulin that can confound *in vitro* studies utilizing antibodies. For example, anti-CD 9 antibodies nonspecifically activate platelets through the $F_c\gamma RII$ (77). This activation pathway may contribute to increased platelet clearance in immune thrombocytopenias (78). Platelet $F_c$ and $C1_q$ receptors may also be involved in immune complex formation and complement activation on the platelet surface. The complement membrane attack complex ($C_{5b-9}$) can directly activate platelets, probably by allowing extracellular calcium entry, and this leads to calcium activated, protease (calpain)–mediated membrane shedding with the formation of platelet microparticles (79). These microparticles, which were first discovered when flow cytometry histograms revealed unexpectedly small particles, express prothrombinase activity (80), suggesting that they are prothrombotic in clinical conditions (81). The platelet also binds specifically to IgE, possibly through GP IIb-IIIa (82), but the significance of this *in vivo* is unknown.

The platelet also has receptors for certain growth factors and cytokines, such as interferon γ, interleukin-1β, and thrombopoietin (TPO). These transmembranous proteins send "priming" signals following binding their ligand. The physiologic importance of these receptors is uncertain, but it is possible that pharmacologic doses of TPO administered to individuals with underproduction thrombocytopenias may be accompanied by *in vivo* platelet activation (see Chapter 8). This is due to TPO lowering the threshold at which platelet agonists induced aggregation (83). The mechanism of action of TPO involves the activation of nonreceptor tyrosine kinases (see below) (84, 85).

Platelets have receptors for plasminogen (86) and tissue plasminogen activator (t-PA) (87), which permit assembly of the fibrinolytic apparatus on the platelet surface in areas of thrombosis. This local generation of plasmin will directly activate platelets during exposure times of a few minutes (88). When platelets are subjected to prolonged exposure to plasmin (e.g., during pharmacologic fibrinolysis), platelets become inhibited, in part because of the generation of inhibitory signals (feedback inhibition by protein kinase C; see below) (89) and in part because of digestion of GP Ibα and GP IIb-IIIa. Plasmin, primarily through its proteolytic effect on plasma vWf, inhibits shear stress induced platelet aggregation (90). Plasmin also causes platelet disaggregation, even in plasma containing various anti-plasmins, by degrading cohesive fibrinogen connecting individual platelets within the platelet thrombus (89).

LDL and lipoprotein Lp(a) bind to platelets, and this interaction may lead to changes in platelet responsiveness to chemical agonists. LDL "primes" platelets and enhances their responsiveness to chemical stimuli, while Lp(a) is inhibitory (91). The precise binding site for LDL is uncertain, but it appears, based on antibody blocking experiments, that Lp(a) binds to GP IIb-IIIa (91).

P-selectin (PADGEM, GMP 140, or CD 62) is an $M_r$-140,000 member of the "selectin" family that is expressed on activated platelets and mediates their binding to leukocytes (92). When platelets bind to neutrophils through P-selectin, no P-selectin–mediated activation signals are generated. Rather, the platelet-neutrophil juxtaposition allows platelet-stimulatory neutrophil proteases to be relatively protected from the neutralizing activity of plasma anti-proteases (93). The neutrophil protease that is most important is cathepsin G, which activates platelet secretion and up-regulates the number and function of GP IIb-IIIa (94). The mechanism by which cathepsin G initiates these responses is unknown, but it does not involve cleavage of the hepta-helical thrombin receptor (95). Cathepsin G paradoxically renders platelets relatively nonadhesive by digesting the vWf binding site from GP Ibα (96). Other neutrophil proteases, such as elastase and gelatinase, synergize with cathepsin G to effect platelet activation (97). Gelatinase is also secreted directly by activated platelets and may be an important extracellular signal for platelet recruitment and amplification (98).

Platelets also express a membrane adhesion receptor of the immunoglobulin gene superfamily. PECAM-1 (CD 31) is an $M_r$-130,000 protein that is constitutively expressed on platelets and is involved in platelet-endothelial interactions (99). There is some evidence that PECAM-1 initiates signals, but the molecules involved and functional importance of this in platelets is unknown at this time.

## ACTIVATION-INDUCED CHANGES IN PLATELET RECEPTORS

Using immunodetection techniques coupled to flow cytometry, many activation-dependent, platelet membrane epitopes can be measured (100). Such epitopes include activation-induced conformational changes of a surface protein such as monoclonal antibody PAC-1 binding to activated GP IIb-IIIa; ligand-induced changes of receptor conformation such as conformational changes induced in GP IIb-IIIa on fibrinogen binding that are recognized by monoclonal antibody ligand-induced binding site-1 (LIBS-1) (101); or receptor-induced changes in ligand conformation such as changes in fibrinogen conformation induced by its binding to GP IIb-IIIa and identified by monoclonal antibody 9F9 specific for this unique, receptor-induced binding site (RIBS) (102).

Activated platelets can also be identified by proteins that are expressed on the membrane as a result of exocytosis, such as lysosomal membrane proteins, α granule membrane proteins like P-selectin (CD 62), or dense granule membrane proteins. Some of these have important functions that can be measured by flow cytometry such as P-selectin which mediates platelet-leukocyte interactions. Leukocyte-platelet complexes can be measured *ex vivo* by flow cytometry, and their formation implies platelet activation (and perhaps associated neutrophil activation) that could be clinically relevant. For example, P-selectin-dependent, leukocyte-platelet complexes develop following cardiopulmonary bypass (103) and have been associated with syndromes of active coronary artery stenosis (104). Activated platelets are very important in regulating the generation of insoluble fibrin (see below), and platelet procoagulant activities (for example, the binding of factors V and VIII) can be detected by flow cytometry.

## G PROTEINS

Guanine nucleotide binding (G) proteins are poised at the inner plasma membrane in preparation for receiving activation signals from heptahelical receptors altered by ligand engagement. Nine different heterotrimeric G pro-

tein α subunits have been identified in human platelets. These are divided into three functionally distinct, G protein families in platelets (25, 105): (a) $G_q$ and $G_{11}$ couple activating ligand–receptor interactions (involving thrombin, $PGG_2$/$PGH_2$/$TXA_2$, PAF, and vasopressin) to the stimulation of phosphoinositide-specific PLCβ1; (b) $G_s$ couples inhibitory prostaglandin-receptor interactions (involving $PGI_2$ and $PGD_2$) to the stimulation of adenylyl cyclase; and (c) $G_{i1}$, $G_{i2}$, and $G_{i3}$ couple some agonist-receptor interactions (involving thrombin, epinephrine, and ADP) to the inhibition of adenylyl cyclase. In addition, there is a functionally characterized $G_{"p"}$ that is inhibited by pertussis toxin-mediated ADP-ribosylation and couples the thrombin receptor to activation of PLCβ1. The $G_i\alpha$ subunits are also inhibited by pertussis toxin, suggesting that $G_{"p"}$ may be a $G_i$ homologue. The $G_s\alpha$ subunit is activated by cholera toxin-mediated ADP-ribosylation. $G_{11}\alpha$ and $G_q\alpha$ are unaffected by ADP-ribosylation. The other G proteins that have been identified in human platelets are $G_z\alpha$, $G_{12}\alpha$, and $G_{13}\alpha$; no functions have been ascribed to these G proteins.

Each of these G proteins is a heterotrimeric complex (comprised of α, β, and γ subunits) that has GDP tightly bound to the α subunit in the basal state (Fig. 12.3). They are tethered to the membrane through "lipidic feet ($G_\alpha$

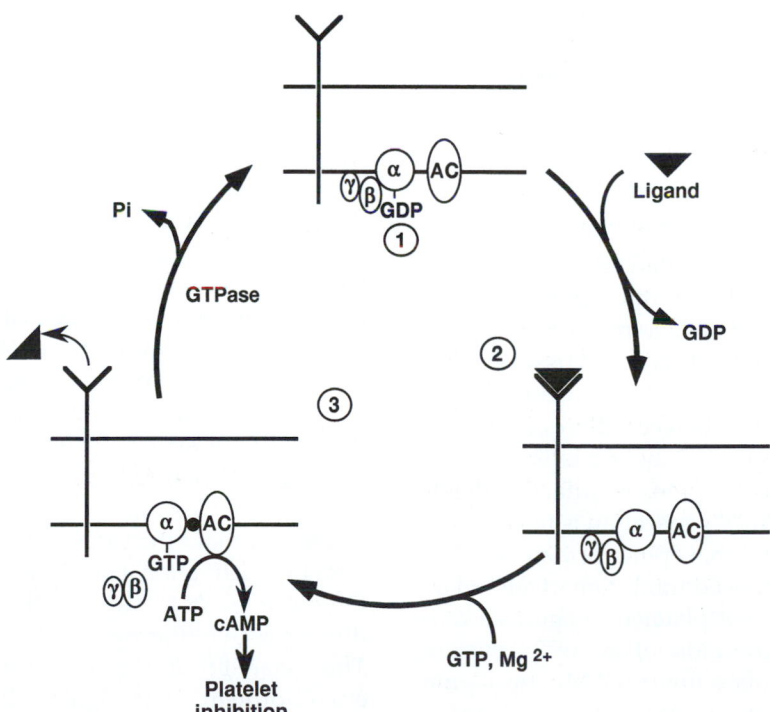

**FIGURE 12.3.** General theoretical model by which G proteins transduce an extracellular stimulus into an intracellular response: (1) in the basal state, GDP is bound to the heterotrimeric G protein (in this case $G_s$) through a binding site on the α subunit; (2) an extracellular ligand binding to the G protein-linked receptor (e.g., the $PGI_2$ receptor linked to $G_s$) causes the hydrolysis of GDP from the α subunit; and (3) in the presence of $Mg^{2+}$, GTP occupies the open guanine nucleotide binding site, resulting in the dissociation of the α subunit from the G protein complex. $G_{s\alpha}$-GTP activates adenylyl cyclase, which converts ATP to cAMP. The intrinsic GTPase activity of the G protein converts GTP to GDP, resulting in the reassociation of the heterotrimer and the cyclic restoration of the basal state (see text for further details).

subunits may be myristoylated and palmitoylated; $G_\gamma$, of the $G_\beta$ dimer, subunits may be farnesylated or geranylgeranylated) (106)." Following receptor-ligand coupling, GDP dissociates from the complex. With normal levels of cytoplasmic GTP and $Mg^{2+}$, GTP binds to the open guanine nucleotide binding site on the $\alpha$ subunit. This binding of GTP to the $\alpha$ subunit results in the dissociation of the $\alpha$ subunit from the $\alpha\beta\gamma$ complex. The dissociated $G_\alpha \cdot GTP$ then undergoes a conformational change permitting its interaction with the enzyme "signal amplifier" within the inner leaflet of the plasma membrane to convert phosphorylated precursors into second messenger molecules. In platelets there are ~10 receptors coupled to six functional G proteins activating at least three different effectors: phospholipase C$\beta$, adenylyl cyclase, and phospholipase $A_2$. Throughout the human genome, however, there exist at least 1000 receptors coupled to at least 20 $G_\alpha$, 5 $G_\beta$, and 12 $G_\gamma$ subunits activating countless effectors (106).

The heterotrimeric structure of G proteins provides them with additional versatility through the $\beta\gamma$ component that remains a single functional unit after dissociation from the $\alpha$ subunit. The $\beta\gamma$ subunit reassociates with the $\alpha$ subunit as the intrinsic-GTPase activity of the $\alpha$ subunit hydrolyzes GTP to GDP, thus terminating the G protein-mediated signal (Fig. 12.3). In addition, the $\beta\gamma$ subunit may also be the functionally relevant molecular unit regulating many important effectors (107). The $\beta\gamma$ subunit may be involved in activating an isoform of phosphoinositide 3-kinase in human platelets (108).

## $G_s$, $G_i$

G proteins in platelets that regulate adenylyl cyclase represent the prototypical system that operates to control cAMP generation in response to many different extracellular stimuli in a variety of cells and tissues. Platelet antagonists that operate through the metabolism of $G_s$ include $PGI_2$ and $PGD_2$. The activation of adenylyl cyclase can be counterbalanced by platelet agonist–induced inhibition of the enzyme. In intact platelets, prostaglandin-induced cAMP generation is inhibited by pretreatment with thrombin, epinephrine, or ADP (109–111). This agonist-induced inhibition of adenyl cyclase is mediated by $G_i$; thus platelet antagonists raise cAMP by $G_s$-directed activation of adenylyl cyclase, while some platelet agonists lower cAMP by $G_i$-mediated inhibition of adenylyl cyclase.

The function of $G_s$ and $G_i$ can be altered by modifying their $\alpha$ subunits with microbial toxins that function as ADP-ribosyltransferases to transfer a minor ADP-ribose modification group (from a NAD donor to $a_s$ or $a_i$) (112–113). Cholera toxin ADP ribosylates $\alpha_s$ causing its activation by preventing the hydrolysis of bound GTP to GDP. Pertussis toxin ADP-ribosylates $\alpha_i$, result-

ing in an impairment in its ability to interact with the receptor to which it is coupled and, thereby, blocking agonist-mediated inhibition of adenylyl cyclase.

## $G_{p,q,11}$

The activation of phosphoinositide-specific PLC in platelets involves at least two functionally separate G proteins, $G_p$ or $G_{q/11}$. $G_p$ mediates pertussis toxin-inhibited platelet activation in response to thrombin and possibly also PAF, vasopressin, and collagen. $G_{q/11}$ mediates pertussis toxin–insensitive platelet activation in response to $TXA_2$ and thrombin. $G_{q/11}$ is designated as such because it appears that $G_q$ functions as the predominant, but not the sole, signal-transducing heterotrimeric G protein coupled to the platelet $TXA_2$ and thrombin receptors. Because it is also present in platelets, pertussis toxin–insensitive, and highly homologous to $G_q$ (most antibodies cannot distinguish the two), $G_{11}$ may also be involved in receptor-mediated activation of PLC.

The important function of these G proteins in platelet PLC activation is supported by data demonstrating that $AlF_4$ and nonhydrolyzable analogs of GTP (GTP$_\gamma$S, $G_{pp}NH_p$), which bypass receptors and cause direct activation of G proteins, stimulate the hydrolysis of $PIP_2$ in permeabilized platelets, platelet membrane preparations, or intact platelets (114, 115). Furthermore, a nonhydrolyzable analog of GDP (GDP$\beta$S), which maintains $G_p$ in its nondissociated and therefore inactive state, inhibits $PIP_2$ hydrolysis in response to agonist stimulation. There is also evidence from platelet reconstitution studies that supports the existence of a functional $G_p$; PLC activity from platelet membrane preparations can be induced by the addition of exogenous G proteins (115).

The physiologic significance of the functional and structural heterogeneity of G proteins mediating PLC activation is an enigma. As stated above, there is good evidence that a unique G protein can affect PLC in a ligand-dependent manner (e.g., $G_q$ and $TXA_2$), indicating the possibility that the heterotrimeric G protein is the switch for specific signal routing. There is also evidence that supports the hypothesis that a platelet $G_p$ is the same as $G_i$, suggesting that ligand binding results in a signal that bifurcates at a G protein "node" toward both PLC activation *and* adenylyl cyclase inhibition. Furthermore, as stated above, the intact $\beta\gamma$ subunit has a direct role in initiating *and* abrogating activation signals. This versatility in signaling function of the heterotrimeric G proteins that regulate PLC will be more clearly defined as their structural interactions with receptors and signal-generating proteins undergo continued investigation.

## LOW-MOLECULAR-WEIGHT G PROTEINS

In addition to the heterotrimeric, GTP-binding proteins found in human platelets, there are several distinct GTP-binding proteins with molecular weights between 21,000 and 31,000 daltons, all of which are members of the *ras* family of GTPases. These include *ras, rho, rac, ral, rap, rab,* CDC42H, and G25K. Like the heterotrimeric G proteins, these low-molecular-weight (LMW) G proteins are predominantly membrane-associated. Their membrane association is due to posttranslational carboxymethylation and lipidation. LMW G proteins function generally as molecular switches in the following way. In the basal state GDP is bound. On activation by an upstream stimulus, GTP is exchanged for GDP; this reaction is catalyzed by a guanine nucleotide exchanging factor (GEF). Following GTP binding, the LMW G protein assumes its active conformation, thereby activating an effector molecule and/or triggering a new molecular association or dissociation. Its activity is attenuated and halted by GTP hydrolysis, for which a new association with a GTPase activating protein (GAP) is required. Unlike the α subunit of heterotrimeric G proteins, LMW G proteins have no intrinsic GTPase activity (116).

The function of these proteins in platelet physiology or pathophysiology is not established. Based on immunoblotting, the predominant groups of LMW G proteins are the 27,000 dalton *ral* species (perhaps 5) and a 25,000 dalton protein designated G25K. Other LMW G proteins detectable by immunoblotting are *rap* 1A, *rap* 1B, *rac* 1, *rho, rab* 3B, *rab* 6, *rab* 8, and the yeast homologue designated CDC42Hs.

There is currently no evidence for LMW G protein-mediated GDP/GTP exchange or GTP hydrolysis in intact platelets. Activity is therefore measured using the surrogate of identifying new molecular associations that the LMW G protein develops during platelet activation. The most commonly reported association is between the LMW G protein and the triton-insoluble cytoskeleton. Following platelet activation by any stimulus, actin polymerizes, trapping a variety of proteins in the "activated cytoskeleton," which is defined by the material that pellets at 14,000 to 15,000 x g following platelet lysis in triton-X detergent. *Rap1b, rap2b, rac, rho,* and CDC42Hs all translocate from the membrane fraction to the activated cytoskeleton (117–119). Within the cytoskeleton, *rap1b* also associates with a phospholipase Cγ (see below) and a GAP (120); *rap2b* associates with GP IIb-IIIa (118). *Rap2b, rac,* and CDC42Hs translocate from the membrane fraction to the activated cytoskeleton in a GP IIb-IIIa–dependent manner (i.e., after activation of GP IIb-IIIa) (118, 119). *Rho* associates with a phosphatidylinositol (PI) 3-kinase in the activated cytoskeleton (121).

Another presumed surrogate for LMW G protein activation is identifying the protein as a substrate of a kinase reaction. The *rab* proteins are phosphorylated by activating stimuli, such as thrombin (122), while an unidentified *ras* protein is phosphorylated by inhibitory stimuli that activate cyclic 5′,3′ adenosine monophosphate (cAMP)-dependent protein kinase (123). The actual functional consequences of the presence and state of phosphorylation of these platelet LMW G proteins are unknown. In other cells *rab* 3 is involved in exocytosis; its state of phosphorylation has no known effect on its activity.

The function of a few platelet LMW G proteins has been demonstrated in cell-free systems or in permeabilized platelets. Their role in intact platelets is unknown. In permeabilized platelets, two well documented conclusions are presented: (a) *Rho* signals PI 3-kinase activation, and PI 3-kinase activity contributes to thrombin-induced platelet aggregation (see below) (121); (b) *Rac* signals F actin uncapping that is required for activation-dependent cytoskeletal reorganization establishing shape changes and secretion (124). This latter activity can also be implied for the *rho*-like LMW G protein CDC42H, which serves this function in other cell types (125).

# INTRACELLULAR SIGNAL PATHWAYS

## PHOSPHOLIPASE C

The importance of phosphoinositide (PI) metabolism in the regulation of cellular stimulus-response coupling was first suggested by Hokin and Hokin in 1953 (126). The turnover of platelet phosphoinositides in association with agonist stimulation was first observed in 1961 by Firkin and Williams (127), but it took almost 20 more years before it became clear that PI metabolism is an important mechanism of platelet activation (128–130). It is now established that human platelets contain several isozymes of phospholipase C (PLC) that hydrolyze phosphatidylinositol 4,5 bisphosphate ($PIP_2$) to the two stimulatory second messengers, inositol 1,4,5-trisphosphate ($IP_3$) and *sn*-1,2-diacylglycerol (DAG) (Fig. 12.4). There are at least six forms of PLC found in human platelets: PLCβ2 > PLCγ2 > PLCβ3 > PLCγ1 > PLCβ1 > PLCβ4 (131, 132). In general, PLC catalyzes the hydrolysis of three common phosphoinositides: phosphatidylinositol, phosphatidyl-inositol 4-phosphate, and $PIP_2$. Platelet PLCs differ in their substrate affinities, rates of catalysis, and requirements for $Ca^{2+}$ (133).

$PIP_2$ is a quantitatively minor platelet membrane phospholipid that is the primary substrate for stimulus-evoked PLC activity (134). The predominant molecular species of platelet $PIP_2$ hydrolyzed by PLC contains the fatty acyl substituents stearoyl-(C18:0) and arachidonoyl-(C20:4) at the C-1 and C-2 positions, respectively. The glycerol backbone of this phosphoinositide structure, including its *sn*-1,2 substituents, undergoes recycling (135). Mass changes in the substrates and products of PLC have been determined, but their correlation with

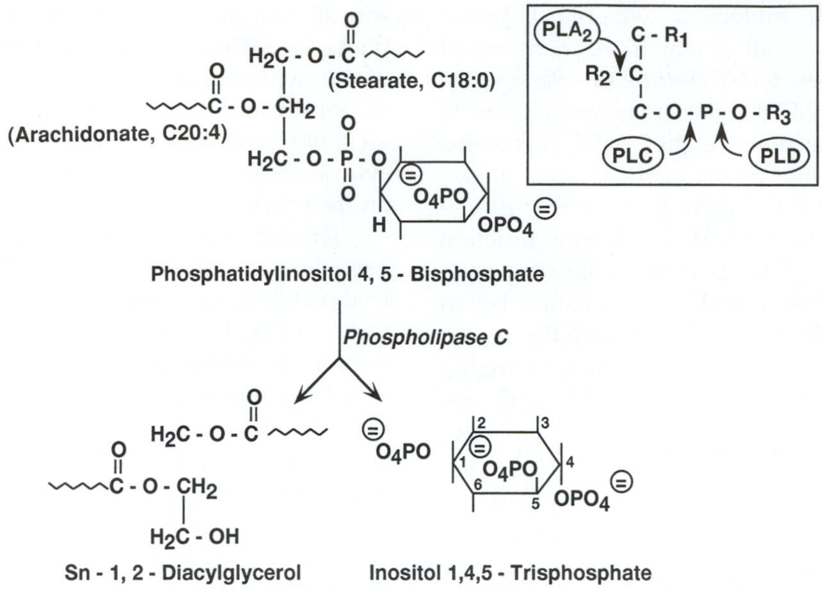

**FIGURE 12.4.**    Primary structure of the predominant molecular species of human platelet phosphatidylinositol 4,5-bisphosphate, and the products of its enzymatic cleavage by phosphoinositide-specific phospholipase C. The boxed insert demonstrates the sites of action of different phospholipases. $R_1$ and $R_2$ represent the C-1 and C-2 fatty acyl substituents, respectively. $R_3$ represents the polar group linked to the glycerol backbone by a phosphodiester bond (e.g., inositol with phosphatidylinositol, choline with phosphatidylcholine, etc.). $PLA_2$, phospholipase $A_2$; PLC, phospholipase C; PLD, phospholipase D.

the magnitude of any particular cellular response is not known.

The mechanisms by which platelet PLC isozymes are activated following receptor engagement by ligand have been partially worked out. PLCβ2 appears to be the major PLC activated by the heptahelical receptor/heterotrimeric G protein systems. Of note, PLCβ2 is activated by both Gα and Gβγ·PLCγ2 (like all PLCγ isoforms) is an SH2-containing protein activated by tyrosine phosphorylation following its engagement by a tyrosine kinase. PLCγ2 appears to be preferentially activated following collagen/platelet interactions, possibly through the GP Ia-IIa complex (integrin $\alpha_2\beta_1$) or GP VI (136). Through its *src* homology 2 (SH2) domain, PLCγ2 binds to activated (tyrosine phosphorylated), nonreceptor tyrosine kinases such as *src*, *syc*, or JAK (137, 138). PLCγ2 activation is triggered by the specific phosphorylation of a single tyrosine residue catalyzed by the nonreceptor tyrosine kinase to which the PLC is docked.

To some extent all of the major PLC isozymes translocate to the cytoskeleton following platelet activation (131). The significance of this is unclear. Many signal molecules move to the cytoskeleton on platelet activation, and this translocation is often assumed to relate to the formation of new molecular complexes that in some way regulate the activity of a signal molecule. In the case of PLC, two points can be made about their association with the cytoskeleton. First, PLCβ3 becomes activated following a PLCγ2- or PLCβ2-initiated signal cascade, and PLCβ3 becomes associated with GP IIb-IIIa in the cytoskeleton and activated following GP IIb-IIIa engaging ligand (131, 139). This is a "postaggregation" event that is of unknown functional consequences. The second point is that the PLC substrate PIP$_2$ is physically associated with the cytoskeletal protein profilin. This association may decrease PIP$_2$ available for background PLC activity present in resting cells, thus maintaining platelet activation signals at a subthreshold level (140). Following PLC activation, including translocation to the cytoskeleton, this idle on the activation machinery is released, allowing for the stimulation reaction to proceed full force. Additionally, the effect of PLC on PIP$_2$/profilin complexes is to cause the release of profilin bound to sequestered actin monomers. The release of sequestered actin permits actin polymerization to develop (see Chapter 10).

The activation of platelet phosphoinositide-specific PLC results in the generation of IP$_3$ and DAG. These molecules effect divergent pathways of platelet activation: IP$_3$ causes elevations of cytosolic ionized calcium concentration ($[Ca^{2+}]_i$) and DAG causes the activation of PKC. $Ca^{2+}$ mobilization or PKC activation independently results in platelet activation; together, they synergistically stimulate a diversity of platelet responses, including granule secretion, the release of arachidonic acid from membrane phospholipids, and the activation of GP IIb-IIIa.

## IP$_3$ AND CALCIUM

Intracellular IP$_3$ regulates agonist-induced platelet cytosolic ionized calcium responses (141). The resting platelet has a $[Ca^{2+}]_i$ of approximately 100 nM. On agonist stimulation, $[Ca^{2+}]_i$ increases to >1000 nM. There are two pools of calcium in the resting platelet: (a) a cytosolic pool demonstrating rapid turnover ($t_{1/2}$ 17 minutes) regulated by a plasma membrane $Ca^{2+}$-ATPase; and (b) a slowly exchanging pool ($t_{1/2}$ 300 minutes), which is driven into and sequestered within the platelet's dense tubular system by the activity of a $Ca^{2+}/Mg^{2+}$ ATPase (142, 143). It is from this latter storage pool that calcium is released into the cytosol following agonist stimulation. Plasma membrane exchange of $Ca^{2+}$ is important for loading the $Ca^{2+}$ storage organelle and, as will be discussed further below, may play a role in agonist-induced changes of $[Ca^{2+}]_i$.

Experiments in which inositol phosphates are introduced into permeabilized platelets show that IP$_3$ in physiologic concentrations causes calcium to be released from its internal storage organelles (144, 145) and that elevated $[Ca^{2+}]_i$ is associated with platelet shape change, secretion, and aggregation. IP$_3$ binds to specific receptors on the dense tubular system. The IP$_3$ receptor from smooth endoplasmic reticulum has been characterized as a tetramer of 260,000 dalton glycoprotein subunits whose activity may be regulated by tyrosine phosphorylation (146–148). The IP$_3$ receptor is coupled to a calcium pump (together forming the calcium channel), which is inactivated by IP$_3$ when it is in conjunction with the increased $[Ca^{2+}]_i$ following channel activation (149, 150). Quantal $Ca^{2+}$ release is an intrinsic property of the receptor. Recent studies of IP$_3$ binding to human-platelet, dense, tubular membranes reveal that there may be two conformational states of the IP$_3$ receptor with a shift from the low affinity state ($K_d \geqslant 13.2$ nM) to the high affinity state ($K_d \geqslant 0.32$ nM) caused by $[Ca^{2+}]_i$ (151). In addition, IP$_3$ binding to its platelet receptor is modulated by pH, monovalent cations, other divalent cations, and guanosine triphosphate (GTP). The regulatory influence of pH may be particularly important since small increases of pH, such as those that accompany platelet activation, dramatically increase the binding of IP$_3$ to its platelet receptor.

Inositol 1,2-(cyclic)-4,5-trisphosphate may also regulate $[Ca^{2+}]_i$. This is formed within 10 seconds of thrombin-induced platelet activation (152). Its capacity to provoke $^{45}Ca$ release when injected into permeabilized platelets (as does IP$_3$) suggests that it may be functionally important in intact platelets (153).

$Ca^{2+}$ influx from the extracellular space across the plasma membrane contributes to the rise of $[Ca^{2+}]_i$ that develops following platelet activation. Both the magnitude of the peak and the duration of $[Ca^{2+}]_i$ responses to platelet activation are increased in the presence of extracellular $Ca^{2+}$. Experiments using "strong agonists" (thrombin, TXA$_2$, PAF, serotonin) and a "weak agonist" (ADP) show divalent cation movement into platelets. ADP appears to activate a receptor-operated channel, while other agonists effect $Ca^{2+}$ influx through a capacitative calcium channel activated in response to IP$_3$-mediated discharge of stored $Ca^{2+}$ (154–156).

Of note is that both inositol 1,4,5-trisphosphate and inositol 1,2-(cyclic)-4,5-trisphosphate are metabolized by a 5'-phosphomonoesterase to inactive compounds (157). A significant quantity of inositol 1,4,5-trisphosphate is also immediately phosphorylated by a 3' kinase to inositol 1,3,4,5-tetrakisphosphate [I(1, 3, 4, 5)P$_4$] (158, 159). In other cell types, this molecule has been shown to cause $Ca^{2+}$ influx across the plasma membrane followed by sequestration into storage pools, a process that reverses IP$_3$-stimulated elevations of $[Ca^{2+}]_i$ (160, 161). This suggests that the phosphorylation of platelet IP$_3$ to I(1, 3, 4, 5)P$_4$ may activate capacitative $Ca^{2+}$ entry. I(1, 3, 4, 5)P$_4$ is also metabolized by a 5' phosphomonoesterase to inositol 1,3,4-trisphosphate, the levels of which peak 60 seconds following platelet activation and persist for up to 10 minutes. Inositol 1,3,4-trisphosphate may function to maintain $[Ca^{2+}]_i$, perhaps by effecting transmembranous $Ca^{2+}$ movement through a specific channel (162). I(1, 3, 4, 5)-P$_4$ can also be metabolized back to IP$_3$, and thereby maintain the platelet $Ca^{2+}$ response, by the activity of a 3' phosphomonoesterase (163).

ADP has been reported to cause a rapid rise (<1 sec) of $[Ca^{2+}]_i$ in cyclooxygenase-inhibited platelets unable to hydrolyze PIP$_2$ to IP$_3$ (164). The ADP-induced $Ca^{2+}$ response is biphasic, with this initial rise being independent of *both* IP$_3$ and extracellular $Ca^{2+}$, suggesting the existence of a third pool of mobilizable $Ca^{2+}$ (165). This could represent a plasma membrane–bound $Ca^{2+}$ compartment that is important in weak, agonist-induced activation of phospholipase A$_2$ (see below). Most data point to GP IIb-IIIa as a component of this compartment (166).

The major binding site for $Ca^{2+}$ on unstimulated platelets is the GP IIb-IIIa complex (167). This has led to the hypothesis that GP IIb-IIIa is involved in the transmembranous influx of $Ca^{2+}$ that occurs during platelet activation (168). Experiments using monoclonal antibodies to block GP IIb-IIIa of platelets (168), or monoclonal antibodies (169) or synthetic ligand peptides (170) to block GP IIb-IIIa in liposomes, demonstrate an associated inhibition of transmembranous $Ca^{2+}$ influx. In human erythroleukemia (HEL) cells (a cell line with many features of megakaryocytes), GP IIb-IIIa appears not to participate directly in agonist-induced changes of $[Ca^{2+}]_i$ (171). It is likely that GP IIb-IIIa plays an indirect role in agonist-induced changes of $[Ca^{2+}]_i$ by regulating a plasma-membrane $Ca^{2+}$ channel (172).

The mechanisms by which $Ca^{2+}$ regulates cellular

responses are understood in some detail (173). $[Ca^{2+}]_i$ contributes to platelet activation through several effector pathways, including the activation of $Ca^{2+}$/calmodulin-dependent protein kinases, $Ca^{2+}$-dependent proteases, phospholipases C and $A_2$, and protein kinase C. Platelet $[Ca^{2+}]_i$ is measured by cytosol-trapped fluorophores or photoproteins which exhibit distinct spectral characteristics when bound to $Ca^{2+}$. These reagents not only allow measurement of $[Ca^{2+}]_i$, but may help detect different pools of $[Ca^{2+}]_i$. Experiments employing these reagents demonstrate that "strong agonists" cause direct elevation of platelet $[Ca^{2+}]_i$, that the rise of $[Ca^{2+}]_i$ in response to ADP and serotonin is inhibited by blocking cyclooxygenase metabolism, and that the $[Ca^{2+}]_i$ response to epinephrine can be measured only with the photoprotein aequorin (174, 175).

The platelet contains $Ca^{2+}$/calmodulin-dependent protein kinases that are activated by elevated $[Ca^{2+}]_i$. One of these is myosin light chain kinase. Myosin light chain is a 20,000 dalton protein that is the major $Ca^{2+}$/calmodulin-dependent protein kinase substrate of platelets; its phosphorylation following platelet activation is observed by gel electrophoresis of radiophosphorus-labeled platelets. The phosphorylation of myosin light chain is directly involved in platelet shape change, contraction, and secretion. Platelet myosin light chain kinase has been partially purified (176, 177). $Ca^{2+}$ induces the binding of calmodulin to the kinase, with consequent enzyme activation resulting in the phosphorylation of myosin light chain. The diphosphorylation of myosin light chain permits the myosin hexamer to be activated by actin, and this activation generates the forces required for shape change and secretion (178). Myosin light chain kinase may also regulate agonist-stimulated $Ca^{2+}$ influx pathways in platelets (179, 180). Phosphorylase kinase is also a $Ca^{2+}$/calmodulin-dependent protein kinase that contributes to these events by activating phosphorylase, leading to increased cytosolic ATP used to fuel the activation of the contractile apparatus (181).

In addition to the $Ca^{2+}$/calmodulin-dependent responses of activated platelets, other important $Ca^{2+}$-dependent biochemical reactions contribute to platelet function. There are two $Ca^{2+}$-dependent proteases in human platelets (calpain I and II) that may play a role in platelet activation. $Ca^{2+}$-dependent protease cleavage of actin-binding protein and talin contributes to platelet cytoskeletal reorganization that is required for platelet aggregation (182, 183). Both calpains also cleave platelet vitronectin, resulting in the loss of vitronectin's heparin- and cell-binding functions (184). Calpains may also be involved in the regulation of PLCβ3; calpain-mediated proteolysis of this PLC isoform is a prerequisite for its activation by heterotrimeric G protein βγ subunits (185). As discussed above, calpains contribute to

agonist-induced platelet procoagulant activity and the shedding of procoagulant-rich microparticles.

Both platelet PLC and $PLA_2$, which cleaves the ester-linked C-2 position fatty acyl group from phospholipids, are regulated by $Ca^{2+}$ (186–188). Platelet PLC activation is $Ca^{2+}$-dependent, and the level of $[Ca^{2+}]_i$ may affect substrate specificity. Activation of $PLA_2$ is $Ca^{2+}$-dependent, and this results in the release and metabolism of arachidonic acid (see below). The activation of protein kinase C is also dependent on $[Ca^{2+}]_i$ (see below).

Specific intraplatelet inhibitory signals counterbalance $Ca^{2+}$-mediated platelet activation. The most important of these are cAMP and cGMP, which antagonize all $Ca^{2+}$-dependent reactions through the activation of their cognate kinases (see below). In addition, the 5′ phosphomonoesterase discussed above inactivates the $IP_3$ signal for $Ca^{2+}$ release from intracellular stores by converting $IP_3$ (inositol 1,4,5-trisphosphate) to $IP_2$ (inositol 1,4-bisphosphate). There is evidence that PKC regulates the activity of the 5′ phosphomonoesterase through the phosphorylation of the 47,000 dalton platelet protein termed "pleckstrin" (platelet leukocyte c-kinase substrate), which forms a complex and thereby activates the 5′ phosphomonoesterase (189). PKC may also cause feedback inhibition of another important $Ca^{2+}$-mediated response by phosphorylating myosin light chain and thereby inhibiting the activation of the contractile apparatus (177).

## PROTEIN KINASE C

Protein kinase C (PKC) is a closely related family of serine/threonine kinases of $M_r \sim 80,000$ that require phosphatidylserine for their activation (190). There are 11 mammalian isoforms of PKC coded for by distinct genes located on different chromosomes. These isoforms are grouped into three types: the conventional (c) PKCα, βI, βII, and γ; the new (n) PKC δ, ε, η (L), θ, and μ; and the atypical (a) PKCζ and λ. The cPKCs generally require diacylglycerol (DG), $Ca^{2+}$, and phosphatidylserine (PS). The nPKCs require only DG and PS and do not require $Ca^{2+}$. The aPKCs are activated in the absence of both $Ca^{2+}$ and DG; they are activated by free fatty acids and polyphosphoinositides.

PKCα, βI, βII, and δ are the major isoforms, and ε, η, and ζ are the minor isoforms, identified by immunoblotting platelet lysates (191–194). In stimulated human platelets, PLC-generated sn-1,2-DG is released into the matrix of the plasma membrane and then rapidly recycled back into the phosphoinositides via its phosphorylation to phosphatidic acid catalyzed by the enzyme diacylglycerol kinase. Membrane-bound DG triggers the translocation of inactive PKC from the cytosol to the membrane; PKC translocated to the membrane is then activated in the presence of $Ca^{2+}$ and phosphatidylserine (195). DG increases the affinity of inactive PKC for $Ca^{2+}$ such that only small increases of $[Ca^{2+}]_i$ are required to effect PKC activation. In agonist-stimulated platelets, however, both DG and elevated $[Ca^{2+}]_i$ synergistically activate PKC. Agonist-stimulated accumulation of platelet DG may be delayed and multiphasic, possibly as a consequence of the sequential hydrolysis of different membrane phospholipids, and this might contribute to the continued activation of PKC and secondary aggregation and secretion (196).

Human platelets contain a large amount of PKC, and the cPKC and nPKC isoforms are primarily activated as a direct consequence of agonist-induced $PIP_2$ hydrolysis. Platelet PKCα, βI, and βII may also be activated in the cytosol by free fatty acids (197), and one free fatty acid (oleic acid) selectively translocates and activates the nPKCs (194). The physiologic importance of these observations is not known. Phosphatidylinositol 3,4,5-trisphosphate, generated when platelet PI 3-kinase is activated by agonist stimulation (99), may induce the slow activation of nPKC and aPKC that contributes to the maintenance phase of aggregation (198, 199). Complement proteins $C_{5b-9}$ (200) and endotoxic lipopolysaccharides (201) also directly activate platelet PKC and may contribute to the pathogenesis of disorders such as disseminated intravascular coagulation. PKC is also activated independently of phospholipase C by phorbol esters or synthetic membrane–permeable diacylglycerols.

Studies using direct pharmacologic stimulation of PKC demonstrate that PKC activation is associated with platelet aggregation (without shape change) and secretion and the release and metabolism of arachidonic acid. In combination with $Ca^{2+}$ ionophores, direct PKC activators cause synergistic platelet responses. The mechanisms by which PKC causes platelet aggregation and secretion are incompletely understood. PKC leads to $Ca^{2+}$-independent modification of the membrane GP IIb-IIIa complex, which allows it to bind fibrinogen and support platelet aggregation (202, 203). Platelet secretion could potentially result from PKC-mediated effects on $[Ca^{2+}]_i$, but there is ambiguous evidence for phorbol ester–induced elevations of $[Ca^{2+}]_i$ (204, 205). PKC may also affect platelet responses by modulating the $Ca^{2+}$-induced activation of $PLA_2$. The release of arachidonic acid (AA) is primarily dependent on $Ca^{2+}$-mediated $PLA_2$ activation, but PKC cooperates with $Ca^{2+}$ in this process (206). This latter effect could involve lipocortins (or annexins), a group of $Ca^{2+}$ and phospholipid binding proteins with anti-$PLA_2$ activity (207). It has been suggested that PKC phosphorylates and thereby inhibits platelet lipocortin, thus enhancing $Ca^{2+}$-dependent, $PLA_2$-mediated AA release (208).

Other functions of PKC that have been observed in platelets *in vitro* include signaling GP IIb-IIIa–initiated, focal-adhesion-kinase (FAK) (see below) phosphorylation that is involved in platelet spreading on a fibrinogen substrate (209). It has also been demonstrated that cytokine stimulation of platelets results in the association of PKCδ with PI 3-kinase (210). These two observations suggest that PKC can effect "rebound" or bidirectional signaling between a receptor molecule (GP IIb-IIIa) or a signal molecule (PI 3-kinase): PKC activates these molecules, which then further activate PKC. This phenomenon may serve to maintain or amplify a triggering stimulus. Platelet PKC also activates mitogen-activated-protein (MAP) kinase and may be involved in regulating $Na^+/H^+$ exchange through MAP kinase or by direct phosphorylation of the $Na^+/H^+$ exchanger (see below) (211).

Physiologic and pharmacologic activation of PKC is associated with the phosphorylation of a 47,000 dalton platelet protein, pleckstrin, which has served as a useful marker for platelet PKC activation. The identity of this substrate of PKC is uncertain. Platelet pleckstrin has been cloned and expressed (212). The identification of pleckstrin cDNA has allowed for functional analyses in heterologous cells. There is indirect evidence that phosphorylated pleckstrin inhibits the accessibility of polyphosphoinositides to hydrolysis by PLCβ and PLCγ (213). As described above, there is also evidence that phosphorylated pleckstrin binds to and activates inositol polyphosphate 5'-phosphatase (189). Additionally, there is evidence that phosphorylated pleckstrin inhibits βγ-activated PI 3-kinase γ (214).

Preincubating platelets with phorbol esters or synthetic DG results in the partial inhibition of subsequent responses to thrombin. $PIP_2$ turnover, $IP_3$ generation, and $Ca^{2+}$ mobilization and secretion are attenuated when PKC is activated prior to thrombin stimulation (215), and relatively selective inhibitors of PKC eliminate this effect of phorbol esters on thrombin-induced PLC activity (216). These data indicate that PKC causes feedback inhibition of platelet activation. More recent observations of the biology of platelet pleckstrin in heterologous systems are consistent with this concept (198, 211, 214). Experiments in intact megakaryocyte lineage (HEL) cells (217) and intact platelets (218) suggest that PKC (perhaps PKCβ) effects feedback inhibition by inhibiting $Ca^{2+}$ influx. Thus, PKC is an important branchpoint for the flow of positive and negative signals discharged from an initiating stimulus, with the activation of PKC contributing initially to platelet activation and subsequently leading to distinct activation-dampening responses.

The activity of PKC is primarily controlled by the metabolism of DG. PKC activity decreases in parallel with the decline in intracellular DG following platelet stimulation, and this is accompanied by dephosphorylation of pleckstrin. DG is predominantly converted to phosphatidic acid (PA) by the action of DG kinase, and

PA is then recycled into the phosphoinositide pool. A smaller amount of DG is converted to monoacylglycerols by the action of specific lipases. In addition to DG-mediated PKC regulation, PKC activity is inhibited by elevated levels of platelet cAMP (219). Sphingosine and lysosphingolipids may be physiologic inhibitors of platelet PKC (220, 221). 14-3-3 proteins, which are present in human platelets, may regulate PKC activity; the addition of peptides containing a PKC pseudosubstrate domain of 14-3-3 to permeabilized platelets inhibited the activation (but not translocation) of PKC in response to thrombin or phorbol esters (222). Finally, calpain cleavage of PKC may serve to turn PKC off (223).

## PHOSPHOLIPASE $A_2$ (PLA$_2$)

The group of phospholipases collectively termed PLA$_2$ plays a pivotal role in platelet stimulus-response coupling. There are two groups of PLA$_2$ in human platelets. Group (or type) II PLA$_2$ is a secreted enzyme of ~ 14,000 daltons. It requires millimolar $Ca^{2+}$ for activation (as is present in extracellular fluids). It has no preference for phosphatidylcholine as a substrate, nor does it prefer arachidonic acid (AA) in the *sn*-2 position (224, 225). Group IV cytosolic (c) PLA$_2$ comprises the predominant, functional PLA$_2$ of platelets. cPLA$_2$ is an 85,000 dalton protein that preferentially hydrolyzes AA from the *sn*-2 position of phosphatidylcholine, which is the predominant plasma membrane phospholipid. It becomes activated when $[Ca^{2+}]_i$ reaches micromolar concentrations following PLC activation. The activation of cPLA$_2$ in platelets also involves its phosphorylation (226). In other cell types, and perhaps platelets, this phosphorylation results from PKC-dependent activation of a MAP kinase (see below) (227). PLA$_2$ may also be activated directly by a heterotrimeric G protein independent of PLC (225). Both of these latter activation mechanisms could potentially bypass the $Ca^{2+}$ requirement.

The major physiologic effect of platelet PLA$_2$ activity is the release of endogenous arachidonic acid (AA) from membrane phospholipid pools. With the release of AA, PLA$_2$ activity simultaneously generates a lysophospholipid that is the substrate for the formation of platelet activating factor (PAF).

Almost all of the AA released following platelet activation is derived from cPLA$_2$-mediated phospholipid hydrolysis. Phosphatidylcholine is the preferred substrate (probably related simply to its larger quantity), but PLA$_2$ also hydrolyzes AA from phosphatidylethanolamine, phosphatidylserine, and, to a lesser extent, phosphatidylinositol. Some AA is also released from the C-2 position of DAG or phosphatidic acid, but these are minor sources of the free fatty acid.

Following deacylation, AA is rapidly metabolized to a diverse group of 20-carbon biologically active products (termed eicosanoids) through the cyclooxygenase and lipoxygenase pathways (Fig. 12.5). In human platelets, cyclooxygenase oxygenates AA to the prostaglandin endoperoxides PGG$_2$ and PGH$_2$, which are then converted to thromboxane A$_2$ (TXA$_2$) by thromboxane synthase. These highly labile AA derivatives are potent platelet agonists that bind to specific platelet receptors and, through G$_q$, directly activate phospholipase C. Small amounts of AA are also converted to PGD$_2$, PGF$_{2a}$, and PGE$_2$, less potent inhibitory eicosanoids that may serve to dampen the platelet response. AA is also oxygenated via platelet 12-lipoxygenase to quantitatively significant 12-monohydroperoxy and 12-monohydroxy fatty acids (12-HPETE and 12-HETE, respectively). *In vitro*, these products inhibit a number of platelet responses to AA and its derivatives, but their physiologic relevance is minor.

Platelets supply eicosanoid substrates to endothelium and vascular smooth muscle, which convert them to biologically important PGI$_2$ (105). Conversely, platelets can convert neutrophil-derived leukotrienes into proinflammatory lipoxins (228). "Packages" of AA are delivered via microparticles from activated platelets. These AA-rich microparticles are metabolized by adjacent platelets, resulting in an amplification scheme mediated by their conversion to TXA$_2$ (229).

PLA$_2$ has a broad specificity for different phospholipids having diverse, acyl chain structures. This is particularly relevant to the biologic consequences of dietary supplementation with fish oils enriched in $\omega$-3 fatty acids, including eicosapentaenoic acid (EPA). Platelet PLA$_2$ hydrolyzes EPA from the C-2 position of membrane phospholipids, and its subsequent metabolism to inactive triene cyclooxygenase products (including TXA$_3$ rather than TXA$_2$) accounts in part for its antiplatelet effects. PLA$_2$ is also important in the synthesis of PAF (1-O-alkyl-2-acetyl-*sn*-glyceryl-3-phosphocholine) because it hydrolyzes 1-alkyl-2-acyl-phosphocholine to lyso-PAF, which is then converted to PAF by an acetyltransferase. Platelet levels of PAF probably contribute little to the state of platelet activation, but released PAF may be important in the recruitment of circulating blood cells, particularly neutrophils, to sites of vascular injury (230).

The regulation of platelet PLA$_2$ is not completely understood. Activation depends on elevations of $[Ca^{2+}]_i$ and phosphorylation by PKC, MAP kinase, or another kinase (226) and is independent of calmodulin. There is some evidence that Na$^+$/H$^+$ exchange provides membrane-level regulation of PLA$_2$ independent of $[Ca^{2+}]_i$ (see below). PLA$_2$ activation may be opposed by the endogenous protein inhibitor(s) termed lipocortin, and this effect of lipocortin may be blocked by PKC-mediated phosphorylation (208). Direct, G protein–induced, PLA$_2$ activation may also be turned off by PKC (231).

## OTHER SIGNAL PATHWAYS
### Na$^+$/H$^+$ Exchange

The platelet Na$^+$/H$^+$ countertransporter maintains basal cytosolic pH (pH$_i$) and becomes activated follow-

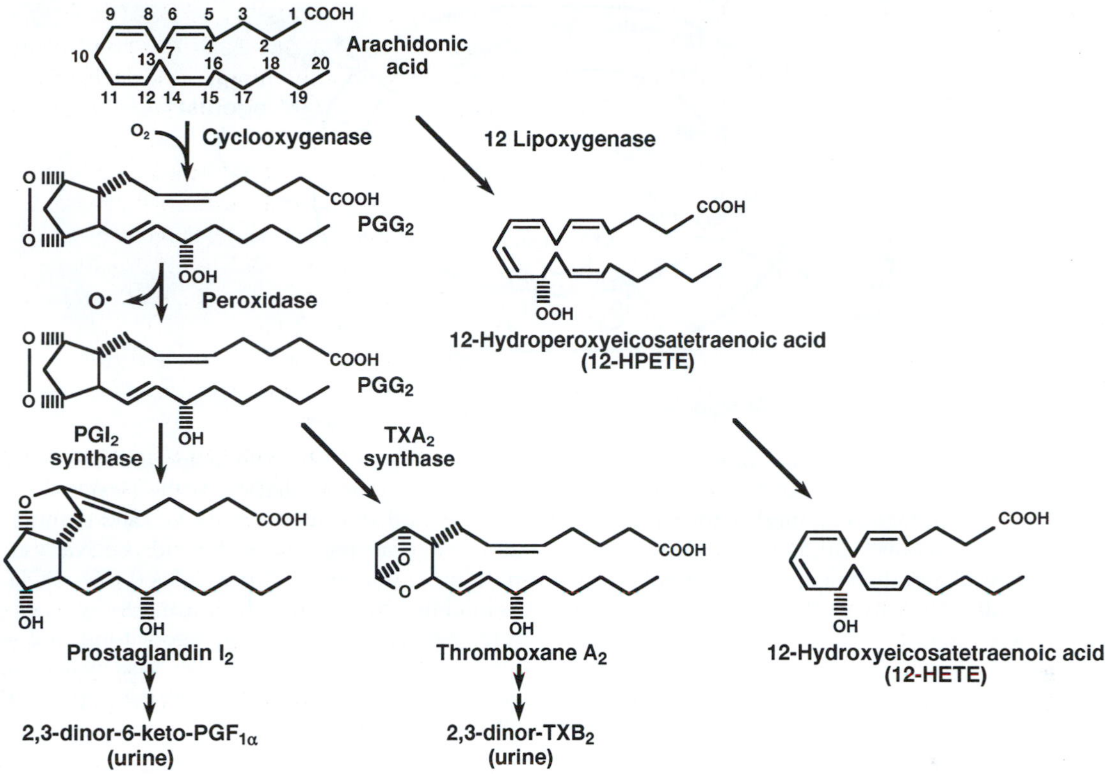

**FIGURE 12.5.** Pathways of arachidonic acid (AA) metabolism in platelets and endothelial cells. AA is liberated from membrane phospholipid and converted by prostaglandin (PG) $G_2/H_2$ synthase to prostaglandin endoperoxides (cyclooxygenase pathway). This pathway is inhibited by aspirin. The endoperoxides are then metabolized in different cells to products with opposite functions: platelet thromboxane $A_2$ (TXA$_2$) is proaggregatory and vasoconstricting, while endothelial cell prostacyclin (PGI$_2$) is antiaggregatory and vasodilatory. These eicosanoids are then nonenzymatically metabolized to stable 2,3 dinor end-products. Platelets also contain 12-lipoxygenase that converts AA to 12-HETE, the function of which is uncertain.

ing platelet stimulation. One observes a resting $pH_i$ of approximately 7.2 and a 0.1 to 0.5 pH unit rise above resting $pH_i$ occurring in platelets following agonist stimulation (232). The platelet membrane $Na^+/H^+$ counter-transporter is 110,000 dalton glycoprotein regulated by $pH_i$, $[Ca^{2+}]_i$, and PKC (233). A number of important platelet responses may be regulated by $pH_i$, including the activation of PLA$_2$, GP IIb-IIIa function, $[Ca^{2+}]_i$, and phosphoinositide metabolism.

$Na^+/H^+$ exchange may be involved in the mechanism by which "weak agonists" (such as ADP or epinephrine) activate platelet PLA$_2$. This concept is based on the observations that AA release does not occur without cytosolic alkalinization, that inhibition of $Na^+/H^+$ exchange prevents PLC activation in response to weak agonists, and that this inhibition is overcome by a synthetic prostaglandin endoperoxide (234, 235). Weak agonists initiate $Na^+/H^+$ exchange–dependent activation of PLA$_2$ resulting in the release of minute quantities of AA metabolized to prostaglandin endoperoxides and TXA$_2$ that then activate PLC (Fig. 12.6). This may involve the $Na^+/H^+$ exchange–mediated release of membrane-bound $Ca^{2+}$ (IP$_3$-independent), that directly activates

PLA$_2$ (236). It has also been observed that blocking fibrinogen binding to GP IIb-IIIa inhibits epinephrine-induced cytoplasmic alkalinization, suggesting that a functional GP IIb-IIIa complex regulates $Na^+/H^+$ exchange and that fibrinogen binding to GP IIb-IIIa may be a prerequisite for $Na^+/H^+$ exchange–dependent, PLA$_2$ activation (237).

As previously stated, IP$_3$-mediated $Ca^{2+}$ release is pH-dependent. Activation-dependent changes in $pH_i$ "fine-tunes" IP$_3$-mediated $Ca^{2+}$ release in response to thrombin (238). On the other hand, platelet $[Ca^{2+}]_i$ responses to ADP or the synthetic prostaglandin endoperoxide U46619 are inhibited by at least 50% when platelet $Na^+/H^+$ exchange and resulting cytosolic alkalinization is blocked, indicating that $Na^+/H^+$ exchange plays an important role in regulating $[Ca^+]_i$ under some conditions (239). $Na^+/H^+$ exchange may also regulate platelet signal-transduction pathways by affecting the "phosphoinositide cycle." This cycle is the pathway by which DG is recycled to PIP$_2$ through the following intermediates: phosphatidic acid (PA), phosphatidylinositol and phosphatidylinositol 4-phosphate. $pH_i$ regulates the enzyme DG kinase (which converts DG to PA),

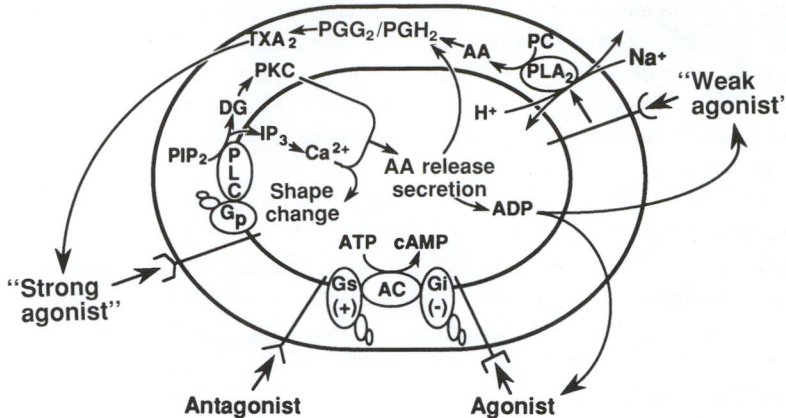

**FIGURE 12.6.** The different pathways of platelet activation. A "strong agonist" binds to a specific receptor and, through a $_{GP}$-mediated process, activates $PIP_2$-specific PLC. This results in second messengers that cause the elevation of $[Ca^{2+}]_i$ and the activation of PKC, which together stimulate the release of membrane-bound arachidonic acid (AA) and granule constituents (such as ADP). A "weak agonist" binds to a specific receptor and, through a process that depends on $Na^+/H^+$ exchange, activates $PLA_2$. This results in the release of AA and its metabolism to prostaglandin endoperoxides ($PGG_2/PGH_2$) and $TXA_2$ that then feedback to directly activate PLC. The metabolism of AA is inhibited by aspirin, which irreversibly blocks the activity of $PGG_2/PGH_2$ synthase ("cyclooxygenase"), and this is the reason for aspirin's effect on weak agonist-induced secretion and secondary aggregation. Certain platelet agonists (e.g., ADP) also inhibit the activation of adenylyl cyclase by activating $G_i$. PLC, phospholipase C; $PIP_2$, phosphatidylinositol 4,5-bisphosphate; DG, diacylglycerol; $IP_3$, inositol 1,4,5-trisphosphate; PKC, protein kinase C; $PLA_2$, phospholipase $A_2$; AC, adenylyl cyclase; PC, phosphatidylcholine.

thereby permitting the platelet phosphoinositide cycle to proceed and contributing to thrombin-induced aggregation and secretion (240).

## Phospholipase D

Platelets contain a third phospholipase that contributes to platelet activation. Phospholipase D (PLD) cleaves the terminal phosphodiester bond of membrane phospholipids, with phosphatidylcholine as its preferred substrate. There is evidence that thrombin activates PLD after PLC is activated and that elevated $[Ca^{2+}]_i$ and/or PKC mediates PLD activation (241, 242). PLD causes the direct release of PA, which may be an important signal controlling the activation of $PLA_2$ (243, 244), perhaps by inducing a conformational change in platelet GP IIb-IIIa (245). Platelet PA is, however, primarily synthesized following $PIP_2$ breakdown by the activity of the enzyme DG kinase, converting DG to PA, and it is generally accepted that PLD-initiated signal generation contributes little to the state of platelet activation (246).

## Tyrosine Kinases

Platelets contain many proteins modified by phosphorylated tyrosine, indicating the presence of tyrosine kinases and tyrosine phosphatases often involved in signaling (137). Platelets contain large amounts of the protein tyrosine kinase pp60$^{c-src}$, as well as other tyrosine kinases, and these become activated and phosphorylate many substrates (247, 248). Their functional im-

portance and the functional importance of platelet phosphatases are poorly understood, primarily because of poor pharmacologic probes. Nonetheless, experiments with tyrosine kinase or tyrosine phosphatase inhibitors generally support the hypothesis that tyrosine kinases are involved in platelet activation.

The tyrosine kinases in platelets are nonreceptor tyrosine kinases. There are four groups: (a) the *src*-related kinases; (b) focal adhesion kinase (FAK); (c) syc kinase; and (d) the Janus kinases (JAK). C-*src* and the related *fyn, lyn, hyc,* and *yes* are the predominant kinases. They are ~60,000 daltons and contain homologous *src* homology SH2 and SH3 domains that effect intermolecular interactions (phosphotyrosine and polyproline recognition, respectively), sites for tyrosine phosphorylation that switches them "on," and lipid anchors that mediate membrane associations. These kinases become tyrosine phosphorylated rapidly, translocate to the cytoskeleton, and develop many new molecular associations, including associations with GP IIb-IIIa and FAK, following platelet activation with chemical agonists and collagen. They may be involved early in the activation of PLCγ (138) and later in the attachment of ligand-engaged GP IIb-IIIa to the cytoskeleton, resulting in the activation of FAK, platelet spreading, and platelet-mediated fibrin clot retraction (65, 249). Their activity is in large part terminated by tyrosine phosphatases.

FAK is a 125,000 dalton protein that interacts with platelet GP IIb-IIIa. It is the major signal transducer originating from fibrinogen binding to GP IIb-IIIa. It is activated when resting platelets are placed on insoluble fibrinogen, or after activated platelets bind cohesive soluble fibrinogen. It has binding domains for the cytoplasmic domain of β integrins, *src,* cytoskeletal proteins, PI 3-kinases and adaptor proteins coupled to the *ras*/MAP kinase signaling system. FAK can also be phosphorylated (and presumably activated) by the platelet FcγRII (250). FAK activation influences cytoskeletal changes that permit platelet spreading and clot retraction. FAK phosphorylation in response to ligand binding GP IIb-IIIa, or by crosslinking the Fc receptors, is mediated in part by PKC, implying that it can be regulated by both serine/threonine and *src*-related tyrosine kinases (209, 250). FAK activity is terminated by a calpain.

Syc is a 72,000 dalton cytosolic protein with two SH2 domains. Unlike *src* and FAK, it is expressed only in hematopoietic cells. Syc deficiency in mice is associated with lethal embryonic bleeding, suggesting that it may be a relatively important platelet signal molecule. Of note, mouse deficiencies of *src* and its related kinases have no obvious effect on the platelets. Syc is rapidly phosphorylated and translocates to the cytoskeleton in response to thrombin, TXA$_2$, collagen binding to GP VI, FcγRII crosslinking, or ligand binding to GP IIb-IIIa (51, 136, 251). It associates with the platelet Fc receptor and PI 3-kinase (99). Its regulation and functional effects in human platelets are not yet known.

The JAKS in platelets are JAK2, TYK1, and TYK2. These are cytosolic kinases that generally interact directly with cytokine receptors to effect nuclear signaling (252). Thrombin induces a delayed Ca$^{2+}$ and PKC-dependent phosphorylation of JAK2 (137). In platelets activated by thrombopoietin (TPO), JAK2 and TYK2 are phosphorylated and activated, and they catalyze the tyrosine phosphorylation of STAT (signal transducers and activators of transcription) 3 and STAT5 (84, 85). This may represent a vestigial signaling system relevant only to the megakaryocyte, although TPO synergizes with other platelet agonists to activate platelets *in vitro.*

There are three cytosolic tyrosine phosphatases in platelets: protein tyrosine phosphatase (PTP) 1B, SH2-containing phosphatase (SHP)-1, and SHP-2. Many substrates for tyrosine phosphorylation in platelets have been identified, and because the state of tyrosine phosphorylation reflects a balance between kinase and phosphatase activities, some data are available about platelet tyrosine phosphatases and how they might affect platelet activation. This is in contrast to the paucity of information about serine or threonine phosphatases.

Inhibitors of tyrosine phosphatases are, like tyrosine kinase inhibitors, relatively nonspecific, but give fairly consistent data in support of the hypothesis that tyrosine phosphatases terminate platelet activation signals. Their mechanism of action is not understood. In stimulated platelets, PTP1B is activated slowly by calpain cleavage

and translocates to the cytoskeleton (253). SHP-1 becomes rapidly phosphorylated (on one tyrosine and one threonine) and translocates to the cytoskeleton following thrombin receptor activation (254). Prolonged SHP-1 activation requires ligand-occupied GP IIb-IIIa. Activated SHP-1 associates with *src* through its SH2 domain (255). In immune cells this deactivates tyrosine phosphorylated *src* and inhibits its activation of PLCγ (256). Platelets may also have SH2-containing inositol phosphatases (SHIP), which dampen stimulation by cleaving phosphates from the inositol ring of soluble inositol polyphosphates or membrane-bound phosphatidylinositol polyphosphates (257).

## Phosphatidylinositol 3-Kinases

The best studied PI 3-kinase in platelets is a heterodimeric protein containing a regulatory 85,000 dalton subunit (with two SH2 and one SH3 domains) and a catalytic 110,000 dalton subunit. There is also a 110,000 dalton protein that contains a pleckstrin homology domain (that may localize the protein to phospholipid-containing structures) and a catalytic domain; this molecule is designated PI 3-kinase γ (99). PI 3-kinases phosphorylate the 3 position of the inositol ring (Fig. 12.4). They use all phosphoinositides as substrate, but have a preference for phosphatidylinositol 4,5 bisphosphate, resulting in the synthesis of PI 3,4,5 tetrakisphosphate.

Platelet PI 3-kinase p85/p110 is activated by ligands that activate PKC (258). Platelet PI 3-kinase γ is activated by heterotrimeric, G protein βδ subunits released by thrombin receptor (and perhaps other heptahelical receptor) activation (259). In both cases, the PI 3-kinase translocates to the cytoskeleton and develops new molecular associations. Neither kinase is phosphorylated. The relevant associations for p85/p110 PI 3-kinase include cytoskeletal proteins (α-actinin and vinculin), signal molecules (*src,* syc, and PKC), and surface receptors (FcγRII and GP IIb-IIIa) (99, 260).

The regulation of PI 3-kinase activity is uncertain. For the p85/p110 PI 3-kinase, PKC is involved in the initiation of its activation. GP IIb-IIIa and the low-molecular-weight, GTP binding protein Rho are involved in maintaining activation (99). This PI 3-kinase has intrinsic serine kinase activity that is stimulated along with its lipid kinase activity. This catalyses the phosphorylation of the regulatory p85 subunit, resulting in the inhibition of lipid kinase activity. Phosphopleckstrin inhibits βδ-stimulated PI 3-kinase γ activation (261). Little else is known about the regulation of PI 3-kinase. Time course data suggest an early peak in the production of PI 3,4,5-P$_3$, followed by a rapid decline to basal levels. The majority of 3 phosphorylated product is actually PI 3,4-P$_2$ (262), suggesting that PI 3,4,5-P$_3$ is rapidly broken down by a 5-phosphatase (i.e., SHIP described above).

The effects of these phosphorylation events on platelet activation are incompletely understood. It is nearly certain that PI 3,4,5-$P_3$ signals the activation of PKC and, through this, contributes to secretion and aggregation (198, 199). It is also clear that PI 3-kinase activity, perhaps initiated by ligand engagement by this receptor, maintains GP IIb-IIIa in an active conformation and promotes continued, cohesive, platelet-platelet interactions (i.e., aggregation) (262).

## Mitogen Activated Protein Kinases

Platelets contain at least three MAP kinases, including extracellular receptor activated kinase (ERK) 1, ERK 2, and p38 MAP kinase (263). These kinases are activated by phosphorylation of both threonine and tyrosine residues by MAP kinase kinases, whose activity is present in platelets (264). Platelet MAP kinase activation is probably coupled to G protein receptor activation by PKC, perhaps through activation of MAP kinase kinase (265). Platelet MAP kinases catalyze serine and threonine phosphorylations of both cPLA$_2$ and the Na$^+$/H$^+$ exchanger, but these phosphorylations are minor signals for the activation of these signal molecules (211, 226, 227). Inhibitor studies suggest that platelet MAP kinases are functionally insignificant (266).

## Ion Channels

For years electrophysiologists dismissed all blood cells as electrically "nonexcitable." In 1978 this concept was challenged by Miller et al (267), who impaled guinea pig megakaryocytes with paired electrodes and showed that these cells, like myocytes and neurons, underwent action potentials when injected with small depolarizing currents. With the development and refinement of the patch-clamp technique came the ability to isolate and study ion channels in the plasma membranes of single blood cells (268, 269). Using this powerful technology, a number of laboratories have now provided clear evidence that megakaryocytes and platelets contain an impressive array of ion channels that permit them to harness electricity to carry out a variety of functions. Voltage-dependent (270) and Ca$^{2+}$-dependent (271–273) K$^+$ channels, nonselective cation channels (274–277), and Ca$^{2+}$-dependent Cl$^-$ channels (278) have been described in human platelets. These channels regulate a variety of biophysical properties of the cells, including cell volume, membrane potential, and cytosolic pH. They also contribute to the transient elevations in cytosolic Na$^+$ and Ca$^{2+}$ which participate in platelet secretion and aggregation.

On exposure to hypoösmolar stress, platelets initially swell, but then shrink toward their original volume in a process referred to as *regulatory volume decrease* (RVD) (279). In most cells RVD results from simultaneous increases in K$^+$ and Cl$^-$ conductances, which then permit nonelectrogenic efflux of K$^+$ and Cl$^-$ ions together with osmotically obligated water molecules (280). The specific ion channels that accommodate the K$^+$ and Cl$^-$ conductances under these conditions have not been clarified (279, 281). In response to hypertonic stress, platelets shrink and Na$^+$/H$^+$ exchange is activated (279).

Platelets maintain a resting membrane potential of $-48$ to $-70$ mV. In response to activation by agonists such as ADP or thrombin, depolarization of variable degree occurs (282). Thrombin-induced depolarization of the platelet's plasma membrane depends on Na$^+$ in the external medium (283), a finding that strongly implicates electrogenic Na$^+$ influx in the depolarization process. Thrombin-mediated activation of platelets results in a doubling of the cytosolic Na$^+$ concentration ([Na$^+$]$_i$), (284, 285). This elevation of [Na$^+$]$_i$ that accompanies thrombin activation may result from the action of Na$^+$/H$^+$ or Na$^+$/Ca$^{2+}$ antiporters or from inhibition of the Na$^+$/K$^+$ pump. Alkalinization of the cytosol follows elevations in [Na$^+$]$_i$ owing to increased Na$^+$/H$^+$ exchange. Elevation in [Na$^+$]$_i$ has also been shown to increase Ca$^{2+}$ influx via electrogenic Na$^+$/Ca$^{2+}$ exchange in platelets (286–288). Elevations of [Na$^+$]$_i$ have also been postulated to modulate receptor-coupled activation of heterotrimeric G proteins (289).

Following platelet stimulation, [Ca$^{2+}$]$_i$ briefly rises to near micromolar levels from both IP$_3$-mediated release of Ca$^{2+}$ from intracellular stores and Ca$^{2+}$ influx across the plasma membrane (see above). By introducing membrane vesicles from human platelets into planar lipid bilayers, Zschauer et al identified a 10 pS, divalent cation channel in thrombin-activated platelets that was absent in control platelet membranes (156). They proposed that channels highly selective for Ca$^{2+}$ opened in the plasma membrane of platelets in response to thrombin activation. Mahaut-Smith et al also proposed that Ca$^{2+}$ influx in response to thrombin occurred through Ca$^{2+}$-selective channels too small to be detected by the patch clamp technique (274). The molecular identity of these divalent cation channels in platelets remains undiscovered.

## Histamine

Histamine is a molecule that has pleiotropic biologic effects. Recent studies suggest that histamine may be an important *intra*cellular signal molecule in human platelets mediating aggregation, although its mechanism of action is not known (290). Platelets contain the enzyme responsible for the synthesis of histamine (histidine decarboxylase), and it appears that PKC stimulates (and Ca$^{2+}$ inhibits) its activity (291). Histamine is also an *extra*cellular signal for platelet activation *in vitro*, although its physiologic significance is unknown. Histamine binds to a platelet H$_1$ receptor and activates PLA$_2$ through a heterotrimeric G protein-mediated mechanism (292).

# SHEAR STRESS–INDUCED PLATELET ACTIVATION

As described in Chapter 20, blood flow generates wall shear stresses (4). Shear stress is described as "the force per unit area between laminae"; blood flow can be described as an "infinite number of infinitesimal laminae sliding across one another, each lamina suffering some frictional interaction with its neighbors" (293). In humans, physiologic levels of shear stress in the arterial circuit reach 25 to 30 dyne/cm$^2$ (shear rate of 625 to 750 sec$^{-1}$), and pathologic levels (e.g., as in a stenosed coronary artery) may reach >350 dyne/cm$^2$ (shear rate of 8750 sec$^{-1}$) (see Chapter 20).

Each of the triad of platelet functional responses has been observed to occur as a function of shear stress (Fig. 12.7). Shear stress affects the rate and magnitude of platelet adhesion to artificial and biologic surfaces, and it induces platelet secretion, the activation of GP IIb-IIIa, and aggregation (4, 294). High-shear platelet responses (> ~ 25 to 30 dyne/cm$^2$) depend only on vWf and platelet GP Ib-IX-V and GP IIb-IIIa, but not on plasma fibrinogen (4, 294, 295). ADP, whether released from platelets or derived from red blood cells, contributes substantially to shear stress–induced platelet responses (295). Elevations of platelet cAMP or cGMP inhibit shear stress–induced platelet aggregation (296, 297), but inhibition of cyclooxygenase metabolism with aspirin has no effect on the initiation of aggregation in response to shear stress (295).

The vWf-platelet interaction is the *sine qua non* of shear stress–induced aggregation. vWf is a multivalent, multimeric plasma protein that is essential for platelet adhesion to the subendothelium of damaged blood vessels (see Chapter 16). vWf has binding sites for platelet GP Ibα and GP IIb-IIIa, as well as sites for various suben-

dothelial constituents, including collagen. vWf bridging platelet GP Ib-IX-V to the subendothelium leads to adhesion *in vivo*, and vWf bridging GP Ib-IX-V on adjacent platelets leads to the cohesive interplatelet interactions induced by ristocetin *in vitro*. Under shear stresses *in vitro* and *in vivo*, vWf binding to GP Ib-IX-V is critically important for platelet adhesion and aggregation (298). In the plasma milieu under static conditions, vWf binding to GP IIb-IIIa is minimal (299), but when shear stress is applied to platelets, vWf binds to GP IIb-IIIa, as well as to GP Ib-IX-V, and this binding contributes substantially to platelet aggregate formation (Fig. 12.7) (300).

Activation signals play an important role in shear stress–induced platelet aggregation. $[Ca^{2+}]_i$ rises in platelets subjected to pathologic shear stress (>30 dynes/cm$^2$), and this depends on vWf binding to platelet GP Ib-IX-V and on extracellular $Ca^{2+}$ (301). Of particular note is that these changes of $[Ca^{2+}]_i$ contribute greatly to the initiation and maintenance of shear-induced aggregation. Platelet PKC is also activated by shear stress (302). As with shear stress–induced elevations of $[Ca^{2+}]_i$, PKC activation depends on vWf binding to GP Ib-IX-V, and the activation of PKC contributes to the maintenance, but not the initiation, of shear-induced platelet aggregation. There is also evidence for functionally significant shear-induced activation of tyrosine kinases and PI 3-kinase (303, 304).

Although little is known of the mechanism by which vWf binding to GP Ibα switches signals "on," recent information using a divalent snake venom protein indicates that receptor crosslinking is required for GP Ib-IX-V-initiated signaling (305). This suggests that vWf receptor clustering or tethering occurs, and this induces a conformational change in the receptor leading to platelet activation. The molecules that couple vWf binding to platelet signaling are not yet elucidated. Of note, how-

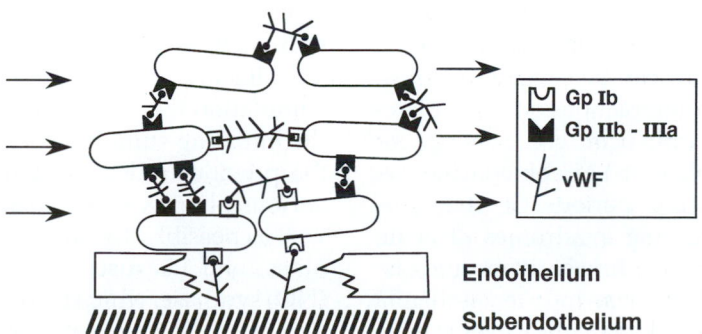

**FIGURE 12.7.** Shear stress induces platelet adhesion, release, and aggregation. Platelet adhesion is dependent on von Willebrand factor (vWf) bridging the subendothelium to platelet glycoprotein (GP) Ibα. Shear stress-induced platelet aggregation, which can occur independent of adhesion, depends on plasma vWf and platelet GP Ib-IX-V and GP IIb-IIIa, but not on plasma fibrinogen. vWf is a multivalent, multimeric plasma protein that has binding sites for platelet GP Ib-IX-V, GP IIb-IIIa and various subendothelial constituents, including collagen. It is not known whether vWf bound to GP Ib-IX-V on one platelet can bind to GP IIb-IIIa on adjacent platelets (see text for additional details).

ever, is that the cytoplasmic domain of GP Ibα binds to a 14-3-3 adaptor protein that has been implicated in coupling transmembranous receptors to signal molecules, including PKC (222, 306–309). It also appears that shear stress–induced platelet signaling differs from signaling in response to other agonists in two ways: the $[Ca^{2+}]_i$ response depends entirely on transmembranous influx, and PKC activity is not associated with the activation of PLC. These observations support the hypothesis that novel signal pathways are activated in pathological shear stress fields. If this hypothesis is true, it suggests the feasibility of developing "lesion-specific" treatments for arterial thrombosis.

# AMPLIFICATION, SYNERGY, AND COAGULATION PROTEIN INTERACTIONS

Platelet activation results in amplification events that contribute to physiologic or pathologic thrombus formation. Amplification occurs by the release of preformed platelet constituents (e.g., stored in granules) or by the *de novo* production of bioactive molecules. In either case the platelet-derived amplifier molecule acts as a platelet agonist and recruits circulating platelets into the developing thrombus. Dense granule–derived serotonin and ADP amplify the initial platelet response by activating nearby platelets. Through surface effects, the α granule constituents fibrinogen and thrombospondin contribute to the formation of a stable platelet aggregate, and fibrinogen and vWf binding platelets may be directly stimulatory (as previously described). The *de novo* production of eicosanoids, PAF, histamine, and phosphatidic acid also serves to amplify the platelet response to an initiating stimulus by affecting both autocrine and paracrine signal transduction pathways.

Synergy among platelet agonists is observed when the response of platelets to two different stimuli is greater than the arithmetic sum of the response to the individual stimuli. Synergism can be considered an *in vitro* correlate of the complex interactions between platelets and their extracellular milieu *in vivo*. Synergy involving ADP (released by platelets) or epinephrine (secreted into the blood during periods of stress) is probably important in triggering syndromes of acute coronary artery thrombosis, including early morning ischemia and infarction, and exercise-induced ischemia (310–312). A number of platelet biochemical events have been hypothesized as contributing to the phenomenon of synergy, including agonist-induced phosphoinositide turnover, protein kinase C and $Ca^{2+}$ responses, AA release and metabolism, and agonist-induced stimulation of the inhibitory G protein ($G_i$) of the adenylyl cyclase system (311–314). The mechanism(s) by which these sig-

nals contribute to synergistic responses is unknown, although there is evidence that functionally trivial rises of $[Ca^{2+}]_i$ in response to a "weak agonist," perhaps signaled by eicosanoids, "primes" the platelet aggregation response to stimulation by a second agonist. This priming could result from the generation of progressively accumulating second messenger "quanta," as has been demonstrated for the thrombin receptor (315). Presumably there is a quantum level, which can be reached by independent but converging ligand-induced signal pathways, above which full cellular activation develops.

Activated platelets are very important in regulating the generation of insoluble fibrin (316). Activated platelets express specific surface binding sites for soluble clotting factors and thereby promote critically important coagulation reactions: the activation of factor X by the factor IXa/factor VIIIa complex and the activation of prothrombin by the factor Xa/factor Va complex (317). The presence of platelet procoagulant activities can be detected by flow cytometry. Activated platelets also regulate natural anticoagulant mechanisms by promoting the inactivation of factor Va by activated protein C and by releasing two proteins, a 112,000 dalton protein that inhibits factor XIa and a low-molecular-weight protein (8500 daltons) that also inhibits factor XIa (318–320). In addition to reactions that take place on intact activated platelets or result from platelet secretion, activated platelets shed "microparticles" that may either stimulate (by binding factor V and factor VIII and promoting prothrombin activation) or inhibit (by promoting factor Va inactivation) fibrin generation (321, 322).

## Inhibitory Signals

Platelet activation is regulated by intracellular signal pathways that attenuate or prevent agonist-induced responses. The major inhibitory pathways of physiologic and pharmacologic importance that are intrinsic to the platelet and activated by extrinsic factors are mediated by elevated cytosolic cAMP or cGMP (Fig. 12.8). In addition, there are a number of inhibitory intracellular signals that are produced endogenously following platelet stimulation that may function to attenuate or terminate the initiating stimulus. These inhibitory signals include the previously described $IP_3$ 5'-phosphomonoesterase, various phophatases, calpains, and protein kinase C, as well as possibly lipocortin, platelet lipoxygenase metabolites, and (as discussed below), platelet nitric oxide (NO) synthase, which mediates the endogenous production of NO. Platelets also are affected by receptor desensitization. This is described best for the thrombin receptor, which undergoes endocytosis following proteolytic cleavage and whose activity is turned "down" by a G protein receptor kinase that phosphorylates its cytoplasmic domain (323, 324). Platelets are also inhibited when the soluble agonist ADP is broken down by an ec-

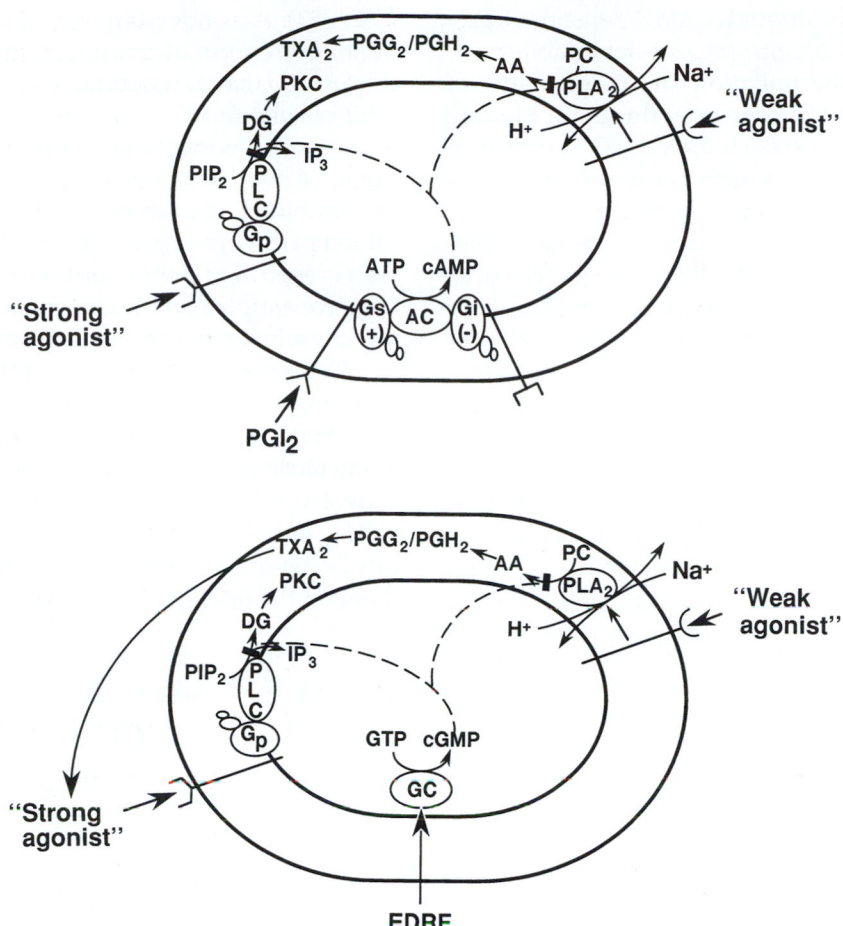

**FIGURE 12.8.**    The major inhibitory pathways in platelets are mediated by cAMP (top) or cGMP (bottom). cAMP is synthesized when extracellular eicosanoids, the most important of which may be endothelial cell-derived $PGI_2$, bind to specific platelet receptors and activate adenylyl cyclase. cGMP is synthesized when nitrovasodilators, including the endogenous nitrovasodilator nitric oxide (or endothelium-derived relaxing factor [EDRF]), diffuse through the platelet plasma membrane and activate soluble (cytosolic) guanylyl cyclase. Both cAMP and cGMP inhibit the activity of PLC and $PLA_2$, thereby blocking the proximal pathways of agonist-induced signal generation and inhibiting aspirin-insensitive mechanisms of platelet activation.

toADPase (identical to CD39) present on the adjacent vascular endothelial surface. This "prereceptor" inhibition may be an important third pathway (the first two being prostacyclin and NO production) by which vascular endothelium modulates platelet thrombus formation (325).

cAMP is synthesized when extracellular eicosanoids, the most important of which may be endothelial cell-derived $PGI_2$, bind to specific platelet receptors and activate adenylyl cyclase. cAMP probably does not regulate the state of platelet activation under physiologic conditions, but it becomes important in areas of endothelial cell injury where it functions as a "natural" antithrombotic molecule. Pharmacologic agents that elevate intraplatelet cAMP are potent platelet inhibitors (326). cGMP is synthesized when nitrovasodilators, including the "endogenous nitrovasodilator" NO (or endothelium-derived relaxing factor [EDRF]), diffuse through the platelet plasma membrane and activate soluble (cytosolic)

guanylyl cyclase (327). The basal release of NO may regulate the state of platelet activation under physiologic conditions (297), and NO production in areas of vascular injury (by both endothelium and smooth muscle) probably modulates the extent of platelet thrombus formation (328). Pharmacologic doses of nitrovasodilators cause elevations of platelet cGMP insufficient to effect platelet inhibition, but the coadministration of a reduced thiol donor, such as $N$-acetylcysteine, produces levels of platelet cGMP that inhibit platelet function *in vivo* (329).

cAMP and cGMP inhibit each component of the triad of platelet functional responses: adhesion, aggregation, and secretion (330–333). cAMP is a relatively more potent inhibitor of secretion and aggregation, and cGMP is a relatively more potent inhibitor of adhesion. The molecular mechanisms of cAMP-mediated inhibition are perhaps best studied. The generation of elevated cytosolic concentrations of cAMP, which inhibits platelet responses primarily through cAMP-dependent protein kinases, results in pleiotropic platelet inhibitory effects involving both the initiation and maintenance of platelet activation. cAMP decreases thrombin binding to platelets and inhibits PLC-mediated DG and $IP_3$ formation, DG signalling of PKC activation and the activity of PKC (334–338). cAMP inhibits many platelet responses that are distal to PKC, such as fibrinogen receptor expression, which may actually undergo "closure" when $PGI_2$ is added to stimulated platelets (336, 337). cAMP also inhibits agonist-induced polymerization of actin. This latter effect is mediated by cAMP-dependent protein kinase phosphorylation of the β subunit of GP Ib (339, 340).

The most important mechanism by which cAMP inhibits platelets is its antagonism of $Ca^{2+}$-mediated responses. PLC is the most proximal point in the common pathway leading to changes of platelet $[Ca^{2+}]_i$, and platelets treated with activators of adenylyl cyclase demonstrate no $Ca^{2+}$ response to agonists primarily because PLC-mediated generation of $IP_3$ is inhibited (338, 341). In addition, cAMP influences both the release and uptake of $Ca^{2+}$ from the dense tubular system (DTS). $IP_3$-mediated release of $Ca^{2+}$ from the DTS may be inhibited by the direct effect of the catalytic subunit of cAMP-dependent protein kinase on the DTS (342). Based on observations that adenylyl cyclase stimulators cause a rapid fall in $[Ca^{2+}]_i$ when they are added after a dose of thrombin has initiated a $Ca^{2+}$ response, it appears that cAMP stimulates the reuptake of $Ca^{2+}$ into the DTS (343). The mechanism by which this resequestration occurs may also involve the cAMP-dependent phosphorylation of a DTS structure regulating this process (343, 344). Through its effect on $[Ca^{2+}]_i$, cAMP inhibits a number of other platelet responses, including $PLA_2$-mediated release of AA (as previously described), cytoskeletal assembly (independent of GP Ibα), and the activity of myosin light chain kinase (345, 346). In this last case there is also a direct inhibitory effect of cAMP independent of $[Ca^{2+}]_i$; myosin light chain kinase is inhibited when it is phosphorylated by a cAMP-dependent protein kinase (347).

The molecular mechanisms by which cGMP inhibits platelet activation are less well understood. Elevated platelet cGMP can be induced by nitrovasodilators, nitrosothiol compounds, EDRF, or nonhydrolyzable analogs of cGMP, and this is associated with the inhibition of $PIP_2$ hydrolysis and all consequent distal signal pathways, suggesting that cGMP directly inhibits phospholipase C (348, 349). cGMP has also been shown to inhibit $PLA_2$-mediated AA release in human platelets (350).

cAMP functions synergistically with cGMP to effect the inhibition of agonist-induced platelet aggregation (351), and this may be due to the effect of cGMP on inhibiting the low $K_m$ cAMP phosphodiesterase of platelets (352, 353). An understanding of the synergistic platelet inhibitory effects of prostaglandins and nitrovasodilators *in vitro* may be useful in developing therapies to inhibit platelet function *in vivo*. Individually, these drugs demonstrate serious side effects or relative inefficacy that might be overcome when the two classes of compounds are combined. The advantage of these agents is that they inhibit pathways of platelet activation that bypass the effects of aspirin, and therefore one might be able to achieve effective antiplatelet therapy in the large number of individuals who do not respond to aspirin.

Platelet production of cGMP by an endogenous route may also contribute to the state of platelet activation. Platelets contain the constitutive form of the enzyme nitric oxide (NO) synthase, and this may become activated following agonist stimulation of platelets, resulting in the synthesis of platelet NO and the activation of platelet guanylyl synthase, which could function to dampen the aggregation response (354).

# BIOCHEMICAL PHARMACOLOGY OF ANTIPLATELET DRUGS

Antiplatelet agents, either currently available or undergoing development and clinical investigation, interfere with some steps in the activation process, including adhesion, release, and/or aggregation (Fig. 12.9). The most commonly prescribed and best known agent is aspirin, which was discovered serendipitously and whose mechanism of action (the irreversible inhibition of platelet cyclooxygenase) was elucidated long after its efficacy was established. It is clear that there are many aspirin-insensitive pathways of platelet activation, and their participation in clinical thrombosis limits the efficacy of aspirin and demands that alternative antiplatelet drugs be made available.

General inhibitors of platelet activation such as prostacyclin or organic nitrates lack specificity, resulting in dangerous nonplatelet side effects that outweigh their beneficial antiplatelet effects. The development of new agents based on an understanding of platelet activation pathways has resulted in drugs with increased specificity. The drug ReoPro® has already become an established adjunct to angioplasty for the treatment of coronary artery stenosis (see Chapter 54). ReoPro® and all of the newer agents do not, however, selectively block platelet-dependent thrombosis, and their inhibitory effect on hemostasis therefore results in bleeding complications. The next step in the development of clinically useful agents to treat arterial thrombosis is identifying antiplatelet agents that inhibit thrombosis without causing serious defects in hemostasis.

## Adhesion ("trigger")

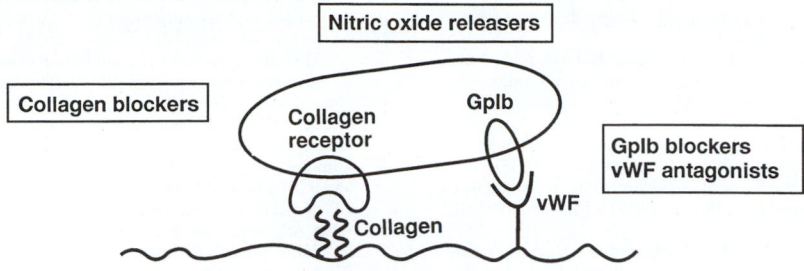

## Release ("Amplification and Recruitment")

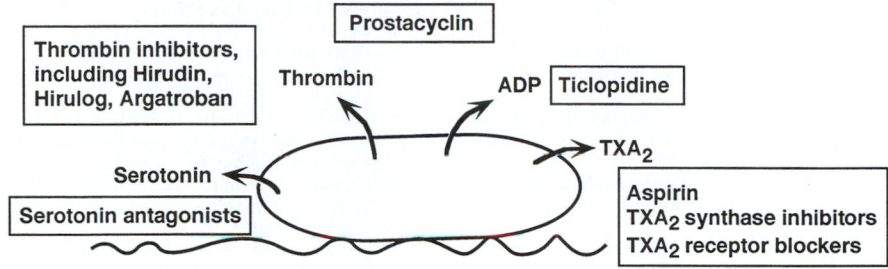

## Aggregation ("final common pathway")

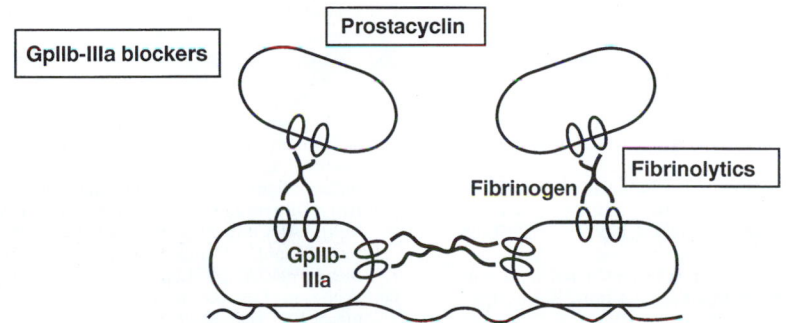

**FIGURE 12.9.**   Antiplatelet agents and their mechanisms of action. See Chapter 54 for additional details.

# REFERENCES

1. Kroll MH, Schafer AI. The analysis of ligand-receptor interactions in platelet activation. In: Joseph M, ed. Immunopharmacology of platelets. London: Academic Press, 1995; pp. 31–65.
2. Sherman CT, Litvack F, Grundfest W et al. Coronary angioscopy in individuals with unstable angina pectoris. N Engl J Med 1986;315:913–919.
3. Phillips DR, Shuman MA. Biochemistry of platelets. Orlando: Academic Press, 1986.
4. Kroll MH, Hellums JD, McIntire LV et al. Platelets and shear stress. Blood 1996;88:1525–1541.
5. Santoro SA. Identification of a 160,000 dalton platelet membrane protein that mediates the initial divalent cation-dependent adhesion of platelets to collagen. Cell 1986;46:913–920.
6. Halushka PV, Mais DE, Saussy DL Jr. Platelet and vascular smooth muscle thromboxane $A_2$/prostaglandin $H_2$ receptors. Fed Proc 1987;46:149–153.
7. Hwang SB, Lee CS, Cheah MJ et al. Specific receptor sites for 1-O-alkyl-2-O-acetyl-Sn-glycero-3-phosphocholine (platelet activating factor) on rabbit platelet and guinea pig smooth muscle membranes. Biochemistry 1983;22:4756–4763.
8. Siess W, Stifel M, Binder H et al. Activation of $V_1$-receptors by vasopressin stimulates inositol phospholipid hydrolysis and arachidonate metabolism in human platelets. Biochem J 1986;233:83–91.
9. de Chaffoy de Courcelles D, Leysen JE, de Clerck F et al. Evidence that phospholipid turnover is the signal transducing system coupled to serotonin-$S_2$ receptor sites. J Biol Chem 1985;260:7603–7608.
10. Bennett JS, Colman RF, Colman RW. Identification of adenine nucleotide binding proteins in human platelet membranes by affinity labeling with 5'-p-fluorosulfonylbenzoyl adenosine. J Biol Chem 1978;253:7346–7354.
11. Adler JR, Handin RI. Solubilization and characterization of a platelet membrane ADP-binding protein. J Biol Chem 1979;254:3866–3872.
12. Alexander RW, Cooper B, Handin RI. Characterization of the human platelet α-adrenergic receptor. Correlation of [3H] dihydroergocryptine binding with aggregation and adenylate cyclase inhibition. J Clin Invest 1978;61:1136–1144.
13. Schafer AI, Cooper B, O'Hara D et al. Identification of platelet receptors for prostaglandin $I_2$ and $D_2$. J Biol Chem 1979;254:2914–2917.
14. Dutta-Roy AK, Sinha AK. Purification and properties of prostaglandin $E_1$/prostacyclin receptor of human blood platelets. J Biol Chem 1987;262:12685–12691.
15. Eidt JF, Allison P, Noble S et al. Thrombin is an important mediator of platelet aggregation in stenosed canine coronary arteries with endothelial injury. J Clin Invest 1989;84:18–27.

16. Vu TK, Hung DT, Wheaton VI et al. Molecular cloning of a functional thrombin receptor reveals a novel proteolytic mechanism of receptor activation. Cell 1991;64:1057–1068.

17. Vu TK, Wheaton VI, Hung DT et al. Domains specifying thrombin-receptor interaction. Nature 1991;353:674–677.

18. Brass LF, Vassallo RR Jr., Belmonte E et al. Structure and function of the human platelet thrombin receptor. Studies using monoclonal antibodies directed against a defined domain within the receptor N terminus. J Biol Chem 1992;267:13795–13798.

19. Coughlin SR, Vu TK, Hung DT et al. Characterization of a functional thrombin receptor. Issues and opportunities. J Clin Invest 1992;89:351–355.

20. Dohlman HG, Thorner J, Caron MG et al. Model systems for the study of seven-transmembrane-segment receptors. Annu Rev Biochem 1991;60:653–688.

21. Brass LF, Manning DR, Shattil SJ. GTP-binding proteins and platelet activation. In: Coller BS, ed. Progress in hemostasis and thrombosis. Vol. 10. Philadelphia: WB Saunders, 1991; pp. 127–174.

22. Benka ML, Lee M, Wang GR et al. The thrombin receptor in human platelets is coupled to a GTP binding protein of the G alpha q family. FEBS Lett 1995;363:49–52.

23. Jamieson GA, Okumura T. Reduced thrombin binding and aggregation in Bernard-Soulier platelets. J Clin Invest 1978;61:861–864.

24. Greco NJ, Tandon NN, Jones GD et al. Contributions of glycoprotein Ib and the seven transmembrane domain receptor to increases in platelet cytoplasmic [Ca2+] induced by alpha-thrombin. Biochemistry 1996;35:906–914.

25. Liu L, Freedman J, Hornstein A et al. Binding of thrombin to the G protein-linked receptor, and not to glycoprotein Ib, precedes thrombin-mediated platelet activation. J Biol Chem 1997;272:1997–2004.

26. Jackson DA, López JA, Dong JF et al. Role of glycoprotein V in the formation of the platelet high-affinity thrombin binding site [Abstract]. Blood 1995;86:454a.

27. Connolly AJ, Ishihara H, Kahn ML et al. Role of the thrombin receptor in development and evidence for a second receptor. Nature 1996;381:516–519.

28. Hanasaki K, Arita H. Recent aspects of $TXA_2$ action on platelets and blood vessels. Platelets 1991;1:69–76.

29. Shenker A, Goldsmith P, Unson CG et al. The G protein coupled to the thromboxane $A_2$ receptor in human platelets is a member of the novel Gq family. J Biol Chem 1991;266:9309–9313.

30. Takahara K, Murray R, Fitzgerald GA et al. The response to thromboxane $A_2$ analogues in human platelets. Discrimination of two binding sites linked to distinct effector systems. J Biol Chem 1990;265:6836–6844.

31. Hirata T, Ushikubi F, Kakizuka A et al. Two thromboxane $A_2$ receptor isoforms in human platelets. Opposite coupling to adenylyl cyclase with different sensitivity to $Arg^{60}$ to Leu mutation. J Clin Invest 1996;97:949–956.

32. Lapetina EG, Siegel FL. Shape change induced in human platelets by platelet-activating factor. Correlation with the formation of phosphatidic acid and phosphorylation of a 40,000-dalton protein. J Biol Chem 1983;258:7241–7244.

33. Honda ZI, Nakamura M, Miki I et al. Cloning by functional expression of platelet-activating factor receptor from guinea-pig lung. Nature 1991;349:342–346.

34. Kunz D, Gerard NP, Gerard C. The human leukocyte-platelet-activating factor receptor. cDNA cloning, cell surface expression, and construction of a novel epitope-bearing analog. J Biol Chem 1992;267:9101–9106.

35. Hwang SB, Lee CS, Cheah MJ et al. Specific receptor sites for 1-O alkyl-2-O-acetyl-sn-glycero-3-phosphocholine (platelet activating factor) on rabbit platelet and guinea pig smooth muscle membranes. Biochemistry 1983;22:4756–4763.

36. Staatz WD, Walsh JJ, Pexton T et al. The a2b1 integrin cell surface collagen receptor binds to the α1(I)-CB3 peptide of collagen. J Biol Chem 1990;265:4778–4781.

37. Karniguian A, Grelac F, Levy-Toledano S et al. Collagen-induced platelet activation mainly involves the protein kinase C pathway. Biochem J 1990;268:325–331.

38. Tandon NN, Kralisz U, Jamieson GA. Identification of glycoprotein IV (CD36) as a primary receptor for platelet-collagen adhesion. J Biol Chem 1989;264:7576–7583.

39. Moroi M, Jung SM, Okuma M et al. A individual with platelets deficient in glycoprotein VI that lack both collagen-induced aggregation and adhesion. J Clin Invest 1989;84:1440–1445.

40. Deckmyn H, Van Houtte E, Vermylen J. Disturbed platelet aggregation to collagen associated with an antibody against an 85- to 90-Kd platelet glycoprotein in a individual with prolonged bleeding time. Blood 1992;79:1466–1471.

41. Takada Y, Hemler ME. The primary structure of the VLA-2/collagen receptor for α2 subunit (platelet GP Ia): homology to other integrins and the presence of a possible collagen-binding domain. J Cell Biol 1989;109:397–407.

42. Nieuwenhuis HK, Akkerman JW, Houdijk WP et al. Human blood platelets showing no response to collagen fail to express surface glycoprotein Ia. Nature 1985;318:470–472.

43. Kainoh M, Ikeda Y, Nishio S et al. Glycoprotein Ia-IIa-mediated activation-dependent platelet adhesion to collagen. Thromb Res 1992;65:165–176.

44. Aiken ML, Ginsberg MH, Byers-Ward V et al. Effects of OKM5, a monoclonal antibody to glycoprotein IV, on platelet aggregation and thrombospondin surface expression. Blood 1990;76:2501–2509.

45. Huang MM, Bolen JB, Barnwell JW et al. Membrane glycoprotein IV (CD36) is physically associated with the Fyn, Lyn, and Yes protein-tyrosine kinases in human platelets. Proc Natl Acad Sci U S A 1991;88:7844–7848.

46. Yamamoto N, Ikeda H, Tandon NN et al. A platelet membrane glycoprotein (GP) deficiency in healthy blood donors: Nak$^a$-platelets lack detectable GP IV (CD36). Blood 1990;76:1698–1703.

47. Asch AS, Nachman RL. Thrombospondin: phenomenology to function. In: Coller BS, ed. Progress in hemostasis and thrombosis. Philadelphia: WB Saunders, 1989; pp. 157–176.

48. Sugiyama T, Okuma M, Ushikubi F et al. A novel platelet aggregating factor found in a individual with defective collagen-induced platelet aggregation and autoimmune thrombocytopenia. Blood 1987;69:1712–1720.

49. Smith JB, Dangelmaier C. Determination of platelet adhesion to collagen and the associated formation of phosphatidic acid and calcium mobilization. Anal Biochem 1990;187:173–178.

50. Coller BS, Beer JH, Scudder LE et al. Collagen-platelet interactions: evidence for a direct interaction of collagen with platelet GP Ia-IIa and an indirect interaction with platelet GP IIb-IIIa mediated by adhesive proteins. Blood 1989;74:182–192.

51. Ichinohe T, Takayama H, Ezumi Y et al. Cyclic AMP-insensitive activation of c-Src and Syk protein-tyrosine kinases through platelet membrane glycoprotein VI. J Biol Chem 1995;270:28029–28036.

52. Gibbins J, Asselin J, Farndale R et al. Tyrosine phosphorylation of the Fc receptor gamma-chain in collagen-stimulated platelets. J Biol Chem 1996;271:18095–18099.

53. Thibonnier M. The human platelet vasopression receptor: identification by direct ultraviolet photoaffinity labeling. J Biol Chem 1987;262:10960–10964.

54. Morel A, O'Carroll AM, Brownstein MJ et al. Molecular cloning and expression of a rat $V_1$a arginine vasopression receptor. Nature 1992;356:523–526.

55. Kobilka BK, Matsui H, Kobilka TS et al. Cloning, sequencing and expression of the gene coding for the human platelet $α_2$-adrenergic receptor. Science 1987;238:650–656.

56. Colman RW. Aggregin: a platelet ADP receptor that mediates activation. FASEB J 1990;4:1425–1435.

57. Greco NJ, Yamamoto N, Tandon NN et al. Identification of a nucleotide-binding site on glycoprotein IIb. Relationship to ADP-induced platelet activation. J Biol Chem 1991;266:13627–13633.

58. Gachet C, Cattaneo M, Ohlmann P et al. Purinoceptors on blood platelets: further pharmacological and clinical evidence to suggest the presence of two ADP receptors. Br J Haematol 1995;91:434–444.

59. Murgo AJ, Contrera JG, Sistare FD. Evidence for separate calcium-signaling P2T and P2U purinoceptors in human megakaryocytic Dami cells. Blood 1994;83:1258–1267.

60. Willerson JT. Serotonin and thrombotic complications. J Cardiovasc Pharmacol 1991;17:S13-S20.

61. Wirz-Justice A. Platelet research in psychiatry. Experientia 1988;44:145–152.

62. Saltzman AG, Morse B, Whitman MM et al. Cloning of the human serotonin 5-HT2 and 5-HT1C receptor subtypes. Biochem Biophys Res Commun 1991;181:1469–1478.

63. Pritchett DB, Bach AW, Wozny M et al. Structure and functional expression of cloned rat serotonin 5HT-2 receptor. EMBO J 1988;7:4135–4140.

64. Kroll MH, Harris TS, Moake JL et al. von Willebrand factor binding to platelet GP Ib initiates signals for platelet activation. J Clin Invest 1991;88:1568–1573.

65. Shattil SJ. Function and regulation of the $β_3$ integrins in hemostasis and vascular biology. Thromb Haemost 1995;74:149–155.

66. Du XP, Plow EF, Frelinger AL III et al. Ligands "activate" integrin alpha IIb beta 3 (platelet GP IIb-IIIa). Cell 1991;65:409–416.

67. Fox JE, Shattil SJ, Kinlough-Rathbone RL et al. The platelet cytoskeleton stabilizes the interaction between alpha IIb-beta 3 and its ligand and induces selective movements of ligand-occupied integrin. J Biol Chem 1996;271:7004–7011.

68. Savage B, Ruggeri ZM. Selective recognition of adhesive sites in surface-bound fibrinogen by glycoprotein IIb-IIIa on nonactivated platelets. J Biol Chem 1991;266:11227–11233.

69. Haimovich B, Lipfert L, Brugge JS et al. Tyrosine phosphorylation and cytoskeletal reorganization in platelets are triggered by interaction of integrin receptors with their immobilized ligands. J Biol Chem 1993;268:15868–15877.

70. Shattil SJ, Ginsberg MH, Brugge JS. Adhesive signaling in platelets [Review]. Curr Opin Cell Biol 1994;6:695–704.

71. Golden A, Brugge JS, Shattil SJ. Role of platelet membrane glycoprotein

IIb-IIIa in agonist-induced tyrosine phosphorylation of platelet proteins. J Cell Biol 1990;111:3117–3127.

72. Law DA, Nannizzi-Alaimo L, Phillips DR. Outside-in integrin signal transduction. Alpha II-beta 3-(GP IIb-IIIa) tyrosine phosphorylation induced by platelet aggregation. J Biol Chem 1996;271:10811–10815.

73. Clark EA, Brugge JS. Integrins and signal transduction pathways: the road taken. Science 1995;268:233–239.

74. Daniel JL, Dangelmaier C, Smith JB. Evidence for a role for tyrosine phosphorylation of phospholipase C gamma 2 in collagen-induced platelet cytosolic calcium mobilization. Biochem J 1994;302:617–622.

75. Yanaga F, Poole A, Asselin J et al. Syk interacts with tyrosine-phosphorylated proteins in human platelets activated by collagen and crosslinking of the Fc gamma-IIA receptor [published erratum appears in Biochem J 1996;313:1047]. Biochem J 1995;311:471–478.

76. Robinson A, Gibbins J, Rodriguez-Liñares B et al. Characterization of Grβ 2-binding proteins in human platelets activated by Fcγ RIIA crosslinking. Blood 1996;88:522–530.

77. Worthington RE, Carroll RC, Boucheix C. Platelet activation by CD9 monoclonal antibodies is mediated by the FcgII receptor. Br J Haematol 1990;74:216–222.

78. Horsewood P, Hayward CP, Warkentin TE et al. Investigation of the mechanisms of monoclonal antibody-induced platelet activation. Blood 1991;78:1019–1026.

79. Wiedmer T, Sims PJ. Participation of protein kinases in complement C5b-9-induced shedding of platelet plasma membrane vesicles. Blood 1991;78:2880–2886.

80. Sims PJ, Faioni EM, Wiedmer T. Complement proteins C5b-9 cause release of membrane vesicles from the platelet surface that are enriched in the membrane receptor for coagulation factor Va and express prothrombinase activity. J Biol Chem 1988;263:18205–18212.

81. Siljander P, Carpen O, Lassila R. Platelet-derived microparticles associate with fibrin during thrombosis. Blood 1996;87:4651–4663.

82. Ameisen JC, Joseph M, Caen JP et al. A role for glycoprotein IIb-IIIa complex in the binding of IgE to human platelets and platelet IgE-dependent cytotoxic functions. Br J Haematol 1986;64:21–32.

83. Oda A, Miyakawa Y, Druker BJ et al. Thrombopoietin primes human platelet aggregation induced by shear stress and by multiple agonists. Blood 1996;87:4664–4670.

84. Oda A, Miyakawa Y, Druker BJ et al. Thrombopoietin induces tyrosine phosphorylation of Stat3 and Stat5 in human blood platelets [Review]. Blood 1996;87:439–446.

85. Rodriguez-Linares B, Watson SP. Thrombopoietin potentiates activation of human platelets in association with JAK2 and TYK2 phosphorylation. Biochem J 1996;316:93–98.

86. Miles LA, Plow EF. Binding and activation of plasminogen on the platelet surface. J Biol Chem 1985;260:4303–4311.

87. Vaughan DE, Mendelsohn ME, Declerck PJ et al. Characterization of the binding of human tissue-type plasminogen activator to platelets. J Biol Chem 1989;264:15869–15874.

88. Schafer AI, Maas AK, Ware JA et al. Platelet protein phosphorylation, elevation of cytosolic calcium, and inositol phospholipid breakdown in platelet activation induced by plasmin. J Clin Invest 1986;78:73–79.

89. Pasche B, Loscalzo J. Platelets and fibrinolysis. Platelets 1991;3:125–134.

90. Kamat SG, Michelson AD, Benoit SE et al. Fibrinolysis inhibits shear stress-induced platelet aggregation. Circulation 1995;92:1399–1407.

91. Pedreño J, Fernández R, Cullaré C et al. Platelet integrin αIIbβ3 (GP IIb-IIIa) is not implicated in the binding of LDL to intact resting platelets. Arterioscler Thromb Vasc Biol 1997;17:156–163.

92. McEver RP, Beckstead JH, Moore KL et al. GMP-140, a platelet alpha-granule membrane protein, is also synthesized by vascular endothelial cells and is localized in Weibel-Palade bodies. J Clin Invest 1989;84:92–99.

93. Evangelista V, Piccardoni P, White JG et al. Cathepsin G-dependent platelet stimulation by activated polymorphonuclear leukocytes and its inhibition by antiproteinases: role of P-selectin-mediated cell-cell adhesion. Blood 1993;81:2947–2957.

94. LaRosa CA, Rohrer MJ, Benoit SE et al. Human neutrophil cathepsin G is a potent platelet activator. J Vasc Surg 1994;19:306–318.

95. Molino M, Blanchard N, Belmonte E et al. Proteolysis of the human platelet and endothelial cell thrombin receptor by neutrophil-derived cathepsin G. J Biol Chem 1995;270:11168–11175.

96. LaRosa CA, Rohrer MJ, Benoit SE et al. Neutrophil cathepsin G modulates the platelet surface expression of the glycoprotein (GP) Ib-IX complex by proteolysis of the von Willebrand factor binding site on GP Ibα and by a cytoskeletal-mediated redistribution of the remainder of the complex. Blood 1994;84:158–168.

97. Renesto P, Chignard M. Enhancement of cathepsin G-induced platelet activation by leukocyte elastase: consequence for the neutrophil-mediated platelet activation. Blood 1993;82:139–144.

98. Sawicki G, Salas E, Murat J et al. Release of gelatinase A during platelet activation mediates aggregation. Nature 1997;386:616–619.

99. Newman PJ. The biology of PECAM-1. J Clin Invest 1997;99:3–8.

100. Michelson, AD. Flow cytometry: a clinical test of platelet function [Review]. Blood 1996;87:4925–4936.

101. Plow EF, D'Sousa SE, Ginsberg MH. Consequences of the interaction of platelet membrane glycoprotein GP IIb-IIIa (αIIbβ3) and its ligands. J Lab Clin Med 1992;120:198–204.

102. Ugarova TP, Budzynski AZ, Shattil SJ et al. Conformational changes in fibrinogen elicited by its interaction with platelet membrane glycoprotein GP IIb-IIIa. J Biol Chem 1993;268:21080–21087.

103. Rinder CS, Bonan JL, Rinder HM et al. Cardiopulmonary bypass induces leukocyte-platelet adhesion. Blood 1992;79:1201–1205.

104. Mickelson JK, Lakkis NM, Villarreal-Levy G et al. Leukocyte activation with platelet adhesion after coronary angioplasty: a mechanism for recurrent disease? J Am Coll Cardiol 1996;28:345–353.

105. Marcus AJ. Platelets and their disorders. In: Ratnoff OD, Forbes CD, eds Disorders of hemostasis. Philadelphia: WB Saunders, 1996; pp. 79–137.

106. Clapham DE. The G protein nanomachine. Nature 1996;379:297–299.

107. Birnbaumer L. Receptor-to-effector signaling through G proteins: roles for βγ dimers as well as α subunits. Cell 1992;71:1069–1072.

108. Rittenhouse, SE. Phosphoinositide 3-kinase activation and platelet function. Blood 1996;88:4401–4414.

109. Houslay MD, Bojanic D, Gawler D et al. Thrombin, unlike vasopressin, appears to stimulate two distinct guanine nucleotide regulatory proteins in human platelets. Biochem J 1986;238:109–113.

110. Brass LF, Woolkalis MJ, Manning DR. Interactions in platelets between G proteins and the agonists that stimulate phospholipase C and inhibit adenylyl cyclase. J Biol Chem 1988;263:5348–5355.

111. Cooper DM, Rodbell M. ADP is a potent inhibitor of human platelet plasma membrane adenylate cyclase. Nature 1979;282:517–518.

112. Lapetina EG, Reep B, Chang KJ. Treatment of human platelets with trypsin, thrombin, or collagen inhibits the pertussis toxin–induced ADP-ribosylation of a 41-kDa protein. Proc Natl Acad Sci U S A 1986;83:5880–5883.

113. Ueda K, Hayaishi O. ADP-ribosylation. Annu Rev Biochem 1985;54:73–100.

114. Hrbolich JK, Culty M, Haslam RJ. Activation of phospholipase C associated with isolated rabbit platelet membranes by guanosine 5'-[γ-thio] triphosphate and by thrombin in the presence of GTP. Biochem J 1987;243:457–465.

115. Banno Y, Nagao S, Katada T et al. Stimulation by GTP-binding proteins (Gi, Go) of partially purified phospholipase C activity from human platelet membranes. Biochem Biophys Res Commun 1987;146:861–869.

116. Boguski MS, McCormick F. Proteins regulating Ras and its relatives. Nature 1993;366:643–654.

117. Fischer TH, Gatling MN, McCormick F et al. Incorporation of Rap 1b into the platelet cytoskeleton is dependent on thrombin activation and extracellular calcium. J Biol Chem 1994;269:17257–17261.

118. Torti M, Ramaschi G, Sinigaglia F et al. Glycoprotein IIb-IIIa and the translocation of Rap2B to the platelet cytoskeleton. Proc Natl Acad Sci U S A 1994;91:4239–4243.

119. Dash D, Aepfelbacher M, Siess W. Integrin αIIbβ3-mediated translocation of CDC42Hs to the cytoskeleton in stimulated human platelets. J Biol Chem 1995;270:17321–17326.

120. Torti M, Lapetina EG. Role of rap1B and p21ras GTPase-activating protein in the regulation of phospholipase c-γ1 in human platelets. Proc Natl Acad Sci U S A 1992;89:7796–7800.

121. Zhang J, Zhang J, Benovic JL et al. Sequestration of a G protein βγ subunit or ADP-ribosylation of Rho can inhibit thrombin-induced activation of platelet phosphoinositide 3-kinases. J Biol Chem 1995;270:6589–6594.

122. Karniguian A, Zahraoui A, Tavitian A. Identification of small GTP-binding rab proteins in human platelets: thrombin-induced phosphorylation of rab3B, rab6, and rab8 proteins. Proc Natl Acad Sci U S A 1993;90:7647–7651.

123. Lapetina EG, Lacal JC, Reep BR et al. A ras-related protein is phosphorylated and translocated by agonists that increase cAMP levels in human platelets. Proc Natl Acad Sci U S A 1989;86:3131–3134.

124. Hartwig JH, Bokoch GM, Carpenter CL et al. Thrombin receptor ligation and activated Rac uncap actin filament barbed ends through phosphoinositide synthesis in permeabilized human platelets. Cell 1995;82:643–653.

125. Symons M, Derry JM, Karlak B et al. Wiskott-Aldrich syndrome protein, a novel effector for the GTPase CDC42Hs, is implicated in actin polymerization. Cell 1996;84:723–734.

126. Hokin MR, Hokin LE. Enzyme secretion and the incorporation of P32 into phospholipids of pancreas slices. J Biol Chem 1953;203:967–977.

127. Firkin BG, Williams WJ. The incorporation of radioactive phosphorus into the phospholipids of human leukemic leukocytes and platelets. J Clin Invest 1961;40:423–432.

128. Rittenhouse-Simmons S. Production of diglyceride from phosphatidylinositol in activated human platelets. J Clin Invest 1979;63:580–587.

129. Mauco G, Chap H, Douste-Blazy L. Characterization and properties of a phosphatidylinositol phosphodiesterase (phospholipase C) from platelet cytosol. FEBS Lett 1979;100:367–370.

130. Bell RL, Majerus PW. Thrombin-induced hydrolysis of phosphatidylinositol in human platelets. J Biol Chem 1980;255:1790–1792.

131. Banno Y, Nakashima S, Ohzawa M et al. Differential translocation of phospholipase C isozymes to integrin-mediated cytoskeletal complexes in thrombin-stimulated human platelets. J Biol Chem 1996;271:14989–14994.

132. Lee SB, Rao AK, Lee KH et al. Decreased expression of phospholipase C-β2 isozyme in human platelets with impaired function. Blood 1996;88:1684–1691.

133. Rhee SG, Choi KD. Regulation of inositol phospholipid-specific phospholipase C isozymes. J Biol Chem 1992;267:12393–12396.

134. Marcus AJ, Ullman HL, Safier LB. Lipid composition of subcellular particles of human blood platelets. J Lipid Res 1969;10:108–114.

135. Huang EM, Detwiler TC. Stimulus-response coupling mechanisms. In: Phillips DR, Shuman MA, eds. Biochemistry of platelets. Orlando: Academic Press, 1986; pp. 1–68.

136. Ichinohe T, Takayama H, Ezumi Y et al. Cyclic AMP-insensitive activation of c-Src and Syk protein-tyrosine kinases through platelet membrane glycoprotein VI. J Biol Chem 1995;270:28029–28036.

137. Jackson SP, Schoenwaelder SM, Yuan Y et al. Non-receptor protein tyrosine kinases and phosphatases in human platelets. Thromb Haemost 1996;76:640–650.

138. Dhar A, Shukla SD. Electrotransjection of pp60$^{v-src}$ monoclonal antibody inhibits activation of phospholipase C in platelets. A new mechanism for platelet-activating factor response. J Biol Chem 1994;269:9123–9127.

139. Gironcel D, Racaud-Sultan C, Payrastre B et al. α$_{IIb}$β$_3$-integrin mediated adhesion of human platelets to a fibrinogen matrix triggers phospholipase C activation and phosphatidylinositol 3′,4′-biphosphate accumulation. FEBS Lett 1996;389:253–256.

140. Sohn RH, Goldschmidt-Clermont PJ. Profilin: at the crossroads of signal transduction and the actin cytoskeleton. Bioessays 1994;16:465–472.

141. Berridge MJ. Inositol trisphosphate and calcium signaling. Nature 1993;361:315–325.

142. Brass LF. Ca$^{2+}$ homeostasis in unstimulated platelets. J Biol Chem 1984;259:12563–12570.

143. Brass LF, Shattil SJ. Changes in surface-bound and exchangeable calcium during platelet activation. J Biol Chem 1982;257:14000–14005.

144. O'Rourke FA, Halenda SP, Zavoico GB et al. Inositol 1,4,5-trisphosphate releases Ca$^{2+}$ from a Ca$^{2+}$-transporting membrane vesicle fraction derived from human platelets. J Biol Chem 1985;260:956–962.

145. Authi KS, Evenden BJ, Crawford N. Metabolic and functional consequences of introducing inositol 1,4,5-trisphosphate into saponin-permeabilized human platelets. Biochem J 1986;233:707–718.

146. Ross CA, Meldolesi J, Milner TA et al. Inositol 1,4,5-trisphosphate receptor localized to endoplasmic reticulum in cerebellar Purkinje neurons. Nature 1989;339:468–470.

147. Ferris CD, Huganir Rl, Supattapone S et al. Purified inositol 1,4,5-trisphosphate receptor mediates calcium flux in reconstituted lipid vesicles. Nature 1989;342:87–89.

148. Jayaraman T, Ondrias K, Ondriasova E et al. Regulation of the inositol 1,4,5-trisphosphate receptor by tyrosine phosphorylation. Science 1996;272:1492–1494.

149. Papp B, Paszty K, Kovacs T et al. Characterization of the inositol trisphosphate-sensitive and insensitive calcium stores by selective inhibition of the endoplasmic reticulum-type calcium pump isoforms in isolated platelet membrane vesicles. Cell Calcium 1993;14:531–538.

150. Hajnóczky G, Thomas AP. The inositol trisphosphate calcium channel is inactivated by inositol trisphosphate. Nature 1994;370:474–477.

151. Hwang SB. Specific binding of tritium-labeled inositol 1,4,5-trisphosphate to human platelet membranes: ionic and GTP regulation. Biochim Biophys Acta 1991;1064:351–359.

152. Ishii H, Connolly TM, Bross TE et al. Inositol cyclic trisphosphate [inositol 1,2-(cyclic)-4,5-triphosphate] is formed upon thrombin stimulation of human platelets. Proc Natl Acad Sci U S A 1986;83:6397–6401.

153. Wilson DB, Connolly TM, Bross TE et al. Isolation and characterization of the inositol cyclic phosphate products of polyphosphoinositide cleavage by phospholipase C. Physiological effects in permeabilized platelets and limulus photoreceptor cells. J Biol Chem 1985;260:13496–13501.

154. Hallam TJ, Rink TJ. Agonists stimulate divalent cation channels in the plasma membrane of human platelets. FEBS Lett 1985;186:175–179.

155. Berridge MJ. Capacitative calcium entry. Biochem J 1995;312:1–11.

156. Zschauer A, van Breemen C, Buhler FR et al. Calcium channels in thrombin-activated human platelet membrane. Nature 1988;334:703–705.

157. Connolly TM, Bross TE, Majerus PW. Isolation of a phosphomonoesterase from human platelets that specifically hydrolyzes the 5-phosphate of inositol 1,4,5-trisphosphate. J Biol Chem 1985;260:7868–7874.

158. Irvine RF, Letcher AJ, Heslop JP et al. The inositol tris/tetrakisphosphate pathway-demonstration of Ins(1, 4, 5)P$_3$-kinase activity in animal tissues. Nature 1986;320:631–634.

159. Choi KY, Kim HK, Lee SY et al. Molecular cloning and expression of a complementary DNA for inositol 1,4,5-trisphosphate 3-kinase. Science 1990;248:64–66.

160. Irvine RF, Moor RM. Micro-injection of inositol 1,3,4,5-tetrakisphosphate activates sea urchin eggs by a mechanism dependent on external Ca$^{2+}$. Biochem J 1986;240:917–920.

161. Hill TD, Dean NM, Boynton AL. Inositol 1,3,4,5-tetrakisphosphate induces Ca$^{2+}$ sequestration in rat liver cells. Science 1988;242:1176–1178.

162. Daniel JL, Dangelmaier CA, Smith JB. Formation and metabolism of inositol 1,4,5-trisphosphate in human platelets. Biochem J 1987;246:109–114.

163. Oberdisse E, Nolan RD, Lapetina EG. Thrombin and phorbol ester stimulate inositol 1,3,4,5-tetrakisphosphate 3-phosphomonoesterase in human platelets. J Biol Chem 1990;265:726–730.

164. Fisher GJ, Bakshian S, Baldassare JJ. Activation of human platelets by ADP causes a rapid rise in cytosolic free calcium without hydrolysis of phosphatidylinositol-4,5-bisphosphate. Biochem Biophys Res Commun 1985;129:958–964.

165. Jones GD, Gear AR. Subsecond calcium dynamics in ADP-and thrombin-stimulated platelets: a continuous-flow approach using indo-1. Blood 1988;71:1539–1543.

166. Ariyoshi H, Salzman EW. Association of localized Ca$^{2+}$ gradients with redistribution of glycoprotein IIb-IIIa and F-actin in activated human blood platelets. Arterioscler Thromb Vasc Biol 1996;16:230–235.

167. Brass LF, Shattil SJ. Identification and function of the high affinity binding sites for Ca$^{2+}$ on the surface of platelets. J Clin Invest 1984;73:626–632.

168. Powling MJ, Hardisty RM. Glycoprotein IIb-IIIa complex and Ca$^{2+}$ influx into stimulated platelets. Blood 1985;66:731–734.

169. Rybak ME, Renzulli LA, Bruns MJ et al. Platelet glycoproteins IIb and IIIa as a calcium channel in liposomes. Blood 1988;72:714–720.

170. Rybak ME, Renzulli LA. Ligand inhibition of the platelet glycoprotein IIb-IIIa complex function as a calcium channel in liposomes. J Biol Chem 1989;264:14617–14620.

171. Suldan Z, Brass LF. Role of the glycoprotein IIb-IIIa complex in plasma membrane Ca$^{2+}$ transport: a comparison of results obtained with platelets and human erythroleukemia cells. Blood 1991;78:2887–2893.

172. Fujimoto T, Fujimura K, Kuramoto A. Electrophysiological evidence that glycoprotein IIb-IIIa complex is involved in calcium channel activation on human platelet plasma membrane. J Biol Chem 1991;266:16370–16375.

173. Salzman EW, Ware JA. Ionized calcium as an intracellular messenger in blood platelets. Prog Hemost Thromb 1989;9:177–202.

174. Rink TJ, Smith SW, Tsien RY. Cytoplasmic free Ca$^{2+}$ in human platelets: Ca$^{2+}$ thresholds and Ca$^{2+}$-independent activation for shape-change and secretion. FEBS Lett 1982;148:21–26.

175. Ware JA, Johnson PC, Smith M et al. Effect of common agonists on cytoplasmic ionized calcium concentration in platelets. Measurement with 2-methyl-6-methoxy 8-nitroquinoline (quin2) and aequorin. J Clin Invest 1986;77:878–886.

176. Hathaway DR, Adelstein RS. Human platelet myosin light chain kinase requires the calcium binding protein calmodulin for activity. Proc Natl Acad Sci U S A 1979;76:1653–1657.

177. Higashihara M, Takahata K, Kurokawa K. Effect of phosphorylation of myosin light chain by myosin light chain kinase and protein kinase C on conformational change and ATPase activities of human platelet myosin. Blood 1991;78:3224–3231.

178. Itoh K, Hara T, Shibata N. Diphosphorylation of platelet myosin by myosin light chain kinase. Biochim Biophys Acta 1992;1133:286–292.

179. Hashimoto Y, Ogihara A, Nakanishi S et al. Two thrombin-activated Ca$^{2+}$ channels in human platelets. J Biol Chem 1992;267:17078–17081.

180. Hashimoto Y, Watanabe T, Kinoshita M et al. Ca$^{2+}$ entry pathways activated by the tumor promoter thapsigargin in human platelets. Biochim Biophys Acta 1993;1220:37–41.

181. Gear AR, Schneider W. Control of platelet glycogenolysis. Activation of phosphorylase kinase by calcium. Biochim Biophys Acta 1975;392:111–120.

182. Fox JE, Goll DE, Reynolds CC et al. Identification of two proteins (actin-binding protein and P235) that are hydrolyzed by endogenous Ca$_{2+}$-dependent protease during platelet aggregation. J Biol Chem 1985;260:1060–1066.

183. O'Halloran T, Beckerle MC, Burridge K. Identification of talin as a major cytoplasmic protein implicated in platelet activation. Nature 1985;317:449–451.

184. Seiffert D. Hydrolysis of platelet vitronectin by calpain. J Biol Chem 1996;271:11170–11176.

185. Banno Y, Nakashima S, Hachiya T et al. Endogenous cleavage of phospholipase C-β3 by agonist-induced activation of calpain in human platelets. J Biol Chem 1995;270:4318–4324.

186. Billah MM, Lapetina EG, Cuatrecasas P. Phospholipase A$_2$ and phospholipase C activities of platelets. Differential substrate specificity, Ca$^{2+}$ requirement, pH dependence, and cellular localization. J Biol Chem 1980;255:10227–10231.

187. Rittenhouse-Simmons S. Differential activation of platelet phospholipases by thrombin and ionophore A23187. J Biol Chem 1981;256:4153–4155.

188. Rittenhouse SE, Horne WC. Ionomycin can elevate intraplatelet Ca$^{2+}$ and activate phospholipase A$_2$ without activating phospholipase C. Biochem Biophys Res Commun 1984;123:393–397.

189. Auethavekiat V, Abrams CS, Majerus PW. Phosphorylation of platelet pleckstrin activates inositol polyphosphate 5-phosphatase I. J Biol Chem 1997;272:1786–1790.

190. Nishizuka Y. Protein kinase C and lipid signaling for sustained cellular responses. FASEB J 1995;9:484–496.

191. Crabos M, Imber R, Woodtli T et al. Different translocation of three distinct PKC isoforms with tumor-promoting phorbol ester in human platelets. Biochem Biophys Res Commun 1991;178:878–883.

192. Grabarek J, Raychowdhury M, Ravid K et al. Identification and functional characterization of protein kinase C isozymes in platelets and HEL cells. J Biol Chem 1992;267:10011–10017.

193. Baldassare JJ, Henderson PA, Burns D et al. Translocation of protein kinase C isozymes in thrombin-stimulated human platelets. Correlation with 1,2-diacylglycerol levels. J Biol Chem 1992;267:15585–15590.

194. Khan WA, Blobe G, Halpern A et al. Selective regulation of protein kinase C isoenzymes by oleic acid in human platelets. J Biol Chem 1993;268:5063–5068.

195. Bell RM, Burns DJ. Lipid activation of protein kinase C. J Biol Chem 1991;266:4661–4664.

196. Werner MH, Hannun YA. Delayed accumulation of diacylglycerol in platelets as a mechanism for regulation of onset of aggregation and secretion. Blood 1991;78:435–444.

197. Khan WA, Blobe GC, Hannun YA. Activation of protein kinase C by oleic acid. Determination and analysis of inhibition by detergent micelles and physiologic membranes: requirement for free oleate. J Biol Chem 1992;267:3605–3612.

198. Zhang J, Falck JR, Reddy KK et al. Phosphatidylinositol (3, 4, 5)-trisphosphate stimulates phosphorylation of pleckstrin in human platelets. J Biol Chem 1995;270:22807–22810.

199. Toker A, Bachelot C, Chen CS et al. Phosphorylation of the platelet p47 phosphoprotein is mediated by the lipid products of phosphoinositide 3-kinase. J Biol Chem 1995;270:29525–29531.

200. Wiedmer T, Ando B, Sims PJ. Complement C5b-9-stimulated platelet secretion is associated with a $Ca^{2+}$-initiated activation of cellular protein kinases. J Biol Chem 1987;262:13674–13681.

201. Romano M, Hawiger J. Interaction of endotoxic lipid A and lipid X with purified human platelet protein kinase C. J Biol Chem 1990;265:1765–1770.

202. Shattil SJ, Brass LF. Induction of the fibrinogen receptor on human platelets by intracellular mediators. J Biol Chem 1987;262:992–1000.

203. Gabbeta J, Yang X, Sun L et al. Abnormal inside-out signal transduction-dependent activation of glycoprotein IIb-IIIa in a individual with impaired pleckstrin phosphorylation. Blood 1996;87:1368–1376.

204. Rink TJ, Sanchez A, Hallam TJ. Diacylglycerol and phorbol ester stimulate secretion without raising cytoplasmic free calcium in human platelets. Nature 1983;305:317–319.

205. Ware JA, Johnson PC, Smith M et al. Aequorin detects increased cytoplasmic calcium in platelets stimulated with phorbol ester or diacylglycerol. Biochem Biophys Res Commun 1985;133:98–104.

206. Halenda SP, Rehm AG. Thrombin and C-kinase activators potentiate calcium-stimulated arachidonic acid release in human platelets. Biochem J 1987;248:471–475.

207. Crompton MR, Moss SE, Crumpton MJ. Diversity in the lipocortin/calpactin family. Cell 1988;55:1–3.

208. Touqui L, Rothhut B, Shaw AM et al. Platelet activation-a role for a 40k anti-phospholipase A$_2$ protein indistinguishable from lipocortin. Nature 1986;321:177–180.

209. Haimovich B, Kaneshiki N, Ji P. Protein kinase C regulates tyrosine phosphorylation of pp125FAK in platelets adherent to fibrinogen. Blood 1996;87:152–161.

210. Ettinger SL, Lauener RW, Duronio V. Protein kinase C delta specifically associates with phosphatidylinositol 3-kinase following cytokine stimulation. J Biol Chem 1996;271:14514–14518.

211. Aharonovitz O, Granot Y. Stimulation of mitogen-activated protein kinase and Na$^+$/H$^+$ exchanger in human platelets. Differential effect of phorbol ester and vasopressin. J Biol Chem 1996;271:16494–16499.

212. yers M, Rachubinski RA, Stewart MI et al. Molecular cloning and expression of the major protein kinase C substrate of platelets. Nature 1988;333:470–473.

213. Abrams CS, Wu H, Zhao W et al. Pleckstrin inhibits phosphoinositide hydrolysis initiated by G protein-coupled and growth factor receptors. A role for pleckstrin's pH domains. J Biol Chem 1995;270:14485–14492.

214. Abrams CS, Zhang J, Downes CP et al. Phosphopleckstrin inhibits Gβγ-activatable platelet phosphatidylinositol-4,5 biphosphate 3-kinase. J Biol Chem 1996;271:25192–25197.

215. Zavoico GB, Halenda SP, Sha'afi RI et al. Phorbol myristate acetate inhibits thrombin-stimulated Ca$^{2+}$ mobilization and phosphatidylinositol 4,5-bisphosphate hydrolysis in human platelets. Proc Natl Acad Sci U S A 1985;82:3859–3862.

216. Watson SP, McNally J, Shipman LJ et al. The action of the protein kinase C inhibitor, staurosporine, on human platelets. Evidence against a regulation role for protein kinase C in the formation of inositol trisphosphate by thrombin. Biochem J 1988;249:345–350.

217. Xu Y, Ware JA. Selective inhibition of thrombin receptor-mediated Ca$^{2+}$ entry by protein kinase C beta. J Biol Chem 1995;270:23887–23890.

218. Murphy CT, Bullock AJ, Westwick J. A role for protein phosphorylation in modulating Ca$^{2+}$ elevation in rabbit platelets treated with thapsigargin. Biochem J 1996;313:83–89.

219. Kroll MH, Zavoico GB, Schafer AI. Control of platelet protein kinase C activation by cyclic AMP. Biochim Biophys Acta 1988;970:61–67.

220. Hannun YA, Bell RM. Functions of sphingolipids and sphingolipid breakdown products in cellular regulation. Science 1989;243:500–507.

221. Buehrer BM, Bell RM. Inhibition of sphingosine kinase *in vitro* and in platelets. Implications for signal transduction pathways. J Biol Chem 1992;267:3154–3159.

222. Wheeler-Jones CP, Learmonth MP, Martin H et al. Identification of 14-3-3 proteins in human platelets: effects of synthetic peptides on protein kinase C activation. Biochem J 1996;315:41–47.

223. Patel Y, Kakkar VV, Authi KS. Calpain-induced down-regulation of protein kinase C inhibits dense-granule secretion in human platelets. Inhibition of platelet aggregation or calpain activity preserves protein kinase C and restores full secretion. Biochim Biophys Acta 1994;1224:480–488.

224. Dennis EA. Diversity of group types, regulation, and function of phospholipase A$_2$. J Biol Chem 1994;269:13057–13060.

225. Mayer RJ, Marshall LA. New insights on mammalian phospholipase A$_2$(s); comparison of arachidonoyl-selective and-nonselective enzymes. FASEB J 1993;7:339–348.

226. Borsch-Haubold AG, Kramer RM, Watson SP. Cytosolic phospholipase A$_2$ is phosphorylated in collagen and thrombin-stimulated human platelets independent of protein kinase C and mitogen-activated protein kinase. J Biol Chem 1995;270:25885–25892.

227. Kramer RM, Roberts EF, Hyslop PA et al. Differential activation of cytosolic phospholipase A$_2$ (cPLA$_2$) by thrombin and thrombin receptor agonist peptide in human platelets. Evidence for activation of cPLA2 independent of the mitogen-activated protein kinases ERK1/2. J Biol Chem 1995;270:14816–14823.

228. Serhan CN, Sheppard KA. Lipoxin formation during human neutrophil-platelet interactions. Evidence for the transformation of leukotriene A$_4$ by platelet 12-lipoxygenase *in vitro*. J Clin Invest 1990;85:772–780.

229. Barry OP, Pratico D, Lawson JA et al. Transcellular activation of platelets and endothelial cells by bioactive lipids in platelet microparticles. J Clin Invest 1997;99:2118–2127.

230. Zimmerman GA, McIntyre TM, Prescott SM. Adhesion and signaling in vascular cell-cell interactions. J Clin Invest 1996;98:1699–1702.

231. Iorio P, Gresele P, Stasi M et al. Protein kinase C inhibitors enhance G protein induced phospholipase A$_2$ activation in intact human platelets. FEBS Lett 1996;381:244–248.

232. Zavoico GB, Cragoe EJ Jr, Feinstein MB. Regulation of intracellular pH in human platelets. Effects of thrombin A23187, and ionomycin and evidence for activation of Na$^+$/H$^+$ exchange and its inhibition by amiloride analogs. J Biol Chem 1986;261:13160–13167.

233. Sardet C, Counillon L, Franchi A et al. Growth factors induce phosphorylation of the Na$^+$/H$^+$ antiporter, a glycoprotein of 110 Kd. Science 1990;247:723–726.

234. Sweatt JD, Johnson SL, Cragoe EJ et al. Inhibitors of Na$^+$/H$^+$ exchange block stimulus-provoked arachidonic acid release in human platelets. Selective effects on platelet activation by epinephrine, ADP, and lower concentrations of thrombin. J Biol Chem 1985;260:12910–12919.

235. Sweatt JD, Blair IA, Cragoe EJ et al. Inhibitors of Na$^+$/H$^+$ exchange block epinephrine- and ADP-induced stimulation of human platelet phospholipase C by blockade of arachidonic release at a prior step. J Biol Chem 1986;261:8660–8666.

236. Sweatt JD, Connolly TM, Cragoe EJ et al. Evidence that Na$^+$/H$^+$ exchange regulates receptor-mediated phospholipase A$_2$ activation in human platelets. J Biol Chem 1986;261:8667–8673.

237. Banga HS, Simons ER, Brass LF et al. Activation of phospholipases A and C in human platelets exposed to epinephrine: role of glycoproteins IIb-IIIa and dual role of epinephrine. Proc Natl Acad Sci U S A 1986;83:9197–9201.

238. Zavoico GB, Cragoe EJ Jr. Ca$^{2+}$ mobilization can occur independent of acceleration of Na$^+$/H$^+$ exchange in thrombin-stimulated human platelets. J Biol Chem 1988;263:9635–9639.

239. Siffert W, Siffert G, Scheid P et al. Na$^+$/H$^+$ exchange modulates Ca$^{2+}$ mobilization in human platelets stimulated by ADP and the thromboxane mimetic U 46619. J Biol Chem 1990;265:719–725.

240. Luzzatto G, Kroll MH, Zavoico GB et al. Regulation of the phosphoinositide cycle by Na$^+$/H$^+$ exchange and intracellular pH in human platelets. Biochim Biophys Acta 1991;1084:78–86.

241. Huang R, Kucera GL, Rittenhouse SE. Elevated cytosolic Ca$^{2+}$ activates phospholipase D in human platelets. J Biol Chem 1991;266:1652–1655.

242. Martinson EA, Scheible S, Greinacher A et al. Platelet phospholipase D is activated by protein kinase C via an integrin alpha IIb beta 3-independent mechanism. Biochem J 1995;310:623–628.

243. Kroll MH, Zavoico GB, Schafer AI. Second messenger function of phosphatidic acid in platelet activation. J Cell Physiol 1989;139:558–564.

244. Hashizume T, Taniguchi M, Sato T et al. Arachidonic acid liberation induced by phosphatidic acid endogenously generated from membrane phospholipids in rabbit platelets. Biochim Biophys Acta 1994;1221:179–184.

245. Smyth SS, Hillery CA, Parise LV. Phosphatidic and lysophosphatidic acid modulate the fibrinogen binding activity of purified platelet glycoprotein IIb-IIIa. Blood 1991;78(Suppl):278a.

246. Haslam RJ, Coorssen JR. Evidence that activation of phospholipase D can mediate secretion from permeabilized platelets. Adv Exp Med Biol 1993;344:149–164.

247. Golden A, Brugge JS. Thrombin treatment induces rapid changes in tyro-

sine phosphorylation in platelets. Proc Natl Acad Sci U S A 1989;86: 901–905.

248. Cichowski K, McCormick F, Brugge JS. P21^ras^GAP association with Fyn, Lyn, and Yes in thrombin-activated platelets. J Biol Chem 1992;267: 5025–5028.

249. Schoenwaelder SM, Jackson SP, Yuan Y et al. Tyrosine kinases regulate the cytoskeletal attachment of integrin alpha IIb beta 3 (platelet glycoprotein IIb-IIIa) and the cellular retraction of fibrin polymers. J Biol Chem 1994;269:32479–32487.

250. Haimovich B, Regan C, DiFazio L et al. The FcgRII receptor triggers pp125FAK phosphorylation in platelets. J Biol Chem 1996;271: 16332–16337.

251. Clark EA, Shattil SJ, Ginsberg MH et al. Regulation of the protein tyrosine kinase pp72^syk^ by platelet agonists and the integrin $\alpha_{IIb}\beta_3$. J Biol Chem 1994;269:28859–28864.

252. Taniguchi T. Cytokine signaling through nonreceptor protein tyrosine kinases. Science 1995;268:251–255.

253. Frangioni JV, Oda A, Smith M et al. Calpain-catalyzed cleavage and subcellular relocation of protein phosphotyrosine phosphatase 1B (PTP-1B) in human platelets. EMBO J 1993;12:4843–4856.

254. Ezumi Y, Takayama H, Okuma M. Differential regulation of protein-tyrosine phosphatases by integrin $\alpha_{IIb}\beta_3$ through cytoskeletal reorganization and tyrosine phosphorylation in human platelets. J Biol Chem 1995;270: 11927–11934.

255. Falet H, Ramos-Morales F, Bachelot C et al. Association of the protein tyrosine phosphatase PTP1C with the protein tyrosine kinase c-Src in human platelets. FEBS Lett 1996;383:165–169.

256. Scharenberg AM, Kinet JP. The emerging field of receptor-mediated inhibitory signaling: SHP or SHIP? Cell 1996;87:961–964.

257. Jackson SP, Schoenwaelder SM, Matzaris M et al. Phosphatidylinositol 3,4,5-triphosphate is a substrate for the 75 Kda inositol polyphosphate 5-phosphatase and a novel 5-phosphatase which forms a complex with the p85/p110 form of phosphoinositide 3-kinase. EMBO J 1995;14:4490–4500.

258. Zhang J, Zhang J, Shattil SJ et al. Phosphoinositide 3-kinase gamma and p85/phosphoinositide 3-kinase in platelets. Relative activation by thrombin receptor or beta-phorbol myristate acetate and roles in promoting the ligand-binding function of $\alpha$IIβ3 integrin. J Biol Chem 1996;271: 6265–6272.

259. Thomason PA, James SR, Casey PJ et al. A G protein $\beta\gamma$-subunit-responsive phosphoinositide 3-kinase activity in human platelet cytosol. J Biol Chem 1994;269:16525–16528.

260. Chacko GW, Brandt JT, Coggeshall KM et al. Phosphoinositide 3-kinase and p72^syk^ noncovalently associate with the low affinity Fc receptor on human platelets through an immunoreceptor tyrosine-based activation motif. Reconstruction with synthetic phosphopeptides. J Biol Chem 1996; 271:10775–10781.

261. Abrams CS, Zhang J, Downes CP et al. Phosphopleckstrin inhibits G$\beta\gamma$-activable platelet phosphatidylinositol-4,5-bisphosphate 3-kinase. J Biol Chem 1996;271:25192–25197.

262. Kovacsovics TJ, Bachelot C, Toker A et al. Phosphoinositide 3-kinase inhibition spares actin assembly in activating platelets but reverses platelet aggregation. J Biol Chem 1995;270:11358–11366.

263. Kramer RM, Roberts EF, Strifler BA et al. Thrombin induces activation of p38 MAP kinase in human platelets. J Biol Chem 1995;270:27395–27398.

264. Charest DL, Mordret G, Harder KW et al. Molecular cloning, expression, and characterization of the human-mitogen-activated protein kinase p44erk1. Mol Cell Biol 1993;13:4679–4690.

265. Qiu ZH, Leslie CC. Protein kinase C-dependent and -independent pathways of mitogen-activated protein kinase activation in macrophages by stimuli that activate phospholipase $A_2$. J Biol Chem 1994;269:19480–19487.

266. Borsch-Haubold AG, Kramer RM, Watson SP. Inhibition of mitogen-activated protein kinase does not impair primary activation of human platelets. Biochem J 1996;318:207–212.

267. Miller JL, Sheridan JD, White JG. Electrical responses by guinea pig megakaryocytes. Nature 1978;272:643–645.

268. Neher E, Sakmann B. Single-channel currents recorded from membrane of denervated frog muscle fibres. Nature 1976;260:799–802.

269. Hamill OP, Marty A, Neher E et al. Improved patch-clamp techniques for high-resolution current recording from cells and cell-free membrane patches. Pflügers Arch 1981;391:85–100.

270. Mahaut-Smith MP, Rink TJ, Collins SC et al. Voltage-gated potassium channels and the control of membrane potential in human platelets. J Physiol 1990;428:723–735.

271. Fine BP, Hansen KA, Salcedo JR et al. Calcium-activated potassium channels in human platelets. Proc Soc Exp Biol Med 1989;192:109–113.

272. Kimura M, Lasker N, Aviv A. Thapsigargin-evoked changes in human platelet $Ca^{2+}$, $Na^+$, pH and membrane potential. J Physiol 1993;464:1–13.

273. Mahaut-Smith MP. Calcium-activated potassium channels in human platelets. J Physiol 1995;484:15–24.

274. Mahaut-Smith MP, Sage SO, Rink TJ. Receptor-activated single channels in intact human platelets. J Biol Chem 1990;265:10479–10483.

275. Mahaut-Smith MP, Sage SO, Rink TJ. Rapid ADP-evoked currents in

human platelets recorded with the nystatin permeabilized patch technique. J Biol Chem 1992;267:3060–3065.

276. Sage SO, Rink TJ, Mahaut-Smith MP. Resting and ADP-evoked changes in cytosolic free sodium concentration in human platelets loaded with the indicator SBFI. J Physiol 1991;441:559–573.

277. MacIntyre DE, Rink TJ. The role of platelet membrane potential in the initiation of platelet aggregation. Thromb Haemost 1982;47:22–26.

278. Mahaut-Smith MP. Chloride channels in human platelets: evidence for activation by internal calcium. J Membr Biol 1990;118:69–75.

279. Livne A, Grinstein S, Rothstein A. Volume-regulating behavior of human platelets. J Cell Physiol 1987;131:354–363.

280. Lang F, Busch GL, Völkl H et al. Cell volume: a second message in regulation of cellular function. News Physiol Sci 1995;10:18–22.

281. Szirmai M, Sarkadi B, Szász I et al. Volume regulatory mechanisms of human platelets. Haematologia 1988;21:33–40.

282. Horne WC, Simons ER. Probes of transmembrane potentials in platelets: changes in cyanine dye fluorescence in response to aggregation stimuli. Blood 1978;51:741–749.

283. Greenberg-Sepersky SM, Simons ER. Cation gradient dependence of the steps in thrombin stimulation of human platelets. Studies with the novel fluorescent cytosolic $Na^+$ indicator sodium-binding benzofuran isophthalate. J Biol Chem 1984;259:1502–1508.

284. Borin M, Siffert W. Stimulation by thrombin increases the cytosolic free $Na^+$ concentration in human platelets. Studies with the novel fluorescent cytosolic $Na^+$ indicator sodium-binding benzofuran isophthalate. J Biol Chem 1990;265:19543–19550.

285. Borin M, Siffert W. Further characterization of the mechanisms mediating the rise in cytosolic free $Na^+$ in thrombin-stimulated platelets. Evidence for inhibition of the $Na^+$, $K(+)$-ATPase and for Na+ entry via a $Ca^{2+}$ influx pathway. J Biol Chem 1991;266:13153–13160.

286. Rengasamy A, Feinberg H. Sodium-calcium exchange in platelet plasma membrane vesicles. Adv Exp Med Biol 1988;232:105–108.

287. Rengasamy A, Soura S, Feinberg H. Platelet $Ca^{2+}$ homeostasis: $Na^+$–$Ca^{2+}$ exchange in plasma membrane vesicles. Thromb Haemost 1987;57: 337–340.

288. Schaeffer J, Blaustein MP. Platelet free calcium concentrations measured with fura-2 are influenced by the transmembrane $Na^+$ gradient. Cell Calcium 1989;10:101–113.

289. Gierschik P, McLeish K, Jakobs KH. Regulation of G protein-mediated signal transfer by ions. J Cardiovasc Pharmacol 1988;12:S20–S24.

290. Saxena SP, Brandes LJ, Becker AB et al. Histamine is an intracellular messenger mediating platelet aggregation. Science 1989;243:1596–1599.

291. Saxena SP, Robertson C, Becker AB et al. Synthesis of intracellular histamine in platelets is associated with activation of protein kinase C, but not with mobilization of $Ca^{2+}$. Biochem J 1991;273:405–408.

292. Murayama T, Kajiyama Y, Nomura Y. Histamine-stimulated and GTP-binding proteins-mediated phospholipase $A_2$ activation in rabbit platelets. J Biol Chem 1990;265:4290–4295.

293. Bird RB, Stewart WE, Lightfoot EN. Transport phenomena. New York: John Wiley, 1960.

294. Savage B, Saldivar E, Ruggeri ZM. Initiation of platelet adhesion by arrest onto fibrinogen or translocation on von Willebrand factor. Cell 1996;84: 289–297.

295. Moake JL, Turner NA, Stathopoulos NA et al. Shear-induced platelet aggregation can be mediated by vWf released from platelets, as well as by exogenous large or unusually large vWf multimers, requires adenosine diphosphate, and is resistant to aspirin. Blood 1988;71:1366–1374.

296. Hardwick RA, Hellums JD, Peterson DM et al. The effect of $PGI_2$ and theophylline on the response of platelets subject to shear stress. Blood 1981;58:678–681.

297. Durante W, Schafer AI, Hrbolich JK et al. Endothelium-derived relaxing factor inhibits shear stress-induced platelet aggregation. Platelets 1993;4: 135–140.

298. Strony J, Phillips M, Brands D et al. Aurintricarboxylic acid in a canine model of coronary artery thrombosis. Circulation 1990;81:1106–1114.

299. Schullek J, Jordan J, Montgomery RR. Interaction of von Willebrand factor with human platelets in the plasma milieu. J Clin Invest 1984;73:421–428.

300. Weiss HJ, Hawiger J, Ruggeri ZM et al. Fibrinogen-independent platelet adhesion and thrombus formation on subendothelium mediated by glycoprotein IIb-IIIa complex at high shear rate. J Clin Invest 1989;83:288–297.

301. Chow TW, Hellums JD, Moake JL et al. Shear stress-induced von Willebrand factor binding to platelet glycoprotein Ib initiates calcium influx associated with aggregation. Blood 1992;80:113–120.

302. Kroll MH, Hellums JD, Guo Z et al. Protein kinase C is activated in platelets subjected to pathological shear stress. J Biol Chem 1993;268:3520–3524.

303. Razdan K, Hellums JD, Kroll MH. Shear stress-induced von Willebrand factor binding to platelets causes the activation of tyrosine kinase(s). Biochem J 1994;302:681–686.

304. Kroll MH, Dong JF, Francis K et al. Shear stress activates a functionally important phosphatidylinositol 3-kinase in intact human platelets. Blood 1995;86(Suppl):612a.

305. Andrews RK, Kroll MH, Ward CM et al. Binding of a novel 50-kilodalton alboaggregin from *Trimeresurus albolabris* and related viper venom pro-

teins to the platelet membrane glycoprotein Ib-IX-V complex. Effect on platelet aggregation and glycoprotein Ib-mediated platelet activation. Biochemistry 1996;35:12629–12639.

306. Du X, Harris SJ, Tetaz TJ et al. Association of a phospholipase $A_2$ (14-3-3 protein) with the platelet glycoprotein Ib-IX complex. J Biol Chem 1994; 269:18287–18290.

307. Du X, Fox JE, Pei S. Identification of a binding sequence for the 14-3-3 protein within the cytoplasmic domain of the adhesion receptor, platelet glycoprotein Ibα. J Biol Chem 1996;271:7362–7367.

308. Muslin AJ, Tanner JW, Allen PM et al. Interaction of 14-3-3 with signaling proteins is mediated by the recognition of phosphoserine. Cell 1996;84: 889–897.

309. Bonnefoy-Berard N, Liu YC, von Willebrand M et al. Inhibition of phosphatidylinositol 3-kinase activity by association with 14-3-3 protein in T cells. Proc Natl Acad Sci U S A 1995;92:10142–10146.

310. Hjemdahl P, Chronos NA, Wilson DJ et al. Epinephrine sensitizes human platelets in vivo and in vitro as studied by fibrinogen binding and P-selectin expression. Arterioscler Thromb 1994;14:77–84.

311. Wagner CT, Kroll MH, Chow TW et al. Epinephrine and shear stress synergistically induce platelet aggregation via a mechanism that partially bypasses vWf-GP Ib interactions. Biorheology 1996;33:209–229.

312. Kestin AS, Ellis PA, Barnard MR et al. Effect of strenuous exercise on platelet activation state and reactivity. Circulation 1993;88:1502–1511.

313. Steen VM, Tysnes OB, Holmsen H. Synergism between thrombin and adrenaline (epinephrine) in human platelets. Marked potentiation of inositol phospholipid metabolism. Biochem J 1988;253:581–586.

314. Ware JA, Smith M, Salzman EW. Synergism of platelet aggregating agents. Role of elevation of cytoplasmic calcium. J Clin Invest 1987;80:267–271.

315. Ishii K, Hein L, Kobilka B et al. Kinetics of thrombin receptor cleavage on intact cells. Relation to signaling. J Biol Chem 1993;268:9780–9786.

316. Walsh PN. Platelet-mediated trigger mechanisms in the contact phase of blood coagulation. Semin Thromb Hemost 1987;13:86–94.

317. Ahmad SS, Rawala-Sheikh R, Ashby B et al. Platelet receptor-mediated factor X activation by factor Ixa. High-affinity factor IXa receptors induced by factor VIII are deficient on platelets in Scott syndrome. J Clin Invest 1989;84:824–828.

318. Solymoss S, Tucker MM, Tracy PB. Kinetics of inactivation of membrane-bound factor Va by activated protein C. Protein S modulates factor Xa protection. J Biol Chem 1988;263:14884–14890.

319. Smith RP, Higuchi DA, Broze GJ Jr. Platelet coagulation factor XIα-inhibitor, a form of Alzheimer amyloid precursor protein. Science 1990;248: 1126–1128.

320. Cronlund AL, Walsh PN. A low-molecular-weight platelet inhibitor of factor XIa: purification, characterization, and possible role in blood coagulation. Biochemistry 1992;31:1685–1694.

321. Abrams CS, Ellison N, Budzynski AZ et al. Direct detection of activated platelets and platelet-derived microparticles in humans. Blood 1990;75: 128–138.

322. Tans G, Rosing J, Thomassen MC et al. Comparison of anticoagulant and procoagulant activities of stimulated platelets and platelet-derived microparticles. Blood 1991;77:2641–2648.

323. Brass LF, Pizarro S, Ahuja M et al. Changes in the structure and function of the human thrombin receptor during receptor activation, internalization, and recycling. J Biol Chem 1994;269:2943–2952.

324. Ishii K, Chen J, Ishii M et al. Inhibition of thrombin receptor signaling by a G protein coupled receptor kinase. Functional specificity among G protein coupled receptor kinases. J Biol Chem 1994;269:1125–1130.

325. Marcus AJ, Broekman MJ, Drosopoulos JH et al. The endothelial cell ecto-ADPase responsible for inhibition of platelet function is CD39. J Clin Invest 1997;99:1351–1360.

326. Vane JR, Anggard EE, Botting RM. Regulatory functions of the vascular endothelium. N Engl J Med 1990;323:27–36.

327. Brenner BM, Troy JL, Ballermann BJ. Endothelium-dependent vascular responses. Mediators and mechanisms. J Clin Invest 1989;84:1373–1378.

328. Durante W, Schini VB, Scott-Burden T et al. Platelet inhibition by an L-arginine–derived substance released by IL-1 β-treated vascular smooth muscle cells. Am J Physiol 1991;261:H2024–H2030.

329. Horowitz JD, Antman EM, Lorell BH et al. Potentiation of the cardiovascular effects of nitroglycerin by N-acetylcysteine. Circulation 1983;68: 1247–1253.

330. Radomski MW, Palmer RM, Moncada S. Endogenous nitric oxide inhibits human platelet adhesion to vascular endothelium. Lancet 1987;2: 1057–1058.

331. Mendelsohn ME, O'Neill S, George D et al. Inhibition of fibrinogen binding to human platelets by S-nitroso-N-acetylcysteine. J Biol Chem 1990;265: 19028–19034.

332. Lieberman EH, O'Neill S, Mendelsohn ME. S-nitrosocysteine inhibition of human platelet secretion is correlated with increases in platelet cGMP levels. Circ Res 1991;68:1722–1728.

333. Broekman MJ, Eiroa AM, Marcus AJ. Inhibition of human platelet reactivity by endothelium-derived relaxing factor from human umbilical vein endothelial cells in suspension: blockade of aggregation and secretion by an aspirin-insensitive mechanism. Blood 1991;78:1033–1040.

334. Lerea KM, Glomset JA, Krebs EG. Agents that elevate cAMP levels in platelets decrease thrombin binding. J Biol Chem 1987;262:282–288.

335. Knight DE, Scrutton MC. Cyclic nucleotides control a system which regulates $Ca^{2+}$ sensitivity of platelet secretion. Nature 1984;309:66–68.

336. Siess W, Lapetina EG. Prostacyclin inhibits platelet aggregation induced by phorbol ester or $Ca^{2+}$ ionophore at steps distal to activation of protein kinase C and $Ca^{2+}$ dependent protein kinases. Biochem J 1989;258:57–65.

337. van Willigen G, Akkerman W. Regulation of glycoprotein IIb-IIIa exposure on platelets stimulated with α-thrombin. Blood 1992;79:82–90.

338. Liu M, Simon MI. Regulation of cAMP-dependent protein kinease of a G protein-mediated phospholipase C. Nature 1996;382:83–87.

339. Fox JE, Reynolds CC, Johnson MM. Identification of glycoprotein $Ib_β$ as one of the major proteins phosphorylated during exposure of intact platelets to agents that activate cyclic AMP-dependent protein kinase. J Biol Chem 1987;262:12627–12631.

340. Fox JE, Berndt MC. Cyclic AMP-dependent phosphorylation of glycoprotein Ib inhibits collagen-induced polymerization of actin in platelets. J Biol Chem 1989;264:9520–9526.

341. Zavoico GB, Feinstein MB. Cytoplasmic $Ca^{2+}$ in platelets is controlled by cyclic AMP: antagonism between stimulators and inhibitors of adenylate cyclase. Biochem Biophys Res Commun 1984;120:579–585.

342. Enouf J, Bredoux R, Bourdeau N et al. Relationship between cAMP and $Ca^{2+}$ fluxes in human platelet membranes. Biochimie 1987;69:297–304.

343. Käser-Glanzmann R, Jakabova M, George JN et al. Stimulation of calcium uptake in platelet membrane vesicles by adenosine 3′,5′-cyclic monophosphate and protein kinase. Biochim Biophys Acta 1977;466:429–440.

344. Enouf J, Giraud F, Bredoux R et al. Possible role of a cAMP-dependent phosphorylation in the calcium release mediated by inositol 1,4,5-trisphosphate in human platelet membrane vesicles. Biochim Biophys Acta 1987; 928:76–82.

345. Cox AC, Carroll RC, White JG et al. Recycling of platelet phosphorylation and cytoskeletal assembly. J Cell Biol 1984;98:8–15.

346. Feinstein MB, Egan JJ, Opas EE. Reversal of thrombin-induced myosin phosphorylation and the assembly of cytoskeletal structures in platelets by the adenylate cyclase stimulants prostaglandin $D_2$ and forskolin. J Biol Chem 1983;258:1260–1267.

347. Hathaway DR, Eaton CR, Adelstein RS. Regulation of human platelet myosin light chain kinase by the catalytic subunit of cAMP-dependent protein kinase. Nature 1981;291:252–256.

348. Durante W, Kroll MH, Vanhoutte PM et al. Endothelium-derived relaxing factor inhibits thrombin-induced platelet aggregation by inhibiting platelet phospholipase C. Blood 1992;79:110–116.

349. Nguyen BL, Saitoh M, Ware JA. Interaction of nitric oxide and cGMP with signal transduction in activated platelets. Am J Physiol 1991;261: H1043–H1052.

350. Sane DC, Bielawska A, Greenberg CS et al. Cyclic GMP analogs inhibit gamma thrombin-induced arachidonic acid release in human platelets. Biochem Biophys Res Commun 1989;165:708–714.

351. MacDonald PS, Read MA, Dusting GJ. Synergistic inhibition of platelet aggregation by endothelium-derived relaxing factor and prostacyclin. Thromb Res 1988;49:437–449.

352. Grant PG, Mannarino AF, Colman RW. cAMP-mediated phosphorylation of the low-$K_m$ cAMP phosphodiesterase markedly stimulates its catalytic activity. Proc Natl Acad Sci U S A 1988;85:9071–9075.

353. Maurice DH, Haslam RJ. Molecular basis of the synergistic inhibition of platelet function by nitrovasodilators and activators of adenylate cyclase: inhibition of cyclic AMP breakdown by cyclic GMP. Mol Pharmacol 1990; 37:671–681.

354. Radomski MW, Palmer RM, Moncada S. An L-arginine/nitric oxide pathway present in human platelets regulates aggregation. Proc Natl Acad Sci U S A 1990;87:5193–5197.

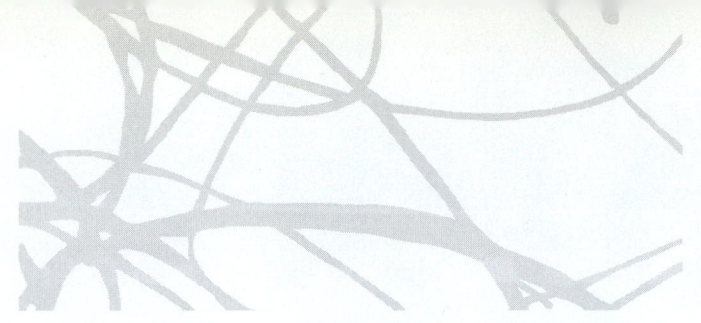

# SECTION 3

# VESSEL WALL

# CHAPTER 13

# OVERVIEW OF THE ENDOTHELIUM

Savvas C. Makrides and Una S. Ryan

## INTRODUCTION

With its vast surface area and strategic interposition between the blood and tissues, the endothelium interacts with and affects the activities of numerous cells and molecules. Endothelial cells participate in multiple physiologic processes, including the control of blood pressure, regulation of vessel tone, the growth of vascular smooth muscle cells, adhesion and infiltration of leukocytes into inflamed tissues, signal transduction, regulation of coagulation and thrombosis, and the highly regulated metabolism and transport of a multitude of blood-borne substances into subendothelial tissues (1, 2). In addition, the endothelium is involved in the pathogenesis of hypertension and atherosclerosis, and it interacts closely with the inflammatory, immune, and complement systems. Thus, the importance of the endothelium in homeostasis cannot be overstated. In recent years the application of new techniques, ranging from improved cell-culture methods to powerful cellular- and molecular-biology techniques, has led to much progress in our understanding of the complex functions of endothelial cells. In this review, we examine recent progress in several areas of endothelial biology, including cell-culture systems, metabolism, hemodynamic regulation of gene expression, and the interaction of endothelium with the complement system. Other areas, including vasoactive and coagulation factors, endothelial interactions with leukocytes, and the fibrinolytic system, are discussed in detail elsewhere in this volume and are mentioned here only briefly to provide more complete coverage of specific developments in endothelial research.

## ENDOTHELIAL BARRIER AND MORPHOLOGY

The structural organization of the endothelium serves to maintain vascular integrity and selective permeability to numerous substances, including leukocytes. Early studies of the structure-function relationships underlying the metabolic activities of endothelium have been reviewed (3), and they indicated that a variety of enzymes are situated on endothelial cells poised for interaction with the appropriate substrates delivered by the blood. Electron micrographs of the luminal side of endothelial cells of the pulmonary artery show a surface covered with fingerlike projections (Fig. 13.1). These structures increase the surface area available for processing of blood solutes by enzymes situated on the plasma membrane. Projections are also evident on pulmonary endothelial cells in culture and are therefore independent of contractions of the vessel wall. Other endothelial structures seen in large numbers in thin sections of pulmonary vessels are caveolae (Fig. 13.2), which, like endothelial projections, vastly increase surface area. Caveolae are positioned in direct communication with the vascular lumen, and this location facilitates the rapid return of the products of specific metabolic reactions to the circulation. The luminal stoma of the caveola is spanned by a thin diaphragm that may provide a specialized microenvironment for processing vasoactive substances. Both projections and caveolae stain prominently with anti–angiotensin-converting-enzyme (ACE) conjugates (4), and the relationship of caveolae to the pulmonary processing of adenine nucleotides, bradykinin, and angiotensin I has been demonstrated (5).

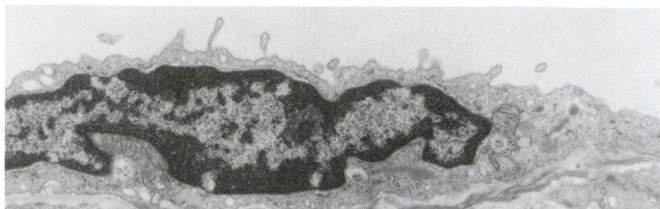

**FIGURE 13.1.** Endothelial cell from a pulmonary artery of the rat showing endothelial projections arising from the main body of the cell. Endothelial projections increase the luminal surface area of the blood vessels and favor interactions between blood-borne substrates and endothelial enzymes.

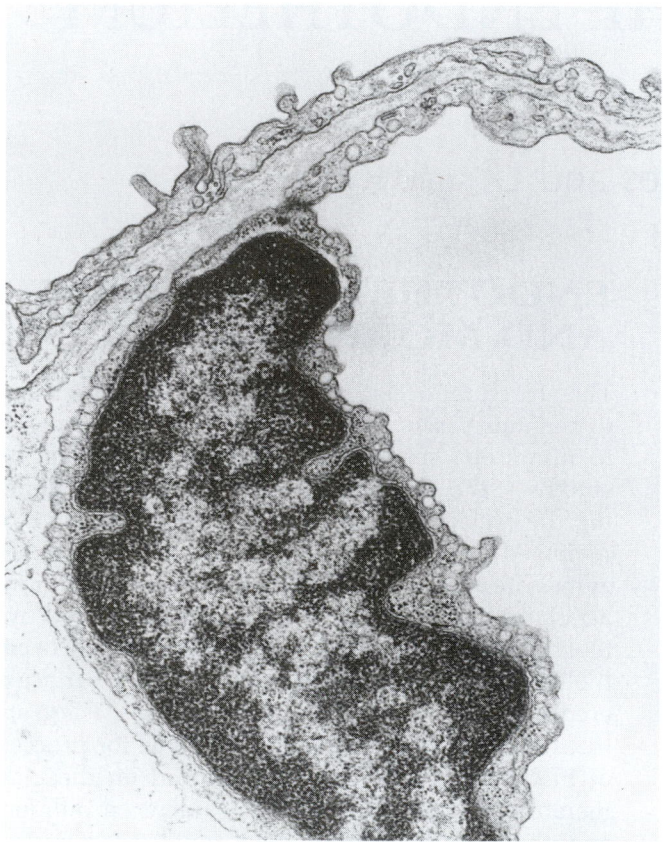

**FIGURE 13.2.** Pulmonary capillary endothelial cell showing large numbers of caveolae, covered on their luminal surfaces by a delicate diaphragm. Together with endothelial projections (Fig. 13.1), caveolae increase surface area and provide an environment for processing of biologically active substances by endothelial plasma membrane–bound enzymes.

In all organs the endothelium regulates transport of solutes, nutrients, lipids, and hormones to the interstitium via intracellular routes or via intercellular junctions. These complex organelles are formed by transmembrane proteins linked to cytoplasmic and cytoskeletal proteins (6, 7). Four types of junctions are known to exist between endothelial cells: tight junctions (8–10), adherence junctions (11), gap junctions (12), and syndesmos (13). In the continuous vascular endothelial monolayer, gap junctions predominate, whereas in regenerating endothelium there is a decrease in both gap junctions and tight junctions (14). In contrast, tight (occluding) junctions predominate in the brain and retina (15) where the development of edema can be dangerous. The close association of the endothelium with smooth muscle cells allows for the bidirectional passage of ions and small molecules via cell junctions. In this case cytoplasmic bridges of smooth muscle cells extend through fenestrations in the internal elastic lamina to contact the endothelium (16). In addition, some endothelial factors freely penetrate smooth muscle cells directly, independent of cell junctions. Other molecules bind to surface receptors to effect signal transduction via second messengers. The transmission of stress-induced signals is linked to cytoskeletal proteins (2, 7). Thus, actin filaments act in concert with a host of proteins, including integrins, actinin, talin, vinculin, and others, to provide the link between hemodynamic forces and biochemical signaling (2). The endothelium is also capable of transducing molecular stimuli into mechanical responses.

## CULTURE OF ENDOTHELIAL CELLS

The development of techniques for the isolation and reproducible culture of endothelial cells (17–21) has facilitated structural and functional studies of the endothelium. However, as several investigators have demonstrated (22–25), the up-regulation of many endothelial genes *in vitro* indicates that care needs to be exercised when extrapolating from cell culture systems to *in vivo* situations.

The limited life span of human primary cells *in vitro* (26) and the difficulties involved in obtaining and propagating primary cultures of endothelial cells have provided the impetus to establish transformed, permanent lines of endothelial cells. Such cell lines have been obtained by a variety of methods, including tumor-derived cell lines, transformation by viral genes, spontaneous transformation, and cell fusion (27). Unfortunately, most of these approaches have been unsatisfactory, as the transformed cells may lose differentiation markers or stop proliferating. An immortalized endothelial cell line has been obtained by microinjection of a gene construct containing a portion of the human vimentin gene promoter plus SV40 sequences encoding the large T and small t antigens (27). Cells immortalized by this method retained many differentiated properties and the morphologic organization of endothelium, alalthough some responses of the transformed cells to exogenous physiologic agonists differed from those of primary endothelial cells. Another problem associated with the use of cultured cells is morphologic or functional variability due to different culture conditions. Human umbilical-vein endothelial cells (HUVECs) are usually propagated under standard culture conditions (28). The availability of commercial sources of HUVECs maintained under different culture conditions has at times produced conflicting results (29, 30).

On the other hand, it is possible that the heteromorphology of endothelial cells observed in culture may not reflect a culture-dependent artifact, but rather may represent phenotypic heterogeneity of different endothelial cell strains. For example, five phenotypically different endothelial cell types were mechanically isolated from the microvascular bed of a single organ, the bovine corpus luteum, and the persistence of the phenotypic differences was demonstrated in cell culture (31). The heterogeneity of endothelial cells in terms of their growth rate and responsiveness to vasoactive agonists was recently demonstrated in a detailed study (32). Thus, endothelial cells derived from different sites of the vasculature exhibit marked differences in their growth rates, endothelin-1 release, and responsiveness to agonists, indicating that it may not be appropriate to generalize the functional properties of endothelial cells irrespective of their vascular bed of origin (32).

## IDENTIFICATION AND CHARACTERIZATION OF ENDOTHELIAL PROTEINS

The identification and characterization of endothelium-specific proteins is important for the elucidation of endothelial structure and function, for the establishment of animal models, and for potential therapeutic intervention in diseases of the vascular system, such as atherosclerosis and restenosis. Thus, the availability of methods for the modification of cells in the vessel wall holds promise for the application of gene therapy to vascular disease (33, 34). The endothelium is an attractive target for the expression of genes *in vivo* (35). Because of their contiguity with the bloodstream, endothelial cells are ideally situated for the release of therapeutic proteins directly into the blood, or, in the case of nonsecreted proteins, for the inactivation of toxic substances in the blood. In addition, endothelial cells present in a capillary bed with a high surface:volume ratio could be engineered to secrete pharmacologic levels of therapeutic substances into the circulation.

The targeting of genes (33) or proteins (36) for the disruption of ligand-receptor interactions requires high specificity to avoid untoward effects. Therefore, it is critical to identify protein components that are both tissue-specific, as well as disease-specific. However, it has been difficult to isolate some of these proteins to homogeneity in sufficient quantity for subsequent characterization and cloning by molecular genetic methods, which themselves are not without limitations (37–40). A recently developed biochemical method (41) can be used to purify the luminal plasma membrane from endothelial cells located in the vascular wall of both normal and diseased tissue. This technique uses positively charged colloidal silica particles to create a positively charged surface. After cell-surface binding, cationic sites are neutralized and crosslinked with a negatively charged polymer to form a laminate that coats the cell surface by multiple ionic interactions. Subsequent removal and homogenization of the silica-coated membrane facilitates the isolation of proteins from the endothelial cell luminal membrane. This method, described in detail elsewhere (42), has already been used to identify several endothelium-specific proteins (41–43).

## ENDOTHELIAL HEMOSTATIC FUNCTIONS

The pluripotent functions of the endothelium are perhaps best exemplified by the ability of endothelial cells to maintain either an anticoagulant surface or, in the activated state, to mount a procoagulant response. The biochemical events that lead to inhibition or promotion of thrombus formation *in vivo* are remarkable, and involve the sequential interaction of numerous agonists and their receptors or specific inhibitors, as well as the coagulation, fibrinolytic, complement, and other systems (44–52).

### ANTITHROMBOTIC ACTIVITIES OF ENDOTHELIUM

The antithrombotic state of the endothelium (Fig. 13.3*A*) is maintained by the interaction of both secreted, as well as membrane-bound, molecules. Secreted substances that have antithrombotic activity include prostacyclin, nitric oxide, and t-PA (tissue-type plasminogen activator), a component of the plasminogen or fibrinolytic pathway. t-PA converts plasminogen to plasmin, which degrades fibrinogen and fibrin into soluble products (47), and it reduces platelet activation by degrading receptors on the platelet surface (53, 54). Prostacyclin release by endothelium is induced by thrombin, histamine, bradykinin, thromboxane, or ATP and stimulates the increased production of platelet intracellular cAMP, which inhibits platelet activation (52). Similarly, nitric oxide increases platelet intracellular cGMP, which also inhibits platelet activation. Anticoagulant proteins include antithrombin III, which binds and inactivates thrombin and other activated coagulation factors, and

## A. Quiescent endothelium

Barrier function maintained
Anticoagulant, antithrombotic surface
Non-adhering surface for leukocytes

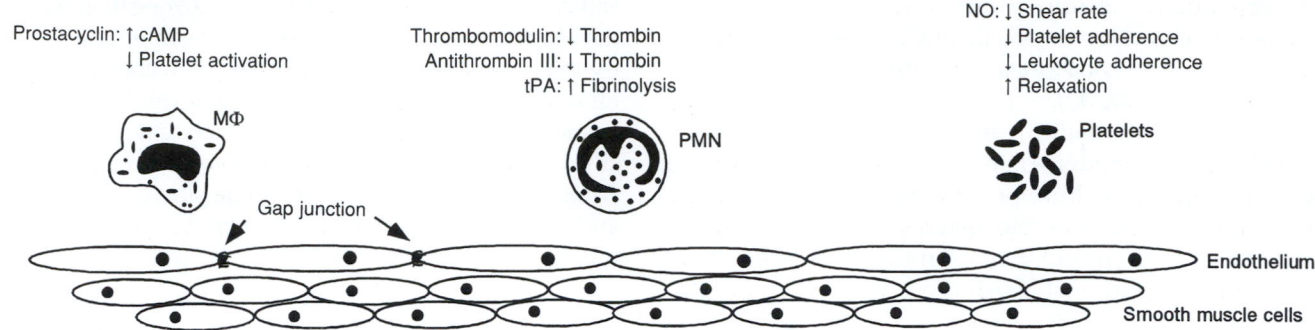

Prostacyclin: ↑ cAMP
    ↓ Platelet activation

Thrombomodulin: ↓ Thrombin
Antithrombin III: ↓ Thrombin
    tPA: ↑ Fibrinolysis

NO: ↓ Shear rate
    ↓ Platelet adherence
    ↓ Leukocyte adherence
    ↑ Relaxation

MΦ      PMN      Platelets

Gap junction

Endothelium

Smooth muscle cells

## B. Activated endothelium

Injury, infection, endothelial denudation
Activation of complement and coagulation pathways

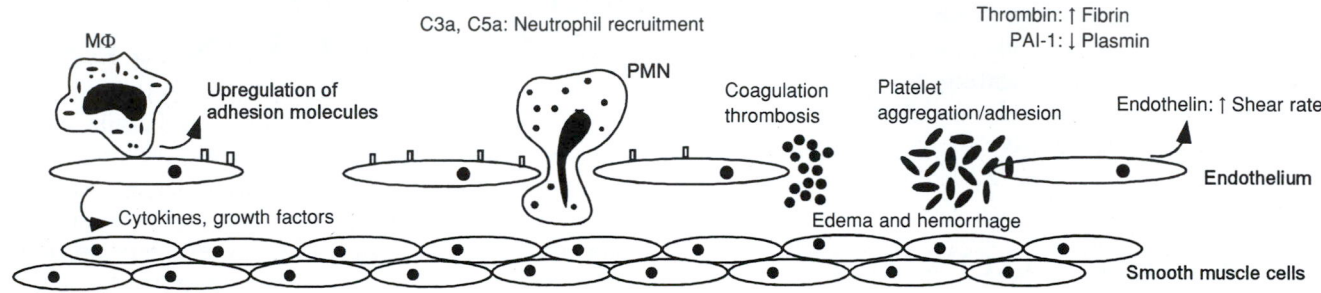

C3a, C5a: Neutrophil recruitment

Thrombin: ↑ Fibrin
PAI-1: ↓ Plasmin

MΦ      PMN

Upregulation of
adhesion molecules

Coagulation
thrombosis

Platelet
aggregation/adhesion

Endothelin: ↑ Shear rate

Endothelium

Cytokines, growth factors

Edema and hemorrhage

Smooth muscle cells

**FIGURE 13.3.** Metabolic events in quiescent (**A**) and activated (**B**) endothelium. **A,** NO causes vasodilatation, reduces shear rate in vessels, attenuates the binding and thrombotic activity of platelets, and inhibits the P-selectin–mediated attachment of leukocytes on the endothelial wall. t-PA converts plasminogen to plasmin, which degrades fibrinogen and fibrin into soluble products, and it reduces platelet activation by degrading receptors on the platelet surface. Prostacyclin release causes increased production of platelet intracellular cAMP, which inhibits platelet activation. Antithrombin III binds and inactivates thrombin. **B,** Procoagulant activities are effected by denudation of the endothelial layer and activation of the complement pathway. The exposed subendothelial surface interacts with blood components to promote coagulation. Thrombin production is elevated concomitant with the increased synthesis and release of the cofactors necessary for its synthesis, that is, factor V, factor VII, tissue factor, and high-molecular-weight kininogen. Thrombin converts soluble fibrinogen to insoluble fibrin, activates platelets, and inhibits vessel-wall fibrinolytic activity. The antifibrinolytic plasminogen activator inhibitor-1 (PAI-1) binds tissue-type plasminogen activator (tPA) and blocks the conversion of plasminogen to plasmin, thus inhibiting the solubilization of fibrin. The binding of platelets to the subendothelium is aided by the increased production of the vasoconstrictor endothelins, which cause an enhanced shear rate. MΦ, macrophage; PMN, polymorphonuclear leukocyte.

TFPI (tissue-factor pathway inhibitor), previously known as LACI (lipoprotein-associated coagulation inhibitor) (55) (see Chapter 4). The primary site of TFPI synthesis is the pulmonary endothelium, and the majority of TFPI is retained in the endothelium, whereas a small fraction (~15%) is secreted into the blood (56, 57). TFPI complexed with lipoprotein binds to heparin and functions as a key regulator of the tissue-factor (extrinsic) pathway of coagulation by its ability to inhibit factor Xa. In addition to soluble substances, endothelial membrane-bound molecules play key roles in the maintenance of the antithrombotic surface. These include ecto-

ADPase, which inactivates ADP released from activated platelets (58); thrombomodulin, which binds and internalizes thrombin, thus inhibiting platelet activation (50); and heparin, which accelerates thrombin inactivation by antithrombin III and binds TFPI-lipoprotein complexes that inhibit factor Xa (52).

## PROCOAGULANT ACTIVITIES OF ENDOTHELIUM

The procoagulant activities of endothelium (Fig. 13.3B) are activated by denudation of the endothelial layer by mechanical or chemical means, or by injury from bacterial endotoxins, thrombin, tumor necrosis factor-$\alpha$, interleukin-1, infection, complement activation, or other inflammatory stimuli. Consequently, the exposed subendothelial surface interacts with blood components to promote coagulation through the increased production of procoagulant, antifibrinolytic, and vasoconstrictor substances (48, 51, 52, 59). Thrombin generation is increased concomitant with the increased synthesis of the cofactors necessary for its synthesis, that is, factor V, factor VII, tissue factor, and high-molecular-weight kininogen. Tissue factor activity may be developed through blood (intrinsic) or tissue (extrinsic) systems. It interacts with factor VII to activate factor X, initiating the tissue factor (extrinsic) pathway of coagulation, and potentiates the cleavage of factor IX, activating the intrinsic pathway as well. von Willebrand factor (vWf) stabilizes factor VIII, which interacts with activated factor IX to activate further factor X. The activated factor X, formed via either the intrinsic or extrinsic pathways, converts prothrombin to thrombin in the presence of factor V. Thrombin then converts soluble fibrinogen to insoluble fibrin, activates platelets, and inhibits vessel-wall fibrinolytic activity. The activated endothelium also synthesizes the antifibrinolytic PAI-1 (plasminogen activator inhibitor), which is activated by binding to vitronectin. In its activated state, PAI-1 binds t-PA and blocks the conversion of plasminogen to plasmin, thus inhibiting the solubilization of fibrin. The binding of platelets to the subendothelium is aided by the increased production of endothelins, which act as potent vasoconstrictors and cause an enhanced shear rate (see below).

# ENDOTHELIAL CONTROL OF VASCULAR-WALL FUNCTION

Numerous substances produced by endothelial cells affect vascular remodeling and vasomotor tone. A diffusible substance, EDRF (endothelium-derived relaxing factor), was shown to mediate the acetylcholine-induced relaxation of rabbit aorta (60) (see Chapter 19). This substance was subsequently demonstrated to be NO or a related oxide species (61, 62). Since then, NO has been demonstrated to be an important signal molecule in the regulation of the cardiovascular, nervous, and immune systems (52, 63, 64). Endothelial NO has several properties: it causes vasodilation by acting on vascular smooth muscle, and it also reduces shear in vessels, thereby attenuating the binding of platelets to subendothelial components and thus reducing platelet thrombotic activity (52). Indeed, inhibition of NO synthesis promotes platelet adhesion to the vessel wall (65). In addition, NO inhibits the P-selectin–mediated attachment of platelets to leukocytes (66).

Another vasodilator is bradykinin (BK), so called for its slow onset of biologic activity ("bradys," slow + "kinein," to move), as contrasted with the faster-acting tachykinins. BK is a member of the kinin family of regulatory peptides, exerting multiple biologic effects in different tissues and organs. It causes vasodilation and enhances vascular permeability, lowers systemic blood pressure, stimulates phospholipase $A_2$ to release arachidonic acid for the synthesis of prostaglandins and leukotrienes, causes smooth muscle contraction in the respiratory and gastrointestinal tracts and the uterus, and mediates immune-cell stimulation and activation of sensory and sympathetic neurons (67, 68). The recently developed, improved BK receptor antagonists (69) and the cloning of rat (70) and human (71) BK receptors provide powerful, new tools for the study of BK metabolism. BK is synthesized by the action of plasma and tissue kallikreins on kininogen precursors and is cleaved by the endothelial membrane–bound ACE (4). BK exerts its effects through at least two types of receptors, $B_1$ and $B_2$. BK is although to mediate most of its physiologic activity through the $B_2$ receptor, whereas $B_1$ receptors may be involved in inflammation and other pathophysiologic conditions (67). Recent work has demonstrated up-regulation of $B_1$ receptors that mediate tone-dependent vasoconstrictor and vasodilator responses in the pulmonary vascular bed of the cat (72).

$PGI_2$ (prostacyclin, prostaglandin $I_2$) is a potent, endothelium-derived vasodilator that can be up-regulated by hemodynamic forces such as shear stress and pulsatile pressure, as well as by chemical mediators, including thrombin, bradykinin, angiotensin II, histamine, PDGF (platelet-derived growth factor), IL-1, $TXA_2$ (thromboxane $A_2$), and adenine nucleotides (73–76). $PGI_2$ is a product of arachidonic-acid metabolism (76a–76c) (Fig. 13.4), and it acts by binding to a G protein–coupled receptor linked to adenylyl cyclase, causing an increase in the intracellular level of cAMP. Unlike NO, which inhibits both adhesion and aggregation of activated platelets partly via a cGMP-dependent mechanism, $PGI_2$ only inhibits platelet aggregation and has no effect on adhesion (52).

In addition to vasodilator substances, the endothelium also releases vasoconstrictors in response to a variety of stimuli (see Chapter 19). A potent vasoconstrictor is endothelin (77), which is produced by a wide variety of cells and organs in the body (78). Endothelin has been shown to be a member of a family of isopeptides, referred to as ET-1, ET-2, and ET-3, which bind with different affinity to three distinct endothelin receptors designated $ET_A$, $ET_B$, and $ET_C$ (79). In the lungs, stimulation of $ET_A$ receptors effects vasoconstriction, release of thromboxane $A_2$, and bronchodilation, whereas stimulation of $ET_B$ receptors results in vasodilatation, release of prostacyclin, and bronchoconstriction (80). The renin-

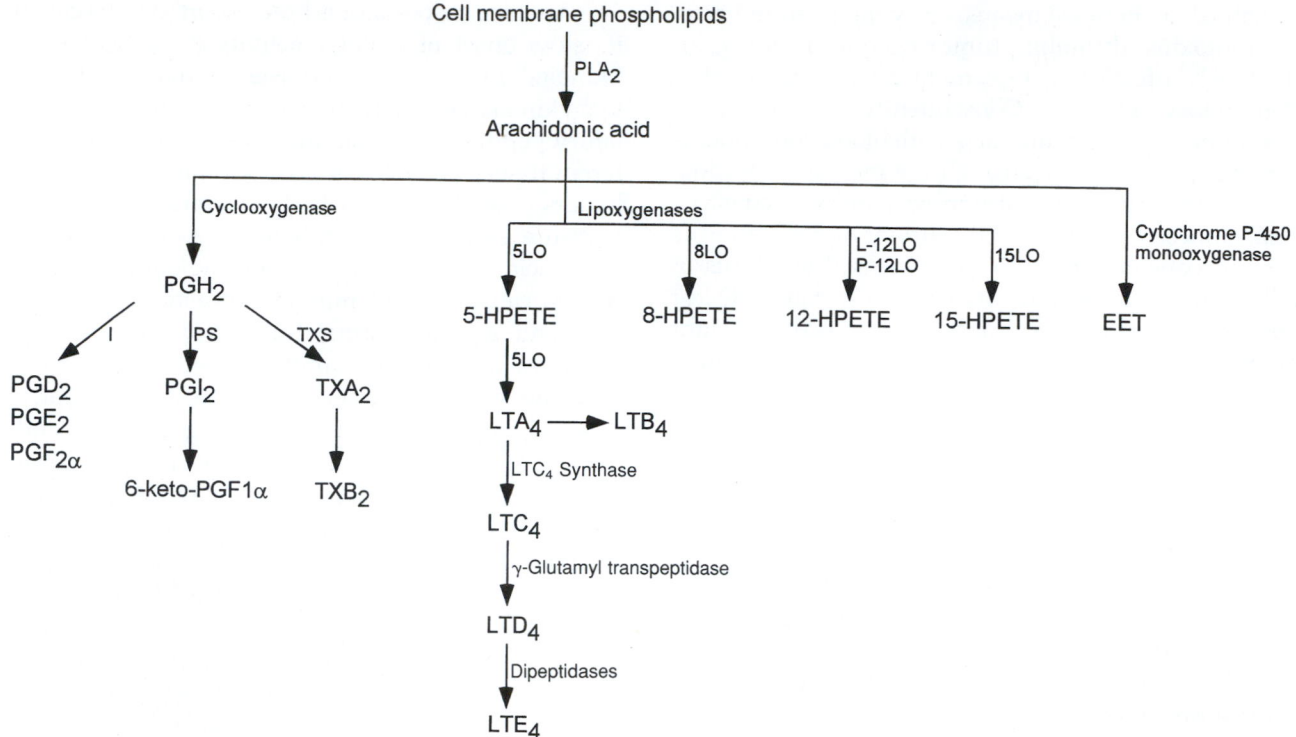

**FIGURE 13.4.** Pathways of arachidonic acid metabolism. The initial step in the production of oxygenation products is the release of arachidonic acid from storage sites in membrane phospholipids, the result of the activity of phospholipases. Following release, arachidonate is oxygenated via three major pathways catalyzed by cyclooxygenase, lipoxygenase (LO), and cytochrome P-450 monooxygenase. EET, epoxyeicosatetraenoic acid; HPETE, hydroperoxy-eicosatetraenoic acid; I, isomerase; L-12LO, leukocyte-type 12 lipoxygenase; LT, leukotriene; P-12LO, platelet-type 12 lipoxygenase; PGH$_2$, prostaglandin H$_2$ endoperoxide; PGI$_2$, prostacyclin; PLA$_2$, phospholipase A$_2$; PS, prostacyclin synthetase; TX, thromboxane; TXS, thromboxane synthetase.

angiotensin system is known to play an important role in blood-pressure regulation and vascular remodeling (4, 81–83). Similarly, the localization of ACE (angiotensin-converting enzyme) on endothelial cells (4) established a role for endothelium in the control of blood pressure. Angiotensin II is synthesized from angiotensin I by the action of the endothelium-bound ACE (83). Angiotensin II binds to receptors on vascular smooth-muscle cells to cause vasoconstriction.

# HEMODYNAMIC REGULATION OF ENDOTHELIAL GENE EXPRESSION (SEE CHAPTER 20)

The endothelium is a *dynamic* interface between the blood and the underlying tissues. As such, it is capable of a range of physical and functional alterations in response to acute, as well as chronic, changes in hemodynamic forces. These changes in blood flow may result from rapidly fluctuating metabolic needs or from

chronic disease–related demands. In either case, mechanical forces act on the endothelial wall to effect changes in cytoskeletal morphology and vasomotor tone and to release numerous substances from endothelial cells. Flow-induced changes may be classified into three temporal categories (84): immediate (seconds to minutes), intermediate (minutes to hours), and delayed (hours to days). Events that are relatively rapid, such as changes in vasoconstriction or vasodilatation, activation of adenylyl cyclase, and increases in the intracellular concentration of calcium and other "second messenger" molecules, are regulated by substrate availability, the activity of rate-limiting enzymes, signal transduction processes, and the proximity of ligand-receptor interactions. For example, when the endothelium is intact, activated platelets cause vasodilatation through the release of NO, but if the endothelium is denuded, platelets cause vasoconstriction. On the other hand, delayed responses to shear stress, such as the production of certain transcription factors, growth factors, and endothelin, are mediated by regulation of gene expression (2, 84, 85).

The first genes shown to be regulated by shear stress were those encoding endothelin-1 (77) and t-PA (86, 87). Subsequently, the effects of hemodynamic forces on en-

**TABLE 13.1.** Hemodynamic Regulation of Gene Expression in the Endothelium

| Gene | Expression Change[a] | Response Type[b] | Reference |
|---|:---:|:---:|---|
| c-fos | ↑ | I | (156) |
| c-myc | ↑ | I | (156) |
| c-jun | ↑ | I | (156) |
| PDGF-A | ↑ | I | (157) |
| ERK1/2 | ↑ | I | (158) |
| tPA | ↑ | II | (85) |
| eNOS | ↑ | II | (95, 159) |
| bFGF | ↑ | II | (160) |
| TGF-β1 | ↑ | II | (161) |
| ICAM-1 | ↑ | II | (95,162) |
| Cyclooxygenase-2 | ↑ | II | (95) |
| Mn-SOD | ↑ | II | (95) |
| Cu/Zn-SOD | ↑ | II | (163) |
| Endothelin-1 | ↑ | III | (164–166) |
| PDGF-B | ↑ | III | (95,157) |
| Thrombomodulin | ↑ | III | (167) |
| VCAM-1 | ↑ | III | (168) |
| MCP-1 | ↑ | III | (92, 93) |
| Egr-1 | ↑ | III | (169) |
| PAI-1 | ↑ | | (2) |
| Tissue factor | ↑ | | (2) |

[a] *The change in gene expression refers to the initial activation of the specified gene. Thereafter, the expression pattern may vary for each gene, depending on its response type.*
[b] *Gene expression responses to flow-induced stress are classified into three types (85): type I is an early transient increase, type II is a continued increase above baseline, and type III is a transient increase followed by a sustained decrease below baseline.*

dothelial gene expression have been documented for many genes (Table 13.1). Flow-induced gene responses have been grouped into three (85) or four (84) temporal patterns. Type I gene regulation (Table 13.1) is characterized by an early and transient response to shear stress, ranging from 1 to 4 hours (85). Type II response exhibits a continuously increasing up-regulation, and type III is characterized by a biphasic pattern of an early, transient up-regulation followed by a sustained decrease in gene expression. The mechanisms that govern these events are unknown. The demonstration that flow-induced gene activation involves a transcriptional component fueled efforts to identify DNA sequences and their associated transcription factors that might be linked to gene activation (2, 84, 85, 88–90). Studies using deletion mutants of the PDGF-B promoter identified a six-base pair sequence that mediated shear-induced gene up-regulation (91). This sequence, termed SSRE (shear-stress response element), was shown to impart shear responsive-

ness to other promoters. In addition, the SSRE sequence GAGACC, or its complementary sequence GGTCTC, was found to be present in the promoters of other shear-responsive genes (84).

However, the initial excitement was tempered by several observations. First, the SSRE sequence does not ipso facto prove its participation in shear-induced gene up-regulation. Thus, for example, the human MCP-1 gene uses a TRE sequence (TPA-responsive element) rather than the SSRE sequence, which is also present in its promoter (92, 93). Second, other shear-inducible genes do not contain this SSRE (94). Third, the GAGACC sequence is also responsive to NFkB, suggesting that shear may only indirectly activate transcription by inducing an oxidative stress. Moreover, an additional level of regulation became apparent with the discovery of a negative shear-responsive element in the preproendothelin-1 gene (85). Besides the complexity of promoter activation *per se* during shear stress, little is known about the specific transduction pathways responsible for the transmission of flow signals to the nucleus. The phosphorylation of mitogen-activated protein kinases is involved in this process (93).

Gimbrone et al (95) identified three genes that display differential responsiveness to different fluid mechanical stimuli. Thus manganese superoxide dismutase, cyclooxygenase-2, and the endothelial isoform of nitric oxide synthase were activated by uniform laminar shear stress (LSS), but not by a nonlaminar or turbulent mechanical stimulus. These three genes exhibit potential antiatherosclerotic activities (antioxidant, antithrombotic, and antiadhesive). The topographic pattern of early atherosclerotic lesions suggests the involvement of hemodynamic forces in the development of such lesions. Thus it was hypothesized that LSS associated with lesion-protected areas selectively induces the expression of atheroprotective genes in the endothelium, and these genes act locally to counteract the effects of atherogenic factors (95). This is an exciting possibility with implications for therapeutic intervention in cardiovascular disease.

Clearly, the modulation of gene activity by shear stress is a complex phenomenon that may require the interaction of transcriptional, translational, and protein-stability mechanisms. For example, the degradation of von Willebrand factor (vWf) is enhanced by shear stress in normal plasma (96). The different types of hemodynamic forces, such as laminar or nonlaminar shear stress, tangential stress, or stretch force (see Chapter 20), may likely use a combination of different elements in effecting gene regulation. Moreover, different genes may use unique signal transduction pathways in response to the same shear forces. Thus, it is doubtful that a single mechanism will emerge in these processes.

# INTERACTION OF ENDOTHELIUM WITH COMPLEMENT

Evidence indicates that complement activation may compromise endothelial function (97, 98). The complement system serves to initiate an inflammatory response, as well as to enhance the primary immune response (99). Alalthough the cytolytic properties of serum were first described more than a century ago (100), it is only in recent years that we are witnessing a much greater understanding of the mechanisms of complement activation and its deleterious effects on the integrity and function of the vascular wall when inappropriately activated (97, 98, 101, 102). Surface-bound proteins on endothelial cells play a key role in the activation of complement and in the localization of immune complexes in vascular injury (103, 104). The receptor-mediated deposition of C1q on endothelium is well documented (105–107) and more recent studies have demonstrated different molecular species of C1q receptors on human endothelial cells (108, 109).

The complement system and its regulators consist of two, linked, biochemical cascades, the classical and alternative pathways (Fig. 13.5). The classical pathway is usually initiated when a complex of antigen and IgM or IgG antibody binds to the first component of complement, C1. The initiation step of the classical pathway is controlled by the C1 inhibitor, which binds to C1r and C1s and dissociates them from C1q (110). Activated C1 cleaves both C4 and C2 to generate C4a and C4b, as well as C2a and C2b. The C4b and C2a fragments bind to form the C3 convertase, which, in turn, cleaves the third component of complement, C3, to form C3a and C3b. The binding of C3b to the C3 convertase yields the C5 convertase, which cleaves C5 into C5a and C5b. The latter becomes part of the MAC (membrane attack complex). The anaphylatoxins C3a, C4a, and C5a, released in this enzymatic cascade, play a key role in the inflammatory response, as they mediate smooth muscle contraction, changes in vascular permeability, chemotaxis, and many other processes (111). The anaphylatoxins differ in their relative potencies. C5a, the most potent one (110), acts as a chemotactic factor for neutrophils (112) and interacts directly with endothelial cells to activate xanthine oxidase (113), an enzyme that produces oxygen metabolites that are toxic to tissues (114). The alternative pathway of complement is triggered by microbial surfaces and a variety of complex polysaccharides. C3b, formed by the spontaneous low-level cleavage of C3, binds to nucleophilic targets on cell surfaces and forms a complex with factor B, which is subsequently cleaved by factor D to form the C3 convertase. The cleavage of C3 and the binding of an additional C3b to the C3 convertase gives rise to the C5 convertase of the alternative pathway (Fig. 13.5). In the subsequent reactions, which are common to both pathways, the C5 convertases in the classical and alternative pathways cleave C5 to produce C5a and C5b. Thereafter, C5b sequentially binds to C6, C7, and C8 to form C5b-8, which catalyzes the polymerization of C9 to form the MAC (115). This structure inserts into endothelial and other target membranes and causes cell lysis (116, 117). However, deposition of low amounts of MAC on cell membranes of nucleated cells does not cause cell lysis. Thus, in addition to its

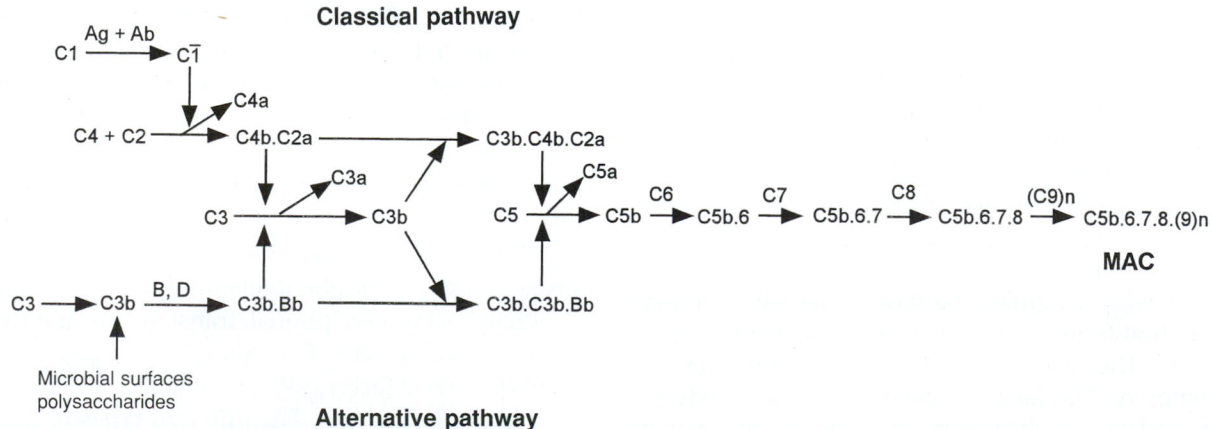

**FIGURE 13.5.** The complement pathway. The classical pathway is activated by immune complexes of antigen (Ag) and IgM or IgG antibody (Ab) subclasses. The alternative pathway is activated by complex polysaccharides, for example, yeast cell walls, endotoxins, lipopolysaccharides, and viral particles. The C3 convertases in both the classical and alternative pathways convert C3 into C3b, whereas the C5 convertases in both complement pathways convert C5 into C5b as shown. The anaphylatoxins C3a, C4a, and C5a are shown. The sequential addition of C6, C7, C8, and the polymerized form of C9 to C5b effect the formation of the membrane attack complex (MAC) C5b-9. The complement system is subject to regulation by both soluble, as well as surface-bound, proteins (see text), including members of the regulators of complement activation family.

cytolytic properties, the MAC is a mediator of a range of cellular processes, including the production of oxygen metabolites, eicosanoids (arachidonic acid metabolites), cytokines, the activation of enzymes, the release of polypeptide mitogens, and stimulation of cellular proliferation (118–120).

Systemic activation of complement and the generation of C5a stimulate neutrophils and cause their sequestration within capillaries, followed by damage to endothelial cells, the result of the generation of toxic oxygen metabolites by neutrophils (121, 122). The involvement of complement activation in ischemia/reperfusion injury is indicated by the deposition of C5b-9 in infarcted tissue (123) and by the fact that human sCR1 (soluble complement receptor type 1) administered prior to ischemia or prior to reperfusion can inhibit tissue damage (98). To date no therapeutic blocker of complement activation is available. The development of a recombinant, soluble form of human CR1 (sCR1) lacking the transmembrane and cytoplasmic domains has provided a potential therapeutic agent for the suppression of tissue injury in ischemia and reperfusion (98, 124) and in other clinical situations that are mediated by inappropriate complement activation (125). The complement-inhibitory activity of sCR1, its safety profile, and its long half-life in clinical trials (126) hold promise for sCR1 as an effective, anticomplement, therapeutic agent.

# LEUKOCYTE INTERACTIONS WITH THE ENDOTHELIUM

Leukocyte traffic through the endothelium is essential for the maintenance of immune surveillance and for the protection of tissues from injury caused by foreign antigens. The adhesion molecules involved in cell-cell and cell-matrix interactions are members of the four families of receptors: the selectins, integrins, the immunoglobulin (Ig) superfamily, and the cadherins (127–130) (see Chapter 15). These families of adhesion receptors orchestrate the complex series of events that ultimately leads to the infiltration of leukocytes into inflamed tissue (131). The L-, P-, and E-selectins are involved in the initial "rolling" adhesions, bringing the circulating leukocytes into close proximity with chemoattractants released from endothelial cells of the vessel wall. Chemoattractants bind to G protein–coupled receptors on leukocytes, signaling the activation of integrins, which, together with members of the Ig superfamily, effects the arrest and subsequent migration of leukocytes into the tissue (128). Among the molecules participating in the directed migration of leukocytes are the chemokines, which are althought to be sequestered on the endothelial cell surface (132–134). The chemokines comprise a fam-

ily of chemoattractant cytokines classified according to sequence homology and a cysteine signature motif: CXC, CC, and C (135–138). The CXC chemokine family acts predominantly on neutrophils and nonhematopoietic cells, and the CC family acts mainly on monocytes, eosinophils, and lymphocytes. A fourth chemokine class with a $CX_3C$ motif has recently been discovered (139). This protein exists as a membrane-bound form on endothelial cells and as a soluble glycoprotein. The latter form has potent chemoattractant activity for T cells and monocytes, whereas the anchored protein induces adhesion of the same leukocytes (139).

The selectins bind carbohydrate ligands containing fucose, including sialyl Lewis$^x$ (SLe$^x$) (140–142); furthermore, SLe$^x$ can inhibit neutrophil adhesion mediated by both E- and P-selectins (127, 140). Alalthough the "true" ligands for selectins are still under investigation (143), the above observations suggested that the disruption of the selectin-SLe$^x$ interaction might be therapeutically beneficial in inflammatory conditions. Indeed, several studies have demonstrated the protective effects of SLe$^x$ synthetic analogs in feline (144) and canine (145, 146) models of myocardial ischemia/reperfusion, as well as in a rat model of lung injury (147). More recently, the *in vivo* administration of an anti-SLe$^x$ monoclonal antibody was shown to have a cardioprotective effect in a rat model of myocardial reperfusion injury (148).

Complement activation (see above) plays a key role in the directed migration of neutrophils to sites of inflammation and in the expression of receptors on leukocytes and platelets that mediate adhesion and aggregation at sites of tissue injury (149, 150). In an effort to control the damaging effects of both complement and neutrophil activation during inflammation, sCR1 has recently been produced in a mammalian cell line capable of SLe$^x$ glycosylation (151–153). It was shown that sCR1 purified from conditioned media possessed SLe$^x$ moieties on the *N*-linked oligosaccharides of sCR1. Since sCR1 has 25 nominal *N*-linked glycosylation sites (154), it is expected that sCR1-SLe$^x$ would be extensively decorated with SLe$^x$ moieties. In addition to blocking complement activation, the potential multivalent interactions between sCR1-SLe$^x$ and its selectin counterligands might render this molecule particularly effective at inhibiting neutrophil activation and recruitment to sites of inflammation on the endothelial surface. This possibility is supported by a recent study (155) indicating that multivalency enhances the saccharide binding to L-selectin. Thus a synthetic SLe$^x$ analog was tested as an inhibitor of L-selectin–mediated lymphocyte-endothelial cell interactions in rejecting rat-kidney transplants. Whereas the nonfucosylated *O*-glycosidic oligosaccharide did not possess any inhibitory activity, the monovalent SLe$^x$ molecule prevented the binding significantly, and the divalent SLe$^x$ saccharide was the most potent inhibitor (155).

# SUMMARY AND CONCLUSIONS

The endothelium is much more than a gatekeeper for blood and blood-borne components. Its complexity is underscored by the numerous functions it performs in coordination with the renin-angiotensin, coagulation, fibrinolytic, complement, and immune systems of the body. In its intact state it maintains an anticoagulant surface; it regulates the transport of nutrients, leukocytes, and many other substances; it participates in the modulation of vasomotor tone and plays a key role in the control of blood pressure; and it forms new vessels in response to angiogenic stimuli. When injured, the endothelium manifests prothrombotic properties; it secretes mediators of vasoconstriction; and up-regulates surface receptors involved in coagulation, complement activation, and leukocyte migration. In recent years the mechanisms employed by the endothelium to effect some of its pluripotent functions in both health and disease are rapidly becoming unraveled. Leukocyte adhesion to activated endothelium, the key role of complement activation in inflammation, and the hemodynamic control of gene up-regulation are examples of areas of remarkable progress. While much remains to be done, the prospect of this knowledge leading to the realization of effective therapeutic interventions is indeed an exciting one.

# REFERENCES

1. Ryan US. Endothelial cells. In: Barker JH, Anderson GL, Menger MD, eds. Clinically applied microcirculation research. Boca Raton, FL: CRC Press, 1995; pp. 407–418.
2. Griendling KK, Alexander RW. Endothelial control of the cardiovascular system: recent advances. FASEB J 1996;10:283–292.
3. Ryan US. Structural bases for metabolic activity. Annu Rev Physiol 1982; 44:223–239.
4. Ryan US, Ryan JW, Whitaker C et al. Localization of angiotensin converting enzyme (kininase II). II. Immunocytochemistry and immunofluorescence. Tissue Cell 1976;8:125–145.
5. Ryan JW, Ryan US. Pulmonary endothelial cells. Fed Proc 1977;36: 2683–2691.
6. Caveda L, Corada M, Martin-Padura I et al. Structural characteristics and functional role of endothelial cell to cell junctions. Endothelium 1994;2: 1–10.
7. Dejana E, Corada M, Lampugnani MG. Endothelial cell-to-cell junctions. FASEB J 1995;9:910–918.
8. Gumbiner BM. Breaking through the tight junction barrier. J Cell Biol 1993; 123:1631–1633.
9. Anderson JM, Balda MS, Fanning AS. The structure and regulation of tight junctions. Curr Opin Cell Biol 1993;5:772–778.
10. Risau W. Differentiation of endothelium. FASEB J 1995;9:926–933.
11. Rubin LL. Endothelial cells: adhesion and tight junctions. Curr Opin Cell Biol 1992;4:830–833.
12. Beyer EC. Gap junctions. Int Rev Cytol 1993;137C:1–37.
13. Schmelz M, Franke WW. Complexus adhaerentes, a new group of desmoplakin-containing junctions in endothelial cells: the syndesmos connecting retothelial cells of lymph nodes. Eur J Cell Biol 1993;61:274–289.
14. Spagnoli LG, Pietra GG, Villaschi S et al. Morphometric analysis of gap junctions in regenerating arterial endothelium. Lab Invest 1982;46: 139–148.
15. Risau W, Wolburg H. Development of the blood-brain barrier. Trends Neurosci 1990;14:14–15.
16. Ryan US, Ryan JW. Vital and functional activities of endothelial cells. In: Nossel HL, Vogel HJ, eds. Pathobiology of the endothelial cell. New York: Academic Press, 1982; pp. 455–469.
17. Jaffe EA, Hoyer LW, Nachman RL. Synthesis of antihemophilic factor antigen by cultured human endothelial cells. J Clin Invest 1973;52:2757–2764.
18. Jaffe EA, Nachman RL, Becker CG et al. Culture of human endothelial cells derived from umbilical veins. Identification by morphologic and immunologic criteria. J Clin Invest 1973;52:2745–2756.
19. Gimbrone MA Jr, Cotran RS, Folkman J. Human vascular endothelial cells in culture. Growth and DNA synthesis. J Cell Biol 1974;60:673–684.
20. Gimbrone MA Jr. Culture of vascular endothelium. In: Spaet T, ed. Progress in hemostasis and thrombosis. Vol. 3. New York: Grune & Stratton; 1976; pp. 1–28.
21. Ryan US, Maxwell G. Isolation, culture, and subculture of bovine pulmonary artery endothelial cells: mechanical methods. J Tissue Culture Methods 1986;1:3–5.
22. Seulberger H, Lottspeich F, Risau W. The inducible blood-brain barrier specific molecule HT7 is a novel immunoglobulin-like cell surface glycoprotein. EMBO J 1990;9:2151–2158.
23. Frey A, Meckelein B, Weiler-Guttler H et al. Pericytes of the brain microvasculature express gamma-glutamyl transpeptidase. Eur J Biochem 1991; 202:421–429.
24. Meyer J, Rauh J, Galla HJ. The susceptibility of cerebral endothelial cells to astroglial induction of blood-brain barrier enzymes depends on their proliferative state. J Neurochem 1991;57:1971–1977.
25. Wolburg H, Neuhaus J, Kniesel U et al. Modulation of tight junction structure in blood-brain barrier endothelial cells. Effects of tissue culture, second messengers and cocultured astrocytes. J Cell Sci 1994;107:1347–1357.
26. Hayflick L, Moorhead PS. The serial cultivation of human diploid cell strains. Exp Cell Res 1961;25:585–621.
27. Vicart P, Testut P, Schwartz B et al. Cell adhesion markers are expressed by a stable human endothelial cell line transformed by the SV40 large T antigen under vimentin promoter control. J Cell Physiol 1993;157:41–51.
28. Thornton SC, Mueller SN, Levine EM. Human endothelial cells: use of heparin in cloning and long-term serial cultivation. Science 1983;222: 623–625.
29. Watson CA, Camera-Benson L, Palmer-Crocker R et al. Variability among human umbilical vein endothelial cultures. Science 1995;268:447–448.
30. Koch AE, Polverini PJ, Kunkel SL et al. Variability among human umbilical vein endothelial cultures. Science 1995;268:448.
31. Spanel-Borowski K, Fenyves A. The heteromorphology of cultured microvascular endothelial cells. Arzneimittel-Forschung 1994;44:385–391.
32. Thorin E, Shatos MA, Shreeve SM et al. Human vascular endothelium heterogeneity: a comparative study of cerebral and peripheral cultured vascular endothelial cells. Stroke 1997;28:375–381.
33. Finkel T, Epstein SE. Gene therapy for vascular disease. FASEB J 1995;9: 843–851.
34. Carmeliet P, Collen D. Gene targeting and gene transfer studies of the plasminogen/plasmin system: implications in thrombosis, hemostasis, neointima formation, and atherosclerosis. FASEB J 1995;9:934–938.
35. Zwiebel JA, Freeman SM, Newman K et al. Drug delivery by genetically engineered cell implants. Ann N Y Acad Sci 1991;618:394–404.
36. Kiely JM, Cybulsky MI, Luscinskas FW et al. Immunoselective targeting of an anti-thrombin agent to the surface of cytokine-activated vascular endothelial cells. Arterioscler Thromb Vasc Biol 1995;15:1211–1218.
37. Debouck C. Differential display or differential dismay? Curr Opin Biotechnol 1995;6:597–599.
38. Wang X, Ruffolo RR Jr, Feuerstein GZ. mRNA differential display: application in the discovery of novel pharmacologic targets. Trends Pharmacol Sci 1996;17:276–279.
39. Schwartz LM, Milligan CE, Bielke W et al. Cloning cell death genes. Methods Cell Biol 1995;46:107–138.
40. Wan JS, Sharp SJ, Poirier GMC et al. Cloning differentially expressed mRNAs. Nat Biotechnol 1996;14:1685–1691.
41. Schnitzer JE, Oh P, Jacobson BS et al. Caveolae from luminal plasmalemma of rat lung endothelium: microdomains enriched in caveolin, $Ca^{2+}$-ATPase, and inositol trisphosphate receptor. Proc Natl Acad Sci U S A 1995;92:1759–63.
42. Jacobson BS, Stolz DB, Schnitzer JE. Identification of endothelial cell-surface proteins as targets for diagnosis and treatment of disease. Nat Med 1996;2:482–484.
43. Schnitzer JE, Liu J, Oh P. Endothelial caveolae have the molecular transport machinery for vesicle budding, docking, and fusion including VAMP, NSF, SNAP, annexins, and GTPases. J Biol Chem 1995;270:14399–14404.
44. Rösen P, Schwippert B, Tschöpe D. Adhesive proteins in platelet-endothelial interactions. Eur J Clin Invest 1994;24(Suppl l):21–24.
45. Herbert JM, Dupuy E, Laplace MC et al. Thrombin induces endothelial cell growth via both a proteolytic and a non-proteolytic pathway. Biochem J 1994;303:227–231.
46. Woolkalis MJ, DeMelfi TM Jr, Blanchard N et al. Regulation of thrombin receptors on human umbilical vein endothelial cells. J Biol Chem 1995; 270:9868–9875.
47. Plow EF, Herren T, Redlitz A et al. The cell biology of the plasminogen system. FASEB J 1995;9:939–945.
48. Hawiger J. Mechanisms involved in platelet vessel wall interaction. Thromb Haemost 1995;74:369–372.

49. Furie B, Furie BC. The molecular basis of platelet and endothelial cell interaction with neutrophils and monocytes: role of P-selectin and the P-selectin ligand, PSGL-1. Thromb Haemost 1995;74:224–227.

50. Esmon CT. Thrombomodulin as a model of molecular mechanisms that modulate protease specificity and function at the vessel surface. FASEB J 1995;9:946–955.

51. Ruggeri ZM. The role of von Willebrand factor and fibrinogen in the initiation of platelet adhesion to thrombogenic surfaces. Thromb Haemost 1995; 74:460–463.

52. Body SC. Platelet activation and interactions with the microvasculature. J Cardiovasc Pharmacol 1996;27(Suppl 1,):13–25.

53. Adelman B, Michelson AD, Loscalzo J et al. Plasmin effect on platelet glycoprotein Ib-von Willebrand factor interactions. Blood 1985;65:32–40.

54. Schafer AI, Adelman B. Plasmin inhibition of platelet function and of arachidonic acid metabolism. J Clin Invest 1985;75:456–461.

55. Broze GJ Jr. The role of tissue factor pathway inhibitor in a revised coagulation cascade. Semin Hematol 1992;29:159–169.

56. Ameri A, Kuppuswamy MN, Basu S et al. Expression of tissue factor pathway inhibitor by cultured endothelial cells in response to inflammatory mediators. Blood 1992;79:3219–3226.

57. Sabharwal AK, Bajaj SP, Ameri A et al. Tissue factor pathway inhibitor and von Willebrand factor antigen levels in adult respiratory distress syndrome and in a primate model of sepsis. Am J Respir Crit Care Med 1995; 151:758–767.

58. Marcus AJ, Broekman MJ, Drosopoulos JHF et al. The endothelial cell ecto-ADPase responsible for inhibition of platelet function is CD39. J Clin Invest 1997;99:1351–1360.

59. Ware JA, Heistad DD. Seminars in medicine of the Beth Israel Hospital, Boston. Platelet-endothelium interactions. N Engl J Med 1993;328:628–635.

60. Furchgott RF, Zawadzki JV. The obligatory role of endothelial cells in the relaxation of arterial smooth muscle by acetylcholine. Nature 1980;288: 373–376.

61. Ignarro LJ, Byrns RE, Buga GM et al. Endothelium-derived relaxing factor from pulmonary artery and vein possesses pharmacologic and chemical properties identical to those of nitric oxide radical. Circ Res 1987;61: 866–879.

62. Palmer RM, Ferrige AG, Moncada S. Nitric oxide release accounts for the biologic activity of endothelium-derived relaxing factor. Nature 1987;327: 524–526.

63. Moncada S, Palmer RMJ, Higgs EA. Nitric oxide: physiology, pathophysiology and pharmacology. Pharmacol Rev 1991;43:109–142.

64. Nathan C, Xie QW. Regulation of biosynthesis of nitric oxide. J Biol Chem 1994;269:13725–13728.

65. Radomski MW, Palmer RM, Moncada S. Endogenous nitric oxide inhibits human platelet adhesion to vascular endothelium. Lancet 1987;2: 1057–1058.

66. Dembinska-Kiec A, Zmuda A, Wenhrynowicz O et al. Selectin-P-mediated adherence of platelets to neutrophils is regulated by prostanoids and nitric oxide. Int J Tissue React 1993;15:55–64.

67. Bhoola KD, Figueroa CD, Worthy K. Bioregulation of kinins: kallikreins, kininogens, and kininases. Pharmacol Rev 1992;44:1–80.

68. Dray A, Perkins M. Bradykinin and inflammatory pain. Trends Neurosci 1993;16:99–104.

69. Hall JM. Bradykinin receptors: pharmacologic properties and biologic roles. Pharmacol Ther 1992;56:131–190.

70. McEachern AE, Shelton ER, Bhakta S et al. Expression cloning of a rat B2 bradykinin receptor. Proc Natl Acad Sci U S A 1991;88:7724–7728.

71. Hess JF, Borkowski JA, Young GS et al. Cloning and pharmacologic characterization of a human bradykinin (BK-2) receptor. Biochem Biophys Res Commun 1992;184:260–268.

72. DeWitt BJ, Cheng DY, McMahon TJ et al. Analysis of responses to bradykinin in the pulmonary vascular bed of the cat. Am J Physiol 1994;266: H2256–H2267.

73. Marcus AJ, Weksler BB, Jaffe EA et al. Synthesis of prostacyclin from platelet-derived endoperoxides by cultured human endothelial cells. J Clin Invest 1980;66:979–986.

74. Bhagyalakshmi A, Frangos JA. Mechanism of shear-induced prostacyclin production in endothelial cells. Biochem Biophys Res Commun 1989;158: 31–37.

75. Baenziger NL, Fogerty FJ, Mertz LF et al. Regulation of histamine-mediated prostacyclin synthesis in cultured human vascular endothelial cells. Cell 1981;24:915–923.

76. Crutchley DJ, Ryan JW, Ryan US et al. Effects of bradykinin and its homologs on the metabolism of arachidonate by endothelial cells. Adv Exp Med Biol 1983;156:527–532.

76a. Holtzman MJ. Arachidonic acid metabolism in airway epithelial cells. Annu Rev Physiol 1992;54:303–329.

76b. Lewis RA, Austen KF, Soberman RJ. Leukotrienes and other products of the 5-lipoxygenase pathway. Biochemistry and relation to pathobiology in human diseases. N Engl J Med 1990;323:645–655.

76c. Funk CD. The molecular biology of mammalian lipoxygenases and the quest for eicosanoid functions using lipoxygenase-deficient mice. Biochim Biophys Acta 1996;1304:65–84.

77. Yanagisawa M, Kurihara H, Kimura S et al. A novel potent vasoconstrictor peptide produced by vascular endothelial cells. Nature 1988;332:411–415.

78. McMillen MA, Sumpio BE. Endothelins: polyfunctional cytokines. J Am Coll Surg 1995;180:621–637.

79. Masaki T, Yanagisawa M, Goto K. Physiology and pharmacology of endothelins. Med Res Rev 1992;12:391–421.

80. Uhlig S, Von Bethmann AN, Featherstone RL et al. Pharmacologic characterization of endothelin receptor responses in the isolated perfused rat lung. Am J Respir Crit Care Med 1995;152:1449–1460.

81. Dzau VJ. Vascular renin-angiotensin system and vascular protection. J Cardiovasc Pharmacol 1993;22 (Suppl 5):S1–S9.

82. Fukamizu A, Murakami K. New aspects of the renin-angiotensin system in blood pressure regulation. Trends Endocrinol Metab 1995;6:279–284.

83. Ryan US. Processing of angiotensin and other peptides by the lungs. In: Fishman AP, ed. Handbook of physiology. Vol. 1. Bethesda, Maryland: American Physiologic Society; 1985; pp. 351–364.

84. Resnick N, Gimbrone MA Jr. Hemodynamic forces are complex regulators of endothelial gene expression. FASEB J 1995;9:874–882.

85. Malek AM, Izumo S. Control of endothelial cell gene expression by flow. J Biomech 1995;28:1515–1528.

86. Diamond SL, Eskin SG, McIntire LV. Fluid flow stimulates tissue plasminogen activator secretion by cultured human endothelial cells. Science 1989; 243:1483–1485.

87. Diamond SL, Sharefkin JB, Dieffenbach C et al. Tissue plasminogen activator messenger RNA levels increase in cultured human endothelial cells exposed to laminar shear stress. J Cell Physiol 1990;143:364–371.

88. Ando J, Kamiya A. Flow-dependent regulation of gene expression in vascular endothelial cells. Jpn Heart J 1996;37:19–32.

89. Patrick CW Jr, McIntire LV. Shear stress and cyclic strain modulation of gene expression in vascular endothelial cells. Blood Purif 1995;13:112–124.

90. Davies PF. Flow-mediated endothelial mechanotransduction. Physiol Rev 1995;75:519–560.

91. Resnick N, Collins T, Atkinson W et al. Platelet-derived growth factor B chain promoter contains a cis-acting fluid shear-stress-responsive element [published erratum appears in Proc Natl Acad Sci U S A 1993 Aug 15; 90(16):7908]. Proc Natl Acad Sci U S A 1993;90:4591–4595.

92. Shyy YJ, Hsieh HJ, Usami S et al. Fluid shear stress induces a biphasic response of human monocyte chemotactic protein 1 gene expression in vascular endothelium. Proc Natl Acad Sci U S A 1994;91:4678–4682.

93. Shyy JY, Lin MC, Han J et al. The cis-acting phorbol ester "12-O-tetradecanoylphorbol 13-acetate"-responsive element is involved in shear stress-induced monocyte chemotactic protein 1 gene expression. Proc Natl Acad Sci U S A 1995;92:8069–8073.

94. Halnon NJ, Collins T, Gimbrone MA Jr et al. Regulation of the endothelial PDGF-A gene by shear stress [Abstract]. Circulation 1994;90:I88.

95. Topper JN, Cai J, Falb D et al. Identification of vascular endothelial genes differentially responsive to fluid mechanical stimuli: cyclooxygenase-2, manganese superoxide dismutase, and endothelial cell nitric oxide synthase are selectively up-regulated by steady laminar shear stress. Proc Natl Acad Sci U S A 1996;93:10417–10422.

96. Tsai HM, Sussman II, Nagel RL. Shear stress enhances the proteolysis of von Willebrand factor in normal plasma. Blood 1994;83:2171–2179.

97. Ryan US. Complement and endothelium: novel complement inhibitory therapeutics. In: Rubanyi GM, ed. Endothelium in clinical practice. New York: Marcel Dekker, 1997; pp. 291–310.

98. Makrides SC, Ryan US. Complement inhibition in ischemia reperfusion injury. In: Grace PA, Mathie RT, eds. Ischaemia reperfusion syndrome. Oxford: Blackwell Science, 1997, in press.

99. Fearon DT. Anti-inflammatory and immunosuppressive effects of recombinant soluble complement receptors. Clin Exp Immunol 1991;86 (Suppl 1):43–46.

100. Bordet J. Sur le mode d'action des sérums préventifs. Annales De L'Institut Pasteur 1896;10:193–219.

101. Homeister JW, Lucchesi BR. Complement activation and inhibition in myocardial ischemia and reperfusion injury. Annu Rev Pharmacol Toxicol 1994;34:17–40.

102. Morgan BP. Complement regulatory molecules: application to therapy and transplantation. Immunol Today 1995;16:257–259.

103. Daha MR, Miltenburg AM, Hiemstra PS et al. The complement subcomponent C1q mediates binding of immune complexes and aggregates to endothelial cells in vitro. Eur J Immunol 1988;18:783–787.

104. Peerschke EI, Ghebrehiwet B. Platelet interactions with C1q in whole blood and in the presence of immune complexes or aggregated IgG. Clin Immunol Immunopathol 1992;63:45–50.

105. Andrews BS, Shadforth M, Cunningham P et al. Demonstration of a C1q receptor on the surface of human endothelial cells. J Immunol 1981;127: 1075–1080.

106. Linder E. Binding of C1q and complement activation by vascular endothelium. J Immunol 1981;126:648–658.

107. Zhang SC, Schultz DR, Ryan US. Receptor-mediated binding of C1q on pulmonary endothelial cells. Tissue Cell 1986;18:13–18.

108. Peerschke EI, Malhotra R, Ghebrehiwet B et al. Isolation of a human endothelial cell C1q receptor (C1qR). J Leukoc Biol 1993;53:179–184.

109. Peerschke EI, Smyth SS, Teng EI et al. Human umbilical vein endothelial cells possess binding sites for the globular domain of C1q. J Immunol 1996;157:4154–4158.
110. Liszewski MK, Farries TC, Lublin DM et al. Control of the complement system. Adv Immunol 1996;61:201–283.
111. Morgan EL. Modulation of the immune response by anaphylatoxins. Complement 1986;3:128–136.
112. Gerard C, Gerard NP. C5a anaphylatoxin and its seven transmembrane-segment receptor. Annu Rev Immunol 1994;12:775–808.
113. Friedl HP, Till GO, Ryan US et al. Mediator-induced activation of xanthine oxidase in endothelial cells. FASEB J 1989;3:2512–2518.
114. Fantone JC, Ward PA. Role of oxygen-derived free radicals and metabolites in leukocyte-dependent inflammatory reactions. Am J Pathol 1982;107:395–418.
115. Tschopp J, Müller-Eberhard HJ, Podack ER. Formation of transmembrane tubules by spontaneous polymerization of the hydrophilic complement protein C9. Nature 1982;298:534–538.
116. Hu VW, Esser AF, Podack ER et al. The membrane attack mechanism of complement: photolabeling reveals insertion of terminal proteins into target membrane. J Immunol 1981;127:380–386.
117. Podack ER, Müller-Eberhard HJ, Horst H et al. Membrane attack complex of complement (MAC): three-dimensional analysis of MAC-phospholipid vesicle recombinants. J Immunol 1982;128:2353–2357.
118. Morgan BP. Effects of the membrane attack complex of complement on nucleated cells. Curr Top Microbiol Immunol 1992;178:115–140.
119. Nicholson-Weller A, Halperin JA. Membrane signaling by complement C5b-9, the membrane attack complex. Immunol Res 1993;12:244–257.
120. Benzaquen LR, Nicholson-Weller A, Halperin JA. Terminal complement proteins C5b-9 release basic fibroblast growth factor and platelet-derived growth factor from endothelial cells. J Exp Med 1994;179:985–992.
121. Mulligan MS, Schmid E, Till GO et al. C5a-dependent up-regulation in vivo of lung vascular P-selectin. J Immunol 1997;158:1857–1861.
122. Mulligan MS, Schmid E, Beck-Schimmer B et al. Requirement and role of C5a in acute lung inflammatory injury in rats. J Clin Invest 1996;98:503–512.
123. Hugo F, Hamdoch T, Mathey D et al. Quantitative measurement of SC5b-9 and C5b-9(n) in infarcted areas of human myocardium. Clin Exp Immunol 1990;81:132–136.
124. Weisman HF, Bartow T, Leppo MK et al. Soluble human complement receptor type 1: in vivo inhibitor of complement suppressing post-ischemic myocardial inflammation and necrosis. Science 1990;249:146–151.
125. Morgan BP. Clinical complementology: recent progress and future trends. Eur J Clin Invest 1994;24:219–228.
126. Dellinger RP, Zimmerman J, Metzler MH et al. Phase I trial of soluble complement receptor I (sCR1, TP10) in acute lung injury. Chest 1995;108(Suppl):R.
127. Lasky LA. Selectins: interpreters of cell-specific carbohydrate information during inflammation. Science 1992;258:964–969.
128. Springer TA. Traffic signals for lymphocyte recirculation and leukocyte emigration: the multistep paradigm. Cell 1994;76:301–314.
129. Tedder TF, Steeber DA, Chen A et al. The selectins: vascular adhesion molecules. FASEB J 1995;9:866–873.
130. Butcher EC, Picker LJ. Lymphocyte homing and homeostasis. Science 1996;272:60–66.
131. Malik AB, Lo SK. Vascular endothelial adhesion molecules and tissue inflammation. Pharmacol Rev 1996;48:213–229.
132. Webb LM, Ehrengruber MU, Clark-Lewis I et al. Binding to heparan sulfate or heparin enhances neutrophil responses to interleukin 8. Proc Natl Acad Sci U S A 1993;90:7158–7162.
133. Tanaka Y, Adams DH, Shaw S. Proteoglycans on endothelial cells present adhesion-inducing cytokines to leukocytes. Immunol Today 1993;14:111–115.
134. Witt DP, Lander AD. Differential binding of chemokines to glycosaminoglycan subpopulations. Curr Biol 1994;4:394–400.
135. Schall TJ, Bacon KB. Chemokines, leukocyte trafficking, and inflammation. Curr Opin Immunol 1994;6:865–873.
136. Clore GM, Gronenborn AM. Three-dimensional structures of alpha and beta chemokines. FASEB J 1995;9:57–62.
137. Wells TN, Power CA, Lusti-Narasimhan M et al. Selectivity and antagonism of chemokine receptors. J Leukoc Biol 1996;59:53–60.
138. Kelner GS, Kennedy J, Bacon KB et al. Lymphotactin: a cytokine that represents a new class of chemokine. Science 1994;266:1395–1399.
139. Bazan JF, Bacon KB, Hardiman G et al. A new class of membrane-bound chemokine with a CX(3)C motif. Nature 1997;385:640–644.
140. Phillips ML, Nudelman E, Gaeta FCA et al. ELAM-1 mediates cell adhesion by recognition of a carbohydrate ligand, Sialyl-Le$^x$. Science 1990;250:1130–1132.
141. Polley MJ, Phillips ML, Wayner E et al. CD62 and endothelial cell-leukocyte adhesion molecule 1 (ELAM-1) recognize the same carbohydrate ligand, sialyl-Lewis x. Proc Natl Acad Sci U S A 1991;88:6224–6228.
142. Foxall C, Watson SR, Dowbenko D et al. The three members of the selectin receptor family recognize a common carbohydrate epitope, the sialyl Lewis$^x$ oligosaccharide. J Cell Biol 1992;117:895–902.
143. Varki A. Selectin ligands: will the real ones please stand up? J Clin Invest 1997;99:158–162.
144. Buerke M, Weyrich AS, Zheng Z et al. Sialyl Lewis$^x$-containing oligosaccharide attenuates myocardial reperfusion injury in cats. J Clin Invest 1994;93:1140–1148.
145. Lefer DJ, Flynn DM, Phillips ML et al. A novel sialyl Lewis$^x$ analog attenuates neutrophil accumulation and myocardial necrosis after ischemia and reperfusion. Circulation 1994;90:2390–2401.
146. Flynn DM, Buda AJ, Jeffords PR et al. A sialyl Lewis$^x$-containing carbohydrate reduces infarct size: role of selectins in myocardial reperfusion injury. Am J Physiol 1996;271:H2086–H2096.
147. Mulligan MS, Paulson JC, DeFrees S et al. Protective effects of oligosaccharides in P-selectin-dependent lung injury. Nature 1993;364:149–151.
148. Seko Y, Enokawa Y, Tamatani T et al. Expression of sialyl Lewis$^x$ in rat heart with ischaemia/reperfusion and reduction of myocardial reperfusion injury by a monoclonal antibody against sialyl Lewis$^x$. J Pathol 1996;180:305–310.
149. Tonnesen MG, Smedly LA, Henson PM. Neutrophil-endothelial cell interactions. Modulation of neutrophil adhesiveness induced by complement fragments C5a and C5a des arg and formyl-methionyl-leucyl-phenylalanine in vitro. J Clin Invest 1984;74:1581–1592.
150. Lehrer RI, Ganz T, Selsted ME et al. Neutrophils and host defense. Ann Intern Med 1988;109:127–142.
151. Picard MD, Pettey CL, Marsh HC Jr et al. Sequence analysis of N-linked oligosaccharides bearing sialyl Lewis x moieties on soluble complement receptor type 1 (sCR1) [Abstract]. Glycobiology 1996;6:766.
152. Sen AC, Picard MD, Mealey R et al. Monosaccharide composition indicates presence of Lewis antigen in oligosaccharides in an alternatively glycosylated form of soluble complement receptor 1 [Abstract]. Glycobiol 1966;6:766.
153. Bertino A, Rittershaus C, Miller D et al. Soluble complement receptor type 1 in Lec11 cells is decorated with the carbohydrate ligand, sialyl Lewis$^x$ [Abstract]. Mol Biol Cell 1996;7(Suppl):449.
154. Klickstein LB, Bartow TJ, Miletic V et al. Identification of distinct C3b and C4b recognition sites in the human C3b/C4b receptor (CR1, CD35) by deletion mutagenesis. J Exp Med 1988;168:1699–1717.
155. Maaheimo H, Renkonen R, Turunen JP et al. Synthesis of a divalent sialyl Lewis x O-glycan, a potent inhibitor of lymphocyte-endothelium adhesion. Evidence that multivalency enhances the saccharide binding to L-selectin. Eur J Biochem 1995;234:616–625.
156. Hsieh HJ, Li NQ, Frangos JA. Pulsatile and steady flow induces c-fos expression in human endothelial cells. J Cell Physiol 1993;154:143–151.
157. Hsieh HJ, Li NQ, Frangos JA. Shear stress increases endothelial platelet-derived growth factor mRNA levels. Am J Physiol 1991;260:H642–H646.
158. Takahashi M, Berk BC. Mitogen-activated protein kinase (ERK1/2) activation by shear stress and adhesion in endothelial cells. Essential role for a herbimycin-sensitive kinase. J Clin Invest 1996;98:2623–2631.
159. Noris M, Morigi M, Donadelli R et al. Nitric oxide synthesis by cultured endothelial cells is modulated by flow conditions. Circ Res 1995;76:536–543.
160. Malek AM, Gibbons GH, Dzau VJ et al. Fluid shear stress differentially modulates expression of genes encoding basic fibroblast growth factor and platelet-derived growth factor B chain in vascular endothelium. J Clin Invest 1993;92:2013–2021.
161. Ohno M, Cooke JP, Dzau VJ et al. Fluid shear stress induces endothelial transforming growth factor beta-1 transcription and production. Modulation by potassium channel blockade. J Clin Invest 1995;95:1363–1369.
162. Nagel T, Resnick N, Atkinson WJ et al. Shear stress selectively upregulates intercellular adhesion molecule-1 expression in cultured human vascular endothelial cells. J Clin Invest 1994;94:885–891.
163. Inoue N, Ramasamy S, Fukai T et al. Harrison DG. Shear stress modulates expression of Cu/Zn superoxide dismutase in human aortic endothelial cells. Circ Res 1996;79:32–37.
164. Malek A, Izumo S. Physiological fluid shear stress causes down-regulation of endothelin-1 mRNA in bovine aortic endothelium. Am J Physiol 1992;263:C389–C396.
165. Malek AM, Greene AL, Izumo S. Regulation of endothelin 1 gene by fluid shear stress is transcriptionally mediated and independent of protein kinase C and cAMP. Proc Natl Acad Sci U S A 1993;90:5999–6003.
166. Wang DL, Wung BS, Peng YC et al. Mechanical strain increases endothelin-gene expression via protein kinase C pathway in human endothelial cells. J Cell Physiol 1995;163:400–406.
167. Malek AM, Jackman R, Rosenberg RD et al. Endothelial expression of thrombomodulin is reversibly regulated by fluid shear stress. Circ Res 1994;74:852–860.
168. Ando J, Tsuboi H, Korenaga R et al. Shear stress inhibits adhesion of cultured mouse endothelial cells to lymphocytes by down-regulating VCAM-1 expression. Am J Physiol 1994;267:C679–C687.
169. Khachigian LM, Lindner V, Williams AJ et al. Egr-1-induced endothelial gene expression: A common theme in vascular injury. Science 1996;271:1427–1431.

# CHAPTER 14

# THE VASCULAR RESPONSE TO INJURY

Gary H. Gibbons

The vasculature is a complex and dynamic organ capable of undergoing a wide spectrum of physiologic and pathophysiologic responses. Vascular cells have the capacity to sense biomechanical and humoral stimuli within the microenvironment and alter the function and structure of the blood vessel in response to both physiologic and pathophysiologic stimuli. Ross and others have proposed that the development of vascular diseases such as atherosclerosis and restenosis after angioplasty reflects a pathologic response to a noxious stimulus or injury. This chapter will focus on the problem of restenosis as a paradigm for understanding the vascular response to injury (1, 2). A deeper understanding of emerging concepts on the pathobiology of vascular injury after angioplasty should foster the development of more effective therapeutic strategies for preventing one of the most vexing clinical problems in cardiovascular medicine.

## THE RESPONSE TO ANGIOPLASTY INJURY: THE CLINICAL CONTEXT

One of the most challenging aspects of elucidating the pathobiological basis of restenosis after angioplasty injury is the lack of an animal model of restenosis that truly reflects the process in humans. Thus, our understanding must be based on careful clinical observations. Fortunately, emerging insights into the process of restenosis have been facilitated by the advent of new technologies, such as intravascular ultrasound (IVUS) (3) and molecular analyses of autopsy and atherectomy specimens.

One of the fundamental features of angioplasty injury involves the stretch of the vessel to the point of creating a tear that breaches the integrity of the intima and allows blood to dissect into the intimal and medial layers of the vessel. Angiographic and IVUS studies have documented substantial increases in lumen dimensions in response to this acute stretch and laceration of the vessel wall. This expansion of the lumen and reduction in the severity of the lesion stenosis are due primarily to increases in overall vessel dimensions with relatively minor changes in the dimensions of the plaque itself. The creation of one or more dissection planes has been well documented by IVUS studies. A subacute response of the vessel to stretch induced by angioplasty involves elastic recoil in which the intrinsic viscoelastic properties of the vessel attempt to restore lumen dimensions to the preprocedural state. This acute elastic recoil of the vessel can be seen as a failure of the intervention in a manner similar to acute closure due to thrombosis or a dissection flap. In addition to relatively passive responses such as elastic recoil, follow-up studies indicate that the vasculature undergoes an active, ongoing process of structural alteration in which the areas of distension and dissections created by the angioplasty become less evident, and the vessel wall architecture achieves a new postprocedure equilibrium. The critical questions are, how does this new equilibrium structure become established, and what determines how much of the acute gain in lumen dimensions that occurs immediately after angioplasty is lost after intervention?

The process of restenosis is best represented as a continuous rather than a dichotomous response. Restenosis can be defined as the late loss of lumen size relative to the acute gain in lumen dimension induced by angioplasty. It is important to emphasize that restenosis is not an inevitable consequence of balloon angioplasty injury, as the response-to-injury hypothesis infers. The spectrum of responses to angioplasty ranges from a time-dependent increase in lumen size that occurs over weeks and extends the immediate postprocedure gain, to maintenance of the acute postintervention gain without any further net changes in lumen area, to a structural loss in lumen dimensions from the acute postintervention gain back toward the pretreatment baseline, to an actual worsening of the stenosis compared to preangioplasty status. It is intriguing that despite the severity of the injury induced by angioplasty, most individuals maintain a net increase in overall lumen dimensions after the procedure. In contrast to many animal models in which balloon injury induces a net loss in lumen area, only a small minority of individuals exhibits an actual worsening of vascular disease in response to balloon angioplasty compared to the preangioplasty baseline status. The clinical data derived from angiographic studies suggest that, in addition to the response to injury that promotes lesion progression, the vasculature also has the countervailing capacity to remodel itself and thereby limit the narrowing of the lumen induced by vessel injury or progressive vascular disease (4).

Serial studies using IVUS appear to confirm the hypothesis that the response to angioplasty injury involves a spectrum from adaptive increases in overall vessel dimensions that preserve the acute gain postprocedure to maladaptive shrinkage remodeling and/or intimal lesion expansion that results in clinically evident restenosis (3). This hypothesis predicts that the response observed in individuals may be heterogeneous. The relative contribution of lesion expansion vs. remodeling may vary from lesion to lesion or individual to individual. Although these processes are often inaccurately conceptualized as dichotomous, in fact they are interrelated and both occur in the vast majority of individuals. In certain individual subsets with restenosis, intimal lesion expansion is a prominent component of the reduction in lumen dimensions; in others, the plaque area is relatively unchanged, but the overall dimensions of the vessel appear to be reduced back toward the original preprocedure baseline. The relative contribution of these processes to the development of a restenotic lesion may be influenced by factors such as lesion characteristics (e.g., calcification, plaque burden), individual-dependent risk factors (e.g., diabetes), or the nature of the angioplasty intervention (atherectomy vs. stent).

Unfortunately, the resolution of IVUS does not provide precise characterization of the histomorphology of the restenotic vessels. In some cases, this has resulted in the overinterpretation of the implications of these studies. For example, most IVUS studies are unable to resolve changes at the intima-media interface given the echolucency of the medial layer. This site is among the most vulnerable for the development of a dissection plane in response to distension injury. It is conceivable that a linear tear at the intima-media interface would allow for stretching of the vessel and a postprocedure increase in overall vessel dimensions without a significant change in plaque-media thickness. It is possible that a reparative process involving cell replication and matrix production that seals a linear rent in the wall may not result in an overall increase in intima-medial dimensions that can be readily quantitated by IVUS. These events within the echolucent areas of the wall may be beyond the resolution of this technique. The expression of these parameters as simple ratios that relate the relative changes in the areas of the external dimensions vs. the intima-medial area obfuscates the fact that small changes in the mass of tissue within the intima-medial population could have profound influences on the overall vessel dimensions. The observation that the intima-medial area does not change as dramatically as the vessel circumference does not exclude the possibility that events within the intima-media may play a critical role in the restenosis process. In short, the recent results of serial IVUS studies must be interpreted carefully. These studies have helped elucidate the role of overall changes in vessel dimensions as a determinant of restenosis. However, studies based on ultrasound tissue analysis do not allow us to draw substantive conclusions about the cellular processes that are involved in the loss of the acute gain in dimensions induced by the angioplasty procedure.

A rigorous dissection of the process would correlate the changes observed on angiography and IVUS with histomorphologic and molecular analyses. Unfortunately, such detailed longitudinal data do not exist in the clinical context. Despite these methodologic limitations, analyses of atherectomy and autopsy specimens have noted several prominent features of the restenotic process, including thrombus formation and organization, intimal hyperplasia, matrix expansion and modification, inflammatory cell infiltration within the intima and adventitia, and overall changes in vessel dimensions consistent with vascular remodeling. In addition, *in situ* analyses have documented critical cellular processes such as the activation of genes involved in thrombosis, cell growth, phenotypic modulation, cell migration, matrix modification, and programmed cell death. The inherent methodologic problems of sampling bias, the limitations of tissue sampling throughout the thickness of the vessel wall, the lack of a longitudinal time course assessment, and the heterogeneity of the pathobiological responses among individual subsets make it difficult to correlate these features precisely with changes noted by IVUS. Thus, the relative role of specific cellular pro cesses and molecular mediators remains an active area of ongoing research and continued debate.

# ANIMAL MODELS OF RESTENOSIS

An ideal model system would be generated quickly and at low expense, and accurately recapitulate the pathobiological processes defined in clinical studies. It would include a matured atherosclerotic plaque that creates an occlusive stenosis, and an angioplasty injury response that results in thrombus formation and organization, intimal hyperplasia, matrix expansion and modification, inflammatory cell infiltration within the intima and adventitia, and overall changes in vessel dimensions consistent with vascular remodeling. Unfortunately, such a model does not exist. Each animal model system has its advantages and limitations and differs in the relative prominence of a given pathobiological process (e.g., cell migration or vascular remodeling). Thus, an important caveat to the study of animal models of restenosis (most of which are simple vascular injury models) involves the recognition that these experimental systems provide useful mechanistic insights, but may fail to predict which therapeutic strategies will be the most effective in preventing restenosis in the clinical context.

Perhaps the simplest and most extensively characterized model is the rat carotid balloon injury system (5). The strengths of this model relate to its simplicity, reproducibility, and low cost. The advantages created by the simplicity of the model are counterbalanced by a number of limitations, such as: 1) the lack of a pre-existent neointimal lesion; 2) the absence of superimposed atherogenesis; 3) the severity and extent of distension injury created by the Fogarty balloon within an elastic artery compared to the injury induced by a clinical angioplasty balloon within a muscular coronary artery; 4) the relative lack of re-endothelialization; and 5) a minimal remodeling response. The failure of this model system to predict therapeutic efficacy of interventions is also cited as a major limitation. Nevertheless, the data derived from this experimental approach have played a critical role in advancing our understanding of vascular biology and established many of the current pathobiological concepts about the restenotic process.

The power of mouse molecular genetics has spurred interest in the development of murine models of vascular injury. Given its size, however, the mouse is generally not amenable to balloon catheter techniques of angioplasty. Therefore, several strategies have been used, including trauma induced by an intraluminal wire, external clamp trauma, electrocautery injury, adventitial cuffs, arterial transplants, and vessel occlusion (6). The strength of mouse models is the ability to elucidate further the molecular mechanisms of lesion formation by gene ablation experiments or gene-targeting strategies. However, there are methodologic concerns about the reproducibility of certain techniques, as well as difficulty extrapolating vessel injury in these models to the clinical context. Also, the small size of the vessels creates the problem of thrombotic occlusion as a prominent feature of the models under study that may not accurately simulate the actual role of thrombus in the clinical context. Despite these problems, the ability to manipulate these systems and superimpose injury upon atherosclerotic lesions that resemble human specimens is an exciting prospect worthy of ongoing investigation.

The rabbit model system has several advantages over the rat model. It is amenable to interventions similar to the human context, such as stents and clinical angioplasty catheters in vessels with pre-existent neointimal lesions. However, the models of atheroma formation typically used in the rabbit fail to simulate accurately the relatively hypocellular and sclerotic lesions observed in the clinical context. The sequential double-injury approach used by many investigators appears to induce two sequential and superimposed stimuli of vascular remodeling. This contrasts with the clinical context in which the development of the atherosclerotic lesion and the adaptive remodeling response to the atherosclerotic plaque is separated from the superimposed angioplasty injury by a time frame measured in decades. The double-injury model used by many investigators truncates this time course and, in essence, duplicates the influence of a balloon injury on the adaptive remodeling response to the first injury. This may explain why restenosis in this model system is influenced so dramatically by overall changes in vessel dimensions consistent with constrictive remodeling rather than neointimal hyperplasia. Indeed, this model often exhibits an exaggerated loss of the acute gain that fails to adequately simulate successful angioplasty observed in the clinical context. Again, the observation that certain therapeutic strategies shown to be effective in rabbits did not exhibit clinical efficacy has been cited as a limitation of this model.

Porcine models have been heralded recently as important models for restenosis relevant to the clinical context (7). The advantages of this system include a focus on the process in muscular coronary arteries using catheter systems similar to those used in humans with vascular disease. The porcine system also appears to combine many of the key pathogenic features noted in human disease, including thrombus formation/organization, cell migration, matrix production and modification, and vascular remodeling. However, cost is a major limitation of this model, especially for studies in which the goal is to superimpose angioplasty on pre-existent atherosclerotic lesions. Similarly, a primate model of restenosis has been described and appears to be rather promising

(8). It is intriguing that one of the limitations of this model is that it is difficult to observe the production of a stenotic lesion in some vascular beds due to the high capacity of the vessels to undergo compensatory enlargement in response to atheroma formation. The restenosis rate in this model in certain beds appears to be lower than other species due to a great capacity for enlargement remodeling. In the same manner that the rabbit model may exhibit an exaggerated constrictive remodeling response to double injury, the primate model may manifest a prominent enlargement remodeling response. Whether the logistical limitations in developing and maintaining this model will mitigate its widespread use is still unknown.

Once it is recognized that each model system has its own strengths and weaknesses, it becomes clear that each contributes to a complementary set of observations that advances our understanding of the overall response to vascular injury. Perhaps more important than the strengths and weaknesses of each model are the common fundamental cellular processes in lesion formation and remodeling after injury. The observation that certain cellular processes form part of a recurring theme clearly indicates the ubiquity of some basic features of the vascular response to injury that transcends the evolutionary distance in these model systems. Based on the evidence that the response in humans is heterogeneous, it is likely that each of these model systems captures some of the prominent features in given individual subsets. It is worthwhile to integrate pathobiological findings derived from the various model systems as a means of approximating the events observed in the clinical context.

# THE VASCULAR RESPONSE IN INJURY: MOLECULAR AND CELLULAR MECHANISMS

The cellular mechanisms involved in the vascular response to injury can be conceptualized as an overlapping, interconnected group of events. Each evolves in a particular temporospatial sequence, yet the precise onset and completion of one event may merge imperceptibly with another. Many of the events of cell fate determination, such as cell-cycle progression, apoptosis, and phenotypic modulation, are distinct processes, yet are linked and often regulated in a coordinate fashion. Although the prominence of each process may vary as part of the heterogeneity of the response to injury, each appears to be a fundamental feature of many models and will be reviewed as a means of gaining insight into the problem of restenosis.

| **TABLE 14.1.** | Molecular and Cellular Determinants of the Response to Vascular Injury |
|---|---|
| Thrombus | Inflammatory Cells |
| Platelets | Matrix Components |
| Thrombin | Endothelial Products |
| Fibrin | Nitric oxide |
| Plasmin | Prostacyclin |
| Apoptotic Cell Death | Heparan sulfates |
| Cell Proliferation | Endothelin |

## THROMBUS FORMATION AND ORGANIZATION

Perhaps the first event that accompanies the response to injury is the onset of thrombus formation. Angioplasty injury removes the endothelial cell surface that generates factors that prevent platelet activation/aggregation and promotes fibrinolysis (see Chapter 13). Moreover, denudation injury unveils a proadhesive surface of matrix proteins, such as collagen, fibronectin, von Willebrand factor, and phospholipids that bind to platelets and promote the generation of a fibrin clot. In particular, the creation of dissection planes exposes the lipid-rich core of the atherosclerotic plaque. The admixture of phospholipids and matrix proteins within this region of the atheroma is thrombogenic. The formation of multiple flaps and dissection planes within the vessel wall creates stagnant channels and areas of disturbed flow fields that promote thrombus formation. Clinical studies involving angiography and angioscopy, as well as analyses of atherectomy and autopsy specimens, have clearly documented the acute onset of thrombus formation after balloon angioplasty as common to angioplasty injury.

There are many mediators that contribute to thrombus formation after vascular injury. The generation of thrombus is facilitated by the loss of endothelium-derived generation of antithrombotic factors, such as nitric oxide, prostacyclin, ectoADPase, heparan sulfate, and tissue-type plasminogen activator (9). Also, the atherosclerotic plaque exhibits increased expression of prothrombotic mediators, such as the thrombin receptor and plasminogen activator inhibitor. One of the acute events in the response to injury involves an up-regulation in the gene expression of tissue factor after balloon distension. Thus, the increased exposure to plasma coagulation factors created by denudation of the endothelium, combined with the prothrombotic platforms created by matrix proteins and lipids within the plaque and activation of procoagulant factors within the vessel wall conspire to promote platelet activation/adherence, fibrin deposition, and the organization of a thrombus.

There are several cellular mechanisms by which platelet activation and thrombus formation may stimulate the process of restenosis. Studies in the rat model of neointima formation have documented that platelets play a critical role in promoting lesion formation by the local release of factors such as platelet-derived growth factor (PDGF) (10) that induce the migration of vascular smooth muscle cells into the neointima and may also provoke the movement of myofibroblasts from the adventitia into the vessel wall. The initial phase of platelet activation/adherence is followed by a phase of increased thrombin activity. Thrombin perpetuates the process of fibrin deposition and thrombus organization. The chemoattractant properties of thrombin favor the migration of vascular smooth muscle cells into the neointima and the infiltration of myofibroblasts into the fibrin gel matrix. The vascular smooth muscle cells and myofibroblasts that migrate into the fibrin scaffolding elaborate a collagen matrix that further fortifies the organization of the thrombus and matrix expansion. In addition to its effect on the extracellular constituents of the vessel, thrombin also stimulates an increase in vascular smooth muscle growth by activating tyrosine kinases, such as mitogen-activated protein kinase, in a manner analogous to PDGF (11). This growth response is mediated in part via the activation of autocrine-paracrine growth factors such as PDGF and transforming growth factor $\beta$1 (TGF-$\beta$1). Thus the process of thrombus formation induced by angioplasty gives rise to a cascade of events that may contribute to restenosis by activating processes such as cell growth, cell migration, and matrix modification.

The formation of a clot in response to a breach in the integrity of the blood vessel is one of the fundamental processes necessary to ensure the survival of the organism in response to injury. It is not surprising that there are powerful and redundant systems in place to ensure that this reparative mechanism becomes activated after vascular injury. One of the difficulties in defining the role of thrombus formation in restenosis relates to the problem of achieving a complete abrogation of this process within the vessel wall without having deleterious effects on systemic hemostatic mechanisms. The prominence of thrombus formation as a pathogenic mechanism of postinjury vessel stenosis varies in the different animal models under study. For example, in the rat carotid artery model, blockade experiments have documented that the thin carpet of platelets that adhere to the vessel wall during the first few days after balloon injury are sufficient to promote lesion formation (12). In contrast, strategies targeted against thrombin rather than platelets appear to have less profound effects on lesion formation in this model system (13). In the rabbit model of angioplasty injury, the inhibition of thrombin

appears to have more substantial effects on the process of restenosis (14). Antagonists developed against factor Xa inhibit lesion formation in rabbit models of vascular injury (15).

In addition to the use of pharmacologic probes, the powerful techniques of molecular genetics in mice are being used to dissect the relative contributions of prothrombotic mechanisms in lesion formation after vascular injury. Studies focused on the fibrinolytic system have documented that genetically engineered mice lacking plasminogen or plasminogen activators exhibit an impairment in lesion formation after vascular injury (see Chapter 22). These results appear to refute the idea that factors that promote thrombosis will enhance vascular lesion formation in response to injury. However, the fibrinolytic system also delivers proteases that promote the degradation of the matrix proteins and/or modulate integrin-matrix interactions. These interactions allow cells to migrate into the neointima. These data further emphasize that the lesion-promoting effects of fibrin and platelet deposition depend on a subsequent organization of the residual clot by the migration of vascular smooth muscle cells and myofibroblasts into the lesion. Recent studies using P-selectin knockout mice have observed a similar attenuation of vascular lesion formation in a mouse model of vascular injury (16). Blockade of platelet-leukocyte interactions observed during the early phase of the response to injury mitigates the activation of cell growth and migration necessary for lesion formation. These studies emphasize that a component of the lesion formation response to vascular injury involves a process of clot formation and organization within the vessel wall. Although the prominence of each component may vary with each model system, a common theme of the response to vascular injury involves a coordinate cascade of events in which platelet activation/aggregation, fibrin deposition, leukocyte influx, fibrinolysis, vascular myocyte and myofibroblast infiltration, and matrix modification promote changes in vessel structure that contribute to stenotic lesion formation.

There is obvious variance in the role of prothrombotic factors in lesion formation in different model systems. There are several variables that may explain this apparent discrepancy, including species differences in hemostatic mechanisms, the difference between the injury to a normal vessel vs. injury to a vessel with a preexistent neointima, and the adequacy of local blockade of prothrombotic activity. The challenge of addressing this question in animal models may be predictive of the difficulties in developing antithrombotic strategies to prevent restenosis in humans.

## APOPTOTIC CELL DEATH

The classic response-to-injury hypothesis has focused on aberrant cell growth as a fundamental pathobiological process of vascular lesion formation. However, emerging evidence suggests that it is the balance between cell proliferation and programmed cell death that governs organ structure during the process of organogenesis throughout ontogeny as well as the maintenance and repair of organ structure during adulthood. The original descriptions of the balloon injury model by Baumgartner (17) noted that medial cell death is one of the early consequences of balloon injury to the vessel wall. Recent studies in our laboratory and others suggest that this initial loss of medial cells after balloon angioplasty injury involves the induction of medial vascular smooth muscle cell apoptosis (18, 19). This response to mechanical distension injury was observed in a variety of species and vascular beds. These medial smooth muscle cells exhibit all of the morphologic and biochemical hallmarks of cell death by apoptosis. This distinction between apoptotic vs. necrotic cell death may be important, because apoptosis infers an active process of cell suicide that is governed by intrinsic cellular mechanisms. The precise stimulus that triggers the induction of cell death after balloon injury must still be defined.

In addition to the initial induction of apoptosis during the acute phase after injury, several laboratories have documented ongoing apoptotic cell death during the ensuing days and weeks. The well-described burst of medial cell replication after vessel injury is accompanied by ongoing apoptotic cell death (18). The persistent cell replication that occurs within the neointima is accompanied by neointimal cell apoptosis. Thus, net changes in the cell population of the vessel wall reflect a balance between parallel activation of cell death vs. cell replication. The cellular mediators that govern whether these cells survive or die remain to be defined. Studies performed in *in vitro* model systems indicate that factors involved in stimulating vascular smooth muscle cell growth, such as PDGF and angiotensin II, are also capable of increasing cellularity by inhibiting apoptotic cell death. Recent studies suggest that the susceptibility of vascular smooth muscle cells to undergo apoptosis may be predetermined by factors that result in phenotypic subsets. For example, the propensity of intimal cells to undergo apoptosis may be different from the inclination of medial cells to commit cell suicide.

The precise role of medial cell apoptosis in the pathogenesis of vascular lesion formation is unclear. It is conceivable that cell death may either promote lesion formation or have a countervailing influence on the disease process. For example, medial cell death may promote the release of cell-associated growth factors such as basic fibroblast growth factor (bFGF) or the generation of thrombin and thereby trigger cell proliferation. Alternatively, a decline in medial cell mass may play a role in the process of either shrinkage or enlargement remodeling after vascular injury. Although the prominence of apoptosis after angioplasty injury in both ani-

mal models and human specimens is clear, one of the important research questions in understanding the pathobiology of restenosis will involve further characterization of the actual role of apoptosis in this process.

## CELL PROLIFERATION

The process of cell replication is a prominent feature of tissue repair in a variety of contexts. In all of the animal models studied to date, it is well documented that angioplasty injury induces increased replication of vascular smooth muscle cells, monocyte/macrophages and fibroblasts. These data are consistent with both autopsy and atherectomy specimen data that have demonstrated the high cellularity of restenotic lesions as compared to the relatively hypocellular and fibrotic characteristics of the primary advanced atherosclerotic plaque. However, the use of *in situ* markers of cell replication in human specimens to further verify evidence of ongoing cell replication in restenotic lesions has yielded conflicting results. The reasons for these apparent discrepancies are numerous and include: differences in analytical techniques of immunohistochemistry; heterogeneity of the individual populations under study; limitations of atherectomy samples as representative of events throughout the vessel wall; the limited time-course analysis that may miss asynchronous and circumscribed periods of high levels of active cell replication; and the greater importance of changes in vascular remodeling, cell migration, matrix modification, and programmed cell death as determinants of intimal lesion volume. It is likely that cell replication remains an important determinant of lesion formation and restenosis in many individuals after angioplasty. Studies using serial IVUS have documented that certain individual subsets, such as individuals with diabetes, exhibit an apparent increase in intimal/medial lesion mass as a critical component of the restenotic process. The process of restenosis after angioplasty involving intravascular stents results in an expansion of the intimal/medial area rather than significant shrinkage remodeling. Histologic analyses of these poststent restenotic lesions have documented hyperplastic lesions reminiscent of those noted in many studies after balloon angioplasty. *In situ* analyses using a variety of markers have documented evidence of increased cell replication in these lesions. Taken together, these data are consistent with the notion that cell proliferation is a prominent component of restenosis after angioplasty.

The process of vascular cell replication after injury has been a universal observation in most models of vascular injury. In simple model systems in which a normal vessel is injured, there is an initial wave of medial cell injury followed by neointima formation and ongoing replication in the neointimal cells. In more complex models with pre-existent intimal lesions, intimal cell replication is also stimulated by vascular injury. Also, myofibroblasts that are prominent in the periadventitial regions of the vessels also undergo cell replication in response to the distension injury. Finally, the leukocytes within the neointima are another cellular component that undergoes replication in this setting.

The cellular processes that govern cell replication after angioplasty injury need further study. The regulation of cell replication involves an interplay between various stimuli within the cellular milieu that either promote or inhibit cell-cycle progression. Studies in the simplest model—the rat carotid artery—indicate that the release of basic fibroblast growth factor after the initial wave of medial cell death stimulates the initial phase of medial cell replication (5). Other blood-borne or locally generated factors, such as angiotensin II, thrombin, insulin-like growth factor I, transforming growth factor β1, and perhaps platelet-derived growth factor, may also play a role. In the simplest models that involve injury to a normal vessel that lack a pre-existent neointima, the potential contribution of resident inflammatory cells is often discounted. Monocytes and leukocytes are major constituents of the primary atherosclerotic lesion. When activated, they express a variety of growth factors and cytokines, such as PDGF and TGF-β1, that may promote the process of lesion formation by stimulating the replication of both leukocytes and vascular cells within the lesion.

In addition to the plethora of growth stimulatory factors that are generated in the setting of vascular injury, antiproliferative factors may also be expressed. The interplay between these locally generated growth factors as determinants of cell growth and lesion formation has been extensively reviewed. Although the activation of growth factors is often emphasized in the description of the response to injury, under normal circumstances, the vessel wall is rather quiescent with rare cell replication even in primary atherosclerotic lesions. This observation is consistent with the notion that vascular cells are tonically exposed to antiproliferative stimuli that maintain the quiescent state. According to this theory, the vascular response to injury involves a decline in a tonic inhibitory signal that unmasks the potential for a reparative response characterized by increased cell replication. It has been a long-standing observation that cell replication ensues after the loss of the endothelium, and the vessel wall achieves a more quiescent state once the integrity of the endothelium is restored. Interventions that enhance the process of re-endothelialization inhibit vascular lesion formation after injury. The implantation of endothelial cells into the periadventitial space using a novel delivery device inhibits lesion formation after vascular injury. The nature of the endothelium-derived factor(s) that inhibits lesion formation is not defined. The candidate mediators of this response include hepa-

rin sulfates, nitric oxide, prostacyclin and C-type natriuretic peptides. Each of these factors can inhibit vascular smooth muscle cell proliferation and migration. Studies involving local delivery of heparin have documented its efficacy in inhibiting vascular lesion formation in animal models. Studies involving *in vivo* gene transfer of the endothelial cell-type nitric oxide synthase gene have demonstrated a substantial inhibition of lesion formation *in vivo* (20). Supporting these findings, the administration of either systemic or locally delivered nitric oxide-donor drugs induces a similar inhibitory effect on lesion formation (21). Thus, factors generated by the endothelium appear to function as endogenous inhibitors of lesion formation. The loss of endothelial integrity after balloon injury may therefore play an important permissive role in the process of restenosis.

Although humoral factors play an important role in regulating cell fate determinations such as cell-cycle progression, other components of the extracellular milieu such as integrin-matrix interactions may be equally important. Cell replication in response to mitogenic stimuli is influenced by the nature of the cell matrix. Recent studies indicate that the nature of the collagen that vascular smooth muscle cells adhere to has dramatic effects on cell-cycle progression. Plating vascular smooth muscle cells on intact polymerized collagen promotes increased activity of the endogenous cell cycle inhibitory gene p21 as compared to denatured collagen. Given that the matrix composition within an atherosclerotic plaque is altered compared to a normal vessel, the regulation of the vascular cell replication in response to injury in this context may be markedly different from analyses of cell replication in the context of a normal vessel. This is yet another limitation in extrapolating from studies in animal models of angioplasty injury to the clinical context in humans.

The induction of cell replication by humoral factors such PDGF and thrombin via tyrosine kinase- and G-protein coupled receptors involves the activation of signaling cascades mediated by factors such as *ras-*, *src-*, and mitogen activated protein kinase. These signals are coupled to cell cycle regulatory genes such as the cyclins (e.g., cyclin D1) and cyclin-dependent kinases (e.g., cdk2). The activation of the multimeric complexes involving cyclins and cdks that stimulate cell cycle progression is counterbalanced by endogenous inhibitors such as p21 and p27 (22). A major checkpoint in the initial G-1 phase of the cell cycle is governed by retinoblastoma protein, which binds to and sequesters the transcription factor, E2F. Phosphorylation of the retinoblastoma protein by the cyclin-cdk complex causes it to release E2F, which in turn activates the gene expression of several essential cell cycle regulatory genes in a coordinate fashion. *In vivo* studies have shown that the acute response to vascular injury involves a release from the inhibitory influences imposed on cell cycle progression (23). There is a decrease in the expression of the inhibitory phosphatase that serves as a brake on the growth stimulatory signaling pathway mediated by the mitogen-activated protein kinase. Cell cycle progression is promoted by the initial decline in p27 activity that accompanies vascular injury. There is a fall in the expression of the growth inhibitory genes APEG-1 and the homeobox gene gax after balloon injury. The disinhibition or release of these braking mechanisms on the cell cycle, coupled with the increase in cyclin and cdk activity, mediates the initial wave of cell replication after balloon injury. Studies using antisense oligonucleotides to inactivate cell cycle regulatory genes such as cdk2, cdc2, cyclins, or transcription factor decoys directed at inhibiting the capacity of E2F to transactivate cell cycle regulatory genes have documented that the inhibition of cell cycle progression prevents lesion formation in various models of vascular injury (24, 25). Targeted overexpression of the endogenous inhibitors p21, p27, or mutant retinoblastoma protein that induces the sequestration of E2F has a similar inhibitory effect on lesion formation. Thus, the activation of cell cycle progression is a fundamental cellular event in the reparative response to vascular injury.

## INFLAMMATION

It is already well established that inflammatory cells, such as monocyte-macrophages and T-lymphocytes, are prominent components of atherosclerotic lesions in animal models as well as human vascular lesions (26). These resident inflammatory cells may also participate in the response to injury induced by angioplasty in addition to their role in atherogenesis. In most of the animal models studied to date, the infiltration of inflammatory cells into the intimal, medial, and adventitial layers of the vessel wall is a ubiquitous finding. The presence of inflammatory cells is also a prominent feature noted in human specimens of restenotic lesions. Given that these cells express cytokines and growth factors capable of modulating cell proliferation, programmed cell death, migration, and matrix modification, it has been postulated that the process of inflammation after injury may play an important role in restenotic lesion formation. Studies in animal models have documented increased expression of adhesion molecules and chemoattractants within the vessel wall that may promote the influx of leukocytes into the vessel wall (see Chapter 15). Studies using antibodies to block leukocyte adhesion in animal models of vascular injury suggest that the inflammatory response contributes to neointima formation. Models of immune-mediated vascular injury in the absence of mechanical distension have documented that activation of the inflammatory response is a sufficient condition for inducing vascular lesion formation. The perturbation in the integrity of the endothelium, the induction of locally generated adhesion molecules and chemoattractants, and the chronic inflammatory state that characterizes the atherosclerotic lesion create a cellular milieu in which inflammatory cells become important contributors to the process of restenosis after angioplasty. Although animal model studies are suggestive, it remains to be demonstrated whether or not therapeutic strategies targeted at the local inflammatory response will also modify all aspects of the response to injury that result in restenosis.

## MATRIX MODIFICATION

An inherent and prominent component of the wound-healing response involves the elaboration of connective tissue to restore the structural integrity of the injured organ. Matrix production by vascular smooth muscle cells and myofibroblasts is a feature of vascular lesion formation in human specimens of restenotic lesions as well as in every animal model studied to date (27). Perhaps 50 to 70% of lesion volume involves noncellular protein components. Increased synthesis of interstitial collagens, fibronectin, elastin, glycosaminoglycans, and osteopontin begins during the acute phase, within days of the initial injury, and continues during the ensuing phases of lesion formation. Changes in the synthesis of matrix proteins are modulated in part by the expression of locally generated growth factors, such as TGF-β1 (28). The modification of the extracellular matrix is a dynamic process involving increased degradation of matrix proteins by plasmin and metalloproteinases as a complement to the increased synthesis. The net volume of the extracellular compartment reflects the balance between synthesis and degradation.

In addition to contributing to the overall volume of vascular tissue, extracellular matrix proteins appear to play a vital biological role by communicating to the cell signals that modulate all aspects of its behavior. The integrin-matrix interactions serve as a platform for transducing extracellular stimuli to the intracellular signaling apparatus. The interplay between matrix proteins and these cell surface receptors regulates each of the cellular processes involved in the cell biology of restenosis, including cell proliferation, apoptosis, cell migration, matrix production, inflammation, and phenotypic modulation. The generation of increased extracellular matrix and its modification is integral to the response to vascular injury. The nature of the signals imposed on vascular cells by the extracellular matrix depends on the expression of specific integrins on the cell surface as well as the particular composition of the matrix that activates these receptors.

Experimental studies indicate that increased expression of matrix proteins such as tenascin and osteopontin and their association with integrins such as αvβIII may tend to promote cell migration and lesion formation. In model systems that accentuate the role of migration in neointima formation, blockade of these matrix-integrin interactions substantially reduces lesion formation. An emerging body of evidence indicates that proteolytic cleavage of certain matrix proteins may unmask cryptic integrin binding sites that contribute to changes in cell behavior. Thus, matrix proteases may also play a critical role in modulating integrin-matrix interactions and contributing to changes in migration and other behaviors. Studies using genetically engineered mice with deficiencies in the capacity to generate plasmin indicate that a decrease in proteolysis impairs cell migration and lesion formation (see Chapter 22). Pharmacologic blockade of proteases also appears to inhibit cell migration and lesion formation. The process of matrix modification after vascular injury is exceedingly complex. The balance between matrix protein production vs. degradation that determines the contribution of extracellular proteins to the overall volume of the lesion is one mechanism by which matrix proteins contribute to restenosis. Ongoing research on the role of integrin-matrix interactions in the regulation of cell proliferation, apoptosis, phenotypic modulation, and migration is an exciting new frontier of matrix biology that is likely to provide important new insights into the mechanisms of restenosis.

## PHENOTYPIC MODULATION

Vascular smooth muscle cells in culture exhibit morphologic features ranging from a contractile to synthetic phenotype (Fig. 14.1). Cultured cells typically lose the spindle shape, and abundant contractile proteins manifest *in situ* within the vessel wall and develop a more elaborate endoplasmic reticulum in association with the synthesis of noncontractile proteins. This process of phenotypic modulation has been associated with alterations in cell growth, matrix production, and different profiles in gene expression. These *in vitro* observations are paralleled by *in vivo* studies that have described striking differences between intimal smooth muscle cells vs. medial cells in the regulation of cell growth, apoptosis, migration, and contractile protein gene expression (29). Thus, in contrast to terminally differentiated muscle cells, vascular smooth muscle cells retain a plasticity that allows transitions from differentiated cells in G-0 arrest to relatively de-differentiated cells capable of proliferation yet maintaining the capacity to revert from one phenotypic state to another.

In addition to the capacity of a single cell to exhibit these phenotypic transitions, evidence indicates that there is heterogeneity within the vascular smooth muscle cell population in the vessel wall. It appears likely that subpopulations of cells exist that are genotypically distinct. During ontogeny, the blood vessel is created by the investment of the endothelial tube by a muscle cell coat. This muscle layer is derived from local mesenchymal cells within primordial organ beds. It is postulated that different pools of mesenchymal progenitor cells may exhibit different genotypic characteristics. That atherosclerotic lesions may be composed of one to several clonal populations of cells may be consistent with the notion of vascular smooth muscle cell heterogeneity and expansion of certain pools of cells as a fundamental feature of intima formation. The response of these intimal cells to angioplasty injury may be distinct from normal medial cells. Indeed these cells have a distinct pattern of expression of autocrine-paracrine

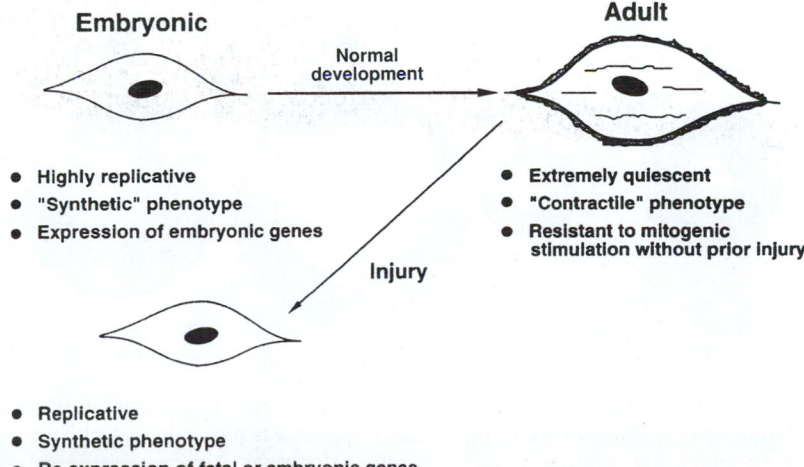

**FIGURE 14.1.**   Conceptual figure demonstrating the dramatic changes that occur in SMC phenotype during development. In response to injury, a reiteration of specific developmental processes is observed. SMCs responding to injury express genes or gene products characteristic of earlier developmental states. (Reprinted with permission from Stenmark KR, Mecham RP. Cellular and molecular mechanisms of pulmonary vascular remodeling [review]. Ann Rev Physiol 1997;59:89–144.)

growth factors, matrix proteins, adhesion molecules, apoptosis regulatory genes, and differentiation markers. This altered pattern of gene expression correlates with altered regulation of cell proliferation, apoptosis, and migration. Animal models that fail to recapitulate the unique character of the intimal cell population may fail to provide insights into the determinants of intimal lesion formation in the clinical context.

It is also unclear to what extent restenosis reflects an expansion of a clonal intimal population vs. an expansion of a polyclonal, phenotypically modified cell population. It is conceivable that the efficacy of therapeutic strategies may depend on special phenotypic characteristics of these cellular targets.

## VASCULAR REMODELING

The process of vascular remodeling (Fig. 14.2) involves the intrinsic capacity of the vasculature to alter its geometry as an adaptive or maladaptive response to its microenvironment (30–32). This process can be defined as an alteration in vessel architecture that involves changes in overall vessel dimensions. This restructuring involves changes in the outer circumference, lumen dimensions, wall thickness:lumen ratio, or intima:media ratio. The process of vascular remodeling is involved in the pathogenesis of a variety of vascular disorders, such as atherosclerosis and hypertension, as well as restenosis. Although vascular remodeling occurs in a wide spectrum of vascular disorders, this process is not necessarily pathologic. Indeed, vascular remodeling is a critical biological process during the normal ontogeny of the circulatory system.

The molecular basis of vascular remodeling remains to be characterized. Vascular remodeling involves four fundamental cellular processes: cell growth, programmed cell death, migration, and modification of the extracellular matrix with associated changes in cell-matrix interactions. The regulation of these processes appears to involve an intriguing interactive balance between endogenous stimulators and inhibitors of each activity. Locally generated humoral factors and matrix constituents regulate the changes in cell growth, death, migration, and cell-matrix interactions in a coordinate fashion necessary for altering vessel structure.

This plasticity of the vasculature is best exemplified by the observation that a chronic increase in blood flow induced by placement of an arteriovenous shunt induces a structural increase in vessel dimensions. Conversely, Langille and his colleagues have shown in adult

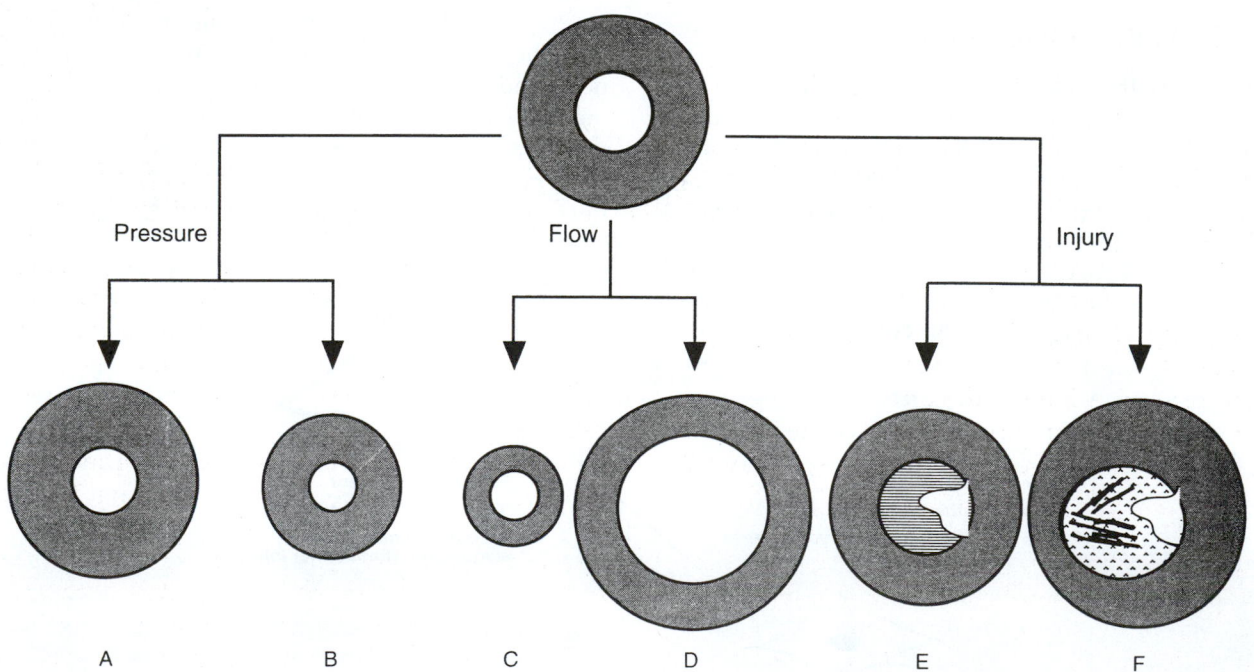

**FIGURE 14.2.** The spectrum of vascular remodeling. Vessel A represents hypertensive vascular disease with vascular hypertrophy, in which the medial layer is thickened and the luminal diameter is reduced; vessel B, hypertensive vascular disease without medial hypertrophy, in which the luminal diameter is reduced; vessel C, decreased vessel dimensions in response to a long-term decrease in flow; vessel D, increased vessel dimensions in response to a long-term increase in flow; vessel E, neointimal hyperplasia (migration and proliferation of vascular smooth muscle cells) in response to a long-term increase in flow; vessel E, neointimal hyperplasia (migration and proliferation of vascular smooth muscle cells) in response to vascular injury; and vessel F, atherosclerosis in response to vascular injury of conduit vessels. (Reprinted with permission from Gibbons GH, Dzau VJ. The emerging concept of vascular remodeling [review]. N Engl J Med 1994;330:1431–1438.)

animals that an artery undergoes a process of shrinkage remodeling in response to a chronic decrease in flow (33). The integrity of the endothelium is a necessary condition for the shrinkage remodeling response, because structural changes can be abolished by denudation of the intimal surface. The capacity of the vasculature to enlarge or shrink is related to the capacity of the endothelium to serve as a mechanotransducer of hemodynamic stimuli (see Chapter 20) and involves the generation of endothelium-derived autocrine-paracrine factors that mediate this process. As we attempt to understand why angioplasty succeeds or fails, we must consider these inherent properties of the vasculature to remodel itself. Shear stress (the tractive force exerted by blood flow) is directly proportional to flow velocity and inversely proportional to the vessel radius to the third power. The phenomena of shrinkage and of enlargement remodeling appear to be adaptive responses of the vasculature that occur in accordance with a bioengineering principle that attempts to maintain a constant level of shear stress throughout the circulation.

Although *in vitro* models and studies with animal models are compelling, it could be argued that these findings are irrelevant in the pathogenesis of human diseases such as atherosclerosis and restenosis after angioplasty. However, the careful studies of human autopsy specimens of vascular disease performed by Glagov et al provide important confirmatory evidence in support of this paradigm (34). These investigators observed a striking direct relationship between atherosclerotic intimal lesion dimensions and the overall dimension of the internal elastic membrane. These studies suggested that the vasculature has an intrinsic capacity to undergo an apparent ''compensatory enlargement'' in which the overall vessel size increases such that lumen dimensions can be maintained despite the encroachment of the expanding intimal lesion. These investigators also noted an apparent critical threshold at which the capacity to enlarge reached a limit and expansion of the intimal lesion produced a significant stenosis of the lumen. Although the mechanism of this response is not clear, this remodeling may be related to the capacity of the endothelium to sense changes in hemodynamic stimuli and modulate overall vessel dimensions. The expansion of the intimal lesion initially may reduce vessel radius, thereby increasing the shear stress sensed by the endothelium. In response to this initial increase in shear stress, the vessel undergoes a compensatory remodeling response to increase overall vessel dimensions so that shear stress is normalized back to a preset level. Recent studies with intravascular ultrasound have confirmed that this phenomenon appears to occur *in situ* in the context of human atherosclerosis as well as in restenosis after angioplasty. Thus, the striking parallel between flow-induced enlargement remodeling and compensa-

tory enlargement in atherosclerosis further substantiates the thesis that the vasculature has the intrinsic capacity to inhibit the deleterious consequences of intimal lesion expansion.

The molecular events that link changes in shear stress with these dramatic alterations in vessel structure must be characterized further. However, it is interesting that cultured endothelial cells exposed to shear stress acutely generate increased quantities of nitric oxide (NO) and the endothelial cell-type nitric oxide synthase (NOS) gene is up-regulated by this flow stimulus (35). It has also been observed that vessels chronically exposed to increased flow have an increased capacity to generate NO (36). These findings suggest a striking association between increased flow, the up-regulation of NO-generating capacity and flow-stimulated vascular remodeling. Although this association was well established, the causal link between increased NO and enlargement remodeling remained to be defined. Blockade of NO generation by the administration of NOS inhibitors significantly attenuates the flow-induced vascular remodeling response to chronic increases in flow. Taken together, these data suggest that the increased generation of NO induced by increased shear stress plays a critical mediator role in promoting the process of enlargement remodeling.

The cellular processes that are activated during flow-induced vascular remodeling are not fully understood. As the vessel enlarges and lumen surface area expands, there should be an increase in the endothelial cell population. Shrinkage remodeling should be characterized by a decrease in the cellularity of the endothelium. Cowan and Langille (32) postulated that shrinkage remodeling and the associated decrease in the cellularity of the endothelium may involve an increase in apoptotic cell death relative to cell replication. Indeed, recent *in vivo* studies have documented that shrinkage remodeling in response to a decrease in flow appears to be initiated by the induction of endothelial cell programmed cell death.

The link between vascular remodeling and the regulation of vascular cell apoptosis is intriguing. The factors that initiate the cell death program in response to decreases in shear stress must still be identified. Using an *in vitro* model system, Zeiher et al demonstrated that shear stress is a potent biomechanical stimulus that prevents endothelial cell apoptosis in response to cytotoxic stimuli (37). In a separate series of experiments using pharmacologic donors of NO, they documented that NO is a potent inhibitor of endothelial cell apoptosis (38). Given that shear stress induces increased generation of NO, they reconciled these two lines of evidence by documenting that NO appears to mediate a significant component of the inhibitory effect of shear stress on endothelial cell programmed cell death. These findings suggest the following working hypothesis: shrinkage remodeling is initiated by a decline in the expression factors that inhibit endothelial cell apoptosis, such as NO; this decrease in survival-promoting stimuli activates endothelial cell death; and the resultant decline in the cellularity of the endothelium promotes the eventual reduction in lumen dimensions.

In attempting to understand the cellular mechanisms of vascular remodeling, our working hypothesis may be guided by insights gained from the wound healing model of tissue repair and remodeling. In response to injury, a skin wound is closed by a sequence of events that includes fibroblast migration and proliferation, phenotypic modulation of fibroblasts into myofibroblasts, the elaboration of extracellular matrix with concomitant degradation and reshaping of matrix structure, a decrease in cellularity at the wound site secondary to apoptosis, and final closure of the wound by a process of matrix contracture. There are many striking parallels between the injury response within the vasculature and other tissues. In particular, the process of wound contracture appears to be a prominent determinant of the final tissue architecture.

The prominence of wound contracture vs. cell proliferation or matrix production as the principle element mediating wound closure varies with the species under study, the nature of the wound, and the tissue context. The importance of wound contracture as a critical determinant of tissue architecture is most graphically illustrated by pathologic circumstances in which an excessive degree of wound contracture induces dramatic cases of tissue disfigurement. Although the molecular mechanisms of wound contracture have not been defined, several lines of evidence indicate that biomechanical forces generated by cell-matrix interactions mediate the changes in tissue structure that accompany the reparative process. The nature of the biomechanical force is related to several processes including: 1) the cellularity of the wound (i.e., the balance of fibroblast proliferation vs. apoptosis); 2) the matrix composition (i.e., the balance of matrix production and degradation); 3) the phenotypic modulation of fibroblasts into myofibroblasts that have enhanced capabilities in promoting force generation; and 4) the cell-matrix interaction mediated by integrins that transmits forces generated by myofibroblasts to the matrix scaffolding and thereby promotes the alteration in overall tissue architecture.

Although extrapolating from the response to injury in cutaneous tissue to the vessel wall must be done with caution, it is intriguing to consider that similar processes may be involved in vascular remodeling after injury. It is already clear that myofibroblast invasion into the media and intima accompanies the response to injury and these myofibroblasts, in conjunction with vascular smooth muscle cells, have the capacity to alter vessel shape by imposing mechanical forces. *In vitro* model studies have documented that vascular cells exhibit behavior similar to fibroblasts in the ability to promote the contraction of collagen gels. These cell-matrix interactions that govern the overall dimensions of the matrix gel scaffold are modulated by the influence of vasoactive substances such as angiotensin II as well as integrins such as $\alpha v\beta III$. Modulating these cell-matrix interactions by specific inhibitors of integrin receptors can acutely alter overall vessel dimensions and vascular tone. Taken together, data suggest that changes in the cell-matrix interactions that impose a biomechanical force on the matrix scaffolding of the blood vessel may be a determinant of vessel structure and the process of vascular remodeling.

Although a growing body of evidence indicates that vascular remodeling plays a critical role in restenosis in individuals after angioplasty, the molecular basis of this process remains elusive. The process of vascular remodeling may involve a complex interplay between several cellular mechanisms. Events within the cellular component of the vessel wall influence the extracellular component and vice versa. It is simplistic to presume that wound contracture reflects an imbalance between matrix production and degradation leading to pathologic fibrosis. In fact, biomechanical models based upon studies of skin wounds indicate that the biomechanical force generated varies in accordance with the extent of myofibroblast proliferation and infiltration as well as variations in the composition of the matrix itself. Thus, therapeutic strategies focused on modifying cellular migration, proliferation, apoptosis, contractile tone, or integrin binding could have as powerful an influence on contracture and vascular remodeling as interventions focused on the relative balance of matrix production vs. degradation. The complexity of the remodeling process may necessitate the development of therapeutic interventions that influence more than one of the several cellular mechanisms involved in determining overall vessel structure. Further investigation is necessary to identify which factors determine whether the vessel undergoes the enlargement remodeling that confers the success of angioplasty vs. factors that promote the process of constrictive remodeling associated with restenosis.

# CLINICAL IMPLICATIONS OF PATHOBIOLOGICAL INSIGHTS

Although each animal model has its strengths and weaknesses, one theme that emerges is the complex interplay between mediators and cellular processes that characterize the response to injury. Many of these cellular processes represent double-edged swords that may either promote salutary responses that mediate the success of angioplasty or doom it to failure. Changes in the balance between matrix synthesis and degradation may be important cellular processes in enlargement remodeling as well as constrictive remodeling. Cell proliferation and/or apoptosis may be necessary components of the reparative process that maintains the acute postintervention gain. They may also help promote the late loss of that acute gain. More investigation is needed to define the regulatory mechanisms governing these processes. The missing link is our understanding of what defines the set point of each of these processes. As we gain greater insight into the molecular mechanisms governing vessel architecture, we will make greater progress toward developing strategies for inducing the adaptive changes in cell growth, death, migration, matrix modification, and cell-matrix interactions that promote enlargement remodeling and maintenance of the acute gain after angioplasty.

Despite the limitations of our current understanding of restenosis, certain therapeutic strategies can be formulated as working models to be tested. One strategy is to use interventions that are pleiotropic in modulating several cellular processes that may contribute to restenosis. This multipronged strategy may have greater efficacy in pathologic processes as complex as restenosis. Therapeutic interventions that have pleiotropic effects may promote a coordinated modification of the response to injury that results in a greater likelihood of a successful outcome. For example, augmenting the local generation of NO may prevent restenosis by inhibiting adverse sequelae such as smooth muscle cell hyperplasia, smooth muscle cell migration, leukocyte infiltration, and matrix production, while stimulating salutary responses such as re-endothelialization, the process of enlargement remodeling, and increased blood flow. A recent clinical trial using an NO donor confirms the potential utility of this approach as more effective NO-donor drugs and/or delivery modalities are developed. Similarly, modifying certain cell-matrix interactions could modulate thrombus formation, cell proliferation, apoptosis, migration, and matrix production and contracture and thereby prevent restenosis. The preliminary observations regarding the reduction of clinical restenosis after the acute use of the anti-integrin antibody 7E3 raises the possibility that more chronic and targeted anti-integrin strategies may have antirestenosis efficacy. Strategies that affect signaling pathways such as those mediated by reactive oxygen species may influence several cellular processes such as the regulation of cell growth, cell death, inflammation, matrix modification, and vascular remodeling. Recent clinical studies agree with the notion that modulating the vascular redox state may be an effective means of preventing restenosis. Adjunctive approaches that combine intravascular stents to minimize constrictive remodeling can be complemented with a therapeutic intervention that inhibits cell proliferation or promotes intimal apoptosis. The use of radiation therapy or antisense oligonucleotides directed against either cell cycle regulatory genes or antiapoptotic genes is an exciting new area of biotechnology development for restenosis. One of the next frontiers will involve the development of strategies that influence the process of vascular remodeling.

Overall, the clinical observations derived from new diagnostic modalities, such as intravascular ultrasound, and the greater breadth and fidelity of the animal models under study have resulted in a better understanding of the cell biology of restenosis. These new pathobiological insights into the response to injury, coupled with advances in biotechnology, will result in new drugs and treatment modalities designed to enhance the success rate of angioplasty procedures.

# REFERENCES

1. Ross R. The pathogenesis of atherosclerosis: A perspective for the 1990s [Review]. Nature 1993;362:801–809.
2. Gibbons GH, Dzau VJ. Molecular therapies for vascular diseases [Review]. Science 1996;272:689–693.
3. Mintz GS, Kent KM, Pichard AD et al. Intravascular ultrasound insights into mechanisms of stenosis formation and restenosis [Review]. Cardiol Clin 1997;15:17–29.
4. Kimura T, Yokoi H, Nakagawa Y et al. Three-year follow-up after implantation of metallic coronary-artery stents. N Engl J Med 1996;334:561–566.
5. Lindner V, Olson NE, Clowes AW et al. Inhibition of smooth muscle cell proliferation in injured rat arteries. Interaction of heparin with basic fibroblast growth factor. J Clin Invest 1992;90:2044–2049.
6. Iafrati MD, Karas RH, Aronovitz M et al. Estrogen inhibits the vascular injury response in estrogen receptor α-deficient mice. Nat Med 1997;3:545–548.
7. Grinstead WC, Rodgers GP, Mazur W et al. Comparison of three porcine restenosis models: The relative importance of hypercholesterolemia, endothelial abrasion, and stenting. Coron Artery Dis 1994;5:425–434.
8. Ryan MJ, Emig LL, Hicks GW et al. Localization of lipoprotein(a) in a monkey model of rapid neointimal growth. Arterioscler Thromb Vasc Biol 1997;17:181–187.
9. Schafer AI. Vascular endothelium: In defense of blood fluidity [Editorial]. J Clin Invest 1997;99:1143–1144.
10. Lindner V, Reidy MA. Platelet-derived growth factor ligand and receptor expression by large-vessel endothelium in vivo. Am J Pathol 1995;146:1488–1497.
11. Molloy CJ, Pawlowski JE, Taylor DS et al. Thrombin receptor activation elicits rapid protein tyrosine phosphorylation and stimulation of the raf-1/MAP kinase pathway preceding delayed mitogenesis in cultured rat aortic smooth muscle cells: Evidence for an obligate autocrine mechanism promoting cell proliferation induced by G protein-coupled receptor agonist. J Clin Invest 1996;97:1173–1183.
12. Vemulapalli S, Chiu PJ, Kurowski S et al. In vivo inhibition of platelet adhesion by a cGMP-mediated mechanism in balloon catheter injured rat carotid artery. Pharmacology 1996;52:235–242.
13. Hamelink JK, Tang DB, Barr CF et al. Inhibition of platelet deposition by combined hirulog and aspirin in a rat carotid endarterectomy model. J Vasc Surg 1995;21:492–498.
14. Barry WL, Gimple LW, Humphries JE et al. Arterial thrombin activity after angioplasty in an atherosclerotic rabbit model: Time course and effect of hirudin. Circulation 1996;94:88–93.
15. Kornowski R, Eldor A, Werber MM et al. Enhancement of recombinant tissue-type plasminogen activator thrombolysis with a selective factor Xa inhibitor derived from the leech Hirudo medicinalis: Comparison with heparin and hirudin in a rabbit thrombosis model. Coron Artery Dis 1996;7:903–909.
16. Johnson RC, Chapman SM, Dong ZM et al. Absence of P-selectin delays fatty streak formation in mice. J Clin Invest 1997;99:1037–1043.
17. Baumgartner HR, Studer A. Folgen des Gefässkatheterismus am normo- und hypercholesterinaemischen Kaninchen. Pathol Microbiol 1966;29:393–405.

18. Perlman H, Maillard L, Krasinski K et al. Evidence for the rapid onset of apoptosis in medial smooth muscle cells after balloon injury. Circulation 1997;95:981–987.

19. Pollman MJ, Yamada T, Horiuchi M et al. Vasoactive substances regulate vascular smooth muscle cell apoptosis. Countervailing influences of nitric oxide and angiotensin II. Circ Res 1996;79:748–756.

20. von der Leyen HE, Gibbons GH, Morishita R et al. Gene therapy inhibiting neointimal vascular lesion: *In vivo* transfer of endothelial cell nitric oxide synthase gene. Proc Natl Acad Sci U S A 1995;92:1137–1141.

21. Lee JS, Adrie C, Jacob HJ et al. Chronic inhalation of nitric oxide inhibits neointimal formation after balloon-induced arterial injury. Circ Res 1996;78:337–342.

22. Chen D, Krasinski K, Sylvester A et al. Downregulation of cyclin-dependent kinase 2 activity and cyclin A promoter activity in vascular smooth muscle cells by p27 (KIP1), an inhibitor of neointima formation in the rat carotid artery. J Clin Invest 1997;99:2334–2341.

23. Wei GL, Krasinski K, Kearney M et al. Temporally and spatially coordinated expression of cell cycle regulatory factors after angioplasty. Circ Res 1997;80:418–426.

24. Morishita R, Gibbons GH, Ellison KE et al. Intimal hyperplasia after vascular injury is inhibited by antisense cdk 2 kinase oligonucleotides. J Clin Invest 1994;93:1458–1464.

25. Morishita R, Gibbons GH, Horiuchi M et al. A gene therapy strategy using a transcription factor decoy of the E2F binding site inhibits smooth muscle cell proliferation *in vivo*. Proc Natl Acad Sci U S A 1995;92:5855–5859.

26. Boyle JJ. Association of coronary plaque rupture and atherosclerotic inflammation. J Pathol 1997;181:93–99.

27. Chen YH, Chen YL, Lin SJ et al. Electron microscopic studies of phenotypic modulation of smooth muscle cells in coronary arteries of individuals with unstable angina pectoris and postangioplasty restenosis. Circulation 1997;95:1169–1175.

28. McCaffrey TA, Consigli S, Du B et al. Decreased type II/type I TGF-β receptor ratio in cells derived from human atherosclerotic lesions. Conversion from an antiproliferative to profibrotic response to TGF-β1. J Clin Invest 1995;96:2667–2675.

29. Holifield B, Helgason T, Jemelka S et al. Differentiated vascular myocytes: Are they involved in neointimal formation? J Clin Invest 1996;97:814–825.

30. Gibbons GH, Dzau VJ. The emerging concept of vascular remodeling [Review]. N Engl J Med 1994;330:1431–1438.

31. Stenmark KR, Mecham RP. Cellular and molecular mechanisms of pulmonary vascular remodeling [Review]. Annu Rev Physiol 1997;59:89–144.

32. Cowan DB, Langille BL. Cellular and molecular biology of vascular remodeling [Review]. Curr Opin Lipidol 1996;7:94–100.

33. Langille BL. Arterial remodeling: Relation to hemodynamics [Review]. Can J Physiol Pharmacol 1996;74:834–841.

34. Zarins CK, Lu CT, Gewertz BL et al. Arterial disruption and remodeling following balloon dilatation. Surgery 1982;92:1086–1095.

35. Nishida K, Harrison DG, Navas JP et al. Molecular cloning and characterization of the constitutive bovine aortic endothelial cell nitric oxide synthase. J Clin Invest 1992;90:2092–2096.

36. Nadaud S, Philippe M, Arnal JF et al. Sustained increase in aortic endothelial nitric oxide synthase expression *in vivo* in a model of chronic high blood flow. Circ Res 1996;79:857–863.

37. Dimmeler S, Haendeler J, Rippmann V et al. Shear stress inhibits apoptosis of human endothelial cells. FEBS Lett 1996;399:71–74.

38. Dimmeler S, Haendeler J, Nehls M et al. Suppression of apoptosis by nitric oxide via inhibition of interleukin-1β-converting enzyme (ICE)-like and cysteine protease protein (CPP)-32-like proteases. J Exp Med 1997;185:601–607.

# CHAPTER 15

# INTERACTIONS OF LEUKOCYTES WITH THE VESSEL WALL

## Rodger P. McEver

Leukocytes interact with the blood vessel wall in response to tissue injury. Various leukocyte subsets adhere to endothelial cells prior to their migration into tissues at sites of inflammation. Lymphocytes bind to endothelial cells before moving through lymphatic tissues as part of the process of immune surveillance. Leukocytes also bind to other leukocytes and to activated platelets. The realization that inflammation and coagulation can be linked responses has led to increasing interest in the participation of leukocytes in hemostasis. This chapter describes our current understanding of how leukocytes adhere to endothelial cells, to other leukocytes, and to platelets, and then discusses how these interactions, when dysregulated, may promote tissue destruction in inflammatory or thrombotic disorders.

## ENDOTHELIAL CELL-LEUKOCYTE INTERACTIONS

The inflammatory process involves the accumulation of fluid and leukocytes in extravascular tissues at sites of infection or physical injury. Leukocytes first adhere to endothelial cells lining the intimal surface of blood vessels and then diapedese between adjacent endothelial cells into underlying tissues (Fig. 15.1). Migration of leukocytes from the blood stream into the extravascular space is tightly regulated. Subsets of leukocytes accumulate with characteristic time courses in response to specific stimuli. In acute inflammation neutrophils rapidly

exit the circulation in response to bacterial invasion. In chronic inflammation lymphocytes enter tissues in a more delayed and sustained fashion, where they destroy viruses and other pathogens through specific immunologic recognition. Allergic responses require the preferential entry of eosinophils into tissues. A specialized form of leukocyte extravasation is the continuous recirculation of subsets of lymphocytes through lymph nodes and other lymphoid structures. This process allows "naive" lymphocytes to encounter exogenous agents that have been processed for recognition by antigen-presenting cells. Lymphocytes stimulated in this fashion acquire immunologic "memory," which favors their subsequent migration into nonlymphoid tissues that have been invaded by specific pathogens.

Although much remains to be learned, there has been a recent explosion of information regarding the molecular mechanisms of leukocyte-endothelial interactions. Four major events appear to operate sequentially to promote leukocyte adhesion and emigration:

1. Hemodynamic changes leading to vascular leakage and altered blood flow.
2. Expression of receptors on the surface of activated endothelial cells that promote reversible leukocyte adhesion.
3. Release of signaling molecules that activate the loosely adherent leukocytes.
4. Expression of receptors by the activated leukocytes that strengthen adhesion to the endothelium and then facilitate emigration.

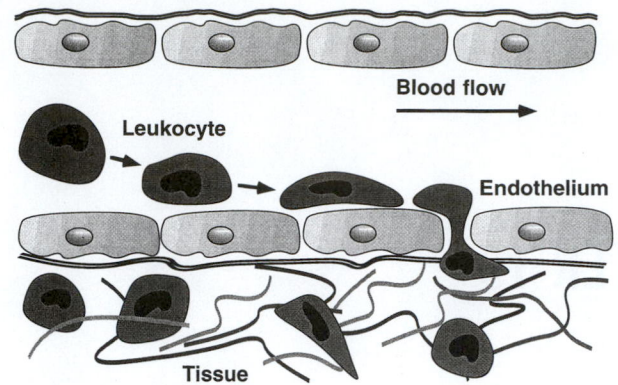

**FIGURE 15.1.** Migration of leukocytes from the circulation into tissues during inflammation. Leukocytes first adhere to the endothelial cells lining the intimal surface of blood vessels, then move between adjacent endothelial cells into extravascular sites of infection or injury.

## HEMODYNAMIC CHANGES

The earliest event observed during acute inflammation is extensive dilation of blood vessels accompanied by vascular leakage of plasma proteins and fluid (1). Most of the dilation occurs in postcapillary venules, where shear rates in the circulation are lowest (see Chapter 20). The vasodilation and fluid leakage further decrease shear forces, thus promoting more extensive contacts between circulating leukocytes and venular endothelium. Rapid release of vasodilators from endothelial cells occurs in response to agonists such as thrombin or histamine (see Chapter 19). These vasodilators, which directly relax vascular smooth muscle, include prostacyclin, a metabolite of arachidonic acid synthesized through the cyclooxygenase pathway, and endothelium-derived relaxing factor (EDRF), a labile substance

identical or closely related to nitric oxide (2). Early vascular leakage results from contraction of endothelial cells in response to thrombin, histamine, or leukotriene C4 (3). Delayed and sustained leakage results from additional cytoskeletal rearrangements of the endothelium induced by inflammatory cytokines such as interleukin-1β (IL-1β), tumor necrosis factor α (TNF-α), and interferon-γ (4).

## REVERSIBLE LEUKOCYTE ADHESION TO ACTIVATED ENDOTHELIUM

During inflammation, flowing leukocytes initially tether to and roll on the endothelial surface. The rolling process, which was first observed in experimental animals over a century ago (1), requires changes in the endothelium, as rolling occurs only on the side of the blood vessel adjacent to an inflammatory challenge. This reversible adhesion is mediated primarily by a group of receptors known as selectins (Fig. 15.2) (Table 15.1). Each of the three selectins contains an aminoterminal domain homologous to a family of $Ca^{2+}$-dependent (C-type) lectins, followed by an epidermal-growth-factor (EGF)–like motif, a variable number of short consensus repeats (SCRs), a transmembrane domain, and a short cytoplasmic tail (5–9). The genes encoding all three proteins are clustered on chromosome 1 (10). Exons encode specific structural domains, suggesting that the selectin genes arose through exon duplication and rearrangement (11–13).

P-selectin is synthesized by megakaryocytes, where it is incorporated into platelets, and by endothelial cells. It is stored in membranes of secretory granules—the α-granules of platelets and the Weibel-Palade bodies of endothelial cells. Following stimulation by rapid activators such as thrombin or histamine, P-selectin is trans-

---

| | **TABLE 15.1.** The Selectin Family of Adhesion Molecules | | | |
|---|---|---|---|---|
| **Selectin** | **CD Nomenclature** | **Previous Names** | **Expressed By** | **Target Cell** |
| L-selectin | CD62L | LAM-1 LECAM-1 | PMNs, monocytes, lymphocyte subsets | Activated ECs, HEVs of PLN and ML, other leukocytes, hematopoietic stem cells |
| E-selectin | CD62E | ELAM-1 | Cytokine-activated ECs | PMNs, monocytes, eosinophils, lymphocyte subsets, some tumor cells |
| P-selectin | CD62P | GMP-140 PADGEM | Thrombin-activated platelets and ECs, cytokine-activated ECs | PMNs, monocytes, eosinophils, lymphocyte subsets, some tumor cells, HEVs, activated ECs? |

*EC, endothelial cell; ELAM, endothelial leukocyte adhesion molecule; GMP, granule membrane protein; HEV, high endothelial venule; LAM, leukocyte adhesion molecule; LECAM, leukocyte-endothelial cell adhesion molecule; ML, mesenteric lymphoid tissue; PLN, peirpheral lymph node; PADGEM, platelet activation–dependent granule external membrane protein; PMN, polymorphonuclear cell or neutrophil.*

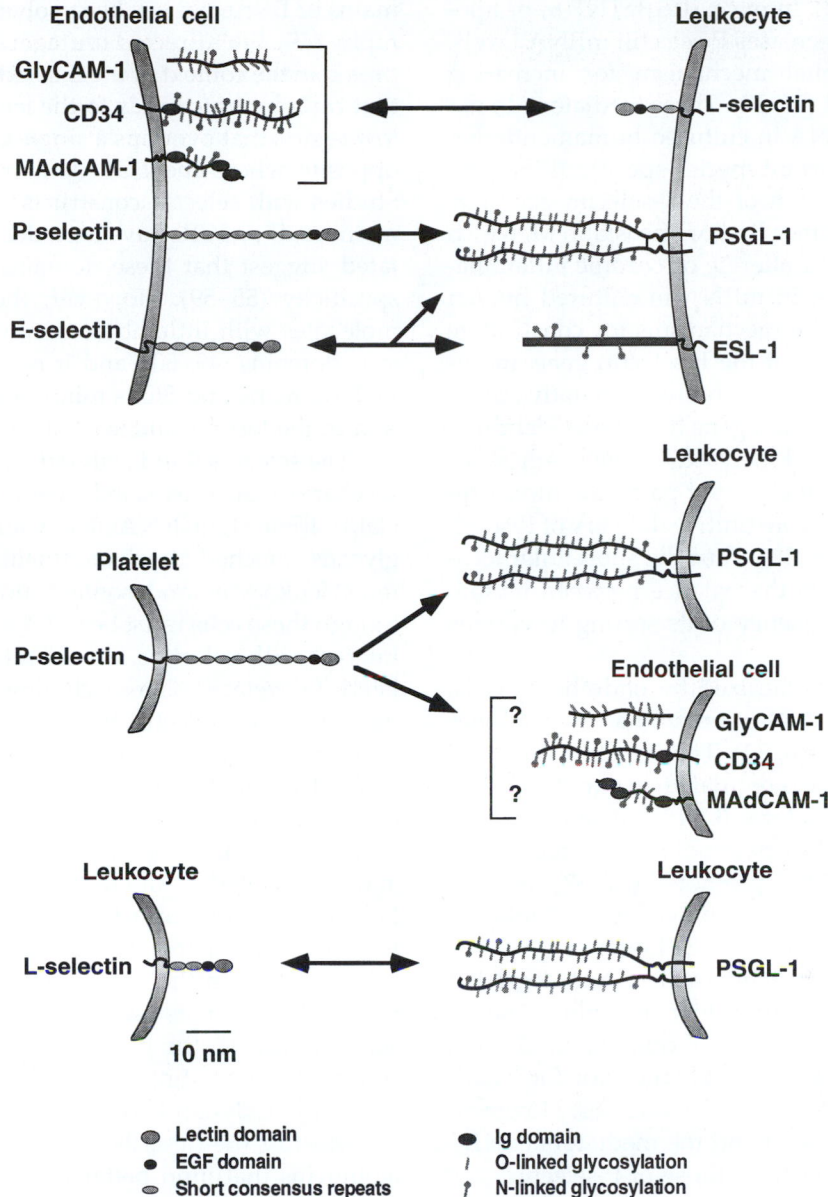

**FIGURE 15.2.** Selectins and their glycoprotein ligands. The domain organization of each protein is shown. The estimated lengths of the selectins (60, 215, 216) and of PSGL-1 (108) are based on hydrodynamic data and electron microscopy. The lengths of GlyCAM-1, CD34, and MAdCAM-1 are modeled from the dimensions of another sialomucin, CD43 (217). Not shown are less well characterized selectin ligands: a 260 Kda bovine leukocyte ligand for E-selectin (218), a 160 Kda murine leukocyte ligand for P-selectin (219), a 200 Kda murine endothelial cell ligand for L-selectin (67), and CD24, a leukocyte ligand for P-selectin (220). ESL-1, E-selectin ligand-1; GlyCAM-1, glycosylated cell adhesion molecule-1; MAdCAM-1, mucosal addressin cell adhesion molecule-1; PSGL-1, P-selectin glycoprotein ligand-1.

located within minutes to the cell surface as granule membranes fuse with the plasma membrane (14–18). P-selectin binds to neutrophils, monocytes, eosinophils, memory T lymphocytes, and subsets of natural killer cells (19–22). Thus P-selectin is a rapidly inducible receptor for leukocytes on activated platelets and endothelial cells. Peak surface expression of P-selectin occurs 5 to 10 minutes after stimulation of endothelial cells with thrombin or histamine, then declines over the next 30 to 60 minutes as a result of endocytosis of the protein (18). The cytoplasmic domain of P-selectin contains signals that mediate sorting into secretory storage granules (23), endocytosis in clathrin-coated pits (24), and rapid movement from endosomes to lysosomes, where the protein is degraded (25). In mice, IL-1β, TNF-α, or lipo-polysaccharide (LPS) increases P-selectin mRNA levels, suggesting an additional mechanism for increasing expression of P-selectin (26, 27). These mediators do not increase P-selectin mRNA in cultured human endothelial cells, implying important species-specific differences in the inducible expression of the P-selectin gene (28, 29). However, the cytokines IL-4 or oncostatin M, which are elaborated at sites of allergic or chronic inflammation, do increase P-selectin mRNA in cultured human endothelial cells (29). The mechanisms for constitutive and inducible expression of the P-selectin gene are incompletely understood, although several putative regulatory elements in the human gene have been identified (30, 31). Cytokine-induced increases in the synthesis of P-selectin may saturate the sorting pathway into secretory granules, leading to constitutive delivery of P-selectin to the cell surface (29, 32). Thus the subcellular location of P-selectin reflects the balance between its rate of synthesis and the efficiency of its sorting to various vesicular compartments.

E-selectin is also synthesized by endothelial cells, but only in response to LPS or inflammatory cytokines such as IL-1β or TNF-α (6, 33). Transcriptional regulation of the E-selectin gene is regulated, in part, by inducible binding of nuclear factor κ-B (NF-κB) and activated transcription factor 2/Jun heterodimers to regulatory elements in the E-selectin promoter (34–37). Surface expression peaks 4 hours after exposure to cytokines, then declines over the next 12 to 24 hours as synthesis ceases and surface protein is internalized and degraded in lysosomes. E-selectin binds to neutrophils, monocytes, eosinophils, and memory T cells (6, 33, 38–40). Thus E-selectin is also an inducible receptor for leukocytes on activated, endothelial cell surfaces. However, the kinetics of its expression and the mediators that induce its expression differ from those of P-selectin.

L-selectin is expressed on the surfaces of all neutrophils and monocytes and on about 70% of lymphocytes, although the density of its distribution on subsets of lymphocytes may vary (41). L-selectin binds to cytokine-activated endothelial cells and to specialized high endothelial venules (HEV) of peripheral lymph nodes (42–45). Thus it has been implicated in leukocyte adhesion to endothelium at sites of inflammation and in the recirculation of subsets of lymphocytes through peripheral lymph nodes. Following activation of neutrophils or lymphocytes, L-selectin is rapidly shed by proteolytic cleavage from the cell surface (41, 42). A novel cell-surface metalloproteinase cleaves L-selectin, which may serve to down-regulate L-selectin–mediated adhesion (46, 47).

Like other C-type lectins, the selectins bind to carbohydrate ligands in a $Ca^{2+}$-dependent manner (48). The three-dimensional structure of the lectin and EGF do-mains of E-selectin has been solved by x-ray crystallography (49). Site-directed mutagenesis of selectins, interpreted in the context of the E-selectin structure, suggests that carbohydrate binds to the lectin domain on a shallow region that overlaps a single $Ca^{2+}$ coordination site opposite where the EGF domain is attached (49–54). Studies with selectin constructs in which the EGF domains and/or SCRs have been deleted, switched, or mutated suggest that these domains contribute to ligand specificity (55–59). However, the selectins are linear molecules with little obvious contact between the various domains (49, 60), and it remains unclear how the EGF domains and SCRs might affect the binding function of the lectin domain.

The selectins bind sialylated and fucosylated oligo-saccharides such as sialyl Lewis x (sLe$^x$; Neu5Acα2,3-Galβ1,4[Fucα1,3]GlcNAc-R), a terminal component of glycans attached to glycoproteins and glycolipids on most leukocytes and some endothelial cells (61). Although these cells must be sialylated and fucosylated to interact with selectins, the affinity of selectins for isolated sLe$^x$-related oligosaccharides is very low. Furthermore, L- and P-selectin, but not E-selectin, bind sulfated molecules such as heparin and sulfatides (61). It has become clear that the selectins bind with higher affinity to only a few glycoproteins on leukocytes or endothelial cells (Fig. 15.2). These glycoproteins must be sialylated and fucosylated to interact with the selectins (62–65). Furthermore, they must be sulfated to bind optimally to L- or P-selectin (66–71). Studies of these glycoproteins have focused on the specific nature of the posttranslational modifications that confer high-affinity binding to selectins and on the potential functions of these glycoproteins in mediating selectin-dependent cell adhesion under hydrodynamic flow.

Most of the described glycoprotein ligands are sialomucins that bind better to L- and/or P-selectin, although they bind to E-selectin under some conditions. Binding requires sialylated and fucosylated O-glycans; the limited number of N-glycans on these molecules does not appear to be essential for binding. The fucosylated glycans on glycosylated, cell-adhesion molecule 1 (GlyCAM-1) from murine HEV are short core-2 structures that lack polylactosamine (72–74). In contrast, most fucosylated O-glycans on P-selectin glycoprotein ligand 1 (PSGL-1) from human myeloid cells are core-2 structures that have a β1,6-linked, trifucosylated polylactosamine terminating in sLe$^x$ (75). Only 14% of the O-glycans of PSGL-1 are fucosylated (75). These data suggest that unique O-glycan structures are created at restricted sites on specific proteins. Sulfate esters are attached to the C-6 position of Gal and GlcNAc residues in the O-glycans of GlyCAM-1 (72–74). In contrast, the O-glycans of PSGL-1 are not sulfated (75). Instead, sulfate is attached to a group of three clustered tyrosines near the aminoterminus (68–71). High-affinity binding of P- or L-selectin to GlyCAM-1 may require appropriate spacing of two or more sialylated, fucosylated, and sulfated O-glycans. High affinity binding to PSGL-1 may require appropriate presentation of one or more tyrosine sulfates located near one or more aminoterminal, sialylated and fucosylated O-glycans. Selectins may bind to specific composite recognition sites on other sialomucins, including some derived from malignant cells (76).

E-selectin, but not P- or L-selectin, binds to E-selectin ligand 1 (ESL-1), a glycoprotein on leukocytes with up to five N-glycans but no demonstrated O-glycans (63, 64). The structures of the N-glycans have not been elucidated.

Many *in vitro* and *in vivo* studies have demonstrated that leukocytes use selectins to tether to and roll on the vessel wall under the shear forces characteristic of postcapillary venules (48, 77–79). Leukocytes roll on the endothelium through interactions of L-selectin with constitutively or inducibly expressed ligands on the endothelial cell surface, and through interactions of E- and P-selectin on the activated endothelium with ligands on the leukocytes. The physiologic functions of the selectins have been confirmed in many animal models in which blocking monoclonal antibodies (mAbs) to selectins were employed (80, 81). The importance of selectins in humans is underscored by the discovery of a congenital disorder of fucose metabolism, termed leukocyte adhesion deficiency 2 (LAD-2) (82–84). Because individuals with LAD-2 lack fucosylated glycoconjugates, they do not express functional selectin ligands on leukocytes or, presumably, on endothelial cells. Leukocytes from these individuals do not tether to and roll on P- or E-selectin surfaces. Clinically, the individuals have more infectious diseases, supporting the concept that the selectins have an important function in initiating recruitment of leukocytes.

Mice made genetically deficient in each of the three selectins appear healthy, but they have obvious defects in leukocyte trafficking in response to specific challenges (85–87). Lymphocytes from L-selectin–deficient mice home less efficiently to peripheral lymph nodes (87). Mice lacking L- or P-selectin demonstrate impaired rolling of leukocytes in venules of exteriorized mesentery (85, 87). The defect in rolling is observed earlier after tissue exteriorization in P-selectin-deficient mice, consistent with the rapid mobilization of P-selectin to the endothelial cell surface after trauma (88). Comparison of the kinetics and degree of leukocyte rolling among wild-type, L-selectin–deficient and P-selectin–deficient mice suggests that L- and P-selectin function cooperatively during acute inflammatory responses (81, 88). This may reflect the overlapping expression of both P-selectin and an L-selectin ligand on the endothelial cell surface (89). In addition, L-selectin–dependent leukocyte-leukocyte contacts and P-selectin–dependent

platelet-leukocyte contacts may significantly amplify the number of flowing cells that attach to the vessel wall (see below) (90–94). Mice deficient in either L- or P-selectin have impaired leukocyte recruitment in models of acute and chronic inflammation (85, 95, 96). Such defects are less obvious in E-selectin–deficient mice, but can be elicited by blocking P-selectin function by infusion of a monoclonal antibody (mAb) (86). Mice lacking both E- and P-selectins have frequent, severe infections and shortened survival (97, 98). Mice lacking Fuc-TVII, a key fucosyltransferase for making selectin ligands, also manifest defects in leukocyte rolling and leukocyte recruitment into sites of infection or injury (99).

Under flow, selectin-ligand interactions must form rapidly to facilitate tethering of leukocytes and then dissociate rapidly to facilitate rolling. Furthermore, shear forces must not significantly accelerate the rate of dissociation (100). L-selectin-ligand interactions have faster rates of association and dissociation than P- or E-selectin-ligand interactions. Leukocytes interacting through L-selectin require a threshold shear force to support rolling, because faster rotation is required to bring L-selectin molecules at the leading edge in proximity to new ligands on the substrate before the bonds at the trailing edge of the cell dissociate (101). Other factors also regulate the efficiency of selectin-dependent tethering and rolling under flow conditions. Cell-cell contact may induce proteolytic shedding of L-selectin, accelerating rolling velocity by reducing the number of effective L-selectin-ligand bonds (102). L-selectin is clustered on the tips of microvilli, which markedly enhances its ability to contact ligands on a surface under shear forces (103). Flowing neutrophils attach and roll poorly on transfected cells expressing P-selectin molecules that are shortened by deletion of some of the SCRs (104).

Of the described glycoprotein ligands for selectins, PSGL-1 has the most clearly demonstrated function in tethering and rolling of leukocytes under flow conditions. PL1, a mAb to human PSGL-1, prevents binding of purified PSGL-1 to purified P-selectin (105). The mAb also blocks tethering and rolling of leukocytes on P-selectin substrates *in vitro* (105, 106) and *in vivo* (107). The PL1 epitope is near the aminoterminus of PSGL-1; it overlaps the tyrosine sulfation sites and includes a threonine to which a critical O-glycan may be attached (108). This supports the concept that P-selectin binds to a composite, aminoterminal recognition site. Like P-selectin, PSGL-1 is a highly extended molecule, which projects its binding site well above the cell surface (108). Like L-selectin, PSGL-1 is concentrated on the tips of microvilli (105). Thus the structure and orientation of PSGL-1 are ideally suited for efficient interactions with P-selectin under flow conditions.

It is clear that leukocytes need not be activated to bind to endothelium through selectins. Rather, endothelial cells must be activated to allow surface expression of E-selectin, P-selectin, and/or ligand(s) for L-selectin. This requirement for endothelial cell, rather than leukocyte, activation provides a means for localizing leukocyte adhesion to blood vessels in the immediate vicinity of an infectious or antigenic challenge. In turn, the transient, selectin-mediated adherence of leukocytes exposes them to activators released from the stimulated endothelium or the underlying tissues.

## RELEASE OF SIGNALING MOLECULES THAT ACTIVATE LEUKOCYTES

A variety of molecules can stimulate specific subsets of leukocytes. The ability of these molecules to bind to target cells requires that they be expressed at the same time and at the same location where leukocytes adhere loosely to endothelium at inflammatory sites. A well-documented example is the phospholipid signaling molecule, platelet-activating factor (PAF), which stimulates neutrophils as well as platelets (109). Thrombin or histamine induces the rapid, transient synthesis and surface expression of PAF on endothelial cells (110). The kinetics of expression are indistinguishable from those of P-selectin. In this "juxtacrine" system of adhesion and activation, P-selectin tethers the neutrophil to the activated, endothelial cell surface, positioning it for activation by PAF through interaction with the PAF receptor on the neutrophil. The activated neutrophil then up-regulates other adhesion molecules (see next section) that strengthen adhesion (Fig. 15.3). A second neutrophil activator is the chemokine IL-8, which is secreted by endothelial cells previously stimulated by IL-1β, TNF-α, or li-

popolysaccharide (111). The kinetics of secretion of IL-8 are similar to those of E-selectin. Furthermore, IL-8 and other chemokines may bind to proteoglycans on the apical surface of the endothelium, preventing their diffusion in the bloodstream (112). Thus E-selectin tethers the neutrophil to the activated endothelium, positioning it for subsequent activation by IL-8 through interactions with the IL-8 receptor (Fig. 15.4).

Neutrophils are also activated by complement protein C5a, the bacterial chemoattractant formyl-methionyl-leucyl-phenylalanine, and leukotriene B₄. Macrophages, endothelial cells, or other cells at sites of chronic or allergic inflammation secrete chemokines such as monocyte chemoattractant protein-1 or eotaxin that activate specific subsets of mononuclear cells or eosinophils (113–117). *In vivo*, flowing leukocytes must first tether to the endothelial cell surface before they are exposed to such regionally elaborated mediators.

Selectin-ligand interactions may themselves transmit signals into leukocytes. Most studies suggest that adhesion of leukocytes to purified E- or P-selectin does not cause overt activation, as defined by changes in cell shape; up-regulation of integrin function; secretion of granule contents; or release of oxygen-derived radicals, cytokines, or other molecules (110, 118–122). However, such interactions may produce signals that are integrated with those produced by chemokines or lipid autacoids to fully activate leukocytes. For example, P-selectin potentiates the ability of PAF and other agonists to stimulate neutrophils (110, 118). Monocytes mobilize the transcription factor NF-κB and secrete cytokines when incubated with P-selectin and PAF, but not with either individual molecule (119). Crosslinking of L-se-

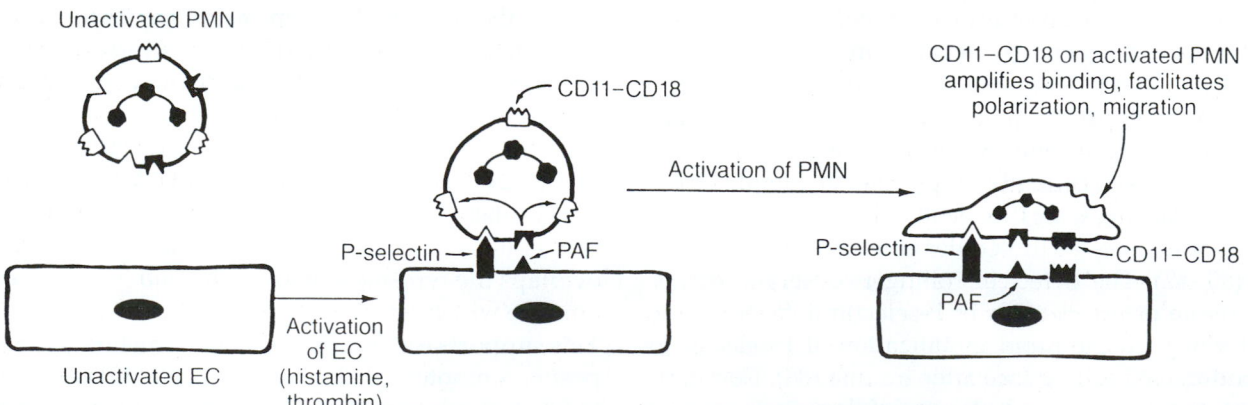

**FIGURE 15.3.** Neutrophil (polymorphonuclear cell [PMN]) adhesion to endothelial cells (EC) activated with histamine or thrombin. P-selectin is rapidly translocated from secretory granules to the plasma membrane, where it mediates reversible adhesion of PMNs. Platelet-activating factor (PAF) is coexpressed with P-selectin on the endothelial cell. PAF ligates a receptor on the PMN, signaling an activation-dependent alteration in the CD11/CD18 molecules (β2 integrins) that allows them to strengthen adhesion by binding to endothelial cell counterreceptors (probably members of the immunoglobulin superfamily). (From Zimmerman GA, Prescott SM, McIntyre TM. Endothelial cell interactions with granulocytes: tethering and signaling molecules. Immunol Today 1992;13:93–100.)

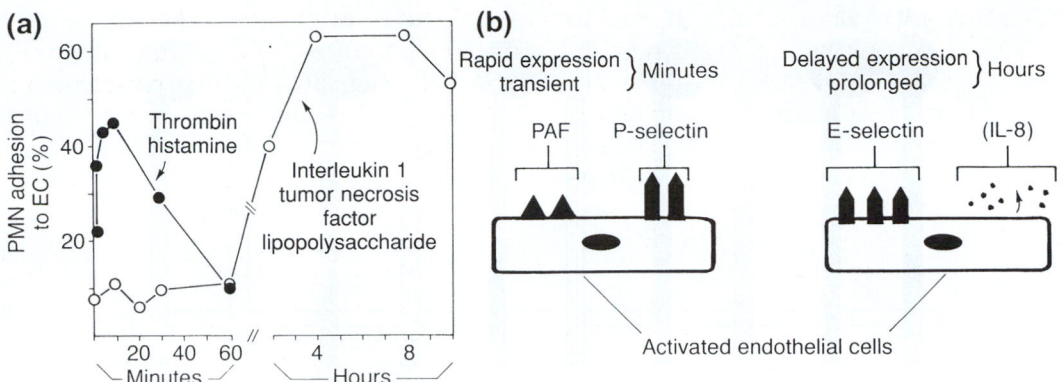

**FIGURE 15.4.** Time-dependent expression of selected adhesion and signaling molecules by activated endothelial cells (EC). (a) Time course of rapid, transient neutrophil (polymorphonuclear cell [PMN]) adhesion to EC activated with thrombin or histamine is compared with delayed, sustained adhesion to EC activated by cytokines or lipopolysaccharide. (b) Expression of adhesion molecules (P- and E-selectin) and signaling molecules (platelet-activating factor [PAF] and interleukin-8 [IL-8]) is correlated with time-dependent alterations in PMN adhesion. Other adhesion and signaling molecules are described in the text. IL-1, interleukin-1; TNF, tumor necrosis factor. (From Zimmerman GA, Prescott SM, McIntyre TM. Endothelial cell interactions with granulocytes: tethering and signaling molecules. Immunol Today 1992;13:93–100.)

lectin on neutrophils with antibodies or with sulfatides (a sulfated carbohydrate ligand for L-selectin) triggers an increase in cytosolic free calcium (123, 124) and potentiates the oxidative burst in response to the bacterial peptide formyl-methionyl-leucyl-phenylalanine (124). The requirement for costimulatory signals may limit the activation of leukocytes to sites where a conventional agonist is coexpressed with a selectin or a selectin ligand.

## EXPRESSION OF ADHESION RECEPTORS BY ACTIVATED LEUKOCYTES

Integrins, which are heterodimeric molecules consisting of noncovalently associated $\alpha$- and $\beta$-subunits, are broadly distributed receptors that mediate a variety of cell-cell and cell-matrix interactions (125). Leukocytes express certain specific members of the integrin family on their cell surfaces that play important roles in adhesion to endothelial cells and other cells (Fig. 15.5) (Table 15.2). The three $\beta_2$-integrins, or CD11/CD18 molecules, are found only on leukocytes and consist of a common $\beta_2$-chain associated with one of three distinct $\alpha$-chains (126). Lymphocyte function-associated antigen 1 (LFA-1) (CD11a/CD18) is present on all leukocytes. Mac-1 (CD11b/CD18) and p150/95 (CD11c/CD18) are expressed on myeloid cells. The importance of these molecules is emphasized in individuals with leukocyte-adhesion deficiency 1 (LAD-1), a genetic defect of the common $\beta_2$-subunit that results in lack of expression of all three $\beta_2$-integrins (127). These individuals have life-threatening bacterial infections because of defective neutrophil accumulation at these sites. Two members of the $\alpha_4$-integrin family, $\alpha_4\beta_1$ (very late antigen 4 or VLA-4)

and $\alpha_4\beta_7$ (lymphocyte Peyer's patch adhesion molecule or LPAM), are present on eosinophils and mononuclear cells but not on neutrophils (128–131). The presence of these integrins may explain why lymphocytes, but not neutrophils, accumulate in inflammatory sites in individuals with LAD-1. T cells from mice deficient in $\alpha_4$-integrins do not home to Peyer's patches, but do home to other secondary lymphoid organs such as spleen and lymph nodes (132).

Like some other integrins, notably $\alpha_{IIb3}$ on platelets (see Chapter 11), the $\beta_2$-integrins support adhesive interactions only when the cells expressing them have been activated (126). Cellular activation also up-regulates the adhesive functions of the $\alpha_4$-integrins, although some cells express constitutively active forms of these molecules (133). "Inside-out" signaling increases the binding avidity of the integrins through both conformational changes and changes in cell-surface distribution mediated by cytoskeletal interactions (125, 126). Some mAbs bind to epitopes on integrins that become accessible only after the leukocytes are activated (126). The I domain of the $\alpha$-chain expresses activation epitopes and is important for binding (134–138). Only a small percentage of the total Mac-1 integrins on leukocytes express an activation epitope; an mAb to this epitope blocks Mac-1–mediated adhesion, suggesting that only this subpopulation of "activated" integrins mediates adhesion (138). Activation of the adhesive competency of the activated $\beta_2$-integrins is rapid and transient, occurring within 1 to 5 minutes after stimulation and declining within 30 minutes (139).

Integrins on activated leukocytes interact with endothelial cell counterreceptors that are members of the immunoglobulin (Ig) superfamily (Fig. 15.6) (see Table

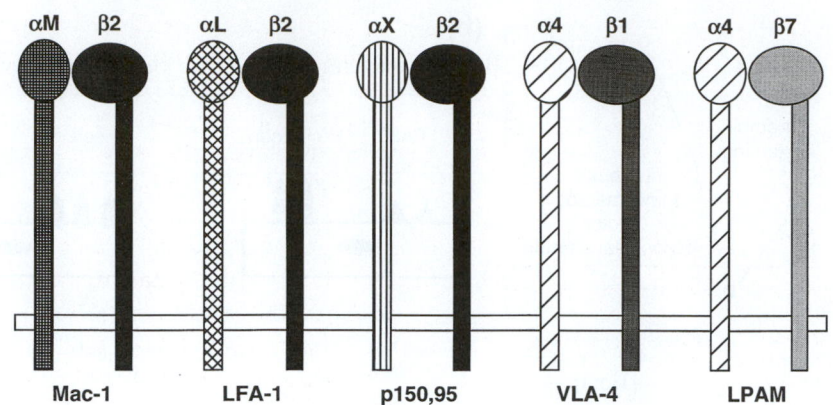

**FIGURE 15.5.** Integrins involved in adhesion of activated leukocytes to endothelial cells. Each molecule is a heterodimer consisting of a noncovalently linked α- and β-chain. Three of the integrins share a common $\beta_2$-chain, but have distinct α-chains. Each integrin is constitutively expressed on the surface of one or more subsets of leukocytes. However, activation of the leukocyte is usually required for optimal binding of the integrin to its counterreceptor on the endothelial cell. LFA-1, lymphocyte function-associated antigen 1; VLA-4, very late antigen 4; LPAM, lymphocyte Peyer's patch adhesion molecule.

**TABLE 15.2.** Integrins That Mediate Adhesion of Activated Leukocytes to Endothelial Cells

| Name | Integrin Nomenclature | CD Nomenclature | Expressed By | Endothelial Cell Counterreceptor |
|---|---|---|---|---|
| LFA-1 | $\alpha L\beta_2$ | CD11a/CD18 | All leukocytes | ICAM-1<br>ICAM-2 |
| Mac-1 | $\alpha M\beta_2$ | CD11b/CD18 | PMN, monocytes, eosinophils | ICAM-1<br>Others? |
| p150, 95 | $\alpha X\beta_2$ | CD11c/CD18 | PMN, monocytes, eosinophils | ? |
| VLA-4 | $\alpha_4\beta_1$ | CD49d/CD29 | Monocytes, eosinophils, lymphocyte subsets | VCAM-1 |
| LPAM | $\alpha_4\beta_7$ | CD49d/CD??[a] | Lymphocyte subsets | VCAM-1<br>MAdCAM-1 |

*ICAM, intercellular ahesion molecule; LFA-1, lymphocyte function–associated antigen 1; LPAM, lymphocyte Peyer's patch adhesion molecule; MAdCAM-1, mucosal addressin cell adhesion molecule 1; PMN, polymorphonuclear cell or neutrophil; VCAM-1, vascular cell adhesion molecule 1; VLA-4, very late antigen 4.*

[a] *The $\beta_7$-integrin subunit has not yet received a CD designation.*

15.2). These proteins have a series of Ig-like domains, each containing 90 to 100 amino acids (77). LFA-1 binds to two, related, Ig-like proteins, intercellular adhesion molecules 1 and 2 (ICAM-1 and ICAM-2). Mac-1 binds to ICAM-1 and to one or more unknown counterreceptors, but not to ICAM-2. The endothelial cell counterreceptors for p150,95 have not been defined, but are likely to be members of the Ig superfamily. VLA-4 and $\alpha_4\beta_7$ bind to vascular-cell adhesion molecule 1 (VCAM-1). $\alpha_4\beta_7$ binds to the Ig domains of mucosal addressin-cell adhesion molecule 1 (MAdCAM-1), an endothelial cell protein with a separate mucinlike region that may serve as a binding site for L-selectin (140–142). Leukocyte integrins also bind to ligands other than Ig molecules. Fibrinogen binds simultaneously to both Mac-1 on leukocytes and ICAM-1 on endothelial cells, serving as a

molecular bridge for leukocyte adhesion (143–145). VLA-4 binds to the connecting segment-1 (CS-1) region of fibronectin, which may be presented on the apical surface of the endothelium (146, 147). Adhesion of activated leukocytes to endothelial cells through $\beta_2$-integrins does not require activation of endothelial cells. Basal levels of ICAM-1 are present on the endothelial cell surface, although the levels increase 6 to 12 hours after stimulation by IL-1β or TNF-α. ICAM-2 is constitutively expressed on the endothelial cell surface and is not up-regulated by cytokines. However, activated leukocytes expressing VLA-4 bind to VCAM-1 only after synthesis of the latter is induced by cytokine activation of the endothelial cells. Peak expression of VCAM-1 occurs 12 to 24 hours after stimulation and persists for at least 3 days (129).

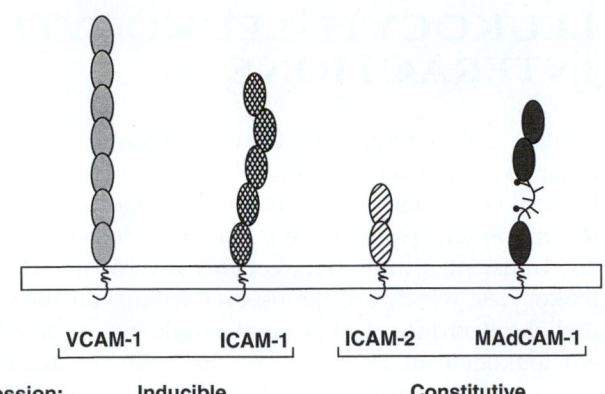

**FIGURE 15.6.** Endothelial cell members of the immunoglobulin (Ig) superfamily that serve as counterreceptors for leukocyte integrins. Each protein contains a series of Ig-like domains, of which some are binding sites for leukocyte integrins and others may position the binding sites at the optimal distance from the cell surface. Intercellular adhesion molecule 1 (ICAM-1), ICAM-2, and mucosal addressin cell adhesion molecule 1 (MAdCAM-1) are constitutively synthesized by endothelial cells in some vascular beds. Synthesis of ICAM-1 is also increased by certain cytokines. Vascular adhesion molecule 1 (VCAM-1) is synthesized only in response to inflammatory mediators. There may be other still uncharacterized Ig counterreceptors for integrins.

Under static conditions, binding of the $\beta_2$-integrins to their Ig-like counterreceptors promotes strong adhesion of activated leukocytes to endothelium. However, $\beta_2$-integrins alone do not support cell adhesion under flow conditions. Activated neutrophils, for example, do not adhere to immobilized purified ICAM-1 at venular shear rates. In contrast, unstimulated neutrophils roll over a surface coated with P-selectin and ICAM-1 and then form stable attachments after they are activated (121). Neutrophils roll on cytokine-activated, cultured endothelium by binding to E-selectin and then form tight, $\beta_2$-integrin–mediated contacts after neutrophil activation (148). Blockade of the E-selectin step with mAbs prevents stable attachment by the integrins (149). *In vivo*, inhibitors of selectin function prevent rolling of leukocytes in inflamed venules, whereas inhibitors of $\beta_2$-integrins prevent stable neutrophil attachment, but have no effect on rolling (80). Thus selectins must first support transient interactions of leukocytes with the endothelium, allowing adequate time for leukocytes to be activated and to form stable contacts through $\beta_2$-integrin–dependent recognition (Fig. 15.7).

Surprisingly, $\alpha_4$-integrins mediate tethering and rolling of flowing leukocytes on VCAM-1 or MAdCAM-1 1 (150, 151). Depending on the "activation" state of the $\alpha_4$-integrins, some flowing cells tether and then abruptly arrest on the surface. Thus, some integrins, like selectins, can mediate the initial tethering of leukocytes under

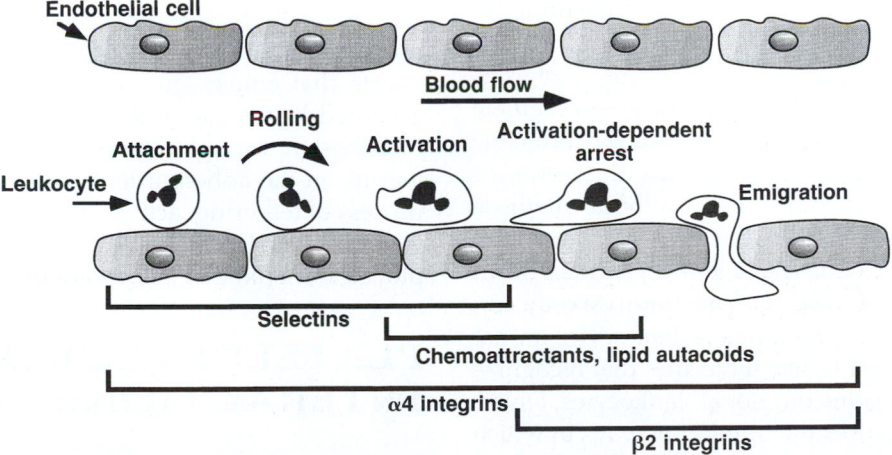

**FIGURE 15.7.** Multistep model of leukocyte recruitment. Free-flowing leukocytes attach to and then roll on postcapillary venules at inflammatory sites or on high endothelial venules of lymphoid tissues. The rolling leukocyte is activated by chemoattractants or lipid autacoids expressed on or near the endothelial cell surface. The activated leukocyte then arrests, spreads, and finally emigrates between endothelial cells into the underlying tissues. Selectins mediate the initial attachment and rolling of leukocytes, whereas $\beta_2$ leukocyte integrins mediate arrest, spreading, and emigration. Under some conditions, $\alpha_4$ integrins expressed on mononuclear cells and eosinophils, but not on neutrophils, mediate both rolling and arrest. Not illustrated are selectin- and integrin-mediated adhesive interactions of leukocytes with other leukocytes or with activated platelets, which may amplify leukocyte recruitment to the endothelial cell surface.

shear forces (Fig. 15.7). Even in this case, however, $\alpha_4$-integrins function best in concert with selectins, and the sequential process of tethering, rolling, and firm adhesion is a key mechanism for recruiting leukocytes to the vessel wall.

Following firm adhesion to the endothelium, leukocytes migrate between adjacent endothelial cells into tissues. The mechanisms underlying emigration are incompletely characterized (152). Migration may first require lessening of the adhesive bonds to the endothelium. After leukocytes are activated, L-selectin is shed (41, 42), and PSGL-1 is redistributed from microvilli to the uropods (153). P-selectin may be cleared from the endothelial cells by rapid endocytosis (18, 24). The increased binding avidity of leukocyte integrins is transient, leading to further weakening of adhesion (139). Rearrangement of functional integrins to the leading edge of the cells through membrane flow and linkages with cytoskeletal proteins may then promote migration along chemotactic gradients (154). The importance of integrins in transendothelial emigration is suggested by the decreased influx of neutrophils into infected tissues in individuals deficient in $\beta_2$-integrins (127) and by the ability of anti-$\beta_2$ antibodies to inhibit leukocyte emigration *in vivo* (80). Adherence of activated leukocytes to cultured endothelium triggers the disorganization of endothelial cell-to-cell adherens junctions, facilitating emigration (155). Homotypic interactions of the Ig-like molecule, platelet–endothelial cell adhesion molecule 1 (PECAM-1), on leukocytes and endothelial cells also promote emigration (156). Migration may require the controlled proteolytic dissolution of the subendothelial matrix to allow passage into the underlying tissues (157).

The differential expression of selectins, integrins, and their respective counterreceptors serves to regulate leukocyte recruitment into tissues (77, 78). The inducible endothelial cell expression of P-selectin, E-selectin, or the ligand(s) for L-selectin limits initial adhesion to those tissues where the endothelium has been activated. Stable adhesion of specific subsets of leukocytes may result from the generation of agonists that stimulate only certain leukocytes or certain integrins on leukocytes or that up-regulate endothelial Ig-like molecules that recognize integrins present on some but not all leukocytes. Diversity at each step increases the number of ways in which subsets of leukocytes can bind to endothelium. Furthermore, the type and quantity of chemotactic stimulus released by tissues may dictate whether an activated leukocyte adherent to the endothelial cell surface actually leaves the circulation. This multistep control system may allow responses as diverse as rapid neutrophil influx into tissues where bacteria have invaded, eosinophil emigration in response to allergic mediators, and sustained lymphocyte emigration into areas infected with intracellular pathogens such as viruses.

# LEUKOCYTE-LEUKOCYTE INTERACTIONS

During inflammation leukocytes interact with each other as well as with the endothelial cell surface. Flowing leukocytes tether to leukocytes already adherent to the endothelial cell surface (158). These tethers are usually transient, although leukocytes also roll on adherent leukocytes, which are themselves rolling on the endothelial cell surface. Tethering of a leukocyte to an adherent leukocyte markedly slows its velocity, making it much easier for the tethered leukocyte to move to the vessel wall, where it then tethers to and rolls on the endothelial cell surface (90, 92). Thus leukocyte-leukocyte interactions may serve as a major mechanism for amplifying leukocyte recruitment to the vessel wall. Selectins initiate leukocyte-leukocyte contacts under shear forces. L-selectin on the flowing leukocyte or the adherent leukocyte can bind to ligands on the other leukocyte, providing a bidirectional mechanism for rapid tethering under flow conditions (90–92, 158). Studies with anti-PSGL-1 mAbs indicate that L-selectin initiates tethering, in part, through interactions with the same aminoterminal region of PSGL-1 that P-selectin recognizes (57, 90, 159). Other ligands for L-selectin may also contribute to leukocyte-leukocyte contacts under shear forces (90, 92). In suspension, neutrophil aggregation is initiated by interactions of L-selectin with PSGL-1 and perhaps with other ligands (94). The addition of a neutrophil agonist such as formyl-methionyl-leucyl-phenylalanine allows stable formation of neutrophil aggregates through interactions of the $\beta_2$-integrin Mac-1 with a ligand on the opposing cell (94). In analogous fashion, a flowing leukocyte that tethers through L-selectin to an adherent, activated leukocyte on the vessel wall may strengthen its adhesion through interactions with functional $\beta_2$-integrins on the adherent leukocyte. Thus the sequential process of tethering, activation, and firm adhesion used for endothelial cell-leukocyte interactions is also employed for leukocyte-leukocyte interactions.

# PLATELET-LEUKOCYTE INTERACTIONS

In response to vascular injury, platelets adhere to subendothelial structures, form platelet plugs, and present membrane surfaces that support thrombin and fibrin generation (see Chapters 11 and 12). In some cases neutrophils and monocytes also associate with platelet aggregates at sites of hemorrhage (160, 161). *In vitro*, platelets bind to myeloid cells and subsets of lymphocytes but only after platelets have been activated by agonists such as thrombin (162). Platelet activation is required for P-selectin to be mobilized from $\alpha$-granules to the cell surface, where it promotes cell-cell contact by binding to PSGL-1 on the leukocyte surface (19, 21). Under shear forces, flowing neutrophils tether to and roll on adherent platelets (163). The addition of a neutrophil agonist causes the rolling leukocytes to arrest firmly on the platelet surface through interactions of the $\beta_2$-integrin Mac-1 with still uncharacterized ligands on the platelets (164, 165). Platelets express ICAM-2, a ligand for the $\beta_2$-integrin LFA-1, but interactions between these two proteins do not strengthen platelet-neutrophil adhesion (165, 166). In some instances the rolling leukocytes spontaneously arrest, suggesting that activated platelets may express signaling molecules that activate the neutrophils (167). Thus platelet-leukocyte interactions also proceed through the sequential process of tethering, activation, and firm adhesion observed in endothelial cell-leukocyte and leukocyte-leukocyte interactions.

The physiologic significance of platelet-leukocyte interactions is not fully appreciated. *In vivo*, P-selectin on activated platelets binds both to L-selectin ligands on endothelial cells and to PSGL-1 on circulating leukocytes (93). Thus activated platelets serve as a bridge that delivers leukocytes to the vessel wall, another mechanism for augmenting leukocyte recruitment to lymphoid tissues or to sites of infection or tissue injury. Leukocytes may also carry platelets into sites of inflammation (168), a mechanism for delivery of platelet factor 4, platelet-derived growth factor, regulated on activation normal T cell expressed presumed secreted (RANTES), and other platelet-derived chemokines. Close contact between platelets and leukocytes may facilitate transcellular metabolism of leukotrienes and lipoxins (169–171). Some of these products induce translocation of P-selectin to the surface of endothelial cells (172). Adhesion of activated platelets to leukocytes enhances secretion of cytokines, tissue factor, or other mediators by the leukocytes (119, 173–175). Such interactions may amplify both inflammation and hemostasis (176, 177).

# PATHOLOGIC INTERACTIONS OF LEUKOCYTES

There is increasing evidence that dysregulated leukocyte recruitment potentiates tissue destruction in a variety of inflammatory or thrombotic disorders. Excessive accumulation of leukocytes contributes to the pathogenesis of inflammatory diseases such as ischemia-reperfusion injury, Gram-negative shock, and rheumatoid arthritis (178, 179). Tissue injury results from the release of oxygen-derived radicals, proteases, and other mediators. Adhesion molecules are major participants in these processes.

Activated complement and oxygen radicals, which are frequently present during the early stages of sepsis or ischemia-reperfusion syndromes, mobilize P-selectin to the surface of endothelial cells *in vitro* (180–183). Oxygen radicals prolong the expression of P-selectin on the cell surface, perhaps by inhibiting endocytosis (181). Endothelial dysfunction decreases formation of nitric oxide, an oxygen-radical scavenger that may normally dampen the expression of P-selectin (184). Hypoxia also translocates P-selectin to the surface of endothelial cells (185, 186). Consistent with these observations, ischemia-reperfusion induces expression of P-selectin on endothelial cells *in vivo* (187–189). Furthermore, mAbs and other P-selectin inhibitors significantly reduce neutrophil accumulation and tissue injury in many ischemia-reperfusion models (187, 190–197). Antibodies to P-selectin decrease neutrophil accumulation in the tissues of rats injected with LPS (198) and in some models of acute lung injury in rats (199). Antibodies to L-selectin also reduce tissue injury in models of ischemia-reperfusion (200, 201) and in some models of acute lung injury (202). Thus, just as L- and P-selectin function cooperatively in physiologic leukocyte recruitment, they may cooperatively enhance leukocyte-mediated tissue injury in some acute inflammatory disorders. Selectins have been less well studied in models of chronic inflammatory disease. However, their contributions to pathogenesis may be inferred from their observed expression on venular endothelial cells from individuals with some chronic or allergic inflammatory disorders (203–205).

Oxidized, low-density lipoprotein activates both platelets and endothelial cells, promoting P-selectin–dependent platelet-leukocyte aggregates and leukocyte adhesion to the arterial endothelium *in vitro* and *in vivo* (206). Cigarette smoke, which causes release of oxygen radicals, produces similar effects *in vivo* (207). Some viral infections prolong the expression of P-selectin on the surface of cultured endothelial cells (208). These insults may allow monocytes and other leukocytes to emigrate beneath the endothelium during the early stages of atherosclerosis. P-selectin is observed on the apical surface of the endothelium overlying atheromas (205), perhaps because of the local synthesis of IL-4 or oncostatin M by subendothelial macrophages or T cells (29). The endothelially expressed P-selectin may promote recruitment of additional monocytes, particularly in areas of arterial bifurcation where shear stresses are lower. Rupture of advanced atherosclerotic plaques promotes platelet aggregation and thrombin formation. Leukocytes accumulating on adherent platelets may express tissue factor, further augmenting thrombin and fibrin generation (176). Consistent with this notion, mAbs to P-selectin accelerate pharmacologic thrombolysis in a primate model of arterial thrombosis (209). Anti–P-selectin mAbs reduce infiltration of inflammatory cells in a rat model of venous thrombosis (177).

*In vivo*, antibodies to the $\beta_2$-leukocyte integrins reduce tissue damage in a variety of animal models of ischemia-reperfusion injury, clearly indicating the importance of these molecules in the disease process (80, 179, 210). Antibodies to ICAM-1, one of the endothelial cell counterreceptors for the $\beta_2$-integrins, reduce tissue injury in models of ischemia-reperfusion (211), allergic asthma (211), and organ transplantation (212). Antibodies to $\alpha_4$-integrins decrease tissue damage in models of chronic and allergic inflammation (210).

The potential importance of leukocyte interactions in promoting inflammatory and thrombotic injury has generated intense interest in strategies to interrupt pathologic leukocyte accumulation. Antiadhesive drugs might include mAbs, peptides, soluble recombinant proteins, or oligosaccharides, variously designed to block adhesion molecules on endothelium, leukocytes, or platelets. Such agents might be used in conjunction with other therapies. In acute coronary artery occlusion, for example, treatment might include a thrombolytic agent to restore blood flow, a drug that blocks platelet aggregation to prevent acute reocclusion, and an agent that prevents leukocyte adhesion to minimize reperfusion injury. A potential risk of such agents is interference with the physiologic recruitment of leukocytes required to combat infections. However, antibodies to P- or L-selectin do not significantly increase infections in some experimental models, suggesting that other adhesion molecules may suffice for this purpose (213, 214). Furthermore, infections are relatively uncommon in LAD-2 individuals (82). The limited number of infections may result from the ability of $\alpha_4$-integrins to tether flowing mononuclear leukocytes and eosinophils to the endothelium (150, 151).

# REFERENCES

1. Cohnheim J. Lectures in general pathology (translated by McKee AD from the second German edition, vol. 1). London: New Sydenham Society, 1889.
2. Brenner BM, Troy JL, Ballermann BJ. Endothelium-dependent vascular responses. Mediators and mechanisms. J Clin Invest 1989;84:1373–1378.
3. Majno G, Shea SM, Leventhal M. Endothelial contraction induced by histamine-type mediators: an electron microscopic study. J Cell Biol 1969;42:647–672.
4. Stolpen AH, Guinan EC, Fiers W et al. Recombinant tumor necrosis factor and immune interferon act singly and in combination to reorganize human vascular endothelial cell monolayers. Am J Pathol 1986;123:16–24.
5. Johnston GI, Cook RG, McEver RP. Cloning of GMP-140, a granule membrane protein of platelets and endothelium: sequence similarity to proteins involved in cell adhesion and inflammation. Cell 1989;56:1033–1044.
6. Bevilacqua MP, Stengelin S, Gimbrone MA Jr et al. Endothelial leukocyte adhesion molecule 1: an inducible receptor for neutrophils related to complement regulatory proteins and lectins. Science 1989;243:1160–1165.
7. Tedder TF, Isaacs CM, Ernst TJ et al. Isolation and chromosomal localization of cDNAs encoding a novel human lymphocyte cell surface molecule, LAM-1. Homology with the mouse lymphocyte homing receptor and other human adhesion proteins. J Exp Med 1989;170:123–133.
8. Lasky LA, Singer MS, Yednock TA et al. Cloning of a lymphocyte homing receptor reveals a lectin domain. Cell 1989;56:1045–1055.
9. Siegelman MH, van de Rijn M, Weissman IL. Mouse lymph node homing receptor cDNA clone encodes a glycoprotein revealing tandem interaction domains. Science 1989;243:1165–1172.
10. Watson ML, Kingsmore SF, Johnston GI et al. Genomic organization of the selectin family of leukocyte adhesion molecules on human and mouse chromosome 1. J Exp Med 1990;172:263–272.
11. Johnston GI, Bliss GA, Newman PJ et al. Structure of the human gene encoding granule membrane protein-140, a member of the selectin family of adhesion receptors for leukocytes. J Biol Chem 1990;265:21381–21385.
12. Collins T, Williams A, Johnston GI et al. Structure and chromosomal location of the gene for endothelial-leukocyte adhesion molecule 1. J Biol Chem 1991;266:2466–2473.
13. Ord DC, Ernst TJ, Zhou LJ et al. Structure of the gene encoding the human leukocyte adhesion molecule-1 (TQ1, Leu-8) of lymphocytes and neutrophils. J Biol Chem 1990;265:7760–7767.
14. Stenberg PE, McEver RP, Shuman MA et al. A platelet alpha-granule membrane protein (GMP-140) is expressed on the plasma membrane after activation. J Cell Biol 1985;101:880–886.
15. Berman CL, Yeo EL, Wencel-Drake JD et al. A platelet alpha granule membrane protein that is associated with the plasma membrane after activation. Characterization and subcellular localization of platelet activation-dependent granule-external membrane protein. J Clin Invest 1986;78:130–137.
16. McEver RP, Beckstead JH, Moore KL et al. GMP-140, a platelet alpha-granule membrane protein, is also synthesized by vascular endothelial cells and is localized in Weibel-Palade bodies. J Clin Invest 1989;84:92–99.
17. Bonfanti R, Furie BC, Furie B et al. PADGEM (GMP 140) is a component of Weibel-Palade bodies of human endothelial cells. Blood 1989;73:1109–1112.
18. Hattori R, Hamilton KK, Fugate RD et al. Stimulated secretion of endothelial von Willebrand factor is accompanied by rapid redistribution to the cell surface of the intracellular granule membrane protein GMP-140. J Biol Chem 1989;264:7768–7771.
19. Larsen E, Celi A, Gilbert GE et al. PADGEM protein: a receptor that mediates the interaction of activated platelets with neutrophils and monocytes. Cell 1989;59:305–312.
20. Geng JG, Bevilacqua MP, Moore KL et al. Rapid neutrophil adhesion to activated endothelium mediated by GMP-140. Nature 1990;343:757–760.
21. Hamburger SA, McEver RP. GMP-140 mediates adhesion of stimulated platelets to neutrophils. Blood 1990;75:550–554.
22. Moore KL, Thompson LF. P-selectin (CD62) binds to subpopulations of human memory T lymphocytes and natural killer cells. Biochem Biophys Res Commun 1992;186:173–181.
23. Disdier M, Morrissey JH, Fugate RD et al. Cytoplasmic domain of P-selectin (CD62) contains the signal for sorting into the regulated secretory pathway. Mol Biol Cell 1992;3:309–321.
24. Setiadi H, Disdier M, Green SA et al. Residues throughout the cytoplasmic domain affect the internalization efficiency of P-selectin. J Biol Chem 1995;270:26818–26826.
25. Green SA, Setiadi H, McEver RP et al. The cytoplasmic domain of P-selectin contains a sorting determinant that mediates rapid degradation in lysosomes. J Cell Biol 1994;124:435–448.
26. Sanders WE, Wilson RW, Ballantyne CM et al. Molecular cloning and analysis of *in vivo* expression of murine P-selectin. Blood 1992;80:795–800.
27. Weller A, Isenmann S, Vestweber D. Cloning of the mouse endothelial selectins. Expression of both E- and P-selectin is inducible by tumor necrosis factor alpha. J Biol Chem 1992;267:15176–15183.
28. Burns SA, DeGuzman BJ, Newburger JW et al. P-selectin expression in myocardium of children undergoing cardiopulmonary bypass. J Thorac Cardiovasc Surg 1995;110:924–933.
29. Yao L, Pan J, Setiadi H et al. Interleukin 4 or oncostatin M induces a prolonged increase in P-selectin mRNA and protein in human endothelial cells. J Exp Med 1996;184:81–92.
30. Pan J, McEver RP. Characterization of the promoter for the human P-selectin gene. J Biol Chem 1993;268:22600–22608.
31. Pan J, McEver RP. Regulation of the human P-selectin promoter by Bcl-3 and specific homodimeric members of the NF-kappa B/Rel family. J Biol Chem 1995;270:23077–23083.
32. Hahne M, Jäger U, Isenmann S et al. Five tumor necrosis factor–inducible cell adhesion mechanisms on the surface of mouse endothelioma cells mediate the binding of leukocytes. J Cell Biol 1993;121:655–664.
33. Bevilacqua MP, Pober JS, Mendrick DL et al. Identification of an inducible endothelial-leukocyte adhesion molecule. Proc Natl Acad Sci U S A 1987;84:9238–9242.
34. Hooft van Huijsduijnen R, Whelan J, Pescini R et al. A T-cell enhancer cooperates with NF-kappa B to yield cytokine induction of E-selectin gene transcription in endothelial cells. J Biol Chem 1992;267:22385–22391.
35. Montgomery KF, Osborn L, Hession C et al. Activation of endothelial-leukocyte adhesion molecule 1 (ELAM-1) gene transcription. Proc Natl Acad Sci U S A 1991;88:6523–6527.
36. Whelan J, Ghersa P, Van Huijsduijnen RH et al. An NF kappa B-like factor is essential but not sufficient for cytokine induction of endothelial leukocyte adhesion molecule 1 (ELAM-1) gene transcription. Nucleic Acids Res 1991;19:2645–2653.
37. Read MA, Whitley MZ, Williams AJ et al. NF-kappa B and I kappa B alpha: an inducible regulatory system in endothelial activation. J Exp Med 1994;179:503–512.

38. Hession C, Osborn L, Goff D et al. Endothelial leukocyte adhesion molecule 1: direct expression cloning and functional interactions. Proc Natl Acad Sci U S A 1990;87:1673–1677.

39. Picker LJ, Kishimoto TK, Smith CW et al. ELAM-1 is an adhesion molecule for skin-homing T cells. Nature 1991;349:796–799.

40. Shimizu Y, Shaw S, Graber N et al. Activation-independent binding of human memory T cells to adhesion molecule ELAM-1. Nature 1991;349: 799–802.

41. Tedder TF, Penta AC, Levine HB et al. Expression of the human leukocyte adhesion molecule, LAM1. Identity with the TQ1 and Leu-8 differentiation antigens. J Immunol 1990;144:532–540.

42. Jutila MA, Rott L, Berg EL et al. Function and regulation of the neutrophil Mel-14 antigen *in vivo*: comparison with LFA-1 and Mac-1. J Immunol 1989;143:3318–3324.

43. Watson SR, Fennie C, Lasky LA. Neutrophil influx into an inflammatory site inhibited by a soluble homing receptor-IgG chimaera. Nature 1991; 349:164–167.

44. Gallatin WM, Weissman IL, Butcher EC. A cell surface molecule involved in organ-specific homing of lymphocytes. Nature 1983;304:30–34.

45. Watson SR, Imai Y, Fennie C et al. A homing receptor-IgG chimera as a probe for adhesive ligands of lymph node high endothelial venules. J Cell Biol 1990;110:2221–2229.

46. Kishimoto TK, Jutila MA, Berg EL et al. Neutrophil Mac-1 and MEL-14 adhesion proteins inversely regulated by chemotactic factors. Science 1989; 245:1238–1241.

47. Kahn J, Ingraham RH, Shirley F et al. Membrane proximal cleavage of L-selectin: identification of the cleavage site and a 6-kD transmembrane peptide fragment of L-selectin. J Cell Biol 1994;125:461–470.

48. McEver RP, Moore KL, Cummings RD. Leukocyte trafficking mediated by selectin-carbohydrate interactions. J Biol Chem 1995;270:11025–11028.

49. Graves BJ, Crowther RL, Chandran C et al. Insight into E-selectin/ligand interaction from the crystal structure and mutagenesis of the lec/EGF domains. Nature 1994;367:532–538.

50. Erbe DV, Watson SR, Presta LG et al. P- and E-selectin use common sites for carbohydrate ligand recognition and cell adhesion. J Cell Biol 1993; 120:1227–1235.

51. Erbe DV, Wolitzky BA, Presta LG et al. Identification of an E-selectin region critical for carbohydrate recognition and cell adhesion. J Cell Biol 1992;119:215–227.

52. Hollenbaugh D, Bajorath J, Stenkamp R et al. Interaction of P-selectin (CD62) and its cellular ligand: analysis of critical residues. Biochemistry 1993;32:2960–2966.

53. Bajorath J, Hollenbaugh D, King G et al. CD62/P-selectin binding sites for myeloid cells and sulfatides are overlapping. Biochemistry 1994;33: 1332–1339.

54. Revelle BM, Scott D, Kogan TP et al. Structure-function analysis of P-selectin-sialyl Lewis[x] binding interactions. Mutagenic alteration of ligand binding specificity. J Biol Chem 1996;271:4289–4297.

55. Kansas GS, Saunders KB, Ley K et al. A role for the epidermal growth factor–like domain of P-selectin in ligand recognition and cell adhesion. J Cell Biol 1994;124:609–618.

56. Gibson RM, Kansas GS, Tedder TF et al. Lectin and epidermal growth factor domains of P-selectin at physiologic density are the recognition unit for leukocyte binding. Blood 1995;85:151–158.

57. Tu L, Chen A, Delahunty MD et al. L-selectin binds to P-selectin glycoprotein ligand-1 on leukocytes. Interactions between the lectin, epidermal growth factor, and consensus repeat domains of the selectins determine ligand binding specificity. J Immunol 1996;157:3995–4004.

58. Kolbinger F, Patton JT, Geisenhoff G et al. The carbohydrate-recognition domain of E-selectin is sufficient for ligand binding under both static and flow conditions. Biochemistry 1996;35:6385–6392.

59. Revelle BM, Scott D, Beck PJ. Single amino acid residues in the E- and P-selectin epidermal growth factor domains can determine carbohydrate binding specificity. J Biol Chem 1996;271:16160–16170.

60. Ushiyama S, Laue TM, Moore KL et al. Structural and functional characterization of monomeric soluble P-selectin and comparison with membrane P-selectin. J Biol Chem 1993;268:15229–15237.

61. Varki A. Selectin ligands. Proc Natl Acad Sci U S A 1994;91:7390–7397.

62. Moore KL, Stults NL, Diaz S et al. Identification of a specific glycoprotein ligand for P-selectin (CD62) on myeloid cells. J Cell Biol 1992;118:445–456.

63. Levinovitz A, Mühlhoff J, Isenmann S et al. Identification of a glycoprotein ligand for E-selectin on mouse myeloid cells. J Cell Biol 1993;121:449–459.

64. Steegmaier M, Levinovitz A, Isenmann S et al. The E-selectin-ligand ESL-1 is a variant of a receptor for fibroblast growth factor. Nature 1995;373: 615–620.

65. Sako D, Chang XJ, Barone KM et al. Expression cloning of a functional glycoprotein ligand for P-selectin. Cell 1993;75:1179–1186.

66. Imai Y, Lasky LA, Rosen SD. Sulphation requirement for GlyCAM-1, an endothelial ligand for L-selectin. Nature 1993;361:555–557.

67. Hemmerich S, Butcher EC, Rosen SD. Sulfation-dependent recognition of high endothelial venules (HEV)-ligands by L-selectin and MECA 79, an adhesion-blocking monoclonal antibody. J Exp Med 1994;180:2219–2226.

68. Wilkins PP, Moore KL, McEver RP et al. Tyrosine sulfation of P-selectin glycoprotein ligand-1 is required for high affinity binding to P-selectin. J Biol Chem 1995;270:22677–22680.

69. Pouyani T, Seed B. PSGL-1 recognition of P-selectin is controlled by a tyrosine sulfation consensus at the PSGL-1 aminoterminus. Cell 1995;83: 333–343.

70. Sako D, Comess KM, Barone KM et al. A sulfated peptide segment at the aminoterminus of PSGL-1 is critical for P-selectin binding. Cell 1995;83: 323–331.

71. Li F, Wilkins PP, Crawley S et al. Post-translational modifications of recombinant P-selectin glycoprotein ligand-1 required for binding to P- and E-selectin. J Biol Chem 1996;271:3255–3264.

72. Hemmerich S, Bertozzi CR, Leffler H et al. Identification of the sulfated monosaccharides of GlyCAM-1, an endothelial-derived ligand for L-selectin. Biochemistry 1994;33:4820–4829.

73. Hemmerich S, Rosen SD. 6'-sulfated sialyl Lewis x is a major capping group of GlyCAM-1. Biochemistry 1994;33:4830–4835.

74. Hemmerich S, Leffler H, Rosen SD. Structure of the O-glycans in GlyCAM-1, an endothelial-derived ligand for L-selectin. J Biol Chem 1995;270: 12035–12047.

75. Wilkins PP, McEver RP, Cummings RD. Structures of the O-glycans on P-selectin glycoprotein ligand-1 from HL-60 cells. J Biol Chem 1996;271: 18732–18742.

76. Crottet P, Kim YJ, Varki A. Subsets of sialylated, sulfated mucins of diverse origins are recognized by L-selectin. Lack of evidence for unique oligosaccharide sequences mediating binding. Glycobiology 1996;6:191–208.

77. Springer TA. Traffic signals on endothelium for lymphocyte recirculation and leukocyte emigration. Annu Rev Physiol 1995;57:827–872.

78. Butcher EC, Picker LJ. Lymphocyte homing and homeostasis. Science 1996; 272:60–66.

79. Kansas GS. Selectins and their ligands: current concepts and controversies. Blood 1996;88:3259–3287.

80. Granger DN, Kubes P. The microcirculation and inflammation: modulation of leukocyte-endothelial cell adhesion. J Leukoc Biol 1994;55:662–675.

81. Ley K, Tedder TF. Leukocyte interactions with vascular endothelium. New insights into selectin-mediated attachment and rolling. J Immunol 1995; 155:525–528.

82. Etzioni A, Frydman M, Pollack S et al. Brief report: recurrent severe infections caused by a novel leukocyte adhesion deficiency. N Engl J Med 1992; 327:1789–1792.

83. Von Andrian UH, Berger EM, Ramezani L et al. *In vivo* behavior of neutrophils from two individuals with distinct inherited leukocyte adhesion deficiency syndromes. J Clin Invest 1993;91:2893–2897.

84. Phillips ML, Schwartz BR, Etzioni A et al. Neutrophil adhesion in leukocyte adhesion deficiency syndrome type 2. J Clin Invest 1995;96:2898–2906.

85. Mayadas TN, Johnson RC, Rayburn H et al. Leukocyte rolling and extravasation are severely compromised in P selectin-deficient mice. Cell 1993; 74:541–554.

86. Labow MA, Norton CR, Rumberger JM et al. Characterization of E-selectin-deficient mice: demonstration of overlapping function of the endothelial selectins. Immunity 1994;1:709–720.

87. Arbonés ML, Ord DC, Ley K et al. Lymphocyte homing and leukocyte rolling and migration are impaired in L-selectin-deficient mice. Immunity 1994;1:247–260.

88. Ley K, Bullard DC, Arbonés ML et al. Sequential contribution of L- and P-selectin to leukocyte rolling *in vivo*. J Exp Med 1995;181:669–675.

89. Ley K, Zakrzewicz A, Hanski C et al. Sialylated O-glycans and L-selectin sequentially mediate myeloid cell rolling *in vivo*. Blood 1995;85:3727–3735.

90. Walcheck B, Moore KL, McEver RP et al. Neutrophil-neutrophil interactions under hydrodynamic shear stress involve L-selectin and PSGL-1. A mechanism that amplifies initial leukocyte accumulation on P-selectin *in vitro*. J Clin Invest 1996;98:1081–1087.

91. Fuhlbrigge RC, Alon R, Puri KD et al. Sialylated, fucosylated ligands for L-selectin expressed on leukocytes mediate tethering and rolling adhesions in physiologic flow conditions. J Cell Biol 1996;135:837–848.

92. Alon R, Fuhlbrigge RC, Finger EB et al. Interactions through L-selectin between leukocytes and adherent leukocytes nucleate rolling adhesions on selectins and VCAM-1 in shear flow. J Cell Biol 1996;135:849–865.

93. Diacovo TG, Puri KD, Warnock RA et al. Platelet-mediated lymphocyte delivery to high endothelial venules. Science 1996;273:252–255.

94. Guyer DA, Moore KL, Lynam EB et al. P-selectin glycoprotein ligand-1 (PSGL-1) is a ligand for L-selectin in neutrophil aggregation. Blood 1996; 88:2415–2421.

95. Subramaniam M, Saffaripour S, Watson SR et al. Reduced recruitment of inflammatory cells in a contact hypersensitivity response in P-selectin-deficient mice. J Exp Med 1995;181:2277–2282.

96. Tedder TF, Steeber DA, Pizcueta P. L-selectin-deficient mice have impaired leukocyte recruitment into inflammatory sites. J Exp Med 1995;181: 2259–2264.

97. Bullard DC, Kunkel EJ, Kubo H et al. Infectious susceptibility and severe deficiency of leukocyte rolling and recruitment in E-selectin and P-selectin double mutant mice. J Exp Med 1996;183:2329–2336.

98. Frenette PS, Mayadas TN, Rayburn H et al. Susceptibility to infection and

altered hematopoiesis and mice deficient in both P- and E-selectin. Cell 1996;84:563–574.

99. Maly P, Thall A, Petryniak B et al. The (1, 3)fucosyltransferase Fuc-TVII controls leukocyte trafficking through an essential role in L-, E-, and P-selectin ligand biosynthesis. Cell 1996;86:643–653.

100. Alon R, Hammer DA, Springer TA. Lifetime of the P-selectin-carbohydrate bond and its response to tensile force in hydrodynamic flow. Nature 1995;374:539–542.

101. Finger EB, Puri KD, Alon R et al. Adhesion through L-selectin requires a threshold hydrodynamic shear. Nature 1996;379:266–269.

102. Walcheck B, Kahn J, Fisher JM et al. Neutrophil rolling altered by inhibition of L-selectin shedding in vitro. Nature 1996;380:720–723.

103. Von Andrian UH, Hasslen SR, Nelson RD et al. A central role for microvillous receptor presentation in leukocyte adhesion under flow. Cell 1995;82:989–999.

104. Patel KD, Nollert MU, McEver RP. P-selectin must extend a sufficient length from the plasma membrane to mediate rolling of neutrophils. J Cell Biol 1995;131:1893–1902.

105. Moore KL, Patel KD, Bruehl RE et al. P-selectin glycoprotein ligand-1 mediates rolling of human neutrophils on P-selectin. J Cell Biol 1995;128:661–671.

106. Patel KD, Moore KL, Nollert MU et al. Neutrophils use both shared and distinct mechanisms to adhere to selectins under static and flow conditions. J Clin Invest 1995;96:1887–1896.

107. Norman KE, Moore KL, McEver RP et al. Leukocyte rolling in vivo is mediated by P-selectin glycoprotein ligand-1. Blood 1995;86:4417–4421.

108. Li F, Erickson HP, James JA et al. Visualization of P-selectin glycoprotein ligand-1 as a highly extended molecule and mapping of protein epitopes for monoclonal antibodies. J Biol Chem 1996;271:6342–6348.

109. Prescott SM, Zimmerman GA, McIntyre TM. Platelet-activating factor. J Biol Chem 1990;265:17381–17384.

110. Lorant DE, Patel KD, McIntyre TM et al. Coexpression of GMP-140 and PAF by endothelium stimulated by histamine or thrombin: a juxtacrine system for adhesion and activation of neutrophils. J Cell Biol 1991;115:223–234.

111. Baggiolini M. Interleukin-8 and related chemotactic cytokines. In: Gallin JI, Goldstein IM, Snyderman R, eds. Inflammation: basic principles and clinical correlates. New York: Raven Press, 1992; pp. 247–255.

112. Rot A. Endothelial cell binding of NAP-1/IL-8: role in neutrophil emigration. Immunol Today 1992;13:291–294.

113. Bokoch GM. Chemoattractant signaling and leukocyte activation. Blood 1995;86:1649–1660.

114. Carr MW, Alon R, Springer TA. The C-C chemokine MCP-1 differentially modulates the avidity of 1 and 2 integrins on T lymphocytes. Immunity 1996;4:179–187.

115. Campbell JJ, Qin S, Bacon KB et al. Biology of chemokine and classical chemoattractant receptors: differential requirements for adhesion-triggering versus chemotactic responses in lymphoid cells. J Cell Biol 1996;134:255–266.

116. Weber C, Alon R, Moser B et al. Sequential regulation of 41 and 51 integrin avidity by CC chemokines in monocytes: implications for transendothelial chemotaxis. J Cell Biol 1996;134:1063–1073.

117. Rothenberg ME, Ownbey R, Mehlhop PD et al. Eotaxin triggers eosinophil-selective chemotaxis and calcium flux via a distinct receptor and induces pulmonary eosinophilia in the presence of interleukin 5 in mice. Mol Med 1996;2:334–348.

118. Lorant DE, Topham MK, Whatley RE et al. Inflammatory roles of P-selectin. J Clin Invest 1993;92:559–570.

119. Weyrich AS, McIntyre TM, McEver RP et al. Monocyte tethering by P-selectin regulates monocyte chemotactic protein-1 and tumor necrosis factor-α secretion. J Clin Invest 1995;95:2297–2303.

120. Abbassi O, Kishimoto TK, McIntire LV et al. E-selectin supports neutrophil rolling in vitro under conditions of flow. J Clin Invest 1993;92:2719–2730.

121. Lawrence MB, Springer TA. Leukocytes roll on a selectin at physiologic flow rates: distinction from and prerequisite for adhesion through integrins. Cell 1991;65:859–873.

122. Lawrence MB, Springer TA. Neutrophils roll on E-selectin. J Immunol 1993;151:6338–6346.

123. Laudanna C, Constantin G, Baron P et al. Sulfatides trigger increase of cytosolic free calcium and enhanced expression of tumor necrosis factor-α and interleukin-8 mRNA in human neutrophils. Evidence for a role of L-selectin as a signaling molecule. J Biol Chem 1994;269:4021–4026.

124. Waddell TK, Fialkow L, Chan CK et al. Potentiation of the oxidative burst of human neutrophils. A signaling role for L-selectin. J Biol Chem 1994;269:18485–18491.

125. Hynes RO. Integrins: versatility, modulation, and signaling in cell adhesion. Cell 1992;69:11–25.

126. Diamond MS, Springer TA. The dynamic regulation of integrin adhesiveness. Curr Biol 1994;4:506–517.

127. Anderson DC, Springer TA. Leukocyte adhesion deficiency: an inherited defect in the Mac-1, LFA-1, and p150,95 glycoproteins. Annu Rev Med 1987;38:175–194.

128. Elices MJ, Osborn L, Takada Y et al. VCAM-1 on activated endothelium interacts with the leukocyte integrin VLA-4 at a site distinct from the VLA-4/fibronectin binding site. Cell 1990;60:577–584.

129. Lobb RR. Integrin-immunoglobulin superfamily interactions in endothelial-leukocyte adhesion. In: Harlan JM, Liu DY, eds. Adhesion: its role in inflammatory disease. New York: WH Freeman, 1992; pp. 1–18.

130. Holzmann B, McIntyre BW, Weissman IL. Identification of a murine Peyer's patch–specific lymphocyte homing receptor as an integrin molecule with an alpha chain homologous to human VLA-4 alpha. Cell 1989;56:37–46.

131. Ruegg C, Postigo AA, Sikorski EE et al. Role of integrin 47/4P in lymphocyte adherence to fibronectin and VCAM-1 and in homotypic cell clustering. J Cell Biol 1992;117:179–189.

132. Arroyo AG, Yang JT, Rayburn H et al. Differential requirements for 4 integrins during fetal and adult hematopoiesis. Cell 1996;85:997–1008.

133. Yednock TA, Cannon C, Vandevert C et al. $\alpha_4\beta_1$-Integrin–dependent cell adhesion is regulated by a low-affinity receptor pool that is conformationally responsive to ligand. J Biol Chem 1995;270:28740–28750.

134. Randi AM, Hogg N. I domain of $\beta_2$ integrin lymphocyte function-associated antigen-1 contains a binding site for ligand intercellular adhesion molecule-1. J Biol Chem 1994;269:12395–12398.

135. Michishita M, Videm V, Arnaout MA. A novel divalent cation-binding site in the A domain of the β2 integrin CR3 (CD11b/CD18) is essential for ligand binding. Cell 1993;72:857–867.

136. Landis RC, Bennett RI, Hogg N. A novel LFA-1 activation epitope maps to the I domain. J Cell Biol 1993;120:1519–1527.

137. Diamond MS, Garcia-Aguilar J, Bickford JK et al. The I domain is a major recognition site on the leukocyte integrin Mac-1 (CD11b/CD18) for four distinct adhesion ligands. J Cell Biol 1993;120:1031–1043.

138. Diamond MS, Springer TA. A subpopulation of Mac-1 (CD11b/CD18) molecules mediates neutrophil adhesion to ICAM-1 and fibrinogen. J Cell Biol 1993;120:545–556.

139. Lo SK, Van Seventer GA, Levin SM et al. Two leukocyte receptors (CD11a/CD18 and CD11b/CD18) mediate transient adhesion to endothelium by binding to different ligands. J Immunol 1989;143:3325–3329.

140. Berlin C, Berg EL, Briskin MJ et al. $\alpha_4\beta_7$-integrin mediates lymphocyte binding to the mucosal vascular addressin MAdCAM-1. Cell 1993;74:185–195.

141. Berg EL, McEvoy LM, Berlin C et al. L-selectin-mediated lymphocyte rolling on MAdCAM-1. Nature 1993;366:695–698.

142. Briskin MJ, McEvoy LM, Butcher EC. MAdCAM-1 has homology to immunoglobulin and mucin-like adhesion receptors and to IgA1. Nature 1993;363:461–464.

143. Languino LR, Plescia J, Duperray A et al. Fibrinogen mediates leukocyte adhesion to vascular endothelium through an ICAM-1-dependent pathway. Cell 1993;73:1423–1434.

144. Languino LR, Duperray A, Joganic KJ et al. Regulation of leukocyte-endothelium interaction and leukocyte transendothelial migration by intercellular adhesion molecule 1-fibrinogen recognition. Proc Natl Acad Sci U S A 1995;92:1505–1509.

145. Sriramarao P, Languino LR, Altieri DC. Fibrinogen mediates leukocyte-endothelium bridging in vivo at low shear forces. Blood 1996;88:3416–3423.

146. Chan BM, Elices MJ, Murphy E et al. Adhesion to vascular cell adhesion molecule 1 and fibronectin. Comparison of $\alpha_4\beta_1$ (VLA-4) and $\alpha_4\beta_7$ on the human B cell line JY. J Biol Chem 1992;267:8366–8370.

147. Elices MJ, Tsai V, Strahl D et al. Expression and functional significance of alternatively spliced CS1 fibronectin in rheumatoid arthritis microvasculature. J Clin Invest 1994;93:405–416.

148. Lawrence MB, Smith CW, Eskin SG et al. Effect of venuous shear stress on CD18-mediated neutrophil adhesion to cultured endothelium. Blood 1990;75:227–237.

149. Kishimoto TK, Warnock RA, Jutila MA et al. Antibodies against human neutrophil LECAM-1 (LAM-1/Leu-8/DREG-56 antigen) and endothelial cell ELAM-1 inhibit a common CD18-independent adhesion pathway in vitro. Blood 1991;78:805–811.

150. Berlin C, Bargatze RF, Campbell JJ et al. $\alpha_4$ integrins mediate lymphocyte attachment and rolling under physiologic flow. Cell 1995;80:413–422.

151. Alon R, Kassner PD, Carr MW et al. The integrin VLA-4 supports tethering and rolling in flow on VCAM-1. J Cell Biol 1995;128:1243–1253.

152. Smith CW. Transendothelial migration. In: Harlan JM, Liu DY, eds. Adhesion: its role in inflammatory disease. New York: WH Freeman, 1992; pp. 83–116.

153. Lorant DE, McEver RP, McIntyre TM et al. Activation of polymorphonuclear leukocytes reduces their adhesion to P-selectin and causes redistribution of ligands for P-selectin on their surfaces. J Clin Invest 1995;96:171–182.

154. Hughes BJ, Hollers JC, Crockett-Torabi E et al. Recruitment of CD11b/CD18 to the neutrophil surface and adherence-dependent cell locomotion. J Clin Invest 1992;90:1687–1696.

155. Del Maschio A, Zanetti A, Corada M et al. Polymorphonuclear leukocyte adhesion triggers the disorganization of endothelial cell-to-cell adherens junctions. J Cell Biol 1996;135:497–510.

156. Muller WA, Weigl SA, Deng X et al. PECAM-1 is required for transendothelial migration of leukocytes. J Exp Med 1993;178:449–460.

157. Huber AR, Kunkel SL, Todd RF III et al. Regulation of transendothelial neutrophil migration by endogenous interleukin-8. Science 1991;254:99–102.

158. Bargatze RF, Kurk S, Butcher EC et al. Neutrophils roll on adherent neutrophils bound to cytokine-induced endothelial cells via L-selectin on the rolling cells. J Exp Med 1994;180:1785–1792.

159. Spertini O, Cordey AS, Monai N et al. P-selectin glycoprotein ligand is a ligand for L-selectin on neutrophils, monocytes and CD34$^+$ hematopoietic progenitor cells. J Cell Biol 1996;135:523–531.

160. Henry RL. Leukocytes and thrombosis. Thromb Diath Haemorrh 1961;13:35–46.

161. Wester J, Sixma JJ, Geuze JJ et al. Morphology of the hemostatic plug in human skin wounds. Transformation of the plug. Lab Invest 1979;41:182–192.

162. Jungi TW, Spycher MO, Nydegger UE et al. Platelet-leukocyte interaction: selective binding of thrombin-stimulated platelets to human monocytes, polymorphonuclear leukocytes, and related cell lines. Blood 1986;67:629–636.

163. Buttrum SM, Hatton R, Nash GB. Selectin-mediated rolling of neutrophils on immobilized platelets. Blood 1993;82:1165–1174.

164. Lalor P, Nash GB. Adhesion of flowing leucocytes to immobilized platelets. Br J Haematol 1995;89:725–732.

165. Diacovo TG, Roth SJ, Buccola JM et al. Neutrophil rolling, arrest, and transmigration across activated, surface-adherent platelets via sequential action of P-selectin and the $\beta_2$-integrin CD11b/CD18. Blood 1996;88:146–157.

166. Diacovo TG, DeFougerolles AR, Bainton DF et al. A functional integrin ligand on the surface of platelets: intercellular adhesion molecule-2. J Clin Invest 1994;94:1243–1251.

167. Yeo EL, Sheppard JA, Feuerstein IA. Role of P-selectin and leukocyte activation in polymorphonuclear cell adhesion to surface adherent activated platelets under physiologic shear conditions (an injured vessel wall model). Blood 1994;83:2498–2507.

168. Issekutz AC, Ripley M, Jackson JR. Role of neutrophils in the deposition of platelets during acute inflammation. Lab Invest 1983;49:716–724.

169. Murphy RC, Maclouf J, Henson PM. Interaction of platelets and neutrophils in the generation of sulfidopeptide leukotrienes. Adv Exp Med Biol 1991;314:91–101.

170. Serhan CN, Sheppard KA. Lipoxin formation during human neutrophil-platelet interactions. Evidence for the transformation of leukotriene A$_4$ by platelet 12-lipoxygenase in vitro. J Clin Invest 1990;85:772–780.

171. Marcus AJ. Eicosanoid interactions between platelets, endothelial cells, and neutrophils. Methods Enzymol 1990;187:585–599.

172. Datta YH, Romano M, Jacobson BC et al. Peptido-leukotrienes are potent agonists of von Willebrand factor secretion and P-selectin surface expression in human umbilical vein endothelial cells. Circulation 1995;92:3304–3311.

173. Weyrich AS, Elstad MR, McEver RP et al. Activated platelets signal chemokine synthesis by human monocytes. J Clin Invest 1996;97:1525–1534.

174. Celi A, Pellegrini G, Lorenzet R et al. P-selectin induces the expression of tissue factor on monocytes. Proc Natl Acad Sci U S A 1994;91:8767–8771.

175. Nagata K, Tsuji T, Todoroki N et al. Activated platelets induce superoxide anion release by monocytes and neutrophils through P-selectin (CD62). J Immunol 1993;151:3267–3273.

176. Palabrica T, Lobb R, Furie BC et al. Leukocyte accumulation promoting fibrin deposition is mediated in vivo by P-selectin on adherent platelets. Nature 1992;359:848–851.

177. Wakefield TW, Strieter RM, Downing LJ et al. P-selectin and TNF inhibition reduce venous thrombosis inflammation. J Surg Res 1996;64:26–31.

178. Albelda SM, Smith CW, Ward PA. Adhesion molecules and inflammatory injury. FASEB J 1994;8:504–512.

179. Sharar SR, Winn RK, Harlan JM. The adhesion cascade and anti-adhesion therapy: an overview. Springer Semin Immunopathol 1995;16:359–378.

180. Hattori R, Hamilton KK, McEver RP et al. Complement proteins C5b-9 induce secretion of high molecular weight multimers of endothelial von Willebrand factor and translocation of granule membrane protein GMP-140 to the cell surface. J Biol Chem 1989;264:9053–9060.

181. Patel KD, Zimmerman GA, Prescott SM et al. Oxygen radicals induce human endothelial cells to express GMP-140 and bind neutrophils. J Cell Biol 1991;112:749–759.

182. Foreman KE, Vaporciyan AA, Bonish BK et al. C5a-induced expression of P-selectin in endothelial cells. J Clin Invest 1994;94:1147–1155.

183. Vischer UM, Jornot L, Wollheim CB et al. Reactive oxygen intermediates induce regulated secretion of von Willebrand factor from cultured human vascular endothelial cells. Blood 1995;85:3164–3172.

184. Murohara T, Parkinson SJ, Waldman SA et al. Inhibition of nitric oxide biosynthesis promotes P-selectin expression in platelets. Role of protein kinase C. Arterioscler Thromb Vasc Biol 1995;15:2068–2075.

185. Rainger GE, Fisher A, Shearman C et al. Adhesion of flowing neutrophils to cultured endothelial cells after hypoxia and reoxygenation in vitro. Am J Physiol Heart Circ Physiol 1995;269:H1398–H1406.

186. Pinsky DJ, Naka Y, Liao H et al. Hypoxia-induced exocytosis of endothelial cell Weibel-Palade bodies. A mechanism for rapid neutrophil recruitment after cardiac preservation. J Clin Invest 1996;97:493–500.

187. Winn RK, Liggitt D, Vedder NB et al. Anti-P-selectin monoclonal antibody attenuates reperfusion injury to the rabbit ear. J Clin Invest 1993;92:2042–2047.

188. Weyrich AS, Buerke M, Albertine KH et al. Time course of coronary vascular endothelial adhesion molecule expression during reperfusion of the ischemic feline myocardium. J Leukoc Biol 1995;57:45–55.

189. Okada Y, Copeland BR, Mori E et al. P-selectin and intercellular adhesion molecule-1 expression after focal brain ischemia and reperfusion. Stroke 1994;25:202–211.

190. Weyrich AS, Ma XY, Lefer DJ et al. In vivo neutralization of P-selectin protects feline heart and endothelium in myocardial ischemia and reperfusion injury. J Clin Invest 1993;91:2620–2629.

191. Davenpeck KL, Gauthier TW, Albertine KH et al. Role of P-selectin in microvascular leukocyte-endothelial interaction in splanchnic ischemia-reperfusion. Am J Physiol 1994;267:H622–H630.

192. Mulligan MS, Paulson JC, De Frees S et al. Protective effects of oligosaccharides in P-selectin-dependent lung injury. Nature 1993;364:149–151.

193. Gauthier TW, Davenpeck KL, Lefer AM. Nitric oxide attenuates leukocyte-endothelial interaction via P-selectin in splanchnic ischemia-reperfusion. Am J Physiol 1994;267:G562–G568.

194. Chen LY, Nichols WW, Hendricks JB et al. Monoclonal antibody to P-selectin (PB1.3) protects against myocardial reperfusion injury in the dog. Cardiovasc Res 1994;28:1414–1422.

195. Winn RK, Paulson JC, Harlan JM. A monoclonal antibody to P-selectin ameliorates injury associated with hemorrhagic shock in rabbits. Am J Physiol 1994;267:H2391–H2397.

196. Lee WP, Gribling P, De Guzman L et al. P-selectin-immunoglobulin G chimera is protective in a rabbit ear model of ischemia-reperfusion. Surgery 1995;117:458–465.

197. Lefer DJ, Flynn DM, Buda AJ. Effects of a monoclonal antibody directed against P-selectin after myocardial ischemia and reperfusion. Am J Physiol 1996;270:H88–H98.

198. Coughlan AF, Hau H, Dunlop LC et al. P-selectin and platelet-activating factor mediate initial endotoxin-induced neutropenia. J Exp Med 1994;179:329–334.

199. Mulligan MS, Polley MJ, Bayer RJ et al. Neutrophil-dependent acute lung injury. Requirement for P-selectin (GMP-140). J Clin Invest 1992;90:1600–1607.

200. Ma XL, Weyrich AS, Lefer DJ et al. Monoclonal antibody to L-selectin attenuates neutrophil accumulation and protects ischemic reperfused cat myocardium. Circulation 1993;88:649–658.

201. Mihelcic D, Schleiffenbaum B, Tedder TF et al. Inhibition of leukocyte L-selectin function with a monoclonal antibody attenuates reperfusion injury to the rabbit ear. Blood 1994;84:2322–2328.

202. Mulligan MS, Miyasaka M, Tamatani T et al. Requirements for L-selectin in neutrophil-mediated lung injury in rats. J Immunol 1994;152:832–840.

203. Grober JS, Bowen BL, Ebling H et al. Monocyte-endothelial adhesion in chronic rheumatoid arthritis: in situ detection of selectin and integrin-dependent interactions. J Clin Invest 1993;91:2609–2619.

204. Symon FA, Walsh GM, Watson SR et al. Eosinophil adhesion to nasal polyp endothelium is P-selectin-dependent. J Exp Med 1994;180:371–376.

205. Johnson-Tidey RR, McGregor JL, Taylor PR et al. Increase in the adhesion molecule P-selectin in endothelium overlying atherosclerotic plaques. Coexpression with intercellular adhesion molecule-1. Am J Pathol 1994;144:952–961.

206. Lehr HA, Olofsson AM, Carew TE et al. P-selectin mediates the interaction of circulating leukocytes with platelets and microvascular endothelium in response to oxidized lipoprotein in vivo. Lab Invest 1994;71:380–386.

207. Lehr HA, Frei B, Arfors KE. Vitamin C prevents cigarette smoke–induced leukocyte aggregation and adhesion to endothelium in vivo. Proc Natl Acad Sci U S A 1994;91:7688–7692.

208. Etingin OR, Silverstein RL, Hajjar DP. Identification of a monocyte receptor on herpes virus–infected endothelial cells. Proc Natl Acad Sci U S A 1991;88:7200–7203.

209. Toombs CF, DeGraaf GL, Martin JP et al. Pretreatment with a blocking monoclonal antibody to P-selectin accelerates pharmacological thrombolysis in a primate model of arterial thrombosis. J Pharmacol Exp Ther 1995;275:941–949.

210. Carlos TM, Harlan JM. Leukocyte-endothelial adhesion molecules. Blood 1994;84:2068–2101.

211. Harlan JM, Winn RK, Vedder NB et al. In vivo models of leukocyte adherence to endothelium. In: Harlan JM, Liu DY, eds. Adhesion: its role in inflammatory disease. New York: WH Freeman, 1992; pp. 117–150.

212. Isobe M, Yagita H, Okumura K et al. Specific acceptance of cardiac allograft after treatment with antibodies to ICAM-1 and LFA-1. Science 1992;255:1125–1127.

213. Sharar SR, Sasaki SS, Flaherty LC et al. P-selectin blockade does not impair

leukocyte host defense against bacterial peritonitis and soft tissue infection in rabbits. J Immunol 1993;151:4982–4988.

214. Sharar SR, Chapman NN, Flaherty LC et al. L-selectin (CD62L) blockade does not impair peritoneal neutrophil emigration or subcutaneous host defense to bacteria in rabbits. J Immunol 1996;157:2555–2563.

215. Moore KL, Eaton SF, Lyons DE et al. The P-selectin glycoprotein ligand from human neutrophils displays sialylated, fucosylated, O-linked poly-N-acetyllactosamine. J Biol Chem 1994;269:23318–23327.

216. Hensley P, McDevitt PJ, Brooks I et al. The soluble form of E-selectin is an asymmetric monomer. Expression, purification, and characterization of the recombinant protein. J Biol Chem 1994;269:23949–23958.

217. Cyster JG, Shotton DM, Williams AF. The dimensions of the T lymphocyte glycoprotein leukosialin and identification of linear protein epitopes that can be modified by glycosylation. EMBO J 1991;10:893–902.

218. Walcheck B, Watts G, Jutila MA. Bovine gamma/delta T cells bind E-selectin via a novel glycoprotein receptor: first characterization of a lymphocyte/E-selectin interaction in an animal model. J Exp Med 1993;178:853–863.

219. Lenter M, Levinovitz A, Isenmann S et al. Monospecific and common glycoprotein ligands for E- and P-selectin on myeloid cells. J Cell Biol 1994;125:471–481.

220. Aigner S, Ruppert M, Hubbe M et al. Heat stable antigen (mouse CD24) supports myeloid cell binding to endothelial and platelet P-selectin. Int Immunol 1995;7:1557–1565.

# CHAPTER 16

# VON WILLEBRAND FACTOR

Zaverio M. Ruggeri, Jerry Ware, and David Ginsburg

## HISTORICAL BACKGROUND

In 1926, Erich von Willebrand described the congenital bleeding disorder that is named after him (see Chapter 34). In 1971, Zimmerman et al (1) identified the protein that typically is decreased in von Willebrand disease, now known as von Willebrand factor (vWf). The newly discovered molecule initially was designated as "AHF-like antigen," and subsequently "factor VIII-related antigen," because the antiserum used for its immunochemical characterization was althought to be specific for factor VIII, which is the antihemophilic factor (AHF). Unknown at the time, however, the immunogen used to prepare the antiserum contained vWf in great molar excess over factor VIII, and this gave rise to precipitating antibodies against the former but not the latter.

Two contrasting opinions developed after the initial discovery (2–5). Both opinions, however, arose from the observation that factor VIII-related antigen (i.e., vWf) normally is present in hemophilic plasma with absent factor VIII activity, but that it is decreased concurrently with factor VIII in most individuals with von Willebrand disease (1). The first explained this situation by considering factor VIII and vWf as being associated but distinct entities. Accordingly, hemophilia was althought to result from primary abnormalities of factor VIII and von Willebrand disease from defects of vWf. The second considered factor VIII and vWf as being two activities of the same protein. In this case, von Willebrand disease was althought to result from quantitative defects in the molecule and hemophilia A from qualitative abnormalities causing a loss of clotting activity. It now is established, however, that factor VIII and vWf are products of two unrelated genes, but, as discussed in more detail later (and in Chapter 34), they circulate in blood as a tightly associated, noncovalent complex. Thus, even although the concept of one molecule with two activities is wrong, the association between vWf and factor VIII does create a functional unit that allows factor VIII to perform its function (6).

## NOMENCLATURE

Considering the confusing, yet historically justified, terminology used for many years when referring to factor VIII and vWf, the International Committee on Thrombosis and Hemostasis has suggested guidelines for an appropriate nomenclature (7) (see Table 34.1 in Chapter 34). The proteins factor VIII and von Willebrand factor should be identified as such; the corresponding abbreviations are FVIII and vWf, respectively. Factor VIII-related antigen (abbreviated as VIIIR:Ag) should not be used when referring to vWf; rather, VIII:Ag and vWf:Ag are the suggested abbreviations to be used in connection with immunological detection, measurement, or both of factor VIII and vWf, respectively. The procoagulant (i.e., clotting) activity of factor VIII is abbreviated as VIII:C. There are no suggested abbreviations for any biological function of vWf. In particular, the Subcommittee has discouraged use of VIIIR:RCo to indicate the ristocetin cofactor activity of vWf, namely the *in vitro* activity supporting platelet agglutination with the antibiotic ristocetin. Some authors use vWf:RCo as an abbreviation for this activity.

Nucleotides in the vWf complementary DNA (cDNA) are numbered from the major transcription cap site, which is located 250 nucleotides before the first nucleotide in the ATG codon for the initiating methionine (8, 9). Amino acid residues may be numbered either according to the sequence of pre-pro-vWf, in which case residue 1 is the initiating Met, or according to the sequence of the mature vWf subunit, in which case residue 1 is Ser at position 764 of pre-pro-vWf. Thus, residue numbers in the mature vWf subunit correspond to those in pre-pro-vWf after adding 763, which accounts for the 22 residues of the signal peptide and the 741 residues of the vWf propeptide (10, 11).

# STRUCTURE

## GENE STRUCTURE AND EXPRESSION

Isolation of vWf cDNA clones and elucidation of the gene organization have contributed greatly to our understanding of vWf biosynthesis, structure, and function (12–15). The original cDNA clones for vWf were prepared from endothelial cell messenger RNA (mRNA) and identified using anti-vWf antibodies to detect the translated product. Later studies used the polymerase chain reaction and demonstrated the presence of vWf mRNA in platelets (16).

## cDNA and Protein Structure

The primary translation product predicted from the cloned cDNA of vWf is a 2813-residue precursor polypeptide, which is referred to as "pre-pro-vWf" (Fig. 16.1) and consists of a 22-residue signal peptide, an unu-

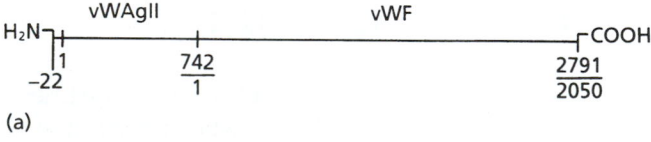

(a)

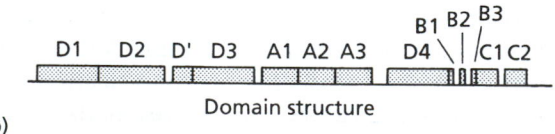

(b)

**FIGURE 16.1.** Structure of pre-pro-von Willebrand factor (vWf). **(a)** The linear amino acid sequence of pre-pro-vWf comprises the signal peptide beginning at position -22 (i.e., 22 residues upstream from the aminoterminus of pro-vWf). The first 741 residues of pro-vWf represent von Willebrand antigen II (vWAgII, the vWf propeptide); residue 742 in the sequence of pro-vWf corresponds to residue 1 (i.e., the aminoterminus) of the 2050-residue mature vWf subunit. Altogether, pro-vWf contains 2791 residues. Note that pro-vWf, the precursor of the mature molecule comprising vWAgII as well as the mature vWf subunit, should not be confused with the propeptide of vWf (vWAgII). **(b)** Location of the four types of repeated domains (A through D) relative to the linear sequence of pro-vWf.

sually large 741-residue propeptide, and a 2050-residue mature subunit (10, 17). Cloning the vWf cDNA demonstrated that the vWf propeptide is identical to a previously characterized protein, von Willebrand antigen II (vWAgII) (18), present in normal plasma and platelets as a species immunologically distinct from mature vWf. As with mature vWf, the level of vWAgII is decreased in individuals with von Willebrand disease (19).

The propeptide and mature subunit of vWf, which together represent pro-vWf, are composed almost entirely of four types of repeating domains, which are designated as A through D and arranged from amino to carboxyterminal in the following order: D1-D2-D'-D3-A1-A2-A3-D4-B1-B2-B3-C1-C2 (Fig. 16.1) (20). The four D domains are approximately 360 residues in length, and each contains between 32 and 36 Cys residues. The vWf propeptide is composed of two D domains, D1 and D2, and is contiguous with the aminoterminus of the mature vWf subunit, which is composed of a truncated D' domain (residues 1–102) followed by a complete D3 domain (residues 103–478). The D domains demonstrate significant sequence similarity with each other, and the location of most Cys residues is preserved, thereby suggesting their tertiary structures may be similar. Cys residues in the D3 domain, however, participate in the intermolecular disulfide bonds necessary for multimer formation, whereas those in D1, D', D2, and D4 are involved exclusively in intramolecular bonds (21, 22). Sequences homologous to vWf type D domains appear in regions of invertebrate vitellogenin (23) and in mucins (24). In the latter multimeric molecules, the common D domain structural motif, which is characterized by several conserved Cys residues, may mediate homodimerization as an early biosynthetic event (analogous to the role played in vWf). Conserved Cys residues in the D domain sequence motif Cys-Gly-Leu-Cys-Gly are similar to those at the active site of disulfide isomerase and correspond to the residues that have been proposed to mediate the multimerization of pro-vWf (discussed later) (25).

The three homologous A domains span residues 497–1111 of the mature vWf subunit. The presence of vWf type A-like domains identifies a superfamily of proteins (26) that are active in hemostasis, cellular adhesion, defense mechanisms, and provide essential components of extracellular matrices. Among the members of this group are integrin $\alpha$ subunits, notably $\alpha_1$ and $\alpha_2$ in the $\beta_1$ integrins and $\alpha_L$, $\alpha_M$, and $\alpha_X$ in the $\beta_2$ integrins; collagens containing non–triple helical domains, such as types VI, VII, and XIV; components of the complement system C2 and Factor B; the dihydropyridine-sensitive calcium channel (27); inter-$\alpha$-trypsin inhibitor (27); and matrix proteins, such as cartilage matrix protein and matrilin-2 (28). Moreover, a vWf type A-like domain within the ligand binding region of integrin $\beta$ subunits is predicted

(29) on the basis of the known crystallographic structure of the A-like I domains of $\alpha_L$ (30) and $\alpha_M$ (31). The vWf type A-like domains in all these molecules are key for establishing specific interactions with appropriate substrates, which in some cases depend on divalent cations but in others (e.g., in vWf) do not. As shown by three-dimensional structural analysis, metal coordination (when present) involves contribution of an Asp-Xxx-Ser-Xxx-Ser motif and an additional Ser and Asp residue, all from noncontiguous regions. vWf type A-like domains also occur in the thrombospondin-related anonymous protein of *Plasmodium falciparum* (27).

Whether and how sequence similarities within and between A domains can support analogous functions in distinct proteins is not known. The A1 domain of vWf contains an intramolecular disulfide bond between Cys$^{509}$-Cys$^{695}$ that forms a 187-residue loop (32, 33), and the A3 domain contains an intramolecular disulfide bond between Cys$^{923}$-Cys$^{1109}$ that generates a loop of identical length to that in the A1 domain (21). Moreover, there is linear sequence homology between the A1 and A3 disulfide loops. The vWf A2 domain is similar to the A1 and A3 domains at the primary sequence level, but it lacks the conserved disulfide loop. Considering the functional similarities related to collagen binding (34), these sequence similarities suggest that A domains may represent a common adhesive motif within vWf and other molecules. For example, among proteins containing at least one A-like domain, the $\alpha_2$ subunit of $\alpha_2\beta_1$ is part of a heterodimeric receptor complex, also known in platelets as glycoprotein (GP) Ia-IIa and in lymphocytes as VLA-2, that, like vWf, interacts with collagen (35). Moreover, collagen type VI, which contains several copies of an A-like domain in the $\alpha3$(VI) chain (26), may use these structures to interact with other types of collagen. Despite these functional similarities, however, the A-like domains within different proteins have evolved additional, diverse recognition specificities.

The C domains of vWf have sequence similarity to thrombospondin and $\alpha$-procollagen types I and III (36). Domain C1 in vWf contains the sequence Arg-Gly-Asp, the signature recognition site for adhesion receptors of integrin superfamily members that may also interact with thrombospondin and collagen (37, 38). Additional sequence homologies with vWf domains probably will be found as the primary sequences of new proteins are determined.

## Gene Structure

The large size of the vWf gene (~180 kb) reflects the complex structural organization of the corresponding protein. The gene, which contains 52 exons (39), is located at the tip of the short arm of chromosome 12, region 12p12-12pter (12). Approximately 19% of its sequence has been determined, including all of the intron–exon boundaries (39). The first exon contains only 5′ untranslated sequence, and the initiation codon is in the second exon. The vWf signal peptide and pro-peptide are encoded by exons 2 through 18, with the remainder of the exons coding for the mature subunit. Repetitive domains identified within the vWf polypeptide sequence (discussed earlier) suggest that duplication events, exon shuffling mechanisms, or both may have played important roles in the origin of the vWf gene. The intron–exon boundaries, however, show only limited similarities between homologous repeats, thus indicating a complex evolutionary history.

An additional sequence that is highly homologous to the vWf gene has been identified on chromosome 22 through cross-hybridization with an internal fragment of vWf cDNA (40). By genomic cloning and sequence analysis, this DNA has been identified as a nonprocessed pseudogene representing a partial duplication of the region spanning exons 23 through 34 of the vWf gene. The two DNA sequences are 97% identical, thus indicating a recent evolutionary origin for the pseudogene.

## Regulation of Gene Expression

Expression of the vWf gene is restricted to endothelial cells and megakaryocytes. The genetic elements supporting expression by endothelial cells have been examined, but no similar studies have been performed on megakaryocytes. The characterization of 2.2 kb of vWf gene sequence upstream of the transcription initiation site has revealed a typical "TATA" box, but without the consensus "CCAAT" or "GC" box elements typical of other promoters (8, 9). The gene contains a small "core" promoter extending 90 nucleotides upstream of the transcription initiation site and capable of initiating transcription in all cell types (41, 42). Endothelial cell expression of the vWf gene depends on at least two positive regulatory domains, the first approximately 200 nucleotides upstream of the transcription start site and the second within the first untranslated exon of the gene (41, 42). These positive regulatory regions can support restricted expression in endothelial cells because of an Nuclear Factor (NF) 1-like protein that binds further upstream from the positive regulatory domains and functions as a negative regulator of activity in nonendothelial cells (43). The positive regulatory domains contain potential binding sites for GATA and SP1 transcription factors, and mutation of the GATA binding site abolishes promoter activity in endothelial cells (42). The GATA family of proteins interacts with a specific element of the promoter ($^{5'}$[A/T]GATA[A/G]$^{3'}$), and these proteins are related by a high degree of sequence similarity throughout their zinc-finger-binding domains (44). GATA-1 primarily is expressed by mature erythroid cells, megakaryocytes, and mast cells; GATA-2 by a wide variety of cell types, including endothelial cells; GATA-3 by T lymphocytes; and GATA-4 by endodermal-derived tissues and heart (44–46). The specific GATA protein interacting with the vWf promoter is not known, but GATA-2 in both endothelial cells and megakaryocytes may be crucial in gene expression.

The studies mentioned here have examined vWf promoter activity by transfecting cultured human or bovine endothelial cells. Indeed, vWf gene expression may change when the cell is transferred from an *in vivo* to an *in vitro* environment (47), thereby suggesting that studies examining vWf gene activity *in vivo* may assess more accurately the elements conferring tissue-specific expression. Aird et al (48) have generated transgenic mice containing fragments of the vWf promoter driving expression of the bacterial LacZ protein. Cells expressing the latter can be identified through the vascular tree as "blue cells," because they develop the color after reaction with the substrate 5-bromo-4-chloro-3-indolylβ-D-galactopyranoside. Mice containing only 487 nucleotides 5′ to the transcription start site display restricted expression to a subpopulation of endothelial cells in the yolk sac and adult brain (48). These results suggest a regional heterogeneity for vWf expression that depends on specific genetic elements within the vWf promoter, possibly contributing to the vascular diversity documented by immunohistochemical and mRNA analyses (49, 50).

## THE CONSTITUENT SUBUNIT OF vWf MULTIMERS

Mature vWf molecules contain a varying number of subunits, from a minimum of two to a maximum that may be of the order of 50 to 100. Each subunit contains several discrete functional sites responsible for the known biological activities of vWf involving interactions with other molecules. The corresponding binding domains appear to exist in each subunit in a functional state independent of multimer assembly. Nevertheless, the molecular organization of vWf into larger structures provides the potential for multivalent contacts that may be important to the biologic role of vWf in platelet thrombus formation.

The mature vWf subunit contains 2050 amino acid residues and as many as 22 carbohydrate side chains, 10 of which are *O*-linked to Ser or Thr residues and 12 of which are *N*-linked to Asn residues (51). The estimated carbohydrate content of vWf varies between 10 and 19% of the total mature subunit mass, which is calculated as approximately 278 Kda (51). Different types of carbohydrate chains are present in the vWf subunit. Structural studies of the *N*-linked chains have shown that approximately 78% are the monosialylated and monofucosylated biantennary type (52, 53), with a smaller number being the uncommon monosialylated and monofucosy-

lated tetraantennary type (≈2%) (53, 54), monoantennary (0.4%) and triantennary (12%) complex type, and high-mannose type (53). Blood group H (O), A, and B structures have been found on biantennary complex-type oligosaccharide chains, and H (O) structures have been found on the triantennary chains (53). This may be relevant in the treatment of individuals with congenital bleeding disorders who require replacement therapy with blood products containing vWf, because antibody production against protein containing an incompatible blood group A, B, or AB structure is possible.

The primary structure of the major *O*-linked carbohydrate in human vWf also has been determined (55). Some investigators had suggested the carbohydrate moiety could have a direct role in maintaining integrity of the multimeric structure of vWf (56) and in mediating interaction with platelets through a function of the penultimate galactose (57). It appears, however, that any such effect is indirect and exerted by protecting the molecule from proteolytic degradation (58).

A characteristic structural feature of vWf is the high content of Cys residues (169 of 2050 residues in the mature subunit). These Cys residues are essential in the structure of vWf because they link subunits into higher order structure (21). That the multimeric pattern of plasma vWf is resistant to boiling in 2% sodium dodecyl sulfate, yet dissociation to the constitutive subunits is readily observed with reducing agents, demonstrates the role of intermolecular disulfide bonds in forming vWf oligomers (59). Analysis of fragments generated through limited proteolysis of multimeric vWf with *Staphylococcus aureus* V8 protease has led to identification of intermolecular disulfide bonds within two regions of the mature subunit: an aminoterminal region (residues 283–695) and a carboxyterminal region (residues 1908–2050) containing 30 and 18 Cys residues, respectively (21). There are no detectable free sulfhydryl groups in vWf, so it is assumed that Cys residues not forming intermolecular disulfide bridges are matched in intramolecular disulfide bonds. Some intramolecular Cys pairings have been identified (21) and demonstrate a complex disulfide bond-dependent conformation that appears important for normal vWf function.

## THE MULTIMERIC PROTEIN

Mature vWf has a typical multimeric structure (4, 60, 61). It exists as a series of oligomers (Fig. 16.2) containing a variable number of mature subunits and ranging in molecular mass from approximately 550 to more than 10,000 Kda, one of the largest known for soluble plasma proteins. The degree of polymerization in different body compartments appears to be regulated, as indicated by the multimers found in storage granules of endothelial cells and platelets being larger than those in plasma (62,

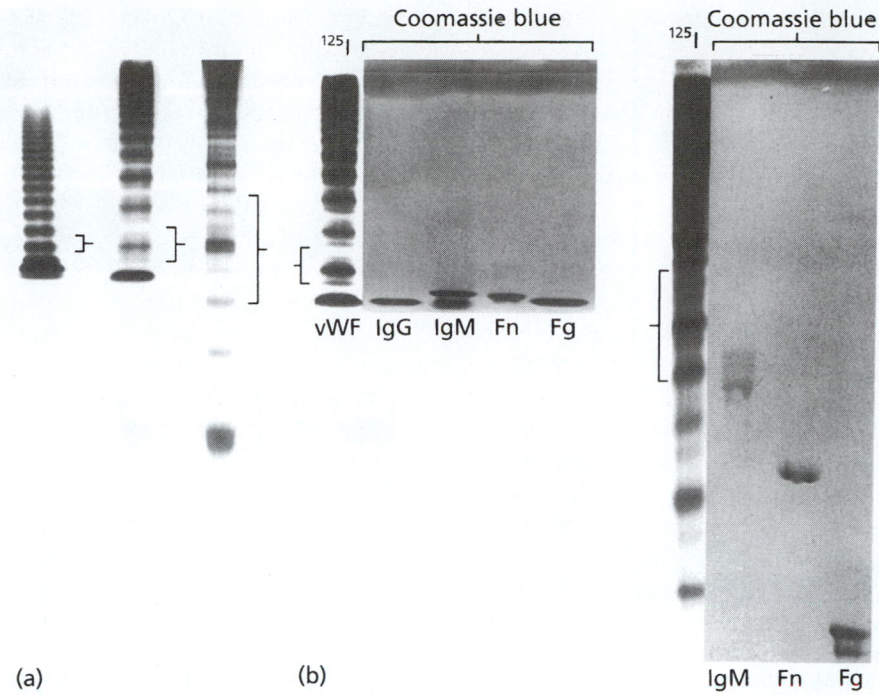

**FIGURE 16.2.**   Multimeric structure of plasma von Willebrand factor (vWf). Multimers were separated by electrophoresis in agarose gels containing the detergent sodium dodecyl sulfate, then visualized with a monospecific anti-vWf antibody labeled with $^{125}$I. All native disulfide bonds in the molecules were left intact (i.e., electrophoresis was performed under nonreducing conditions). **(a)** Three lanes derived from gels prepared with agarose at different concentrations, from lower (left lane) to higher (right lane). The right lane gel also was of greater length. Direction of the electrophoretic migration was from top to bottom; thus, oligomers of larger mass are toward the top. Note increasing resolution of the structure of individual oligomers seen in gels of higher agarose concentration. All the bands comprised in the bracket to the right appear as one band in the gel to the left; the lane in the middle shows the results obtained with a gel of intermediate resolution. Larger multimers, however, are resolved better in gels of lower agarose concentration; thus, studying the structure of vWf multimers in detail requires a combined approach. **(b)** Multimers of vWf were identified with a radiolabeled antibody ($^{125}$I) as described earlier and are shown next to markers of molecular mass stained by Coomassie Blue: immunoglobulin (Ig) G, 166 Kda; IgM (top band in the corresponding lane), 900 Kda; fibronectin (Fn), 450 Kda; fibrinogen (Fg), 340 Kda. The left gel is of intermediate resolution (corresponding to the middle lane in (a); the gel to the right is of high resolution (corresponding to the right lane in (a). Brackets enclose corresponding species in different gels. (Modified with permission from Dent JA, Galbusera M, Ruggeri ZM. Heterogeneity of plasma von Willebrand factor multimers resulting from proteolysis of the constituent subunit. J Clin Invest 1991;88:774–782; and Ruggeri ZM. Classification of von Willebrand disease. In: Thrombosis and haemostasis. In: Verstraete M, Vermylen J, Lijnen R, Arnout J, eds. Leuven: Leuven University Press, 1987:419–445.)

63). This size heterogeneity is complicated by proteolysis (discussed later in this chapter), which is partly responsible for the clusters of bands enclosed by brackets in Fig. 16.2.

Electron microscopic analysis of purified vWf by rotary shadowing (64) has demonstrated filamentous structures with a diameter of 2 to 3 nm and a length as great as 1300 nm, and loosely coiled molecules with an apparent diameter of 200 to 300 nm (Fig. 16.3). These different shapes suggest the extended forms represent "uncoiled" molecules as they appear after being subjected to shear forces in the circulation. This hypothesis has found convincing support in experiments based on the visualization by atomic force microscopy of vWf exposed to defined shear stress, which directly showed

the unfolding of globular molecules with acquisition of an extended-chain shape oriented in the direction of the shear-stress field (65). The threshold shear stress that caused the change in vWf three-dimensional structure was on the order of 35 dyn/cm$^2$, which is well within physiologic levels encountered in the arterial circulation (66). The longest vWf molecules approach the diameter of platelets in length and offer a clear impression of their repeating structure, consisting of two elongated globules connected to a small, central nodule by thin rods (Fig. 16.3C). The repeating unit, the protomer, is composed of two mature subunits linked at the center through their carboxyterminal ends (i.e., the COOH termini), whereas the globules at the two extremes of the protomer represent the aminoterminal ends (i.e., the NH$_2$ termini). The

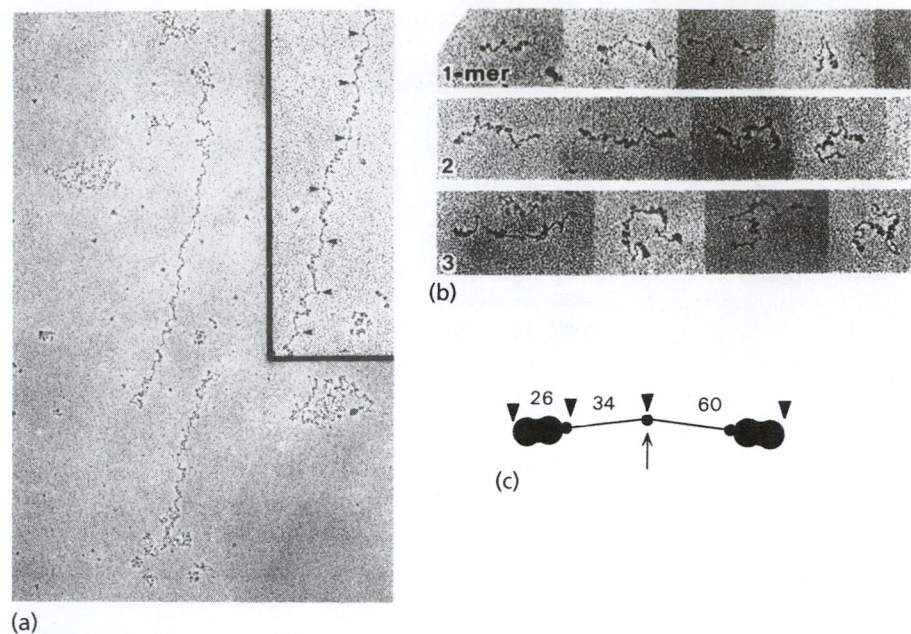

**FIGURE 16.3.** Electron photomicrograph of rotary shadowed von Willebrand factor (vWf) multimers. **(a)** Two multimer configurations: extended, and coiled. The inset shows part of one of the extended multimers at higher magnification in which several arrowheads mark repeats of one structural feature. In the lower-right corner of the inset, a trinodular fibrinogen molecule and a radially symmetric immunoglobulin M molecule can be seen for comparison. **(b)** Photomicrographs of vWf multimers selected from preparations containing predominantly smaller oligomers: single protomers or ''1-mers'' (top row), ''2-mers'' (middle row), and ''3-mers'' (bottom row). To avoid confusion, note that each ''protomer'' (i.e., the building block of all oligomers of greater molecular mass) is composed of two vWf subunits and, thus, is itself a dimer. Therefore, a ''2-mer'' is composed of four subunits (i.e., a tetramer regarding subunit composition), a ''3-mer'' of six subunits (i.e., a hexamer regarding subunit composition), and so on. **(c)** Structure of the vWf protomer based on consistent morphologic and structural features, with the maximum measured dimensions in nanometers (not corrected for thickness of metal replica). The large arrow indicates a twofold axis of symmetry. (Modified with permission from Fowler WE, Fretto LJ. Electron microscopy of von Willebrand factor. In: Zimmerman TS, Ruggeri ZM, eds. Coagulation and bleeding disorders. New York: Marcel Dekker, 1989:181–193; and Fowler WE, Fretto LJ, Hamilton KK et al. Substructure of human von Willebrand factor. J Clin Invest 1985;76:1491–1500.)

molecular mass of the protomer is 550 Kda. Larger oligomers are created by linking protomeric units through aminoterminal interactions, so the minimal progressive increment in molecular mass is 550 Kda (67).

# BIOSYNTHESIS

## ENDOTHELIAL CELLS

Most of our knowledge about biosynthesis of vWf derives from experiments using cultured endothelial cells and transfected heterologous cells. These studies should be considered critically, however, because endothelial cells from different segments of the vasculature may exhibit distinct functional properties, as exemplified by not all endothelial cells synthesizing vWf (49, 50). The concepts presented here probably apply to all endothelial cells. The data on rate of synthesis, storage, and polarity of secretion probably are influenced most by experimental conditions *in vitro* and by anatomic location of the endothelial cell *in vivo*.

Following translation of the mRNA, removal of signal peptide, and initial glycosylation, pro-vWf undergoes extensive posttranslational processing to produce multimeric vWf (Fig. 16.4). As currently understood (68), the process is initiated by association of pro-vWf monomers into dimers through intermolecular disulfide bridges within their carboxyterminal regions (69). The last 151 residues in the vWf subunit, following the C2 domain and without any other obvious internal homologous sequence, are the only structures required for dimerization (70). At this stage, pro-vWf dimers are modified by carbohydrate processing, which leads to development of 12 *N*-linked and 10 *O*-linked carbohydrate side chains within the sequence of the mature subunit. Specific *N*-linked carbohydrate structures are additionally modified by sulfation (71), which is a posttranslational event whose significance in vWf function is not known. There is limited heterogeneity in the carbohydrate structure of vWf. Such variability may explain generation of the closely spaced doublet of 52/48 Kda seen after reduction of a dimeric 116 Kda tryptic fragment encompassing the vWf A1 domain (72); the latter contains eight of the ten *O*-linked carbohydrate side chains of vWf. By analogy with other plasma proteins, the vWf carbohydrate side chains are presumed to be important for stability of the molecule in the circulation (58).

Concurrent with carbohydrate processing in the Golgi apparatus, or soon after transit through it, or both, the propeptide drives the association of pro-vWf dimers into higher order structures linked through Cys residues in the aminoterminal domain of each mature subunit (Fig. 16.4). Multimer formation requires domains D1 and D2, which form the propeptide sequence, and domains D' and D3 at the aminoterminus of the mature subunit (73). Domain D3 contains interchain disulfide bonds in mature vWf. Studies using heterologous cells transfected with recombinant vWf plasmids have dem-

onstrated that molecules without the propeptide but with the whole, mature vWf sequence are assembled only to the dimer stage and presumably linked through their carboxytermini (74, 75). Coexpression of propeptide and mature vWf on separate plasmids can give rise to multimers (75), thus highlighting the critical, independent role of the propeptide in this process even when it is not a continuous part of the same polypeptide containing the mature vWf sequence. The mechanism whereby vWf propeptide promotes multimerization is not defined, but relevant information in this regard has been obtained. This function may be facilitated initially by an intrinsic ability of D domains to self-associate. Nevertheless, multimerization in the acidic trans- and post-Golgi compartments is an unusual feature because spontaneous formation of disulfide bonds is optimal at basic pH. In most proteins, these bonds form in the en-

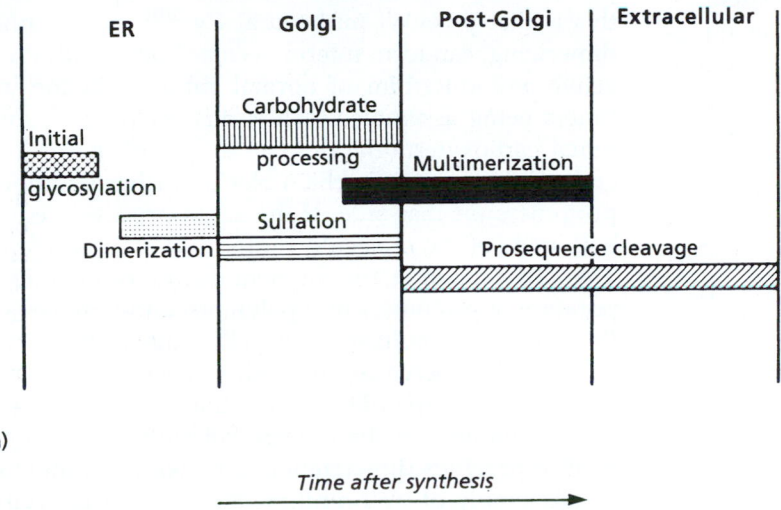

(a)

*Time after synthesis*

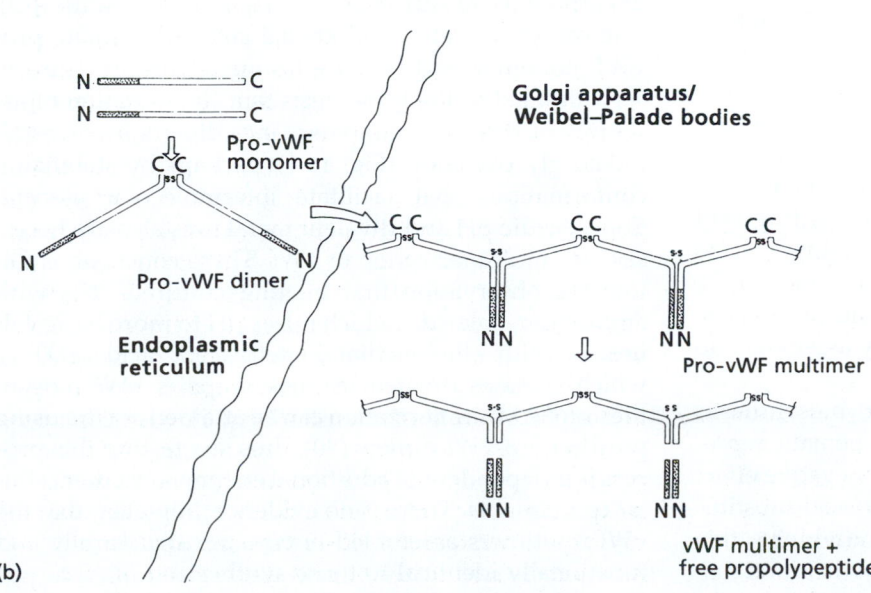

(b)

**FIGURE 16.4.** Processing and assembly of pro-von Willebrand factor (vWf) into multimers. **(a)** Sequence of events (from left to right) occurring from synthesis of pro-vWf to secretion of mature vWf. **(b)** The process of multimer assembly, which occurs in distinct, successive steps (from left to right). First, pro-vWf monomers form disulfide-linked dimers in the endoplasmic reticulum, soon after translation and synthesis of pro-vWf. Then, during or after transit in the Golgi apparatus, these dimers (i.e., the "protomers" of vWf multimers; see Fig. 16.3) are linked through disulfide bonds at their aminotermini and assembled into larger molecules. The latter process presumably is driven by self-assembly of propeptides into noncovalent dimers, which persist as such after the propeptide sequence is cleaved from mature vWf. (Modified with permission from Mayadas TN, Wagner DD. Von Willebrand factor biosynthesis and processing (review). Ann N Y Acad Sci 1991; 614:153–166; and Handin RI, Wagner DD. Molecular and cellular biology of von Willebrand Factor. In: Coller BS, ed. Progress in hemostasis and thrombosis. Philadelphia: WB Saunders 1989; 9:233–259.)

doplasmic reticulum through disulfide interchange, which is catalyzed by disulfide isomerase. The process involves labile disulfide bonds within the active site of the enzyme formed by Cys residues separated by two amino acids (i.e., vicinal Cys residues). The vWf propeptide contains two identical sequences with vicinal Cys pairs, one each in domains D1 and D2 ($Cys^{159}$-Gly-Leu-$Cys^{162}$ and $Cys^{521}$-Gly-Leu-$Cys^{524}$, respectively; note that residue numbering in this case is from the initiating methionine in pre-pro-vWf.) Experiments on site-directed mutagenesis have provided direct evidence that the vicinal Cys residues in the vWf propeptide do play a role in multimer assembly (25). Thus, the propeptide may endow pro-vWf with endogenous disulfide isomerase-like activity, which promotes interdimer disulfide bond formation at the aminoterminus of the mature subunit between pairs of D3 domains.

Expression of variously truncated vWf molecules provides important information on the independent assembly of isolated domains and, consequently, on multimerization. For example, a recombinant molecule containing the vWf propeptide (i.e., domains D1 and D2) and residues 1–479 of the mature subunit (i.e., domains D' and D3) forms covalent dimers linked through interchain disulfide bonds in the D3 region (73). The propeptide sequence, however, is not strictly required to form disulfide-linked dimers of isolated, mature vWf aminoterminal domains. Expression in mammalian cells (i.e., Chinese hamster ovary) of a vWf fragment spanning residues 445–733, representing the carboxyterminal portion of domain D3 (residues 445–479, containing five Cys residues) and the entire domain A1, resulted in secretion of dimeric structures (22, 76). This indicates that independent folding of isolated domains in the mature subunit may be sufficient, under appropriate circumstances, to promote assembly of vWf multimers. It also demonstrates that a small portion of the D3 domain is sufficient to establish key interchain bonds. Therefore, the propeptide sequence is crucial in promoting multimer assembly in the physiologic environment of endothelial cells, but it is not strictly required for dimerization of vWf aminoterminal domains, at least during overexpression in heterologous cells. Moreover, expression in eukaryotic cells of a carboxyterminal fragment composed of mature vWf residues $Glu^{1366}$-$Lys^{2050}$ also leads to production of disulfide-linked dimers (77), thereby confirming that isolated amino and carboxyterminal domains of vWf can independently assemble into covalent dimers (22, 70, 73).

The complexity of vWf multimer biosynthesis, which is not fully explained by current schematic representations, is illustrated by the dominant negative effect exerted on the process by the single amino acid substitution $Cys^{2010}$→Arg (77). In heterozygous individuals, this mutation is responsible for type IID von Willebrand disease (see Chapter 34), which is characterized by abnormal vWf structure without the largest multimers. Introducing the mutation in the isolated carboxyterminal vWf fragment $Glu^{1366}$-$Lys^{2050}$ prevented the spontaneous dimerization seen with the wild-type counterpart (77). As discussed, the protomeric unit of vWf polymers is assumed to be a dimer in which the two subunits are linked at the carboxytermini. Thus, subunits that cannot dimerize in this manner should not be incorporated into vWf polymers or interfere with multimer assembly. Indeed, even accepting that dimers of such abnormal subunits may form through N-terminal domains (22, 73, 78), their incorporation into multimers should be prevented by the inability to form disulfide bridges through C-terminal domains. The dominant negative nature of the phenotype caused by the $Cys^{2010}$→Arg mutation, however, indicates that molecules unable to dimerize at their C-termini still may be incorporated into nascent polymers as individual subunits. One explanation for this is that pro-vWf mutated at $Cys^{2010}$, even without dimerizing, can form intermolecular bonds with the reactive amino-termini of normal subunits in the multimers being assembled. When this occurs, a dysfunctional carboxyterminal domain at one of the growing ends of the polymeric chain blocks further addition of protomers on that side. If the same process occurs at both ends of the molecule, multimerization is arrested. This can happen at any moment during random incorporation of protomers into polymers, and it makes synthesis of large multimers virtually impossible in these individuals. Therefore, the pathogenesis of von Willebrand disease type IID indicates that even *in vivo*, individual subunits may become part of multimers independent of previous dimerization at carboxytermini (73).

Assembly of vWf multimers in endothelial cells is sensitive to changes in pH and to treatment with tunicamycin, which is an antibiotic that prevents attachment of carbohydrate side chains to asparagine residue (79). Tunicamycin-treated endothelial cells accumulate pro-vWf monomers in the endoplasmic reticulum. This observation led to the hypothesis that the initiation of assembly of pro-vWf monomers into dimers involves N-linked glycosylation (Fig. 16.4), perhaps by stabilizing conformations that facilitate intermolecular associations. Acidic pH and divalent metal ions also are necessary for multimerization of vWf. These conclusions follow the observation that treating cultured cells with ammonium chloride, which raises pH to more basic values, or with ethylenediaminetetraacetic acid (EDTA), which chelates divalent cations, impairs vWf biosynthesis (68). Multimerization can be attained *in vitro* using purified pro-vWf dimers (80), thus suggesting this process is independent of additional enzymes or other cellular components. There is no evidence, however, that the vWf multimers assembled *in vitro* are structurally and functionally identical to those synthesized *in vivo*.

Toward the end of the process leading to mature vWf multimers but apparently before secretion, a specific endoproteolytic event removes the propeptide sequence, which then is released independently into circulating blood and is known as von Willebrand antigen II (vWAgII) (18). Initially, cleavage of the propeptide sequence was proposed to occur in Weibel-Palade bodies because the stoichiometry of vWf and vWAgII in the organelles is 1:1 (81). This concept was modified after evidence suggested that multimerization and propeptide processing precede the appearance of storage organelles (82). That vWf released constitutively, and thus never stored in Weibel-Palade bodies, also is processed with removal of the propeptide, even although vWf multimers with persistence of the propeptide may be found in the circulation, favors this conclusion (18, 62). The "candidate" processing enzyme for cleavage of the vWf propeptide is furin/PACE, which is a calcium-dependent serine protease acting on precursor polypeptides at paired basic amino acid residues (83). The location of this enzyme in the trans-Golgi network, which carries vWf destined for storage in Weibel-Palade bodies (82), also indicates that propeptide proteolytic processing may precede formation of the storage organelles.

A final modification after endothelial cell-derived vWf is released into the circulation is noncovalent association (84, 85) with coagulation factor VIII. This complex is essential for normal survival of factor VIII in the circulation (6), and binding to the aminoterminal domain of vWf confers on factor VIII protection from degradation by activated protein C (86, 87). Where the initial interaction between the two proteins occurs, however, is not known. Endothelial cells in culture do not synthesize factor VIII; the same is true for endothelial cells *in vivo*. The major *in vivo* site of factor VIII production has not been defined, but factor VIII mRNA has been detected in the liver, spleen, and kidney (88–90). Because the respective sites of synthesis are although to differ, it generally is considered to be unlikely that the factor VIII–vWf complex forms inside a cell. Rather, the two proteins probably interact after release from their respective cells of origin, possibly at sites where the latter are in proximity. These issues remain open to further investigation.

The binding of factor VIII to vWf depends on residues 1–272 at the aminoterminus of the mature vWf subunit (discussed later). The propeptide of vWf (i.e., vWAgII) is important in the formation of a functional factor VIII-binding site, as shown by dimeric vWf molecules synthesized without propeptide failing to associate with factor VIII (91). This may result from the propeptide being necessary for posttranslational processes conferring the appropriate conformation to the aminoterminal domain of vWf, perhaps through correct intrachain disulfide bonding. Persistence of the un-

cleaved propeptide, however, impairs the ability of vWf to bind factor VIII (92), perhaps because the propeptide masks the factor VIII-binding site by steric hindrance. Alternatively, cleavage of the propeptide may lead to a conformational modification of the aminoterminal domain of vWf necessary to express the factor VIII-binding function.

## MEGAKARYOCYTES

Synthesis of vWf by megakaryocytes (93, 94) has not been studied in detail because of unsolved problems with culturing these platelet progenitors *in vitro* (see Chapter 8). The protein they make, however, is assumed to be identical to that produced by endothelial cells. Whether megakaryocytes, like endothelial cells, have a constitutive secretion pathway for vWf, even although secretion into the culture medium has been demonstrated *in vitro* (94), is not known. Results from experiments with bone marrow transplantation from normal pigs into pigs with severe von Willebrand disease (95) argue against a physiologic mechanism for vWf release from megakaryocytes. In these studies, the affected animals had extremely low levels of both plasma and platelet vWf before the procedure. After engraftment, platelets containing vWf in the α-granules (96) became visible, but levels of plasma vWf remained low, thus suggesting that normal megakaryocytes producing vWf and storing it in platelets do not significantly increase the amount of vWf released into the blood. Moreover, because platelets do not acquire their vWf from blood, as they may other proteins like fibrinogen (97–99), it appears that vWf in the α-granules of platelets is an isolated compartment that becomes available for hemostasis only when platelets are activated and the release reaction occurs (63, 100). Platelet-derived vWf is structurally similar to that stored within the Weibel-Palade bodies of endothelial cells, and it is composed of the largest multimeric species (discussed later). Whether other aspects of the posttranslational processing of vWf in megakaryocytes differ from those in endothelial cells is not known.

# STORAGE AND SECRETION

Unlike most proteins, vWf can follow more than one pathway of secretion from endothelial cells (101): a constitutive pathway directly linked to synthesis (i.e., molecules are released once their synthesis is completed) and a regulated pathway involving storage of mature molecules in appropriate granules for release after stimulation by secretagogues (102). Regulated secretion yields multimers of higher molecular mass than those originating from constitutive secretion (103), which may have biologic relevance as larger multimers are more effective hemostatically. In megakaryocytes, only the regulated pathway may be effectively operative *in vivo* (discussed earlier). In contrast, it has been suggested that most of the vWf synthesized by cultured endothelial cells may be secreted through the constitutive pathway (104), and only approximately 5% of the newly synthesized vWf is stored inside endothelial cells. This proportion does not change after secretion is induced from storage sites, thus suggesting the lack of a regulatory mechanism affecting the amount of vWf stored inside endothelial cells in response to accumulation or rapid release (104). This phenomenon may occur because formation of storage organelles in endothelial cells is an intrinsically independent process.

Studies using *in vitro* cultures have provided discordant results regarding the amount of vWf constitutively secreted into circulating blood (i.e., apical or luminal secretion) as opposed to that incorporated into the subendothelial matrix (i.e., basolateral or abluminal secretion). Estimated values range from those indicating a nonpolar process, with 50:50 partition between apical and basolateral secretion (105), to a highly polarized process, with assessments varying from three times as much basolateral as apical secretion (106) to preferential apical secretion (107). These conclusions should be viewed critically, however, because the conditions under which cells are cultured can influence experimental results. The modality of constitutive vWf secretion *in vivo* is essentially unknown, and whether polarity of secretion varies in different areas of the vasculature or under various stimuli affecting the endothelium is not established. For example, investigators conducting an immunohistologic survey of the human body concluded that subendothelial deposition of vWf occurs only in arteries, arterioles, and large veins (89). Another group showed that secretion of vWf toward the basal membrane of capillary endothelial cells *in vivo* occurs only after stimulation (108). Regarding regulated secretion, the identified storage organelles for vWf are the Weibel-Palade body in endothelial cells (102, 109) and the α-granule in megakaryocytes and platelets (110, 111).

## WEIBEL-PALADE BODIES

Weibel-Palade bodies are rod-shaped structures that are unique to endothelial cells (112) and that presumably derive from the Golgi apparatus. On electron micrographs, they are composed of longitudinally oriented tubules surrounded by a membrane. These tubules probably represent multimeric vWf organized in a longitudinal array (102). The vWf propeptide is responsible for the formation of organelles similar to Weibel-Palade bodies in heterologous cells, but initially, this was althought possible only in cells with independent, specific machinery effecting regulated secretion (113). This con-

cept has been debated (114), however, and experimental data support the view that formation of storage organelles similar to proper Weibel-Palade bodies can be driven by intrinsic features of the vWf molecule, even in cells otherwise lacking a specific regulated pathway for protein secretion (107). The mechanisms determining whether a newly synthesized vWf molecule is destined for constitutive secretion or a storage granule are not known. It is assumed, although not demonstrated, that mature subunits are identical in molecules secreted through either the constitutive or the regulated pathway. The vWf propeptide sequence is important in formation of Weibel-Palade bodies, but there is no definitive agreement on why. The vWf propeptide may act directly as a routing signal for storage (113), but the importance of the propeptide in this regard also may be an indirect consequence of its role in multimerization. In the latter view, mutant vWf molecules lacking domains D1 and D2, and thus the propeptide moiety of pro-vWf, cannot be stored and are secreted constitutively because they are unable to multimerize, not because they lack a specific routing signal harbored in the missing sequence (107). Thus, multimerization itself is considered to be the triggering event in formation of organelles similar to Weibel-Palade bodies in cells expressing vWf, regardless of any specific signals recognized by specific cellular structures (107). If this hypothesis is correct, multimer size could be the intrinsic property that determines whether a vWf molecule undergoes constitutive or regulated secretion, thereby justifying why larger multimers are released in a regulated manner.

In addition to vWf and vWAgII, with the latter being present as a distinct molecule after cleavage from vWf multimers, only one other protein exists in Weibel-Palade bodies: P-selectin (115, 116). Referred to previously as GMP-140 or PADGEM, this is a cell adhesion molecule that may be involved in the interactions of leukocytes with endothelial cells and platelets (see Chapter 15). Reasons for this association and the possible contribution of P-selectin to the formation and morphology of Weibel-Palade bodies are not known.

As discussed, it generally is assumed that vWf stored within Weibel-Palade bodies is composed of the largest multimeric species (104, 117), whereas protein secreted through the constitutive pathway does not multimerize to the same extent (104). In one study, however, vWf released by cultured endothelial cells, either constitutively or after stimulation, was composed of a homogeneous species larger than any multimer found in plasma (117). Reasons for the discordant results obtained by different investigators are not known, but the latter finding raises the possibility that heterogeneity of vWf multimers always is generated after secretion from endothelial cells (117). The largest vWf multimers stored inside endothelial cells, however, are "unusually large" in the sense they usually are not seen in the blood of normal individuals (118). Indeed, controlled release at the time of injury probably limits the unusually large, most thrombogenic forms of vWf at sites of tissue damage. Moreover, physiologic mechanisms are althought to cause their disappearance from the circulation (discussed later). Unusually large vWf multimers can be detected in normal plasma only transiently, after secretion is induced from endothelial storage sites with the therapeutic agent 1-deamino-8-D-arginine vasopressin (DDAVP) (119) (see Chapter 53). They may occur in the blood of neonates but tend to disappear by the eighth week of life (120, 121).

Regulated secretion of stored vWf from endothelial cells occurs in response to several agonists of potential physiologic relevance, including histamine, estrogens, thrombin, and fibrin (68, 103, 122). The effect of the latter two suggests that secretion of vWf from Weibel-Palade bodies probably occurs whenever the hemostatic mechanism is activated, thus making the largest vWf multimers available locally, where they may be needed for their potent prothrombotic effects. The action of fibrin on release of vWf is mediated by specific sequences in the $\beta$ chain, including its aminoterminus (123). Local endothelial secretion of vWf also may occur in areas of inflammation, as shown by mechanical injury to the endothelium (124), endotoxin (125), *Rickettsia rickettsii* infection (126), complement proteins (127), and products of mononuclear cell activation such as interleukin-1 (128) increasing synthesis or release (or both) of endothelial vWf. In contrast, $\gamma$-interferon and tumor necrosis factor may modulate this endothelial response by decreasing the synthesis, storage, and secretion of vWf during inflammatory or immunologic processes (129), thus helping to balance the pro-thrombotic effects of the stimuli identified previously.

A number of vasoactive substances cause acute release of vWf into the circulation. The prototype is epinephrine, the activity of which is recognized *in vivo* but initially was althought to be negligible on cultured endothelial cells (102). Now, however, it is apparent this agonist induces a small increase in vWf release *in vitro* and potentiates the action of other effective substances, such as thrombin (130). The mechanism of action for epinephrine is distinct from that of other secretagogues, involving adenylyl cyclase-coupled $\beta$-adrenergic receptors that increase the cytoplasmic levels of cyclic adenosine monophosphate without raising $[Ca^{2+}]_i$ (130).

A substance with important activity on vWf release *in vivo*, but without a clear activity *in vitro*, is the synthetic hormone DDAVP (131), which is now used widely in the treatment of selected individuals with decreased circulating levels of vWf and factor VIII (see Chapter 53). The origin of vWf released by DDAVP is assumed to be the vessel wall endothelium. Consequently, it is postulated the effect of this agonist is achieved through one or more unknown intermediates that are not found *in vitro*. Peripheral blood monocytes may be the intermediary target cells, responding to stimulation by the peptide with release of a factor or factors that, in turn, induce vWf secretion from endothelial cells (132). This concept is not definitively accepted, however. Fluid mechanical forces also are potentially important in regulating release from storage organelles, but apparently not in regulating synthesis, as demonstrated by vWf being more abundant in the medium and the matrix when cultured endothelial cells are exposed to shear stress as opposed to being grown under static conditions (133).

The vWf released from storage in the Weibel-Palade bodies is directed toward the lumen and the subendothelial matrix. As with constitutive secretion from cultured endothelial cells, there is debate about the polarity of release. The concept initially proposed—that regulated secretion occurs predominantly in the basolateral direction (103)—has been challenged by evidence that as much as 80% of vWf released from storage organelles is directed toward the apical side of the cell (107). These differing results may be explained by unknown effects of different experimental conditions. The polarity of vWf secretion from both the constitutive and the regulated pathways simply may be more complex than presently understood, both *in vitro* and *in vivo*, and may be influenced by the nature of the release-inducing stimulus. Thrombin, for example, which because it is generated early in the hemostatic response is a secretagogue with probable pathophysiologic relevance, causes cultured endothelial cells to release into the luminal compartment a significant amount of "unusually" large multimers originating from storage organelles. Moreover, studies in humans have demonstrated that administration of epinephrine, as well as of DDAVP, results in redistribution of vWf in endothelial cells of the oral mucosa, with localization in the basement membrane and the surrounding interstitium (108).

## PLATELET $\alpha$-GRANULES

The second storage site for vWf is in the platelet $\alpha$-granules (96) (see Chapter 10) that may contain as much as 20% of the total vWf present in the blood. Unlike Weibel-Palade bodies, which primarily are composed of vWf, $\alpha$-granules of platelets contain additional molecules, some of which are important for hemostasis, including fibrinogen, thrombospondin, fibronectin, and platelet factor 4 (134). A proportion of the proteins in $\alpha$-granules is not synthesized by megakaryocytes; rather, it is acquired from the circulating blood although endocytosis (97, 99). Nevertheless, virtually all the vWf in platelets is of megakaryocytic origin and, like the vWf in Weibel-Palade bodies, characteristically contains the unusually large vWf multimers not seen in any appreciable amount in the circulation of normal individuals under basal conditions (63, 119). Examination of platelet α-granules with electron microscopy demonstrates tubular structures reminiscent of those in the Weibel-Palade bodies of endothelial cells (111). There is evidence these tubules are vWf multimers tightly packed in ordered longitudinal arrays, as shown by their absence in platelets from pigs with severe von Willebrand disease (135). In the α-granules, however, unlike in the Weibel-Palade bodies, these structures represent only a small part of the organelle and usually are placed at the periphery, in accordance with the notion that vWf is only one of many proteins stored there. A small amount of the total platelet vWf content (≈5%) may be present outside the α-granules, presumably associated with the membrane of the surface-connected canalicular system (136). This pool may represent a normal redistribution of molecules originally stored in the α-granules, and this redistribution may occur in parallel with, or because of, events leading to changes in the buoyant density of platelets during their life span in the circulation (136).

Platelet α-granules release their contents on stimulation by agonists, including adenosine diphosphate (ADP), collagen, and thrombin (100), thus representing another source of unusually large vWf multimers at a site of vascular injury early during hemostasis. As mentioned, unusually large vWf multimers normally are sequestered within storage sites in endothelial cells and platelets, but they can become available locally at sites of injury, thereby providing maximal efficacy in arresting hemorrhage. Release from both platelets and endothelial cells ensures that the largest vWf multimers are present in the subendothelial matrix and the soluble compartment surrounding the vascular lesion. The former may provide an effective anchorage for the initial adhesion of platelets; the latter, by quickly binding to the membrane of activated platelets, may promote the platelet-platelet interactions (i.e., aggregation) necessary for thrombus growth. It should be noted that vWf acutely released from storage sites, unlike that circulating in blood, probably does not have factor VIII bound to it. Indeed, factor VIII is activated to factor VIII$_a$ early in the response to a hemostatic challenge and, in the process, is modified so that its continued association with vWf is precluded. The initial binding to circulating vWf may localize factor VIII at a site of vascular injury, but the subsequent detachment from vWf may be a requisite for factor VIII$_a$ binding to platelets and its cofactor function in thrombin generation (137).

## REGULATION OF CIRCULATORY vWf MULTIMER SIZE

Regulation of plasma vWf multimer size, which is a molecular property that probably affects interaction with platelets (138, 139), may be important in preventing pathologic thrombus formation. The largest multimers, which are althought to be the most thrombogenic, are present only in cellular compartments (i.e., endothelial cell and platelet storage sites) separated from circulating blood, and they become available only during regulated secretion at sites of a vascular lesion. The enhanced thrombogenic potential of the larger vWf multimers may relate to the presence of multiple interaction sites for both platelets and structures in the vessel wall because of a greater number of constituent subunits. Such multivalency may result in more efficient binding to other molecules (138). When unusually large vWf multimers appear in plasma, such as after infusion of DDAVP, their presence is transient and their clearance rapid (119). Along with unusually large plasma vWf multimers in individuals with certain pathologic conditions (118), this suggests the existence of physiologic regulatory processes that normally limit accumulation of the largest vWf molecules in the circulation. These mechanisms may become operative only after birth, as shown by the presence of unusually large multimers in fetal and neonatal blood (120, 121).

Regulation of vWf multimer size is based on the occurrence of proteolytic modifications of the subunit, which probably occur at or soon after secretion into the bloodstream (Fig. 16.5). This type of subunit proteolytic processing should not be confused with that leading to removal of the entire propeptide sequence from the mature protein. Invariably, vWf stored in platelet α-granules is composed of intact subunits, all identical in size (140), whereas a defined proportion of smaller fragments can be found along with the prevalent intact subunit in the plasma-derived vWf of all normal individuals (141). Consequently, because of the presence of subunits of different molecular mass, vWf multimers in blood are more heterogeneous than those in storage compartments (140). The cleavage responsible for this heterogeneity, a single event that can separate vWf multimers into two smaller species, each having a cleaved subunit at the amino or carboxyterminal end of the polymeric chain, involves the peptide bond between residues Tyr$^{842}$-Met$^{843}$ (140, 142). The two corresponding subunit fragments have an apparent molecular mass of 176 and 140 Kda, respectively (Fig. 16.5), the sum of which is greater than the apparent molecular mass of the intact subunit (225 Kda) probably indicating that size estimates are erroneous because of aberrant electrophoretic migration in gels containing sodium dodecyl sulfate (140). The presence of additional minor fragments of slightly different size than the major ones probably results from heterogeneity in the cleavage site (140, 142), the occurrence of additional proteolytic events after the first one, or both. Models have been proposed to explain how cleavage of the single Tyr$^{842}$-Met$^{843}$ bond results in

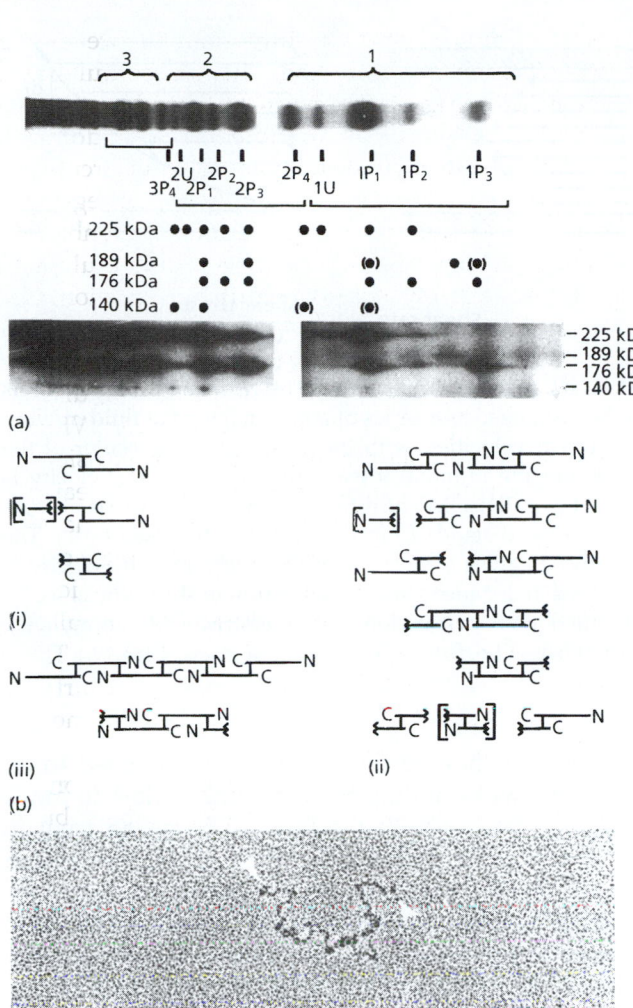

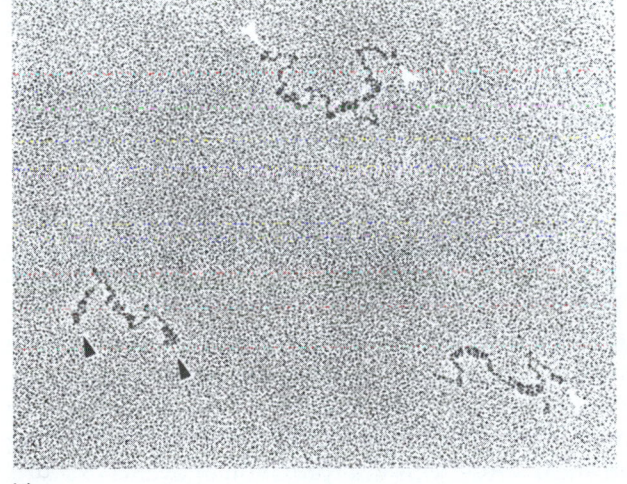

(c)

**FIGURE 16.5.** Analysis of the subunit composition of individual plasma von Willebrand factor (vWf) multimers. **(a)** Electrophoresis of nonreduced plasma vWf in agarose gel leads to separation of vWf multimers according to their size (top gel; direction left to right). The second-dimension electrophoresis in polyacrylamide gel, performed after reduction of disulfide bonds in each of the bands separated in the first dimension, leads to definition of the subunit composition of individual multimers and the demonstration they may contain cleaved subunits (bottom gel; direction top to bottom). Bands corresponding to vWf protein are identified by reactivity with specific, radiolabeled monoclonal antibodies and detected by autoradiography. A repeating pattern of five bands can be identified in nonreduced plasma vWf. The three fastest migrating sets are indicated by brackets above the top gel; each contains

the diversity of species seen on high-resolution electrophoretic analysis of plasma vWf (140), and to explain the "end" heterogeneity seen on electron microscopic studies of the molecule (Fig. 16.5). Accordingly, proteolytic cleavage of the subunit is the main, if not the only, physiologic mechanism responsible for reducing the size of the largest vWf multimers, both by generating smaller species from larger ones and by modifying the aminoterminal ends of the subunits by removal of the 140-kDa fragment. This region of vWf contains numerous cysteine residues, and its removal may prevent multimer reassembly via new interchain disulfide bond formation (Fig. 16.5).

Definitively identifying the protease responsible for specific cleavage of vWf at $Tyr^{842}$-$Met^{843}$ has proved to be difficult. Initially, and despite some ambiguities, the sequence surrounding this bond suggested the protease involved was calpainlike (140). Under experimental conditions, an activity in the cryosupernatant from both normal and von Willebrand disease plasma prevented accumulation of unusually large multimers in the culture medium of endothelial cells, but it did not interfere with release of the same largest multimers toward the subendothelial matrix (143). This effect was althought to be associated with a protein having a molecular mass of between 140 and 200 Kda, but the initial studies could not define whether proteolytic activity was involved

◀──────────

**FIGURE 16.5**   *(Continued)*

five species. After reduction of disulfide bonds, each vWf multimer, except for the bands identified with the letter U (for unproteolyzed), is composed of a variable proportion of intact 225 Kda subunit and proteolytic fragments of 189, 176, and 140 Kda. These markers of molecular mass are indicated on the right of the bottom gel. The subunit composition of each band is shown in the space separating the two gels. A new proposed terminology for identification of vWf multimers is shown below the top gel; this is based on the identification of unproteolyzed bands (U) composed of intact subunit only and listed in order of increasing molecular mass. Bands containing proteolyzed subunit fragments are indicated with the letter P and listed in progressive order below the unproteolyzed band preceding them. **(b)** Different molecular species that can derive from a vWf subunit dimer (i), tetramer (ii), or hexamer (iii) through cleavage of the bond between residues 842–843 in the vWf subunit. **(c)** Electron photomicrograph of "end" heterogeneity of vWf molecules, showing either large globular ends corresponding to intact subunits (black arrowheads) or smaller globular ends corresponding to cleaved subunits (white arrowheads). (Modified with permission from Dent JA, Galbusera M, Ruggeri ZM. Heterogeneity of plasma von Willebrand factor multimers resulting from proteolysis of the constituent subunit. J Clin Invest 1991;88:774–782; and Fowler WE, Fretto LJ, Hamilton KK et al. Substructure of human von Willebrand factor. J Clin Invest 1985;76:1491–1500.)

(143). Other investigators suggested that endothelial cell-derived vWf initially is a homogeneous species of large molecular mass (117), then converted by a granulocyte protease into the polydisperse series of multimers normally seen in plasma (144). Considering this, it is important to note that several proteases, including some in leukocytes as well as in plasmin, cleave the vWf subunit and reduce the size of large vWf multimers. However, these enzymes are not likely to be responsible for the physiologic mechanism controlling vWf multimer size because the resulting subunit fragments differ from those in normal individuals (145, 146). Two independent studies have provided strong evidence that normal plasma contains a metalloproteinase that acts specifically on vWf multimers, cleaving the subunit at Tyr[842]-Met[843] (147, 148). Estimates for the molecular mass of this enzyme vary from 200 Kda (148) to 300 Kda (147), and its action is greatly facilitated by partial denaturation of vWF in vitro, which may have an in vivo counterpart in the shear forces that change the three-dimensional structure of vWf (65) and may expose the susceptible peptide bond. The relevance of the initial characterization of this protease, which apparently is vWf specific, is illustrated by the finding of decreased vWf cleaving activity (149) in the plasma of individuals with chronic relapsing thrombocytopenic purpura (see Chapter 27), which results from diffuse thrombotic occlusion of small-vessels variably associated with unusually large vWf multimers in plasma (118). Thus, control of the size of circulating vWf multimers appears to be an important physiologic regulatory process in vivo, that may contribute to the mechanisms responsible for complex pathologic conditions involving thrombosis.

# BIOLOGIC FUNCTION

## BLOOD VISCOSITY, SHEAR STRESS, AND PLATELET FUNCTION

The complex series of events determining the occurrence of a normal hemostatic response, including chemical reactions involving cells, the vessel wall, and molecules in solution, are influenced by the flow of blood. Rheology is the science that deals with flow and deformation of structures under flow conditions (see Chapter 20). Blood near the vessel wall moves more slowly than blood toward the center of the vessel. This difference in velocity creates a shearing effect between adjacent layers of blood, which is greatest near the vessel wall and decreases progressively toward the center of the vessel. Shear stress is the force per unit area that can be viewed as the underlying cause of the shearing motion of blood. The shear rate, as measured in reciprocal seconds ($s^{-1}$), is directly proportional to the shear stress and inversely proportional to the fluid viscosity (Fig. 16.6).

The role of platelets in hemostasis and thrombosis

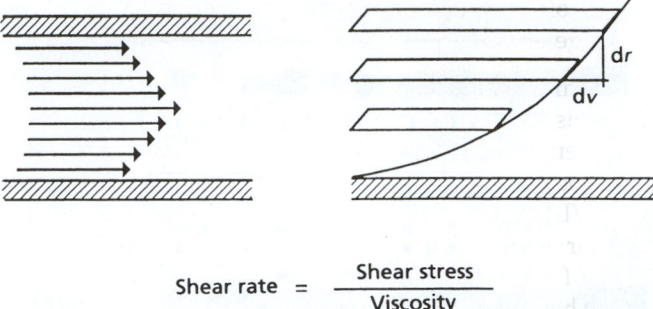

$$\text{Shear rate} = \frac{\text{Shear stress}}{\text{Viscosity}}$$

**FIGURE 16.6.** Shear flow. The flow of blood in vessels can be visualized as a series of adjacent layers of fluid moving at different velocities, with the maximal at the center of the vessel and the minimal toward the vessel wall. (Velocity is zero at the wall itself.) The difference in velocity (dv) is proportional to the distance from the center of the vessel (dr). The ratio dv/dr gives a measure of the shear rate; if velocity is measured in distance *per second*, the unit of shear rate is $sec^{-1}$. (Modified with permission from Verstraete M, Vermylen J. Thrombosis. Elmsford, NY: Pergamon Press, 1984:49.)

requires that they become irreversibly attached to an injury site, withstanding the tendency of flow to move adhering platelets with the layer of blood adjacent to the surface (150). The force opposing stable adhesion and aggregation is greater with an increased shear rate. The role of vWf in supporting these processes appears to be most significant at high shear rates (151), presumably because of its unique molecular architecture. Thus, under the effect of high shear forces, vWf molecules may take the shape of extended filaments (Fig. 16.3). The repeating subunit structure in these large multimers offers an array of interaction sites capable of binding in a multivalent manner to receptors on the platelet membrane, thus increasing the number of contact points and the affinity (i.e., strength) of the interaction (138). As a result, the overall force linking platelets to the surface, to one another, or to both is increased, effectively opposing fluid shear stress. This interpretation of events explains why the role of vWf is less relevant at lower shear rates, because other adhesive molecules may provide sufficient force of interaction to withstand shear forces of lesser magnitude.

## THE ROLES OF vWf IN HEMOSTASIS

Normal hemostasis requires vWf for two reasons:

1. The protein is necessary for platelet adhesion to thrombogenic surfaces and for platelet aggregation under conditions of high shear stress, and

2. The protein is necessary as a carrier for the procoagulant factor VIII molecule, which

performs an essential cofactor function in factor $X_a$ generation.

In the first instance, vWf is directly involved in the mechanisms of platelet thrombus formation. In the second, even without a direct role in coagulation, vWf fulfills important supporting functions, such as stabilizing factor VIII in blood, delivering factor VIII to the sites of vascular injury at which vWf binds, and protecting factor VIII from inactivation. Diminished vWf function results in bleeding tendency, and presumably, abnormally increased function could result in thrombotic complications.

Confusion may remain regarding the terminology of "agglutination" and "aggregation" of platelets mediated by vWf. Agglutination is an experimental event, and it refers to close contact between several platelets mediated by vWf bound to GP Ibα, typically (but not exclusively) with ristocetin. Agglutination may have no correlate *in vivo*, as it also occurs with fixed, metabolically inactive platelets, but may be useful in studying the interaction between vWf and GP Ibα. Aggregation reflects the ability of vWf to support platelet thrombus formation; as such, it relates more directly to important *in vivo* events. It requires active platelet metabolism and involves vWf binding to both its platelet receptors, GP

Ibα and integrin $\alpha_{IIb}\beta_3$, which also is known as the GP IIb-IIIa complex (152–154). Platelet aggregation dependent on vWf can be demonstrated with the traditional aggregometer, but only when fibrinogen is not present (153), or even in platelet-rich plasma as aggregation induced by high shear stress (155–158).

Participation of vWf in thrombogenesis probably follows a temporal sequence, with the molecule performing distinct functions at different topographic locations in the area of the vascular injury (Fig. 16.7). The first step involves establishing platelet contact with exposed, damaged tissue, either subendothelial structures or altered endothelial cells. This role is performed by subendothelial matrix vWf and plasma vWf rapidly adsorbed onto exposed structures of the damaged vessel, such as collagen. The second step may involve generating a signal that activates platelets; indeed there is clear experimental evidence that vWf is not just a biologic "glue" that allows platelets to adhere to surfaces, but upon binding to GP Ibα, acts also as a platelet agonist (159–165). The third step is establishing irreversible platelet adhesion with spreading (162), which is followed by recruitment of additional platelets through aggregation (i.e., platelet–platelet contact). This latter role probably is performed by soluble vWf (166), either circu-

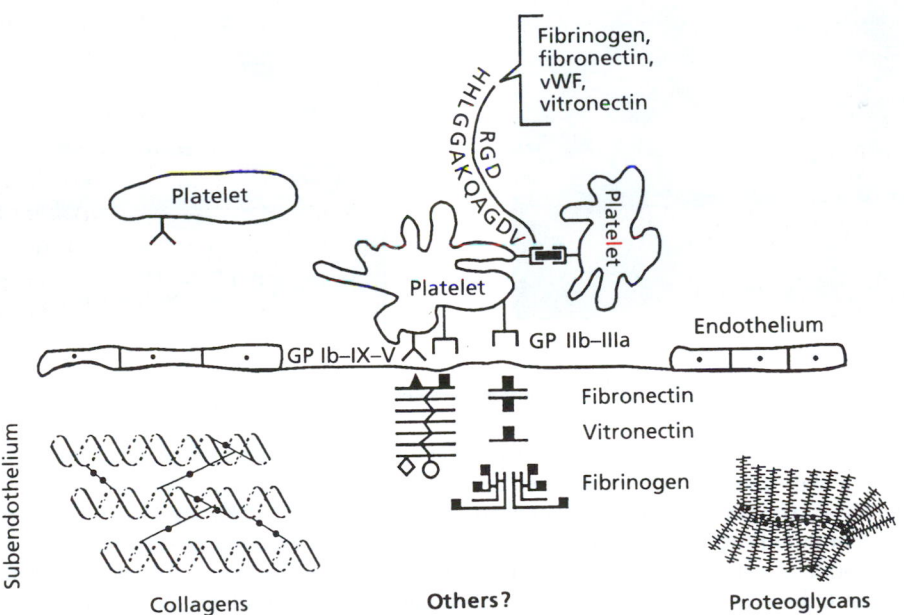

**FIGURE 16.7.** The multiple roles of von Willebrand factor (vWf) in hemostasis. A nonactivated platelet (the discoid one on the left) carries the functional glycoprotein (GP) Ibα receptor for vWf; thus, it can interact with the molecule exposed on the subendothelium and expressing the GP Ibα-binding site. Platelets adhering to vWf become activated and express a functional $\alpha_{IIb}\beta_3$ receptor that can interact with vWf, either surface-bound or in solution. The former mediates platelet spreading; the latter mediates platelet aggregation. Alternative platelet ligands that can mediate both adhesion and aggregation are indicated. The two short sequences known to be $\alpha_{IIb}\beta_3$-recognition signatures are indicated with the one letter abbreviation for amino acids. The respective roles of different adhesive substrates may vary depending on hemodynamic conditions, and vWf may be the only effective mediator of adhesion and aggregation under conditions of high shear stress (high blood flow in small caliber vessels).

efforts undoubtedly will aim at expanding our knowledge on the atomic structure of this complex molecule, spurred by initial findings derived from successful crystallization of two key domains. Targeting vWf-dependent activities for the design of antithrombotic compounds has proceeded slowly thus far, but the coming years should see concerted efforts to evaluate definitively potential therapeutic opportunities offered by this approach. Basic and clinical research will continue to provide exciting discoveries regarding the physiologic and pathologic significance of vWf in hemostasis and thrombosis.

# REFERENCES

1. Zimmerman TS, Ratnoff OD, Powell AE. Immunologic differentiation of classic hemophilia (factor VIII deficiency) and von Willebrand's disease, with observations on combined deficiencies of antihemophilic factor and proaccelerin (factor V) and on an acquired circulating anticoagulant against antihemophilic factor. J Clin Invest 1971;50:244–254.
2. Weiss HJ, Hoyer IW. Von Willebrand factor: dissociation from antihemophilic factor procoagulant activity. Science 1973;182:1149–1151.
3. Bouma BN, van Mourik JA, Sixma JJ et al. Von Willebrand factor and antihemophilic factor A (factor VIII). Thromb Diath Haemorrh 1973;54:191–196.
4. Van Mourik JA, Bouma BN, La Bruyer WT et al. Factor VIII, a series of homologous oligomers and a complex of two proteins. Thromb Res 1974;4:155–164.
5. McKee PA. Observations on structure-function relationships of human antihemophilic/von Willebrand factor protein [Review]. Ann N Y Acad Sci 1981;370:210–226.
6. Weiss HJ, Sussman II, Hoyer LW. Stabilization of factor VIII in plasma by the von Willebrand factor. Studies on posttransfusion and dissociated factor VIII and in individuals with von Willebrand's disease. J Clin Invest 1977;60:390–404.
7. Marder VJ, Mannucci PM, Firkin BG et al. Standard nomenclature for factor VIII and von Willebrand factor: a recommendation by the International Committee on Thrombosis and Haemostasis. Thromb Haemost 1985;54:871–872.
8. Bonthron D, Orkin SH. The human von Willebrand factor gene. Structure of the 5' region. Eur J Biochem 1988;171:51–57.
9. Assoulin Z, Kerbiriou-Nabias DM, Piétu G et al. The human gene for von-Willebrand factor. Identification of repetitive Alu sequences 5' to the transcription initiation site. Biochem Biophys Res Commun 1988;153:1159–1166.
10. Bonthron DT, Handin RI, Kaufman RJ et al. Structure of pre-pro-von Willebrand factor and its expression in heterologous cells. Nature 1986;324:270–273.
11. Bonthron D, Orr EC, Mitsock LM et al. Nucleotide sequence of pre-pro-von Willebrand factor cDNA. Nucleic Acids Res 1986;14:7125–7127.
12. Ginsburg D, Handin RI, Bonthron DT et al. Human von Willebrand factor (vWf): isolation of complementary DNA (cDNA) clones and chromosomal localization. Science 1985;228:1401–1406.
13. Lynch DC, Zimmerman TS, Collins CJ et al. Molecular cloning of cDNA for human von Willebrand factor: authentication by a new method. Cell 1985;41:49–56.
14. Sadler JE, Shelton-Inloes BB, Sorace JM et al. Cloning and characterization of two cDNAs coding for human von Willebrand factor. Proc Natl Acad Sci U S A 1985;82:6394–6398.
15. Verweij CL, de Vries CJ, Distel B et al. Construction of cDNA coding for human von Willebrand factor using antibody probes for colony-screening and mapping of the chromosomal gene. Nucleic Acids Res 1985;13:4699–4717.
16. Ginsburg D, Konkle BA, Gill JC et al. Molecular basis of human von Willebrand disease: Analysis of platelet von Willebrand factor mRNA. Proc Natl Acad Sci U S A 1989;86:3723–3727.
17. Verweij CL, Diergaarde PJ, Hart M et al. Full-length von Willebrand factor (vWf) cDNA encodes a highly repetitive protein considerably larger than the mature vWf subunit. EMBO J 1986;5:1839–1847.
18. Fay PJ, Kawai Y, Wagner DD et al. Propolypeptide of von Willebrand factor circulates in blood and is identical to von Willebrand antigen II. Science 1986;232:995–998.
19. Montgomery RR, Zimmerman TS. Von Willebrand's disease antigen II. A new plasma and platelet antigen deficient in severe von Willebrand's disease. J Clin Invest 1978;61:1498–1507.
20. Shelton-Inloes BB, Titani K, Sadler JE. cDNA sequences for human von Willebrand factor reveal five types of repeated domains and five possible protein sequence polymorphisms. Biochemistry 1986;25:3164–3171.
21. Marti T, Rosselet SI, Titani K et al. Identification of disulfide-bridged substructures within human von Willebrand factor. Biochemistry 1987;26:8099–8109.
22. Azuma H, Dent JA, Sugimoto M et al. Independent assembly and secretion of a dimeric adhesive domain of von Willebrand factor containing the glycoprotein Ib-binding site. J Biol Chem 1991;266:12342–12347.
23. Baker ME. Invertebrate vitellogenin is homologous to human von Willebrand factor. Biochem J 1988;256:1059–1061.
24. Joba W, Hoffman W. Similarities of integumentary mucin B.1 from Xenopus laevis and prepon-von Willebrand factor at their aminoterminal regions. J Biol Chem 1997;272:1805–1810.
25. Mayadas TN, Wagner DD. Vicinal cysteines in the prosequence play a role in von Willebrand factor multimer assembly. Proc Natl Acad Sci U S A 1992;89:3531–3535.
26. Colombatti A, Bonaldo P. The superfamily of proteins with von Willebrand factor type A-like domains: one theme common to components of extracellular matrix, hemostasis, cellular adhesion, and defense mechanisms. Blood 1991;77:2305–2315.
27. Bork P, Rohde K. More von Willebrand factor type A domains? Sequence similarities with malaria thrombospondin-related anonymous protein, dihydropyridine-sensitive calcium channel and inter-α-trypsin inhibitor [Letter]. J Biol Chem 1997;279:908–910.
28. Deak F, Piecha D, Bachrati C et al. Primary structure and expression of matrilin-2, the closest relative of cartilage matrix protein with in the von Willebrand factor type A-like module superfamily. J Biol Chem 1997;272:9268–9274.
29. Tuckwell DS, Humphries MJ. A structure prediction for the ligand-binding region of the integrin β subunit: evidence for the presence of a von Willebrand factor A domain. FEBS Lett 1997;400:297–303.
30. Qu A, Leahy DJ. Crystal structure of the I-domain from the CD11a/CD18(LFA-1, $\alpha_1\beta_2$) integrin. Proc Natl Acad Sci U S A 1995;92:10277–10281.
31. Lee JO, Rieu P, Arnaout MA et al. Crystal structure of the A domain from the α subunit of integrin CR3 (CD11b/CD18). Cell 1995;80:631–638.
32. Andrews RK, Gorman JJ, Booth WJ et al. Crosslinking of a monomeric 39/34-kDa dispase fragment of von Willebrand factor (Leu-480/Val-481-Gly—18) to the N-terminal region of the α chain of membrane glycoprotein Ib on intact platelets with bis(sulfosuccinimidyl) suberate. Biochemistry 1989;28:8326–8336.
33. Mohri H, Fujimura Y, Shima A et al. Structure of the von Willebrand factor domain interacting with glycoprotein Ib. J Biol Chem 1988;263:17901–17904.
34. Roth GJ, Titani K, Hoyer LW et al. Localization of binding sites within human von Willebrand factor for monomeric type III collagen. Biochemistry 1986;25:8357–8361.
35. Kunicki TJ, Nugent DJ, Staats SJ et al. The human fibroblast class II extracellular matrix receptor mediates platelet adhesion to collagen and is identical to the platelet glycoprotein Ia-IIa complex. J Biol Chem 1988;263:4516–4519.
36. Hunt LT, Barker WC. Von Willebrand Factor shares a distinctive cysteine-rich domain with thrombospondin and procollagen. Biochem Biophys Res Commun 1987;144:876–882.
37. Ginsberg MH, Loftus JC, Plow EF. Cytoadhesins, integrins, and platelets [Review]. Thromb Haemost 1988;59:1–6.
38. Hynes RO. Integrins: versatility, modulation, and signaling in cell adhesion. Cell 1992;69:11–25.
39. Mancuso DJ, Tuley EA, Westfield LA et al. Structure of the gene for human von Willebrand factor. J Biol Chem 1989;264:19514–19527.
40. Mancuso DJ, Tuley EA, Westfield LA et al. Human von Willebrand factor gene and pseudogene: structure analysis and differentiation by polymerase chain reaction. Biochemistry 1991;30:253–269.
41. Ferreira V, Assouline Z, Schwachtgen JL. The role of the 5'-flanking region in the cell-specific transcription of the human von Willebrand factor gene. Biochem J 1993;293:641–648.
42. Jahroudi N, Lynch DC. Endothelial cell-specific regulation of von Willebrand factor gene expression. Mol Cell Biol 1994;14:999–1008.
43. Jahroudi N, Ardekani AM, Greenberger JS. An NF1-like protein functions as a repressor of the von Willebrand factor promoter. J Biol Chem 1996;271:21413–21421.
44. Orkin SH. Transcription factors and hematopoietic development. J Biol Chem 1995;270:4955–4958.
45. Orkin SH. GATA-binding transcription factors in hematopoietic cells [Review]. Blood 1992;80:575–581.
46. Leonard M, Brice M, Engel JD et al. Dynamics of GATA transcription factor expression during erythroid differentiation. Blood 1993;82:1071–1079.
47. Liaw L, Schwartz SM. Comparison of gene expression in bovine aortic endothelium *in vivo* versus *in vitro*. Differences in growth regulatory molecules. Arterioscler Thromb 1993;13:985–993.
48. Aird WC, Jahroudi N, Weiler-Guettler H et al. Human von Willebrand

factor gene sequences target expression to a subpopulation of endothelial cells in transgenic mice. Proc Natl Acad Sci U S A 1995;92:4567–4571.

49. Wu QY, Drouet L, Carrier JL et al. Differential distribution of von Willebrand factor in endothelial cells. Comparison between normal pigs and pigs with von Willebrand Disease. Arteriosclerosis 1987;7:47–54.

50. Bahnak BR, Wu QY, Coulombel L et al. Expression of von Willebrand factor in porcine vessels: heterogeneity at the level of von Willebrand factor mRNA. J Cell Physiol 1989;138:305–310.

51. Titani K, Kumar S, Takio K et al. Amino acid sequence of human von Willebrand factor Biochemistry 1986;25:3171–3184.

52. Debeire P, Montreuil J, Samor B et al. Structure determination of the major asparagine-linked sugar chain of human factor VIII-von Willebrand factor. FEBS Lett 1983;151:22–26.

53. Matsui T, Titani K, Mizuochi T. Structures of the asparagine-linked oligosaccharide chains of human von Willebrand factor. J Biol Chem 1992;267: 8723–8731.

54. Samor B, Michalski JC, Debray H et al. Primary structure of a new tetraantennary glycan of the N-acetyllactosaminic type isolated from human factor VIII/von Willebrand factor. Eur J Biochem 1986;158:295–298.

55. Samor B, Michalski JC, Mazurier C et al. Primary structure of the major O-glycosidically linked carbohydrate unit of human von Willebrand Factor. Glycoconj J 1989;6:263–270.

56. Gralnick HR, Williams SB, Rick ME. Role of carbohydrate in multimeric structure of factor VIII/von Willebrand factor protein. Proc Natl Acad Sci U S A 1983;80:2771–2774.

57. Gralnick HR. Factor VIII/von Willebrand factor protein. Galactose. A cryptic determinant of von Willebrand factor activity. J Clin Invest 1978; 62:496–499.

58. Federici AB, Elder JH, De Marco L et al. Carbohydrate moiety of von Willebrand factor is not necessary for maintaining multimeric structure and ristocetin cofactor activity but protects from proteolytic degradation. J Clin Invest 1984;74:2049–2055.

59. Counts RB, Paskell SL, Elgee SK. Disulfide bonds and the quaternary structure of factor VIII/von Willebrand factor. J Clin Invest 1978;62:702–709.

60. Ruggeri ZM, Zimmerman TS. Variant von Willebrand's disease: characterization of two subtypes by analysis of multimeric composition of factor VIII/von Willebrand factor in plasma and platelets. J Clin Invest 1980;65: 1318–1325.

61. Hoyer LW, Shainoff JR. Factor VIII-related protein circulates in normal human plasma as high molecular weight multimers. Blood 1980;55: 1056–1059.

62. Sporn LA, Marder VJ, Wagner DD. Inducible secretion of large, biologically potent von Willebrand factor multimers. Cell 1986;46:185–190.

63. Fernandez MF, Ginsberg MH, Ruggeri ZM et al. Multimeric structure of platelet factor VIII/von Willebrand factor: the presence of larger multimers and their reassociation with thrombin-stimulated platelets. Blood 1982;60:1132–1138.

64. Fowler WE, Fretto LJ. Electron microscopy of von Willebrand factor. In: Zimmerman TS, Ruggeri ZM, eds. Coagulation and bleeding disorders. New York: Marcel Dekker, 1989:181–193.

65. Siediecki CA, Lestini BJ, Kottke-Marchant KK et al. Shear-dependent changes in the three-dimensional structure of human von Willebrand Factor. Blood 1996;88:2939–2950.

66. Tangelder GJ, Slaaf DW, Arts T et al. Wall shear rate in arterioles in vivo: least estimates from platelet velocity profiles. Am J Physiol 1988;254: H1059–H1064.

67. Perret BA, Furlan M, Beck EA. Studies on factor VIII-elated protein. II. Estimation of molecular size differences between factor VIII oligomers. Biochim Biophys Acta 1979;578:164–174.

68. Mayadas TN, Wagner DD. Von Willebrand factor biosynthesis and processing [Review]. Ann N Y Acad Sci 1991;614:153–166.

69. Wagner DD, Lawrence SO, Ohlsson-Wilhelm BM et al. Topology and order of formation of interchain disulfide bonds in von Willebrand factor. Blood 1987;69:27–32.

70. Voorberg J, Fontijn R, Calafat J et al. Assembly and routing of von Willebrand factor variants: the requirements for disulfide-linked dimerization reside within the carboxyterminal 151 amino acids. J Cell Biol 1991;113: 195–205.

71. Carew JA, Browning PJ, Lynch DC. Sulfation of von Willebrand Factor. Blood 1990;76:2530–2539.

72. Fujimura Y, Titani K, Holland LZ. Von Willebrand factor. A reduced and alkylated 52/48-kDa fragment beginning at amino acid residue 449 contains the domain interacting with platelet glycoprotein Ib. J Biol Chem 1986;261:381–385.

73. Voorberg J, Fontijn R, van Mourik JA et al. Domains involved in multimer assembly of von Willebrand factor (vWf): multimerization is independent of dimerization. EMBO J 1990;9:797–803.

74. Verweij CL, Hart M, Pannekoek H. Expression of variant von Willebrand factor (vWf) cDNA in heterologous cells: requirement of the pro-polypeptide in vWf multimer formation. EMBO J 1987;6:2885–2890.

75. Wise RJ, Pittman DD, Handin RI et al. The propeptide of von Willebrand factor independently mediates the assembly of von Willebrand multimers. Cell 1988;52:229–236.

76. Azuma H, Hayashi T, Dent JA et al. Disulfide bond requirements for assembly of the platelet glycoprotein Ib-binding domain of von Willebrand factor. J Biol Chem 1993;268:2821–2877.

77. Schneppenheim R, Brassard J, Krey S et al. Defective dimerization of von Willebrand factor subunits due to a Cys→Arg mutation in type IID von Willebrand disease. Proc Natl Acad Sci U S A 1996;93:3581–3586.

78. Ware J, Dent JA, Azuma H et al. Identification of a point mutation in Type IIB von Willebrand disease illustrating the regulation of von Willebrand factor affinity for the platelet membrane glycoprotein Ib-IX receptor. Proc Natl Acad Sci U S A 1991;88:2946–2950.

79. Wagner DD, Mayadas T, Marder VJ. Initial glycosylation and acidic pH in the Golgi apparatus are required for multimerization of von Willebrand factor. J Cell Biol 1986;102:1320–1324.

80. Mayadas TN, Wagner DD. In vitro multimerization of von Willebrand factor is triggered by low pH. Importance of the propolypeptide and free sulfhydryls. J Biol Chem 1989;264:13497–13503.

81. Wagner DD, Fay PJ, Sporn LA. Divergent fates of von Willebrand factor and its propolypeptide (von Willebrand antigen II) after secretion from endothelial cells. Proc Natl Acad Sci U S A 1987;84:1955–1959.

82. Vischer UM, Wagner DD. Von Willebrand factor proteolytic processing and multimerization precede the formation of Weibel-Palade bodies. Blood 1994;83:3536–3544.

83. Wise RJ, Barr PJ, Wong PA et al. Expression of a human proprotein processing enzyme: correct cleavage of the von Willebrand factor precursor at a paired basic amino acid site. Proc Natl Acad Sci U S A 1990;87:9378–9382.

84. Vehar GA, Davie EW. Preparation and properties of bovine factor VIIII (antihemophilic factor) Biochemistry 1980;19:401–410.

85. Foster PA, Fulcher CA, Marti T et al. A major factor VIII binding domain resides within the aminoterminal 272 amino acid residues of von Willebrand factor. J Biol Chem 1987;262:8443–8446.

86. Fay PJ, Coumans JV, Walker FJ. Von Willebrand factor mediates protection of factor VIII from activated protein C-catalyzed inactivation. J Biol Chem 1991;266:2172–2177.

87. Koppelman SJ, van Hoeij M, Vink T et al. Requirements of von Willebrand factor to protect factor VIII from inactivation by activated protein C. Blood 1996;87:2292–2300.

88. Zelechowska MG, van Mourik JA, Brodniewicz-Proba T. Ultrastructural localization of factor VIII procoagulant antigen in human liver hepatocytes. Nature 1985;317:729–730.

89. Van der Kwast TH, Stel HV, Cristen E et al. Localization of factor VIII-procoagulant antigen: an immunohistological survey of the human body using monoclonal antibodies. Blood 1986;67:222–227.

90. Wion KL, Kelly D, Summerfield JA et al. Distribution of factor VIII mRNA and antigen in human liver and other tissues. Nature 1985;317:726–729.

91. Leyte A, Voorberg J, Van Schijndel HB et al. The pro-polypeptide of von Willebrand factor is required for the formation of a functional factor VIII-inding site on mature von Willebrand factor. Biochem J 1991;274:257–261.

92. Wise RJ, Dorner AJ, Krane M et al. The role of von Willebrand Factor multimers and propeptide cleavage in binding and stabilization of factor VIII. J Biol Chem 1991;266:21948–21955.

93. Nachman RL, Levine R, Jaffe EA. Synthesis of factor VIII antigen by cultured guinea pig megakaryocytes. J Clin Invest 1977;60:914–921.

94. Sporn LA, Chavin SI, Marder VJ et al. Biosynthesis of von Willebrand protein by human megakaryocytes. J Clin Invest 1985;76:1102–1106.

95. Bowie EJ, Solberg LA Jr, Fass N et al. Transplantation of normal bone marrow into a pig with severe von Willebrand disease. J Clin Invest 1986; 78:26–30.

96. Cramer EM, Breton-Gorius J, Beesley JE et al. Ultrastructural demonstration of tubular inclusions coinciding with von Willebrand factor in pig megakaryocytes. Blood 1988;71:1533–1538.

97. Harrisonn P, Wilbourn B, Debili N et al. Uptake of plasma fibrinogen into the alpha granules of human megakaryocytes and platelets. J Clin Invest 1989;84:1320–1324.

98. Cramer EM, Debili N, Martin JF et al. Uncoordinated expression of fibrinogen compared with thrombospondin and von Willebrand factor in maturing human megakaryocytes. Blood 1989;73:1123–1129.

99. Louache F, Debili J, Cramer E et al. Fibrinogen is not synthesized by human megakaryocytes. Blood 1991;77:311–316.

100. Koutts J, Walsh PN, Plow EF et al. Active release of human platelet factor VIII-related antigen by adenosine diphosphate, collagen and thrombin. J Clin Invest 1978;62:1255–1263.

101. Loesberg C, Gonsalves MD, Zandbergen J et al. The effect of calcium on the secretion of factor VIII-related antigen by cultured human endothelial cells. Biochim Biophys Acta 1983;763:160–168.

102. Wagner DD. Storage and secretion of von Willebrand factor. In: Zimmerman TS, Ruggeri ZM, eds. Coagulation and bleeding disorders. The role of factor VIII and von Willebrand factor. New York: Marcel Dekker, 1989: 161–180.

103. Wagner DD. Cell biology of von Willebrand factor. Annu Rev Cell Biol 1990;6:217–246.

104. Wagner DD, Marder VJ. Biosynthesis of von Willebrand protein by human endothelial cells: processing steps and their intracellular localization. J Cell Biol 1984;99:2123–2130.

105. Sporn LA, Marder VJ, Wagner DD. Differing polarity of the constitutive and regulated secretory pathways for von Willebrand factor in endothelial cells. J Cell Biol 1989;108:1283–1289.

106. Van Buul-Wortelboer MF, Brinkman HJ, Reinders JH et al. Polar secretion of von Willebrand factor by endothelial cells. Biochim Biophys Acta 1989;1011:129–133.

107. Hop C, Fontijn R, Van Mourik JA et al. Polarity of constitutive and regulated von Willebrand factor secretion by transfected MDCK-II cells. Exp Cell Res 1997;230:352–361.

108. Takeuchi M, Nagura H, Kaneda T. DDAVP and epinephrine-induced changes in the localization of von Willebrand factor antigen in endothelial cells of human oral mucosa. Blood 1988;72:850–854.

109. Ewensteinn BM, Warhol MJ, Handin RI et al. Composition of the von Willebrand factor storage organelle (Weibel-Palade body) isolated from cultured human umbilical vein endothelial cells. J Cell Biol 1987;104:1423–1433.

110. Zucker MB, Broekman, MJ, Kaplan KL. Factor VIII related antigen in human blood platelets: localization and release by thrombin and collagen. J Lab Clin Med 1979;94:675–682.

111. Cramer EM, Meyer D, le Menn R et al. Eccentric localization of von Willebrand factor in an internal structure of platelet alpha-granule resembling that of Weibel-Palade bodies. Blood 1985;66:710–713.

112. Weibel ER, Palade GE. New cytoplasmic components in arterial endothelia. J Cell Biol 1964;23:101–112.

113. Wagner DD, Saffaripour S, Bonfanti R et al. Induction of specific storage organelles by von Willebrand factor propolypeptide. Cell 1991;64:403–413.

114. Voorberg J, Fontijn R, van Mourik JA et al. Multimeric von Willebrand Factor directs storage in non-endothelial transfected monkey kidney CV-1 cells (abstract). Thromb Haemost 1991;65:969.

115. McEver RP, Beckstead JH, Moore KL et al. GMP-140, a platelet α-granule membrane protein is also synthesized by vascular endothelial cells and is localized in Weibel-Palade bodies. J Clin Invest 1989;84:92–99.

116. Koedam JA, Cramer EM, Briend E et al. P-selectin, a granule membrane protein of platelets and endothelial cells, follows the regulated secretory pathway in AτT-20 cells. J Cell Biol 1992;116:617–625.

117. Tsai HM, Nagel RL, Hatcher VB et al. Multimeric composition of endothelial cell-derived von Willebrand factor. Blood 1989;73:2074–2076.

118. Moake JL, Rudy CK, Troll JH et al. Unusually large plasma factor VIII: von Willebrand factor multimers in chronic relapsing thrombotic thrombocytopenic purpura. N Engl J Med 1982;307:1432–1435.

119. Ruggeri ZM, Mannucci PM, Federici AB et al. Multimeric composition of factor VIII/von Willebrand factor following administration of DDAVP: implications for pathophysiology and therapy of von Willebrand's disease subtypes. Blood 1982;59:1272–1278.

120. Katz JA, Moake JL, McPherson PD et al. Relationship between human development and disappearance of unusually large von Willebrand factor multimers from plasma. Blood 1989;73:1851–1858.

121. Weinsteinn MJ, Blanchard R, Moake JL et al. Fetal and neonatal von Willebrand factor (vWf) is unusually large and similar to the vWf in individuals with thrombotic thrombocytopenic purpura. Br J Haematol 1989;72:68–72.

122. Harrison RL, McKee PA. Estrogen stimulates von Willebrand factor production by cultured endothelial cells. Blood 1984;63:657–664.

123. Ribes JA, Ni F, Wagner DD et al. Mediation of fibrin-induced release of von Willebrand factor from cultured endothelial cells by the fibrin β chain. J Clin Invest 1989;84:435–442.

124. Reidy MA, Chopek M, Chao S et al. Injury induces increase of von Willebrand factor in rat endothelium. Am J Pathol 1989;134:857–864.

125. Gralnick HR, McKeown LP, Wilson OM et al. Von Willebrand factor release induced by endotoxin. J Lab Clin Med 1989:113:118–122.

126. Sporn LA, Shi RJ, Lawrence SO et al. Rickettsia rickettsii infection of cultured endothelial cells induces release of large von Willebrand factor multimers from Weibel-Palade bodies. Blood 1991;78:2595–2602.

127. Hattori R, Hamilton KK, McEver RP et al. Complement proteins C5b-9 induce secretion of high molecular weight multimers of endothelial von Willebrand factor and translocation of granule membrane protein GMP-140 to the cell surface. J Biol Chem 1989;264:9053–9060.

128. Breit SN, Green I. Modulation of endothelial cell synthesis of von Willebrand factor by mononuclear cell products. Haemostasis 1988;18:137–145.

129. Tannenbaum SH, Gralnick HR. Gamma-interferon modulates von Willebrand factor release by cultured human endothelial cells. Blood 1990;75:2177–2184.

130. Vischer UM, Wollheim CB. Epinephrine induces von Willebrand factor release from cultured endothelial cells: involvement of cyclic AMP-dependent signalling in exocytosis. Thromb Haemost 1997;77:1182–1188.

131. Mannucci PM. The role of Willebrand factor in haemostasis and atherosclerosis. Eur J Clin Invest 1978;8:201–203.

132. Hashemi S, Tackaberry ES, Palmer DS et al. DDAVP-induced release of von Willebrand factor from endothelial cells in vitro: the effect of plasma and blood cells. Biochim Biophys Acta 1990;1052:63–70.

133. Galbusera M, Zoja C, Donadelli R et al. Fluid shear stress modulates von Willebrand factor release from human vascular endothelium. Blood 1997;90:1558–1564.

134. Wencel-Drake JD, Painter RG, Zimmerman TS et al. Ultrastructural locali-

135. Cramer EM, Caen JP, Drouet L et al. Absence of tubular structures and immunolabeling for von Willebrand factor in the platelet alpha-granules from porcine von Willebrand disease. Blood 1986;68:774–778.

136. Parker RI, Shafer BC, Grallnick HR. Platelet density-dependent partition of platelet-von Willebrand Factor between alpha granule and non-alpha granule pools. Thromb Haemost 1987;58:911–914.

137. Nesheim M, Pittman DD, Giles AR et al. The effect of plasma von Willebrand factor on the binding of human factor VIII to thrombin-activated human platelets. J Biol Chem 1991;266:17815–17820.

138. Federici AB, Bader R, Pagani S et al. Binding of von Willebrand factor to glycoproteins Ib and IIb-IIIa complex: affinity is related to multimeric size. Br J Haematol 1989;73:93–99.

139. Sixma JJ, Sakariassen KS, Beeser-Visser NH et al. Adhesion of platelets to human artery subendothelium: effect of factor VIII-von Willebrand factor of various multimeric composition. Blood 1984;63:128–139.

140. Dent JA, Galbusera M, Ruggeri ZM. Heterogeneity of plasma von Willebrand factor multimers resulting from proteolysis of the constituent subunit. J Clin Invest 1991;88:774–782.

141. Zimmerman TS, Dent JA, Ruggeri ZM et al. Subunit composition of plasma von Willebrand factor. Cleavage is present in normal individuals, increased in IIA and IIB von Willebrand disease, but minimal in variants with aberrant structure of individual oligomers (types IIC, IID and IIE). J Clin Invest 1986;77:947–951.

142. Dent JA, Berkowitz SD, Ware J et al. Identification of a cleavage site directing the immunochemical detection of molecular abnormalities in type IIA von Willebrand factor. Proc Natl Acad Sci U S A 1990;87:6306–6310.

143. Frangos JA, Moake JL, Nolasco L et al. Cryosupernatant regulates accumulation of unusually large vWf multimers from endothelial cells. Am J Physiol 1989;256:H1635–H1644.

144. Tsai HM, Nagel RL, Hatcher VB et al. Endothelial cell-derived high molecular weight von Willebrand factor is converted into the plasma multimer pattern by granulocyte proteases. Biochem Biophys Res Commun 1989;158:980–985.

145. Berkowitz SD, Nozaki H, Titani K et al. Evidence that calpains and elastase do not produce the von Willebrand factor fragments present in normal plasma and IIA von Willebrand disease. Blood 1988;72:721–727.

146. Federici AB, Berkowitz SD, Zimmerman TS et al. Proteolysis of von Willebrand factor after thrombolytic therapy in individuals with acute myocardial infarction. Blood 1992;79:38–44.

147. Furlan M, Robles R, Lämmle B. Partial purification and characterization of a protease from human plasma cleaving von Willebrand factor to fragments produced by in vivo proteolysis. Blood 1996;87:4223–4234.

148. Tsai HM. Physiologic cleavage of von Willebrand factor by a plasma protease is dependent on its conformation and requires calcium ion. Blood 1996;87:4235–4244.

149. Furlan M, Robles R, Solenthaler M et al. Deficient activity of von Willebrand factor–cleaving protease in chronic relapsing thrombotic thrombocytopenic purpura. Blood 1997;89:3097–3103.

150. Kroll MH, Hellums JD, McIntire LV et al. Platelets and shear stress [Review]. Blood 1996;88:1525–1541.

151. Weiss HJ, Turitto VT, Baumgartner HR. Effect of shear rate on platelet interaction with subendothelium in citrated and native blood. I. Shear rate-dependent decrease of adhesion in von Willebrand's disease and the Bernard-Soulier syndrome. J Lab Clin Med 1978;92:750–764.

152. Fujimoto T, Hawiger J. Adenosine diphosphate induces binding of von Willebrand factor to human platelets. Nature 1982;297:154–156.

153. De Marco L, Girolami A, Zimmerman TS et al. Von Willebrand factor interaction with the glycoprotein IIb-IIIa complex. Its role in platelet function as demonstrated in individuals with congenital afibrinogenemia. J Clin Invest 1986;77:1272–1277.

154. De Marco L, Mazzucato M, Grazia Del Ben M et al. Type IIB von Willebrand factor with normal sialic acid content induces platelet aggregation in the absence of ristocetin. Role of platelet activation, fibrinogen, and two distinct membrane receptors. J Clin Invest 1987;80:475–482.

155. Anderson GH, Hellums JD, Moake JL et al. Platelet lysis and aggregation in shear fields. Blood Cells 1978;4:499–511.

156. Moake JL, Turner NA, Stathopoulos NA et al. Involvement of large plasma von Willebrand factor (vWf) multimers and unusually large vWf forms derived from endothelial cells in shear stress-induced platelet aggregation. J Clin Invest 1986;78:1456–1461.

157. Peterson DM, Stathopoulos NA, Giorgio TD et al. Shear-induced platelet aggregation requires von Willebrand factor and platelet membrane glycoproteins Ib and IIb-IIIa. Blood 1987;69:625–628.

158. Ikeda Y, Handa M, Kawano K et al. The role of von Willebrand factor and fibrinogen in platelet aggregation under varying shear stress. J Clin Invest 1991;87:1234–1240.

159. De Marco L, Girolami A, Russell S et al. Interaction of asialo von Willebrand factor with glycoprotein Ib induces fibrinogen binding to the glycoprotein IIb-IIIa complex and mediates platelet aggregation. J Clin Invest 1985;75:1198–1203,

160. De Marco L, Girolami A, Zimmerman TS et al. Interaction of purified IIB

von Willebrand factor with the platelet membrane glycoprotein Ib induces fibrinogen binding to the glycoprotein IIb-IIIa complex and initiates aggregation. Proc Natl Acad Sci U S A 1985;82:7424–7428.

161. Kroll MH, Harris TS, Moake JL et al. Von Willebrand factor binding to platelet Gp Ib initiates signals for platelet activation. J Clin Invest 1991; 88:1568–1573.

162. Savage B, Shattil SJ, Ruggeri ZM. Modulation of platelet function through adhesion receptors: A dual role for glycoprotein IIb-IIIa (integrin $\alpha_{IIb}\beta_3$) mediated by fibrinogen and glycoprotein Ib-von Willebrand factor. J Biol Chem 1992;267:11300–11306.

163. Ozaki Y, Satoh K, Yatomi Y et al. Protein tyrosine phosphorylation in human platelets induced by interaction between glycoprotein Ib and von Willebrand factor. Biochim Biophys Acta 1995;1243:482–488.

164. Francesconi M, Casonato A, Pontara E et al. Type IIB von Willebrand factor induces phospholipase A2 activation and cytosolic $Ca^{2+}$ increase in platelets. Biochem Biophys Res Commun 1995;214:102–109.

165. Mazzucato M, De Marco L, Pradella P et al. Porcine von Willebrand factor binding to human platelet GP 1b induces transmembrane calcium influx. Thromb Haemost 1996;75:655–660.

166. Goto S, Salomon DR, Ikeda Y et al. Characterization of the unique mechanism mediating the shear-dependent binding of soluble von Willebrand factor to platelets. J Biol Chem 1995;270:23352–23361.

167. Weiss HJ, Hawiger J, Ruggeri ZM et al. Fibrinogen-independent platelet adhesion and thrombus formation on subendothelium mediated by glycoprotein IIb-IIIa complex at high shear rate. J Clin Invest 1989;83:288–297.

168. Savage B, Saldivar E, Ruggeri ZM. Initiation of platelet adhesion by arrest onto fibrinogen or translocation on von Willebrand factor. Cell 1996;84: 289–297.

169. Savage B, Ruggeri ZM. Selective recognition of adhesive sites in surface-bound fibrinogen by glycoprotein IIb-IIIa on nonactivated platelets. J Biol Chem 1991;266:11227–11233.

170. Weiss HJ, Hoffmann T, Yoshioka A et al. Evidence that the arg[1744] gly[1745] asp[1746] sequence in the GP IIb-IIIa-binding domain of von Willebrand factor is involved in platelet adhesion and thrombus formation on subendothelium. J Lab Clin Med 1993;122:324–332.

171. Takagi J, Fujisawa T, Sekiya F et al. Collagen-binding domain within bovine propolypeptide of von Willebrand Factor. J Biol Chem 1991;266: 5575–5579.

172. Takagi J, Sekiya F, Kasahara K et al. Inhibition of platelet-collagen interaction by propolypeptide of von Willebrand Factor. J Biol Chem 1989;264: 6017–6020.

173. Isobe T, Hisaoka T, Shimizu A et al. Propolypeptide of von Willebrand factor is a novel ligand for very late antigen-4 integrin. J Biol Chem 1997; 272:8447–8453.

174. Stel HV, Sakariassen KS, de Groot PG et al. Von Willebrand factor in the vessel wall mediates platelet adherence. Blood 1985;65:85–90.

175. Turitto VT, Weiss HJ, Zimmerman TS et al. Factor VIII/von Willebrand factor in subendothelium mediates platelet adhesion. Blood 1985;65: 823–831.

176. Sakariassen KS, Bolhuis PA, Sixma JJ. Human blood platelet adhesion to artery subendothelium is mediated by factor VIII-von Willebrand factor bound to the subendothelium. Nature 1979;279:636–638.

177. Nyman D. Interaction of collagen with the factor VIII antigen-activity–von Willebrand factor complex. Thromb Res 1977;11:433–438.

178. Legrand YJ, Rodriguez-Zeballos A, Kartalis G et al. Adsorption of factor VIII antigen-activity complex by collagen. Thromb Res 1978;13:909–911.

179. Scott DM, Griffin B, Pepper DS et al. The binding of purified factor VIII/ von Willebrand factor to collagens of differing type and form. Thromb Res 1981;24:467–472.

180. Rand JH, Patel ND, Schwartz E et al. 150-kD von Willebrand factor binding protein extracted from human vascular subendothelium is type VI collagen. J Clin Invest 1991;88:253–259.

181. Wu XX, Gordon RE, Glanville RW et al. Morphological relationships of von Willebrand factor, type VI collagen, and fibrillin in human vascular subendothelium. Am J Pathol 1996;149:283–291.

182. Bonaldo P, Russo V, Bucciotti F et al. Alpha-1 chain of chick type VI collagen. The complete cDNA sequence reveals a hybrid molecule made of one short collagen and three von Willebrand factor type A-like domains. J Biol Chem 1989;264:5575–5580.

183. Legrand YJ, Fauvel F, Gutman N et al. Microfibrils (MF) platelet interaction: requirement of von Willebrand factor. Thromb Res 1980;19:737–739.

184. Fauvel F, Grant ME, Legrand YJ et al. Interaction of blood platelets with a microfibrillar extract from adult bovine aorta: requirement for von Willebrand factor. Proc Natl Acad Sci U S A 1983;80:551–554.

185. Wagner DD, Urban-Pickering M, Marder VJ. Von Willebrand protein binds to extracellular matrices independently of collagen. Proc Natl Acad Sci U S A 1984;81:471–475.

186. Ross JM, McIntire LV, Moake JL et al. Platelet adhesion and aggregation on human type VI collagen surfaces under physiological flow conditions. Blood 1995;85:1826–1835.

187. de Groot PG, Ottenhof-Rovers M, van Mourik JA et al. Evidence that the primary binding site of von Willebrand factor that mediates platelet adhesion on subendothelium is not collagen. J Clin Invest 1988;82:65–73.

188. Denis C, Baruch D, Kielty CM et al. Localization of von Willebrand factor binding domains to endothelial extracellular matrix and to type VI collagen. Arterioscler Thromb 1993;13:398–406.

189. Fujimura Y, Titani K, Holland LZ et al. A heparin-binding domain of human von Willebrand factor. Characterization and localization to a tryptic fragment extending from amino acid residue Val[449] to Lys[728]. J Biol Chem 1987;262:1734–1739.

190. Fretto LJ, Fowler WE, McCaslin DR et al. Substructure of human von Willebrand factor. Proteolysis by V8 and characterization of two functional domains. J Biol Chem 1986;261:15679–15689.

191. Pareti FI, Fujimura Y, Dent JA et al. Isolation and characterization of a collagen binding domain in human von Willebrand factor. J Biol Chem 1986;261:15310–15315.

192. Pareti FI, Niiya K, McPherson JM et al. Isolation and characterization of two domains of human von Willebrand factor that interact with fibrillar collagen types I and III. J Biol Chem 1987;262:13835–13841.

193. Ruoslahti E. Proteoglycans in cell regulation [Review]. J Biol Chem 1989; 264:13369–13372.

194. Christophe O, Obert B, Meyer D et al. The binding domain of von Willebrand factor to sulfatides is distinct from those interacting with glycoprotein Ib, heparin, and collagen and resides between amino acid residues Leu 512 and Lys 673. Blood 1991;78:2310–2317.

195. Sobel M, McNeill PM, Carlson PL et al. Heparin inhibition of von Willebrand factor-dependent platelet function *in vitro* and *in vivo*. J Clin Invest 1991;87:1787–1793.

196. Sobel M, Bird KE, Tyler-Cross R et al. Heparins designed to specifically inhibit platelet interactions with von Willebrand factor. Circulation 1996; 93:992–999.

197. Ruggeri ZM, De Marco L, Gatti L et al. Platelets have more than one binding site for von Willebrand factor. J Clin Invest 1983;72:1–12.

198. Sakariassen KS, Nievelstein PF, Coller BS et al. The role of platelet membrane glycoproteins Ib and IIb-IIIa in platelet adherence to human artery subendothelium. Br J Haematol 1986;63:681–691.

199. Howard MA, Firkin BG. Ristocetin–a new tool in the investigation of platelet aggregation. Thromb Diath Haemorrh 1971;26:362–369.

200. Read MS, Smith SV, Lamb MA et al. Role of botrocetin in platelet agglutination: formation of an activated complex of botrocetin and von Willebrand factor. Blood 1989;74:1031–1035.

201. Sugimoto M, Mohri H, McClintock RA et al. Identification of discontinuous von Willebrand factor sequences involved in complex formation with botrocetin. A model for the regulation of von Willebrand factor binding to platelet glycoprotein Ib. J Biol Chem 1991;266:18172–18178.

202. Fujimoto T, Ohara S, Hawiger J. Thrombin-induced exposure and prostacyclin inhibition of the receptor for factor VIII/von Willebrand factor on human platelets. J Clin Invest 1982;69:1212–1222.

203. Ruggeri ZM, Bader R, de Marco L. Glanzmann thrombasthenia: deficient binding of von Willebrand factor to thrombin-stimulated platelets. Proc Natl Acad Sci U S A 1982;79:6038–6041.

204. Pietu G, Cherel G, Marguerie G et al. Inhibition of von Willebrand factor-platelet interaction by fibrinogen. Nature 1984;308:648–649.

205. Coller BS, Peerschke EI, Scudder LE et al. A murine monoclonal antibody that completely blocks the binding of fibrinogen to platelets produces a thrombasthenic-like state in normal platelets and binds to glycoproteins IIB and/or IIIa. J Clin Invest 1983;72:325–338.

206. McCrary JK, Nolasco LH, Hellums JD et al. Direct demonstration of radiolabeled von Willebrand factor binding to platelet glycoprotein Ib and IIb-IIIa in the presence of shear stress. Ann Biomed Eng 23:787–793.

207. Chow TW, Hellums JD, Moake JL et al. Shear stress-induced von Willebrand factor binding to platelet glycoprotein Ib initiates calcium influx associated with aggregation. Blood 1992;80:113–120.

208. Ikeda Y, Handa M, Kamata T et al. Transmembrane calcium influx associated with von Willebrand factor binding to GP Ib in the initiation of shear-induced platelet aggregation. Thromb Haemost 1993;69:496–502.

209. Oda A, Yokoyama K, Murata M et al. Protein tyrosine phosphorylation in human platelets during shear stress-induced platelet aggregation (SIPA) is regulated by glycoprotein (GP) Ib-IX as well as GP IIb-IIIa and requires intact cytoskeleton and endogenous ADP. Thromb Haemost 1995;74: 736–742.

210. Roberts DD, Williams SB, Gralnick HR et al. Von Willebrand factor binds specifically to sulfated glycolipids. J Biol Chem 1986;261:3306–3309.

211. Loscalzo J, Inbal A, Handin RI. Von Willebrand protein facilitates platelet incorporation in polymerizing fibrin. J Clin Invest 1986;78:1112–1119.

212. Parker RI, Gralnick HR. Fibrin monomer induces binding of endogenous platelet von Willebrand factor to glycocalicin portion of platelet glycoprotein Ib. Blood 1987;70:1589–1594.

213. Ribes JA, Francis CW. Multimer size dependence of von Willebrand factor binding to crosslinked or noncrosslinked fibrin. Blood 1990;75:1460–1465.

214. Hada M, Kaminski M, Bockenstedt P et al. Covalent crosslinking of von Willebrand Factor to fibrin. Blood 1986;68:95–101.

215. Hantgan RR, Hindriks G, Taylor RG et al. Glycoprotein Ib von Willebrand factor and glycoprotein IIb:IIIa are all involved in platelet adhesion to fibrin in flowing whole blood. Blood 1990;76:345–353.

216. Hill-Eubanks DC, Lollar P. von Willebrand factor is a cofactor for throm-

bin-catalyzed cleavage of the factor VIII light chain. J Biol Chem 1990;265: 17854–17858.

217. Mohri H, Yoshioka A, Zimmerman TS et al. Isolation of the von Willebrand factor domain interacting with platelet glycoprotein Ib, heparin, and collagen and characterization of its three distinct functional sites. J Biol Chem 1989;264:17361–17367.

218. Cruz MA, Yuan H, Lee JR et al. Interaction of the von Willebrand factor (vWf) with collagen. Localization of the primary collagen-binding site by analysis of recombinant vWf a domain polypeptides. J Biol Chem 1995; 270:10822–10827.

219. Hoylaerts MH, Yamamoto H, Nuyts K et al. Von Willebrand factor binds to native collagen VI primarily via its A1 domain. Biochem J 1997;324: 185–191.

220. Amador E, Zimmerman TS, Wacher WEC. Urinary alkaline phosphatase activity. I. Elevated urinary LDH and Alkaline phosphatase activities for the diagnosis of renal adenocarcinomas. JAMA 1963;185:769–775.

221. Kessler CM, Floyd CM, Frantz SC et al. Critical role of the carbohydrate moiety in human von Willebrand factor protein for interactions with type I collagen. Thromb Res 1990;57:59–76.

222. Sobel M, Soler DF, Kermode JC et al. Localization and characterization of a heparin binding domain peptide of human von Willebrand factor. J Biol Chem 1992;267:8857–8862.

223. Matsushita T, Sadler JE. Identification of amino acid residues essential for von Willebrand factor binding to platelet glycoprotein Ib. Charged-to-alanine scanning mutagenesis of the A1 domain of human von Willebrand factor. J Biol Chem 1995;270:13406–13414.

224. Ruggeri ZM, Pareti FI, Mannucci PM et al. Heightened interaction between platelets and Factor VIII/von Willebrand factor in a new subtype of von Willebrand's disease. N Engl J Med 1980;302:1047–1051.

225. Randi AM, Rabinowitz I, Mancuso DJ. Molecular basis of von Willebrand disease type IIB. Candidate mutations cluster in one disulfide loop between proposed platelet glycoproteins Ib binding sequences. J Clin Invest 1991;87:1220–1226.

226. Cooney KA, Nichols WC, Bruck ME et al. The molecular defect in type IIB von Willebrand disease. Identification of four potential missense mutations within the putative GP Ib binding domain. J Clin Invest 1991;87: 1227–1233.

227. Ribba AS, Lavergne JM, Bahnak BR et al. Duplication of a methionine within the glycoprotein Ib binding domain of von Willebrand factor detected by denaturing gradient gel electrophoresis in an individual with type IIB von Willebrand disease. Blood 1991;78:1738–1743.

228. Miyata S, Goto S, Federici AB et al. Conformational changes in the A1 domain of von Willebrand factor modulating the interaction with platelet glycoprotein Ibα. J Biol Chem 1996;271:9046–9053.

229. Scott JP, Montgomery RR, Retzinger GS. Dimeric ristocetin flocculates proteins, binds to platelets, and mediates von Willebrand factor-dependent agglutination of platelets. J Biol Chem 1991;266:8149–8155.

230. Berndt MC, Ward CM, Booth WJ et al. Identification of aspartic acid 514 through glutamic acid 542 as a glycoprotein Ib-IX complex receptor recognition sequence in von Willebrand factor. Mechanisms of modulation of von Willebrand factor by ristocetin and botrocetin. Biochemistry 1992;31: 11144–11151.

231. Knott HM, Berndt MC, Kralicek AV et al. Determination of the solution structure of a platelet-adhesion peptide of von Willebrand factor. Biochemistry 1992;31:11152–11158.

232. Sugimoto M, Ricca G, Hrinda ME et al. Functional modulation of the isolated glycoprotein Ib-binding domain of von Willebrand factor expressed in Escherichia coli. Biochemistry 1991;30:5202–5209.

233. Prior CP, Chu V, Cambou B et al. Optimization of a recombinant von Willebrand factor fragment as an antagonist of the platelet glycoprotein Ib receptor. Biotechnology (N Y) 1993;11:709–713.

234. Pierschbacher MD, Ruoslahti E. Cell attachment activity of fibronectin can be duplicated by small synthetic fragments of the molecule. Nature 1984; 309:30–33.

235. Ruoslahti E, Pierschbacher MD. New perspectives in cell adhesion: RGD and integrins (review). Science 1987;238:491–497.

236. Hynes RO. Integrins: a family of cell surface receptors [Review]. Cell 1987; 48:549–554.

237. Plow EF, Srouji AH, Meyer D et al. Evidence that three adhesive proteins interact with a common recognition site on activated platelets. J Biol Chem 1984;259:5385–5391.

238. Berliner S, Niiya K, Roberts JR et al. Generation and characterization of peptide-specific antibodies that inhibit von Willebrand factor binding to glycoprotein IIb-IIIa without interacting with other adhesive molecules. Selectivity is conferred by Pro1743 and other amino acid residues adjacent to the sequence Arg1744–Gly1745–Asp1746. J Biol Chem 1988;263: 7500–7505.

239. Beacham DA, Wise RJ, Turci SM et al. Selective inactivation of the Arg-Gly-Asp-Ser (RGDS) binding site in von Willebrand factor by site-directed mutagenesis. J Biol Chem 1992;267:3409–3415.

240. Dejana E, Lampugnani MG, Giorgi M et al. Von Willebrand factor promotes endothelial cell adhesion via an Arg-Gly-Asp-dependent mechanism. J Cell Biol 1989;109:367–375.

241. Bahou WF, Ginsburg D, Sikkink R et al. A monoclonal antibody to von Willebrand factor (vWf) inhibits factor VIII binding. Localization of its antigenic determinant to a nonadecapeptide at the aminoterminus of the mature vWf polypeptide. J Clin Invest 19889;84:56–61.

242. Ginsburg D, Bockenstedt PL, Allen EA. Fine mapping of monoclonal antibody epitopes on human von Willebrand factor using a recombinant peptide library. Thromb Haemost 1992;67:166–171.

243. Tuley EA, Gaucher C, Jorieux S et al. Expression of von Willebrand factor "Normandy": an autosomal mutation that mimics hemophilia A. Proc Natl Acad Sci U S A 1991;88:6377–6381.

244. Gaucher C, Mercier B, Jorieux S et al. Identification of two point mutations in the von Willebrand factor gene of three families with the 'Normandy' variant of von Willebrand disease. Br J Haematol 1991;78:506–514.

245. Cacheris PM, Nichols WC, Ginsburg D. Molecular characterization of a unique von Willebrand disease variant. A novel mutant affecting von Willebrand factor/factor VIII interaction. J Biol Chem 1991;266:13499–13502.

246. Kroner PA, Friedman KD, Fahst SA et al. Abnormal binding of Factor VIII is linked with the substitution of glutamine for arginine 91 in von Willebrand factor in a variant form of von Willebrand disease. J Biol Chem 1991;266:19146–19149.

247. Gu J, Jorieux S, Lavergne JM et al. A individual with type 2N von Willebrand disease is heterozygous for a new mutation: Gly22Glu. Demonstration of a defective expression of the second allele by the use of monoclonal antibodies. Blood 1997;89:3263–3269.

248. Celikel R, Varughese KI, Madhusudan A et al. Crystal structure of von Willebrand factor A1 domain in complex with the function blocking NMC-4 Fab [Abstract]. Thromb Haemost 1997;94(Suppl):I-217A–I-218A.

249. Bienkowska J, Cruz MA, Handlin RI et al. The von Willebrand factor A3 domain does not contain a metal ion-dependent adhesion site motif. J Biol Chem 1997;272:25162–25167.

250. Huizinga EG, van der Plas RM, Kroon J et al. Crystal structure of the A3 domain of human von Willebrand factor: implications for collagen binding. Structure 1997;5:1147–1156.

251. Ruggeri ZM. Classification of von Willebrand disease. In: Thrombosis and haemostasis. In: Verstraete M, Vermylen J, Lijnen R, Arnout J, eds. Leuven: Leuven University Press, 1987:419–445.

252. Fowler WE, Fretto LJ, Hamilton KK et al. Substructure of human von Willebrand factor. J Clin Invest 1985;76:1491–1500.

253. Handin RI, Wagner DD. Molecular and cellular biology of von Willebrand Factor. In: Coller BS, ed. Progress in hemostasis and thrombosis. Philadelphia: WB Saunders 1989;9:233–259.

254. Verstraete M, Vermylen J. Thrombosis. Elmsford, NY: Pergamon Press, 1984:49.

255. Ruggeri ZM. von Willebrand factor [Review]. J Clin Invest 1997;99: 559–564.

# CHAPTER 17

# INTERACTION OF COAGULATION FACTORS WITH THE VESSEL WALL

Ann Marie Schmidt, David J. Pinsky, Charles A. Lawson,
and David M. Stern

## INTRODUCTION

It has long been althought that endothelial cells formed an inert surface of blood vessels that did not interact with blood components. Over the last two decades, however, it has become clear that endothelium actively participates in a set of complex processes to maintain the fluidity of blood. The extremely high cell surface: volume ratio, which is found in the majority of the vasculature (1), provides optimal conditions for intensive interactions between endothelial-membrane components and blood constituents. The active interaction of endothelial cells in blood processes is illustrated by the observation that endothelial cells are capable of synthesizing and secreting proteins that function in diverse regulatory mechanisms (see Chapter 13). For example, endothelium is capable of synthesizing prostacyclin (2), endothelium-derived relaxing factor or nitric oxide (3), and the vitamin K-dependent anticoagulant cofactor protein S (4). Moreover, endothelium participates in fibrinolysis by the production and secretion of tissue-type plasminogen activator (5) and plasminogen activator inhibitor type 1 (6, 7), as well as by providing critical binding sites for assembly of fibrinolytic complexes on the cell surface.

Generally, activation of the coagulation mechanism occurs in a regulated and localized manner. Endothelial cells clearly act in a multifunctional way to modulate the coagulant response. Endothelial cells are able to bind activated coagulation factors to obtain a localized and persistent effect. In addition, the endothelial cell membrane contains proteins that function as cofactors in the coagulation process. If the integrity of the endothelial cell monolayer is lost by injury, the exposed subendothelium, which is largely synthesized by endothelium, forms a highly reactive surface for the initiation of the coagulant response. In this chapter we will discuss several of the interactions between coagulation factors and endothelium/subendothelium to illustrate the complex nature of this interaction. Two specific examples will be outlined in some detail: cellular interactions that underlie activation of coagulation associated with oxygen deprivation, and cellular and coagulation interactions in a model of electric current–induced arterial thrombosis.

## ACTIVATION PATHWAYS OF THE COAGULATION MECHANISM

In the traditional cascade arrangement of the blood coagulation mechanism (8, 9), two possible mechanisms of activation of coagulation exist: contact activation or tissue factor (TF)–mediated activation (Fig. 17.1) (see Chapter 1). Both activation pathways ultimately lead to the activation of factor X following which, via a common pathway, thrombin is formed. Thrombin, in turn, has multiple substrates and cellular interaction sites (thrombin receptor, surface-bound protease inhibitors, throm-

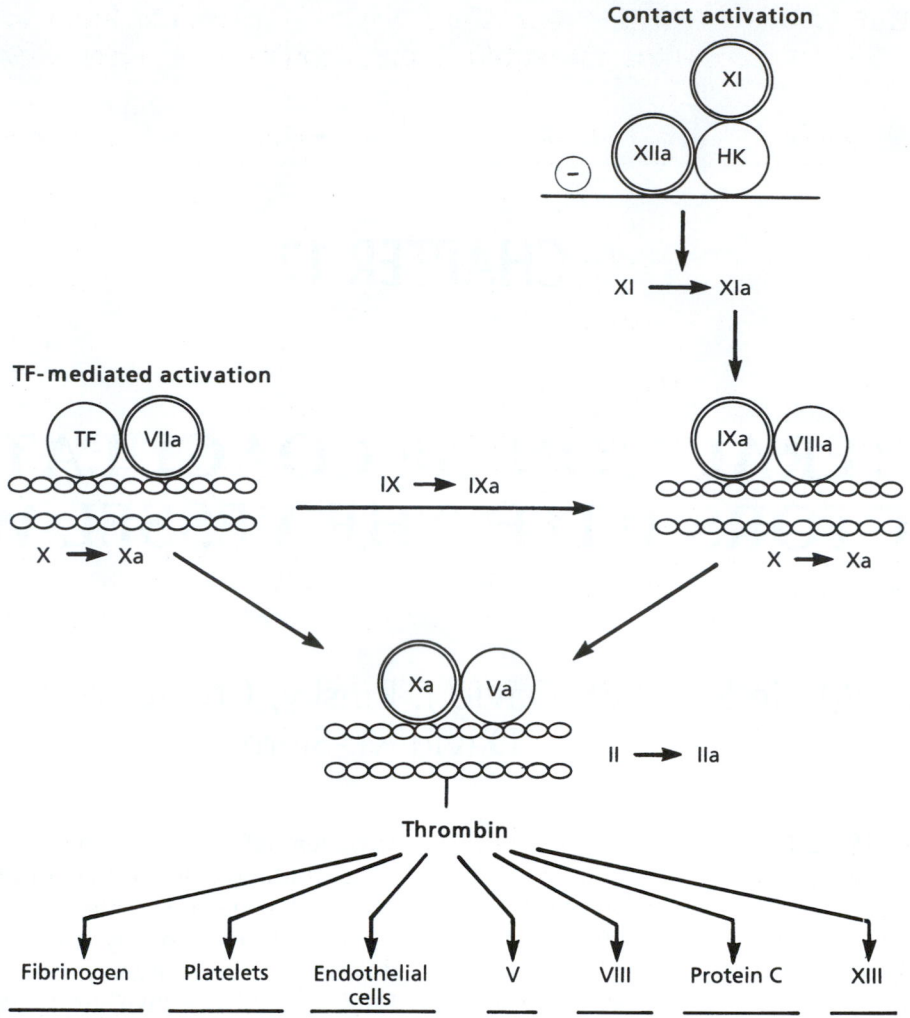

**FIGURE 17.1.** Schematic representation of the interaction of the classic coagulation mechanism with the vessel wall. Each protease is shown in association with the appropriate cofactor protein on a negatively charged surface or a membrane surface. HK, high-molecular-weight kininogen; TF, tissue factor.

bomodulin, etc.) and is responsible for a great number of the phenomena triggered by activation of coagulation (see Fig. 17.1). In this context site-specific regulation of activation of coagulation likely occurs in the setting of high versus low levels of TF. Earlier studies indicated that TF-factor VIIa–mediated activation of factor IX versus factor X is about tenfold more effective in the presence of low amounts of TF, compared with favored activation off factor X at higher levels of TF (10). These data led to the hypothesis that selective blockade of the participation of factor IX/IXa in the clotting cascade would prevent thrombosis in a low-TF environment; however, in settings of high TF, such as that in the extravascular space or surgical wound, direct activation of factor X would occur by the TF-factor VIIa–mediated pathway of coagulation, thus ensuring protective hemostasis. This hypothesis was supported by studies performed in a canine model of electric current–induced coronary thrombosis (11). In this model an electrode was placed in the lumen of the left circumflex coronary artery. Application of electric current results in a local burn and the exposure of TF present in the subendothelial layers of the vessel wall. As a normal vessel wall contains only small amounts of TF (except at the adventia) (12), selective blockade of factor IX/IXa should prevent intravascular thrombosis. An active-site–blocked factor IXa, prepared by inactivation of the native enzyme with dansyl-glutamyl-glycinyl-arginine chloromethylketone, is devoid of procoagulant activity (13). The product, IXai, is a competitive inhibitor for the assembly of factor IXai into the factor IXa-VIIIa-X complex. In this model of electric current-induced thrombosis, administration of IXai, either by intracoronary route or by a single dose into a peripheral vein, provided complete protection from fibrin-induced occlusion of the vessel in a dose-dependent manner (Table 17.1). The protective effect of

**TABLE 17.1.**  Effect of Factors IX and IXai on Coronary Occlusion in the Electric Current-Induced Coronary Thrombosis Model[a]

| n | Agent | Dose | Occlusion | Time to Occlusion (mean ± SD) |
|---|-------|------|-----------|-------------------------------|
| | | | | *min* |
| 36 | Saline | — | 36/36 | 70 ± 11 |
| 3 | IXai | 460 µg/kg i.c. | 0/3 | >180[b] |
| 5 | IXai | 460 µg/kg i.v. | 0/5 | >180[b] |
| 5 | IXai | 300 µg/kg i.v. | 0/5 | >180[b] |
| 6 | IXai | 150 µg/kg i.v. | 3/6 | 102 ± 31[c] |
| 5 | IX | 460 µg/kg i.v. | 5/5 | 79 ± 13 |
| 8 | Heparin | 200 U/kg per min i.v. | 0/8 | >180[b] |
| 5 | Heparin | 100 U/kg per min i.v. | 5/5 | 58 ± 14 |

[a] *The indicated number of dogs (n) were infused with saline alone (8 mL), factor IX, or IXai in saline (volume: 8 mL), or heparin (5000-U bolus followed by the indicated rate of infusion). The number of animals that developed coronary artery occlusion (complete cessation of flow) is shown divided by the total number of animals in that group. Time required for total coronary occlusion to develop is shown. i.c., direct infusion into the left circumflex artery just proximal to the needle electrode; i.v., infusion via peripheral vein (extremity).*

[b] *P <.001 compared with controls infused with saline or factor IX.*

[c] *Time required for occlusion in three of the dogs in this group (remaining three did not develop coronary artery occlusion in >180 min).*

IXai, with respect to thrombosis, was comparable with that observed with heparin. However, concentrations of IXai with antithrombotic efficacy neither elevated the activated partial thromboplastin time (aPTT) nor increased blood loss following a standardized abdominal incision. In marked contrast, levels of heparin that provided protection from thrombosis increased both the aPTT and blood loss in parallel. Thus it can be hypothesized that, whereas factors IX–VIII make an important contribution to activation of coagulation in the presence of lower levels of TF, direct TF-factor VIIa–mediated activation of factor Xa, bypassing factors IX–VIII, predominates at higher levels of TF characteristic of protective situations, as in cutaneous wounds. To further test these predictions, experiments were performed using active site–blocked Xa or Xai, a competitive inhibitor of the assembly of factor Xa into the prothrombinase complex. Since factor Xa is present in the final common pathway of the procoagulant mechanism, its inhibition should block, in parallel, a procoagulant stimulus within the intravascular space and the protective hemostatic response. Administration of Xai blocked occlusive thrombosis in the canine left circumflex electric current model (14). However, levels of Xai required to block thrombosis were identical to those that elevated the prothrombin time and increased blood loss following an abdominal incision. Thus preventing assembly of the prothrombinase complex with Xai does not distinguish between protective hemostasis and antithrombotic protection. Therefore the potential utility of preventing par-

ticipation of factor IX/IXa in the procoagulant pathway, as a future antithrombotic strategy in low-TF situations, is predicted by these studies.

# TISSUE FACTOR–MEDIATED ACTIVATION OF COAGULATION

The extrinsic pathway of the coagulation mechanism is activated on exposure of tissue factor (TF) to blood. This system is discussed in detail in Chapter 4. The TF-VIIa complex is capable of activating factors IX and X (10, 15). Kinetic studies in well-defined systems with purified coagulation factors and phospholipids indicated that the activation rate of factor X exceeds the activation rate of factor IX (15, 16), suggesting that factor IX could be bypassed (as noted in the section above). This is, however, difficult to understand in view of the situation *in vivo* where the TF-factor VIIa complex, in combination with factors VIII and IX, is a most important mechanism for arresting bleeding (17, 18). Such considerations suggested the possibility that in certain situations, a low-TF environment might be present at sites in which thrombosis is initiated. In contrast to rupture of a coronary atheroma or subcutaneous wound, where TF is abundant, within the intravascular space much lower levels of TF are present on monocytes and in certain situations on the endothelium. In contrast to the high constitutive expression of TF by cells in subendothelial

Hypoxia                          Normoxia

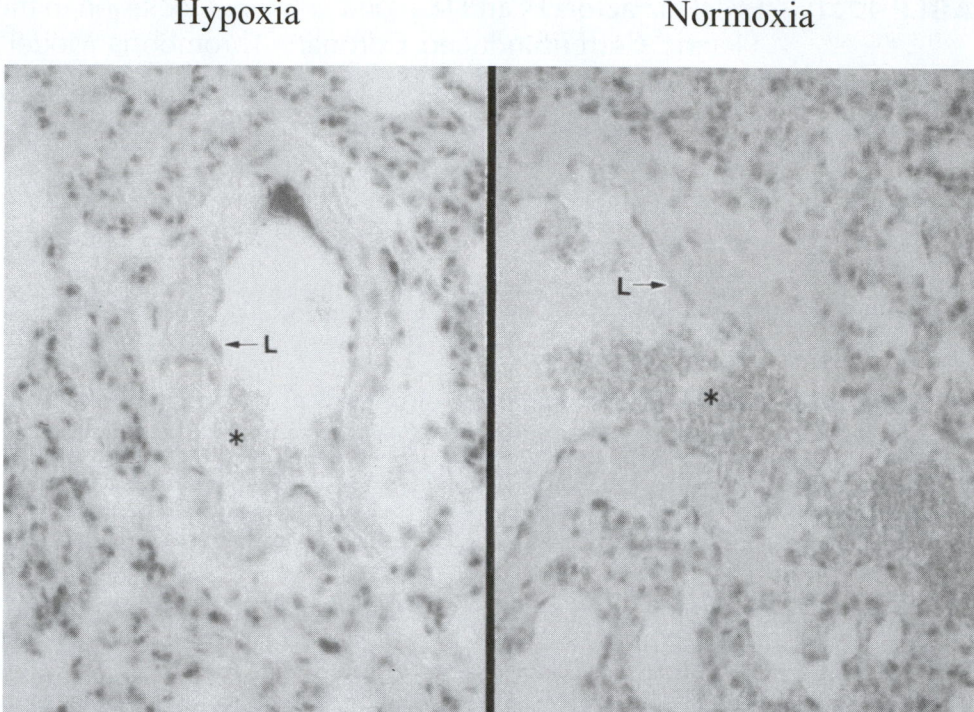

**FIGURE 17.2.** Fibrin accumulation in the pulmonary vasculature of mice exposed to hypoxia or normoxia. Mice were exposed to hypoxia ($F_iO_2$ of 6%) or maintained in normoxia for 8 hours, followed by administration of heparin prior to sacrifice. Tissue was immunostained with a rabbit antibody raised to rat fibrin monomer. Intravascular fibrin formation can be observed in the hypoxic, but not the normoxic lung. L, vascular lumen; arrows, vascular endothelium; *, red blood cells. (Adapted from Lawson CA, Yan SD, Yan SF et al. Monocytes and tissue factor promote thrombosis in a murine model of oxygen deprivation. J Clin Invest 1997;99:1729–1738.)

layers of the vessel wall (especially atheromas) and by mesenchymal/parenchymal cells, the levels of TF achieved by local stimulation of circulating monocytes or endothelial cell surfaces are much lower. These considerations have stimulated studies to delineate relevant, pathophysiologic stimuli triggering intravascular clotting. One series of events likely to be involved in inflammatory settings is the induction of TF in monocytes and endothelial cells by bacteria-derived lipopolysaccharide or proinflammatory cytokines. Another possibility is the increase in vascular smooth muscle cell TF following their exposure to growth factors, chemokines, vasoactive agonists, and thrombin (19).

## TRIGGERING OF VASCULAR FIBRIN DEPOSITION BY OXYGEN DEPRIVATION

An association between hypoxemia and thrombosis has been recognized for some time, especially in the setting of venous thrombosis in the lower extremity. Blood sta-

sis rapidly results in hypoxemia following immobilization of a canine extremity, and fibrin deposition on venous valve leaflets is observed at hypoxemic sites. However, mechanisms through which oxygen deprivation triggers coagulation are only now being defined. Experiments with cultured endothelial cells subjected to oxygen deprivation have shown suppression of thrombomodulin, although only after 24 hours, and changes in expression of fibrinolytic components were not dramatic compared with cytokine induction of plasminogen-activator inhibitor-1 (PAI-1). Hypoxic endothelial cells did not express increased amounts of TF. To analyze mechanisms contributing to fibrin deposition in settings where hypoxemia could have a central role, mice were subjected to an environment with 5.0 to 6.5% oxygen, and pulmonary vascular fibrin deposition was studied. Immunostaining with an antibody to fibrin demonstrated the presence of the antigen in the vessel wall of hypoxic but not normoxic vasculature (Fig. 17.2). That this immunoreactive material represented fibrin was confirmed by electron microscopy; it demonstrated the characteristic 22.5-nm periodicity of fibrin (20). Furthermore, immunoblotting of mouse-tissue extracts, with antibody raised to the gamma-gamma chain dimer present in crosslinked fibrin, showed the presence of antigen in hypoxic lung versus its virtual absence in normoxic controls (20).

Hypoxia triggers endothelial exocytosis of Weibel-Palade bodies translocating P-selectin onto the cell surface (21). As these events could support a wave of leukocyte adhesion to hypoxic endothelium, it can be speculated that polymorphonuclear leukocytes (PMNs) might induce vascular damage and trigger thrombosis. However, pathologic examination of vascular fibrin deposits in hypoxic lung vasculature did not show PMNs to be present at these sites. Furthermore, antibody-mediated depletion of PMNs did not suppress fibrin formation in mice exposed to hypoxia. However, histologic studies of hypoxic lung displayed monocytes associated with hypoxic vasculature, and these monocytes expressed TF. (Fig. 17.3 shows double-staining of the same section with an antibody to the murine monocyte antigen F4/80 and TF.) Consistent with these results, Northern analysis of hypoxic lung displayed a significant increase in TF mRNA after only 4 hours of hypoxia (20).

These data suggest a novel pathway through which hypoxia potentially triggers activation of coagulation: hypoxic vasculature attracts monocytes; the latter become activated and modulate expression of procoagu-

lant cofactors underlying the observed fibrin deposition. Insights into the possible mechanisms involved derives from our pilot work in which hypoxic endothelium expresses the monocyte chemoattractant protein-1 (MCP-1) or the murine homologue (JE), and hypoxic monocytes express TF and increased levels of plasminogen activator inhibitor-1 (PAI-1) (22). These observations suggest a mechanism involving the interaction of vascular cells in mediating local fibrin formation in the setting of oxygen deprivation.

## ANTICOAGULANT FUNCTIONS OF ENDOTHELIUM

The data discussed above indicate that hypoxia-stimulated endothelium can set in motion events supporting the initiation and propagation of the procoagulant pathway. On the other hand, endothelium has a critical role in the negative regulation of blood coagulation by virtue of its membrane components. For example, cell-surface, heparin-like molecules accelerate the inactivation of coagulation proteases by antithrombin III (23, 24). The cell surface also possesses a thrombin-binding protein,

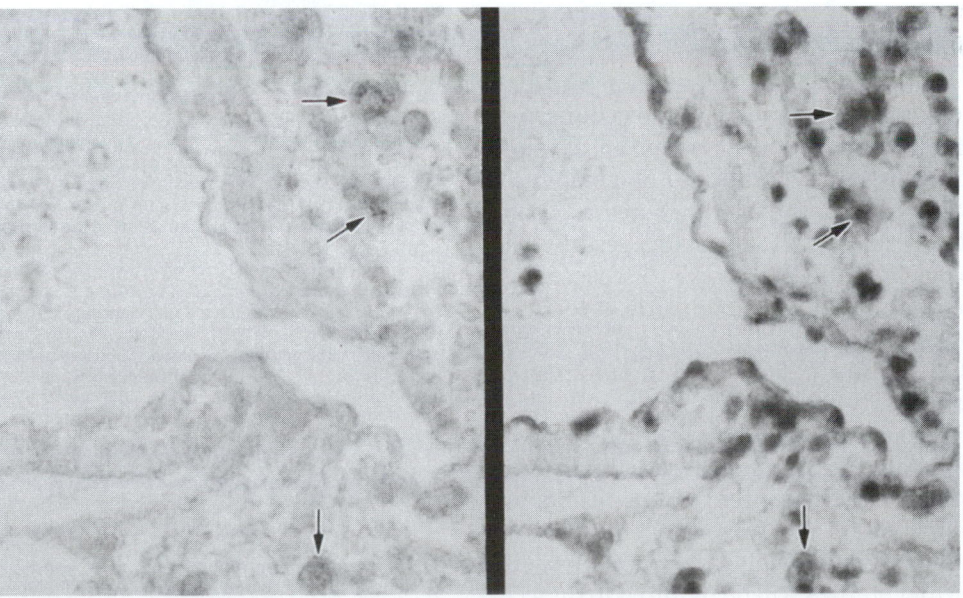

## F4/80 Immunostaining

## Tissue Factor Immunostaining

**FIGURE 17.3.** Expression of tissue factor (TF) during hypoxia. Mice were exposed to either normoxia or to 6 hours of hypoxia, after which lung tissue was immunostained with a cross reacting goat anti-rabbit TF IgG. TF is most prominent in cells in the hypoxic lung, which immunostain for the MP antigen F4/80 (arrows) (Magnification × 600). (Adapted from Lawson CA, Yan SD, Yan SF et al. Monocytes and tissue factor promote thrombosis in a murine model of oxygen deprivation. J Clin Invest 1997;99:1729–1738.)

thrombomodulin (TM), that participates in an intriguing anticoagulant process (25). Binding of thrombin to TM virtually inhibits the ability of thrombin to catalyze clot formation and, at the same time, converts thrombin into a potent activator of protein C (26–28). Activated protein C is capable of functioning as an anticoagulant, and its anticoagulant activity is enhanced by the cofactor protein S. Activated protein C may form a complex with protein S (4, 29) on the endothelial cell surface (30) and function as an anticoagulant by catalyzing the inactivation of the two cofactors of the coagulation pathway, factors Va and VIIIa.

TM is synthesized and expressed by endothelial cells (approximately 100,000 molecules per cell), except those in the microcirculation of the brain. It is clear that a major component of endothelial anticoagulant activity is determined by expression of TM. For example, exposure of endothelium to cytokines, such as TNF, reduces TM expression on the surface of cultured endothelium at the mRNA level (29, 31). The molecular mechanisms involved are of special interest, as suppression of TM expression is correlated with enhanced levels of TF. Thus TNF potentially switches the phenotype of endothelium from the quiescent anticoagulant state to a potentially prothrombotic surface. Although it is tempting to speculate that such changes could underlie intravascular fibrin formation observed in sepsis, in view of the multiple mechanisms involved *in vivo*, further studies will be required to understand the contribution of cytokine-mediated perturbation of endothelial properties to the coagulopathy.

## GENERAL REMARKS

The vessel wall can actively orchestrate the cellular response underlying activation of coagulation in physiologic and pathophysiologic conditions. Hypoxia-mediated perturbation of endothelial function has been shown to modulate a range of homeostatic, vessel-wall properties. These include the production of vasoactive mediators such as endothelin and nitric oxide, cytokines such as interleukins 1 and 6, and JE/MCP-1. The example of hypoxia-induced fibrin deposition in pulmonary vasculature is particularly relevant in that the principal initial role of the endothelium may be in drawing monocytes to the vessel wall. Their subsequent activation in a milieu with limited oxygen concentrations results in enhanced expression of TF and plasminogen activator inhibitor-1, both of which ultimately favor fibrin deposition. Although further studies will be required to dissect precise cause-and-effect relationships *in vivo*, these studies demonstrate the cellular stress response to hypoxia and suggest a mechanism through which these changes determine the response of the coagulation mechanism.

Taken together, these findings indicate that understanding how the vessel wall interacts with the clotting mechanism is essential for further analysis of the host response to changes in the vascular microenvironment.

## ACKNOWLEDGMENT

The authors gratefully acknowledge the contributions of Dr. P.M.N. Tijburg in this work.

## REFERENCES

1. Gimbrone MA Jr. Vascular endothelium in hemostasis and thrombosis. Edinburgh: Churchill Livingstone, 1986.
2. Weksler BB, Marcus AJ, Jaffe EA. Synthesis of prostaglandin $I_2$ (prostacyclin) by cultured human and bovine endothelial cells. Proc Natl Acad Sci U S A 1977;74:3922–3926.
3. Ignarro LJ, Buga GM, Wood KS et al. Endothelium-derived relaxing factor produced and released from artery and vein is nitric oxide. Proc Natl Acad Sci U S A 1987;84:9265–9269.
4. Walker FJ. The regulation of activated protein C by a new protein: a possible function for bovine protein S. J Biol Chem 1980;255:5521–5524.
5. Loskutoff DJ, Edgington TS. Synthesis of fibrinolytic activator and inhibitor by endothelial cells. Proc Natl Acad Sci U S A 1977;74:3903–3907.
6. Bevilacqua MP, Schleef RR, Gimbrone MAJ et al. Regulation of the fibrinolytic system of cultured human vascular endothelium by interleukin 1. J Clin Invest 1986;78:587–591.
7. Nachman RL, Hajjar KA, Silverstein RL et al. Interleukin 1 induces endothelial cell synthesis of plasminogen activator inhibitor. J Exp Med 1986;163:1595–1600.
8. McFarlane RG. An enzyme cascade in the blood clotting mechanism, and its function as a biochemical amplifier. Nature 1964;202:498–499.
9. Davie EW, Ratnoff OD. Waterfall sequence for intrinsic blood clotting. Science 1964;145:1310–1312.
10. Osterud B, Rapaport SI. Activation of Factor IX by the reaction product of tissue factor and factor VII: additional pathway for initiating blood coagulation. Proc Natl Acad Sci U S A 1977;74:5260–5264.
11. Benedict CR, Ryan J, Wolitzky B et al. Active site-blocked Factor IXa prevents intravascular thrombus formation in the coronary vasculature without inhibiting extravascular coagulation in a canine thrombosis model. J Clin Invest 1991;88:1760–1765.
12. Drake T, Morrissey J, Edgington T. Selective cellular expression of tissue factor in human tissues. Am J Pathol 1988;134:1087–1097.
13. Lollar P, Fass D. Inhibition of activated porcine Factor IX with dansyl-glutamyl-glycyl-arginyl chloromethylketone. Arch Biochem Biophys 1984;233:438–446.
14. Benedict CR, Ryan J, Todd J et al. Active site-blocked Factor Xa prevents thrombus formation in the coronary vasculature in parallel with inhibition of extravascular coagulation in a canine thrombosis model. Blood 1993;81:2059–2066.
15. Silverberg SA, Nemerson Y, Zur M. Kinetics of the activation of bovine coagulation factor X by components of the extrinsic pathway. J Biol Chem 1977;252:8481–8488.
16. Zur M, Nemerson Y. Kinetics of factor IX activation via the extrinsic pathway. J Biol Chem 1980;255:5703–5707.
17. Nemerson Y. Tissue factor and hemostasis. Blood 1988;71:1–8.
18. Bauer KA, Kass BL, ten Cate H et al. Factor IX is activated *in vivo* by the tissue factor mechanism. Blood 1990;76:731–736.
19. Taubman MB, Marmur JD, Rosenfield CL et al. Agonist-mediated tissue factor expression in cultured vascular smooth muscle cells. Role of $Ca^{2+}$ mobilization and protein kinase C activation. J Clin Invest 1993;91:547–552.
20. Lawson CA, Yan SD, Yan SF et al. Monocytes and tissue factor promote thrombosis in a murine model of oxygen deprivation. J Clin Invest 1997;99:1729–1738.
21. Pinsky DJ, Naka Y, Liao H et al. Hypoxia-induced exocytosis of endothelial cell Weibel-Palade bodies. A mechanism for rapid neutrophil recruitment after cardiac preservation. J Clin Invest 1996;97:493–500.
22. Lawson CA, Loskutoff DJ, Stern DM et al. Hypoxia-mediated expression of plasminogen activator inhibitor-1 triggers pulmonary fibrin deposition [Abstract]. Circulation 1995;92:I-375a.
23. Marcum JA, McKenney JB, Rosenberg RD. Acceleration of thrombin-antithrombin complex formation in rat hindquarters via heparinlike molecules bound to the endothelium. J Clin Invest 1984;74:341–350.
24. Stern D, Nawroth P, Marcum J et al. Interaction of antithrombin III with bovine aortic segments: role of heparin in binding and enhanced anticoagulant activity. J Clin Invest 1985;75:272–279.

25. Esmon CT, Owen WG. Identification of an endothelial cell cofactor for thrombin-catalyzed activation of protein C. Proc Natl Acad Sci U S A 1981;78:2249–2252.

26. Esmon CT, Esmon NL, Harris KW. Complex formation between thrombin and thrombomodulin inhibits both thrombin catalyzed fibrin formation and factor V activation. J Biol Chem 1982;257:7944–7947.

27. Esmon NL, Carrol RC, Esmon CT. Thrombomodulin blocks the ability of thrombin to activate platelets. J Biol Chem 1983;258:12238–12242.

28. Maruyama I, Salem HH, Ishii H et al. Human thrombomodulin is not an efficient inhibitor of the procoagulant activity of thrombin. J Clin Invest 1985;75:987–991.

29. Walker FJ. Regulation of activated protein C by protein S. J Biol Chem 1981;256:11128–11131.

30. Stern DM, Nawroth PP, Harris KW et al. Cultured bovine aortic endothelial cells promote activated protein C-protein S-mediated inactivation of factor Va. J Biol Chem 1986;261:713–718.

31. Koga S, Morris S, Ogawa S et al. TNF modulates endothelial properties by decreasing cAMP. Am J Physiol 1995;268:C1104–C1113.

# CHAPTER 18

# INTERACTION OF THE FIBRINOLYTIC SYSTEM WITH THE VESSEL WALL

Edward F. Plow, Tatiana Ugarova, and Lindsey A. Miles

## INTRODUCTORY CONSIDERATIONS

As emphasized in the chapters dealing with thrombolysis (Chapters 7 and 8), the regulation of the plasminogen system is sophisticated, multifaceted, and crucial for homeostasis. Plasminogen activators (t-PA and u-PA) and inhibitors of these activators (PAI-1 and PAI-2) and of plasmin ($\alpha_2$-antiplasmin) play critical roles in the initiation, propagation, and regulation of fibrinolysis. Additionally, the fibrin surface, *per se*, is an important regulator of its own degradation by providing specific binding sites for many fibrinolytic proteins (e.g., plasminogen, t-PA, $\alpha_2$-antiplasmin). Aberrations in any of these control mechanisms can upset the delicate balance between thrombus formation and dissolution and result in thrombotic or bleeding tendencies. Studies reported in the mid 1980s provided the groundwork for an additional mechanism for the regulation of fibrinolysis, namely, the existence and function of specific binding sites for components of the fibrinolytic system on cell surfaces and in extracellular matrices. This chapter will consider the interrelationships between cell surfaces, cell matrices, and fibrinolysis. As a component of this section on the "vessel wall," the interaction of fibrinolytic proteins with endothelial cells will be emphasized.

As schematically depicted in Fig. 18.1, endothelial cells express specific binding sites for t-PA (1–3), u-PA (4–8), and plasminogen (4, 9, 10). The proximity of endothelial cells to intravascular thrombi suggests that the interaction of these fibrinolytic "ligands" with

the surface of these cells may be particularly relevant in the regulation of thrombolysis. The capacity of endothelial cells to synthesize and secrete plasminogen activators in a responsive fashion allows for autocrine or paracrine saturation and adds to the potential role of receptors for these activators in the regulation of fibrinolysis. While endothelial cells do not synthesize plasminogen, the luminal surface of the cells is continuously exposed to plasminogen within the blood. Based on the affinity considerations, occupancy of the cell surface with high levels of the zymogen is predicted.

While the above considerations emphasize the significance of the fibrinolytic receptors on endothelial cells, receptors with similar properties and functions are present on many other cell types. This statement is important from three perspectives. First, conclusions drawn from studies of the fibrinolytic receptors on other cell types are directly applicable to endothelium. Second, the receptors on other cell types also may contribute to fibrinolysis, particularly those on cells that accumulate within thrombi such as platelets and neutrophils. Third, the binding of fibrinolytic proteins to cells may have functional consequences that extend beyond fibrinolysis *per se*. These receptors, in fact, provide cells with a means of harnessing proteolytic activity, which they utilize to modify their local environment. Migration is a general behavior of cells that depends on such local proteolysis, and expression and occupancy of receptors for fibrinolytic proteins have been directly implicated in many of the physiologic and pathophysiologic processes that involve cell migration such as angiogenesis, fertili-

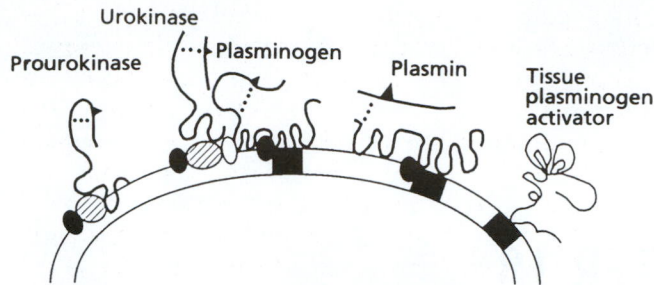

**FIGURE 18.1.**   Schematic model depicting the interaction and assembly of the fibrinolytic system on the surface of endothelial cells. The cells are capable of binding both plasminogen activators, t-PA and u-PA, and plasminogen. Cell-bound zymogens, single chain u-PA or plasminogen, may be converted to active enzymes, urokinase, or plasmin; these may also be retained on the cell surface.

zation, tumor cell invasion and metastasis, and tissue injury in the inflammatory response. While these generalizations stress the roles of the fibrinolytic system and its receptors, other proteolytic systems, either independently or by networking with the fibrinolytic system, contribute to these biologic events. As specific examples, alternative fibrinolytic systems are associated with neutrophils and monocytes (11, 12), and the interplay between the fibrinolytic system and metalloproteinases is key to many physiologic and pathophysiologic responses involving tissue remodeling (13–15).

Endothelial cell injury leads to exposure of the subendothelial matrix. The matrix contains many thrombogenic components and supports thrombus formation. Fibrinolytic components also interact with constituents of the subendothelial matrix, and these associations may play a significant role in regulating the stability of thrombi to lysis. The matrix produced by cultured human umbilical vein endothelial cells has the capacity to bind plasminogen (16), and several individual matrix proteins, including fibronectin, thrombospondin, and certain types of collagen, have been identified as plasminogen-binding proteins (17–21). PAI-1 also accumulates in the matrix of cultured cells (22–24). While the binding of a profibrinolytic molecule, plasminogen, and an antifibrinolytic molecule, PAI-1, could result in a significant regulatory role for the subendothelium in fibrinolysis, the occurrence of these interactions is supported primarily by *in vitro* observations. Thus the significance of these interactions remains conjectural. The recent generation of mice deficient in fibrinolytic proteins (25) and the matrix proteins, which bind plasminogen and PAI-1 (26–28), affords the opportunity to examine directly the biologic significance of these interactions.

As a final introductory comment, it must be emphasized that the interaction of fibrinolytic components with vascular endothelium remains an area of continuing and active research. Even with the extrapolation of data from other cell types and matrices, gaps in information remain large, generalizations are still limited, and consensus views are only beginning to emerge.

# PLASMINOGEN RECEPTORS

## GENERAL CHARACTERISTICS

The general characteristics of plasminogen binding to cells are summarized in Table 18.1, and are discussed individually below.

One of the most striking features of plasminogen receptors is their broad cellular distribution (Table 18.2).

**TABLE 18.1.**   Characteristics of Plasminogen Binding to Cells

Broad cellular distribution
Very high density on cells
Low affinity ($K_d \approx 1 \mu mol/1$)
Various forms of plasmin(ogen) are bound
Recognition is mediated by lysine-binding sites of plasminogen
Plasmin formation is enhanced on cell surfaces
Multiple receptors mediate plasminogen binding to cells

**TABLE 18.2.**   Binding Characteristics and Cellular Distribution of Plasminogen Receptors

| Cell Type | $K_d$ ($\mu mol/l$) | Sites/Cell (x $10^5$) |
|---|---|---|
| Blood cells | | |
| Unstimulated platelets | 1.9 | 0.37 |
| Thombin-stimulated platelets | 2.6 | 1.9 |
| Monocytes | 0.9 | 4.4 |
| Granulocytes | 1.4 | 1.6 |
| Lymphocytes (whole) | 0.9 | 49 |
| T-lymphocyes | 0.4 | 43 |
| B-lymphocytes | 1.3 | 45 |
| Endothelial cells | 2.8 | 210 |
| Erythrocytes | ND[a] | <0.02 |
| Cultured cells | | |
| U937 monocytoid | 0.8 | 160 |
| THP-1 monocytoid | 1.8 | 240 |
| RPMI-1788 lymphoblastoid | 0.3 | 140 |
| GM1380 fibroblasts | 0.9 | 310 |
| Hepatocytes | 0.6 | 141 |

*From Plow EF, Miles LA. Plasminogen receptors in the mediation of pericellular proteolysis. Cell Differ Dev 1990;32:293–298.*

[a] *Not determined.*

With the exception of erythrocytes, the major types of circulating blood cells—platelets (29), neutrophils, monocytes, and lymphocytes (30)—bind plasminogen. The binding is specific (not inhibited by unrelated proteins) and saturable, indicative of the presence of a discrete number of binding sites on these cells. Indeed, as discussed below, most cells exhibit a very high capacity for binding plasminogen. Tissue-fixed cells such as hepatocytes (31) and fibroblasts (32) also bind plasminogen. Many transformed cell lines bind plasminogen when analyzed *in vitro* (33), and plasmin(ogen) has been localized on the surface of tumors *in situ* (34–36). While the identity of the plasminogen receptors (see below) on the many cell types from diverse anatomic origins may be different, the characteristics and functional consequences of ligand binding are similar.

A second notable feature of plasminogen receptors is their very high density (see Table 18.2). Despite its small size, each platelet, when stimulated with thrombin, can bind approximately 200,000 plasminogen molecules on its surface (29). It is not uncommon for larger cells, including endothelial cells, to bind $10^6$ to $10^7$ plasminogen molecules on their surface (33). Many tumor cell lines also exhibit very high plasminogen binding capacities (33, 36, 37), which could contribute to their invasive and metastatic properties. Monocytes bind less plasminogen than U937 and THP-1 monocytoid cell lines (30, 32), suggesting that differentiation and/or transformation can influence plasminogen receptor expression.

The dissociation constant ($K_d$) of glu-plasminogen, the native form of the zymogen that circulates in blood, is approximately 1 μM for cells (see Table 18.2). Based on this affinity, cells exposed to the blood, both circulating blood cells and endothelial cells, should have more than 50% of their plasminogen-binding sites occupied, and experimental measurements support this deduction (38, 39).

Although cells are capable of binding glu-plasminogen, certain forms of the molecule—carbohydrate variants (40), lys-plasminogen (a proteolytically modified form of glu-plasminogen) (9, 38) and plasmin (41, 42)—bind to cells with higher affinity than glu-plasminogen. Such preferential interactions may be of significance in influencing the rate of plasmin generation and the retention of plasmin activity on cell surfaces. The conversion of cell-bound glu-plasminogen to lys-plasminogen occurs on certain cell types (43). This conversion may be of physiologic significance because lys-plasminogen is more rapidly activated to plasmin than glu-plasminogen.

Plasminogen binding to cells is mediated by its lysine binding sites associated with its kringles (38). Kringles are disulfide-looped structures of approximately 90 amino acids and are basic building blocks within many fibrinolytic and coagulation proteins. There are five kringles in plasminogen. By virtue of their capacity to interact with specific lysyl residues in proteins, the kringles mediate the binding of plasminogen to fibrin, $\alpha_2$-antiplasmin, and cell surfaces. Kringle 1, which contains the highest-affinity, lysine-binding site, and kringle 5, which contains the lowest-affinity, lysine-binding site, have both been implicated in the binding of plasminogen to cells (38).

Binding of plasminogen to cells has functional consequences. As illustrated in Fig. 18.2, plasminogen binding to cells accelerates plasminogen activation to plasmin (29, 44, 45). Furthermore, cell-bound plasmin is protected from inactivation by $\alpha_2$-antiplasmin (32, 46). These effects are common consequences of plasminogen binding to all cell types. The identity (t-PA or u-PA) and the source (soluble or cell-surface bound) of the plasminogen activator are cell-type specific and also may influence the rate of plasmin formation.

The high density of plasminogen receptors on some cell types suggests that multiple cell-surface components serve as binding sites. Among the candidate plasminogen receptors are both protein and nonprotein cell membrane constituents. Gangliosides, glycolipids in the outer membrane of cells, are capable of binding plasminogen and inhibiting plasminogen binding to cells. Therefore gangliosides are candidate plasminogen-binding sites (47). Treatment of cells with carboxypeptidases, en-

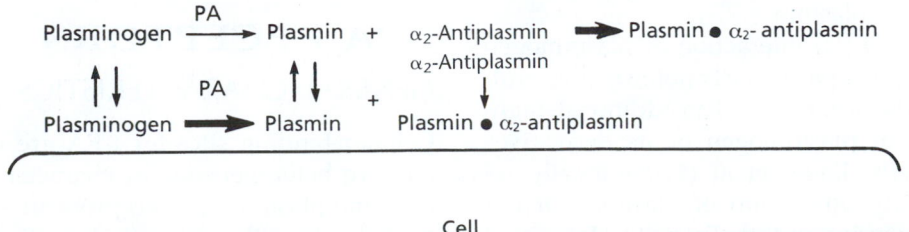

**FIGURE 18.2.**   Reactions of plasminogen on the cell surface and in the fluid phase. Plasminogen exists in an equilibrium between the cell surface and fluid phase. Cell-bound plasminogen is more rapidly activated to plasmin than in the fluid phase by plasminogen activators (PA). Soluble plasmin is neutralized more rapidly by its inhibitor, $\alpha_2$-antiplasmin, than cell-bound plasmin. (From Plow EF, Miles LA. Plasminogen receptors in the mediation of pericellular proteolysis. Cell Differ Dev 1990;32: 293–298.)

zymes that remove carboxyterminal lysyl residues from proteins, reduces plasminogen binding to cells (37, 48, 49). Thus proteins with carboxyterminal lysines also are candidate plasminogen receptors. In addition, certain proteins lacking carboxyterminal lysines appear capable of binding to the lysine-binding sites of plasminogen (39, 50–57). These proteins may present an internal lysine or arginine in an appropriate configuration for recognition by the lysine-binding sites of plasminogen. It is unknown whether any of these candidate receptors, either protein or glycolipid, impart distinct properties to plasminogen such as to influence its proteolytic functions. However, it has been reported that only those plasminogen-binding sites with carboxyterminal lysines are responsible for the acceleration of plasminogen activation on cell surfaces (58). Indeed, on certain cell types the functional effects of plasminogen binding have been ascribed primarily to single plasminogen receptors (36, 59).

## PLASMINOGEN RECEPTORS ON ENDOTHELIAL CELLS

*In vitro* studies indicate that the interaction of plasminogen with endothelial cells conforms to the general characteristics described above. In several independent studies using cultured, human, umbilical-vein endothelial cells, $K_d$ values fell within a tenfold range of 0.3 to 2.0 $\mu M$ (4, 9, 10). The number of plasminogen binding sites was extraordinarily high, ranging from 1.4 to 12.4 $\times 10^6$ plasminogen molecules bound per cell. Comparative studies with endothelial cells derived from arteries and capillaries yielded similar binding parameters with respect to affinity and number of sites (10). The binding of plasminogen to endothelial cells is inhibited by 6-aminohexanoic acid (a lysine analog), implicating the lysine-binding sites within the kringles of plasminogen in mediating recognition (4, 9). Endothelial cell–bound plasminogen is more readily activated than fluid-phase plasminogen (9). Since binding of plasminogen to endothelial cells involves the lysine-binding sites of the molecule, it can be anticipated that interaction of plasmin with endothelial cells also will protect the enzyme from inactivation by $\alpha_2$-antiplasmin.

Several features of the interaction of plasminogen with endothelial cells are particularly noteworthy. Studies have suggested the occurrence of an additional, high-affinity interaction of plasminogen or its derivatives with endothelial cells. Bauer et al (41) originally reported a high-affinity interaction of plasmin but not plasminogen with porcine endothelial cells. Hajjar et al (9) noted a higher affinity of lys-plasminogen than glu-plasminogen for endothelial cells and also observed a conversion of cell-bound glu-plasminogen to the lys form (43). Ganz et al (10) detected a higher-affinity binding ($K_d$ = 0.07 $\mu M$ with 6.2 $\times 10^6$ sites/cell) of plasmin-

ogen to vein endothelial cells, as well as the typical, lower-affinity interaction ($K_d$ = 0.4 $\mu M$ with 12.4 $\times 10^6$ sites/cell). A proteolytic derivative of plasminogen, angiostatin, has been identified that suppresses angiogenesis and thereby influences tumor neovascularization (60, 61). It is likely that angiostatin exerts this activity by binding to an endothelial cell receptor that reacts poorly with plasminogen. While the high capacity of endothelial cells for plasminogen suggests the existence of multiple binding sites, the contribution of proteins within the 40,000- to 50,000-molecular-weight range may be of particular importance. Several studies have identified proteins in this molecular-weight range as plasminogen-binding molecules (48, 62, 63). Cesarman et al (62) isolated one such protein, annexin II, and showed that it also bound t-PA. The colocalization of a plasminogen activator and the zymogen on a single molecule could lead to efficient activation of plasminogen, with fibrin being the prototype for this prediction. Intact annexin II does not have a carboxyterminal lysine and does not bind plasminogen. However, with limited proteolysis it acquires a carboxyterminal lysine- and plasminogen-binding capacity. A 50,000-molecular-weight protein, which binds plasminogen, is related to $\alpha$-enolase. Enolase, which has a naturally occurring carboxyterminal lysine, is found in endothelial cells (48), and a portion is expressed at the cell surface. Actin (57) is an additional endothelial cell protein that has been shown to bind plasminogen. It is not known whether cytokeratin 8, which was identified as a prominent plasminogen binding protein in tumor cells (36), contributes to the plasminogen binding capacity of endothelial cells. A perplexing issue that applies to all of the candidate plasminogen receptors is the absence of classical signal peptide sequences. Thus the mechanisms for their expression at cell surfaces, including the endothelial cell surface, remains unexplained at this time. Additionally, naturally occurring basic carboxypeptidases are present in blood and may rapidly "neutralize" the plasminogen-binding capacity of these receptors by removing their carboxyterminal lysines as they are expressed at the cell surface (49).

## t-PA RECEPTORS

### GENERAL CHARACTERISTICS

Cellular binding sites for t-PA are widely distributed and are heterogeneous in character. In these respects t-PA and plasminogen receptors are similar; and, as discussed below, these two fibrinolytic ligands do indeed share certain binding sites. Of the circulating blood cells, t-PA binding sites are found on platelets (64), monocytes, and neutrophils (65). The t-PA binding sites on platelets are distinct from those on leukocytes (as well as from those on endothelial cells). The presence of

**TABLE 18.3.** Classes of Tissue-Type Plasminogen Activator (t-PA) Binding Sites on Endothelial Cells

| Class | $K_d$ (nmol/l) | Approximate Number of Sites Per Cell ($\times 10^5$) | Role of PAI-1[a] |
|---|---|---|---|
| High-affinity | 1 | Variable | PAI-1–dependent |
| Intermediate-affinity | 18 | 8 | PAI-1–independent |
| Low-affinity | 500 | 100 | PAI-1–independent |

[a] *PAI-1, plasminogen activator inhibitor 1.*

t-PA binding sites on monocytes may be of particular importance, as these cells can be stimulated to synthesize t-PA in response to certain cytokines (66, 67).

The interaction of t-PA with hepatocytes and hepatoma cell lines has been a major focus of interest, as t-PA is rapidly and efficiently cleared by the liver (68–70). If the receptor(s) involved in hepatic clearance were known, it might be possible to create a mutant t-PA with improved pharmacokinetic properties. Both liver parenchymal cells and hepatic endothelial cells contribute to t-PA clearance by the liver (71–73). Binding of t-PA to cultured hepatocytes depends in part on its interaction with its inhibitor, PAI-1 (74, 75). The liver is a site of PAI-1 synthesis, and the inhibitor accumulates within the extracellular matrix of cultured hepatocytes. When t-PA is added to hepatocytes in culture, it can complex with matrix-associated PAI-1; and the t-PA: PAI-1 complexes formed then can bind to the cells (75). These binding sites have been partially characterized (76). An additional and major pathway for t-PA clearance by the liver involves recognition of its carbohydrate side chains. The mannose receptor has been identified as a receptor involved in carbohydrate-mediated recognition (77). In addition, a carbohydrate-independent mechanism for t-PA binding to hepatic cells also has been demonstrated (78). It may be that the next generation of therapeutic t-PA derivatives will be engineered to reduce hepatic clearance, thereby allowing for bolus administration.

## t-PA RECEPTORS ON ENDOTHELIAL CELLS

t-PA is synthesized by and secreted from endothelial cells (79). Thus, while the blood concentration of t-PA is relatively low, its concentration at the endothelial cell surface may be high, allowing for the occupancy of even low-affinity receptors. Accordingly, the interaction of t-PA with endothelial cells has been the subject of analysis by several groups of investigators (1–3, 80, 81). The cells used in these studies have been derived primarily from human umbilical veins. A composite of the information derived from these studies would suggest the existence of three distinct classes of t-PA binding sites

on endothelial cells (although all three classes of sites have not been demonstrated in any single study). The three classes of sites are distinguished on the basis of their affinity for t-PA (Table 18.3).

The highest-affinity interaction of t-PA with endothelial cells can be ascribed to its binding to PAI-1 (3, 82, 83). PAI-1 is synthesized by endothelial cells. It accumulates within the matrix of cultured endothelial cells by virtue of its binding to the matrix protein, vitronectin (84, 85). Vitronectin, however, is not synthesized by endothelial cells, but deposits in the subendothelial matrix from the serum used to culture the cells (86). As vitronectin is a major plasma protein, its incorporation into the subendothelial matrix may be operative *in vivo*, particularly at sites of vascular injury. PAI-1 is a member of the serpin family of protease inhibitors. As such, it forms a very tight complex with t-PA. In general, serpins interact with the active sites of proteases, but there is evidence to suggest an additional mechanism of PAI-1–t-PA interaction that does not require an enzymatically active t-PA molecule (82, 83). Accordingly, not all of the PAI-1–mediated interactions of t-PA with cultured endothelial cells depend on the active site of t-PA. Although the majority of PAI-1 in endothelial cell cultures is secreted into the medium or deposits onto the substratum, a portion also becomes cell-surface associated and contributes to t-PA binding to the cells (80). While the binding of t-PA to either cell- or matrix-associated PAI-1 should not be viewed as a ligand-receptor interaction, this pathway of binding is likely to be of physiologic and pathophysiologic significance in regulating proteolysis at the vascular wall.

A second class of t-PA binding sites with an intermediate affinity for the ligand has been identified and characterized by Hajjar and associates (2, 5, 87). The affinity of this site for t-PA is 18 nM and as many as 800,000 copies of this receptor may exist on the surface of each endothelial cell. The endothelial cell constituent contributing to this interaction has been isolated and identified as annexin II. It is a protein with a molecular weight of 48,000 (87). Interestingly, as noted above, this same protein also binds plasminogen, although the two ligands do not compete with one another for binding to annexin II. Further characterization of this molecule as a discrete t-PA/plasminogen receptor should provide new insights into endothelial cell biology.

The third class of t-PA binding sites on endothelial cells is of low affinity but of very high capacity. This interaction has been demonstrated in several independent studies (3, 65, 81, 88). Binding to this class of sites does involve the cell surface, as it has been demonstrated with the endothelial cells in suspension, as well as in monolayer cultures (65). The $K_d$ values for this class of site fall within the 0.1- to 2-$\mu$M range, and the number of binding sites exceeds $10^6$ per cell. This particular category of t-PA–binding sites on endothelial cells appears to be capable of binding plasminogen as well (89). Moreover, related binding sites are also present on monocytes and neutrophils (65). Thus the above discussion on the identity of plasminogen receptors is pertinent to this class of t-PA–binding sites. Tubulin is an additional endothelial cell protein that has been shown to bind t-PA (90). While t-PA and plasminogen can compete with each other for these shared sites, based on the large number of such sites, their relatively low affinity for both ligands, and the low physiologic concentration of t-PA, competition is calculated to have rather a minimal effect on receptor occupancy. At pharmacologic concentrations of t-PA, competition between t-PA and plasminogen does become germane. Nevertheless, even although plasminogen is present at much higher concentrations than t-PA, several hundred thousand molecules of t-PA are still predicted to occupy these low-affinity binding sites on each endothelial cell during therapeutic administration of the thrombolytic agent.

## FUNCTION OF t-PA RECEPTORS

Plasminogen activation by t-PA in the presence of endothelial cells is greatly enhanced. Compared with the kinetics of fluid-phase activation, this enhancement is more than tenfold (2). Because both plasminogen and t-PA bind to the cells, the acceleration may depend on the effects on one of the ligands or on the colocalization of both ligands on the cell surface. As discussed in Chapter 7, the condensation of t-PA and plasminogen on the fibrin surface results in a marked enhancement of plasmin generation. The cell surface and the fibrin surface serve similar but not identical mechanistic roles in enhancing plasminogen activation (91). Fibrin is still more favorable than cell surfaces for increasing the catalytic efficiency of plasminogen activation (58).

# UROKINASE (u-PA) RECEPTORS

## GENERAL CHARACTERISTICS

In contrast to the interactions of t-PA and plasminogen with cells, which involve multiple classes of binding sites for each ligand, u-PA binding is mediated predominantly by a single molecular entity, the u-PA receptor (u-PAR). This receptor was identified first on cells of the monocytoid lineage (92) and now has been shown to exist on many cell types (93, 94), including endothelial cells (4, 6). Of the circulating blood cells, u-PA receptors are present on neutrophils (30), monocytes (30, 92), and NK cells (95). Platelets bind u-PA (96), but the characteristics of the interaction are sufficiently different from those of other cells to suggest that a different binding mechanism is involved. u-PA receptors are expressed by a variety of tumor cells and play an important role in determining their invasive and metastatic phenotype (97–101).

The u-PA receptors on the various cell types bind u-PA with similar characteristics. The interaction with the ligand is of high affinity; determined $K_d$ values have ranged from <0.1 to >2 nM (93). Modulation of the affinity of the receptor for u-PA has been demonstrated on several cell types in response to various stimuli (102–104). Such alterations may be associated with tenfold or greater decreases in affinity and are frequently accompanied by an increase in the number of receptors on the cell surface (105). The number of u-PA receptors on many cell types fall within the range of 50,000 to 200,000 sites per cell (e.g., monocytoid cells, endothelial cells, fibroblasts). Some species specificity is an additional characteristic of the u-PA receptor. Human u-PA fails to bind to the mouse u-PA receptor, and mouse u-PA does not bind to the human u-PA receptor (105, 106). However, both rat and hamster u-PARs recognize human u-PA (107). Recognition of u-PA by its receptor does not depend on the enzymatic activity of the ligand. Single-chain u-PA (pro u-PA), the zymogen, and two-chain, high-molecular-weight ($M_r$ = 55,000) u-PA, the primary form of the active enzyme, react with the receptor with similar affinity (108). On the other hand, two-chain, low-molecular-weight ($M_r$ = 33,000) u-PA, which is formed by proteolytic removal of the aminoterminal aspects of u-PA, fails to bind to the receptor (32, 92, 109). Thus the conversion of high-molecular-weight to low-molecular-weight u-PA, a transition that occurs *in vivo*, may play a role in regulating receptor occupancy. Complexes of u-PA with its naturally occurring inhibitors, PAI-1 and PAI-2, are also recognized by the u-PA receptor (110). However, the fate of receptor-bound u-PA and u-PA-inhibitor complexes differs. While bound u-PA remains surface associated, binding of the u-PA–inhibitor complexes leads to internalization (111, 112). Such internalization provides a mechanism for clearing enzymatically inactive u-PA from the cell surface. The clearance of u-PA–serpin complexes involves their interaction with LDL receptor–related protein (LRP) (25, 113), which also can bind u-PA directly, but exhibits a preference for its complexes (114). Internalization of u-PA:

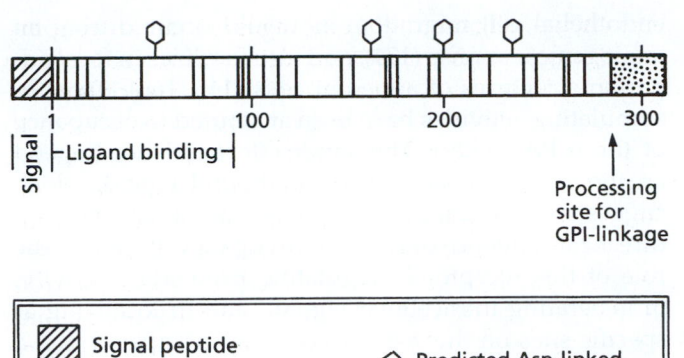

**FIGURE 18.3.** Schematic depiction of the urokinase receptor. The mature protein consists of 313 amino acids and is preceded by a 21 amino acid signal peptide. The receptor is processed at its carboxyterminus to remove approximately 30 amino acids and acquires a glycosyl-phosphatidylinositol (GP I) moiety for membrane anchoring. The vertical lines indicate cysteine residues, and the predicted Asn-linked glycosylation sites are marked. The urokinase ligand binds to the aminoterminal aspects of the receptor.

PAI-1 complexes can also occur via two receptors related to LRP, glycoprotein 330 (115) and the very low density lipoprotein receptor (116).

The structure within u-PA recognized by the u-PA receptor resides in epidermal growth factor–like domain of u-PA. This disulfide-looped sequence resides in the aminoterminal aspect of the molecule and is absent in low-molecular-weight u-PA. A proteolytic fragment of u-PA, the aminoterminal fragment, which contains the first 135 amino acids, binds to the receptor with an affinity similar to that of intact u-PA (102). A synthetic peptide, which corresponds to amino acid residues 12–35 within the growth-factor domain of u-PA, also binds to the receptor, albeit with a considerably lower affinity (106).

The cell-surface protein that serves as the u-PA receptor (u-PAR) has been isolated (117, 118), and its full amino acid sequence has been deduced by cDNA cloning (119). It is composed of 313 amino acids and is cysteine-rich (Fig. 18.3). Glycosylation is extensive, resulting in a cell-surface form of the receptor of $M_r = 55,000$ to 60,000 (105, 120). Changes in glycosylation may contribute to affinity modulation of the receptor. A notable feature of the u-PAR is the nature of its linkage to the cell membrane. The receptor does not contain a typical transmembrane domain, but rather falls into the family of proteins that are linked to the cell surface via a glycosyl-phosphatidylinositol (GP I)-anchor (121). Consequently, the u-PAR is released when cells are treated with phosphatidylinositol-specific phospholipase C.

Certain forms of paroxysmal nocturnal hemoglobinuria (PNH) are associated with a deficiency of GP I-anchored proteins from cell surfaces. The leukocytes from such individuals are deficient in u-PA receptors (122). It is interesting to speculate that the deficiency of the u-PAR may contribute to the thrombotic tendencies in PNH individuals. The ligand-binding domain of the u-PAR resides in the disulfide-rich, aminoterminal aspects of the molecule (121), although additional domains may modulate ligand affinity (123).

Despite the absence of a transmembrane region, there are clear examples of intracellular signaling pathways and events being activated by engagement of u-PAR (124–136). This suggests that u-PAR must be complexed to transmembrane proteins. Evidence has been developed that directly or indirectly links u-PAR to members of the integrin family of adhesion receptors (11, 134, 137–146). Integrins are heterodimeric receptors in which each subunit contains a transmembrane domain (147) (see Chapters 12 and 15). Integrins bind matrix or cell-surface proteins via their extracellular domains and cytoskeletal and signaling molecules via their intracellular domains. Cell-surface complexes of u-PAR and certain integrins have been demonstrated. Additionally, u-PAR has been shown to be a receptor for vitronectin (148–150). Vitronectin is a major plasma protein that deposits within extracellular matrices (151, 152), where it mediates cell adhesion by serving as a ligand for several different integrins (153). Vitronectin also is the major PAI-1 binding protein within extracellular matrices (154). The various intramolecular recognition sites for the above-described interactions are not identical. Thus u-PAR binds u-PA and vitronectin to distinct sites so that both ligands can bind to the same receptor (148, 149). Indeed, u-PA can enhance vitronectin binding to u-PAR (148, 149). The site within vitronectin that is recognized by integrins is distinct from its u-PAR binding site (141). Thus it is possible for a macromolecular complex of u-PAR/u-PA/vitronectin/integrin to organize on cell surfaces. u-PA and u-PAR may shift recognition of vitronectin from one integrin to another (141), thereby influencing cell adhesion. Moreover, PAI-1 binds to a site in *vitro*nectin in close proximity to its integrin recognition site (142) and can interfere with the integrin-vitronectin interaction (142). As a consequence, cells are released from their adhesive substratum, and their migration is initiated (142, 155). Plasminogen bound to the cell surface in proximity to bound u-PA is efficiently activated (45), and the plasmin that is formed facilitates cell migration by degrading matrix proteins and matrix or by activating degrading enzymes. Thus a complex series of intermolecular interactions link the fibrinolytic system to the control of cell migration.

## u-PA RECEPTORS ON ENDOTHELIAL CELLS

u-PA binds to endothelial cells in a time- and temperature-dependent manner. This interaction is of high affinity (4, 7, 8, 156); the $K_d$ of the interaction is <2 nM. The capacity of human endothelial cells has varied from less than 20,000 to more than 200,000 u-PA molecules bound per cell (4, 156). Analyses at both the protein and the mRNA levels indicate that the authentic u-PA receptor (u-PAR) is present in endothelial cells and mediates the binding of u-PA to these cells (6). Accordingly, the characteristics of the u-PAR described above are applicable to the endothelial cell form of the receptor. The molecular mass of the u-PAR on the surface of endothelial cells was determined to be $M_r$ = 42,000 to 46,000 (6, 156), smaller than the cell-surface form of the protein from monocytoid cells ($M_r$ = 55,000). Glycosylation differences are likely to account for these size differences. Expression of the u-PARs by endothelial cells is responsive to various agonists and cytokines. Thrombin causes a modest but statistically significant down-regulation in the number of u-PARs expressed by human umbilical-vein endothelial cells (4). In contrast, PMA stimulation of these cells is associated with a significant increase in receptor number (157). Stimulation of endothelial cells with bFGF, an angiogenic growth factor, leads to a five-fold decrease in the affinity of u-PA for the cells and a tenfold increase in the number of receptors (156). Proteases play a significant role in angiogenesis (14, 15), and modulation of the u-PARs in response to this growth factor may be of major importance in regulating blood-vessel growth and development.

## FUNCTION OF u-PA RECEPTORS

An understanding of the functional consequences of u-PA binding to its receptor continues to evolve. From a kinetic standpoint, the colocalization of u-PA and plasminogen on cell surfaces enhances the efficiency of plasmin formation (128, 158, 159). Certain studies have suggested that binding of prourokinase to the u-PAR imparts enzymatic activity to the zymogen (159), but this point remains controversial. Once small amounts of plasmin are formed on the cell surface, it can catalyze the conversion of receptor-bound prourokinase to u-PA, which, in turn, can catalyze the formation of more plasmin on the cell surface.

Numerous studies have now documented how cells utilize receptor-bound u-PA. Tumor-cell invasion and metastasis are markedly influenced by the occupancy of the u-PAR on the cells (98–100, 160). As many tumors produce u-PA, autocrine saturation of the receptors may occur (161, 162). However, it also has been shown that tumors and other cells that do not synthesize u-PA may acquire the ligand from their environment and utilize the bound enzyme to instigate local proteolysis (163). Receptor-bound u-PA has been implicated in the migration of monocytes in the inflammatory response (128, 164), and myeloid differentiation is influenced by occupancy of the u-PAR (127). Cell-bound u-PA stimulates endothelial cell migration, as would occur during an angiogenic response (124), and also localizes in focal adhesion structures of adherent cells (165, 166). Growth-stimulating activities have been attributed to occupancy of the u-PAR (129). This latter effect did not depend on the enzymatic activity of the bound ligand, which suggests that intracellular signals may be elicited as a direct consequence of receptor occupancy. Based on the role of this receptor in regulating proteolytic activity, in generating intracellular signals, and in localizing at specific sites on the cell surface, it is anticipated that a widening circle of biologic functions and responses will be ascribed to this ligand-receptor system. As noted above, a complex series of intermolecular interactions link this ligand-receptor system to the regulation of cell migration. Nevertheless, initial descriptions of the inactivation of the gene for u-PAR in mice have failed to identify a major phenotype (167, 168). Indeed, these mice have behaved similarly to wild-type animals even under conditions where inactivation of u-PA itself has resulted in abnormalities (169). The latter observations suggest that u-PA can exert at least some of its functions independent of its receptor (170).

# THE MATRIX METALLOPROTEASES AND THE VESSEL WALL

While this chapter has focused on the plasminogen system, it is important to recognize that other proteolytic systems play important roles in vascular biology. A prime example is the matrix metalloprotease (MMP) family. These enzymes are involved in the turnover of extracellular matrix constituents, including the collagens, elastin, glycoproteins, and proteoglycans, and are implicated in physiologic, matrix-remodeling events such as embryogenesis, morphogenesis, and wound healing. Alterations in MMP activity can result in excessive matrix destruction or accumulation and have been associated with pathophysiologic remodeling events such as atherosclerosis and restenosis.

The MMP constitute a family of zinc-dependent endopeptidases, optimally active at neutral pH (Table 18.4). These enzymes share a similar domain structure with a signal peptide domain, a propeptide domain that is cleaved during activation; a catalytic domain that contains a thermolysin-type, zinc-binding region; and a hinge region connected to a carboxyterminal domain that has homology to hemopexin and vitronectin (this last domain is absent in MMP-7, matrilysin). Two matrix metalloproteases (MMP-2, gelatinase A and MMP-9, gelatinase B) have an additional domain inserted into the catalytic domain that has homology to the gelatin-binding domains of fibronectin.

**TABLE 18.4.**   The Matrix Metalloprotease (MMP) Family

| Enzyme | Molecular Weight, Kd | MMP Number | Substrates |
|---|---|---|---|
| Gelatinases | | | Denatured collagens |
|   Gelatinase A | 72 | MMP-2 | Native collagen types IV, V, VII, X |
|   Gelatinase B | 92 | MMP-9 | Elastin, fibronectin |
| | | | Fibrinogen/fibrin (MMP-2) |
| Collagenases | | | |
|   Interstitial collagenase | 52 | MMP-1 | Collagen types I, II, III, VII, VIII, X |
|   Collagenase 3 | 52 | MMP-13 | Gelatin, proteoglycans |
|   Neutrophil collagenase | 75 | MMP-8 | |
| Stromelysins | | | |
|   Stromelysin-1 | 55 | MMP-3 | Proteoglycan core protein |
|   Stromelysin-2 | 55 | MMP-10 | Fibronectin, laminin, elastin |
| | | | Collagen types IV, V, IX, X |
|   Stromelysin-3 | 61 | MMP-11 | Fibrinogen/fibrin (MMP-3) |
|   Metalloelastase | 54 | MMP-12 | Elastin |
| Matrilysin (PUMP-1) | 28 | MMP-7 | Fibronectin, laminin, collagen type IV, proteoglycan core protein, urokinase |
| Membrane-type MMP | | | |
|   MT-MMP-1 | 63 | MMP-14 | Progelatinase A, collagen type IV |
|   MP-MMP 2 | | MMP-15 | Gelatin |

The MMP are all secreted as latent proenzymes, which are subsequently activated in the pericellular and extracellular environment, resulting in liberation of propeptide. The physiologic mechanism of activation is not fully understood and can occur by a plasmin/u-PA-dependent mechanism or by interaction with other MMP. The physiologic mechanism of activation of at least one metalloprotease, MMP-2 (progelatinase A), has been identified and includes the activation of MMP-2 by membrane-bound metalloprotease, MT-MMP-2, thus localizing the proteolytic activation to the cell surface (171).

The metalloproteases are inhibited by a family of naturally occurring specific inhibitors (TIMPs) and also by $\alpha_2$-macroglobulin and heparin (172). To date, three TIMPs have been well-characterized: TIMP-1, TIMP-2, and TIMP-3. TIMPs bind with high affinity in a 1:1 molar ratio to active MMPs and inhibit their proteolytic activity.

MMP expression is tightly controlled by cytokines, growth factors, and hormones. Among them, IL-1, PDGF, and TNF-$\alpha$ induce the synthesis of MMP, whereas TGF-$\beta$, IL-4, heparin, and corticosteroids repress transcription of MMP genes (173). Interestingly, these cytokines do not augment the production of TIMP. Many of these cytokines and growth factors have been identified as mediators in atherogenesis and restenosis.

There is considerable evidence that MMPs are expressed in atherosclerotic plaques and induced in response to mechanical injury in vascular smooth muscle cells (VSMC). In rat and rabbit models of VSMC migra-tion, both migration and proliferation depend on the secretion of gelatinase A (MMP-2) and gelatinase B (MMP-9) from VSMC (174). Endothelial cells are known to express collagenase (MMP-1), gelatinase A (MMP-2), and TIMP constitutively (14). Inflammatory cytokines up-regulate the production of these proteins and induce the expression of stromelysin (MMP-3) and gelatinase B (MMP-2). Both macrophages, which play an important role in the development of atherosclerosis, and VSMC can express stromelysin; in fact, this MMP has been found in atherosclerotic plaques (174). It has been suggested that in the late stages of atherosclerosis, MMPs derived from macrophages and VSMC may contribute to plaque rupture (175). In addition, collagenase, stromelysin, and gelatinase B are induced, and gelatinase A is up-regulated in response to mechanical injury. The relevance of these findings in models of restenosis to VSMC migration and proliferation is confirmed by a reduction in the early migration of VSMC into the intima following systemic administration of a metalloprotease inhibitor. Thus the MMP family plays a key role in the maintenance of vascular integrity.

Linkages between the MMP and fibrinolytic systems are multiple. The following are specific examples: (a) as noted above, the two systems cooperate to mediate vascular remodeling events (14, 15, 176); (b) plasmin and urokinase can activate several MMPs (173); and (c) a specific MMP matrilysin can convert high-molecular-weight u-PA to a low-molecular-weight form. This transition results in the formation of u-PA that can no longer bind to the u-PA receptor (177).

# REFERENCES

1. Beebe DP. Binding of tissue plasminogen activator to human umbilical vein endothelial cells. Thromb Res 1987;46:241–254.
2. Hajjar KA, Hamel NM, Harpel PC et al. Binding of tissue plasminogen activator to cultured human endothelial cells. J Clin Invest 1987;80:1712–1719.
3. Barnathan ES, Kuo A, Van der Keyl H et al. Tissue–type plasminogen activator binding to human endothelial cells. Evidence of two distinct binding sites. J Biol Chem 1988;263:7792–7799.
4. Miles LA, Levin EG, Plescia J et al. Plasminogen receptors, urokinase receptors, and their modulation on human endothelial cells. Blood 1988;72:628–635.
5. Hajjar KA, Hamel NM. Identification and characterization of human endothelial cell membrane binding sites for tissue plasminogen activator and urokinase. J Biol Chem 1990;265:2908–2916.
6. Barnathan ES, Kuo A, Karikó K et al. Characterization of human endothelial cell urokinase-type plasminogen activator receptor protein and messenger RNA. Blood 1990;76:1795–1806.
7. Barnathan ES, Kuo A, Rosenfeld L et al. Interaction of single-chain urokinase-type plasminogen activator with human endothelial cells. J Biol Chem 1990;265:2865–2872.
8. Haddock RC, Spell ML, Baker CDIII et al. Urokinase binding and receptor identification in cultured endothelial cells. J Biol Chem 1991;266:21466–21473.
9. Hajjar KA, Harpel PC, Jaffe EA et al. Binding of plasminogen to cultured human endothelial cells. J Biol Chem 1986;261:11656–11662.
10. Ganz PR, Dupuis D, Dudani AK et al. Characterization of plasminogen binding to human capillary and arterial endothelial cells. Biochem Cell Biol 1991;69:442–448.
11. Simon DI, Ezratty EM, Francis SA et al. Fibrin(ogen) is internalized and degraded by activated human monocytoid cells via Mac-1 (CD11b/CD18): a nonplasmin fibrinolytic pathway. Blood 1993;82:2414–2422.
12. Plow EF. The major fibrinolytic proteases of human leukocytes. Biochim Biophys Acta 1980;630:47–56.
13. Lee E, Vaughan DE, Parikh SH et al. Regulation of matrix metalloproteinases and plasminogen activator inhibitor-1 synthesis by plasminogen in cultured human vascular smooth muscle cells. Circ Res 1996;78:44–49.
14. Mignatti P, Rifkin DB. Plasminogen activators and matrix metalloproteinases in angiogenesis. Enzyme Protein 1996;49:117–137.
15. Pepper MS, Montesano R, Mandriota SJ et al. Angiogenesis: a paradigm for balanced extracellular proteolysis during cell migration and morphogenesis. Enzyme Protein 1996;49:138–162.
16. Knudsen BS, Silverstein RL, Leung LLK et al. Binding of plasminogen to extracellular matrix. J Biol Chem 1986;261:10765–10771.
17. Salonen EM, Zitting A, Vaheri A. Laminin interacts with plasminogen and its tissue-type activator. FEBS Lett 1984;172:29–32.
18. Stack MS, Moser TL, Pizzo SV. Binding of human plasminogen to basement-membrane (type IV) collagen. Biochem J 1992;284:103–108.
19. Salonen EV, Saksela O, Vartio T et al. Plasminogen and tissue-type plasminogen activator bind to immobilized fibronectin. J Biol Chem 1985;260:12302–12307.
20. Preissner KT. Specific binding of plasminogen to vitronectin. Evidence for a modulatory role of vitronectin on fibrin(ogen)-induced plasmin formation by tissue plasminogen activator. Biochem Biophys Res Commun 1990;168:966–971.
21. Silverstein RL, Leung LL, Harpel PC et al. Complex formation of platelet thrombospondin with plasminogen. Modulation of activation by tissue activator. J Clin Invest 1984;74:1625–1633.
22. Murata T, Nakashima Y, Yasunage C et al. Extracellular and cell-associated localizations of plasminogen activators and plasminogen activator inhibitor-1 in cultured endothelium. Exp Mol Pathol 1991;55:105–118.
23. Levin EG, Santell L. Association of a plasminogen activator inhibitor (PAI-1) with the growth substratum and membrane of human endothelial cells. J Cell Biol 1987;105:2543–2549.
24. Schleef RR, Podor TJ, Dunne E et al. The majority of type 1 plasminogen activator inhibitor associated with cultured human endothelial cells is located under the cells and is accessible to solution-phase tissue-type plasminogen activator. J Cell Biol 1990;110:155–163.
25. Carmeliet P, Collen D. Targeted gene manipulation and transfer of the plasminogen and coagulation systems in mice. Fibrinolysis 1996;10:195–213.
26. George EL, Georges-Labouesse EN, Patel-King RS et al. Defects in mesoderm, neural tube and vascular development in mouse embryos lacking fibronectin. Development 1993;119:1079–1091.
27. Zheng X, Saunders TL, Camper SA et al. Vitronectin is not essential for normal mammalian development and fertility. Proc Natl Acad Sci U S A 1995;92:12426–12430.
28. Noakes PG, Gautam M, Mudd J et al. Aberrant differentiation of neuromuscular junctions in mice lacking s-laminin/laminin beta 2. Nature 1995;374:258–262.
29. Miles LA, Plow EF. Binding and activation of plasminogen on the platelet surface. J Biol Chem 1985;260:4303–4311.
30. Miles LA, Plow EF. Receptor mediated binding of the fibrinolytic components, plasminogen and urokinase, to peripheral blood cells. Thromb Haemost 1987;58:936–942.
31. Gonias SL, Braud LL, Geary WA et al. Plasminogen binding to rat hepatocytes in primary culture and to thin slices of rat liver. Blood 1989;74:729–736.
32. Plow EF, Freaney DE, Plescia J et al. The plasminogen system and cell surfaces: evidence for plasminogen and urokinase receptors on the same cell type. J Cell Biol 1986;103:2411–2420.
33. Miles LA, Plow EF. Plasminogen receptors: ubiquitous sites for cellular regulation of fibrinolysis. Fibrinolysis 1988;2:61–71.
34. Burtin P, Chavanel G, Andre-Bougaran J et al. The plasmin system in human adenocarcinomas and their metastases. A comparative immunofluorescence study. Int J Cancer 1987;39:170–178.
35. Durliat M, Komano O, Correc P et al. Plasminogen receptors on rat colon carcinoma cells. Br J Cancer 1992;66:51–56.
36. Hembrough TA, Li L, Gonias SL. Cell-surface cytokeratin 8 is the major plasminogen receptor on breast cancer cells and is required for the accelerated activation of cell-associated plasminogen by tissue-type plasminogen activator. J Biol Chem 1996;271:25684–25691.
37. Camacho M, Fondanèche MC, Burtin P. Limited proteolysis of tumor cells increases their plasmin-binding ability. FEBS Lett 1989;245:21–24.
38. Miles LA, Dahlberg CM, Plow EF. The cell-binding domains of plasminogen and their function in plasma. J Biol Chem 1988;263:11928–11934.
39. Adelman B, Rizk A, Hanners E. Plasminogen interactions with platelets in plasma. Blood 1988;72:1530–1535.
40. Edelberg JM, Enghild JJ, Pizzo SV et al. Neonatal plasminogen displays altered cell surface binding and activation kinetics: correlation with increased glycosylation of the protein. J Clin Invest 1990;86:107–112.
41. Bauer PI, Machovich R, Buki KG et al. Interaction of plasmin with endothelial cells. Biochem J 1984;218:119–124.
42. Burtin P, Fondanèche MC. Receptor for plasmin on human carcinoma cells. J Natl Cancer Inst 1988;80:762–765.
43. Hajjar KA, Nachman RL. Endothelial cell-mediated conversion of Glu-plasminogen to Lys-plasminogen. J Clin Invest 1988;82:1769–1778.
44. Stephens RW, Pollanen J, Tapiovaara H et al. Activation of pro-urokinase and plasminogen on human sarcoma cells: a proteolytic system with surface-bound reactants. J Cell Biol 1989;108:1987–1995.
45. Ellis V, Behrendt N, Dano K. Plasminogen activation by receptor-bound urokinase. A kinetic study with both cell-associated and isolated receptor. J Biol Chem 1991;266:12752–12758.
46. Hall SW, Humphries JE, Gonias SL. Inhibition of cell surface receptor-bound plasmin by $\alpha_2$-antiplasmin and $\alpha_2$-macroglobulin. J Biol Chem 1991;266:12329–12336.
47. Miles LA, Dahlberg CM, Levin EG et al. Gangliosides interact directly with plasminogen and urokinase and may mediate binding of these fibrinolytic components to cells. Biochemistry 1989;28:9337–9343.
48. Miles LA, Dahlberg CM, Plescia J et al. Role of cell-surface lysines in plasminogen binding to cells: identification of alpha-enolase as a candidate plasminogen receptor. Biochemistry 1991;30:1682–1691.
49. Redlitz A, Tan AK, Eaton DL et al. Plasma carboxypeptidases as regulators of the plasminogen system. J Clin Invest 1995;96:2534–2538.
50. Miles LA, Ginsberg MH, White JG et al. Plasminogen interacts with human platelets through two distinct mechanisms. J Clin Invest 1986;77:2001–2009.
51. Merenmies J, Pihlaskari R, Laitinen J et al. 30-kDa heparin-binding protein of brain (amphoterin) involved in neurite outgrowth. Amino acid sequence and localization in the filopodia of the advancing plasma membrane. J Biol Chem 1991;266:16722–16729.
52. Parkkinen J, Rauvala H. Interactions of plasminogen and tissue plasminogen activated (t-PA) with amphoterin. Enhancement of t-PA-catalyzed plasminogen activation by amphoterin. J Biol Chem 1991;266:16730–16735.
53. Kanalas JJ, Makker SP. Identification of the rat Heymann nephritis autoantigen (GP330) as a receptor site for plasminogen. J Biol Chem 1991;266:10825–10829.
54. Kanalas JJ. Analysis of plasmin binding and urokinase activation of plasminogen bound to the Heymann nephritis autoantigen, gp330. Arch Biochem Biophys 1992;299:255–260.
55. Parkkinen J, Raulo E, Merenmies J et al. Amphoterin, the 30-kDa protein in a family of HMG1-type polypeptides. Enhanced expression in transformed cells, leading edge localization, and interactions with plasminogen activation. J Biol Chem 1993;268:19726–19738.
56. Hajjar KA, Jacovina AT, Chacko J. An endothelial cell receptor for plasminogen/tissue plasminogen activator. I. Identity with annexin II. J Biol Chem 1994;269:21191–21197.
57. Dudani AK, Ganz PR. Endothelial cell surface actin serves as a binding

site for plasminogen, tissue plasminogen activator and lipoprotein(a). Br J Haematol 1996;95:168–178.

58. Felez J, Miles LA, Fabregas P et al. Characterization of cellular binding sites and interactive regions within reactants required for enhancement of plasminogen activation by t-PA on the surface of leukocytic cells. Thromb Haemost 1996;76:577–584.

59. Lopez-Alemany R, Longstaff C, Fabregas P et al. Inhibition of plasmin generation on cell surfaces by monoclonal antibodies against a 55-60 Kda plasminogen receptor [Abstract]. Fibrinolysis 1996;10:5.

60. O'Reilly MS, Holmgren L, Shing Y et al. Angiostatin: a novel angiogenesis inhibitor that mediates the suppression of metastases by a Lewis lung carcinoma. Cell 1994;79:315–328.

61. Cao YH, Ji RW, Davidson D et al. Kringle domains of human angiostatin. Characterization of the anti-proliferative activity on endothelial cells. J Biol Chem 1996;271:29461–29467.

62. Cesarman GM, Guevara CA, Hajjar KA. An endothelial cell receptor for plasminogen/tissue plasminogen activator (t-PA). II. Annexin II-mediated enhancement of t-PA-dependent plasminogen activation. J Biol Chem 1994;269:21198–21203.

63. Dudani AK, Hashemi S, Aye MT et al. Identification of an endothelial cell surface protein that binds plasminogen. Mol Cell Biochem 1991;108:133–140.

64. Vaughan DE, Mendelsohn ME, Declerck PJ et al. Characterization of the binding of human tissue-type plasminogen activator to platelets. J Biol Chem 1989;264:15869–15874.

65. Felez J, Chanquia CJ, Levin EG et al. Binding of tissue plasminogen activator to human monocytes and monocytoid cells. Blood 1991;78:2318–2327.

66. Hart PH, Vitti GF, Burgess DR et al. Human monocytes can produce tissue-type plasminogen activator. J Exp Med 1989;169:1509–1514.

67. Hart PH, Burgess DR, Vitti GF et al. Interleukin-4 stimulates human monocytes to produce tissue-type plasminogen activator. Blood 1989;74:1222–1225.

68. Emeis JJ, Van den Hoogen CM, Jense D. Hepatic clearance of tissue-type plasminogen activator in rats. Thromb Haemost 1985;54:661–664.

69. Bounameaux H, Stassen JM, Seghers C et al. Influence of fibrin and liver blood flow on the turnover and the systematic fibrinogenolytic effects of recombinant human tissue-type plasminogen activator in rabbits. Blood 1986;67:1493–1497.

70. Garabedian HD, Gold HK, Leinbach RC et al. Dose-dependent thrombolysis, pharmacokinetics and hemostatic effects of recombinant human tissue–plasminogen activator for coronary thrombosis. Am J Cardiol 1986;58:673–679.

71. Einarsson M, Smedsrod B, Pertoft H. Uptake and degradation of tissue plasminogen activator in rat liver. Thromb Haemost 1988;59:474–479.

72. Kuiper J, Otter M, Rijken DC et al. Characterization of the interaction *in vivo* of tissue-type plasminogen activator with liver cells. J Biol Chem 1988;263:18220–18224.

73. Smedsrod B, Einarsson M. Clearance of tissue plasminogen activator by mannose and galactose receptors in the liver. Thromb Haemost 1990;63:60–66.

74. Owensby DA, Sobel BE, Schwartz AL. Receptor-mediated endocytosis of tissue-type plasminogen activator by the human hepatoma cell line Hep G2. J Biol Chem 1988;263:10587–10594.

75. Morton PA, Owensby DA, Wun TC et al. Identification of determinants involved in binding of tissue-type plasminogen activator-plasminogen activator inhibitor type 1 complexes to HepG2 cells. J Biol Chem 1990;265:14093–14099.

76. Bu G, Morton PA, Schwartz AL. Identification and partial characterization by chemical crosslinking of a binding protein for tissue-type plasminogen activator (t-PA) on rat hepatoma cells. A plasminogen activator inhibitor type 1-independent t-PA receptor. J Biol Chem 1992;267(22):15595–15602.

77. Otter M, Zocková P, Kuiper J et al. Isolation and characterization of the mannose receptor from human liver potentially involved in the plasma clearance of tissue-type plasminogen activator. Hepatology 1992;16:54–59.

78. Nguyen G, Self SJ, Camani C et al. Demonstration of a specific clearance receptor for tissue-type plasminogen activator on rat Novikoff hepatoma cells. J Biol Chem 1992;267:6249–6256.

79. Loskutoff DJ. The fibrinolytic system of cultured endothelial cells: deciphering the balance between plasminogen activation and inhibition. In: Davidson JF, Donati MB, Coccheri S, eds. Progress in fibrinolysis. 7th ed. New York: Churchill Livingstone, 1985; pp. 15–22.

80. Sakata Y, Okada M, Noro A et al. Interaction of tissue–type plasminogen activator and plasminogen activator inhibitor 1 on the surface of endothelial cells. J Biol Chem 1988;263:1960–1969.

81. Aerts RJ, Gillis K, Pannekoek H. Single-chain and two-chain tissue-type plasminogen activator (t-PA) bind differently to cultured human endothelial cells. Thromb Haemost 1989;62:699–703.

82. Russell ME, Quertermous T, Declerck PJ et al. Binding of tissue-type plasminogen activator with human endothelial cell monolayers. Characterization of the high affinity interaction with plasminogen activator inhibitor-1. J Biol Chem 1990;265:2569–2575.

83. Ramakrishnan V, Sinicropi DV, Dere R et al. Interaction of wild-type and catalytically inactive mutant forms of tissue-type plasminogen activator

with human umbilical vein endothelial cell monolayers. J Biol Chem 1990;265:2755–2762.

84. Salonen EM, Vaheri A, Pollanen J et al. Interaction of plasminogen activator inhibitor (PAI-1) with vitronectin. J Biol Chem 1989;264:6339–6343.

85. Mimuro J, Loskutoff DJ. Purification of a protein from bovine plasma that binds to type 1 plasminogen activator inhibitor and prevents its interaction with extracellular matrix. Evidence that the protein is vitronectin. J Biol Chem 1989;264:936–939.

86. Seiffert D, Wagner NN, Loskutoff D. Serum-derived vitronectin influences the pericellular distribution of type 1 plasminogen activator inhibitor. J Cell Biol 1990;111:1283–1291.

87. Hajjar KA. The endothelial cell tissue plasminogen activator receptor. Specific interaction with plasminogen. J Biol Chem 1991;266:21962–21970.

88. Beebe DP, Miles LA, Plow EF. A linear amino acid sequence involved in the interaction of t-PA with its endothelial cell receptor. Blood 1989;74:2034–2037.

89. Felez J, Chanquia CJ, Fabregas P et al. Competition between plasminogen and t-PA for cellular binding sites. Blood 1993;82:2433–2441.

90. Beebe DP, Wood LL, Moos M. Characterization of tissue plasminogen activator binding proteins isolated from endothelial cells and other cell types. Thromb Res 1990;59:339–350.

91. Plow EF, Felez J, Miles LA. Cellular regulation of fibrinolysis. Thromb Haemost 1991;66:32–36.

92. Vassalli JD, Baccino D, Belin D. A cellular binding site for the $M_r$ 55,000 form of the human plasminogen activator, urokinase. J Cell Biol 1985;100:86–92.

93. Blasi F. Surface receptors for urokinase plasminogen activator. Fibrinolysis 1988;2:73–84.

94. Blasi F, Stoppelli MP, Cubellis MV. The receptor for urokinase-plasminogen activator. J Cell Biochem 1986;32:179–186.

95. Nykjaer A, Moller B, Andreasen P et al. The urokinase receptor: an activation antigen coexpressed with the human t-cell specific serine proteinase (HTUSP-1) in activated t-lymphocytes [Abstract]. Fibrinolysis 1992;6:249.

96. Vaughan DE, Van Houtte EC, Collen D. Urokinase binds to platelets through a specific saturable, low affinity mechanism. Fibrinolysis 1990;4:141–146.

97. Needham GK, Nicholson S, Angus B et al. Relationship of membrane-bound-tissue type and urokinase type plasminogen activators in human breast cancers to estrogen and epidermal growth factor receptors. Cancer Res 1988;48:6603–6607.

98. Cohen RL, Xi XP, Crowley CW et al. Effects of urokinase receptor occupancy on plasmin generation and proteolysis of basement membrane by human tumor cells. Blood 1991;78:479–487.

99. Hollas W, Blasi F, Boyd D. Role of the urokinase receptor in facilitating extracellular matrix invasion by cultured colon cancer. Cancer Res 1991;51:3690–3695.

100. Schlechte W, Murano G, Boyd D. Examination of the role of the urokinase receptor in human colon cancer mediated laminin degradation. Cancer Res 1989;49:6064–6069.

101. Ossowski L, Clunie G, Masucci MT et al. *In vivo* paracrine interaction between urokinase and its receptor: effect on tumor cell invasion. J Cell Biol 1991;115:1107–1112.

102. Stoppelli MP, Corti A, Soffientini A et al. Differentiation-enhanced binding of the aminoterminal fragment of human urokinase plasminogen activator to a specific receptor on U937 monocytes. Proc Natl Acad Sci U S A 1985;82:4939–4943.

103. Picone R, Kajtaniak EL, Nielsen LS et al. Regulation of urokinase receptors in monocyte-like U937 cells by phorbol ester phorbol myristate acetate. J Cell Biol 1989;108:693–702.

104. Lund LR, Ronne E, Roldan AL et al. Urokinase receptor mRNA level and gene transcription are strongly and rapidly increased by phorbol myristate acetate in human monocyte-like U937 cells. J Biol Chem 1991;266:5177–5181.

105. Estreicher A, Wohlwend A, Belin D et al. Characterization of the cellular binding site for the urokinase-type plasminogen activator. J Biol Chem 1989;264:1180–1189.

106. Appella E, Robinson EA, Ullrich SJ et al. The receptor-binding sequence of urokinase. A biological function for the growth-factor module of proteases. J Biol Chem 1987;262:4437–4440.

107. Fowler BJ, Mackman N, Parmer RJ et al. Molecular basis for the species specificity of single chain urokinase (Scu-PA) binding to the urokinase receptor (u-PAR) [Abstract]. Circulation 1996;94:I-512.

108. Cubellis MV, Nolli ML, Cassani G et al. Binding of single-chain prourokinase to the urokinase receptor of human U937 cells. J Biol Chem 1986;261:15819–15822.

109. Bajpai A, Baker JB. Urokinase binding sites on human foreskin cells. Evidence for occupancy with endogenous urokinase. Biochem Biophys Res Commun 1985;133:994–1000.

110. Cubellis MV, Andreasen P, Ragno P et al. Accessibility of receptor-bound urokinase to type-1 plasminogen activator inhibitor. Proc Natl Acad Sci U S A 1989;86:4828–4832.

111. Cubellis MV, Wun TC, Blasi F. Receptor-mediated internalization and deg-

radation of urokinase is caused by its specific inhibitor PAI-1. EMBO J 1990;9:1079–1085.

112. Olson D, Pollanen J, Hoyer-Hansen G et al. Internalization of the urokinase-plasminogen activator inhibitor type-1 complex is mediated by the urokinase receptor. J Biol Chem 1992;267:9129–9133.

113. Conese M, Olson D, Blasi F. Protease nexin-1-urokinase complexes are internalized and degraded through a mechanism that requires both urokinase receptor and $\alpha_2$-macroglobulin receptor. J Biol Chem 1994;269:17886–17892.

114. Kounnas MZ, Henkin J, Argraves WS et al. Low density lipoprotein receptor-related protein/$\alpha_2$-macroglobulin receptor mediates cellular uptake of pro-urokinase. J Biol Chem 1993;268:21862–21867.

115. Moestrup SK, Holtet TL, Etzerodt M et al. $\alpha_2$-macroglobulin proteinase complexes, plasminogen activator inhibitor type-1-plasminogen activator complexes, and receptor-associated protein bind to a region of the $\alpha_2$-macroglobulin receptor containing a cluster of eight complement-type repeats. J Biol Chem 1993;268:13691–13696.

116. Heegaard CW, Simonsen AC, Oka K et al. Very low density lipoprotein receptor binds and mediates endocytosis of urokinase-type plasminogen activator-type-1 plasminogen activator inhibitor complex. J Biol Chem 1995;270:20855–20861.

117. Behrendt N, Ronne E, Ploug M et al. The human receptor for urokinase plasminogen activator. NH2 terminal amino acid sequence and glycosylation variants. J Biol Chem 1990;265:6453–6460.

118. Behrendt N, Ploug M, Patthy L et al. The ligand-binding domain of the cell surface receptor for urokinase-type plasminogen activator. J Biol Chem 1991;266:7842–7847.

119. Roldan AL, Cubellis MV, Masucci MT et al. Cloning and expression of the receptor for human urokinase plasminogen activator, a central molecule in cell surface, plasmin dependent proteolysis. EMBO J 1990;9:467–474.

120. Nielsen LS, Kellerman GM, Behrendt N et al. A 55,000-60,000 Mr receptor protein for urokinase-type plasminogen activator. Identification in human tumor cell lines and partial purification. J Biol Chem 1988;263:2358–2363.

121. Ploug M, Ronne E, Behrendt N et al. Cellular receptor for urokinase plasminogen activator. Carboxylterminal processing and membrane anchoring by glycosyl-phosphatidylinositol. J Biol Chem 1991;266:1926–1933.

122. Ploug M, Plesner T, Ronne E et al. The receptor for urokinase-type plasminogen activator is deficient on peripheral blood leukocytes in individuals with paroxysmal nocturnal hemoglobinuria. Blood 1992;79:1447–1455.

123. Behrendt N, Ronne E, Dano K. Domain interplay in the urokinase receptor. Requirement for the third domain in high affinity ligand binding and demonstration of ligand contact sites in distinct receptor domains. J Biol Chem 1996;271:22885–22894.

124. Fibbi G, Ziche M, Morbidelli L et al. Interaction of urokinase with specific receptors stimulates mobilization of bovine adrenal capillary endothelial cells. Exp Cell Res 1988;179:385–395.

125. Kirchheimer JC, Wojta J, Christ G et al. Mitogenic effect of urokinase on malignant and unaffected adjacent human renal cells. Carcinogenesis 1988;9:2121–2123.

126. Rabbani SA, Desjardins J, Bell AW et al. An aminoterminal fragment of urokinase isolated from a prostate cancer cell line (PC-3) is mitogenic for osteoblast-like cells. Biochem Biophys Res Commun 1990;173:1058–1064.

127. Nusrat AR, Chapman HA Jr. An autocrine role for urokinase in phorbol ester-mediate differentiation of myeloid cell lines. J Clin Invest 1991;87:1091–1097.

128. Kirchheimer JC, Remold HG, Wanivenhaus A et al. Increased proteolytic activity on the surface of monocytes from individuals with rheumatoid arthritis. Arthritis Rheum 1991;34:1430–1433.

129. Rabbani SA, Mazar AP, Bernier SM et al. Structural requirements for the growth factor activity of the aminoterminal domain of urokinase. J Biol Chem 1992;267:14151–14156.

130. Odekon LE, Sato Y, Rifkin DB. Urokinase-type plasminogen activator mediates basic fibroblast growth factor–induced bovine endothelial cell migration independent of its proteolytic activity. J Cell Physiol 1992;150:258–263.

131. Del Rosso M, Anichini E, Pedersen N et al. Urokinase–urokinase receptor interaction: non-mitogenic signal transduction in human epidermal cells. Biochem Biophys Res Commun 1993;190:347–352.

132. Dumler I, Petri T, Schleuning WD. Interaction of urokinase-type plasminogen activator (u-PAR) with its cellular receptor (u-PAR) induces phosphorylation on tyrosine 18 Kda protein. FEBS Lett 1993;322:37–40.

133. Dumler I, Petri T, Schleuning WD. Induction of c-fos gene expression by urokinase-type plasminogen activator in human ovarian cancer cells. FEBS Lett 1994;343:103–106.

134. Gyetko MR, Todd RF,III, Wilkinson CC et al. The urokinase receptor is required for human monocyte chemotaxis in vitro. J Clin Invest 1994;93:1380–1387.

135. Anichini E, Fibbi G, Pucci M et al. Production of second messengers following chemotactic and mitogenic urokinase-receptor interaction in human fibroblasts and mouse fibroblasts transfected with human urokinase receptor. Exp Cell Res 1994;213:438–448.

136. Rao NK, Shi GP, Chapman HA. Urokinase receptor is a multifunctional protein: influence of receptor occupancy on macrophage gene expression. J Clin Invest 1995;96:465–474.

137. Xue W, Kindzelskii A, Todd RF III et al. Physical association of complement receptor type 3 and urokinase-type plasminogen activator receptor in neutrophil membranes. J Immunol 1994;152:4630–4640.

138. Cao D, Mizukami IF, Garni-Wagner BA et al. Human urokinase-type plasminogen activator primes neutrophils for superoxide anion releases. Possible roles of complement receptor type 3 and calcium. J Immunol 1995;154:1817–1829.

139. Bohuslav J, Horejsí V, Hansmann C et al. Urokinase plasminogen activator receptor, $\beta2$-integrins, and Src-kinases within a single receptor complex of human monocytes. J Exp Med 1995;181:1381–1390.

140. Reinartz J, Schafer B, Batrla R et al. Plasmin abrogates alpha beta$_3$ mediated adhesion of a human keratinocyte cell line (HaCaT) to vitronectin. Exp Cell Res 1995;220:274–282.

141. Wei Y, Lukashev M, Simon DI et al. Regulation of integrin function by the urokinase receptor. Science 1996;273:1551–1555.

142. Stefansson S, Lawrence DA. The serpin PAI-1 inhibits cell migration by blocking integrin alpha v beta$_3$ binding to vitronectin. Nature 1996;383:441–443.

143. Bianchi E, Ferrero E, Fazioli F et al. Integrin-dependent induction of functional urokinase receptors in primary T lymphocytes. J Clin Invest 1996;98:1133–1141.

144. Simon DI, Rao NK, Xu H et al. Mac-1 (CD11b/CD18) and the urokinase receptor (CD87) form a functional unit on monocytic cells. Blood 1996;88:3185–3194.

145. Wong WSF, Simon DI, Rosoff PM et al. Mechanisms of pertussis toxin–induced myelomonocytic cell adhesion: role of Mac-1 (CD11b/CD18) and urokinase receptor (CD87). Immunology 1996;88:90–97.

146. Sitrin RG, Todd RF,III, Albrecht E et al. The urokinase receptor (CD87) facilitates CD11b/CD18-mediated adhesion of human monocytes. J Clin Invest 1996;97:1942–1951.

147. Haas TA, Plow EF. Integrin-ligand interactions: a year in Review. Curr Opin Cell Biol 1994;6:656–662.

148. Waltz DA, Chapman HA. Reversible cellular adhesion to vitronectin linked to urokinase receptor occupancy. J Biol Chem 1994;269:14746–14750.

149. Wei Y, Waltz DA, Rao N et al. Identification of the urokinase receptor as an adhesion receptor for vitronectin. J Biol Chem 1994;269:32380–32388.

150. Kanse SM, Kost C, Wilhelm OG et al. The urokinase receptor is a major vitronectin-binding protein on endothelial cells. Exp Cell Res 1996;224:344–353.

151. Loridon-Rosa B, Vielh P, Cuadrado C et al. Comparative distribution of fibronectin and vitronectin in human breast and colon carcinomas. An immunofluorescence study. J Clin Pathol 1988;90:7–16.

152. Niculescu F, Rus HG, Porutiu D et al. Immunoelectron-microscopic localization of S-protein/vitronectin in human atherosclerotic wall. Atherosclerosis 1989;78:197–203.

153. Felding-Habermann B, Cheresh DA. Vitronectin and its receptors. Curr Opin Cell Biol 1993;5:864–868.

154. Mimuro J, Loskutoff DJ. Binding of type 1 plasminogen activator inhibitor to the extracellular matrix of cultured bovine endothelial cells. J Biol Chem 1989;264:5058–5063.

155. Deng G, Curriden SA, Wang SJ et al. Is plasminogen activator inhibitor-1 the molecular switch that governs urokinase receptor-mediated cell adhesion and release? J Cell Biol 1996;134:1563–1571.

156. Mignatti P, Mazzieri R, Rifkin DB. Expression of the urokinase receptor in vascular endothelial cells is stimulated by basic fibroblast growth factor. J Cell Biol 1991;113:1193–1202.

157. Barnathan ES. Characterization and regulation of the urokinase receptor of human endothelial cells. Fibrinolysis 1992;6(1):1–9.

158. Ellis V, Scully MF, Kakkar VV. Plasminogen activation initiated by single-chain urokinase-type plasminogen activator. J Biol Chem 1989;264:2185–2188.

159. Manchanda N, Schwartz BS. Single chain urokinase. Augmentation of enzymatic activity upon binding to monocytes. J Biol Chem 1991;266:14580–14584.

160. Bruckner A, Filderman AE, Kirchheimer JC et al. Endogenous receptor-bound urokinase mediates tissue invasion of the human lung carcinoma cell lines A549 and Calu-1. Cancer Res 1992;52:3043–3047.

161. Bajpai A, Baker JB. Cryptic urokinase binding sites on human foreskin fibroblasts. Biochem Biophys Res Commun 1985;133:475–482.

162. Stoppelli MP, Tacchetti C, Cubellis MV et al. Autocrine saturation of pro-urokinase receptors on human A431 cells. Cell 1986;45:675–684.

163. Huarte J, Belin D, Bosco D et al. Plasminogen activator and mouse spermatozoa: urokinase synthesis in the male genital tract and binding of the enzyme to the sperm cell surface. J Cell Biol 1987;104:1281–1289.

164. Estreicher A, Mühlhauser J, Carpentier JL et al. The receptor for urokinase type plasminogen activator polarizes expression of the protease to the leading edge of migrating monocytes and promotes degradation of enzyme inhibitor complexes. J Cell Biol 1990;111:783–792.

165. Hebert CA, Baker JB. Linkage of extracellular plasminogen activator to

the fribroblast cytoskeleton: colocalization of cell surface urokinase with vinculin. J Cell Biol 1988;106:1241–1247.

166. Pollanen J, Hedman K, Nielsen LS et al. Ultrastructural localization of plasma membrane-associated urokinase–type plasminogen activator at focal contacts. J Cell Biol 1988;106:87–95.

167. Bugge TH, Suh TT, Flick MJ et al. The receptor for urokinase-type plasminogen activator is not essential for mouse development or fertility. J Biol Chem 1995;270:16886–16894.

168. Dewerchin M, Nuffelen AV, Wallays G et al. Generation and characterization of urokinase receptor-deficient mice. J Clin Invest 1996;97:870–878.

169. Carmeliet P, Schoonjans L, Kieckens L et al. Physiological consequences of loss of plasminogen activator gene function in mice. Nature 1994;368:419–424.

170. Bugge TH, Flick MJ, Danton MJS et al. Urokinase-type plasminogen activator is effective in fibrin clearance in the absence of its receptor or tissue-type plasminogen activator. Proc Natl Acad Sci U S A 1996;93:5899–5904.

171. Birkedal-Hansen H. Proteolytic remodeling of extracellular matrix. Curr Opin Cell Biol 1995;7:728–735.

172. Willenbrock F, Murphy G. Structure-function relationships in the tissue inhibitors of metalloproteinases. Am J Respir Crit Care Med 1994;150:165–170.

173. Woessner JF Jr. The family of matrix metalloproteinases [Review]. Ann NY Acad Sci 1994;732:11–21.

174. Dollery CM, McEwan JR, Henney AM. Matrix metalloproteinases and cardiovascular disease. Circ Res 1995;77:863–868.

175. Libby P, Sukhova G, Lee RT et al. Cytokines regulate vascular functions related to stability of the atherosclerotic plaque. J Cardiovasc Pharmacol 1995;25(Suppl 2)9–12.

176. Brooks PC. Cell adhesion molecules in angiogenesis. Cancer Metastasis Rev 1996;15:187–194.

177. Marcotte PA, Kozan IM, Dorwin SA et al. The matrix metalloproteinase pump-1 catalyzes formation of low-molecular-weight (pro)urokinase in cultures of normal human kidney cells. J Biol Chem 1992;267:13803–13806.

# CHAPTER 19

# ENDOTHELIUM-DERIVED VASOACTIVE FACTORS

Richard A. Cohen

## INTRODUCTION

It has been known for more than a century that blood vessels play an active role in the regulation of blood flow to the organs of the body. Cardiovascular research has established that neural, humoral, and local control mechanisms play a role in that regulation. An understanding of neural control of the vasculature grew out of early studies of the effects of denervation on blood flow to skin and other organs. Using pharmacologic antagonists, subsequent studies of the adrenal gland hormone, epinephrine; the neurotransmitter, norepinephrine; and the renin-angiotensin axis led to an understanding of the balance between neural reflexes and humoral agents that regulate blood pressure. Aside from these neural and humoral mechanisms, studies of exercising skeletal and cardiac muscle indicated that local tissue metabolism had an overriding influence on vascular resistance and blood flow.

Through the 1970s the endothelium was considered to be an inactive cell with respect to regulation of blood flow, despite the evidence that an intact endothelial lining prevented platelet aggregation (1). Indeed, it was recognized that injury of the endothelial cell with resultant platelet aggregation and release of platelet vasoconstrictor factors was an important hemostatic mechanism. However, through the work of Robert Furchgott, it became evident in 1980 that the endothelial cell plays a major role in local control of blood flow (2). He discovered that mechanical denudation of the endothelium from isolated arteries eliminated the relaxation to many humoral agents such as acetylcholine (Fig. 19.1), 5-hydroxytryptamine (Fig. 19.2), and bradykinin (Tables 19.1 and 19.2). Furchgott made the important observation that an artery with intact endothelium could relax another artery from which the endothelium had been denuded, simply by apposing the intimal surfaces of the two arteries or by superfusing the perfusate of the intact artery onto the denuded artery. Thus he demonstrated the existence of a diffusible endothelium-derived vasodilator substance that he termed "endothelium-derived relaxing factor." Furchgott (3), Ignarro et al (4, 5), and Palmer et al (6) characterized the chemical and physical properties of this relaxing factor as being identical to those of nitric oxide. These properties include a half-life of about 5 seconds under physiologic conditions, inactivation by superoxide anion, prolongation of half-life by superoxide dismutase, scavenging by hemoglobin, and the ability to stimulate soluble guanylyl cyclase. It was then found that nitric oxide was synthesized in macrophages and endothelial cells from the amino acid, L-arginine. The physiologic importance of nitric oxide became apparent following the observation that L-arginine analogs such as L-N$^G$-monomethyl arginine (L-NMMA), which competitively inhibit substrate utilization by the enzyme, cause vasoconstriction and increase blood pressure (7–10). These studies indicated that a tonic, local production of nitric oxide is a major mechanism regulating blood flow (Fig. 19.3). Since these original observations, it has become evident that nitric oxide participates in other far-ranging physiologic functions, including regulating proliferation of vascular

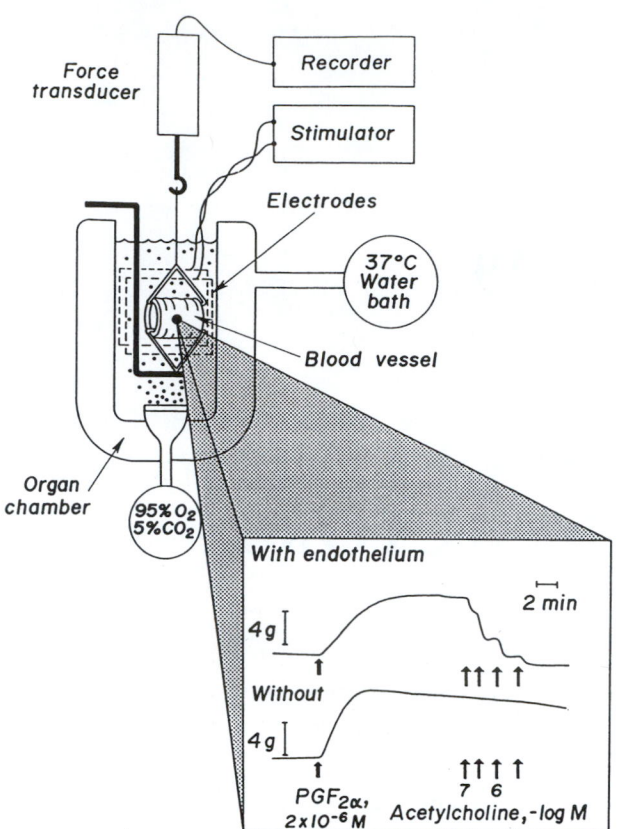

**FIGURE 19.1.** Apparatus for measurement of physiologic responses of isolated ring segments of blood vessels. The recording shows an experiment like that of Furchgott and Zawadski (2) in which it is demonstrated in a ring of dog coronary artery contracted with prostaglandin $F_{2\alpha}$ ($PGF_{2\alpha}$) that the concentration-dependent relaxation caused by acetylcholine depends on an intact endothelial cell layer. The lower ring, which was denuded of endothelium prior to mounting in the organ chamber, does not relax. (From Vanhoutte PM, Cohen RA. Effects of acetylcholine on the coronary artery. Fed Proc 1984;43:2878–2880, by permission of the Federation of American Societies of Experimental Biology.)

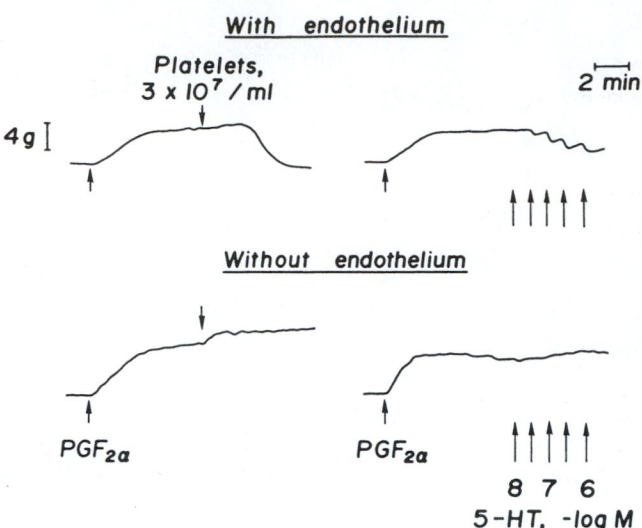

**FIGURE 19.2.** Recordings of dog coronary artery rings mounted in a chamber like that shown in Fig. 19.1, which show responses to aggregating platelets and 5-hydroxytryptamine (5-HT) in rings contracted with $PGF_{2\alpha}$. In a ring with intact endothelium, platelets cause relaxation, which as shown in the ring without endothelium below, is endothelium-dependent. In the ring without endothelium (lower), contraction occurs. The response to platelets may be attributable, in part, to the release by the platelets of 5-HT. As shown in the rings at the right, 5-HT also causes endothelium-dependent relaxation, as well as contraction of the ring denuded of endothelium. (From Cohen RA, Shepherd JT, Vanhoutte PM. Inhibitory role of the endothelium in the response of isolated coronary arteries to platelets. Science 1983;221:273–274; and Cohen RA, Shepherd JT, Vanhoutte PM. 5-Hydroxytryptamine can mediate endothelium-dependent relaxation of coronary arteries. Am J Physiol 1983;245:H1077–H1080, by permission of the American Association for the Advancement of Science and the American Physiological Society.)

**TABLE 19.1.** Endothelium-Derived Vasoactive Factors

Nitric Oxide
Arachidonic-Acid Metabolites
  $PGH_2$
  $PGI_2$
  HETEs
  EETs
EDHF
Endothelin
Angiotensin II
Bradykinin

*$PGH_2$, prostaglandin endoperoxide; $PGI_2$, prostacyclin; HETE, hydroxyeicosatetraenoic acid; EET, epoxyeicosatrienoic acid; EDHF, endothelium-derived hyperpolarizing factor.*

**TABLE 19.2.** Humoral Stimuli of Endothelial Cell Vasoactive Factors

| Stimulus | Endothelial Cell Receptor | References |
|---|---|---|
| Acetylcholine | $M_2$ | (200, 201) |
| Histamine | $H_{1,2}$ | (202–204) |
| Arginine vasopressin | $VP_1$ | (74) |
| Norepinephrine/ epinephrine | Alpha$_2$ | (205) |
| Bradykinin | $B_2$ | (206, 207) |
| Adenosine di-, triphosphate | $P_{2y}$ | (208, 209) |
| 5-Hydroxytryptamine | $5\text{-}HT_1$ | (210, 211) |
| Thrombin | T | (212) |
| Endothelin | $ET_B$ | (213) |
| Insulin | I | (214, 215) |

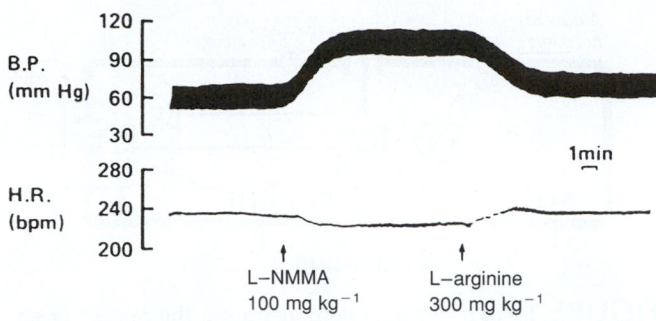

**FIGURE 19.3.** Recording of blood pressure and heart rate in the anesthetized rat demonstrating the hypertensive response to the nitric oxide synthase inhibitor, L-N$^G$-monomethyl arginine (100 mg/kg i.v.). The nitric oxide synthase inhibitor increases blood pressure and causes a reflex decrease in heart rate. The effect is reversed by infusion of the substrate for nitric oxide synthase, L-arginine (300 mg/kg iv). (From Rees DD, Palmer RM, Moncada S. Role of endothelium-derived nitric oxide in the regulation of blood pressure. Proc Natl Acad Sci U S A 1989;86:3375–3378, by permission of the Proceedings of the National Academy of Science.)

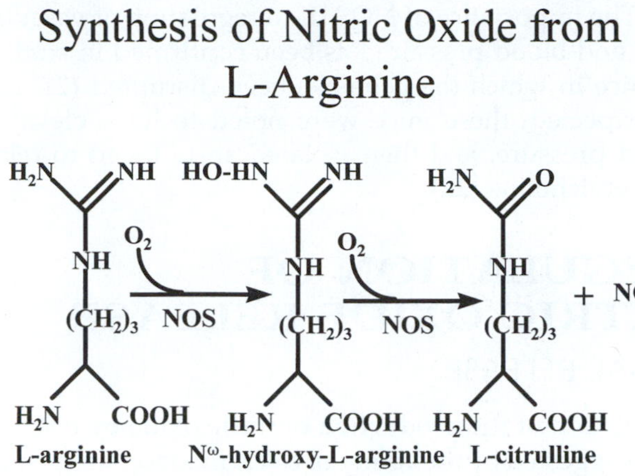

cells, platelet aggregation, and immune responses, and also that it can act as a neurotransmitter. The purpose of this chapter is to review the vasoactive functions of the endothelium, the mechanisms of production and action of nitric oxide, and the role of other vasoactive factors (Table 19.1). Because of the present context, special emphasis has been placed on the interplay among the endothelium, other cells within the vascular wall, and circulating blood platelets and leukocytes (11).

# ENDOTHELIAL-CELL SYNTHESIS OF NITRIC OXIDE

## NITRIC-OXIDE SYNTHASE

Nitric oxide is a free radical with an unpaired electron and is produced by a family of three enzymes (12). These three isoforms share about 50% amino acid homology and are encoded by three different genes residing on different chromosomes. In addition to the endothelial isoform (eNOS or NOS III), neuronal (nNOS or NOS I) and inducible isoforms (iNOS or NOS II) also exist. Although all three isoforms may exist in blood vessels, NOS III in endothelial cells accounts for the majority of nitric oxide production in normal arteries. Each of the synthases catalyze a five-electron oxidation of one of the two basic guanidino nitrogen atoms of L-arginine to nitric oxide, leaving L-citrulline (Fig. 19.4). N$^\omega$-hydroxy-L-arginine is althought to be an intermediate (12). NOS III, like the other isoforms, bears homology to cytochrome P$_{450}$ reductases that require flavin nucleotides (FMN and FAD), NADPH, and oxygen for activity. The

## Synthesis of Nitric Oxide from L-Arginine

**FIGURE 19.4.** Diagram of nitric oxide synthesis by nitric oxide synthase (NOS) showing the chemical structures of the substrate L-arginine, the proposed intermediate N$^\omega$-hydroxy-L-arginine, and the products, nitric oxide and L-citrulline.

enzymes require the cofactor, tetrahydrobiopterin (13), and their activity may be under negative feedback control by nitric oxide itself (14). NOS III in endothelium is doubly acetylated, being both myristoylated and palmitoylated. N-myristoylation is necessary for its membrane association in the Golgi apparatus (15). Palmitoylation is involved in targeting the enzyme to plasma membrane structures termed caveoli (15, 16). Tyrosine phosphorylation of the enzyme was found to lead to association with caveolin in these structures and to affect the activity of the enzyme (17). In addition, NOS III is rapidly phosphorylated at serine residues during hormone-induced activation. Accompanying this chemical change, the enzyme, which is normally associated with the plasma membrane of endothelial cells under basal conditions, is translocated to the cytoplasm (18). In addition to these metabolic factors, NOS III is regulated by virtue of its requirement for calmodulin and its resultant responsiveness to intracellular-calcium levels (see below).

Over the longer term, NOS III protein expression may be regulated, leading to chronic changes in endothelial cell function. For instance, increased shear stress, which regulates endothelial cell calcium and nitric oxide synthesis acutely (see below), also up-regulates enzyme expression chronically (13) and accounts for enhanced, endothelium-dependent vasodilation associated with exercise training (19). In addition, inflammatory cytokines have dual effects on NOS III activity. During the first 24 hours of exposure under culture conditions, cytokines increase GTP cyclohydrolase I, which is the rate-limiting enzyme for the synthesis of tetrahydrobiopterin, and thus enhances enzyme activity (20). Simultaneously, there is an increased degradation of NOS III mRNA, leading to decreased enzyme activity in 48 to 72 hours (20).

The importance of NOS III to regulation of vascular tone and blood pressure has been confirmed in studies of mice in which the gene has been disrupted (21, 22). As expected, these mice were noted to have elevated blood pressure, and their isolated aorta failed to relax to acetylcholine (22).

# REGULATION OF NITRIC OXIDE RELEASE

## BASAL RELEASE

Regulation of the production of nitric oxide by calcium was suggested by the ability of calcium ionophores, such as A23187, to mimic hormone-stimulated nitric oxide production, as well as by the regulation of NOS III by calmodulin. Even in the absence of hormonal stimulation, nitric oxide is released from endothelial cells. This basal release of the vasodilator attenuates contractions of smooth muscle accounting for the fact that isolated arteries from which the endothelium has been removed, or in which NOS III has been inhibited, contract to a greater degree (23–26). This basal release of nitric oxide probably occurs as a result of the fact that calmodulin binds to the enzyme even at resting intracellular-calcium levels (27).

As in all cells, intracellular-calcium levels in the endothelium are maintained under resting conditions by a balance that exists between the influx of calcium into the cell and transport mechanisms that remove calcium, either by pumping it into intracellular storage compartments or out of the cell. Of therapeutic importance is the fact that endothelial cells lack L-type calcium channels. Therefore the common, clinically used, L-type calcium-channel antagonists do not block the calcium-conducting ion channels in endothelium. This allows for their therapeutic use without interfering with a vital vasodilator function. The basal level of intracellular calcium, and therefore nitric oxide release, depends on the electro-physiologic properties of the calcium-conducting ion channels in the endothelium which dictate that a greater influx of calcium occurs at more negative membrane potentials (28). Thus hyperpolarization of the endothelial cell membrane promotes calcium influx and increases intracellular-calcium levels (Fig. 19.5) (29).

## SHEAR STRESS

Control of membrane potential is a key mechanism whereby shear and stretch forces on the endothelial cell surface increase the release of nitric oxide (see Chapter 20). By poorly understood molecular mechanisms, shear stress activates the opening of potassium channels, which results in hyperpolarization, increases influx of calcium, and increases intracellular-calcium levels (30, 31). The greater nitric oxide production, in part, explains

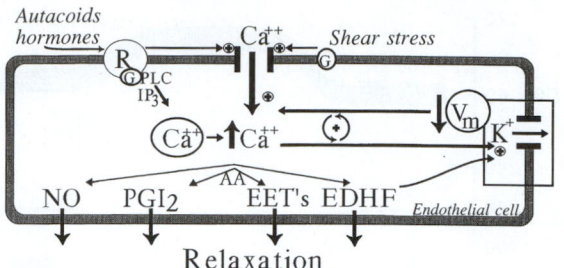

**FIGURE 19.5.** Scheme demonstrating the release of endothelium-derived vasoactive factors, including nitric oxide (NO), prostacyclin (PGI$_2$), and epoxyeicosatrienoic acids (EETs), as well as endothelium-derived hyperpolarizing factor(s) (EDHF). Hormones and autacoids, acting at endothelial membrane receptors (R), or shear stress causes G protein (G)–mediated increases in calcium (Ca$^{++}$) influx and phospholipase C (PLC)–mediated hydrolysis of phosphotidyl inositol bisphosphate, yielding inositol triphosphate (IP$_3$), which releases calcium from intracellular stores. The resulting increase in calcium activates nitric oxide synthase to produce nitric oxide and phospholipase A$_2$ to release arachidonic acid (AA). The released arachidonic acid is converted to PGI$_2$ and EETs. The endothelial cell membrane potential (Vm) is hyperpolarized possibly due to activation of calcium-dependent potassium (K$^+$) channels, either by the rise in calcium or by the vasoactive factors acting in an autocrine manner. The resulting hyperpolarization accentuates calcium influx due to the increased electrochemical gradient for calcium and thereby, through positive feedback, potentiates the release of endothelium-derived mediators. (From Cohen RA, Vanhoutte PM. Endothelium-dependent hyperpolarization. Beyond nitric oxide and cyclic GMP. Circulation 1995;92:3337–3349; reproduced by permission of the American Heart Association.)

the vasodilation accompanying increased blood flow or pulsations (32–37). This is a sensitive mechanism that can account for an increase in nitric oxide release associated with small changes in shear stress introduced by a small increase in viscosity of the arterial perfusate (Fig. 19.6) (35). It is therefore likely that changes in shear stress associated with anemia or polycythemia exert effects on endothelial cells.

Small resistance vessels in exercising muscle dilate to admit more oxygen-carrying blood in response to the increased metabolism within the muscle. The resulting increased blood flow increases shear forces in upstream arteries, thereby causing vasodilation via the local release of nitric oxide. This positive-feedback mechanism in feeder arteries, termed "flow-mediated vasodilation," may account for a substantial portion of the increased blood flow to exercising or ischemic muscle (38, 39). In exercising forearm muscle, blood flow is decreased and oxygen extraction increased by 15 to 25% when nitric oxide synthase inhibitors are infused (40). Ischemic hyperemia is decreased by about 25% by the inhibitors (41). These findings infer that nitric oxide re-

**Effect of Dextran on Endothelium-derived Relaxing Factor**

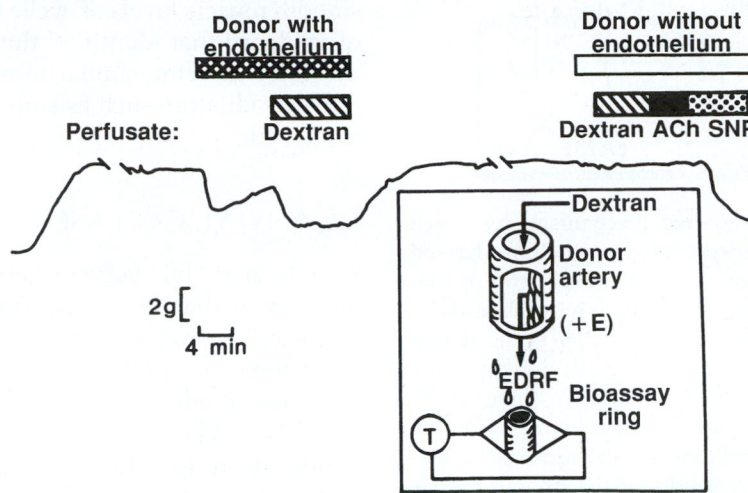

**FIGURE 19.6.**   The effect of shear stress on the release of nitric oxide. A recording of tension (T) is shown of a rabbit carotid artery ring without endothelium (inset) on which nitric oxide (EDRF) is superfused from a donor segment of carotid artery with intact endothelium. After the ring is contracted with phenylephrine, the perfusate of the donor artery is shown to relax the ring due to the basal release of nitric oxide. The release of nitric oxide and the associated relaxation is increased by raising the viscosity of the artery perfusate with dextran and causing a threefold increase in shear stress. The release of nitric oxide and the effect of dextran is then shown to be endothelium-dependent by showing that dextran or acetylcholine (ACh) has no effect when perfused through a donor without endothelium. The artery relaxes to sodium nitroprusside (SNP), a nitric oxide do not.

lease normally contributes significantly to the physiologic function of exercising muscle.

## HUMORAL STIMULATION

Many substances stimulate receptors on endothelial cells to increase the release of nitric oxide (Table 19.2). Stimulation of these receptors increases intracellular calcium by two mechanisms. The first is the result of receptor, G protein–dependent activation of phospholipase C; elaboration of inositol triphosphate; and release of calcium from endoplasmic reticulum stores (42). The second mechanism results from the calcium influx that occurs in response to calcium-store depletion (43). Although hormone stimulation of endothelial cells by agents such as acetylcholine or bradykinin has been the most commonly used tool in the study of endothelium-dependent vasodilation, there is actually no conclusive evidence that these agents activate endothelial cells under normal physiologic circumstances. Thus the neurotransmitter, acetylcholine, has not yet been demonstrated conclusively to activate endothelial cells after its release from cholinergic nerves. An important, relevant physiologic role for such a mechanism might be vasodilation by acetylcholine released at motor endplates in skeletal muscle where it might cause an increase in blood flow to meet the metabolic requirement of the working muscle (44, 45). Also, little evidence exists that endogenous bradykinin stimulates endothelial cells

under ordinary physiologic conditions. However, the clinically relevant vasodilator response to angiotensin-converting enzyme inhibitors in individuals with heart failure or hypertension may be the result of the accumulation of bradykinin, which is normally degraded by the kininase activity of angiotensin-converting enzyme (see below) (46).

# REGULATION OF VASCULAR TONE BY NITRIC OXIDE

The vasodilatory action of nitric oxide depends on the contractile state of the vascular smooth muscle (Fig. 19.7). This is dictated primarily by the intracellular-calcium level, which, in turn, regulates contractile protein activity. In resting smooth muscle there is little if any effect of nitric oxide on intracellular-calcium levels or contractile tone. The principle action of nitric oxide is to reduce an already elevated intracellular-calcium level or to prevent a rise in the level caused by contractile agents or myogenic mechanisms (47). Although reduction of intracellular-calcium levels can largely account for vasodilation to nitric oxide, an additional mechanism of relaxation is the reduction of calcium sensitivity of smooth muscle contractile proteins (48). Nitric oxide relaxes smooth muscle whether it is contracted as a result of depolarization-induced activation of L-type calcium

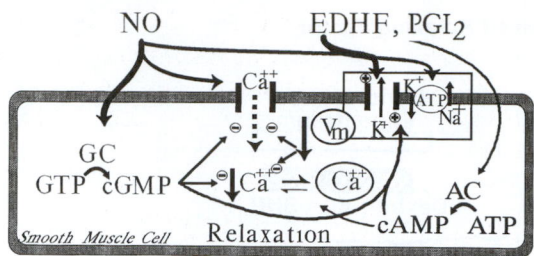

**FIGURE 19.7.** Scheme showing mechanisms by which vascular smooth muscle cells respond to endothelium-derived vasoactive factors, including nitric oxide, EDHF, and prostacyclin (PGI$_2$). Nitric oxide stimulates guanylyl cyclase (GC), which converts guanosine triphosphate (GTP) to cyclic guanosine monophosphate (cGMP). The cyclic nucleotide phosphorylates kinases, which favor reuptake of calcium, increase calcium extrusion from the cell and inhibit calcium influx, all leading to a decrease in intracellular free calcium and relaxation. Cyclic GMP may also hyperpolarize the smooth muscle cell by activating potassium channels. Nitric oxide may also have direct calcium inhibitory effects, as well as direct hyperpolarizing actions via activation of potassium channels or the Na$^+$/K$^+$ ATPase. EDHF may hyperpolarize smooth muscle cells by activating potassium channels or possibly Na$^+$/K$^+$ ATPase. The resulting hyperpolarization decreases smooth cell calcium levels by inhibiting influx through voltage-dependent calcium channels and favoring the reuptake of calcium into intracellular stores and extrusion of calcium from the cell, resulting in a decrease in intracellular free calcium levels and relaxation. Cyclic AMP (cAMP) generated by adenylate cyclase (AC) from adenosine triphosphate (ATP) in response to PGI$_2$ or other mediators may also regulate ion channels and intracellular calcium to mediate relaxation. (From Cohen RA, Vanhoutte PM. Endothelium-dependent hyperpolarization. Beyond nitric oxide and cyclic GMP. Circulation 1995;92: 3337–3349; reproduced by permission of the American Heart Association.)

channels or by activation of receptors for mediators such as angiotensin II, endothelin, or norepinephrine. In the later case, these mediators cause contraction by G protein–mediated, phospholipase C activation and the inositol triphosphate–induced rise in intracellular calcium. The ability of nitric oxide to inhibit diverse contractile mechanisms suggests that the effects of nitric oxide in vascular smooth muscle are diverse and redundant. Furthermore, the early phylogenetic appearance of endothelium-dependent vasodilation (49) suggests the primordial importance of this mechanism.

# THE ROLE OF CYCLIC GMP

The relationship between endothelium-dependent relaxation and cyclic GMP was actually noted before the mediator of relaxation was identified as nitric oxide. The observations that inhibitors of soluble guanylyl cyclase such as methylene blue and LY83583 decrease endothe-

lium-dependent relaxations and that endothelium-dependent relaxations are accompanied by a rise in smooth muscle levels of cyclic GMP were the key pieces of evidence that identified the endogenous endothelial mediator as being similar to nitric oxide released from nitrovasodilators such as sodium nitroprusside and nitroglycerin.

## GUANYLYL CYCLASE

Soluble guanylyl cyclase is a ubiquitous heme-containing enzyme that has a high affinity for nitric oxide. Activation of the enzyme depends only on the diffusion distance and concentration of nitric oxide and in fact occurs in the endothelial cell itself when nitric oxide is synthesized (50). When nitric oxide reacts with the iron-containing heme moiety of the enzyme, the rate of enzymatic conversion of GTP to cyclic GMP increases dramatically. The ultimate intracellular level of the cyclic nucleotide is determined by the activity of a variety of phosphodiesterases (51). These enzymes, which degrade the cyclic nucleotide, represent only one of many types of intracellular target molecules for cyclic GMP. The most important target in terms of mediating actions of nitric oxide is cyclic GMP-dependent protein kinase.

## CYCLIC GMP–DEPENDENT PROTEIN KINASE (PROTEIN KINASE G)

Cyclic GMP activates a cyclic GMP–dependent protein kinase that is responsible for phosphorylating multiple intracellular targets, which are ultimately responsible for regulating intracellular-calcium levels. The sequence of guanylyl cyclase activation by nitric oxide, followed by protein kinase G activation, and its phosphorylation of calcium regulatory proteins provides for a signaling mechanism that is both redundant and sensitive. Thus this signaling mechanism targets proteins that accomplish the same tasks by differing mechanisms and amplifies the response to low levels of nitric oxide. Protein kinase G exists in mammalian cells as two isoforms: type I is the form present in smooth muscle, endothelium, and blood cells, including platelets; type II is expressed in intestinal epithelium and the brain (52). The smooth muscle isoform exists as a cytosolic enzyme, although it may be associated with intracellular structures (52). Of importance is the fact that the specificity for activation of the protein kinase by cyclic GMP is low enough that cyclic AMP also activates the enzyme. Activation of protein kinase G, in fact, is more important for cyclic AMP–induced smooth muscle relaxation than is activation of authentic, cyclic AMP–dependent protein kinase (protein kinase A) (52).

The targets of protein kinase G include calcium ion

transporters, which decrease cytosolic calcium by either pumping calcium from the cell or into intracellular stores. These include the plasma membrane calcium ATPase and the sodium-calcium exchanger, as well as the sarcoplasmic reticulum calcium ATPase. The activation of the sarcoplasmic calcium ATPase pump occurs indirectly following phosphorylation of phospholamban by protein kinase G. Phospholamban, when unphosphorylated, is bound to and inhibits the activity of the calcium ATPase, thereby limiting sequestration of calcium into the intracellular storage pool (53). On phosphorylation, phospholamban dissociates from the ATPase and its activity increases. In addition, it is possible that protein kinase G interferes with the agonist-induced signal to empty stores by inhibiting both the generation of inositol triphosphate by phospholipase C, as well as the sensitivity of its receptor on the sarcoplasmic reticulum. The protein kinase also inhibits the activity of L-type calcium channels. This is accomplished either by directly inhibiting the calcium channels or maybe by activating calcium-dependent potassium channels, which mediate membrane hyperpolarization and thereby inhibit L-type calcium channels that depend on depolarization for their activation. In addition to these effects on calcium-transport mechanisms, protein kinase G may also regulate the activity of myosin light-chain kinase, which catalyzes the phosphorylation of the light chain of myosin leading to contraction. The effect of protein kinase G on myosin light-chain kinase is primarily mediated indirectly through its effects on calcium levels (54). In addition, an increase in myosin light-chain phosphatase activity has been attributed to protein kinase G (55). These latter effects thus down-regulate the sensitivity of the contractile apparatus to calcium, favoring relaxation. Most evident from the above is the redundancy of the multiple mechanisms that ensure that nitric oxide accomplishes a reduction in intracellular calcium and relaxation of vascular smooth muscle.

# MECHANISMS OF NITRIC OXIDE ACTION INDEPENDENT OF CYCLIC GMP

As noted above, the amplifying nature of signaling by nitric oxide through cyclic GMP is likely responsible for major actions of nitric oxide, allowing for responses to concentrations of nitric oxide below the nanomolar level. Nevertheless, cyclic GMP–independent mechanisms do exist that are capable of responding to somewhat higher concentrations of nitric oxide near the micromolar range. Because the concentration of nitric oxide released after stimulating endothelial cell receptors reaches this concentration range (56, 57), cyclic GMP may not account for all the actions of nitric oxide (58). Indeed, in an experimental model of atherosclerosis, endothelium-dependent relaxation can occur without a measurable rise in cyclic-GMP content (58). These responses have been ascribed to direct activation by nitric oxide of calcium-dependent potassium channels (59), which causes relaxation by hyperpolarizing the smooth muscle cell membrane. This effect of nitric oxide was attributed to S-nitrosation of a redox-sensitive protein thiol group associated with the ion channel. Another hyperpolarizing, ion-transport mechanism, sodium-potassium ATPase, which also contains redox-sensitive thiol groups, also may be activated by nitric oxide independently of cyclic GMP (60).

There are additional potential effects of nitric oxide on cellular proteins, although the functional effects of these reactions are not well understood. These include reduction of the activity of enzymes containing ferrous-sulfhydryl groups (61), ADP ribosylation of proteins (62), and actions mediated by the formation of nitrotyrosine (63).

# FATE OF NITRIC OXIDE RELEASED BY VASCULAR CELLS

Nitric oxide is released from endothelial cells luminally, where it may interact with blood cells, as well as abluminally, where it interacts with cells within the vascular wall. It may form nitrosothiols on extracellular or intracellular proteins (64). Some of these nitrosothiols may be formed on functional target molecules such as guanylyl cyclase or ion channels (mentioned above), while others may represent temporary storage or transfer forms such as albumin in the plasma (65) or intracellular glutathione (66). In addition, it has been proposed that hemoglobin in red blood cells may act as a transport form of nitric oxide (67).

Nitric oxide is also oxidized by both oxygen and superoxide anion, accounting for its short half-life and the relatively short distance over which the active molecule can exert its effects. Superoxide anion is produced by endothelial and other vascular cells in the normal course of aerobic metabolism. Endogenous superoxide dismutase, which scavenges the superoxide anion, normally prevents significant decomposition of released nitric oxide. However, in the course of several disease states, superoxide-anion levels increase and decomposition of nitric oxide can account significantly for reduced endothelium-dependent relaxations (68, 69). The ultimate oxidization products of nitric oxide are nitrite and nitrate; the formation of the latter product depends on

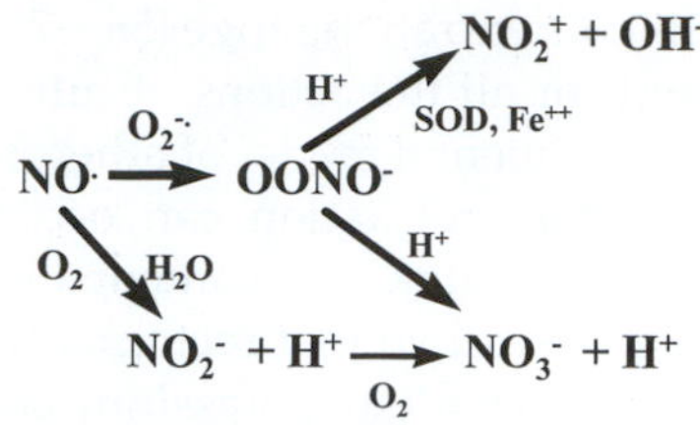

$$NO\cdot \longrightarrow OONO^- \xrightarrow[\text{SOD, Fe}^{++}]{H^+} NO_2^+ + OH^-$$

**FIGURE 19.8.** Degradation of nitric oxide by oxygen and superoxide anion. Nitric oxide reacts with oxygen to form nitrite ($NO_2^-$) and with superoxide anion to form peroxynitrite ($OONO^-$). Nitrate ($NO_3^-$) forms from nitrite or peroxynitrite in oxidizing conditions and $NO_2^+$ forms from peroxynitrite under reducing conditions in the presence of superoxide dismutase (SOD) or ferrous iron ($Fe^{++}$).

oxygen or heme iron (Fig. 19.8). The immediate product of the reaction of nitric oxide with superoxide anion is peroxynitrite anion ($OONO^-$). Peroxynitrite is highly reactive and is capable of causing lipid peroxidation and nitrosating protein tyrosines and thiols. In pathologic states the concentrations of both nitric oxide and superoxide may rise. For instance, immunohistochemical studies with antinitrotyrosine antibodies have demonstrated formation of peroxynitrite in atherosclerotic lesions where it may contribute to abnormal cell function or growth (70).

# INTERACTIONS OF NITRIC OXIDE WITH OTHER VASCULAR AND BLOODS CELLS

## ENDOTHELIAL CELLS RELEASE NITRIC OXIDE IN RESPONSE TO VASOACTIVE FACTORS FROM PLATELETS AND LEUKOCYTES

An important situation in which endothelial cell receptors may be physiologically activated by humoral agents is during platelet aggregation and thrombosis (Table 19.3). The integrity of endothelial cells normally prevents platelet aggregation through the release of nitric oxide and prostacyclin (see below). Additionally, the presence of normal endothelium accounts for vasodilation when platelet products and coagulation factors are released during blood clotting (Table 19.3). Aggregating platelets themselves cause endothelium-dependent relaxation of isolated blood vessels and dilation of normal vascular beds (71, 72). The vasodilation caused by platelets (Fig. 19.2) is accounted for primarily by platelet-released adenosine 5'-diphosphate and 5-hydroxytryptamine (47) interacting with their respective endothelial cell receptors (Table 19.3) (Fig. 19.2). Also, the proteolytic activity of thrombin formed as a result of activity of

the clotting cascade activates an endothelial cell receptor that increases nitric oxide release. Platelet-derived growth factor (73) and vasopressin (74), which are released from human platelets, may also mediate endothelium-dependent vasodilation during coagulation. The importance of the vasodilation that occurs in response to these platelet-released substances is all the more striking if one considers that the same substances constrict arteries when the endothelium is injured or removed or when nitric oxide release is impaired by inhibitors or disease (47). It is also possible that red-blood-cell lysis and release of hemoglobin in the region of a clot inhibits vasodilation by scavenging nitric oxide.

The endothelium also likely plays a role in the vascular response to leukocytes. Intraarterial injection of leukocyte activators, the chemotactic peptide, C5a, or N-formyl-methionyl-leucyl-phenylalanine causes vasodilation in normal vascular beds, but vasoconstriction in atherosclerotic disease (75, 76). The response may involve release of vasoactive factors from both leukocytes and platelets. The primary platelet mediators, adenosine 5'-diphosphate and 5-hydroxytryptamine, discussed above, are important in mediating the vasodilation. The vasoconstriction is mediated by thromboxane $A_2$ released from both activated platelets and leukocytes, as well as by leukotrienes, superoxide anion, and prostaglandin $E_2$ released from the leukocytes. The two cell types may interact; adenosine diphosphatase on the leukocyte or endothelial cell membrane (ecto-ADPase) apparently limits the response to ADP released by the platelets (77).

# EFFECT OF NITRIC OXIDE ON OTHER VASCULAR AND BLOOD CELLS AND RELEASE OF NITRIC OXIDE BY OTHER VASCULAR CELLS

Nitric oxide is synthesized by other vascular cells, including platelets, leukocytes, macrophages, smooth muscle cells, neurons, and fibroblasts. Platelets and leukocytes possess a constitutive NOS similar to that in endothelial cells, whereas in other cells nitric oxide synthesis occurs as a result of the induction of NOS II.

## PLATELETS

Cytosol of washed platelets can convert L-arginine to nitric oxide in a calcium-dependent manner (78). L-NMMA, but not D-NMMA, inhibits the conversion. Furthermore, during *in vitro* platelet aggregation initiated by adenosine 5'-diphosphate, calcium ionophore,

**TABLE 19.3.**   Vasoactive Factors Released During Hemostasis/Thrombosis[a]

| Substance | Source | Target Cell | Tone | Reference |
|---|---|---|---|---|
| ADP | platelet | endo($P_{2y}$, $\uparrow$ NO) | – | (216) |
| | | SMC ($P_{2x}$, $\uparrow$ $Ca^{++}$) | + | (217) |
| 5-HT | platelet | endo (5-$HT_1$, $\uparrow$ NO) | – | (71) |
| | | SMC (5-$HT_2$, $\uparrow$ $Ca^{++}$) | + | (71, 218) |
| Thromboxane $A_2$ | platelet | SMC ($TxA_2$, $\uparrow$ $Ca^{++}$) | + | (217) |
| $PGH_2$ | platelet | endo ($\uparrow$ $PGI_2$) | – | (219) |
| | | SMC ($TxA_2$, $\uparrow$ $Ca^{++}$) | + | (220) |
| Thrombin | plasma | endo ($\uparrow$ NO) | – | (212) |
| | | SMC (T, $\uparrow$ $Ca^{++}$) | + | (221) |
| Hemoglobin | red blood cell | endo ($\downarrow$ NO) | + | (23, 222) |

[a] *During thrombosis vasoactive factors are released from aggregating platelets, plasma clotting factors (in the case of thrombin), and lysed red blood cells (in the case of hemoglobin). Thrombin and platelet-drived substances activate specific receptors indicated on endothelial (endo) or smooth muscle (SMC) cells, in which they release nitric oxide (NO) and increase calcium ($Ca^{++}$), respectively, resulting in decreases ($-$) or increases ($+$) in tone.*

*$P_{2y}$, $P_{2x}$, 5-$HT_1$, 5-$HT_2$, $TxA_2$, T refer to membrane receptors for purines (ADP, adenosine diphosphate), 5-hydroxytryptamine, thromboxane $A_2$, and thrombin, respectively; $PGH_2$, prostaglandin endoperoxide.*

thrombin, arachidonic acid, or collagen there is a calcium-dependent increase in platelet cyclic GMP that is inhibited by L-NMMA (79). This indicates that platelets contain a constitutive nitric oxide synthase. Its physiologic significance is suggested by the fact that, accompanying the inhibition of nitric oxide synthesis caused by L-NMMA, platelet aggregation induced by collagen is augmented (78). Thus it may be that platelet activation is moderated by nitric oxide released by the endothelium and by the platelet itself.

## NEUTROPHILS

Neutrophils release nitric oxide, and the vasodilation caused by leukocytes mentioned above may be mediated in part by this mechanism. Neutrophils relax isolated arteries and can inhibit platelet aggregation (80–83). Neutrophil cytosol contains a nitric oxide synthase that, although it is not dependent on calmodulin, resembles in other respects the characteristics of the endothelial cell enzyme, including a sensitivity to calcium (84). Nitric oxide plays an important role in the killing of bacteria by neutrophils. This is indicated by the fact that L-NMMA decreases chemotaxis of neutrophils (85) and the accumulation and killing of staphylococci (86).

## MACROPHAGES

The inducible form of nitric oxide synthase, NOS II, was first described in macrophages exposed to endotoxin or cytokines. It was noted that following a time delay an L-arginine–dependent production of nitric oxide occurred that was dependent on new protein synthesis (87–89). NOS II produces higher concentrations of nitric oxide because the enzyme is induced and because, unlike the endothelial cell enzyme, the catalytic activity is not calcium dependent. This allows the enzymatic activity to be governed by the availability of L-arginine and other cofactors, especially tetrahydrobiopterin. Nitric oxide production by the inducible enzyme is involved in the ability of macrophages to kill bacteria and tumor cells (90–93).

## SMOOTH MUSCLE CELLS AND FIBROBLASTS

The contractile tone of the rat aorta decreases spontaneously within several hours after its isolation from the animal. This effect is exaggerated if the blood vessel is treated with endotoxin or the cytokine interleukin-1 and can be prevented in each case by inhibiting new RNA or protein synthesis (94–96) or by glucocorticoids (97–101). Endotoxin or cytokines have been shown to induce NOS II rapidly in cultured smooth muscle cells and fibroblasts and to produce large amounts of nitric oxide from L-arginine, which can be prevented by nitric oxide synthase inhibitors (102–107). The inhibition of vascular tone may occur as a result of the production of nitric oxide in both smooth muscle cells and fibroblasts in the vascular wall (107). This mechanism has been implicated in the hypotension accompanying bacterial-endotoxin release during sepsis and in the reversal of hypotension by nitric oxide synthase inhibitors (108). In addition, enough nitric oxide is produced by cytokine-stimulated, smooth muscle cells to inhibit their own growth (109), as well as platelet aggregation (110). The induction of NOS II in vascular cells likely plays a role in pathologic situations other than sepsis. Balloon injury of the rat carotid artery is followed by the growth of neointima, which is modulated by growth factors (e.g., PDGF, TGF-β, and thrombin) and cytokines (111). The cytokines are probably responsible for the presence of NOS II found in the neointima, which has been implicated in decreased vascular tone (112). The growth factors have been shown to inhibit the expression of NOS II (113–115) in cells in culture, suggesting that part of their growth-stimulation effect may depend on limiting nitric oxide production in the lesion (11). Release of cytokines by leukocytes has been implicated in NOS II induction in a variety of inflammatory conditions, including arthritis (116, 117). The high amounts of nitric oxide that NOS II is capable of producing may by itself, or through the formation of peroxynitrite, participate in inflammation and tissue damage (117). The ability of glucocorticoids, as well as salicylates (118), to inhibit expression of NOS II has been implicated in their antiinflammatory properties.

## NERVES

In some blood vessels, including coronary and cerebral arteries, the gut, and human penile erectile tissue, autonomic nerves mediate vasodilation by releasing catecholamines, which activate beta-adrenoceptors; acetylcholine, which activates smooth muscle and possibly endothelial muscarinic receptors; peptides such as the vasoactive intestinal polypeptide and the calcitonin gene–related peptide, as well as nitric oxide. In some cases nitric oxide is the principle neurotransmitter, while in others it plays a supplemental role (119–121). In human or rabbit penile erectile tissue, stimulation of the nerves within the microvasculature causes vasodilation, which is inhibited by L- but not D-arginine analogs (119). Nitric oxide may be made by the calcium-calmodulin–dependent NOS I present in neurons.

## OTHER ENDOTHELIUM-DERIVED VASOACTIVE FACTORS

A wide variety of endothelium-derived factors have been described, both before and after the discovery of nitric oxide, but none have as prominent a physiologic role as nitric oxide. These other factors may participate in the regulation of vascular tone, as well as in interactions with other vascular cells. Also, factors other than nitric oxide may assume a more important role in the setting of vascular diseases.

## ENDOTHELIUM-DERIVED HYPERPOLARIZING FACTOR(S)

Before acetylcholine was known to relax arteries by releasing endothelium-derived vasodilators, it was known to hyperpolarize arterial smooth muscle. The hyperpolarization is althought to reduce the intracellular-calcium concentration and cause relaxation by inhibiting L-type calcium channels, which are activated by depolarization (29). The response can be explained by activation of potassium channels either directly by nitric oxide or by cyclic GMP through the action of protein kinase G (Fig. 19.7). Because hyperpolarizing responses to endothelium-dependent vasodilators are poorly inhibited by L-arginine analogs of nitric oxide synthase, it has been proposed that several other endothelial cell factors contribute to the hyperpolarizing response. These have included prostacyclin (122) and arachidonic-acid products of cytochrome $P_{450}$ (123), although recent studies would indicate that nitric oxide can account for the majority of the response (29, 56). With the realization that nitric oxide released from the endothelium accounts primarily for endothelium-dependent relaxation through multiple mechanisms affecting intracellular-calcium levels, it has been estimated from pharmacologic studies that smooth muscle cell hyperpolarization accounts for about 20% of the relaxant response to some endothelium-dependent vasodilators. The most prominent of these is bradykinin, which strongly hyperpolarizes coronary arteries, including those of human origin (124). It is possible that endothelium-dependent hyperpolarization contributes to the therapeutic effects of angiotensin-converting enzyme inhibitors (see below).

## ARACHIDONIC-ACID METABOLITES

Increases in the endothelial intracellular calcium concentration are accompanied by activation of nitric oxide synthase and several enzyme systems dependent on calcium. These include phospholipase $A_2$, which cleaves arachidonic acid from the *sn*-2 position of membrane phospholipids (125). The liberated free fatty acid may reach concentrations where it exerts effects of its own, and is metabolized by cyclooxygenase, lipoxygenase, and cytochrome $P_{450}$ enzymes to more potent vasoactive products (eicosanoids).

### PROSTAGLANDINS

Prostacyclin ($PGI_2$) was the first vasoactive product discovered to be released from endothelial cells and is usually the predominant prostaglandin synthesized by these cells (1). It was quickly realized that the effects of $PGI_2$ on platelet aggregation were more important than its effects on vascular tone (1). This prostaglandin is a major, but not the only, product of arachidonic acid. When cleaved from phospholipids, arachidonic acid is metabolized by cyclooxygenase to the endoperoxide, prostaglandin $H_2$ ($PGH_2$). $PGH_2$ is a substrate for a series of prostaglandin synthetic enzymes that form $PGI_2$, $PGE_2$, and $PGF_{2\alpha}$ as major products in vascular endothelial and smooth muscle cells.

All the prostaglandins are vasoactive, although their potency varies according to species and blood vessel. $PGI_2$ exerts its effects on smooth muscle cells via a receptor and increases the intracellular concentration of cyclic AMP. In turn, protein kinase A, like protein kinase G, influences calcium regulatory mechanisms, resulting in decreased intracellular-calcium concentrations. Important among these mechanisms is the activation of ATP-dependent potassium channels leading to hyperpolarization and relaxation by that mechanism (126, 127). Thus $PGI_2$ has been proposed as an EDHF (29, 122, 128). $PGI_2$ is believed to contribute to endothelium-dependent vasodilation in a number of vascular beds (129–136). Although $PGI_2$ mediates vasodilation of the rabbit heart (135), the rabbit aorta does not relax in response to $PGI_2$, but rather only contracts in response to high concentrations via a thromboxane $A_2$–like receptor (134). Thus the vascular effects of $PGI_2$ vary even in the same animal. Its physiologic role as an important vasodilator is probably restricted to the microcirculation, but even there its role is overshadowed by nitric oxide. This conclusion is made evident by the fact that inhibition of the synthesis of prostanoids by cyclooxygenase inhibitors leads to no reproducible change in blood pressure, in contradistinction to the hypertension associated with nitric oxide inhibition.

$PGI_2$ inhibits the aggregation of platelets and promotes their disaggregation (137–139) (see also Chapter 12). This action on platelets is mediated by increases in intracellular cyclic-AMP levels (1). The physiologic role of $PGI_2$ in preventing platelet activation, like its vasodilator role, is likely restricted to a synergistic relationship with nitric oxide (140–142). Furthermore, the most important effect of normal endothelial cells, that of preventing adhesion of platelets to blood vessels, is unaffected by aspirin, which inhibits the production of $PGI_2$.

Other prostaglandins may be produced in high enough concentrations to contribute to vascular homeostasis. $PGH_2$, by virtue of the fact that it is the precursor for all prostaglandins, is made in the highest amounts. It is a potent vasoconstrictor, indicating that vasodilation by arachidonic-acid products such as prostacyclin depends on rapid conversion of $PGH_2$ by prostaglandin synthases (1). In a variety of vascular diseases such as diabetes mellitus and hypertension the conversion of $PGH_2$ to prostacyclin may be impaired, leading to endothelium-dependent contractions by the precursor prostaglandin endoperoxide (143, 144). It has also been suggested that activated platelets release extracellular $PGH_2$, which can be used by endothelial cells as a substrate to convert it to $PGI_2$, accounting in part for the antiaggregatory actions of the endothelium (145). Thus the conversion of $PGH_2$ to $PGI_2$ in endothelial cells may be a key event on which rests the balance between endothelium-dependent vasodilation and constriction, particularly that associated with vascular diseases (146).

Cyclooxygenase exists as two enzymes. A constitutive form, termed cyclooxygenase I (COX-1) is present in most cells, including endothelial cells. In addition, another form of cyclooxygenase, COX-2, is induced by cytokines in endothelial and other cells (147). The induction of COX-2 and the increased formation of prostanoids that are derived from it, may play a role in inflammatory conditions such as arthritis (148).

## LIPOXYGENASE AND EPOXYGENASE PRODUCTS OF ARACHIDONIC ACID

Lipoxygenase activity in endothelial cells leads to the synthesis of several vasoactive species, including the hydroperoxy- and hydroxyeicosatetraenoic fatty acids (HETEs), leukotrienes, and lipoxins (149, 150). Lipoxygenase products were first althought to be the principal endothelium-dependent vasodilators from experiments showing that inhibitors of the enzyme system blocked acetylcholine-induced relaxation (2, 131, 151). The production of these arachidonic-acid metabolites are considered to be important in leukocyte and platelet interactions with the endothelium (131, 151–155). Indeed, it is althought that some of the toxic effects of cyclooxygenase inhibitors may result from shunting of arachidonic-acid metabolism from cyclooxygenase to lipoxygenase.

Cytochrome $P_{450}$ epoxygenases produce epoxyeicosatrienoic fatty acids from arachidonic acid, which are also vasoactive. These products of arachidonic acid exert various activities on ion channels and may regulate nitric oxide release from endothelial cells (156, 157). In addition, it has been proposed that these products of arachidonic acid act as endothelium-derived, smooth muscle cell, hyperpolarizing factors (123). The precise role of arachidonic-acid metabolites is often difficult to discern because the metabolites and inhibitors of their production and action may nonspecifically decrease production, increase the breakdown, or interfere with the action of nitric oxide.

## ENDOTHELINS

The endothelins (ET) are a group of three distinct peptides, ET-1, ET-2, and ET-3, which are encoded by three separate genes (158). Endothelin was originally identified (159) in studies of the vasoconstrictor properties of conditioned media from cultured endothelial cells (160). The vasoconstrictor activity was extremely potent and produced long-lasting contractions of vascular smooth muscle that could be prevented by proteases and inhibitors of protein synthesis (160). From the purified-peptide amino acid sequence, three distinct genes were cloned from animal and human endothelial cells, although only ET-1 is known to be synthesized by endothelial cells. Each of the peptides consists of 21 amino acids. ET is synthesized by a two-step process. A prepropolypeptide is cleaved by a furin-like protease into a biologically inactive intermediate, termed big ET-1. Big ET-1 is subsequently cleaved to the active peptide by a specific endopeptidase, termed endothelin-converting enzyme (158). The latter enzymatic activity is prevented by phosphoramidon or metal chelators, characteristic of a metalloproteinase. The production of ET-1 is known to be regulated only at the level of transcription; there is no known storage or calcium-dependent stimulation of the release of the peptide. Big endothelin is several orders of magnitude less potent in producing vasoconstriction, indicating that only the mature peptide is physiologically active. The synthesis of the peptide is up-regulated by thrombin and vasoactive substances released by platelets (161) and is inhibited by nitric oxide (162).

Like the other vasoactive factors discussed in this chapter, ET-1 is althought to exert its effects primarily on target cells within the same tissue. Circulating plasma levels are affected by clearance through the lungs and are themselves not high enough to be vasoactive. The potency of the vasoconstrictor suggested that ET-1 might be a physiologic vasoconstrictor or might be involved in mediating hypertension; however, this hypothesis was dealt a major setback by the discovery that a mouse in which the ET gene was knocked out was in fact hypertensive (163). This apparent contradiction is likely due to the fact that ET mediates its actions through two classes of receptors, $ET_A$ and $ET_B$ which mediate diverse cellular responses. The hypertension of the ET knockout mouse may be explained by the fact that endothelial cells possess $ET_B$ receptors, which mediate increases in endothelial cell calcium and the release of nitric oxide and prostacyclin, leading to vasodilation (158). $ET_B$ receptors and the release of nitric oxide and prostacyclin also mediate the initial hypotensive response to intravenously injected ET, relaxation of some isolated blood vessels with intact endothelium, and inhibition of *in vivo* platelet aggregation caused by endothelin (164–166). The hypertension observed in the ET knockout mouse may also be due to other diverse physiologic roles for ET, which were made evident by the fact that these mice had craniofacial developmental abnormalities. Nevertheless, the most pronounced and long-lasting effect of high doses of ET administered *in vivo* or *in vitro* is vasoconstriction, mediated primarily by $ET_A$ receptors on smooth muscle cells.

The analysis of the physiologic role of ET is further complicated by the fact that both $ET_B$ and $ET_B$ receptors

mediate vasoconstriction in a variety of blood vessels and vascular beds with a large degree of heterogeneity among different species (158). Pharmacologic studies designed to block $ET_A$ receptors in a variety of pathologic animal models have nonetheless shown amelioration of ischemia- and cyclosporine-induced acute renal failure (167–170), hypertensive proliferative renal disease (170), myocardial infarction (171–173), cerebrovascular vasospasm associated with subarachnoid hemorrhage (174), and hypertension (167, 175–177). These studies have promoted further research into the effects of blocking ET receptors or endothelin-converting enzyme in a variety of disease states (158).

# ANGIOTENSIN AND BRADYKININ

The endothelium is a major site of localization of the angiotensin-converting enzyme, which converts angiotensin I to angiotensin II, the primary humoral mediator of the renin-angiotensin system. In this system angiotensinogen produced in the liver circulates and is converted to angiotensin I by renin in the kidney and elsewhere (178). Angiotensin I, which is not vasoactive, is converted to angiotensin II by the angiotensin-converting enzyme (ACE) (Table 19.4) found in the kidneys and lungs, as well as other tissues (178, 179). Angiotensin II is by far a more potent vasoconstrictor so that its conversion from angiotensin I by endothelial cell ACE results in endothelium-dependent contractions (144, 180, 181).

ACE also possesses the activity of kininase II, a dipeptidase responsible for the breakdown of the nonapeptide, bradykinin, to inactive hepta- and penta-peptides (182). Because bradykinin stimulates endothelial cells to produce nitric oxide via stimulation of type 2 bradykinin receptors, ACE activity decreases its vasodilator action. Bradykinin is formed by tissue and circulating kallikreins from kininogens (183) (see Chapter 5), and exogenous kininogen can cause endothelium-dependent relaxation of isolated arteries owing to endothelial cell-dependent conversion to bradykinin (184). Thus bradykinin is both synthesized and metabolized by endothelial cells. Bradykinin produced within endothelial cells contributes to flow-induced and shear stress–induced vasodilation and may account for the vasodilator effects of ACE inhibitors (185).

Until the recent development of selective angiotensin II and bradykinin (type 2) receptor antagonists, the dual activities of ACE have made it difficult to determine its precise physiologic role (179). The pharmacologic and therapeutic effects of ACE inhibitors, the most notable of which is to decrease blood pres-

**TABLE 19.4.** Metabolism of Vasoactive Factors[a] by the Endothelium

| Vasoactive Factors | Enzyme | Metabolite | Reference |
|---|---|---|---|
| Angiotensin I | ACE →→→ | Angiotensin II (active) | (178) |
| Bradykinin | Kininase II →→→ | Bradykinin 1–7, 1–5 (inactive) | (182) |
| 5-Hydroxytryptamine | MAO →→→ | 5-Hydroxyindole acetic acid (inactive) | (223) |
| Nor-, epinephrine | MAO →→→ | DOPEG (inactive) | (223) |
| ATP, ADP | Nucleotidases →→→ | AMP, adenosine (less active) | (224) |

[a] *Endothelial cell metabolism activates and inactivates many vasoactive factors.*

*ACE, angiotensin-converting enzyme; MAO, monoamine oxidase; DOPEG, 3,4-dihydroxyphenylglycol.*

sure, could be explained by either decreased effects of angiotensin II or increased effects of bradykinin. It is now considered that both activities of ACE are important. This is suggested by the fact that both angiotensin II receptor antagonists and ACE inhibitors reduce blood pressure and ameliorate congestive heart failure (179). Nevertheless, the effects of the ACE inhibitors are more potent, perhaps as a consequence of the stimulation of nitric oxide production by bradykinin. Through the use of nitric oxide synthase inhibitors and specific bradykinin (type 2) receptor antagonists, there is growing evidence that a major portion of the beneficial therapeutic effects of ACE inhibitors in myocardial infarction, atherosclerosis, and cardiac hypertrophy is mediated by bradykinin via nitric oxide (46, 186–188).

# CONCLUSION

The normal endothelium is responsible for vasodilation, inhibition of platelet and leukocyte activation, and control of growth and proliferation of vascular cells. Nitric oxide is the major mediator of these effects. Many other factors, either synthesized or converted in the endothelium, including arachidonic-acid products, bradykinin, angiotensin II, and endothelin, may play a role, but their effects are most pronounced when nitric oxide function is disturbed either by pharmacologic agents or by vascular disease. Indeed, many pathologic events in the vasculature may depend on upsetting the balance between nitric oxide and the other factors produced by endothelial and circulating blood cells (68, 78, 189, 190). The aggregation of platelets, which is althought to be a key pathophysiologic event mediating acute cardiovascular syndromes of coronary and cerebral ischemia, is a good example of the complex relationship between substances released from the endothelium and platelets. Not only do both normal endothelial cells and platelets release nitric oxide to inhibit adhesion and aggregation, but endothelial cells synthesize $PGI_2$ directly from platelet-derived $PGH_2$, thereby promoting the antiaggregating effects. Furthermore, the vasoactive response to platelet-derived substances depends strongly on the nitric oxide released from endothelial cells or, in the absence of normally functioning endothelial cells, on smooth muscle receptors, which mediate vasoconstriction (Fig. 19.9).

The development of vascular disease may also depend on the balance between vasoactive factors because all known risk factors for cardiovascular disease disturb endothelial cell function long before any structural changes or clinical events occur (68) (see Chapter 41). Because hypertension (7), platelet aggregation (78), leukocyte infiltration (191), and atherosclerotic lesions (192) can be promoted by pharmacologic inhibition of nitric oxide, it is likely that interference of this vital function by cardiovascular risk factors is important in the progression of those features in vascular disease. Because of the knowledge that risk factors for vascular disease such as hypertension, diabetes, and hypercholesterolemia all rapidly and adversely influence endothelial function, physicians should understand the function of the endothelium and should treat risk factors aggressively. Recent studies indicate that the impaired endothelial cell function in vascular disease is not irretrievably lost, but may be restored by risk factor management, exercise, and antioxidants (19, 193–199). These improvements in endothelial cell function occur well before any benefit is seen on the size of vascular lesions, suggesting that endothelial cell function may be an important endpoint for physicians to monitor in the effort to reduce the development or progression of vascular disease.

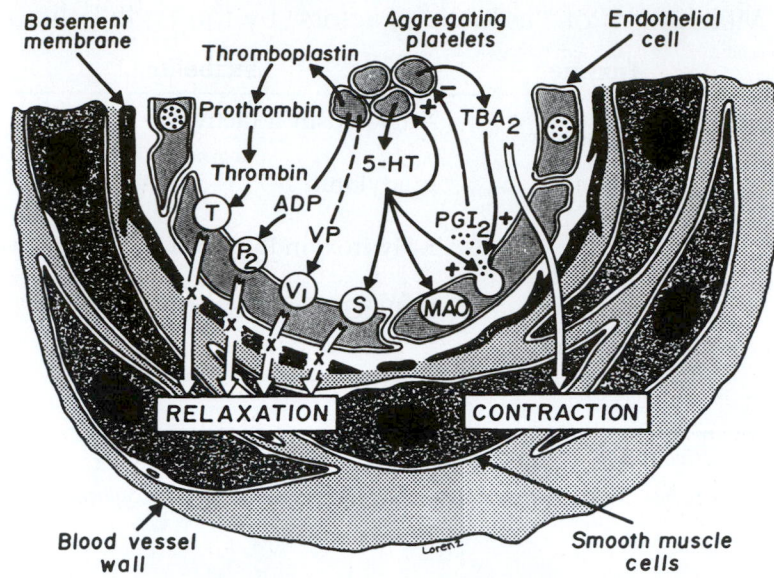

**FIGURE 19.9.** Mediators released or formed during thrombosis normally cause endothelium-dependent vasodilation. 5-Hydroxytryptamine (5-HT) and adenosine diphosphate (ADP) released from platelets and thrombin formed during coagulation stimulate endothelial receptors to release nitric oxide and cause relaxation. Vasopressin (VP) is also released from human platelets and can stimulate nitric oxide release. Release of thromboxane A₂ (TBA₂) can counter the vasodilatory effects of platelet-released products by contracting smooth muscle. Monoamine oxidase (MAO) contributes to the protective effect of the endothelium by metabolizing 5-HT. Prostacyclin (PGI₂) synthesized in the endothelium contributes to the anti-aggregatory role of the endothelium together with nitric oxide. (From Cohen RA, Vanhoutte PM. Platelets, serotonin, and endothelial cells. In: Vanhoutte PM, ed. Serotonin and the cardiovascular system. New York: Raven Press, 1985; reproduced by permission of Raven Press.)

# REFERENCES

1. Moncada S, Vane JR. Pharmacology and endogenous roles of prostaglandin endoperoxides, thromboxane A₂, and prostacyclin. Pharmacol Rev 1978;30:293–331.
2. Furchgott RF, Zawadzki JV. The obligatory role of the endothelial cells in the relaxation of arterial smooth muscle by acetylcholine. Nature 1980; 288:373–376.
3. Furchgott RF. Studies on relaxation of rabbit aorta by sodium nitrate: basis for the proposal that the acid-activatable component of the inhibitory factor from retractor penis is inorganic nitrate and the endothelium-derived relaxing factor is nitric oxide. In: Vanhoutte PM, ed. Vasodilation: vascular smooth muscle, peptides, autonomic nerves, and endothelium. New York: Raven Press, 1988; pp. 401–414.
4. Ignarro LJ, Byrns RE, Wood KS. Biochemical and pharmacologic properties of endothelium-derived relaxing factor and its similarity to nitric oxide radical. In: Vanhoutte PM, ed. Mechanisms of vasodilatation. New York: Raven Press, 1988; pp. 427–435.
5. Ignarro LJ, Buga GM, Wood KS et al. Endothelium-derived relaxing factor produced and released from artery and vein is nitric oxide. Proc Natl Acad Sci U S A 1987;84:9265–9269.
6. Palmer RM, Ferrige AG, Moncada S. Nitric oxide release accounts for the biologic activity of endothelium-derived relaxing factor. Nature 1987;327: 524–526.
7. Rees DD, Palmer RM, Moncada S. Role of endothelium-derived nitric oxide in the regulation of blood pressure. Proc Natl Acad Sci U S A 1989; 86:3375–3378.
8. Fozard JR, Part ML. Haemodynamic responses to Nᴳ-monomethyl-L-arginine in spontaneously hypertensive and normotensive Wistar-Kyoto rats. Br J Pharmacol 1991;102:823–826.
9. Aisaka K, Gross SS, Griffith OW et al. Nᴳ-methylarginine, an inhibitor of endothelium-derived nitric oxide synthesis, is a potent pressor agent in the guinea pig: does nitric oxide regulate blood pressure *in vivo*? Biochem Biophys Res Commun 1989;160:881–886.
10. Vallance P, Collier J, Moncada S. Effects of endothelium-derived nitric oxide on peripheral arteriolar tone in man. Lancet 1989;2:997–1000.
11. Schini VB, Vanhoutte PM. Endothelium-derived vasoactive factors. In: Loscalzo J, Schafer AI, eds. Thrombosis and hemorrhage. 1st ed. Boston: Blackwell Scientific, 1994; pp. 349–367.
12. Schini-Kerth VB, Vanhoutte PM. Nitrix oxide synthases in vascular cells. Exp Physiol 1995;80:885–905.
13. Nishida K, Harrison DG, Navas JP et al. Molecular cloning and characterization of the constitutive bovine aortic endothelial cell nitric oxide synthase. J Clin Invest 1992;90:2092–2096.
14. Buga GM, Griscavage JM, Rogers NE et al. Negative feedback regulation of endothelial cell function by nitric oxide. Circ Res 1993;73:808–812.
15. Liu J, Garcia-Cardena G, Sessa WC. Palmitoylation of endothelial nitric oxide synthase is necessary for optimal stimulated release of nitric oxide: implications for caveolae localization. Biochemistry 1996;35:13277–13281.
16. Garcia-Cardena G, Oh P, Liu J et al. Targeting of nitric oxide synthase to endothelial cell caveolae via palmitoylation: implications for nitric oxide signaling. Proc Natl Acad Sci U S A 1996;93:6448–6453.
17. Garcia-Cardena G, Fan R, Stern DF et al. Endothelial nitric oxide synthase is regulated by tyrosine phosphorylation and interacts with caveolin-1. J Biol Chem 1996;271:27237–27240.
18. Michel T, Li GK, Busconi L. Phosphorylation and subcellular translocation of endothelial nitric oxide synthase. Proc Natl Acad Sci U S A 1993;90: 6252–6256.
19. Sessa WC, Pritchard K, Seyedi N et al. Chronic exercise in dogs increases coronary vasuclar nitric oxide production and endothelial cell nitric oxide synthase gene expression. Circ Res 1994;74:349–353.
20. Rosenkranz-Weiss P, Sessa WC, Milstein S et al. Regulation of nitric oxide synthesis by proinflammatory cytokines in human umbilical vein endothelial cells. J Clin Invest 1994;93:2236–2243.
21. Shesely EG, Maeda N, Kim HS et al. Elevated blood pressures in mice lacking endothelial nitric oxide synthase. Proc Natl Acad Sci U S A 1996; 93:13176–13181.
22. Huang PL, Huang Z, Mashimo H et al. Hypertension in mice lacking the gene for endothelial nitric oxide synthase. Nature 1995;377:239–242.
23. Martin W, Villani GM, Jothianandan D et al. Selective blockade of endothelium-dependent and glyceryl trinitrate–induced relaxation by hemoglobin and by methylene blue in rabbit aorta. J Pharmacol Exp Ther 1985;232(3): 708–716.
24. Martin W, Furchgott RF, Villani GM et al. Depression of contractile responses in rat aorta by spontaneously released endothelium-derived relaxing factor. J Pharmacol Exp Ther 1986;237:529–538.
25. Cohen RA, Zitnay KM, Weisbrod RM et al. Influence of the endothelium on tone and the response of isolated pig coronary artery to norepinephrine. J Pharmacol Exp Ther 1988;244:550–555.
26. Tesfamariam B, Weisbrod RM, Cohen RA. Endothelium inhibits responses

of rabbit carotid artery to adrenergic nerve stimulation. Am J Physiol 1987; 253:H792–H798.

27. Schmidt HH, Pollock JS, Nakane M et al. $Ca^{2+}$/calmodulin-regulated nitric oxide synthases. Cell Calcium 1992;13:427–434.

28. Nilius B, Droogmans G, Gericke M et al. Nonselective ion pathways in human endothelial cells. In: Siemen D, Hescheler J, eds. Nonselective cation channels: pharmacology, physiology and biophysics. Basel/Switzerland: Birkhauser Verlag, 1993; pp. 269–280.

29. Cohen RA, Vanhoutte PM. Endothelium-dependent hyperpolarization. Beyond nitric oxide and cyclic GMP. Circulation 1995;92:3337–3349.

30. Luckhoff A, Busse R. Calcium influx into endothelial cells and formation of endothelium-derived relaxing factor is controlled by the membrane potential. Pflugers Arch 1990;416:305–311.

31. Cooke JP, Rossitch E Jr, Andon NA et al. Flow activates an endothelial potassium channel to release an endogenous nitrovasodilator. J Clin Invest 1991;88:1663–1671.

32. Tesfamariam B, Halpern W. Modulation of adrenergic responses in pressurized resistance arteries by flow. Am J Physiol 1987;253:H1112–H1119.

33. Kaiser L, Sparks HV Jr. Mediation of flow-dependent arterial dilation by endothelial cells. Circ Shock 1986;18:109–114.

34. Lansman JB. Endothelial mechanosensors. Going with the flow. Nature 1988;331:481–482.

35. Tesfamariam B, Cohen RA. Inhibition of adrenergic vasoconstriction by endothelial cell shear stress. Circ Res 1988;63:720–725.

36. Rubanyi GM, Lorenz RR, Vanhoutte PM. Bioassay of endothelium-derived relaxing factor(s): inactivation by catecholamines. Am J Physiol 1985;249: H95–H101.

37. Laurent S, Brunel P, Lacolley P et al. Flow-dependent vasodilation of the brachial artery in essential hypertension: preliminary report. J Hypertens Suppl 1988;6:S182–S184.

38. Meredith IT, Currie KE, Anderson TJ et al. Postischemic vasodilation in human forearm is dependent on endothelium-derived nitric oxide. Am J Physiol 1996;270:H1435–1440.

39. Yamabe H, Okumura K, Ishizaka H et al. Role of endothelium-derived nitric oxide in myocardial reactive hyperemia. Am J Physiol 1992;263: H8–H14.

40. Gilligan DM, Panza JA, Kicoyne CM et al. Contribution of endothelium-derived nitric oxide to exercise-induced vasodilation. Circulation 1994;90: 2853–2858.

41. Tagawa T, Imaizumi T, Endo T et al. A. Role of nitric oxide in reactive hyperemia in human forearm vessels. Circulation 1994;90:2285–2290.

42. Freay AD, Johns A, Adams DJ et al. Bradykinin and inositol 1,4,5-triphosphate-stimulated calcium release from intracellular stores in cultured bovine endothelial cells. Pflugers Arch 1989;414:377–384.

43. Gericke M, Droogmans G, Nilius B. Thapsigargin discharges intracellular calcium stores and induces transmembrane currents in human endothelial cells. Pflugers Arch 1993;422:552–557.

44. Gath I, Closs EI, Godtel-Ambrust U et al. Inducible NO synthase II and neuronal NO synthase I are constitutively expressed in different structures of guinea pig skeletal muscle: implications for contractile function. FASEB J 1996;10:1614–1620.

45. Welsh DG, Segal SS. Acetylcholine release from motor nerves triggers vasodilation. FASEB J 1996;10:A55.

46. Mombouli JV, Vanhoutte PM. Heterogeneity of endothelium-dependent vasodilator effects of angiotensin-converting enzyme inhibitors: role of bradykinin generation during ACE inhibition. J Cardiovasc Pharmacol 1992;20:S74–S82.

47. Cohen RA, Vanhoutte PM. Platelets, serotonin, and endothelial cells. In: Vanhoutte PM, ed. Serotonin and the cardiovascular system. New York: Raven Press, 1985.

48. McDaniel NL, Chen XL, Singer HA et al. Nitrovasodilators relax arterial smooth muscle by decreasing $[Ca^{2+}]_i$ and uncoupling stress from myosin phosphorylation. Am J Physiol 1992;263:C461–467.

49. Miller VM, Vanhoutte PM. Endothelium-dependent responses in isolated blood vessels of lower vertebrates. Blood Vessels 1986;23:225–235.

50. Schini V, Grant NJ, Miller RC et al. Morphologic characterization of cultured bovine aortic endothelial cells and the effects of atriopeptin II and sodium nitroprusside on cellular and extracellular accumulation of cyclic GMP. Eur J Cell Biol 1988;47:53–61.

51. Beltman J, Sonnenburg WK, Beavo JA. The role of protein phosphorylation in the regulation of cyclic nucleotide phosphodiesterases. Mol Cell Biochem 1993;128:239–253.

52. Lincoln TM, Cornwell TL, Komalavilas P et al. The nitric oxide-cyclic GMP signaling system. In: Biochemistry of smooth muscle contraction. New York: Academic Press, 1996; pp. 257–268.

53. Karczewski P, Kelm M, Hartmann M et al. Role of phospholamban in NO/EDRF-induced relaxation in rat aorta. Life Sci 1992;51:1205–1210.

54. Taylor DA, Bowman BF, Stull JT. Cytoplasmic $Ca^{2+}$ is a primary determinant for myosin phosphorylation in smooth muscle cells. J Biol Chem 1989; 264:6207–6213.

55. Wu X, Somlyo AV, Somlyo AP. Cyclic GMP–dependent stimulation reverses G protein–coupled inhibition of smooth muscle myosin light chain phosphate. Biochem Biophys Res Commun 1996;220:658–663.

56. Cohen RA, Plane F, Najibi S et al. Nitric oxide is the mediator of both endothelium-dependent relaxation and hyperpolarization of the rabbit carotid artery. Proc Natl Acad Sci U S A 1997;94:4193–4198.

57. Malinski T, Taha Z, Grunfeld S et al. Diffusion of nitric oxide in the aorta wall monitored *in situ* by porphyrinic microsensors. Biochem Biophys Res Commun 1993;193(3):1076–1082.

58. Cohen RA, Najibi S, Bolotina VM. The other role of nitric oxide as an endothelium-derived hyperpolarizing factor. In: Vanhoutte PM, ed. Endothelium-derived hyperpolarizing factor. Reading, U.K.: Harwood Academic, 1996:161–172.

59. Bolotina VM, Najibi S, Palacino JJ et al. Nitric oxide directly activates calcium-dependent potassium channels in vascular smooth muscle cells. Nature 1994;368:850–853.

60. Gupta S, McArthur C, Grady C et al. Stimulation of vascular $Na^+$-$K^+$-ATPase activity by nitric oxide: a cGMP-independent effect. Am J Physiol.1994;266:H2146–H151.

61. Lancaster JR Jr, Hibbs JB Jr. EPR demonstration of iron-nitrosyl complex formation by cytotoxic activated macrophages. Proc Natl Acad Sci U S A 1990;87:1223–1227.

62. Kwon NS, Stuehr DJ, Nathan CF. Inhibition of tumor cell ribonucleotide reductase by macrophage-derived nitric oxide. J Exp Med 1991;174: 761–767.

63. Koppenol WH, Moreno JJ, Pryor WA et al. Peroxynitrite, a cloaked oxidant formed by nitric oxide and superoxide. Chem Res Toxicol 1992;5:834–842.

64. Stamler JS, Simon DI, Jaraki O. S-nitrosylation of proteins with nitric oxide: synthesis and characterization of biologicly active compounds. Proc Natl Acad Sci U S A 1992;89:8087–8091.

65. Stamler JS, Jaraki O, Osborne J et al. Nitric oxide circulates in mammalian plasma primarily as an S-nitroso adduct of serum albumin. Proc Natl Acad Sci U S A 1992;89:7674–7677.

66. Boesgaard S, Poulsen HE, Aldershvile J et al. Acute effects of nitroglycerin depend on both plasma and intracellular sulfhydryl compound levels *in vivo*. Effect of agents with different sulfhydryl-modulating properties. Circulation 1993;87:547–553.

67. Jia L, Bonaventura J, Stamler JS. S-nitrosohaemoglobin: a dynamic activity of blood involved in vascular control. Nature 1996;380:221–226.

68. Cohen RA. The role of nitric oxide and other endothelium-derived vasoactive substances in vascular disease. Prog Cardiovasc Dis 1995;38:105–128.

69. Cohen RA, Pagano PJ. Other factors in endothelial cell dysfunction in hypertension and diabetes. In: Vallance P, Webb D, eds. The endothelium in hypertension. Heidelberg: Springer Verlag; 1997, 39–51.

70. White CR, Brock TA, Chang LY et al. Superoxide and peroxynitrite in atherosclerosis. Proc Natl Acad Sci U S A 1994;91:1044–1048.

71. Cohen RA, Shepherd JT, Vanhoutte PM. Inhibitory role of the endothelium in the response of isolated coronary arteries to platelets. Science 1983;221: 273–274.

72. Lopez JA, Armstrong ML, Piegors DJ et al. Effect of early and advanced atherosclerosis on vascular responses to serotonin, thromboxane $A_2$, and ADP. Circulation 1989;79:698–705.

73. Cunningham LD, Brecher P, Cohen RA. Platelet-derived growth factor receptors on macrovascular endothelial cells mediate relaxation via nitric oxide in rat aorta. J Clin Invest 1992;89:878–882.

74. Katusic ZS, Shepherd JT, Vanhoutte PM. Vasopressin causes endothelium-dependent relaxations of the canine basilar artery. Circ Res 1984;55: 575–579.

75. Mugge A, Lopez JA, Heistad DD et al. Vasoconstriction in response to activated leukocytes: implications for vasospasm. Eur Heart J 1993;14: 87–92.

76. Kaul S, Padgett RC, Heistad DD. Role of platelets and leukocytes in modulation of vascular tone. Ann NY Acad Sci 1994;714:122–135.

77. Marcus AJ, Broekman MJ, Drosopoulos JHF et al. The endothelial cell ecto-ADPase responsible for inhibition of platelet function is CD39. J Clin Invest 1997;99:1351–1360.

78. Radomski MW, Palmer RM, Moncada S. An L-arginine/nitric oxide pathway present in human platelets regulates aggregation. Proc Natl Acad Sci U S A 1990;87:5193–5197.

79. Radomski MW, Palmer RM, Moncada S. Characterization of the L-arginine: nitric oxide pathway in human platelets. Br J Pharmacol 1990;101: 325–328.

80. Rimele TJ, Sturm RJ, Adams LM et al. Interaction of neutrophils with vascular smooth muscle: identification of a neutrophil-derived relaxing factor. J Pharmacol Exp Ther 1988;245:102–111.

81. McCall TB, Boughton-Smith NK, Palmer RM et al. Synthesis of nitric oxide from L-arginine by neutrophils. Biochem J 1989;261:293–296.

82. Salvemini D, deNucci G, Gryglewski RJ et al. Human neutrophils and mononuclear cells inhibit platelet aggregation by releasing a nitric oxide-like factor. Proc Natl Acad Sci U S A 1989;86:6328–6332.

83. Wright CD, Mulsch A, Busse R et al. Generation of nitric oxide by human neutrophils. Biochem Biophys Res Commun 1989;160:813–819.

84. Yui Y, Hattori R, Kosuga K et al. Calmodulin-independent nitric oxide synthase from rat polymorphonuclear neutrophils. J Biol Chem 1991;266: 3369–3371.

85. Kaplan SS, Billiar T, Curran RD et al. Inhibition of cemotaxis with N^G-monomethyl-L-arginine: a role for cyclic GMP. Blood 1989;74:1885–1887.

86. Malawista SE, Montgomery RR, van Blaricom G. Evidence for reactive nitrogen intermediates in killing of staphylococci by human neutrophil cytoplasts. A new microbial pathway for polymorphonuclear leukocytes. J Clin Invest 1992;90:631–636.

87. Stuehr DJ, Marletta MA. Mammalian nitrate biosynthesis: mouse macrophages produce nitrite and nitrate in response to *Escherichia coli* lipopolysaccharide. Proc Natl Acad Sci U S A 1985;82:7738–7742.

88. Stuehr DJ, Marletta MA. Induction of nitrite/nitrate synthesis in murine macrophages by BCG infection, lymphokines, or interferon-gamma. J Immunol 1987;139:518–525.

89. Iyengar R, Stuehr DJ, Marletta MA. Macrophage synthesis of nitrite, nitrate, and *N*-nitrosamines: precursors and role of the respiratory burst. Proc Natl Acad Sci U S A 1987;84:6369–6373.

90. Granger DL, Hibbs JB Jr, Perfect JR et al. Metabolic fate of L-arginine in relation to microbiostatic capability of murine macrophages. J Clin Invest 1990;85:264–273.

91. Granger DL, Hibbs JB Jr, Perfect JR et al. Specific amino acid (L-arginine) requirement for the microbiostatic activity of murine macrophages. J Clin Invest 1988;81:1129–1136.

92. Keller R. Cytostatic elimination of syngeneic rat tumor cells *in vitro* by nonspecifically activated macrophages. J Exp Med 1973;138:625–644.

93. Drapier JC, Hibbs JB Jr. Differentiation of murine macrophages to express nonspecific cytotoxicity for tumor cells results in L-arginine–dependent inhibition of mitochondrial iron-sulfur enzymes in the macrophage effector cells. J Immunol 1988;140:2829–2838.

94. Beasley D, Cohen RA, Levinsky NG. Endotoxin inhibits contraction of vascular smooth muscle *in vitro*. Am J Physiol 1990;258:H1187–H1192.

95. Beasley D, Cohen RA, Levinsky NG. Interleukin-1 inhibits contraction of vascular smooth muscle. J Clin Invest 1989;83:331–335.

96. Beasley D, Schwartz JH, Brenner BM. Interleukin-1 induces prolonged L-arginine–dependent cyclic guanosine monophosphate and nitrite production in rat vascular smooth muscle cells. J Clin Invest 1991;87:602–608.

97. Szabo C, Thiemermann C, Wu CC et al. Attenuation of the induction of nitric oxide synthase by endogenous glucocorticoids accounts for endotoxin tolerance *in vivo*. Proc Natl Acad Sci U S A 1994;91:271–275.

98. Knowles RG, Salter M, Brooks SL et al. Anti-inflammatory glucocorticoids inhibit the induction by endotoxin of nitric oxide synthase in the lung, liver and aorta of the rat. Biochem Biophys Res Commun 1990;172:1042–1048.

99. Palmer RM, Bridge L, Foxwell NA et al. The role of nitric oxide in endothelial cell damage and its inhibition by glucocorticoids. Br J Pharmacol 1992; 105:11–12.

100. Wright CE, Rees DD, Moncada S. Protective and pathologic roles of nitric oxide in endotoxin shock. Cardiovasc Res 1992;26:48–57.

101. Geller DA, Nussler AK, DiSilvio M et al. Cytokines, endotoxin, and glucocorticoids regulate the expression of inducible nitric oxide synthase in hepatocytes. Proc Natl Acad Sci U S A 1993;90:522–526.

102. Marsden PA, Ballermann BJ. Tumor necrosis factor α activates soluble guanylate cyclase in bovine glomerular mesangial cells via an L-arginine–dependent mechanism. J Exp Med 1990;172:1843–1852.

103. Werner-Felmayer G, Werner ER, Fuchs D et al. Tetrahydrobiopterin-dependent formation of nitrite and nitrate in murine fibroblasts. J Exp Med 1990;172:1599–1607.

104. Kilbourn RG, Belloni P. Endothelial cell production of nitrogen oxides in response to interferon gamma in combination with tumor necrosis factor, interleukin-1, or endotoxin. J Natl Cancer Inst 1990;82:772–776.

105. Busse R, Mulsch A. Induction of nitric oxide synthase by cytokines in vascular smooth muscle cells. FEBS Lett 1990;275:87–90.

106. Schini VB, Junquero DC, Scott-Burden T et al. Interleukin-1 β induces the production of an L-arginine–derived relaxing factor from cultured smooth muscle cells from rat aorta. Biochem Biophys Res Commun 1991;176:114–121.

107. Zhang H, Chobanian AV, Brecher P. Aortic adventitia is a source of nitric oxide: a possible paracrine role. Hypertension 1995;26:569

108. Nava E, Palmer RM, Moncada S. Inhibition of nitric oxide synthesis in septic shock: how much is beneficial? Lancet 1991;338:1555–1557.

109. Scott-Burden T, Schini VB, Vanhoutte PM. Induction by interleukin-β of nitric oxide synthase leads to inhibition of mitogen-stimulated DNA synthesis in cultured vascular smooth muscle cells. In: Moncada S, Marletta JB, Hibbs JB Jr, eds. Biology of nitric oxide. New York: Elsevier, 1992; pp. 48–52.

110. Durante W, Schini VB, Scott-Burden T et al. Platelet inhibition by an L-arginine–derived substance released by IL-1β–treated vascular smooth muscle cells. Am J Physiol 1991;261:H2024–H2030.

111. Walker LN, Bowen-Pope DF, Ross R et al. Production of platelet-derived growth factor–like molecules by cultured arterial smooth muscle cells accompanies proliferation after arterial injury. Proc Natl Acad Sci U S A 1986;83:7311–7315.

112. Major TC, Overhiser RW, Panek RL. Evidence for NO involvement in regulating vascular reactivity in balloon-injured rat carotid artery. Am J Physiol 1995;269:H988–H996.

113. Ding A, Nathan CF, Graycar J et al. Macrophage deactivating factor and

114. Lazzarino G, Tavazzi B, DiPierro D et al. Ischemia and reperfusion: effect of fructose-1,6-bisphosphate. Free Radic Res Commun 1992;16:325–339.

115. Schini VB, Durante W, Catovsky S et al. Thrombin inhibits the induction of nitric oxide synthase in cultured vascular smooth muscle cells. Am J Physiol 1993;264:H611–H616.

116. Sakurai H, Kohsaka H, Liu MF et al. Nitric oxide production and inducible nitric oxide synthase expression in inflammatory arthritides. J Clin Invest 1995;96:2357–2363.

117. Ialenti A, Moncada S, DiRosa M. Modulation of adjuvant arthritis by endogenous nitric oxide. Br J Pharmacol 1993;110:701–706.

118. Farivar RS, Brecher P. Salicylate is a transcriptional inhibitor of the inducible nitric oxide synthase in cultured cardiac fibroblasts. J Biol Chem 1996; 271:31585–31592.

119. Kim N, Azadzoi KM, Goldstein I et al. A nitric oxide–like factor mediates nonadrenergic-noncholinergic neurogenic relaxation of penile corpus cavernosum smooth muscle. J Clin Invest 1991;88:112–118.

120. Cellek S, Kasakov L, Moncada S. Inhibition of nitrergic relaxations by a selective inhibitor of the soluble guanylate cyclase. Br J Pharmacol 1996; 118:137–140.

121. Klimaschewski L, Kummer W, Mayer B et al. Nitric oxide synthase in cardiac nerve fibers and neurons of rat and guinea pig heart. Circ Res 1992;71:1533–1537.

122. Parkington HC, Tare M, Tonta MA et al. Stretch revealed three components in the hyperpolarization of guinea-pig coronary artery in response to acetylcholine. J Physiol 1993;465:459–476.

123. Campbell WB, Gebremedhin G, Pratt PF et al. Identification of epoxyeicosatrienoic acids as endothelium-derived hyperpolarizing factors. Circ Res 1996;78:415–423.

124. Nakashima M, Mombouli JV, Taylor AA et al. Endothelium-dependent hyperpolarization caused by bradykinin in human coronary arteries. J Clin Invest 1993;92:2867–2871.

125. Alonso MJ, Salaices M, Sanchez-Ferrer CF et al. Predominant role for nitric oxide in the relaxation induced by acetylcholine in cat cerebral arteries. J Pharmacol Exp Ther 1992;261:12–20.

126. Jackson WF, Konig A, Dambacher T et al. Prostacyclin-induced vasodilation in rabbit heart is mediated by ATP-sensitive potassium channels. Am J Physiol 1993;264:H238–H243.

127. Siegel G, Carl A, Adler A et al. Effect of the prostacyclin analogue iloprost on K^+ permeability in the smooth muscle cells of the canine carotid artery. Eicosanoids 1989;2:213–222.

128. Nakashima M, Vanhoutte PM. Isoproterenol causes hyperpolarization through opening of ATP-sensitive potassium channels in vascular smooth muscle of the canine saphenous vein. J Pharmacol Exp Ther 1995;272:379–384.

129. Forstermann U, Goppelt-Strube M, Frolich JC et al. Inhibitors of acyl-coenzyme A: lysolecithin acyltransferase activate the production of endothelium-derived vascular relaxing factor. J Pharmacol Exp Ther 1986;238:352–359.

130. Holtz J, Forstermann U, Pohl U et al. Flow-dependent, endothelium-mediated dilation of epicardial coronary arteries in conscious dogs: effects of cyclooxygenase inhibition. J Cardiovasc Pharmacol 1984;6:1161–1169.

131. Forstermann U, Hertting G, Neufang B. The role of endothelial and non-endothelial prostaglandins in the relaxation of isolated blood vessels of the rabbit induced by acetylcholine and bradykinin. Br J Pharmacol 1986; 87:521–532.

132. Gordon JL, Martin W. Stimulation of endothelial prostacyclin production plays no role in endothelium-dependent relaxation of the pig aorta. Br J Pharmacol 1983;80:179–186.

133. Forstermann U, Hertting G, Neufang B. The importance of endogenous prostaglandins other than prostacyclin, for the modulation of contractility of some rabbit blood vessels. Br J Pharmacol 1984;81:623–630.

134. Vegesna RV, Diamond J. Elevation of cyclic AMP by prostacyclin is accompanied by relaxation of bovine coronary arteries and contraction of rabbit aortic rings. Eur J Pharmacol 1986;128:25–31.

135. Lamontagne D, Konig A, Bassenge E et al. Prostacyclin and nitric oxide contribute to the vasodilator action of acetylcholine and bradykinin in the intact rabbit coronary bed. J Cardiovasc Pharmacol 1992;20:652–657.

136. Domae M, Kuriyama H. Effects of prostaglandin I_2 synthesized in the endothelium and in the smooth muscle on mechanical properties of the canine thoracic aorta. Naunyn Schmiedebergs Arch Pharmacol 1986;333:294–302.

137. Gorman RR, Bunting S, Miller OV. Modulation of human platelet adenylate cyclase by prostacyclin (PGX). Prostaglandins 1977;13:377–388.

138. Tateson JE, Moncada S, Vane JR. Effects of prostacyclin (PGX) on cyclic AMP concentrations in human platelets. Prostaglandins 1977;13:389–397.

139. Kinlough-Rathbone RL, Packham MA et al. The effect of prostaglandin E_1 on platelet function *in vitro* and *in vivo*. Br J Haematol 1970;19:559–571.

140. Levin RI, Weksler BB, Jaffe EA. The interaction of sodium nitroprusside with human endothelial cells and platelets: nitroprusside and prostacyclin synergistically inhibit platelet function. Circulation 1982;66:1299–1307.

141. Radomski MW, Palmer RM, Moncada S. The anti-aggregating properties

of vascular endothelium: interactions between prostacyclin and nitric oxide. Br J Pharmacol 1987;92:639–646.

142. Stamler JS, Vaughan DE, Loscalzo J. Synergistic disaggregation of platelets by tissue-type plasminogen activator, prostaglandin E₁, and nitroglycerin. Circ Res 1989;65:796–804.

143. Cohen RA. Dysfunction of vascular endothelium in diabetes mellitus. Circulation 1993;87:V67–76.

144. Luscher TF, Boulanger CM, Dohi Y et al. Endothelium-derived contracting factors. Hypertension 1992;19:117–130.

145. Marcus AJ, Broekman MJ, Weksler BB et al. Interactions between stimulated platelets and endothelial cells *in vitro*. Philos Trans R Soc Lond [Biol] 1981;294:343–353.

146. Dusting GJ, Macdonald PS. Prostacyclin and vascular function: implications for hypertension and atherosclerosis. Pharmacol Ther 1990;48: 323–344.

147. Habib A, Creminon C, Frobert Y et al. Demonstration of an inducible cyclooxygenase in human endothelial cells using antibodies raised against the carboxylterminal region of the cyclooxygenase-2. J Biol Chem 1993; 268:23448–23454.

148. Anderson GD, Hauser SD, McGarity KL et al. Selective inhibition of cyclooxygenase (COX)-2 reverses inflammation and expression of COX-2 and interleukin-6 in rat adjuvant arthritis. J Clin Invest 1996;97:2672–2679.

149. Pace-Asciak CR, Asotra S. Biosynthesis, catabolism, and biologic properties of HPETEs, hydroperoxide derivatives of arachidonic acid. Free Radic Biol Med 1989;7:409–433.

150. Pfister SL, Spitzbarth N, Edgemond W et al. Vasorelaxation by an endothelium-derived metabolite of arachidonic acid. Am J Physiol 1996;270: H1021–H1030.

151. Diamond J. Effects of LY83583, nordihydroguaiaretic acid, and quinacrine on cyclic GMP elevation and inhibition of tension by muscarinic agonists in rabbit aorta and left atrium. Can J Physiol Pharmacol 1987;65:1913–1917.

152. Setty BN, Stuart MJ. 15-hydroxy-5,8,11,13-eicosatetraenoic acid inhibits human vascular cyclooxygenase: potential role in diabetic vascular disease. J Clin Invest 1986;77:202–211.

153. Creese BR, Temple DM. The effect of indomethacin on anaphylactic contraction and histamine release in guinea-pig lung parenchymal strips. Arch Int Pharmacodyn Ther 1986;281:265–276.

154. Billah MM, Bryant RW, Siegel MI. Lipoxygenase products of arachidonic acid modulate biosynthesis of platelet-activating factor (1-O-alkyl-2-acetyl-sn-glycero-3-phosphocholine) by human neutrophils via phospholipase A2. J Biol Chem 1985;260:6899–6906.

155. Schafer AI, Takayama H, Farrell S et al. Incorporation of platelets and leukocyte lipoxygenase metabolites by cultured vascular cells. Blood 1986; 67:373–378.

156. Graier WF, Simecek S, Sturek M. Cytochrome P₄₅₀ mono-oxygenase–regulated signalling of Ca²⁺ entry in human and bovine endothelial cells. J Physiol 1995;482:259–274.

157. Harder DR, Gebremedhin D, Narayanan J et al. Formation and action of a P-450 4A metabolite of arachidonic acid in cat cerebral microvessels. Am J Physiol 1994;266:H2098–2107.

158. Yanagisawa M. The endothelin system. A new target for therapeutic intervention. Circulation 1994;89:1320–1322.

159. Yanagisawa M, Kurihara H, Kimura S et al. A novel potent vasoconstrictor peptide produced by vascular endothelial cells. Nature 1988;332:411–415.

160. Hickey KA, Rubanyi G, Paul RJ et al. Characterization of a coronary vasoconstrictor produced by cultured endothelial cells. Am J Physiol 1985;248: C550–556.

161. Ohlstein EH, Storer BL, Butcher JA et al. Platelets stimulate expression of endothelin mRNA and endothelin biosynthesis in cultured endothelial cells. Circ Res 1991;69:832–841.

162. Boulanger C, Luscher TF. Release of endothelin from the porcine aorta. Inhibition by endothelium-derived nitric oxide. J Clin Invest 1990;85: 587–590.

163. Kurihara Y, Kurihara H, Suzuki H et al. Elevated blood pressure and craniofacial abnormalities in mice deficient in endothelin-1. Nature 1994; 368:703–710.

164. Herman F, Magyar K, Chabrier PE et al. Prostacyclin mediates antiaggregatory and hypotensive actions of endothelin in anesthetized beagle dogs. Br J Pharmacol 1989;98:38–40.

165. Lidbury PS, Thiemermann C, Korbut R et al. Endothelins release tissue plasminogen activator and prostanoids. Eur J Pharmacol 1990;186: 205–212.

166. Thiemermann C, Lidbury P, Thomas R et al. Endothelin inhibits *ex vivo* platelet aggregation in the rabbit. Eur J Pharmacol 1988;158:181–182.

167. Clozel M, Breu V, Burri K et al. Pathophysiologic role of endothelin revealed by the first orally active endothelin receptor antagonist. Nature 1993;365:759–761.

168. Warner TD, Allcock GH, Corder R et al. Use of the endothelin antagonist BQ-123 and PD 142893 to reveal three endothelin receptors mediating smooth muscle contraction and the release of EDRF. Br J Pharmacol 1993; 110:777–782.

169. Kon V, Badr KF. Biologic actions and pathophysiologic significance of endothelin in the kidney. Kidney Int 1991;40:1–12.

170. Benigni A, Zoja C, Coma D et al. A specific endothelin subtype A receptor antagonist protects against injury in renal disease progression. Kidney Int 1993;44:440–444.

171. Watanabe T, Suzuki N, Shimamoto N et al. Contribution of endogenous endothelin to the extension of myocardial infarct size in rats. Circ Res 1991;69:370–377.

172. Kusumoto K, Awane Y, Fujiwara S et al. Role of endogenous endothelin in extension of rabbit myocardial infarction. J Cardiovasc Pharmacol 1993; 22:S339–S342.

173. Grover GJ, Dzwonczyk S, Parham CS. The endothelin-1 receptor antagonist BQ-123 reduces infarct size in a canine model of coronary occlusion and reperfusion. Cardiovasc Res 1993;27:1613–1618.

174. Itoh S, Sasaki T, Ide K et al. A novel endothelin ETₐ receptor antagonist, BQ-485, and its preventive effect on experimental cerebral vasospasm in dogs. Biochem Biophys Res Commun 1993;195:969–975.

175. Ohlstein EH, Douglas SA, Ezekiel M et al. Antihypertensive effects of the endothelin receptor antagonist BQ-123 in conscious spontaneously hypertensive rats. J Cardiovasc Pharmacol 1993;22:S321–S324.

176. Nishikibe M, Tsuchida S, Okada M et al. Antihypertensive effect of a newly synthesized endothelin antagonist, BQ-123, in a genetic hypertensive model. Life Sci 1993;52:717–724.

177. Clozel M, Clozel JP, Hesse P. Endothelin receptor antagonism: a new therapeutic approach in experimental hypertension. Circulation 1993;88:I316.

178. Schunkert H, Ingelfinger JR, Dzau VJ. Evolving concepts of the intrarenal renin-angiotensin system in health and disease: contributions of molecular biology. Renal Physiol Biochem 1991;14:146–154.

179. Smith RD, Chiu AT, Wong PC et al. Pharmacology of nonpeptide angiotensin II receptor antagonists. Annu Rev Pharmacol Toxicol 1992;32:135–165.

180. Feletou M, Germain M, Teisseire B. Modulation of angiotensin-peptide-induced contraction by the vascular endothelium. J Vasc Med Biol 1990;2:18–25.

181. Manabe K, Shirahase H, Usui H et al. Endothelium-dependent contractions induced by angiotensin I and angiotensin II in canine cerebral artery. J Pharmacol Exp Ther 1989;251:317–320.

182. Drapeau G, Rhaleb NE, Dion S et al. [Phe8psi(Ch2-NH)Arg9]bradykinin, a B₂ receptor selective agonist which is not broken down by either kininase I or kininase II. Eur J Pharmacol 1988;155:193–195.

183. Vanhoutte PM, Boulanger CM, Mombouli JV. Endothelium-derived relaxing factors and converting enzyme inhibition. Am J Cardiol 1995;76: 3E–12E.

184. Mombouli JV, Vanhoutte PM. Kinins mediate kallikrein-induced endothelium-dependent relaxations in isolated canine coronary arteries. Biochem Biophys Res Commun 1992;185:693–697.

185. Mombouli JV, Vanhoutte PM. Kinins and endothelium-dependent relaxations to converting enzyme inhibitors in perfused canine arteries. J Cardiovasc Pharmacol 1991;18:926–927.

186. Martorana PA, Kettenbach B, Breipohl G et al. Reduction of infarct size by local angiotensin-converting enzyme inhibition is abolished by a bradykinin antagonist. Eur J Pharmacol 1990;182:395–396.

187. Linz W, Schölkens BA. A specific B₂-bradykinin receptor antagonist HOE 140 abolishes the antihypertrophic effect of ramipril. Br J Pharmacol 1992; 105:771–772.

188. Farhy RD, Carretero OA, Ho KH et al. Role of kinins and nitric oxide in the effects of angiotensin-converting enzyme inhibitors on neointima formation. Circ Res 1993;72:1202–1210.

189. De Caterina R, Libby P, Peng HB et al. Nitric oxide decreases cytokine-induced endothelial activation. J Clin Invest 1995;96:60–68.

190. Garg UC, Hassid A. Nitric oxide-generating vasodilators and 8-bromocyclic guanosine monophosphate inhibit mitogenesis and proliferation of cultured rat vascular smooth muscle cells. J Clin Invest 1989;83:1774–1777.

191. Gaboury J, Woodman RC, Granger DN et al. Nitric oxide prevents leukocyte adherence: role of superoxide. Am J Physiol 1993;265:H862–H867.

192. Cayatte AJ, Palacino JJ, Horten K et al. Chronic inhibition of nitric oxide production accelerates neointima formation and impairs endothelial function in hypercholesterolemic rabbits. Arterioscler Thromb 1994;14: 753–759.

193. Kamata K, Sugiura M, Kojima S et al. Preservation of endothelium-dependent relaxation in cholesterol-fed and streptozotocin-induced diabetic mice by the chronic administration of cholestyramine. Br J Pharmacol 1996; 118:385–391.

194. Delp MD, McAllister RM, Laughlin MH. Exercise training alters endothelium-dependent vasoreactivity of rat abdominal aorta. J Appl Physiol 1993; 75:1354–1363.

195. Chen H, Li HT. Physical conditioning can modulate endothelium-dependent vasorelaxation in rabbits. Arterioscler Thromb 1993;13:852–856.

196. Keaney JF Jr, Gaziano JM, Xu A et al. Dietary antioxidants preserve endothelium-dependent vessel relaxation in cholesterol-fed rabbits. Proc Natl Acad Sci U S A 1993;90:11880–11884.

197. Kunisaki M, Bursell SE, Umeda F et al. Normalization of diacylglycerol-protein kinase C activation by vitamin E in aorta of diabetic rats and cultured rat smooth muscle cells exposed to elevated glucose levels. Diabetes 1994;43:1372–1377.

198. Stephens NG, Parsons A, Schofield PM et al. Randomised controlled trial of vitamin E in individuals with coronary disease. Lancet 1996;347: 781–786.

199. Ting HH, Timimi FK, Boles KS et al. Vitamin C improves endothelium-dependent vasodilation in individuals with non–insulin-dependent diabetes mellitus. J Clin Invest 1996;97:22–28.

200. Tsukahara T, Hongo K, Kassell NF et al. Characterization of muscarinic cholinergic receptors on the endothelium and the smooth muscle of the rabbit thoracic aorta. J Cardiovasc Pharmacol 1989;13:870–878.

201. Hynes MR, Banner W, Yamamura HI et al. Characterization of muscarinic receptors of the rabbit ear artery smooth muscle and endothelium. J Pharmacol Exp Ther 1986;238:100–105.

202. Niimi N, Noso N, Yamamoto S. The effect of histamine on cultured endothelial cells. A study of the mechanism of increased vascular permeability. Eur J Pharmacol 1992;221:325–331.

203. Hide M, Fukui H, Watanabe T et al. Histamine $H^1$-receptor in endothelial and smooth muscle cells of guinea-pig aorta. Eur J Pharmacol 1988;148: 161–169.

204. Van de Voorde J, Leusen I. Influence of prostaglandin-synthesis inhibitors on carbachol- and histamine-induced vasodilatation in perfused rat hindquarters. Pflugers Arch 1983;397:290–294.

205. Miller VM, Vanhoutte PM. Endothelial alpha-2-adrenoceptors in canine pulmonary and systemic blood vessels. Eur J Pharmacol 1985;118:123–129.

206. Keravis TM, Nehlig H, Delacroix MF et al. High-affinity bradykinin $B_2$ binding sites sensitive to nucleotides in bovine aortic endothelial cells. Eur J Pharmacol 1991;207:149–155.

207. Sung CP, Arleth AJ, Shikano K et al. Characterization and function of bradykinin receptors in vascular endothelial cells. J Pharmacol Exp Ther 1988;247:8–13.

208. Boeynaems JM, Pearson JD. $P_2$ purinoceptors on vascular endothelial cells: physiologic significance and transduction mechanisms. Trends Pharmacol Sci 1990;11:34–37.

209. Houston DA, Burnstock G, Vanhoutte PM. Different $P_2$-purinergic receptor subtypes of endothelium and smooth muscle in canine blood vessels. J Pharmacol Exp Ther 1987;241:501–506.

210. Houston DS, Vanhoutte PM. Comparison of serotonergic receptor subtypes on the smooth muscle and endothelium of the canine coronary artery. J Pharmacol Exp Ther 1988;244:1–10.

211. Schoeffter P, Hoyer D. 5-Hydroxytryptamine (5-HT)–induced endothelium-dependent relaxation of pig coronary arteries is mediated by 5-HT receptors similar to the 5-HT$_{1D}$ receptor subtype. J Pharmacol Exp Ther 1990;252:387–395.

212. Hollenberg MD, Laniyonu AA, Saifeddine M et al. Role of the amino- and carboxylterminal domains of thrombin receptor–derived polypeptides in biologic activity in vascular endothelium and gastric smooth muscle: evidence for receptor subtypes. Mol Pharmacol 1993;43:921–930.

213. Karaki H, Sudjarwo SA, Hori M et al. $ET_B$ receptor antagonist, IRL 1038, selectively inhibits the endothelin-induced endothelium-dependent vascular relaxation. Eur J Pharmacol 1993;231:371–374.

214. Zeng G, Quon MJ. Insulin-stimulated production of nitric oxide is inhibited by wortmannin. J Clin Invest 1996;98:894–898.

215. Hu RM, Levin ER, Pedram A et al. Insulin stimulates production and secretion of endothelin from bovine endothelial cells. Diabetes 1993;42: 351–358.

216. Houston DS, Shepherd JT, Vanhoutte PM. Adenine nucleotides, serotonin, and endothelium-dependent relaxations to platelets. Am J Physiol 1985; 248:H389–H395.

217. Houston DS, Shepherd JT, Vanhoutte PM. Aggregating human platelets cause direct contraction and endothelium-dependent relaxation of isolated canine coronary arteries. J Clin Invest 1986;78:539–544.

218. Cohen RA, Shepherd JT, Vanhoutte PM. 5-Hydroxytryptamine can mediate endothelium-dependent relaxation of coronary arteries. Am J Physiol 1983;245:H1077–H1080.

219. Rittenhouse-Simmons S, Deykin D. Release and metabolism of arachidonate in human platelets. In: Gordon, ed. Platelets in biology and pathology. Holland: 1981:349–372.

220. Mukhopadhyay A, Navran SS, Amin HM et al. Effect of trimetoquinol analogs for antagonism of endoperoxide/thromboxane $A_2$–mediated response in human platelets and rat aorta. J Pharmacol Exp Ther 1985;232: 1–9.

221. Madhane P, Saifeddine M, Green FHY et al. Contractile actions of thrombin receptor–derived polypeptides in rat and guinea pig lung parenchymal smooth muscle. Proc West Pharmacol Soc 1995;38:93–96.

222. Salvemini D, Radziszewski W, Korbut R et al. The use of oxyhaemoglobin to explore the events underlying inhibition of platelet aggregation induced by NO or NO-donors. Br J Pharmacol 1990;101:991–995.

223. Gillis CN. Measurement of endothelial metabolic functions *in vivo*. Ann Biomed Eng 1987;15:183–188.

224. Marcus AJ, Safier LB, Hajjar KA et al. Inhibition of platelet function by an aspirin-insensitive endothelial cell ADPase. Thromboregulation by endothelial cells. J Clin Invest 1991;88:1690–1696.

# CHAPTER 20

# RHEOLOGY

Julia Myers Ross, Barbara Rita Alevriadou, and Larry Vern McIntire

## INTRODUCTION

By definition, rheology is the study of the flow and deformation of matter and thus encompasses the classic theories of fluid mechanics and elasticity. Applied to the cardiovascular system, rheologic considerations involve the flow properties of blood as well as the deformation of soft tissues, including the blood cells and vessel walls. As blood flows through a blood vessel, several mechanical forces are generated. These forces include a tangential shear stress (acting in a plane parallel to the fluid flow) caused by blood flow over the endothelial cells, a normal (perpendicular) stress caused by the blood pressure, and a tensile stress caused by vessel wall deformations (Fig. 20.1). In addition, local fluid dynamics control the access of platelets and leukocytes to the blood vessel wall and can greatly alter cellular responses to a biochemical stimulus. For example, thrombi formed under high flow rate conditions (arteries and arterioles) consist primarily of platelets and are called "white thrombi." In contrast, those formed under low flow (veins and venules) include more fibrin and erythrocytes and are called "red thrombi." Such observations demonstrate that rheologic principles are critical to elucidating the complex dynamic molecular mechanisms of thrombosis and hemostasis.

## INTRODUCTION TO FLUID DYNAMICS

Blood flows through vessels and artificial organs in response to imposed pressure differences and boundary wall movements generated in the vascular system. The simplest mathematical description of blood flow is the case of pressure-driven steady flow of an incompressible Newtonian fluid through a long cylindrical tube of constant cross-sectional area. The velocity profile is given by the equation:

$$v_z = 2\langle v_z\rangle[1 - (r/R)^2] \tag{20.1}$$

where $v_z$ is the axial velocity at a radial position r, R is the vessel radius, and $\langle v_z\rangle$ is the mass average velocity given by:

$$\langle v_z\rangle = -R^2/8\mu(\Delta P/L) \tag{20.2}$$

where $\Delta P/L$ is the local vessel pressure gradient (pressure drop per unit length) and $\mu$ is the fluid viscosity. The velocity profile is a parabolic function of the radial distance from the tube axis (Fig. 20.2). Fluid motion obeying equation 20.1 is referred to as Poiseuille flow (1, 2).

Poiseuille flow exists when the fluid flow rate is relatively low, or more precisely, the Reynolds number is less than about 2300. In this flow regime, termed laminar flow, the fluid is characterized by smooth motion in laminae, or layers. The Reynolds number ($N_{Re}$) is a dimensionless parameter defined for tube flow as:

$$N_{Re} = \rho\langle v_z\rangle D/\mu \tag{3}$$

where $\rho$ is the fluid density, $\mu$ the fluid viscosity, and $D$ the vessel diameter. $N_{Re}$ is a measure of the importance of fluid momentum or inertial forces relative to viscous forces. At low $N_{Re}$, viscous forces dominate, and at high $N_{Re}$, inertial forces are of greater importance in momentum transfer. For very high $N_{Re}$ (>2300), steady

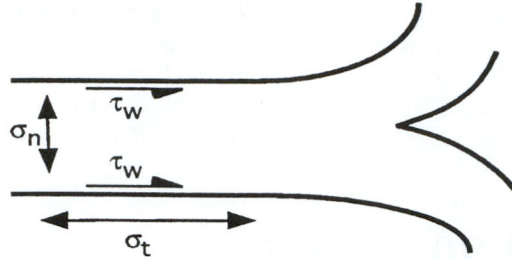

**FIGURE 20.1.** Hemodynamic forces of the vasculature. $\tau_w$ is the wall shear stress and results from viscous drag of the blood flowing across the endothelial cell surface. Physiologic levels of shear stress range from 1–60 dyn/cm$^2$, with higher shear stresses in the arterial circulation than in the venous circulation. $\sigma_n$ is a normal force that results from blood pressure. $\sigma_t$ is a tensile stress caused by dilation and contraction of the blood vessel. (Modified from Patrick CW, McIntire LV. Bioengineering contributions in vascular biology at the cellular and molecular level. Trends Cardiovasc Med 1996;6:122–129.)

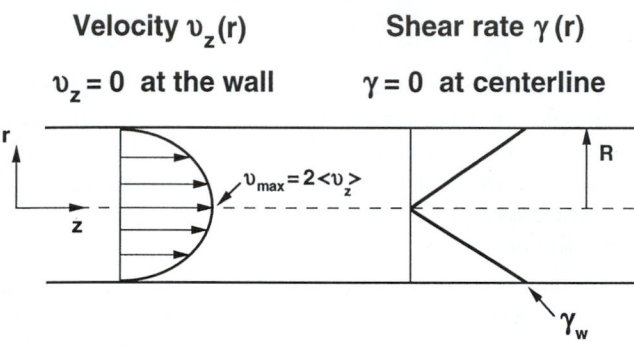

**FIGURE 20.2.** Velocity and shear rate as a function of radial distance for pressure-driven flow of a Newtonian liquid in a cylindrical tube (Poiseuille flow). The velocity profile is parabolic and is calculated by equation 20.1. The maximum fluid velocity, $v_{max}$, occurs along the vessel center line and is twice the mass average velocity $\langle v_z \rangle$. The shear rate (equation 20.4) becomes zero at the tube axis and is maximum at the tube wall, $\gamma_w$ (equations 20.5 and 20.7).

laminar Poiseuille flow is replaced by very complex, locally time-dependent turbulent flow, characterized by random three-dimensional motions of the fluid particles. Local Reynolds numbers are less than 2300 almost everywhere in normal human blood vessels, so truly turbulent flow is unusual.

A commonly used term in fluid dynamics is the shear rate, $\gamma$. It is a measure of how rapidly adjacent fluid layers slide past each other (velocity gradient) and is expressed in inverse seconds (/s). For our model flow, the shear rate is given by:

$$\gamma = -dv_z/dr = 4\langle v_z \rangle r/R^2 \qquad (20.4)$$

and is a linear function of radial position. The shear rate is zero at the tube axis and becomes maximum at the

**TABLE 20.1.** Typical Ranges of Wall Shear Rates and Wall Shear Stresses

| Blood Vessel | Mean Wall Shear Rate (s$^{-1}$) | Mean Wall Shear Stress (dyn/cm$^2$) |
|---|---|---|
| Large arteries | 300–800 | 11.4–30.4 |
| Arterioles | 500–1600 | 19.0–60.8 |
| Veins | 20–200 | 0.76–7.6 |
| Stenotic vessels | 800–10,000 | 30.4–380 |

*Shear stresses are calculated assuming that whole blood has a viscosity of approximately 0.038 poise. Local shear rate values in the microcirculation can be quite high, but flow there can no longer be treated as if blood were a continuum, because blood cell diameters are of the same order of magnitude as vessel diameter.*

vessel wall (see Fig. 20.2). The wall shear rate, $\gamma_w$, is found by setting $r = R$ in equation 20.4:

$$\gamma_w = 4\langle v_z \rangle/R = 8\langle v_z \rangle/D \qquad (20.5)$$

where $D$ is the vessel diameter. The wall shear rate is often expressed in terms of the volumetric flow rate, $Q$:

$$Q = \pi R^2 \langle v_z \rangle = \frac{\pi D^2}{4} \langle v_z \rangle \qquad (20.6)$$

as:

$$\gamma_w = 4Q/\pi R^3 = 32Q/\pi D^3 \qquad (20.7)$$

Using equation 20.7, the time-average wall shear rates can be calculated for various parts of the vascular system from the known vessel diameters and volumetric flow rates (2, 3). Wall shear rates were estimated to be below 200/s in veins and venules, and to vary from 300/s (in arteries) up to 1600/s (in high-flow arterioles) in the arterial circulation. Values of wall shear rates in pathophysiologic situations, in atherosclerotic or vasospastic arteries and arterioles, or in the vicinity of some cardiovascular prosthesis can attain local magnitudes of the order of $10^5$/s (Table 20.1).

The wall shear stress, $\tau_w$, is a measure of the force exerted on the vessel surface per unit area by the viscous fluid, as it flows at a constant flow rate in the vessel. For a Newtonian fluid, the shear stress, $\tau$, is linearly related to the shear rate, $\gamma$, with the constant of proportionality called the fluid viscosity, $\mu$. Therefore, at the wall:

$$\tau_w = \mu\gamma_w = 4\mu\langle v_z \rangle/R = 4\mu Q/\pi R^3 \qquad (20.8)$$

The wall shear stress is thus independent of axial position. The viscosity is a measure of the resistance to deformation of a fluid. In the case of whole blood, the viscosity is a function of plasma viscosity, red cell concentration, red cell aggregation, and red cell deformability. If viscosity is in units of poise ($\mu$ of water at room temperature is approximately 1 centipoise = 0.01 poise = 0.01 g cm$^{-1}$ s$^{-1}$), then shear stress is in dyn/cm$^2$ (1 dyn = 1 g cm s$^{-2}$). Thus, a vessel containing normal whole blood with a hematocrit of 45% at 37°C ($\mu$ = 0.038 poise) flowing at a wall shear rate of 1500/s would experience a wall shear stress of approximately 57 dyn/cm$^2$.

The Hagen-Poiseuille equation relates the pressure drop along the vessel to the average fluid velocity or the volumetric flow rate:

$$\Delta P/L = 8\mu\langle v_z\rangle/R^2 = 8\mu Q/\pi R^4 \qquad (20.9)$$

where $\Delta P/L$ is the local vessel pressure gradient (pressure drop per unit length).

The above simplified analysis of fluid dynamics does not strictly apply to the circulation for reasons (2, 4) that include the following: 1) flow is not steady, but pulsatile throughout the arterial tree, and the vessel walls are not rigid; 2) flow, although nonturbulent (because $N_{re} < 2300$), is often complex, including recirculation regions and secondary flows due to branching and vessel curvature; 3) in severely stenotic and topologically distorted atherosclerotic vessels, jetting and actual turbulence may occur locally, coupled with complex secondary flows; 4) in the smallest arterioles and venules and in the capillaries (regions where vessel diameter approximates blood cell diameter), blood does not behave as a homogeneous Newtonian fluid, and one must consider multiphasic behavior; and 5) at shear rates less than 100/s, blood exhibits non-Newtonian behavior and the apparent viscosity increases with a decrease in shear rate (shear thinning). In addition, for capillary tubes with a diameter less than 150 $\mu$m, blood viscosity decreases with decreasing tube diameter (the Fahraeus-Lindquist effect). Due to these non-Newtonian aspects of the flow behavior of blood , the equations described do not apply in the venous circulation nor in the microcapillaries. However, the equations presented above are a reasonable starting point if interpreted in terms of local time-average velocities, wall shear rates, and wall shear stresses in arterial vessels.

# MASS TRANSFER CONSIDERATIONS

Access of blood cellular components and plasma proteins to vascular surfaces can be an important step in the formation of mural thrombi, embolization, platelet activation, hemolysis, and leukocyte-surface interactions. Transfer of material within a fluid occurs both by molecular diffusion (due to Brownian motion) and fluid convection (due to bulk flow). The diffusion process in liquids is extremely slow (molecular diffusion coefficients on the order of $10^{-5}$ to $10^{-8}$ cm$^2$/s), so convection, if present, will dominate mass transport. This class of mass transfer problems is called the large Peclet number limit. The Peclet number, $N_{Pe}$, is a dimensionless parameter that measures the importance of convection relative to diffusion ($N_{Pe} = \langle v\rangle 2R/\mathscr{D}$, where $\mathscr{D}$ is the molecular diffusion coefficient). In steady Poiseuille flow, the only fluid velocity component is in the axial direction. Thus, mass transport is by axial fluid convection and radial molecular diffusion (much slower). Because blood components must move radially to contact the vessel surface, creation of a radial velocity component would greatly enhance radial mass transport and blood-vessel wall interaction. This process occurs in regions of curved or branched vessels or under conditions of high transmural flow, where secondary convective radial flows are superimposed on the main axial flow. Pulsatility can also engender secondary radial convective flows that enhance mass transport.

The steady-state mass conservation equation of cells or solutes in blood flowing in a cylindrical tube (assuming Poiseuille flow), is given by:

$$v_z\frac{\partial C}{\partial z} = \frac{1}{r}\frac{\partial}{\partial r}\left(r\mathscr{D}\frac{\partial C}{\partial r}\right) \qquad (20.10)$$

where C is the concentration and $\mathscr{D}$ the effective diffusion coefficient of a blood cell type or plasma protein (5, 6).

The continued collisions between and deformation of the erythrocytes in flowing blood lead to an enhanced radial mixing of platelets and large protein or lipoprotein molecules. The movement induced by this mixing can be described by diffusion coefficients 2–3 orders of magnitude higher than those determined by Brownian motion alone. The diffusion coefficient, due to red cell motions, becomes a function of the local shear rate and hematocrit, and has been found to have the form:

$$\mathscr{D} = \alpha\gamma^n \qquad (20.11)$$

where $\alpha$ is a proportionality constant, and n a power-law constant (5, 7). In the case of the platelet, the consequence of increased radial dispersion is an increase in the frequency of encounters with the vessel wall, which is of significant importance for thrombosis. In addition to causing increased platelet diffusion constants, red blood cells demonstrate a radial hematocrit gradient leading to a drift force on platelets toward the region of lower hematocrit at the wall (8). This effect further increases platelet concentration in the vicinity of the blood vessel wall. Similarly, the white blood cell is led to outward displacement (called margination), which may be accompanied at low flow rates (<200/s) by adhesion of granulocytes to the wall followed by extravasation and migration to a site of inflammation (9). Because of the radial dispersion, large plasma proteins, such as von Willebrand factor (vWf) and fibrinogen, may also have much greater access to damaged blood vessel surfaces, where they are rapidly adsorbed.

For mass transfer in liquids (high Peclet number),

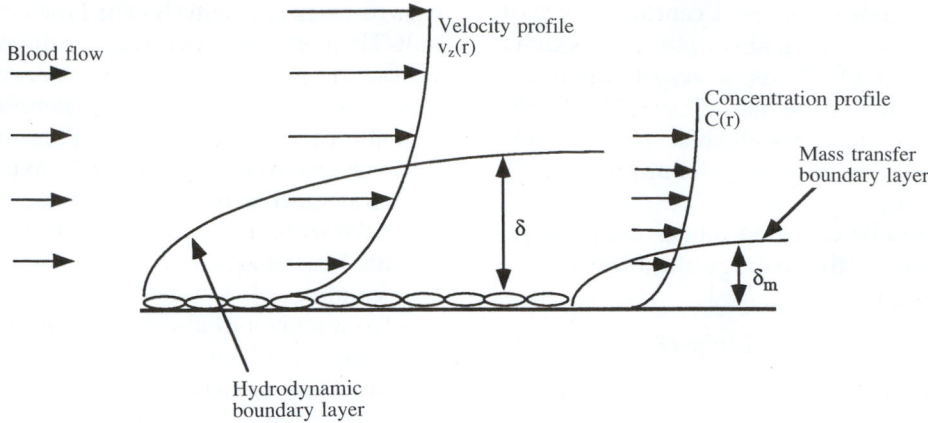

**FIGURE 20.3.** The development of a hydrodynamic boundary layer (the region over which the velocity profile develops from zero at the wall to 99% of its free stream value) at the entry of a vessel and a mass transfer boundary layer (the region over which the concentration profile develops to 99% of its free stream value) where endothelial cells have been denuded. For platelets the mass transfer boundary layer thickness is very small (<0.4%) compared to the hydrodynamic boundary layer thickness. This leads to simplification of the mathematical analysis of platelet diffusion. $V_z$, velocity; C, concentration; $\delta$, hydrodynamic boundary layer thickness; $\delta_m$, mass boundary layer thickness. (Modified from Goldsmith HL, Turitto VT. Rheological aspects of thrombosis and haemostasis: basic principles and applications. Thromb Haemost 1986;55:415–435.)

the thickness of the mass boundary layer (the distance over which the concentration profile develops from zero at the wall to 99% of its maximum-free stream value) is small compared to the momentum boundary layer thickness (the distance over which the velocity profile develops from zero at the wall to 99% of its maximum-free stream value) (Fig. 20.3). In the case of platelets, the mass transfer boundary layer thickness, $\delta_m$, is less than 0.4% of the fluid dynamic boundary layer, $\delta$, and for plasma proteins, $\delta_m$ is 2 to 3% of $\delta$ (2). This means that the material exchange that occurs between the blood and the vessel surface occurs in a region very close to the wall. Outside the mass transfer boundary layer, there is no concentration gradient and cells or solutes beyond the boundary layer will never interact with the surface, regardless of the velocity gradient. Therefore, the value of the diffusion constant is essentially that at the wall, and the velocity profile near the wall can be considered a linear function of the distance from the wall. Equation 20.10 becomes the boundary layer mass transfer equation and is solved using the boundary conditions (6):

$$C = C_\infty \text{ at } r \leq \delta_m$$

$$-\mathcal{D}\frac{\partial C}{\partial r} = kC \text{ at } r = R \quad (20.12)$$

where $\delta_m$ is the mass boundary layer thickness. In case of the platelet, the assumptions implicit in these boundary conditions are that the platelet concentration is considered homogeneous outside the boundary layer; and that there is a balance of mass flux to the wall with the reaction rate, where k is a reaction rate constant and the reaction rate is first order with respect to platelet concentration. At high degrees of surface saturation, the second boundary condition may not be applicable be-

cause platelet reactivity with the surface can become dependent on available surface area.

The general solution for the steady-state mass flux (mass/unit surface area/unit time) of platelets at any point on the reactive surface is given by equation 20.13:

$$j_z = [-\mathcal{D}_w \frac{\partial C}{\partial r}]_{r=R} =$$

$$\frac{C_\infty}{\dfrac{1}{k} + \dfrac{1.48}{\left(\dfrac{4\langle v_z \rangle \mathcal{D} w^2}{Dz}\right)^{1/3}}} \quad (20.13)$$

where $C_\infty$ is the bulk platelet concentration, k the reaction (adhesion) rate constant, $\langle v_z \rangle$ the average blood velocity, $\mathcal{D}_w$ the platelet diffusion coefficient near the vessel wall, D the vessel diameter, and z the axial distance along the vessel segment.

In the limiting case where the reaction rate is much slower than the diffusional transport (reaction-controlled transport:nonthrombogenic surface), k << $\mathcal{D}$, equation 20.13 becomes:

$$j_z = kC_\infty$$

which implies that the transport rate does not depend on axial position and flow parameters, but only on reaction rate and bulk concentration.

In the most general case, where the two transport rates are of the same order of magnitude, k ≈ $\mathcal{D}$, the fluid dynamic and reaction rate processes are coupled and the solution for the concentrations of blood components requires prior solution of the equations of motion. For laminar flow in a tube (Poiseuille flow), the solution is the parabolic velocity profile (equation 20.1). However, in channels of complex geometry, where the flow pattern may show a finite velocity component perpendicular to the wall, both the equations of motion and of mass conservation need to be solved simultaneously, which cannot be done analytically.

In the limiting case of very reactive surfaces, when $k >> \mathscr{D}$ (diffusion-controlled transport), the platelet flux to the surface from equation 20.13 becomes a function of flow parameters, axial position, geometric system characteristics and bulk concentration:

$$j_z = 0.67C_\infty[4\langle v_z\rangle\mathscr{D}w^2/Dz]^{1/3} \qquad (20.14)$$

Substituting equation 20.5 into equation 20.14 leads to an expression for the platelet flux in diffusion-controlled transport:

$$j_z = 0.67 C_\infty[\gamma_w Dw^2/2z]^{1/3} \qquad (20.15)$$

which depends only on the wall shear rate, platelet diffusivity, axial position, and platelet concentration (10). It is shown that the platelet flux is an explicit function of the wall shear rate. However, recall that the platelet diffusivity is also a power function of the wall shear rate, according to equation 20.11. Thus, platelet deposition on the vessel wall should increase with the wall shear rate at a rate substantially greater than the one-third power. Platelet flux is inversely proportional to the third root of the axial distance. Thus, platelet deposition will decrease along the axis of the flowing blood.

Data of platelet deposition from flowing normal whole blood on to exposed subendothelium or collagen-coated surfaces (10–12) fit the theoretically predicted dependence on axial position and on wall shear rate reasonably well (for wall shear rates up to 1500/s), according to diffusion-controlled kinetics. For wall shear rates above 2000/s, deposition rates on subendothelium were found to be decreased compared to what would be expected at such flow rates by diffusion-controlled transport (10), perhaps due to some shear-induced embolization.

# MODEL EXPERIMENTAL SYSTEMS

In order to elucidate the molecular mechanisms of coagulation and thrombosis, it is necessary to examine the dynamic interactions among blood components, the vessel wall, and the mechanical environment. Various experimental models have been developed, taking into account the rheologic principles described above, allowing *in vitro* experimentation in a fluid dynamic environment similar to that found *in vivo*. Several such devices and methodologies recently have been reviewed in the literature (13, 14). Model experimental systems have been used in investigating the role of wall shear stress and/or mass transport on the molecular mechanisms of platelet attachment to surfaces (adhesion), platelet cohesion to

each other (aggregation, either mural or bulk) and endothelial cell metabolism. The model systems that have been used most frequently fall into two distinct categories: 1) devices in which the local fluid effects are controlled and well defined at the solid-liquid interface, such as parallel-plate, annular, and tubular flow chambers; and 2) devices in which the entire fluid phase is subjected to uniform shear forces, such as viscometers of various configurations (14). Each of these devices has the advantage that the fluid dynamics are well understood and well characterized. Therefore, the forces generated by the fluid can be controlled precisely. In the following section, these experimental devices will be discussed, including a brief description of the types of information that can be acquired from each.

## MURAL THROMBOSIS AND PERFUSION SYSTEMS

One possibility for initiating the formation of mural platelet thrombi is the adhesion of blood platelets onto the subendothelium of injured blood vessels (or on ruptured atherosclerotic plaque surfaces) containing collagen and other matrix proteins, with subsequent platelet aggregation. During the past decade, engineering principles have been used to design experimental models that simulate the fluid mechanical conditions in injured blood vessels or narrowed arteries and arterioles. Whole-blood perfusion studies using annular (15) or parallel-plate (12) perfusion chambers simulate the events of mural thrombus formation *in vivo* that may occur as a result of adhesion and aggregation on an injured, exposed subendothelial or atherosclerotic plaque surface.

A typical parallel plate flow chamber (Fig. 20.4) consists of a polycarbonate plate, a silicon gasket (the thickness of which determines the height of the flow path), a glass coverslip and a metallic base plate. The glass coverslip forms one side of the parallel-plate flow chamber and can be coated with proteins, cells, or biomaterials of interest. The wall shear rate is a function of the flow chamber geometry (16) and is calculated from the following equation (1):

$$\dot{\gamma} = \frac{1.5\,Q}{b^2w} \qquad (20.16)$$

where $Q$ is the volumetric flow rate, $b$ is half the height of the flow path, and $w$ is the width of the flow channel. Assuming Newtonian behavior of whole blood, the wall shear stress can be calculated as described above using the viscosity of whole blood.

A parallel-plate flow chamber can be combined with epifluorescence video microscopy and a microphotometric measurement technique for real-time visualization and high-resolution endpoint measurement of

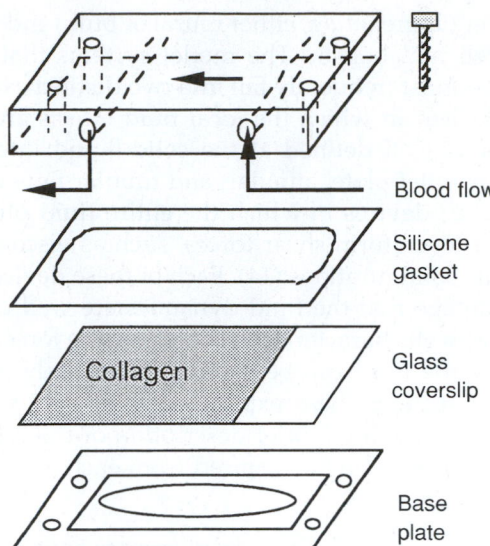

**FIGURE 20.4.** Schematic of a parallel-plate flow chamber (12). Collagen or other protein-coated surfaces or cellular monolayers form one wall of the parallel plate geometry. The gap thickness between the plates is determined by the gasket and is usually on the order of 200 μm. Even at high wall shear rates, this is a low Reynolds number problem, and the entry length is very short (16). Thus, essentially all of the collagen-coated surface (except very close to the gasket walls) experiences the same wall shear stress.

platelet deposition from flowing whole blood with fluorescently labeled platelets onto surfaces as a function of axial distance (12). Blood is aspirated from a test tube via the flow chamber by a syringe pump at a known constant flow rate, corresponding to a known wall shear rate. The flow chamber is mounted on an inverted-stage microscope maintained at 37°C and equipped with an epifluorescent illumination attachment and a video camera suitable for very low light levels (silicone intensified target or CCD camera) to directly visualize platelet adhesion and subsequent aggregation throughout the perfusion period. Platelets can be fluorescently labeled with mepacrine (12, 17) or using fluorescently-labeled platelet-specific monoclonal antibodies (18).

Macroscopic measurement of platelet accumulation at the end of the perfusion period may be accomplished by scanning along the center line of the coverslip and continuously recording the locally averaged fluorescence intensity over the microscope field of view using a motorized microscope stage and a computerized microphotometric measurement system. The local-averaged fluorescence intensity is divided by an intensity-per-platelet constant and is converted to local-averaged platelet density, in millions per square centimeter, along the surface. Fig. 20.5 shows a typical curve generated by this type of measurement of platelet deposition from whole blood onto bovine collagen type I. By integrating the platelet density vs. distance curve up to any length of the coated surface, the number of platelets accumu-

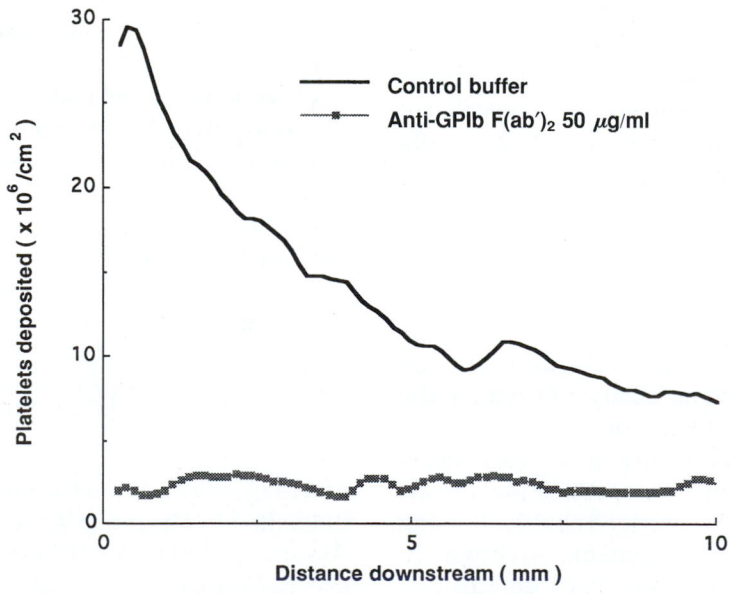

**FIGURE 20.5.** A typical platelet density profile (in millions per square centimeter) at the center line of a parallel-plate flow chamber along the first 10 mm of collagen type I-coated glass surfaces (coating density 20 mg/cm²). At zero axial distance is the beginning of the collagen coating. Citrated whole blood was preincubated with either control buffer or 50 mg/ml of the F(ab')₂ portion of the antiglycoprotein (GP) Ib monoclonal antibody for 5 minutes before perfusion at 37°C for 1 minute at a wall shear rate of 1500/s (approximately 57 dyn/cm² shear stress).

lated on a portion of the surface can be estimated. Division of the number of platelets deposited by the surface area provides an average platelet deposition per unit surface area.

Digital image processing can be used for quantitative off-line local measurement of the growth of individual thrombi (12, 19, 20). Videotape images taken during and at the end of the perfusion period are digitized and processed by a digital image processor. The analysis provides information on the morphologic characteristics of each thrombus at each time point and enables the reconstruction of three-dimensional models of thrombi formed on the surface included in the microscope field of view (Fig. 20.6; see plate 20.6). The percentage of the surface covered by thrombi is a measurement of platelet adhesion. The average number of platelets per thrombus for all the thrombi in the digitized frame, as well as the average thrombus height, can be used as a measure of platelet aggregation (20).

In summary, the macroscopic analysis (epifluorescence video microscopy and the microphotometric measurement system) can provide information on platelet mass transport and reaction kinetics with the surface, whereas the microscopic analysis (digital image processing) allows dynamic real-time study of cell surface and intracellular interactions. Such a technology enables the study of key molecules involved in mural thrombus formation, such as vWf. In addition, tests of antithrombotic agents (21, 22) and investigation of the thrombogenicity of various purified components of the vessel wall or polymeric biomaterials (23) can be performed with this system.

Other techniques used for monitoring platelet deposition on reactive surfaces include perfusion of reconstituted blood with [$^{111}$In]- or [$^{51}$Cr]-radiolabeled platelets, sectioning the surfaces into pieces and either measuring radioactivity directly or using $\gamma$-camera imaging to estimate total platelet deposition (24–27); and fixation and staining of the thrombi at the end of the perfusion for morphometric evaluation by *en face* light microscopy or with an image analyzer (26–31).

## COMPLEX FLOW GEOMETRIES

To elucidate the possible connection between blood flow and the localization of thrombosis in more complex geometries, the flow patterns and wall adhesion of platelets from suspensions of platelets and red cells have been investigated in the annular vortex formed at a sudden tubular expansion, serving as a model of axisymmetric stenosis; dog saphenous vein bileaflet valves; and the human carotid artery bifurcation, at steady and pulsatile flow, using flow visualization techniques (32–35). In the expansion tube, the platelet deposition profile exhibited a peak within the vortex and just downstream of the reattachment point. The localization of platelet adhesion

peaks was explained by the curved streamlines carrying platelets with a velocity component perpendicular to the wall on either side of the reattachment point. In the case of the venous valves, flow separation at the edges of valve leaflets resulted in the formation of a vortex in each valve pocket and of a stagnant region deeper in the valve pocket, which is the place of venous thrombi formation. The flow patterns in a human carotid artery bifurcation showed the existence of a recirculation zone on the distal wall of the internal carotid artery, the preferential site for atherosclerotic lesions (36). Laser-Doppler anemometry was used to determine fluid flow velocity profiles and shear stresses in fixed postmortem specimens of the human carotid bifurcation. After comparing the flow pattern and the position of the intimal plaques obtained at autopsy, it was concluded that atherosclerosis and thrombosis develop in regions of flow separation and departure from the axially aligned laminar flow (disturbed flow), which are areas of low shear stresses, close to stasis (37).

## BULK PHASE AGGREGATION SYSTEMS

A second mechanism for initiating the formation of arterial platelet thrombi is shear-induced aggregation of platelets in areas of the arterial circulation partially constricted by atherosclerosis or vasospasm. In these regions, platelets are transiently exposed to elevated levels of shear stress that may exceed 200 dyn/cm$^2$ (38). Rotational viscometers have been widely used to study the direct effect of bulk shear stress on platelet reactions *in vitro*, mimicking arterial stenosis in the presence of an intact endothelium (38). The most common types of viscometers are the couette viscometer (Fig. 20.7), which consists of a rotating concentric cylinder, and the cone-and-plate viscometer (Fig. 20.8), in which a rotating cone is placed near a stationary platen. Each type of viscometer provides a constant uniform shear stress within the suspension, which is proportional to the rotational rate of the system. The shear stress generated in the suspension can therefore be held constant by maintaining constant revolutions per minute. To study the effects of bulk shear stress on platelets independently of platelet-surface reactions, it is common to coat the viscometer surfaces with silicone or other nonthrombogenic materials. Many rotational viscometers have been designed to study bulk phase platelet aggregation (39–42) based on modifications of the above types of viscometers (43, 44). In addition to investigating platelet responses to shear stress, rotational viscometers have been used to study the mechanisms of shear stress-induced platelet activation. Coupled with flow cytometry, the use of a rotational viscometer also allows the study of the effect of shear stress on adhesion molecule expression and number (45).

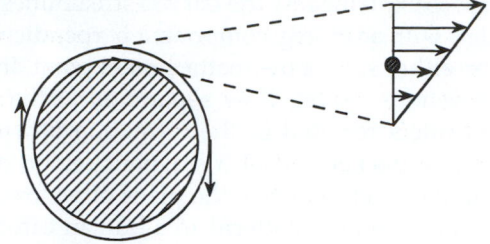

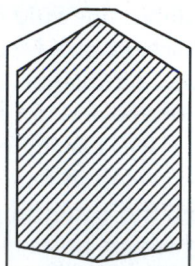

Cross section through couette region

Transverse section

**FIGURE 20.7.** Schematic of the Rice University concentric cylinder viscometer. The platen geometry (61) consists of a long concentric cylinder section in the middle, flanked by a cone-and-plate section at the bottom and a cone-and-plate section at the top. The gaps and cone angles for specific platen pairs are machined such that the shear rate (and therefore the shear stress) in the entire fluid region is essentially constant at fixed rates of rotation. In studying the molecular mechanisms of stress effects on blood cells, this uniformity of stress history is crucial for data interpretation and is dramatically different from what is found in an aggregometer.

# HEMODYNAMIC MODULATION OF THROMBOSIS

## FLOW MODULATION OF MURAL THROMBUS FORMATION

The formation of mural thrombi depends on a cascade of events that includes platelet adhesion onto exposed subendothelial surfaces and subsequent platelet aggregation. These events take place in a dynamic environment in which wall shear stress caused by the viscous nature of flowing blood is a key element. For a thrombus to form on the denuded vessel wall, platelets must be transported to the location, be able to adhere to the surface and to one another, and resist detachment due to shear forces. These processes depend on mechanical shear forces (38). For this reason, the effects of shear stress on the mechanisms involved in mural thrombus formation have been well studied.

### Mass Transfer Effects

The subendothelium may be considered to be a reactive surface for platelets in which the adhesion rate constant,

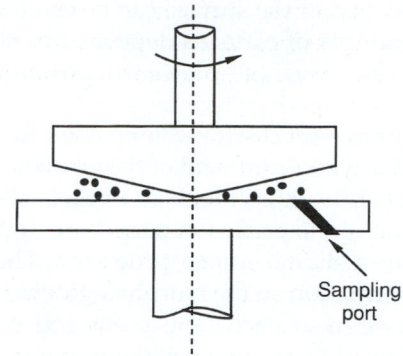

Sampling port

**FIGURE 20.8.** Schematic of a cone-and-plate viscometer. Normally, the plate is held stationary and the cone is rotated. For small cone angles (normally less than 2 degrees) and for relatively low rates of rotation, the shear rate is constant throughout the fluid volume. Therefore, shear stresses are also uniform everywhere within the fluid and all cellular elements experience the same stress history. Also shown is a sampling port in the lower platen that allows specimen withdrawal under shear. (From Jen CJ, McIntire LV. Characteristics of shear-induced aggregation in whole blood. J Lab Clin Med 1984;103:115–124.)

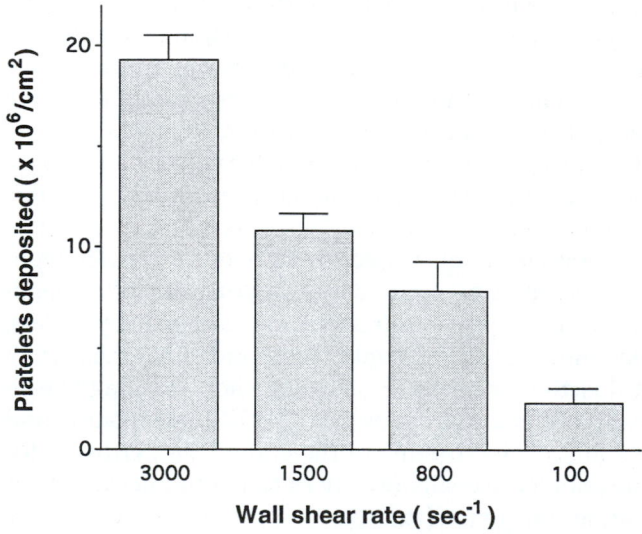

**FIGURE 20.9.** Shear rate dependence of platelet accumulation from flowing citrated whole blood onto collagen-coated (type I; 20 mg/cm²) glass surfaces. Experiments were carried out in a parallel-plate flow chamber at 37°C. The number of platelets deposited increases with increasing shear rate, demonstrating diffusion-controlled kinetics. The data are consistent with the theoretically predicted model for adhesion to a very reactive surface (equations 20.14 and 20.15).

k, is much greater than the diffusion constant, $\mathcal{D}$. As mentioned above, platelet deposition onto exposed subendothelium is a diffusion-controlled process in which the level of platelet deposition is proportional to the shear rate. Fig. 20.9 demonstrates this result, showing a typical trend of platelet deposition from whole blood onto a bovine type I collagen surface as a function of shear rate. The range of shear rates encompasses the physiologic and pathophysiologic relevant range of shear rates from veins to partially constricted arterioles and produces wall shear stresses of approximately 4, 32, 60, and 120 dynes/cm$^2$, respectively (equation 20.8; blood viscosity ~0.04 poise). The number of platelets that accumulated onto collagen I paralleled the increase in wall shear rate, in good agreement with the theoretical predictions (equation 20.15) demonstrating diffusion-controlled kinetics. Whereas platelet deposition onto collagen I demonstrates diffusion-controlled kinetics, care must be taken when considering other isolated components of the subendothelium. For example, platelet deposition onto collagen type VI surfaces does not follow this prediction, giving higher levels of deposition at low shear rates (20, 46). Similar results were recently shown on surface-bound fibrinogen surfaces (47).

## von Willebrand Factor

vWf has been found to be crucial in thrombus formation after vessel wall injury under conditions of high wall shear rates, normally encountered in the arterial circulation (48). It has been shown that vWf mediates platelet adhesion to the injured vessel wall by forming a bridge between insolubilized type I or type III collagen fibrils and platelet surface membrane glycoproteins (49–53). Platelet aggregate formation follows platelet adhesion and requires fibrinogen, vWf, and other adhesive proteins to bind to the platelet surface and bridge the gap between adjacent circulating platelets and the initially adherent ones (29, 31, 54). The importance of vWf is shown qualitatively (see Fig. 20.6; see color plate 20.6) in three-dimensional reconstructions of thrombi formed at the end of a perfusion (1500/s wall shear rate; ~57 dyn/cm$^2$ wall shear stress) over collagen I using severe von Willebrand disease blood in the presence (right) or absence (left) of vWf (19). In addition to collagen types I and III, vWf has also been shown to bind collagen type VI (55, 56), which is known to colocalize with vWf in the subendothelium (57). Platelet adhesion and aggregation on collagen type VI at low wall shear stress depends on vWf (20). The source of vWf can be subendothelial matrix (51), plasma (48), or platelet α-granules (29, 54). However, insoluble vWf in the extracellular matrix appears to be most reactive in initiating platelet adhesion under flow (53). In the absence of shear forces, insoluble vWf alone does not support platelet adhesion.

In perfusion studies using blood from normal subjects: 1) individuals with von Willebrand disease (deficient in vWf; [58]), individuals with Bernard-Soulier syndrome (deficient in platelet membrane GP Ib), or individuals with Glanzmann's thrombasthenia (deficient in platelet membrane GP IIb-IIIa); 2) monoclonal antibodies directed against either platelet GP Ib or IIb-IIIa; and 3) proteolytic fragments of vWf possessing one or two of the epitopes involved in binding to platelets, it was found that both GP Ib and IIb-IIIa interactions with vWf are required for normal platelet thrombus formation on exposed subendothelium or purified collagens under the high wall shear rates normally encountered in the arterial circulation (27–31, 54).

The insolubilization of vWf multimers onto exposed subendothelium or purified collagens may induce a conformational change in the GP Ib binding domain of vWf monomers, allowing platelet adhesion via vWf-GP Ib interactions (27, 29–31, 54). Alternatively, or in addition, it is possible that the arginine-glycine-aspartate sequence (RGD), that is an essential part of the GP IIb-IIIa binding site in the vWf monomeric subunit, might mediate the adhesion between activated GP IIb-IIIa complexes on flowing platelets and vWf multimers insolubilized onto the reactive surface (29, 59). The subsequent cohesion of additional platelets from flowing blood onto those initially adherent may be mediated by GP IIb-IIIa, GP Ib, or both. The precise mechanisms used by the platelet to adhere and subsequently aggregate most likely depend both on the specific surface investigated (i.e., subendothelium, a specific type of collagen, etc.) and the hemodynamics of the shear environment (19, 20, 46).

## SHEAR SRESS-INDUCED PLATELET AGGREGATION

In a rotational cone-and-plate concentric or cylinder viscometer at high shear rates in which platelet-surface interactions are of minimal importance (60, 61), platelets aggregate from platelet-rich plasma (PRP) or from whole blood under conditions of abnormally high fluid shear stress in the presence of large or unusually large vWf multimers, ADP, and Ca$^{2+}$ (62, 63). These components may either be in the fluid exogenous to the platelets or, alternatively, released from the platelet granules themselves. Epinephrine acts synergistically with shear stress to produce platelet aggregation, demonstrating that the effects of shear stress on platelets can be modulated by chemical agonists (64–66). Platelet aggregation can be quantified by measuring the percent decrease in singlet platelets compared to unsheared controls (62, 63), by measuring the actual size distribution of aggregates using an electronic particle counter (60, 61) or flow cytometry (45). High shear rate-induced, vWf-mediated platelet aggregation requires both platelet GP Ib and GP IIb-IIIa receptors (60, 61, 67, 68). These viscometric studies may serve as a model for platelet aggregation and thrombus formation under very high wall shear stresses on the order of $10^2$–$10^5$ dyn/cm$^2$, which may be encountered in atherosclerotic (partially occluded) or vasospastic arteries and arterioles *in vivo*.

# FLOW MODULATION OF ENDOTHELIAL CELL METABOLISM

The production of many bioactive substances by endothelial cells is affected by the local fluid dynamics of their environment (69). This has led to the hypothesis that endothelial cells may act as a "flow sensor" for mechanical forces in the vascular system (70–72). The effects of shear stress and cyclical stain on the cellular function of endothelial cells have been recently reviewed (13, 73, 74) and will be summarized here (Table 20.2). Wall shear stress, in particular, is known to affect numerous endothelial cell functions, including the synthesis and release of a variety of vasoactive and antithrombotic substances. Parallel-plate flow chambers have been used to investigate the effect of shear stress on the gene expression and secretion of many of these substances.

Prostacyclin (PGI$_2$) is a potent vasodilator and endogenous inhibitor of platelet aggregation. Both its pro-

**TABLE 20.2.** Hemodynamic Modulation of Endothelial Cell Gene Expression

| | Cell Type | Hemodynamics | | Response | References |
| --- | --- | --- | --- | --- | --- |
| | | **Force** | **Magnitude** | | |
| PGI$_2$ | HUVEC | SS | Arterial | ⇑ | 16, 75 |
| | BAEC | SS | Arterial | ⇑ | 76 |
| | HUVEC | CS | 10%, 1 Hz | ⇑ | 97 |
| NO | HUVEC | SS | Arterial | ⇑ | 77, 78 |
| tPA | HUVEC | SS | Arterial | ⇑ | 80 |
| | HUVEC | CS | 24%, 1 Hz | ⇑ | 96 |
| | HUVEC | CS | 10%, 1 Hz | NC | 97 |
| PAI-1 | HUVEC | SS | Arterial | NC | 80 |
| ET-1 | BAEC | SS | Arterial | ⇓ | 82, 83 |
| | HUVEC | SS | Arterial | ⇓ | 84 |
| | PAEC | SS | Venous | ⇑ | 85 |
| | HUVEC | CS | 20%, 1 Hz | ⇑ | 98 |
| | BAEC | CS | 20%, ⅓ Hz | NC | 82 |
| PDGF-B | BAEC | SS | Arterial | ⇓ | 83 |
| | | | | ⇑ | 88, 90 |
| | HUVEC | SS | Arterial | ⇑ | 89 |
| | BAEC | CS | 20%, ⅓ Hz | NC | 83 |
| PDGF-A | BAEC | SS | Arterial | NC | 90 |
| | | | | ⇑ | 91 |
| ICAM-1 | HUVEC | SS | Venous | ⇑ | 94 |
| | | | Arterial | ⇑ | 94 |
| VCAM-1 | HUVEC | SS | Venous | ⇓ | 94 |
| | | | Arterial | ⇓ | 94 |
| ELAM-1 | HUVEC | SS | Venous | ⇓ | 94 |
| | | | Arterial | ⇓ | 94 |
| HB-EGF | HUVEC | SS | Arterial | ⇑ | 92 |
| bFGF | HUVEC | SS | Arterial | NC | 81 |
| | BAEC | SS | Arterial | ⇑ | 88 |
| | BAEC | CS | 20%, ⅓ Hz | NC | 83 |
| TGF-β1 | BAEC | SS | Arterial | ⇑ | 93 |
| c-fos | HUVEC | SS | Arterial | ⇑ | 112 |
| | | CS | 20%, 1 Hz | ⇑ | 119 |
| c-jun | HUVEC | SS | Arterial | ⇑ | 112 |
| | | CS | 20%, 1 Hz | ⇑ | 119 |
| c-myc | HUVEC | SS | Arterial | ⇑ | 112 |

SS, shear stress; CS, cyclic strain (% elongation and cycling rate); HUVEC, human umbilical vein endothelial cells; BAEC, bovine aorta endothelial cells; ⇑, increased synthesis or release; ⇓, decreased synthesis or release; NC, no change. (Modified from Patrick CW Jr, McIntire LV. Shear stress and cyclic strain modulation of gene expression in vascular endothelial cells. Blood Purif 1995;13:112–124.)

duction and release are increased by laminar arterial wall shear stress of approximately 10–25 dyn/cm$^2$ in human umbilical vein endothelial cells (HUVEC) or bovine aortic endothelial cells (BAEC) (16, 75, 76). This response is doubled in the presence of pulsatile flow (76). Wall shear stress also increases the release of endothelium-derived relaxing factor or nitric oxide (NO), another inhibitor of platelet aggregation and vasodilator (77, 78). In addition, thrombomodulin (surface receptor that binds thrombin and activates the protein C anticoagulant pathway) mRNA may be upregulated initially, followed by a net decrease in response to arterial levels of wall shear stress (15–36 dyn/cm$^2$) (79). There is also increased production of tissue-type plasminogen activator (t-PA), an antithrombotic glycoprotein and serine protease, but not of plasminogen activator inhibitor type 1 (PAI-1) by HUVEC (80) at these wall shear stress levels. The changes in secretion rate of t-PA with wall shear stress are accompanied by parallel alterations in the messenger RNA levels (81).

In contrast, endothelin-1 (ET-1), a smooth muscle cell (SMC) mitogen and vasoconstrictor, shows decreased release and mRNA expression in response to sustained arterial levels of shear stress (15–25 dyn/cm$^2$) in both BAEC (82, 83) and HUVEC (84). The downregulation is sensitive to the shear stress level in a dose-dependent manner, with maximal inhibition occurring at 15 dyn/cm$^2$. However, venous levels of shear stress have been shown to cause a transient increase in ET-1 mRNA expression, which peaked at 4 hours and returned to basal level at 12–24 hours (85) in porcine aortic endothelial cells (PAEC). Similarly, Kuchan and Frangos demonstrated that sustained levels of low shear stress (1.8 dyn/cm$^2$) or brief exposure (<1 hour) to 10 dyn/cm$^2$ caused an increase in ET-1 release from HUVEC (86). Platelet-derived growth factor (PDGF) is another SMC mitogen and vasoconstrictor that is regulated at the mRNA level by wall shear stress. PDGF is a dimer that is made of two subunits: PDGF-A and PDGF-B. Conflicting results on PDGF-B mRNA expression in response to shear stress have been reported for BAEC. In one case, arterial levels of wall shear stress (15–36 dyn/cm$^2$) were shown to decrease mRNA levels over a 9-hour period (87). Conversely, wall shear stresses of 10–30 dyn/cm$^2$ have been shown to increase mRNA expression (88). In support of the latter finding, Hsieh et al have reported up-regulation of PDGF-B mRNA in HUVEC in the presence of 16 dyn/cm shear stress (89). There are also conflicting reports regarding the expression of PDGF-A in response to shear stress, with one study demonstrating no change in mRNA expression upon exposure to arterial shear stress (90) and another showing a shear-dependent increase from 0–6 dyn/cm$^2$ that plateaus from 6–51 dyn/cm$^2$ (91).

The mRNA expression of several growth factors has also been shown to be regulated by wall shear stress. Specifically, heparin binding epidermal growth factor (HB-EGF), an SMC mitogen, and transforming growth factor β1 (TGF-β1) are both upregulated in response to arterial levels of shear stress (92, 93). The response of basic fibroblast growth factor (bFGF) mRNA expression is not clear, with arterial levels of shear stress causing an increase in expression in BAEC and no change in HUVEC (81, 88).

Wall shear stress has also been shown to modulate the mRNA expression of several adhesion molecules in endothelial cells (94). Endothelial cell intercellular adhesion molecule-1 (ICAM-1) binds leukocytes, monocytes, and granulocytes (see Chapter 15). Arterial (10–25 dyn/cm$^2$) as well as venous (2 dyn/cm$^2$) levels of shear stress cause transient up-regulation of ICAM-1. Conversely, vascular cell adhesion molecule-1 (VCAM-1), which binds lymphocytes and monocytes, and E-selectin (ELAM-1), which binds sialylated carbohydrate molecules on leukocytes, both show decreased mRNA expression upon exposure to either venous or arterial levels of shear stress. These results suggest that endothelial cell response to shear stress may play a role in modulating the inflammatory response.

The above findings of endothelial cell response to shear stress are consistent with the observations that atherosclerotic plaques develop in regions of relatively low wall shear stress. In these regions, high secretion of endothelin and low secretion of t-PA by the endothelial cells on the vessel wall could lead to smooth muscle cell proliferation and to problems with clot formation. The observations that blood vessels constrict in response to decreased flow (95) could be explained by the increase in endothelin secretion with decreased wall shear stress (69). Flow-modulated vessel dilation and constriction can also be explained by the coupling of changes in local wall shear stress and the production of NO (77) and prostacyclin (16, 75).

## CYCLIC STRAIN MODULATION OF ENDOTHELIAL CELL METABOLISM

In addition to wall shear stress caused by flowing blood, endothelial cells are exposed to cyclic strain due to transmural pressure changes that cause deformation (dilation or constriction) of the vessel wall (38). The ensuing tensile stress produces strain, which is the force that would tear a cell from its normal position in the vessel wall. This force is a measure of the change of vessel circumference generated by the dilation or constriction of a blood vessel. One effect of the tensile stress is to stretch cells that are anchored in the vessel wall. A physiologic level of cyclic strain is 10% elongation at a cycling rate of 1 Hz.

As with shear stress, endothelial cell gene expression and function may be affected by cyclic stretch. Specifically, t-PA mRNA has been shown to be upregulated in response to a cyclic strain of 24% at 1 Hz (96); however, a cyclic strain of 10% at 1 Hz yielded no change in t-PA production (97). Similar to the effect of shear stress, cyclic strain has been shown to increase prostacyclin release (HUVEC, 10% stretch at 1 Hz) (97) and to upregulate endothelial NO synthase mRNA (BAEC, 6–10% stretch at 1 Hz). Interestingly, endothelial cells in the presence of cyclic stretch demonstrate an opposite response than to shear stress with respect to ET-1 and PAI-1. The mRNA level of ET-1 has been shown to increase in response to a cyclic stretch of 20% at 1 Hz in HUVEC (98). However, BAEC show no response in ET-1 mRNA regulation in response to a cyclic stretch of 20% at 1/3 Hz (82). This difference could be a result of the cycling rate or difference in cell source. Cyclic strain has also been shown to increase PAI-1 secretion in endothelial cells (97) that is mediated by an increase in reactive oxygen species (99). Endothelial cells (BAEC) show no change in expression of PDGF-B or bFGF mRNA in response to a cyclic strain of 20% at 1/3 Hz (87, 88).

## MECHANOTRANSDUCTION IN ENDOTHELIAL CELLS

At the interface between the flowing blood and vessel wall, endothelial cells are in a physiologic position to "sense" shear stress and cyclic strain and to convert the mechanical signal to an intracellular response. The mechanisms of "mechanotransduction" have not yet been elucidated and are currently poorly understood (100). The result that endothelial cells are able to respond differently to shear stress vs. cyclic strain (such as in the cases of ET-1 and PAI-1) supports the concept that different mechanical stimuli act as different mechanical signals or "agonists" (72). This implies a high level of sophistication not only in sensing mechanical signals, but also in differentiating between them.

Endothelial cell responses to mechanical "agonists" can either be very rapid or delayed (reflecting up-regulation of gene expression) and may involve both second messengers and cytoskeletal reorganization in the signal transduction. Second messengers are important components of various signal transduction schemes and, when elevated, activate metabolic and regulatory pathways in endothelial cells. Hemodynamic forces, including shear stress (and the resultant mass transfer) and cyclic strain, are known to affect many second messengers (73, 101), including: 1) increasing cytosolic free calcium ion ($Ca^{2+}$) concentration (102–106); 2) inositol 1,4,5-triphosphate ($IP_3$) (107–109); 3) diacylglycerol (DAG) (107, 110); 4) cyclic adenosine monophosphate (cAMP); 5) cyclic guanosine monophosphate (cGMP) (86, 111); 6) protein kinase C (PKC) (86, 89, 112); 7) pH (113); and 8) adenylyl cyclase (114). There is substantial evidence that the PKC signal transduction pathway may be important in trans-

mitting mechanical signals into altered gene expression. The PKC pathway has been shown to be involved in several endothelial cell responses. Examples include PKC involvement in the increase in ET-1 in response to cyclic strain (98) and in the PDGF gene expression in response to shear stress (89). In addition, hemodynamic forces may also modulate cell behavior by transducing the signal into cytoskeletal reorganization or by direct transmission of the force via the cytoskeleton (115). Muller et al recently demonstrated that inhibition of integrin binding to the RGD sequence in extracellular matrix proteins blunts shear stress-induced vasodilation of coronary arterioles, suggesting that integrin binding and focal adhesion formation between endothelial cells and the ECM are important in mechanotransduction (116).

The mechanism by which endothelial cell gene transcription is modulated by mechanical forces may also include transcriptional factors ("third messengers"), which are proteins that are typically located in the cytosol or plasma membrane (117). These molecules, upon activation by second messengers, bind to the DNA and play an active role in mediating signal transduction (73, 100, 118). Several transcriptional factors shown to be upregulated in response to shear stress and cyclic strain are protein products of proto-oncogenes (112, 119). The transcription factors in endothelial cells can be grouped into two families: nuclear activator protein 1 (AP-1) and nuclear factor kappa B (NFκB) (100, 120) (Table 20.3). AP-1 complex is formed through the dimerization of Fos/Jun families of proteins (118) and can bind to cis-acting elements TRE (tumor-promoting agent response element) and CRE (cAMP response element) found in certain gene promoters (121, 122). To date, only the monocyte chemotactic protein 1 (MCP-1) gene has been

**TABLE 20.3.** Transcription Factors Involved in Shear Stress-Induced Gene Regulation and their DNA Binding Sequences

| DNA Binding Factor | DNA Binding Sequence |
|---|---|
| AP-1 (*c-fos/c-jun* or *c-jun/c-jun*) | TRE: TGACTCA |
| | CRE: TGACGTCA |
| NFκB (p50/p65) | NFκB: GGAAGATCCCT |
| NFκB, others (p50/p65, others) | SSRE: GAGACC |

AP-1, activator protein-1; TRE, tumor-promoting agent response element; CRE, cAMP response element; NFκB, nuclear factor kappa B; SSRE, shear stress response element.
(From Papadaki M, Eskin SG. Effects of fluid shear stress on gene regulation of vascular cells. Biotech Proc 1997;13:209–221.)

shown to respond to shear stress through AP1-DNA binding in endothelial cells (122). NFκB is a pluripotent transcription factor that exists as a heterodimer of p50 and p65 proteins (120). NFκB/DNA binding sites are found on inducible genes in vascular cells, including VCAM-1 (vascular cell adhesion molecule 1), E-selectin, tissue factor, IL-1, IL-6, IL-8 and *c-myc* (123). In addition, it has been proposed that shear stress can initiate molecular signaling events through a "stress sensitive" response element (73, 88, 100, 121, 124). There is experimental evidence of a shear stress response element (SSRE) in the promoter the PDGF-B gene (88) and this sequence is found in several other shear sensitive genes, including *c-fos, c-jun*, NO synthase III, MCP-1, t-PA, TGF-β1, and ICAM-1 (88, 121). Interestingly, the transcription factor that appears to interact with the SSRE in the promoter of the PDGF-B gene is NFκB (125).

The mechanisms by which platelet behavior and thrombosis are modulated by endothelial cells are complex. Whereas high levels of shear stress can activate platelets, the same mechanical force acting on endothelial cells causes the release of antithrombotic agents such as prostacyclin and NO. These endothelial cell products may act synergistically to inhibit platelet aggregation, as has been shown with prostacyclin and NO (126). Thus a complex and delicate balance is struck in maintaining the fluidity of blood. Perturbing this balance may lead to platelet adhesion, subsequent aggregation, and thrombus formation.

## FLOW MODULATION OF SMOOTH MUSCLE CELL GROWTH AND METABOLISM

Vascular smooth muscle cells are not typically exposed to fluid shear stresses caused by flowing blood because they lie beneath the endothelium. However, if the endothelial cell layer is damaged, such as in the case of percutaneous transluminal angioplasty or atherosclerosis, smooth muscle cells will be directly subjected to shear stresses. In contrast to endothelial cells that elongate in the direction of flow *in vitro* (127, 128), human aortic smooth muscle cell (hASMC) orientation is not affected by shear stresses of the level 5-25 dyn/cm$^2$ (129). However, Papadaki et al recently showed that exposure to hydrodynamic forces caused hASMC to alter their population dynamics, resulting in a decreased growth rate due to shear stress exposure *in vitro* (129). Previous work by Sterpetti et al with bovine smooth muscle cells demonstrated a similar trend of reduced SMC growth rate with increasing levels of shear stress (130, 131). However, in the case of bSMC, growth was arrested at shear stresses above 3 dyn/cm$^2$.

In addition to the shear stress generated by blood flow at the site of a denuding endothelial cell injury, smooth muscle cells are exposed to significant levels of fluid shear stress that are predicted to be on the order of 1 dyn/cm$^2$ due to normal transmural flow (132). As mentioned above, this level of shear stress is known to affect endothelial cell biology, including the secretion of eicosanoids. In particular, arachidonic acid metabolites prostaglandin I$_2$ (PGI$_2$) and prostaglandin E$_2$ (PGE$_2$) have been shown to be potent vasoactive substances that regulate vasomotor tone and intimal thickness (133). A recent study by Alshihabi et al demonstrated that there is a direct effect of fluid shear stress (0.5–20 dyn/cm$_2$) on the production of both PGI$_2$ and PGE$_2$ in rat aortic smooth muscle cells (134). Two distinct dynamic patterns of secretion were observed. The SMC production of PGI$_2$ progressed more rapidly and was more sensitive to shear stress than the production of PGE$_2$, with a level of 0.5 dyn/cm$^2$ producing maximal PGI$_2$ release. These results suggest that a low level of shear stress, such as that associated with transmural flow, may be sufficient to influence arterial wall remodeling. Inasmuch as production of PGI$_2$ is known to inhibit the proliferation of arterial SMC (135), these results are consistent with the results presented above in which increased fluid shear stress caused a decrease in SMC proliferation. Wagner et al have also shown that shear stress, as well as cyclic stretch, induces heme-oxygenase-1 gene expression and resultant carbon monoxide production by SMC (136). Finally, intimal thickening in vascular proliferative diseases is known to be correlated with regions of low wall shear stress (137, 138). The recent studies on the effect of shear stress on smooth muscle cell metabolism and growth further support the notion that mechanical forces are important in the hyperproliferative response of the vascular wall.

## FLOW MODULATION OF COAGULATION

Pathologic interactions among blood lipids, platelets, leukocytes, and vascular cells can damage the endothelium (via neutrophil-derived substances) and induce thrombosis at the injury site (via released procoagulants) (139). Exposed subendothelial fibrillar collagen activates the intrinsic pathway, and tissue factor from damaged cells triggers the extrinsic pathway of the coagulation cascade, both leading to thrombin production, fibrin deposition, and thrombus formation (140).

Several important reactions in the coagulation cascade that lead to the production of thrombin and generation of fibrin involve the formation of catalytic complexes consisting of a circulating component and a component bound to cell membranes (141). Formation of these enzyme complexes and the rates of product formation from the reactions they catalyze will depend on the delivery (mass transport) of the circulating factor by flowing blood to the immobilized factor (142). Gemmell et al demonstrated this to be the case for the complex composed of circulating factor VII and membrane-bound tissue factor, which activates factor X (143). Similarly, Schoen et al (144) studied the implication of flow in the formation of the prothrombinase complex, which consists of circulating factor Xa and phospholipid-bound factor Va and converts prothrombin to thrombin (see Chapter 1). The results of the study were consistent with the assembly of prothrombinase being dependent on the flux of factor Xa to the phospholipid-bound factor Va.

In addition to enhancing the transport of reactants and products to and from the vessel wall, fluid flow may also have a direct effect on the enzyme kinetics involved in thrombosis. For example, a recent numerical analysis of the activation of factor X by surface-bound tissue factor-factor VIIa demonstrated that fluid flow has a direct effect on the kinetics of factor X activation, with $K_m$ decreasing and $V_{max}$ increasing with increasing shear rate (145). These results demonstrate that some coagulation processes are accelerated in the presence of shear.

In contrast, analysis of fibrin deposition on exposed subendothelial surfaces to normal flowing whole blood showed an inverse relationship between fibrin formation and shear rate. Because convective mass transport increases as the wall shear rate increases, it follows that the concentration of activated coagulation factors produced by complexes at the vessel wall will decrease, with a subsequent decrease in thrombin and fibrin formation (146). Flow-induced increase in the secretion of t-PA by endothelial cells could also lead to the same result, by enhancing the breakdown of any fibrin polymer formed.

## ARTERIAL VS. VENOUS THROMBOSIS

In the arterial circulation, vascular injury can occur by hemodynamic stresses, oxidized cholesterol and neutrophil-released substance, rupture of an atherosclerotic plaque by activated macrophages, or during surgery, leading to endothelial denudation and, if severe, to exposure of flowing blood to fibrillar collagens from the intima or media of the subendothelial layers. The combination of high flow rates with the platelet-subendothelium adhesive interactions mediated by vWf (48, 49) could lead to the formation of arterial platelet-rich thrombi. Vascular injury with superimposed occlusive thrombus formation is the most common mechanism leading to the acute coronary syndromes in humans (unstable angina, acute myocardial infarction, and sudden death). It also appears to be a critical event in coronary vein graft disease and in postangioplasty restenosis (16).

Badimon and Badimon (25) evaluated the location of the growing thrombus in a stenotic injured vessel within an extracorporeal perfusion chamber in the swine model, simulating the mechanism of platelet deposition after plaque rupture in atherosclerotic coronary

arteries *in vivo*. Significantly, higher platelet accumulation occurred at the top of the stenosis (area of high wall shear rate) compared to the areas proximal or distal to the stenosis, in contrast to the preferential sites of thrombosis observed in the absence of severe vascular injury (areas of low wall shear rate). They concluded that vWf-mediated platelet adhesion and vWf-mediated, shear-induced platelet aggregation are the determinant factors for thrombosis in injured stenosed arteries (147).

In the venous circulation, venous wall damage is often due to monocyte and neutrophil adherence, and the release of lysosomal enzymes by leukocytes at inflammatory sites. Because the wall shear rates are low, the residence time of circulating cells and macromolecules near the injured vessel wall is prolonged. This facilitates the interaction of platelets and clotting factors with the subendothelium. It also prevents the mixing of activated coagulation factors with their inhibitors. Thrombi, which form in regions of stasis to low flow, usually in the venous system of the legs, are composed of entrapped red blood cells with a large amount of interspersed fibrin and a smaller component of aggregated platelets. It seems that the major mechanism for venous thrombosis is the activation of the coagulation cascade, and that molecular mechanisms used for cellular adhesion may be quite different in venous vs. arterial flows.

## REFERENCES

1. Bird RB, Stewart WE, Lightfoot EN. Transport phenomena. New York: John Wiley and Sons, Inc., 1960:42.
2. Goldsmith HL, Turitto VT. Rheological aspects of thrombosis and haemostasis: basic principles and applications. Thromb Haemost 1986;55: 415–435.
3. Turitto VT, Baumgartner HR. Platelet-surface interactions. In: Colman RW, Hirsh J, Marder VJ, Saltzman EW, eds. Hemostasis and thrombosis: basic principles and clinical practice. Philadelphia: J.B. Lippincott, 1982.
4. Errill EW. Rheology of blood. Physiol Rev 1969;49:863–888.
5. Grabowski EF, Friedman LI, Leonard EF. Effects of shear rate on the diffusion and adhesion of blood platelets to a foreign surface. Ind Eng Chem Fundam 1972;11:224–232.
6. Turitto VT, Baumgartner HR. Platelet deposition on subendothelium exposed to flowing blood: mathematical analysis of physical parameters. Trans Am Soc Artif Intern Organs 1975;21:593–610.
7. Wang N-HL, Keller KH. Augmented transport of extracellular solutes in concentrated erythrocyte suspensions in couette flow. J Colloid Interface Sci 1985;103:210–225.
8. Eckstein EC, Belgacem F. Model of platelet transport in flowing blood with drift and diffusion terms. Biophys J 1991;60:53–69.
9. McIntire LV, Eskin SG. Mechanical and biochemical aspects of leukocyte interactions with model vessel walls. In: Meiselman HJ, Lichtman MA, Celle PLL, eds. White cell mechanics: Basic science and clinical aspects. New York: Alan R. Liss, 1984.
10. Turitto VT, Muggli R, Baumgartner HR. Physical factors influencing platelet deposition on subendothelium: importance of blood shear rate. Ann N Y Acad Sci 1977;283:284–292.
11. Baumgartner HR, Sakariassen KS. Factors controlling thrombus formation on arterial lesions. Ann N Y Acad Sci 1985;454:162–177.
12. Hubbell JA, McIntire LV. Technique for visualization and analysis of mural thrombogenesis. Rev Sci Instrum 1986;57:892–897.
13. Patrick CW, Sampath R, McIntire LV. Fluid shear stress effects on cellular function. In: Bronzino JD, ed. Biomedical engineering handbook. Boca Raton: CRC Press, 1995:1636–1655.
14. Slack SM, Turitto VT. Flow chambers and their standardization for use in studies of thrombosis. Thromb Haemost 1994;72:771–781.
15. Baumgartner HR, Haudenschild C. Adhesion of platelets to subendothelium. Ann N Y Acad Sci 1972;201:22–36.

16. Frangos JA, McIntire LV, Eskin SG. Shear stress induced stimulation of mammalian cell metabolism. Biotechnol Bioeng 1988;32:1053–1060.

17. Dise CA, Burch JW, Goodman DB. Direct interaction of mepacrine with erythrocyte and platelet membrane phospholipid. J Biol Chem 1982;257:4701–4704.

18. Grabowski EF. Platelet aggregation in flowing blood at a site of injury to an endothelial cell monolayer: quantitation and real-time imaging with the TAB monoclonal antibody. Blood 1990;75:390–398.

19. Alevriadou BR, Moake JL, Turner NA et al. Real-time analysis of shear-dependent thrombus formation and its blockade by inhibitors of von Willebrand factor binding to platelets. Blood 1993;81:1263–1276.

20. Ross JM, McIntire LV, Moake JL et al. Platelet adhesion and aggregation on human type VI collagen surfaces under physiological flow conditions. Blood 1995;85:1826–1835.

21. Folie BJ, McIntire LV, Lasslo A. Effects of a novel antiplatelet agent in mural thrombogenesis on collagen-coated glass. Blood 1988;72:1393–1400.

22. Turner NA, Moake JL, Kamat SG et al. Comparative real-time effects on platelet adhesion and aggregation under flowing conditions of in vivo aspirin, heparin, and monoclonal antibody fragment against glycoprotein IIb-IIIa. Circulation 1995;91:1354–1362.

23. Hubbell JA, McIntire LV. Visualization and analysis of mural thrombogenesis on collagen, polyurethane and nylon. Biomaterials 1986;7:354–363.

24. Hanson SR, Kotze HF, Savage B et al. Platelet interactions with Dacron vascular grafts: a model of acute thrombosis in baboons. Arteriosclerosis 1985;5:595–603.

25. Badimon L, Badimon JJ. Mechanisms of arterial thrombosis in nonparallel streamlines: platelet thrombi grow on the apex of stenotic severely injured vessel wall. Experimental study in the pig model. J Clin Invest 1989;84:1134–1144.

26. Sixma JJ, Nievelstein PF, Houdijk WP et al. Adhesion of blood platelets to isolated components of the vessel wall. Ann N Y Acad Sci 1987;509:103–117.

27. Fressinaud E, Baruch D, Girma JP et al. von Willebrand factor-mediated platelet adhesion to collagen involves platelet membrane glycoprotein IIb-IIIa as well as glycoprotein Ib. J Lab Clin Med 1988;112:58–67.

28. Sakariassen KS, Fressinaud E, Girma JP et al. Mediation of platelet adhesion to fibrillar collagen in flowing blood by a proteolytic fragment of human von Willebrand factor. Blood 1986;67:1515–1518.

29. Weiss HJ, Turitto VT, Baumgartner HR. Platelet adhesion and thrombus formation on subendothelium in platelets deficient in glycoproteins IIb-IIIa, Ib, and storage granules. Blood 1986;67:322–330.

30. Sakariassen KS, Fressinaud E, Girma JP et al. Role of platelet membrane glycoproteins and von Willebrand factor in adhesion of platelets to subendothelium and collagen. Ann N Y Acad Sci 1987;516:52–65.

31. Meyer D, Fressinaud E, Sakariassen KS et al. Role of von Willebrand factor in platelet vessel-wall interactions. Ann N Y Acad Sci 1987;509:118–130.

32. Karino T, Motomiya M. Flow visualization in isolated transparent natural blood vessels. Biorheology 1983;20:119–127.

33. Karino T, Goldsmith HL. Role of blood cell-wall interactions in thrombogenesis and atherogenesis: a microrheological study. Biorheology 1984;21:587–601.

34. Motomiya M, Karino T. Flow patterns in the human carotid artery bifurcation. Stroke 1984;15:50–56.

35. Karino T, Goldsmith HL, Motomiya M et al. Flow patterns in vessels of simple and complex geometries. Ann N Y Acad Sci 1987;516:422–441.

36. Zarins CK, Giddens DP, Bharadaj BK et al. Carotid bifurcation atherosclerosis. Quantitative correlation of plaque localization with flow velocity profiles and wall shear stress. Circ Res 1983;53:502–514.

37. Ku DN, Giddens DP, Zarins CK et al. Pulsatile flow and arteriosclerosis in the human carotid bifurcation. Positive correlation between plaque location and low oscillating shear stress. Arteriosclerosis 1985;5:293–302.

38. Kroll MH, Hellums JD, McIntire LV et al. Platelets and shear stress. Blood 1996;88:1525–1541.

39. MacCallum RN, O'Bannon W, Hellums JD et al. Viscometric instruments for studies on red blood cell damage. In: Gabelnick HL, Litt M, eds. Rheology of biological systems. Springfield, IL: Charles C Thomas, 1973:70.

40. Belval T, Hellums JD, Solis RT. The kinetics of platelet aggregation induced by fluid-shearing stress. Microvasc Res 1984;28:279–288.

41. Giorgio TD, Hellums JD. A cone and plate viscometer for the continuous measurement of blood platelet activation. Biorheology 1988;25:605–624.

42. Fukuyama M, Sakai K, Itagaki I et al. Continuous measurement of shear-induced platelet aggregation. Thromb Res 1989;54:253–260.

43. Joist JH, Zeffren DJ, Bauman JE. A programmable, computer-controlled cone-plate viscometer for the application of pulsatile shear stress to platelet suspensions. Biorheology 1988;25:449–459.

44. Chow TW, Hellums JD, Moake JL et al. Shear stress-induced von Willebrand factor binding to platelet glycoprotein Ib initiates calcium influx associated with aggregation. Blood 1992;80:113–120.

45. Konstantopoulos K, Wu KK, Udden MM et al. Flow cytometric studies of platelet responses to shear stress in whole blood. Biorheology 1995;32:73.

46. Saelman EU, Nieuwenhuis HK, Hese KM et al. Platelet adhesion to collagen types I through VIII under conditions of stasis and flow is mediated by GP Ia/IIa (a2b1—integrin). Blood 1994;83:1244–1250.

47. Zaidi TN, McIntire LV, Farrell DH et al. Adhesion of platelets to surface-bound fibrinogen under flow. Blood 1996;88:2967–2972.

48. Weiss HJ, Turitto VT, Baumgartner HR. Effect of shear rate on platelet interaction with subendothelium in citrated and native blood. I. Shear rate-dependent decrease of adhesion in von Willebrand's disease and the Bernard-Soulier syndrome. J Lab Clin Med 1978;92:750–764.

49. Sakariassen KS, Bolhuis PA, Sixma JJ. Human blood platelet adhesion to artery subendothelium is mediated by factor VIII-von Willebrand factor bound to the subendothelium. Nature 1979;279:636–638.

50. Bolhuis PA, Sakariassen KS, Sander HJ et al. Binding of factor VIII-von Willebrand factor to human arterial subendothelium precedes increased platelet adhesion and enhances platelet spreading. J Lab Clin Med 1981;97:568–576.

51. Stel HV, Sakariassen KS, de Groot PG et al. von Willebrand factor in the vessel wall mediates platelet adherence. Blood 1985;65:85–90.

52. Turitto VT, Weiss HJ, Zimmerman TS et al. Factor VIII/von Willebrand factor in subendothelium mediates platelet adhesion. Blood 1985;65:823–831.

53. Baruch D, Denis C, Marteaux C et al. Role of von Willebrand factor associated to extracellular matrices in platelet adhesion. Blood 1991;77:519–527.

54. Sakariassen KS, Nievelstein PF, Coller BS et al. The role of platelet membrane glycoproteins Ib and IIb-IIIa in platelet adherence to human artery subendothelium. Br J Haematol 1986;63:681–691.

55. Pareti FI, Fujimura Y, Dent JA et al. Isolation and characterization of a collagen binding domain in human von Willebrand factor. J Biol Chem 1986;261:15310–15315.

56. Rand JH, Patel ND, Schwartz E et al. 150-kD von Willebrand factor binding protein extracted from human vascular subendothelium is type VI collagen. J Clin Invest 1991;88:253–259.

57. Rand JH, Wu XX, Uson RR et al. Co-localization of von Willebrand factor and type VI collagen in human vascular subendothelium. Am J Pathol 1993;142:843–850.

58. Ruggeri ZM, Zimmerman TS. von Willebrand factor and von Willebrand disease. Blood 1987;70:895–904.

59. Sheppeck RA, Bentz M, Dickson C et al. Examination of the roles of glycoprotein Ib and glycoprotein IIb-IIIa in platelet deposition on an artificial surface using clinical antiplatelet agents and monoclonal antibody blockade. Blood 1991;78:673–680.

60. Jen CJ, McIntire LV. Characteristics of shear-induced aggregation in whole blood. J Lab Clin Med 1984;103:115–124.

61. Dewitz TS, Martin RR, Solis RT et al. Microaggregate formation in whole blood exposed to shear stress. Microvasc Res 1978;16:263–271.

62. Moake JL, Turner NA, Stathopoulos NA et al. Involvement of large plasma von Willebrand factor (vWf) multimers and unusually large vWf forms derived from endothelial cells in shear stress-induced platelet aggregation. J Clin Invest 1986;78:1456–1461.

63. Moake JL, Turner NA, Stathopoulos NA et al. Shear-induced platelet aggregation can be mediated by vWf released from platelets, as well as by exogenous large or unusually large vWf multimers, requires adenosine diphosphate, and is resistant to aspirin. Blood 1988;71:1366–1374.

64. Goto S, Ikeda Y, Murata M et al. Epinephrine augments von Willebrand factor-dependent shear-induced platelet aggregation. Circulation 1992;86:1859–1863.

65. Goto S, Handa S, Takahashi E et al. Synergistic effect of epinephrine and shearing on platelet activation. Thromb Res 1996;84:351–359.

66. Wagner CT, Kroll MH, Chow TW et al. Epinephrine and shear stress synergistically induce platelet aggregation via a mechanism that partially bypasses vWf-GP Ib interactions. Biorheology 1996;33:209–229.

67. Peterson DM, Stathopoulos NA, Giorgio TD et al. Shear-induced platelet aggregation requires von Willebrand factor and platelet membrane glycoproteins Ib and IIb-IIIa. Blood 1987;69:625–628.

68. Ikeda Y, Handa M, Kawano K et al. The role of von Willebrand factor and fibrinogen in platelet aggregation under varying shear stress. J Clin Invest 1991;87:1234–1240.

69. Nollert MU, Diamond SL, McIntire LV. Hydrodynamic shear stress and mass transport modulation of endothelial cell metabolism. Biotechnol Bioeng 1991;38:588–602.

70. Glagov S. Intimal hyperplasia, vascular modeling, and the restenosis problem. Circulation 1994;89:2888–2891.

71. Reinhart WH. Shear-dependence of endothelial functions. Experientia 1994;50:87–93.

72. Ziegler T, Nerem RM. Tissue engineering a blood vessel: regulation of vascular biology by mechanical stresses. J Cell Biochem 1994;56:204–209.

73. Patrick CW Jr, McIntire LV. Shear stress and cyclic strain modulation of gene expression in vascular endothelial cells. Blood Purif 1995;13:112–124.

74. Patrick CW, McIntire LV. Bioengineering contributions in vascular biology at the cellular and molecular level. Trends Cardiovasc Med 1996;6:122–129.

75. Frangos JA, Eskin SG, McIntire LV et al. Flow effects on prostacyclin production by cultured human endothelial cells. Science 1985;227:1477–1479.

76. Grabowski EF, Jaffe EA, Weksler BB. Prostacyclin production by cultured endothelial cell monolayers exposed to step increases in shear stress. J Lab Clin Med 1985;105:36–43.

77. Rubanyi GM, Romero JC, Vanhoutte PM. Flow-induced release of endothelium-derived relaxing factor. Am J Physiol 1986;250:H1145–H1149.

78. Taylor WR, Harrison DG, Nerem RM et al. Characterization of the release of endothelium-derived nitrogen oxides by shear stress [Abstract]. FASEB J 1991;5:A1727.

79. Malek AM, Jackman R, Rosenberg RD et al. Endothelial expression of thrombomodulin is reversibly regulated by fluid shear stress. Circ Res 1994;74:852–860.

80. Diamond SL, Eskin SG, McIntire LV. Fluid flow stimulates tissue plasminogen activator secretion by cultured human endothelial cells. Science 1989;243:1483–1485.

81. Diamond SL, Sharefkin JB, Dieffenbach C et al. Tissue plasminogen activator messenger RNA levels increase in cultured human endothelial cells exposed to laminar shear stress. J Cell Physiol 1990;143:364–371.

82. Malek A, Izumo S. Physiological fluid shear stress causes downregulation of endothelin-1 mRNA in bovine aortic endothelium. Am J Physiol 1992;263:C389–C396.

83. Malek AM, Greene AL, Izumo S. Regulation of endothelin-1 gene by fluid shear stress is transcriptionally mediated and independent of protein kinase C and cAMP. Proc Natl Acad Sci U S A 1993;90:5999–6003.

84. Sharefkin JB, Diamond SL, Eskin SG et al. Fluid flow decreases preproendothelin mRNA levels and suppresses endothelin-1 peptide release in cultured human endothelial cells. J Vasc Surg 1991;14:1–9.

85. Yoshizumi M, Kurihara H, Sugiyama T et al. Hemodynamic shear stress stimulates endothelin production by cultured endothelial cells. Biochem Biophys Res Commun 1989;161:859–864.

86. Kuchan MJ, Frangos JA. Shear stress regulates endothelin-1 release via protein kinase C and cGMP in cultured endothelial cells. Am J Physiol 1993;264:H150–H156.

87. Malek AM, Gibbons GH, Dzau VJ et al. Fluid shear stress differentially modulates expression of genes encoding basic fibroblast growth factor and platelet-derived growth factor B chain in vascular endothelium. J Clin Invest 1993;92:2013–2021.

88. Resnick N, Collins T, Atkinson W et al. Platelet-derived growth factor B chain promoter contains a cis-acting fluid shear-stress-responsive element. Proc Natl Acad Sci U S A 1993;90:4591–4595.

89. Hsieh HJ, Li NQ, Frangos JA. Shear induced platelet-derived growth factor gene expression in human endothelial cells is mediated by protein kinase C. J Cell Physiol 1992;150:552–558.

90. Mitsumata M, Fishel RS, Nerem RM et al. Fluid shear stress stimulates platelet-derived growth factor expression in endothelial cells. Am J Physiol 1993;265:H3–H8.

91. Hsieh HJ, Li NQ, Frangos JA. Shear stress increases endothelial platelet-derived growth factor mRNA levels. Am J Physiol 1991;260:H642–H646.

92. Morita T, Yoshizumi M, Kurihara H et al. Shear stress increases heparin-binding epidermal growth factor-like growth factor mRNA levels in human vascular endothelial cells. Biochem Biophys Res Commun 1993;197:256–262.

93. Ohno M, Cooke J, Dzau V et al. Fluid shear stress induces endothelial transforming growth factor β-1 transcription and production. Modulation by potassium channel blockade. J Clin Invest 1995;95:1363–1369.

94. Sampath R, Kukielka G, Smith CW et al. Shear stress-mediated changes in the expression of leukocyte adhesion receptors on human umbilical vein endothelial cells in vitro. Ann Biomed Eng 1995;23:247–256.

95. Rubanyi GM, Freay AD, Kauser K et al. Mechanoreception by the endothelium: Mediators and mechanisms of pressure- and flow-induced vascular responses. Blood Vessels 1990;27:246–257.

96. Iba T, Shin T, Sonoda T et al. Stimulation of endothelial secretion of tissue-type plasminogen activator by repetitive stretch. J Surg Res 1991;50:457–460.

97. Carosi JA, McIntire LV. Modulation of secretion of vasoactive materials from human and bovine endothelial cells by cyclic strain. Biotechnol Bioeng 1994;43:615–621.

98. Wang DL, Tang CC, Wung BS et al. Cyclical strain increases endothelin-1 secretion and gene expression in human endothelial cells. Biochem Biophys Res Commun 1993;195:1050–1056.

99. Cheng JJ, Chao YJ, Wung BS et al. Cyclic strain-induced plasminogen activator inhibitor-1 (PAI-1) release from endothelial cells involves reactive oxygen species. Biochem Biophys Res Commun 1996;225:100–105.

100. Papadaki M, Eskin SG. Effects of fluid shear stress on gene regulation of vascular cells. Biotech Prog 1997;13:209–221.

101. Davies PF, Tripathi SC. Mechanical stress mechanism and the cell. An endothelial paradigm. Circ Res 1993;72:239–245.

102. Ando J, Komatsuda T, Kamiya A. Cytoplasmic calcium response to fluid shear stress in cultured vascular endothelial cells. In Vitro Cell Dev Biol 1988;24:871–877.

103. Mo M, Eskin SG, Schilling WP. Flow-induced changes in Ca2+ signaling of vascular endothelial cells: effect of shear stress and ATP. Am J Physiol 1991;260:H1698–H1707.

104. Dull RO, Davies PF. Flow modulation of agonist (ATP)-response (Ca++) coupling in vascular endothelial cells. Am J Physiol 1991;261:H149–H154.

105. Nollert MU, McIntire LV. Convective mass transfer effects on the intracellular calcium response of endothelial cells. J Biomech Eng 1992;114:321–326.

106. Shen J, Luscinskas FW, Connolly A et al. Fluid shear stress modulates cytosolic free calcium in vascular endothelial cells. Am J Physiol 1992;262:C384.

107. Bhagyalakshmi A, Frangos JA. Mechanism of shear-induced prostacyclin production in endothelial cells. Biochem Biophys Res Commun 1989;158:31–37.

108. Nollert MU, Eskin SG, McIntire LV. Shear stress increases inositol triphosphate levels in human endothelial cells. Biochem Biophys Res Commun 1990;170:281–287.

109. Bhagyalakshmi A, Berthiaume F, Reich KM et al. Fluid shear stress stimulates membrane phospholipid metabolism in cultured human endothelial cells. J Vasc Res 1992;29:443–449.

110. Rosales OR, Sumpio BE. Changes in cyclic strain increase inositol triphosphate and diacylglycerol in endothelial cells. Am J Physiol 1992;262:C956–C962.

111. Ohno M, Gibbons GH, Dzau VJ et al. Shear stress elevates endothelial cGMP. Role of a potassium channel and G protein coupling. Circulation 1993;88:193–197.

112. Hsieh H, Li NQ, Frangos JA. Pulsatile and steady flow induces c-fos expression in human endothelial cells. J Cell Physiol 1993;154:143–151.

113. Ziegelstein RC, Chang L, Capogrossi MC. Flow-dependent cytosolic acidification of vascular endothelial cells. Science 1992;258:656–659.

114. Letsou GE, Rosales O, Maitz S et al. Stimulation of adenylate cyclase activity in cultured endothelial cells subjected to cyclic stretch. J Cardiovasc Surg 1990;31:634–639.

115. Davies PF. Endothelium as a signal transduction interface for flow forces: cell surface dynamics. Thromb Haemost 1993;70:124–128.

116. Muller JM, Chilian WM, Davis MJ. Integrin signaling transduces shear stress-dependent vasodilation of coronary arterioles. Circ Res 1997;80:320–326.

117. Davies PF. Flow-mediated endothelial mechanotransduction. Physiol Rev 1995;75:519–560.

118. Nollert MU, Panaro NJ, McIntire LV. Regulation of genetic expression in shear stress-stimulated endothelial cells. Ann N Y Acad Sci 1992;665:94–104.

119. Du W, Xu WJ, Sumpio BE. Proto-oncogenes c-fos, c-jun, and transcription factors AP-1 and NF-kB are activated in endothelial cells (EC) exposed to cyclic strain [Abstract]. FASEB J 1993;7:A2.

120. Lan Q, Mercurius KO, Davies PF. Stimulation of transcription factors NFkB and AP1 in endothelial cells subjected to shear stress. Biochem Biophys Res Commun 1994;201:950–956.

121. Malek AM, Izumo S. Control of endothelial cell gene expression by flow. J Biomech 1995;28:1515–1528.

122. Shyy JY, Lin MC, Han J et al. The cis-acting phorbol ester "12-O-tetradecanoylphorbol 13-acetate" -responsive element is involved in shear stress-induced monocyte chemotactic protein 1 gene expression. Proc Natl Acad Sci U S A 1995;92:8069–8073.

123. Read MA, Whitley MZ, Williams AJ et al. NF-kB and IkBa: an inducible regulatory system in endothelial activation. J Exp Med 1994;179:503–512.

124. Resnick N, Gimbrone MA Jr. Hemodynamic forces are complex regulators of endothelial gene expression. FASEB J 1995;9:874–882.

125. Khachigian LM, Resnick N, Gimbrone MA Jr et al. Nuclear factor-kB interacts functionally with the platelet-derived growth factor B-chain shear stress response element in vascular endothelial cells exposed to fluid shear stress. J Clin Invest 1995;96:1169–1175.

126. MacDonald PS, Read MA, Dusting GJ. Synergistic inhibition of platelet aggregation by endothelium-derived relaxing factor and prostacyclin. Thromb Res 1988;49:437–449.

127. Eskin SG, McIntire LV, Navarro LT. Response of cultured endothelial cells to steady flow. Microvasc Res 1984;28:87–94.

128. Levesque MJ, Nerem RM. The elongation and orientation of cultured endothelial cells in response to shear stress. J Biomech Eng 1985;107:341–347.

129. Papadaki M, McIntire LV, Eskin SG. Effects of shear stress on the growth kinetics of human aortic smooth muscle cells in vitro. Biotechnol Bioeng 1996;50:555–561.

130. Sterpetti AV, Cucina A, D'Angelo LS et al. Response of arterial smooth muscle cells to laminar flow. J Cardiovasc Surg 1992;33:619–624.

131. Sterpetti AV, Cucina A, D'Angelo LS et al. Shear stress modulates the proliferation rate, protein synthesis, and mitogenic activity of arterial mooth muscle cells. Surgery 1993;113:691–699.

132. Wang DM, Tarbell JM. Modeling interstitial flow in an artery wall allows estimation of wall shear stress on smooth muscle cells. J Biomech Eng 1995;117:358–363.

133. Dusting GJ, Moncada S, Vane JR. Prostaglandins, their intermediates and precursors: cardiovascular actions and regulatory roles in normal and abnormal circulatory systems. Prog Cardiovasc Dis 1979;21:405–430.

134. Alshihabi SN, Chang YS, Frangos JA et al. Shear stress-induced release of PGE2 and PGI2 by vascular smooth muscle cells. Biochem Biophys Res Comm 1996;224:808–814.

135. Sinzinger H, Zidek T, Fitscha P et al. Prostaglandin I2 reduces activation

of human arterial smooth muscle cells in-vivo. Prostaglandins 1987;33:915–918.

136. Wagner CT, Durante W, Christodoulides N et al. Hemodynamic forces induce the expression of heme oxygenase in cultured vascular smooth muscle cells. J Clin Invest 1997;100:589–596.

137. Gibson CM, Diaz L, Kandarpa K et al. Relation of vessel wall shear stress to atherosclerosis progression in human coronary arteries. Arterioscler Thromb 1993;13:310–315.

138. Nerem RM, Cornhill JF. The role of fluid mechanics in atherogenesis. J Biomech Eng 1980;102:181–189.

139. Dinerman JL, Mehta JL. Endothelial, platelet and leukocyte interactions in ischemic heart disease: insights into potential mechanisms and their clinical relevance. J Am Coll Cardiol 1990;16:207–222.

140. Jackson CM, Nemerson Y. Blood coagulation. Ann Rev Biochem 1980;49:765–811.

141. Mann KG, Jenny RJ, Krishnaswamy S. Cofactor proteins in the assembly and expression of blood clotting enzyme complexes. Annu Rev Biochem 1988;57:915–956.

142. Nemerson Y, Turitto VT. The effect of flow on hemostasis and thrombosis. Thromb Haemost 1991;66:272–276.

143. Gemmell CH, Turitto VT, Nemerson Y. Flow as a regulator of the activation of factor X by tissue factor. Blood 1988;72:1404–1406.

144. Schoen P, Lindhout T, Willems G et al. Continuous flow and the prothrombinase-catalyzed activation of prothrombin. Thromb Haemost 1990;64:542–547.

145. Gir S, Slack SM, Turitto VT. A numerical analysis of factor X activation in the presence of tissue factor–factor VIIa complex in a flow reactor. Ann Biomed Eng 1996;24:394–399.

146. Weiss HJ, Turitto VT, Baumgartner HR. Role of shear rate and platelets in promoting fibrin formation on rabbit subendothelium. Studies utilizing individuals with quantitative and qualitative platelet defects. J Clin Invest 1986;78:1072–1082.

147. Badimon L, Badimon JJ, Turitto VT et al. Platelet thrombus formation on collagen type I. A method of deep vessel injury. Influence of blood rheology, von Willebrand factor, and blood coagulation. Circulation 1988;78:1431–1442.

148. Ip JH, Stein B, Fuster V, Badimon L. Antithrombotic therapy in cardiovascular diseases. Future directions based on pathogenesis and risk. Ann N Y Acad Sci 1991;614:289–311.

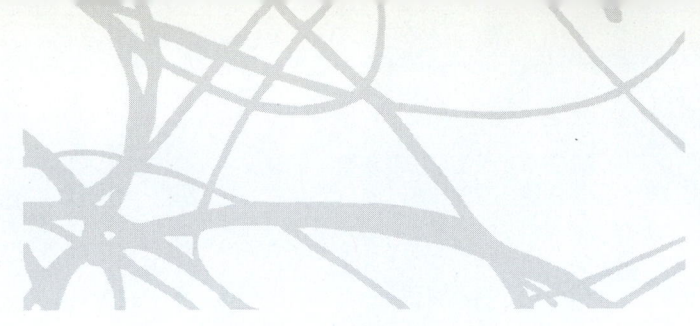

# SECTION 4

# EXPERIMENTAL MODELS

# CHAPTER 21

# EXPERIMENTAL MODELS OF THROMBOSIS AND THROMBOLYSIS

## H. Vernon Anderson, James T. Willerson

Thrombotic occlusion of a coronary artery, with subsequent acute myocardial infarction or sudden lethal arrhythmia, is the most common cause of death in Western industrial countries. Thrombotic occlusive disease of cerebral and peripheral arteries is responsible for further significant amounts of morbidity and mortality in these populations. Effective therapies for thrombotic disorders requires the development of animal models. These models can allow testing of hypotheses regarding thrombus initiation, thrombus growth and dissolution, effects of pharmaceutical agents, responses of arterial walls, and responses of perfused organs. At present, there are no ideal models for the human situation, i.e., an atherosclerotic plaque with an ulcerated endothelial surface and superimposed thrombosis. However, six different and extremely useful models of arterial thrombosis have been developed. These are: 1) electrical injury; 2) copper coil; 3) Folts (cyclic flow) model; 4) thrombin injection; 5) vessel eversion; and 6) arteriovenous (AV) shunt graft. Each of these models will be described in this chapter. Any one of them could theoretically be used for any arterial system, and they have been used for carotid, coronary, aorta, and iliofemoral arteries. Because the *coronary* arterial system is of greatest clinical interest, it will be the one described in most detail here. Venous thrombosis models will be discussed briefly at the end of this chapter.

## ELECTRICAL INJURY MODEL

In the early 1950s, Sawyer and Pate noted that abnormal electrical potentials developed at aortic wall sites that suffered crush injury (1, 2). They found that the normal electrical potential across the wall of the aorta was −3 to −15 mV, with the lumen being more negative than the adventitial surface. Crush injury reversed the electrical potential at the injury site, and the injured luminal surface rose to 2 to 5 mV. The injury and this new electrical potential were associated with localized thrombus development. With these observations as background, Sawyer and Pate constructed a needle electrode that they advanced through the walls of aortas and positioned in the lumens (Fig. 21.1). The exterior end of the electrode was connected to the positive pole of a 9-volt battery. Small metal rings were placed around the aorta and connected through potentiometers to the negative battery pole. Using this setup, they could simulate the effects of crush injury by establishing a positive electrical potential on the inner surface of an otherwise normal artery. This reversed electrical potential difference also caused thrombosis, if sufficient current was applied. The smallest current that would cause complete thrombosis of an aorta was 50 μA and required 270 minutes. Histologic examination revealed that the electrically induced thrombus was no different from that which developed after crush injury.

In 1961, Salazar described a modification of this technique that did not require surgery (3). A catheter was introduced in a dog via a carotid artery and positioned under fluoroscopic guidance in the left coronary ostium. A wire electrode was advanced out of the tip of the catheter into one of the major coronary branches. This wire, which extended the length of the

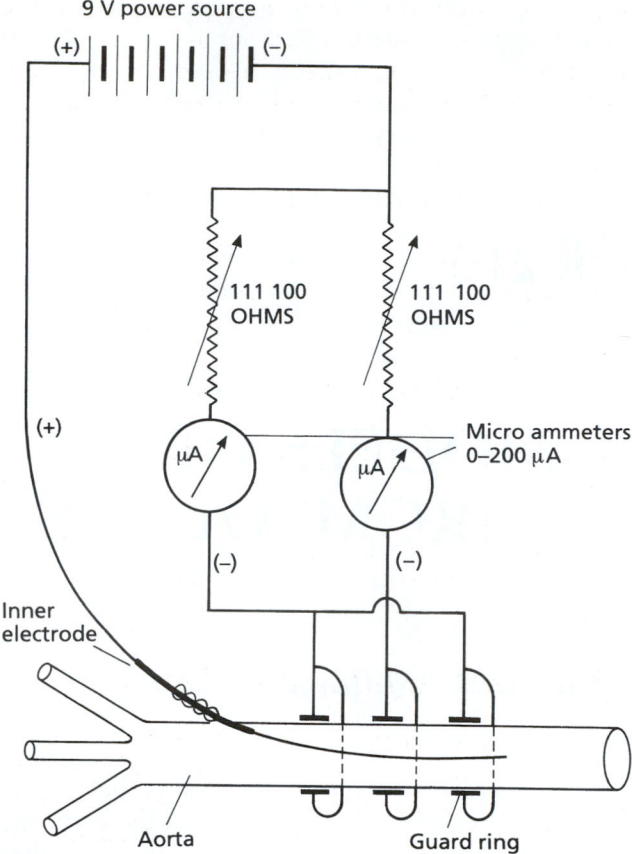

**FIGURE 21.1.** Schematic diagram of animal model for studying the effects of reversed electrical potentials on thrombus formation in aortas. This was originally developed as a model of crush injury. When connected to a 9-volt battery, the needle electrode introduced into the lumen of the aorta, along with the metal rings surrounding a portion of the aorta, made the lumen positive in charge compared to the adjacent wall. Thrombosis occurred if sufficient current was delivered. Adapted with permission from Sawyer PN, Pate JW. Bioelectric phenomena as an etiologic factor in intravascular thrombosis. Am J Physiol 1953;175:103–107.)

catheter, was connected at its proximal end to a positive voltage source. The negative pole of the voltage source was connected through potentiometers to the chest wall of the dog. The coronary artery lumen could then be made positive in charge compared to the adventitial surface. Currents of 200 to 300 μA for 2 to 3 hours were required to produce thrombosis. Currents less than 200 μA caused thrombosis only inconsistently, whereas currents greater than 500 μA caused a burn injury on the endothelial surface of the lumen. This catheter technique was quickly adopted and used by many investigators for acute (nonsurvival) studies in anesthetized animals (4).

In 1980, Romson et al (5) described another modification of the electrical injury model that has become one of the most commonly used methods for acute as well as some chronic (survival) studies. In this experimental preparation (Fig. 21.2), a 25-gauge stainless steel hypodermic needle is inserted directly through the coronary arterial wall so that the tip protrudes into the vessel lumen. Two or three shallow sutures in the epicardium secure the needle tip and prevent its dislodgement during cardiac motion. To this needle tip, a 28- or 30-gauge silver-coated copper wire with Teflon insulation is attached. (Usually the wire and needle tip are assembled into a unit prior to the procedure.) The coronary artery just proximal to the needle insertion site is gently dissected free from surrounding epicardial tissue over a length of several millimeters. Either an electromagnetic or Doppler ultrasound flow probe is attached around the exposed artery proximal to the needle tip. Occasionally, a snare or clamp is placed around the coronary artery just distal to the needle tip to impede flow selectively through the vessel (Fig. 21.3). For acute studies, the needle tip wire is connected immediately to the positive pole of a 9-volt battery via a potentiometer. The negative terminal of the battery is connected with a wire

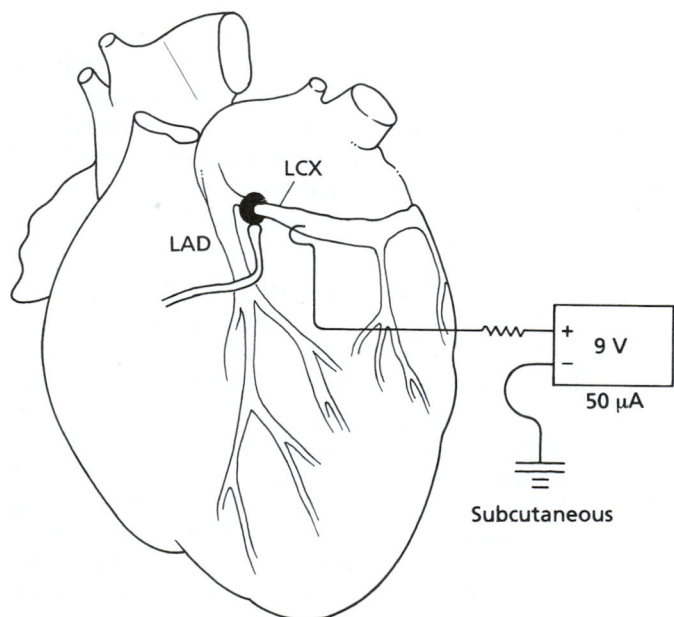

**FIGURE 21.2.** Schematic diagram of electrical injury model for producing acute coronary artery thrombosis. A 25-gauge stainless steel needle attached to a 28- or 30-gauge wire is inserted through the arterial wall into the lumen. The needle/wire is anchored with a shallow epicardial suture. An electromagnetic or Doppler ultrasound flow probe is placed on the coronary artery proximal to the needle. The wire from the needle is connected to the positive terminal of a 9-volt battery. The negative battery terminal is connected with another wire to any subcutaneous site. Abbreviations: LAD, left anterior descending artery; LCX, left circumflex artery. Adapted with permission from Shea MJ, Driscoll EM, Romson JL, et al. The beneficial effects of nafazatrom (BAYg6575) on experimental coronary thrombosis. Am Heart J 1984;107:629–637.)

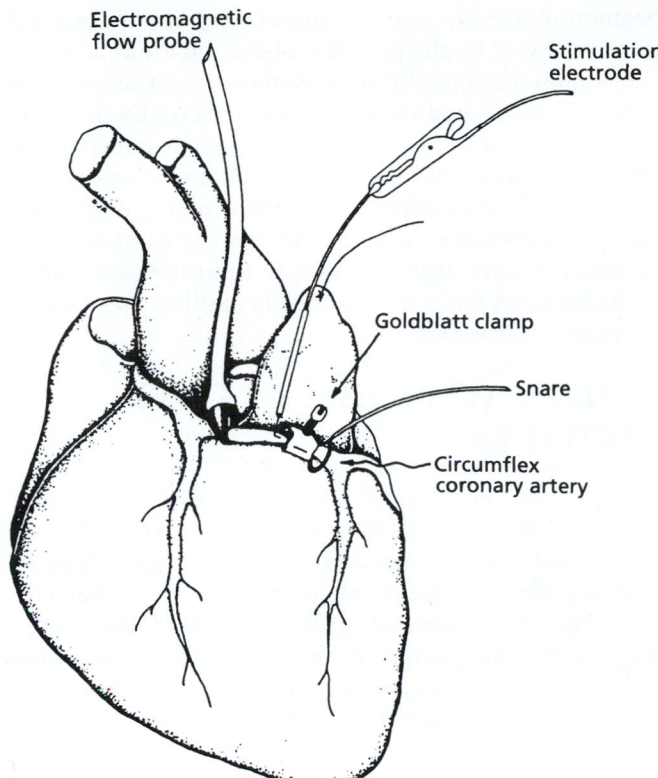

**FIGURE 21.3.** Schematic diagram of one variation of electrical injury animal model for producing acute coronary artery thrombosis. In addition to the flow probe and an electrode, a clamp and a snare are added distally. The snare can be used to occlude blood flow transiently, thereby hastening development of thrombus at the needle tip electrode. The clamp can be used to add a fixed stenosis to the artery, mimicking more closely the usual human coronary situation. Adapted with permission from Bush LR, Shebuski RJ. *In vivo* models of arterial thrombosis and thrombolysis [Review]. FASEB J 1990;4:3087–3098.)

to any subcutaneous site. The potentiometer is adjusted to deliver 50 to 200 μA current. Blood flow in the artery is continuously monitored by the flow probe. Several parameters related to arterial thrombosis can be studied, including: 1) documenting occurrence of complete thrombotic occlusion (flow signal to zero); 2) measuring elapsed time until occlusion; 3) documenting restoration of vessel patency (flow returns nearly to preocclusion value); 4) documenting occurrence and time of vessel reocclusion; and 5) documenting cyclic declines and restorations of blood flow due to repetitive accumulation and dislodgement of platelet aggregates (the so-called cyclic flow variations) (6–13). In general, rapidity of initial thrombus development in this model is a function of two factors: first, the amount of electric current delivered, and second, the degree of constriction by a clamp or snare. Higher currents and more tightly constricted arteries develop thrombus more quickly (about 30 min-

utes), whereas lower currents and lesser or no constriction will require longer times (about 3–4 hours). Part of the rationale for use of a clamp or snare, in addition to the time savings, is that it more closely mimics the human situation of a stenotic coronary artery with some stimulus to acute thrombosis.

One advantage of this model over most of the others described later is that it can also be used for chronic studies (6, 8). After placing the flow probe, the needle electrode, and a constrictor (if this addition is desired), the wires can be exteriorized and connected to appropriate monitoring equipment. Animals can then have their chests closed and be recovered until they are ambulatory. When the investigator is ready, the coronary artery electrode can be connected to a current source and thrombosis initiated. Acute coronary thrombosis in awake, unsedated animals can be modeled with this technique. In addition to coronary arterial thrombosis, the electrical injury method has been applied to model carotid (14–16) as well as femoral (17, 18) arterial thrombosis.

## COPPER COIL MODEL

In the early 1950s, as Sawyer and Pate were investigating the altered electrical potentials associated with crush injury of blood vessels and the influence this had on vessel thrombosis, other investigators were studying the thrombotic influence of metal alloys. At the time, this was althought to have some use for treating saccular aortic aneurysms. In 1951, Stone and Lord (19) published an account of the superior thrombogenic effects of magnesium and magnesium-aluminum wire coils in dog aortas. In 1964, Blair et al (20) described a modification of Stone and Lord's technique that advanced the model into coronary arteries. Anesthetized dogs had their hearts exposed by thoracotomy. A short segment of the left anterior descending coronary artery in each dog was gently dissected free from surrounding epicardial tissue. A short, spiral-shaped coil of wire was inserted directly into the exposed coronary artery by twisting it in like a screw. The two advantages of this technique were that no fluoroscopy equipment was required and occlusive thrombosis occurred gradually over 7 to 10 days. The gradual formation of thrombus was an advantage over then-popular coronary artery ligation models because it avoided the high incidence of fatal ventricular fibrillation that often accompanied acute coronary ligation.

In 1972, Kordenat et al (21) described another modification of the coil method, which, with minor adaptations, has become the standard technique. This method involves formation of small coils of wire around an 18-gauge needle. Magnesium and magnesium-aluminum alloy were used originally, but subsequently these were replaced by copper wire. The wrapping of the coil can be varied to achieve different lengths with selected num-

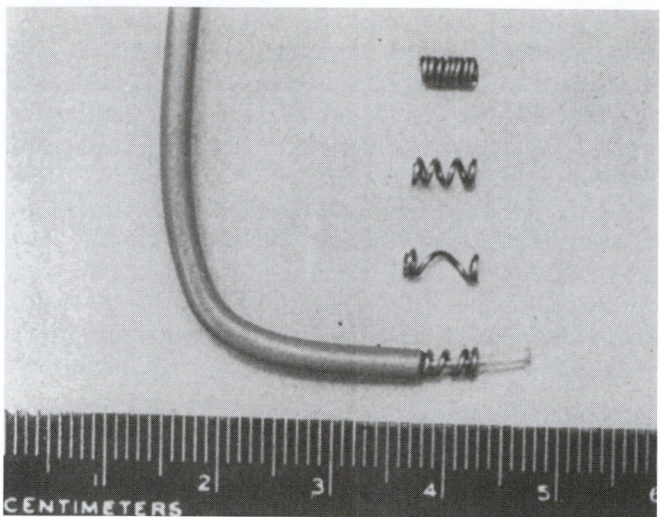

**FIGURE 21.4.** Photograph of copper coils and other items used to produce acute coronary artery thrombosis. The coils can be made with various numbers of turns of wire. A large guiding catheter contains both a coil and a small central tube or guidewire. The guiding catheter is positioned under fluoroscopic control in the coronary ostium, then the smaller guidewire is directed out of the larger catheter into the desired coronary artery. Finally, the coil slides into the coronary artery over the guidewire and lodges at the level where the outer diameter of the coil matches the inner diameter of the artery. The smaller guidewire and larger catheter are then removed. Adapted with permission from Kordenat RK, Kezdi T, Stanley EL. A new catheter technique for producing experimental coronary thrombosis and selective coronary visualization. Am Heart J 1972;83:360–364.)

bers of turns (Fig. 21.4). The coil must be inserted under fluoroscopic guidance. A large-bore catheter is inserted into the anesthetized animal via either the carotid or femoral arteries. This catheter is directed to the ostium of the left coronary artery. A small inner catheter or coronary guidewire is then advanced out of this larger catheter and manipulated into the desired coronary artery, typically being placed quite far distally. The coil slides out of the larger catheter over the smaller wire and lodges in the coronary artery. The catheters and wire are then taken out. A common and useful adaptation has been to put a Doppler or electromagnetic flow probe on the artery to monitor flow.

This copper coil model has been used extensively to evaluate and compare thrombolytic agents (22, 23). Thrombus formation is rapid, and complete arterial occlusion usually occurs within 10 to 20 minutes. Therefore, the copper coil model is used for acute studies only. A clamp or snare is not usually added to the artery, because the metallic coil alone is such a powerful stimulus to thrombosis. Although the thickness of the wire does create some degree of stenosis of the arterial lumen, this is not considered to be an important mechanism in promoting thrombosis. The amount of local endothelial trauma caused by the presence of the coil is likewise not considered a major stimulus. Rather, the existence of a relatively large area of positive charges on the metallic coil surface is apparently the mechanism by which platelets, fibrin, and other blood elements are attracted and adhere. This resembles the electrical injury and crush injury phenomena discussed in the previous section. Turbulence and stasis of blood flow in the deep interstices between the coil windings is another mechanism promoting thrombosis.

# FOLTS (CYCLIC FLOW) MODEL

In 1976, Folts et al (24) made the seminal observation that repetitive cycles of blood flow reduction, followed by sudden restorations to full flow, would occur in partially obstructed canine coronary arteries that had been injured by squeezing or pinching. These cycles (Fig. 21.5) were presumed to be due to the repetitive accumulation and dislodgement of platelet aggregates at the site of an arterial stenosis where there also was endothelial injury. Subsequent research has shown that this indeed is the process generating cyclic flow reductions (25–27). The exact rheologic conditions required to produce cyclic flows involve both the turbulence and stasis produced by partial arterial constriction of significant length (i.e., at least 3 mm), along with exposure of subendothelial elements by arterial injury at or very near the constricted region. The model is created by exposing the heart and gently dissecting free from surrounding tissue a length of one major coronary artery. The left anterior descending and left circumflex coronary arteries are the ones most commonly used. An electromagnetic or Doppler flow probe is placed on the proximal portion of the exposed length of artery. Cushioned forceps are used to pinch several times the artery just distal to the flow probe. A hard, plastic disk with a center hole and slit is used. Disks with central holes of various sizes must be made ahead of time. Variation in size between individual arteries requires the experimenter to try first one and then another of these disks as a constrictor. Eventually one is found that reduces flow appropriately. Other methods to achieve appropriate partial constriction involve using either a length of tapered nylon fishing line or an angioplasty catheter balloon positioned between a loose plastic collar and the external arterial surface. The plastic collar provides support while the tapered nylon line is manipulated backward or forward and then is fixed when the experimenter achieves the desired degree of arterial narrowing. With the second system, the angioplasty balloon is partially inflated between the collar and the artery, compressing the artery slightly and producing the narrowing (25).

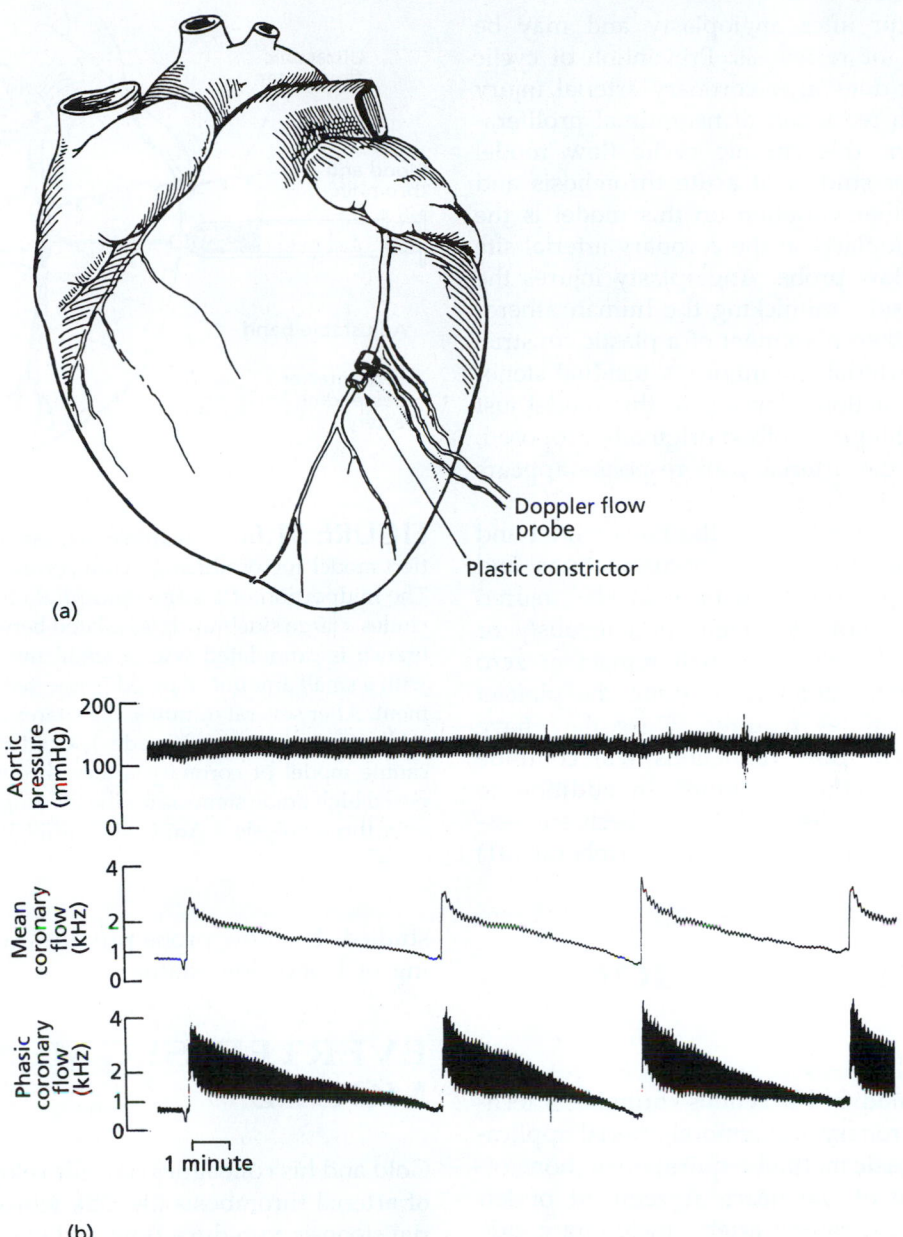

**FIGURE 21.5.**   **(a)** Schematic diagram of the Folts model for producing coronary artery cyclic flow variations. The midportion of a large epicardial coronary artery is injured by pinching or squeezing. A plastic constrictor that reduces but does not occlude coronary blood flow is placed on the artery at the injured zone. **(b)** Representative tracings from a Folts model in a canine coronary artery. The upper tracing is aortic pressure. The middle tracing is mean or average coronary flow velocity from the Doppler ultrasound flow probe. The lower tracing is phasic or instantaneous coronary flow velocity. These cycles of gradual decline in blood flow over several minutes followed by sudden restorations of flow are due to repetitive accumulation and dislodgement of platelet aggregates at sites of coronary artery stenosis with endothelial injury.

Recently, the Folts model has been extended to a chronic, awake, and unsedated canine preparation. With properly applied mild injury, cyclic flow reductions develop immediately after injury but then fade away. Animals are recovered and returned to their housing. Several days later, cyclic flow reductions may return, but this can be prevented by administration of effective antiplatelet agents. This new model may offer some additional insights into chronic influences of platelets and platelet aggregates on injured arterial walls. In particular, platelets adhering to arterial walls at sites of injury are known to release various mediators that may play a role in the proliferation of medial smooth muscle cells and elaboration of extracellular matrix, which occur after angioplasty and may be partly responsible for restenosis. Prevention of cyclic flow reductions in dogs after coronary arterial injury does correlate with reduction of neointimal proliferation (28). However, this chronic cyclic flow model is likely limited for studies of acute thrombosis and thrombolysis. Another variation on this model is the use of balloon angioplasty at the coronary arterial site just distal to the flow probe. Angioplasty injures the artery from the inside, mimicking the human atherosclerotic situation, then placement of a plastic constrictor at the injured arterial site mimics a residual stenosis. Cyclic flow reductions develop in this model just as with the external injury method originally proposed, and histologically the arterial wall response appears to be similar (29).

The cyclic flow reductions in the Folts model and its variants are due to periodic accumulations and dislodgements of platelet aggregates at the injured and stenotic site. If not dislodged spontaneously or manually, occasionally the flow will remain at zero and not be restored. Therefore, shaking the platelet plug loose is sometimes required. Once they have developed, the cyclic flow reductions will continue undiminished for 3 hours or more. In addition to coronary arteries, the Folts method has been successfully applied in carotid (25, 30) and peripheral (31) arteries.

# THROMBIN INJECTION MODEL

Gold and Collen modified a venous thrombosis technique to include coronary and femoral arterial applications (32–34). The basic method requires open thoracotomy and exposure of the heart. A segment of left anterior descending coronary artery, including a side branch, is gently dissected free from surrounding tissue (Fig. 21.6). An electromagnetic or Doppler flow probe is placed on the artery proximal to the side branch. A variable constrictor is placed on the distal portion of the exposed segment. The side branch is cannulated with a small-bore plastic tube attached to a needle. The exposed segment of artery is injured by pinching it with forceps. Snares are then placed to isolate the entire exposed segment temporarily and occlude flow. Using the cannulated side branch, a mixture of whole blood and thrombin (10 U) is injected into the injured and static segment of artery. After approximately 5 minutes of occlusion, the proximal snare is released, and about 2 minutes later the distal snare is released. This leaves an injured and stenotic coronary artery with occlusive thrombus present. The effects of various agents on restoration of flow can be

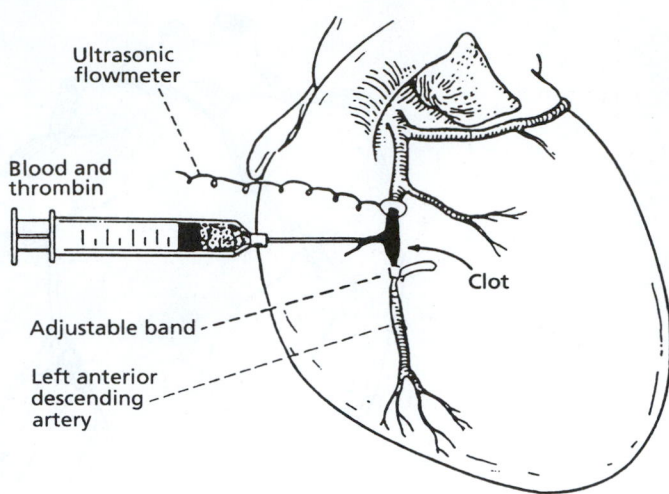

**FIGURE 21.6.** Schematic diagram of the thrombin injection model for producing acute coronary artery thrombosis. The midportion of a large epicardial coronary artery that includes a large sidebranch is isolated between snares. The sidebranch is cannulated with a small needle. Thrombin mixed with a small amount of blood is injected into the isolated segment. After several minutes, the snares are released. Adapted with permission from Yasuda T, Gold HK, Fallon JT, et al. A canine model of coronary artery thrombosis with superimposed high grade stenosis for the investigation of rethrombosis after thrombolysis. J Am Coll Cardiol 1989;13:1409–1414.)

studied. The flow probe provides continuous monitoring of blood flow status.

# EVERTED SEGMENT MODEL

Gold and his colleagues have developed another model of arterial thrombosis (34, 35), which relies on an arterial stenosis to reduce flow and exposure to the bloodstream of nonendothelial tissues (Fig. 21.7). The heart is exposed by thoracotomy. A segment of left circumflex coronary artery is gently dissected free from surrounding tissue. An electromagnetic or Doppler flow probe is placed on the proximal portion of the exposed segment. A plastic snare is placed around the distal portion of the exposed segment to create partial obstruction. A 1-cm section of artery between the flow probe and snare is isolated with microvascular clamps, excised, everted inside out, and then reattached in position using nylon sutures. The microvascular clamps are then removed. This procedure places the adventitial surface of the everted section into contact with blood flowing through the artery. The combination of reduced blood flow due to the snare, along with the abnormal nonendothelial surface creates total thrombotic occlusion within about 5 minutes. In addition to

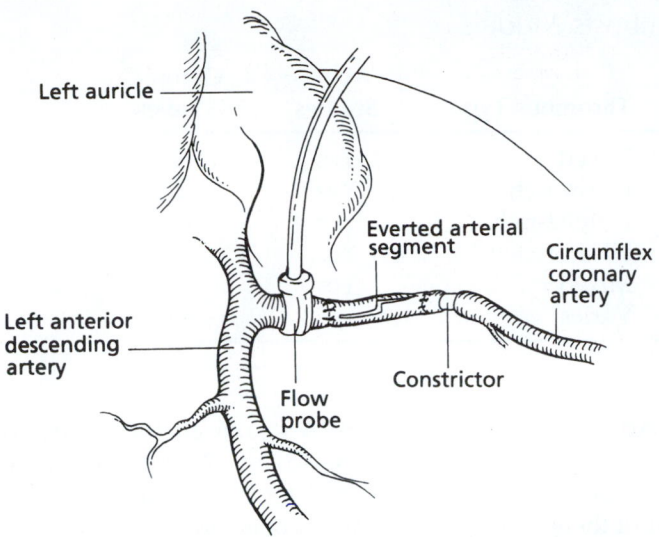

**FIGURE 21.7.** Schematic diagram of the everted vessel segment model for producing acute coronary artery thrombosis. A large epicardial coronary artery is isolated between microvascular snares. A 1-cm-long section between the snares is cut out, everted inside out, and reattached. The adventitial surface is therefore placed into the lumen of the vessel. The microvascular snares are then released. Adapted with permission from Gold HK, Yasuda T, Jang IK, et al. Animal models for arterial thrombolysis and prevention of reocclusion. Circulation 1991;83(suppl IV):26–40.)

coronary arteries, the everted vessel segment method has been used in femoral arteries (34).

# ARTERIOVENOUS SHUNT-GRAFT MODEL

In 1985, Hanson et al described a standardized arteriovenous shunt system for thrombosis studies (36). This model is created by exposing surgically the vessels of the upper leg. One length of 3.0-mm-diameter silicone rubber tubing is grafted to the femoral artery; a second is grafted to the femoral vein. In between these two arms, various materials in tubular shapes can be placed, and as blood flows through the shunt circuit from artery to vein, the effects on platelets and thrombosis can be studied. In baboons, similar to humans hematologically, the shunt circuit itself does not meaningfully increase platelet or fibrinogen removal rates from blood, nor produce measurable activation of platelets or coagulation factors (36–38). The shunt can be exteriorized and the skin closed, so that chronic models can be developed if desired. Numerous materials have been studied as inserts into the shunt arms, including synthetic woven polyester meshes (Dacron), other biopolymers, explanted and/or endarterectomized arterial segments, and collagen-coated tubes (36, 37, 39–41). Inasmuch as the variety of

materials that can be inserted into the shunt circuit is so broad, this model offers a great deal of flexibility. The disadvantage is that it is mainly a model of blood-material interactions and not one of clinically relevant organ system or disease response.

# MODELS OF THROMBOSIS AND THROMBOLYSIS

The six experimental animal models of arterial thrombosis described here have a number of similar features, although the arteriovenous shunt graft model is slightly different from the other five. In all six models, an electromagnetic or Doppler ultrasound flow probe can be arranged to provide continuous monitoring of flow within the subject artery. They are all basically acute models requiring open thoracotomy or other surgical exposure with monitoring of continuously anesthetized animals. The electrical injury, Folts, and arteriovenous shunt models can be closed and the animals recovered, with thrombosis created later in awake and unsedated animals. This, however, may or may not have substantial relevance for studies dealing with acute thrombosis and thrombolysis.

The major difference between these models appears to be related to the character of the occluding thrombus that forms. Because thrombus is a combination of both aggregating platelets and insoluble fibrin polymers generated by the coagulation cascade, these two elements (platelets and fibrin) can be present in differing proportions. Some of the models produce relatively platelet-rich thrombi, whereas others produce relatively fibrin-rich thrombi (Table 21.1). Of the first five, the Folts cyclic flow model is probably the most platelet-rich thrombus model of the group, whereas the copper coil and thrombin injection models are probably the most fibrin-rich. The other two models (electrical injury and everted vessel segment) are probably intermediate in platelet-rich and fibrin-rich compositions. The relative simplicity of the electrical injury model along with its balanced mixture of thrombus components has made it one of the most popular methods of studying thrombolytic agents (7, 42–44). It is also one of the most popular models for studying the roles of antithrombins, antiplatelet agents, and their combinations in conjunction with thrombolytics (45–48). The last model, arteriovenous shunt graft, can have a wide variety of thrombus types developed, given that the kinds of materials placed into the shunt circuit are so variable. This distinction between thrombus types likely is quite important. Because thrombolytic agents achieve their effects by activating the enzyme plasminogen, thereby lysing strands of fibrin, they are highly effective in fibrin-rich models but less effective in platelet-rich models. For example,

**TABLE 21.1.**   Characteristics of Thrombosis Models

| Model | Fluoroscopy Required | Thrombus Type | Acute Studies | Chronic Studies |
|---|---|---|---|---|
| Electrical injury | No | Mixed | Yes | Yes |
| Copper coil | Yes | Fibrin-rich | Yes | No |
| Folts | No | Platelet-rich | Yes | Yes |
| Thrombin injection | No | Fibrin-rich | Yes | No |
| Everted vessel | No | Mixed | Yes | No |
| Arteriovenous shunt graft | No | Varies | Yes | Yes |

in one study (17) using both the relatively platelet-rich electrical injury model in one group of dogs and the relatively fibrin-rich copper coil model for another, the fibrinolytic agent recombinant tissue-type plasminogen activator (rt-PA) was given to both groups of animals. Successful reperfusion was achieved in 100% (18 of 18) of the copper coil arteries (fibrin rich), but in only 79% (19 of 24) of the electrically injured arteries (platelet rich). On the other hand, agents that interfere with platelet function, such as thromboxane receptor antagonists (49), serotonin receptor antagonists (50), glycoprotein IIb-IIIa receptor antagonists (10, 51), and others, are more effective in platelet-rich models but less effective in fibrin-rich models. Furthermore, it has been demonstrated that reocclusion of an artery after successful thrombolysis, in all models, is usually preceded by a period of cyclic flow variations, which appears to be predominantly a platelet-mediated process (34). Histologic studies of the reoccluding thrombus that forms after thrombolysis have confirmed their platelet-rich composition (35, 52). Antiplatelet agents, when they are added to thrombolytic agents, are able to attenuate or eliminate these cyclic flows and delay or prevent reocclusion.

Another important and related topic is that of thrombus age. Platelet-rich thrombi, which predominate early in thrombus development, gradually accumulate more fibrin as the coagulation process becomes activated and progresses (53). What begins as a platelet-rich thrombus, perhaps at that phase more sensitive to antiplatelet agents but less sensitive to fibrinolytics, might gradually shift in its responsiveness as its character changes. Furthermore, even fibrin-rich thrombi change as they age as factor XIII-dependent cross-linkages form between recently deposited fibrin strands (54). In one study, using a copper coil (fibrin-rich) model of canine coronary thrombosis, significant differences related to thrombus age were found (55). In dogs with occlusive thrombi present for 30 minutes prior to treatment with rt-PA, 5 of 6 (83%) could be successfully reperfused. However, when occlusive thrombi were present for 180 minutes prior to treatment, only 1 of 7 (15%, $P < 0.05$) could be reperfused.

Addition of heparin to rt-PA equalized the ability to successfully lyse thrombi—5 of 7 for 30-minute thrombi compared to 4 of 7 for 180-minute thrombi. But there still was a significant delay in time to successful reperfusion using rt-PA and heparin—15 ± 3 minutes for 30-minute thrombi compared to 38 ± 5 minutes for 180-minute thrombi; ($P < 0.01$). In another study, using the Folts cyclic flow model (platelet-rich), time-related effects were also observed (56). When cyclic flow variations had been established in canine coronary arteries for only 30 minutes, either heparin or a specific thrombin antagonist (MCI-9038) were equally effective in abolishing them (12 of 18 = 66% vs. 5 of 7 = 71%). When the cyclic flows had been established for 180 minutes before treatment, 0 of 7 dogs treated with heparin and only 1 of 7 dogs treated with MCI-9038 had cyclic flows abolished. The mechanisms responsible for this age-related decline in sensitivity to thrombolytic and antithrombin agents are not known and require further study. Furthermore, whether these findings apply only to these particular models or to other models with more equally mixed thrombus types is not known.

These animal models have highlighted the complex and important interactions that occur between platelet activation and coagulation pathways. Arterial thrombosis begins with the deposition, activation, and aggregation of platelets. Platelet aggregates serve as substrates to initiate and accelerate thrombin activation, ultimately producing fibrin. Whereas thrombolysis can degrade the fibrin meshwork of a mature clot, platelets and platelet aggregates, if left uninhibited, can remain active and activate more platelets, interfere with the fibrinolytic state, and cause rethrombosis (57, 58). Thrombin and factor Xa appear to play critical roles in this process (45). Appreciation of these phenomena in recent years has led to an explosion of combination therapies directed both at fibrinolysis as well as antiplatelet and antithrombin activities. Further research studies using the animal models of arterial thrombosis described here should continue to expand our knowledge of these important mechanisms and lead to additional improvements and refinements in therapies.

# VENOUS THROMBOSIS MODELS

Deep venous thrombosis, particularly in pelvic and peripheral veins, and the morbidity and mortality associated with its most serious sequela—pulmonary embolism—have led to interest in models of venous thrombosis. Because of the lower pressures and slower flow rates that exist within the venous system (see Chapter 20), thrombi developing there are particularly fibrin rich. These models are, therefore, especially useful for testing fibrinolytic agents.

In 1974, Nowak and Gurewich reported a method for developing venous thrombi by injecting small amounts of thrombin into a jugular vein of a rabbit (59). The thrombus was then deliberately dislodged, creating a pulmonary embolism, the subject of their study of fibrinolytics. In 1981, Dupe and his colleagues extended this model by creating stationary venous thrombi in the inferior vena cava of a rabbit (60, 61). During open laparotomy, a 3-cm section of the infrarenal vena cava was isolated with loose snares. Vascular clamps were then attached and a woolen thread was introduced into the vena cava lumen. A small amount of rabbit thromboplastin was injected into the isolated and static segment. Ten minutes later, the clamps were released. Reproducible, nonmigratory thrombi developed with this method and were used to study fibrinolysis with streptokinase. Collen's group, at about the same time, reported a similar method for producing stationary venous thrombi in a dog femoral vein (62), as well as in a rabbit jugular vein (63). They have more recently extended the method to a model of primate femoral vein thrombosis using baboons (64). The basic technique involves isolating a short segment of vein between vascular clamps and injecting into the isolated segment a small fluid volume containing several hundred units of thrombin. No anchoring thread is used. The vein is kept clamped for 30 minutes before release. This model has been used extensively to evaluate thrombolytic agents and has also sparked the development of an arterial thrombosis model using similar techniques.

# REFERENCES

1. Sawyer PN, Pate JW. Bioelectric phenomena as an etiologic factor in intravascular thrombosis. Am J Physiol 1953;175:103–107.
2. Sawyer PN, Pate JW, Weldon CS. Relations of abnormal and injury electric potential differences to intravascular thrombosis. Am J Physiol 1953;175:108–112.
3. Salazar AE. Experimental myocardial infarction: Induction of coronary thrombosis in the intact closed-chest dog. Circ Res 1961;9:1351–1356.
4. Moschos CB, Lahiri K, Lyons M et al. Relation of microcirculatory thrombosis to thrombus in the proximal coronary artery: Effect of aspirin, dipyridamole, and thrombolysis. Am Heart J 1973;86:61–68.
5. Romson JL, Haack DW, Lucchesi BR. Electrical induction of coronary artery thrombosis in the ambulatory canine: A model for *in vivo* evaluation of anti-thrombotic agents. Thromb Res 1980;17:841–853.
6. Shea MJ, Driscoll EM, Romson JL et al. The beneficial effects of nafazatrom (BAYg6575) on experimental coronary thrombosis. Am Heart J 1984;107:629–637.
7. Bush LR, Shebuski RJ. *In vivo* models of arterial thrombosis and thrombolysis [Review]. FASEB J 1990;4:3087–3098.
8. Schumacher WA, Lee EC, Lucchesi BR. Augmentation of streptokinase-induced thrombolysis by heparin and prostacyclin. J Cardiovasc Pharmacol 1985;7:739–746.
9. Fitzgerald DJ, Fitzgerald GA. Role of thrombin and thromboxane A2 in reocclusion following coronary thrombolysis with tissue-type plasminogen activator. Proc Natl Acad Sci U S A 1989;86:7585–7589.
10. Mickelson JK, Simpson PJ, Cronin M et al. Antiplatelet antibody (7E3 F[ab']2) prevents rethrombosis after recombinant tissue-type plasminogen activator-induced coronary artery thrombosis in a canine model. Circulation 1990;81:617–627.
11. Jackson CV, Crowe VG, Craft TJ et al. Thrombolytic activity of a novel plasminogen activator, LY 210825, compared with recombinant tissue-type plasminogen activator in a canine model of coronary artery thrombosis. Circulation 1990;82:930–940.
12. Shebuski RJ, Stabilito IJ, Sitko GR et al. Acceleration of recombinant tissue-type plasminogen activator-induced thrombolysis and prevention of reocclusion by the combination of heparin and a Arg-Gly-Asp-containing peptide bitistatin in a canine model of coronary thrombosis. Circulation 1990;82:169–177.
13. Demrow HS, Slane PR, Folts JD. Administration of wine and grape juice inhibits *in vivo* platelet activity and thrombosis in stenosed canine coronary arteries. Circulation 1995;91:1182–1188.
14. Buchanan MR, Dejana E, Gent M et al. Enhanced platelet accumulation onto injured carotid arteries in rabbits after aspirin treatment. J Clin Invest 1981;67:503–508.
15. Dougherty JH Jr, Levy DE, Rawlinson DG et al. Experimental cerebral ischemia produced by extracranial vascular injury: protection with indomethacin and prostacyclin. Neurology 1982;32:970–974.
16. Benedict CR, Refino CJ, Keyt BA et al. New variant of human tissue type plasminogen activator (TPA) with enhanced efficacy and lower incidence of bleeding compared with recombinant human TPA. Circulation 1995;92:3032–3040.
17. Haskel EJ, Adams SP, Feigen LP et al. Prevention of reoccluding platelet-rich thrombi in canine femoral arteries with a novel peptide antagonist of platelet glycoprotein IIb-IIIa receptors. Circulation 1989;80:1775–1782.
18. Mousa SA, Bozarth JM, Forsythe MS et al. Antiplatelet and antithrombotic efficacy of DMP 728, a novel platelet GP IIb-IIIa receptor antagonist. Circulation 1994;89:3–12.
19. Stone P, Lord JW. An experimental study of thrombogenic properties on magnesium and magnesium-aluminum wire in the dog's aorta. Surgery 1951;30:987–993.
20. Blair E, Nygren E, Cowley RA. A spiral wire technique for producing gradually occlusive coronary thrombosis. J Thorac Cardiovasc Surg 1964;48:476–485.
21. Kordenat RK, Kezdi T, Stanley EL. A new catheter technique for producing experimental coronary thrombosis and selective coronary visualization. Am Heart J 1972;83:360–364.
22. Bergmann SR, Fox KA, Ter-Pogossian MM et al. Clot-selective coronary thrombolysis with tissue-type plasminogen activator. Science 1983;220:1181–1183.
23. Cercek B, Lew AS, Hod H et al. Enhancement of thrombolysis with tissue-type plasminogen activator by pre-treatment with heparin. Circulation 1986;74:583–587.
24. Folts JD, Crowell EB Jr, Rowe GG. Platelet aggregation in partially obstructed vessels and its elimination with aspirin. Circulation 1976;54:365–370.
25. Folts JD. An *in vivo* model of experimental arterial stenosis, intimal damage, and periodic thrombosis. Circulation 1991;83(suppl IV):3–14.
26. Willerson JT, Golino P, Eidt J et al. Specific platelet mediators and unstable coronary artery lesions. Experimental evidence and potential clinical implications. Circulation 1989;80:198–205.
27. Maalej N, Folts JD. Increased shear stress overcomes the antithrombotic platelet inhibitory effect of aspirin in stenosed dog coronary arteries. Circulation 1996;93:1201–1205.
28. Willerson JT, McNatt J, Yao SK et al. Frequency and severity of cyclic flow alterations and platelet aggregation predict the severity of neointimal proliferation following experimental coronary stenosis and endothelial injury. Proc Natl Acad Sci U S A 1991;88:10624–10628.
29. Anderson HV, Yao SK, Murphree SS et al. Cyclic coronary artery flow in dogs after coronary angioplasty. Coron Artery Dis 1990;1:717–723.
30. Cook JJ, Sitko GR, Bednar B et al. An antibody against the exosite of the cloned thrombin receptor inhibits experimental arterial thrombosis in the African green monkey. Circulation 1995;91:2961–2971.
31. Torr SR, Haskel EJ, VonVoigtlander PF et al. Inhibition of cyclic flow variations and reocclusion after thrombolysis in dogs by a novel antagonist of platelet activating factor. J Am Coll Cardiol 1991;18:1804–1810.
32. Flameng W, Vanhaecke J, Stump DC et al. Coronary thrombolysis by intravenous infusion of recombinant single chain urokinase-type plasminogen activator or recombinant urokinase in baboons: Effect on regional blood flow, infarct size and hemostasis. J Am Coll Cardiol 1986;8:118–124.

33. Yasuda T, Gold HK, Fallon JT et al. A canine model of coronary artery thrombosis with superimposed high grade stenosis for the investigation of rethrombosis after thrombolysis. J Am Coll Cardiol 1989; 13:1409–1414.

34. Gold HK, Yasuda T, Jang IK et al. Animal models for arterial thrombolysis and prevention of reocclusion. Circulation 1991;83(suppl IV):26–40.

35. Jang IK, Gold HK, Ziskind AA et al. Differential sensitivity of erythrocyte-rich and platelet-rich arterial thrombi to lysis with recombinant tissue-type plasminogen activator. Circulation 1989;79:920–928.

36. Hanson SR, Kotze HF, Savage B et al. Platelet interactions with Dacron vascular grafts. A model of acute thrombosis in baboons. Arteriosclerosis 1985;5:595–603.

37. Savage B, McFadden PR, Hanson SR et al. The relation of platelet density to platelet age: Survival of low- and high-density 111-indium-labelled platelets in baboons. Blood 1986;68:386–393.

38. Harker LA, Kelly AB, Hanson SR. Experimental arterial thrombosis in nonhuman primates. Circulation 1991;83(suppl IV):IV41–IV55.

39. Schneider PA, Hanson SR, Price TM et al. Confluent durable endothelialization of endarterectomized baboon aorta by early attachment of cultured endothelial cells. J Vasc Surg 1990;11:365–372.

40. Krpski WC, Bass A, Kelly AB et al. Heparin-resistant thrombus formation by endovascular stents in baboons. Circulation 1990;82:570–577.

41. Bode C, Hanson SR, Schmedtje JF et al. Antithrombotic potency of hirudin is increased in nonhuman primates by fibrin targeting. Circulation 1997; 95:800–804.

42. Martin U, Sponer G, Strein K. Evaluation of thrombolytic and systemic effects of the novel recombinant plasminogen activator BM 06.022 compared with alteplase, anistreplase, streptokinase and urokinase in a canine model of coronary artery thrombosis. J Am Coll Cardiol 1992;19:433–440.

43. Nicolini FA, Nichols WW, Mehta JL et al. Sustained reflow in dogs with coronary thrombosis with K2P, a novel mutant of tissue-plasminogen activator. J Am Coll Cardiol 1992;20:228–235.

44. Markland FS, Friedrichs GS, Pewitt SR et al. Thrombolytic effects of recombinant fibrolase or APSAC in a canine model of carotid artery thrombosis. Circulation 1994;90:2448–2456.

45. Eisenberg PR. The role of thrombin in coronary artery thrombosi [Review]. Coronary Artery Dis 1996;7:400–408.

46. Martin U, Fischer S, Sponer G. Influence of heparin and systemic lysis on coronary blood flow after reperfusion induced by the novel recombinant plasminogen activator BM 06.022 in a canine model of coronary thrombosis. J Am Coll Cardiol 1993;22:914–920.

47. Lefkovits J, Malycky JL, Rao JS et al. Selective inhibition of factor Xa is more efficient than Factor VIIa-tissue factor complex blockade at facilitating coronary thrombolysis in the canine model. J Am Coll Cardiol 1996; 28:1858–1865.

48. Shetler TJ, Crowe VG, Bailey BD et al. Antithrombotic assessment of the effects of combination therapy with the anticoagulants efegatran and heparin and the glycoprotein IIb-IIIa platelet receptor antagonist 7E3 in a canine model of coronary artery thrombosis. Circulation 1996;94:1719–1725.

49. Ashton JH, Ogletree ML, Michel IM et al. Cooperative mediation by serotonin S2 and thromboxane A2/prostagladin H2 receptor activation of cyclic flow variations in dogs with severe coronary artery stenoses. Circulation 1987;76:952–959.

50. Golino P, Buja LM, Ashton JH et al. Effect of thromboxane and serotonin receptor antagonists on intracoronary platelet deposition in dogs with experimentally stenosed coronary arteries. Circulation 1988;78:701–711.

51. Yasuda T, Gold HK, Leinbach RC et al. Lysis of plasminogen activator-resistant platelet-rich coronary artery thrombus with combined bolus injection of recombinant tissue-type plasminogen activator and antiplatelet GP IIb-IIIa antibody. J Am Coll Cardiol 1990;16:1728–1735.

52. Gold HK, Leinbach RC. Strategy of thrombolytic therapy. In: Haber E, Braunwald E, eds. Thrombolysis: Basic contributions and clinical progress. St Louis: Mosby-Year Book, 1991;207–223.

53. Coller BS. Role of platelets in thrombolytic therapy. In: Haber E, Braunwald E, eds. Thrombolysis: Basic contributions and clinical progress. St Louis: Mosby-Year Book, 1991;155–178.

54. Verstraete M. Biology and chemistry of thrombosis. In: Haber E, Braunwald E, eds. Thrombolysis: Basic contributions and clinical progress. St Louis: Mosby-Year Book, 1991;3–16.

55. Yao SK, McNatt J, Anderson HV et al. Thrombin inhibition enhances tissue-type plasminogen activator-induced thrombolysis and delays reocclusion. Am J Physiol 1992;262:H374–H379.

56. Eidt JF, Allison P, Noble S et al. Thrombin is an important mediator of platelet aggregation in stenosed canine coronary arteries with endothelial injury. J Clin Invest 1989;84:18–27.

57. Coller BS. Platelets and thrombolytic therapy. N Engl J Med 1990;322: 33–42.

58. Fujii S, Abendschein DR, Sobel BE. Augmentation of plasminogen activator inhibitor type 1 activity in plasma by thrombosis and thrombolysis. J Am Coll Cardiol 1991;18:1547–1554.

59. Nowak A, Gurewich V. Thrombolysis with streptokinase in rabbits. Dose-response, fibrin-clot specificity and laboratory evaluation of fibrinolytic effect. Thromb Diath Haemorrh 1974;31:265–272.

60. Dupe RJ, English PD, Smith RAG et al. The evaluation of plasmin and streptokinase activator complexes in a new rabbit model of venous thrombosis. Thromb Haemost 1981;46:528–534.

61. English PD, Smith RA, Dupe RJ et al. The thrombolytic activity of streptokinase in the rabbit. Thromb Haemost 1981;46:535–537.

62. Korninger C, Matsuo O, Suy R et al. Thrombolysis with human extrinsic (tissue type) plasminogen activator in dogs with femoral vein thrombosis. J Clin Invest 1982;69:573–580.

63. Collen D, Stassen JM, Verstraete M. Thrombolysis with human extrinsic (tissue type) plasminogen activator in rabbits with experimental jugular vein thrombosis. Effect of molecular form and dose of activator, age of the thrombus, and route of administration. J Clin Invest 1983;71:368–376.

64. Collen D, Lu HR, Lijnen HR et al. Thrombolytic and pharmacokinetic properties of chimeric tissue-type and urokinase-type plasminogen activators. Circulation 1991;84:1216–1234.

# CHAPTER 22

# GENETIC MODELS OF THROMBOSIS AND HEMORRHAGE

Peter Carmeliet and Désiré Collen

## INTRODUCTION

The blood coagulation and the fibrinolytic (or plasminogen/plasmin) systems determine the balance between the formation and dissolution of blood clots and contribute to the pathogenesis of various cardiovascular disorders such as thrombosis, atherosclerosis, and restenosis. Furthermore, they participate in many other biological and pathobiological processes such as reproduction, wound healing, cancer, and brain function. A surprising development in the molecular biology of these systems is that the coagulation system is involved in developmental processes beyond fibrin-dependent hemostasis, for example, in the formation and integrity of an intact vasculature. Two recently developed technologies, gene targeting and gene transfer, which allow manipulation of the genetic balance of these proteinase systems in a controllable manner, have provided the opportunity to elucidate the biological role of these systems. This chapter summarizes the insights that have been obtained from the gene-targeting studies and discusses the use of adenovirus-mediated transfer of fibrinolytic genes to study and, possibly, to develop novel strategies for the treatment of arterial stenosis and thrombosis.

## THE COAGULATION SYSTEM (SEE CHAPTER 1)

Preservation of vascular integrity following traumatic or infectious challenges is essential for survival of multi-cellular organisms. A major defense mechanism involves the formation of hemostatic plugs by activation of platelets and polymerization of fibrin. Initiation of the plasma coagulation system upon exposure of blood to nonvascular cells is triggered by tissue factor (TF), which is expressed by a variety of cells surrounding the vasculature as a hemostatic envelope, and which functions as a cellular receptor and cofactor for activation of the zymogen factor VII to the serine proteinase factor VIIa (1). This complex activates factor X directly or indirectly via activation of factor IX, resulting in the generation of thrombin and the conversion of fibrinogen to fibrin (2, 3). Thrombin and factor Xa produce a positive feedback stimulation of coagulation by activating factor VIII and factor V, which serve as membrane-bound receptors/cofactors for the proteolytic enzymes, factor IXa and factor Xa, respectively (2, 3).

In contrast, thrombin, when bound to its cellular receptor thrombomodulin, also functions as an anticoagulant by activating the protein C anticoagulant system (4, 5). Activated protein C in the presence of its cofactor protein S inactivates factor Va and factor VIIIa, thereby reducing thrombin generation (4, 5). Anticoagulation is provided further by antithrombin, which binds to and inactivates thrombin, factor IXa, and factor Xa in a reaction that is greatly enhanced by heparin (6). Anticoagulation is further secured by TF pathway inhibitor, which directly inhibits factor Xa and, in a factor Xa-dependent manner, produces feedback inhibition of the factor VIIa/TF catalytic complex (7). A revised hypothesis of coagulation has been suggested in which factor VIIa/

435

TF is responsible for the initiation of coagulation but, owing to TF pathway inhibitor-mediated feedback inhibition, amplification of the procoagulant response through the actions of factor VIII, factor IX, and factor XI is required for sustained coagulation (7). Deficiencies of anticoagulant factors or aberrant expression of procoagulant factors have been implicated in hemostasis during inflammation, sepsis, atherosclerosis, and cancer (1, 6), whereas deficiencies of procoagulant factors have been related to increased bleeding tendencies (8, 9).

Evidence has been provided that the coagulation system may also be involved in other functions beyond coagulation, including cellular migration and proliferation, the immune response, angiogenesis, embryonic development, cancer, and brain function (1, 10, 11). Its precise role and relevance in these processes *in vivo* remain, however, largely unknown.

## THE PLASMINOGEN SYSTEM (SEE CHAPTER 7)

The plasminogen system is composed of an inactive pro-enzyme plasminogen that can be converted to plasmin by either of two plasminogen activators (PA): tissue-type PA (t-PA) or urokinase-type PA (u-PA) (12–14). This system is controlled at the level of plasminogen activators by plasminogen activator inhibitors (PAIs), of which PAI-1 is believed to be physiologically the most important (15–17), and at the level of plasmin by $\alpha_2$-antiplasmin (13). Vitronectin stabilizes PAI-1 in its active conformation and may also localize PAI-1 to specific sites in the extracellular matrix (17). Other inhibitors include PAI-2, PAI-3, proteinase nexin-1, and $\alpha_2$-macro-globulin (13, 18). Owing to its fibrin-specificity, t-PA is primarily involved in clot dissolution, although it is said also to be involved in ovulation, bone remodeling, and brain function (14, 19). Cellular receptors for t-PA and plasminogen have been identified, which can localize plasmin proteolysis to the cell surface (20, 21). Urokinase-type PA also binds a cellular receptor, the urokinase receptor (u-PAR), and has been implicated in pericellular proteolysis during cell migration and tissue remodeling in a variety of normal and pathologic processes including ovulation, trophoblast invasion, angiogenesis, keratinocyte migration, inflammation, wound healing, and cancer (22–24). The urokinase plasminogen activator receptor binds to vitronectin, whereas PAI-1 controls recognition of vitronectin by u-PAR or the $\alpha_v\beta_3$-integrin receptor, suggesting a role in coordinating cell adhesion (25, 26). It is not clear whether or in which conditions binding of u-PA to u-PAR is required *in vivo*. Plasmin can degrade fibrin and extracellular matrix proteins, but it can also activate or liberate growth factors from the extracellular matrix, including latent transforming growth factor β, basic fibroblast growth factor,

and vascular endothelial growth factor, and activate other matrix-degrading proteinases, such as the metallo-proteinases (27). Cell-specific clearance of plasminogen activators or of complexes with their inhibitors by low-density lipoprotein receptor-related protein (LRP) or gp330 may modulate pericellular plasmin-mediated proteolysis (28).

## TARGETED MANIPULATION AND ADENOVIRUS-MEDIATED TRANSFER OF GENES IN MICE

New gene technologies that were developed over the last decade have permitted the manipulation of the genetic balance of candidate molecules in mice in a controllable manner. Targeting of genes via homologous recombination in embryonic stem cells permits the study of the consequences of deficiencies, mutations, and conditional or tissue-specific expression of gene products in transgenic mice (29). Using a novel embryonic stem cell technology (aggregation of embryonic stem cells with tetraploid embryos), it has become possible to generate and phenotype embryonic stem cell-derived embryos in a single step (30). Indeed, the tetraploid embryos will preferentially develop into extraembryonic support tissues, whereas the embryonic stem cells will develop into the embryo proper. When embryonic stem cells are generated, which are homozygous for the desired genetic inactivation or mutation, it is possible to phenotype immediately the homozygous mutant embryos generated via this technology. Thus, this technology saves considerable time, inasmuch as the need for conventional germline transmission and the time-consuming breeding of chimeric and heterozygous deficient/mutant animals can be bypassed. In addition, the technology permits the study of homozygous deficiency (using homozygous-deficient embryonic stem cells) when heterozygous-deficient phenotypes of genes cause embryonic lethality (30, 31).

Viral gene transfer can also be used to manipulate the expression of genes, for example, via implantation of retrovirally transduced cells (32) or via adenoviral-mediated gene transfer *in vivo* (33). In fact, intravenous administration of a recombinant adenovirus in mice results in infection of hepatocytes with resultant increased expression of target genes to plasma levels above 10 μg/ml (34). Although adenoviral gene transfer using first generation vectors is transient, use of second-generation vectors, perinatal adenovirus infection, and appropriate tissue-specific control elements may significantly pro-

**TABLE 22.1.** Phenotypes Resulting from Targeted Gene Deletions in Mice and Spontaneous Mutations in Humans

| Deficiency | Mouse | Man |
|---|---|---|
| **I. Coagulation System** | | |
| Tissue factor (TF) | Embryonic lethality due to defective blood vessel formation | Unknown |
| Factor VII (fVII) | —Normal embryonic development | Bleeding |
| | —Perinatal lethality due to bleeding | |
| Thrombomodulin (TM) | Embryonic lethality possibly due to defective feto-material interaction | Unknown |
| Factor V (fV) | Postnatal lethality due to severe spontaneous bleeding | Bleeding |
| Fibrinogen (Fbg) | —Bleeding associated with trauma | Bleeding |
| | —Abnormal wound healing | |
| | —Abortion due to maternal bleeding | |
| Factor XI (fXI) | Normal[1] | Minor bleeding |
| Factor VIII (fVIII) | Bleeding | Bleeding |
| **II. Fibrinolytic System** | | |
| Tissue-type plasminogen activator (t-PA) | —Increased thrombotic susceptibility | Unknown |
| | —Mild glomerulonephritis | |
| | —Reduced neurotoxicity | |
| | —Abnormal long term potentiation | |
| | —Impaired neuronal migration | |
| | —Aneurysm formation in atherosclerotic vessels | |
| Urokinase-type plasminogen activator (u-PA) | —Increased thrombotic susceptibility | Unknown |
| | —Impaired neointima formation | |
| | —Mild glomerulonephritis | |
| | —Impaired macrophage function | |
| | —Reduced decidual vascularization | |
| | —Reduced trophoblast invasion | |
| | —Reduced platelet activation and trapping | |
| | —Reduced tumor invasion | |
| | —Protection against atherosclerotic aneurysm formation | |
| t-PA:u-PA | —Severe spontaneous thrombosis | Unknown |
| | —Impaired neointima formation | |
| | —Reduced ovulation and fertility | |
| | —Cachexia and shorter survival | |
| | —Severe glomerulonephritis | |
| | —Abnormal tissue remodeling | |
| Urokinase receptor (u-PAR) | Normal | Unknown |
| t-PA:u-PAR | Normal | Unknown |
| Plasminogen (Plg) | —Severe spontaneous thrombosis | Thombosis |
| | —Reduced ovulation and fertility | |
| | —Cachexia and shorter survival | |
| | —Severe glomerulonephritis | |
| | —Reduced neurotoxicity | |
| | —Impaired skin healing | |
| | —Reduced macrophage and keratinocyte migration | |
| | —Impaired transplant atherosclerosis | |
| Plasminogen activator inhibitor-1 (PAI-1) | —Reduced thrombotic incidence | Bleeding |
| | —No bleeding | |
| | —Accelerated neointima formation | |
| | —Reduced lung inflammation and fibrosis | |
| | —Reduced atherosclerosis | |
| Plaminogen activator inhibitor-2 (PAI-2) | Normal[1] | Unknown |
| Vitronectin (VN) | Normal[1] | Unknown |
| Alpha$_2$-macroglobulin | —Reduced lung inflammation | Unknown |
| | —Severe pancreatitis | |
| | —Increased resistance to endotoxin shock | |
| Proteinase nexin-1 (PN-1) | Reduced fertility | Unknown |
| LDL receptor-related protein (LRP) | Embryonic lethality due to bleeding | Unknown |

[1] *Initial phenotypic analyses have not revealed any major abnormalities thus far.*

*Only those genetic deficiencies in man that correspond to published genetic deficiencies in mice are summarized. The table only displays the abnormal phenotypes, which are described in more detail in the text; the possible lack of a phenotype is discussed in the text.*

long target gene expression. Another attractive strategy to manipulate gene expression in mice is based on the transplantation of transgenic donor bone marrow stem cells into a wild type recipient host, allowing reconstitution of the wild type host hematopoietic cells with transgenic cells. Such studies allow generation and rescue of disease models and evaluation of possible gene-transfer therapies. Table 22.1 summarizes the phenotypes associated with genetic alterations in the fibrinolytic or coagulation systems that result from targeted inactivation in mice as compared to those that occur spontaneously in humans.

# EMBRYONIC DEVELOPMENT AND REPRODUCTION

## COAGULATION SYSTEM

### Tissue Factor and Factor VII

Limited information is available on the expression of coagulation factors during embryonic development. Tissue factor expression has been identified in the visceral endoderm of the yolk sac, embryonic epithelia, the heart, the nervous system, and vascular smooth muscle cells (35). Intriguingly, expression of prothrombin and factor VII is undetectable in the early embryo, raising the question of whether these molecules might act independently of their currently known ligands (36). Because deficiency of TF in man has not been reported, it was althought that it might cause embryonic lethality. In contrast, individu-

als with low to undetectable factor VII plasma levels are born, but may suffer severe bleeding (9).

After initial differentiation of stem cells into endothelial cells and their assembly into endothelial cell-lined channels (vasculogenesis), the embryonic vasculature develops further via sprouting of new channels from pre-existing vessels (angiogenesis) (Fig.22.1). Once the endothelial cells are assembled into vascular channels, they become surrounded by smooth muscle cells/pericytes that may affect maturation of the blood vessels, not only by providing the fragile primitive blood vessels with the structural support required to accommodate the increased blood pressure, but also by controlling endothelial cell proliferation, vascular permeability, and vascular tone (37) (see Fig. 22.1).

Targeted inactivation of the TF gene resulted in increased fragility of the endothelial cell-lined channels in the yolk sac, which are essential for transferring maternally derived nutrients from the yolk sac to the rapidly growing embryo (38) (Fig. 22.2A). At a time when the blood pressure increased during embryogenesis (day 9 of gestation), the immature TF-deficient blood vessels ruptured, formed microaneurysms and "blood lakes," and failed to sustain proper circulation between the yolk sac and embryo. As a result, the embryo became wasted and died due to generalized necrosis. Only in advanced stages of deterioration did the immature blood vessels become leaky, resulting in bleeding into the extracoelomic cavity. Because hematopoiesis at 8.5 days of gestation in TF-deficient embryos appeared normal, and the proliferation and differentiation potential of TF-deficient hematopoietic stem cells *in vitro* was normal, pallor

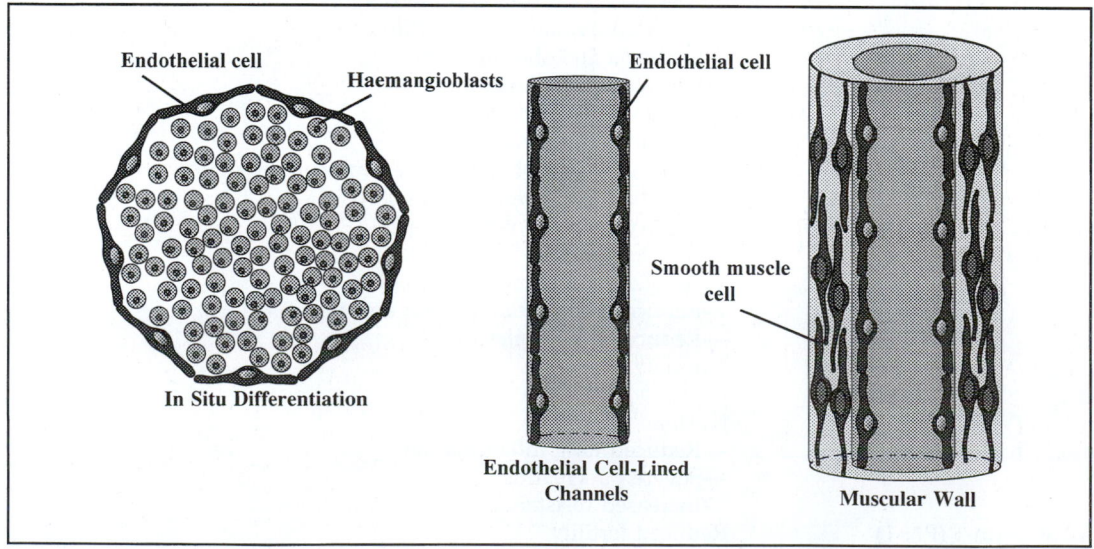

**FIGURE 22.1.** Formation of blood vessels. Early endothelial stem cells (hemangioblasts) differentiate *in situ* into endothelial cells (*left panel*) and become organized into a primitive vascular plexus consisting of endothelial cell-lined channels (*middle panel*). Subsequently, these primitive blood vessels acquire a muscular wall to accommodate the increased blood pressure during further embryonic development (*right panel*).

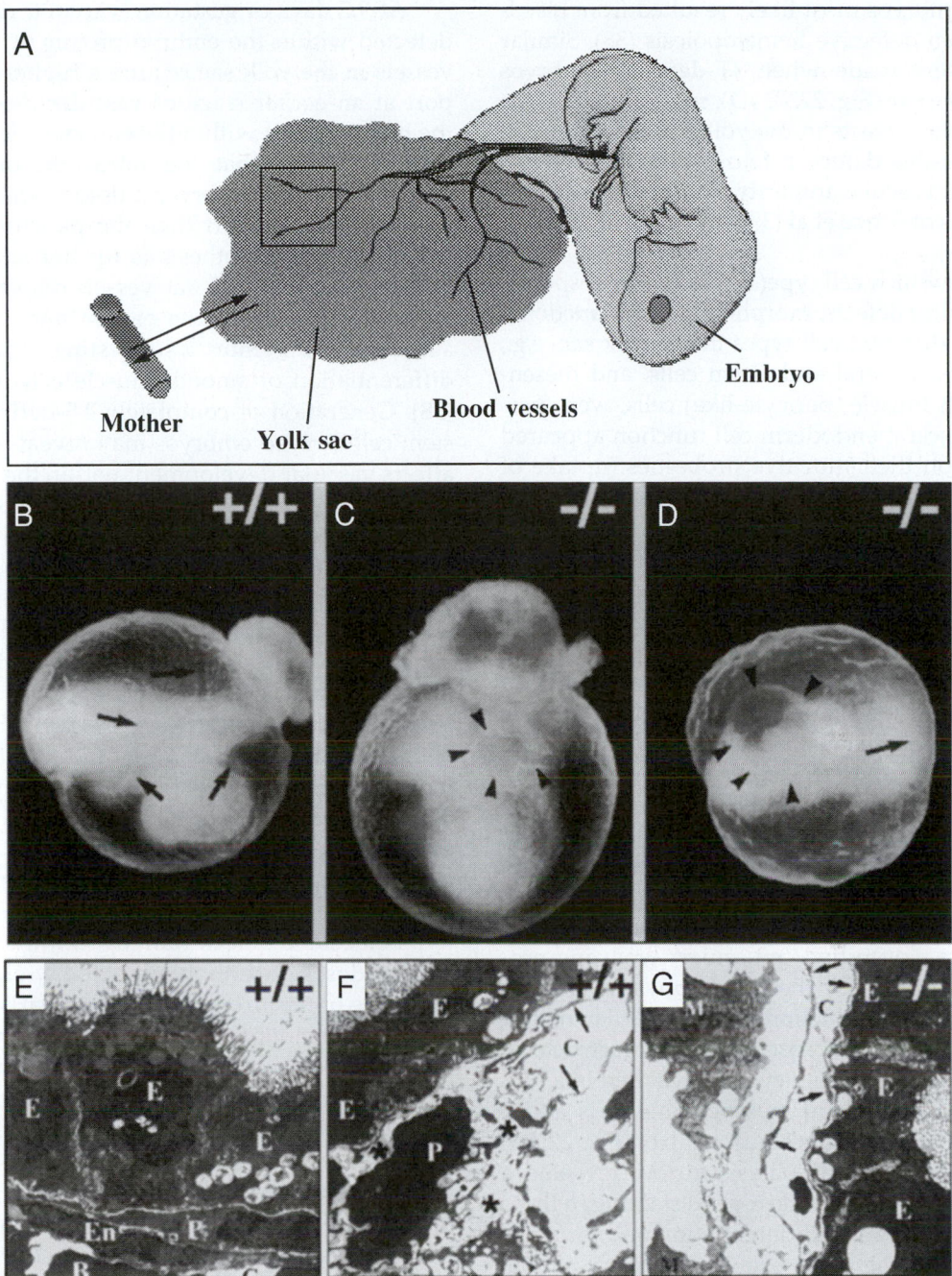

**FIGURE 22.2.**  **A,** Schematic representation of the yolk sac connected to the embryo via the vitello-embryonic blood vessels, mediating transfer of maternally derived nutrients to the embryo proper. **B–D,** The yolk sac of wild type tissue factor (TF$^{+/+}$) embryos at 9.5 days of age, cultured *in vitro* from 8.5 days of age, contains large blood-filled vitello-embryonic vessels (*arrows*) interconnected with a capillary-like vascular plexus in the yolk sac (**B**). In contrast, the yolk sac in homozygous TF deficient (TF$^{-/-}$) embryos reveals significant vascular defects, ranging from microaneurysmatic "vascular blood lakes" in an early stage (**C**), to complete disintegration of the whole vascular plexus and vitelline vessels and leakage of blood in the extracoelomic cavity (*arrow*) ("vascular bleeding") in a preterminal stage (**D**). Note the enlarged pericardial cavity (*arrowheads*) in the mutant embryo, indicative of defective vitello-embryonic circulation. **E–G,** Ultrastructural analysis of the yolk sac of TF$^{+/+}$ (**E, F**) and TF$^{-/-}$ (**G**) embryos, revealing the presence of normal visceral endoderm cells (**E**), endothelial cell, *En,* and an interposed pericyte, *P* (**E**). Note the abundant extracellular matrix between the visceral endoderm cells and the endothelium (*arrows* in **F**). In contrast, in the mutant yolk sac, pericytes are absent and there is a paucity of extracellular matrix. *C* indicates the lumen of the vascular channels.

of the mutant embryos most likely resulted from bleeding and not from defective hematopoiesis (38). Similar observations were made when TF-deficient embryos were cultured *in vitro* (Fig. 22.2B–D), suggesting that the observed vascular defects in the yolk sac were not due merely to a possible defect in feto-maternal exchange. A role for TF in vascular integrity is also suggested by the observations of Broze et al (39 and personal communication).

To evaluate which cell type(s) was (were) responsible for the vascular defects, morphologic and functional analyses of the different cell types in the yolk sac, e.g., endothelial cells, visceral endoderm cells, and mesenchymal (smooth muscle/pericyte-like) cells, were performed (38). Visceral endoderm cell function appeared normal, based on their nutritive properties (uptake of horseradish peroxidase), expression of specific markers (hepatocyte nuclear factor 4, E-cadherin, α-fetoprotein, VEGF), ultrastructure, and normal proliferation and apoptosis rates. Microaneurysms also did not result from increased plasmin proteolysis by visceral endoderm cells, as evidenced by *in situ* zymographic analysis of yolk sac sections (38). Endothelial cells were not likely to be the primary cause of the vascular defect, because expression of endothelial cell specific markers (Flt, Flk, PECAM, TIE, TEK, and VE-cadherin), as well as their ultrastructural and growth properties, were normal.

In contrast, defective development and/or maturation of mesenchymal cells (smooth muscle cell/pericyte-like cells) appeared to be the likely reason for the vascular defects. These cells surround the endothelium in yolk sac vessels, form a primitive "muscular" wall, and provide structural support by their close physical association and increasing production of extracellular matrix proteins (Fig. 22.2E, F). Microscopic and ultrastructural analysis revealed that deficiency of TF resulted in a 75% reduction of the number of mesenchymal cells and a diminished amount of extracellular matrix (Fig. 22.2G) (38). Immunocytochemical analysis further revealed a reduced level of smooth muscle α-actin staining in these cells, suggesting impaired differentiation and/or accumulation (38). Because these primitive smooth muscle cells provide structural support for the endothelium, the vessels in the mutant embryos are too fragile and break open at a time during development when the blood pressure is increased due to more vigorous heart contractions and increased blood cell viscosity (Fig. 22.3A). Inappropriate vascular fragility as a result of peri-endothelial mesenchymal cell/pericyte defects, sometimes resulting in bleeding, has also been observed in mice deficient in platelet derived growth factor (PDGF) (40), transforming growth factor β (41) and angiopoietin-1 (42). Pericytes have also been implicated in adult diabetic retinopathy, where pericyte "drop out" results in the formation and rupture of microaneurysms and blindness (37).

At 9.5 days of gestation, vascular defects were not detected within the embryo proper. It is possible that vessels in the yolk sac require a higher structural support at an earlier stage of vascular development than the blood vessels within the embryo. One simple explanation may be that the intraembryonic vessels are embedded within embryonic tissue, which provides better structural support than the paucity of cells in the yolk sac. This hypothesis is further supported by the observations that yolk sac vessels display smooth muscle α-actin staining at an earlier stage than the dorsal aorta within the embryo, suggesting earlier maturation/differentiation of smooth muscle cells in the yolk sac (38). Generation of completely TF-deficient embryonic stem cell-derived embryos may reveal whether TF also affects vascular development within the embryo proper at later stages during embryonic development.

Unresolved are how TF exerts this morphogenic action, that is, via intracellular signaling as suggested previously (43), and/or whether fibrin formation occurs and is essential during early vascular development, as suggested by others (44). Thus far, there is no conclusive evidence that coagulation factors pass the feto-maternal barrier and that the early-stage embryo has a functional clotting system (45). Indeed, factor VII levels in the plasma from 11.5-day-old wild type embryos are less than 0.5% of those during adulthood. There is also no evidence for fibrin deposits in the visceral yolk sac from ultrastructural analysis of wild type embryos (38, 45), as would be expected if TF-deficient embryos died due to a hemostatic defect. Moreover, intracardial injection of high doses of thrombin in 9.5-day-old embryos fails to induce fibrin thrombi (45). Thus, early embryonic hemostasis may depend less on fibrin formation than anticipated. Because the yolk sac contains TF-mediated procoagulant activity, which, by immunostaining, is localized in the visceral endoderm cells and possibly in the mesenchymal periendothelial cells (38), it is possible that TF provides spatial migratory cues for recruitment of mesenchymal cells to envelope the endothelial cells, provides a signal for mesenchymal cells to differentiate into pericytes/smooth muscle cells, and/or affects their growth (Fig. 22.4). Although it could do so by generation of downstream coagulation molecules (including factor Xa and thrombin, which both can affect migration/proliferation of vascular cells [10, 11]), recent analysis that the factor VIIa inhibitor rNAPc2 fails to induce the typical TF deficient-like vascular fragility in cultured embryos suggests that TF may act via alternative pathways, for example, by acting as a cellular adhesion molecule, or by affecting novel cellular mechanisms (for example, the production of a mesenchymal recruitment signal), or via interaction with another ligand/receptor (Fig. 22.3B). Although analysis revealed no endothelial cell abnormalities and normal expression of VEGF, a possi-

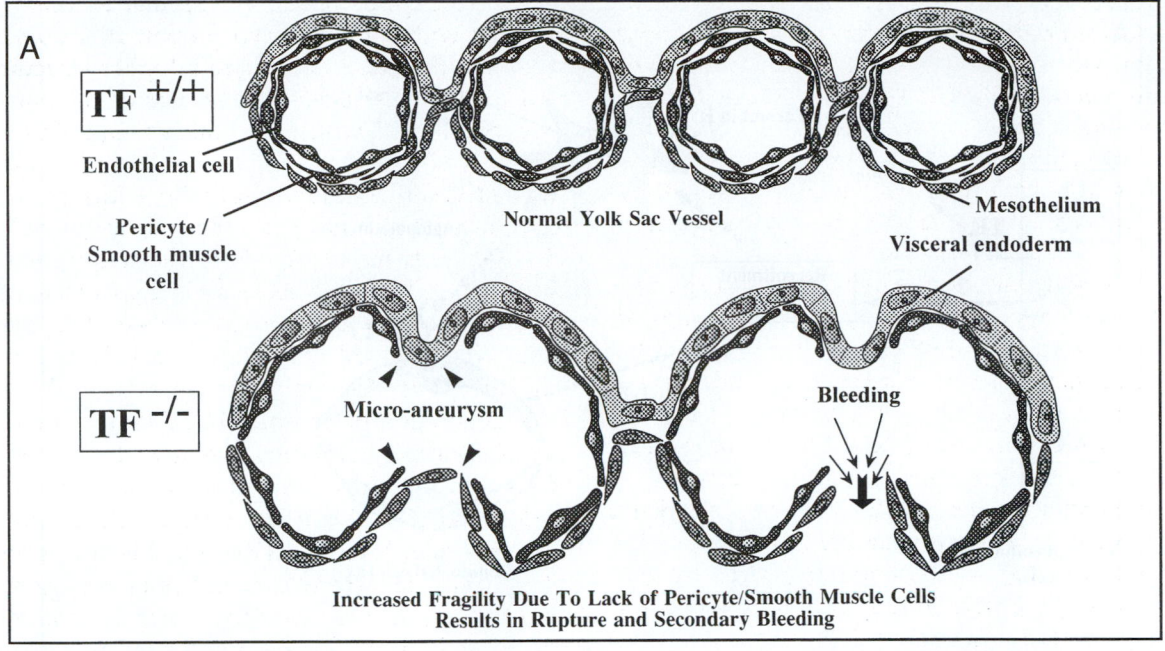

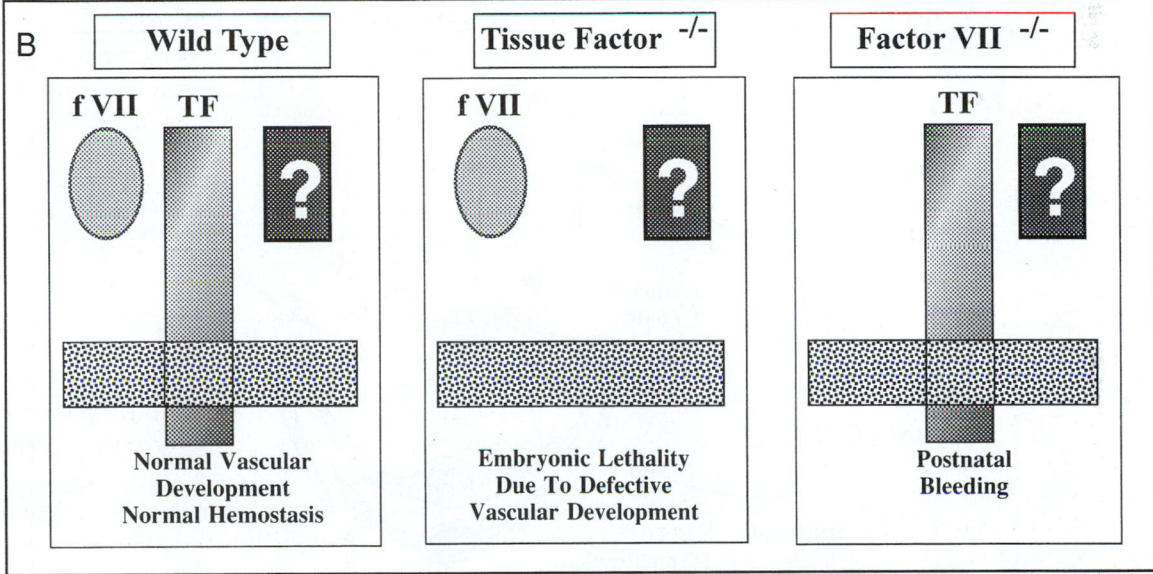

**FIGURE 22.3.** **A,** Vascular defects induced by tissue factor deficiency. Smooth muscle cell/pericyte-like mesenchymal cells accumulate and differentiate around endothelial cell-lined capillaries in the yolk sac from a wild type (TF$^{+/+}$) embryo beyond 9 days of gestation to sustain the increased blood pressure load. In the TF deficient (TF$^{-/-}$) yolk sac, these mesenchymally derived smooth muscle cell/pericyte-like cells fail to accumulate and differentiate around the endothelial cells. As a result, the visceral endoderm and mesothelial cell layers detach (*arrowheads* in left capillaries), and the fragile capillaries rupture and form microaneurysms and "blood lakes" that ultimately leak blood into the extravascular, extracoelomic cavity (*arrows* in right capillaries). As a result of the vascular defects, blood circulation from the yolk sac to the rapidly growing embryo is compromised, inducing wasting of the embryo due to deprivation of essential nutrients. Notably, leakage of blood from defective vessels ("vascular" bleeding) only occurs at a final stage of necrosis and deterioration. **B,** Targeting studies of the coagulation system. Tissue factor is a membrane receptor, the extracellular domain of which is sufficient and required for initiation of the coagulation cascade and fibrin formation. The intracellular domain has been implicated in intracellular signaling. It remains to be determined whether TF interacts with factor VII or an unidentified factor to mediate its morphogenic properties during embryogenesis and whether this involves intracellular signal transduction. Indeed, factor VII-deficient embryos develop normally until birth, after which they die due to massive bleeding, suggesting that, in these embryos, TF either interacts with another ligand or acts independently. Alternatively, placental transfer of factor VII might rescue factor VII-deficient embryogenesis, but transfer of human factor VIIa across mouse placenta was undetectable. TF, tissue factor; f, factor.

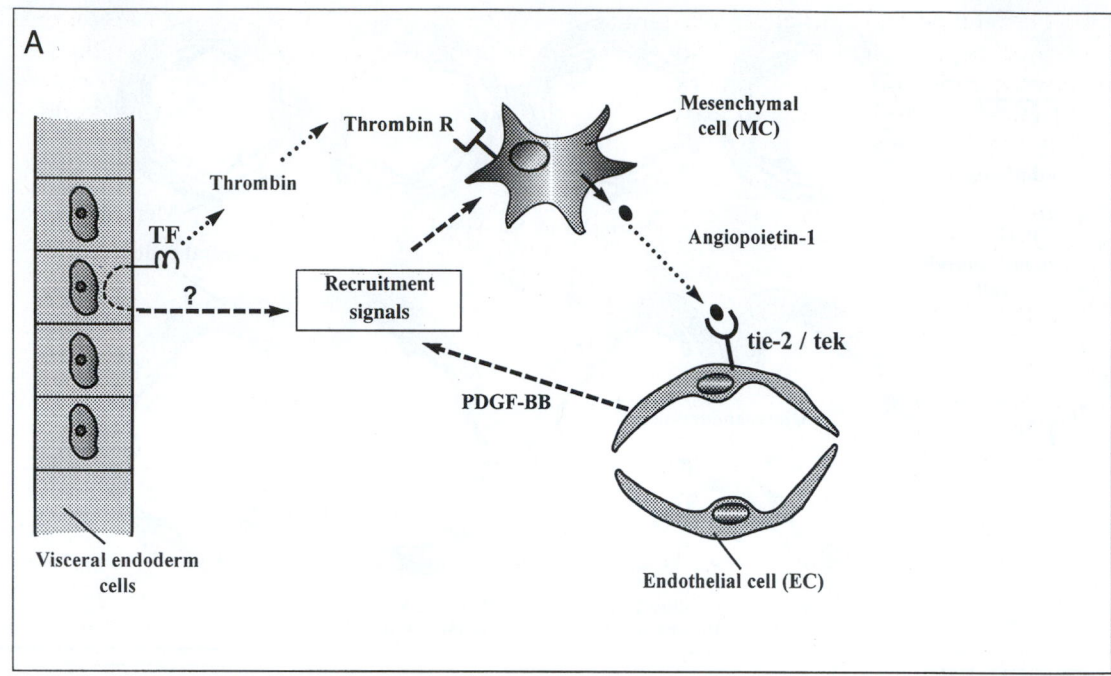

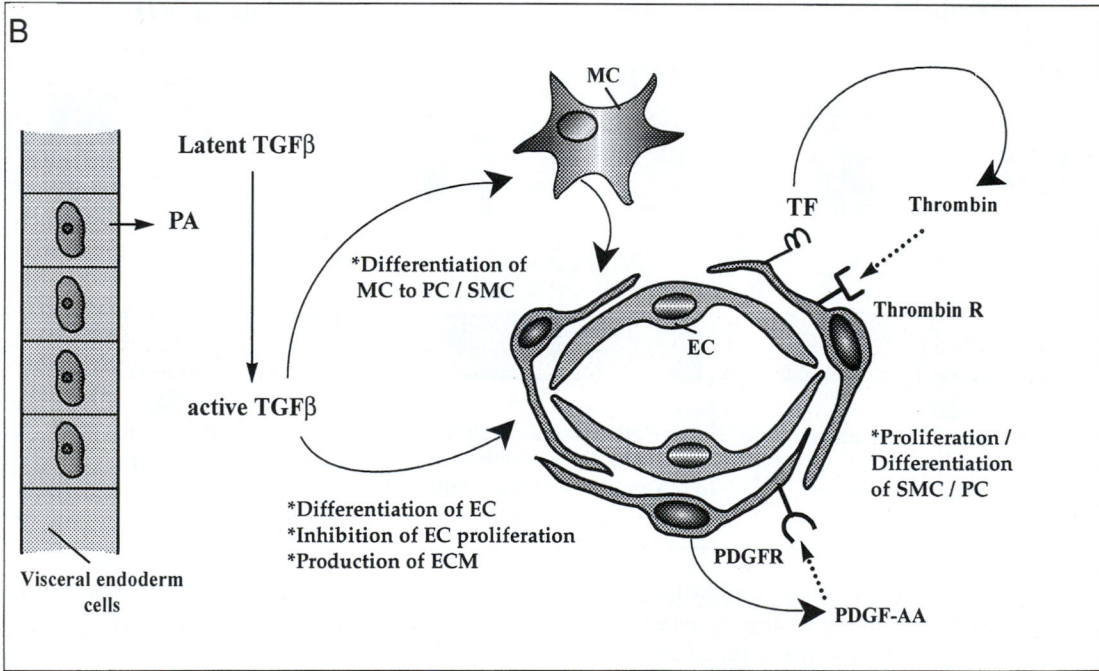

**FIGURE 22.4.** Schematic representation of a molecular model of the development of a smooth muscle cell layer around the endothelial cell-lined channels during the recruitment (**A**) and maturation (**B**) phase. Vascular development in the yolk sac is shown as an example. **A,** Undifferentiated mesenchymal cells (MC) produce angiopoietin-1 that, via interaction with the TIE-2/TEK receptor on early endothelial cells (EC), induces the production of recruitment signal(s), possibly PDGF-BB. In addition, the cellular TF receptor, present on neighboring cells (for example, on visceral endoderm cells [VE] in the yolk sac), may act as a chemotactic recruitment signal or differentiation factor by itself, or induce the generation of downstream coagulation factors such as thrombin, that can interact with its receptor on mesenchymal cells. **B,** Once mesenchymal cells are in close contact with the endothelial cells, TGF-β1, produced by the mesenchymal or endothelial cells, may become activated by plasmin, that is converted from plasminogen by the action of plasminogen activator (PA), produced by the visceral endoderm, endothelial, or mesenchymal cells. Active TGF-β1 may then induce differentiation of mesenchymal cells to pericytes/smooth muscle cells (PC/SMC), control production of extracellular matrix (ECM), inhibit endothelial cell growth, and regulate their differentiation. PDGF-AA, produced by smooth muscle cells, and TF (possibly via generation of thrombin) may control proliferation and differentiation of SMC in an autocrine loop. TF, tissue factor.

ble indirect effect of TF on endothelial cells cannot be excluded in view of the close structural and functional relationship between endothelial cells and pericytes.

In contrast to the severe embryonic TF-deficient lethality, factor VII-deficient mice develop normally until birth and die early postnatally due to massive hemorrhaging (45). Interestingly, factor VII levels in the plasma from 11.5-day-old factor VII deficient embryos are undetectable (< 0.05%) during the entire development. Moreover, intravenous injection of human recombinant factor VIIa into pregnant mice induces supraphysiologic plasma levels in the mother but only background levels in early stage embryos, indicating that the transfer of maternal factor VII is exceedingly low. The TF and factor VII targeting studies suggest that hemostasis during early embryonic development (around 9.5 to 10.5 days of gestation) may depend less on TF-dependent fibrin formation than anticipated, and that TF-mediated vascular integrity may relate to other morphogenic processes, the nature of which is unknown. That hemostasis during early embryogenesis may differ from that during adulthood is further supported by previous gene-inactivation studies revealing that embryos deficient in platelets develop normally without bleeding, but that inactivation of genes involved in function or assembly of periendothelial cells is the most frequent cause of bleeding and defective hemostasis during embryonic development.

## Thrombomodulin

In mouse embryos, thrombomodulin is present in the parietal endoderm (day 7.5 of gestation). Later, the antigen is present in the developing vasculature and in nonvascular structures, including the lung buds and the developing central nervous system. Thrombomodulin is found on all endothelial cells of the blood vessels and lymphatics, except on the high endothelium of postcapillary venules, and hepatic sinusoids. Thrombomodulin is also present on megakaryocytes, platelets, syncytiotrophoblasts, synovium, meningeal cells, mononuclear phagocytes, and mesothelium of the pleura and peritoneum. However, its function in these nonendothelial cells remains unknown.

Transgenic embryos bearing a single copy of the *LacZ* gene, targeted into the endogenous thrombomodulin gene locus via homologous recombination (46), express this marker gene in the parietal endoderm, trophoblast, mesoderm of the yolk sac, and the embryo (7 days of gestation), in the cardiogenic mesoderm, angioblastic head mesenchyme, dorsal aorta, and yolk sac vessels (8.5 days), and in all intra- and extraembryonic vessels (9.5 days). *LacZ* staining was also prominent in nonvascular structures including the leptomeninges, neuroepithelium, and lung of 9.5 day old embryos. In the adult mouse, *LacZ* stained the endothelial cells in

the heart, lung, and spleen and, less intensely, in the brain, liver, skin, body wall, bones, retina, skeletal muscle, gastrointestinal tract, choroid plexus, kidney, and aorta. Reporter gene activity was also documented in nonvascular structures, such as brain meninges, interstitium of testes, and the skin. Thus, targeting of transgenes to the thrombomodulin gene reproduces in most tissues a temporospatial pattern indistinguishable from the endogenous thrombomodulin gene.

Gene inactivation of thrombomodulin resulted in overall growth retardation and embryonic death around 9.0 to 9.5 days postcoitum (47). This may explain why loss of thrombomodulin has not been observed in man. Notably, removal of thrombomodulin-deficient embryos from the maternal decidua rescued the arrested organogenesis, suggesting that defective feto-maternal interactions might compromise the development of the embryo proper (47). Increased fibrin deposition did not seem to affect the barrier function of the Reichert's membrane or the parietal endoderm (47). Whether the embryonic lethality might be related to defective trophoblast function is unknown. Initial studies (in collaboration with E. Conway, unpublished observations) suggest that mutant mice expressing a mutant thrombomodulin lacking its cytosolic domain develop normally during embryogenesis and appear macroscopically normal.

## Thrombin Receptor and Factor V

Thrombin has been implicated in processes beyond hemostasis (11). Indeed, the molecule is mitogenic for fibroblasts and vascular smooth muscle cells, chemotactic for monocytes, induces neurite outgrowth, and activates endothelial cells. Many of the cell-signaling activities of thrombin appear to be mediated by the thrombin receptor (11). Expression studies have further suggested that the thrombin receptor participates in inflammatory, proliferative, or reparative responses such as restenosis, atherosclerosis, neovascularization, and tumorigenesis. In addition, *in situ* analysis indicated that the thrombin receptor is expressed during early embryogenesis in the developing heart and blood vessels, in the brain, and in several epithelial tissues (36).

Targeting of the thrombin receptor resulted in block of embryonic development in approximately 50% of the homozygous-deficient embryos around a similar developmental stage, as in TF-deficient embryos, presumably resulting from impaired yolk sac vascular integrity (48). Although the cellular defect was not characterized in detail, vitelline vessels appeared to be defective, resulting in increased fragility of blood vessels with secondary rupture, blood leakage, and pallor of the embryo. Enlarged pericardial cavities in the thrombin receptor-deficient embryos suggested compromised vitello-embryonic blood circulation. A putative role of thrombin in early blood vessel formation is represented in Fig. 22.4.

Similar to the thrombin receptor-deficient phenotype, deficiency of factor V resulted in embryonic lethality in approximately half of the homozygously deficient embryos, possibly due to vascular defects in the yolk sac (49). The leakage of blood from the defective blood vessels in TF, thrombin receptor, and factor V-deficient embryos ("vascular" bleeding) contrasts with the postnatal bleeding in mice deficient of factor VII, factor VIII (50), and fibrinogen (51), and in the surviving fraction of factor V-deficient mice, which occurs due to defective clot formation after trauma of normally developed blood vessels ("hemostatic" bleeding). Bleeding in the latter mice occurred shortly after birth (factor V, factor VII, and fibrinogen) or was associated with injury (factor VIII). Thus, these target studies show that several coagulation factors (tissue factor, factor V, thrombin receptor) participate in morphogenic processes beyond control of hemostasis, whereas other coagulation factors (factor VII, factor VIII, fibrinogen) play a predominant role in hemostasis via clot formation. This raises an interesting question of whether TF and the thrombin receptor, which are expressed during restenosis, atherosclerosis, and neovascularization, also play a similar (nonhemostatic) role in these processes. If so, this could open an attractive therapeutic avenue by which to inhibit selectively the hemostatic or morphogenic properties of these molecules.

## Fibrinogen

Ovulation, embryo implantation, and placentation involve tissue remodeling and breaching of intact vessels, requiring proper hemostasis. Somewhat surprisingly, intraovarian bleeding did not occur after ovulation in fibrinogen-deficient mice (51). However, deficiency of fibrinogen significantly affected embryogenesis (51). Indeed, development of fibrinogen-deficient embryos in homozygous fibrinogen-deficient females was arrested 9 to 10 days postcoitum due to severe intrauterine bleeding. There was no evidence of bleeding within developing embryos or their amniotic or yolk sacs as long as the placentas were intact. Rather, the location, volume, and absence of nucleated (embryonic) red blood cells within the hemorrhagic areas suggest that hemorrhaging was from a maternal source. It is possible that bleeding was caused by the invasion of embryonic trophoblasts into and disruption of maternal vasculature within the placenta. Abortion was not observed in heterozygous fibrinogen-deficient females mated to heterozygous or homozygous fibrinogen-deficient males, indicating the importance of maternal fibrinogen during embryonic development (51).

## FIBRINOLYTIC SYSTEM

The plasminogen system has been proposed to be involved in ovulation, spermatocyte migration, fertiliza-

tion, embryo implantation, and embryogenesis, and in the associated remodeling of the ovary, prostate, and mammary gland (12, 14). Because homozygous deficiencies of several fibrinolytic system components, including t-PA and u-PA have not been observed, it was anticipated that inactivation of these genes might cause embryonic lethality. However, transgenic mice overexpressing PAI-1 (52, 53), u-PA (54), or the aminoterminal fragment of u-PA (55), and mice with single or combined deficiencies of t-PA and/or u-PA (56, 57), t-PA and u-PAR (58), PAI-1 (59, 60), u-PAR (61, 62), plasminogen (63, 64), PAI-2 (65), vitronectin (66), or $\alpha_2$-macroglobulin (67) survived embryonic development and were viable at birth. Thus far, u-PA deficiency has only been found to reduce the rate of trophoblast migration during early embryogenesis and the formation of blood lacunae in late pregnancies, possibly due do impaired endothelial cell function (Teesalu, Blasi, and Tallerico, personal communication). The normal embryonic development of mice with inactivated fibrinolytic genes was not anticipated, inasmuch as deficiency of t-PA, u-PA, u-PAR in man had not been reported previously and only individuals with low to undetectable levels of PAI-1 or plasminogen were known.

Inactivation of the low-density lipoprotein receptor-related protein (LRP) gene resulted in embryonic lethality at midgestation, secondary to abdominal bleeding (68). It is not clear at present to what extent lethality in these mice is caused by abnormal plasmin proteolysis, since LRP is a multifunctional clearance receptor not only for fibrinolytic system components but also for other unrelated molecules (28). Another interesting but unresolved question is why homozygous, but not heterozygous proteinase nexin-1-deficient mice are unable to sire offspring (Botteri and Vander Putten, personal communication).

Mice with single deficiency of t-PA or u-PA (56, 57), u-PAR (61, 62), PAI-1 (59, 60), vitronectin (66), or $\alpha_2$-macroglobulin (67) are fertile. Normal fertility was also observed in a transgenic mouse strain expressing an antisense t-PA mRNA with reduction of t-PA activity in the oocytes by more than 50% (69). Both plasminogen activators appeared to cooperate, because plasminogen-deficient and combined t-PA:u-PA-deficient mice were less fertile than wild type mice or mice with a single deficiency of t-PA or u-PA (56, 63). In part, this could be due to poor general health and fibrin deposits in the gonads once they became sick and cachectic. However, gonadotropin-induced ovulation was also significantly reduced in healthy 25-day-old female mice lacking both plasminogen activators (70) or plasminogen (Ny et al, personal communication). The observation that combined t-PA:u-PAR-deficient mice are fertile (58) suggests that u-PA can still mediate sufficient pericellular proteolysis in the absence of u-PAR to rescue the defective ovulation of combined t-PA:u-PA-deficient mice (56). Thus, ovulation can occur in the absence of t-PA, u-PA, u-PAR, PAI-1, or $\alpha_2$-macroglobulin, but is reduced in mice with plasminogen deficiency or combined t-PA and u-PA deficiency.

## INTEGRATED VIEW OF A ROLE FOR THE COAGULATION AND FIBRINOLYTIC SYSTEM IN VASCULAR DEVELOPMENT

It is apparent from the gene targeting studies that the coagulation system participates in vascular develop-

ment and integrity during embryogenesis. The following discussion presents a hypothetical model of the possible role of the coagulation and fibrinolytic factors in vessel formation during embryonic development and their relationship with other vascular growth factors (Fig. 22.5). Differentiation of endothelial cells, their organization in vascular tubes and assembly into a network, and the sprouting of new blood vessels are mediated in large part by vascular endothelial growth factor (VEGF) interacting with its cellular receptors Flk-1 and Flt-1 (71–73). However, once endothelial cell-lined channels are formed, vascular integrity is maintained by organization of a primitive muscular wall, providing the re-

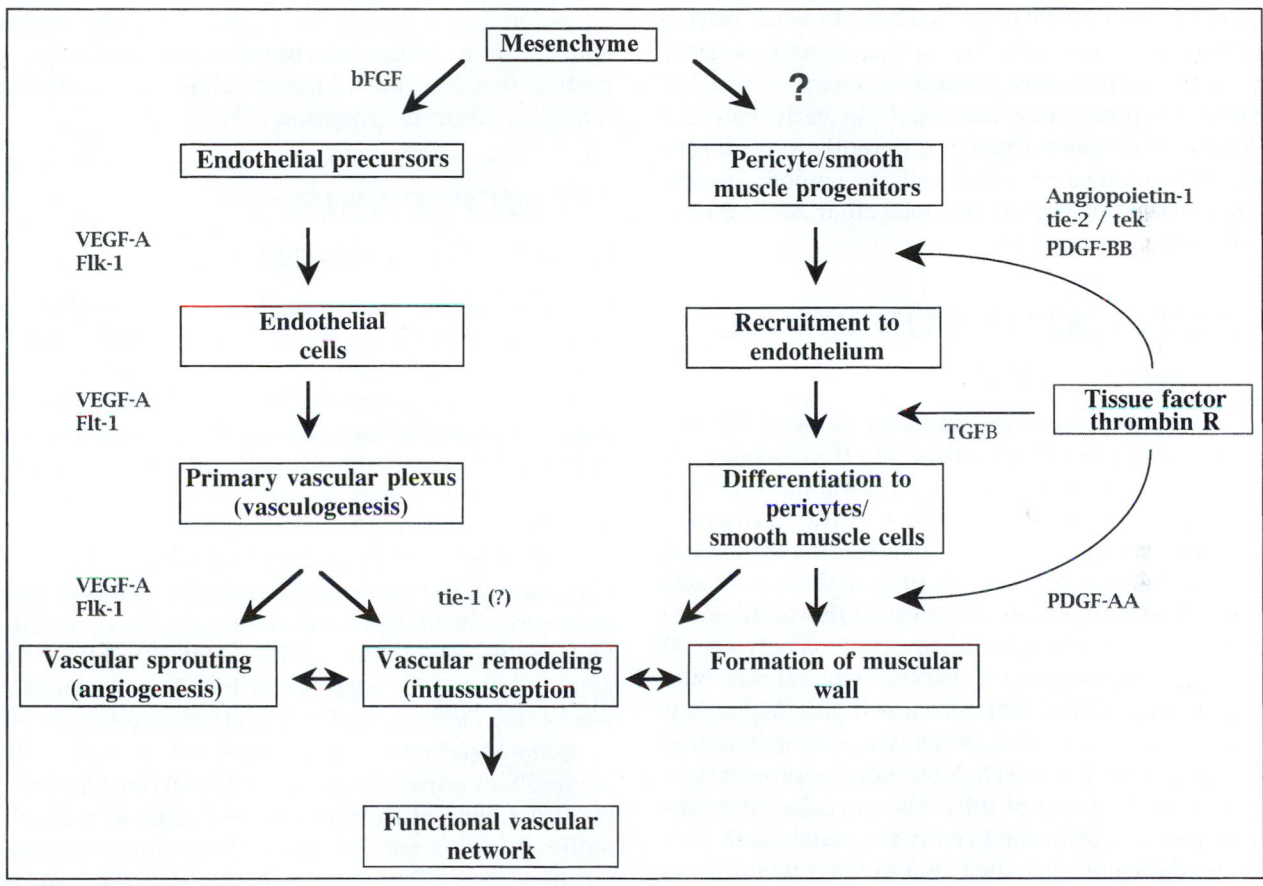

**FIGURE 22.5.** Integrated view of early blood vessel development during embryogenesis. *Mesenchymal cells differentiate* to hemangioblasts, in part by the action of basic fibroblast growth factor (bFGF). Further *in situ* differentiation into endothelial cells is mediated by VEGF-A, through interaction with VEGFR-2/Flk-1, whereas formation of the endothelial cell-lined channels and organization into a primitive vascular plexus (vasculogenesis) is dependent on VEGF-A and its receptor Flt-1. VEGF-A and Flk-1 are further involved in the process of angiogenesis, or the sprouting of neovessels from pre-existing vessels, in lumen formation and in mediating correct vascular connections. Tissue factor, and possibly the thrombin receptor and factor V, participate in the formation of a primitive smooth muscle cell sheet around the fragile endothelial cell-lined channels, possibly by acting as a recruitment signal or as a differentiation/proliferation factor for mesenchymal cells. Angiopoietin-1 and its receptor TEK play a somewhat similar role in recruiting mesenchymal cells and the remodeling of early blood vessels by intussusception. PDGF-BB might be one of the recruitment signals for the mesenchymal cells, whereas TGF-β1 could participate in differentiation of the mesenchymal cells to pericytes/smooth muscle cells, inhibition of endothelial cell growth and production of extracellular matrix. The role of TIE-1 is less defined, but may relate to maturation and integrity of the microvasculature. PDGF is not essential for embryonic vascular development, but appears to be required for neovascularization during adulthood, for example during wound healing.

quired structural support against increased blood pressure and modulating endothelial cell function. The recently cloned angiopoietin-1, via interaction with its TIE-2/TEK receptor, may activate endothelial cells to produce a recruitment factor for mesenchymal cells, possibly PDGF-BB (40, 41). Once the mesenchymal cells contact the endothelium, transforming growth factor β1 (TGF-β1) may be activated and induce differentiation of the mesenchymal cells into pericytes and smooth muscle cells, inhibit endothelial cell proliferation, and stimulate extracellular matrix (ECM) deposition (42). Activation of latent TGF-β1 may occur via plasmin, generated from plasminogen by the action of plasminogen activators, which can be produced by endothelial, mesenchymal, and visceral endoderm (VE) cells (27). Smooth muscle cells may further control their own growth via autocrine production of PDGF-AA. Tissue factor, and possibly other coagulation factors (including factor V and the thrombin receptor), may participate in early vascular development via recruitment, differentiation, and/or proliferation of mesenchymal cells to smooth muscle cells/pericytes, but the precise molecular mechanisms have not been determined.

# HEALTH AND SURVIVAL
## COAGULATION SYSTEM

Deficiencies of the procoagulant factor V, factor VII, factor VIII, and fibrinogen significantly affect survival of mutant mice due to bleeding complications. Within 2 days after birth, approximately 30% of the fibrinogen-deficient offspring developed overt intra-abdominal bleeding but surprisingly, only 10% of these neonates died (51). A second period of increased risk of developing fatal intra-abdominal bleeding occurred between 30 and 60 days, resulting in a 50 to 60% survival rate. Survival of fibrinogen-deficient mice was highly dependent on the genetic background, possibly due to differences in general activity level (51). A fraction (approximately 50%) of factor V-deficient mice also revealed intra-abdominal bleeding resulting in early postnatal death (49). Factor VII-deficient mice died due to massive intra-abdominal bleeding within the first 3 days postnatally, whereas the remainder of the factor VII-deficient neonates died due to intracranial bleeding within 2 to 3 weeks (45). In contrast, factor VIII-deficient mice did not bleed spontaneously, but displayed life-threatening bleeding when challenged with trauma during tail cutting (50).

## FIBRINOLYTIC SYSTEM

No effects on health and survival were observed in t-PA-, u-PAR-, PAI-1-, vitronectin- or α₂-macroglobulin-deficient mice (56–67). A small percentage of u-PA-defi-cient mice developed chronic (nonhealing) ulcerations and rectal prolapse but without effect on survival (56). Plasminogen-deficient (63, 64) and combined t-PA:u-PA-deficient (56), but not combined t-PA:u-PAR-deficient (58) mice developed chronic ulcerations and rectal prolapse, suggesting that sufficient u-PA-mediated plasmin proteolysis can occur in the absence of u-PAR. In addition, these mice suffered significant growth retardation, developed a wasting syndrome with anemia, dyspnea, lethargy, and cachexia, and had a significantly shorter life span (Fig. 22.6). Generalized thrombosis in the gastrointestinal tract, lungs, and other organs (including gonads, liver, and kidney) might, at least in part, explain their increased morbidity and mortality. Crossbreeding of the plasminogen-deficient mice with fibrinogen-deficient mice rescued the increased morbidity and mortality of the plasminogen-deficient mice, suggesting that the role of plasminogen is primarily mediated by fibrin degradation (74).

# HEMOSTASIS
## COAGULATION SYSTEM

Deficiency of tissue factor and loss of the thrombin receptor and factor V (in approximately 50% of the embryos) resulted in bleeding due to vascular defects ("vascular bleeding"). This section describes the bleeding, resulting from defects in clot formation in the absence of vascular defects ("hemostatic bleeding"). Inactivation of the intrinsic (contact activation) pathway by deletion of factor XI had little effect as mutant animals showed normal survival, fertility, and fecundity, but no signs of bleeding (75). Factor VII-deficient mice died due to massive intra-abdominal bleeding within the first 3 days postnatally, whereas the remainder of the factor VII-deficient neonates died due to intracranial bleeding within 2 to 3 weeks (45). Deficiency of factor VII in individuals results in severe bleeding when plasma levels of factor VII are below 2% of normal plasma levels (76) (see Chapter 36). However, lack of early postnatal deaths in individuals with reduced factor VII plasma levels may relate to the fact that factor VII was not completely absent, compared with the factor VII-deficient mice, which completely lack this factor. Factor V-deficient mice appeared to suffer a severe bleeding phenotype (resulting in early postnatal death), suggesting critical hemostatic functions of thrombin activation beyond fibrin generation (49). The more severe phenotype of factor V deficiency in mice than in humans is consistent with the detection of residual factor V activities in most individuals (77). Deficiency of factor VIII (hemophilia A) in individuals predisposes to spontaneous and trauma-induced bleeding into joints and soft tissues (2) (see Chapter 35). Mice deficient in factor VIII suffered life-threatening bleeding in association with tail injury, but did not appear to bleed spontaneously (50).

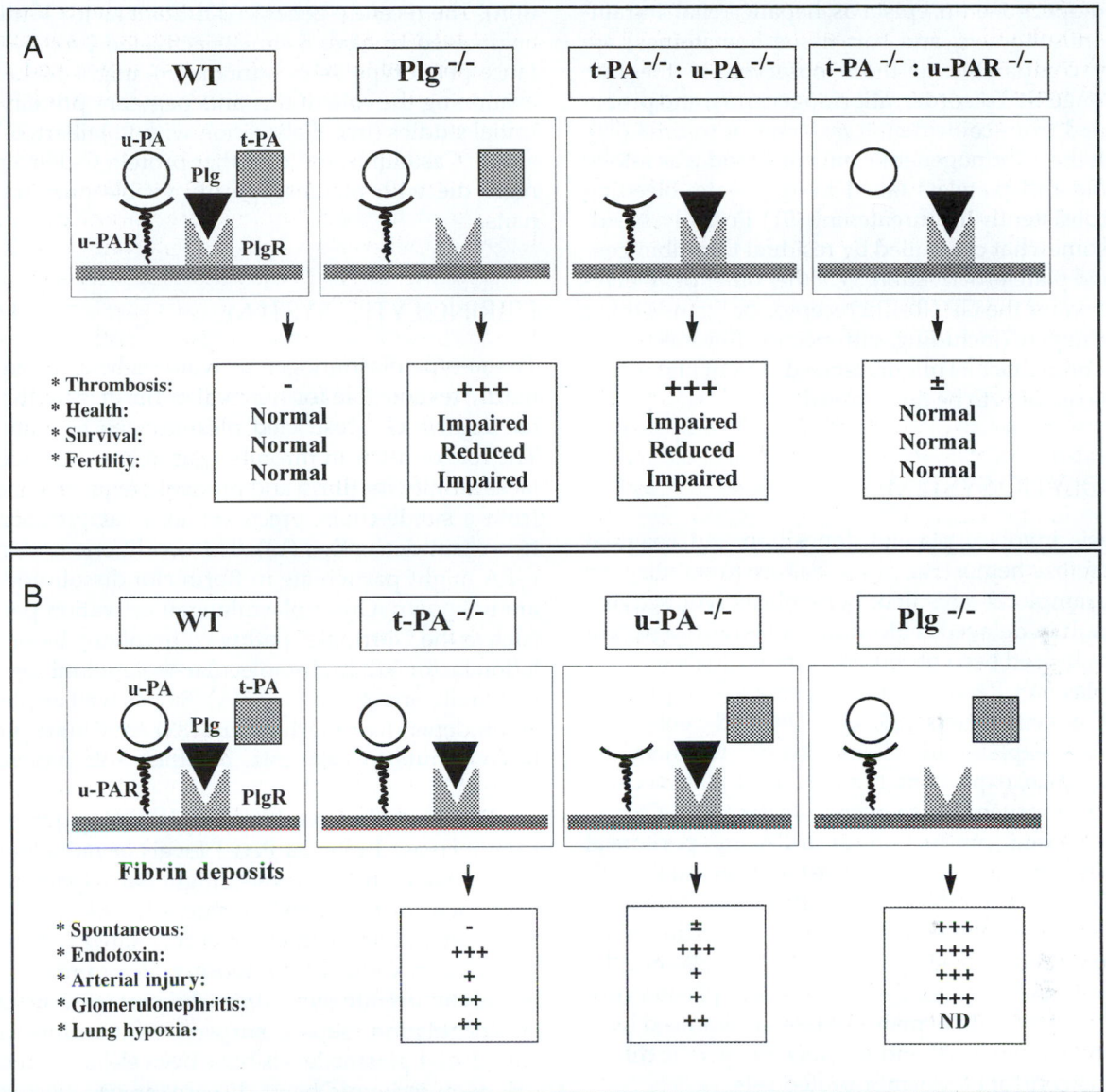

**FIGURE 22.6.**   Role of the plasminogen system in fibrin surveillance. Fibrin deposits in plasminogen system knockout mice before and after experimental challenges. **A,** Fibrin deposits during unchallenged conditions were occasionally observed in u-PA-deficient mice and more extensively in plasminogen-deficient or combined t-PA:u-PA-deficient mice, indicating that both plasminogen activators cooperate in prevention of fibrin deposition. Inflammatory and/or traumatic challenges, including local injection of proinflammatory endotoxin in the footpad, skin wounding, experimental glomerulonephritis, lung hypoxia, and arterial injury induce extravascular fibrin deposits and intravascular thrombosis in veins or capillaries (endotoxin, lung hypoxia, skin wounding, glomerulonephritis) and arteries (arterial injury). **B,** Combined deficiency of t-PA and u-PA, but not of t-PA and u-PAR, results in widespread fibrin deposition, reduced fertility, multiorgan dysfunction with dyspnea, lethargy, and cachexia, ultimately leading to premature death, indicating that sufficient pericellular plasmin proteolysis occurs in the absence of binding of u-PA to its cellular receptor.

The factor VIII-deficient mice may constitute useful models for studying the immune response that limits recombinant factor VIII substitution in hemophilic individuals as well as for designing possible gene therapy strategies. Surprisingly, the thrombin receptor-deficient mice that developed properly did not reveal signs of bleeding, suggesting that other related thrombin receptors may play a significant role in platelet activation and hemostasis (48). Deficiency of fibrinogen resulted in overt intraabdominal, subcutaneous, joint, or periumbilical bleeding in the neonatal period (51). These are the common sites of spontaneous bleeding events in humans with acquired or congenital coagulation disorders (78). The bleeding manifestations in adult fibrinogen-deficient mice (hemoperitoneum, epistaxis, hepatic, renal, intraintestinal, intrathoracic, and soft tissue hematomas) are generally comparable to those observed in the rare human congenital disorder, afibrinogenemia, and probably resulted from coincidental mechanical trauma (79). Although the afibrinogenemic murine blood was totally unclottable and platelets failed to aggregate, bleeding was not consistently life threatening (51). Possibly, bleeding was somewhat controlled by residual thrombin generation and platelet activation. Whether other platelet receptors beyond the GP IIb-IIIa receptor or ligands other than fibrinogen (including vitronectin, fibronectin, or von Willebrand factor) might rescue deficient platelet interactions remains to be determined.

## FIBRINOLYTIC SYSTEM

Hemostasis involves platelet deposition and coagulation to stabilize hemostatic plugs. Failure to stabilize the clot, for example, as a result of hyperfibrinolytic activity, might result in delayed rebleeding. A hemorrhagic tendency has indeed been observed in individuals with increased plasma t-PA or reduced plasma $\alpha_2$-antiplasmin or PAI-1 activity levels (80, 81). Delayed rebleeding might also explain the hemorrhagic tendency in transgenic mice, expressing high levels of plasma u-PA (54) and in transgenic mice overexpressing GM-CSF, in which increased production of u-PA by peritoneal macrophages occurs (82). In contrast to individuals with low or absent plasma PAI-1 levels, PAI-1 deficient mice did not exhibit spontaneous or delayed rebleeding, even after trauma (60). Lower plasma PAI-1 levels and the occurrence of alternative PAIs in murine plasma (unpublished data) might explain the less pronounced hyperfibrinolytic phenotype and the species-specific difference in the control of plasmin proteolysis.

# THROMBOSIS AND THROMBOLYSIS

## COAGULATION SYSTEM

Deficiencies of coagulation inhibitors in humans predispose to an increased risk for thrombosis (6). Heterozygous thrombomodulin-deficient mice were viable and did not appear to develop spontaneous thrombosis, possibly indicating that the mice need to be challenged either genetically (by cross-breeding them with other thrombosis-prone transgenic mice) or physiologically (by administration of proinflammatory reagents, injury, etc.). However, recently generated transgenic mice with a mutated thrombomodulin$^{Q387P}$ gene, which reduces interaction with protein C, survived embryonic development and revealed an increased spontaneous thrombotic incidence (Rosenberg et al, personal communica-

tion). The recently generated mutant factor V mice (83), engineered to have a similar activated protein C-resistance phenotype as in humans (5), might be useful for examining the role of this anticoagulant protein *in vivo*. Initial studies (in collaboration with L. Jalbert, E. Rosen, and F. Castellino) indicate that protein C-deficient neonates die with macroscopically visible purpura fulminans.

## FIBRINOLYTIC SYSTEM

Tissue-type plasminogen activator is believed to be primarily responsible for removal of fibrin from the vascular tree via clot-restricted plasminogen activation (13). The role of u-PA in thrombolysis is less well defined. It lacks affinity for fibrin and probably requires conversion from a single-chain precursor to a catalytically active two-chain derivative (13). The conditions under which u-PA might participate in fibrin clot dissolution *in vivo* are unknown. Other plasminogen activation pathways, such as the "intrinsic" pathway (involving blood coagulation factor XII, high-molecular-weight kininogen, prekallikrein, and possibly u-PA) (84), as well as plasminogen-independent mechanisms (85) have been proposed to contribute to clot lysis, but their role has not been defined.

Deficient fibrinolytic activity resulting, for example, from increased plasma PAI-1 levels or reduced plasma t-PA or plasminogen levels, might participate in the development of thrombotic events (81). Elevated plasma PAI-1 levels have indeed been correlated with a higher risk of deep venous thrombosis and thrombosis during hemolytic uremic syndrome, disseminated intravascular coagulation, sepsis, surgery, and trauma (15, 16). Also, PAI-1 plasma levels have been elevated in individuals with ischemic heart disease, angina pectoris, and recurrent myocardial infarction (86). However, the acute-phase reactant behavior of PAI-1 does not permit deduction of whether increased PAI-1 levels are a cause or consequence of thrombosis. To date, abnormal fibrin clot surveillance resulting from genetic deficiencies of t-PA or u-PA has not been reported in humans, but quantitative and qualitative deficiencies of plasminogen have been associated with an increased thrombotic tendency (81, 87).

## FIBRIN DEPOSITS AND PULMONARY PLASMA CLOT LYSIS IN TRANSGENIC MICE

Microscopic analysis of tissues from u-PA-deficient mice revealed occasional minor fibrin deposits in liver and intestines and excessive fibrin deposition in chronic nonhealing skin ulcerations, whereas in t-PA-deficient mice, no spontaneous fibrin deposits were observed

(56). Mice with a single deficiency of plasminogen or a combined deficiency of t-PA and u-PA, however, revealed extensive fibrin deposits in several organs (including the liver, lung, gastrointestinal tract, reproductive organs, etc.) associated with ischemic necrosis, possibly resulting from thrombotic occlusions (56, 63, 64). Fibrin deposits were observed at the same predilection sites and around the same age in plasminogen-deficient as in combined t-PA:u-PA-deficient mice, suggesting that t-PA and u-PA are the only physiologically significant plasminogen activators *in vivo*. These fibrin deposits were absent in mice with a combined deficiency of plasminogen and fibrinogen (74). Interestingly, mice with a combined deficiency of t-PA and u-PAR did not display such excessive fibrin deposits, suggesting that sufficient plasmin proteolysis can occur in the absence of u-PA binding to u-PAR (Fig. 22.6) (58). Transgenic mice overexpressing human PAI-1 under the control of the metallothionein promoter displayed cell-, fibrin-, and platelet-rich venous occlusions in the tail and hind-legs (52), whereas mice overexpressing murine PAI-1 under the control of the cytomegalous virus promoter did not suffer such complications (53 and Ginsburg et al, personal communication). The reason for this discrepancy is not yet clear. Mice with a single deficiency of t-PA or u-PA were significantly more susceptible to the development of venous thrombosis after local injection of proinflammatory endotoxin in the footpad (56). Hypoxia also induced [$^{125}$I]-labeled fibrin deposition in t-PA- or u-PA-deficient mice, but not in wild type or PAI-1-deficient mice (Pinsky et al, personal communication). The increased susceptibility of t-PA-deficient mice to endotoxin and the severe spontaneous thrombotic phenotype of combined t-PA:u-PA or plasminogen-deficient mice could be explained by their significantly reduced rate of spontaneous lysis of [$^{125}$I]-fibrin-labeled plasma clots, injected via the jugular vein and embolized into the pulmonary arteries (56, 63). In contrast, PAI-1-deficient mice were virtually protected against the development of venous thrombosis after injection of endotoxin, consistent with their ability to lyse [$^{125}$I]-fibrin labeled plasma clots at a significantly higher rate than wild type mice (60). The increased susceptibility of u-PA-deficient mice to thrombosis associated with inflammation or injury might be due to their impaired macrophage function. Indeed, thioglycollate-stimulated macrophages (which are known to express cell-associated u-PA) isolated from u-PA-deficient mice, lacked plasminogen-dependent breakdown of [$^{125}$I]-labeled fibrin (fibrinolysis) or of [$^{3}$H]-labeled subendothelial matrix (mostly collagenolysis), whereas macrophages from t-PA-deficient or PAI-1-deficient mice did not (56, 57).

Lipoprotein(a) contains the lipid and protein components of low-density lipoprotein plus apolipoprotein(a) (88). Extensive homology of apolipoprotein(a) to plasminogen has prompted the proposal that apolipoprotein(a) forms a link between thrombosis and atherosclerosis, but *in vitro* studies have not yielded conclusive evidence. Transgenic mice overexpressing apolipoprotein(a) displayed reduced thrombolytic potential, but only after administration of pharmacologic doses of recombinant t-PA, suggesting a mild hypofibrinolytic condition (89). Studies using transgenic mice overexpressing lipoprotein(a) extended these findings and revealed that spontaneous lysis of [$^{125}$I]-fibrin labeled pulmonary plasma clots (thus not lysis induced by exogenous administration of recombinant t-PA) was also reduced (Carmeliet et al, unpublished observations).

## ADENOVIRUS-MEDIATED TRANSFER OF t-PA OR PAI-1

More recently, adenoviral-mediated transfer of fibrinolytic system components in these "knockout" mice has been used in an attempt to revert their phenotypes. Intravenous injection of adenoviruses, expressing a recombinant PAI-1 resistant human t-PA (rt-PA) gene, in t-PA-deficient mice increased plasma rt-PA levels 100- to 1000-fold above normal and restored their impaired thrombolytic potential in a dose-related way (34). Notably, adenoviral t-PA gene transfer increased thrombolysis to significant levels as early as within 4 hours and was sustained for more than 1 week, suggesting that it might be useful for restoring deficient thrombolysis in subacute conditions. Conversely, adenovirus-mediated transfer of recombinant human PAI-1 in PAI-1-deficient mice resulted in 100- to 1000-fold increased plasma PAI-1 levels above normal and efficiently reduced the increased thrombolytic potential of PAI-1-deficient mice (Carmeliet et al, unpublished observations).

Collectively, these gene-targeting and gene-transfer studies confirm the importance of the plasminogen system in maintaining vascular patency and indicate that t-PA and u-PA are the only physiologically significant plasminogen activators *in vivo* that appear to cooperate significantly in fibrin surveillance. Interestingly, u-PA plays a more significant role than previously anticipated in the prevention of fibrin deposition during conditions of inflammation or injury, possibly through cell-associated plasmin proteolysis. A surprising finding is that u-PA can still exert its biological role (pericellular proteolysis) in the absence of u-PAR. Whether the marginal role of u-PAR is related to the ability of u-PA to become *localized around*, but not *bound to* the cell surface via interaction with other macromolecules such as fibrin, plasminogen, vitronectin, or proteoglycans must still be determined.

# NEOINTIMA FORMATION

Vascular interventions for the treatment of atherothrombosis, such as bypass surgery, percutaneous transluminal balloon angioplasty, atherectomy, or the *in situ* application of vascular stents, restore blood flow and improve tissue oxygenation but induce "restenosis" of the vessel within 3 to 6 months in 30 to 50% of treated individuals (90). This may result from remodeling of the vessel wall and/or accumulation of cells and extracellular matrix in the intimal or adventitial layer. Several mechanisms are believed to participate in the intimal thickening as part of a hyperactive wound healing response, including thrombosis, proliferation, apoptosis, and migration of smooth muscle cells (91, 92). Proteases participate in the degradation of the extracellular basement membrane surrounding the smooth muscle cells, allowing them to migrate to distant sites. Two protease systems have been implicated, the plasminogen (or fibrinolytic) system and the metalloproteinase system, which in concert can degrade most extracellular matrix proteins.

In contrast to the constitutive expression of t-PA by quiescent endothelial cells (13) and of PAI-1 by uninjured vascular smooth muscle cells (93), u-PA and t-PA activity in the vessel wall are significantly increased after injury, coincident with the time of smooth muscle cell proliferation and migration (94–96). This increase in plasmin proteolysis is counterbalanced by increased expression of PAI-1 in injured smooth muscle and endothelial cells and by its release from accumulating platelets (97). Expression of components of the fibrinolytic system is also induced in cultured endothelial cells, smooth muscle cells, or macrophages as a result of wounding or treatment with growth factors and cytokines that are released after injury (22, 98). Tissue-type plasmingen activator has been proposed to act as an autocrine mitogen after injury (99). The precise and causative role of the plasminogen system in matrix remodeling, passivation of the injured luminal vessel surface, migration, or proliferation of vascular cells is unknown.

To examine the molecular mechanisms of neointima formation in mice deficient in fibrinolytic system components, an experimental model based on the use of an electric current in addition to a mechanical injury model has been used (100). The electric current injury model differs from mechanical injury models in that it induces a more severe injury across the vessel wall, resulting in necrosis of all smooth muscle cells. This necessitates wound healing to initiate from the adjacent uninjured borders and to progress into the central necrotic region. Microscopic and morphometric analysis revealed that the rate and degree of neointima formation and the neointimal cell accumulation after injury was similar in wild type, t-PA-deficient and u-PAR-deficient arteries (101, 102). However, neointima formation in PAI-1 deficient arteries occurred at earlier times postinjury (103). In contrast, both the degree and the rate of arterial neointima formation in u-PA-deficient, plasminogen-deficient and combined t-PA:u-PA-deficient arteries were significantly reduced until 6 weeks after injury (101, 104). Evaluation of the mechanisms responsible for these genotype-specific differences in neointima formation revealed marginal differences in proliferation of medial and neointimal smooth muscle cells between the genotypes (101–104). Impaired migration of smooth muscle cells could be a significant cause of reduced neointima formation in mice lacking u-PA-mediated plasmin proteolysis, because smooth muscle cells migrate over a shorter distance from the uninjured border into the central injured region in plasminogen-deficient than in wild type arteries (101–104).

A surprising observation was that deficiency of u-PA, but not of u-PAR, reduced neointima formation *in vivo*. Because u-PAR is expressed by smooth muscle (102) and endothelial cells (22), and u-PAR is the only currently known receptor for u-PA (22–24), binding of u-PA to its cellular receptor appears to be more neglible for the role of u-PA than anticipated. Such a conclusion is supported by previous observations that an increase in soluble (not membrane-bound) human u-PA in murine tumor cells enhances their invasiveness (105), and that scavenging of soluble u-PA by a truncated (non-membrane-anchored) u-PAR impairs cellular invasion (106). Furthermore, a membrane-anchored form of u-PA catalyzes plasminogen activation on the cell surface with characteristics comparable to those of u-PAR-bound u-PA (107), suggesting that *cell surface localization* rather than *binding to* u-PAR is important. Possibly, the kinetic advantage resulting from u-PAR-accelerated plasminogen activation may be irrelevant for certain u-PA-dependent phenomena that develop over long periods, or that are compensated by the increased extracellular accumulation of u-PA in u-PAR-deficient mice (probably resulting from defective clearance of u-PA) (62). Alternatively, u-PA may be localized to the cell surface via binding to other molecules such as fibrin, plasminogen, extracellular matrix, or cell adhesion molecules (21, 25, 102, 108). Our results also suggest that pericellular proteolysis can still occur in the absence of u-PAR. This is confirmed by the observation that degradation of [$^{125}$I]-labeled fibrin or subendothelial matrix over 8 hours is only transiently affected by u-PAR deficiency (61, 102) and that thrombosis, sterility, and organ dysfunction in combined t-PA:u-PAR-deficient mice is significantly less severe than in combined t-PA:u-PA-deficient mice (56, 58). Fig. 22.7 schematically represents a hypothetical model of smooth muscle cell function and neointima formation in the absence of u-PA or u-PAR. However, the lack of an appreciable effect on neointima formation in u-PAR knockout mice does not exclude a role for this receptor in other biological processes (such as in cancer), inasmuch as the relevance of u-PAR may

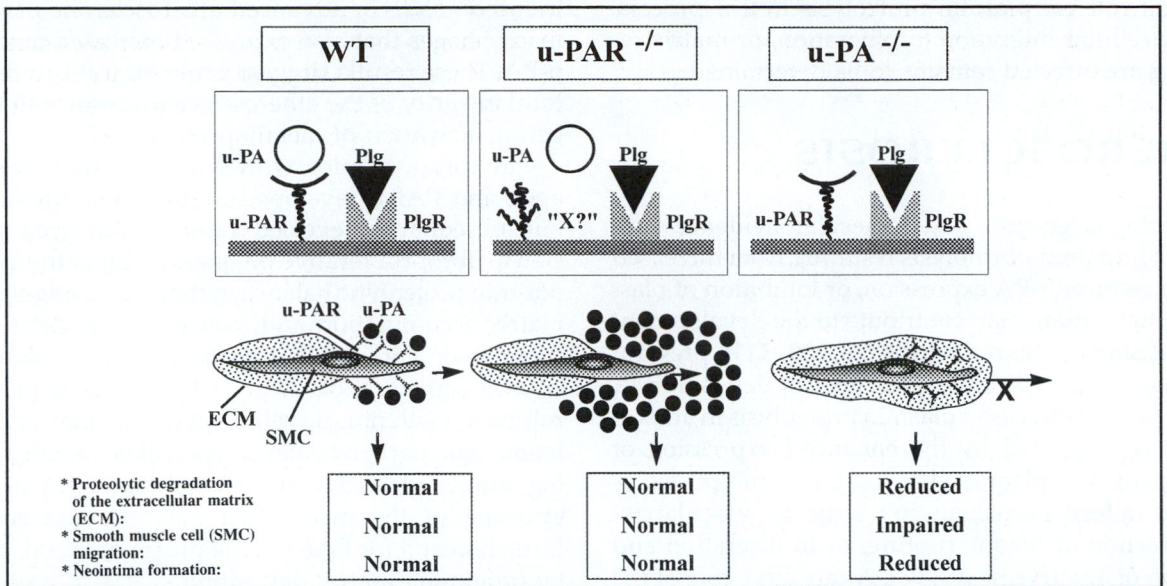

**FIGURE 22.7.** Hypothetical model of the role of receptor-independent u-PA-mediated plasminogen activation in neointima formation. The smooth muscle cell (SMC) is surrounded by an extracellular matrix (ECM) that needs to be proteolytically degraded to allow cellular migration. In the wild type (WT) smooth muscle cells, u-PA is bound to u-PAR, mediating plasminogen activation and plasmic degradation of the extracellular matrix such that the cell can migrate. In the u-PAR-deficient SMC, u-PA becomes localized to the cell surface, possibly via interaction with other matrix molecules (denoted as "X"), allowing sufficient pericellular plasmin proteolysis for the cells to migrate. u-PA might also accumulate to increased levels due to deficient u-PAR-mediated clearance. In contrast, SMC that lack u-PA have reduced pericellular plasmin proteolysis and fail to migrate efficiently, resulting in reduced neointima formation. The proposed impairment of SMC migration in mice lacking u-PA-mediated plasminogen activation is indirectly suggested by the observations that proliferation of u-PA-deficient cells was similar to that in wild type and that SMC migrated over a shorter distance in the plasminogen (Plg)-deficient than in wild type arteries.

depend on the amount and the cell-specific, temporal, and spatial expression of u-PAR. Whether, to what extent, and under which conditions u-PAR may be more important in other u-PA-dependent phenomena, such as cancer or angiogenesis, remains to be determined.

## INHIBITION OF NEOINTIMA FORMATION BY ADENOVIRUS-MEDIATED PAI-1 GENE TRANSFER

The involvement of plasmin proteolysis in neointima formation was supported by intravenous injection in PAI-1-deficient mice of a replication-defective adenovirus expressing human PAI-1 at a time when neointimal thickening occurred. After intravenous injection, the human PAI-1 gene was expressed by transduced hepatocytes resulting in more than 1000-fold increased plasma PAI-1 levels and subsequent deposition of PAI-1 in the developing intima. This resulted in a similar degree of inhibition of neointima formation as observed in u-PA-deficient mice (102). Protease inhibitors have been suggested as anti-restenosis drugs. Our studies suggest that strategies aimed at reducing u-PA-mediated plasmin proteolysis may reduce intimal thicken-

ing. However, antifibrinolytic strategies should be targeted at inhibiting plasmin proteolysis and not at preventing the interaction of u-PA with its receptor.

## TRANSPLANT ATHEROSCLEROSIS IN PLASMINOGEN-DEFICIENT MICE

More recently, (in a collaboration with V. Shi and E. Haber), the role of the plasminogen system in a mouse model of transplant arteriosclerosis, which mimics in many ways the accelerated arteriosclerosis in coronary arteries of transplanted cardiac allografts in men, was analyzed. In this model, host-derived leukocytes infiltrate beneath the endothelium and form a predominantly leukocyte-rich neointima by 15 days after transplantation, whereas, at later times, smooth muscle cells, derived from the donor graft, accumulate in the neointima. Because previous targeting studies have shown that migration of leukocytes and smooth muscle cells is dependent on plasmin proteolysis, carotid arteries from B.10A(2R) wild type mice were transplanted in C57Bl6:129 plasminogen-deficient mice. Initial analysis suggests that neointima formation within 45 days after transplantation is reduced in these mice, suggesting a significant role for plasmin proteolysis in this process. Whether cellular migration, proliferation, or matrix remodeling are affected remains to be determined.

# ATHEROSCLEROSIS

Epidemiologic, genetic, and molecular evidence suggests that impaired fibrinolysis resulting from increased PAI-1, or reduced t-PA expression, or inhibition of plasminogen activation, may contribute to the development or progression of atherosclerosis (16, 109–111), presumably by promoting thrombosis or matrix deposition. A possible role for increased plasmin proteolysis in atherosclerosis is suggested by the enhanced expression of t-PA and u-PA in plaques (112–114). Plasmin proteolysis might indeed participate in plaque neovascularization, induction of plaque rupture, or in ulceration and formation of aneurysms (97, 98). A causative role of the plasminogen system in these processes has not been conclusively demonstrated.

Atherosclerosis was studied in mice deficient in apolipoprotein E (apoE) and in t-PA, u-PA, or PAI-1, and fed a cholesterol-rich diet for 5 to 25 weeks. No differences in the size or predilection site of plaques were observed between mice with a single deficiency of apoE or with a combined deficiency of apoE and t-PA or of apoE and u-PA. However, significant genotypic differences were observed in the destruction of the media with resultant erosion, transmedial ulceration, medial smooth muscle cell loss, dilatation of the vessel wall, and microaneurysm formation. At the ultrastructural level, elastin fibers were eroded, fragmented, and completely degraded, whereas collagen bundles and glycoprotein-rich matrix were totally disorganized and scattered. Although both apoE-deficient and apoE:t-PA-deficient mice developed severe media destruction, apoE:u-PA-deficient mice were virtually completely protected. Plaque macrophages expressed abundant amounts of u-PA mRNA, antigen, and activity at the base of the plaque and in the media, similar to the atherosclerotic, aneurysmatic arteries in individuals (112, 113). Macrophages cross the elastin fibers, but only after proteolytic digestion of the elastin, a process that was remarkably enhanced by u-PA. Urokinase-plasminogen activator-mediated plasmin increased degradation by macrophages of [$^3$H] fucose-labeled glycoproteins. Because glycoproteins surround elastin fibers in the aortic wall, their degradation will increase exposure of the highly insoluble elastin to elastases, thereby facilitating *in vivo* elastolysis. In addition, plasmin promoted degradation of elastin and collagen via activation of matrix metalloproteinases (MMPs), such as stromelysin-1 (MMP-3), gelatinase-B (MMP-9), the macrophage metalloelastase (MMP-12), and collagenase-3 (MMP-13). The expression of several of these metalloproteinases was induced *in situ* in advanced atherosclerotic plaques by macrophages that also expressed increased amounts of u-PA. These results suggest a role for u-PA in the structural integrity of the atherosclerotic vessel wall via triggering activation of metalloproteinases.

In contrast, mice with a combined deficiency of apoE and PAI-1 developed normal fatty streak lesions but subsequently revealed a transient delayed progression to fibroproliferative plaques. Whether the increased plasmin proteolytic balance in these mice might prevent matrix accumulation and, consequently, delay plaque progression, or whether more abundant plasmin increased activation of latent TGF-β1 with its pleiotropic role on smooth muscle cell function and matrix accumulation, remains to be determined. Taken together, targeting studies identify a specific role for u-PA in the destruction of the media that may precede aneurysm formation and for PAI-1 in plaque progression, possibly by promoting matrix deposition.

Lipoprotein(a) has been proposed to reduce plasminogen activation and to predispose to atherosclerosis by reducing clot lysis (88). Alternatively, reduced plasmin proteolysis could diminish activation of latent TGF-β1, thereby providing a growth stimulus for smooth muscle cells (114). A significant correlation between high levels of apolipoprotein(a) and reduced *in situ* plasmin activity was observed in atherosclerotic vessels of transgenic mice overexpressing apolipoprotein(a) (114). Ongoing experiments in mice deficient in t-PA, u-PA, PAI-1, u-PAR, or plasminogen will demonstrate whether plasmin is a significant activator of latent TGF-β1 *in vivo*.

# TISSUE REMODELING ASSOCIATED WITH WOUND HEALING

Impaired fibrinolysis, resulting from reduced U-PA or increased PAI-1 activity, has been implicated in the deposition of fibrin and of extracellular matrix components in the kidney and the lung during inflammation (115, 116). Electron microscopic analysis demonstrated that adult combined t-PA:u-PA-deficient mice developed fibrin deposition not only in the intravascular lumen but also in extravascular compartments such as the alveoli of the lung, the mesangium in the kidney, and in the subendothelial space of Disse in the liver (Carmeliet et al, unpublished observations). Furthermore, severe tissue remodeling, such as fusion of the podocytes in the glomerulus and endothelial cell necrosis in adjacent capillaries, was frequently observed. Notably, extravascular fibrin deposition appeared to precede intravascular thrombosis, possibly suggesting that the triggering event for abnormal fibrin deposition and tissue remodeling is located in the extracellular compartment. These pathologic findings are reminiscent of those observed in glomerulonephritis and in the acute respiratory distress syndrome in individuals (115, 116). The involvement of the plasminogen system in inflammation and wound healing was further extended by the observations that plasminogen-deficient and combined t-PA:u-PA-deficient mice, and to a lesser extent t-PA-deficient or u-PA-deficient mice, suffered severe experimental glomerulonephritis characterized by increased formation of fibrin-rich glomerular crescents after challenge with antiglomerular membrane antibodies (117). In addition, PAI-1 overexpressing mice suffered a more severe lung injury and deposition of fibrin and collagen-rich matrix after bleomycin challenge (53) or hyperoxia (118), whereas PAI-1-deficient (53) or $\alpha_2$-macroglobulin-deficient (67) mice were protected against such fibrotic reaction. Deficiency of $\alpha_2$-macroglobulin also increased the mortality associated with experimentally induced acute pancreatitis, possibly because of uncontrolled proteolysis (67). Plasminogen-deficient mice also displayed fibrin-rich gastric ulcerations, in association with infection by pathogenic *Helicobacter* (63, 64). In addition, they suffered delayed and impaired closure of skin wounds (119). Notably, keratinocyte migration appeared to be reduced, but surprisingly, the granulation tissue was normal except for the more abundant presence of fibrinogen and fibronectin at the wound edges (119). In fact, plasminogen-deficient mice, like their wild type controls, had abundant infiltration of macrophages, neutrophilic granulocytes, and fibroblast-like cells, and pronounced neovascularization. However, wound healing in combined plasminogen:fibrinogen-deficient mice was not impaired, indicating that fibrin mediates, to a large degree, the effects of plasminogen deficiency (74). The plasminogen system appears to play a significant role in tissue remodeling during wound healing, in part mediated by its role in fibrin surveillance. This notion is supported by the observation that fibrinogen-deficient mice had an unusual wound healing response in which the migrating and proliferating cells (primarily fibroblasts) form a thick layer *encapsulating* but *not infiltrating* hematomas (51). It is thus possible that fibrin provides a critical initial matrix for the movement of cells into sites of injury.

Depending on the environmental conditions and infectious challenges, different degrees of wound healing responses have been reported. The most significant phenotype occurred in u-PA-deficient mice after infection with botryomycosis (120). In contrast to their wild type littermates, although housed in the same environmental conditions, u-PA-deficient mice developed a suppurative infection of the skin characterized by the presence of abscesses and granulomas containing large numbers of polymorphonuclear leukocytes and histiocytes surrounded by a capsule of fibrous connective tissue. Such destructive tissue remodeling is indeed more severe than observed in combined t-PA:u-PA-deficient or plasminogen-deficient mice (56, 63), indicating that the phenotypes observed in these knockout mice is determined by the infectious or inflammatory challenge.

# CONCLUSIONS

Studies with transgenic mice over- or underexpressing components of the coagulation or fibrinolytic system not only confirmed the important role of these protease systems in hemostasis and fibrin clot surveillance but have also revealed novel insights into the precise role and interaction of the individual molecules. The coagulation system, not the fibrinolytic system, appeared to play a more essential role in embryonic development than anticipated. Although life without plasminogen is possible, health and survival are severely compromised. Both systems are involved in infection, inflammation, and wound healing such as in arterial neointima formation, glomerulonephritis, skin ulcerations, pancreatitis, and lung inflammation. The lack of an appreciable effect of a specific gene deletion does not rule out its possible involvement in pathologic processes when inappropriately expressed and warrants examination for compensatory mechanisms. These transgenic mice may not only provide suitable models for further elucidation of the relevance of the plasminogen system in other pathophysiologic processes such as atherosclerosis or malignancy, but they may also serve as models for the evaluation of new gene therapies.

# REFERENCES

1. Edgington TS, Mackman N, Brand K et al. The structural biology of expression and function of tissue factor [Review]. Thromb Haemost 1991;66:67–79.
2. Furie B, Furie BC. The molecular basis of blood coagulation [Review]. Cell 1988;53:505–518.
3. Davie EW. Biochemical and molecular aspects of the coagulation cascade. Thromb Haemost 1995;74:1–6.
4. Esmon CT. The protein C anticoagulant pathway [Review]. Arterioscler Thromb 1992;12:135–145.
5. Dahlbäck B. New molecular insights into the genetics of thrombophilia. Resistance to activated protein C caused by Arg506 to Gln mutation in factor V as a pathogenic risk factor for venous thrombosis [Review]. Thromb Haemost 1995;74:139–148.
6. Bick RL, Pegram M. Syndromes of hypercoagulability and thrombosis: A Review. Semin Thromb Hemost 1994;20:109–132.
7. Broze GJ. Tissue factor pathway inhibitor and the revised hypothesis of blood coagulation. Trends Cardiovasc Med 1992;2:72–77.
8. Hoyer LW. Hemophilia A. N Engl J Med 1994;330:38–47.
9. Bolton-Maggs PH, Hill FG. The rarer inherited coagulation disorders: A Review. Blood Rev 1995;9:65–76.
10. Altieri DC. Xa receptor EPR-1 [Review]. FASEB J 1995;9:860–865.
11. Coughlin SR. Molecular mechanisms of thrombin signaling [Review]. Semin Hematol 1994;31:270–277.
12. Astrup T. In: Davidson JF, Rowan RM, Samama MM, Desnoyers PC, eds. Progress in chemical fibrinolysis and thrombolysis. New York: Raven Press, 1978;1–57.
13. Collen D, Lijnen HR. Basic and clinical aspects of fibrinolysis and thrombolysis [Review]. Blood 1991;78:3114–3124.

14. Vassalli JD, Sappino AP, Belin D. The plasminogen activator/plasmin system [Review]. J Clin Invest 1991;88:1067–1072.
15. Schneiderman J, Loskutoff DJ. Plasminogen activator inhibitors. Trends Cardiovasc Med 1991;1:99–102.
16. Wiman B. Plasminogen activator inhibitor 1 (PAI-1) in plasma: Its role in thrombotic disease [Review]. Thromb Haemost 1995;74:71–76.
17. Lawrence DA, Ginsburg D. Plasminogen activator inhibitors. In: High KA, Roberts HR, eds. Molecular basis of thrombosis and hemostasis. New York: Marcel Dekker, 1995;517–543.
18. Bachmann F. The enigma PAI-2. Gene expression, evolutionary and functional aspects. Thromb Haemost 1995;74:172–179.
19. Martin TJ, Allan EH, Fukumoto S. The plasminogen activator and inhibitor system in bone remodelling [Review]. Growth Regul 1993;3:209–214.
20. Hajjar KA. Cellular receptors in the regulation of plasmin generation [Review]. Thromb Haemost 1995;74:294–301.
21. Plow EF, Herren T, Redlitz A et al. The cell biology of the plasminogen system [Review]. FASEB J 1995;9:939–945.
22. Vassalli JD. The urokinase receptor. Fibrinolysis 1994;8(Suppl 1):172–181.
23. Blasi F, Conese M, Moller LB et al. The urokinase receptor: Structure, regulation and inhibitor-mediated internalization. Fibrinolysis 1994; 8(Suppl 1):182–188.
24. Dano K, Behrendt N, Brünner N et al. The urokinase-receptor. Protein structure and role in plasminogen activation and cancer invasion. Fibrinolysis 1994;8(Suppl 1);189–203.
25. Wei Y, Lukashev M, Simon DI et al. Regulation of integrin function by the urokinase receptor. Science 1996;273:1551–1555.
26. Stefansson S, Lawrence DA. The serpin PAI-1 inhibits cell migration by blocking integrin $\alpha_v\beta_3$ binding to vitronectin. Nature 1996;383:441–443.
27. Saksela O, Rifkin DB. Cell-associated plasminogen activation: Regulation and physiological functions [Review]. Annu Rev Cell Biol 1988;4:93–126.
28. Andreasen PA, Sottrup-Jensen L, Kjoller L et al. Receptor-mediated endocytosis of plasminogen activators and activator/inhibitor complexes. FEBS Lett 1994;338:239–245.
29. Nagy A. Engineering the mouse genome. Methods Enzymol (In press).
30. Nagy A, Rossant J. Targeted mutagenesis: Analysis of phenotype without germ line transmission. J Clin Invest 1996;98:S31–S35.
31. Carmeliet P, Ferreira V, Breier G et al. Abnormal blood vessel development and lethality in embryos lacking a single VEGF allele. Nature 1996;380:435–439.
32. Mulligan RC. The basic science of gene therapy [Review]. Science 1993;260:926–932.
33. Schneider MD, French BA. The advent of adenovirus. Gene therapy for cardiovascular disease. Circulation 1993;88:1937–1942.
34. Carmeliet P, Stassen JM, Collen D et al. Adenovirus-mediated gene transfer of rt-PA restores thrombolysis in t-PA deficient mice. (Submitted for publication).
35. Luther T, Flössel C, Mackman N et al. Tissue factor expression during human and mouse development. Am J Pathol 1996;149:101–113.
36. Soifer SJ, Peters KG, O'Keefe J et al. Disparate temporal expression of the prothrombin and thrombin receptor genes during mouse development. Am J Pathol 1994;144:60–69.
37. Nelhs V, Drenckhan D. The versatility of microvascular pericytes: From mesenchymal cell to smooth muscle cell? Histochemistry 1993;99:1–12.
38. Carmeliet P, Mackman N, Moons L et al. Role of tissue factor in embryonic blood vessel development. Nature 1996;383:73–75.
39. Toomey JR, Kratzer KE, Lasky NM et al. Targeted disruption of the murine tissue factor gene results in embryonic lethality. Blood 1996;88:1583–1587.
40. Levéen P, Pekny M, Gebre-Medhin S et al. Mice deficient for PDGF B show renal, cardiovascular, and hematological abnormalities. Genes Dev 1994;8:1875–1887.
41. Suri C, Jones PF, Patan S et al. Requisite role of angiopoietin-1, a ligand for the TIE2 receptor, during embryonic angiogenesis. Cell 1996;87:1171–1180.
42. Dickson MC, Martin JS, Cousins FM et al. Defective haematopoiesis and vasculogenesis in transforming growth factor-β1 knock out mice. Development 1995;121:1845–1854.
43. Rottingen JA, Enden T, Camerer E et al. Binding of human factor VIIa to tissue factor induces cytosolic Ca2+ signals in J82 cells, transfected COS-1 cells, Madin-Darby canine kidney cells and in human endothelial cells induced to synthesize tissue factor. J Biol Chem 1995;270:4650–4660.
44. Bugge TH, Xiao Q, Kombrinck KW et al. Fatal embryonic bleeding events in mice lacking tissue factor, the cell-associated initiator of blood coagulation. Proc Natl Acad Sci U S A 1996;93:6258–6263.
45. Rosen E, Chan JY, Idusohe E et al. Factor VII deficient mice develop normally but suffer fatal perinatal bleeding. Nature (in press).
46. Weiler-Guettler H, Aird WC, Husain M et al. Targeting of transgene expression to the vascular endothelium of mice by homologous recombination at the thrombomodulin locus. Circ Res 1996;78:180–187.
47. Healy AM, Rayburn HB, Rosenberg RD et al. Absence of the blood-clotting regulator thrombomodulin causes embryonic lethality in mice before development of a functional cardiovascular system. Proc Natl Acad Sci U S A 1995;92:850–854.
48. Connolly A, Ishihara H, Kahn ML et al. Role of the thrombin receptor in

development and evidence for a second receptor. Nature 1996;381:516–519.
49. Cui J, O'Shea KS, Purkayastha A et al. Fatal haemorrhage and incomplete block to embryogenesis in mice lacking coagulation factor V. Nature 1996;384:66–68.
50. Bi L, Lawler AM, Antonarakis SE et al. Targeted disruption of the mouse factor VIII gene produces a model of haemophilia A [Letter]. Nat Genet 1995;10:119–121.
51. Suh TT, Holmbäck K, Jensen NJ et al. Resolution of spontaneous bleeding events but failure of pregnancy in fibrinogen deficient mice. Genes Dev 1995;9:2020–2033.
52. Erickson LA, Fici GJ, Lund JE et al. Development of venous occlusions in mice transgenic for the plasminogen activator inhibitor-1 gene. Nature 1990;346:74–76.
53. Eitzman DT, McCoy RD, Zheng X et al. Bleomycin-induced pulmonary fibrosis in transgenic mice that either lack or overexpress the murine plasminogen activator inhibitor-1 gene. J Clin Invest 1996;97:232–237.
54. Heckel JL, Sandgren EP, Degen, JL et al. Neonatal bleeding in transgenic mice expressing urokinase-type plasminogen activator. Cell 1990;62:447–456.
55. Sidenius N. Expression of the aminoterminal fragment of urokinase-type plasminogen activator in transgenic mice [Thesis]. Copenhagen, Denmark: University of Copenhagen, 1993.
56. Carmeliet P, Schoonjans L, Kieckens L et al. Physiological consequences of loss of plasminogen activator gene function in mice. Nature 1994;368:419–424.
57. Carmeliet P, Bouche A, De Clercq C et al. Biological effects of disruption of the tissue-type plasminogen activator, urokinase-type plasminogen activator and plasminogen activator inhibitor-1 genes in mice. Ann N Y Acad Sci 1995;748:367–381.
58. Bugge TH, Flick MJ, Danton MJ et al. Urokinase-type plasminogen activator is effective in fibrin clearance in the absence of its receptor or tissue-type plasminogen activator. Proc Natl Acad Sci U S A 1996;93:5899–5904.
59. Carmeliet P, Kieckens L, Schoonjans L et al. Plasminogen activator inhibitor-1 gene deficient mice. I. Generation by homologous recombination and characterization. J Clin Invest 1993;92:2746–2755.
60. Carmeliet P, Stassen JM, Schoonjans L et al. Plasminogen activator inhibitor-1 gene deficient mice. II. Effects on hemostasis, thrombosis, and thrombolysis. J Clin Invest 1993;92:2756–2760.
61. Dewerchin M, Nuffelen AV, Wallays G et al. Generation and characterization of urokinase receptor-deficient mice. J Clin Invest 1996;97:870–878.
62. Bugge TH, Suh TT, Flick, MJ et al. The receptor for urokinase-type plasminogen activator is not essential for mouse development or fertility. J Biol Chem 1995;270:16886–16894.
63. Ploplis VA, Carmeliet P, Vazirzadeh S et al. Effects of disruption of the plasminogen gene on thrombosis, growth and health in mice. Circulation 1995;92:2585–2593.
64. Bugge TH, Flick MJ, Daugherty CC et al. Plasminogen deficiency causes severe thrombosis but is compatible with development and reproduction. Genes Dev 1995;9:794–807.
65. Dougherty K, Yang A, Harris J et al. Targeted deletion of the murine plasminogen activator inhibitor-2 (PAI-2) gene by homologous recombination [Abstract]. Blood 1995;86(suppl 1):455a.
66. Zheng X, Saunders TL, Camper SA et al. Vitronectin is not essential for normal mammalian development and fertility. Proc Natl Acad Sci 1995;92:12426–12430.
67. Umans L, Serneels L, Overbergh L et al. Targeted inactivation of the mouse α2-macroglobulin gene. J Biol Chem 1995;270:19778–19785.
68. Herz J, Clouthier DE, Hammer RE. LDL receptor-related protein internalizes and degrades u-PA-PAI-1 complexes and is essential for embryo implantation. Cell 1992;71:411–421.
69. Richards WG, Carroll PM, Kinloch RA et al. Creating maternal effect mutations in transgenic mice: Antisense inhibition of an oocyte gene product. Dev Biol 1993;160:543–553.
70. Leonardsson G, Peng XR, Liu K et al. Ovulation efficiency is reduced in mice that lack plasminogen activator gene function: Functional redundancy among physiological plasminogen activators. Proc Natl Acad Sci U S A 1995;92:12446–12450.
71. Carmeliet P, Ferreira V, Breier G et al. Abnormal blood vessel development and lethality in embryos lacking a single VEGF allele. Nature 1996;380:435–439.
72. Shalaby F, Rossant J, Yamaguchi TP et al. Failure of blood-island formation and vasculogenesis in Flk-1 deficient mice. Nature 1995;376:62–66.
73. Fong GH, Rossant J, Gertsenstein M et al. Role of the Flt-1 receptor tyrosine kinase in regulating the assembly of vascular endothelium. Nature 1995;376:66–70.
74. Bugge TH, Kombrinck KW, Flick MJ et al. Loss of fibrinogen rescues mice from the pleiotropic effects of plasminogen deficiency. Cell 1996;87:709–719.
75. Gailani D, Laskey N, Broze GJ. A murine model of factor XI deficiency [Abstract]. Blood 1996;88:469a.
76. Tuddenham EG, Pemberton S, Cooper DN. Inherited factor VII deficiency:

Genetics and molecular pathology [Review]. Thromb Haemost 1995;74: 313–321.

77. White GC. Coagulation factors V and VIII: Normal function and clinical disorders. In: Handin RI, Lux SE, Stossel TP, eds. Blood. Principles and practice of hematology. Philadelphia: JB Lippincott, 1995;1151–1180.

78. Montgomery RR, Scott JP. Hemostasis: Diseases of the fluid phases. In: Nathan GD, Oski FA, eds. Haematology of infancy and childhood. Philadelphia: WB Saunders Co., 1993;1605–1650.

79. al-Mondhiry H, Ehmann WC. Congenital afibrinogenemia. Am J Hematol 1994;46:343–347.

80. Fay WP, Shapiro AD, Shih JL et al. Brief report: Complete deficiency of plasminogen-activator inhibitor type 1 due to a frameshift mutation. N Engl J Med 1992;327:1729–1733.

81. Aoki N. Hemostasis associated with abnormalities of fibrinolysis [Review]. Blood Rev 1989;3:11–17.

82. Elliott MJ, Faulkner-Jones BE, Stanton H et al. Plasminogen activator in granulocyte-macrophage-CSF transgenic mice. J Immunol 1992;149: 3678–3681.

83. Cui J, Saunders TL, Ginsburg D. Analysis of factor V function by gene targeting in embryonic stem cells [Abstract]. Blood 1995;86(suppl 1):449a.

84. Kluft C, Dooijewaard G, Emeis JJ. Role of the contact system in fibrinolysis [Review]. Semin Thromb Hemost 1987;13:50–68.

85. Plow EF, Edgington TS. An alternative pathway for fibrinolysis. I. The cleavage of fibrinogen by leukocyte proteases at physiologic pH. J Clin Invest 1975;56:30–38.

86. Hamsten A, de Faire U, Walldius G et al. Plasminogen activator inhibitor in plasma: Risk factor for recurrent myocardial infarction. Lancet 1987; 2:3–9.

87. Robbins KC. Dysplasminogenemias [Review]. Enzyme 1988;40:70–78.

88. Liu AC and Lawn RM. Lipoprotein(a) and atherogenesis. Trends Cardiovasc Med 1994;4:40–44.

89. Palabrica TM, Liu AC, Aronovitz MJ et al. Antifibrinolytic activity of apolipoprotein(a) in vivo: Human apolipoprotein(a) transgenic mice are resistant to tissue plasminogen activator-mediated thrombolysis. Nat Med 1995;1:256–259.

90. Forrester JS, Fishbein M, Helfant R et al. A paradigm for restenosis based on cell biology: Clues for the development of new preventive therapies [Review]. J Am Coll Cardiol 1991;17:758–769.

91. Libby P, Schwartz D, Brogi E et al. A cascade model for restenosis. A special case of atherosclerotic progression [Review]. Circulation 1992; 86(suppl III);47–52.

92. Clowes AW, Reidy MA. Prevention of stenosis after vascular reconstruction: Pharmacologic control of intimal hyperplasia–a Review. J Vasc Surgery 1991;13:885–891.

93. Simpson AJ, Booth NA, Moore NR et al. Distribution of plasminogen activator inhibitor (PAI-1) in tissues. J Clin Pathol 1991;44:139–143.

94. Clowes AW, Clowes MM, Au YP et al. Smooth muscle cells express urokinase during mitogenesis and tissue-type plasminogen activator during migration in injured rat carotid artery. Circ Res 1990;67:61–67.

95. Jackson CL, Reidy MA. The role of plasminogen activation in smooth muscle cell migration after arterial injury. Ann N Y Acad Sci 1992;667: 141–150.

96. Jackson CL, Raines EW, Ross R et al. Role of endogenous platelet-derived growth factor in arterial smooth muscle cell migration after balloon catheter injury. Arterioscler Thromb 1993;13:1218–1226.

97. Sawa H, Fujii S, Sobel BE. Augmented arterial wall expression of type-1 plasminogen activator inhibitor induced by thrombosis. Arterioscler Thromb 1992;12:1507–1515.

98. Carmeliet P, Collen D. Physiological consequences of over- or underexpression of fibrinolytic system components in transgenic mice. In: Vadas M, Harlan J, eds. Vascular control of hemostasis: Advances of vascular biology. (In press).

99. Herbert JM, Lamarche I, Prabonnaud V et al. Tissue-type plasminogen

activator is a potent mitogen for human aortic smooth muscle cells. J Biol Chem 1994;269:3076–3080.

100. Carmeliet P, Stassen JM, Declercq C et al. A model for arterial neointima formation using perivascular electric injury in mice. Am J Pathol 1997; 150:761–777.

101. Carmeliet P, Moons L, Herbert JM et al. Urokinase-type but not tissue-type plasminogen activator mediates arterial neointima formation in mice. Circ Res (in press).

102. Carmeliet P, Moons L, Dewerchin M et al. Receptor-independent role of urokinase-type plasminogen activator during vascular wound healing in mice. J Cell Biol (under revision).

103. Carmeliet P, Moons L, Lijnen R et al. Inhibitory role of plasminogen activator inhibitor-1 in arterial wound healing and neointima formation. A gene targeting and gene transfer study in mice. Circulation (in press).

104. Carmeliet P, Moons L, Ploplis V et al. Impaired arterial neointima formation in mice with a disruption of the plasminogen gene. J Clin Invest 1997; 99:200–208.

105. Yu HR, Schultz RM. Relationship between secreted urokinase plasminogen activator activity and metastatic potential in murine B16 cells transfected with human urokinase sense and antisense genes. Cancer Res 1990;50:7623–7633.

106. Wilhelm O, Weidle U, Hohl S et al. Recombinant soluble urokinase receptor as a scavenger for urokinase-type plasminogen activator (uPA). Inhibition of proliferation and invasion of human ovarian cancer cells. FEBS Lett 1994;337:131–134.

107. Lee SW, Kahn ML, Dichek DA. Expression of an anchored urokinase in the apical endothelial cell membrane. Preservation of enzymatic activity and enhancement of cell surface plasminogen activation. J Biol Chem 1992; 267:13020–13029.

108. Stephens RW, Bokman AM, Myöhänen HT et al. Heparin binding to the urokinase kringle domain. Biochemistry 1992;31:7572–7579.

109. Hamsten A, Eriksson P. Fibrinolysis and atherosclerosis: An update. Fibrinolysis 1994;8(Suppl 1);253–262.

110. Juhan-Vagut I, Collen D. On the role of coagulation and fibrinolysis in atherosclerosis [Review]. Ann Epidemiol 1992;2:427–438.

111. Schneiderman J, Sawdey MS, Keeton MR et al. Increased type 1 plasminogen activator inhibitor gene expression in atherosclerotic human arteries. Proc Natl Acad Sci U S A 1992;89:6998–7002.

112. Schneiderman J, Bordin GM, Engelberg I et al. Expression of fibrinolytic genes in atherosclerotic abdominal aortic aneurysm wall. A possible mechanism for aneurysm expansion. J Clin Invest 1995;96:639–645.

113. Lupu F, Heim DA, Bachmann F et al. Plasminogen activator expression in human atherosclerotic lesions. Arterioscler Thromb Vasc Biol 1995;15: 1444–1455.

114. Grainger DJ, Kemp PR, Liu AC et al. Activation of transforming growth factor-$\beta$ is inhibited in transgenic apolipoprotein(a) mice. Nature 1994; 370:460–462.

115. Bertozzi P, Astedt B, Zenzius L et al. Depressed bronchoalveolar urokinase activity in individuals with adult respiratory distress syndrome. N Engl J Med 1990;322:890–897.

116. Tomooka S, Border WA, Marshall BC et al. Glomerular matrix accumulation in linked to inhibition of the plasmin protease system. Kidney Int 1992;42:1462–1469.

117. Kitching R, Carmeliet P, Ploplis V et al. Glomerulonephritis in mice with genetic deficiencies of the plasminogen system. J Exp Med 1997;185: 963–968.

118. Barazzone C, Belin D, Piguet PF et al. Plasminogen activator inhibitor-1 in acute hyperoxic mouse lung injury. J Clin Invest 1996;98:2666–2673.

119. Romer J, Bugge TH, Piguet PF et al. Impaired wound healing in mice with a disrupted plasminogen gene. Nat Med 1996;2:287–292.

120. Shapiro RL, Duquette JG, Nunes I et al. Urokinase-type plasminogen activator-deficient mice are predisposed to staphylococcal botryomycosis, pleuritis and effacement of lymphoid follicles. Am J Pathol 1997;150: 359–369.

# SECTION 5

# CLINICAL APPROACH TO BLEEDING AND THROMBOSIS

# CHAPTER 23

# APPROACH TO BLEEDING

Andrew I. Schafer

The evaluation of individuals with a possible, systemic, bleeding diathesis is usually undertaken in one of three general clinical settings. First, individuals with active or past histories of unexpected bleeding require diagnostic studies. Second, individuals may be found incidentally to have abnormalities of screening laboratory tests of hemostasis, the significance of which requires explanation. Finally, individuals without previous coagulation problems frequently undergo routine testing for bleeding risk prior to the performance of invasive procedures or surgery. This chapter focuses primarily on the clinical approach to individuals presenting with the first two of these situations, but a brief discussion of preoperative screening is also presented.

In the evaluation of individuals with a history of unexplained or excessive bleeding, the first question that must be addressed is whether the bleeding is most likely caused by a systemic coagulopathy or by an anatomic or mechanical abnormality of the vasculature. This problem is most urgently encountered in individuals who bleed excessively and unexpectedly after surgical procedures. In most cases a careful history and physical examination will yield vital diagnostic information. In general, individuals who bleed from multiple sites and on multiple occasions are more likely to have an underlying systemic defect of hemostasis, while those whose bleeding is restricted to a single, traumatized site are more likely to have an anatomic cause of bleeding. However, even this generalization is sometimes violated. For example, individuals with the vascular anomalies of hereditary hemorrhagic telangiectasia (see Chapter 43) may have lifelong problems of recurrent bleeding from the respiratory and gastrointestinal tracts

that may strongly suggest a systemic hemorrhagic diathesis unless a careful physical examination is performed. Conversely, isolated bleeding from a surgical site may be the first manifestation of a mild defect of hemostasis that had not been sufficiently challenged prior to surgery.

In the approach to individuals who have an abnormal coagulation test on incidental laboratory studies, it is important to question whether the finding is clinically relevant. Again, in most cases, a thorough history will often provide the answer. For example, individuals with a hereditary deficiency of one of the contact activation coagulation factors (factor XII, prekallikrein, high-molecular-weight kininogen) typically have an extraordinarily prolonged activated partial thromboplastin time (aPTT), often considerably more prolonged than that found even in the most severe hemophiliacs, and yet bleeding problems do not occur. Individuals with the lupus anticoagulant also characteristically have prolongations of the aPTT, sometimes accompanied by an increased prothrombin time (PT), without an associated bleeding tendency. In fact, individuals with contact activation factor deficiencies or lupus anticoagulants may actually develop thrombotic complications despite these abnormalities of the aPTT and PT that are expected to be associated with bleeding. Likewise, individuals with severe thrombocytopenia caused by an idiosyncratic response to heparin present with thrombotic manifestations more commonly than with bleeding manifestations.

These examples illustrate the critical importance of considering the history, physical examination, and screening laboratory tests as complementary facets of the clinical approach to individuals with suspected systemic coagulopathies. Each part alone is inadequate and may actually be misleading.

Although it is now recognized that platelet activation and activation of the coagulation proteins are not independent processes and that complex reciprocal interactions occur between these systems, it is still clinically expedient to separate the processes of primary and secondary hemostasis. In the discussion of the clinical approach to individuals with suspected systemic coagulopathies, this chapter will therefore refer to the interaction between platelets and the vessel wall as the process of "primary" hemostasis and to the formation of fibrin by the reactions of the coagulation cascade as the process of "secondary" hemostasis.

# HISTORY AND PHYSICAL EXAMINATION

When a systemic coagulopathy is suspected in a individual, several aspects of the history can provide important clues to its presence and to its possible causes. It is critical to probe systematically for the individual's hemostatic responses to specific challenges to the coagulation system that may occur throughout life. Many of these challenges are commonly encountered traumatic events such as circumcision, tonsillectomy, menses, labor and delivery, minor trauma, dental procedures, vaccinations, and inoculations. Oral surgery (including simple dental procedures) provides a particularly good "stress test" of hemostasis, possibly because of the locally high concentration of fibrinolytic activity in the oral cavity (1, 2). Individuals with mild systemic coagulation abnormalities may bleed excessively after oral surgical procedures but not after surgery or trauma at other sites. In some cases individuals can provide additional information about hemostasis following major surgery or trauma. The history of normal hemostasis following such events is just as important to record as episodes of excessive bleeding. The finding that a individual has recently withstood surgery without bleeding complications in many ways constitutes a better test of systemic hemostasis than any laboratory test could possibly provide.

A careful history of drug use and coexisting systemic diseases must be taken. Aspirin and a variety of nonsteroidal antiinflammatory drugs, often contained in over-the-counter medications that individuals may fail to report without specific questioning, can cause platelet dysfunction by inhibiting platelet thromboxane $A_2$ production. Other drugs, including certain antibiotics, may also cause abnormalities of platelet function or immune-mediated thrombocytopenia. Acquired hemostatic defects may be caused by some specific underlying systemic diseases. For example, renal failure is characteristically associated with impaired platelet–vascular interactions and prolongation of the bleeding time. Liver disease can be associated with thrombocytopenia, coagulation factor deficiencies, disseminated intravascular coagulation, and dysfibrinogenemia. Connective tissue diseases, such as systemic lupus erythematosus, and lymphoproliferative disorders may be associated with immune thrombocytopenia and circulating anticoagulants. Abnormal platelet function may occur with myeloproliferative disorders, while disseminated intravascular coagulation and thrombocytopenia may complicate the course of sepsis or cancer. In most of these cases, the underlying systemic illness is apparent and dominates the clinical picture.

According to the ancient Talmud, "if two children of the same mother or one child each of two sisters died as a result of circumcision, circumcision of the third child must be omitted." This opinion was based on the Talmudic recognition that there are some families in which the blood is loose (*raphi*) and others in which the blood is held fast (*kamit*, or easily congealed). It represents the earliest observations concerning the X-linked inheritance of classic hemophilia (3). The importance of obtaining a family history of bleeding has certainly not diminished over the 1500 years since these writings. It should be noted, however, that while a positive family history of bleeding problems is helpful in elucidating the nature of a suspected coagulopathy, a negative family history does not exclude the possibility of a hereditary bleeding disorder. For example, since the spontaneous mutation rate for classic hemophilia may be as high as 20%, many such individuals provide a completely negative family history of bleeding problems. Even in the absence of a positive family history, a individual who has had a lifelong problem of recurrent bleeding complications should be suspected of having an inherited coagulopathy.

The characteristics of the bleeding events, particularly as they relate to the sites and timing following injury, often reveal the general type of coagulopathy involved (Table 23.1). In general, individuals with defects of primary hemostasis (e.g., thrombocytopenia, or abnormal platelet function and platelet–vessel wall interactions) tend to exhibit superficial hemorrhage into the skin or mucous membranes that occurs either spontaneously or immediately after trauma. Petechiae (characteristically seen in individuals with severe thrombocytopenia), ecchymoses, purpura, gastrointestinal or genitourinary tract bleeding, hemoptysis, or epistaxis are typical manifestations of defective primary hemostasis. "Easy bruising" is a common symptom of disorders of primary hemostasis, but as many as 10% of men and 20% of women may report this problem if the interviewer asks leading questions, such as "Do you think you bruise more easily than others when you hurt your-

**TABLE 23.1.**    Patterns of Clinical Bleeding in Disorders of Hemostasis

| | Disorders of Primary Hemostasis (Platelet-Vascular Problem) | Disorders of Secondary Hemostasis (Coagulation Factor Problem) |
|---|---|---|
| Onset of bleeding | Spontaneous or immediately after trauma | Delayed after trauma |
| Sites of bleeding | Superficial surfaces | Deep tissues |
|   Skin | Petechiae, ecchymoses | Hematomas |
|   Mucous membranes | Common (nasal, oral, gastrointestinal, genitourinary) | Rare |
|   Other sites | Rare | Common (joint, muscle, retroperitoneal) |
| Clinical examples | Thrombocytopenia, functional platelet defect, vascular fragility | Congenital coagulation factor deficiency, acquired inhibitor, anticoagulation |
| | Disseminated intravascular coagulation, liver failure | Disseminated intravascular coagulation, liver failure |

self?'' (4). In contrast, individuals with abnormalities of secondary hemostasis (e.g., coagulation factor deficiencies) characteristically develop extensive, deep-tissue hemorrhage such as hemarthroses, hematomas, or retroperitoneal bleeding that may be delayed in onset for up to 24 to 48 hours after surgery or trauma. Delayed bleeding is also characteristic of hyperfibrinolytic disorders. The additional history of delayed wound healing may suggest factor XIII deficiency. Individuals with complex coagulopathies (e.g., disseminated intravascular coagulation, liver failure) may exhibit mixed patterns of bleeding that are associated with both primary and secondary hemostatic defects.

# LABORATORY TESTS

Two general categories of laboratory tests of hemostasis are performed in individuals who are evaluated for the presence of a systemic bleeding disorder. The methodology of these tests is described in detail in Chapter 26.

Screening tests are simple and rapid studies that are performed in general clinical laboratories, although each is susceptible to artifacts and pitfalls in interpretation that must be recognized by the coagulation consultant. In this discussion the four basic screening tests are considered to be (a) platelet count, (b) bleeding time, (c) PT, and (d) aPTT. The first two tests measure the integrity of primary hemostasis, while the second two are measurements of secondary hemostasis. With a few notable exceptions (see below), normal results for all four of these tests essentially rule out any clinical, significant, systemic coagulopathy.

Specialized tests of hemostasis are generally performed to follow up the screening tests for one of two reasons. First, specialized tests may be ordered as diagnostic studies when one or more of the screening tests

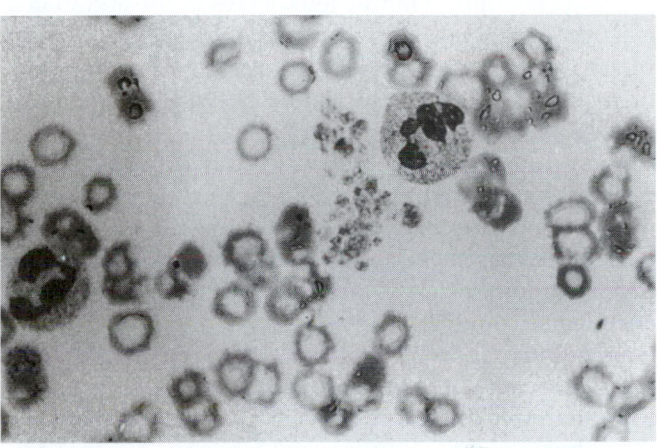

**FIGURE 23.1.**    Peripheral smear of blood anticoagulated with ethylenediaminetetraacetic acid, showing clumps of platelets (pseudothrombocytopenia).

is abnormal. Second, certain specialized tests may be indicated when the screening tests are normal but the clinical index of suspicion for an unusual systemic coagulopathy is high. These specialized tests are also discussed in detail in Chapter 26.

## PLATELET COUNT

The report of a low platelet count determined by electronic counting machines must always be followed by examination of the peripheral blood smear. This may reveal diagnostic abnormalities in other blood cells (e.g., red cell fragments in thrombotic thrombocytopenic purpura, blasts in acute leukemia, etc.) or the presence of platelet clumps that are characteristic of certain forms of pseudothrombocytopenia (Fig. 23.1). Pseudothrombocytopenia (5) is the phenomenon of a spuriously low platelet count that may be due to a variety of laboratory

**TABLE 23.2.** Causes of Pseudothrombo-cytopenia

Improper blood-sampling technique
Giant platelets
Platelet satellitism
*Ex vivo* platelet clumping
    EDTA-dependent and other anticoagulant-dependent agglutinins[a]
Cold agglutinins

---

[a] *EDTA, ethylenediaminetetraacetic acid.*

artifacts (Table 23.2). The phenomenon should be suspected when an unexpectedly low platelet count is reported in a individual who has had no clinical bleeding problems. It is occasionally associated with pseudoleukocytosis (6), when the platelet clumps formed *ex vivo* are large enough to mimic leukocytes in the automated electronic counter, or with pseudoleukopenia, when platelet–leukocyte adherence (heterotypic aggregates), or satellitism (7, 8), causes gating out of the large platelet–leukocyte masses by the counter (9).

Spuriously low platelet counts can be caused by improper blood sampling technique, when partial clotting of the blood sample occurs due to problems with venipuncture or an inadequate amount of anticoagulant. In certain conditions giant platelets are excluded by gated, automated counters, and artifactual thrombocytopenia is therefore reported. Abnormally large platelets are found in several hematologic disorders, including myeloproliferative disorders (see Chapter 33) and immune thrombocytopenic purpura (see Chapter 30). In addition, there are a number of rare, hereditary "giant platelet disorders" that are also characterized by low platelet counts and clinical bleeding of variable severity (10); these include Bernard-Soulier syndrome, May-Hegglin anomaly, gray platelet syndrome, and Montreal platelet syndrome.

Ethylenediaminetetraacetic acid (EDTA)–induced platelet clumping is probably the most common cause of pseudothrombocytopenia (5), with reported incidences ranging from 1 of 50 to 1 of 1000 hospitalized individuals (6). It has been reported to be the second most frequent cause of isolated thrombocytopenia in referrals to a hematology practice (11). It is due to the presence of agglutinating antiplatelet antibodies that react with platelets in the presence of the EDTA anticoagulant used in tubes for routine blood counts. More recently, the phenomenon has been reported to occur in the presence of virtually all anticoagulants, although it is most pronounced with EDTA. It was therefore proposed that the phenomenon is more accurately referred to as "anticoagulant-induced pseudothrombocytopenia" (12). Membrane components of platelets exposed to EDTA *ex vivo* may

undergo conformational change, exposing neoantigens to which the agglutinating antibodies bind (13). In many cases the agglutinating antibody may be directed against the platelet membrane glycoprotein IIb or IIb-IIIa complex (12, 14, 15). The phenomenon of EDTA-dependent pseudothrombocytopenia appears more frequently in hospitalized, severely ill individuals (16, 17), although it often occurs in healthy individuals and is devoid of pathologic significance in most cases (18). Pseudothrombocytopenia has been found to be frequently associated with antiphospholipid antibodies (19) and with the administration of monoclonal antibody to platelet glycoprotein IIb-IIIa (20). It is diagnosed by the findings (a) of platelet clumps in the peripheral smear of an EDTA-anticoagulated blood sample and (b) of normal platelet counts in blood samples simultaneously obtained by fingerstick using an ammonium oxalate Unopette and counting platelets by phase-contrast microscopy (5). Some platelet agglutinins react optimally at temperatures below 37°C (cold agglutinins) and therefore cause pseudothrombocytopenia by *ex vivo* clumping in blood samples that await counting in tubes maintained at room temperature for prolonged periods (21–23). When this phenomenon is suspected, a discrepancy should be found in the platelet counts of blood samples drawn simultaneously from the individual, one of which is allowed to stand at room temperature while the other is counted immediately or maintained at 37°C.

## BLEEDING TIME

The bleeding time is widely recognized as the best screening test of *in vivo* primary hemostasis (24–29). Although it remains a useful test in the diagnostic evaluation of individuals with suspected systemic bleeding disorders, its role as a routine preoperative screening test to predict surgical hemorrhage has been seriously challenged (see below). Furthermore, the bleeding time is fraught with potential technical artifact and its results are susceptible to misinterpretations that must be recognized.

The standard Ivy method (30) has been modified to improve sensitivity and reproducibility. Semiautomated template devices (31) have been largely supplanted by newer disposable automated products (32–34). These latter devices permit an incision of standardized width, but differences in pressure exerted by the operator produce variability in wound depth (35). Bleeding times are traditionally performed by making a standardized incision over the volar aspect of the forearm while a blood pressure cuff is inflated to between systolic and diastolic pressures proximal to the incision (Fig. 23.2). However, the bleeding time may be equally valid over the medial aspect of the calf (36). The reproducibility of bleeding times is influenced by several variables, including the direction (37), size, and depth of the

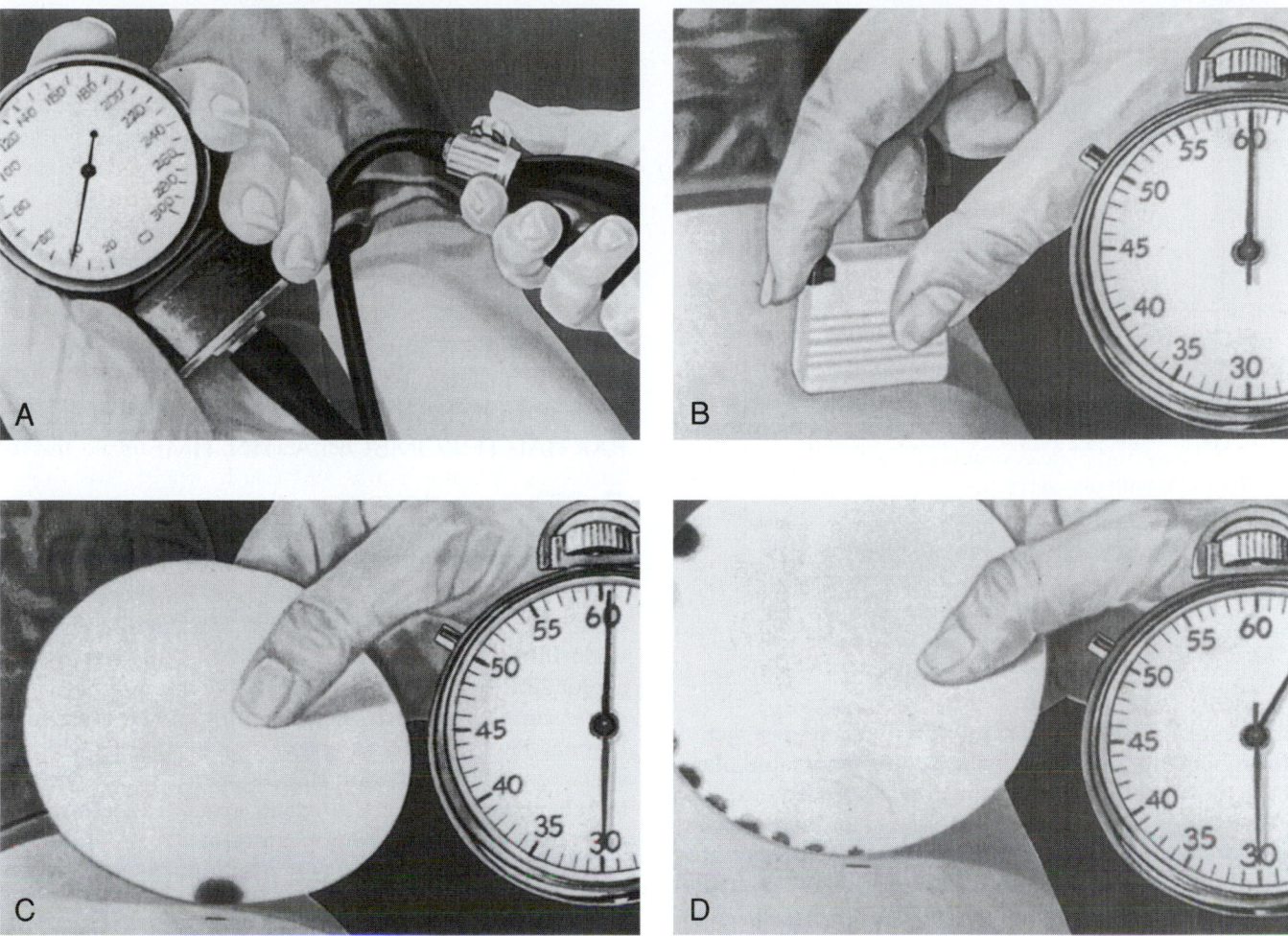

**FIGURE 23.2.** Technique of the bleeding time. **A,** A sphygmomanometer cuff on the upper arm is inflated to 40 mm Hg. **B,** A standardized incision is made over the volar aspect of the forearm, parallel to the antecubital crease, in an area free of superficial veins or scars. **C,** Timing is started with the incision. **D,** The flow of blood from the incision is wicked with filter paper at regular intervals, with care taken to avoid touching the filter paper directly to the interior of the incision or its margins. The bleeding time is taken as the time to complete cessation of free blood flow from the incision. (Reprinted with permission from International Technidyne Corporation.)

incision, as well as the skin temperature and vascularity at the wound site (24, 38). Results may vary among subjects as a function of age, sex, ethnic origin, skinfold thickness, and anxiety (29). In general, bleeding times obtained in children are significantly shorter than those obtained in adults (39).

The bleeding time has been considered to provide a test of the integrity of systemic primary hemostasis. It cannot be assumed, however, that a skin bleeding time necessarily correlates with bleeding times at other anatomic sites (40). For example, prolongation of the skin bleeding time by aspirin may not be associated with a prolonged gastric bleeding time as determined by endoscopic biopsy of the stomach (41). Lack of correlation between gastric bleeding time and skin bleeding time was recently confirmed (42).

In general, prolongation of the bleeding time indi-

cates a quantitative or qualitative abnormality of platelets, a defect in platelet–vessel wall interaction (e.g., von Willebrand disease), or a primary vascular disorder (e.g., vasculitis, Cushing syndrome, amyloidosis, scurvy, and connective-tissue disorders such as Ehlers-Danlos syndrome and pseudoxanthoma elasticum). Thrombocytopenia prolongs the bleeding time when the platelet count drops below $100,000/mm^3$. Under this platelet level, there is generally a direct, inverse correlation between the degree of thrombocytopenia and the degree of prolongation of the bleeding time until the platelet count falls below about $10,000/mm^3$, where the bleeding time becomes an inaccurate index of the severity of the thrombocytopenia (Fig. 23.3) (24). While this linear relationship between platelet count and bleeding time has been widely cited, studies published subsequently have shown more broadly scattered data that suggest a curvi-

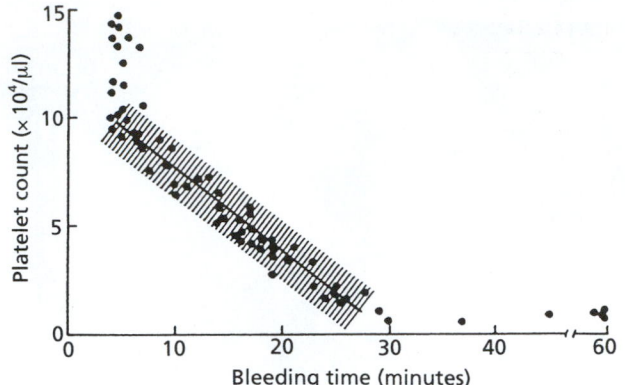

**FIGURE 23.3.** Relationship between the bleeding time and the platelet count, as determined in 70 individuals with marrow failure and platelet counts of less than 150,000/mm³. In individuals with platelet counts between 10,000 and 100,000/mm³, there was a direct, inverse relationship between bleeding time and platelet count. At platelet counts less than 10,000/mm³, bleeding time was greater than 30 minutes. (Adapted with permission from Harker LA, Slichter SJ. The bleeding time as a screening test for evaluation of platelet function. N Engl J Med 1972;287:155–159.)

linear relationship (28). Individuals with destructive thrombocytopenias that are characterized by rapid platelet turnover (e.g., immune thrombocytopenic purpura) may exhibit bleeding times that are shorter than those expected for the degree of thrombocytopenia, presumably because the circulating platelet population is enriched in young, hemostatically more effective cells (43). Conversely, the coexistence of a functional platelet defect (e.g., the use of aspirin) with thrombocytopenia may cause a disproportionate prolongation of the bleeding time for any given platelet count.

Severe anemia also causes prolongation of the bleeding time (44–47). The inverse relationship between the bleeding time and the hematocrit is particularly well established in renal failure (see Chapter 33), where correction of the anemia by transfusion or by recombinant erythropoietin therapy tends to normalize the bleeding time (48–51). Red cells may affect the bleeding time by rheologic mechanisms, displacing platelets laterally from the axial stream to the periphery of the flowing blood and thereby promoting platelet–vessel wall interactions, or by directly enhancing platelet reactivity (52). Hypertension and hyperbilirubinemia may also influence the bleeding time by less well understood mechanisms (53). Exaggerated prolongations of the bleeding time are observed following the ingestion of aspirin in individuals who have mild underlying disorders of primary hemostasis (the so-called aspirin tolerance test) (54, 55) or who are simultaneously drinking alcohol—conditions that by themselves do not generally affect the bleeding time (56).

Finally, the sensitivity and specificity of the bleeding time as a test of primary hemostasis have been challenged. For example, the bleeding time may vary considerably in individuals with von Willebrand disease who are studied repeatedly (57) and may be normal even in individuals with type I von Willebrand disease who have had clinical bleeding complications (58). Conversely, the bleeding time may be prolonged not only in disorders of primary hemostasis but also in some cases of hemophilia (59–61) and other coagulation factor deficiencies (62–66). These latter observations may reflect the complex interrelationships between the activation of platelets and the coagulation enzymes.

## PROTHROMBIN TIME AND ACTIVATED PARTIAL THROMBOPLASTIN TIME

The PT measures the activity of the extrinsic and common pathways of coagulation. The aPTT assesses the integrity of the intrinsic and common pathways of coagulation (Figs. 23.4 and 23.5). False-positive prolongations of either the PT or the aPTT (68, 69) may occur as a result of underfilling the test tube; the aPTT may also be falsely prolonged in individuals with polycythemia or when blood samples drawn from indwelling catheters are contaminated with even trace amounts of heparin (70). Blood specimens for coagulation studies should always be obtained by clean venipuncture from arms without intravenous lines, since coagulation times may be lengthened not only by heparin but also by dilutional factors caused by the admixture of intravenous fluids with blood (71).

The sensitivity of the PT and the aPTT in detecting coagulation factor deficiencies may vary with the reagents used to perform these tests. Thromboplastins prepared from human brain are generally more responsive to reduction in the coagulation factors affected by the PT than those prepared from rabbit brain. It was because of this marked variability of responses to different thromboplastins between laboratories that the international normalized ratio was adopted to standardize reporting of the PT in individuals receiving oral anticoagulation (72) (see Chapter 55). Similarly, various aPTT reagents differ in their sensitivity to detect mild deficiencies of intrinsic pathway coagulation factors (4, 73–75). Various manufacturers' aPTT reagents, and even reagent lots from the same manufacturer, show considerable variation in response to heparin, and it has been suggested that measurements of protamine titration heparin levels may be more reliable than aPTT in following heparin anticoagulant response (76). The aPTT is also the most commonly used assay to screen for the presence of a lupus anticoagulant, but marked variation in the sensitivity of the aPTT reagents to the lupus anticoagulant has been documented (77–79). This variability is due to differences in the choice of PTT activator, as well as in the amount, type, and physical properties of the phospholipid used in the assay (80, 81).

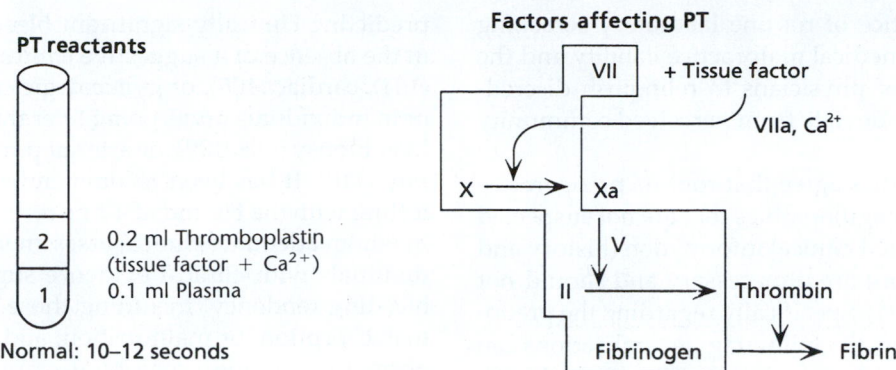

**FIGURE 23.4.** The prothrombin time (PT) is sensitive to isolated or combined deficiencies of factors VII, X, V, and II (prothrombin) and fibrinogen. (Adapted with permission from Burns ER, ed. Laboratory tests of hemostasis. In: Clinical management of bleeding and thrombosis. Boston: Blackwell Scientific, 1987; pp. 43–56.)

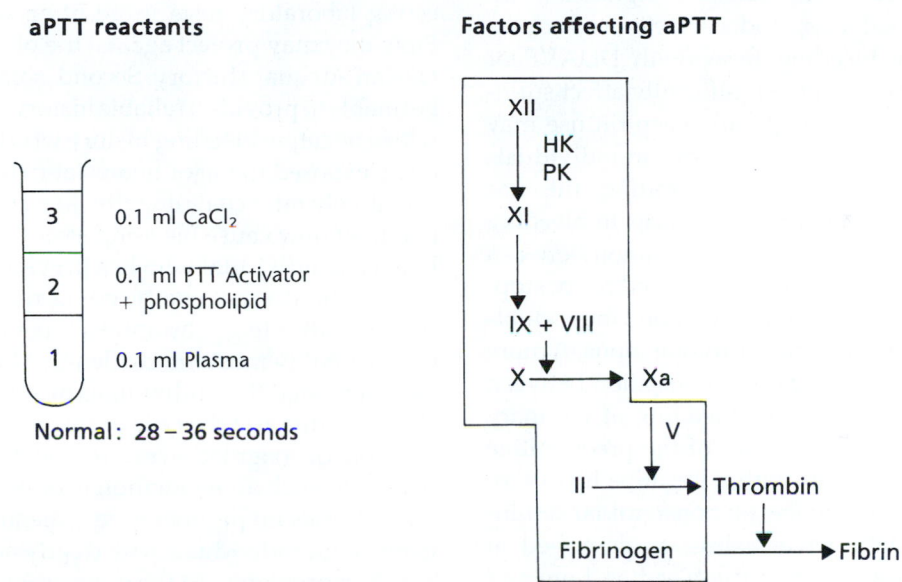

**FIGURE 23.5.** The activated partial thromboplastin time (aPTT) is sensitive to isolated or combined deficiencies of all of the coagulation factors except VII and XIII. HK, high-molecular-weight kininogen; PK, prekallikrein. (Adapted with permission from Burns ER, ed. Laboratory tests of hemostasis. In: Clinical management of bleeding and thrombosis. Boston: Blackwell Scientific, 1987; pp. 43–56.)

In view of these considerations, every coagulation laboratory must determine its own reference standard times for the PT and aPTT and must perform mixing studies to establish the sensitivities of the reagents used to detect specific factor deficiency states. The aPTT is variably prolonged with deficiencies of all coagulation factors except factor VII. In general, factor VIII or factor IX activities of less than 30% should be detectable on screening by clear prolongations of the aPTT. The PT, which is variably prolonged with deficiencies of factors VII, X, V, prothrombin, and fibrinogen, is significantly affected by factor VII levels of less than 50% or by more severe deficiencies (less than 30% levels) of the other factors.

# PREOPERATIVE COAGULATION SCREENING

Laboratory evaluation of adult general surgery individuals prior to elective surgery traditionally includes a coagulation panel, usually consisting of the four screening tests discussed above (platelet count, bleeding time, PT, and aPTT). Mounting evidence indicates, however, that such routine screening of all preoperative cases is uninformative and may even be counterproductive when it causes unnecessary expense of follow-up testing or delay involving the surgery. Factors that contribute to the continued practice of routine laboratory screening include the fear of medical malpractice liability and the general reluctance of physicians to relinquish discredited practices and to deviate from perceived community standards (82).

Most recent studies agree that routine preoperative screening tests for coagulopathies that are not suspected on the basis of detailed clinical information (history and physical examination) are unnecessary and should not be done (28, 69, 82–94). Specifically regarding the preoperative bleeding time, the following generalizations can be drawn from critical review of the literature (28, 29, 93, 95). With respect to cardiac surgery, it has been found that surgical "bleeders" and "nonbleeders" have no significant differences in mean preoperative bleeding times; a prolonged preoperative bleeding time is not necessarily associated with clinically significant increased surgical blood loss; and correction of a prolonged preoperative bleeding time (with DDAVP or platelet transfusions) does not significantly affect surgical blood loss. Although preoperative aspirin use may increase surgical bleeding complications in individuals undergoing coronary-artery bypass grafting, this has not been consistently related to differences in bleeding times (96, 97). One report found a correlation between the preoperative bleeding time and the need for postoperative blood transfusions (98), but included individuals with drug-induced bleeding time prolongations. A more recent prospective study found no association between perioperative and postoperative bleeding at coronary bypass surgery and any parameter of the preoperative bleeding time in individuals with a negative history of bleeding and no recent intake of nonsteroidal antiinflammatory drugs (99). Nevertheless, as described in Chapter 50, in studies in which the bleeding time and post-cardiopulmonary bypass blood loss were measured carefully, the *postoperative* bleeding time correlated with the magnitude of postoperative blood loss.

With respect to the bleeding time as a predictor of hemorrhagic complications of noncardiac surgery, a prolonged preoperative bleeding time has not been associated with clinically significant increased blood loss in either elective or emergency general, hip, cataract, or vascular surgery (93) or in multiple surgical services (100). The most extensive retrospective study of 1941 noncardiac surgery cases concluded that a prolonged bleeding time does not correlate with clinically significant perioperative bleeding (101), a finding supported by many other studies (102). The bleeding time also does not predict complications from percutaneous renal biopsy (103).

Similarly, it has been found that the preoperative PT and aPTT cannot predict surgical bleeding complications in individuals who are not found to be at increased risk on clinical grounds alone (68, 84, 85, 90). Specifically, the preoperative PT and aPTT are not useful in predicting clinically significant bleeding complications in the absence of a suggestive clinical history in general (104), cardiac (105), or gynecologic cancer (106) surgery or in individuals undergoing liver transplantation (107), liver biopsy (108, 109), or arterial puncture for angiography (110). It has been recommended that preoperative testing with the PT and aPTT be reserved for individuals in whom adequate clinical assessment is impossible; individuals with clinical evidence suggesting a possible bleeding tendency, including those with liver disease, malabsorption, or malnutrition; and individuals whose normal coagulation may be disrupted by the planned procedure itself (e.g., prostatectomy, cardiopulmonary bypass, insertion of peritoneovenous shunt, etc.) (69).

Since a thorough clinical assessment should serve as the guide for obtaining preoperative screening coagulation tests, Rapaport has suggested four reasons for advocating laboratory tests in addition to the history (89). First, they may protect against the physician who fails to take an adequate history. Second, some individuals may be unable to provide a reliable history. Third, a individual with a negative bleeding history who has not been previously exposed to major hemostatic challenges may have a relatively mild coagulopathy (e.g., factor XI deficiency) that may now cause bleeding after the planned surgery. Finally, a individual who has previously withstood surgery without excessive bleeding may have acquired a coagulopathy (e.g., thrombocytopenia) since his or her most recent hemostatic challenge. Therefore it has been recommended that individuals be stratified according to clinical status and the type of surgery planned for the indication for coagulation evaluation (89). A suggested approach to such an evaluation is outlined in Fig. 23.6. At one extreme, no preoperative screening tests are recommended for individuals with clearly negative histories of bleeding problems. At the opposite extreme, individuals whose bleeding histories are very suspicious for a serious hemostatic abnormality should certainly undergo screening tests and, if this evaluation is not diagnostic, should probably be subjected to further definitive testing with specialized assays (see below) prior to surgery. Individuals between these extremes, including those whose histories raise the possibility of defective hemostasis or those with negative histories who are to undergo procedures that may impair hemostasis or procedures in which even minimal postoperative hemorrhage could be hazardous (e.g., neurosurgery), should have screening laboratory tests.

# EVALUATION OF ABNORMAL SCREENING TESTS OF HEMOSTASIS
## THROMBOCYTOPENIA

As shown in Fig. 23.7, the two major mechanisms of thrombocytopenia are decreased production and in-

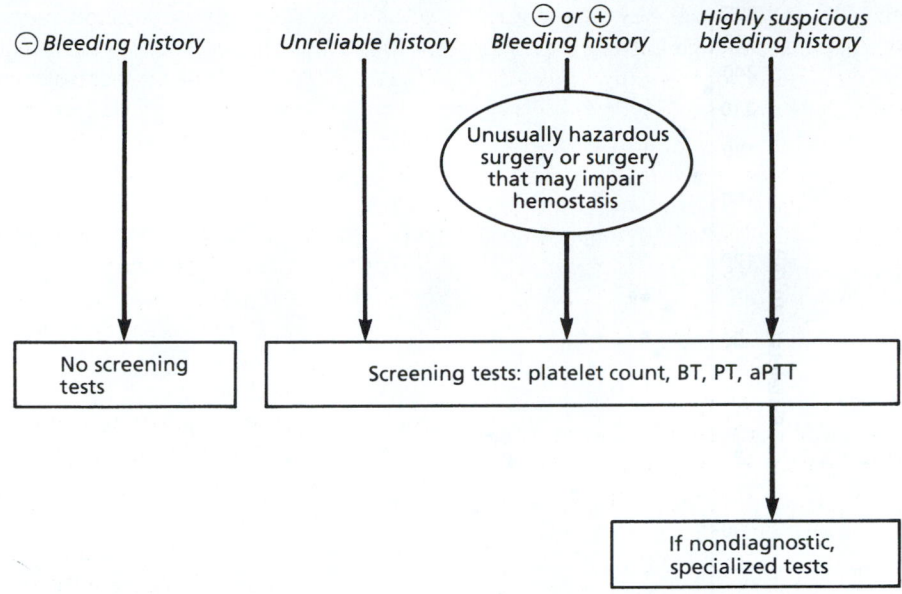

**FIGURE 23.6.**    Indications for preoperative coagulation screening. The extent of preoperative testing is determined by the individual's clinical history of bleeding and by the type of surgery to be performed. aPTT, activated partial thromboplastin time; BT, bleeding time; PT, prothrombin time.

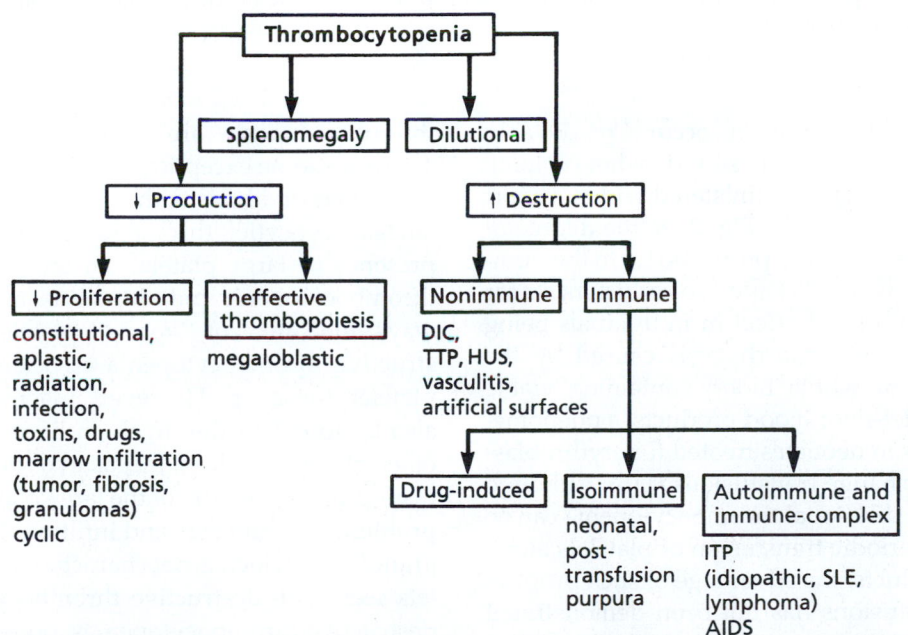

**FIGURE 23.7.**    Causes of thrombocytopenia. The major mechanisms of thrombocytopenia are (a) decreased production by the marrow (which can be due to either decreased proliferation or ineffective thrombopoiesis); and (b) increased destruction (which can be due to either nonimmune or immune causes). Other etiologies of thrombocytopenia are splenomegaly (hypersplenism) and dilution. DIC, disseminated intravascular coagulation; HUS, hemolytic–uremic syndrome; ITP, immune thrombocytopenic purpura; SLE, systemic lupus erythematosus; TTP, thrombotic thrombocytopenic purpura.

creased destruction of platelets. In addition, splenomegaly and dilutional effects may also cause thrombocytopenia. Splenic sequestration of platelets may be due to any congestive or infiltrative cause of splenomegaly and is characteristically associated with the physical findings of an enlarged spleen and/or signs of portal hypertension. Hypersplenism is discussed in further detail in Chapter 45.

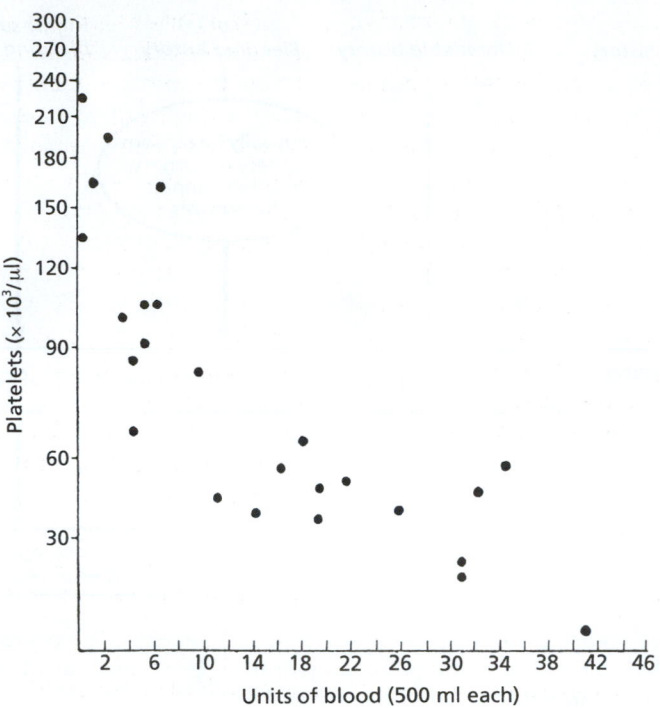

**FIGURE 23.8.**    Dilutional thrombocytopenia. Platelet counts in 37 individuals with massive blood loss who were transfused platelet-poor blood. (Adapted with permission from Krevans JR, Jackson DP. Hemorrhagic disorder following massive whole blood transfusions. JAMA 1955;159:171–177.)

Dilutional thrombocytopenia occurs predictably after massive transfusions of stored whole blood, plasma, or packed red cells administered within a short period (111–114). As shown in Fig. 23.8, the degree of thrombocytopenia is generally proportional to the number of transfusions given (111) and typically persists for 3 to 5 days. This dilutional effect in individuals being transfused for massive hemorrhage is caused by the acute replacement of whole blood containing viable platelets with platelet-poor blood products, a phenomenon that also occurs in neonates treated for erythroblastosis fetalis with exchange transfusions (115). Although the development of dilutional thrombocytopenia can be prevented by the periodic transfusion of platelets along with the blood products, the advantage of such prophylactic platelet transfusions has not been demonstrated (21, 116). The thrombocytopenia associated with hemodialysis and extracorporeal circulation is discussed in Chapters 42 and 50.

Several clues may be useful in distinguishing between thrombocytopenia caused by decreased production and increased destruction of platelets (117). In general, individuals who have a selective, severe thrombocytopenia (i.e., without accompanying anemia or leukopenia) probably have a destructive type of thrombocytopenia. Most bone marrow disorders (e.g., aplasia, fibrosis, infiltrative processes) that interfere with platelet production sufficiently to cause severe thrombocytopenia are likely to cause pancytopenia. There are some exceptions to this generalization, particularly in individuals with congenital, acquired, or cyclic amegakaryocytic thrombocytopenia (118–122). The presence of large platelets in the peripheral smear of thrombocytopenic individuals is usually, but not always, indicative of "young" platelets and thus a destructive thrombocytopenia associated with increased platelet turnover. However, macrothrombocytes can also be found in the myeloproliferative disorders and other abnormalities of megakaryocyte fragmentation. A distinguishing feature of the large platelets of the myeloproliferative disorders and infiltrated marrows is hypogranularity, which is not characteristic of the large platelets seen with destructive thrombocytopenias (123). In destructive thrombocytopenias, bone marrow aspirates reveal normal or increased numbers of megakaryocytes, the margins of which are largely free of adherent platelets. In contrast, thrombocytopenias caused by impaired platelet production are often associated with characteristic or even diagnostic bone marrow abnormalities. Finally, although formal radiolabeled platelet-survival studies are almost never indicated in clinical practice to determine platelet kinetics, the response of nonalloimmunized, thrombocytopenic individuals to platelet transfusions, specifically with respect to the initial increment in platelet count and the subsequent survival, can indicate whether a hypoproliferative or a destructive process is operative (124).

The thrombocytopenia of impaired platelet production may be caused either by decreased proliferation or by ineffective thrombopoiesis (see Fig. 23.7). Constitutional amegakaryocytic thrombocytopenia may be the initial manifestation of Fanconi's aplastic anemia, usually appearing in early childhood (125). Neonatal amegakaryocytic thrombocytopenia is often associated with congenital skeletal, renal, and cardiac malformations, including the syndrome of thrombocytopenia with absent radii (126, 127). Fatal hemorrhage occurs early in life in most of these individuals, but some individuals with less severe neonatal thrombocytopenia may recover as they approach adulthood. Sex-linked hereditary thrombocytopenias include the Wiskott-Aldrich syndrome, which is associated with a functional platelet defect (128, 129), and sex-linked recessive thrombocytopenia (130). Autosomal dominant hereditary thrombocytopenias include the May-Hegglin anomaly, which is associated with giant platelets and inclusions (Döhle bodies) in granulocytes (131, 132); Alport syndrome or macrothrombocytopenia with nerve deafness and nephritis (133, 134); and other less well characterized thrombocytopenias. Autosomal recessive thrombocytopenias have also been reported (135).

Acquired thrombocytopenias caused by decreased megakaryocyte proliferation include aplastic anemia; megakaryocytic aplasia; ionizing radiation and myelosuppressive drugs; other drugs and toxins (including thiazide diuretics and alcohol); viral infections; and marrow infiltration by malignant cells (e.g., carcinoma, leukemia), Gaucher cells, granulomas, or fibrosis. Most of these diagnoses are readily made on analyses of bone marrow aspirates and biopsies. The marrow infiltrative processes are characteristically accompanied by myelophthisic changes in the peripheral blood smear, including nucleated and teardrop-shaped red cells and immature white cell precursors.

Cyclic thrombocytopenia is a rare disorder that is characterized by regular, predictable oscillations in the platelet count (136, 137). The major mechanism has been considered to be periodic failure of effective platelet production, although accelerated platelet destruction may also be operative. An immunologic basis for the disorder in some cases has been suggested by the finding of platelet-reactive autoantibodies (138, 139) or antibody blocking the hematopoietic action of granulocyte macrophage colony-stimulating factor (120).

Ineffective thrombopoiesis (140) occurs in individuals with vitamin $B_{12}$ and folic acid deficiency, occasionally causing sufficiently severe thrombocytopenia to lead to clinical bleeding complications. In more advanced cases of megaloblastic anemias, bone marrow megakaryocytes may even be markedly reduced in number (141).

The various types of destructive thrombocytopenias are discussed in depth in chapters to follow. In contrast to the thrombocytopenias of decreased platelet production, bone marrow examination is rarely diagnostic in these cases. The destructive thrombocytopenias can be broadly divided into nonimmunologically and immunologically mediated groups (see Fig. 23.7). Among the immune thrombocytopenias, drug-induced, isoimmune, or autoimmune mechanisms may be operative. In these cases, platelet surface-associated immunoglobulin is usually detected by a variety of antiplatelet-antibody assays that have been developed (see Chapters 26 and 30). Drug-induced thrombocytopenia (Chapter 29) should be considered when a careful medication history is taken. Specific laboratory tests to confirm the role of certain drug-dependent antibodies (e.g., for quinine, quinidine, heparin) are available, using *in vitro* mixtures of the individual's plasma (or serum), normal target platelets, and the implicated offending drug (see Chapter 29). The diagnosis of isoimmune thrombocytopenia can be confirmed by acute-phase serologic testing for alloantibodies specific for different platelet alloantigens (most commonly anti-Pl[A1]) and platelet alloantigen typing after recovery (see Chapters 26 and 28). The diagnosis of autoimmune thrombocytopenia (ITP) in adults should be followed by testing for specific underlying systemic diseases (e.g., human immunodeficiency virus infection, connective tissue disease, lymphoma), unless the diagnosis of such diseases has antedated the development of ITP.

Postoperative thrombocytopenia is a frequently encountered, special circumstance (142). Major considerations for differential diagnosis in this setting include infection; drug-induced immune thrombocytopenia, including heparin-induced thrombocytopenia; disseminated intravascular coagulation; and posttransfusion purpura.

## PROLONGED BLEEDING TIME

The finding of a prolonged bleeding time in the absence of thrombocytopenia indicates a defect in platelet function, abnormal microvascular integrity, or impaired platelet–vessel wall interaction. One approach to the further evaluation of this abnormality is depicted in Fig. 23.9.

In many cases the cause of a prolonged bleeding time can be attributed to the ingestion of aspirin or an aspirin-containing medication, nonsteroidal antiinflammatory drugs, or other medications that may interfere with platelet function. On close questioning, some individuals admit to being unsure about whether they might have taken aspirin during the week prior to the bleeding time. In such cases the simplest procedure is to discontinue all implicated medications for at least 1 week before repeating the bleeding time.

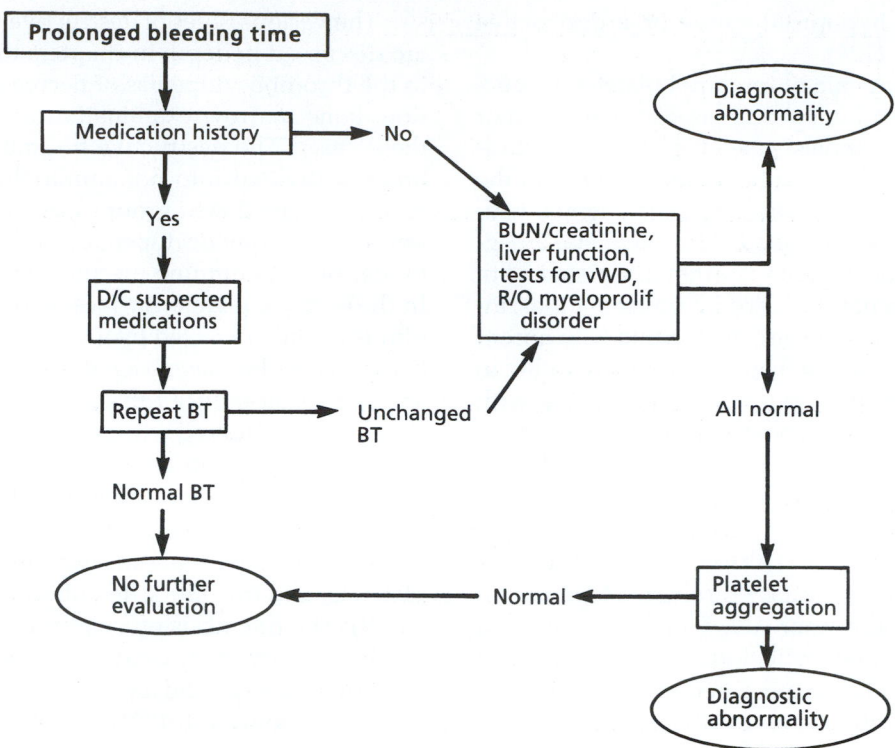

**FIGURE 23.9.**    A diagnostic approach to further evaluation of a prolonged bleeding time (BT). vWd, von Willebrand disease.

If no medications are suspected by careful history, or if the bleeding time fails to correct after discontinuation of suspected offending agents, further laboratory testing is required to determine the cause. As discussed in Chapters 33 and 34, uremia, liver disease, the myeloproliferative disorders, and von Willebrand disease are among the most common defects of primary hemostasis. Therefore individuals with unexplained prolongations of the bleeding time should have blood tests of renal and liver function. If any abnormalities of blood counts or the presence of splenomegaly suggests the possibility of a myeloproliferative disorder, this evaluation should be pursued. Finally, the diagnosis of von Willebrand disease should be excluded by assays for von Willebrand factor.

If all of these tests are unrevealing, platelet aggregation studies (see Chapter 26) should be performed to determine if one of the rare qualitative abnormalities of platelet function (unrelated to drugs) is present (143). While platelet aggregation studies have traditionally occupied a front-line position in the workup of the prolonged bleeding time, they are in fact rarely useful in the diagnosis of specific bleeding disorders after a careful drug history and the tests noted above have excluded the more common causes of a prolonged bleeding time (144, 145). An occasional case of platelet storage pool disease, Glanzmann's thrombasthenia, or Bernard–Sou-

lier syndrome may be diagnosed by this test (Fig. 23.10), but about 75% of individuals with abnormal bleeding times have normal platelet aggregation studies (144). Platelet aggregation studies may even be completely normal (despite a prolonged bleeding time) in some individuals with storage pool disease (146). Furthermore, many variables affect platelet aggregation, including venipuncture and centrifugation technique, platelet concentration, time of study after blood collection, and individual day-to-day and circadian variability of platelet reactivity (144, 147–149). Therefore this relatively costly and labor-intensive test should generally not be used in the initial evaluation of individuals with a prolonged bleeding time (144).

## ABNORMAL PT AND aPTT

Prolongation of the PT and/or the aPTT indicates an abnormality of secondary hemostasis, which may be caused by a deficiency or an inhibitor of one or more coagulation factors. However, not all individuals with abnormalities of these tests have a clinical bleeding disorder.

Fig. 23.11 is a matrix of coagulopathies that are detected by combinations of abnormal or normal PT and aPTT results. Isolated deficiencies of intrinsic pathway factors (prekallikrein, high-molecular-weight kininogen, factors XII, XI, IX, and VIII) cause an isolated pro-

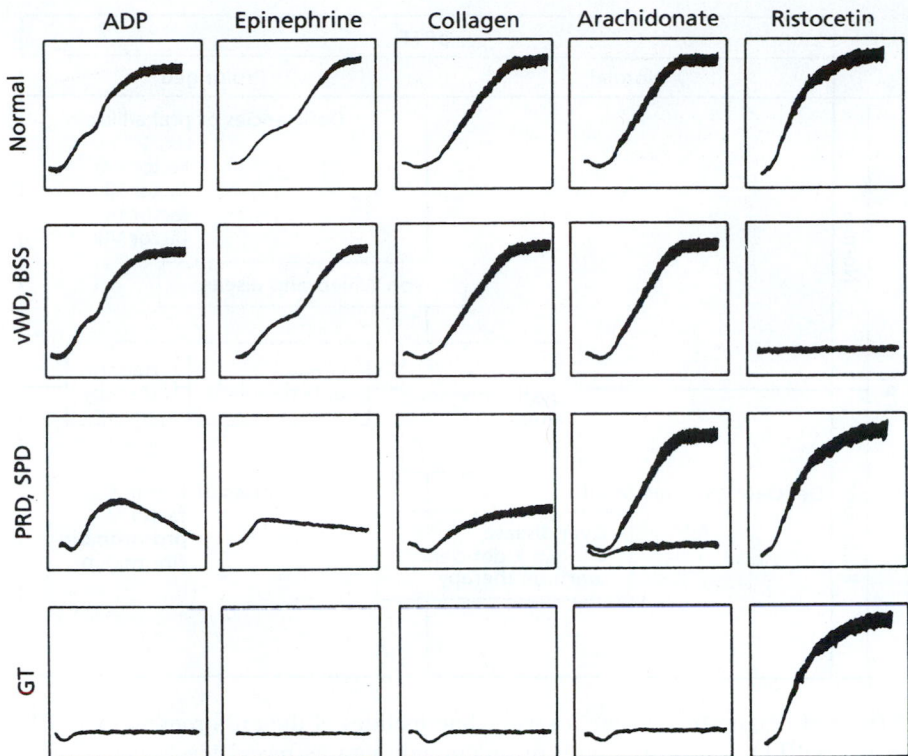

**FIGURE 23.10.**   Normal and abnormal patterns of platelet aggregation in response to adenosine diphosphate (ADP), epinephrine, collagen, arachidonate, and ristocetin. In classic (type I) von Willebrand disease (vWd) and Bernard–Soulier syndrome (BSS), platelet aggregation is normal with all agents except ristocetin. In platelet release defects (PRD) and storage pool disease (SPD), only first-wave aggregation occurs in response to ADP and epinephrine, and collagen-induced aggregation is markedly blunted; arachidonate-induced aggregation may or may not be abnormal, but is always lost following aspirin ingestion. In Glanzmann's thrombasthenia (GT), the initial shape-change remains normal, but aggregation is completely inhibited in response to all agents except ristocetin. (Adapted with permission from Schafer AI. Thrombocytopenia and disorders of platelet function. In: Stein JH, ed. Internal medicine. 3rd ed. Boston: Little, Brown, 1990; pp. 1041–1048.)

longation of the aPTT, while deficiency of the only extrinsic pathway factor (factor VII) causes an isolated prolongation of the PT. Deficiencies of the common pathway factors (factor X, V, prothrombin, and fibrinogen) cause prolongations of both the aPTT and PT. Individuals with von Willebrand disease characteristically have a prolonged aPTT, but this test may also be normal. The lupus anticoagulant typically prolongs the aPTT, but it may also affect the PT to a lesser extent in some cases.

Although dysfibrinogenemias would be expected to prolong both the PT and the aPTT, they tend to affect most prominently the PT; any combination of abnormalities of these two screening tests (including entirely normal values for both) can be found. Liver disease, early vitamin K deficiency, and therapeutic anticoagulation with warfarin typically cause prolongation of the PT but not the aPTT. Conversely, therapeutic anticoagulation with heparin prolongs the aPTT but not the PT. Nevertheless, advanced liver failure or vitamin K deficiency and overanticoagulation with either warfarin or heparin may be associated with prolongations of both screening

tests, as would be expected in conditions that cause inhibitory effects on multiple coagulation factors, including those involved in the common pathway.

The finding of a prolonged aPTT, with or without a prolonged PT, should be followed up with a mixing study to screen for the presence of an inhibitor in the individual's plasma. The premise of this simple test is that if the abnormal aPTT in the individual is caused by even the most severe deficiency of a coagulation factor, a 50% mix of individual plasma with normal plasma should completely correct the aPTT. For example, assuming that normal plasma contains 100% levels of all coagulation factors, the 1:1 mix of normal plasma with the plasma of a hemophiliac individual with a factor VIII level of 0% should raise the factor VIII level in the mixture to 50%, which is sufficient to correct the aPTT completely. Failure to correct the aPTT after the 50% mix indicates that the individual's plasma contains an inhibitor (usually an antibody) that indiscriminately interferes with fibrin formation in both the individual's plasma and in the normal plasma with which it is mixed. In the inhibitor screen the aPTT should be measured

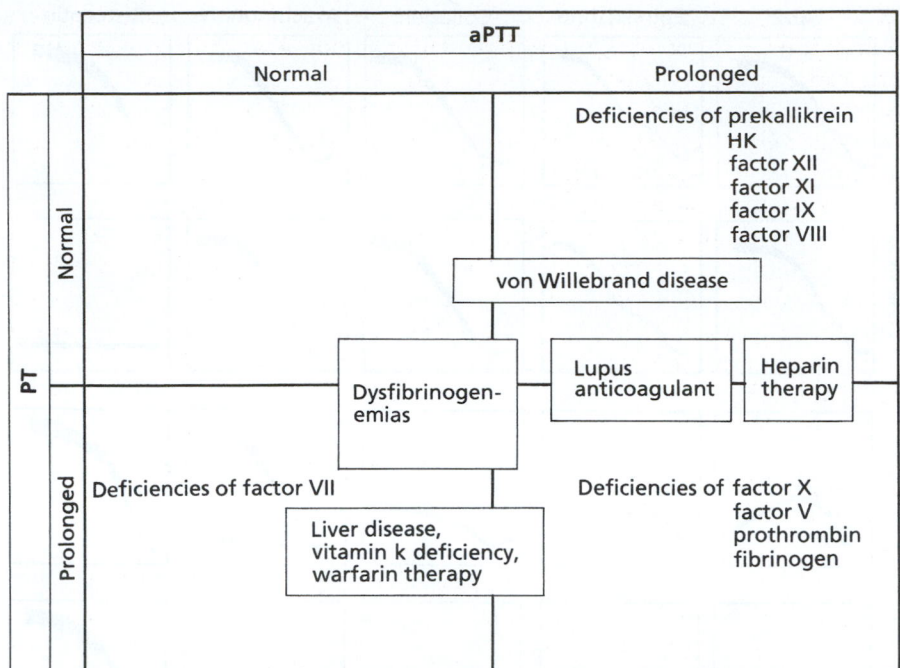

**FIGURE 23.11.** Matrix of diagnostic possibilities with abnormalities of the prothrombin time (PT) and/or the activated partial thromboplastin time (aPTT). Individuals with disorders indicated as boxed insets may exhibit different patterns of abnormalities of the PT and/or aPTT. For example, in von Willebrand disease, the PT is normal, but the aPTT may be either prolonged or normal. In the lupus anticoagulant or in individuals receiving heparin, the usual pattern is a prolonged aPTT and a normal PT; however, in some cases the PT may also be prolonged. In individuals with liver disease, vitamin K deficiency, or on warfarin therapy, the usual pattern is a prolonged PT and a normal aPTT; however, in more severe cases the aPTT may also be prolonged. Any combination of results of the PT and aPTT may be seen in dysfibrinogenemias. HK, high-molecular-weight kininogen.

immediately after the mix, as well as after a 2-hour incubation of the mixed plasma at 37°C. Lupus anticoagulants will demonstrate immediate failure of normal plasma to correct the aPTT. However, the presence of specific antibodies to factor VIII or factor IX in the individual's plasma may cause only delayed prolongation for the aPTT after the mix, following an apparent immediate correction of the aPTT with the addition of normal plasma.

If both the immediate and incubated mixing studies demonstrate complete correction of the aPTT, a specific coagulation factor deficiency is likely to be the cause of the individual's prolonged aPTT. The diagnosis is then made by performing individual factor assays. The sequence of factor assays to be performed should be dictated by the individual's clinical history and by the pattern of abnormalities of the screening PT and aPTT (see Fig. 23.11). In individuals with isolated prolongations of the aPTT who have had no bleeding problems even after surgery or trauma, determination of levels of factor XII, prekallikrein, and high-molecular-weight kininogen are likely to be of the highest yield. In women with isolated prolongations of the aPTT who have had a significant bleeding history, assays of factor VIII (only as part

of the evaluation for von Willebrand disease) and factor XI would be indicated, since female carrier states for classic hemophilia or factor IX deficiency are very rarely associated with factor levels low enough to cause hemorrhagic complications (150). In individuals with isolated prolongations of the PT, who have no clinical evidence of liver disease or vitamin K deficiency, a factor VII level should be determined.

In individuals with prolongations of both the PT and the aPTT, a quantitative or qualitative abnormality of fibrinogen should first be excluded by performing a thrombin time. The thrombin time directly measures the conversion of fibrinogen to fibrin. If the thrombin time is normal, levels of factors X and V should be assayed. If the thrombin time is prolonged, an immunologic assay of fibrinogen should be performed; concordant abnormalities of both the thrombin time and the fibrinogen level indicates hypofibrinogenemia or afibrinogenemia, while a prolonged thrombin time with a simultaneously normal immunologic fibrinogen level indicates the presence of dysfibrinogenemia.

An important factor that might artifactually prolong the thrombin time (as well as the PT and aPTT) is the presence of even trace amounts of heparin in the collected blood sample. This is most frequently encountered in hospitalized individuals whose blood is drawn through an indwelling catheter that is kept open with heparin, even when several milliliters of blood are initially discarded before collecting a sample for coagulation studies (151). The presence of heparin in the blood specimen can be excluded by protamine neutralization *in vitro*. Alternatively, a reptilase time can be performed with the thrombin time. Reptilase converts fibrinogen to fibrin by a direct mechanism that is insensitive to heparin, and therefore the simultaneous finding of a prolonged thrombin time and a normal reptilase time indicates the presence of heparin.

## FURTHER EVALUATION OF PATIENTS WITH NORMAL SCREENING TESTS OF COAGULATION

As noted above, the finding of normal values for the platelet count, bleeding time, PT, and aPTT excludes almost all clinically significant, systemic coagulopathies. Nevertheless, when the clinical history of bleeding is a compelling one and particularly when there is a strongly positive family history, additional specialized tests (see Chapter 26) are indicated to exclude more unusual causes.

Factor XIII deficiency (Chapters 6 and 36) is associated with delayed bleeding and impaired wound healing after surgery or trauma. However, since non-cross-linked fibrin formation is normal in this disease, the PT and aPTT are normal. An assay for factor XIII activity, such as clot stability in 5 mol/l urea, should be performed in such suspected cases.

Rare familial disorders of primary fibrinolysis may also cause hemophilia-like bleeding without affecting the screening laboratory tests of coagulation. Hyperfibrinolytic disorders are characterized by delayed bleeding because a normal hemostatic plug is formed that is later more susceptible to breakdown as a result of increased fibrinolytic activity. Examples of hyperfibrinolytic disorders, which may be either inherited or acquired, include decreased type-1 plasminogen activator inhibitor (PAI-1) activity (due to quantitative or qualitative deficiency of PAI-1 or autoantibody against PAI-1) and $\alpha_2$-antiplasmin deficiency (152). The possibility of $\alpha_2$-antiplasmin deficiency should be considered if a euglobulin lysis time is performed and found to be shortened.

Mild coagulation factor deficiencies, such as classic hemophilia, may be associated with plasma factor levels that are not sufficiently low to prolong the aPTT but may cause clinical bleeding problems under certain provocative conditions (e.g., oral surgery); if this is considered, specific factor levels should be determined even in the presence of normal screening tests. Finally, mild

heterozygous von Willebrand disease (particularly type I) may not be associated with either a prolonged bleeding time or a prolonged aPTT, and its diagnosis may require full von Willebrand factor testing (see Chapters 26 and 34). The problem of diagnosis of von Willebrand disease is further complicated by physiologic variations in plasma levels of von Willebrand factor (e.g., after exercise or during late pregnancy, adrenergic stimuli, stress, or hypoglycemia), which may transiently raise factor levels to the normal range in congenitally deficient individuals (153). When the diagnosis is strongly suspected, normal von Willebrand factor assays may have to be repeated.

## REFERENCES

1. Sindet-Pederson S, Gram J, Jespersen J. The possible role of oral epithelial cells in tissue-type plasminogen activator-related fibrinolysis in human saliva. J Dent Res 1990;69:1283–1286.
2. Sindet-Pederson S, Gram J, Jespersen J. Characterization of plasminogen activators in unstimulated and stimulated human whole saliva. J Dent Res 1987;66:1199–1203.
3. Rosner F. Julius Preuss' Biblical and Talmudic medicine. New York: Sanhedrin Press, 1978.
4. Bachmann F. Diagnostic approach to mild bleeding disorders. Semin Hematol 1980;17:292–305.
5. Payne BA, Pierre RV. Pseudothrombocytopenia: a laboratory artifact with potentially serious consequences. Mayo Clin Proc 1984;59:123–125.
6. Lombarts AJ, de Kieviet W. Recognition and prevention of pseudothrombocytopenia and concomitant pseudoleukocytosis. Am J Clin Pathol 1988; 89:634–639.
7. Kjeldsberg CR, Swanson J. Platelet satellitism. Blood 1974;43:831–836.
8. Larson JH, Pierre RV. Platelet satellitism as a cause of abnormal hemalog D differential results. Am J Clin Pathol 1977;68:758–759.
9. Savage RA. Pseudoleukocytosis due to EDTA-induced platelet clumping. Am J Clin Pathol 1984;81:317–322.
10. Jantunen E. Inherited giant platelet disorders. Eur J Haematol 1994;53: 191–196.
11. Silvestri F, Virgolini L, Savignano C et al. Incidence and diagnosis of EDTA-dependent pseudothrombocytopenia in a consecutive outpatient population referred for isolated thrombocytopenia. Vox Sang 1995;68: 35–39.
12. Schrezenmeier H, Müller H, Gunsilius E et al. Anticoagulant-induced pseudothrombocytopenia and pseudoleucocytosis. Thromb Haemost 1995;73:506–513.
13. Onder O, Weinstein A, Hoyer LW. Pseudothrombocytopenia caused by platelet agglutinins that are reactive in blood anticoagulated with chelating agents. Blood 1980;56:177–182.
14. Pegels JG, Bruynes EC, Engelfriet CP et al. Pseudothrombocytopenia: an immunologic study on platelet antibodies dependent on ethylene diamine tetra-acetate. Blood 1982;59:157–161.
15. van Vliet HH, Kappers-Klunne MC, Abels J. Pseudothrombocytopenia: a cold autoantibody directed against platelet glycoprotein GP II$^b$. Br J Haematol 1986;62:501–511.
16. Berkman N, Michaeli Y, Or R et al. EDTA-dependent pseudothrombocytopenia: a clinical study of 18 individuals and a Review of the literature. Am J Hematol 1991;36:195–201.
17. Edelman B, Kickler T. Sequential measurement of anti-platelet antibodies in a individual who developed EDTA-dependent pseudothrombocytopenia. Am J Clin Pathol 1993;99:87–89.
18. Bizzaro N. EDTA-dependent pseudothrombocytopenia: a clinical and epidemiological study of 112 cases, with 10-year follow-up. Am J Hematol 1995;50:103–109.
19. Bizzaro N, Brandalise M. EDTA-dependent pseudothrombocytopenia. Association with antiplatelet and antiphospholipid antibodies. Am J Clin Pathol 1995;103:103–107.
20. Christopoulos CG, Machin SJ. A new type of pseudothrombocytopenia: EDTA-mediated agglutination of platelets bearing Fab fragments of a chimaeric antibody. Br J Haematol 1994;87:650–652.
21. Watkins SP Jr, Shulman NR. Platelet cold agglutinins. Blood 1970;36: 153–158.
22. Greipp PR, Didisheim P, Brigden M. Platelet cold agglutinins. Lancet 1975; 2:814–815.
23. De Caterina M, Fratellanza G, Grimaldi E et al. Evidence of a cold immuno-

globulin-autoantibody against 78-kD platelet glycoprotein in a case of EDTA-dependent pseudothrombocytopenia. Am J Clin Pathol 1993;99:163–167.

24. Harker LA, Slichter SJ. The bleeding time as a screening test for evaluation of platelet function. N Engl J Med 1972;287:155–159.

25. Bowie EJW, Owen CA Jr. The bleeding time. Prog Hemost Thromb 1974;2:249–271.

26. Levine PH. Platelet function tests: predictive value. N Engl J Med 1975;292:1346–1347.

27. Lind SE. Prolonged bleeding time. Am J Med 1984;77:305–312.

28. Burns ER, Lawrence C. Bleeding time. A guide to its diagnostic and clinical utility. Arch Pathol Lab Med 1989;113:1219–1224.

29. Rodgers RPC, Levin J. A critical reappraisal of the bleeding time. Semin Thromb Hemost 1990;16:1–20.

30. Ivy AC, Nelson D, Bucher MS. The standardization of certain factors in the cutaneous "venostasis" bleeding time technique. J Lab Clin Med 1941;26:1812–1822.

31. Mielke CH Jr, Kaneshiro MM, Maher IA et al. The standardized normal Ivy bleeding time and its prolongation by aspirin. Blood 1969;34:204–215.

32. Babson SR, Babson AL. Development and evaluation of a disposable device for performing simultaenous duplicate bleeding time determinations. Am J Clin Pathol 1978;70:406–408.

33. Burns ER. The Hemalet bleeding time device. Lab Med 1986;17:745–747.

34. Smith C. Surgicutt: a device for modified template bleeding times. J Med Tech 1986;3:29–31.

35. Buchanan GR, Holtkamp CA. A comparative study of variables affecting the bleeding time using two disposable devices. Am J Clin Pathol 1989;91:45–51.

36. Hertzendorf LR, Stehling L, Kurec AS et al. Comparison of bleeding times performed on the arm and the leg. Am J Clin Pathol 1987;87:393–396.

37. Mielke CH Jr. Aspirin prolongation of the template bleeding time: influence of venostasis and direction of incision. Blood 1982;60:1139–1142.

38. Valeri CR, MacGregor H, Cassidy G et al. Effects of temperature on bleeding time and clotting time in normal male and female volunteers. Crit Care Med 1995;23:698–704.

39. Aversa LA, Vázquez A, Peñalver JA et al. Bleeding time in normal children. J Pediatr Hematol Oncol 1995;17:25–28.

40. McGurk M, Dinsdale RC. A comparison of template bleeding time with mucosal petechiometry as a measure of the platelet function defect induced by aspirin. Br J Oral Maxillofac Surg 1991;29:173–175.

41. O'Laughlin JC, Hoftiezer JW, Mahoney JP et al. Does aspirin prolong bleeding from gastric biopsies in man? Gastrointest Endosc 1981;27:1–5.

42. Jalan R, Grose R, Dillon JF et al. Gastric mucosal bleeding time in cirrhosis. Gastrointest Endosc 1994;40:599–602.

43. Shulman NR, Watkins SP Jr, Itscoitz SB et al. Evidence that the spleen retains the youngest and hemostatically most effective platelets. Trans Assoc Am Physicians 1968;81:302–313.

44. Hellem AJ, Borchgrevink CF, Ames DB. The role of red cells in haemostasis: the relation between haematocrit, bleeding time and platelet adhesiveness. Br J Haematol 1961;7:42–50.

45. Small M, Lowe GDO, Cameron E et al. Contribution of the haematocrit to the bleeding time. Haemostasis 1983;13:379–384.

46. Soltani G, Fernandez F, Pris J et al. Prolonged bleeding time in severe anemia. Presse Med 1986;15:745–747.

47. Anand A, Feffer SE. Hematocrit and bleeding time: an update. South Med J 1994;87:299–301.

48. Livio M, Gotti E, Marchesi D et al. Uraemic bleeding: role of anaemia and beneficial effect of red cell transfusions. Lancet 1982;2:1013–1015.

49. Fernandez F, Goudable C, Sie P et al. Low haematocrit and prolonged bleeding time in uraemic individuals: effect of red cell transfusions. Br J Haematol 1985;59:139–148.

50. Moia M, Mannucci PM, Vizzotto L et al. Improvement in the haemostatic defect of uraemia after treatment with recombinant human erythropoietin. Lancet 1987;2:1227–1229.

51. Vigano G, Benigni A, Mendogni D et al. Recombinant human erythropoietin to correct uremic bleeding. Am J Kidney Dis 1991;18:44–49.

52. Santos MT, Valles J, Marcus AJ et al. Enhancement of platelet reactivity and modulation of eicosanoid production by intact erythrocytes. A new approach to platelet activation and recruitment. J Clin Invest 1991;87:571–580.

53. Editorial. The bleeding time. Lancet 1991;337:1447–1448.

54. Czapek EE, Deykin D, Salzman E et al. Intermediate syndrome of platelet dysfunction. Blood 1978;52:103–113.

55. Stuart MJ, Miller ML, Davey FR et al. The post-aspirin bleeding time: a screening test for evaluating haemostatic disorders. Br J Haematol 1979;43:649–659.

56. Deykin D, Janson P, McMahon L. Ethanol potentiation of aspirin-induced prolongation of the bleeding time. N Engl J Med 1982;306:852–854.

57. Abildgaard CF, Suzuki Z, Harrison J et al. Serial studies in von Willebrand's disease: variabililty versus "variants." Blood 1980;56:712–716.

58. Gralnick HR, Rick ME, McKeown LP et al. Platelet von Willebrand factor: an important determinant of the bleeding time in type I von Willebrand's disease. Blood 1986;68:58–61.

59. Buchanan GR, Holtkamp CA. Prolonged bleeding time in children and young adults with hemophilia. Pediatrics 1980;66:951–955.

60. Eyster ME, Gordon RA, Ballard JO. The bleeding time is longer than normal in hemophilia. Blood 1981;58:719–723.

61. Smith PS, Baglini R, Meissner GF. The prolonged bleeding time in hemophilia A: comparison of two measuring technics and clinical associations. Am J Clin Pathol 1985;83:211–215.

62. Breederveld K, van Royen EA, Ten Cate JW. Severe factor V deficiency with prolonged bleeding time. Thromb Diath Haemorrh 1974;32:538–548.

63. Ly B, Solum NO, Vennerod AM et al. A syndrome of factor VII deficiency and abnormal platelet release reaction. Scand J Haematol 1978;21:206–214.

64. Brody JI. Prolonged bleeding times with factor IX and XI deficiency (von Willebrand syndromes). Am J Med Sci 1975;269:19–24.

65. Edgin RA, Metz EN, Fromkes JJ et al. Acquired factor X deficiency with associated defects in platelet aggregation. A response to corticosteroid therapy. Am J Med 1980;69:137–139.

66. Winter M, Needham J, Barkhan P. Factor XI deficiency and a platelet defect. Haemostasis 1983;13:83–88.

67. Burns ER. Laboratory tests of hemostasis. In: Burns ER, ed. Clinical management of bleeding and thrombosis. Boston: Blackwell Scientific, 1987; pp. 43–56.

68. Peterson P, Gottfried EL. The effects of inaccurate blood sample volume on prothrombin time (PT) and activated partial thromboplastin time (aPTT). Thromb Haemost 1982;47:101–103.

69. Suchman AL, Griner PF. Diagnostic uses of the activated partial thromboplastin time and prothrombin time. Ann Intern Med 1986;104:810–816.

70. Bark CJ. Coagulation nondisease. N Engl J Med 1970;282:1214.

71. Czapek EE. Iatrogenic prolonged aPTT: a nondisease state. JAMA 1974;227:1304.

72. Hirsh J, Poller L, Deykin D et al. Optimal therapeutic range for oral anticoagulants. Chest 1989;95(Suppl 2):5S–11S.

73. Sibley C, Singer JW, Wood RJ. Comparison of activated partial thromboplastin reagents. Am J Clin Pathol 1973;59:581–586.

74. Hoffman JJ, Meulendijk PN. Comparison of reagents for determining the activated partial thromboplastin time. Thromb Haemost 1978;39:640–645.

75. Hathaway WE, Assmus SL, Montgomery RR et al. Activated partial thromboplastin time and minor coagulopathies. Am J Clin Pathol 1979;71:22–25.

76. Brill-Edwards P, Ginsberg JS, Johnston M et al. Establishing a therapeutic range for heparin therapy. Ann Intern Med 1993;119:104–109.

77. Mannucci PM, Canciani MT, Mari D et al. The varied sensitivity of partial thromboplastin and prothrombin time reagents in the demonstration of lupus-like anticoagulant. Scand J Haematol 1979;22:423–432.

78. Green D, Hougie C, Kazmier FJ et al. Report of the working party on acquired inhibitors of coagulation: studies of the "lupus" anticoagulant. Thromb Haemost 1983;49:144–146.

79. Brandt JT, Triplett DA, Musgrave K et al. The sensitivity of different coagulation reagents to the presence of lupus anticoagulants. Arch Pathol Lab Med 1987;111:120–124.

80. Stevenson KJ, Easton AC, Curry A et al. The reliability of activated partial thromboplastin time methods and the relationship to lipid composition and ultrastructure. Thromb Haemost 1986;55:250–258.

81. Triplett DA, Brandt J. Laboratory identification of the lupus anticoagulant. Br J Haematol 1989;73:139–142.

82. Mozes B, Lubin D, Modan B et al. Evaluation of an intervention aimed at reducing inappropriate use of preoperative blood coagulation tests. Arch Intern Med 1989;149:1836–1838.

83. Eika C, Havig O, Godal HC. The value of preoperative hemostatic screening. Scand J Haematol 1978;21:349–354.

84. Robbins JA, Rose SD. Partial thromboplastin time as a screening test. Ann Intern Med 1979;90:796–797.

85. Eisenberg JM, Clarke JR, Sussman SA. Prothrombin and partial thromboplastin times as preoperative screening tests. Arch Surg 1982;117:48–51.

86. Kaplan EB, Sheiner LB, Boeckmann AJ et al. The usefulness of preoperative laboratory screening. JAMA 1985;253:3576–3581.

87. Barber A, Green D, Galluzzo T et al. The bleeding time as a preoperative screening test. Am J Med 1985;78:761–764.

88. Koutts J. Clinching the diagnosis: assessment of hemostatic function. Pathology 1985;17:643–647.

89. Rapaport SI. Preoperative hemostatic evaluation: which tests, if any? Blood 1983;61:229–231.

90. Suchman AL, Mushlin AI. How well does the activated partial thromboplastin time predict postoperative hemorrhage? JAMA 1986;256:750–753.

91. Rohrer MJ, Michelotti MC, Nahrwold DL. A prospective evaluation of the efficacy of preoperative coagulation testing. Ann Surg 1988;208:554–557.

92. Bushick JB, Eisenberg JM, Kinman J et al. Pursuit of abnormal coagulation screening tests generates modest hidden preoperative costs. J Gen Intern Med 1989;4:493–497.

93. Lind SE. The bleeding time does not predict surgical bleeding. Blood 1991;77:2547–2552.

94. Macpherson CR, Jacobs P, Dent DM. Abnormal peri-operative haemorrhage in asymptomatic individuals is not predicted by laboratory testing. S Afr Med J 1993;83:106–108.

95. De Rossi SS, Glick M. Bleeding time: an unreliable predictor of clinical hemostasis. J Oral Maxillofac Surg 1996;54:1119–1120.

96. Sethi GK, Copeland JG, Goldman S et al. Implications of preoperative administration of aspirin in individuals undergoing coronary artery bypass grafting. J Am Coll Cardiol 1990;15:15–20.

97. Goldman S, Copeland J, Moritz T et al. Starting aspirin therapy after operation. Effects on early graft patency. Circulation 1991;84:520–526.

98. Ferraris VA, Berry WR, Klingman RR. Comparison of blood reinfusion techniques used during coronary artery bypass grafting. Ann Thorac Surg 1993;56:433–439.

99. De Caterina R, Lanza M, Manca G et al. Bleeding time and bleeding: an analysis of the relationship of the bleeding time test with parameters of surgical bleeding. Blood 1994;84:3363–3370.

100. Gewirtz AS, Miller ML, Keys TF. The clinical usefulness of the preoperative bleeding time. Arch Pathol Lab Med 1996;120:353–356.

101. Barber A, Green D, Galluzzo T et al.The bleeding time as a preoperative screening test. Am J Med 1985;78:761–764.

102. Gewirtz AS, Kottke-Marchant K, Miller ML. The preoperative bleeding time test: assessing its clinical usefulness. Cleve Clin J Med 1995;62:379–382.

103. Marwah DS, Korbet SM. Timing of complications in percutaneous renal biopsy: what is the optimal period of observation? Am J Kidney Dis 1996;28:47–52.

104. Rohrer MJ, Michelotti MC, Nahrwold DL. A prospective evaluation of the efficacy of preoperative coagulation testing. Ann Surg 1988;208:554–557.

105. Gravlee GP, Arora S, Lavender SW et al. Predictive value of blood clotting tests in cardiac surgical individuals. Ann Thorac Surg 1994;58:216–221.

106. Myers ER, Clarke-Pearson DL, Olt GJ et al. Preoperative coagulation testing on a gynecologic oncology service. Obstet Gynecol 1994;83:438–444.

107. Ritter DM, Owen CA Jr, Bowie EJ et al. Evaluation of preoperative hematology-coagulation screening in liver transplantation. Mayo Clin Proc 1989;64:216–223.

108. Friedman EW, Sussman II. Safety of invasive procedures in individuals with the coagulopathy of liver disease. Clin Lab Haematol 1989;11:199–204.

109. McVay PA, Toy PT. Lack of increased bleeding after liver biopsy in individuals with mild hemostatic abnormalities. Am J Clin Pathol 1990;94:747–753.

110. Darcy MD, Kanterman RY, Kleinhoffer MA et al. Evaluation of coagulation tests as predictors of angiographic bleeding complications. Radiology 1996;198:741–744.

111. Krevans JR, Jackson DP. Hemorrhagic disorder following massive whole blood transfusions. JAMA 1955;159:171–177.

112. Counts RB, Haisch C, Simon TL et al. Hemostasis in massively transfused trauma individuals. Ann Surg 1979;190:91–99.

113. Noe DA, Graham SM, Luff R et al. Platelet counts during rapid massive transfusion. Transfusion 1982;22:392–395.

114. Harvey MP, Greenfield TP, Sugrue ME et al. Massive blood transfusion in a tertiary referral hospital. Clinical outcomes and haemostatic complications. Med J Aust 1995;163:356–359.

115. Desforges JF, O'Connell LG. Hematologic observations of the course of erythroblastosis fetalis. Blood 1955;10:802–811.

116. Reed RL, Ciavarella D, Heimbach DM et al. Prophylactic platelet administration during massive transfusion. A prospective, randomized, double-blind clinical study. Ann Surg 1986;203:40–48.

117. Rutherford CJ, Frenkel EP. Thrombocytopenia. Issues in diagnosis and therapy. Med Clin North Am 1994;78:555–575.

118. Boggs DR. Amegakaryocytic thrombocytopenia. Am J Hematol 1985;20:413–416.

119. Manoharan A, Williams NT, Sparrow R. Acquired amegakaryocytic thrombocytopenia: report of a case and Review of literature. Q J Med 1989;70:243–252.

120. Hoffman R, Briddell RA, van Besien K et al. Acquired cyclic amegakaryocytic thrombocytopenia associated with an immunoglobulin blocking the action of granulocyte-macrophage colony-stimulating factor. N Engl J Med 1989;321:97–102.

121. Freedman MH, Estrov Z. Congenital amegakaryocytic thrombocytopenia: an intrinsic hematopoietic stem cell defect. Am J Pediatr Hematol Oncol 1990;12:225–230.

122. Trimble MS, Glynn MF, Brain MC. Amegakaryocytic thrombocytopenia of 4 years duration: successful treatment with antithymocyte globulin. Am J Hematol 1991;37:126–127.

123. Zeigler Z, Murphy S, Gardner FH. Microscopic platelet size and morphology in various hematologic disorders. Blood 1978;51:479–486.

124. Slichter SJ. Platelet transfusion therapy. Hematol Oncol Clin North Am 1990;4:291–311.

125. McIntosh S, Breg WR, Lubiniecki AS. Fanconi's anemia: the preanemic phase. Am J Pediatr Hematol Oncol 1979;1:107–110.

126. Hall JG. Thrombocytopenia and absent radium (TAR) syndrome. J Med Genet 1987;24:79–83.

127. Homans AC, Cohen JL, Mazur EM. Defective megakaryocyteopoiesis in the syndrome of thrombocytopenia with absent radii. Br J Haematol 1988;70:205–210.

128. Perry GS, Spector BD, Schuman LM et al. The Wiskott–Aldrich syndrome in the United States and Canada (1892–1979). J Pediatr 1980;97:72–78.

129. Ochs HD, Slichter SJ, Harker LA et al. The Wiskott–Aldrich syndrome: studies of lymphocytes, granulocytes, and platelets. Blood 1980;55:243–252.

130. Thompson AR, Wood WG, Stamatoyannopoulos G. X-linked syndrome of platelet dysfunction, thrombocytopenia, and imbalanced globin chain synthesis with hemolysis. Blood 1977;50:303–316.

131. Lusher JM, Schneider J, Mizukami I et al. The May-Hegglin anomaly: platelet function, ultrastructure, and chromosome studies. Blood 1968;32:950–961.

132. Godwin HA, Ginsburg AD. May-Hegglin anomaly: a defect in megakaryocyte fragmentation? Br J Haematol 1974;26:117–128.

133. Parsa KP, Lee DB, Zamboni L et al. Hereditary nephritis, deafness and abnormal thrombopoiesis: study of a new kindred. Am J Med 1976;60:665–672.

134. Bernheim J, Dechavanne M, Bryon PA et al. Thrombocytopenia, macro-thrombocytopathia, nephritis, and deafness. Am J Med 1976;61:145–150.

135. Murphy S, Oski FA, Naiman JL et al. Platelet size and kinetics in hereditary and acquired thrombocytopenia. N Engl J Med 1972;286:499–504.

136. Pepper H, Liebowitz D, Lindsay S. Cyclical thrombocyoptenic purpura related to the menstrual cycle. Arch Pathol 1956;61:1–5.

137. Cohen T, Cooney DP. Cyclic thrombocytopenia: case report and Review of literature. Scand J Haematol 1974;12:9–17.

138. Menitove JE, Anderson T, Hoffman R et al. Cyclic autoimmune thrombocytopenic purpura. Blood 1983;62(Suppl 1):245a.

139. Tomer A, Schreiber AD, McMillan R et al. Menstrual cyclic thrombocytopenia. Clin Res 1988;36:615a.

140. Smith MD, Smith DA, Fletcher M. Haemorrhage associated with thrombocytopenia in megaloblastic anaemia. Br Med J 1963;1:982–986.

141. Ghosh K, Sarode R, Varma N et al. Amegakaryocytic thrombocytopenia of nutritional vitamin $B_{12}$ deficiency. Trop Geogr Med 1988;40:158–160.

142. Chang JC. Review: Postoperative thrombocytopenia: with etiologic, diagnostic, and therapeutic consideration. Am J Med Sci 1996;311:96–105.

143. Bick RL. Platelet function defects associated with hemorrhage or thrombosis. Med Clin North Am 1994;78:577–607.

144. Remaley AT, Kennedy JM, Laposata M. Evaluation of the clinical utility of platelet aggregation studies. Am J Hematol 1989;31:188–193.

145. Schafer AI. Thrombocytopenia and disorders of platelets function. In: Stein JH, ed. Internal medicine. 3rd ed. Boston: Little, Brown, 1990; pp. 1041–1048.

146. Nieuwenhuis HK, Akkerman JW, Sixma JJ. Individuals with a prolonged bleeding time and normal aggregation tests may have storage pool deficiency: studies on one hundred six individuals. Blood 1987;70:620–623.

147. Malpass TW, Harker LA. Acquired disorders of platelet function. Semin Hematol 1980;17:242–258.

148. MacMillan DC, Sim AK. A comparative study of platelet aggregation in man and laboratory animals. Thromb Diath Haemorrh 1970;24:385–389.

149. Tofler GH, Brezinski D, Schafer AI et al. Concurrent morning increase in platelet aggregability and the risk of myocardial infarction and sudden cardiac death. N Engl J Med 1987;316:1514–1518.

150. Nisen P, Stamberg J, Ehrenpreis R et al. The molecular basis of severe hemophilia B in a girl. N Engl J Med 1986;315:1139–1142.

151. Bark CJ. Coagulation nondisease. N Engl J Med 1970;282:1214.

152. Lee MH, Vosburgh E, Anderson K et al. Deficiency of plasma plasminogen activator inhibitor 1 results in hyperfibrinolytic bleeding. Blood 1993;81:2357–2362.

153. Bloom AL. Von Willebrand factor: clinical features of inherited and acquired disorders. Mayo Clin Proc 1991;66:743–751.

# CHAPTER 24

# APPROACH TO THROMBOSIS

## Kenneth A. Bauer

## INTRODUCTION

Major advances have been made in our understanding of the natural anticoagulant and fibrinolytic systems that regulate the activity of the hemostatic mechanism. However, only during the last few years has this information been translated into the ability to diagnose clinically relevant risk factors in substantial numbers of individuals presenting with thrombosis. The impact of these clinical diagnostic advances has been most dramatic in younger individuals with idiopathic (without identifiable precipitating factors, such as cancer, recent surgery, etc.) venous thrombosis, in more than 50% of whom hereditary defects can be identified. Important strides have also been made in delineating the contribution of thrombotic risk factors to arterial thrombosis, but identification of the common risk factors for atherogenesis (e.g., smoking, hyperlipidemia, diabetes mellitus) retains primacy in the evaluation of such individuals.

This chapter will focus on the clinical approach to individuals with thrombosis and will complement Chapter 40, "Inherited and Acquired Hypercoagulable States." Although there has been little solid evidence that individuals with genetic defects predisposing to venous thrombosis should be managed differently from those without identifiable defects, data are emerging that such individuals are at higher risk for recurrent thromboembolic events. This, coupled with our newly acquired ability to identify such risk factors, frequently increases the relevance of such an evaluation.

## DIFFERENTIAL DIAGNOSIS

When approaching individuals suspected of having an active thrombotic process or a thrombotic diathesis, it is useful to place them in one of two major categories. The first group has characteristics that suggest the presence of an inherited thrombotic disorder or a primary hypercoagulable state (Table 24.1). These disorders result from mutations in single genes encoding a plasma protein component of one of the major natural anticoagulant mechanisms. The anticoagulant systems most frequently involved in the inherited (primary) hypercoagulable states include antithrombin III in the heparan sulfate-antithrombin III mechanism, and protein C, protein S, and factor V (substitution of the amino acid Gln for Arg at amino acid 506 [1], termed factor V Leiden) in the protein C anticoagulant pathway (Fig. 24.1). Elevation in plasma prothrombin levels in association with a G to A transversion at position 20210 in the 3'-untranslated region of the prothrombin gene is a newly identified genetic risk factor for venous thrombosis (2). The second category, the acquired or secondary hypercoagulable states, consists of a heterogeneous group of disorders in which there appears to be an increased risk for developing thrombotic complications as compared to the general population (Table 24.2). The pathophysiologic basis for the hypercoagulable state in most of these situations is complex and multifactorial. Hyperhomocysteinemia is a common laboratory abnormality that results in an increased risk in venous as well as arterial thrombosis. Plasma homocysteine levels are determined by genetic as well as environmental factors, the latter primarily including dietary intake of folic acid and vitamins $B_{12}$ and $B_6$. It is listed separately from the inherited thrombotic disorders because it may result from defects in several genes encoding different enzymes involved in the metabolism of the amino acid.

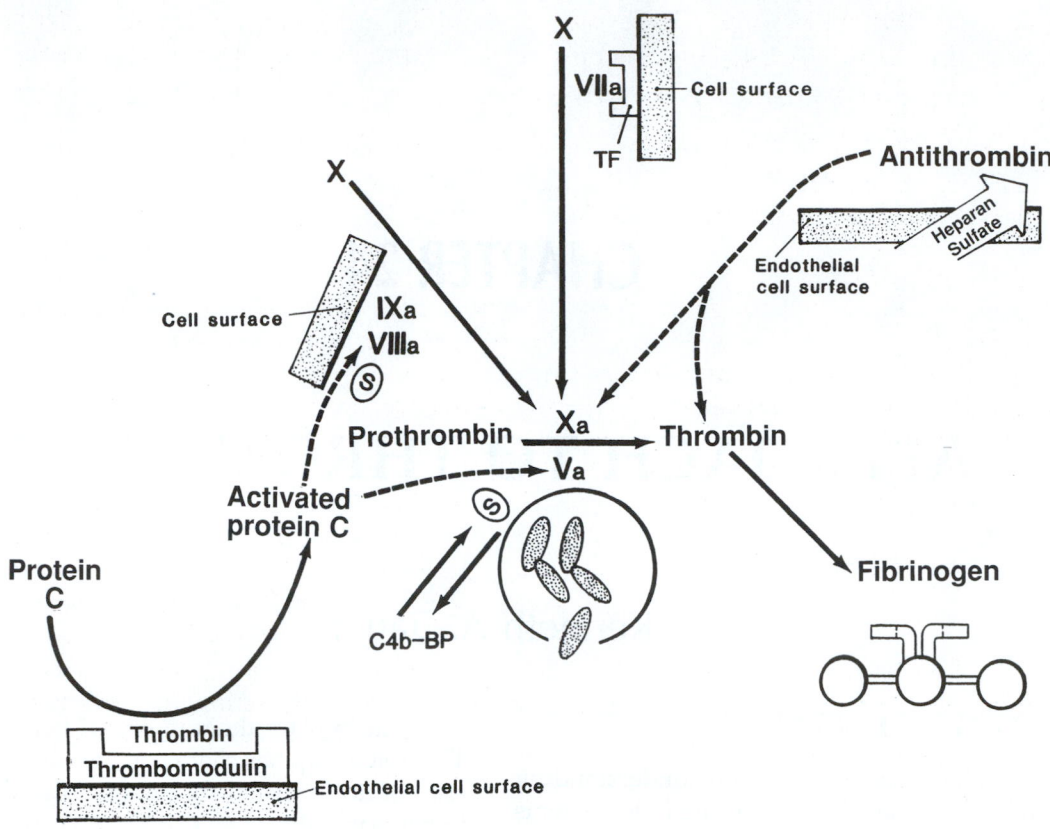

**FIGURE 24.1.** A schematic diagram of the pathways that generate factor Xa and thrombin, and the natural anticoagulant mechanisms that regulate the activity of these enzymes.

Factor X can be activated by factor VIIa-tissue factor (TF) complex or the factor IXa-VIIIa-activated cell surface complex. Factor Xa binds to the factor Va on activated platelets and mediates the conversion of prothrombin to thrombin under physiologic conditions. During this process, the inactive $F_{1+2}$ fragment is released from the aminoterminus of prothrombin. Thrombin is then able to act upon fibrinogen to form a fibrin clot; the initial step in this conversion results in the liberation of fibrinopep-tide A.

Thrombin and factor Xa are inactivated by antithrombin III bound to heparan sulfate molecules associated with the vascular endothelium, resulting in the formation of factor Xa-antithrombin III and thrombin-antithrombin III complexes. Protein C is activated by thrombin bound to the endothelial cell receptor thrombomodulin. Once activated, protein C functions as a potent anticoagulant by inactivating factors VIIIa and Va. Protein S enhances the binding of activated protein C to phospholipid-containing membranes and is able to accelerate the inactivation of factors VIIIa and Va by this enzyme. The complement component, C4b-binding protein (C4b-BP), forms complexes with protein S, which neutralizes its ability to serve as a cofactor for activated protein C in inactivating factors VIIIa and Va. Adapted with permission from Fig. 41.1 in Bauer KA. Inherited hypercoagulable states. In: Loscalzo J, Schafer AI, eds. Thrombosis and hemorrhage. Boston: Blackwell Scientific Publications, 1994;809–834 [96].)

The inherited thrombotic disorders (Table 24.1) have been almost exclusively associated with venous thrombosis. Whereas hereditary deficiencies of antithrombin III, protein C, or protein S will be found in fewer than 5% of unselected individuals with venous thromboembolism (Table 24.3), the likelihood of identifying these defects is increased several-fold by screening individuals with initial thrombosis occurring before age 50, by a family history of venous thromboembolism, and by recurrent venous thrombosis (3). Resistance to activated protein C (due to factor V Leiden), the prothrombin gene mutation, and hyperhomocysteinemia are more prevalent defects that can also be found in signifi-

cant numbers of individuals with first episodes of idiopathic venous thrombosis (that is, no apparent precipitating factor such as recent surgery or active malignancy) after age 50 in the absence of a positive family history (4–8). Testing for the presence of factor V Leiden, the prothrombin gene mutation, and hyperhomocysteinemia should be considered in such individuals.

Women with thrombosis in association with oral contraceptive use or pregnancy should also undergo thorough evaluation, because a significant percentage will have an inherited disorder, especially the factor V Leiden mutation (9–13). Individuals with venous thrombosis in uncommon sites such as the portal, hepatic, mes-

**TABLE 24.1.** Differential Diagnosis of the Individual Presenting with Thrombosis or a Thrombotic Diathesis

Inherited (primary) hypercoagulable states
  Activated protein C resistance due to factor V Leiden mutation
  Antithrombin III deficiency
  Protein C deficiency
  Protein S deficiency
  Prothrombin gene mutation (G to A transversion at position 20210 in the 3'-untranslated region)
  Dysfibrinogenemia (rare)
Acquired (secondary) hypercoagulable states
  In association with physiologic or thrombogenic stimuli
  Pregnancy (especially the postpartum period)
  Immobilization
  Trauma
  Postoperative state
  Advancing age
  Estrogen use
  Antiphospholipid syndrome or lupus anticoagulant
  In association with other clinical disorders (see Table 24.2)
Hyperhomocysteinemia

**TABLE 24.2.** Acquired Conditions and Disorders Associated with Hypercoagulable States

Pregnancy (and the postpartum period)
Immobilization
Trauma
Postoperative state
Advancing age
Estrogen administration associated with oral contraceptives, postmenopausal estrogens, treatment of prostate cancer with diethylstilbestrol
"Antiphospholipid syndrome" with or without overt systemic lupus erythematosus
Malignancy
  Disease-related includes migratory superficial thrombophlebitis (Trousseau's syndrome), nonbacterial thrombotic endocarditis, thrombosis associated with chronic disseminated intravascular coagulation, thrombotic microangiopathy
  Treatment-related associated with the administration of various chemotherapeutic agents (L-asparaginase, mitomycin, adjuvant programs for breast cancer)
Infusion of prothrombin complex concentrates
Nephrotic syndrome
Heparin-induced thrombocytopenia
Thrombotic thrombocytopenic purpura
Myeloproliferative disorders
Paroxysmal nocturnal hemoglobinuria
Hyperlipidemia
Diabetes mellitus
Hyperviscosity
Congestive heart failure

enteric, and cerebral veins should also undergo a complete laboratory evaluation. Interestingly, individuals with axillary vein thrombosis appear to have a low prevalence of hereditary defects, even in the absence of triggering risk factors (14). The presence of indwelling venous catheters is the most common risk factor today for upper extremity venous thrombosis, and individuals with this complication generally do not warrant evaluation for an underlying hypercoagulable state.

Although the aforementioned classification of individuals into hereditary or acquired categories is useful in directing the laboratory evaluation for hypercoagulability, it is simplistic in the sense that thrombosis frequently results from an interplay of genetic and acquired factors. Individuals with hereditary defects are at lifelong risk of developing thrombosis, and acquired stimuli (pregnancy, estrogen use, surgery) trigger thrombotic episodes in perhaps 50% of individuals. Also, defects in more than one coagulation protein are now being found in individuals with venous thrombosis due to the high background frequency in the general population of abnormalities such as factor V Leiden (6% in U.S. caucasians) (15) and the prothrombin gene mutation (2% in the Netherlands) (2). Such individuals have a more severe thrombotic diathesis than those with a

**TABLE 24.3.** Prevalence of Defects in Individuals with Venous Thrombosis

| | |
|---|---|
| Activated protein C resistance (factor V Leiden) | 12–40% |
| Deficiencies of antithrombin III, protein C, protein S | 5–15% |
| Prothrombin gene mutation (G to A transversion at position 20210 in the 3'-untranslated region) | 6–18% |
| Hyperhomocysteinemia | 10–20% |
| Unknown | ~15–66% |

**FIGURE 24.2.** Venous thrombosis can be viewed as a multigene disorder in which susceptible individuals will have one or more genetic mutations. Clinical events often occur when they are exposed to exogenous prothrombotic stimuli. (Modified from Fig. 2 in Schafer AI. Hypercoagulable states: Molecular genetics to clinical practice [Review]. Lancet 1994;344:1739–1742.)

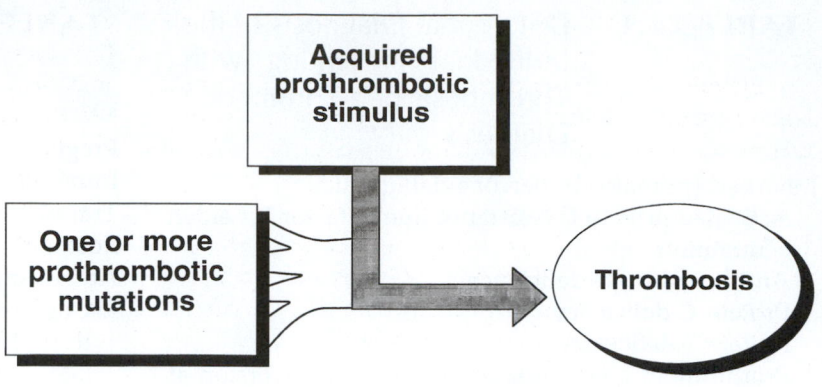

single identifiable mutation (8, 16–21). Thus, thrombosis can be viewed as a multigene disorder in which susceptible individuals will have one or more genetic mutations, with clinical events occurring when they are exposed to exogenous prothrombotic stimuli (22) (Fig. 24.2). In many cases however, the inciting precipitant to thrombosis is not reported by the individual and is therefore subclinical.

## HISTORY AND PHYSICAL EXAMINATION

A complete history is mandatory in evaluating individuals with a recent or remote history of thrombosis. Details should be obtained regarding the age of onset, location of prior thromboses, and results of objective diagnostic studies documenting thrombotic episodes. The latter is critical, as the clinical diagnosis of deep vein thrombosis, in particular, is notoriously inaccurate (see Chapter 25 ). The individual should be carefully questioned about circumstances near the time of thrombosis that might have precipitated the event. These include surgical procedures, trauma, pregnancy, immobility, or estrogen administration. Women should be questioned carefully regarding prior use of oral contraceptives or hormone replacement therapy and obstetric history. An increased risk of recurrent fetal loss is associated with the presence of lupus anticoagulants or antiphospholipid antibodies, as well as the hereditary thrombotic disorders (23–26). A family history is particularly important, as a well-documented history of venous thrombosis in one or more first-degree relatives strongly suggests the presence of a hereditary defect. The initial manifestation of a malignancy can be a thrombotic event, so inquiry should be made regarding the presence of constitutional symptoms (such as diminished appetite, weight loss, fatigue), pain, hematochezia, hemoptysis, or hematuria. It should be ascertained whether the individual has an underlying disease (cancer, collagen-vascular disease, a myeloproliferative disorder, atherosclerotic disease, nephrotic syndrome), or takes medications (synthetic or natural estrogens, or drugs that can induce lupus antico-

agulants such as hydralazine, procainamide, and phenothiazines). Recurrent thrombosis in spite of therapeutic anticoagulation with oral anticoagulants is common in individuals with an occult neoplasm or recurrent cancer.

In the general physical examination, special attention should be directed to the vascular system, extremities (for example, looking for signs of superficial or deep venous thrombosis), chest, heart, abdominal organs, and skin (necrosis, livedo reticularis). As venous thromboembolism may be the first manifestation of an underlying malignancy, rectal examination and stool testing for occult blood should be done and women should undergo a pelvic examination.

The hereditary thrombotic disorders include deficiencies of antithrombin III, protein C or protein S, resistance to activated protein C due to factor V Leiden, the prothrombin gene mutation, and rare dysfibrinogenemias. The most common sites of thrombosis in such individuals are the deep leg veins, iliac veins, and pulmonary arteries. Thrombosis in mesenteric, portal, and cerebral veins as well as superficial thrombophlebitis has been described in some series of individuals with these disorders. Typical precipitating factors for thrombosis in such individuals include the postoperative state, immobilization, trauma, pregnancy, oral contraceptive use, and advancing age.

Individuals with thrombosis should be questioned regarding their ethnic background. Factor V Leiden is not found in aboriginal African, American Indian, or Asian populations (27), and a recent study determined that this mutation only arose approximately 30,000 years ago among caucasians in Europe (28). This information should be considered when determining whether individuals should be tested for this abnormality.

## LABORATORY EVALUATION

### ROUTINE LABORATORY TESTS

The initial laboratory evaluation for individuals with thrombosis should include a complete blood count, review of the peripheral blood smear, and serum chemistries including liver and renal function tests, and urinalysis.

Elevations in hematocrit or platelet count should lead to consideration of polycythemia vera and essential thrombocythemia in the differential diagnosis. These myeloproliferative disorders clearly predispose individuals to venous as well as arterial thrombotic events, particularly when the hematocrit or platelet count is not controlled by therapy. In addition, secondary polycythemia or secondary (reactive) thrombocytosis may provide a clue to an underlying occult neoplasm that may itself be the predisposing factor to thrombosis. Leukopenia and thrombocytopenia are often found in paroxysmal nocturnal hemoglobinuria, a rare hematologic disorder characterized by chronic intravascular hemolysis with episodes of gross hematuria and a unique constellation of thrombotic complications. These occur almost exclusively in the abdominal venous network, including the mesenteric, hepatic, portal, splenic, and renal veins, and the cerebral venous circulation. The development of thrombosis and thrombocytopenia concurrent with heparin administration should always prompt consideration of the diagnosis of heparin-induced thrombocytopenia.

If the blood smear shows evidence of red cell fragmentation or schistocytes, the differential diagnosis includes disseminated intravascular coagulation (DIC) and the thrombotic microangiopathies (thrombotic thrombocytopenic purpura/hemolytic-uremic syndrome). Although bleeding is the most common coagulation problem in DIC, individuals with malignancy can have a low-grade consumptive coagulopathy and can develop venous or arterial thrombosis. The latter can result from emboli arising from fibrin vegetations on the mitral or aortic valves (nonbacterial thrombotic endocarditis). A leukoerythroblastic picture with nucleated red blood cells or immature white cells on the peripheral smear should suggest the possibility of bone marrow involvement by tumor.

Individuals with Budd-Chiari syndrome, which occurs when there is obstruction of the hepatic venous circulation, have ascites and hepatomegaly along with abnormal liver function tests. The nephrotic syndrome is characterized by large amounts of protein in the urine, hypoalbuminemia, and hyperlipidemia. Renal vein thrombosis can complicate the course of up to one-third of such individuals, but individuals with nephrotic syndrome are prone as well to venous thrombosis in distant, common sites (such as leg veins and pulmonary arteries).

Individuals with thrombosis should routinely undergo baseline coagulation tests, including prothrombin time and activated partial thromboplastin time (aPTT). If the reagent used for the latter test is sensitive to the presence of lupus anticoagulants, this will provide an initial screen for this acquired abnormality. If the aPTT is normal, the use of additional specialized clotting assays (e.g., dilute Russell viper venom time, kaolin clotting time, and the tissue thromboplastin inhibition test) may facilitate making this diagnosis in individuals clinically suspected of having a lupus anticoagulant (see Chapters 26 and 38). Some, but not all, individuals with lupus anticoagulants have elevated titers of anticardiolipin antibodies, and this serologic test should be ordered in individuals suspected of having this acquired defect. Individuals with abnormal test results should be re-evaluated, as lupus anticoagulants or elevated anticardiolipin antibody levels are generally considered to be risk factors for thrombosis only if the abnormalities persist over several months.

## TESTS FOR SPECIFIC BIOLOGICAL RISK FACTORS

Based on the history and physical examination, a decision must be made as to whether testing should be performed to identify specific biological risk factors predisposing to thrombosis. Clinical judgment must be exercised with regard to the scope of the evaluation as well as the optimal time for its performance. The decision regarding which tests should be ordered is determined partly by the type of thrombotic event (Table 24.4). Hereditary deficiencies of antithrombin III, protein C, and protein S and activated protein C resistance due to the factor V Leiden mutation have been shown to predispose principally to venous thrombosis. Although anecdotal reports suggest an association between arterial thrombosis and the inherited thrombotic disorders (particularly protein S deficiency), it is generally not recommended to test for these defects in such individuals. The presence of a lupus anticoagulant/elevated antiphospholipid antibody titer and hyperhomocysteinemia are risk factors for venous as well as arterial thrombosis. Therefore, testing for these two defects is warranted in the latter group of individuals, particularly when other factors predisposing to arterial thrombosis are absent.

Additional factors will guide the extent of the labora-

**TABLE 24.4.**   Sites of Thrombosis According to Coagulation Defect

| Abnormality | Arterial | Venous |
|---|---|---|
| Factor V Leiden | − | + |
| Antithrombin III deficiency | − | + |
| Protein C deficiency | − | + |
| Protein S deficiency | − | + |
| Prothrombin gene mutation | ? | + |
| Hyperhomocysteinemia | + | + |
| Lupus anticoagulant/ antiphospholipid syndrome | + | + |

tory evaluation (see Differential Diagnosis, above). As discussed above, clinical features that increase the likelihood of identifying individuals with deficiencies of antithrombin III, protein C, and protein S include an initial venous thrombotic event before age 50, recurrent thrombosis, or positive family history. These features also increase the chances of identifying individuals with factor V Leiden and the prothrombin gene mutation, although these genetic defects frequently can be identified in older individuals with an initial episode of deep venous thrombosis who do not have acquired risk factors or a positive family history. It is also warranted to screen for all of these defects, hyperhomocysteinemia, and antiphospholipid syndrome/lupus anticoagulant in individuals with thrombosis in unusual vascular beds, for example, portal, hepatic, or mesenteric vein thrombosis or cerebral venous thrombosis.

Some clinical features have been associated with individual hereditary thrombotic disorders. Approximately one-third of individuals who sustain the rare complication of warfarin-induced skin necrosis will have underlying protein C deficiency; however, this syndrome has also been reported in individuals with protein S deficiency (29) and factor V Leiden (30). In newborn infants, the development of skin necrosis and visceral thrombosis (neonatal purpura fulminans) indicates a likely diagnosis of severe hereditary protein C deficiency, although cases have been reported in association with homozygous protein S deficiency as well (31, 32). Both conditions require emergent therapy if major morbidity or mortality in neonatal purpura fulminans is to be averted (see below). Although resistance to heparin's anticoagulant effect, as measured by the aPTT, often leads to consideration of antithrombin III deficiency, congenital antithrombin III deficiency is infrequently diagnosed in such individuals.

Table 24.5 gives a list of tests useful in screening individuals suspected of having a biological defect predisposing to thrombosis. These tests are described in further detail in Chapter 26. Coagulation assays with high sensitivity and specificity for the factor V Leiden mutation are now widely available and are based on the resistance of the mutant factor Va molecule to inactivation by activated protein C. Testing for the factor V Leiden mutation can also be done by analyzing DNA obtained from peripheral blood mononuclear cells. Testing for hyperhomocysteinemia should be done after an overnight fast when the individual is consuming a normal diet. Measuring increments in total plasma homocysteine 4–8 hours after an oral methionine load as well as fasting levels facilitates the identification of approximately 10% more hyperhomocystinemic individuals and improves discrimination of affected subjects from controls. The homocysteine measurements are performed using ion-exchange chromatography, gas chromatography-mass

**TABLE 24.5.** Screening Laboratory Evaluation for Individuals Suspected of Having a Biological Defect Predisposing to Thrombosis

Test for resistance to activated protein C
    Clotting assay*
    Genetic test for factor V-Arg506Gln (factor V Leiden)
Measurement of total plasma homocysteine
Genetic test for prothrombin gene mutation (G to A transversion at position 20210 in the 3'-untranslated region)
Functional assay of antithrombin III (heparin-cofactor assay)*
Functional assays of protein C*
Functional assay of protein S/immunological assays of total and free protein S*
Screen for dysfibrinogenemias (immunologic and functional assays of fibrinogen, thrombin time)*
Clotting assay for lupus anticoagulant*/serologic tests for antiphospholipid antibodies

*Coagulation assays are performed on platelet-poor plasma obtained from blood samples drawn into a solution containing 3.8% (wt/vol) sodium citrate. The ratio of anticoagulant to blood is 0.1:0.9 (vol/vol). In the absence of an accompanying clinical history for the individual, the performance of a prothombin time will help to exclude the ingestion of warfarin, which will affect the measurements of protein C, protein S, and "first generation" aPTT-based assays for activated protein C-resistance. Performance of a thombin time, as well as an aPTT, will help to exclude the administration of heparin.*

spectrometry, or high-performance liquid chromatography with electrochemical or fluorescent detection.

The best screening tests for deficiencies of antithrombin III, protein C, and protein S are functional assays that detect both quantitative and qualitative defects. Immunologic (antigenic) assays detect only quantitative deficiencies of these proteins. For plasma antithrombin III, convenient functional assays are available that measure the heparin cofactor activity of the molecule. Among protein C assays, coagulation assays provide a more complete evaluation of the functional activity of the molecule than amidolytic assays. However, coagulation assays for protein C as well as protein S can give falsely low values if the factor V Leiden mutation is present, and reliable application of these assays must initially assess whether this mutation is present (33). Because factor V Leiden is much more commonly encountered than deficiencies of protein C or protein S, clinical laboratories often resort to measuring protein C activity by amidolytic assay and only perform immunoassays for total and free protein S. It is important to measure free protein S, as some individuals with hereditary protein S deficiency have low free levels with normal or borderline total protein S levels. To screen for a dysfibrinogenemia, the thrombin time is recommended along with measurements of plasma fibrinogen by clotting and immunologic assay.

## TIMING OF LABORATORY TESTING

An important consideration in the laboratory evaluation of individuals with a suspected deficiency of antithrombin III, protein C, or protein S is the timing of testing. Erroneous diagnoses can be made due to the influence of acute thrombosis, comorbid illness, or anticoagulant therapy on the levels of these plasma proteins. Table 24.6 provides a list of some of the common causes of acquired deficiencies of antithrombin III, protein C, or protein S.

Acute thrombosis by itself can result in transiently reduced levels of antithrombin III and, occasionally, protein C and protein S. Heparin therapy can be associated with an up to 30% decline in plasma antithrombin III levels over several days, whereas warfarin produces a drop in the functional activity of protein C and protein S and a lesser decline in immunologic levels. Warfarin has also been shown rarely to elevate antithrombin III levels significantly, sometimes into the normal range, in individuals with a hereditary deficiency of this inhibitor. For these reasons, it is optimal to test for these deficiency states at least 2 weeks after completing the initial 3- to 6-month course of oral anticoagulant therapy after a thrombotic event. If, upon acute presentation, levels of

antithrombin III, protein C, or protein S are obtained that are well within the normal range, diagnosis of these deficiency states will have been excluded from consideration. However, the finding of a low level during this period will need to be confirmed by repeat testing after anticoagulation is discontinued. The investigation of first degree family members is useful to document the hereditary nature of the deficiency. Confirmation of a deficiency state in first degree family members is particularly helpful diagnostically in individuals in whom the risks of recurrent thrombosis are too great to temporarily discontinue anticoagulation. In such individuals, a diagnosis of protein C or protein S can be confirmed by carrying out testing after warfarin has been discontinued for 2 weeks under the cover of intravenous or subcutaneous heparin at therapeutic doses.

The original ("first generation") aPTT-based activated protein C resistance tests were sensitive to the choice of reagents (aPTT reagent, activated protein C, $CaCl_2$ concentration), instrument used for clot detection, and preanalytical conditions (centrifugation, plasma storage conditions, fresh or frozen samples). Based on the choice of methodology, certain acquired conditions (for example, elevated factor VIII levels, pregnancy, oral contraceptive use) could result in the phenotype of activated protein C resistance, although it is not known whether this confers an increased risk of thrombosis. The original tests also could not be used to test individuals with lupus anticoagulants or those receiving heparin or oral anticoagulants because of the increased sensitivity of such plasmas to activated protein C. The discovery that the activated protein C resistance phenotype is frequently due to the factor V Leiden mutation led to modifications in the original aPTT-based activated protein C resistance tests and prediluted individual's plasma in factor V-deficient plasma. Such "second generation" clotting assays have high sensitivity and specificity for the factor V Leiden mutation and can be used reliably in individuals taking anticoagulants as well as for most of the acquired conditions noted above.

## OTHER COAGULATION ABNORMALITIES

There has been renewed interest in elevated plasma factor VIII coagulant activity (VIII:C) as an independent marker of increased thrombotic risk. In a population-based case control study performed in the Netherlands, 25% of individuals had levels of factor VIII coagulant activity (VIII:C) that were greater than 150% of normal, and they had an adjusted odds ratio of 4.8 for a first episode of venous thrombosis event as compared to individuals with levels under 100% (34). Elevated VIII:C levels were also found in a similar proportion of English individuals referred for evaluation of unexplained thrombosis (35). This laboratory abnormality could not be attributed to overt inflammation, as fewer than 10%

---

**TABLE 24.6.**   Causes of Acquired Deficiencies in Antithrombin III, Protein C, and Protein S

| Antithrombin III | Protein C | Protein S |
|---|---|---|
| Neonatal period | Neonatal period | Neonatal period |
| Pregnancy | | Pregnancy |
| Liver disease | Liver disease | Liver disease |
| DIC | DIC | DIC |
| Nephrotic syndrome | Chemotherapy (CMF)* | |
| Major surgery | | Inflammatory states |
| Acute thrombosis | Acute thrombosis | Acute thrombosis |
| *Treatment with:* | | |
| Heparin | Warfarin | Warfarin |
| L-asparaginase | L-asparaginase | L-asparaginase |
| Estrogens | Estrogens | Estrogens |

\* *CMF, cyclophosphamide, methotrexate, 5-fluorouracil.*

of individuals with VIII:C levels greater than 150% had elevations in acute phase reactants such as C-reactive protein, fibrinogen, and erythrocyte sedimentation rate. The levels of VIII:C were in reasonable concordance with factor VIII antigen concentrations, and it was postulated that the elevations result from a constitutive increase in synthesis or an exaggerated response to minimal inflammation (35). Additional studies are required to determine the molecular basis underlying increased VIII:C concentrations and the clinical utility of measuring this parameter in individuals with thrombosis.

There have been reports of thrombosis in association with abnormalities in other coagulation or fibrinolytic system proteins. These include heparin cofactor II deficiency, plasminogen deficiency (either hypoplasminogenemias or dysplasminogenemias), factor XII deficiency, thrombomodulin mutations, and elevations in histidine-rich glycoprotein or plasminogen activator inhibitor-1. However, causal associations between these abnormalities and an increased risk of thrombosis have not been clearly defined. Thus, it is not currently recommended to test for these components.

# THROMBOSIS IN ASSOCIATION WITH MALIGNANCY

Cancer is one of the most common acquired risk factors for venous or arterial thrombosis (Table 24.2). The clinical manifestations that are attributable to the underlying neoplasm include deep venous thrombosis/pulmonary embolism, migratory superficial thrombophlebitis (Trousseau's syndrome), nonbacterial thrombotic endocarditis with arterial emboli, or thrombosis in the presence of chronic disseminated intravascular coagulation. Thrombosis can also be associated with the administration of various chemotherapeutic agents. The occurrence of a clinical picture of a thrombotic microangiopathy can be due to the cancer itself or antineoplastic treatment, especially mitomycin-C.

Although thrombosis is most commonly encountered in the setting of advanced disease, deep venous thrombosis or pulmonary embolism can be the first sign of malignancy. In previously healthy individuals presenting with a first episode of venous thrombosis, one should have a high index of suspicion for cancer as 10 to 20% of such individuals will have cancer diagnosed at presentation or within the ensuing 24 months (36–38). The most common sites of origin of cancer are the gastrointestinal tract, genitourinary organs, and lung. A complete medical history, physical examination including digital rectal examination and testing for fecal occult blood, pelvic examination in women, routine laboratory testing (complete blood count, chemistry panel including electrolytes, renal function tests, liver function tests, calcium, urinalysis), and chest radiograph should be performed in all individuals presenting with thrombosis. The presence of constitutional symptoms (weight loss, fatigue), unusual pain or bleeding, change in cough or hoarseness, or alterations in bowel or bladder habits warrants further diagnostic testing. It is controversial whether individuals with none of the aforementioned symptoms or signs of neoplasia should undergo more detailed investigation, including computed tomography or endoscopic evaluation. Although the literature contains studies indicating that up to 10% of individuals with initial venous thrombotic episodes will have early stage cancers that were not detected by routine testing, there are no current data showing that more aggressive diagnostic evaluation either leads to improved survival or is cost effective. The development of recurrent idiopathic thrombosis after an adequate initial course of anticoagulant therapy is even more worrisome for an underlying cancer and warrants a thorough diagnostic evaluation (37).

Although the treatment of acute thrombosis with heparin is usually effective in cancer individuals, some will have recurrences when they are switched to oral anticoagulants despite a therapeutic international normalized ratio (INR). This scenario is particularly characteristic of cancer individuals with metastatic or locally advanced disease that is refractory to antineoplastic therapy. Long-term anticoagulation with subcutaneous heparin at therapeutic doses is recommended to reduce the morbidity and mortality of thrombotic complications in such individuals.

# INDIVIDUALS WITH RECURRENT THROMBOSIS BUT NORMAL LABORATORY TESTS

Despite recent advances, there remains a substantial fraction of individuals in whom we cannot uncover hereditary or acquired risk factors predisposing to thrombosis even after detailed laboratory evaluation (Table 24.3). It is sometimes helpful for the clinician caring for such individuals to refer the individual to an appropriate specialist for review of the laboratory results and consideration of additional workup. Additional prothrombotic mutations will certainly be discovered in the next several years. Specialists will be knowledgeable as to the availability and relevance of new diagnostic developments before their commercial and wide clinical availability. In addition, some assays measure the extent of coagulation enzyme generation in the blood *in vivo* (for example, prothrombin activation fragment $F_{1+2}$, thrombin-antithrombin III complex, [Fig. 24.1]), although these assays do not give information regarding the specific type of hypercoagulable state that is present (39). Studies are ongoing to determine whether such markers will improve our ability to identify individuals who are destined to develop a clinically relevant hypercoagulable state.

# APPROACH TO MANAGEMENT AND TREATMENT OF ACUTE THROMBOSIS

The acute management of venous thrombosis or pulmonary embolism in individuals with biological risk factors for thrombosis is generally not different from that of other individuals. Thrombolytic therapy should be seriously considered in individuals with massive acute venous thrombosis or pulmonary embolism. Unfractionated heparin should be initiated, with an intravenous bolus of 5,000 U, followed by an infusion of 1400 U/hour (40), or if a weight-adjusted regimen is used, a bolus of 80 U/kg/body weight followed by an infusion of 18 U/kg/hour (41). The aPTT should be performed approximately 6 hours after therapy is initiated, and at least daily thereafter to maintain the aPTT in the therapeutic range. For many commercial aPTT reagents, this corresponds to an aPTT that is 1.8 to 3.0 times the mean of the normal range, or an antifactor Xa heparin level of 0.3 to 0.7 U/mL (42). For less sensitive aPTT reagents, the therapeutic aPPT ratio is 1.5 to 2.0 times normal (43). Alternatively low-molecular-weight heparin in therapeutic doses can be administered, which obviates the need for monitoring the aPTT. Warfarin can be started within the first 24 hours. Heparin, or low-molecular-weight heparin, is continued for at least 5 days (44) or until the prothrombin time is in the therapeutic range, namely an INR of 2.0 to 3.0. The principles of anticoagulation are described in further detail in Chapter 55.

Individuals with antithrombin III deficiency can usually be treated successfully with intravenous heparin (45), although in some situations higher than usual doses of the drug are required to achieve adequate anticoagulation. In antithrombin III-deficient individuals receiving heparin for the treatment of acute thrombosis, the adjunctive role of antithrombin III concentrate purified from human plasma (see Chapter 52) is not clearly defined, as controlled trials have not been done (45, 46). This product should probably be administered when difficulty is encountered in achieving adequate heparinization, or when recurrent thrombosis is observed despite adequate anticoagulation. It is also reasonable to treat antithrombin III-deficient subjects with concentrate before major surgeries or in obstetrical situations when the risks of bleeding from anticoagulation are unaccept-

able. The manufacturing processes used to prepare antithrombin III concentrate result in a product that is more than 95% pure; they also inactivate the hepatitis B virus and human immunodeficiency virus-I (47, 48). Hence, it is preferable to administer antithrombin III concentrate rather than fresh frozen plasma.

The infusion of 50 U of antithrombin III concentrate per kilogram of body weight (1 U is defined as the amount of antithrombin III in 1 mL of pooled normal human plasma) will usually raise the plasma antithrombin III level to approximately 120% in a congenitally deficient individual with a baseline level of 50% (48–52). Plasma levels should be monitored to ensure that they remain above 80%; the administration of 60% of the initial dose at 24-hour intervals is recommended to maintain inhibitor levels in the normal range (52).

Due to the infrequent occurrence of warfarin-induced skin necrosis, it may be advisable to take special precautions when initiating oral anticoagulant treatment in a individual who is previously known or likely to have protein C deficiency. Warfarin should be started when the individual is fully heparinized, and the dose of the drug should be increased gradually, starting from a relatively low level (for example, 2 mg for the first 3 days, then in increasing amounts of 2 to 3 mg until therapeutic anticoagulation is achieved). Individuals with heterozygous protein C deficiency and a history of warfarin-induced skin necrosis have been successfully retreated with oral anticoagulants. Here, protein C administration, either in the form of fresh frozen plasma or protein C concentrate, provides protection against the development of recurrent skin necrosis until a stable level of anticoagulation is achieved (53, 54).

# LONG-TERM MANAGEMENT

After an initial episode of venous thrombosis or pulmonary embolism, individuals are usually continued on oral anticoagulants for 3 to 6 months at an INR of 2.0 to 3.0, as clinical trials have established the efficacy of this regimen for preventing early recurrences. Recent data indicate that the risk of recurrence is greater in individuals with permanent as opposed to temporary risk factors for thrombosis (55, 56). In individuals with inherited thrombophilia, it is reasonable to continue warfarin for at least 6 months for those without an identifiable exogenous triggering insult (such as surgery, pregnancy, etc.) for thrombosis.

After 6 months of anticoagulant treatment for an acute thrombotic event, an assessment must be made as to the relative benefit conferred by long-term anticoagulant therapy in preventing future thromboembolic complications vs. the potential side effects, cost, and inconvenience for the individual. Unfortunately, there are little reliable data regarding the true magnitude of the thrombotic risk in unselected individuals with deficiencies of antithrombin III, protein C, or protein S, as these are relatively uncommon disorders.

Cross-sectional studies of selected kindreds with thrombosis in association with heterozygous deficiencies of antithrombin III, protein C, and protein S have given estimates of the cumulative risk of thrombosis as a function of age. The risk is extremely low until about age 15, and then occurs at a rate of approximately 2 to 4% per year. Cross-sectional studies of family members of unselected individuals with these defects indicate that the rate of spontaneous and induced venous thrombosis is lower at 0.41% and 0.52% per year, respectively (57). Many clinicians with experience in managing individuals with these disorders feel that individuals with congenital antithrombin III deficiency (particularly type I defects) are at higher thrombotic risk than those with other defects.

Due to the relatively high frequency of the factor V Leiden mutation in individuals with a first episode of venous thrombosis, reliable data have recently shown their recurrence risk. Two studies have found a significant increase. Among 77 men in the Physicians' Health Study with a first episode of idiopathic venous thromboembolism followed up for an average of 68 months, the rate of recurrent venous thromboembolism in factor V Leiden heterozygotes was fourfold to fivefold higher than in genetically unaffected men (4/14 = 29%, incidence rate of 7.5%/year vs. 7/63 = 11%, incidence rate of 1.82%/year, respectively) (58). In a second study of 251 Italian individuals with a first episode of deep vein thrombosis proven by venography, the cumulative incidence of recurrent venous thromboembolism after 8 years of follow-up was over twofold higher among 41 heterozygotes with factor V Leiden than in those without the mutation (39.7% vs. 18.3%) (59). Rintelen et al (60) and Eichinger et al (61) have not found an increased recurrence risk in heterozygotes with factor V Leiden, but the former study was retrospective and the latter included individuals who were followed up for shorter periods.

Although some of the aforementioned data indicate that recurrent venous thromboembolism occurs much more frequently in individuals with factor V Leiden and an initial idiopathic event, this does not necessarily imply that oral anticoagulant treatment should be prolonged beyond 3–6 months; its benefits may be counterbalanced by its hemorrhagic risk. Indeed, a recent trial of long-term warfarin therapy (INR 2–2.85) in individuals with a second venous thrombotic episode found that the drug was highly effective in preventing recurrences, as compared with 6 months of therapy (2.6% vs. 21% over 4 years), but there was a considerable price to pay in terms of major hemorrhage (8.6% vs. 2.3%, respectively) (62).

Prospective data are not currently available regarding the utility of extending oral anticoagulation beyond 3–6 months in individuals with biological risk factors for thrombosis. Therefore, only general guidelines for managing and treating such individuals can be offered (Table 24.7).

When a heterozygous individual with one of the hereditary thrombotic disorders is identified, family studies should be conducted, because approximately half of his or her first-degree relatives will be affected. Affected asymptomatic individuals should receive counseling regarding the implications of the diagnosis and advice regarding symptoms that require immediate medical attention. In women of childbearing age, oral contraceptives are contraindicated in view of the increased thrombotic risk associated with the use of these medications. Recent data indicate that estrogen replacement therapy can increase the risk of venous thrombosis by twofold to fourfold in perimenopausal and postmenopausal women (63–65), but there are not yet data available for women with specific hereditary thrombotic disorders. Thus, in making a decision as to whether to prescribe hormone replacement therapy to women with thrombotic histories, the potential for recurrence must be weighed against the benefits of the medication.

All individuals with biological risk factors for thrombosis should be carefully evaluated before surgical, medical, or obstetric procedures. They should then

**TABLE 24.7.**   Management of Biological Defects Predisposing to Thrombosis

| Risk Classification | Management |
|---|---|
| High risk | Indefinite anticoagulation |
| • Two or more spontaneous thromboses | |
| • One spontaneous life-threatening thrombosis | |
| • One spontaneous thrombosis at an unusual site (mesenteric or cerebral venous) | |
| • One spontaneous thrombosis in the presence of more than a single biological defect | |
| Moderate risk | Vigorous prophylaxis during high-risk situations |
| • One thrombosis with a prothrombotic stimulus | |
| • Asymptomatic | |

receive appropriate prophylactic anticoagulation regimens. If specific concentrates are available for the individual's deficiency state, these can also be administered to raise the plasma levels of the protein to the normal range during the perioperative period.

In individuals with or without an inherited thrombotic disorder, the occurrence of two or more spontaneously occurring thromboembolic episodes often leads to the continuation of oral anticoagulants for life. Chronic warfarin therapy is usually not recommended until an individual has had at least one documented thrombotic episode.

With regard to the issue of long-term warfarin therapy in other individuals with thrombosis recommendations must be individualized. The clinical features that should be considered along with the presence of biological risk factors include:

1. The severity and site of thrombosis; for example, a individual who previously sustained a massive pulmonary embolus is more likely to receive long-term warfarin than one who developed deep venous thrombosis in a calf vein, unless there are symptoms or signs of a significant postphlebitic syndrome; individuals with mesenteric, portal, or cerebral venous thrombosis are frequently anticoagulated indefinitely after diagnosis due to the potential morbidity or mortality of a recurrence at these sites.

2. Whether the thrombotic episodes were spontaneous, or whether triggering factors were present; for instance, if a precipitant such as a major abdominal operation was present, it would be reasonable to manage the individual without long-term oral anticoagulation after the acute episode was adequately treated.

3. Resolution of thrombosis; for example, if ultrasound was used to diagnose deep venous thrombosis, a follow-up study after 3–6 months of anticoagulant therapy can indicate whether the initial thrombus has completely resolved. The presence of persistent abnormalities suggests incomplete fibrinolysis of the clot and may prompt the physician to consider long-term anticoagulation. A baseline study after therapy is also useful in case the individual returns with symptoms of phlebitis in the same leg and ultrasound is to be used to document the recurrence.

4. In individuals with hereditary defects, a history of thromboembolism in other biochemically affected members of the family; for instance, although marked intrafamilial and interfamilial heterogeneity has been observed in the phenotypic expression of the inherited thrombotic disorders, it is not unreasonable to place asymptomatic, biochemically affected individuals from severely affected kindreds on oral anticoagulants starting at puberty.

5. The sex and lifestyle of the individual; situations where these factors may influence the decision-making process include: women of childbearing age planning to conceive, occupations that entail prolonged periods of immobilization that might be associated with an increased risk of thromboembolism, and jobs with a higher than average chance of trauma that might lead to thrombotic or bleeding complications.

# LUPUS ANTICOAGULANTS (SEE CHAPTER 38)

The management of acute venous thromboembolism in individuals with lupus anticoagulants is similar to that of individuals without this laboratory abnormality. However, the initial treatment is complicated by the fact that the baseline aPTT is often prolonged and cannot be used reliably to monitor unfractionated heparin dosing unless proper *in vitro* calibration studies are done by adding known amounts of heparin into plasma samples and measuring the dose response. Thus, it is preferable to monitor anticoagulant therapy in such individuals by measuring plasma heparin levels using either factor Xa or thrombin with an appropriate chromogenic substrate. Alternatively, low-molecular-weight heparin can be used in therapeutic doses, which will obviate the need for monitoring. The presence of lupus anticoagulants can also interfere with heparin monitoring during cardiac surgery (66). Warfarin is effective in this population, but the literature suggests that a higher than usual INR (3.0 to 4.5) is required to prevent recurrent thromboembolism (67, 68). The concurrent use of aspirin does not improve antithrombotic efficacy.

The clinical heterogeneity of the individual populations that develop lupus anticoagulants makes it difficult to generalize regarding their long-term antithrombotic management. Whereas the relationship between thrombosis and the lupus anticoagulant appears to be strong in individuals with systemic lupus erythematosus (69), the significance of the association in individuals without this disorder is more ambiguous (70). Indeed, individuals who develop transient lupus anticoagulants in association with infections do not usually sustain thromboembolic episodes, and it is unclear whether drug-associated lupus anticoagulants are associated with thrombosis. Thus, the presence of persistent lupus anticoagulant, a high-titer antiphospholipid antibody, or both in an asymptomatic individual with no prior thrombotic history is not currently an indication for anticoagulant or antiplatelet medications. However, inasmuch as it is not possible to determine reliably the risk of thrombosis in an asymptomatic individual with these laboratory abnormalities, all such individuals should receive appropriate prophylaxis in conjunction with major surgical procedures (71), prolonged immobilization, pregnancy, and the postpartum period unless there is a strong contraindication to such treatment. Corticosteroids can normalize clotting assay times or reduce antiphospholipid antibody titers in individuals with lupus anticoagulants. However, these and other immunosuppressive medications have not been proven to prevent recurrent thrombosis.

# MANAGEMENT OF PREGNANCY (SEE CHAPTER 46)

The management of pregnancies in women with thrombotic histories or hereditary thrombotic disorders poses special problems (72). The incidence of thrombotic complications during pregnancy and the postpartum period appears to be greater in women with antithrombin III deficiency than in those with deficiencies of protein C or protein S (73). The factor V Leiden mutation is frequently identified in Caucasian women with venous thromboembolism during pregnancy and the puerperium (11–13), but the thrombotic risk in asymptomatic women from the general population has not been defined. Pregnant women with factor V Leiden and a personal or familial history of thrombosis should, therefore, be considered for anticoagulant prophylaxis. Routine screening for the mutation in women of childbearing age is not recommended because the potential risks of anticoagulation may equal or exceed its benefits (74). During pregnancy, adjusted-dose unfractionated heparin administered by the subcutaneous route is the anticoagulant of choice because its efficacy and safety for the fetus are established (75). Low-molecular-weight heparin should prove an attractive alternative to unfractionated heparin in these individuals due to its better bioavailability and longer half-life. Individuals with a previous history of thrombotic episodes should definitely receive treatment throughout pregnancy, whereas affected women with antithrombin III deficiency who have not yet experienced such events should probably also receive treatment. Treatment of asymptomatic women with other hereditary thrombotic disorders should be considered on an individual basis.

The dose and duration of heparin therapy in pregnancy is uncertain, as appropriately designed clinical trials have not been performed in these individual populations. Individuals considered to be at high risk should receive full-dose heparin by subcutaneous injection every 12 hours for the duration of pregnancy. The dose of heparin should be adjusted to maintain the 6-hour postinjection-aPTT at 1.5 times the control value. In women considered to be at intermediate risk, lower doses of heparin can be used (5, 000 to 10, 000 U subcutaneously every 12 hours) and therapy can be started during the second or third trimester and continued for approximately 6 weeks into the postpartum period. Low-risk individuals can be observed closely throughout the pregnancy with duplex ultrasound imaging of the leg veins at regular intervals.

In women who are planning pregnancy while taking oral anticoagulants, several approaches can be taken to minimize the risk of both thrombotic complications and warfarin embryopathy. One is to stop warfarin and commence subcutaneous heparin therapy; this potentially exposes the individual to many months of heparin therapy and the risk of dose-related osteoporosis while she is trying to conceive. An approach in women with antithrombin III deficiency is to use antithrombin III concentrates until conception. This product, however, is costly and needs to be administered intravenously at frequent intervals. Finally, warfarin therapy could be continued with the performance of pregnancy tests on a frequent basis. As soon as pregnancy is diagnosed, and prior to the sixth week of gestation, oral anticoagulants must be discontinued and heparin therapy initiated. Although the risk of warfarin embryopathy appears to be small during the first 6 weeks of pregnancy (76), even so small a risk makes this the least preferable of the three approaches.

# MANAGEMENT OF WARFARIN-INDUCED SKIN NECROSIS AND NEONATAL PURPURA FULMINANS

An association has been established between the rare complication of warfarin-induced skin necrosis and hereditary protein C deficiency (53, 77–80) (see Chapters 43 and 55). About one-third of individuals with warfarin-induced skin necrosis will prove to have hereditary protein C deficiency (81). This complication has also been described in individuals with heterozygous protein S deficiency (29) and factor V Leiden (30).

Because warfarin-induced skin necrosis is a rare complication, therapy has been guided primarily by knowledge regarding its pathogenesis. The diagnosis should be suspected in individuals with painful, red skin lesions developing within a few days after the initiation of the drug, and immediate intervention is required to prevent rapid progression and to minimize complications. Therapy should consist of immediate discontinua tion of warfarin, administration of vitamin K, and infusion of heparin at therapeutic doses. Lesions, however, have been reported to progress despite adequate anticoagulation with heparin. In individuals with hereditary pro tein C deficiency, the administration of a source of protein C should be seriously considered. It may also be appropriate in other individuals with warfarin-induced skin necrosis, as they invariably have reduced plasma levels of functional protein C when the skin lesions first appear. Fresh frozen plasma has been used, but improved results can be expected with the administration of a highly purified protein C concentrate, which facilitates the rapid and complete normalization of plasma protein C levels (82).

The management of neonatal purpura fulminans in association with homozygous or doubly heterozygous protein C deficiency is more complicated, and heparin therapy as well as antiplatelet agents have not been shown to be effective (83–88) (see Chapter 47). The administration of a source of protein C appears to be critical in the initial treatment of these individuals. Fresh frozen plasma has been used with success to treat these infants. However, the half-life of protein C in the circulation is only about 6 to 16 hours (89, 90), and the administration of plasma on a frequent basis is limited by the development of hyperproteinemia, hypertension, loss of venous access, and the potential for exposure to infectious viral agents. A highly purified concentrate of protein C has been developed and is efficacious in treating neonatal purpura fulminans (91). Warfarin has been administered to these infants without the redevelopment of skin necrosis during the phased withdrawal of fresh frozen plasma infusions (83, 86, 92–94), and this medication has been used chronically to control the thrombotic diathesis. Successful liver transplantation undertaken in a child with liver failure and homozygous protein C deficiency resulted in normalization of the plasma protein C level and resolution of the thrombotic diathesis (95).

# REFERENCES

1. Dahlbäck B. Physiological anticoagulation. Resistance to activated protein C and venous thromboembolism [Review]. J Clin Invest 1994;94:923–927.
2. Poort SR, Rosendaal FR, Reitsma PH et al. A common genetic variation in the 3′-untranslated region of the prothrombin gene is associated with elevated plasma prothrombin levels and an increase in venous thrombosis. Blood 1996;88:3698–3703.
3. Heijboer H, Brandjes DP, Buller HR et al. Deficiencies of coagulation-inhibiting and fibrinolytic proteins in outindividuals with deep-vein thrombosis. N Engl J Med 1990;323:1512–1516.
4. Koster T, Rosendaal FR, de Ronde H et al. Venous thrombosis due to poor anticoagulant response to activated protein C: Leiden Thrombophilia Study. Lancet 1993;342:1503–1506.
5. Ridker PM, Glynn RJ, Miletich JP et al. Age-specific incidence rates of venous thromboembolism among heterozygous carriers of factor V Leiden mutation. Ann Intern Med 1997;126:528–531.
6. Selhub J, Jacques PF, Wilson PW et al. Vitamin status and intake as primary determinants of homocysteinemia in an elderly population. JAMA 1993;270:2693–2698.
7. Den Heijer M, Koster T, Blom HJ et al. Hyperhomocysteinemia as a risk factor for deep-vein thrombosis. N Engl J Med 1996;334:759–762.
8. Ridker PM, Hennekens CH, Selhub J et al. Interrelation of hyperhomocyst(e)inemia, factor V Leiden, and risk of future venous thromboembolism. Circulation 1997;95:1777–1782.
9. Vandenbroucke JP, Koster T, Bri't E et al. Increased risk of venous thrombosis in oral-contraceptive users who are carriers of factor V Leiden mutation. Lancet 1994;344:1453–1457.
10. Bloemenkamp KW, Rosendaal FR, Helmerhorst FM et al. Enhancement by factor V Leiden mutation of risk of deep-vein thrombosis associated with oral contraceptives containing a third-generation progestagen. Lancet 1995;346:1593–1596.
11. Hellgren M, Svensson PJ, Dahlbäck B. Resistance to activated protein C as a basis for venous thromboembolism associated with pregnancy and oral contraceptives. Am J Obstet Gynecol 1995;173:210–213.
12. De Stefano V, Mastrangelo S, Paciaroni K et al. Thrombotic risk during pregnancy and puerperium in women with APC-resistance-effective subcutaneous heparin prophylaxis in a pregnant individual [Letter]. Thromb Haemost 1995;74:793–794.
13. Bokarewa MI, Bremme K, Blombäck M. Arg$^{506}$-Gln mutation in factor V and risk of thrombosis during pregnancy. Br J Haematol 1996;92:473–478.
14. Martinelli I, Cattaneo M, Panzeri D et al. Risk factors for deep venous thrombosis of the upper extremities. Ann Intern Med 1997;126:707–711.
15. Ridker PM, Hennekens CH, Lindpaintner K et al. Mutation in the gene coding for coagulation factor V and the risk of myocardial infarction, stroke, and venous thrombosis in apparently healthy men. N Engl J Med 1995;332:912–917.
16. Koeleman BP, Reitsma PH, Allaart CF et al. Activated protein C resistance as an additional risk factor for thrombosis in protein C-deficient families. Blood 1994;84:1031–1035.
17. Gandrille S, Greengard JS, Alhenc-Gelas M et al. Incidence of activated protein C resistance caused by the ARG 506 GLN mutation in factor V in 113 unrelated symptomatic protein C-deficient individuals. The French Network on the behalf of INSERM. Blood 1995;86:219–224.
18. Koeleman BP, van Rumpt D, Hamulyak K et al. Factor V Leiden: An additional risk factor for thrombosis in protein S deficient families? Thromb Haemost 1995;74:580–583.
19. Zöller B, Berntsdotter A, Garcia de Frutos P et al. Resistance to activated protein C as an additional genetic risk factor in hereditary deficiency of protein S. Blood 1995;85:3518–3523.
20. van Boven HH, Reitsma PH, Rosendaal FR et al. Factor V Leiden (FV R506Q) in families with inherited antithrombin deficiency. Thromb Haemost 1996;75:417–421.
21. Cattaneo M, Tsai MY, Bucciarelli P et al. A common mutation in the methylenetetrahydrofolate reductase gene (C677T) increases the risk for deep-vein thrombosis in individuals with mutant factor V (Factor V:Q$^{506}$). Arterioscler Thromb Vasc Biol 1997;17. In press.
22. Schafer AI. Hypercoagulable states: Molecular genetics to clinical practice [Review]. Lancet 1994;344:1739–1742.
23. Preston FE, Rosendaal FR, Walker ID et al. Increased fetal loss in women with heritable thrombophilia. Lancet 1996;348:913–916.
24. Rai R, Regan L, Hadley E et al. Second-trimester pregnancy loss is associated with activated protein C resistance. Br J Haematol 1996;92:489–490.
25. Sanson BJ, Friederich PW, Simioni P et al. The risk of abortion and stillbirth in antithrombin-, protein C-, and protein S-deficient women. Thromb Haemost 1996;75:387–388.
26. Grandone E, Margaglione M, Colaizzo D et al. Factor V Leiden is associated with repeated and recurrent unexplained fetal losses. Thromb Haemost 1997;77:822–824.
27. Rees DC, Cox M, Clegg JB. World distribution of factor V Leiden. Lancet 1995;346:1133–1134.
28. Zivelin A, Griffin JH, Xu X et al. A single genetic origin for a common Caucasian risk factor for venous thrombosis. Blood 1997;89:397–402.
29. Friedman KD, Marlar RA, Houston JG et al. Warfarin-induced skin necrosis in a individual with protein S deficiency [Abstract]. Blood 1986;68 (suppl 1):333a.
30. Makris M, Bardhan G, Preston FE. Warfarin induced skin necrosis associated with activated protein C resistance [Letter]. Thromb Haemost 1996;75:523–524.
31. Mahasandana C, Suvatte V, Chuansumrit A et al. Homozygous protein S deficiency in an infant with purpura fulminans. J Pediatr 1990;117:750–753.
32. Pegelow CH, Ledford M, Young JN et al. Severe protein S deficiency in a newborn [Review]. Pediatrics 1992;89:674–676.
33. Faioni EM, Franchi F, Asti D et al. Resistance to activated protein C in nine thrombophilic families: Interference in a protein S functional assay. Thromb Haemost 1993;70:1067–1071.
34. Koster T, Blann AD, Bri't E et al. Role of clotting factor VIII in effect of von Willebrand factor on occurrence of deep-vein thrombosis. Lancet 1995;345:152–155.
35. O'Donnell J, Tuddenham EGD, Manning R et al. High prevalence of elevated factor VIII levels in individuals referred for thrombophilia screening: Role of increased synthesis and relationship to the acute phase reaction. Thromb Haemost 1997;77:825–828.
36. Monreal M, Lafoz E, Casals A et al. Occult cancer in individuals with deep venous thrombosis. A systematic approach. Cancer 1991;67:541–545.
37. Prandoni P, Lensing AW, Buller HR et al. Deep-vein thrombosis and the incidence of subsequent symptomatic cancer. N Engl J Med 1992;327:1128–1133.
38. Cornuz J, Pearson SD, Creager MA et al. Importance of findings on the initial evaluation for cancer in individuals with symptomatic idiopathic deep venous thrombosis. Ann Intern Med 1996;125:785–793.
39. Bauer KA, Weitz JI. Laboratory markers of coagulation and fibrinolysis.

In: Colman RW, Hirsh J, Marder V, Salzman E, eds. Hemostasis and thrombosis. Basic principles and practice. 3d ed. Philadelphia: J.B. Lippincott Company, 1994;1197–1210.

40. Cruickshank MK, Levine MN, Hirsh J et al. A standard heparin nomogram for the management of heparin therapy. Arch Intern Med 1991;151: 333–337.

41. Raschke RA, Reilly BM, Guidry JR et al. The weight-based heparin dosing nomogram compared with a "standard care" nomogram. A randomized controlled trial. Ann Intern Med 1993;119:874–881.

42. Brill-Edwards P, Ginsberg JS, Johnston M et al. Establishing a therapeutic range for heparin therapy. Ann Intern Med 1993;119:104–109.

43. Bjornsson TD, Nash PV. Variability in heparin sensitivity of APTT reagents. Am J Clin Pathol 1986;86:199–204.

44. Hull RD, Raskob GE, Rosenbloom D et al. Heparin for 5 days as compared with 10 days in the initial treatment of proximal venous thrombosis. N Engl J Med 1990;322:1260–1264.

45. Schulman S, Tengborn L. Treatment of venous thromboembolism in individuals with congenital deficiency of antithrombin III. Thromb Haemost 1992;68:634–636.

46. Lechner K, Kyrle PA. Antithrombin III concentrates-are they clinically useful [Review]? Thromb Haemost 1995;73:340–348.

47. Hoffman DL. Purification and large-scale preparation of antithrombin III. Am J Med 1989;87:23S–26S.

48. Menache D, O'Malley JP, Schorr JB et al. Evaluation of the safety, recovery, half-life, and clinical efficacy of antithrombin III (human) in individuals with hereditary antithrombin III deficiency. Cooperative Study Group. Blood 1990;75:33–39.

49. Mannucci PM, Boyer C, Wolf M et al. Treatment of congenital antithrombin III deficiency with concentrates. Br J Haematol 1982;50:531–535.

50. Winter JH, Fenech A, Bennett B et al. Transfusion studies in individuals with familial antithrombin III (ATIII) deficiency: Half disappearance time of infused ATIII and influence of such infusion on platelet life-span. Br J Haematol 1981;49:449–453.

51. Brandt P. Observations during the treatment of antithrombin III deficient women with heparin and antithrombin concentrate during pregnancy, parturition, and abortion. Thromb Res 1981;22:15–24.

52. Schwartz RS, Bauer KA, Rosenberg RD et al. Clinical experience with antithrombin III concentrate in treatment of congenital and acquired deficiency of antithrombin. The Antithrombin III Study Group [Review]. Am J Med 1989;87:53S–60S.

53. Zauber NP, Stark MW. Successful warfarin anticoagulation despite protein C deficiency and a history of warfarin necrosis. Ann Intern Med 1986;104: 659–660.

54. De Stefano V, Mastrangelo S, Schwarz HP et al. Replacement therapy with a purified protein C concentrate during initiation of oral anticoagulation in severe protein C congenital deficiency. Thromb Haemost 1993;70:247–249.

55. Schulman S, Rhedin AS, Lindmarker P et al. A comparison of six weeks with six months of oral anticoagulant therapy after a first episode of venous thromboembolism. Duration of Anticoagulation Trial Study Group. N Engl J Med 1995;332:1661–1665.

56. Levine MN, Hirsh J, Gent M et al. Optimal duration of oral anticoagulant therapy: A randomized trial comparing four weeks with three months of warfarin in individuals with proximal deep vein thrombosis. Thromb Haemost 1995;74:606–611.

57. Friederich PW, Scudeller A, Sanson BJ et al. The incidence of venous thromboembolism and superficial-vein thrombosis in ATIII-, protein S, and protein C-deficient subjects [Abstract]. Thromb Haemost 1995;73:1262.

58. Ridker PM, Miletich JP, Stampfer MJ et al. Factor V Leiden and risks of recurrent idiopathic venous thromboembolism. Circulation 1995;92: 2800–2802.

59. Simioni P, Prandoni P, Lensing AW et al. The risk of recurrent venous thromboembolism in individuals with an Arg$^{506}$Gln mutation in the gene for factor V (factor V Leiden). N Engl J Med 1997;336:399–403.

60. Rintelen C, Pabinger I, Knöbl P et al. Probability of recurrence of thrombosis in individuals with and without factor V Leiden. Thromb Haemost 1996;75:229–232.

61. Eichinger S, Pabinger I, Schneider B et al. The risk of recurrent venous thromboembolism in individuals with and without factor V Leiden. Thromb Haemost 1997;77:624–628.

62. Schulman S, Granqvist S, Holmström M et al. The duration of oral anticoagulant therapy after a second episode of venous thromboembolism. The Duration of Anticoagulation Trial Study Group. N Engl J Med 1997;336: 393–398.

63. Daly E, Vessey MP, Hawkins MM et al. Risk of venous thromboembolism in users of hormone replacement therapy. Lancet 1996;348:977–980.

64. Jick H, Derby LE, Myers MW et al. Risk of hospital admission for idiopathic venous thromboembolism among users of postmenopausal oestrogens. Lancet 1996;348:981–983.

65. Grodstein F, Stampfer MJ, Goldhaber SZ et al. Prospective study of exogenous hormones and risk of pulmonary embolism in women. Lancet 1996; 348:983–987.

66. Wanger GP, Roberts W, Brandt J. Misleading heparin monitoring leading

67. Rosove MH, Brewer PM. Antiphospholipid thrombosis: Clinical course after the first thrombotic event in 70 individuals. Ann Intern Med 1992; 117:303–308.

68. Khamashta MA, Cuadrado MJ, Mujic F et al. The management of thrombosis in the antiphospholipid-antibody syndrome. N Engl J Med 1995;332: 993–997.

69. Long AA, Ginsberg JS, Brill-Edwards P et al. The relationship of antiphospholipid antibodies to thromboembolic disease in systemic lupus erythematosus: A cross-sectional study. Thromb Haemost 1991;66:520–524.

70. Love PE, Santoro SA. Antiphospholipid antibodies: Anticardiolipin and the lupus anticoagulant in systemic lupus erythematosus (SLE) and in non-SLE disorders. Prevalence and significance [Review]. Ann Int Med 1990;112:682–698.

71. Ahn SA, Kalunian K, Rosove M et al. Postoperative thrombotic complications in individuals with the lupus anticoagulant: Increased risk after vascular procedures. J Vasc Surg 1988;7:749–756.

72. Hirsh J, Piovella F, Pini M. Congenital antithrombin III deficiency. Incidence and clinical features [Review]. Am J Med 1989;87:34S–38S.

73. Conard J, Horellou MH, Van Dreden P et al. Thrombosis and pregnancy in congenital deficiencies in ATIII, protein C or protein S: Study of 78 women. Thromb Haemost 1990;63:319–320.

74. Vandenbroucke JP, van der Meer FJM, Helmerhorst FM et al. Factor V Leiden: Should we screen oral contraceptive users and pregnant women? BMJ 1996;313:1127–1130.

75. Ginsberg JS, Hirsh J. Anticoagulants during pregnancy [Review]. Annu Rev Med 1989;40:79–86.

76. Iturbe-Alessio I, Fonseca MC, Mutchinik O et al. Risks of anticoagulant therapy in pregnant women with artificial heart valves. N Engl J Med 1986;315:1390–1393.

77. Broekmans AW, Bertina RM, Loeliger EA et al. Protein C and the development of skin necrosis during anticoagulant therapy [Letter]. Thromb Haemost 1983;49:244–251.

78. McGehee WG, Klotz TA, Epstein DJ et al. Coumarin necrosis associated with hereditary protein C deficiency. Ann Intern Med 1984;101:59–60.

79. Samama M, Horellou MH, Soria J et al. Successful progressive anticoagulation in a severe protein C deficiency and previous skin necrosis at the initiation of oral anticoagulant treatment [Letter]. Thromb Haemost 1984; 51:132–133.

80. Bauer KA. Coumarin-induced skin necrosis [Editorial; comment]. Arch Dermatol 1993;129:766–768.

81. Broekmans AW, Teepe RG, van der Meer FJM et al. Protein C (PC) and coumarin-induced skin necrosis [Abstract]. Thromb Res 1986;69(suppl): 137.

82. Schramm W, Spannagl M, Bauer KA et al. Treatment of coumarin-induced skin necrosis with a monoclonal antibody purified protein C concentrate. Arch Dermatol 1993;129:753–756.

83. Branson HE, Katz J, Marble R et al. Inherited protein C deficiency and coumarin-responsive chronic relapsing purpura fulminans in a newborn infant. Lancet 1983;2:1165–1168.

84. Estelles A, Garcia-Plaza I, Dasi A et al. Severe inherited "homozygous" protein C deficiency in a newborn infant. Thromb Haemost 1984;52:53–56.

85. Sills RH, Marlar RA, Montgomery RR et al. Severe homozygous protein C deficiency. J Pediatr 1984;105:409–413.

86. Yuen P, Cheung A, Lin HJ et al. Purpura fulminans in a Chinese boy with congenital protein C deficiency. Pediatrics 1986;77:670–676.

87. Rappaport ES, Speights VO, Helbert B et al. Protein C deficiency. South Med J 1987;80:240–242.

88. Marciniak E, Wilson HD, Marlar RA. Neonatal purpura fulminans: A genetic disorder related to the absence of protein C in blood. Blood 1985;65: 15–20.

89. Vigano D'Angelo S, Comp PC, Esmon CT et al. Relationship between protein C antigen and anticoagulant activity during oral anticoagulation and in selected disease states. J Clin Invest 1986;77:416–425.

90. Vigano S, Mannucci PM, Solinas S et al. Decrease in protein C antigen and formation of an abnormal protein soon after starting oral anticoagulant therapy. Br J Haematol 1984;57:213–220.

91. Dreyfus M, Magny JF, Bridey F et al. Treatment of homozygous protein C deficiency and neonatal purpura fulminans with a purified protein C concentrate. N Engl J Med 1991;325:1565–1568.

92. Peters C, Casella JF, Marlar RA et al. Homozygous protein C deficiency: Observations on the nature of the molecular abnormality and the effectiveness of warfarin therapy. Pediatrics 1988;81:272–276.

93. Garcia-Plaza I, Jimenez-Astorga C, Borrego D et al. Coumarin prophylaxis for fulminant purpura syndrome due to homozygous protein C deficiency [Letter]. Lancet 1985;1:634–635.

94. Hartman KR, Manco-Johnson M, Rawlings JS et al. Homozygous protein C deficiency: Early treatment with warfarin. Am J Pediatr Hematol Oncol 1989;11:395–401.

95. Casella JF, Lewis JH, Bontempo FA et al. Successful treatment of homozygous protein C deficiency by hepatic transplantation. Lancet 1988;1: 435–438.

# CHAPTER 25

# ASSESSMENT OF ARTERIAL AND VENOUS THROMBOSIS

## Mark A. Creager and Joshua A. Beckman

## ARTERIAL THROMBOSIS

Thrombotic occlusion of arteries contributes to the pathophysiology of many vascular disorders affecting the limb, coronary, mesenteric, and cerebral arteries. As discussed elsewhere in this text, thrombosis most often occurs in a vessel affected by atherosclerosis, but may also develop in arteries affected by vasculitis. Thrombi form at sites of plaque rupture, arterial injury, and within arterial aneurysms. Disorders of primary hemostasis, coagulation, or fibrinolysis may cause arterial thrombi to develop in a vessel that is otherwise normal. As opposed to chronic arterial disorders, the symptoms and clinical consequences of arterial thrombi are usually acute and potentially catastrophic. This section will review the clinical presentation and diagnosis of clinical disorders caused by arterial thrombosis.

### PERIPHERAL (LIMB) ARTERIAL THROMBOSIS

Atherosclerosis is the most common cause of limb arterial occlusive disease. The prevalence of limb atherosclerosis increases with age, ranging from 3 to 4% in those younger than age 60 to at least 20% in individuals older than age 75 (1–3). In institutionalized elderly individuals, the prevalence of limb atherosclerosis is even higher (4–6). Many individuals with peripheral atherosclerosis are asymptomatic. The onset of symptoms of claudication depends on the severity of the underlying atherosclerosis and the presence of collateral vessels. The overall incidence of claudication ranges from 1 to 6% (8–10),

developing in approximately 1 to 2% of men aged 40–60 years, and in 6% of men and 2% of women older than 60 years of age (2, 10).

Arterial thrombi usually occur in atherosclerotic vessels. Rarely, arterial thrombi form *in situ* in morphologically normal arteries. Acute occlusion of an artery by thrombus is likely to produce symptoms if there is insufficient collateral blood supply. The symptoms range from claudication, often severe and disabling, to ischemic pain, skin ulceration, and necrosis. An arterial thrombus superimposed on a stenotic atherosclerotic lesion may not affect the individual's symptoms of claudication. If, however, thrombus were to form in a normal vessel or one mildly affected by atherosclerosis, it is likely that the onset of symptoms would be rapid and severe.

The causes of arterial thrombosis are listed in Table 25.1. The most common predisposing risk factor for arterial thrombosis is atherosclerosis. The many well-established risk factors for coronary artery disease, such as tobacco use, diabetes mellitus, dyslipidemias, hypertension, and hyperhomocystenemia also confer an increased risk for limb arterial atherosclerotic disease (11–19). In addition to atherosclerosis, other obstructive arterial diseases are associated with intraluminal thrombus formation. These include several vasculitides, endothelial injury, trauma, extrinsic compression or entrapment, and arterial dissection causing obstruction of the true lumen. Disorders of coagulation and fibrinolysis are usually associated with venous thrombosis, but arterial thrombi may also occur. Synthetic and saphenous

**TABLE 25.1.** Causes of Arterial Thrombosis

Atherosclerosis
Hypercoagulable states
   Deficiencies of protein C or S
   Antithrombin III deficiency
   Myeloproliferative disorders
   Antiphospholipid syndrome (anticardiolipin antibody, lupus anticoagulant)
Endotheliopathies
   Homocysteinuria/hyperhomocysteinemia
   Radiation
   Chemotherapy (5-fluorouracil)
Vasculitides
   Thromboangiitis obliterans
   Takayasu arteritis
   Giant cell arteritis
   Systemic lupus erythematosus
   Rheumatoid arthritis
   Scleroderma
Miscellaneous disorders
   Extrinsic compression (tumor, trauma)
   Popliteal entrapment syndrome
   Aortic dissection
   Heparin-induced thrombocytopenia and thrombosis (HITT)

vein bypass grafts are also subject to acute thrombus formation.

Embolism constitutes the other major cause of acute arterial occlusion. Emboli originating from the heart occur in individuals with atrial fibrillation, valvular heart disease, acute myocardial infarction, ventricular aneurysm, and dilated cardiomyopathy. Deep venous thrombi may embolize to limb or other arteries via a patent foramen ovale or other atrial septal defects, ventricular septal defects, or a patent ductus arteriosus, producing a so-called paradoxical embolism. Rarely, acute arterial occlusions are caused by embolism of an atrial myxoma. Thrombus or atherosclerotic debris may embolize from the aorta or other large arteries to distal, smaller vessels.

## CLINICAL PRESENTATION

Intermittent claudication is the cardinal symptom of arterial occlusive disease of a limb. Leg claudication is much more common than arm claudication, since atherosclerosis preferentially affects the lower extremities. Intermittent claudication is defined as a pain, ache, heaviness, fatigue, or numbness that occurs in the limb with exercise, such as walking, and is relieved within a few minutes of rest. The location of the symptom reflects the site of stenosis or occlusion. The triad of buttock or thigh claudication, impotence, and diffuse atrophy of the lower extremity characterizes a classic presentation of aorto-iliac disease known as Leriche's syndrome. Individuals with aortic or iliac artery obstructions tend to develop buttock or thigh claudication. Individuals with femoral and popliteal artery disease typically will have calf claudication. Arterial occlusive disease affecting the tibial and peroneal arteries, as frequently occurs in diabetics, may cause ankle or foot pain while walking.

Subclavian, axillary, or brachial artery occlusive disease causes arm claudication with activities as diverse as carrying bundles, shampooing, or painting. If a subclavian artery stenosis occurs proximal to the origin of the vertebral artery, subclavian steal syndrome may occur. In this situation, the perfusion requirements of the exercising arm are met by blood flowing retrograde down the vertebral artery into the distal subclavian artery, thereby "stealing" blood from the brainstem and causing light-headedness or dizziness.

Critical limb ischemia occurs when a severe reduction in limb blood flow, as may occur with acute arterial occlusion caused by thrombus or embolism, fails to meet even the minimal nutritional requirements of the resting limb. Limb ischemia resulting from an acute arterial occlusion is characterized by pain, pallor, paresthesias, pulselessness, and paralysis, the so-called "five Ps" (Table 25.2). A proximal occlusion, such as occurs at the

**TABLE 25.2.** Distinguishing Features of Acute and Chronic Limb Ischemia

Acute limb ischemia
   Pain
   Diminished or absent pedal pulses
   Skin pallor or mottling
   Cool skin
   Paresthesias
   Impaired sensation (hypesthesia)
   Weakness or paralysis
Chronic limb ischemia
   Claudication
   ± Resting pain
   Diminished or absent pulses
   Subcutaneous atrophy
   Hair loss
   Petechiae
   Cool skin
   Brittle toenails
   ± Pallor or cyanosis of foot and hand
   Pallor with limb elevation
   Dependent rubor
   ± Hypesthesia

aortic bifurcation, may be much more catastrophic than one that occurs distally. The limb becomes pale and mottled. There is often a clearly demarcated area of decreased skin temperature. The resulting ischemic neuropathy causes hypesthesia and weakness or paralysis. Even distal acute occlusion may threaten the viability of the limb. Chronic severe limb ischemia also causes severe pain at rest, particularly in the cutaneous tissues of the foot. Ischemic foot pain is typically worse at night when individuals are in bed and the legs are in a horizontal position. The ischemic pain often improves with standing because of the beneficial perfusion effects of gravity. Individuals frequently remark that their toes are numb and cold.

Physical examination is fundamental to the diagnosis of limb arterial occlusion. The appearance of the extremities gives insight into the nature and severity of the arterial occlusion. The limb may appear entirely normal if the stenosis is chronic, adequate collaterals have developed, and resting ischemia has not occurred. Chronic low-grade ischemia is characterized by subcutaneous atrophy, hair loss, cool skin, brittle toenails, pallor with elevation, and dependent rubor (Table 25.2). With severe ischemia, petechiae develop and the skin appears smooth and shiny (Fig. 25.1). The distal aspects of the limb are cold and appear pale or cyanotic. Ischemia can induce a sensory-motor neuropathy characterized by decreased perception of vibration and touch, weakness, and diminished deep tendon reflexes. Chronic, severe ischemia ultimately induces skin ulceration, particularly at the tips of digits, in the web space between toes, or at points of pressure, such as the heel, or over interphalangeal joints. Arterial ulcers may begin as fissures and range in size from 3–5 mm to several centimeters in diameter. The border may be irregular or have well-demarcated edges. A thick black eschar often covers a pale base that has little granulation tissue. The ulcers are exquisitely painful to touch.

The most useful information is obtained by careful palpation of the pulses. In the lower extremity, the femoral, popliteal, posterior tibial, and dorsalis pedis pulses are normally palpable. In 5% of the population, the dorsalis pedis pulses are congenitally absent; this is usually indicative of an aberrant pathway of the distal anterior tibial artery. Axillary, brachial, radial, and ulnar pulses can be palpated in the upper extremities. Diminution or absence of femoral pulses suggests the presence of aortic or iliac artery stenosis or occlusion. If the femoral pulse is present and the popliteal pulse is absent, the occlusion can be localized to the superficial femoral or proximal popliteal artery. Similarly, a palpable axillary pulse combined with an absent brachial pulse suggests that a stenosis or occlusion is present in the brachial artery.

An Allen test is helpful in evaluating occlusion of the arteries supplying the hand, including the distal radial and ulnar arteries, and the palmar arches. To perform this test, the examiner compresses the radial and ulnar arteries simultaneously as the individual blanches the hand by clenching and then opening the fist. Release of compression over either artery should result in the prompt restoration of color to the hand. Persistent pallor after release of compression is indicative of arterial occlusion in the territory of the relevant artery or of an interrupted palmar arch.

## NONINVASIVE DIAGNOSTIC TESTING

The diagnosis of acute arterial occlusion should be evident from the history and physical examination. Noninvasive tests provide confirmatory and quantitative information. The tests used to diagnose arterial occlusive disease are the same whether the problem is an atherosclerotic lesion, vasculitis, or a new thrombus. These tests include pulse volume analysis, extremity blood pressure measurements, Doppler ultrasonography, duplex ultrasonography, and magnetic resonance imaging (MRI).

Pulse volume recordings are useful to evaluate limb arterial obstruction (Fig. 25.2). A variety of plethysmographic techniques are used to measure changes in limb volume with each pulse. These include strain gauge, air, impedance, and photo plethysmography. In many laboratories, a strain gauge is used to evaluate the pulse volume. As the circumference of the limb alters the length of the strain gauge, its electrical resistance is affected. The variation in the voltage drop across the strain gauge can be detected with a Wheatstone bridge from

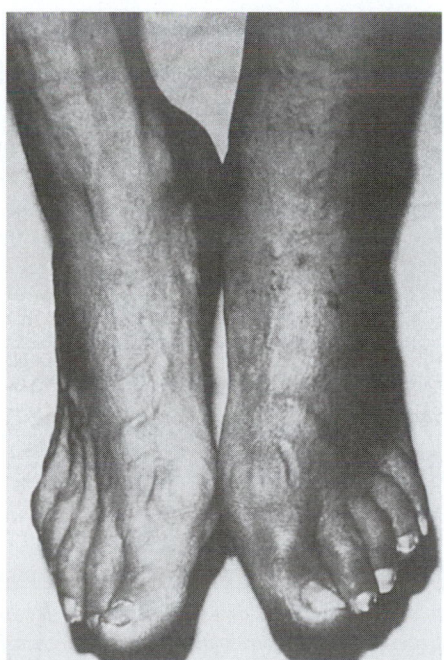

**FIGURE 25.1.**  Chronic severe ischemia of the left foot. The skin is smooth and shiny and the nails are thickened.

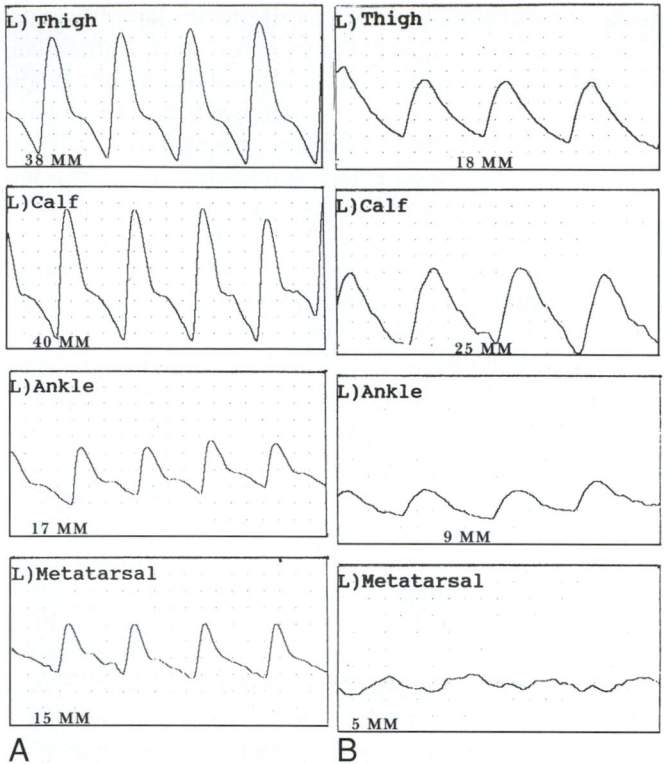

**FIGURE 25.2.** **A,** Normal pulse volume recording. The tracing is derived from the thigh, upper calf, ankle, and metatarsal segments. The pulse volume contour displays a normal upstroke, dicrotic notch, and downstroke at each level. **B,** Pulse volume recording from a individual with arterial occlusive disease. The amplitude of the pulse volume is diminished, the upstroke is delayed, and there is no dicrotic notch. (Reprinted with permission from Loscalzo J, Creager MA, Dzau VJ, eds. Vascular medicine. Boston: Little, Brown and Co., 1996.)

which the signal is amplified and recorded. The pulse volume recording is graphically displayed for interpretation. With air plethysmography, the limb segment of interest is enclosed in an airtight chamber. Increases in the volume of the limb segment decrease the surrounding air volume and increase the pressure within the chamber. The pressure changes are transduced and graphically illustrated. Impedance plethysmography relates blood volume in the limb to electrical impedance. Impedance can be determined by applying a current across a segment of the limb while measuring the change in voltage. The voltage change is demonstrated on a graphic recorder. Photoplethysmography uses a light source that emits red or near-infrared light and a photosensor. Blood reflects and scatters light emitted from the source. As blood volume increases, there is greater dispersion of light; therefore less reflected light is received by the sensor. Electrical signals from the photosensor can be amplified and displayed graphically. Laser flowmeters can also be used to measure red cell

velocity. Laser light, emitted from a probe, undergoes a shift in wave frequency when encountering moving blood cells. The reflected light is detected by optical fibers on the probe.

The normal pulse volume recording resembles a blood pressure waveform and is composed of a systolic upstroke with a sharp peak and downslope that includes a dicrotic wave that is concave toward the baseline (Fig. 25.2). The pulse volume is recorded at multiple levels in the limb. In the leg, this would include the upper and lower thigh, the upper and lower calf, and the digits. In the upper extremity, detecting devices are placed along the upper arm, forearm, and fingers. A significant arterial obstruction will alter the appearance of the pulse volume waveform. The pulse volume may be entirely absent in the presence of severe ischemia caused by an acute arterial occlusion. Nonobstructive lesions causing less severe ischemia induce abnormalities in the pulse volume waveform that include loss of the dicrotic wave, a flattened systolic peak, and decreased amplitude. The location of the obstruction is implicated by the site at which the pulse volume waveform becomes abnormal.

The most frequently used noninvasive test to detect the presence of significant arterial obstruction is measurement of systolic blood pressure in the extremities (20–23) (Table 25.3). This is a more extensive evaluation of limb pressure measurements than that used during the bedside evaluation. To evaluate the leg, pneumatic cuffs are placed serially on the upper and lower thigh, below the knee, and above the ankle. Flow is usually detected with a Doppler ultrasound probe that is placed over the posterior tibial, dorsalis pedis, and peroneal

**TABLE 25.3.** Leg Segmental Blood Pressure Measurements in a Individual with Peripheral Arterial Occlusion

|  | Segmental Pressure Measurments (mm Hg) | |
|---|---|---|
|  | Right | Left |
| Arm blood pressure | 154/94 | 150/94 |
| Cuff location |  |  |
|     Upper thigh | 160 | 158 |
|     Lower thigh | 162 | 110 |
|     Upper calf | 162 | 108 |
|     Lower calf | 158 | 108 |
| Ankle/brachial index | 1.0 | 0.7 |

*Note the fall in systolic blood pressure in the left leg between the upper and lower thigh measurements. This difference indicates a significant stenosis or occlusion in the left superficial femoral artery. All pressure measurements in the leg are made with the Doppler probe positioned over the dorsalis pedis pulse.*

arteries. To assess arterial obstruction in the upper extremity, cuffs are placed on the upper arm, on the forearm just below the elbow, and at the wrist. The Doppler probe is placed at the brachial artery in the antecubital fossa or over the radial or ulnar arteries at the wrist. Each segment's arterial pressure is determined by inflating the cuff to suprasystolic pressure. Systolic pressure is defined as the pressure at which blood flow resumes during cuff deflation. Systolic blood pressure in the lower extremities should be the same as, or even greater than, that in the upper extremities. This is because the amplitude of the pressure wave increases as the wave travels distally. A limb arterial stenosis producing more than 70% cross-sectional narrowing of the lumen is sufficient to decrease blood pressure. A pressure gradient higher than 20 mm Hg between sequential cuffs is suggestive of a significant stenosis. Calculation of the ankle/brachial systolic blood pressure ratio provides insight into the severity of ischemia. A ratio less than 1.0 is abnormal. Individuals with modest leg claudication secondary to chronic arterial occlusive disease typically have ankle/brachial systolic pressure indices of 0.5– to 0.8, whereas individuals with significant ischemia at rest have indices less than 0.5 (23–25). Healing of foot ulcers is poor if the ankle pressure is less than 55 mm Hg. Determination of segmental pressures in the extremity will not distinguish acute from chronic arterial obstruction, but will provide important information regarding the severity of ischemia.

Doppler ultrasonography may provide additional information. Doppler ultrasound transducers use a piezoelectric crystal that emits and receives an ultrasound signal (20, 26, 27). If the transmitted ultrasound signal of fixed frequency strikes a moving target, such as blood cells, the frequency of the reflected signal will be shifted by an amount proportional to the velocity of the target. This is termed the Doppler shift. Therefore, blood flow through a vessel can be detected and evaluated by auditory assessment or graphic display of the Doppler signal.

In the lower extremities, the Doppler probe is positioned at a 60 degree angle over the common femoral, superficial femoral, popliteal, dorsalis pedis, and posterior tibial pulses. In the upper extremity, it is placed over the subclavian artery in the supraclavicular fossa, over the brachial artery in its location near the axilla, as well as in the antecubital fossa, and over the radial and ulnar arteries on the volar aspect of the wrist. The Doppler probe can evaluate the presence of blood flow in the palmar arch and along the digital arteries. The Doppler frequency shift is proportional to the velocity of blood flow.

The normal Doppler velocity waveform has three components: rapid forward flow during systole, transient flow reversal during early diastole, and slower for-

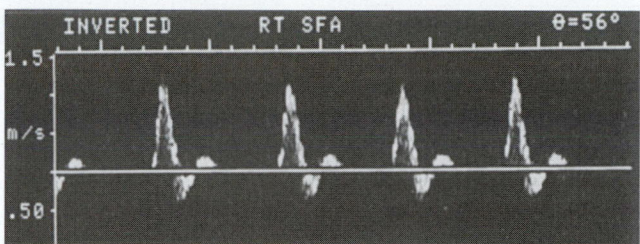

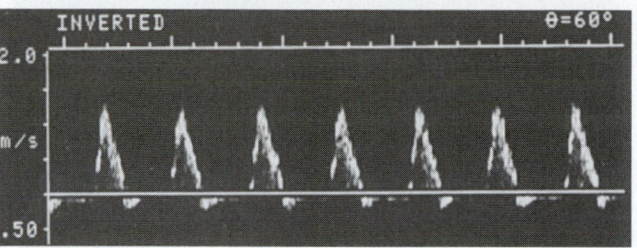

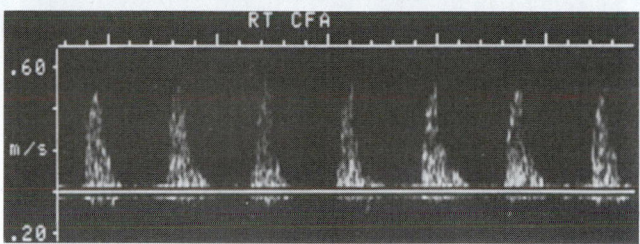

**FIGURE 25.3.**   Doppler velocity profile in: **A,** Normal superficial femoral artery in which there is a triphasic wave form; **B,** Atherosclerotic superficial femoral artery distal to a mild stenosis in which there is an absence of flow reversal during early diastole; and **C,** severely obstructed common femoral artery distal to occlusion in which there is a delayed rate of rise and decreased amplitude. Note that the peak velocity is only 0.5 m/sec whereas in the normal artery it is 1.3 m/sec.

ward flow during late diastole (Fig. 25.3). When the probe is placed distal to an arterial stenosis or occlusion, the normal triphasic appearance is altered. With acute arterial occlusion causing severe ischemia, no flow may be detected. If some collateral flow is present, a severe stenosis or occlusion will cause a dampened waveform, characterized by a delayed rate of rise and a lower systolic peak. In the presence of a severe stenosis, the reverse flow component disappears. If the probe is positioned directly over a nonobstructive stenosis, the signal will be high pitched and turbulent. Thus, by sampling the Doppler frequency waveform over multiple sites of the limb's vessels, it is possible to detect the location and assess the severity of arterial obstruction. This technique is limited by time. To accurately assess the 30 to 40 cm of the femoral and popliteal arteries generally requires 1 to 2 hours.

Duplex ultrasonography combines both B-mode ultrasound imaging and pulse Doppler velocity analysis to study the morphology and hemodynamic signifi-

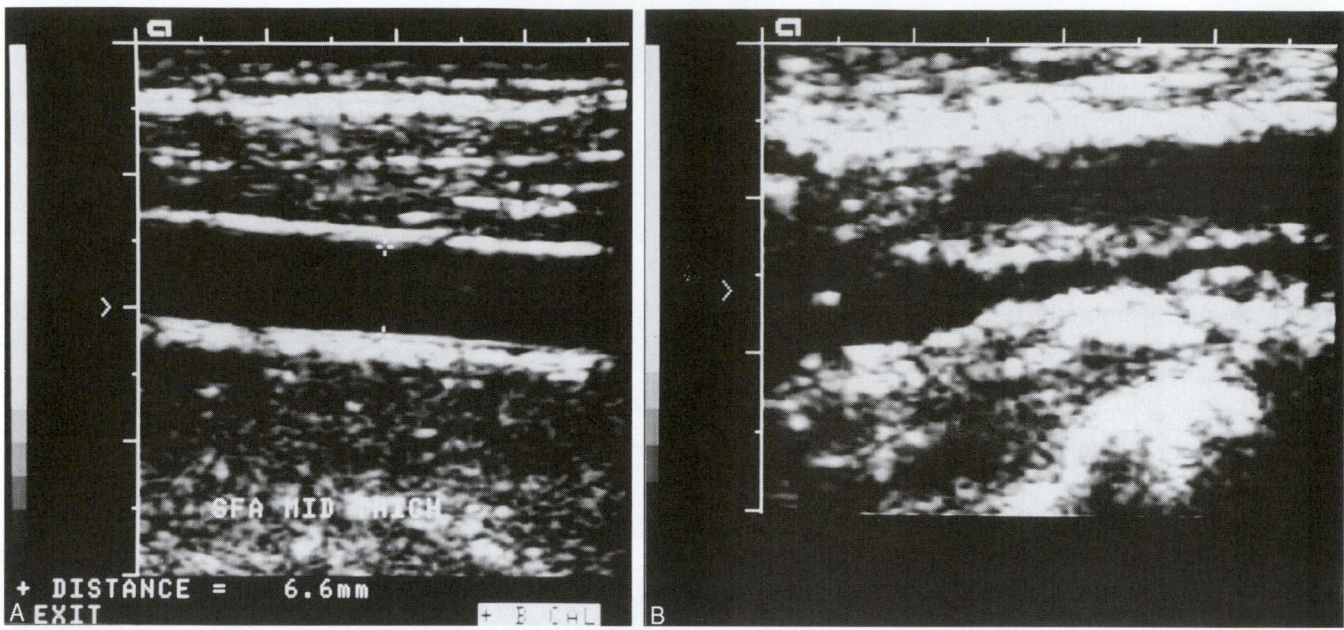

**FIGURE 25.4.**  B-mode ultrasound images of the superficial femoral artery. **A,** Normal artery. The intima is delineated as a thin echogenic line (*cursors*). **B,** Atherosclerotic artery. The intima is thickened and disrupted by plaque.

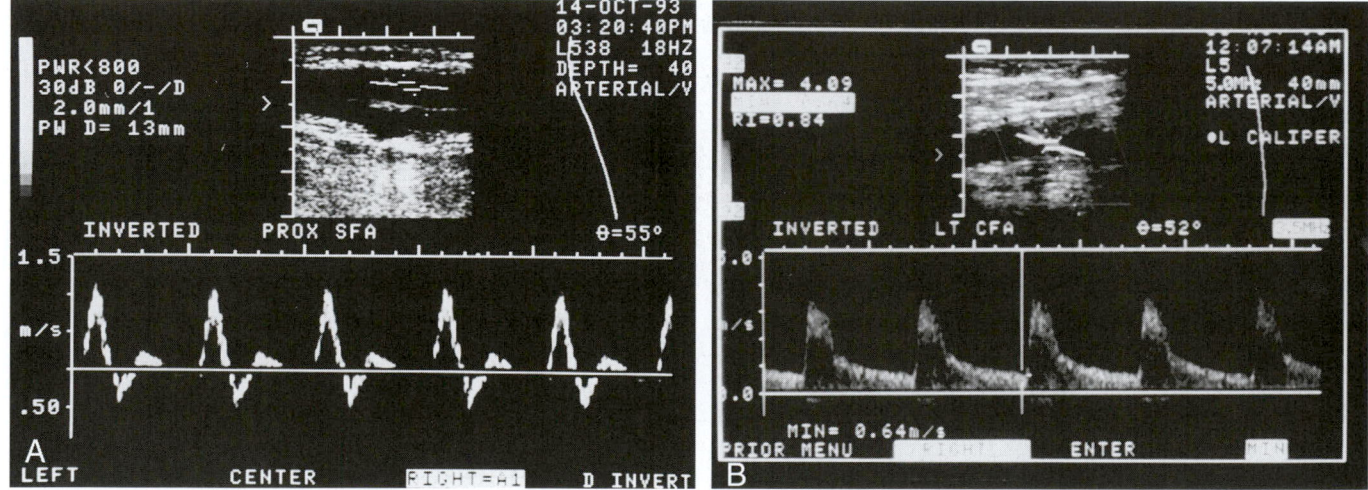

**FIGURE 25.5.**  Pulse Doppler velocity measurements made in the superficial femoral artery just beyond the common femoral artery bifurcation. **A,** Normal artery. The velocity profile is triphasic. There is a distinct envelope indicating uniform movement of cells. **B,** Atherosclerotic femoral artery with critical stenosis. The velocity is considerably increased at 4 m/sec. No distinct envelope is apparent because turbulent flow through the stenosis causes cells to move at varying speeds.

cance of arterial obstructions. The B-mode image provides information regarding the appearance of the vessel wall, particularly the intima, and the nature of intraluminal filling defects (Fig. 25.4). Images are constructed from high frequency sound waves that "echo" at tissue interfaces. The brightness of the image is related to the intensity of the reflected wave. It is often possible to distinguish dense, or calcific, atherosclerotic plaque from intraluminal thrombus. The pulse Doppler, guided

by the ultrasound image, samples blood velocity at specific arterial sites. Flow through a stenotic vessel is accelerated and turbulent. Accordingly, the pulse Doppler detects a high peak velocity and spectral broadening of the velocity profile owing to the turbulence (Fig. 25.5).

The velocity, amplitude, and direction of blood flow can also be assessed by Doppler color flow imaging (28–30). The frequency shift information is processed in real time to form a color velocity display within the blood vessel. Color assignment is arbitrary, but typical units used are red and blue, assigning the former to arteries and the latter to veins. With increasing velocity, the hue and intensity of the display causes progressive desaturation of the color toward white at the highest detectable velocities (Fig. 25.6; see color plate 25.6). An arterial occlusion, such as that caused by acute thrombus formation, would cause cessation of flow (Fig. 25.7; see color plate 25.7). Use of color-assisted Doppler imaging can improve the diagnostic accuracy of ultrasound, yielding sensitivities of more than 80% and specificities higher than 90%, as compared to the gold standard examination of contrast angiography (31, 32).

The ultrasound imaging procedure is performed with the individual supine. To evaluate the lower extremities, the aorta is imaged in the midline below the level of the xiphoid and traced to its iliac bifurcation. The iliac artery is examined to the groin. Thereafter, the common and superficial femoral arteries are imaged, including the latter's location in the adductor canal. To examine the popliteal artery, the individual is placed in a prone position. It is often possible to examine the origin of the anterior tibial artery and the tibioperoneal trunk. It may be difficult to examine the distal tibial and peroneal arteries. Ultrasound penetration of the soft tissues may be limited by the presence of gas or calcification. Trying to scan areas with these items would generate artifact instead of a reliable image. Duplex ultrasonography has advantages over other noninvasive measurements. It is more sensitive than segmental blood pressure measurements for detecting mildly stenotic lesions. It also provides information regarding the morphologic characteristics of the obstructing lesion. There are some limitations; for example, multiple stenoses impair this modality's ability to assess serial lesions because of the altered waveform distally (33, 34).

Magnetic resonance imaging develops images by measuring the electromagnetic energy from the body's atoms. Most commonly, hydrogen is used in its water form. Electromagnetic pulses from a large magnet alter the alignment of the hydrogen atoms. When the atoms return to baseline, energy is released and measured, and an image is developed. Magnetic resonance angiography (MRA) generates images in which the vascular structures appear bright compared to the surrounding tissues. The peripheral arterial tree can be assessed by two methods: time-of-flight MRA, which uses flow-sensitive pulses, and contrast-enhanced MRA (Fig. 25.8). Time-of-flight MRA uses electromagnetic pulses to saturate the stationary tissues, rendering them dark in contrast to the light flowing blood. Arterial stenoses are diagnosed through imaged luminal narrowing. In the assessment of the arterial tree below the aortic bifurcation, time-of-flight MRA concurs with conventional contrast angiography from 57 to 100% of the time (35, 36).

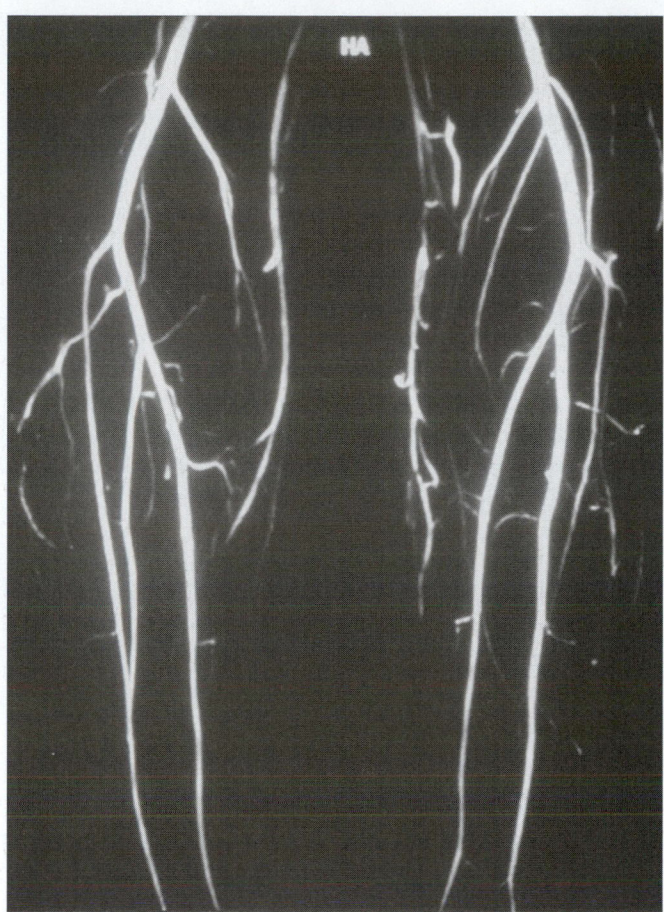

**FIGURE   25.8.**   Contrast-enhanced   two-dimensional MRA of the right and left popliteal, tibial, and peroneal arteries.

Several groups have demonstrated time-of-flight MRA's superiority to contrast angiography in the runoff vessels (37–39). A multicenter, randomized trial of 155 individuals demonstrated 83% sensitivity for contrast angiography and 85% sensitivity for MRA in distinguishing patent from occluded vessels (40). In this study, time-of-flight MRA was more sensitive but less specific than contrast angiography in determining segments suitable for insertion of bypass grafts.

Magnetic resonance angiography, using the time-of-flight technique, does have some limitations. It is still not an accurate method to gauge the severity of a stenosis (41, 42). Time-of-flight MRA is also limited by the required study period of 40 to 80 minutes, respiratory variation that affects the imaging of the aortoiliac vessels, its inability to discern the vasculature in the setting of surgical clips, the exclusion of individuals with pacemakers, and the high rate of individuals unable to be studied because of claustrophobia. In addition, although MRA compares favorably to conventional contrast angiography, it still lags behind digital subtraction angiography (43). Several modifications are being developed to address these issues. New types and placements of coils are being tested (44). Three-dimensional imaging and high-speed systems are improving images while decreasing scan times to minutes.

The development of contrast-enhanced MRA of the arterial tree is at a less advanced state. There have been no large or multicenter trials. Investigations have been limited to pilot and small group studies to set up standard protocols and demonstrate the possible efficacy of the technique (45–49). Gadolinium chelate contrast is administered by intravenous bolus and the correct timing is developed to obtain images of the arterial tree without concomitant venous images (Fig. 25.8). With the advent of faster machines, it is becoming possible to acquire three-dimensional images in less than a minute. This time is crucial, for it allows individuals to hold their breath and decreases the motion artifact of the study. Motion artifact is a significant limitation of the longer studies, especially in the abdominal cavity when evaluating the renal and iliac arteries. This technique is less affected by the poor signal intensity caused by complex flow patterns in stenotic regions or from the lateral flow of the iliac arteries than time-of-flight MRA.

## ARTERIOGRAPHY

Arteriography is performed to define arterial anatomy before a revascularization procedure. It is rarely used solely for diagnostic purposes, because the presence of arterial occlusive disease can usually be diagnosed from history, physical examination, and noninvasive vascular diagnostic tests. Occasionally, arteriography is useful for distinguishing atherosclerosis from other causes of arterial occlusion, such as dissection, entrapment, and vasculitis.

Arteriography requires specialized imaging equipment, catheters, and contrast agents (50). Individuals undergoing angiography are placed on a specially designed "stepping" table that enables precise movement of the individual during the study. After sterile preparation and draping, polyethylene or polyurethane catheters are placed percutaneously into the arterial system and advanced proximal to the area of interest. Often, catheters are inserted via groin puncture into the femoral artery in a retrograde manner and localized under fluoroscopic guidance to the ipsilateral external iliac artery or aorta, or manipulated in a retrograde manner into the contralateral external iliac or common femoral artery. The catheter can be selectively placed in most vessels of interest, including the branches of the aortic arch and branch arteries feeding the abdominal and pelvic viscera. On occasion, the catheter is inserted percutaneously via the brachial or axillary arteries, or directly into the aorta via a translumbar approach.

The contrast agents used in angiography generally are organic iodine compounds. Carbon dioxide ($CO_2$) is

undergoing investigation as a contrast agent. Automated injector systems set to deliver a selected amount of contrast at a predetermined rate are used to administer the radiopaque contrast agents into the arteries via the catheter. An x-ray generator, x-ray tube, and image intensifier system are used to image and photograph the arterial anatomy during contrast injection. Digital subtraction angiography is a computer-assisted angiographic technique that enhances the appearance of the contrast-filled vessels. It is used in selected situations when it is advantageous to the individual to reduce the amount of the contrast agent.

The primary indications for arteriography are those conditions requiring revascularization. These include disabling claudication and severe limb ischemia portending limb loss. It is useful in individuals with acute thrombotic occlusion of peripheral arteries to determine the nature and severity of the occlusion and plan a revascularization procedure. Angiographic definition of an arterial thrombus includes an abrupt cut-off of an otherwise normal-appearing vessel, an intraluminal filling defect outlined by contrast material, or a segmental occlusion beginning just after a patent branch vessel (Fig. 25.9).

Arteriography is done to determine the type of intervention required to restore blood flow to the involved limb. This may include thrombolysis, percutaneous transluminal angioplasty, surgical thromboembolectomy, or surgical bypass. Catheters used for diagnostic angiography may also be used to administer thrombolytic agents in the vicinity of the thrombus. Arteriography is used to guide and monitor the response to percutaneous transluminal balloon angioplasty as well. In the operating room, angiography is used to assess the response to thrombectomy, as well as to ensure technical success of infrainguinal bypass grafts.

## INTRAVASCULAR IMAGING

Intravascular ultrasound combines some of the advantages of angiography with those of transcutaneous ultrasound. As with angiography, intravascular ultrasound enables definition of the vascular lumen and severity of stenosis. Unlike angiography, however, it also provides an opportunity to examine the morphologic appearance of the vascular wall. A potential advantage of this technique over transcutaneous ultrasound is that the proximity of the intravascular ultrasound unit to the lesion enhances resolution.

Intravascular ultrasound devices include imaging catheters that incorporate ultrasound crystals and transducers placed at the tip of the catheter. Available intravascular ultrasound catheters range in size from 2.9 French (outer diameter = 1.0 mm) to 8 French (outer diameter = 2.7 mm). They emit frequencies of 10 to 50 MHz. The most practical frequencies range from 20 to

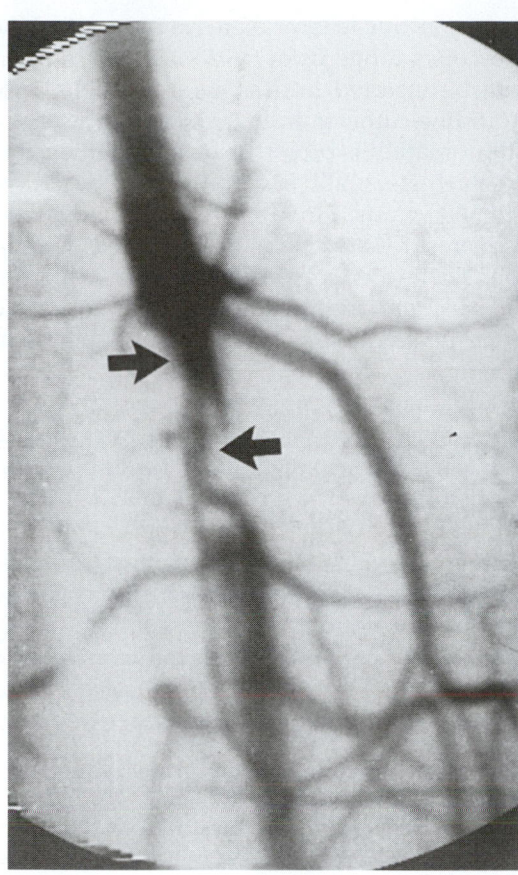

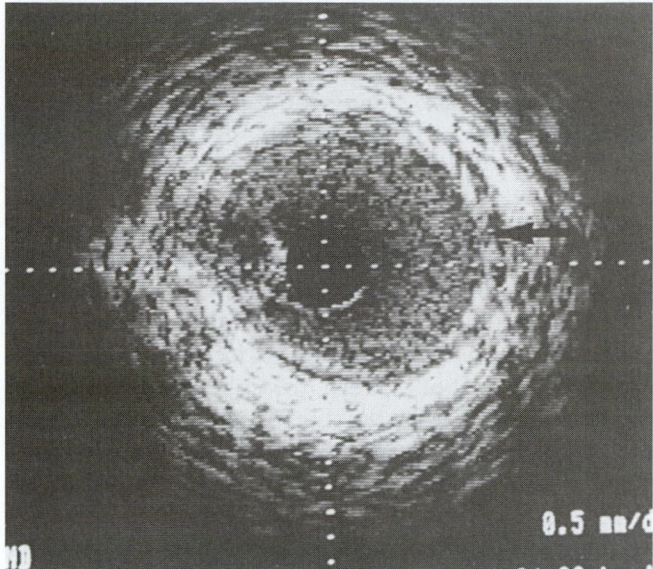

**FIGURE 25.10.**   Intravascular ultrasound image of a coronary artery. The intima-media layer (*arrow*) is thin. (Courtesy of Drs. Ian Meredith and Alan Yeung, Brigham and Women's Hospital, Boston, MA.)

**FIGURE 25.9.**   Arteriogram of the right superficial femoral artery demonstrates an acute arterial occlusion by thrombus. There is an abrupt cutoff of an otherwise normal-appearing artery. Arrows indicate intraluminal filling defect. (Courtesy of Drs. Joseph Polak and Ram Chaturvedi.)

30 MHz. Both mechanical and phased-array ultrasound transducers are available and provide a 360 degree tomographic image of the artery. Through the reflectivity of the wall, characterizations of its composition and disease state may be elucidated.

The intravascular ultrasound appearance of a normal large artery consists of a halo comprising one or two layers that include intima-media and adventitia. The intravascular ultrasound appearance of a normal smaller, muscular artery often comprises three layers (51–53) (Fig. 25.10). The intima is a thin echogenic layer, surrounded by a thicker echolucent layer, althought to represent the media. The outer layer is echogenic and most likely represents the interface between media and adventitia. The nature of an atherosclerotic plaque may be inferred from its echo characteristics. Lipid rich plaques often have echolucent zones; fibrous plaques often produce homogeneous bright echo signals; and calcified plaques are very echogenic and are associated with acoustic shadowing, that is, an area of echo dropout caused by the failure of the ultrasound signal to

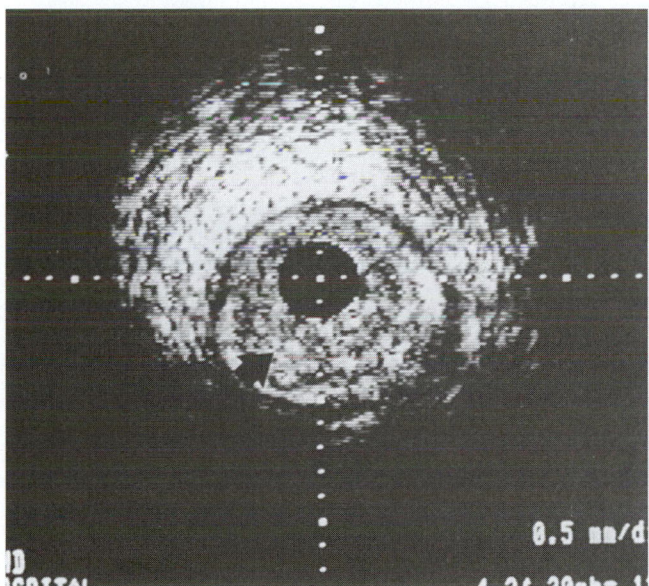

**FIGURE 25.11.**   Intravascular ultrasound of a coronary artery with thick, concentric plaque deposition (*arrow*) disrupting the normal intimal appearance. (Courtesy of Drs. Ian Meredith and Alan Yeung, Brigham and Women's Hospital, Boston, MA.)

permeate the calcified area (Fig. 25.11). Intravascular ultrasound can be used to calculate how much of the vascular lumen has been compromised by plaque formation. This technique can also distinguish concentric from eccentric plaque.

In its ability to estimate lumenal size and the nature of vessel wall plaque burden, intravascular ultrasound is being used as an adjunct to angiography, angioplasty, stent placement, and atherectomy. By accurately gauging vessel size, determining the amount of lumen expansion, the size of the induced vessel wall dissection, the adequacy of intravascular stent placement and the reduction in plaque burden, intravascular ultrasound is finding a role in assessing the success of interventional procedures (54–56).

Intravascular ultrasound, however, may not be as useful in diagnosing thrombus as it is in defining and imaging plaque (57). Fresh thrombus may have the acoustic properties of flowing blood and may not be detected by ultrasound. Alternatively, old thrombus may impart echogenic characteristic comparable to plaque, making distinction between these two entities difficult. A thrombus that is only partially adherent to the vessel wall may be diagnosed because its mobile nature is more easily detected by ultrasound (57) (Fig. 25.12). Adherent wall thrombus, in contrast, is difficult to distinguish from atherosclerotic plaque. The specificity of intravascular ultrasound for detecting thrombus is high, often exceeding 90% (58, 59). Its sensitivity to detect thrombus is relatively low, approximately 60% (57–59).

Angioscopy is a technique that enables direct visualization of the vascular lumen. An angioscope comprises a fiber illumination system, a high intensity light source, an objective lens, and an eye piece (60). Fiberoptic angioscopes range from 0.8 to 3.0 mm in diameter. They can be inserted into a larger diameter balloon-tipped guiding catheter and advanced to the area of interest. Illumination is provided by a high intensity light source, which is usually a xenon-arc lamp with power of 300 to 1000 watts. Blood must be removed from the area of interest for structures to be viewed with the angioscope. Therefore, collateral irrigation with a saline solution is usually provided through an irrigation channel within the angioscope or through a separate irrigation catheter.

An advantage of angioscopy over other imaging techniques, such as angiography and intravascular ultrasound, is its ability to distinguish thrombus from atherosclerosis (Fig. 25.13; see color plate 25.13). The flexible characteristics of the angioscope enable it to be positioned in coronary arteries, peripheral arteries, and in infrainguinal bypass grafts. Its sensitivity for detecting coronary thrombosis approaches 100% (59). It is being used more frequently for intraoperative monitoring of infrainguinal bypass grafting and for intraoperative guidance of thromboembolectomy (61–63).

## CORONARY ARTERY THROMBOSIS

Whereas coronary atherosclerosis with flow-limiting lesions contributes importantly to anginal syndromes and myocardial ischemia, acute myocardial infarction has been attributed to abrupt occlusion of a coronary artery by thrombosis. Approximately 80 years ago, Herrick argued in his now classic treatise that fatal and nonfatal myocardial infarction was caused by sudden obstruction of the coronary arteries (64). Results of some, but not all, autopsy studies confirmed the presence of occlusive coronary thrombosis in many individuals who succumbed to myocardial infarction, particularly those who died within 48 hours of acute infarction (65–67). The high prevalence of occlusive coronary thrombosis in individuals with acute myocardial infarction was confirmed by DeWood et al, who used coronary arteriography to study individuals presenting within 24 hours of acute myocardial infarction (68–69). They reported that 80% of individuals evaluated within 4 hours of the onset of symptoms had total coronary occlusion caused by thrombus. The major angiographic feature of coronary thrombosis was defined as a persistent staining of intraluminal material by the radiopaque contrast agent. The presence of thrombus was confirmed in the majority of these individuals after retrieval by a Fogarty catheter (68). Importantly, in individuals studied 12 to 24 hours after the onset of symptoms, the prevalence of thrombus decreased to 65%. These findings suggested that partial recanalization of an occlusive thrombus may occur in individuals surviving acute myocardial infarction. The incidence of occlusive coronary thrombosis appears to be less in individuals with nontransmural (non–Q-

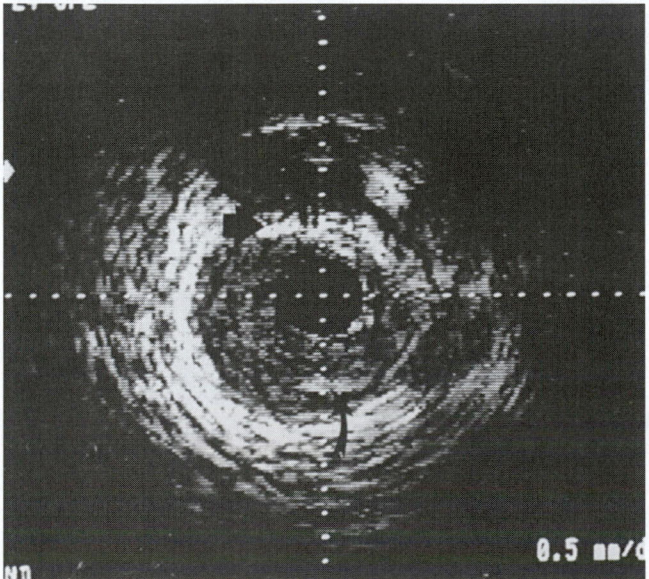

**FIGURE 25.12.** Intravascular ultrasound of a coronary artery demonstrating eccentric plaque (*thick arrow*) and echogenic thrombus (*curved arrow*) that is partially adherent to the vessel wall; it appeared mobile on real-time imaging. (Courtesy of Drs. Ian Meredith and Alan Yeung, Brigham and Women's Hospital, Boston, MA.)

wave) myocardial infarctions (70). In a small series, however, Mandelkorn et al did find evidence of coronary thrombosis in the majority of individuals who presented with nontransmural myocardial infarction (71). Mizuno et al found variation in the type and rate of complete occlusion of the lumen by thrombosis in myocardial infarctions and unstable angina. Myocardial infarctions had erythrocyte-rich reddish thrombi whereas in unstable angina, the thrombi, were red blood cell-poor, whitish plaques (72, 73).

Coronary artery thrombus has also been implicated as a contributing factor in individuals with unstable angina. In an autopsy study, Falk reported that the majority of individuals with unstable angina culminating in infarction or sudden death had evidence of coronary thrombosis (74). Other investigators, using angiography, have demonstrated coronary artery thrombosis in many, albeit not all, individuals with unstable angina (71, 75–76). Sherman et al used coronary angioscopy to assess the presence of coronary thrombus in individuals with unstable angina and in those with stable coronary artery disease (77). None of the arteries in individuals with stable coronary disease had thrombus, whereas the majority of those with unstable angina had evidence of thrombus. Bresnahan found thrombi in 40% of individuals with unstable angina at rest and in only 2.5% of those with stable angina (78). Rehn et al observed thrombus in 42% of individuals with unstable rest angina vs. 17% of those with stable angina (79), whereas Vetrovec et al found thrombi in 85% (80) and Capone found thrombi in 52% of individuals with unstable angina (81).

The genesis of thrombosis in the acute coronary syndromes depends on the disruption of an atherosclerotic plaque and exposure of its inner, lipid core. Mature plaques consist primarily of two components: a soft, lipid-rich core and a hard, collagen-rich fibrous cap. Plaques causing moderate stenosis are more often the site of plaque rupture than severely stenotic fibrous plaque.

The tendency or vulnerability of a plaque to rupture is, in large part, related to the size of the atheromatous core, the thickness and collagen content of the fibrous cap, and the inflammation in the cap. Atheromatous cores, rich in cholesterol and its esters, covered by thin fibrous caps infiltrated with macrophages, are particularly at risk. After plaque disruption, three factors are related to the severity of the thrombosis: the character of the lipid components exposed; the degree of stenosis and surface irregularities that activate platelets; and the systemic thrombotic tendency at the time. The process is affected by cellular elements including macrophages, endothelial cells, vascular smooth muscle cells, and T-lymphocytes; and by vasoactive stimuli such as sympathetic tone (83–85).

A detailed discussion of the clinical presentation and diagnosis of coronary artery syndromes is beyond the scope of this chapter. Salient features of the clinical presentation of individuals with acute myocardial infarction and unstable angina will be discussed. The classic symptoms of individuals with acute myocardial infarction include severe, often crushing, chest discomfort, frequently located in the retrosternal area or over the precordium, and at times radiating to the jaw, back, shoulder, or arm. Individuals variably describe their discomfort using qualitative terms such as heavy, pressure-like, burning, or "indigestion." Symptoms of chest discomfort may be accompanied by a sense of dyspnea as well as diaphoresis. Depending on the location and severity of the myocardial infarction, individuals may be hypertensive or hypotensive. Many are tachycardic, particularly those with anterior wall infarctions causing substantial compromise in left ventricular function. However, individuals with inferior and posterior myocardial infarction, as well as those with conduction disturbances, may have low heart rates. Signs of congestive heart failure, including neck vein distention, gallop rhythms, and rales, depend on the extent of ventricular damage.

The diagnosis of myocardial infarction is often, although not always, confirmed by electrocardiogram (86–87). An acute transmural (Q-wave) myocardial infarction is heralded by ST segment elevation. Thereafter, the appearance of new, significant Q-waves that persist in one or more tracings is diagnostic of an acute, evolving myocardial infarction. Other electrocardiographic findings that are consistent with, but by themselves not diagnostic of myocardial infarction include new ST segment depression and/or T-wave inversion that persist on several tracings. Myocardial necrosis is confirmed by increased serum concentrations of cardiac enzymes including creatine phosphokinase (CPK) particularly CPK MB, aspartate transaminase (AST), and lactate dehydrogenase (LDH).

Another chemical marker has come into use for the confirmation and assessment of myocardial infarction: components of troponin. Troponin is part of the regulatory mechanism of actin and myosin interaction. It has three components: I, the inhibitory subunit; T, the domain that regulates actin/myosin attachment; and C, the calcium-binding regulatory protein. Troponin I and troponin T have been found to be elevated in myocardial, but not skeletal muscle necrosis (88–90). Elevations have also been found to carry prognostic significance concerning future events, procedures, and mortality (91–94).

Coronary angiography is indicated in selected cases to guide therapeutic interventions. The typical angiographic features of coronary artery thrombus include the following: abrupt occlusion of an artery with no antegrade appearance of radiopaque contrast beyond the occlusion, or subtotal occlusion enabling contrast to outline the thrombus, which usually appears to have irregular, hazy margins, and opacify the artery distal to the obstruction. Coronary angioscopy and intravascular ultrasound imaging have been used on an investigational basis to diagnose coronary artery thrombus. The principles of these techniques are described above.

## MESENTERIC ARTERY THROMBOSIS

Mesenteric artery occlusion is one of the three major causes of acute mesenteric ischemia. The others include mesenteric vein occlusion (discussed below) and nonobstructive mesenteric ischemia. Mesenteric arterial occlusion results from either thrombus formation *in situ* or as a consequence of embolism from a proximal source. The major vessels supplying the small and large intestines include the celiac, superior mesenteric, and inferior mesenteric arteries. A collateral network of communicating arteries connects the celiac and superior mesenteric arteries and the superior and inferior mesenteric arteries. Acute mesenteric artery thrombosis most often occurs in a vessel affected by atherosclerosis (95–97). Other less common causes include vasculitides, such as polyarteritis nodosa, giant cell arteritis, and thromboangiitis obliterans (98–101). A vessel affected by fibromuscular dysplasia is an unusual site of thrombus formation (102).

Acute mesenteric ischemia is heralded by the onset of severe abdominal pain located most frequently in the periumbilical area and associated with vomiting and occasionally diarrhea. Initially, there may be few, if any, physical findings. As ischemia progresses and peritonitis develops, individuals develop abdominal distention, marked abdominal tenderness, and loss of bowel sounds. Gastrointestinal bleeding occurs in the majority of individuals.

Patients with mesenteric atherosclerosis may also have symptoms of intestinal angina. This is althought to occur if at least two of the three major visceral vessels are obstructed (103, 104). Symptoms of chronic visceral ischemia include abdominal pain 15 to 30 minutes after meals, a fear of eating, and weight loss. Most of these individuals have evidence of atherosclerosis elsewhere, including coronary artery disease and atherosclerosis of the extremity vasculature. Examination of the abdomen may detect a bruit.

Submucosal hemorrhage and edema of the large intestinal wall may give the appearance of "thumbprinting" on the abdominal x-ray in cases of ischemic colitis. Plain x-rays of the abdomen are also useful to exclude other causes of acute abdominal pain. Angiography is used to confirm the diagnosis. Aortography is performed in the anteroposterior and lateral projections. Thereafter, selected images of the celiac artery, superior mesenteric artery, and inferior mesenteric artery are ob-

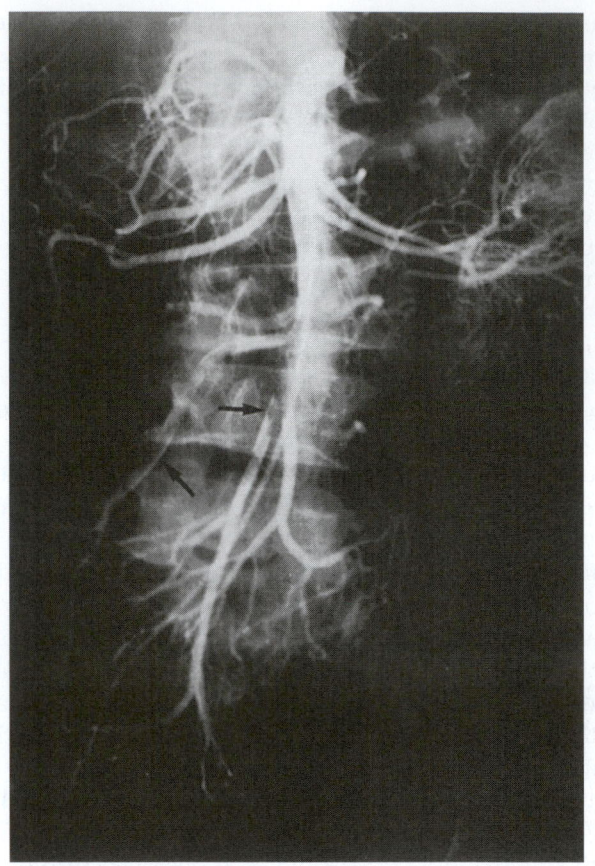

**FIGURE 25.14.**   Superior mesenteric arteriogram of a individual with acute mesenteric ischemia. The arrows denote the site of thrombus formation. (Courtesy of Drs. Joseph Polak and Ram Chaturvedi.)

tained. Acute arterial occlusion is suggested by an abrupt occlusion of the affected vessel (Fig. 25.14).

## RENAL ARTERY THROMBOSIS

Renal artery thrombosis is an uncommon cause of obstruction. It can occur as a result of atherosclerotic plaque rupture or by extension of thrombus from the aorta. Antiphospholipid antibodies have also been described as a cause of renal artery thrombosis (105). Individuals may have back pain or hypertension. The diagnosis is usually made by arteriography. Duplex Doppler ultrasonography, helical computed tomography (CT) scanning, and MRA may be helpful in making the diagnosis but are not as accurate as arteriography (106–113).

# VENOUS THROMBOSIS (SEE CHAPTER 61)

Venous thrombosis afflicts approximately 10 per 10,000 people in the United States each year (114–116). Approximately 300,000 individuals are hospitalized and treated annually (114, 116). The most common location of venous thrombus is in the veins of the lower extremities, but thrombus may also affect veins of the upper extremities, kidneys, intestines, spleen, and liver. The clinical presentation of individuals with venous thrombosis depends on the location and extent of thrombotic occlusion. This section will focus primarily on the clinical presentation and diagnosis of deep venous thrombosis of the limb. Salient features of other venous thrombotic disorders also will be reviewed.

## LIMB VENOUS THROMBOSIS

The factors associated with limb venous thrombosis were initially described by Virchow and include the triad: stasis, vascular damage, and hypercoagulability (117) (see Chapter 25). One or more of these factors occur in clinical situations that predispose to venous thrombosis. The conditions associated with venous thrombosis are listed in Table 25.4. Several individual populations are at a very increased risk for venous thrombosis, as discussed in detail in Chapter 25. Surgery, for example, is associated with venous thrombosis because individuals are usually at bed rest during the perioperative period and their legs are relatively immobile. The normal ''milking'' of veins by active leg muscles is limited and the venous blood velocity is reduced compared to the ambulatory state. Individuals undergoing orthopedic and neurosurgical procedures are at particularly high risk. The incidence of asymptomatic deep venous thromboses, in the absence of prophylaxis, ranges from 20 to 50% of individuals with these underlying problems (118–125).

Nonsurgical individuals with vascular disease also have an increased frequency of deep venous thrombosis. In studies from 1971 to 1980, 20 to 35% of hospitalized individuals with myocardial infarction developed venous thrombosis (126–128). Cerebrovascular accidents predisposed individuals to venous thrombosis. Deep venous thromboses were diagnosed in 10 to 75% of individuals, depending on the diagnostic modality used (129–131). Congestive heart failure is associated with venous thrombosis, probably as a consequence of bed rest. Hospitalization itself is associated with an increased risk for venous thrombosis, likely as a surrogate for other risk factors for thrombosis (132). The incidence of venous thrombosis may correlate with severity of illness. Approximately 12 to 33% of individuals admitted to the medical intensive care unit developed deep vein thrombosis (133–134).

Neoplasms are associated with venous thrombosis for reasons that have not been clearly defined except in the most general terms of a hypercoagulable state. Trauma may precipitate venous thrombosis by injuring blood vessels and also by causing the individual to be relatively immobile.

Disorders of coagulation are associated with an increased incidence of venous thrombosis (see Chapter 40). The most common hereditary abnormality associated with venous thrombosis is resistance to activated protein C caused by factor V Leiden (135–138). A single amino acid substitution in factor V decreases the affinity of activated protein C for factor V and decreases its degradation, thus potentiating coagulation. Of idiopathic venous thromboses, 21 to 33% have had activated protein C resistance documented in association with the event (136, 139, 140). The prevalence increases as the age of the studied population decreases. Factor V Leiden may also act synergistically with high estrogen states like pregnancy or oral contraceptive use (141) and with homocystinuria (142) to increase the risk of thrombosis. Hyperhomocysteinemia itself is an independent risk for thrombosis (143). Increasing factor VIII concentration is related in a dose-dependent relative risk for venous thrombosis (144). Deficiencies of antithrombin III, protein C, protein S, and plasminogen cause a hypercoagulable state and have been demonstrated to account for 8.3% of outpatients presenting with deep venous thrombosis (145). These deficiencies also leave individuals at increased risk for recurrent events. The presence of antiphospholipid antibodies are associated with an increased incidence of venous thrombosis (146, 147) (see Chapter 38).

---

## TABLE 25.4.   Venous Thrombosis: Associated Conditions

Surgery
 Orthopedic, thoracic, abdominal, and genitourinary procedures
Neoplasms
 Pancreas, lung, genitalia, urinary tract, breast, stomach
Trauma
 Fractures of spine, pelvis, femur, tibia
Immobilization
 Acute myocardial infarction, congestive heart failure, stroke, postoperative convalescence
Pregnancy
Estrogen use
Hypercoagulable states
 Resistance to activated protein C (Factor V Leiden); Deficiencies of antithrombin III, protein C or protein S; lupus anticoagulant; myeloproliferative disorders, dysfibrinogenemia; disseminated intravascular coagulation
Venulitis
 Thromboangiitis obliterans, Behcet's disease, hyperhomocysteinemia, previous deep vein thrombosis

Venous thrombosis occurs during pregnancy (see Chapter 46), but the overall incidence is low, approximately 1 per 2000 pregnancies (148–150); this occurs most frequently in the third trimester and postpartum. The gravid uterus may compress the left iliac vein, particularly when the woman is lying on her left side, thereby causing venous stasis. Venous thrombosis, however, can occur on the right side and in the postpartum period, implicating a hypercoagulable state as the cause of venous thrombosis. The use of oral contraceptives is accompanied by increased risk of venous thrombosis (151, 152). Also, the use of hormone replacement therapy is associated with an additional case of deep venous thrombosis for every 5000 users (153). A recent prospective study of the risk factors for pulmonary embolism in women indicated that obesity, cigarette smoking, and hypertension are associated with an increased risk of pulmonary embolism.

Intimal damage provides a substrate for venous thrombosis. Damage to the intima also may lead to venous thrombosis as a sequela to the venulitis that occurs in thromboangiitis obliterans and Behcet's syndrome (154, 155). Previous thrombosis itself may alter the endothelial surface to provide a site for recurrent venous thrombosis.

## Clinical Presentation

The veins of the extremities are broadly categorized as deep or superficial. In the legs, the deep veins are subclassified as distal—the calf, and proximal—the thigh and pelvis. The distal deep venous system of the legs comprises the soleus and gastrocnemius venous plexi and the paired posterior tibial, anterior tibial, and peroneal veins of the calf. The proximal deep leg veins include the popliteal, superficial femoral, deep femoral, common femoral, and external iliac veins. The external iliac vein is joined by the internal iliac vein, draining the pelvis, to form the common iliac vein as it courses into the inferior vena cava. The superficial veins of the legs include the greater and lesser saphenous veins and their tributaries. The superficial and deep venous systems are connected by a series of perforating veins that direct blood from the surface to the deeper vessels. The deep veins in the upper extremity include the radial, ulnar, brachial, axillary, and subclavian veins. The superficial veins are composed of the basilar and cephalic veins and their tributaries. It is important to distinguish thrombosis of superficial from deep veins because the presentation, potential consequences, and treatment modalities are very different.

The clinical features of superficial vein thrombosis include pain, erythema, heat, and tenderness at the site of the affected vein. Careful inspection reveals a red streak over the affected area. Palpation elicits tenderness and enables the examiner to appreciate a subcutaneous cord-like structure. Palpation is one of the best means to determine the extent of the superficial vein thrombosis. Thrombi of superficial veins rarely embolize unless they have propagated into the deep system. Therefore, it is important that the examiner be aware of the proximal extent of the thrombus, particularly if it is present in the greater saphenous vein of the thigh. The greater saphenous vein anastomoses to the common femoral vein, providing a site of entry of a superficial vein thrombus into the deep system. It is for this reason that anti-inflammatory drugs should be used cautiously, because they may obscure the physical findings of an ascending superficial vein thrombosis. Edema is usually confined to the area immediately surrounding the affected vein.

The importance of recognizing deep venous thrombosis is underscored by the potentially fatal consequence of this disorder, pulmonary embolism. In addition, deep venous thrombosis damages the delicate venous valves, and predisposes the individual to chronic venous insufficiency. Deep venous thrombosis of the extremities should be identified as proximal or distal, that is, the calf. The risk of pulmonary embolism is easier to predict when one distinguishes proximal from calf deep vein thrombosis. Pulmonary embolism occurs in approximately 50% of untreated individuals with proximal deep vein thrombosis and in 5 to 20% of untreated individuals with distal (calf) deep vein thrombosis (156–158). Approximately 10 to 20% of calf vein thrombi propagate into the proximal veins from which they are more likely to embolize (159, 160).

Deep venous thrombosis of the iliac, femoral, or popliteal veins, so-called proximal veins, is suggested by unilateral leg swelling, warmth, and erythema (Fig. 25.15). Tenderness may be present along the course of the involved veins and a cord may be palpable. Additional signs include increased tissue turgor, distention of superficial veins, and the appearance of prominent venous collaterals (Table 25.5). Thrombotic occlusion of the inferior vena cava occurs as a consequence of proximal propagation of iliofemoral vein thrombosis, extrinsic compression caused by pelvic and abdominal masses, or intrinsic obstruction caused by inferior vena cava filters. Individuals develop bilateral leg swelling that is often quite severe and uncomfortable. Superficial venous collaterals are often present along both sides of the pelvis and lower abdomen.

The diagnosis of deep vein thrombosis of the calf is often difficult at the bedside because only one of the multiple veins may be involved, allowing adequate venous return via the remaining patent vessels. The most common complaint is calf pain. Examination may reveal posterior calf tenderness, warmth, increased tissue turgor, modest swelling, and rarely, a cord. Homans' sign, which is the perception of pain during active dorsiflexion of the foot, is sensitive but nonspecific.

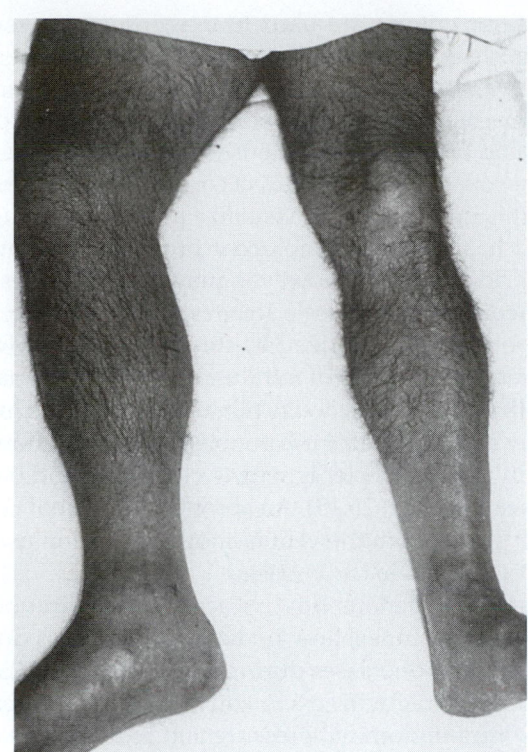

**FIGURE 25.15.**  Patient with acute proximal deep vein thrombosis of the right leg. Note that the swelling involves the thigh as well as the calf.

**TABLE 25.5.**  Clinical Features of Deep Venous Thrombosis

Proximal deep vein thrombosis
  Unilateral calf or thigh discomfort
  Edema
  Warmth
  Erythema
  Tenderness along course of involved veins
  Cord
  Distension of superficial veins
  Prominent superficial collateral veins
Calf deep vein thrombosis
  Calf pain
  Posterior calf tenderness
  Increased tissue turgor
  ± Edema
  Cord, rarely palpable

Deep vein thrombosis of the upper extremity occurs much less frequently but is also subject to the consequences of pulmonary embolism and venous insufficiency. The most common cause of upper extremity deep vein thrombosis is venous catheterization, particularly into the subclavian vein. Trauma, such as may occur with a crutch in the axilla and with shoulder injuries, may precipitate deep vein thrombosis. Vigorous arm exercise rarely causes subclavian or axillary vein thrombosis. The features of upper extremity proximal deep vein thrombosis include arm swelling and the appearance of prominent superficial venous collaterals in the periclavicular area. A cord may be palpable in the axilla. Superficial vein thrombosis of the upper extremity is caused frequently by the placement of intravenous cannulas. The physical findings include local erythema, swelling, and tenderness. These are readily visualized or palpable during examination.

Paget-Schroetter syndrome is a thrombotic variant of thoracic outlet syndrome. The syndrome is characterized by effort-related or spontaneous thrombosis of the axillosubclavian vein in otherwise healthy individuals. The etiology of the thrombosis is a mechanical abnormality at the costoclavicular segment of the axillosubclavian vein. The vein is compressed between a hypertrophied scalene or subclavius tendon and the first rib. Frequently, a large bony projection is found at the costoclavicular junction. The acute thrombosis is almost always in the area of the chronic compression (161). Typical individuals, generally young athletes or those who perform physical work, report the sudden onset of severe, unilateral, upper extremity swelling in the absence of trauma. The swelling dissipates with rest. Chronically, the individuals may be asymptomatic at rest, but complain of swelling, tightness, heaviness, or easy fatigability with associated pallor or sweating at various levels of exertion. Physical examination may demonstrate mild rubor or cyanosis, prominence of upper extremity, shoulder, or lateral pectoral veins, and tenderness in the axilla over the axillary vein. If untreated, the swelling will usually resolve over the course of days to weeks. With the development of collateral circulation, physical findings may be difficult to define. Maneuvers, including examination after exercise or complaints of pain when the arm is used in the outstretched or overhead position, may bring out the expected symptoms and signs. The rapid resolution of symptoms after these manuevers excludes acute thrombosis (161).

## NONINVASIVE DIAGNOSTIC TESTS

A variety of noninvasive tests have been used to evaluate individuals for deep vein thrombosis (Table 25.6). These include duplex ultrasonography, impedance plethysmography, and [125I] fibrinogen scanning.

Venous duplex ultrasonography is the principal noninvasive test used to diagnose deep vein thrombosis. It uses both B-mode imaging and pulse wave Doppler techniques to examine the veins of the limb (162–164). With newer, high-resolution ultrasound units, it is possible to image the proximal and distal deep veins of most individuals (Fig. 25.16). In the legs, the scanner is used

**TABLE 25.6.** Noninvasive Testing for Deep Venous Thrombosis: Sensitivity and Specificity

|  | Sensitivity | Specificity |
| --- | --- | --- |
| Proximal deep vein thrombosis | | |
| Continuous wave Doppler ultrasonography | 85% | 90% |
| Impedance plethysmography | 90% | 90% |
| Phleborrheography | 90% | 90% |
| Duplex ultrasonography | 92–100% | 95–100% |
| Calf deep vein thrombosis | | |
| [125I] Fibrinogen scanning | 88–97% | 95% |
| Duplex ultrasonography | 80% | 75% |

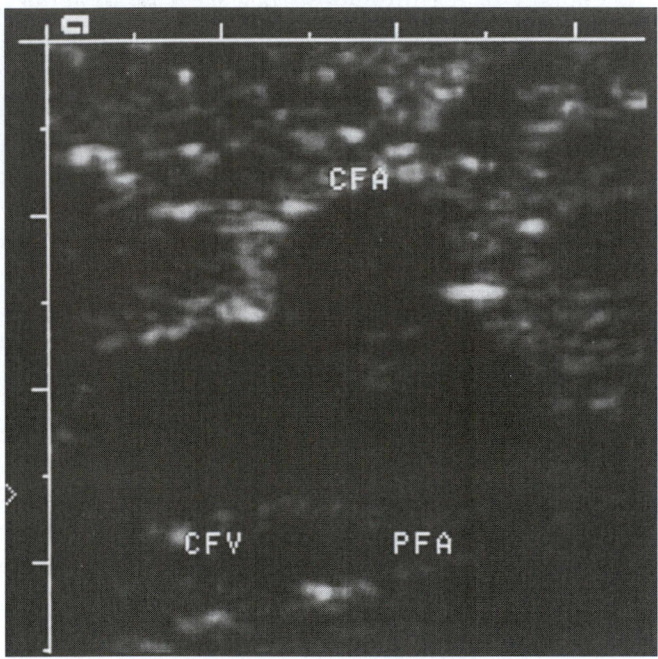

**FIGURE 25.16.** Transverse B-mode image of common femoral vein (CFV), superficial femoral artery (SFA), and profunda femoral artery (PFA).

to visualize the proximal veins, including the common femoral, proximal deep femoral, superficial femoral, and popliteal veins. In many individuals, it is also possible to scan the paired anterior tibial, posterior tibial, and peroneal veins as well as the muscular veins comprising the gastrocnemius and soleus venous plexi. In the neck and upper extremities, it is possible to visualize the internal jugular, subclavian, axillary, and brachial veins. The pulse Doppler is used to sample venous flow in each of these vessels. Color Doppler enhances the usefulness of pulse Doppler and provides a visual image of venous flow (27, 165), although alone, color Doppler has limited clinical utility (166).

Several criteria are used to diagnose deep venous thrombosis by ultrasound. Normally, the examiner can cause a vein to collapse simply by applying pressure on the probe, because a low venous pressure is easy to overcome (Fig. 25.17). If a thrombus is present in the vein, it will not collapse during a direct compressive maneuver. Often it is not possible to visualize a new thrombus because it has the same echolucent properties as flowing blood. Older thrombi, however, may impart echoes that are detected on gray scale images. Chronic deep vein thrombosis is characterized by thickened venous walls, increased echogenicity of intraluminal thrombus, partial recanalization, and venous collateral channels. Thrombus may be diagnosed if it is nonobstructive and flow detected by color Doppler is seen to course around it (Fig. 25.18; see color Fig. 25.18). An absent or abnormal Doppler shift signal from the vein is another criterion used to diagnose deep vein thrombosis.

Normally, venous flow varies with respiration. In the lower extremities, flow in the veins increases during expiration and decreases during inspiration (Fig. 25.19), because diaphragmatic excursion during inspiration increases intra-abdominal pressure and reduces transmural pressure in the inferior vena cava. Conversely, changes in intrathoracic pressure cause venous flow to increase in the upper extremities during inspiration and decrease during expiration. If a thrombus is present in a vein proximal to the location of the ultrasound probe, respiratory variation diminishes or ceases. The absence of flow from a large vein is evidence of occlusion. Doppler ultrasound can also be used to detect increases in flow that accompany manual compression of the foot, calf, or forearm. During this maneuver, flow accelerates in the veins. If a thrombus is present between the site of compression and the location of the probe, flow acceleration will not occur.

Using contrast venography as a gold standard, the sensitivity of venous ultrasound testing for diagnosing proximal deep vein thrombosis has been reported to range from 92 to 100%, whereas its specificity approaches 100% (128, 163, 164). There is less information available regarding the predictive value of venous ultrasonography for diagnosing deep calf vein thrombosis. It is more difficult to visualize all of the calf veins than it is to image the proximal veins. In two small studies, the specificity of venous ultrasound for deep calf vein thrombosis was reported to be 94 to 96%; sensitivity was 88 to 97% (165, 167). The experience in the literature concerning the use of ultrasound in the diagnosis of axillary and subclavian vein thrombosis or Paget-Schroetter syndrome is conflicting, with sensitivity rates of 50 to 100% (168–172).

Impedance plethysmography is a technique that detects changes in limb volume during maneuvers designed to affect venous flow. With this technique, small

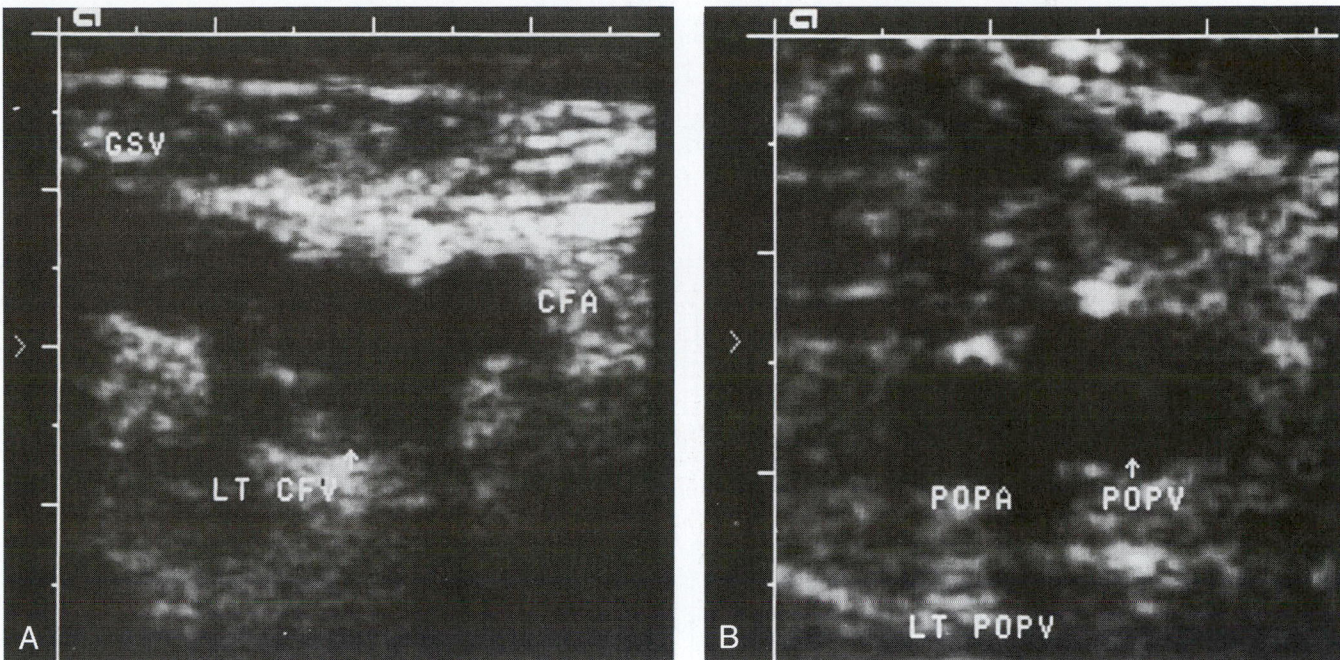

**FIGURE 25.17.** Venous ultrasound imaging to detect deep vein thrombosis. Normally, manual compression overcomes venous pressure, causing the vein to collapse. If the vein is obstructed by thrombus, the vein will not collapse during a compression maneuver. **A,** Left common femoral vein thrombus; **B,** Popliteal vein thrombus. Neither vein collapsed during compression.

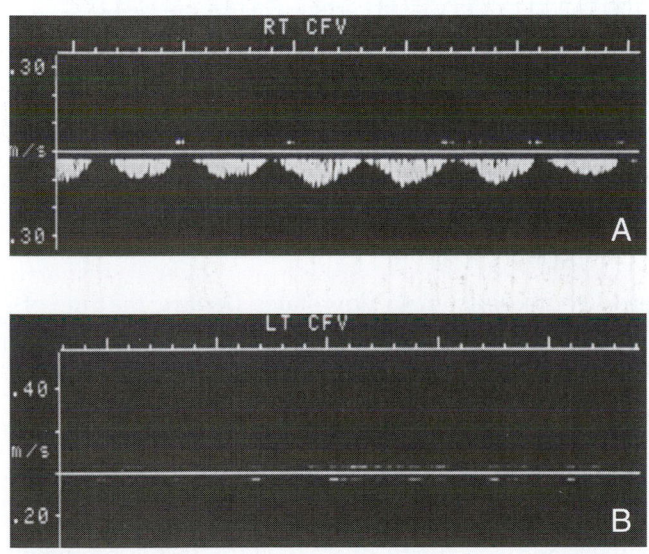

**FIGURE 25.19.** Doppler ultrasound assessment of deep vein thrombosis. **A,** Normal recording demonstrating respiratory variation in the venous velocity pattern. **B,** Deep vein thrombosis demonstrating absence of variation in Doppler velocity recording during respiration.

amounts of electrical current are transmitted to electrodes placed on the limb. The change in voltage across two electrodes is measured, and impedance is determined. Typically, this technique uses a sphygmomanometric cuff that is placed on the thigh and inflated to a

pressure that impairs venous flow, causing calf volume to increase (Fig. 25.20). With cuff deflation, calf volume normally decreases as blood exits through a patent venous system. If there is a proximal deep vein thrombosis, thigh cuff inflation and subsequent deflation cause only a modest increase and decrease in calf volume, respectively. Impedance plethysmography has a sensitivity and specificity of approximately 90% for diagnosis of proximal deep vein thrombosis; it is not a reliable test for deep calf vein thrombosis (173).

[125I] fibrinogen scanning is based on the principle that fibrinogen is incorporated into a propagating thrombus (174, 175). Thus, by labeling fibrinogen with a radioisotope, a growing thrombus can be detected by nuclear scanning. The radiolabeled fibrinogen will be incorporated into a propagating thrombus, detected as a focal increase in isotope counts over the affected area. False-positive tests occur if [125I] fibrinogen localizes to areas of inflammation or hematoma, as may develop after orthopedic surgery or leg trauma. [125I] fibrinogen scanning is particularly useful in the diagnosis of deep calf vein thrombosis; its sensitivity and specificity are approximately 80% and 75%, respectively (174, 175). It is less specific for the diagnosis of proximal deep vein thrombosis, because the large blood volume in the proximal part of the thigh causes elevated counts and false-positive tests. The use of [125I] fibrinogen scanning has declined with the increased attendant risks of the use of blood products.

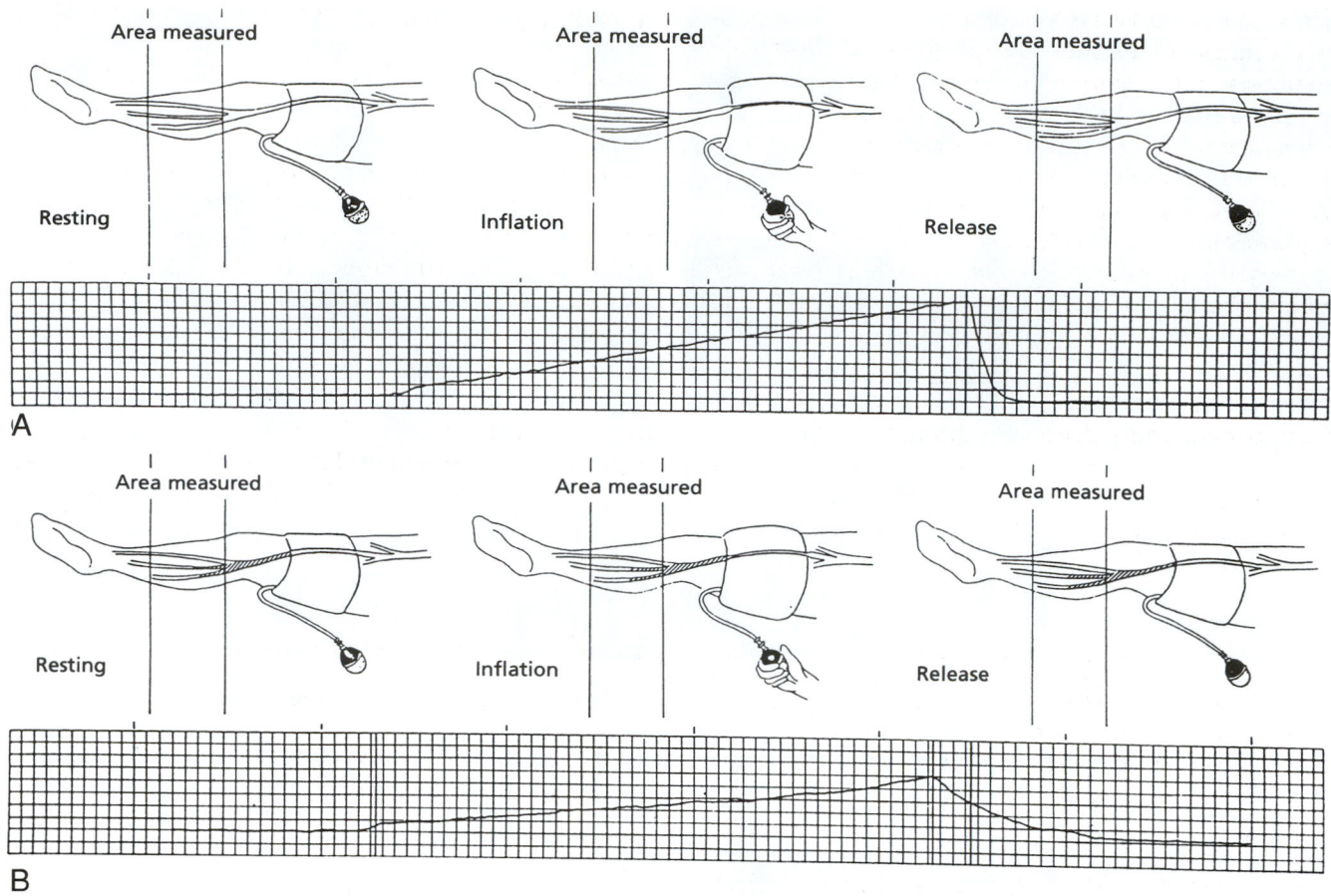

**FIGURE 25.20.** Impedance plethysmography. **A,** A normal tracing. Note the rate of rise with thigh cuff inflation and the rapid decline that occurs after thigh cuff deflation. **B,** An abnormal tracing indicating deep vein thrombosis. The rate of rise during thigh cuff inflation is slow, and there is a delayed decline after thigh cuff deflation. (Reproduced with permission from Hirsh J, Genten E, Hull R. Venous thromboembolism. New York: Grune and Stratton, 1981.)

## MAGNETIC RESONANCE VENOGRAPHY

Magnetic resonance venography is a further refinement of MRA. As in the assessment of arterial disease, magnetic resonance venography depicts the vascular structures on the basis of flow characteristics. To remove the arteries from the field of view, a two-pulse method is used. The first pulse is for the two-dimensional slice in consideration and the second to presaturate the arterial flow, yielding only a discernible venous tree. Patent veins are bright structures, whereas areas of no flow or thrombosis are dark.

There are several potential advantages of magnetic resonance venography over other methods of imaging. It has the ability to image the entire vascular system below the bifurcation in contrast to the limited imaging of the pelvic veins by ultrasound. It also provides an opportunity to assess lumen size and vessel wall characteristics. Potential etiologies may also be investigated by examining nearby soft tissue disease. One of the limitations of magnetic resonance venography is its poor ability to dis-

cern thrombosis from no-flow states. Because the time-of-flight method depends on the direction of flow, regions of turbulent flow that occur distal to a bifurcation, beyond a severe stenosis, or by compression by adjacent arteries limit the accuracy of this method.

Using contrast venography as a gold standard in diagnosing a deep venous thrombosis, magnetic resonance venography has demonstrated a sensitivity of 88 to 100% and specificity of 92 to 100% in the proximal venous system (176–178). In the calf, the sensitivity for diagnosing deep venous thrombosis is 87% and the specificity is 97% (178). New techniques to improve diagnostic accuracy are in development, such as calf vein flow amplification (179) and three-dimensional imaging. Breath-holding techniques with high speed imaging machines are also under investigation. The cost and time of the examinations are limiting factors at present.

## CONTRAST VENOGRAPHY

Venography is still considered the gold standard for diagnosing venous thrombosis. It is indicated in individuals in whom noninvasive vascular studies fail to definitively confirm or exclude the presence of deep vein thrombosis. It is performed using a modification of the approach described by Rabinov and Paulin (180). A 23- to 25-gauge needle is used to cannulate a dorsal pedal vein. A dilute radiopaque contrast agent is injected under fluoroscopic guidance. Posteroanterior and lateral views are obtained at the levels of the calf, the knee, and the pelvis to the level of the anastomosis of the iliac vein into the inferior vena cava. A venogram is judged positive for venous thrombosis if a discrete filling defect or an abrupt vessel cutoff is seen (Fig. 25.21). Nonfilling of venous segments is classified as equivocal. To diagnose upper extremity deep vein thrombosis, contrast is injected via a hand or forearm vein and images are obtained of the upper arm and upper thorax to visualize the brachial, axillary, and subclavian veins.

## PULMONARY EMBOLISM

Estimates of the annual incidence of pulmonary embolism in the United States range from 120,000 to more than 500,000 cases (114–116). Lower estimates are derived from databases using hospital discharge codes (114, 116). Approximately 15 to 30% of these individuals die, many before they receive medical attention. The incidence of pulmonary embolism rises with age, affects men more than women, and blacks more than whites (181). Predisposing conditions for pulmonary embolism are similar to those causing deep venous thrombosis. The most common cause of pulmonary embolism is deep venous thrombosis, 80 to 90% of which are located in the proximal veins of the legs (182, 183). Other sources include the deep veins of the calves, the pelvic veins, and the proximal veins (brachiocephalic, subclavian) of

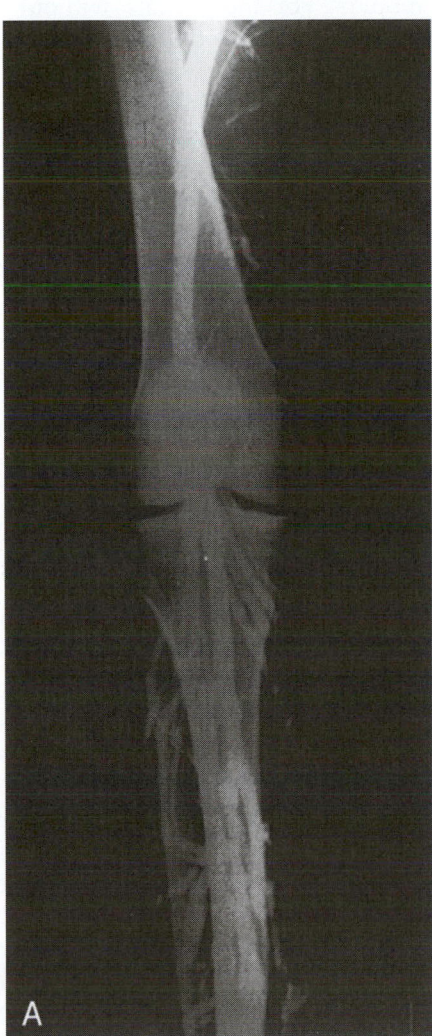
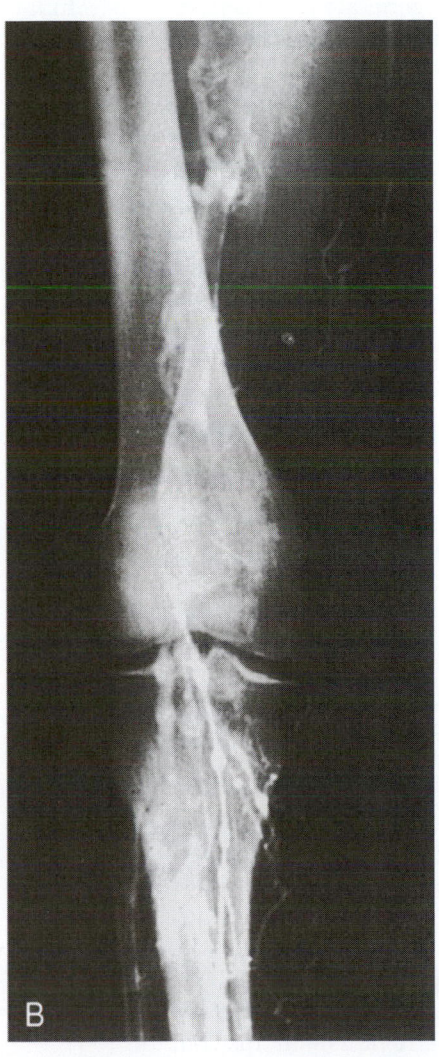

**FIGURE 25.21.**   Venography is the gold standard to diagnose deep vein thrombosis. **A,** Normal venogram. **B,** Deep vein thrombosis. There is absence of filling of multiple calf veins. In the thigh, an extensive thrombus is outlined by contrast material in the superficial femoral vein.

the upper extremities. Pulmonary thromboembolism can also originate on the right side of the heart and is known to occur in individuals with atrial fibrillation or right ventricular failure. Nonthrombotic forms of pulmonary embolism include fat embolism, as might occur after a bone fracture; amniotic fluid embolism, associated with childbirth; mycotic embolism, resulting from tricuspid or pulmonic native and prosthetic valve endocarditis; air embolism, as a complication of an intravenous cannula; and foreign particle embolism, such as may occur in intravenous drug abusers.

As discussed previously, comorbid conditions like surgery, stroke, fractures, malignancy, and myocardial infarction are associated with stasis, thrombosis, and hypercoagulability. They provide an environment permissive for the development of thromboembolism and are associated with increased event rates compared to controls. Reduction in endogenous anticoagulants like antithrombin III, protein C, and protein S, or activated protein C resistance, generate increased risk (184). Individuals with antiphospholipid antibodies (185) and hyperhomocysteinemia (186) are also at increased risk. In addition, in the Nurses Health Study, women who were obese, smoked cigarettes, had hypertension, or used oral contraceptives had an increased risk of pulmonary embolism (187, 188). Postmenopausal women taking hormone replacement therapy were at a mildy increased risk (189). Women with activated protein C resistance were found to be at increased risk while pregnant or taking oral contraceptives (190).

The cardinal symptoms of pulmonary embolism are chest pain and dyspnea. Chest pain occurs in approximately 90% of individuals (183, 191–193). Characteristically, the pain is sharp and pleuritic. Dyspnea occurs in approximately 85%, cough in 50%, and hemoptysis in 30% of individuals. Individuals often are apprehensive and occasionally diaphoretic. Syncope is an unusual, albeit important, symptom of pulmonary embolism. Physical findings are often related to the extent of pulmonary embolism. More than 90% of individuals are tachypneic. Chest examination may reveal rales, wheezing, evidence of a pleural effusion, and/or a pleural friction rub. Extensive pulmonary embolism may cause signs of pulmonary hypertension, including neck vein distention with prominent 'a' waves, a right ventricular lift, an accentuated pulmonic component of the second heart sound, and a murmur of tricuspid regurgitation. Individuals with pulmonary embolism may be hypotensive and cyanotic. Evidence of deep vein thrombosis should be sought in individuals with symptoms and signs of pulmonary embolism. The clinical features of deep vein thrombosis have been described previously in this chapter.

Several laboratory tests are useful to assist decision analysis but are not diagnostic. The electrocardiogram may show sinus tachycardia, atrial arrhythmias, and nonspecific repolarization abnormalities (192). If pulmonary hypertension occurs from massive pulmonary embolism, there may be evidence of right heart strain. Abnormalities on chest x-ray include atelectasis, an elevated hemidiaphragm, a wedge-shaped infiltrate (Hampton's hump), and pleural effusion (193). Arterial blood gases often indicate hypoxia; however, this is neither a specific nor sensitive finding (194). Neither a normal partial pressure of arterial oxygen nor a normal alveolar-arterial oxygen gradient excludes the possibility of pulmonary embolism (195, 196). Regional right ventricular dysfunction, in which the apex is spared, as demonstrated by transthoracic echocardiography, had a 77% sensitivity and 94% specificity in one study (197).

D-dimers are the products of plasmin fibrinolysis of a crosslinked fibrin clot. They are increased during disseminated intravascular coagulation. Measurement by an ELISA of the level of D-dimers in the blood has been helpful in excluding the likelihood of a pulmonary embolus. For individuals without a high-probability ventilation perfusion scan, D-dimers below 500 ng/mL have a negative predictive value of 91 to 100% (198–200). Latex assays are not as reliable (201).

The ventilation:perfusion (V/Q) lung scan is the principal screening test for diagnosing pulmonary embolism. The rationale of performing perfusion and ventilation scans in tandem is based on the fact that pulmonary emboli obstruct blood flow to pulmonary capillaries but do not directly affect alveolar function. Perfusion lung scanning uses the injection of macroaggregates of albumin labeled with technetium 99m. These particles are trapped in the pulmonary capillary bed. A gamma scintillation camera is positioned over the lungs and images are obtained in the anterior, posterior, lateral, and left and right posterior oblique projections. Perfusion abnormalities are detected on the scans as isotope-free zones. Ventilation scanning is performed by having the individual inhale an inert gas labeled with a radioisotope, such as xenon 133. The gamma camera is used to scan the lungs in a manner similar to that described for perfusion scanning. Localized abnormalities in ventilation, as may occur in individuals with parenchymal infiltrates or chronic obstructive lung disease, will cause abnormalities on the ventilation scan.

By convention, the V/Q lung scan is interpreted as "normal" or "low probability," "intermediate probability," or "high probability" for pulmonary embolism (202). A perfusion scan is normal if no perfusion defects are present and the perfusion outlines exactly the shape of the lungs as seen on the chest x-ray. The diagnosis of pulmonary embolism can be excluded if the perfusion lung scan is normal. A V/Q lung scan is designated as "very low probability" if there are fewer than three small segmental perfusion defects with a normal chest x-ray. A V/Q lung scan is designated as "low probability" if there are subsegmental defects on the perfusion scan and a normal ventilation scan, a single moderate, mismatched segmental perfusion defect with a normal chest x-ray, any perfusion defect with a substantially larger chest x-ray abnormality, or matched defects on both the ventilation and perfusion scans. The V/Q scan is considered "high probability" for pulmonary embolism if there is more than one large segmental perfusion defect without corresponding ventilation or chest x-ray abnormalities, more than one moderate segment and one large mismatched segment, or more than three moderate segmental perfusion defects without ventilation scan or chest radiographic abnormality. A V/Q scan is interpreted as "intermediate" or "indeterminate" probability if it does not fall into any of the other categories or is difficult to characterize (202).

If the diagnosis of pulmonary embolus is suspected from the clinical presentation, a "high probability" V/Q lung scan is usually sufficient to confirm the diagnosis. Neither "low probability" nor "intermediate probability" scans are adequate to confirm the diagnosis of pulmonary embolism. However, they are useful in assisting clinical decision making. If there is a low index of suspicion for pulmonary embolism based upon the clinical presentation, a "low probability" scan is reassuring and one need not pursue additional diagnostic testing. If, however, the clinical presentation is consistent with pulmonary embolism, neither "low" nor "moderate probability" scans are adequate to exclude nor confirm the diagnosis of pulmonary embolism. A pulmonary angiogram (see below) would be indicated as the gold standard diagnostic study.

Two large studies evaluated the predictive value of V/Q lung scans in individuals suspected of having pulmonary embolism (202, 203). Each indicated that "high probability" lung scans identified only one-half the individuals with pulmonary embolism. The Prospective Investigation of Pulmonary Embolism Diagnosis trial (PIOPED) examined the predictive value of ventilation perfusion lung scanning in 931 individuals suspected of having a pulmonary embolism (202). Of 116 individuals with "high probability" scans, 88% had pulmonary embolism confirmed by angiography, yielding a sensitivity of 41% and a specificity of 97%. Of 322 individuals with "intermediate probability" scans, 33% had pulmonary embolism confirmed by angiography; of those with "low probability" scans, 12% had angiographic evidence of pulmonary embolism.

Pulmonary angiography is used to definitively confirm or exclude the diagnosis of pulmonary embolism. It is important that pulmonary angiography be performed within 48 to 72 hours of presentation, because lysis and recanalization of a thromboembolism may obviate the diagnostic accuracy of this test. The procedure is performed in a specially designed angiography laboratory. A 6 to 8

French pigtail catheter is inserted into the individual percutaneously via the femoral vein. The catheter is initially placed in the main pulmonary artery to look for a large proximal thromboembolism. The catheter is then placed in the pulmonary artery of the lung with the most significant perfusion scan abnormality. Iodinated contrast material is injected and x-ray images are acquired. Pulmonary embolism is diagnosed if there is an intraluminal filling defect, or if obstruction in a pulmonary artery is identified on at least two projections.

Spiral CT and MRA are undergoing investigation as other noninvasive means to diagnose pulmonary emboli. Spiral CT can acquire volumetric image data and allow acquisition of an entire image during a single breath-hold. The ability to scan continuously during a single breath allows peak contrast opacification of the vasculature and better imaging (204). This technique allows for the reconstruction of overlying sections and multiplanar and three-dimensional imaging. The sensitivity for diagnosing pulmonary emboli ranges from 63 to 97% and the specificity from 89 to 100% (205–206). It is not yet as accurate as pulmonary angiography. Causes of false-positive scans include hilar lymph nodes, perivascular edema in heart failure, and partial opacification of pulmonary veins (204). The efficacy of gadolinium-contrast enhanced MRA in the diagnosis of pulmonary embolism showed promise in one recent clinical trial (207).

## SUPERIOR VENA CAVA SYNDROME

Superior vena cava syndrome is rarely caused by *in situ* development of thrombosis. More frequently, obstruction of the superior vena cava occurs as a consequence of extrinsic compression or invasion by tumors of the superior mediastinum, including lung neoplasms and lymphoma (208–210). Ascending aortic aneurysms, sclerosing mediastinitis, tuberculosis, fungal infections, and sarcoidosis are uncommon causes of superior vena cava syndrome (211–213). Central venous catheters may incite thrombus formation causing obstruction of the superior vena cava (210). Rarely, subclavian vein thrombus propagates to the innominate vein and, subsequently, into the superior vena cava. Symptoms include dyspnea, dysphagia, hoarseness, cough, headache, and visual disturbances. Lethargy and stupor may develop in severe cases. The physical findings include facial, neck, and arm swelling, jugular venous distention, and a prominent venous pattern on the upper chest.

Superior vena cava syndrome is suggested by the clinical presentation. Venography is used to demonstrate the presence of thrombus or extrinsic compression of the superior vena cava (214). Computerized tomographic imaging with contrast can detect the presence of extrinsic masses and superior vena cava obstruction (215, 216). The underlying cause of extrinsic compression or invasion can be evaluated further by bronchoscopy, mediastinoscopy, or thoracotomy (213).

## VENOUS THROMBOSIS OF ABDOMINAL VISCERA

Budd-Chiari syndrome refers to the clinical condition that occurs when the hepatic venous circulation is obstructed (217–219). Hepatic vein thrombosis, one cause of the Budd-Chiari syndrome, may occur from *in situ* thrombosis of the hepatic vein or propagation of thrombus from the inferior vena cava. Budd-Chiari syndrome can also be caused by occlusion of the suprahepatic vena cava by thrombus or membranous webs, and by nonthrombotic veno-occlusive disease of the sublobular branches of the hepatic veins and venules (219). Clinical conditions associated with thrombosis of the hepatic vein and suprahepatic vena cava include: myeloproliferative disorders, particularly polycythemia vera; paroxysmal nocturnal hemoglobinuria; oral contraceptive use; pregnancy; previous hepatitis; hepatocellular, renal cell, and adrenal carcinomas; leiomyosarcoma of the inferior vena cava; parasitic infection of the liver such as amebic cysts; and trauma (217, 220). Deficiencies of antithrombin III, protein C, and protein S, and the presence of factor V Leiden have been associated with Budd-Chiari syndrome as a sequela of hepatic vein thrombosis (221–225). Thirty percent of cases are idiopathic (217). The clinical features of Budd-Chiari syndrome include abdominal pain, ascites, hepatomegaly, and right upper quadrant tenderness. Individuals with portal hypertension may have jaundice, splenomegaly, and esophageal varices. Terminal manifestations of liver failure include encephalopathy and hepatorenal syndrome.

The diagnosis of hepatic vein thrombosis is confirmed by selective hepatic venography. Several noninvasive tests are useful in the diagnostic evaluation of individuals suspected of having Budd-Chiari syndrome. Duplex ultrasonography may be suggestive of hepatic vein thrombosis if pulse wave Doppler interrogation reveals abnormal venous flow patterns (226–230). Contrast-assisted CT and MRI may demonstrate hepatic or suprahepatic vena cava obstruction (231, 232). Hepatic scintigraphy may show decreased isotope uptake in the right lobe and central accumulation of isotope in the caudate lobe (233, 234). Liver biopsy of individuals with Budd-Chiari syndrome typically demonstrates central lobular congestion and hepatocellular atrophy (217).

Portal vein and splenic vein thromboses can cause extrahepatic portal venous hypertension. Clinical conditions associated with portal and splenic vein thromboses include intra-abdominal infections, biliary surgery, splenectomy, myeloproliferative disorders, pregnancy, oral contraceptive drugs, and malignant neoplasms. Nonthrombotic causes of portal and splenic vein obstruction include tumor invasion from hepatocellular carcinoma or extrinsic compression from neoplasms, abscesses, or retroperitoneal fibrosis (235). The clinical features of portal and splenic vein obstruction are those typically associated with portal hypertension and include gastrointestinal hemorrhage, usually from esophageal or gastric varices, splenomegaly, and rarely, ascites. In contrast to hepatic causes of portal hypertension, these individuals do not have features of liver dysfunction and therefore do not develop jaundice or encephalopathy. The diagnosis of portal vein thrombosis can be suggested by abdominal ultrasonography (236–239), CT imaging (240), or MRI (240–243). The diagnosis is confirmed by portal venography. Two techniques are used to visualize the portal venous system. The first involves imaging the venous phase of a selective mesenteric arteriogram. The second involves direct administration of radiocontrast into the portal vein via a transhepatic approach.

Mesenteric vein thrombosis is one of the three causes of acute mesenteric ischemia, as discussed earlier in the chapter. Causes of mesenteric vein thrombosis are broadly divided into primary, or idiopathic, and secondary. The most common secondary cause is intra-abdominal infection (95). Other causes include disorders of coagulation, such as thrombocytosis, polycythemia vera, and deficiencies of antithrombin III, protein C, or protein S (244–247). The clinical presentation is similar to that of acute mesenteric ischemia secondary to arterial thrombus. This includes severe abdominal pain, vomiting, and diarrhea. Physical findings result from peritonitis and include abdominal distention, tenderness, and loss of bowel sounds. The venous phase of selective superior mesenteric arteriography is examined to diagnose mesenteric vein thrombosis. Recently, MRI has been used successfully to diagnose venous thrombi affecting abdominal viscera (248, 249).

Renal vein thrombosis occurs most commonly in individuals with nephrotic syndrome (250). It may occur also as a consequence of extension of thrombus from the inferior vena cava. Individuals may present with severe lower back pain and hematuria. Bilateral renal vein thrombosis can cause renal failure. The diagnosis is confirmed by renal venography.

# REFERENCES

1. Criqui MH, Fronek A, Barrett-Connor E et al. The prevalence of peripheral arterial disease in a defined population. Circulation 1985;71:510–515.
2. Smith GD, Shipley MJ, Rose G. Intermittent claudication, heart disease risk factors, and mortality. Circulation 1990;82:1925–1931.
3. Schroll M, Munck O. Estimation of peripheral arteriosclerotic disease by ankle blood pressure measurements in a population study of 60-year-old men and women. J Chronic Dis 1981;34:261–269.
4. Gofin R, Kark JD, Friedlander Y et al. Peripheral vascular disease in a middle-aged population sample. Isr J Med Sci 1987;28:157–167.
5. Postiglione A, Cicerano U, Gallotta G et al. Prevalence of peripheral arterial disease and related risk factors in elderly institutionalized subjects. Gerontology 1992;38:330–337.
6. Paris BE, Libow LS, Halperin J et al. The prevalence and one-year outcome of limb arterial obstructive disease in a nursing home population. J Am Geriatr Soc 1988;36:607–612.

7. Rose G. The diagnosis of ischaemic heart pain and intermittent claudication in field surveys. Bull WHO 1962;27:645–658.
8. Hughson WG, Mann JI, Garrod A. Intermittent claudication: Prevalence and risk factors. Br Med J 1978;1:1379–1381.
9. Fowkes FG, Housley E, Cawood EH et al. Edinburgh Artery Study: Prevalence of asymptomatic and symptomatic peripheral arterial disease in the general population. Int J Epidemiol 1991;20:384–392.
10. Kannel WB, Skinner JJ Jr, Schwartz MJ et al. Intermittent claudication. Incidence in the Framingham study. Circulation 1970;41:875–883.
11. Kannel WB, McGee DL. Update on some epidemiologic features of intermittent claudication: The Framingham Study. J Am Geriatr Soc 1985;33:13–18.
12. Brand FN, Abbott RD, Kannel WB. Diabetes, intermittent claudication, and the risk of cardiovascular events. The Framingham study. Diabetes 1989;38:504–509.
13. Kannel WB, Shurtleff D. The Framingham study. Cigarettes and the development of intermittent claudication. Geriatrics 1973;28:61–68.
14. Thomas M. Smoking and vascular surgery. Br J Surg 1981;68:601–604.
15. Pomrehn P. The association of dyslipoproteinemia with symptoms and signs of peripheral arterial disease. The Lipid Research Clinics Program Prevalence Study. Circulation 1986;73(Suppl I):I100–I107.
16. Clarke R, Daly L, Robinson K et al. Hyperhomocystinemia: An independent risk factor for vascular disease. N Engl J Med 1991;324:1149–1155.
17. Fryer RH, Wilson BD, Gubler DB et al. Homocysteine, a risk factor for premature vascular disease and thrombosis, induces tissue factor activity in endothelial cells. Arterioscler Thromb 1993;13:1327–1333.
18. Malinow MR, Kang SS, Taylor LM et al. Prevalence of hyperhomocystinemia in individuals with peripheral arterial occlusive disease. Circulation 1989;79:1180–1188.
19. Rees MM, Rodgers GM. Homocysteinemia: Association of a metabolic disorder with vascular disease and thrombosis [Review]. Thromb Res 1993;71:337–359.
20. Creager M, O'Leary D, Doubilet P. Noninvasive vascular testing. In: Loscalzo J, Creager M, Dzau V, eds. Vascular medicine. Boston: Little, Brown, 1996;415–443.
21. Kempczinski RF. Segmental volume plethysmography in the diagnosis of lower extremity arterial occlusive disease. J Cardiovasc Surg 1982;23:125–129.
22. Carter SA. Clinical measurement of systolic pressures in limbs with arterial occlusive disease. JAMA 1969;207:1869–1874.
23. Yao ST, Hobbs JT, Irvine WT. Ankle systolic pressure measurements in arterial disease affecting the lower extremities. Br J Surg 1969;56:676–679.
24. Cutajar CL, Marston A, Newcombe JF. Value of cuff occlusion pressures in assessment of peripheral vascular disease. Br Med J 1973;2:392–395.
25. Lezack JD, Carter SA. The relationship of distal systolic pressures to the clinical and angiographic findings in limbs with arterial occlusive disease. Scand J Clin Lab Invest Suppl 1973;31:97–101.
26. Wells P. Basic principles and Doppler physics. In: Taylor K, Burns P, Wells P, eds. Clinical applications of Doppler ultrasound. New York: Raven Press, 1988;1–25.
27. Polak JF. Peripheral vascular sonography. Baltimore: Williams & Wilkins, 1992.
28. Merritt CR. Doppler color flow imaging. J Clin Ultrasound 1987;15:591–597.
29. Zierler RE, Phillips DJ, Beach KW et al. Noninvasive assessment of normal carotid bifurcation hemodynamics with color-flow ultrasound imaging. Ultrasound Med Biol 1987;13:471–476.
30. Middleton WD, Foley WD, Lawson TL. Color-flow Doppler imaging of carotid artery abnormalities. AJR Am J Roentgenol 1988;150:419–425.
31. Hatsukami TS, Primozich JF, Zierler RE et al. Color Doppler imaging of infrainguinal arterial occlusive disease. J Vasc Surg 1992;16:527–531.
32. Cossman DV, Ellison JE, Wagner WH et al. Comparison of contrast arteriography to arterial mapping with color-flow duplex imaging in the lower extremities. J Vasc Surg 1989;10:522–529.
33. Allard L, Cloutier G, Durand LG et al. Limitations of ultrasonic duplex scanning for diagnosing lower limb arterial stenoses in the presence of adjacent segment disease. J Vasc Surg 1994;19:650–657.
34. Bergamini TM, Tatum CM Jr, Marshall C et al. Effect of multilevel sequential stenosis on lower extremity arterial duplex scanning. Am J Surg 1995;169:564–566.
35. Quinn SF, Demlow TA, Hallin RW et al. Femoral MR angiography versus conventional angiography: preliminary results. Radiology 1993;189:181–184.
36. Cambria RP, Yucel EK, Brewster DC et al. The potential for lower extremity revascularization without contrast arteriography: Experience with magnetic resonance angiography. J Vasc Surg 1993;17:1050–1057.
37. Carpenter JP, Owen RS, Baum RA et al. Magnetic resonance angiography of peripheral runoff vessels. J Vasc Surg 1992;16:807–813.
38. Hertz SM, Baum RA, Owen RS et al. Comparison of magnetic resonance angiography and contrast arteriography in peripheral arterial stenosis. Am J Surg 1993;166:112–116.
39. Owen RS, Carpenter JP, Baum RA et al. Magnetic resonance angiography

of angiographically occult runoff vessels in peripheral arterial occlusive disease. N Engl J Med 1992;326:1577–1581.
40. Hoch JR, Tullis MJ, Kennell TW et al. Use of magnetic resonance angiography for the preoperative evaluation of individuals with infrainguinal arterial occlusive disease. J Vasc Surg 1996;23:792–801; discussion 801.
41. Masui T, Caputo GR, Bowersox JC et al. Assessment of popliteal arterial occlusive disease with 2D time-of-flight MRA. J Comput Assist Tomogr 1995;19:449–454.
42. Baum RA, Rutter CM, Sunshine JH et al. Multicenter trial to evaluate vascular magnetic resonance angiography of the lower extremity. American College of Radiology Rapid Technology Assessment Group. JAMA 1995;274:875–880.
43. Krug B, Kugel H, Harnischmacher U et al. Diagnostic performance of digital subtraction angiography (DSA) and magnetic resonance angiography (MRA): Preliminary results in vascular occlusive disease of the abdominal and lower-extremity arteries. Eur J Radiol 1995;19:77–85.
44. Kojima KY, Szumowski J, Sheley RC et al. Lower extremities: MR angiography with a unilateral telescopic phased-array coil. Radiology 1995;196:871–875.
45. Douek PC, Revel D, Chazel S et al. Fast MR angiography of the aortoiliac arteries and arteries of the lower extremity: Value of bolus-enhanced, whole-volume subtraction technique. AJR Am J Roentgenol 1995;165:431–437.
46. Adamis MK, Li W, Wielopolski PA et al. Dynamic contrast-enhanced subtraction MR angiography of the lower extremities: Initial evaluation with a multisection two-dimensional time-of-flight sequence. Radiology 1995;196:689–695.
47. Prince MR, Narasimham DL, Stanley JC et al. Breath-hold gadolinium-enhanced MR angiography of the abdominal aorta and its major branches. Radiology 1995;197:785–792.
48. Snidow JJ, Johnson MS, Harris VJ et al. Three-dimensional gadolinium-enhanced MR angiography for aortoiliac inflow assessment plus renal artery screening in a single breath hold. Radiology 1996;198:725–732.
49. Rofsky NM, Purdy DE, Johnson G et al. Suppression of venous signal in time-of-flight MR angiography of the lower extremities after administration of gadopentetate dimeglumine. Radiology 1997;202:177–182.
50. Bettmann MA. Principles of angiography. In: Loscalzo J, Creager MA, Dzau VJ, eds. Vascular medicine. A textbook of vascular biology and diseases. 1st ed. Boston: Little, Brown, 1992;483–507.
51. Waller BF, Pinkerton CA, Slack JD. Intravascular ultrasound: A histological study of vessels during life. Circulation 1992;85:2305–2310.
52. Meyer CR, Chiang EH, Fechner KP. Feasibility of high resolution intravascular ultrasonic imaging catheters. Radiology 1988;168:113–116.
53. Yock PG, Linker DT, Angelsen BA. Two-dimensional intravascular ultrasound: Technical development and initial clinical experience. J Am Soc Echocardiogr 1989;2:296–304.
54. Gussenhoven EJ, van der Lugt A, Pasterkamp G et al. Intravascular ultrasound predictors of outcome after peripheral balloon angioplasty. Eur J Vasc Endovasc Surg 1995;10:279–288.
55. Klauss V, Blasini R, Regar E. Deployment of the Palmaz-Schatz intracoronary stents with an imaging balloon catheter results in an improvement of acute luminal gain. Circulation 1993;88:3215.
56. Tielbeek AV, Vroegindeweij D, Buth J et al. Comparison of intravascular ultrasonography and intraarterial digital subtraction angiography after directional atherectomy of short lesions in femoropopliteal arteries. J Vasc Surg 1996;23:436–445.
57. Coy KM, Maurer G, Siegel R. Intravascular ultrasound imaging: A current perspective. J Am Coll Cardiol 1991;181:1811–1823.
58. Pandian NG, Kreis A, Brockway B et al. Detection of intra-arterial thrombus by high frequency two-dimensional ultrasound imaging in vitro and in vivo studies. Am J Cardiol 1990;65:1280–1283.
59. Siegel RJ, Ariani M, Fishbein MC et al. Histopathologic validation of angioscopy and intravascular ultrasound. Circulation 1991;84:109–117.
60. Smith P, Prevosti L, Underhill D, Leon M. Angioscopy: Basic principles of operation and performance characteristics. In: White G, White R, eds. Angioscopy: Vascular and coronary applications. Chicago: Yearbook Medical Publisher, 1989;6–19.
61. Miller A, Stonebridge PA, Jepsen SJ et al. Continued experience with intraoperative angioscopy for monitoring infrainguinal bypass grafting. Surgery 1991;109:286–293.
62. Gilbertson JJ, Walsh DB, Swolak RM et al. A blinded comparison of angiography, angioscopy, and duplex scanning in the intraoperative evaluation of in situ saphenous vein bypass grafts. J Vasc Surg 1991;15:121–129.
63. Segalowitz J, Grundfest WS, Treeman RL et al. Angioscopy for intraoperative management of thromboembolectomy. Arch Surg 1990;125:1357–1362.
64. Herrick JB. Clinical features of sudden obstruction of the coronary arteries. JAMA 1912;59:2015–2020.
65. Roberts WC, Buja LM. The frequency and significance of coronary arterial thrombi and other observations in fatal acute myocardial infarction. Am J Med 1972;52:425–443.
66. Eherlich JC, Shinohara Y. Low incidence of coronary thrombosis in myo-

cardial infarction: A restudy by serial block technique. Arch Pathol 1964; 78:432–445.

67. Ridolfi RL, Hutchins GM. The relationship between coronary artery lesions and myocardial infarcts: Ulceration of atherosclerotic plaques precipitating coronary thrombosis. Am Heart J 1977;93:468–486.

68. DeWood MA, Spores J, Watske R et al. Prevalence of total coronary occlusion during the early hours of transmural myocardial infarction. N Engl J Med 1980;303:897–902.

69. DeWood MA, Spores J, Hensley GR et al. Coronary arteriographic findings in acute transmural myocardial infarction. Circulation 1983;68:I39–I49.

70. Laffel GL, Braunwald E. Thrombolytic therapy. A new strategy for the treatment of acute myocardial infarction [Review]. Part I. N Engl J Med 1984;311:710–717.

71. Mandelkorn JB, Wolf NM, Singh S et al. Intracoronary thrombus in non-transmural myocardial infarction and in unstable angina pectoris. Am J Cardiol 1983;52:1–6.

72. Mizuno K, Satomura K, Miyamoto A et al. Angioscopic evaluation of coronary-artery thrombi in acute coronary syndromes. N Engl J Med 1992;326: 287–291.

73. Mizuno K. Angioscopic coronary macromorphology in individuals with acute coronary disorders. Lancet 1991;337:809–812.

74. Falk E. Unstable angina with fatal outcome: Dynamic coronary thrombosis leading to infarction and/or sudden death. Autopsy evidence of recurrent mural thrombosis with peripheral embolization culminating in total vascular occlusion. Circulation 1985;71:699–708.

75. Gotoh K, Minamino T, Katoh O et al. The role of intracoronary thrombus in unstable angina: Angiographic assessment and thrombolytic therapy during ongoing anginal attacks. Circulation 1988;77:526–534.

76. Ambrose JA, Winters SL, Stern A et al. Angiographic morphology and the pathogenesis of unstable angina pectoris. J Am Coll Cardiol 1985;5: 609–616.

77. Sherman CT, Litvack F, Grundfest W et al. Coronary angioscopy in individuals with unstable angina pectoris. N Engl J Med 1986;315:913–919.

78. Bresnahan DR, Davis JL, Holmes DR Jr et al. Angiographic occurrence and clinical correlates of intraluminal coronary artery thrombus: Role of unstable angina. J Am Coll Cardiol 1985;6:285–289.

79. Rehr R, Disciascio G, Vetrovec G et al. Angiographic morphology of coronary artery stenosis in prolonged rest angina: Evidence of intracoronary thrombus. J Am Coll Cardiol 1989;14:1429–1437.

80. Vetrovec GW, Leinbach RC, Gold HK et al. Intracoronary thrombolysis in syndromes of unstable ischemia: Angiographic and clinical results. Am Heart J 1982;104:946–952.

81. Capone G, Wolf NM, Meyer B et al. Frequency of intracoronary filling defects by angiography in angina pectoris at rest. Am J Cardiol 1985;56: 403–406.

82. Ambrose JA, Tannenbaum MA, Alexopoulos D et al. Angiographic progression of coronary artery disease and the development of myocardial infarction. J Am Coll Cardiol 1988;12:56–62.

83. Fuster V, Fallon JT, Nemerson Y. Coronary thrombosis. Lancet 1996; 348(Suppl 1):S7–S10.

84. Libby P. Atheroma: More than mush. Lancet 1996;348(Suppl 1):S4–S7.

85. Falk E, Shah PK, Fuster V. Coronary plaque disruption. Circulation 1995; 92:657–671.

86. Gillum RF, Folsom A, Leupker RV et al. Sudden death and acute myocardial infarction in a metropolitan area, 1970–1980. The Minnesota heart survey. N Engl J Med 1983;309:1353–1358.

87. Burke GL, Edlavitch SA, Crow RS. The effects of diagnostic criteria on trends in coronary heart disease morbidity: The Minnesota heart Survey. J Clin Epidemiol 1989;42:17–24.

88. Adams JE 3d, Bodor GS, Davila-Roman VG et al. Cardiac troponin I. A marker with high specificity for cardiac injury. Circulation 1993;88: 101–106.

89. Fitzgerald RL, Frankel WL, Herold DA. Comparison of troponin-T with other cardiac markers in a VA hospital. Am J Clin Pathol 1996;106:396–401.

90. de Winter RJ, Koster RW, Sturk A et al. Value of myoglobin, troponin T, and CK-MB mass in ruling out an acute myocardial infarction in the emergency room. Circulation 1995;92:3401–3407.

91. Antman EM, Tanasijevic MJ, Thompson B et al. Cardiac-specific troponin I levels to predict the risk of mortality in individuals with acute coronary syndromes. N Engl J Med 1996;335:1342–1349.

92. Stubbs P, Collinson P, Moseley D et al. Prognostic significance of admission troponin T concentrations in individuals with myocardial infarction. Circulation 1996;94:1291–1297.

93. Stubbs P, Collinson P, Moseley D et al. Prospective study of the role of cardiac troponin T in individuals admitted with unstable angina. Br Med J 1996;313:262–264.

94. Ohman EM, Armstrong PW, Christenson RH et al. Cardiac troponin T levels for risk stratification in acute myocardial ischemia. GUSTO IIA Investigators. N Engl J Med 1996;335:1333–1341.

95. Hansen KJ, Connelly DP, Stoney RJ. Visceral ischemia syndromes. In: Loscalzo J, Creager MA, Dzau VJ, eds. Vascular medicine. A textbook of vascular biology and diseases. 1st ed. Boston: Little, Brown, 1992;887–902.

96. Pierce GE, Brockenbrough EC. The spectrum of mesenteric infarction. Am J Surg 1970;119:233–239.

97. Ottinger LW. Mesenteric ischemia. N Engl J Med 1982;307:535–537.

98. Gorton M, John JF Jr. Polyarteritis overlap syndrome with extensive bowel infarction. Am J Gastroenterol 1980;74:153–156.

99. Edwards WH Jr, Martin RS 3d, Edwards WH Sr et al. Surviving gastrointestinal infarction due to polyarteritis nodosa: A rare event. Am J Surg 1992;58:167–172.

100. Smith JA, O'Sullivan M, Gough J et al. Small intestinal perforation secondary to localized giant-cell arteritis of the mesenteric vessels. Br J Rheumatol 1988;27:236–238.

101. Wolf EA Jr, Sumner DS, Strandness DE Jr. Disease of the mesenteric circulation in individuals with thromboangiitis obliterans. Vasc Surg 1972;6: 218–223.

102. Ripley HR, Levin SM. Abdominal angina associated with fibromuscular hyperplasia of the celiac and superior mesenteric arteries. Angiology 1966; 17:297–310.

103. Rogers DM, Thompson JE, Garrett WV et al. Mesenteric vascular problems. A 26-year experience. Ann Surg 1982;195:554–565.

104. Stanton PE Jr, Hollier PA, Seidel TW et al. Chronic intestinal ischemia: Diagnosis and therapy. J Vasc Surg 1986;4:338–344.

105. Hernandez D, Dominguez ML, Diaz F et al. Renal infarction in a severely hypertensive individual with lupus erythematosus and antiphospholipid antibodies. Nephron 1996;72:298–301.

106. Van Hoe L, Vandermeulen D, Gryspeerdt S et al. Assessment of accuracy of renal artery stenosis grading in helical CT angiography using maximum intensity projections. Eur Radiol 1996;6:658–664.

107. Dawson DL. Noninvasive assessment of renal artery stenosis. Semin Vasc Surg 1996;9:172–181.

108. Spies KP, Fobbe F, El-Bedewi M et al. Color-coded duplex sonography for noninvasive diagnosis and grading of renal artery stenosis. Am J Hypertens 1995;8:1222–1231.

109. Bass JC, Prince MR, Londy FJ et al. Effect of gadolinium on phase-contrast MR angiography of the renal arteries. AJR Am J Roentgenol 1997;168: 261–266.

110. Baxter GM, Aitchison F, Sheppard D et al. Colour Doppler ultrasound in renal artery stenosis: Intrarenal waveform analysis. Br J Radiol 1996;69: 810–815.

111. Loubeyre P, Trolliet P, Cahen R et al. MR angiography of renal artery stenosis: Value of the combination of three-dimensional time-of-flight and three-dimensional phase-contrast MR angiography sequences. AJR Am J Roentgenol 1996;167:489–494.

112. Bass JC, Prince MR, Londy FJ et al. Effect of gadolinium on phase-contrast MR angiography of the renal arteries. AJR Am J Roentgenol 1997;168: 261–266.

113. Rene PC, Oliva VL, Bui BT et al. Renal artery stenosis: Evaluation of Doppler US after inhibition of angiotensin-converting enzyme with captopril. Radiology 1995;196:675–679.

114. Anderson FA Jr, Wheeler HB, Goldberg RJ et al. A population-based perspective of the hospital incidence and case-fatality rates of deep vein thrombosis and pulmonary embolism. The Worcester DVT Study. Arch Intern Med 1991;151:933–938.

115. Dalen JE, Alpert JS. Natural history of pulmonary embolism. Prog Cardiovasc Dis 1975;17:257–270.

116. Gillum RF. Pulmonary embolism and thrombophlebitis in the United States. Am Heart J 1987;114:1262–1264.

117. Virchow R. Gesammelte abhandlungen zur wissenschafflichen medizin. Frankfurt-am-Main: Von Meidinger Sohn, 1856.

118. Ascani A, Radicchia S, Parise P et al. Distribution and occlusiveness of thrombi in individuals with surveillance detected deep vein thrombosis after hip surgery. Thromb Haemost 1996;75:239–241.

119. Potyk D, Tabbarah HJ. The pathogenesis and prevention of thromboembolic complications in individuals undergoing total hip replacement. J Gen Intern Med 1993;8:213–219.

120. Hodge WA. Prevention of deep vein thrombosis after total knee arthroplasty. Clin Orthop 1991;271:101–105.

121. Swann KW, Black PM, Baker MF. Management of symptomatic deep venous thrombosis and pulmonary embolism on a neurosurgical service. J Neurosurg 1986;64:563–567.

122. Turpie AG, Gent M, Doyle DJ et al. An evaluation of suloctidil in the prevention of deep vein thrombosis in neurosurgical individuals. Thromb Res 1985;39:173–181.

123. Nurmohamed MT, van Riel AM, Henkens CM et al. Low-molecular-weight heparin and compression stockings in the prevention of venous thromboembolism in neurosurgery. Thromb Haemost 1996;75:233–238.

124. Davidson HC, Mazzu D, Gage BF et al. Screening for deep venous thrombosis in asymptomatic postoperative orthopedic individuals using color Doppler sonography: Analysis of prevalence and risk factors. AJR Am J Roentgenol 1996;166:659–662.

125. Planes A, Vochelle N, Darmon JY et al. Risk of deep-venous thrombosis after hospital discharge in individuals having undergone total hip replacement: double-blind randomised comparison of enoxaparin versus placebo. Lancet 1996;348:224–228.

126. Maurer BJ, Wray R, Shillingford JP. Frequency of venous thrombosis after myocardial infarction. Lancet 1971;2:1385–1387.

127. Warlow C, Beattie AG, Terry G et al. A double-blind trial of low doses of subcutaneous heparin in the prevention of deep-vein thrombosis after myocardial infarction. Lancet 1973;2:934–936.

128. Pitt A, Anderson ST, Habersberger PG et al. Low dose heparin in the prevention of deep-vein thromboses in individuals with acute myocardial infarction. Am Heart J 1980;99:574–578.

129. McCarthy ST, Turner JJ, Robertson D et al. Low-dose heparin as a prophylaxis against deep-vein thrombosis after acute stroke. Lancet 1977;2:800–801.

130. Gelmers HJ. Effects of low-dose subcutaneous heparin on the occurrence of deep vein thrombosis in individuals with ischemic stroke. Acta Neurol Scand 1980;61:313–318.

131. Oczkowski WJ, Ginsberg JS, Shin A et al. Venous thromboembolism in individuals undergoing rehabilitation for stroke. Arch Phys Med Rehabil 1992;73:712–716.

132. Lechler E, Schramm W, Flosbach CW. The venous thrombotic risk in non-surgical individuals: Epidemiological data and efficacy/safety profile of a low-molecular-weight heparin (Enoxaparin). The Prime Study Group. Haemostasis 1996;26(Suppl 2):49–56.

133. Marik PE, Andrews L, Maini B. The incidence of deep venous thrombosis in ICU individuals. Chest 1997;111:661–664.

134. Hirsch DR, Ingenito EP, Goldhaber SZ. Prevalence of deep venous thrombosis among individuals in medical intensive care. JAMA 1995;274:335–337.

135. Dahlbeck B, Carlsson M, Svensson PJ. Familial thrombophilia due to a previously unrecognized mechanism characterized by poor anticoagulant response to activated protein C: Prediction of a cofactor to activated protein C. Proc Natl Acad Sci U S A 1993;90:1004–1008.

136. Koster T, Rosendaal FR, de Ronde H et al. Venous thrombosis due to poor anticoagulant response to activated protein C: Leiden Thrombophilia Study. Lancet 1993;342:1503–1506.

137. Griffin JH, Evatt B, Wideman C et al. Anticoagulant protein C pathway defective in majority of thrombophilic individuals. Blood 1993;82:1989–1993.

138. Dahlbeck B, Hildebrand B. Inherited resistance to activated protein C is corrected by anticoagulant cofactor activity found to be a property of factor V. Proc Natl Acad Sci U S A 1994;91:1396–1400.

139. Svensson PJ, Dahlback B. Resistance to activated protein C as a basis for venous thrombosis. N Engl J Med 1994;330:517–522.

140. Simioni P, Prandoni P, Lensing AW et al. The risk of recurrent venous thromboembolism in individuals with an Arg506 Gln mutation in the gene for factor V (factor V Leiden). N Engl J Med 1997;336:399–403.

141. Rintelen C, Mannhalter C, Ireland H et al. Oral contraceptives enhance the risk of clinical manifestation of venous thrombosis at a young age in females homozygous for factor V Leiden. Br J Haematol 1996;93:487–490.

142. Mandel H, Brenner B, Berant M et al. Coexistence of hereditary homocystinuria and factor V Leiden—Effect on thrombosis. N Engl J Med 1996;334:763–768.

143. den Heijer M, Koster T, Blom HJ et al. Hyperhomocystinemia as a risk factor for deep-vein thrombosis. N Engl J Med 1996;334:759–762.

144. Koster T, Blann AD, Bri't E et al. Role of clotting factor VIII in effect of von Willebrand factor on occurrence of deep-vein thrombosis. Lancet 1995;345:152–155.

145. Heijboer H, Buller HR, Brandjes DP et al. Deficiencies of coagulation-inhibiting and fibrinolytic proteins in outpatients with deep-vein thrombosis. N Engl J Med 1990;323:1512–1516.

146. Ginsberg JS, Wells PS, Brill-Edwards P et al. Antiphospholipid antibodies and venous thromboembolism. Blood 1995;86:3685–3691.

147. Ginsburg KS, Liang MH, Newcomer L et al. Anticardiolipin antibodies and the risk for ischemic stroke and venous thrombosis. Ann Intern Med 1992;117:997–1002.

148. Jeffries WS, Bochner F. Thromboembolism and its management in pregnancy. Med J Aust 1991;155:253–258.

149. Aaro LA, Juergens JL. Thrombophlebitis associated with pregnancy. Am J Obstet Gynecol 1971;109:1128–1136.

150. Tawes RL Jr, Kennedy PA, Harris EJ et al. Management of deep venous thrombosis and pulmonary embolism during pregnancy. Am J Surg 1982;144:141–146.

151. Grodstein F, Stampfer MJ, Goldhaber SZ et al. Prospective study of exogenous hormones and risk of pulmonary embolism in women. Lancet 1996;348:983–987.

152. Jick H, Derby LE, Myers MW et al. Risk of hospital admission for idiopathic venous thromboembolism among users of postmenopausal oestrogens. Lancet 1996;348:981–983.

153. Daly E, Vessey MP, Hawkins MM et al. Risk of venous thromboembolism in users of hormone replacement therapy. Lancet 1996;348:977–980.

154. Olin JW, Young JR, Graor RA et al. The changing clinical spectrum of thromboangiitis obliterans (Buerger's disease). Circulation 1990;82:IV3–IV8.

155. Lie JT. Vascular involvement in Behcet's disease: Arterial and venous and vessels of all sizes. J Rheumatol 1992;19:341–343.

156. Moser KM, LeMoine JR. Is embolic risk conditioned by location of deep venous thrombosis? Ann Intern Med 1981;94:439–444.

157. Doyle DJ, Turpie AG, Hirsh J et al. Adjusted subcutaneous heparin or continuous intravenous heparin in individuals with acute deep vein thrombosis. A randomized trial. Ann Intern Med 1987;107:441–445.

158. Huisman MV, Buller HR, ten Cate JW et al. Unexpected high prevalence of silent pulmonary embolism in individuals with deep venous thrombosis. Chest 1989;95:498–502.

159. Kakkar VV, Flanc C, Howe CT et al. Natural history of postoperative deep-vein thrombosis. Lancet 1969;2:230–232.

160. Hirsh J, Genten E, Hull R. Venous thromboembolism. New York: Grune and Stratton, 1981.

161. Machleder H. Neurovascular compression syndromes of the thoracic outlet. In: Loscalzo J, Creager M, Dzau V, eds. Vascular medicine. Boston: Little, Brown, 1996;1187–1208.

162. White RH, McGahan JP, Daschbach MM et al. Diagnosis of deep-vein thrombosis using duplex ultrasound. Ann Intern Med 1989;111:297–304.

163. O'Leary DH, Kane RA, Chase BM. A prospective study of the efficacy of B-scan sonography in the detection of deep venous thrombosis in the lower extremities. J Clin Ultrasound 1988;16:1–8.

164. Lensing AW, Prandoni P, Brandjes D et al. Detection of deep-vein thrombosis by real-time B-mode ultrasonography. N Engl J Med 1989;320:342–345.

165. Polak JF, Culter SS, O'Leary DH. Deep veins of the calf: Assessment with color Doppler flow imaging. Radiology 1989;171:481–485.

166. Davidson BL, Elliott CG, Lensing AW. Low accuracy of color Doppler ultrasound in the detection of proximal leg vein thrombosis in asymptomatic high-risk individuals. The RD Heparin Arthroplasty Group. Ann Intern Med 1992;117:735–738.

167. Yucel EK, Fisher JS, Egglin TK et al. Isolated calf venous thrombosis: Diagnosis with compression US. Radiology 1991;179:443–446.

168. Seminow GM, Friedell ML, Buchbinder D et al. The efficacy of ultrasonic venography in the detection of calf vein thrombosis. J Vasc Tech 1988;12:240–244.

169. Haire WD, Lynch TG, Lund GB et al. Limitations of magnetic resonance imaging and ultrasound-directed (duplex) scanning in the diagnosis of subclavian vein thrombosis. J Vasc Surg 1991;13:391–397.

170. Longley DG, Yedlicka JW, Molina EJ et al. Thoracic outlet syndrome: Evaluation of the subclavian vessels by color duplex sonography. AJR Am J Roentgenol 1992;158:623–630.

171. Haire WD, Lynch TG, Lieberman RP et al. Utility of duplex ultrasound in the diagnosis of asymptomatic catheter-induced subclavian vein thrombosis. J Ultrasound Med 1991;10:493–496.

172. Baxter GM, Kincaid W, Jeffrey RF et al. Comparison of colour Doppler ultrasound with venography in the diagnosis of axillary and subclavian vein thrombosis. Br J Radiol 1991;64:777–781.

173. Hull R, Taylor DW, Hirsh J et al. Impedance plethysmography: The relationship between venous filling and sensitivity and specificity for proximal vein thrombosis. Circulation 1978;58:898–902.

174. Browse NL, Clapham WF, Croft DN et al. Diagnosis of established deep vein thrombosis with the [125]I-fibrinogen uptake test. Br Med J 1971;4:325–328.

175. Kakkar VV, Nicolaides AN, Raney JT et al. [125]I-labelled fibrinogen test adapted for routine screening for deep vein thrombosis. Lancet 1970;1:540–542.

176. Carpenter JP, Holland GA, Baum RA et al. Magnetic resonance venography for the detection of deep venous thrombosis: Comparison with contrast venography and duplex Doppler ultrasonography. J Vasc Surg 1993;18:734–741.

177. Spritzer CE, Norconk JJ Jr, Sostman HD et al. Detection of deep venous thrombosis by magnetic resonance imaging. Chest 1993;104:54–60.

178. Evans AJ, Sostman HD, Knelson MH et al. 1992 ARRS Executive Council Award. Detection of deep venous thrombosis: Prospective comparison of MR imaging with contrast venography. AJR Am J Roentgenol 1993;161:131–139.

179. Holtz DJ, Debatin JF, McKinnon GC et al. MR venography of the calf: Value of flow-enhanced time-of-flight echoplanar imaging. AJR Am J Roentgenol 1996;166:663–668.

180. Rabinov K, Paulin S. Roentgen diagnosis of venous thrombosis in the leg. Arch Surg 1972;104:134–144.

181. Kniffin WD Jr, Baron JA, Barrett J et al. The epidemiology of diagnosed pulmonary embolism and deep venous thrombosis in the elderly. Arch Intern Med 1994;154:861–866.

182. Dalen JE, Paraskos JA, Ockene IS et al. Venous thromboembolism. Scope of the problem. Chest 1986;89(Suppl):370S–373S.

183. Moser KM. Venous thromboembolism [Review]. Am Rev Respir Dis 1990;141:235–249.

184. Pabinger I, Schneider B. Thrombotic risk in hereditary antithrombin III, protein C, or protein S deficiency. A cooperative, retrospective study. Gesellschaft fur Thrombose- und Hamostaseforschung (GTH) Study Group on Natural Inhibitors. Arterioscler Thromb Vasc Biol 1996;16:742–748.

185. Ginsberg JS, Wells PS, Brill-Edwards P et al. Antiphospholipid antibodies and venous thromboembolism. Blood 1995;86:3685–3691.

186. Falcon CR, Cattaneo M, Panzeri D et al. High prevalence of hyperhomo-

cyst(e)inemia in individuals with juvenile venous thrombosis. Arterioscler Thromb 1994;14:1080–1083.

187. Goldhaber SZ, Grodstein F, Stampfer MJ et al. A prospective study of risk factors for pulmonary embolism in women. JAMA 1997;277:642–645.

188. Grodstein F, Stampfer MJ, Goldhaber SZ et al. Prospective study of exogenous hormones and risk of pulmonary embolism in women. Lancet 1996; 348:983–987.

189. Daly E, Vessey MP, Hawkins MM et al. Risk of venous thromboembolism in users of hormone replacement therapy. Lancet 1996;348:977–980.

190. Hirsch DR, Mikkola KM, Marks PW et al. Pulmonary embolism and deep venous thrombosis during pregnancy or oral contraceptive use: Prevalence of factor V Leiden. Am Heart J 1996;131:1145–1148.

191. Anonymous. The urokinase pulmonary embolism trial. A national cooperative study. Circulation 1973;47(Suppl):1–108.

192. Stein PD, Dalen JE, McIntyre KM et al. The electrocardiogram in acute pulmonary embolism. Prog Cardiovasc Dis 1975;17:247–257.

193. Talbot S, Worthington BS, Roebuck EJ. Radiographic signs of pulmonary embolism and pulmonary infarction. Thorax 1973;28:198–203.

194. Stein PD, Terrin ML, Hales CA et al. Clinical, laboratory, roentgenographic, and electrocardiographic findings in individuals with acute pulmonary embolism and no pre-existing cardiac or pulmonary disease. Chest 1991;100:598–603.

195. Stein PD, Goldhaber SZ, Henry JW et al. Arterial blood gas analysis in the assessment of suspected acute pulmonary embolism. Chest 1996;109:78–81.

196. Stein PD, Goldhaber SZ, Henry JW. Alveolar-arterial oxygen gradient in the assessment of acute pulmonary embolism. Chest 1995;107:139–143.

197. McConnell MV, Solomon SD, Rayan ME et al. Regional right ventricular dysfunction detected by echocardiography in acute pulmonary embolism. Am J Cardiol 1996;78:469–473.

198. Harrison KA, Haire WD, Pappas AA et al. Plasma D-dimer: A useful tool for evaluating suspected pulmonary embolus [published erratum appears in J Nucl Med 1993;34:1409]. J Nucl Med 1993;34:896–898.

199. Goldhaber SZ, Simons GR, Elliott CG et al. Quantitative plasma D-dimer levels among individuals undergoing pulmonary angiography for suspected pulmonary embolism. JAMA 1993;270:2819–2822.

200. Ginsberg JS, Brill-Edwards PA, Demers C et al. D-dimer in individuals with clinically suspected pulmonary embolism. Chest 1993;104:1679–1684.

201. Bounameaux H, de Moerloose P, Reber G et al. Plasma measurement of D-dimer as diagnostic aid in suspected venous thromboembolism: An overview [Review]. Thromb Haemost 1994;71:1–6.

202. Anonymous. Value of the ventilation/perfusion scan in acute pulmonary embolism: Results of the prospective investigation of pulmonary embolism diagnosis (PIOPED). The PIOPED Investigators. JAMA 1990;263: 2753–2759.

203. Hull RD, Hirsh J, Carter CJ et al. Diagnostic value of ventilation-perfusion lung scanning in individuals with suspected pulmonary embolism. Chest 1985;88:819–828.

204. Gefter WB, Hatabu H, Holland GA et al. Pulmonary thromboembolism: Recent developments in diagnosis with CT and MR imaging [Review]. Radiology 1995;197:561–574.

205. Remy-Jardin M, Remy J, Wattinne L et al. Central pulmonary thromboembolism: Diagnosis with spiral volumetric CT with the single-breath-hold technique—Comparison with pulmonary angiography. Radiology 1992; 185:381–387.

206. Goodman LR, Curtin JJ, Mewissen MW et al. Detection of pulmonary embolism in individuals with unresolved clinical and scintigraphic diagnosis: Helical CT versus angiography. AJR Am J Roentgenol 1995;164: 1369–1374.

207. Meaney JF, Weg JG, Chenevert TL et al. Diagnosis of pulmonary embolism with magnetic resonance angiography. N Engl J Med 1997;336:1422–1427.

208. Perez-Soler R, McLaughlin P, Velasquez WS et al. Clinical features and results of management of superior vena cava syndrome secondary to lymphoma. J Clin Oncol 1984;2:260–266.

209. Citron ML, Fossieck BE Jr, Krasnow SH et al. Superior vena cava syndrome due to non-small-cell lung cancer. Resolution with chemotherapy alone. JAMA 1983;250:71–72.

210. Parish JM, Marschke RF Jr, Dines DE et al. Etiologic considerations in superior vena cava syndrome. Mayo Clin Proc 1981;56:407–413.

211. Kahn SE, Kotler MN, Goldman AP et al. Superior vena caval obstruction secondary to acute dissecting aneurysm of the aorta. Am Heart J 1986; 111:606–608.

212. Phillips PL, Amberson JB, Libby DM. Syphilitic aortic aneurysm presenting with the superior vena cava syndrome. Am J Med 1981;71:171–173.

213. Helms SR, Carlson MD. Cardiovascular emergencies [Review]. Semin Oncol 1989;16:463–470.

214. Stanford W, Doty DB. The role of venography and surgery in the management of individuals with superior vena cava obstruction. Ann Thorac Surg 1986;41:158–163.

215. Bechtold RE, Wolfman NT, Karstaedt N et al. Superior vena caval obstruction: Detection using CT. Radiology 1985;157:485–487.

216. Schwartz EE, Goodman LR, Haskin ME. Role of CT scanning in the superior vena cava syndrome. Am J Clin Oncol 1986;9:71–78.

217. Mitchell MC, Boitnott JK, Kaufman S et al. Budd-Chiari syndrome: Etiology, diagnosis, and management [Review]. Medicine 1982;61:199–218.

218. Murphy FB, Steinberg HV, Shires GT 3d et al. The Budd-Chiari syndrome: A Review. AJR Am J Roentgenol 1986;147:9–15.

219. Klein AS, Cameron JL. Diagnosis and management of the Budd-Chiari syndrome [Review]. Am J Surg 1990;160:128–133.

220. Valla D, Casadevall N, Lacombe C et al. Primary myeloproliferative disorder and hepatic vein thrombosis. A prospective study of erythroid colony formation in vitro in 20 individuals with Budd-Chiari syndrome. Ann Intern Med 1985;103:329–334.

221. McClure S, Dincsoy HP, Glueck H. Budd-Chiari syndrome and antithrombin III deficiency. Am J Clin Pathol 1982;78:236–241.

222. Bourliere M, Le Treut YP, Arnoux D et al. Acute Budd-Chiari syndrome with hepatic failure and obstruction of the inferior vena cava as presenting manifestations of hereditary protein C deficiency. Gut 1990;31:949–952.

223. Couffinhal T, Bonnet J, Benchimol D et al. A case of the Budd-Chiari syndrome attributed to a deficit in protein C. Eur Heart J 1991;12:266–269.

224. Blanshard C, Pasi J, Rolles K et al. Acute Budd-Chiari syndrome treated by liver transplantation in a woman homozygous for factor V Leiden. Eur J Gastroenterol Hepatol 1996;8:925–927.

225. Fickert P, Ramschak H, Kenner L et al. Acute Budd-Chiari syndrome with fulminant hepatic failure in a pregnant woman with factor V Leiden mutation. Gastroenterology 1996;111:1670–1673.

226. Hosoki T, Kuroda C, Tokunaga K et al. Hepatic venous outflow obstruction: Evaluation with pulsed duplex sonography. Radiology 1989;170:733–737.

227. Ralls PW, Johnson MB, Radin DR et al. Budd-Chiari syndrome: detection with color Doppler sonography. AJR Am J Roentgenol 1992;159:113–116.

228. Bolondi L, Gaiani S, Li Bassi S et al. Diagnosis of Budd-Chiari syndrome by pulsed Doppler ultrasound. Gastroenterology 1991;100:1324–1331.

229. Hosoki T, Kuroda C, Tokunaga K et al. Hepatic venous outflow obstruction: Evaluation with pulsed duplex sonography. Radiology 1989;170: 733–737.

230. Grant EG, Schiller VL, Millener P et al. Color Doppler imaging of the hepatic vasculature. AJR Am J Roentgenol 1992;159:943–950.

231. Stark DD, Hahn PF, Trey C et al. MRI of the Budd-Chiari syndrome. AJR Am J Roentgenol 1986;146:1141–1148.

232. Mathieu D, Vasile N, Menu Y et al. Budd-Chiari syndrome: Dynamic CT. Radiology 1987;165:409–413.

233. Meindok H, Langer B. Liver scan in Budd-Chiari syndrome. J Nucl Med 1976;17:365–368.

234. Tavill AS, Wood EJ, Kree L et al. The Budd-Chiari syndrome: Correlation between hepatic scintigraphy and the clinical, radiological and pathological findings in nineteen cases of hepatic venous outflow obstruction. Gastroenterology 1975;68:509–518.

235. Sherlock S. Extrahepatic portal venous hypertension in adults. Clin Gastroenterol 1985;14:1–19.

236. Bach AM, Hann LE, Brown KT et al. Portal vein evaluation with US: Comparison to angiography combined with CT arterial portography. Radiology 1996;201:149–154.

237. Letourneau JG, Carlson JE, Longley DG et al. Portal vein reflectors: Duplex sonographic appearance. Gastrointest Radiol 1992;17:141–144.

238. Nordback I, Sisto T. Ultrasonography and computed tomography in the diagnosis of portomesenteric vein thrombosis. Int Surg 1991;76:179–182.

239. Fidler H, Booth A, Hodgson HJ et al. Portal vein thrombosis in myeloproliferative disease. Uses of thrombolytic and antiplatelet treatment. Br Med J 1990;300:590–592.

240. Zirinsky K, Markisz JA, Rubenstein WA et al. MR imaging of portal venous thrombosis: Correlation with CT and sonography. AJR Am J Roentgenol 1988;150:283–288.

241. Kashitani N, Kimoto S, Tsunoda M et al. Portal blood flow in the presence or absence of diffuse liver disease: Measurement by phase contrast MR imaging. Abdom Imaging 1995;20:197–200.

242. Taylor CR, McCauley TR. Magnetic resonance imaging in the evaluation of the portal venous system. J Clin Gastroenterol 1992;14:268–273.

243. Levy HM, Newhouse JH. MR imaging of portal vein thrombosis. AJR Am J Roentgenol 1988;151:283–286.

244. Edmondson HT. Mesenteric vein thrombosis secondary to polycythemia vera. J Med Assoc Ga 1972;61:159–161.

245. De Stefano V, Leone G, Teofili L et al. Mesenteric vein thrombosis in protein S congenital deficiency. Thromb Res 1990;57:935–944.

246. Gruenberg JC, Smallridge RC, Rosenberg RD. Inherited antithrombin-III deficiency causing mesenteric venous infarction: a new clinical entity. Ann Surg 1975;181:791–794.

247. Pabinger I, Schneider B. Thrombotic risk in hereditary antithrombin III, protein C, or protein S deficiency. A cooperative, retrospective study. Gesellschaft fur Thrombose-und Hamostaseforschung (GTH) Study Group on Natural Inhibitors. Arterioscler Thromb Vasc Biol 1996;16:742–748.

248. Gehl HB, Bohndorf K, Klose KC et al. Two-dimensional MR angiography in the evaluation of abdominal veins with gradient refocused sequences. J Comput Assist Tomogr 1990;14:619–624.

249. Haddad MC, Clark DC, Sharif HS et al. MR, CT, and ultrasonography of splanchnic venous thrombosis. Gastrointest Radiol 1992;17:34–40.

250. Llach F, Arieff AI, Massry SG. Renal vein thrombosis and nephrotic syndrome. A prospective study of 36 adult individuals. Ann Intern Med 1975; 83:8–14.

# CHAPTER 26

# LABORATORY METHODS IN HEMOSTASIS

## Paula L. Bockenstedt

The laboratory assessment of hemostatic components has evolved from the assays of the early 1900s, in which the rate and physical characteristics of clot formation and dissolution were observed, to a wide variety of immunologic, functional, and DNA-based assays of individual components of the hemostatic system. This explosion in technology was fostered by the careful observations of early coagulation specialists on the effect of mixing blood from individuals with hemostatic disorders with normal blood and observing the effect on the clotting time. In this manner, components of the coagulation and fibrinolytic systems were dissected for further analysis by biochemists and enzymologists. These early studies were performed manually in glass test tubes. Later, with the advent of the fibrometer, plasma samples could be collected and assays performed with more precise endpoint determination. The modern coagulation laboratory currently uses many methodologies and instrumentation to perform chromogenic, clot-based, immunologic, electrophoretic, aggregation and radioisotope-based assays. With the cloning, sequencing, and identification of molecular defects in most of these hemostatic factors, polymerase chain reaction (PCR) based technologies and specific genetic probes have become available for identification of congenital deficiencies of these factors, although most DNA-based testing in the United States is still confined to the research laboratory. For the majority of coagulation abnormalities, which are due to acquired and not inherited defects, the routine coagulation assays will still be necessary. Interpretation of these laboratory results for use in individual management requires a fundamental understanding of the sensitivity and specificity of each assay and how the result may be affected by medications, associated diseases, or defects in other parts of the hemostatic system not tested. Most importantly, these results depend on adequate sample preparation and handling, with strict adherence to methods proven to result in a minimum of *ex vivo* disturbance of the hemostatic factors (1, 2). The individual's hemostatic defect should not be diagnosed solely on the basis of a laboratory test without correlation with a careful, complete medical history.

The following discussion includes a compendium of clinical laboratory hemostasis assays available in routine and reference laboratories with an emphasis on laboratory interpretation.

## HISTORICAL PERSPECTIVES

### LEE-WHITE WHOLE BLOOD CLOTTING TIME

The whole blood clotting time (WBCT), developed in 1913, is no longer used, but the principle of measuring the time to visible clot formation as an assessment of the overall status of the coagulation system forms the basis for many of the modern assays of hemostasis. In the WBCT, fresh blood is collected sequentially into three separate glass tubes, labeled 3, 2, and 1, while monitoring time (3). After 3 minutes, tube 1 is carefully tilted to 45 degrees every 30 seconds until a clot forms. The same procedure is followed for tube 2, then for tube 3, at which point the elapsed time is recorded. The range of normal values is 4 to 8 minutes at 37°C or 8 to 15 minutes at room temperature. No control assay is performed. The test is affected by factors in the intrinsic, extrinsic, and common pathways, but is insensitive to extrinsic pathway defects. Unfortunately, the test is affected by the diameter of the test tube, material composition of the test tube, temperature, and tilting technique (3). It was often used as a bedside monitor of heparin therapy, where the goal was to prolong the clotting time to twice that of the individual's baseline value.

## RECALCIFICATION TIME

The recalcification time is a modification of the WBCT, devised to eliminate dependence of the results on hematocrit (4, 5). In this case, the blood is centrifuged to produce platelet-rich plasma (PRP). Calcium chloride is added to the PRP and the time to clot formation recorded. The normal recalcification time is 100 to 150 seconds. Results of this assay are inversely related to the platelet count and are affected by platelet function. Thus, in the presence of platelet dysfunction, the recalcification time will be prolonged regardless of whether there is a true factor deficiency, and little information is gained.

# SCREENING TESTS IN HEMOSTASIS (SEE ALSO CHAPTER 23)

## ACTIVATED COAGULATION TIME

To minimize the effect of variable degrees of contact activation upon exposure to glass blood collection tubes, a modification of the WBCT, the activated coagulation

time (ACT), was developed in 1966 (6). Blood is drawn into tubes containing a particulate activator of the contact activation system, such as diatomaceous earth, kaolin, or celite. Exposure to these negatively charged surfaces activates the contact activation system maximally and more uniformly. Typical values are slightly below 100 seconds. The ACT is sensitive to heparin therapy and yields results of 150 to 190 seconds on therapeutic doses. Controversy exists as to whether the ACT is a better monitor of heparin therapy than the activated partial thromboplastin time (aPTT) or thrombin clotting time (TCT). It is simpler and more linear than the aPTT and may be performed at the bedside, but it is influenced by the presence of platelets and requires an alert, skilled observer (6–8). The ACT is most often used as a monitor during regional heparinization.

## PROTHROMBIN TIME

The prothrombin time (PT), developed by Quick et al in 1935, is a measure of extrinsic and common pathway factors (Fig. 26.1) (9). In this assay, blood is collected into sodium citrate anticoagulant and the sample is centrifuged to produce citrated plasma. Tissue thromboplastin, usually rabbit, bovine, or human cadaver brain, or lipidated recombinant tissue factor, suspended in calcium chloride, forms the commercial PT reagent. Prewarmed PT reagent is added to the test plasma sample and time to clot formation recorded. Thus, the added tissue thromboplastin activates factor VII to VIIa and forms a complex to catalyze the conversion of factor X to Xa. Factors Xa and Va and the phospholipid present in the rabbit brain extract, together, form the prothrombinase complex. The prothrombinase complex converts prothrombin to thrombin in the presence of calcium. The last step in the reaction, the conversion of fibrinogen to

**FIGURE 26.1.** Schematic diagram of the coagulation cascade. The dotted lines encircle the factors measured by the prothrombin time assay. HK, high-molecular-weight kininogen.

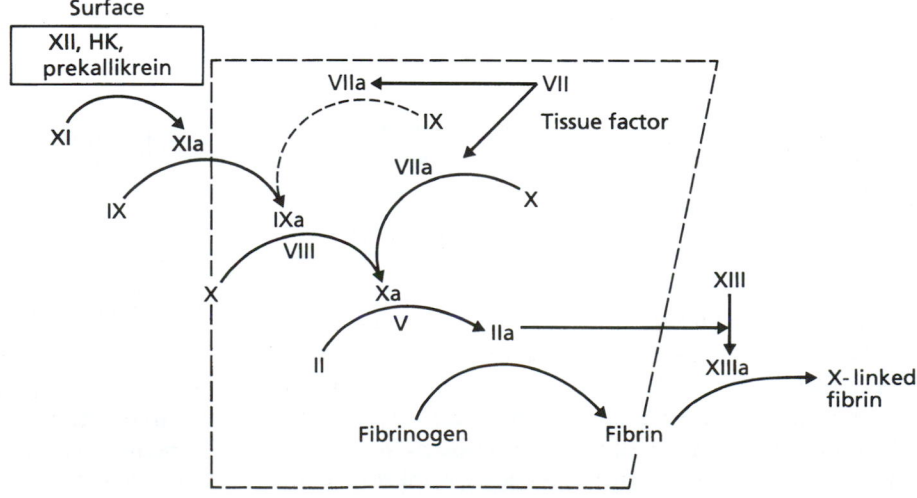

fibrin by thrombin is detected visually, photo-optically or by electrical impedance (4, 10).

## Interpretation

The PT is prolonged in deficiencies of fibrinogen, prothrombin, and factors V, VII, or X (Fig. 26.1). It is also prolonged by disseminated intravascular coagulation (DIC), vitamin K deficiency, liver disease, heparin therapy and, to variable degrees, by lupus anticoagulants and high levels of fibrin degradation products (FDPs) (4, 11). After anticoagulation with warfarin, the initial PT prolongation is due predominantly to a decline in factor VII levels. Factor VII activity is reduced after 6 hours, factor X in 40 hours, and prothrombin in 60 hours (Fig. 26.2). This PT prolongation is due not only to the decline in antigenic levels of vitamin K-dependent clotting factors, but also to the presence of incompletely γ-carboxylated forms of the vitamin K-dependent factors that do not bind normally to phospholipid within the PT reagent.

The PT is affected by the source of thromboplastin used, which is of particular concern in monitoring individuals being given oral anticoagulation (12–18). Attempts to develop synthetic PT reagents with more uniform lipid and recombinant tissue factor content in order to reduce interlaboratory variability has not been entirely successful (15–16). Recombinant tissue factor-based reagents tend to be more sensitive to factor VII levels and to incompletely γ-carboxylated forms of vitamin K-dependent factors than rabbit or human cadaver brain thromboplastin. The increased sensitivity of recombinant thromboplastin to decreased coagulant factor levels, as well as γ-carboxylated forms of vitamin K-dependent factors, may lead to higher PT values when compared to values obtained with the more traditional rabbit brain thromboplastin (15). Commercial thromboplastins are now standardized for activity against an international reference thromboplastin. At a minimum, results should be reported as a PT ratio or, preferably, in international normalized ratio (INR) units in warfarinized individual samples (10, 18–24). The INR value, designed for use in standardizing the PT in warfarin monitoring, should not be used when evaluating individuals with liver disease (19, 25). Monitoring of warfarin therapy using the PT is further discussed in Chapter 55.

## ACTIVATED PARTIAL THROMBOPLASTIN TIME

The PTT and aPTT are measures of components of the contact activation, intrinsic, and common pathways (4). Thus, the aPTT provides information on all clotting factors but factor VII. A chloroform extract of human, rabbit, or bovine brain, containing variable types of phospholipid, serves as the surface for elaboration of the prothrombinase complex (26). In the aPTT, an activator of the contact activation system is also added in the form of diatomaceous earth, celite, kaolin, ellagic acid, or micronized silica particles (Table 26.1). This allows for full and standardized activation of the contact activation system. Test plasma is added to 100 μL of the partial thromboplastin/activator mix (aPTT reagent) and incubated for 3 minutes at 37°C. Calcium chloride is then added to the preactivated mix and the time to clot formation recorded as described for the PT assay.

**TABLE 26.1.** Components of Various Thromboplastin Reagents

| Platelet Substitute | Activator |
| --- | --- |
| Rabbit brain | Aluminum-coated silica |
| Rabbit brain phospholipid | Micronized kaolin |
| Rabbit brain cephalin | Ellagic acid |
| Bovine brain | $Mg^{2+}$, $Al^{2+}$ silicate |
| Bovine brain | Celite |

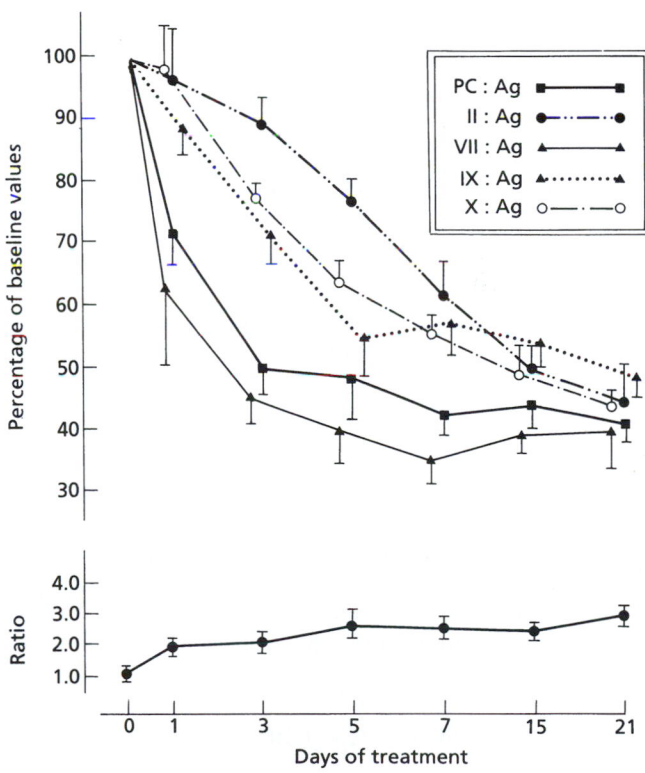

**FIGURE 26.2.** Changes in the thrombotest (**lower panel**) and vitamin K-dependent proteins (**upper panel**) in 10 individuals at the initiation of oral anticoagulant therapy. PC:Ag, protein C antigen. (Adapted with permission from Vigano S, Mannucci PM, Solinas S. Decrease in protein C antigen and formation of an abnormal protein soon after starting oral anticoagulant therapy. Br J Haematol 1984;57:213–220.)

**FIGURE 26.3.** Schematic diagram of the coagulation cascade. The dotted lines encircle the factors measured by the partial thromboplastin time assay.

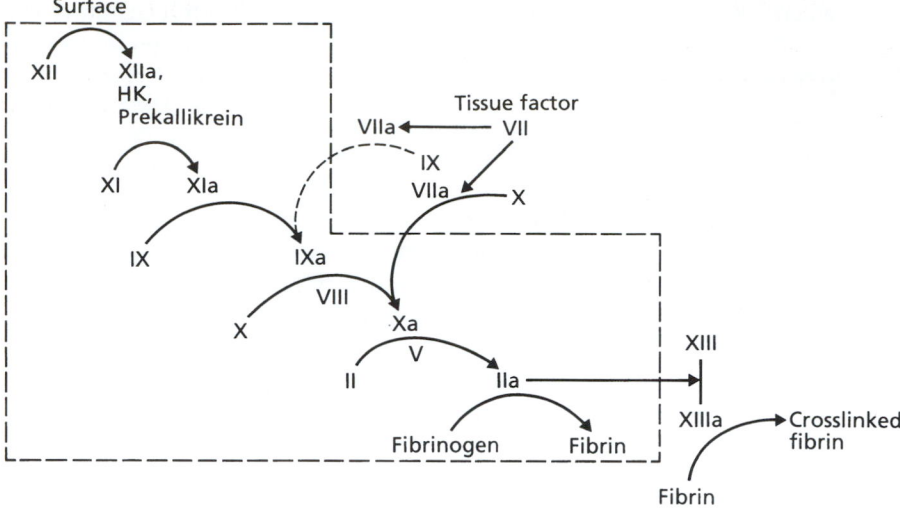

## Interpretation

The normal ranges for the PTT and aPTT depend on the reagents used by individual laboratories. Typical normal ranges for the aPTT and PTT are 21 to 29 and 68 to 82 seconds, respectively. The aPTT is prolonged in deficiencies of fibrinogen, and factors II, V, VIII, IX, X, XI, or XII, prekallikrein and high-molecular-weight kininogen (HK) (Fig. 26.3). It is also prolonged in DIC, vitamin K deficiency, and with warfarin or heparin therapy (8). Lupus anticoagulants may interfere with the prothrombinase complex assembly on the phospholipid extract, resulting in prolongation of the aPTT (see Acquired Coagulation Inhibitors, below). Sensitivity of the aPTT to mild factor deficiencies is directly related to the thromboplastin reagent used (26–28). The aPTT may be prolonged due to interference by paraproteins with fibrin polymerization (11, 26), and artifactually prolonged in markedly icteric, lipemic, or hemolyzed specimens in optical clot detection instruments (4). The aPTT may be artifactually shortened by exposure of blood to glass, resulting in activation of the contact system prior to assay (29). The aPTT is sensitive to the effects of heparin (30) and is the most frequently used test for monitoring heparin anticoagulation (8, 28, 30).

## PROTHROMBIN CONSUMPTION TEST

The prothrombin consumption test is a generalized screening test that detects, but does not identify, a deficiency in either factor V, VIII, IX, XI, or XII (8). The test blood sample is allowed to clot for 1 hour at 37°C. The serum is collected and added to adsorbed rabbit plasma containing a source of factor V and fibrinogen but deficient in factors II, VII, IX, and X (Simplastin). A PT is

|  | Serum | Adsorbed rabbit plasma |
|---|---|---|
| Factor present | VII, IX, X, XI, XII | I, V, VII, XI, XII, XIII |
| Factor absent | I, II, V, VIII, XIII | II, VII, IX, X |

(a)

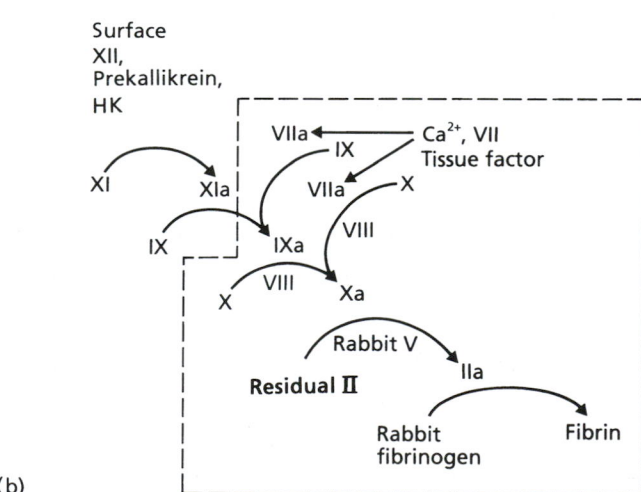

(b)

**FIGURE 26.4.** Prothrombin consumption test. **a,** Factors present and absent in serum and absorbed plasma. **b,** The dotted lines encircle the coagulation factors affecting the prothrombin consumption test.

then performed on the test mixture (Fig. 26.4). If there is a factor deficiency in the test sample, then prothrombin will not have been as effectively consumed in the original clotting process. Hence the serum will contain increased prothrombin levels, compared to control serum. This residual prothrombin will be detected by a shortening of the PT compared to control values ob-

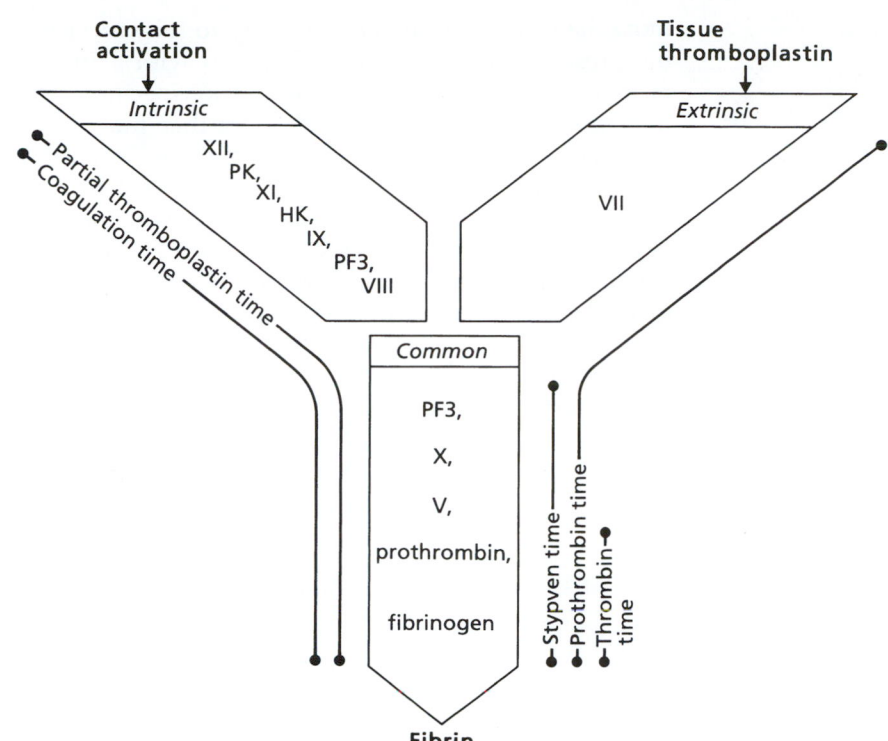

**FIGURE 26.5.** Diagrammatic relationship of common screening tests of blood coagulation. The major pathways of coagulation are enclosed in the arrow-shaped boxes. The screening tests are indicated at the side of the boxes in relation to the pathways and coagulation factors measured by each. (Adapted with permission from Wintrobe M et al, eds. Clinical haematology. Philadelphia: Lea & Febiger, 1981;1056.)

tained from normal serum. The test does not identify factor VII or factor X deficiency, because the PT will be prolonged (that is, normal) because of decreased activation of factor V. This cannot be distinguished from the normal decreased prothrombin level expected in serum; consequently the test sample result will be normal (4). The prothrombin consumption test is also used in screening for platelet defects when coagulation factors are known to be normal (31, 32). (See Fig. 26.5 for the relationship between the prothrombin consumption test and other screening tests of coagulation (33).)

## THROMBOPLASTIN GENERATION TEST

The thromboplastin generation test measures both the amount and rate of thrombin generation using a two-stage method (32, 34). In the first stage, calcium chloride is added to the test plasma. At certain intervals, an aliquot of the test plasma is removed and added, in the second stage, to a solution of fibrinogen; the time to clot formation is then measured. The time of fibrinogen cleavage and polymerization to fibrin is a function of the amount of thrombin present. Both the rate of formation and the decay rate of thrombin produced in the test plasma can be monitored. The time to peak thrombin production is an indicator of the clotting activity of the plasma.

## THROMBOTEST

The Thrombotest (35) evaluates the extrinsic pathway and has been used predominantly in monitoring indi-

viduals taking oral anticoagulants. The Thrombotest reagent consists of adsorbed bovine plasma containing factor V and fibrinogen, and bovine brain tissue thromboplastin. Addition of a maximal amount of factor V and fibrinogen ensures that these common pathway factors are not rate limiting in the formation of thrombin and detectable clot. The assay has longer result times than the one stage PT. The test is particularly sensitive to factors VII and X, as well as to factor IX. It is most accurate at factor levels below 50%. The therapeutic range for anticoagulation is 5 to 15%.

## THROMBIN CLOTTING TIME

The TCT, or thrombin time, is the most sensitive screening test for decreases or abnormalities in fibrinogen. The assay is based on the original procedure by Clauss (36) and measures the rate of fibrin formation (37). It is a measure of clottable fibrinogen and, therefore, provides qualitative information on fibrinogen function. The time to clot formation is measured when dilute thrombin (5 to 10 U/mL) is added to undiluted test plasma.

### Interpretation

The assay is affected by the presence of heparin, hirudin, FDPs, and paraproteins (4, 8, 36–39). The normal range for the neonatal TCT is different from the normal adult values owing to the presence of fetal fibrinogen, which is biochemically different from adult fibrinogen (40–42). The TCT is also useful in monitoring heparin anticoagu-

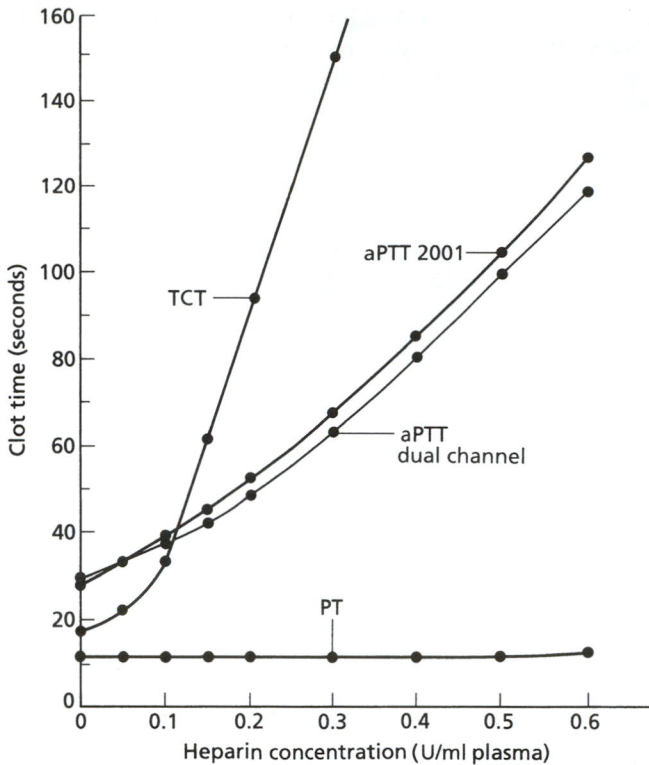

**FIGURE 26.6.** Sensitivity of various tests to heparin concentration. (Adapted with permission from Palkuti HS. Laboratory monitoring of anticoagulant therapy. J Med Tech 1985; 2:81–86.)

lation, especially in the setting of lupus anticoagulants (37, 38). (See Fig. 26.6 for the relationship between the aPTT, TCT, PT, and plasma heparin concentration.) Like the aPTT, it is also affected by low levels of antithrombin III (ATIII) (39).

# EVALUATION OF A PROLONGED PROTHROMBIN OR ACTIVATED PARTIAL THROMBOPLASTIN TIME (SEE ALSO CHAPTER 23)

## MIXING STUDIES

The first step in identification of the cause of a prolonged PT or aPTT is to determine whether addition of normal plasma can correct the deficit (4, 43). The PT and aPTT assays do not reliably detect single factor deficiencies until an individual factor level falls below approximately 40%. Failure to correct the prolonged laboratory study by addition of 50% normal plasma is suggestive of the presence of a specific or nonspecific inhibitor in the individual's plasma. A PT or aPTT prolongation of

more than 2 or 3 seconds is necessary to fully ascertain the presence of an inhibitor compared with a simple factor deficiency. Because specific and nonspecific inhibitors more frequently involve the aPTT than the PT, the discussion will be focused on analysis of mixing studies using the aPTT assay (Table 26.2). In plasma mixing studies, the effect of mixing individual with normal plasma in ratios of 0:1, 1:0, 4:1, 1:1, and 1:4 are analyzed. If mixing test plasma and control normal plasma in a 1:1 mix results in correction of the aPTT, a plasma factor(s) deficiency is to be suspected. Based on clinical history, specific factor assays can be performed to identify the deficient factor (see Factor Assays, below). If the aPTT remains prolonged, either a nonspecific inhibitor, such as a lupus anticoagulant inhibitor (LA) or parapro-

**TABLE 26.2.** Evaluation of an Abnormal Activated Partial Thromboplastin Time Using Mixing Studies

| | | Time (seconds) | |
|---|---|---|---|
| N | P | Immediate | 1 Hour Incubation at 37°C |
| *Factor deficiency* | | | |
| 1 | 0 | 20.2 | 20.6 |
| 0 | 1 | 33.1 | 33.4 |
| 4 | 1 | 22.5 | 22.8 |
| 1 | 1 | 20.4 | 20.7 |
| 1 | 4 | 25.1 | 25.3 |
| *Factor inhibitor* | | | |
| 1 | 0 | 20.5 | 21.1 |
| 0 | 1 | 33.5 | 38.2 |
| 4 | 1 | 23.8 | 29.3 |
| 1 | 1 | 30.2 | 37.1 |
| 1 | 4 | 29.3 | 35.1 |
| *Lupus inhibitor* | | | |
| 1 | 0 | 24.1 | 24.4 |
| 0 | 1 | 60.2 | 60.1 |
| 4 | 1 | 28.1 | 28.5 |
| 1 | 1 | 38.3 | 37.9 |
| 1 | 4 | 47.1 | 47.3 |

N, *normal pooled plasma*; P, *individual's plasma.*

*Note that in the case of the simple factor deficiency the activated partial thromboplastin time corrects to normal upon 1:1 mix of normal and test plasma. In the case of a specific factor inhibitor, the 1:1 mix does not fully correct to normal. With incubation for 1 hour, the activated partial thromboplastin time prolongs even further at all mixes of normal and test plasma, demonstrating progressive neutralization of clotting factor. In the case of the lupus inhibitor, the activated partial thromboplastin time is prolonged at all mixes of normal and test plasma but does not prolong significantly further with incubation, suggesting the presence of a lupus inhibitor.*

tein, or a specific inhibitor, most commonly to factor VIII, is present (44, 45). However, some low-titer inhibitors may be sufficiently diluted as to correct with the 1:1 mix of test plasma and normal plasma (45). Thus, to increase sensitivity of mixing studies to low titer LA or factor inhibitors, a dilution of 4 parts test plasma to 1 part normal plasma is also assayed. Low-titer inhibitors will generally prolong the aPTT in the 4:1 mix (46–49).

Having determined that the 1:1 normal plasma mix did not correct the aPTT, the difference in time-dependence characteristics between coagulation factor inhibitors, such as antifactor VIII antibodies and LA, can be used. The more common factor inhibitors, such as those against factor VIII and factor IX, progressively neutralize coagulation factors present in the normal plasma with time. Thus, control normal plasma, individual test plasma, and 4:1, 1:1, and 1:4 mixes of test plasma with normal plasma are incubated for 30 to 60 minutes at 37°C, after which an aPTT is again performed. If the aPTT prolongs with incubation, a specific coagulation factor inhibitor should be suspected. However, if the prolonged aPTT remains unchanged with incubation, then a nonspecific inhibitor is more likely.

## Interpretation

Caution must be taken in interpreting these mixing studies because some less common factor inhibitors, such as antifactor V and antiprothrombin antibodies, may not prolong with incubation (50). Similarly, 10 to 15% of LAs show time-dependent inhibition and another 15 to 20% may be borderline (51). Clinical correlation is important because individuals with coagulation factor inhibitors tend to have hemorrhagic symptoms, whereas those with LA are asymptomatic or prone to thrombosis (see Chapters 37 and 38).

Mixing studies should be done on fresh test samples. The presence of residual platelets in centrifuged plasma causes shortening of the aPTT owing to the presence of platelet lysate in the frozen thawed plasma sample (43, 46). If the use of frozen samples is necessary, the test sample should be centrifuged at 15,000 g for 10 minutes or filtered before freezing. Mixing studies are sensitive, but not specific, and can only be used as a screening test (52). Thus, additional testing is required to confirm the diagnosis of LA, specific factor inhibitor, or factor deficiency.

# ACQUIRED COAGULATION INHIBITORS

## NONSPECIFIC INHIBITORS

Nonspecific inhibitors include increased titers of fibrin dehydration products, paraproteins associated with monoclonal gammopathies, especially high levels of im-

munoglobulin M (IgM), and LAs. These nonspecific inhibitors do not exhibit classic antibody-antigen-type interactions with clotting factors. Therapy is directed at the underlying disease process. The LAs and antiphospholipid antibodies are of increasing interest because of their association with a prothrombotic rather than a hemorrhagic state (53–59).

## EVALUATION OF LUPUS ANTICOAGULANTS (SEE CHAPTER 38)

Lupus anticoagulants are antiphospholipid antibodies, which characteristically prolong the aPTT, minimally prolong the PT, and generally do not affect the thrombin time. This prolongation is due to binding of LA antibodies to phospholipid in the thromboplastin and partial thromboplastin reagents, resulting in interference with assembly of the prothrombinase complex *in vitro*. No single test system will identify all antiphospholipid antibodies or LAs (59–63). Controversy exists as to which tests are most reliable in identifying LAs. Lupus anticoagulant activity should not be equated with anticardiolipin antibodies, inasmuch as these two tests identify related, but not necessarily identical, antibodies (53, 61–66).

In addition to the potential problems in interpretation of mixing studies in the diagnosis of LA, the ability to detect LA activity relies strongly on the source of thromboplastin (14, 46, 67), amounts of various phospholipids, configuration of phospholipid present (46, 47, 68, 69), and the type of surface activator used (46). Rabbit brain and recombinant human tissue thromboplastin are generally more sensitive, and bovine brain thromboplastin the least sensitive, in identifying LA-induced prolongation of the aPTT (14, 63). Similarly, the activator, ellagic acid, is less sensitive to the presence of LA activity (46). To add to the confusion in identifying LA activity, the degree of aPTT prolongation with any combination of contact activator or thromboplastin reagent is not well correlated with LA titer measured immunologically (61, 62, 64, 70, 71). Thus, additional tests have been devised in an attempt to more accurately and reliably identify LA-type inhibitory activity (Fig. 26.7). Because LA activity is heterogenous, and the conventional aPTT identifies only 50% of affected individuals, it is recommended that at least two coagulation-based tests be performed, increasing the diagnostic sensitivity of coagulation-based tests to 88% (71–76).

## TISSUE THROMBOPLASTIN INHIBITION TEST

The tissue thromboplastin inhibition (TTI) test (69) is based on the principle of augmenting the effect of LA activity by further diluting the thromboplastin reagent,

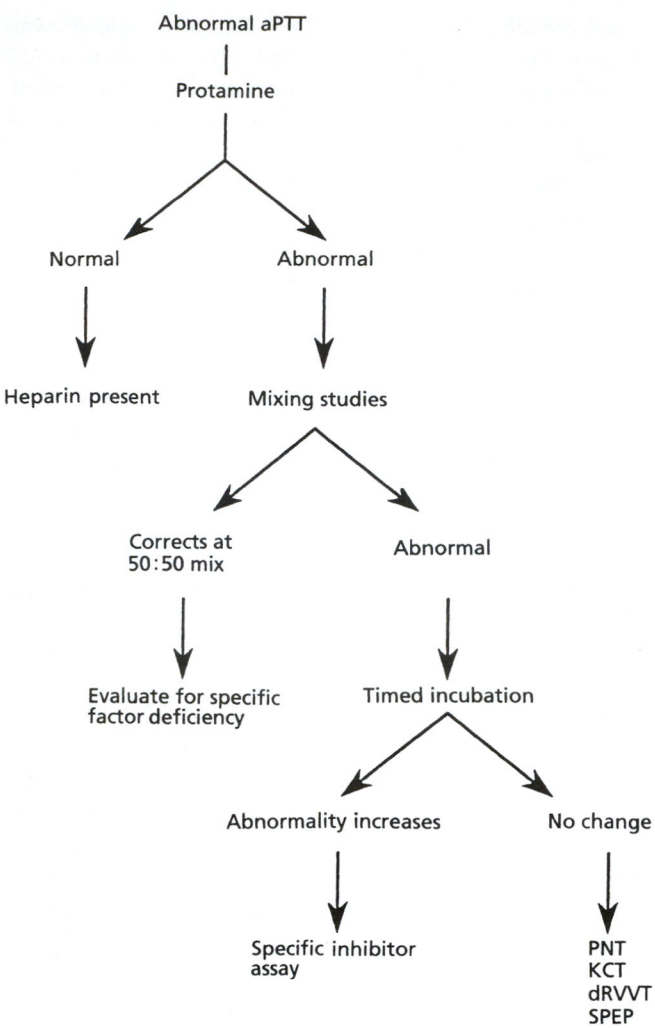

**FIGURE 26.7.** Suggested schema for laboratory evaluation of a prolonged aPTT. dRVVT, dilute Russell's viper venom time; KCT, kaolin clotting time; PNT, platelet neutralization test; SPEP, serum protein electrophoresis.

thereby enhancing the ability of LA to interfere with assembly of the prothrombinase complex. In this test, thromboplastin is diluted 1:50 and 1:500 with saline. The diluted thromboplastin is then incubated 1:1 with normal or test plasma for 3 minutes, after which calcium chloride is added and time to clot formation recorded. A ratio of result for test sample PT to control plasma PT is then made.

## Interpretation

A PT ratio higher than 1.3 suggests an LA. A ratio of 1.1 or less is considered normal. This test must also be interpreted with caution, because individuals with factor VIII or IX levels of less than 10%, abnormal levels of fibrinogen, and individuals with factor VIII inhibitors, have been shown to have PT ratios of 1.3 or higher and hence are serious false positives in this assay (67, 75,

76). In addition, in centers where aPTT prolongation is frequently seen in critically ill individuals, as many as 40% of individuals who do not have an LA may have a positive TTI result (46, 69, 60, 75). Thus, as a single test, a positive TTI is not diagnostic of LA and other tests may be more useful (63, 69, 75, 77).

## KAOLIN CLOTTING TIME

The kaolin clotting time (KCT) was designed in an effort to eliminate the problem of variable sensitivity of the aPTT assay to lupus inhibitor activity due to varying thromboplastin reagent characteristics. Two hundred μs of test plasma and a 1:1 mix of test plasma and control plasma are incubated individually with 0.1 mL of kaolin at 37°C. Calcium chloride is added and time to clot formation is recorded. A KCT index is then derived according to the formula:

$$\frac{\text{KCT 1:1 Mix} - \text{Control KCT}}{\text{Test KCT}} \times 100\% \qquad (1)$$

## Interpretation

The control index range is 5% ± 2 standard deviations. A sample is considered positive if the index is greater than 17% (43, 67). This test is somewhat limited in utility, inasmuch as it is not universally automated and is adversely affected by the presence of increased phospholipids in the test plasma (67, 69, 78–80). Further studies are needed to determine the sensitivity and specificity of the KCT (52, 65, 67).

## DILUTE RUSSELL'S VIPER VENOM TIME

The dilute Russell's viper venom time (dRVVT) is based on the ability of the snake venom, RVV, directly to activate factor X to Xa (69). Consequently the dRVVT measures the rate of formation and activity of the prothrombinase complex in producing thrombin. A 1:1 mix of RVV and diluted rabbit brain phospholipid is added to 100 μL of test plasma and incubated at 37°C for 2 minutes. Calcium chloride is then added and the time to clot formation measured in a fibrometer.

## Interpretation

The normal range for the dRVVT is 24–37 seconds. The dRVVT is prolonged in the presence of an LA. In international studies of the sensitivity of the dRVVT to LA, the assay method was not standardized among laboratories, and no clear statement of its diagnostic value could be made (75). The dRVVT varies with the type of thromboplastin and the ionic strength of buffers used in the assay system, with low ionic strength buffers of 0.01 mol/L producing greater assay sensitivity (69).

## PLATELET NEUTRALIZATION TEST

This test is based on the principle that the addition of an increased amount of phospholipid, or phospholipid of a specific conformational complex, will bypass or neutralize LA activity (43, 52, 77). Platelet lysate prepared by freeze-thawing followed by dialysis, or commercial frozen, lyophilized platelet lysate is added to the test plasma and prewarmed aPTT reagent for 3 minutes at 37°C. After this incubation, calcium chloride is added and the time to clot formation recorded.

### Interpretation

The prolonged aPTT will shorten in the presence of the platelet extract by a range of 3 to 63 seconds, with a mean shortening of approximately 17 seconds (43, 75, 77). The assay is very specific and sensitive, but the results are not linear with respect to the amount of LA activity present (75). In the presence of true coagulation factor inhibitors, the aPTT does not shorten with the addition of platelet extract. Commercial freeze-dried platelet extract is somewhat less sensitive than freshly prepared, noncommercial platelet extract. As in all other lupus anticoagulant assays, the individual's plasma should be centrifuged twice to remove residual platelets before freezing or testing (79, 80).

## ASSAYS USING HEXAGONAL (II) PHASE PHOSPHOLIPIDS

Some studies indicate that monoclonal lupus anticoagulants are inhibited by hexagonal (II) phase phospholipids, whereas lamellar phase phospholipids have no effect in clot-based lupus anticoagulant assays. The Staclot LA system uses hexagonal (II) phase phosphatidyletha-nolamine in an aPTT-based assay as a confirmatory test for lupus anticoagulants. In this assay, 50 μL of test plasma is incubated with an equal volume of buffer in tube 1 at 37°C. In tube 2, a similar volume of test plasma is incubated with 50 μL of hexagonal phase phospholipid. After 9 minutes, reconstituted lyophilized human plasma is added to tubes 1 and 2 to correct any possible factor deficiencies in the test sample. The reconstituted human plasma also contains polybrene to neutralize up to 1 U/mL of heparin in heparinized test samples. After 1 minute, the aPTT reagent consisting of rabbit brain cephalin and micronized silica is added and incubated for 5 minutes. Then, $CaCl_2$ is added and the time to clot formation is recorded. When compared to the results from tube 1, a shortening of the clotting time in tube 2 by more than 8 seconds is considered positive for LA (81).

### Interpretation

Concentrations of heparin of more than 1 U/mL will yield false negative results. In one test of the Staclot sys-tem, no false positives were obtained from warfarinized samples. Samples from individuals with acquired factor V inhibitors, which had previously yielded false positive results in the platelet neutralization procedure, were not false positives in the Staclot system. One sample from a hemophilia individual with an allo factor VIII inhibitor had a false positive test result (81, 82). Further studies are required to determine the sensitivity and specificity of the hexagonal (II) phase phospholipid system.

## TEXTARIN/ECARIN RATIO

In this assay, prothrombinase activity of the test plasma is measured in the presence and absence of phospholipid, using the procoagulant activating properties of two different snake venoms. The snake venom Textarin has prothrombinase activity in the presence of exogenous sources of phospholipid, calcium, and factor V. The snake venom Ecarin activates prothrombin directly without the need for cofactors. The time to clot formation of 0.1 mL of individual's plasma activated with 0.1 mL of Textarin reagent in the presence of calcium is compared to the rate of clot formation of 0.2 mL of individual's plasma mixed with 0.1 mL of Ecarin solution. An increased ratio of the time to clot formation in the Textarin and Ecarin assays suggests the presence of LA. Only very preliminary information is available on the usefulness of this assay system for evaluating LA activity. The assay can be done in heparinized samples if they are treated with polybrene (82, 83).

## IMMUNOLOGIC ASSAYS FOR ANTIPHOSPHOLIPID ANTIBODIES

Antiphospholipid antibodies of varying subclass and specificity can be measured in test plasma. The presence of antiphospholipid activity does not necessarily mean that LA activity (defined by the presence of a prolonged PT or aPTT as described above) is present and vice versa (54, 59–64). Moreover, some subsets of anticardiolipin antibodies require the presence of $\beta_2$ glycoprotein I for binding (70, 84, 85). Several different enzyme-linked immunosorbent assays (ELISAs) have been described using cardiolipin (64, 65), phosphatidyl serine (53, 65), and a commercial partial thromboplastin reagent, such as Thrombofax (86), as the antigen. Variations in sensitivity and reproducibility are directly related to the type of plastic used in the microtiter wells, the solvent used in application of the phospholipid, and the type of blocking agent used to coat nonspecific binding sites in the wells, and the presence or absence of $\beta_2$ glycoprotein I in the assay (70, 85, 87). Blocking agents such as bovine serum, bovine serum albumin, or fetal calf serum are considered the most reliable. Results are reported as a range of activity of high positive, moderately positive, low positive, or negative (see Chapter 38) (70).

A specific ELISA assay for measurement of antibodies to $\beta_2$ glycoprotein I measurement is available for research purposes (88).

## SPECIFIC FACTOR INHIBITORS (SEE CHAPTER 37)

Specific factor inhibitors are suspected when plasma mixing studies fail to correct after addition of 50% normal plasma, and when incubation of the test plasma with normal plasma results in even further prolongation of the clotting time. Inhibitors with strong activity will neutralize an equivalent amount of clotting factor. Weak inhibitors have complex reactivity with clotting factors, and the inhibitor-clotting factor complex frequently retains some clotting activity.

Two distinct assays are used in quantification of factor inhibitors. The results of these assays are not interchangeable (45).

## NEW OXFORD ASSAY

The new Oxford assay was developed in England as a modification of the original Oxford method (89, 90). In the Oxford assay, the test plasma containing the inhibitor is incubated with a source of factor VIII concentrate (45, 49). One part of factor VIII concentrate, containing 10 to 20 U factor VIII/mL, is incubated with 9 parts of test plasma for 4 hours at 37°C. The comparison control is 1 part factor VIII concentrate incubated with 9 parts factor VIII-deficient plasma from a hemophiliac. The residual factor VIII activity is then measured in a standard one-stage or two-stage aPTT-based factor VIII assay. The ratio of factor VIII present in test plasma-to-factor VIII in control is calculated. Using a linear scale, the percentage of residual factor VIII is plotted against plasma dilution. The 50% residual factor VIII point can thus be ascertained (Fig. 26.8). The inhibitor level is then calculated from the formula:

$$\text{Factor VIII inhibitor (IU/mL)} = a \times b \times c \quad (2)$$

where $a$ = reciprocal of the plasma dilution giving 50% residual factor VIII derived from the graph, $b$ = plasma dilution factor, and $c$ = factor VIII concentration in the control mixture. One international new Oxford unit is defined as that activity that destroys 0.5 U of factor VIII.

Assay of factor IX inhibitors using the new Oxford assay is performed in the same manner, except that the incubation period is shortened to 10 minutes.

## BETHESDA ASSAY

The Bethesda assay is based on the ability of test plasma to inactivate the factor VIII present in normal pooled plasma (89, 91, 92). Normal pooled plasma is incubated

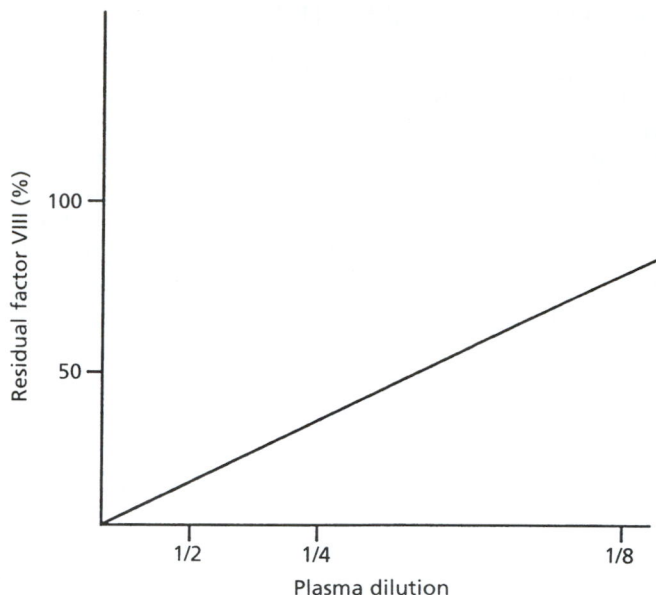

**FIGURE 26.8.** Graph of plasma dilution versus residual factor VIII activity in the New Oxford method of factor VIII inhibitor measurement.

with either serial dilutions of test plasma or buffer for 2 hours at 37°C. The residual factor VIII is measured in a standard one-stage factor VIII assay. The observed test factor VIII activity is divided by the activity in the control plasma. Percentage residual factor VIII is plotted on a logarithmic scale, and units of inhibitor on a linear scale (Fig. 26.9 and Table 26.3). One international unit is the amount of antibody that destroys 0.5 U of factor VIII in 2 hours at 37°C. For example, if the control factor VIII is 60% and the test plasma value is 30%, then the ratio is 0.5 (U/mL). Hence, one Bethesda unit inhibitor is present in the test plasma. If the residual factor VIII activity does not fall between 25 and 75%, then the test plasma must be further diluted to find the 50% residual factor VIII activity point.

## AGAROSE GEL METHOD

Normal pooled plasma is mixed 1:1 with 2% agarose and poured onto a glass plate (45, 93). Holes are then punched in the gel and dilutions of individual plasma are added along with dilutions of a standard antibody to the clotting factor in question as control. The gels are incubated in a vapor chamber for 16 to 20 hours to allow the antibody to diffuse into the gel. The gel is then immersed in a calcium chloride solution for 3 minutes. After removal from the solution, fibrin forms. The gel is fixed in a 4% formaldehyde solution and the diameter of the clear zones of inhibition is measured. This diameter is compared to the standard curve derived from the diameter of the zones of inhibition plotted against the known concentrations of the antibody standards.

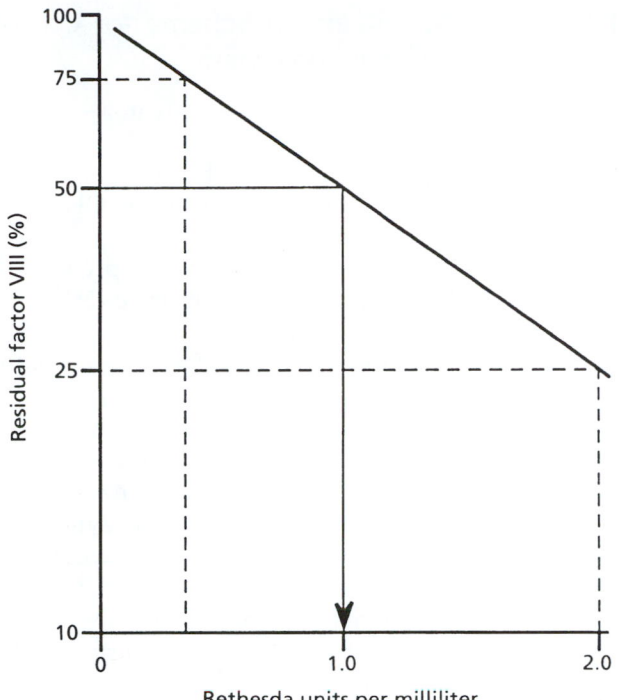

**FIGURE 26.9.** Relationship between the corrected residual factor VIII level and the units of inhibitor present in the Bethesda assay. Inhibitor units can be interpreted from the graph if the corrected residual factor VIII is between 25 and 75% (*dashed lines*) and the inhibitor exhibits simple reaction kinetics. One Bethesda unit is defined by a corrected residual factor VIII of 50% in the assay (*line with arrows*).

**TABLE 26.3.** Factor VIII Inhibitor Calculations in the Bethesda Assay

| Plasma | Plasma Dilution | Residual Factor VIII | Units from Graph × Dilution | Bethesda Units |
|--------|-----------------|----------------------|-----------------------------|----------------|
| A | 1:10 | 30 | 1.75 × 10 | 17.5 |
|   | 1:20 | 55 | 0.87 × 20 | 17.4 |
|   | 1:40 | 70 | 0.45 × 40 | 18.0 |
| B | 1:10 | 50 | 1.00 × 10 | 10 |
|   | 1:20 | 47 | 1.10 × 20 | 22 |
|   | 1:40 | 45 | 1.20 × 40 | 48 |

*Plasma A contains an inhibitor with simple reaction kinetics. The unitage is assigned based on the dilution with residual corrected factor VIII nearest to 50%. Hence plasma A is assigned the value 17.4.*

*Plasma B contains an inhibitor with complex reaction kinetics. Both 1:10 and 1:20 dilutions gave residual factor VIII levels of equal or close to 50%. The lesser dilution (1:10) is used to assign the Bethesda unitage.*

**TABLE 26.4.** Classification of Specific Inhibitors

| Neutralizing | Nonneutralizing |
|--------------|-----------------|
| Factor V | Factor II |
| Factor VIII | Factor VIII |
| Factor IX | Factor X |
| Factor XI | von Willebrand factor |
| Factor XIII | |
| von Willebrand factor | |

## Interpretation

The Bethesda assay may be somewhat more sensitive than the new Oxford assay. However, the Bethesda assay is more prone to errors arising from assignment of an arbitrary factor level of 1 U/mL for the normal pooled plasma (45). The agarose gel technique is more time consuming. Zones of inhibition are not specific for a certain inhibitor, because anything that inhibits fibrin formation will create a zone of inhibition. Ten percent of individuals with hemophilia (see Chapter 35) develop inhibitors upon exposure to plasma sources of factor VIII or IX (45, 92). Acquired factor inhibitors (see Chapter 37) occur in a variety of conditions, but inhibitors to factor VIII are the most common (92). Factor VIII and IX inhibitors are seen postpartum, after prolonged antibiotic therapy, and with autoimmune disorders (92). Inhibitors to factors II, X, and XI may be seen in systemic lupus erythematosus (93, 94). Factor V inhibitors may be seen postoperatively, and, in some cases are due to development of antibodies to bovine thrombin (present in surgical glue) cross reactive with human factor V (95). Such inhibitors are also observed with certain infections (48). Antibodies to von Willebrand factor (vWf) (see Chapter 34) may occur in autoimmune disease, lymphoma, and Wilms' tumor (48, 96). Factor XIII inhibitors may occur after treatment with isoniazid (48, 97) (Table 26.4).

# METHODS IN COAGULATION FACTOR ASSAYS
## SYNTHETIC SUBSTRATE ASSAYS IN HEMOSTASIS

Clot-based assays of many of the procoagulant and anticoagulant factors involved in hemostasis often require multiple steps. Analysis of the activity of one factor requires normal amounts and activity of all other participating factors so that they do not become rate-limiting. For example, when measuring factor Xa activity in a clot-based assay, fibrinogen levels must be normal to produce sufficient clot. Most importantly, clot-based factor assays require a suitable factor-deficient substrate plasma, which may be difficult to obtain in rare factor deficiencies. Thus, considerable interest has evolved in the design of synthetic substrates useful in measuring the enzymatic activity of each individual clotting factor or endogenous inhibitor present in plasma, independent of the level and activity of other participating factors. A synthetic chromogenic substrate is a 3–5 amino acid peptide sequence attached to a chromophore, which mimics the cleavage site on the natural substrate for the enzyme to be tested. One of the first synthetic substrates was based on the amino acid sequence of the thrombin cleavage site on fibrinogen, Phe-Val-Arg. One of the first chromogenic substrates used the tripeptide Phe-Val-Arg coupled to paranitroanilide (pNA) for analysis of thrombin activity. In this enzymatic reaction thrombin cleaves Phe-Val-Arg, releasing pNA, which has a measurably different optical activity than the parent molecule. The amount of thrombin can then be calculated by comparison with amounts of pNA released by thrombin standards. Because many of these factors are serine proteases recognizing arginyl peptide bonds, specificity of a substrate for a particular enzyme is conferred by modification of the particular amino acid sequence adjacent to the Arg-pNA bond. Chromogenic and, more recently, flourigenic assays have been developed for a variety of hemostatic factors (98–104).

Chromogenic assays have the potential for being highly sensitive and specific, but limitations do exist. Enzyme/chromogenic substrate assays may be measured kinetically, as in a centrifugal analyzer, or by end-point analysis after termination of the reaction by addition of acid. In some cases, addition of acetic acid to the test plasma specimen may cause precipitation of plasma proteins, obscuring optical density readings. A second problem is that many synthetic substrates may be competitive inhibitors of activated clotting factors participating in production of a particular enzymatic activity measured effectively by the substrate. An example of this is the inhibition of factor Xa produced by synthetic thrombin substrates (104). Such inhibition will ultimately slow down the rate of thrombin production in a sample and lead to artifactually low levels for thrombin activity. Lastly, synthetic substrates only approximate the *in vivo* interaction of the enzyme with the site of cleavage on the natural substrate. Synthetic substrates do not take into account the effects of tertiary protein structure or conformation of the natural substrate and, thus, may not duplicate slow reaction kinetics between abnormal enzyme or substrate that may occur *in vivo*. In such circumstances the enzyme may appear to be normal in chromogenic substrate assays but is found to have subnormal activity in clot-based assays in which the enzyme and substrate may exhibit abnormal interaction.

| **TABLE 26.5.** | Reaction Schema for Chromogenic Assay |
| --- | --- |
| Procoagulant assay | Procoagulant + activator → coagulant |
| | Coagulant + substrate:pNA → coagulant + substrate-OH + free pNA |
| Coagulant assay | Coagulant + substrate:pNA → coagulant + substrate-OH + free pNA |
| Cofactor assay | Proenzyme + cofactor + activator → enzyme |
| | Enzyme + substrate:pNA → substrate-OH + free pNA |
| Inhibitor assay | Known quantity pure enzyme + plasma inhibitor → enzyme-inhibitor complex + excess enzyme |
| | Remaining enzyme + substrate:pNA → substrate-OH + free pNA |

pNA, *paranitroanilide.*

Examples of this discordance occur in many inherited genetic abnormalities of clotting factor enzymes or natural inhibitors of clotting, but are most seriously evident in testing samples from individuals anticoagulated with warfarin. Activity of factors II, VII, IX, or X will appear to be normal in chromogenic substrate assays because the incompletely γ-carboxylated vitamin K-dependent factors are still able to cleave synthetic substrates, although they are nonfunctional in producing detectable clots in the routine PT or aPTT clot-based assays (98, 99, 104). The latter situation appears to reflect more directly the *in vivo* interactions of des-γ-carboxy clotting factors with natural substrates in subjects anticoagulated with warfarin.

The principles of the methodologies devised to analyze procoagulants, activated coagulation factors, cofactors, and inhibitors are described in the simplified reaction schema in Table 26.5.

## IMMUNOLOGIC METHODS

Immunologic assays provide important quantitative information in analysis of hemorrhagic and thrombotic states (105). Immunologic assays are based on the principles of antibody recognition of antigen. Specificity of the assay will consequently be directly affected by the specificity of the antibody for the desired antigen. Immunologic assays in general have the capacity for determining antigenic levels as low as 1 ng/mL. The information provided, however, is only representative of the

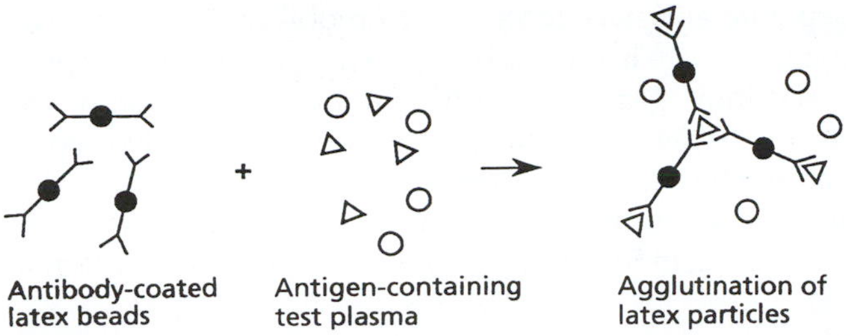

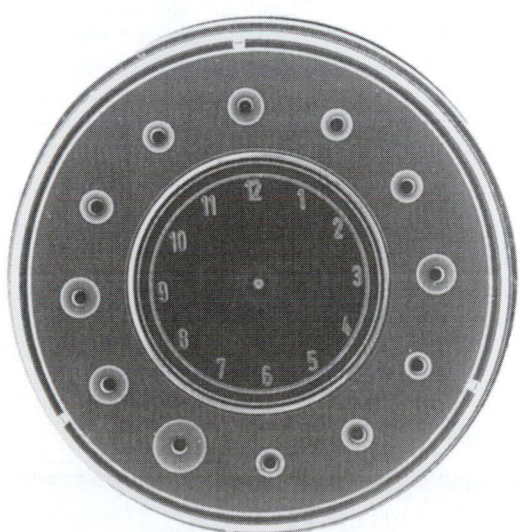

**FIGURE 26.10.** Latex agglutination. Antibody-coated latex beads are mixed with dilutions of test plasma containing the antigen to be measured. Binding of the antibody to antigen induces visible agglutination of the latex beads.

quantitative presence of the antigen in the test sample, and only in certain circumstances is the antibody fortuitously specific enough to provide qualitative information. An example of functionally informative antibodies is monoclonal antifibrinogen antibodies directed at sites in the α-chain that are specific for thrombin cleavage sites. These antibodies are informative in dysfibrinogenemias where mutations have occurred at thrombin cleavage sites, because these monoclonal antibodies, unlike polyclonal antifibrinogen antibodies, do not recognize the mutant fibrinogen. Also, immunologic analysis has been an important diagnostic tool in prenatal analysis of fetal samples in detection of factor VIII or IX deficiency, when clot-based analysis is subject to interference by contamination with amniotic fluid (106). A variety of techniques are available, some more easily implemented in routine coagulation laboratories than others (105).

## LATEX AGGLUTINATION

Latex agglutination assays are used clinically in semiquantitative measurement of a variety of proteins. Using the example of the fibrinogen assay, latex particles coated with specific polyclonal or monoclonal antibodies to fibrinogen are incubated for 2 to 3 minutes with increasing dilutions of plasma sample on individual glass slides. Complex formation between fibrinogen antigen and antibody causes agglutination of the beads, which can be visually ascertained. The highest plasma dilution at which agglutination occurs is used to quantify the antigen concentration when compared to standard curves generated from dilutions of normal pooled plasma or purified reference standard. The latex agglutination method is rapid and inexpensive, but only semiquantitative, and is subject to false positives due to the presence of rheumatoid factor, cold agglutinins, or cryoglobulins (Fig. 26.10) (105).

## NEPHELOMETRY

Nephelometry is based on the ability of antigen-antibody complexes to scatter light (107). Dilutions of test sample are incubated with antigen-specific antibody in a photo-optical cell and the amount of light scatter quantitated kinetically or by fixed time point analysis. Results are affected by the presence of plasma lipids (101). Nephelometry has the advantage that it is not affected by varying mobility of different plasma forms of the antigen; however, it may yield spuriously high values because many of the antibodies do not distinguish between degraded forms of the antigen (101). Laser nephelometric analysis is used in quantitation of ATIII, α₁-antitrypsin, α₂-macroglobulin, plasminogen, fibrinogen, fibrin(ogen) degradation products, vWf, and protein C.

## RADIAL IMMUNODIFFUSION

Radial immunodiffusion (RID) is based on the Ouchterlony principle that the concentration of antigen is proportional to the rate of precipitation of antigen-antibody complexes during diffusion of antigen in an agarose gel containing specific polyclonal antibody (108, 109). The rate of precipitation is determined directly by measurement of the diameter of the precipitate ring formed in the gel and this measurement is compared with known standards. Radial immunodiffusion (RID) generally requires up to 48 hours for complete formation of antigen-antibody complexes, and consequently many more rapid immunological assays are used when possible. Radial immunodiffusion analysis has been used in determination of ATIII, fibrinogen, α₂-antiplasmin, α₂-macroglobulin, α₁-antitrypsin, and plasminogen (Fig. 26.11).

## ELECTROIMMUNODIFFUSION (EID, EIA, OR LAURELL ROCKET ASSAY)

The Laurell rocket assay is one of the most widely used assays of immunologic levels of antigens (110–112). The

**FIGURE 26.11.** Fibrinogen measurement by radial immunodiffusion. Ring diameters are proportional to fibrinogen concentration.

technique is based on the same principles as RID but is considerably shortened by the use of an electric current to move antigens through an agarose gel containing specific polyclonal antibody. The height of the rocket peak is directly proportional to the amount of antigen present in the sample. A reference curve is generated by making serial dilutions of pooled plasma standards and plotting the concentration versus the height of the rocket. The assay requires 1 to 2 hours for electrophoresis and variable time for Coomassie staining and destaining for visualization of the rocket peaks. The Laurell assay is sensitive to approximately 5% antigen levels (Fig. 26.12).

In some instances, proteins may exist in different molecular weight forms or in complex with other plasma factors, resulting in multiple peaks in a single sample lane on Laurell assay and making quantification impossible. Two-dimensional counter immunoelectrophoresis (2DCIE), a variation of the Laurell assay, is useful in separating different molecular weight forms or complexes of the same antigen. The test sample is electrophoresed in an agarose gel in the first dimension to

separate antigens according to mobility (111, 112). The agarose plate is then turned 90 degrees and electrophoresed into agarose containing antibody specific for the desired antigen. Multiple peaks are then detected representing the differing forms of antigens (Fig. 26.13). This technique has been useful in the analysis of free protein S and protein S bound to C4b-binding protein in plasma.

## RADIOIMMUNOASSAY

Radioimmunoassay (RIA) is based on competition between radiolabeled antigen and unlabeled test sample antigen for binding to monospecific antibody. After the complexes of antigen and antibody are separated from unbound material, the remaining radiolabeled free antigen is quantitated (Fig. 26.14). For each test sample antigen bound to the antibody, a radiolabeled antigen remains free in solution (113). Thus, unbound radiolabeled antigen is directly related to the amount of bound antigen from the unknown sample. Radioimmunoassay is a very sensitive method that is used frequently in research laboratories, but it is less clinically preferable because of the use of radiochemicals and the need for purified antigen to radiolabel. The sensitivity of the assay depends on the quantity of added radiolabeled antigen. Too much or too little radiolabeled antigen decreases the sensitivity of the assay.

## IMMUNORADIOMETRIC ASSAY

Two basic types of immunoradiometric assay (IRMA) are available. In one assay, a radiolabeled antibody is added to the test assay in fluid phase, and antigen bound to the antibody is precipitated from unbound antibody in solution with ammonium sulfate or polyethylene glycol. In the two-site method, a polyclonal capture antibody is coated on a microtiter well or plastic tube. The antigen-containing solution is incubated in the wells. After removal of the antigen, radiolabeled antibody is

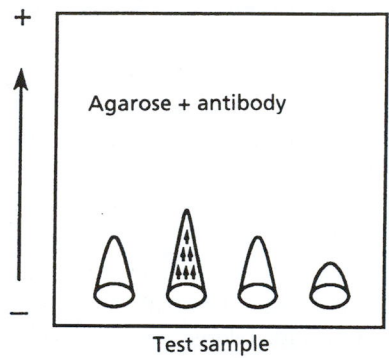

**FIGURE 26.12.** Electroimmunodiffusion. Dilutions of test plasma are placed in sample wells and electrophoresed into agarose containing specific antibody. Antigen-antibody complex formation results in a line of precipitation, the height of which is proportional to the amount of antigen present.

**FIGURE 26.13.** Two-dimensional counter immunoelectrophoresis. **a,** The test sample is placed in a sample well and electrophoresed horizontally into an agarose gel, separating the proteins according to their size and mobility. **b,** The agarose is then removed and replaced with agarose containing specific antibody. **c,** The gel is then rotated 90 degrees and the samples are electrophoresed into the antibody-containing agarose. Antigen-antibody complexes form precipitation lines visible after staining with Coomassie blue.

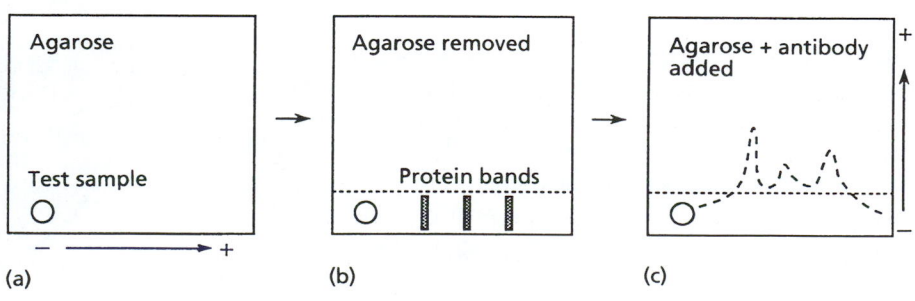

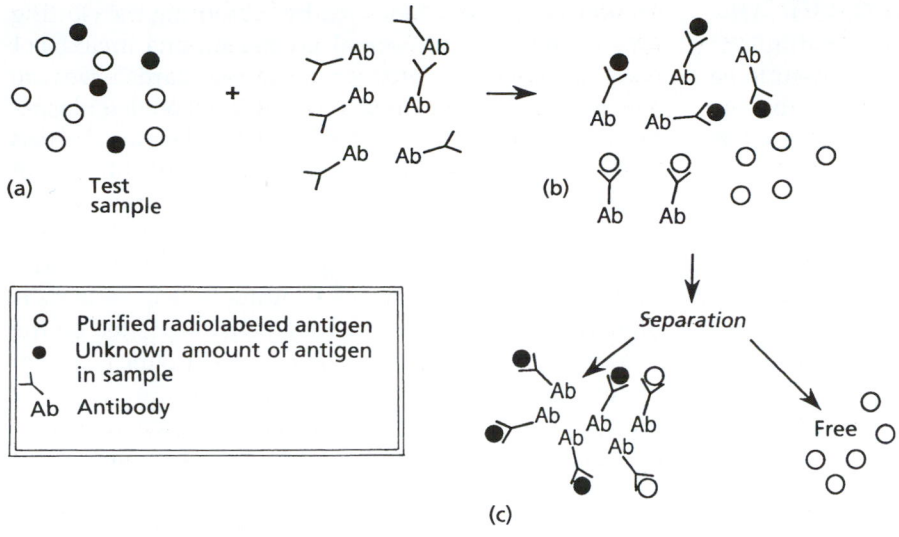

**FIGURE 26.14.** Radioimmunoassay. **a,** A known quantity of purified radiolabeled antigen is added to the test sample containing an unknown amount of antigen. **b,** Antibody (Ab) is added and antibody combines stoichiometrically with antigen. **c,** Antibody-antigen complexes are separated from the remaining free radiolabeled antigen, which is then measured.

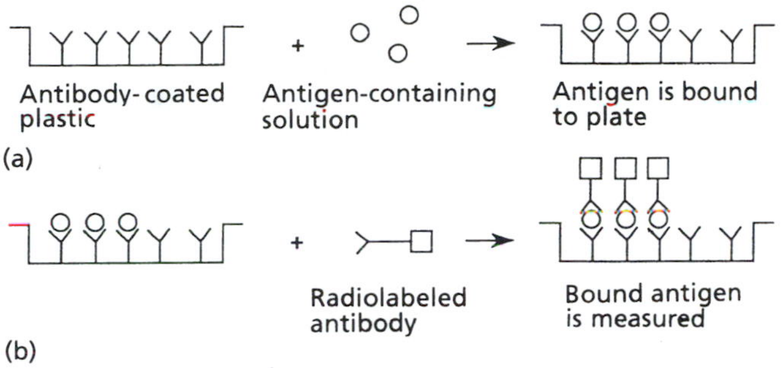

**FIGURE 26.15.** Two-site immunoradiometric assay. **a,** Antigen-containing solution is added to wells precoated with specific antibody. **b,** Antigen bound to antibody is detected by addition of radiolabeled antibody. After removal of the excess unbound radiolabeled antibody, bound radioactivity is measured.

added. After a second incubation, excess unbound antibody is removed by wash, and radioactivity in the wells is counted in a γ counter (Fig. 26.15). Immunoradiometric assay is more sensitive than RIA in general and does not require purified antigen for radiolabeling (114).

## ENZYME-LINKED IMMUNOASSAY (ELISA)

Enzyme-linked immunoassay methodology, although more complicated and requiring more steps than RIA, eliminates the need for radioisotopes or a purified antigen standard. In an ELISA, microtiter plate wells are coated with a polyclonal antibody directed against the desired antigen (108, 115). Test sample is added and incubated for periods of 1 hour or overnight, depending on the antigen. Unbound reactants are then washed away and a second antigen-specific antibody which has been chemically coupled to an enzyme-based detection system is added. Typical enzymes include horseradish

peroxidase or alkaline phosphatase. The unbound antibody is again washed away and the amount of antigen detected by the second antibody is then quantitated by incubating the microtiter wells with a colorimetric substrate. The reaction is quenched by addition of acid at a specific time interval and the color absorbance generated is measured (Fig. 26.16). The amount of protein can be determined from curves generated from the absorbance of known concentrations of antigens.

Variations of the assay have also been described that allow for the greater specificity inherent to monoclonal antibodies. Enzyme-linked immunoassay allows for the use of very small amounts of test sample and has the capacity to detect 50 to 100 ng of antigen.

## NEUTRALIZATION INHIBITION ASSAY

This assay combines both immunologic and clot-based techniques of measuring coagulation factors and has been used in determination of immunologic levels of factors XIII, XI, IX, and VIII (116, 117). In the first step, test plasma is incubated with excess homologous antibody against the desired factor, usually derived from a individual with an inhibitor. The reaction mix is then added to normal plasma and an aPTT performed. The degree of prolongation of the aPTT is directly related to the amount of excess antibody remaining which, in turn, is indirectly related to the amount of antigen in the original test plasma (Fig. 26.17) (116). Unfortunately, these assays lack sensitivity and are less reproducible than the methodologies mentioned previously.

## FACTOR ASSAYS

Activity levels of clotting factors II to XII may be measured using plasma deficient in the factor in question in a standard PT-based or aPTT-based assay (4, 45, 48, 118). In a typical one-stage assay of a clotting factor, dilutions of test plasma are mixed 1:1 with plasma known to be deficient in that factor (termed deficient substrate plasma) and a routine aPTT or PT assay is performed. A

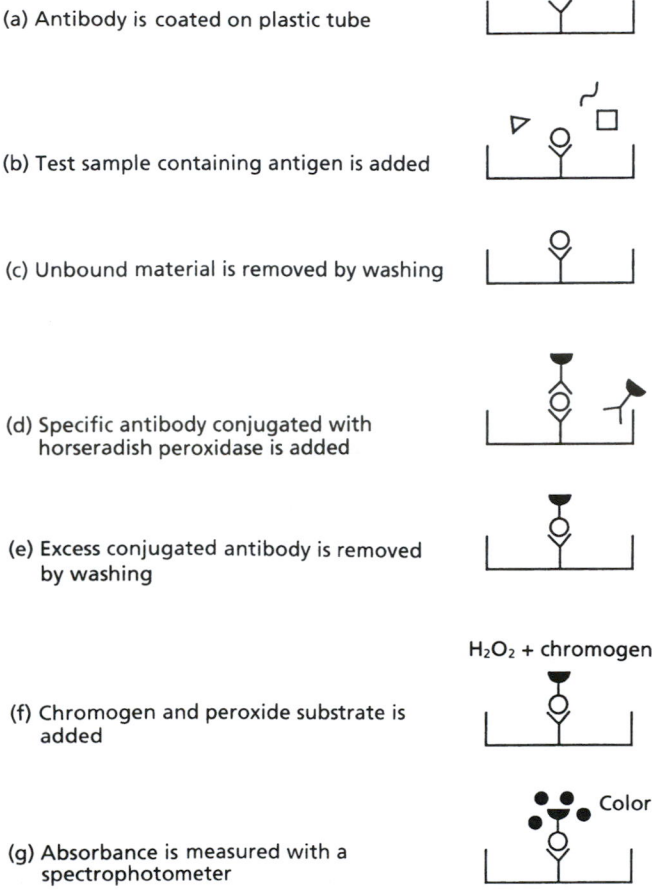

(a) Antibody is coated on plastic tube

(b) Test sample containing antigen is added

(c) Unbound material is removed by washing

(d) Specific antibody conjugated with horseradish peroxidase is added

(e) Excess conjugated antibody is removed by washing

H₂O₂ + chromogen

(f) Chromogen and peroxide substrate is added

Color

(g) Absorbance is measured with a spectrophotometer

**FIGURE 26.16.**    Steps in the measurement of an antigen in solution using an enzyme-linked immunoassay.

standard curve is established by measuring the clotting time of dilutions of normal pooled plasma mixed 1:1 with the deficient substrate plasma. Standard curves are generated using 1:10 dilutions of normal pooled plasma to increase sensitivity. A 100% activity level is defined arbitrarily as the time required for a 1:10 dilution of normal plasma to clot. Thus, a 1:20 dilution of normal plasma will yield a 50% activity level, a 1:40 dilution a 25% activity level, a 1:80 dilution a 12.5% level, and a 1:160 dilution a 6.25% level. Clotting time in seconds is plotted on the *y-axis* and factor activity is plotted on the *x-axis* using log-log graph paper. A best-fit line is drawn or calculated by computer. The clotting time result of the test plasma is then plotted on the line generated and the corresponding factor activity level recorded. Only values falling within the linear portion of the standard curve may be used. Using the PT assay, factor activity levels can be performed for factors II, V, VII, and X. Using the aPTT assay, all factors with the exception of VII can be measured (Fig. 26.18).

Measurement of the factor activity using several dilutions of the test plasma also allows for identification of a possible inhibitor, because dilution decreases the immediate effect of an inhibitor. Thus, the apparent factor level measured will increase as the effect of the inhibitor is decreased at successively higher dilution.

A two-stage clotting factor assay is used in some laboratories for the measurement of factor VIII levels. The two-stage assay is althought to be more precise, but requires more steps (119).

## Interpretation

One-stage assays are subject to a variety of technical problems that could result in imprecise results. Overestimates of factor levels occur because of poor quality, factor-deficient substrate. Some deficient substrates still have as much as 5% factor activity (120, 121). A second

**FIGURE 26.17.**    Inhibitor neutralization assay. **a,** Antibody is added to the test plasma and the clotting factor to be assayed is neutralized by complex formation. **b,** After incubation, the test plasma is mixed with fresh normal plasma. **c,** The residual unbound antibody in the test plasma further neutralizes additional clotting factor antigen in the fresh normal plasma. **d,** An aPTT assay is performed. The degree of prolongation of the aPTT is directly correlated with the amount of residual antibody present in the test sample, which is inversely related to the amount of clotting factor antigen in the original test plasma.

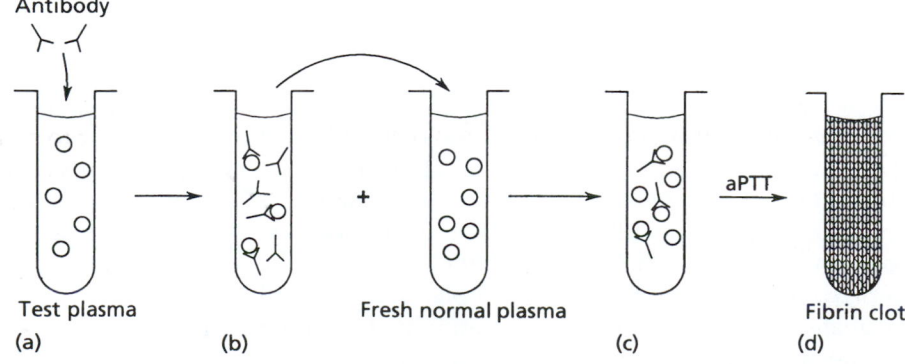

Antibody

Test plasma
(a)

Fresh normal plasma

+

(b)

(c)

aPTT

Fibrin clot
(d)

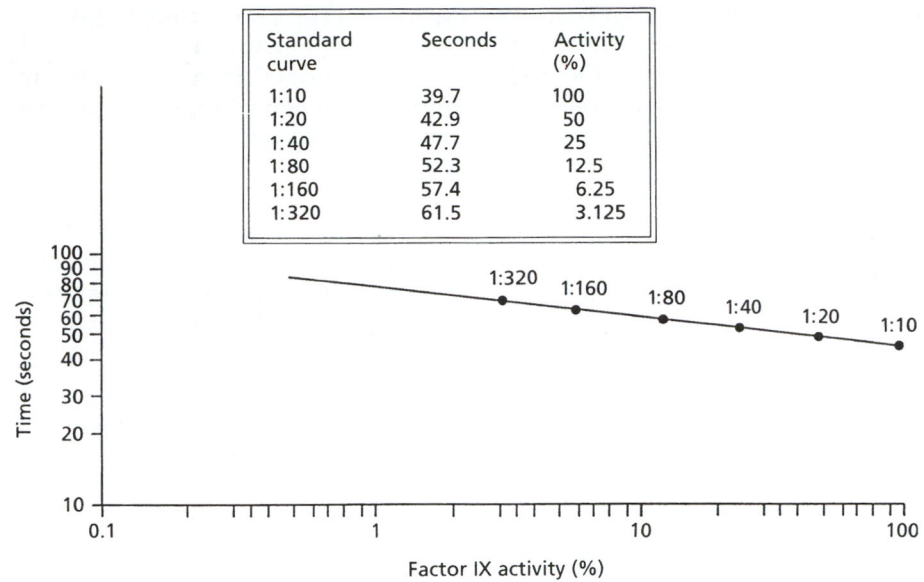

| Standard curve | Seconds | Activity (%) |
|---|---|---|
| 1:10 | 39.7 | 100 |
| 1:20 | 42.9 | 50 |
| 1:40 | 47.7 | 25 |
| 1:80 | 52.3 | 12.5 |
| 1:160 | 57.4 | 6.25 |
| 1:320 | 61.5 | 3.125 |

**FIGURE 26.18.** Assay of factor IX activity using the aPTT assay. A standard curve is generated using dilutions of normal plasma in an aPTT assay. The log of the clotting time of each dilution ($y$-axis) is plotted against the log of the dilution ($x$-axis).

source of error in clot-based factor assays is the type of normal pooled plasma used. Surveys of the factor VIII activity level in the normal pooled plasma used to generate standard curves have revealed ranges from 63 to 135% of the mean (122, 123). Activity levels between laboratories using different normal pooled plasma preparations may not be comparable. Thus, international reference plasmas are being developed for measurement of factors VIII and IX, as well as other clotting factors, as an index against which local pooled normal plasmas may be assayed for standardization of clotting factor activity levels (123, 124). A 20% error is not unusual for measuring factor VIII levels. This degree of variability, when measuring plasma samples with factor VIII activity levels in the range of 40%, makes the diagnosis of mild hereditary deficiencies more difficult. Results as divergent as 27 to 78% have occurred in international laboratory proficiency studies (124–126).

Because of these inherent technical problems of clot-based factor assays, considerable effort has been devoted to utilization of chromogenic substrates to determine functional activity levels of specific clotting factors. Additional information is obtained by also measuring the antigenic level of clotting factors. The following is a description of chromogenic and immunologic assay techniques for clotting factors.

## FACTOR XII

Factor XII is most frequently measured in a clot-based assay. In the chromogenic assay, factor XII is measured indirectly by the measurement of kallikrein activity (127, 128). Factor XII in the test plasma is activated to XIIa by incubation with kaolin, ellagic acid, or micronized silica. Kallikrein produced from the test plasma prekallikrein

(PK) is inactivated by incubation for 1 hour. The test sample containing activated factor XIIa is then mixed with a known amount of exogenous PK. When kallikrein substrate is added, the amount of factor XIIa can be quantitated chromogenically. Factor XII is also measured by standard immunologic methods (128, 129).

## Interpretation

Factor XII levels vary by ethnic background, with Orientals having lower levels of both antigen and activity when compared with Caucasians (44% versus 100%) (130, 131). In those older than age 65, factor XII levels are slightly higher in women compared to men (132). Low levels of factor XII may be associated with an increased predilection to thrombosis and coronary artery disease (133, 134). Factor XII levels are decreased in the neonate and do not reach normal adult levels until 2 weeks of age (135). Factor XII levels are also decreased in septic shock (128, 129), in type II hyperlipoproteinemia (136, 137), and in severe liver disease (levels 40 ± 28%) (128, 138). Factor XII functional activity is low in nephrotic syndrome, and this has been reported to be due to excess excretion with nephrotic-range proteinuria (50, 137) or to an apparent functionally abnormal factor XII molecule (139). Factor XII levels may be artifactually decreased by the presence of lupus anticoagulants (140–144). Factor XII levels are increased in pregnancy and with oral contraceptive use (145). True genetic deficiency of factor XII is inherited as an autosomal recessive trait (see Chapter 36). Levels of antigen and activity are 40 to 60% in the heterozygous state and are undetectable in the homozygous state. Variants of factor XII have been reported in which the antigen, measured by RIA (128, 129, 134), is higher than the activity level; in some cases this is due to slow activation of factor XII when bound to negatively charged surfaces (146).

## PREKALLIKREIN

Prekallikrein (PK) is quantified by activation to kallikrein. Test plasma is incubated with dextran, ellagic acid, micronized silica, or kaolin. Chromogenic substrate H-D-Pro-Phe-Arg-pNA (S2302) is then added, and released pNA is quantitated by endpoint assay at 1 minute (98, 147–149). Some laboratories use an activator consisting of factor XI, ellagic acid, and phospholipid to ensure that factor XII levels are of sufficient concentration and do not thereby influence the quantitative conversion of PK to kallikrein (149, 150). Kallikrein adsorbs to plastics, so transfer of the assay to a new tube after PK activation may yield falsely low levels (149).

Prekallikrein antigen may be quantitated using RID techniques (149). An RIA has been described for PK and kallikrein that is highly sensitive and specific but requires access to purified $^{125}$I-kallikrein. Consequently, it is generally performed only in research settings (149, 151, 152). Prekallikrein can also be measured using immunoelectrophoresis (149). Because PK migrates as a complex with high-molecular-weight kininogen (HK) at pH 8.6 and does not migrate alone owing to its high isoelectric point, care must be taken that sufficient HK is present in the test plasma, or falsely low antigenic levels may occur (152).

### Interpretation

Frozen samples may lose PK activity and fresh samples or samples snap frozen at $-20°C$ are preferred (153). The aPTT-based assay of PK is sensitive to incubation time, with apparent levels of PK increasing with incubation time with contact activator (153, 154). The clot-based assay also tends to yield varying results depending on the activator used. Ellagic acid is a contact activator that is insensitive to plasma deficiencies in PK and cannot be used as the activator in determination of PK levels (147, 154, 155). For these reasons, amidolytic and antigenic assays are preferred. Prekallikrein levels are decreased postpartum (156), in DIC (128), septic shock (128), carcinoid tumor (157), and type II hyperlipoproteinemia (158). Prekallikrein is more strikingly depressed than other contact activation factors in cirrhosis and other liver diseases (128). Congenital deficiency states are heterogenous in expression and autosomal (some recessive and some dominant) inheritances have been reported (128, 149). Congenital deficiencies with absent functional and antigenic PK are found in American blacks, and deficiencies associated with absent function, but with 10 to 30% antigenic levels, are found in Mediterranean and Japanese individuals (128, 152, 159).

## HIGH-MOLECULAR-WEIGHT KININOGEN

High-molecular-weight kininogen may be measured in a standard clot-based aPTT assay using deficient substrate plasma. The rarity of the deficiency state limits the availability of the assay.

The chromogenic assay requires HK in factor XI activation to XIa by factor XIIa and a reactive surface (160, 161). Thus, in the chromogenic assay, a factor XIa assay is performed under conditions in which HK is rate limiting. Dilutions of plasma previously acidified to inactivate inhibitors are added to purified factor XI, factor XIIa, kaolin, and soybean trypsin inhibitor to inactivate generated kallikrein. The process is stopped by the addition of corn trypsin inhibitor to inactivate factor XIIa, and XIa is measured using the chromogenic substrate S2366.

### Interpretation

In clot-based assays, the aPTT may shorten upon prolonged incubation of test plasma with contact activators (151). As in PK deficiencies, amidolytic and immunologic assays are preferred over clot-based assays for diagnosis of deficiency states. Antisera against heavy-chain precipitates both high-molecular-weight and low-molecular-weight forms of kininogen. Consequently, when measuring HK, antilight-chain antisera is used (125, 160, 162). The Laurell rocket assay is the most routinely used assay of HK antigenic levels. A hemagglutination assay is also available (163). Radioimmunoassay is limited to research settings.

In addition to artifactual decreases in HK activity due to exposure to cold, artifactual increases due to shortening of the aPTT-based assay with increased incubation time occur. High-molecular-weight kininogen is decreased postpartum (156), in DIC, liver disease, and more markedly in septic shock (128).

## FACTOR XI

Most routine and hemophilia treatment center laboratories measure factor XI with a modified aPTT assay (149, 164–166). Two synthetic substrate assays are available for measurement of factor XIa. To date, no chromogenic substrates that are specific for XIa activity alone have been identified. The test plasma is incubated with kaolin to activate XI, XII, and PK. Kallikrein and XIIa are inhibited by the addition of corn and soybean trypsin inhibitors and the remaining factor XIa activity can be measured with S2366 (167). Some simulation of factor XIa activity occurs due to incompletely inhibited kallikrein, accounting for 14 to18% of the measured activity (149). A fluorigenic substrate assay (Boc-Phe-Ser-Arg-MCA) is also available (168).

Immunologic levels of factor XI can be determined

by RIA (167), rocket immunoelectrophoresis (149), and radial immunodiffusion (149). The RIA method requires access to radiolabeled purified factor XI and is typically performed only in a research setting. Factor XI requires special handling for analysis by immunoelectrophoresis because, owing to its isoelectric point of 9.1, it does not migrate in the gel (149). In the presence of HK, factor XI forms a complex that will then migrate in the electrophoretic field and form a rocket using specific antifactor XI antibodies. The height of the rocket correlates with the level of factor XI, provided HK is not at subnormal levels.

Factor XI antigen can be measured by immunodiffusion. An increased sample volume must be used in the assay, because the plasma concentration of factor XI antigen is below the visual detection limits with Coomassie Brilliant Blue. An incubation time of 8 days is required to form a visible precipitate (149).

## Interpretation

Factor XI levels are low at birth and reach adult levels by 2 months of age (169–171). Like factor XII, factor XI levels are significantly lower in the Asian population when compared with Caucasians (128). Factor XI levels decrease during the second and third trimesters of pregnancy (172). Factor XI activity and antigen levels do not correlate very well with a clinical bleeding tendency. Levels of less than 20% are associated with a greater predilection to bleeding; 20 to 60% levels correlate with a minor tendency to bleed (149, 155). In most congenital deficiencies, activity and antigen levels correlate. Rare cases of congenital deficiency are associated with antigen levels that are higher than activity levels (155, 173).

## FACTOR X

Factor X may be measured using coagulant assays based on the PT, aPTT, or dRVVT (173, 174). In the amidolytic assay, RVV is added to the test plasma with calcium in the first step. After activation, factor Xa is measured by its ability to cleave a specific chromogenic or fluorogenic substrate (168, 175).

## Interpretation

Presence of incompletely γ-carboxylated forms of factor X, which can be activated by RVV, may yield falsely high levels of factor X in plasma of warfarin-anticoagulated individuals when compared to results obtained with conventional clot-based assays (98–100). Acquired deficiencies in factor X are associated with liver disease (48), and vitamin K deficiency (48). Absorption of factor X on amyloid fibrils has been reported to be a cause of depressed factor X levels in amyloidosis (176). Congenital deficiency of factor X may be subdivided into as

many as ten different types depending on abnormalities observed using amidolytic, snake venom, immunologic and clot-based assays (162). Factor X levels are depressed to 6 to 10% in homozygous and to 40 to 67% in heterozygous deficiency states (174, 177).

## FACTOR IX

Factor IX levels are most commonly measured using an aPTT-based method and factor IX-deficient substrate plasma. In amidolytic assays, factor IX is measured as a rate limiting factor in the production of factor Xa using Xa-specific substrate (98). Therefore, the routine chromogenic assay conditions for factor X are adjusted so that IXa limits the rate of factor Xa formation to be directly correlated with factor IX levels in the test plasma. Factor IX is activated by kaolin, silica, or exogenous purified factor XIa. In the presence of factor VIIIa, calcium, and phospholipid, factor IXa catalyzes the conversion of factor X to Xa. Factor Xa then cleaves a specific chromogenic or fluorogenic substrate (178). Factor IX levels may be measured antigenically by IRMA, RIA, or inhibitor neutralization assay (106, 179–183). Discrepancies between antigenic and functional activities form the basis for the CRM + and coagulant reactive material (CRM) − nomenclatures for hereditary factor IX deficiency states or hemophilia B (155). Additionally, variant factor IX molecules have been reported, which exhibit different activity levels in bovine compared with rabbit thromboplastin-based factor assays (179, 184).

## Interpretation

Factor IX antigenic levels tend to be normal with chronic warfarin anticoagulation, but activity levels are decreased (185). Factor IX levels are 40 to 50% of normal in the newborn (169, 170). Factor IX has been found to be decreased in nephrotic syndrome, where it is lost from plasma through glomerular capillary protein leak (185). Factor IX activity is reduced and factor IX antigen may be concomitantly absent, decreased, or normal in congenital deficiency (155, 179, 184).

## FACTOR VIII

Two types of factor VIII assays based on the aPTT method are available. In practice, most laboratories use the one-stage assay. In the one-stage assay, test plasma is diluted with plasma deficient in factor VIII, as described above (118, 186). The two-stage assay is based on the generation of factor Xa activity, which is then measured in the aPTT assay. Factor VIII levels are very sensitive to the thromboplastin reagent used in the aPTT assay. Some thromboplastin reagents do not detect mild reductions in factor VIII levels to 25% (157). Factor VIII levels measured by the two-stage method may also be 20%

higher than activity levels measured by the one-stage method, when assaying factor VIII activity in commercial factor VIII concentrates. For unknown reasons, this difference in assay results is also apparent when measuring plasma levels of factor VIII in individuals transfused with factor VIII concentrates (187). Discrepancies in factor activities between the two methods are less apparent when plasma samples are assayed against plasma standards, rather than against dilutions of purified factor VIII. The two-stage assay is not sensitive to thrombin-activated forms of factor VIII (122, 123).

Chromogenic and flourigenic assays are based on the generation of factor Xa in test specimens under conditions in which factor VIIIa is a limiting factor (178, 188). A commercially available reagent cocktail consisting of purified factor IXa, factor X, and phospholipid is added to dilutions of normal pooled plasma or test plasma and incubated for 30 minutes. During this time, factor VIIIa in the test sample acts as cofactor for factor IXa conversion of factor X to Xa. Factor Xa produced is measured using a specific factor Xa chromogenic substrate.

A variety of immunologic assays exist for measurement of factor VIII antigen levels (189–194). Until recently, most immunologic assays used homologous antibodies derived from individuals with factor VIII inhibitors (189, 190). Currently, with better techniques of separation and purification of factor VIII from VWf, monoclonal antibodies have been prepared to factor VIII (191, 192). Factor VIII antigen may also be measured by IRMA (193). For routine purposes, factor VIII levels are better measured functionally than by immunologic assay.

## Interpretation

Factor VIII levels are elevated as acute-phase reactants in liver disease (50, 194), systemic rheumatic disease (195), pregnancy (196), and in response to desmopressin acetate (DDAVP) (197) and prolonged venous occlusion (1). Factor VIII levels are decreased in DIC, in hemophilia A, and vWd Willebrand's disease (vWd). Factor VIII activity levels correlate well with antigen levels.

## FACTOR VII

There is no synthetic substrate available for direct measurement of factor VIIa, and the assay is based on measurement of generated factor Xa activity (198–200). Factor VII is activated to VIIa in the presence of thromboplastin (200). Factor VIIa is used in the presence of calcium to activate factor X to Xa, and the amount of factor Xa generated is quantitated by cleavage of factor Xa-specific substrate.

## Interpretation

In clot-based assays, measured factor VII activity may vary with the species of thromboplastin used. The tendency to clinical bleeding may correlate best with factor VII activity levels from human thromboplastin-based assays (173, 201, 202). Chromogenic assay may not be used in samples from individuals anticoagulated with warfarin (98). Factor VII levels are significantly increased in the elderly compared to levels seen in 20 year olds (203). Factor VII levels are decreased in liver disease, vitamin K deficiency, and disorders of bilirubin metabolism, such as Dubin-Johnson, Rotor, and Gilbert's syndromes (204), and in homocystinuria, in which levels as low as 20 to 50% may be found (205); in this latter prothrombotic disorder, reduced levels may reflect increased factor consumption. Factor VII levels are decreased in the neonate (169, 170) and increased with pregnancy (206). In 10% of individuals with congenital factor VII deficiency, the antigenic level is normal (207).

## FACTOR V

Factor V is usually measured in clot-based assay using factor V-deficient substrate (208). In the chromogenic assay, factor V functional activity is measured by generation of thrombin amidolytic activity (209). Test plasma is incubated with excess prothrombin, Xa, calcium, Va, and phospholipid to produce thrombin. Thrombin is then measured by specific chromogenic substrate.

## Interpretation

Factor V levels are decreased in liver failure (194), chronic myelogenous leukemia, and in DIC (210). Factor V can be decreased due to inhibitors seen with pancreatitis (97), tuberculosis (211), cholecystitis (212), and autoimmune reactions. Similarly, decreased factor V levels are reported postoperatively due to antibodies produced against residual bovine thrombin present in surgical glue that cross react with human factor V (95). Heterozygous congenitally deficient individuals have factor V activity levels of approximately 50% and congenital homozygous deficiency results in levels of less than 10%. Antigenic levels of 45 to 70% antigen may occur in some of these individuals (155).

## FACTOR II

Prothrombin levels are measured amidolytically after activation in a two-stage assay, because factor Xa is inhibited by synthetic thrombin substrates (100). Activation of prothrombin can be carried out using a factor Xa/Va and phospholipid mixture. Alternatively, staphcoagulase or *Echis carinatus* snake venom may be used to activate prothrombin directly without the need for factor Xa and Va (212). The thrombin generated is measured by addition of a specific thrombin substrate.

## Interpretation

The staphcoagulase and snake venom activate factor II in warfarin-anticoagulated or vitamin K-deficient plasma, leading to artificially high levels of prothrombin activity (100). Dysprothrombinemias have been described in which the antigen level (155) is disparate from the low functional activity observed.

# VON WILLEBRAND FACTOR

von Willebrand disease is one of the most common congenital bleeding disorders and can be difficult to diagnose in its milder forms (see Chapter 34). The antigenic and functional activities of vWf fluctuate normally and may be grossly altered in some unrelated pathologic states, such that the diagnosis of vWd may be masked. The functional tests available are relatively crude compared with those available for other clotting factors, and they are highly reliant on fortuitous observations of the effects of addition of nonphysiologic agents on the ability by vWf to agglutinate platelets. Tests for vWf abnormalities are divided into tests for functional platelet agglutinating activity, functional platelet or receptor-specific binding, total antigenic level, and multimer distribution analysis. The diagnosis of vWd requires, at a minimum, an assessment of vWf functional activity in agglutinating platelets, an antigenic measurement, and measurement of factor VIII activity. Classification of the subtype of vWd requires additional 2DCIE or, preferably, vWf multimeric analysis.

## ANTIGENIC ASSAY OF VON WILLEBRAND FACTOR

The most common method of assessment of vWf antigenic levels is the Laurell rocket assay. Low dilutions of test plasma are compared with results of standard curves generated with normal pooled plasma. Because the Laurell rocket assay depends on the mobility of antigen within a field of agarose containing specific polyclonal antibody, the height of the rocket depends on both the quantity of antigen present as well as the amounts of various molecular weight species. Thus, a low amount of an abnormally fast-migrating array of vWf multimer species, as seen in type II vWd, may appear quantitatively normal by the Laurell rocket assay. Antigenic levels of vWf may also be measured by nephelometry, IRMA, or RIA (110, 213–216).

## TWO-DIMENSIONAL IMMUNOELECTROPHORESIS

To determine whether a variant-type vWd is present, vWf may be electrophoresed under nonreducing conditions. The gel is turned 90 degrees and the sample is then electrophoresed into agarose gel containing polyclonal antibody to vWf. The shift of the peak of vWf antigen to more anodal forms implies that vWf multimers are smaller than normal, and a type II variant vWd may be suspected (217). Two-dimensional electrophoresis is more readily available in routine laboratories than vWf multimeric analysis, but subtyping of vWd is optimally performed using multimer analysis techniques (Fig. 26.19).

## VON WILLEBRAND FACTOR MULTIMER ANALYSIS

von Willebrand factor multimeric forms may be visualized directly by electrophoresis on 1 to 2% agarose gels containing variable concentrations of acrylamide. The protein bands are then transferred directly to nitrocellulose and visualized by a Western blot technique using polyclonal rabbit anti-vWF antibody (218). The antibody is either radiolabeled with $Na^{125}I$ or conjugated with peroxidase for enzymatic detection. More recently, a chemiluminescent assay has been developed that is highly sensitive, more rapid than the enzymatic methods, and does not require the use of radioisotopes (219).

## Interpretation

Interpretation of vWf multimer patterns requires experience. In general, the gels are analyzed for the presence of all multimeric forms from 500 Kda to over 10,000 to 20,000 Kda, and for the presence of satellite bands around each major multimeric subunit. Each multimeric subunit on high-resolution agarose gel electrophoresis typically contains one major and four to six minor bands (Fig. 26.20). Deviations from the normal pattern, as well as the functional assay profile, are used in the definition of vWd types I and IIA, B, M, and N, and type III (see Chapter 34). Improper sample handling prior to multimeric analysis may lead to vWf proteolysis *ex vivo*, and a spurious type II vWd result may thus be obtained.

## VON WILLEBRAND FACTOR AGGLUTINATING MEASUREMENTS

Two reagents are available to assess the ability of vWf to agglutinate platelets. Ristocetin is an antibiotic glycopeptide that, when added to platelet-rich plasma containing vWf, results in agglutination detectable by a platelet aggregometer (220, 221). This agglutination process also occurs when platelets have been previously formalin fixed, indicating that this is not an interaction that depends on metabolic energy (222, 223). In the ristocetin cofactor assay, test plasma is added to formalin-fixed platelets and incubated in an aggregometer cuvette. Ristocetin is then added at a final concentration of 1 to 2 mg/mL. The extent of agglutination is recorded and compared to that obtained from dilutions of normal

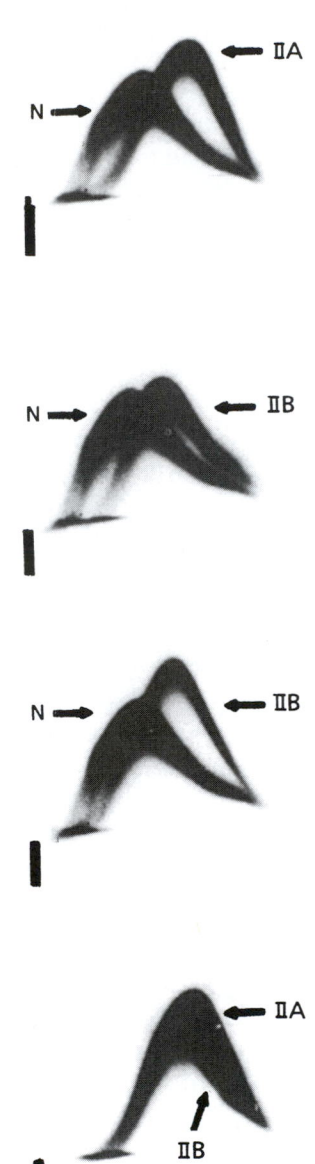

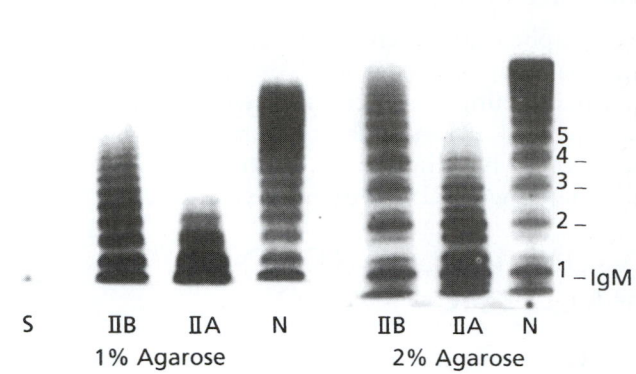

**FIGURE 26.20.** Sodium dodecyl sulfate agarose gel electrophoresis of plasma sample. After electrophoresis, the gels were then reacted with radiolabeled anti-vWf antibody and the bands identified by autoradiography. Normal plasma (N) consists of a broad array of vWf polymers. In severe (S) type III vWd, no mulitmers can be seen. In type IIA, only the smallest vWf multimers are present. In 2% agarose, there is a reduction in the highest-molecular-weight forms in type IIB vWd, which is much less pronounced than that seen in type IIA vWd, but the normal triplet repeating unit of satellite bands is different. (Adapted with permission from Zimmerman TS, Ratnoff OD, Powell AE. Immunologic differentiation of classic hemophilia (factor VIII deficiency) and von Willebrand's disease, with observations of combined deficiencies of antihemophilic factor and proaccelerin (factor V) and on an acquired circulating anticoagulant against antihemophilic factor. J Clin Invest 1971;50:244–254.)

**FIGURE 26.19.** Crossed immunoelectrophoresis of vWf antigen in normal plasma and types IIA and IIB vWd. The direction of electrophoresis of the test sample is from the left to right (anode) in the first dimension and vertically in the second dimension. The patterns of electrophoresis for types IIA and IIB vWd have been superimposed for comparison. In the case of both types IIA and IIB disease, the highest-molecular-weight multimers (the slowest migrating multimers) are diminished compared to normal. No difference is observed in the migration pattern between types IIA and IIB vWf multimers in this system. (Adapted with permission from Ruggeri ZM, Pareti FI, Mannucci PM et al. Heightened interaction between platelets and factor VIII/von Willebrand factor in a new subtype of von Willebrand's disease. N Engl J Med 1980;302:1047–1051.)

pooled plasma. Erroneous results in the ristocetin cofactor assay are obtained after infusion of Haemaccel, or in conditions in which there is a markedly elevated plasma protein level, particularly fibrinogen or paraproteins, which may inhibit platelet agglutination (224–226). Moreover, ristocetin cofactor activity is markedly pH dependent (227). Heightened sensitivity to ristocetin at concentrations of less than 1 mg/mL is suggestive of type IIB vWd (227, 228).

A second agglutinating agent, which is less frequently used or required in routine laboratories, is the snake venom-derived glycopeptide, botrocetin. Botrocetin activity generally parallels ristocetin cofactor activity in classic vWd. However, in some forms of variant vWd, there is no ristocetin cofactor activity and botrocetin activity remains normal (228).

Ristocetin cofactor assays, using fresh platelets, are sensitive to levels as low as 1% vWf activity, and, using formalin-fixed platelets, to levels of 5% vWf activity. A reference curve is generated by diluting normal pooled plasma with buffer at pH 7.4 containing 4% albumin. Both the extent or percentage aggregation and the rate of aggregation may be recorded, with the latter possibly more directly associated with clinical severity of the disease.

## MACROSCOPIC AGGLUTINATION ASSAYS

In this assay, dilutions of test plasma, platelets, and ristocetin are mixed on a glass slide and observed with a magnifier for time to agglutination. The test is rapid, requires only 40 μL of plasma, and several samples can be tested at once. It is sensitive to levels of vWf ristocetin cofactor activity of 5% (223, 229). A platelet-counting method for assaying the degree of ristocetin-dependent agglutination induced by a test plasma is also available and results are comparable to the macroscopic agglutination method (230, 231).

## FACTOR VIII BINDING ASSAY

To differentiate type IIN vWd, or vWd Normandy, from mild hemophilia, it is necessary to demonstrate decreased binding of normal factor VIII to the individual's defective vWf. In this assay, polyclonal rabbit anti-vWF antibody bound to microtiter wells is used to capture the vWf present in dilutions of the individual's plasma incubated in the microtiter wells. The factor VIII present on the bound vWf is then removed by incubation of the plates with high salt concentrations. The wells are washed, recombinant factor VIII is added, and the wells are incubated for 1 hour. The vWf-bound factor VIII is then quantitated by ELISA using a peroxidase-conjugated antifactor VIII antibody, or by chromogenic coagulant assay. The amount of factor VIII bound is normalized for the amount of vWf bound per well determined by incubation with peroxidase conjugated anti-vWF antibodies. Factor VIII binding is normally 60 to 170% (232–234). The abnormality in factor VIII binding is associated most frequently with genetic mutations Arg(53)Trp or Arg(91)Gln in the factor VIII binding region on vWf (232, 235). At present, in the United States, both the factor VIII binding assay and the genetic analysis for the factor VIII binding mutations are performed in research laboratories, although it is expected that a factor VIII binding assay will soon be commercially available.

Radioreceptor and immunoradiometric assays are also available for analysis of ristocetin-dependent and other platelet-binding and collagen-binding functions of vWf. The assays are quite complex and are beyond the scope of most routine hemostasis laboratories.

### Interpretation

von Willebrand factor levels are elevated in diabetes, pregnancy, rheumatologic diseases, and cirrhosis, and vWf rises with other acute-phase reactants (194, 196, 236, 237). Levels increase after exercise and with estrogens (238, 239). von Willebrand factor antigenic, ristocetin cofactor, and factor VIII levels rise in response to DDAVP. Because of the association of vWf and factor VIII, some forms of vWd in which factor VIII levels are less than 40% may be associated with a prolonged aPTT. The laboratory distinction between milder forms of factor VIII deficiency and vWd can be difficult without molecular biological techniques (213, 233–235) (Table 26.6). Levels of ristocetin cofactor activity vary with blood group and race (240–242). (For review of vWd subtypes, see Chapter 34 and [242–245].) In general, the ristocetin cofactor activity is more predictive of vWd than are vWf antigenic levels (243).

## FIBRINOGEN ASSAYS

The routine screening tests of PT, aPTT, and thrombin time are variably prolonged in hypofibrinogenemia, dysfibrinogenemia, or afibrinogenemia (246). The thrombin time is most sensitive to decreases or abnormalities in fibrinogen, especially with fibrinogen levels of less than 100 mg/dL. The assay can be performed

**TABLE 26.6.** Comparison of Assay Results in Hemophilia A and von Willebrand Disease (vWd)

| Assay | Hemophilia A | Hemophilia Carrier | vWd Type I | vWd Type II | vWd Type III |
|---|---|---|---|---|---|
| VIII:C | D | D | D | N–D | D |
| VIIIC Ag | D (except CRM+) | D (except CRM+) | D | N–D | D |
| VIIIR:Ag | N | N | D | N–D | A |
| Multimers | N | N | N | Abn | |
| RiCoF | N | N | D | D | A |

A, *absent;* Abn, *abnormal;* CRM+, *crossreacting material is present;* D, *decreased;* N, *normal;* RiCoF, *ristocetin cofactor activity.* VIII:C, *factor VIII;* VIIIC:Ag, *factor VIII antigen;* VIIIR:Ag, *factor VIII-related antigen.* (For new nomenclature see Chapter 34.)

(CRM+ indicates a factor deficiency state in which the factor's functional activity is disproportionately low compared to the level of antigen as detected by immunologic techniques.)

**TABLE 26.7.** Fibrinogen Assays

| Method | Information Provided | | Affected by | |
|--------|:---:|:---:|:---:|:---:|
| | Quantitative | Qualitative | Heparin | FDPs |
| Thrombin time | + | + | Yes | Yes |
| Turbidometry | + | + | No | Yes |
| Precipitation | + | − | No | Yes |
| Total clottable | + | + | Yes | No |
| Latex agglutination | + | − | Yes | Yes |
| Reptilase time | + | + | No | No |
| RIA | + | − | No | Yes |
| RID | + | − | No | Yes |

FDPs, *fibrin degradation products;* RIA, *radioimmunoassay;* RID, *radial immunodiffusion.*

manually by tilt tube methods. However, it is subject to excessive tilt dislodging the clot and to be reproducible it depends heavily on experienced, alert technicians. Hence, assays are now generally performed in a fibrometer. There are several types of fibrinogen assays that measure the amount by physical or immunologic methods or that measure functional activity (36, 247, 248) (Table 26.7).

## MODIFIED THROMBIN TIME

This assay is based on the TCT, but is modified to enhance sensitivity to small changes in fibrinogen concentration (37, 249). Plasma is diluted 1:10 so that fibrinogen concentrations are effectively 20 to 40 mg/dL. Thrombin (100 U/mL) is added and the time to clot formation recorded in a fibrometer. If the modified thrombin time result is too long or too short to be read on the linear portion of the standard curve derived from normal pooled plasma, then the plasma dilution is repeated at either 1:5 or 1:20 dilution with buffer, respectively. The test reflects changes in the first two stages of fibrin formation: the release of fibrinopeptide A and the formation of detectable fibrin polymers. The use of a high thrombin concentration with a low fibrinogen substrate concentration provides a linear assessment of plasma fibrin(ogen) levels between 10 and 400 mg/dL. Dilution of the test plasma also minimizes the effects of ATIII, heparin, and FDPs on the assay for fibrinogen. The modified thrombin time is reliable as a measure of fibrinogen with heparin levels up to 0.6 U/mL and FDPs of 100 μg/dL. Commercial fibrinogen references are available, but they may be highly variable in true clottable fibrinogen content (250, 251).

## TURBIDOMETRIC ASSAY

Turbidometric assessments of fibrinogen are based on the optical changes induced by polymerization of fibrinogen in a test sample. As originally described by Ellis and Stransky (252), one drop of a mixture of thrombin (50 U/mL) and 0.025 mol/L CaCl$_2$ is added to 3 mL of plasma diluted 1:10 in saline. A flocculent precipitate will form over 20 minutes. The turbidity is measured in a spectrophotometer against a blank of diluted plasma. Results are influenced by high fibrinogen concentrations. The assay provides only quantitative information and does not identify qualitative defects (dysfibrinogenemias).

## PRECIPITATION TECHNIQUES

Fibrinogen may be precipitated from plasma using heat (253) or salts such as ammonium sulfate (254–256). The protein content is then measured spectrophotometrically. Because other proteins are frequently precipitated with fibrinogen, and only 80 to 85% of the fibrinogen is precipitable (253), the method is only semiquantitative. It is also influenced by heparin, FDPs, and lipids (37, 249). It is inaccurate at low concentrations of fibrinogen and cannot detect abnormalities in fibrinogen function (249).

## TOTAL CLOTTABLE FIBRINOGEN

In this assay, plasma is completely clotted with an excess of thrombin. The clot is then removed and the total protein content of the clot is assayed either by weight, colorimetric protein assay (257), or by dissolution in urea and measuring UV absorbance (256). In the method of Ratnoff and Menzie (257), plasma is allowed to clot on glass beads. The beads are removed and the adherent fibrin is washed and dissolved in NaOH. The total tyrosine content is then measured with Folin's reagent or by the Biuret reaction. These methods are inaccurate because of other proteins, lipids, and salts that may lead to artifactually increased levels of fibrinogen, depending on the assays used (258). These methods are also time consuming and not practical for most routine labs.

## IMMUNOLOGIC ASSAYS

Immunologic methods are used to determine the amount of fibrinogen antigen present in a sample. They have been supplanted by the use of the more popular TCT-based methods because of the lack of functional information provided by the antigenic assay. They are, however, useful when confirming the suspicion of a dys-fibrinogenemia in which there is generally a clear discrepancy between fibrinogen antigenic levels and results obtained from clot-based assays (246).

Fibrinogen levels can be semiquantitatively measured by observing the agglutination of latex particles coated with antifibrinogen antisera in the presence of dilutions of test plasma and control pooled plasma. Falsely high results may occur depending on the specificity of the antibodies to fibrinogen. This is frequently observed when FDPs are high, because many of the fibrinogen antigenic sites are retained on FDPs. Fibrinogen levels can also be measured by RIA (259) or RID (260). Immunologic methods have the advantage that they are usually not influenced by the presence of heparin.

## SNAKE VENOM ASSAYS OF FIBRINOGEN

Snake venoms contain enzymes capable of activating many clotting factors as well as cleaving fibrinopeptides A or B from fibrinogen directly (261). The venoms from *Agkistrodon rhodostoma* (ancrod), *Bothrops atrox* (batroxobin), and *Bothrops jararaca* (botropase) hydrolyze only fibrinopeptide A from fibrinogen. *Agkistrodon contortrix contortrix* cleaves fibrinopeptide B. Upon incubation of these enzymes with fibrinogen, additional clues may be provided as to the molecular defects accounting for abnormal fibrinogen function.

Clinically, the reptilase time is performed to provide a functional assessment of the ability of fibrinopeptide A to be cleaved from fibrinogen proteolytically. In this assay, reptilase is added to the test plasma instead of thrombin, and time to clot formation is monitored (262).

In general, both the TCT and the reptilase time are prolonged in most dysfibrinogenemias (42, 263). A few dysfibrinogenemias exhibit an abnormal TCT and normal reptilase time (42, 263, 264). The reptilase time is also affected by the presence of increased levels of FDPs and paraproteins, and by low but functionally normal fibrinogen concentrations (42, 263, 264). A normal reptilase time in the setting of an unexplained PTT can be associated with a dysfibrinogenemia, but it is more often due to the presence of occult heparin in the sample (264). (For a review of snake venoms available for analysis of dysfibrinogenemias, see [261].)

## ASSAYS OF FIBRIN/ FIBRINOGEN DEGRADATION PRODUCTS

Fibrinogen degradation products are generally measured in the assessment of ongoing clot formation and lysis *in vivo*. A variety of assays are available for measurement of FDPs. An understanding of the specificity of each of these assays requires a basic knowledge of the differences between the thrombin and plasmin-derived proteolytic fragments of fibrinogen and the plasmin-derived fragments of factor XIIIa crosslinked and non-crosslinked fibrin, as shown in Fig. 26.21 (265).

## PARACOAGULANT ASSAYS

Paracoagulants are soluble fibrin monomers that are predominantly the earlier plasmin degradation products X and Y observed in conditions of unchecked fibrinolysis. The ethanol gelation and protamine sulfate pre-

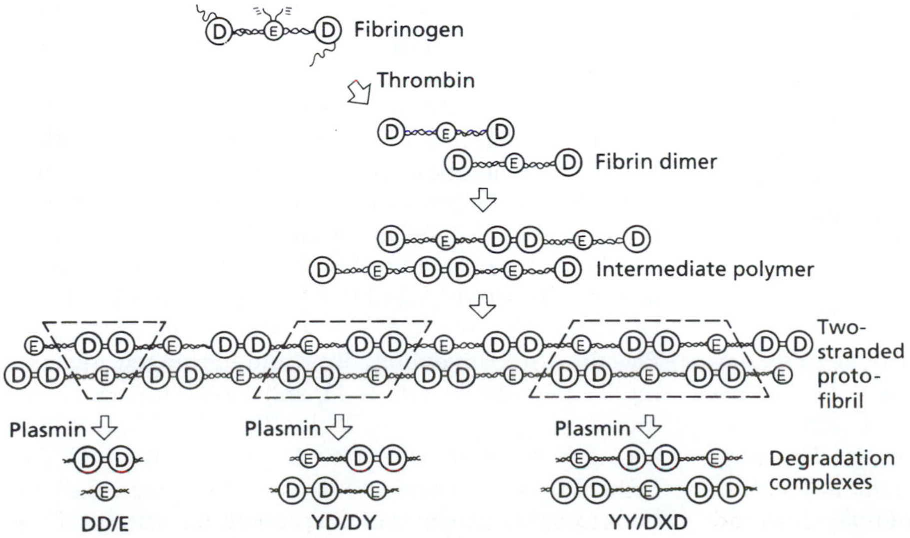

**FIGURE 26.21.** Schematic drawing of the formation of fibrin polymers from fibrinogen (*first three arrows*). The next arrow shows the array of fibrin degradation products produced after plasmin degradation of fibrin. (Adapted with permission from Francis CW, Marder VJ. Mechanisms of fibrinolysis. In: Williams WJ, Beutler E, Erslev AJ, Lichtman MA, eds. Hematology. 4th ed. New York: McGraw-Hill, 1990;1313–1321.)

cipitation assays are simple; however, with more specific FDP assays now available, they have been replaced in most hospital laboratories.

## ETHANOL GELATION

Ethanol is added to test plasma that is then manually observed for the development of fibrin strands or gel (266). Ethanol dissociates and alters the conformation of fibrin monomer complexes and allows the monomers to polymerize. Normal plasma containing no fibrin monomer complexes is negative for strand or gel formation.

## PROTAMINE SULFATE TEST

This test is similar to the ethanol gelation test. One hundred $\mu$ s of 1% protamine sulfate is added to 12 mL of test plasma and observed for formation of a gel (267, 268). A normal result is the absence of gel formation. The test will often give false positive results when blood is not promptly anticoagulated with citrate, when platelet debris are present, and if the reaction is not conducted at 37°C.

## LATEX AGGLUTINATION ASSAY (THROMBO-WELLCO ASSAY)

Blood is collected into a special tube containing bovine thrombin and 3600 U of soybean trypsin inhibitor (STI) (269–272). Because antibodies used in this assay cross react with native fibrinogen, the fibrinogen must be completely removed from the test sample before assay for FDPs. The thrombin present in the collection tube completely and rapidly consumes all clottable fibrinogen into fibrin clot. The STI inhibits plasmin cleavage of the formed fibrin. The supernatant serum then contains only FDPs produced by *in vivo* clotting and lytic activity. In the presence of heparin, which inhibits thrombin activity, reptilase can be used to form clot from test plasma fibrinogen (273). Dilutions of 1:5 and 1:20 of the test serum are made and a drop of each is placed on a slide with a preformed circle. Latex beads coated with antifragment D and antifragment E antibody are then added and the slides gently rocked and observed for agglutination compared with negative and positive controls. The results are reported based on the highest dilution resulting in agglutination of the latex particles.

### Interpretation

The assay is limited in that most polyclonal antibodies used in this assay are still cross reactive with epitopes on fibrinogen (269, 274), and it does not differentiate between fibrinolysis and fibrinogenolysis. The most common false positive in this assay is due to the presence of unneutralized heparin in the sample (263). The

FDPs are elevated with vigorous exercise, DIC, pulmonary embolus, deep venous thrombosis, states with increased lytic activity, and postoperatively where levels may be as high as 10 to 40 $\mu$g/mL in the absence of deep venous thrombosis (275). Urinary FDP levels may also be similarly measured and are increased in active glomerulonephritis (276) and with renal transplant rejection (277). In cases of very high FDPs, a prozone effect may occur and FDPs may falsely be recorded as negative. In the case of dysfibrinogenemias, the FDP assay may be falsely elevated due to the inability of thrombin to effectively clot the abnormal fibrinogen (42, 246). Thus, the abnormal fibrinogen will be incorrectly detected in the FDP agglutination assay as FDP. Falsely low FDPs may be recorded if a significant amount of FDP is due to X and Y (soluble) oligomer fibrin peptides that are still clottable with thrombin. Hence, the X and Y degradation products will not be detected as FDPs.

## TANNED RED CELL HEMAGGLUTINATION INHIBITION IMMUNOASSAY

The tanned red cell hemagglutination inhibition immunoassay assay (TRCHII) detects both fibrin and fibrinogen degradation products, X, Y, D, and E. Serum is incubated with antifibrinogen antiserum and then fibrinogen-coated tanned red cells are added (269–273). If FDPs are present in the test serum, they will bind to the antifibrinogen antiserum and prevent agglutination of the fibrinogen-coated red cells.

## STAPHYLOCOCCUS CLUMPING ASSAY

A select strain of coagulase negative *Staphylococcus aureus* forms clumps in the presence of fibrinogen, fibrin monomer, and FDPs X and Y. Dilutions of the serum are mixed with the suspension and observed for clumping (278, 279).

## FIBRINOPEPTIDE ASSAY

Thrombin cleaves fibrinopeptide A, followed by fibrinopeptide B, from fibrinogen during fibrin clot formation. Thrombin generation *in vivo* can be monitored by measurement of the amount of fibrinopeptide A or B in a test sample (280–282). Sensitivity and specificity of these assays are directly related to the antibodies used to detect fibrinopeptide A and B. Fibrinopeptide A levels can be measured using RIA or ELISA techniques (283, 284). Plasmin also cleaves both fibrin and fibrinogen, generating B$\beta$ peptides 1–118, 1–42, and 15–42, for which immunologic assays are available (108, 282, 285). Antibodies have been generated to fragments B$\beta$15–42 and B$\beta$1–118. When fragments B$\beta$15–42 and B$\beta$1–118 are both elevated, without an increase in fibrinopeptide A,

**TABLE 26.8.**   Fibrinopeptide Levels in Disseminated Intravascular Coagulation and Primary Fibrinolysis

| Fibrinopeptides | Thrombin-derived | Plasmin-derived | DIC | Primary Fibrinolysis |
|---|:---:|:---:|:---:|:---:|
| A | + | | + | − |
| B | + | | + | − |
| Bβ1–13 | + | | + | − |
| Bβ1–42 | | + | + | − |
| Bβ15–42 | + | + | + | + |
| Bβ1–118 | | + | + | + |

DIC, *disseminated intravascular coagulation.*

this is suggestive evidence of primary fibrinolysis. When both fibrinopeptide A and Bβ related fragments are elevated, DIC with secondary fibrinolysis is most likely (Table 26.8).

## Interpretation

The combined results of both fibrinopeptide A and Bβ peptide assays are helpful in distinguishing primary from secondary fibrinolysis (282). Fibrinopeptide A levels are increased in systemic lupus erythematosus, DIC, pulmonary embolus, deep venous thrombosis, burns (283), and when blood has been in contact with artificial surfaces such as during bypass procedures, hemodialysis and with prosthetic heart valves (286–288). There is a 10 to 15% rate of both false positives and false negatives. It is more sensitive to states of increased thrombin activity than fibrin monomer assays and is more than one hundred times more sensitive than levels of β-thromboglobulin or platelet factor 4 (PF4) levels (288). Careful venipuncture technique is necessary to achieve a valid result because levels of fibrinopeptide A increase with duration of veno-occlusion (289).

## FIBRIN MONOMER ASSAYS

The release of FPA from fibrinogen by thrombin exposes neo-epitopes on fibrin molecules that can be detected by specific monoclonal antibodies. These neo-epitopes are due to exposure of the cleavage site and to conformational changes in fibrin induced by the removal of FPA. Enzyme-linked immunosorbent assays have been developed to detect these fibrin monomers that may not be detected by D-dimer and FPA assays. Fibrin monomers are indicators of thrombin cleavage of fibrinogen, but the clinical utility of these assays in either diagnosis of deep vein thrombosis or monitoring of anticoagulation remains to be proven (290, 291).

## D-DIMER ASSAY

The D-dimer assay is currently the most widely used method of measuring FDPs specifically. In this assay, a monoclonal antibody directed against a neoantigen found on a late plasmin digestion product of crosslinked fibrin (D-dimer), and not present on fibrinogen or noncrosslinked fibrin fragments, is used in the detection of crosslinked fibrin fragments (292, 293). The D-dimer assay, like other FDP assays, also uses latex beads that are coated with antibody directed against D-dimer. The test requires only 10 μL of plasma. Because of the high antibody specificity for the plasmin fragment of digested factor XIIIa crosslinked fibrin, D-dimer, and the lack of cross reactivity with fibrinogen or non crosslinked fibrin fragments, the test can be performed on serum samples as well as on plasma samples anticoagulated with ethylenediaminetetraacetic acid (EDTA) or sodium citrate.

## Interpretation

Increased D-dimer levels are found in DIC, deep venous thrombosis, pulmonary embolism, postoperatively, after myocardial infarction, during thrombolytic therapy, and during vaso-occlusive crisis in sickle cell disease (294–299). Although the D-dimer latex assay is more readily performed than the D-dimer ELISA, it is less sensitive and more subject to observer error (300, 301).

## D-DIMER ENZYME LINKED IMMUNOSORBENT ASSAY

Two forms of the D-dimer ELISA assay are available (299–303). In the first, monoclonal antibody to D-dimer is used as the surface-bound capture antibody for test plasma. Captured D-dimer is then recognized and quantitated by antibody to fragment E coupled to peroxidase or alkaline phosphatase. In the second procedure, a less specific capture antibody that recognizes fibrinogen, FDPs, and fibrinogen degradation products is used, and bound fibrin degradation products are detected and quantitated by the more specific anti-D-dimer monoclonal antibody. The D-dimer ELISA is more time consuming than the latex assay, but it is more sensitive (304).

## D-DIMER AGGLUTINATION ASSAY

This new assay combines the sensitivity of the ELISA assay with the rapidity of the latex agglutination method. In this test, a drop of individual's blood is mixed with a bispecific antibody that is formed by conjugation of a monoclonal antibody that reacts with a high affinity site on the $\gamma$-chain of D-dimer with an anti-red cell antibody. With increased levels of D-dimer in the test blood specimen, the antibody induces agglutination of the individual's own red cells. The test is read as either positive or negative and has a high sensitivity and negative predictive value for pulmonary embolus (305, 306).

## FACTOR XIII

Factor XIII (see Chapter 6) is a transpeptidase that, when activated by thrombin cleavage to factor XIIIa, catalyzes covalent bond formation between fibrin strands in the presence of calcium (Fig. 26.22). Most laboratories perform a screening assay, such as the urea clot solubility assay, for factor XIII activity and only a few reference laboratories actually quantitate factor XIIIa activity (307–309).

## CLOT SOLUBILITY

This assay is based on the difference in chemical solubility characteristics between factor XIIIa crosslinked and non-crosslinked fibrin clot (310–312). Plasma is recalcified and fibrin clot is formed over 1 hour. The clot is then dislodged from the side of the tube and incubated with 5 mol/L urea or 1% monochloroacetic acid. The clot is observed for signs of dissolution at 1, 2, 4, and 24 hours.

### Interpretation

Decreasing size of the clot over time, fragmentation, and increased turbidity indicate dissolution. Clot lysis in less than 24 hours is indicative of poorly crosslinked fibrin and, consequently, factor XIII levels of less than 1%. Only 2% levels of factor XIII are required to maintain a normal clot stability. Exact quantitation is seldom necessary. Results are generally recorded as factor XIII pres-

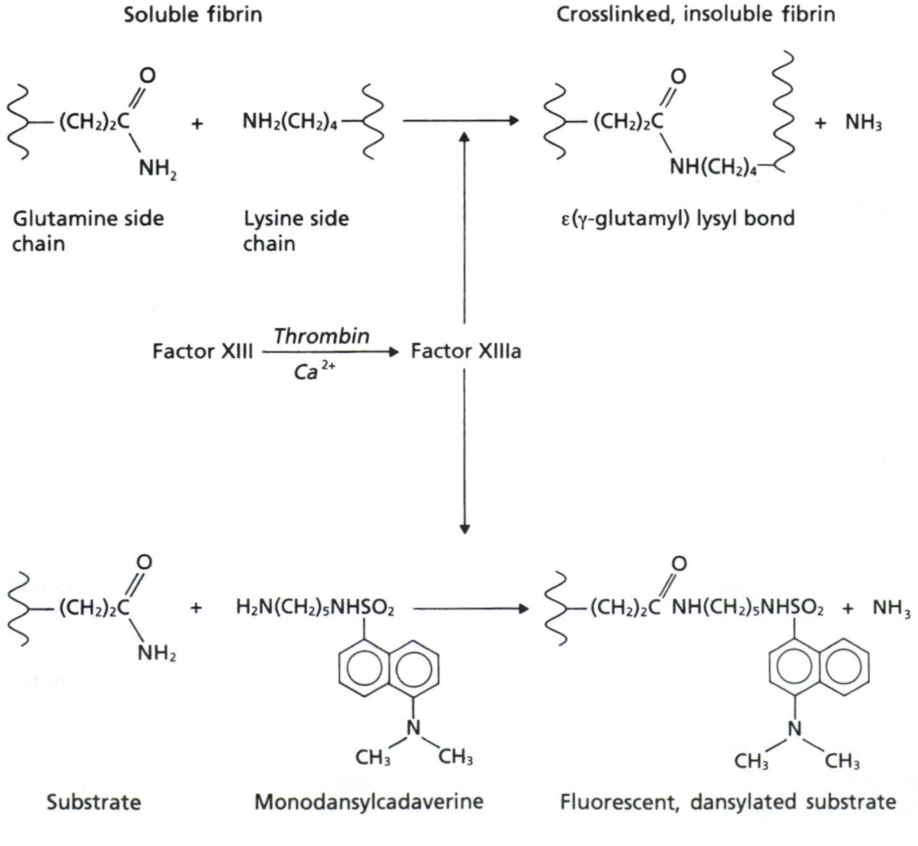

**FIGURE 26.22.** Schematic representation of the covalent crosslinking of glutamine and lysine residues in fibrin by factor XIIIa (**upper reaction**). Factor XIIIa-dependent incorporation of monodansylcadaverine into a substrate protein (**lower reaction**). Curved lines represent protein, with relevant glutamine and lysine residues shown. (Adapted with permission from McDonagh J. Structure and function of factor XIII. In: Colman RW, Mirsh J, Marder VJ Salzman EW, eds. Hemostasis and thrombosis: Basic principles and clinical practice. Philadelphia: JB Lippincott, 1987:292.)

ent or absent. Because factor XIII has a very long half-life of 10 to 14 days, detection of a true deficiency requires attention to the timing of transfusion of plasma products prior to assay (307, 308). The presentation of factor XIII deficiency in adulthood is highly suspicious for an inhibitor of factor XIII (307, 308).

Factor XIII activity can be assessed by measuring factor XIIIa-dependent incorporation of labeled amines into a suitable substrate such as fibrinogen or casein (309).

## SYNTHETIC PEPTIDE ASSAY

This assay is based on measurement of the ammonia released upon incorporation of glycine-ethylester into a specific factor XIII synthetic substrate (313). A factor XIIIa activating cocktail is added to an undiluted plasma specimen, and the decline in absorbance is measured at 340 nm for 10 minutes. The decrease in optical density is directly proportional to factor XIIIa activity. The reagent cocktail used consists of bovine thrombin, calcium chloride, polybrene, gly-pro-arg-pro-ala-amide, specific peptide substrate and glycine-ethylester, NADH, $\alpha$-ketoglutarate, adenosine diphosphate, glutamate dehydrogenase, and bovine serum albumin in buffer. Two hundred $\mu$ s of this reagent cocktail is added to 20 $\mu$L of plasma and the linear phase of absorbance is monitored.

## FACTOR XIII ANTIGENIC ASSAY

Factor XIII can be measured by electroimmunodiffusion assay (EIA) and inhibition neutralization assays (309). The Laurell method is more sensitive and can be used to measure factor XIII A and B subunits separately. The ratio of B:A subunits may be useful in carrier detection of factor XIII deficiency. Deficiency states have been defined where the A subunit is totally absent and B is normal to slightly decreased (307, 308).

# ENDOGENOUS NATURAL INHIBITORS TO COAGULATION FACTORS

## PROTEIN C

Protein C, when activated by thrombin in the presence of thrombomodulin, inactivates phospholipid-bound factors Va and VIIIa (314). Protein S serves as a cofactor in these activities (see Chapter 3). Protein C levels can be determined using a variety of assays that measure either antigenic levels of protein C or protein C functional activity. Each of these methods is limited by very specific problems due to the assay system. In general, measurement of protein C should include a measurement of the amount of plasma antigenic protein C and an assessment of the functional activity.

## PROTEIN C FUNCTIONAL ASSAYS

Measurement of protein C functional activity is inherently subject to experimental error. To measure functional activity, protein C must be activated to protein Ca by removal of the activation peptide. The ability of protein Ca to inactivate factor Va or VIIIa must then be quantitated before inactivation by endogenous plasma inhibitors of protein Ca occurs. In general, this requires separation of protein C from plasma by one of several methods, including absorption of protein C on aluminum hydroxide (315) or barium citrate (316, 317), or by removal of protein C from plasma by immunoabsorption (Fig. 26.23) (318). Unfortunately, absorption techniques do not remove all of the protein C from plasma. Aluminum hydroxide removes only 26% of the protein C and this percentage is even lower when des-$\gamma$-carboxy forms are present in samples from individuals receiving warfarin anticoagulation (319). Consequently, meticulous care is required in performing these assays to ensure that plasma absorption time is uniform and standard controls are used. Antibody absorption techniques have the same possibility for error and depend on the affinity of the antibody for protein C in various states of carboxylation.

Once the protein C has been isolated from plasma, its functional activity can be measured in an amidolytic assay using the substrate BCP 300, Behring (320), or in a clot-based method (316, 320). Both techniques require activation of protein C. This can be accomplished by using thrombin or thrombin complexed with thrombomodulin (319). The activated protein C is then added to either a normal reference plasma deficient in protein C or to a chromogenic substrate, and time to clot formation or absorbance is measured respectively. Snake venom from *Agkistrodon contortrix contortrix*, Protac, is now used to directly activate protein C in whole plasma, eliminating complicated absorption and activation steps (321).

## PROTEIN C ANTIGENIC ASSAYS

Protein C levels may be measured by EIA, ELISA, and RIA (320, 322, 323). In the standard EIA, all forms of protein C, including activated protein C (protein Ca), noncarboxylated forms of protein C, and protein Ca complexed to inhibitors, are measured. As in all EIA methods, this assay is less sensitive to very low levels of protein C. The ELISA assays are 50% less sensitive to low protein C levels, especially in individuals receiving warfarin. This is due to the inability of the antiprotein C antibodies used to recognize des-$\gamma$-carboxyprotein C molecules (315). The RIA sensitivity falls even further when using monoclonal antiprotein C antibodies that generally react with activation peptide that is absent in

**FIGURE 26.23.** Schematic diagram of available methods for assessment of protein C functional activity.

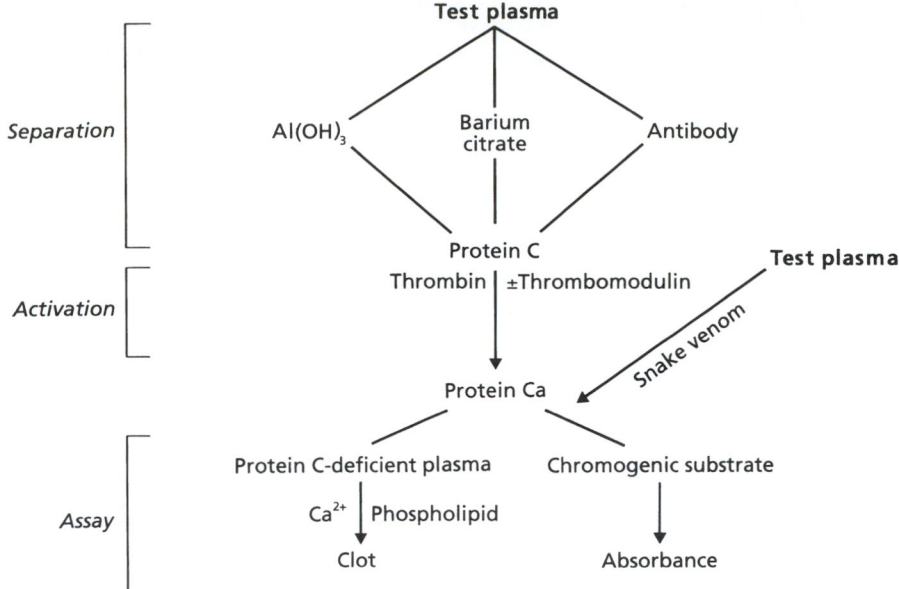

protein Ca or with the protein C inhibitor-binding region on protein Ca heavy chain (324).

## Interpretation

Clot-based functional assays are affected by the presence of heparin, and most laboratories neutralize heparin with polybrene before assay (315, 320, 323). Measurement of protein C antigenic and functional activities should be interpreted with careful assessment of the clinical picture. Protein C is transiently consumed during thrombosis, pulmonary embolism, and DIC, and heterozygous deficiency states should not be diagnosed based on laboratory values obtained during an acute thrombotic event (318). Levels of both protein C antigen and functional activity are elevated in pregnancy, estrogen use, nephrotic syndrome, and ischemic heart disease (318, 320, 324, 325). Functional levels of protein C are increased with danazol use (326). Levels are low in oral contraceptive users (324, 327–329), preeclampsia and postoperatively, and are very depressed in DIC and liver disease (317, 327, 330). In systemic lupus erythematosus, functional activity may be low despite a normal antigen level (Table 26.9) (331). Furthermore, when evaluating protein C functional activity, care must be taken to exclude the presence of an LA because this falsely prolongs the aPTT, resulting in spuriously high levels of protein C activity in clot-based methods (332, 333). Congenital protein C deficiency (see Chapter 40) has been classified into type I, in which the antigen and functional activities are both depressed, and type II, in which defective protein C molecules are produced and the functional activity is lower than the antigenic level (315, 318, 333, 334). Protein C levels are very low (27 to 40 IU)

in neonates and are even more depressed in the preterm infant; 50% of premature infants have levels of less than 20 IU/dL (335–340). Congenital heterozygous deficiency states cannot be diagnosed in that setting. Protein C levels increase approximately 4% with each decade of life beyond age 30 (318, 339).

## Interpretation of Protein C Levels in Individuals Receiving Oral Anticoagulants

Patients should be given stable oral anticoagulation for at least 4 weeks before determination of protein C levels. Under these conditions, protein C determination is best performed using a clot-based assay rather than an amidolytic assay, because the des-γ-carboxy forms still cleave the chromogenic substrate (320, 341, 342). Protac does not recognize the des-γ-carboxy forms of protein C present in warfarin-anticoagulated plasma and, thus, will result in lower levels of protein C activity than those determined by amidolytic assays using other modes of activation. Consequently, in the presence of oral anticoagulants, measurement of protein C functional activity should be performed in a clot-based method (320, 341, 342). All methods should have an established laboratory control range for individuals without congenital protein C deficiency anticoagulated with warfarin.

Protein C functional activity is more depressed than antigenic levels due to the presence of des-γ-carboxy forms of protein C, which are immunologically detectable but nonfunctional (341, 343). In individuals who are not congenitally deficient in protein C and who are receiving oral anticoagulants, functional protein C levels correlate with prothrombin or factor X levels when tested using clot-based assays (Table 26.10) (315, 341).

**TABLE 26.9.**   Protein C and Protein S in Various Diseases

| | Protein C | | Protein S | |
|---|---|---|---|---|
| | **Antigen** | **Activity** | **Free** | **Bound** |
| Liver disease | DD | DD | DD | DD |
| Disseminated intravascular coagulation | DD | DD | DD | DD |
| Oral contraceptives | N–D | N–D | D | D |
| Warfarin | DD | D | D | N–D |
| Pregnancy | N–I | N–I | D | D |
| Nephrotic syndrome | I | I | N–D | N–D |
| Systemic lupus erythematosus | N | D | D | N–I |
| Postoperative | N–D | D | D | I |
| Pulmonary embolus | D | D | N–D | N–D |
| Deep venous thrombosis | D | D | N–D | N–D |
| Preeclampsia | D | D | D | D |

D, *decreased*; DD, *markedly decreased*; I, *increased*; N, *normal*.

**TABLE 26.10.**   The Effects of Anticoagulant Therapy on the Assay Values of Protein C, Protein S, Factors II, IX, and X in Individuals with Heterozygous Protein C and Protein S Deficiency and in Nondeficient Individuals. From George [344]

| | Protein C (IU/dL) | | Protein S (U/dL) | | Factor II (U/dL) | | Factor IX (IU/dL) | | Factor X (U/dL) | |
|---|---|---|---|---|---|---|---|---|---|---|
| | **C** | **Ag** | **C** | **Ag** | **C** | **Ag** | **C** | **Ag** | **C** | **Ag** |
| *No anticoagulation* | | | | | | | | | | |
| Nondeficient | 95 | 98 | 101 | 106 | 94 | 97 | 98 | 105 | 96 | 98 |
| Protein C deficient | 45 | 50 | 100 | 105 | 95 | 97 | 96 | 99 | 96 | 102 |
| Protein S deficient | 93 | 97 | 37 | 56 | 93 | 99 | 101 | 103 | 98 | 103 |
| *INR 2.0–2.5* | | | | | | | | | | |
| Nondeficient | 40 | 54 | 65 | 87 | 44 | 63 | 55 | 61 | 42 | 44 |
| Protein C deficient | 26 | 29 | 64 | 86 | 46 | 64 | 52 | 60 | 43 | 46 |
| Protein S deficient | 40 | 55 | 28 | 50 | 45 | 62 | 51 | 59 | 42 | 45 |
| *INR 2.5–3.5* | | | | | | | | | | |
| Nondeficient | 34 | 43 | 50 | 70 | 28 | 55 | 38 | 54 | 29 | 42 |
| Protein C deficient | 18 | 22 | 54 | 68 | 27 | 51 | 37 | 50 | 28 | 42 |
| Protein S deficient | 35 | 40 | 24 | 40 | 28 | 53 | 37 | 51 | 27 | 40 |
| *INR 3.5–4.5* | | | | | | | | | | |
| Nondeficient | 22 | 39 | 43 | 66 | 23 | 47 | 29 | 46 | 24 | 38 |
| Protein C deficient | 11 | 16 | 44 | 65 | 24 | 44 | 27 | 49 | 23 | 37 |
| Protein S deficient | 23 | 36 | 19 | 33 | 22 | 48 | 26 | 47 | 24 | 37 |

Ag, *antigenic level*; C, *coagulant activity*; INR, *international normalized ratio*.

Antigen levels of less than 30 IU/dL are rarely seen in stable individuals on routine anticoagulation, and functional and antigenic levels of less than 20 IU/dL strongly suggest inherited deficiency.

## PROTEIN S

Protein S is a natural anticoagulant protein that serves as a cofactor for protein Ca to degrade factors Va and VIIIa enzymatically (344). Laboratory analysis of protein S is complicated by the presence of two forms of protein S in plasma. Forty percent of protein S is free and fully active as a cofactor for protein Ca, and 60% circulates bound to the complement regulatory protein C4b-binding protein (C4bBp) and is inactive as cofactor (344, 345). Assays of protein S are, therefore, complicated by an equilibrium between bound and free forms that may be disturbed during the assay procedure. In general, protein S is measured as an antigenic level (346). Although functional assays have been described, because of their complexity these determinations are still limited to research laboratories (347–349). Antigenic assays for total protein S include the Laurell rocket (EIA), ELISA, and 2DCIE, with the latter assay providing the most information on bound versus free protein S forms (350, 351). The Laurell assay uses polyclonal antiprotein S antisera that recognize both bound and free forms of protein S (350). Because of the difference in molecular weight between the free and complexed forms of protein S, estimation of the height of the protein S rocket may be complicated by multiple peaks and underestimation of total protein S (350–353). Slow electrophoresis at room temperature to allow maximal dissociation of protein S from C4bBp for quantitation may not completely resolve this problem. A two-site IRMA of total protein S antigen using an antibody that reacts with all forms of protein S, including cleaved and des-γ-carboxy forms of protein S, is also available (353).

## MEASUREMENT OF FREE PROTEIN S

Free protein S may be measured by EIA if the plasma is first precipitated with polyethylene glycol (PEG) to remove C4bBp complexed forms (354, 355). Some free protein S may also be precipitated if strict adherence to PEG precipitation time does not occur (324, 354). The normal range for free protein S is lower in women than in men (356). A one step ELISA for direct measurement of free protein S in plasma is also available. This assay uses two monoclonal antibodies against distinct epitopes on the free form of protein S (356). Free protein S levels are a better marker of a predilection to thrombosis (354, 355, 357).

## TWO-DIMENSIONAL COUNTER IMMUNOELECTROPHORESIS OF PROTEIN S

Two-dimensional counter immunoelectrophoresis allows for separation of free from bound protein S on the basis of differences in electrophoretic mobility. Agarose electrophoresis is first performed in the horizontal direction, followed by electrophoresis vertically into agarose containing polyclonal antiprotein S antibody. Two major precipitin peaks of protein S are visualized, one of free protein S and the other of protein S complexed to C4bBp. This technique allows for assessment of relative amounts of free functional and inactive, complexed forms of protein S (350).

## FUNCTIONAL ASSAYS OF PROTEIN S

In these assays, the cofactor activity of protein S is assessed by measuring its ability to catalyze protein Ca

inhibition of factor Va (347–350). The assay is sensitive to levels of protein S functional activity of 5%. It is not suitable for individuals receiving oral anticoagulants and is very pH dependent (349).

## Interpretation

Protein S levels are decreased in liver disease (358, 359), although to a lesser extent than those of prothrombin and ATIII, presumably because of extrahepatic sources of protein S synthesis (359). Both free and bound forms of protein S are low in pregnancy (324), preeclampsia, nephrotic syndrome (360), and with estrogen therapy (324). Protein S is decreased with oral contraceptive use, but to levels not generally less than 35 U/dL found in oral anticoagulant use (358). Both levels are extremely depressed with bound forms virtually absent in sick preterm infants and in healthy full-term infants (169, 170, 361), DIC, and liver disease (359). The pattern of depressed free protein S and elevated or normal protein S bound to C4bBp is seen in systemic lupus erythematosus (362), HIV infection (363), in the presence of lupus anticoagulants (364), and postoperatively (Table 26.9). Although attempts have been made to draw ratios between plasma protein S levels and other vitamin K-dependent factors during oral anticoagulant therapy, no reliable correlation has been found, and it is not advisable to make a diagnosis in the presence of oral anticoagulants (346, 355). Spuriously low levels of protein S activity are obtained when factor V Leiden containing the Arg506Gln mutation conferring activated protein C resistance is present in the individual's plasma (365). To overcome this potential artifact, the test also now includes an excess of exogenously added factor Va.

## THROMBOMODULIN

Measurement of thrombomodulin levels is generally only available in a research setting. Assay of thrombomodulin is performed using an RIA on plasma or urine specimens. Recently a two site ELISA has been developed using monoclonal antibodies to human thrombomodulin (366, 367). Thrombomodulin levels are increased in antiphospholipid syndrome, DIC, thrombotic thrombocytopenic purpura, collagen vascular disease, dialysis, and diabetes mellitus, and are believed to be elevated due to vascular damage.

## ACTIVATED PROTEIN C RESISTANCE

In initial biochemical studies of protein C, it was noted that addition of activated protein C (aPC) to plasma caused a prolongation of the aPTT assay. Occasionally, however, a donor plasma appeared resistant to this anticoagulant effect (368). The majority of individuals who exhibit this aberrant response to addition of aPC to the plasma aPTT assay have been shown to have a mutation in factor V (Arg506Gln), which confers resistance to cleavage of factor Va by activated protein C. Individuals who are heterozygous for this mutation in factor V (termed factor V Leiden) have a predilection to thrombosis. Those who are homozygous have a substantially increased risk of significant thromboembolic events (369–372). In this test, the ability of activated protein C to prolong the aPTT is measured. A ratio between the aPTT obtained in the presence and absence of exogenous aPC is obtained. When the individual's plasma factors, typically factor Va, are resistant to proteolytic degradation by aPC, the baseline aPTT fails to prolong significantly upon the addition of exogenous aPC. The normal aPC/aPTT to aPTT ratio is 2.4 to 4.0 (373, 374).

## Interpretation

The individual's baseline aPTT must be normal to reliably interpret the aPC resistance assay. Hence, samples from individuals receiving warfarin therapy or heparin cannot be used. Proper preparation of the blood sample is critical, because contamination with residual platelets will result in shortening of the aPTT response to aPC and, consequently, a shortened aPC ratio. This is most noticeable when the plasma is frozen and thawed before analysis. The assay is affected by decreased levels of prothrombin, factor X, and protein S. Low levels of factor V, VIII, and IX result in increased aPC ratios (373). Activated protein C ratios are decreased in women compared to men and by birth control pill use (375). The aPC ratio is higher for infants younger than 6 months of age (376, 377). Performance of the aPC resistance assay in factor V deficient plasma may improve assay sensitivity (374). Recently a new assay based on the PT has been developed. In this assay, a diluted plasma specimen is incubated with thrombin to activate factor V. Activated protein C is added. Residual factor Va is then measured by addition of a chromogenic substrate, S2238. A ratio between factor Va activities in the presence and absence of aPC is obtained (378, 379). The advantage of this system compared to the aPTT-based assay remains to be demonstrated.

Not all individuals with aPC resistance have been shown to have the mutation in factor V. In one study, 57% of heterozygous individuals had an abnormal aPC ratio, whereas 12 without any known mutation had abnormal ratios (380–384). Conversely, some individuals with the Arg506Gln mutation in factor V have an aPC resistance assay ratio in the lower range of normal. For these reasons, it is recommended that suspected aPC resistance due to the Arg506Gln mutation of the factor V gene (the factor V Leiden mutation) be confirmed by PCR analysis (380–384).

## ANTITHROMBIN III

Antithrombin III (ATIII) is the major thrombin inhibitor in plasma (see Chapter 3). When heparin binds to ATIII, it catalyzes ATIII-dependent inhibition of thrombin and other serine proteases. Antithrombin III assays include antigenic assays and assays that measure its ability to bind to heparin and to inhibit thrombin (Table 26.11). Antigenic assays include Laurell (110), nephelometry (110), RID (109), ELISA (115), and RIA (113). The Laurell assay, the most commonly used method, is affected by the presence of heparin, because heparin causes a conformational change in ATIII that alters its electrophoretic mobility when compared to control ATIII standards (384) (Fig. 26.24). Enzyme-linked immunosorbent assay and RIA offer the advantage that they are not affected by heparin and extend sensitivity down to microgram-per-milliliter levels of ATIII (384, 385).

Functional ATIII assays are divided into more cumbersome clot-based methods and amidolytic assays.

## INHIBITION OF MODIFIED THROMBIN CLOTTING TIME

Thrombin is added to the test plasma, and the ability of ATIII in the presence of heparin to prolong the thrombin clotting time is measured (385). This requires the removal of fibrinogen from the test specimen. Serum, which is devoid of fibrinogen, may be used instead of plasma; however there is a 20 to 30% loss of ATIII in serum samples (100). Fibrinogen can be precipitated from plasma by careful heating at 65°C, but residual fibrinogen may still be present. Heparin cofactor II levels

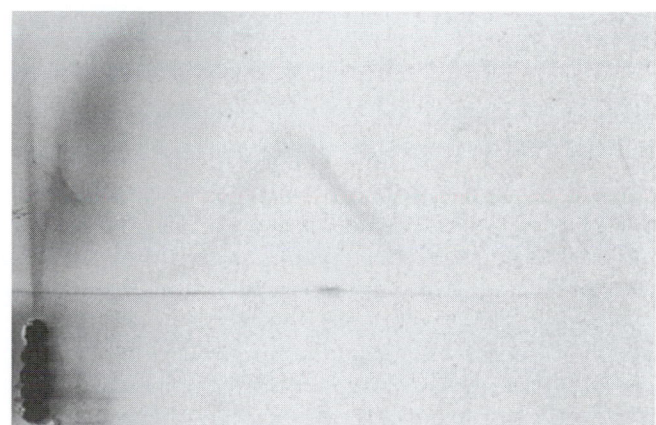

**FIGURE 26.24.** Two-dimensional crossed immunoelectrophoresis of AT III in plasma. The test plasma sample was placed in the well in the lower left and electrophoresis was carried out in agarose with the anode at the right. After removal of the upper portion of agarose and replacement with agarose containing anti-AT III antibody, the sample was then electrophoresed vertically.

**TABLE 26.11.** Methods of Assessment of Antithrombin III Abnormalities

| | Assay | Type I | Type II | Type III |
|---|---|---|---|---|
| Antigen | EIA<br>RID<br>RIA<br>ELISA<br>Nephelometry | Abnormal | Normal | Normal |
| Functional | Modified thrombin<br>Clotting time<br>(−heparin) | Abnormal | Abnormal | Normal |
| | Amidolytic assay<br>Factor Xa inhibition<br>Thrombin inhibition<br>(−heparin) | Abnormal | Abnormal | Normal |
| | Modified thrombin<br>Clotting time<br>(+heparin) | Abnormal | Abnormal | Abnormal |
| | Amidolytic activity<br>Factor Xa inhibition<br>Thrombin inhibition<br>(+heparin) | Abnormal | Abnormal | Abnormal |
| Heparin sepharose affinity chromatography | | | Normal | Abnormal |
| Two-dimensional counter immunoelectrophoresis<br>in the presence of heparin | | | Normal | Abnormal |

EIA, *electroimmunodiffusion assay;* ELISA, *enzyme-linked immunosorbent assay;* RIA, *radioimmunoassay;* RID, *radial immunodiffusion.*

may influence results in thrombin-based ATIII assays (386). Lastly, snake venoms such as ancrod have been used to defibrinate the plasma, but resulting FDPs may interfere with fibrinogen clotting in the final assay system, thereby resulting in artifactually high levels of ATIII.

## AMIDOLYTIC ASSAYS OF ANTITHROMBIN III

Amidolytic assays overcome many of the technical problems caused by the presence of fibrinogen. Test plasma containing ATIII is incubated with heparin for 3 minutes (198, 386–389). An excess of thrombin or factor Xa and chromogenic substrate is then added and absorbance measured in a fixed endpoint analysis after addition of monochloroacetic acid. Bovine thrombin is preferred in this assay because heparin cofactor II, which may account for a portion of the thrombin-neutralizing activity of the test sample, reacts more readily with human thrombin than with bovine thrombin (390, 391).

## MEASUREMENTS OF HEPARIN AFFINITY

Antithrombin III functional activity may also be impaired by decreased affinity for heparin (392, 393). The

ability of ATIII to bind to heparin is measured by 2DCIE. Plasma to which heparin is added is electrophoresed in the first dimension on agarose. Antithrombin III peaks are then detected by electrophoresis into the second dimension containing polyclonal antibody to ATIII.

## Interpretation

Antithrombin III levels may be as low as 20% in severe liver disease and chronic hepatitis (329, 394). In protein-losing conditions, such as protein-losing enteropathy and nephrotic syndrome, ATIII levels may also be low due to loss into stool or urine (395). Antithrombin III levels have also been shown to fall as much as 15% during acute bolus administration of heparin (396) and may be subnormal during DIC, acute pulmonary embolism, and deep venous thrombosis due to ongoing consumption (397, 398). Levels are low in the newborn. Maternal levels of ATIII decrease in the third trimester and for a few days postpartum. Antithrombin III levels are slightly higher in postmenopausal women (397, 399). Three general types of congenital deficiencies of ATIII have been recognized (see Chapter 40). In type I, both antigen and functional activity are decreased. In type II, the antigenic level is normal, but the defective molecule has poor functional activity. In type III, the antigenic level is normal, as is the amidolytic ATIII assay, but the heparin cofactor activity is decreased (386, 392, 400).

## HEPARIN COFACTOR II

The mode of action of heparin cofactor II (HC II) is similar to that of ATIII. Like ATIII, in the absence of heparin, the catalytic rate of thrombin inactivation by complex formation with HC II is slow. In the presence of heparin, this rate is catalyzed 1000-fold (401). The concentration of heparin required to catalyze this activity is higher than with ATIII and, unlike ATIII, HC II inactivation of factor Xa is much slower and not catalyzed by heparin (390). In addition, HC II activity is also catalyzed 1300-fold by dermatan sulfate, whereas dermatan sulfate has no effect on ATIII (401, 402). Thus, in measuring activity of HC II, either ATIII must be removed from the test sample, or its selective catalysis with dermatan sulfate must be exploited. In the assay described by Tollefsen and Pestka (403), dermatan sulfate is used as the activator of HC II activity in a two-stage chromogenic assay (404). The concentrations of activator and thrombin must be optimal and consistent to obtain reproducible results. Test plasma is mixed with an excess of thrombin and dermatan sulfate. The residual thrombin is then measured by using a thrombin-specific chromogenic substrate (401, 402).

Immunodepletion assays have been used for measuring HC II activity. In the method of Tran and Duckert, interfering ATIII is removed by immunoabsorption of the test plasma on an anti-AT III immunoaffinity column (391). The HC II activity is then measured in the column eluate in a two-stage chromogenic assay for residual thrombin activity. A second method is to add saturating concentrations of neutralizing antibody to AT III to the test plasma. The test plasma is then assayed for thrombin inhibition by addition of heparin in a two-stage chromogenic assay. Both immunodepletion-type assays depend highly on the affinity and concentrations of the antibodies used to remove AT III activity in order for measurements to truly reflect HC II activity.

## Interpretation

Congenital deficiencies in HC II are associated with decreased functional and antigenic levels (386). However, functional and antigenic levels may be disparate in DIC (403), because complexes of HC II and thrombin measured by immunologic methods may give falsely high antigenic levels and low functional levels (403). The HC II levels are increased with oral contraceptive use and are depressed during renal allograft rejection and in HIV infection (405–408). The HC II levels normally increase somewhat with age (404).

## TISSUE FACTOR PATHWAY INHIBITOR

Tissue factor pathway inhibitor (TFPI) is a plasma factor that, in the presence of factor Xa, inhibits factor VII (see Chapter 4). A chromogenic assay is available for the measurement of this activity in plasma. Test plasma diluted 1:50 is incubated with a mixture of thromboplastin, factor VII, factor X, and calcium chloride for 10 minutes, during which time the test plasma TFPI inhibits factor VII. Residual thromboplastin-factor VII activity is then measured by the addition of 0.4 U/mL of factor X. After a 10 minute incubation period, the amount of factor Xa activity generated is quantitated by the addition of factor Xa chromogenic substrate (407, 409). An ELISA assay is also available (410, 411). TFPI levels are normal in liver disease and depressed postoperatively and in thrombotic thrombocytopenic purpura (412). The TFPI levels are increased by heparin therapy and increased cholesterol levels (413). No congenital deficiency states of TFPI have yet been described.

## $\alpha_2$-MACROGLOBULIN

$\alpha_2$-Macroglobulin has a wide specificity of protease-inhibiting activity and forms complexes with thrombin, plasmin, and kallikrein, in addition to other proteases such as elastase, collagenase, and cathepsin D. The chromogenic analysis of $\alpha_2$-macroglobulin is based on formation of a trypsin-$\alpha_2$-macroglobulin complex when a known quantity of trypsin is added to the test sample (100, 413, 414). Residual trypsin is then measured by adding a fixed, known concentration of the trypsin inhibitor, aprotinin. Any residual trypsin is then measured using a specific trypsin chromogenic substrate. Thus, residual trypsin is inversely related to the amount of $\alpha_2$-macroglobulin in the test plasma. An alternate method of chromogenic analysis uses plasmin, instead of trypsin, and plasmin-specific chromogenic substrate.

## Interpretation

$\alpha_2$-Macroglobulin levels are markedly elevated in neonates and progressively decline up to age 25 (415). Levels are normally increased in women compared to men. Pathologic increases are detected in nephrosis and hepatic cirrhosis (416). Decreases occur in response to thrombolytic therapy (417). Functional levels of $\alpha_2$-macroglobulin are markedly decreased in sepsis and DIC, the functional activity being more depressed than the antigenic level in sepsis associated with shock (413).

## C1 ESTERASE INHIBITOR

C1 esterase inhibitor is an inhibitor of C1 esterase as well as of factors XIa, XIIa, kallikrein, and plasmin. C1 esterase inhibitor is measured by incubating test plasma with a known amount of C1 esterase, thereby forming a complex. Residual C1 esterase is then measured by specific chromogenic substrate (418).

## $\alpha_1$-ANTITRYPSIN

$\alpha_1$-Antitrypsin is a weak inhibitor of thrombin and also inhibits plasmin, factor XIa, and protein C. The test for $\alpha_1$-antitrypsin involves mixing test plasma with trypsin and measuring residual trypsin in a specific trypsin substrate based chromogenic assay (418). One mutant $\alpha_1$-antitrypsin has been reported in association with a fatal bleeding disorder (104).

## MARKERS OF THROMBIN ACTIVATION *IN VIVO*

One problem with the assessment of ongoing thrombosis using current assays and methodologies concerns the inability to detect low, but significant, coagulation factor enzyme activation by measurement of clotting factor zymogen. A more specific indicator of activation of zymogen would be the presence of a marker of activated enzyme that is relatively stable (419). The presence of activation peptides of prothrombin ($F_{1+2}$) (419–422), protein C (PCP) (292, 423), and the irreversible complex of thrombin and AT III (TAT) (424) in blood samples indicates activation of the clotting system *in vivo*. Radioimmunoassays and ELISAs are available for detection of $F_{1+2}$, PCP, and TAT complexes. These assays are sensitive and correlate well with active thrombosis. Normal ranges for endogenous $F_{1+2}$ and PCP levels tend to increase with age (339). The $F_{1+2}$ levels are increased in malignancy, DIC, and pregnancy. The TAT complexes are elevated in DIC, trauma, sepsis, inflammation, deep venous thrombosis, myocardial infarction, non-insulin dependent diabetes mellitus, active hemolytic anemia, graft-versus-host disease, and preeclampsia (416, 425). Results for $F_{1+2}$ are sometimes higher in samples collected in heparin when compared with those collected in citrate anticoagulant (426–430) and are seriously affected by the quality of the venipuncture in obtaining the test sample (428). Results have not been standardized, making interlaboratory comparison impossible (427, 429, 430).

# MEASUREMENTS OF THE FIBRINOLYTIC SYSTEM

## WHOLE BLOOD CLOT LYSIS TIME

The whole blood clot lysis time (WBCLT) is the simplest of all fibrinolytic screening tests, but it is very limited in the information it provides. Consequently, it has been largely supplanted by screening tests such as the euglobulin lysis time. In this assay, 2 mL of blood is drawn into a glass tube and the formed clot is incubated at 37°C with periodic inspection for clot formation followed by clot lysis. Normal clot lysis occurs after 48 hours. When hyperfibrinolysis is present, the clot lyses more rapidly. Risk of hemorrhage is correlated with lysis times of less than 6 hours. The test is clearly influenced by plasma fibrinogen and plasminogen levels and the equilibrium between lytic factors and inhibitors. It is not useful in the evaluation of hypofibrinolytic states (4).

## DILUTE WHOLE BLOOD CLOT LYSIS TIME

The influence of inhibitors of fibrinolysis may be reduced by diluting whole blood 1:10 in a cooled buffer. Addition of thrombin induces immediate clotting (431). The clot tube is then transferred to a 37°C water bath and the time to clot dissolution observed. A very wide range of normal results is obtained in normal individuals. Lysis times of less than 2 hours suggest hyperfibrinolysis and lysis times of over 20 hours suggest hypofibrinolysis. Although endpoints in the dilute whole blood clot lysis test are shorter, it is subject to the same interpretation constraints as the whole blood clot lysis assay (4).

## EUGLOBULIN LYSIS TIME

Test plasma is diluted and acidified with 1% acetic acid until the solution reaches a pH of 5.35 to 5.4. The plasma is then refrigerated and the precipitate (the euglobulin fraction) that forms contains fibrinogen, plasminogen, active plasmin, and plasminogen activators (431). The euglobulin fraction is collected by centrifugation and the remaining drops of supernatant solution, which contain inhibitors of plasmin such as $\alpha_2$-antiplasmin, are removed. The precipitate is redissolved and thrombin is added to form a fibrin clot immediately. The clot is then observed visually or, less typically, with an automated clot lysis timer (Fig. 26.25) (4).

### Interpretation

Normal fibrinolysis usually proceeds slowly and, depending on the assay system, a firm clot is normally present after 90 minutes. More recently, it has been recognized that variable amounts of inhibitors of plasminogen and plasminogen activators such as C1 esterase inhibitor and plasminogen activation inhibitor 1 (PAI-1) are also partially precipitated (431, 432). Thus, results reflect both fibrinolytic and inhibitor capacity. The assay system is influenced by ionic strength, pH, and the type of buffers used. Caution must be used in attempting to interrelate values obtained between different laboratories (433). Lysis times of less than 30 minutes indicate a hyperfibrinolytic state. Prolongation of the lysis time could be due to a decrease in plasminogen activator (PA)

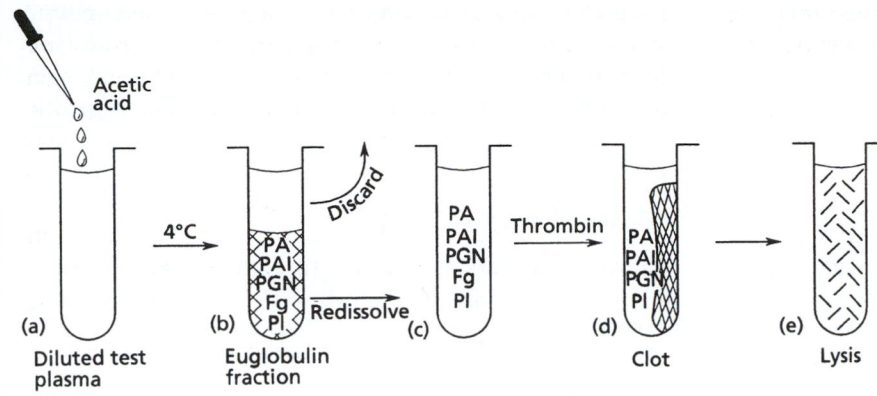

**FIGURE 26.25.** Pictorial diagram of the steps in the euglobulin lysis time assay. **a,** Acetic acid is added to diluted test plasma and the plasma is then incubated at 4°C. **b,** A precipitate forms, called the euglobulin fraction. The precipitate is removed by centrifugation and resuspended in buffer. **c,** Thrombin is added to the resuspended euglobulin fraction. **d,** The euglobulin forms a fibrin clot. The clot liquor contains plasminogen (PGN), plasmin (PI), plasminogen activator (PA) and plasminogen activator inhibitors (PAI). **e,** The time to lysis of the euglobulin clot is then measured. *Fg,* fibrinogen.

**TABLE 26.12.**  Assays of Fibrinolytic Activity

| Assay | Length of Assay | Factors Affecting Results | | | |
|---|---|---|---|---|---|
| | | Fibrinogen | Factor XIII | PAI | Antiplasmin |
| Whole blood clot lysis | 24–48 hours | + | + | + | + |
| Dilute whole blood clot lysis | 2–20 hours | + | + | + | + |
| Euglobulin clot lysis | 2 hours | + | + | + | − |
| Fibrin plate | 18 hours | − | − | + | − |
| Plasmin(ogen) chromogenic | Minutes | − | − | − | − |
| Plasmin(ogen) caseinolytic | Minutes | − | − | − | − |

PAI, *plasminogen activator inhibitor.*

and an increase in PA-PAI complex formation or, less commonly, to a plasminogen defect. Euglobulin lysis time is affected by liver disease, and also by pregnancy, where increases in plasminogen and fibrinogen as well as PAI occur. The euglobulin lysis time normally shortens during pregnancy (434). A control individual euglobulin fraction to which streptokinase is added should also be performed to ensure that a normal value obtained for lysis time is not an artifact due to the absence of plasminogen, as seen in prolonged DIC. The test also depends on fibrinogen concentration. When fibrinogen concentration is below normal, only a small clot may form in the euglobulin fraction, and consequently, the time to lysis will be falsely short. If the fibrinogen concentration is above 600 mg/dL, then the fibrin clot formed provides excessive substrate for the formed plasmin, and the time to full lysis will increase. Thus, alternative methods of analysis should be used in the case of abnormal fibrinogen levels. The euglobulin lysis time is also shortened in factor XIII deficiency, because the fibrin clot formed is poorly crosslinked and dissolution will be more rapid (4). Controversy exists as to the relationship between plasma tissue-type plasminogen activator levels (t-PA) and euglobulin lysis time, because the inhibitor, PAI-1, variably precipitates with the euglo-

bulin fraction (435). Some studies suggest an inverse correlation of PAI-1 level with euglobulin lysis time (see Table 26.12 for a comparison of available assays of fibrinolysis) (436).

## FIBRIN PLATE METHODS

The ability of a euglobulin fraction to lyse a standardized plasminogen-rich fibrin plate can also be measured (437–439). Although this method is technically more difficult to perform because the fibrin-rich plates must be prepared within 4 days of use, it has the advantage of being unaffected by the levels of plasminogen and fibrinogen in the test plasma. The plates must be incubated undisturbed for 18 hours at 37°C. The diameter of the lysis area is measured in two directions perpendicular to each other. Linearity is lost at low concentrations of PA activity. The assay can be modified to analyze plasmin activity in test plasma or euglobulin fractions by heating plates. Automated fibrin plate assays have been developed for use with microtiter plates and ELISA readers, with decrease in turbidity measured (440, 441). Because the fibrin plate assay depends on the quality and uniformity of fibrin produced on the plates, as well as the variable amount of plasminogen present in the fibrin clot, care must be taken to use only the highest grade clottable fibrinogen. Significant fluctuation of factor XIII levels contaminating commercial fibrinogen, which promotes crosslinks in the fibrin, can cause the assay to vary as much as 15 to 200%.

## PLASMINOGEN ASSAYS

Plasminogen activity can be measured using a variety of substrates including casein, chromogenic substrates, or fibrin (442, 443). Several plasminogen antigenic assays are also available, but they may give an overestimate of functionally active plasminogen.

## CASEINOLYTIC ASSAY

Test plasma is first treated with hydrochloric acid to neutralize antiplasmins. Streptokinase is then added and the generated plasmin activity is measured by addition of casein (442). Aliquots of the reaction mix are removed at 2 and 62 minutes and precipitated with 10% trichloracetic acid to remove residual proteins and casein. The supernatant, containing tyrosine released by plasmin cleavage of casein, is mixed with sodium hydroxide, then phenol reagent is added. The difference between absorbance at 650 nm at 2 and 62 minutes is an indicator of tyrosine generated. Plasmin activity of a test plasma sample is measured similarly, but without the need for addition of hydrochloric acid or streptokinase. The assay must be highly standardized, because variations in the amount of casein, streptokinase, or incubation time will result in artefactual fluctuations in plasmin levels.

## CHROMOGENIC ASSAY

A variety of substrates have been developed for the measurement of plasmin and plasminogen (98). In a typical assay, an excess of streptokinase is added to ensure complete and rapid activation of plasminogen to plasmin to minimize effects of endogenous inhibitors. The kinetics of interaction of purified plasmin and streptokinase-activated plasminogen with the chromogenic substrate differ, so appropriate standard curves must be generated using dilutions of normal plasma and not purified plasmin when assaying plasminogen in a test blood sample. Plasminogen can only be reliably measured to levels of 25% because the sensitivity and linearity of the assay is grossly altered below this level (98).

## FIBRIN SUBSTRATE ASSAY

Plasminogen-free bovine fibrinogen or human fibrinogen is allowed to form fibrin on a tissue culture plate. Test plasma, pretreated by addition of acid or acetone to destroy natural inhibitors of plasmin, is then spotted on the plate and the area of lysis is correlated with lysis areas generated by plasma standards (435, 438, 443, 444). The fibrin plate technique is most reliably performed in a research setting.

## IMMUNOLOGIC ASSAYS

Multiple assays exist for antigenic determination of plasminogen and plasmin, including EIA, RID, ELISA, and RIA (445, 446).

## Interpretation

Plasminogen levels are low in hyaline membrane disease in premature infants, in DIC, and with acute promyelocytic leukemia (447, 448). Synthesis of plasminogen is reduced in liver disease, particularly in cirrhosis. Plasminogen levels may be low for up to 1 week after thrombolytic therapy (449). Falsely high values for plasminogen occur in the setting of high FDPs or high fibrinogen levels due to their potentiating effects on plasmin activity (450). Congenital deficiency is most often expressed as a dysplasminogenemia with normal antigenic level and decreased functional activity (446).

## $\alpha_2$-ANTIPLASMIN

$\alpha_2$-Antiplasmin may be measured amidolytically (98, 451) or immunochemically (108). The amidolytic assay is based on the ability of test plasma to inhibit the plasmin activity of a fixed concentration of added plasmin. Residual plasmin is then measured chromogenically using S2251 as a substrate. The amount of antiplasmin present in the test sample is inversely related to the amount of residual plasmin present.

## Interpretation

A blank derived from the individual plasma must be used in analyzing individuals with severe jaundice, in that hyperbilirubinemia may interfere with chromogenic readings, giving a falsely high value. Antiplasmin levels decrease during obstetrical delivery and later increase to normal. Levels of $\alpha_2$-antiplasmin are reduced in severe liver disease and may even be undetectable in pretransplant individuals (452). It is also reduced in DIC and during thrombolytic therapy (449). Congenital deficiency of $\alpha_2$-antiplasmin is very rare and is associated with a hemorrhagic tendency (453).

## TISSUE-TYPE PLASMINOGEN ACTIVATOR ASSAYS

Tissue-type PA assays are very much influenced by PAI levels, which may vary as much as 40-fold in test samples (454). Moreover t-PA levels are influenced by the length of veno-occlusion during venipuncture and require special processing to obtain reliable levels. Functional t-PA assays and, to a lesser extent, t-PA antigen levels are affected by the storage conditions of plasma samples. Plasma should be immediately acidified upon collection for no less than 15 minutes and then analyzed or snap frozen. Unless precautions are taken, t-PA levels can be decreased by as much as 25% by incorrect sample handling.

## IMMUNOLOGIC METHODS

Highly specific antisera to t-PA are now available, and several sensitive IRMAs and ELISAs are available for t-PA measurement (455–457). The ELISA is based on the same two-site antibody method as the IRMA technique, but has the advantage of using a stable enzyme label and not an isotope. However, the IRMA is more sensitive than the ELISA.

## BIOIMMUNOASSAY

This technique is based on the immunoabsorption of t-PA from plasma and does not depend on the presence of fibrin fragments for the stimulation of t-PA activity. It can also be used to measure fast-acting anti-t-PA activity (432). Plasma is incubated in microtiter wells coated with anti-t-PA antibody. Residual plasma is then washed away. The activity of the bound t-PA is then measured by addition of plasminogen and the chromogenic substrate S2251. Liberated pNA is quantitated. Results are compared to dilutions of a t-PA standard or pooled normal plasma. Use of a recombinant t-PA as a reference standard yields inaccurate results when compared to normal pooled plasma (458).

## AMIDOLYTIC ASSAY

Several different assays are available, but all are based on the principle of adding a stimulator of t-PA, such as fibrin, sufficient plasminogen, and acidified plasma. The Wiman assay uses diluted acidified plasma and solubilized fibrin as a stimulator of fibrinolysis, and S2251 as a plasmin substrate (459). Alternate methods use soluble fibrinogen fragments (460). The assay requires incubation at 37°C for 3 hours.

### Interpretation

Because t-PA normally exists in plasma complexed with PAI-1, measurement of functional t-PA is actually an assessment of free t-PA dissociated from complex with PAI-1. Measurement of t-PA antigen gives a more reliable assessment of the total t-PA present. Functional assays of t-PA are affected by the presence of streptokinase

and other lytic drugs in the circulation (449). Levels of t-PA are increased by diethylstilbestrol and heparin, which induce its release from endothelium. Both PAI-1 and t-PA activity and antigen are increased in sepsis. Both t-PA and PAI levels increase slightly with age, and t-PA levels are slightly lower in men than in women (461). The t-PA levels exhibit a diurnal variation in plasma, with peak antigen levels in the morning and the lowest levels in the late afternoon (462–464). For that reason, careful timing of analysis may be important when comparing samples.

## ASSESSMENT OF RECOMBINANT T-PA ACTIVITY

Recombinant t-PA activity (rt-PA) can be analyzed in a purified system using an automated coagulation analyzer (440). In this assay system, 20 mL of rt-PA to be analyzed is mixed with 20 mL of thrombin and 200 mL of a 50:1 (v/v) solution of fibrinogen and plasmin. An insoluble clot is formed within 40 seconds, which increases turbidity. The typical time at the beginning of lysis is approximately 140 seconds, and the lysis is complete at 300 seconds. The rate of change can be monitored every 3 seconds, and the rate of lysis determined and compared to known international rt-PA standards (458). The assay is 99.5% accurate and has a precision level of 5%. The rt-PA levels can be measured in a range of 40 to 1000 ng/mL.

## PLASMINOGEN ACTIVATOR INHIBITORS

There are several inhibitors of plasminogen activator, including PAI-1, PAI-2, and PAI-3, $\alpha_2$-antiplasmin and $\alpha_2$-macroglobulin, but only PAI-1 and PAI-2 are of importance in plasma t-PA inhibition clinically (461, 463). All of the assays described below measure both PAI-1 and PAI-2.

## FUNCTIONAL ASSAY

The most common test involves the addition of a fixed amount of t-PA to the plasma sample, allowing t-PA and PAI complexes to form (464, 465). The residual excess t-PA present is then measured. Standardized reference preparations are available for t-PA for calibration of local laboratory t-PA standards. The result of the assay is expressed as the quantity of exogenously added t-PA neutralized by the assayed plasma. Lyophilized plasma is available with predetermined PAI activity to generate a control standard curve. Because assays of t-PA activity depend on plasminogen conversion to plasmin, the test sample should be treated to remove inhibitors of plasmin activity. One method is to dilute standards and test plasma in reference plasma from which PAI has been immunoabsorbed. The blank includes the endogenous t-PA activity, which is subtracted. Unfortunately the immune depleted reference plasma has been shown in at least one laboratory to contain as much as 6 IU/dL of PAI, possibly accounting for the very large discrepancy in results between laboratories in measuring low levels of PAI, not observed when the same laboratories were measuring samples with higher PAI levels (458, 466, 467).

A second method uses the ability of PAI to inhibit urokinase (465). An excess amount of urokinase is added to a plasma sample that has been treated to inactivate antiplasmin. The PAI present inactivates a portion of the urokinase. The residual urokinase activates the endogenous plasminogen to plasmin, which can be measured by specific chromogenic substrate assays. The amount of plasmin activity generated as measured by absorbance is inversely proportional to the amount of PAI in the test sample.

## Interpretation

All of these assays measure only active forms of PAI. No information is provided about t-PA complexed to PAI or to nonactivatable forms of PAI. Plasminogen activator inhibitor-1 is present in platelet α-granules, and spurious levels of PAI can be obtained by incomplete centrifugation of platelets from platelet-poor plasma. The PAI-1 levels are affected by phenformin, metformin, stanozol, and antiplatelet drugs (468, 469). Plasminogen activator inhibitor activity is increased in individuals taking warfarin. The PAI-1 levels exhibit a diurnal variation and samples should be obtained at a consistent time in the morning, with fasting, to decrease the effect of lipids on the assay (463, 469, 470). The PAI-1 levels increase somewhat with age (461, 462). The PAI-2 levels, which are at subdetection levels in normal plasma, are increased dramatically to 25 μg/dL in pregnancy and for 7 days postpartum (324, 471). Specific assays of PAI-1 and PAI-2 may be useful as an early indicator of placental dysfunction in certain obstetric diseases.

## IMMUNOLOGIC ASSAYS

Immunologic assays variably measure all forms of PAI, including complexed and latent forms, depending on the specificity of the antibody used (472–474). Solid-phase immunoabsorption techniques have allowed for discrimination of active and latent forms. Most assays use a polyclonal PAI antibody that recognizes both free and complexed forms of PAI bound to microtiter wells to adsorb PAI from test plasma specimens (474, 475). The bound PAI is then recognized by peroxidase conjugated anti-PAI antibody followed by a peroxidase-sensitive chromogenic substrate. Unlike other ELISAs, because of the very low concentrations of PAI in plasma, more pro-

longed incubations of test plasma with microtiter wells are required for detection and the assay generally requires overnight incubation. Radioimmunoassays have been described for PAI that can recognize both active and inactive forms, or simply active forms alone, but are not generally available in clinical laboratories. No international reference plasma is available for PAI-1, but immunologic assays may be standardized against pooled normal plasma.

## Interpretation

Plasminogen activator inhibitor-1 is elevated as an acute-phase reactant and rises to a lesser extent after venous occlusion than does t-PA (476, 477). The PAI-1 levels also vary significantly in the normal population (478). Plasminogen activator inhibitor-1 is higher in men than women before age 50 years. It rises immediately postoperatively and for 5 days thereafter (478). The PAI-1 levels also rise significantly in individuals with septic shock (479) and in thrombotic thrombocytopenic purpura, malignancy, pancreatitis, hyperlipoproteinemia and hypertriglyceridemia, growth hormone deficiency, obesity, non-insulin dependent diabetes mellitus and cardiovascular disease (455, 460, 480–482). Results are not easily interpreted in the setting of liver disease because of the complicated interrelationship of low or abnormal fibrinogen, plasminogen, and α₂-antiplasmin and the impaired clearance of t-PA. A recent multicenter evaluation of commercially available methods of assay concluded that results are comparable if care is taken to use a universal standard (483, 484). Discrepancies between functional and immunologic assay results for PAI may reflect high levels of t-PA-PAI complexes, although some consideration must be made for the possibility of latent or inactive forms of PAI alone (479). Erickson et al have developed an assay for t-PA and PAI complexes (423). The t-PA and t-PA complexes are first absorbed from test plasma using microtiter wells coated with polyclonal antibody to t-PA. The t-PA-PAI complex present is then quantitated by measuring PAI with rabbit antihuman PAI. The assay is sensitive to 1 ng/mL.

## EFFECTS OF LYTIC AGENTS ON CLOTTING ASSAYS

The presence of any lytic agent such as streptokinase, urokinase, or t-PA in a test plasma sample can lead to *ex vivo* prolongation of the clotting time. Without careful sample handling, the presence of active t-PA within plasma specimens will permit lysis to continue, *in vitro* and measured levels of plasminogen, fibrinogen, and α₂-antiplasmin, as well as factors V, VIII, and XIII will be artifactually low and not reflective of *in vivo* levels (423, 449). Therefore, samples must be drawn into protease inhibitor cocktails such as Phe-Pro-Arg-CH₂Cl

(PPACK), anti-rt-PA antibody or aprotinin (485–488). Phe-Pro-Arg-CH$_2$Cl is useful in obtaining correct fibrinogen levels in samples containing rt-PA and will prevent loss of rt-PA by coupling with $\alpha_2$-macroglobulin (399, 485). Phe-Pro-Arg-CH$_2$Cl does not interfere with measurement of components of the lytic system; however, it interferes with all coagulometric assays (489, 490). Aprotinin interferes with plasminogen and antiplasmin chromogenic assays (489). Increased levels of D-dimer observed in samples from individuals on lytic therapy are althought to be reflective of degraded fibrin clot *in vivo*.

## TESTING WITH A FIBRINOLYTIC CHALLENGE

Blood samples for analysis of total fibrinolytic activity and components of the fibrinolytic system require special handling. It has been shown that fibrinolytic activity increases substantially at the site of venipuncture when blood flow is interrupted by veno-occlusion (476, 477, 491). In normal individuals, a fourfold rise in t-PA antigen occurs at 10 minutes, with a peak increase to eightfold at 20 minutes of veno-occlusion between systolic and diastolic blood pressure. Thus, the cuff pressure and length of occlusion time must be standardized when obtaining blood for t-PA levels. A similar standardized challenge to assess total fibrinolytic potential can be performed by intravenous infusion of DDAVP 0.4 $\mu$/kg over 10 to 12 minutes in 50 to 100 $\mu$L saline, with measurement of t-PA and PAI levels at 30 and 60 minutes (197).

# PLATELET FUNCTION TESTING

## BLEEDING TIME

The bleeding time is a screening test of primary hemostasis. The reliability of the bleeding time in the screening of clinical bleeding disorders, particularly preoperatively, has come under critical scrutiny and is the subject of several reviews (492, 493). The bleeding time depends on platelet count and function, vessel wall characteristics and vWf activity. Several different bleeding time methods are available. In general, with all of these methods, the incision should be deep enough to incise only capillary loops and small-vessels. The Duke method measures the bleeding time from an earlobe incision (494). Most laboratories prefer to use the lateral aspect of the volar surface of the forearm in the Ivy technique (495–497). As illustrated in Chapter 23, a blood pressure cuff is inflated to 40 mm Hg and a small incision is made on the forearm with a lancet. The blood is dabbed with cotton wool or filter paper at regular times and the time for the bleeding to stop is recorded. To standardize re-

sults, commercial devices, the simplate and template bleeding time instruments, are used to provide a standardized incision (498, 499). The simplate and template devices produce vertical and horizontal incisions, respectively. The normal range for bleeding times is slightly different depending on the direction of the incision, with a horizontal incision producing a longer bleeding time.

## Interpretation

The Ivy bleeding time is longer in women than men, but the response to aspirin is greater in men than in women (499). One incision provides as much information as multiple incisions. Incisions are most reproducible over the 5 cm below the antecubital crease laterally. Without venostasis, the horizontal bleeding time is shortened and sensitivity to aspirin is reduced (500). When the incision size is reduced to 3 mm, the mean bleeding time is shortened compared to that obtained with 5 mm and 9 mm incisions. The bleeding time may be prolonged in type III collagen defects, such as Ehlers-Danlos syndrome, and is also prolonged in some individuals with factor V, VIII, or IX deficiency. It is also prolonged to a variable degree in vWd, thrombocytopenia, and platelet function defects (501–503). The bleeding time may be prolonged by a variety of medications, most notably salicylates, as well as by cold temperature and anesthesia (504). Diabetes and hyperlipidemia shorten the bleeding time (Table 26.13). It has been noted that the bleeding time may also be affected by blood group, independently of the level of vWf antigen or ristocetin cofactor

**TABLE 26.13.    Bleeding Time Abnormalities**

| Prolonged | Shortened |
| --- | --- |
| Thrombocytopenia | Diabetes mellitus |
| Platelet qualitative defects | Hyperlipidemia |
| Drugs, e.g., salicylates, heparin | Estrogens |
| von Willebrand disease | DDAVP |
| Collagen defects | |
| Uremia | |
| Vasculitis | |
| Factor VIII, IX, or V deficiency (occasionally) | |
| Technical causes | Technical causes |
|   Skin edema |   Degree of venostasis |
|   Body temperature decreased |   Incision length |
|   Incision depth | |
|   Anesthesia | |

activity (240). The bleeding time is not a method for assessing hypercoagulability.

## RUMPEL-LEEDE TEST

This test of capillary fragility (505) is no longer performed in routine clinical practice.

## PLATELET ADHESION STUDIES

Most of the routine tests for platelet adhesion actually measure a combination of platelet-platelet (i.e., aggregation) as well as platelet-nonplatelet interactions. The tests are usually complicated and are highly influenced by the method used. In the platelet retention test, anticoagulated blood is forced through a narrow plastic tube containing fine glass beads. The difference in concentration of platelets entering and exiting the column has been considered to be a measure of platelet adherence to the glass beads (506, 507).

## Interpretation

Decreased platelet retention has been most clinically useful in the preliminary diagnosis of vWd (506). The results depend highly on the anticoagulant used, the rate of perfusion, the diameter and the material of the tubing, and the size of the glass beads (507). For these

reasons, this test is seldom used in clinical practice today.

## PLATELET AGGREGATION STUDIES

Uniform measurement of platelet aggregation using an optical instrument was initially described by O'Brien (508) and Born and Cross (509) (see Chapter 23). Freshly drawn blood is centrifuged to prepare platelet-rich plasma (PRP) and allowed to stand for 30 minutes at room temperature (510). The platelet concentration is adjusted to 200,000 to 300,000/mm$^3$ by the addition of autologous platelet-poor plasma (PPP). An aliquot of PRP is placed in a cuvette and stirred at 800 to 1200 rpm at 37°C. Aggregation is monitored with a spectrophotometer set at wavelength 600 nm and a photoelectric cell connected to a recorder with the chart speed at 1 to 2 cm/min. Baseline (or 0%) light transmission is established with the PRP and 100% transmission is established with PPP from the same individual. Observation of the PRP for several minutes, with stirring at 37°C before the addition of any stimulus, rules out spontaneous aggregation. Several different agonists are available to initiate platelet aggregation. Correlations have been drawn between the type of response to thrombin, adenosine diphosphate, epinephrine, collagen, ristocetin, and abnormalities of platelet function (Table 26.14) (503, 511–514).

During platelet aggregation, there is often an initial

**TABLE 26.14.** Hereditary Disorders of Platelet Function: Diagnosis [503]

| Disorder | Platelet Count | Platelet Size | Platelet Aggregation | | | | Release of 5HT/ADP by Thrombin | Heredity | Associated Abnormalities |
|---|---|---|---|---|---|---|---|---|---|
| | | | ADP | Collagen | Arachidonic Acid | Ristocetin | | | |
| Thrombasthenia | N | N | O | O | O | (1) | N | Autosomal recessive | |
| Bernard-Soulier syndrome | ↓ (or N) | ↑ | N | N | N | O | N or ↓ | Autosomal recessive | |
| Hermansky-Pudlak syndrome | N | N | (1) | ↓ | N | (1) | ↓ | Autosomal recessive | Albinism Pigmented macrophages in bone marrow |
| Storage pool disease | N | N or ↓ | (1) | ↓ | N | (1) | ↓ | Autosomal dominant | |
| Wiskott-Aldrich syndrome | ↓ | ↓ | | ↓ | | | ↓ | X-borne recessive | Eczema Recurrent infections |
| Chédiak-Higashi syndrome | N or ↓ | N | (1) | ↓ | | | ↓ | Autosomal recessive | Partial albinism Recurrent infections Lysosomal abnormality of granulocytes |
| Cyclooxygenase deficiency Thromboxane synthesis deficiency | N | N | (1) | ↓ | ↓ | | ↓ | ? | |
| Gray platelet syndrome | ↓ | ↑ | ↓ | ↓ | N | N | ↓ | Autosomal dominant | |

*(1), First phase aggregation only.*

ADP, *adenosine diphosphate;* 5HT, *serotonin;* N, *normal;* O, *absent.*

depression in the baseline tracing associated with decreased light transmission. This deflection reflects the initial shape change that follows platelet stimulation. This is followed by a rapid rise, the primary wave of aggregation, during which there is an increase in light transmission (Fig. 26.26). There may then be a slight pause before the platelets fully aggregate during the second wave of aggregation. Exceptions to this pattern occur with strong agonists like collagen, in which there may be immediate irreversible aggregation without the intermediate pause. With submaximal doses of an agonist, there may be only a primary wave of aggregation, followed by disaggregation (Fig. 26.27).

## ADENOSINE 5'-DIPHOSPHATE

At adenosine diphosphate (ADP) concentrations of $1 \times 10^{-6}$ mol/L, aggregation is usually biphasic. Some variation may occur due to pH of the plasma, presence of inhibitors, and to sample temperature (515–518). If the ADP concentration is too low, disaggregation will occur. When aggregation is optimal, a full deflection of 60 to 80% is observed. A primary wave, followed by disaggregation, suggests an aspirin-like defect or storage pool disease. When no response occurs, Glanzmann's thrombasthenia may be present.

## EPINEPHRINE

Epinephrine response is the most variable in the normal donor pool (519). At a concentration of $1.2 \times 10^{-5}$ mol/L, epinephrine induces a primary wave followed by a secondary wave of aggregation due to the release of endogenous ADP. Aspirin ingestion may cause loss of the second wave of aggregation. Myeloproliferative disorders may be associated with the complete loss of even the first wave of epinephrine-induced aggregation. Epinephrine response is temperature dependent, with only a primary wave followed by disaggregation observed in response to 0.5 μmol/L epinephrine at 25°C.

## COLLAGEN

Lyophilized bovine tendon collagen induces a brief lag, during which increased optical density is observed by downward deflection of the pen, followed by complete aggregation within 30 to 60 seconds (520). No primary wave is observed. In Glanzmann's thrombasthenia, the initial shape change may be observed, but there is no aggregation response. Defective collagen response is also seen with release defects and storage pool diseases.

## ARACHIDONIC ACID

Arachidonic acid is added at a final concentration of 500 μg/mL and stimulates a monophasic aggregation

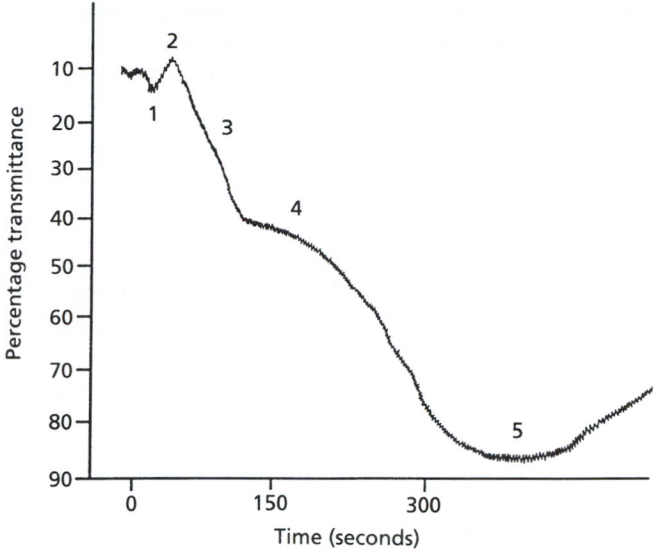

**FIGURE 26.26.**  Changes in light transmittance during platelet aggregation with adenosine diphosphate. (1) Slight increase in transmittance due to dilution upon addition of aggregating agent. (2) Decrease in light transmittance due to platelet shape change. (3) Progressive increase in light transmittance as platelet aggregates form. (4) Release reaction followed by secondary wave of aggregation. (5) Maximal irreversible aggregation.

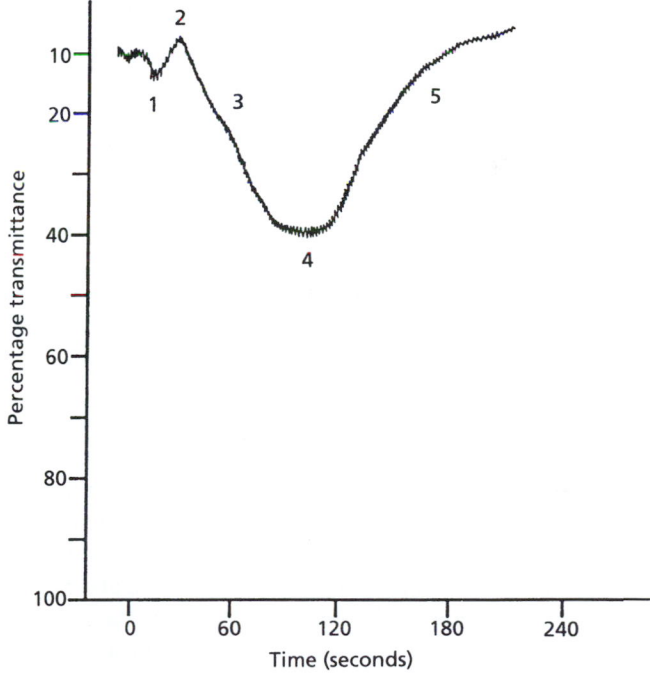

**FIGURE 26.27.**  Platelet aggregation tracing. Changes in transmittance during aggregation followed by disaggregation. (1) Slight increase in transmittance due to addition of aggregating agent. (2) Slight decrease in transmittance due to platelet shape change. (3) Progressive increase in transmittance as platelet aggregates form. (4) Maximal platelet aggregation. (5) Decrease in transmittance due to platelet disaggregation.

pattern (521). Abnormalities in the cyclooxygenase pathway are thus detected. Most frequently, arachidonic acid response defects are due to aspirin and nonsteroidal anti-inflammatory agents.

## RISTOCETIN

Ristocetin-induced aggregation is not a true active metabolic process, but is a monophasic agglutination reaction of vWf binding to its glycoprotein Ib receptor on platelets. Response is highly variable in the general population and is markedly affected by increases in plasma pH. Because the pH of PRP rises on exposure to air, ristocetin agglutination should be performed first in the panel of aggregation assays. A decreased agglutination response to ristocetin maybe seen in Bernard-Soulier syndrome and vWd (522).

## Interpretation

Platelet aggregability is influenced by a number of variables including calcium concentration, temperature, and pH of the PRP. Because platelet aggregation patterns may also be affected by the type of anticoagulant used in preparation of PRP, routine platelet aggregation studies are performed on blood that has been drawn into sodium citrate anticoagulant and maintained at room temperature. The length of time between venipuncture and performance of platelet aggregation studies is critical because the pH of plasma rises with time, resulting in variable platelet aggregation patterns. Finally, diurnal variations in platelet aggregability have been reported (523). Platelet aggregation tests are usually performed using uniform conditions because the aggregation response is directly a function of speed of stirring, temperature, and stir bar size (513–515). A minimal starting whole blood platelet count of 80,000 to 100,000/mm$^3$ is required for aggregation studies. Results are not reliable with counts of less than 50,000/mm$^3$. Many disease states can cause abnormal platelet function testing (514, 524). The congenital and acquired platelet disorders that can affect aggregation are discussed in detail in Chapters 32 and 33. High fat diet, oral contraceptives, diabetes, exercise, and stress may enhance platelet aggregation. Aggregation studies have not generally been shown to be useful in the diagnosis of a prothrombotic state, although spontaneous platelet aggregation has been noted in some individuals with myeloproliferative disorders that are associated with thrombotic complications.

## ALTERNATE METHODS OF PLATELET AGGREGOMETRY

Platelet aggregation studies are usually performed after separation of platelets from whole blood. It is now known that leukocytes and red blood cells may play a role in modulating platelet responsiveness. Considerable interest has, therefore, arisen in monitoring platelet function in the presence of these other cell types and with the minimum of manipulation that may alter platelet response to agonists. The whole blood aggregometer uses an electrical impedance detection system to measure deposition of platelet aggregates on an electrode placed in the whole blood sample. Aggregation patterns in whole blood differ from the traditional biphasic responses seen in aggregometry using PRP (Fig. 26.28). Whole blood aggregation is increased in the setting of polycythemia (525–531). Smoking within 30 minutes before venipuncture for platelet aggregation studies may result in an abnormal response to ADP in the aggregation assay (532).

# MEASUREMENTS OF THE PLATELET RELEASE REACTION

The platelet release reaction can be measured as an assessment of specific platelet functional and metabolic defects, such as storage pool disease. In general, the release reaction is measured by assaying the quantity of a platelet granule constituent, such as adenosine diphosphate, adenosine triphosphate, or serotonin that is released after platelet stimulation with an agonist (Table 26.15). Analysis of plasma samples can be performed as a measurement of ongoing platelet activation *in vivo*. When measuring the release of platelet granule constituents in plasma, it is important to be certain that release has not occurred *in vitro* during blood sampling and processing. This can be controlled by the addition of inhibitors of platelet aggregation such as prostaglandin E$_1$, calcium chelators, and theophylline to the anticoagulant cocktail (533).

## PLATELET FACTOR 4

Functional assays of PF4 measure its ability to neutralize heparin or to induce nonenzymatic polymerization of fibrinogen. Antiheparin activity may be measured using a modification of the heparin-thrombin clotting time in either a clot-based or chromogenic assay, or by measuring residual heparin in an anti-Xa clotting method (534, 535). Functional assays are nonspecific, because not all antiheparin activity in plasma is due to PF4 (535). Therefore, antigenic measurement of PF4 is the preferred assay method. Platelet factor 4 released from platelets during platelet aggregation experiments may be measured in a Laurell assay. Measurement of PF4 in plasma requires detection limits as low as 10 ng/mL. Commercial RIA and a double antibody sandwich ELISA, with

**Platelet-rich plasma**

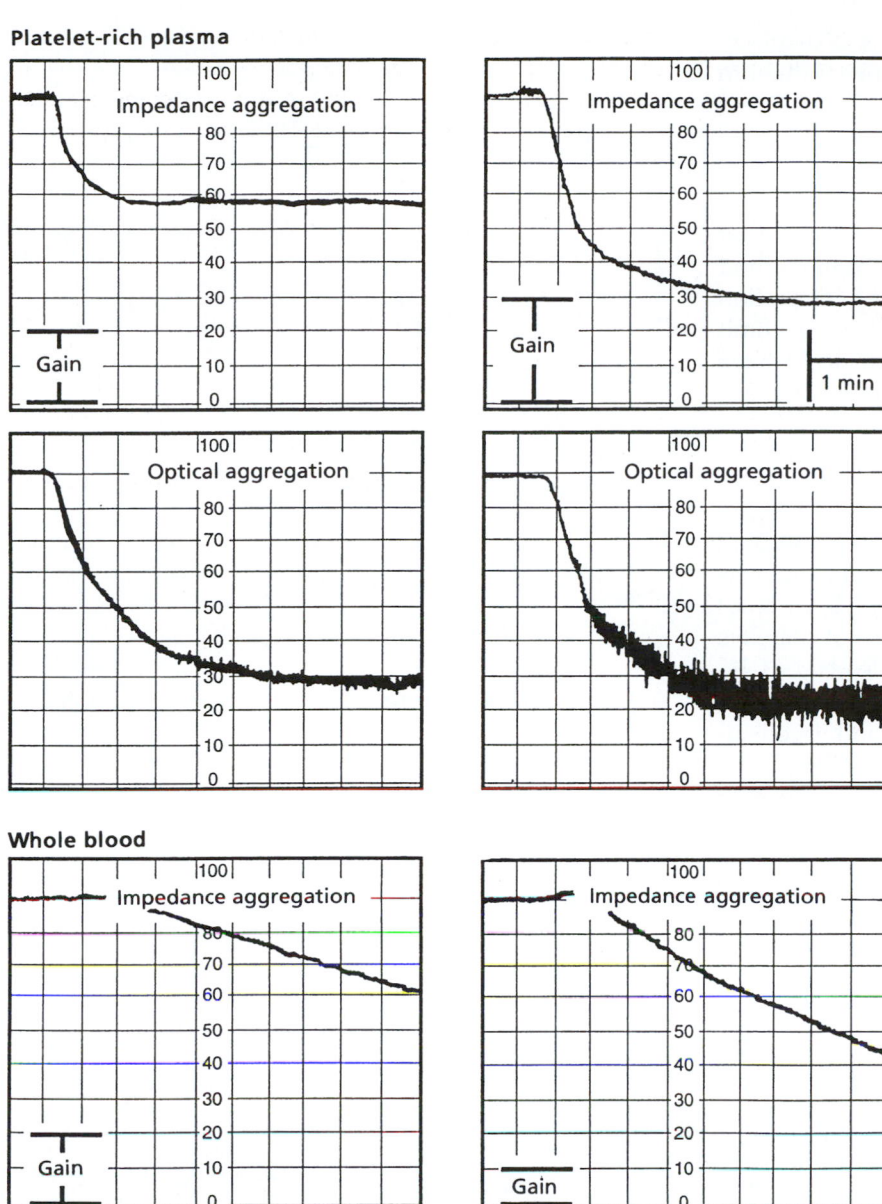

**FIGURE 26.28.** Comparison of platelet aggregation tracings using optical and impedance aggregation. **Top two panels:** Impedance aggregation tracings of PRP using adenosine diphosphate (**left**) and collagen (**right**) as agonists. **Middle panels:** Aggregation tracings of PRP using an optical detection system. **Bottom two panels:** Whole blood aggregation tracings using an impedance detection system. Adapted with permission from Chrono-Lag Corporation, Havertown, PA.

**Whole blood**

ADP 10 μmol/l

Collagen 2 μg/ml

---

**TABLE 26.15.** Laboratory Assessment of Platelet Release

| Granule Constituent | Assay Method |
| --- | --- |
| Platelet factor 4 | RIA |
|  | ELISA |
| β-Thromboglobulin | RIA |
|  | ELISA |
| Adenine nucleotides | Lumiaggregometry |
| Serotonin | $^{14}$C-serotonin uptake and release |

ELISA, *enzyme-linked immunosorbent assay; RIA, radioimmunoassay.*

a sensitivity of less than 2 ng/mL and requiring only 2 to 3 hours, are now available (536). The blood sample must be collected, without venostasis, into an anticoagulant containing EDTA, PGE$_1$, and theophylline to avoid *ex vivo* release of PF4 from platelets.

### Interpretation

Artifactual results may be obtained if the sample is not processed within 4 hours due to the leak of PF4 from residual platelets (533). Platelet-rich plasma contains 1000 times more PF4 than does plasma. Artifactually low results may also be obtained in the presence of plasmin or other proteases that may destroy PF4 antigenic reactivity with antibodies (533). Normal plasma concentrations of PF4 are 2 to 8 ng/mL. The PF4 levels rise after the administration of heparin due to displacement of PF4 from binding sites on vascular endothelium (537).

## β-THROMBOGLOBULIN

Several methods are available for measurement of β-thromboglobulin (β-TG). The most common method is by RIA, which requires an initial 3 day incubation phase of plasma with antibody and has a detection limit of 700 pg/mL (538). Some nonequilibrium RIAs have also been developed using only 1 to 24 hour incubations, with detection levels of 140 to 630 pg/mL.

### Interpretation

As in the case of PF4 measurement, sample handling is critical because the release of β-TG from platelets increases progressively to a 20-fold level if samples are not maintained at 4°C, and persistence of platelets in samples will lead to artifactually elevated β-TG levels. β-Thromboglobulin is elevated in conditions associated with platelet release reactions and is considered a more sensitive indicator of *in vivo* platelet activation than PF4 (539, 540). Elevated levels are also seen in renal failure due to decreased renal clearance. Increased levels of both β-thromboglobulin and PF4 are not in themselves indicators of any specific prothrombotic disease (537).

## PLATELET DENSE GRANULE CONTENTS

Dense granule secretion can be evaluated by measuring extraplatelet adenosine diphosphate and adenosine triphosphate after platelet stimulation. The most common method of measurement uses chemiluminescence (541). Firefly luciferin, in the presence of a source of adenosine triphosphate, emits a measurable luminescence and can be used to quantitate directly the amount of adenosine triphosphate present. Adenosine diphosphate is measured by phosphorylating adenosine diphosphate to adenosine triphosphate in the presence of phosphoenolpyruvate and pyruvate kinase. Direct measurement of adenosine diphosphate and adenosine triphosphate in PRP samples requires chelation of calcium and precipitation of plasma proteins with ethanol to prevent inhibition of luminescence. Excess ethanol itself can reduce luminescence. Most laboratories find it more convenient to use a lumiaggregometer for the measurement of both aggregation and chemiluminescence due to adenosine triphosphate and adenosine diphosphate release (Fig. 26.29). Because luciferase enhances platelet aggregation, this assay is generally performed on a second sample not being used for the interpretation of aggregation tracings. An alternate method measures total adenosine content by forming a

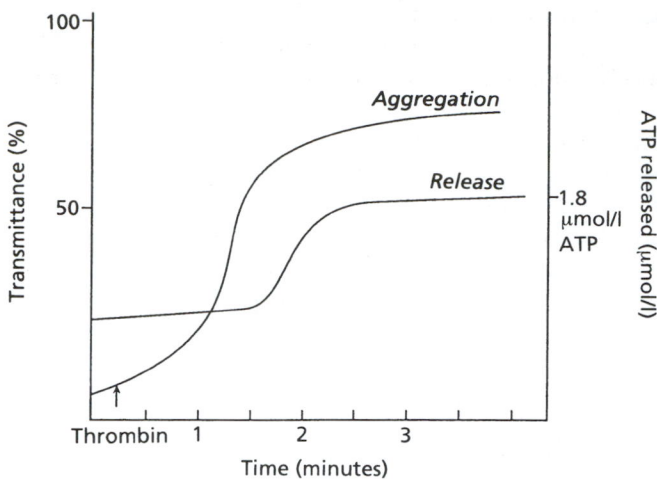

**FIGURE 26.29.** Lumiaggregometry tracing showing simultaneous aggregation and release. *ATP*, adenosine triphosphate.

stable fluorescent product between chloroacetaldehyde and adenine and its derivatives.

## SEROTONIN UPTAKE AND RELEASE

Platelets have a transport mechanism for serotonin uptake and storage within dense granules. Thus, the extent of the release reaction can be measured by measuring the uptake and release of [14C]-serotonin by platelets in PRP (542). Platelet-rich plasma is incubated with [14C]-serotonin for 1 hour at room temperature. The release reaction is then evoked by the addition of an aggregating agent, such as epinephrine or collagen, after which EDTA is added. A control nonaggregated PRP specimen previously labeled with [14C]-serotonin is also incubated with EDTA and triton. The blank consists of PRP labeled with [14C]-serotonin that has been centrifuged to produce PPP. Aliquots of all three reaction samples are then placed on glass fiber filter paper and immersed in scintillation fluid, then released radioactivity is counted in a scintillation counter. The percentage of serotonin uptake and release can then be calculated. Abnormal serotonin uptake and release has been found in high frequency in the setting of a prolonged bleeding time and normal routine platelet aggregation studies (543). A modification of the serotonin release assay can be used in the evaluation of drug-induced immune thrombocytopenia.

# RETICULATED PLATELET COUNT

Young platelets, like erythrocytes, are larger and have increased RNA content compared to older platelets.

Platelet RNA can be quantitated by staining with a flourochrome, such as thiazole orange, which becomes intensely fluorescent when it binds to RNA. The flourochrome is then excited by a laser and the emitted light is detected and quantitated by a flow cytometer. Fluorescent staining of platelet RNA allows for the detection of platelet subpopulations with differing RNA content using flow cytometric analysis. The percentage of platelets rich in RNA, and consequently having high intensity staining, is calculated using either stained or unstained formalin fixed platelets as the threshold control value for fluorescence (544–546).

## INTERPRETATION

The mean percentage of reticulated platelets in normal control individual blood samples is about 5 to 12%, depending on the technique used for establishing control fluorescence ranges. The percentage of reticulated platelets is elevated threefold in immune thrombocytopenia where adequate marrow megakaryocytes are present. The reticulated platelet count is normal *in situ*ations in which a decrease in peripheral blood platelet count is associated with a decrease in bone marrow megakaryocytes, such as after treatment with chemotherapy, or in primary bone marrow disorders such as myelodysplasia. Selection of the optimal dye for RNA, which shows saturable, stable binding to RNA, and adherence to a specified incubation period of blood sample with the dye are important factors in assay reproducibility. The sensitivity and specificity of the reticulated platelet count for distinguishing between thrombocytopenic individuals with increased or normal numbers of megakaryocytes and those with decreased megakaryocytes is higher than 95% (544, 545).

## PLATELET FACTOR 3 (PLATELET PHOSPHOLIPID)

Exposure of platelet phospholipids on platelet membrane surfaces after activation is involved in the conversion of factor X to Xa and prothrombin to thrombin. Platelet membrane procoagulant activity, referred to in the past as "PF3," is decreased in thrombocytopathies resulting in decreased platelet activation as well as in thrombocytopenia. The serum prothrombin consumption test is a clot-based assay that may be used as an indicator of abnormal platelet procoagulant activity. A normal aPTT result on test plasma is important for this test to reflect abnormal PF3 availability. Platelet factor 3 activity is decreased in myeloproliferative diseases and uremia as well as in primary platelet disorders (524). Other similar tests include the kaolin-activated PRP clot-

ting time, the RVV PRP clotting time and the thromboplastin generation test. These tests are limited by problems with reproducibility. Because PF3 deficiency itself is exceedingly rare, the diagnosis of platelet function disorders resulting in defective release of PF3 is probably better made with alternative tests (547).

## PLATELET INTRACELLULAR IONIZED CALCIUM MEASUREMENT

Movement of ionized calcium into the platelet cytosol is important in the regulation of platelet activation (see Chapter 12). Whole blood lumiaggregometry can be adapted to measure fluxes of calcium in select platelet intracellular compartments by use of the calcium sensitive photoprotein aequorin. Fluxes in signals generated from this molecule incorporated within PRP fractions can be correlated with aggregation response to selected stimuli in the lumiaggregometer (548, 549).

## PLATELET ARACHIDONIC ACID METABOLISM

Stimulation of platelet aggregation with a variety of agonists results in release of membrane-bound stores of arachidonic acid and subsequent conversion of the free arachidonic acid to thromboxanes $A_2$ and $B_2$ and a variety of additional eicosanoid derivatives by cyclooxygenase and thromboxane synthetase (Fig. 26.30) (550). Radioimmunoassays are commercially available for the measurement of many of these eicosanoid intermediates as well as the stable breakdown product of thromboxane $A_2$, thromboxane $B_2$ (551). In addition, total end product of the thromboxane pathway can be measured by a simple chromogenic assay for malonyldialdehyde (552). Thromboxane measurements are of particular importance in the diagnosis of congenital or drug-induced defects in cyclooxygenase and thromboxane synthetase manifest by variable bleeding time prolongation and platelet aggregation abnormalities (553).

## PLATELET MEMBRANE GLYCOPROTEINS

Several distinct clinical disorders of platelet membrane glycoproteins have been described in association with characteristic aggregation abnormalities, such as Glanzmann's thrombasthenia and the Bernard-Soulier syndrome (see Chapter 32). To further identify and confirm the presence or absence of specific glycoprotein receptors on platelets exhibiting abnormal function, platelets have been radiolabeled with $Na^{125}I$ by the lactoperoxi-

**FIGURE 26.30.** Diagram of the platelet thromboxane and vascular prostacyclin synthesis pathways. *PG*, prostaglandin; *TX*, thromboxane. (Adapted with permission from Akkerman JW, Nieuwenhuis HK, Sixma JJ. Thrombosis and atherosclerosis II. Laboratory diagnosis. Parkville, MO: Boehringer Ingelheim, 1986:203.)

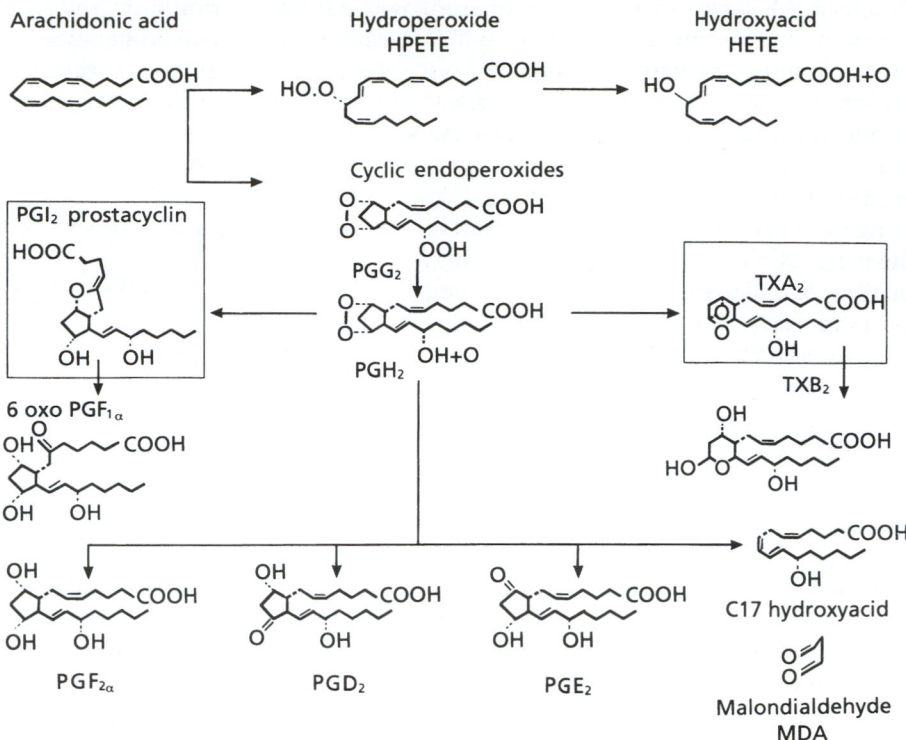

dase method or with tritiated sodium borohydride. After isolation and solubilization of the membranes, proteins are separated on one-dimensional or two-dimensional gels, and the bands corresponding to the known platelet glycoproteins are identified (554, 555). More recently, with the development of numerous monoclonal antibodies identifying platelet glycoproteins GP Ib, IIb-IIIa, IX, and V, flow cytometric techniques have been adapted to platelet membrane glycoprotein analysis (556).

## PLATELET SURVIVAL STUDIES (SEE CHAPTER 9)

Platelets can be radiolabeled with [$^{51}$chromium], [$^{14}$C]-serotonin, or [$^{111}$indium] oxine and injected intravenously. The rate of disappearance of isotope in serial blood samplings can be correlated with platelet survival *in vivo* (557, 558). Platelet kinetic studies may be of use in determining the etiology of observed thrombocytopenias, defining whether the process is due to peripheral destruction or ineffective thrombopoiesis. Platelet-labeling techniques are also used in nuclear medicine imaging for localization of active thrombosis (559). External γ radiation counting, particularly over the spleen, may provide additional information about the site of platelet sequestration (560, 561) (Fig. 26.31). The major drawback to labeling of platelets with [$^{14}$C]-serotonin has been that it is not maintained irreversibly within the platelets and

it can be released and taken up by other serotonin pools within the body. Radiolabeled platelet survival studies are infrequently used now in clinical practice to determine the cause of thrombocytopenia, except in evaluation of pediatric disorders.

## ANTIPLATELET ANTIBODIES

A variety of tests are available for the measurement of IgG associated with platelets and are generally divided into those that measure total platelet-associated IgG, both intracellular and surface bound, and those that measure only surface-bound IgG (562). In addition, assays are available for measuring antiplatelet antibodies in the serum. These assays include the $^{125}$I-Fab-anti-Fab assay, the complement lysis inhibition test, the radioactive Coombs' test, competitive RIA, a radioactive anti-immunoglobulin test, an ELISA, and new flow cytometric techniques (562–569). A few of these assays will be discussed to illustrate technical principles. However, antiplatelet antibody assays are not considered essential in making or excluding the diagnosis of immune thrombocytopenia purpura (ITP) (570). In the solid phase radioimmunoassay, washed platelets are lysed by freeze-thawing and sonication and aliquots of lysate are added to microtiter wells to which the proteins adhere. The amount of adherent protein is then quantitated by reaction with rabbit antihuman IgG and detected by the addition of $^{125}$I *Staph* protein A. The ELISA-based method is essentially the same, measuring total intracellular immunoglobulin. It offers the advantage of not requiring radioactivity inasmuch as the amount of IgG present is quantitated by addition of a peroxidase or alkaline phosphatase conjugated secondary antibody reactive with human IgG (571).

In the RIA, a radiolabeled monoclonal antibody to the Fc portion of human IgG or a radiolabeled *Staph* protein A is used to quantitate the surface-bound IgG or complement present on platelets. Washed test platelets are incubated with 200 ng of $^{125}$I-labeled antibody or *Staph* protein A for 60 minutes, after which the platelets are separated from the unbound radioactive material. The total platelet-associated radioactivity is then counted in a γ counter.

Platelet surface-bound immunoglobulin can be rapidly measured using fluorescein conjugated goat antihuman IgG and washed test platelets in a spectrofluorometer (562). This assay is readily adapted for indirect study of antiplatelet antibodies in the serum.

Finally, using flow cytometric techniques, the amount of antiplatelet antibody bound to the platelet surface may be directly measured (572, 573). In a new method, designed to use only a very limited amount of blood—a feature particularly important when analyzing pediatric specimens—PRP is gel filtered to separate plasma components and lymphocytes from platelets. The gel filtered platelets are then centrifuged to produce a platelet pellet, and fluorescein-conjugated goat anti F(ab')$_2$ antihuman IgG is added. A control platelet pellet is included, to which no antibody is added. The platelets are then washed and resuspended in buffer containing paraformaldehyde and subjected to flow cytometric analysis. A fluorescence index is then obtained by multiplying the mean intensity of fluorescence by the number of fluorescent platelets, and subtracting the endogenous fluorescence of the untreated control platelets. An index of more than 10.4 is considered positive (Fig. 26.32) (573).

## INTERPRETATION

Antiplatelet antibody studies are complicated by the tendency for immunoglobulin to associate with platelets nonspecifically. In immune thrombocytopenias, there is no correlation between the intensity of fluorescence or number of platelet-associated IgG molecules, as measured by RIA or ELISA, and the degree of thrombocyto-

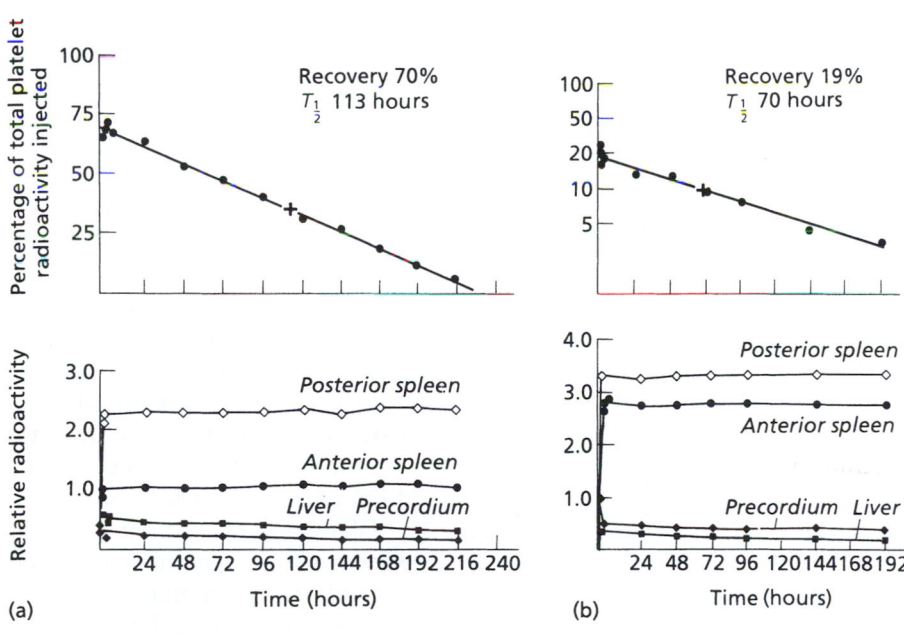

(a)

(b)

**FIGURE 26.31.** $^{51}$Cr autologous platelet survival studies. $^{51}$Cr-labeled platelets were infused (a) into a normal subject (**left**) and (b) into a individual with splenomegaly and massive platelet pooling (**right**). In normal individuals, the percentage recovery of infused platelets in a blood sample taken 10 to 12 minutes after injection is only 70%, owing to entry of 30% of infused platelets initially into the splenic compartment (**upper left**). This is evidenced by the rapid rise in radioactivity over the spleen (**lower left**). In the individual with splenomegaly, only 20% of the infused platelets are recoverable in the peripheral blood sample (**upper right**) with the majority of radioactivity entering the splenic compartments (**lower right**). The survival of platelets in the individual with splenomegaly is shorter. (Note that the normal percent recovery of platelets is plotted on an arithmetic graph and platelet survival in splenomegaly is plotted on a semilog graph.) (Adapted with permission from Ries CA, Price DC. [$^{51}$Cr] Platelet kinetics in thrombocytopenia. Correlation between splenic sequestration of platelets and response to splenectomy. Ann Intern Med 1974;80:702–707.)

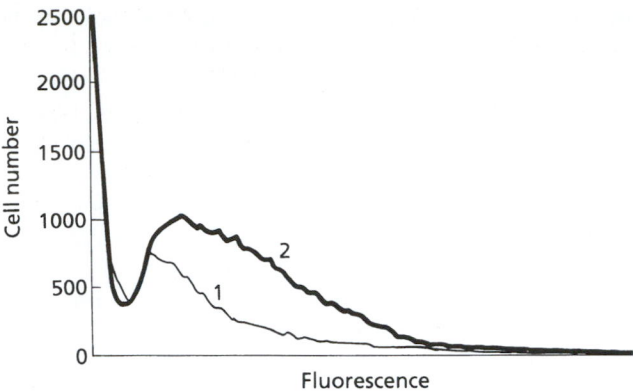

**FIGURE 26.32.** Demonstration of platelet-associated immunoglobulin G (PAIgG) on platelets from normal donors and ITP individuals. Cells were incubated with FITC-conjugated goat F(ab')₂ antihuman IgG and analyzed by flow cytometry. (1) Fluorescence histogram showing PAIgG on platelets from a normal donor; (2) Fluorescence histogram showing PAIgG on platelets from a individual with ITP. (Adapted with permission from Helm MC, Peterson BH. Detection of platelet-associated immunoglobulin in immune thrombocytopenia by flow cytometry. Diagn Clin Immunol 1988;5:309–313.)

penia. In addition, most assays have high background fluorescence due to the presence of contaminating white blood cells that bear immunoglobulin (see [562] for comparison of different assays). The flow cytometric method effectively reduces the problem of contaminating white blood cells, because only a specific cell size is selected for analysis by specific instrument programming, excluding the larger white cells. (A review of the sensitivity and specificity of each of these methods is found in [562].) False-positive results occur in the setting of rheumatic diseases, paraproteinemias, heparin anticoagulation, and infections. A negative direct or indirect antiplatelet antibody test by any of these methods does not exclude the diagnosis of immune thrombocytopenia.

# PLATELET FLOW CYTOMETRY

Flow cytometry is useful in diagnosis of a number of disorders affecting platelet function and number (547, 574–578). Flow cytometry has been used to determine surface-bound and intracellular antiplatelet antibody in immune thrombocytopenia (572). It has most recently been used to determine the percentage of young platelets in conditions associated with thrombocytopenia by measuring the number of circulating platelets with high concentrations of RNA (see Reticulated Platelet Count, above). In the research setting, flow cytometric analysis has been used to study specific characteristics of a large number of individual populations of cells, as in the case

of immunophenotypic analysis of peripheral blood leukocytes in malignant and nonmalignant disorders (576). Using an adaptation of these techniques, platelet flow cytometry can be used to study surface-bound and intracellular platelet antigens in both resting and activated states. In these studies, citrated washed platelets, PRP, or whole blood is labeled with a fluorescently conjugated monoclonal antibody directed to a platelet antigen such as the GP IIb-IIIa complex (CD41/61), the receptor for fibrinogen, vWf, fibronectin, and vitronectin that mediates platelet aggregation. The platelets are then fixed in glutaraldehyde or formalin and diluted for analysis. In the flow cytometer, the suspended cells pass through a flow chamber at a rate of 1,000 to 10,000 cells per minute through a focused laser beam. After fluorescent activation of the flurophore, a detector processes the fluorescent and light scattering properties of each cell. The intensity of fluorescence of each population of cells can be translated into quantitative amounts of antibody bound per cell. Several monoclonal antibodies have been developed for research on platelet membrane glycoprotein structure and function. Some monoclonal antibodies, such as PAC1, have been found to bind only to activated platelets. Other monoclonal antibodies are directed against ligand-induced conformation sites on the GP IIb-IIIa complex or to receptor-induced binding sites in fibrinogen bound to its receptor on the platelet (575). Using a battery of such monoclonal antibodies, it is possible to determine whether circulating platelets are activated, degranulated, or in a resting state. The importance of such information lies in the fact that the current methodologies to assess platelet function, such as aggregometry, are only able to identify whether the total mass of circulation platelets have altered reactivity, but do not provide insight into the mechanism by which altered reactivity has occurred. Platelet activation can be identified and correlated with clinical conditions, such as unstable coronary syndromes, recurrent arterial thrombosis, stroke, and eclampsia, in which ongoing platelet activation may directly relate to disease activity. Flow cytometry of platelet membranes can be used to rapidly identify abnormal or absent platelet membrane glycoproteins in hereditary diseases such as Bernard-Soulier syndrome or Glanzmann's thrombasthenia without the need to perform the more cumbersome gel electrophoretic analysis of platelet membranes. Platelet storage pool disorders can also be diagnosed by staining of platelet intracellular adenine nucleotide pools with the fluorescent dye mepacrine (579).

## INTERPRETATION

Flow cytometry has the advantage of being able to perform studies directly in whole blood using only μ volumes. Both the presence of activated platelets and the ability of the platelets to react to selected agonists can be analyzed. Samples must be prepared within 45 minutes of venipuncture to reduce artifactual results. Once samples have been formalin fixed, flow cytometric analysis may be done at a later time. Unfortunately not all hospital laboratories have a flow cytometer due to its expense and the technical expertise required to process and interpret sample results.

# TESTS FOR HEPARIN-ASSOCIATED THROMBOCYTOPENIA

Several tests are available for the diagnosis of heparin-associated thrombocytopenia (579–583) (see Chapter 29). Platelet-associated IgG is increased in heparin-associated thrombocytopenia but is not diagnostic of the disorder (564). The recovery-phase plasma of individuals with heparin-associated thrombocytopenia contains a factor that causes platelets to agglutinate in the presence of heparin. This observation serves as the basis for a test that uses individuals' serum or plasma added to normal control platelets in the presence of heparin. An aggregation response is considered a positive result, consistent with, but not diagnostic of, the diagnosis of heparin-associated thrombocytopenia. The test has a relatively low sensitivity due, at least in part, to variability in donor platelet response to heparin-associated antibodies present in the test plasma. The phenotype of the platelet FγRIIa influences the aggregation response with the His/His$^{131}$ phenotype showing virtually no reactivity to heparin-associated antibodies, whereas the Arg/Arg$^{131}$ phenotype is the most reactive (579). Interestingly, individuals with the His/His$^{131}$ phenotype have the greatest predilection to produce heparin-associated antibodies. It is recommended that laboratories use donors who consistently exhibit a strongly positive aggregation response to plasma containing heparin-associated antibodies. With this modification in testing, the heparin-induced aggregation assay has been shown to have an improved sensitivity to heparin-associated antibodies (579, 584, 585).

The heparin-induced platelet aggregation assay has been modified to increase its sensitivity by measuring the release reaction induced by the plasma of affected individuals in the presence of low concentrations of heparin (579, 580). An assay has been devised for demonstrating activation of the release reaction by heparin in those individuals with heparin-associated thrombocytopenia. The assay is based on the [14C]-serotonin release test (see above) with certain modifications (542). Recovery phase plasma from individuals with heparin-associated thrombocytopenia is incubated with fresh normal PRP from a normal donor. Five μ s each of 0.1 U/mL heparin and 100 U/mL heparin is added to separate tubes containing test PRP. The tubes are stirred for 60 minutes, after which the reaction is terminated by the addition of 0.5% EDTA. The samples are centrifuged and the supernatants counted for released [14C]-serotonin. The percentage release is calculated, as in the standard serotonin release assay. The test is considered positive for heparin-associated thrombocytopenia if there is greater than 20% release at 0.1 U/mL and less than 20% release at 100 U/mL heparin. Most false-positive results are due to platelet-associated antibody, as in immune thrombocytopenia.

In some cases of heparin-associated thrombocytopenia, antibodies to PF4-heparin complexes have been found. An ELISA has been developed in which heparin/PF4 complexes are bound to microtiter wells (586). Dilutions of test plasma are incubated with the microtiter wells. Immunoglobulin bound to the heparin/PF4 complexes is then detected using peroxidase-conjugated anti-human immunoglobulin. In one series all individuals with heparin-associated thrombocytopenia had antibodies to heparin/PF4 complexes; however, some individuals without thrombocytopenia who had been given heparin for 7 days were also noted to have positive test results. Further studies are necessary to determine the sensitivity and specificity of this assay system.

# MOLECULAR GENETIC STUDIES IN HEMOSTASIS

The cloning and detailed analysis of the genes encoding proteins involved in hemostasis has provided important information on the effect of abnormalities in structure and function resulting from various types of mutations. For the majority of coagulation defects that are acquired, genetic analysis is neither indicated nor useful in diagnosis or treatment of the coagulation disorder. However, for individuals with hereditary hypercoagulable or hemorrhagic diseases, molecular biological study of the individual's DNA may be crucial in diagnosis of a mutated gene, as in the factor V Leiden defect (382, 383), or in identifying an asymptomatic carrier of an abnormal gene, as in female carriers of hemophilia. A variety of techniques are available in the research setting for the study of mutations in nearly all hemostatic proteins. In practice, however, clinical laboratories are able to provide, at most, genetic studies for defects in factors VIII, IX, and XI, or for the factor V Leiden mutation, with the bulk of genetic studies on other disorders confined to research laboratories with interests in specific hemostatic factors.

## CARRIER DETECTION IN HEMOPHILIA
### Bioassays

Prior to the availability of gene based family studies to determine carrier status in hemophilia, bioassays were the sole means of determining the probability of a female carrying an abnormal factor VIII gene in a family with affected male individuals (587, 588). The principle of carrier detection by bioassay is that for any given somatic cell, the Lyon hypothesis dictates that one of the two possible X chromosomes is randomly inactivated. Thus, the cells in which the chromosome carrying the normal factor VIII gene is activated will produce normal amounts of factor VIII. Those cells in which the X chromosome carrying the abnormal hemophilic factor VIII gene is activated will produce low to absent factor VIII levels. Thus, on average, a female carrier of hemophilia A will have half the amount of factor VIII compared with a normal female. Because factor VIII activity assumes a gaussian distribution in the normal population, there is overlap in factor VIII levels between normal females and carriers. In determining carrier status for hemophilia A, both factor VIII activity and vWf antigen levels are measured on two separate occasions and compared to control ranges present in normal populations of the same blood group to allow for normal differences in factor VIII and VWF antigen levels between blood groups. Using bivariate analysis, the probability of carrier status may be calculated with an accuracy of 90% (587–589).

## Genetic Assays

### Factor VIII Carrier Testing

Because of the large size of the factor VIII gene, pedigree analysis by direct sequencing to identify a potential mutation is not practical. Almost 50% of severe hemophilia A cases result from inversion of a portion of intron 22 (590, 591). In pedigree analysis for severe hemophilia, the initial analysis involves detection of intron 22 inversion in BclI digested genomic DNA by southern blot analysis (592).

When the genetic defect in a family is known, direct genetic probes can be constructed and used to identify carriers within the family pedigree. Factor VIII RNA analysis can be performed by rt-PCR from residual ectopic mRNA found in peripheral blood leukocytes (593). Carrier identification is performed using a labeled oligomer probe specific for the defect. If the defect involves a restriction enzyme site, then restriction site analysis may be used (594). The second, and more commonly used approach, restriction enzyme polymorphism analysis (RFLP) does not require knowledge of the specific genetic mutation resulting in hemophilia in a family pedigree. Changes in DNA sequence within a gene result in either a polymorphism or a mutation. The latter results in an abnormal gene product. A compendium of polymorphisms occurring with high frequency within various populations has been described for various hemostatic proteins. For factor VIII, at least ten useful polymorphisms have been described (595, 596). The two most useful polymorphisms are the variable number

tandem repeat (VNTR) CA repeats found within introns 1 and 22 (597). Multiplex PCR of the intron 13 and 22 CA repeats results in an informative pattern in 90% of families studied (598). Nucleotide substitution polymorphisms are detected either by RFLP or by allele specific oligonucleotide hybridization (ASO). The DNA probes used to identify RFLPs within, or closely linked to a particular gene, can be used to trace the gene through a family pedigree. The chance of misidentifying the inheritance of a particular gene using intragenic polymorphisms is less than 1%, whereas the use of polymorphisms flanking the gene results in a theoretical 5% error due to inherent DNA recombination events. Crossovers occurring between the commonly used DNA probes BglII-DXs15 or TaqI-DxS52 and the factor VIII gene have resulted in erroneous carrier status reporting (599). Hence a combination of intragenic and flanking RFLP probes are used. Restriction enzyme polymorphism analysis is not useful in carrier testing when the female is homozygous for the polymorphic marker, because it is not possible to determine on which of the alleles the defective gene lies. Limitations of polymorphism analysis also relate to the necessity of studying several family members, nonpaternity issues, and the ability to exclude the diagnosis of carrier status only where there are other affected members. Moreover, RFLP analysis is not useful in isolated or sporadic cases of hemophilia due to both gonadal and somatic mosaicism that have been described in hemophilia and can result in incorrect identification of carrier status (600, 601).

### Factor IX Carrier Testing

Hemophilia B results from a large number of different mutations in the factor IX gene (602). Direct DNA sequencing techniques are available for identification of factor IX mutations. However, these methods are generally not applied until a screening assay, such as amplification mismatch detection (AMD), denaturing gradient gel electrophoresis (DGGE), or single stranded conformation polymorphism (SSCP), has identified and localized a potential mutation (602–607). In these techniques a difference between individual and normal DNA sequence for a gene is detected. In conjunction with PCR amplification of genomic DNA or rt-PCR amplification from mRNA, followed by direct sequencing of the PCR fragments where a mismatch is observed, many mutations can be identified. When adequate numbers of affected and unaffected family members are available for linkage analysis, more than 80% of family studies are informative using the 5'MseI RFLP, plus the 3'HhaI RFLP and the DdeI polymorphisms in Caucasian populations. In Asian and American black populations, only the HhaI and MseI RFLPs are informative (595, 608, 609).

# APPENDIX

Reference Values for Inhibitors of Coagulation in Infants, Children, and Adults. Adapted from Andrew et al [170, 610]

|  | 1 Day | 1 Month | 6 Months | 1–5 Years | 6–10 Years | 11–16 Years | Adult |
|---|---|---|---|---|---|---|---|
| ATIII | 0.63 ± 0.12 | 0.78 ± 0.15 | 1.04 ± 0.10 | 1.11 (0.82–1.39) | 1.11 (0.9–1.31) | 1.05 (0.77–1.32) | 1.0 (0.74–1.26) |
| $\alpha_2$M | 1.39 ± 0.22 | 1.50 ± 0.22 | 1.91 ± 0.21 | 1.69 (1.14–2.23) | 1.69 (1.28–2.09) | 1.56 (0.98–2.12) | 0.86 (0.52–1.20) |
| C1INH | 0.72 ± 0.18 | 0.89 ± 0.21 | 1.41 ± 0.26 | 1.35 (0.85–1.83) | 1.14 (0.88–1.54) | 1.03 (0.68–1.50) | 1.0 (0.71–1.31) |
| $\alpha_1$AT | 0.93 ± 0.22 | 0.62 ± 0.13 | 0.77 ± 0.15 | 0.93 (0.39–1.46) | 1.00 (0.69–1.30) | 1.01 (0.65–1.37) | 0.93 (0.55–1.30) |
| HCII | 0.43 ± 0.25 | 0.47 ± 0.20 | 1.20 ± 0.35 | 0.88 (0.48–1.28) | 0.86 (0.4–1.32) | 0.91 (0.53–1.29) | 1.08 (0.66–1.26) |
| PC | 0.35 ± 0.09 | 0.43 ± 0.11 | 0.59 ± 0.11 | 0.66 (0.4–0.92) | 0.69 (0.45–0.93) | 0.83 (0.55–1.11) | 0.96 (0.64–1.28) |
| PS$_T$ | 0.36 ± 0.12 | 0.50 ± 0.14 | 0.87 ± 0.16 | 0.86 (0.54–1.18) | 0.78 (0.41–1.14) | 0.72 (0.52–0.92) | 0.81 (0.60–1.13) |
| PS$_F$ |  |  |  | 0.45 (0.21–0.69) | 0.42 (0.22–0.62) | 0.38 (0.26–0.55) | 0.45 (0.27–0.61) |

ATIII, antithrombin III; $\alpha_2$M, $\alpha_2$-macroglobulin; $\alpha_2$AT, $\alpha_1$-antitrypsin; C1INH, C1 inhibitor; HCII, heparin cofactor II; PC, protein C; PS$_F$, protein S free, PS$_T$, protein S total.

Values are expressed as the mean ± 1 SD for ages 1 day to 6 months and as the mean followed by the range encompassing 95% of normal controls for ages 1 year to adult. All values are expressed as units per milliliter based on a value of 1 U/mL in normal plasma.

Reference Values for Coagulation Screening Tests in Infants, Children, and Adults. Adapted from Andrew et al [170, 610]

|  | 1 Day | 1 Month | 6 Months | 1–5 Years | 6–10 Years | 11–16 Years | Adult |
|---|---|---|---|---|---|---|---|
| PT | 13.0 ± 1.43 | 11.8 ± 1.25 | 12.3 ± 0.79 | 11.0 (10.6–11.4) | 11.1 (10.1–12.1) | 11.2 (10.2–12.0) | 12.0 (11.0–14.0) |
| INR |  |  |  | 1.0 (0.96–1.04) | 1.01 (0.91–1.11) | 1.02 (0.93–1.10) | 1.10 (1.0–1.3) |
| TCT | 23.5 ± 2.38 | 24.3 ± 2.44 | 25.5 ± 2.86 |  |  |  | 25.0 ± 2.66 |
| aPTT | 42.9 ± 5.80 | 40.4 ± 7.42 | 35.5 ± 3.71 | 30.0 (24–36) | 31 (26–36) | 32 (26–37) | 33 (27–40) |
| BT |  |  |  | 6 (2.5–10) | 7 (2.5–13) | 5 (3–8) | 4 (1–7) |

aPTT, activated partial thromboplastin time; BT, bleeding time; INR, international normalized ratio; PT, prothrombin time; TCT, thrombin clotting time.

All values are expressed in seconds, with the exception of the bleeding time, which is expressed in minutes. Values are expressed as the mean ± 1 SD for ages 1 day to 6 months and as the mean followed by the range encompassing 95% of normal controls for ages 1 year to adult.

Reference Values for Coagulation Factor Assays in Infants, Children, and Adults. Adapted from Andrew et al [170, 610]

|  | 1 Day | 1 Month | 6 Months | 1–5 Years | 6–10 Years | 11–16 Years | Adult |
|---|---|---|---|---|---|---|---|
| I | 2.83 ± 0.58 | 2.7 ± 0.54 | 25.1 ± 0.68 | 2.76 (1.70–4.05) | 2.79 (1.57–4.0) | 3.0 (1.54–4.48) | 2.78 (1.56–4.0) |
| II | 0.48 ± 0.11 | 0.68 ± 0.17 | 0.88 ± 0.14 | 0.94 (0.71–1.16) | 0.88 (0.67–1.07) | 0.83 (0.61–1.04) | 1.08 (0.7–1.46) |
| V | 0.72 ± 0.18 | 0.98 ± 0.18 | 0.91 ± 0.18 | 1.03 (0.79–1.27) | 0.90 (0.63–1.16) | 0.77 (0.55–0.99) | 1.06 (0.62–1.50) |
| VII | 0.66 ± 0.19 | 0.90 ± 0.24 | 0.87 ± 0.20 | 0.82 (0.55–1.16) | 0.85 (0.52–1.2) | 0.83 (0.58–1.15) | 1.05 (0.67–1.43) |
| VIII | 1.0 ± 0.39 | 0.91 ± 0.33 | 0.73 ± 0.18 | 0.90 (0.59–1.42) | 0.95 (0.58–1.32) | 0.92 (0.53–1.31) | 0.99 (0.50–1.49) |
| IX | 0.53 ± 0.19 | 0.51 ± 0.15 | 0.86 ± 0.25 | 0.73 (0.47–1.01) | 0.75 (0.63–0.89) | 0.82 (0.59–1.22) | 1.09 (0.55–1.63) |
| X | 0.40 ± 0.14 | 0.59 ± 0.14 | 0.78 ± 0.20 | 0.88 (0.58–1.16) | 0.75 (0.55–1.01) | 0.79 (0.50–1.17) | 1.06 (0.70–1.52) |
| XI | 0.38 ± 0.14 | 0.53 ± 0.13 | 0.86 ± 0.24 | 0.97 (0.56–1.50) | 0.86 (0.52–1.20) | 0.74 (0.50–0.97) | 0.97 (0.67–1.27) |
| XII | 0.53 ± 0.20 | 0.49 ± 0.16 | 0.77 ± 0.19 | 0.93 (0.64–1.29) | 0.92 (0.60–1.40) | 0.81 (0.34–1.37) | 1.08 (0.52–1.64) |
| PK | 0.37 ± 0.16 | 0.57 ± 0.17 | 0.86 ± 0.15 | 0.95 (0.65–1.30) | 0.99 (0.66–1.31) | 0.99 (0.53–1.45) | 1.12 (0.62–1.62) |
| HK | 0.54 ± 0.24 | 0.77 ± 0.22 | 0.82 ± 0.23 | 0.98 (0.64–1.32) | 0.93 (0.60–1.30) | 0.91 (0.63–1.19) | 0.92 (0.50–1.36) |
| XIIIa | 0.79 ± 0.26 | 0.93 ± 0.27 | 1.04 ± 0.29 | 1.08 (0.72–1.43) | 1.09 (0.65–1.51) | 0.99 (0.57–1.40) | 1.05 (0.55–1.55) |
| XIIIs | 0.76 ± 0.23 | 1.11 ± 0.36 | 1.10 ± 0.30 | 1.13 (0.69–1.56) | 1.16 (0.77–1.54) | 1.02 (0.60–1.43) | 0.97 (0.57–1.37) |
| vWf | 1.53 ± 0.67 | 1.28 ± 0.59 | 1.07 ± 0.45 | 0.82 (0.60–1.20) | 0.95 (0.44–1.44) | 1.00 (0.46–1.53) | 0.92 (0.50–1.58) |

HK, high molecular weight kininogen; PK, prekallikrein; vWf, von Willebrand factor.

All of the above factors are expressed as units per milliliter based on a value of 1 U/mL in normal plasma except for factor I (fibrinogen), which is expressed as grams per liter.

Reference Values for Fibrinolytic Screening Tests in Infants, Children, and Adults. Adapted from Andrew et al [170, 610]

|  | 1 Day | 1 Month | 6 Months | 1–5 Years | 6–10 Years | 11–16 Years | Adult |
|---|---|---|---|---|---|---|---|
| PGN | 1.95 ± 0.35 | 1.98 ± 0.36 | 3.0 ± 0.4 | 0.98 (0.78–1.18) | 0.92 (0.75–1.08) | 0.86 (0.68–1.03) | 0.99 (0.77–1.22) |
| t-PA |  |  |  | 2.15 (1.0–4.5) | 2.42 (1.0–5.0) | 2.16 (1.0–4.0) | 4.90 (1.4–8.4) |
| $\alpha_2$AP | 0.85 ± 0.15 | 1.00 ± 0.12 | 1.11 ± 0.21 | 1.05 (0.93–1.17) | 0.99 (0.89–1.10) | 0.98 (0.78–1.18) | 1.02 (0.68–1.36) |
| PAI |  |  |  | 5.42 (1.0–10.0) | 6.79 (2.0–12.0) | 6.07 (2.0–10.0) | 3.6 (0–11.0) |

$\alpha_2$AP, $\alpha_2$-antiplasmin; PAI, plasminogen activator inhibitor; PGN, plasminogen; t-PA, tissue-type plasminogen activator.

Values are expressed as the mean followed by the range encompassing 95% of the normal controls for ages 1 year to adult, and as the mean ± 1 SD for ages 1 day to 6 months. PGN and $\alpha_2$AP are expressed as units per milliliter, where pooled normal plasma contains 1.0 U/mL t-PA values are expressed as nanograms per milliliter. Values for PAI are given as units per milliliter, where 1 U of PAI activity is the amount of PAI that inhibits I IU of human single-chain t-PA.

# CONCLUSIONS

Great advances have occurred during the past 50 years in our understanding of the factors that affect normal hemostasis. The complete array of factors that play a role in controlling the evolution of pathologic thrombosis remains elusive, as evidenced by the inability to identify an abnormal factor in half the individuals with recurrent arterial and venous thrombosis. Within the next several years, more sophisticated tests of new hemostatic factors will be developed and studied for their relevance in the prethrombotic individual population. Lastly, the powerful analytic tools provided by molecular biological techniques soon will be available outside the research laboratory for the identification and classification of suspected congenital hemostatic disorders.

# REFERENCES

1. Palkuti AS. Specimen collection and quality control. In: Corriveau DM, Fritsma GA, eds. Hemostasis and thrombosis in the clinical laboratory. Philadelphia: JB Lippincott, 1988:67–91.
2. Ray MJ. An artefact related to the ratio of sample volume to the blood collection vial size which effects the APTTs of specimens taken to monitor heparin therapy [Review]. Thromb Haemost 1991;66:387–388.
3. Quick AJ. Haemorrhagic diseases and thrombosis. Philadelphia: Lea & Febiger, 1966.
4. Fritsma GA. Clot-based assays of coagulation. In: Corriveau DM, Fritsma GA, eds. Hemostasis and thrombosis in the clinical laboratory. Philadelphia: JB Lippincott, 1988:92–127.
5. Hougie C. Recalcification time test and its modifications (partial thromboplastin time, activated partial thromboplastin time, and expanded partial thromboplastin time). In: Williams J, Beutler E, Erslev J, eds. Hematology. New York: McGraw-Hill, 1977:1642.
6. Hattersley PG. Activated coagulation time of whole blood. JAMA 1966; 196:436–440.
7. Bode AP, Castellani WJ, Hodges ED et al. The effect of lysed platelets on neutralization of heparin *in vitro* with protamine as measured by the activated coagulation time (ACT). Thromb Haemost 1991;66:213–217.
8. Palkuti HS. Laboratory monitoring of anticoagulant therapy. J Med Tech 1985;2:81–86.
9. Quick AJ, Stanley-Brown M, Bancroft FW. A study of the coagulation defect in hemophilia and in jaundice. Am J Med Sci 1935;190:501–511.
10. National Committee for Clinical Laboratory Standards NCCCLS H28-P. Proposed guidelines for the one-stage prothrombin time test (PT). Villanova: NCCLS, 1980.
11. Lackner H. Hemostatic abnormalities associated with dysproteinemias. Semin Hematol 1973;10:125–133.
12. Vigano S, Mannucci PM, Solinas S. Decrease in protein C antigen and formation of an abnormal protein soon after starting oral anticoagulant therapy. Br J Haematol 1984;57:213–220.
13. Hirsh J, Levine M. Confusion over the therapeutic range for monitoring oral anticoagulant therapy in North America. Thromb Haemost 1988;59:129–132.
14. Arnout J, Vanrusselt M, Huybrechts E et al. Optimization of the dilute prothrombin time for the detection of the lupus anticoagulant by use of a recombinant tissue thromboplastin. Br J Haematol 1994;87:94–99.
15. Kitchen S, Jennings I, Woods TA et al. Two recombinant tissue factor reagents compared to conventional thromboplastins for determination of international normalised ratio: a thirty-three-laboratory collaborative study. The Steering Committee of the UK National External Quality Assessment Scheme for Blood Coagulation. Thromb Haemost 1996;76:372–376.
16. Tripodi A, Chantarangkul V, Braga M et al. Results of a multicenter study assessing the status of standardization of a recombinant thromboplastin for the control of oral anticoagulant therapy. Thromb Haemost 1994;72:261–267.
17. Roussi J, Drouet L, Samama M et al. French multicentric evaluation of recombinant tissue factor (recombiplastin) for determination of prothrombin time. Thromb Haemost 1994;72:698–704.
18. Kazama M, Suzuki S, Abe T et al. Evaluation of international normalized ratios by a controlled field survey with 4 different thromboplastin reagents. Thromb Haemost 1990;64:535–541.
19. Kovacs MJ, Wong A, MacKinnon K et al. Assessment of the validity of the INR system for individuals with liver impairment. Thromb Haemost 1994;71:727–730.
20. Loeliger EA, van den Besselaar AM, Bertina RM. Critical appraisal, clinical usefulness and implementation of the thromboplastin concept of prothrombin-time standardization. Scand J Haematol Suppl 1980;37:34–48.
21. Miale JB. The use of reference plasmas in the control of oral anticoagulant therapy. Scand J Haematol Suppl 1980;37:21–33.
22. Kirkwood TB. Calibration of reference thromboplastins and standardisation of the prothrombin time ratio. Thromb Haemost 1983;49:238–244.
23. Peters RH, van den Besselaar AM, Olthuis FM. Determination of the mean normal prothrombin time for assessment of international normalized ratios. Usefulness of lyophilized plasma. Thromb Haemost 1991;66:442–445.
24. Ray MJ, Smith IR. The dependence of the International Sensitivity Index on the coagulometer used to perform the prothrombin time. Thromb Haemost 1990;63:424–429.
25. Denson KW, Reed SV, Haddon ME. Validity of the INR system for individuals with liver impairment. Thromb Haemost 1995;73:162.
26. Poller L. Standardization of the APTT test. Current status. Scand J Haematol Suppl 1980;37:49–63.
27. D'Angelo A, Seveso MP, D'Angelo SV et al. Effect of clot-detection methods and reagents on activated partial thromboplastin time (APTT). Implications in heparin monitoring by APTT. Am J Clin Pathol 1990;94:297–306.
28. Van der Velde EA, Poller L. The APTT monitoring of heparin—the ISTH/ICSH collaborative study. Thromb Haemost 1995;73:73–81.
29. Hattersley PG, Hayse D. The effect of increased contact activation time on the activated partial thromboplastin time. Am J Clin Pathol 1976;66:479–482.
30. Brill-Edwards P, Ginsberg JS, Johnston M et al. Establishing a therapeutic range for heparin therapy. Ann Intern Med 1993;119:104–109.
31. Quick AJ, Favre-Gilly JE. The prothrombin consumption test: its clinical and theoretic implications. Blood 1949;4:1281–1289.
32. Owen CA Jr, Thompson JH Jr. Soybean phosphatides in prothrombin-consumption and thromboplastin-generation tests: their use in recognizing "thrombasthenic hemophilia." Am J Clin Pathol 1960;33:197–208.
33. Wintrobe M et al, eds. Clinical haematology. Philadelphia: Lea & Febiger, 1981;1056.
34. Biggs R, Douglas AS. The thromboplastin generation test. J Clin Pathol 1953;6:23–29.
35. Duckert F, Fluckiger P, Isenschmid H et al. A modification of the thromboplastin generation test. Acta Haematol 1954;12:197–202.
36. Clauss VA. Gerinnungsphysiologische Schnellmethode zur Bestimmung des Fibrinogens. Acta Haematol 1957;17:237–246.
37. Jim RTS. A study of the plasma thrombin time. J Lab Clin Med 1957;50:45–60.
38. Penner JA. Experience with a thrombin clotting time assay for measuring heparin activity. Am J Clin Pathol 1974;61:645–653.
39. Delorme MA, Inwood MJ, O'Keefe B. Sensitivity of the thrombin clotting time and activated partial thromboplastin time to low level of antithrombin III during heparin therapy. Clin Lab Haematol 1990;12:433–436.
40. Exner T, Burridge J, Power P et al. An evaluation of currently available methods for plasma fibrinogen. Am J Clin Pathol 1979;71:521–527.
41. Witt I, Muller H, Kunzer W. Evidence for the existence of foetal fibrinogen. Thromb Diath Haemorrh 1969;22:101–109.
42. Dang CV, Bell WR, Shuman M. The normal and morbid biology of fibrinogen. Am J Med 1989;87:567–576.
43. Triplett DA. Laboratory diagnosis of lupus anticoagulants. Semin Thromb Hemost 1990;16:182–192.
44. Bellotti V, Gamba G, Merlini G et al. Study of three individuals with monoclonal gammopathies and "lupus-like" anticoagulants. Br J Haematol 1989;73:221–227.
45. Kasper CK, Ewing NP. Acquired inhibitors of plasma coagulation factors. J Med Tech 1986;3:431–439.
46. Kaczor DA, Bickford NN, Triplett DA. Evaluation of different mixing study reagents and dilution effect in lupus anticoagulant testing. Am J Clin Pathol 1991;95:408–411.
47. Lesperance B, David M, Rauch J et al. Relative sensitivity of different tests in the detection of low titer lupus anticoagulants. Thromb Haemost 1988;60:217–219.
48. Ewing NP, Kasper CK. *In vitro* detection of mild inhibitors to factor VIII in hemophilia. Am J Clin Pathol 1982;77:749–752.
49. White KS, Dombrose FA, Blatt PM. A rapid screening method to increase efficiency in assaying plasma levels of clotting factor VIII:C inhibitors. Am J Clin Pathol 1982;78:450–456.
50. Weiss AE. Acquired coagulation disorders. In: Corriveau DM, Fritsma GA, eds. Hemostasis and thrombosis in the clinical laboratory. Philadelphia: JB Lippincott, 1988;169–205.
51. Clyne LP, White PF. Time dependency of lupus like anticoagulants. Arch Intern Med 1988;148:1060–1063.
52. Forastiero RR, Falcon CR, Carreras LO. Comparison of various screening and confirmatory tests for the detection of the lupus anticoagulant. Haemostasis 1990;20:208–214.
53. Harris EN. Antiphospholipid antibodies. Br J Haematol 1990;74:1–9.

54. Mackworth-Young CG, Loizou S, Walport MJ. Primary antiphospholipid syndrome: features of individuals with raised anticardiolipin antibodies and no other disorder. Ann Rheum Dis 1989;48:362–367.
55. McHugh NJ, Maymo J, Skinner RP et al. Anticardiolipin antibodies, livedo reticularis, and major cerebrovascular and renal disease in systemic lupus erythematosus. Ann Rheum Dis 1988;47:110–115.
56. Petri M, Rheinschmidt M, Whiting-O'Keefe Q et al. The frequency of lupus anticoagulant in systemic lupus erythematosus. A study of sixty consecutive individuals by activated partial thromboplastin time, Russell viper venom time, and anticardiolipin antibody level. Ann Intern Med 1987;106:524–531.
57. Duhrsen U, Paar D, Brittinger G. Lupus anticoagulant associated syndrome in benign and malignant systemic disease. Klin Wochenschr 1987;65:818–822.
58. Gastineau DA, Kazmier FJ, Nichols WL et al. Lupus anticoagulant: an analysis of the clinical and laboratory features of 219 cases. Am J Hematol 1985;19:265–275.
59. Roubey RA. Immunology of the antiphospholipid antibody syndrome. Arthritis Rheum 1996;39:1444–1454.
60. McLucus E, Harrison RL. The lupus anticoagulant. J Med Tech 1986;3:440–442.
61. Alving BM, Barr CF, Tang DB. Correlation between lupus anticoagulants and anticardiolipin antibodies in individuals with prolonged activated partial thromboplastin times. Am J Med 1990;88:112–116.
62. Love PE, Santoro SA. Antiphospholipid antibodies: anticardiolipin and the lupus anticoagulant in systemic lupus erythematosus (SLE) and in non-SLE disorders. Prevalence and clinical significance. Ann Intern Med 1990;112:682–698.
63. Anonymous. Comparison of a standardized procedure with current laboratory practices for the detection of lupus anticoagulant in France. Working Group on Hemostasis of the Société Française de Biologie Clinique. Thromb Haemost 1993;70:781–786.
64. Derksen RH, Hasselaar P, Blokzijl L et al. Coagulation screen is more specific than the anticardiolipin antibody ELISA in defining a thrombotic subset of lupus individuals. Ann Rheum Dis 1988;47:364–371.
65. Colaco CB, Male DK. Anti-phospholipid antibodies in syphilis and a thrombotic subset of SLE: distinct profiles of epitope specificity. Clin Exp Immunol 1985;59:449–456.
66. Permpikul P, Rao LV, Rapaport SI. Functional and binding studies of the roles of prothrombin and β₂-glycoprotein I in the expression of lupus anticoagulant activity. Blood 1994;83:2878–2892.
67. Rosove MH, Ismail M, Koziol BJ et al. Lupus anticoagulants: improved diagnosis with a kaolin clotting time using rabbit brain phospholipid in standard and high concentrations. Blood 1986;68:472–478.
68. Rauch J, Tannenbaum M, Janoff AS. Distinguishing plasma lupus anticoagulants from anti-factor antibodies using hexagonal (II) phase phospholipids. Thromb Haemost 1989;62:892–896.
69. Brandt JT, Triplett DA. The effect of phospholipid on the detection of lupus anticoagulants by the dilute Russell viper venom time. Arch Pathol Lab Med 1989;113:1376–1378.
70. Reber G, Arvieux J, Comby E et al. Multicenter evaluation of nine commercial kits for the quantitation of anticardiolipin antibodies. The Working Group on Methodologies in Haemostasis from the GEHT (Groupe d'Etudes sur l'Hemostase et la Thrombose). Thromb Haemost 1995;73:444–452.
71. Forastiero RR, Cerrato GS, Carreras LO. Evaluation of recently described tests for detection of the lupus anticoagulant. Thromb Haemost 1994;72:728–733.
72. Johns AS, Chamley L, Ockelford PA et al. Comparison of tests for the lupus anticoagulant and antiphospholipid antibodies in systemic lupus erythematosus. Clin Exp Rheumatol 1994;12:523–526.
73. Anonymous. Laboratory heterogeneity of the lupus anticoagulant: a multicentre study using different clotting assays on a panel of 78 samples. Hemostasis Committee of the "Société Française de Biologie Clinique." Thromb Res 1992;66:349–364.
74. Anonymous. Guidelines on testing for the lupus anticoagulant. Lupus Anticoagulant Working Party on behalf of the BCSH Haemostasis and Thrombosis Task Force. J Clin Pathol 1991;44:885–889.
75. Exner T, Triplett DA, Taberner DA et al. Comparison of test methods for the lupus anticoagulant: international survey on lupus anticoagulants-I (ISLA-1). Thromb Haemost 1990;64:478–484.
76. Eschwege V, Seddiki S, Robert A. The tissue thromboplastin inhibition test in the detection of lupus anticoagulants: importance of a correction factor eliminating the influence of fibrinogen level. Thromb Haemost 1996;76:65–68.
77. Triplett DA, Brandt JT, Kaczor D et al. Laboratory diagnosis of lupus inhibitors: a comparison of the tissue thromboplastin inhibition procedure with a new platelet neutralization procedure. Am J Clin Pathol 1983;79:678–682.
78. O'Neill AI, Ibrahim KM, Des Parkin J. Automation of the kaolin clotting time. Pathology 1992;24:12–14.
79. Sletnes KE, Gravem K, Wisloff F. Preparation of plasma for the detection

of lupus anticoagulants and antiphospholipid antibodies. Thromb Res 1992;66:43–53.
80. Brien WF, Schaus MR, Cooper KE et al. Lupus anticoagulant testing: effect of the platelet count on the activated partial thromboplastin time. Br J Biomed Sci 1993;50:114–116.
81. Triplett DA, Barna LK, Unger GA. A hexagonal (II) phase phospholipid neutralization assay for lupus anticoagulant identification. Thromb Haemost 1993;70:787–793.
82. Rooney AM, McNally T, Mackie IJ et al. The Taipan snake venom time: a new test for lupus anticoagulant. J Clin Pathol 1994;47:497–501.
83. Triplett DA, Stocker KF, Unger GA et al. The Textarin/Ecarin ratio: a confirmatory test for lupus anticoagulants. Thromb Haemost 1993;70:925–931.
84. McNeil HP, Simpson RJ, Colin NC et al. Anti-phospholipid antibodies are directed against a complex antigen that includes a lipid-binding inhibitor of coagulation: β₂-glycoprotein I (apolipoprotein H). Proc Natl Acad Sci U S A 1990;87:4120–4124.
85. Exner T. Some recent developments with lupus anticoagulants. Blood Coagul Fibrinolysis 1994;5:281–289.
86. Arnout J, Huybrechts E, Vanrusselt M et al. Detection of lupus-like anticoagulants by an enzyme-linked immunosorbent assay using a partial thromboplastin as antigen: A comparative study. Thromb Haemost 1990;64:26–31.
87. Arvieux J, Roussel B, Ponard D et al. IgG2 subclass restriction of anti-β₂-glycoprotein I antibodies in autoimmune individuals. Clin Exp Immunol 1994;95:310–315.
88. Martinuzzo ME, Forastiero RR, Carreras LO. Anti β₂-glycoprotein I antibodies: detection and association with thrombosis. Br J Haematol 1995;89:397–402.
89. Lossing TS, Kasper CK, Feinstein DI. Detection of factor VIII inhibitors with the partial thromboplastin time. Blood 1977;49:793–797.
90. Biggs R, Bidwell E. A method for the study of antihaemophilic globulin inhibitors with reference to six cases. Br J Haematol 1959;5:379–395.
91. Anonymous. A more uniform measurement of factor VIII inhibitors [letter]. Thromb Diath Haemorrh 1975;34:869–872.
92. Kasper CK. Treatment of factor VIII inhibitors. Prog Hemost Thromb 1989;9:57–86.
93. Bird P. Coagulation in an agarose gel and its application to the detection and measurement of factor VIII antibodies. Br J Haematol 1975;29:329–340.
94. Angles-Cano E, Sultan Y, Clauvel JP. Predisposing factors to thrombosis in systemic lupus erythematosus: possible relation to endothelial cell damage. J Lab Clin Med 1979;94:312–323.
95. Nichols WL, Daniels TM, Fisher PK et al. Inhibitors of coagulation factor V and thrombin associated with surgical use of topical bovine thrombin or fibrin "glue" [Abstract]. Blood 1991;78(Suppl 1):63a.
96. Zimmerman TS, Ruggeri ZM. von Willebrand's disease. Clin Haematol 1983;12:175–200.
97. Shapiro SS. Antibodies to blood coagulation factors. Clin Haematol 1979;8:207–214.
98. Fareed J, Messmore HL, Walenga JM et al. Diagnostic efficacy of newer synthetic-substrates methods for assessing coagulation variables: a critical overview. Clin Chem 1983;29:225–236.
99. Mitchell GA. Development and clinical use of automated synthetic substrate methods for the evaluation of coagulation and fibrinolysis. Semin Thromb Hemost 1983;9:268–280.
100. Svendsen LG, Fareed J, Walenga JM et al. Newer synthetic peptide substrates in coagulation testing: some practical considerations for automated methods. Semin Thromb Hemost 1983;9:250–262.
101. Martinoli JL, Amiral J. The impact of automation in the development of reagents and kits for automated methods in coagulation testing. Semin Thromb Hemost 1983;9:194–205.
102. Aiach M, Leon M, Michaud A et al. Adaptation of synthetic peptide substrate-based assays on a discrete analyzer. Semin Thromb Hemost 1983;9:206–216.
103. Bartl K, Becker U, Lill H. Application of several chromogenic substrate assays to automated instrumentation for coagulation analysis. Semin Thromb Hemost 1983;9:301–308.
104. Walenga JM. Molecular and automated assessments of coagulation. In: Corriveau DM, Fritsma GA, eds. Hemostasis and thrombosis in the clinical laboratory. Philadelphia: JB Lippincott, 1988;367–416.
105. Williams CE, Short PE, George AJ et al. Immunological study of coagulation factors. In: Williams CE, Short PE, George AJ, Entwistle MBP, eds. Critical factors in haemostasis. Chichester: Ellis Horwood, Ltd, 1988;34–66.
106. Thompson AR. Factor IX and prothrombin in amniotic fluid and fetal plasma: constraints on prenatal diagnosis of hemophilia B and evidence of proteolysis. Blood 1984;64:867–874.
107. Seiber A. Gross determination of proteins by laser nephelometer. In: Peters H, ed. Proteins of biological fluids. Oxford: Pergamon Press, 1975;295–298.
108. Gidding JC, Peake IR. Principles of immunoassays of haemostatic components. In: Bloom AL, Thomas DP, eds. Haemostasis and thrombosis. Edinburgh: Churchill Livingstone, 1991;824–831.
109. Mancini G, Carbonara AO, Heremans JF. Immunochemical quantitation

of antigens by single radial immunodiffusion. Immunochemistry 1965;2: 235–254.

110. Laurell CB. Quantitative estimation of proteins by electrophoresis in agarose gel containing antibodies. Anal Biochem 1966;15:45–52.

111. Laurell CB. Antigen-antibody crossed electrophoresis. Anal Biochem 1965; 10:358–361.

112. Ganrot PO. Crossed immunoelectrophoresis. Scand J Clin Lab Invest Suppl 1972;124:39–47.

113. Miles LE, Hales CN. Labelled antibodies and immunological assay systems. Nature 1968;219:186–189.

114. Woodhead JS, Addison GM, Hales CN. Radioimmunoassay and saturation analysis. The immunoradiometric assay and related techniques. Br Med Bull 1974;30:44–49.

115. Engvall E, Perlman P. Enzyme-linked immunosorbent assay (ELISA). Quantitative assay of immunoglobulin G. Immunochemistry 1971;8: 871–874.

116. Hoyer LW. Immunologic studies of antihemophilic factor (AHF, factor VIII). IV. Radioimmunoassay of AHF antigen. J Lab Clin Med 1972;80: 822–833.

117. Bertina RM, van der Linden IK. Inhibitor-neutralisation assay and electroimmuno assay of human factor IX (Christmas factor). Clin Chim Acta 1977;77:275–286.

118. Langdell RD, Wagner RH, Brinkhous KM. Effect of antihemophilic factor on one-stage clotting tests. J Lab Clin Med 1953;41:637–647.

119. Biggs R, Eveling J, Richards G. The assay of anti-haemophilic-globulin activity. Br J Haematol 1955;1:20–34.

120. Brandt JT, Triplett DA, Fair DS. Characterization and comparison of immune-depleted and hereditary factor VII-deficient plasmas as substrate plasmas for factor VII assays. Am J Clin Pathol 1986;85:583–589.

121. Rothschild C, Amiral J, Adam M et al. Preparation of factor VIII-depleted plasma with antibodies and its use for the assay of factor VIII. Haemostasis 1990;20:321–328.

122. Brandt JT, Triplett DA, Musgrave K et al. Factor VIII assays. Assessment of variables. Arch Pathol Lab Med 1988;112:7–12.

123. Barrowcliffe TW. Standards for Factor VIII. Scand J Haematol Suppl 1980; 37:104–109.

124. Kirkwood TB. Problems in the standardization of factor VIII assays. Scand J Haematol Suppl 1980;37:110–115.

125. Triplett DA, Kocoshis TA, Harms CS. Factor assay (VIII and IX) results in the College of American Pathologists Survey Program (1976-1979). Scand J Haematol Suppl 1980;37:116–129.

126. Ingram GI, O'Brien PF, North WR. The ICTH/WFH study of the partial thromboplastin time in mild haemophilia. Scand J Haematol Suppl 1980; 37:64–72.

127. Vinazzer H. Assay of total factor XII and of activated factor XII in plasma with a chromogenic substrate. Thromb Res 1979;14:155–166.

128. Saito H. Contact factors in health and disease. Semin Thromb Hemost 1987;13:36–49.

129. Saito H, Ratnoff OD, Pensky J. Radioimmunoassay of human Hageman factor (factor XII). J Lab Clin Med 1979;88:506–514.

130. Gordon EM, Donaldson VH, Saito H et al. Reduced titers of Hageman factor (factor XII) in Orientals. Ann Intern Med 1981;95:697–700.

131. Biland L, Duckert F. Coagulation factors of the newborn and his mother. Thromb Diath Haemorrh 1973;29:644–651.

132. Halbmayer WM, Haushofer A, Schön R et al. The prevalence of moderate and severe F XII (Hageman factor) deficiency among the normal population: evaluation of the incidence of F XII deficiency among 300 healthy blood donors. Thromb Haemost 1994;71:68–72.

133. Winter M, Gallimore M, Jones DW. Should factor XII assays be included in thrombophilia screening? Lancet 1995;346:52.

134. Lammle B, Wuillemin WA, Huber I et al. Thromboembolism and bleeding tendency in congenital factor XII deficiency–A study on 74 subjects from 14 Swiss families. Thromb Haemost 1991;65:117–121.

135. Kurkcuoglu M, McElfresh AE. The Hageman factor: determinations of its concentration during the neonatal period and presentation of a case of Hageman factor deficiency. J Pediatr 1960;57:61–65.

136. Carvalho AC, Lees RS, Vaillancourt RA et al. Intravascular coagulation in hyperlipidemia. Thromb Res 1976;8:843–857.

137. Hruby MA, Honig GR, Shapira E. Immunoquantitation of Hageman factor in urine and plasma of children with nephrotic syndrome. J Lab Clin Med 1980;96:501–510.

138. Martinez J, Palascak JE. Hemostatic alterations in liver disease. In: Zakisom D, Poyer TD, eds. Hepatology: a textbook of liver disease. Philadelphia: WB Saunders, 1982;546.

139. Saito H, Goodnough LT, Makker SP et al. Urinary excretion of Hageman factor (factor XII) and the presence of nonfunctional Hageman factor in the nephrotic syndrome. Am J Med 1981;70:531–534.

140. Jones DW, Gallimore MJ, Winter M. Pseudo factor XII deficiency and phospholipid antibodies. Thromb Haemost 1996;75:696–697.

141. Jaeger U, Kapiotis S, Pabinger I et al. Transient lupus anticoagulant associated with hypoprothrombinemia and factor XII deficiency following adenovirus infection. Ann Hematol 1993;67:95–99.

142. Endo Y. Congenital factor XII deficiency and lupus anticoagulant. Intern Med 1994;33:188.

143. Brookfield C, Malia RG, Cooper SM et al. Factor XII levels and the lupus anticoagulant [Abstract]. Thromb Haemost 1995;73:1441.

144. Halbmayer WM, Haushofer A, Angerer V et al. The discrimination of factor XII deficiency and lupus anticoagulant [Letter]. Thromb Haemost 1996;75:698–699.

145. Gordon EM, Ratnoff OD, Saito H et al. Rapid fibrinolysis, augmented Hageman factor (factor XII) titers and decreased C1 esterase inhibitor titers in women using oral contraceptives. J Lab Clin Med 1980;96:762–769.

146. Berrettini M, Lammle B, Ciavarella G et al. Functional and immunological studies of abnormal factor XII in a cross reacting material positive (CRM+) factor XII deficiency [Abstract]. Thromb Haemost 1985;54:120.

147. Stormorken H, Baklund A, Gallimore M et al. Chromogenic substrate assay of plasma prekallikrein. With a note on its site of biosynthesis. Haemostasis 1978;7:69–75.

148. Kluft C. Determination of prekallikrein in human plasma: optimal conditions for activating prekallikrein. J Lab Clin Med 1978;91:83–95.

149. Mannhalter CH. Biochemical and functional properties of factor XI and prekallikrein. Semin Thromb Hemost 1987;13:25–35.

150. Alving BM, Tankersley DL, Mason BL. Plasma prekallikrein: quantitative determination by direct activation with Hageman factor fragment (β-XIIa). J Lab Clin Med 1983;101:226–241.

151. Bagdasarian A, Lahiri B, Talamo RC et al. Immunochemical studies of plasma kallikrein. J Clin Invest 1974;54:1444–1454.

152. Saito H, Poon MC, Vicic W. Human plasma prekallikrein (Fletcher factor) clotting activity and antigen in health and disease. J Lab Clin Med 1978; 92:84–95.

153. Czendlik C, Lammle B, Duckert F. Cold promoted activation and factor XII, prekallikrein and C1-inhibitor. Thromb Haemost 1985;53:242–244.

154. LaDuca FM, Tourbaf KD. Fletcher factor deficiency, source of variations of the activated partial thromboplastin time test. Am J Clin Pathol 1981; 75:626–628.

155. Giddings JC. The nature of procoagulants. In: Molecular genetics and immunoanalysis in blood coagulation. New York: Ellis Horwood, 1988; 27–119.

156. Alving BM, Niebyl JR, Proud D et al. Human plasma prekallikrein and high molecular weight kininogen decrease during parturition. Thromb Res 1984;34:473–477.

157. Oates JA, Melmon K, Sjoerdsma A et al. Release of a kinin peptide in the carcinoid syndrome. Lancet 1964;1:514–517.

158. Carvalho AC, Lees RS, Vaillancourt RA et al. Activation of the kallikrein system in hyperbetalipoproteinemia. J Lab Clin Med 1978;91:117–122.

159. Saito H, Goodnough LT, Soria J et al. Heterogeneity of human prekallikrein deficiency (Fletcher trait): evidence that five of 18 cases are positive for cross reacting material. N Engl J Med 1981;305:910–914.

160. Van Iwaarden F, Bouma BN. Role of high molecular weight kininogen in contact activation. Semin Thromb Hemost 1987;13:15–24.

161. Scott CF, Pixley RA, Colman RW. A new assay for high molecular weight kininogen in human plasma using a chromogenic substrate. Thromb Res 1987;48:685–700.

162. Kerbiriou DM, Griffin JH. Human high-molecular weight kininogen. Studies of structure-function relationships and of proteolysis of the molecule occurring during contact activation of plasma. J Biol Chem 1979;254: 12020–12027.

163. Kleniewski I, Donaldson VH. Quantification of human high-molecular weight kininogen (HMW-KGN) by specific hemagglutination inhibition reaction (39887). Proc Soc Exp Biol Med 1977;156:113–117.

164. Kociba GJ, Ratnoff OD, Loeb WF et al. Bovine plasma thromboplastin antecedent (factor XI) deficiency. J Lab Clin Med 1969;74:37–41.

165. Forbes CD, Ratnoff OD. Studies on plasma thromboplastin antecedent (factor XI), PTA deficiency and inhibition of PTA by plasma: pharmacologic inhibitors and specific antiserum. J Lab Clin Med 1972;79:113–127.

166. Rapaport SI, Schiffman S, Patch MJ et al. A simple, specific one-stage assay for plasma thromboplastin antecedent activity. J Lab Clin Med 1961;57: 771–780.

167. Scott CF, Sinha D, Seaman FS et al. Amidolytic assay of human factor XI in plasma: comparison with a coagulant assay and a new rapid radioimmunoassay. Blood 1984;63:42–50.

168. Morita T, Kato H, Iwanaga S et al. New fluorogenic substrates for α-thrombin, factor Xa, kallikreins, and urokinase. J Biochem 1977;82: 1495–1498.

169. Zipursky A, deSa D, Hsu E et al. Clinical and laboratory diagnosis of hemostatic disorders in newborn infants. Am J Pediatr Hematol Oncol 1979;1:217–226.

170. Andrew M, Paes B, Milner R et al. Development of the human coagulation system in the full-term infant. Blood 1987;70:165–172.

171. Hilgartner MW, Smith CH. Plasma thromboplastin antecedent (factor XI) in the neonate. J Pediatr 1965;66:747–752.

172. Nossel HL, Lanzkowsky P, Levy S et al. A study of coagulation factor levels in women during labour and in their newborn infants. Thromb Diath Haemorrh 1966;16:185–197.

173. Denson KW. The specific assay of Prower-Stuart factor and factor VII. Acta Haematol 1961;25:105–120.

174. Girolami A, Coser P, Brunetti A et al. Classical factor X deficiency. Report of a further case. Acta Haematol 1975;53:118–127.

175. Egberg N, Heedman PA. Simplified performance of amidolytic factor X assay. Thromb Res 1982;25:437–440.

176. Bernhardt B, Valletta M, Brook J et al. Amyloidosis with factor X deficiency. Am J Med Sci 1972;264:411–414.

177. Mammen EF. Factor X abnormalities. Semin Thromb Hemost 1983;9: 31–33.

178. Mitchell GA, Abdullahad CM, Ruiz JA et al. Fluorogenic substrate assays for factors VIII and IX: introduction of a new solid phase fluorescent detection method. Thromb Res 1981;21:573–584.

179. Hamaguchi M, Matsushita T, Tanimoto M et al. Three distinct point mutations in the factor IX gene of three Japanese CRM + hemophilia B individuals (factor IX B$_m$Nagoya 2, factor IX Nagoya 3 and 4). Thromb Haemost 1991;65:514–520.

180. Thompson AR. Factor IX antigen by radioimmunoassay. Abnormal factor IX protein in individuals on warfarin therapy and with hemophilia B. J Clin Invest 1977;59:900–910.

181. Yang HC. Immunologic studies of factor IX (Christmas Factor). II. Immunoradiometric assay of factor IX antigen. Br J Haematol 1978;39:215–224.

182. Thompson AR. Monoclonal antibody to an epitope on the heavy chain of factor IX missing in three hemophilia-B individuals. Blood 1983;62: 1027–1034.

183. Ljung R, Holmberg L. Genetic variants of haemophilia B detected by immunoradiometric assay: implications for prenatal diagnosis. Pediatr Res 1982;16:256–258.

184. Kidd P, Denson KWE, Biggs R. The thrombotest reagent and Christmas disease. Lancet 1963;2:522.

185. Natelson EA, Lynch EC, Hettig RA et al. Acquired factor IX deficiency in the nephrotic syndrome. Ann Intern Med 1970;73:373–378.

186. Pool JG, Robinson J. Assay of plasma antihaemophilic globulin (AHG). Br J Haematol 1959;5:17–23.

187. Kasper CK, Kim HC, Gomperts ED et al. In vivo recovery and survival of monoclonal-antibody-purified factor VIII concentrates. Thromb Haemost 1991;66:730–733.

188. Rosen S, Friberger P, Anderson M et al. A new chromogenic assay for determination of human factor VIII:C activity. In: Triplett DA, ed. Standardization of coagulation assays: an overview. Skokie: College of American Pathologists, 1982;255–260.

189. Hoyer LW. Immunologic properties of antihemophilic factor. In: Brown EB, ed. Progress in hematology. New York: Grune & Stratton, 1973; 191–221.

190. Holmberg L, Borge L, Ljung R et al. Measurement of antihaemophilic factor A antigen (VIII:CAg) with a solid phase immunoradiometric method based on homologous non-haemophilic antibodies. Scand J Haematol 1979;23:17–24.

191. Dinesen B, Feddersen C. An enzyme immunoassay (ELISA) for the quantitation of human factor VIII coagulant antigen (VIII:CAg). Thromb Res 1983;31:707–718.

192. Goodall AH, Jarvis J, Chand S et al. An immunoradiometric assay for human factor VIII/von Willebrand factor (VIII:vWF) using a monoclonal antibody that defines a functional epitope. Br J Haematol 1985;59:565–577.

193. Hoyer LW, Trabold NC. Immunoradiometric assays for factor VIII antigens: coagulant protein (antihemophilic factor) and factor VIII-related protein (von Willebrand factor). Methods Enzymol 1982;84:51–60.

194. Kelly DA, O'Brien FJ, Hutton RA et al. The effect of liver disease on factors V, VIII and protein C. Br J Haematol 1985;61:541–548.

195. Rose PE, Struthers GS, Robertson M et al. Factor VIII von Willebrand protein in haemolytic uraemic syndrome and systemic vasculitides. Lancet 1990;335:500–502.

196. Bonnar J. Hemostasis and coagulation disorders in pregnancy. In: Haemostasis and thrombosis. New York: Churchill Livingstone, 1981:454–471.

197. Aberg M, Nilsson IM, Vilhardt H. The release of fibrinolytic activator and factor VIII after injection of DDAVP. In: Progress in chemical fibrinolysis and thrombolysis. 4th ed. Edinburgh: Churchill Livingstone, 1979;92–97.

198. Hills LP, Lorenzi-Anderson M, Huey EE et al. Use of a centrifugal analyzer in coagulation testing. Semin Thromb Hemost 1983;9:217–227.

199. Seligsohn U, Osterud B, Rapaport SI. Coupled amidolytic assay for factor VII: its use with a clotting assay to determine the activity state of factor VII. Blood 1978;52:978–988.

200. Avvisati G, ten Cate JW, Van Wijk EM et al. Evaluation of a new chromogenic assay for factor VII and its application in individuals on oral anticoagulant treatment. Br J Haematol 1980;45:343–352.

201. Poggio M, Tripodi A, Mariani G et al. Factor VII clotting assay: influence of different thromboplastins and factor VII-deficient plasmas. CISMEL Study Group. Thromb Haemost 1991;65:160–164.

202. Koller F, Loeliger A, Duckert F. Experiments on a new clotting factor (factor VII). Acta Haematol 1951;6:1–18.

203. Kario K, Matsuo T, Nakao K. Factor VII hyperactivity in the elderly. Thromb Haemost 1991;65:25–27.

204. Roberts HR, Cederbaum AI. The liver and blood coagulation: physiology and pathology. Gastroenterology 1972;63:297–320.

205. Dautzenberg MD, Saudubray JM, Girot R et al. Factor VII deficiency in homocystinuria [Abstract]. Thromb Haemost 1983;50:409.

206. Fadel HE, Krauss JS. Factor VII deficiency and pregnancy. Obstet Gynecol 1989;73:453–454.

207. Mariani G, Mazzucconi MG, Hermans J et al. Factor VII deficiency: immunological characterization of genetic variants and detection of carriers. Br J Haematol 1981;48:7–14.

208. Quick AJ. The assay and properties of labile factor (factor V). J Clin Pathol 1960;13:457–462.

209. Nishibe H. The assay of factor V in plasma using a synthetic chromogenic substrate. Clin Chim Acta 1980;106:301–307.

210. Feinstein DI. Acquired inhibitors of factor V. Thromb Haemost 1978;39: 663–674.

211. Feinstein DI, Rapaport SI, McGehee WG et al. Factor V anticoagulants: clinical, biochemical, and immunological observations. J Clin Invest 1970; 49:1578–1588.

212. Franza BR Jr, Aronson DL. Detection and measurement of low levels of prothrombin. Use of a procoagulant from Echis carinatus venom. Thromb Res 1976;8:329–336.

213. Zimmerman TS, Ratnoff OD, Powell AE. Immunologic differentiation of classic hemophilia (factor VIII deficiency) and von Willebrand's disease, with observations of combined deficiencies of antihemophilic factor and proaccelerin (factor V) and on an acquired circulating anticoagulant against antihemophilic factor. J Clin Invest 1971;50:244–254.

214. Giddings JC, Evans DJ, Bloom AL. Quantitation of factor VIII related antigen (FVIIIRAg) using a laser nephelometer. Thromb Res 1979;15:847–855.

215. Peake IR, Bloom AL. The use of an immunoradiometric assay for factor VIII related antigen in the study of atypical von Willebrand's disease. Thromb Res 1977;10:27–32.

216. Counts RB. Solid-phase immunoradiometric assay of factor VIII protein. Br J Haematol 1975;31:429–436.

217. Ruggeri ZM, Pareti FI, Mannucci PM et al. Heightened interaction between platelets and factor VIII/von Willebrand factor in a new subtype of von Willebrand's disease. N Engl J Med 1980;302:1047–1051.

218. Ruggeri ZM, Zimmerman TS. The complex multimeric composition of factor VIII/von Willebrand factor. Blood 1981;57:1140–1143.

219. Budde U, Schneppenheim R, Plendl H et al. Luminographic detection of von Willebrand factor multimers in agarose gels and on nitrocellulose membranes. Thromb Haemost 1990;63:312–315.

220. MacFarlane DE, Stibbe J, Zucker MB et al. A method for assaying von Willebrand factor (ristocetin cofactor) [Letter]. Thromb Diath Haemorrh 1975;34:306–308.

221. Olson JD, Brockway WJ, Fass DN et al. Evaluation of ristocetin-Willebrand factor assay and ristocetin-induced platelet aggregation. Am J Clin Pathol 1975;63:210–218.

222. Kelton JG, Bishop J, Carter CJ et al. A comparison of the quantitative ristocetin von Willebrand factor assay by using fresh and fixed platelets. Thromb Res 1980;18:477–483.

223. Wright RD, Krauss JS. A comparison of two macroscopic platelet agglutination assays for von Willebrand factor. Ann Clin Lab Sci 1990;20:73–78.

224. Stibbe J, Kirby EP. The influence of Haemaccel, fibrinogen and albumin on ristocetin-induced platelet aggregation. Relevance to the quantitative measurement of the ristocetin cofactor. Thromb Res 1976;8:151–165.

225. Baugh RF, Brown JE, Hougie C. Plasma components which interfere with ristocetin-induced platelet aggregation. Thromb Diath Haemorrh 1975;33: 540–546.

226. Weiss HJ, Meyer D, Rabinowitz R et al. Pseudo-von Willebrand's disease. An intrinsic platelet defect with aggregation by unmodified human factor VIII/von Willebrand factor and enhanced adsorption of its high-molecular-weight multimers. N Engl J Med 1982;306:326–333.

227. Coller BS, Franza JR, Gralnick BR Jr. The pH dependence of quantitative ristocetin-induced platelet aggregation: theoretical and practical implications—A new device for maintenance of platelet-rich plasma pH. Blood 1976;47:841–854.

228. Howard MA, Salem HH, Thomas KB et al. Variant von Willebrand's disease type B-revisited. Blood 1982;60:1420–1428.

229. Brinkhous KM, Graham JE, Cooper HA et al. Assay of von Willebrand factor in von Willebrand's disease and hemophilia: use of a macroscopic platelet aggregation test. Thromb Res 1975;6:267–272.

230. Evans RJ, Austen DE. Assay of ristocetin co-factor using fixed platelets and a platelet counting technique. Br J Haematol 1977;37:289–294.

231. Bird AR, Sacks R, Smith A. Assay of ristocetin cofactor: experience with a platelet counting technique. Med Lab Sci 1984;41:38–45.

232. Schneppenheim R, Budde U, Krey S et al. Results of a screening for von Willebrand disease type 2N in individuals with suspected haemophilia A or von Willebrand disease type 1. Thromb Haemost 1996;76:598–602.

233. Nishino M, Girma JP, Rothschild C et al. New variant of von Willebrand disease with defective binding to factor VIII. Blood 1989;74:1591–1599.

234. Mazurier C, Dieval J, Jorieux S et al. A new von Willebrand factor (VWf) defect in a individual with factor VIII (FVIII) deficiency but with normal

levels and multimeric patterns of both plasma and platelet vWf. Characterization of abnormal vWf/FVIII interaction. Blood 1990;75:20–26.

235. Nesbitt IM, Goodeve AC, Guilliatt AM et al. Characterisation of type 2N von Willebrand disease using phenotypic and molecular techniques. Thromb Haemost 1996;75:959–964.

236. Sarji KE, Nair RMG, Chambers AL. Increased levels of von Willebrand Factor (vWF) and platelet aggregation in diabetes mellitus. Diabetes 1985; 25(suppl 2):398.

237. Maisonneuve P, Sultan Y. Modification of factor VIII complex properties in individuals with liver disease. J Clin Pathol 1977;30:221–227.

238. Harrison RL, McKee PA. Estrogen stimulates von Willebrand factor production by cultured endothelial cells. Blood 1984;63:657–664.

239. Sarji KE, Graves JM, Colwell JA. von Willebrand factor activity in normal subjects: sex difference and variability. Thromb Res 1975;7:885–895.

240. Caekebeke-Peerlinck KM, Koster T, Bri't E. Bleeding time, blood groups and von Willebrand factor. Br J Haematol 1989;73:217–220.

241. Buchanan GR, Holtkamp CA, Levy EN. Racial differences in ristocetin-induced platelet aggregation. Br J Haematol 1981;49:455–464.

242. Bloom AL. von Willebrand factor: clinical features of inherited and acquired disorders. Mayo Clin Proc 1991;66:743–751.

243. Rodeghiero F, Castaman G, Tosetto A. von Willebrand factor antigen is less sensitive than ristocetin cofactor for the diagnosis of type I von Willebrand disease—Results based on an epidemiological investigation. Thromb Haemost 1990;64:349–352.

244. Sadler JE, Matsushita T, Dong Z et al. Molecular mechanism and classification of von Willebrand disease. Thromb Haemost 1995;74:161–166.

245. Miller JL. Sorting out heightened interactions between platelets and von Willebrand factor. "IIB or not IIB?" is becoming an increasingly answerable question in the molecular era. Am J Clin Pathol 1991;96:681–683.

246. Mammen EF. Fibrinogen abnormalities. Semin Thromb Hemost 1983;9: 1–9.

247. Goodwin JF. An evaluation of techniques for the separation and estimation of plasma fibrinogen. Clin Chem 1965;11:63–73.

248. Rampling MW, Gaffney PJ. Measurement of fibrinogen in plasma. In: Davidson JF, Samama MM, Desnoyers PC, eds. Progress in chemical fibrinolysis and thrombolysis. New York: Raven Press, 1976;91–105.

249. National Committee for Clinical Laboratory Standards NCCLS H30-P. Proposed guidelines for a standardization procedure for the determination of fibrinogen in biological samples. Villanova: NCCLS, 1982.

250. Furlan M, Felix R, Escher N et al. How high is the true fibrinogen content of fibrinogen standards? Thromb Res 1989;56:583–592.

251. Palareti G, Maccaferri M, Manotti C et al. Fibrinogen assays: a collaborative study of six different methods. C.I.S.M.E.L. Comitato Italiano per la Standardizzazione dei Metodi in Ematologia e Laboratorio. Clin Chem 1991; 37:714–719.

252. Ellis BC, Stransky A. A quick and accurate method for the determination of fibrinogen in plasma. J Lab Clin Med 1961;58:477–488.

253. Millar HR, Simpson JC, Stalker AL. An evaluation of the heat precipitation method for plasma fibrinogen estimation. J Clin Pathol 1971;24:827–830.

254. Parfentjev IA, Johnson ML, Cliffton EE. The determination of plasma fibrinogen by turbidity with ammonium sulfate. Arch Biochem Biophys 1953;46:470–440.

255. Rampling MW, Gaffney PJ. The sulphite precipitation method for fibrinogen measurement: its use on small samples in the presence of fibrinogen degradation products. Clin Chim Acta 1976;67:43–52.

256. Blomback B. On the properties of fibrinogen and fibrin. Arkiv Kemi 1958; 12:99.

257. Ratnoff OD, Menzie C. A new method for the determination of fibrinogen in small samples of plasma. J Lab Clin Med 1951;37:316–320.

258. Koepke JA. Standardization of fibrinogen assays. Scand J Haematol Suppl 1980;37:130–138.

259. Catt KJ, Hirsh J, Castelan DJ et al. Radioimmunoassay of fibrinogen and its proteolysis products. Thromb Diath Haemorrh 1968;20:1–6.

260. Brittin GM, Rafinia H, Raval D et al. Evaluation of single radial immunodiffusion for quantitation of plasma fibrinogen. Am J Clin Pathol 1972;57: 89–94.

261. Markland FS Jr. Inventory of α and β fibrinogenases from snake venoms. For the Subcommittee on Nomenclature of Exogenous Hemostatic Factors of the Scientific and Standardization Committee of the International Society of Thrombosis and Haemostasis. Thromb Haemost 1991;65:438–443.

262. Funk C, Gmür J, Herold R et al. Reptilase–R-a new reagent in blood coagulation. Br J Haematol 1971;21:43–52.

263. Capel P, Roose A, Vanderpas JB. Discordance between reptilase time measured by the hook manual method and the optical method in individuals with high fibrinogen level. Thromb Haemost 1989;62:1143.

264. Latallo ZS, Teisseyre E. Evaluation of Reptilase R and thrombin clotting time in the presence of fibrinogen degradation products and heparin. Scand J Haematol Suppl 1971;13:261–266.

265. Francis CW, Marder VJ. Mechanisms of fibrinolysis. In: Williams WJ, Beutler E., Erslev AJ, Lichtman MA, eds. Hematology. 4th ed. New York: McGraw-Hill, 1990;1313–1321.

266. Godal HC, Abildgaard U. Gelation of soluble fibrin in plasma by ethanol. Scand J Haematol 1966;3:342–350.

267. Kidder WR, Logan LJ, Rapaport SI et al. The plasma protamine paracoagulation test: clinical and laboratory evaluation. Am J Clin Pathol 1972;58: 675–686.

268. Sanfelippo MJ, Stevens DJ, Koenig RR. Protamine sulfate test for fibrin monomers. Am J Clin Pathol 1971;56:166–173.

269. Merskey C, Kleiner GJ, Johnson AJ. Quantitative estimation of split products of fibrinogen in human serum: Relation to diagnosis and treatment. Blood 1966;28:1–18.

270. Mertens BF, McDuffie FC, Bowie EJ et al. Rapid sensitive method for measuring fibrinogen split-products in human serum. Mayo Clin Proc 1969;44:114–120.

271. Arocha-Piñango CL. A comparison of the TRCII and latex-particle tests for the titration of FR-antigen. J Clin Pathol 1972;25:757–761.

272. Garvey MB, Black JM. The detection of fibrinogen/fibrin degradation products by means of a new antibody-coated latex particle. J Clin Pathol 1972;25:680–682.

273. Connaghan DG, Francis CW, Ryan DH et al. Prevalence and clinical implications of heparin-associated false positive tests for serum fibrin(ogen) degradation products. Am J Clin Pathol 1986;86:304–310.

274. Hedner U. Immunochemical methods for determination of fibrin/fibrinogen degradation products. In: Davidson JF, Samama MM, Desnoyer PC, eds. Progress in chemical fibrinolysis and thrombolysis. New York: Raven Press, 1976;107–125.

275. Smith RT, Ts'ao CH. Fibrin degradation products in the postoperative period. Evaluation of a new latex agglutination method. Am J Clin Pathol 1973;60:644–647.

276. Clarkson AR, MacDonald MK, Petrie JJ et al. Serum and urinary fibrin-fibrinogen degradation products in glomerulonephritis. Br Med J 1971;3: 447–451.

277. Clarkson AR, Morton JB, Cash JD. Urinary fibrin-fibrinogen degradation products after renal homotransplantation. Lancet 1970;2:1220–1223.

278. Allington MJ. Fibrinogen and fibrin degradation products and the clumping of staphylococci by serum. Br J Haematol 1967;13:550–567.

279. Hawiger J, Niewiarowski S, Gurewich V et al. Measurement of fibrinogen and fibrin degradation products in serum by staphylococcal clumping test. J Lab Clin Med 1970;75:93–108.

280. Leeksma OC, Meijer-Huizinga F, Stoepman-van Dalen EA et al. Fibrinopeptide A and the phosphate content of fibrinogen in venous thromboembolism and disseminated intravascular coagulation. Blood 1986;67: 1460–1467.

281. Kockum C, Frebelius S. Rapid radioimmunoassay of human fibrinopeptide A—Removal of cross reacting fibrinogen with bentonite. Thromb Res 1980;19:589–598.

282. Owen J. The utility of plasma fibrinopeptide assays. Thromb Haemost 1989;62:807–810.

283. Alkjaersig N, Fletcher AP. Catabolism and excretion of fibrinopeptide-A. Blood 1982;60:148–156.

284. Nossel HL, Yudelman I, Canfield RE et al. Measurement of fibrinopeptide A in human blood. J Clin Invest 1974;54:43–53.

285. Walenga JM, Fareed J, Mariani G et al. Diagnostic efficacy of a simple radioimmunoassay test for fibrinogen/fibrin fragments containing the Bβ15-42 sequence. Semin Thromb Hemost 1984;10:252–263.

286. Nossel HL. Fibrinopeptide A measurements in the study of thrombosis [Abstract]. Thromb Haemost 1977;38:171.

287. Davies GC, Sobel M, Salzman EW. Plasma thromboxane B$_2$ (TXB$_2$) and fibrinopeptide A (FpA) in individuals with thrombosis and during contact of blood with artificial surfaces [Abstract]. Thromb Haemost 1979;42:72.

288. Dudczak R, Niessner H, Thaler E et al. Beta thromboglobulin (βTG), platelet factor 4 (PF4) and fibrinopeptide A (FPA) in individuals with porcine (PO) and prosthetic (PR) heart valves [Abstract]. Thromb Haemost 1979; 42:72.

289. Miller GJ, Bauer KA, Barzegar S et al. The effects of quality and timing of venepuncture on markers of blood coagulation in healthy middle-aged men. Thromb Haemost 1995;73:82–86.

290. Dempfle CE, Pfitzner SA, Dollman M et al. Comparison of immunological and functional assays for measurement of soluble fibrin. Thromb Haemost 1995;74:673–679.

291. Wieding JU, Hosius C. Determination of soluble fibrin: a comparison of four different methods. Thromb Res 1992;65:745–756.

292. Grau E, Linares M, Estany A et al. Utility of D dimer in the diagnosis of deep venous thrombosis in outpatients [Letter]. Thromb and Haemost 1991;66:510.

293. Gormsen J, Feddersen C. Demonstration of different D- and E-antigenic intermediates during plasmin digestion of non-stabilized and stabilized fibrin clots. Scand J Haematol 1973;10:337–348.

294. Chang-Liem GS, Lustermans FA, van Wersch JW. Comparison of the appropriateness of the latex and Elisa plasma D-dimer determination for the diagnosis of deep venous thrombosis. Haemostasis 1991;21:106–110.

295. Rowbotham BJ, Carroll P, Whitaker AN et al. Measurement of crosslinked fibrin derivatives—Use in the diagnosis of venous thrombosis. Thromb Haemost 1987;57:59–61.

296. Speiser W, Mallek R, Koppensteiner R et al. D-dimer and TAT measurement in individuals with deep venous thrombosis: utility in diagnosis and

judgment of anticoagulant treatment effectiveness. Thromb Haemost 1990; 64:196–201.

297. Boneu B, Bes G, Pelzer H et al. D-dimers, thrombin anithrombin III complexes and prothrombin fragments 1 + 2: diagnostic value in clinically suspected deep vein thrombosis. Thromb Haemost 1991;65:28–31.

298. Greenberg CS, Devine DV, McCrae KM. Measurement of plasma fibrin D-dimer levels with the use of a monoclonal antibody coupled to latex beads. Am J Clin Pathol 1987;87:94–100.

299. Chapman CS, Akhtar N, Campbell S et al. The use of D-Dimer assay by enzyme immunoassay and latex agglutination techniques in the diagnosis of deep vein thrombosis. Clin Lab Haematol 1990;12:37–42.

300. van Beek EJ, van den Ende B, Berckmans RJ et al. A comparative analysis of D-dimer assays in individuals with clinically suspected pulmonary embolism. Thromb Haemost 1993;70:408–413.

301. Charles LA, Edwards T, Macik BG. Evaluation of sensitivity and specificity of six D-Dimer latex assays. Arch Pathol Lab Med 1994;118:1102–1105.

302. Eisenberg PR, Jaffe AS, Stump DC et al. Validity of enzyme-linked immunosorbent assays of crosslinked fibrin degradation products as a measure of clot lysis. Circulation 1990;82:1159–1168.

303. Koppert PW, Hoegee-de Nobel E, Nieuwenhuizen W. A monoclonal antibody-based enzyme immunoassay for fibrin degradation products in plasma. Thromb Haemost 1988;59:310–315.

304. Elias A, Aptel I, Huc B et al. D-Dimer test and diagnosis of deep vein thrombosis: a comparative study of 7 assays. Thromb Haemost 1996;76: 518–522.

305. Ginsberg JS, Wells PS, Brill-Edwards P et al. Application of a novel and rapid whole blood assay for D-Dimer in individuals with clinically suspected pulmonary embolism. Thromb Haemost 1995;73:35–38.

306. John MA, O'Reilly EJ, Rylatt DB et al. The simpliRED D-dimer test: a novel assay for the detection of crosslinked fibrin degradation products in whole blood. Thromb Res 1990;58:273–281.

307. McDonagh J. Structure and function of factor XIII. In: Colman RW, Mirsh J, Marder VJ, Salzman EW, eds. Hemostasis and thrombosis: basic principles and clinical practice. Philadelphia: JB Lippincott, 1987:292.

308. Mammen EF. Factor XIII deficiency. Semin Thromb Hemost 1983;9:10–12.

309. Francis JL. The detection and measurement of factor XIII activity: a Review. Med Lab Sci 1980;37:137–147.

310. Losowsky MS, Hall R, Goldie W. Congenital deficiency of fibrin stabilising factor. Lancet 1965;2:156–158.

311. Duckert F, Jung E, Shmerling DH. A hitherto undescribed congenital haemorrhagic diathesis probably due to fibrin stabilizing factor deficiency. Thromb Diath Haemorrh 1960;5:179–186.

312. Ikkala E, Nevanlinna HR. Congenital deficiency of fibrin stabilizing factor. Thromb Diath Haemorrh 1962;7:567–571.

313. Fickenscher K, Aab A, Stuber W. A photometric assay for blood coagulation factor XIII. Thromb Haemost 1991;65:535–540.

314. La Croix KA, Davis GL. A Review of protein C and its role in hemostasis. J Med Technol 1985;2:95–98.

315. Bertina RM, Broekmans AW, Krommenhoek-van Es C et al. The use of a functional and immunologic assay for plasma protein C in the study of the heterogeneity of congenital protein C deficiency. Thromb Haemost 1984;51:1–5.

316. Francis RB Jr, Patch MJ. A functional assay for protein C in human plasma. Thromb Res 1983;32:605–613.

317. Sala N, Owen WG, Collen D. Functional assay of protein C in human plasma. Thromb Haemost 1984;63:671–675.

318. Miletich JP. Laboratory diagnosis of protein C deficiency. Semin Thromb Hemost 1990;16:169–176.

319. Comp PC, Nixon RR, Esmon CT. Determination of functional levels of protein C, an antithrombotic protein, using thrombin-thrombomodulin complex. Blood 1984;63:15–21.

320. Mannucci PM, Boyer C, Tripodi A. Multicenter comparison of five functional and two immunological assays for protein C. Thromb Haemost 1987;57:44–48.

321. Martinolli JL, Stocker K. Fast functional protein C assay using protac, a novel protein C activator. Thromb Res 1986;43:253–264.

322. Vukovich TC, Knobl PN, Bauer K et al. Quantitative determination of human protein C. Evaluation of a "fast" functional assay in comparison to a "traditional" functional and an immunological assay. Thromb Res 1988;49:169–179.

323. Bertina RM. An international collaborative study on the performance of protein C antigen assays. Report of the ICTH subcommittee on protein C. International Committee on Thrombosis and Haemostasis. Thromb Haemost 1987;57:112–117.

324. Gonzalez R, Alberca I, Vicente V. Protein C levels in late pregnancy, postpartum and in women on oral contraceptives. Thromb Res 1985;39: 637–640.

325. Mannucci PM, Vigano S, Bottasso B et al. Protein C antigen during pregnancy, delivery and puerperium [Letter]. Thromb Haemost 1984;52:217.

326. Ford I, Li TC, Cooke ID et al. Changes in haematological indices, blood viscosity and inhibitors of coagulation during treatment of endometriosis and Danazol. Thromb Haemost 1994;72:218–221.

327. Granata A, Sobbrio GA, D'Arrigo F et al. Changes in the plasma levels of

328. Bauer KA. Management of individuals with hereditary defects predisposing to thrombosis including pregnant women. Thromb Haemost 1995;74: 94–100.

329. Vigano S, Mannucci PM, Solinas SB et al. Decrease in protein C antigen and formation of an abnormal protein soon after starting oral anticoagulant therapy. Br J Haematol 1984;57:213–220.

330. Rodeghiero F, Mannucci PM, Vigano S et al. Liver dysfunction rather than intravascular coagulation as the main cause of low protein C and antithrombin III in acute leukemia. Blood 1984;63:965–969.

331. Freyssinet JM, Cazenave JP. Lupus-like anticoagulants, modulation of the protein C pathway and thrombosis [Review]. Thromb Haemost 1987;58: 679–681.

332. Francis RB, Patch MJ. A comparative study of commercial PTT reagents in a PTT-based functional protein C assay. Thromb Res 1984;36:481–483.

333. Girault C, Gufflet V, Robert A. The effect of lupus anticoagulant (LA) on clotting assay for plasma protein C (PC) [Letter]. Thromb Haemost 1991; 66:389.

334. Marlar RA, Adcock DM, Madden RM. Hereditary dysfunctional protein C molecules (type II): assay characterization and proposed classification. Thromb Haemost 1990;63:375–379.

335. Marlar RA, Montgomery RR, Broekmans AW. Report on the diagnosis and treatment of homozygous protein C deficiency. Thromb Haemost 1989;61: 529–531.

336. Karpatkin M, Mannuccio Mannucci P, Bhogal M et al. Low protein C in the neonatal period. Br J Haematol 1986;62:137–142.

337. Marlar RA, Neumann A. Neonatal purpura fulminans due to homozygous protein C or protein S deficiencies. Semin Thromb Hemost 1990;16: 299–309.

338. Melissari E, Scully MF, Ellis V et al. Severe antigenic deficiency of protein C associated with moderate deficiency of protein C activity. Thromb Res 1985;39:641–644.

339. Bauer KA, Weiss LM, Sparrow D et al. Aging-associated changes in indices of thrombin generation and protein C activation in humans. J Clin Invest 1987;80:1527–1534.

340. Harper PL, Edgar PF, Luddington RJ. Protein C deficiency and portal thrombosis in liver transplantation in children. Lancet 1988;2:924–927.

341. Pabinger I, Kyrle PA, Speiser W et al. Diagnosis of protein C deficiency in individuals on oral anticoagulant treatment: comparison of three different functional protein c assays. Thromb Haemost 1990;63:407–412.

342. Han P, Fung KP, Rahdakrishnan U. Lack of agreement of chromogenic and clotting assays for factor X and protein C in warfarinised plasma. Thromb Haemost 1991;65:360–363.

343. Schofield KP, Thomson JM, Poller L. Protein C response to induction and withdrawal of oral anticoagulant treatment. Clin Lab Haematol 1987;9: 255–262.

344. George AJ. The laboratory investigation of thrombotic disorders. Part 2. The protein C pathway. In: Williams CE, Short G, Entwistle MBP, eds. Critical factors in haemostasis. Chichester: Ellis Horwood, 1988:144.

345. Hessing M. The interaction between complement component C4b-binding protein and the vitamin K-dependent protein S forms a link between blood coagulation and the complement system. Biochemistry 1991;277:581–592.

346. Comp PC. Measurement of the natural anticoagulant protein S. How and when. Am J Clin Pathol 1990;94:242–243.

347. Wolf M, Boyer-Neumann C, Martinolli JL et al. A new functional assay for human protein S activity using activated factor Va as substrate. Thromb Haemost 1989;62:1144–1145.

348. Han P, Pradham M. A simple functional protein S assay using PROTAC. Clin Lab Haematol 1990;12:201–208.

349. Suzuki K, Nishioka J. Plasma protein S activity measured using Protac, a snake venom derived activator of protein C. Thromb Res 1988;49:241–251.

350. Comp PC. Laboratory evaluation of protein S status. Semin Thromb Hemost 1990;16:177–181.

351. Krachmalnicoff A, Tombesi S, Valsecchi C et al. A monoclonal antibody to human protein S used as the capture antibody for measuring total protein S by enzyme immunoassay. Clin Chem 1990;36:43–46.

352. Girolami A, Simioni P, Lazzaro AR. Peculiar rocket profile in the electroimmunoassay of protein-S-deficient plasma: a clue to diagnosis? [Letter]. Clin Lab Haematol 1990;12:109–111.

353. Bertina RM, van Wijngaarden A, Reinalda-Poot J et al. Determination of plasma protein S: the protein cofactor of activated plasma protein C. Thromb Haemost 1985;53:268–272.

354. Woodhams BJ. The simultaneous measurement of total and free protein S by ELISA. Thromb Res 1988;50:213–220.

355. Edson JR, Vogt JM, Huesman DA. Laboratory diagnosis of inherited protein S deficiency. Am J Clin Pathol 1990;94:176–186.

356. Aillaud MF, Pouymayou K, Brunet D et al. New direct assay of free protein S antigen applied to diagnosis of protein S deficiency. Thromb Haemost 1996;75:283–285.

357. Taylor FB Jr. Protein S, C4b binding protein and the hypercoagulable state. J Lab Clin Med 1992;119:596–597.

358. Pui CH, Chesney CM, Bergum PW et al. Lack of pathogenetic role of

proteins C and S in thrombosis associated with asparaginase-prednisone-vincristine therapy for leukaemia. Br J Haematol 1986;64:283–290.

359. D'Angelo A, Vigano-D'Angelo S, Esmon CT et al. Acquired deficiencies of protein S. Protein S activity during oral anticoagulation, in liver disease, and in disseminated intravascular coagulation. J Clin Invest 1988;81:1445–1454.

360. Vigano-D'Angelo S, D'Angelo A, Kaufman CE Jr. Protein S deficiency occurs in the nephrotic syndrome. Ann Intern Med 1987;107:42–47.

361. Malm J, Bennhagen R, Holmberg L et al. Plasma concentrations of C4b-binding protein and vitamin K-dependent protein S in term and preterm infants: low levels of protein S-C4b-binding protein complexes. Br J Haematol 1988;68:445–449.

362. Comp PC, Vigano S, D'Angelo A et al. Acquired protein S deficiency occurs in pregnancy, the nephrotic syndrome and acute systemic lupus erythematosus. Blood 1985;66(S):348a.

363. Gris JC, Toulon P, Brun S et al. The relationship between plasma microparticles, protein S and anticardiolipin antibodies in individuals with human immunodeficiency virus infection. Thromb Haemost 1996;76:38–45.

364. Crowther MA, Johnston M, Weitz J et al. Free protein S deficiency may be found in individuals with antiphospholipid antibodies who do not have systemic lupus erythematosus. Thromb Haemost 1996;76:689–691.

365. Faioni EM, Boyer-Neumann C, Franchi F et al. Another protein S functional assay is sensitive to resistance to activated protein C [Letter]. Thromb Haemost 1994;72:648.

366. van der Velden PA, Krommenhoek-Van Es T, Allaart CF et al. A frequent thrombomodulin amino acid dimorphism is not associated with thrombophilia. Thromb Haemost 1991;65:511–513.

367. Martinuzzo ME, Forastiero RR, Carreras LO. Increased plasma thrombomodulin in different subgroups of individuals with antiphospholipid and anti $\beta_2$ glycoprotein I antibodies [Letter]. Thromb Haemost 1996;75:971–973.

368. Dahlbäck B, Carlsson M, Svensson PJ. Familial thrombophilia due to a previously unrecognized mechanism characterized by poor anticoagulant response to activated protein C: prediction of a cofactor to activated protein C. Proc Natl Acad Sci U S A 1993;90:1004–1008.

369. Dahlbäck B. Physiological anticoagulation. Resistance to activated protein C and venous thromboembolism. J Clin Invest 1994;94:923–927.

370. Bertina RM, Koeleman BPC, Koester T et al. Mutation in blood coagulation factor V associated with resistance to activated protein C. Nature 1994;369:64–67.

371. Lane DA, Mannucci PM, Bauer KA et al. Inherited thrombophilia: Part 1 [Review]. Thromb Haemost 1996;76:651–662.

372. de Ronde H, Bertina RM. Laboratory diagnosis of APC-resistance: a critical evaluation of the test and the development of diagnostic criteria. Thromb Haemost 1994;72:880–886.

373. Freyburger G, Bilhou-Nabera C, Dief S et al. Technical and biological conditions influencing the functional APC resistance test. Thromb Haemost 1996;75:460–465.

374. Denson KWE, Reed SV, Haddon ME. The modified APC resistance test [Letter]. Thromb Haemost 1995;74:995.

375. Henkens CM, Bom VJ, Seinen AJ et al. Sensitivity to activated protein C: Influence of oral contraceptives and sex. Thromb Haemost 1995;73:402–404.

376. Uttenreuther-Fischer MM, Ziemer S, Gaedicke G. Resistance to activated protein C (APCR): reference values of APC-ratios for children [Letter]. Thromb Haemost 1996;76:813–814.

377. Nowak-Göttl U, Kohlhase B, Vielhaber H et al. APC resistance in neonates and infants: adjustment of the APTT-based method. Thromb Res 1996;81:665–670.

378. Kraus M, Noah M, Fickenscher K. The PCAT—a simple screening assay for assessing the functionality of the protein C anticoagulant pathway. Thromb Res 1995;79:217–222.

379. Nicolaes GA, Thomassen CL, van Oerle R et al. A prothrombinase-based assay for detection of resistance to activated protein C. Thromb Haemost 1996;76:404–410.

380. Blasczyk R, Ritter M, Thiede C et al. Simple and rapid detection of factor V Leiden by allele-specific PCR amplification. Thromb Haemost 1996;75:757–759.

381. Dahlbäck B. Resistance to activate protein C, the Arg[506] to Gln mutation in the factor V gene, and venous thrombosis. Functional tests and DNA-based assays, pros and cons. Thromb Haemost 1995;73:739–742.

382. Corral J, Iniesta JA, González-Conejero R et al. Detection of factor V Leiden from a drop of blood by PCR-SSCP. Thromb Haemost 1996;76:735–737.

383. Kirschbaum NE, Foster PA. The polymerase chain reaction with sequence specific primers for the detection of the factor V mutation associated with activated protein C resistance. Thromb Haemost 1995;74:874–878.

384. Nagy I, Losonczy H. Three types of antithrombin III deficiency. Thromb Haemost 42:187a.

385. Bick RL, Kovacs I, Fekete LF. A new two-stage functional assay for antithrombin III (heparin cofactor): clinical and laboratory evaluation. Thromb Res 1976;8:745–756.

386. Tollefsen DM. Laboratory diagnosis of antithrombin and heparin cofactor II deficiency [Review]. Semin Thromb Hemost 1990;16:162–168.

387. Savidge GF, Kesteven PJ, AL-Hasani SF et al. Rapid quantitation of plasma heparin and antithrombin III levels for cardiopulmonary bypass monitoring, using fluorometric substrate assays. Thromb Haemost 1983;50:745–748.

388. Bick RL, Wheeler A, Camposano N. A comparative study of the DuPont antithrombin III and fibrinogen assay systems. Am J Clin Pathol 1985;83:541–546.

389. Mitchell GA, Hudson PM, Huseby RM. Fluorescent substrate assay for antithrombin III. Thromb Res 1978;12:219–225.

390. Friberger P, Egberg N, Holmer E et al. Antithrombin assay—the use of bovine thrombin and the observation of a "second" heparin cofactor. Thromb Res 1982;25:433–436.

391. Tran TH, Duckert F. Influence of heparin cofactor II (HCII) on the determination of antithrombin III (AT). Thromb Res 1985;40:571–576.

392. Hultin MB, McKay J, Abildgaard U. Antithrombin Oslo: type Ib classification of the first reported antithrombin-deficient family, with a Review of hereditary antithrombin variants [Review]. Thromb Haemost 1988;59:468–473.

393. Murayama H, Matsuda M. Abnormal properties and behaviors of antithrombin III found in a thrombophilic individual: defective biological functions and dissimilar antigenic determinants. Thromb Haemost 1986;56:165–171.

394. Knot E, Ten Cate JW, Drijfhout HR et al. Antithrombin III metabolism in individuals with liver disease. J Clin Pathol 1984;37:523–530.

395. Kauffmann RH, Veltkamp JJ, van Tilburg NH et al. Acquired antithrombin III deficiency and thrombosis in the nephrotic syndrome. Am J Med 1978;65:607–613.

396. Marciniak E, Gockerman JP. Heparin-induced decrease in circulating antithrombin-III. Lancet 1977;2:581–584.

397. Fagerhol MK, Abildgaard U. Immunological studies on human antithrombin III: influence of age, sex, and use of oral contraceptives on serum concentration. Scand J Haematol 1970;7:10–17.

398. Wessler S, Gitel SN. Thrombotic complications of oral contraceptives. In: Colman RW, Hirsh J, Marder VJ, Salzman EW, eds. Hemostasis and thrombosis: basic principles and clinical practice. Philadelphia: JB Lippincott, 1987;1158–1164.

399. Rodeghiero F, Tosetto A. The VITA project: population-based distributions of protein C, antithrombin III, heparin-cofactor II and plasminogen–relationship with physiological variables and establishment of reference ranges. Thromb Haemost 1996;76:226–233.

400. Lane DA, Ireland H, Olds RJ et al. Antithrombin III: a database of mutations. Thromb Haemost 1991;66:657–661.

401. Abildgaard U, Larsen ML. Assay of dermatan sulfate cofactor (heparin cofactor II) activity in human plasma. Thromb Res 1984;35:257–266.

402. Tollefsen DM. Insight into the mechanism of action of heparin cofactor II. Thromb Haemost 1995;74:1209–1214.

403. Tollefsen DM, Pestka CA. Heparin cofactor II activity in individuals with disseminated intravascular coagulation and hepatic failure. Blood 1985;66:769–774.

404. Andersson TR, Larsen ML, Handeland GF et al. Heparin cofactor II activity in plasma: application of an automated assay method to the study of a normal adult population. Scand J Haematol 1986;36:96–102.

405. Toulon P, Bardin JM, Blumenfeld N. Increased heparin cofactor II levels in women taking oral contraceptives. Thromb Haemost 1990;64:365–368.

406. Toulon P, Moulonguet-Doleris L, Costa JM et al. Heparin cofactor II deficiency in renal allograft recipients: no correlation with the development of thrombosis. Thromb Haemost 1991;65:20–24.

407. Abildgaard U, Sandset PM, Andersson TR et al. The inhibitor of F VIIa in plasma measured with a sensitive chromogenic substrate assay: comparison with antithrombin, protein C and heparin cofactor II in a clinical material. Folia Haematol Int Mag Klin Morph Blutforsch 1988;115:274–277.

408. Toulon P, Lamine M, Ledjev I et al. Heparin cofactor II deficiency in individuals infected with the human immunodeficiency virus. Thromb Haemost 1993;70:730–735.

409. Abbink JJ, Nuijens JH, Eerenberg AJ et al. Quantification of functional and inactivated $\alpha_2$-macroglobulin in sepsis. Thromb Haemost 1991;65:32–39.

410. Sandset PM, Abildgaard U, Pettersen M. A sensitive assay of extrinsic pathway inhibitor (EPI) in plasma and plasma fractions. Thromb Res 1987;47:389–400.

411. Abumiya T, Yamaguchi T, Terasaki T et al. Decreased plasma tissue factor pathway inhibitor activity in ischemic stroke individuals. Thromb Haemost 1995;74:1050–1054.

412. Pedersen AH, Nordfang O, Norris F et al. Recombinant human extrinsic pathway inhibitor. Production, isolation, and characterization of its inhibitory activity on tissue factor-initiated coagulation reactions. J Biol Chem 1990;265:16786–16793.

413. Kobayashi M, Wada H, Wakita Y et al. Decreased plasma tissue factor pathway inhibitor levels in individuals with thrombotic thrombocytopenic purpura. Thromb Haemost 1995;73:10.

414. Ganrot PO. Determination of $\alpha_2$ macroglobulin as trypsin-protein esterase. Clin Chim Acta 1966;14:493–501.

415. Ganrot PO, Schersten B. Serum $\alpha_2$ macroglobulin concentration and its variation with age and sex. Clin Chim Acta 1967;15:113–120.

416. Giddings JC. Naturally occurring inhibitors. In: Giddings JC, ed. Molecular genetics and immunoanalysis in blood coagulation. Chichester: Ellis Horwood, 1988:143–162.

417. Arnesen H, Fagerhol MK. $\alpha_2$-Macroglobulin, $\alpha_1$-antitrypsin and antithrombin III in plasma and serum during fibrinolytic therapy with urokinase. Scand J Clin Lab Invest 1972;29:259–263.

418. Harpel PC. C$_1$ Inactivator. In: Lorand L, ed. Methods in enzymology. New York: Academic Press, 1976;751–760.

419. Pelzer H, Stuber W, Dati F et al. New trends in the field of coagulation diagnosis—new possibilities to improve monitoring of antithrombotic therapy. Folia Haematol Int Mag Klin Morphol Blutforsch 1989;116: 867–871.

420. Pelzer H, Schwarz A, Stuber W. Determination of human prothrombin activation fragment 1 + 2 in plasma with an antibody against a synthetic peptide. Thromb Haemost 1991;65:153–159.

421. Lau HK, Rosenberg JS, Beeler DL et al. The isolation and characterization of a specific antibody population directed against the prothrombin activation fragments F$_2$ and F$_{1+2}$. J Biol Chem 1979;254:8751–8761.

422. Mannucci PM, Bottasso B, Tripodi A et al. Prothrombin fragment 1 + 2 and intensity of treatment with oral anticoagulants. Thromb Haemost 1991;66:741.

423. Erickson LA, Schleef RR, Ny T et al. The fibrinolytic system of the vascular wall. Clin Haematol 1985;14:513–530.

424. Hoek JA, Nurmohamed MT, ten Cate JW et al. Thrombin-antithrombin III complexes in the prediction of deep vein thrombosis following total hip replacement. Thromb Haemost 1989;62:1050–1052.

425. Shimizu H, Ohtani KI, Tanaka Y et al. Increased plasma thrombin-antithrombin III complex levels in non-insulin dependent diabetic individuals with albuminuria are reduced by ethyl icosapentatenoate. Thromb Haemost 1995;74:1231–1234.

426. Gaffney PJ. Standards in fibrinolysis—current status and future challenges. Thromb Haemost 1995;74:1389–1397.

427. Tripodi A, Chantarangkul V, Bottasso B et al. Poor comparability of prothrombin fragment 1 + 2 values measured by two commercial ELISA methods: influence of different anticoagulants and standards. Thromb Haemost 1994;71:605–608.

428. Leroy-Mathurin C, Gouault-Heilmann M. Influence of conditions of blood sampling on coagulation activation markers (prothrombin fragment 1 + 2, thrombin-antithrombin complexes and D-dimers) measurements. Thromb Res 1994;74:399–407.

429. D'Angelo A, Della Valle P, Calori G et al. Harmonization of commercial ELISA methods for the measurement of prothrombin fragment 1.2: is it feasible? [Letter]. Thromb Haemost 1995;73:548.

430. Tripodi A, Chantarangkul V, Braga M et al. Comparison of commercial ELISA methods for the measurement of prothrombin fragment 1 + 2—rebuttal [Letter]. Thromb Haemost 1995;73:549–550.

431. von Kaulla KN, von Kaulla E. Remarks on the euglobulin lysis time. In: Davidson JF, Samama MM, Desnoyers PC, eds. Progress in chemical fibrinolysis and thrombolysis. New York: Raven Press, 1975:131–149.

432. Mahmoud M, Gaffney PJ. Bioimmunoassay (BIA) of tissue plasminogen activator (tPA) and its specific inhibitor (tpa/INH). Thromb Haemost 1985;53:356–359.

433. Westlund LE, Andersson LO. Studies on the influence of reactants and buffer environment on clot lysis induced by human plasminogen activators. Thromb Res 1985;37:213–223.

434. Bonnar J, McNicol GP, Douglas AS. Coagulation and fibrinolytic systems in pre-eclampsia and eclampsia. Br Med J 1971;2:12–16.

435. Kluft C, Brakman P, Veldhuyzen-Stolk EC. Screening of fibrinolytic activity in plasma euglobulin fractions on the fibrin plate. In: Davidson JF, Samama MM, Desnoyers PC, eds. Progress in chemical fibrinolysis and thrombolysis. New York: Raven Press, 1976:57–65.

436. Urano T, Sakakibara K, Rydzewski A, Urano S. Relationships between euglobulin clot lysis time and the plasma levels of tissue plasminogen activator and plasminogen activator inhibitor. Thromb Haemost 1990;63: 82–86.

437. Marsh NA, Arocha-Pinango CL. Evaluation of the fibrin plate method for estimating plasminogen activators. Thromb Diath Haemorrh 1972;28: 75–88.

438. Brakman P, Traas DW. Assay of plasminogen in blood on fibrin plates. In: Davidson JF, Samama MM, Desnoyers PC, eds. Progress in chemical fibrinolysis and thrombolysis. New York: Raven Press, 1976:79–82.

439. Astrup T, Mullertz S. The fibrin plate method for estimating fibrinolytic activity. Arch Biochem 1952;40:346–351.

440. Carlson RH, Garnick RL, Jones AJ et al. The determination of recombinant human tissue-type plasminogen activator activity by turbidimetry using a microcentrifugal analyzer. Anal Biochem 1988;168:428–435.

441. Jones AJ, Meunier AM. A precise and rapid microtitre plate clot lysis assay: methodology, kinetic modeling and measurement of catalytic constants for plasminogen activation during fibrinolysis. Thromb Haemost 1990;64:455–463.

442. Alkjaersig N, Fletcher AP, Sherry S. The mechanism of clot dissolution by plasmin. J Clin Invest 1959;38:1086–1095.

443. Knos M, Friberger P. Methods for plasminogen determination in human

444. Lassen M. Heat denaturation of plasminogen in the fibrin plate method. Acta Physiol Scand 1952;27:371–376.

445. Rabiner SF, Goldfine ID, Hart A et al. Radioimmunoassay of human plasminogen and plasmin. J Lab Clin Med 1969;74:265–273.

446. Robbins KC. Classification of abnormal plasminogens: dysplasminogenemias. Semin Thromb Hemost 1990;16:217–220.

447. Prentice CR. Acquired coagulation disorders. Clin Haematol 1985;14: 413–422.

448. Ekelund H, Hedner U, Nilsson IM. Fibrinolysis in newborns. Acta Paediatr Scand 1970;59:33–43.

449. Yang G, Green D. Plasminogen, alpha$_2$-antiplasmin, and protein C decline following infusions of recombinant tissue plasminogen activator. Semin Thromb Hemost 1990;16:242–244.

450. Gram J, Munkvad S, Jespersen J. Elevated plasma concentrations of fibrinogen may cause an overestimation of functional plasminogen [Letter]. Thromb Haemost 1989;61:154.

451. Lawson DE, Mitchell GA, Huseby RM. A sensitive fluorescent assay for determining $\alpha_2$-plasmin inhibitor using a synthetic substrate. Thromb Res 1979;14:323–332.

452. Aoki N, Yamanaka T. The $\alpha_2$-plasmin inhibitor levels in liver diseases. Clin Chim Acta 1978;84:99–105.

453. Aoki N, Saito H, Kamiya T et al. Congenital deficiency of a $\alpha2$-plasmin inhibitor associated with severe hemorrhagic tendency. J Clin Invest 1979; 63:877–884.

454. Nicoloso G, Hauert J Kruithof EK et al. Fibrinolysis in normal subjects—comparison between plasminogen activator inhibitor and other components of the fibrinolytic system. Thromb Haemost 1988;59:299–303.

455. Juhan-Vague I, Moerman B, De Cock F et al. Plasma levels of a specific inhibitor of tissue plasminogen activator (and urokinase) in normal and pathological conditions. Thromb Res 1984;33:523–530.

456. Rijken DC, Juhan-Vague I, DeCock F et al. Measurement of human tissue-type plasminogen activator by a two site immunoradiometric assay. J Lab Clin Med 1983;101:274–284.

457. Bergsdorf N, Nilsson T, Wallén P. An enzyme linked immunosorbent assay for determination of tissue plasminogen activator applied to individuals with thromboembolic disease. Thromb Haemost 1983;50:740–744.

458. Gaffney PJ, Curtis AD. A collaborative study of a proposed international standard for tissue plasminogen activator (t-PA). Thromb Haemost 1985; 53:134–136.

459. Wiman B, Mellbring G, Ranby M. Plasminogen activator release during venous stasis and exercise as determined by a new specific assay. Clin Chim Acta 1983;127:279–288.

460. Kruithof EK, Nicoloso G, Gudinchet A et al. Plasminogen activator inhibitor (PAI) activity as well as PAI-1 and PAI-2 antigen in healthy individuals and hospitalized individuals [Abstract 12]. Thromb Haemost 1987;58:3.

461. Krishnamurti C, Tang DB, Barr CF et al. Plasminogen activator and plasminogen activator inhibitor activities in a reference population. Am J Clin Pathol 1988;89:747–752.

462. Ranby M, Bergsdorf N, Nilsson T et al. Age dependence of tissue plasminogen activator concentrations in plasma, as studied by an improved enzyme-linked immunosorbent assay. Clin Chem 1986;32:2160–2165.

463. Kluft C, Jie AF, Rijken DC et al. Daytime fluctuations in blood of tissue-type plasminogen activator (t-PA) and its fast-acting inhibitor (PAI-1). Thromb Haemost 1988;59:329–332.

464. Fearnley GR, Balmforth G, Fearnley E. Evidence of a diurnal fibrinolytic rhythm: With a simple method of measuring natural fibrinolysis. Clin Sci 1957;16:645–650.

465. Chmielewska J, Ranby M, Wiman B. Evidence for a rapid inhibitor to tissue plasminogen activator in plasma. Thromb Res 1983;31:427–433.

466. Variel EG, Baye B, Toulemond F. Increase of plasminogen activator release by heparins and other sulphated polysaccharides. In: Davidson JF, Bachmann F., Bouvier CA et al, eds. Progress in fibrinolysis. Edinburgh: Churchill Livingstone, 1983;577–580.

467. Gram J, Declerck PJ, Sidelmann J et al. Multicentre evaluation of commercial kit methods: plasminogen activator inhibitor activity. Thromb Haemost 1993;70:852–857.

468. Mannucci PM, Kluft C, Traas DW et al. Congenital plasminogen deficiency associated with venous thromboembolism: therapeutic trial with stanozolol. Br J Haematol 1986;63:753–759.

469. Hessel LW, Kluft C. Advances in clinical fibrinolysis. Clin Haematol 1986; 15:443–463.

470. Landin K, Tengborn L, Chimielewska J et al. The acute effect of insulin on tissue plasminogen activator and plasminogen activator inhibitor in man. Thromb Haemost 1991;65:130–133.

471. Kruithof EK, Gudinchet A, Bachmann F. Plasminogen activator inhibitors 1 and plasminogen activator inhibitor 2 in various disease states. Thromb Haemost 1988;59:7–12.

472. Erickson LA, Hekman CM, Loskutoff DJ. The primary plasminogen activator inhibitor in endothelial cells, platelets, serum and plasma are immunologically related. Proc Natl Acad Sci U S A 1985;82:8710–8714.

plasma and for streptokinase standardisation. In: Davidson JF, Cepelak V, Samama MM, Desnoyers PC, eds. Progress in chemical fibrinolysis and thrombolysis. Edinburgh: Churchill Livingstone, 1979;154–158.

473. Ranby M, Norrman IB, Wallen P. A sensitive assay for tissue plasminogen activator. Thromb Res 1982;27:743–749.

474. MacGregor IR, Booth NA. An enzyme-linked immunosorbent assay (ELISA) used to study the cellular secretion of endothelial plasminogen activator inhibitor (PAI-1). Thromb Haemost 1988;59:68–72.

475. Speiser W, Bowry S, Anders E et al. Method for the determination of fast acting plasminogen activator inhibitor capacity (PAI-CAP) in plasma, platelets and endothelial cells. Thromb Res 1986;44:503–515.

476. Keber D, Blinc A, Fettich J. Increase of tissue plasminogen activator in limbs during venous occlusion: a simple haemodynamic model. Thromb Haemost 1990;64:433–437.

477. Jennings I, Luddington RJ, Harper PL. Changes in endothelial-related coagulation proteins in response to venous occlusion. Thromb Haemost 1991;65:374–376.

478. Lijnen HR, Collen D. Natural inhibitors of fibrinolysis. In: Bloom AL, Thomas DP, eds. Haemostasis and thrombosis. Edinburgh: Churchill Livingstone, 1981:255–266.

479. Philippe J, Offner F, Declerck PJ. Fibrinolysis and coagulation in individuals with infectious disease and sepsis. Thromb Haemost 1991;65:291–295.

480. Johansson JO, Landin K, Tengborn L et al. High fibrinogen and plasminogen activator inhibitor activity in growth hormone-deficient adults. Arterioscler Thromb 1994;14:434–437.

481. Mansfield MW, Stickland MH, Grant PJ. Environmental and genetic factors in relation to elevated circulating levels of plasminogen activator inhibitor-1 in Caucasian individuals with non-insulin-dependent diabetes mellitus. Thromb Haemost 1995;74:842–847.

482. Malm J, Laurell M, Nilsson IM et al. Thromboembolic disease—Critical evaluation of laboratory investigation. Thromb Haemost 1992;68:7–13.

483. Declerck PJ, Moreau H, Jespersen J et al. Multicenter evaluation of commercially available methods for the immunological determination of plasminogen activator inhibitor-1 (PAI-1). Thromb Haemost 1993;70:858–863.

484. Gaffney PJ, Edgell TA. The international standard for plasminogen activator inhibitor-1 (PAI-1) activity. Thromb Haemost 1996;76:80–83.

485. Hermelin LI, Eichelberger JW. Monitoring thrombolytic therapy: the new laboratory challenge. J Med Tech 1985;2:89–93.

486. Garabedian HD, Gold HK, Leinbach RC. Laboratory monitoring of hemostasis during thrombolytic therapy with recombinant human tissue-type plasminogen activator. Thromb Res 1988;50:121–133.

487. Holvoet P, Lijnen HR, Collen D. A monoclonal antibody preventing binding of tissue-type plasminogen activator to fibrin: useful to monitor fibrinogen breakdown during t-PA infusion. Blood 1986;67:1482–1487.

488. Stump DC, Topol EJ, Chen AB et al. Monitoring of hemostasis parameters during coronary thrombolysis with recombinant tissue-type plasminogen activator. Thromb Haemost 1988;59:133–137.

489. Seifried E, Tanswell P. Comparison of specific antibody, D-Phe-Pro-Arg-CH₂Cl and aprotinin for prevention of in vitro effects of recombinant tissue-type plasminogen activator on haemostasis parameters. Thromb Haemost 1987;58:921–926.

490. Mohler MA, Refino CJ, Chen SA et al. D-Phe-Pro-Arg-chloromethylketone: its potential use in inhibiting the formation of in vitro artifacts in blood collected during tissue-type plasminogen activator thrombolytic therapy. Thromb Haemost 1986;56:160–164.

491. Brommer EJ, Verheijen JH, Chang GT et al. Masking of fibrinolytic response to stimulation by an inhibitor of tissue-type plasminogen activator in plasma. Thromb Haemost 1984;52:154–156.

492. Rodgers RP, Levin J. A critical reappraisal of the bleeding time. Semin Thromb Hemost 1990;16:1–20.

493. Burns ER, Lawrence C. Bleeding time. A guide to its diagnostic and clinical utility. Arch Pathol Lab Med 1989;113:1219–1224.

494. Duke WW. The pathogenesis of purpura haemorrhagica with especial reference to the part played by the blood platelets. Arch Intern Med 1912;10:445–469.

495. Kessels H, Kester AD, Hemker HC. Intrinsic and method-induced variation of the bleeding time and related parameters [Letter]. Thromb Haemost 1994;71:798–799.

496. Mielke CH. Measurement of the bleeding time. Thromb Haemost 1984;52:210–211.

497. Ivy AC, Nelson D, Brecher G. The standardization of certain factors in the cutaneous "venostasis" bleeding time technique. J Lab Clin Med 1940;26:1812–1822.

498. Macherel P, Sulzer I, Furlan M et al. Warning: simplate II—lack of standardization in standardized bleeding time devices. Thromb Haemost 1990;64:605.

499. Bowie EJ, Owen CA Jr. Standardization of the bleeding time. Scand J Haematol Suppl 1980;37:87–94.

500. Mielke CH Jr. Aspirin prolongation of the template bleeding time: influence of venostasis and direction of incision. Blood 1982;60:1139–1142.

501. Schulman S, Johnsson H. Heparin, DDAVP and the bleeding time. Thromb Haemost 1991;65:242–244.

502. ten Cate JW. Platelet function tests. Clin Haematol 1972;1:283–294.

503. Hardisty RM. Hereditary disorders of platelet function. Clin Haematol 1983;12:153–173.

504. Triplett DA, ed. Platelet function, laboratory evaluation and clinical application. Chicago: American Society of Clinical Pathology, 1978.

505. Leede C. Zur beurteilung des rumpel-leedeschen scharlach-phanomens. Mnch Med Wochenschr 1911;58:1673.

506. Bowie EJ, Owen CA Jr, Thompson JH et al. Platelet adhesiveness in von Willebrand's disease. Am J Clin Pathol 1969;52:69–77.

507. Bowie EJW, Owen CA. Some factors influencing platelet retention in glass bead columns including the influence of plastics. Am J Clin Pathol 1971;56:479–483.

508. O'Brien JR. Platelet aggregation. Part II. Some results from a new method of study. J Clin Pathol 1962;15:452–456.

509. Born GV, Cross MJ. The aggregation of blood platelets. J Physiol 1963;168:178–195.

510. Warlow C, Corina A, Ogston D. The relationship between platelet aggregation and time interval after venepuncture. Thromb Diath Haemorrh 1974;31:133–141.

511. Kirchhof B, Kirchhof U, Etscheid G. Attempts to standardize platelet aggregation measurements: simplified screening tests. Haemostasis 1990;20:169–180.

512. Fritsma GA. Tests of platelet number and function. In: Corriveau DM, Fritsma JB, eds. Hemostasis and thrombosis in the clinical laboratory. Philadelphia: JB Lippincott, 1988:278–304.

513. Thompson SG, Vickers MV. Methods in dose response platelet aggregometry. Thromb Haemost 1985;53:216–218.

514. Ludlam CA. Assessment of platelet Function. In: Bloom AL, Thomas DP, eds. Haemostasis and thrombosis. Edinburgh: Churchill Livingstone, 1988:933–952.

515. Vickers MV, Thompson SG. Sources of variability in dose response platelet aggregometry. Thromb Haemost 1985;53:219–220.

516. Scrutton MC, Clare KA, Hutton RA et al. Depressed responsiveness to adrenaline in platelets from apparently normal human donors: a familial trait. Br J Haematol 1981;49:303–314.

517. Born GV. Aggregation of blood platelets by adenosine diphosphate and its reversal. Nature 1962;194:927–929.

518. MacFarlane DE, Mills DCB. The effects of ATP on platelets: evidence against the central role of released ADP in primary aggregation. Blood 1975;46:309–320.

519. Owen NE, Feinberg H, Le Breton GC. Epinephrine induces calcium uptake in human blood platelets. Am J Physiol 1980;239:H483–H488.

520. Muggli R, Baumgartner HR. Collagen induced platelet aggregation: requirement for tropocollagen aggregates. Thromb Res 1973;3:715.

521. Marcus AJ. The role of lipids in platelet function: with particular reference to the arachidonic acid pathway. J Lipid Res 1978;19:793–826.

522. Coller BS. Biochemical and electrostatic considerations in primary platelet aggregation. Ann N Y Acad Sci 1983;416:693–708.

523. Tofler GH, Brezinski D, Schafer AI. Concurrent morning increase in platelet aggregability and the risk of myocardial infarction and sudden death. N Engl J Med 1987;316:1514–1518.

524. Rao AK, Walsh PN. Acquired qualitative platelet disorders. Clin Haematol 1983;12:201–238.

525. Sharp DS, Benowitz NL, Bath PM et al. Cigarette smoking sensitizes and desensitizes impedance-measured ADP-induced platelet aggregation in whole blood. Thromb Haemost 1995;74:730–735.

526. Sweeney JD, Labuzzetta JW, Michielson CE et al. Whole blood aggregation using impedance and particle counter methods. Am J Clin Pathol 1989;92:794–797.

527. Sweeney JD, Hoernig LA, Fitzpatrick JE. Whole blood aggregation in von Willebrand disease. Am J Haematol 1989;32:190–193.

528. Elwood PC, Beswick AD, Sharp DS. Whole blood impedance platelet aggregometry and ischemic heart disease. The caerphilly collaborative heart disease study. Arteriosclerosis 1990;10:1032–1036.

529. Abbate R, Favilla S, Boddi M et al. Factors influencing platelet aggregation in whole blood. Am J Clin Pathol 1986;86:91–96.

530. Sharp DS, Beswick AD, O'Brian JR. The association of platelet and red cell count with platelet impedance changes in whole blood and light-scattering changes in platelet rich plasma: evidence from the caerphilly collaborative heart disease study. Thromb Haemost 1990;64:211–215.

531. Hett DA, Walker D, Pilkington SN et al. Sonoclot analysis. Br J Anaesth 1995;75:771–776.

532. Ingerman-Wojenski CM, Smith JB, Silver MJ. Difficulty in detecting inhibition of platelet aggregation by the impedance method. Thromb Res 1982;28:427–432.

533. Randi ML, Fabris F, Casonato A et al. The effect of anticoagulant mixtures on btG and PF₄ levels. Thromb Haemost 1981;46:569.

534. Fuster V, Kazmier FJ, Cash JD. Assay of platelet factor 4 in plasma. Mayo Clin Proc 1973;48:103–106.

535. Vinazzer H. A simplified assay method for PF4 in plasma and in platelets with a chromogenic substrate. Haemostasis 1978;7:352–358.

536. Bolton AE, Ludlam CA, Pepper DS. A radioimmunoassay for platelet factor 4. Thromb Res 1976;8:51–58.

537. Dawes J, Smith RC, Pepper DS. The release, distribution, and clearance of human β-thromboglobulin and platelet factor 4. Thromb Res 1978;12:851–861.

538. Bolton AE, Ludlam CA, Moore S et al. Three approaches to the radioimmunoassay of human β-thromboglobulin. Br J Haematol 1976;33:233–238.

539. Ludlam CA, Cash JD. Studies on the liberation of β-thromboglobulin from human platelets *in vitro*. Br J Haematol 1976;33:239–247.

540. Kaplan KL, Owen J. Plasma levels of β-thromboglobulin and platelet factor 4 as indices of platelet activation *in vivo*. Blood 1981;57:199–202.

541. Holmsen H, Holmsen I, Bernhardsen A. Microdetermination of adenosine diphosphate and adenosine triphosphate in plasma with the firefly luciferase system. Anal Biochem 1966;17:456–473.

542. David JL, Herion F. Method for measurement of [14]C-HT uptake and release by platelets. In: Mannucci PM, Gorini S, eds. Platelet functions and thrombosis: a review of methods. New York: Plenum Press, 1972;335.

543. Israels SJ, McNicol A, Robertson C et al. Platelet storage pool deficiency: diagnosis in individuals with prolonged bleeding times and normal platelet aggregation. Br J Haematol 1990;75:118–121.

544. Tàssies D, Reverter JC, Cases A et al. Reticulated platelets in uremic individuals: effect of hemodialysis and continuous ambulatory peritoneal dialysis. Am J Hematol 1995;50:161–166.

545. Romp KG, Peters WP, Hoffman M. Reticulated platelet counts in individuals undergoing autologous bone marrow transplantation: an aid in assessing marrow recovery. Am J Hematol 1994;46:319–324.

546. Peng J, Friese P, Wolf RF et al. Relative reactivity of platelets from thrombopoietin- and interleukin-6- treated dogs. Blood 1996;87:4158–4163.

547. Weiss HJ. Platelet aggregation, adhesion and adenosine diphosphate release in thrombopathia (platelet factor 3 deficiency). A comparison with Glanzmann's thrombasthenia and von Willebrand's disease. Am J Med 1967;43:570–578.

548. Mackie IJ, Machin SJ. Platelet aggregation measurement. Med Lab World 1984;19:22.

549. Johnson PC, Ware JA, Salzman EW. Concurrent measurement of platelet ionised calcium concentration and aggregation: studies with the lumiaggregometer. Thromb Res 1985;40:435–443.

550. Akkerman JW, Nieuwenhuis HK, Sixma JJ. Thrombosis and atherosclerosis II. Laboratory diagnosis. Parkville, MO: Boehringer Ingelheim, 1986:203.

551. Marcus AJ. Transcellular metabolism of eicosanoids. In: Spate TH, ed. Progress in hemostasis and thrombosis. New York: Grune & Stratton, 1986;127.

552. Defreyn G, Machin SJ, Carreras LO et al. Familial bleeding tendency with partial platelet thromboxane synthetase deficiency: reorientation of cyclic endoperoxidase metabolism. Br J Haematol 1981;49:29–41.

553. Pant SS, Levine L. Prostaglandin biosynthesis and metabolism measured by radioimmunoassay. Prostaglandins 1977;3:41–76.

554. Berndt MC, Caen JP. Platelet glycoproteins. In: Spate TH, ed. Progress in hemostasis and thrombosis. New York: Grune & Stratton, 1984;111.

555. Kunicki TJ, Nurden AT, Pidard D et al. Characterization of human platelet glycoprotein antigens giving rise to individual immunoprecipitates in crossed-immunoelectrophoresis. Blood 1981;58:1190–1197.

556. Hourdillé P, Heilmann E, Combrié R et al. Thrombin induces a rapid redistribution of glycoprotein Ib-IX complexes within the membrane systems of activated human platelets. Blood 1990;76:1503–1513.

557. Heyssel RM. Determination of human platelet survival utilizing [14]C labeled serotonin. J Clin Invest 1961;40:2134–2142.

558. Aas KA, Gardner FH. Survival of blood platelets labeled with chromium. J Clin Invest 1958;37:1257–1268.

559. Ezekowitz MD, Wilson DA, Smith EO et al. Comparison of I[111] platelet scintigraphy and two-dimensional echocardiography in the diagnosis of left ventricular thrombi. N Engl J Med 1982;306:1509–1513.

560. Aster RH, Jandl JH. Platelet sequestration in man: I. Methods. J Clin Invest 1964;43:843.
Ries CA, Price DC. [[51]Cr] Platelet kinetics in thrombocytopenia. Correlation between splenic sequestration of platelets and response to splenectomy. Ann Intern Med 1974;80:702–707.

562. Schwartz KA. Platelet antibody: review of detection methods. Am J Haematol 1988;29:106–114.

563. Cines DB, Schreiber AD. Immune thrombocytopenia. Use of a Coombs' antiglobulin test to detect IgG and C3 on platelets. N Engl J Med 1979;300:106–111.

564. Kelton JG, Powers PJ, Carter CJ. A prospective study of the usefulness of the measurement of platelet associated IgG for the diagnosis of idiopathic thrombocytopenic purpura. Blood 1982;60:1050–1053.

565. Sugiura K, Steiner M, Baldini MG. Platelet antibody in idiopathic thrombocytopenic purpura and other thrombocytopenias. J Lab Clin Med 1980;96:640–653.

566. LoBuglio AF, Court WS, Vinocur L et al. Immune thrombocytopenic purpura. Use of a [125]I-labeled antihuman IgG monoclonal antibody to quantify platelet-bound IgG. N Engl J Med 1983;309:459–463.

567. Dixon R, Rosse W, Ebbert L. Quantitative determination of antibody in idiopathic thrombocytopenic purpura. Correlation of serum and platelet-bound antibody with clinical response. N Engl J Med 1975;292:229–235.

568. Luiken GA, McMillan R, Lightsey AL. Platelet-associated IgG immune thrombocytopenic purpura. Blood 1977;50:317–325.

569. Soulier JP, Patereau C, Drouet J. Platelet indirect radioactive Coombs test. Its utilization for Pla1 grouping. Vox Sang 1975;29:253–268.

570. Anonymous. Diagnosis and treatment of idiopathic thrombocytopenic purpura: recommendations of the American Society of Hematology. The American Society of Hematology ITP Practice Guideline Panel. Ann Intern Med 1997;126:319–326.

571. Tate DY, Sorenson RL, Gerrard JM et al. An immunoenzyme histochemical technique for the detection of platelet antibodies from the serum of individuals with idiopathic (autoimmune) thrombocytopenic purpura (ITP). Br J Haematol 1977;37:265–275.

572. Rosenfeld CS, Nichols G, Bodensteiner DC. Flow cytometric measurement of antiplatelet antibodies. Am J Clin Pathol 1987;87:518–522.

573. Heim MC, Petersen BH. Detection of platelet-associated immunoglobulin in immune thrombocytopenia by flow cytometry. Diagn Clin Immunol 1988;5:309–313.

574. Michelson AD. Flow cytometry: a clinical test of platelet function. Blood 1996;87:4925–4936.

575. Ruf A, Patscheke H. Flow cytometric detection of activated platelets: comparison of determining shape change, fibrinogen binding, and P-selectin expression. Semin Thromb Hemost 1995;21:146–151.

576. Orfao A, Ruiz-Arguelles A, Lacombe F et al. Flow cytometry: its applications in hematology. Haematologica 1995;80:69–81.

577. Wall JE, Buijs-Wilts M, Arnold JT et al. A flow cytometric assay using mepacrine for study of uptake and release of platelet dense granule contents. Br J Haematol 1995;89:380–385.

578. Gordon N, Thom J, Cole C et al. Rapid detection of hereditary and acquired platelet storage pool deficiency by flow cytometry. Br J Haematol 1995;89:117–123.

579. Brandt JT, Isenhart CE, Osborne JM et al. On the role of platelet FcRIIa phenotype in heparin-induced thrombocytopenia. Thromb Haemost 1995;74:1564–1572.

580. Warkentin TE, Kelton JG. Heparin-induced thrombocytopenia. Annu Rev Med 1989;40:31–44.

581. Sheridan D, Carter C, Kelton JG. A diagnostic test for heparin-induced thrombocytopenia. Blood 1986;67:27–30.

582. Ansell J, Deykin D. Heparin induced thrombocytopenia and recurrent thromboembolism. Am J Hematol 1980;8:325–332.

583. Greinacher A, Michels I, Kiefel V et al. A rapid and sensitive test for diagnosing heparin-associated thrombocytopenia. Thromb Haemost 1991;66:734–736.

584. Chong BH. Heparin-induced thrombocytopenia. Aust N Z J Med 1992;22:145–152.

585. Chong BH, Burgess J, Ismail F. The clinical usefulness of the platelet aggregation test for the diagnosis of heparin-induced thrombocytopenia. Thromb Haemost 1993;69:344–350.

586. Amiral J, Bridey F, Wolf M et al. Antibodies to macromolecular platelet factor 4-heparin complexes in heparin-induced thrombocytopenia: a study of 44 cases. Thromb Haemost 1995;73:21–28.

587. Duncan BM, Tubridge LJ, Duncan EM et al. Detection of haemophilia carriers: multivariate analysis compared with discriminant analysis using up to five factor VIII variates. Br J Haematol 1984;57:113–121.

588. Ault KA, Mitchell J. Analysis of platelets by flow cytometry. Methods Cell Biol 1994;42:275–294.

589. Rudzki Z, Rodgers SE, Sheffield LJ et al. Detection of carriers of haemophilia A: use of bioassays and restriction fragment length polymorphisms (RFLP). Aust N Z J Med 1996;26:195–205.

590. Levinson B, Kenwrick S, Lakich D et al. A transcribed gene in an intron of the human factor VIII gene. Genomics 1990;7:1–11.

591. Higuchi M, Kazazian HH Jr, Kasch L et al. Molecular characterisation of severe haemophilia A suggests that about half the mutations are not within the coding regions and splice junctions of the factor VIII gene. Proc Natl Acad Sci U S A 1991;88:7405–7409.

592. Windsor S, Taylor SA, Lillicrap D. Direct detection of a common inversion mutation in the genetic diagnosis of severe hemophilia A. Blood 1994;84:2202–2205.

593. Orita M, Suzuki Y, Sekiya T et al. Rapid and sensitive detection of point mutations and DNA polymorphisms using the polymerase chain reaction. Genomics 1989;5:874–879.

594. Higuchi M, Kochhan L, Schwaab R et al. Molecular defects in hemophilia A: identification and characterization of mutations in the factor VIII gene and family analysis. Blood 1989;74:1045–1051.

595. Peake I. Molecular genetics and counselling in haemophilia. Thromb Haemost 1995;74:40–44.

596. Tuddenham EG, Schwaab R, Seehafer J et al. Haemophilia A: database of nucleotide substitutions, deletions, insertions and rearrangements of the factor VIII gene. 2nd ed. Nucleic Acids Res 1994;22:4851–4868.

597. Lalloz MR, Schwaab R, McVey JH et al. Haemophilia A diagnosis by simultaneous analysis of two variable dinucleotide tandem repeats within the factor VIII gene. Br J Haematol 1994;86:804–809.

598. Windsor S, Taylor SAM, Lillicrap D. Multiplex analysis of two intragenic microsatellite repeat polymorphisms in the genetic diagnosis of haemophilia A. Br J Haematol 1994;86:810–815.

599. Lehesjoki AE, de la Chapelle A, Rasi V. Haemophilia A: two recombinations detected with probe St14. Lancet 1986;2:280.

600. Rossiter JP, Young M, Kimberland ML et al. Factor VIII gene inversions causing severe hemophilia A originate almost exclusively in male germ cells. Hum Mol Genet 1994;3:1035–1039.

601. Lebo RV, Koerper MA, Kim JH et al. Prenatal diagnosis of hemophilia involving grandpaternal mosaicism. Am J Med Genet 1993;47:401–404.

602. Giannelli F, Green PM, High KA et al. Haemophilia B: database of point mutations and short additions and deletions. 3rd ed. Nucleic Acids Res 1992;20(Suppl):2027–2063.

603. Fraser BM, Poon MC, Hoar DI. Identification of factor IX mutations in haemophilia B: application of polymerase chain reaction and single strand conformation analysis. Hum Genet 1992;88:426–430.

604. Ghanem N, Costes B, Martin J et al. Twenty-four novel hemophilia B mutations revealed by rapid scanning of the whole factor IX gene in a French population sample. Eur J Hum Genet 1993;1:144–155.

605. Attree O, Vidaud D, Vidaud M et al. Mutations in the catalytic domain of human coagulation factor IX: rapid characterization by direct genomic sequencing of DNA fragments displaying an altered melting behavior. Genomics 1989;4:266–272.

606. Montandon AJ, Green PM, Giannelli F et al. Direct detection of point mutations by mismatch analysis: application to haemophilia B. Nucleic Acids Res 1989;17:3347–3358.

607. Martinez PA, Romey MC, Schved JF et al. Direct carrier testing of haemophilia B by SSCP. Clin Lab Haematol 1994;16:15–20.

608. Weinmann AF, Reiner AP, Thompson AR. A polymorphic MseI site 5′ to the factor IX gene varies among ethnic groups. Hum Mol Genet 1993;2:486.

609. Ketterling RP, Bottema CD, Koeber DD et al. T296M, a common mutation causing mild hemophilia B in the Amish and others: founder effect, variability in factor IX activity assays and rapid carrier detection. Hum Genet 1991;2:333–337.

610. Andrew M, Vegh P, Johnston M et al. Maturation of the hemostatic system during childhood. Blood 1992;80:1998–2005.

611. Helm MC, Peterson BH. Detection of platelet-associated immunoglobulin in immune thrombocytopenia by flow cytometry. Diagn Clin Immunol 1988;5:309–313.

# SECTION 6

# QUANTITATIVE PLATELET DISORDERS

# CHAPTER 27

# THROMBOTIC MICROANGIOPATHIES: THROMBOTIC THROMBOCYTOPENIC PURPURA AND THE HEMOLYTIC-UREMIC SYNDROME

## Joel L. Moake

## INTRODUCTION

First described by Moschcowitz in 1924 (1), thrombotic thrombocytopenic purpura (TTP) has fascinated physicians with its dramatic clinical presentations, high mortality rate, and during the past 2 decades the effectiveness of empirical therapy (2, 3).

Platelet aggregates in the microcirculation in TTP produce fluctuating ischemia or infarction in various organs, including the brain in 50 to 71% of episodes (4–6). In the closely related hemolytic-uremic syndrome (HUS), initially reported by Gasser et al (7) in 1955, the ischemia is predominantly renal. Thrombocytopenia and erythrocyte fragmentation (Fig. 27.1; see color plate 27.1), along with intravascular hemolysis and tissue damage that result in increased serum levels of lactate dehydrogenase (LDH), are usually less extreme in HUS. However, the variability of organ dysfunction in TTP, including renal abnormalities in 50 to 75% of episodes (4, 5), and the occasional extrarenal manifestations in HUS can make the two syndromes difficult to distinguish (5, 8). If these clinical observations are combined with the fact that TTP and HUS are sometimes associated with similar inciting cofactors (e.g., infection, pregnancy, immune disorders, and chemotherapy), then it is no wonder that many hematologists consider TTP and HUS to be different clinical manifestations of a common mechanism for intravascular platelet aggregation.

Subsequent to the initial description of TTP, the most important therapeutic advance was the discovery by Byrnes et al (2) and Bukowski et al (3), and subsequently confirmed by studies in more than 200 individuals (4, 5), that plasma infusion combined with plasmapheresis (plasma exchange) allows most individuals to survive an episode of TTP. In the majority of these individuals the disorder neither recurs nor produces persistent organ damage (5).

Truly recurrent TTP, as opposed to a single protracted episode with brief intervening periods of incomplete remission (5), occurs in at least 11 to 28% of TTP individuals (4, 5). HUS usually occurs as a single episode. In adults, HUS may follow the administration of mitomycin, cyclosporin, total body irradiation, or multiple chemotherapeutic agents (8). In children HUS is often associated with gastroenteritis caused by cytotoxin-producing serotypes of *Escherichia coli* (e.g., 0157:H7) or *Shigella* (9). TTP and HUS are likely to be the result of the intrusion of platelet-aggregating agents into the systemic or renal circulation, respectively. This probably accounts for observations that TTP can often be aggravated by platelet transfusions (5, 10).

This chapter will discuss the histopathology, possible pathophysiologic mechanisms, clinical manifestations, laboratory features, differential diagnosis, and current therapy of TTP and HUS.

# EPIDEMIOLOGY AND ETIOLOGY OF TTP AND HUS

## TTP

Perhaps 500 to 1000 new cases of TTP occur each year in the United States, with women affected about twice as often as men. Most individuals are in the 20- to 60-year age range, with occasional case reports in infants and the elderly. No racial or seasonal predisposition is obvious. With the exception of one description of TTP in a husband and wife within an 8-month period (11), case clustering is rare (in contrast to HUS). The majority of individuals who develop TTP have no identifiable associated risk factor, although TTP during pregnancy or the postpartum period accounts for a small percentage of cases. Neame (12) suggested that abnormal immune modulation might contribute to etiology in these circumstances.

TTP has been associated occasionally with diseases characterized by autoimmune or other types of abnormal immune responses, including systemic lupus erythromatosus (SLE) (13, 14), rheumatoid arthritis (15), ankylosing spondylitis (16), Sjögren's syndrome (17), polyarteritis (18), polymyositis (19), Graves' disease (20), autoimmune ''idiopathic'' thrombocytopenic purpura (ITP) (21, 22), and the acquired immunodeficiency syndrome (AIDS) (23, 24). TTP has been reported rarely following the use of various drugs, including chlorpropamide (25), procainamide (25), oxophenarsine (26), diphenylhyantoin (27), penicillin (28), sulfonamides (29), oral contraceptives (27), penicillamine (28), and more commonly in association with ticlopidine therapy (29–31). Some individuals with TTP have a prodromal illness suggesting viral infection (25), although this is one of the least specific pieces of information in a clinical history. The syndrome has been reported rarely following influenza or polio vaccinations (32, 33) and in association with infections by Coxsackie B (34), influenza (12), or the herpes simplex virus (20). The role, if any, of viral infections in triggering TTP is unknown.

A variety of observations suggest that endothelial cells may be functionally altered by components in the blood of TTP individuals. As examples, the following have been reported:

1. Endothelial cells contain the p24 antigenic marker of human immunodeficiency virus–type 1 (HIV-1) in individuals with HIV-1–related TTP (35).
2. TTP serum stimulates tissue-factor production by cultured, human, umbilical-vein endothelial cells (36).

3. Autoantibodies in the plasma of some TTP individuals react with endothelial cell and platelet-surface glycoprotein (GP) IV molecules (also known as CD36) (37).
4. Autoantibodies in the plasma of some TTP individuals react with an internal, endothelial cell, 43-kDa antigen that, presumably, could only have been exposed by previous endothelial cell injury or alteration (38).
5. Antiphospholipid antibodies are found in occasional TTP individuals (39), and these antibodies may recognize endothelial cell phospholipids.
6. Apoptosis is induced in cultured, microvascular, endothelial cells, but not in HUVECs, by exposure to the serum of some TTP individuals. The mechanism of this latter phenomenon is presently unknown, but does not require endothelial cell GP IV or the presence of tumor necrosis factor-$\alpha$ (TNF-$\alpha$) or other toxic cytokines (40).

The possibility of endothelial cell perturbation in TTP is supported by observations that levels of thrombomodulin, P-selectin (GMP-140), tissue plasminogen activator (tPA), and plasminogen activator inhibitor-1 (PAI-1) are increased in the plasma of some TTP individuals. Plasma levels of tissue factor pathway inhibitor (TFPI) are sometimes decreased in TTP (41–49). These various compounds are found in platelets or other tissue cells, in addition to endothelial cells. Observations that levels of one or more of these substances are abnormal in the plasma of some TTP individuals is not, therefore, conclusive evidence for endothelial cell involvement. Discussion of another endothelial cell and platelet component, von Willebrand factor (vWf), is included in the section on Pathophysiology of Intravascular Platelet Aggregation in TTP and HUS.

The possibility that immunologic events are involved in any endothelial cell disturbance in TTP is supported by studies that suggest macrophage/lymphocyte activation in some TTP individuals (36, 50, 51). Elevated levels of interleukin (IL)-1, IL-6, the soluble IL-2 receptor, TNF-$\alpha$, and transforming growth factor-$\beta$ (TGF-$\beta$) have all been reported in the disorder. There is also preliminary evidence that individuals lacking the class II HLA antigen, DR53, may be more susceptible to thrombotic microangiopathy (52).

## HUS

Although first described and most often encountered in children, HUS is also seen in adults (in association with pregnancy, chemotherapy, and bone marrow transplantation) (53, 54). There is one strong relationship that represents a profound clue to etiology. This is the observation that the predominant type of childhood HUS is usually preceded by gastroenteritis and may be related to cytotoxin-producing strains of *E. coli* or *Shigella* (9).

## Diarrhea-Associated HUS

Most cases of childhood HUS occur after the age of 6 months following a bout of bloody diarrhea caused by either *Shigella dysenteriae* serotype I or various *E. coli* serotypes (7–9, 55–59). Enterohemorrhagic *E. coli* are endemic to Buenos Aires and Calgary, among other locales, where HUS is a relatively common cause of acute renal failure in children (56, 57). The bacteria produce one or more structurally similar forms of a powerful exotoxin detectable in fecal material (56–58). The prototype of this 70 Kda protein is Shiga-toxin (ST) that is encoded in *S. dysenteriae* DNA (60). Shiga-like toxin-1 (SLT-1) and shiga-like toxin-2 (SLT-2) are closely-related exotoxins encoded in the DNA of bacteriophages that become incorporated into the genome of a restricted number of *E. coli* OH serotypes (60). Normal individuals generate increasing titers of Shiga toxin–neutralizing

antibodies in response to infection (56–58). *E. coli* 0157: H7 is associated with about 50% of HUS cases (57–59).

Shiga toxin is composed of one A subunit (31.5 Kda) and five B subunits (7.7 Kda each) (57, 58, 60) (Fig. 27.2). The structural genes for one A and one B subunit are adjacent to one another in the DNA of *S. dysenteriae* and in the incorporated bacteriophage DNA of enterohemorrhagic *E. coli*. Each of the B subunits is capable of binding with high affinity to an unusual disaccharide linkage (galactose α1-4 galactose). This disaccharide is found in the terminal trisaccharide sequence of the predominant membrane glycosphingolipid receptor for the Shiga toxins, globotriosyl ceramide (Gb$_3$) (Fig. 27.2) (60, 61). Gb$_3$ is a component of the membranes of renal glomerular capillary endothelial cells, especially those of children under 3 years of age (62), as well as the membranes of other types of endothelial cells (60).

The A subunit of ST is then internalized by endocy-

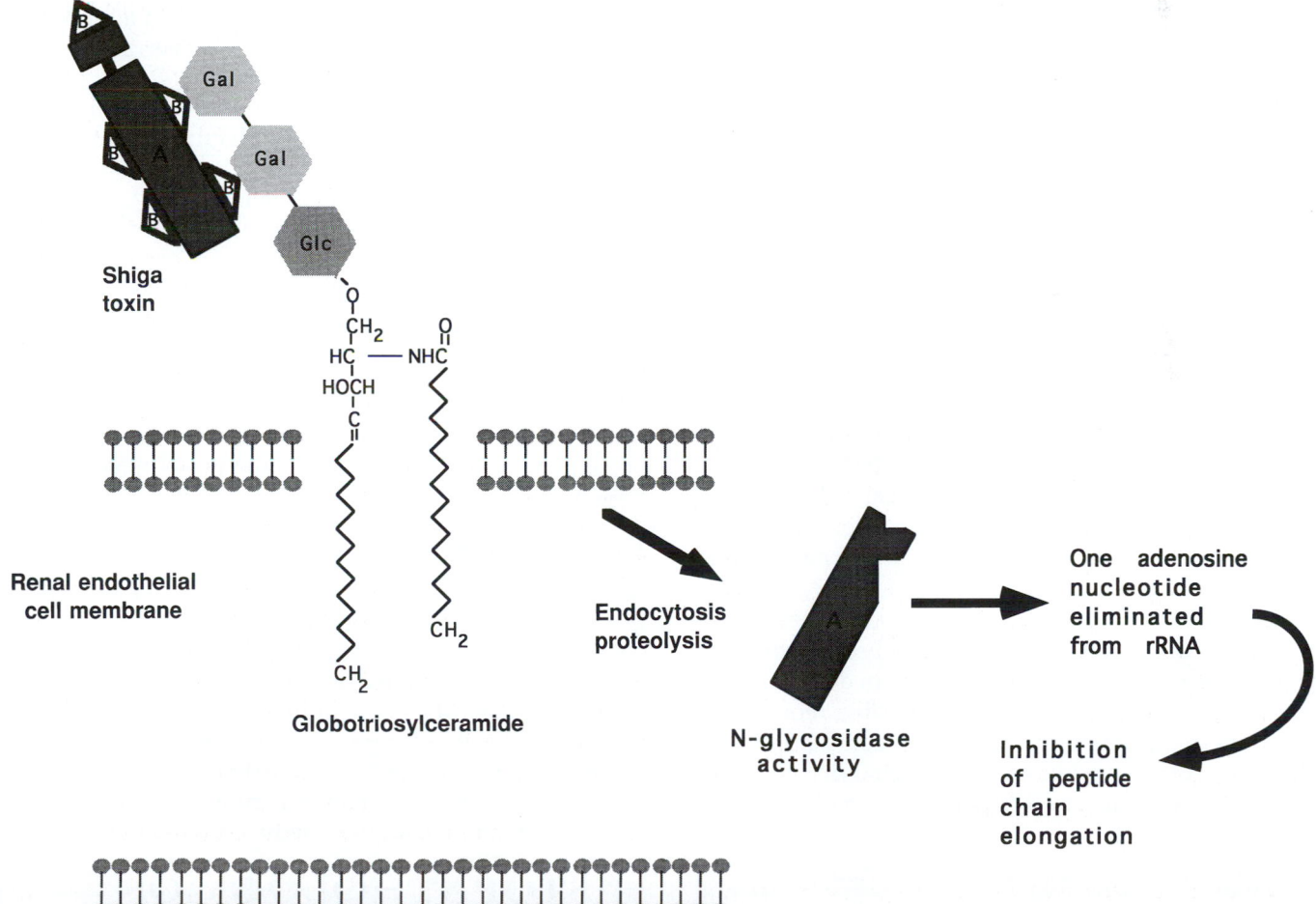

**FIGURE 27.2.** Binding of Shiga toxins to renal endothelial cells. The B subunits of Shiga toxin (and Shiga-like toxins) attach to the terminal disaccharide portion of globotriosyl ceramide (Gb3) receptors on renal microvascular endothelial cells. After attachment of the toxin, the A subunit enters the endothelial cell, undergoes activation, and inhibits protein synthesis. (Adapted with permission from Moake JL. Science and practice. Haemolytic-uraemic syndrome: basic science. Lancet 1994;343:393–397.)

tosis, partially proteolyzed and subjected to disulfide bond reduction (Fig. 27.2). These processes generate an active intracellular enzyme (27 Kda) capable of cleaving an adenosine from ribosomal RNA subunits (60). The elongation factor–dependent attachment to ribosomes of aminoacyl-bound transfer RNA molecules is inhibited, and peptide-chain elongation is blocked (60).

ST-producing *S. dysenteriae,* or an *E. coli* serotype that produces SLT-1 and/or SLT-2, can be ingested in contaminated meat, milk, cheese, or other insufficiently cooked or pasteurized food (56, 57, 63). The enterohemorrhagic *Shigella* or *E. coli* then adhere to mucosal epithelial cells of the large intestine and invade, replicate, and destroy colonic cells. Exotoxin and, possibly, endotoxin (56, 57, 60) damage the underlying tissue and vasculature. The result is bloody diarrhea. ST from *S. dysenteriae,* or SLT-1, SLT-2, or both from enterohemorrhagic *E. coli,* enter the circulation and attach to $Gb_3$ molecules on renal glomerular capillary endothelial cells. In some individuals the toxins may also attach to some endothelial cell $Gb_3$ receptors in other organs (57, 60, 64, 65). The involved endothelial cells swell and are likely to release intracellular components. *In vitro*, ST, SLT-1, and SLT-2 are directly cytotoxic to proliferating human umbilical vein endothelial cells (60).

Other substances may up-regulate $Gb_3$ levels and, therefore, the extent of toxin binding onto renal endothelial cells, or they may potentiate by other mechanisms the injurious effects *in vivo* of the Shiga toxins (66). Substances that have been implicated in causing these accentuating effects include (a) endotoxin lipopolysaccharide, which is a component of both *S. dysenteriae* and enterohemorrhagic *E. coli* (60, 66); (b) IL-1; and (c) TNF-α, which is released from monocytes and macrophages and possibly from renal mesangial cells exposed to endotoxin (60, 66); and (d) complement-fixing antibodies produced against antigens that have been altered in structure or exposure on injured renal endothelial cells. These altered antigens may be suppressed by interferon-γ (67). Compounds released from IL-8-activated neutrophils, including oxygen-derived free radicals, $H_2O_2$, elastase, and other proteases (68, 69), may also contribute to endothelial cell damage and account for the observed relationship between the extent of neutrophilia in diarrhea-associated HUS and the degree of irreversible renal injury (70). Superoxide anions released from activated neutrophils may combine with renal endothelial-derived nitric oxide (NO) to form cytotoxic peroxynitrite (71).

### HUS Nonassociated with Diarrhea

Mitomycin C (72), cyclosporine (73), FK506 (tacrollimus) (74), chemotherapeutic agents in combination, and total-body irradiation have been associated with the subsequent development of thrombotic microangiopathy (54, 75). The syndrome often more closely resembles HUS than TTP and usually develops weeks to months after exposure (54, 75). Individuals who have been treated for various illnesses by bone marrow transplantation make up a relatively large subgroup (54). HUS has also been reported after kidney, liver, heart, and lung transplants (76). It is not known if free radicals or other drug metabolites are involved in the putative initial direct damage to the endothelial cells of renal arteries and arterioles that is characteristic of this type of HUS. It is also not known if the delayed development of thrombotic microangiopathy is somehow related to therapy-associated alterations in antigenic expression on renal and other types of endothelial cells, with subsequent anti–endothelial cell antibody production in the individuals.

HUS occurs during the postpartum period (77); rarely, however, does it occur *during* pregnancy. (In contrast, TTP does occur during pregnancy, especially during the last trimester.) Endothelial cell autoantibody formation associated with putative immune dysregulation during pregnancy or oral contraceptive use might explain the occasional association between these conditions and thrombotic microangiopathy. Whether either enteropathogenic *E. coli* or antiphospholipid antibodies are involved in pathogenesis in these cases is not yet known (57).

Quinine-induced immune thrombocytopenia (see Chapter 29) has been associated with HUS in some individuals (78). In this syndrome individuals produce antibodies against components of platelet glycoprotein (GP) Ib-IX-V or platelet GP IIb-IIIa complexes that may be antigenically altered by the attachment of quinine. In the subgroup of individuals with quinine-induced immune thrombocytopenia who also develop HUS, it is possible that the antibodies may cross react with quinine-altered GP IIIa molecules (79) on renal endothelial cell membranes.

Patients with HUS not associated with diarrhea may be more prone to recurrence (18% of individuals in one series) (80).

### Familial HUS

Rare individuals with HUS have the disorder on a congenital basis (55). A few of these individuals have been studied and found to be severely deficient in factor H, a control protein for the alternative pathway of complement activation (81). These individuals, as a result, have low serum levels of complement component C3 and complement factor B. It is possible that these individuals are more susceptible than normal individuals to autoantibody or immune complex-mediated renal injury.

# HISTOPATHOLOGY OF TTP AND HUS
## TTP

TTP was first described (1) in a 16-year-old girl who had the abrupt onset of fever, anemia, renal dysfunction, central nervous system impairment, and cardiac failure. She died within 2 weeks. At necropsy, hyaline thrombi were found in terminal arterioles and capillaries. It was subsequently determined (2, 82) that thrombocytopenia with increased marrow megakaryocytes is characteristic of the disorder and that the microvascular thrombi characterized by Moschcowitz as "hyaline" (1) are composed of aggregated platelets with little fibrin (Figs. 27.3 and 27.4; for Fig. 27.3 see color plate 27.3).

Microvascular occlusions are seen in most organs, including the lungs and eyes. Most frequently involved are the brain, heart, spleen, kidneys, pancreas, and adrenals. Harkness et al (10) found that early vascular lesions in the brain consist almost exclusively of platelet thrombi without evidence of perivascular inflammation or other vessel wall pathology. TTP may, therefore, be a disease of *direct* platelet aggregation in the

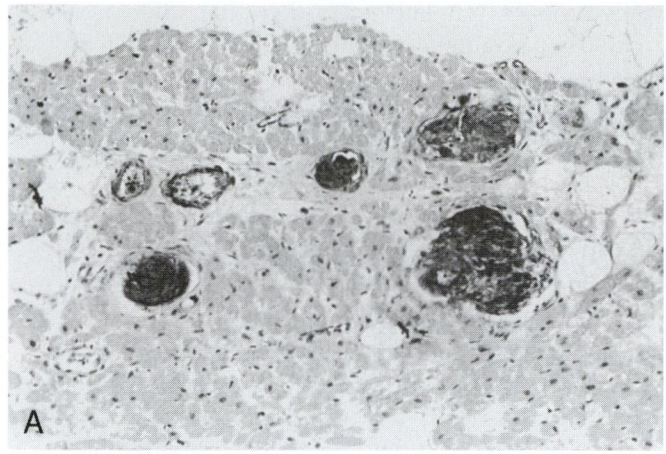

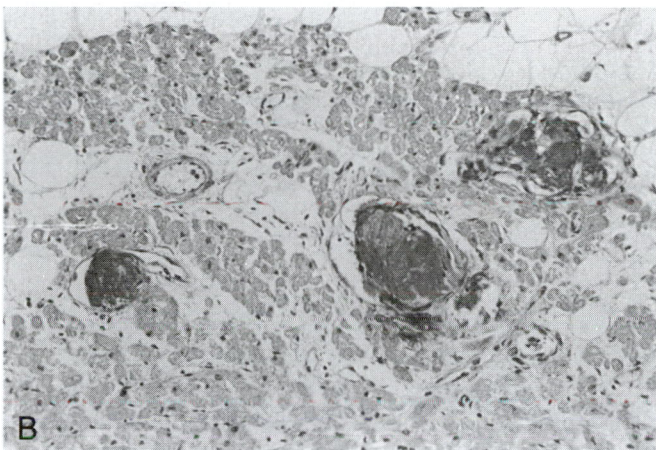

**FIGURE 27.5.** Immunohistochemical staining of thrombotic thrombocytopenic purpura thrombi in the myocardium. The lesions stain strongly positive for von Willebrand factor antigen **(A)**, but only weakly for fibrinogen/fibrin **(B)**. (Adapted with permission from Asada Y, Sumiyoshi A, Hayashi T et al Immunohistochemistry of the vascular lesion in thrombotic thrombocytopenic purpura, with special reference to factor VIII-related antigen. Thromb Res 1985;38:469–479; and Asada Y, Sumiyoshi A. Pathological features of thrombotic thrombocytopenic purpura. In: Kaplan BS, Trompeter RS, Moake JL, eds. Hemolytic-uremic syndrome and thrombotic thrombocytopenic pupura. New York: Marcel Dekker, 1992; pp. 491–498.)

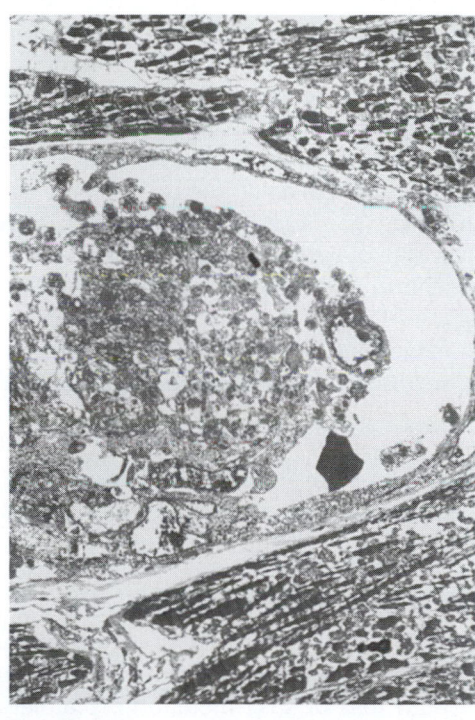

**FIGURE 27.4.** Electron micrograph of a thrombotic thrombocytopenic purpura thrombus in a myocardial arteriole. The occluding thrombus, which consists predominantly of packed platelets interspersed with amorphous material, is becoming covered with endothelial cells. (Adapted with permission from Asada Y, Sumiyoshi A, Hayashi T et al. Immunohistochemistry of the vascular lesion in thrombotic thrombocytopenic purpura, with special reference to factor VIII-related antigen. Thromb Res 1985;38:469–479; and Asada Y, Sumiyoshi A. Pathological features of thrombotic thrombocytopenic purpura. In: Kaplan BS, Trompeter RS, Moake JL, eds. Hemolytic-uremic syndrome and thrombotic thrombocytopenic pupura. New York: Marcel Dekker, 1992; pp. 491–498.)

microcirculation of the brain and other organs that is not preceded by endothelial desquamation and platelet adherence to exposed subendothelium. This supposed direct platelet aggregation is potentially reversible by effective therapeutic intervention. Immunohistochemical study of early TTP lesions has revealed an abundance of vWf with little fibrinogen present (Fig. 27.5) (83–85). The opposite findings are characteristic of thrombotic lesions in disseminated intravascular coagulation (DIC) (83–85). vWf multimers within these thrombi may function as polymeric bridges promoting platelet-platelet cohesion (aggregation). The relative predominance of platelets (rather than fibrin) as the occlusive component in microvessels, as well as the paucity of coagulation abnormalities, also distinguishes TTP from DIC (see Chapter 44).

## HUS

Renal endothelial cell injury is likely to be the primary etiologic event in HUS. Swollen endothelial cells, widened subendothelial spaces, and hypertrophy of the mesangial cells between glomerular capillaries result in the narrowing of the lumina of glomerular capillaries. Intraluminal platelet thrombi, accompanied by some fibrin polymers, occlude the narrowed glomerular capillaries and afferent arterioles in diarrhea-associated HUS (86). In the type of HUS that is not associated with diarrhea, thrombi form in renal arterioles and small arteries (86).

The histopathology and thrombocytopenia of HUS suggest that renal endothelial cell perturbation may result predominantly in *direct* platelet aggregation in the renal microvasculature. This direct platelet aggregation is likely to differ only in extent from the systemic microvascular platelet aggregation in TTP. The absence of consistent clotting abnormalities in HUS indicates that activation of coagulation and fibrin generation is secondary and limited in extent. Complete obstruction of renal microvessels in this disorder may produce glomerular and tubular necrosis, hypertension, and end-stage renal failure.

Thrombi may be mostly intraglomerular if renal biopsies are obtained early in the course of HUS. The characteristic lesion later in the clinical course is granular eosinophilic material in the subendothelium, which may represent endothelial growth over degenerating platelet thrombi (86). In some HUS individuals other organs may be affected by microvascular thrombosis and local infarction (86).

TTP and HUS are clinical diagnoses. Tissue obtained from the biopsy of bone marrow, gingiva, or kidney may be obtained at a time when there are few (or no) arterial thrombi in the microvessels of the area sampled. This may account for the finding of characteristic microvascular hyaline thrombi in only about 50% of gingival biopsies obtained from individuals considered on the basis of clinical evidence to have TTP (87). Biopsy samples are usually not necessary for diagnosis. In some circumstances it is not even safe to do the procedure. It is likely that TTP and HUS are manifestations of a similar mechanism of microvascular platelet aggregation. If the platelet aggregation is systemic and extensive, and especially if the central nervous system is involved, the disorder is called "TTP." If platelet aggregation is relatively less extensive and predominantly involves the kidneys, the individual is considered to have "HUS."

# PATHOPHYSIOLOGY OF INTRAVASCULAR PLATELET AGGREGATION IN TTP AND HUS

## TTP

TTP is likely to be the result of the intrusion into the circulation of one or more platelet-aggregating agents. It has been suggested that the aggregating substance is a protein of 59 Kda (88) or a 37-kDa protein capable of binding to platelet GP IV and inducing clumping (89–92). Others have reported that TTP individuals have defects in production or plasma binding of the potent, endothelial cell-derived, aggregation-inhibitor prostaglandin $I_2$ (PGI$_2$ or prostacyclin) (93). It is possible that PGI$_2$-related findings reflect an underlying alteration of endothelial function in TTP. Therapeutic infusions of PGI$_2$ derivatives have led to conflicting results (93–95).

As mentioned previously, the histopathologic and clinical findings suggest that organ ischemia and thrombocytopenia in TTP may be caused by direct, potentially reversible, platelet aggregation in the microcirculation of multiple organs concurrently. Any conclusions about the pathophysiology of platelet aggregation in TTP must be reconciled with the immunohistochemical studies of TTP thrombi that reveal an abundance of vWf with little fibrinogen/fibrin (83–85), implying that vWf is involved in microvascular platelet aggregation in TTP.

Some experimental findings support a relationship between some TTP episodes and the presence in individual plasma of either a $Ca^{2+}$-dependent, cysteine protease (calpain) (96–98) or a lysosomal-derived, non-$Ca^{2+}$-dependent, cathepsin-type, cysteine protease (99). It is possible that proteases may enter the bloodstream of some TTP individuals from injured (or apoptotic) tissue sources. Calpain is reported to bind to GP IX components of GP Ib-IX-V and to GP IIb-IIIa sites on platelets and platelet microparticles. Calpain may also be capable of cleaving vWf multimers into fragments that can clump platelets (96–98). This latter possibility is an unusual one, because the proteolysis of vWf multimers is commonly associated with loss of vWf-mediating, platelet-aggregating activity.

Animal studies indicate that the binding of intact vWf multimers to the GP Ib component of platelet GP Ib-IX-V receptors may induce thrombotic thrombocytopenia. In the rat, dog, or pig, *in vivo* platelet clumping can be initiated by the binding to animal platelets of animal plasma vWf multimers in complexes with the injected snake-venom protein, botrocetin (100–102). The intravascular platelet thrombi in these short-term animal experiments were found in the microcirculation of the lungs and spleen, but not in the brain or kidneys. Circulating vWf, rather than any vWf released from the α-granules of animal platelets, was required for the intravascular platelet aggregation in these animal models of thrombotic thrombocytopenia (102).

vWf monomers are linked by disulfide bonds into multimers of varying sizes that range into the millions of Daltons (103) (see Chapter 16). vWf multimers are produced within megakaryocytes and endothelial cells and are stored within the α-granules of platelets and the Weibel-Palade bodies of endothelial cells. The predominant sources of plasma vWf multimers are endothelial cells. The entire constellation of vWf multimers found in the normal circulation is produced within both megakaryocytes and endothelial cells (103). Additionally, both cell types construct vWf multimeric forms that are even larger in size than those found in normal plasma (Fig. 27.6) (104–105). These unusually large (UL) vWf multimers probably consist of an increased number of mature vWf subunits. ULvWf forms are not composed of the pro-vWf monomers that have a molecular mass greater than mature vWf monomeric subunits. ULvWf forms may be more effective than the largest, plasma

vWf forms at binding under the influence of elevated, fluid-shear stresses to the GP Ib component of platelet GP Ib-IX-V receptors and GP IIb-IIIa complexes, and at inducing aggregation (104–107).

Serial studies of plasma samples from individuals during single episodes of TTP have often shown either the presence of ULvWf multimers or, alternatively, the absence of the largest, plasma vWf forms (Figs. 27.6 and 27.7) (108–112). The presence of ULvWf forms in TTP individual plasma may reflect systemic, endothelial cell perturbation, resulting in the outpouring of ULvWf multimers from endothelial cells that may overwhelm plasma ULvWf "reductase" (106, 107) and vWf protease (113–115) activities. It is also possible that some individuals may develop TTP as a result of producing autoantibodies against one or the other of these activities.

Platelet aggregation and α-granule release either *in vivo* or *in vitro* do not account for the appearance of ULvWf multimeric forms in the plasma. This may be either because the quantity of released ULvWf forms from platelets is relatively low or because any released ULvWf multimers attach tenaciously to the GP Ib component of GP Ib-IX-V and/or GP IIb-IIIa vWf receptors on the external surface of platelet membranes (105).

It has been suggested that the absence of the largest plasma vWf multimers might be related to proteolysis of large vWf multimeric forms by plasma vWf protease in the high-shear environment of the arterial circulation (Fig. 27.7) (113–115). Another explanation is that both ULvWf forms and the largest plasma vWf multimers may bind to platelets and cause aggregation (Fig. 27.7C) (116–118).

If a TTP individual survives an initial episode and suffers no subsequent relapse, vWf multimeric forms in recovery samples are almost always normal (109). In contrast, ULvWf multimers found in individual plasma samples after recovery may indicate persistent ULvWf "seepage" from perturbed endothelial cells or continuing interference with ULvWf processing. Whatever the precise explanation, detection of ULvWf forms in individual plasma after recovery indicates that the individual is likely to have recurrent episodes of TTP (108, 109, 119–122). During recurrences of the intermittent or chronic relapsing types of TTP, ULvWf forms (and sometimes also the largest plasma vWf multimers) may disappear from individual plasma (108, 109).

Several chronic relapsing TTP individual plasmas have recently been found to be deficient in the vWf protease activity capable of cleaving ULvWf forms (123). This finding is compatible with the suggestion that ULvWf multimers are involved in pathologic platelet aggregation in TTP. In chronic relapsing TTP the accumulation of ULvWf forms in the circulation may periodically (about every 3 to 4 weeks) exceed a threshold level required for intravascular aggregation.

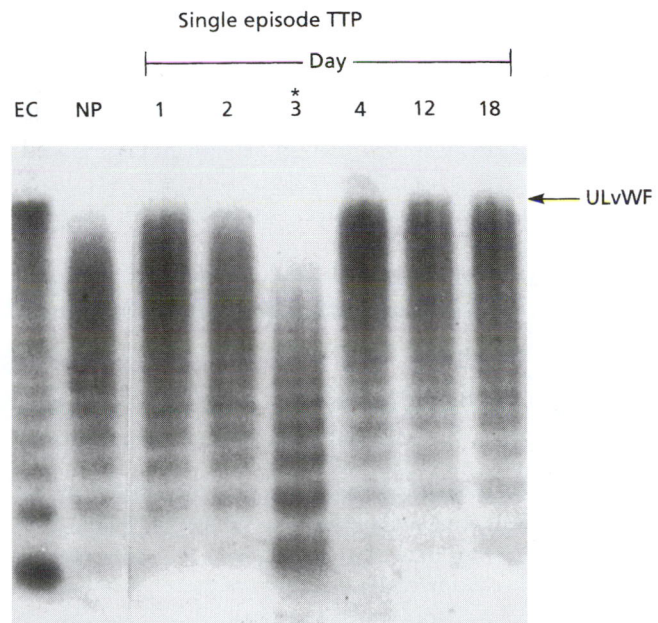

**FIGURE 27.6.** Unusually large (UL) von Willebrand factor (vWf) multimers (indicated by arrow), similar to a portion of those released from human endothelial cells (EC) in culture and larger than vWf multimers found in normal plasma (NP), were present in EDTA-anticoagulated, platelet-poor plasma samples obtained on days 1, 2, 4, 12, and 18 from this individual with a single episode of thrombotic thrombocytopenic purpura. On day 3 (*), the largest, plasma vWf multimers were relatively decreased. vWf forms are displayed by sodium dodecyl sulfate (SDS)-1% agarose gel electrophoresis, followed by overlay with polyclonal rabbit [125]I-anti-human vWf antibody and autoradiography. The fastest migrating vWf forms are dimers.

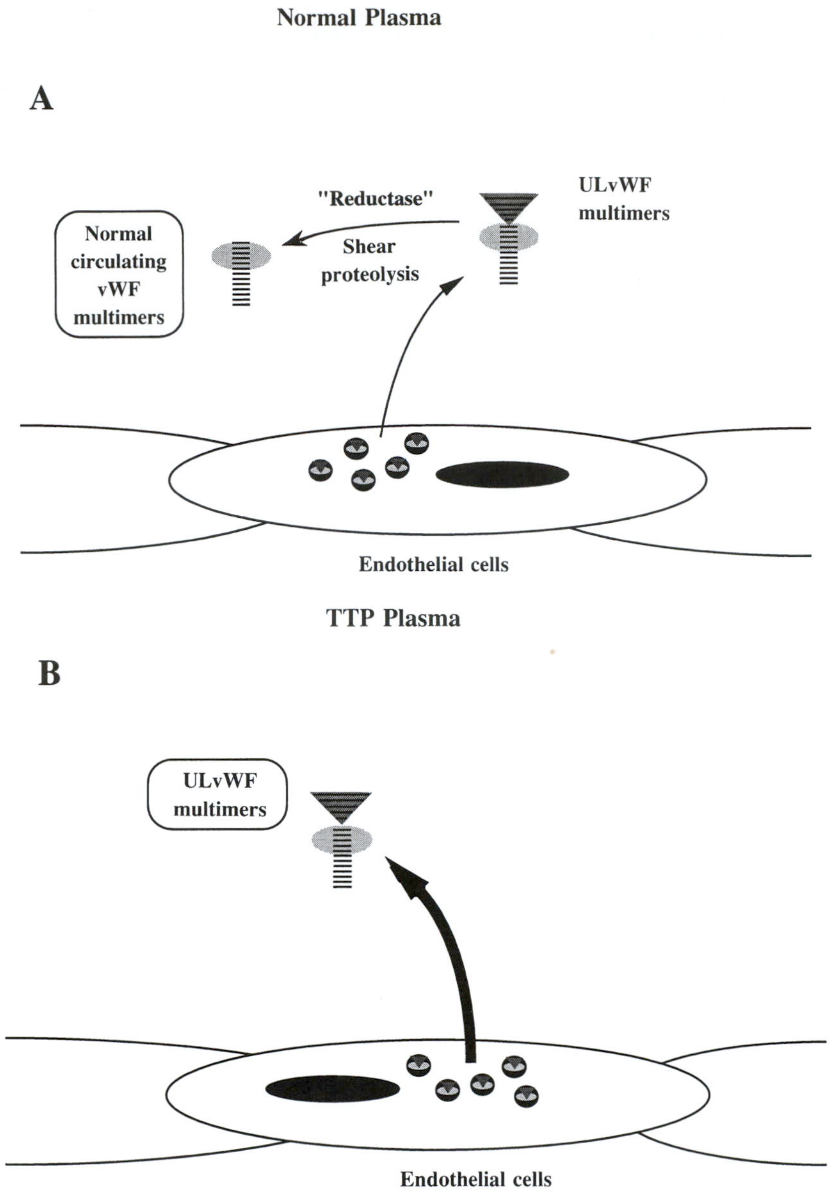

**Normal Plasma**

**A**

**TTP Plasma**

**B**

**FIGURE 27.7.**   Possible explanation for von Willebrand factor (vWf) involvement in the pathophysiology of intravascular platelet aggregation in thrombotic thrombocytopenic purpura (TTP). **A,** Normal processing of unusually large (UL) vWf multimers by a putative UlvWf "reductase" following the release of ULvWf forms from Weibel-Palade bodies of endothelial cells. A vWf protease may also cleave ULvWf multimers in the presence of fluid shear stresses in the circulation. **B,** Excessive release of ULvWf multimers from perturbed endothelial cells in TTP (or interference with ULvWf breakdown), resulting in the presence of ULvWf forms in individual plasma.

Fluid-shear stresses (i.e., the relative parallel motion between fluid planes during flow) in the microcirculation may be important during episodes of TTP of all types in inducing the association of ULvWf multimers and the largest plasma vWf forms with shear-altered vWf receptors (121). Shear-induced platelet aggregation (see Chapters 12 and 20) can be induced *in vitro* in normal blood at abnormally elevated levels of fluid shear stress. This phenomenon requires only a small amount of vWf binding to platelets to initiate aggregation. Most

evidence indicates that the initial attachment of large and unusually large vWf multimers is to the shear-altered GP Ib component of platelet GP Ib-IX-V receptors, and then subsequently to activated platelet GP IIb-IIIa (104, 105, 124–128). If the formation of platelet thrombi in TTP is analogous to shear-induced platelet aggregation *in vitro*, then vWf binding to platelets would be expected to be absolutely required for the direct microvascular aggregation process (121, 129). This type of vWf-mediated, shear-induced platelet aggregation may

**TTP Plasma**

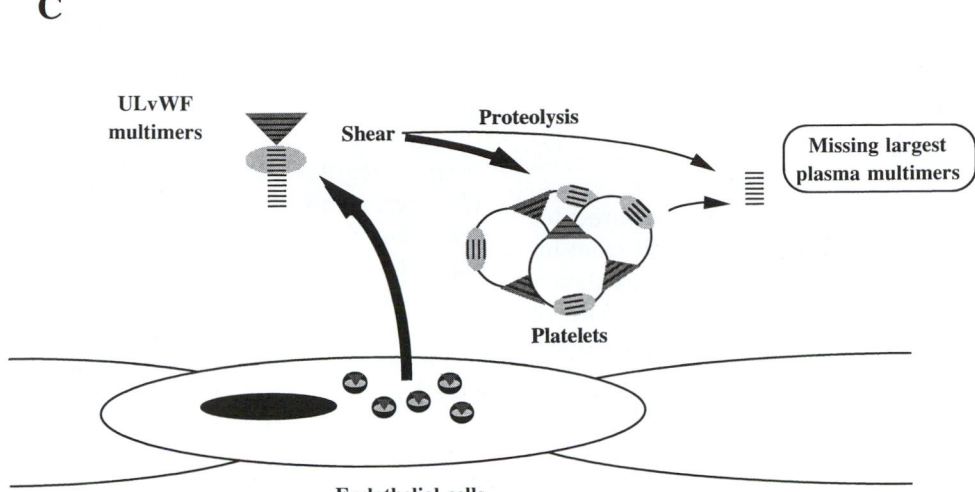

**FIGURE 27.7.** *(Continued)* **C,** Binding of ULvWf forms and the largest plasma vWf multimers to platelet vWf receptors altered by shear stresses in the circulation of TTP individuals. This binding results in the aggregation of platelets and the absence of ULvWf and the largest plasma vWf multimers from individual plasma. Some proteolysis of ULvWf forms and large, plasma vWf multimers in the presence of fluid shear stresses in the circulation may also occur. (Adapted with permission from Moake JL. Studies on pathophysiology of TTP. [Review]. Semin Hematol 1997;34:83–89.)

account for the vWf-positive/fibrinogen (fibrin)-negative platelet thrombi obtained from TTP individuals (83–85). The initial formation of small thrombi in the microcirculation during TTP episodes may further increase shear stresses on platelets in flowing blood, thereby potentiating and perpetuating *in vivo* shear-induced platelet aggregation (104).

## HUS

More than half of the children and adults with HUS thus far evaluated have had a relative decrease in the largest plasma vWf forms during the period when platelet counts were lowest (109, 130–133). A few HUS individuals have had ULvWf forms in their plasma during episodes. These two types of vWf multimeric abnormalities are similar to those observed in plasma samples obtained serially from most individuals during episodes of TTP (Figs. 27.6 and 27.7).

Renal arterial endothelial cell injury or intense stimulation may result in the outpouring into the renal circulation of ULvWf multimers in excess of their capacity to be processed by the ULvWf "reductase" or vWf protease activities in plasma. Exposure of cultured human umbilical-vein endothelial cells to purified Shiga toxin for 30 minutes results in the release of vWf multimers, including ULvWf forms, even in the absence of cell lysis (8). It is possible that ULvWf

multimers, along with the largest plasma vWf forms, may then be induced to attach *in vivo* to platelet GP Ib-IX-V and GP IIb-IIIa receptors that have been altered by elevated fluid-shear stresses in glomerular capillaries and arterioles narrowed by the swelling of endothelial cells, subendothelial spaces, and mesangial cells. In this hypothetical series of events, the result would be aggregated platelets in the renal microcirculation (8, 104).

The pathophysiologic importance in HUS of the following findings is not clear: a relative reduction in renal endothelial cell production of PGI$_2$ (134), which normally suppresses platelet aggregation induced by either chemical agonists or shear stress; an increase in tissue factor exposure on renal endothelial cell surfaces, followed by local coagulation activation and fibrin polymer formation; or the release of renal endothelial cell plasminogen-activator inhibitor-type 1 in excess of tissue-type plasminogen activator and urokinase, possibly impairing local renal microvascular fibrinolysis (135). Platelet activating factor (PAF, 1-O-alkyl, 2-O-acetyl, glycerol-3-phosphorylchorine), which is released from injured renal endothelial cells, is excreted in increased amounts in the urine of some children during the acute phase of HUS (136). PAF promotes platelet activation and impairs renal function. It is not yet known if PAF release from renal vascular endothelial cells is unique and important in HUS or if excessive PAF excretion also occurs in other glomerulopathies as a marker of renal endothelial cell damage.

# ERYTHROCYTE FRAGMENTATION IN TTP AND HUS

It has been presumed that the fragmented erythrocytes characteristic of TTP and HUS episodes result from injury to red cells traversing areas of the microcirculation partially occluded by platelet aggregates. It is not known whether this is the entire explanation. GP Ib-like and/or GP IIb-IIIa receptors may be present in the membranes of young erythrocytes with the capacity to bind endothelial cell-derived ULvWf multimers (137). The membranes of young red cells contain GP IV-like molecules that bind thrombospondin, a compound secreted from platelet α-granules (138). Endothelial cell membranes contain GP Ib and GP IIb-IIIa, as well as the vitronectin receptor, which is also capable of binding thrombospondin. Young red cells in the circulation during TTP or HUS episodes may attach to perturbed renal or systemic microvascular endothelial cells via molecular bridges of ULvWf multimers and thrombospondin that link the young erythrocytes to endothelial cells (137, 138). The young red cells attached momentarily to endothelial cells may then be dissociated by elevated fluid-shear stresses in microvessels. A portion of the red cell membranes may be left behind, and the resealed young erythrocytes may circulate as schistocytes.

# CLINICAL MANIFESTATION OF TTP AND HUS

## TTP

Severe thrombocytopenia and intravascular hemolytic anemia with serum LDH elevation and many schistocytes on the blood smear, along with neurologic symptoms and signs, constitute the characteristic clinical triad. The neuropathy may range in severity from transient bizarre mentation and behavior to sensory-motor deficits, aphasia, seizures, or coma. The peripheral blood smear typically shows reticulocytosis (polychromatic large erythrocytes) and nucleated red blood cells, both of which are responses to the intense hemolysis. A minority of individuals also have fever and some have renal dysfunction. The latter usually includes proteinurea and hematuria, as well as azotemia. Symptoms and signs of ischemia in the retinal (visual defects), coronary (conduction abnormalities), and abdominal circulation (abdominal pain) may be present. Pulmonary vascular occlusion may result in lung infiltrates.

Since the general application of plasma manipulation therapy, many individuals have survived episodes of TTP. It has become apparent that there are several types of the disorder (53). Single-episode TTP never recurs if the individual recovers. Intermittent TTP is characterized by occasional episodes at irregular intervals. In the rarest type, chronic relapsing TTP, frequent episodes occur at regular (approximately 3- to 4-week) intervals. Children are more likely than adults to develop chronic relapsing TTP (121–123, 129). Two siblings have been reported with infection-associated, recurrent TTP that developed in childhood (129). It is not yet known if this is a variant of chronic relapsing TTP. HUS almost always occurs as a single, nonrecurrent episode (8, 9, 55–58).

## HUS

This is a triad of thrombocytopenia, acute renal failure, and intravascular hemolytic anemia with schistocytosis and elevated serum LDH. Renal dysfunction is severe in HUS, in contrast to TTP. Proteinurea and hematuria are present in most HUS individuals, and renal failure often requires dialysis. Oliguria, anuria, chronic renal failure, and hypertension sometimes complicate HUS, whereas this is uncommon in individuals who recover from episodes of TTP. Although the microvascular platelet aggregation is usually predominantly renal, other organs may sometimes also be involved (55–58). The occasional extra-renal manifestations in HUS can sometimes make the distinction between HUS and TTP enigmatic. This distinction has therapeutic implications, as discussed under "Treatment and Prognosis."

# LABORATORY FINDINGS

In both TTP and HUS the degree of thrombocytopenia reflects the extent of intravascular platelet clumping. Platelet counts are often less than 10,000/μl during acute episodes of TTP. Erythrocyte fragmentation occurs in both disorders, and schistocytes on peripheral blood films are characteristic (Fig. 27.1). Occasionally, schistocytes do not appear until a day or two following the initial clinical presentation. The hemolysis is predominantly intravascular and, along with tissue damage, results in increased serum levels of LDH. Thrombocytopenia, hemolytic anemia, schistocytosis, and LDH elevations are almost always less extreme in HUS than during episodes of TTP.

Clotting studies are usually normal in the early stages of a TTP or HUS episode. However, if there is considerable tissue necrosis (as during an especially severe or protracted episode of TTP), secondary disseminated intravascular coagulation (DIC) may occur as a result of overactivation of the coagulation pathway (see Chapter 44). This overactivation probably occurs because of the binding of factor VIIa to exposed tissue factor on injured tissue cells. The ominous development of secondary DIC can be detected by the appearance of elevated levels of D-dimers or fibrin degradation products, prolongation of the prothrombin or partial thromboplastin times, and a declining fibrinogen level.

# DIFFERENTIAL DIAGNOSIS OF TTP AND HUS

The constellation of thrombocytopenia, hemolysis, and schistocytosis also occurs (to an extent that is usually less extreme than in TTP or HUS) in the following:

1. DIC.
2. Preeclampsia/eclampsia.
3. The HELLP syndrome (preeclampsia-associated *h*emolytic anemia with *e*levated *l*iver *e*nzymes and *l*ow *p*latelets).
4. Malignant hypertension.
5. Severe vasculitis.
6. Scleroderma with associated hypertension and renal failure (characterized pathologically by intimal thickening, medial hypertrophy, and perivascular inflammatory infiltrates, in contrast to the thrombosed but otherwise relatively normal appearing microvessels in TTP).
7. Evans's syndrome (concurrent autoimmune thrombocytopenia and direct Coombs' test-positive autoimmune hemolysis).
8. Patients with a malfunctioning prosthetic cardiac valve.

Of these, the most frequently troublesome diagnostic dilemma is between TTP or HUS and DIC.

Heparin-associated thrombocytopenia/thrombosis (HITT) is a common complication of heparin use (see Chapter 29). As platelet counts decline over a period of days, individuals are prone to develop arterial and venous thrombi. The relatively slow decline in circulating platelets, along with the absence of intravascular hemolysis, schistocytosis, and extreme elevation of LDH values, distinguishes HITT from TTP and HUS. Occasional individuals, however, develop HITT as they recover from an acute episode of TTP. This possibility should be considered in a TTP individual who is responding well to therapy and then worsens in association with exposure to heparin by any route or in any dosage (e.g., via "keep-open" intravenous line or during plasma exchange).

# TREATMENT AND PROGNOSIS

## TTP

In many individuals with TTP episodes, nearly 90% in some series (4, 5), the process can be reversed by inten-

## TABLE 27.1.   Treatment of TTP

Immediate infusion of fresh frozen plasma (30 mL/kg/day)
Daily exchange transfusion with fresh frozen plasma (3 to 4 L/day) to commence as soon as possible, and not to be interrupted before complete remission
Glucocorticoids (e.g., intravenous prednisolone, 200 mg per day)
Red cell transfusions as needed
Platelet transfusions only for intracerebral (or other life-threatening) hemorrhage

### Refractory Individuals

Vincristine (≤2 mg on day 1, then 1 mg on days 4, 7, and 10)
Exchange transfusions with 3 to 4 L/day of cryosupernatant (plasma minus vWf-rich cryoprecipitate)
Splenectomy
Azathioprine (Imuran, 100 to 150 mg/day)

sive plasma manipulation (2–5, 53, 139–141) (Table 27.1). This is best done using daily plasma exchanges, that is, the combination of plasmapheresis and plasma infusion with normal platelet–poor, fresh frozen plasma (FFP) (3-4 liters). Skipping even 1 day prior to complete remission may lead to rapid relapse. Cryoprecipitate-poor plasma (cryosupernatant) is at least as effective as FFP in plasma exchange procedures (142, 143). Compared with FFP, cryosupernatant is relatively deficient in fibrinogen and fibronectin. Perhaps even more important, cryosupernatant does not contain the largest vWf forms that are present in normal FFP and in the cryoprecipitate fraction of FFP.

It is presumed that platelet-aggregating substances (ULvWf multimers; other aggregating proteins or enzymes?) are being removed by plasmapheresis. It is also presumed that infused normal plasma is providing supplemental quantities of some plasma antiaggregating agent (ULvWf reductase or protease some other type of aggregation inhibitor?). If plasmapheresis is not immediately available, infusion of normal FFP at the rate of about 30 mL per kilogram per day can be used initially until plasma exchange can be arranged. This should be within 24 to 48 hours in most circumstances, because plasma infusion alone is less effective than plasma exchange (4) and may result in volume overload. TTP individuals with coma, cardiac failure, or renal dysfunction should receive plasma exchange commencing immediately after diagnosis, if possible. Relapses in children with chronic relapsing TTP often respond to, or are prevented by, the transfusion of normal FFP alone (in quantities varying from one to several units) without the need for concurrent plasmapheresis (2, 53, 121–123, 140).

Although some individuals have recovered from

TTP episodes without receiving glucocorticoids, in a recent series a subset of TTP individuals recovered in association with glucocorticoid therapy alone (5). On the basis of this study by Bell et al, it is probably prudent to institute glucocorticoid therapy in all adult individuals with initial or recurrent TTP episodes unless there is a strong contraindication. The apparent effectiveness of glucocorticoids may relate to an underlying autoimmune pathogenesis (e.g., production by the individual of autoantibodies to endothelial cells or to ULvWf reductase or protease). One approach is to begin prednisolone intravenously immediately following diagnosis in a dosage of about 200 mg per day and to continue it until the individual recovers (5).

Depending on the hemoglobin level and intensity of hemolysis, red blood cell transfusions may be required. If the platelet count is very low and bleeding is a primary problem, or if intracranial bleeding is demonstrated by computerized tomography or magnetic resonance imaging, then platelet transfusions will be necessary. Otherwise, it is probably better to withhold platelet transfusions because they have been temporally associated with exacerbation of the microcirculatory thrombotic process in the central nervous system (10, 53, 144).

Plasma exchange should be continued for more than 3 days after individuals attain complete remission (i.e., a normal neurologic status, a platelet count of 150,000 to 200,000/μl, a rising hemoglobin value, and a normal serum LDH level). Schistocytes in declining numbers often persist for many days on peripheral blood films (5). At least five additional exchanges are currently recommended. Otherwise, incomplete remission with relapse is likely (5). Then, the exchanges are stopped, and the tapering of the glucocorticoid dosage is begun. Platelet counts should be monitored regularly thereafter. Individuals with a protracted initial episode, as well as individuals with the chronic relapsing form of TTP, may have a recurrence within a few weeks of the discontinuation of therapy. If there is subsequent relapse, the same treatment protocol should be repeated.

In individuals who achieve only a partial response without deterioration in clinical condition, plasma exchange should be continued for a period of a few to many additional days in an effort to achieve a complete remission. In these individuals concomitant HITT should also be suspected, especially if LDH values have declined to (or are near) normal, and all exposure of the individual to heparin eliminated.

If a individual responds minimally within the first 5 days of therapy, or deteriorates within the first 3 days, other forms of therapy should be tried (Table 27.1). Options include the following:

1. The addition of vincristine, which may depolymerize cellular microtubules and thereby alter antigenic exposure on endothelial cells or the availability of GP Ib-IX-V or GP IIb-IIIa receptors on platelet surfaces (1.4 mg per meter, but not exceeding 2 mg total dosage, given as an intravenous bolus on day 1, followed by 1 mg on days 4, 7, and 10) (145).
2. The substitution for FFP in the plasma exchange procedures with vWf-poor cryosupernatant (120, 142).
3. Splenectomy (removal of immunologic cells involved in the production of autoantibodies against endothelial cells or ULvWf reductase or protease?) (53, 131, 146).
4. The addition of other immunosuppressive agents to suppress production of putative autoantibodies that may be involved in pathogenesis (e.g., azathioprine [Imuran] or cyclophosphamide [Cytoxan]) (53, 147).

The use of aspirin and dipyridamole during TTP episodes is controversial (139, 148–150). If shear stress-induced, vWf-mediated platelet aggregation *in vivo* is important in the pathogenesis of platelet aggregation, then aspirin may not be helpful. Aspirin does not inhibit shear-induced aggregation *in vitro* and may actually exacerbate hemorrhagic complications in some individuals (148), especially those who are severely thrombocytopenic. Neither aspirin nor dipyridamole has been unequivocally demonstrated to be useful. The same comments pertain to intravenous $PGI_2$ derivatives, dextran, and fibrinolytic agents (53). Heparin in therapeutic dosages is contraindicated. Transfusions or exchange transfusions with fluids other than plasma or its cryosupernatant fraction are usually ineffective (e.g., albumin alone; concentrated immunoglobulin) (53).

In some individuals who turn out to have intermittent TTP, the disorder may not recur for months to years after an initial TTP episode. This cohort of TTP individuals has been estimated to be 36% of adults with the disorder (151). A recent small study suggested that frequent relapses in some adult TTP individuals may be controlled by splenectomy (151). Detection of ULvWf multimers in individual plasma samples after recovery from an initial episode of TTP may indicate the propensity for recurrence (108, 109, 131).

## HUS

There has been considerable controversy concerning the management of individuals with HUS (53). The variability of the disorder in etiology and severity explains the difficulty in determining the effectiveness of any specific form of therapy. The extent of renal involvement, reflected by the duration of oliguria, generally correlates with the rate of recovery in both adults and children. In mildly affected children in whom anuria is present for less than 24 hours, attention to fluid and electrolytes is usually sufficient. In children with more severe HUS, dialysis is frequently required. Early dialysis improves survival in this situation. HUS in children is, nevertheless, associated with some mortality and often residual renal dysfunction. Additional forms of therapy have therefore been investigated. There is no consensus on the value of anticoagulant therapy (53). Fibrinolytic therapy and antiplatelet agents have been used with conflicting results (53).

Management of HUS in adults has generally been similar to that in children. Renal impairment is often more severe in adults, and hemodialysis is generally required. Heparin therapy has been extensively used, especially in postpartum HUS, without general agreement about its effectiveness (53).

Based on the utility of plasma therapy in TTP, this form of treatment has been tried in HUS. The results do not provide clear guidelines for the management of HUS (150–154). Individuals have been treated by the initial infusion of 30 to 40 mL/kg, followed by 15 to 20 mL/kg daily (152). Some severe HUS individuals have received plasma exchange (154). Hemodialysis has also been used in association with plasma infusion, providing a variant of plasma exchange. A recent trial of plasma exchange using cryosupernatant alternating with plasma adsorption over staphylococcal protein A columns (which adsorb the Fc portions of IgG antibodies in immune complexes) suggests that this approach may be useful in some individuals who develop thrombotic microangiopathy following bone marrow transplantation (155) or treatment with mitomycin C (156). It is presently not known if γ-interferon might be effective *in vivo* in suppressing any interaction between autoantibodies (67) and renal endothelial cells in HUS.

# POSSIBLE NEW APPROACHES TO THERAPY OF TTP AND HUS

Aurin tricarboxylic acid (ATA) is a polyphenolic, polycarboxylated compound that may ultimately prove useful in the treatment of TTP and HUS episodes and in the prophylaxis of relapsing TTP. ATA reversibly binds to vWf multimers (157) and prevents ULvWf and plasma vWf forms from attaching to the GP Ib component of platelet GP Ib-IX-V complexes (157, 158). The binding of ULvWf or large vWf forms to platelet GP Ib, followed by vWf binding to GP IIb-IIIa complexes, is required for platelet aggregation in fluid shear fields (104, 105, 124–128).

ATA is capable of inhibiting platelet thrombosis *in vivo* in the Folts dog model of unstable angina (159), platelet-mediated rethrombosis following fibrinolytic therapy (160), and excessive vWf-mediated shear aggregation *in vitro* using the platelet-rich plasma of chronic relapsing TTP individuals (122). Investigation of ATA *in vitro* and *in vivo* in arterial thrombotic models may lead ultimately to a trial of some non-toxic derivative of ATA in refractory TTP, relapsing TTP, HUS, myocardial infarction, and stroke.

Other new agents that are likely to be tried sooner than a derivative of ATA in the treatment of HUS and refractory TTP, and in the prophylaxis of relapsing TTP, include the following:

1. A recombinant fragment of the human vWf monomer that contains the platelet GP Ib–binding site, binds to the GP Ib component of platelet GP Ib-IX-V in the absence of any modulator, and competes with large vWf multimers for binding to GP Ib (158).
2. A monoclonal antibody directed against the arginine-glycine-aspartate (RGD) sequence of the vWf monomer, which is important in binding vWf multimers to platelet GP IIb-IIIa (e.g., ReoPro or abciximab [Eli Lilly and Co., Indianapolis, IN], a chimeric mouse/human 7E3Fab used to prevent coronary thrombosis or restenosis after angioplasty) (161).
3. A cyclic heptapeptide, integrelin, containing the lysine-glycine-aspartate (KGD) sequence that is also capable of blocking the binding of vWf to platelet GP IIb-IIIa (162).

Each of these compounds could cause life-threatening hemorrhage in a severely thrombocytopenic individual, and so any initial trials will likely be confined to thrombotic microangiopathy individuals whose lives are threatened because they are unresponsive to the usual therapeutic interventions.

# REFERENCES

1. Moschcowitz E. Hyaline thrombosis of the terminal arterioles and capillaries: a hitherto undescribed disease. Proc N Y Pathol Soc 1924;24:21–24.
2. Byrnes JJ, Khurana M. Treatment of thrombotic thrombocytopenic purpura with plasma. N Engl J Med 1977;297:1386–1389.
3. Bukowski RM, Hewlett JS, Reimer RR et al. Therapy of thrombotic thrombocytopenic purpura: an overview. Semin Thromb Hemost 1981;7:1–8.
4. Rock GA, Sumak KH, Buskard NA et al. Comparison of plasma exchange with plasma infusion in the treatment of thrombotic thrombocytopenic purpura. Canadian Apheresis Study Group. N Engl J Med 1991;325:393–397.
5. Bell WR, Braine HG, Ness PM et al. Improved survival in thrombotic thrombocytopenic purpura–hemolytic-uremic syndrome. Clinical experience in 108 individuals. N Engl J Med 1991;325:398–403.
6. Baehr G, Klemperer P, Schifrin A. An acute febrile anemia with thrombocytopenic purpura and diffuse platelet thrombosis of capillaries and arterioles. Trans Assoc Am Phys 1936;51:43–58.
7. Gasser C, Gautier E, Steck A et al. Hemolytic-uremic syndrome: bilateral kidney cortex necrosis in acute acquired hemolytic anemia. Schweiz Med Wochenschr 1955;125:2528–2532.
8. Moake JL. Science and practice. Haemolytic-uraemic syndrome: basic science. Lancet 1994;343:393–397.
9. Karmali MA, Petric M, Lim C et al. The association between idiopathic hemolytic uremic syndrome and infection by verotoxin-producing *Escherichia coli*. J Infect Dis 1985;151:775–782.
10. Harkness DR, Byrnes JJ, Lian EC et al. Hazard of platelet transfusion in thrombotic thrombocytopenic purpura. JAMA 1981;246:1931–1933.

11. Watson CG, Copper WM. Thrombotic thrombocytopenic purpura. Concomitant occurrence in husband and wife. JAMA 1971;215:1821–1822.

12. Neame PB. Immunologic and other factors in thrombotic thrombocytopenic purpura (TTP). Semin Thromb Hemost 1980;6:416–429.

13. Dekker A, O'Brien ME, Cammarata RJ. The association of thrombotic thrombocytopenic purpura with systemic lupus erythematosus: a report of two cases with successful treatment of one. Am J Med Sci 1974;267:243–249.

14. Nesher G, Hanna VE, Moore TL et al. Thrombotic microangiopathic hemolytic anemia in systemic lupus erythematosus. Semin Arthritis Rheum 1994;24:165–172.

15. Anonymous. Case records of the Massachusetts General Hospital. N Engl J Med 1963;269:1195–1206.

16. Morey DA, White JB, Daily WM. Thrombotic thrombocytopenic purpura diagnosed by random lymph node biopsy. Arch Intern Med 1956;98:821–823.

17. Steinberg AD, Green WT Jr, Talal N. Thrombotic thrombocytopenic purpura complicating Sjogren's syndrome. JAMA 1971;215:757–761.

18. Benitez L, Mathews M, Mallory GK. Platelet thrombosis with polyarteritis nodosa: report of a case. Arch Pathol 1964;77:116–125.

19. McLeod BC, Wu KK, Knospe WH. Plasmapheresis in thrombotic thrombocytopenic purpura. Arch Intern Med 1980;140:1059–1060.

20. Myers TJ, Wakem CJ, Ball ED et al. Thrombotic thrombocytopenic purpura: combined treatment with plasmapheresis and antiplatelet agents. Ann Intern Med 1980;92:149–155.

21. Zacharski LR, Lusted D, Glick JL. Thrombotic thrombocytopenic purpura in a previously splenectomized individual. Am J Med 1976; 60:1061–1063.

22. Yospur LS, Sun NC, Figueroa P et al. Concurrent thrombotic thrombocytopenic pupura and immune thrombocytopenic purpura in an HIV-positive individual: case report and Review of the literature. Am J Hematol 1996;51:73–78.

23. Leaf AN, Laubenstein LJ, Raphael B et al. Thrombotic thrombocytopenic purpura associated with human immunodeficiency virus type I (HIV-1) infection. Ann Intern Med 1988;109:194–197.

24. Nair JM, Bellevue R, Bertoni M et al. Thrombotic thrombocytopenic purpura in individuals with the acquired immunodeficiency syndrome (AIDS)-related complex: a report of two cases. Ann Intern Med 1988;109:209–212.

25. Amorosi EL, Ultmann JE. Thrombotic thrombocytopenic purpura: report of 16 cases and Review of the literature. Medicine 1966;45:139–159.

26. Symmers WC. Thrombotic microangiopathy (thrombotic thrombocytopenic purpura) associated with acute haemorrhagic leukoencephalitis and sensitivity to oxophenarsine. Brain 1956;79:511–521.

27. Cuttner J. Thrombotic thrombocytopenic purpura: a ten year experience. Blood 1980;56:301–306.

28. Speth PA, Boerbooms AM, Holdrinet RS et al. Thrombotic thrombocytopenic purpura associated with D-penicillamine treatment in rheumatoid arthritis. J Rheumatol 1982;9:812–813.

29. Page Y, Tardy B, Zeni F et al. Thrombotic thrombocytopenic purpura related to ticlopidine. Lancet 1991;337:774–776.

30. Kovacs MJ, Soong PY, Chin-Yee IH. Thrombotic thrombocytopenic purpura associated with ticlopidine. Ann Pharmacother 1993;27:1060–1061.

31. Kupfer Y, Tessler S. Ticlopidine and thrombotic thrombocytopenic purpura. N Engl J Med 1997;337:1245.

32. Brown RC, Blecher TE, French EA et al. Thrombotic thrombocytopenic purpura after influenza vaccination. BMJ 1973;2:303.

33. Blecher TE, Raper AB. Early diagnosis of thrombotic microangiopathy by paraffin sections of aspirated bone marrow. Arch Dis Child 1967;42:158–162.

34. Berberich FR, Cuene SA, Chard RL Jr et al. Thrombotic thrombocytopenic purpura. Three cases with platelet and fibrinogen survival studies. J Pediatr 1974;84:503–509.

35. del Arco A, Martinez MA, Pena JM et al. Thrombotic thrombocytopenic purpura associated with human immunodeficiency virus infection: demonstration of p24 antigen in endothelial cells. Clin Infect Dis 1993;17:360–363.

36. Wada H, Minami N, Shirakawa S. Cytokine levels in individuals with thrombotic thrombocytopenic purpura. Nippon Rinsho 1993;51:151–154.

37. Tandon NN, Rock G, Jamieson GA. Anti-CD36 antibodies in thrombotic thrombocytopenic purpura. Br J Haematol 1994;88:816–825.

38. Koenig DW, Barley-Maloney L, Daniel TO. A Western blot assay detects autoantibodies to cryptic endothelial antigens in thrombotic microangiopathies. J Clin Immunol 1993;13:204–211.

39. Umibe T, Nawata Y, Mori N et al. Thrombotic thrombocytopenic purpura (TTP) observed in a individual with primary antiphospholipid antibody syndrome. Ryumachi 1994;34:981–987.

40. Laurence J, Mitra D, Steiner M et al. Plasma from individuals with idiopathic and human immunodeficiency virus-associated thrombotic thrombocytopenic purpura induces apoptosis in microvascular endothelial cells. Blood 1996;87:3245–3254.

41. Nagaya S, Wada H, Oka K et al. Hemostatic abnormalities and increased vascular endothelial cell markers in individuals with red cell fragmentation syndrome induced by mitomycin C. Am J Hematol 1995;50:237–243.

42. Kobayashi M, Wada H, Wakita Y et al. Decreased plasma tissue factor pathway inhibitor levels in individuals with thrombotic thrombocytopenic purpura. Thromb Haemost 1995;73:10–14.

43. Chong BH, Murray B, Berndt MC et al. Plasma P-selectin is increased in thrombotic consumptive platelet disorders. Blood 1994;83:1535–1541.

44. Koyama T, Nishida K, Ohdama S et al. Determination of plasma tissue factor antigen and its clinical significance. Br J Haematol 1994;87:343–347.

45. Katayama M, Handa M, Araki Y et al. Soluble P-selectin is present in normal circulation and its plasma level is elevated in individuals with thrombotic thrombocytopenic purpura and the haemolytic uraemic syndrome. Br J Haematol 1993;84:702–710.

46. Wada H, Kaneko T, Ohiwa M et al. Increased levels of vascular endothelial cell markers in thrombotic thrombocytopenic purpura. Am J Hematol 1993;44:101–105.

47. Hirosawa S, Koyama T. Thrombomodulin as a clinical marker in thrombotic thrombocytopenic purpura. Japan TTP Study Group. Nippon Rinsho 1993;51:129–134.

48. Wada H, Ohiwa M, Kaneko T et al. Plasma thrombomodulin as a marker of vascular disorders in thrombotic thrombocytopenic purpura and disseminated intravascular coagulation. Am J Hematol 1992;39:20–24.

49. Handa M, Katayama M, Ikeda Y. Detection of soluble forms of platelet membrane glycoproteins and its clinical significance. Nippon Rinsho 1992;50:360–365.

50. Zauli G, Gugliotta L, Catani L et al. Increased serum levels of transforming growth factor beta-1 in individuals affected by thrombotic thrombocytopenic purpura (TTP): its implications on bone marrow haematopoiesis. Br J Haematol 1993;84:381–386.

51. Wada H, Kaneko T, Ohiwa M et al. Plasma cytokine levels in thrombotic thrombocytopenic purpura. Am J Hematol 1992;40:167–170.

52. Joseph G, Smith KJ, Hadley TJ et al. HLA-DR53 protects against thrombotic thrombocytopenic purpura/adult hemolytic uremic syndrome. Am J Hematol 1994;47:189–193.

53. Byrnes JJ, Moake JL. Thrombotic thrombocytopenic purpura and the haemolytic-uraemic syndrome: evolving concepts of pathogenesis and therapy. Clin Haematol 1986;15:413–442.

54. Moake JL, Byrnes JJ. Thrombotic microangiopathies associated with drugs and bone marrow transplantation. Hematol Oncol Clin North Am 1996;10:485–497.

55. Kaplan BS, Proesmans W. The hemolytic uremic syndrome of childhood and its variants. Semin Hematol 1987;24:148–160.

56. Cleary TG. Cytotoxin producing *Escherichia coli* and the hemolytic uremic syndrome. Pediatr Clin North Am 1988;35:485–501.

57. Karmali MA. The association of verotoxins and the classical hemolytic uremic syndrome. In: Kaplan BS, Trompeter RS, Moake JL, eds. Hemolytic-uremic syndrome and thrombotic thrombocytopenic purpura. New York: Marcel Dekker, 1992; pp. 99–212.

58. Ashkenazi S. Role of bacterial cytotoxins in hemolytic uremic syndrome and thrombotic thrombocytopenic purpura. Annu Rev Med 1993;44:11–18.

59. Kovacs MJ, Roddy J, Gregoire S et al. Thrombotic thrombocytopenic purpura following hemorrhagic colitis due to *Escherichia coli* 0157:H7. Am J Med 1990;88:177–179.

60. Obrig TG. Pathogenesis of Shiga toxin (verotoxin)-induced endothelial cell injury. In: Kaplan BS, Trompeter RS, Moake JL, eds. Hemolytic-uremic syndrome and thrombotic thrombocytopenic purpura. New York: Marcel Dekker, 1992; pp. 405–419.

61. Lindberg AA, Brown JE, Stromberg N et al. Identification of the carbohydrate receptor for Shiga toxin produced by *Shigella dysenteriae* type I. J Biol Chem 1987;262:1779–1785.

62. van de Kar NC, Heuvelink AE, de Boer E et al. Infections with verocytotoxin-producing *Escherichia coli* and hemolytic-uremic syndrome. Ned Tijdschr Geneeskd 1996;140:134–137.

63. Deschenes G, Casenave C, Grimont F et al. Cluster of cases of haemolytic uraemic syndrome due to unpasteurized cheese. Pediatr Nephrol 1996;10:203–205.

64. Boyd B, Lingwood C. Verotoxin receptor glycolipid in human renal tissue. Nephron 1989;51:207–210.

65. Taylor CM, Milford DV, Rose PE et al. The expression of blood group P1 in post-enteropathic hemolytic uremic syndrome. Pediatr Nephrol 1990; 4:59–61.

66. van de Kar NC, Monnens LA, Karmali MA et al. Tumor necrosis factor and interleukin-1 induce expression of the verocytotoxin receptor globotriaosylceramide on human endothelial cells: implications for the pathogenesis of the hemolytic uremic syndrome. Blood 1992;80:2755–2764.

67. Leung DY, Moake JL, Havens PL et al. Lytic anti-endothelial cell antibodies in haemolytic-uraemic syndrome. Lancet 1988;2:183–186.

68. Milford DV, Taylor CM, Rafaat F et al. Neutrophil elastases and haemolytic uraemic syndrome. Lancet 1989;2:1153.

69. Fitzpatrick MM, Shah V, Trompeter RS et al. Interleukin-8 and polymorphoneutrophil leukocyte activation in hemolytic-uremic syndrome of childhood. Kidney Int 1992;42:951–956.

70. Walters MD, Matthei IU, Kay R et al. The polymorphunuclear leukocyte

count in childhood haemolytic uraemic syndrome. Pediatr Nephrol 1989; 3:130–134.

71. Noris M, Ruggenenti P, Todeschini M et al. Increased nitric oxide formation in recurrent thrombotic microangiopathies: a possible mediator of microvascular injury. Am J Kidney Dis 1996;27:790–796.

72. Rabadi SJ, Khandekar JD, Miller HJ. Mitomycin-induced hemolytic uremic syndrome: case presentation and Review of literature. Cancer Treat Rep 1982;66:1244–1247.

73. Atkinson K, Biggs JC, Hayes J et al. Cyclosporin A-associated nephrotoxicity in the first 100 days after allogeneic bone marrow transplantation: three distinct syndromes. Br J Haematol 1983;54:59–67.

74. Mach-Pascual S, Samii K, Beris P. Microangiopathic hemolytic anemia complicating FK506 (tacrolimus) therapy. Am J Hematol 1996;52:310–312.

75. Charba D, Moake JL, Harris MA et al. Abnormalities of von Willebrand factor multimers in drug-associated thrombotic microangiopathies. Am J Hematol 1993;42:268–277.

76. Singh N, Gayowski T, Marino IR. Hemolytic uremic syndrome in solid-organ transplant recipients. Transpl Int 1996;9:68–75.

77. Martinez-Roman S, Gratacos E, Torne A et al. Successful pregnancy in a individual with hemolytic-uremic syndrome during the second trimester of pregnancy. J Reprod Med 1996;41:211–214.

78. Gottschall JL, Elliot W, Lianos E et al. Quinine-induced immune thrombocytopenia associated with hemolytic-uremic syndrome: a new clinical entity. Blood 1991;77:306–310.

79. Pfueller SL, Bilston RA, Jane S et al. Expression of the drug-dependent antigen for quinine-dependent antiplatelet antibodies on GP IIIa, but not on GP Ib, IIb or IX on human endothelial cells. Thromb Haemost 1990; 63:279–281.

80. Siegler RL, Pavia AT, Hansen FL et al. Atypical hemolytic-uremic syndrome: a comparison with postdiarrheal disease. J Pediatr 1996;128:505–511.

81. Pichette V, Querin S, Schurch W et al. Familial hemolytic-uremic syndrome and homozygous factor H deficiency. Am J Kidney Dis 1994;24:936–941.

82. Neame PB, Lechago J, Ling ET et al. Thrombotic thrombocytopenic purpura: report of a case with disseminated intravascular platelet aggregation. Blood 1973;42:805–814.

83. Asada Y, Sumiyoshi A, Hayashi T et al. Immunohistochemistry of the vascular lesion in thrombotic thrombocytopenic purpura, with special reference to factor VIII-related antigen. Thromb Res 1985;38:469–479.

84. Asada Y, Sumiyoshi A. Histopathology of thrombotic thrombocytopenic purpura. Nippon Rinsho 1993;51:159–162.

85. Asada Y, Sumiyoshi A. Pathological features of thrombotic thrombocytopenic purpura. In: Kaplan BS, Trompeter RS, Moake JL, eds. Hemolytic-uremic syndrome and thrombotic thrombocytopenic pupura. New York: Marcel Dekker, 1992; pp. 491–498.

86. Habib R. Pathology of the hemolytic-uremic syndrome. In: Kaplan BS, Trompeter RS, Moake JL, eds. Hemolytic-uremic syndrome and thrombotic thrombocytopenic purpura. New York: Marcel Dekker, 1992; pp. 315–353.

87. Goodman A, Ramos R, Petrelli M et al. Gingival biopsy in thrombotic thrombocytopenic purpura. Ann Intern Med 1978;89:501–504.

88. Chen S, Lian EC. Purification and some properties of a 59KDa platelet-aggregating protein from the plasma of a individual with thrombotic thrombocytopenic purpura. Blood 1988;72(Suppl):318.

89. Siddiqui FA, Lian EC. Novel platelet-agglutinating protein from a thrombotic thrombocytopenic purpura plasma. J Clin Invest 1985;76:1330–1337.

90. Siddiqui FA, Lian EC. Characterization of platelet agglutinating protein p37 purified from the plasma of a individual with thrombotic thrombocytopenic purpura. Biochem Mol Biol Int 1993;30:385–395.

91. Siddiqui FA, Lian EC. Platelet-agglutinating protein p37 from a thrombotic thrombocytopenic purpura plasma forms complexes with platelet membrane glycoprotein IV (CD36). Biochem Int 1992;27:485–496.

92. Lian EC, Siddiqui FA, Chen SH et al. Platelet agglutinating/aggregating proteins from the plasma of individuals with thrombotic thrombocytopenia purpura. In: Kaplan BS, Trompeter RS, Moake JL, eds. Hemolytic-uremic syndrome and thrombotic thrombocytopenic pupura. New York: Marcel Dekker, 1992; pp. 473–481.

93. Wu KK. Role of prostacyclin in the pathogenesis and therapy of thrombotic thrombocytopenic purpura. In: Kaplan BS, Trompter RS, Moake JL, eds. Hemolytic-uremic syndrome and thrombotic thrombocytopenic pupura. New York: Marcel Dekker, 1992; pp. 483–489.

94. Bobbio-Pallavicini E, Porta C, Tacconi F et al. Intravenous prostacyclin (as epoprostenol) infusion in thrombotic thrombocytopenic purpura. Four case reports and Review of the literature. Italian Cooperative Group for Thrombotic Thrombocytopenic Purpura. Haematologica 1994;79:429–437.

95. Kurosawa S, Nagata M, Saito T et al. Thrombotic thrombocytopenic purpura (TTP) with a low level of apolipoprotein A-1 (Apo A-1) which responded to combination of vincristine and beraprost. Rinsho Ketsueki 1994;35:704–709.

96. Moore JC, Murphy WG, Kelton JG. Calpain proteolysis of von Willebrand factor enhances its binding to platelet membrane glycoprotein IIb-IIIa:

an explanation for platelet aggregation in thrombotic thrombocytopenic purpura. Br J Haematol 1990;74:457–464.

97. Kelton JG, Warkentin TE, Hayward CP et al. Calpain activity in individuals with thrombotic thrombocytopenic purpura is associated with platelet microparticles. Blood 1992;80:2246–2251.

98. Kelton JG, Moore JC, Warkentin TE et al. Isolation and characterization of cysteine proteinase in thrombotic thrombocytopenic purpura. Br J Haematol 1996;93:421–426.

99. Consonni R, Falanga A, Barbui T. Further characterization of platelet-aggregating cysteine proteinase activity in thrombotic thrombocytopenic purpura. Br J Haematol 1994;87:321–324.

100. Sanders WE, Read MS, Reddick RL et al. Thrombotic thrombocytopenia with von Willebrand factor deficiency induced by botrocetin. An animal model. Lab Invest 1988;59:443–452.

101. Sanders WE, Brinkhous KM, Read MS. An Animal model of thrombotic thrombocytopenia with von Willebrand factor deficiency: the role of botrocetin in studies of human TTP. In: Kaplan BS, Trompeter RS , Moake JL, eds. Hemolytic-uremic syndrome and thrombotic thrombocytopenic pupura. New York: Marcel Dekker, 1992; pp. 499–512.

102. Sanders WE Jr, Reddick RL, Nichols TC et al. Thrombotic thrombocytopenia induced in dogs and pigs. The role of plasma and platelet vWf in animal models of thrombotic thrombocytopenic purpura. Arterioscler Thromb Vasc Biol 1995;15:793–800.

103. Wagner DD, Ginsburg D. Structure, biology, and genetics of von Willebrand factor. In: Hoffman R, Benz EJ, Shattil SJ et al., eds. Hematology: basic principles and practice. 2nd ed. London: Churchill Livingstone, 1995; pp. 1717–1725.

104. Moake JL, Turner NA, Stathopoulos NA et al. Involvement of large plasma von Willebrand factor (vWf) multimers and unusually large vWf forms derived from endothelial cells in shear stress-induced platelet aggregation. J Clin Invest 1986;78:1456–1461.

105. Moake JL, Turner NA, Stathopoulos NA et al. Shear-induced platelet aggregation can be mediated by vWf released from platelets, as well as by exogenous large or unusually large vWf multimers, requires adenosine diphosphate, and is resistant to aspirin. Blood 1988;71:1366–1374.

106. Frangos JA, Moake JL, Nolasco L et al. Cryosupernatant regulates accumulation of unusually large vWf multimers from endothelial cells. Am J Physiol 1989;256:H1635–H1644.

107. Phillips MD, Moake JL, Nolasco L et al. Plasma von Willebrand factor processing activity functions like a disulfide bond reductase: reversible decrease of multimer size. Thromb Haemost 1993;69:1199.

108. Moake JL, Rudy CK, Troll JH et al. Unusually large plasma factor VIII: von Willebrand factor multimers in chronic relapsing thrombotic thrombocytopenic purpura. N Engl J Med 1982;307:1432–1435.

109. Moake JL, McPherson PD. Abnormalities of von Willebrand factor multimers in thrombotic thrombocytopenic purpura and the hemolytic-uremic syndrome. Am J Med 1989;87:9N–15N.

110. Pereira A, Monteagudo J, Bono A et al. Effect of splenectomy on von Willebrand factor multimeric structure in thrombotic thrombocytopenic purpura refractory to plasma exchange. Blood Coagul Fibrinolysis 1993; 4:783–786.

111. Ruggenenti P, Galbusera M, Cornejo RP et al. Thrombotic thrombocytopenic purpura: evidence that infusion rather than removal of plasma induces remission of disease. Am J Kidney Dis 1993;21:314–318.

112. Tatewaki W. Multimeric composition of von Willebrand factor in thrombotic thrombocytopenic purpura. Japanese TTP Study Group. Nippon Rinsho 1993;51:146–150.

113. Tsai HM, Sussman II, Nagel RL. Shear stress enhances the proteolysis of von Willebrand factor in normal plasma. Blood 1994;83:2171–2179.

114. Tsai HM. Physiologic cleavage of von Willebrand factor by a plasma protease is dependent on its conformation and requires calcium ion. Blood 1996;87:4235–4244.

115. Furlan M, Robles R, Lämmle B. Partial purification and characterization of a protease from human plasma cleaving von Willebrand factor to fragments produced by *in vivo* proteolysis. Blood 1996;87:4223–4234.

116. Chow TW, Turner NA, Chintagumpala M et al. Direct quantification of increased von Willebrand factor binding to platelets in chronic thrombotic thrombocytopenic purpura. Blood 1995;86(Suppl):88.

117. Moake JL. Thrombotic thrombocytopenic purpura. Thromb Haemost 1995; 74:240–245.

118. Chow TW, Turner NA, McPherson P et al. Platelet-bound von Willebrand factor (vWf) is consistently elevated during acute episodes of adult thrombotic thrombocytopenic purpura (TTP). Blood 1996;88(Suppl):518.

119. Moake JL, Byrnes JJ, Troll JH et al. Effects of fresh frozen plasma and its cryosupernatant fraction on von Willebrand factor multimeric forms in chronic relapsing thrombotic thrombocytopenic purpura. Blood 1985;65:1232–1236.

120. Chintagumpala MM, Hurwitz RL, Moake JL et al. Chronic relapsing thrombotic thrombocytopenic purpura in infants with large von Willebrand factor multimers during remission. J Pediatr 1992;120:49–53.

121. Moake J, Chintagumpala M, Turner N et al. Solvent/detergent-treated plasma suppresses shear-induced platelet aggregation and prevents episodes of thrombotic thrombocytopenic purpura. Blood 1994;84:490–497.

122. Daghistani D, Jimenez JJ, Moake JL et al. Familial infantile thrombotic thrombocytopenic purpura. J Pediatr Hematol Oncol 1996;18:171–174.
123. Furlan M, Robles R, Solenthaler M et al. Deficient activity of von Willebrand factor-cleaving protease in chronic relapsing thrombotic thrombocytopenic purpura. Blood 1997;89:3097–3103.
124. Peterson DM, Stathopoulos NA, Giorgio TD et al. Shear-induced platelet aggregation requires von Willebrand factor and platelet membrane glycoproteins Ib and IIb-IIIa. Blood 1987;69:625–628.
125. Chow TW, Hellums JD, Moake JL et al. Shear stress-induced von Willebrand factor binding to platelet glycoprotein Ib initiates calcium influx associated with aggregation. Blood 1992;80:113–120.
126. McCrary JK, Nolasco LH, Hellums JD et al. Direct demonstration of radiolabeled von Willebrand factor binding to platelet glycoprotein Ib and IIb-IIIa in the presence of shear stress. Ann Biomed Eng 1995;23:787–793.
127. Goto S, Salomon DR, Ikeda Y et al. Characterization of the unique mechanism mediating the shear-dependent binding of soluble von Willebrand factor to platelets. J Biol Chem 1995;270:23352–23361.
128. Konstantopoulos K, Chow TW, Turner NA et al. Shear stress–induced binding of von Willebrand factor to platelets. Biorheology 1997;34:57–71.
129. Karpman D, Holmberg L, Jirgard L et al. Increased platelet retention in familial recurrent thrombotic thrombocytopenic purpura. Kidney Int 1996;49:190–199.
130. Moake JL, Byrnes JJ, Troll JH et al. Abnormal VIII: von Willebrand factor patterns in the plasma of individuals with the hemolytic-uremic syndrome. Blood 1984;64:592–598.
131. Moake JL, McPherson PD. von Willebrand factor in thrombotic thrombocytopenic purpura and the hemolytic-uremic syndrome. Transfus Med Rev 1990;4:163–168.
132. Rose PE, Enayat SM, Sunderland R et al. Abnormalities of factor VIII-related protein multimers in the haemolytic-uraemic syndrome. Arch Dis Child 1984;59:1135–1140.
133. Mannucci PM, Lombardi R, Lattuada A et al. Enhanced proteolysis of plasma von Willebrand factor (vWf) in thrombotic thrombocytopenic purpura (TTP) and the hemolytic-uremic syndrome. Blood 1989;74:978–983b.
134. Noris M, Benigni A, Siegler R et al. Renal prostacyclin biosynthesis is reduced in children with hemolytic-uremic syndrome in context of systemic platelet activation. Am J Kidney Dis 1992;20:144–149.
135. Bergstein JM, Kuederli U, Bang NU. Plasma inhibitor of glomerular fibrinolysis in the hemolytic-uremic syndrome. Am J Med 1982;73:322–327.
136. Benigni A, Boccardo P, Noris M et al. Urinary excretion of platelet-activating factor in haemolytic-uraemic syndrome. Lancet 1992;339:835–836.
137. Wick TM, Moake JL, Udden MM et al. Unusually large von Willebrand factor multimers preferentially promote young sickle and non-sickle young erythrocyte adhesion to endothelial cells. Am J Hematol 1993;42:284–292.
138. Sugihara K, Sugihara T, Mohandas N et al. Thrombospondin mediates adherence of CD36+ sickle reticulocytes to endothelial cells. Blood 1992;80:2634–2642.
139. Shepard KV, Bukowski RM. The treatment of thrombotic thrombocytopenic purpura with exchange transfusions, plasma infusions, and plasma exchange. Semin Hematol 1987;24:178–193.
140. Byrnes JJ. Plasma infusion in the treatment of thrombotic thrombocytopenic purpura. Semin Thromb Hemost 1981;7:9–14.
141. Moake JL. TTP—desperation, empiricism, progress. N Engl J Med 1991;325:426–428.
142. Byrnes JJ, Moake JL, Klug P et al. Effectiveness of the cryosupernatant fraction of plasma in the treatment of refractory thrombotic thrombocytopenic purpura. Am J Hematol 1990;34:169–174.
143. Rock G, Shumack KH, Sutton DM et al. Cryosupernatant as replacement fluid for plasma exchange in thrombotic thrombocytopenic purpura. Members of the Canadian Apheresis Group. Br J Haematol 1996;94:383–386.
144. Gordon LI, Kwaan HC, Rossi EC. Deleterious effects of platelet transfusions and recovery thrombocytosis in individuals with thrombotic microangiopathy. Semin Hematol 1987;24:194–201.
145. Gutterman LA, Stevenson TD. Treatment of thrombotic thrombocytopenic purpura with vincristine. JAMA 1982;247:1433–1436.
146. Rowe JM, Francis CW, Cyran EM et al. Thrombotic thrombocytopenic purpura: recovery after splenectomy associated with persistence of abnormally large von Willebrand factor multimers. Am J Hematol 1985;20:161–168.
147. Moake JL, Rudy CK, Troll JH et al. Therapy of chronic relapsing thrombotic thrombocytopenic purpura with prednisone and azathioprine. Am J Hematol 1985;20:73–79.
148. Rosove MH, Ho WG, Goldfinger D. Ineffectiveness of aspirin and dipyridamole in the treatment of thrombotic thrombocytopenic purpura. Ann Intern Med 1982;96:27–33.
149. del Zoppo GJ. Antiplatelet therapy in thrombotic thrombocytopenic purpura. Semin Hematol 1987;24:130–139.
150. Phillips MD. Antiplatelet agents in thrombotic thrombocytopenic purpura. In: Kaplan BS, Trompeter RS, Moake JL, eds. Hemolytic-uremic syndrome and thrombotic thrombocytopenic purpura. New York: Marcel Dekker, 1992; pp. 531–540.
151. Shumak KH, Rock GA, Nair RC. Late relapses in individuals successfully treated for thrombotic thrombocytopenic purpura. Canadian Apheresis Group. Ann Intern Med 1995;122:569–572.
152. Misiani R, Appiani AC, Edefonti A et al. Haemolytic uraemic syndrome: therapeutic effect of plasma infusion. BMJ 1982;285:1304–1306.
153. Sheth KJ, Gill JC, Hanna J et al. Failure of fresh frozen plasma infusions to alter the course of hemolytic-uremic syndrome. Child Nephrol Urol 1988–89;9:38–41.
154. Slavicek J, Puretic Z, Novak M et al. The role of plasma exchange in the treatment of severe forms of hemolytic-uremic syndrome in childhood. Artif Organs 1995;19:506–510.
155. Zeigler ZR, Shadduck RK, Nath R et al. Pilot study of combined cryosupernatant and protein A immunoadsorption exchange in the treatment of grade 3–4 bone marrow transplant-associated thrombotic microangiopathy. Bone Marrow Transplant 1996;17:81–86.
156. Korec S, Schein PS, Smith FP et al. Treatment of cancer-associated hemolytic-uremic syndrome with staphylococcal protein A immunoperfusion. J Clin Oncol 1986;4:210–215.
157. Phillips MD, Moake JL, Nolasco L et al. Aurin tricarboxylic acid: a novel inhibitor of platelet-von Willebrand factor association. Blood 1988;72:1898–1903.
158. Sugimoto M, Ricca G, Hrinda ME et al. Functional modulation of the isolated glycoprotein Ib-binding domain on von Willebrand factor expressed in *Escherichia coli*. Biochemistry 1991;30:5202–5209.
159. Strony J, Phillips M, Brands D et al. Aurin tricarboxylic acid in a canine model of coronary artery thrombosis. Circulation 1990;81:1106–1114.
160. Strony J, Brands D, Hanners E et al. Platelet thrombus formation following fibrinolytic therapy is dependent upon shear stress and von Willebrand factor. Clin Res 1990;38:470.
161. Turner NA, Moake JL, Kamat SG et al. Comparative real-time effects on platelet adhesion and aggregation under flowing conditions of *in vivo* aspirin, heparin and monoclonal antibody fragment against glycoprotein IIb-IIIa. Circulation 1995;91:1354–1362.
162. Kamat SG, Turner NA, Konstantopoulos K et al. Effects of integrelin on platelet function in flow models of arterial thrombosis. J Cardiovas Pharmacol 1997;29:156–163.

# CHAPTER 28

# THE ALLOIMMUNE THROMBOCYTOPENIAS

Peter J. Newman, Janice G. McFarland, and Richard H. Aster

## INTRODUCTION AND CLINICAL SIGNIFICANCE

The human platelet plasma membrane contains over 100 proteins that can be recognized biochemically as individual discrete spots on two-dimensional SDS polyacrylamide gels. During the past 15 to 20 years, the biochemical basis for platelet function has advanced greatly as the structures and functions for many of these membrane components have been solved at the molecular level. With the realization that platelet membrane glycoproteins control crucial platelet functions such as platelet activation, adhesion to sites of vessel-wall damage, aggregation, and clot retraction (see Chapter 11 for a thorough treatment of platelet membrane receptors), we have also come to appreciate that many of these same glycoprotein receptors are polymorphic within the human gene pool; that is, there exist two or more perfectly functional allelic forms for several of these key platelet membrane glycoprotein receptors. The clinical consequences of these molecular variations are not unlike that found in other cellular and organ systems in that, broadly defined, these polymorphisms can be, and are recognized as, immunologic targets in a transplant setting. Such settings can include organ transplantation, blood transfusion, and pregnancy.

Recent advances in biochemical and molecular biologic techniques have made it possible to localize and precisely define at the molecular level several of the most clinically important platelet membrane glycoprotein polymorphisms. A detailed understanding of the molecular variations that are responsible for forming these polymorphic structures on the platelet surface has, not surprisingly, led to important new insights regarding the immunologic basis for alloimmune recognition and subsequent destruction of circulating platelets. This chapter will review the antigenic composition of those platelet membrane glycoproteins that are known to be polymorphic in man at the serologic, biochemical, and molecular biologic levels. Clinically relevant alloimmune thrombocytopenic disorders that directly result from platelet membrane glycoprotein variability will be discussed, focusing on the pathophysiology and mechanisms of platelet destruction, current methods of treatment, and both current and future methods of laboratory evaluation.

## PLATELET MEMBRANE GLYCOPROTEINS AS CARRIERS OF ALLOANTIGENIC DETERMINANTS

Molecular definition of the primary structures of many of the functionally important platelet membrane glycoproteins has been brought about in large part by the advent of molecular cloning techniques. As a result, we now appreciate that many of these glycoproteins are members of large, broadly distributed protein families, members of which are found on many other cell types.

Members of these protein families participate variously in cell-cell recognition, adhesion, cell migration, inflammation, and hemostasis. The important structural and functional features of platelet membrane glycoproteins are described in detail in Chapter 11, but it is important to point out that although many platelet surface receptors are invariant from individual to individual, an increasing number have been found, largely through serologic analysis, to contain clinically relevant polymorphisms that can result in platelet alloimmune and isoimmune disorders.

The first indications that the platelet surface was polymorphic appeared in the late 1950s and early 1960s, when alloantibodies that developed in individuals with posttransfusion purpura (PTP) and neonatal alloimmune thrombocytopenic purpura (NATP) were shown to discriminate antigen-positive from antigen-negative platelets (1–4). Since that time serologic studies have continued to provide important population frequency data for the currently recognized human platelet antigen systems, which now number at least four. Because serologic evidence for human platelet membrane glycoprotein polymorphisms has historically been indepen-

dently discovered in a number of different laboratories throughout the world, there have been attempts of late to unify and standardize the somewhat complex platelet antigen nomenclature that has evolved over the past 30 years (5, 6). For example, the human platelet $Pl^{A1}/Pl^{A2}$ polymorphism was independently discovered in the Netherlands and given the designation Zw. Currently recognized polymorphic forms of platelet membrane glycoproteins that can induce an alloimmune response can be found in Table 28.1. As shown, five platelet membrane glycoproteins have been shown to be encoded by multiple allelic forms that result in the expression of antigenic variants on the platelet surface. Of these, two immunogenic alleles each have been identified for GP Ia and GP Ibβ, while GP IIb is tri-allelic, GP Ibα has five alleles, and GP IIIa is encoded by more than seven allelic forms within the human gene pool. To date, no selective functional advantage to inheriting one allele versus another has been demonstrated, although the adhesive properties of only the Arg143Gln polymorphism in GP IIIa have been examined in any detail (7).

The human genome is continually subjected to environmental, chemical, and biologic factors that can, infre-

**TABLE 28.1.**    Naturally Occurring Allelic Forms of Platelet Membrane Glycoproteins That Can Induce Alloimmune Thrombocytopenia[a]

| Allelic Form | Gene Frequency | Serologic Designation |
|---|---|---|
| GP Ia Glu$_{505}$ | 0.89 | Br$^b$ (HPA-5a) |
| GP Ia Lys$_{505}$ | 0.11 | Br$^a$ (HPA-5b) |
| GP Ibα Thr$_{145}$—D (short) isoform | 0.11 (0.296) | Ko$^b$/Sib$^b$ (HPA-2a) |
| GP Ibα Thr$_{145}$—C isoform | 0.82 (0.539) | Ko$^b$/Sib$^b$ (HPA-2a) |
| GP Ibα Met$_{145}$—C isoform | <0.01 (<0.01) | Ko$^a$/Sib$^a$ (HPA-2b) |
| GP Ibα Met$_{145}$—B isoform | 0.07 (0.010) | Ko$^a$/Sib$^a$ (HPA-2b) |
| GP Ibα Met$_{145}$—A (long) isoform | <0.01 (0.155) | Ko$^a$/Sib$^a$ (HPA-2b) |
| GP Ibβ Gly$_{15}$ | .99 | Iy$^b$ |
| GP Ibβ Glu$_{15}$ | < .01 | Iy$^a$ |
| GP IIb Val$_{837}$, Ile$_{843}$ | 0.61 | Bak$^a$, Max$^b$ (HPA-3a, Max$^b$) |
| GP IIb Val$_{837}$, Ser$_{843}$ | 0.36 | Bak$^b$, Max$^b$ (HPA-3b, Max$^b$) |
| GP IIb Met$_{837}$, Ser$_{843}$ | 0.03 | Bak$^b$, Max$^a$ (HPA-3b, Max$^a$) |
| GP IIIa Leu$_{33}$ Leu$_{40}$ Arg$_{62}$ Arg$_{143}$ Pro$_{407}$ Arg$_{489}$ Arg$_{636}$ | 0.85 | Pl$^{A1}$, Pen$^a$, Mo$^b$, Ca/Tu$^b$, Sr$^b$ (HPA-1a, 4a, 6a, 7a, 8a) |
| GP IIIa *Pro*$_{33}$ Leu$_{40}$ Arg$_{62}$ Arg$_{143}$ Pro$_{407}$ Arg$_{489}$ Arg$_{636}$ | 0.15 | Pl$^{A2}$ (HPA-1b) |
| GP IIIa *Pro*$_{33}$ *Arg*$_{40}$ Arg$_{62}$ Arg$_{143}$ Pro$_{407}$ Arg$_{489}$ Arg$_{636}$ | 0.005 | Pl$^{A2}$ variant |
| GP IIIa Leu$_{33}$ Leu$_{40}$ *Gln*$_{62}$ Arg$_{143}$ Pro$_{407}$ Arg$_{489}$ Arg$_{636}$ | <0.001 | La$^a$ (HPA-10wb) |
| GP IIIa Leu$_{33}$ Leu$_{40}$ Arg$_{62}$ *Gln*$_{143}$ Pro$_{407}$ Arg$_{489}$ Arg$_{636}$ | <0.01 | Pen$^b$ (HPA-4b) |
| GP IIIa Leu$_{33}$ Leu$_{40}$ Arg$_{62}$ Arg$_{143}$ *Ala*$_{407}$ Arg$_{489}$ Arg$_{636}$ | <0.001 | Mo$^a$ (HPA-7b) |
| GP IIIa Leu$_{33}$ Leu$_{40}$ Arg$_{62}$ Arg$_{143}$ Pro$_{407}$ *Gln*$_{489}$ Arg$_{636}$ | <0.001 | Ca/Tu (HPA-6b) |
| GP IIIa Leu$_{33}$ Leu$_{40}$ Arg$_{62}$ Arg$_{143}$ Pro$_{407}$ Arg$_{489}$ *Cys*$_{636}$ | <0.001 | Sr$^a$ (HPA-8b) |

[a] *Gene frequencies shown are for the Caucasian population. Significant differences in the prevalence of glycoprotein alleles often exist in African and Asian populations. One example of this is provided for the gene frequencies of the allelic forms of GP Ibα present in the Japanese population (shown in parentheses).*

quently, cause nucleotide substitutions in the germ line that are not repaired and therefore become inherited. This phenomenon is undoubtedly the cause of the molecular polymorphisms in platelet membrane glycoproteins that have led, over a long period, to the existence of the currently recognized distribution of allelic variants of human platelet membrane glycoproteins. Statistically, it is likely that the clinically most important alloantigenic determinants among Caucasians have already been recognized and at least partially characterized. However, low-frequency alleles, as well as those that may exist among Asian, African, Indian, and other less well-studied population groups, remain to be described or fully characterized. Historically, glycoprotein alleles found in only one family (i.e., produced as a result of a recent mutagenic event and not yet disseminated outside one particular family, extended or otherwise) have been classified as "private" antigen systems. With further comparative serologic or molecular biologic evaluation, some of these alleles have been found in one or more unrelated families, at which point they become merely low-frequency allelic isoforms. Examples of both high- and low-frequency variants of platelet membrane glycoproteins that have been found to be immunogenic in man will be discussed below.

## MOLECULAR VARIANTS OF GP IIIa (THE INTEGRIN $\beta_3$ SUBUNIT)—PI$^{A1}$/PI$^{A2}$ AS A PARADIGM FOR INVESTIGATING THE IMMUNOBIOLOGY OF THE PLATELET SURFACE

Human platelet membrane glycoprotein IIIa (GP IIIa) constitutes the $\beta$-subunit of the major platelet integrin, $\alpha_{IIb}\beta_3$, which functions as the fibrinogen receptor that mediates platelet-platelet interactions (see Chapter 11). Excluding Class I histocompatibility antigens, GP IIIa is the most polymorphic molecule on the platelet surface with more than seven allelic isoforms having been described to date. The ancestral allele of GP IIIa, and that which occurs with the highest frequency in all human populations, will be referred to as GP IIIa-01. GP IIIa-01 encodes the amino acid residues Leu$_{33}$, Leu$_{40}$, Arg$_{62}$, Arg$_{143}$, Pro$_{407}$, Arg$_{489}$, and Arg$_{636}$ (see Table 28.1).

The polymorphism underlying the formation of the PI$^{A1}$/PI$^{A2}$ alloantigenic determinants is most frequently responsible for eliciting an immune response in both PTP and NATP in the Caucasian population, and, as such, a great deal of attention has been applied to solving its molecular structure. Consequently, this section will review in some detail the recent biochemical and molecular biologic approaches that have been used to examine the PI$^{A1}$ and PI$^{A2}$ epitopes, as the strategies employed in studies of the PI$^A$ polymorphism have served

as a prototype for solving the polymorphisms of the other platelet antigen systems as well.

In the late 1970s Kunicki and Aster (8, 9) reported the association of PI$^{A1}$ with GP IIIa, and Newman et al (10) later used a combination of one-dimensional peptide mapping and enzymatic deglycosylation of the GP IIb-IIIa complex to show that the PI$^{A1}$ antigenic determinant was present on a 17 Kda polypeptide portion of GP IIIa. High resolution protein fingerprint analysis further showed that the migration of two small polypeptide fragments derived from GP IIIa migrated differently depending on the PI$^A$ phenotype of the individual from which the GP IIIa was isolated, suggesting that subtle, amino acid sequence differences were most likely responsible for the PI$^{A1}$/PI$^{A2}$ polymorphism.

Progress on the molecular characterization of the PI$^A$ alloantigenic determinants was hampered by the formidable task of obtaining amino acid sequence information from both PI$^{A1}$ and PI$^{A2}$ forms of the 100 Kda GP IIIa molecule. However, with the demonstration that human platelets contain sufficient levels of residual mRNA to be amplified using the polymerase chain reaction (PCR), it became possible for the first time to directly compare platelet-specific cDNA sequences derived from single individuals of known serologic phenotype (11). Shortly thereafter, platelet RNA-PCR technology was used to amplify the NH$_2$-terminal region of platelet GP IIIa mRNA from 12 serologically defined individuals: five PI$^{A1/A1}$ homozygotes, three PI$^{A1/A2}$ heterozygotes, and three PI$^{A2/A2}$ homozygotes. Nucleotide sequence analysis of GP IIIa-derived PCR products proved that a single cytosine $\leftrightarrow$ thymidine base change at nucleotide 196 of the GP IIIa mRNA transcript correlated perfectly with the PI$^{A1}$-PI$^{A2}$ phenotype of the individual (12). This represented the first platelet-specific polymorphism to be solved at the molecular level and, as discussed below, has opened up significant new diagnostic and therapeutic approaches for the detection and management of alloimmune thrombocytopenias.

The single nucleotide base change associated with the PI$^A$ polymorphism is also able to explain the alloimmunogenicity of GP IIIa, as this nucleotide difference results in a leucine proline$\leftrightarrow$polymorphism at amino acid 33 of the mature GP IIIa glycoprotein molecule. A two-dimensional model of the aminoterminal region of GP IIIa is shown in Fig. 28.1 and, as can be seen, residue 33 is positioned in the middle of a small, 11 amino acid loop formed by the pairing of Cys$_{26}$ and Cys$_{38}$. Molecular modeling of this highly constrained protein loop (Fig. 28.2; see color plate of Fig. 28.2), shows that the shape of the leucine$_{33}$ form of the loop (left side) differs considerably from the proline$_{33}$ form, shown on the right. This amino acid residue has been shown to directly control the formation of the PI$^{A1}$ and PI$^{A2}$ alloantigenic determinants, as recombinant GP IIIa molecules containing a

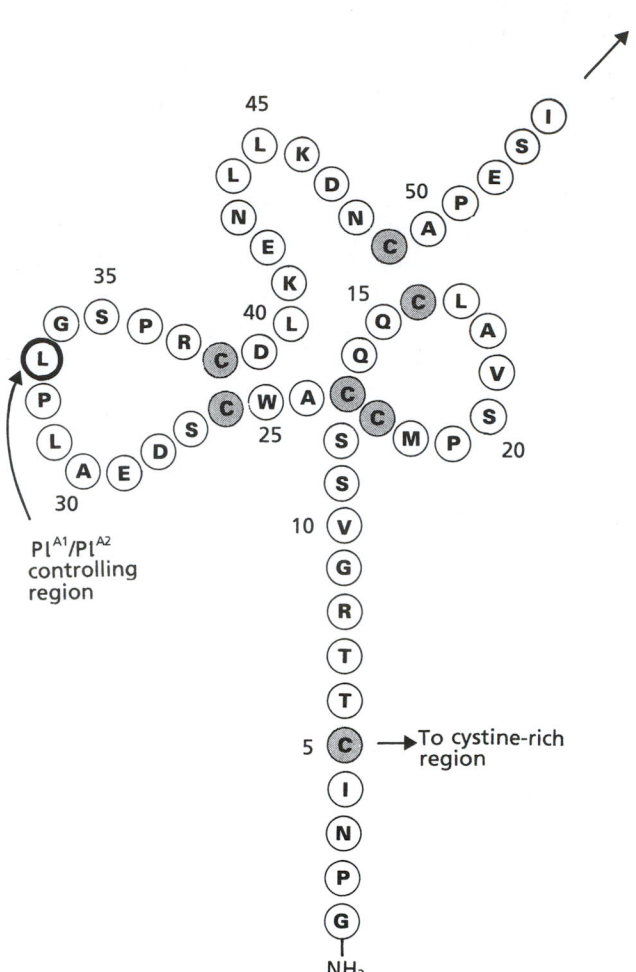

**FIGURE 28.1.** Hypothetical model of the secondary structure of the first 54 amino acids of GP IIIa. This region is extremely cysteine-rich, containing 7 Cys within the first 49 residues. Disulfide bond pairing within this region of the molecule has been partially established by Calvete et al (13). The cysteine at residue 5 is portrayed as the residue involved in the formation of the large loop known to exist in GP IIIa (see text), and pairs with cysteine 435 further down on the GP IIIa polypeptide chain. Disulfide bonds between residues 13–23, 26–39, and 16–49 result in the formation of 3 small highly constrained loops, and probably account for both the stability of this antigenic determinant following treatment with organic acids or 100°C temperatures, as well as the known sensitivity of the conformationally-dependent Pl$^{A1}$ epitope to disulfide bond reduction. The 13 amino acid loop bounded by Cys$_{26}$ and Cys$_{38}$ contains the polymorphic Leu$_{33}$ ↔ Pro$_{33}$ polymorphism that is responsible for the formation of the Pl$^{A1}$ and Pl$^{A2}$ alloantigenic determinants. (Adapted with permission from Newman PJ. Platelet GP IIb-IIIa: molecular variations and alloantigens [Review]. Thromb Haemost 1991;66:111–118, and from Newman PJ, Goldberger A. Molecular genetic aspects of human platelet antigen systems [Review]. Baillieres Clin Haematol 1991;4:869–888.

leucine at amino acid residue 33 bind anti-Pl$^{A1}$, but not anti-Pl$^{A2}$ human alloantibodies, while the Pro$_{33}$ form of GP IIIa reacts with anti-Pl$^{A2}$, but not anti-Pl$^{A1}$ serum (15). More recently, Valentin et al showed that immune recognition of this polymorphic region may be more complex than originally thought, as the anti-Pl$^{A1}$ antibodies derived from some alloimmunized individuals appear to recognize polymorphic amino acid residue 33 in combination with one or more sequences derived from the cysteine-rich domain of GP IIIa (16). The clinical significance of this newly appreciated heterogeneity in the humoral response to the Pl$^{A}$ polymorphism is not yet known.

Evidence suggests that the production of anti-Pl$^{A1}$ alloantibodies depends on the contribution of specific T-lymphocytes. First, anti-Pl$^{A1}$ alloantibodies are IgG, rather than IgM, in subclass—an event that requires T-cell help. Second, the alloimmune response to the Pl$^{A1}$ epitope is one of most highly HLA-associated disorders in man (17); only individuals expressing HLA-DR52a (DRB3*0101 using the nomenclature of the World Health Organization) on the surface of their antigen-presenting cells are able to produce anti-Pl$^{A1}$ antibodies (18, 19). Interestingly, Kuijpers et al showed that, unlike anti-Pl$^{A1}$ antibody production, the immune response to Pl$^{A2}$ (i.e., the Pro$_{33}$ form of GP IIIa) is not at all HLA-linked (20). Together, these findings suggest that specific T-cell clones respond to GP IIIa-derived peptides on the surface of antigen-presenting cells only when (a) the peptides contain leucine at position 33, and (b) the peptide is presented within the context of the DR52a allele. They further predict that the Pro$_{33}$-containing GP IIIa peptide might not be presented efficiently by *any* particular DR molecule—consistent with the observation that anti-Pl$^{A2}$ alloantibodies are encountered so rarely. Direct experimental evidence for the involvement of specific T-cell help during the development of the alloimmune response to Pl$^{A1}$ has recently been provided by Maslanka et al (21), who analyzed the T-cell repertoire of a woman with a child affected by NATP and found predominant T-cell clonotypes having the shared motif L-P-S/T within the complementarity-determining 3 (CDR3) region of the T-cell receptor (TCR) β-chain. These specific T-cells were found to be in high abundance immediately after delivery of the affected child, and their frequency dropped at later times. Further insight into the molecular mechanism by which Leu$_{33}$-containing GP IIIa peptide fragments are able to stimulate T-cells has been provided by Wu et al (22), who employed *in vitro* peptide binding assays to show that Leu$_{33}$ actually serves as a specific anchor residue that directly contacts the restricting DR52a allele. Importantly, this group further demonstrated that Leu$_{33}$-containing GP IIIa peptides are able to interact with a recombinant soluble form of DR52a, while the Pro$_{33}$-containing peptides are not (22), providing a molecular explanation for the relative paucity of an alloimmune response to the Pl[A2] epitope. Improved understanding of the B- and T-cell epitopes that are responsible for the development of the alloimmune response to Pl[A1] should facilitate the development of sensitive and predictive diagnostic assays and make possible therapeutic regimens that employ antagonistic peptides.

## PEN[a]/PEN[b]

Although the Pl[A1]/Pl[A2] polymorphisms are most often implicated in causing NATP and PTP in the Caucasian population, the Pl[A2] form of GP IIIa occurs much less frequently in the black population (23) and was not found at all in 300 Oriental individuals examined (24). Thus anti-Pl[A1] antibodies rarely pose a clinical problem within these populations. Rather, the Pen[a]/Pen[b] polymorphism is more frequently the cause of PTP and NATP among Orientals. Like the other human platelet membrane glycoprotein polymorphisms, this molecular variation was independently discovered serologically in two different laboratories (24, 25) and given two different designations, Pen (25) and Yuk (24).

Shibata and Mori (26) and Furihata et al (27) demonstrated that the Pen epitopes, like Pl[A1], are associated with the GP IIIa molecule. Anti-Pen alloantibodies completely inhibit ADP-induced platelet aggregation (27), indicating that the region of GP IIIa containing the Pen epitope probably lies within a functionally important region of this membrane glycoprotein complex. Biochemical studies have provided evidence that there is a large disulfide-bonded loop in GP IIIa that is cleaved by chymotrypsin at residues 121 and 348 (28, 29). This loop contains the Arg-Gly-Asp (RGD) binding domain on the receptor that recognizes fibrinogen, von Willebrand factor, and other adhesive ligands of the GP IIb-IIIa integrin complex (30). Analysis of chymotryptic fragments of GP IIIa also showed that the Pen[a] determinant is lost from GP IIIa, coincident with the removal of part of this large loop (31). Taken together with the ability of anti-Pen antibodies to inhibit the binding of fibrinogen to platelets, these data suggested that the Pen epitopes are located within this region of the GP IIIa molecule. In this regard Wang et al (32, 33) found an Arg143Gln amino acid polymorphism in GP IIIa, located directly in the middle of the RGD binding domain, that is responsible for the formation of the Pen[a] and Pen[b] alloantigenic determinants, consistent with the above predictions. Despite its positioning within the ligand-binding domain, the $Gln_{143}$ form of GP IIIa has retained full adhesive capabilities (7). The location of the Pen polymorphism relative to Pl[A] is shown in Fig. 28.3.

## LOW-FREQUENCY ALLELIC FORMS OF GP IIIa

The Pl[A] and Pen polymorphisms are by far the most frequent cause of an alloimmune response to GP IIIa. However, a number of low-frequency allelic isoforms of this glycoprotein have been detected serologically, all having been implicated in cases of NATP. These include the Sr[a] epitope resulting from an Arg636Cys dimorphism (34, 35), Mo (Pro407Ala) (36), Ca/Tu (Arg489Gln) (37–39), and La (Arg62Gln) (40). All of these represent relatively recent point mutations of GP IIIa-01—the high-frequency ancestral allele (41)—and are therefore not widespread outside of the region in which they were first discovered. They are therefore expected to be of less clinical significance. One exception may be the $Gln_{489}$ form of GP IIIa (Ca/Tu), which has been found in Canada, Finland, and the Philippines. In addition to these GP IIIa-01 variants, the Pl[A2] ($Pro_{33}$) allelic form of GP IIIa has been subjected to an independent mutational event, as three different groups have reported a variant allele having a Leu40Arg polymorphism just downstream from $Pro_{33}$ (42–44). The Pl[A2] variant allele, however, has not been found to be immunogenic. As would be expected, $Arg_{40}$ has not been found on the $Leu_{33}$ (Pl[A1]) form of GP IIIa. The currently recognized allelic forms of GP IIIa are summarized in Table 28.1, and the putative location of many of their epitopes are shown schematically in Fig. 28.3.

## ALLELIC FORMS OF PLATELET GP Ia (THE INTEGRIN $\alpha_2$ SUBUNIT)

The human GP Ia-IIa complex, also known as VLA-2 or the integrin $\alpha_2\beta_1$, serves as a major receptor for collagen in platelets and other cell types (see Chapter 11). In the mid-1980s, Mueller-Eckhardt et al identified serologically a platelet polymorphism of GP Ia that may be responsible for up to 5% of the cases of NATP in Germany (45). Termed the Br[a]/Br[b] alloantigen system (HPA-5a and -5b according to the HPA nomenclature [46]), Santoso et al (47, 48), Smith et al (49), and Woods et al (50) all used immunochemical techniques to localize the Br alloantigenic epitopes to GP Ia. Unlike the more abundant GP IIb-IIIa integrin complex, only 2000 to 5000 $\alpha_2\beta_1$ complexes exist per platelet (51); consequently, NATP caused by GP Ia incompatibility tends to be rather mild, which may explain why this alloantigen system went largely undetected prior to 1988. Santoso et al amplified GP Ia mRNA from the platelets of Br[a] and Br[b] homozygous individuals and showed that an A1648G nucleotide substitution, which results in a Lys505Glu amino acid polymorphism, is responsible for the formation of the Br[a] and Br[b] epitopes (52).

## Platelet Membrane Glycoprotein Epitopes in Alloimmune Thrombocytopenia

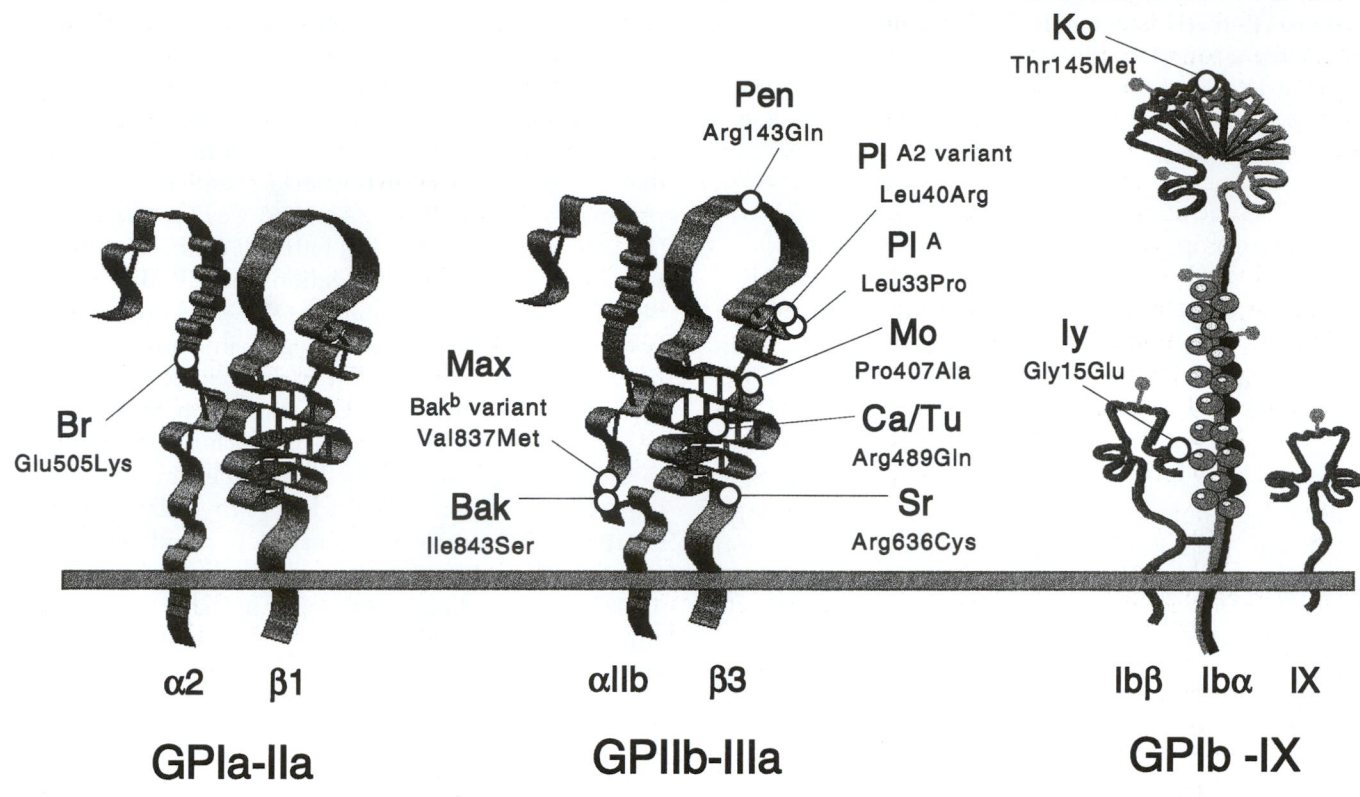

**FIGURE 28.3.**   Physical location of the human platelet alloantigenic epitopes. Shown are schematics of three membrane glycoprotein complexes found on the platelet surface. The circles represent polymorphic residues that can be recognized by the human immune system in a transfusion or transplantation setting. (Artwork generously provided by Chris Ward, M.D., Ph.D.)

## POLYMORPHISMS OF GP Ib

As described in detail in Chapter 11, platelet membrane glycoprotein Ib is actually a complex of four different subunits: GP Ibα, GP Ibβ, GPV, and GP IX, all of which are members of a larger family of proteins characterized by the presence of one or more leucine-rich motifs (53–55). Together, this glycoprotein complex serves as the major platelet receptor for the adhesive ligand, von Willebrand factor, and plays an important role in the adhesion of platelets to the vessel wall following vascular injury.

The GP Ibα subunit has two different types of polymorphism—both of which affect its phenotype. The first, known as $Ko^a/Ko^b$, was first described in the early 1960s in association with posttransfusion platelet refractoriness (2, 56, 57). An identical polymorphism responsible for platelet transfusion refractoriness was independently described in the Japanese population by Saji et al in 1989 (58) and given the designation $Sib^a/Sib^b$. The molecular basis of the Ko/Sib polymorphism was

solved by Kuijpers et al (59, 60) and by Murata et al (61), who showed that a Thr145Met polymorphism in the GP Ibα subunit segregated with Ko/Sib phenotype. The $Thr_{145}$ form of GP Ib (=$Ko^b$ = $Sib^b$ = HPA-2a) has a gene frequency of 93% in the Caucasian population, while the $Met_{145}$ form of GP Ib (=$Ko^a$ = $Sib^a$ = HPA-2b) has a gene frequency of approximately 7%. Thus anti-$Sib^a$ and anti-$Ko^a$ alloantibodies are formed by $Thr_{145}$ individuals upon exposure to the low-frequency $Met_{145}$ form of GP Ibα during platelet transfusion. Interestingly, human alloantibodies that bind the $Met_{145}$ form of GP Ibα have been shown to inhibit ristocetin-induced platelet agglutination, most likely due to the location of this polymorphic amino acid residue within the N-terminal globular von Willebrand factor binding domain (60).

In 1984 Moroi et al described four polymorphic *size* variants of the GP Ibα subunit that they termed A, B, C, and D (ranging from largest to smallest), having gene frequencies of 0.073, 0.11, 0.561, and 0.355, respectively, in the Japanese population (62). This size polymorphism was later shown to be due to a difference in the number of 13-amino acid (39 base pair) tandem repeats present within the macroglycopeptide region of the GP Ibα chain (63)—the D isoform of GP Ibα contains one such repeat, the C form two tandem repeats, and so on. Interestingly, human alloantibodies directed against the Sib$^a$ epitope on the Met$_{145}$ form of GP Ib were shown to react with only the larger (A or B) forms of GP Ibα (64), providing serologic evidence for genetic linkage between the Thr143Met dimorphism and GP Ibα size variants. This relationship was formally established by Simsek et al (65) and Ishida et al (66), who showed that this amino acid dimorphism is in nearly complete linkage disequilibrium with the molecular-weight polymorphism. They showed that the larger A and B forms of GP Ibα contain a methionine at residue 145 and therefore express the Ko$^a$ (= Sib$^a$) epitope, while the more commonly inherited shorter C and D isoforms of GP Ibα contain Thr$_{145}$. The C isoform appears to have been the target for the Thr$_{145}$ → Met mutagenic event. Thus *five* different allelic isoforms of the GP Ibα subunit are now known to exist in the human gene pool: Shorter D and C forms encoding Thr$_{145}$, a rare transitional C form containing Met$_{145}$, and larger B and A size variants that contain Met at residue 145. It is important to note that the gene frequencies of these alleles vary significantly among different ethnic and geographic populations. The allelic forms of GP Ibα and their frequencies in the Caucasian versus Japanese populations are summarized in Table 28.1.

In addition to molecular variations of GP Ibα, two allelic forms of the smaller GP Ibβ subunit have also been described. Termed Iy$^a$ (67), this low-frequency allele of GP Ibβ was responsible for a case of severe NATP and is not restricted to a single family. Santoso et al have recently shown that a G141A mutation, resulting in a Gly15Glu amino acid substitution within the extracellular domain of GP Ibβ, is associated with the presence of Iy$^a$ epitope (68).

## GP IIb (THE INTEGRIN $\alpha_{IIb}$ SUBUNIT)

The α-subunit of the integrin GP IIb-IIIa ($\alpha_{IIb}$) is also polymorphic in man, with three allelic isoforms characterized to date. The Bak polymorphism was first described by von dem Borne et al (69) when they reported a new specificity present in a maternal alloantibody in a case of NATP. Subsequently, an alloantibody isolated from the serum of a individual with PTP, termed anti-Lek$^a$, was described by Wautier and his associates, and the antigenic determinant for this antibody localized to 76- and 60-kDa fragments of the heavy chain of GP IIb (70, 71). Shortly thereafter, the Bak$^a$ antigen was also localized to GP IIb (72), and the Bak$^a$ and Lek$^a$ antigenic determinants were shown to be identical (73, 74). Their allelic counterpart, Bak$^b$ (Lek$^b$), is also immunogenic (75).

The polymorphism underlying Bak/Lek was shown

by Lyman et al (76) to be due to an isoleucine ↔ serine polymorphism at residue 843 of the GP IIb heavy chain. Interestingly, Take et al showed that anti-Bak$^a$ antibodies produced by different alloimmunized individuals vary in their reactivity with asialo-GP IIb (77), suggesting some role for carbohydrate moieties in contributing to the actual alloantibody recognition site. The role of carbohydrate residues in the formation of the Bak epitopes was formally shown in studies performed using allele-specific recombinant forms of the GP IIb molecule, in which it was shown that anti-Bak alloantibodies are not able to bind to the recombinant precursor form of the GP IIb molecule, pre-GP IIb (15). Pre-GP IIb differs from the mature form in two important ways. First, it is not cleaved into heavy and light chains, and second, its high mannose carbohydrate residues have not yet been modified into complex sugar moieties within the Golgi apparatus. From this information and the data of Take et al (77), it appears that carbohydrate residues added posttranslationally to the GP IIb polypeptide chain contribute to the antibody combining site on the mature GP IIb molecule to which many anti-Bak$^a$ and anti-Bak$^b$ alloantibodies bind. This was formally shown by the combined studies of Djaffar et al (78), who localized the antigenic epitope to a 29-amino acid fragment of the GP IIb heavy chain, and by Calvete and Muniz-Diaz (79), who identified Ser$_{847}$ as bearing the O-linked oligosaccharide moiety that contributes to the alloantibody combining site.

The Ser$_{843}$ form of GP IIb has been proposed to represent the ancestral form of this glycoprotein in primates (41) and appears to have been subjected to an additional mutational event at nearby residue 837. Thus, Noris et al have recently reported that a Ser837Met dimorphism in the GP IIb heavy chain is immunogenic, having been responsible for a case of NATP in which the neonatal platelet count dropped to 6000/μl (80). Termed the Max$^a$ epitope, this variant form of the Ser$_{843}$ (Bak$^b$) allele of GP IIb has an apparent gene frequency of approximately 3% in Caucasians of Western European ancestry (Table 28.1).

## THE NaK ISOANTIGEN—GP IV (CD36) DEFICIENCY

Ikeda et al reported the presence of antibodies to a platelet antigen, termed Nak$^a$, in a thrombocytopenic individual with refractoriness to HLA-matched platelet transfusions (81). Tomiyama et al (82) later showed that anti-Nak$^a$ antibodies reacted specifically with GP IV (CD36), an 88-kDa membrane glycoprotein reported to serve variously as a collagen (83) and thrombospondin (84) receptor (see Chapter 11). GP IV deficiency has been subdivided into type I, where GP IV is absent from the surface of *all* cells, and the more commonly found type II, where GP IV is absent from the platelet surface only (e.g., monocyte surface expression is positive). It is the type I (but not type II) individuals who develop *iso* (not *allo*) antibodies, that is, a polyclonal response to an entire protein not previously seen by the immune system when they receive GP IV-positive platelet transfusions.

Platelet GP IV deficiency is present in about 3% of the Japanese population and in 0.3% of the United States population (85). To date, four different molecular variants of GP IV responsible for this genetic defect have been identified, including (a) an Ser478Pro substitution that results in the production of an unstable protein that is degraded in the cytoplasm (86, 87); (b) a mutant form harboring a dinucleotide deletion (residues 539 and 540) that results in a frameshift and premature termination of the GP IV polypeptide chain (88); (c) a form missing base 1159, leading to a frameshift and premature termination (89); and (d) an incompletely characterized allele whose mRNA transcript is either not made or is selectively degraded in platelets but not other cell types (90). It is inheritance of the latter allele together with any of the other three mutant forms (normally the unstable $Ser_{478}$ allele of GP IV) that leads to type II deficiency.

Interestingly, GP IV-deficient (Nak[a] negative) platelets exhibit normal to near-normal adhesion to types I, III, and IV collagen (91, 92), normal platelet aggregation to type I and III collagen (93, 94), and normal thrombospondin binding (91). They are markedly deficient, however, in their ability to initially adhere to fibrillar collagen (91) and show reduced aggregation to collagen type V (94), suggesting that GP IV functions primarily in type V collagen-induced platelet aggregation and may also play a role in initial attachment to fibrillar collagen.

# POSTTRANSFUSION PURPURA (PTP)

## CLINICAL COURSE AND PROGNOSIS

Posttransfusion purpura (PTP) is characterized by acute, usually severe, thrombocytopenia occurring 5 to 10 days, typically 7 days, after a blood transfusion. The condition was first defined as a distinct syndrome by Shulman et al in 1961 (3). Serum from most individuals with PTP contains a potent alloantibody, usually specific for the antigen Pl[A1], induced by platelets or platelet fragments contained in the transfused blood. In the acute stage, petechial hemorrhages, ecchymoses, and hemorrhagic bullae are typically seen in the skin and mucous membranes, and bleeding from the urinary and gastrointestinal tracts is often severe. Most cases of PTP occur in multiparous women following receipt of their first blood transfusion. However, the syndrome can occur in nulliparous and previously transfused women (95) and in men (95–97). It can be induced by whole blood, red blood cells, or plasma. It is common for the provocative transfusion to be associated with a febrile reaction, often

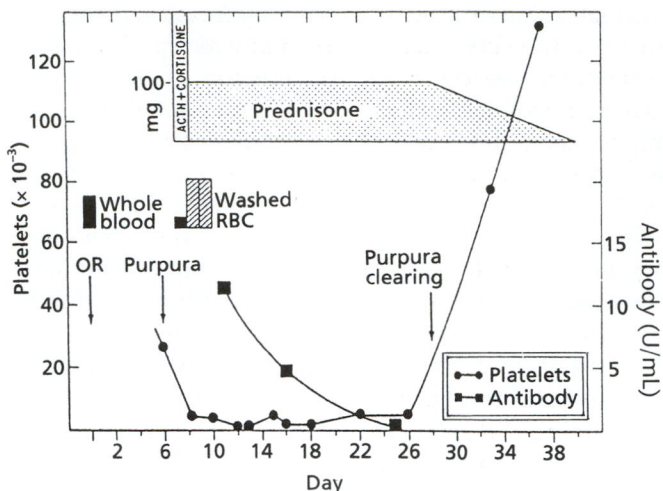

**FIGURE 28.4.** Clinical course of a 43-year-old woman who developed PTP 6 days after receiving whole blood during surgery. Thrombocytopenia lasted for 3 weeks, despite treatment with prednisone. Recovery occurred after disappearance of anti-Pl[A1] antibodies from the individual's plasma. (Adapted with permission from Shulman NR, Aster RH, Leitner A et al. Immunoreactions involving platelets. V. Post-transfusion purpura due to a complement-fixing antibody against a genetically controlled platelet antigen. A proposed mechanism for thrombocytopenia and its relevance in "autoimmunity." J Clin Invest 1961;40:1597–1620, with permission.)

accompanied by chills. About 10% of the reported cases of PTP suffered an intracranial hemorrhage, which was fatal in most instances. Individuals who did not experience this complication recovered completely within 1 to 4 weeks.

The course of a typical individual with PTP treated only with corticosteroids and transfusions of washed red cells is shown in Fig. 28.4. PTP associated with active immunization against platelet alloantigens should be distinguished from thrombocytopenia occurring acutely after transfusion of blood unexpectedly containing anti-Pl[A1] antibody to a Pl[A1]-positive recipient (98).

## PATHOGENESIS

Alloantibodies associated with PTP have been shown to react with three different platelet membrane glycoproteins: the Pl[A1] and Pl[A2] epitopes on GP IIIa (3, 97, 99), the Bak[a] and Bak[b] epitopes on GP IIb (73, 75, 100, 101), the Pen[a] epitope on GP IIIa (102), and the Br[a] antigenic determinant on GP Ia (103). In addition, a case of probable PTP associated with immunization against the Nak[a] isoantigen (GP IV) has also been reported (104).

The individuals' platelets, typed following recovery, are invariably found to be negative for the antigens with which their alloantibodies react. How an alloantibody can promote destruction of autologous platelets lacking the alloantigen for which it is specific has puzzled clinical investigators for many years. From early studies, it was clear that alloantibody alone is not responsible for destruction of $Pl^{A1}$-negative platelets in the transfusion recipient because alloantibody can still be detected at significant levels after recovery (3, 105) and because reinfusion of plasma obtained during the acute phase to individuals after recovery did not affect platelet levels (3, 105, 106). Shulman et al originally suggested that transfused, platelet-specific alloantigen survives in the circulation, forms immune complexes with subsequently produced alloantibody, and then binds to autologous platelets to promote their destruction (3). Material containing $Pl^{A1}$ antigen that did not sediment after ultracentrifugation was detected in plasma from blood stored for several weeks at 4°C and could be passively transferred to $Pl^{A1}$-negative platelets. The $Pl^{A1}$-containing material was althought to be particulate because it could be removed by a 0.3-micron filter. Kickler et al also found that plasma from stored blood contained nonsedimentable material that could transfer $Pl^{A1}$ antigen to $Pl^{A1}$-negative platelets (107). The demonstration of anti-$Pl^{A1}$ in eluates from platelets obtained following recovery from PTP was althought to be consistent with nonspecific adsorption of immune complexes to platelets (108). As noted, however, anti-$Pl^{A1}$ antibody usually persists after recovery, and it seems likely that the anti-$Pl^{A1}$ detected in these eluates was derived from IgG released from platelet storage granules (109).

Studies by Shulman provided further evidence that membrane-associated GP IIIa bearing the $Pl^{A1}$ antigenic determinant exists in normal plasma and can be transferred to and expressed by $Pl^{A1}$-negative platelets with which it is incubated (110). Up to 1% of the total $Pl^{A1}$ antigen present in the circulation may exist in this form—a quantity that would be sufficient to transfer $Pl^{A1}$ antigen sites to platelets of a $Pl^{A1}$-negative recipient and to allow their destruction by subsequently formed anti-$Pl^{A1}$ alloantibody (110). This mechanism could explain acute destruction of autologous platelets in individuals with PTP. How thrombocytopenia could persist for 3 or 4 weeks in some individuals on this basis in the face of new platelet production is less certain, however. Probably only a few hundred anti-$Pl^{A1}$ IgG molecules bound to the surface of a platelet are sufficient to cause its destruction by anti-$Pl^{A1}$ antibody (110, 111). Conceivably, $Pl^{A1}$ antigen can be recycled to newly produced $Pl^{A2}$ homozygous platelets in quantities sufficient to allow destruction by alloantibody, but it is more difficult to envision weakly expressed glycoproteins such as GP Ia (bearing the Br epitopes) behaving in this way. An important, but unanswered, question is whether GP IIIa or other passively acquired alloantigens can also transfer to endothelial cells, priming them for destruction by alloantibody and precipitating hemorrhage.

A third proposal for a mechanism for posttransfusion purpura is that a true autoantibody reactive with a individual's own platelets is produced in parallel with the alloantibody. Support for this proposal was provided by studies in which injection of one species of marmoset with platelets from another was followed by acute, severe thrombocytopenia associated with platelet-reactive autoantibody production (112). In several studies eluates obtained from $Pl^{A1}$-negative platelets during the acute stage of PTP were found to be capable of binding to autologous platelets obtained following recovery and to $Pl^{A1}$-negative platelets from other persons (113, 114). This was althought to reflect transfer of antigen-antibody complexes, but it seems equally possible that autoantibodies were being detected. The possibility that some cases of PTP are induced by this mechanism gains credence from observations in individuals with delayed hemolytic transfusion reactions in which destruction of transfused red cells by alloantibodies was accompanied by destruction of autologous red cells by simultaneously formed autoantibodies (115, 116). Destruction of autologous red cells is self-limited in such individuals, as with platelets in individuals with PTP.

The three mechanisms proposed to explain posttransfusion purpura are summarized in Table 28.2. PTP is a rare condition, although nearly all transfusions are

**TABLE 28.2.** Mechanisms Proposed for the Etiology of Posttransfusion Purpura

| | |
|---|---|
| Immune complexes | Alloantigens transfused in the form of platelet fragments or microparticles in plasma combine complexes with subsequently formed alloantibody to produce immune complexes that bind with high affinity to autologous platelets. |
| Acquired antigens | Alloantigens transfused with plasma or released from platelets after transfusion attach to autologous platelets, allowing them to be sensitized by subsequently formed alloantibody. |
| Autoantibody formation | In addition to stimulating an alloantigen-specific antibody, transfused platelets or platelet fragments induce an *auto*antibody specific for a site on autologous platelets. |

*Adapted from Aster RH. Post-transfusion purpura. In: Engelfreit CP, von dem Borne AE, eds. Baillieres clinical immunology. London: WB Saunders, 1987; pp. 453–461.*

mismatched for one or more of the recognized platelet-specific alloantigens and at least 2% of transfusions are mismatched for Pl$^{A1}$. In part, the rarity of this condition may reflect a requirement for the histocompatibility antigen HLA-DRw52a to mount an immune response to Pl$^{A1}$ (19, 118). The need for prior exposure to platelet-specific antigens as a result of pregnancy or previous transfusions is another limiting factor. It is uncertain whether blood from only certain donors can induce the condition.

## LABORATORY EVALUATION

Thrombocytopenia is usually very severe, with platelet levels less than 10,000 per μl. Megakaryocytes are found in normal or increased numbers in bone marrow aspirates. Platelet-reactive alloantibodies, usually specific for Pl$^{A1}$, but sometimes for other platelet-specific alloantigens (see above), can be detected by a number of currently available assays. Since high-titer, HLA-reactive alloantibodies are often present (95, 97, 119), it is best to use methods that are specific for determinants carried on the GP IIb-IIIa or Ia-IIa complexes, such as modified antigen capture ELISA (120), monoclonal antibody-specific immobilization of platelet antigen (MAIPA) test (121), or antigen capture ELISA (ACE) (27). Unexpected red cell-specific alloantibodies are also found in some individuals (119). PTP occurring in the context of allogeneic bone marrow transplantation can present an especially difficult challenge (122).

Pl$^{A1}$-reactive alloantibodies characteristic of PTP are usually complement-fixing in the acute stage, in contrast to the alloantibodies that cause neonatal alloimmune thrombocytopenic purpura (123). Platelets obtained from individuals in early stages of PTP have been shown to carry IgG and IgM (113, 124) and, rarely, IgA (114) immunoglobulins. The failure of anti-Pl$^{A1}$ antibodies obtained after recovery to fix complement may reflect disappearance of alloantibody of the IgG$_3$ subclass, typical of the acute phase (125, 126).

## TREATMENT

As noted, untreated individuals with PTP usually recover spontaneously within 1 to 4 weeks of the onset of symptoms. Intracranial hemorrhage, often fatal, has occurred in about 10% of cases described in the literature (95, 117, 127). Therapeutic intervention should therefore be considered in all cases with severe thrombocytopenia and hemorrhagic symptoms. Nearly all individuals with PTP have been treated with prednisone or other corticosteroids. Improvement has been attributed to this therapy in a few instances (119, 128, 129), but it is uncertain whether corticosteroids influence the clinical course.

The first case of PTP described by Shulman et al (3) was treated empirically by whole blood exchange

transfusion and regained normal platelet levels a few days thereafter. Subsequently, numerous individuals have been treated successfully with plasma exchange. Although controlled studies have not been performed, the association between plasma exchange and recovery from PTP is often striking, and a cause and effect relationship seems certain. The effectiveness of plasma exchange cannot be explained by removal of platelet-specific alloantibody alone because antibody can often be detected several years following recovery (3, 105, 106).

Intravenous (IV) immunoglobulin, 0.4 g per kg daily for 5 days, has been used to treat PTP in recent years (95, 117, 129–131). In most cases, platelet levels have risen within a few days after treatment was begun. A consensus is developing that IV immunoglobulin therapy is the treatment of choice for PTP and that plasma exchange should be undertaken only in individuals who fail to respond. Individuals with autoimmune thrombocytopenia sometimes improve rapidly after a single infusion of 1 g per kg of IV immunoglobulin (see Chapter 30). This treatment regimen deserves evaluation in PTP. Splenectomy was effective in one individual unresponsive to other therapy (132).

Platelet transfusions are usually ineffective in PTP and are sometimes accompanied by severe, fever-chill reactions, possibly triggered by reactions of HLA-specific alloantibodies with the transfused blood components. If platelets are administered because of severe bleeding symptoms, reactions of this nature should be anticipated. Pl$^{A1}$-negative platelets were ineffective when transfused to one reported individual during the acute phase of the disease (133), but did elevate platelet levels in another case when given a few days before recovery (134).

Pl$^{A1}$-positive blood has been transfused without complication several years later to individuals who recovered from an earlier episode of PTP associated with anti-Pl$^{A1}$ antibody (95, 105, 110). In several instances, however, PTP recurred in association with later transfusions (135–137). The suggestion has been made that relapse is more likely to be triggered by transfusions given many years after the original event, possibly because residual anti-Pl$^{A1}$ alloantibody is protective for a few years (110). When individuals with a history of PTP require transfusions, it is reasonable to use platelet-poor products such as washed red cells or Pl$^{A1}$-negative blood, if available. However, a recurrence of PTP apparently triggered by frozen-thawed red cells has also been described (137).

# NEONATAL ALLOIMMUNE THROMBOCYTOPENIA

Neonatal alloimmune thrombocytopenic purpura (NATP) is a syndrome characterized by thrombocytopenia in the neonate developing at or shortly after birth due to passively transmitted maternal antibody directed against a fetal platelet antigen that is inherited from the father and that is lacking on the mother's platelets. The incidence of NATP is about 1 in 2500 live births (138). Maternal antibody is usually raised against the Pl[A1] epitope on GP IIIa (see Table 28.1). This incompatibility is implicated in 46 to 83% of all cases (95, 138–140). The Pro[33] form of GP IIIa, bearing the Pl[A2] epitope, has also been linked to NATP (141, 142). Many other platelet-specific alloantigenic determinants have been implicated in NATP cases as well (4, 24, 25, 45, 69, 143–147). Immunization to HLA class I antigens may also cause NATP (139, 148), although a true cause-and-effect relationship between the presence of anti-HLA antibodies, which are quite common in pregnancy, and neonatal thrombocytopenia is unproven.

## PATHOPHYSIOLOGY

The mechanism of platelet destruction in NATP is analogous to that of the red-blood cell destruction in hemolytic disease of the newborn (HDN). Transplacental passage of the immunizing antigen (e.g., GP IIIa) occurs as early as 14 weeks of gestation (149). In turn, maternal IgG is produced, crosses the placenta, coats fetal platelets, and ultimately causes their sequestration. Although there are some striking similarities in the pathogenesis of NATP and HDN, NATP is distinguished from the latter by a high rate of affected first pregnancies. In reported series, between 20 and 59% of cases occur in primiparae (4, 95, 139). Therefore immunization of mothers to platelet antigens must occur more readily than to the usual red cell antigens implicated in HDN.

The existence of an incompatibility for a platelet-specific antigen between fetus and mother is necessary, but insufficient, for clinical NATP to develop. Since 98% of the Caucasian population is positive for the Pl[A1] antigenic determinant, fetuses of 2% of women are at risk for developing NATP. However, far fewer than 2% of normal pregnancies are affected by this disorder. The lower-than-expected rate of NATP does not appear to be due to underreporting, since prospective and retrospective studies of pregnancies arrive at about the same incidence (138, 150). It is probable that a specific immune response gene(s) is required for a Pl[A2] homozygous mother to produce anti-Pl[A1] alloantibodies. Indeed, there are several studies describing significant associations between anti-Pl[A1] production and specific HLA phenotypes (118, 151–154). To date, the strongest link is with the DR52a allele found in nearly 100% of Pl[A2] mothers who produce anti-Pl[A1] antibodies (19).

The severity of NATP may vary according to the specificity of maternal antibody. The most severe cases, those with *in utero* intracranial hemorrhage (IUICH), for instance, are usually related to incompatibilities for Pl[A1].

Anti-Pen[a], although a less commonly implicated antibody in NATP, has also been reported to cause IUICH. Similarly, the Bak[b] and Pl[A2] epitopes have been linked to severe NATP with perinatal ICH. To date, ICH has not been reported to occur in anti-Br[b] mediated-NATP, despite the fact that this allele of GP Ia is the second most commonly implicated incompatibility in NATP cases (146). The apparent difference in the clinical severity of NATP according to antigen involved may relate to the relative density of target molecules on the fetal platelets. The most densely represented glycoprotein on the platelet surface is GP IIIa (bearing the Pl[A] and Pen epitopes), with approximately 40,000 antigenic determinants each per platelet in the heterozygote, in this case the affected fetus. The same number of GP IIb molecules (bearing the Bak and Max epitopes) are present on each heterozygous platelet. In contrast, the GP Ia-IIa integrin complex is present at only 1000 to 2000 sites per platelet (51). If antigen density is related to clinical severity, it follows that it must also be inversely related to platelet count in the affected fetus. This has not been adequately studied to date, but there are at least three cases of severe fetal thrombocytopenia (<10,000 per μl) in NATP related to Br (146, 147). Therefore severe NATP, although less likely when a specific antigen is implicated (e.g., Br[a] or Br[b]), cannot be ruled out on that basis alone.

## CLINICAL FEATURES

As many as 81% of affected infants have petechiae, purpura, or overt bleeding at birth (140). It has been recently shown that fetal alloimmune thrombocytopenia occurs early in gestation, with initial platelet counts of ≤20,000 per μl in almost 50% of fetuses studied before 24 weeks of gestation (154). Since approximately half of the cases of NATP occur in first pregnancies, many of these infants are delivered vaginally; hence bleeding symptoms may be associated with forceps trauma or cephalohematomas. By one estimate, 28% of affected infants diagnosed in the neonatal period have evidence of central-nervous-system hemorrhage (140). Up to one-half of the intracranial hemorrhages occur prenatally (155, 156). These *in utero* intracranial hemorrhages (IUICH) are characterized by severe neurologic sequelae, porencephaly and optic hypoplasia (157). An additional complication of NATP is late-onset neurologic deficits that are not noted clinically in the neonatal period (158). If untreated, the thrombocytopenia in NATP normally lasts 2 to 3 weeks and then resolves spontaneously. There are cases, however, in which the thrombocytopenia is unusually prolonged (144, 145).

## LABORATORY DIAGNOSIS

Neonatal platelet counts are uniformly low and hemoglobin concentrations are occasionally decreased secondary to bleeding. The *maternal* platelet count, however, is normal, distinguishing NATP from neonatal thrombocytopenia caused by the presence of maternal *auto*antibodies. After 72 to 96 hours the serum bilirubin may be elevated due to passive resorption of extravasated blood. A bone marrow aspirate is occasionally performed to determine the source of severe thrombocytopenia, and megakaryocytes are usually found to be present in normal numbers. In at least three cases, however, decreased megakaryocytes have been reported (139, 145, 159). Cranial ultrasound examination prenatally and postnatally occasionally shows sonolucent areas in the brain or intraventricular hemorrhage (160). Computerized tomographic (CT) scans can confirm an abnormal ultrasound.

Once NATP is suspected on the basis of both clinical and routine laboratory studies, specialized platelet antigen and antiplatelet antibody studies can confirm the diagnosis. Platelet antigen typing of the parents can reveal whether the mother's platelets lack a platelet-specific antigen present on the father's cells. If the infant's platelets are available for typing, the paternal antigen will likewise be found on these cells. In more than 85% of cases, antibodies specific for the implicated platelet antigen are detected in the mother's serum (69, 143, 161).

A variety of platelet antibody assays have been used for platelet typing and to detect platelet antibody in maternal serum. The indirect immunofluorescence test of von dem Borne was once the most widely used test for clinical diagnosis of NATP (141, 143, 162), but has been largely replaced by ELISA-based, antigen-capture assays that test the mother's serum against immobilized platelet glycoprotein targets (45, 163). These methods provide the advantage of excluding interfering HLA antibodies to more clearly delineate the presence of platelet-specific alloantibodies.

Because of the limitations associated with serologically based methods, an increasing number of laboratories are turning to DNA-based genotyping as a supplementary technique for determining the allelic forms of the platelet membrane glycoproteins that have been inherited. Several approaches are currently used for platelet genotyping—all based on the polymerase chain reaction (PCR). Initially, restriction fragment length polymorphism (RFLP) analysis of restriction enzyme-digested PCR products spanning polymorphic sites (12, 164) and allele-specific probes (76, 163, 165) were used to distinguish platelet glycoprotein variants, but more recently a variety of more efficient methods have been adopted, including allele-specific PCR (166, 167). These are useful for initial screening, as well as for diagnosis of fetal genotypes in mothers who have previously given birth to infants affected with NATP.

## DIAGNOSIS OF SECOND OR SUBSEQUENT AFFECTED INFANTS

The prediction of the likelihood of second and subsequent affected infants developing NATP can be greatly facilitated by knowledge of gene frequencies of the alleles involved (Table 28.1). In the case of $Pl^{A1}$, the gene frequency data predict that about 87% of subsequent pregnancies will be affected, that is, would have the relevant antigen incompatibility. Typing the father's platelets for both alleles of the implicated antigen system enables one to determine if he is either homozygous or heterozygous for this system. If the father is found to be a heterozygote, there is a good chance that he will pass the incompatible allele to a subsequent offspring, resulting in an affected neonate. However, a *homozygous* father will always pass the incompatible antigen to the fetus. Identifying the phenotype of a potentially affected fetus can be difficult in cases where the father is found to be heterozygous for the implicated antigen, as the amount of fetal blood that can be obtained is often inadequate for classical platelet antigen typing assays. However, the recent discovery of the genetic polymorphisms associated with the allelic differences in most of the clinically important alloantigen systems (see Table 28.1) now allows the determination of fetal genotypes. Using as little as 1 mL of fetal blood or 5 to 10 mL of amniotic fluid, the platelet alloantigen genotypes for these systems can be determined using any of the DNA-based methods described in the last section. This approach allows early detection of the alleles that have been inherited by the fetus and allows one to determine whether the second and subsequent fetuses may be at risk for developing NATP so that prenatal treatment or preparations can be considered, if appropriate.

Predicting the actual severity of NATP is difficult. *In utero* intracranial hemorrhage is especially devastating, and efforts should be directed at predicting this particular subset of affected infants. Prenatal serum testing of the mother is useful in some cases (69, 139, 140, 162, 168), but is not always reliable (163, 169). A recent study of maternal antibody characteristics found a correlation between the ability of the antibody to fix complement (the titer of anti-HPA-1a as measured in an antigen capture ELISA) and the occurrence of fetal or neonatal intracranial hemorrhage (170).

Percutaneous umbilical vein sampling (PUBS) allows clinicians to assess fetal platelet count early in pregnancy. PUBS can be performed as early as 20 weeks gestation of an at-risk pregnancy to obtain fetal platelets for counting or platelet antigen typing (171–173). If early PUBS indicates that the fetus is affected, subsequent PUBS can be done to monitor the efficacy of prenatal therapy in the mother. Another application of PUBS is quantification of fetal platelets following transfusion of maternal platelets to the fetus during the pregnancy (174, 175).

## TREATMENT

The major treatment goal in NATP is to increase the neonate's platelet count. In a severely thrombocytopenic neonate, a platelet transfusion should be given. Platelets compatible with the maternal antibody are ideal, since they will not be destroyed by antibody in the neonate's serum (140, 159, 176). Maternal platelets washed free of antibody-containing plasma are commonly used (95). Alternatively, donors with compatible platelets may be found among the mother's siblings, or, for some cases, regional blood centers maintain files of donors known to be negative for the antigens commonly implicated in NATP. Compatible platelets in a first pregnancy are usually provided as soon as possible after the diagnosis of NATP is made. In second or subsequent pregnancies, caesarian section is recommended to prevent birth trauma (177, 178), and maternal platelets can be obtained the day before planned delivery for transfusion to the neonate. Responses to random donor platelets may be adequate, albeit temporary, and therefore emergent use of these products is warranted in severely affected neonates if compatible platelets are not on hand (95, 176).

Results of NATP treatment with high dose intravenous immunoglobulin (IVIG) are variable. The platelet count usually increases within the first 24 to 48 hours; however, in some cases up to 8 days are required for response (145, 179–181). IVIG should not be used as a sole therapy for NATP if there is serious risk of hemorrhage, since the rate of platelet count correction is unpredictable. The mechanism of action of IVIG in this disorder is unknown. It is possible either that reticuloendothelial cell blockade prevents antibody-coated platelets from being consumed or that antibodies in the IVIG interfere with the binding of the maternally derived antiplatelet antibodies to neonatal platelets.

## PRENATAL TREATMENT

Since second or subsequent affected fetuses in a family are rarely if ever *less* severely affected than the first affected child (173), it is reasonable to provide prenatal treatment in pregnancies following a severely affected NATP infant. If the father is heterozygous, fetal platelet type should be determined from amniocytes using PCR-based methods, as described above. PUBS can also be considered as early as 20 weeks gestation to document fetal platelet count and to obtain fetal blood to verify the fetal platelet antigen type. If fetal thrombocytopenia is present, maternal IVIG treatment can be given in weekly doses of 1 g/kg until delivery. At approximately

4 to 5 weeks after IVIG therapy is begun, a repeat PUBS should be considered to assess treatment success. If there has been no response, low-dose dexamethasone treatment should be added according to the results of one ongoing clinical trial. Although these studies are still in progress, overall a 75% response rate to maternal IVIG with or without corticosteroids might be expected in such pregnancies (182). It is still too early to assess the benefit of adding steroids to the IVIG therapy, but the current clinical trial should answer this question.

An alternative approach to treating NATP is to give the fetus repeated transfusions of antigen-negative platelets throughout the pregnancy. This treatment is more complex than that used in its counterpart, hemolytic disease of the newborn, where the survival of transfused compatible RBCs can be expected to be about 3 weeks. In the case of transfused platelets, 5 to 7 days is about the maximum survival that can be anticipated. This then obligates the mother to receive weekly intrauterine platelet transfusions to maintain safe levels of fetal platelet count. The transfusion of platelets must be done rapidly, often before the platelet count can be determined from a PUBS sample, to minimize risk to the fetus from the procedure. The platelets must be volume-reduced and washed if they are derived from the mother (approximately $0.4 \times 10^{11}$ in 5–10 mL) and gamma-irradiated prior to infusion to the fetus (173).

## PROGNOSIS

The prognosis of NATP is generally good. Initially, the reported overall mortality was between 12 and 14% (139). A more recent review reported a mortality rate of 9% (140). Intracranial hemorrhage occurs in between 15 and 28% of all cases reported (140, 152, 155). Up to one-half of these intracranial events may occur prenatally. Second and subsequent siblings often have a better prognosis than first affected children, probably due to the ability to take preventive measures (e.g., elective caesarian deliveries) and to provide immediate compatible platelet transfusions that were not able to be made immediately available to their older siblings (140). It is estimated that roughly 400 cases of ICH due to NATP continue to occur each year in the United States (183), and over half of these new cases of NATP are recognized only after a thrombocytopenic infant is born. In this regard, recently developed prenatal screening options designed to detect potentially affected fetuses, described above, are now available. This, together with the advent of effective prenatal treatment, will hopefully result in a reduction in the incidence of IUICH caused by NATP.

## REFERENCES

1.  van Loghem JJ Jr, Dorfmeijer H, van der Hart M et al. Serological and genetical studies on a platelet antigen (Zw). Vox Sang 1959;4:161–169.

2. van der Weerdt CM, Veenhoven-von Riesz LE, Nijenhuis LE et al. The Zw blood group system in platelets. Vox Sang 1963;8:513–530.

3. Shulman NR, Aster RH, Leitner A et al. Immunoreactions involving platelets. V. Post-transfusion purpura due to a complement-fixing antibody against a genetically controlled platelet antigen. A proposed mechanism for thrombocytopenia and its relevance in "autoimmunity." J Clin Invest 1961;40:1597–1620.

4. Shulman NR, Marder VJ, Hiller MC et al. Platelet and leukocyte isoantigens and their antibodies: serologic, physiologic, and clinical studies. Prog Haemo 1964;4:222–304.

5. von dem Borne AE, Decary F. ICSH/ISBT Working Party on platelet serology. Nomenclature of platelet-specific antigens. Vox Sang 1990;58:176.

6. von dem Borne AE, Decary F. Nomenclature of platelet-specific antigens. Hum Immunol 1990;29:1–2.

7. Wang R, Newman PJ. Adhesive properties of a naturally occurring allele of GP IIIa having an amino acid substitution within the ligand binding domain—the Pen$^a$/Pen$^b$ alloantigenic epitopes [Abstract]. Blood 1996;88:467a.

8. Kunicki TJ, Aster RH. Deletion of the platelet-specific alloantigen Pl$^{A1}$ from platelets in Glanzmann's thrombasthenia. J Clin Invest 1978;61:1225–1231.

9. Kunicki TJ, Aster RH. Isolation and immunologic characterization of the human platelet alloantigen, Pl$^{A1}$. Mol Immunol 1979;16:353–360.

10. Newman PJ, Martin LS, Knipp MA et al. Studies on the nature of the human platelet alloantigen, Pl$^{A1}$: localization to a 17,000-dalton polypeptide. Mol Immunol 1985;22:719–729.

11. Newman PJ, Gorski J, White GC II et al. Enzymatic amplification of platelet-specific messenger RNA using the polymerase chain reaction. J Clin Invest 1988;82:739–743.

12. Newman PJ, Derbes RS, Aster RH. The human platelet alloantigens, Pl$^{A1}$ and Pl$^{A2}$, are associated with a leucine$_{33}$/proline$_{33}$ amino acid polymorphism in membrane glycoprotein IIIa, and are distinguishable by DNA typing. J Clin Invest 1989;83:1778–1781.

13. Calvete JJ, Henschen A, Gonzalez-Rodriguez J. Assignment of disulphide bonds in human platelet GP IIIa. A disulphide pattern for the beta-subunits of the integrin family. Biochem J 1991;274:63–71.

14. Newman PJ. Platelet GP IIb-IIIa: molecular variations and alloantigens [Review]. Thromb Haemost 1991;66:111–118.

15. Goldberger A, Kolodziej M, Poncz M et al. Effect of single amino acid substitutions on the formation of the Pl$^A$ and Bak alloantigenic epitopes. Blood 1991;78:681–687.

16. Valentin N, Visentin GP, Newman PJ. Involvement of the cysteine-rich domain of glycoprotein IIIa in the expression of the human platelet alloantigen, Pl$^{A1}$: evidence for heterogeneity in the humoral response. Blood 1995;85:3028–3033.

17. Reznikoff-Etievant MF, Muller JY, Julien F et al. An immune response gene linked to MHC in man. Tissue Antigens 1983;22:312–314.

18. de Waal LP, van Dalen CM, Engelfriet CP et al. Alloimmunization against the platelet-specific Zwa antigen, resulting in neonatal alloimmune thrombocytopenia or posttransfusion purpura, is associated with the supertypic DRw52 antigen including DR3 and DRw6. Hum Immunol 1986;17:45–53.

19. Valentin N, Vergracht A, Bignon JD et al. HLA-DRw52a is involved in alloimmunization against Pl$^{A1}$ antigen. Hum Immunol 1990;27:73–79.

20. Kuijpers RW, Von dem Borne AE, Kiefel V et al. Leucine$^{33}$-proline$^{33}$ substitution in human platelet glycoprotein IIIa determines HLA-DRw52a (Dw24) association of the immune response against HPA-1a (Zw$^a$/Pl$^{A1}$) and HPA-1b (Zw$^b$/Pl$^{A2}$). Hum Immunol 1992;34:253–256.

21. Maslanka K, Yassai M, Gorski J. Molecular identification of T cells that respond in a primary bulk culture to a peptide derived from a platelet glycoprotein implicated in neonatal alloimmune thrombocytopenia. J Clin Invest 1996;98:1802–1808.

22. Wu S, Maslanka K, Gorski J. An integrin polymorphism that defines reactivity with alloantibodies generates an anchor for MHC class II peptide binding: a model for unidirectional alloimmune responses. J Immunol 1997;158:3221–3226.

23. Ramsey G, Salamon DJ. Frequency of Pl$^{A1}$ in blacks. Transfusion 1986;26:531–532.

24. Shibata Y, Matsuda I, Miyaji T et al. Yuk$^a$, a new platelet antigen involved in two cases of neonatal alloimmune thrombocytopenia. Vox Sang 1986;50:177–180.

25. Friedman JM, Aster RH. Neonatal alloimmune thrombocytopenic purpura and congenital porencephaly in two siblings associated with a "new" maternal antiplatelet antibody. Blood 1985;65:1412–1415.

26. Shibata Y, Mori H. A new platelet-specific alloantigen system, Yuk$^a$/Yuk$^b$ is located on platelet membrane glycoprotein IIIa. Proc Japan Acad 1987;63:36–38.

27. Furihata K, Nugent DJ, Bissonette A et al. On the association of the platelet-specific alloantigen, Pen$^a$, with glycoprotein IIIa. Evidence for heterogeneity of glycoprotein IIIa. J Clin Invest 1987;80:1624–1630.

28. Niewiarowski S, Norton KJ, Eckardt A et al. Structural and functional characterization of major platelet membrane components derived by limited proteolysis of glycoprotein IIIa. Biochim Biophys Acta 1989;983:91–99.

29. Beer J, Coller BS. Evidence that platelet glycoprotein IIIa has a large disul-fide-bonded loop that is susceptible to proteolytic cleavage. J Biol Chem 1989;264:17564–17573.

30. D'Souza SE, Ginsberg MH, Lam SC et al. Chemical crosslinking of arginyl-glycyl-aspartic acid peptides to an adhesion receptor on platelets. J Biol Chem 1988;263:3943–3951.

31. Santoso S, Shibata Y, Kiefel V et al. Identification of the Yuk$^b$ alloantigen on platelet glycoprotein IIIa. Vox Sang 1987;53:48–51.

32. Wang L, Juji T, Shibata Y et al. Sequence variation of human platelet membrane glycoprotein IIIa associated with the Yuk$^a$/Yuk$^b$ alloantigen system. Proc Japan Acad 1991;67:102–196.

33. Wang R, Furihata K, McFarland JG et al. An amino acid polymorphism within the RGD binding domain of platelet membrane glycoprotein IIIa is responsible for the formation of the Pen$^a$/Pen$^b$ alloantigen system. J Clin Invest 1992;90:2038–2043.

34. Kroll H, Kiefel V, Santoso S et al. Sr$^a$, a private platelet antigen on glycoprotein IIIa associated with neonatal alloimmune thrombocytopenia. Blood 1990;76:2296–2302.

35. Santoso S, Kalb R, Kroll H et al. A point mutation leads to an unpaired cysteine residue and a molecular weight polymorphism of a functional platelet β3 integrin subunit. The Sr$^a$ alloantigen system of GP IIIa. J Biol Chem 1994;269:8439–8444.

36. Kuijpers RW, Simsek S, Faber NM et al. Single point mutation in human glycoprotein IIIa is associated with a new platelet-specific alloantigen (Mo) involved in neonatal alloimmune thrombocytopenia. Blood 1993;81:70–76.

37. Kekomäki R, Jouhikainen T, Ollikainen J et al. A new platelet alloantigen, Tu$^a$, on glycoprotein IIIa associated with neonatal alloimmune thrombocytopenia in two families. Br J Haematol 1993;83:306–310.

38. McFarland JG, Blanchette V, Collins J et al. Neonatal alloimmune thrombocytopenia due to a new platelet-specific alloantibody. Blood 1993;81:3318–3323.

39. Wang R, McFarland JG, Kekomaki R et al. Amino acid 489 is encoded by a mutational "hot spot" on the β3 integrin chain: the CA/TU human platelet alloantigen system. Blood 1993;82:3386–3391.

40. Peyruchaud O, Bourre F, Morel-Kopp MC et al. HPA-10w$^b$ (La$^a$): genetic determination of a new platelet-specific alloantigen on glycoprotein IIIa and its expression in COS-7 cells. Blood 1997;89:2422–2428.

41. Newman PJ, Valentin N. Human platelet alloantigens: recent findings, new perspectives. Thromb Haemost 1995;74:234–239.

42. Unkelbach K, Kalb R, Santoso S et al. New polymorphism on platelet glycoprotein IIIa gene recognized by endonuclease Msp I: implications for typing by allele-specific restriction analysis. Transfusion 1994;34:592–595.

43. Perichon B, Clemenceau S, Romand A et al. An additional HpaII polymorphism in exon 2 of the human platelet membrane glycoprotein IIIa gene. Hum Genet 1994;93:353–354.

44. Walchshofer S, Ghali D, Fink M et al. A rare leucine$^{40}$/arginine$^{40}$ polymorphism on platelet glycoprotein IIIa is linked to the human platelet antigen 1b. Vox Sang 1994;67:231–234.

45. Kiefel V, Santoso S, Katzmann B et al. A new platelet-specific alloantigen Br$^a$. Report of 4 cases with neonatal alloimmune thrombocytopenia. Vox Sang 1988;54:101–106.

46. Newman PJ. Nomenclature of human platelet alloantigens: a problem with the HPA system? Blood 1994;83:1447–1451.

47. Santoso S, Kiefel V, Mueller-Eckhardt C. Human platelet alloantigens Br$^a$/Br$^b$ are expressed on the very late activation antigen 2 (VLA-2) of T lymphocytes. Hum Immunol 1989;25:237–246.

48. Santoso S, Kiefel V, Mueller-Eckhardt C. Immunochemical characterization of the new platelet alloantigen system Br$^a$/Br$^b$. Br J Haematol 1989;72:191–198.

49. Smith JW, Kelton JG, Horsewood P et al. Platelet specific alloantigens on the platelet glycoprotein Ia/IIa complex. Br J Haematol 1989;72:534–538.

50. Woods VL Jr, Pischel KD, Avery ED et al. Antigenic polymorphism of human very late activation protein-2 (platelet glycoprotein Ia-IIa). Platelet alloantigen Hca. J Clin Invest 1989;83:978–985.

51. Kiefel V, Santoso S, Katzmann B et al. The Br$^a$/Br$^b$ alloantigen system on human platelets. Blood 1989;73:2219–2223.

52. Santoso S, Kalb R, Walka M et al. The human platelet alloantigens Br$^a$ and Br$^b$ are associated with a single amino acid polymorphism on glycoprotein Ia (integrin subunit a2). J Clin Invest 1993;92:2427–2432.

53. Roth GJ. Developing relationships: arterial platelet adhesion, glycoprotein Ib, and leucine-rich glycoproteins [Review]. Blood 1991;77:5–19.

54. Lopez JA, Leung B, Reynolds CC et al. Efficient plasma membrane expression of a functional platelet glycoprotein Ib–IX complex requires the presence of its three subunits. J Biol Chem 1992;267:12851–12859.

55. Modderman PW, Admiraal LG, Sonnenberg A et al. Glycoproteins V and Ib-IX form a noncovalent complex in the platelet membrane. J Biol Chem 1992;267:364–369.

56. van der Weerdt CM, van de Wiel-Dorfmeyer H, Engelfriet CP et al. A new platelet antigen. Proceedings of the 8th Congress of the European Society of Haematology. Basel: S Karger, 1961; p. 379.

57. Dausset J, Berg P. Un nouvel exemple d'anticorps anti-plaquettaire Ko. Vox Sang 1963;8:341–347.

58. Saji H, Maruya E, Fujii H et al. New platelet antigen, Sib[a], involved in platelet transfusion refractoriness in a Japanese man. Vox Sang 1989;56:283–287.

59. Kuijpers RW, Faber NM, Cuypers HT et al. NH[2]-terminal globular domain of human platelet glycoprotein Ibα has a methionine[145]/threonine[145] amino acid polymorphism, which is associated with the HPA-2 (Ko) alloantigens. J Clin Invest 1992;89:381–384.

60. V Kuijpers RW, Ouwehand WH, Bleeker PM et al. Localization of the platelet-specific HPA-2 (Ko) alloantigens on the N-terminal globular fragment of platelet glycoprotein Ibα. Blood 1992;79:283–288.

61. Murata M, Furihata K, Ishida F et al. Genetic and structural characterization of an amino acid dimorphism in glycoprotein Ibα involved in platelet transfusion refractoriness. Blood 1992;79:3086–3090.

62. Moroi M, Jung SM, Yoshida N. Genetic polymorphism of platelet glycoprotein Ib. Blood 1984;64:622–629.

63. Lopez JA, Ludwig EH, McCarthy BJ. Polymorphism of human glycoprotein Ibα results from a variable number of tandem repeats of a 13-amino acid sequence in the mucin-like macroglycopeptide region. Structure/function implications. J Biol Chem 1992;267:10055–10061.

64. Ishida F, Saji H, Maruya E et al. Human platelet-specific antigen, Sib[a], is associated with the molecular weight polymorphism of glycoprotein Ibα. Blood 1991;78:1722–1729.

65. Simsek S, Bleeker PM, van der Schoot CE et al. Association of a variable number of tandem repeats (VNTR) in glycoprotein Ibα and HPA-2 alloantigens. Thromb Haemost 1994;72:757–761.

66. Ishida F, Furihata K, Ishida K et al. The largest variant of platelet glycoprotein Ibα has four tandem repeats of 13 amino acids in the macroglycopeptide region and a genetic linkage with methionine[145]. Blood 1995;86:1356–1360.

67. Kiefel V, Vicariot M, Giovangrandi Y et al. Alloimmunization against Iy, a low-frequency antigen on platelet glycoprotein Ib/IX as a cause of severe neonatal alloimmune thrombocytopenic purpura. Vox Sang 1995;69:250–254.

68. Santoso S, Bohringer M, Sachs U et al. Point mutation in human platelet glycoprotein Ibβ is associated with the new platelet specific alloantigen Iy [Abstract]. Blood 1996;88:319a.

69. von dem Borne AE, von Riesz E, Verheugt FW et al. Bak[a], a new platelet-specific antigen involved in neonatal allo-immune thrombocytopenia. Vox Sang 1980;39:113–120.

70. Boizard B, Wautier JL. Lek[a], a new platelet antigen absent in Glanzmann's thrombasthenia. Vox Sang 1984;46:47–54.

71. Kieffer N, Boizard B, Didry D et al. Immunochemical characterization of the platelet-specific alloantigen Lek[a]: a comparative study with the PlA alloantigen. Blood 1984;64:1212–1219.

72. van der Schoot CE, Wester M, von dem Borne AE et al. Characterization of platelet-specific alloantigens by immunoblotting: localization of Zw and Bak antigens. Br J Haematol 1986;64:715–723.

73. Keimowitz RM, Collins J, Davis K et al. Post-transfusion purpura associated with alloimmunization against the platelet-specific antigen, Bak[a]. Am J Hematol 1986;21:79–88.

74. von dem Borne AE, van der Plas-van Dalen CM. Bak-a and Lek-a are identical antigens [Letter]. Br J Haematol 1986;62:404–405.

75. Kickler TS, Herman JH, Furihata K et al. Identification of Bak[b], a new platelet-specific antigen associated with posttransfusion purpura. Blood 1988;71:894–898.

76. Lyman S, Aster RH, Visentin GP et al. Polymorphism of human platelet membrane glycoprotein IIb associated with the Bak[a]/Bak[b] alloantigen system. Blood 1990;75:2343–2348.

77. Take H, Tomiyama Y, Shibata Y et al. Demonstration of the heterogeneity of epitopes of the platelet-specific alloantigen, Bak[a]. Br J Haematol 1990;76:395–400.

78. Djaffar I, Vilette D, Pidard D et al. Human Platelet Antigen 3 (HPA-3): localization of the determinant of the alloantibody Lek[a] (HPA-3a) to the C-terminus of platelet glycoprotein IIb heavy chain and contribution of O-linked carbohydrates. Thromb Haemost 1993;69:485–489.

79. Calvete JJ, Muñiz-Diaz E. Localization of an O-glycosylation site in the α-subunit of the human platelet integrin GP IIb-IIIa involved in Bak[a] (HPA-3a) alloantigen expression. FEBS Lett 1993;328:30–34.

80. Noris P, Simsek S, De Bruijne-Admiraal LG et al. Max[a], a new low-frequency platelet-specific antigen localized on glycoprotein IIb, is associated with neonatal alloimmune thrombocytopenia. Blood 1995;86:1019–1026.

81. Ikeda H, Mitani T, Ohnuma M et al. A new platelet-specific antigen, Nak[a] involved in the refractoriness of HLA-matched platelet transfusion. Vox Sang 1989;57:213–217.

82. Tomiyama Y, Take H, Ikeda H et al. Identification of the platelet-specific alloantigen, Nak[a], on platelet membrane glycoprotein IV. Blood 1990;75:684–687.

83. Tandon NN, Kralisz U, Jamieson GA. Identification of glycoprotein IV (CD36) as a primary receptor for platelet-collagen adhesion. J Biol Chem 1989;264:7576–7583.

84. Asch AS, Barnwell J, Silverstein RL et al. Isolation of the thrombospondin membrane receptor. J Clin Invest 1987;79:1054–1061.

85. Yamamoto N, Ikeda H, Tandon NN et al. A platelet membrane glycoprotein (GP) deficiency in healthy blood donors: Nak[a]-platelets lack detectable GP IV (CD36). Blood 1990;76:1698–1703.

86. Kashiwagi H, Honda S, Tomiyama Y et al. A novel polymorphism in glycoprotein IV (replacement of proline-90 by serine) predominates in subjects with platelet GP IV deficiency. Thromb Haemost 1993;69:481–484.

87. Kashiwagi H, Tomiyama Y, Honda S et al. Molecular basis of CD36 deficiency. Evidence that a [478]C → T substitution (proline90 → serine) in CD36 cDNA accounts for CD36 deficiency. J Clin Invest 1995;95:1040–1046.

88. Kashiwagi H, Tomiyama Y, Kosugi S et al. Identification of molecular defects in a subject with type I CD36 deficiency. Blood 1994;83:3545–3552.

89. Kashiwagi H, Tomiyama Y, Nozaki S et al. A single nucleotide insertion in codon 317 of the CD36 gene leads to CD36 deficiency. Arterioscler Thromb Vasc Biol 1996;16:1026–1032.

90. Kashiwagi H, Tomiyama Y, Kosugi S et al. Family studies of type II CD36 deficient subjects: linkage of a CD36 allele to a platelet-specific mRNA expression defect(s) causing type II CD36 deficiency. Thromb Haemost 1995;74:758–763.

91. Tandon NN, Ockenhouse CF, Greco NJ et al. Adhesive functions of platelets lacking glycoprotein IV (CD36). Blood 1991;78:2809–2813.

92. McKeown L, Vail M, Williams S et al. Platelet adhesion to collagen in individuals lacking glycoprotein IV. Blood 1994;83:2866–2871.

93. Yamamoto N, Akamatsu N, Yamazaki H et al. Normal aggregations of glycoprotein IV (CD36)-deficient platelets from seven healthy Japanese donors. Br J Haematol 1992;81:86–92.

94. Kehrel B, Kronenberg A, Rauterberg J et al. Platelets deficient in glycoprotein IIIb aggregate normally to collagens type I and III but not to collagen type V. Blood 1993;82:3364–3370.

95. Shulman NR, Jordan JV. Platelet immunology. In: Coleman RW, Hirsh J, Marder VJ, Salzman EW, eds. Hemostasis and thrombosis. Philadelphia: JB Lippincott, 1987; pp. 452–529.

96. Seidenfeld AM, Owen J, Glynn MF. Post-transfusion purpura cured by steroid therapy in a man. Can Med Assoc J 1978;118:1285–1286.

97. Aster RH. The immunologic thrombocytopenias. In: Kunicki TJ, George JN, eds. Platelet immunobiology. Philadelphia: Lippincott, 1989; pp. 387–435.

98. Ballem PJ, Buskard NA, Decary F et al. Post-transfusion purpura secondary to passive transfer of anti-Pl[A1] by blood transfusion. Br J Haematol 1987;66:113–114.

99. Taaning E, Morling N, Ovesen H et al. Posttransfusion purpura and anti-Zw[b] (-Pl[A2]). Tissue Antigens 1985;26:143–146.

100. Kiefel V, Santoso S, Glockner WM et al. Posttransfusion purpura associated with an anti-Bak[b]. Vox Sang 1989;56:93–97.

101. McCrae KR, Herman JH. Posttransfusion purpura: two unusual cases and a literature Review [Review]. Am J Hematol 1996;52:205–211.

102. Simon TL, Collins J, Kunicki TJ et al. Posttransfusion purpura associated with alloantibody specific for the platelet antigen, Pen[a]. Am J Hematol 1988;29:38–40.

103. Christie DJ, Pulkrabek S, Putnam JL et al. Posttransfusion purpura due to an alloantibody reactive with glycoprotein Ia/IIa (anti-HPA-5b). Blood 1991;77:2785–2789.

104. Bierling P, Godeau B, Fromont P et al. Posttransfusion purpura-like syndrome associated with CD36 (Nak[a]) isoimmunization. Transfusion 1995;35:777–782.

105. Lau P, Sholtis CM, Aster RH. Post-transfusion purpura: an enigma of alloimmunization. Am J Hematol 1980;9:331–336.

106. Cimo PL, Aster RH. Post-transfusion purpura: successful treatment by exchange transfusion. N Engl J Med 1972;287:290–292.

107. Kickler TS, Ness PM, Herman JH et al. Studies on the pathophysiology of posttransfusion purpura. Blood 1986;68:347–350.

108. Taaning E, Skov F. Elution of anti-Zwa (-PIA1) from autologous platelets after normalization of platelet count in post-transfusion purpura. Vox Sang 1991;60:40–44.

109. George JN. Platelet immunoglobulin G: its significance for the evaluation of thrombocytopenia and for understanding the origin of α-granule proteins [Review]. Blood 1990;76:859–870.

110. Shulman NR. Post-transfusion purpura. In: Nance ST, ed. Clinical and basic science aspects of immunohematology. Arlington: American Association of Blood Banks, 1991; pp. 137–154.

111. Shulman NR. Mechanism of blood cell damage by adsorption of antigen-antibody complexes. Immunopathology III international symposium. Basel: Schwabe, 1963; pp. 338–352.

112. Gengozian N, McLaughlin CL. IgG+ platelets in the marmoset: their induction, maintenance, and survival. Blood 1980;55:885–890.

113. Pegels JG, Bruynes EC, Engelfriet CP et al. Post-transfusion purpura: a serological and immunochemical study. Br J Haematol 1981;49:521–530.

114. von dem Borne AEGK, van der Plas-van Dalen CM. Further observation on post-transfusion purpura (PTP) [Letter]. Br J Haematol 1985;61:374–375.

115. Polesky HF, Bove JR. A fatal hemolytic transfusion reaction with acute autohemolysis. Transfusion 1964;4:285–292.

116. Shirey RS, Ness PM. New concepts of delayed hemolytic transfusion reac-

tions. In: Nance SJ, ed. Clinical and basic science aspects of immunohematology. Arlington: American Association of Blood Banks, 1991; pp. 179–197.

117. Aster RH. Post-transfusion purpura. In: Engelfreit CP, von dem Borne AE, eds. Baillieres clinical immunology. London: WB Saunders, 1987; pp. 453–461.

118. deWaal LP, van Dalen CM, Engelfriet CP et al. Alloimmunization against the platelet specific Zw<sup>a</sup> antigen, resulting in neonatal alloimmune thrombocytopenia or posttransfusion purpura, is associated with the supertypic DRw52 antigen including DR3 and DRw6. Hum Immunol 1986;17:45–53.

119. Slichter SJ. Post-transfusion purpura: response to steroids and association with red blood cell and lymphocytotoxic antibodies. Br J Haematol 1982; 50:599–605.

120. Menitove JE, Pereira J, Hoffman R et al. Cyclic thrombocytopenia of apparent autoimmune etiology. Blood 1989;73:1561–1569.

121. Kiefel V, Santoso S, Weisheit M et al. Monoclonal antibody-specific immobilization of platelet antigens (MAIPA): a new tool for the identification of platelet-reactive antibodies. Blood 1987;70:1722–1726.

122. Evenson DA, Stroncek DF, Pulkrabek S et al. Posttransfusion purpura following bone marrow transplantation. Transfusion 1995;35:688–693.

123. Kunicki TJ, Aster RH. Qualitative and quantitative tests for platelet alloantibodies and drug-dependent antibodies. In: McMillan R, ed. Methods in hematology—immune cytopenias. 9th ed. New York: Churchill-Livingston, 1983; pp. 49–67.

124. Becker T, Panzer S, Maas D et al. High-dose intravenous immunoglobulin for post-transfusion purpura. Br J Haematol 1985;61:149–155.

125. Taaning E, Killmann SA, Morling N et al. Post-transfusion purpura (PTP) due to anti-Zw<sup>b</sup> (-Pl<sup>A2</sup>): the significance of IgG3 antibodies in PTP. Br J Haematol 1986;64:217–225.

126. Abramson N, Eisenberg PD, Aster RH. Post-transfusion purpura: immunologic aspects and therapy. N Engl J Med 1974;291:1163–1166.

127. Mueller-Eckhardt C. Post-transfusion purpura. Br J Haematol 1986;64: 419–424.

128. Weisberg LJ, Linker CA. Prednisone therapy of post-transfusion purpura. Ann Intern Med 1984;100:76–77.

129. Glud TK, Rosthoj S, Jensen MK et al. High-dose intravenous immunoglobulin for post-transfusion purpura. Scand J Haematol 1983;31:495–500.

130. Berney SI, Metcalfe P, Wathen NC et al. Post-transfusion purpura responding to high dose intravenous IgG: further observations on pathogenesis. Br J Haematol 1985;61:627–632.

131. Chong BH, Cade J, Smith JA et al. An unusual case of post-transfusion purpura: good transient response to high-dose immunoglobulin. Vox Sang 1986;51:182–184.

132. Cunningham CC, Lind SE. Apparent response of refractory post-transfusion purpura to splenectomy. Am J Hematol 1989;30:112–113.

133. Gerstner JB, Smith MJ, Davis KD et al. Posttransfusion purpura: therapeutic failure of PlAl-negative platelet transfusion. Am J Hematol 1979;6: 71–75.

134. Brecher ME, Moore SB, Letendre L. Posttransfusion purpura: the therapeutic value of Pl<sup>A1</sup>-negative platelets. Transfusion 1990;30:433–435.

135. Soulier JP, Patereau C, Gobert N et al. Posttransfusional immunologic thrombocytopenia. A case report. Vox Sang 1979;37:21–29.

136. Budd JL, Wiegers SE, O'Hara JM. Relapsing post-transfusion purpura. A preventable disease. Am J Med 1985;78:361–362.

137. Godeau B, Fromont P, Bettaieb A et al. Relapse of posttransfusion purpura after transfusion with frozen-thawed red cells [Letter]. Transfusion 1991; 31:189–190.

138. Blanchette VS, Peters MA, Pegg-Feige K. Alloimmune thrombocytopenia. Review from a neonatal intensive care unit. Curr Stud Hematol Blood Transfus 1986;52:87–96.

139. Pearson HA, Shulman NR, Marder VJ et al. Isoimmune neonatal thrombocytopenic purpura: clinical and therapeutic considerations. Blood 1964;23: 154–177.

140. Deaver JE, Leppert PC, Zaroulis CG. Neonatal alloimmune thrombocytopenic purpura [Review]. Am J Perinatol 1986;3:127–131.

141. Mueller-Eckhardt C, Becker T, Weisheit M et al. Neonatal alloimmune thrombocytopenia due to fetomaternal Zw<sup>b</sup> incompatibility. Vox Sang 1986;50:94–96.

142. Maslanka K, Lucas GF, Gronkowska A et al. A second case of neonatal alloimmune thrombocytopenia associated with anti-Pl<sup>A2</sup> (Zw<sup>b</sup>). Haematologia 1989;22:109–113.

143. von dem Borne AEGK, van Leeuwen EF, von Riesz LE et al. Neonatal alloimmune thrombocytopenia: detection and characterization of the responsible antibodies by the platelet immunofluorescence test. Blood 1981; 57:649–656.

144. Miller DT, Etzel RA, McFarland JG et al. Prolonged neonatal alloimmune thrombocytopenic purpura associated with anti-Bak<sup>a</sup> Two cases in siblings [published erratum appears in Am J Perinatol 1987(Apr);4(2):177]. Am J Perinatol 1987;4:55–58.

145. Bizzaro N, Dianese G. Neonatal alloimmune **amegakaryocytosis** Case report. Vox Sang 1988;54:112–114.

146. Mueller-Eckhardt C, Kiefel V, Grubert A et al. 348 cases of suspected neonatal alloimmune thrombocytopenia. Lancet 1989;1:363–366.

147. Kiefel V, Shechter Y, Atias D et al. Neonatal alloimmune thrombocytopenia due to anti-Br<sup>b</sup> (HPA-5a). Report of three cases in two families [Letter]. Vox Sang 1991;60:244–245.

148. Sternbach MS, Malette M, Nadon F et al. Severe alloimmune neonatal thrombocytopenia due to specific HLA antibodies. Curr Stud Hematol Blood Transfus 1986;52:97–103.

149. Morales WJ, Stroup M. Intracranial hemorrhage *in utero* due to isoimmune neonatal thrombocytopenia. Obstet Gynecol 1985;65(Suppl):20s–21s.

150. Blanchette VS, Chen L, de Friedberg ZS et al. Alloimmunization due to the Pl<sup>A1</sup> platelet antigen: results from a prospective study. Br J Haematol 1990;74:209–215.

151. Mueller-Eckhardt C, Mueller-Eckhardt G, Willen-Ohff H et al. Immunogenicity of and immune response to the human platelet antigen Zw<sup>a</sup> is strongly associated with HLA-B8 and DR3. Tissue Antigens 1985;26: 71–76.

152. Reznikoff-Etievant MF, Muller JY, Kaplan C et al. L'immunisation contre l'antigene plaquettaire Zw<sup>a</sup> (Pl<sup>A1</sup>): groupe a risque prevention des complications. Pathol Biol 1986;34:783–787.

153. Reznikoff-Etievant MF, Dangu C, Lobet R. HLA-B8 antigens and anti-Pl<sup>A1</sup> allo-immunization. Tissue Antigens 1981;18:66–68.

154. Bussel JB, Zabusky MR, Berkowitz RL et al. Fetal alloimmune thrombocytopenia. N Engl J Med 1997;337:22-26.

155. Bussel JB. Neonatal alloimmune thrombocytopenia (NAIT): a prospective case accumulation study [Abstract]. Pediatr Res 1988;23(Suppl):337a.

156. Herman JH, Jumbelic MI, Ancona RJ et al. *In utero* cerebral hemorrhage in alloimmune thrombocytopenia. Am J Pediatr Hematol Oncol 1986;8: 312–317.

157. Davidson JE, McWilliam RC, Evans TJ et al. Porencephaly and optic hypoplasia in neonatal isoimmune thrombocytopenia. Arch Dis Child 1989;64: 858–860.

158. Sitarz AL, Driscoll JM Jr, Wolff JA. Management of isoimmune neonatal thrombocytopenia. Am J Obstet Gynecol 1976;124:39–42.

159. Adner MM, Fisch GR, Starobin SG et al. Use of "compatible" platelet transfusions in treatment of congenital isoimmune thrombocytopenic purpura. N Engl J Med 1969;280:244–247.

160. Lam AH, Shulman LA. Ultrasound in congenital intracranial haemorrhage secondary to isoimmune thrombocytopaenia. Pediatr Radiol 1985;15:8–11.

161. Mueller-Eckhardt C, Kayser W, Forster C et al. Improved assay for detection of platelet-specific Pl<sup>A1</sup> antibodies in neonatal alloimmune thrombocytopenia. Vox Sang 1982;43:76–81.

162. Naidu S, Messmore H, Caserta V et al. CNS lesions in neonatal isoimmune thrombocytopenia. Arch Neurol 1983;40:552–554.

163. McFarland JG, Aster RH, Bussel JB et al. Prenatal diagnosis of neonatal alloimmune thrombocytopenia using allele-specific oligonucleotide probes. Blood 1991;78:2276–2282.

164. Simsek S, Faber NM, Bleeker PM et al. Determination of human platelet antigen frequencies in the Dutch population by immunophenotyping and DNA (allele-specific restriction enzyme) analysis. Blood 1993;81:835–840.

165. Bray PF, Jin Y, Kickler T. Rapid genotyping of the five major platelet alloantigens by reverse dot-blot hybridization. Blood 1994;84:4361–4367.

166. Metcalfe P, Waters AH. HPA-1 typing by PCR amplification with sequence-specific primers (PCR-SSP): a rapid and simple technique. Br J Haematol 1993;85:227–229.

167. Skogen B, Bellissimo DB, Hessner MJ et al. Rapid determination of platelet alloantigen genotypes by polymerase chain reaction using allele specific primers. Transfusion 1994;34:955–960.

168. Sia CG, Amigo NC, Harper RG et al. Failure of caesarian section to prevent intracranial hemorrhage in siblings with isoimmune neonatal thrombocytopenia. Am J Obstet Gynecol 1985;153:79–81.

169. McFarland JG, Frenzke M, Aster RH. Testing of maternal sera in pregnancies at risk for neonatal alloimmune thrombocytopenia. Transfusion 1989; 29:128–133.

170. Bussel JB, McFarland JG, NAIT working party. The chromium release assay correlates with intracranial hemorrhage (ICH) in neonatal alloimmune thrombocytopenia (NAIT). Pediatr Res 1990;27(Suppl):139a.

171. Daffos F, Forestier F, Muller JY et al. Prenatal treatment of alloimmune thrombocytopenia [Letter]. Lancet 1984;2:632.

172. Bussel JB, Berkowitz RL, McFarland JG et al. Antenatal treatment of neonatal alloimmune thrombocytopenia. N Engl J Med 1988;319:1374–1378.

173. Reznikoff-Etievant MF. Management of alloimmune neonatal and antenatal thrombocytopenia [Review]. Vox Sang 1988;55:193–201.

174. Kaplan C, Daffos F, Forestier F et al. Management of alloimmune thrombocytopenia: antenatal diagnosis and *in utero* transfusion of maternal platelets. Blood 1988;72:340–343.

175. Kaplan C. Prenatal treatment in neonatal alloimmune thrombocytopenia. Curr Stud Hematol Blood Transfus 1988;55:142–147.

176. Katz J, Hodder FS, Aster RS et al. Neonatal isoimmune thrombocytopenia. The natural course and management and the detection of maternal antibody. Clin Pediatr 1984;23:159–162.

177. Mennuti M, Schwarz RH, Gill F. Obstetric management of isoimmune thrombocytopenia. Am J Obstet Gynecol 1974;118:565–566.
178. Pearson HA, McIntosh S. Neonatal thrombocytopenia. Clin Haematol 1978;7:111–122.
179. Suarez CR, Anderson C. High dose intravenous gamma globulin (IVG) in neonatal immune thrombocytopenia. Am J Hematol 1987;26:247–253.
180. Derycke M, Dreyfus M, Ropert JC et al. Intravenous immunoglobulin for neonatal isoimmune thrombocytopenia. Arch Dis Child 1985;60:667–669.
181. Sidiropoulos D, Straume B. The treatment of neonatal isoimmune thrombocytopenia with intravenous immunoglobulin. Blut 1984;48:383–386.
182. Bussel JB, McFarland JG, Lynch L et al. Antenatal treatment of alloimmune thrombocytopenia [Abstract]. Blood 1991;78(Suppl):387a.
183. Bussel JB, McFarland JG, Berkowitz RL. Antenatal management of fetal alloimmune and autoimmune thrombocytopenia. Transfus Med Rev 1990;4:149–162.

# CHAPTER 29

# DRUG-INDUCED THROMBOCYTOPENIAS

Keith R. McCrae and Douglas B. Cines

## INTRODUCTION

In recent years drug-induced thrombocytopenia has become one of the more common diagnostic problems encountered by hematologists caring for hospitalized individuals. Drug-induced thrombocytopenia has been estimated to occur in approximately one per 100,000 inhabitants of developed countries per year (1–3), but the actual incidence is likely to be much higher (4). The rising frequency with which this condition is encountered reflects the dramatic increase in the number of conditions treated with medication, the large number of new drugs introduced into clinical practice, and the advent of automated platelet counts as part of routine individual care. These developments have led to a marked increase in the number of reported cases of drug-induced thrombocytopenia and a better appreciation of the immunologic specificity and complexity of these syndromes. Nevertheless, many of the pieces of information needed by the clinician to diagnose and manage this diverse group of disorders optimally have not yet been clarified.

In this chapter we will discuss the general approach to the individual in whom a diagnosis of drug-induced thrombocytopenia is entertained. We have chosen not to provide an exhaustive compendium of citations for all drugs reported to cause thrombocytopenia in isolated individuals (Table 29.1). Such lists are available in previous reviews of this topic and are readily obtained by most physicians through computer-based literature searches. Rather, we will examine in detail several of the more common syndromes of drug-associated thrombocytopenia, emphasizing their distinctive characteristics with respect to clinical presentation, pathogenesis, natural history, and management.

The traditional criteria used to diagnose drug-induced thrombocytopenia have remained constant for decades. First, the onset of thrombocytopenia should relate temporally to the initiation of therapy. Second, there should be no reasonable alternative explanation for the thrombocytopenia based on history, physical examination, evaluation of the peripheral blood film, coagulation tests, and other relevant laboratory studies. Third, the platelet count should return to normal or to its baseline level after the drug in question has been discontinued. Fourth, the diagnosis should be confirmed through *in vitro* testing or rechallenge, when indicated. The drugs that had been confirmed to cause thrombocytopenia using these criteria through 1982, for example, have been the subject of a comprehensive review (5). However, several changes in medical practice, described below, have made it difficult to apply these criteria to most individuals currently evaluated for drug-induced thrombocytopenia.

First, prior to the introduction of automated platelet counts, the vast majority of individuals who developed verified drug-induced thrombocytopenia presented with the rapid onset of bleeding associated with platelet counts <20,000/μL, and often <10,000/μL. Most individuals were ingesting a limited number of drugs capable of producing thrombocytopenia and recovered rapidly once the suspected drug was discontinued. While it is likely that such clinical situations still occur with similar frequency, this classic presentation represents a diminishing fraction of the total number of cases of drug-induced thrombocytopenia the hematologist is

**TABLE 29.1.** Drugs That Have Been Implicated as Causing Antibody-Mediated Thrombocytopenia[a]

Acetaminophen
Acetylsalicylic acid
Amrinone
Alpha-methyldopa
Carbamazepine
Chlorthalidone
Chlorthiazine
Cimetidine
Cocaine
Digitoxin
Diphenylhydantoin
Furosemide
Gold salts
Heparin
Heroin
Ibuprofen and other nonsteroidal antiinflammatory drugs
Interferons
Indomethacin
Measles-mumps-rubella vaccine
Noraminopyrine
Penicillin and beta-lactam-containing antibiotics
Penicillamine
Procainamide
Quinidine/quinine
Ranitidine
Rifampin
Sulfonamides
Valproic acid

[a] *Criteria for inclusion include >5 separate reports and immunologic confirmation or in vivo rechallenge.*

asked to evaluate today. Currently, many consultations involve very ill individuals with several potential causes of thrombocytopenia who present with platelet counts that span the entire range of thrombocytopenia. For example, the extent to which infection *per se* versus the numerous agents used in its management contributes to thrombocytopenia is a common problem. As a second example, individuals treated with thiazides or heparin may be referred with moderate thrombocytopenia (platelet counts 50,000 to 100,000/μL) detected as part of an incidentally obtained, automated blood count. In the case of thiazides the natural history of continued drug ingestion in this setting has not been well described, and the need to change therapy is uncertain. In the case of heparin the natural history of the disease in this setting has not been fully explored because the assumed risk of continuing heparin has become appreciated more widely. Similar considerations apply to the

difficulty of establishing maternal drug ingestion as the cause of neonatal thrombocytopenia (6, 7).

Second, many individuals with thrombocytopenia are taking multiple drugs reported either in the peer-reviewed literature or in the *Physicians Desk Reference* to cause thrombocytopenia. Increasingly, such reports are also found within the unpublished files of the drug manufacturers themselves, although these files often consist primarily of individuals with thrombocytopenia in similarly complex and unverifiable clinical situations, and the causal relationship between a particular drug and thrombocytopenia often remains unproven. In addition, individuals are frequently taking newly released medications for which a relationship to thrombocytopenia might not yet have become apparent, assuming a typical frequency of this complication of one in 10,000 to one in 100,000 courses of treatment of newly released drugs.

Third, multiple drugs are often introduced or withdrawn simultaneously because of the complexity of the underlying conditions. Indeed, the hematologist's recommendation in this setting is often to discontinue all unnecessary medications. Although generally successful, the physician is left unsure of which medications should be avoided in the future. The issue of rechallenge with the potential offending agent is rarely considered in current practice because it is possible in most cases to substitute equally effective drugs that differ in their chemical compositions for the drug or drugs in question.

A fourth complicating feature has been the development of numerous assays to measure antiplatelet antibodies that have been adapted to the diagnosis of drug-dependent thrombocytopenia. Two general classifications of assays have been introduced. The first are the modifications of the indirect antiglobulin test used to measure antierythrocyte antibodies. This test demonstrates whether the addition of drug to the patient's serum or plasma increases the deposition of immunoglobulin or complement on normal donor platelets. The second type of assay depends on the capacity of drug-dependent antibodies to alter one of several platelet functions such as aggregation, release of the contents of the dense granules, release of cytoplasmic contents, or alteration in platelet procoagulant activity.

These assays have been especially useful in helping to elucidate the pathogenesis of immune platelet destruction caused by various drugs. Indeed, the mechanism(s) by which drug-dependent antibodies bind to platelets have been the subject of considerable investigation and controversy (Fig. 29.1). The nature of these interactions has been delineated most clearly in the case of antibodies that require quinidine or quinine to bind to platelets. The controversy as to whether preformed drug-antibody complexes bind to platelets, or whether the epitope responsible for antibody binding forms on the cell surface after drug binding has been resolved in merely to concentrate the drug (Model B), alters the three-dimensional structure of the drug (Model C), is itself altered by binding of the drug (Model D), or becomes part of a neoepitope composed of both drug and a component from the platelet (Model E). Platelets may also express certain products on the cell surface on activation that become part of the antigen (see section on Heparin-Induced Thrombocytopenia), and, rarely, drug-independent autoantibodies may develop coincident with drug-dependent antibodies (see section on Quinidine-Induced Thrombocytopenia). These various models are not mutually exclusive and a range of interactions with various affinities could exist in the same or in different individuals, as well as for different drugs and metabolites.

Despite the utility of these assays in helping to elucidate the mechanism of immune platelet injury *in vitro*, the appropriate use of these assays in diagnosing or excluding a drug-dependent thrombocytopenia in the clinical setting is considerably more complex. The following issues should be considered before the results of such tests are used as the basis for clinical decision making.

The sensitivity of the assays have been defined for very few drugs. Therefore the clinical significance of a negative test is generally unclear and the utility of performing additional types of assays is unknown. In some cases, the sensitivity of the assay is decreased because a drug metabolite, rather than the drug itself, may be the inciting antigen. The importance of drug metabolites has been defined most clearly with respect to certain drug-dependent red cell antibodies (8). Recently, several drug-dependent, platelet-reactive antibodies directed at drug metabolites have also been identified (9, 10), and it is likely that others will be identified in the future. However, the possibility of metabolite-dependent antibodies is rarely taken into consideration when these tests are designed or interpreted. Although urine may suffice as a source of antigen in some situations, in the case of other drugs the concentration of specific metabolites in the urine may be insufficient. Theoretically, serum from unaffected individuals taking the drug in question may be more likely to contain the relevant metabolites and can be used as a source of antigen. Testing may also be complicated by difficulties that include failure to identify potentially antigenic substances not commonly recognized as drugs (11, 12) and by exposure to complex substances of undefined composition such as illicit drugs (13–15). It has also been reported that polymorphic determinants involved in the binding of drug and/or antibody to platelets may allow some normal platelets, and especially platelets from affected individuals, to be more suitable targets for drug-dependent antibodies than others (15–18). In other cases, drug-dependent antibodies may be directed at a marrow precursor (19). Furthermore, drugs such as alpha-methyldopa and

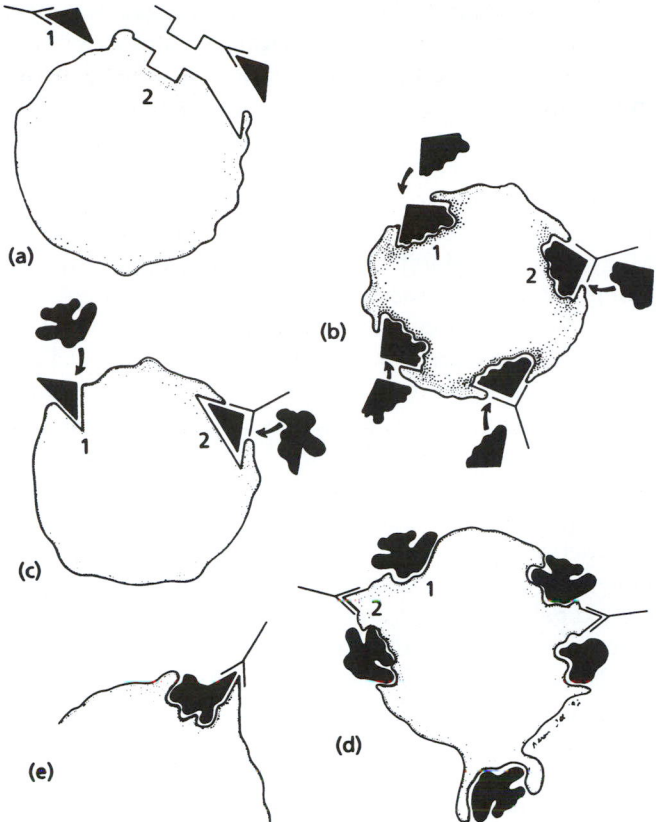

**FIGURE 29.1.** Potential mechanisms by which drug-dependent antibodies may bind to platelets. **a,** The antibody may bind to the drug in plasma to form circulating immune complexes. Formation of the complex may induce a conformational change in the IgG molecule recognized by platelet Fc receptors. **b,** The antibody may bind directly to the drug, which is concentrated on the platelet surface relative to its plasma concentration. **c,** When the drug binds to the platelet, it may undergo a conformational change recognized by antibody. **d,** Binding of the drug may induce a conformational change in a platelet component recognized by antibody. **e,** The antibody may recognize one or more neoepitopes comprised of both platelet-derived and drug-derived determinants.

favor of the latter hypothesis. It is likely that the experimental data interpreted as favoring the hypothesis that preformed immune complexes bound to platelets (Model A) may have been based on the low avidity of binding of either drug or antibody to the platelet. Because of the low avidity, stable interactions between the antibody or drug with the platelet surface were not maintained when the cells were washed. Furthermore, direct evidence in favor of circulating immune complexes composed of drug and specific antibody has been lacking. In contrast, the cell specificity of the majority of drug-dependent antibodies argues against simple binding of immune complexes to platelet Fcγ receptors. However, it is not clear whether the platelet serves

L-dopa may induce either drug-dependent antibodies (20) or antibodies that react with platelets in the absence of added drugs (21, 22). In some cases both drug-dependent and drug-independent autoreactive (22, 23) or alloreactive (24, 25) antibodies may coexist in the same sample.

The specificity of most assays for drug-dependent, antiplatelet antibodies has rarely been assessed. In only a few studies has the effect of adding the drug to plasma from individuals with other established causes of immune thrombocytopenia been determined (26). Even more importantly, few studies have examined the effect of adding drug to the plasma of other, unaffected individuals who have received comparable courses of therapy (27, 28). The consequence of adding combinations of drugs comparable to the actual therapy received by the individual has rarely been considered or tested. All these factors become matters of concern when the physician has to decide how to apply the results of a particular assay to individual individuals, since it is often observed that the concentration of drug needed to elicit a positive assay *in vitro* greatly exceeds that attained in plasma (14).

Since neither the positive nor the negative predictive value of most tests for drug-dependent antibodies have been defined, and since there are few situations in which rechallenge with a suspected, offending drug is medically indicated, the diagnosis of drug-induced thrombocytopenia remains a clinical judgment in most situations encountered in practice. This is not to deny the importance of *in vitro* studies that provide insight into the pathogenesis of specific drug-induced thrombocytopenias. Rather, thorough familiarity with the typical and atypical presentations of the more common causes of drug-induced thrombocytopenia remains essential for proper management of affected individuals. The specialized tests described below cannot yet be used to substitute for such clinical judgments.

# THROMBOCYTOPENIA DUE TO DRUG-INDUCED INHIBITION OF THROMBOPOIESIS

Several drugs have been reported to inhibit megakaryocytopoiesis, leading to diminished platelet production and peripheral thrombocytopenia. While suppression of platelet production by drugs or drug-dependent antibodies occurs much less frequently than thrombocytopenia caused by enhanced platelet destruction, the contribution of this mechanism may be underestimated because of two factors: first, the assumption that the presence of megakaryocytes in a bone marrow sample can be used as a surrogate marker of platelet production and,

second, the relative difficulty in studying megakaryocytopoiesis *in vitro*. The same technical limitations have impaired identification of the mechanisms by which drug-induced megakaryocyte toxicity may develop.

There are a number of steps in the production of platelets (Chapter 8) that represent potential sites of drug toxicity. First, the drug may be directly toxic to pluripotential (CFU-GEMM) or committed stem cells (CFU-Meg) or may inhibit their subsequent differentiation along the megakaryocytic pathway. A drug might also inhibit megakaryocyte differentiation or the production of platelets from the mature megakaryocyte (29, 30). Each step in this process is influenced by one or more specific growth factors (29, 30), as well as by cytokines released by marrow accessory cells (30). Theoretically, thrombopoiesis may be inhibited via direct effects of a drug on the megakaryocyte or indirectly through an effect on the production of factors important in megakaryocytopoiesis. There is also evidence to indicate, as will be discussed below, that several drugs alter both megakaryocyte development and platelet survival.

Unfortunately, little definitive information exists concerning the effects of specific drugs on megakaryocyte physiology. In the absence of these data, several drugs have been assumed to cause thrombocytopenia by inhibiting megakaryocytopoiesis, although on careful review, other mechanisms are more likely. It has generally been assumed that a drug exerts its effect on platelet production based on a relative paucity of megakaryocytes in bone marrow biopsies and the time course of platelet recovery following drug withdrawal, rather than specific, clinically validated, *in vitro* assays of megakaryocyte development.

Although drugs such as chemotherapeutic agents universally inhibit megakaryocytopoiesis if used in high enough doses (31), this review will focus on the effects of more commonly used drugs that have been reported to inhibit megakaryocyte development.

## ETHANOL

The association between thrombocytopenia and alcohol was first reported by Jandl, who described the development of severe thrombocytopenia and gastrointestinal bleeding in two individuals who had ingested large amounts of alcohol for several weeks (32). Platelet counts in both individuals recovered within several days of abstention, although additional studies were not performed to document unequivocally that alcohol was the actual cause of the thrombocytopenia. Thrombocytopenia was noted, but not commented on, by Sullivan and Herbert, who demonstrated a direct suppressant effect of alcohol on erythropoiesis, even when folic acid was administered simultaneously (33). The first detailed description of thrombocytopenia in individuals with alcohol abuse was published by Lindenbaum and Hargrove in 1968 (34). These investigators described the cases of five chronic alcoholics who presented with platelet counts ranging from 45,000/μL to 115,000/μL. The platelet counts rose to normal or elevated levels after a period of abstinence, even without folate or B12 supplementation, and in four instances before food was given. Bone marrow examination performed in these individuals within 24 hours of admission showed striking alterations in the appearance of pronormoblasts in the absence of typical megaloblastic changes.

## Clinical Presentation

The clinical characteristics of individuals who develop alcohol-induced thrombocytopenia have been described in detail in many studies. The incidence of this complication after heavy ingestion of ethanol ranges from 3% in chronic stable alcoholics (35) to as high as 81% after acute intoxication (36). Although individuals usually present with mild to moderate thrombocytopenia, with platelet counts ranging from 40,000/μL to 150,000/μL (35–40), some individuals may develop severe thrombocytopenia with platelet counts as low as 14,000/μL reported (37). Platelet size is generally normal to small on initial presentation, an observation attributed to diminished thrombopoiesis with a resultant increase in the percentage of older platelets in the circulation (39). The wide variation in the reported incidence of purpura and bleeding manifestations in individuals with moderate thrombocytopenia may reflect the effects of additional coagulopathies due to hepatic dysfunction (see Chapter 45) and other underlying medical illnesses (34, 36, 37). Bone marrow examination in alcoholic individuals often reveals toxic vacuolization of pronormoblasts (41), which resembles that described in the setting of chloramphenicol toxicity (42, 43). Thrombopoiesis may be megaloblastic (33, 36, 41) or normoblastic (34, 37, 44), depending primarily on the patient's folate status. However, serum and erythrocyte folate levels do not correlate closely with the extent of thrombocytopenia (36), suggesting that individual differences exist either in the sensitivity of the enzymes involved in folate metabolism to the effect of alcohol or in the variation in folate use by megakaryocytes in the presence of ethanol or its metabolites. Megakaryocyte numbers are generally mildly increased, normal, or slightly decreased (34, 36), with significant megakaryocytopenia occurring only in rare cases (45).

## Pathophysiology

It is most likely that the most important mechanism by which ethanol causes thrombocytopenia is by inhibiting megakaryocyte development and platelet production. Studies performed prior to the development of techniques for assessing megakaryocyte colony formation *in vitro* demonstrated that ingestion of ethanol by human subjects could inhibit the production of platelets. The thrombokinetic studies performed by Cowan in both folate deficient and folate replete individuals were the first to indicate that ethanol induced a state of "ineffective thrombopoiesis" (46). Cowan detected increases in total megakaryocyte number and mass in individuals who developed thrombocytopenia after 4 weeks of controlled ethanol intake; these increases were greater in individuals in whom folate deficiency had been induced simultaneously. Although total megakaryocyte mass in these individuals increased, platelet production was reduced in comparison with baseline values. Cowan also detected decrements in platelet survival in individuals ingesting, but not infused with, ethanol, and concluded that alcohol-induced thrombocytopenia resulted from the combined effects of diminished platelet survival and decreases in effective thrombopoiesis (46). These findings are supported by those of Sullivan et al, who noted significant delays in the rate of recovery of peripheral platelet counts after thrombopheresis in individuals ingesting alcohol compared to the rate of recovery in the same individuals during abstinence (47). These delays were not accompanied by diminished numbers of megakaryocytes in the bone marrow.

The results of *in vitro* studies, which employed techniques previously developed for study of the effects of ethanol on erythroid (48) or granulocyte-macrophage (48, 49) colony formation, offer direct evidence that ethanol can suppress megakaryocyte development. Gewirtz and Hoffman analyzed the bone marrow of a individual with alcohol-induced thrombocytopenia (45), observing a paucity of megakaryocytes on routine histology. However, immunostaining of this marrow with an antiserum raised against platelet glycoproteins revealed an increased number of small, morphologically unrecognizable megakaryocyte precursors. Megakaryocyte colony-stimulating activity (Meg-CSA) in the patient's serum increased dramatically during the period of severe thrombocytopenia, falling before an increase in the number of circulating platelets was observed (45). These observations are of interest in light of the recently described, inverse correlation between plasma thrombopoietin levels and megakaryocyte mass (50), suggesting that the levels of this cytokine may also depend on the state of megakaryocyte differentiation. These investigators also observed that ethanol concentrations as high as 450 mg/dL did not suppress megakaryocyte colony formation in plasma clot culture, leading to the conclusion that ethanol has little direct effect on the development of committed megakaryocyte progenitors, but instead may arrest megakaryocyte development and differentiation at the stage of a more mature precursor (45). This postulate is in accord with the time course of platelet recovery in most individuals with ethanol-induced thrombocytopenia (47) and has since been confirmed by other investigators using similar marrow culture systems (28, 51). The latter studies have shown that megakaryocyte colony formation is directly suppressed by ethanol when added at the initiation of marrow cultures only at concentrations above those achievable *in vivo*. In contrast, when ethanol is added to marrow cultures 7 days after their initiation, colony formation is suppressed at concentrations of only 500 mg/dL, suggesting that a more differentiated cell than the megakaryocyte progenitor (CFU-Meg) is most susceptible to ethanol toxicity at or near ethanol concentrations attainable *in vivo* (51).

The preferential effects of ethanol on more differentiated megakaryocytic cells is also suggested by studies in which its effects on megakaryocytopoiesis in the guinea pig have been studied. Earlier reports confirmed that concentrations of ethanol and/or its metabolite, acetaldehyde, greater than those achievable *in vivo* were required to suppress megakaryocyte colony formation (52). However, although the viability of cultured, guinea-pig megakaryocytes was unaltered at ethanol concentrations as high as 500 mg/dL, protein synthesis by these cells was inhibited at concentrations as low as 120 mg/dL (52). Furthermore, thrombocytopenia developed in these animals in the absence of megakaryocytopenia after 11 days of ethanol ingestion. These results support the hypothesis that ethanol may affect the function of more differentiated megakaryocytes, leading to ineffective thrombopoiesis, without affecting the viability of primitive megakaryocyte progenitors, as initially suggested by the thrombokinetic studies of Cowan (46). Additional support for such effects has been provided by recent studies in the guinea pig in which modest ethanol consumption, insufficient to yield detectable blood levels, caused only mild thrombocytopenia but significant alterations in platelet morphology with a striking decrease in the number of circulating, elongated, platelet forms (53). This morphologic alteration was accompanied by a marked increase in the rigidity of mature megakaryocytes, as determined by measuring their deformability when aspirated into micropipettes (53).

Finally, it has been suggested that much of the ethanol-associated damage to megakaryocytes, as well as other hematopoietic elements, may be induced by its metabolites, particularly acetaldehyde (52, 54). The potential role of bone marrow macrophages in the metabolism of ethanol and in the production of such toxic metabolites has recently been demonstrated (55).

Ethanol may also affect the survival of circulating platelets. A decrease in platelet survival and a transient drop in the platelet count occur within 3 hours of the acute ingestion (38) or infusion (37, 56) of alcohol. The pathogenesis of shortened platelet survival is uncertain, but has been attributed to ethanol-induced platelet aggregation and sequestration (37, 38, 56). The actual site of such sequestration has not been determined, although the acute fall in circulating preinfused [$^{51}$Cr]-labeled platelets after ethanol infusion is not accompanied by the expected increase in radioactivity over the liver and spleen that occurs in other platelet destructive disorders (56). These observations suggest that a more diffuse, perhaps vascular, site of transient sequestration may exist, although it is unlikely that such a mechanism contributes to the stable depression in platelet counts observed in association with ethanol ingestion in the clinical setting.

There is some evidence that ethanol may alter platelet function as well (see Chapter 33) (57). Abnormalities in the second wave of platelet aggregation in response to adenosine diphosphate (ADP) and epinephrine (40), deficient generation of platelet factor 3 (PF3), and prolongation of the bleeding time have been reported in some alcoholic individuals with adequate numbers of platelets (40, 57). The mechanism accountable for these changes is uncertain, although a variety of abnormalities have been described (58, 59). Since these abnormalities were induced more readily by ethanol ingestion than by exposure of normal platelets to ethanol *in vitro*, the changes in platelet function may reflect biochemical changes in the megakaryocytes (40). This hypothesis is supported by the reported morphologic abnormalities in megakaryocyte maturation induced by ethanol, as well as by abnormalities in the ultrastructure of platelets obtained from alcoholic individuals (60). The latter include unusually large azurophilic granules, poor definition of the circumferential band of microtubules observed in normal platelets, and the presence of large, unidentified, rod-shaped structures in some cells (60). However, the relationship between alterations in platelet production, metabolic activity, function, and structure to clinical bleeding has not been established, and impaired platelet function by itself is generally not a major source of morbidity in individuals with moderate thrombocytopenia.

## Management

Treatment of ethanol-induced thrombocytopenia consists of supportive measures only. Alternative causes of thrombocytopenia such as folate deficiency (44) and hypersplenism should be considered, and individuals should be provided with adequate nutrition and folic acid as needed. Thrombocytopenic individuals should receive platelet transfusions in the presence of bleeding, although the physician should be cognizant that concurrent vitamin K deficiency, liver dysfunction, and unrecognized trauma may also contribute to purpura and bleeding in alcoholic individuals. In the absence of other conditions, ethanol-induced thrombocytopenia generally begins to improve within 3 days of abstinence, with complete recovery achieved within 10 days (36, 38, 47,

61). Platelet counts commonly exceed the normal range for several days during recovery (61).

## THIAZIDES

Thiazide diuretics were implicated as causing thrombocytopenia soon after their introduction for the treatment of hypertension and congestive heart failure in 1958. The first individual reported with this syndrome presented with mild thrombocytopenia (platelet count of 94,000/μL), which resolved after discontinuation of the drug and recurred on rechallenge (62). Several additional cases were reported soon thereafter (63–66).

The overall incidence of thiazide-induced thrombocytopenia has been estimated to be approximately one in 15,000 courses; the prevalence of this syndrome has been reported to be higher in the elderly (1). Individuals with thiazide-induced thrombocytopenia generally present with mild to moderate thrombocytopenia (platelet counts of 30,000 to 100,000/μL) (1, 67); however, occasional individuals have presented with platelet counts below 10,000/μL (66). A surprising number of individuals present with purpura, despite only modest reductions in platelet counts (67). It is possible that in some individuals purpura reflects secondary bleeding into areas affected by superficial vasculitis (64). Examination of the peripheral blood in individuals with thiazide-induced thrombocytopenia generally demonstrates only reduced numbers of platelets. Occasionally, individuals present with concomitant neutropenia. Bone marrow examination may reveal diminished or absent megakaryocytes (63), although just as frequently megakaryocyte numbers are normal or increased (64).

Although several prominent hematology texts list thiazides among the drugs that impair platelet production, there is only limited experimental evidence to support the contention that direct, bone marrow toxicity occurs. Rather, the pathogenesis of thiazide-induced thrombocytopenia appears to be heterogeneous. In many of the initial cases in which thrombocytopenia was attributed to impaired production, bone marrow examination was not performed (62, 65, 66, 68). The toxicity of thiazides on megakaryocytes has been assumed because of the relatively long interval between drug withdrawal and platelet recovery and between drug rechallenge and recurrence of thrombocytopenia in a few reported cases (65, 69). Postmortem examination of the bone marrow in one individual did reveal severe hypoplasia and replacement by fibrogelatinous tissue (63).

A syndrome of thrombocytopenia in neonates born to women receiving thiazides has been reported by Rodriguez et al (70). These investigators described seven infants with severe thrombocytopenia (platelet counts 8,000 to 28,000/μL). Platelet counts of all of the mothers were normal, and no isoantibodies were detected. Two of the infants had concurrent neutropenia, two had

moderate reticulocytopenia, and another had pancytopenia. Examination of bone marrow from five infants revealed decreased or absent megakaryocytes in four infants. The time to recovery of neonatal platelet counts ranged from 1 week to as long as 3 months. Since thiazides cross the placenta (71), the authors postulated that toxicity of these drugs to the fetal marrow was responsible for the induction of thrombocytopenia. However, no correlation between the duration or intensity of thiazide ingestion by the mother and the degree of neonatal thrombocytopenia was observed. Moreover, the incidence of this syndrome is extremely low, since the authors state that these seven cases were derived from analysis of several thousand deliveries (72). The incidence of preeclampsia in these women, a potential cause of neonatal thrombocytopenia and a common indication for thiazide therapy during the years when these cases were observed, is not stated (70). Furthermore, no difference in mean platelet counts between healthy term and premature infants and those neonates born to mothers treated with thiazide therapy was detected in a subsequent, retrospective analysis by another group (73). In another study no cases of neonatal thrombocytopenia were detected in over 3000 mothers treated with thiazides. The authors of this report conclude that the incidence of this syndrome must be exceptionally low (73).

Most adult individuals with thiazide-associated thrombocytopenia have normal bone marrow examinations (64). In addition, evidence from several, more recent studies suggests that the most cases of thiazide-induced thrombocytopenia may actually result from drug-induced immune platelet destruction (65, 68, 74).

Management of the individual with thiazide-induced thrombocytopenia is supportive. In most cases, platelet counts generally recover within 5 to 14 days of discontinuation of the drug (1, 31, 62, 66, 68), and corticosteroid therapy has not been shown to hasten recovery. The risk of rechallenge with thiazides themselves or with related drugs is unknown, but any risk seems excessive given the multiple alternative forms of diuretic and antihypertensive therapies currently available.

## ESTROGENS

Administration of conjugated estrogens to several species of animals causes thrombocytopenia that is accompanied by striking decreases in megakaryocyte number (75, 76). The mechanism of this effect may be secondary to direct and selective toxicity of these compounds to megakaryocyte progenitors (77) or to disruption of the function of marrow accessory cells (78). However, the relevance of these observations to the development of thrombocytopenia in humans is uncertain, as the effects of estrogens on thrombopoiesis appear to be species specific. Only isolated cases of estrogen-associated thrombocytopenia have been reported in humans, although purpura associated with estrogen therapy may occasionally occur in the absence of significant hematologic abnormalities (79). Furthermore, little evidence is available to suggest that cases of estrogen-associated thrombocytopenia have occurred as a result of drug-induced megakaryocyte suppression. For example, Watson et al reported the development of purpura in five individuals treated with estrone, estradiol, or stilbesterol (79), which could be attributed to severe thrombocytopenia in only three of the individuals. Bone marrow examination in the latter group revealed essentially no abnormalities in two of the individuals, while the marrow of the third revealed trilineage hypoplasia, which did not resolve following discontinuation of estrogen therapy.

Thrombocytopenia responsive to estrogen withdrawal that recurred on rechallenge has been well documented in only one case, occurring in a individual treated with diethylstilbestrol (DES) (80). Although it was suggested that thrombocytopenia in this individual occurred as a result of DES-induced marrow suppression, the rapid recurrence of thrombocytopenia after drug reexposure suggests that a mechanism other than impaired platelet production, such as a hypersensitivity reaction leading to the destruction of circulating platelets, may have been involved. This latter hypothesis is supported by reports implicating estrogen in the induction of some cases of cyclic thrombocytopenia, perhaps by enhancing the clearance of antibody-coated platelets by the reticuloendothelial system (81). Furthermore, a recent report has described the occurrence of thrombocytopenia accompanied by the appearance of drug-dependent antiplatelet antibodies in a individual treated with the antiestrogenic compound, tamoxifen (82). Several cases of thrombocytopenia secondary to thrombotic thrombocytopenia purpura have also been recently observed in individuals treated with the progestational agent, levonorgestrel (Norplant) (83), suggesting another mechanism by which estrogen or related compounds may potentially induce accelerated destruction of circulating platelets.

## INTERFERONS

The interferons are a family of proteins with diverse biologic effects. The antiproliferative effects of these proteins have been used to advantage in several neoplastic diseases (84), and their immunomodulatory effects have proven effective in diminishing the activity and progression of chronic, active hepatitis (85–87). Since the introduction of recombinant interferon in 1981 (88), the interferons' effects on granulocyte (84, 89, 90) and erythrocyte production (89) have been well described.

Thrombocytopenia is a prominent manifestation of interferon therapy. Typically, thrombocytopenia develops gradually over several weeks after the initiation of interferon therapy and is generally mild to moderate in severity, although platelet counts below 50,000/$\mu$L may occasionally occur (87, 89). The incidence and severity of thrombocytopenia is dose-related (84) and may vary depending on the specific disease state for which interferon is being administered (84, 89). For example, thrombocytopenia develops in only 10% of individuals with solid tumors who receive interferon therapy (89), while approximately 30 to 50% of individuals with multiple myeloma (84, 91) and 25% of individuals with chronic lymphocytic leukemia (92) develop this complication, presumably reflecting preexisting, bone marrow compromise. Indeed, individuals with thrombocytopenia prior to initiation of therapy and those who have been heavily pretreated with chemotherapy are at increased risk to develop more severe thrombocytopenia. Despite the high incidence of thrombocytopenia noted in conjunction with interferon therapy, bleeding is unusual.

Several studies have addressed the pathogenesis of interferon-mediated thrombocytopenia. Human multipotential progenitor cells (CFU-GEMM) and BFU-E are equally suppressed by interferons $\alpha$, $\beta$, and $\gamma$, although CFU-GM are more sensitive to interferon $\gamma$ (93). Both interferon $\alpha$ and $\gamma$ also have direct antiproliferative activity against CFU-Meg (94), with interferon $\alpha$ more potent in this regard. The presence of bone marrow accessory cells is necessary for the maximal antiproliferative effects of interferon $\gamma$ to be expressed, perhaps through their elaboration of additional cytokines acting in concert with interferon $\gamma$ to suppress hematopoiesis. However, megakaryocytic cell lines have been shown to express receptors for interferon (95), and it is likely that many interferon-mediated effects, particularly those involving interferon $\alpha$, occur secondary to its effects on normal hematopoietic progenitor cells, similar to its therapeutic effects on hematopoietic progenitor cells in individuals with myelofibrosis, myeloid metaplasia (96), and chronic myelogenous leukemia (97–99).

In addition to its direct antiproliferative activity on megakaryocyte progenitor cells, interferon may occasionally exacerbate or induce the onset of immune thrombocytopenia purpura (35). Although this syndrome may be difficult to distinguish from that resulting from the antiproliferative effects of interferon on megakaryocytes, its onset tends to be more rapid, platelet counts may fall to levels as low as 10,000/$\mu$L, and the disorder responds rapidly to standard therapeutic interventions such as prednisone or intravenous immunoglobulin (100). Interestingly, the induction of immune-mediated thrombocytopenia (ITP) has been reported primarily in individuals receiving therapy for chronic hepatitis B (85–87) or C (100, 101) and is in marked contrast to its efficacy in the treatment of preexisting thrombocytopenia in some individuals with refractory (102, 103) or HIV-associated (104) ITP. The reasons for these discrepant responses are not understood, but likely reflect differences in the nature of the underlying immune dysregulation.

# DRUGS THAT CAUSE IMMUNE PLATELET DESTRUCTION

## HEPARIN-INDUCED THROMBOCYTOPENIA (HIT)

### Clinical Presentation

The association of heparin with thrombocytopenia and thrombosis was first described almost 40 years ago and has been repeatedly confirmed since that time (105–109). Approximately 1% of individuals treated with intravenous heparin for a minimum of 1 week develop thrombocytopenia (110, 111), making this the most common cause of drug-induced immune thrombocytopenia. Individuals generally present with moderate thrombocytopenia (platelet count 20,000 to 100,000/μL), which first appears 3 to 7 days after the initiation of a continuous infusion of heparin if there has been no history of prior drug exposure, but may develop more rapidly, in some cases after a single dose (27), in individuals who have received heparin previously. Thrombocytopenia developing more than 14 days after initiation of heparin therapy, while described, is more likely to have another cause. Thrombocytopenia and/or thrombosis (see below) has been described in occasional individuals who have been exposed to only minimal amounts of heparin, for example during angioplasty procedures, infusion of parenteral hyperalimentation solutions, or after prophylactic subcutaneous administration (112–118). Exposure of sensitized individuals to even a few units of heparin eluted from bonded catheters is sufficient to sustain the disorder (119, 120). Thrombocytopenia has also been reported after the administration of low-molecular-weight heparin, heparinoids, and other anionic mucopolysaccharides (see below).

When platelet counts are monitored frequently, most individuals are asymptomatic at the time thrombocytopenia is first noted. Bleeding from surgical wounds occurs infrequently, unless there are additional disturbances of coagulation (116). However, the most severe clinical complication of HIT is the paradoxical development of thrombosis (heparin-induced thrombocytopenia and thrombosis or HITT) that occurs in a subset of affected individuals. Therefore thrombocytopenia serves primarily as a warning of impending thrombosis, a complication that is associated with a mortality approaching 10% (116). Arterial thrombosis occurs most commonly in individuals with atherosclerosis, especially in peripheral arteries that have been manipulated surgically or that contain prosthetic grafts (116, 121) (Fig.

29.2). Less commonly, individuals present with occlusion of large or medium sized central arteries resulting in stroke, myocardial or mesenteric infarction, renal or spinal artery occlusion, or adrenal infarction and hemorrhage (105, 106, 122–127). Skin necrosis caused by occlusion of dermal vessels has also been reported (123, 128). Thrombi developing in the deep venous system of the legs and pulmonary emboli also occur commonly, especially after orthopedic or other types of surgery (129, 130). Since venous thromboses and pulmonary emboli are common in this setting, it is important to measure the platelet count to determine whether heparin may be a predisposing cause. In any of these settings, thrombi may be multiple and can recur at the same or other sites if the affected individual continues to be exposed to heparin (105, 106).

Although platelet counts are generally less than 100,000/μL at the time thrombi become evident clinically, it should not be assumed that heparin can be continued safely with values above this level. Platelet counts may fall precipitously within 24 hours preceding overt thrombosis, and thrombi may occur in the absence of thrombocytopenia (121, 131–136). Thus it is often difficult to decide when to discontinue heparin in individuals with either mild thrombocytopenia (platelet counts >100,000/μL) or in whom the platelet count is falling but is still within the normal range, since the proportion of individuals who will develop HITT if heparin is continued is uncertain. Several investigators consider the gradual development of mild thrombocytopenia to be common and to have a pathogenesis distinct from that of HITT, since the platelet count may recover even if heparin is continued (137–140). It has been speculated that platelets from affected individuals are more susceptible to aggregation in the presence of heparin, leading to transient sequestration (141). However, a diagnosis of benign, transient, type I HIT can neither be made nor excluded using currently identified clinical criteria or laboratory tests (26, 139, 140). Therefore there is no method to distinguish individuals whose platelet counts will recover without interruption of therapy from those who are at risk of developing more severe thrombocytopenia and thrombosis if heparin is continued.

### Incidence

Meta-analyses indicate the incidence of HIT to be 1.1 to 1.3% (111, 142) (platelet count <100,000/μL) in individuals who received "therapeutic" doses of porcine heparin by intravenous administration for a minimum of 1 week. The incidence of thrombocytopenia is approximately fivefold greater with bovine heparin (142, 143), less with low-molecular-weight heparin (144), and minimal in individuals receiving only "prophylactic doses" of heparin (112, 142). However, the clinical utility of these estimates must be qualified by the wide variation

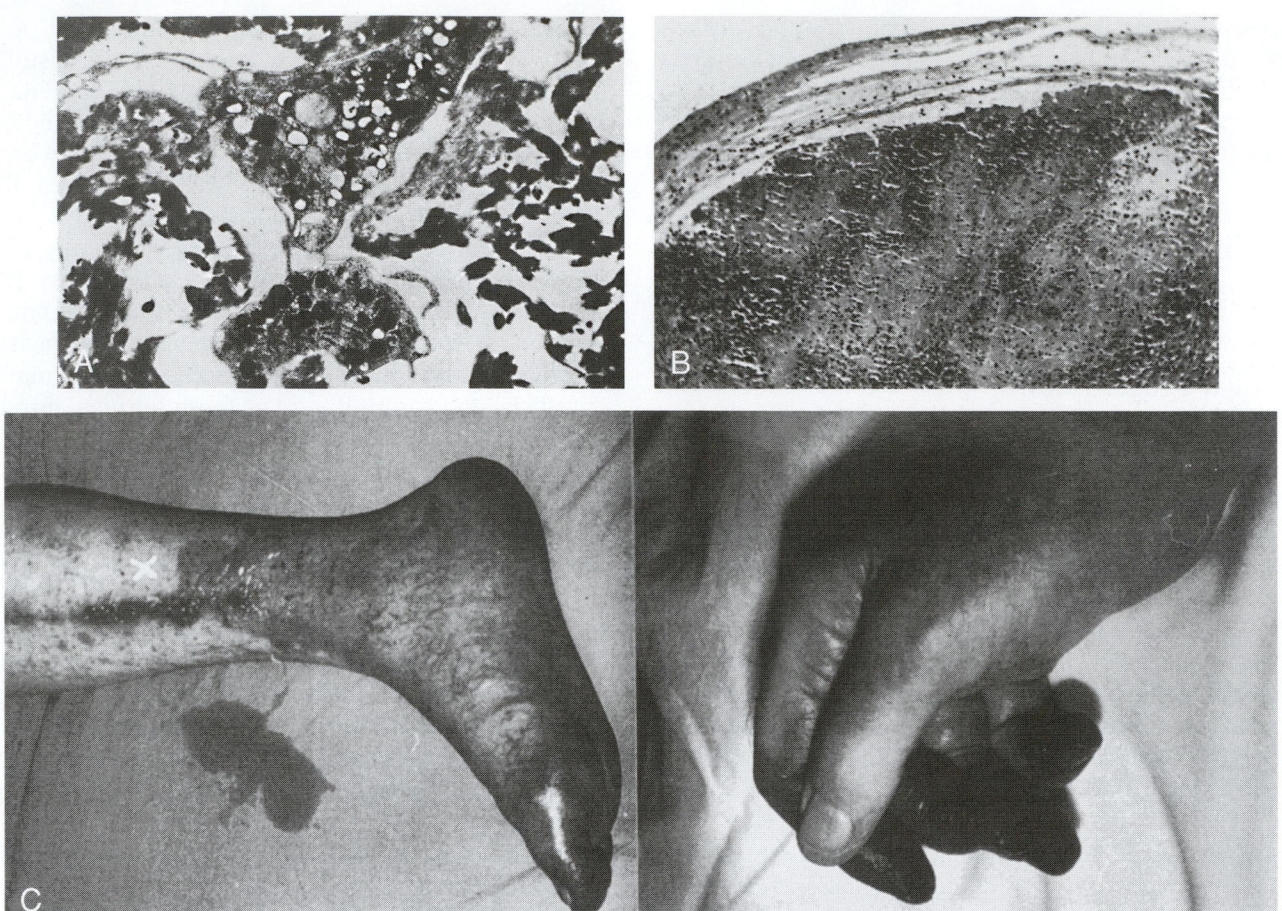

**FIGURE 29.2.** Thrombotic complications of heparin-associated thrombosis and thrombocytopenia (HITT). **A,** Electron micrograph of a platelet-rich thrombus from a individual with HITT. (Reproduced with permission from Towne JB, Bernhard VM, Hussey C et al. White clot syndrome. Peripheral vascular complication of heparin therapy. Arch Surg 1979;114:372–377.) **B,** Thrombus removed from radial artery of a individual with HITT. (Adapted with permission from Roberts B, Rosato FE, Rosato EF. Heparin—a cause of arterial emboli? Surgery 1964;55:803–811.) **C,** Thrombotic vascular occlusion in a individual with HITT causing ischemic necrosis of extremities. (Courtesy of Dr. Kelly A. Spratt.)

in the reported incidence of HIT (0 to 30%) (reviewed in Ref. 142). Thrombocytopenia occurs more frequently in individuals with underlying cardiovascular disease (145), especially after coronary bypass or other forms of vascular surgery (146) either as a result of repetitive drug exposure or concomitant events such as platelet activation on extracorporeal surfaces or at sites of vascular trauma. However, the variation in the incidence and the reported clustering of cases (143, 147) cannot be fully explained by these factors and is unlikely to have occurred solely on the basis of chance. To some extent differences in drug formulation may account for variations in the incidence of HIT/HITT, since heparin is biochemically heterogeneous (148) and standardization is based on net anticoagulant activity rather than chemical purity. There is no currently available method to compare the antigenicity of heparin from different sources.

The incidence of thrombosis is also a matter of uncertainty. In studies published before 1990, thrombotic complications were reported in approximately 20% of the individuals with HIT (149). However, this figure may represent an overestimation since platelet counts were not routinely monitored before the prevalence of HITT was appreciated. Furthermore, prior to a broader awareness of HITT, most physicians attributed the failure to resolve preexisting thrombi or the appearance of new thrombi in individuals on heparin therapy to preexisting disease and were reluctant to discontinue heparin until after the development of additional complications. Therefore HITT was often diagnosed only after new arterial or recurrent venous thrombi developed, and it is likely that the true incidence of thrombosis in association with HITT is appreciably lower if platelet counts are surveyed appropriately and corrective action is taken in all individuals receiving heparin.

## Pathogenesis

### Thrombocytopenia

HIT is caused by heparin-dependent antiplatelet antibodies (150). Although platelets from normal donors adhere to each other after brief exposure to heparin at concentrations somewhat higher than those attained *in vivo* (141, 151, 152), the observation that thrombocytopenia develops only after several days of heparin administration in the absence of previous exposure (27, 153) argues for the role of antibodies in the pathogenesis of HIT. Heparin-dependent platelet-reactive antibodies can be demonstrated in plasma from most individuals with HIT based on tests that measure platelet activation. The addition of heparin to individual plasma initiates the binding of antibody and complement to normal donor platelets (27, 154–156), causing them to aggregate and release their dense granule contents, including the platelet agonist and vasoconstrictor thromboxane $A_2$ (154, 155, 157–159). Both the $F(ab')_2$ and Fc portions of isolated IgG molecules are required for platelet activation to occur *in vitro* (157, 160–162). It has been proposed that binding of the $F(ab')_2$ portion of the immunoglobulin molecule to the platelet permits the exposed IgG Fc domain to crosslink FcγRIIA receptors within and between platelets, thereby stimulating second messenger systems that initiate platelet activation (163–165). High concentrations of heparin inhibit serum-induced platelet injury, presumably by blocking antibody binding (26, 156, 157). There is a histidine/arginine polymorphism at position 131 in FcγRIIA, and it has been reported that only platelets on which the phenotype representative of the histidine allele is expressed are susceptible to activation *in vitro* (166). However, the relationship between expression of this permissive allele and susceptibility to developing HIT/HITT is uncertain (166–169).

Recent studies indicate that plasma from approximately 90% of individuals with HIT contains antibodies that recognize complexes between heparin and platelet factor 4 (PF4) (170–173). Antibodies to complexes containing other heparin-binding proteins such as neutrophil-activating peptide-2 and interleukin-8 have been reported in some of the remaining cases (174). It is hypothesized that PF4 released from activated platelets forms complexes with heparin in the circulation and/or on platelet surfaces (Fig. 29.3). The contribution of PF4 (175) and the glycosaminoglycan (176, 177) to the autoantigen is currently under study. Antibodies to heparin/PF4 are readily measured by ELISA (170, 173). However, such antibodies are quite common after drug exposure, whether assessed by ELISA (178–180) or platelet activation assays (27, 139, 140), and it is unclear whether differences in titer, isotype, avidity, specificity, or platelet responsiveness explain why only a small fraction of individuals with demonstrable antibodies develop HIT.

### Thrombosis

HIT/HITT is unique among the drug-induced thrombocytopenias in the prevalence of thrombosis, yet even less is known about the pathogenesis of this complication. The effect of heparin-dependent antibodies on platelet aggregation or secretion *in vitro* does not differ in an obvious way from that of quinidine-dependent antibodies or complement-fixing anti-HLA or anti-Pl$^{A1}$ antibodies, for example. Thus, any purported mechanism must explain how platelets sensitized by some antibodies cause thrombocytopenia and bleeding, while those sensitized by heparin-dependent antibodies lead to thrombosis. "Heparin resistance" (i.e., a sudden shortening of the aPTT) has been noted in a small number of individuals (63, 109, 122, 124, 126, 181, 182). HIT plasma promotes the release of platelet microparticles with procoagulant activity (183), although it is uncertain whether this effect is unique to this disorder or correlates with thrombosis.

Sera from individuals with HIT/HITT also contain antibodies that recognize endothelial cell-bound complexes consisting of PF4 and heparin or heparan sulfate; these antibodies promote platelet adhesion and lead to the expression of endothelial cell procoagulant activity *in vitro* (127, 184), a finding that has not been associated with most other drug-dependent antibodies to date. Although this observation cannot by itself account for the selective involvement of specific vessels, concurrent activation of platelets and disruption of endothelial cell anticoagulant function by HIT antibody may accelerate platelet-vessel wall interactions and thereby promote thrombosis.

A syndrome resembling DIC (see also Chapter 44) has been observed in a few individuals with HITT (109, 142, 185–187). In addition to thrombocytopenia and thrombosis, these antibodies may have low plasma concentrations of fibrinogen and elevated concentrations of fibrin/fibrinogen degradation products. Acute reductions in the plasma concentration of antithrombin III, heparin cofactor II, and protein C have also been observed in a high proportion of individuals with HITT (145). Such manifestations may represent only the extreme end of the spectrum of disruption in anticoagulant functions, and the clinical course of individuals with heparin-associated "DIC" does not differ significantly from that in which heparin-dependent platelet antibodies are detected. Nevertheless, recognition of this atypical presentation is important to ensure that the individuals are not inappropriately treated with heparin.

## Diagnosis

The development of thrombocytopenia or thrombosis in any individual receiving heparin should alert the clinician to the possibility of HIT and the attendant need to discontinue heparin. The diagnosis should also be

Pathogenesis of Heparin-Induced Thrombocytopenia

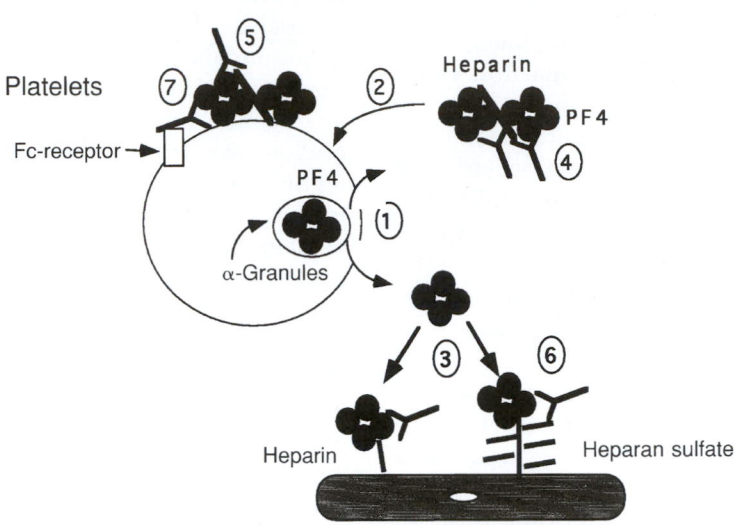

**FIGURE 29.3.** Pathogenesis of HITT. Proposed model outlining possible steps in the pathophysiology of the thrombocytopenia and thrombosis. Activated platelets secrete platelet factor 4 tetramers (PF4) from their alpha granules (Step 1). PF4 binds to the surface of the activated platelets (Step 2). PF4 also binds to heparin-like components in the matrix of endothelial cells and to therapeutic heparin that binds to the endothelium (Step 3). Antibodies form to heparin-PF4 complexes in the circulation (Step 4), on the surface of platelets (Step 5), and/or on the endothelium (Step 6). HITT antibodies induce endothelial cell procoagulant reactions and stimulate platelet activation either directly or via the platelet Fc receptor (Step 7). Platelet activation by antibody or on injured vessels releases additional PF4 and promotes platelet-vessel wall interaction setting up a cycle leading to platelet consumption that eventuates in thrombosis. (Adapted with permission from the Rockefeller University Press.)

suspected when there has been a 50% reduction in the platelet count unexplained by other events (121, 134–136). The diagnosis depends primarily on clinical recognition, including the recognition that the syndrome can be sustained by small amounts of heparin, such as those used to flush catheters or to coat central venous catheters (113, 114, 116–119).

However, HIT/HITT is one of the few immune platelet disorders in which laboratory testing can be of use to help affirm or to refute the clinical impression. Heparin-dependent platelet antibodies can be detected by measuring the release of serotonin from normal donor platelets incubated with individual plasma and heparin (26, 27, 155, 159). Two variations of this assay have been validated clinically (26, 27). In one, the test becomes positive at therapeutic heparin concentrations (0.1 U/ml), but reverts to negative at suprapharmacologic concentrations (100 U/ml), which are reported not to affect platelet secretion induced by other agonists, although somewhat different findings have also been reported (188). In the other assay (27) residual heparin is removed from plasma using a cationic bead, and heparin is added back at concentrations within or below the therapeutic range. The test is considered to be positive when individual plasma causes serotonin release at heparin concentrations below

0.5 U/ml but is generally positive at concentrations several orders of magnitude lower. Approximately 90% of individuals in whom the diagnosis of HIT is highly probable by clinical criteria will have a positive serotonin release assay (189). False-positive tests have not been noted in individuals with other forms of immune thrombocytopenia, but may occur at heparin concentrations above those attained therapeutically in treated individuals who are not thrombocytopenic (27, 139). Therefore a positive test using either assay strongly supports a clinical diagnosis of HIT/HITT, while a negative test cannot, by itself, be used to exclude the diagnosis. Heparin-induced platelet aggregation is a less sensitive and less specific endpoint than the serotonin release assay, but has been used successfully in some settings (189, 190).

Several additional factors should be considered in evaluating these *in vitro* tests. First, concurrent administration of drugs that inhibit platelet function may prevent aggregation or secretion in response to antibody (see below). Second, platelets from normal individuals vary in their sensitivity to HIT sera (16, 17, 188). Third, platelet activation has been reported to occur when heparin is added directly to platelet-rich plasma from some affected individuals but not when added to individual plasma and normal platelets (15–17). Fourth, occasional individuals have heparin-induced DIC rather than antibody-mediated thrombocytopenia. Fifth, the utility of the heparin/PF4 ELISA remains to be determined, since positive tests may occur after treatment with heparin in the absence of thrombocytopenia (173, 178, 179).

## Management

Once a diagnosis of HIT-HITT has been made, heparin must be discontinued immediately since it cannot be assumed that gradually progressive thrombocytopenia will precede the development of thrombosis. Further, failure to appreciate that thrombosis can be caused by exposure to even minute concentrations of heparin, such as those used to flush arterial catheters, is a common cause of mismanagement. Acute arterial thromboses may result from transfusion of platelets (191, 192), which should only be used to treat profound bleeding (193, 194).

In many clinical situations there is no substitute for heparin that is readily available. Simply discontinuing heparin may leave the individual at risk for recurrent thrombosis due to a preexisting condition, as well as HITT itself. Since thrombocytopenia generally occurs 5 to 6 days after heparin has been started, the frequency of this dilemma may be lessened by initiating warfarin early during the course of heparin therapy. Most individuals will therefore be at least partially anticoagulated by the time HITT develops, in which case it may be preferable simply to discontinue heparin if there is no evidence of recent thrombosis. In other cases dextran or aspirin may be used for several days if the risk of recurrent thrombosis is high such as in individuals with artificial heart valves, although there are no controlled studies documenting the efficacy of this approach.

Management is more difficult in individuals with life-threatening or limb-threatening thrombosis or when HITT develops before the initial thrombotic event has been treated adequately. Several general principles concerning treatment can be offered. First, the therapeutic option chosen should be based on the site of thrombosis and the magnitude of the threat of ongoing or incipient vascular occlusion. Second, in no situation should heparin be continued under the assumption that the syndrome will be transient. Third, an alternative source of heparin should not be substituted unless the indications for heparin therapy are critical and lack of cross reactivity can be documented. Fourth, decisions concerning the management of HITT should be made with the knowledge that thrombi can recur within the first 36 to 48 hours after heparin is discontinued. In the experience of the authors, such events are infrequent in the absence of inadvertent drug exposure, but a much higher rate of recurrence has recently been reported (130).

Thrombi in peripheral arteries may be managed by thrombectomy or bypass surgery (153, 195). Addition of dextran, aspirin, or warfarin may decrease the risk of local recurrence (87, 153, 195), although amputation of the affected extremity remains a common outcome (153). Intraarterial (196, 197), as well as systemic, thrombolytic therapy has been used successfully to treat limb-threatening arterial occlusion, myocardial infarction, and life-threatening pulmonary embolism and represents a viable alternative to surgery in select cases (198–201). Mechanical interruption of the vena cava has also been used to treat life-threatening pulmonary emboli (195).

Several alternatives to unfractionated heparin have been used in individuals who require prolonged anticoagulation for disorders in which aspirin, dextran, or coumadin are of unproven value. The most extensive experience has been with heparinoids such as Orgaran, a combination of heparan sulfate, chondroitin sulfate, and dermatan sulfate, which cross reacts with heparin in only 7 to 10% of cases (165, 202–208). There is appreciably less experience with other heparinoids, and thrombocytopenia has been reported in occasional individuals treated exclusively with these drugs (209–213). Individuals with HIT/HITT have also been treated successfully with hirudin (214), hirulog (215), and the synthetic thrombin inhibitor argatroban (66). Ancrod, a defibrinating agent, may be given as an intravenous bolus followed by a continuous infusion adjusted to maintain the serum fibrinogen concentration between 0.2 to 0.4 g/L (216–219). Unfortunately, only Orgaran is available for this indication in the United States to date. Low-molecular-weight (LMW) heparin has a reported success rate exceeding 80% (220–223), but persistent thrombocytopenia and recurrent thrombi have developed in some individuals due to antibody cross reactivity (219–222, 224–226). Unfortunately, in the experience of the authors and others (207, 227, 228), heparin-dependent antibodies from almost all individuals with HIT induced by unfractionated heparin cross react with LMW heparin *in vitro*. Plasmapheresis has been reported to decrease antibody titer with apparent benefit, although other modalities were used concurrently (87, 229). Intravenous immunoglobulin, which may contain antiidiotypic antibodies (230), has been used in a few individuals (193), although the merit of acutely raising the platelet count to treat a thrombotic disorder in the absence of bleeding has not been established.

Two interrelated management problems that occur with some frequency are the risk of re-exposing individuals with HIT to heparin and the management of individuals during extracorporeal bypass. These issues arise not infrequently because HIT is prevalent in individuals with atherosclerosis, particularly after vascular surgery, and because recurrent vascular and thrombotic problems are common in this population. There are no prospective studies that establish the risk of reexposure, but readministration of heparin to individuals with demonstrable antibodies can be followed by the rapid development of thrombocytopenia and thrombosis (27, 115, 127, 146, 231). Antibody production and thrombosis has been reported within days of reexposure even 2 years after the initial episode, and persistence of antibodies for years has been reported in a few cases (115, 132, 146, 231). However, heparin-dependent antibodies are no longer detected in most individuals within 3 months after heparin has been discontinued (27, 115, 145). In view of this, it is prudent to delay reexposure to heparin for as long as possible, preferably until the disappearance of heparin-dependent antibodies can be documented. Exposure of individuals to heparin only during extracorporeal circulation has been accomplished safely in this setting (115, 125, 207). Heparin must be omitted from intravenous catheters for this approach to succeed. Plasmapheresis has also been used to reduce antibody titers rapidly before surgery (229). Coronary bypass and other forms of vascular surgery have also been accomplished using LMW heparin or heparinoids as a substitute (205, 231–234). Dextran or warfarin have been used as the sole anticoagulant in a few individuals (195), and several individuals have been given aspirin or Iloprost to inhibit platelet activation prior to heparin administration (15, 21, 133, 195, 231, 235).

## QUINIDINE/QUININE PURPURA

### Clinical Presentation

Quinidine or quinine are second only to heparin as causes of life-threatening, drug-induced, immune thrombocytopenia. The incidence of thrombocytopenia in individuals taking these drugs has been estimated to be as high as one in 1000 (236). Individuals with quinidine/quinine-induced thrombocytopenia usually present with petechiae and purpura within 2 months of beginning therapy, although thrombocytopenia has been noted within the first 2 weeks of treatment (237). In individuals previously sensitized to the drugs, thrombocytopenia may develop within hours of reexposure (238) (Fig. 29.4). However, bleeding may not be noted until months to years after initiation of therapy, especially when the exposure has been intermittent (236, 239). Neonatal thrombocytopenia has been reported to develop acutely after ingestion of quinine by a sensitized nursing mother (6, 240). Exposure to either drug may also be inadvertent (241, 242) or surreptitious (243). In one study bleeding attributable to a qualitative platelet defect was reported in individuals taking quinidine and aspirin concurrently (244).

Platelet counts at presentation are generally less than 20,000/μL, and often less than 10,000/μL, but mild chronic thrombocytopenia has been reported (14). Leukopenia (236, 245–248), immune hemolytic anemia (249), manifestations of a drug-induced "lupuslike"

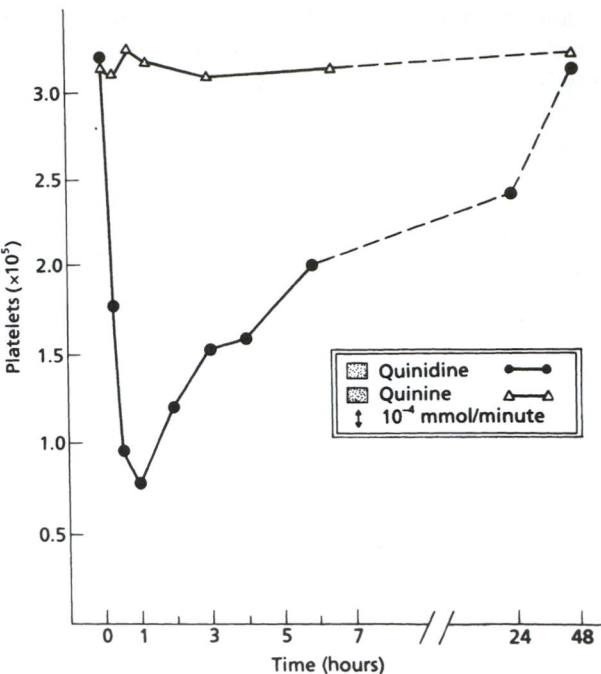

**FIGURE 29.4.** Acute thrombocytopenia induced by *in vivo* rechallenge of a individual with a history of quinine-associated thrombocytopenia with either quinidine or quinine. (Adapted with permission from Shulman NR. Immunoreactions involving platelets. I. A steric and kinetic model for formation of a complex from a human antibody, quinidine as a haptene, and platelets; and for fixation of complement by the complex. J Exp Med 1958;107:665–690.)

syndrome (250), or a syndrome resembling hemolytic uremic syndrome may coexist in some individuals (251). Disseminated intravascular coagulation, accompanied by intravascular hemolysis, acute renal failure, respiratory distress syndrome, and manifestations of anaphylaxis, has also been reported (252–254). Whether this presentation represents an extreme example of intravascular platelet lysis or has another pathophysiology such as endothelial cell injury (251) has not been determined.

### Pathophysiology and Diagnosis

Quinidine-dependent and quinine-dependent antiplatelet antibodies can be demonstrated in the serum of most thrombocytopenic individuals using one of several *in vitro* assays. Rarely, antibody cannot be detected during the acute phase of thrombocytopenia, presumably due to its total consumption; however, in these situations the *in vitro* tests may become positive several days later at a time when the platelet count begins to rise (254, 255).

The mechanism by which quinidine- and quinine-dependent antibodies bind to platelets has received considerable investigation, but uncertainties remain. Quinidine and quinine do not act as typical haptens; high concentrations of drug augment, rather than inhibit, antibody binding to platelets (14, 256). However, platelets preincubated with quinidine or quinine, and then washed, do not form suitable targets for drug-dependent antibodies, and soluble drug must be added to optimize antibody binding (256, 257). Although both drugs bind directly to platelets (257, 258), and in high concentrations alter platelet shape and function (244, 258, 259), such binding is reversible and of low affinity in the absence of antibody (256, 257, 259). These results suggest that quinidine- and quinine-dependent antibodies do not bind directly to either drug with high affinity, making it unlikely that the platelet becomes a target merely as a result of providing a surface on which the drug may become concentrated. Rather, there is strong experimental evidence indicating that both quinidine and quinine bind to specific platelet surface proteins, which subsequently become integral parts of the epitope (see below). This concept gains further support from the observation that in individuals who also develop hemolytic anemia or neutropenia, the quinidine-dependent antibodies that bind to platelets can be physically separated from those that bind to erythrocytes or leukocytes (246, 249). Quinidine- and quinine-dependent anti-platelet antibodies are heterogeneous with respect to the structural features of the drug and the platelet glycoprotein(s) required for antibody binding to occur. They also vary in their affinity, stoichiometry, and concentration of drug required for optimal antibody binding to the drug-platelet complex (260–263). Indeed, low-affinity antibodies have been detected in individuals receiving quinidine in whom thrombocytopenia did not develop (28). Although the parent compounds are generally 10 to 300 times as potent as drug analogs or metabolites in mediating antibody binding, there is wide variability in the extent of this cross reactivity (264–266). While some non-cross-reactive antibodies recognize a specific configuration at the C(9)-hydroxyl position or other sites within the quinoline ring, cross reactive antibodies generally recognize the quinoline ring itself (which is common to all drug analogs) (266). However, even the cross reactive antibodies require a specific configuration at C(9) for maximal avidity.

The serologic heterogeneity of quinidine/quinine antibodies for the parent drugs and their metabolites extends to the platelet glycoproteins that comprise the antibody binding site. Most clinically significant quinine- or quinidine-dependent antibodies bind to epitopes within either the glycoprotein Ib/IX (239, 262, 267–273) or IIb-IIIa complexes (261, 270–272, 274), perhaps because these are the most prevalent surface glycoproteins on the platelet, and therefore antibodies that recognize these determinants are most likely to produce clinically significant disease. Some antibodies recognize determinants on the individual proteins (262, 270, 271, 273, 274), but in other cases the epitope is complex-dependent (262, 270, 272). Sera may contain several drug-dependent, platelet-reactive antibodies with varying specificities (261, 262, 270–272). Antibodies that bind directly to glycoprotein V (270, 275) or other undetermined surface components (23, 237, 239) in the absence of added drug have also been reported. These results have been interpreted as suggesting that these antibodies recognize an altered conformation of the platelet glycoprotein induced by the drug (275). Some sera contain autoreactive antibodies not dependent on the presence of drugs for platelet reactivity (239). Some quinidine-dependent antibodies also recognize antigens expressed by cultured endothelial cells, and it has been speculated that immune vascular injury could contribute to the bleeding tendency (276). However, to date, only one report indicates that serologic diversity of quinidine- and quinine-dependent platelet antibodies may be of clinical significance (239).

Quinidine- and quinine-dependent antibodies bind through the F(ab)' portion of the molecule to a drug-platelet complex, thereby forming a ternary complex necessary to stabilize the epitope (260, 262, 263). *In vitro*, the Fc portion of the cell-bound antibody may further stabilize this complex (23, 263, 277), interact with platelet FcγRII receptors, initiate platelet crosslinking (163, 164), or activate complement (256). *In vivo*, cell-bound antibody may be recognized by FcγR receptors on tissue macrophages (260), thereby accelerating platelet clearance. However, the relative importance of platelet lysis versus activation and extravascular clearance has not been determined.

## Management

Emergent therapy for quinidine/quinine-induced thrombocytopenia consists of immediately discontinuing the responsible drug and instituting supportive therapy for thrombocytopenic bleeding. Bleeding generally resolves within 2 days after the drug is stopped. It may be prudent to administer corticosteroids and/or intravenous immunoglobulin in individuals with severe thrombocytopenia and bleeding (14, 239, 278), although proof of their benefit is lacking. Corticosteroids may benefit the unusual individual with drug-induced lupus (250). Transfused platelets are unlikely to have a prolonged intravascular survival in severely affected individuals, but may be administered in the setting of uncontrolled bleeding (239). Plasma exchange is indicated in individuals with hemolytic uremic syndrome (251), but no specific therapy for drug-induced DIC has been reported. Thrombocytopenia usually begins to resolve within 3 to 5 days, and recovery is usually complete by 1 week (238, 239, 255, 279), although more protracted courses have been reported (14, 238, 239, 255, 279). Platelet antibodies may persist for years (6, 242, 254, 255, 279), and their significance can be inferred from rechallenge of previously treated individuals (6, 252). However, the utility of using platelet antibody tests to decide whether quinine or quinidine can be reinstituted has not been formally determined.

## SULFA-CONTAINING DRUGS

Sulfa-containing drugs are a common cause of severe thrombocytopenia (280–286), with a reported incidence of between one per thousand to one per million courses of therapy (283–285). In some studies, the incidence of thrombocytopenia has been reported to be higher in children (287–289), the elderly (283, 285), individuals with impaired renal function (284), individuals expressing the slow acetylator phenotype (290), and in those previously exposed to chemically related drugs such as thiazides and furosemide (283). However, the increased incidence of this disorder in children (289) and the elderly remains controversial (286). Recently, individuals with HIV-related disorders (291, 292) and those receiving concomitant therapy with azathioprine have also been reported to be at increased risk for developing sulfa-induced thrombocytopenia (293, 294).

Two forms of thrombocytopenia related to sulfa-containing drugs have been reported. Most commonly, severe thrombocytopenia develops suddenly in an otherwise healthy individual, typically occurring within 1 to 2 weeks after the initiation of therapy (285, 286). Some individuals present with similar clinical findings after having taken sulfa-containing drugs for as long as 2 months (285, 286). In either setting, individuals present with platelet counts below 20,000/μL, and often below 10,000/μL (285, 286). The onset of thrombocytopenia may be more rapid in individuals previously sensitized through prior drug exposure or diet (285, 286). Platelet survival is impaired (295), and fatalities have occurred, especially when additional cytopenias are present (281, 285, 286). The bone marrow typically appears normal (295). Drug-dependent platelet antibodies have been demonstrated (18, 296–302), which may react against either component of trimethoprim-sulfamethoxazole (TMX-SMX) (18, 296, 297, 299, 301), while antibodies against a drug metabolite have been implicated in a few cases (296, 303). The mechanism of drug-platelet-antibody interaction is uncertain. In one study, platelets from some but not all donors could serve as targets for drug-dependent antibodies, raising a question about the involvement of polymorphic platelet determinants in drug or antibody binding (18). The sensitivity, specificity, and clinical utility of antibody testing for this drug-induced thrombocytopenia has not been established.

Thrombocytopenia typically begins to resolve within 72 hours after the drug is discontinued (285). The use of prednisone in the acute phase has been reported

(286), but the usefulness of this or other drugs effective in treating comparably severe ITP has not been established. Thrombocytopenia and other systemic effects can recur within 1 hour of rechallenge in individuals previously sensitized to sulfa (291, 297). There is no information available concerning how long sulfa-dependent antibodies persist, and the risk of rechallenge with the same or with related compounds has not been established.

Other individuals, generally those taking TMP-SMX, may present with the gradual onset of moderate thrombocytopenia (286). This presentation is more common in children (287, 288), individuals with HIV-infection (291, 292), and allograft recipients receiving azathioprine (293, 294). The mechanism by which thrombocytopenia develops in such individuals is uncertain, and the role of drug-dependent antibodies has neither been demonstrated nor excluded. It has been suggested that TMP-SMX may impair platelet production through its capacity to inhibit dihydrofolate reductase (DHFR). However, this explanation remains controversial, since the affinity of these antibiotics for the human DHFR enzyme is several orders of magnitude below that for the microbial and parasitic counterparts. Furthermore, serum and presumably tissue levels of folate do not fall in normal individuals during a typical course of therapy (295). Although TMP-SMX and related drugs have been reported to act synergistically to impair thrombopoiesis in vitro (293, 304) and to impair the response to therapy in established megaloblastic disorders (298, 305), development of megaloblastic thrombopoiesis responsive to withdrawal of the antibiotic or addition of folate or folinic acid, although reported, is exceedingly unusual (288, 291, 306–309).

## PENICILLINS

Thrombocytopenia is encountered rarely in individuals receiving beta-lactam ring containing antibiotics such as penicillin (310, 311), ampicillin (14, 312–314), methicillin (315–317), other synthetic penicillins (18, 316–318), and a variety of cephalosporins (319–321). The incidence of thrombocytopenia related to treatment with these medications is too low to establish relative risk estimates for individual drugs, although in one study thrombocytopenia occurred more commonly after prolonged use of ureidopenicillins than after comparable courses of carbenicillin (316). Thrombocytopenia may be more common when high doses of penicillin are administered (311, 316), and it has been reported to recur after administration of a cephalosporin to penicillin-sensitive individuals (322, 323), although the incidence of cross reactivity has not been established.

The clinical presentation of penicillin-related thrombocytopenia has been somewhat variable. Most individuals with this disorder present with severe thrombocytopenia, often accompanied by bleeding, beginning 1 to 2 weeks after initiation of therapy. However, thrombocytopenia has also occurred within 24 to 48 hours in individuals in whom prior sensitization to penicillin was suspected (311, 319), and within 4 hours of rechallenge in individuals with documented penicillin sensitivity (321). In other individuals the onset of thrombocytopenia has been delayed for several weeks (311). The frequency and severity of bleeding in this syndrome may be exacerbated by the well-described ability of penicillins to inhibit platelet function and prolong the bleeding time (see Chapter 33) (324). In most cases penicillin administration has been associated with isolated thrombocytopenia in the absence of other hematologic disorders or additional evidence of hypersensitivity. However, a single case of penicillin-associated, microangiopathic, hemolytic anemia has been reported (322). The appearance of the bone marrow is normal in most individuals (311).

Drug-dependent antibodies reactive with platelets and erythrocytes have been identified in a few cases of penicillin-associated thrombocytopenia (18, 311, 320, 321, 325). Relatively little is known about the serologic specificity of these antibodies, and it is unclear whether the mechanism by which they bind to platelets and erythrocytes is similar. Penicillins bind tightly to the erythrocyte membrane and are not readily removed by washing (323). Immune hemolytic anemia is believed to result from the formation of high-affinity IgG antibodies that are reactive with the benzylpenicilloyl (BPO) group (323). Sera from over 90% of individuals treated with penicillin have been reported to contain antibodies reactive with this moiety. However, these antibodies are generally of the IgM class or, less commonly, IgG class that are readily neutralized by soluble drug and thus differ serologically from antibodies involved in the pathogenesis of hemolytic anemia (323). In contrast to antierythrocyte antibodies, exogenous penicillin must be present to demonstrate penicillin-dependent platelet antibodies *in vitro* (14, 311, 320, 321, 325), presumably due to a lower affinity of the drug with the platelet compared with the erythrocyte surface. However, in one study, absorption of serum with penicillin-coated erythrocytes reduced the binding of antibody to platelets as well (321). In addition, in one report, an eluate from penicillin-coated platelets showed cross reactivity with erythrocytes (321). Platelets from normal donors may vary in their capacity to serve as *in vitro* targets for penicillin-associated antibodies (18). The clinical utility of testing for penicillin-dependent antibodies has not been established, and neither the sensitivity nor specificity of *in vitro* assays has been determined using sera from unaffected individuals receiving a comparable course and dose of antibiotics. The utility of testing for cross reactivity with other beta-lactam containing antibiotics is also unknown (320). Management generally involves discontinuation of the penicillin or related drug. This generally leads to resolution of thrombocytopenia within 48 hours, although more gradual responses to drug withdrawal are not unusual (14). Prednisone and platelet transfusions have been administered when individuals present with significant bleeding.

## VALPROIC ACID

An unusually high incidence of thrombocytopenia was recognized in individuals treated with valproic acid soon after the drug was introduced (326–329). The reported incidence of thrombocytopenia approaches 25% in some series (330), but varies widely (331–335), probably because thrombocytopenia typically resolves spontaneously despite continuation of the drug (see below). Platelet counts may fall as early as the second week of therapy, although the nadir may not be reached for an additional 2 weeks. Occasionally, thrombocytopenia develops months after treatment is started (330). Thrombocytopenia is generally mild to moderate in severity (332, 334–337). However, profound thrombocytopenia has been reported in sporadic cases (328, 338–340). Transient neutropenia is a common accompaniment (334, 341). Rarely, individuals may develop a drug-dependent, lupuslike syndrome (339); unexplained red cell macrocytosis (342, 343); marrow dysplasia (343); or aplasia (344).

Valproic acid has also been reported to cause platelet dysfunction (see Chapter 33) and in some individuals a coagulopathy characterized by impaired platelet aggregation, prolongation of the bleeding time in the absence of thrombocytopenia, prolonged prothrombin and partial thromboplastin times, and a mild reduction in plasma fibrinogen (326, 331, 336, 345–348). The qualitative platelet defects are not generally of clinical significance in the absence of thrombocytopenia, although occasional individuals have been reported to have experienced bruising and postoperative bleeding (329, 331). The explanation for these phenomena remains obscure but may involve a direct effect of valproic acid on cell membranes (342, 343).

The mechanism by which valproic acid causes thrombocytopenia is likewise poorly understood and more than one mechanism may be involved. Valproic acid may directly impair platelet production in most affected individuals, although morphologic evidence of bone marrow toxicity is infrequent (340, 344, 346, 348, 349). Thrombocytopenia is more common and more severe in individuals on higher doses of the drug (330, 335), and a reduction in drug dosage is often associated with a return of the platelet count (330, 332, 333, 336, 340, 350, 351). Indeed, thrombocytopenia may remit on occasion even when the dosage has not been changed (334).

However, the relationship between plasma levels and platelet counts is an inconstant finding (329, 334, 336), and there is evidence suggesting a destructive, possibly antibody-mediated cause of thrombocytopenia in some individuals, especially those with severe thrombocytopenia in whom the bone marrow appears normal (335). Acute, reversible thrombocytopenia may be associated with a febrile illness (328, 337, 351), and platelet counts generally rise within several days after the drug has been discontinued (328, 335, 336). In one study increased platelet-associated IgG was detected in 12 of 15 thrombocytopenic individuals during the acute episode, as well as in more than half the individuals who did not develop thrombocytopenia (334). This observation has been cited as evidence in favor of the possibility that the return in platelet count despite continuation of valproic acid is due to the development of a compensated state of increased platelet destruction (334). However, comparative studies of platelet kinetics during the acute and convalescent periods have not been reported. Also unresolved is the issue of why antibody formation would be so common (352). However, there have been few formal demonstrations of valproic acid-dependent, platelet reactive or neutrophil reactive antibodies, and little is known about the interaction between the drug and platelets at a biochemical or molecular level. Nor is it clear why persistent exposure to valproic acid does not generally lead to progressive thrombocytopenia.

Platelet counts should be documented in individuals taking valproic acid during the first month of treatment, with intercurrent infection, before surgery, and periodically thereafter. When thrombocytopenia is discovered, the major clinical decision lies in whether to lower the dose of the drug, discontinue the drug, or assume that the fall in platelet count will be transient (334, 353, 354). Reducing the dose of valproic acid, when possible, may or may not be sufficient to hasten the resolution of thrombocytopenia (330, 332, 333, 336, 340, 351–354), but seems to be a reasonable first step, especially when individuals have been receiving exceptionally high doses and when other causes of thrombocytopenia such as coincident administration of other antiepileptic medications have been excluded. However, stopping the drug should be considered in the setting of clinical bleeding or if the platelet count falls below 20,000/μL. There is little information to indicate that treatment of thrombocytopenia with drugs useful in ITP is of benefit if valproic acid is continued (333). In one reported case thrombocytopenia as part of a lupus-like illness persisted despite treatment with prednisone, intravenous immunoglobulin, vincristine, and plasmapheresis (339).

## GOLD

### Clinical Presentation

Approximately 1 to 3% of individuals treated with a conventional course of gold compounds develop thrombocytopenia (355–360). Thrombocytopenia occurs with equal frequency after parenteral administration of sodium aurothiomalate, thioglucose, or thiosulfate (361), as well as after administration of auranofin orally (356–359, 362). In some but not all reports, thrombocytopenia has occurred more commonly in individuals who have the extended HLA haplotype B8, Dr3, DQA2.1, DQB2.1 (363–366).

In the vast majority of individuals the onset of thrombocytopenia is acute, occurring within 1 month after documentation of a normal platelet count (367, 368). Thrombocytopenia may and often does precede other, more common, gold-associated toxicities (363, 368, 369). Therefore, the absence of dermatologic complications, eosinophilia, etc., is not a useful negative predictor for hematologic toxicity. Moreover, serum levels of gold are generally within the therapeutic range at the time thrombocytopenia develops (367, 370, 371).

Thrombocytopenia is generally severe, as reflected in the observation that as of 1972 sodium aurothiomalate was the drug with the highest reported ratio of deaths/annum/number of prescriptions written in one large series (372). On occasion, thrombocytopenia may be moderate in severity and the onset more gradual (363, 372). In most individuals thrombocytopenia is the only hematologic abnormality, although neutropenia may occasionally occur concomitantly (367). The appearance of the bone marrow is usually normal, although infrequently it may be hypoplastic (365, 369). Isolated thrombocytopenia may precede the development of aplastic anemia (365, 373), and several cases of gold-associated DIC have been reported (374).

There is wide variation in the extent of exposure to gold that has occurred before thrombocytopenia develops (356, 363, 365, 367). In several large series thrombocytopenia was first detected after individuals received an average dose of approximately 600 to 900 mg of gold (363, 365, 367). However, platelet counts have fallen in some individuals who received only 50 mg of gold (375), while other individuals developed thrombocytopenia after receiving several grams of gold compounds over many years (356, 363, 365, 367, 369, 376). In contrast to other drugs, severe thrombocytopenia has also developed weeks to months after the last administration of gold (375, 377–379) because of the persistence of the metal in tissues (see below) (263, 380).

### Pathogenesis

Gold accumulates in multiple tissues, including the bone marrow (381), and this metal may remain deposited in these sites for months to years. Gold depresses the production of hematopoietic progenitors *in vitro* in a concentration-dependent manner (382), and direct toxicity to hematopoietic progenitors may play a role in the pathogenesis of aplastic anemia (369, 370, 373, 383).

Removal of gold from these sites by chelation or providing unaffected hematopoietic precursors by bone marrow transplantation has been effective in some individuals with direct marrow toxicity.

However, it is more likely that isolated thrombocytopenia is caused most commonly by antiplatelet antibodies. Until recently, it has been difficult to demonstrate gold-dependent antibodies. In the absence of suitable *in vitro* assays to identify such antibodies, the evidence in favor of an immune etiology has consisted of the following: (a) the blastogenic response of individual lymphocytes exposed to gold *in vitro* (367, 384, 385); (b) the shortened survival of autologous platelets (14, 384, 386); (c) the appearance of the bone marrow, which is generally more consistent with shortened survival than impaired platelet production (365, 367); and (d) the response to therapy. Gold-dependent platelet antibodies have been demonstrated in some individuals (14, 384), while serum from others may contain gold-induced, autoreactive antibodies that bind to normal platelets in the absence of gold. This binding is unlikely to result from immune complexes (384), since the antibodies did not bind to platelets from a individual with Glanzmanns thrombasthenia (387) and gold was not detected in platelet eluates using atomic absorption spectroscopy.

There are several ways in which gold may bind to the platelet surface. After parenteral administration, a portion of the gold taken up by the marrow is released back into the blood bound to cells (388, 389). Gold may be taken up by megakaryocytes and stored in granules until the platelets reach the circulation. Platelets may be persistently exposed to gold that has been slowly released by tissue macrophages into the interstitial fluid and plasma. It is also possible that gold may bind directly to exposed sulfhydryl groups on platelet or megakaryocyte membranes, although this has not been demonstrated to date (388, 390). At high concentrations, gold rapidly forms adducts with serum proteins, including immunoglobulin and complement components (391). Adducts between gold and platelet membrane proteins may form more slowly *in vivo* since the plasma concentration of gold is much lower. The delay in onset and the persistence of thrombocytopenia months after therapy has been stopped suggest that low concentrations of gold are sufficient to sustain antibody production and binding to platelets. Slow formation of the epitope *in vivo* may also contribute to the apparent discrepancy between the concentration of gold needed to demonstrate platelet antibodies *in vitro* (14, 384) and those attained clinically (388). Chelation therapy, which is efficacious in some individuals, removes gold primarily from plasma and possibly interstitial fluid, which together represent only a small percentage of the total tissue burden (376, 387, 392). Therefore, it is likely that the beneficial effect of chelation depends on removing gold from

plasma or other labile pools that suffice to permit antibody binding to platelets. Chelation may also remove gold from cell membranes directly since it may remain detectable in serum or urine despite clinical remission (393). The accessibility and lability of the gold-platelet bond may explain why chelation therapy can be effective without significantly depleting total tissue stores (see below).

## Management

Treatment of gold-induced thrombocytopenia is based on three principals: (a) severe, potentially life-threatening thrombocytopenia occurs abruptly and generally without warning; (b) thrombocytopenia can be prolonged, consistent with slow release of gold from tissue stores; and (c) treatment may have to be given for many months, or occasionally years, since thrombocytopenia often recurs without reexposure.

Unlike most drugs, it is not sufficient simply to discontinue gold. As noted above, gold persists in tissues for years, providing a source for its gradual release into plasma (380, 392, 394, 395). Continuous exposure of the immune system to low concentration of antigen accounts both for the delayed onset of thrombocytopenia in some individuals and its persistence for months to years in others (394). Because most individuals present with or may develop severe thrombocytopenia, prednisone is generally begun as soon as thrombocytopenia is detected. Most but not all individuals with gold-induced thrombocytopenia respond to prednisone given in doses of 1 to 1.5 mg/kg/day (363, 366, 367, 393, 396). Occasional individuals have been treated successfully with vincristine (367), intravenous immunoglobulin (397, 398), or cyclophosphamide (399). Splenectomy has been successful in some individuals (14, 358, 384). Since gold-induced thrombocytopenia ultimately remits, splenectomy should be restricted to the atypical individual who fails to respond to therapy, who requires a long course of intensive therapy or who experiences severe therapy-related side effects precluding further treatment.

The role of chelation therapy has become less certain with the advent of several other effective forms of treatment. Individuals with isolated thrombocytopenia and other hematologic complications of gold therapy, including some who have failed to respond to corticosteroids, have been treated successfully with BAL, penicillamine, and N-acetyl-L-cysteine (296, 366, 367, 373, 375–377, 379, 393, 399–401). However, it is not clear whether chelation shortens the course or reduces the incidence of complications in the typical individual with gold-induced thrombocytopenia, and each chelating agent has its own side effects. Therefore chelation should be restricted to individuals with severe thrombocytopenia who do not respond to or cannot tolerate prednisone and to those with multiple recurrences.

## COCAINE

Several cases of severe thrombocytopenia attributable to cocaine have been reported (402–406). Cocaine was the only illicit drug used by some of these individuals, and adulterants were not detected. Typically, the most recent ingestion of cocaine occurred within several days of presentation, although occasional individuals reported no drug exposure for several weeks (403, 404). Exposure is generally intravenous, although exceptions have been noted (403). Most of the individuals reported were HIV-negative (407).

Most individuals have been symptomatic at presentation with platelet counts frequently below 10,000/μL. The remainder of the blood counts and the appearance of the bone marrow have usually been normal, with no other cause of severe thrombocytopenia evident. A single individual with severe thrombocytopenia as part of a preeclampsia-like illness has been reported (406).

The pathophysiology of cocaine-associated thrombocytopenia has not been completely defined. In sheep, acute thrombocytopenia has been induced following administration of cocaine (408). In this model cocaine has been reported to stimulate platelet aggregation directly, and the thrombocytopenia was associated with vasospasm due to potentiation by cocaine of the sympathomimetic effects of norepinephrine (408, 409). However, the clinical presentation in the reported individuals is more consistent with a drug-induced immune thrombocytopenia, although the presence of drug-dependent platelet antibodies has not been formally documented. The duration between the most recent exposure to cocaine and the seemingly prolonged duration of the disorder in a few of the reported individuals is somewhat atypical for drug-induced thrombocytopenia, but evaluation of these phenomena assumes the accuracy of the drug history provided.

Therapy has generally consisted of hospitalization (i.e., drug withdrawal), corticosteroids (403, 404), or intravenous immunoglobulin (402). Responses have been noted in all individuals within several days. Platelet transfusions have been used emergently with success in one individual (405). Splenectomy has been used to manage recurrences due to repeat drug ingestion and relapse following corticosteroid withdrawal (402, 403).

# REFERENCES

1. Bottiger LE, Westerholm B. Thrombocytopenia. II. Drug-induced thrombocytopenia. Acta Med Scand 1973;191:541–548.
2. Bottiger LE, Bottiger B. Incidence and cause of aplastic anemia, hemolytic anemia, agranulocytosis and thrombocytopenia. Acta Med Scand 1981;210:475–479.
3. Pedersen-Bjergaard U, Andersen M, Hansen PB. Thrombocytopenia induced by noncytotoxic drugs in Denmark 1968–91. J Intern Med 1996;239:509–515.
4. Classen DC, Pestotnik SL, Evans RS et al. Computerized surveillance of adverse drug events in hospital individuals. JAMA 1991;266:2847–2851.
5. Hackett T, Kelton JG, Powers P. Drug-induced platelet destruction. Semin Thromb Hemost 1982;8:116–137.
6. Mauer AM, DeVaux W, Lehyer ME. Neonatal and maternal thrombocytopenic purpura due to quinine. Pediatrics 1957;19:84–87.
7. Jerker K, Kutti K, Victorin L. Platelet counts in mothers and their newborns with respect to ante-partum administration of oral diuretics. Acta Med Scand 1973;194:473–475.
8. Salama A, Santoso S, Mueller-Eckhardt C. Antigenic determinants responsible for the reactions of drug-dependent antibodies with blood cells. Br J Haematol 1991;78:535–539.
9. Eisner EV, Kaspar K. Immune thrombocytopenia due to a metabolite of paraminosalicylic acid. Am J Med 1972;53:790–796.
10. Kiefel V, Santoso S, Schmidt S et al. Metabolite-specific (IgG) and drug-specific antibodies (IgG, IgM) in two cases of trimethoprim-sulfamethoxazole–induced immune thrombocytopenia. Transfusion 1987;27:262–265.
11. Hammerschmidt DE. Szechwan purpura. N Engl J Med 1980;302:1191–1193.
12. Michelson AD. Thrombocytopenia associated with environmental exposure to polyurethane. Am J Hematol 1991;38:145–146.
13. Adams WH, Rufo RA, Talrico L et al. Thrombocytopenia and intravenous heroin use. Ann Intern Med 1978;89:207.
14. Kelton JG, Meltzer D, Moore J et al. Drug-induced thrombocytopenia is associated with increasing binding of IgG to platelets both *in vivo* and *in vitro*. Blood 1981;58:525–529.
15. Kappa JR, Fisher CA, Berkowitz HD et al. Heparin-induced platelet activation in sixteen surgical individuals: diagnosis and management. J Vasc Surg 1987;5:101–109.
16. Pfueller SL, David R. Different platelet specificities of heparin-dependent platelet aggregating factors in heparin-induced associated immune thrombocytopenia. Br J Haematol 1986;64:149–159.
17. Salem HH, van der Weyden. Heparin induced thrombocytopenia. Variable platelet-rich plasma reactivity to heparin-dependent platelet aggregating factor. Pathology 1983;15:297.
18. Class FHJ, Langerak J, van Rood JJ. Drug-induced antibodies with restricted specificity. Immunol Lett 1981;2:323–326.
19. Kelton JG, Huang AT, Mold N et al. The use of *in vitro* techniques to study drug-induced pancytopenia. N Engl J Med 1979;301:621–624.
20. Marcus GJ, Stevenson M, Brown T. Alpha-methyldopa–induced immune thrombocytopenia. Am J Clin Pathol 1975;64:113–115.
21. Wanamaker WM, Wanamaker SJ, Celesia GG et al. Thrombocytopenia associated with long-term levodopa therapy. JAMA 1976;235:2217–2219.
22. Beenvaad AH, Schoenaker AH. Thrombocytopenia after the use of methyldopa. Lancet 1965;2:292.
23. Lerner W, Caruso R, Faig D et al. Drug-dependent and non–drug-dependent antiplatelet antibody in drug-induced immunologic thrombocytopenic purpura. Blood 1985;66:306–311.
24. Christie DJ, van Byren N, Lennon SS et al. Vancomycin-dependent antibodies associated with thrombocytopenia and refractoriness to platelet transfusion in individuals with leukemia. Blood 1991;75:518–523.
25. Bepler G, Hoffman SE, Thompson BP et al. Captopril-enhanced binding of PI^A1 (HPA-1a) antibodies in post-transfusion purpura. Tranfusion 1991;31:752–755.
26. Sheridan D, Carter C, Kelton JG. A diagnostic test for heparin-induced thrombocytopenia. Blood 1986;67:27–30.
27. Cines DB, Kaywin P, Bina M et al. Heparin-associated thrombocytopenia. N Engl J Med 1980;303:788–795.
28. Okuno T, Crockatt D. Anti-drug-related antibodies in non-thrombocytopenic cardiac individuals. Am J Clin Pathol 1976;65:523–527.
29. Gewirtz AM. Human megakaryocytopoieses. Semin Hematol 1986;23:27–42.
30. Hoffman R. Regulation of megakaryocytopoieses. Blood 1989;74:1196–1212.
31. Miescher PA. Drug-induced thrombocytopenia. Semin Hematol 1973;10:311–325.
32. Jandl JH. Hematologic changes in chronic liver disease. Am J Gastroenterol 1958;30:46–50.
33. Sullivan LW, Herbert V. Suppression of hematopoiesis by ethanol. J Clin Invest 1964;43:2048–2061.
34. Lindenbaum J, Hargrove RL. Thrombocytopenia in alcoholics. Ann Intern Med 1968;68:526–532.
35. Eichner ER, Buchanon B, Smith JW et al. Variations in the hematologic and medical status in alcoholics. Am J Med Sci 1972;263:35–42.
36. Cowan DH, Hines JD. Thrombocytopenia of severe alcoholism. Ann Intern Med 1971;74:37–43.
37. Post RM, Desforges JF. Thrombocytopenia and alcoholism. Ann Intern Med 1968;68:1230–1236.
38. Ryback R, Desforges J. Alcoholic thrombocytopenia in three inpatient drinking alcoholics. Arch Intern Med 1970;125:475–477.
39. Sahud MA. Platelet size and number in alcoholic thrombocytopenia. N Engl J Med 1972;286:355–356.
40. Haut MJ, Graham DH. The effect of ethanol on hemostatic properties of human blood platelets. Am J Med 1974;56:22–33.

41. McCurdy PR, Pierce LE, Rath CE. Abnormal bone marrow morphology in acute alcoholism. N Engl J Med 1962;266:505–507.
42. Saidi P, Wallerstein RO, Aggeler PM. Effect of chloramphenicol on erythropoiesis. J Lab Clin Med 1961;57:247–256.
43. McCurdy PR. Chloramphenicol bone marrow toxicity. JAMA 1961;176:588–593.
44. Eichner E. The hematologic disorders of alcoholism. Am J Med 1973;54:621–630.
45. Gewirtz AM, Hoffman R. Transitory hypomegakaryocytic thrombocytopenia: aetiological association with ethanol abuse and implications regarding regulation of human megakaryocytopoiesis. Br J Haematol 1986;62:333–344.
46. Cowan DH. Thrombokinetic studies in alcohol-related thrombocytopenia. J Lab Clin Med 1973;81:64–76.
47. Sullivan LW, Adams WH, Yang KL. Induction of thrombocytopenia in man: patterns of recovery in normal subjects during ethanol ingestion and abstinence. Blood 1977;49:197–207.
48. Meagher RC, Sieber F, Spivak J. Suppression of hematopoietic progenitor cell proliferation by ethanol and acetaldyhye. N Engl J Med 1982;307:845–849.
49. Tisman G, Herbert V. In vitro myelosuppression and immunosuppression by ethanol. J Clin Invest 1973;52:1410–1414.
50. Emmons RVZB, Reid DM, Cohen RL et al. Human thrombopoeitin levels are high when thrombocytopenia is due to megakaryocyte deficiency and low when due to increased platelet destruction. Blood 1996;87:4068–4071.
51. Clark DA, Krantz SB. Effects of ethanol on cultured human megakaryocyte progenitors. Exp Hematol 1986;14:951–954.
52. Levine RF, Spivak JL, Meagher RC et al. Effect of ethanol on thrombopoiesis. Br J Haematol 1986;62:345–354.
53. Smith CM, Tobin JD, Burris SM et al. Alchohol consumption in the guinea pig is associated with reduced megakaryocyte deformability and platelet size. J Lab Clin Med 1992;120:699–706.
54. Korsten MA, Matsuzaki S, Feinman L et al. High blood acetaldehyde levels after ethanol administration. N Engl J Med 1975;292:386–389.
55. Wickramasinghe SN, Hasan R. Possible role of macrophages in the pathogenesis of ethanol-induced bone marrow damage. Br J Haematol 1993;83:574–579.
56. Post RM, Desforges JF. Thrombocytopenic effect of ethanol infusion. Blood 1968;31:344–347.
57. Mikhailidis DP, Barradas MA, Jeremy Y. The effect of ethanol on platelet function and vascular prostanoids. Alcohol 1990;7:171–180.
58. Cowan DH, Kitka M, Baunach D. Alteration of platelet cyclic AMP (cAMP) by ethanol. Thromb Haemost 1977;38:270.
59. Cowan DH. Effect of alcoholism on hemostasis. Semin Hematol 1980;17:137–147.
60. Cowan DH, Graham RC. Studies on the platelet defect in alcoholism. Thromb Diath Haemorrh 1975;33:310–327.
61. Haselager EM, Vreeken J. Rebound thrombocytosis after alcohol abuse: a possible factor in the pathogenesis of thromboembolic disease. Lancet 1977;1:774–775.
62. Jaffe MO, Kierland RR. Purpura due to chlorothiazide (Diuril). JAMA 1958;168:2264–2265.
63. Zuckerman AJ, Chazan AA. Agranulocytosis with thrombocytopenia following chlorothiazide therapy. Br Med J 1958;2:13–38.
64. Dinon LR, Kim YS, Vander Veer JB. Clinical experience with chlorothiazide (Diuril) with particular emphasis on untoward responses. Am J Med Sci 1958;236:533–545.
65. Gesink MH, Bradfors HA. Thrombocytopenic purpura associated with hydrochlorothiazide. JAMA 1960;172:556–559.
66. Ball P. Thrombocytopenia and purpura in individuals receiving chlorothiazide and hydrochlorothiazide. JAMA 1960;173:663–665.
67. Lundh B, Hasselgren KH. Hematologlical side effects from antihypertensive drugs. Acta Med Scand 1979;628:73–75.
68. Nordqvist P, Cramer G, Bjorntorp P. Thrombocytopenia during chlorothiazide treatment. Lancet 1959;1:272.
69. Kutti J, Weinfeld A. The frequency of thrombocytopenia in individuals with heart disease treated with oral diuretics. Acta Med Scand 1968;183:245–250.
70. Rodriguez SU, Leikin SL, Hiller MC. Neonatal thrombocytopenia associated with antepartum administration of thiazide drugs. N Engl J Med 1964;270:881–884.
71. Garnet JD. Placental transfer of chlorothiazide. Obstet Gynecol 1963;21:123–125.
72. Leikin SL. Maternal thiazides and platelet counts of neonates. J Pediatr 1970;77:1097–1098.
73. Merenstein GB, O'Loughlin EP, Plunket DC. Effects of maternal thiazides on platelet counts of newborn infants. J Pediatr 1970;76:766–767.
74. Eisner EV, Crowell EB. Hydrochlorothiazide-dependent thromboytopenia due to IgM antibody. JAMA 1971;215:480–482.
75. von Haam E, Hammel MA, Rardin TE et al. Experimental studies on the activity and toxicity of stilbesterol. Endocrinology 1941;28:253–273.
76. Castrodale D, Bierbaum O, Helwig EB et al. Comparative studies of the

77. Fried W, Tickler T, Dennenber I et al. Effects of estrogens on hematopoietic stem cells and on hematopoiesis of mice. J Lab Clin Med 1974;83:807–815.
78. Crandall TL, Joyce RA, Boggs DR. Estrogens and hematopoiesis: characization and studies on the mechanism of neutropenia. J Lab Clin Med 1980;95:857–867.
79. Watson CJ, Schultz AL, Wikoff HM. Purpura following estrogen therapy with particular reference to hypersensitivity to (diethyl) stilbesterol and with a note on the possible relationship of purpura to endogenous estrogens. J Lab Clin Med 1947;32:606–617.
80. Cooper BA, Bigelow FS. Thrombocytopenia associated with the administration of diethylstilbesterol in man. Ann Intern Med 1960;52:907–909.
81. Friedman D, Schreiber AD. Effect of estradiol and steroid analogues on the clearance of IgG-coated erythrocytes. J Clin Invest 1985;75:162–167.
82. Candido A, Bussa A, Tartaglione R et al. Tamoxifen-induced immune-mediated platelet destruction. A case report. Tumori 1993;79:231–234.
83. Fraser JL, Millenseon M, Malynn ER et al. Possible association between the Norplant contraceptive system and thrombotic thrombocytopenic purpura. Obstet Gynecol 1996;87:860–863.
84. Quesada JR, Hawkins M, Horning S et al. Collaborative phase I-II study of recombinant DNA-produced leukocyte interferon (cone A) in metastatic breast cancer, malignant lymphoma, and multiple myeloma. Am J Med 1984;77:427–432.
85. Alexander GJM, Brahm J, Fagan EA et al. Loss of HbsAg with interferon therapy in chronic hepatitis B virus infection. Lancet 1987;2:66–69.
86. Perillo RP, Schiff ER, Davis GL et al. A randomized controlled trial of interferon alfa-2b alone and after prednisone withdrawal in individuals with chronic hepatitis B: a prospective randomized treatment trial. Mayo Clin Proc 1990;65:1330–1335.
87. Rakela J, Wood JR, Czaja AJ et al. Long-term versus short-term treatment with recombinant interferon alfa-2a in individuals with chronic hepatitis B: a prospective reandomized treatment trial. Mayo Clin Proc 1990;65:1330–1335.
88. Pestka S. The human interferons—from protein purification and sequence to cloning and expression in bacteria. Arch Biochem Biophys 1983;221:1–37.
89. Quesada JR, Talpaz M, Rios A et al. Clinical toxicity of interferons in cancer individuals: a review. J Clin Oncol 1986;4:234–243.
90. Spitzer VD, Zander A, Gutterman JU. Human leukocyte interferon preparation—mediated block of granulopoietic differentiation in vitro. Exp Hematol 1981;9:63–66.
91. Costanzi JJ, Cooper MR, Scarffe JH et al. Phase II study of recombinant alpha-2 interferon in resistant multiple myeloma. J Clin Oncol 1985;3:654–659.
92. Foon KA, Bottino CC, Abrams PG et al. Phase II trial of recombinant leukocyte A interferon in individuals with advanced chronic lymphocytic leukemia. Am J Med 1985;78:216–220.
93. Broxmeyer HE, Lu L, Platzer E et al. Comparative analysis of the influence of human gamma, alpha and beta interferons on human multipotential (CFU-GEMM), erythroid (BFU-E) and granulocyte-macrophage (CFU-GM) progenitor cells. J Immunol 1983;131:1300–1305.
94. Ganser A, Carlo-Stella C, Greher J et al. Effects of recombinant interferons alpha and gamma on human bone marrow progenitor cells. Blood 1987;70:1173–1179.
95. Monte D, Wietzerbin J, Pancre V et al. Identification and characterization of a functional receptor for interferon gamma on a megakaryocytic cell line. Blood 1991;78:2060–2069.
96. Carlo-Stella C, Cazzola M, Gasner A et al. Effects of recombinant alpha and gamma interferons on the in vitro growth of circulating hematopoietic progenitor cells (CFU-GEMM, CFU-MK, BFU-E, and CFU-GM) from individuals with myelofibrosis with myeloid metaplasia. Blood 1987;70:1014–1019.
97. Oladilupo-Williams Ck, Svet-Moldavskaya I, Vilcek J et al. Inhibitory effect of human leukocyte and fibroblast interferons on normal and chronic myelogenous leukemic granulocytic progenitor cells. Oncology 1981;38:356–362.
98. Carlo-Stella C, Cazzola M, Ganser A et al. Synergistic antiproliferative effect of recombinant interferon-γ with recombinant interferon-α on chronic myelogenous leukemia hematopoietic progenitor cells (CFU-GEMM, CRU-Mk, BFU-E, and CFU-GM). Blood 1988;72:1293–1299.
99. Talpaz M, McCredie KB, Mavligit GM et al. Leukocyte interferon-induced myeloid cytoreduction in chronic myelogenous leukemia. Blood 1983;62:689–692.
100. Shrestha R, McKinley C, Bilir BM, Everson GT. Possible idiopathic thrombocytopenic purpura associated with natural alpha interferon therapy for chronic hepatitis C. Am J Gastroenterol 1995;90:1146–1147.
101. Lopez-Morante AJ, Seaz-Royuela F, Casanova-Valero F. Immune thrombocytopenia after alpha interferon in a individual with chronic hepatitis C. Am J Gastroenterol 1992;87:809–810.
102. Proctor SJ, Jackson G, Carey P et al. Improvement of platelet counts in steroid-unresponsive idiopathic immune thrombocytopenic purpura after

short-course therapy with recombinant (α-2b interferon. Blood 1989;74: 1894–1897.

103. Fujimura K, Takafuta T, Kuriya S et al. Recombinant human interferon (α-2b (rh IFN α-2b) therapy for steroid resistant idiopathic thrombocytopenic purpura (ITP). Am J Hematol 1996;51:37–44.

104. Marroni M, Gresele P, Landonio G et al. Interferon-α is effective in the treatment of HIV-1-related, severe, zidovudine-resistant thromobcytopenia. Ann Intern Med 1994;121:423.

105. Weissman RE, Tobin RW. Arterial embolism during systemic heparin therapy. Arch Surg 1958;76:219–227.

106. Roberts B, Rosato FE, Rosato EF. Heparin—a cause of arterial emboli? Surgery 1964;55:803–811.

107. Gollub S, Ulin AWL. Heparin-induced thrombocytopenia in man. J Lab Clin Med 1962;59:430–435.

108. Bell WR, Tomasulo PA, Alving BM et al. Thrombocytopenia occurring during the administration of heparin: a prospective study in 52 individuals. Ann Intern Med 1976;85:155–160.

109. Rhodes GR, Dixon RH, Silver D. Heparin-induced thrombocytopenia with thrombotic and hemorrhagic manifestations. Surg Gynecol Obstet 1973; 136:409–416.

110. Hirsh J. Heparin. N Engl J Med 1991;324:1565–1574.

111. Schmitt BP, Adelman B. Heparin-associated thrombocytopenia: a critical review and pooled analysis. Am J Med Sci 1993;305:208–215.

112. Hrushesky WJ. Subcutaneous heparin-induced thrombocytopenia. Arch Intern Med 1978;138:1489–1491.

113. Galle PC, Muss HB, McGrath KM et al. Thrombocytopenia in two individuals treated with low-dose heparin. Obstet Gynecol 1978;52 (Suppl): 9S–11S.

114. van der Weyden MB, Hunt H, McGrath K et al. Delayed-onset heparin-induced thrombocytopenia. A potentially malignant syndrome. Med J Aust 1983;2:132–135.

115. Laster J, Cikrit D, Walker N, Silver D. The heparin-induced thrombocytopenia syndrome: an update. Surgery 1987;102:763–770.

116. Rizzoni WE, Miller K, Rick M et al. Heparin-induced thrombocytopenia in the postoperative period. Surgery 1988;103:470–476.

117. Doty JR, Alving BM, McDonnell DE et al. Heparin-associated thrombocytopenia in the neurosurgical individual. Neurosurgery 1986;19:69–72.

118. Heeger PS, Backstrom JR. Heparin flushes and thrombocytopenia. Ann Intern Med 1986;105:143.

119. Laster J, Silver D. Heparin-coated catheters and heparin-induced thrombocytopenia. J Vasc Surg 1988;7:667–672.

120. Pelouze GA, Coste B, Rassam TH et al. Thrombocytopenia immunoallergique declenchee par le revetement heparine d'un catheter. Presse Med 1989;18:1481–1482.

121. Singer RL, Mannion JD, Bauer TL et al. Complications from heparin-induced thrombocytopenia in individuals undergoing cardiopulmonary bypass. Chest 1993;104:1436–1440.

122. Towne JB, Bernhard VM, Hussey C et al. White clot syndrome. Peripheral vascular complication of heparin therapy. Arch Surg 1979;114:372–377.

123. CPC. N Engl J Med 1989;321:1595–1603.

124. Kapsch DN, Adelstein EH, Rhodes GR et al. Heparin-induced thrombocytopenia, thrombosis and hemorrhage. Surgery 1979;86:148–155.

125. Olinger GN, Hussey CV, Olive JA et al. Cardiopulmonary bypass for individuals with previously documented heparin-induced platelet aggregation. J Thorac Cardiovasc Surg 1984;87:673–677.

126. Herring WB, Shelburne PF. Heparin-induced thrombosis. N C Med J 1984; 45:149–152.

127. Cines DB, Tomaski A, Tannenbaum S. Immune endothelial cell injury in heparin-associated thrombocytopenia. N Engl J Med 1987;316:581–589.

128. White PW, Sadd JR, Nensel RE. Thrombotic complications of heparin therapy. Including six cases of heparin-induced skin necrosis. Ann Surg 1979; 190:595–608.

129. Boshkov LK, Warkentin TE, Hayward CPM et al. Heparin-induced thrombocytopenia and thrombosis: clinical and laboratory studies. Br J Haematol 1993;84:322–328.

130. Warkentin TE, Kelton JG. A 14-year study of heparin-induced thrombocytopenia. Am J Med 1996;101:502–507.

131. Phelan BK. Heparin-associated thrombosis without thrombocytopenia. Ann Intern Med 1983;99:637–638.

132. Chesney CM, Lands RH. Thrombosis in individuals with heparin-induced thrombocytopenia. Thromb Haemost 1987;308:58a.

133. Kappa JR, Cottrell ED, Berkowitz HD et al. Carotid endarterectomy in individuals with heparin-induced platelet activation: comparative efficacy of aspirin and iloprost (ZK36374). J Vasc Surg 1987;5:693–701.

134. Klement D, Rammos S, von Kreis R et al. Heparin as a cause of thrombus progression. Heparin-associated thrombocytopenia is an important differential diagnosis in paediatric individuals even with normal platelet counts. Eur J Pediatr 1996;155:11–14.

135. Hache-Wunderle V, Kainer K, Krug B et al. Heparin-associated thrombosis despite normal platelet counts. Lancet 1994;344:469–470.

136. Atkinson JLD, Sundt TMJ, Kazmier FJ et al. Heparin-induced thrombocytopenia and thrombosis in ischemic stroke. Mayo Clin Proc 1988;63: 353–361.

137. Saffle JR, Russo J Jr, Dukes GE Jr et al. The effect of low-dose heparin therapy on human platelet and transamidase levels. J Surg Res 1980;28: 297–305.

138. Schwartz KA, Royer G, Kaufman DB et al. Complications of heparin administration in normal individuals. Am J Hematol 1985;19:355–363.

139. Nelson JC, Lerner RG, Golstein R et al. Heparin-induced thrombocytopenia. Arch Intern Med 1978;138:548–552.

140. Ansell J, Slepchusch N Jr, Kumar R et al. Heparin induced thrombocytopenia: a prospective study. Thromb Haemost 1980;43:61–65.

141. Brace LD, Fareed J. An objective assessment of the interaction of heparin and its fractions with human platelets. Semin Thromb Hemost 1985;11: 190–198.

142. Warkentin TE, Kelton JG. Heparin-induced thrombocytopenia. Annu Rev Med 1989;40:31–44.

143. Bell WR, Royall RM. Heparin-associated thrombocytopenia: a comparison of three heparin preparations. N Engl J Med 1980;303:902–907.

144. Warkentin TE, Levine MN, Hirsh J et al. Heparin-induced thrombocytopenia in individuals treated with low-molecular-weight heparin or unfractionated heparin. N Engl J Med 1995;332:1330–1335.

145. Boshkov LK, Warkentin TE, Hayward C et al. Heparin-induced thrombocytopenia and thrombosis: clinical and laboratory studies. Blood 1990; 76(S):447a.

146. Walls JT, Curtis JJ, Silver D et al. Heparin-induced thrombocytopenia in individuals who undergo open heart surgery. Surgery 1990;108:686–693.

147. Stead RB, Schafer AI, Rosenberg RD et al. Heterogeneity of heparin lots associated with thrombocytopenia and thromboembolism. Am J Med 1984;77:185–188.

148. Walton PL, Ricketts CR, Bangham DR. Heterogeneity of heparin. Br J Haematol 1966;12:310–325.

149. King DJ, Kelton JG. Heparin-associated thrombocytopenia. Ann Intern Med 1984;100:535–540.

150. Bell WR. Heparin-associated thrombocytopenia and thrombosis. J Lab Clin Med 1988;111:600–605.

151. Salzman EW, Rosenberg RD, Smith MH et al. The effect of heparin and heparin fractions on platelet aggregation. J Clin Invest 1980;65:64–71.

152. Chong BH, Castaldi PA. Platelet proaggregating effect of heparin: possible mechanisms for non-immune heparin-associated thrombocytopenia. Aust N Z J Med 1986;16:715–717.

153. Silver D, Kapsch DN, Tsoi EKM. Heparin-induced thrombocytopenia, thrombosis, and hemorrhage. Ann Surg 1983;198:301–306.

154. Green D, Harris K, Reynolds N et al. Heparin immune thrombocytopenia: evidence for a heparin-platelet complex as the antigenic determinant. J Lab Clin Med 1978;91:167–175.

155. Kelton JG, Sheridan D, Brain H et al. Clinical usefulness of testing for a heparin-dependent platelet-aggregating factor in individuals with suspected heparin-associated thrombocytopenia. J Lab Clin Med 1984;103: 606–612.

156. Gruel Y, Rupin A, Darnige L et al. Specific quantification of heparin-dependent antibodies for the diagnosis of heparin-associated thrombocytopenia using an enzyme-linked immunosorbent assay. Thromb Res 1991; 62:377–387.

157. Kelton JG, Sheridan D, Santos A et al. Heparin-induced thrombocytopenia: laboratory studies. Blood 1988;72:925–930.

158. Frantantoni JC, Pollet RM, Gralnick HR. Heparin-induced thrombocytopenia: confirmation of diagnosis with *in vitro* methods. Blood 1975;45: 395–401.

159. Chong BH, Pitney WR, Castaldi PA. Heparin-induced thrombocytopenia: association of thrombotic complications with heparin-dependent IgG antibody that induces thromboxane synthesis and platelet aggregation. Lancet 1982;2:1246–1249.

160. Adelman B, Sobel M, Fujimura Y et al. Heparin-associated thrombocytopenia: observations on the mechanism of platelet aggregation. J Lab Clin Med 1989;113:204–210.

161. Chong BH, Fawaz I, Chesterman CN et al. Heparin-induced thrombocytopenia: mechanism of interaction of the heparin-dependent antibody with platelets. Br J Haematol 1989;73:235–240.

162. Horne III MK, Alkins BR. Platelet binding of IgG from individuals with heparin-induced thrombocytopenia. J Lab Clin Med 1996;127:435–442.

163. Horsewood P, Hayward CPM, Warkentin TE et al. Investigation of the mechanisms of monoclonal antibody-induced platelet activation. Blood 1991;78:1019–1026.

164. Anderson GP, Anderson CL. Signal transduction by the platelet Fc receptor. Blood 1990;76:1165–1172.

165. Chong BH. Heparin-induced thrombocytopenia. Aust N Z J Med 1992;22: 145–152.

166. Brandt JT, Isenhart CE, Osborne JM et al. On the role of platelet Fcγ(RIIa phenotype in heparin-induced thrombocytopenia. Thromb Haemost 1995; 74:1564–1572.

167. Burgess JK, Lindeman R, Chesterman CN et al. Single amino acid mutation of Fcγ(R receptor is associated with the development of heparin-associated thrombocytopenia. Br J Haematol 1995;91:761–766.

168. Amiral J, Wolf M, Fischer A et al. Pathogenicity of IgA and/or IgM anti-

bodies to heparin-PF4 complexes in individuals with heparin-induced thrombocytopenia. Br J Haematol 1996;92:954–959.

169. Arepally G, McKenzie SE, Joang X et al. FcγRIIA H/R¹³¹ polymorphism, subclass-specific IgG anti-heparin/PF4 antibodies and clinical course in individuals with heparin-indcued thrombocytopenia and thrombosis. Blood 1997;89:370–375.

170. Amiral J, Bridey F, Dreyfus M et al. Platelet factor 4 complexed to heparin is the target for antibodies generated in heparin-induced thrombocytopenia. Thromb Haemost 1992;68:95–96.

171. Greinacher A, Potzsch B, Amiral J et al. Heparin-associated thrombocytopenia: isolation of the antibody and characterization of a multimolecular PF4-heparin complex as the major antigen. Thromb Haemost 1994;71:247–251.

172. Amiral J, Bridey F, Wolf M et al. Antibodies to macromolecular platelet factor 4-heparin complexes in heparin-induced thrombocytopenia: a study of 44 cases. Thromb Haemost 1995;73:21–28.

173. Arepally G, Reynolds C, Tomaski A et al. Comparison of PF4/ELISA with the ¹⁴C-serotonin release assay in the diagnosis of heparin-associated thrombocytopenia/thrombosis. Am J Clin Pathol 1995;104:648–654.

174. Amiral J, Marfaing-Koka A, Wolf M et al. Presence of autoantibodies to interleukin-8 or neutrophil-activating-peptide-2 in individuals with heparin-associated thrombocytopenia. Blood 1996;88:410–416.

175. Horsewood P, Warkentin TE, Hayward CP et al. The epitope specificity of heparin-induced thrombocytopenia. Br J Haematol 1996;95:161–167.

176. Greinacher A, Alban S, Dummel V et al. Characterization of the structural requirements for a carbohydrate based anticoagulant with a reduced risk of inducing the immunologic type of heparin-associated thrombocytopenia. Thromb Haemost 1995;74:886–892.

177. Kelton JG, Smith JW, Warkentin TE et al. Immunoglobulin G from individuals with heparin-induced thrombocytopenia binds to a complex of heparin and platelet factor 4. Blood 1994;83:3232–3239.

178. Visentin GP, Malik M, Cyganiak KA et al. Individuals treated with unfractionated heparin during open heart surgery are at high risk to form antibodies reactive with heparin:platelet 4 complexes. J Lab Clin Med 1996;128:376–383.

179. Amiral J, Peynaud-Debayle E, Wolf M et al. Generation of antibodies to heparin-PF4 complexes without thrombcytopenia in individuals treated with unfractionated or low-molecular-weight heparin. Am J Hematol 1996;52:90–95.

180. Bauer TL, Arepally G, Konkle BA et al. Prevalence of heparin-associated antibodies without thrombosis in individuals undergoing cardiopulmonary bypass. Circulation 1997;95:1242–1246.

181. Ansell J, Deykin D. Heparin-induced thrombocytopenia and recurrent thromboembolism. Am J Hematol 1980;8:325–332.

182. Benhamou AC, Gruel Y, Barsotti J et al. The white clot syndrome or heparin-associated thrombocytopenia and thrombosis (WCS or HATT): 26 cases. Int Angiol 1986;4:303–310.

183. Warkentin T, Hayward CPM, Boshkov LK et al. Sera from individuals with heparin-induced thrombocytopenia generate platelet-derived microparticles with procoagulant activity: an explanation for the thrombotic complications of heparin-associated thrombocytopenia. Blood 1994;84:3691–3699.

184. Visentin GP, Ford SE, Scott JP et al. Antibodies from individuals with heparin-induced thrombocytopenia/thrombosis are specific for platelet factor 4 complexed with heparin or bound to endothelial cells. J Clin Invest 1994;93:81–88.

185. Bell WR, Tomasulo PA, Alving BM et al. Heparin thrombocytopenia. Ann Intern Med 1976;85:155–160.

186. Zalcberg JR, McGrath K, Dauer R et al. Heparin-induced thrombocytopenia with associated disseminated intravascular coagulation. Br J Haematol 1990;54:655–660.

187. Kapsch D, Silver D. Heparin-induced thrombocytopenia with thrombosis and hemorrhage. Arch Surg 1990;116:1423–1427.

188. Isenhart CE, Brandt JT. Platelet aggregation studies for the diagnosis of heparin-induced thrombocytopenia. Am J Clin Pathol 1993;99:324–339.

189. Chong BH, Burgess J, Ismail F. The clinical usefulness of the platelet aggregation test for the diagnosis of heparin-induced thrombocytopenia. Thromb Haemost 1993;69:344–350.

190. Greinacher A, Michels I, Kiefel V et al. A rapid and sensitive test for diagnosing heparin-associated thrombocytopenia. Thromb Haemost 1991;66:734–736.

191. Cimo PL, Moake JL, Weinger RS et al. Heparin-induced thrombocytopenia: association with a platelet-aggregating factor and arterial thromboses. Am J Hematol 1979;6:125–133.

192. Babcock RB, Dumper CW, Scharfman WB. Heparin-induced thrombocytopenia. N Engl J Med 1976;295:237–241.

193. Frame JN, Mulvey KP, Phares JC et al. Correction of severe heparin-associated thrombocytopenia with intravenous immunoglobulin. Ann Intern Med 1989;111:946–947.

194. Grau E, Linares M, Olaso MA et al. Heparin-induced thrombocytopenia—response to intravenous immunoglobulin *in vivo* and *in vitro*. Am J Hematol 1992;39:312–313.

195. Sobel M, Adelman B, Szentpetry S et al. Surgical management of heparin-associated thrombocytopenia. Strategies for treatment of venous and arterial thromboembolism. J Vasc Surg 1988;8:395–401.

196. Greisler H, Baker W, Nand S et al. Heparin induced thrombosis with peripheral arterial occlusion. Treatment wtih intra-arterial urokinase. Thromb Haemost 1985;54:100–101.

197. Fiessinger JN, Aich M, Roncato M et al. Critical ischemia during heparin-induced thrombocytopenia: treatment by intra-arterial streptokinase. Thromb Res 1984;33:235–238.

198. Krueger SK, Andres E, Weinand E. Thrombolysis in heparin-induced thrombocytopenia with thrombosis. Ann Intern Med 1991;159:198.

199. Cohen JL, Cooper MR, Greenberg CS. Streptokinase therapy of pulmonary emboli with heparin-associated thrombocytopenia. Arch Intern Med 1985;145:1725–1726.

200. Cummings JM, Mason TJ, Chomka EV et al. Fibrinolytic therapy of acute myocardial infarction in the heparin thrombosis syndrome. Am Heart J 1986;122:407–409.

201. Clifton JD, Smith MD. Thrombolytic therapy in heparin-associated thrombocytopenia with thrombosis. Clin Pharmacol 1986;5:597–601.

202. Magnani HN. Heparin-induced thrombocytopenia (HIT): an overview of 230 individuals treated with Orgaran (Org 10172). Thromb Haemost 1993;70:554–561.

203. Harenberg J, Zimmermann R, Schwarz F et al. Treatment of heparin-induced thrombocytopenia by a new heparinoid. Lancet 1983;1(8831)986–987.

204. Kiers L, Grigg LE, Cade JF et al. Use of Org 10172 in the treatment of heparin-induced thrombocytopenia and thrombosis. Aust N Z Med J 1991;21:52–54.

205. Rowlings PA, Mansberg R, Rozenberg MC et al. The use of a low-molecular-weight heparinoid (Org 10172) for extracorporal procedures in individuals with heparin dependent thrombocytopenia and thrombosis. Aust N Z Med J 1991;21:52–54.

206. Greinacher A, Michels I, Mueller-Eckhardt C. Heparin-associated thrombocytopenia: the antibody is not heparin specific. Thromb Haemost 1992;67:545–549.

207. Makhoul RG, Greenberg CS, McCann RL. Heparin-associated thrombocytopenia and thrombosis: a serious clinical problem and potential solution. J Vasc Surg 1987;4:522–528.

208. Chong B, Ismail F, Cade J et al. Heparin-induced thrombocytopenia: studies with a new low-molecular-weight heparinoid, Org 10172. Blood 1989;73:1592–1596.

209. Goualt-Heilmann M, Payen D, Conant G et al. Thrombocytopenia related to synthetic heparin analogue therapy. Thromb Haemost 1985;54:577.

210. Follen G, Hamandijian I, Treciah MC et al. Pentostan polysulphate (Sp 54)–induced thrombocytopenia. Thromb Haemost 1985;54:94–95.

211. Maiza D, Derlon A, Khayat MC et al. Role du polysulfate de pentusane dans le declenchement de deux accidents thrombopeniques. Presse Med 1985;14:1290–1291.

212. Manchon ND, Flechet B, Borg JY et al. Demonstration du role polysulfate de pentosane a l'origine d'un accident thrombopenique. Presse Med 1986;15:38–39.

213. Rosenthal E, Tiger F, Benoit P et al. Thrombopenic et hemorrhagie intracerebrale mortelle induites par le polysulfate de pentosane. Presse Med 1988;17:126.

214. Schiele F, Vuillemenot A, Kramarz P et al. Use of recombinant hirudin as antithrombotic treatment in individuals with heparin-induced thrombocytopenia. Am J Hematol 1995;50:20–25.

215. Reid III T, Alving BM. Hirulog therapy for heparin-associated thrombocytopenia and deep venous thrombosis. Am J Hematol 1993;43:352–353.

216. Cole CW, Fournier LM, Bormanis J. Heparin-associated thrombocytopenia and thrombosis: optimal therapy with Ancrod. Can J Surg 1990;33:207–210.

217. Demers C, Ginsberg JS, Brill-Edwards P et al. Rapid anticoagulation using Ancrod for heparin-induced thrombocytopenia. Blood 1991;78:2194–2197.

218. Cole CW, Bormanis J. Ancrod: a practical alternative to heparin. J Vasc Surg 1988;8:59–63.

219. Boon DMS, Kappers-Klunne MC, Michiels JJ et al. Heparin-induced thrombocytopenia and thrombosis: a potential fatal complication in a routine treatment. Neth J Med 1995;146:152.

220. Leroy L, Leclerc MH, Delahousse B et al. Treatment of heparin-associated thrombocytopenia and thrombosis with low-molecular-weight heparin (CY 216). Semin Thromb Hemost 1985;11:326–329.

221. Goualt-Heilmann M, Huet Y, Adnot S et al. Low-molecular-weight heparin fractions as an alternative in heparin-induced thrombocytopenia. Haemostasis 1987;17:134–140.

222. Vitoux J-F, Mathieu J-F, Roncato M et al. Heparin induced thrombocytopena treatment with low-molecular-weight heparin. Thromb Haemost 1986;55:37–39.

223. Laprevote-Heully MC, Bollaert PE, Bauer P et al. Thrombogenic thrombopenia related to heparin. Clinical, biological, and therapeutical results. Apropos of 32 cases. J Mal Vasc 1987;12:133–137.

224. Lecrubier C, Lecompte T, Potevin F et al. Test d'agregation plaquettaire dan 26 cas de thrombopenies induites par l'heparine (TUH). J Mal Vasc 1987;12:128–132.

225. Horellou MH, Conard J, Lecrubier C et al. Persistent heparin induced

thrombocytopenia despite therapy with low-molecular-weight heparin [Letter]. Thromb Haemost 1984;51:134.

226. Bauer P, Vidrequin A, Laprevote-Heully L. Persisting thrombocytopenia due to heparin despite its replacement by low-molecular-weight heparin. Ann Fr Anesth Reanim 1985;4:383–384.

227. Messmore HL, Fareed J, Corey J et al. *In vitro* assessment of low-molecular-weight heparin in individual with thrombocytopenia. Blood 1984;64(S):5a.

228. Eichinger S, Kryle PA, Brenner B et al. Thrombocytopenia associated with low-molecular-weight heparin. Lancet 1991;37:1435–1436.

229. Nand S, Robinson JA. Plasmapheresis in the management of heparin-associated thrombocytopenia with thrombosis. Am J Hematol 1988;28:204–206.

230. Greinacher A, Liebenhoff U, Kiefel V et al. Heparin-associated thrombocytopenia: the effects of various intravenous IgG preparations on antibody mediated platelet activation—a possible new indication for high dose i.v. IgG. Thromb Haemost 1994;71:641–645.

231. Laster J, Elfrink R, Silver D. Reexposure to heparin of individuals with heparin-associated antibodies. J Vasc Surg 1989;9:677–682.

232. Touchot B, Berthelot A, Boizard B et al. Major thrombocytopenia induced by heparin: a practical attitude in cardiac surgery under cardiopulmonary bypass. Arch Mal Coeur Vaiss 1987;80:93–95.

233. Ortel TL, Gockerman JP, Califf RM et al. Parenteral anticoagulation with the heparinoid Lomoparan (Org 10172) in individuals with heparin-induced thrombocytopenia and thrombosis. Thromb Haemost 1992;67:292–296.

234. Wilhelm MJ, Schmid C, Kececioglu D et al. Cardiopulmonary bypass in individuals with heparin-induced thrombocytopenia using Org 10172. Ann Thorac Surg 1996;61:920–924.

235. Addonizio VP Jr, Fisher CA, Kappa JR et al. Prevention of heparin-induced thrombocytopenia during open heart surgery with iloprost (2K36374). Surgery 1987;102:796–807.

236. Danielson DA, Douglas SW, Herzog P et al. Drug-induced blood disorders. JAMA 1984;252:3257–3260.

237. Garty M, Ilfeld D, Kelton JG. Correlation of a quinidine-induced platelet-specific antibody with the development of thrombocytopenia. Am J Med 1985;79:253–255.

238. Bishop RC, Spencer HH, Bethell FH. Quinidine purpura: report of six cases. Ann Intern Med 1959;50:1227–1240.

239. Nieminen U, Kekomaki R. Quinidine-induced thrombocytopenic purpura: clinical presentation in relation to drug-dependent and drug-independent antibodies. Br J Haematol 1992;80:77–82.

240. Posner AC. Purpura hemorrhagica complicating the puerperium. Am J Obstetr Gynecol 1937;34:155–158.

241. Belkin GA. Cocktail purura: an unusual case of quinine sensitivity. Ann Intern Med 1967;66:583–586.

242. Christie DJ, Waker RH, Kolins MD et al. Quinine-induced thrombocytopenia following intravenous use of heroin. Arch Intern Med 1983;143:1174–1175.

243. Reid DM, Shulman NR. Drug purpura due to surreptitious quinidine intake. Ann Intern Med 1988;108:206–208.

244. Lawson D, Mehta P, Lipman BC et al. Cumulative effects of quinine and aspirin on bleeding time and platelet a2-adrenoreceptors: potential mechanism of bleeding diarthesis in individuals receiving this combination. J Lab Clin Med 1986;108:581–586.

245. Castro O. Quinidine leukopenia and thrombocytopenia with a drug-induced leukoagglutinin. N Engl J Med 1977;296:572.

246. Chong BH, Berndt MC, Koutts J et al. Quinidine-induced thrombocytopenia and leukopenia: demonstration and characterization of distinct antiplatelet and antileukocyte antibodies. Blood 1983;62:1218–1223.

247. Freiman JP. Fatal quinine-induced thrombocytopenia. Ann Intern Med 1990;112:308–309.

248. Stroncek DF, Vercellotti GM, Hammerschmidt DE et al. Characterization of multiple quinine-dependent antibodies in a individual with episodic hemolytic uremic syndrome and immune agranulocytosis. Blood 1992;80:241–248.

249. Ziegler Z, Shadduck RK, Winkelstein A et al. Immune hemolytic anemia and thrombocytopenia secondary to quinidine: *in vitro* studies of the quinidine-dependent red cell and platelet antibodies. Blood 1979;53:396–402.

250. Lavie CJ, Biundo J, Quinet RJ et al. Systemic lupus erythimatosus (SLE) induced by quinidine. Arch Intern Med 1985;145:446–448.

251. Gottschall JL, Neahring B, McFarland JG et al. Quinine-induced immune thrombocytopenia with hemolytic uremic syndrome: clinical and serological findings in nine individuals and review of the literature. Am J Hematol 1994;47:283–289.

252. Elliot HL, Trash DB. Intravascular coagulation induced by quinine. Scott Med J 1979;24:244–245.

253. Barr E, Douglas JF, Hill CM. Recurrent acute hypersensitivity to quinine. Br Med J 1990;301:323.

254. Spearling RL, Hickton CM, Sizeland P et al. Quinine-induced disseminated intravascular coagulation. Lancet 1990;336:1535–1537.

255. van der Weerdt CM. Thrombocytopenia due to quinidine or quinine. Report on a series of 28 individuals. Vox Sang 1967;12:265–272.

256. Shulman NR. Immunoreactions involving platelets. I. A steric and kinetic

257. model for formation of a complex from a human antibody, quinidine as a haptene, and platelets; and for fixation of complement by the complex. J Exp Med 1958;107:665–690.

257. Christie DJ, Aster RD. Drug-antibody-platelet interaction in quinine- and quinidine-induced thrombocytopenia. J Clin Invest 1982;70:989–998.

258. Boullin DJ, O'Brien RA. Accumulation of quinidine by human blood platelets: effects on platelet ultrastructure and 5-hydroxytryptamine. Br J Pharmacol 1971;42:114–126.

259. Davis JW, Wilson SJ. The effect of quinidine on the uptake and release of serotonin by platelets *in vitro*. Proc Soc Exp Biol Med 1969;131:1107–1110.

260. Christie DJ, Mullen PC, Aster RH. Fab-mediated binding of drug-dependent antibodies to platelets in quinidine- and quinine-induced thrombocytopenia. J Clin Invest 1985;75:310–314.

261. Christie DJ, Mullen PC, Aster RH. Quinine- and quinidine-platelet antibodies can react with GP IIb/IIIa. Br J Haematol 1987;67:213–219.

262. Viscentin GP, Newman PJ, Aster RH. Characteristics of quinine- and quinidine-induced antibodies specific for platelet glycoproteins IIb and IIIa. Blood 1991;77:2668–2676.

263. Smith ME, Reid DM, Jones CE et al. Binding of quinine- and quinidine-dependent drug antibodies to platelets is mediated by the Fab domain of the immunlogbulin G and is not Fc dependent. J Clin Invest 1987;79:912–917.

264. Shulman NR. Immunologic reactions to drugs. N Engl J Med 1972;287:408–412.

265. Christie DJ, Diaz-Arauzo H, Cook JM. Antibody-mediated platelet destruction by quinine, quinidine, and their metabolites. J Lab Clin Med 1988;112:92–98.

266. Christie DJ, Weber RW, Mullen PC et al. Structural features of the quinidine and quinine molecules necessary for binding of drug-induced antibodies to human platelets. J Lab Clin Med 1984;104:730–740.

267. van Leeuwen EF, Engelfriet CP, von dem Borne AE. Studies on quinine- and quinidine-dependent antibodies against platelets and their reaction with platelets in the Bernard-Soulier syndrome. Br J Haematol 1982;51:551–560.

268. Kunicki TJ, Johnson MM, Aster RH. Absence of the platelet receptor for drug-dependent antibodies in the Bernard-Soulier syndrome. J Clin Invest 1978;62:716–719.

269. Kunicki TJ, Russu J, Nurden AT et al. Further studies of the human platelet receptor for quinine- and quinidine-dependent antibodies. J Immunol 1981;126:398–402.

270. Chong BH, Du X, Berndt MC et al. Characterization of the binding domains on platelet glycoproteins Ib-IX and IIb-IIIa complexes for the quinine/quinidine-dependent antibodies. Blood 1991;77:2190–2199.

271. Pfueller SL, Bilston RA, Logan D et al. Heterogeneity of drug-dependent platelet antigens and their antibodies in quinine- and quinidine-induced thrombocytopenia: involvement of glycoproteins Ib, IIb, IIIa, IX. Blood 1988;72:1155–1162.

272. Berndt MC, Chong BH, Bull HA et al. Molecular charcterization of quinine/quinidine drug dependent antibody platelet interaction using monoclonal antibodies. Blood 1985;66:1292–1301.

273. Lopez JA, Li CQ, Weisman S et al. The glycoprotein Ib-IX complex–specific monoclonal antibody SZ1 binds to a conformation-sensitive epitope on glycoprotein IX: implications for the target antigen of quinine/quinidine-dependent autoantibodies. Blood 1995;85:1254–1258.

274. Pfueller SL, Contizo F, Gibson J et al. Location of the quinine-dependent epitope on platelet glycoprotein IIIa. Haemostasis 1991;21:293–299.

275. Stricker RB, Shuman MA. Quinidine purpura: evidence that glycoprotein V is a target platelet antigen. Blood 1986;67:1377–1381.

276. Pfueller SL, Bilston RA, Jane S et al. Expression of the drug-dependent antigen for quinidine-dependent antiplatelet antibodies of gp IIIa but not that on gp Ib, IIb, or IX on human endothelial cells. Thromb Haemost 1990;63:279–281.

277. Nieminen U, Kekomaki R. Quinidine-induced thrombocytopenic purpura: clinical presentation in relation to drug-dependent and drug-independent antibodies. Br J Haematol 1992;80:77–82.

278. Rendell MA, Moore BR, Fass L. Use of i.v. immunoglobulin for presumed quinidine-induced thrombocytopenia. Clin Pharmacol 1989;8:89.

279. Shulman NR. Mechanisms of immunologic drug effects of blood cells. Physiol Pharmacol 1974;5:237–249.

280. Hammett JF. Thrombocytopenia following administration of Bactrim. Med J Aust 1970;2:200.

281. Adverse effects of drugs commonly used in the treatment of urinary tract infection. A report from the Australian drug evaluation committee. Med J Aust 1972;1:435–438.

282. McPherson VJ, Raik E. Thrombocytopenia following administration of Septrin. Med J Aust 1970;2:755.

283. Frisch JM. Clinical experience with adverse reactions to trimethoprim-sulfamethoxazole. J Infect Dis 1973;128:S607–S611.

284. Jick H. Adverse reactions to trimethoprim-sulfamethoxazole in hospitalized individuals. Rev Infect Dis 1982;4:426–428.

285. Keisu M, Wilhom BE, Palblad J. Trimethoprim-sulphamethoxazole–associated blood dyscrasias. Ten years experience of the Swedish spontaneous reporting system. J Intern Med 1990;228:353–360.

286. Dickson HG. Trimethoprim-sulfamethoxazole and thrombocytopenia. Med J Aust 1978;2:5–7.

287. Bose W, Karama A, Linzmeier G et al. Controlled trial of cotrimoxazole in children with urinary-tract infection. Bacteriological efficacy and haematologic toxicity. Lancet 1974;2:614–616.

288. Asmar BI, Maqbool S, Dajani AS. Hematologic abnormalities after oral trimethoprim-sulfamethoxazole therapy in children. Am J Dis Child 1981; 135:1100–1103.

289. Feldman S, Doolittle M, Lott L et al. Similar hematologic changes in children receiving trimethoprim-sulfamethoxazole or amoxacillin for otitis media. J Pediatr 1985;106:995–1000.

290. Shear NH, Speilberg SP, Grant DM et al. Differences in metabolism of sulfonamides predisposing to idosyncratic toxicity. Ann Intern Med 1992; 194:179–183.

291. Jaffe HS, Abrams DI, Ammann AJ et al. Complications of cotrimoxazole in treatment of AIDS-associated *Pneumocystis carinii* pneumonia in homosexual men. Lancet 1983;2:1109–1111.

292. Gordin FM, Simon GL, Wofsy CB et al. Adverse reactions to trimethoprim-sulfamethoxazole in parients with the acquired immunodeficiency syndrome. Ann Intern Med 1984;100:495–499.

293. Bradley PP, Warden GD, Maxwell JG et al. Neutropenia and thrombocytopenia in renal allograft recipients treated with trimethoprim-sulfamethoxazole. Ann Intern Med 1980;93:560–562.

294. Ballardie FW, Winearls CG, Cohen J et al. *Pneuomcystis carinii* pneumonia in renal transplant recipients—clinical and radiographic features, diagnosis and complications of treatment. Q J Med 1985;223:729–747.

295. Bateson MC, Hayes JPLA, Pendharker P. Cotrimoxazole and folate metabolism. Lancet 1976;2:339–340.

296. Lockie LM, Norcross BM, George CW. Treatment of two reactions due to gold. JAMA 1947;163:754–755.

297. Hamilton HE, Sheets RF. Sulfisoxazole-induced thrombocytopenia purpura. JAMA 1978;239:2586–2587.

298. Claas FHJ, van der Meer J, Langerak J. Immunological effect of co-trimoxazole on platelets. Br Med J 1970;2:898–899.

299. Karpatkin M, Siskind GW, Karpatkin S. The platelet factor 3 immunoinjury technique re-evaluated. Development of a rapid test for antiplatelet antibody. Detection in various clinical disorders, including immunologic drug–induced and neonatal thrombocytopenia. J Lab Clin Med 1977;89: 400–408.

300. Schwartz RH, Rodriguez WJ, Luban NLC. Thrombocytopenia association with PF3 antiplatelet activity against the sulfa component of trimethoprim-sulfamethoxazole. South Med J 1981;74:640–641.

301. Barr AL, Whineray M. Immune thrombocytopenia induced by cotrimoxazole. Aust N Z J Med 1980;10:54–55.

302. Curtis BR, McFarland JG, Wu G-G et al. Antibodies in sulfonamide-induced immune thrombocytopenia recognize calcium-dependent epitopes on the glycoprotein IIb-IIIa complex. Blood 1994;84:175–183.

303. Claas FHJ, Langerak J, van Rood JJ. Metabolite-specific (IgG) and drug-specific antibodies (IgG, IgM) in two cases of trimethoprim-sulfamethoxazole–induced immune thrombocytopenia. Transfusion 1987;27:262–265.

304. Golde DW, Bersch N, Quan SG. Trimethoprim and sulphamethoxazole inhibition of haematopoiesis *in vitro*. Br J Haematol 1978;40:363–367.

305. Chanarin I, England JM. Toxicity of trimethoprim-sulphamethoxazole in individuals with megaloblastic haemopoiesis. Br Med J 1972;1:651–653.

306. Rickard KA, Uhr E. Acute thrombocytopenia associated with Spectrin. Med J Aust 1971;1:769–770.

307. Jenkins GC, Hughes DTD, Hall PC. A haematological study of individuals receiving long-term treatment with trimethoprim and sulphonamide. J Clin Pathol 1970;23:392–396.

308. Kobrinsky NL, Ramsey NKC. Acute maegaloblastic anemia induced by high-dose trimethoprim-sulphamethoxazole. Ann Intern Med 1981;94: 780–781.

309. Jewkes RF, Edwards MS, Grant BJB. Haematological changes in a individual on long-term treatment with a trimethoprim-sulphonamide combination. Postgrad Med J 1970;46:723–726.

310. Hsi Y-J, Kuo H-Y, Ouyand A. Thrombocytopenia following administration of penicillin. Chin Med J 1966;85:249–251.

311. Murphy MR, Riordan T, Minchinton RM et al. Demonstration of an immune-mediated mechanism of penicillin-induced neutropenia and thrombocytopenia. Br J Haematol 1983;55:155–160.

312. Brooks AP. Thrombocytopenia during treatment with ampicillin. Lancet 1974;2:723.

313. Bottinger LE, Westerholm B. Thrombocytopenia. Drug-induced thrombocytopenia. Acta Med Scand 1972;191:541–548.

314. Hughes G. Ampicillin and hematologic effects. Ann Intern Med 1983;99: 573.

315. Schiffer CA, Weinstein HJ, Wiernick PH. Methicillin-associated thrombocytopenia. Ann Intern Med 1976;338:339.

316. Lang G, Lishner M, Ravid M. Adverse reactions to prolonged treatment with high doses of carbenicillin and ureidopencillins. Rev Infect Dis 1992; 13:68–72.

317. Drusano G, Schimpff S, Hewitt W. The acylampicillins: mezlocillin, piperacillin, and azlocillin. Rev Infect Dis 1984;6:13–32.

318. Lee M, Sharifi R. Severe thrombocytopenia due to apalcillin. Urol Int 1987; 42:313–315.

319. Sheiman L, Spielvogel AR, Horowitz HI. Thrombocytopenia caused by cepthalothin sodium. Occurrence in a penicillin-sensitive individual. JAMA 1968;203:601–603.

320. Christie DJ, Lennon SS, Drew RL. Cefotetan-induced immunologic thrombocytopenia. Br J Haematol 1988;70:423–426.

321. Gralnick HR, McGinniss M, Halterman R. Thrombocytopenia with sodium cephalothin therapy. Ann Intern Med 1972;77:401–444.

322. Parker JC, Barrett DA II. Microangiopathic hemolysis and thrombocytopenia related to penicillin drugs. Arch Intern Med 1971;127:474–477.

323. Garratty G, Petz LD. Drug-induced immune hemolytic anemia. Am J Med 1975;58:398–407.

324. Bang NU, Kammer RB. Hematologic complications associated with β-lactam antibiotics. Rev Infect Dis 1983;5:S80–S393.

325. Salaman DJ, Nusbacher J, Stroupe T et al. Red cell and platelet-bound IgG antibodies in a individual with thrombocytopenia. Transfusion 1984;24: 395–398.

326. Sutor AH, Jedkinsky-Bucher C. Coagulation changes caused by dipropylacetic acid. Med Welt 1974;25:447–449.

327. Eastham RD, Jancar J. Sodium valproate and platelet counts. Br Med J 1980;1:186.

328. Winfield DA, Benton P, Espir ML et al. Sodium valproate and thrombocytopenia. Br Med J 1976;2:981.

329. Raworth RE, Birchall G. Sodium valproate and platelet count. Lancet 1978; 1:670–671.

330. Delgado MR, Riela AR, Mills J et al. Thrombocytopenia secondary to high valproate levels in children with epilepsy. J Child Neurol 1994;9:311–314.

331. Loiseau P. Sodium valproate and platelet counts. Epilepsia 1981;22: 141–146.

332. Erenberg G, Rothner D, Henry CE et al. Valproic acid in the treatment of intractable absence seizures in children. Am J Dis Child 1982;136:526–529.

333. Drug Ther Bull 1984;22:23–24.

334. Barr RD, Copeland SA, Stockwell ML et al. Valproic acid and immune thrombocytopenia. Arch Dis Child 1982;57:681–684.

335. Neophytides AN, Nutt JG, Lodish JR. Thrombocytopenia associated with sodium valproate treatment. Ann Neurol 1978;5:389–390.

336. Prats JM, Garaizar C, Rua MJ et al. Infantile spasms treated with high doses of sodium valproate: initial response and followup. Dev Med Child Neurol 1991;33:617–625.

337. Cole AP. Transient thrombocytopenia in a child on sodium valproate. Dev Med Child Neurol 1978;20:487–490.

338. Sandler RM, Emberson C, Roberts GE et al. IgM platelet autoantibody due to sodium valproate. Br Med J 1978;2:1683–1685.

339. Bleck TP, Smith MC. Possible induction of systemic lupus erythematosus by valproate. Epilepsia 1990;31:343–345.

340. Ganick DJ, Sunder T, Finley JL. Severe hematologic toxicity of valproic acid. A report of four individuals. Am J Ped Hematol Oncol 1990;12:80–85.

341. Coulter DL, Wu H, Allen RJ. Valproic acid in childhood epilepsy. JAMA 1980;244:785–788.

342. Ozkara C, Dreifuss FE, Apperson Hansen C. Changes in red blood cells with valproate therapy. Acta Neurol Scand 1993;88:210–212.

343. May RB, Sunder TR. Hematologic manifestations of long-term valporate therapy. Epilepsia 1993;34:1098–1101.

344. Brichard B, Vermylen C, Scheiff JM et al. Haematological disturbances during long-term valproate therapy. Eur J Pediatr 1994;153:378–380.

345. Richardson SG, Fletcher DJ, Jeavons PM et al. Sodium valproate and platelet function. Br Med J 1976;1:221–222.

346. Monnet P, David M, Phillips N. Alterations de l'hemostase lors des traitements au dipropylacetate de sodium. Pediatrics 1979;34:603–620.

347. Dale BM, Puride GH, Rischbieth RH. Fibrinogen depletion with sodium valproate. Lancet 1978;1:1316–1317.

348. Boutellier L, DeLumley L, Saura R et al. Aplasie medullaire transitoire au cours d'un traitement par le depropulacetate de sodium. Nouv Presse Med 1979;8:611–614.

349. Smith FR, Boots M. Sodium valproate and bone marrow suppression. Ann Neurol 1980;8:197–199.

350. Hoffman LM. Sodium valproate and thrombocytopenia. Can Med Assoc J 1982;126:358–359.

351. Siemes J, Spohr HL, Michael TH et al. Therapy of infantile spasms with valproate: results of a prospective study. Epilepsia 1988;29:533–560.

352. Bruni J, Wilder BJ. Valproic acid—review of a new epileptic drug. Arch Neurol 1979;36:393–398.

353. Miyake S, Honda K, Kimura S et al. Sodium valproate and thrombocytopenia. Brain Dev 1979;1:319–322.

354. Armour DJ, Veitch GBA. Is valproate monotherapy a practical possibility in chronically uncontrolled epilepsy. J Clin Pharm Ther 1988;13:53–64.

355. Hartfall SJ, Garland HG, Goldie W. Gold treatment of arthritis. Lancet 1937;2:744-88–838-42.

356. Lockie LM, Smith DM. Forty-seven years experience with gold therapy in 1019 rheumatoid arthritis individuals. Semin Arthritis Rheum 1985;17: 238–246.

357. Price AE, Leichtentritt B. Gold therapy in rheumatoid arthritis. Ann Intern Med 1943;19:70–80.

358. Mettier SR, McBride A, Li J. Thrombocytopenic purpura complicating gold therapy for rheumatoid arthritis. Report of three cases with spontaneous recovery and one case with recovery following aspenectomy. Blood 1948;3:1705–1717.

359. Cecil RI, Kammerer W, DePrume FJ. Gold salts in the treatment of rheumatoid arthritis: a study of 245 cases. Ann Intern Med 1942;10:817–827.

360. Cervi PL, Wright P, Casey EB. Audit of full blood count monitoring in individuals on long-term gold therapy for rheumatoid arthritis. Ir J Med Sci 1992;16:73–74.

361. Rothermich NO, Philips VK, Bergen W et al. Chrysotherapy. A prospective study. Arthritis Rheum 1991;19:1621–1627.

362. Oral gold approval for some arthritis individuals. FDA Drug Bulletin 1985;15:15–16.

363. Coblyn JS, Weinblatt M, Holdsworth D et al. Gold-induced thrombocytopenia. A clinical and immunogenetic study of twenty-three individuals. Ann Intern Med 1981;95:188–191.

364. Singal DO, Reid B, Green D et al. Polymorphism of major histocompatibility complex extended haplotypes bearing HLA-DR3 in individuals with rheumatoid arthritis and gold-induced thrombocytopenia or proteinuria. Ann Rheum Dis 1990;49:582–586.

365. Adachi JD, Bensen WG, Kassam Y et al. Gold-induced thrombocytopenia: 18 cases and a review of the literature. Semin Arthritis Rheum 1987;10:287–293.

366. Adachi JD, Bensen WG, Singal DP et al. Gold-induced thrombocytopenia: platelet associated IgG and HLA typing in three individuals. J Rheumatol 1984;17:355–357.

367. Harth M, Hickey JP, Coulter WK et al. Gold-induced thrombocytopenia. J Rheumatol 1978;5:105–172.

368. Gibbons RB. Complications of chrysotherapy. A review of recent studies. Arch Intern Med 1979;169:343–346.

369. Kay AG. Myelotoxicity of gold. Br Med J 1976;1:1886–1888.

370. Baldwin JL, Storb RT, Thomas ED et al. Bone marrow transplantation in individuals with gold-induced marrow aplasia. Arthritis Rheum 1977;20:1743–1748.

371. Gottlieb NL, Smith PM, Smith EM. Pharmacodynamics of $^{197}$Au- and $^{195}$Au-labeled aurothromalate in blood. Correlation with course of rheumatoid arthritis, gold toxicity and gold excretion. Arthritis Rheum 1974;18:181–183.

372. Girdwood RH. Death after taking medicaments. Br Med J 1984;1:501–504.

373. Godfrey NF, Peter A, Simon TM et al. N-acetylcysteine treatment of hematologic reactions to chrysotherapy. J Rheumatol 1982;9:519–526.

374. Bray VJ, Singleton JD. Disseminated intravascular coagulation in Still's disease. Semin Arthritis Rheum 1994;222:229.

375. Saphir JR, Ney RG. Delayed thrombocytopenic purpura after diminutive gold therapy. JAMA 1966;195:782–784.

376. Hansen RM, Csuka ME, McCarty DJ et al. Gold-induced aplastic anemia. Complete response to corticosteroids, plasmapheresis, and N-acetylcysteine infusion. J Rheumatol 1985;18:794–797.

377. Stafford BT, Crosby WH. Late onset of gold-induced thrombocytopenia with a practical note on the injections of dimercaprol. JAMA 1978;239:50–51.

378. Cook DJ, Bensen WG, Adachi JD. Late-onset gold-induced thrombocytopenia. J Rheumatol 1988;18:1750–1751.

379. Hazlett BE, Yendt ER. Thrombocytopenia following gold therapy with successful treatment. Can Med Assoc J 1958;79:31–33.

380. Cox AJ, Marich KW. Gold in the dermis following gold therapy for rheumatoid arthritis. Arch Dermatol 1973;108:655–657.

381. Gottlieb NL, Smith PM, Smith EM. Tissue gold concentration in a rheumatoid arthritic receiving crysotherapy. Arthritis Rheum 1972;18:10–22.

382. Howell A, Gumpel JM, Watts RWE. Depression of bone marrow colony formation in gold-induced neutropenia. Br Med J 1975;1:432–434.

383. McCarty DJ, Brill JM, Harrop D. Aplastic anemia secondary to gold-salt therapy. Report of a fatal case and a review of the literature. JAMA 1962;189:655–657.

384. Levin HA, McMillan R, Tavossoli M et al. Thrombocytopenia associated with gold therapy. Observations on the mechanism of platelet destruction. Am J Med 1975;59:274–280.

385. Denman EJ, Denman AM. The lymphocytic transformation test and gold hypersensitivity. Ann Rheum Dis 1968;27:582–589.

386. Walker DJ, Saunders P, Griffiths ID. Gold-induced thrombocytopenia. J Rheumatol 1986;16:225–226.

387. von dem Borne AE, Pegels JG, van der Stadt RJ et al. Thrombocytopenia associated with gold therapy: a drug-induced autoimmune disease. Br J Haematol 1986;63:509–516.

388. Smith PM, Smith EM, Gottlieb NL. Gold distribution in whole blood during cryotherapy. J Lab Clin Med 1973;82:930–937.

389. Lorber A, Chandor SB, Simon TM et al. Immunosuppressive action of gold salts in rheumatoid arthritis. Abstracts of the VIth Pan-American Congress on Rheumatoid Diseases 1974;208a:

390. Stavem P, Stromme J, Bull O. Immunological studies in a case of gold salt–induced thrombocytopenia. Scand J Haematol 1968;5:271–277.

391. Lorber A, Bovy RA, Chang CC. The relationship between serum gold content and distribution to serum immunoglobulins and complement. Nature 1972;236:250–252.

392. Rubin M, Silwinski A, Photias M et al. Influence of chelation on gold metabolism in rats. Proc Soc Exp Med Biol 1967;184:290–296.

393. England JM, Smith DS. Gold-induced thrombocytopenia and response to dimercaprol. Br Med J 1972;2:748–749.

394. Herbst KD, Stone WH, Flannery EP. Chronic thrombocytopenia following gold therapy [Letter]. Arch Intern Med 1975;135:1622.

395. Hartung EF, Cotter J, Gannon C. The excretion of gold following the administration of gold sodium thiomalate in rheumatoid arthritis. J Lab Clin Med 1941;26:1850–1855.

396. Deren B, Masi R, Weksler M et al. Gold-associated thrombocytopenia. Report of six cases. Arch Intern Med 1974;134:1012–1015.

397. Goldstein R, Blanchette VS, Huebsch LB et al. Treatment of gold-induced thrombocytopenia by high-dose intravenous gamma globulin. Arthritis Rheum 1986;29:426–430.

398. Stein M, Miller KB. Treatment of gold-induced thrombocytopenia with high-dose gamma globulin [Letter]. Arthritis Rheum 1988;31:454–455.

399. Kozloff M, Votaw M, Penner JA. Gold-induced thrombocytopenia responsive to cyclophosphamide. South Med J 1979;72:1490–1492.

400. Thompson M, Sinclair RJG, Duthie JJR. Thrombocytopenic purpura after administration of gold. Comparison of treatment with dimercaprol, ACTH, and cortisone. Br Med J 1954;1:899–902.

401. Bluhm GB, Sigler JW, Winsign DC et al. d-Penicillamine therapy of thrombocytopenia secondary to chrysotherapy: a case report. Arthritis Rheum 1968;5:638a.

402. Burday MJ, Martin SE. Cocaine-associated thrombocytopenia. Am J Med 1991;91:656–660.

403. Leissinger CA. Severe thrombocytopenia associated with cocaine use. Ann Intern Med 1990;112:708–710.

404. Koury MJ. Thrombocytopenic purpura in HIV-seronegative users of intravenous cocaine. Am J Hematol 1990;35:134–135.

405. Orser B. Thrombocytopenia and cocaine abuse. Anesthesiology 1991;74:195–196.

406. Abramowicz JS, Sherer DM, Woods JR. Acute transient thrombocytopenia associated with cocaine abuse in pregnancy. Obstet Gynecol 1991;78:499–500.

407. Kain ZN, Mayes LC, Pakes J et al. Thrombocytopenia in pregnant women who use cocaine. Am J Obstetr Gynecol 1995;173:885–890.

408. Weaver K. Effect of magnesium on cocaine-induced, catecholamine-mediated platelet and vascular response in term pregnant ewes. Am J Obstetr Gynecol 1989;5:133–137.

409. Togna G, Tempesta E, Togna AR et al. Platelet responsive and biosynthesis of thromboxane and prostacyclin in response to in vitro cocaine treatment. Haemostasis 1985;15:100–107.

# CHAPTER 30

# IMMUNE THROMBOCYTOPENIC PURPURA

## Robert McMillan and Paul Imbach

Immune thrombocytopenic purpura (ITP) occurs in a group of disorders with the common manifestation of immune-mediated destructive thrombocytopenia (Table 30.1). This process may be acute and self-limited (acute ITP) or chronic, and it may occur as a primary autoimmune disorder (chronic ITP) or be related to a variety of diseases such as collagen vascular disease, lymphoproliferative disorders, or infection. Immune thrombocytopenia due to alloimmune platelet destruction (posttransfusion purpura, neonatal purpura) or drug-dependent antibodies is covered in Chapters 28 and 29, respectively.

The symptoms, signs, and laboratory findings seen in individuals with immune thrombocytopenia are similar regardless of the disorder (Tables 30.2 and 30.3). Individuals may be asymptomatic with thrombocytopenia being noted during routine blood studies. However, most individuals seek medical attention because they have noted a skin rash (petechiae or purpura) or have developed mucosal bleeding from the nose, gastrointestinal tract, or genitourinary tract. Women often note prolonged or heavy menstrual bleeding. Occasionally, central nervous system (CNS) bleeding occurs but usually only as a late manifestation in a individual with severe mucosal bleeding. Symptoms are rare if the platelet count is >50,000/μL. Purpura with minor trauma is noted with platelet counts of 30,000 to 50,000/μL and spontaneous purpura with counts <30,000/μL. Serious mucosal bleeding or CNS bleeding is rare unless the platelet count is <5,000 to 10,000/μL. Symptoms may be exaggerated by certain medications (e.g., aspirin) or if the antibody is directed against a functional site on the platelet. If thrombocytopenia is associated with another disease process, symptoms of the primary disease may dominate.

Laboratory findings, unless influenced by an associated disease, reflect the peripheral platelet destruction and the attempt of the bone marrow to respond. The blood count shows a normal hematocrit (unless significant bleeding has occurred), normal leukocyte and differential counts, and thrombocytopenia. A greater percentage of the platelets are large (1). Bone marrow aspirates show normal granulocytic and erythroid elements. Megakaryocytes, if counted, are increased when compared with normal marrows, and in general they are larger and less mature and show little or no platelet budding.

Intravascular platelet survival is usually shortened, although, as will be discussed, there is now evidence that decreased platelet production is also important in some instances. Increased platelet-associated IgG (PAIgG) is usually noted, and antigen-specific antiplatelet antibodies can often be demonstrated.

## CHRONIC ITP

Chronic ITP (2–6) is an autoimmune disorder characterized by platelet destruction due to an antiplatelet autoantibody or to autoantibodies most often directed to one or more of the major platelet surface glycoproteins (GP). Autoantibody binding results in platelet phagocytosis by the reticuloendothelial system (RES) and, possibly in some instances, complement-mediated platelet lysis.

The frequency of chronic ITP has been estimated in two ways. From a 5 year Swedish study of a general hospitalized population (age >14), the incidence of thrombocytopenia was 123 cases per million population per year; 47% of these (58 individuals per million per year) were due to chronic ITP (7). If the frequency is similar in the United States, with a population of about 250 million, 14,500 new chronic ITP individuals should be diagnosed per year. From European studies the average incidence of acute ITP in children is 50 individuals per million population per year (6). Using the ratio of adult (chronic ITP):acute ITP, it was calculated that 66 new chronic ITP individuals per million would occur each year or 16,500 new chronic ITP individuals per year in the United States. Chronic ITP is most common in women in the third and fourth decade, with a female: male ratio of 3 to 4:1, and is uncommon in children.

## ETIOLOGY AND PATHOPHYSIOLOGY

Chronic ITP is an autoimmune disorder in which surface membrane proteins become antigenic for unknown reasons, leading to the synthesis and binding of autoantibody to platelets that result in their destruction.

**TABLE 30.1.** Immune Thrombocytopenia

Chronic autoimmune thrombocytopenic purpura
Acute immune thrombocytopenic purpura
Disease-associated
  Collagen vascular disease
  Lymphoproliferative disorders
  Solid tumors
  Infection
    Viral
    Bacterial
    Parasitic
Alloimmune
  Posttransfusion
  Neonatal
Drug-induced

## PLATELET KINETICS AND THROMBOPOIESIS IN CHRONIC ITP (SEE CHAPTERS 8 AND 9)

Although earlier kinetic studies used the [$^{51}$Cr] labeling technique, [$^{111}$In]-oxine has become the platelet label of choice because its high labeling efficiency allows the study of autologous platelets in individuals with low platelet counts and its high energy, gamma emitting properties permit quantitative imaging of the *in vivo* label distribution. International recommendations describing these methods have been published (8, 9). For more detail on the methods of evaluating platelet kinetics and turnover see Chapter 9.

### Initial Recovery and the Splenic Platelet Pool

A portion of the injected radioactivity disappears rapidly after platelet infusion due to equilibration with unlabeled circulating platelets and the exchangeable splenic platelet pool. The initial recovery in normal and splenectomized subjects averages about 60 and 90%, respectively; the difference reflects the size of the exchangeable splenic platelet pool (10, 11). In individuals with splenomegaly, this pool is proportionally larger (10).

Since recovery values based on equilibration may be influenced by early platelet destruction, it is impossible to calculate accurately the splenic platelet pool in

**TABLE 30.3.** Laboratory Findings in Immune Thrombocytopenia

Thrombocytopenia with increased percentage of large platelets (>2.5 μm)
Increased numbers and size of megakaryocytes
Reduced intravascular platelet survival
Elevated levels of platelet-associated immunoglobulin G
Demonstrable antigen-specific autoantibodies in some individual groups

**TABLE 30.2.** Clinical Features of Immune Thrombocytopenia

| Platelet Count | Symptoms | Physical Findings |
|---|---|---|
| >50,000/μL | None | None |
| 30,000–50,000/μL | Bruising with minor trauma | Scattered bruises at trauma site |
| 10,000–30,000/μL | Spontaneous bruising, menorrhagia | Generalized purpura, more prominent on extremities |
| <10,000/μL | Spontaneous bruising, mucosal bleeding, central nervous system bleeding risk | Generalized purpura, epistaxis, gastrointestinal/genitourinary bleeding, central nervous system signs |

chronic ITP using this method. However, measurement of the splenic platelet pool in chronic ITP individuals, using epinephrine infusion, gives similar results to those of normal subjects (12).

## Intravascular Platelet Survival

Platelet survival in normal subjects is essentially linear with a total survival of 8 to 10 days (11, 13–16). In individuals with chronic ITP, platelet survival is decreased (11, 14, 17–20). Survival curves are exponential, reflecting random platelet destruction, and in many cases correlate with the individual's platelet count. [$^{51}$Cr]-labeled homologous platelets have a shorter mean life span in chronic ITP individuals than those using [$^{111}$In]-labeled autologous platelets (18, 19, 21).

In most individuals platelet destruction occurs mainly in the spleen (17, 20), while liver sequestration is seen in more severe disease (17, 22). Although individuals with a splenic sequestration pattern have less severe disease and are more likely to respond to splenectomy than those with liver sequestration, results vary widely, and kinetic studies should not be used to decide therapy.

## Platelet Production

Two approaches have been used to quantitate platelet production: platelet turnover and megakaryocyte mass. Platelet turnover is calculated from the platelet count and intravascular life span and is corrected for the exchangeable platelet pool using the following formula:

$$\text{Platelet turnover (plts/}\mu\text{L/day)}$$

$$= [\text{platelet count (per }\mu\text{L)/life span (days)}]$$

$$\times\ [90\%/\text{initial recovery}]$$

Ninety percent is the platelet recovery in asplenic normal subjects; the initial recovery is determined from survival curves by some investigators, while others use the average normal recovery since they consider the ITP exchangeable pool to be equivalent.

Earlier studies, using chromium-labeled homologous platelets (low counts prohibited the use of autologous platelets), showed uniformly increased platelet turnover, which averaged 4.9 times normal in one study (23) and 2.25 times normal in another (11). However, platelet turnover, using labeled autologous platelets, may be decreased, normal, or increased. Using combined data from four studies of 55 untreated chronic ITP individuals (18, 20, 21, 24), the following turnover results were calculated: decreased—21 (38.2%), normal—24 (43.6%), and increased—10 (18.2%). Interpretation of these discordant results is difficult since either may be correct. It is possible that homologous platelets are destroyed more rapidly than autologous platelets. If so, platelet turnover based on homologous platelets

would be falsely increased. Conversely, circulating autologous platelets in chronic ITP individuals may be a selected population particularly resistant to immune destruction; this would result in a falsely low platelet turnover. Platelet turnover studies in ITP should be evaluated with these reservations in mind.

Megakaryocyte mass is the product of the total number of megakaryocytes and the average megakaryocyte volume. Total megakaryocytes are calculated by multiplying the ratio of megakaryocytes to nucleated erythroid cells, determined from marrow sections, by the total number of marrow erythroid cells, as estimated from plasma iron turnover studies (14). Mean megakaryoctye volume is calculated from the mean megakaryocyte diameter.

Increased megakaryocyte mass was noted in all chronic ITP individuals studied by one group with an average of 4.8 times control values (range 2.2 to 8.4) (23). Another group estimated megakaryocyte mass by relating the megakaryocyte area in tissue sections to total marrow area. A 2.2-fold increase in megakaryocyte mass was noted in chronic ITP (25).

The relationship between platelet turnover and megakaryocyte mass is important since platelet turnover is a measure of platelet delivery into the circulation and the megakaryocyte mass reflects platelet production capacity. Harker (23) reported a proportional increase suggesting effective thrombopoiesis, while Branehog et al (25) showed platelet turnover to be about one-half the megakaryocyte mass suggesting reduced platelet delivery. However, both of these studies employed labeled homologous platelets, which, as noted above, result in shorter platelet survival times and proportionately increased turnovers when compared with labeled autologous platelets.

As noted above, studies using labeled autologous platelets suggest that most individuals with chronic ITP have either normal or decreased platelet turnover values (18, 20, 21, 24). These findings, which suggest that the bone marrow in many chronic ITP individuals responds suboptimally to the increase in platelet destruction, are compatible with either antibody-induced inhibition of thrombopoiesis or intramedullary platelet destruction.

## Effect of Therapy on Platelet Kinetics

Conflicting results have been obtained depending on whether homologous or autologous platelets were studied. When [$^{51}$Cr]-labeled homologous platelets were used, a steroid response was accompanied by an increase in the initial recovery and platelet life span, while platelet turnover was unchanged (26). It was concluded that steroids affected the platelet removal mechanism, but did not alter production. Conversely, more recent studies using labeled autologous platelets gave the opposite result. No significant change in the initial recovery or platelet life span was noted, but there was a significant increase in platelet production as measured by turnover. It was concluded that steroids worked by increasing platelet production (27).

The effect of splenectomy on platelet kinetics has been studied by the same two groups (26, 27). Each noted, in responding individuals, an increase in platelet recovery (reflecting removal of the splenic pool) and platelet survival but no change in platelet turnover. They concluded that the major effect of splenectomy was reduced platelet destruction.

## Thrombopoietin

The major platelet growth factor, thrombopoietin, has recently been purified and cloned. For details about this growth factor, refer to Chapter 8. Mean blood levels of endogenous thrombopoietin (TPO) are mildly elevated in chronic ITP when compared with normal subjects, although a significant number of the ITP values fall within the normal range. In addition, the TPO levels in ITP are lower for a given platelet count than those seen in cases of thrombocytopenia due to decreased platelet production such as aplastic anemia (28, 29). These seemingly out-of-proportion TPO levels are probably due to its removal by the rapid turnover of the platelet compartment and the expanded megakaryocytic mass.

## THE IMMUNE SYSTEM IN CHRONIC ITP

The immune system normally responds to antigenic challenge by producing specific antibody and by activating cell-mediated immunity (CMI) with production of cytotoxic killer cells and lymphokines. Humoral immunity plays a central role in chronic ITP; the importance of CMI is unknown.

## Antiplatelet Antibody

Harrington et al reported that the infusion of blood or plasma from individuals with chronic ITP into normal recipients resulted in thrombocytopenia (30). Subsequent studies by Shulman et al showed the following: the effect was dose-dependent and was less marked in splenectomized individuals and in individuals pretreated with corticosteroids or RES blockade; the factor reacted with both autologous and homologous platelets, was in the IgG-rich fraction after serum fractionation, and could be removed by adsorption with platelets (31, 32). These *in vivo* studies suggested that the antiplatelet factor was an IgG antibody.

Further support for this was provided by the studies from many laboratories showing an increase in platelet-associated IgG (PAIgG) in most individuals with chronic ITP (see later section for details). In addition, IgG synthesized *in vitro* by washed ITP splenic lymphocytes

binds to washed homologous and autologous platelets (33, 34) and megakaryocytes (35).

The characteristics of the surface Ig (presumed to be antibody) in chronic ITP has been further defined (36). In 95% of individuals, IgG antibodies were detected either alone or in combination with IgM, IgA, or both. In 5%, only IgM antibodies were detected. Of 48 individuals with IgG antibodies, 45 had IgG1 either alone or with IgG3 (22 individuals), IgG4 (14 individuals), or IgG2 (one individual). A few individuals had either IgG3 or IgG4 alone.

Van Leeuwen et al (37) provided the first evidence for autoantibodies in chronic ITP. They reported that 32 of 42 eluates from ITP platelets would bind to normal but not to thrombasthenic platelets. Since these latter platelets are deficient in glycoproteins (GP) IIb and IIIa, they postulated that these ITP individuals had autoantibodies to one of these glycoproteins. Subsequent studies from several laboratories provided direct evidence for this (38–40). In 1987 two new assays were described that are more sensitive and can detect both platelet-associated and plasma autoantibodies: the immunobead assay and the monoclonal antibody-specific immobilization of platelet antigens (MAIPA) assay (41, 42). Using the former assay, positive platelet-associated and plasma autoantibody results were noted in 79.7 and 43.2% of 74 chronic ITP individuals, respectively (43). In 81.3% of the cases the autoantibody was against GP IIb/IIIa, while in the remainder it was toward GP Ib/IX. Similar plasma autoantibody results were reported using the MAIPA assay, although the incidence of anti-GP Ib/IX antibodies was greater (44).

The autoantibody in chronic ITP may also bind to the megakaryocyte and affect thrombopoiesis. Early immunofluorescent studies showed increased megakaryocyte-associated immunoglobulins (45, 46), although negative results were also seen (47). More recent studies show that autoantibodies can bind to megakaryocytes (35) and inhibit megakaryocyte colony formation *in vitro* (48). Whether autoantibodies affect thrombopoiesis remains unclear, but, as noted above, platelet turnover studies showing normal or reduced thrombopoiesis despite increased platelet destruction are consistent with intramedullary antibody effects (18, 20, 21, 24).

## Immune Complexes

Circulating immune complexes in chronic ITP have been described by some investigators (49–51) but not by others (52, 53). One group noted platelet proteins in the immune complexes, but found no correlation between the level of complexes and the platelet count (51), although others noted such a correlation (49, 50). Although it seems likely that immune complexes occur in chronic ITP, it is unlikely that they are important in the pathogenesis.

## Sites of Antibody Production

The spleen is an important site of antiplatelet antibody production in chronic ITP (33, 34). Splenic cells from ITP individuals produce 5 to 6 times more IgG in culture than control cells; a portion of the IgG produced binds specifically to both autologous and homologous platelets (33). The production of IgG by marrow cells from individuals with chronic ITP is also increased, and platelet-specific IgG could be detected in nine of the 20 chronic ITP marrow samples studied (54).

## Cell-Mediated Immunity (CMI)

Studies are sparse in this area. Two groups noted blastic transformation of ITP lymphocytes after exposure to autologous platelets and interpreted these results as evidence for CMI activation (55, 56). Since normal lymphocytes transform when incubated with normal platelets sensitized with ITP serum (57), this transformation may be due to ITP lymphocytes reacting to immune complexes on the ITP platelets rather than CMI.

Migration inhibition factor (MIF) as a manifestation of CMI has also been studied. Clancy noted that autologous platelets inhibited migration of ITP lymphocytes from capillary tubes suggesting MIF production (58). Morimoto et al provided the best evidence for CMI in chronic ITP. They incubated ITP lymphocytes with and without platelets and then studied the inhibition properties of the supernatant fluid. Samples from platelet-containing cultures of six of nine individuals with severe ITP inhibited macrophage migration, while samples from individuals with mild ITP, heavily transfused individuals, or control subjects did not (59).

Activation of CMI may also result in T cell–dependent cytotoxicity of target platelets; attempts by two groups to demonstrate this have given variable results (60, 61).

## Platelet Antigens

Approximately 75% of platelet autoantigens lie on either the platelet GP IIb/IIIa or GP Ib/IX complexes (41, 62); in the other 25% it seems likely that other membrane proteins are involved since alloantibodies bind to antigens localized to other proteins (e.g., Br antigen on GP Ia-IIa [63]). There is also evidence that some ITP antibodies bind to glycolipids (64).

Localization of the antigenic epitopes has only recently been investigated. Earlier studies showed that plasma anti-GP IIb/IIIa autoantibodies, from about 15% of ITP individuals, react with the carboxyterminal region (C-terminus) of GP IIIa (65). Since this region of GP IIIa is probably in the cytoplasm, these antibodies are more likely the result of platelet destruction by antibodies directed to surface antigens with resulting exposure of cytoplasmic antigens to the immune system. This

hypothesis is supported by subsequent studies showing that autoantibodies eluted from the individuals' platelets (platelet-associated autoantibodies), including individuals with plasma anti–C-terminus autoantibody, react with epitopes located on other areas of the GP IIb/IIIa complex (66). These platelet-associated antibodies could be directed to antigens located on GP IIb or GP IIIa or to antigenic sites on the GP IIb/IIIa complex.

Other laboratories have also evaluated epitope location. Kekomaki et al have reported that plasma autoantibodies from 14 of 31 chronic ITP individuals would bind to a 50-kD cysteine-rich region of GP IIIa. They also noted positive results in six of 18 plasma samples from individuals with nonimmune thrombocytopenia (67). He et al also studied plasma antibodies from ITP individuals. Of 50 ITP plasmas, they found 83, 81, 38, and 28% were positive against GP Ib/IX, GP IIb/IIIa, GP IV, and GP Ia/IIa, respectively. Of the positive individuals, 51% had IgG and IgA antibodies, 13% had IgG alone, 17% had IgA alone, and the remainder had IgM antibody with either IgG, IgA, or both. Using adsorption techniques, they determined that there were antibodies against both extracellular and cytosolic regions of GP IIb/IIIa or GP Ib (68).

More recent studies show that most platelet-associated anti-GP IIb/IIIa autoantibodies from chronic ITP individuals depend on a conformationally intact GP IIb/IIIa complex for maximal binding. In these studies antibodies were preincubated with purified intact GP IIb/IIIa, EDTA-dissociated GP IIb/IIIa, GP IIIa, or GP IIb, and then residual antibody was measured in an antigen capture assay. In every case, intact GP IIb/IIIa resulted in greater inhibition of antibody binding than the EDTA-dissociated complex and little inhibition was noted using either GP IIb or GP IIIa. These results suggested that platelet-associated anti-GP IIb/IIIa autoantibodies in chronic ITP are frequently directed to cation-dependent conformational antigens (69). These conformational antigens could be dependent on a conformationally intact complex or located near the calcium-binding sites on either GP IIb or GP IIIa. The latter possibility seems less likely in view of studies evaluating antibody binding to a panel of large recombinant peptides that span the GP IIIa molecule. Only one of 33 ITP platelet-associated autoantibodies showed binding to any region of GP IIIa (70). These results suggest that GP IIb/IIIa antigenic epitopes that react with platelet-associated antibodies from ITP individuals are rarely localized to GP IIIa alone but probably require a conformationally intact GP IIb/IIIa complex or bind to antigens near the calcium binding sites on GP IIb.

## The Immune Response

The proposed immune response sequence is shown in Fig. 30.1. The initial antigenic response should occur either in the spleen, which monitors the intravascular

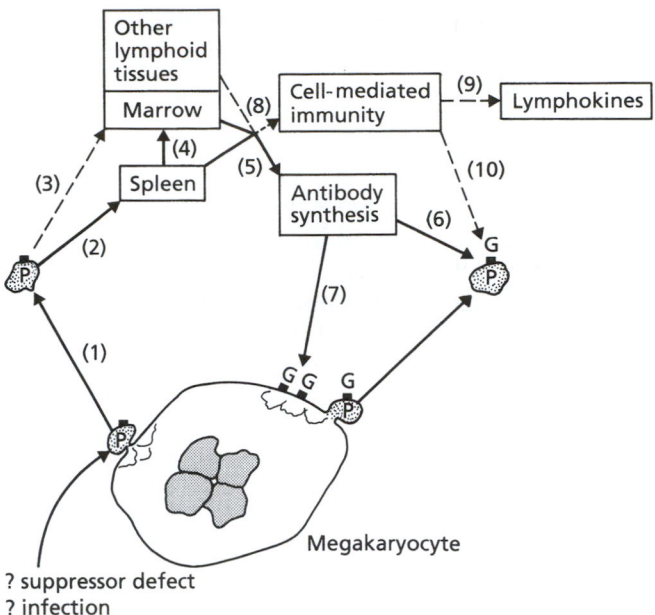

**FIGURE 30.1.** The immune response in chronic immune thrombocytopenic purpura. A platelet-associated antigen—solid rectangle attached to platelet (P)—develops; this antigen may be either a platelet autoantigen or a tightly adherent native or foreign molecule (1). Since the platelet is intravascular, the initial antigenic stimulation and lymphoid proliferation occur in the spleen (2) and conceivably the bone marrow (3). In time, antigen-specific memory cells develop, circulate, and allow a more generalized response (4). Antiplatelet antibody synthesis occurs initially in the spleen and later in the bone marrow and possibly other lymphoid organs (5). The IgG antiplatelet antibody (G) binds to platelet-associated antigen (6), causing platelet destruction. In addition, the antibody binds to megakaryocyte-associated antigen (solid rectangle attached to megakaryocyte) (7) and may suppress thrombopoiesis. Concurrent activation of cell-mediated immunity may occur (8), with resultant lymphokine production (9) and possible cell-mediated toxicity to platelet (10). Solid lines represent reactions with solid experimental support; broken lines show proposed reactions with either preliminary or no experimental support. (Adapted with permission from McMillan R. Chronic idiopathic thrombocytopenic purpura [Review]. N Engl J Med 1981;304:1135–1147.)

space, or in the bone marrow where megakaryocytes or intramedullary platelets could stimulate a response. Initially, the spleen is probably more important since, in animal studies, it is the primary organ involved in responding to intravascular antigens, while the marrow assumes greater importance later in the immune response (71). These animal studies are consistent with the observations in chronic ITP where the spleen is a major antibody production site (33, 34, 72); in some cases it may be the only site in view of the permanent return of platelet-associated IgG (73–75), antigen-specific anti-

body (76), and platelet kinetic values (77) to normal in some individuals after surgery.

Obviously, there must be other antibody production sites since antibody may persist postsplenectomy (75, 76). The bone marrow is the most likely site of residual antibody production (54). The observation that individuals with long-standing ITP are less likely to respond to splenectomy (78) suggests that circulating memory cells have permitted a more generalized immune response.

## Immune Regulation (79)

Since chronic ITP is an autoimmune disorder manifested by production of antiplatelet autoantibodies, defective immunoregulation must be present. Normally, the immune system is carefully regulated. Two antigenically distinct T cell populations, CD4+ helper-inducer cells and CD8+ suppressor-cytotoxic cells, permit a controlled antigenic response. These two cell types and their subpopulations are formed during the course of T-cell maturation in the thymus. Immature T cells (CD4-CD8), produced in the bone marrow, migrate to the thymus, and during their maturation they gain or lose a variety of surface proteins and synthesize a functional T cell receptor capable of responding to antigen if presented by the appropriate major histocompatibility complex (MHC) molecule. Immature T cells containing self-reactive receptors are either eliminated (thymic deletion) (80) or rendered tolerant (thymic anergy) (81) during the CD4+ CD8+ intermediate thymic maturation stage. During the final stage of maturation, T cells lose either the CD8 or CD4 antigen and are released into the circulation as either CD4+ inducer cells or CD8+ suppressor-cytotoxic cells.

In the periphery, CD4+ inducer T cells react with processed antigen bound to MHC class II molecules on antigen presenting cells (macrophages, B cells). Once activated, one population of these cells (helper-inducer cells) stimulates both the proliferation and differentiation of antigen-specific B cells into antibody-producing plasma cells and the expansion of CD8+ cytotoxic T cells, which are activated by antigen bound to MHC class I molecules. Another CD4+ population (suppressor-inducer cells) stimulates expansion of antigen-MHC class I activated CD8+ suppressor cells, which suppress both humoral and cell-mediated immune responses, preventing overreaction to a stimulus. In addition, the development of anti-idiotypic antibodies to the variable region of specific antibodies is also althought to be involved in the down-regulation of the immune response (82). Autoimmunity results from a breakdown at some level of this immunoregulatory network (83).

Over the past few years, there have been several studies on immunoregulation in chronic ITP; these have been recently reviewed (84). Interpretation of the results is somewhat difficult because of the following: (a) the relatively small numbers of individuals studied, (b) the variability of individual ages and disease severity, (c) the inclusion of treated and untreated individuals in some studies, and (d) the drawing of conclusions from the study of peripheral blood cells which may not reflect what is happening throughout the immune system.

Early studies, showing increased *in vitro* immunoglobulin production by ITP splenic (72) and blood (85–87) cells, suggested defective regulation of antibody synthesis. There is mounting evidence that this defect is in suppressor T cell activity. Trent et al reported that T lymphocytes from most chronic ITP individuals show decreased suppressor cell activity when cultured with either autologous or homologous B cells; conversely, ITP B lymphocytes respond to suppression by normal T cells (85). More recent studies (87) show that *in vitro* incubation of ITP lymphocytes with platelets results in lymphocyte activation, manifested by [³H] incorporation, and increased production of IL-2. Examination of the circulating lymphocyte phenotypes in this same group of individuals showed a reduction of CD4 + suppressor-inducer cells and an increase in CD4 + helper-inducer cells, DR + activated T cells, and B cells. The decrease in CD4 + suppressor-inducer cells is consistent with observations showing a diminished autologous, mixed lymphocyte reaction in chronic ITP (88–90). Other studies have shown reduced suppression of pokeweed mitogen–induced IgG production by T cells stimulated in the AMLR reaction or by concanavalin A (90).

Additional studies, which may shed light on the pathogenesis of ITP, show the following: increased numbers of circulating double labeled (CD4 + CD8 +) lymphocytes (91, 92), consistent with imperfect thymic deletion of self-reactive cells; increased numbers of both blood and splenic CD5 + B cells (87, 93), which in two individuals produced platelet-bindable IgM (93), and the presence of clonal B-cell populations in 10 of 11 individuals (94). The natural-killer cell subset (CD56 + CD3-) was found increased by one group (95) and normal by another (96); however, the latter group noted a marked decrease in killer cell activity. The relevance of this to disease pathogenesis is presently not known although these cells may be involved in B cell regulation (suppression of antibody production) (86).

Multiple other studies have evaluated T cells, B cells, T cell:B cell ratios, and T or B cell subsets with variable results, although three studies show an increased number of activated T cells (DR + or CD25 +) (87, 89, 97). Most studies show a normal response to polyclonal mitogens such as phytohemagglutinin (PHA), although one group noted a decreased response to the membrane stimulators PHA and anti-CD3 monoclonal antibody, as well as to the intracytoplasmic stimulator phorbol myristate acetate (98).

## Platelet Destruction

Platelet destruction in chronic ITP is due to antibody binding to the platelet autoantigen, with or without complement activation, followed by platelet phagocytosis or lysis (Fig. 30.2). Platelet phagocytosis has been demonstrated by electron microscopy (99, 100) and by *in vitro* studies (101–103) and has been supported by *in vivo* studies employing reticuloendothelial blockade using either red cell stroma (32) or monoclonal anti–Fc receptor antibody (104). Macrophage-mediated platelet destruction in ITP may be modulated by macrophage colony–stimulating factor (M-GCSF); plasma levels of this factor are increased in individuals with ITP (105).

Phagocytosis may be triggered by either the Fc portion of the IgG molecule or by complement activation with C3b fixation to the cell surface (106). The Fc mechanism is clearly important in ITP since increased PAIgG (4) and antigen-specific antibody (41) are demonstrable on ITP platelets and the quantity correlates with both platelet survival (22) and the degree of thrombocytopenia (73, 74, 76).

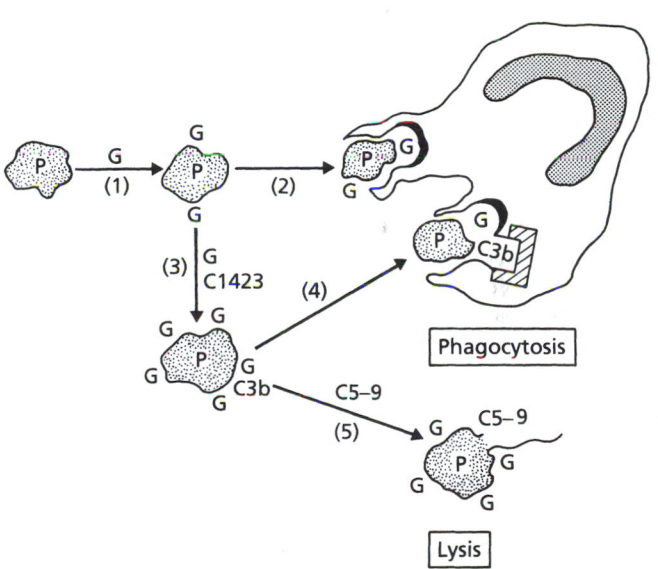

**FIGURE 30.2.** Antiplatelet-antibody–induced destruction of platelets (P) in chronic immune thrombocytopenic purpura. IgG antibody (G) binds to platelet-associated antigen (1), resulting in phagocytosis by means of the macrophage Fc receptor (2). With further IgG binding, an IgG doublet is formed, permitting complement activation with fixation of C3b to the platelet surface (3). This process permits more efficient phagocytosis through both the macrophage Fc and C3b receptors (4). In individuals with severe disease, complement-induced lysis may also occur (5). Solid areas of the macrophage indicate Fc receptors, the hatched area indicates a C3b receptor, and figures without parentheses indicate complement components. (Adapted with permission from McMillan R. Chronic idiopathic thrombocytopenic purpura [Review]. N Engl J Med 1981;304:1135–1147.)

It seems likely that complement also has a role. Hauch and Rosse reported increased platelet-associated C3 on ITP platelets; the amount correlated with antibody levels (107). This was confirmed by other groups (108, 109), and, more recently, increased platelet-associated C4 and C9 have been reported (109). *In vitro* studies show binding of C4 and C3 followed by platelet lysis after incubation of platelets with individual plasma followed by fresh serum (110). These *in vivo* and *in vitro* results suggest a role for complement in some ITP individuals. If so, the degree of complement activation may be important since, in experimental systems using anti-RBC antibodies, the fixation of only a few molecules of C3 on the cell surface markedly increases phagocyte efficiency (111).

For optimal platelet destruction there must be sufficient antigen (platelets), autoantibody, and phagocytic cells under conditions that allow time for antibody binding and phagocytosis. The splenic milieu is optimal for all these functions (72). About one-third of the platelet mass is present in the spleen at all times (11), and the local production of antiplatelet antibody (72) would subject the intrasplenic platelets to antibody concentrations much higher than those in the plasma. These sensitized platelets would then circulate slowly through the dense reticular network of the spleen, which is rich in phagocytic cells.

By contrast, the liver, although a more efficient phagocytic organ (112), contains no intraorgan platelet pool, produces little or no local antibody, and has a rapid circulation. The liver assumes importance in severe disease, which results in heavily sensitized platelets that can be removed by the liver's efficient reticuloendothelial system (17, 32).

Finally, the bone marrow has a resident megakaryocyte and platelet population and is a likely source of local antibody production (54). Since the antibody binds to platelets and megakaryocytes (35), both inhibition of thrombopoiesis and intramedullary platelet destruction could be expected. Recent platelet kinetic studies, showing decreased platelet delivery into the blood stream, as measured by platelet turnover, in a large percentage of ITP individuals suggest that intramedullary events may be important in many individuals (18, 20, 21, 24).

## CLINICAL COURSE

The diagnosis of chronic ITP is one of exclusion and is based on the following criteria described by the ITP Practice Guidelines Panel of the American Society of Hematology: individuals must have thrombocytopenia without associated leukocyte abnormalities or anemia (unless due to bleeding secondary to thrombocytopenia) and absence of diseases associated with immune thrombocytopenia such as collagen vascular disease, lymphoproliferative disorders, HIV positivity, etcetera (113).

Patients with chronic ITP most commonly present with a history of bruising and petechiae, but may also bleed from mucosal surfaces or be asymptomatic. Symptoms at presentation may be acute, but have usually been present for some time and occasionally for years. Petechiae and purpuric lesions may occur anywhere, although they are most commonly on the distal extremities. Mucosal bleeding, except for menorrhagia (epistaxis, oral hemorrhagic bullae, gastrointestinal or genitourinary bleeding) suggests extremely low platelet counts and the danger of central nervous system (CNS) bleeding. Physical examination is normal except for petechiae and purpura. Significant splenomegaly is unusual in chronic ITP; its presence suggests an alternate diagnosis.

## LABORATORY EVALUATION

The initial evaluation of thrombocytopenic individuals requires a complete blood count, a platelet count, and examination of the blood smear. In individuals with chronic ITP, the blood counts are normal except for thrombocytopenia. Anemia, if present is due either to blood loss or to an associated Coombs-positive hemolytic anemia. The blood smear shows an increased percentage of large platelets that can be quantitated by measuring diameter or volume (1). In addition, examination of the blood smear allows other conditions such as pseudothrombocytopenia, thrombotic thrombocytopenic purpura, etc., to be ruled out.

As recommended by the ITP Practice Guidelines Panel of the American Society of Hematology, bone marrow evaluation is not necessary for diagnosis, unless the individual has an atypical presentation or is older (>60 years old) to rule out myelodysplasia (113). Bone marrow examination in ITP individuals shows normal granulocytic and erythroid elements. Megakaryocytes, if counted, are increased when compared with normal marrows; in general they are larger and less mature and show little or no platelet budding.

The spleen in chronic ITP contains large numbers of lymphatic nodules with reactive germinal centers and marginal zones with large numbers of vessels surrounded by plasma cells consistent with active antibody production. Platelets, in varying stages of degradation are seen in the cords, particularly in the marginal zone, and are present both extracellularly and within the cytoplasm of macrophages (100).

## EVALUATION OF ANTIPLATELET ANTIBODY

Antiplatelet antibodies can be demonstrated in most individuals with ITP. However, as recommended by the ITP Practice Guidelines Panel of the American Society of Hematology, their measurement is not required for diagnosis, but their evaluation is not inappropriate (113). Platelet-associated IgG (PAIgG) is increased in about 90% of chronic ITP individuals, and plasma antibodies measured by indirect PAIgG are increased in about one-half (4, 114). However, PAIgG is also increased in many individuals with thrombocytopenia of other causes and is not a specific diagnostic test for chronic ITP (115, 116). Antigen-specific tests for platelet-associated and plasma anti-GP IIb/IIIa and/or anti-GP Ib/IX autoantibodies are positive in 75 and 45%, respectively, and appear more specific for autoantibodies (41, 42, 44, 62). However, they are also positive in other disorders such as collagen vascular disease and lymphoproliferative disorders with immune thrombocytopenia, which may also be due to autoantibodies (117). In the individual ITP individual, these antiglycoprotein autoantibodies reflect the therapeutic response (76, 118).

## DIFFERENTIAL DIAGNOSIS

The diagnosis of chronic ITP is one of exclusion. Disorders associated with decreased platelet production or marrow infiltration (e.g., aplastic anemia, acute leukemia) can be ruled out by blood counts and marrow evaluation, and diseases of abnormal platelet distribution (e.g., congestive splenomegaly) manifest with splenomegaly. Thrombocytopenia due to drugs (e.g., quinine, quinidine), sepsis, thrombotic thrombocytopenic purpura, and disseminated intravascular coagulation, as well as secondary thrombocytopenia related to collagen vascular disease, lymphoproliferative disorders, and infections (particularly HIV), can be ruled out by careful evaluation of the individual's history and performing the appropriate laboratory studies.

## PROGNOSIS

Some individuals either have stable disease with a platelet count >40,000 to 50,000/μL or remit spontaneously. This occurred in 58 of 1212 individuals (4.8%) (119). No treatment is indicated in these individuals. Approximately 75% of individuals attain a complete remission with either corticosteroids or splenectomy (see below). The mortality rate has been estimated from two large individual groups as 3.7% (119) and 4.5% (120). In individuals refractory to both corticosteroids and splenectomy, the mortality rate was 16.5% (119).

## THERAPY (113, 119, 121–124)

The results of the commonly used treatments are summarized in Table 30.4, and the doses and side effects of therapy are summarized in Table 30.5.

### Emergency Treatment

In individuals with severe mucosal bleeding or suspected CNS bleeding or in those who require urgent surgery, a rapid increase in the platelet count can be obtained with platelet transfusion (6 to 8 random units or a plateletpheresis) combined with either intravenous gamma globulin (IVIgG) or "industrial strength" corticosteroids.

### Intravenous Gammaglobulin

Give 0.5 to 1.0 g/kg i.v. followed by a platelet transfusion; this therapy can be repeated (125). Side effects are rare and limited to headache and local phlebitis. HIV conversion has not been reported with IVIgG use, although there have been cases of hepatitis C. IVIgG is extremely expensive and should be used judiciously. Oral corticosteroids (see below) should be given concomitantly.

### Methylprednisolone

Give 1.0 g i.v. daily for 3 days (126) followed by a platelet transfusion after the first dose. The serum potassium must be normal before using this treatment. Osteoporosis with compression fractures may be a problem if used frequently, particularly in young individuals.

When high-dose steroids, IVIgG, and standard-dose steroids were compared, high-dose steroids were as effective as IVIgG in both the frequency and speed of response. Oral steroids, although initially less effective, gave comparable results at 3 and 4 weeks (126). Since the ultimate response rate with IVIgG and high-dose steroids was no better than that of standard-dose steroids, they are only indicated for the emergency management of a life-threatening situation.

### Plasmapheresis

Plasma exchange (3 liter exchange daily for 3 to 5 days) may occasionally be useful, although this is both expensive and technically difficult in a severely thrombocytopenic individual. It is rarely indicated.

### Splenectomy

Rarely, severe bleeding persists despite the above measures. In this situation emergency splenectomy is indicated. It is recommended prior to craniotomy if CNS bleeding has occurred.

### Therapy for CNS Bleeding

If CNS bleeding is suspected, a CT scan or sonogram (young children) should be obtained to localize the bleeding site. If bleeding into the posterior compartment is noted, IgG infusion (1 g/kg) and platelet transfusions should be given and an emergency splenectomy followed by a craniotomy should be performed. Periodic IVIgG and platelet transfusions should be continued for at least 7 days postoperatively with the aim of a platelet count >50,000/μL. If bleeding is hemispheric, the need

**TABLE 30.4.** Response to Therapy in Individuals With Chronic Immune Thrombocytopenic Purpura

| Treatment | No. Individuals | Response[a] | | | Follow-Up (years) |
|---|---|---|---|---|---|
| | | CR/Excellent | PR/Good | NR/Poor | |
| Corticosteroids | 1420 | 418 (29.5) | 216 (15)[b] | 788 (55.5) | 0.5–20 |
| Splenectomy | 669 | 401 (59.9)[c] | 82 (12.3) | 186 (27.8) | 0.5–20 |
| Vinca Alkaloids | | | | | |
|   Pulse therapy | 96 | 11 (11.5) | 35 (36.4)[b] | 50 (52.1) | 0.5–6 |
|   Slow infusion | 59 | 17 (28.8) | 31 (52.5)[b] | 11 (18.7) | 0.5–2 |
| Danazol | 125 | 30 (24.0) | 21 (16.8) | 74 (59.2) | 0.1–1.2 |
| Cyclophosphamide | 145 | 54 (37.2) | 39 (26.9) | 52 (35.9) | 1.0–9 |
| Azathioprine | 127 | 40 (31) | 30 (23) | 58 (45) | 0.5–4 |

*Adapted with permission from Berchtold P, McMillan R. Therapy of chronic idiopathic thrombocytopenic purpura in adults. Blood 1989; 74:2309–2317.*

[a] *Data are expressed as number of individuals responding (percent response). CR, complete response, normal platelet count for the duration of observation; PR, partial response, platelet count >50,000/μL for any duration; NR, no response, platelet count <50,000/μL. In the case of danazol, different criteria are used: Excellent, platelet count >100,000/μL for more than 2 months; Good, platelet count >50,000/μL for more than 2 months; and Poor (all others).*

[b] *Most responses were transient, and relapse occurred on tapering the drug (corticosteroids) or with time (vinca alkaloids).*

[c] *Splenectomy resulted in a normal platelet count in 468 of 669 (66.7%) individuals with chronic ITP; 67 of these relapsed resulting in a stable remission rate of 59.9%.*

for surgery depends on the neurologic status and response to treatment.

## Initial Specific Treatment

Initial treatment is aimed at obtaining a complete response. If this is unsuccessful, subsequent therapy is directed to the maintenance of "safe" platelet counts (>20,000 to 30,000/μL). Table 30.4 summarizes the results, which will be discussed. The following responses are defined: complete—platelet count becomes normal; partial—platelet count increases to >50,000/μL; no response—platelet count increases to <50,000/μL.

## Stable Disease or Spontaneous Remission

About 5% of individuals have stable disease with platelet counts >30,000 to 50,000/μL or remit spontaneously (119). These individuals require no treatment.

## Corticosteroids

Corticosteroids are advised as the initial therapy in chronic ITP. About one-half of the individuals who attain normal platelet counts do so within 4 weeks and 90% within 6 weeks. One report noted that all individuals who obtained a permanent remission with steroids had platelet counts >50,000/μL within 4 weeks (127). If relapse occurs after an initial response, subsequent therapy is unlikely to induce a complete response. Persistent complete and partial response rates in 1420 individuals (119, 124) averaged 29.5 and 15.0%, respectively,

with follow-up ranging from >6 months to more than 5 years (see Table 30.4). Higher remission percentages were noted in reports with shorter follow-up intervals. The true long-term complete remission rate is probably about 5 to 10%, and many people in the field believe that complete responders may have other causes of thrombocytopenia (e.g., drugs, viral illness).

Prednisone, 1 mg/kg/day, is given initially. If the platelet count is <50,000/μL at 4 weeks or is less than normal at 6 weeks, a complete response is unlikely and other treatment should be given. In individuals who develop normal counts, prednisone should be tapered over several weeks (e.g., decrease 20 mg/day until dose is 40 mg/day; decrease by 10 mg/day until dose is 20 mg/day; and decrease 5 mg/day until off therapy). If relapse occurs, additional therapy is required. Prophylactic antacids or H2 blockers should be given, and the serum potassium should be monitored. Side effects include cushingoid facies, fluid retention, gastric hyperacidity, steroid psychosis, osteoporosis, and the risk of infection.

A recent alternative method of giving corticosteroids has been reported (128). Pulsed dexamethasone (40 mg/day for 4 days every 4 weeks for 6 cycles) was given to four individuals prior to splenectomy. All individuals achieved platelet counts >100,000/μL, which persisted for the follow-up period. A larger study is needed to confirm these findings.

## Splenectomy

Splenectomy results in the highest cure rate and is indicated early in the disease if steroids do not result in a

**TABLE 30.5.**  Characteristics of the Treatments Used in Chronic ITP

| Therapy | Dose | Side Effects |
| --- | --- | --- |
| **Initial/emergency therapy** | | |
| Gammaglobulin emergency | 1.0 g/kg/day plus platelets × 1–2 | Headache, fever, rare fatal thrombosis in elderly individuals; hepatitis C is reported. |
| Corticosteroids | | |
|   Emergency | Methylprednisolone 1.0 g/day × 3 plus platelets | Hypokalemia, gastric upset, sodium and fluid retention, weight gain, hyperglycemia, hypertension, myopathy, osteoporosis, increased infection risk, psychosis. |
|   Standard | Prednisone 1 mg/kg/day—taper | Hypokalemia, gastric upset, sodium and fluid retention, weight gain, hyperglycemia, hypertension, myopathy, osteoporosis, increased infection risk, psychosis. |
| Splenectomy | | Overwhelming sepsis (rare). |
| **Refractory individuals**[a] | | |
| *Level 1 therapy* | | |
|   Prednisone | 1 mg/kg p.o. qd—taper | Hypokalemia, gastric upset, sodium and fluid retention, weight gain, hyperglycemia, hypertension, myopathy, osteoporosis, increased infection risk, psychosis. |
|   Dexamethasone | 40 mg p.o. qd × 4 days every 4 weeks × 6 cycles | Same as for prednisone. |
|   Vincristine | 1–2 mg i.v./week × 4–6 doses | Peripheral neuropathy, alopecia, constipation, local corrosive effects if extravasated. |
|   Danazol | 200 mg p.o. qid | Weight gain, fluid retention, seborrhea, hirsutism, vocal changes, amenorrhea, acne, headache, liver toxicity, thrombocytopenia, erythema multiforme. |
|   Colchicine | 0.6 mg p.o. tid | Diarrhea (may limit therapy), nausea, vomiting. |
|   Dapsone | 75–100 mg p.o. qd | Hemolysis, agranulocytosis, aplastic anemia, exfoliative dermatitis, toxic hepatitis, choleostatic jaundice, peripheral neuropathy. |
| *Level 2 therapy* | | |
|   Staph A column | 6 treatments | Generalized pain, fever, chills, rash, nausea, vomiting, respiratory distress, hives, diarrhea, dizziness, tachycardia, and severe generalized vasculitis. |
|   Cyclophosphamide | 150 mg p.o. qd | Cytopenias, hemorrhagic cystitis, GI symptoms, sterility, secondary malignancies.[b] |
|   Azathioprine | 150 mg p.o. qd | Cytopenias, GI symptoms, secondary malignancies.[b] |
| *Level 3 therapy* | | |
|   High-dose cyclophosphamide | 1.0–1.5 g/m² i.v. every 4 weeks | Cytopenias, hemorrhagic cystitis, GI symptoms, alopecia, sterility, myocardiopathy, secondary malignancies.[b] |
|   Combination chemotherapy | See below[c] | Cytopenias, hemorrhagic cystitis, alopecia, dermatitis, analphalaxis, GI symptoms, sterility, myocardiopathy, mucusitis, secondary malignancies.[b] |
| *Level 4 therapy* | | |
|   Interferon alpha-2b | 3 million units s.c. three times a week for 12 doses | "Flu like" symptoms, fever, cytopenias, cardiomyopathy, hypotension, tachycardia, depression, confusion, hepatotoxicity, respiratory insufficiency. |
|   Gamma globulin | 0.5–1.0 g/kg i.v. as needed | Headache, fever, rare fatal thrombosis in elderly individuals; hepatitis C is reported. |
|   Vinblastine | 5–10 mg i.v./week | Leukopenia, alopecia, constipation, local corrosive effects if extravasated. |
|   Cyclosporine | 1.25–2.5 mg/kg p.o. bid | Renal insufficiency, hepatotoxicity, hypertension, tremor, hirsutism, gum hyperplasia, hypomagnesemia, secondary malignancies.[b] |

p.o., by mouth; i.v., intravenous; s.c., subcutaneously; qd, daily; bid, 2 times daily; tid, 3 times daily; qid, 4 times daily.

[a] Refractory individuals: individuals who have failed to respond to standard dose prednisone and splenectomy.

[b] Lymphoproliferative disorders or acute leukemia have occurred in individuals receiving these drugs.

[c] Cyclophosphamide 750 mg/m² i.v. (days 1 and 8); prednisone 40 mg/m² (days 1–14); and etoposide 100 mg/m² (days 14, 15, and 16).

remission. Splenectomy induced a complete response in 468 of 669 (66.7%) individuals; 67 (14.3%) of these relapsed giving a stable remission rate of 59.9%. An additional 12.3% of individuals achieved a stable partial response (seeTable 30.4) (119, 124). Therefore 72.2% of the individuals required no additional treatment. After surgery, the platelet count increases rapidly with normal counts appearing within 2 weeks in most responding individuals. Most relapses occur within a few months after surgery. Youth, a short disease duration, and an increase in the platelet count to >400,000/μL are good prognostic signs. Some groups have noted a correlation between steroid and splenectomy response (129); other groups have not (127, 130). Prior to surgery, individuals should be immunized with pneumococcal, *Haemophilus influenzae*, and meningococcal vaccines (131). In individuals with severe thrombocytopenia, the steroid dose should be increased or IVIgG should be given to increase the platelet count prior to surgery. Platelet transfusions should not be given prophylactically or during surgery unless undue bleeding occurs. Laparoscopic splenectomy may be preferable in experienced hands (132).

Surgical mortality in skilled hands should approach zero. Although overwhelming sepsis in splenectomized individuals occurs frequently in young children (see below), this is rare in adults and should not influence the recommendation of surgery.

### Accessory Spleens

Some ITP individuals, who fail splenectomy, have an accessory spleen; this is not ruled out by the presence of Howell-Jolly bodies. Of 28 individuals in 4 reports, 13 attained a complete remission after removal of the accessory spleen. Follow-up ranged from a few months to several years (119). A late relapse is more often associated with successful accessory splenectomy. All individuals with a postsplenectomy relapse should be evaluated for an accessory spleen.

## Management of Refractory Individuals

Studies to support a treatment approach in refractory individuals are unsatisfactory (113), and the approach described here is based on the author's experience and biases (124). Therapy is arbitrarily divided into four levels depending on either the severity of treatment-related side effects (levels 1–3) or the level of demonstrable effectiveness and the expense of the treatment (level 4).

### Level 1 Therapy

These treatments have moderate risk; they should be tried in the order listed. Criteria for continuing or stopping the therapy are discussed.

### Corticosteroids

Prednisone (1 mg/kg/day followed by tapering) is the drug of choice if safe counts can be maintained on doses

acceptable for long-term use (5 to 10 mg/day). If this is not possible, pulsed dexamethasone, 40 mg/day for 4 days every 28 days for 6 cycles should be given. Preliminary results of small studies report results ranging from excellent to poor (128, 133, 134). Individuals should be given at least 4 cycles before abandoning therapy and responding individuals should receive all 6 courses even if counts become normal. Individuals who fail corticosteroids and require treatment should receive one of the following treatments. Many require concomitant corticosteroids to help maintain their platelet counts while the other agents are tried. If a response occurs, steroids should be tapered.

### Vinca Alkaloids (119, 135)

Of 96 individuals receiving vincristine or vinblastine by bolus injection, 11.5% achieved a complete response lasting from 0.5 to 6 years. A transient response was noted in 36.4% and no response in 52.1% (see Table 30.4) (119).

More recently, two other methods of administration have been tried: "vinca-loaded" platelets (136) and slow infusion (137). Since vinca alkaloids are taken up by platelets, platelets were incubated *in vitro* with vincristine or vinblastine and then infused. It was postulated that these "vinca-loaded" platelets would be sensitized with the individual's antibody and then be phagocytosed by the reticuloendothelial system (RES) with resulting macrophage and/or antigen-reactive lymphocyte destruction. Two studies noted good responses, with 11 of 25 individuals attaining complete remissions lasting from 5 to 18 months. Three other groups obtained different results with only 3 of 26 obtaining a complete remission (119). Moreover, serious side effects were noted, including severe hypotension and fever (probably related to platelet alloantibodies), neuropathy, agranulocytosis, and hepatitis. In one case, etoposide-loaded platelets resulted in a complete remission lasting >40 months (138).

Slow infusion of vinca alkaloids over 4 to 8 hours was introduced with the aim of coupling the drug and platelets *in vivo*. Two groups, whose results are included in Table 30.4, reported complete remissions in 11 of 34 individuals. In one of these studies all responding individuals had been recently diagnosed and were not truly refractory. However, in another report on 16 individuals (also included in the Table 30.4 results), only two of 12 individuals with refractory ITP (17%) obtained prolonged complete responses (one of these relapsed in 8 months), while three of four individuals with recent disease entered a remission (119). A randomized study comparing continuous infusion and pulsed vincristine showed no difference in responses (139).

For bolus therapy, vincristine 0.02 mg/kg (1 to 2 mg, maximum 2 mg) or vinblastine 0.1 mg/kg (5 to 10 mg) is given i.v. every 7 days for 4 to 6 weeks. Infusions use the same dose given over 6 to 8 hours. If a complete response does not occur over this time, therapy should be abandoned to prevent peripheral neuropathy (vincristine). Peripheral neuropathy is a serious and limiting side effect of vincristine. Other side effects include alopecia, constipation, leukopenia (vinblastine) and corrosive effects if extravasated.

## Danazol (140)

Several small studies, summarized in Table 30.4, have been published with different results. Three of the studies, included in Table 30.4 summary, have shown excellent (platelet count >100,00/μL for >2 months) or good responses (>50,000/μL) in 26 of 42 (61.9%) individuals. Conversely, four other studies included in the Table 30.4 summary noted excellent or good responses in only 14 of 54 (25.9%) individuals (119). A recent review of the Miami experience (96 individuals) reported 61.2% excellent or good responses with a mean response time of 2.7 months (range 1 week to 20 months) with 85% of responses within 4 months. This group recommended treatment for at least 10 months. Unmaintained remissions were commonly seen (23 of 30) in responders treated for greater than 1 year, while relapse was common (7 of 10) in responders receiving <6 months of treatment. Responses were more likely in older women, in individuals responsive to corticosteroids, and in individuals who had undergone splenectomy (141).

Danazol is given orally at a dose of 200 mg three or four times daily for at least 4 months, although one group advises therapy for 10 months (141). Prednisone should be given concomitantly (1 mg/kg/day) and tapered as a response occurs. Responses may occur slowly. In responders, therapy should be given for at least 1 year. Danazol causes androgenic side effects, including weight gain, seborrhea, and acne. Headache, lethargy, gastric intolerance, liver toxicity (liver function should be monitored monthly), and erythema multiforme are less commonly seen.

## Colchicine

Only one study on the use of colchicine in ITP has been published. Of 14 individuals refractory to steroids and splenectomy, three maintained normal platelet counts for 14 to 18 months with continued therapy, and one had a partial response lasting 6 months (142). Responses occurred within 8 weeks, and drug withdrawal resulted in relapse.

The initial dose is 0.6 mg orally daily; the dose should be increased by 0.6 mg/day every two weeks to a maximum of 0.6 mg p.o. three times daily. In responding individuals the dose should be tapered to the lowest dose resulting in safe platelet counts. The major side effects are gastrointestinal with diarrhea often limiting the tolerated dose. Rarely, granulocytopenia, myopathy, and neuropathy are seen.

## Dapsone

Dapsone was first used in five older individuals (68 to 87 years old) (143); each individual had received some prior form of therapy, but none had been splenectomized. All individuals responded within 45 days with peak platelet counts of 71,000 to 124,000/μL. Responses persisted for 2 to 48 months, but required that therapy be continued. There have been two subsequent reports using dapsone in 36 individuals with ITP (seven postsplenectomy) (144, 145). Of these, seven achieved platelet counts >100,000/μL and eight >50,000/μL. Follow-up in both series was less than a year in most individuals.

The recommended dose of dapsone is 75 to 100 mg p.o. daily; responses generally occur within 2 months. Hemolysis is the major side effect and is dose-dependent; this required stopping therapy in three individuals in the latter two series. Hemolysis may be severe in individuals deficient in red cell glucose-6-phosphate dehydrogenase so all individuals should be screened for this prior to therapy.

## Level 2 Therapy

Since these treatments have more serious toxicities, they should be given only when potentially dangerous platelet counts (10, 000 to 15, 000/μL) and/or mucosal bleeding are present. The role of staphylococcal-A immunoadsorption remains controversial, and some physicians feel strongly that its side effects outweigh the benefits (146). If used, it should be tried prior to cyclophosphamide and azathioprine since the best results are reported to occur in individuals with more recent disease onset and higher platelet counts.

## Staphylococcal Protein A-Immunoadsorption Column

A single, large, multiinstitutional study has been published (147). Of 72 individuals (68 with chronic ITP and four with HIV-ITP), 18 good responses (>100,000/μL) and 15 fair responses (>50,000/μL) were seen; two of the good and five of the fair responses were transient. A durable response rate (mean follow-up of 8 months) was noted in 36%. Responses occurred within 4 weeks. Forty-nine of the chronic ITP individuals had a splenectomy prior to therapy. In this group 12 achieved a good response (none relapsed) and eight a fair response (two relapsed) for a response rate of 36.7%. Individuals with higher pretherapy counts (>20,000/μL) did better than those with low counts.

Side effects include generalized pain (26%), fever (21%), chills (16%), and rash (11%); less commonly noted are nausea, vomiting, respiratory distress, hives, diarrhea, dizziness, and tachycardia. In the large series described above, treatment of three of 72 individuals was stopped due to side effects. Another group (146) reported severe generalized vasculitis in two of five individuals treated and only one remission and concluded that "protein A silica column treatment of chronic AITP is of questionable benefit and has an unacceptably high rate of severe, generalized adverse effects."

## Cyclophosphamide (119, 148)

Four early studies reported complete, unmaintained remissions in 27 of 60 (45%) individuals with follow-up of 10 to 96 months. Recent reports have been less favorable with complete responses in only 17 of 72 individuals (23.6%) (119). Responses are more likely after splenectomy and in individuals with the recent onset of disease. For best results it should be given postsplenectomy and early in the course of the disease.

Cyclophosphamide is given orally at a dose of 1 to 2 mg/kg/day (100 to 200 mg), and the dose is adjusted to cause mild neutropenia. Responses occur within 3 months or are unlikely to occur. If a complete response is attained, the drug should be given at full dosage for 2 to 3 more months and then stopped. One group used cyclophosphamide i.v. in doses of 300 to 600 mg/m² every 3 weeks (149). Individuals treated with cyclophosphamide should drink at least 2 quarts of liquid daily to prevent hemorrhagic cystitis.

Side effects include marrow suppression (which may cause anemia or neutropenia or may accentuate the thrombocytopenia), alopecia, hemorrhagic cystitis, hepatic toxicity, and sterility. The development of secondary malignancy, particularly acute leukemia, due to therapy with alkylating agents is a well recognized complication. Although this has been reported only rarely in chronic ITP, individuals should be aware of this infrequent but usually lethal complication.

## Azathioprine (119, 150, 151)

Complete remission rates with azathioprine (31.2%) are similar to those seen with cyclophosphamide, although continued therapy is required in some cases (see Table 30.4). A recent large study of 53 individuals (151) reported 22 complete remissions (12 off drug and 10 on drug) and two partial remissions (both on drug). Responses to this agent are slow, and this same study concluded that therapy at full doses (150 mg/day) should be continued for at least 4 months before abandoning treatment. They also advised that therapy be stopped after 18 months unless no other reasonable options are available.

Initial doses are 1 to 4 mg/kg/day (200 to 400 mg) orally; the dose should be adjusted to cause mild neutropenia. The dose should be tapered slowly to the lowest dose that maintains safe platelet counts. Relapse may occur on stopping the drug. Continuation of therapy beyond 18 months should be based on considering the risk:benefit ratio.

Marrow suppression is the only common side effect, although anorexia, nausea, or vomiting is seen on occa-

sion. Secondary malignancies, particularly lymphomas, are reported using this agent for other disorders, and at least one case of acute nonlymphocytic leukemia has been described in an ITP individual.

## Level 3 Therapy

These treatments are reserved for individuals who are unresponsive to the above treatments and who have life-threatening symptoms or extremely low platelet counts (<5,000 to 10,000/μL). One approach is to give the high-dose cyclophosphamide first because it is easier and less expensive; if unsuccessful, combination chemotherapy is indicated. Toxicities and response rates of the two modalities, in the few individuals treated, are similar (152, 153).

## High-Dose Cyclophosphamide (152)

A recent report describes the use of one to four cycles of high-dose intravenous cyclophosphamide (1.0–1.5 g/m² every 4 weeks) in 20 refractory individuals (152). Of these, 10 obtained a complete response that either persisted after initial therapy (8 individuals) or after retreatment (2 individuals) with follow-up ranging from 7 months to 7 years. In addition, four had a partial response, and three of these persist (two after initial therapy and one after retreatment).

Give 1.0 to 1.5 g/m² i.v.; repeat at 4-week intervals for three to four cycles. If no response after two cycles, stop therapy. Maintain a high fluid intake (3 to 4 liters daily either p.o. or i.v. for 3 days after treatment) to prevent hemorrhagic cystitis. Monitor blood counts frequently during the first 2 weeks and at least weekly thereafter.

## Combination Chemotherapy (153)

There are no data to recommend any specific drug combination. One approach is to use the following: cyclophosphamide 750 mg/m² i.v. on days 1 and 8; prednisone 40 mg/m² on days 1 to 14; and etoposide 100 mg/m² i.v. on days 14, 15, and 16. If there is no response after two cycles, therapy should be stopped. In responding individuals six cycles should be administered even if the platelet count becomes normal with earlier cycles. At least 2 quarts of fluid should be given daily for 3 days after each cyclophosphamide dose to prevent hemorrhagic cystitis; antacids or H₂ blockers should be given during and for a week after prednisone. Blood counts should be monitored weekly. If neutropenia is severe, the etoposide dose should be reduced in subsequent cycles. Other combinations have been successful (153).

## Level 4 Therapy

These treatments are used last because either there is limited experience with their use, response rates are low, or their expense and frequency of administration weigh against their use. Many individuals require concomitant steroids.

## Interferon α-2b

Several small studies have been reported with a total of 51 individuals (154–158). Of these, 8 individuals attained normal platelet counts and 18 attained platelet counts >50,000/μL. The great majority of the responses occurred within 4 to 8 weeks, and all but a few were transient. In some cases responses occurred after completion of treatment.

Interferon α-2b is given at a dose of 3 million units s.c. three times a week for 4 weeks. There is some evidence that long-term treatment may be beneficial (159). Side effects include mild fever, flulike symptoms, and marrow suppression. One report described a individual whose thrombocytopenia worsened on interferon, and following interferon treatment she was resistant to therapy to which she had previously responded. She subsequently died of CNS bleeding (160).

## IVIgG

IVIgG is of unquestioned use in emergency situations or when a rapid, temporary increase in the platelet count is needed (161). Although most individuals obtain only a temporary response to this agent, one study reported that five of 40 individuals with refractory ITP receiving monthly maintenance IVIgG (mean total infusion of 606 g per individual) achieved a complete response, and 11 individuals developed stable disease. Responses persisted after stopping treatment with follow-up averaging 12 months (162). Although this approach is appealing due to the safety of this agent, the high cost hampers its widespread use. Before maintenance IgG can be recommended, these findings will require confirmation.

However, it is clear that some individuals, who fail all other treatments, continue to respond to IVIgG (0.5 to 1.0 g/kg as needed to prevent mucosal bleeding). Responses are transient lasting up to a few weeks. This treatment is extremely expensive and inconvenient, but it may be the only option.

Adverse effects are uncommon other than mild headache and occasionally local phlebitis. Fatal thrombotic events after IVIgG therapy have been reported in elderly individuals with severe atherosclerotic disease (163). The development of AIDS or HIV seroconversion has not occurred with IgG use (164), although hepatitis C transmission has been reported (165). However, since the introduction of solvent/detergent-treated products, this is unlikely to be a future problem.

## Vinblastine

Occasionally, in vinca-responsive individuals, vinblastine (5 to 10 mg i.v. every 1 to 4 weeks) can be used with benefit for long intervals. The side effects have been described above.

## Cyclosporine

The experience with cyclosporine is limited to case reports (166–168). Brief responses were noted in 1 to 4 weeks in three individuals, but relapse occurred shortly thereafter in each individual. Cyclosporine should be used only as an ancillary agent in severe refractory individuals.

Cyclosporine is given orally, 1.25 to 2.5 mg/kg twice daily (total dose 2.5 to 5.0 mg/kg/day). Side effects include renal insufficiency, hepatic damage, hirsutism, and secondary malignancies. Periodic serum creatinine and cyclosporine levels must be obtained and the dose adjusted as needed. In view of the serious side effects, this drug should be used cautiously and only when there are no good alternatives.

# ACUTE ITP

Acute idiopathic thrombocytopenic purpura (ITP) is a transient, mostly postinfectious disorder that is characterized by increased peripheral platelet destruction; it occurs almost exclusively in children, although a similar clinical picture is rarely seen in adults. There are several excellent reviews of this disorder (169–172). Individuals present with the abrupt onset of bruising, petechiae, and often mucosal bleeding in a previously well child. At diagnosis, epistaxis or other mucosal bleeding occurs in 10 to 30%, while hematuria or gastrointestinal bleeding is seen in <10%. Rarely, life-threatening CNS bleeding is present. In most children, thrombocytopenia occurs within 1 to 3 weeks of an infectious disease. Most commonly, the infection is a nonspecific viral (upper respiratory or gastrointestinal) or bacterial infection, but it may occur after rubella, rubeola, chickenpox, or other documented viral illnesses or may follow live virus vaccination. The incidence of acute ITP is estimated at about four per 100,000 children. The peak age is between 2 and 5 years, and there is no sex predilection. Chronic ITP, defined as thrombocytopenia persisting for more than 6 months, occurs in 10 to 15% of children althought initially to have acute ITP. The risk of chronic ITP increases with the age of the child, and, unlike acute ITP, the female:male ratio is 3:1 (169–172). Initially, there are no differentiating features between acute and chronic ITP, although the latter tends to occur more insidiously and without antecedent infection. Chronic ITP in children is an autoimmune disease comparable to the adult disorder described earlier.

## ETIOLOGY AND PATHOPHYSIOLOGY

There are few experimental data available. The observation that acute ITP often follows a viral illness suggests that the child responds to the viral antigens by antibody production and immune complex formation. Platelet destruction could result from adsorption of viral antigens onto the platelet surface followed by antibody binding or to the binding of preformed immune complexes to the platelet surface via the platelet Fc receptors. The increased PAIgG values, noted in these individuals (173) and the observation that intravenous gammaglobulin and anti-D antibody will reverse the thrombocytopenia in acute ITP (see below) are compatible with either hypothesis. The observation that individuals with ITP may respond to splenectomy (although this is rarely employed as therapy) suggests that the spleen is involved in the pathogenesis.

Alternative theories are possible. Infection could alter the platelet surface resulting in autoantibody formation against "hidden antigens," or antibodies produced against the infectious agent may cross react with constituents on the individual's platelets. There are several lines of evidence arguing for an immune-mediated mechanism operative in ITP: increased HLA-DR expression (174), defects in cellular and humoral immunity (84, 175), and specific autoantibody production (176, 177).

## LABORATORY EVALUATION

Patients have decreased platelet counts ($<30,000/\mu L$) usually in the absence of other blood abnormalities. Large, mean, platelet volume—routinely available by automated analysis—supports the diagnosis (178). Anemia, unless due to blood loss, suggests another diagnosis. Additional blood testing may be required to rule out other disorders (see differential diagnosis). If the clinical diagnosis is compelling and a rapid increase in the platelet count is noted after one infusion of IVIgG, bone marrow examination is unnecessary (179). However, if corticosteroids are considered for primary therapy, bone marrow examination is mandatory. Marrow evaluation in acute ITP shows normal or increased numbers of megakaryocytes as in chronic ITP. PAIgG levels are uniformly increased in acute ITP and tend to be higher than those in children or adults with chronic ITP with the same degree of thrombocytopenia (173). As noted earlier, PAIgG is a nonspecific assay that may reflect the presence of young platelets rather than antiplatelet antibody or immune complexes. Recent studies suggest that antigen-specific assays may be capable of distinguishing acute from chronic ITP, although additional confirmation will be required (176, 177). Neither of these studies is required for differential diagnosis or treatment decisions. Platelet survival is invariably shortened. The bleeding time may occasionally be helpful in deciding whether to observe or to treat the individual.

## DIFFERENTIAL DIAGNOSIS

The clinical picture of thrombocytopenia in a child following a recent febrile illness suggests the diagnosis of acute ITP immediately. In atypical cases, other disorders must be ruled out (Table 30.6). A decreased mean platelet volume suggests marrow hypoplasia or the Wiskott-Aldrich syndrome. If there is anemia or leukocyte abnormalities, a bone marrow examination will be required to rule out marrow diseases such as acute leukemia, aplastic anemia, myelodysplasia, lymphoma, or metastatic disease. Autoimmune hemolysis, if suspected, can be confirmed by a Coombs test. If risk factors are present for human immunodeficiency virus (HIV), antibody

---

**TABLE 30.6.**    Differential Diagnosis in Childhood Thrombocytopenia

| | Onset | MPV | -PAIgG | Coagulation | Marrow | Other |
|---|---|---|---|---|---|---|
| Destructive thrombocytopenia | | | | | | |
|   ITP | Sudden | Increased | Increased | ND | ND | |
|   Wiskott-Aldrich | Insidious | Decreased | Increased | ND | ND | |
|   HIV-ITP | Variable | Increased | Increased | ND | ND | HIV-positive |
|   DIC, TTP, HUS | Sudden | Increased | Increased | Diagnostic | ND | |
|   Hypersplenism | Insidious | Increased | ND | ND | ND | Splenomegaly |
| Decreased production | | | | | | |
|   Amegakaryocytic | Insidious | Decreased | ND | ND | Diagnostic | ± Radius |
|   Aplastic anemia | Insidious | Decreased | ND | ND | Diagnostic | |
|   Myelodysplasia | Insidious | Decreased | ND | ND | Diagnostic | |
|   Acute leukemia | Insidious | Decreased | ND | ND | Diagnostic | |
|   Lymphoma | Insidious | Decreased | ND | ND | Diagnostic | |
|   Metastatic disease | Insidious | Decreased | Variable | ND | Diagnostic | |

*DIC, disseminated intravascular coagulation; HIV, human immunodeficiency virus; HUS, hemolytic uremic syndrome; ITP, immune thrombocytopenic purpura; MPV, mean platelet volume; ND, nondiagnostic; PAIgG, platelet-associated immunoglobulin; TTP, thrombotic thrombocytopenic purpura.*

testing must be pursued. Thrombotic thrombocytopenic purpura and hemolytic uremic syndrome can be distinguished by the presence of hemolysis, a negative Coombs test, and microangiopathic red cell changes. Disseminated intravascular coagulation is associated with characteristic coagulation abnormalities. Hypersplenism is associated with splenomegaly.

## CLINICAL COURSE AND PROGNOSIS

The complete remission rate of children with ITP, with or without treatment, is 80 to 90% after 6 months and above 90% after 3 to 37 years (169–172, 180, 181). Three to five percent of these children develop chronic ITP (excluding HIV-related ITP). The children who develop chronic ITP are mostly over 7 years of age and are rarely those with postinfectious ITP. Recurrent ITP, defined as periodic episodes of thrombocytopenia at intervals of greater than 3 months, occurs in 1 to 4% of children with acute ITP (172, 182).

Intracranial hemorrhage occurs in 0.5 to 1% of hospitalized children with ITP and is fatal in one third. The complication is limited to individuals with platelet counts less than 20,000/μL (172, 183). The risk is greater during the initial days of thrombocytopenia, but can occur at any time in persistent ITP with platelet counts <20,000/μL despite treatment with corticosteroids (183) or IVIgG (184). Salicylate-containing medications or antihistamines may increase the risk (183). The other cause of death in children with ITP is postsplenectomy sepsis.

## THERAPY

The rationale for treating ITP is to increase the platelet count by interfering with platelet phagocytosis or by suppressing production of antiplatelet antibodies or immune complexes. Before 1980, corticosteroids were the conventional form of treatment. Since then, IVIgG has become an alternative possibility (184–188), especially in children with severe bleeding.

Whether to observe or treat the individual depends on the severity of the disease. The following children with acute ITP require treatment: (a) children with platelet counts <20,000/μL and those with either severe mucosal bleeding or other emergency circumstances (e.g., requiring surgery, CNS bleeding), and (b) children with higher platelet counts with special circumstances (sports, vaccinations, etc.). Children with no bleeding symptoms (petechiae and few bruises only), platelet counts >20,000/μL, and a normal bleeding time may be carefully observed without treatment (172).

## RECOMMENDED THERAPY

Treatment is indicated in children at risk of or with overt signs of bleeding. Hospitalization is required for severe bleeding regardless of the platelet count. It is also necessary for a child with mucosal bleeding and platelet counts below 20,000/μL and for a child with mild bleeding and platelet counts below 10,000/μL. Therapeutic measures in the acute management of ITP should be maintained until cessation of bleeding has occurred and the platelet counts have reached hemostatic levels (i.e., more than 20,000/μL). However, continued treatment beyond this defined point is not indicated. Moreover, it also seems unnecessary to treat individuals without signs of bleeding and with platelet counts above 20,000/μL.

The therapy of ITP focuses on measures modulating the immune response and includes intravenous immunoglobulins (IVIgG) or anti Rh (D) immunoglobulin (113, 185–190). Immunosuppressive treatment with corticosteroids (128, 191) or cytostatic agents is used as an alternative treatment strategy. In life-threatening situations the combination of IVIgG (1 g/kg per day for 1 to 2 days) and/or high-dose corticosteroids (methylprednisolone 10 to 20 mg/kg/day x 3 days) with platelet transfusion may provide rapid control of bleeding (see chronic ITP, emergency treatment, above). If the individual with long-term ITP does not respond or continues to relapse for more than 2 months after a satisfactory initial response, further workup is indicated to reevaluate the diagnosis (see Chapter 49).

The recently published practice guidelines of the American Society of Hematology (ASH) (113) are generally in accordance with these recommendations for the diagnosis and treatment of ITP (187).

## CHRONIC ITP IN CHILDREN

The approach to children with chronic ITP differs somewhat from that of the adult. Splenectomy in children before the end of puberty should be avoided because of the risk of postsplenic sepsis (172). One possible exception is severe menstrual bleeding in teenage girls with chronic ITP. Treatment in childhood chronic ITP should be limited, if possible, to either corticosteroids, IVIgG (192), or anti-D (193, 194). If splenectomy is required because of uncontrollable clinical circumstances, the individuals should receive pneumococcal vaccination and prophylactic antibiotics (195).

# DISEASE-ASSOCIATED THROMBOCYTOPENIA

Immune thrombocytopenia is associated with a variety of diseases (see Table 30.1). In some individuals thrombocytopenia is a major symptomatic feature, but in most individuals symptoms and signs of the primary disease dominate.

## COLLAGEN VASCULAR DISEASE

Systemic lupus erythematosus (SLE) is the major disease in this category, with thrombocytopenia noted in 14 to 26% of individuals (196, 197). Clinical features related to the thrombocytopenia are similar to those in chronic ITP and mirror the level of platelet reduction. Splenomegaly is not unusual. Laboratory findings show increased numbers of megakaryocytes on marrow aspirates and shortened platelet survival (1). Increased PAIgG levels are reported in SLE individuals both with and without thrombocytopenia (73, 74, 116, 198). More recently, specific autoantibodies against a variety of platelet proteins, particularly the GP IIb/IIIa complex (117, 199), and against cardiolipin (200) have been reported.

Since individuals with SLE produce a variety of autoantibodies (antinuclear, anti-DNA, anti-RBC), it seems likely that in most individuals the thrombocytopenia is another manifestation of their altered immune system. This hypothesis is supported by the presence of multiple autoantibodies in some individuals and by human-human hybridoma studies showing that immunoglobulin synthesized *in vitro* by SLE splenic cells binds to platelets (201). Therapy is similar to that of chronic ITP, although the response to splenectomy varies among investigators with some finding it quite useful (202, 203) while others report it to be less effective (204). Danazol is particularly useful both presplenectomy and postsplenectomy (205, 206). Intermittent pulsed cyclophosphamide has been found useful in individuals unresponsive to the other approaches (202, 207).

## LYMPHOPROLIFERATIVE DISORDERS AND SOLID TUMORS

Thrombocytopenia is commonly seen in individuals with lymphoproliferative disorders. In most cases this is due to decreased platelet production resulting from marrow infiltration or to the effects of treatment. However, immune thrombocytopenia is seen in some individuals, particularly individuals with chronic lymphocytic leukemia and indolent non-Hodgkin's lymphomas (208–210). Immune thrombocytopenia is also reported in Hodgkin's disease (211) and in solid tumors (212), but this is rare. Symptoms and signs reflect the severity of both the primary disease and the degree of thrombocytopenia. Splenomegaly is common. Bone marrow aspirates show adequate or increased numbers of megakaryocytes, as well as findings of the primary disease, and platelet survival is shortened (208). Platelet-associated IgG is increased in about one-quarter of individuals with lymphoproliferative disorders and thrombocytopenia, and this has been recommended as a means of diagnosing this condition (210). Recent studies have shown platelet-associated and plasma autoantibodies against platelet GP IIb/IIIa and GP Ib/IX (117).

The mechanism of the immune thrombocytopenia is not known, but the association of autoimmune hemolytic anemia with these disorders and the demonstration of antiglycoprotein autoantibodies in some of these individuals suggest an autoimmune etiology.

Therapy is similar to that of chronic ITP, although in some individuals thrombocytopenia responds to the treatment used for the primary disease.

## INFECTION

Thrombocytopenia is associated with a variety of infectious diseases (see Table 30.1).

### Viral Infection

Commonly reported infections associated with immune thrombocytopenia include rubella (213), mumps (214), mononucleosis (215), cytomegalovirus (216), and human immunodeficiency virus (HIV). Hematologic abnormalities associated with HIV infection are discussed in Chapter 48 and will not be commented on here.

Symptoms of the primary viral disease are usually well established (7 to 10 days) prior to the onset of thrombocytopenia. Thrombocytopenia is often acute and severe with symptoms of generalized purpura and severe mucosal bleeding; occasional deaths have been reported. Splenomegaly may be seen, particularly in individuals with mononucleosis and CMV infection. Increased megakaryocytes are usually noted in aspirates, although reduced or absent megakaryocytes are also reported. Thrombocytopenia usually remits spontaneously in 2 to 4 weeks, although in occasional individuals it may persist for months before remitting.

The pathogenesis is unknown, but the most reasonable explanation is either that antiviral antibody binds to either platelet-bound viruses or viral proteins, resulting in platelet destruction, or that the antibody and circulating viral antigens form complexes that bind and cause platelet destruction. These mechanisms are similar to those postulated for acute ITP and probably reflect the same syndrome. Thrombocytopenia in this setting is usually self-limited and should be treated as described with acute ITP.

### Other Infections

Thrombocytopenia is commonly seen in septicemic individuals due to either Gram-positive or Gram-negative organisms (217). The relative role of intravascular coagulation and the immune system in producing this thrombocytopenia is unknown, although increased PAIgG has been noted in these individuals and attributed to the formation of complexes composed of antibody and bacterial antigens. A similar syndrome is associated with malarial infection (218).

# REFERENCES

1. Garg SK, Amorosi EL, Karpatkin S. Use of the megathrombocyte as an index of megakaryocyte number. N Engl J Med 1971;284:11–17.
2. Mueller-Eckhardt C. Idiopathic thrombocytopenic purpura (ITP): clinical and immunologic considerations. Semin Thromb Hemost 1977;3:125–159.
3. Karpatkin S. Autoimmune thrombocytopenic purpura. Blood 1980;56:329–343.
4. McMillan R. Chronic idiopathic thrombocytopenic purpura. N Engl J Med 1981;304:1135–1147.
5. Kelton JG, Gibbons S. Autoimmune platelet destruction: idiopathic thrombocytopenic purpura. Semin Thromb Hemost 1982;8:83–104.
6. George JN, El-Harake MA, Aster RH. Thrombocytopenia due to enhanced platelet destruction by immunologic mechanisms. In: Beutler E, Lichtman MA, Coller BS, Kipps TJ, eds. Williams hematology. 5th ed. New York: McGraw-Hill, 1995; pp. 1315–1355.
7. Bottiger LE, Westerholm B. Thrombocytopenia. I. Incidence and aetiology. Acta Med Scand 1972;191:535–540.
8. The panel on Diagnostic Application of Radioisotopes in Hematology, International Committee for Standardization in Hematology. Recommended methods for radioisotope platelet survival studies. Blood 1977;50:1137–1144.
9. The panel on Diagnostic Applications of Radionuclides, International Committee for Standardization in Hematology. Recommended method for Indium-111 platelet survival studies. J Nucl Med 1988;29:564–566.
10. Aster RH. Pooling of platelets in the spleen: role of the pathogenesis of ''hypersplenic'' thrombocytopenia. J Clin Invest 1966;45:645–657.
11. Branehog I, Kutti J, Weinfeld A. Platelet survival and platelet production in idiopathic thrombocytopenic purpura (ITP). Br J Haematol 1974;27:127–143.
12. Branehog I, Weinfeld A, Roos B. The exchangeable splenic platelet pool studied with epinephrine infusion in idiopathic thrombocytopenic purpura and in individuals with splenomegaly. Br J Haematol 1973;25:239–248.
13. Aster RH, Jandl JH. Platelet sequestration in man. I. Methods. J Clin Invest 1964;43:843–855.
14. Harker LA, Finch CA. Thrombokinetics in man. J Clin Invest 1969;48:963–974.
15. Heyns AD, Lotter MG, Badenhorst PN et al. Kinetics, distribution and sites of destruction of Indium-labelled human platelets. Br J Haematol 1980;44:269–280.
16. Wadenvik H, Kutti J. The in vivo kinetics of 111-In– and 51-Cr–labelled platelets: a comparative study using both stored and fresh platelets. Br J Haematol 1991;78:523–528.
17. Aster RH, Keene WR. Sites of platelet destruction in idiopathic thrombocytopenic purpura. Br J Haematol 1969;16:61–73.
18. Heyns AP, Lotter MG, Badenhorst PN et al. Kinetics and sites of destruction of 111-Indium-oxine–labeled platelets in idiopathic thrombocytopenic purpura: a quantitative study. Am J Hematol 1982;12:167–177.
19. Schmidt KG, Rasmussen JW. Kinetics and distribution in vivo of 111-In–labelled autologous platelets in idiopathic thrombocytopenic purpura. Scand J Haematol 1985;34:47–56.
20. Ballem PJ, Segal GM, Stratton JR et al. Mechanisms of thrombocytopenia in chronic autoimmune thrombocytopenic purpura. Evidence for both impaired platelet production and increased platelet clearance. J Clin Invest 1987;80:33–40.
21. Heyns AP, Badenhorst PN, Lotter MG et al. Platelet turnover and kinetics in immune thrombocytopenic purpura: results with autologous 111-In–labeled and homologous 51-Cr–labeled platelets differ. Blood 1986;67:86–92.
22. Kernoff LM, Blake KCH, Shackleton D. Influence of the amount of platelet-bound IgG on platelet survival and site of sequestration in autoimmune thrombocytopenia. Blood 1980;55:730–733.
23. Harker LA. Thrombokinetics in idiopathic thrombocytopenic purpura. Br J Haematol 1970;19:95–104.
24. Stoll D, Cines DB, Aster RH et al. Platelet kinetics in individuals with idiopathic thrombocytopenic purpura and moderate thrombocytopenia. Blood 1985;65:584–588.
25. Branehog I, Kutti J, Ridell B et al. The relation of thrombokinetics to bone marrow megakaryocytes in idiopathic thrombocytopenic purpura (ITP). Blood 1975;45:551–562.
26. Branehog I, Weinfeld A. Platelet survival and platelet production in idiopathic thrombocytopenic purpura (ITP) before and during treatment with corticosteroids. Scand J Haematol 1974;12:69–79.
27. Gernsheimer T, Stratton J, Ballem PJ et al. Mechanisms of response to treatment in autoimmune thrombocytopenic purpura. N Engl J Med 1989;320:974–980.
28. Kosugi S, Kurata Y, Tomiyama Y et al. Circulating thrombopoietin level in chronic immune thrombocytopenic purpura. Br J Haematol 1996;93:704–706.
29. Emmons RVB, Reid DM, Cohen RL et al. Human thrombopoietin levels are high when thrombocytopenia is due to megakaryocyte deficiency and low when due to increased destruction. Blood 1996;87:4068–4071.
30. Harrington WJ, Sprague CC, Minnich V et al. Immunologic mechanisms in idiopathic and neonatal thrombocytopenic purpura. Ann Intern Med 1953;38:433–469.
31. Shulman NR, Marder VJ, Weinrach RS. Similarities between known antiplatelet antibodies and the factor responsible for thrombocytopenia in idiopathic purpura. Physiologic, serologic, and isotopic studies. Ann NY Acad Sci 1965;124:499–542.
32. Shulman NR, Weinrach RS, Libre EP et al. The role of the reticuloendothelial system in the pathogenesis of idiopathic thrombocytopenic purpura. Trans Assoc Am Phys 1965;78:374–390.
33. McMillan R, Longmire RL, Yelenosky R et al. Immunoglobulin synthesis in vitro by ITP splenic tissue. N Engl J Med 1972;286:681–684.
34. Karpatkin S, Strick N, Siskind GW. Detection of splenic anti-platelet antibody synthesis in idiopathic autoimmune thrombocytopenic purpura (ATP). Br J Haematol 1972;23:167–176.
35. McMillan R, Luiken GA, Levy R et al. Antibody against megakaryocytes in idiopathic thrombocytopenic purpura. JAMA 1978;239:2460–2462.
36. von dem Borne AEG, Helmerhorst FM, van Leeuwen EF et al. Autoimmune thrombocytopenia: detection of platelet autoantibodies with the suspension immunofluorescence test. Br J Haematol 1980;45:319–327.
37. van Leeuwen EF, van der Ven JTH, Engelfriet CP et al. Specificity of autoantibodies in autoimmune thrombocytopenia. Blood 1982;59:23–26.
38. Woods VL, Oh EH, Mason D et al. Autoantibodies against the platelet glycoprotein IIb-IIIa complex in individuals with chronic ITP. Blood 1984;63:368–375.
39. Woods VL, Kurata Y, Montgomery RR et al. Autoantibodies against platelet glycoprotein Ib in individuals with chronic idiopathic thrombocytopenic purpura. Blood 1984;64:156–160.
40. Beardsley DS, Spiegel JE, Jacobs MM et al. Platelet membrane glycoprotein IIIa contains target antigens that bind antiplatelet antibodies in immune thrombocytopenias. J Clin Invest 1984;74:1701–1707.
41. McMillan R, Tani P, Millard F et al. Platelet-associated and plasma antiglycoprotein autoantibodies in chronic ITP. Blood 1987;70:1040–1045.
42. Kiefel V, Santoso S, Weisheit M et al. Monoclonal antibody-specific immobilization of platelet antigens (MAIPA): a new tool for the identification of platelet-reactive antibodies. Blood 1987;70:1722–1726.
43. Tani P, Berchtold P, McMillan R. Autoantibodies in chronic ITP. Blut 1989;59:44–46.
44. Kiefel V, Santoso S, Kaufmann E et al. Autoantibodies against platelet glycoprotein Ib/IX: a frequent finding in autoimmune thrombocytopenic purpura. Br J Haematol 1991;79:256–262.
45. McKenna JL, Pisciotta AV. Fluorescence of megakaryocytes in idiopathic thrombocytopenic purpura (ITP) stained with fluorescent antiglobulin serum. Blood 1962;19:664–674.
46. Koepke JA, Jobe MG, Braunstein H. Platelet histiocytosis of the spleen. J Reticuloendothel Soc 1968;5:378–383.
47. Corn M, Upshaw JD Jr. Evaluation of platelet antibodies in idiopathic thrombocytopenic purpura. Arch Intern Med 1962;109:157–167.
48. Hoffman R, Zaknoen S, Yang HH et al. An antibody cytotoxic to megakaryocyte progenitor cells in a individual with immune thrombocytopenic purpura. N Engl J Med 1985;312:1170–1174.
49. Fiasse R, Lurhuma AZ, Cambiaso CL et al. Circulating immune complexes and disease activity in Crohn's disease. Gut 1978;19:611–617.
50. Trent RJ, Clancy RL, Danis V et al. Immune complexes in thrombocytopenic individuals: cause or effect? Br J Haematol 1980;44:645–654.
51. Kurata Y, Hayashi S, Aochi H et al. Analysis of antigen involved in circulating immune complexes in individuals with idiopathic thrombocytopenic purpura. Clin Exp Immunol 1987;67:293–299.
52. Ercilla MG, Borche L, Vives J et al. Circulating immune complexes in immune thrombocytopenic purpura (ITP). Br J Haematol 1982;52:679–682.
53. Kiefel V, Spaeth P, Mueller-Eckhardt C. Immune thrombocytopenic purpura: autoimmune or immune complex disease? Br J Haematol 1986;64:57–68.
54. McMillan R, Yelenosky RJ, Longmire RL. Antiplatelet antibody production by the spleen and bone marrow in immune thrombocytopenic purpura. In: Battisto JR, Streinlein JW, eds. Immunoaspects of the spleen. Amsterdam: North Holland Biomedical Press, 1976.
55. Piessens WF, Wybran J, Manaster J, Strijckmans PA. Lymphocyte transformation induced by autologous platelets in a case of thrombocytopenic purpura. Blood 1970;36:421–427.
56. Wybran J, Fudenberg HH. Cellular immunity to platelets in idiopathic thrombocytopenic purpura. Blood 1972;40:856–861.
57. Handin RI, Piessens WF, Moloney WC. Stimulation of nonimmunized lymphocytes by platelet-antibody complexes in idiopathic thrombocytopenic purpura. N Engl J Med 1973;289:714–718.
58. Clancy R. Cellular immunity to autologous platelets and serum-blocking factors in idiopathic thrombocytopenic purpura. Lancet 1972;1:6–9.
59. Morimoto C, Abe T, Hara M et al. Cell-mediated immune response in idiopathic thrombocytopenic purpura. In vitro cellular response to autologous and homologous platelet and platelet membrane by macrophage inhibitory test. Clin Immunol Immunopathol 1977;8:181–189.

60. Quagliata F, Karpatkin S. Impaired lymphocyte transformation and capping in autoimmune thrombocytopenic purpura. Blood 1979;53:341–349.
61. Wautier JL, Boizard B, Rendu F, Caen JP. Vinca alkaloids and platelets. N Engl J Med 1978;299:310–311.
62. McMillan R. Antigen-specific assays in immune thrombocytopenia. Transfus Med Rev 1990;4:136–143.
63. Kiefel V, Santoso S, Katzmann B et al. A new platelet-specific alloantigen Bra. Report of 4 cases with neonatal alloimmune thrombocytopenia. Vox Sang 1988;54:101–106.
64. Koerner TAW, Weinfeld HM, Bullard LSB et al. Antibodies against platelet glycosphingolipids: detection in serum by quantitative HPTLC-autoradiography and association with autoimmune and alloimmune processes. Blood 1989;74:274–284.
65. Fujisawa K, O'Toole TE, Tani P et al. Autoantibodies to the presumptive cytoplasmic domain of platelet glycoprotein IIIa in individuals with chronic immune thrombocytopenic purpura. Blood 1991;77:2207–2213.
66. Fujisawa K, Tani P, O'Toole TE et al. Different specificities of platelet-associated and plasma autoantibodies to platelet GP IIb-IIIa in individuals with chronic ITP. Blood 1992;79:1441–1446.
67. Kekomaki R, Dawson B, McFarland J et al. Localization of human platelet autoantigens to the cysteine-rich region of glycoprotein IIIa. J Clin Invest 1991;88:847–854.
68. He R, Reid DM, Jones CE et al. Spectrum of Ig classes, specificities, and titers of serum antiglycoproteins in chronic idiopathic thrombocytopenic purpura. Blood 1994;83:1024–1032.
69. Fujisawa K, McMillan R. Platelet-associated antibody to glycoprotein IIb-IIIa from chronic immune thrombocytopenic purpura individuals often binds to divalent cation-dependent antigens. Blood 1993;81:1284–1289.
70. Bowditch RD, Tani P, McMillan R. Reactivity of autoantibodies from chronic ITP individuals with recombinant glycoprotein IIIa peptides. Br J Haematol 1995;91:178–184.
71. Askonas BA, Humphrey JH. Formation of specific antibodies and γ-globulin in vitro: a study of the synthetic ability of various tissues from rabbits immunized by different methods. Biochem J 1958;68:252–261.
72. McMillan R, Longmire RL, Yelenosky R et al. Quantitation of platelet-binding IgG produced in vitro by spleens from individuals with idiopathic thrombocytopenic purpura. N Engl J Med 1974;291:812–817.
73. Dixon R, Rosse W, Ebbert L. Quantitative determination of antibody in idiopathic thrombocytopenic purpura: correlation of serum and platelet-bound antibody with clinical response. N Engl J Med 1975;292:230–236.
74. Hegde UM, Gordon-Smith EC, Worlledge S. Platelet antibodies in thrombocytopenic individuals. Br J Haematol 1977;35:113–122.
75. Luiken GA, McMillan R, Lightsey AL et al. Platelet-associated IgG in immune thrombocytopenic purpura. Blood 1977;50:317–325.
76. Fujisawa K, Tani P, Piro L et al. The effect of therapy on platelet-associated autoantibody in chronic immune thrombocytopenic purpura. Blood 1993;81:2872–2877.
77. Branehog I. Platelet kinetics in idiopathic thrombocytopenic purpura (ITP) before and at different times after splenectomy. Br J Haematol. 1975;29:413–426.
78. Carpenter AF, Wintrobe MM, Fuller EA et al. Treatment of idiopathic thrombocytopenic purpura. JAMA 1959;171:103–108.
79. Anonymous. Immunology. In: Federman DD, Rubenstein E, eds. Medicine. New York: Scientific American, 1996; Section 6, Chapters: I–VI.
80. Von Boehmer H, Kisielow P. Self-nonself discrimination by T cells. Science 1990;248:1369–1372.
81. Ramsdell F, Fowlkes BJ. Clonal deletion versus clonal anergy: the role of the thymus in inducing self-tolerance. Science 1990;248:1342–1348.
82. Geha RS. Current concepts in immunology. Regulation of the immune response by idiotypic-antiidiotypic interactions. N Engl J Med 1981;305:25–28.
83. Sinha AA, Lopez MT, McDevitt HO. Autoimmune diseases: the failure of self-tolerance. Science 1990;248:1380–1388.
84. Semple JW, Freedman J. Abnormal cellular immune mechanisms associated with autoimmune thrombocytopenia. Trans Med Rev 1995;9:327–338.
85. Trent RJ, Clancy RL, Danis V, Basten A. Disordered immune homeostasis in chronic idiopathic thrombocytopenic purpura. Clin Exp Immunol 1981;45:9–17.
86. Hymes KB, Karpatkin S. In vitro suppressor T lymphocyte dysfunction in autoimmune thrombocytopenic purpura associated with a complement-fixing antibody. Br J Haematol 1990;74:330–335.
87. Semple JW, Freedman J. Increased antiplatelet T helper lymphocyte reactivity in individuals with autoimmune thrombocytopenia. Blood 1991;78:2619–2625.
88. Zinberg M, Francus T, Weksler ME et al. Abnormal autologous mixed lymphocyte reaction in autoimmune thrombocytopenic purpura. Blood 1982;59:148–151.
89. Mizutani H, Tsubakio T, Tomiyama Y et al. Increased circulating Ia-positive cells in individuals with idiopathic thrombocytopenic purpura. Clin Exp Immunol 1987;67:191–197.
90. Furubayashi T, Mizutani H, Take H et al. Impaired suppressor function of T cells induced by autologous mixed lymphocyte reaction in individuals with idiopathic thrombocytopenic purpura. Acta Haematol 1992;87:32–36.
91. Mizutani H, Katagiri S, Uejima K et al. T-cell abnormalities in individuals with idiopathic thrombocytopenic purpura: the presence of OKT4 + 8 + cells. Scand J Haematol 1985;35:233–239.
92. Campana D, Bergui L, Camussi G et al. Immune-complexes and antiplatelet antibodies in idiopathic thrombocytopenic purpura. Haematologica 1983;68:157–166.
93. Mizutani H, Furubayashi T, Kashiwagi H et al. B cells expressing CD5 antigen are markedly increased in peripheral blood and spleen lymphocytes from individuals with immune thrombocytopenic purpura. Br J Haematol 1991;78:474–479.
94. Van der Harst D, de Jong D, Limpens J et al. Clonal B-cell populations in individuals with idiopathic thrombocytopenic purpura. Blood 1990;76:2321–2326.
95. Garcia-Suarez J, Prieto A, Reyes E et al. Severe chronic autoimmune thrombocytopenic purpura is associated with an expansion of CD56+ CD3-natural killer cells subset. Blood 1993;82:1538–1545.
96. Semple JW, Bruce S, Freedman J. Suppressed natural killer cell activity in individuals with chronic autoimmune thrombocytopenic purpura. Am J Hematol 1991;37:258–262.
97. Garcia-Suarez J, Prieto A, Reyes E et al. The clinical outcome of autoimmune thrombocytopenic purpura individuals is related to their T cell immunodeficiency. Br J Haematol 1993;84:464–470.
98. Garcia-Suarez J, Prieto A, Manzano L et al. T lymphocytes from autoimmune thrombocytopenic purpura show a defective activation and proliferation after cytoplasmic membrane and intracytoplasmic mitogenic signals. Am J Hematol 1993;44:1–8.
99. Firkin BG, Wright R, Miller S et al. Splenic macrophages in thrombocytopenia. Blood 1969;33:240–245.
100. Tavassoli M, McMillan R. Structure of the spleen in idiopathic thrombocytopenic purpura. Am J Clin Pathol 1975;64:180–191.
101. Handin RI, Stossel TP. Phagocytosis of antibody-coated platelets by human granulocytes. N Engl J Med 1974;290:989–993.
102. McMillan R, Longmire RL, Tavassoli M et al. In vitro platelet phagocytosis by ITP splenic leukocytes in idiopathic thrombocytopenic purpura. N Engl J Med 1974;290:249–251.
103. Tsubakio T, Kurata Y, Kanayama Y et al. In vitro platelet phagocytosis in idiopathic thrombocytopenic purpura. Acta Haematol 1983;70:250–256.
104. Clarkson SB, Bussel JB, Kimberly RP et al. Treatment of refractory immune thrombocytopenic purpura with anti-Fcg-receptor antibody. N Engl J Med 1986;314:1236–1239.
105. Zeigler ZR, Rosenfeld CS, Nemunaitis JJ et al. Increased macrophage colony-stimulating factor levels in immune thrombocytopenic purpura. Blood 1993;81:1251–1254.
106. Stossel TP. Phagocytosis (first of three parts). N Engl J Med 1974;290:717–723.
107. Hauch TW, Rosse WF. Platelet-bound complement (C3) in immune thrombocytopenia. Blood 1977;50:1129–1136.
108. Cines DB, Schreiber AD. Immune thrombocytopenia: use of a Coombs antiglobulin test to detect IgG and C3 on platelets. N Engl J Med 1979;300:106–111.
109. Kurata Y, Curd JG, Tamerius JD, McMillan R. Platelet-associated complement in chronic ITP. Br J Haematol 1985;60:723–733.
110. Tsubakio T, Tani P, Curd JG et al. Complement activation in vitro by antiplatelet antibodies in chronic immune thrombocytopenic purpura. Br J Haematol 1986;63:293–300.
111. Frank MM, Schreiber AD, Atkinson JP et al. Pathophysiology of immune hemolytic anemia. Ann Intern Med 1977;87:210–222.
112. Saba TM. Physiology and physiopathology of the reticuloendothelial system. Arch Intern Med 1970;126:1031–1052.
113. George JN, Woolf SH, Raskob GE et al. Idiopathic thrombocytopenic purpura: a practice guideline developed by explicit methods for the American Society of Hematology. Blood 1996;88:3–40.
114. LoBuglio AF, Court WS, Vinocur L et al. Immune thrombocytopenic purpura. Use of a $^{125}$I-labeled antihuman IgG monoclonal antibody to quantify platelet-bound IgG. N Engl J Med 1983;309:459–463.
115. Kelton JG, Powers PJ, Carter CJ. A prospective study of the usefulness of the measurement of platelet-associated IgG for the diagnosis of idiopathic thrombocytopenic purpura. Blood 1982;60:1050–1053.
116. Mueller-Eckhardt C, Kayser W, Mersch-Baumert K et al. The clinical significance of platelet-associated IgG: a study on 298 individuals with various disorders. Br J Haematol 1980;46:123–131.
117. Berchtold P, Harris JP, Tani P et al. Autoantibodies to platelet glycoproteins in individuals with disease-related immune thrombocytopenia. Br J Haematol 1989;73:365–368.
118. Berchtold P, Wenger M. Autoantibodies against platelet glycoproteins in autoimmune thrombocytopenic purpura: their clinical significance and response to treatment. Blood 1993;81:1246–1250.
119. Berchtold P, McMillan R. Therapy of chronic idiopathic thrombocytopenic purpura in adults. Blood 1989;74:2309–2317.
120. Doan CA, Bouroncle BA, Wiseman BK. Idiopathic and secondary thrombocytopenic purpura: clinical study and evaluation of 381 cases over a period of 28 years. Ann Intern Med 1960;53:861–876.

121. Ahn YS, Harrington WJ. Treatment of idiopathic thrombocytopenic purpura (ITP). Annu Rev Med 1977;28:299–309.

122. Rosse W. Management of chronic immune thrombocytopenia. Clin Haematol 1983;12:267–284.

123. Lacey JV, Penner JA. Management of idiopathic thrombocytopenic purpura in the adult. Semin Thromb Hemost 1977;3:160–174.

124. McMillan R. Therapy for adults with refractory chronic immune thrombocytopenic purpura. Ann Intern Med 1997;126:307–314.

125. Baumann MA, Menitove JE, Aster RH et al. Urgent treatment of idiopathic thrombocytopenic purpura with single-dose gammaglobulin infusion followed by platelet transfusion. Ann Intern Med 1986;104:808–809.

126. von dem Borne AE, Vos JJ, Pegels JG et al. High dose intravenous methylprednisolone or high dose intravenous gammaglobulin for autoimmune thrombocytopenia. BMJ (London) 1988;296:249–250.

127. DiFino SM, Lachant NA, Kirshner JJ, Gottlieb AJ. Adult idiopathic thrombocytopenic purpura. Clinical findings and response to therapy. Am J Med 1980;69:430–442.

128. Andersen JC. Response of resistant idiopathic thrombocytopenic purpura to pulsed high-dose dexamethasone therapy. N Engl J Med 1994;330:1560–1564.

129. Thompson RL, Moore RA, Hess CE et al. Idiopathic thrombocytopenic purpura. Long-term results of treatment and the prognostic significance of response to corticosteroids. Arch Intern Med 1972;130:730–734.

130. Jacobs P, Wood L, Dent DM. Results of treatment in immune thrombocytopenia. Q J Med 1986;58:153–165.

131. Centers for Disease Control and Prevention. Recommendations of the advisory committee on immunization practices: use of vaccines and immune globulins in persons with altered immunocompetence. Morbidity and Mortality Weekly Report 1993;42:1–18.

132. Lefor AT, Melvin S, Bailey RW et al. Laparoscopic splenectomy in the management of immune thrombocytopenia purpura. Surgery 1993;114:613–618.

133. Caulier MT, Rose C, Roussel MT et al. Pulsed high-dose dexamethasone (DXM) in refractory chronic idiopathic thrombocytopenic purpura (ITP): a report of 10 cases [Abstract]. Blood 1995;86:3380.

134. Young RR, Marchioli CC, Basmajian JH et al. Pulsed high-dose dexamethasone therapy in individuals with idiopathic thrombocytopenic purpura [Abstract]. Blood 1995;86:252.

135. Ahn YS, Harrington WJ, Seelman RC et al. Vincristine therapy of idiopathic and secondary thrombocytopenias. N Engl J Med 1974;291:376–380.

136. Ahn YS, Byrnes JJ, Harrington WJ et al. The treatment of idiopathic thrombocytopenic purpura with vinblastine-loaded platelets. N Engl J Med 1978;298:1101–1107.

137. Ahn YS, Harrington WJ, Mylvaganam R et al. Slow infusion of vinca alkaloids in the treatment of idiopathic thrombocytopenic purpura. Ann Intern Med 1984;100:192–196.

138. Wood L, Jacobs P. Durable response to etoposide-loaded platelets in refractory immune thrombocytopenic purpura: a case report. Am J Hematol 1988;27:63–64.

139. Facon T, Caulier MT, Wattel E et al. A randomized trial comparing vinblastine in slow infusion and by bolus i.v. injection in idiopathic thrombocytopenic purpura: a report on 42 individuals. Br J Haematol 1994;86:678–680.

140. Ahn YS, Harrington WJ, Simon SR et al. Danazol for the treatment of idiopathic thrombocytopenic purpura. N Engl J Med 1983;308:1396–1399.

141. Ahn YS, Rocha R, Mylvaganam R et al. Long-term Danazol therapy in autoimmune thrombocytopenia: unmaintained remission and age-dependent response in women. Ann Intern Med 1989;111:723–729.

142. Strother SV, Zuckerman KS, LoBuglio AF. Colchicine therapy for refractory idiopathic thrombocytopenic purpura. Arch Intern Med 1984;144:2198–2200.

143. Durand JM, Lefevre P, Hovette P et al. Dapsone for idiopathic autoimmune thrombocytopenic purpura in elderly individuals. Br J Haematol 1991;78:459–463.

144. Godeau B, Oksenhendler E, Bierling P. Dapsone for autoimmune thrombocytopenic purpura. Am J Hematol 1993;44:70–72.

145. Hernandez F, Linares M, Colomina P et al. Dapsone for refractory chronic idiopathic thrombocytopenic purpura. Br J Haematol 1995;90:473–475.

146. Kabisch A, Kroll H, Wedi B et al. Severe adverse effects of protein A immunoadsorption [Letter]. Lancet 1994;343:116.

147. Snyder HW, Cochran SK, Balint JP et al. Experience with protein A–immunoadsorption in treatment-resistant adult immune thrombocytopenic purpura. Blood 1992;79:2237–2245.

148. Laros RK, Penner JA. "Refractory" thrombocytopenic purpura treated successfully with cyclophosphamide. JAMA 1971;215:445–449.

149. Weinerman B, Maxwell I, Hryniuk W. Intermittent cyclophosphamide treatment of autoimmune thrombocytopenia. Can Med Assoc J 1974;111:1100–1102.

150. Bouroncle BA, Doan CA. Treatment of refractory idiopathic thrombocytopenic purpura. JAMA 1969;207:2049–2052.

151. Quiquandon I, Fenaux P, Canlier MT et al. Reevaluation of the role of azathioprine in the treatment of adult chronic idiopathic thrombocytopenia purpura: a report on 53 cases. Br J Haematol 1990;74:223–229.

152. Reiner A, Gernsheimer T, Slichter SJ. Pulse cyclophosphamide therapy for refractory autoimmune thrombocytopenic purpura. Blood 1995;85:351–358.

153. Figueroa M, Gehlsen J, Hammond D et al. Combination chemotherapy in refractory immune thrombocytopenic purpura. N Engl J Med 1993;328:1226–1229.

154. Proctor SJ, Jackson G, Carey P et al. Improvement of platelet counts in steroid-unresponsive idiopathic immune thrombocytopenic purpura after short-course therapy with recombinant α-2b interferon. Blood 1989;74:1894–1897.

155. Bellucci S, Bordessoule D, Coiffier B, Tabah I. Interferon alpha-2b therapy in adult chronic thrombocytopenic purpura (ITP). Br J Haematol 1989;73:578–579.

156. Hurtado R, Pita L, Karpovitch XL et al. Recombinant interferon alpha-2B in refractory idiopathic immune thrombocytpenia. Blood 1990;75:1744–1745.

157. Molica S, Santoro R, Muleo G. Recombinant interferon alpha-2B in refractory idiopathic immune thrombocytopenia. Am J Hematol 1991;36:297–298.

158. Dubbeld P, Hillen HFP, Schouten HC. Interferon treatment of refractory idiopathic thrombocytopenic purpura (ITP). Eur J Haematol 1994;52:233–235.

159. Proctor SJ. Alpha interferon therapy in the treatment of idiopathic thrombocytopenic purpura. Eur J Cancer 1991;27:S63–S68.

160. Matthey F, Ardeman S, Jones L et al. Bleeding in immune thrombocytopenic purpura after alpha-interferon. Lancet 1990;335:471–472.

161. Bussel JB, Pharm LC. Intravenous treatment with gammaglobulin in adults with immune thrombocytopenic purpura: Review of the literature. Vox Sang 1987;52:206–211.

162. Bussel JB, Pham LC, Aledrot L et al. Maintenance treatment of adults with chronic refractory immune thrombocytopenic purpura using repeated intravenous infusions of gammaglobulin. Blood 1988;72:121–127.

163. Woodruff RK, Griff AP, Firkin FC et al. Fatal thrombotic events during treatment of autoimmune thrombocytopenia with intravenous immunoglobulin in elderly individuals [Letter]. Lancet 1986;2:217–218.

164. Delfraissy JF, Tertian G, Dreyfus M et al. Intravenous gammaglobulin, thrombocytopenia, and the acquired immunodeficiency syndrome. Ann Intern Med 1985;103:478–479.

165. Bjorkander J, Cunningham-Rundles C, Lundin C et al. Intravenous immunoglobulin prophylaxis causing liver damage in 16 of 77 individuals with hypogammaglobulinemia or IgG subclass deficiency. Am J Med 1988;84:107–111.

166. Matsumura O, Kawashima Y, Kato S et al. Therapeutic effect of cyclosporine in thrombocytopenia associated with autoimmune disease. Transplant Proc 1988;20(Suppl 4):317–322.

167. Velu TJ, Debusscher L, Stryckmans PA. Cyclosporine for the treatment of refractory idiopathic thrombocytopenic purpura [Letter]. Eur J Haematol 1987;38:95.

168. Kelsey PR, Schofield KP, Geary CG. Refractory idiopathic thrombocytopenic purpura (ITP) treated with cyclosporine. Scand J Haematol 1985;60:197–198.

169. Walker RW, Walker W. Idiopathic thrombocytopenia, initial illness and long-term follow-up. Arch Dis Child 1984;59:316–322.

170. Lusher JM, Enami A, Ravindranath Y et al. Idiopathic thrombocytopenic purpura in children. The case for management without corticosteroids. Am J Pediatr Hematol Oncol 1984;6:149–157.

171. Lilleyman JS. Idiopathic thrombocytopenic purpura—where do we stand? [Editorial]. Arch Dis Child 1984;59:701–703.

172. Beardsley DS. Platelet abnormalities in infancy and childhood. In: Nathan DG, Oski FA, eds. Hematology of infancy and childhood. 4th ed. Philadelphia: WB Saunders, 1993; p. 1561.

173. Lightsey AL. Thrombocytopenia in children. Pediatr Clin North Am 1980;27:293–308.

174. Boshkov LK, Kelton JG, Halloran PF. HLA-DR expression by platelets in acute idiopathic thrombocytopenic purpura. Br J Haematol 1992;81:552–557.

175. Semple JW, Milev Y, Cosgrave D et al. Differences in serum cytokine levels in acute and chronic autoimmune thrombocytopenic purpura: relationship to platelet phenotype and antiplatelet T-cell reactivity. Blood 1996;87:4245–4254.

176. Berchtold P, Muller D, Beardsley D et al. International study to compare antigen-specific methods used for the measurement of antiplatelet autoantibodies. Br J Haematol 1997;96:477–483.

177. Imbach P, Tani P, Berchtold W. Different forms of chronic childhood thrombocytopenic purpura defined by antiplatelet autoantibodies. J Pediatr 1991;118:535–539.

178. Dumoulin-Lagrange M, Capelle C. Evaluation of automated platelet counters for the enumeration and sizing of platelets in the diagnosis and management of hemostatic problems. Semin Thromb Hemost 1983;9:235–244.

179. Halperin DS, Doyle JJ. Is bone marrow examination justified in idiopathic thrombocytopenic purpura? Am J Dis Child 1988;142:508–511.

180. Ramos ME, Newman AJ, Gross S. Chronic thrombocytopenia in childhood. J Pediatr 1978;92:584–586.

181. Venetz U, Willi P, Hirt A et al. Chronic idiopathic thrombocytopenic purpura in childhood. Helv Paediatr Acta 1982;37:27–33.

182. Dameshek W, Ebbe S. Recurrent acute idiopathic thrombocytopenic purpura. N Engl J Med 1963;269:647.

183. Woerner SJ, Abildgaard CF. Intracranial hemorrhage in children with idiopathic thrombocytopenic purpura. Pediatrics 1981;67:453–460.

184. Imbach P, Berchtold W, Hirt A et al. Intravenous immunoglobulin versus oral corticosteroids in acute immune thrombcytopenic purpura in childhood. Lancet 1985;2:464–468.

185. Imbach P, Barandun S, d'Apuzzo V et al. High-dose intravenous gammaglobulin for idiopathic thrombocytopenic purpura in childhood. Lancet 1981;1:1228–1231.

186. NIH Consensus Conference. Intravenous immunoglobulin: prevention and treatment of disease. JAMA 1990;264:3189–3193.

187. Imbach P, Kuhne T, Hollander G. Immunologic aspects in pathogenesis and treatment of immune thrombocytopenic purpura ITP in children. Curr Opin Pediatr 1997;9:35–40.

188. Imbach P, Blanchette V, Nugent D et al. Immune thrombocytopenic purpura: immediate and longterm effects in intravenous immunoglobulin. In: Kazatchkine M, ed. Intravenous Immunoglobulin-research and therapy. New York, London: The Parthenon Publishing Group, 1996;135–141.

189. Imbach P, Blanchette V, Nugent D et al. Immune thrombocytopenic purpura: immediate and longterm effects in intravenous immunoglobulin. In: Kazatchkine M, ed. Intravenous immunoglobulin-research and therapy. New York, London: The Parthenon Publishing Group, 1996:135–141.

190. Andrew M, Blanchette V, Adams M et al. A multicenter study of the treatment of childhood chronic idiopathic thrombocytopenic purpura with anti-D. J Pediatr 1992;120:522–527.

191. Ozsoylu S, Sayli TR, Ozturk G. Oral megadose methylprednisolone versus intravenous immunoglobulin for acute childhood idiopathic thrombocytopenic purpura. Pediatr Hematol Oncol 1993;10:317–321.

192. Bussel JB, Schulman I, Hilgartner MW, Barandun S. Intravenous use of gammaglobulin in the treatment of chronic immune thrombocytopenic purpura as a means to defer splenectomy. J Pediatr 1983;103:651–654.

193. Bussel JB, Graziano JN, Kimberly RP et al. Intravenous anti-D treatment of immune thrombocytopenic purpura: analysis of efficacy, toxicity, and mechanism of effect. Blood 1991;77:1884–1893.

194. Becker T, Kuenzlen E, Salama A et al. Treatment of childhood idiopathic thrombocytopenic purpura with Rhesus antibodies (anti-D). Eur J Pediatr 1986;145:166–169.

195. Dickerman JD. Splenectomy and sepsis: a warning. Pediatrics 1979;63:938–941.

196. Budman DR, Steinberg AD. Haematologic aspects of systemic lupus erythematosus. Ann Intern Med 1977;86:220–229.

197. Keeling DM, Isenberg DA. Haematological manifestations of systemic lupus erythematosus. Blood Rev 1993;7:199–207.

198. Pujol M, Ribera A, Vilardell M et al. High prevalence of platelet autoantibodies in individuals with systemic lupus erythematosus. Br J Haematol 1995;89:137–141.

199. Kurata Y, Hayashi S, Kosugi S et al. Elevated platelet-associated IgG in SLE individuals due to anti-platelet autoantibody: differentiation between autoantibodies and immune complexes by ether elution. Br J Haematol 1993;85:723–728.

200. Harris EN, Asherson RA, Gharavi AE et al. Thrombocytopenia in SLE and related autoimmune disorders: association with anticardiolipin antibody. Br J Haematol 1985;59:227–230.

201. Shoenfeld Y, Rauch J, Massicotte H et al. Polyspecificity of monoclonal lupus autoantibodies produced by human-human hybridomas. N Engl J Med 1983;308:414–420.

202. Boumpas DT, Barez S, Klippel JH et al. Intermittent cyclophosphamide for the treatment of autoimmune thrombocytopenia in systemic lupus erythematosus. Ann Intern Med 1990;112:674–677.

203. Coon WW. Splenectomy for cytopenias associated with systemic lupus erythematosus. Am J Surg 1988;155:391–394.

204. Hall S, McCormick JL, Greipp PR et al. Splenectomy does not cure the thrombocytopenia of systemic lupus erythematosus. Ann Intern Med 1985;102:325–328.

205. West SG, Johnson SC. Danazol for the treatment of refractory autoimmune thrombocytopenia in systemic lupus erythematosus. Ann Intern Med 1988;108:703–706.

206. Cervera H, Jara LJ, Pizarro S et al. Danazol for systemic lupus erythematosus with refractory autoimmune thrombocytopenia or Evans' syndrome. J Rheumatol 1995;22:1867–1871.

207. Roach BA, Hutchinson GJ. Treatment of refractory systemic lupus erythematosus–associated thrombocytopenia with intermittent low-dose intravenous cyclophosphamide. Arthritis Rheum 1993;36:682–684.

208. Ebbe S, Wittels B, Dameshek W. Autoimmune thrombocytopenic purpura (ITP type) with chronic lymphocyte leukemia. Blood 1962;19:23–37.

209. Carey RW, McGinnis A, Jacobson BM et al. Idiopathic thrombocytopenic purpura complicating chronic lymphocytic leukemia. Management with sequential splenectomy and chemotherapy. Arch Intern Med 1976;136:62–66.

210. Kaden BR, Rosse WF, Hauch TW. Immune thrombocytopenia in lymphoproliferative disease. Blood 1979;53:545–551.

211. Waddell CC, Cimo PL. Idiopathic thrombocytopenic purpura occurring in Hodgkin Disease after splenectomy: report of two cases and Review of the literature. Am J Hematol 1979;7:381–387.

212. Schwartz KA, Slichter SJ, Harker LA. Immune-mediated platelet destruction and thrombocytopenia in individuals with solid tumours. Br J Haematol 1982;51:17–24.

213. Morse EE, Zinkham WH, Jackson DP. Thrombocytopenic purpura following rubella infection in children and adults. Arch Intern Med 1966;117:573–579.

214. Graham DY, Brown CH, Benrey J et al. Thrombocytopenia: a complication of mumps. JAMA 1974;227:1162–1164.

215. Mazza JJ, Magnin GE. Severe thrombocytopenia in infectious mononucleosis. Report of two cases and Review of the literature. Wis Med J 1975;74:124–127.

216. Chanarin I, Walford DM. Thrombocytopenic purpura in cytomegalovirus mononucleosis. Lancet 1973;2:238–239.

217. Wilson JJ, Neame PB, Kelton JG. Infection-induced thrombocytopenia. Semin Thromb Hemost 1982;8:217–233.

218. Kelton JG, Keystone J, Moore J et al. Immune-mediated thrombocytopenia of malaria. J Clin Invest 1983;71:832–836.

# CHAPTER 31

# THROMBOCYTOSIS

## Tiziano Barbui and Guido Finazzi

## DEFINITION

The definition of thrombocytosis as an elevation of the concentration of platelets in the blood is deceptively simple. By convention (1), the normal range for the platelet concentration in humans has been taken to be 150 to $400 \times 10^9/l$, with some studies showing an upper limit of $450 \times 10^9/l$. This would seem to be an unusually broad normal range. There are several reasons for this. There is some evidence (2, 3) that mean platelet volume varies inversely with the platelet concentration in normal individuals and that therefore the concentration of platelet mass per cubic millimeter may be controlled in a much narrower range than is the numeric concentration. Furthermore, the percentage of the body's platelets residing in the splenic platelet pool may also vary among normal individuals (3). Thus the normal range for the total body platelet mass may be far narrower than that for the numeric concentration in the blood. These concepts must also be kept in mind when assessing individuals with marked splenomegaly and platelet counts in the normal range. Because of the expanded splenic platelet pool, the total body platelet mass may be greatly increased.

In addition, some published normal ranges may include fundamentally healthy individuals who have modest degrees of reactive thrombocytosis such as young women with iron deficiency secondary to excessive menstrual blood loss. Thus, although this is not well documented, the upper limit of the normal range in truly healthy people may be less than $400 \times 10^9/l$. Finally, as will be discussed in the next section, reactive thrombocytosis is common in many clinical settings. Therefore clinicians may tend to disregard elevations in the range of 400 to $600 \times 10^9/l$, and $600 \times 10^9/l$ has generally been listed as the level above which the diagnosis of essential thrombocythemia can be considered (4). These points are stressed simply to indicate that one must interpret a given platelet concentration within its clinical context and against a background of knowledge concerning normal and abnormal platelet physiology.

## DIFFERENTIAL DIAGNOSIS

Platelet survival is normal or somewhat shortened in all types of thrombocytosis (5–6), and the cause of thrombocytosis is an increased rate of production of platelets. A corresponding increase in the mass of megakaryocytes in the marrow can be demonstrated (7).

There are many synonyms that have appeared in the literature to identify the thrombocytotic processes to be discussed. Thrombocythemia has been used interchangeably with thrombocytosis. Conceptually, thrombocytotic individuals can be divided into two major groups, based primarily on analogy with better-defined processes in the granulocytic and erythroid lines. The production of granulocytes is stimulated in a variety of inflammatory and toxic states. The same is true for platelet production, although there is no direct correlation between the diseases associated with leukocytosis and those associated with thrombocytosis. These thrombocytoses have been referred to as reactive or secondary. Reactive thrombocytosis (RT) will be the term used in this chapter.

In polycythemia vera (PV) there is strong evidence that the production of erythrocytes can occur at extremely low levels of the regulating hormone, erythropoietin, and also in its absence. Erythropoiesis is excessive, but erythropoietin cannot be detected in plasma, suggesting some degree of autonomy of erythropoiesis. Furthermore, as will be discussed in greater detail subsequently, hematopoiesis in PV is clonal (8, 9). This term indicates that a single hematopoietic precursor or stem cell and its progeny gain a growth advantage over their normal counterparts, so that the proliferation of the latter is suppressed. This growth advantage is derived, at least in part, from increased sensitivity of erythroid progenitors to the stimulatory effects of several growth factors such as granulocyte-macrophage colony-stimulating factor (GM-CSF), interleukin (IL)-3, and insulin-like growth factor I (IGF-I) (10, 11). Thus we refer to the second group of thrombocytotic individuals as having clonal thrombocytosis. This occurs in several myelodysplastic syndromes (MDSs) and myeloproliferative diseases (MPDs).

Within the MPDs there is a disease process in which the overproduction of platelets is relatively isolated, with less involvement of the granulocytic and erythroid lines. By convention, this process has been referred to as primary or essential thrombocythemia (thrombocytosis). Essential thrombocythemia (ET) will be the term used in this chapter.

The control of megakaryocyte proliferation is discussed in detail in Chapter 8. It has now become clear that thrombopoietin (TPO) is the primary regulator of megakaryocyte development (12). TPO is able to drive megakaryocytes to full maturation as evidenced by the generation of the entire spectrum of normal murine megakaryocytopoiesis in mouse bone marrow cultures grown in the presence of TPO alone (13). Among other cytokines, IL-3, IL-6, IL-11, leukemia inhibitory factor (LIF), and kit ligand (KL) have also been reported to promote megakaryocyte proliferation *in vitro* and to increase the peripheral blood platelet count in rodents, dogs, and nonhuman primates (14–21). However, the coordination of these many factors *in vivo* remains to be elucidated. It is also unknown which, if any, of the factors described above have a unique role in producing RT, and whether the factors function by circulating as hormones or locally after release in the marrow.

## REACTIVE THROMBOCYTOSIS

Patients with RT are rather frequently encountered (22). Even when extreme thrombocytosis (i.e., platelet counts greater than or equal to $1000 \times 10^9/l$) is considered, RT is far more common than clonal thrombocytosis. Thus in a recent study of 280 cases (166 males, 114 females; mean age 37 years, range 12 days to 100 years) with extreme thrombocytosis, 231 (82%) had RT and only 38 (14%) had a myeloproliferative disorder (23). Characteristically, in this study the proportion of individuals with

| **TABLE 31.1.**    Classification of Thrombocytosis |
| --- |
| Reactive thrombocytosis |
|     Infectious or inflammatory diseases |
|     Malignancy |
|     Iron-deficiency anemia, hemolytic anemia, acute blood loss |
|     Splenectomy |
|     Rebound effect after chemotherapy or immune thrombocytopenia |
| Clonal thrombocytosis |
|     Essential thrombocythemia |
|     Polycythemia vera |
|     Idiopathic myelofibrosis |
|     Chronic granulocytic leukemia |
|     Myelodysplastic syndromes |
|         5q- syndrome |
|         Idiopathic refractory sideroblastic anemia |

clonal thrombocytosis increased with age, and a peak was reached in the highest age groups.

In children the incidence and causes of RT were investigated by Vora et al (24). During a 12-month period, over 16,000 platelet counts were performed on 7916 individuals attending a children's hospital. Of these individuals 36 (0.5%) produced at least one count of $>800 \times 10^9/l$ and seven (0.1%) had platelet counts $>1000 \times 10^9/l$. Most of them had an acute infection, although two were also recovering from antineoplastic chemotherapy and one was concomitantly iron deficient.

Table 31.1 lists the categories of disease that are associated with thrombocytosis. Although RT is associated with many specific pathologic states, there are four major groups into which most of these individuals can be placed.

## Inflammatory Disease and Malignancy

Thrombocytosis has long been recognized to accompany acute and chronic infections and noninfectious inflammatory states as well. Early reviews stressed that thrombocytosis was commonly present during the course of bacterial pneumonia, pyelonephritis, osteomyelitis, pyogenic arthritis, chronic wound infections, and other bacterial infections (25). More recently (26), 76% of individuals with active pulmonary tuberculosis were reported to have elevated platelet counts, with 11% having platelet counts greater than $1000 \times 10^9/l$. In contrast, thrombocytosis is rare during the course of viral infections. In fact, the platelet count often falls to some degree along with the leukocyte count.

A similar degree of thrombocytosis accompanies a wide variety of noninfectious, inflammatory illnesses such as rheumatoid arthritis (27), vasculitis (including polyarteritis nodosa and polymyalgia rheumatica) (25), inflammatory bowel disease (28), hepatic cirrhosis (25), and nephritis (25). In general, the degree of thrombocytosis parallels the activity of disease, and the elevated platelet count returns to normal levels with effective therapy. In all of these situations, the platelet count can be viewed as an acute-phase reactant. One generally finds an accompanying anemia of inflammation (29), along with a decrease in serum iron, iron-binding capacity, and albumin and an increase in fibrinogen, ferritin, and haptoglobin. The elevated fibrinogen correlates with an increase in the erythrocyte sedimentation rate that is out of proportion to the degree of anemia.

In one series of individuals with active tuberculosis (26), the degree of thrombocytosis correlated with the degree of inflammation as reflected in increases in the erythrocyte sedimentation rate and the serum C-reactive protein concentration.

A similar increase in platelet count is seen in individuals with advanced malignancy (25, 30–32). Ninety percent of individuals with thrombocytosis secondary to malignancy have platelet counts in the range of 400 to $1000 \times 10^9/l$; occasional individuals have been reported (31) with counts as high as $6000 \times 10^9/l$. The pathophysiologic mechanisms of the thrombocytosis of malignancy and inflammation may be similar. In a study of individuals with carcinoma of the lung and colon (32), the platelet count correlated directly with the leukocyte count and the fibrinogen level and inversely with the hemoglobin, again suggesting that the platelet count may be regarded as an acute-phase reactant. Recently, it has been pointed out that the modest, nonspecific anemia that is seen in many individuals with malignancy has all of the characteristics of the anemia of inflammation (29), and it has been hypothesized that anemia (and, by inference, the thrombocytosis) is a reflection of the host's inflammatory response to the tumor.

Thrombocytosis has been reported with most types of tumors. The literature has stressed its frequency in carcinoma of the lung (32) and in mesothelioma (30). In a recent series, thrombocytosis was more common in carcinoma of the lung than in carcinoma of the colon. However, the extent of disease in the different tumor types in such series is not always clear.

## Splenectomy

The relationship between the spleen, the platelet count, and the rate of platelet production is complex. Approximately one-third of the total-body platelet mass normally resides in a pool in the spleen. Therefore the platelet count should theoretically rise by approximately 50% after splenectomy. The inflammation related to surgery might transiently increase the platelet count by approximately another 50%. However, if splenectomy is performed in a hematologically normal person, the platelet

count often rises far in excess of that predicted by these two considerations, sometimes reaching in excess of $1000 \times 10^9/l$. Therefore the removal of the spleen may stimulate platelet production. Thrombocytosis generally subsides over weeks to months and rarely persists for more than 2 years following splenectomy. Thus the stimulation must be transient or compensated for in some circulating factor that suppresses platelet production (33), but this is not well established. It is generally accepted that such transient, self-limited postsplenectomy thrombocytosis is not associated with thrombotic or hemorrhagic complications (34) and that therapy for it is not necessary. Following splenectomy (even many years later) infectious or inflammatory thrombocytosis may be exaggerated considerably.

Postsplenectomy thrombocytosis can be expected to persist under two circumstances. A individual with MPD who has splenomegaly and a normal platelet count may, in fact, have a marked increase in the rate of platelet production that is masked by an increase in the size of the pool of platelets in the spleen. If the spleen is removed under these circumstances, there may be a massive increase in the platelet count, often to 10 times the presplenectomy value. There are many reports of thrombotic complications in this situation (35). The second circumstance occurs when the spleen is removed in individuals with anemia secondary to hemolysis or ineffective erythropoiesis and the splenectomy does not completely correct the anemia (36). Typical situations in which this might occur are hereditary, nonspherocytic, hemolytic anemia and thalassemia major. In such individuals it is typical for the platelet count to persist indefinitely in the range of 600 to $1000 \times 10^9/l$. In addition, such individuals have an increased incidence of deep vein thrombosis (36).

Autosplenectomy and hyposplenism may occur in the course of several hereditary and acquired disorders. The best example is sickle cell anemia in which repeated infarctions cause the organ to be dramatically reduced in size by the time the individual reaches adulthood. Since these individuals have a hemolytic anemia, persistent thrombocytosis is expected. In one series (37) the mean platelet count was $525 \times 10^9/l$ with some counts reaching $1000 \times 10^9/l$. These levels were significantly higher than the mean for sickle-hemoglobin C (SC) disease, which is $275 \times 10^9/l$. In the latter condition, there is a brisk, hemolytic anemia, but the spleen is generally enlarged rather than infarcted.

Functionally, hyposplenism without shrinkage of the organ may also occur in a variety of states, including inflammatory bowel disease (38). Such hyposplenism may contribute to the marked thrombocytosis seen in these cases.

## Iron-Deficiency Anemia

Patients with anemia secondary to simple iron deficiency typically have an elevated platelet count, not uncommonly to levels in excess of $1000 \times 10^9/l$. In adults in the Western world, blood loss is the most common cause of iron deficiency, and, as will be discussed below, bleeding itself can cause thrombocytosis. However, in experimental animals iron deficiency produced by an iron-deficient diet also leads to thrombocytosis (39). The mechanism is not known, and there is no explanation for the observation that some individuals develop marked thrombocytosis while others with equally severe anemia have only modest elevations in platelet count. The platelet count falls rapidly as soon as iron replacement is begun, so that normal or even low levels may be reached within 7 to 10 days (40). Thus the increased rate of platelet production appears to be secondary to iron deficiency *per se* and not to the erythroid hyperplasia in the marrow, which continues until the anemia is corrected. Although there have been case reports of thrombotic complications in this setting (40), the response of the thrombocytosis to iron replacement is so rapid that no other therapy is required.

## Miscellaneous, Transitory Thrombocytosis

If a individual has been thrombocytopenic and recovers, either due to therapy as in the treatment of megaloblastic anemia or spontaneously after removal of a myelosuppressive process such as chemotherapy for malignancy, a rebound thrombocytosis occurs and may persist for 1 to 2 weeks (41). A transitory thrombocytosis may also be seen with acute bleeding, hemolysis, exercise (42), after administration of epinephrine (43) and the vinca alkaloids (44), and during alcohol withdrawal (45); this transitory increase may be exaggerated in asplenic or hyposplenic individuals.

## CLONAL THROMBOCYTOSIS

As mentioned above it can be shown that hematopoiesis is clonal in many cases of MPD and MDS. This was originally shown for all of the MPDs and acute myelogenous leukemia (46–49) by studying glucose-6-phosphate dehydrogenase (G6PD) isoenzymes in females who were coincidentally heterozygous at this X-linked locus. More recently, molecular probes for restriction fragment length polymorphism (RFLP) of other X-linked genes have made it possible to assess clonality in the nucleated cells of up to 50% of women with these illnesses (50).

RFLP analyses have confirmed the previous G6PD studies in most instances, but there have been exceptions. The G6PD studies suggested that all circulating red cells, granulocytes, and platelets were derived from the clone in PV and essential thrombocythemia (48). The RFLP technique, which has allowed the study of a larger number of individuals, has found a minority of individuals with these two diseases whose leukocytes were not derived or were variably derived from the clone (50–52).

Thus in these cases it is presumed that the abnormal clonal progenitor had very little capacity to differentiate into some leukocyte lineages.

At least two hypotheses can explain the variable features of hematopoiesis in different individuals (53). It is possible that the transformation event may affect stem cells at different levels of commitment in different individuals as demonstrated in other hematopoietic disorders, such as acute myelogenous leukemia, Philadelphia chromosome-positive leukemia, and lymphoma. Alternatively, it is possible that the transformation originates from a multipotent stem cell in all ET individuals, but that the selective advantage of the abnormal clone over polyclonal hematopoiesis is initially restricted to the megakaryocytic lineage. Additional mutagenic events could extend this advantage to other lineages or an inhibition of polyclonal hematopoiesis might occur during the evolution of the disease.

As mentioned above, the concept of autonomous hematopoiesis arose from studies of individuals with PV, in whom erythropoietin cannot be detected in plasma. Furthermore, erythroid colony-forming units can grow *in vitro* to form colonies in the absence of added erythropoietin (so-called endogenous erythroid colonies, EEC) (54). EEC can also be seen in individuals with otherwise typical ET (55, 56). Similarly, in *in vitro* studies of blood and marrow from individuals with ET and other MPD, megakaryocytic colony-forming units increased in number and were able to develop without added growth factors (endogenous megakaryocytic colonies, EMC) (55–59).

Clonogenic assays for EEC and EMC have been advocated as diagnostic markers of PV and ET (55, 58–59). However, the specificity of these assays is not clearly demonstrated (54). Furthermore, clonogenic culture techniques are not amenable to external quality assurance, are technically demanding, and are unlikely to be available in most clinical hematology laboratories. Thus, for diagnostic use, EEC and EMC assays remain to be exhaustively validated using clinically appropriate controls.

## Polycythemia Vera

Approximately two-thirds of these individuals (60) have an elevated platelet count, with about 5% having a value over $1000 \times 10^9/l$. For the past 25 years, the most commonly used criteria for this diagnosis have been those of the Polycythemia Vera Study Group (PVSG) (61). The PVSG criteria have proved to be reasonably reliable, but some new and more specific techniques are becoming available. While awaiting a precise diagnostic marker for PV, some modifications of the original PVSG criteria have been proposed (62). These are listed in Table 31.2.

These modified criteria have a similar structure to the original PVSG criteria. The major criteria in combi-

**TABLE 31.2.**  Proposed Modified Criteria for the Diagnosis of Polycythemia Vera[a]

| | |
|---|---|
| A1. Raised red cell mass (>25% above mean normal predicted value) | B1. Thrombocytosis (platelet count >400 × 10⁹/l) |
| A2. Absence of causes of secondary polycythemia | B2. Neutrophil leukocytosis (neutrophil count >10 × 10⁹/l) |
| A3. Palpable splenomegaly | B3. Splenomegaly on isotope or ultrasound scanning |
| A4. Clonality marker (e.g., abnormal marrow karyotype) | B4. Characteristic BFU-E growth or reduced serum erythropoietin |

*Adapted with permission from Pearson TC, Messinezy M. The diagnostic criteria of polycythemia rubra vera. Leuk Lymphoma 1996;22(Suppl 1):87–94.*

[a] *Diagnosis of polycythemia vera is acceptable if the following combinations are present: A1 + A2 + A3 or A4, or A1 + A2 + any two from category B.*

nation have a sensitivity/specificity of virtually 100% (62). The minor criteria are less specific for the diagnosis of PV. The original criteria included the measurement of the red cell mass (RCM) in milliliters per kilogram body weight. However, RCM is more closely correlated with lean body mass rather than total body weight, since adipose tissue is considerably less vascular than lean tissue and therefore does not contribute equally to the RCM. The radionuclide panel of the International Council for Standardization in Hematology has addressed this problem and recently put forward prediction formulas for mean normal RCM (63). The normal ranges for these predictions were examined, and it was proposed that an absolute polycythemia was present when the measured RCM was greater than 25% above the mean normal predicted value for that individual. In practice this measurement can be omitted if the hematocrit is greater than 60% or less than 40%, since it is almost always increased in the former circumstance and almost never increased in the latter. However, in the range of 40 to 60% the red cell mass may or may not be elevated (60, 61), and it is impossible to distinguish PV from ET in this hematocrit range without the direct measurement. Increased splenic size demonstrated by scanning techniques and reduced serum erythropoietin/characteristic burst-forming units-erythroid (BFU-E) growth are more specific than the raised serum $B_{12}$ and leukocyte alkaline phosphatase (LAP) score. Thus serum $B_{12}$ and LAP have been omitted from the minor criteria.

## Agnogenic Myeloid Metaplasia

This syndrome, which is also often associated with and referred to as idiopathic myelofibrosis, is characterized by splenomegaly (characteristically massive), anemia with ineffective erythropoiesis and teardrop changes of red cell morphology on peripheral blood smear, and the appearance of immature red cell and white cell precursors in the smear, the so-called leukoerythroblastic blood picture (64).

Thrombocytosis may be present in approximately

one-third of individuals. In most cases it is impossible to obtain a bone marrow aspirate because of increased marrow reticulin and fibrous tissue, which can be visualized on the bone marrow biopsy. Typical, fully expressed cases are easily identified, but occasional individuals present with marked thrombocytosis and only modest anemia and splenomegaly. Therefore full evaluation with bone marrow biopsy is crucial in most cases in which clonal thrombocytosis is suspected. The course of the disease is highly variable. One quarter of individuals are asymptomatic at diagnosis. Forty percent experience progressive splenomegaly with worsening of anemia. A wide variety of complications and associated medical problems emerge during follow-up such as infection, heart failure, bleeding, and cerebrovascular accidents. As compared with other myeloproliferative disorders, individuals with myelofibrosis tend to have more hemorrhagic problems (65). In a recent analysis of 71 splenectomized individuals (66), new hemorrhagic or thrombotic complications occurred in 17% of surviving individuals; these were predicted by age lower than 50 years, a normal to high platelet count (>200 × 10⁹/1), and massive splenomegaly (>16 cm below the costal margin). Median survival time from diagnosis ranges from 1.4 to 9.1 years, and most individuals die from infections, hemorrhages, or evolution to acute leukemia.

## Chronic Myelogenous Leukemia (CML)

Two-thirds of these individuals have thrombocytosis at diagnosis (67, 68). The diagnosis is not a problem if the thrombocytosis is accompanied by the typical anemia, splenomegaly, leukocytosis with marked left shift in the granulocytic series, and low leukocyte alkaline phosphatase (69), as well as the presence of the Philadelphia (Ph) chromosome in the bone marrow karyotype. However, there are cases in which marked thrombocytosis and the Ph chromosome are seen together in individuals without the typical anemia, splenomegaly, leukocytosis, and low leukocyte alkaline phosphatase (70). In one series (70) such individuals developed acute leukemia (blast crisis) at essentially the same rate as individuals with classic CML, and it was argued that all individuals with the Ph chromosome should be considered to have CML. Others (71) have proposed that a separate category of Ph-positive ET be retained. Furthermore, it is now known that some individuals with clinically typical CML lack the Ph chromosome on karyotypic analysis, but have the *bcr/abl* gene rearrangement at the DNA level. The same finding has now been reported in individuals with the clinical picture of ET (71). Complete study of a individual with a clonal thrombocytosis should include karyotype analysis and search for the *bcr/abl* gene rearrangement.

## Myelodysplastic Syndromes

This group of diseases is characterized by anemia and an increased red cell mean corpuscular volume (MCV) associated with megaloblastic changes and evidence of dysmelopoiesis on examination of the bone marrow. There may be monocytosis and ringed sideroblasts in the bone marrow and abnormalities of the bone marrow karyotype. The platelet count may be low, normal, or high. Myelodysplastic syndromes with thrombocytosis are often associated with specific karyotypic abnormalities. These include (a) the 5q- syndrome, which predominantly occurs in elderly females and is characterized by the presence of megakaryocytes with nonlobulated nuclei in the bone marrow (72); (b) abnormalities involving bands 3q21 and 3q26, usually characterized by overexpression of the Evi-1 proto-oncogene and atypical megakaryopoiesis; and (c) deletion of the p34 region of chromosome 1 (73). In ET one very rarely sees a hemoglobin concentration less than 10 g%, an increased red cell MCV, ringed sideroblasts, or an abnormal karyotype. The distinction is important, since leukemic transformation is common in the MDS and rare in ET.

## Essential Thrombocythemia

There is no single clinical or laboratory finding that permits a positive diagnosis of ET. Rather, many clinicians have concluded that the diagnosis in a individual with thrombocytosis must be reached by excluding the conditions listed above that are associated with an elevated platelet count. The principle was used in the development of the criteria of the PVSG (60) that has been recently updated (74) (Table 31.3). Reference to Fig. 31.1 allows one to work through the reactive and clonal causes of thrombocytosis listed in Table 31.1. Clinical evaluation and laboratory studies designed to detect iron deficiency and occult inflammatory or malignant disease are generally sufficient to exclude RT. In addition, a recent study (75) suggested that most individuals with RT have elevated serum levels of interleukin-6 and C-reactive protein, while individuals with MPD and thrombocytosis have normal levels.

If the individual's hematocrit is above 60%, the total-body red cell mass is almost always elevated (61), and, by convention, the diagnosis should be PV. If the hematocrit is in the range of 40 to 60%, the total body red cell mass may or may not be elevated (60, 61), and it should be measured directly. If it is elevated, the diagnosis should be PV. If the red cell mass is not elevated, the possibility of PV, masked by bleeding or iron deficiency, should be considered. For practical purposes, a normal or increased serum ferritin level along with a normal red blood cell mean corpuscular volume suffices to exclude both reactive thrombocytosis secondary to iron deficiency and the possibility that one may be dealing with PV masked by iron deficiency. When iron-deficiency erythropoiesis is present or cannot be excluded, the distinction between PV and ET cannot be made with certainty until revaluation is performed after 1 to 2 months of iron replacement therapy. During the initial evaluation of a individual suspected of having ET, it is advisable to perform a bone marrow aspiration, biopsy, and karyotype analysis. The iron stain of the bone marrow aspirate helps to establish the presence or absence of iron deficiency. If there is frank fibrosis present on the bone marrow biopsy, the diagnosis of AMM can be made, particularly if the individual also has marked splenomegaly on physical examination and teardrop poikilocytosis and a leukoerythroblastic reaction in the peripheral blood smear.

The bone marrow karyotype is critical to exclude

---

**TABLE 31.3.**   Updated Diagnostic Criteria for Essential Thrombocythemia

I   Platelet count $>600 \times 10^9$/l

II   Hematocrit <40% or normal RBC mass (males <36 mL/kg, females <32 mL/kg)

III   Stainable iron in marrow or normal serum ferritin or normal RBC mean corpuscular volume[a]

IV   No Philadelphia chromosome or *bcr/abl* gene rearrangement

V   Collagen fibrosis of marrow
   A.   Absent or
   B.   <1/3 biopsy area without both marked splenomegaly and leukoerythroblastic reaction

VI   No cytogenetic or morphologic evidence for a myelodysplastic syndrome

VII   No cause for reactive thrombocytosis

*Adapted with permission from Murphy S, Peterson P, Iland H et al. Experience of the Polycythemia Vera Study Group with essential thrombocythemia: a final report on diagnostic criteria, survival and leukemic transition by treatment. Semin Hematol 1997;34:29–39.*

*[a] If these measurements suggest iron deficiency, PV cannot be excluded unless a trial of iron therapy fails to increase the RBC mass into the polycythemic range.*

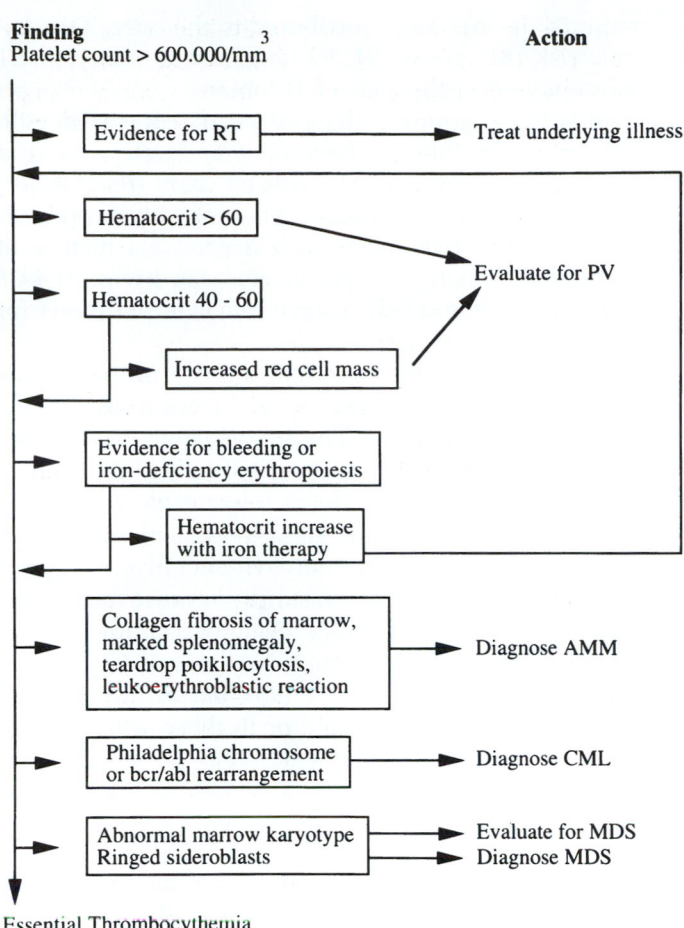

**Finding**
Platelet count > 600.000/mm³          **Action**

Essential Thrombocythemia

**FIGURE 31.1.** Flow diagram for the diagnosis of essential thrombocythemia. See text for details. AMM, agnogenic myeloid metaplasia; CML, chronic myelogenous leukemia; MDS, myelodysplastic syndrome; PV, polycythemia vera; RT, reactive thrombocytosis.

the Ph chromosome and therefore atypical CML. If the clinical picture is atypical for ET, the *bcr/abl* rearrangement diagnostic of CML should be sought by either DNA analysis by Southern blotting and hybridization with a *bcr* probe or RNA analysis by reverse amplification of the *bcr-abl* fusion transcript. As mentioned above, it is now known that MDS may present with thrombocytosis. Karyotypic abnormalities may be present in ET, but in no more than 5% of cases (76). Therefore a clonal karyotypic abnormality, particularly 5q-, or the presence of ringed sideroblasts on an iron stain of the marrow would place the individual in the MDS category.

This approach to ET as a diagnosis of exclusion is intrinsically unsatisfactory, and positive criteria that would distinguish ET from RT have been proposed (22, 77). Findings favoring the diagnosis of ET were vascular occlusive phenomena by history; splenic enlargement by physical examination or splenic scanning; the growth of autonomous, erythroid colony-forming units from bone marrow aspirates or peripheral blood; increased platelet distribution width on platelet sizing with a Coulter counter; and increased ratio of the concentrations of platelet adenosine triphosphate (ATP) and adenosine diphosphate (ADP) (ATP:ADP). However, all of these findings may be found in any of the clonal thrombocytoses, and they are not specific for ET. In addition, it has been proposed (78) that ET can be distinguished from RT and other MPD by careful, quantitative examination of the bone marrow biopsy. Typical clustering of enlarged megakaryocytes with multilobated nuclei has been advocated to represent the hallmark feature of ET (78). Histologic background of hematopoiesis in ET is featured by a discrete pattern of minimal or no prominence of erythropoiesis, no change in granulopoiesis, almost no fibrosis and reduction of stainable iron (78). However, an experienced observer is required to diagnose ET by examination of the bone marrow biopsy.

## CLINICAL FEATURES AND RISK FACTORS FOR BLEEDING AND THROMBOSIS

The clinical features of individuals with thrombocytosis vary with the cause. Individuals with RT do not have an increased incidence of hemorrhage. Individuals with postsplenectomy thrombocytosis associated with ongoing hemolytic anemia are prone to thrombotic complications, as described above. However, other types of postsplenectomy thrombocytosis, and RT in general, are not associated with an excess incidence of thrombosis, even when the increase in the platelet count is dramatic. Thus in these cases thrombocytosis is simply a laboratory marker for the underlying state.

Within the category of clonal thrombocytosis, it is clear that PV and ET are closely related to MPD, and in fact the finding of autonomous erythroid colony formation in some individuals with ET suggests that the stem-cell defect may be similar if not identical. However, when large series are compared and contrasted, clear clinical differences emerge. PV is most frequent in upper middle age with a male to female ratio of approximately 1.2:1. Within ET there is a subset of individuals with a similar age and sex distribution. However, several series indicate that there is an additional population of young women with ET not found in PV (4, 79–82). Unexplained pruritis is found in 40% of individuals with PV (61) but in only 10% of individuals with ET (83). Palpable enlargement of the spleen is found in two-thirds and one-third of individuals with PV and ET, respectively. Furthermore, if the spleen is enlarged in ET, it is rarely more than 2 to 4 cm below the costal margin, while much more pronounced splenomegaly may be seen at the onset of PV.

The clinical features of PV and ET that are of the greatest concern are those of hemorrhage and thrombosis. The frequency and severity of these complications have been reviewed in a large number of publications (79–92). Hemorrhage is seen in approximately 5 to 20% of cases and is generally of the type seen in individuals with thrombocytopenia and disorders of platelet function. Ecchymoses and bleeding from superficial mucosal sites are most common, whereas deep tissue and joint bleeding is rare. Such hemorrhage is rarely life-threatening. Several authors have concluded that the risk of hemorrhage is related to the height of the platelet count, being rare unless the platelet count is greater than 1000 $\times$ $10^9$/l (79, 80, 86). This bleeding tendency may be related to a reduction of large von Willebrand factor multimers (93, 94) and can be reduced by lowering the platelet count with myelosuppressive therapy (79, 80, 86). Bleeding complications in the MPD are reviewed in detail in Chapter 33.

Several generalizations can be made concerning thrombotic complications in PV and in ET. In PV the frequencies of venous and arterial thrombosis are similar (95), but arterial thrombosis accounts for more than 80% of fatal thrombotic events (96). In ET, reports of venous thrombosis are relatively less frequent than arterial and arteriolar thrombosis. In both PV and ET, advanced age and history of previous thrombosis were the main risk factors that contributed to the overall thrombotic risk (81, 87–89, 91, 92, 96). In one study in ET individuals (87) the rate of thrombosis was 1.7%/pt-yr in subjects younger than 40 years, compared with 6.3%/pt-yr in those between 40 and 60 years and 15.1%/pt-yr in individuals over 60 years ($P<.001$ versus individuals $<40$ years). The rate of thrombosis was also higher in those with a previous history of vascular occlusion (3.4%/pt-yr compared with 31.4%/pt-yr). These clinical data have major implications for therapy (see below).

There also is consensus that the risk of thrombosis in both PV (95) and ET (82, 86, 92) is not related to the height of platelet count. Thrombosis may occur when the platelet count is in the range of only 600 to 900 $\times$ $10^9$/l, while many individuals tolerate platelet counts well over 1000 $\times$ $10^9$/l for many years without complications. Therefore it is uncertain whether myelosuppressive therapy should be given simply because the platelet count exceeds some arbitrary level, for example 1000 $\times$ $10^9$/l. However, myelosuppressive therapy does reduce the risk of thrombosis in PV (95) and in high-risk ET individuals over 60 years old or in those who have already had a thrombotic episode (97).

## TYPES OF THROMBOSIS IN PV AND ET

The most characteristic clinical manifestation of small, arterial, vascular occlusion in ET and PV is the syndrome of erythromelalgia, as shown in Figs. 31.2 and 31.3 (see color plates 31.2 and 31.3) (98–101). Individuals experience episodic or continuing pain and burning, accompanied by redness and warmth of one or more digits. Involvement is asymmetric and generally includes one or more toes or, less commonly, fingers. There may be progression to coldness, cyanosis, and eventually gangrene. There is considerable evidence suggesting that these manifestations result from inflammation, intimal proliferation, and thrombotic occlusion of arterioles resulting from the toxic effect of metabolites of arachidonic acid produced locally by platelets. Aspirin and other nonsteroidal antiinflammatory agents that interrupt arachidonic acid metabolism generally relieve these symptoms dramatically, often within several hours, although several days may be required for complete resolution. The syndrome may precede the hematologic abnormalities by several years. It may be seen in clinical settings other than the clonal thrombocytoses (102). However, within the clonal thrombocytoses it is essentially unique to PV and ET, and occasionally AMM. There are only case reports of its occurrence in CML and MDS (101). It has not been described in RT.

Occlusion of other arteriolar beds may also produce symptoms. Neurologic manifestations include transient ischemic attacks, visual disturbances, headaches, dizziness, and seizures (103). Angina and myocardial infarction may occur even in the absence of coronary atherosclerosis (104). Recurrent spontaneous abortion and *in utero* growth retardation associated with placental infarction have been described in individuals with ET (89, 105–108). Therapy with aspirin, subcutaneous heparin (109), or α-interferon (110) in subsequent pregnancies has been associated with successful outcome, although at least an equal number of successful pregnancies without therapy have been described (108, 111). Apparently, only a subset of individuals with ET are subject to arteriolar occlusive complications.

Thrombosis of hepatic (112) and portal (113) veins occurs with increased frequency in individuals with PV and perhaps also with ET, although the latter association is less clear. There is no correlation between the frequency of these complications and the height of the platelet count. In fact, there is an increased frequency of autonomous, erythroid-colony formation in individuals with hepatic and portal vein thrombosis who have no clinical evidence for MPD (112, 113). Thus, as with erythromelalgia, the thrombotic tendency may precede recognizable hematologic disease. Priapism (114) and pyoderma gangrenosum (115) have also been described in individuals with ET.

It is less common for thrombocytosis to be associated with clinical manifestations of thrombosis and hemorrhage in individuals with AMM, MDS, and CML (65, 91, 92). In these entities hemorrhagic manifestations are common, but are more frequently related to thrombocytopenia and disorders of platelet function than to thrombocytosis.

## NATURAL HISTORY

Life expectancy in most of these illnesses is unrelated to the thrombocytosis. In one study in PV and ET, survival was similar to an age-matched, normal population (116). However, in a more recent analysis of 1213 Italian individuals with PV, the age- and gender-standardized mortality rate of PV individuals was 1.7 times greater than that of the general Italian population (96). Survival is shortened substantially in CML because of the tendency to transform into acute leukemia; in MDS because of the tendency to develop severe bone marrow failure and acute leukemia; and in AMM because of infection, complications of massive splenomegaly, and bone marrow failure.

At least 10% (95) and perhaps as many as 50% of individuals with PV evolve into the clinical picture of postpolycythemic myeloid metaplasia. Such transformation is far less frequent in ET, occurring in perhaps less than 5% of cases (79, 80, 88, 89). This represents a noteworthy difference between the two illnesses. The risk of acute leukemic transformation, particularly after myelosuppressive therapy, is substantial in PV (95), but is also present in ET (79–81, 88, 117–120). Murphy et al

(74) analyzed the experience of the PVSG in ET individuals and reported a 20% risk for development of acute leukemia during 10 years of study. Subgroups of individuals at high risk for acute leukemia were identified by myelofibrotic features, such as mild marrow fibrosis, splenomegaly, and leukoerythroblastosis, and by failure of hydroxyurea to control thrombocytosis. Finally, 5 to 10% of individuals who initially present with ET subsequently develop rises in hematocrit and red cell mass into the polycythemic range.

## TREATMENT

There are no risk-free therapies for individuals with thrombocytosis. Therefore one has to assess the risk of no treatment and balance that risk against the known or possible risks of therapy. It is now accepted that a category of individuals at particularly higher risk of thrombosis is defined by age over 60 years and a previous history of thrombotic events. Therefore myelosuppressive treatment for the thrombocytosis should be focused on these individuals, whereas a different policy should be considered for the remainder (Fig. 31.4).

### MANAGEMENT OF "LOWER-RISK" ET PATIENTS

The natural history of "lower-risk" ET individuals not given myelosuppressive therapy was evaluated in two cohorts followed in France (Paris) and in Italy (Bergamo) (121). The French series consisted of 20 asymptomatic cases (9 males and 11 females; median age 40 years, range 7 to 64 years; median platelet count $909 \times 10^9/l$, range 600 to $1470 \times 10^9/l$) observed for a median of 6.7 years. The rates of major and total thrombotic complications in this cohort were 3 and 5.1%/pt-yr, respectively. The Italian lower-risk ET cohort consisted of 40 asymptomatic ET subjects (22 males and 18 females; median age 37 years, range 4 to 55 years; median platelet count $808 \times 10^9/l$, range 600 to $1350 \times 10^9/l$) followed for a median of 4.3 years. Seven individuals suffered thrombotic complications during the follow-up, including two strokes and one each of TIA, myocardial infarction, unstable angina, deep vein thrombosis, and superficial thrombophlebitis. The rate of vascular occlusion was 4.1%/pt-yr, in good agreement with the French cohort. None of the complications observed in these two cohorts was fatal. Even although thrombotic deaths have been occasionally reported in young individuals with ET (88), they seem very rare in lower-risk subjects, and data showing that fatalities can be prevented by starting cytoreductive drugs early have not been produced. Therefore one can conclude that withholding cytoreductive therapy might be justifiable in asymptomatic, young ET individuals with a platelet count below $1000 \times 10^9/l$,

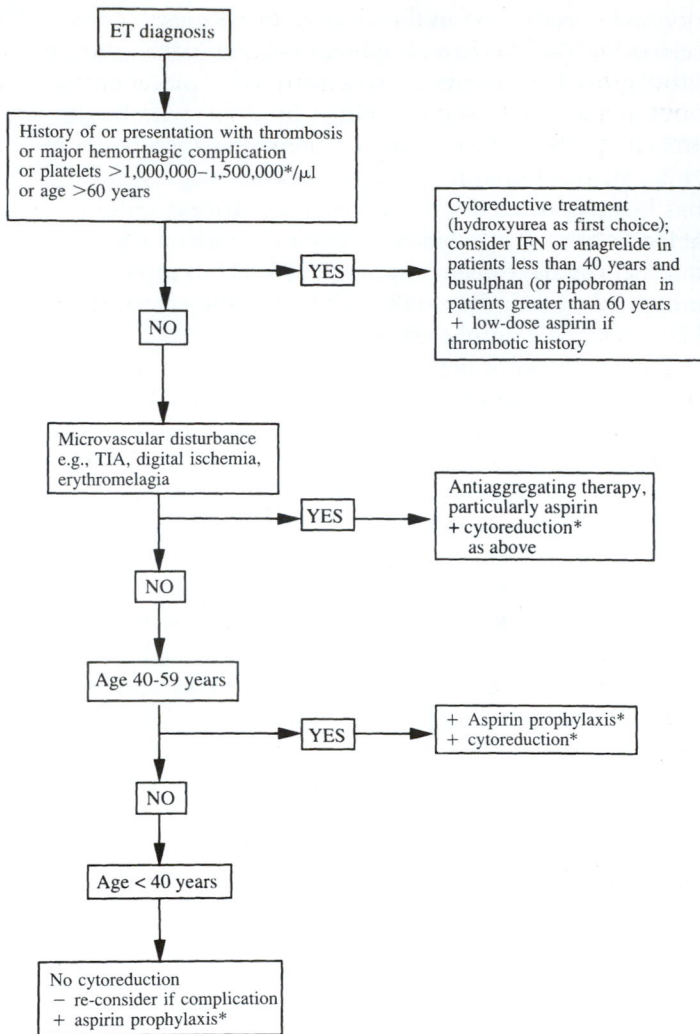

**FIGURE 31.4.** Flow-chart of recommended treatment for individuals with essential thrombocythemia (ET). Areas of uncertainty are marked with the asterisk (*). IFN, interferon; TIA, transient ischemic attack.

based on their very low risk of developing fatal thrombotic or bleeding events and for the concern about the potential leukemogenicity of cytotoxic drugs (see below).

Having made this generalization concerning myelosuppressive therapy, it may be rational to propose a primary antithrombotic prophylaxis with aspirin for reducing the rate of vascular complications in these asymptomatic individuals. Aspirin has received wide acknowledgment for efficacy in ET individuals with microvascular disturbances such as erythromelalgia or transient cerebral or ocular ischemia (122). In the absence of contraindications and/or side effects, a dose of 100 to 300 mg/day is required in the acute management of these individuals. Cytoreduction usually relieves these symptoms, and the continued use of aspirin is indicated when a recurrence of symptoms is observed with a normal platelet count. Aspirin at a dose of 75 to 100 mg/day is also recommended as secondary prophylaxis for major arterial thrombosis (123). However, in the absence of clinical trials in the specific setting of ET,

this recommendation is largely based on the assumption that the use of platelet antiaggregating agents is associated with a risk reduction comparable with that achievable in other clinical conditions (124).

In prescribing antiaggregating agents one should consider the risk of bleeding, an issue particularly important in ET individuals, who very often have platelet functional defects (125). In normal subjects a recent case-control study showed that the use of enteric-coated or buffered aspirin at average daily doses of 325 mg or less carried a twofold to threefold relative increase in the risk of major upper-gastrointestinal hemorrhages (126) indicating that the risk of bleeding is increased even with low-dose aspirin. However, it should be stressed that such complication is very rarely associated with life-threatening morbidity or mortality.

Pregnancy and elective surgery in asymptomatic ET individuals deserve special consideration. Approximately 50% of pregnancies develop obstetric complications, including recurrent abortion, particularly in the first trimester, premature delivery, fetal growth retardation, and abruptio placenta. The likely mechanism of these complications is placental infarction, so that some authors recommend the use of aspirin (127) or subcutaneous heparin (109), particularly in individuals who have had previous fetal losses. By reviewing the relevant literature, it would appear that aspirin was associated with a more successful outcome of pregnancy than in those managed without the drug (127). However, in a recent single institutional analysis from Mayo Clinic, Beressi et al (111) were unable to substantiate the benefit of specific therapy during pregnancy or delivery of 34 pregnancies occurring in 18 women with ET. Consequently, they do not recommend any prophylactic therapy in asymptomatic pregnant women with ET. In symptomatic individuals the use of α-interferon (see also below) has been proposed (110), but only very few anecdotal reports are available so far. Thus some uncertainty still remains in treating pregnant individuals with ET, and it is likely that therapy should be considered on an individual basis.

An exception to the generalization that cytoreductive therapy should not be given to lower-risk asymptomatic individuals applies to those individuals with ET who have to undergo major surgery. It is recognized that individuals with uncontrolled PV and ET have an increased risk of thrombosis and hemorrhage in the postoperative period. Based on this rationale, a course of myelosuppressive therapy to lower the platelet count is recommended prior to elective surgery. Myelosuppressive therapy is particularly indicated in individuals with myeloproliferative disorders who require splenectomy, since thrombohemorrhagic complications associated with massive postsplenectomy thrombocytosis might occur.

## MANAGEMENT OF "HIGH-RISK" ET PATIENTS—BENEFITS AND RISKS OF CYTOREDUCTIVE DRUGS

Patients aged more than 60 years or with platelet counts exceeding $1000 \times 10^9/l$ or those with a previous history of thrombosis or major bleeding are candidates to receive a cytoreductive drug.

### Conventional Cytotoxic Agents

Hydroxyurea (HU) has emerged as the treatment of choice in individuals with ET because of its efficacy and only rare acute toxicity (121, 128–130). The drug is given at an initial dose of 15 to 20 mg/kg/day, with adjustments to maintain reduced platelet values, ideally to less than $400 \times 10^9/l$ without excessive lowering of the neutrophil count. Continuous treatment with HU has been shown to reduce the platelet count to below $500 \times 10^9/l$ within 8 weeks in 80% of individuals.

Lowering the platelet count by HU is associated with significant improvement in acute ischemic or hemorrhagic symptoms. In a randomized clinical trial, the efficacy of HU in preventing thrombosis in ET individuals aged >60 years or with a history of previous thrombosis or with a platelet count above $1500 \times 10^9/l$ has been shown (97). One hundred and fourteen individuals (35 males and 79 females; median age 68 years, range 40 to 85 years; median platelet count $788 \times 10^9/l$, range 533 to $1240 \times 10^9/l$) were randomized to long-term treatment with HU (n = 56) or to no cytoreductive treatment (n = 58). During a median follow-up of 27 months, two thromboses (one stroke and one myocardial infarction) were recorded in the HU-treated group (1.6%/pt-yr) compared with 14 (one stroke, five transient ischemic attacks, five peripheral arterial occlusions, one deep vein thrombosis, and two individuals with superficial thrombophlebitis) in the control group (10.7%/pt-yr; $P = .003$) (Fig. 31.5).

Hematopoietic impairment, leading to neutropenia and macrocytic anemia, is the major, short-term, toxic effect of HU. Neutropenia is dose-related and generally quickly reversible if the drug is discontinued for a few days. Withdrawal is followed by a rebound of platelet counts, so that continuous treatment is necessary. Failure of HU to provide adequate control of the platelet count was reported in five out of 29 (17%) individuals included in a PVSG protocol (74) and in nine of 79 (11%) in a French series (121).

Although it is likely that ET individuals have an intrinsic likelihood of acute leukemic transformation, the precise incidence in untreated individuals is not known. A recent review of the literature from 1981 to 1994 (118) identified a total of 40 Ph-negative ET cases transformed into acute leukemia after a mean time from presentation of 6.5 years. Three major factors are associated with the risk of, or possibly facilitate, blastic transformation: cytogenetic abnormalities (131), myelofibrotic features (74), and the use of cytotoxic agents (74). The role of cytotoxic drugs in enhancing the risk of leukemic transformations is one of the major issues currently under discussion in the question of using chemotherapy for ET. HU, a nonalkylating agent, is generally although to be nonmutagenic (120); however, long-term, follow-up studies of HU-treated individuals with PV and ET revealed that some cases developed acute leukemia (117, 131).

These reports cast doubts on the innocence of HU in the process of leukemogenicity. Even when used as a single agent in the treatment of PV and ET, the reported rate of acute leukemia is 5 to 10% and this fatal complication is encountered 4 to 10 years after the start of treatment. The incidence of acute leukemic transformation might be enhanced in individuals given multiple cytotoxic drugs with different mechanisms of action (antimetabolites, alkylating agents). An alternative ex-

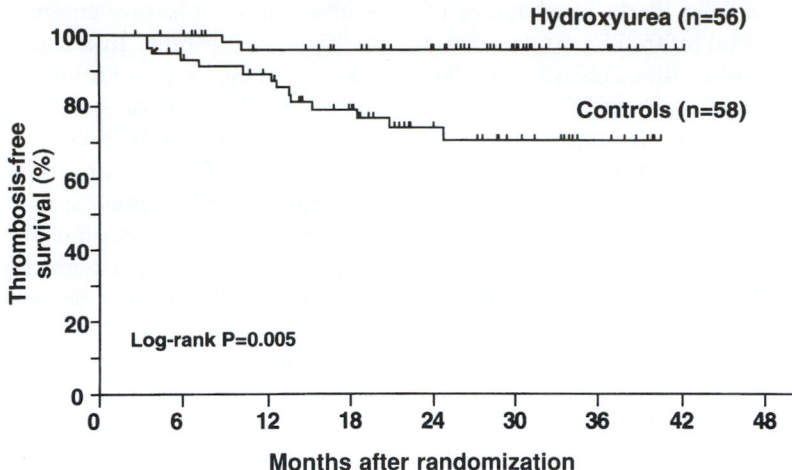

**FIGURE 31.5.** Probability of thrombosis-free survival in 114 individuals with essential thrombocythemia treated with hydroxyurea or left untreated. The *P* value is for the difference between the two groups (by the log rank test). The median follow-up was 27 months. Tick marks indicate surviving individuals who were continuously free of thrombosis. (Adapted with permission from Cortelazzo S, Finazzi G, Ruggeri M, et al. Hydroxyurea in the treatment of individuals with essential thrombocythemia at high risk of thrombosis: a prospective randomized trial. N Engl J Med 1995;332:1132–1136.)

planation for the higher risk of developing leukemia when individuals are exposed to several cytotoxic drugs is that these individuals represent a selected population in which the underlying disease is poorly controlled and more likely to undergo genetic transformations (74).

When balancing benefits and risks, one can conclude that there is convincing evidence for giving HU to ET individuals at higher risk for major thrombotic complications. In contrast, the risk of acute leukemia associated with the use of HU is more difficult to accept in young individuals at low risk for thrombosis. In these cases vascular occlusive complications are expected to occur in 4 to 5% of individuals yearly with only occasional fatal events, and no data are available on the effectiveness of HU or other cytotoxic drugs in reducing this rate. Thus recommendations in this group of ET individuals remain uncertain. Concerning the place of other drugs in the management of ET, it will essentially depend on whether they can be proven to be equally effective and associated with a lower incidence of leukemic transformation than HU.

Busulfan is an alkylating agent with a specific action on megakaryocyte proliferation (132). The recommended dose is 2 to 4 mg daily, according to hematologic response, under weekly control of platelet count. After normalization of the platelet count, adequate long-term control of thrombocytosis can be obtained with intermittent courses, allowing long intervals without the need for therapy. Busulfan is particularly useful for elderly individuals where the convenience of its use outweighs the leukemogenic risk, which is no higher than with HU therapy (122, 123).

Pipobroman, a piperazine derivative, is another ef-

fective drug for treating ET. In two series representing 45 individuals (133, 134), at a dose of 0.7 to 1 mg/kg/day, it was shown to give a complete hematologic response in about 90% of the cases in a median time of 1.5 to 3 months. However, the chemical structure of the drug suggests that it is an alkylating agent and its safety in terms of risk of leukemia in ET remains to be established in further studies with longer follow-up and a greater number of individuals.

## Interferon-α

Recombinant interferon-α (IFN) is an active agent in MPDs virtually devoid of mutagenic risk (135–138). The rationale for this drug includes its myelosuppressive activity and its ability to antagonize the action of platelet-derived growth factor (PDGF), a product of megakaryopoiesis that initiates fibroblast proliferation. This observation would suggest that IFN could, theoretically, modify the natural history of MPDs and reduce or delay the development of myelofibrosis.

In ET individuals, IFN has been evaluated in some phase II studies, and overall results indicate that an initial hematologic response can be obtained in about 90% of cases with an average dose of about 3 million IU daily. During maintenance the dose could be tapered, but if IFN is suspended the platelet count rebounds in the majority of individuals. Side effects are a major problem with this drug. Apart from the immediate side effects experienced by most individuals, signs of chronic IFN toxicity, including weakness, myalgia, weight and hair loss, severe depression, and gastrointestinal and cardiovascular toxicity, occur in some cases. A recent review of 273 cases (138) showed that IFN therapy had to be interrupted in 67 individuals (25%). The rate of withdrawal ranged between 0 and 66% among studies. This wide range is partly explained by the difference in the observation time lasting from 1 month to 4 years in the reported individuals. The most common reasons for withdrawal were IFN-related side effects in 55% and individual refusal or loss to follow-up in the other 20% of cases. Thus far, no leukemogenic effects have been reported.

## Anagrelide

This quinazolin derivative was initially developed as an inhibitor of platelet function. In normal volunteers, doses sufficient to inhibit platelet function also produced substantial cardiovascular side effects. However, a lowering of the platelet count was noted. In individuals with MPD, 0.5 to 1.0 mg orally four times daily lowers the platelet count to less than $600 \times 10^9/l$ in 2 to 4 weeks in 90% cases. At these doses, there is no measurable effect on platelet function. In contrast to $^{32}$P, alkylating agents, hydroxyurea, and the interferons, the drug does not lower the white cell count, although its use is associated with a mild anemia. Discontinuation of the drug results in a rapid return of thrombocytosis. Like the interferons, anagrelide does not reduce the number of megakaryocytes in the bone marrow, but interferes in some way with their maturation. Approximately 25% of individuals treated with anagrelide develop fluid retention and some develop frank congestive heart failure. Two cases of sudden death were described in the initial series of 577 individuals. Side effects result in discontinuation of treatment in 15% of cases (139–141).

Although it is extremely promising, the ultimate place of anagrelide in the management of thrombocytosis is not yet known. It should clearly be used with caution in individuals with known or suspected heart disease. It has been used for too short a period to be certain about its ability to control thrombotic and hemorrhagic complications and to judge its potential for toxicity over years or decades.

## CONCLUSIONS AND FUTURE TRENDS

Thrombocytosis can be a reactive phenomenon associated with other diseases or the manifestation of a clonal, bone marrow disorder. Clonal thrombocytosis, as typically seen in essential thrombocythemia, is due to an abnormal response of megakaryocytic progenitors to thrombopoietin and other hematopoietic growth factors. The molecular bases for this abnormal behavior are now under investigation in many laboratories. If a molecular marker for essential thrombocythemia is

identified, this would be of great interest to clinicians who currently lack a specific and sensitive diagnostic test for this disease. More reliable diagnostic criteria would allow a more precise knowledge of the natural history of the disease and a more accurate identification of individuals at different risk for bleeding and thrombosis.

Available evidence in the literature shows that the treatment of ET individuals should be based primarily on the expected risk of major thrombotic complications. Young, asymptomatic subjects with platelet counts in the range of 600 to $1000 \times 10^9/l$ are at lower risk and can be followed untreated. Nevertheless, it should be emphasized that major thrombotic events can also occur in a small percentage of these lower-risk cases. Future studies should be directed toward identifying other parameters useful for predicting the vascular risk in this particular subset of individuals. Furthermore, the risk/benefit of low-dose aspirin in the primary prevention of thrombosis should be tested in appropriate clinical trials. As far as higher-risk individuals are concerned, HU (plus aspirin in the case of ischemia and/or thrombosis) is the treatment of choice because its efficacy in preventing thrombotic complications has been clearly proven. However, the possible long-term leukemogenicity of this drug, as well as that of other effective cytoreductive agents such as busulfan and pipobroman, remains a major concern. Anagrelide and interferon could overcome this problem, but their efficacy has been hitherto demonstrated only in lowering the platelet count, and clinical studies aimed at documenting additional clinical benefit in ET are urgently needed.

## REFERENCES

1. Williams WJ. Secondary thrombocytosis. In: Williams WJ, Beutler E, Lichtman MA et al., eds. Hematology. 5th ed. New York: McGraw-Hill, 1995; pp. 1361–1363.
2. Levin J, Bessman JD. The inverse relation between platelet volume and platelet number. J Lab Clin Med 1983;101:295–307.
3. Thompson CB, Jakubowski JA. The pathophysiology and clinical relevance of platelet heterogeneity. Blood 1988;72:1–8.
4. Schafer AI. Essential (primary) thrombocythemia. In: Williams WJ, Beutler E, Lichtman MA et al., eds. Hematology. 5th ed. New York: McGraw-Hill, 1995; pp. 340–348.
5. Bautista AP, Buckler PW, Towler et al. Measurement of platelet life-span in normal subjects and individuals with myeloproliferative disease with indium oxine labelled platelets. Br J Haematol 1984;58:679–687.
6. Tranum BL, Haut A. Thrombocytosis: platelet kinetics in neoplasia. J Lab Clin Med 1974;84:615–619.
7. Murphy S. Thrombocytosis and thrombocythaemia. Clin Haematol 1983; 12:89–106.
8. Adamson JW, Fialkow PJ, Murphy S et al. Polycythemia vera stem-cell and probable clonal origin of the disease. N Engl J Med 1976;295:913–916.
9. Prchal JF, Adamson JW, Murphy S et al. Polycythemia vera. The in vitro response of normal and abnormal stem cell lines to erythropoietin. J Clin Invest 1978;61:1044–1047.
10. Prchal JT, Prchal JF. Evolving understanding of the cellular defect in polycythemia vera: implications for its clinical diagnosis and molecular pathophysiology. Blood 1994;83:1–4.
11. Green AR. Pathogenesis of polycythemia vera. Lancet 1996;347:844–845.
12. Levin J. Thrombopoietin—clinically realized? N Engl J Med 1997; 336: 434–436.
13. Zucker-Franklin D, Kaushansky K. Effect of thrombopoietin on the devel-

opment of megakaryocytes and platelets: an ultrastructural analysis. Blood 1996;88:1632–1638.

14. Long MW, Huthinson RJ, Gragowski LL et al. Synergistic regulation of human megakaryocyte development. J Clin Invest 1988;82:1779–1786.

15. Mazur EM, Cohen JL, Newton J et al. Human serum megakaryocyte colony-stimulating activity appears to be distinct from interleukin-3, granulocyte-macrophage colony-stimulating factor, and lymphocyte-conditioned medium. Blood 1990;76:290–297.

16. Debili N, Hegyi E, Navarro S et al. In vitro effects of hematopoietic growth factors on the proliferation, endoreplication, and maturation of human megakaryocyte. Blood 1991;77:2326–2338.

17. Briddell RA, Burno E, Cooper RJ. Effect of c-kit ligand on in vitro human megakaryocytopoiesis. Blood 1991;78:2854–2859.

18. Han ZC, Bellucci S, Caen JP. Megakaryocytopoiesis: characterization and regulation in normal and pathologic states. Int J Hematol 1991;54:3–14.

19. Kimura H, Ishibashi T, Shikama Y et al. Interleukin-1β (IL-1β) induces thrombocytosis in mice: possible implication of IL-6. Blood 1990;76:2493–2500.

20. Metcalf D, Nicola NA, Gearing DP. Effects of injected leukemia inhibitory factor on hematopoietic and other tissues in mice. Blood 1990;76:50–56.

21. Neben TY, Loebelenz J, Hayes L et al. Recombinant interleukin-11 stimulates megakaryocytopoiesis and increases peripheral platelets in normal and splenectomized mice. Blood 1993;81:901–908.

22. Kutti J, Wadenvik H. Diagnostic and differential criteria of essential thrombocythemia and reactive thrombocytosis. Leuk Lymphoma 1996;22(Suppl 1):41–45.

23. Buss DH, Cashell AW, O'Connor ML et al. Occurrence, etiology, and clinical significance of extreme thrombocytosis: a study of 280 cases. Am J Med 1994;96:247–253.

24. Vora AJ, Lilleyman JS. Secondary thrombocytosis. Arch Dis Child 1993;68:88–90.

25. Selroos O. Thrombocytosis. Acta Med Scand 1973;193:431–436.

26. Baynes RD, Bothwell TH, Flax H et al. Reactive thrombocytosis in pulmonary tuberculosis. J Clin Pathol 1987;40:676–679.

27. Ghosh P. Thrombocytosis in rheumatoid arthritis. Br J Clin Pract 1986;40:388–389.

28. Morowitz DA, Allen LW, Kirsner JB. Thrombocytosis in chronic inflammatory bowel disease. Ann Intern Med 1968;68:1013–1021.

29. Schilling RF. Anemia of chronic disease: a misnomer. Ann Intern Med 1991;115:572–573.

30. Chahinian AP, Pajak TF, Holland JF et al. Diffuse malignant mesothelioma. Prospective evaluation of 69 individuals. Ann Intern Med 1982;96:746–755.

31. Spigel SC, Mooney LR. Extreme thrombocytosis associated with malignancy. Cancer 1977;39:339–341.

32. Constantini V, Zacharski LR, Moritz TE et al. The platelet count in carcinoma of the lung and colon. Thromb Haemost 1990;64:501–505.

33. Bessler H, Notti I, Djaldetti M. The effect of partial splenectomy on platelet production in mice. Thromb Haemost 1981;46:602–603.

34. Boxer MA, Braun J, Ellman L. Thromboembolic risk of postsplenectomy thrombocytosis. Arch Surg 1978;113:808–809.

35. Gordon DH, Schaffner D, Bennett JM et al. Postsplenectomy thrombocytosis: its association with mesenteric, portal, and/or renal vein thrombosis in individuals with myeloproliferative disorders. Arch Surg 1978;113:713–715.

36. Hirsh J, Dacie JV. Persistent post-splenectomy thrombocytosis and thrombo-embolism: a consequence of continuing anaemia. Br J Haemat 1966;12:44–53.

37. Ballas SK, Lewis CN, Noone AM et al. Clinical, hematological, and biochemical features of Hb SC disease. Am J Hematol 1982;13:37–51.

38. Marsh GW, Stewart JS. Splenic function in adult coeliac disease. Br J Haematol 1970;19:445–457.

39. Schloesser LL, Kipp MA, Wenzel FJ. Thrombocytosis in iron-deficiency anemia. J Lab Clin Med 1965;66:107–114.

40. Knizley H, Noyes WD. Iron deficiency anemia, papilledema, thrombocytosis and transient hemiparesis. Arch Intern Med 1972;129:483–486.

41. Ogston D, Dawson AA. Thrombocytosis following thrombocytopenia in man. Postgrad Med J 1969;45:754–756.

42. Dawson AA, Ogston D. Exercise-induced thrombocytosis. Acta Haematol 1969;42:241–246.

43. Libre EP, Cowan DH, Watkins SP Jr et al. Relationships between spleen, platelets and factor VIII levels. Blood 1968;31:358–368.

44. Robertson JH, McCarthy GM. Periwinkle alkaloids and the platelet count. Lancet 1969;2:353–355.

45. Lindenbaum J. Hematologic complications of alcohol abuse. Semin Liver Dis 1987;7:169–181.

46. Fialkow PJ, Gartler SM, Yoshida A. Clonal origin of chronic myelocytic leukemia in man. Proc Natl Acad Sci U S A 1967;58:1468–1471.

47. Jacobson RJ, Salo A, Fialkow PJ. Agnogenic myeloid metaplasia: a clonal proliferation of hematopoietic stem cells with secondary myelofibrosis. Blood 1978;51:189–194.

48. Fialkow PJ, Faguet GB, Jacobson RJ et al. Evidence that essential thrombocythemia is a clonal disorder with origin in a multipotent stem cell. Blood 1981;58:916–919.

49. Fialkow PJ, Singer JW, Adamson JW et al. Acute nonlymphocytic leukemia: expression in cells restricted to granulocytic and monocytic differentiation. N Engl J Med 1979;301:1–5.

50. Gilliland DG, Blanchard KL, Bunn HF. Clonality in acquired hematologic disorders. Annu Rev Med 1991;42:491–506.

51. Janssen JW, Anger BR, Drexler HG et al. Essential thrombocythemia in two sisters originating from different stem cell levels. Blood 1990;75:633–1636.

52. Yan L, El Kassar N, Gardin C et al. Clonality assays and megakaryocyte culture techniques in essential thrombocythemia. Leuk Lymphoma 1996;22(Suppl 1):31–40.

53. El Kassar N, Hetet G, Li Y et al. Clonal analysis of haemopoietic cells in essential thrombocythemia. Br J Haematol 1995;90:131–137.

54. Westwood NB, Pearson TC. Diagnostic applications of haemopoietic progenitor culture techniques in polycythaemias and thrombocythaemias. Leuk Lymphoma 1996;22(Suppl 1):95–103.

55. Shih LY, Lee CT. Identification of masked polycythemia vera from individuals with idiopathic marked thrombocytosis by endogenous erythroid colony assay. Blood 1994;83:744–748.

56. Mazur EM, Cohen JL, Bogart L. Growth characteristics of circulating hematopoietic progenitor cells from individuals with essential thrombocythemia. Blood 1988;71:1544–1550.

57. Battegay EJ, Thomssen C, Nissen C et al. Endogenous megakaryocyte colonies from peripheral blood in precursor cell cultures of individuals with myeloproliferative disorders. Eur J Haematol 1989;42:321–326.

58. Juvonen E, Ikkala E, Oksanen K et al. Megakaryocyte and erythroid colony formation in essential thrombocythemia and reactive thrombocytosis: diagnostic value and correlation to complications. Br J Haematol 1993;83:192–197.

59. Rolovic Z, Basara N, Gotic M et al. The determination of spontaneous megakaryocyte colony formation is an unequivocal test for discriminating between essential thrombocythemia and reactive thrombocytosis. Br J Haematol 1995;90:326–331.

60. Murphy S, Iland H, Rosenthal D et al. Essential thrombocythemia: an interim report from the Polycythemia Vera Study Group. Semin Hematol 1986;23:177–182.

61. Berlin NI. Diagnosis and classification of the polycythemias. Semin Hematol 1975;12:339–351.

62. Pearson TC, Messinezy M. The diagnostic criteria of polycythemia rubra vera. Leuk Lymphoma 1996;22(Suppl 1):87–94.

63. Pearson TC, Guthrie DL, Simpson J et al. Interpretation of measured red cell mass and plasma volume in adults: Expert Panel on Radionuclides of the International Council for Standardization in Haematology. Br J Haematol 1995;89:748–756.

64. Barbui T, Finazzi G, Barosi G. Chronic myeloid disorders other than CML. In: Degos L, Herrmann F, Linch D, Lowenberg B, eds. Textbook of malignant haematology. London: Martin Dunitz, 1997 (in press).

65. Schafer AI. Bleeding and thrombosis in the myeloproliferative disorders. Blood 1984;64:1–12.

66. Barosi G, Ambrosetti A, Buratti A et al. Splenectomy for individuals with myelofibrosis with myeloid metaplasia: pretreatment variables and outcome prediction. Leukemia 1993;7:200–206.

67. Mason JE Jr, DeVita VT, Canellos GP. Thrombocytosis in chronic granulocytic leukemia: incidence and clinical significance. Blood 1974;44:483–487.

68. The Italian Cooperative Study Group on Chronic Myeloid Leukemia. Interferon alfa-2a as compared with conventional chemotherapy for the treatment of chronic myeloid leukemia. N Engl J Med 1994;330:820–825.

69. Rambaldi A, Masuhara K, Borleri GM et al. Flow cytometry of leucocyte alkaline phosphatase in normal and pathologic haemopoietic cells. Br J Haematol 1997;96 (in press).

70. Stoll DB, Peterson P, Exten R et al. Clinical presentation and natural history of individuals with essential thrombocythemia and the Philadelphia chromosome. Am J Hematol 1988;27:77–83.

71. LeBrun DP, Pinkerton PH, Sheridan BL et al. Essential thrombocythemia with the Philadelphia chromosome and BCR-ABL gene rearrangement. An entity distinct from chronic myeloid leukemia and Philadelphia chromosome-negative essential thrombocythemia. Cancer Genet Cytogenet 1991;54:21–25.

72. Boultwood J, Lewis S, Wainscoat JS. The 5q-syndrome. Blood 1994;84:3253–3260.

73. Jondeau K, Bouscary D, Viguie F et al. Thrombocythemia and abnormal megakaryopoiesis associated with abnormality of chromosome 1p34 in myelodysplastic syndromes. Leukemia 1996;10:1692–1695.

74. Murphy S, Peterson P, Iland H et al. Experience of the Polycythemia Vera Study Group with essential thrombocythemia: a final report on diagnostic criteria, survival and leukemic transition by treatment. Semin Hematol 1997;34:29–39.

75. Tefferi A, Ho TC, Ahmann GJ et al. Plasma interleukin-6 and C-reactive protein levels in reactive versus clonal thrombocytosis. Am J Med 1994;97:374–378.

76. Third International Workshop on Chromosomes in Leukemia, 1980. Re-

port on essential thrombocythemia. Cancer Genet Cytogenet 1981;4: 138–142.

77. Dudley JM, Messinezy M, Eridani S et al. Primary thrombocythaemia: diagnostic criteria and a simple scoring system for positive diagnosis. Br J Haematol 1989;71:331–335.

78. Georgii A, Buhr T, Buesche G et al. Classification and staging of Ph-negative myeloproliferative disorders by histopathology from bone marrow biopsies. Leuk Lymphoma 1996;22(Suppl 1):15–29.

79. Bellucci S, Janvier M, Tobelem G et al. Essential thrombocythemia. Clinical evolutionary and biological data. Cancer 1986;58:2440–2447.

80. Fenaux P, Simon M, Caulier MT et al. Clinical course of essential thrombocythemia in 147 cases. Cancer 1990;66:549–556.

81. McIntyre KJ, Hoagland HC, Silverstein MN et al. Essential thrombocythemia in young adults. Mayo Clin Proc 1991;66:149–154.

82. Barbui T, Cortelazzo S, Viero P et al. Thrombohaemorrhagic complications in 101 cases of myeloproliferative disorders: relationship to platelet number and function. Eur J Cancer Clin Oncol 1983;191:593–1599.

83. Iland HJ, Laszlo J, Peterson P et al. Essential thrombocythemia: clinical and laboratory characteristics at presentation. Trans Assoc Am Physicians 1983;96:165–174.

84. Randi ML, Casonato A, Fabris F et al. The significance of thrombocytosis in old age. Acta Haematol 1987;78:41–44

85. Lahuerta-Palacios JJ, Bornstein R, Fernandez-Debora FJ et al. Controlled and uncontrolled thrombocytosis. Its clinical role in essential thrombocythemia. Cancer 1988;61:1207–1212.

86. Hehlmann R, Jahn M, Baumann B et al. Essential thrombocythemia. Clinical characteristics and course of 61 cases. Cancer 1988;61:2487–2496.

87. Cortelazzo S, Viero P, Finazzi G et al. Incidence and risk factors for thrombotic complications in a historical cohort of 100 individuals with essential thrombocythemia. J Clin Oncol 1990;8:556–562.

88. Mitus AJ, Barbui T, Shulman LN et al. Hemostatic complications in young individuals with essential thrombocythemia. Am J Med 1990;88:371–375.

89. Millard FE, Hunter CS, Anderson M et al. Clinical manifestations of essential thrombocythemia in young adults. Am J Hematol 1990;33: 27–31.

90. Colombi M, Radaelli F, Zocchi L et al. Thrombotic and hemorrhagic complications in essential thrombocythemia. Cancer 1991;67:2926–2930.

91. Randi ML, Fabris F, Girolami A. Thrombocytosis in young people: evaluation of 57 cases diagnosed before the age of 40. Blut 1990;60:233–237.

92. Wehmeier A, Daum I, Jamin H et al. Incidence and clinical risk factors for bleeding and thrombotic complications in myeloproliferative disorders. Ann Hematol 1991;63:101–106.

93. Budde U, Scharf RE, Franke P et al. Elevated platelet count as a cause of abnormal von Willebrand factor multimer distribution in plasma. Blood 1993;82:1749–1757.

94. van Genderen PJ, Budde U, Michiels JJ et al. The reduction of large von Willebrand factor multimers in plasma in essential thrombocythemia is related to the platelet count. Br J Haematol 1996;93:962–965.

95. Berk PD, Goldberg JD, Donovan PB et al. Therapeutic recommendations in polycythemia vera based on Polycythemia Vera Study Group protocols. Semin Hematol 1986;23:132–143.

96. Gruppo Italiano Studio Policitemia (GISP). Polycythemia vera: the natural history of 1213 individuals followed for 20 years. Ann Intern Med 1995; 123:656–664.

97. Cortelazzo S, Finazzi G, Ruggeri M et al. Hydroxyurea in the treatment of individuals with essential thrombocythemia at high risk of thrombosis: a prospective randomized trial. N Engl J Med 1995;332:1132–1136.

98. Michiels JJ, Abels J, Steketee J et al. Erythromelalgia caused by platelet-mediated arteriolar inflammation and thrombosis in thrombocythemia. Ann Intern Med 1985;102:466–471.

99. van Genderen PJ, Lucas IS, van Strik R et al. Erythromelagia in essential thrombocythemia is characterized by platelet activation and endothelial cell damage but not by thrombin generation. Thromb Haemost 1996;76: 333–338.

100. van Genderen PJ, Michiels JJ, van Strik R et al. Platelet consumption in thrombocythemia complicated by erythromelalgia: reversal by aspirin. Thromb Haemost 1995;73:210–214.

101. Michiels JJ, van Joost T. Erythromelalgia and thrombocytosis: a causal relation. J Am Acad Dermatol 1990;22:107–111.

102. Drenth JP, Michiels JJ. Three types of erythromelagia. BMJ 1990;301: 454–455.

103. Jabaily J, Iland HJ, Laszlo J et al. Neurologic manifestations of essential thrombocythemia. Ann Intern Med 1983;99:513–518.

104. Scheffer MG, Michiels JJ, Simoons ML et al. Thrombocythemia and coronary artery disease. Am Heart J 1991;122:573–576.

105. Johnson PM, Davies JM. Thrombocythaemia and recurrent miscarriage. Br J Obstet Gynaecol 1989;96:1231–1232.

106. Falconer J, Pineo G, Blahey W et al. Essential thrombocythemia associated with recurrent abortions and fetal growth retardation. Am J Hematol 1987; 25:345–347.

107. Frezzato M, Rodeghiero F. Pregnancy in women with essential thrombocythaemia [Letter]. Br J Haematol 1996;93:977.

108. Beard J, Hillmen P, Anderson CC et al. Primary thrombocytopenia in pregnancy. Br J Haematol 1991;77:371–374.

109. Pagliaro P, Arrigoni L, Muggiasca ML et al. Primary thrombocyhthemia

110. Shpilberg O, Shimon I, Sofer O et al. Transient normal platelet counts and decreased requirement for interferon during pregnancy in essential thrombocythemia. Br J Haematol 1996;93:491–493.

111. Beressi AH, Tefferi A, Silverstein MN et al. Outcome analysis of 34 pregnancies in women with essential thrombocythemia. Arch Intern Med 1995; 155:1217–1222.

112. Valla D, Casadevall N, Lacombe C et al. Primary myeloproliferative disorders and hepatic vein thrombosis. A prospective study of erythroid colony formation *in vitro* in 20 individuals with Budd-Chiari syndrome. Ann Intern Med 1985;103:329–334.

113. Cohen J, Edelman RR, Chopra S. Portal vein thrombosis: a review. Am J Med 1992;92:173–182.

114. Welford C, Spies SM, Green D. Priapism in primary thrombocythemia. Arch Intern Med 1981;141:807–808.

115. Shepherd P, Liddell K. Pyoderma gangrenosum associated with primary thrombocythaemia. BMJ (London) 1982;285:837–838.

116. Rozman C, Giralt M, Feliu E et al. Life expectancy of individuals with chronic nonleukemic myeloproliferative disorders. Cancer 1991;67: 2658–2663.

117. Weinfeld A, Swolin B, Westin J. Acute leukaemia after hydroxyurea therapy in polycythemia vera and allied disorders: prospective study of efficacy and leukaemogenicity with therapeutic implications. Eur J Haematol 1994;52:134–139.

118. Shibata K, Shimamoto Y, Suga K et al. Essential thrombocythemia terminating in acute leukemia with minimal myeloid differentiation—a brief Review of recent literature. Acta Haematol 1994;91:84–88.

119. Brandt L, Anderson H. Survival and risk of leukemia in polycythaemia vera and essential thrombocythaemia treated with oral radiophosphorus: are safer drugs available? Eur J Haematol 1995;54:21–26.

120. Nand S, Stock W, Godwin J et al. Leukemogenic risk of hydroxyurea therapy in polycythemia vera, essential thrombocythemia and myeloid metaplasia with myelofibrosis. Am J Hematol 1996;52:42–46.

121. Barbui T, Finazzi G, Dupuy E et al. Treatment strategies in essential thrombocythemia. Leuk Lymphoma 1996;22(Suppl 1):149–160.

122. Michiels JJ, Koudstaal PJ, Mulder AH, van Vliet HH. Transient neurologic and ocular manifestations in primary thrombocythemia. Neurology 1993; 43:1107–1110.

123. Pearson TC. Primary thrombocythaemia: diagnosis and management. Br J Haematol 1991;78:145–148.

124. Antiplatelet Trialists' Collaboration. Collaborative overview of randomized trials of antiplatelet therapy. I. Prevention of death, myocardial infarction, and stroke by prolonged antiplatelet therapy in various categories of individuals. BMJ 1994;308:81–106.

125. Finazzi G, Budde U, Michiels JJ. Bleeding time and platelet function in essential thrombocythemia and other myeloproliferative syndromes. Leuk Lymphoma 1996;22(Suppl 1):71–78.

126. Kelly JP, Kaufman DW, Jurgelon JM et al. Risk of aspirin-associated major upper-gastrointestinal bleeding with enteric-coated or buffered product. Lancet 1996;348:1413–1416.

127. Griesshammer M, Heimpel H, Pearson TC. Essential thrombocythemia and pregnancy. Leuk Lymphoma 1996;22(Suppl 1):57–63.

128. Löfvenberg E, Wahlin A. Management of polycythaemia vera, essential thrombocythaemia and myelofibrosis with hydroxyurea. Eur J Haematol 1988;41:375–381.

129. Schafer AI. Essential thrombocythemia. Prog Hemost Thromb 1991;10:69–96.

130. Tefferi A, Silverstein MN, Hoagland HC. Primary thrombocythemia. Semin Oncol 1995;22:334–340.

131. Löfvenberg E, Nordenson I, Wahlin A. Cytogenetic abnormalities and leukemic transformation in hydroxyurea-treated individuals with Philadelphia chromosome negative chronic myeloproliferative disease. Cancer Genet Cytogenet 1990;49:57–67.

132. Van de Pette JE, Prochazka AV, Pearson TC et al. Primary thrombocythemia treated with busulfan. Br J Haematol 1986;62:229–237.

133. Brusamolino E, Canevari A, Salvaneschi L et al. Efficacy trial of pipobroman in essential thrombocythemia: a study of 24 individuals. Cancer Treat Rep 1984;68:1339–1342.

134. Mazzucconi MG, Francesconi M, Chistolini A et al. Pipobroman therapy of essential thrombocythemia. Scand J Haematol 1986;37:306–309.

135. Silver RT. Interferon in the treatment of myeloproliferative diseases. Semin Hematol 1990;27(Suppl 4):6–14.

136. Gisslinger H, Chott A, Scheithauer W et al. Interferon in essential thrombocythemia. Br J Haematol 1991;79(Suppl 1):42–47.

137. Wadenvik H, Kutti J, Ridell B et al. The effect of alpha-interferon on bone marrow megakaryocytes and platelet production rate in essential thrombocythemia. Blood 1991;77:2103–2108.

138. Lengfelder E, Griesshammer M, Hehlmann R. Interferon-alpha in the treatment of essential thrombocythemia. Leuk Lymphoma 1996;22(Suppl 1):135–142.

139. Silverstein MN, Petitt RM, Solberg LA Jr et al. Angrelide: a new drug for treating thrombocytosis. N Engl J Med 1988;318:1292–1294.

140. Anagrelide Study Group. Anagrelide, a therapy for thrombocythemic states: experience in 577 individuals. Am J Med 1992;92:69–76.

141. Mazur EM, Rosmarin AG, Sohl PA et al. Analysis of the mechanism of anagrelide-induced thrombocytopenia in humans. Blood 1992;79: 1931–1937.

# SECTION 7

# QUALITATIVE PLATELET DISORDERS

# CHAPTER 32

# CONGENITAL DISORDERS OF PLATELET FUNCTION

Lindsay C. Dunlop, Robert K. Andrews, José A. López,
and Michael C. Berndt

## INTRODUCTION

In normal vasculature, blood platelets circulate freely and do not adhere to the endothelial cells lining the blood vessel wall. However, in response to vascular injury blood platelets rapidly adhere to exposed elements of the subendothelial matrix. This adhesion depends in part on von Willebrand factor (vWf) and a specific vWf receptor on platelets, the platelet membrane glycoprotein (GP) Ib-IX-V complex, and in part on adhesion to collagen. The adherent platelets spread on the subendothelial surface and become activated. Arachidonic acid is mobilized from platelet phospholipid pools and is metabolized by cyclooxygenase and thromboxane synthase to form thromboxane $A_2$, a potent platelet-aggregating substance. Activated platelets also release the contents of their storage organelles (e.g., adenosine 5'-diphosphate [ADP] from the platelet dense bodies), some of which act in the recruitment of additional platelets leading to the formation of a platelet aggregate or primary hemostatic plug. In a plasma milieu, platelet aggregation is mediated primarily by fibrinogen, which bridges activated platelets by binding to a specific receptor, the platelet membrane GP IIb-IIIa complex. An abnormality in any of the stages of platelet adhesion, activation, secretion, or aggregation can result in a bleeding diathesis and prolonged skin bleeding time (Table 32.1). These abnormalities may be associated with an intrinsic platelet defect (of cytoplasmic components or surface recep-

tors) or with defective extracellular ligands (such as vWf or fibrinogen).

In this chapter platelet-related congenital bleeding disorders will be discussed in the context of adhesion, secretion, activation, and aggregation, with particular emphasis on recent advances in understanding their underlying genetic defects. The therapy of congenital platelet bleeding disorders is discussed in the final section of the chapter.

## CLINICAL MANIFESTATIONS AND APPROACH TO CLINICAL DIAGNOSIS

The clinical manifestations of congenital platelet disorders related to adhesion, activation, secretion, or aggregation may often be indistinguishable. A family history of a bleeding diathesis can give a guide to the mode of inheritance of the bleeding diathesis, and this, combined with the association of other clinical manifestations of the disorder, may allow the underlying platelet abnormality to be identified (e.g., Hermansky-Pudlak syndrome or Wiskott-Aldrich syndrome). The initial laboratory assessment would normally involve measurement of blood cell counts and examination of a peripheral blood smear. These investigations could indicate thrombocytopenia on the blood count, as well as revealing

**TABLE 32.1.** Congenital Platelet-Related Bleeding Abnormalties

| Stage and Disease | Defect(s) | Comments |
|---|---|---|
| *Adhesion* | | |
| von Willebrand disease | Types 1 and 3. Partial quantitative deficiency (type 1) or virtual absence (type 3) of von Willebrand factor | Prolonged SBT |
| | Type 2A. von Willebrand factor with decreased affinity for platelets, lack of high-molecular-weight multimers | Prolonged SBT |
| | Type 2B. von Willebrand factor binds spontaneously to platelets, loss of high-molecular-weight multimers | Prolonged SBT and may be associated with thrombocytopenia |
| Pseudo–von Willebrand disease | von Willebrand factor spontaneously binds GP Ib-IX-V | Marginally prolonged SBT, intermittent thrombocytopenia |
| Bernard-Soulier syndrome | GP Ib-IX-V is absent or dysfunctional as a receptor for von Willebrand factor | Prolonged SBT, large platelets, and thrombocytopenia |
| Collagen receptor defect | GP Ia-IIa ($\alpha2\beta1$) deficiency due to low GP Ia ($\alpha2$) expression | Prolonged SBT (>30 minutes) |
| | GP IV deficiency on platelets associated with absence (type I) or presence (type II) of GP IV on monocytes | No apparent phenotype |
| | GP VI expression markedly decreased | Purpura and marginally prolonged SBT |
| *Secretion* | | |
| Gray platelet syndrome | Abnormal function of $\alpha$-storage granules and deficiency of $\alpha$-granule components | Normal to prolonged SBT; large, poorly stained platelets on peripheral blood smear; thrombocytopenia; "Swiss-cheese" morphology; and fibrotic marrow |
| $\delta$-Storage pool disease | Dense-body deficiency | Inherited or acquired. Also in Hermansky-Pudlak, Chediak-Higashi, and Wiskott-Aldrich syndromes |
| $\alpha\delta$-Storage pool disease | Defective, variable deficiencies of both $\alpha$- and $\delta$-granules | |
| *Activation* | | |
| Release defect | Arachidonic acid and prostaglandin pathway abnormal. May be related to cyclooxygenase, thromboxane synthase, or thromboxane $A_2$ receptor deficiencies | Normal to prolonged SBT. Classically occurs with aspirin and other drugs |
| Signal-transduction defect | Failure to mobilize arachidonic acid | Normal to prolonged SBT |
| *Aggregation* | | |
| Glanzmann's thrombasthenia | GP IIb-IIIa is absent, present in markedly decreased amounts, or dysfunctional | Prolonged SBT |

*GP, glycoprotein; SBT, skin bleeding time.*

morphologic abnormalities of platelets (e.g., gray platelet syndrome) or of leukocytes (e.g., May-Hegglin anomaly or Chediak-Higashi syndrome). The type of bleeding abnormality, however, can usually be readily differentiated experimentally by functional analysis of stirred platelet suspensions in an aggregometer (Table 32.2) (Chapter 23). In many instances, however, this provisional diagnosis needs to be confirmed by additional specialized tests, which may include flow cytometry to assess surface glycoprotein expression by platelets or mepacrine staining to assess dense bodies. Electron microscopy is useful in assessing platelet storage granules or leukocyte granulation. Ultimately, however, the final diagnosis for deficiency of one or more surface glycoproteins requires biochemical analysis involving either surface-labeling of washed platelets, followed by SDS-polyacrylamide gel electrophoresis and autoradiography, or immunologic probing with specific antiplatelet glycoprotein antibodies analyzed by Western blotting. Secretion defects of platelets may require characterization by SDS-polyacrylamide gel electrophoresis of supernatants of stirred, washed platelet suspensions. Finally, the establishment of an abnormal genotype by molecular studies should allow precise definition of the abnormality causing the platelet defect. The way in which these techniques can be used to unequivocally

establish individual disorders in particular cases is evident from the more detailed discussion of congenital platelet defects in the ensuing sections.

# CONGENITAL PLATELET ADHESION DEFECTS

## BERNARD-SOULIER SYNDROME

One rare but important congenital platelet disorder is the Bernard-Soulier syndrome, characterized, in part, by prolonged skin bleeding time, normal clot retraction, morphologically enlarged platelets, and thrombocytopenia (1, 2). The main clinical symptoms, evident from early childhood, include frequent episodes of epistaxis and hemorrhage associated with cutaneous bleeding or trauma.

The major functional defect of Bernard-Soulier syn-

**TABLE 32.2.**  Platelet Function Analysis

| Disease | ADP (5 μmol/L) | Collagen (2 μg/ml) | Arachidonic Acid (1 mmol/L) | Ristocetin (1.5 mg/ml) | Ristocetin (0.5 mg/ml) | Comments |
|---|---|---|---|---|---|---|
| von Willebrand disease | | | | | | |
| Types 1 and 3[a] | Normal | Normal | Normal | Absent | Absent | Platelets aggregate in response to bovine plasma |
| Type 2A | Normal | Normal | Normal | Decreased | Absent | Confirm by platelet and plasma vWf multimer analysis |
| Type 2B[b] | Normal | Normal | Normal | Normal | Aggregation | Confirm by platelet and plasma vWf multimer analysis |
| Pseudo-von Willebrand disease[b] | Normal | Normal | Normal | Normal | Aggregation | Confirm by platelet and plasma vWf multimer analysis |
| Bernard-Soulier syndrome[a] | Normal | Normal | Normal | Absent | Absent | Platelets fail to aggregate in response to bovine plasma |
| Collagen receptor defect | Normal | Absent | Normal | Normal | Absent | Very rare |
| Release defect[c] | Primary wave only | Decreased | Absent | Normal | Absent | Always suspect aspirin or antiinflammatory drug |
| Storage pool deficiency[cd] | Primary wave only | Decreased | Variable | Normal | Absent | Perform mepacrine labeling |
| Signal transduction defect[d] | Primary wave only | Decreased | Normal | Normal | Absent | |
| Glanzmann's thrombasthenia | Absent (shape change only) | Absent (shape change only) | Absent (shape change only) | Normal | Absent | |

ADP, adenosine diphosphate; vWf, von Willebrand factor.

[a] Type 1 and 3 von Willebrand disease differentiated from Bernard-Soulier syndrome by response to bovine plasma.

[b] Platelets aggregate to factor VIII concentrate or cryoprecipitate in pseudo- but not type 2B von Willebrand disease.

[c] Differentiated by response to arachidonic acid.

[d] Differentiated by mepacrine labeling and/or release studies.

drome platelets is impaired adhesion to the vascular subendothelium, associated with an absence or dysfunctional expression of the GP Ib-IX-V complex. As discussed above, adhesion of circulating platelets to the vessel wall is the first step in normal hemostasis. This process can be modeled *in vitro* using a Baumgartner chamber, where whole blood or platelet-rich plasma is perfused at different shear rates over a subendothelial section (3). The extent of platelet adhesion is determined by microscopic examination of the subendothelium. Compared with normal platelets, Bernard-Soulier platelets show greatly reduced adhesion in the high range of physiologic shear flow rates (>650/second), whereas essentially normal levels of adhesion are seen at low shear rates (4, 5). Those platelets that do adhere are able to spread over the matrix surface, although to a lesser extent than control platelets, indicating that poor initial adhesion is the main defect in Bernard-Soulier platelets. Adhesion of normal platelets at high shear has been shown to depend on vWf bound to the subendothelial matrix; platelet adhesion can be blocked by certain anti-vWf monoclonal antibodies and is absent or diminished in von Willebrand disease individuals where vWf is either missing or dysfunctional (6, 7). The defective platelet adhesion at high shear associated with Bernard-Soulier syndrome is therefore consistent with an absence or nonfunctional expression of the platelet vWf receptor, the GP Ib-IX-V complex, a conclusion supported by *in vitro* aggregation experiments. Although stirred suspensions of Bernard-Soulier platelets aggregate normally in response to platelet stimuli such as ADP, collagen, and adrenaline, there is no vWf-dependent agglutination. Unlike platelets from von Willebrand disease individuals, Bernard-Soulier platelets fail to agglutinate in the presence of normal vWf and the vWf activators, ristocetin and botrocetin (Table 32.2). In addition, they do not agglutinate in the presence of bovine vWf, which does not require a modulator (1, 8). Finally, vWf from the plasma of Bernard-Soulier individuals is functionally normal since it supports the agglutination of normal platelets. Taken together, these findings are consistent with Bernard-Soulier platelets lacking a functional vWf adhesion receptor. Further, the GP Ib-IX-V complex also binds α-thrombin (1) (see Chapter 11), and recent evidence suggests that both GP Ib-IX-V and the seven-transmembrane thrombin receptor are involved in the optimal response of platelets to thrombin (9, 10). Supporting this view, Bernard-Soulier platelets show markedly impaired responsiveness to α-thrombin (11, 12).

Biochemical analysis of Bernard-Soulier platelets demonstrates a marked deficiency or absence of the surface glycoproteins, GP Ib, GP IX, and GP V (Fig. 32.1) (13, 14). The disulfide-linked GP Ib α-subunit (135 Kda) and β-subunit (25 Kda) form a noncovalently linked heterodimeric complex with GP IX (22 Kda) (15). GP V (82 Kda) forms a 1:2 complex with GP Ib-IX on the platelet mem-

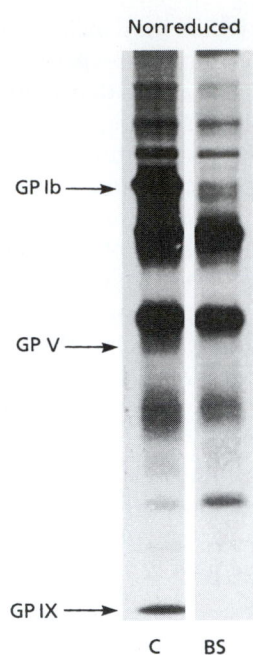

**FIGURE 32.1.** Autoradiogram of surface [³H]–labeled control (C) and Bernard-Soulier syndrome (BS) platelets electrophoresed on sodium dodecyl sulfate polyacrylamide gels under nonreducing conditions. The positions of GP Ib (GP Ibα disulfide-linked to GP Ibβ), GP V, and GP IX, which are deficient in Bernard-Soulier syndrome platelets, are indicated by the arrows.

brane surface (16), such that the GP Ib-IX-V complex consists of seven transmembrane polypeptides that may associate to form even larger complexes (15). Interestingly, GP Ibα, GP Ibβ, GP IX, and GP V are all members of the leucine-rich protein family and contain a variable number of ~24-residue, leucine-rich, repeat domains (seven, one, one, and fifteen, respectively) and conserved aminoterminal and carboxylterminal flanking sequences in their extracellular domains (8, 15). The vWf binding site on the GP Ib-IX-V complex is contained within an ~40-kDa globular domain ($His_1$–$Glu_{282}$) at the aminoterminal region of GP Ibα (8) (see Chapters 11 and 16). vWf interacts with an anionic stretch of amino acid residues ($Tyr_{276}$–$Glu_{282}$) (17–19) containing three sulfated tyrosines ($Tyr_{276}$, $Tyr_{278}$, and $Tyr_{279}$) (17, 19) and at least one other site within the sequence $His_1$–$Leu_{275}$ that contains the leucine-rich repeats and flanking sequences (19). The $Tyr_{276}$–$Glu_{282}$ sequence also constitutes a binding site for α-thrombin (18, 19). Binding of vWf to the GP Ib-IX-V complex on platelets induces intracellular signaling that mediates subsequent post-adhesion events (20–24). These include the cytoskeletal rearrangement, associated with shape change, spreading, and secretion, and activation of the platelet fibrinogen receptor, GP IIb-IIIa, that mediates platelet-platelet associations through fibrinogen binding. The signaling pathway(s) involved in GP Ib-

IX-V–dependent platelet activation are unknown, but may be at least partly regulated by the 14-3-3 ($\zeta$) signaling molecule that is directly associated with the cytoplasmic domain of the receptor (25) and is implicated in the regulation/activation of a range of signaling molecules such as raf-1, protein kinase C, and phosphatidyl inositol 3-kinase (26).

In the resting platelet, the cytoplasmic region of the GP Ib-IX-V complex is attached to cytoplasmic filamentous actin via actin-binding protein. There is increasing evidence that this interaction establishes the surface distribution of the GP Ib-IX-V complex, enhances the avidity of the receptor for vWf, and anchors the plasma membrane to the cytoskeleton to maintain cell shape and membrane stability (27, 28). The loss of the normally rigid, disk-like shape and decreased membrane stability found in Bernard-Soulier platelets may be explained by disruption of normal cytoskeletal associations. Cyclic adenosine monophosphate-dependent activation of protein kinase A, which inhibits platelet activation, results in phosphorylation of $Ser_{166}$ on the cytoplasmic region of GP Ib$\beta$, an event that regulates actin polymerization and thus, presumably, the reorganization of the actin cytoskeleton (29, 30).

While it has been known for some time that Bernard-Soulier platelets lack functional GP Ib-IX-V complex, recent studies have provided new insights into the specific genetic defects underlying the disease. Each polypeptide chain comprising the receptor complex is the product of a separate gene, and the regions encoding each mature polypeptide are contained within a single exon within their respective genes. It has been demonstrated that, like other membrane complexes such as GP IIb-IIIa (see below), the stable surface expression of GP Ib$\alpha$, GP Ib$\beta$, GP IX, and GP V probably requires the presence of all of the components of the complex (31–33). This suggests that genetic lesions associated with any component of the GP Ib-IX complex, and possibly GP V, or with related regulatory elements could potentially prevent normal posttranslational modification, assembly, and/or membrane insertion and lead to Bernard-Soulier syndrome. In virtually all cases where it has been assessed, Bernard-Soulier syndrome shows an autosomal recessive inheritance pattern and is almost always associated with consanguinity.

It has now been established that Bernard-Soulier syndrome arises from a heterogeneous array of genetic defects (Table 32.3). Bernard-Soulier syndrome can be broadly categorized in two ways. First, classification may be based on the localization of the defect to (a) the GP Ib$\alpha$ gene (chromosome 17ptr-p12), (b) the GP Ib$\beta$ gene (chromosome 22q11.2), (c) the GP IX gene (chromosome 3), and possibly (d) the GP V gene (chromosome 3). Second, the abnormality may be either (1) a biosynthetic defect, affecting synthesis, processing, or expression, or (2) a

functional defect, where GP Ib$\alpha$ is expressed in a dysfunctional form that fails to bind ligand. Thus the syndrome might be classified as type 1a, for example, to indicate a defect of the GP Ib$\alpha$ gene that results in a biosynthetic defect. Most of the reported defects arise from missense, nonsense, or deletion mutations of the GP Ib$\alpha$ (34–43) or GP IX (43–46) genes that produce truncated, unstable, or dysfunctional polypeptides. In both proteins a number of the amino acid substitutions/deletions are clustered within the leucine-rich repeats or flanking sequences (Table 32.3), emphasizing the importance of these domains in ligand binding (GP Ib$\alpha$) and/or assembly and surface expression of a functional receptor complex. In this regard each of the $Asp_{21}$ to Gly and $Asn_{45}$ to Ser Bernard-Soulier mutations introduced into recombinant GP IX abolished the ability of GP IX to support stable surface expression of cotransfected GP Ib in Chinese hamster ovary cells (50). This was related to the diminished ability of the mutants to form a stable complex with GP Ib. Diminished surface expression of the entire GP Ib-IX-V complex following truncation of GP Ib$\alpha$ (36, 42, 43) or GP IX (43) is generally consistent with findings from expression studies using recombinant components of the receptor, alone or in combination, in transfected cell lines (31–33). Correlating with the variability in genetic defects, there is considerable variation in the levels of different components of the GP Ib-IX-V complex expressed in Bernard-Soulier platelets and in the amounts of each protein that appear on the membrane surface (which may be as high as 40 to 50% of normal for individual polypeptides) (13, 14, 51–53). In several cases of Bernard-Soulier syndrome, family members heterozygous for the Bernard-Soulier mutation express about half of the normal levels of GP Ib$\alpha$ on their platelets with a corresponding decrease in vWf binding, but with no substantial bleeding disorder (41, 52). This finding indicates that GP Ib$\alpha$ is probably the polypeptide of the receptor complex present in limiting amounts.

A variant form of Bernard-Soulier syndrome showed autosomal-dominant inheritance in three generations of one family (35). In this family a woman with a long history of prolonged bleeding, menorrhagia, and epistaxis had a son and a daughter from different fathers, and both children had Bernard-Soulier syndrome. Her father, although not studied in detail, showed increased susceptibility to bruising and excessive bleeding following trauma, while her two other daughters (the affected daughter's sisters), her mother, and the son's father showed no or very mild bleeding abnormalities. All of the affected individuals in this family showed increased mean platelet volume, thrombocytopenia, and variable but characteristically decreased ristocetin-dependent agglutination that was not corrected by normal vWf. Genomic amplification and sequencing indicated that the affected members of the family were heterozygous for a

**TABLE 32.3.** Platelet Glycoprotein (GP) Ib-IX-V Complex Defects

| Location of Mutation in the GP Ib-IX-V Complex | Disease | Abnormality | Genetic Defect(s) | Inheritance | Ref. |
|---|---|---|---|---|---|
| | Bernard-Soulier syndrome | 1 $Lys_{19}$/Arg | GP Ibα codon AAG ($Lys_{19}$) to AGA (Arg) following A deletion, frameshift and premature stop after codon 21. No surface GP Ibα | AR | [34] |
| | | 2 $Leu_{57}$/Phe | GP Ibα codon CTC ($Leu_{57}$) to TTC (Phe) in one allele, wild type allele is not expressed. Mutant is expressed in dysfunctional form. | AD | [35] |
| | | 3 $Leu_{76}$/Arg | GP Ibα deletion of T in codon 76 causing frameshift and truncation after 20 residues. | AR | [36] |
| | | 4 $Leu_{129}$/Pro | GP Ibα codon CTC ($Leu_{129}$) to CCC (Pro), normal GP V expression. | AR | [37] |
| | | 5 $Ala_{156}$/Val | GP Ibα codon GCT ($Ala_{156}$) to GTT (Val), associated with apparently inconsequential ACG ($Thr_{145}$) to ATG (Met) mutation. | AR | [38] |
| | | 6 $Leu_{179}$ deletion | GP Ibα codon TCC ($Leu_{179}$) deleted (Nancy I variant). | AR | [39] |
| | | 7 $Cys_{209}$/Ser | GP Ibα codon TGC ($Cys_{209}$) to AGC (Ser). | AR | [40] |
| | | 8 $Trp_{343}$/stop | GP Ibα mutation is in one allele, unidentified defect in another allele. | AR | [41] |
| | | 9 $Ser_{444}$/stop | GP Ibα codon TCA ($Ser_{444}$) to TAA (stop), normal GP Ibβ and IX. | AR | [42] |
| | | 10 Frame shift | GP Ibα nucleotide deletion within a seven A repeat sequence resulting in $Thr_{452}$ to Pro followed by a 58-residue frameshift and early stop. | AR | [43] |
| | | 11 $Asp_{21}$/Gly | GP IX codon GAC ($Asp_{21}$) to GGC (Gly), combined with $Asn_{45}$/Ser. | AR | [44] |
| | | 12 $Asn_{45}$/Ser | GP IX codon AAC ($Asn_{45}$) to AGC (Gly). | AR | [45] |
| | | 13 $Cys_{73}$/Tyr | GP IX codon TGT ($Cys_{73}$) to TAT (Tyr). | AR | [46] |
| | | 14 $Trp_{126}$/stop | GP IX codon TGG ($Trp_{126}$) to TGA (stop), no GP IX expression. | AR | [43] |
| | | 15 Complex | C to G mutation at -133 in the GP Ibβ promoter of one allele, other allele missing due to deletion within chromosome 22q11.2. | AR | [47] |
| | Pseudo–von Willebrand disease | 16 $Gly_{233}$/Val | GP Ibα codon GGT ($Gly_{233}$) to GTT (Val), plus wild type allele. | AD | [48] |
| | | 17 $Met_{239}$/Val | GP Ibα codon ATG ($Met_{239}$) to GTG (Val). | AD | [49] |

☐, leucine-rich repeat; ■, anionic/sulfated tyrosine sequence; ♯, glycosylation sites; ▨, plasma membrane (the upper surface is extracytoplasmic). Disulfide bonds in leucine-rich domain flanking sequences are not shown. AD, autosomal dominant; AR, probably autosomal recessive.

single base mutation in the coding region of GP Ibα predicting a single amino acid substitution, $Leu_{57}$ to Phe. Why the wild-type GP Ibα was not expressed in functional form is unknown. This interesting, possibly dominant-negative mutation suggests that a functional GP Ib-IX-V complex may be composed of more than one functional GP Ibα polypeptide. In this case the product of the mutant allele may inhibit the function of wild-type GP Ibα, or the mutant GP Ibα may show greater than normal susceptibility to proteolysis that disrupts normal complex function.

Only one case of Bernard-Soulier syndrome has so far been attributed to a mutation in the GP Ibβ gene (47). One allele of the GP Ibβ gene was missing, in association with a deletion in the DiGeorge/velo-cardio-facial region of chromosome 22q11.2, while the other allele contained a C to G mutation at position −133 in the promoter region of the GP Ibβ gene (47). The spectrum of phenotypic manifestations of mutations to members of the GP Ib-IX-V complex also includes disorders with milder clinical features. For example, one case of giant platelet syndrome without marked bleeding has recently been described associated with compound heterozygous mutations of GP Ibβ (54). In platelets from these individuals, expressed GP Ibβ is not disulfide-linked to GP Ibα, indicating that this linkage may be important for the cytoskeletal linkage of the entire complex.

In addition to the examples of Bernard-Soulier syndrome listed in Table 32.3, individuals have also been described with bleeding disorders resembling Bernard-Soulier syndrome, but which are not caused by congenital defects of the GP Ib-IX-V complex. Devine et al have reported a individual with normal-sized platelets, but absent ristocetin-induced agglutination, who had acquired antiplatelet HLA and anti-GP Ib-IX-V complex autoantibodies following procainamide therapy (55). Another individual had a severe acquired bleeding disorder associated with juvenile myelodysplastic syndrome. The genetic basis of this disorder is not clear, but was associated with monosomy 7 (56).

## PSEUDO–VON WILLEBRAND DISEASE

Pseudo-von Willebrand disease (or platelet-type von Willebrand disease) is a congenital bleeding disorder of platelets associated with an increased skin bleeding time, intermittent thrombocytopenia, morphologically normal platelets, and decreased levels of high-molecular-weight vWf multimers in plasma (57–59). Compared with normal platelets, there is a marked decrease in adhesion of platelets from pseudo-von Willebrand disease individuals to the subendothelium under conditions of high shear (3300/second) (58). The poor adhesion of platelets at high shear and the absence of high-molecular-weight vWf multimers in the plasma are also features of type 2A and type 2B von Willebrand disease (6)

(see Chapter 34). In type 2A von Willebrand disease, a number of specific-point mutations in vWf have been identified (involving the region of the gene that encodes amino acid residues between $Ser_{743}$ and $Glu_{875}$), which result in an almost total absence of medium- and high-molecular-weight multimers and a decreased affinity for platelet binding. In type 2B von Willebrand disease, amino acid substitutions within the GP Ib-IX-V-binding A1 domain (8) activate vWf, enhance its binding to platelets, and lead to its clearance from the circulation. Platelet-rich plasma from individuals with type 2B von Willebrand disease shows increased sensitivity to ristocetin-dependent platelet agglutination. Platelets of individuals with pseudo-von Willebrand disease are also more sensitive than normal to ristocetin-induced vWf-dependent agglutination. In contrast to normal and type 2B von Willebrand disease platelets, however, platelets from individuals with pseudo-von Willebrand disease aggregate spontaneously when exposed to high-molecular-weight vWf multimers from normal plasma (57, 58). Normal levels of the whole range of vWf multimers are found in the α-granules of pseudo-von Willebrand disease platelets (57). Rather than an abnormality in vWf, these findings are consistent with a defect associated with the vWf receptor, the GP Ib-IX-V complex. The lack of high-molecular-weight vWf multimers in the plasma of individuals with pseudo-von Willebrand disease is therefore probably a consequence of clearance through spontaneous binding of these multimers to platelets.

Unlike Bernard-Soulier syndrome, which is usually autosomal recessive, pseudo-von Willebrand disease showed autosomal dominant inheritance in four individuals representing four generations of one family (48). Interestingly, the severity of the bleeding disorder in these individuals increased in each successive generation, although the reason for this is not known. Two genetic defects underlying pseudo-von Willebrand disease have been determined (Table 32.3) (48, 49). Both single amino acid substitution mutations ($Gly_{233}$ to Val and $Met_{239}$ to Val) are within the disulfide-bonded loop structure C-terminal to the leucine-rich repeats in GP Ibα, and separating these repeat domains from the anionic/sulfated tyrosine sequence implicated in binding vWf (17–19). Either of these mutations conceivably alters the orientation of the anionic/sulfated tyrosine motif and a second vWf-binding site within the amino-terminal domain, allowing the receptor to spontaneously bind vWf without the usual requirement for conformational activation of either the receptor or vWf (8, 15). In the circulation, the poor adhesion of pseudo-von Willebrand disease platelets at high-shear flow can probably be attributed to the absence of high-molecular-weight vWf multimers rather than being directly related to the platelet GP Ibα defect, which would otherwise be expected to increase adhesion.

## COLLAGEN RECEPTOR DEFICIENCY

As discussed in the preceding sections, both vWf and the platelet membrane GP Ib-IX-V complex are necessary for adhesion of platelets to vascular subendothelium at high-shear flow. They are not, however, critical for platelet adhesion at low-shear rates (3–5). Under low-shear conditions (<500/second), other platelet proteins such as the collagen receptors may mediate platelet adhesion. At high shear, secondary receptors may also play a role in stabilizing adhered platelets after initial GP Ib-IX-V-mediated contact (60, 61). Although precise physiologic roles have not been defined, there are three surface receptors on platelets that have been identified as potential collagen receptors: GP Ia-IIa, GP IV, and GP VI (see Chapter 12).

GP Ia-IIa (VLA-2) is a noncovalently linked heterodimer of the integrin superfamily of adhesion receptors and consists of an α2 subunit (GP Ia) and a β1 subunit (GP IIa). Other integrins found on platelets include GP Ic-IIa (α5β1; VLA-5) and α6β1 (VLA-6), the vitronectin receptor (αvβ3), and GP IIb-IIIa (αIIbβ3). Like the GP Ib-IX-V complex, GP Ia-IIa is also able to transmit intracellular signals when engaged by ligand, in the latter case by a mechanism that is linked to phosphorylation of the focal adhesion kinase pp125[fak] and activation of p72[syk] (62, 63). GP Ia-IIa was implicated as a collagen adhesion receptor by the finding that an anti-GP Ia-IIa monoclonal antibody blocked the adhesion of platelets to collagen-coated plastic, although this antibody did not inhibit collagen-induced platelet aggregation (64). Purified GP Ia-IIa has been shown to bind specifically to collagen (65). A congenital GP Ia deficiency has been reported in a individual with a normal platelet count and a very long skin bleeding time of >30 minutes (66). Platelets from this individual contained only ~20% of normal levels of GP Ia on their surface and showed impaired adhesion to fibrillar collagen. There was no collagen-dependent aggregation of either platelet-rich plasma or gel-filtered platelets (67). The individual's platelets adhered poorly to subendothelial matrix at both low- and high-shear flow rates. Those platelets that did adhere spread poorly, and there was a defect in the formation of microthrombi (67).

GP IV (GP IIIb; CD36) is an ~88-kDa transmembrane glycoprotein of 471 amino acid residues, which also mediates the adhesion of platelets to collagen-coated surfaces (68). GP IV also transmits an intracellular signal in response to ligand binding by a pathway that involves the src-related kinases, pp60[fyn], pp62[yes], and pp54/58[lyn] (69, 70). It has recently been found that platelet antigen Nak[a]-negative platelets from healthy donors are deficient in GP IV expression, despite the presence of GP IV mRNA (71, 72). The Nak[a]-negative phenotype occurs in ~3% of the Japanese and African populations and in ~0.3% of the United States Caucasian population. These platelets show impaired adhesion to fibrillar collagen in vitro, although there is no associated bleeding abnormality. The platelet GP IV deficiency may be associated with the absence (type I) or presence (type II) of GP IV on monocytes (73). The molecular defects related to type I or type II GP IV deficiency are summarized in Table 32.4. The type I deficiency appears to result from unstable mRNA and/or defective post-translational processing (74–76), while type II deficiency in two families may be associated with a platelet-specific lesion of the GP IV gene (77).

GP VI is a platelet glycoprotein of ~62 Kda that has not been well characterized. A individual has been reported with autoimmune thrombocytopenia who developed an anti-GP VI antibody (78, 79). Platelets from this individual aggregate poorly to collagen, and individual IgG-containing serum blocks the interaction of normal platelets with collagen. Subsequently, a individual was described whose platelets had significantly decreased levels of GP VI, aggregated normally in response to all platelet agonists except collagen, and failed to adhere to collagen fibrils (79). More recently, it was shown that under flow conditions, GP VI-deficient platelets exhib-

**TABLE 32.4.** Molecular Defects Associated With GP IV (CD36) Deficiency on Platelets

| Type | Abnormality/Defect(s) | Reference |
|------|----------------------|-----------|
| Type I | One form of mRNA with 161 base-pair deletion (331–491) corresponding to loss of exon 4, plus a dinucleotide deletion (539–540) in exon 5 of both deleted and normal-sized mRNA. | [74] |
| Type I | Nucleotide insertion at position 1159 in codon 317, leading to frameshift and premature stop. Also heterozygous for the 539–540 dinucleotide deletion. | [75] |
| Type I | C to T mutation at position 478 within codon 90 causing Pro$_{90}$ to Ser substitution, impaired posttranslational modification to 88-kDa mature form of GP IV. | [76] |
| Type II | Heterozygous for Pro$_{90}$ to Ser mutation in one allele plus unidentified platelet-specific defect in other allele associated with microsatellite sequence in GP IV gene. | [77] |

*GP, glycoprotein.*

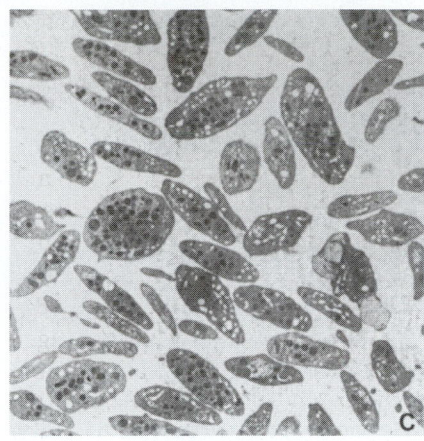 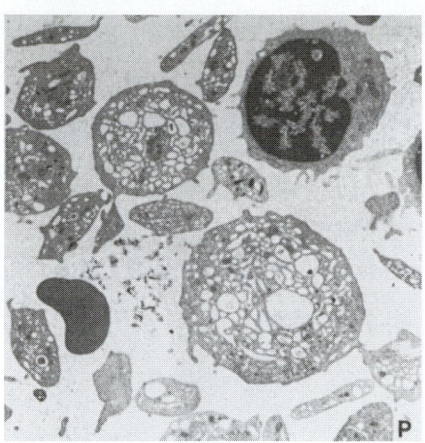

**FIGURE 32.2.** Electron micrographs of control platelets (C) and gray platelet syndrome platelets (P) showing that gray platelets are larger than normal platelets (compare with lymphocyte in upper right quadrant of panel P), have a marked deficiency of α-granules (dark electron-dense granules in panel C), and have a highly vacuolized "Swiss-cheese" appearance.

ited defective secondary adhesion following initial GP Ib-IX-V-dependent contact with a thrombogenic surface (60). These findings suggested that GP VI may be a collagen receptor. The GP VI-deficient individual had purpura and a marginally prolonged bleeding time (8.5 minutes). Both parents showed ~ 50% of normal levels of platelet GP VI, were not related, and had no obvious functional abnormality of their platelets. It has also been demonstrated that both human anti-GP VI antibody and the related F(ab')₂ fragments induced intracellular signaling involving activation of pp60$^{src}$ and p72$^{syk}$ in normal but not GP VI-deficient platelets (80).

# CONGENITAL PLATELET SECRETION DEFECTS

Platelet storage pool deficiencies are a heterogeneous group of abnormalities in which there is a deficiency of one or more platelet granules and/or granule contents (see Chapter 10). These abnormalities include the gray platelet syndrome (GPS), where platelets are deficient in α-granules; δ-storage-pool deficiency (δ-SPD), where platelets lack dense bodies; and αδ-storage-pool deficiency (αδ-SPD), where platelets lack both α-granules and dense bodies to a variable degree. Acquired forms of platelet-storage-pool deficiency are described in Chapter 33.

## THE GRAY PLATELET SYNDROME

The gray platelet syndrome was initially described by Raccuglia in 1971 (81). It is characterized by a morphologic abnormality of platelets and megakaryocytes in which these cells appear gray when a peripheral blood smear or bone marrow aspirate is stained with Romanowsky stains. This appearance has been shown to result from the absence of α-granules in the megakaryocyte and platelet cytoplasm (Fig. 32.2) (82, 83). Other characteristic features of this syndrome are a clinical bleeding

diathesis, which is usually mild to moderate, a prolonged skin bleeding time, morphologically large platelets, and mild to moderate thrombocytopenia (84–87). Normal α-granules are absent from megakaryocytes and platelets, although other platelet granules, including dense bodies and lysosomes, are present in normal amounts (88). As a result, the platelets demonstrate a severe deficiency, although not complete absence, of megakaryocyte synthesized α-granule proteins such as vWf, fibronectin, platelet factor 4, platelet-derived growth factor (PDGF), thrombospondin, and β-thromboglobulin (Fig. 32.3) (89–91). However, the α-granule membrane protein P-selectin (GMP-140) is present in GPS platelets, consistent with the α-granule membranes being present (92). Proteins gaining entry into platelets by pinocytosis, for example, albumin and IgG, are found in normal quantities, although secretion during stimulation and aggregation is deficient (91–94). As would be expected with the morphologic findings of normal amounts of dense bodies, secretion of serotonin and ATP by platelets is normal (95). Ultrastructural studies have demonstrated small granules up to 0.1 μm diameter in gray platelet syndrome megakaryocytes, which are althought to be precursors of α-granules (88). Further, P-selectin has been found to be localized to these granule membranes, consistent with these being α-granule derivatives (92). Other studies have been able to localize other membrane proteins, including GP Ib, GP IX, and GP V, as well as PECAM-1 and GP IV to these abnormal granules, further supporting these being α-granule derivatives (96–98). It would therefore appear that the primary defect in the gray platelet syndrome is the abnormal packaging of megakaryocyte-derived proteins into α-granules before the platelets are released from the bone marrow. This is supported by the finding of increased reticulin in the marrow of individuals with gray platelet syndrome, consistent with local release of PDGF by megakaryocytes (83, 89). Furthermore, gray platelet syndrome plasma has increased levels of

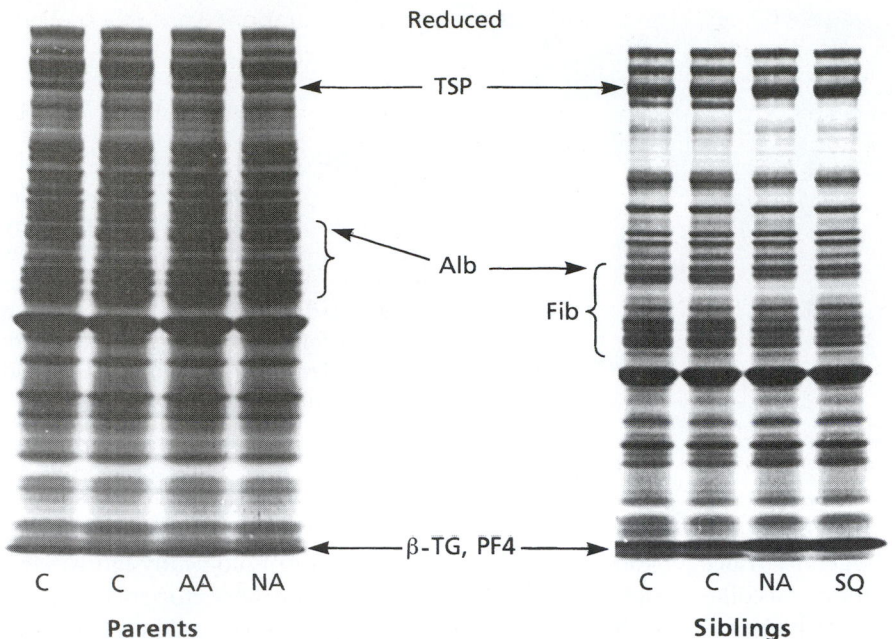

**FIGURE 32.3.** Platelets from siblings with gray platelet syndrome (NA and SQ, right panel) electrophoresed on sodium dodecyl sulfate polyacrylamide gels under reducing conditions and stained with Coomassie blue showing a deficiency of thrombospondin (TSP), albumin (Alb), fibrinogen (Fib), β-thromboglobulin (β-TG), and platelet factor 4 (PF4), compared with control platelets (C). The parents (AA and NA, left panel), presumably heterozygous for gray platelet syndrome, are indistinguishable from controls.

β-thromboglobulin and platelet factor 4, both megakaryocyte products found in α-granules. It would appear that the fundamental targeting defect in the gray platelet syndrome is specific to the megakaryocyte cell line, since the endothelial cell equivalent storage granule, the Weibel-Palade bodies, of individuals with gray platelet syndrome contain normal vWf and P-selectin (99).

The cause of the bleeding diathesis in the gray platelet syndrome is related to the deficiency of the α-granule contents, as all other granules and their contents are normal, with no known deficiency of any platelet membrane glycoprotein such as GP Ib-IX-V or GP IIb-IIIa. The mechanism of the bleeding diathesis is not clearly defined at the molecular level. It has, however, been suggested that bleeding is caused by the lack of high local concentrations of the α-granule contents such as vWf, fibronectin, and thrombospondin, which are necessary for cell contact, thrombin generation, and subsequent development of platelet aggregates (84).

Autosomal inheritance is likely in the few families in whom gray platelet syndrome has been reported since in these instances both male and female siblings have been affected (83, 90, 100). The particular genetic abnormality has not been identified. Individuals with gray platelet syndrome have a variable bleeding diathesis, characterized by easy bruising and petechiae, epistaxis, menorrhagia, and particularly postoperative and posttraumatic bleeding (101–103), although individuals may be asymptomatic throughout life (104). A case report in which pulmonary fibrosis occurred simultaneously with gray platelet syndrome suggested a role for the abnormal megakaryocytes in its etiology (105). The bleeding time is characteristically prolonged, and there is usually

an associated moderate thrombocytopenia. Platelet counts may vary from $20 \times 10^9$/L to the normal range (86), although the mechanism of the thrombocytopenia is poorly understood and probably multifactorial. There is evidence of shortened platelet survival in this syndrome (106), although the inability of abnormal megakaryocytes to mature normally has also been suggested as a contributing factor (87). On Romanowsky staining of the peripheral blood film, the platelets appear large and gray. However, other causes of apparently "gray" platelets have been described, including treatment of the blood sample with EDTA (102). Bone marrow examination reveals apparently normal numbers of megakaryocytes with increased reticulin fibers, particularly around megakaryocytes (89, 94, 96).

Platelet aggregation studies most commonly show an aggregation defect to threshold concentrations of thrombin (89, 93, 107), with a similar defect to threshold concentrations of collagen also common (87, 105, 106, 108). However, normal responses to all platelet-aggregating agents have also been reported (100).

In normal platelets, thrombin causes release of platelet-associated immunoglobulin. However, in gray platelet syndrome platelets there is no thrombin-induced release, even although these platelets contain normal levels of immunoglobulin. This would be consistent with immunoglobulin entering storage sites in gray platelet syndrome platelets separate from those of normal platelets (94).

## δ-STORAGE-POOL DEFICIENCY

δ-Storage-pool deficiency (δ-SPD) is defined as a deficiency of dense bodies in megakaryocytes and circulating platelets. It was first described as a deficiency of dense granule substances (109), although later specifically used to describe deficiency of dense granules (110). The clinical syndrome of δ-SPD is characterized by a variable bleeding diathesis, prolonged skin bleeding time, normal morphology of platelets when stained by Romanowsky stains, and a normal platelet count. δ-SPD may occur as a sole abnormality or may be associated with a variety of other congenital disorders.

In δ-SPD, α-granules are normal; however, dense bodies are absent (103, 111–113). Dense bodies are normally identifiable either by their electron opaque nature when viewed on unfixed, unstained whole preparations (114), which is although to be due to their high calcium content (115, 116), or by their affinity for uranyl ions (uranaffin reaction) or the fluorescent dye mepacrine (117–119). In normal platelets these dense bodies are a metabolically inert storage pool, containing ATP, ADP, serotonin, calcium ion, and pyrophosphate, all of which are secreted in response to platelet activation (120). However in δ-SPD, where these dense bodies are absent, the platelet content of these granule components is reduced (110). The basis for the deficiencies of dense granules in humans with δ-SPD has not been established. Normally, when platelets are incubated with [$^{14}$C]-serotonin, it is taken up and stored in the platelet dense bodies where it is protected from platelet monoamine oxidases (121). As a result serotonin remains in the platelet over periods of 4 to 6 hours. If, however, δ-SPD platelets are incubated with [$^{14}$C]-serotonin, then, although initial uptake into the platelet is normal, the serotonin is rapidly metabolized by platelet enzymes to 5-hydroxyindoleacetic acid (122) and 5-hydroxytryptophol (123). This process can be simulated in normal platelets by incubation with [$^{14}$C]-serotonin in the presence of reserpine, which blocks incorporation into dense bodies (122).

In δ-SPD, the ATP:ADP ratio in platelets tends toward that of the metabolically active pool (10:1) and increases from a ratio of <2.5:1 in normal platelets to >3:1 (109, 110, 123, 124). Although the role of the components of the storage pool is not entirely known, it has been found that the granule ADP contents correlate best with the bleeding time in individuals with δ-SPD (125). δ-SPD platelets lack the granule contents that are important in platelet aggregation, that is, ADP and, to a lesser extent, serotonin. The decreased release of ADP in δ-SPD may result in decreased vWf-dependent and fibrinogen-dependent aggregation of platelets involving GP IIb-IIIa (126) and may partly mediate the bleeding diathesis. In addition, *in vitro* adhesion assays at high shear (2600/second) have shown that δ-SPD platelets have reduced thrombus formation in proportion to the magnitude of the dense granule deficit (5).

δ-SPD is characterized by a mild to moderate bleeding diathesis, with mucosal bleeding such as epistaxis, bruising and petechiae, menorrhagia, and prominent posttraumatic bleeding, including postsurgical bleeding. Other clinical associations reported with δ-SPD include a family in which the occurrence of δ-SPD was associated with acute myeloid leukemia (127) and the possible association of δ-SPD with primary pulmonary hypertension, suggesting a role for the high plasma serotonin found in δ-SPD in its etiology (128).

δ-SPD has been associated with other congenital abnormalities (Table 32.5). The **Hermansky-Pudlak syndrome** is characterized by tyrosinase-positive oculocutaneous albinism and reticuloendothelial deposits of ceroid in macrophages in association with gastrointestinal lesions (129). Additionally, pulmonary fibrosis can

**TABLE 32.5.** Syndromes Associated with δ-Storage Pool Deficiency

| Disease | Inheritance | Clinical and Laboratory Findings |
|---|---|---|
| δ-Storage pool deficiency (with no other associations) | Autosomal dominant | Mild to moderate bleeding diathesis, absent dense bodies in platelets[a] |
| Hermansky-Pudlak syndrome | Autosomal recessive | Tyrosinase positive oculocutaneous albinism, restrictive lung disease, granulomatous gastrointestinal lesions, reticuloendothelial deposits of ceroid, granulophysin deficiency |
| Chediak-Higashi syndrome | Autosomal recessive | Oculocutaneous albinism, frequent pyogenic infections, abnormal granules in hemopoietic and nonhemopoietic cells |
| Thrombocytopenia and absent radii syndrome | Autosomal recessive | Radial hypoplasia, hypomegakaryocytic thrombocytopenia |
| Wiskott-Aldrich syndrome | X-linked | Thrombocytopenia, small platelets, eczema, severe T-cell deficiency, defective O-linked oligosaccharide biosynthesis in lymphocytes and platelets |

[a] Applies to all syndromes in which δ-storage pool deficiency occurs.

occur in Hermansky-Pudlak syndrome. This may mimic cryptogenic fibrosing alveolitis (130) with one group proposing that PDGF from macrophages plays an important role in the initiation of alveolar remodeling (131). The Hermansky-Pudlak syndrome has been described in Swiss and Puerto Rican cohorts, with the latter cases exhibiting a shortened life expectancy due to the systemic manifestations above and also renal failure, although the Swiss kindred had a normal life expectancy (132). The gene for both groups has been localized to an interval in chromosome segment 10q23.1-q23.3 (133, 134). Individuals with Hermansky-Pudlak syndrome have been found to be deficient in a 40-kDa platelet dense granule membrane protein, granulophysin (135). The protein appears identical to CD63 (136) and has also been found to be low in other forms of δ-SPD associated with albinism (137).

The **Chediak-Higashi syndrome** is characterized by oculocutaneous albinism, abnormal granules in a variety of hemopoietic and nonhematopoietic cells, a clinical course punctuated by frequent pyogenic infections, and deficient natural killer cell activity (138). The genetic locus for the Chediak-Higashi syndrome has recently been mapped to the chromosome segment 1q42-44 (138, 139). The underlying mechanism is postulated to relate to a lack of primary lysosomes (140, 141). The syndrome may also be associated with diffuse atrophy of the brain, as well as other neurologic findings, which can be detected by CT and MRI (141, 142).

**Thrombocytopenia and absent radii syndrome (TAR)** is a syndrome in which there is hypomegakaryocytic thrombocytopenia with variable degrees of radial hypoplasia in association with δ-SPD. The syndrome can be diagnosed *in utero* via ultrasound (143) or by other methods such as fetal radiography and fetoscopy (144). Interestingly, TAR is one of the inherited, impaired-DNA repair disorders and forms part of the newly described radiation sensitivity syndromes (145). Finally, δ-SPD may also be associated with the **Wiskott-Aldrich syndrome** (described in detail below) (146).

In the absence of other congenital abnormalities or an associated α-granule deficiency, δ-SPD is inherited as an autosomal dominant trait (147). The other forms of δ-SPD coincident with other congenital abnormalities such as Hermansky-Pudlak syndrome, the Chediak-Higashi syndrome, and the thrombocytopenia and absent radii syndrome are inherited as autosomal recessive traits. δ-SPD has been associated with acute leukemia, with one suggestion for this association being the deletion of a gene coding for a protein necessary for dense granule formation and the deletion of an adjacent tumor suppressor gene (148). In δ-SPD the bleeding time is typically prolonged, although the platelets on peripheral blood smear appear normal both qualitatively and quantitatively. The absence of dense bodies can be confirmed by electron microscopy or, more conveniently, by mepacrine staining (111, 112, 149). Platelet aggregation studies typically show the lack of a secondary wave of aggregation when stimulated with ADP, adrenaline, or low concentrations of thrombin. In addition, the response to collagen may also be markedly impaired (85). In some cases aggregation to all agonists may be normal (150). Because of the variability of platelet-aggregation studies and the lack of convenience of electron microscopy, a reliable, mepacrine, flow-cytometry method suitable for the routine laboratory to detect dense granule deficiency has been described. This should provide a rapid and reliable screening method for δ-SPD (149, 151). Other tests reveal reduced levels of platelet granule ADP, total platelet ADP, and serotonin and decreased [14C]-serotonin uptake. In addition, since diadenosine 5′,5′′-P1,P4-tetraphosphate (Ap4A) is found only in dense granules, a method for diagnosing δ-SPD has been suggested that involves measuring whole blood levels of Ap4A (152).

## αδ-STORAGE-POOL DEFICIENCY

αδ-Storage-pool deficiency is characterized by a deficiency of platelet dense granules and a variable deficiency of platelet α-granules. As a result, depending on the degree of α-granule deficiency, the platelets may have a similar gray morphologic appearance to those in the gray platelet syndrome. Unlike gray platelet syndrome, where P-selectin has been reported to be present in normal quantities (92), the P-selectin content in αδ-SPD may be diminished (153). In flow-chamber experiments, αδ-SPD platelet thrombus formation is reduced when compared with pure δ-SPD platelets (5). Clinically, individuals with αδ-SPD have a similar bleeding diathesis to that described in the gray platelet syndrome and δ-SPD. The occurrence of acute leukemia in two members of a family with αδ-SPD was reported to suggest a deficit in a proto-oncogene that regulates the maturation of granulocytes and megakaryocytes (153, 154). Platelet function abnormalities are similar to those described for δ-SPD (103).

# CONGENITAL PLATELET ACTIVATION DEFECTS

Following stimulation of normal platelets with appropriate agonists, membrane phospholipids are hydrolyzed by phospholipases $A_2$ and C, both calcium-dependent enzymes, and by diglyceride lipase to liberate arachidonic acid. Endoperoxides and prostaglandins $G_2$ and $H_2$ are formed by the action of cyclooxygenase (prostaglandin $H_2$ synthase-1) on arachidonic acid, and subsequently thromboxane synthase acts on these metabolites to form thromboxane $A_2$. Thromboxane $A_2$ is necessary for a secretion response to occur. Congenital defects at several stages in thromboxane $A_2$ production and action have been described, most of which present clinically with a mild bleeding diathesis.

## DEFECTS IN ARACHIDONIC ACID MOBILIZATION

Individuals with this defect have impaired aggregation and secretion responses to ADP, epinephrine, platelet activating factor, and collagen, with a normal response to arachidonic acid, in the presence of normal, dense-granule ADP and ATP (155).

## CYCLOOXYGENASE DEFICIENCY (PROSTAGLANDIN $H_2$ SYNTHASE-1 DEFICIENCY)

Clinically, individuals with this disorder have a slightly prolonged skin bleeding time, with impaired aggregation in response to ADP, epinephrine, collagen, and arachidonic acid, although a normal response to natural endoperoxide, for example, prostaglandin $G_2$ (156, 157). Cyclooxygenase activity has recently been identified and characterized to be expressed by two isoforms. The type 1 isoform is expressed in most mammalian cells (158), while the type 2 (prostaglandin $H_2$ synthase-2) enzyme is inducible (159). The active sites of these enzymes are conserved at the amino acid level (160), with each having a similar molecular weight and sharing ~60% sequence identity. Cyclooxygenase deficiency in platelets is caused by lack of the type 1 enzyme, which is the only isoform normally present in platelets. Deficiency of cyclooxygenase has been found to be due to both a deficiency in expression, as well as a deficiency in functional enzyme activity despite normal enzyme quantities being present in some individuals (161, 162).

## THROMBOXANE SYNTHASE DEFICIENCY

The bleeding diathesis in thromboxane synthase deficiency has been found to be variable in the few individuals that have been described. The mode of inheritance appears to be autosomal (163, 164). Since thromboxane $A_2$ is not formed in these individuals' platelets, there is more prostaglandin $E_2$ and prostaglandin $D_2$ production, as well as increased, natural endoperoxide–induced aggregation (147, 163–165).

## DEFECTS IN SENSITIVITY TO THROMBOXANE $A_2$

Several mechanisms have been described for the lack of sensitivity of platelets to thromboxane $A_2$ stimulation (103). These include defects in mobilization of intracellu-

lar calcium ion, consistent with thromboxane $A_2$ acting as a calcium-dependent ionophore (166); increased platelet cyclic AMP (167); or an abnormal thromboxane $A_2$ receptor (168). The mode of inheritance of specific genetic defects for this group of disorders is unclear.

# GLANZMANN'S THROMBASTHENIA

Glanzmann's thrombasthenia is a congenital platelet bleeding abnormality with autosomal recessive inheritance (169, 170), first described by Glanzmann in 1918 (171). The disorder is frequently associated with consanguinity (172). It is characterized by a prolonged skin bleeding time, normal platelet count, moderately defective to absent clot retraction, and a profound defect of platelet aggregation to platelet agonists such as ADP, collagen, arachidonic acid, and thrombin (103, 173). Ristocetin-induced platelet aggregation, a measure of GP Ib-IX-V complex–vWf interaction, is normal (103). These aggregometry findings are consistent with flow studies that have assessed the interaction of Glanzmann's thrombasthenic platelets with subendothelial matrix. These studies suggest that, while the initial contact adhesion of Glanzmann's thrombasthenic platelets to subendothelial matrix is probably near normal or normal, there is a pronounced defect in the ability of these platelets to spread on the subendothelium and an inability to form subendothelium-associated microthrombi (174–176). Clinically, Glanzmann's thrombasthenia usually manifests in early childhood. Common features are purpura, epistaxis, gingival hemorrhage, menorrhagia, and prolonged bleeding from superficial cuts (172).

Like Bernard-Soulier syndrome, the clinical manifestations of Glanzmann's thrombasthenia are due to the absence, reduction, or dysfunction of a specific platelet membrane receptor, in this case the GP IIb-IIIa complex (Fig. 32.4) (103, 173). GP IIb-IIIa ($\alpha$IIb$\beta$3 in the integrin nomenclature) is a member of the integrin superfamily of cell adhesion receptors that frequently recognize the arginine-glycine-aspartic acid (RGD) peptide sequence in their respective ligands (174). When platelets are activated in plasma, the GP IIb-IIIa complex undergoes one or more conformational changes leading to the binding of fibrinogen, which is a bivalent ligand that bridges adjacent activated platelets (177, 178). This binding of fibrinogen to GP IIb-IIIa may involve recognition of an RGD sequence in the $\alpha$-chain of fibrinogen; however, a dodecapeptide sequence at the C-terminus of the $\gamma$ chain of fibrinogen is crucial (179, 180). In this regard recombinant fibrinogen containing RGD to RGE amino acid substitution supported platelet aggregation to a similar extent as plasma fibrinogen (181). At least one sequence in GP IIb, 296–306, and two sequences in GP IIIa, 109–171 and 211–222, are althought to be important in fibrinogen

Reduced

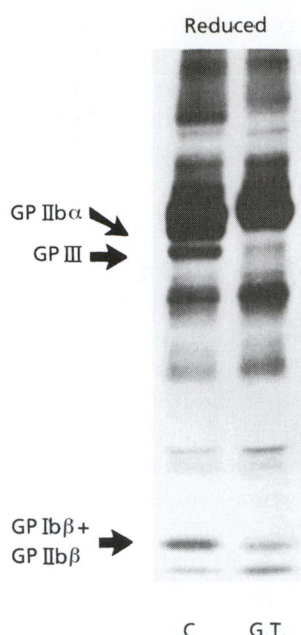

GP IIbα →
GP III →

GP Ibβ + →
GP IIbβ

C    G.T.

**FIGURE 32.4.** Autoradiograms of surface [$^{125}$I]–labeled control (C) and Glanzmann's thrombasthenia (G.T.) platelets electrophoresed on sodium dodecyl sulfate polyacrylamide gels under reducing conditions. The positions of GP IIbα, GP III, and GP IIbβ (which co-migrates with GP Ibβ), which are deficient in Glanzmann's thrombasthenia platelets, are indicated by the arrows.

recognition (182–184). The structure and function of GP IIb-IIIa are discussed in detail in Chapter 11.

## TYPE I GLANZMANN'S THROMBASTHENIA

Type I Glanzmann's thrombasthenia is characterized by the lack of surface-detectable GP IIb-IIIa complex, very low levels of platelet α-granule fibrinogen, and a profound defect of platelet aggregation and clot retraction. Recent evidence has identified a specific mechanism for uptake of plasma fibrinogen into the α-granules of both platelets and megakaryocytes, a mechanism that involves GP IIb-IIIa (185, 186). Although it is difficult to detect GP IIb-IIIa on the surface of type I Glanzmann's thrombasthenic platelets, trace amounts (1 to 5%) of GP IIb, pro-GP IIb, GP IIIa, or GP IIb-IIIa can be detected in most individuals with this type of thrombasthenia (187–189). This diversity of expression and similar molecular and functional variability in other types of thrombasthenia (see below) suggest that there must exist multiple genetic and molecular defects that are capable of causing the clinical entity of Glanzmann's thrombasthenia. This conclusion has now been borne out by molecular genetic studies on individuals with Glanzmann's thrombas-

thenia, with the disease phenotype resulting from a wide variety of genetic defects, including deletions, insertions, inversions, and point mutations in the genes encoding both the GP IIb and GP IIIa subunits (Tables 32.6 and 32.7, respectively).

The largest cohort of individuals with type I Glanzmann's thrombasthenia that have been extensively studied belongs to the Iraqi-Jewish and Arab populations in Israel. Restriction enzyme analyses identified no gross abnormalities in either the gene for GP IIb or for GP IIIa in either group of individuals (212). Individuals belonging to the Iraqi-Jewish population have no immunodetectable GP IIIa, and hence their platelets lack both the GP IIb-IIIa complex (αIIbβ3) and the related β3 integrin, the vitronectin receptor (αvβ3) (188, 213). Although platelets express αvβ3 in only trace quantities (~100 copies/platelet), it is a major integrin on other cell types such as endothelial cells (214). Glanzmann's thrombasthenia, however, is solely a disease of platelets. One explanation for this is that on other cell types the lack of β3 expression can be compensated for by the association of αv with other β subunits (215). In contrast to the lack of GP IIIa, the platelets of Iraqi-Jewish thrombasthenics have immunodetectable pro-GP IIb, and some have detectable GP IIb (189). Newman et al (190) have shown an 11-base deletion within exon 12 of the GP IIIa gene in six of six Iraqi-Jewish families. This results in a reading frame shift leading to premature termination of transcribed GP IIIa protein shortly before the transmembrane domain. Since no form of GP IIIa can be immunologically detected in the platelets of these individuals (188), the truncated GP IIIa must either be secreted from the megakaryocyte or degraded. In contrast to the Iraqi-Jewish thrombasthenics, the Arab thrombasthenics have immunodetectable GP IIIa (β3) and normal to above-normal levels of vitronectin receptor (αvβ3) (188, 209). Trace amounts of pro-GP IIb can be detected by Western blot analysis (189). In three of five Arab families with thrombasthenia, a 13-base deletion was detected that removed the normal splice acceptor site at the start of exon 4 of the GP IIb gene (190). Alternative splicing to an AG splice acceptor site 16 nucleotides downstream leads to the in-frame deletion of amino acids 106 to 111 of the heavy-chain region of pro-GP IIb, Ala-Cys-Ala-Pro-Trp-Gln. Since only trace amounts of pro-GP IIb transcript can be detected in the individuals' platelets, this hexapeptide sequence, including Cys$_{17}$, must be important for the normal folding of pro-GP IIb and/or for normal complex formation with GP IIIa.

## TYPE II GLANZMANN'S THROMBASTHENIA

In contrast to the platelets from type I Glanzmann's thrombasthenia, the platelets of individuals with type II Glanzmann's thrombasthenia have detectable, but markedly reduced, GP IIb-IIIa on their surface, ~10 to 20% of normal levels (172). The level of α-granule fibrin-

## TABLE 32.6.   Platelet Glycoprotein (GP) IIb Defects

| Location of Mutation on GP IIb | | Abnormality/Genetic Defect(s) | % Surface Expression | Reference |
|---|---|---|---|---|
| | 1 | 13 base-pair deletion in exon 4 of GP IIb gene, deletion of amino acids 106–111 in pro-GP IIb | <5 | [190] |
| | 2 | 4.5 kilobase deletion, including exons 2–9 of GP IIb gene | <5 | [191] |
| | 3 | Single nucleotide mutation G to A at position 819 in exon 8, $Gly_{242}$ to Asp within the first $Ca^{2+}$-binding domain | <5 | [192] |
| | 4 | Single nucleotide mutation G to A at position 1074 in exon 12, $Arg_{327}$ to His near the $Ca^{2+}$-binding region; some clot retraction (type II Glanzmann's thrombasthenia) | <10 | [193] |
| | 5 | Single nucleotide mutation G to A at position 1347 in exon 13, $Gly_{418}$ to Asp near the fourth $Ca^{2+}$-binding domain | <5 | [194] |
| | 6 | 6 base-pair deletion in exon 13, deletion of amino acids $Val_{425}$ and $Asp_{426}$ | <5 | [195] |
| | 7 | Single nucleotide mutation G to A within intron 15, frameshift of amino acids 482–582 and premature stop | <5 | [196] |
| | 8 | Single nucleotide mutation C to T at position 1751 in exon 17, $Arg_{553}$ to stop; unstable mRNA | <5 | [197–200] |
| | 9 | 6 base-pair deletion/31 base-pair insertion in exon 25, in frame substitution of amino acids 817–826 | <5 | [201] |
| | 10 | Single nucleotide mutation C to G near splice acceptor site of intron 25/26, 42 amino acid deletion, including the heavy/light-chain cleavage site | <5 | [197] |
| | 11 | Single nucleotide mutation C to T at position 2942 in exon 28, $Gln_{950}$ to stop, deletion of exon 28 | <5 | [202] |

▨, *transmembrane domain*; ▬, *$Ca^{2+}$-binding domains*; ▨, *plasma membrane (the upper surface is extracytoplasmic)*; ●, *potential N-linked glycosylation site.*

ogen is near normal, and clot retraction is only moderately impaired (170). The platelets have sufficient GP IIb-IIIa to allow microaggregate formation, although there is still a profound defect in the ability to form large aggregates (216). Although type II probably represents a milder form of Glanzmann's thrombasthenia, severe hemorrhagic complications can still occur (172). Since heterozygotes for type I Glanzmann's thrombasthenia are asymptomatic, it is probable that there needs to be a critical level of surface-expressed GP IIb-IIIa for normal hemostasis to occur and that this level is between 15 and 50% of the normal level.

## GLANZMANN'S THROMBASTHENIA VARIANTS

In the past decade individuals have been described with the clinical and laboratory features of Glanzmann's thrombasthenia where the level of the GP IIb-IIIa complex is low to normal, but is dysfunctional in that the platelets, when activated, can neither aggregate nor bind fibrinogen. From a basic research viewpoint, the detailed structural and functional analysis of these variant forms of Glanzmann's thrombasthenia are of major interest because they provide important insights into the normal structure and function of the GP IIb-IIIa complex and the mechanism of receptor-ligand interaction.

Ginsberg et al (205, 217, 218) initially described a variant form of Glanzmann's thrombasthenia, which they termed the Cam variant, in two male and one female siblings from Guam. The platelets of the affected individuals did not aggregate to either ADP or α-thrombin, nor did they support clot retraction. The levels of GP IIb-IIIa complex were near normal, but platelet α-granule fibrinogen levels were markedly decreased.

**TABLE 32.7.** Platelet Glycoprotein (GP) IIIa Defects

| Location of Mutation on GP IIIa | | Abnormality/Genetic Defect(s) | % Surface Expression | Reference |
|---|---|---|---|---|
| | 1 | 1 kilobase deletion/15 kilobase inversion in exons 1–5 | <5 | [203] |
| | 2 | 3 point mutations at exon 1/intron 1 boundary, exon 1 sequence deletion, frameshift, and truncation | <5 | [204] |
| | 3 | Single nucleotide mutation C to T in codon 33 in exon II resulting in $Arg_{62}$ to stop, early truncation | <5 | [200] |
| | 4 | Single nucleotide substitution T to G at position 453 in exon 3 resulting in $Asp_{119}$ to Tyr substitution within RGD domain | 100[a] | [205] |
| | 5 | Single nucleotide mutation G to A at position 739 in exon 4 resulting in $Arg_{214}$ to Gln substitution within GP IIIa regulatory domain | 100[a] | [206] |
| | 6 | Single nucleotide mutation C to T at position 738 in exon 4 resulting in $Arg_{214}$ to Trp substitution, complex dissociates | 65[a] | [207, 208] |
| | 7 | Single nucleotide mutation G to A at position 1219 in exon 8 resulting in $Cys_{374}$ to Tyr substitution, signaling defect, only 30–35% GP IIb expression | 10[a] | [209, 210] |
| | 8 | Insertion in exon 8 | | [211] |
| | 9 | 11 base-pair deletion in exon 12 at position 2051–2061 resulting in a frameshift and premature stop at amino acid 654 before the transmembrane domain | <5 | [190] |
| | 10 | Single nucleotide mutation T to C at position 2352 in exon 13 resulting in $Ser_{752}$ to Pro substitution, signaling defect | 50[a] | [209] |

▨, *transmembrane domain;* ▧, *Cys-rich domain;* ▦, *plasma membrane (the upper surface is extracytoplasmic);* ●, *potential N-linked glycosylation site.*

[a] *Variant Glanzmann's thrombasthenia.*

In contrast to normal platelets, the thrombin-activated individual platelets did not bind fibrinogen, fibronectin, or vWf or the Arg-Gly-Asp–containing peptides. The defect is due to a point mutation that changes an aspartic acid to a tyrosine residue at position 119 in mature GP IIIa (205). The $Asp_{119}$ residue in GP IIIa (β3) is highly conserved in other β-subunits and throughout evolution, and is near $Lys_{125}$, the presumptive residue to which Arg-Gly-Asp–containing peptide becomes covalently bound in the presence of bifunctional, crosslinking reagents. This suggests that in individuals with the Cam mutation, Glanzmann's thrombasthenia is due to the inability of the GP IIb-IIIa to bind fibrinogen because of a point mutation within the Arg-Gly-Asp recognition sequence of GP IIIa. Another individual with variant Glanzmann's thrombasthenia originally described by Fournier et al (219), has also been characterized at the molecular genetic level by Ginsberg et al (206). The platelets of this individual did not support clot retraction; did not aggregate in response to ADP, collagen, epinephrine, or α-thrombin; and had normal levels of GP IIb-IIIa but with very low fibrinogen levels (219). The individual's GP IIb-IIIa complex was unstable and showed a markedly increased sensitivity to EDTA dissociation (219). This GP IIb-IIIa did not bind fibrinogen and had a markedly reduced capacity to bind either Arg-Gly-Asp–containing peptide or a dodecapeptide sequence corresponding to the carboxyterminus of the γ-chain of fibrinogen. The individual's GP IIIa gene contained a single identified point mutation that altered $Arg_{214}$ in mature GP IIIa to a glutamine residue (206). This point mutation occurred within a peptide sequence $Ser_{211}$ to $Gly_{222}$ previously identified to be important in fibrinogen binding to the GP IIb-IIIa complex (184). Similarly, Lanza et al have identified a functionally defective GP IIb-IIIa complex containing an $Arg_{214}$ to tryptophan mutation within GP IIIa resulting in a form of Glanzmann's thrombasthenia named Strasbourg I variant (207). Most variant Glanzmann's thrombasthenia individuals, so far characterized, have been associated with point mutations in the GP IIIa subunit (Table 32.6).

# FUNCTIONAL DEFECTS OF PLATELETS ASSOCIATED WITH CYTOSKELETAL ABNORMALITIES

One congenital disorder in platelets characterized by defects of the cytoskeleton is the **Wiskott-Aldrich syndrome.** Individuals with this syndrome display variable abnormalities of platelet function. This rare disorder is inherited as an X-linked trait and therefore affects boys almost exclusively. The clinical manifestations of the disorder result from the two blood cells that are most affected, T lymphocytes and platelets, and they include thrombocytopenia with small platelets, eczema, and immunodeficiency (220). This disorder is closely related to X-linked thrombocytopenia (XLT) in which the platelets are similarly affected but the immunodeficiency is absent or greatly attenuated compared with full-blown Wiskott-Aldrich syndrome (221). The hemostatic abnormality has at least three potential causes: thrombocytopenia that can be profound (platelet counts may be as low as 15,000/$\mu$l), an adhesive defect of platelets secondary to abnormalities of GP Ib$\alpha$ brought about either by defective oligosaccharide synthesis (222) or by enhanced proteolysis by calpain released into the plasma by the destruction of platelets (223), and a very abnormal platelet cytoskeleton (224). The thrombocytopenia seen in the Wiskott-Aldrich syndrome appears to be caused by accelerated platelet destruction resulting from an intrinsic defect of the platelets. The fact that the abnormality resides in the platelets and is not secondary to other cellular or plasma defects is supported by the observation that transfused platelets survive normally in Wiskott-Aldrich syndrome individuals (225) and by the improvements in platelet counts and platelet volume experienced by those individuals who have undergone splenectomy (226).

Recently, the genetic lesion in Wiskott-Aldrich syndrome was identified by positional cloning of a gene that resides on the X-chromosome (Xpll.22) (227). The gene encodes a protein named WASP (Wiskott-Aldrich syndrome protein) that contains 502 amino acid residues without a hydrophobic signal peptide for export from the cell. This protein has several regions rich in proline, suggesting that it may associate with signaling proteins and adaptors that contain SH3 domains, and may thereby be involved in signaling pathways. WASP has, in fact, been demonstrated to interact with p47[nck], an SH3-containing adaptor protein (228). In addition, WASP was recently shown to interact with a member of the Rho family of GTPases, cdc42 (229, 230), which is involved in regulating actin polymerization, providing insight into WASP's role in the cytoskeletal abnormalities of Wiskott-Aldrich-syndrome platelets and lymphocytes. The WASP genes from nearly 80 Wiskott-Aldrich syndrome families have been sequenced, and all reveal defects (231). In addition, X-linked thrombocytopenia also appears to be due to defects in the WASP gene (232). Why defects of the same gene lead to two diseases of different clinical severity is not clear. However, mutations in XLT are much more likely to be missense mutations, and frameshift and nonsense mutations are more common in Wiskott-Aldrich syndrome (224), which indicates that some mutations may allow WASP to retain partial function, consistent with the assignment of different interactive domains to different regions of the protein (228, 230). Nevertheless, disease severity is also dependent on other environmental or genetic factors because some XLT individuals have been found to carry the same mutations that cause Wiskott-Aldrich syndrome in other individuals (224). Interestingly, the platelets and T cells of Wiskott-Aldrich syndrome individuals are deficient in related membrane sialomucins. The membrane content of platelet GP Ib and of T-cell CD43 (leukosialin) have both been reported to be deficient. These proteins, while not homologous, are very similar to each other, each containing elongated extracellular regions rich in serine, threonine, and proline residues that are heavily *O*-glycosylated and rich in sialic acid. The common defect in the membrane sialomucins may reflect an inherent defect in *O*-glycosylation or sialylation (222), or it may be a secondary consequence of increased plasma levels of calpain, a cysteine proteinase normally present in the platelet cytoplasm that is released into the plasma in Wiskott-Aldrich syndrome individuals and to which both of these proteins are sensitive (223). Treatment of Wiskott-Aldrich syndrome is designed to correct the defect in blood cell function. In individuals in whom the immunodeficiency is not profound, splenectomy has been demonstrated to increase the platelet count and to result in a normalization of platelet size (226, 232, 233). If both immunodeficiency and platelet dysfunction are severe, bone marrow transplantation should be considered (234, 235).

# OTHER CONGENITAL PLATELET DEFECTS

Other qualitative and quantitative congenital platelet defects have been described. In most cases the specific defect producing these abnormalities is yet to be elucidated. The **Montreal platelet syndrome,** which has autosomal dominant inheritance, is characterized by a prolonged skin bleeding time, moderate thrombocytopenia, formation of artifactually giant platelets on physical or biochemical stimulation (236, 237), spontaneous platelet aggregation with a reduced response to thrombin-induced aggregation (238, 239), and normal platelet-surface glycoproteins. A defect involving calpain (calcium-activated neutral protease) has been found in Montreal platelets, which is although to be the etiologic cause of this syndrome (239). **Epstein's syndrome** is the association of hereditary macrothrombocytopenia with nerve deafness and nephritis. This syndrome has autosomal-dominant inheritance with the bleeding tendency being attributed to the thrombocytopenia (240–242), although a platelet function defect has been reported (243). The **Sebastian platelet syndrome** has autosomal-dominant inheritance and the features of macrothrombocytopenia and neutrophil inclusions. The neutrophil inclusions consist of dispersed filaments, clusters of ribosomes, and a few segments of rough endoplasmic reticulum (244). Light and electron microscopic assessment of platelets is similar to the Fechtner syndrome, although the clinical associations are absent (245). The **Fechtner syndrome** is defined by the association of nephritis, congenital deafness and cataracts, macrothrombocytopenia, and polymorphonuclear inclusions distinct from toxic Döhle bodies and the inclusions found in the May-Hegglin anomaly (246). These polymorphonuclear inclusions can be distinguished from those of the May-Hegglin anomaly by electron microscopy (247, 248). The **May-Hegglin anomaly** also has autosomal-dominant inheritance, with the anomaly appearing to be a defect in megakaryocyte maturation and/or fragmentation, resulting in macrothrombocytopenia, and a defect in leukocytes that leads to RNA-containing, Döhle-like bodies in polymorphonuclear leukocytes and monocytes (249). The underlying defect has not been defined. Although thrombocytopenia and increased platelet size are common laboratory findings, platelet morphology is otherwise normal. Ultrastructural studies show normal platelet structure but an increased amount of disorganized tubules (250). The bleeding diathesis in individuals with this anomaly varies from asymptomatic to a significant hemorrhagic diathesis, and it varies according to the degree of thrombocytopenia. Platelets aggregate normally in response to various agonists with platelet-surface glycoproteins being normal (87, 147, 249, 251–253). Isolated **platelet factor 3 deficiency** has been reported (254–257). Platelet factor 3 is the overall contribution of platelets to the acceleration of clot formation. It is the platelet contribution to the interaction of factors Xa, Va, and calcium ion to prothrombin activation. This activity is apparently mediated by a lipoprotein complex on the activated platelet surface. Clinically, individuals have a bleeding diathesis, and with rare exceptions, a normal skin bleeding time. This normal skin bleeding time is although to reflect a defect in the ability of the platelet factor 3 to accelerate thrombin production rather than a defect in platelet plug formation. A bleeding diathesis associated with a defect in mobilizing intracellular calcium ion has been described; however, the site of the defect in platelets has not been determined (258). **Medi-**terranean macrothrombocytopenia** is an asymptomatic disorder with moderate thrombocytopenia and large platelets (259, 260). The mode of inheritance is unclear.

# THERAPY OF CONGENITAL PLATELET BLEEDING DISORDERS

The therapeutic approaches to the management of individuals with congenital platelet bleeding disorders can be subdivided into general supportive measures, specific measures for bleeding episodes, and other therapeutic modalities. General measures include education of the individual about their bleeding diathesis and informing individuals that the use of antiplatelet medications is contraindicated (113, 147). All individuals should carry identification to indicate their hemorrhagic diathesis. Adequate dental hygiene should be maintained to prevent gingival disease and to avoid the necessity for dental procedures. Iron deficiency may result from general gum oozing, as well as menorrhagia. The hormonal control of menses may therefore be of benefit to premenopausal women. As a result, iron therapy may be necessary, especially during rapid growth in infancy and adolescence. Specific treatment of bleeding episodes or as prophylaxis for the prevention of bleeding during surgical procedures is based on the use of platelet transfusions (113, 147, 261) (see Chapter 51). Local measures to obtain hemostasis and minimize or obviate the need for platelet transfusions include arterial embolization, which may be effective in, for example, severe epistaxis (103, 113, 147).

As well as the potential in Glanzmann's thrombasthenia and the Bernard-Soulier syndrome for alloimmunization by HLA antigens following platelet transfusion, the risk of which can be reduced by the use leukocyte-depleted platelet concentrates (262), there is also the risk of developing antibodies directed against the specifically deficient platelet-surface glycoproteins, GP IIb-IIIa and GP Ib-IX-V, respectively (263–265). This can result in ineffectiveness of subsequent platelet transfusions (113). The development of specific antiglycoprotein antibodies, however, is rare in both diseases and is not a reason to withhold the transfusion of platelets when therapeutically indicated. In all individuals, the ideal, whenever possible, is the use of HLA-matched, single-donor transfusions of platelets with a leukocyte filter irrespective of the underlying congenital platelet disorder. Other measures although to be of use in Glanzmann's thrombasthenia include using the antifibrinolytic drug, $\epsilon$-aminocaproic acid (see Chapter 53), concurrently with platelet transfusions in managing tooth extractions (261). The roles of other systemic measures although to be of use in Glanzmann's thrombasthenia have not been proven. DDAVP (see Chapter 53) has been shown to shorten the bleeding time in some (266), although not all (267), individuals with the Bernard-Soulier syndrome. DDAVP's place in managing individuals with the Bernard-Soulier syndrome is therefore presently unclear. The use of cryoprecipitate (see Chapter 52) in storage-pool deficiency has been shown to shorten the bleeding time and prevent bleeding during surgery (268). In addition, DDAVP has also been shown to be effective in shortening the bleeding time in some individuals with storage-pool deficiency, as well as in some individuals with other intrinsic platelet defects (269–275). The use of DDAVP in individuals with storage-pool deficiency may therefore decrease the need to use platelets or cryoprecipitate. A role for correction of a low hematocrit toward normal levels, althought to be due to an ADP effect, may be of benefit in $\delta$-SPD (276). Disorders in which the use of other plasma factors may supplement platelet transfusion therapy include platelet factor 3 deficiency, where therapy with prothrombin complex has also been reported to be effective (255), and pseudo-von Willebrand disease, where platelet transfusion may need to be given with cryoprecipitate if the plasma factor VIII/vWf level is markedly decreased (147). By itself, however, cryoprecipitate can cause thrombocytopenia (277), as can the use of DDAVP in this condition (278).

# REFERENCES

1. Berndt MC, Fournier DJ, Castaldi PA. Bernard-Soulier syndrome. Baillières Clin Haematol 1989;2:585–607.
2. Nurden AT. Polymorphisms of human platelet membrane glycoproteins: structure and clinical significance. Thromb Haemost 1995;74:345–351.
3. Weiss HJ, Tschopp TB, Baumgartner HR et al. Decreased adhesion of giant (Bernard-Soulier) platelets to subendothelium. Further implications on the role of von Willebrand factor in haemostasis. Am J Med 1974;57:920–925.
4. Weiss HJ, Turitto VT, Baumgartner HR. Effect of shear rate on platelet interaction with subendothelium in citrated and native blood. Shear-dependent decrease of adhesion in von Willebrand's disease and the Bernard-Soulier syndrome. J Lab Clin Med 1978;92:750–764.
5. Weiss HJ, Turitto VT, Baumgartner HR. Platelet adhesion and thrombus formation on subendothelium in platelets deficient in glycoproteins IIb-IIIa, Ib and storage granules. Blood 1986;67:322–330.
6. Sadler JE. von Willebrand Factor. J Biol Chem 1991;266:22777–22780.
7. Sakariassen KS, Bolhuis PA, Sixma JJ. Human blood platelet adhesion to artery subendothelium is mediated by factor VIII-von Willebrand Factor bound to the subendothelium. Nature 1979;279:636–638.
8. Andrews RK, López JA, Berndt MC. Molecular mechanisms of platelet adhesion and activation [Review]. Int J Biochem Cell Biol 1997;29:91–105.
9. Greco NJ, Tandon NN, Jones GD et al. Contributions of glycoprotein Ib and the seven transmembrane domain receptor to increases in platelet cytoplasmic $[Ca^{2+}]$ induced by $\alpha$-thrombin. Biochemistry 1996;35:906–914.
10. Connolly AJ, Ishihara H, Kahn ML et al. Role of the thrombin receptor in development and evidence for a second receptor. Nature 1996;381:516–519.
11. Berndt MC, Gregory C, Dowden G et al. Thrombin interactions with platelet membrane proteins. Ann N Y Acad Sci 1986;485:374–386.
12. Harmon JT, Jamieson GA. The glycocalicin portion of platelet glycoprotein Ib expresses both high and moderate affinity receptor sites for thrombin. A soluble radio-receptor assay for interaction of thrombin with platelets. J Biol Chem 1986;261:13224–13229.
13. Berndt MC, Gregory C, Chong BH et al. Additional glycoprotein defects in Bernard-Soulier's syndrome: confirmation of genetic basis by parental analysis. Blood 1983;62:800–807.
14. Clemetson KJ, McGregor JL, James E et al. Characterization of the platelet

15. López JA. The platelet glycoprotein -IX complex. Blood Coagul Fibrinolysis 1994;5:97–119.
16. Modderman PW, Admiraal LG, Sonnenberg A et al. Glycoproteins V and -IX form a noncovalent complex in the platelet membrane. J Biol Chem 1992;267:364–369.
17. Dong JF, Li CQ, López JA. Tyrosine sulfation of the glycoprotein -IX complex: identification of sulfated residues and effect on ligand binding. Biochemistry 1994;33:13946–13953.
18. Marchese P, Murata M, Mazzucato M et al. Identification of three tyrosine residues of glycoprotein Ib with distinct roles in von Willebrand factor and $\alpha$-thrombin binding. J Biol Chem 1995;270:9571–9578.
19. Ward CM, Andrews RK, Smith AI et al. Mocarhagin, a novel cobra venom metalloproteinase, cleaves the platelet von Willebrand factor receptor glycoprotein Ib$\alpha$. Identification of the sulfated tyrosine/anionic sequence Tyr-276–Glu-282 of glycoprotein Ib$\alpha$ as a binding site for von Willebrand factor and $\alpha$-thrombin. Biochemistry 1996;35:4929–4938.
20. De Marco L, Shapiro SS. Properties of human asialo-factor VIII. A ristocetin-independent platelet-aggregating agent. J Clin Invest 1981;68:321–328.
21. Kroll MH, Harris TS, Moake JL et al. von Willebrand factor binding to platelet Gp initiates signals for platelet activation. J Clin Invest 1991;88:1568–1573.
22. Ikeda Y, Handa M, Kamata T et al. Transmembrane calcium influx associated with von Willebrand factor binding to GP Ib in the initiation of shear-induced platelet aggregation. Thromb Haemost 1993;69:496–502.
23. Clemetson KJ. Platelet activation: signal transduction via membrane receptors [Review]. Thromb Haemost 1995;74:111–116.
24. Ozaki Y, Satoh, K, Yatomi Y et al. Protein tyrosine phosphorylation in human platelets induced by interaction between glycoprotein Ib and von Willebrand factor. Biochim Biophys Acta 1995;1243:482–488.
25. Du X, Harris SJ, Tetaz TJ et al. Association of a phospholipase A$_2$ (14-3-3 protein) with the platelet glycoprotein -IX complex. J Biol Chem 1994;269:18287–18290.
26. Aitken A. 14-3-3 proteins on the MAP. Trends Biochem Sci 1995;20:95–97.
27. Fox JE. The platelet cytoskeleton. Thromb Haemost 1993;70:884–893.
28. Hartwig JH, DeSisto M. The cytoskeleton of the resting human platelet: structure of the membrane skeleton and its attachment to actin filaments. J Cell Biol 1991;112:407–425.
29. Wardell MR, Reynolds CC, Berndt MC et al. Platelet glycoprotein Ib$\beta$ is phosphorylated on serine 166 by cyclic AMP–dependent protein kinase. J Biol Chem 1989;264:15656–15661.
30. Fox JE, Berndt MC. Cyclic AMP–dependent phosphorylation of glycoprotein Ib inhibits collagen-induced polymerization of actin in platelets. J Biol Chem 1989;264:9520–9526.
31. López JA, Leung B, Reynolds CC et al. Efficient plasma membrane expression of a functional platelet glycoprotein -IX complex requires the presence of its three subunits. J Biol Chem 1992;267:12851–12859.
32. Li CQ, Dong JF, Lanza F et al. Expression of platelet glycoprotein (GP) V in heterologous cells and evidence for its association with GP Ib$\alpha$ in forming a GP Ib-IX-V complex on the cell surface. J Biol Chem 1995;270:16302–16307.
33. Meyer SC, Fox JE. Interaction of platelet glycoprotein V with glycoprotein -IX regulates expression of the glycoproteins and binding of von Willebrand factor to glycoprotein -IX in transfected cells. J Biol Chem 1995;270:14693–14699.
34. Li C, Pasquale DN, Roth GJ. Bernard-Soulier syndrome with severe bleeding: absent platelet glycoprotein Ib alpha due to a homozygous one-base deletion. Thromb Haemost 1996;76:670–674.
35. Miller JL, Lyle VA, Cunningham D. Mutation of leucine-57 to phenylalanine in a platelet glycoprotein Ib$\alpha$ leucine tandem repeat occurring in individuals with an autosomal dominant variant of Bernard-Soulier disease. Blood 1992;79:439–446.
36. Simsek S, Admiraal LG, Modderman PW et al. Identification of a homozygous single base pair deletion in the gene coding for the human platelet glycoprotein Ib$\alpha$ causing Bernard-Soulier syndrome. Thromb Haemost 1994;72:444–449.
37. Li C, Martin SE, Roth GJ. The genetic defect in two well-studied cases of Bernard-Soulier syndrome: a point mutation in the fifth leucine-rich repeat of platelet glycoprotein Ib$\alpha$. Blood 1995;86:3805–3814.
38. Ware J, Russell SR, Marchese P et al. Point mutation in a leucine-rich repeat of platelet glycoprotein Ib$\alpha$ resulting in the Bernard-Soulier syndrome. J Clin Invest 1993;92:1213–1220.
39. de la Salle C, Baas MJ, Lanza F et al. A three-base deletion removing a leucine residue in a leucine-rich repeat of platelet glycoprotein Ib$\alpha$ associated with a variant of Bernard-Soulier syndrome (Nancy I). Br J Haematol 1995;89:386–396.
40. Simsek S, Noris P, Lozano M et al. Cys209 Ser mutation in the platelet membrane glycoprotein Ib$\alpha$ gene is associated with Bernard-Soulier syndrome. Br J Haematol 1994;88:839–844.
41. Ware J, Russell SR, Vicente V et al. Nonsense mutation in the glycoprotein

Ibα coding sequence associated with Bernard-Soulier syndrome. Proc Natl Acad Sci U S A 1990;87:2026–2030.

42. Kunishima S, Miura H, Fukutani H et al. Bernard-Soulier syndrome Kagoshima: Ser 444→stop mutation of glycoprotein (GP) Ibα resulting in circulating truncated GP Ibα and surface expression of GP Ibβ and GP IX. Blood 1994;84:3356–3362.

43. Noda M, Fujimura K, Takafuta T et al. Heterogenous expression of glycoprotein, IX and V in platelets from two individuals with Bernard-Soulier syndrome caused by different genetic abnormalities. Thromb Haemost 1995;74:1411–1415.

44. Wright SD, Michaelides K, Johnson DJ et al. Double heterozygosity for mutations in the platelet glycoprotein IX gene in three siblings with Bernard-Soulier syndrome. Blood 1993;81:2339–2347.

45. Clemetson JM, Kyrle PA, Brenner B et al. Variant Bernard-Soulier syndrome associated with a homozygous mutation in the leucine-rich domain of glycoprotein IX. Blood 1994;84:1124–1131.

46. Noda M, Fujimura K, Takafuta T et al. A point mutation in glycoprotein IX coding sequence (Cys73[TGT] to Tyr[TAT]) causes impaired surface expression of GP Ib-IX-V complex in two families with Bernard-Soulier syndrome. Thromb Haemost 1996;76:874–878.

47. Budarf ML, Konkle BA, Ludlow LB et al. Identification of a individual with Bernard-Soulier syndrome and a deletion in the DiGeorge/velocardio-facial chromosomal region in 22q11.2. Hum Mol Genet 1995;4:763–766.

48. Miller JL, Cunningham D, Lyle VA et al. Mutation in the gene encoding the α-chain of platelet glycoprotein Ib in the platelet type von Willebrand disease. Proc Natl Acad Sci U S A 1991;88:4761–4765.

49. Takahashi H, Murata M, Moriki T et al. Substitution of Val for Met at residue 239 of platelet glycoprotein Ibα in Japanese individuals with platelet-type von Willebrand disease. Blood 1995;85:727–733.

50. Sae-Tung G, Dong JF, López JA. Biosynthetic defect in platelet glycoprotein IX mutants associated with Bernard-Soulier syndrome. Blood 1996;87:1361–1367.

51. Drouin J, McGregor JL, Parmentier S et al. Residual amounts of glycoprotein Ib concomitant with near-absence of glycoprotein IX in platelets of Bernard-Soulier individuals. Blood 1988;72:1086–1088.

52. Hourdillé P, Pico M, Jandrot-Perrus M et al. Studies on the megakaryocytes of a individual with the Bernard-Soulier syndrome. Br J Haematol 1990;76:521–530.

53. Arai M, Yamamoto N, Akamatsu N et al. Substantial expression of glycoproteins IX and V on the platelet surface from a individual with Bernard-Soulier syndrome. Br J Haematol 1994;87:185–188.

54. Kunishima S, López JA, Kobayashi S et al. Missense mutations of the glycoprotein (GP) Ibβ gene impairing the GP Ib α/β disulfide linkage in a family with giant platelet disorder. Blood 1997;89:2404-2412.

55. Devine DV, Currie MS, Rosse WF et al. Pseudo–Bernard-Soulier syndrome: thrombocytopenia caused by auto-antibody to platelet glycoprotein. Blood 1987;70:428–431.

56. Berndt MC, Kabral A, Grimsley P et al. An acquired Bernard-Soulier–like platelet defect associated with juvenile myelodysplastic syndrome. Br J Haematol 1988;68:97–101.

57. George JN, Nurden AT, Phillips DR. Molecular defects in interactions of platelets with the vessel wall. N Engl J Med 1984;311:1084–1098.

58. Weiss HJ, Meyer D, Rabinowitz R et al. Pseudo–von Willebrand's disease. An intrinsic platelet defect with aggregation by unmodified human factor VIII/von Willebrand factor and enhanced absorption of its high-molecular-weight multimers. N Engl J Med 1982;306:326–333.

59. Miller JL, Castella A. Platelet-type von Willebrand's disease: characterization of a new bleeding disorder. Blood 1982;60:790–794.

60. Moroi M, Jung SM, Shinmyozu K et al. Analysis of platelet adhesion to a collagen-coated surface under flow conditions: the involvement of glycoprotein VI in the platelet adhesion. Blood 1996;88:2081–2092.

61. Savage B, Saldivar E, Ruggeri ZM. Initiation of platelet adhesion by arrest onto fibrinogen or translocation on von Willebrand factor. Cell 1996;84:289–297.

62. Clark EA, Brugge JS. Integrins and signal transduction pathways: the road taken. Science 1995;268:233–239.

63. Asazuma N, Yatomi Y, Ozaki Y et al. Protein-tyrosine phosphorylation and p72syk activation in human platelets stimulated with collagen is dependent upon glycoprotein Ia/IIa and actin polymerization. Thromb Haemost 1996;75:648–654.

64. Coller BS, Beer JH, Scudder LE et al. Collagen-platelet interactions: evidence for a direct interaction of collagen with platelet GP Ia-IIa and an indirect interaction with platelet GP I/IIIa mediated by adhesive proteins. Blood 1989;74:182–192.

65. Staatz WD, Rajpara SM, Wayner EA et al. The membrane glycoprotein Ia-IIa (VLA-2) complex mediates the Mg++-dependent adhesion of platelets to collagen. J Cell Biol 1989;108:1917–1924.

66. Nieuwenhuis HK, Akkerman JW, Houdijk WP et al. Human blood platelets showing no response to collagen fail to express surface glycoprotein Ia. Nature 1985;318:470–472.

67. Nieuwenhuis HK, Sakariassen KS, Houdijk WP et al. Deficiency of platelet membrane glycoprotein Ia associated with a decreased platelet adhesion to subendothelium: a defect in platelet spreading. Blood 1986;68:692–695.

68. Tandon NN, Kralisz U, Jamieson GA. Identification of glycoprotein IV (CD36) as a primary receptor for platelet-collagen adhesion. J Biol Chem 1989;264:7576–7583.

69. Bull HA, Brickell PM, Dowd PM. Src-related protein tyrosine kinases are physically associated with the surface antigen CD36 in human dermal microvascular endothelial cells. FEBS Lett 1994;351:41–44.

70. Huang MM, Bolen JB, Barnwell JW et al. Membrane glycoprotein IV (CD36) is physically associated with the Fyn, Lyn, and Yes protein-tyrosine kinases in human platelets. Proc Natl Acad Sci U S A 1991;88:7844–7848.

71. Tandon NN, Ockenhouse CF, Greco NJ et al. Adhesive functions of platelets lacking glycoprotein IV (CD36). Blood 1991;78:2809–2813.

72. Kashiwagi H, Honda S, Take H et al. Presence of the entire coding region of GP IV mRNA in Nak(a)-negative platelets. Int J Hematol 1993;57:153–161.

73. Yamamoto N, Akamatsu N, Sakuraba H et al. Platelet glycoprotein IV (CD36) deficiency is associated with the absence (type I) or the presence (type II) of glycoprotein IV on monocytes. Blood 1994;83:392–397.

74. Kashiwagi H, Tomiyama Y, Kosugi S et al. Identification of molecular defects in a subject with type I CD36 deficiency. Blood 1994;83:3545–3552.

75. Kashiwagi H, Tomiyama Y, Nozaki S et al. A single nucleotide insertion in codon 317 of the CD36 gene leads to CD36 deficiency. Arterioscler Thromb Vasc Biol 1996;16:1026–1032.

76. Kashiwagi H, Tomiyama Y, Honda S et al. Molecular basis of CD36 deficiency. Evidence that a 478C→T substitution (proline90→serine) in CD36 cDNA accounts for CD36 deficiency. J Clin Invest 1995;95:1040–1046.

77. Kashiwagi H, Tomiyama Y, Kosugi S et al. Family studies of type II CD36 deficient subjects: linkage of a CD36 allele to a platelet-specific mRNA expression defect(s) causing type II CD36 deficiency. Thromb Haemost 1995;74:758–763.

78. Sugiyama T, Okuma M, Ushikubi F et al. A novel platelet aggregating factor found in a individual with defective collagen–induced platelet aggregation and autoimmune thrombocytopenia. Blood 1987;69:1712–1720.

79. Moroi M, Jung SM, Okuma M et al. A individual with platelets deficient in glycoprotein VI that lack both collagen-induced aggregation and adhesion. J Clin Invest 1989;84:1440–1445.

80. Ichinohe T, Takayama H, Ezumi Y et al. Cyclic AMP-insensitive activation of cSrc and Syk protein-tyrosine kinases through platelet membrane glycoprotein VI. J Biol Chem 1995;270:28129–28036.

81. Raccuglia G. Gray platelet syndrome. A variety of qualitative platelet disorder. Am J Med 1971;51:818–828.

82. White JG. Ultrastructural studies of the gray platelet syndrome. Am J Pathol 1979;95:445–462.

83. Breton-Gorius J, Vainchenke W, Nurden A et al. Defective alpha-granule production in megakaryocytes from gray platelet syndrome: ultrastructural studies of bone marrow cells and megakaryocytes growing in culture from blood precursors. Am J Pathol 1981;102:10–19.

84. George JN, Nurden AT, Phillips DR. Molecular defects in interaction of platelets with the vessel wall. N Engl J Med 1984;311:1084–1098.

85. Rao AK. Congenital disorders of platelet function. Haematol Oncol Clin North Am 1990;4:65–86.

86. Jantunen E, Hanninen A, Naukkarinen A et al. Gray platelet syndrome with splenomegaly and signs of extramedullary hematopoiesis: a case report with Review of literature. Am J Haematol 1994;46:218–224.

87. Jantunen E. Inherited giant platelet disorders. Eur J Haematol 1994;53:191–196.

88. Cramer EM, Vainchenker W, Vinci G et al. Gray platelet syndrome: immunoelectron microscopic localization of fibrinogen and von Willebrand factor in platelets and megakaryocytes. Blood 1985;66:1309–1316.

89. Levy-Toledano S, Caen JP, Breton-Gorius J et al. Gray platelet syndrome: α-granule deficiency. Its influence on platelet function. J Lab Clin Med 1981;98:831–848.

90. Nurden AT, Kunicki TJ, Dupuis D et al. Specific protein and glycoprotein deficiencies in platelets isolated from two individuals with the gray platelet syndrome. Blood 1982;59:709–718.

91. Harrison P, Cramer EM. Platelet α-granules. Blood Rev 1993;7:52–62.

92. Rosa JP, George JN, Bainton DF et al. Gray platelet syndrome. Demonstration of alpha granule membranes that can fuse with the cell surface. J Clin Invest 1987;80:1138–1146.

93. Gerrard JM, Phillips DR, Rao GH et al. Biochemical studies of two individuals with the gray platelet syndrome. Selective deficiency of the platelet α-granules. J Clin Invest 1980;66:102–109.

94. Pfueller SL, David R. Platelet-associated immunoglobulins G, A and M are secreted during platelet activation: normal levels but deficient secretion in grey platelet syndrome. Br J Haematol 1988;68:235–241.

95. Vermylen C, Vermylen J, Hoet B et al. Grey platelet syndrome: evidence for alpha-granule localization of the platelet plasminogen activator inhibitor-1 pool. Pediatr Hematol Oncol 1991;8:111–120.

96. Berger G, Masse JM, Cramer EM. Alpha-granule membrane mirrors the platelet plasma membrane and contains glycoproteins Ib, IX and V. Blood 1996;87:1385–1395.

97. Cramer EM, Berger G, Berndt MC. Platelet α-granule and plasma mem-

brane share two new components: CD9 and PECAM-1. Blood 1994;84: 1722–1730.

98. Berger G, Caen JP, Berndt MC et al. Ultrastructural demonstration of CD36 in the α-granule membrane of human platelets and megakaryocytes. Blood 1993;82:3034–3044.

99. Gebrane-Younes S, Cramer EM, Orcel L et al. Gray platelet syndrome. Dissociation between abnormal sorting in megakaryocyte alpha-granules and normal sorting in Weibel-Palade bodies of endothelial cells. J Clin Invest 1993;92:3023–3028.

100. Berndt MC, Castaldi PA, Gordon S et al. Morphological and biochemical confirmation of gray platelet syndrome in two siblings. Aust N Z J Med 1983;13:387–390.

101. Rao AK, Holmsen H. Congenital disorders of platelet function. Semin Hematol 1986;23:102–118.

102. Cockbill SR, Burmester HB, Heptinstall S. Pseudo grey platelet syndrome—grey platelets due to degranulation in blood collected into EDTA. Eur J Haematol 1988;41:326–333.

103. Coller BS. Platelets and their disorders. In: Ratnoff OD, Forbes CD, eds. Disorders of haemostasis. Orlando: Grune & Stratton, 1984; pp. 73–177.

104. Berrebi A, Klepfish A, Varon D et al. Gray platelet syndrome in the elderly. Am J Hematol 1988;28:270–272.

105. Facon T, Goudemand J, Caron C et al. Simultaneous occurrence of gray platelet syndrome and idiopathic pulmonary fibrosis: a role for abnormal megakaryocytes in the pathogenesis of pulmonary fibrosis. Br J Haematol 1990;74:542–543.

106. Kohler M, Hellstern P, Morgenstern E et al. Gray platelet syndrome: selective alpha-granule deficiencies and thrombocytopenia due to increased platelet turnover. Blut 1985;50:331–340.

107. Srivastava PC, Powling MJ, Nokes TJ et al. Grey platelet syndrome: studies on platelet alpha-granules, lysosomes and defective response to thrombin. Br J Haematol 1987;65:441–446.

108. Pfueller SL, Howard MA, White JG et al. Shortening of bleeding time by 1-desamino-8-D-arginine vasopressin (DDAVP) in the absence of platelet von Willebrand Factor in gray platelet syndrome. Thromb Haemost 1987; 58:1060–1063.

109. Holmsen H, Weiss HJ. Further evidence of a deficient storage pool of adenine nucleotides in platelets from individuals with thrombocytopathia—"storage pool disease." Blood 1972;39:179–209.

110. Weiss HJ, Witte LD, Kaplan KL et al. Heterogeneity in storage pool deficiency: studies on granule-bound substances in 18 individuals including variants deficient in α-granules, platelet factor 4, β-thromboglobulin and platelet derived growth factor. Blood 1979;54:1296–1319.

111. Weiss HJ, Ames RP. Ultrastructural findings in storage pool disease and aspirin like defects of platelets. Am J Pathol 1973;71:447–466.

112. White JG, Edson JR, Desnick SJ et al. Studies of platelets in a variant of the Hermansky-Pudlak syndrome. Am J Pathol 1971;63:319–329.

113. Bellucci S, Tobelem G, Caen JP. Inherited platelet disorders. Prog Haematol 1983;13:223–263.

114. Witkop CJ, Krumwiede M, Sedano HO et al. Reliability of absent platelet dense bodies as a diagnostic criterion for Hermansky-Pudlak syndrome. Am J Hematol 1987;26:305–311.

115. Skaer RJ, Peters PD, Emmines JP. Platelet dense bodies: a quantitative microprobe analysis. J Cell Sci 1976;20:441–457.

116. Costa JL, Fay DD, McGill M. Electron probe microanalysis of calcium and phosphorus in dense bodies isolated from human platelets. Thromb Res 1981;22:399–405.

117. Richards JG, DaPrada M. Uranaffin reaction: a new cytochemical technique for the localization of adenine nucleotides in organelles storing biogenic amines. J Histochem Cytochem 1977;25:1322–1336.

118. Payne CM. A quantitative ultrastructural evaluation of the cell organelle specificity of the uranaffin reaction in normal human platelets. Am J Clin Pathol 1984;81:62–70.

119. Lorez HP, DaPrada M, Rendu F et al. Mepacrine, a tool for investigating the 5-hydroxytryptamine organelles of blood platelets by fluorescence microscopy. J Lab Clin Med 1977;89:200–206.

120. Holmsen H, Weiss HJ. Secretable storage pools in platelets. Annu Rev Med 1979;30:119–134.

121. Weiss HJ. Congenital disorders of platelet function. Semin Hematol 1980; 17:228–241.

122. Weiss HJ, Tschopp TB, Brand H et al. Studies of platelet 5-hydroxytryptamine (serotonin) in storage pool disease and albinism. J Clin Invest 1974; 74:421–433.

123. Pareti FI, Day HJ, Mills DC. Nucleotide and serotonin metabolism in platelets with defective secondary aggregation. Blood 1974;44:789–800.

124. Bennett JS, Shattil SJ. Congenital qualitative platelet disorders. In: Williams WJ, Beutler E, Erslev AJ, Lichtman MA, eds. Haematology. 4th ed. New York: McGraw-Hill, 1990; pp. 1407–1418.

125. Akkerman JW, Nieuwenhuis HK, Mommersteeg-Leautaud ME et al. ATP-ADP compartmentation in storage pool deficient platelets: correlation between granule-bound ADP and the bleeding time. Br J Haematol 1983;55: 135–143.

126. Timmons S, Kloczewiak M, Hawiger J. ADP-dependent common receptor

127. mechanism for binding of von Willebrand factor and fibrinogen to human platelets. Proc Natl Acad Sci U S A 1984;81:4935–4939.

127. Gerrard JM, Israels ED, Bishop AJ et al. Inherited platelet storage pool deficiency associated with a high incidence of acute myeloid leukaemia. Br J Haematol 1991;79:246–255.

128. Herve P, Drouet L, Dosquet C et al. Primary pulmonary hypertension in a individual with a familial platelet storage pool disease: role of serotonin. Am J Med 1990;89:117–120.

129. Witkop CJ, Townsend D, Bitterman PB et al. The role of ceroid in lung and gastrointestinal disease in Hermansky-Pudlak syndrome. Adv Exp Med Biol 1989;266:283–296.

130. Reynolds SP, Davies BH, Gbs AR. Diffuse pulmonary fibrosis and the Hermansky-Pudlak syndrome: clinical course and postmortem findings. Thorax 1994;49:617–618.

131. Harmon KR, Witkop CJ, White JG et al. Pathogenesis of pulmonary fibrosis: platelet derived growth factor precedes structural alterations in the Hermansky-Pudlak syndrome. J Lab Clin Med 1994;123:617–627.

132. Schallreuter KU, Frenk E, Wolfe LS et al. Hermansky-Pudlak syndrome in a Swiss population. Dermatology 1993;187:248–256.

133. Fukai K, Oh J, Frenk E et al. Linkage disequilibrium mapping of the gene for Hermansky-Pudlak syndrome to chromosome 10q23.1-q23.3. Hum Mol Genet 1995;4:1665–1669.

134. Wildenberg SC, Oetting WS, Almodovar C et al. A gene causing Hermansky-Pudlak syndrome in a Puerto Rican population maps to chromosome 10q2. Am J Hum Genet 1995;57:755–765.

135. Gerrard JM, Lint D, Sims PJ et al. Identification of a platelet dense granule membrane protein that is deficient in a individual with Hermansky-Pudlak syndrome. Blood 1991;77:101–112.

136. Nishori M, Cham B, McNicol A et al. The protein CD63 is in platelet dense granules, is deficient in a individual with Hermansky-Pudlak syndrome, and appears identical to granulophysin. J Clin Invest 1993;91:1775–1782.

137. Shalev A, Michaud G, Israels SJ et al. Quantifiation of a novel dense granule protein (granulophysin) in platelets of individuals with dense granule storage pool deficiency. Blood 1992;80:1231–1237.

138. Barrat FJ, Auloge L, Pastural E et al. Genetic and physiological mapping of the Chediak-Higashi syndrome on chromosome 1q42-43. Am J Hum Genet 1996;59:625–632.

139. Fukai K, Oh J, Karim MA et al. Homozygosity mapping of the gene for Chediak-Higashi syndrome to chromosome 1q42-q44 in a segment conserved synteny that includes the mouse beige locus (bg). Am J Hum Genet 1996;59:620–624.

140. Baetz K, Isaaz S, Griffiths GM. Loss of cytotoxic T lymphocyte function in Chediak-Higashi syndrome arises from a secretory defect that prevents lytic granule exocytosis. J Immunol 1995;154:6122–6131.

141. Ballard R, Tier RD, Nohria V et al. The Chediak-Higashi syndrome: CT and MR findings. Pediatr Radiol 1994;24:266–267.

142. Uyama E, Hirano T, Ito K et al. Adult Chediak-Higashi syndrome presenting as parkinsonism and dementia. Acta Neurol Scand 1994;89:175–183.

143. Weinblatt M, Petrikovsky B, Bialer M et al. Prenatal evaluation and *in utero* platelet transfusion for thrombocytopenia absent radii syndrome. Prenat Diagn 1994;14:892–896.

144. Labrune P, Pons JC, Khalil M et al. Antenatal thrombocytopenia in three individuals with TAR (thrombocytopenia with absent radii) syndrome. Prenat Diagn 1993;13:463–466.

145. Symonds RP, Clark BJ, George WD et al. Thrombocytopenia with absent radii (TAR) syndrome: a new increased cellular radiosensitivity syndrome. Clin Oncol (R Coll Radiol) 1995;7:56–58.

146. Parkman R, Remold-O'Donnell E, Kenney DM et al. Surface protein abnormalities in lymphocytes and platelets from individuals with Wiskott-Aldrich syndrome. Lancet 1981;2:1387–1389.

147. Bellucci S, Caen JP. Congenital platelet disorders. Blood Rev 1988;2:16–26.

148. Gerrard JM, McNicol A. Platelet storage pool deficiency, leukemia, and myelodysplastic syndromes. Leuk Lymphoma 1992;8:277–281.

149. Gordon N, Thom J, Cole C et al. Rapid detection of hereditary and acquired platelet storage pool deficiency by flow cytometry. Br J Haematol 1995; 89:117–123.

150. Nieuwenhuis HK, Akkerman JW, Sixma JJ. Individuals with a prolonged bleeding time and normal aggregation tests may have storage pool deficiency: studies on one hundred six individuals. Blood 1987;70:620–623.

151. Wall JE, Buijs-Wilts M, Arnold JT et al. A flow cytometric assay using mepacrine for study of uptake and release of platelet dense granule contents. Br J Haematol 1995;89:380–385.

152. Flodgaard H, Zamecnik PC, Meyers K et al. Diagnosis of storage pool deficiency by determination of diadenosine 5',5'''-P1,P4-tetraphosphate in whole blood. Thromb Res 1986;41:345–351.

153. Lages B, Shattil SJ, Bainton DF et al. Decreased content and surface expression of α-granule membrane protein GMP-140 in one of two types of platelet αδ-storage pool deficiency. J Clin Invest 1991;87:919–929.

154. Weiss HJ, Lages B, Vicic W et al. Heterogeneous abnormalities of platelet dense granule ultrastructure in 20 individuals with congenital storage pool deficiency. Br J Haematol 1993;83:282–295.

155. Rao AK, Koike K, Willis J et al. Platelet secretion defect associated with

impaired liberation of arachidonic acid and normal myosin light chain phosphorylation. Blood 1984;64:914–921.

156. Malmsten C, Hamberg M, Svensson J et al. Physiological role of an endoperoxide in human platelets: haemostatic defect due to platelet cyclooxygenase deficiency. Proc Natl Acad Sci U S A 1975;72:1446–1450.

157. Lagarde M, Byron PA, Vargaftig BB et al. Impairment of platelet thromboxane $A_2$ generation and of platelet release reaction in two individuals with congenital deficiency of platelet cyclooxygenase. Br J Haematol 1978; 38:251–266.

158. Funk CD, Funk LB, Kennedy ME et al. Human platelet/erythroleukemia cell prostaglandin G/H synthase: cDNA cloning, expression and gene chromosomal assignment. FASEB J 1991;5:2304–2312.

159. Jones DA, Carlton DP, McIntyre TM et al. Molecular cloning of human prostaglandin endoperoxide synthase type II and demonstration of expression in response to cytokines. J Biol Chem 1993;268:9049–9054.

160. Shimokawa T, Kulmacz RJ, DeWitt DL et al. Tyrosine 385 of prostaglandin endoperoxide synthase is required for cyclooxygenase catalysis. J Biol Chem 1990;265:20073–20076.

161. Roth GJ, Machuga ET. Radioimmune assay of human platelet prostaglandin synthetase. J Lab Clin Med 1982;99:187–196.

162. Matijevic-Aleksic N, McPhedran P, Wu KK. Bleeding disorder due to platelet prostaglandin H synthase-1 (PGHS-1) deficiency. Br J Haematol 1996;92:212–217.

163. Machin SJ, Carreras LO, Chamone DAF et al. Familial deficiency of thromboxane synthase [Abstract]. Br J Haematol 1981;47:629.

164. Mestel F, Oetliker O, Beck E et al. Severe bleeding associated with defective thromboxane synthetase. Lancet 1980;1:157.

165. Defreyn G, Machin SJ, Carreras LO et al. Familial bleeding tendency with partial platelet thromboxane synthetase deficiency: reorientation of cyclic endoperoxide metabolism. Br J Haematol 1981;49:29–41.

166. Lages B, Malmsten C, Weiss HJ, Samuelsson B. Impaired platelet response to thromboxane $A_2$ and defective calcium mobilization in a individual with a bleeding disorder. Blood 1981;49:545–552.

167. Samama M, Lecrubier C, Conard J et al. Constitutional thrombocytopathy with subnormal response to thromboxane $A_2$. Br J Haematol 1981;48: 293–303.

168. Wu KK, Le Breton GC, Tai HH, Chen YC. Abnormal platelet response to thromboxane $A_2$. J Clin Invest 1981;67:1801–1804.

169. Bray PF. Inherited diseases of platelet glycoproteins: considerations for rapid molecular characterization. Thromb Haemost 1994;72:492–502.

170. Caen JP. Glanzmann's thrombasthenia. Baillières Clin Haematol 1989;2: 609–625.

171. Glanzmann E. Hereditäre hämorrhagische thrombasthenie. Ein beitrag znr pathologie der blutplättchen. Jahr Kinderheilk 1918;88:1–42.

172. George JN, Caen JP, Nurden AT. Glanzmann's thrombasthenia: the spectrum of clinical disease. Blood 1990;75:1383–1395.

173. Berndt MC, Caen JP. Platelet glycoproteins. Prog Hemost Thromb 1984; 7:111–150.

174. Weiss HJ, Turitto VT, Baumgartner HR. Further evidence that glycoprotein IIb-IIIa mediates platelet spreading on subendothelium. Thromb Haemost 1991;65:202–205.

175. Weiss HJ, Hawiger J, Ruggeri ZM et al. Fibrinogen-independent platelet adhesion and thrombus formation on subendothelium mediated by glycoprotein IIb-IIIa complex at high shear rate. J Clin Invest 1989;83:288–297.

176. Lawrence JB, Gralnick HR. Monoclonal antibodies to the glycoprotein IIb-IIIa epitopes involved in adhesive protein binding: effects on platelet spreading and ultrastructure on human arterial subendothelium. J Lab Clin Med 1987;109:495–503.

177. Phillips DR, Charo IF, Scarborough RM. GP IIb-IIIa: the responsive integrin. Cell 1991;65:359–362.

178. Plow EF, Ginsberg MH. Cellular adhesion: GP IIb-IIIa as a prototypic adhesion receptor. Prog Hemost Thromb 1988;9:117–156.

179. Smith JW, Ruggeri ZM, Kunicki TJ et al. Interaction of integrins $\alpha v\beta 3$ and glycoprotein IIb-IIIa with fibrinogen. Differential peptide recognition accounts for distinct binding sites. J Biol Chem 1990;265:12267–12271.

180. Kloczewiak M, Timmons S, Hawiger J. Localization of a site interacting with human platelet receptor on carboxyterminal segment of human fibrinogen γ-chain. Biochem Biophys Res Commun 1982;107:181–187.

181. Farrell DH, Thiagarajan P, Chung DW et al. Role of fibrinogen alpha and gamma chain sites in platelet aggregation. Proc Natl Acad Sci U S A 1992; 89:10729–10732.

182. D'Souza SE, Ginsberg MH, Burke TA et al. The ligand binding site of the platelet integrin receptor GP IIb-IIIa is proximal to the second calcium binding domain of its α-subunit. J Biol Chem 1990;265:3440–3446.

183. D'Souza SE, Ginsberg MH, Burke TA et al. Localization of an Arg-Gly-Asp recognition site within an integrin adhesion receptor. Science 1988; 242:91–93.

184. Charo IF, Nannizzi L, Phillips DR et al. Inhibition of fibrinogen binding to GP IIb-IIIa by a GP IIIa peptide. J Biol Chem 1991;266:1415–1421.

185. Harrison P, Wilbourn B, Debili N et al. Uptake of plasma fibrinogen into the -granules of human megakaryocytes and platelets. J Clin Invest 1989; 84:1320–1324.

186. Coller BS, Seligsohn U, West SM et al. Platelet fibrinogen and vitronectin

187. in Glanzmann thrombasthenia: evidence consistent with specific roles for glycoprotein IIb-IIIa and $\alpha v\beta 3$ integrins in platelet protein trafficking. Blood 1991;78:2603–2610.

187. Nurden AT, Didry D, Kieffer N et al. Residual amounts of glycoproteins IIb and IIIa may be present in the platelets of most individuals with Glanzmann's thrombasthenia. Blood 1985;65:1021–1024.

188. Coller BS, Seligsohn U, Little PA. Type I Glanzmann thrombasthenia individuals from the Iraqi-Jewish and Arab populations in Israel can be differentiated by platelet glycoprotein IIIa immunoblot analysis. Blood 1987;69: 1696–1703.

189. Seligsohn U, Coller BS, Zivelin A et al. Immunoblot analysis of platelet glycoprotein IIb in individuals with Glanzmann thrombasthenia in Israel. Br J Haematol 1989;72:415–423.

190. Newman PJ, Seligsohn U, Lyman S et al. The molecular genetic basis of Glanzmann thrombasthenia in the Iraqi-Jewish and Arab populations in Israel. Proc Natl Acad Sci U S A 1991;88:3160–3164.

191. Burk CD, Newman PJ, Lyman S et al. A deletion in the gene for glycoprotein IIb associated with Glanzmann's thrombasthenia. J Clin Invest 1991; 87:270–276.

192. Poncz M, Rifat S, Coller BS et al. Glanzmann thrombasthenia secondary to a Gly273→Asp mutation adjacent to the first calcium-binding domain of platelet glycoprotein I. J Clin Invest 1994;93:172–179.

193. Wilcox DA, Paddock CM, Lyman S et al. Glanzmann thrombasthenia resulting from a single amino acid substitution between the second and third calcium-binding domains of GP I. Role of the GP I aminoterminus in integrin subunit association. J Clin Invest 1995;95:1553–1560.

194. Wilcox DA, Wautier JL, Pidard D et al. A single amino acid substitution flanking the fourth calcium binding domain of αIIB prevents maturation of the αIIβ3 integrin complex. J Biol Chem 1994;269:4450–4457.

195. Basani RB, Vilaire G, Shattil SJ et al. Glanzmann thrombasthenia due to a two amino acid deletion in the fourth calcium-binding domain of αIIb: demonstration of the importance of calcium-binding domains in the conformation of αIIbβ3. Blood 1996;88:167–173.

196. Schlegel N, Gayet O, Morel-Kopp MC et al. The molecular genetic basis of Glanzmann's thrombasthenia in a gypsy population in France: identification of a new mutation on the αIIb gene. Blood 1995;86:977–982.

197. Kato A, Yamamoto K, Miyazaki S et al. Molecular basis for Glanzmann's thrombasthenia (GT) in a compound heterozygote with glycoprotein IIb gene: a proposal for the classification of GT based on the biosynthetic pathway of glycoprotein IIb-IIIa complex. Blood 1992;79:3212–3218.

198. Gu JM, Xu WF, Wang XD et al. Identification of a nonsense mutation at amino acid 584-arginine of platelet glycoprotein IIb in individuals with type I Glanzmann thrombasthenia. Br J Haematol 1993;83:442–449.

199. Tomiyama Y, Kashiwagi H, Kosugi S et al. Abnormal processing of the glycoprotein IIb transcript due to a nonsense mutation in exon 17 associated with Glanzmann's thrombasthenia. Thromb Haemost 1995;73: 756–762.

200. Vinciguerra C, Trzeciak MC, Phillippe N et al. Molecular study of Glanzmann thrombasthenia in 3 individuals issued from 2 different families. Thromb Haemost 1995;74:822–827.

201. Peretz H, Rosenberg N, Usher S et al. Glanzmann's thrombasthenia associated with deletion-insertion and alternative splicing in the glycoprotein IIb gene. Blood 1995;85:414–420.

202. Iwamoto S, Nishiumi E, Kajii E et al. An exon 28 mutation resulting in alternative splicing of the glycoprotein IIb transcript and Glanzmann's thrombasthenia. Blood 1994;83:1017–1023.

203. Li L, Bray PF. Homologous recombination among three intragene Alu sequences causes an inversion-deletion resulting in the hereditary bleeding disorder Glanzmann thrombasthenia. Am J Hum Genet 1993;53: 140–149.

204. Simsek S, Heyboer H, de Bruijne-Admiraal LG et al. Glanzmann's thrombasthenia caused by homozygosity for a splice defect that leads to deletion of the first coding exon of the glycoprotein IIIa mRNA. Blood 1993;81: 2044–2049.

205. Loftus JC, O'Toole TE, Plow EF et al. A β3 integrin mutation abolishes ligand binding and alters divalent cation-dependent conformation. Science 1990;249:915–918.

206. Bajt ML, Ginsberg MH, Frelinger AL 3d et al. A spontaneous mutation of integrin αIIβ3 (platelet glycoprotein IIb-IIIa) helps define a ligand binding site. J Biol Chem 1992;267:3789–3794.

207. Lanza F, Stierle A, Fournier D et al. A new variant of Glanzmann's thrombasthenia (Strasbourg I). Platelets with functionally defective glycoprotein IIb-IIIa complexes and a glycoprotein IIIa 214Arg–214Trp mutation. J Clin Invest 1992;89:1995–2004.

208. Djaffar I, Rosa JP. A second case of variant of Glanzmann's thrombasthenia due to substitution of platelet glycoprotein IIIa (integrin β3) Arg214 by Trp. Hum Mol Genet 1993;2:2179–2181.

209. Chen YP, Djaffar I, Pidard D et al. Ser-752-Pro mutation in the cytoplasmic domain of integrin B3 subunit and defective activation of platelet integrin αIIβ3 (glycoprotein IIb-IIIa) in a variant of Glanzmann thrombasthenia. Proc Natl Acad Sci U S A 1992;89:10169–10173.

210. Grimaldi CM, Chen F, Scudder LE et al. A Cys374Tyr homozygous muta-

tion of platelet glycoprotein IIIa (β3) in a Chinese individual with Glanzmann's thrombasthenia. Blood 1996;88:1666–1675.

211. Djaffer I, Caen JP, Rosa JP. A large alteration in the human platelet glycoprotein IIIa (integrin β3) gene associated with Glanzmann's thrombasthenia. Hum Mol Genet 1993;2:2183–2185.

212. Russell ME, Seligsohn U, Coller BS et al. Structural integrity of the glycoprotein IIb and IIIa genes in Glanzmann thrombasthenia individuals from Israel. Blood 1988;72:1833–1836.

213. Coller BS, Cheresh DA, Asch E et al. Platelet vitronectin receptor expression differentiates Iraqi-Jewish from Arab individuals with Glanzmann thrombasthenia in Israel. Blood 1991;77:75–83.

214. Fitzgerald LA, Phillips DR. Structure and function of platelet membrane glycoproteins. In: Kunicki TJ, George JN, eds. Platelet immunobiology: molecular and clinical aspects. Philadelphia: JB Lippincott, 1989; pp. 9–30.

215. Krissansen GW, Elliott MJ, Lucas CM et al. Identification of a novel integrin β-subunit expressed on cultured monocytes (macrophages). Evidence that one α-subunit can associate with multiple β-subunits. J Biol Chem 1990;265:823–830.

216. Burgess-Wilson ME, Cockbill SR, Johnston GI et al. Platelet aggregation in whole blood from individuals with Glanzmann's thrombasthenia. Blood 1987;69:38–42.

217. Ginsberg MH, Lightsey A, Kunicki TJ et al. Divalent cation regulation of the surface orientation of platelet membrane glycoprotein I. Correlation with fibrinogen binding function and definition of a novel variant of Glanzmann's thrombasthenia. J Clin Invest 1986;78:1103–1111.

218. Ginsberg MH, Frelinger AL, Lam SCT et al. Analysis of platelet aggregation disorders based on flow cytometric analysis of membrane glycoprotein IIb-IIIa with conformation-specific monoclonal antibodies. Blood 1990;76:2017–2023.

219. Fournier DJ, Kabral A, Castaldi PA et al. A variant of Glanzmann's thrombasthenia characterized by abnormal glycoprotein IIb-IIIa complex formation. Thromb Haemost 1989;62:977–983.

220. Rosen FS, Cooper MD, Wedgwood RJ. The primary immunodeficiencies. N Engl J Med 1995;333:431–440.

221. Canales ML, Mauer AM. Sex-linked hereditary thrombocytopenia as a variant of Wiskott-Aldrich syndrome. N Engl J Med 1967;277:899–901.

222. Higgins EA, Siminovitch KA, Zhuang DL et al. Aberrant O-linked oligosaccharide biosynthesis in lymphocytes and platelets from individuals with the Wiskott-Aldrich syndrome. J Biol Chem 1991;266:6280–6290.

223. Kenney DM, Reid R, Parent DW et al. Evidence implicating calpain (Ca[2+])-dependent neutral protease) in the destructive thrombocytopenia of the Wiskott-Aldrich syndrome. Br J Haematol 1994;87:773–781.

224. Remold-O'Donnell E, Rosen FS, Kenney DM. Defects in Wiskott-Aldrich syndrome blood cells. Blood 1996;87:2621–2631.

225. Murphy S, Oski FA, Naiman JL et al. Platelet size and kinetics in hereditary and acquired thrombocytopenia. N Engl J Med 1972;286:499–504.

226. Mullen CA, Anderson KD, Blaese RM. Splenectomy and/or bone marrow transplantation in the management of Wiskott-Aldrich syndrome: long-term follow-up of 62 cases. Blood 1993;82:2961–2966.

227. Derry JM, Ochs HD, Francke U. Isolation of a novel gene mutated in Wiskott-Aldrich syndrome. Cell 1994;78:635–644.

228. Rivero-Lezcano OM, Marcilla A, Sameshima JH et al. Wiskott-Aldrich syndrome protein physically associates with Nck through Src homology 3 domains. Mol Cell Biol 1995;15:5725–5731.

229. Kolluri R, Tolias KF, Carpenter CL et al. Direct interaction of the Wiskott-Aldrich syndrome protein with the GTPase Cdc42. Proc Natl Acad Sci U S A 1996;93:5615–5618.

230. Symons M, Derry JMJ, Karlak B et al. Wiskott-Aldrich syndrome protein, a novel effector for the GTPase cdc42hs, is implicated in actin polymerization. Cell 1996;84:723–734.

231. Zhu Q, Zhang M, Blaese RM et al. The Wiskott-Aldrich syndrome and X-linked congenital thrombocytopenia are caused by mutations of the same gene. Blood 1995;86:3797–3804.

232. Corash L, Shafer B, Blaese RM. Platelet-associated immunoglobulin, platelet size and the effect of splenectomy in the Wiskott-Aldrich syndrome. Blood 1985;65:1439–1443.

233. Lum LG, Tubergen DG, Corash L et al. Splenectomy in the management of the thrombocytopenia of the Wiskott-Aldrich syndrome. N Engl J Med 1980;302:892–896.

234. Ozsahin H, Le Deist F, Benkerrou M et al. Bone marrow transplantation in 26 individuals with Wiskott-Aldrich syndrome from a single center. J Pediatr 1996;129:238–244.

235. Brochstein JA, Gillio AP, Ruggiero M et al. Marrow transplantation from human leukocyte antigen-identical or haploidentical donors for correction of Wiskott-Aldrich syndrome. J Pediatr 1991;119:907–912.

236. Milton JG, Hutton RA, Tuddenham EG et al. Platelet size and shape in hereditary giant platelet syndromes on blood smear and in suspension: evidence for two types of abnormalities. J Lab Clin Med 1985;106:326–335.

237. Milton JG, Frojmovic MM. Shape-changing agents produce abnormally large platelets in a hereditary "giant platelet syndrome (MPS)." J Lab Clin Med 1979;93:154–161.

238. Milton JG, Frojmovic MM, Tang SS et al. Spontaneous platelet aggregation in a hereditary giant platelet syndrome (MPS). Am J Pathol 1984;114:336–345.

239. Okita JR, Frojmovic MM, Kristopeit S et al. Montreal platelet syndrome: a defect in calcium-activated neutral proteinase (calpain). Blood 1989;74:715–721.

240. Epstein CJ, Sahud MA, Piel CF et al. Hereditary macrothrombocytopathia, nephritis and deafness. Am J Med 1972;52:299–310.

241. Eckstein JD, Filip DJ, Watts JC. Hereditary thrombocytopenia, deafness and renal disease. Ann Intern Med 1975;82:639–645.

242. Bernheim J, Dechavanne M, Bryon PA et al. Thrombocytopenia, macro-thrombocytopathia, nephritis and deafness. Am J Med 1976;61:145–150.

243. Turi S, Kobor J, Erdos A et al. Hereditary nephritis, platelet disorders and deafness—Epstein's syndrome. Pediatr Nephrol 1992;6:38–43.

244. Khalil SH, Qari MH. The Sebastian platelet syndrome. Report of the first native Saudi Arabian individual. Pathology 1995;27:197–198.

245. Greinacher A, Nieuwenhuis HK, White JG. Sebastian platelet syndrome: a new variant of hereditary macrothrombocytopenia with leukocyte inclusions. Blut 1990;61:282–288.

246. Peterson LC, Roa KV, Crosson JT et al. Fechtner syndrome—a variant of Alport's syndrome with leukocyte inclusions and macrothrombocytopenia. Blood 1985;65:397–406.

247. Gershoni-Baruch R, Baruch Y, Viener A et al. Fechtner syndrome: clinical and genetic aspects. Am J Med Genet 1988;31:357–367.

248. Heynen MJ, Blockmans D, Verwilghen RL et al. Congenital macrothrombocytopenia, leukocyte inclusions, deafness and proteinuria: functional and electron microscopic observations on platelets and megakaryocytes. Br J Haematol 1988;70:441–448.

249. Godwin HA, Ginsburg AD. May-Hegglin anomaly: a defect in megakaryocyte fragmentation. Br J Haematol 1974;26:117–128.

250. Greinacher A, Mueller-Eckhardt C. Hereditary types of thrombocytopenia with giant platelets and inclusion bodies in the leukocytes. Blut 1990;60:53–60.

251. Hamilton RW, Shilkh BS, Ottie JN et al. Platelet function, ultrastructure and survival in the May-Hegglin anomaly. Am J Clin Pathol 1980;74:663–668.

252. Djaldetti M, Creter D, Bujanover Y et al. Ultrastructural and functional studies of the platelets in individuals with May-Hegglin anomaly. Haematologica 1982;67:530–538.

253. Coller BS, Zarrabi MH. Platelet membrane studies in the May-Hegglin anomaly. Blood 1981;58:279–284.

254. Girolami A, Brunetti A, Fioretti D et al. Congenital thrombocytopathy (platelet factor 3 defect) with prolonged bleeding time but normal platelet adhesiveness and aggregation. Acta Haematol 1973;50:116–123.

255. Sultan Y, Brouet JC, Devergie A. Isolated platelet factor 3 deficiency [Letter]. N Engl J Med 1976;294:1121.

256. Minkoff IM, Wu KK, Walasek J et al. Bleeding disorders due to an isolated platelet factor 3 deficiency. Arch Intern Med 1980;140:366–367.

257. Weiss HJ, Vicic WJ, Lages BA et al. Isolated deficiency of platelet procoagulant activity. Am J Med 1979;67:206–213.

258. Hardisty RM, Machin SJ, Nokes TJ et al. A new congenital defect of platelet secretion: impaired responsiveness of the platelets to cytoplasmic free calcium. Br J Haematol 1983;53:543–557.

259. von Behrens WE. Splenomegaly, macrothrombocytopenia and stomatocytosis in healthy Mediterranean subjects (splenomegaly in Mediterranean macrothrombocytopenia). Scand J Haematol 1975;14:258–267.

260. Paulus JM, Casals FJ. Platelet formation in Mediterranean macrothrombocytosis. Nouv Rev Fr Hematol 1978;20:151–154.

261. George JN, Caen JP, Nurden AT. Glanzmann's thrombasthenia: the spectrum of clinical disease. Blood 1990;75:1383–1395.

262. Handa M, Ikeda Y, Kurata Y et al. Efficacy of leukocyte-depleted platelet concentrates for prevention of HLA-alloimmunization in individuals with frequent platelet transfusions: a prospective multi-institutional study using a polyester platelet filter [in Japanese]. Rinsho Ketsueki 1992;33:451–460.

263. Degos L, Dautigny A, Brouet JC et al. A molecular defect in thrombasthenic platelets. J Clin Invest 1975;56:236–240.

264. Degos L, Tobelem G, Lethielleux P et al. Molecular defect in platelets from individuals with Bernard-Soulier syndrome. Blood 1977;50:899–903.

265. Levy-Toledano S, Tobelem G, Legrand C et al. Acquired IgG antibody occurring in a thrombasthenic individual: its effect on human platelet function. Blood 1978;51:1065–1071.

266. Cuthbert RJ, Watson HH, Handa SI et al. DDAVP shortens the bleeding time in Bernard-Soulier syndrome. Thromb Res 1988;49:649–650.

267. Mant MJ. DDAVP in Bernard-Soulier syndrome [Letter]. Thromb Res 1988;52:77–78.

268. Gerritsen SW, Akkerman JW, Sixma JJ. Correction of the bleeding time in individuals with storage pool deficiency by infusion of cryoprecipitate. Br J Haematol 1978;40:153–160.

269. Kobrinsky NL, Israels ED, Gerrard JM et al. Shortening of bleeding time by 1-deamino-8-D-arginine vasopressin in various bleeding disorders. Lancet 1984;1:1145–1148.

270. Mannucci PM, Vicente V, Vianello L et al. Controlled trial of desmopressin

in liver cirrhosis and other conditions associated with a prolonged bleeding time. Blood 1987;67:1148–1153.

271. Nieuwenhuis HK, Sixma JJ. 1-Desamino-8-D-arginine vasopressin (desmopressin) shortens the bleeding time in storage pool deficiency. Ann Intern Med 1988;108:65–67.

272. Schulman S, Johnsson H, Egberg N et al. DDAVP-induced correction of prolonged bleeding time in individuals with congenital platelet function defects. Thromb Res 1987;45:165–174.

273. Pfueller SL, Howard MA, White JG et al. Shortening of bleeding time by 1-deamino-8-arginine vasopressin (DDAVP) in the absence of platelet von Willebrand factor in gray platelet syndrome. Thromb Haemost 1987;58:1060–1063.

274. Cattaneo M, Pareti FI, Zighetti M et al. Platelet aggregation at high shear is impaired in individuals with congenital defects of platelet secretion and is corrected by DDAVP: correlation with the bleeding time. J Lab Clin Med 1995;125:540–547.

275. Rao AK, Ghosh S, Sun L et al. Mechanisms of platelet dysfunction and response to DDAVP in individuals with congenital platelet function defects. A double-blind placebo-controlled trial. Thromb Haemost 1995;74:1071–1078.

276. Weiss HJ, Lages B, Hoffmann T et al. Correction of the platelet adhesion defect in δ-storage pool deficiency at elevated haematocrit—possible role of adenosine diphosphate. Blood 1996;87:4214–4222.

277. Takahashi H, Handa M, Watanabe K et al. Further characterization of platelet-type von Willebrand's disease in Japan. Blood 1984;64:1254–1262.

278. Takahashi H, Nagayama R, Hattori A et al. Platelet aggregation induced by DDAVP in platelet-type von Willebrand's disease [Letter]. N Engl J Med 1984;310:722–723.

# CHAPTER 33

# ACQUIRED DISORDERS OF PLATELET FUNCTION

Andrew I. Schafer

Unlike many of the inherited disorders of platelet function discussed in the previous chapter, which have clearly defined molecular mechanisms, most acquired, qualitative, platelet abnormalities involve uncertain or multifactorial defects. In some cases it is not even clear if the disorder is intrinsic to the platelets or is due to a humoral or vascular abnormality that secondarily inhibits platelet function. As noted elsewhere (see Chapters 23 and 43), some bleeding diatheses that are characterized by prolonged bleeding time and normal platelet count are probably due to primary vessel wall disorders. Major causes of acquired platelet dysfunction include uremia, liver failure, dysproteinemias, myeloproliferative disorders, and the use of a variety of drugs that are either designed to act as antiplatelet agents or coincidentally interfere with platelet function. While the molecular basis of platelet dysfunction is poorly characterized in most of these cases, this heterogeneous group represents some relatively common disorders that may cause clinically significant bleeding.

## UREMIA

Bleeding has been recognized as a major complication of renal failure since at least 1764, when Morgagni reported a uremic individual with gastrointestinal hemorrhage and epistaxis (1, 2). In 1827 Bright described purpura as a frequent presentation of individuals with renal failure (2, 3). In 1907 Reisman proposed that the bleeding tendency of uremia is caused by the actions of a "toxin" on blood and the vessel wall (4, 5). This general hypothe-

sis has largely withstood the subsequent scrutiny of a large body of fragmented experimental evidence, which has implicated abnormalities of platelet function, vascular metabolism, platelet-vessel wall interactions, and rheology in the hemostatic defect of uremia. No simple, unifying pathogenetic mechanism has yet been established. In fact a variety of successful, empiric, therapeutic interventions for uremic bleeding have preceded and anticipated experimental evidence regarding pathophysiology.

## CLINICAL FEATURES

The advent of dialysis has greatly reduced the problem of bleeding as a major cause of morbidity and mortality in renal failure. Nevertheless, fatal hemorrhagic complications of surgery and invasive procedures still occur. The bleeding manifestations are characteristic of defects of primary hemostasis (see Chapter 23), predominantly involving the skin and mucous membranes (2, 5). Purpura, ecchymoses, bleeding at venipuncture sites, epistaxis, and gastrointestinal bleeding occur most commonly. Upper gastrointestinal bleeding can be particularly severe, frequently originating in anatomic lesions such as ulcers (6, 7) and telangiectasia (8).

More unusual hemorrhagic manifestations of uremia have also been reported. Retroperitoneal bleeding may occur spontaneously in a variety of renal diseases (9–12) or may be a complication of percutaneous femoral catheterization for hemodialysis (13). Subdural hematoma occurs in 6 to 16% of uremic individuals on hemodialysis (14–16). Head trauma, hypertension, and anticoagulation are predisposing factors to this frequently fatal bleeding complication in these individuals. The formerly common problems of hemorrhagic pericarditis, sometimes with cardiac tamponade (17–19) and pleural effusion (20), are now rarely seen since the advent of dialysis. Spontaneous subcapsular hematoma of the liver has also been reported in hemodialysis individuals (21).

Paradoxically, some individuals with renal failure may actually have hypercoagulable (22) manifestations. Thrombotic complications include shunt clotting, as well as both arterial and venous thromboembolism (23–25). The association between thrombosis and the nephrotic syndrome is discussed in Chapter 40.

## LABORATORY FINDINGS

The clinical laboratory hallmark of the hemostatic defect of renal failure is the prolonged bleeding time. Clinical bleeding symptoms are best correlated with this test (26–28), even although no significant relationship can be found between the bleeding time and either the BUN or creatinine (27, 29). Platelet counts are generally normal, although mild thrombocytopenia is sometimes noted (5). This latter finding cannot explain the bleeding diathesis and can usually be attributed to coexisting conditions such as infection, disseminated intravascular coagulation, or the use of certain drugs. While the prolonged bleeding time is the most reproducible and consistent laboratory abnormality of hemostasis in uremia, the results of platelet aggregation studies are highly variable and unpredictable; they range from global defects in response to all agonists to entirely normal or even hyperreactive responses (29–37). While plasma coagulation factor activities are usually normal (38), a variety of coagulation and fibrinolytic defects may be found occasionally in these individuals (5); these are unlikely to be causally associated with clinical bleeding complications.

## PATHOGENESIS

### Uremic Toxins

The clinical bleeding tendency of individuals with renal failure is generally ameliorated by dialysis. Therefore uremic toxins have been implicated as important mediators of the bleeding diathesis. Nevertheless, the general experience has been that dialysis only incompletely corrects the prolonged bleeding time and abnormal platelet function, and that even partial improvements in these tests of primary hemostasis may not be achieved in some cases (28, 39–43).

The search for specific uremic toxins that interfere with primary hemostasis has been elusive. Urea (44), guanidinosuccinic acid (45), and phenols (46) inhibit

platelet aggregation *in vitro* at concentrations found in uremic plasma. Uremic retention products, referred to as "middle molecules" with molecular weights ranging from 500 Da to 3 Kda (47, 48), have been demonstrated to inhibit platelet aggregation and release (48, 49) and to stimulate vascular $PGI_2$ production (50). These molecules are difficult to remove from, and tend therefore to accumulate in, dialysis individuals (37). More recently, it has been demonstrated that fibrinogen degradation products containing the RGD amino acid sequence accumulate in the plasma of renal failure individuals. These low-molecular-weight products can inhibit platelet aggregation by blocking the binding of fibrinogen to its platelet membrane GP IIb-IIIa receptors (51). Other studies have likewise reported a reversibly impaired defect in platelet membrane GP IIb-IIIa function in uremia (52, 53), which is associated with decreased platelet aggregation in response to chemical stimuli and shear stress (54). It now appears that several types of uremic retention products may contribute to the hemostatic defect of renal failure.

### Hemostatic Defect

Despite a substantial body of experimental evidence in the literature showing that the hemostatic defect of uremia involves abnormalities of several facets of primary hemostasis, no single unifying pathogenetic mechanism has yet been established. Previous studies can be divided into the following overlapping and converging lines of investigation: (a) defects of platelet function and metabolism; (b) defects of vascular endothelial cell metabolism; (c) defects of platelet–vessel wall interactions; and (d) the anemia of renal failure. These are summarized in Table 33.1 and in Fig. 33.1. The finding of the

**TABLE 33.1.** Possible Hemostatic Defects in Uremia[a]

*Defects of platelet function and metabolism*
Abnormal aggregability
Decreased thromboxane $A_2$ production
Abnormal intracellular calcium mobilization
Increased intracellular cAMP, cGMP

*Defects of vascular endothelial cell metabolism*
Increased $PGI_2$ (prostacyclin) release
Increased nitric oxide release

*Defects of platelet–vessel wall interactions*
Decreased platelet adhesion
Decreased von Willebrand factor activity

*Anemia of renal failure*

cAMP, cyclic adenosine monophosphate; cGMP, cyclic guanosine monophosphate.

[a] *Several of these mechanisms have been disputed by contradictory data (see discussion in text). None of the defects listed provides an exclusive explanation of the clinical bleeding tendency.*

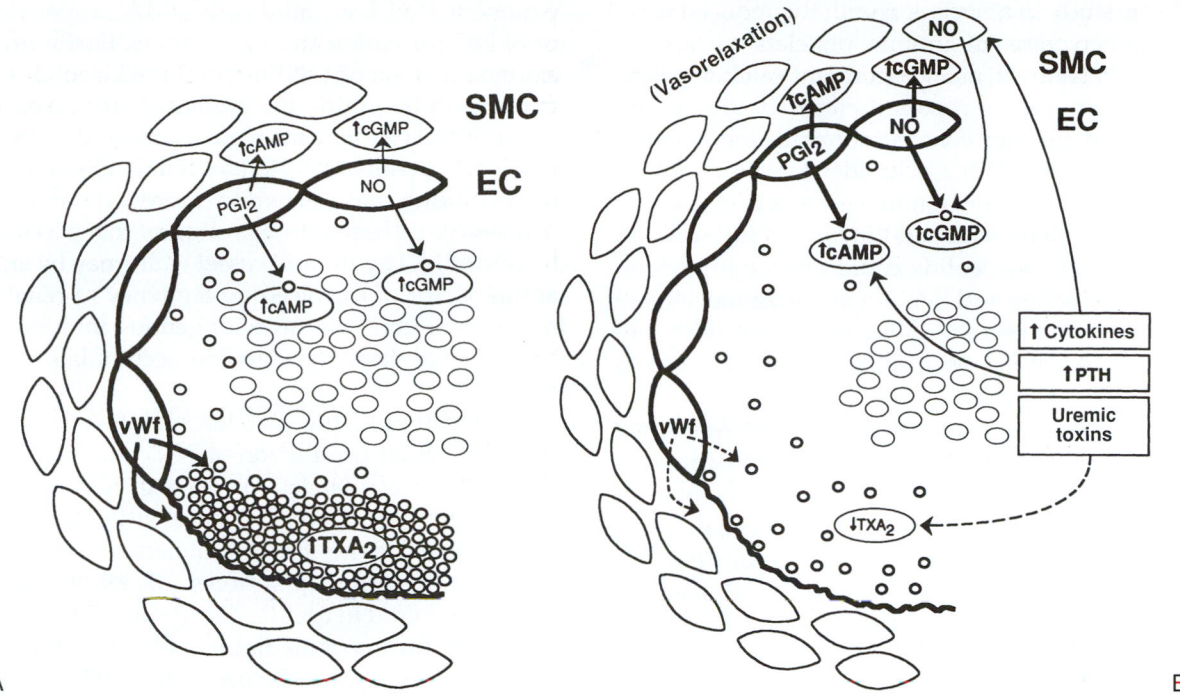

**FIGURE 33.1.**   Under normal circumstances (panel **A**), platelets adhere and aggregate at a site of vascular injury to form an occlusive hemostatic plug. Platelet adhesion is mediated by von Willebrand factor (vWf) released from adjacent endothelial cells (EC), as well as from the activated platelets themselves. Platelet aggregation is initiated by the release of thromboxane $A_2$ ($TXA_2$) and other platelet products and is mediated by vWf and other proteins. Blood fluidity and vascular tone are normally maintained in the presence of intact EC by their release of autocoids such as nitric oxide (NO) and $PGI_2$, which inhibit platelet activation and promote vasorelaxation by raising the intracellular levels of cGMP and cAMP, respectively, in both platelets and vascular smooth muscle cells (SMC). In renal failure (panel **B**), abnormal hemostasis has been considered to occur as a result of the following: (a) abnormalities of the vessel wall that lead to increased release of vasodilatory and platelet inhibitory NO and $PGI_2$; (b) defective platelet adhesion and aggregation due to impaired platelet $TXA_2$ production and possibly functionally abnormal vWf; (c) increased plasma levels of parathormone (PTH), which may further increase platelet cAMP, cytokines, which may induce NO production by SMC (and macrophages), and uremic toxins, which may interfere with platelet–vessel wall interactions; and (d) anemia in which the decreased number of red cells may rheologically reduce physical platelet interactions with the vessel wall and metabolically diminish platelet reactivity.

efficacy of certain empiric treatments for uremic bleeding has sometimes preceded basic studies and has provided important leads in elucidating the causes of hemorrhage in renal failure.

Numerous studies have failed to determine a consistent intrinsic defect of platelet function that can be causally linked to the bleeding tendency of uremia. The high variability of *in vitro* platelet aggregability in response to various stimuli is probably due in part to platelet activation induced by dialysis membranes (55) and by the use of heparin (56) (see below). An acquired form of storage pool deficiency may cause a platelet secretion defect in renal failure. The findings of low levels of platelet adenosine 5'-diphosphate (ADP) and serotonin have suggested dense body deficiency in some (36, 57), but not in all (58, 59), studies. Platelet α-granule deficiency and elevated plasma levels of α-granule contents have also been reported in renal failure (60–62). Activation and degranulation of platelets during pas-

sage across the membrane dialyzer may partly explain these findings in hemodialyzed individuals (63). The increased release of platelet α-granule mitogens could theoretically accelerate the development of arteriosclerosis in renal failure. Hemodialysis may also contribute to the uremic platelet defect by altering platelet turnover and causing selective elimination of the younger and more active platelets (64).

Several groups have reported that uremic platelets produce significantly less thromboxane $A_2$ than normal platelets, but the mechanism of this observation has been disputed. Original studies suggested that uremic plasma may induce a dysfunction of platelet cyclooxygenase (65–67). Subsequent work has indicated that the reduced platelet thromboxane $A_2$ production is due to impairment of endogenous arachidonic acid release in uremia (36, 59, 68). A defect in intracellular mobilization of calcium, leading to decreased levels of free cytoplasmic calcium after platelet stimulation, has been noted in one study in association with the reduced functional responsiveness of uremic platelets to various stimuli (69). In contrast, using a different calcium probe, a subsequent study has reported elevated resting and stimulated free calcium concentrations in the platelets of uremic individuals (32). Cyclic adenosine monophosphate (cAMP) is a major inhibitory second messenger in platelets (see Chapter 12), and increased intracellular levels of this cyclic nucleotide could block both thromboxane $A_2$ production and calcium mobilization, as well as aggregation and secretion. Indeed, the platelet concentration of cAMP has been found to be increased in individuals with renal failure (70–73).

It is possible that many of the platelet functional and metabolic activities that are found to be impaired in uremia are caused by primary alterations in the platelet inhibitory properties of vascular endothelium; this represents the second major line of investigations into the hemostatic defect(s) of uremia referred to above. The most potent physiologic activators of platelet adenylyl cyclase (leading to increased levels of cAMP) and guanylyl cyclase (leading to increased levels of cGMP) are prostacyclin ($PGI_2$) and nitric oxide (NO), respectively. Vascular $PGI_2$ production has been found to be increased in both individuals with severe renal failure and in nephrectomized rats. The finding of increased $PGI_2$ release by vessel walls in uremia (74) has been attributed to abnormally high $PGI_2$ stimulatory activity (75, 76) of uremic plasma (77), now considered to be a plasma component that protects vascular $PGI_2$ synthetic enzymes from exhaustion during persistent stimulation (78). In agreement with these findings in human studies, increased generation of vascular $PGI_2$ has been noted in uremic rats that have undergone bilateral nephrectomy or extensive renal mass ablation (79, 80). The clinical relevance of these observations is still unclear, however, since (a) complete inhibition of vascular $PGI_2$ formation with aspirin actually markedly increases (rather than corrects) the prolonged bleeding time of uremic individuals (81, 82), (b) there is no correlation between the bleeding time and vascular $PGI_2$ in rats with renal failure (79), and (c) correction of the bleeding time with estrogens in uremic rats does not affect the abnormal vascular $PGI_2$ production (80).

Parathyroid hormone (PTH) likewise stimulates platelet adenylyl cyclase and is consistently elevated in uremia. Therefore, this hormone has also been proposed to play a role both in the elevation of platelet cyclic AMP and in the bleeding defect (83, 84). However, a correlation between alterations in PTH levels and the bleeding diathesis has not been always observed (85).

Increased vascular NO synthesis and release have likewise been found in uremic rats and in individuals with renal failure. The prolonged bleeding time of uremic rats can be completely normalized by the injection of

$N$-monomethyl-L-arginine (L-NMMA), a specific inhibitor of NO formation from L-arginine. Furthermore, the shortening effect of L-NMMA on the bleeding time can be reversed by giving the animals L-arginine, the precursor of NO (86). Plasma from uremic individuals stimulates NO synthesis by endothelial cells, and human uremic individuals generate more NO than control platelets (87). These findings suggest that excessive production of NO by uremic vessel walls may be an important mediator of the bleeding tendency of renal failure. In apparent contrast, an endogenous inhibitor of NO synthesis has been reported to accumulate in uremia (88).

In addition to the platelet inhibitory action of enhanced vascular production of $PGI_2$ and NO in uremia, other defects of platelet–vessel wall interactions have been sought. Impaired platelet retention to glass beads and abnormal adhesion of platelets to subendothelial structures in perfusion systems (37, 89, 90) have been repeatedly found in uremia. Since von Willebrand factor is normally the major mediator of platelet adhesion, considerable attention has focused on possible abnormalities of this adhesive protein in renal failure. This line of investigation has been fueled by the clinical observations of striking improvement in the hemostatic defect of uremia by therapeutic interventions that raise plasma von Willebrand factor levels, including cryoprecipitate, DDAVP, and estrogens. However, no consistent and clear defects involving von Willebrand factor have been identified in individuals with uremia. Studies have reported normal or increased plasma levels of von Willebrand factor antigen (39, 91–95) in renal failure. Both normal (94) and abnormal (95–97) von Willebrand factor multimer distribution patterns have been reported, the latter studies demonstrating loss of the largest multimeric forms. Furthermore, high plasma von Willebrand factor antigen levels have been associated with disproportionately low ristocetin cofactor activity in some reports (95, 97, 98). It has been reported that a relative adhesion defect of uremic blood platelets to vascular subendothelial structures is compensated for by the high plasma levels of von Willebrand factor found in individuals with renal failure; normalization of the von Willebrand factor levels by dilution with von Willebrand factor depleted uremic plasma unmasks the impaired platelet interaction with artery segments (90) that is caused by an unknown factor in uremic plasma. Surface expression of the platelet membrane von Willebrand factor receptor (GP Ib) and binding of von Willebrand factor to platelet GP Ib have been reported to be either normal (52, 54, 99) or impaired (95, 100) in uremia. An abnormality of factor VIII coagulant antigen has also been found in uremia and has been attributed to proteolysis (101).

The fourth major line of investigation of the pathogenesis of uremic bleeding has focused on the role of the anemia that is characteristic of this disorder (102, 103). A negative correlation has been demonstrated between the hematocrit and the bleeding time in progressive renal failure and in hemodialysis individuals. Correction of the anemia of renal failure with either red cell transfusions (104, 105) or recombinant erythropoietin (89, 106–108) reduces the clinical bleeding symptoms and normalizes the bleeding time. The threshold hematocrit that must be reached with either type of treatment to achieve a normal or near-normal bleeding time is 27 to 32% (104, 105, 108). Red cells may enhance hemostasis by several mechanisms. They promote platelet-vascular interactions in flowing blood by causing the radial displacement of platelets from the axial stream toward the vessel wall (109–111) (Chapter 20). Furthermore, red cells (which contain ADP) may directly augment platelet activation (112) or bind and inactivate platelet inhibitory $PGI_2$ (113). However, anemia is unlikely to be the sole cause of the abnormal bleeding time of renal failure; although non-uremic anemia is also associated with prolongation of the bleeding time (114), the bleeding time for any given hematocrit is significantly longer in uremic than in non-uremic individuals.

## TREATMENT (SEE TABLE 33.2)

### Dialysis

The mainstay of treatment of the bleeding diathesis of uremia (115) has been dialysis, although it is not consistently effective (5). While dialysis reduces clinical complications, its effects on normalizing the bleeding time and platelet function are only partial (27, 36, 39, 40, 43, 116, 117). Improvement in hemostasis depends in part on the frequency of dialysis, being more effective when it is performed three times weekly rather than twice weekly (30, 39). The improvement in hemostatic parameters generally persists for 1 to 2 days after dialysis (5, 116).

Although some have found that hemodialysis and peritoneal dialysis are comparably effective in improving the hemostatic abnormality of uremia (39), other reports have suggested that peritoneal dialysis is more effective in this respect (40, 116, 118). However, both forms of dialysis can actually produce adverse effects on hemostasis. Peritoneal dialysis is associated with platelet hyperreactivity, which may be caused by the hypoalbuminemia that results from this procedure (43, 116, 119). On the other hand, hemodialysis is also accompanied by transient platelet activation (120–123) that may be mediated by the complement activation of certain cuprophane dialyzer membranes (see Chapter 42); platelet activation has not been observed during hemodialysis with noncomplement-activating dialyzer membranes such as polymethylmethacrylate (55). The heparin that is used to maintain patency of the extracorporeal circuit may also contribute to hemodialysis-associated platelet activation (56, 124). Platelet activation and degranulation may play a role in the accelerated atherosclerotic and vascular complications of hemodialysis individuals, as well as in the

**TABLE 33.2.**   Therapeutic Regimens for the Correction of Impaired Hemostasis in Uremia

| Treatment | Regimen | Onset and Duration of Action | Limitations and Complications |
|---|---|---|---|
| Red cell transfusions | Maintain hematocrit of 27–32% | Onset within 1 hour of achieving target hematocrit | Isoimmunization, risk of HIV and hepatitis, iron overload |
| Recombinant human erythropoietin | Maintain hematocrit of 27–32%; usually requires 150–400 U/kg/week | When target hematocrit is achieved | Hypertension, encephalopathy, thrombosis, hyperkalemia |
| Cryoprecipitate | 10 bags | Onset within 1 hour; maximum action at 4–12 hours; duration of action 24–36 hours | Inconsistent response; risk of HIV and hepatitis |
| DDAVP | 0.3–0.4 μg/kg i.v. or s.c.; or 2.0–3.0 μg/kg intranasal | Onset within 1 hour; maximum action at 2–4 hours; duration of action 4–8 hours | Rapid tachyphylaxis; minor side effects of flushing, headache or dizziness; ? rare thrombosis |
| Conjugated estrogens | 0.6 mg/kg per day i.v. for 4–5 days; or Premarin 50 mg p.o. daily; or transdermal 17β-estradiol 50 or 100 μg/24 hours, applied as a patch every 3.5 days | Onset at 6 hours after 1st infusion; maximum action after 1–2 weeks; duration of action 14 days | Hot flashes, fluid retention, hypertension, abnormal liver function tests |

*HIV, human immunodeficiency virus; i.v., intravenous; p.o., per os (oral); subcutaneous.*

pulmonary and neurologic syndromes that occur due to microembolization of platelet and leukocyte aggregates (125) or their activation products during the treatment.

## Correction of Anemia

Correction of the anemia of renal failure, together with dialysis, has now been established as primary management for the prevention and treatment of uremic bleeding. Initial studies that demonstrated improvement in clinical bleeding complications and the abnormal bleeding time with correction of the anemia were conducted with red cell transfusions (104, 105). Because of complications (e.g., isoimmunization, transmission of HIV and hepatitis, iron overload), the regular use of transfusions has now been largely supplanted by recombinant erythropoietin (89, 106–108). Erythropoietin has been demonstrated to be effective in improving the bleeding problem in children with renal failure (126, 127), as well as in adults. Since complete correction of the anemia of chronic renal failure may lead to risks of hypertension, encephalopathy, thrombosis, and hyperkalemia, it has been determined that raising the hematocrit to only about 27 to 32%, which requires erythropoietin doses ranging from 150 to 300 U/kg per week, is sufficient to normalize the bleeding time in almost all individuals (108). This is comparable with the hematocrit levels required to achieve normal bleeding times by red cell transfusions as well. Raising the hematocrit to correct the prolonged bleeding time of renal failure may (126, 128, 129) or may not (107) be accompanied by improvement in platelet function.

With the advent of regular dialysis and erythropoietin therapy, it can be predicted that the general problem of uremic bleeding will become markedly reduced in the future. Nevertheless, some of the following additional therapeutic modalities may be considered as ancillary treatment for the management of bleeding.

## Cryoprecipitate

Shortening of the bleeding time and improvement in clinical bleeding complications for up to 24 to 36 hours after infusion of cryoprecipitate have been reported (24, 93, 94). Nevertheless, administration of cryoprecipitate has failed to shorten the bleeding time in at least half of the individuals with renal failure (130).

## Desmopressin (DDAVP)

The synthetic vasopressin derivative, 1-deamino-8-D-arginine vasopressin (desmopressin or DDAVP) (see Chapter 53), has been shown to shorten the bleeding time rapidly and improve clinical bleeding in uremia (94). Although not proven, the mechanism of action of DDAVP has been considered to be mediated by the release of larger von Willebrand factor multimers from endothelial cells. DDAVP may also improve hemostasis in von Willebrand disease, hemophilia, qualitative platelet disorders and liver failure. The drug is infused intravenously at a dose of 0.3 or 0.4 µg/kg bodyweight over 15 to 30 minutes. It improves the bleeding time within 1 hour, an effect that may continue for only up to 4 to 8 hours (94, 131). Thus, repeated infusion after 8 hours may be necessary to maintain its hemostatic action. Rapid tachyphylaxis occurs with DDAVP, however, so that it produces a reduced response after only two or three infusions in 1 day (132). The improvement in the bleeding time is only partial in many individuals (133).

Administration of DDAVP subcutaneously rather than intravenously has been shown to be equally effective, making self-administration at home a possibility (131, 134). Furthermore, intranasal administration at a dose of 2 µg/kg bodyweight has been reported to shorten the bleeding time of uremic individuals within 2 hours (135). Side effects of DDAVP are unusual and generally minor, including facial flushing, headache, and dizziness (5, 94). However, cerebral thrombosis has been reported immediately after DDAVP infusion in an elderly uremic individual with vascular disease, prompting some caution in the use of this drug in individuals with advanced atherosclerotic cardiovascular disease (136).

## Estrogens

In contrast to cryoprecipitate and DDAVP, which produce very prompt, short-term effects on the hemostatic defect of uremia, conjugated estrogens have a more delayed but also more sustained action (80, 117, 137–140). Estrogens have been specifically reported to be effective in controlling bleeding from gastrointestinal telangiectasias in individuals with chronic renal failure (141). Intravenous infusion of conjugated estrogen, at a dose of approximately 0.6 mg/kg daily for 4 to 5 days, causes detectable improvement in the bleeding time of most individuals 6 hours after the first infusion, maximal improvement between the first and second week of treatment, and effects that persist for about 14 days (137, 139, 140). The bleeding time returns to baseline by day 16 in most cases (140). The improvement in bleeding times is accompanied by increased platelet reactivity, as measured by thromboxane $A_2$ and β-thromboglobulin release (137). More recently, it has been found that orally administered conjugated estrogens (Premarin 50 mg daily) normalize or markedly improve the bleeding time and the clinical bleeding tendency of most individuals with renal failure (138). Transdermal 17β-estradiol (Estraderm, 50 to 100 µg/day, applied as a patch every 3.5 days) has also been found to be effective in shortening the bleeding time and is possibly devoid of the potential disadvantages of first-pass liver metabolism of oral preparations (142). Hot flashes, fluid retention, hypertension, and abnormal liver function tests may occur in some individuals receiving conjugated estrogens.

# LIVER DISEASE

Individuals with liver failure are at high risk of bleeding complications for a variety of reasons (see Chapter 45). Anatomic abnormalities such as esophageal varices, gastritis, and hemorrhoids can predispose to gastrointestinal hemorrhage. Hypersplenism secondary to portal hypertension characteristically causes mild to moderate thrombocytopenia. Derangements of the coagulation and fibrinolytic systems in liver failure include impaired synthesis of coagulation factors, dysfibrinogenemia, and disseminated intravascular coagulation (143).

Qualitative platelet defects may also contribute to the bleeding tendency of individuals with liver disease (144). The bleeding time is frequently prolonged in individuals with cirrhosis (145, 146), even when other coagulation abnormalities may be relatively mild (147). Abnormal platelet function has been found to be generally related to the severity of liver disease (148, 149), and a correlation of the bleeding time with the bilirubin concentration has been specifically found (146). As in renal failure, results of platelet aggregation studies are highly variable and no characteristic pattern of abnormalities has been identified.

Several causes of defective platelet function in liver disease have been proposed. An uncharacterized plasma inhibitor of platelet aggregation has been found in some individuals (148). Increased platelet-associated immunoglobulin, possibly due to the polyclonal hypergammaglobulinemia associated with liver disease, may interfere with platelet function. Changes in platelet membrane lipid composition (with a decreased content of arachidonic acid) are related to impaired platelet function and to the severity of cirrhosis (149). The frequently elevated levels of fibrin(ogen) degradation production (FDP) in advanced liver disease can inhibit platelet aggregation (150, 151), although no correlation between platelet aggregation abnormalities and plasma levels of FDP has been found in these individuals (146). Finally, the synthesis of qualitatively abnormal fibrinogen (acquired dysfibrinogenemia) in some individuals with hepatic failure (152) could prevent normal platelet-platelet interactions. However, none of these possible factors has yet been directly linked to the cause of platelet dysfunction in liver disease.

Treatment is difficult because of the complexity of the coagulopathy of liver failure. Rapid and transient shortening of the prolonged bleeding time has been reported in some (but not all) cirrhosis individuals with the intravenous (153) or subcutaneous (154) administration of DDAVP. However, shortening of the bleeding time is usually only partial, and its clinical correlation with improved hemostasis has not been demonstrated.

# DYSPROTEINEMIAS

Bleeding in individuals with dysproteinemias, such as multiple myeloma and Waldenström's macroglobulinemia may be occasionally due to structural abnormalities such as amyloid angiopathy (155) or plasmacytoma (156). However, many individuals with these disorders may exhibit complex and multiple, systemic, coagulation abnormalities. The bleeding diathesis of dysproteinemia is related in part to qualitative platelet defects, but other coagulopathies are also frequently operative. Monoclonal immunoglobulins may interact with coagulation proteins to induce bleeding (157), sometimes acting as circulating inhibitors to specific factors (158). The paraprotein can inhibit fibrin polymerization (159, 160). Acquired factor X deficiency can develop in amyloidosis as a result of binding of factor X to amyloid fibrils, leading to its clearance from the circulation (161). Acquired von Willebrand disease can also develop as a rare complication of Waldenström's macroglobulinemia (162). A circulating heparin-like anticoagulant has been reported in multiple myeloma (163).

Mild thrombocytopenia is not unusual in these individuals, most frequently caused by myelosuppression from bone marrow infiltration or from the chemotherapy used to treat the disease. Several studies have demonstrated abnormalities of the bleeding time, platelet adhesion, platelet aggregation, and platelet procoagulant activity in dysproteinemias (158, 160, 164–166). Prolonged bleeding times and abnormalities of platelet aggregation are poor predictors of clinical bleeding risk in these disorders (167). Impaired platelet function has been found to correlate with serum paraprotein levels (168, 169) and to improve after plasmapheresis (170) in some studies, but not in others (167). However, some studies have reported normal or even increased platelet reactivity in these individuals, particularly when platelet function is studied in whole blood (171). The mechanism of the impairment of platelet function by paraproteins is not well understood, but has been considered to be due to nonspecific adherence of the immunoglobulin to the platelet surface. In one individual with multiple myeloma, a fatal bleeding disorder was caused by specific paraprotein binding to platelet membrane glycoprotein IIIa, inducing an acquired thrombasthenic-like state (172); the antibody in this case was comparable in activity with those isolated from transfused individuals with Glanzmann's thrombasthenia (173, 174) or from individuals with immune thrombocytopenia purpura (175, 176).

The treatment of the bleeding diathesis of dysproteinemias depends on the underlying mechanism of the coagulopathy. Platelet transfusions are generally ineffective, except in unusual cases of severe thrombocytopenia due to myelosuppression. Plasmapheresis, however, usually improves platelet function, as well as the other coagulation abnormalities (42).

# MYELOPROLIFERATIVE DISORDERS

The myeloproliferative disorders (MPD) are a group of related bone marrow diseases of the pluripotent hematopoietic stem cell and include the clinical entities of polycythemia vera (PCV), chronic myelogenous leukemia (CML), essential thrombocythemia (ET), and myeloid metaplasia with or without myelofibrosis. Although their clinical manifestations vary and overlap, sometimes involving transition from one MPD to another during the natural history of the disease and making precise classification difficult in some individuals, their pathogenic origin as clonal stem cell disorders is now incontrovertible (177–181). Apparently paradoxically, both bleeding and thrombosis are major causes of morbidity and mortality in the MPD. The thrombotic complications of MPD are further discussed in Chapter 40, while ET is specifically reviewed in Chapter 31. This section focuses on the role of qualitative platelet defects in the pathogenesis of bleeding complications in the MPD.

## CLINICAL FEATURES

The sites of hemorrhage in the MPD are characteristic of those of other platelet-vascular disorders. Superficial bleeding involving mucocutaneous surfaces is most commonly seen, including ecchymoses and purpura, epistaxis, and gastrointestinal and genitourinary tract bleeding. Deep-seated bleeding into joints, soft tissues, and the retroperitoneum is rare. The use of aspirin may unpredictably precipitate or exacerbate bleeding complications in some individuals with MPD (182, 183). Thrombocytopenia, which may develop particularly in the course of CML or myeloid metaplasia and myelofibrosis as a result of bone marrow replacement or chemotherapy, compounds the bleeding problems caused by the qualitative platelet abnormalities in some cases. While many individuals with MPD exhibit a clinical pattern of predominantly either bleeding or thrombotic events, others have hemostatic complications of both types occurring unpredictably during the course of their disease. On physical examination the primary finding of a MPD is the presence of splenomegaly; this is detected in most individuals with MPD, but varies from typically minimal enlargement of the spleen in ET to a frequently enormous spleen size in myeloid metaplasia.

## LABORATORY FINDINGS

In individuals who present with a bleeding or thrombotic problem in association with clinical findings that suggest a MPD (e.g., erythrocytosis, leukocytosis, thrombocytosis, splenomegaly), it is first critical to establish the diagnosis of MPD. Reactive or secondary elevations in blood counts (e.g., due to underlying inflammatory, infectious, or neoplastic processes) generally do not cause clinical hemostatic complications. When bleeding occurs in such cases, it is usually coincidental and cannot be attributed to the high blood counts *per se*. Therefore, the correct diagnosis and control of the MDP are crucial in managing the related bleeding problem. Detailed discussion of the diagnosis of MPD is beyond the scope of this chapter. In general, however, the diagnosis of PCV is made by establishing that the red cell mass is absolutely increased and then ruling out secondary causes of polycythemia; the diagnosis of CML is made by finding the cytogenetic abnormality of the Philadelphia chromosome (or the *bcr-abl* rearrangement on DNA analysis); the diagnosis of myelofibrosis is made pathologically by the finding of fibrosis on bone marrow biopsy. Diagnostic criteria have been published for PCV (184) and for ET (185).

Except for some cases of acquired von Willebrand disease (see below), no deficiencies of coagulation factors or abnormalities of fibrinolysis are associated with the MPD. The PT and aPTT are characteristically normal. The plasma fibrinogen and von Willebrand factor antigen levels are elevated in many cases (186, 187). Although the bleeding tendency of the MPD has been predominantly attributed to a disorder of primary hemostasis, the bleeding time is actually normal in most individuals (188). Even when the bleeding time is prolonged, it does not correlate with an increased risk of hemorrhage (188–191). Thus, the test has practically no clinical utility in the diagnosis or management of individuals with MPD. The results of platelet aggregation studies are highly variable. In some cases hyperaggregability or even spontaneous platelet aggregation is found (192, 193), although these findings are not diagnostic of a MPD. More frequently, various patterns of impaired aggregation responses to ADP, collagen, and epinephrine are noted (188, 194). The platelets of individuals with MPD are more hyperreactive when studied in whole blood than in platelet-rich plasma (194). The most common and characteristic abnormality of platelet aggregation in the MPD is complete loss of responsiveness to epinephrine (195). The finding of the absence of even primary wave aggregation in response to epinephrine, with normal aggregation responses to other agonists, is virtually diagnostic of a MPD; however, a familial bleeding tendency, caused by reduction in platelet membrane $\alpha_2$-adrenergic receptors and the resultant isolated loss of epinephrine responsiveness, has been recently reported (196).

## PATHOGENESIS

### Polycythemia and Thrombocytosis

In PCV the increased whole blood viscosity caused by the erythrocytosis is directly related to the risk of thrombosis (197); its relationship to bleeding risk is less clear. However, individuals with comparably elevated hematocrits due to secondary polycythemia are much less prone to hemostatic complications, and therefore increased blood viscosity cannot be the sole causal determinant of these clinical problems in PCV. Thrombocytosis is most pronounced in ET, but it may accompany the other MPD as well. While some studies have suggested an association between the degree of thrombocytosis and either thrombotic (198) or bleeding (199, 200) complications, others have been unable to support this relationship (201–204). Furthermore, individuals without MPD who have secondary or reactive thrombocytosis do not have a significant increase in bleeding or thrombotic complications. The weight of evidence in the literature, based entirely on retrospective analysis, thus fails to demonstrate a simple correlation between the platelet count and the incidence of hemostatic complications in the MPD (188). Nevertheless, extreme thrombo-

cytosis (platelet counts generally >2,000,000/mm³) has been associated with an increased risk of bleeding (205–207). Furthermore, isolated case reports have shown that lowering the platelet count (by chemotherapy or plateletpheresis) in some individuals with MPD who have active bleeding or thrombosis can result in symptomatic improvement (208–214) and in improvement in platelet function (211, 214, 215).

## Specific Qualitative Platelet Abnormalities

A wide variety of specific morphologic, biochemical, and metabolic platelet defects have been identified in individuals with MPD, as summarized in Fig. 33.2 (216–218). Some of these abnormalities are specific for MPD, while others are also seen in other unrelated conditions.

Striking morphologic abnormalities of circulating platelets have been noted. Giant, agranular or hypo-

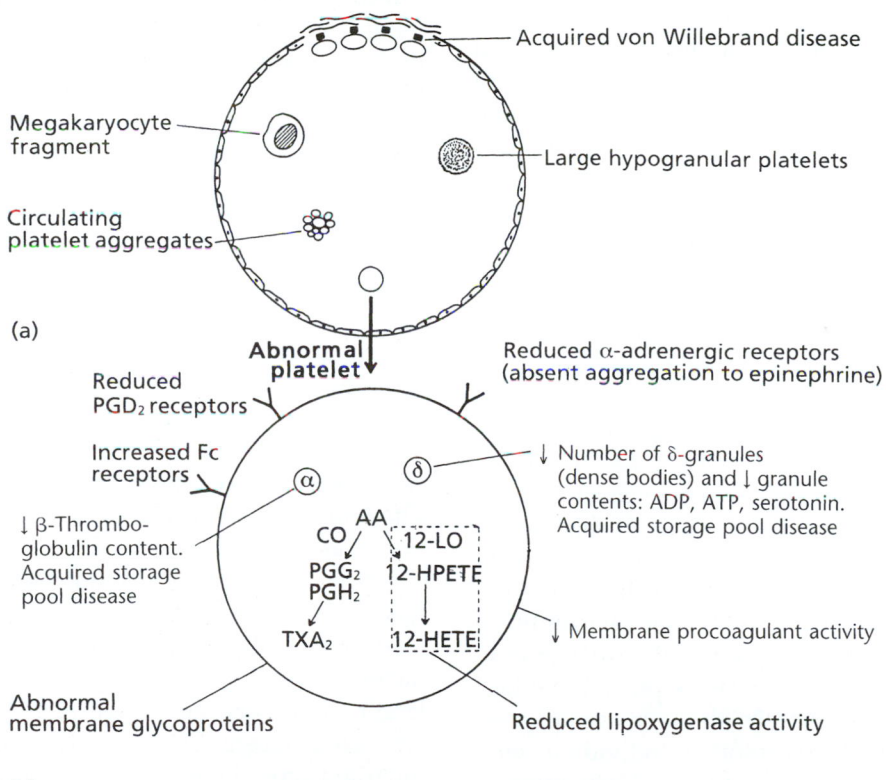

**FIGURE 33.2.** Structural, biochemical, and metabolic abnormalities of platelets in the myeloproliferative disorders. Upper panel (**a**): Morphologic abnormalities may include circulating megakaryocyte fragments and large, hypogranular platelets; defective platelet adhesion due to acquired von Willebrand disease; and circulating platelet aggregates. Lower panel (**b**): Specific platelet defects may include loss of α-adrenergic receptors (correlating with loss of epinephrine responsiveness in platelet aggregation studies); loss of prostaglandin D$_2$ (PGD$_2$) receptors; increased expression of Fc receptors; abnormal membrane procoagulant activity; abnormal membrane glycoproteins; acquired storage pool deficiency; and deficiency of lipoxygenase activity. AA, arachidonic acid; ADP, adenosine diphosphate; ATP, adenosine triphosphate; CO, cyclooxygenase; 12-HPETE, 12-hydroperoxytetraenoic acid; 12-HETE, 12-hydroxytetraenoic acid; 12-LO, 12-lipoxygenase; PG, prostaglandin; PGG$_2$, prostaglandin G$_2$; PGH$_2$, prostaglandin H$_2$; TXA$_2$, thromboxane A$_2$. (Adapted with permission from Schafer AI. Essential thrombocythemia. Prog Hemost Thromb 1991;10:69–96.)

granular platelets that appear "clear blue" are often seen on routine Wright's stain on the peripheral blood smear of individuals with MPD. Circulating megakaryocytes may also be found, presumably as a result of the dysmegakaryocytopoiesis that is characteristic of MPD (219–222). These cells sometimes appear like lymphocytes or lymphoblasts by light microscopy of routinely stained blood smears and are identified as megakaryocytes only by special immunohistochemical or electron microscopic studies.

A number of specific platelet surface membrane and receptor abnormalities have been reported in MPD. There may be decreases in platelet GP IIb-IIIa and, to a lesser extent, in GP Ib (223) in MPD. The decreases in GP Ib and GP IIb-IIIa have been associated with a loss of binding sites for their respective ligands, that is, von Willebrand factor (223) and fibrinogen (223, 224), respectively. Flow cytometric analysis has demonstrated that the platelets of individuals with MPD and myelodysplastic syndromes have an agonist-specific defect in the activation of the GP IIb-IIIa receptor and/or its ligand binding function (225). Complete loss of collagen-induced platelet aggregation and adhesion, with normal responses to other agonists, has been associated with absence of surface expression of the platelet collagen receptor in the GP Ia-IIa complex of an individual with MPD (226). The platelet membranes of individuals with MPD have also been shown to have defective platelet procoagulant activity (227), impaired binding and uptake of serotonin (228), and reduced content of arachidonic acid (229).

Other platelet membrane abnormalities in MPD involve specific surface receptors. As noted above, absence of functional responsiveness to epinephrine as an aggregating agent corresponds to a decreased number of $\alpha$-adrenergic receptors (195, 230). Loss of platelet prostaglandin $D_2$ receptors leads to a selective platelet resistance to the antiaggregating activity of this prostaglandin, while the platelet inhibitory response to $PGI_2$, which binds to separate receptors on the platelet surface (231), remains intact (232, 233). A similar platelet $PGD_2$ receptor defect has been subsequently identified in individuals without MPD during the acute phase of venous thromboembolism (234). Finally, the increased expression of platelet surface Fc receptors in individuals with MPD has been correlated with enhanced activation in response to immunoglobulin aggregates (235). While the loss of platelet $\alpha$-adrenergic and collagen receptors might be expected to cause a bleeding tendency, whereas the loss of $PGD_2$ receptors and the increased expression of Fc receptors would be expected to cause a thrombotic tendency on a theoretical basis, such clinical correlations have not been consistently found.

MPD may be associated with an acquired platelet storage pool deficiency. Both dense body (215, 236–244) and $\alpha$-granule (219, 245–249) deficiency have been found. The finding that depletion of platelet $\beta$-thromboglobulin (246) is associated with increased plasma levels of the same platelet granule protein (246, 250) has suggested the possibility that storage pool deficiency in the MPD is acquired as a result of *in vivo* degranulation. This has been confirmed by the finding of circulating activated platelets in some individuals with MPD, as detected by surface expression of activation-dependent epitopes (251). It has been hypothesized that myelofibrosis develops in certain individuals with MPD because of inappropriate platelet secretion in the bone marrow, which releases $\alpha$-granule mitogens such as platelet-derived growth factor (PDGF); transforming growth factor-$\beta$ (TGF-$\beta$), acting to stimulate fibroblast proliferation and collagen synthesis (252); and platelet factor 4 (PF4), which inhibits collagenase activity (253, 254). Support for such a mechanism comes from the observations that individuals with gray platelet syndrome, or selective $\alpha$-granule storage pool deficiency, are found to have fibrosis on bone marrow biopsy (255, 256). Nevertheless, clinical correlations in the different MPD indicate that intramedullary degranulation of platelets is not sufficient by itself to account for the development of myelofibrosis (247).

Abnormalities of platelet arachidonic acid metabolism are also known to occur in individuals with MPD. A selective deficiency of 12-lipoxygenase activity (257, 258), with an accompanying increase in cyclooxygenase-derived thromboxane $A_2$ formation (258), has also been found. Despite the enhanced production of platelet proaggregatory thromboxane $A_2$ in these MPD individuals, clinical correlations indicated a bleeding rather than a thrombotic tendency (258). A defect in nitric oxide–stimulated protein phosphorylation and calcium flux has been observed in cGMP-dependent protein kinase–deficient platelets from some individuals with CML (259). The role of this abnormality in clinical platelet dysfunction is as yet unknown.

Acquired von Willebrand disease (see Chapter 34) has been associated with MPD, particularly ET (260–264). Multimer analysis of plasma von Willebrand factor in these cases usually shows a reduction in the larger multimers, and there is a disproportionate decrease of ristocetin cofactor activity, most resembling the inherited type IIA form of this disease (265–267). Both the clinical bleeding tendency and the laboratory abnormalities have been observed to improve by lowering the platelet count or by treatment with DDAVP. The mechanism of acquired von Willebrand disease in the MPD has been considered to be either adsorption of the high-molecular-weight multimers of von Willebrand factor onto the surfaces of the abnormal platelets, resulting in a plasma deficiency of these multimers, or proteolytic degradation of the protein. Binding of von Willebrand factor to its receptors on platelet membrane GP

Ib has been found to be normal, but elevated plasma levels of glycocalicin and impaired ristocetin-induced platelet aggregation have been found in some individuals with MPD (266).

## Causes of Qualitative Platelet Abnormalities in the MPD

It has been generally assumed that the various qualitative platelet defects described above in the MPD result from the dysmegakaryocytopoiesis of the stem cell disorder and the release of morphologically and functionally abnormal platelets into the circulation. This is supported by cases of correction of platelet lipoxygenase deficiency (268) and α-adrenergic receptor deficiency (188) by bone marrow transplantation. Nevertheless, as noted above, it has been suggested that some of the platelet abnormalities (e.g., storage pool deficiency) in the MPD may be acquired during hemostatic encounters in the circulation, leading to in vivo platelet release and exhaustion (269). These "spent" platelets would then recirculate with a relatively normal life span, giving rise to the various platelet abnormalities detected in vitro (217). Thus various platelet abnormalities in the MPD may have different pathogenetic mechanisms.

## Clinical Correlations

It has been difficult to clinically correlate any of the platelet abnormalities described above with a clear predisposition to either bleeding or thrombosis (188, 270). There may be several explanations for this lack of clinical correlations. First, some of the morphologic, functional, and biochemical defects described in these cases may be clinically irrelevant to the control of hemostasis. Second, several defects may coexist simultaneously in the same platelet population, exerting functionally offsetting actions on hemostasis. Third, as demonstrated in a longitudinal study (271), multiple platelet defects may change with time during the natural history of the MPD or as a result of treatment. Thus, platelet abnormalities identified at any given point in time may not correlate with past clinical history or predict future hemostatic complications. Finally, other, as yet poorly defined hemostatic abnormalities may be involved in MPD individuals, including endothelial dysfunction (272).

## TREATMENT

### Cytoreduction

It is established that thrombotic and vascular complications in PCV can be prevented by maintaining the hematocrit below 45%. However, there has been controversy about the indications for reducing elevated platelet counts in individuals with ET and other MPD associated with thrombocytosis. In general, retrospective studies had suggested that there is little rationale for platelet cytoreduction in asymptomatic individuals with MPD, regardless of the degree of thrombocytosis. However, a prospective study of 114 individuals with essential thrombocythemia, who were randomly assigned to receive hydroxyurea or no platelet-lowering therapy and followed for a median of 27 months, showed that treated individuals had significantly fewer thrombotic episodes (207). Furthermore, in individuals with recurrent hemostatic complications, suppression of the platelet count with plateletpheresis, [$^{32}$P], chemotherapy, α-interferon or anagrelide (see Chapter 31) may be effective in abrogating clinical complications and improving in vitro platelet function.

### Antiplatelet Drugs

There is likewise dispute about the indications and contraindications for the use of aspirin and other antiplatelet agents in the MPD. Laboratory tests alone (e.g., bleeding time, platelet aggregation studies) have been found to be unreliable in predicting the risk of hemorrhage or thrombosis in these individuals. Therefore, the clinical history should largely dictate the use of antiplatelet drugs. Several reports have noted serious bleeding complications or exaggerated prolongations of the bleeding time with the use of aspirin in some MPD individuals (182, 183); therefore the risks and benefits of the use of aspirin should be carefully weighed and periodically reassessed in each individual individual.

# DRUGS

Certain drugs are designed to interfere with platelet function as antithrombotic agents. Aspirin and nonsteroidal antiinflammatory drugs inhibit platelet (and endothelial cell) cyclooxygenase activity, produce a platelet release defect, and prolong the bleeding time. Omega-3 fatty acids (fish oils containing eicosapentaenoic acid) cause similar antiplatelet effects, at least in part by competing with the arachidonic acid substrate for cyclooxygenase. The mechanisms of action of dipyridamole in prolonging platelet survival and reducing platelet turnover in various thrombotic and vascular disorders are poorly defined and are probably multifactorial. Unlike aspirin, this drug does not prolong the bleeding time or inhibit platelet aggregation at pharmacologic concentrations. Sulfinpyrazone, a uricosuric drug structurally similar to phenylbutazone, is an incomplete and reversible platelet cyclooxygenase inhibitor that usually produces a release defect on aggregation studies. Ticlopidine and clopidogrel are thienopyridine derivatives with potent platelet inhibitory effects, which selectively inhibit platelet aggregation induced by ADP (273) and block shear-induced platelet aggregation

(274). These drugs are described in greater detail in Chapter 54.

## Antimicrobial Agents

Platelet functional abnormalities caused by certain antimicrobial agents, particularly β-lactam antibiotics, may lead to severe bleeding problems, particularly when the clinical risks are compounded by coexisting illnesses that require the use of the antibiotics, such as renal or hepatic disease, sepsis, and malignancy, or the concomitant use of anticoagulants which by themselves independently cause a bleeding diathesis (275). Individuals with chronic illness and malnutrition are particularly prone to bleeding complications with the administration of β-lactam antibiotics. Penicillins, including penicillin G (276–278), carbenicillin (279, 280), ticarcillin (281), and ampicillin (276), have been reported to inhibit platelet function and to cause a clinically significant bleeding tendency when administered in high doses (279). Some of the newer semisynthetic penicillins such as piperacillin have less potent antiplatelet effects (282). Cephalosporins, including moxalactam (283, 284), nitrofurantoin (285), and hydroxychloroquine (286), can likewise interfere with platelet function.

The actual clinical bleeding complications may appear anywhere from 1 day to 4 weeks after starting β-lactam antibiotics (275). Platelet dysfunction is characteristically noted within hours of starting the offending antimicrobial agent, is maximal after 3 to 4 days, and resolves within days of discontinuation of the drug (287). Antibiotics cause prolongation of the bleeding time (Fig. 33.3), inhibition of platelet aggregation and secretion in response to several agonists, decreased ristocetin-induced platelet agglutination, and impaired platelet adhesion to subendothelial and collagen sur-

faces (288). The exact mechanism of the platelet inhibitory actions of these drugs is not completely understood. High doses of the penicillins block the binding of different agonists (epinephrine, ADP, von Willebrand factor) to the platelet surface (289), thereby interfering with the initiation of signal transduction. Penicillin also inhibits agonist stimulated modulation of platelet membrane (290, 291). It has also been suggested that these antibiotics inhibit platelets by an irreversible mechanism involving postreceptor impairment of signal transduction in response to various agonists (292). The β-lactam antibiotics may not act directly on platelet membrane receptors but rather by binding to and causing deformation of platelet membranes, thus making the receptors inaccessible to the agonists (293). The platelet effects of β-lactam antibiotics are inversely related to the serum albumin concentration (294), an *in vitro* finding that may partly explain the clinical observation that hypoalbuminemic individuals with chronic illness or malnutrition are particularly prone to antibiotic-related bleeding complications. The carboxyl group of the acyl side-chain of antibiotics has been considered to be involved in their platelet inhibitory effects (292), but it has been found that all antibiotics containing an *N*-methyltetrazolethiol group in their structure (e.g., moxalactam, cefoperazone, cefamandole) show inhibitory activity on platelet aggregation (293, 295); the semisynthetic cephalosporin cefonicid, which is similar to cefamandole except that its substitution at position 3 on the dihydrothiazine ring is an *N*-sulfomethyltetrazolethiol group, does not affect platelet aggregation at therapeutic doses (296).

## Alcohol

Several studies have demonstrated an inhibitory effect of ethanol on platelet function (297). However, the clinical relevance of these observations has been difficult to establish because a number of other factors may contribute to the bleeding tendencies of alcoholics, including anatomic vascular abnormalities, thrombocytopenia, and coagulation factor deficiencies. Inhibition of platelet function has been considered to be one possible factor accounting for the epidemiologic observations on the effect of moderate consumption of alcohol in protection from atherosclerotic cardiovascular disease (298–301).

Although alcohol by itself does not affect the bleeding time, it can potentiate the prolongation of the bleeding time caused by aspirin (Fig. 33.4) or nonsteroidal antiinflammatory drugs, particularly when alcohol ingestion occurs simultaneously with or following aspirin ingestion (302). Alcohol can likewise potentiate aspirin-induced fecal blood loss (303, 304). Physiologic concentrations of ethanol variably inhibit platelet aggregation and release *in vitro* in response to several agonists, including ADP, collagen, thrombin, arachidonic acid, and platelet-activating factor (305–309). The physi-

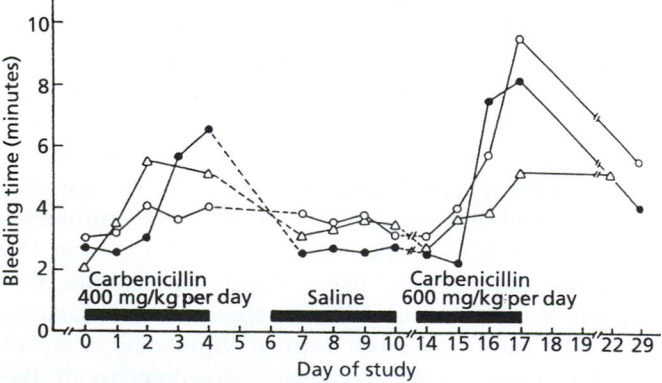

**FIGURE 33.3.** Bleeding times in three volunteers receiving carbenicillin, 400 and then 600 mg/kg per day, each dose for 4 days. (Adapted with permission from Brown CH III, Natelson EA, Bradshaw MW et al. The hemostatic defect produced by carbenicillin. N Engl J Med 1974;291:265–270.)

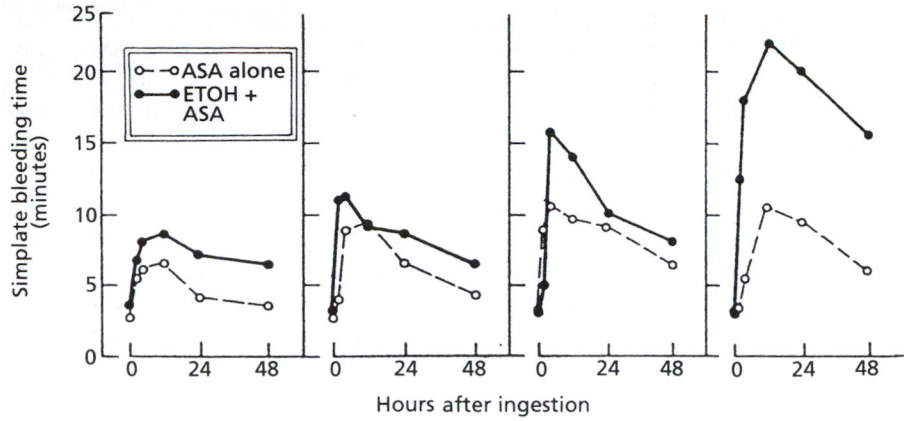

**FIGURE 33.4.**  Effects of ethanol (ETOH, 50 g) and aspirin (ASA, 325 mg) on the bleeding time in four different subjects. (Adapted with permission from Deykin D, Janson P, McMahon L. Ethanol potentiation of aspirin-induced prolongation of the bleeding time. N Engl J Med 1982;306: 852–854.)

ologic relevance of these studies is suggested by the finding that platelets obtained from alcoholics are hyporesponsive to agonists *ex vivo* (308), gradually return to normal after several days of abstinence, and may even become hyperreactive during withdrawal (297, 310). Nevertheless, moderate alcohol consumption in otherwise healthy individuals has no acute effects on *ex vivo* platelet aggregability (311). The inhibition of platelet function *in vivo* by the administration of alcohol has been observed in a dog model of shear-induced coronary thrombosis (312), in a rabbit model of thrombus formation induced by indwelling aortic catheters (313), and in hypercholesterolemic rabbits (314). More recently, red wine and grape juice, but not white wine, were found to inhibit *in vivo* platelet reactivity in stenosed dog coronary arteries, suggesting that some naturally occurring compounds in the former solutions (such as quercetin and resveratrol), other than ethanol, might also contribute to abnormal primary hemostasis induced by some alcoholic beverages (315).

The mechanism of ethanol-induced platelet dysfunction remains unclear. However, there is evidence that ethanol exerts a major inhibitory action on phospholipase $A_2$-mediated arachidonic acid release (306, 307, 316). Ethanol may also directly interfere with the function of the platelet secretory apparatus (316), unrelated to its effects on phospholipase signaling.

## Miscellaneous Agents

β-Adrenergic blocking agents reduce the "hyperreactivity" of platelets in individuals with coronary artery disease (317), but are weak and inconsistent direct inhibitors of *in vitro* platelet function (318, 319). The mechanism of the antiplatelet actions of β-blockers is unknown, but has been considered to involve binding to membrane phospholipids (320) to interfere with phospholipase $A_2$–mediated arachidonic acid release (321, 322). These drugs can also inhibit intracellular calcium mobilization in platelets (323). β-Adrenergic blocking agents have not been shown to cause a clinical bleeding tendency.

Local and general anesthetics act as membrane stabilizing agents to inhibit platelet responses *in vitro*, and general anesthesia with halothane has been found to cause a prolongation of the bleeding time (324). Tricyclic antidepressants (e.g., imipramine, amitriptyline) and phenothiazines (e.g., chlorpromazine, trifluoperazine) may likewise interfere with platelet function by their membrane stabilizing actions, although effects of these drugs on clinical hemostasis are questionable (325–327). *Ex vivo* platelet aggregability has been found to be variably impaired in response to different agonists in individuals treated with neuroleptics of the phenothiazine, butyrophenone, and benzamide classes (328). However, it has also been reported that platelet aggregation is abnormal even in unmedicated schizophrenic individuals (329). As noted in Chapter 29, valproic acid can cause not only thrombocytopenia but also qualitative platelet defects (330).

Dextrans cause prolongation of the bleeding time and inhibit platelet aggregation (331, 332). The onset of these effects on primary hemostasis is within hours of starting an intravenous infusion. It has been postulated that dextrans adsorb to platelets causing their activation *in vivo* and resulting in the circulation of "spent" platelets that are refractory to subsequent stimulation (333). In a similar manner, the higher-molecular-weight, non-anticoagulant fractions of commercial heparin preparations may cause *in vivo* platelet activation, resulting in impaired *ex vivo* responsiveness of the refractory platelets (56, 334). The antifibrinolytic agent ε-aminocaproic acid (EACA) causes prolongation of the bleeding time when it is administered at a dose of ≥24 g/day. The effect on the bleeding time correlates with the duration of EACA therapy and returns to normal within 72 hours of discontinuation of the drug (335). Although EACA inhibits ADP-induced and collagen-induced platelet aggregation and release *in vitro*, this effect is not considered to be its mechanism of action in prolonging the bleeding time, because these platelet functional abnormalities are not found in blood drawn from individuals receiving the drug.

Dietary constituents such as onions (336, 337), garlic (338, 339), black tree fungus (associated with the syndrome of "Szechwan purpura") (340), and vitamin E (341) may inhibit *in vitro* platelet function under certain conditions, but the clinical relevance of these findings has not been determined.

# REFERENCES

1. Morgagni GB. Opera Omnia. 1764.
2. Remuzzi G. Bleeding in renal failure. Lancet 1988;1:1205–1208.
3. Bright R. Reports of medical cases. 1827.
4. Reisman D. Hemorrhages in the course of Bright's disease with special reference to the occurrence of hemorrhagic diathesis of nephritic origin. Am J Med Sci 1907;134:709–716.
5. Zachée P, Vermylen J, Boogaerts MA. Hematologic aspects of end-stage renal failure. Ann Hematol 1994;69:33–40.
6. Margolis DM, Saylor JL, Geisse G et al. Upper gastrointestinal disease in chronic renal failure. A prospective evaluation. Arch Intern Med 1978;138: 1214–1217.
7. Alvarez L, Puleo J, Balint JA. Investigation of gastrointestinal bleeding in individuals with end-stage renal disease. Am J Gastroenterol 1993;88: 30–33.
8. Kang JY. The gastrointestinal tract in uremia. Dig Dis Sci 1993;38:257–268.
9. Shaw RE. Spontaneous rupture of the kidney. Br J Surg 1957;45:68–71.
10. Horner BA, Hunt JC, Kincaid OW et al. Perirenal hematoma secondary to intrarenal microaneurysms of periarteritis nodosa demonstrated radiographically. Mayo Clin Proc 1966;41:169–178.
11. Link GS. Spontaneous bilateral perirenal hematoma. J Urol 1953;69:13–18.
12. Howalt JS, Squires JW. Spontaneous rupture of the kidney. A case of atraumatic retroperitonal bleeding. Am J Surg 1972;123:484–488.
13. Kjellstrand CM, Merino GE, Mauer SM et al. Complications of percutaneous femoral vein catheterization for hemodialysis. Clin Nephrol 1975;4: 37–40.
14. Pan A, Rogers AG, Pearlman D. Subdural hematoma complicating anticoagulant therapy. Can Med Assoc J 1960;82:1162–1164.
15. Maher JF, Schreiner GE. Hazards and complications of dialysis. N Engl J Med 1966;272:370–372.
16. Bechar M, Lakke JP, Hem GK van der et al. Subdural hematoma during long-term hemodialysis. Arch Neurol 1972;26:513–516.
17. Giuld WR, Bray G, Merrill JP. Hemopericardium with cardiac tamponade in chronic uremia. N Engl J Med 1957;257:230–231.
18. Symmons HS, Wrong OM. Uremic pericarditis with cardiac tamponade: a report of four cases. Br Med J 1964;1:605–606.
19. Alfrey AC, Goss JE, Ogden DA et al. Uremic hemopericardium. Am J Med 1968;45:391–400.
20. Berger HW, Rammohan G, Neff MS et al. Uremic pleural effusion. A study in 14 individuals on chronic dialysis. Ann Intern Med 1975;82:362–364.
21. Borra S, Kleinfeld M. Subcapsular liver hematomas in a individual on chronic hemodialysis. Ann Intern Med 1980;93:574–575.
22. Nakamura S, Chida Y, Tomura S. Enhanced coagulation—fibrinolysis in individuals on regular hemodialysis treatment. Nephron 1991;58:201–204.
23. Panicucci F, Sagripanti A, Vispi M et al. Comprehensive study of haemostasis in nephrotic syndrome. Nephron 1983;33:9–13.
24. Jubelirer SJ. Hemostatis abnormalities in renal disease. Am J Kidney Dis 1985;5:219–225.
25. Sagripanti A, Barsotti G. Bleeding and thrombosis in chronic uremia [Editorial]. Nephron 1997;75:125–139.
26. Rabiner SF. Uremic bleeding. In: Spaet TH, ed. Progress in hemostasis and thrombosis. Orlando: Grune & Stratton, 1972;1:233–250.
27. Steiner RW, Coggins C, Carvalho AC. Bleeding in uremia: a useful test to assess clinical bleeding. Am J Hematol 1979;7:107–117.
28. Livio M, Benigni A, Remuzzi G. Coagulation abnormalities in uremia. Semin Nephrol 1985;5:82–90.
29. Gordge MP, Faint RW, Rylance PB et al. Platelet function and the bleeding time in progressive renal fialure. Thromb Haemost 1988;60:83–87.
30. Lindsay RM, Moorthy AV, Koens F et al. Platelet function in dialyzed and non-dialyzed individuals with chronic renal failure. Clin Nephrol 1975;4: 52–57.
31. Evans EP, Branch RA, Bloom AL. A clinical and experimental study of platelet function in chronic renal failure. J Clin Pathol 1972;25:745–753.
32. Moosa A, Greaves M, Brown CB et al. Elevated platelet-free calcium in uremia. Br J Haematol 1990;74:300–305.
33. Castaldi PA, Rozenberg MC, Stewart JH. The bleeding disorder of uraemia. A qualitative platelet defect. Lancet 1966;2:66–69.
34. Salzman EW, Neri LL. Adhesiveness of blood platelets in uremia. Thromb Diath Haemorrh 1966;15:84–92.
35. Ballard HS, Marcus AJ. Primary and secondary platelet aggregation in uraemia. Scand J Haematol 1972;9:198–203.
36. Di Minno G, Martinez J, McKean ML et al. Platelet dysfunction in uremia. Multifaceted defect partially corrected by dialysis. Am J Med 1985;79: 552–559.
37. Zwaginga JJ, Ijsseldijk MJ, de Groot PG et al. Defects in platelet adhesion and aggregate formation in uremic bleeding disorder can be attributed to factors in plasma. Arterioscler Thromb 1991;11:733–744.
38. Larsson SO, Hedner U, Nilsson IM. On coagulation and fibrinolysis in conservatively treated chronic uraemia. Acta Med Scand 1971;189: 433–441.
39. Stewart JH, Castaldi PA. Uraemic bleeding: a reversible platelet defect corrected by dialysis. Q J Med 1967;36:409–423.
40. Lindsay RM, Friesen M, Koens F et al. Platelet function in individuals on long term peritoneal dialysis. Clin Nephrol 1976;6:335–339.
41. Remuzzi G, Livio M, Marchiaro G et al. Bleeding in renal failure: altered platelet function in uraemia only partially corrected by haemodialysis. Nephron 1978;22:347–353.
42. Harker LA. Acquired disorders of platelet function. Ann N Y Acad Sci 1987;509:188–204.
43. Knudsen F, Dyerburg J. Platelets and antithrombin III in uraemia: the acute effect of hemodialysis. Scand J Clin Lab Invest 1985;45:341–347.
44. Eknoyan G, Wacksman SJ, Glueck HI et al. Platelet function in renal failure. N Engl J Med 1969;280:677–681.
45. Horowitz HI, Stein IM, Cohen BD et al. Further studies on the platelet inhibitory effect of guanidinosuccinic acid and its role in uremic bleeding. Am J Med 1970;49:336–345.
46. Rabiner SF, Molinas F. The role of phenol and phenolic acids on the thrombocytopathy and defective platelet aggregation of individuals with renal failure. Am J Med 1970;49:346–351.
47. Schoots A, Mikkers F, Cramers C et al. Uremic toxins and the elusive middle molecules. Nephron 1984;38:1–8.
48. Bazilinski N, Shaykh M, Dunea G et al. Inhibition of platelet function by uremic middle molecules. Nephron 1985;40:423–428.
49. Lindsay RM, Bolton CF, Clark WF et al. The effect of alterations of uremic retention products upon platelet and peripheral nerve function. Clin Nephrol 1983;19:110–115.
50. Sinzinger H, Leithner C. Eicosanoids of platelets and vascular wall in chronic renal insufficiency. Am J Nephrol 1987;7:212–220.
51. Walkowiak B, Michalak E, Borkowska E et al. Concentration of RGDS-containing degradation products in uremic plasma is correlated with progression in renal failure. Thromb Res 1994;76:133–144.
52. Benigni A, Boccardo P, Galbusera M et al. Reversible activation defect of the platelet glycoprotein IIb-IIIa complex in individuals with uremia. Am J Kidney Dis 1993;22:668–676.
53. Gawaz MP, Dobos G, Späth M et al. Impaired function of platelet membrane glycoprotein IIb-IIIa in end-stage renal disease. J Am Soc Nephrol 1994;5:36–46.
54. Sreedhara R, Itagaki I, Hakim RM. Uremic individuals have decreased shear-induced platelet aggregation mediated by decreased availability of glycoprotein IIb-IIIa receptors. Am J Kidney Dis 1996;27:355–364.
55. Hakim RM, Schafer AI. Hemodialysis-associated platelet activation and thrombocytopenia. Am J Med 1985;78:575–580.
56. Salzman EW, Rosenberg RD, Smith MH et al. Effect of heparin and heparin fractions on platelet aggregation. J Clin Invest 1980;65:64–73.
57. Eknoyan G, Brown CH. Biochemical abnormalities of platelets in renal failure. Evidence for decreased platelet serotonin, adenosine diphosphate and Mg-dependent adenosine triphosphatase. Am J Nephrol 1981;1:17–23.
58. Komarnicki M, Twardowski T. Platelet glycoprotein concentrations in individuals with chronic uraemia. Folia Haematol (Leipz) 1987;114:642–645.
59. Rao AK. Uraemic platelet [Letter]. Lancet 1986;1:913–914.
60. Green D, Santhanam S, Krumlovsky FA et al. Elevated beta-thromboglobulin in individuals with chronic renal failure: effect of hemodialysis. J Lab Clin Med 1980;95:679–685.
61. Guzzo J, Niewiarowski S, Musial J et al. Secreted platelet proteins with antiheparin and mitogenic activities in chronic renal fialure. J Lab Clin Med 1980;96:102–113.
62. Kubisz P, Parizek M, Seghier F et al. Relationship between platelet aggregation and plasma beta-thromboglobulin levels in arteriovascular and renal diseases. Atherosclerosis 1985;55:363–368.
63. Reverter JC, Escolar G, Sanz C et al. Platelet activation during hemodialysis measured through exposure of P-selectin: analysis by flow cytometric and ultrastructural techniques. J Lab Clin Med 1994;124:79–85.
64. Tàssies D, Reverter JC, Cases A et al. Reticulated platelets in uremic individuals: effect of hemodialysis and continuous ambulatory peritoneal dialysis. Am J Hematol 1995;50:161–166.
65. Remuzzi G, Marchesi D, Livio M et al. Altered platelet and vascular prostaglandin generation in individuals with chronic renal failure and prolonged bleeding times. Thromb Res 1978;13:1007–1015.
66. Smith MC, Dunn M. Impaired thromboxane production in renal failure. Nephron 1981;29:133–137.
67. Remuzzi G, Benigni A, Dodesini P et al. Reduced platelet thromboxane formation in uremia. Evidence for functional cyclooxygenase defect. J Clin Invest 1983;71:762–768.

68. Bloom A, Greaves M, Preston FE et al. Evidence against a platelet cyclooxy-genase defect in uraemic subjects on chronic haemodialysis. Br J Haematol 1986;62:143–149.
69. Ware JA, Clark BA, Smith M et al. Abnormalities of cytoplasmic Ca$^{2+}$ in platelets from individuals with uremia. Blood 1989;73:172–176.
70. von Kaulla KN, von Kaulla E, Wasantapruck S et al. Blood coagulation in uremia before and after hemodialysis and transplantation of the kidney. Arch Surg 1966;92:184–191.
71. Benigni A, Livio M, Dodesini P et al. Inhibition of human platelet aggrega-tion by parathyroid hormone. Is cyclic AMP implicated? Am J Nephrol 1985;5:243–247.
72. Mannhalter CH, Deutsch E, Kopsa E. Clotting activities and antigen con-centrations of contact factors in kidney disease. Thromb Res 1985;39: 475–484.
73. Vlachoyannis J, Schoeppe W. Adenylate cyclase activity and cAMP content of human platelets in uraemia. Eur J Clin Invest 1982;12:379–381.
74. Remuzzi G, Cavenaghi AE, Mecca G et al. Prostacyclin-like activity and bleeding in renal failure. Lancet 1977;2:1195–1197.
75. MacIntyre DE, Pearson JD, Gordon JL. Localization and stimulation of prostacyclin production in vascular cells. Nature 1978;271:549–551.
76. Deckmyn H, Zoja C, Arnout J et al. Partial isolation and function of the prostacyclin regulating plasma factor. Clin Sci 1985;69:383–393.
77. Defreyn G, Dauden MV, Machin SJ et al. A plasma factor in uraemia which stimulates prostacyclin release from cultured endothelial cells. Thromb Res 1980;19:695–699.
78. Remuzzi G. Bleeding disorders in uremia: pathophysiology and treatment. Adv Nephrol Necker Hosp 1989;18:171–186.
79. Leithner CH, Winter M, Silbauer K et al. Enhanced prostacyclin availabil-ity of blood vessels in uraemic humans and rats. In: Robinson RHB, Hawk-ins JB, eds. Dialysis transplantation nephrology. Proceedings of the 15th Congress of European Dialysis and Transplant Association. Tunbridge Wells: Pitman Medical Publishing, 1978; p. 418.
80. Zoja C, Vigano G, Bergamelli A et al. Prolonged bleeding time and in-creased vascular prostacyclin in rats with chronic renal failure: effects of conjugated estrogens. J Lab Clin Med 1988;112:380–386.
81. Livio M, Benigni A, Vigano G et al. Moderate doses of aspirin and risk of bleeding in renal failure. Lancet 1986;1:414–416.
82. Gaspari F, Vigano G, Orisio S et al. Aspirin prolongs bleeding time in uremia by a mechanism distinct from platelet cyclooxygenase inhibition. J Clin Invest 1987;79:1788–1797.
83. Remuzzi G, Benigni A, Dodesini P et al. Parathyroid hormone inhibits human platelet function. Lancet 1981;2:1321–1323.
84. Benigni A, Livio M, Dodesini P et al. Inhibition of human platelet aggrega-tion by parathyroid hormone. Is cyclic AMP implicated? Am J Nephrol 1985;5:243–247.
85. Docci D, Turci F, Delvecchio C et al. Lack of evidence for a role of second-ary hyperparathyroidism in the pathogenesis of uremic thrombocytopa-thy. Nephron 1986;43:28–32.
86. Remuzzi G, Perico N, Zoja C et al. Role of endothelium-derived nitric oxide in the bleeding tendency of uremia. J Clin Invest 1990;86:1768–1771.
87. Noris M, Benigni A, Boccardo P et al. Enhanced nitric oxide synthesis in uremia: implications for platelet dysfunction and dialysis hypotension. Kidney Int 1993;44:445–450.
88. Vallance P, Leone A, Calver A et al. Accumulation of an endogenous inhibitor of nitric oxide synthesis in chronic renal failure. Lancet 1992;339: 572–575.
89. Moia M, Mannucci PM, Vizzotto L. Improvement in the haemostatic defect of uraemia after treatment with recombinant human erythropoietin. Lan-cet 1987;2:1227–1229.
90. Zwaginga JJ, Ijsseldijk MJ, Beeser-Visser N et al. High von Willebrand factor concentration compensates a relative adhesion defect in uremic blood. Blood 1990;75:1498–1508.
91. Willoughby MLN, Crouch SG. An investigation of the hemorrhagic ten-dency in renal failure. Br J Haematol 1971;7:315–326.
92. Remuzzi G, Livio M, Roncaglion MC et al. Bleeding in renal failure: is von Willebrand factor implicated? Br Med J 1977;2:359–361.
93. Janson PA, Jubelirer SJ, Weinstein MJ et al. Treatment of the bleeding tendency in uremia with cryoprecipitate. N Engl J Med 1980;303: 1318–1322.
94. Mannucci PM, Remuzzi G, Pusineri F et al. Deamino-8-d-arginine vaso-pressin shortens the bleeding time in uremia. N Engl J Med 1983;308:8–12.
95. Yoshida E, Fujimura Y, Ikeda Y et al. Impaired high-shear-stress-induced platelet aggregation in individuals with chronic renal failure undergoing haemodialysis. Br J Hematol 1995;89:861–867.
96. Winter M, Seghatchian MJ, Cameron JS. An abnormal factor VIII molecular in uremia? Lancet 1983;1:1112.
97. Gralnick HR, McKeown LP, Williams SB et al. Plasma and platelet von Willebrand's factor defects in uremia. Am J Med 1988;85:806–810.
98. Kazatchkine M, Sultan Y, Caen JP et al. Bleeding in renal failure: a possible cause. Br Med J 1976;2:612–615.
99. Rabelink TJ, Zwaginga JJ, Koomans HA et al. Thrombosis and hemostasis in renal disease. Kidney Int 1994;46:287–296.
100. Sloand EM, Sloand JA, Prodouz K et al. Reduction of platelet glycoprotein Ib in uraemia. Br J Haemotol 1991;77:375–381.

101. Weinstein MJ, Chute LE, Schmitt GW et al. Abnormal factor VIII coagulant antigen in individuals with renal dysfunction and in those with dissemi-nated intravascular coagulation. J Clin Invest 1985;76:1406–1411.
102. Loge JR, Lange RD, Moore CV. Characterization of the anemia associated with chronic renal insufficiency. Am J Med 1958;24:4–18.
103. Eschbach JW, Adamson JW. Anemia of end-stage renal disease. Kidney Int 1985;28:1–5.
104. Livio M, Gotti E, Marchesi D et al. Uraemic bleeding: role of anaemia and beneficial effect of red cell transfusions. Lancet 1982;2:1013–1015.
105. Fernandez F, Goudable C, Sie P et al. Low haematocrit and prolonged bleeding time in uraemic individuals: effect of red cell transfusions. Br J Haematol 1985;59:139–148.
106. Moia M, Mannucci PM, Vizzotto L et al. Improvement in the haemostatic defect of uraemia after treatment with recombinant human erythropoietin. Lancet 1987;2:1227–1229.
107. Gordge MP, Leaker B, Patel A et al. Recombinant human erythropoietin shortens the uraemic bleeding time without causing intravascular haemo-static activation. Thromb Res 1990;57:171–182.
108. Vigano G, Benigni A, Mendogni D et al. Recombinant human erythropoie-tin to correct uremic bleeding. Am J Kidney Dis 1991;18:44–49.
109. Turitto VT, Baumgartner HR. Platelet interaction with subendothelium in a perfusion system: physical role of red blood cells. Microvasc Res 1975; 9:335–344.
110. Aarts PA, Heethaar RM, Sixma JJ. Red blood cell deformability influences platelet–vessel wall interaction in flowing blood. Blood 1984;64: 1228–1233.
111. Goldsmith HL, Turitto VT. Rheological aspects of thrombosis and haemo-stasis: basic principles and applications. Thromb Haemost 1986;55: 415–435.
112. Valles J, Santos MT, Aznar J et al. Erythrocytes metabolically enhance collagen-induced platelet responsiveness via increased thromboxane pro-duction, adenosine diphosphate release, and recruitment. Blood 1991;78: 154–162.
113. Willems C, Stel HV, van Aken WG et al. Binding and inactivation of prosta-cyclin (PGI$_2$) by human erythrocytes. Br J Haematol 1983;54:43–52.
114. Hellem AJ, Borchrevink ChrF, Ames SB. The role of red cells in haemosta-sis: the relation between haematocrit, bleeding time and platelet adhesive-ness. Br J Haematol 1961;7:42–50.
115. Gordge MP, Faint RW, Rylance PB et al. Platelet function and the bleeding time in progressive renal fialure. Thromb Haemost 1988;60:83–87.
116. Nenci GG, Berrettini M, Agnelli G et al. Effect of peritoneal dialysis, hemo-dialysis, and kidney transplantation on blood platelet function. Nephron 1979;23:287–292.
117. Liu YK, Kosfeld RE, Marcum SG. Treatment of uraemic bleeding with conjugated oestrogen. Lancet 1984;2:887–889.
118. Arends JP, Krediet RT, Boeschoten EW et al. Improvement of bleeding time, platelet aggregation and platelet count during CAPD treatment. Proc Eur Dial Transplant Assoc 1981;18:280–285.
119. Sloand EM, Bern MM, Kaldany A. Effect on platelet function of hypoal-buminemia in peritoneal dialysis. Thromb Res 1986;44:419–425.
120. Lindsay RM, Prentice CR, Ferguson D et al. A method for the measurement of platelet adhesiveness by use of dialysis membranes in a test cell. Br J Haematol 1973;24:377–389.
121. Lindsay RM, Prentice CR, Burton JA et al. The role of the platelet-dialysis membrane interaction in thrombus formation and blood loss during hemo-dialysis. Trans Am Soc Artif Intern Organs 1973;19:487–491.
122. Adler AJ, Berlyne GM. β-Thromboglobulin and platelet factor-4 levels during hemodialysis with polyacrylonitrile. Trans Am Soc Artif Intern Organs 1981;4:100–102.
123. Buccianti G, Pogliani E, Miradoli R et al. Reduction of plasma levels of betathromboglobulin and platelet factor 4 during hemodialysis: a possible role for a short acting inhibitor of platelet aggregation. Clin Nephrol 1982; 18:204–208.
124. Flicker W, Milthorpe BK, Schindhelm K et al. Platelet factor release follow-ing heparin administration and during extracorporeal circulation. Trans Am Soc Artif Intern Organs 1982;28:431–436.
125. Jacob HS. Complement-mediated leucoembolization: a mechanism of tis-sue damage during extracorporeal perfusions, myocardial infarction and in shock—a review. Q J Med 1983;52:289–296.
126. Fabris F, Cordiano I, Randi ML et al. Effect of human recombinant erythro-poietin on bleeding time, platelet number and function in children with end-stage renal disease maintained by haemodialysis. Pediatr Nephrol 1991;5:225–228.
127. Montini G, Zacchello G, Beraldi E et al. Benefits and risks of anemia correc-tion with recombinant human erythropoietin in children maintained by hemodialysis. J Pediatr 1990;117:556–560.
128. Cases A, Escolar G, Reverter JC et al. Effect of the treatment with human recombinant erythropoietin on primary hemostasis in uremic individuals. Med Clin (Barc) 1990;95:644–647.
129. van Geet C, Hauglustaine D, Verresen L et al. Haemostatic effects of re-combinant human erythropoietin in chronic haemodialysis individuals. Thromb Haemost 1989;61:117–121.
130. Triulzi DJ, Blumberg N. Variability in response to cryoprecipitate treat-ment for hemostatic defects in uremia. Yale J Biol Med 1990;63:1–7.

131. Vigano GL, Mannucci PM, Lattuada A et al. Subcutaneous desmopressin (DDAVP) shortens the bleeding time in uremia. Am J Hematol 1989;31:32–35.

132. Canavese C, Salomone M, Pacitti A. Reduced response of uraemic bleeding time to repeated doses of desmopressin. Lancet 1985;1:867–868.

133. Malyszko J, Pietraszek M, Buczko W et al. Study on mechanisms of haemostatic effect of 1-deamino-8-d-arginine vasopressin (desmopressin) in uraemic individuals. Folia Haematol (Leipz) 1990;117:319–324.

134. Kohler M, Hellstern P, Tarrach H et al. Subcutaneous injection of desmopressin (DDAVP): evaluation of a new, more concentrated preparation. Haemostasis 1989;19:38–44.

135. Rydzewski A, Rowinski M, Mysliwiec M. Shortening of bleeding time after intranasal administration of 1-deamino-8-d-arginine vasopressin to individuals with chronic uremia. Folia Haematol (Leipz) 1986;113:823–830.

136. Byrnes JJ, Larcada A, Moake JL. Thrombosis following desmopressin for uremic bleeding. Am J Hematol 1988;28:63–65.

137. Heistinger M, Stockenhuber F, Schneider B et al. Effect of conjugated estrogens on platelet function and prostacyclin generation in CRF. Kidney Int 1990;38:1181–1186.

138. Shemin D, Elnour M, Amarantes B et al. Oral estrogens decrease bleeding time and improve clinical bleeding in individuals with renal failure. Am J Med 1990;89:436–440.

139. Vigano G, Gaspari F, Locatelli M et al. Dose-effect and pharmacokinetics of estrogens given to correct bleeding time in uremia. Kidney Int 1988;34:853–858.

140. Livio M, Mannucci PM, Vigano G et al. Conjugated estrogens for the management of bleeding associated with renal failure. N Engl J Med 1986;315:731–735.

141. Bronner MH, Pate MB, Cunningham JT et al. Estrogen-progesterone therapy for bleeding gastrointestinal telangiectasias in chronic renal failure. An uncontrolled trial. Ann Intern Med 1986;105:371–374.

142. Sloand JA, Schiff MJ. Beneficial effect of low-dose transdermal estrogen on bleeding time and clinical bleeding in uremia. Am J Kidney Dis 1995;26:22–26.

143. Mammen EF. Coagulation abnormalities in liver disease. Hematol Oncol Clin North Am (Review) 1992;6:1247–1257.

144. Glassman AB. Platelet abnormalities in hepatobiliary diseases. Ann Clin Lab Sci 1990;20:119–122.

145. Thomas DP. Abnormalities of platelet aggregation in individuals with alcoholic cirrhosis. Ann NY Acad Sci 1972;201:243–250.

146. Ballard HS, Marcus AJ. Platelet aggregation in portal cirrhosis. Arch Intern Med 1976;136:316–319.

147. Blake JC, Sprengers D, Grech P et al. Bleeding time in individuals with hepatic cirrhosis. Br Med J 1990;301:12–15.

148. Rubin MH, Weston MJ, Langley PG et al. Platelet function in chronic liver disease: relationship to disease severity. Dig Dis Sci 1979;24:197–202.

149. Owens JS, Hutton RA, Day RC et al. Platelet lipid composition and platelet aggregation in human liver disease. J Lipid Res 1981;22:423–430.

150. Jerushalmy Z, Zucker MB. Some effects of fibrinogen degradation products (FDP) on blood platelets. Thromb Diath Haemorrh 1966;15:413–419.

151. Stachurska J, Latallo Z, Kopec M. Inhibition of platelet aggregation by dialysable fibrinogen degradation products (FDP). Thromb Diath Haemorrh 1970;23:91–98.

152. Martinez J, Palascak JE, Kwasniak D. Abnormal sialic acid content on the dysfibrinogenemia associated with liver disease. J Clin Invest 1978;61:535–538.

153. Mannucci PM, Vicente V, Vianello L et al. Controlled trial of desmopressin in liver cirrhosis and other conditions with a prolonged bleeding time. Blood 1986;67:1148–1153.

154. Cattaneo M, Tenconi PM, Alberca I et al. Subcutaneous desmopressin (DDAVP) shortens the prolonged bleeding time in individuals with liver cirrhosis. Thromb Haemost 1990;64:358–360.

155. Rapoport S, Yona R, Kaufman S et al. Unusual bleeding manifestations of amyloidosis in individuals with multiple myeloma. Clin Lab Haemat 1994;16:349–353.

156. Shpilberg O, Raviv G, Ramon J et al. Massive hematuria due to extramedullary plasmacytoma invading the bladder. Med Pediatra Oncol 1993;21:67–69.

157. Patterson WP, Caldwell CW, Doll DC. Hyperviscosity syndromes and coagulopathies. Semin Oncol 1990;17:210–216.

158. Lackner H. Hemostatic abnormalities associated with dysproteinemias. Semin Hematol 1973;10:125–133.

159. Coleman M, Vigliano EM, Weksler ME. Inhibition of fibrin monomer polymerization by lambda myelomas globulins. Blood 1972;39:210–223.

160. Perkins HA, MacKenzie MR, Fundenberg HH. Hemostatic defects in dysproteinemias. Blood 1970;35:695–707.

161. Furie B, Greene E, Furie BC. Syndrome of acquired factor X deficiency and systemic amyloidosis. N Engl J Med 1977;297:81–85.

162. Mazurier C, Parquet-Gernez A, Descamps J et al. Acquired von Willebrand's syndrome in the course of Waldenström's disease. Thromb Haemost 1980;44:115–118.

163. Khoory MS, Nesheim ME, Bowie EJ et al. Circulating heparin sulfate proteoglycan anticoagulant from a individual with a plasma cell disorder. J Clin Invest 1980;65:666–674.

164. Saraya AK, Kasturi J, Kishan R. A study of haemostasis in macroglobulinaemia. Acta Haematol 1972;47:33–42.

165. Malpass TW, Harker LA. Acquired disorders of platelet function. Semin Hematol 1980;17:242–258.

166. Penny R, Castaldi PA, Whitsed HM. Inflammation and haemostasis in paraproteinemias. Br J Haematol 1971;20:35–44.

167. Robert F, Mignucci M, McCurdy SA et al. Hemostatic abnormalities associated with monoclonal gammopathies. Am J Med Sci 1993;306:359–366.

168. McGrath KM, Stuart JJ, Richards F. Correlation between serum IgG, platelet membrane IgG, and platelet function in hypergammaglobulinemia states. Br J Haematol 1979;42:585–591.

169. Czestochowska E, Tyminski W, Gorski J et al. Disturbances of platelet function in individuals with multiple myeloma. Folia Haematol (Leipz) 1987;114:845–851.

170. Wallace MR, Simon SR, Ershler WB et al. Hemorrhagic diathesis in multiple myeloma. Acta Haematol 1984;72:340–342.

171. Schinco PC, Fusaro A, Marranca R et al. Paraproteinaemias and platelet aggregation: role of whole blood aggregometry. Thromb Res 1989;55:265–277.

172. DiMinno G, Coraggio F, Cerbone AM et al. A myeloma paraprotein with specificity for platelet glycoprotein IIIa in a individual with a fatal bleeding disorder. J Clin Invest 1986;77:157–164.

173. Levy-Toledano S, Tobelem G, Legrand C et al. Acquired IgG antibody occurring in thrombasthenic individuals: its effects on human platelet function. Blood 1978;51:1065–1071.

174. Lee H, Nurden AT, Thomaidis A et al. Relationship betweeen fibrinogen binding and platelet glycoprotein deficiencies in Glanzmann's thrombasthenia type I and type II. Br J Haematol 1981;48:47–57.

175. Woods VL Jr, Oh EH, Mason D et al. Autoantibodies against the platelet glycoprotein IIb–IIIa complex in individuals with chronic ITP. Blood 1984;63:368–375.

176. Beardsley DS, Spiegel JE, Jacobs MM et al. Platelet membrane glycoprotein IIIa contains antigens that bind anti-platelet antibodies in immune thrombocytopenias. J Clin Invest 1984;74:1701–1707.

177. Adamson JW, Fialkow PJ, Murphy S et al. Polycythemia vera: stem-cell and probably clonal origin of the disease. N Engl J Med 1976;295:913–916.

178. Fialkow PJ, Faquet GB, Jacobson RJ et al. Evidence that essential thrombocythemia is a clonal disorder with origin in a multipotent stem cell. Blood 1981;58:916–919.

179. Gialkow PJ, Gartler SM, Yoshida A. Clonal origin of chronic myelocytic leukemia in man. Proc Natl Acad Sci U S A 1967;58:1468–1471.

180. Gaetani GF, Ferraris AM, Galiano S et al. Primary thrombocythemia: clonal origin of platelets, erythrocytes, and granulocytes in a $Gd^B/Gd^{Mediterranean}$ subject. Blood 1982;59:76–79.

181. Jacobson RJ, Salo A, Fialkow PJ. Agnogenic myeloid metaplasia: a clonal proliferation of hematopoietic stem cells with secondary meylofibrosis. Blood 1978;51:189–194.

182. Tartaglia AP, Goldberg JD, Berk PD et al. Adverse effects of antiaggregating platelet therapy in the treatment of polycythemia vera. Semin Hematol 1986;23:172–176.

183. Barbui T, Buelli M, Cortelazzo S et al. Aspirin and risk of bleeding in individuals with thrombocythemia. Am J Med 1987;83:265–268.

184. Wasserman LR. Annotation: the management of polycythaemia vera. Br J Haematol 1971;21:371–376.

185. Iland HJ, Laszlo J, Peterson P et al. Essential thrombocythemia: clinical and laboratory characteristics at presentation. Trans Assoc Am Phys 1983;96:165–174.

186. Takahasi H, Hattori A, Shibata A. Profile of blood coagulation and fibrinolysis in chronic myeloproliferative disorders. Tohoku J Exp Med 1982;138:71–80.

187. Majer RV, Dawe A, Weir P et al. Which tests are most useful in distinguishing between reactive thrombocytosis and the thrombocytosis of myeloproliferative disease? Clin Lab Haematol 1991;13:9–15.

188. Schafer AI. Bleeding and thrombosis in the myeloproliferative disorders. Blood 1984;64:1–12.

189. Murphy S, Davis JL, Walsh PN et al. Template bleeding time and clinical hemorrhage in myeloproliferative disease. Arch Intern Med 1978;138:1251–1253.

190. Boneu B, Nouvel C, Sie P et al. Platelets in myeloproliferative disorders. I. A comparative evaluation with certain platelet function tests. Scand J Haematol 1980;25:214–220.

191. Barbui T, Cortelazzo S, Viero P et al. Thrombohaemorrhagic complications in 101 cases of myeloproliferative disorders: relationship to platelet number and function. Eur J Cancer Clin Oncol 1983;19:1593–1599.

192. Waddell CC, Brown JA, Repinecz YA. Abnormal platelet function in myeloproliferative disorders. Arch Pathol Lab Med 1981;105:432–435.

193. Wu KK-Y. Platelet hyperaggregability and thrombosis in individuals with thrombocythemia. Ann Intern Med 1978;88:7–11.

194. Balduini CL, Bertolino G, Noris P et al. Platelet aggregation in platelet-rich plasma and whole blood in 120 individuals with myeloproliferative disorders. Am J Clin Pathol 1991;95:82–86.

195. Kaywin P, McDonough M, Insel PA et al. Platelet function in essential thrombocythemia. Decreased epinephrine responsiveness associated with a deficiency of platelet α-adrenergic receptors. N Engl J Med 1978;299: 505–509.

196. Rao AK, Willis J, Kowalska MA et al. Differential requirements for platelet aggregation and inhibition of adenylate cyclase by epinephrine. Studies of a familial platelet alpha₂-adrenergic receptor defect. Blood 1988;71: 494–501.

197. Pearson TC, Wetherley-Mein G. Vascular occlusive episodes and venous haematocrit in primary proliferative polycythaemia. Lancet 1978;2: 1219–1222.

198. Lahuerta-Palacios JJ, Bornstein R, Fernandez-Debora FJ et al. Controlled and uncontrolled thrombocytosis: its clinical role in essential thrombocythemia. Cancer 1988;61:1207–1212.

199. Bellucci S, Janvier M, Tobelem G et al. Essential thrombocythemias. Clinical evolutionary and biological data. Cancer 1986;58:2440–2447.

200. Buss DH, Stuart JJ, Lipscomb GE. The incidence of thrombotic and hemorrhagic disorders in association with extreme thrombocytosis: an analysis of 129 cases. Am J Hematol 1985;20:365–372.

201. Berk PD, Goldberg JD, Donovan PB et al. Therapeutic recommendations in polycythemia vera based on Polycythemia Vera Study Group protocols. Semin Hematol 1986;23:132–143.

202. Grossi A, Rosseti S, Vannucchi AM et al. Occurrence of haemorrhagic and thrombotic events in myeloproliferative disorders: a retrospective study of 108 individuals. Clin Lab Haematol 1988;10:167–175.

203. Hehlmann R, Jahn M, Baumann B et al. Essential thrombocythemia. Clinical characteristics and course in 61 cases. Cancer 1988;61:2487–2496.

204. Kessler CM, Klein HG, Havlik RJ. Uncontrolled thrombocytosis in chronic myeloproliferative disorders. Br J Haematol 1982;50:157–167.

205. Tefferi A, Silverstein MN, Hoagland HC. Primary thrombocythemia. Semin Oncol 1995;22:334–340.

206. Tefferi A, Hoagland HC. Issues in the diagnosis and management of essential thrombocythemia. Mayo Clin Proc 1994;69:651–655.

207. Cortelazzo S, Finazzi G, Ruggeri M et al. Hydroxyurea for individuals with essential thrombocythemia and a high risk of thrombosis. N Engl J Med 1995;332:1132–1136.

208. Bensinger TA, Logue GL, Rundles RW. Hemorrhagic thrombocythemia; control of postsplenectomy thrombcytosis with melphalan. Blood 1970;36: 61–69.

209. Frick PG. Primary thrombocythemia. Clinical, hematological, and chromosomal studies of 13 individuals. Helv Med Acta 1969;35:20–29.

210. Hussain S, Schwartz JM, Friedman SA et al. Arterial thrombosis in essential thrombocythemia. Am Heart J 1978;96:31–36.

211. Orlin JB, Berkman EM. Improvement of platelet function following plateletpheresis in individuals with myeloproliferative diseases. Transfusion 1980;20:540–545.

212. Singh AK, Wetherly-Mein G. Microvascular occlusive lesions in primary thrombocythaemia. Br J Haematol 1977;36:553–564.

213. Taft EG, Babcock RB, Scharfman WB et al. Plateletpheresis in the management of thrombocytosis. Blood 1977;50:927–933.

214. Zucker S, Mielke CH. Classification of thrombocytosis based on platelet function tests: correlation with hemorrhagic and thrombotic complications. J Lab Clin Med 1972;80:385–394.

215. Spaet TH, Gaynor E, Goldstein ML et al. Defective platelets in essential thrombocythemia. Arch Intern Med 1969;124:135–141.

216. Mitus AJ, Schafer AI. Thrombocytosis and thrombocythemia. Hematol Oncol Clin North Am 1990;4:157–178.

217. Schafer AI. Essential thrombocythemia. Prog Hemostas Thromb 1991;10: 69–96.

218. Landolfi R, Marchioli R, Patrono C. Mechanisms of bleeding and thrombosis in myeloproliferative disorders [Review]. Thromb Haemost 1997;78: 617–621.

219. Maldonado JE. Dysplastic platelets and circulating megakaryocytes in chronic myeloproliferative diseases. II. Ultrastructure of circulating megakaryocytes. Blood 1974;43:811–820.

220. Thiele J, Holgado S, Choritz H et al. Density distribution and size of megakaryocytes in inflammatory reactions of the bone marrow (myelitis) and chronic myeloproliferative disease. Scand J Haematol 1983;31:329–341.

221. Matolcsy A, Majdic O. Circulating megakaryoblasts in chronic myeloproliferative diseases. An immunoelectron-microscopic study. Acta Haematol 1990;84:57–63.

222. Pedersen N, Laursen B. Megakaryocytes in cubital venous blood in individuals with chronic myeloproliferative diseases. Scand J Haematol 1983; 30:50–58.

223. Mazzucato M, De Marco L, De Angelis V et al. Platelet membrane abnormalities in myeloproliferative disorders: decrease in glycoproteins Ib and IIb-IIIa complex is associated with deficient receptor function. Br J Haematol 1989;73:369–374.

224. Landolfi R, De Critofaro RD, Castagnolo M et al. Increased platelet-fibrinogen affinity in individuals with myeloproliferative disorders. Blood 1988; 71:978–982.

225. Scharf RE, del Zoppo GJ, Figueroa M et al. Platelet dysfunction in individuals with myeloproliferative disorders (MPD) or myelodysplastic syndrome (MDS): flow cytometric analysis of defective membrane glycoprotein (GP) IIb/IIIa [Abstract]. Blood 1991;78(Suppl 1):138a.

226. Handa M, Watanabe K, Kawai Y. Platelet unresponsiveness to collagen: involvement of glycoprotein Ia-IIa (alpha 2 beta 1 integrin) deficiency associated with a myeloproliferative disorder. Thromb Haemost 1995;73: 521–528.

227. Walsh PN, Murphy S, Barry WWE. The role of platelets in the pathogenesis of thrombosis and hemorrhage in individuals with thrombocytosis. Thromb Haemost 1977;38:1085–1096.

228. Carbone C, Sie P, Fernandez F et al. Abnormal platelet serotonin uptake and binding sites in myeloproliferative disorders. Thromb Haemost 1984; 51:349–353.

229. Leoncini G, Maresca M, Balestrero F et al. Platelet membrane fatty acids in thrombocytosis due to myeloproliferative disorders. Cell Biochem Funct 1984;2:23–25.

230. Johnson GJ, Leis LA. Epinephrine-induced human platelet aggregation is dependent upon alpha₂ adrenergic receptor density: evidence from myeloproliferative disorders [Abstract]. Blood 1991;78(Suppl 1):141a.

231. Schafer AI, Cooper B, O'Hara D et al. Identification of platelet receptors for prostaglandin I₂ and D₂. J Biol Chem 1979;254:2914–2917.

232. Cooper B, Schafer AI, Puchalsky D et al. Platelet resistance to prostaglandin D₂ in individuals with myeloproliferative disorders. Blood 1978;52: 618–626.

233. Cooper B, Ahren D. Characterization of the platelet prostaglandin D₂ receptor: loss of prostaglandin D₂ receptors in platelets of individuals with myeloproliferative disorders. J Clin Invest 1979;64:586–590.

234. Cooper B. Diminished platelet adenylate cyclase activation by prostaglandin D₂ in acute thrombosis. Blood 1979;54:684–693.

235. Moore A, Nachman RL. Platelet Fc receptor. Increased expression in myeloproliferative disease. J Clin Invest 1981;67:1064–1071.

236. Ts'ao CH, Rossi EC, Lestina FC. Abnormalities in platelet function and morphology in a case of thrombocythaemia. Arch Pathol Lab Med 1977; 101:526–533.

237. Gerrard JM, Stoddard SF, Shapiro RS et al. Platelet storage pool deficiency and prostaglandin synthesis in chronic granulocytic leukaemia. Br J Haematol 1978;40:597–607.

238. Nishimura J, Okamoto S, Ibayashi H. Abnormalities of platelet adenine nucleotides in individuals with myeloproliferative disorders. Thromb Haemost 1979;41:787–795.

239. Russell NH, Salmon J, Keenan JP et al. Platelet adenine nucleotides and arachidonic acid metabolism in the myeloproliferative disorders. Thromb Res 1981;22:389–397.

240. Pareti FI, Gugliotta L, Mannucci L et al. Biochemical and metabolic aspects of platelet dysfunction in chronic myeloproliferative disorders. Thromb Haemost 1982;47:84–89.

241. Carbone C, Sie P, Nouvel C et al. Platelets in myeloproliferative disorders. II. Serotonin uptake and storage: correlations with mepacrine labelled dense bodies and with platelet density. Scand J Haematol 1980;25:289–295.

242. Burkhardt R, Bartl R, Jager K et al. Working classification of chronic myeloproliferative disorders based on histological, haematological and clinical findings. J Clin Pathol 1986;39:237–252.

243. Löfvenberg E, Nilsson TK. Qualitative platelet defects in chronic myeloproliferative disorders: evidence for reduced ATP secretion. Eur J Haematol 1989;43:435–440.

244. Leoncini G, Maresca M, Buzzi E et al. Platelet of individuals affected with essential thrombocythaemia are abnormal in plasma membrane and adenine nucleotide content. Eur J Haematol 1990;44:116–120.

245. Zeigler Z, Murphy S, Gardner FH. Microscopic platelet size and morphology in various hematologic disorders. Blood 1978;51:479–486.

246. Boughton BJ, Allington MJ, King A. Platelet and plasma β-thromboglobulin in myeloproliferative syndromes and secondary thrombocytosis. Br J Haematol 1978;40:125–132.

247. Rueda F, Pinol G, Marti F et al. Abnormal levels of platelet-specific proteins and mitogenic activity in myeloproliferative disease. Acta Haematol 1991;85:12–15.

248. Meschengieser S, Blanco A, Woods A et al. Intraplatelet levels of vWf: Ag and fibrinogen in myeloproliferative disorders. Thromb Res 1987;48: 311–319.

249. Burstein SA, Malpass TW, Yee E et al. Platelet factor-4 excretion in myeloproliferative disease: implications for the aetiology of myelofibrosis. Br J Haematol 1984;57:383–392.

250. Cortelazzo S, Viero P, Barbui T. Platelet activation in myeloproliferative disorders. Thromb Haemost 1981;45:211–213.

251. Wehmeier A, Tschöpe D, Esser J et al. Circulating activated platelets in myeloproliferative disorders. Thromb Res 1991;61:271–278.

252. Roberts AB, Sporn MB, Assoian RK. Transforming growth factor type β: rapid induction of fibrosis and angiogenesis in vivo and stimulation of collagen formation in vitro. Proc Natl Acad Sci U S A 1986;83:4167–4171.

253. Hiti-Harper J, Wohl H, Harper E. Platelet factor 4: an inhibitor of collagenase. Science 1978;199:991–992.

254. Groopman JE. The pathogenesis of myelofibrosis in myeloproliferative disorders. Ann Intern Med 1980;92:857–858.

255. Levy-Toledano S, Caen JP, Breton-Gorius J et al. Gray platelet syndrome:

α-granule deficiency. Its influence on platelet function. J Lab Clin Med 1981;98:831–848.

256. Breton-Gorius J, Vanchenker W, Nurden A et al. Defective α-granule production in megakaryocytes from gray platelet syndrome: ultrastructural studies of bone marrow cells and megakaryocytes growing in culture from blood precursors. Am J Pathol 1981;102:10–19.

257. Okuma M, Uchino H. Altered arachidonate metabolism by platelets in individuals with myeloproliferative disorders. Blood 1979;54:1258–1271.

258. Schafer AI. Deficiency of platelet lipoxygenase activity in myeloproliferative disorders. N Engl J Med 1982;306:381–386.

259. Eigenthalen M, Ullrich H, Geiger J et al. Defective nitro-vasodilation–stimulated protein phosphorylation and calcium regulation in cGMP-dependent protein kinase–deficient human platelets of chronic myelocytic leukemia. J Biol Chem 1993;268:13526–13531.

260. Bloom AL. von Willebrand factor: clinical features of inherited and acquired disorders. Mayo Clin Proc 1991;66:743–751.

261. Budde U, Schaefer G, Mueller N et al. Acquired von Willebrand's disease in the myeloproliferative syndromes. Blood 1984;64:981–985.

262. Budde U, Dent JA, Berkowitz SD et al. Subunit composition of plasma von Willebrand factor in individuals with the myeloproliferative syndrome. Blood 1986;68:1213–1217.

263. Fabris F, Casonats A, Del Ben MG. Abnormalities of von Willebrand factor in myeloproliferative disease: a relationship with bleeding diathesis. Br J Haematol 1986;63:75–83.

264. Jakway JL. Acquired von Willebrand's disease. Hematol Oncol Clin North Am (Review) 1992;6:1409–1419.

265. Raman BK, Sawdyk M, Saeed SM. Essential thrombocythemia with acquired von Willebrand's disease. Am J Clin Pathol 1987;88:102–106.

266. Sato K. Plasma von Willebrand factor abnormalities with essential thrombocythemia. Keio J Med 1988;37:54–71.

267. Castaman G, Lattuada A, Ruggeri M et al. Platelet von Willeband factor abnormalities in myeloproliferative syndromes. Am J Hematol 1995;49:289–293.

268. Okuma M, Takayama H, Sawada H et al. Platelet lipoxygenase activity: a possible indicator for marrow engraftment in lipoxygenase-deficient individuals [Letter]. N Engl J Med 1983;308:778–779.

269. Boughton BJ, Corbett WEN, Ginsburg AD. Myeloproliferative disorders: a paradox of in vivo and in vitro platelet function. J Clin Pathol 1977;30:228–234.

270. Holme S, Murphy S. Platelet abnormalities in myeloproliferative disorders. Clin Lab Med 1990;10:873–888.

271. Baker RI, Manoharan A. Platelet function in myeloproliferative disorders: characterization and sequential studies show multiple platelet abnormalities, and change with time. Eur J Haematol 1988;40:267–272.

272. Friedenberg WR, Roberts RC, David DE. Relationship of thrombohemorrhagic complications to endothelial cell function in individuals with chronic myeloproliferative disorders. Am J Hematol 1992;40:283–289.

273. Mills DC, Puri R, Hu CJ et al. Clopidogrel inhibits the binding of ADP analogues to the receptor mediating inhibition of platelet anenylat cyclase. Arterioscler Thromb 1992;12:430–436.

274. Cattaneo M, Lombardi R, Bettega D et al. Shear-induced platelet aggregation is potentiated by desmopressin and inhibited by ticlopidine. Arterioscler Thromb 1993;13:393–397.

275. Fornells J, Grau E, Montserrat S et al. Bleeding diathesis associated with beta-lactam antibiotics. Eur J Haematol 1990;45:272–273.

276. Brown CH III, Bradshaw MJ, Natelson EA et al. Defective platelet function following the administration of penicillin compounds. Blood 1976;47:949–956.

277. Andrassy K, Ritz E, Hasper B et al. Penicillin-induced coagulation disorder. Lancet 1976;2:1039–1041.

278. Cazenave JP, Guccione MA, Packham MA et al. Effects of cephalothin and penicillin G on platelet function in vitro. Br J Haematol 1977;35:135–152.

279. Brown CH III, Natelson EA, Bradshaw MW et al. The hemostatic defect produced by carbenicillin. N Engl J Med 1974;291:265–270.

280. Haburchak DR, Head DR, Everett ED. Postoperative hemorrhage associated with carbenicillin administration. Report of two cases and Review of the literature. Am J Surg 1977;134:630–634.

281. Brown CH III, Natelson EA, Bradshaw MW. Study of the effects of ticarcillin on blood coagulation and platelet function. Antimicrob Agents Chemother 1975;7:652–657.

282. Gentry LO, Jemsek JG, Natelson EA. Effects of sodium piperacillin on platelet function in normal volunteers. Antimicrob Agents Chemother 1981;19:532–533.

283. Pakter RL, Russell TR, Mielke CH et al. Coagulopathy associated with the use of moxalactam. JAMA 1982;248:1100.

284. Weitekamp MR, Aber RC. Prolonged bleeding times and bleeding diathesis associated with moxalactam administration. JAMA 1983;249:69–71.

285. Rossi EC, Levin NW. Inhibition of primary ADP-induced platelet aggregation in normal subjects after administration of nitrofurantoin (furadantin). J Clin Invest 1973;52:2457–2467.

286. Carter AE, Eban R, Perrett RD. Prevention of postoperative deep venous thrombosis and pulmonary embolism. Br Med J 1971;1:312–314.

287. Johnson GJ, Rao GHR, White JG. Platelet dysfunction induced by parenteral carbenicillin and ticarcillin. Studies of the dose-response relationship and mechanism of action in dogs. Am J Pathol 1978;91:85–106.

288. Cazenave JP, Packham MA, Guccione MA et al. Effects of penicillin G on platelet aggregation, release and adherence to collagen. Proc Soc Exp Biol Med 1973;142:159–166.

289. Shattil SJ, Bennett JS, McDonough M et al. Carbenicillin and penicillin G inhibit platelet function in vitro by impairing the interaction of agonists with the platelet surface. J Clin Invest 1980;65:329–337.

290. Pastakia KB, Terle D, Prodouz KN. Penicillin-induced dysfunction of platelet membrane glycoproteins. J Lab Clin Med 1993;121:546–554.

291. Johnson GJ. Platelets, penicillins, and purpura: what does it all mean? J Lab Clin Med 1993;121:531–533.

292. Burroughs SF, Johnson GJ. β-Lactam antibiotic–induced platelet dysfunction: evidence for irreversible inhibition of platelet activation in vitro and in vivo after prolonged exposure to penicillin. Blood 1990;75:1473–1480.

293. Sunakawa K, Akita H, Iwata S et al. The influence of cefotaxime on intestinal flora and bleeding diathesis in infants and neonates, compared with other β-lactams. J Antimicrob Chemother 1984;14(Suppl B):317–324.

294. Sloand EM, Klein HG, Pastakia KB et al. Effect of albumin on the inhibition of platelet aggregation by β-lactam antibiotics. Blood 1992;79:2022–2027.

295. Sunakawa K, Akita H, Iwata S et al. Effects of antibiotics on platelet aggregation. Drugs 1988;35(Suppl 2):205–207.

296. Cazzola M, Santangelo G, Paizis G et al. Effects of cefonicid on platelet aggregation. Drugs Exp Clin Res 1991;17:105–108.

297. Rubin R. Effects of ethanol on platelets. Lab Invest 1990;63:729–732.

298. Renaud S, de Lorgeril M. Wine, alcohol, platelets, and the French paradox for coronary heart disease. Lancet 1992;339:1523–1526.

299. Renaud SC, Beswick AD, Fehily AM et al. Alcohol and platelet aggregation: the Caerphilly Prospective Heart Disease Study. Am J Clin Nutr 1992;55:1012–1017.

300. Renaud SC, Ruf J-C. Effects of alcohol on platelet functions. Clin Chim Acta 1996;246:77–89.

301. Rubin R, Rand ML. Alcohol and platelet function. Alcohol Clin Exp Res 1994;18:105–110.

302. Deykin D, Janson P, McMahon L. Ethanol potentiation of aspirin-induced prolongation of the bleeding time. N Engl J Med 1982;306:852–854.

303. Goulston K, Cooke AR. Alcohol, aspirin, and gastrointestinal bleeding. Br Med J 1968;4:664–665.

304. Fleming JL, Ahlquist DA, McGill DB et al. Influence of aspirin and ethanol on fecal blood levels as determined by using the hemoquant assay. Mayo Clin Proc 1987;62:159–163.

305. Bengmark S, Elmer O, Garansson G et al. In vitro effect of ethanol on ADP and collagen-induced platelet aggregation. Thromb Haemost 1981;46:673–675.

306. Rand ML, Packham MA, Kinlough-Rathbone RL et al. Effects of ethanol on pathways of platelet aggregation in vitro. Thromb Haemost 1988;59:383–387.

307. Rubin R. Ethanol interferes with collagen-induced platelet activation by inhibition of arachidonic acid mobilization. Arch Biochem Biophys 1989;270:99–113.

308. Mikhailidis DP, Barradas MA, Jeremy JY. The effect of ethanol on platelet function and vascular prostanoids. Alcohol 1990;7:171–180.

309. Torres Duarte AP, Dong QS, Young J et al. Inhibition of platelet aggregation in whole blood by alcohol. Thromb Res 1995;78:107–115.

310. Hutton RA, Fink R, Wilson DT et al. Platelet hyperaggregability during alcohol withdrawal. Clin Lab Haematol 1981;3:223–229.

311. Veenstra J, van de Pol H, Schaafsma G. Moderate alcohol consumption and platelet aggregation in healthy middle-aged men. Alcohol 1990;7:547–549.

312. Keller JW, Folts JD. Relative effects of cigarette smoke and ethanol on acute platelet thrombus formation in stenosed canine coronary arteries. Cardiovasc Res 1988;22:73–78.

313. Rand ML, Groves HM, Packham MA et al. Acute administration of ethanol to rabbits inhibits thrombus formation induced by indwelling aortic catheters. Lab Invest 1990;63:742–745.

314. Latta EK, Packham MA, DaCosta SM et al. Effects of chronic administration of ethanol on platelets from rabbits with diet-induced hypercholesterolemia. Unchanged characteristics and responses to ADP but reduction of enhanced thrombin-induced, TxA2-independent platelet responses. Arterioscler Thromb 1994;14:1372–1377.

315. Demrow HS, Slane PR, Folts JD. Administration of wine and grape juice inhibits in vivo platelet activity and thrombosis in stenosed canine coronary arteries. Circulation 1995;91:1182–1188.

316. Benistant C, Rubin R. Ethanol inhibits thrombin-induced secretion by human platelets at a site distinct from phospholipase C or protein kinase C. Biochem J 1990;269:489–497.

317. Frishman WH, Weksler B, Christodoulo JB et al. Reversal of abnormal platelet aggregability and change in exercise tolerance in individuals with angina pectoris following oral propranolol. Circulation 1974;50:887–896.

318. Leon R, Tiarks CY, Pechet L. Some observations on the in vivo effect of propranolol on platelet aggregation and release. Am J Hematol 1978;5:117–121.

319. Weksler BB, Gillick M, Pink J. Effect of propranol on platelet function. Blood 1977;49:185–196.

320. Dachary-Prigent J, Dufourcq J, Lussan C et al. Propranolol, chlorpromazine and platelet membrane: a fluorescence study of the drug-membrane interaction. Thromb Res 1979;14:15–22.

321. Hawiger J, White RB. Propranolol and prostacyclin inhibit human platelet phospholipase A-induced release of arachidonic acid. Circulation 1978;58:II-138.

322. Vanderhoek JY, Feinstein MB. Local anesthetics, chlorpromazine and propranolol inhibit stimulus-activation of phospholipase $A_2$ in human platelets. Mol Pharmacol 1979;16:171–180.

323. Nosál R, Jancinová V, Petríková M. The role of intracellular calcium in A-23187–stimulated and β-adrenoceptor blocking drug–treated blood platelets. Biochem Pharmacol 1994;47:2207–2211.

324. Dalsgaard-Nielsen J, Risbo A, Simmelkjaer P et al. Impaired platelet aggregation and increased bleeding time during general anaesthesia with halothane. Br J Anaesth 1981;53:1039–1042.

325. Jain MF, Eskow E, Kuchibhotla J et al. Correlation of inhibition of platelet aggregation by phenothiazines and local anesthetics with their effects on a phospholipid bilayer. Thromb Res 1978;13:1067–1075.

326. White GC, Raynor ST. The effects of trifluoroperazine, an inhibitor of calmodulin on platelet function. Thromb Res 1980;18:279–284.

327. Warlow C, Ogston D, Douglas AS. Platelet function after the administration of chlorpromazine to human subjects. Haemostasis 1976;5:21–26.

328. Dinan TG. Neuroleptic effects on platelet aggregation: a study in normal volunteers and schizophrenics. Psychol Med 1987;17:875–881.

329. Kaiya JM, Imai H, Muramatsu Y et al. Platelet aggregation response in schizophrenia and prostaglandin E1. Psychiatry Res 1983;9:309–318.

330. Richardson SGN, Fletcher DJ, Jeavans PM et al. Sodium valproate and platelet function. BMJ 1976;1:221–222.

331. Langdell RD, Adelson EA, Furth FW. Dextran and prolonged bleeding time. JAMA 1958;166:346–351.

332. Weiss HJ. The effect of clinical dextran on platelet aggregation, adhesion and ADP release in man: *in vivo* and *in vitro* studies. J Lab Clin Med 1967;69:37–46.

333. Evans RJ, Gordon JL. Mechanism of the antithrombotic action of dextran [Letter]. N Engl J Med 1974;290:748.

334. Zucker MB. Heparin and platelet function. Fed Proc 1977;36:47–49.

335. Green D, Tsao CH, Cerullo L et al. Clinical and laboratory investigation of the effects of epsilon-aminocaproic acid on hemostasis. J Lab Clin Med 1985;105:321–327.

336. Baghurst KI, Raj MJ, Truswell AS. Onions and platelet aggregation [Letter]. Lancet 1977;1:101.

337. Phillips C, Poyser NL. Inhibition of platelet aggregation by onion extracts [Letter]. Lancet 1978;1:1051–1052.

338. Srivastava KC, Tyagi OD. Effects of a garlic-derived principle (ajoene) on aggregation and arachidonic acid metabolism in human blood platelets. Prostagland Leukotr Essen Fatty Acids 1993;49:587–595.

339. Das I, Khan NS, Sooranna SR. Potent activation of nitric oxide synthase by garlic: a basis for its therapeutic applications. Curr Med Res Opin 1995;13:257–263.

340. Hammerschmidt DE. Szechwan purpura. N Engl J Med 1980;302:1191–1193.

341. Steiner M, Anastasi J. Vitamin E: an inhibitor of the platelet release reaction. J Clin Invest 1976;57:732–737.

# SECTION 8

# DISORDERS OF COAGULATION FACTORS AND FIBRINOLYSIS

# CHAPTER 34

# VON WILLEBRAND DISEASE

William C. Nichols, Kathleen A. Cooney, David Ginsburg,
and Zaverio M. Ruggeri

## HISTORICAL PERSPECTIVE

von Willebrand disease (vWd) was first described in 1926 by Erik von Willebrand (1), who identified a hereditary bleeding disorder in a large family from the Åland archipelago in the Gulf of Bothnia. The proband, a 7-year-old girl, suffered from episodes of mucosal bleeding and eventually died of uncontrollable hemorrhage during her fourth menstrual period at age 13. Nine of her eleven siblings also had bleeding problems, including four sisters who died of severe hemorrhage between the ages of 2 and 4 years (2, 3). Family members were found to have prolonged bleeding times but normal coagulation times and platelet counts. Clot retraction in the proband was normal. von Willebrand recognized the autosomal dominant pattern of inheritance of this bleeding diathesis and called the disorder "hereditary pseudohemophilia." He attributed the disease to abnormalities in the vessel wall, as well as to a functional disorder of platelets (2, 4–6). A similar clinical disorder was subsequently reported by four American groups in 1928 (2, 3, 7).

In 1953, Alexander and Goldstein (8) first described the association of decreased factor VIII levels and prolonged bleeding times in two individuals with typical pseudohemophilia or vWd, and others subsequently confirmed this observation. Nilsson et al (9) found that infusion of plasma fraction I-O, containing both factor VIII and von Willebrand factor (vWf), corrected both the prolonged bleeding times and the factor VIII levels of individuals with vWd. Similarly, plasma fraction I-O prepared from a individual with hemophilia was also found to decrease the bleeding time and improve the factor VIII levels in vWd individuals (10). Cornu et al (11) further observed that when individuals with vWd were transfused with plasma from individuals with hemophilia A, there was a paradoxical and sustained rise in the factor VIII level. This pattern was quite distinct from the abrupt rise and fall of the factor VIII level obtained when a individual with hemophilia A was transfused with plasma from a normal individual or a vWd individual (11, 12). This difference in response to plasma infusion was often used to distinguish vWd and hemophilia A.

The immunologic characterization of factor VIII and vWf began in the early 1970s (see below) and paved the way for the cDNA cloning of factor VIII in 1984 (13, 14) and of vWf in 1985 (15–18). The advent of the polymerase chain reaction (PCR) has led to the precise characterization of many of the molecular defects in individuals with hemophilia and vWd. This knowledge has broadened our understanding of the nature of these coagulation disorders.

## TERMINOLOGY OF vWf AND FACTOR VIII

From the time of the initial observation that individuals with vWd also have decreased plasma levels of factor VIII, there has been considerable confusion regarding the specific nature of the interaction between factor VIII and vWf and the terminology used to describe these proteins. Initially, a polyclonal antiserum was prepared using "purified factor VIII" or antihemophilic factor

(AHF) as the immunogen. As a result of the high affinity noncovalent interaction between factor VIII and vWf (see Chapter 16), these early crude preparations, as well as many current factor VIII concentrates, contain large amounts of vWf with a stoichiometry of approximately 50:1 vWf:FVIII (the same ratio as in plasma). Thus, antibodies raised in this way are directed primarily against vWf. Using this antiserum, individuals with hemophilia were found to have normal levels of antigen, whereas individuals with vWd had low levels of antigen (19). Soon it was discovered that AHF or factor VIII and vWf are dissociable (20–23) and new terminology was introduced to describe the various antigen and activity measurements. Factor VIII antihemophilic activity was called VIII:C to denote its coagulant function. The precipitating antigen found to be decreased in individuals with vWd was referred to as factor VIII-related antigen (VIIIR:Ag).

In 1971, Howard and Firkin (24) reported that ristocetin, an antibiotic previously noted to cause thrombocytopenia, was able to aggregate platelets in the presence of normal plasma but not in the presence of plasma from some individuals with vWd. Others confirmed this observation, and the defective platelet aggregation seen with vWd plasma was further shown to be corrected by the addition of normal or hemophiliac plasma (25). Weiss et al (26) developed a quantitative assay of vWf function based on this principle, and the activity measured was subsequently referred to as the ristocetin cofactor activity, or VIII:RCo.

In 1985, the International Committee in Thrombosis and Haemostasis recommended new terminology for factor VIII and vWf (Table 34.1) (27). This nomenclature was introduced to provide distinct names for each protein, because it was clear that factor VIII and vWf were separate molecular entities encoded by two distinct genes (13–18). Using the new system, factor VIII protein is abbreviated as VIII, the coagulant function VIII:C, and the antigen VIII:Ag. von Willebrand factor is abbreviated as vWf with its antigen referred to as vWf:Ag. No specific functional assay was designated by this group as being completely representative of the *in vivo* function of vWf. Although the term VIII:RCo was considered outmoded, no replacement was recommended. Alternative nomenclatures in use, although not officially endorsed by the committee, are vWf activity and vWf ristocetin cofactor activity (vWf:RCo).

# VON WILLEBRAND DISEASE: OVERVIEW

von Willebrand disease is a heterogeneous bleeding disorder with a bewildering array of variants and subtypes, as described in Table 34.2 (28–31). A recently revised classification of vWd merges a number of previously

**TABLE 34.1.**   Factor VIII and von Willebrand Factor Terminology[1]

|  | Original | Current |
|---|---|---|
| *Factor VIII* | | |
| Protein | VIII:C | VIII |
| Antigen | VIIIC:Ag | VIII:Ag |
| Function | | VIII:C |
| *von Willebrand factor* | | |
| Protein | VIIIR:Ag | vWf |
| Antigen | VIIIR:Ag | vWf:Ag |
| Function | VIIIR:RCo | [2] |

[1] As recommended by the International Committee on Thrombosis and Haemostasis. (Adapted with permission from Marder VJ, Mannucci PM, Firkin BG, et al. Standard nomenclature for factor VIII and von Willebrand factor: A recommendation by the International Committee on Thrombosis and Haemostasis. Thromb Haemost 1985; 54:871–872.)

[2] von Willebrand factor ristocetin cofactor activity (vWf:RCo) is often used as a measure of vWf function, although not officially recognized. (Adapted with permission from Marder VJ, Mannucci PM, Firkin BG, et al. Standard nomenclature for factor VIII and von Willebrand factor: A recommendation by the International Committee on Thrombosis and Haemostasis. Thromb Haemost 1985;54: 871–872.)

distinct subtypes, thus reducing the number of subgroups from more than 20 to only 6 (Table 34.3) (32, 33). The subtypes can be divided into two main categories based on whether there is a quantitative (type 1 or type 3) or qualitative (type 2) defect in vWf. Type 1 is the most common form of vWd, accounting for approximately 70% of clinical cases (2, 10, 34). It is inherited as an autosomal dominant disorder and presents as a mild to moderately severe bleeding disorder. By comparison, type 3 vWd is quite rare. The disease is transmitted in an autosomal recessive pattern and presents as a very severe bleeding diathesis. There continues to be debate as to whether type 3 vWd is homozygous type 1 vWd or a distinct recessive genetic disorder (see below).

The type 2 variants (2A, 2B, 2M, and 2N) are distinguished primarily by a defect in vWf function and often an altered plasma vWf multimer pattern, as visualized by agarose gel electrophoresis (Fig. 34.1) or crossed immunoelectrophoresis. Together, the type 2 subtypes account for 20 to 30% of vWd cases (2, 10, 34). Most forms of type 2 vWd are transmitted in an autosomal dominant fashion, with the notable exception of one of the type 2A variants, formerly referred to as vWd type IIC (see Table 34.3), which appears to be recessive (see below).

## PREVALENCE

von Willebrand disease is the most common inherited bleeding disorder in humans. Initial studies in the Swed-

**TABLE 34.2.**   Classification of von Willebrand Disease Subtypes[1]

| Subtype | Frequency | Clinical Features | Diagnosis | Molecular Basis |
|---|---|---|---|---|
| Type 3 | $1-5:10^6$. | Severe bleeding disorder; autosomal recessive inheritance. | Markedly decreased or undetectable vWf:Ag, vWf activity, and VIII:C. | vWf gene deletions; nonsense, missense and frameshift mutations throughout gene; other *cis*-defects in mRNA expression. |
| Type 1 | $1-30:1000$; most common vWd variant (>70% of vWd). | Mild to moderate bleeding disorder; autosomal dominant; incomplete penetrance (approximately 60%). | vWf:Ag, vWf activity, and VIII:C all proportionately decreased (20–50%). Normal multimer distribution. | A few missense mutations reported, presumed to disrupt function; some cases represent heterozygous form of type 3. |
| Type 2A | Approximately 10–15% of clinical vWd cases. | Mild to moderate bleeding disorder; generally autosomal dominant although some autosomal recessive, more complete penetrance than type 1; generally poor response to DDAVP. | Variably decreased vWf:Ag, vWf activity, and VIII:C; absent high and intermediate size vWf multimers with prominent satellite bands. | Missense mutations clustered within vWf A2 repeat. Two subgroups: Group 1—Defect in intracellular transport; group 2—Increased proteolysis in plasma after secretion. |
| Type 2B | Uncommon variant (<5% of clinical vWd). | Mild to moderate bleeding disorder; autosomal dominant, more complete penetrance than type 1; ? DDAVP contraindicated. | Variably decreased vWf antigen and VIII:C; loss of large multimers; enhanced RIPA; thrombocytopenia. | Missense mutations clustered in vWf A1 repeat result in increased or spontaneous binding to platelet GP Ib. |
| Type 2M | Rare (case reports). | Variable bleeding disorder; autosomal dominant. | Variably decreased vWf:Ag and VIII:C. vWf activity decreased relative to antigen despite presence of large and intermediate multimers. | Missense mutations and small in-frame deletions in vWf A1 repeat. |
| Type 2N | Uncommon; heterozygotes may be prevalent in some populations. | Variable bleeding disorder. Homozygotes (or compound heterozygotes) may resemble autosomal hemophilia A. Coinheritance may modify severity of type 1. | Variable vWf:Ag and vWf activity. Disproportionately low VIII:C. Generally normal multimers. Decreased or absent vWf binding to FVIII. | Missense mutations within the N-terminus of mature vWf which interfere with FVIII binding. |

*Adapted with permission from Nichols WC, Ginsburg D. von Willebrand disease [review]. Medicine 1997;76:1–20.*

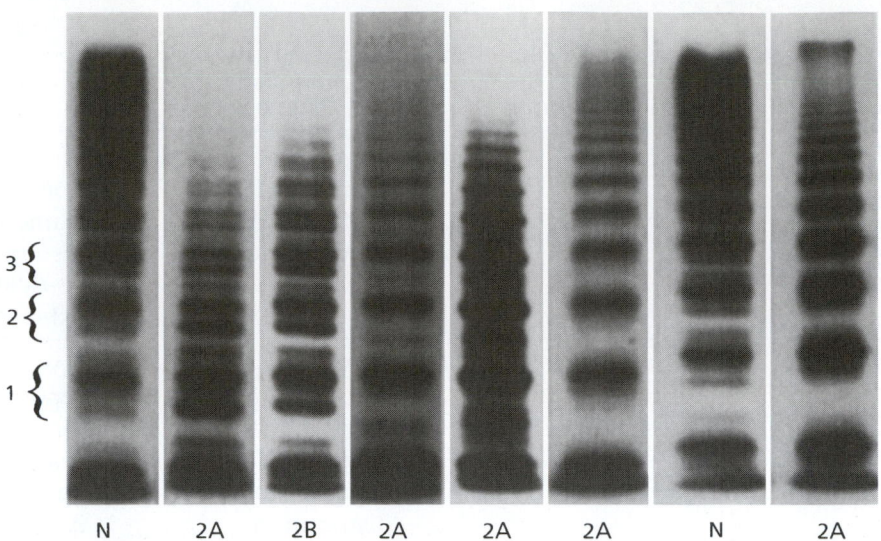

**FIGURE 34.1.** von Willebrand factor multimer analysis of plasma from individuals with various qualitative variants of vWd performed by agarose gel electrophoresis. The brackets encompass three individual multimer subunits including the main band and its associated satellite bands. Note the relatively decreased amount of the largest and intermediate vWf multimers in the type 2A plasma compared to the loss of only the largest multimers in the type 2B plasma. There is also a relative increase in the fastest moving (176 Kda) satellite band in both the type 2A and 2B plasma. Aberrant multimer subunit structure can also be seen in the plasma from individuals with other type 2A variants formerly known as types IIC, IID, IIE, and IIF vWd when compared to normal (N) plasma. (Adapted with permission from Berkowitz SD, Ruggeri ZM, Zimmerman TS. von Willebrand Disease. In: Zimmerman TS, Ruggeri ZM, eds. Coagulation and bleeding disorders. The role of factor VIII and von Willebrand factor. New York: Marcel Dekker, 1989;215–259.)

**TABLE 34.3.** Revised Classification of von Willebrand Disease Subtypes (32)

| Revised Classification | Previous Classification |
|---|---|
| 3 | III |
| 1 | I, I platelet normal, I platelet low, IA, I-1, I-2, I-3 |
| 2A | IIA, IB, I platelet discordant, IIC, IID, IIE, IIF, IIG, IIH |
| 2B | IIB, I New York, I Malmö, I Sydney |
| 2M | B, IC, ID, Vincenza |
| 2N | Normandy |

ish population suggested that the prevalence of vWd is 1 in 10,000, which made vWd twice as common as hemophilia in the same population (3). However, a more recent screening program of school-age children in Italy found the prevalence of vWd to be 0.82% (35). Similar studies in several different populations have been reported with prevalence figures ranging from 1 to 2% or more (36–38). Most of the individuals identified in these studies appear to have type 1 vWd. There are numerous factors that might contribute to the surprisingly high

prevalence figures obtained in screening studies. First, there are no absolute clinical and/or laboratory criteria for identification of vWd cases, and the sensitivity and specificity of available laboratory tests for vWd are low (see below) (39). Furthermore, the disease exhibits significant phenotypic heterogeneity even among members of the same family (39). The explanation for the high degree of variability in laboratory tests and clinical symptoms may be in part due to the effects of blood group antigens (40, 41), estrogen (42), and the changes in vWf levels resulting from stress (see below) (29, 43–45).

By comparison, type 3 vWd has been reported to occur in only 0.1 to 3 per million population (46). These prevalence figures vary greatly around the world, with the most cases reported in the Scandinavian countries and the fewest cases cited in Spain and France. In one survey, however, a remarkably similar incidence of type 3 vWd was reported in the United States and Europe, with 1.38 and 1.51 cases observed per million population, respectively (47). Based on these numbers, the carrier frequency can be estimated to be as high as 1:500.

## CLINICAL DESCRIPTION

von Willebrand's disease is a bleeding disorder that varies in severity depending on the subtype as well as other factors. Because vWf is required for the formation of the

**TABLE 34.4.**   Symptoms Associated with von Willebrand Disease

| | Patients with vWd (n = 264) | Normal Individuals (n = 500) |
|---|---|---|
| Epistaxis | 62.5% | 4.6% |
| Menometrorrhagia[1] | 60.1% | 25.3% |
| Hemorrhage after dental extraction | 51.5% | 4.8% |
| Ecchymoses and hematomas | 49.2% | 11.8% |
| Bleeding from wounds | 36.0% | 0.2% |
| Gingival bleeding | 34.8% | 7.4% |
| Postoperative bleeding | 28.0% | 1.4% |
| Postpartum bleeding[1] | 23.3% | 19.5% |
| Gastrointestinal bleeding | 14.0% | 0.6% |
| Petechiae | 11.5% | 1.2% |
| Joint bleeding | 8.3% | 0% |
| Hematuria | 6.8% | 0.6% |

[1] *Calculated for females older than 15 years of age.*

*(Adapted with permission from Silwer J. von Willebrand's disease in Sweden. Acta Paediatr Scand Suppl 1973; 238:1–159.)*

initial hemostatic plug (see Chapter 16), bleeding in this disease tends to be mucocutaneous in origin. The most common complaints are epistaxis, easy bruising, and heavy menses (Table 34.4). In comparison, intra-articular bleeding, commonly seen in individuals with coagulation factor deficiencies, is much less prevalent and typically seen only in individuals with severe type 3 vWd. Because the symptoms of vWd are frequently mild, the clinician must often combine a careful history with repeated laboratory evaluation. There have been several large population studies examining the frequency of various bleeding problems in individuals with vWd. Silwer (48) compared the bleeding histories from 264 individuals with vWd to those obtained from a large group of normal individuals without documented bleeding disorders (Table 34.4). Interestingly, many normal individuals gave histories of heavy menses, bruising, and postpartum hemorrhage, pointing out the difficulties of assessing mild hemostatic abnormalities by history alone.

von Willebrand's disease exhibits significant phenotypic heterogeneity among individuals with the same type of vWd and even among affected members of the same family (39, 49). Some of this variability can be accounted for by the fact that plasma vWf antigen levels are altered by many factors. The ABO blood group is the best characterized of these factors. Mean vWf antigen levels for type O individuals are approximately 75%; for type AB individuals, they are 123% when compared to a pool of normal donor plasmas (40). Thus, it may be difficult to differentiate between a low-normal vWf antigen level and mild type 1 vWd in blood group O individuals. Accordingly, type 1 vWd is more commonly diagnosed in individuals with blood type O. It has been estimated that 30% of the variance in vWf antigen levels may be accounted for by blood type (41). There may be an additional contribution from the Lewis blood group antigens (41). Estrogen also appears to affect vWf, with plasma vWf levels noted to be elevated during pregnancy, in individuals taking oral contraceptive pills, and in individuals with liver disease (42). von Willebrand factor levels also increase with age (50), and, therefore, mild symptoms often abate over time. Finally, stress and its resultant hormonal alterations can result in an increase in circulating levels of vWf (29, 43–45).

## DIAGNOSIS AND LABORATORY EVALUATION

Accurate diagnosis of vWd depends heavily on laboratory testing and may require repeated analyses of individuals and family members. Five tests (see also Chapter 26) are commonly used to establish the diagnosis and specific subtype of vWd. The recommended panel of tests for the evaluation of possible vWd includes measurement of factor VIII:C, vWf antigen, vWf activity as determined by ristocetin cofactor activity, vWf multimer analysis, and the bleeding time. Factor VIII:C levels are typically determined by a one-stage assay with a normal value in most laboratories within the range of 50 to 150 U/dL (50 to 100%). Test plasmas are compared to a normal reference plasma empirically determined to have a factor VIII level of 100%, which corresponds to a factor VIII:C of 100 units U/dL. von Willebrand factor antigen is quantitated in the laboratory using a polyclonal rabbit anti-vWf antibody, by either the Laurell rocket electroimmunoassay (51) or an enzyme-linked immunoabsorbent assay (ELISA). Normal levels are between 50 and 200 U/dL (50 to 200%). The Laurell method is more sensitive to the number of vWf multimers, regardless of size, whereas the ELISA (or radioimmunoassay) more directly reflects the number of individual vWf monomeric subunits (52). As a result, individuals with qualitative variants of vWd (type 2) will have lower vWf antigen levels measured by ELISA compared to the Laurell technique, because the ELISA is more sensitive to qualitative abnormalities in vWf (52, 53).

Although vWf has many functions that can be studied in the research laboratory, ristocetin cofactor activity, which measures induced binding of vWf to platelet glycoprotein Ib (GP Ib), is the standard functional assay used in the clinical laboratory (25). In this assay, ristocetin is added to formalin-fixed platelets in the presence of individual plasma, and platelet agglutination is measured. The results are typically expressed as a percentage of the activity of a normal pooled plasma standard, and the normal plasma concentration is typically within the range of 50 to 150%. The ristocetin cofactor activity assay is the only widely used clinical measure of vWf functional activity. In individuals with quantitative disorders of vWf (vWd type 1 or 3), the ristocetin cofactor activity is generally decreased in proportion to the decrease in vWf antigen. However, in individuals with qualitative abnormalities in vWf (vWd type 2), the ristocetin cofactor activity is often diminished to a greater degree than vWf antigen.

Crossed immunoelectrophoresis (CIE) or vWf multimer analysis by agarose gel electrophoresis is performed to assess multimer structure. During CIE, plasma proteins are first separated horizontally according to size and charge, then electrophoresed vertically into a gel containing an anti-vWf polyclonal antibody forming a precipitate peak. Qualitative abnormalities in vWf can be detected by an alteration in the symmetry or the mobility of the precipitate peak. von Willebrand factor multimer analysis is performed by fractionating individual plasma on a nonreducing agarose gel and visualizing vWf with a radiolabeled polyclonal anti-vWf antibody (Fig. 34.1). By this technique, normal plasma vWf is seen as a complex series of bands that is typically divided into groups of low, intermediate, and high molecular weight multimers. Each multimer subunit actually consists of five separate bands, but this structure is usually only seen on high resolution (3%) agarose gels (54). These satellite bands have been shown to represent the results of proteolytic degradation (54–56). Alteration of this complex pattern has formed the basis of the identification of many of the vWd type 2 variants. Whereas type 1 vWd is diagnosed by a normal multimer pattern in the presence of decreased vWf antigen and activity, the most common type 2 vWd subtypes (2A and 2B) are characterized by an abnormal multimer pattern, including loss of the high and intermediate molecular weight multimers. When possible, multimer analysis should be performed initially upon diagnosis of vWd in a given family to identify the specific vWd subtype. Correct subclassification of vWd has important therapeutic implications, because 1-deamino 8-D-arginine vasopressin (DDAVP), most effective in classic type 1 vWd, may be contraindicated in type 2B vWd, although this latter point is controversial (see below and Chapter 53).

Bleeding times are often used both in the diagnosis of vWd and in its subsequent management. The bleeding time assesses the formation of the platelet plug *in vivo* by determining the time to cessation of bleeding from a small skin laceration (57). Most laboratories use a standardized template bleeding time in which a small incision is made on the volar aspect of the forearm while a blood pressure cuff maintains a constant pressure of 40 mm Hg (see Chapter 23). This technique has been demonstrated to measure platelet function accurately in a variety of clinical situations (57), although its potential fallibilities have recently been emphasized (58, 59) (see Chapter 23). Historically, there have been reports both of good (60) and poor (61, 62) correlation of the bleeding time with vWf antigen levels. These data were reviewed in tabular form in 1990 by Rodgers (58). Gralnick et al (63) studied 17 individuals with vWd type 1 and found that the bleeding time correlated best with platelet vWf activity and, to a lesser extent, with platelet vWf antigen. Because individuals with vWd type 1 have been reported to differ in their levels of platelet vWf (64, 65), this may explain some of the variability of bleeding times in this disorder. Bleeding times in normal individuals may also depend on platelet vWf levels (66). Whereas a prolonged bleeding time is not specific for vWd, with repeated testing most individuals with symptomatic vWd will at some time exhibit a prolonged bleeding time (49).

There are several other tests that are useful in the diagnosis and subclassification of vWd. The activated partial thromboplastin time (aPTT) is typically prolonged in individuals with moderate to severe vWd due to the low factor VIII:C levels in these disorders (see above). Ristocetin-induced platelet aggregation (RIPA) is similar to the measurement of ristocetin cofactor activity except that the individual's own platelets are used and aggregation is measured rather than agglutination. This test is essential for the diagnosis of type 2B and platelet-type or pseudo-vWd (see below).

Unfortunately, none of the routine tests used for the diagnosis of vWd have high sensitivity or specificity. When bleeding time, vWf antigen, ristocetin cofactor activity, and factor VIII:C levels were all performed on members of two large vWd kindreds, 42% of the obligate heterozygotes had test results within the normal range (39). Thus, the sensitivity of this panel of laboratory tests for type 1 vWd may be as low as 60%. In addition, the results of each of these tests show considerable variability when performed repeatedly in a given individual with vWd over time (39, 49). In a individual suspected of having vWd based on a clinical history of bleeding or a positive family history, repeated testing may be necessary to establish the diagnosis (49). No one test for vWd appears to have more sensitivity than the others for all types of vWd (39, 49). Rodeghiero et al (67), however, reported greater sensitivity of ristocetin cofactor activity compared to vWf antigen in a large screening study of school-age children.

## MOLECULAR CLASSIFICATION

Given the complexity of vWf biosynthesis, secretion, and function (see Chapter 16), defects at a number of genetic loci could potentially result in a vWd phenotype. Although genetic heterogeneity could be partially responsible for the extensive phenotypic heterogeneity ob-

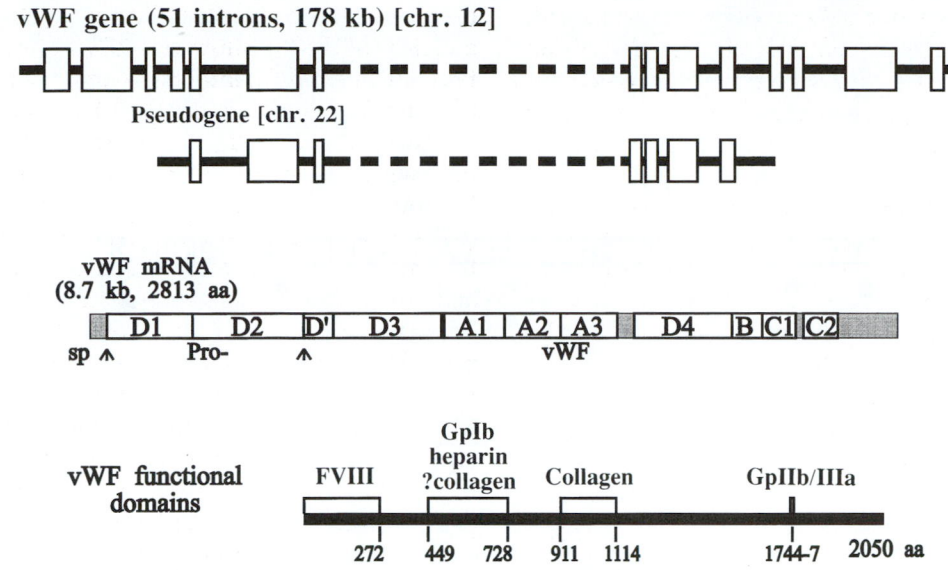

**FIGURE 34.2.**   Schematic of vWf gene, mRNA, and protein. The vWf gene and pseudogene are depicted at the top; boxes represent exons and the solid black lines represent introns. The vWf mRNA encoding the full prepro-vWf subunit is depicted in the middle as the gray bar and lettered boxes. Arrowheads indicate the location of signal peptide (sp) and propeptide (Pro) cleavage sites. The lettered boxes denote the series of repeated homologous segments. The approximate localizations for known vWf functional domains within the mature vWf sequence are indicated at the bottom. Numbers beneath the domains refer to amino acid residues within the mature vWf subunit. (Adapted with permission from Ginsburg D, Bowie EJ. Molecular genetics of von Willebrand disease [Review]. Blood 1992;79:2507–2519.)

served in vWd, all mutations identified in individuals with von Willebrand disease to date have been detected at the vWf locus (Figs. 34.2 and 34.3 and see below) (68–70). A database of known vWd mutations and polymorphisms is maintained by a consortium of vWd investigators and can be accessed through the Internet at *http://mmg2.im.med.umich.edu/vWf*. Individual researchers contribute mutations/polymorphisms as they are identified; thus, some of the information contained in the database has not yet been published.

# TYPE 1 VON WILLEBRAND DISEASE

Accounting for 70% of all cases, type 1 vWd is the most common form of vWd (2, 30, 34, 39, 71). It is inherited in an autosomal dominant pattern. Individuals typically present with a mild to moderately severe bleeding disorder although there is significant phenotypic heterogeneity even among affected members in the same family (39). Laboratory evaluation generally reveals vWf antigen, factor VIII:C, and ristocetin cofactor activity of approximately 30 to 50%, although the full range of vWf multimers is seen on agarose gel analysis.

Whereas the recently revised classification of vWd does not formally subdivide type 1 vWd, analysis of large numbers of individuals with type 1 vWd has previously suggested distinct subgroups among individuals,

and several subclassification schemes have been proposed. Hoyer et al (34) performed plasma vWf multimer analysis on individuals from 33 type 1 vWd kindreds and were able to separate the families into two groups. Individuals with type Ia vWd had a full complement of vWf multimers present with a pattern similar to that detected in normal plasma. In contrast, individuals with type Ib vWd were observed to have a relatively decreased amount of the larger multimeric forms. These differences in vWf multimer patterns were confirmed by densitometry. By this analysis, 18 of 33 type I families were found to have type Ia vWd and the remaining 15 had type Ib vWd (34). Individuals with type Ib vWd were distinguished from individuals with type II vWd, because the highest molecular weight vWf multimers were present in a reduced amount in type Ib individuals and absent in type II individuals. Because type 1 vWd is now constrained to include only purely quantitative disorders, type Ib vWd has been reclassified as type 2A vWd (see below and Tables 34.2 and 34.3) (32).

Weiss et al (64) proposed a subclassification scheme based on quantification of plasma and platelet vWf from type 1 vWd individuals. Individuals with subtype I-1 were described as having a moderate decrease (30 to 45% of control values) in both plasma and platelet vWf. By comparison, individuals with subtype I-2 had decreased plasma but normal platelet vWf antigen levels, and subtype I-3 individuals had the converse. This subclassification strategy was further developed by

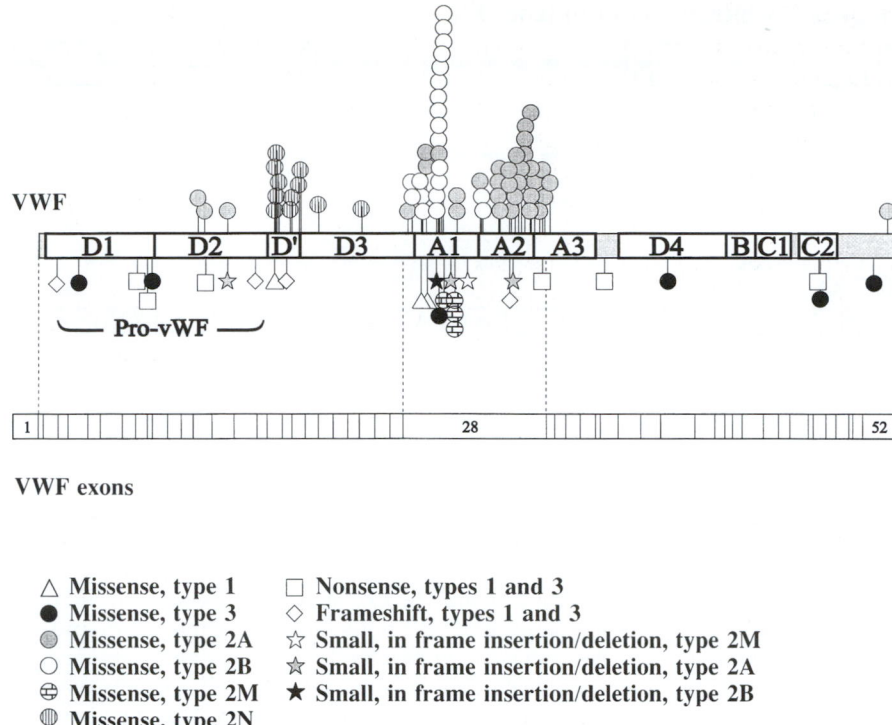

△ Missense, type 1　　□ Nonsense, types 1 and 3
● Missense, type 3　　◇ Frameshift, types 1 and 3
◉ Missense, type 2A　☆ Small, in frame insertion/deletion, type 2M
○ Missense, type 2B　✩ Small, in frame insertion/deletion, type 2A
⊕ Missense, type 2M　★ Small, in frame insertion/deletion, type 2B
⦿ Missense, type 2N

**FIGURE 34.3.** von Willebrand disease mutations. The location of all point mutations and small, in-frame insertions/deletions associated with vWd, as reported to the vWd Database (*http://mmg2.im.med.umich.edu/vWf*), are depicted on the vWf protein. Shown below are all 52 exons, ranging in size from 40 base pairs to 1.4 kilobases (exon 28), of the vWf gene. As seen, the majority of mutations have been identified in exon 28, primarily for vWd types 2A and 2B, which are clustered in specific functional domains. Mutations for vWd type 2N cluster in the D' repeat. (Adapted with permission from Nichols WC, Ginsburg D. von Willebrand disease [review]. Medicine 1997;76:1–20.)

Mannucci et al (65), using the clinical response to DDAVP in addition to the measurement of plasma and platelet vWf. Individuals with the "platelet normal" subtype of type I vWd were found to have normal platelet and decreased plasma vWf, similar to the subtype I-2 described by Weiss et al. These individuals responded to DDAVP with an increase in vWf levels and correction of the bleeding time. Individuals with the "platelet low" subtype were similar to the subtype I-1 of Weiss et al with low plasma and platelet vWf. These individuals did not respond to an infusion of DDAVP. Finally, a group of individuals was identified with decreased plasma and normal platelet vWf levels but with relatively decreased plasma and platelet vWf ristocetin cofactor activities. Multimer analysis of both plasma and platelet vWf revealed a relative decrease in the highest-molecular-weight multimer species, similar to the subgroup Ib defined by Hoyer et al. This group of individuals, referred to as "platelet discordant" by Mannucci et al, demonstrated an increase in vWf antigen after the administration of DDAVP, without correction in the bleeding time (65). Type I "platelet discordant" has been reclassified as type 2A (or type 2M, see below) vWd, because type 1 vWd is constrained to include only purely quantitative disorders, as discussed above (32).

None of these subclassification schemes for type 1 vWd are routinely used in the clinical setting. Because DDAVP does not typically correct the bleeding time in individuals with the "platelet low" and "platelet discordant" subtypes, precise subclassification may eventually obviate the need for a therapeutic DDAVP trial in some type 1 individuals. However, because the response to DDAVP in the setting of type 1 vWd is so variable, DDAVP therapeutic trials should probably be performed in all type 1 individuals prior to the routine use of this drug (see "Treatment of von Willebrand Disease," below) until the predictive value of the type 1 subclassification is confirmed by additional studies. These data also suggest that there may be more than one molecular defect that results in type 1 vWd, a hypothesis that should be addressed by future studies.

## MOLECULAR PATHOGENESIS OF TYPE 1 VON WILLEBRAND DISEASE

Despite the fact that type 1 is the most common form of vWd, little is known about its molecular pathogenesis (72). Linkage analysis of type 1 has been complicated by the variable penetrance as well as the low sensitivity and specificity of available laboratory tests. Restriction fragment length polymorphism (RFLP) analyses of several type 1 pedigrees have been consistent with linkage to the vWf gene, although no single study has reached statistical significance (logarithm of the odds [LOD] score > 3) (73–78). This information suggests that type 1 vWd may be due to a defect within the vWf gene, although a defect in another gene cannot be excluded. As discussed above, the phenotypic heterogeneity of type 1 vWd suggests that more than one molecular mechanism may eventually be identified as the basis for this group of disorders. A subset of vWd type 1 cases are due to heterozygous inheritance of a vWd type 3 defect (see below). Heterozygous carriers of vWf gene deletions, or more subtle defects resulting in loss of vWf mRNA expression, are generally asymptomatic and have normal laboratory values consistent with the autosomal recessive pattern generally ascribed to vWd type 3 (79–83). However, vWd type 1 has been reported in some vWd type 3 heterozygotes, including individuals inheriting nonsense and frameshift mutations (see Fig. 34.3) (84–87).

The reported 1% prevalence for vWd type 1 (35) corresponds to an allele frequency of approximately 0.005, which would translate into a homozygote frequency (i.e., those expected to have type 3 vWd) of 1:40,000. This is much greater than the observed frequency of ~1:1,000,000 for type 3 vWd. This discrepancy could be explained by an overestimation of the prevalence of vWd type 1 or a significant loss of type 3 homozygotes. Alternatively, defects at other genetic loci could potentially result in a vWd phenotype. Linkage analysis in the inbred mouse strain RIIIS/J, an animal model for vWd type 1, has shown that the low vWf level in these mice is not due to a defect at the vWf locus, but rather to a novel locus on mouse chromosome 11 (88, 89).

Although vWf null alleles appear to often be silent in the heterozygote, other defects giving rise to an abnormal vWf protein may result in greater reduction in vWf levels and, thus, symptomatic vWd type 1 in the heterozygote. Eikenboom et al have identified a candidate missense mutation, T3445C, which predicts the substitution of a cysteine residue (Cys386→Arg) known to be part of a disulfide bond (90). Functional studies suggest that this mutation affects secretion of wild-type vWf via involvement of this cysteine in a disulfide bond between vWf monomers, i.e., a dominant-negative mechanism. These same researchers have identified another candidate missense mutation that predicts substitution of Cys367 for Phe, which may act in a similar dominant-negative manner (90). Functional studies have not yet confirmed this hypothesis. In contrast, although heterozygotes for the common vWd type 3 exon 18 frameshift mutation (see below) may have vWd type 1, the misfolded protein does not appear to exert a dominant-negative effect on normal vWf subunits expressed

from the wild-type allele (91). Three additional candidate missense mutations have been identified in individuals with type 1 vWd although functional data have not yet been reported (92) (*http://mmg2.im.med.umich.edu/vWf*).

# TYPE 3 VON WILLEBRAND DISEASE

Type 3 vWd is a severe hemorrhagic disorder manifest by potentially life-threatening episodes of bleeding and the frequent need for blood product support. In addition to more severe mucosal bleeding than commonly encountered in the other forms of vWd, type 3 individuals also suffer from intraarticular and deep tissue bleeding similar to that occurring in individuals with hemophilia A (see Chapter 35). This latter pattern of bleeding is attributed to the markedly decreased factor VIII levels observed in most type 3 individuals. Inheritance is generally autosomal recessive (see below) and the presumably heterozygous parents are typically observed to be phenotypically normal. However, careful laboratory analysis of these obligate heterozygotes has revealed significant heterogeneity (93–95). In one study of 28 obligate heterozygotes for type 3 vWd from 15 unrelated families (93), 11 of 28 individuals were found to have decreased vWf antigen levels and ristocetin cofactor activity in plasma and platelets, 5 of 28 had decreased vWf antigen and ristocetin cofactor activity in plasma but not in platelets, 8 of 28 had decreased vWf antigen and cofactor activity in platelets but not in plasma, and 1 of 28 had all measurements within the normal range. Interestingly, 7 of 28 obligate carriers were found to have mildly prolonged bleeding times and all of these individuals had decreased vWf in plasma and platelets. This variability likely reflects the genetic heterogeneity of type 3 vWd. Similar to other rare recessive human diseases, type 3 individuals sometimes have remote family histories indicating some degree of consanguinity, and these individuals are likely homozygous for the same defective type 3 allele. Several individuals have also been described who appear to be compound heterozygotes for two separate type 3 alleles (76, 80, 81, 96).

## MOLECULAR PATHOGENESIS OF TYPE 3 VON WILLEBRAND DISEASE

Although many type 3 vWd individuals have been screened by Southern blot analysis for gross gene deletions or rearrangements, this seems to be an uncommon mechanism for the disorder (79, 80, 86). Homozygous deletions involving the entire vWf gene have been detected in seven individuals, four from the same family (79, 80). Six vWd type 3 individuals with partial gene deletions have been reported (81, 86, 97), with the smallest being a homozygous deletion for 2.3 kilobases containing exon 42 (81) and the largest a heterozygous deletion for 100 kb at the 3' end of the vWf gene (86). Alloantibodies to vWf have been described in approximately 10% of individuals with severe type 3 vWd. Alloantibodies to transfused vWf developed in 10 of 12 individuals with gene deletions in both alleles (79, 80, 86, 97). In contrast, only one of 47 type 3 vWd individuals with normal Southern blot patterns has had alloantibodies (87, 97). Therefore, although the numbers are small, homozygous vWf gene deletion appears to predispose to alloantibody formation (79). It is possible that small gene deletions may be overlooked by routine Southern blot analysis. The presence of the highly homologous vWf pseudogene on chromosome 22 that duplicates exons 23-34 complicates this analysis, since a heterozygous deletion in this region would result in only a 25% reduction in band intensity (72).

Once gene deletion has been excluded, molecular analysis of type 3 vWd (and type 1 vWd) has been more difficult compared to the type 2 variants (see below) because no specific functional domain can be implicated in this form, and thus, defects may lie anywhere within the approximately 180 kb vWf gene including coding and noncoding regions. Comparative analysis of vWf genomic DNA and platelet vWf mRNA has identified nondeletion defects resulting in complete loss of vWf mRNA expression as a molecular mechanism in some individuals with vWd type 3 (82, 83). A number of nonsense and frameshift mutations that would be predicted to result in loss of vWf protein expression, or expression of a markedly truncated or disrupted protein, have been identified in some type 3 vWd families (see Fig. 34.3) (82, 84, 86, 87, 96, 98) (*http://mmg2.im.med.umich.edu/vWf*). Several vWd type 3 individuals have also been shown to be homozygous or compound heterozygous for missense mutations in the vWf gene (85, 98). The mechanisms whereby these missense mutations confer vWd type 3 are not yet known. Three mutations that result in incorrect splicing of the vWf mRNA have also been identified in three different type 3 families (98, 99) (*http://mmg2.im.med.umich.edu/vWf*).

The most common mutation in vWd type 3 individuals identified to date is a frameshift mutation in exon 18 resulting from a cytosine deletion in a run of six cytosines beginning at nucleotide 2680. In a study of 48 vWf alleles in 24 Swedish vWd type 3 individuals, 50% were shown to carry this mutation (100). This mutation is also common in the German population (86) and has been shown to be the mutation responsible for vWd in the family originally reported by von Willebrand (1, 91, 101). The mutation predicts a protein containing the full vWf propeptide and the first 48 N-terminal amino acids of mature vWf, followed by 30 miscoded residues. Although a frameshift mutation in exon 45 results in an

unstable mRNA (82), this mutation in exon 18 does not alter mRNA expression or stability (91).

## TYPE 3 VON WILLEBRAND DISEASE: HOMOZYGOUS TYPE 1 VON WILLEBRAND DISEASE?

Although type 3 vWd is usually defined as autosomal recessive, this is not a completely consistent finding. Whereas one or both parents of severely affected individuals are frequently clinically asymptomatic and have normal laboratory tests (82, 83), some families have been reported in which one or both parents have classic type 1 vWd (84–87). Thus, in some families, type 3 vWd appears to represent the homozygous form of type 1 vWd, whereas in others it is a true autosomal recessive disorder. Although the apparent recessive inheritance of type 3 in some families may simply result from the incomplete penetrance of type 1 vWd, there may be a fundamental difference in the molecular mechanisms responsible for types 1 and 3 vWd (see vWd type 1 above). There are two distinct animal models of vWd that appear to have different pathogenic mechanisms. Porcine vWd, a severe autosomal recessive bleeding disorder analogous to type 3 vWd, is due to a defect within or near the porcine vWf gene (102). In contrast, the murine model of vWd, described by Sweeney et al, is inherited in an autosomal dominant pattern resembling type 1 human vWd. Interestingly, murine type 1 vWd is a true dominant disorder, with heterozygotes and homozygotes demonstrating a similar mild phenotype (103). As discussed earlier (see type 1 vWd), linkage analysis in the inbred mouse strain RIIIS/J has shown that the low vWf levels in these mice are not due to a defect at the vWf locus, but rather to a novel locus on mouse chromosome 11 (88, 89).

# TYPE 2 VON WILLEBRAND DISEASE

Although no accurate incidence figures are available, type 2 vWd is generally felt to comprise 20 to 30% of all vWd diagnoses (2, 30, 34). Under the new classification system, type 2 vWd includes subtypes 2A, 2B, 2M, and 2N (32, 33). Penetrance of vWd type 2 is generally more complete than for vWd type 1.

## TYPE 2A VON WILLEBRAND DISEASE

Type 2A vWd is the most common qualitative vWd variant, encountered in approximately 5 to 10% of vWd individuals. It is typically transmitted in an autosomal dominant pattern, although recessive inheritance has been described (104). Most individuals have a moderately severe bleeding diathesis characterized by a disproportionately low ristocetin cofactor activity relative to the vWf antigen level and decreased circulating intermediate and high-molecular-weight vWf multimers. In addition, plasma vWf from most individuals with type 2A vWd has a characteristic increase in the small satellite band of each multimer species, as well as an accumulation of a distinct 176 Kd proteolytic fragment of the mature vWf monomer visualized on reducing gels (105).

## MOLECULAR PATHOGENESIS OF TYPE 2A VON WILLEBRAND DISEASE

Evidence supporting the concept that type 2A vWd is due to a defect within the vWf gene was first reported by Verweij et al (106). These investigators established linkage of two vWf RFLPs to type 2A vWd in a 39 member kindred with a LOD score of 5.88. Linkage was similarly demonstrated in an additional type 2A vWd family (107).

Significant heterogeneity has been described among individuals with type 2A vWd (64, 108). Weiss et al (64) originally recognized that platelets from type 2A individuals either contained the full spectrum of vWf multimers or had diminished intermediate and high-molecular-weight multimers similar to that seen in type 2A plasma. Gralnick et al further reported that loss of plasma high-molecular-weight multimers in three individuals with type 2A vWd could be prevented by collection of blood in the presence of protease inhibitors, thus suggesting a role for proteolysis in the pathogenesis of this disease (109). In another study, collection of blood in the presence of protease inhibitors restored the intermediate multimers in some type 2A individuals but not in others (108, 110).

As noted above, an approximately 176 Kda fragment is frequently observed to be increased in the plasma of type 2A individuals. A partial epitope map placed the N-terminus of the 176 Kda fragment between amino acid residues 844 and 947 of the mature protein (111). Because *in vivo* proteolysis had been proposed to be critical in the pathogenesis of type 2A vWd, attention was focused on the apparent protease cleavage site as a potential location for mutations resulting in this disorder. Using PCR to amplify platelet vWf mRNA from individuals with type 2A vWd, Ginsburg et al (112) identified the first two type 2A mutations, Val844→Asp and Arg834→Trp. Subsequently, N-terminal protein sequencing of the 176 Kda subunit, as well as further studies using monoclonal antibodies raised against synthetic peptides constructed from this region, allowed placement of the protease cleavage site, giving rise to the 176 Kda fragment between Tyr842 and Met843 (113). To date, more than 25 point mutations have been identified in a large number of vWd type 2A individuals analyzed, all resulting in single amino acid substitutions (see Figs. 34.2 and 34.3) (107, 112, 114–130) (*http://mmg2.im.med.u-*

*mich.edu/vWf*). Although additional mutations are likely to be identified, the current panel appears to account for the majority of vWd type 2A individuals. All but 9 of these mutations lie within a 134 amino acid segment from Gly742 to Glu875. A number of these mutations have been identified on distinct genetic backgrounds in multiple individuals. The most common mutation, Arg834→Trp, has been identified in 39 vWd type 2A individuals in 15 unrelated families and may account for 1/3 of vWd type 2A (112, 118, 121, 124) (*http://mmg2.im.med.umich.edu/vWf*). In addition to the above point mutations, a duplication of a small segment from Ser589-Ala623 and an in-frame deletion of exons 26–34 have also been reported to result in a type 2A phenotype (131–133).

Expression of mutant vWf sequences by DNA transfection into mammalian cells has provided further important information regarding the pathogenesis of this disorder (112, 117). This work has defined two distinct classes of missense mutations resulting in type 2A vWd (Fig. 34.4). Group 1 mutations result in defective intracellular transport of vWf as demonstrated by transient transfection in tissue culture cells. In contrast, recombinant vWf containing group 2 mutations is normally secreted into the tissue culture medium with the full range of multimers. Analysis of platelet vWf from type 2A individuals suggests that these differences in transport also occur in the megakaryocyte *in vivo* and explain the different platelet vWf patterns originally observed in type 2A vWd by Weiss et al (64). Thus, individuals with group 1 mutations have absent intermediate and high-molecular-weight vWf multimers in platelets, whereas group 2 individuals exhibit the full spectrum of platelet multimers (117) (Fig. 34.5). The absence of high-molecular-weight vWf multimers in the plasma of group 2 individuals is likely the result of *in vivo* proteolysis (54, 108, 109). Dent et al (54) proposed a model for the origin of the type 2A vWf multimer pattern from the single proteolytic cleavage between Tyr842 and Met843. Because there are no intramolecular disulfide bonds bridging this region of the molecule, a single proteolytic cleavage is sufficient to cleave a multimer into two distinct fragments. Recently, a novel protease responsible for cleavage of the peptide bond between Tyr842 and Met843 within the A2-repeat of vWf has been isolated from human plasma in two different laboratories (134, 135). Tsai suggests that some of the mutations responsible for vWd type 2A result in a conformational change in vWf, thus making it more susceptible to cleavage by this novel protease (135).

## RARE TYPE 2A VON WILLEBRAND DISEASE VARIANTS

A number of rare type 2 variants have been reclassified as type 2A (see Table 34.3). These include type IIC, type

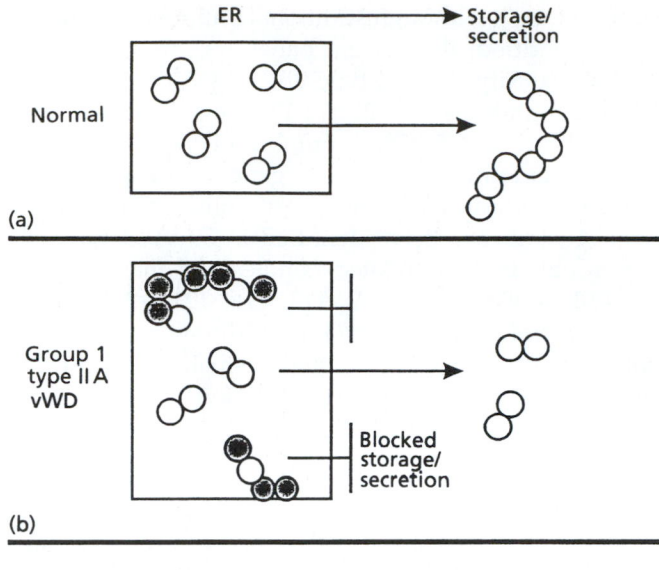

(a)

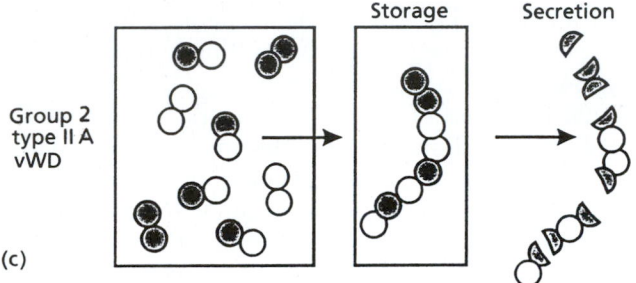

(b)

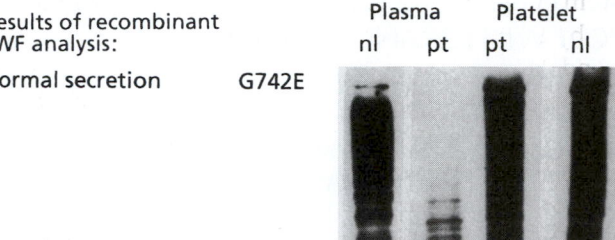

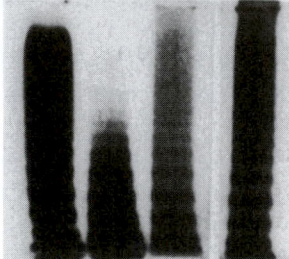

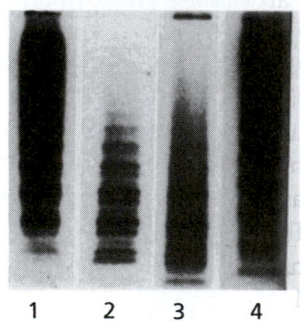

(c)

**FIGURE 34.4.** Schematic of the mechanisms of type 2A vWd. In panel **a,** normal vWf (*white*) is shown forming dimers in the endoplasmic reticulum (ER). The vWf subsequently multimerizes and is secreted into plasma. In panel **b,** mutant vWf containing a group 1 type 2A vWd mutation (*gray*) is shown forming multimers with normal vWf. Multimers containing mutant vWf are retained, whereas multimers containing only normal vWf are secreted into plasma. Because larger multimers have a greater chance of containing mutant vWf monomers, they are preferentially blocked from secretion. Panel **c** illustrates the effect of group 2 type 2A vWd mutations. In this disorder, multimers are stored and secreted normally, but the vWf containing mutant subunits is cleaved by proteases in the plasma. Again, the larger multimers contain more mutant subunits and are preferentially cleaved in the circulation.

IID, type IIE, type IIF, type IIG, and type IIH (28, 136–139). There is a characteristic decrease in the large plasma vWf multimers in individuals with the variant formerly known as type IIC vWd similar to that seen in many of the other type 2 variants (see Fig. 34.1). Additional features of this variant include a relative increase in the fastest migrating multimer band, the absence of satellite bands or triplet structure, and the presence of minor multimer bands in some individuals (136, 140). Studies of several type IIC kindreds have revealed phenotypic heterogeneity both between members of different

kindreds (141, 142) and between individuals in a given family (143). Type IIC has been most often observed to be inherited as an autosomal recessive disorder. However, many or all individuals with type IIC vWd may represent compound heterozygotes, inheriting two unique defective vWf alleles. One allele may result in the specific multimer pattern seen in this variant, with the other allele contributing to a quantitative abnormality in vWf. The

**FIGURE 34.5.** Multimer patterns in plasma and platelets of group 1 (defective transport) and group 2 (normal secretion) type 2A in individuals with vWd. On the left are the results of analysis of recombinant vWf containing the Gly742→Glu (G742E), Gly742→Arg (G742R), and Ser743→Leu (S743L) mutations. Individuals with group 1 or transport defective mutations (G742R and S743L) have decreased or absent intermediate and high-molecular-weight multimers in plasma and platelets. In comparison, individuals with group 2 mutations that result in normal secretion of vWf in COS cells (G742E) have decreased intermediate and high-molecular-weight multimers in plasma but the full spectrum of platelets multimers. *nl*, normal; *pt*, individual. (Adapted with permission from Lyons SE, Bruck ME, Bowie EJ et al. Impaired intracellular transport produced by a subset of type IIA von Willebrand disease mutations. J Biol Chem 1992;267:4424–4430.)

nature of the quantitative defect might thus impact on the specific clinical phenotype and may explain some of the variability seen in this disorder (141, 143). Recent molecular characterization has identified several mutations responsible for this variant in the vWf propeptide (D2-repeat), presumably interfering with proper vWf processing and multimer assembly (119, 144, 145).

Kinoshita et al first described the qualitative vWd variant formerly known as type IID in 1984 (137), and there have now been at least four families described. This dominantly transmitted bleeding disorder is characterized by disproportionately low ristocetin cofactor activity and decreased circulating high molecular weight vWf multimers. However, instead of the usual triplet structure on high resolution agarose gels, a four-band pattern is seen in plasma and in platelets (137, 146, 147). A single mutation (Cys2010→Arg) was recently identified in two unrelated individuals with vWd type IID, and expression studies indicate that this mutation is responsible for defective disulfide bonding of C-terminal domains, thus impairing dimer formation (see Fig. 34.3) (120).

Rare kindreds have been described with unique vWd variants, each characterized by a specific vWf structural abnormality visualized on high resolution agarose gel. In what was formerly type IIE vWd, the individual multimers lack satellite bands, similar to type IIC; however, there is no relative increase in the fastest moving multimer band (56). In type IIF vWd, each plasma vWf multimer contains five, rather than three bands; however, the platelet vWf is structurally normal (138). The single individual with type IIG vWd was found to have absent plasma intermediate and high-molecular-weight vWf multimers. The multimer triplet structure appeared normal, but there was a relative decrease in the intensity of the slowest migrating band compared to the major and fastest migrating band (139). The triplet structure of type IIH vWd is characterized by a broader major and a faster migrating minor band compared to normal plasma vWf (148). The interested reader is referred to the specific original references for detailed descriptions of the unique multimer patterns. It is likely that additional type 2 variants will be described as more individuals are carefully analyzed using high resolution gels to assess specific vWf structural abnormalities. Continued identification of the specific mutations responsible for many of these variants may eventually permit a more biologically consistent and clinically useful subclassification scheme. Although no mutations have yet been identified, vWd type Ib and type I "platelet discordant," both associated with decreased platelet-dependent function and reduction of the large vWf multimers, have also been reclassified as type 2A (34, 64, 65), although type I "platelet discordant" may be more appropriately classified as type 2M since the reduction of the large multimers is very slight (see below).

## TYPE 2B VON WILLEBRAND DISEASE

Type 2B is a unique qualitative vWd variant characterized by increased reactivity of vWf with the platelet receptor GP Ib. Clearance of the resulting vWf-platelet complex leads to thrombocytopenia and the selective loss of the largest vWf multimers from plasma (Fig. 34.6). The original description of type 2B vWd was published in 1980 by Ruggeri et al (149). These authors described 20 individuals from 5 families, each demonstrating enhanced RIPA. Subsequently, numerous individuals with type 2B vWd have been described. These individuals have bleeding disorders of variable severity. The following features, however, appear to be consistent: 1) thrombocytopenia; 2) prolonged bleeding time; 3) low to normal factor VIII:C; 4) low to normal vWf antigen; 5) low ristocetin cofactor activity; 6) decreased high-molecular-weight vWf multimers in plasma but a normal pattern in platelets; and 7) enhanced RIPA. The apparent contradiction between the low ristocetin cofactor activity and enhanced RIPA is explained by the fact that the ristocetin cofactor activity assay is performed at a maximally stimulating dose of 1 mg/mL of ristocetin, and the concentration of vWf, which is reduced in type 2B vWd individuals, becomes the limiting factor. Ristocetin-induced platelet aggregation is examined at several different concentrations of ristocetin and does not depend on the amount of vWf antigen present.

Thrombocytopenia is common in type 2B vWd. In general, the degree of thrombocytopenia is quite mild but pregnancy (150, 151), stress (152), or advanced age (50) can exacerbate it. Type 2B vWd must be distinguished from "pseudo-vWd" or platelet-type vWd,

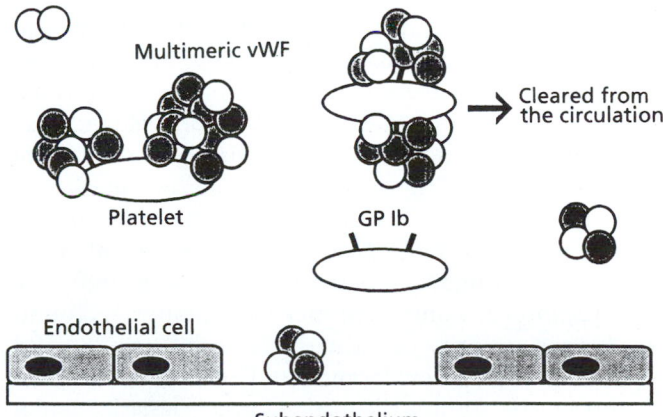

**FIGURE 34.6.** Schematic of type 2B vWd. In type 2B vWd, vWf demonstrates increased reactivity with the platelet receptor GP Ib, which is more marked for the larger vWf multimers. The platelet-vWf complex is subsequently cleared from the circulation resulting in the characteristic loss of high-molecular-weight vWf multimers and thrombocytopenia seen in this disorder.

which is similar in presentation (see Chapter 32) (153–155). Individuals with "pseudo-vWd" have been shown to have a primary platelet defect resulting from mutations in the platelet GP Ib/IX receptor complex (155–157). Platelet-type pseudo vWd and vWd type 2B are distinguished by plasma and platelet mixing experiments between control and individual samples (see below).

## THE MOLECULAR BASIS OF TYPE 2B VON WILLEBRAND DISEASE

It was initially hypothesized that type 2b vWd might be due to a molecular defect in the platelet GP Ib binding domain of vWf. In support of this hypothesis, De Marco et al demonstrated that vWf purified from a individual with type 2B vWd can induce spontaneous platelet aggregation not seen with normal vWf. This spontaneous platelet aggregation was blocked by a monoclonal antibody against platelet GP Ib (158, 159). Furthermore, vWf secreted from type 2B endothelial cells in culture was shown to contain a full range of vWf multimers and to bind spontaneously to platelets (160). Therefore, several groups have analyzed the vWf DNA sequence from individuals with type 2B vWd concentrating on exon 28, which encodes the GP Ib binding domain. Using this approach, 21 missense mutations and one single amino acid insertion have been identified in the vWF A1-repeat containing the glycoprotein Ib (GP Ib) binding domain (161–164) resulting in a unique gain of function (see Figs. 34.2 and 34.3) (116, 128, 130, 165–185) (*http://mmg2.im.med.umich.edu/vWf*). Four of these mutations are particularly common and have arisen independently on multiple genetic backgrounds (167, 168, 175, 176). These four mutations (Arg543→Trp, Arg545→Cys, Val-553→Met, and Arg578→Gln) are clustered within a 35 amino acid stretch and account for more than 80% of vWd type 2B individuals reported to the vWd database (*http://mmg2.im.med.umich.edu/vWf*) (128). Functional analysis of mutant recombinant vWf confirms that these single amino acid substitutions are sufficient to account for increased binding of vWf to GP Ib on the platelet surface, resulting in the characteristic vWd type 2B phenotype of loss of the largest vWf multimers, enhanced RIPA, and thrombocytopenia (170, 178, 186–188). The identification of a limited number of mutations accounting for the majority of individuals with Type 2B vWd should lead to the development of DNA-based diagnostic procedures for this disorder. Correct classification of type 2B vWd may be particularly important because of implications for therapy with DDAVP (see below).

## RARE TYPE 2B VON WILLEBRAND DISEASE VARIANTS

Some rare vWd variants previously classified as type I have been reclassified as vWd type 2B because, despite a normal vWf multimer distribution pattern, they are characterized by enhanced RIPA. These include type I New York, type I Malmö, and type I Sydney (189–191). Type I New York and type I Malmö have been shown to be due to the same substitution of Pro503→Leu located in the same region as the cluster of mutations observed for classic vWd type 2B and resulting in similar increased binding to platelet GP Ib (192).

## TYPE 2M VON WILLEBRAND DISEASE

These variants are characterized by decreased platelet-dependent function that is not caused by absence of the largest vWf multimers (32, 33). Despite normal-sized multimers, the decreased platelet-dependent function indicates the presence of multimers, which are qualitatively abnormal. Most of the vWd type 2M variants were previously classified as type I and include variants with normal multimers, but decreased ristocetin cofactor activity, as well as variants with larger than normal plasma multimers (vWd "Vincenza"), subtle differences from normal multimer structure (types IC and ID), and the presence of large amounts of uncleaved pro-vWf in the multimers (193–198).

von Willebrand disease "Vincenza" was first described in 1988 by Mannucci et al (193). Ten individuals from two families with mild hemostatic defects were described, and each affected family member had reduced vWf antigen and factor VIII:C levels consistent with type I vWd. However, multimer analysis of both plasma and platelet vWf revealed a relative increase in the highest vWf multimer species. The release of "supranormal" vWf multimers has been reported after the administration of DDAVP (199) and in endothelial cell culture systems (200). In addition, these large vWf multimers have also been described in chronic relapsing thrombotic thrombocytopenic purpura (201, 202) (see Chapter 27) and in the plasma of newborns (203).

Lopez-Fernandez et al described the vWd variant that they called type ID vWd. A father and son were reported to have a mild factor XII deficiency as well as laboratory parameters consistent with type 1 vWd, including a prolonged bleeding time. Although plasma and platelet multimers appeared normal on low resolution agarose gels, a distinctive abnormal plasma vWf multimer pattern characterized by decreased satellite bands was seen on high resolution gels. Administration of DDAVP to both of these individuals resulted in the correction of the hemostatic defect, but evidence of possible increased proteolytic degradation was seen on the high resolution gels (195).

In 1985, Ciavarella et al (197) described five individuals from two unrelated families with a mild autosomal dominant inherited bleeding disorder that they termed type IC vWd. The majority of the affected family members had normal vWf antigen levels but decreased ristocetin cofactor activities and prolonged bleeding times. High resolution agarose gel electrophoresis revealed abnormal vWf multimer structure. A DDAVP infusion in two individuals resulted in correction of the vWf antigen levels and normalization of the bleeding times, but the multimer abnormality persisted.

## MOLECULAR BASIS OF TYPE 2M VON WILLEBRAND DISEASE

Several type 2M variants are characterized by decreased ristocetin-induced binding to platelets due to mutations in the GP Ib binding domain of vWf (see Fig. 34.3). Four unrelated individuals with normal vWf multimers and disproportionately low ristocetin cofactor activity were found to have heterozygous mutations in the A1-repeat of vWf: one with a deletion of 11 amino acids (Arg629-Gln639, type 2M:Milwaukee-1) (204), another with a Phe606→Ile substitution (205), and two carrying a deletion of Lys645 (131, 206). A single individual has been described with a form of vWd characterized by normal levels of factor VIII and vWf antigen but undetectable ristocetin cofactor activity (196, 207). The absence of ristocetin cofactor activity could be corrected *in vitro* by the addition of normal plasma, therefore excluding an intrinsic platelet defect (207). Multimer analysis also identified the presence of a unique band not seen in normal plasma vWf (196). Further studies of this individual revealed a normal platelet aggregation response to botrocetin, a protein prepared from snake venom, but no aggregation occurred in the presence of ristocetin. This dissociation between the response to botrocetin and ristocetin appears to be a unique feature of this variant, formerly known as type B vWd. This variant has been shown to be due to a Gly561→Ser substitution also within the A1 domain (208). Hilbert et al have identified two mutations (Arg611→Cys and Arg611→His) in members of three unrelated families with a variant vWd associated with decreased platelet-dependent function and a slight reduction in the high molecular weight vWf multimers (209). The same Arg611→His mutation was also detected in four individuals from two unrelated families classified with the variant previously known as type I "platelet discordant" (210). It is debatable whether these mutations should be classified as type 2M or type 2A. They really fit neither classification as defined by the revised classification, although they are probably more appropriately classified as type 2M, given that the reduction in the largest multimers is slight. Recently, Meyer et al (130) have identified five new mutations in the A1 domain in twelve unrelated individuals with type 2M (or unclassified). Two of these (Gly561→Ala, Arg611→Leu) are at residues already implicated in type 2M. Expression of recombinant vWf containing the substitutions will be necessary for proper classification of the remaining three mutations (Leu513→Pro, Glu596→Lys, Ile662→Phe).

## TYPE 2N VON WILLEBRAND DISEASE

As described in Chapter 35, hemophilia A is due to one of a number of molecular defects in the factor VIII gene. The latter is located on the X chromosome, accounting for the classic X-linked inheritance of this disorder (211). Rare female carriers are affected with mild hemophilia ascribed to unequal lyonization. However, there have been scattered reports in the literature of pedigrees in which hemophilia A appears to be transmitted in an autosomal dominant fashion (212, 213). Several of these individuals were shown to have plasma vWf that is defective in its ability to bind factor VIII (214–216). A potentially similar defect had been identified previously in a group of individuals with type 1 vWd (217). This entity had been called vWd Normandy by Gaucher et al in reference to the province of origin of the first individuals (218). Inherited as an autosomal recessive and sometimes mimicking mild hemophilia A, type 2N vWd is characterized by normal vWf multimers, normal vWf antigen, normal ristocetin cofactor activity, but moderately decreased FVIII activity (generally 5% or less).

## MOLECULAR BASIS OF TYPE 2N VON WILLEBRAND DISEASE

The factor VIII binding domain has been localized to the N-terminus of vWf by studies of proteolytic fragments (see Chapter 16). Epitope-mapping for two anti-vWf monoclonal antibodies that block FVIII/vWf binding suggested a further sublocalization to a region at or near a 19 amino acid segment extending from Thr78 to Thr96 (Fig. 34.2) (219, 220). A DNA sequence analysis in these individuals has identified 11 mutations, all at the N-terminus of vWf in the region of FVIII binding domain (219, 221, 222) (Arg19→Trp, Gly22→Glu, Glu24→Lys, Cys25→Tyr, Thr28→Met, Arg53→Trp, His54→Gln, Arg91→Gln, Cys95→Phe, Asp116→Asn, and Cys297→Arg) (see Figs. 34.2 and 34.3) (86, 128, 130, 216, 223–232) (*http://mmg2.im.med.umich.edu/vWf*). The Arg91→Gln mutation is the most common vWd type 2N mutation accounting for 19 of 28 reported families. In addition, its frequency may be as high as 1% in some populations (92). Expression of recombinant vWf containing each of these mutations confirms the defective FVIII binding (223, 226, 228–230, 233). Interestingly, an amino acid substitution of Gln for Arg at position 89, two amino acids upstream from one of the factor VIII binding mutations, was shown to be a rare sequence polymorphism that did not alter factor VIII binding when expressed in recombinant vWf (228). Type 2N vWd individuals are generally homozygous or compound heterozygous for one of these mutations and present with a mild to moderate hemophilia-like phenotype (216, 227, 234). Although this variant is probably considerably less common than classic hemophilia A, it should be considered in the differential diagnosis of FVIII deficiency, particularly in a female individual, or if other aspects of the pedigree support autosomal recessive inheritance.

In some vWd type 1 individuals, disproportionately low FVIII activity has been noted as compared to vWf antigen and activity. In several cases this has been shown to be due to co-inheritance of vWd type 1 and 2N alleles (86, 92, 225, 228, 230). These results suggest that heterozygosity for a type 2N mutation may contribute to the variable expressivity of vWd type 1, as hypothesized by Eikenboom et al (92). Several individuals carrying a vWd type 2N mutation on one vWf allele and a frameshift mutation on the other allele have been reported (86, 230). A number of symptomatic vWd type 1 individuals have also been shown to be heterozygous for Arg91→Gln, the most common type 2N mutation (92, 225, 228).

# ACQUIRED VON WILLEBRAND DISEASE

There have been at least 50 reported cases in the literature of acquired vWd, sometimes referred to as von Willebrand syndrome. It has been associated with a variety of underlying pathologic conditions (Table 34.5), but a number of common features can be delineated. Typically, individuals develop mucocutaneous bleeding and are found to have a prolonged bleeding time, decreased plasma vWf antigen, and normal plate-

let vWf antigen. Cases consistent with type 1 vWd, demonstrating reduction of all plasma vWf multimers, as well as type 2 vWd, with relative decrease in the high-molecular-weight multimer forms, have been described. Given the high prevalence of vWd, the diagnosis of acquired vWd should only be made in a individual with no prior history of mucocutaneous bleeding and with a negative family history for hemorrhagic diatheses.

There are several distinct pathophysiologic mechanisms responsible for acquired vWd leading to the variable clinical presentation of this disorder and differing responses to therapy. A number of individuals with circulating antibodies directed against vWf have been described (235–238). Several of these antibodies have been shown to inhibit RIPA by vWf (235, 237), whereas others appear to lack significant inhibitory activity (236, 238). The latter antibodies are although to form complexes with vWf *in vivo*, resulting in rapid clearance from plasma by the reticuloendothelial system (236). Most reported cases of antibody-mediated acquired vWd have occurred in individuals with multiple myeloma (239), monoclonal gammopathies (236, 237, 240, 241), or lymphoproliferative disorders (235, 241). However, at least one individual has been described with gastrointestinal telangectasia and acquired vWd with an inhibitory antibody to vWf (242).

Budde et al (243, 244) explored the role of proteolysis in the development of acquired vWd. Individuals with acquired vWd associated with a myeloproliferative disorder were noted to have decreased circulating intermediate and high-molecular-weight vWf multimers, similar to individuals with type 2A vWd. These individuals were also noted to have an alteration in vWf triplet structure, with a relative increase in the fastest migrating satellite band (244). This finding was confirmed in three additional acquired vWd individuals, and felt to be consistent with increased proteolysis (243). However, Budde et al concluded that, although proteolysis likely contributes to the development of acquired vWd in individuals with myeloproliferative syndromes, other mechanisms should also be considered (243).

Several individuals with solid tumors have been described with acquired vWd that often improves with treatment of the underlying neoplasm. Inhibitors to vWf are typically not detected and the mechanism of vWd in these individuals remains unclear. Adherence of vWf to the malignant neoplasm has been proposed (245), although in one individual with Wilm's tumor no specific tumor adsorption could be demonstrated (246). Others have hypothesized that Wilm's tumors secrete a plasma factor that interacts with vWf, resulting in clearance of vWf from the circulation (247). Adherence of large vWf multimers to endothelial cells

---

**TABLE 34.5.**    Causes of Acquired von Willebrand Disease

**Plasma cell diseases**
  Multiple myeloma
  Monoclonal gammopathy
**Lymphoma**
**Myeloproliferative disorders**
  Essential thrombocythemia
  Polycythemia vera
**Angiodysplasia**
**Wilm's tumor**
**Congenital cardiac defects**
**Uremia**
**Hypothyroidism**
**Drugs (valproic acid)**
**Systemic lupus erythematosus**

or activated platelets has also been suggested as the mechanism of acquired vWd associated with noncyanotic congenital cardiac abnormalities, such as ventricular septal defects and aortic stenosis (248). Four of five individuals described had normalization of their vWf multimers after corrective surgery, and the fifth individual was found to have a residual pressure gradient across a previous pulmonary artery banding site.

Acquired vWd has also been associated with uremia. Several groups (249–252) have investigated the role of vWf in the development of uremic bleeding (see Chapter 33). Kazatchkine initially reported high vWf antigen levels in individuals with chronic renal failure but decreased ristocetin cofactor activity (250). This was not confirmed by others (249) and in two studies, vWf antigen and ristocetin cofactor activity appear to be elevated in individuals with renal failure (249, 252). However, there has been a report of two individuals with renal failure on hemodialysis who were evaluated for the new onset of mucocutaneous bleeding (individual 1) and a prolonged aPTT (individual 2). Neither individual had a prior history of hemorrhagic symptoms or a family history of bleeding problems. Individual 1 had a laboratory evaluation consistent with "platelet discordant" or type Ib vWd and individual 2 was found to have increased plasma high molecular weight vWf multimers consistent with vWd "Vincenza" (253). Thus, although uremic bleeding cannot generally be attributed to abnormalities in vWf, forms of acquired vWd may develop in the face of chronic renal failure.

There is a well-described association between hypothyroidism and acquired vWd (254–257). The diagnosis of acquired vWd can precede the recognition of hypothyroidism by months or can be discovered by routine laboratory analysis during the evaluation of hypothyroidism. Acquired vWd in this setting typically resolves with thyroid hormone replacement. The mechanism of hypothyroidism-associated vWd is unclear. It is postulated to result from decreased protein synthesis, although alterations in adrenergic activity have also been proposed (258). Decreased synthesis of other coagulation factors may also be contributory. Thus, bleeding may be more severe than that predicted based on vWf and factor VIII levels alone.

Only one drug currently available, valproic acid, has been associated with the development of vWd. Kreuz et al reported that in a series of 30 children treated with valproic acid for seizures, 19 gave a history of new mucocutaneous bleeding and 7 had prolonged bleeding times. Laboratory evaluation of these individuals appeared to be most consistent with type 1 vWd. Replacement therapy was recommended, if necessary, rather than DDAVP, because one individual given DDAVP developed seizures (259).

# VON WILLEBRAND DISEASE AND OTHER ASSOCIATED DISEASES

## von WILLEBRAND DISEASE AND ATHEROSCLEROSIS

The relationship between vWd and atherogenesis was first noted in the porcine model of vWd, which is analogous to type 3 vWd in humans. Pigs affected with vWd have been described to be resistant to both spontaneous and diet-induced coronary atherosclerosis (260), however there appears to be no protection against atherogenesis in heterozygous animals (261). Furthermore, the risk of coronary and aortic plaque formation appears to differ among vWd pigs (262), perhaps due to the influence of other genetic factors (29). However, severe porcine vWd does seem to afford protection from thrombosis in a vessel-injury model (263). Interestingly, Nichols et al (264) reported the association of a polymorphism within the apolipoprotein B100 gene with the development of dietary-induced hypercholesterolemia and atherosclerosis in the pig model independent of the vWd genotype.

The risk of atherosclerosis in humans with vWd has never been definitively addressed. In 1984, Mannucci et al (46) established a registry of 154 individuals from 137 families with severe vWd with the goal of performing a prospective epidemiologic study addressing the risk of atherogenesis in these individuals. Potential problems in this study, as identified by its authors, were the relatively young age of the individuals and the role of vWf transfusion. Some have suggested that the potential protective effect of vWd against atherosclerotic vascular disease may exert selective pressure and, thus, contribute to the high prevalence of vWd in the population. However, because most vascular disease occurs late in life, any selective advantage would probably be more than counterbalanced by even a mild increase in hemorrhagic risk.

## von WILLEBRAND DISEASE, HEREDITARY HEMORRHAGIC TELANGECTASIA, AND MITRAL VALVE PROLAPSE

Associations between vWd and various mesenchymal disorders have been described since the early 1960s. There have been reports of several families whose members are affected with both vWd and hereditary hemorrhagic telangectasia (HHT) (265, 266). Hereditary hemorrhagic telangectasia is an inherited disorder characterized by excessive bleeding from fragile, angiodysplastic blood vessels (see Chapter 43). The simultaneous occurrence of these two diseases suggested a common pathogenetic mechanism, perhaps resulting from defective endothelial cells. Potential linkage of the HHT locus to the vWf gene (located on the short arm of chromosome 12[15]) was examined in a study by Iannuzzi et al (107). Two large families, one with vWd and HHT and one with HHT alone were studied. Linkage of HHT to the vWf gene was not detected in either family. Subsequently, linkage studies have identified at least three HHT loci: on chromosome 9, the long arm of chromosome 12, and an as-yet unmapped locus (267). The mutated genes have been identified on chromosomes 9 and 12. Both *endoglin* on chromosome 9 and *ALK1* (activin receptor-like kinase) on chromosome 12 encode a transmembrane protein expressed on endothelial cells (267). Any association between vWd and HHT has yet to be explained, although vWd may act as a modifier of the HHT phenotype.

A relationship between mitral valve prolapse and vWd was suggested in 1981 by Pickering et al (268). This association, however, has not been confirmed by other investigators. Kuhsel et al reported that the incidence of mitral valve prolapse in individuals with vWd was 5.3% and not statistically different from that of the normal population (269).

# ANIMAL MODELS OF VON WILLEBRAND DISEASE

## PORCINE von WILLEBRAND DISEASE

Animal models are valuable resources for the study of human disease. The first animal model of vWd was identified in 1941 by Hogan et al (270), who described a hemorrhagic disorder affecting Poland/China swine in Missouri. These animals were noted to suffer from spontaneous hemorrhages as well as excessive bleeding after traumatic injury. The disease affected animals of both sexes and appeared to be recessively inherited (271). The swine were demonstrated to have very low factor VIII levels and infusion of plasma resulted in a sustained rise in the factor VIII level similar to that seen in human vWd (see above) (272). More recent analysis of these pigs has confirmed the near absence of vWf in plasma and platelets (less than 1%), analogous to type 3 vWd in humans (273). The molecular defect resulting in porcine vWd is unknown, but appears to lie within the vWf gene (102).

This porcine model has been used to study the role of plasma and platelet vWf in hemostasis. In 1976, Webster et al (274) successfully performed orthotopic liver transplants on two pigs with vWd. Correction of plasma vWf and factor VIII levels, as well as bleeding times, was achieved presumably via transplantation of endothelial cells releasing normal vWf. Transplantation of normal porcine bone marrow into a pig with vWd resulted in

delayed and variable correction of the bleeding time despite the presence of platelets containing normal amounts of vWf (275). Thus, the porcine model provides an important tool in the analysis of each of these vWf compartments in hemostasis.

## OTHER ANIMAL MODELS OF von WILLEBRAND DISEASE

von Willebrand disease has been recognized in more than 40 species of purebred dogs as well as in cats and rabbits (273). Both quantitative and qualitative forms of canine vWd have been described (276). As already discussed, Sweeney et al have described a murine model that closely resembles type 1 vWd in humans (103). Linkage analysis in the inbred mouse strain RIIIS/J has shown that the low vWf levels in these mice are not due to a defect at the vWf locus, but rather to a novel locus on mouse chromosome 11 (88, 89).

# TREATMENT OF VON WILLEBRAND DISEASE

Accurate diagnosis and subclassification is important for the optimal choice of therapy in vWd. The treatment options in the management of vWd can be divided into two groups, namely replacement and nonreplacement therapy (see Table 34.6). All forms of currently available replacement therapy carry some risk of viral transmission (277). Thus, initial treatment approaches should maximize the use of nonreplacement options, wherever possible.

Individual education can play an important role in the long term management of vWd. Because many of the bleeding problems in these individuals occur after medical procedures, communication between the surgeon/dentist and the hematologist should be encouraged. Individuals should also be cautioned about the use of over-the-counter medications containing aspirin

---

**TABLE 34.6.**    Treatment of von Willebrand Disease[1]

**Nonreplacement therapy**
  DDAVP
  Estrogens
  Antifibrinolytic agents
**Replacement therapy**
  Cryoprecipitate
  Factor VIII concentrates
  Platelet transfusions

[1] *Refer to Chapters 51–53 for specific regimens.*

or nonsteroidal anti-inflammatory drugs due to the inhibition of platelet function by these agents (278).

Additionally, individuals should be familiar with the diagnosis of vWd and especially the genetic risk of transmission to offspring. Formal genetic counseling may be useful for certain individuals with vWd, particularly those with severe or type 3. Prenatal testing by DNA analysis or fetal blood sampling has been performed on types 1, 2A, 2B, and 3 vWd individuals (73, 74, 279, 280). DNA analysis has typically been performed by genetic linkage analysis using the highly polymorphic variable number tandem repeat in intron 40 of the vWf gene, although specific point mutations for some subtypes can also be detected. Given the potential for locus heterogeneity, or defects in genes other than the vWf gene resulting in vWd, caution should be taken in interpreting linkage results.

## 1-DEAMINO 8-D-ARGININE VASOPRESSIN (SEE CHAPTER 53)

1-Deamino 8-D-arginine vasopressin is a synthetic analog of vasopressin that was originally produced for the treatment of diabetes insipidus. Because DDAVP had been shown to increase vWf antigen, factor VIII:C and ristocetin cofactor activity levels in individuals with vWd and mild hemophilia, Mannucci et al performed the first successful therapeutic trial of this agent in 1977 with the goal of decreasing the requirement for blood products (281). Subsequently, DDAVP has become widely used for the treatment of both vWd and mild hemophilia A (282–284). The mode of action of DDAVP is still unknown. Addition of DDAVP to cultured human endothelial cells has no effect on vWf synthesis or secretion and is presumed to act via an as-yet-unknown second messenger.

1-Deamino 8-D-arginine vasopressin is typically administered in the intravenous form at a dose of 0.2–0.4 µg/kg in 50 mL saline over 15 to 30 minutes (285). A rise in vWf antigen, factor VIII:C and ristocetin cofactor activity usually occurs within 30 minutes after infusion and generally lasts for 6 or more hours (283, 286). Recently, an intranasal preparation of DDAVP (concentration 1.5 mg/mL, 0.1 mL per application) has become available, and it may be as effective as the intravenous form (287, 288). An oral form has also recently become available, but has not yet been tested in vWd individuals. The most common side effects of DDAVP include headache, flushing, angioedema, hypotension, and mild tachycardia. These symptoms are attributed to the vasomotor effects of the drug and can often be attenuated by slowing the rate of infusion. The expected incidence of hyponatremia and volume overload due to the antidiuretic effects of the drug appears to be quite low. However, the drug should be used with caution in individuals receiving significant amounts of intravenous fluids

or general anesthesia (289). The most serious complication of DDAVP administration is the risk of thrombosis (256, 290). There have been reports of myocardial infarction (291) and stroke (290) after the use of DDAVP in elderly individuals with significant underlying atherosclerotic vascular disease. This drug should therefore be used with caution in such individuals. The other significant problem with this agent is tachyphylaxis, although this can be lessened by once-daily instead of twice-daily infusions (283, 292–294).

1-Deamino 8-D-arginine vasopressin is most effective in the management of individuals with vWd type 1. Approximately 80% of type 1 individuals respond to DDAVP therapy, and it has been suggested that the ''platelet normal'' pattern may be a useful indicator of favorable response (65, 193, 295). A trial infusion should be performed prior to therapeutic use (294). For type 1 vWd individuals undergoing surgical procedures DDAVP is generally administered at 12-hour intervals.

Approximately 20 to 25% of individuals with vWd do not respond to DDAVP. This includes many of the type 2 variants, individuals with vWd type 3, and individuals with type 1 ''platelet low'' (65). Response to DDAVP therapy is variable in vWd type 2A. Complete hemostatic correction, including the presence of high molecular weight multimers, has been reported in some type 2A individuals. However, in most the response is very transient, and the vWf multimer pattern either does not change significantly or rapidly reverts to the typical type 2A pattern (282, 296). Favorable response to DDAVP may be associated with group 2 mutations, although this hypothesis has not yet been tested. Many experts consider DDAVP to be contraindicated in type 2B vWd, although this view is controversial (297, 298). The release of high molecular weight vWf multimers with increased affinity for GP Ib might exacerbate the spontaneous platelet aggregation and thrombocytopenia (299). Nonetheless, a number of vWd type 2B individuals have been treated successfully with DDAVP without apparent complications (297, 298). Therapy of vWd type 2B with cryoprecipitate or FVIII concentrates (see below) has been effective. 1-Deamino 8-D-arginine vasopressin therapy is of limited utility for vWd type 2N. Although DDAVP increases plasma vWf levels in these individuals, it does not significantly increase FVIII activity levels owing to the inability of the mutant vWf to bind FVIII (300).

## OTHER NONREPLACEMENT THERAPIES FOR von WILLEBRAND DISEASE (SEE CHAPTER 53)

There are several adjunctive therapies that can be used in the management of vWd. Antifibrinolytic agents are often administered after dental procedures to prevent clot lysis since the involved tissues have high fibrinolytic activity (30). The two most commonly used drugs, ε-aminocaproic acid (EACA; Amicar) and *trans-p-aminomethyl-cyclohexanecarboxylic acid* (AMCA; tranexamic acid; Amstat), block the activity of plasmin. Drugs that inhibit the fibrinolytic system may carry a significant risk of thrombosis in individuals with an underlying prothrombotic state, such as disseminated intravascular coagulation (DIC). They are also considered relatively contraindicated in the management of genitourinary bleeding.

Estrogens (see Chapter 53) have been shown to increase vWf levels, although the response is variable and unpredictable. This effect is although to be due to direct endothelial cell stimulation, because estrogen added to endothelial cells in culture has been shown to increase the synthesis of vWf (301). Women with chronic bleeding, particularly menorrhagia, can sometimes be managed with the use of oral estrogens (278). There has also been one report describing the successful use of preoperative estrogen therapy in individuals with type 1 vWd. Three women, each previously requiring plasma or cryoprecipitate to control bleeding, underwent a major surgical procedure without the need for replacement therapy after taking estrogens (either conjugated estrogens or oral contraceptive drugs) preoperatively, followed by 5 mg/day of conjugated estrogens postoperatively for a period of 2 weeks (302).

## REPLACEMENT THERAPY (SEE CHAPTER 52)

For the group of individuals who are unresponsive to DDAVP or for whom DDAVP therapy is contraindicated, the treatment of choice is factor replacement (303, 304). Until recently, cryoprecipitate was the product of choice. However, several purified FVIII concentrates have been shown to be effective. Because these products are heat treated or detergent treated to inactivate viruses including HIV and hepatitis, they are the products currently preferred by most experts. It is important to note that most standard FVIII concentrates are not effective for vWd. Only preparations that contain large quantities of vWf of normal multimer structure are useful as replacement therapy. In a recent survey of an international registry on the treatment of vWd individuals unresponsive to DDAVP, the use of 11 different FVIII concentrates was reported (303). The two most frequently used concentrates were Hemate P (available in the United States) and VHP vWf concentrate. The latter contains low FVIII activity levels and is more properly considered a vWf concentrate. Both of these concentrates have been reported to contain vWf multimers similar in size to those found in normal plasma (304, 305). Whereas most FVIII concentrates in this group seem to be equally effective in correction of the FVIII activity, the effect of concentrates on the bleeding time is variable.

Therapy is largely empiric and is often determined by the response to prior treatments. In instances of serious bleeding or major surgical interventions, treatment may have to be repeated at least once a day. Unfortunately, no clear guidelines have been established for monitoring response. In general, there is a correlation between normal hemostasis and correction of the bleeding time and FVIII activity. Although the bleeding time and FVIII activity are often used to monitor a individual's response to therapy, the value of each of these indicators is unproven. Individuals with thrombocytopenia may also need transfusions of platelets in addition to factor replacement. It is generally recommended that individuals be treated for 7 to 10 days after major surgical procedures and for 3 to 5 days after minor procedures. Postpartum hemorrhage can occur for up to a month or more after delivery, and therapy in this setting may need to be prolonged.

Because most forms of therapy for vWd correct only the plasma vWf levels, attention has been focused on platelet transfusion (see Chapter 51) as a means of correcting deficiencies of platelet vWf that also occur in this disease. It has been suggested that individuals with type 1 vWd "platelet normal" may have shorter bleeding times and respond better to DDAVP than do individuals with the other type 1 subtypes (63, 65). Furthermore, vWf replacement therapy does not always correct the bleeding time in individuals with severe vWd (306). Castillo et al administered cryoprecipitate to five individuals with type 3 vWd and found that, despite correction of the vWf antigen, factor VIII, and ristocetin cofactor activity, bleeding times remained prolonged. However, platelet transfusion performed 1 hour after cryoprecipitate infusion fully corrected the bleeding time, suggesting a role for platelet transfusions in type 3 vWd individuals (307). Because platelet transfusions carry a risk of viral transmission like other blood products, this therapy should be reserved only for type 3 individuals with severe bleeding refractory to standard replacement therapy.

## TREATMENT OF vWf ANTIBODIES

Antibodies against vWf occur in approximately 5 to 10% of individuals with severe vWd, as well as in acquired vWd. Alloantibodies associated with severe vWd can be extremely difficult to manage because many are precipitating antibodies (289). In general, vWf replacement should be avoided in this setting because severe and potentially life threatening reactions to replacement have been reported. These severe reactions have been attributed to the presence of complement-fixing immune complexes (308, 309). Others have described the successful use of pure factor VIII preparations containing much less vWf of a smaller multimeric composition (310).

In the setting of acquired vWd, several other treatment modalities have been used. Antibodies against vWf associated with lymphoproliferative disorders are often improved with treatment of the underlying disease. Corticosteroid therapy, with or without the use of cytotoxic immunosuppressive therapy, has also been tried. In refractory cases, high-dose intravenous gamma-globulin (311, 312), plasma exchange (313), or extracorporeal immunoadsorption (314) can also be considered.

# PREGNANCY IN VON WILLEBRAND DISEASE

In most, but not all, individuals with vWd, vWf antigen and factor VIII levels rise during pregnancy, presumably due to alterations in the hormonal milieu (315, 316). This increase does not occur until the eleventh week of gestation. Therefore, individuals are at risk for serious bleeding during spontaneous abortions occurring during the first trimester (317). Because improvement in the vWf and factor VIII levels during pregnancy is variable, individuals should be monitored closely throughout pregnancy and for several months after delivery when levels fall precipitously. Late hemorrhage has been described, presumably due to this latter phenomenon (316, 318). It has been suggested that normalization of the factor VIII level is the most critical factor determining the risk of bleeding complications during delivery. Abnormalities in primary hemostasis, as reflected by the prolonged bleeding time, may be managed with careful surgical technique. Vaginal deliveries are usually determined to be safe if the factor VIII level is higher 50 U/dL at the time of delivery. A factor VIII level less than 30 U/dL is generally indicative of the need for replacement therapy during delivery (315, 317). Individuals with type 2B vWd have been reported to develop more severe thrombocytopenia during pregnancy. This is presumably due to increased levels of defective plasma vWf binding to platelets, with subsequent clearance of the complexes from the circulation (150, 151, 319). Although it is not clear whether this degree of thrombocytopenia truly exacerbates clinical bleeding, infusion of Hemate-P has been shown to correct the low platelet counts seen in Type 2B vWd individuals during pregnancy (319).

# REFERENCES

1. von Willebrand EA. Hereditär Pseudohemofili. Finska Läkarsällskapetes Handl 1926;67:7–112.
2. Nilsson IM. In memory of Erik Jorpes. von Willebrand's disease from 1926-1983. Scand J Haematol Suppl 1984;40:21–43.
3. Nilsson IM. von Willebrand's disease–Fifty years old. Acta Med Scand 1977;201:497–508.
4. Mammen EF. von Willebrand's disease—History, diagnosis and management. Semin Thromb Hemost 1975;2:61–84.
5. Hoyer LW. von Willebrand's disease [Review]. Prog Hemost Thromb 1976;3:231–287.
6. Bowie EJ, Didisheim P, Thompson JH Jr et al. von Willebrand's disease: A critical review. Hematologic Reviews 1968;1:1–50.
7. Holmberg L, Nilsson IM. von Willebrand's disease. Annu Rev Med 1975; 26:33–44.
8. Alexander B, Goldstein R. Dual hemostatic defect in pseudohemophilia. J Clin Invest 1953;32:551.
9. Nilsson IM, Blombäck M, Jorpes E et al. v Willebrand's disease and its correction with human plasma fraction 1-0. Acta Med Scand 1957;159: 179–188.
10. Nilsson IM, Blombäck M, Blombäck B. von Willebrand's disease in Sweden: Its pathogenesis and treatment. Acta Med Scand 1959;164:263–278.
11. Cornu P, Larrieu MJ, Caen J et al. Transfusion studies in von Willebrand's disease: Effect on bleeding time and factor VIII. Br J Haematol 1963;9: 189–202.
12. Larrieu MJ, Caen JP, Meyer DO et al. Congenital bleeding disorders with long bleeding time and normal platelet count. Am J Med 1968;45:354–372.
13. Gitschier J, Wood WI, Goralka TM et al. Characterization of the human factor VIII gene. Nature 1984;312:326–330.
14. Toole JJ, Knopf JL, Wozney JM et al. Molecular cloning of a cDNA encoding human antihaemophilic factor. Nature 1984;312:342–347.
15. Ginsburg D, Handin RI, Bonthron DT et al. Human von Willebrand factor (vWf): Isolation of complementary DNA (cDNA) clones and chromosomal localization. Science 1985;228:1401–1406.
16. Lynch DC, Zimmerman TS, Collins CJ et al. Molecular cloning of cDNA for human von Willebrand factor: Authentication by a new method. Cell 1985;41:49–56.
17. Sadler JE, Shelton-Inloes BB, Sorace JM et al. Cloning and characterization of two cDNAs coding for human von Willebrand factor. Proc Natl Acad Sci U S A 1985;82:6394–6398.
18. Verweij CL, de Vries CJ, Distel B et al. Construction of cDNA coding for human von Willebrand factor using antibody probes for colony-screening and mapping of the chromosomal gene. Nucleic Acids Res 1985;13: 4699–4717.
19. Zimmerman TS, Ratnoff OD, Powell AE. Immunologic differentiation of classic hemophilia (factor VIII deficiency) and von Willebrand disease, with observations on combined deficiencies of antihemophilic factor and proaccelerin (factor V) and on an acquired circulating anticoagulant against antihemophilic factor. J Clin Invest 1971;50:244–254.
20. Weiss HJ, Phillips LL, Rosner W. Separation of sub-units of antihemophilic factor (AHF) by agarose gel chromatography. Thromb Diath Haemorrh 1972;27:212–219.
21. Rick ME, Hoyer LW. Immunologic studies of antihemophilic factor (AHF, Factor VIII). V. Immunologic properties of AHF subunits produced by salt dissociation. Blood 1973;42:737–747.
22. Zimmerman TS, Edgington TS. Factor VIII coagulant activity and factor VIII-like antigen: Independent molecular entities. J Exp Med 1973;138: 1015–1020.
23. Baugh R, Brown J, Sargeant R et al. Separation of human factor VIII activity from the von Willebrand's antigen and ristocetin platelet aggregating activity. Biochim Biophys Acta 1974;371:360–367.
24. Howard MA, Firkin BG. Ristocetin–A new tool in the investigation of platelet aggregation. Thromb Diath Haemorrh 1971;26:362–369.
25. Weiss HJ, Rogers J, Brand H. Defective ristocetin-induced platelet aggregation in von Willebrand's disease and its correction by factor VIII. J Clin Invest 1973;52:2697–2707.
26. Weiss HJ, Hoyer LW, Rickles FR et al. Quantitative assay of a plasma factor deficient in von Willebrand's disease that is necessary for platelet aggregation. Relationship to factor VIII procoagulant activity and antigen content. J Clin Invest 1973;52:2708–2716.
27. Marder VJ, Mannucci PM, Firkin BG et al. Standard nomenclature for factor VIII and von Willebrand factor: A recommendation by the International Committee on Thrombosis and Haemostasis. Thromb Haemost 1985;54:871–872.
28. Ruggeri ZM, Zimmerman TS. von Willebrand factor and von Willebrand disease [Review]. Blood 1987;70:895–904.
29. Bloom AL. von Willebrand factor: Clinical features of inherited and acquired disorders [Review]. Mayo Clin Proc 1991;66:743–751.
30. Holmberg L, Nilsson IM. von Willebrand Disease. Clin Haematol 1985; 14:461–488.
31. Berkowitz SD, Ruggeri ZM, Zimmerman TS. von Willebrand Disease. In: Zimmerman TS, Ruggeri ZM, eds. Coagulation and bleeding disorders. The role of factor VIII and von Willebrand factor. New York: Marcel Dekker, 1989;215–259.
32. Sadler JE. A revised classification of von Willebrand disease. For the Subcommittee on von Willebrand Factor of the Scientific and Standardization Committee of the International Society on Thrombosis and Haemostasis. Thromb Haemost 1994;71:520–525.
33. Sadler JE, Gralnick HR. Commentary: A new classification for von Willebrand disease. Blood 1994;84:676–679.
34. Hoyer LW, Rizza CR, Tuddenham EG et al. von Willebrand factor multimer patterns in von Willebrand's disease. Br J Haematol 1983;55:493–507.
35. Rodeghiero F, Castaman G, Dini E. Epidemiological investigation of the prevalence of von Willebrand's disease. Blood 1987;69:454–459.

36. Miller CH, Lenzi R, Breen C. Prevalence of von Willebrand's disease among US adults [Abstract]. Blood 1987;70(Suppl):377a.
37. Werner EJ, Broxson EH, Tucker EL et al. Prevalence of von Willebrand disease in children: A multiethnic study [Abstract]. Blood 1991;78(Suppl): 68a.
38. Meriane F, Sultan Y, Arabi H et al. Incidence of a low von Willebrand factor activity in a population of Algerian students [Abstract]. Blood 1991; 78(Suppl):484a.
39. Miller CH, Graham JB, Goldin LR et al. Genetics of classic von Willebrand's disease. I. Phenotypic variation within families. Blood 1979;54: 117–145.
40. Gill JC, Endres-Brooks J, Bauer PJ et al. The effect of ABO blood group on the diagnosis of von Willebrand disease. Blood 1987;69:1691–1695.
41. Orstavik KH, Kornstad L, Reisner H et al. Possible effect of secretor locus on plasma concentration of factor VIII and von Willebrand factor. Blood 1989;73:990–993.
42. Triplett DA. Laboratory diagnosis of von Willebrand's disease [Review]. Mayo Clin Proc 1991;66:832–840.
43. Rickles FR, Hoyer LW, Rick ME et al. The effects of epinephrine infusion in individuals with von Willebrand's disease. J Clin Invest 1976;57: 1618–1625.
44. Takeuchi M, Nagura H, Kaneda T. DDAVP and epinephrine–induced changes in the localization of von Willebrand factor antigen in endothelial cells of human oral mucosa. Blood 1988;72:850–854.
45. Hampton KK, Grant PJ, Primrose J et al. Haemostatic responses and vasopressin release during colonoscopy in man. Clin Sci (Colch) 1991;81: 257–260.
46. Mannucci PM, Bloom AL, Larrieu MJ et al. Atherosclerosis and von Willebrand factor. I. Prevalence of severe von Willebrand's disease in western Europe and Israel. Br J Haematol 1984;57:163–169.
47. Weiss HJ, Ball AP, Mannucci PM. Incidence of severe von Willebrand's disease [Letter]. N Engl J Med 1982;307:127.
48. Silwer J. von Willebrand's disease in Sweden. Acta Paediatr Scand Suppl 1973;238:1–159.
49. Abildgaard CF, Suzuki Z, Harrison J et al. Serial studies in von Willebrand's disease: Variability versus "variants." Blood 1980;56:712–716.
50. Mazurier C, Parquet-Gernez A, Goudemand J et al. Investigation of a large kindred with type IIB von Willebrand's disease, dominant inheritance and age-dependent thrombocytopenia. Br J Haematol 1988;69:499–505.
51. Zimmerman TS, Hoyer LW, Dickson L et al. Determination of the von Willebrand's disease antigen (factor VIII-related antigen) in plasma by quantitative immunoelectrophoresis. J Lab Clin Med 1975;86:152–159.
52. Girma JP, Ardaillou N, Meyer D et al. Fluid-phase immunoradiometric assay for the detection of qualitative abnormalities of factor VIII/von Willebrand factor in variants of von Willebrand's disease. J Lab Clin Med 1979;93:926–939.
53. Weis JW, Nelson D. Factor VIII-related antigen in variant von Willebrand's disease [Letter]. Thromb Res 1984;33:457–459.
54. Dent JA, Galbusera M, Ruggeri ZM. Heterogeneity of plasma von Willebrand factor multimers resulting from proteolysis of the constituent subunit. J Clin Invest 1991;88:774–782.
55. Lynch DC, Zimmerman TS, Ling EH et al. An explanation for minor multimer species in endothelial cell-synthesized von Willebrand factor. J Clin Invest 1986;77:2048–2051.
56. Zimmerman TS, Dent JA, Ruggeri ZM et al. Subunit composition of plasma von Willebrand factor. Cleavage is present in normal individuals, increased in IIA and IIB von Willebrand disease, but minimal in variants with aberrant structure of individual oligomers (types IIC, IID, and IIE). J Clin Invest 1986;77:947–951.
57. Harker LA, Slichter SJ. The bleeding time as a screening test for evaluation of platelet function. N Engl J Med 1972;287:155–159.
58. Rodgers RP. Bleeding time tables. A tabular summary of pertinent literature. Semin Thromb Hemost 1990;16:21–138.
59. Rodgers RP, Levin J. A critical reappraisal of the bleeding time. Semin Thromb Hemost 1990;16:1–20.
60. Weiss HJ. Letter: Relation of the von Willebrand factor to the bleeding time. N Engl J Med 1974;291:420.
61. Anonymous. Spectrum of von Willebrand's Disease: A study of 100 cases. Italian Working Group. Br J Haematol 1977;35:101–112.
62. Ratnoff OD, Bennett B. Clues to the pathogenesis of bleeding in von Willebrand's disease. N Engl J Med 1973;289:1182–1183.
63. Gralnick HR, Rick ME, McKeown LP et al. Platelet von Willebrand factor: An important determinant of the bleeding time in type I von Willebrand's disease. Blood 1986;68:58–61.
64. Weiss HJ, Piétu G, Rabinowitz R et al. Heterogeneous abnormalities in the multimeric structure, antigenic properties, and plasma-platelet content of factor VIII/von Willebrand factor in subtypes of classic (type I) and variant (type IIA) von Willebrand's disease. J Lab Clin Med 1983;101: 411–425.
65. Mannucci PM, Lombardi R, Bader R et al. Heterogeneity of type I von Willebrand disease: Evidence for a subgroup with an abnormal von Willebrand factor. Blood 1985;66:796–802.
66. Rodeghiero F, Castaman G, Ruggeri M et al. The bleeding time in normal subjects is mainly determined by platelet von Willebrand factor and is independent from blood group. Thromb Res 1992;65:605–615.
67. Rodeghiero F, Castaman G, Tosetto A. von Willebrand factor antigen is less sensitive than ristocetin cofactor for the diagnosis of type I von Willebrand disease—Results based on a epidemiological investigation. Thromb Haemost 1990;64:349–352.
68. Sadler JE. von Willebrand disease. In: Scriver CR, Beaudet AL, Sly WS, Valle D, eds. The metabolic basis of inherited disease. 7th ed. New York: McGraw-Hill, 1995;3269–3287.
69. Gralnick HR, Ginsburg D. von Willebrand disease. In: Beutler E, Lichtman MA, Coller BS, Kipps TJ, eds. Williams hematology. 5th ed. McGraw-Hill, 1994;1458–1480.
70. Nichols WC, Ginsburg D. von Willebrand disease [Review]. Medicine 1997;76:1–20.
71. Holmberg L, Nilsson IM. von Willebrand's disease [Review]. Eur J Haematol 1992;48:127–141.
72. Ginsburg D, Bowie EJ. Molecular genetics of von Willebrand disease [Review]. Blood 1992;79:2507–2519.
73. Standen GR, Bignell P, Bowen DJ et al. Family studies in von Willebrand's disease by analysis of restriction fragment length polymorphisms and an intragenic variable number tandem repeat (VNTR) sequence. Br J Haematol 1990;76:242–249.
74. Bignell P, Standen GR, Bowen DJ et al. Rapid neonatal diagnosis of von Willebrand's disease by use of the polymerase chain reaction [Letter]. Lancet 1990;336:638–639.
75. Bernardi F, Guerra S, Patracchini P et al. von Willebrand disease investigated by two novel RFLPs. Br J Haematol 1988;68:243–248.
76. Bahnak BR, Lavergne JM, Verweij CL et al. Carrier detection in severe (type III) von Willebrand disease using two intragenic restriction fragment length polymorphisms. Thromb Haemost 1988;60:178–181.
77. Peake IR, Bowen D, Bignell P et al. Family studies and prenatal diagnosis in severe von Willebrand disease by polymerase chain reaction amplification of a variable number tandem repeat region of the von Willebrand factor gene [Abstract]. Blood 1990;76:555–561.
78. Caekebeke-Peerlinck KM, Bakker E, Briët E. An infrequent DNA polymorphism associated with severe von Willebrand's disease. Br J Haematol 1990;75:78–81.
79. Shelton-Inloes BB, Chehab FF, Mannucci PM et al. Gene deletions correlate with the development of alloantibodies in von Willebrand disease. J Clin Invest 1987;79:1459–1465.
80. Ngo KY, Glotz VT, Koziol JA et al. Homozygous and heterozygous deletions of the von Willebrand factor gene in individuals and carriers of severe von Willebrand disease. Proc Natl Acad Sci U S A 1988;85: 2753–2757.
81. Peake IR, Liddell MB, Moodie P et al. Severe type III von Willebrand's disease caused by deletion of exon 42 of the von Willebrand factor gene: Family studies that identify carriers of the condition and a compound heterozygous individual. Blood 1990;75:654–661.
82. Eikenboom JC, Ploos van Amstel HK, Reitsma PH et al. Mutations in severe, type III von Willebrand's disease in the Dutch population: Candidate missense and nonsense mutations associated with reduced levels of von Willebrand factor messenger RNA. Thromb Haemost 1992;68: 448–454.
83. Nichols WC, Lyons SE, Harrison JS et al. Severe von Willebrand disease due to a defect at the level of von Willebrand factor mRNA expression: Detection by exonic PCR-restriction fragment length polymorphism analysis. Proc Natl Acad Sci U S A 1991;88:3857–3861.
84. Bahnak BR, Lavergne JM, Rothschild C et al. A stop codon in a individual with severe, type III, von Willebrand disease [Letter]. Blood 1991;78: 1148–1149.
85. Zhang Z, Lindstedt M, Blombäck M et al. Effects of the mutant von Willebrand factor gene in von Willebrand disease. Hum Genet 1995;96:388–394.
86. Schneppenheim R, Krey S, Bergmann F et al. Genetic heterogeneity of severe von Willebrand disease type III in the German population. Hum Genet 1994;94:640–652.
87. Zhang ZP, Lindstedt M, Falk G et al. Nonsense mutations of the von Willebrand factor gene in individuals with von Willebrand disease type III and type I. Am J Hum Genet 1992;51:850–858.
88. Nichols WC, Cooney KA, Mohlke KL et al. von Willebrand disease in the RIIIS/J mouse is caused by a defect outside of the von Willebrand factor gene. Blood 1995;83:3225–3231.
89. Mohlke KL, Nichols WC, Westrick RJ et al. A novel modifier gene of plasma von Willebrand factor level maps to distal mouse chromosome II. Proc Natl Acad Sci U S A 1996;93:15352–15357.
90. Eikenboom JC, Matsushita T, Reitsma PH et al. Dominant type 1 von Willebrand disease caused by mutated cysteine residues in the D3 domain of von Willebrand factor. Blood 1996;88:2433–2441.
91. Mohlke KL, Nichols WC, Rehemtulla A et al. A common frameshift mutation in von Willebrand factor does not alter mRNA stability but interferes with normal propeptide processing. Br J Haematol 1996;95:184–191.
92. Eikenboom JC, Reitsma PH, Peerlinck KM et al. Recessive inheritance of von Willebrand's disease type I. Lancet 1993;341:982–986.
93. Mannucci PM, Lattuada A, Castaman G et al. Heterogeneous phenotypes

of platelet and plasma von Willebrand factor in obligatory heterozygotes for severe von Willebrand disease. Blood 1989;74:2433–2436.

94. Sultan Y, Simeon J, Caen JP. Detection of heterozygotes in both parents of homozygous individuals with von Willebrand's disease. J Clin Pathol 1975;28:309–316.

95. Fischer RR, Lerner C, Bandinelli E et al. Inheritance and prevalence of von Willebrand's disease severe form in a Brazilian population. J Inherit Metab Dis 1989;12:293–301.

96. Zhang ZP, Falk G, Blombäck M et al. Identification of a new nonsense mutation in the von Willebrand factor gene in individuals with von Willebrand disease type III. Hum Mol Genet 1992;1:61–62.

97. Mancuso DJ, Tuley EA, Castillo R et al. Characterization of partial gene deletions in type III von Willebrand disease with alloantibody inhibitors. Thromb Haemost 1994;72:180–185.

98. Zhang ZP, Blombäck M, Egberg N et al. Characterization of the von Willebrand factor gene (VWF) in von Willebrand disease type III individuals from 24 families of Swedish and Finnish origin. Genomics 1994;21:188–193.

99. Mertes G, Ludwig M, Finkelnburg B et al. A G+3-to-T donor splice site mutation leads to skipping of exon 50 in von Willebrand factor mRNA. Genomics 1994;24:190–191.

100. Zhang ZP, Falk G, Blombäck M et al. A single cytosine deletion in exon 18 of the von Willebrand factor gene is the most common mutation in Swedish vWd type III individuals. Hum Mol Genet 1992;1:767–768.

101. Zhang ZP, Blombäck M, Nyman D et al. Mutations of von Willebrand factor gene in families with von Willebrand disease in the Åland Islands. Proc Natl Acad Sci U S A 1993;90:7937–7940.

102. Bahou WF, Bowie EJ, Fass DN et al. Molecular genetic analysis of porcine von Willebrand disease: tight linkage to the von Willebrand factor locus. Blood 1988;72:308–313.

103. Sweeney JD, Novak EK, Reddington M et al. The RIIIS/J inbred mouse strain as a model for von Willebrand disease. Blood 1990;76:2258–2265.

104. Asakura A, Harrison J, Gomperts E et al. Type IIA von Willebrand disease with apparent recessive inheritance. Blood 1987;69:1419–1420.

105. Ruggeri ZM, Zimmerman TS. The complex multimeric composition of factor VIII/von Willebrand factor. Blood 1981;57:1140–1143.

106. Verweij CL, Quadt R, Briët E et al. Genetic linkage of two intragenic restriction fragment length polymorphisms with von Willebrand's disease type IIA. J Clin Invest 1988;81:1116–1121.

107. Iannuzzi MC, Hidaka N, Boehnke ML et al. Analysis of the relationship of von Willebrand disease (vWd) and hereditary hemorrhagic telangiectasia and identification of a potential type IIA vWd mutation (IIe865 to Thr). Am J Hum Genet 1991;48:757–763.

108. Batlle J, Lopez-Fernandez MF, Campos M et al. The heterogeneity of type IIA von Willebrand's disease: Studies with protease inhibitors. Blood 1986;68:1207–1212.

109. Gralnick HR, Williams SB, McKeown LP et al. In vitro correction of the abnormal multimeric structure of von Willebrand factor in type IIA von Willebrand's disease. Proc Natl Acad Sci U S A 1985;82:5968–5972.

110. Kunicki TJ, Montgomery RR, Schullek J. Cleavage of human von Willebrand factor by platelet calcium-activated protease. Blood 1985;65:352–356.

111. Berkowitz SD, Dent J, Roberts J et al. Epitope mapping of the von Willebrand factor subunit distinguishes fragments present in normal and type IIA von Willebrand disease from those generated by plasmin. J Clin Invest 1987;79:524–531.

112. Ginsburg D, Konkle BA, Gill JC et al. Molecular basis of human von Willebrand disease: Analysis of platelet von Willebrand factor mRNA. Proc Natl Acad Sci U S A 1989;86:3723–3727.

113. Dent JA, Berkowitz SD, Ware J et al. Identification of a cleavage site directing the immunochemical detection of molecular abnormalities in type IIA von Willebrand factor. Proc Natl Acad Sci U S A 1990;87:6306–6310.

114. Lavergne JM, Ribba AS, Bahnak BR et al. The use of denaturing gradient gel electrophoresis to detect base changes in the von Willebrand factor gene from Type IIA von Willebrand disease individuals [Abstract]. Thromb Haemost 1991;65:738.

115. Gaucher C, Hanss M, Dechavanne M et al. Substitution of fysteine for phenylalanine 751 in mature von Willebrand factor is a novel candidate mutation in a family with type IIA von Willebrand disease. Br J Haematol 1993;83:94–99.

116. Piétu G, Ribba AS, Cherel G et al. Epitope mapping by cDNA expression of a monoclonal antibody which inhibits the binding of von Willebrand factor to platelet glycoprotein IIb-IIIa. Biochem J 1992;284 (Pt 3):711–715.

117. Lyons SE, Bruck ME, Bowie EJ et al. Impaired intracellular transport produced by a subset of type IIA von Willebrand disease mutations. J Biol Chem 1992;267:4424–4430.

118. Inbal A, Seligsohn U, Kornbrot N et al. Characterization of three mutations causing von Willebrand disease type IIA in five unrelated families. Thromb Haemost 1992;67:618–622.

119. Schneppenheim R, Thomas KB, Krey S et al. Identification of a candidate missense mutation in a family with von Willebrand disease type IIC. Hum Genet 1995;95:681–686.

120. Schneppenheim R, Brassard J, Krey S et al. Defective dimerization of von Willebrand factor subunits due to a Cys?Arg mutation in type IID von Willebrand disease. Proc Natl Acad Sci U S A 1996;93:3581–3586.

121. Sugiura I, Matsushita T, Tanimoto M et al. Three distinct candidate point mutations of the von Willebrand factor gene in four individuals with type IIA von Willebrand disease. Thromb Haemost 1992;67:612–617.

122. Inbal A, Englender T, Kornbrot N et al. Identification of three candidate mutations causing type IIA von Willebrand disease using a rapid, non-radioactive allele-specific hybridization method. Blood 1993;82:830–836.

123. Donnér M, Kristoffersson AC, Berntorp E et al. Two new candidate mutations in type IIA von Willebrand's disease (Arg834?Gly,Gly846?Arg) and one polymorphism (Tyr821?Cys) in the A2 region of the von Willebrand factor. Eur J Haematol 1993;51:38–44.

124. Bowen DJ, Standen GR, Bignell P et al. A C-T transition in the gene for von Willebrand factor effects the replacement of ARG 1597 (CGG) with TRP (TGG) in affected members of a family with type IIA von Willebrand's disease [Abstract]. Br J Haematol 1990;76(Suppl 1):36.

125. Hilbert L, Gaucher C, Si P et al. Expression of type 2A von Willebrand disease mutations. Identification of a new mutation: L817P [Abstract]. Br J Haematol 1996;93(Suppl 2):17.

126. Winter PC, Mayne EE. Type IIA von Willebrand's disease associated with A C to T point mutation at nucleotide 4789 of the von Willebrand factor gene [Abstract]. Blood 1992;(Suppl 1) 80:496a.

127. Chang HY, Chen YP, Chediak JR et al. Molecular analysis of von Willebrand factor produced by endothelial cell strains from individuals with type IIA von Willebrand disease [Abstract]. Blood 1989;74(Suppl):482a.

128. Ginsburg D, Sadler JE. von Willebrand disease: A database of point mutations, insertions, and deletions. For the Consortium on von Willebrand Factor Mutations and Polymorphisms, and the Subcommittee on von Willebrand Factor of the Scientific and Standardization Committee of the International Society on Thrombosis and Haemostasis [Review]. Thromb Haemost 1993;69:177–184.

129. Hagiwara T, Inaba H, Yoshida S et al. A novel mutation Gly 1672?Arg in type 2A and a homozygous mutation in type 2B von Willebrand disease. Thromb Haemost 1996;76:253–257.

130. Meyer D, Fressinaud E, Gaucher C et al. Gene defects in 150 unrelated French cases with type 2 von Willebrand disease: From the individual to the gene. Thromb Haemost 1997;78:451–456.

131. Gaucher C, Hilbert L, Meriane F et al. Type 2 von Willebrand disease resulting from an insertion or deletion in the 509-695 disulphide loop of von Willebrand factor [Abstract]. Thromb Haemost 1995;73:1168.

132. Bernardi F, Patracchini P, Gemmati D et al. In-frame deletion of von Willebrand factor A domains in a dominant type of von Willebrand disease. Hum Mol Genet 1993;2:545–548.

133. Bernardi F, Marchetti G, Guerra S et al. A de novo and heterozygous gene deletion causing a variant of von Willebrand disease. Blood 1990;75:677–683.

134. Furlan M, Robles R, Lämmle B. Partial purification and characterization of a protease from human plasma cleaving von Willebrand factor to fragments produced by in vivo proteolysis. Blood 1996;87:4223–4234.

135. Tsai HM. Physiologic cleavage of von Willebrand factor by a plasma protease is dependent on its conformation and requires calcium ion. Blood 1996;87:4235–4244.

136. Ruggeri ZM, Nilsson IM, Lombardi R et al. Aberrant multimeric structure of von Willebrand factor in a new variant of von Willebrand's disease (type IIC). J Clin Invest 1982;70:1124–1127.

137. Kinoshita S, Harrison J, Lazerson J et al. A new variant of dominant type II von Willebrand's disease with aberrant multimeric pattern of factor VIII-related antigen (type IID). Blood 1984;63:1369–1371.

138. Mannucci PM, Lombardi R, Federici AB et al. A new variant of type II von Willebrand disease with aberrant multimeric structure of plasma but not platelet von Willebrand factor (type IIF). Blood 1986;68:269–274.

139. Gralnick HR, Williams SB, McKeown LP et al. A variant of type II von Willebrand disease with an abnormal triplet structure and discordant effects of protease inhibitors on plasma and platelet von Willebrand factor structure. Am J Hematol 1987;24:259–266.

140. Mannucci PM, Lombardi R, Pareti FI et al. A variant of von Willebrand's disease characterized by recessive inheritance and missing triplet structure of von Willebrand factor multimers. Blood 1983;62:1000–1005.

141. Mazurier C, Mannucci PM, Parquet-Gernez A et al. Investigation of a case of subtype IIC von Willebrand disease: Characterization of the variability of this subtype. Am J Hematol 1986;22:301–311.

142. Batlle J, Lopez Fernandez MF, Fernandez Villamor A et al. Multimeric pattern discrepancy between platelet and plasma von Willebrand factor in type IIC von Willebrand disease. Am J Hematol 1986;22:87–88.

143. Batlle J, Lopez Fernandez MF, Lasierra J et al. Von Willebrand disease type IIC with different abnormalities of von Willebrand factor in the same sibship. Am J Hematol 1986;21:177–188.

144. Gaucher C, Dieval J, Mazurier C. Characterization of von Willebrand factor gene defects in two unrelated individuals with type IIC von Willebrand disease. Blood 1994;84:1024–1030.

145. Gaucher C, Mazurier C. Phenotype IIC von Willebrand disease: The expression of three mutant recombinant von Willebrand factors (VWF) confirms the importance of the D2 domain of VWF propeptide in the

multimer assembly process [Abstract]. Br J Haematol 1996;93(Suppl 2): 15–16.

146. Exner T, Hill P, Cleland J et al. Studies on an unusual von Willebrand's variant–type IID. Aust N Z J Med 1990;20:553–557.

147. Hill FG, Enayat MS, George AJ. Investigation of a kindred with a new autosomal dominantly inherited variant type von Willebrand's disease (possible type IID). J Clin Pathol 1985;38:665–670.

148. Federici AB, Mannucci PM, Lombardi R et al. Type IIH von Willebrand disease: New structural abnormality of plasma and platelet von Willebrand factor in a individual with prolonged bleeding time and borderline levels of ristocetin cofactor activity. Am J Hematol 1989;32:287–293.

149. Ruggeri ZM, Pareti FI, Mannucci PM et al. Heightened interaction between platelets and factor VIII/von Willebrand factor in a new subtype of von Willebrand's disease. N Engl J Med 1980;302:1047–1051.

150. Rick ME, Williams SB, Sacher RA et al. Thrombocytopenia associated with pregnancy in a individual with type IIB von Willebrand's disease. Blood 1987;69:786–789.

151. Giles AR, Hoogendoorn H, Benford K. Type IIB von Willebrand's disease presenting as thrombocytopenia during pregnancy. Br J Haematol 1987; 67:349–353.

152. Hultin MB, Sussman II. Postoperative thrombocytopenia in type IIB von Willebrand disease. Am J Hematol 1990;33:64–68.

153. Weiss HJ, Meyer D, Rabinowitz R et al. Pseudo-von Willebrand's disease. An intrinsic platelet defect with aggregation by unmodified human factor VIII/von Willebrand factor and enhanced adsorption of its high-molecular-weight multimers. N Engl J Med 1982;306:326–333.

154. Miller JL, Castella A. Platelet-type von Willebrand's disease: Characterization of a new bleeding disorder. Blood 1982;60:790–794.

155. Miller JL. Platelet-type von Willebrand disease. Thromb Haemost 1996; 75:865–869.

156. Miller JL, Cunningham D, Lyle VA et al. Mutation in the gene encoding the á chain of platelet glycoprotein Ib in platelet-type von Willebrand disease. Proc Natl Acad Sci U S A 1991;88:4761–4765.

157. Russell SD, Roth GJ. A mutation in the platelet glycoprotein (GP) Ib alpha gene associated with pseudo-von Willebrand disease [Abstract]. Blood 1991;1114(Suppl):281a.

158. De Marco L, Girolami A, Zimmerman TS et al. Interaction of purified type IIB von Willebrand factor with the platelet membrane glycoprotein Ib induces fibrinogen binding to the glycoprotein IIb-IIIa complex and initiates aggregation. Proc Natl Acad Sci U S A 1985;82:7424–7428.

159. De Marco L, Mazzucato M, De Roia D et al. Distinct abnormalities in the interaction of purified types IIA and IIB von Willebrand factor with the two platelet binding sites, glycoprotein complexes Ib-IX and IIb-IIIa. J Clin Invest 1990;86:785–792.

160. de Groot PG, Federici AB, de Boer HC et al. von Willebrand factor synthesized by endothelial cells from a individual with type IIB von Willebrand disease supports platelet adhesion normally but has an increased affinity for platelets. Proc Natl Acad Sci U S A 1989;86:3793–3797.

161. Mohri H, Fujimura Y, Shima M et al. Structure of the von Willebrand factor domain interacting with glycoprotein Ib. J Biol Chem 1988;263: 17901–17904.

162. Mohri H, Yoshioka A, Zimmerman TS et al. Isolation of the von Willebrand factor domain interacting with platelet glycoprotein Ib, heparin, and collagen and characterization of its three distinct functional sites. J Biol Chem 1989;264:17361–17367.

163. Vicente V, Houghten RA, Ruggeri ZM. Identification of a site in the alpha-chain of platelet glycoprotein-Ib that participates in von Willebrand factor binding. J Biol Chem 1990;265:274–280.

164. Sugimoto M, Mohri H, McClintock RA et al. Identification of discontinuous von Willebrand factor sequences involved in complex formation with botrocetin. A model for the regulation of von Willebrand factor binding to platelet glycoprotein Ib. J Biol Chem 1991;266:18172–18178.

165. Donnér M, Andersson AM, Kristoffersson AC et al. An Arg545—Cys545 substitution mutation of the von Willebrand factor in type IIB von Willebrand's disease. Eur J Haematol 1991;47:342–345.

166. Hilbert L, Gaucher C, de Romeuf C et al. Identification of "new" type 2B von Willebrand disease mutations: R543Q, R545P and R578L [Abstract]. Br J Haematol 1996;94(Suppl 2):310.

167. Lillicrap D, Murray EW, Benford K et al. Recurring mutations at CpG dinucleotides in the region of the von Willebrand factor gene encoding the glycoprotein Ib binding domain, in individuals with type IIB von Willebrand's disease. Br J Haematol 1991;79:612–617.

168. Cooney KA, Nichols WC, Bruck ME et al. The molecular defect in type IIB von Willebrand disease. Identification of four potential missense mutations within the putative GP Ib binding domain. J Clin Invest 1991;87: 1227–1233.

169. Murray EW, Giles AR, Lillicrap D. Recurring mutations at CpG dinucleotides and germ line mosaicism in the von Willebrand factor (vWf) gene as a cause of type IIB von Willebrand's disease (vWd) [Abstract]. Am J Hum Genet 1991;49:4:199.

170. Randi AM, Jorieux S, Tuley EA et al. Recombinant von Willebrand factor Arg578?Gln. A type IIB von Willebrand disease mutation affects binding

171. Liu X, Scott JP, Mancuso DJ et al. Substitution of Pro or Glu for Arg578 of von Willebrand factor (vWf) differentially affects vWf interaction with platelets [Abstract]. Blood 1992;(Suppl 1) 80:368a.

172. Ribba AS, Lavergne JM, Bahnak BR et al. Duplication of a methionine within the glycoprotein Ib binding domain of von Willebrand factor detected by denaturing gradient gel electrophoresis in a individual with Type IIB von Willebrand disease. Blood 1991;78:1738–1743.

173. Hilbert L, Gaucher C, Mazurier C. Effects of different amino acid substitutions in the leucine 694-proline 708 segment of recombinant von Willebrand factor. Br J Haematol 1995;91:983–990.

174. Hilbert L, Gaucher C, de Romeuf C et al. Leu697?Val mutation in mature von Willebrand factor is responsible for type IIB von Willebrand disease. Blood 1994;83:1542–1550.

175. Murray EW, Giles AR, Lillicrap D. Germ-line mosaicism for a valine-to-methionine substitution at residue 553 in the glycoprotein Ib-binding domain of von Willebrand factor, causing type IIB von Willebrand disease. Am J Hum Genet 1992;50:199–207.

176. Randi AM, Rabinowitz I, Mancuso DJ et al. Molecular basis of von Willebrand disease type IIB. Candidate mutations cluster in one disulfide loop between proposed platelet glycoprotein Ib binding sequences. J Clin Invest 1991;87:1220–1226.

177. Piao YC, Lavergne JM, Boyer-Neumann C et al. Arg578Gln mutations in the von Willebrand factor gene in three unrelated cases of type IIB von Willebrand disease. Blood Coagul Fibrinolysis 1993;4:787–789.

178. Kroner PA, Kluessendorf ML, Scott JP et al. Expressed full-length von Willebrand factor containing missense mutations linked to type IIB von Willebrand disease shows enhanced binding to platelets. Blood 1992;79: 2048–2055.

179. Ware J, Dent JA, Azuma H et al. Identification of a point mutation in type IIB von Willebrand disease illustrating the regulation of von Willebrand factor affinity for the platelet membrane glycoprotein Ib-IX receptor. Proc Natl Acad Sci U S A 1991;88:2946–2950.

180. Rabinowitz I, Randi AM, Shindler KS et al. Type IIB mutation His505?Asp implicates a new segment in the control of von Willebrand factor binding to platelet glycoprotein Ib. J Biol Chem 1993;268:20497–20501.

181. Holmberg L, Donner M, Dahlbäck B et al. Apparently recessive IIB von Willebrand disease (vWd) is caused by de novo mutations (ARG543?TRP; VAL551?LEU) [Abstract]. Blood 1991;78(Suppl 1):150a.

182. Sugiura I, Matsushita T, Tanimoto M et al. The molecular defects in Japanese individuals with type II von Willebrand disease [Abstract]. Thromb Haemost 1991;65:763.

183. Donnér M, Kristoffersson AC, Lenk H et al. Type IIB von Willebrand's disease: Gene mutations and clinical presentation in nine families from Denmark, Germany and Sweden. Br J Haematol 1992;82:58–65.

184. Eikenboom JC, Vink T, Briët E et al. Multiple substitutions in the von Willebrand factor gene that mimic the pseudogene sequence. Proc Natl Acad Sci U S A 1994;91:2221–2224.

185. Wood N, Standen GR, Bowen DJ et al. UHG-based mutation screening in type 2B von Willebrand's disease: detection of a candidate mutation Ser547Phe. Thromb Haemost 1996;75:363–367.

186. Cooney KA, Lyons SE, Ginsburg D. Functional analysis of a type IIB von Willebrand disease missense mutation: increased binding of large von Willebrand factor multimers to platelets. Proc Natl Acad Sci U S A 1992; 89:2869–2872.

187. Ribba AS, Voorberg J, Meyer D et al. Characterization of recombinant von Willebrand factor corresponding to mutations in type IIA and type IIB von Willebrand disease. J Biol Chem 1992;267:23209–23215.

188. Ichinose A, Espling ES, Takamatsu J et al. Two types of abnormal genes for plasminogen in families with a predisposition for thrombosis. Proc Natl Acad Sci U S A 1991;88:115–119.

189. Wylie B, Gibson J, Uhr E et al. von Willebrand's disease characterized by increased ristocetin sensitivity and the presence of all von Willebrand factor multimers in plasma: A new subtype. Pathology 1988;20:62–63.

190. Holmberg L, Berntorp E, Donner M et al. von Willebrand's disease characterized by increased ristocetin sensitivity and the presence of all von Willebrand factor multimers in plasma. Blood 1986;68:668–672.

191. Weiss HJ, Sussman II. A new von Willebrand variant (type I, New York): Increased ristocetin-induced platelet aggregation and plasma von Willebrand factor containing the full range of multimers. Blood 1986;68: 149–156.

192. Holmberg L, Dent JA, Schneppenheim R et al. von Willebrand factor mutation enhancing interaction with platelets in individuals with normal multimeric structure. J Clin Invest 1993;91:2169–2177.

193. Mannucci PM, Lombardi R, Castaman G et al. von Willebrand disease "Vicenza" with larger-than-normal (supranormal) von Willebrand factor multimers. Blood 1988;71:65–70.

194. Montgomery RR, Dent J, Schmidt W et al. Hereditary persistence of circulating pro von Willebrand factor (pro-vWf) [Abstract]. Circulation 1986; 74(Suppl II):II-406–II-406.

195. Lopez-Fernandez MF, Gonzalez-Boullosa R, Blanco-Lopez MJ et al. Abnormal proteolytic degradation of von Willebrand factor after desmopressin

to glycoprotein Ib but not to collagen or heparin. J Biol Chem 1992;267: 21187–21192.

infusion in a new subtype of von Willebrand disease (ID). Am J Hematol 1991;36:163–170.

196. Howard MA, Salem HH, Thomas KB et al. Variant von Willebrand's disease type B–revisited. Blood 1982;60:1420–1428.

197. Ciavarella G, Ciavarella N, Antoncecchi S et al. High-resolution analysis of von Willebrand factor multimeric composition defines a new variant of type I von Willebrand disease with aberrant structure but presence of all size multimers (type IC). Blood 1985;66:1423–1429.

198. Rabinowitz I, Mancuso DJ, Tuley EA et al. von Willebrand disease (vWd) type B, a variant with absent ristocetin- but normal botrocetin-cofactor activity, is caused by a missense mutation in the GP Ib binding domain of von Willebrand factor (vWf) [Abstract]. Blood 1991;78(Suppl 1):179a.

199. Ruggeri ZM, Mannucci PM, Lombardi R et al. Multimeric composition of factor VIII/von Willebrand factor following administration of DDAVP: Implications for pathophysiology and therapy of von Willebrand's disease subtypes. Blood 1982;59:1272–1278.

200. Sporn LA, Marder VJ, Wagner DD. Inducible secretion of large, biologically potent von Willebrand factor multimers. Cell 1986;46:185–190.

201. Moake JL, McPherson PD. Abnormalities of von Willebrand factor multimers in thrombotic thrombocytopenic purpura and the hemolytic-uremic syndrome. Am J Med 1989;87:9N–15N.

202. Moake JL, Rudy CK, Troll JH et al. Unusually large plasma factor VIII: von Willebrand factor multimers in chronic relapsing thrombotic thrombocytopenic purpura. N Engl J Med 1982;307:1432–1435.

203. Weinstein MJ, Blanchard R, Moake JL et al. Fetal and neonatal von Willebrand factor (vWf) is unusually large and similar to the vWf in individuals with thrombotic thrombocytopenic purpura. Br J Haematol 1989;72:68–72.

204. Mancuso DJ, Kroner PA, Christopherson PA et al. Type 2M:Milwaukee-1 von Willebrand disease: An in-frame deletion in the Cys509-Cys695 loop of the von Willebrand factor A1 domain causes deficient binding of von Willebrand factor to platelets. Blood 1996;88:2559–2568.

205. Mancuso DJ, Montgomery RR, Adam P. The identification of a candidate mutation in the von Willebrand factor gene of individuals with a variant form of type I von Willebrand disease [Abstract]. Blood 1991;78(Suppl 1):67a.

206. Jenkins PV, Ononye C, Collins PW et al. Dominant type 1 von Willebrand's disease as a result of a deletion of a single codon in exon 28 of the VWF gene [Abstract]. Br J Haematol 1996;93(Suppl 2):310.

207. Firkin B, Firkin F, Stott L. von Willebrand's disease type B: A newly defined bleeding diathesis. Aust N Z J Med 1973;3:225–229.

208. Rabinowitz I, Tuley EA, Mancuso DJ et al. von Willebrand disease type B: A missense mutation selectively abolishes ristocetin-induced von Willebrand factor binding to platelet glycoprotein Ib. Proc Natl Acad Sci U S A 1992;89:9846–9849.

209. Hilbert L, Gaucher C, Mazurier C. Identification of two mutations (Arg611-Cys and Arg611His) in the A1 loop of von Willebrand factor (vWf) responsible for type 2 von Willebrand disease with decreased platelet-dependent function of vWf. Blood 1995;86:1010–1018.

210. Castaman G, Eikenboom JC, Rodeghiero F et al. A novel candidate mutation (Arg611?His) in type I "platelet discordant" von Willebrand's disease with desmopressin-induced thrombocytopenia. Br J Haematol 1995;89:656–658.

211. White GC, II, Shoemaker CB. Factor VIII gene and hemophilia A [Review]. Blood 1989;73:1–12.

212. Veltkamp JJ, Tilburg NH van. Autosomal Haemophilia: A variant of von Willebrand's disease. Br J Haematol 1974;26:141–152.

213. Graham JB, Barrow ES, Roberts HR et al. Dominant inheritance of hemophilia A in three generations of women. Blood 1975;46:175–188.

214. Nishino M, Girma JP, Rothschild C et al. New variant of von Willebrand disease with defective binding to factor VIII. Blood 1989;74:1591–1599.

215. Mazurier C, Dieval J, Jorieux S et al. A new von Willebrand factor (vWf) defect in an individual with factor VIII (FVIII) deficiency but with normal levels and multimeric patterns of both plasma and platelet vWf. Characterization of abnormal vWf/FVIII interaction. Blood 1990;75:20–26.

216. Mazurier C. von Willebrand disease masquerading as haemophilia A [Review]. Thromb Haemost 1992;67:391–396.

217. Montgomery RR, Hathaway WE, Johnson J et al. A variant of von Willebrand's disease with abnormal expression of factor VIII procoagulant activity. Blood 1982;60:201–207.

218. Gaucher C, Jorieux S, Mercier B et al. The "Normandy" variant of von Willebrand disease: Characterization of a point mutation in the von Willebrand factor gene. Blood 1991;77:1937–1941.

219. Bahou WF, Ginsburg D, Sikkink R et al. A monoclonal antibody to von Willebrand factor (vWf) inhibits factor VIII binding. Localization of its antigenic determinant to a nonadecapeptide at the aminoterminus of the mature vWf polypeptide. J Clin Invest 1989;84:56–61.

220. Ginsburg D, Bockenstedt PL, Allen EA et al. Fine mapping of monoclonal antibody epitopes on human von Willebrand factor using a recombinant peptide library. Thromb Haemost 1992;67:166–171.

221. Foster PA, Fulcher CA, Marti T et al. A major factor VIII binding domain resides within the aminoterminal 272 amino acid residues of von Willebrand factor. J Biol Chem 1987;262:8443–8446.

222. Takahashi Y, Kalafatis M, Girma JP et al. Localization of a factor VIII binding domain on a 34 kilodalton fragment of the N-terminal portion of von Willebrand factor. Blood 1987;70:1679–1682.

223. Wise RJ, Ewenstein BM, Gorlin J et al. Autosomal recessive transmission of hemophilia A due to a von Willebrand factor mutation [Review]. Hum Genet 1993;91:367–372.

224. Lavergne JM, Piao Y, Ribba AS et al. Functional analysis of the Arg 91Gln substitution in the factor VIII binding domain of von Willebrand factor demonstrates variable phenotypic expression. Thromb Haemost 1993;70:691–696.

225. Peerlinck K, Eikenboom JC, Ploos Van Amstel HK et al. A individual with von Willebrand's disease characterized by a compound heterozygosity for a substitution of Arg854 by Gln in the putative factor VIII-binding domain of von Willebrand factor (vWf) on one allele and very low levels of mRNA from the second vWf allele. Br J Haematol 1992;80:358–363.

226. Kroner PA, Friedman KD, Fahs SA et al. Abnormal binding of factor VIII is linked with the substitution of glutamine for arginine 91 in von Willebrand factor in a variant form of von Willebrand disease. J Biol Chem 1991;266:19146–19149.

227. Gaucher C, Mercier B, Jorieux S et al. Identification of two point mutations in the von Willebrand factor gene of three families with the "Normandy" variant of von Willebrand disease. Br J Haematol 1991;78:506–514.

228. Cacheris PM, Nichols WC, Ginsburg D. Molecular characterization of a unique von Willebrand disease variant. A novel mutation affecting von Willebrand factor/factor VIII interaction. J Biol Chem 1991;266:13499–13502.

229. Jorieux S, Tuley EA, Gaucher C et al. The mutation Arg (53)?Trp causes von Willebrand disease Normandy by abolishing binding to factor VIII. Studies with recombinant von Willebrand factor. Blood 1992;79:563–567.

230. Kroner PA, Foster PA, Fahs SA et al. The defective interaction between von Willebrand factor and factor VIII in a individual with type 1 von Willebrand disease is caused by substitution of Arg19 and His54 in mature von Willebrand factor. Blood 1996;87:1013–1021.

231. Nishino M, Miura S, Yoshioka A et al. Variant von Willebrand disease with defective binding to factor VIII: The first case from Japan. Int J Hematol 1993;57:163–173.

232. Gu J, Jorieux S, Lavergne JM et al. A individual with type 2N von Willebrand disease is heterozygous for a new mutation: Gly22Glu. Demonstration of a defective expression of the second allele by the use of monoclonal antibodies. Blood 1997;89:3263–3269.

233. Tuley EA, Gaucher C, Jorieux S et al. Expression of von Willebrand factor "Normandy": An autosomal mutation that mimics hemophilia A. Proc Natl Acad Sci U S A 1991;88:6377–6381.

234. Mazurier C, Gaucher C, Jorieux S et al. Evidence for a von Willebrand factor defect in factor VIII binding in three members of a family previously misdiagnosed mild haemophilia A and haemophilia A carriers: Consequences for therapy and genetic counselling. Br J Haematol 1990;76:372–379.

235. Handin RI, Martin V, Moloney WC. Antibody-induced von Willebrand's disease: A newly defined inhibitor syndrome. Blood 1976;48:393–405.

236. Gan TE, Sawers RJ, Koutts J. Pathogenesis of antibody-induced acquired von Willebrand syndrome. Am J Hematol 1980;9:363–371.

237. Mannucci PM, Lombardi R, Bader R et al. Studies of the pathophysiology of acquired von Willebrand's disease in seven individuals with lymphoproliferative disorders or benign monoclonal gammopathies. Blood 1984;64:614–621.

238. Fricke WA, Brinkhous KM, Garris JB et al. Comparison of inhibitory and binding characteristics of an antibody causing acquired von Willebrand syndrome: An assay for von Willebrand factor binding by antibody. Blood 1985;66:562–569.

239. Mohri H, Noguchi T, Kodama F et al. Acquired von Willebrand disease due to inhibitor of human myeloma protein specific for von Willebrand factor. Am J Clin Pathol 1987;87:663–668.

240. Castaman G, Rodeghiero F, Di Bona E et al. Clinical effectiveness of desmopressin in a case of acquired von Willebrand's syndrome associated with benign monoclonal gammopathy. Blut 1989;58:211–213.

241. Goudemand J, Samor B, Caron C et al. Acquired type II von Willebrand's disease: Demonstration of a complexed inhibitor of the von Willebrand factor-platelet interaction and response to treatment. Br J Haematol 1988;68:227–233.

242. McGrath KM, Johnson CA, Stuart JJ. Acquired von Willebrand disease associated with an inhibitor to factor VIII antigen and gastrointestinal telangiectasia. Am J Med 1979;67:693–696.

243. Budde U, Dent JA, Berkowitz SD et al. Subunit composition of plasma von Willebrand factor in individuals with the myeloproliferative syndrome. Blood 1986;68:1213–1217.

244. Budde U, Schaefer G, Mueller N et al. Acquired von Willebrand's disease in the myeloproliferative syndrome. Blood 1984;64:981–985.

245. Joist JH, Cowan JF, Zimmerman TS. Acquired von Willebrand's disease. Evidence for a quantitative and qualitative factor VIII disorder. N Engl J Med 1978;298:988–991.

246. Scott JP, Montgomery RR, Tubergen DG et al. Acquired von Willebrand's disease in association with Will's tumor: Regression following treatment. Blood 1981;58:665–669.

247. Coppes MJ, Zandvoort SWH, Sparling CR et al. Acquired von Willebrand disease in Wilms' tumor individuals. J Clin Oncol 1992;10:422–427.

248. Gill JC, Wilson AD, Endres-Brooks J et al. Loss of the largest von Willebrand factor multimers from the plasma of individuals with congenital cardiac defects. Blood 1986;67:758–761.

249. Remuzzi G, Livio M, Roncaglioni MC et al. Bleeding in renal failure: Is von Willebrand factor implicated? Br Med J 1977;2:359–361.

250. Kazatchkine M, Sultan Y, Caen JP et al. Bleeding in renal failure: A possible cause. Br Med J 1976;2:612–615.

251. Janson PA, Jubelirer SJ, Weinstein MJ et al. Treatment of the bleeding tendency in uremia with cryoprecipitate. N Engl J Med 1980;303:1318–1322.

252. Warrell RP, Jr., Hultin MB, Coller BS. Increased factor VIII/von Willebrand factor antigen and von Willebrand factor activity in renal failure. Am J Med 1979;66:226–228.

253. Rodeghiero F, Castaman G, Lombardi R et al. von Willebrand factor abnormalities in two individuals with uraemia [Letter]. Lancet 1988;2:1016–1017.

254. Coccia MR, Barnes HV. Hypothyroidism and acquired von Willebrand disease. J Adolesc Health 1991;12:152-154.

255. Tachman ML, Guthrie GP, Jr. Hypothyroidism: Diversity of presentation. Endocr Rev 1984;5:456–465.

256. Dalton RG, Dewar MS, Savidge GF et al. Hypothyroidism as a cause of acquired von Willebrand's disease. Lancet 1987;1:1007–1009.

257. Anonymous. Hypothyroidism and von Willebrand's disease [Letter]. Lancet 1987;1:1314–1315.

258. Rogers JS, Shane SR, Jencks FS. Factor VIII activity and thyroid function. Ann Intern Med 1982;97:713–716.

259. Kreuz W, Linde R, Funk M et al. Induction of von Willebrand disease type I by valproic acid. Lancet 1990;335:1350–1351.

260. Fuster V, Lie JT, Badimon L et al. Spontaneous and diet-induced coronary atherosclerosis in normal swine and swine with von Willebrand disease. Arteriosclerosis 1985;5:67–73.

261. Badimon L, Steele P, Badimon JJ et al. Aortic atherosclerosis in pigs with heterozygous von Willebrand disease. Comparison with homozygous von Willebrand and normal pigs. Arteriosclerosis 1985;5:366–370.

262. Griggs TR, Reddick RL, Sultzer D et al. Susceptibility to atherosclerosis in aortas and coronary arteries of swine with von Willebrand's disease. Am J Pathol 1981;102:137–145.

263. Nichols TC, Bellinger DA, Tate DA et al. von Willebrand factor and occlusive arterial thrombosis. A study in normal and von Willebrand's disease pigs with diet-induced hypercholesterolemia and atherosclerosis. Arteriosclerosis 1990;10:449–461.

264. Nichols TC, Bellinger DA, Davis KE et al. Porcine von Willebrand disease and atherosclerosis. Influence of polymorphism in apolipoprotein B100 genotype. Am J Pathol 1992;140:403–415.

265. Conlon CL, Weinger RS, Cimo PL et al. Telangiectasia and von Willebrand's disease in two families. Ann Intern Med 1978;89:921–924.

266. Ahr DJ, Rickles FR, Hoyer LW et al. von Willebrand's disease and hemorrhagic telangiectasia. Am J Med 1977;62:452–458.

267. Shovlin CL. Molecular defects in rare bleeding disorders: Hereditary haemorrhagic telangiectasia. Thromb Haemost 1997;78:145–150.

268. Pickering NJ, Brody JI, Barrett MJ. von Willebrand syndromes and mitral-valve prolapse: Linked mesenchymal dysplasias. N Engl J Med 1981;305:131–134.

269. Kuhsel LC, Polster J, Rudiger HW. An investigation into the frequency of mitral valve prolapse in von Willebrand disease. Clin Genet 1983;24:128–131.

270. Hogan AG, Muhrer ME, Bogart R. A hemophilia-like disease in swine. Proc Soc Exp Biol Med 1941;48:217–219.

271. Bogart R, Muhrer ME. The inheritance of a hemophilia-like condition in swine. J Hered 1942;33:59–64.

272. Muhrer ME, Lechler E, Cornell CN et al. Antihemophilic factor levels in bleeder swine following infusions of plasma and serum. Am J Physiol 1965;208:508–510.

273. Bowie EJW, Owen CA, Jr, Giles AR. Animal models for the study of Factor VIII and von Willebrand factor. In: Zimmerman TS, Ruggeri ZM, eds. Coagulation and bleeding disorders. The role of factor VIII and von Willebrand factor. New York: Marcel Dekker, 1989;305–324.

274. Webster WP, Mandel SR, Strike LE et al. Factor VIII synthesis: Hepatic and renal allografts in swine with von Willebrand's disease. Am J Physiol 1976;230:1342–1348.

275. Bowie EJ, Solberg LA Jr, Fass DN et al. Transplantation of normal bone marrow into a pig with severe von Willebrand's disease. J Clin Invest 1986;78:26–30.

276. Johnson GS, Turrentine MA, Kraus KH. Canine von Willebrand's disease: A heterogeneous group of bleeding disorders [Review]. Vet Clin North Am Small Anim Pract 1988;18:195–229.

277. Aledort LM. Factor VIII/von Willebrand factor replacement therapy: Problems and challenges. Ann N Y Acad Sci 1987;509:49–52.

278. Logan LJ. Treatment of von Willebrand's disease [Review]. Hematol Oncol Clin North Am 1992;6:1079–1094.

279. Rothschild C, Forestier F, Daffos F et al. Prenatal diagnosis in type IIA von Willebrand disease. Nouv Rev Fr Hematol 1990;32:125–127.

280. Mannhalter C, Kyrle PA, Brenner B et al. Rapid neonatal diagnosis of type IIB von Willebrand disease using the polymerase chain reaction [Letter]. Blood 1991;77:2538–2544.

281. Mannucci PM, Ruggeri ZM, Pareti FI et al. 1-Deamino-8-d-arginine vasopressin: A new pharmacological approach to the management of haemophilia and von Willebrand's' diseases. Lancet 1977;1:869–872.

282. de la Fuente B, Kasper CK, Rickles FR et al. Response of individuals with mild and moderate hemophilia A and von Willebrand's disease to treatment with desmopressin. Ann Intern Med 1985;103:6–14.

283. Aledort LM. Treatment of von Willebrand's disease. Mayo Clin Proc 1991;66:841–846.

284. Mannucci PM. Desmopressin (DDAVP) for treatment of disorders of hemostasis [Review]. Prog Hemost Thromb 1986;8:19–45.

285. Lusher JM. Response to 1-deamino-8-D-arginine vasopressin in von Willebrand disease. Haemostasis 1994;24:276–284.

286. Robertson GL, Harris A. Clinical use of vasopressin analogues [Review]. Hosp Pract (Off Ed) 1989;24:114-118.

287. Rose EH, Aledort LM. Nasal spray desmopressin (DDAVP) for mild hemophilia A and von Willebrand disease. Ann Intern Med 1991;114:563–568.

288. Lethagen S, Harris AS, Nilsson IM. Intranasal desmopressin (DDAVP) by spray in mild hemophilia A and von Willebrand's disease type I. Blut 1990;60:187–191.

289. Mannucci PM, Meyer D, Ruggeri ZM et al. Precipitating antibodies in von Willebrand's disease. Nature 1976;262:141–142.

290. Byrnes JJ, Larcada A, Moake JL. Thrombosis following desmopressin for uremic bleeding. Am J Hematol 1988;28:63–65.

291. Bond L, Bevan D. Myocardial infarction in a individual with hemophilia treated with DDAVP [Letter]. N Engl J Med 1988;318:121.

292. Mannucci PM, Bettega D, Cattaneo M. Patterns of development of tachyphylaxis in individuals with haemophilia and von Willebrand disease after repeated doses of desmopressin (DDAVP). Br J Haematol 1992;82:87–93.

293. Scott JP, Montgomery RR. Therapy of von Willebrand disease [Review]. Semin Thromb Hemost 1993;19:37–47.

294. Rodeghiero F, Castaman G, Di Bona E et al. Consistency of responses to repeated DDAVP infusions in individuals with von Willebrand's disease and hemophilia A. Blood 1989;74:1997–2000.

295. Rodeghiero F, Castaman G, Di Bona E et al. Hyper-responsiveness to DDAVP for individuals with type I von Willebrand's disease and normal intra-platelet von Willebrand factor. Eur J Haematol 1988;40:163–167.

296. Gralnick HR, Williams SB, McKeown LP et al. DDAVP in type IIa von Willebrand's disease. Blood 1986;67:465–468.

297. Casonato A, Sartori MT, de Marco L et al. 1-Desamino-8-D-arginine vasopressin (DDAVP) infusion in type IIB von Willebrand's disease: Shortening of bleeding time and induction of a variable pseudothrombocytopenia. Thromb Haemost 1990;64:117–120.

298. McKeown LP, Connaghan D, Wilson O et al. 1-Desamino-8-arginine-vasopressin corrects the hemostatic defects in type 2B von Willebrand's disease. Am J Hematol 1996;51:158–163.

299. Holmberg L, Nilsson IM, Borge L et al. Platelet aggregation induced by 1-desamino-8-D-arginine vasopressin (DDAVP) in type IIB von Willebrand's disease. N Engl J Med 1983;309:816–821.

300. Mazurier C, Gaucher C, Jorieux S et al. Biological effect of desmopressin in eight individuals with type 2N ("Normandy") von Willebrand disease. Collaborative Group. Br J Haematol 1994;88:849–854.

301. Harrison RL, McKee PA. Estrogen stimulates von Willebrand factor production by cultured endothelial cells. Blood 1984;63:657–665.

302. Alperin JB. Estrogens and surgery in women with von Willebrand's disease. Am J Med 1982;73:367–371.

303. Foster PA. A perspective on the use of FVIII concentrates and cryoprecipitate prophylactically in surgery or therapeutically in severe bleeds in individuals with von Willebrand disease unresponsive to DDAVP: Results of an international survey. Thromb Haemost 1995;74:1370–1378.

304. Mannucci PM, Tenconi PM, Castaman G et al. Comparison of four virus-inactivated plasma concentrates for treatment of severe von Willebrand disease: A cross-over randomized trial. Blood 1992;79:3130–3137.

305. Rodeghiero F, Castaman G, Meyer D et al. Replacement therapy with virus-inactivated plasma concentrates in von Willebrand disease [Review]. Vox Sang 1992;62:193–199.

306. Mannucci PM, Moia M, Rebulla P et al. Correction of the bleeding time in treated individuals with severe von Willebrand disease is not solely dependent on the normal multimeric structure of plasma von Willebrand factor. Am J Hematol 1987;25:55–65.

307. Castillo R, Monteagudo J, Escolar G et al. Hemostatic effect of normal platelet transfusion in severe von Willebrand disease individuals. Blood 1991;77:1901–1905.

308. Mannucci PM, Ruggeri ZM, Ciavarella N et al. Precipitating antibodies to factor VIII/von Willebrand factor in von Willebrand's disease: Effects on replacement therapy. Blood 1981;57:25–31.

309. Mannucci PM, Tamaro G, Narchi G et al. Life-threatening reaction to factor VIII concentrate in a individual with severe von Willebrand disease and alloantibodies to von Willebrand factor. Eur J Haematol 1987;39:467–470.

310. Bloom AL, Peake IR, Furlong RA et al. High potency factor VIII concen-

trate: More effective than cryoprecipitate in a individual with von Willebrand's disease and inhibitor. Thromb Res 1979;16:847–852.

311. Macik BG, Gabriel DA, White GC et al. The use of high-dose intravenous gammaglobulin in acquired von Willebrand syndrome. Arch Pathol Lab Med 1988;112:143–146.

312. Delannoy A, Saillez AC. High-dose intravenous gammaglobulin for acquired von Willebrand's disease [Letter]. Br J Haematol 1988;70:387.

313. Silberstein LE, Abrahm J, Shattil SJ. The efficacy of intensive plasma exchange in acquired von Willebrand's disease. Transfusion 1987;27:234–237.

314. Uehlinger J, Rose E, Aledort LM et al. Successful treatment of an acquired von Willebrand factor antibody by extracorporeal immunoadsorption [Letter]. N Engl J Med 1989;320:254–255.

315. Telfer MC, Chediak J. Factor VIII-related disorders and their relationship to pregnancy. J Reprod Med 1977;19:211–222.

316. Conti M, Mari D, Conti E et al. Pregnancy in women with different types of von Willebrand disease. Obstet Gynecol 1986;68:282–285.

317. Punnonen R, Nyman D, Gronroos M et al. von Willebrand's disease and pregnancy. Acta Obstet Gynecol Scand 1981;60:507–509.

318. Hanna W, McCarroll D, McDonald T et al. Variant von Willebrand's disease and pregnancy. Blood 1981;58:873–879.

319. Ieko M, Sakurama S, Sagawa A et al. Effect of a factor VIII concentrate on type IIB von Willebrand's disease-associated thrombocytopenia presenting during pregnancy in identical twin mothers. Am J Hematol 1990;35:26–31.

# CHAPTER 35

# HEMOPHILIA–FACTOR VIII DEFICIENCY

## Donna M. DiMichele and David Green

"It was the best of times, it was the worst of times," so F. R. Rosendaal (1) quotes from Charles Dickens' *A Tale of Two Cities* to characterize the status of hemophilia in the 1990s. It is the best of times because superb, safe, and efficacious clotting factor concentrates are available to treat hemophilia and its complications. It is the worst of times because many adolescents and adults with hemophilia are infected with the human immunodeficiency virus (HIV), and nearly 10% have already developed the acquired immunodeficiency syndrome (AIDS). Between 65 and 90% of this population have been infected with hepatitis C as well. In addition, whereas survival among all individuals with hemophilia increased to near normal in 1970s, it dropped sharply in the 1980s, so that the median life expectancy at age 30 had decreased from 40.3 to 30.9 years (2). This chapter describes the manifestations of hemophilia A, or factor VIII deficiency, in both children and adults, discusses the appropriate diagnostic procedures, and indicates the currently accepted methods of management.

## INTRODUCTION

Hemophilia is a bleeding disorder resulting from a deficiency of factor VIII or factor IX coagulant activity. The incidence of factor VIII deficiency has been estimated at one in 5000 male births (3). In individuals with a family history of hemophilia, the condition is readily suspected, but in the one-third of individuals without such history, it may not be immediately obvious that clinical signs and symptoms are caused by hemorrhage. Hemophilia should be suspected in any child who presents with prolonged bleeding after circumcision, prolonged

oozing from a small cut on the tongue or tear of the frenulum, or a painful and swollen joint. A complete family history should be recorded for each individual, with inquiries especially focused on the maternal side of the family. Simple laboratory tests such as the partial thromboplastin time also are helpful.

## HISTORY OF HEMOPHILIA

The history of hemophilia has been an 1800 year trek, from the second century Talmud through the advances and setbacks of twentieth century transfusion therapy to the promise of twenty-first century gene transplantation. This history, at least through the 1970s, was eloquently compiled and presented by Professor G. I. Ingram in his opening lecture to the Third European Congress of the World Federation of Hemophilia in 1976 (4). The original gene mutation for hemophilia is postulated to be at least 65 million years old, having been described in humans, the horse (5), and nine breeds of dog (6). These species belong to three orders of placental mammals that probably became distinct in evolutionary history by the end of the Cretaceous Era.

The first description of hemophilia in humans appears in the Talmud, with references to several Rabbinic rulings that exempted newborn males from circumcision if siblings or maternal cousins had previously died of bleeding complications related to that procedure (7, 8). No further attempts were made to define precisely the clinical syndrome of "hemophilia" until the late eighteenth and early nineteenth centuries, when U.S. physicians Otto and Hay each described an extensive family pedigree, which resulted in two important principles governing the heredity of this disorder. First, Otto (9) concluded that even although only males were "bleeders," this tendency was transmitted by unaffected females. It was noted by Hay (10) that "children of bleeders are never subject to this disposition, but their grandsons by their daughters [are]." The sex-linked nature of hemophilia transmission was reiterated as Nasse's Law in 1820, the second such disorder to be described after color blindness (10).

Another historically important pedigree from the Swiss village of Tenna was first described by Thormann in 1837 (10). A critical evaluation of the clinical symptoms associated with hemophilia, as distinguished from those associated with other bleeding disorders, was first presented by Dr. J. Wickham Legg in 1872 in his authoritative treatise (11), in which the author describes hemophilia as "a disease both hereditary and congenital, usually lasting throughout the life of a individual, accompanied by a haemorrhagic diathesis and a tendency to swelling in the joints." The same joints we acknowledge as being most afflicted today were similarly described in this work. In this treatise, bleeding from circumcision was distinguished from umbilical cord stump bleeding as a symptom of hemophilia in newborns, "three well-marked degrees of haemophilia" were accurately described, and the word *haemophilia* (popularized by Schonlein's student Hopff in his 1828 thesis [12] and meaning "love of blood") was described as "barbarous and senseless." The name has endured despite Legg's opinion, but little progress in understanding the disorder was made during the ensuing 83 years. In the next major compendium (10), written by Bulloch and Fildes and published in 1911, hemophilia was still only described clinically and genealogically.

The etiology of hemophilia was ascribed by Schonlein (13) in the early nineteenth century to cyanosis and malformation of the heart. Legg stated in 1872 there was "no unnatural state of hemophilic blood with respect to water content, corpuscles, fibrin, and albumin," but abnormal blood clotting in hemophilia had been described since the 1840s (14). In 1893, Wright (15A) demonstrated the prolonged clotting time of hemophilic blood in the capillary tube, and by the early twentieth century, a prolonged blood clotting time had been added to the definition of hemophilia. On the basis of the classical coagulation theory, as proposed by Morawitz in 1905 (15B), Addis (16) in 1910, and Howell (17) in 1914 demonstrated that the clotting of fibrinogen by thrombin was normal in individuals with hemophilia, and Quick (18) in 1935 determined the prothrombin time of hemophilic blood to be normal as well. During the next 10 years, Patek and Taylor (19) identified "antihemophilic globulin," a plasma fraction that corrected the clotting defect in hemophilic blood and later became known by international convention as factor VIII (20).

In 1952, Biggs et al (21) described Christmas disease, a bleeding disorder distinct from classical hemophilia and resulting from a deficiency in "Christmas factor," so named for the Canadian individual in whom the defect was described. Later called hemophilia B or factor IX deficiency (see Chapter 36), Christmas disease was determined to be the bleeding disorder afflicting the Tenna pedigree first described in 1837, thereby also proving its sex-linked inheritance pattern (22).

With the development of the protein bioassays in the 1950s and 1960s, nearly 100 years after Legg's first attempt at an exclusive definition of the disorder, hemophilia became defined simply as one of two congenital bleeding disorders characterized by a plasma deficiency in either factor VIII or factor IX. In the 1970s, Zimmerman et al (23) complicated this definition by introducing the concept of CRM+ hemophilia A, but they also clarified it by distinguishing classical hemophilia from von Willebrand's disease (23, 24). The 1980s witnessed cloning of the genes for both factor VIII (25, 26) and factor IX (27) as well as remarkable discoveries regarding the posttranslational cellular processing of these proteins (28, 29). Now, as we enter the twenty-first century, hemophilia is defined by a mode of inheritance and set of clinical manifestations as well as by a quantitative and qualitative measure of the clotting protein defect and a heterogeneous collection of abnormalities on the molecular and cellular levels.

# LABORATORY TESTING

## RECOGNITION OF FACTOR VIII DEFICIENCY (SEE CHAPTER 26)

The diagnosis of hemophilia usually begins with a thorough individual history, including specific questions about bleeding disorders on the maternal side of the family. The initial laboratory study is a partial thromboplastin time (see Chapter 23). If an appropriately sensitive thromboplastin reagent is selected and the control is fresh frozen plasma prepared from a pool of at least 20 normal donors, an abnormal test will occur in individuals with less than 30% of the mean normal concentration of factor VIII. In hemophilia, the prothrombin time is invariably normal, and if no inhibitors are present, mixing equal volumes of individual plasma with normal plasma will shorten the partial thromboplastin time to within 4 seconds of the control value. A specific clotting assay for factor VIII, which may be either a one-stage or a two-stage method, is then performed. In the one-stage method, the partial thromboplastin time is performed on a mixture of individual plasma and substrate plasma known to be deficient in factor VIII, and the results are analyzed using a standard curve constructed with known concentrations of factor VIII. In the two-stage method, an incubation mixture is prepared containing the individual plasma and excess amounts of all other relevant clotting factors (i.e., factors II, V, IX, X, phospholipid, calcium). This incubation mixture generates activated factor X and thrombin, which are added to substrate plasma. The clotting times are then noted.

One-stage methods are simple and readily automated. Concentrations of other clotting factors in the individual or substrate plasma, however, may be rate-limiting, and the final result may not reflect the actual factor VIII concentration. In addition, anticoagulants present in the individual plasma, such as heparin or lupuslike inhibitors, may cause falsely low values. The two-stage method does not have these disadvantages, but it is more complicated with respect to preparing the reagents and performing the assay. The relative merits of the two types of assays are ably discussed by Barrowcliffe (30).

Most recently, a chromogenic substrate assay for the measurement of factor VIII has become commercially available (31). This test is based on the principle of factor VIII-dependent factor X activation.

## INHIBITOR (ANTIBODY) DETECTION (SEE CHAPTERS 26 AND 37)

One-stage or two-stage assays of factor VIII may be modified to detect factor VIII antibodies. The Bethesda method calls for the assay of residual factor VIII in an equal mixture of individual plasma and normal, pooled citrated plasma incubated for 2 hours at 37°C (32). One Bethesda unit of antibody is defined as the amount that will inactivate 50% of the factor VIII activity of the normal plasma. A second method, the Oxford assay, uses 0.5 U of factor VIII and a 4 hour incubation period. In this method, one Bethesda unit of antibody corresponds to approximately 0.8 New Oxford units (33). Factor VIII inhibitors are discussed in detail in Chapter 37.

## CARRIER DETECTION

The diagnosis of hemophilia in a family will usually lead to questions about which female relatives may be hemophilia carriers. The first step in carrier detection is a careful history. Surprisingly, a female relative sometimes is assured that she is not a carrier only to subsequently bear a child with severe factor IX deficiency simply because the physician and the laboratory assumed that factor VIII hemophilia was in question. Carrier testing is unnecessary if the individual is an obligate carrier, such as the mother of more than one hemophilic son or the daughter of a hemophiliac. Carriership also becomes less likely if the suspected person has already had normal sons; the greater the number of normal sons, the less likely the woman is a carrier. Thus, a detailed history can provide considerable insight into the likelihood of carriership.

There are two kinds of laboratory testing: analysis of clotting factors, and DNA-based techniques. Analysis of clotting factors depends on a discrepancy between the individual's level of factor VIII clotting activity and the von Willebrand factor, which is a factor VIII-stabilizing protein. There is usually a 1:1 stoichiometry between these two factors. However, when one X chromosome bears the factor VIII gene defect, the cells in which this X chromosome is dominant produce less factor VIII coagulant activity. Thus, the more cells in which this X chromosome is dominant, the lower the ultimate plasma concentration of factor VIII activity (i.e., the Lyon hypothesis [34]). On the other hand, von Willebrand factor is unaffected by these vagaries in factor VIII, and its concentration in carriers will always be higher than that of factor VIII. With rigidly standardized assay techniques for factor VIII and von Willebrand factor as well as discriminant analysis, the 95% confidence limits for carrier detection are 91 to 99% (35, 36). It is generally recommended that suspected carriers be tested at monthly intervals for 3 months, so the consistency of the factor VIII-von Willebrand factor relationship can be established.

Currently, DNA-based techniques are the preferred method for identifying carriers. First cloned in 1984 and 186 kb in size, the factor VIII gene (see Chapter 2) comprises one-thousandth of the X-chromosome DNA and is one of the largest human genes identified to date (25, 26, 37). By 1991, more than 150 different mutations (>70 gene alterations, >80 point mutations) had been identified within the 8 kb coding sequence of its 26 exons (38). As could be predicted from the X-linked genetic nature of this disease and the size of the gene, 70% of families have different mutations (39, 40). Until recently, however, the causative mutation could be detected in 90% of individuals with moderate or mild hemophilia A but in 50 to 60% of individuals with severe disease (40).

In the past, carrier detection was largely performed using intragenic and extragenic linkage analysis of DNA polymorphisms (41). These gene tracking techniques are precise, however, only when an affected male and intervening family members are available for analysis (42–45). For example, direct gene mutation analysis could be useful in some families with limited pedigrees and only one affected male, but for more than 40% of potential carriers in severely affected families, this technique would not be informative.

In 1993, however, an inversion in the factor VIII gene intron 22, resulting from an intrachromosomal recombination, was identified (46, 47). This mutation accounts for 40 to 50% of all severe hemophilia A gene abnormalities (i.e., essentially all previously unidentified mutations in this group of families) (46, 48, 49). Carrier detection and prenatal diagnosis for severe hemophilia A was revolutionized by this discovery. Direct gene mutation analysis for the intron 22 inversion is now recommended as first-line testing for carriership in families with severe hemophilia A, particularly when affected and intervening family members are unavailable (50).

In addition, the techniques used for identifying gene mutations and carrier detection can also be used for prenatal diagnosis.

# PATHOGENESIS

Tissue injury results in the exposure of tissue factor, an integral membrane protein, to flowing blood, in which it binds factor VII (see Chapter 4). The tissue factor-factor VII complex activates factors IX and X, and activated factor X (factor Xa) in turn activates factor VII to VIIa, thereby increasing its own activation by approximately a hundredfold. Because factor Xa is the major component of prothrombinase (see Chapter 1), one would anticipate rapid formation of thrombin, but this does not occur. Instead, as factor Xa forms, it is complexed by tissue factor pathway inhibitor (TFPI), and this complex inhibits the tissue factor-factor VIIa complex (52–54). Some factor Xa probably escapes this inhibitor, and in normal subjects, the thrombin that is generated activates factor VIII to VIIIa. Along with the factor IXa generated by the tissue factor-factor VIIa complex, this factor VIIIa is a potent activator of factor Xa, and the amounts of factor Xa produced are sufficient to generate sufficient thrombin to form fibrin.

Patients with hemophilia, who lack either factor VIII or factor IX, have markedly delayed thrombin generation despite significant tissue injury. Both Nordfang et al (55) and Lewis et al (56) recently showed *in vitro* that if the TFPI of these individuals is neutralized by antibody, the clotting time of hemophilic plasma is corrected almost to normal.

Deficiencies of factors VIII or IX also affect bleeding from skin incisions. Eyster et al (57) reported a prolonged template bleeding time in some individuals, but this did not correlate with the degree of factor deficiency, thus making it unlikely that defective thrombin formation alone explains the abnormal bleeding.

# CLINICAL PRESENTATION

Because of the lurid descriptions of hemophilic hemorrhage, many caregivers are intimidated by any physical contact with such individuals, and they feel reluctant to perform venipunctures, start intravenous infusions, or give routine immunizations. These fears are groundless. If these procedures are performed in the careful manner requisite for any individual, bleeding will be minimal.

Certain characteristics of hemophilic bleeding, however, are unique. These include the tendency to form extensive ecchymoses, to have delayed oozing from lacerations, and to develop large hematomas after even minor trauma. The severity of bleeding relates to the plasma concentration of the clotting factor. Those individuals with a level of factor VIII less than 1% of normal have spontaneous hemorrhages and ecchymoses and develop frequent hemarthroses and eventually crippling joint deformities. Clotting factor levels of from 1 to 5% of normal are associated with severe bleeding after trauma, occasional hemarthroses, and spontaneous hemorrhages. In those with a factor level of 5 to 20% of normal, excessive bleeding after minor injuries or surgery occurs. Those with concentration of 20 to 40% of normal have bleeding problems only after major trauma or surgery and often are unrecognized preoperatively (58).

Severe hemophilia can present during the newborn period. Excessive bleeding from circumcision or heel-stick puncture can be the first clue that a bleeding disorder exists. Following vaginal delivery, a cephalo-hematoma may occur, as might an intracranial hemorrhage. Reported frequencies are 0.2 and 1.8%, respectively (59). Even without a family history of hemophilia, all newborn males with intracranial hemorrhage must be considered to have a bleeding disorder until proven otherwise by appropriate coagulation studies. As children with severe and moderately severe hemophilia begin to ambulate, around the age of 1 year, bleeding episodes occur more frequently and begin to involve primarily the muscles, joints, and oral mucosa. The factors that provoke hemorrhage are poorly understood, however. For example, although it is not recommended, youngsters with severe hemophilia may perform 100 jumps on a trampoline without sustaining a joint hemorrhage, yet these same children may have extensive knee hemarthroses without any history of trauma. Cochran et al (60) evaluated psychologic factors as possible causes of bleeding but found no associations. Specifically, using a battery of psychological tests, they found no significant differences between individuals with high bleeding frequencies and individuals with low bleeding frequencies. Some individuals relate bleeding to time of year, stress of school examinations, and family events, but most often, the onset of hemorrhage is totally unpredictable.

# TREATMENT OF HEMOPHILIA
## HISTORICAL PERSPECTIVE

The treatment of hemophilia has its own fascinating history. Given the treatments available at the time of Legg's treatise in 1872 (11), avoidance of any procedure or activity that could produce trauma was good advice. The therapeutic compendium of the time did include methods still employed today, such as cautery, application of ice, and splinting, but the oral ingestion of lead, antimony, strychnine, and turpentine were also recommended. Not surprisingly, Legg quoted a mortality rate of 90% by the age of 21 years. Even in the first half of the twentieth century, as documented in the second through fourth series volumes of the U.S. Surgeon General's Catalogue, therapy for hemophilia included use of oxygen, bromide extract of egg white, Witte's peptone, and interestingly, female hormone. The topical use of Russell's viper venom and injections of adrenaline were also advocated during this period, and mortality statistics differed little from those of the nineteenth century (61).

The first use of transfusion in the treatment of hemophilic bleeding is attributed to Lane (14), a British physician who in 1840 successfully transfused 12 ounces of blood from a young woman directly into an 11 year old boy who was bleeding after an eye operation. Although used sporadically after that, the relationship between the effectiveness of transfusion and the temporary replacement of a missing blood clotting factor was not generally understood and appreciated until 100 years later (62), and from then on, the goal became development of a concentrated specific factor replacement therapy. The 1950s saw use of fresh frozen plasma and early factor VIII concentrates prepared from plasma by Cohn fractionation (63). The discovery of cryoprecipitate by Pool and Shannon (64) in the 1960s was a major development in factor VIII replacement therapy, and freeze-dried intermediate purity factor VIII and factor IX concentrates in the 1970s enabled individuals with hemophilia to undergo dental and orthopaedic surgery and to transfer their care to the home setting with self-infusion training. Furthermore, capitalizing on the known effect of adrenaline on factor VIII plasma levels, Mannucci et al (65) developed the parameters for effective intravenous use of 1-deamino-8D-arginine vasopressin (DDAVP) for mild hemophilia A (see Chapter 53). Quality of life improved dramatically, as did the average life expectancy of even those with severe hemophilia, which rose from 11 years in 1921 to 60 years in 1980 (66).

The transmission of hepatitis from these concentrates was already well recognized by 1980 (67), but the decimation of the hemophilia population from infection with the HIV-1 virus could not have been anticipated. The 1980s therefore called for purer replacement products and for therapy that was safe from viral contamination. The development of monoclonal antibody affinity chromatography purification (68, 69) allowed the production of factor VIII concentrates nearly devoid of all extraneous protein contamination and of unprecedented specific activity (2000 U per mg of protein before the addition of stabilizers). HIV-1 viral inactivation was accomplished first by dry heat treatment (70) and subsequently by methods such as solvent and detergent treatment as well as pasteurization, which appear to be more effective than dry heat in the inactivation of the hepatitis viruses (71, 72). As the 1990s approached, monoclonal antibody purification technology and improved biochemical purification techniques were applied to produce effective factor IX replacement products of high purity (73). Furthermore, recombinant factor IX was licensed in 1997 (74). The early 1990s also saw an effective recombinant factor VIII replacement therapy, which was licensed a mere 7 years after the factor VIII gene had been cloned (75–77). Clinical trials are now underway to show the efficacy and safety of recombinant products free of human protein stabilizers. With these advances in therapy came the hope for an end to the concerns of both the individuals and caregivers regarding viral transmission through factor replacement products. Of course, no technologic advance during the 1980s and 1990s came without a price: a major increase in the cost of hemophilia care. This effect is discussed further under "Psychosocial and Economic Considerations."

## OVERVIEW

Treatment of hemophilia consists of clotting factor replacement to prevent and control bleeding as well as ancillary therapies to supplement factor replacement and to relieve pain. Without clotting factor replacement, individuals with hemophilia are at constant risk of bleeding and should avoid activities that may lead to hemorrhage. The difficulty is that the factors which cause bleeding are not well understood. Contact sports and hazardous occupations should be discouraged. On the other hand, no evidence suggests that a sedentary lifestyle leads to decreased musculoskeletal bleeding. On the contrary, deconditioning probably enhances the individuals' bleeding tendencies by making joints more vulnerable to the stresses and strains of daily life. Many individuals claim that programs to build muscle strength protect their joints from bleeding, but a formal study to confirm these observations has not been reported. It is well recognized that strict prohibitions on the activities of very young individuals often lead to rebellious behavior and risk-taking during the teenage years. Children need to establish their own boundaries and limitations regarding those activities that may produce hemorrhage. Fortunately, methods to control bleeding are now well developed and effective. Therefore, it is recommended that children with hemophilia be encouraged to ride bicycles, swim, play baseball and tennis, and so on, but to avoid contact sports such as football, rugby, and the like.

## REPLACEMENT THERAPY (SEE CHAPTER 52)

The mainstay of therapy for hemophilia is clotting factor replacement. Clotting factor concentrates are given to prevent bleeding and to limit existing hemorrhage. The amount of clotting factor needed for a particular purpose is easily calculated. One unit of clotting factor is that amount present in 1 mL of pooled normal plasma; thus, an individual with a plasma volume of 3000 mL would have 3000 U of clotting factor in his circulation. If such an individual has severe hemophilia, with less than 1% of the normal concentration of factor VIII in his or her plasma, a dose of 3000 U of factor VIII would raise the plasma level to 100% of normal. In individuals with higher baseline levels of the factor, the plasma level will increase by an estimated 2% of normal for each unit of factor VIII that is given.

Doses of 15 to 20 U/kg body weight can control hemarthroses, but doses of 30 U/kg are required for muscle hematomas or to prevent bleeding associated with dental surgery. Raising clotting factor levels to 100% of normal is indicated for severe bleeding, such as intracranial or intra-abdominal hemorrhage. There is considerable variation in individual responses to particular dosages, however, and trial and error dose finding is common. Laboratory measurement of clotting factor levels immediately after clotting factor administration is helpful in establishing the appropriate dose. For example, a factor VIII concentration of 25% of normal, which is usually achieved with a dose of 15 U/kg, controls joint bleeding, whereas a level of 50% of normal, which is generally obtained with a dose of 30 U/kg, prevents bleeding following tooth extraction. Clotting factor is always given when a individual with hemophilia must undergo an invasive procedure; even such a seemingly innocuous technique as arterial blood gas sampling will provoke serious bleeding if the individual is not protected with clotting factor replacement. Likewise, intramuscular injections should be avoided if possible.

The half-disappearance time of factor VIII from the circulation is approximately 12 hours. Therefore, doses are repeated on a 12-hour basis if maintaining a specific plasma concentration of the factor is necessary. Clotting factor assays are performed near the end of this 12-hour period to ensure that levels adequate for hemostasis have been achieved. Alternatively, concentrate may be given by continuous infusion, which provides more constant blood levels and requires less concentrate than intermittent infusions (78). This method of administration is relevant for individuals undergoing extensive surgical procedures or with major hemorrhages, in whom the danger of rebleeding remains until all bleeding sites are healed. On the other hand, the usual hemarthrosis, especially if treated early, will almost always respond to a single dose of clotting factor. Thus, early treatment of bleeding limits hemorrhage and tissue damage. To ensure early treatment, clotting factor and individuals who are competent in its administration must be readily available. As mentioned, the concentrates must be given intravenously; however, this does not preclude family members or individuals themselves from administering the product (79, 80). Indeed, both parents and individuals can be instructed in sterile technique, preparation of the correct dose, and intravenous infusion. Even children as young as 3 to 4 years can be treated safely at home.

Table 35.1 shows the wide range of products available for treatment of hemophilia A. Random donor cryoprecipitate is no longer recommended, but the regular plasmapheresis of DDAVP-treated (see "Ancillary Therapy") fathers of children with hemophilia generally yields a sufficient amount of product to meet the routine requirements of a small hemophilic child (81). Even although this material does not undergo a viral attenuation process, the designated donor is appropriately screened at each donation. Therefore, when available, directed donor cryoprecipitate is chosen by some families and physicians as a safe, inexpensive alternative to concentrates. For most individuals, however, replacement therapy uses either plasma-derived or recombinant clotting factor concentrates. All such products appear to have similar hemostatic efficacy, and all plasma-derived concentrates undergo a viral attenuation step during purification. Even so, concentrates vary widely regarding final product purity, as defined by units of specific activity per milligram of protein. The choice of factor VIII product is generally based on cost and the relative importance of product purity. There is an approximate fourfold increase in the average wholesale cost between cryoprecipitate and recombinant concentrates, the unit price rising proportionately with the final product purity and the sophistication of the production technology employed.

The relative importance of product purity is still debated. The results of some studies suggest that lower purity products may be immunodepressive in both normal and compromised hosts, possibly because of the high content of extraneous protein or contamination with transforming growth factor–$\beta$ (82–84), but the results of other studies are less clear or contradictory (85, 86). Currently, most pediatric individuals are treated with very high purity (monoclonal antibody-purified plasma derived, or recombinant) products when donated cryoprecipitate is not an option.

## ANCILLARY AGENTS (SEE CHAPTER 53)

Several valuable, ancillary agents in the treatment of hemophilia are shown in Table 35.2. Corticosteroids are ineffective for reducing the frequency of bleeding and they have no role as a maintenance treatment. However, they are helpful in reducing the pain and swelling associated with chronic hemarthroses, especially in a target joint. When used in this way, they are given over a 5 day period at a dose of up to 80 mg daily for 3 days and then 40 mg for 2 days (87). The equivalent pediatric dose is 1 mg/kg/day in two to three divided doses for 5 to 7 days.

**TABLE 35.1.** Factor VIII Treatment Products (Manufacturers) Available in the United States in 1997

| Product | Viral Inactivation Procedure |
| --- | --- |
| Low purity[a] | |
|   Cryoprecipitate (directed donor only) | None |
| Intermediate purity[b] | |
|   Humate-P (Centeon GmbH) | Pasteurization |
| High purity[c] | |
|   Alphanate (Alpha) | Solvent detergent/dry heat |
|   Koate-HP (Bayer) | Solvent detergent |
| Very high (ultra) purity[d] | |
|   *Plasma-derived, monoclonal antibody-purified* | |
|     Monarc-m (American Red Cross) | Solvent detergent |
|     Hemofil-M (Baxter/Hyland) | Solvent detergent |
|     Monoclate-P (Centeon) | Pasteurization |
|   *Recombinant* | |
|     Bioclate (Centeon) | None[e] |
|     Helixate (Centeon) | None[e] |
|     Kogenate (Bayer) | None[e] |
|     Recombinate (Baxter/Hyland) | None[e] |

*Adapted with permission from DiMichele D. Hemophilia 1996. New approaches to an old disease. Pediatr Clin North Am 1996;43:709–736.*
[a] *Specific activity, <5 U/mg protein.*
[b] *Specific activity, 1–10 U/mg protein.*
[c] *Specific activity, 50–1000 U/mg protein.*
[d] *Specific activity, 3000 U/mg protein (before the addition of human albumin to all ultrapure products for stabilization of the final product.*
[e] *Human albumin added as a stabilizer undergoes standard pasteurization.*

**TABLE 35.2.** Ancillary Agents Used in the Treatment of Hemophilia

| Agent | Indication |
| --- | --- |
| Corticosteroids | Brief, high dose for recurrent bleeding into a single joint (target joint) |
|   Prednisone | Chronic (up to 2 weeks) for hemarthropathy |
| Antifibrinolytics | Mucosal bleeding, especially dental and gastrointestinal bleeding |
|   Tranexamic acid | |
|   EACA | |
| DDAVP (desmopressin) | Mild to moderate hemophilia shown to have a rise in factor VIII level with DDAVP |
| | Minor bleeding and surgery (dentistry) |
| Analgesics | Pain management |
|   Acetaminophen with or without codeine | |
|   Ibuprofen | |
|   Nonacetylated salicylates | |
|   Propoxyphene | |

Antifibrinolytic agents likewise are ineffective as maintenance therapy (88), but they may be useful as supplements to clotting factor replacement in individuals with oral mucous membrane bleeding. In individuals requiring tooth extractions, they are given preoperatively and continued postoperatively until all wounds are healed. Such treatment dramatically decreases the need for concentrate. Two agents are available: ε-aminocaproic acid (EACA), which in adults is given orally in doses of 5 g every 6 hours; and tranexamic acid, which is given in doses of 1.5 g every 8 hours. Both drugs may be given intravenously if necessary, EACA in a dose of 5 g every 6 hours and tranexamic acid in a dose of 1 g every 8 hours. In children, EACA is administered orally or intravenously at an initial dose of 200 mg/kg, followed by 100 mg/kg every 6 hours. Tranexamic acid is given at a dose of 25 mg/kg orally or 10 mg/kg intravenously preoperatively. For tranexamic acid, a mouthwash preparation may be prepared by diluting the 10% intravenous solution with an equal volume of saline (89). Therapy is continued until the mucosal lesions are healed, which usually occurs in 2 to 5 days.

Desmopressin (DDAVP) increases the plasma concentrations of von Willebrand factor and raises the levels of factor VIII in mild to moderately severe hemophilia (90). It may be used in such individuals, in combination with an antifibrinolytic agent, to prevent bleeding associated with oral surgery. However, it is prudent to measure factor VIII levels after a test dose of the drug to be certain an adequate response is obtained (usually a fourfold increase in factor level). The customary dose is 0.3 μg/kg diluted in 30 to 50 mL of saline and infused intravenously over 20 minutes. The peak effect occurs in 30 to 60 minutes and is dissipated in 4 hours. A concentrated DDAVP intranasal spray (Stimate) is available as well. It has similar efficacy to the intravenous preparation, but its peak effect is observed 60 to 90 minutes after administration (91, 92). The intranasal dose is 150 μg in one metered dose for individuals weighing less than 50 kg and 300 μg in two metered doses for individuals weighing 50 kg or more (92). Several doses of DDAVP can be infused every 12 to 24 hours before tachyphylaxis is observed (90, 92). Side effects include asymptomatic facial flushing and, in individuals receiving large volumes of fluid or repeated doses, hyponatremia. This is particularly a problem in children younger than 2 years, in whom the hyponatremia may be sufficient to result in seizures (81). Therefore, fluid restriction, avoidance of hyponatremic oral and intravenous solutions, and close monitoring of urine output are mandatory in this age group. With the administration of repeated doses, monitoring of serum electrolytes is highly advisable. Another rare complication of DDAVP administration is thrombosis (86).

Aspirin and most nonsteroidal anti-inflammatory agents, such as naproxen, indomethacin, and piroxicam, are contraindicated in individuals with hemophilia, but a variety of other analgesic drugs are safe. For example, acetaminophen, propoxyphene, and codeine may be given to relieve pain from acute hemarthrosis. For arthritic pain associated with chronic hemophilic arthropathy, several nonacetylated salicylates (i.e., choline magnesium trisalicylate [Trilisate], salsalate [Disalcid], diflunisal) may provide relief. In some individuals, small doses of ibuprofen (400 mg once or twice daily) are well tolerated (93–95), but in others, more frequent bleeding may result. Individuals must always be warned about the risk of gastrointestinal bleeding with salicylates or ibuprofen and regularly check the character of their stools.

# SPECIFIC PROBLEMS

Specific problems are outlined in Table 35.3.

## MUSCULOSKELETAL BLEEDING

One of the most frequent complications of hemophilia, joint and muscle hemorrhage occur infrequently in children with this disorder until some time after the age of 1 year, and their occurrence corresponds to a developmental increase in mobility. When musculoskeletal bleeding begins, prompt therapy at the earliest sign should be initiated to ensure against recurrent bleeds that could lead to joint deformity, muscle atrophy, flexion contracture, and lifelong chronic disability. Detecting early hemorrhage, however, in very young children who are unable to communicate effectively can be difficult. With infants and young toddlers, early signs of musculoskeletal bleeding might include irritability and guarding or decreased use of the affected limb. By about 3 years of age, the child can learn to recognize an early acute hemarthrosis by the peculiar sensation within the joint that occurs before overt manifestations of a bleed, such as pain, swelling, warmth, and restricted mobility (96). Home infusion training should begin as soon as the family situation allows, in order to capitalize on early factor replacement. In preschoolers, enforced rest or splinting of the affected limb is rarely necessary because these children will automatically self-splint as long as there is discomfort. In older children, or in any child with a severe or advanced musculoskeletal hemorrhage, enforced rest, splinting, or both is followed by a program of active range of motion and strengthening exercises as symptoms abate. Analgesics other than acetaminophen are infrequently used in the treatment of early or minor bleeding; the pain associated with acute severe or advanced hemorrhage is usually treated successfully with acetaminophen and codeine.

Prevention of musculoskeletal bleeding is an important part of comprehensive hemophilia care. A general

**TABLE 35.3**   Guidelines Regarding Factor Replacement Therapy for Hemorrhage in Severe Hemophilia[a]

| Site of Bleed | Hemostatic Factor Level[b] | Factor Dosing | Comment |
|---|---|---|---|
| Joint | 40–50% | 20–40 U/kg QD as needed | Rest/immobilization/physical therapy rehabilitation post-bleed. Several doses may be necessary to prevent/treat target joint. |
| Muscle | 40–50% | 25–30 U/kg QD as needed | Calf/forearm bleed is limb-threatening. Significant blood loss with femoral/retroperitoneal bleed. |
| Oral mucosa | Initially 50%, then antifibrinolytic coverage usually suffices | 25 U/kg | Antifibrinolytic therapy is critical. Use cautiously with PCCs or APCCs. |
| Epistaxis | Initially 80–100%, then 30% until healing occurs | 40–50 U/kg, then 30–40 U/kg QD | Local measures: pressure/packing/cautery useful for severe/recurrent bleed. |
| Gastrointestinal | Initially 100%, then 30% until healing occurs | 40–50 U/kg, then 30–40 U/kg QD | Lesion is usually found (endoscopy highly recommended). Antifibrinolytics may be useful. |
| Genitourinary | Initially 100%, then 30% until healing occurs | 40–50 U/kg, then 30–40 U/kg QD | Evaluate for stones/UTI. Lesion usually not found. Prednisone, 1–2 mg/kg/day for 5–7 days is useful. |
| Central nervous system | Initially 100%, then 50–100% for 10–14 days | 50 U/kg, then 25 U/kg every 12 hours or by continuous infusion | Anticonvulsants frequently used preventatively, with neurologic follow-up. Lumbar puncture requires prophylactic factor coverage. |
| Trauma/surgery | Initially 100%, then 50% until wound healing begins, then 30% until wound healing is complete | 50 U/kg, then dose every 12 hours or by continuous infusion | Peri/postoperative management plan must be in place preoperatively; evaluation for inhibitors crucial before elective surgery. |

Adapted with permission from DiMichele D. Hemophilia 1996. New approaches to an old disease. Pediatr Clin North Am 1996;43:709–736.
APCC, activated prothrombin complex concentrate; PCC, prothrombin complex concentrate; UTI, urinary tract infection.
[a] Factor VIII level, <1% of normal.
[b] All percentages are of normal.

physical fitness program is encouraged through a wide range of recreational activity. Its aim is to promote good muscle strength and tone and, consequently, optimal stability of the joint. In severe or moderately severe hemophilia, only those activities involving excessive body contact or joint stress are discouraged. Undue trauma to muscle also should be avoided by refraining from intramuscular injections. Finally, long-term prophylactic infusion therapy has been used historically in Europe, with considerable success, for the reduction of musculoskeletal morbidity (97). The aim of therapy is to prevent spontaneous hemorrhage by converting severe hemophilia to moderate hemophilia by maintaining trough factor VIII levels at or above 1% of normal. In the past, routine use of such therapy in North America has been limited by the availability of a safe replacement product

and a high, unreimbursable cost. In 1994, however, acknowledging the advent of safer clotting factor, the Medical and Scientific Advisory Council of the National Hemophilia Foundation recommended use of primary prophylaxis beginning at between 1 and 2 years of age in children with severe hemophilia (98). Clinical trials are underway to establish the cost/benefit ratio of such therapy regarding both short-term and long-term morbidity.

## ACUTE HEMARTHROSIS

At the first indication of bleeding, which is usually a sensation of joint fullness or tingling, the individual should infuse clotting factor at a dose of 20 to 40 U/kg. The dose required to provide hemostasis varies among individuals (99). Early treatment aborts full-blown hemorrhage. As long as the joint is symptomatic, it should be kept immobilized.

When a joint undergoes repeated hemorrhages, it is called a *target joint*. At the first sign of a target joint, a child is placed on an aggressive regimen of short-term infusion of prophylactic factor and prolonged rest of the affected limb. This is followed by a joint rehabilitation program closely supervised by physical therapists. To prevent further hemorrhage into a developing target joint, secondary prophylactic factor replacement at a dose of 25 to 40 U/kg three to four times a week for several weeks to several months is instituted. In individuals with significant synovial inflammation, the brief, high dose prednisone regimen described previously may be implemented.

In teenagers and adults, one usually must distinguish between an acute hemarthrosis and the arthritic symptoms of a joint that has been ravaged by repeated hemorrhages. Acute joint bleeding is painful. The individual keeps the joint flexed and immobile, and there is warmth, erythema, and swelling. These signs result from an acute inflammatory reaction provoked by exposure of the synovium to blood. Marked vasodilatation and increased blood flow in the tissues adjacent to the acute hemarthrosis occur (100), and secondary to the inflammatory process, the synovium becomes hyperplastic, hyperemic, and thereby, more likely to bleed. Thus, a vicious cycle is initiated, with each bleed increasing the joint's vulnerability to a new hemorrhage. The joint often becomes deformed, has thickened synovium, and may have a chronic effusion. The situation is differentiated from that of acute bleeding by the lack of tenderness and warmth, which are the usual responses to fresh bleeding. The joints most often affected are the elbows, knees, and ankles. Radiographic findings include irregularity of the articular surface, loss of the joint space, formation of exostoses at the joint margins, and subchondral bone destruction, giving a cystic appearance to the articular bone (58).

Joint aspiration has always been controversial. We usually reserve this procedure for individuals with an acutely swollen, distended synovium, in whom the removal of blood results in the prompt relief of pain. Before aspiration, clotting factor levels should be raised to at least 50% of normal by infusing 30 U of clotting factor per kilogram. It is mandatory that individuals have a recent assay for the presence of clotting factor inhibitors before undergoing any invasive procedure, such as a joint aspiration. Should the individual have an inhibitor, treatment is altered as described in Chapter 37. Analgesics are usually necessary for adult individuals with acute hemarthroses. Acetaminophen with codeine, propoxyphene, hydrocodone, meperidine, or other agents not affecting platelet function should be given in doses

sufficient to control the severe pain associated with acute joint hemorrhage.

## CHRONIC HEMARTHROPATHY

Hemophilic arthropathy is a painful disorder, similar to that experienced by individuals with rheumatoid arthritis. There is usually morning stiffness and painful range of motion, and weight-bearing is limited and uncomfortable. Individuals with hemophilia are denied medications that give relief to those with rheumatic diseases, such as aspirin and other nonsteroidal anti-inflammatory drugs, because these drugs aggravate bleeding. Nonacetylated salicylates may bring some relief, however, and as noted, some individuals can tolerate small doses of ibuprofen without excessive bleeding. Short courses of steroids also may be helpful.

When conservative measures fail and effusions and bleeds recur, invasive procedures such as synoviorthesis with radioactive colloid (101) and arthroscopic synovectomy (102, 103) have helped many individuals (104). These procedures destroy or remove the affected synovium. If they are unsuccessful or there is persistent bleeding associated with constant pain, joint deformity, and loss of function, total joint replacement must be considered. With an experienced surgeon and adequate clotting factor replacement, good to excellent results may be anticipated. Long-term follow-up (up to 20 years) has shown that hip and knee prosthetic joints are both durable and serviceable (105, 106). They are usually pain-free and do not bleed. On the downside, however, range of motion at the joint is usually restricted, and they may become infected, requiring removal and a subsequent fusion procedure. Physical therapy plays a major role in the restoration of joint function following surgery and clotting factor replacement is continued for as long as active and passive range-of-motion exercises are performed to prevent bleeding as adhesions are broken and soft tissues are stretched.

## MUSCLE HEMORRHAGE

Bleeding into muscles may occur spontaneously or after trivial trauma. Hematomas may form in any muscle, but the quadriceps, iliopsoas (Fig. 35.1), and forearm muscle groups are usually affected. The clinical signs are pain, swelling, and alterations in sensation and strength if the neurovascular structures are compressed. For example, iliacus bleeding typically presents with vague abdominal, back, and groin pain, as well as flexion of the hip on the involved side (58). Pressure on the femoral nerve results in numbness of the skin over the anterior thigh, weakness of the quadriceps, loss of the patellar reflex, and impaired dorsiflexion of the foot. Bleeding into the forearm muscles or calf typically leads to a compartment

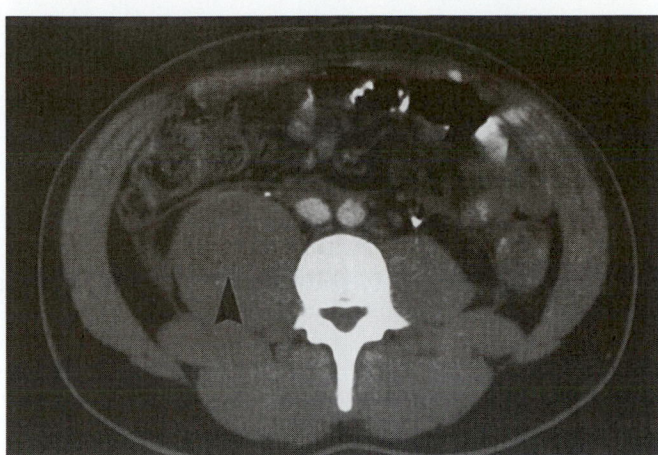

**FIGURE 35.1.** Computed tomography showing extensive iliopsoas hematoma (arrows).

syndrome with eventual loss of peripheral pulses, development of neurologic deficits, and need for fasciotomy. Any vague musculoskeletal pain in a individual with severe hemophilia should be attributed to a muscle hemorrhage, even if there are no outward signs of swelling or discoloration. An ultrasound examination often is helpful in localizing the hemorrhage to a specific muscle group.

Following an untreated or incompletely treated muscle or subperiosteal hemorrhage, a hemophilic pseudotumor may form (107) (Fig. 35.2). A hemophilic pseudotumor is a hematoma encased by a fibrous membrane. Progressive expansion of the hematoma because of rebleeding leads to encroachment on nearby soft tissues and bone as well as compression of adjacent neurovascular structures. Treatment invariably is surgical excision (108).

## ORAL MUCOSAL HEMORRHAGE

Bleeding from the mouth is one of the earliest manifestations of hemophilia in children younger than 1 year. In that age group, hemorrhage usually results from trauma to the tongue, gingiva, or frenula and, rarely, secondary to tooth eruption. Later in life, oral mucosal hemorrhage less often results from trauma and more frequently relates to dental procedures. Such bleeding can be treated or prevented with one dose of factor VIII replacement therapy, to a plasma level of at least 50% of normal, followed by a 2 to 5 day course of oral antifibrinolytic agents, such as tranexamic acid or EACA. Typically, antifibrinolytic therapy is started before dental procedures are performed. In the hands of an experienced dentist, however, dental scaling and minor restoration can often be accomplished with minimal hemostatic therapy.

## EAR, NOSE, AND THROAT

Minor trauma to the external ear canal or the nasal mucosa may produce annoying bleeding. The lesions are often tiny, but the amount of blood loss may be substantial. Barotrauma resulting from airplane flights may cause hemorrhage into the sinuses (Fig. 35.3). Bleeding into the posterior pharynx may occur with coughing or vomiting; the individual complains of a full feeling in the back of the throat. On examination, an ecchymosis or hematoma may be seen on the posterior pharyngeal wall. These hematomas are potentially dangerous, be-

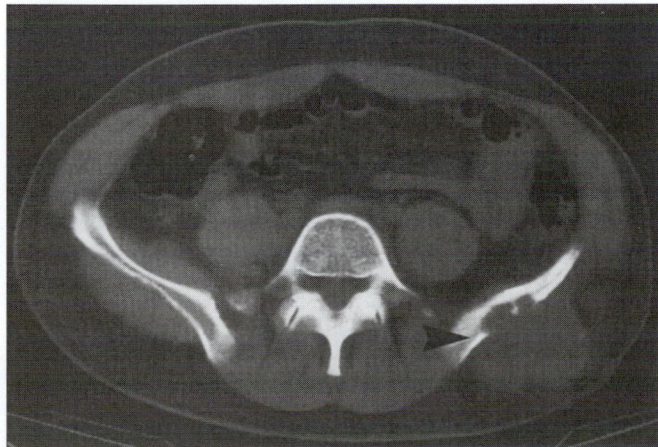

**FIGURE 35.2.** Computed tomography showing a large pseudotumor with erosion of ileum (arrow).

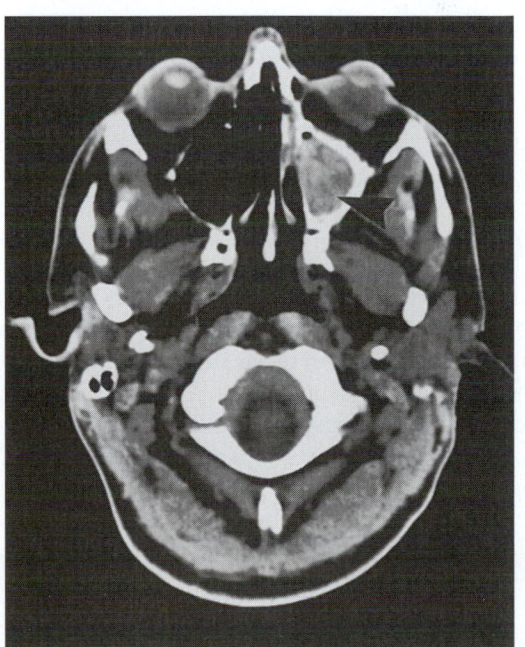

**FIGURE 35.3.** Computed tomography showing bleed into the maxillary sinus (arrow).

cause they may extend inferiorly to involve the larynx and compromise the airway. Thus, prompt and vigorous replacement therapy is required, as discussed in the section "Life-threatening Hemorrhage."

## CENTRAL NERVOUS SYSTEM

Intracranial bleeding may occur with minimal trauma and usually manifests by headache, lethargy, vomiting, or visual defects, which should be taken seriously in these individuals. By the time localizing signs of a brain hemorrhage appear, the bleeding is usually extensive. Therefore, as soon as the individual mentions the onset of new headache, a computed tomographic examination of the brain should be performed. In addition, clotting factor should be administered at a dose of 50 U/kg at the first suggestion of an intracranial bleed, even before diagnostic tests. If hemorrhage is documented, hospitalization is indicated, and a minimum clotting factor level of 50% of normal should be maintained for at least 10 to 14 days. Subsequently, long-term prophylactic factor therapy is usually instituted to prevent the high incidence of recurrence.

## GASTROINTESTINAL TRACT

The appearance of gross blood in the stool, or melena, should prompt a search for a gastrointestinal tract lesion. Investigation in adults usually reveals that bleeding is from esophagitis, gastritis, peptic ulcers, proctitis, or hemorrhoids. Neoplasms, polyps, and diverticuli are much less common in this population. In children, bowel intussusception, Meckel's diverticulum, infectious colitis, esophagitis, hiatal hernia, gastritis, peptic ulcer disease, and swallowed blood following epistaxis must be considered depending on the age of the individual and the associated symptoms. In adolescents, Crohn's disease or ulcerative colitis may cause either hematochezia or melena. Treatment should continue until bleeding has subsided and ulcerations have healed.

## GENITOURINARY TRACT

Hematuria occurs at least once or twice during the lifetime of every individual with moderate or severe hemophilia, but usually, no source for the bleeding is discovered (109). If bleeding is persistent, a hematoma may be observed in the papillary area of the kidney. Recurrent episodes of hematuria may be responsible for the higher than normal incidence of hypertension in individuals with hemophilia. Alternatively, hypertension may be responsible for the kidney bleeding. In children, a urinary tract infection should be ruled out.

## PATIENTS UNDERGOING SURGERY

When contemplating any invasive procedure in a individual with hemophilia, the physician must determine whether the individual has an inhibitor and, therefore, may be refractory to the usual doses of clotting factor. If no inhibitor is present, the initial dose depends on the extent of surgery. Dental extractions require 25 to 30 U/kg, whereas a laparotomy or orthopaedic procedure requires 50 U/kg. The dose is given immediately before the procedure so that surgery is performed at the time of the peak blood level. Additional doses generally are not needed during the operation, and individuals having dental procedures usually do not require additional clotting factor if they are receiving an antifibrinolytic agent. In those individuals undergoing major surgery, one should measure the clotting factor level immediately after the operation and administer additional concentrate to raise the levels to between 50 and 100% of normal. Doses are then given every 12 hours (or continuously infused) to maintain the clotting factor at this level, and assays are performed daily on blood samples drawn before the dose (at the nadir of the previous dose) to confirm that levels of 50 to 100% are being maintained. Treatment must continue until all wounds are healed; for orthopaedic individuals, doses generally are given every day before physical therapy sessions. Thus, one should anticipate at least 2 to 3 weeks of twice daily dosing, and for individuals undergoing major muscle and joint surgery, another 3 to 6 weeks of daily dosing.

## LIFE-THREATENING HEMORRHAGE

Life-threatening bleeding may occur after head injury, abdominal trauma, and major surgery. Whenever such bleeding is suspected, the rule is to treat first and obtain diagnostic tests second. Doses of clotting factor should be at least 50 U/kg and given by the first person to encounter the injured individual. Early treatment can mean the difference between permanent impairment and full recovery. If the diagnostic studies fail to reveal evidence of bleeding, but there has been definite trauma (e.g., striking the head, nonpenetrating abdominal injury), the individual should be kept under observation for 24 hours and additional concentrate infused to maintain clotting factor levels between 50 and 100% of normal. As mentioned, treatment must be continued until all wounds are healed.

# PSYCHOSOCIAL AND ECONOMIC CONSIDERATIONS

The psychosocial impact of a diagnosis of hemophilia on individuals and families is enormous (110). As with other types of chronic disease, its lifelong nature and the limitations it imposes have implications for the individuals' psychologic, emotional, social, and financial well-being.

Beginning in infancy, the diagnosis of hemophilia may affect significantly the mutual development of attachment between infant and parent (111, 112). Then, as children enter the separation and individuation phase of development, the child-parent relationship is further strained by the children's need to explore their world and limitations on their own terms and by the parents' natural tendency to overprotect. The balance between maintaining physical health, as achieved by establishing reasonable limitations, and promoting emotional and psychologic health, as achieved by fostering responsible and independent behavior, is difficult but critical to development of an overall sense of well-being by the person with hemophilia. The disability resulting from acute hemorrhage may cause an inordinate number of absences from school as well, and this greatly interferes with the student's positive perception of the educational experience and excitement about learning. These consequences may have a lifelong impact.

Adolescents are at a developmental stage when peer approval is of primary importance. They are acutely sensitive to and aware of even the slightest differences between themselves and their peers. Therefore, the effect of intermittent or chronic physical disability on the development of a healthy body image and, consequently, on the crucial development of the self-confidence and self-esteem necessary for healthy socialization cannot be overestimated. In addition, the prevalence of HIV infection in this population has complicated the issues of emerging sexuality and precipitated premature confrontation with death at a time when peers are experiencing feelings of immortality. Furthermore, the social stigmata associated with HIV infection isolate the adolescent with hemophilia in a cloak of secrecy and anxiety when peers are actively socializing.

Adulthood traditionally is associated with exploring career interests, achieving sexual identity and independence from parents and other authority figures, and developing one's own family. Before the 1980s, the major concerns of adults with hemophilia centered around the impact of intermittent or chronic physical disability from hemorrhage, hepatitis, or both on job security, medical insurability, and consequently, on the family's financial survival and well-being. Now, with the markedly reduced life expectancy of these individuals from HIV infection, these concerns are greatly intensified. Not infrequently, despite being primarily infected with HIV, adults with hemophilia survive their spouse and children, who die from AIDS.

Never in the history of hemophilia care has the comprehensive treatment center model (discussed later), with its multidisciplinary approach to the treatment of both individuals with hemophilia and the family unit, been so important to the successful delivery of health care to this population. The effectiveness of this intervention is related to collaborative efforts among members of the treatment team as well as the creative use of community resources, such as the medical consumer based hemophilia foundation chapter, local mental health facilities, and community organizations that provide services to specific ethnicities and culture oriented populations.

Despite the enormity of the physical and psychosocial hardships facing these individuals today, optimism about the future is still expressed by both individuals and caregivers. The scourge of HIV infection will most likely be limited, as there has been no further transmission of the retrovirus through factor replacement since 1985. The prospect for future transmission of another, similarly deadly virus through plasma-derived products has been reduced by the arrival of genetically engineered (i.e., recombinant) factor therapy, and the potential for eventual cure through gene therapy now exists. To suggest that future therapy will not involve its own set of risks and complications would be folly, but, as discussed, DNA-based techniques for prenatal diagnosis can, under optimal conditions, detect almost all potential carriers of the hemophilia A gene and all affected males *in utero*. Nevertheless, the results of a 1990 study suggest that despite a diagnosis of even severe hemophilia A in a male fetus *in utero*, most of the involved families opt against therapeutic abortion (113). Persons with hemophilia and their families, given the available and potential therapy, are still anticipating good to excellent quality of life for their affected offspring.

Finally, however, as alluded to earlier, therapeutic advances have not come without a high price. The cost of a unit of factor replacement alone has at least doubled, and in some cases quadrupled, during the last half-decade. Consequently, loss of medical insurability is a constant threat and a frequent reality because of lifetime spending capitation, limitations imposed by managed care, temporary exclusion by preexisting condition clauses, and job insecurity. Alternatives such as state subsidies and catastrophic health insurance programs are severely limited. Furthermore, at a time when they are most needed, hemophilia treatment programs are themselves threatened by shrinking federal subsidies and the inability of hospitals to absorb the cost of caring for this increasingly uninsured population. Issues of affordability may limit access to state-of-the-art hemophilia care as it develops and pose difficult ethical dilemmas for caregivers. To whom do we recommend recombinant factor replacement therapy? Who will have access to gene therapy when the technology becomes available? Even these questions become trivial, however, when placed in the perspective of the state of hemophilia care throughout the world. Indeed, for most individuals, the dilemma for caregivers is who should receive the small amount of available factor replacement. No doubt solving the problems of the cost of health care delivery in this country and of health care access throughout the world will be the major challenge for the hemophilia community in the twenty-first century.

# CONCLUSIONS

Because of the unique requirements of hemophilia care, which include specialized laboratory procedures, genetic counseling, home infusion education, arrangements for the acquisition of and payment for expensive concentrates, and frequent collaborations with specialists in dental, orthopaedic, and psychiatric care, hemophilia treatment centers have been organized throughout the world. Devoted to the unique problems of this individual population, these centers are an important resource for local health care deliverers. When a individual is diagnosed with hemophilia, referral to a treatment center is obligatory to confirm the diagnosis, institute appropriate therapy, provide counseling, and so on. The local physician should remain the primary caregiver, working with the center in the best interests of the individual and family.

Hopefully, persons with hemophilia will never again experience a scourge such as HIV infection (114). For those who have been infected, however, either with this virus or with others such as hepatitis B and C, close collaboration between the primary physician and the infectious disease specialist is essential. The myriad of infectious problems that HIV-positive individuals experience requires constant surveillance and use of potent new antiretroviral therapy and antimicrobial drugs, which are probably best administered by those who are knowledgeable in the risks and benefits of these agents. Furthermore, sexual counseling and psychologic support for the individual and family usually require a team approach using the services of a social worker, nurse clinician, psychologist, and physician.

With the approach of the twenty-first century, technologic advancement is now directed toward a cure. Liver transplantation performed in 1985 for hepatitis-related cirrhosis in a individual with hemophilia A effectively cured the hemophilia (115). The same procedure when first performed on a individual with hemophilia B had the same outcome (116). It is hoped that transplantation of a normal gene for either the factor VIII or factor IX protein will produce much the same outcome. To that end, *in vitro* gene insertion experiments using several mammalian cell lines and *in vivo* gene deficiency trials using selected animal models are currently underway (117–119). In a canine model of hemophilia, infusion of an adenoviral vector expressing human factor VIII cDNA resulted in factor VIII expression for up to 2 weeks (120). Clinical trials in gene therapy are anticipated in humans before the year 2000, thus making a cure for hemophilia a tangible expectation of the next century.

# References

1. Rosendaal FR. Hemophilia—the best of times, the worst of times (doctoral thesis). Leiden: University of Leiden, 1989.
2. Jones PK, Ratnoff OD. The changing prognosis of classic hemophilia (factor VIII "deficiency"). Ann Intern Med 1991;114:641–648.
3. Gitschier J, Kogan S, Diamond C et al. Genetic basis of hemophilia A. Thromb Haemost 1991;66:37–39.
4. Ingram GI. The history of haemophilia. J Clin Pathol 1976;29:469–479.
5. Nossel HL, Archer RK, Macfarlane RG. Equine haemophilia: report of a case and its response to multiple infusions of heterospecific AHG. Br J Haematol 1962;8:335–342.
6. Kaneko JJ, Cordy DR, Carlson G. Canine hemophilia resembling classic hemophilia A. J Am Vet Med Assoc 1967;150:15–21.
7. Rosner F. Hemophilia in the Talmud and rabbinic writings. Ann Intern Med 1969;70:833–837.
8. Seligsohn U. Hemophilia and other clotting disorders. Isr J Med Sci 1973;9:1338–1340.
9. Otto JC. An account of an hemorrhagic disposition existing in certain families. Med Repos 1803;6:1.
10. Bulloch W, Fildes P. Treasury of human inheritance, parts V and VI, section XIVa, haemophilia. London: Dulau & Company Ltd., 1911.
11. Legg JW. A treatise on haemophilia sometimes called the hereditary haemorrhagic diathesis. London: HK Lewis, 1872:158.
12. Hopff F. Ueberdie haemophilie oder die erbliche anlage zu todtlichen blutungen. Wurtzburg: CW Becker, 1828.
13. Schonlein JL. Vorlesungen ueber pathologie und therapie. 3tte Auflage 1837;2:63.
14. Lane S. Successful transfusion of blood. Lancet 1840;i:185.
15A. Wright AE. On a method of determining the condition of blood coagulability for clinical and experimental purposes, and on the effect of the administration of calcium salts in haemophilia and actual or threatened haemorrhage. Br Med J 1893;2:223–225.
15B. Morawitz P. Die chemie der blutgerinnung. Ergebn Physiol 1905;4:307.
16. Addis T. Hereditary haemophilia: deficiency in the coagulability of the blood the only immediate cause of the condition. Q J Med 1910;4:14.
17. Howell WH. The condition of the blood in haemophilia. Am J Physiol 1914;33:13.
18. Quick AJ. The prothrombin in hemophilia and in obstructive jaundice. J Biol Chem 1935;109:23.
19. Patek AJ, Taylor FHL. Hemophilia. Some properties of a substance obtained from normal human plasma effective in accelerating the coagulation of hemophilic blood. J Clin Invest 1937;16:113.
20. Wright IS. The nomenclature of blood clotting factors. Thromb Diath Haemorrh 1962;7:381–386.
21. Biggs R, Douglas AS, Macfarlane RG et al. Christmas disease: a condition previously mistaken for haemophilia. Br Med J 1952;2:1378–1382.
22. Koller F. Is hemophilia a nosologic entity? Blood 1954;9:286–290.
23. Zimmerman TS, Ratnoff OD, Powell AE. Immunologic differentiation of classic hemophilia (factor VIII deficiency) and von Willebrand's disease, with observations on combined deficiencies of antihemophilic factor and proaccelerin (factor V) and on an acquired circulating anticoagulant against antihemophilic factor. J Clin Invest 1971;50:244–254.
24. Zimmerman TS, Ratnoff OD, Littell AS. Detection of carriers of classic hemophilia using an immunologic assay for antihemophilia factor (factor VIII). J Clin Invest 1971;50:225–258.
25. Wood WI, Capon DJ, Simonsen CC et al. Expression of active human factor VIII from recombinant DNA clones. Nature 1984;312:330–337.
26. Toole JJ, Knopf JL, Wozney JM et al. Molecular cloning of a cDNA encoding human antihaemophilic factor. Nature 1984;312:342–347.
27. Kurachi K, Davie EW. Isolation and characterization of a cDNA coding for human factor IX. Proc Natl Acad Sci U S A 1982;79:6461–6464.
28. Kaufman RJ. Structure and biology of factor VIII. In: Hoffman R, Benz EJ, Shattil SJ, Furie B, Cohen HJ, eds. Hematology—basic principles and practice. New York: Churchill Livingstone, 1990;1276–1284.
29. Thompson AR. Structure and biology of factor IX. In: Benz EJ, Cohen JH, Furie B, Hoffman R, Shatil SJ, eds. Hematology—basic principles and practice. New York: Churchill Livingstone, 1990:1308–1316.
30. Barrowcliffe TW. Comparisons of one-stage and two-stage assays of factor VIII:C. Scand J Haematol 1984;33(Suppl 41):39–54.
31. Tripodi A, Mannucci PM. Factor VIII activity as measured by an amidolytic assay compared with a one-stage clotting assay. Am J Clin Pathol 1986;86:341–344.
32. Kasper CK, Aledort L, Aronson D et al. Proceedings: a more uniform measurement of factor VIII inhibitors. Thromb Diath Haemorrh 1975;34:612.
33. Austen DE, Lechner K, Rizza CR et al. A comparison of the Bethesda and New Oxford method of factor VIII antibody assay. Thromb Haemost 1982;47:72–75.
34. Lyon M. Sex chromatin and gene action in the mammalian X chromosome. Am J Hum Genet 1962;14:135–148.
35. Fishman DJ, Jones PK, Menitove JE et al. Detection of the carrier state for

classic hemophilia using an enzyme-linked immunosorbent assay (ELISA). Blood 1982;59:1163–1168.

36. Ratnoff OD, Jones PK. Diagnosis of the carrier state in hemophilia [Letter]. Am J Hematol 1988;28:132.

37. Gitschier J, Wood WI, Goralka TM et al. Characterization of the human factor VIII gene. Nature 1984;312:326–330.

38. Wacey AI, Kemball-Cook G, Kazazian HH et al. The haemophilia A mutation search test and resource site, home page of the factor VIII mutation database: HAMSTeRS. Nucleic Acids Res 1996;24:100–102.

39. Haldane JBS. The rate of spontaneous mutation of a human gene. J Genet 1935;31:317–326.

40. Kazazian HH Jr. The molecular basis of hemophilia A and the present status of carrier and antenatal diagnosis of the disease. Thromb Haemost 1993;70:60–62.

41. Lillicrap DP, White BN, Holden JJ et al. Carrier detection in the hemophilias. Am J Hematol 1987;26:285–296.

42. Janco RL, Phillips JA III, Orlando PJ et al. Detection of hemophilia A carriers using intragenic factor VIII:C DNA polymorphisms. Blood 1987;69:1539–1541.

43. Lalloz MR, McVey JH, Pattinson JK et al. Haemophilia A diagnosis by analysis of a hypervariable dinucleotide repeat within the factor VIII gene. Lancet 1991;338:207–211.

44. Pecorara M, Casarino L, Mori PG et al. Hemophilia A: carrier detection and prenatal diagnosis by DNA analysis. Blood 1987;70:531–535.

45. Suehiro K, Tanimoto M, Hamaguchi M et al. Carrier detection in Japanese hemophilia A by use of three intragenic and two extragenic factor VIII DNA probes: a study of 24 kindreds. J Lab Clin Med 1988;112:314–318.

46. Lakich D, Kazazian H, Antonarakis SE et al. Inversions disrupting the factor VIII gene are a common cause of severe hemophilia A. Nat Genet 1993;5:236–241.

47. Naylor J, Brinke A, Hassock S et al. Characteristic mRNA abnormality found in half the individuals with severe hemophilia A is due to large DNA inversions. Hum Mol Genet 1993;2:1773–1778.

48. Naylor JA, Green PM, Rizza CR et al. Analysis of factor VIII mRNA reveals defects in everyone of 28 haemophilia A individuals. Hum Mol Genet 1993;2:11–17.

49. Windsor S, Taylor SA, Lillicrap D. Direct detection of a common inversion mutation in the genetic diagnosis of severe hemophilia A. Blood 1994;84:2202–2205.

50. Jenkins PV, Collins PW, Goldman E et al. Analysis of intron 22 inversions of the factro VIII gene in severe hemophilia A: implications for genetic counselling. Blood 1994;84:2197–2201.

51. Hemker HC, Kessels H. Feedback mechanisms in coagulation. Haemostasis 1991;21:189–196.

52. Rao LV, Rapaport SI, Bajaj SP. Activation of human factor VII in the initiation of tissue factor-dependent coagulation. Blood 1986;68:685–691.

53. Rao LV, Rapaport SI. Studies of a mechanism inhibitng the initiation of the extrinsic pathway of coagulation. Blood 1987;69:645–651.

54. Broze GJ Jr, Warren LA, Novotny WF et al. The lipoprotein-associated coagulation inhibitor that inhibits the factor VII-tissue factor complex also inhibits factor Xa: insight into its possible mechanism of action. Blood 1988;71:335–343.

55. Nordfang O, Valentin S, Beck TC et al. Inhibition of extrinsic pathway inhibitor shortens the coagulation time of normal plasma and of hemophilia plasma. Thromb Haemost 1991;66:464–467.

56. Lewis RM, Schneider MJ, Fricke W. Neutralization of tissue factor pathway inhibitor corrects the clotting time of hemophilic plasma in vitro [Abstract]. Blood 1991;87:73A.

57. Eyster ME, Gordon RA, Ballard JO. The bleeding time is longer than normal in hemophilia. Blood 1981;58:719–723.

58. Matthews JM, Rizza CR. Clinical features of clotting factor deficiencies. In: Biggs R, Rizza CR, eds. Human blood coagulation, haemostasis and thrombosis. Oxford: Blackwell Scientific Publications, 1984:119–169.

59. Goldsmith JC, Kletzel M. Risk of birth intracranial hemorrhage in hemophilic newborns: results of a North American survey [Abstract]. Blood 1990;76(Suppl 1):421A.

60. Cochran CD, Ahles TA, Weiss AE. Psychological factors and bleeding frequency in hemophilia. Lack of association. Am J Pediatr Hematol Oncol 1987;9:136–139.

61. Kerr CB. The fortunes of haemophiliacs in the nineteenth century. Med Hist 1963;7:359.

62. Biggs CR. Thirty years of haemophilia treatment in Oxford. Br J Haematol 1967;13:429–436.

63. Kekwick RA, Wolf P. A concentrate of human antihaemophilic factor—its use in six cases of haemophilia. Lancet 1957;i:647.

64. Pool JD, Shannon AE. Production of high potency concentrates of antihemophilic globulin in a closed bag system. N Engl J Med 1965;273:1443.

65. Mannucci PM, Pareti FI, Ruggeri ZM et al. 1-Deamino-8-D-arginine vasopressin: a new pharmacological approach to the management of hemophilia and von Willebrand's disease. Lancet 1977;i:869–872.

66. Larsson SA. Life expectancy of Swedish haemophiliacs, 1831–1980. Br J Haematol 1985;59:593–602.

67. Schulman S, Wiechel B. Hepatitis, epidemiology and liver function in hemophiliacs in Sweden. Acta Med Scand 1984;215:249–256.

68. Fulcher CA, Zimmerman TS. Characterization of the human factor VIII procoagulant protein with a heterologous precipitating antibody. Proc Natl Acad Sci U S A 1982;79:1648–1652.

69. Fass DN, Knutson GJ, Katzmann JA. Monoclonal antibodies to porcine factor VIII coagulant and their use in the isolation of active coagulant protein. Blood 1982;59:594–600.

70. McDougal JS, Martin LS, Cort SP et al. Thermal inactivation of the acquired immunodeficiency syndrome virus, human T-lymphotropic virus III/lymphadenopathy-associated virus, with special reference to antihaemophilic factor. J Clin Invest 1985;76:875–877.

71. Prince AM, Horowitz B, Brotman B. Sterilization of hepatitis and HTLV-III viruses by exposure to tri(n-butyl) phosphate and sodium cholate. Lancet 1986;i:706–710.

72. Schimpf K, Mannucci PM, Kreutz W et al. Absence of hepatitis after treatment with a pasteurized factor VIII concentrate in individuals with hemophilia and no previous transfusion. N Engl J Med 1987;316:918–922.

73. Shapiro AD, Ragni MV, Lusher JM et al. Safety and efficacy of monoclonal antibody purified factor IX concentrate in previously untreated individuals with hemophilia B. Thromb Haemost 1996;75:30–35.

74. White G, Pasi J, Lusher J et al. Recombinant factor IX in the treatment of previously-treated individuals with hemophilia B. Thromb Haemost (Suppl) 1997;52A.

75. Bray GL, Gomperts ED, Courter S et al. A multicenter study of recombinant factor VIII (recombinate): safety, efficacy and inhibitor risk in previously untreated individuals with hemophilia A. The Recombinate Study Group. Blood 1994;83:2428–2435.

76. Schwartz RS, Abildgaard CF, Aledort LM et al. Human recombinant DNA-derived antihemophilic factor (factor VIII) in the treatment of haemophilia A. N Engl J Med 1990;323:1800–1805.

77. Schwartz RS, Rousell RH. A summary of the world-wide clinical investigations of recombinant factor VIII. Semin Hematol 1991;28(Suppl 1):53–54.

78. Schulman S, Martinowitz U. Continuous infusion instead of bolus injections of factor concentrate? Haemophilia 1996;2:189–191.

79. Rabiner SF, Telfer MC. Home transfusion for individuals with hemophilia A. N Engl J Med 1970;283:1011–1015.

80. Levine PH. Efficacy of self-therapy in hemophilia. N Engl J Med 1974;291:1381–1384.

81. Smith TJ, Gill JC, Ambruso DR et al. Hyponatremic seizures in young children given DDAVP. Am J Hematol 1989;31:199–202.

82. de Biasi R, Rocino A, Miraglia E et al. The impact of very high-purity factor VIII concentrate on the immune system of human immunodeficiency virus-infected hemophiliacs: a randomized prospective two-year comparison with an intermediate purity concentrate. Blood 1991;78:1919–1922.

83. Seremetis SV, Aledort LM, Bergman GE et al. Three-year randomized study of high-purity or intermediate-purity factor VIII concentrates in symptom-free HIV-seropositive haemophiliacs: effects on immune status. Lancet 1993;342:700–703.

84. Wadhwa M, Dilger P, Tubbs J et al. Identification of transforming growth factor–B as a contaminant in factor VIII concentrates: a possible link with immunosuppressive effects in hemophiliacs. Blood 1994;84:2021–2030.

85. Gjerset GF, Pike MC, Mosley JW et al. Effect a low- and intermediate-purity clotting factor therapy on progression of human immunodeficiency virus infection in congenital clotting disorders. Transfusion Safety Study Group. Blood 1994;84:1666–1671.

86. Mannucci PM, Lusher JM. Desmopressin and thrombosis. Lancet 1989;ii:675–676.

87. Kisker CT, Burke C. Double-blind studies on the use of steroids in the treatment of acute hemarthrosis in individuals with hemophilia. N Engl J Med 1970;282:639–642.

88. Strauss HS, Kevy SV, Diamond LK. Ineffectiveness of prophylactic epsilon aminocaproic acid in severe hemophilia. N Engl J Med 1965;273:301–304.

89. Sindet-Pedersen S, Ingerslev J, Ramstrom G et al. Management of oral bleeding in haemophiliac individuals. Lancet 1989;i:325.

90. Mannucci PM. Desmopressin (DDAVP) for treatment of disorders of hemostasis. Prog Hemost Thromb 1986;8:19–45.

91. Lethagen S, Harris AS, Nilsson IM. Intranasal desmopressin (DDAVP) by spray in mild hemophilia A and von Willebrand's disease type I. Blut 1990;60:187–191.

92. Rose EH, Aledort LM. Nasal spray desmopressin (DDAVP) for mild hemophilia A and von Willebrand disease. Ann Intern Med 1991;114:563–568.

93. McIntyre BA, Philp RB, Inwood MJ. Effect of ibuprofen on platelet function in normal subjects and hemophiliac individuals. Clin Pharmacol Ther 1978;24:616–621.

94. Hasiba U, Scranton PE, Lewis JH et al. Efficacy and safety of ibuprofen for hemophilic arthropathy. Arch Intern Med 1980;140:1583–1585.

95. Inwood MJ, Killackey B, Startup SJ. The use and safety of ibuprofen in the hemophiliac. Blood 1983;61:709–711.

96. Hilgartner MW. The management of recurrent hemarthroses: the hematologist's viewpoint. In: Wiedel JD, Gilbert MS, eds. Management of musculo-

skeletal problems in hemophilia. New York: The National Hemophilia Foundation, 1985:16–19.

97. Nilsson IM, Berntorp E, Lofqvist T. Prophylactic treatment of hemophilia in Sweden. Thromb Haemost 1991;65:823.

98. Hemophilia Information Exchange: Medical and Scientific Advisory Council (MASAC) recommendations concerning prophylaxis. Med Bulletin #193, Chapter Advisory #197, March 11, 1994.

99. Aronstam A, Choudhury DP, Wasssef M et al. Double-blind controlled trial of three dosage regimens in treatment of haemarthroses in haemophilia A. Lancet 1980;i:169–171.

100. Green D, Spies SM, Rana NA et al. Hemophilic bleeding evaluated by blood pool scanning. Thromb Haemost l981;45:208–210.

101. Rivard GE. Synoviorthesis with radioactive colloids in hemophiliacs. Prog Clin Biol Res 1990;324:215–229.

102. Kim HC, Klein K, Hirsch S et al. Arthroscopic synovectomy in the treatment of hemophilic synovitis. Scand J Haematol 1984;33(Suppl 40):271–279.

103. Wiedel JD. Arthroscopic synovectomy for chronic hemophilic synovitis of the knee. Arthroscopy 1985;1:205–209.

104. Kasper CK. Recent advances in hemophilia care. In: Kasper CK, ed. Progress in clinical and biological research. New York: Alan R. Liss, 1990:324–341.

105. Rana NA, Shapiro GR, Green D. Long-term follow-up of prosthetic joint replacement in hemophilia. Am J Hematol 1986;23:329–337.

106. Luck JV, Kasper CK. Surgical management of advanced hemophilic arthropathy. Clin Orthop 1989;242:60–82.

107. Duthie RB, Matthews JM, Rizza CR et al. Haemophilic cysts and pseudotumours. In: Duthie RB, ed. The management of musculoskeletal problems in the haemophilias. Oxford: Blackwell Scientific Publications, 1972:84–100.

108. Tezanos Pinto M, Nieto R, Perez Bianco R. Hemophilic pseudotumor: a report of 25 cases. In: Lusher JM, Kessler CM, eds. Hemophilia and von Willebrand's disease in the 1990's. Amsterdam: Excerpta Medica, 1991:165–178.

109. Prentice CRM, Lindsay RM et al. Renal complications in haemophilia and Christmas disease. Q J Med 1971;40:47–61.

110. Seligman M, Darling RB. Ordinary families, special children, a systems approach to childhood disability. New York: Guild Press, 1989.

111. Stern DN. The interpersonal world of the infant. A view from psychoanalysis and developmental psychology. New York: Basic Books, 1985.

112. Greenspan SI, Lieberman A. The clinical approach to attachment. In: Harvey D, ed. Parent-Infant Relationships. New York:Wiley, 1987.

113. Varekamp I, Suurmeijer TP, Brocker-Vriends AH et al. Carrier testing and prenatal diagnosis for hemophilia: experiences and attitudes of 549 potential and obligate carriers. Am J Med Genet 1990;37:147–154.

114. Ratnoff OD. Some complications of the therapy of classic hemophilia. J Lab Clin Med 1984;103:653–659.

115. Bontempo FA, Lewis JH, Gorenc TJ et al. Liver transplantation in hemophilia A. Blood 1987;69:1721–1724.

116. Merion RM, Delius RE, Campbell DA Jr et al. Orthotopic liver transplantation totally corrects factor IX deficiency in hemophilia B. Surgery 1988;104:929–931.

117. Hoeben RC, Fallaux FJ, Van Tilburg NH et al. Toward gene therapy for hemophilia A: long-term persistence of factor VIII–secreting fibroblasts after transplantation into immunodeficient mice. Hum Gene Ther 1993;4:179–186.

118. Hoeben RC, van der Jagt RC, Schoute F et al. Expression of functional factor VIII in primary human skin fibroblasts after retrovirus-mediated gene transfer. J Biol Chem 1990;265:7318–7323.

119. Zatloukal K, Cotten M, Berger M et al. In vivo production of human factor VII in mice after intrasplenic implantation of primary fibroblasts transfected by receptor-mediated adenovirus-augmented gene delivery. Proc Natl Acad Sci U S A 1994;91:5148–5152.

120. Connelly S, Mount J, Mauser A et al. Complete short-term correction of canine hemophilia A by in vivo gene therapy. Blood 1996;88:3846–3853.

# CHAPTER 36

# OTHER COAGULATION FACTOR DEFICIENCIES

Harold R. Roberts and M. Daniel Bingham

## DISORDERS OF FIBRINOGEN

### QUANTITATIVE FIBRINOGEN ABNORMALITIES (AFIBRINOGENEMIA, HYPOFIBRINOGENEMIA)

Congenital disorders of fibrinogen with quantitative abnormalities include afibrinogenemia and hypofibrinogenemia. Afibrinogenemia is a very rare condition. The first case was reported in 1920 (1); since then, approximately 150 cases have been described (2, 3). Congenital hypofibrinogenemia was first recognized in 1935 (4), but some cases of hypofibrinogenemia are, in fact, cases of dysfibrinogenemia with low circulating levels of clottable fibrinogen.

### Pathogenesis

In congenital afibrinogenemia and hypofibrinogenemia, there is a failure of synthesis, secretion, or intracellular transport of the gene product (5–8). In some cases, the newly synthesized fibrinogen is not secreted. Rather, it accumulates in the rough endoplasmic reticulum of the hepatocyte, where it can cause mild hepatic disease (9–11). True hypofibrinogenemia, in which the fibrinogen has a normal structure, probably represents the heterozygous state of afibrinogenemia. In afibrinogenemia and true hypofibrinogenemia, the fibrinolytic system and other coagulation factors are normal, and there is no evidence of increased fibrinogen use or consumption.

### Genetics

The fibrinogen gene is located on chromosome 4, which contains three separate genes for the α, β, and γ chains, respectively (6, 12–14). In afibrinogenemia, all three genes are present. The inheritance pattern of the disorder is autosomal recessive (3, 5, 6, 13), and affected individuals are homozygotes. Consanguinity is present in over 50% of affected individuals with afibrinogenemia.

### Clinical Manifestations

Individuals with afibrinogenemia may have frequent and dangerous hemorrhages. Their blood is incoagulable, so it is surprising that abnormal bleeding does not occur more frequently. Life-threatening hemorrhage does occur, however, and early death may ensue. Prolonged umbilical bleeding often leads to the diagnosis in early infancy (3, 13–15). Intracranial bleeding is a leading cause of death, again often in infancy or childhood (13, 16–18). Hemorrhage from the gastrointestinal tract and mucosal membranes is common, and menorrhagia is a frequent complication in affected women. Hemarthroses occur in approximately 20% of individuals but usually are not as frequent as hemarthroses in individuals with hemophilia. Many individuals reach adulthood without the crippling joint complications seen in individuals with severe, classic hemophilia. There also is an increased incidence of first trimester abortion, placental abruption, and postpartum hemorrhage (13, 19–21). Fetuses of individuals with afibrinogenemia rarely reach full term unless fibrinogen is replaced throughout pregnancy (22). Paradoxically,

773

afibrinogenemia may be complicated by thromboembolic disease that is precipitated by fibrinogen replacement (23–25).

Individuals with congenital hypofibrinogenemia usually do not have spontaneous bleeding. Spontaneous bleeding may occur, however, if the fibrinogen level is less than 50 mg/dL (3).

## Laboratory Tests

Results of coagulation screening tests, such as prothrombin time (PT), activated partial thromboplastin time (aPTT), and thrombin clotting time (TCT), in individuals with afibrinogenemia are infinitely long. These tests are easily corrected, however, by mixing individual plasma with normal plasma. Specific diagnosis rests on demonstration of (no significant amount can be detected) circulating fibrinogen through clotting or immunologic assays (26). Platelet fibrinogen also is absent. Mild thrombocytopenia has been reported, but the platelet count usually is not lower than 100,000 cells/µl (27). The bleeding time is characteristically prolonged in afibrinogenemia, presumably from absent platelet fibrinogen—even although platelet aggregation has occurred in the absence of fibrinogen (28–30). In individuals with afibrinogenemia, delayed-type hypersensitivity skin tests may show erythema only and no induration, because the latter depends on the deposition of subcutaneous fibrin (31). In true hypofibrinogenemia, the plasma concentration of fibrinogen is about half the normal value, but lower values have been reported.

## Differential Diagnosis

Congenital quantitative defects in fibrinogen must be distinguished from those of congenital hypodysfibrinogenemia (32) and the more common, acquired qualitative and quantitative defects in liver disease and disseminated intravascular coagulation (see Chapters 44 and 45). Acquired hypofibrinogenemia has been associated with sodium valproate (33, 34) and L-asparaginase (35–38), which impairs hepatic synthesis. In addition, individuals with aplastic anemia who are treated with antithymocyte globulin and corticosteroids develop low levels of fibrinogen (39).

## Therapy

Therapy of choice for quantitative disorders of fibrinogen is cryoprecipitate prepared from well-screened human plasma (see Chapter 52). Cryoprecipitates treated by solvent-detergent techniques to inactivate the human immunodeficiency virus (HIV) and hepatitis viruses are preferred. Prophylactic therapy generally is not recommended except during pregnancy, largely because of the danger for developing antifibrinogen antibodies, which not only neutralize infused fibrinogen but may be associated with anaphylaxis.

Replacement therapy is indicated for episodes of active bleeding, preoperatively, and during pregnancy. Fibrinogen levels of 50 to 100 mg/dL are adequate for hemostasis (40); levels greater than 60 mg/dL are recommended for maintenance of pregnancy (22). Each bag of cryoprecipitate contains approximately 300 mg of fibrinogen, so five to 10 bags are required for an initial dose in a 70 kg individual. Subsequent doses of cryoprecipitate can be administered daily in amounts based on the preinfusion fibrinogen level. Remember, however, that each bag of cryoprecipitate raises the fibrinogen level by approximately 10 mg/dL and that the biologic half-life of fibrinogen ranges from 2 to 4 days. 1-Desamino-8-D-arginine vasopressin (DDAVP) has shortened the prolonged bleeding time by improving platelet aggregation (41), but its clinical benefit is not clear.

Complications of replacement therapy include allergic reactions, anaphylaxis, and development of antifibrinogen antibodies (42, 43). Thromboembolic complications, including deep venous thrombosis and pulmonary embolism, have occurred with fibrinogen replacement used in conjunction with fibrinolytic inhibitors or oral contraceptive agents (23–25, 44). Low-molecular-weight heparin has been used to prevent potential thromboembolic side effects (45).

## QUALITATIVE FIBRINOGEN ABNORMALITIES (DYSFIBRINOGENEMIA)

The first familial case of dysfibrinogenemia, defined as presence of a qualitatively abnormal fibrinogen molecule, was described in 1964 (46). Since then, several hundred other cases have been reported. For a complete listing of the many types of dysfibrinogenemia, the reader is referred to several reviews of the subject (6, 47–49). Table 36.1 presents several fibrinogen variants (6, 50–54).

## Pathogenesis

The molecular abnormalities of dysfibrinogenemia are most easily considered from the perspective of normal fibrinogen function (see Chapter 6). Fibrinogen is composed of three pairs of polypeptide chains, Aα, Bβ, and γ, that are joined by disulfide bonds. As described in Chapter 6, conversion of fibrinogen to an insoluble fibrin mesh involves three major steps:

1. Enzymatic cleavage of fibrinopeptides A and B by thrombin, resulting in conversion of fibrinogen to fibrin monomers;
2. Polymerization of fibrin monomers, resulting in a visible fibrin clot; and
3. Fibrin stabilization, resulting from covalent crosslinking of Aα and γ chains by factor XIIIa.

Many dysfibrinogenemias result in a functional defect at one or more steps in the process of converting

**TABLE 36.1.**  Variants of Dysfibrinogemia

| Designation | Clinical Effect | Functional Defect | Structural Defect |
|---|---|---|---|
| Barcelona III | Asymptomatic | Polymerization defect | γ (275) Arg → His |
| Fukuoka II | Asymptomatic | Fibrinopeptide B release defect | Bβ (15) Gly → Cys |
| Bremen I | Hemorrhagic | Polymerization defect | Aα (17) Gly → Val |
| Christ Church II | Hemorrhagic | Fibrinopeptide B release defect | Bβ (14) Arg → Cys |
| Guarenas I | Hemorrhagic | Fibrinopeptide A release defect and polymerization defect | Unknown |
| Kyoto II | Hemorrhagic | Polymerization defect | Aα (18) Pro → Leu |
| Milano VI | Hemorrhagic | Fibrinopeptide A release defect | Aα (16) Arg → His |
| Mitaka II | Hemorrhagic | Fibrinopeptide A release defect | Aα (11) Glu → Gly |
| Date I | Thrombotic | Polymerization defect and t-PA binding defect | Unknown |
| Naples II | Thrombotic | Fibrinopeptide A and B release defect | Bβ (68) Ala → Thr |
| Paris V | Thrombotic | Polymerization defect, decreased binding of plasminogen, and decreased t-PA induced fibrinolysis | Aα (554) Arg → Cys |
| Villa Joyosa I | Thrombotic | Polymerization defect | γ (275) Arg → Cys |
| Vlissingen I | Thrombotic | Polymerization defect | γ (319–320) deletion |

*t-PA, tissue plasminogen activator.*

fibrinogen to fibrin. Most common are those causing abnormal polymerization. Others result in abnormal cleavage of fibrinopeptides. Still others affect stabilization. Some dysfibrinogens result in fibrin clots that are abnormally resistant to fibrinolysis; others result in clots that are abnormally susceptible to fibrinolysis (6).

Dysfibrinogens may be associated with bleeding or thrombosis, or the individual may be clinically asymptomatic. Clinical bleeding results from abnormal clot formation. The tendency for thrombosis is not well understood, but it may be secondary to one or more of the following:

1. Defective interactions with plasminogen, thus leading to abnormal fibrinolysis;
2. Decreased susceptibility to cleavage by plasmin;
3. Poor adsorption of tissue plasminogen activator (t-PA) to fibrin; and
4. Ability to induce platelet aggregation.

Delayed wound healing also is sometimes seen.

Theoretically, 50% of the fibrinogen in heterozygous individuals with dysfibrinogenemia is normal, which should be adequate for hemostasis. The abnormal fibrinogen may inhibit conversion of the normal molecule to fibrin, however, so the functional deficiency is much greater than expected.

Hypodysfibrinogenemia occurs when the abnormality in the fibrinogen molecule results in decreased synthesis, decreased secretion, or increased clearance.

Numerous families with hypodysfibrinogenemia have been described.

## Genetics

With rare exceptions, dysfibrinogenemia is inherited as an autosomal dominant trait with high penetrance. As a result, most affected individuals are heterozygotes. There are a few who are homozygotes, and even fewer who represent compound heterozygotes (6, 55, 56).

## Clinical Manifestations

Of individuals with dysfibrinogenemia, approximately 55% are asymptomatic. Approximately 25% have a bleeding tendency, and 20% have a thrombotic tendency (arterial, venous, or both) (57). A few have both bleeding and thrombotic tendencies. Hemorrhages caused by dysfibrinogenemia usually are mild, but some are severe, including soft-tissue hemorrhage, easy bruising, and menorrhagia. Intraoperative and postoperative bleeding can occur; however, in most cases, hemorrhage is not life-threatening.

Thrombotic complications generally are mild, but they can be fatal. Deep venous thrombosis and pulmonary emboli have been reported, and other complications include recurrent, spontaneous abortions and other obstetric complications (58, 59). Abnormal wound healing is seen as well. Interestingly, different structural defects correlate in a general way with clinical manifestations. Dysfibrinogenemias that lead to simple abnormal polymerization often are asymptomatic, and those associated with abnormal fibrinopeptide cleavage can be associated with bleeding or thrombosis. Those associated with abnormalities of crosslinking usually result in bleeding complications or abnormal wound healing. Most homozygous individuals exhibit hemorrhagic manifestations.

## Laboratory Tests

In dysfibrinogenemia, results of routine coagulation screening tests are usually prolonged. The TCT is the most sensitive screening test, and the PT is more sensitive than the aPTT. Sometimes, visible clot formation is virtually absent, and the reptilase time may be more prolonged than the TCT (60). Some dysfibrinogens exhibit a shortened TCT (61), and these individuals may have thrombotic complications.

The fibrinogen concentration can be normal or low. Most individuals with dysfibrinogenemia have a discrepancy between the level of clottable fibrinogen and that detected by immunologic assays. The specific diagnosis requires demonstration of an abnormal amino acid sequence or characterization of the functional defect (or defects).

## Differential Diagnosis

Hereditary dysfibrinogenemia must be distinguished from hypofibrinogenemia, either congenital or acquired. Acquired dysfibrinogenemias most commonly occur in liver disease (see Chapter 45). Other conditions associated with acquired dysfibrinogenemia include malignancies such as hepatoma (62, 63), renal cell carcinoma (64, 65), and autoimmune diseases. A individual with pseudotumor cerebri with an acquired dysfibrinogenemia has also been described (66). Acquired qualitative abnormalities of fibrinogen usually can be distinguished by the clinical setting and results of family studies.

Acquired inhibitors of the fibrinogen-to-fibrin conversion can be confused with dysfibrinogenemia. These include heparin, fibrin/fibrinogen degradation products, and inhibitory immunoglobulins such as those found in macroglobulinemia, multiple myeloma, and other immunologic disorders (67–70). Acquired antibodies against fibrinogen are rare complications of several diseases (71–76).

## Therapy

Most individuals with dysfibrinogenemia do not require therapy. When present, bleeding complications can be managed through transfusion of plasma or cryoprecipitate (43, 77–79). Antifibrinolytic agents such as aminocaproic acid (80) have been used, but they should be avoided in individuals with thrombotic tendencies. In

dividuals with repeated venous thromboses usually require long-term anticoagulation therapy. Women with dysfibrinogenemia and recurrent, spontaneous abortions can be treated with use of cryoprecipitate (22, 81).

# DISORDERS OF PROTHROMBIN (FACTOR II)

Hereditary prothrombin deficiency is a rare disorder resulting from decreased synthesis of the normal molecule (i.e., hypoprothrombinemia) or synthesis of an abnormal molecule with decreased functional activity (i.e., dysprothrombinemia). More than 30 cases have been reported. Table 36.2 presents several prothrombin variants (82–109).

## PATHOGENESIS

Hemorrhagic manifestations of hypoprothrombinemia or dysprothrombinemia relate to the degree that the abnormality decreases thrombin formation and subsequent fibrin clot. Some dysprothrombinemias affect only the "pro" piece of the molecule; in others, there is defective activation or some defect in the thrombin piece of the molecule (110, 111). In the latter instances, thrombin generation is impaired or the thrombin dysfunctional.

## GENETICS

Both hypoprothrombinemia and dysprothrombinemia are inherited in an autosomal recessive pattern. The prothrombin gene is located on chromosome 11 (112, 113), and affected individuals can be homozygotes, heterozygotes, or compound heterozygotes (Table 36.2). There is no evidence for any racial or ethnic predilection to these abnormalities.

## Clinical Manifestations

There is a rough correlation between prothrombin activity and severity of bleeding. In all individuals with hypoprothrombinemia or dysprothrombinemia, some detectable, functional prothrombin activity is preserved, suggesting that complete absence of prothrombin is incompatible with life. Many heterozygous individuals are asymptomatic or have minimal episodes of bleeding. Homozygous and compound heterozygous individuals are subject to lifelong mild or moderate hemorrhagic symptoms, including easy bruising, epistaxis, soft-tissue hemorrhage, excessive postoperative bleeding, and in females, menorrhagia. Hemarthroses rarely occur (114).

**TABLE 36.2.** Inherited Prothrombin Variants

| Designation | Defect | Genotype | Antigen (%) | Activity (% of normal) | Hemorrhagic Tendency |
|---|---|---|---|---|---|
| Barcelona/Madrid | Arg 271 → Cys | Homozygous | 100 | 10–15 | Yes |
| Brussel | Unknown | Heterozygous | 84 | 25–50 | Yes |
| Cardeza | Impaired F Xa proteolysis | Heterozygous | 100 | 30–50 | No |
| Clamart | Impaired F Xa proteolysis | Heterozygous | 100 | 50 | No |
| Corpus Christi | Arg 382 → Cys | Heterozygous | 25 | 2 | No |
| Denver | Unknown | Homozygous | 13 | <1 | Yes |
| Dharan | Arg 271 → His | Homozygous | 95 | 5 | Yes |
| Frankfurt | Glu 466 → Ala | Homozygous | 91 | 13 | Yes |
| Gainesville | Unknown | Unknown | 75 | 25 | Yes |
| Habana | Unknown | Heterozygous[a] | 50 | <10 | Yes |
| Himi I | Met 337 → Thr | Heterozygous[b] | 100 | 10 | No |
| Himi II | Arg 388 → His | Heterozygous[b] | 100 | 10 | No |
| Houston | Unknown | Heterozygous[a] | 50 | 5–10 | Yes |
| Magdeburg | Unknown | Heterozygous | 100 | 45 | Yes |
| Madrid | Arg 271 → Cys | Homozygous | 100 | 3–5 | Yes |
| Metz | Defective thrombin active site | Heterozygous[a] | 50 | 10 | Yes |
| Mexico City | Unknown | Heterozygous[a] | <10 | <10 | Yes |
| Molise | Defective thrombin active site | Heterozygous[a] | 45 | 10 | Yes |
| Not named | Unknown | Homozygous | 5 | 2 | Yes |
| Obihiro | Arg 271 → Cys | Homozygous | 100 | 18 | Yes |
| Padua | Defective activation | Heterozygous | 100 | 50 | Yes |
| Perija | Unknown | Homozygous | 70 | 2 | Yes |
| Poissy | Defective activation | Homozygous | 50 | 2 | Yes |
| Quick I | Arg 382 → Cys | Heterozygous[b] | 37–40 | <2 | Yes |
| Quick II | Gly 558 → Val | Heterozygous[b] | — | <1 | Yes |
| Salatka | Glu 466 → Ala | Homozygous | 100 | 7–20 | No |
| San Juan I | Defective calcium binding | Heterozygous[b] | 100 | 15–20 | Yes |
| San Juan II | Unknown | Heterozygous[b] | 90 | 15–20 | Yes |
| Segovia | Unknown | Homozygous | 100 | 7–20 | Yes |
| Tokushima | Arg 418 → Tyr | Heterozygous[a] | — | 21 | Yes |

[a] Compound heterozygous state with one gene for hypoprothrombinemia and one gene for dysprothrombinemia.

[b] Compound heterozygous state for two abnormal alleles.

## LABORATORY TESTS

Both the PT and aPTT are prolonged in these individuals, but the TCT and bleeding time are normal. The diagnosis of dysprothrombinemia requires specific assays of prothrombin clotting activity. Levels of prothrombin antigen can be normal or decreased. Some individuals with hypoprothrombinemia actually represent individuals with hypodysprothrombinemia.

## DIFFERENTIAL DIAGNOSIS

Hereditary prothrombin deficiency can be distinguished from acquired hypoprothrombinemia by a lifelong history of bleeding and a family history of hypoprothrombinemia confirmed by specific laboratory tests. Acquired hypoprothrombinemia is common and usually associated with warfarin administration, vitamin K deficiency, liver disease, or some combination. In contrast to congenital hypoprothrombinemia, the acquired disorder is also associated with low levels of the other vitamin K-dependent factors (i.e., factors VII, IX, and X). The severe bleeding tendency reported in individuals who ingest warfarin or the so-called "super warfarins" (brodifacoum) for secondary gain is of particular interest. In these individuals, prothrombin levels can be very low (115). Low levels of prothrombin are frequently reported in individuals treated with third-generation cephalosporins containing the N-methyl-thio-tetrazole (NMTT) side chain (116–119). The NMTT side chain inhibits the vitamin K-dependent γ-carboxylation of glutamic acid residues necessary for production of functional prothrombin and other vitamin K-dependent factors. Hemorrhagic complications from use of NMTT cephalosporins are most likely to occur with malnutrition, renal failure, liver disease, biliary obstruction, and malignancy (120, 121). Prophylactic administration of vitamin K may prevent such complications.

Hereditary deficiency of prothrombin also must be distinguished from congenital combined deficiency of prothrombin and factors VII, IX, and X. The combined deficiency also is referred to as familial multiple factor deficiency, type III (discussed later).

Acquired antibodies to prothrombin have been reported in individuals with lupus anticoagulant or antiphospholipid antibody syndrome, including systemic lupus erythematosus and other conditions (see Chapter 38). The antiprothrombin antibodies recognize epitopes on the molecule, resulting in rapid clearance of the prothrombin–antibody complex by the reticuloendothelial system (122–125). Bleeding in these individuals is similar to that seen in those with hereditary prothrombin deficiency.

## THERAPY

A prothrombin clotting activity 20 to 30% of the normal level usually is sufficient for hemostasis. For minor episodes of bleeding, plasma is used for prothrombin replacement. Based on a prothrombin half-life of 3 days, plasma can be administered in a loading dose of 15 to 20 mL/kg of body weight, followed by 3 mL/kg every 12 to 24 hours, provided the individual has a normal cardiovascular status. Lower doses also may be effective. Prothrombin complex concentrates (PCCs), which contain prothrombin and the other vitamin K-dependent factors (see Chapter 52), can be administered for major episodes of bleeding and for prophylactic treatment before surgery. Care should be taken to choose concentrates that do not transmit HIV or hepatitis viruses. PCCs have been associated with thromboembolic episodes; therefore, the minimal dose required for effective hemostasis should be used. (PCCs are discussed further in the section on hemophilia B [Table 36.7]). Hereditary prothrombin abnormalities do not respond to vitamin K supplementation.

# FACTOR V DEFICIENCY

In 1943, Quick (126) postulated a labile clotting factor, which later became known as factor V. The first factor V-deficient individual was described in 1947 by Owren (127). Factor V also is known as proaccelerin and factor V deficiency as parahemophilia. Approximately 150 cases of congenital factor V deficiency have been described (128), and the incidence is estimated at less than one in 1 million (129).

## PATHOGENESIS

Hemorrhage in individuals with factor V deficiency results from a quantitative deficiency of factor V or dysfunctional factor V in the plasma and platelets (130). Factor V is an essential cofactor in conversion of prothrombin to thrombin by activated factor X. Without factor V, thrombin generation is slowed and fibrin formation delayed. There also is variability between the factor V antigen and activity, thus suggesting that some individuals have dysfunctional factor V molecules (131).

## GENETICS

The factor V gene is found on chromosome 1 (132, 133). Various abnormalities in the gene result in defective factor V molecules, which have decreased function. A genetic variant of factor V resulting in substitution of a glutamyl for an arginyl residue at position 506 of the protein renders factor V resistant to inactivation by activated protein C (134, 135) (see Chapter 40). Congenital factor V deficiency is inherited in an autosomal recessive pattern, and consanguinity is common among affected families. Symptoms usually occur only in homozygous or compound heterozygous individuals, in whom levels of functional factor V range from less than 1 to approximately 20% of normal (129).

## CLINICAL MANIFESTATIONS

Bleeding symptoms in individuals with factor V deficiency vary from mild to severe. Severely affected individuals have less than 1% factor V activity, whereas moderately to mildly affected individuals have 2 to 20% activity. Plasma and platelet levels of factor V do not necessarily correlate, however, and the clinical bleeding tendency may depend more on the level of platelet factor V (130, 136). Approximately 18 to 25% of the body mass of factor V is found in the platelet alpha granules (137). Hemorrhagic manifestations in individuals with less than 1% of normal factor V activity usually are not as severe or frequent as those occurring in individuals with severe, classic hemophilia. There often is excessive bleeding from the umbilical stump allowing early diagnosis, but as many as 50% of individuals are not diagnosed until adulthood. Bleeding from mucous membranes is common and includes epistaxis and gastrointestinal hemorrhage, and menorrhagia is frequent. Hemarthroses occur, but not as frequently as those in individuals with classic hemophilia or hemophilia B. Ecchymoses are frequent as well, and bleeding may occur from any site after trauma. One family with congenital factor V deficiency and recurrent thromboembolic complications has been described (138), as have other congenital abnormalities, including syndactylism and cardiac abnormalities, in these individuals (139).

## LABORATORY TESTS

Screening tests of coagulation show a prolonged PT and aPTT. When individual plasma is mixed with normal plasma, results of both tests are corrected. The TCT is normal, and the diagnosis of factor V deficiency is made on the basis of specific assays for factor V clotting activity. Levels of factor V antigen may be normal or low. In severe factor V deficiency, the bleeding time usually is prolonged, presumably because of decreased or absent platelet factor V (136). One form of deficiency, factor V Quebec (136), has decreased platelet factor V associated with mild hemorrhagic symptoms; in this condition, plasma levels of factor V are relatively normal.

## DIFFERENTIAL DIAGNOSIS

Congenital factor V deficiency can occur in combination with congenital factor VIII deficiency in type I familial multiple coagulation factor deficiency (discussed later) (140). Acquired factor V deficiency is common in individuals with liver disease or disseminated intravascular coagulation, but in these individuals, levels of several other clotting factors also are decreased. Low levels of factor V in individuals with liver disease indicate significant hepatocellular impairment.

An inhibitor (i.e., antibody) to factor V has been described in individuals with congenital factor V deficiency after exposure to normal plasma (141). There also is extensive literature characterizing individuals who develop spontaneous antifactor V antibodies (142–158), which usually are polyclonal immunoglobulin (IgG) but occasionally IgM or IgA. There is no common underlying disease in these individuals, but up to 50% of the spontaneous factor V inhibitors occur in postoperative individuals. Antifactor V antibodies also have been associated with use of antibiotics (i.e., streptomycin, gentamicin, penicillin), previous transfusions, infections (i.e., tuberculosis), topical bovine thrombin that contains bovine factor V (159), and malignancies. Usually, these antibodies are short-lived, persisting for less than 10 weeks in more than 50% of individuals. Hemorrhagic complications in individuals with inhibitors can be severe, however, and even fatal. Bleeding complications in some individuals with factor V antibodies have responded to infusions of platelets, presumably because platelet factor V can be delivered in a milieu protected from circulating antibodies.

## THERAPY

Plasma is used to replace factor V; no concentrates are commercially available. Mild to moderate hemorrhage can be treated by raising the factor V clotting activity to approximately 20% of normal. An initial plasma dose of 15 to 20 mL/kg, followed by 3 to 6 mL/kg every 24 hours, is generally adequate based on a factor V half-life of 36 hours (160). Prophylactic therapy is used preoperatively. Because platelets contain factor V, platelet transfusions sometimes have been used to treat hemorrhagic episodes. This therapy is not ordinarily recommended, however, because of the potential for antiplatelet antibodies.

# FACTOR VII DEFICIENCY

The first case of congenital factor VII deficiency was described in 1951 by Alexander et al (161). Since then, numerous others have been described, and many genetic variants are recognized (162).

## PATHOGENESIS

Factor VII is essential for initiation of the tissue factor pathway of coagulation, and a deficiency or structural defect in the factor VII molecule leads to bleeding symptoms. Factor VII deficiency is a heterogeneous disorder. There may be reduced or absent synthesis of factor VII or synthesis of a dysfunctional molecule (163–167). Several factor VII variants (167, 168) have been distinguished (Table 36.3) (169–172). Recently, however, specific genetic variants have been described (Table 36.3) (173–184). One individual had a missense mutation resulting in substitution of an arginine for a glutamine at position 79 in the first epidermal growth factor–like domain. This individual had severe hemorrhagic manifestations.

## GENETICS

The factor VII gene is located on chromosome 13 adjacent to the factor X gene (162, 185). Expression of factor VII might be regulated by an element on chromosome 8 (186). Factor VII deficiency is inherited in an autosomal recessive pattern (187). Heterozygous individuals usually are asymptomatic, whereas homozygous individuals are clinically affected.

## CLINICAL MANIFESTATIONS

In individuals with congenital deficiency of factor VII, severity of bleeding varies and does not always correlate with the factor VII level. It should be emphasized that individuals with factor VII clotting activity of less than 1% of normal usually have severe bleeding, equivalent to that seen in classic hemophilia, with hemarthroses, chronic arthropathy, hematomas, retroperitoneal bleeding, and fatal cerebral hemorrhage (188). Even low levels of factor VII (10%), however, are effective in controlling hemorrhage, and this may account for the variability in clinical manifestations. Homozygous individuals are most likely to have severe hemorrhages, whereas compound heterozygous individuals usually have moderate

**TABLE 36.3.** Selected Factor VII Variants

| Designation | FVII Antigen (%) | Factor VII Activity (%) | | |
|---|---|---|---|---|
| | | **Rabbit Thromboplastin** | **Ox Thromboplastin** | **Human Thromboplastin** |
| Padua I | 100 | 11 | 105 | 40 |
| Padua II | 50 | 40 | 20 | 40 |
| Verona | 50 | 25 | 45 | 20 |

| | Mutation(s) | Human Factor VII Activity (%) | Factor VII Antigen (%) | Clinical Manifestations |
|---|---|---|---|---|
| Central | Phe 328 → Ser | <1 | 38 | Severe bleeding |
| Charlotte | Arg 79 → Gln | <1 | 100 | Severe bleeding |
| Kansas | Arg 152 → Gln | 4 | 60 | Asymptomatic |
| | Gln 100 → Arg | | | |
| | Arg 304 → Gln | | | |
| Mie | Arg 247 → His | 24 | 26 | Asymptomatic |
| Nagoya | Arg 304 → Trp | <5 | 100 | Asymptomatic |
| Padua I | Arg 304 → Gln | 40 | 100 | Mild bleeding |
| Polish A-H | Ala 294 → Val | <2 | <4 | Moderate to severe bleeding |
| | Arg 353 → Gln | | | |
| | 11125–11128 Frameshift | | | |
| Polish I | Ala 294 → Val | 4 | 17 | Moderate bleeding |
| | 11125–11128 Frameshift | | | |
| Polish J | Ala 294 → Val | 11 | 47 | Moderate bleeding |
| | Arg 353 → Gln | | | |
| Richmond | Arg 304 → Gln | 14 | 120 | Thrombosis |
| Shinjo | Arg 79 → Gln | 11 | 115 | Asymptomatic |
| Undesignated | Arg 353 → Gln | <1 | <1 | Severe bleeding |
| | Thr 359 → Met | | | |
| Undesignated | Thr 359 → Met | <1 | <1 | Severe bleeding |
| Undesignated | Promoter 61 T → G | <1 | <1 | Severe bleeding |

to mild hemorrhages. Hemorrhage is more likely to occur with factor VII levels of less than 10% of normal. Symptomatic individuals commonly have easy bruising, soft-tissue hemorrhage, epistaxis, and menorrhagia. Postoperative bleeding also is common but not predictable, and affected infants have a 16% incidence of intracranial hemorrhage at delivery (189).

Factor VII deficiency does not necessarily protect individuals from thromboembolic disease (190, 191). One affected individual was reported to have thrombosis of the inferior vena cava and fatal pulmonary embolism (192).

## LABORATORY TESTS

Laboratory studies of individuals with factor VII deficiency typically show an isolated, prolonged PT. The aPTT and TCT are normal. This is the only congenital abnormality showing such a pattern. Rarely, the aPTT can also be prolonged. Diagnosis requires a specific assay of factor VII clotting activity. The *in vitro* factor VII activity can vary with different sources of tissue factor, thus allowing for distinction among several variants (Table 36.3). It has been suggested that clinical bleeding best correlates with the PT as determined using human tissue factor.

## DIFFERENTIAL DIAGNOSIS

Hereditary deficiency of factor VII must be distinguished from acquired deficiency. The most common causes of acquired factor VII deficiency are liver disease, vitamin K deficiency, and use of warfarin (193). These individuals have low levels of all vitamin K-dependent factors, but the factor VII level may be lowest because of its short half-life (3–6 hours).

Rarer causes of factor VII deficiency include the familial multiple-factor deficiencies (types III and IV). In type III, there is a combined deficiency of all vitamin K-dependent factors (discussed later). Acquired factor VII deficiency also may occur in individuals with homocystinuria (194), and individuals with acquired factor VII deficiency and aplastic anemia have been described (195). The defect was corrected by successful allogenic bone marrow transplantation in one of these individuals. Acquired factor VII deficiency resulting from an inhibitor to factor VII has been described but is rare (196–198). Decreased factor VII levels have been reported in association with the Dubin-Johnson syndrome, Rotor syndrome, and possibly, Gilbert syndrome (199). The mechanism of factor VII deficiency in these disorders, however, is not understood.

## THERAPY

A factor VII clotting activity approximately 10% of normal usually is adequate for hemostasis, but levels of 15 to 25% have been recommended for individuals undergoing surgery. Individuals with congenital factor VII deficiency do not respond to therapy with vitamin K. Products that can be used for replacement include plasma, PCCs, and recombinant factor VIIa (see Chapter 52). Based on a half-life of 3 to 6 hours, plasma is given at 5 to 10 mL/kg every 6 to 12 hours for 1 to 2 days for minor episodes of bleeding. For surgery, plasma is administered in a loading dose of 15 to 20 mL/kg, followed by maintenance doses of 3 to 6 mL/kg every 12 hours for several days. Replacement therapy with PCCs may be considered for major surgery (200) or for life-threatening bleeding. The amount of factor VII in PCCs varies according to the manufacturer, however, and this must be ascertained before use. PCCs can be obtained that do not transmit HIV or hepatitis viruses; however, thromboembolic complications can still occur, thus necessitating caution and use of the lowest effective dose. Recombinant factor VIIa, which is available in several European countries and is awaiting approval in the United States, would be the agent of choice if available (201).

In severely affected individuals, replacement therapy may be complicated by development of antifactor VII antibodies. It is although this complication more likely occurs in those individuals whose genetic defect precludes expression of any recognizable factor VII antigen. Purified plasma derived factor VII is available in some European countries.

# FACTOR IX DEFICIENCY

Congenital deficiency of coagulation factor IX results in hemophilia B. Hemophilia B was first suspected as being different from hemophilia A in 1947 (202). Further clarification came in 1952, when Aggeler et al (203), Biggs et al (204), and Shulman and Smith (205) characterized factor IX and distinguished it from factor VIII. The incidence of hemophilia B is estimated as approximately one in 30,000 live male births (206, 207).

## PATHOGENESIS

Bleeding occurs in hemophilia B because a quantitative deficiency of factor IX or a defective molecule results in decreased thrombin generation and delayed formation of fibrin clots. Factor IX normally is activated by the factor VIIa-tissue factor complex or by factor XIa. In complex with factor VIIIa, calcium, and phospholipid, factor IXa converts factor X to Xa. Defects in the factor IX molecule, however, lead to delayed activation; defective interaction with factor VIII, X, or both; defective catalytic function; or some combination. Depending on the amount of functional factor IX, hemorrhagic manifestations vary from mild to severe (Table 36.4). In general, there is good correlation between factor IX clotting activity and clinical severity of the disease.

## GENETICS

Hemophilia B is inherited in an X-linked recessive pattern (208), and the sequence of the entire normal gene has been reported (209). It is located near the tip of the long arm of the X chromosome at Xq26-27 (210, 211). Genetic defects resulting in decreased or absent production of the molecule or in production of an abnormal molecule include partial and total deletions, point mutations, frame shifts, and premature stop codons (Table 36.5) (212). Male individuals are clinically affected, and female carriers are usually asymptomatic. Female carriers can be symptomatic, however, and have factor IX levels less than 20% of normal in extreme lyonization or abnormalities of the X chromosome (213, 214). Factor IX deficiency has been reported in one female with a nonrandom inactivation of a structurally abnormal X chromosome that contained the structurally normal factor IX gene (215). In one-third of all individuals, hemophilia B arises by *de novo* mutations in the factor IX gene, many of which occur at C-G dinucleotides. More than 400 different mutations leading to hemophilia B have been described, and these are tabulated yearly in a database maintained by several investigators and published in *Nucleic Acids Research* (216). Some of the more interesting mutations occur in the promoter region of the gene, leading to hemophilia B Leyden. Individuals with this form may be severely affected at birth, but at about the time of adolescence, levels of factor IX begin to rise, presumably in response to androgenic hormones that increase at puberty. Factor IX Leyden mutations occur close to androgen response elements in the promoter region (217).

## CLINICAL MANIFESTATIONS

Clinically, hemophilia B is indistinguishable from hemophilia A. Unless the disease is mild, bleeding symptoms usually are apparent in infancy or early childhood. Excessive bleeding following circumcision may occur,

**TABLE 36.4.   Clinical Classification of Hemophilia B**

|  | Mild | Moderate | Severe |
|---|---|---|---|
| Factor IX level | | | |
| % of normal | 6–50 | 1–5 | <1 |
| U/mL | 0.06–0.50 | 0.01–0.05 | <0.01 |
| Clinical manifestations | Hemorrhage only with trauma or surgery | Occasional hemarthroses; hemorrhage following trauma | Frequent hemarthroses; life- and limb-threatening hemorrhages are common |

**TABLE 36.5.   Factor IX Gene Defects in Hemophilia B**

| Individual Entries | 1535 |
|---|---|
| Point mutations | 1267 |
| Short (<30 nt) mutations | 119 |
| Deletions | 91 |
| Additions | 22 |
| Deletions and additions | 6 |
| Missense mutations | 1046 |
| Double mutations | 21 |
| Triple mutations | 1 |
| Somatic mosaics | 2 |
| Mutation entries in various factor IX regions | |
| Promoter | 46 |
| Signal peptide | 13 |
| Propeptide | 99 |
| Glutamic acid domain | 156 |
| EGF-1 domain | 153 |
| EGF-2 domain | 147 |
| Activation peptide | 120 |
| Catalytic domain | 823 |
| Mutations affecting specific amino acids | |
| γ-Carboxyglutamyl residues with known mutations | 9/12 |
| Cysteinyl residues with known mutations | 22/22 |

*EGF, epidermal growth factor.*

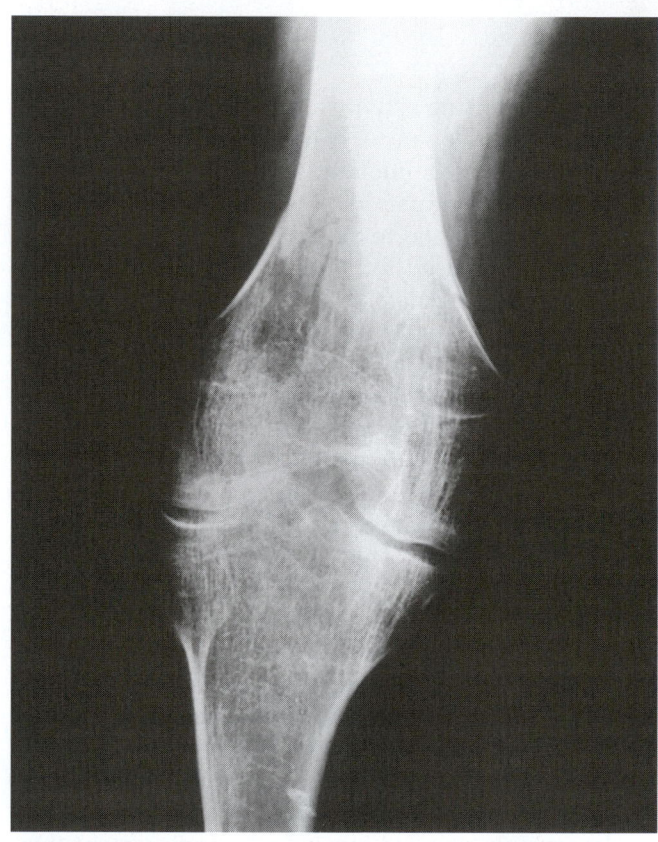

**FIGURE 36.1.**   Advanced hemophilic arthropathy of the knee with narrowing of the joint space and incidental supracondylar fracture.

but afterward, bleeding may not be frequent until the child is old enough to move about.

The most common bleeding manifestations in severely affected individuals are recurrent hemarthroses leading to chronic, crippling arthropathy (Figs. 36.1 to 36.3). The joints most frequently involved are, in decreasing order, the knees, elbows, ankles, shoulders, hips, and wrists. Individuals with hemophilia B, like those with hemophilia A, usually can tell when a hemarthrosis begins. They notice a feeling of "tightness" or burning over the involved joint that soon progresses to swelling and pain. This pain often becomes extremely severe within a matter of hours. Because of the pain and swelling, the joint usually is held in a fixed position,

often in flexion, thus leading to flexion contractures. Movement of an affected joint not only increases the pain but can lead to increased bleeding. Bleeding usually occurs into the synovial tissues of the joints, and this results in synovial hypertrophy and final scarring. This is followed by narrowing of the joint space and, ultimately, osteoporosis and sclerosis. In addition, bone cysts and pseudotumors may form in the latter stages of joint degeneration.

Repeated hemorrhage into joints results in a so-called "target joint" with synovial thickening and chronic synovitis. Target joints bleed more frequently and create a vicious cycle in which small capillaries in

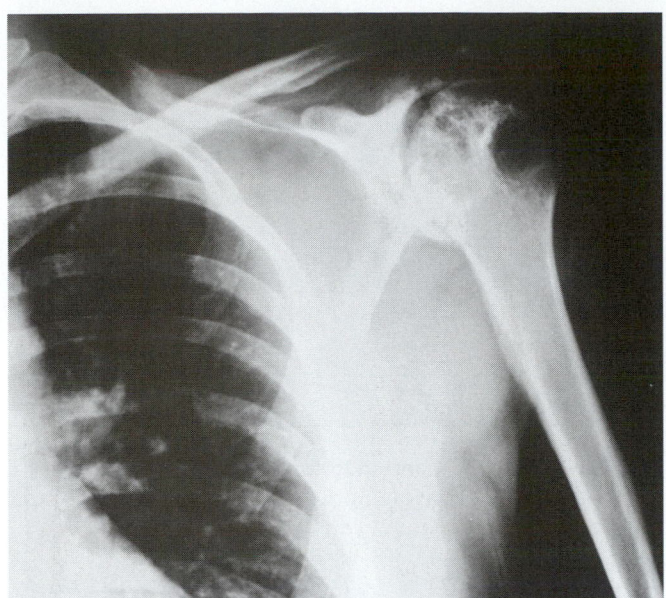

**FIGURE 36.2.** Advanced hemophilic arthropathy of the shoulder with a cyst in the humeral head.

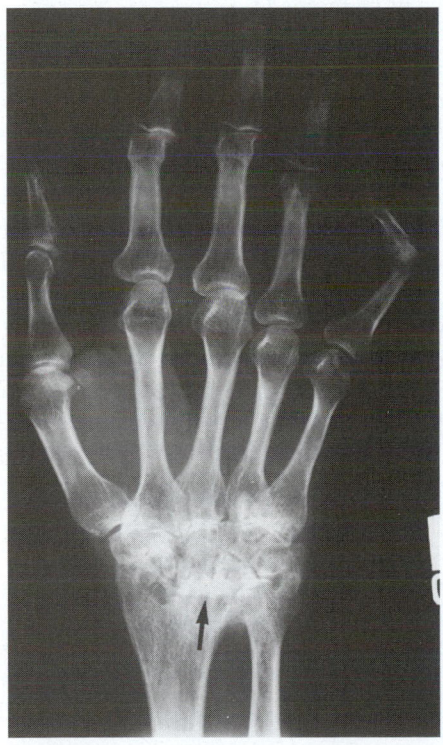

**FIGURE 36.3.** Advanced hemophilic arthropathy of the carpal joints of the right hand with loss of joint space (arrow).

the synovial tissues are easily injured by routine movement, thus resulting in repeated hemorrhages. Without adequate treatment, adults with severe hemophilia B become severely crippled, with valgus deformities of the lower extremities and ankylosis of the weight-bearing

| TABLE 36.6. | Radiographic Staging of Hemophilic Arthropathy |
|---|---|
| Stage 0 | Normal. |
| Stage 1 | Soft-tissue swelling without skeletal changes. |
| Stage 2 | Osteoporosis and epiphyseal overgrowth without bone cysts or joint-space narrowing. |
| Stage 3 | Subchondral bone cysts with minor joint-space irregularities but without narrowing. |
| Stage 4 | Prominent bone cysts and joint-space irregularities with marked narrowing. |
| Stage 5 | Obliteration of joint space with epiphyseal overgrowth. |

joints. Radiographic staging of joints is shown in Table 36.6.

Individuals with factor IX levels as low as 5% of normal have much less joint involvement. They also may not show overt clinical evidence of crippling hemarthroses as adults.

The second most common type of hemorrhage in hemophilia is the formation of hematoma, which is highly characteristic of both severe hemophilia B and classic hemophilia (see Chapter 35). They occur in muscle and other soft tissues, and they tend to dissect into adjacent structures. Bleeding into muscles of the leg and arm may lead to atrophy and contractures of the involved extremities. Hemorrhage may occur "spontaneously," without apparent trauma, although unnoticed trauma probably always is the initiating event. As in classic hemophilia, hemorrhagic manifestations may be delayed for several hours or days after trauma, especially after surgery. Hemorrhages involving the retroperitoneum, retropharynx, and central nervous system are often life-threatening and require prompt recognition and treatment (Figs. 36.4 and 36.5).

The physician should be alert for certain symptoms in severely affected individuals. A individual with an unusual headache should raise suspicion of an intracranial hemorrhage. Individuals with the common cold and coughing should be watched for retropharyngeal bleeding that might impair the airway. Hematuria, often from an unidentified source, is frequently seen. Pseudotumors in bone or soft tissue can form in areas of unresolved hematoma as well, and these can lead to bone destruction and neurovascular compromise (Fig. 36.6).

Individuals with hemophilia should be advised to avoid using aspirin or other agents that interfere with platelet function. Contact sports and other activities that predispose to hemorrhage should be avoided as well.

Because of frequent hemarthroses, chronic pain be-

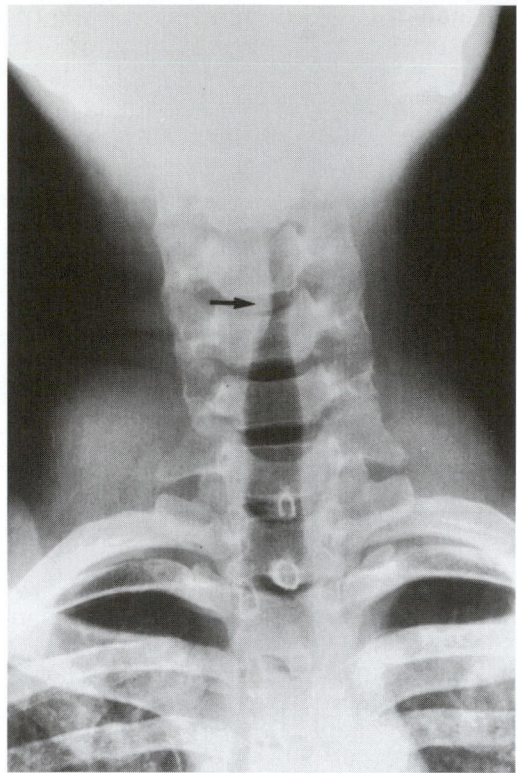

**FIGURE 36.4.**   Severe tracheal narrowing (arrow) resulting from soft-tissue hematoma in a individual with severe hemophilia.

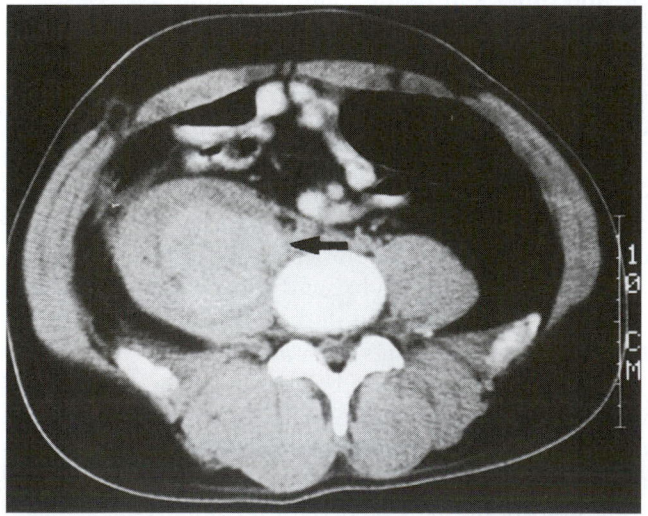

**FIGURE 36.5.**   Computed tomographic scan showing a large hematoma involving the right psoas muscle (arrow).

comes a problem. Thus, both individual and physician should be aware of the dangers of addiction to analgesics.

## LABORATORY TESTS

Typically, individuals with hemophilia B have a prolonged aPTT, but the PT, TCT, and bleeding time are

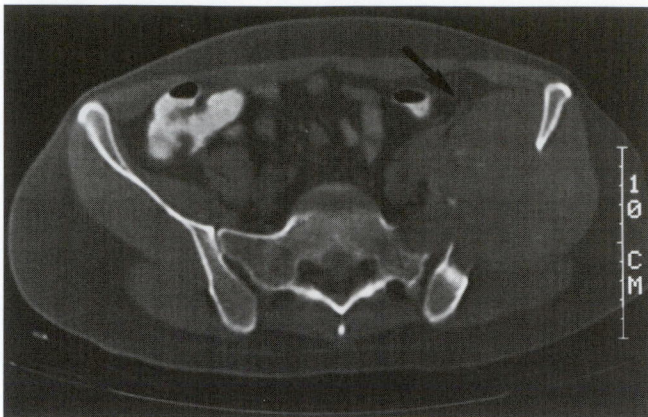

**FIGURE 36.6.**   Computed tomographic scan showing a large pseudotumor involving the left iliac crest and sacrum (arrow).

normal. The aPTT may be normal in individuals with mild disease. A history of unusual or excessive bleeding is a better indicator of mild procoagulant defect than the results of laboratory tests. The diagnosis requires a specific assay of factor IX.

The PT typically is normal in most genetic variants of hemophilia B, but it is characteristically prolonged in some variants, especially when the PT is performed using ox brain tissue factor. Individuals whose plasma exhibits a prolonged PT are designated as having hemophilia Bm (218–223). Hemophilia Bm variants were first described by Hougie and Twomey (219), who based the designation Bm on the surname of the original individual. Such individuals account for approximately 15% of all cases of hemophilia B.

Inhibitor antibodies to factor IX can occur in individuals with hemophilia B as a complication of therapy. They rarely occur in individuals without hemophilia B. Among individuals with hemophilia B, the incidence of inhibitors is 2.5 to 6.0% in severely affected individuals, and these inhibitors may be more likely to develop in individuals with no circulating factor IX antigen (207, 224). Antifactor IX antibodies are alloantibodies usually restricted to IgG₄ heavy chains and kappa light chains, but this is variable (225).

## DIFFERENTIAL DIAGNOSIS

Hemophilia B must be distinguished from classic hemophilia with use of a specific assay. Factor IX also can be congenitally deficient in several of the familial multiple-factor deficiency syndromes, including types II, III, V, and VI (discussed later).

Acquired deficiency of factor IX commonly occurs in hepatic disease, vitamin K deficiency, and after warfarin administration. Other vitamin K-dependent factors are decreased in these conditions as well (see Chapter 45).

Disease states that may be associated with acquired factor IX deficiency include amyloidosis, nephrotic syndrome, and Gaucher disease. In amyloidosis, factor IX as well as factor X are believed to bind to the amyloid fibrils, thus resulting in the deficiency (226–229) (discussed later). Individuals with nephrotic syndrome lose factor IX protein in the urine (230–232). Bleeding complications are unusual in this setting, and the defect can resolve with glucocorticoid therapy and resolution of nephrotic syndrome. In Gaucher disease, the plasma half-life of factor IX is shortened, presumably because of binding and clearance of the protein by the cerebroside deposits (233). Factor IX deficiency in Gaucher disease is not corrected by splenectomy, but bleeding complications rarely occur.

Spontaneously acquired factor IX inhibitors in individuals without hemophilia B are extremely rare. They have been described in individuals with autoimmune disorders, postpartum, and in association with malignancy (234–237). Some inhibitors disappear after 1 to 7 months; some may persist for many years. Immunosuppressive therapy with various combinations of chemotherapy can be used to prevent or reduce the antibody titer.

## THERAPY

The goal of replacement therapy in individuals with hemophilia B depends on the location and severity of hemorrhage (238). Minor bleeds, such as uncomplicated hemarthroses and superficial muscular and soft-tissue bleeds, require a hemostatic level of 20 to 30% of the normal circulating factor IX level. Usually, one or two doses of a factor IX concentrate over 24 to 48 hours is sufficient to stop uncomplicated bleeding. Recurrent hemarthroses in a target joint with chronic synovitis, however, may require daily treatment with factor IX for 6 weeks or longer.

Moderate hemorrhages, such as muscle or soft-tissue bleeds with evidence of dissection and bleeding from mucous membranes, require factor IX levels of 25 to 50% of normal. In these individuals, treatment should continue for several days or until the bleeding stops. Serious hemorrhages, including those involving the airway, retroperitoneum, and central nervous system, require factor IX levels of 50 to 100% of normal for 7 to 10 days or longer. For surgery, factor IX levels should be raised to at least 50% of normal preoperatively and maintained for 7 to 10 days postoperatively. Factor IX levels greater than 50% of normal are not recommended when using PCCs as a source of factor IX because of possible thromboembolic complications. Levels up to 100% of normal can be achieved safely using highly purified factor IX products (discussed later).

Individuals with severe hemophilia require special attention in certain situations. Any bleeding in the central nervous system is especially dangerous. Thus, if a individual with severe hemophilia B presents in the emergency room after an accident, factor IX replacement therapy should be administered even without symptoms. Unusual headaches should be treated with factor IX even before computed tomography of the head. Time-consuming diagnostic procedures should not be performed before administering treatment to individuals with severe hemophilia B who experience hemorrhage in vital areas. Any bleeding in the throat or elsewhere around the airway requires urgent replacement therapy and frequent monitoring until the symptoms subside.

Factor IX replacement therapy is changing after the introduction of highly purified factor IX concentrates. Table 36.7 lists the currently available products, methods of preparation, and side effects (see Chapter 52).

In 1969, PCCs, which contain prothrombin and factors VII, IX, and X, became commercially available in the United States (238–241). Soon thereafter, they became the mainstay of treatment for hemophilia B. These concentrates are significantly purified compared with plasma, thereby allowing large doses of factor IX to be administered in a small volume. Recently, these products have been heated in the dry state or otherwise treated to inactivate HIV and hepatitis viruses. For example, one currently available PCC, commercially known as Konyne 80 (Cutter), is "superheated" to 80°C for 72 hours in the lyophilized state. All other available factor IX products are free of these agents as well.

Doses of PCCs are based on units of factor IX. One unit of factor IX per kilogram of body weight raises the plasma factor IX concentration by 1%. Recovery of infused factor IX is lower than expected, however, presumably because factor IX is adsorbed to sites in the vasculature, recently shown to be collagen IV (242). Thus, in a 70-kg individual, 50 U of factor IX per kg of body weight would raise the circulating factor IX level to 50% of normal. After a loading dose, subsequent doses are administered every 12 hours at 50% of the original dose. Using this regimen, factor IX levels must be monitored immediately before and after administration of the concentrate.

Use of PCCs also can be complicated by arterial or venous thrombosis and by disseminated intravascular coagulation. The exact cause of thromboembolic disease in this situation is not clear, but these products may contain activated factors that induce thrombotic events. Therefore, factor IX levels should not be raised higher than 50% of normal when using PCCs.

Highly purified factor IX concentrates that contain negligible amounts of other factors are available as well (Table 36.7). AlphaNine is almost pure, and Mononine (Rhône-Poulenc Rorer) (243–248), which is prepared by monoclonal antibody immunoaffinity purification, is highly purified. Both products are less likely than PCCs to produce thromboembolic side effects. All factor IX products are apparently safe in terms of HIV and hepatitis viruses.

A recombinant factor IX product, Benefix (Genetics

**TABLE 36.7.** Commercial Clotting Factor Products

| Product (Manufacturer) | Preparation | Factor Units/100 Units of Factor IX | | | |
|---|---|---|---|---|---|
| | | II | VII | IX | X |
| *Prothrombin complex concentrates* | | | | | |
| Konyne 80 (Cutter, USA) | Dry heat at 80°C for 72 hours | 100 | 20 | 100 | 140 |
| Profilnine HT (Alpha, USA) | *n*-Heptane suspension, 60°C for 20 hours | 148 | 11 | 100 | 64 |
| Proplex T (Baxter Hyland, USA) | Dry heat at 60°C for 144 hours | 50 | 400 | 100 | 50 |
| Bebulin VH (Immuno) | | 120 | 13 | 100 | 140 |
| *Highly purified factor IX concentrates* | | | | | |
| AlphaNine (Alpha, USA) | Profilnine HT product; adsorption on barium citrate followed by elution and chromatography | <5 | <5 | 100 | <20 |
| Mononine (Rhône-Poulenc Rorer, USA) | Monoclonal antibody immunoaffinity chromatography, extraction with sodium thiocyanate, ultrafiltration | 0 | 0 | 100 | 0 |
| Benefix (Genetics Institute-Baxter, Hyland, USA) | Recombinant factor IX | 0 | 0 | 100 | 0 |
| *Activated prothrombin complex concentrates* | | | | | |
| Autoplex (Baxter Hyland, USA) | Initial exposure to ethanol, dry heat at 60°C for 144 hours | Variable amounts of factors II, VII, IX, X and activated factors VIIa, IXa, and Xa | | | |
| FEIBA (Immuno, USA) | Heated at 60°C for 10 hours at 1.25 atm, then heated at 80°C for 1 hour at 1.6 atm | Variable amounts of factors II, VII, IX, and X, and activated factors VIIa, IXa, and Xa | | | |
| *Other* | | | | | |
| NovoSeven (Novo Nordisk, USA) | Recombinant factor VIIa | | | | |

Institute-Baxter Hyland) has recently been approved for use in the United States (249). Some clinicians prefer recombinant products on the assumption they are less likely to transmit infectious agents. Recovery of recombinant factor IX is less than that of plasma derived factor IX. Thus, to raise a given individual's plasma concentration by 1%, the recombinant product should be given in doses of 1.2 U/kg.

Prophylactic therapy is recommended for individuals with severely affected hemophilia B. One regimen is to administer highly purified factor IX concentrate twice weekly at 25 to 40 U/kg.

One possible complication of replacement therapy in individuals with hemophilia B is anaphylactic shock, which is more likely to occur in those without detectable factor IX antigen (250). Anaphylactic shock occurs in approximately 50% of severely affected children with antibodies against factor IX.

Individuals with anti-factor IX antibodies but without a history of anaphylaxis can be treated with higher-than-normal doses of factor IX concentrates, but this depends on concentration of the inhibitor during treatment.

Individuals with undetectable inhibitor concentrations at the beginning of treatment can be treated with conventional doses of factor IX for approximately 5 days, at which time an anamnestic response occurs and renders further factor IX replacement therapy useless. If the initial inhibitor titer is greater than 10 B.U., replacement with factor IX concentrate is not recommended; activated PCCs such as Autoplex (Baxter Hyland) or FEIBA (Immuno, USA) can be used (Table 36.7). Recombinant factor VIIa also is effective and may be the agent of choice if available. Immune tolerance to factor IX inhibitors can be induced by daily infusions of factor IX for several weeks to several months. Nephrotic syndrome has been a complication, however, in individuals subjected to immune tolerance regimens in individuals with hemophilia B (251).

# FACTOR X DEFICIENCY

Factor X was discovered in the mid-1950s by two groups working independently (252, 253). Initially, the original individual with factor X deficiency was although to have factor VII deficiency until it was demonstrated his plasma corrected the prolonged PT of the original individual with factor VII deficiency (252).

## PATHOGENESIS

Activated factor X is the enzyme that converts prothrombin to thrombin. When factor X is deficient or defective hemorrhagic episodes occur, thrombin generation is delayed and fibrin formation impaired. Abnormalities of factor X include reduced or absent synthesis of the molecule and synthesis of an abnormal molecule that may be antigenically normal but has reduced activity (168, 254, 255). The exact molecular defect is known in some individuals. These defects include point mutations (256–258) and deletions (259).

## GENETICS

The gene for factor X is located on chromosome 13 at position 13q34, next to the gene for factor VII (260, 261). Factor X deficiency is an autosomal recessive trait, and consanguinity frequently is demonstrated. Specific genetic defects have been identified (Table 36.8).

## CLINICAL MANIFESTATIONS

Individuals with severe factor X deficiency (factor X activity, <1% of normal) can have a clinical course similar to that of individuals with severe hemophilia A, including hemarthroses, soft-tissue hemorrhages, retroperitoneal bleeding, central nervous system hemorrhages, hematuria, and pseudotumors (262, 263). Menorrhagia is frequent in affected women. Those with a factor X activity of 10 to 15% of normal have few problems with spontaneous bleeding, and hemorrhage occurs only in association with surgery or trauma.

## LABORATORY TESTS

Typical laboratory results in individuals with factor X deficiency include prolonged PTs and aPTTs. TCTs and bleeding times, however, are normal, and individuals with normal aPTTs have been reported (Table 36.8) (264). Diagnosis rests on demonstrating isolated factor X deficiency by a specific factor X assay. Characteristic laboratory features of the several variants of factor X are listed in Table 36.8 (252, 253, 256–258, 261, 265–272).

## DIFFERENTIAL DIAGNOSIS

Congenital factor X deficiency is rare, and it must be distinguished from the more common causes of low factor X levels. Because of its hepatic synthesis and vitamin K dependency, low factor X levels commonly are found with liver disease and vitamin K deficiency. In these settings, the other vitamin K-dependent factors will also be reduced to varying degrees. Warfarin results in a sim-

## TABLE 36.8. Factor X Variants

| Designation | Factor X Antigen (%) | PT | aPTT | RVVT | Genetic Defect |
|---|---|---|---|---|---|
| Friuli | 100 | Prolonged | Prolonged | Prolonged | Pro 343 → Ser |
| Ketchikan | 20 | Prolonged | Prolonged | Prolonged | Gla 14 → Gly |
| Malmö | Unknown | Prolonged | Prolonged | Normal/ prolonged | Gla 26 → Asp |
| Marseille | Unknown | Prolonged | Normal | Normal | Ser 334 → Pro |
| Melbourne | 120 | Normal | Prolonged | Normal | Unknown |
| Padua | 100 | Moderately prolonged | Normal | Normal | Unknown |
| Prower | 85 | Prolonged | Prolonged | Prolonged | Unknown |
| Roma | 80 | Moderately prolonged | Prolonged | Normal | Unknown |
| San Antonio | 36 | Prolonged | Normal | Unknown | Cys 366 → Arg |
| Santo Domingo | Unknown | Prolonged | Prolonged | Unknown | Gly 20 → Arg |
| Stockton | 100 | Prolonged | Prolonged | Unknown | Asp 282 → Asn |
| Stuart | <1 | Prolonged | Prolonged | Prolonged | Val 104 → Met |
| Vorarlberg | 20 | Prolonged | Prolonged | Prolonged | Glu 14 → Lys |
| Wenatchee I/II | 35 | Prolonged | Prolonged | Prolonged | Arg 139 → Cys |
| Compound heterozygote | | | | | Asn 57 → Thr |

*RVVT, Russell's viper venom time.*

ilar picture as well. Isolated acquired factor X deficiency is well described in individuals with amyloidosis and occurs transiently in a small number of individuals without amyloid, often associated with respiratory infections (273–275). Selective factor X deficiency has been described in individuals with acute leukemia at presentation (276, 277); this often resolves with treatment of the leukemia. Acquired inhibitors to factor X have been reported and account for some of the individuals described earlier (278–280). Acquired factor X inhibitors have been associated with agricultural chemical exposure, antibiotic exposure, concurrent infectious illness, and in one individual, with adrenal carcinoma.

## THERAPY

Factor X activity levels of 10 to 15% of normal are adequate to control minor bleeding, such as hemarthroses and soft-tissue bleeds. Plasma can be the source of factor X replacement therapy when minimal elevation of the level is required. Based on a factor X half-life of approximately 40 hours, an initial loading dose of 10 to 15 mL/kg is given, followed by approximately 50% of that dose every 24 hours. For serious bleeding or surgery, PCCs that contain factor X (Table 36.7) may be used for replacement. Only those concentrates known to be free of hepatitis and HIV should be used. Care should be taken with these products, however, because the risk of thromboembolic episodes may complicate their use. Thus, factor X levels greater than 50% of normal should be avoided. Activated PCCs also have been used in individuals with hereditary factor X deficiency, but in the absence of an inhibitor, use of such products is not recommended. Individuals with hereditary factor X deficiency rarely develop inhibitors.

# FACTOR XI DEFICIENCY

The first case of congenital factor XI deficiency was described in 1953, in a individual who developed excessive bleeding after dental extractions (281). Since then, numerous other individuals have been reported. Factor XI deficiency occurs with very high frequency among Ashkenazi Jews of Eastern European descent. One study (282) in an Ashkenazi population reported a frequency of homozygotes of 0.1 to 0.3%, a frequency of heterozygotes of 6 to 10%, and an estimated frequency of the gene among this population of 4.3%. Other studies have shown similar findings (283, 284). Approximately 50% of all cases of homozygous or heterozygous factor XI deficiency are reported in individuals not of Jewish background (285–288).

## PATHOGENESIS

Factor XI deficiency, also known as plasma thromboplastin antecedent, most commonly results from decreased or absent synthesis of the factor XI protein. Antigenic and functional factor XI levels usually are concordant (284, 285). Less common are cases of abnormally functioning factor XI molecules (285, 288–292). Factor XIa is necessary for activation of factor IX via the so-called "intrinsic" (i.e., contact activation) pathway, and when levels are deficient, the end result is decreased thrombin generation and poor clot formation.

## GENETICS

In affected Ashkenazi Jews, different point mutations have been identified in the factor XI gene that result in reduced or absent synthesis of the factor XI molecule (293). There is a poor correlation between factor XI functional levels and bleeding complications (282, 285, 294–296). Two of the three identified genotypes are associated with an increased risk of bleeding problems, including the genotypes resulting in synthesis of a truncated molecule and molecules resulting from a missense mutation (289, 297). Platelets have a factor XI-like activity, but it is not known whether this is clinically relevant (298).

The gene for factor XI is located on chromosome 4 (289, 299). Factor XI deficiency is inherited in an autosomal recessive pattern, and men and woman are affected equally. Homozygous, compound heterozygous, and heterozygous individuals may be distinguished by genotype, but they may be indistinguishable by phenotype (283). Three genotypes have been described:

1. Type I, or abnormalities at the intron-exon boundary;
2. Type II, or mutations resulting in a stop codon and premature truncation of translation; and
3. Type III, which results from a missense mutation.

In a large study of Ashkenazi Jews, most individuals, whether heterozygous, compound heterozygous, or homozygous, had either type II or type III factor XI deficiency (288, 289).

## CLINICAL MANIFESTATIONS

Clinical bleeding does not always correlate with factor XI clotting activity, but if one member of an affected kindred has hemorrhagic problems, others will likely experience hemorrhage as well. Those individuals with a factor XI activity less than 10% of normal are most likely to have bleeding complications. In addition, there is suggestive evidence that hemorrhage is more likely when tissues rich in fibrinolytic activity are traumatized. For example, bleeding is more severe after dental extractions and prostatectomy (300–303). Common bleeding problems include bruising, epistaxis, menorrhagia, hematuria, postpartum bleeding, and hematomas. Hemarthroses and intramuscular bleeding rarely occur.

## LABORATORY TESTS

Typical coagulation studies in individuals with factor XI deficiency reveal a prolonged aPTT with a normal PT. Diagnosis requires a specific factor XI assay. Such assays must be performed on fresh plasma collected in plastic containers, however, because results may be affected if the plasma is frozen and thawed or collected in glass.

## DIFFERENTIAL DIAGNOSIS

In addition to the inheritance of factor XI as a single deficiency, congenitally low levels of factor XI are seen in individuals with familial combined factor deficiencies (types V and VI) as well. Congenital factor XI deficiency also has been associated with Noonan's syndrome (304–307), factor VIII deficiency (308, 309), factor IX deficiency, and von Willebrand disease (310).

Hereditary factor XI deficiency must be distinguished from that caused by an acquired inhibitor (i.e., antibody) (311–314). Individuals with an acquired inhibitor often have immunologic diseases such as systemic lupus erythematosus (315, 316).

## THERAPY

Individuals with factor XI deficiency who present with bleeding obviously require replacement therapy. In most instances, however, these individuals only experience hemorrhage following trauma or surgery. Because some individuals, even those with undetectable levels of factor XI, may not bleed under normal circumstances, the question of surgery in such individuals poses a problem. Some individuals with low levels of factor XI do not experience bleeding even after surgery, and if a individual has such a history, surgery may be tried without replacement therapy. In a individual without such a history, however, the wisest course is to pretreat those whose factor XI levels are less than 10 to 20% of normal or any individual with a history of abnormal bleeding. Factor XI levels of 20 to 30% of normal should be adequate for hemostasis, but bleeding complications cannot be predicted on the basis of these levels. It generally is recommended that individuals with factor XI levels less than 20% of normal should have factor XI replaced both preoperatively and for a week to 10 days postoperatively (unless previous history suggests no bleeding has occurred after surgery). Based on the bleeding history, all individuals with factor XI deficiency, even those with levels 50% of normal, should be considered for preoperative replacement therapy, because significant bleeding has occurred in heterozygous individuals with 50% activity (294, 317).

Plasma is used for replacement of factor XI. The usual dose is 15 mL/kg as a loading dose, followed by 3 to 6 mL/kg every 24 hours. The half-life of factor XI is approximately $52 \pm 22$ hours; therefore, the plasma level of factor XI may gradually rise over several days of continuous treatment. With replacement therapy, successful surgery, including prostatectomy, coronary artery bypass graft surgery (318), and cataract surgery (319), can be performed in individuals with factor XI deficiency. It has been suggested that for major surgery, a minimal level of 45% of normal should be obtained, whereas for minor surgery, levels of 30% of normal are sufficient.

Use of antifibrinolytic agents such as $\epsilon$-aminocaproic acid may be a valuable adjunctive treatment after dental extractions and general surgery (320). Antifibrinolytic therapy should not be used in individuals with hematuria or bleeding in the bladder because of possible ureteral or urethral obstruction from clots. Therapy should be maintained for 10 to 14 days after major surgery.

Acquired antibodies (i.e., inhibitors) to factor XI can develop in individuals with congenital deficiency who are treated with replacement therapy (321–324). These individuals have been successfully treated with "factor eight inhibitor bypassing" products such as Autoplex or FEIBA (321). A factor XI concentrate is available in Europe.

# DEFICIENCY OF FACTOR XII AND OTHER CONTACT FACTORS

## FACTOR XII DEFICIENCY

The first case of congenital factor XII deficiency was identified in 1955 in a individual named Hageman (325). This individual had no history of bleeding, and the abnormality was identified during routine preoperative testing. Since then, several hundred other individuals have been described.

### Pathogenesis

Factor XII was originally although to be the physiologic activator of factor XI. More recent evidence, however, suggests that factor XI is activated by thrombin, but activation by factor XIIa has not been excluded completely (326). Factor XII (see Chapter 5) may be more important in inflammatory processes or other host defense mechanisms and play a lesser role in systemic coagulation. This hypothesis would account for the absence of hemorrhagic episodes in individuals with factor XII deficiency. Some cases of factor XII deficiency result from deficient or absent synthesis of the factor XII molecule; others result from synthesis of an abnormal molecule (327).

### Genetics

Factor XII deficiency usually is inherited in an autosomal recessive pattern, but autosomal dominant inherit-

**TABLE 36.9.** Factor XII Variants

| Designation | Surface Binding | Molecular Weight | Limited Proteolysis by Kallikrein | Enzymatic Activity |
|---|---|---|---|---|
| Bari | Normal | Normal | Delayed | Positive |
| Bern | Normal | Normal | Normal | None |
| Locano | Normal | Normal | Delayed | None |
| Toronto | Normal | Normal | Not determined | Not determined |
| Valencia | Not determined | Not determined | Not determined | Not determined |
| Washington | Normal | Normal | Normal | Normal |

*Adapted with permission from Saito H, Scott JG, Movat MZ, et al Molecular heterogeneity of Hageman trait (factor X deficiency): evidence that 2 of 49 cases are cross reacting material positive (CRM + ). J Lab Clin Med 1979;94:256–265.*

ance has been reported in one kindred (328). Heterozygous individuals have factor XII levels 40 to 60% of normal. The gene for factor XII is located on chromosome 5 (329–331), and several variants of factor XII have been described (Table 36.9).

## Clinical Manifestations

Individuals with factor XII deficiency, even those with undetectable activity, do not experience hemorrhagic complications. Even major surgery can be performed on individuals with factor XII deficiency without bleeding complications. Suggested associations between early spontaneous abortion, premature delivery, and thromboembolic disease, including arterial and venous thrombosis, pulmonary embolism, and myocardial infarction, are anecdotal, but there are numerous reports (332–342).

## Laboratory Tests

The aPTT may be markedly prolonged (>100 seconds), but the results of other coagulation screening tests are normal. The diagnosis requires a specific factor XII assay (343). Asian individuals normally have lower factor XII levels than white individuals (344).

## Differential Diagnosis

Rarely, factor XII deficiency results from spontaneous development of an antibody (i.e., inhibitor) to factor XII (345). Such inhibitors have been identified in individuals treated with phenothiazines, chlorpromazine (346, 347), and procainamide (348). Congenital deficiency of factor XII has been described in a individual with von Willebrand disease (349), another with factor IX deficiency (350), and a carrier of hemophilia B who also had von Willebrand disease (351).

## Therapy

No specific therapy is required for individuals with factor XII deficiency, because there are no bleeding complications.

## DEFICIENCY OF PREKALLIKREIN AND HIGH-MOLECULAR-WEIGHT KININOGEN

Prekallikrein, high-molecular-weight kininogen, and factor XII are proteins although to play a role in the "contact" phase of coagulation as well as in activation of the fibrinolytic, kinin, and complement systems (352) (see Chapter 5). Similar to factor XII deficiency, deficiency of prekallikrein or high-molecular-weight kininogen is not associated with excessive bleeding.

## Prekallikrein

Prekallikrein deficiency was first described in 1965 in a family named Fletcher (353). The gene is located on chromosome 4q. Affected individuals exhibited a prolonged aPTT and normal levels of all other clotting factors. No individuals have suffered from bleeding complications. Fletcher factor was later identified as prekallikrein (354), and whereas some affected individuals have a quantitative deficiency, others have a dysfunctional molecule (355, 356). The inheritance pattern for prekallikrein deficiency has not been clearly elucidated, but some cases appear to be autosomal recessive and others autosomal dominant.

Two variants of prekallikrein (PK) have been described. $PK_{Long\ Beach}$ possesses no functional activity. $PK_{Zurich}$ has a similar defect. Whether these two variants are identical is not yet known (331).

Despite the prolonged aPTT, some individuals with prekallikrein deficiency have been reported to have thromboembolic disease. As yet, however, there is no proof of a cause-and-effect relationship between the two (357–359). Because prekallikrein is a proactivator of plasminogen (360), some postulate that a deficiency could result in impaired fibrinolysis (361, 362).

Diagnosis of prekallikrein deficiency requires a specific assay (363). Screening tests of coagulation are normal except for a prolonged aPTT, which can be corrected by addition of normal plasma. The prolonged partial thromboplastin time of prekallikrein-deficient plasma also sometimes is corrected by exposure to glass. Individuals with prekallikrein deficiency do not require specific therapy, and their life expectancy is normal. It must be distinguished from deficiencies of the other "contact factors" by demonstrating that addition of plasma deficient in those other "contact factors" corrects the defect. Acquired prekallikrein deficiency occurs in individuals with hepatic cirrhosis or viral illnesses with decreased hepatic synthesis of prekallikrein (364, 365).

## High-molecular-weight Kininogen

The gene for high-molecular-weight kininogen (HK) is located on chromosome 3q, and genetic variants are known to exist. A missense mutation in exon 5 results in a stop codon with total high-molecular-weight kininogen deficiency (331). A partial deletion of the HK gene has been described as well. HK deficiency, which was first described in a individual named Fitzgerald (366), thus explaining the name "Fitzgerald factor," also is known as Williams factor and Flaujeac factor (367–369). The deficiency is inherited in an autosomal recessive pattern and affected individuals are asymptomatic. Some also are deficient in low-molecular-weight kininogen (367). The diagnosis is established when the prolonged aPTT is corrected by plasma containing HK but is not corrected by plasma deficient in HK. A specific assay is necessary for a definitive diagnosis.

# FACTOR XIII DEFICIENCY

A fibrin-stabilizing factor, now known as factor XIII (see Chapter 6), was first postulated in 1944 by Robbins (370). The first case of factor XIII deficiency was described in 1960, in a individual with severe hemorrhage and poor wound healing (371). Since then, more than 100 cases of congenital factor XIII deficiency have been reported.

## PATHOGENESIS

Factor XIII is found in plasma and platelets. Plasma factor XIII has two A-subunits and two B-subunits; platelet factor XIII consists only of two α subunits. Three types of factor XIII deficiency have been described, differentiated on the basis of these subunits (372–379):

1. Type I, a combined deficiency of subunits A and B;
2. Type II, in which the A-subunit is absent; and
3. Type III, in which the B-subunit is absent.

Factor XIII is responsible for catalyzing the formation of peptide bonds between adjacent molecules of fibrin monomers, which confers mechanical and chemical stability on the fibrin clot (see Chapter 6). Fibrin that is not covalently crosslinked is permeable to blood and exhibits increased susceptibility to fibrinolysis.

## GENETICS

Factor XIII deficiency is inherited in an autosomal recessive fashion (380). Homozygous individuals frequently are the children of consanguineous marriages (381, 382). Heterozygous individuals do not have bleeding symptoms, but heterozygous females may have a higher incidence of spontaneous abortion than normal women. The gene for the α subunit of factor XIII is located on chromosome 6 (383); the gene for the B-subunit is located on chromosome 1 (384). Most individuals with factor XIII deficiency exhibit absent or defective α subunits. One individual without the B-subunit has been described and clinically resembled individuals with α chain abnormalities.

## CLINICAL MANIFESTATIONS

Clinically affected individuals with factor XIII deficiency have plasma levels less than 1% of normal (385, 386). Excessive bleeding usually manifests shortly after birth, typically from the umbilical cord. Other bleeding manifestations include soft-tissue hemorrhages, hemarthroses, and hematomas (387). Surgery is complicated by poor wound healing and excessive bleeding, which may be either immediate or delayed (388, 389). Abnormal scar formation is seen as well. Intracranial hemorrhage, which often is not associated with known trauma, occurs with a higher incidence than such hemorrhage in other inherited bleeding disorders (381, 390); in some series, up to 25% of individuals with congenital factor XIII deficiency experience intracranial bleeding (391). Affected male individuals may have oligospermia, and female individuals commonly have repeated spontaneous abortions (392, 393).

## LABORATORY TESTS

Individuals with factor XIII deficiency have normal coagulation screening tests (i.e., PT, aPTT, TCT) as well as normal platelet count and function. The solubility of a fibrin clot in 5-M urea also is a useful screening test for this disorder (see Chapter 26). Clots formed from factor XIII-deficient plasma are soluble in 5-M urea, usually within minutes, whereas normal clots remain insoluble for at least 24 hours. Clot solubility also can be tested in 2% chloroacetic acetic acid (394). Factor XIII can be specifically assessed by measuring ammonia production through its amidase activity. Activated factor XIII is assayed quantitatively by its ability to catalyze incorporation of fluorescent or radioactive amines into proteins such as casein (395–397). Other assays measure actual fibrin crosslinking (398).

## DIFFERENTIAL DIAGNOSIS

Congenital factor XIII deficiency must be distinguished from acquired deficiency resulting in an autoantibody against the factor. Such antibodies have been described in individuals taking isoniazid (399–401), phenytoin (402, 403) and penicillin (404). In some individuals, the autoantibody is idiopathic (405). Severe hemorrhagic complications have occurred in individuals with acquired antifactor XIII antibodies. Treatment of such individuals is difficult, and the mortality rate from hemorrhage approaches 50% (399). The most useful therapy for factor XIII inhibitors is exchange transfusion with or without immunosuppression from cytotoxic drugs. Platelet infusions sometimes are successful, presumably because of their factor XIII content.

Low levels of factor XIII have been described in individuals with Henoch-Schönlein purpura (406), liver disease, Crohn disease (407), and ulcerative colitis (408). One individual with congenital factor XIII deficiency and von Willebrand disease has been described as well (409).

## THERAPY

Only small amounts of factor XIII are required to normalize hemostasis. Because of its long half-life (9–19 days) (410, 411), prophylactic therapy is both practical and advisable, especially as intracranial hemorrhage can be prevented with this approach. Individuals are routinely given prophylactic fresh frozen plasma in doses of 2 to 3 mL of plasma per kilogram (approximately 1–2 U of fresh frozen plasma) every 4 to 6 weeks (412, 413). Cryoprecipitate also contains factor XIII and can be administered in a dose of 1 bag per 10 to 20 kg every 3 to 4 weeks. Factor XIII concentrates prepared from pooled human plasma are available in Europe (Fibrogammin, Hoechst-Marion Roussel, Switzerland) (414, 415). Factor XIII concentrates have also been prepared from placenta (416). Affected individuals with a history of spontaneous abortions can complete a normal pregnancy when treated with prophylactic fresh frozen plasma every 14 days or with factor XIII concentrate every 21 days (417, 418). In addition to prophylactic therapy, affected individuals who undergo surgery or trauma will require more intensive replacement therapy. Therapy can be complicated by blood-borne infections such as hepatitis, HIV, and other viruses, and antibodies to factor XIII can occur following replacement therapy in individuals with congenital deficiency (419).

# FAMILIAL COMBINED FACTOR DEFICIENCIES

Inherited deficiencies of multiple coagulation factors, or the so-called "familial multiple coagulation factor deficiencies" (FMFD), occur in two situations. First, there can be a different genetic defect associated with each deficient factor, so the simultaneous factor deficiencies are coincidental. Second, a single genetic defect can re-

| TABLE 36.10. | Familial Multiple Coagulation Factor Deficiencies |
|---|---|
| **Type** | **Deficient Factors** |
| I | V and VIII |
| II | VIII and IX |
| III | II, VII, IX, and X |
| IV | VII and VIII |
| V | VIII, IX, and XI |
| VI | IX and XI |

sult in multiple factor deficiencies. The latter situation usually is associated with consanguinity (420).

These deficiencies are classified on the basis of which factors are affected (Table 36.10) (Stafford, unpublished data; 420–430). Type I and type III deficiencies have been extensively characterized. Type I FMFD (i.e., deficiency of factors V and VIII) was first reported in 1954 (431); since then, more than 30 affected families have been identified. Initially, type I FMFD was although to result from deficiency of protein C inhibitor, but this is not the case (422). Levels of factor V and VIII clotting activity usually are 5 to 15% of normal. The specific genetic defect has not been identified, but the combined deficiency results from a single genetic lesion. The locus of the gene controlling combined factor V and VIII deficiency has been localized to a small region on chromosome 18 (432).

Type III FMFD (i.e., deficiency of the vitamin K-dependent factors) was first described in 1966 (424). Since then, six other individuals have been identified. Affected individuals exhibit low levels of prothrombin and factors VII, IX, and X. Levels of proteins C and S also are decreased. The carboxylase gene in five individuals has been examined, but a mutation was identified in only one: an arginine replaced with a leucine residue at position 394 (Stafford, Unpublished data). Of these five individuals, at least two had a defect in the vitamin K reductase gene. A defect in either the carboxylase or epoxide reductase gene could result in impaired gamma carboxylation of the glutamic acid residues in the vitamin K-dependent factors (428, 429), which could in turn result in synthesis of dysfunctional proteins with abnormalities of calcium-dependent lipid binding. Type III FMFD is transmitted in an autosomal recessive pattern; some affected individuals show a partial response to large doses of vitamin K (426, 427).

Clinical manifestations of type I and III defects range from asymptomatic to severe hemorrhage, depending on the degree of factor deficiency or dysfunction. The other types of FMFD are rare and not well understood. FMFD must be distinguished from multiple factor deficiencies in liver disease, disseminated intravascular coagulation, and during the use of certain drugs (e.g., warfarin ingestion, surreptitious or otherwise). Treatment of bleeding episodes requires therapy to replace the deficient factors.

# HEMORRHAGIC MANIFESTATIONS OF MULTIPLE MYELOMA AND MACROGLOBULINEMIA

Individuals with dysproteinemias, including multiple myeloma and macroglobulinemia, often have coagulation abnormalities. These can include deficiency of one or more clotting factors, abnormal platelet function, and excessive fibrinolysis (67, 198, 433–436). Hyperviscosity also may contribute to hemorrhagic manifestations.

In both multiple myeloma and macroglobulinemia, there may be reduced activity of one or more of the following: fibrinogen; prothrombin; factors V, VII, VIII, IX, and X; von Willebrand factor; or protein C (67). The paraprotein is postulated to form a complex with a given clotting factor, thus impairing its function (67, 437, 438). Increased clearance of the clotting factor–paraprotein complexes by the reticuloendothelial system may occur as well (198, 438–440). Myeloma proteins and other paraproteins may act as specific inhibitors of one or more coagulation factors, and in some cases, they may act as inhibitory antibodies.

Myeloma proteins that react with the platelet membrane frequently interfere with normal platelet function; therefore, platelet aggregation is impaired (see Chapter 33). This results in a long bleeding time, petechiae, purpura, and mucosal hemorrhage. In addition to qualitative platelet defects, thrombocytopenia also is a frequent complication of multiple myeloma.

A common hemostatic abnormality in multiple myeloma is a prolonged TCT, which is found in approximately 50% of individuals (198). It has been suggested that fibrin monomers bind to the Fab sites of the monoclonal protein, thus inhibiting fibrin polymerization (441) and resulting in a prolonged TCT (442–445). Coagulation abnormalities are common in individuals with multiple myeloma, but bleeding complications occur in only 10% of individuals. For example, a prolonged TCT is a common finding in individuals with multiple myeloma, but it seldom is associated with hemorrhage. On the other hand, hemorrhagic complications are more likely to occur among individuals in whom myeloma protein inhibits factor VIII or von Willebrand factor (446–450). These episodes usually are mild, but fatal gastrointestinal bleeding has been reported.

Hyperviscosity is more common in Waldenstrom's

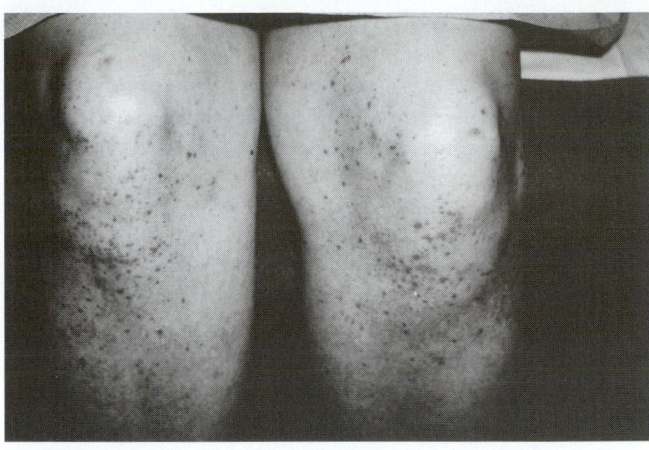

**FIGURE 36.7.** Purpuric lesions on the lower extremities in a individual with Waldenstrom's macroglobulinemia. Similar lesions may be seen in individuals with benign hyperglobulinemic purpura.

macroglobulinemia, in which it occurs secondary to increased plasma concentrations of IgM. Hyperviscosity also occurs in multiple myeloma, however, because of complexes of IgG and, sometimes, IgA immunoglobulins. When viscosity of blood increases three- to fourfold over that of water, sludging of blood occurs. As a result, there is infarction of small blood vessels with extravasation of blood. Clinical manifestations include purpura, which usually are more evident on the lower extremities (Fig. 36.7), and bleeding from the mucous membranes, particularly the nose and nasopharynx. Benign hyperglobulinemic purpura is characterized by a broad-based increase in γ-globulins with complex formation. Lower extremity purpura also are common in this syndrome, and they must be distinguished from those occurring in multiple myeloma or macroglobulinemia.

Bleeding complications of multiple myeloma are best managed by treatment of the underlying disease (452). Specific bleeding episodes, however, may require transfusion, PCCs, or replacement of the affected clotting factors.

## ACQUIRED FACTOR DEFICIENCIES IN AMYLOIDOSIS

Multiple coagulation abnormalities have been described in individuals with systemic amyloidosis. These include hypofibrinogenemia, hyperfibrinolysis (434), dysfibrinogenemia, and inhibited conversion of fibrinogen to fibrin (453). Deficiencies of certain clotting factors, particularly factor X, also are common findings.

Factor X deficiency in individuals with systemic amyloidosis has been reported (226–228, 453–459). In these individuals, levels of factor X range from 2 to 50% of normal, and the circulating factor X may not function normally *in vivo* (460, 461). Factor X deficiency results from a shortened half-life in the circulation (228), most likely because of adsorption of factor X onto amyloid fibrils (227, 462).

Bleeding occurs when factor X levels drop to less than 10% of normal, and this bleeding can be fatal. Treatment of factor X deficiency in amyloidosis is difficult, however, because plasma infusions are ineffective and PCCs are only transiently effective (463). Some individuals have responded dramatically to splenectomy, presumably because of the removal of factor X-binding amyloid deposits (229, 460, 464). Chemotherapy with prednisone, cyclophosphamide, or melphalan, however, has met with minimal success (465). In one individual, plasma exchange was effective in stopping bleeding, and both the PT and circulating factor X levels normalized (466). In addition to factor X, factor IX deficiency also occurs in some individuals with amyloidosis (226).

# $\alpha_2$-PLASMIN INHIBITOR DEFICIENCY

$\alpha_2$-Plasmin inhibitor ($\alpha_2$PI), also called $\alpha_2$-antiplasmin, was described fully in 1976 (467). More than 10 kindreds have been characterized with congenital $\alpha_2$PI deficiency (468). One family has been described with near-normal antigenic levels of $\alpha_2$PI that has essentially no functional activity because of a mutation at the active site (469).

## PATHOGENESIS

$\alpha_2$PI is a serine protease inhibitor with high affinity for plasmin. It inhibits plasmin-mediated fibrinolysis by:

1. Inhibition of the binding of plasmin to fibrin,
2. Direct inhibition of the proteolytic activity of plasmin, and
3. Covalently binding to fibrin (470).

$\alpha_2$PI has a binding site that recognizes the so-called "lysine binding sites" (LBS) on the plasmin molecule. These are the sites where fibrin is noncovalently bound as well. Thus, $\alpha_2$PI interferes with plasmin-fibrin binding. After noncovalent binding of $\alpha_2$PI to the LBS of plasmin, the reactive site of $\alpha_2$PI covalently binds to the active-site serine of plasmin, thus directly inhibiting its proteolytic activity. $\alpha_2$PI also is incorporated into crosslinked fibrin by factor XIIIa, thus contributing to the resistance of crosslinked fibrin to proteolysis by plasmin. Deficiency of $\alpha_2$PI or production of a dysfunctional molecule leads to decreased inhibition of plasmin, thereby resulting in increased fibrinolytic activity.

## GENETICS

The gene for $\alpha_2$PI is found on chromosome 17 at 17p13 (471). The deficiency is inherited as an autosomal recessive disorder, with no demonstrated difference in incidence by sex or ethnic origin. In one family with dysfunctional $\alpha_2$PI, an in-frame insertion of alanine occurs seven positions downstream from the $\alpha_2$PI reactive site. As a result, the altered molecule has only 3% functional activity, but the antigen level is normal.

In other individuals with $\alpha_2$PI deficiency in whom the mutation has been characterized, insertions or deletions within the gene lead to concomitant decreases in both $\alpha_2$PI antigenic and activity levels. In these individuals, homozygotes have essentially no $\alpha_2$PI antigen or activity, and heterozygotes have reduced functional and antigen levels (i.e., 40 to 60% of normal). The deficiency is related to defective intracellular transport with decreased Golgi secretion (472).

## CLINICAL MANIFESTATIONS

Homozygous individuals with $\alpha_2$PI deficiency demonstrate a severe bleeding tendency, which is characterized by easy bruising, epistaxis, hemarthroses, menorrhagia, hematuria, and excessive bleeding following trauma or surgery. Posttraumatic and postsurgical bleeding often are delayed (473–476).

Heterozygous individuals with $\alpha_2$PI deficiency have a variable bleeding tendency, but they usually are only mildly affected, if at all. Severe bleeding in heterozygous individuals generally is associated with trauma. In one such individual, trauma resulted in severe bleeding accompanied by a decrease in $\alpha_2$PI levels from approximately 45 to 20% of normal. When bleeding ceased, $\alpha_2$PI levels returned to the baseline value (477).

Acquired $\alpha_2$PI deficiency has been reported with liver failure, acute promyelocytic leukemia, solid tumors, disseminated intravascular coagulation (478), and thrombolytic therapy (479). The diagnosis of congenital $\alpha_2$PI deficiency should be suspected in any individual with a lifelong history of bleeding and normal coagulation tests.

## LABORATORY TESTS

Individuals with $\alpha_2$PI deficiency exhibit a normal PT, aPTT, and TCT. The bleeding time also is normal. Direct measurement of $\alpha_2$PI antigen and activity demonstrates the deficiency. Clot lysis times are accelerated.

## THERAPY

$\epsilon$-Aminocaproic acid (EACA) preferentially binds the LBS of plasmin and, similar to $\alpha_2$PI, inhibits plasmin binding to fibrin (480). In acute bleeding, EACA is given in a dose of 2 to 3 g intravenously or orally every 6 hours. Comparable doses may be given as a continuous infusion. The dose can be increased to 24 g intravenously or orally during each 24-hour period, either in divided doses or as a continuous infusion. There are no data regarding prophylaxis using EACA in individuals with $\alpha_2$PI deficiency.

# $\alpha_1$-ANTITRYPSIN PITTSBURGH (ANTITHROMBIN III PITTSBURGH)

Two individuals with mutated $\alpha_1$-antitrypsin and a bleeding disorder have been described. In both, the mutation resulted in substitution of arginine for methionine at position 358 (481, 482).

The first individual had a serious bleeding disorder characterized by frequent hospitalizations beginning in childhood (483). Bleeding was primarily posttraumatic, with external bleeding, melena, hematuria, and soft-tissue hematomas. Bleeding tests, including the PT, aPTT, TCT, and bleeding time, were prolonged. Ultimately, the individual died of massive hemorrhage. Extensive studies suggested that substitution of arginine for methionine at position 358 converted $\alpha_1$-antitrypsin into a potent antithrombin. The episodic nature of the bleeding was ascribed to the mutant protein acting as an acute-phase reactant following trauma.

The second individual exhibited similar laboratory findings, but in contrast to the first individual, the bleeding tendency has so far been mild. In addition, the second individual was found to have decreased protein C concentration, to levels as low as 13% of normal. The low protein C level in this individual is although to result from increased protein C turnover, but the precise mechanism is unclear (484). Analysis of the protein C gene showed no abnormalities that could account for the low circulating protein level. Normal $\alpha_1$-antitrypsin inhibits activated protein C and factor XIa (485, 486); the mutant $\alpha_1$-antitrypsin has enhanced inhibitory activity against activated protein C and factor XIa as well as inhibitory activity against plasma kallikrein and the factor XII fragment (487, 488).

# REFERENCES

1. Rabe F, Salomon E. Uber Faserstoffmangel im Blut bei einem Falle von Hämophilie. Dtsch Arch Klin Med 1920;132:240–244.
2. Gralnick HR, Connaghan DG. Hereditary abnormalities of fibrinogen. Williams hematology. New York: McGraw-Hill, 1995:1439–1454.
3. Mammen EF. Fibrinogen abnormalities. Semin Thromb Hemost 1983;9:1–9.
4. Risak E. Fibrinopenie. Arch Klin Med 1935;128:605.
5. Uzan G, Courtois G, Besmond C et al. Analysis of fibrinogen genes in individuals with congenital afibrinogenemia. Biochem Biophys Res Commun 1984;120:376–383.
6. Lord ST. Fibrinogen. In: High KA, Roberts HR, eds. Molecular basis of thrombosis and hemostasis. New York: Marcel Dekker, 1995:51–74.
7. Hardisty RM, Pinninger JL. Congenital afibrinogenemia: further observations on the blood coagulation mechanism. Br J Haematol 1956;2:139–152.
8. Gitlin D, Borges WH. Studies on the metabolism of fibrinogen in two individuals with congenital afibrinogenemia. Blood 1953;8:679–686.
9. Callea F, Tortora O, Kojima T et al. Hypofibrinogenemia and fibrinogen storage disease. In: Mosesson MW, Amrani DL, Siebenlist KR, Diorio JP, eds. Fibrinogen 3: biochemistry, biologic functions, gene regulation and expression. New York: Elsevier Science Publishing, 1988:247.
10. Wehinger H, Klinge O, Alexandrakis E et al. Hereditary hypofibrinogenemia with fibrinogen storage in the liver. Eur J Pediatr 1983;141:109–112.
11. Pfeifer U, Ormanns W, Klinge O. Hepatocellular fibrinogen storage in familial hypofibrinogenemia. Virchows Arch B Cell Pathol Incl Mol Pathol 1981;36:247–255.
12. Kant JA, Fornace AJ Jr, Saxe D et al. Evolution and organization of the fibrinogen locus on chromosome 4: gene duplication accompanied by transposition and inversion. Proc Natl Acad Sci U S A 1985;82:2344–2348.
13. Menaché D. Congenital fibrinogen abnormalities. Ann N Y Acad Sci 1983;408:121–130.
14. Galanakis DK. Fibrinogen anomalies and disease: a clinical update. Hematol Oncol Clin North Am 1992;6:1171–1187.
15. Al-Mondhiry H, Ehmann WC. Congenital afibrinogemia. Am J Hematol 1994;46:343–347.
16. Montgomery R, Natelson SE. Afibrinogenemia with intracerebral hematoma. Report of a successfully treated case. Am J Dis Child 1977;131:555–556.
17. Fried K, Kaufman S. Congenital afibrinogenemia in 10 offspring of uncle-niece marriages. Clin Genet 1980;17:223–227.
18. Fernando PB, Dharmasena BD. A case of congenital afibrinogenemia. Blood 1957;12:474–479.
19. Goodwin TM. Congenital hypofibrinogenemia in pregnancy. Obstet Gynecol Surv 1989;44:157–161.
20. Ness PM, Budzynski AZ, Olexa SA et al. Congenital hypofibrinogenemia and recurrent placental abruption. Obstet Gynecol 1983;61:519–523.
21. Pritchard JA. Chronic hypofibrinogenemia and frequent placental abruption. Obstet Gynecol 1961;18:146–151.
22. Inamoto Y, Terao T. First report of a case of congenital afibrinogenemia with successful delivery. Am J Obstet Gynecol 1985;153:803–804.
23. Soria J, Soria C, Hedner U et al. Episodes of increased fibronectin level observed in a individual suffering from recurrent thrombosis related to congenital hypodysfibrinogenemia (fibrinogen Malmor). Br J Haematol 1985;61:727–738.
24. Mackinnon HH, Fekete JF. Congenital afibrinogenemia. Vascular changes and multiple thromboses induced by fibrinogen infusions and contraceptive medication. Can Med Assoc J 1971;104:597–599.
25. Ingram GI, McBrien DJ, Spencer H. Fatal pulmonary embolus in congenital fibrinopenia. Report of two cases. Acta Haematol 1966;35:56–62.
26. Alexander B, Goldstein R, Rich L et al. Congenital afibrinogenemia: a study of some basic aspects of coagulation. Blood 1954;9:843–865.
27. Yamagata S, Mori K, Kayaba T. A case of congenital afibrinogenemia and Review of reported cases in Japan. Tohoku J Exp Med 1968;96:15–35.
28. Gugler E, Luscher EF. Platelet function in congenital afibrinogenemia. Thromb Diath Haemorrh 1965;14:361–373.
29. Soria J, Soria C, Borg JY et al. Platelet aggregation occurs in congenital afibrinogenemia despite the absence of fibrinogen or its fragments in plasma and platelets, as demonstrated by immunoenzymology. Br J Haematol 1985;60:503–514.
30. Cattaneo M, Kinlough-Rathbone RL, Lecchi A et al. Fibrinogen-independent aggregation and deaggregation of human platelets: studies in two afibrinogenemic individuals. Blood 1987;70:221–226.
31. Colvin RB, Mosesson MW, Dvorak HF. Delayed-type hypersensitivity skin reactions in congenital afibrinogenemia lack fibrin deposition and induration. J Clin Invest 1979;63:1302–1306.
32. Hasselback RB, Marion RB, Thomas JW. Congenital hypofibrinogenemia in five members of a family. Can Med Assoc J 1963;88:19–22.
33. Dale BM, Purdie GH, Rischbieth RH. Fibrinogen depletion with sodium valproate [Letter]. Lancet 1978;i:1316–1317.
34. Majer RV, Green PJ. Neonatal afibrinogenemia due to sodium valproate [Letter]. Lancet 1987;ii:740–741.
35. Gralnick HR, Henderson E. Hypofibrinogenemia and coagulation factor deficiencies with L-asparaginase treatment. Cancer 1971;27:1313–1320.
36. Ramsay NK, Coccia PF, Krivit W et al. The effect of L-asparaginase of plasma coagulation factors in acute lymphoblastic leukemia. Cancer 1977;40:1398–1401.
37. Capizzi RL, Bertino JR, Skeel RT et al. L-Asparaginase: clinical, biochemical, pharmacological, and immunological studies. Ann Intern Med 1971;74:893–901.
38. Whitecar JP Jr, Bodey GP, Harris JE et al. L-Asparaginase. N Engl J Med 1970;282:732–734.
39. Fischer M, Lechner K, Hinterberger W et al. Deficiency of fibrinogen and factor VII following treatment of severe aplastic anemia with antithymocyte globulin and high-dose methylprednisolone. Scand J Haematol 1985;34:312–316.
40. Mason DY, Ingram GI. Management of the hereditary coagulation disorders. Semin Hematol 1971;8:158–188.
41. DeMarco L, Girolami A, Zimmerman TS et al. von Willebrand factor inter-

action with the glycoprotein IIb-IIIa complex: its role in platelet function as demonstrated in individuals with congenital afibrinogenemia. J Clin Invest 1986;77:1272–1277.

42. deVries A, Rosenberg T, Kochwa S et al. Precipitating antifibrinogen antibody appearing after fibrinogen infusions in a individual with congenital afibrinogenemia. Am J Med 1961;30:486–494.

43. Beck EA. Abnormal fibrinogen (fibrinogen "Baltimore") as a cause of familial hemorrhagic disorder. Blood 1964;24:853–854.

44. Cronin C, Fitzpatrick D, Temperley I. Multiple pulmonary emboli in a individual with afibrinogenemia. Acta Haematol 1988;79:53–54.

45. Calenda E, Borg JY, Peillon C et al. Perioperative management of a individual with congenital hypofibrinogenemia [Letter]. Anesthesiology 1989;71:622–623.

46. Menaché D. Constitutional and familial abnormal fibrinogen. Thromb Diath Haemorrh 1964;13(suppl):173–185.

47. Kother M, Egbring R, Fuchs G et al. Bleeding and thrombotic events related to structural variants of fibrinogen. In: Mosesson MW, Amrani DL, Siebenlist KR, Diorio JP, eds. Fibrinogen 3: biochemistry, biologic functions, gene regulation and expression. New York: Elsevier Science Publishing, 1988:333.

48. Ebert R. Index of variant human fibrinogens. Boca Raton: CRC Press, 1994.

49. Haverkate F, Samama M. Familial dysfibrinogenemia and thrombophilia. Report on a study of the SSC subcommittee on fibrinogen. Thromb Haemost 1995;73:151–161.

50. Ieko M, Sawada K, Sakurama S et al. Fibrinogen date: congenital hypodysfibrinogenemia associated with decreased binding of tissue-plasminogen activator. Am J Hematol 1991;37:228–233.

51. Yoshida N, Okuma M, Hirata H et al. Fibrinogen Kyoto II, a new congenitally abnormal molecule, characterized by the replacement of Aα proline-18 by leucine. Blood 1991;78:149–153.

52. Yoshida N, Wada H, Morita K et al. A new congenital abnormal fibrinogen Ise characterized by the replacement of Bβ glycine-15 by cysteine. Blood 1991;77:1958–1963.

53. Bolgi C, Cofrancesco E, Cortellaro M et al. Fibrinogen Milano VI: a heterozygous dysfibrinogenemia (Aα 16 Arg → His) with bleeding tendency. Eur J Haematol 1990;45:26–30.

54. Koopman J, Haverkate F, Bri't E et al. A congenitally abnormal fibrinogen (Vlissingen) with a 6-base deletion in the γ chain gene, causing defective calcium binding and impaired fibrin polymerization. J Biol Chem 1991;266:13456–13461.

55. Mammen EF, Prasad AS, Barnhart MI et al. Congenital dysfibrinogenemia: fibrinogen Detroit. J Clin Invest 1969;48:235–249.

56. Alving BM, Henschen AH. Fibrinogen Giessen I: a congenital homozygously expressed dysfibrinogenemia with Aα 16 Arg → His substitution. Am J Hematol 1987;25:479–482.

57. Francis RB Jr. Clinical disorders of fibrinolysis: a critical review. Blut 1989;59:1–14.

58. Takala T, Oksa H, Rasi V et al. Dysfibrinogenemia associated with thrombosis and third-trimester fetal loss. A case report. J Reprod Med 1991;36:410–412.

59. Caldwell DC, Williamson RA, Goldsmith JC. Hereditary coagulopathies in pregnancy. Clin Obstet Gynecol 1985;28:53–72.

60. Galanakis DK. Dysfibrinogenemia: a current perspective. Clin Lab Med 1984;4:395–418.

61. Gandrille S, Prilollet P, Capron L et al. Association of inherited dysfibrinogenemia and protein C deficiency in two unrelated families. Br J Haematol 1988;68:329–337.

62. Gralnick HR, Givelber H, Abrams E. Dysfibrinogenemia associated with hepatoma: increased carbohydrate content of the fibrinogen molecule. N Engl J Med 1978;299:221–226.

63. von Felten A, Straub PW, Frick PG. Dysfibrinogenemia in a individual with primary hepatoma. First observation of an acquired abnormality of fibrin monomer aggregation. N Engl J Med 1969;280:405–409.

64. Duchosal M, Reber G, Vader JP et al. Acquired dysfibrinogenemia associated with a non-hepatic malignancy without liver involvement [Abstract]. Thromb Haemost 1985;54:166.

65. Dawson NA, Barr CF, Alving BM. Acquired dysfibrinogenemia: paraneoplastic syndrome in renal cell carcinoma. Am J Med 1985;78:682–686.

66. D'Souza L, Coots MC, Glueck HI. An acquired abnormal fibrinogen associated with thromboembolic disease and pseudotumor cerebri. Thromb Haemost 1979;42:994–1008.

67. Lackner H. Hemostatic abnormalities associated with dysproteinemias. Semin Hematol 1973;10:125–133.

68. Coleman M, Vigliano EM, Weksler ME et al. Inhibition of fibrin monomer polymerization by lambda myeloma globulins. Blood 1972;39:210–223.

69. Galanakis DK, Ginzler EM, Fikrig SM. Monoclonal IgG anticoagulants delaying fibrin aggregation in two individuals with systemic lupus erythematosus (SLE). Blood 1978;52:1037–1046.

70. Galanakis DK, Newman J, Summers D. Circulating thrombin time anticoagulant in a procainamide-induced syndrome. JAMA 1978;239:1873–1874.

71. Ruiz-Arguelles A. Spontaneous reversal of acquired autoimmune dysfibrinogenemia probably due to an antiidiotypic antibody directed to an interspecies cross reactive idiotype expressed on antifibrinogen antibodies. J Clin Invest 1988;82:958–963.

72. Ghosh S, McEvoy P, McVerry BA. Idiopathic autoantibody that inhibits fibrin monomer polymerization. Br J Haematol 1983;53:65–72.

73. Hoots WK, Carrell NA, Wagner RH et al. A naturally occurring antibody that inhibits fibrin polymerization. N Engl J Med 1981;304:857–861.

74. Marciniak E, Greenwood MF. Acquired coagulation inhibitor for delaying fibrinopeptide release. Blood 1979;53:81–92.

75. Rosenberg RD, Colman RW, Lorand L. A new haemorrhagic disorder with defective fibrin stabilization and cryofibrinogenaemia. Br J Haematol 1974;26:269–284.

76. Mammen EF, Schmidt KP, Barnhart MI. Thrombophlebitis migrans associated with circulating antibodies against fibrinogen: a case report. Thromb Diath Haemorrh 1967;18:605–611.

77. Gralnick HR, Givelber HM, Shainoff JR et al. Fibrinogen Bethesda: a congenital dysfibrinogenemia with delayed fibrinopeptide release. J Clin Invest 1971;50:1819–1830.

78. Gralnick HR, Coller BS, Fratantoni JC et al. Fibrinogen Bethesda III: a hypodysfibrinogenemia. Blood 1979;53:28–46.

79. Forman WB, Ratnoff OD, Boyer MH. An inherited qualitative abnormality in plasma fibrinogen: fibrinogen Cleveland. J Lab Clin Med 1968;72:455–472.

80. Foreman WB, Kraus J. Transurethral resection in a individual with a dysfibrinogen: fibrinogen Cleveland I. J Urol 1977;118:885.

81. Gilabert J, Reganon E, Vila V et al. Congenital hypofibrinogenemia and pregnancy, obstetric and hematological management. Gynecol Obstet Invest 1987;24:271–276.

82. Josso F, de Sanchez JM, Lavergne JM et al. Congenital abnormality of the prothrombin molecule (factor II) in four siblings: prothrombin Barcelona. Blood 1971;38:9–16.

83. Kahn MJ, Govaerts A. Prothrombin Brussels, a new congenital defective protein. Thromb Res 1974;5:141–156.

84. Shapiro SS, Martinez J, Holburn RR. Congenital dysprothrombinemia: an inherited structural disorder of human prothrombin. J Clin Invest 1969;48:2251–2259.

85. Huisse MG, Dreyfus M, Guillin MC. Prothrombin Clamart: prothrombin variant with defective Arg 320-Ile cleavage by factor Xa. Thromb Res 1986;44:11–21.

86. Montgomery RR, Corrigan JJ, Clarke S et al. Prothrombin Denver—a new dysprothrombinemia [Abstract]. Circulation 1980;III:279.

87. Smith LG, Coone LA, Kitchens CS. Prothrombin Gainesville. A dysprothrombinemia in a pair of identical twins. Am J Hematol 1981;11:223–231.

88. Rubio R, Almagro D, Cruz A et al. Prothrombin Habana: a new dysfunctional molecule of human prothrombin associated with a true prothrombin deficiency. Br J Haematol 1983;54:553–560.

89. Weinger RS, Rudy C, Moake JL et al. Prothrombin Houston: a dysprothrombin identifiable by crossed immunoelectrofocusing and abnormal Echis carinatus venom activation. Blood 1980;55:811–816.

90. Lutze G, Frick U, Topfer G et al. Hereditaire dysprothrombinamie mit geringen Blutunsneigung Prothrombin Magdeburg. Dtsch Med Wochenschr 1989;114:288–292.

91. Bezeaud A, Guillin MC, Olmeda F et al. Prothrombin Madrid: a new familial abnormality of prothrombin. Thromb Res 1979;16:47–58.

92. Josso F, Rio Y, Beguin S. A new variant of human prothrombin, prothrombin Metz: demonstration in a family showing double heterozygosity for congenital hypoprothrombinemia and dysprothrombinemia. Thromb Haemost 1982;12:309–316.

93. Valls-de-Ruiz M, Ruiz-Arguelles A, Ruiz-Arguelles GJ et al. Prothrombin "Mexico City," an asymptomatic autosomal dominant prothrombin variant. Am J Hematol 1987;24:229–240.

94. Girolami A, Coccheri S, Palareti G et al. Prothrombin Molise: a "new" congenital dysprothrombinemia, double heterozygosity with an abnormal prothrombin and "true" prothrombin deficiency. Blood 1978;52:115–125.

95. Girolami A, Bareggi G, Brunetti A et al. Prothrombin Padua: a "new" congenital dysprothrombinemia. J Lab Clin Med 1974;84:654–666.

96. Ruiz-Saez A, Luengo J, Rodriguez A et al. Prothrombin Perija: a new congenital dysprothrombinemia in an Indian family. Thromb Res 1986;44:587–598.

97. Tapon-Bretaudiere J, Dumont MD, Fischer AM et al. Prothrombin Poissy: a new variant of human prothrombin [Abstract]. Thromb Haemost 1983;50:250.

98. Owen CA Jr, Henriksen RA, McDuffie FC et al. Prothrombin Quick. A newly identified dysprothrombinemia. Mayo Clin Proc 1978;53:29–33.

99. Henriksen RA, Mann KG. Substitution of valine for glycine-558 in the congenital dysthrombin prothrombin Quick II alters primary substrate specificity. Biochemistry 1989;28:2078–2082.

100. Bezeaud A, Drouet L, Soria C et al. Prothrombin Salakta: an abnormal prothrombin characterized by a defect in the active site of thrombin. Thromb Res 1984;34:507–518.

101. Shapiro SS, Maldonado NI, Fradera J et al. Prothrombin San Juan: a complex new dysprothrombinemia [Abstract]. J Clin Invest 1974;53:73A.

102. Guillin MC, Bezeaud A, Rabiet MJ et al. Congenitally abnormal prothrombin and thrombin. Ann N Y Acad Sci 1986;485:56–65.

103. Rocha E, Paramo JA, Bascones C et al. Prothrombin Segovia: a new congenital abnormality of prothrombin. Scand J Haematol 1986;36:444–449.

104. Miyata T, Morita T, Inomoto T et al. Prothrombin Tokushima, a replacement of arginine-418 by tryptophan that impairs the fibrinogen clotting activity of derived thrombin Tokushima. Biochemistry 1987;26:1117–1122.

105. Degen SJ, McDowell SA, Sparks LM et al. Prothrombin Frankfurt: a dysfunctional prothrombin characterized by substitution of Glu-466 by Ala. Thromb Haemost 1995;73:203–209.

106. Morishita E, Saita M, Kumabashier I et al. Prothrombin Himi: a compound heterozygote for two dysfunctional prothrombin molecules (Met-337→Thr and Arg-388→His). Blood 1992;80:2275–2280.

107. Poort SR, Michiels JJ, Reitsma PH et al. Homozygosity for a novel missense mutation in the prothrombin gene causing a severe bleeding disorder. Thromb Haemost 1994;72:819–824.

108. Miyata T, Zheng YZ, Kato A et al. A point mutation (Arg-271→Cys) of a homozygote for dysfunctional prothrombin, prothrombin Obihiro, which has a region of high sequence variability. Br J Haematol 1995;90:688–692.

109. O'Marcaigh AS, Nichols WL, Hassinger NL et al. Genetic analysis and functional characterization of prothrombins Corpus Christi (Arg-382→His) Dharan (Arg-271→His), and hypoprothrombinemia. Blood 1996;88:2611–2618.

110. Board PG, Coggan M, Pidcock ME. Genetic heterogeneity of prothrombin (FII). Ann Hum Genet 1982;46:1–9.

111. Shapiro SS, McCord S. Prothrombin. Prog Hemost Thromb 1978;4:177–209.

112. Royle NJ, Irwin DM, Koschinsky ML et al. Human genes encoding prothrombin and ceruloplasmin map to 11p11-q12 and 3q21-24 respectively. Somat Cell Mol Genet 1987;13:285–292.

113. Degen SJF. Prothrombin. In: High KA, Roberts HR, eds. Molecular basis of thrombosis and hemostasis. New York: Marcel Dekker, 1995:75–99.

114. Baudo F, de Cataldo F, Josso F et al. Hereditary hypoprothrombinemia. True deficiency of factor II. Acta Haematol 1972;47:243–249.

115. Hollinger BR, Pastoor TP. Case management and plasma half-life in a case of brodifacoum poisoning. Arch Intern Med 1993;153:1925–1928.

116. Kaiser CW, McAuliffe JD, Barth RJ et al. Hypoprothrombinemia and hemorrhage in a surgical individual treated with Cefotetan. Arch Surg 1991; 126:524–525.

117. Neu HC. Third generation cephalosporins: safety profiles after 10 years of clinical use. J Clin Pharmacol 1990;30:396–403.

118. Lipsky JJ. Antibiotic-associated hypoprothrombinemia. J Antimicrob Chemother 1988;21:281–300.

119. Shearer MJ, Bechtold H, Andrassy K. Mechanism of cephalosporin-induced hypoprothrombinemia: relation to cephalosporin side chain, vitamin K metabolism, and vitamin K status. J Clin Pharmacol 1988;28:88–95.

120. Sattler FR, Weitekamp MR, Sayegh A et al. Impaired hemostasis caused by beta-lactam antibiotics. Am J Surg 1988;155:30–39.

121. Grasela TH Jr, Walawander CA, Welage LS et al. Prospective surveillance of antibiotic-associated coagulopathy in 970 individuals. Pharmacotherapy 1989;9:158–164.

122. Baudo F, Redaelli R, Pezzetti L et al. Prothrombin-antibody coexistent with lupus anticoagulant (LA): clinical study and immunochemical characterization. Thromb Res 1990;57:279–287.

123. Fleck RA, Rapaport SI, Rao LV. Anti-prothrombin antibodies and the lupus anticoagulant. Blood 1988;72:512–519.

124. Bajaj SP, Rapaport SI, Barclay S et al. Acquired hypoprothrombinemia due to nonneutralizing antibodies to prothrombin: mechanism and management. Blood 1985;65:1538–1543.

125. Scully MF, Ellis V, Kakkar VV et al. An acquired coagulation inhibitor to factor II. Br J Haematol 1982;50:655–664.

126. Quick AJ. On the constitution of prothrombin. Am J Physiol 1943;140:212–220.

127. Owren PA. The coagulation of blood. Investigations on a new clotting factor. Acta Med Scand 1947;194:11–41.

128. Girolami A, De Marco L, Dal Bo Zanon R et al. Rarer quantitative and qualitative abnormalities of coagulation. Clin Haematol 1985;14:385–411.

129. Seeler RA. Parahemophilia: factor V deficiency. Med Clin North Am 1972; 56:119–125.

130. Breederveld K, Giddings JC, ten Cate JW et al. The localization of factor V within normal human platelets and the demonstration of a platelet-factor V antigenin congenital factor V deficiency. Br J Haematol 1975;29:405–412.

131. Chiu HC, Whitaker E, Colman RW. Heterogeneity of human factor V deficiency. Evidence for the existence of an antigen-positive variants. J Clin Invest 1983;72:493–503.

132. Wang H, Riddell DC, Guinto ER et al. Localization of the gene encoding human factor V to chromosome 1q 21-25. Genomics 1988;2:324–328.

133. Ortel TL, Keller FG, Kane WH. Factor V. In: High KA, Roberts HR, eds. Molecular basis of thrombosis and hemostasis. New York: Marcel Dekker, 1995:119–146.

134. Dahlback B, Carlsson M, Svensson PJ. Familiar thrombophilia due to a previously unrecognized mechanism characterized by poor anti-coagulant response to activated protein C: prediction of a cofactor to activated protein C. Proc Natl Acad Sci U S A 1993;90:1004–1008.

135. Bertina RM, Koeleman BP, Koster T et al. Mutation in blood coagulation factor V associates with resistance to activated protein C. Nature 1994; 369:64–67.

136. Tracy PB, Giles AR, Mann KG et al. Factor V (Quebec): a bleeding diathesis associated with a qualitative platelet factor V deficiency. J Clin Invest 1984; 74:1221–1228.

137. Tracy PB, Eide LL, Bowie EJ et al. Radioimmunoassay of factor V in human plasma and platelets. Blood 1982;60:59–63.

138. Manotti C, Quintavalla R, Pini M et al. Thromboembolic manifestations and congenital factor V deficiency: a family study. Thromb Haemost 1989; 19:331–334.

139. Forbes CD. Clinical aspects of the genetic disorders of coagulation. In: Ratnoff OD, Forbes CD, eds. Disorder of hemostasis. Philadelphia: WB Saunders, 1996:138–185.

140. Soff GA, Levin J. Familial multiple coagulation factor deficiencies. I. Review of the literature: differentiation of single hereditary disorders associated with multiple deficiencies from coincidental concurrence of single factor deficiency states. Semin Thromb Hemost 1981;7:112–148.

141. Fratantoni JC, Hilgartner M, Nachman RL. Nature of the defect in congenital factor V deficiency: study in a individual with an acquired circulating anticoagulant. Blood 1972;39:751–758.

142. Chediak J, Ashenhurst JB, Garlick I et al. Successful management of bleeding in a individual with a factor V inhibitor by platelet transfusions. Blood 1980;56:835–841.

143. Feinstein DI. Acquired inhibitors of factor V. Thromb Haemost 1978;39:663–674.

144. Grace CS, Wolf P. Proceedings: a high-titre circulating inhibitor of human factor V: clinical, biochemical and immunological features and its treatment by plasmapheresis [Abstract]. Thromb Diath Haemorrh 1975;34:322.

145. Coots MC, Muhleman AF, Glueck HI. Hemorrhagic death associated with a high titer factor V inhibitor. Am J Hematol 1978;4:193–206.

146. Lane TA, Shapiro SS, Burka ER. Factor V antibody and disseminated intravascular coagulation. Ann Intern Med 1978;89:182–185.

147. Crowell EB Jr. A spontaneous factor V inhibitor in an elderly man (abstract). Clin Res 1971;19:664.

148. Feinstein DI, Rapaport SI, McGehee WG et al. Factor V anticoagulants: clinical, biochemical and immunological observations. J Clin Invest 1970; 49:1578–1588.

149. Handley DA, Duncan BM. A circulating anticoagulant specific for factor V. Pathology 1969;1:265–272.

150. Onuora CA, Lindenbaum J, Nossel HL. Massive hemorrhage associated with circulating antibodies to factor V. Am J Med Sci 1973;265:407–417.

151. Chiu HC, Rao AK, Beckett C et al. Immune complexes containing factor V in a individual with an acquired neutralizing antibody. Blood 1985;65:810–818.

152. Chong LL, Wong YC. A case of factor V inhibitor. Am J Hematol 1985; 19:395–399.

153. Vickars LM, Coupland RW, Naiman SC. The response of an acquired factor V inhibitor to activated factor IX concentrate. Transfusion 1985;25:51–53.

154. Brandt JT, Britton A, Kraut E. A spontaneous factor V inhibitor with unexpected laboratory features. Arch Pathol Lab Med 1986;110:224–227.

155. Lazarchick J, Wolff CM, Pepkowitz SH et al. Factor V inhibitor associated with immune complex formation. Arch Pathol Lab Med 1986;110:448–451.

156. Nesheim ME, Nichols WL, Cole TL et al. Isolation and study of an acquired inhibitor of human coagulation factor V. J Clin Invest 1986;77:405–415.

157. Aliaga JL, de Gracia J, Vidal R et al. Acquired factor V deficiency in an individual with pulmonary tuberculosis. Eur Respir J 1990;3:109–110.

158. Grigg AP, Dauer R, Thurlow PJ. Bleeding due to an acquired inhibitor of platelet associated factor V. Aust N Z J Med 1989;19:310–314.

159. Rapaport SI, Zivelin A, Minow RA et al. Clinical significance of antibodies to bovine and human thrombin and factor V after surgical use of bovine thrombin. Am J Clin Pathol 1992;97:84–91.

160. Webster WP, Roberts HR, Penick GD. Hemostasis in factor V deficiency. Am J Med Sci 1964;248:194–202.

161. Alexander G, Goldstein R, Landwehr G et al. Congenital serum prothrombin conversion accelerator deficiency: a new hitherto unrecognized defect with hemorrhage rectified by serum and serum fractions. J Clin Invest 1951;30:596–608.

162. Peterson LC, Hedner U, Wildgoose P. Factor VII. In: High KA, Roberts HR, eds. Molecular basis of thrombosis and hemostasis. New York: Marcel Dekker, 1995:147–165.

163. Mariani G, Mazzucconi MG, Hermans J et al. Factor VII deficiency: immunological characterization of genetic variants and detection of carriers. Br J Haematol 1981;48:7–14.

164. Hall CA, Rapaport SI, Ames SB et al. A clinical and family study of hereditary proconvertin (factor VII) deficiency. Am J Med 1964;37:172–181.

165. Triplett DA, Brandt JT, Batard MA et al. Hereditary factor VII deficiency defined by combined functional and immunochemical analysis. Blood 1985;66:1284–1287.

166. Fujita I, Takahashi Y, Sakaguchi T et al. Congenital factor VII abnormality discovered in an infant at a routine checkup. Am J Pediatr Hematol Oncol 1991;13:47–48.

167. Denson KW, Conard J, Samama M. Genetic variants of factor VII. Lancet 1972;i:1234.

168. Girolami A, De Marco L, Dal Bo Zanon R et al. Rarer quantitative and qualitative abnormalities of coagulation. Clin Haematol 1985;14:385–411.

169. Girolami A, Fabris F, Dal Bo Zanon R et al. Factor VII Padua: a congenital disorder due to an abnormal factor VII with a peculiar activation pattern. J Lab Clin Med 1977;91:387–395.

170. Girolami A, Dal Bo Zanon R, Zanella F et al. Factor VII Padua defect: the heterozygote population. Acta Haematol 1982;68:34–38.

171. Girolami A, Cattarozzi G, Dal Bo Zanon R et al. Factor VII Padua $_2$: another factor VII abnormality with defective ox brain thromboplastin activation and a complex hereditary pattern. Blood 1979;54:46–53.

172. Girolami A, Falezza G, Patrassi G et al. Factor VII Verona coagulation disorder: double heterozygosis with an abnormal factor VII and heterozygous factor VII deficiency. Blood 1977;50:603–610.

173. Chaing S, Clarke B, Sridhara S et al. Severe factor VII deficiency caused by mutations abolishing the cleavage site for activation and altering binding to tissue factor. Blood 1994;83:3524.

174. Arbini AA, Bodkin D, Lopaciuk S et al. Molecular analysis of Polish individuals with factor VII deficiency. Blood 1994;84:2214–2220.

175. Arbini AA, Mannucci M, Bauer KA. A Thr$^{359}$Met mutation in factor VII of a individual with a hereditary deficiency causes defective secretion of the molecule. Blood 1996;87:5085–5094.

176. Takamiya O, Abe S, Yoshioka A et al. Factor VII Shinjo: a dysfunctional factor VII variant homozygous for the substitution Gln for Arg at position 79. Thromb Haemost 1995;25:89–97.

177. Ohiwa M, Hayashi T, Wada H et al. Factor VII Mie: homozygous asymptomatic type I deficiency caused by an amino acid substitution of His (CAC) for Arg (247) (CGC) in the catalytic domain. Thromb Haemost 1994; 71:773–777.

178. Matsushita T, Kojima T, Emi N et al. Impaired human tissue factor mediated activity in blood clotting factor VII Nagoya (Arg 304 → Trp). Evidence that a region in the catalytic domain of factor VII is important for the association with tissue factor. J Biol Chem 1994;269:7355–7363.

179. James HL, Girolami A, Hubbard JG et al. The dysfunction of coagulation factor VII Padua results from substitution of arginine-304 by glutamine. Biochim Biophys Acta 1993;1772:301–305.

180. Sabharwal AK, Kuppuswamy MN, Foster DC et al. Factor VII deficiency (FVII Richmond, R304Q Mutant) associated with thrombosis. Circulation 1992;86:I–679.

181. Kuppuswamy MN, Sabharwal AK, Birktoft JJ et al. Molecular characterization of factor VII Kansas (GK 704): substitution of Gln 100 by Arg in one allele and of Arg 304 by Gln possibly in the other allele [Abstract]. Thromb Haemost 1993;69:1292.

182. Bharadwaj D, Iino M, Kontoyianni M et al. Factor VII central. A novel mutation in the catalytic domain that reduces tissue factor binding, impairs activation of factor Xa, and abolishes amidolytic and coagulant activity. J Biol Chem 1996;271:30685–30691.

183. Arbini AA, Pollak ES, Bayleran JK et al. Severe factor VII deficiency due to a mutation disrupting a hepatocyte nuclear factor 4 binding site in a factor VII promoter. Blood 1997;89:176–182.

184. Cooper ON, Millar DS, Wacey A et al. Inherited factor VII deficiency: Molecular genetics and pathophysiology. Thromb Haemost 1997;78: 151–160.

185. Pfeiffer RA, Ott R, Gilgenkrantz S et al. Deficiency of coagulation factors VII and X associated with deletion of a chromosome 13 (q34). Evidence of two cases with 46 XY, t(13;Y) (q11; q34). Hum Genet 1982;62:358–360.

186. de Grouchy J, Dautzenberg MD, Turleau C et al. Regional mapping of clotting factors VII and X to 13q34. Expression of factor VII through chromosome 8. Hum Genet 1984;66:230–233.

187. Cleton FJ, Leoliger EA. Two typical hereditary charts of congenital factor VII deficiency. Thromb Diath Haemorrh 1961;5:87–92.

188. Briet E, Onvlee G. Hip surgery in a individual with severe factor VII deficiency. Thromb Haemost 1987;17:273–277.

189. Ragni MV, Lewis JH, Spero JA et al. Factor VII deficiency. Am J Hematol 1981;10:79–88.

190. Marder VJ, Shulman NR. Clinical aspects of congenital factor VII deficiency. Am J Med 1964;37:182–194.

191. Zimmermann R, Ehlers G, Ehlers W et al. Congenital factor VII deficiency. Blut 1979;38:119–125.

192. Gershwin ME, Gude JK. Deep vein thrombosis and pulmonary embolism in congenital factor VII deficiency. N Engl J Med 1973;288:141–142.

193. Fair DS. Quantitation of factor VII in the plasma of normal and warfarin-treated individuals by radioimmunoassay. Blood 1983;62:784–791.

194. Dantzenberg MD, Saudubray JM, Girot R et al. Factor VII deficiency in homocysteinuria [Abstract]. Thromb Haemost 1983;50:409.

195. Weisdorf D, Hasegawa D, Fair DS. Acquired factor VII deficiency associated with aplastic anemia: correction with bone marrow transplantation. Br J Haematol 1989;71:409–413.

196. Campbell E, Sanal S, Mattson J et al. Factor VII inhibitor. Am J Med 1980; 68:962–964.

197. Delmer A, Horellou MH, Andreu G et al. Life threatening intracranial bleeding associated with the presence of an antifactor VII antibody. Blood 1989;74:229–232.

198. Perkins HA, MacKenzie MR, Fudenberg HH. Hemostatic defects in dysproteinemias. Blood 1970;35:695–707.

199. Roberts HR, Lefkowitz JB. Inherited disorders of prothrombin conversion. In: Colman RW, Hirsch J, Marder VJ, Salzman EVY, eds. Hemostasis and thrombosis: basic principles and clinical practice. Philadelphia: JB Lippincott, 1994:200–218.

200. Greene WB, McMillan CW. Surgery for scoliosis in congenital factor VII deficiency. Am J Dis Child 1982;136:411–413.

201. Hedner U, Glazer S, Falch J. Recombinant activated factor VII in the treatment of bleeding episodes in individuals with inherited and acquired bleeding disorders. Transfusion Med Rev 1993;7:78–83.

202. Pavlovsky A. Contribution to the pathogenesis of hemophilia. Blood 1947; 2:185–191.

203. Aggeler PM, White SG, Glendenning MB et al. Plasma thromboplastin component (PTC) deficiency: a new disease resembling hemophilia. Proc Soc Exp Biol Med 1952;79:692–694.

204. Biggs R, Douglas AS, Macfarlane RG et al. Christmas disease. Br Med J 1952;2:1378–1382.

205. Schulman I, Smith CH. Hemorrhagic disease in an infant due to deficiency of a previously undescribed clotting factor. Blood 1952;7:794–807.

206. Aledort LM. A safe approach to treatment of factor IX-deficient individuals. Introduction and overview of treatment. Semin Hematol 1991; 28(Suppl 6):1–2.

207. McGraw RA, Davis LM, Lundblad RL et al. Structure and function of factor IX: defects in hemophilia B. Clin Hematol 1985;14:359–383.

208. High KA, Roberts HR. Factor IX. In: High KA, Roberts HR, eds. Molecular basis of thrombosis and hemostasis. New York: Marcel Dekker, 1995: 215–237.

209. Yoshitake S, Schach BG, Foster DC et al. Nucleotide sequence of the gene for human factor IX (antihemophilic factor B). Biochemistry 1985;24: 3736–3750.

210. Camerino G, Grzeschik KH, Jaye M et al. Regional localization on the human X chromosome and polymorphism of the coagulation factor IX gene (hemophilia B locus). Proc Natl Acad Sci U S A 1984;81:498–502.

211. Lawn RM. The molecular genetics of hemophilia: blood clotting factors VIII and IX. Cell 1985;42:405–406.

212. Lozier JM, High KA. Molecular basis of hemophilia. Hematol Pathol 1990; 4:1–26.

213. Lusher JM, McMillan CW. Severe factor VIII and factor IX deficiency in females. Am J Med 1978;65:637–648.

214. Orstavik KH, Stormorken H, Sparr T. Hemophilia Bm in a female. Thromb Res 1985;37:561–566.

215. Nisen P, Stamberg J, Ehrenpreis R et al. The molecular basis of severe hemophilia B in a girl. N Engl J Med 1986;315:1139–1142.

216. Giannelli F, Green PM, Sommer SS et al. Haemophilia B: database of point mutations and short additions and deletions, 7$^{th}$ edition. Nucleic Acids Res 1997;25:133–135.

217. Roberts HR. Molecular biology of hemophilia B. Thromb Haemost 1993; 70:1–9.

218. Hougie C, Twomey JJ. Hemophilia Bm: a new type of factor IX deficiency. Lancet 1967:698–700.

219. Brown PE, Hougie C, Roberts HR. The genetic homogeneity of hemophilia B. N Engl J Med 1970;283:61–64.

220. Bertina RM, van der Linden IK. Factor IX Deventer—evidence for heterogeneity of hemophilia Bm. Thromb Haemost 1982;47:136–140.

221. Usharani P, Warn-Carmer BJ, Kasper CK et al. Characterization of three abnormal factor IX variants (Bm, Lake Elsinore, Long Beach and Los Angeles) of hemophilia B. Evidence for defects affecting the latent catalytic site. J Clin Invest 1985;75:76–83.

222. Huang MN, Kasper CK, Roberts HR et al. Molecular defect in factor IX$_{Hilo}$, a hemophilia Bm variant: Arg → Gln at the carboxyterminal cleavage site of the activation peptide. Blood 1989;73:718–721.

223. Monroe DM, McCord DM, Huang MN. Functional consequences of an arginine 180 to glutamine mutation in factor IX$_{Hilo}$. Blood 1989;73: 1540–1544.

224. Giannelli F, Choo KH, Rees DJ et al. Gene deletions in individuals with haemophilia B and anti-factor IX antibodies. Nature 1983;303:181–182.

225. Pike IM, Yount WJ, Puritz EM et al. Immunochemical characterization of a monoclonal γG4 lambda human antibody to factor IX. Blood 1972;50:1–10.

226. McPherson RA, Onstad JW, Ugoretz RJ et al. Coagulopathy in amyloidosis: combined deficiency of factors IX and X. Am J Hematol 1977;3: 225–235.

227. Furie B, Voo L, McAdam KP et al. Mechanism of factor X deficiency in systemic amyloidosis. N Engl J Med 1981;304:827–830.

228. Furie B, Greene E, Furie BC. Syndrome of acquired factor X deficiency and systemic amyloidosis in vivo studies of the metabolic fate of factor X. N Engl J Med 1977;297:81–85.

229. Greipp PR, Kyle RA, Bowie EJ. Factor X deficiency in amyloidosis. Resolution after splenectomy. N Engl J Med 1979;301:1050–1051.

230. Natelson EA, Lynch EC, Hettig RA et al. Acquired factor IX deficiency in the nephrotic syndrome. Ann Intern Med 1970;73:373–378.

231. Handley DA, Lawrence JR. Factor IX deficiency in the nephrotic syndrome. Lancet 1967;i:1079–1081.

232. Vaziri ND, Branson HE, Ness R. Changes in coagulation factors IX, VIII, VII, X and V in nephrotic syndrome. Am J Med Sci 1980;280:167–171.

233. Boklan BF, Sawitsky A. Factor IX deficiency in Gaucher disease. Arch Intern Med 1976;136:489–492.

234. Castro O, Farber LR, Clyne LP. Circulating anticoagulants against factors IX and XI in systemic lupus erythematosus. Ann Intern Med 1972;77:543–548.

235. Largo R, Sigg P, von Felten A et al. Acquired factor IX inhibitor in a nonhaemophilic individual with autoimmune disease. Br J Haematol 1974; 26:129–140.

236. Collins HW, Gonzalez MF. Acquired factor IX inhibitor in a individual with adenocarcinoma of the colon. Acta Haematol 1984;71:49–52.

237. Miller K, Neely JE, Krivit W et al. Spontaneously acquired factor IX inhibitor in a non-hemophiliac child. J Pediatr 1978;93:232–234.

238. Roberts HR, Eberst ME. Current management of hemophilia B. Hematol Oncol Clin North Am 1993;7:1269–1280.

239. Gilchrist GS, Ekert H, Shanbrom E et al. Evaluation of a new concentrate for the treatment of factor IX deficiency. N Engl J Med 1969;280:291–295.

240. Hoag MS, Johnson FF, Robinson JA et al. Treatment of hemophilia B with a new clotting factor concentrate. N Engl J Med 1969;280:581–586.

241. Nilsson IM, Berntorp E, Zettervall O. Induction of split tolerance and clinical cure in high responding hemophiliacs with factor IX antibodies. Proc Natl Acad Sci U S A 1986;83:9169–9173.

242. Cheung WF, Van Den Born J, Kuhn K et al. Identification of the endothelial cell binding site for factor IX. Proc Natl Acad Sci U S A 1996;93: 11068–11073.

243. Mannucci PM, Bauer KA, Gringeri A et al. Thrombin generation is not increased in the blood of hemophilia B individuals after the infusion of a purified factor IX concentrate. Blood 1990;76:2540–2545.

244. Aledort LM. Discussion. In: A safe approach to treatment of factor IX-deficient individuals. Semin Hematol 1991;28(Suppl 6):20–24.

245. Hrinda ME, Huang C, Tarr GC et al. Preclinical studies of a monoclonal antibody purified factor IX, Mononine. In: A safe approach to treatment of factor IX-deficient individuals. Semin Hematol 1991;28(Suppl 6):15–19.

246. Kim HC, Matts L, Eisele J et al. Monoclonal antibody-purified factor IX-comparative thrombogenicity to prothrombin complex concentrate. In: A safe approach to treatment of factor IX-deficient individuals. Semin Hematol 1991;28(Suppl 6):15–19.

247. Kim HC, McMillan CW, White GC et al. Clinical experience of a new monoclonal antibody purified factor IX: half-life, recovery and safety in individuals with hemophilia B. In: The clinical benefits of ultrapure replacement factor therapy. Semin Hematol 1990;27(Suppl 2):30–35.

248. Smith KJ. Immunoaffinity purification of factor IX from commercial concentrates and infusion studies in animals. Blood 1988;72:1269–1277.

249. White GC, Beebe A, Nielsen, B. Recombinant factor IX. Thromb Haemost 1997;78:261–265.

250. Warrier I, Ewenstein BM, Koerper MA et al. Factor IX inhibitors and anaphylaxis in haemophilia B. Hemophilia 1996;2:259–261.

251. Ewenstein BM, Takemoto C, Warrier I et al. Nephrotic syndrome as a complication of immune tolerance in hemophilia B [Letter]. Hemophilia 1996;2:1115–1116.

252. Hougie C, Barrow EM, Graham JB. Stuart clotting defect. I. Segregation of an hereditary hemorrhagic state from the heterogeneous group heretofore called "stable factor" (SPCA, proconvertin, factor VII) deficiency. J Clin Invest 1957;36:485–496.

253. Telfer TP, Denson KW, Wright DR. A "new" coagulation defect. Br J Haematol 1956;2:308–316.

254. Denson KW, Lurie A, DeCataldo F et al. The factor X defect: recognition of abnormal forms of factor X. Br J Haematol 1970;18:317–327.

255. Porter NR, Malia RG, Cooper PC. The heterogeneity of congenital factor X deficiency. A study of two unrelated individuals [Abstract]. Thromb Haemost 1979;42:58.

256. Watzke HH, Lechner K, Roberts HR et al. Molecular defect (Gla$^{+14}$ → Lys) and its functional consequences in a hereditary factor X deficiency (factor X$_{Vorarlberg}$). J Biol Chem 1990;265:11982–11989.

257. Reddy SV, Zhou ZQ, Rao KJ et al. Molecular characterization of mutations causing human factor X$_{San Antonio}$. Blood 1989;74:1486–1490.

258. Watzke HH, Hilgartner M, Reddy SV. Factor X$_{Santo Domingo}$: a mutation in the signal peptide resulting in a severe bleeding diathesis. Blood 1989;74: 134A.

259. Bernardi F, Marchetti G, Patracchini P et al. Partial gene deletion in a family with factor X deficiency. Blood 1989;73:2123–2127.

260. Scambler PJ, Williamson R. The structural gene for human coagulation factor X is located on chromosome 13q34. Cytogenet Cell Genet 1985;39: 231–233.

261. Watzke HH, High KA. Factor X. In: High KA, Roberts HR, eds. Molecular basis of thrombosis and hemostasis. New York: Marcel Dekker, 1995; 239–255.

262. Machin SJ, Winter MR, Davies SC et al. Factor X deficiency in the neonatal period. Arch Dis Child 1980;55:406–408.

263. Endo Y. Congenital factor X deficiency and incomplete transverse paralysis. JAMA 1981;246:1708.

264. Bertina RM, Alderkamp GJH, de Nooy E. A variant of factor X that is defective only in extrinsic coagulation [Abstract]. Thromb Haemost 1981; 46:88.

265. Fair DS, Revak DJ, Hubbard JG et al. Isolation and characterization of the factor X$_{Friuli}$ variant. Blood 1989;73:2108–2116.

266. Kim DJ, Girolami A, James HL. Characterization of recombinant human coagulation factor X$_{Friuli}$. Thromb Haemost 1996;75:313–317.

267. Parkin JD, Madaras F, Sweet B et al. A further inherited variant of coagulation factor X. Aust N Z J Med 1974;4:561–564.

268. Girolami A, Vicarioto M, Ruzza G et al. Factor X$_{Padua}$: a "new" congenital factor X abnormality with a defect only in the extrinsic system. Acta Haematol 1985;73:31–36.

269. De Stafano V, Leone G, Ferrelli R et al. Factor X$_{Roma}$: a congenital factor X variant defective at different degrees in the intrinsic and extrinsic activation. Br J Haematol 1988;69:387–391.

270. Messier TL, Wong CY, Bovill EG et al. Factor X$_{Stockton}$: a mild bleeding diathesis associates with an active site mutation in factor X. Blood Coagul Fibrinolysis 1996;7:5–14.

271. Kim DJ, Thompson AR, Nash DR et al. Factors X$_{Wenatchee}$ I and II: compound heterozygosity involving 2 variant proteins. Biochim Biophys Acta 1995;1271:327–334.

272. Kim DJ, Thompson AR, James HL. Factor X$_{Ketchikan}$: a variant molecule in which Gly replaces a Gla residue at position 14 in the light chain. Hum Genet 1995;95:212–214.

273. Mulhare PE, Tracy PB, Golden EA et al. A case of acquired factor X deficiency with *in vivo* and *in vitro* evidence of inhibitor activity directed against factor X. Am J Clin Pathol 1991;96:196–200.

274. Currie MS, Stein AM, Rustagi PK et al. Transient acquired factor X deficiency associated with pneumonia. N Y State J Med 1984;84:572–573.

275. Peuscher FW, van Aken WG, van Mourik JA et al. Acquired, transient factor X (Stuart factor) deficiency in a individual with mycoplasma pneumonial infection. Scand J Haematol 1979;23:257–264.

276. Caimi MT, Redaelli R, Cattaneo D et al. Acquired selective factor X deficiency in acute nonlymphocytic leukemia. Am J Hematol 1991;36:65–66.

277. Pabinger I, Bettelheim P, Dudczak R et al. Coincidence of acquired factor X deficiency and disseminated intravascular coagulation in individuals with acute nonlymphoblastic leukemia. Ann Hematol 1991;62:174–179.

278. Rao LV, Zivelin A, Iturbe I et al. Antibody-induced acute factor X deficiency: clinical manifestations and properties of the antibody. Thromb Haemost 1994;72:363–371.

279. Liles DK. Acquired inhibitor to factor X. Submitted for publication.

280. Henson K, Files JC, Morrison FS. Transient acquired factor X deficiency: report of the use of activated clotting concentrate to control a life-threatening hemorrhage. Am J Med 1989;87:583–585.

281. Rosenthal RL, Dreskin OH, Rosenthal N. New hemophilia-like disease caused by deficiency of a third plasma thromboplastin factor. Proc Soc Exp Biol Med 1953;82:171–174.

282. Seligsohn U. High gene frequency of factor XI (PTA) deficiency in Ashkenazi Jews. Blood 1978;51:1223–1228.

283. Kitchens CS. Factor XI: a Review of its biochemistry and deficiency. Semin Thromb Hemost 1991;17:55–72.

284. Rimon A, Schiffman S, Feinstein DI et al. Factor XI activity and factor XI antigen in homozygous and heterozygous factor XI deficiency. Blood 1976; 48:165–174.

285. Ragni MV, Sinha D, Seaman F et al. Comparison of bleeding tendency, factor XI coagulant activity, and factor XI antigen in 25 factor XI-deficient kindreds. Blood 1985;65:719–724.

286. Niskanen EO, Saito M, Cline MJ. Plasma thromboplastin antecedent (factor XI) deficiency in a black family. Arch Intern Med 1981;141:936–937.

287. Aghai E, Yaniv I, David M. Factor XI deficiency in an Arab Moslem family in Israel. Scand J Haematol 1984;32:327–331.

288. Asakai R, Chung DW, Davie EW et al. Factor XI deficiency in Ashkenazi Jews in Israel. N Engl J Med 1991;325:153–158.

289. Fujikawa K, Chung DW. Factor XI. In: High KA, Roberts HR, eds. Molecular basis of thrombosis and hemostasis. New York: Marcel Dekker, 1995: 257–268.

290. Asakai R, Ratnoff OD, Davie EW et al. Factor XI deficiency due to a point mutation in the intron/exon boundary in the gene. Circulation 1988;78: 0471A.

291. Mannhalter C, Hellstern P, Deutsch E. Identification of a defective factor XI cross reacting material in a factor XI deficient individual. Blood 1987; 70:31–39.

292. Hellstern P, Mannhalter C, Kohler M et al. Combined dys-form of homozygous factor XI deficiency and heterozygous factor XII deficiency. Thromb Haemost 1985;15:215–219.

293. Asakai R, Chung DW, Ratnoff OD et al. Factor XI (plasma thromboplastin antecedent) deficiency in Ashkenazi Jews is a bleeding disorder that can result from three types of point mutations. Proc Natl Acad Sci U S A 1989; 86:7667–7671.

294. Bolton-Maggs PH, Young-WanYin B, McGraw AH et al. Inheritance and bleeding in factor XI deficiency. Br J Haematol 1988;69:521–528.

295. Edson JR, White JG, Krivit W. The enigma of severe factor XI deficiency without hemorrhagic symptoms. Distinction from Hageman factor and "Fletcher factor" deficiency, family study, and problems of diagnosis. Thromb Diath Haemorrh 1967;18:342–348.

296. Todd M, Wright IS. Factor XI (PTA) deficiency with no hemorrhagic symptoms. Case report. Thromb Diath Haemorrh 1964;11:187–194.

297. Hancock JF, Wieland K, Pugh RE et al. A molecular genetic study of factor XI deficiency. Blood 1991;77:1942–1948.

298. Lipscomb MS, Walsh PN. Human platelets and factor XI. Localization in platelet membranes of factor XI-like activity and its functional distinction from plasma factor XI. J Clin Invest 1979;63:1006–1014.

299. Kato A, Asakai R, Davie EW et al. Factor XI gene (f11) is located on the distal end of the long arm of chromosome 4. Cytogenet Cell Genet 1989; 52:77–78.

300. Panisko DM, Al-Sheikh T. Transurethral prostatectomy in severe factor XI deficiency without bleeding complications [Letter]. Urology 1990;36: 201.

301. Kirby K, Mesrobian HG, Fried F. Prostatectomy in individuals with bleeding disorders. J Urol 1988;140:87–90.

302. Sidi A, Seligsohn U, Jonas P et al. Factor XI deficiency: detection and management during urological surgery. J Urol 1978;119:528–530.

303. Kaufman JM. Prostatectomy in factor XI deficiency. J Urol 1977;117:75–78.

304. Kitchens CS, Alexander JA. Partial deficiency of coagulation factor XI as a newly recognized feature of Noonan's syndrome. J Pediatr 1983;102: 224–227.

305. Mendez HM, Opitz JM. Noonan syndrome: a review. Am J Med Genet 1985;21:493–506.

306. de Haan M, van de Kamp JJ, Bri't E et al. Noonan syndrome: partial factor XI deficiency. Am J Med Genet 1988;29:277–282.

307. Flick JT, Singh AK, Kizer J et al. Platelet dysfunction in Noonan's syndrome. Am J Clin Pathol 1991;95:739–742.

308. Lian EC, Deykin D, Harkness DR. Combined deficiencies of factor VIII (AHF) and factor XI (PTA). Am J Hematol 1976;1:319–324.

309. De Angelis V, Orazi BM, Santarossa L et al. Combined factor VIII and factor XI congenital deficiency: a case report. Haematologica 1990;75:272–273.

310. Chediak J, Lambert E, Johnson EI et al. Combined severe factor XI deficiency and von Willebrand's disease. Am J Clin Pathol 1980;74:108–114.

311. Reece EA, Clyne LP, Romero R et al. Spontaneous factor XI inhibitors. Arch Intern Med 1984;144:525–529.

312. Goldsmith GH Jr, Silverman P. Inhibitors of plasma thromboplastin antecedent (factor XI): studies on mechanism of inhibition. J Lab Clin Med 1985;106:279–285.

313. Aberg H, Nilsson IM. Recurrent thrombosis in a young woman with a circulating anticoagulant directed against factors XI and XII. Acta Med Scand 1972;192:419–425.

314. Cronberg S, Nilsson IM. Circulating anticoagulant against factors XI and XII together with massive spontaneous platelet aggregation. Scand J Haematol 1973;10:309–314.

315. Krieger H, Breckenridge RT. Circulating anticoagulant interfering with the action of factor XIa in lupus [Abstract]. Blood 1973;42:1002.

316. Poon MC, Saito H, Koopman WJ. A unique precipitating autoantibody against plasma thromboplastin antecedent associated with multiple apparent plasma clotting factor deficiencies in a individual with systemic lupus erythematosus. Blood 1984;63:1309–1317.

317. Litz CE, Swaim WR, Dalmasso AP. Factor XI deficiency: genetic and clinical studies of a single kindred. Am J Hematol 1988;28:8–12.

318. Vander-Woude JC, Milam JD, Walker WE et al. Cardiovascular surgery in individuals with congenital plasma coagulopathies. Ann Thorac Surg 1988;46:283–288.

319. Blatt PM, McFarland DH, Eifrig DE. Ophthalmic surgery and plasma thromboplastin antecedent (factor XI) deficiency. Arch Ophthalmol 1980; 98:863–864.

320. Seligsohn U. Factor XI deficiency. Thromb Haemost 1993;70:68–71.

321. Stern DM, Nossel HL, Owen J. Acquired antibody to factor XI in a individual with congenital factor XI deficiency. J Clin Invest 1982;69:1270–1276.

322. Schnall SF, Duffy TP, Clyne LP. Acquired factor XI inhibitors in congenitally deficient individuals. Am J Hematol 1987;26:323–328.

323. Morgan K, Schiffman S, Feinstein D. Acquired factor XI inhibitors in two individuals with hereditary factor XI deficiency. Thromb Haemost 1984; 51:371–375.

324. Josephson AM, Lisker R. Demonstration of a circulating anticoagulant in plasma thromboplastin antecedent deficiency. J Clin Invest 1958;37: 148–152.

325. Ratnoff OD, Colopy JH. A familial hemorrhagic trait associated with a deficiency of a clot-promoting fraction of plasma. J Clin Invest 1955;34: 602–613.

326. Mosito K, Fuykawa K. Activation of human blood coagulation factor XI independent of factor XII. J Biol Chem 1991;266:7353–7358.

327. Saito H, Scott JG, Movat MZ et al. Molecular heterogeneity of Hageman trait (factor XII deficiency): evidence that 2 of 49 cases are cross reacting material positive (CRM+). J Lab Clin Med 1979;94:256–265.

328. Bennett B, Ratnoff OD, Holt JB et al. Hageman trait (factor XII deficiency):

329. Cool DE, MacGillivray RT. Characterization of the human blood coagulation factor XII gene. Intron/exon gene organization and analysis of the 5'-flanking region. J Biol Chem 1987;262:13662–13673.

330. Cool DE, Edgell CJ, Louie GV et al. Characterization of human blood coagulation factor XII cDNA. Prediction of the primary structure of factor XII and the tertiary structure of beta-factor XIIa. J Biol Chem 1985;260: 13666–13676.

331. Saito H, Kojma T. Factor XII, prekallikrein, and high-molecular-weight kininogen. In: High KA, Roberts HR, eds. Molecular basis of thrombosis and hemostasis. New York: Marcel Dekker, 1995:269–285.

332. Lao TT, Lewinsky RM, Ohlsson A et al. Factor XII deficiency and pregnancy. Obstet Gynecol 1991;78:491–493.

333. Schved JF, Gris JC, Neveu S et al. Factor XII congenital deficiency and early spontaneous abortion. Fertil Steril 1989;52:335–336.

334. Lammle B, Wuillemin WA, Huber I et al. Thromboembolism and bleeding tendency in congenital factor XII deficiency—a study on 74 subjects from 14 Swiss families. Thromb Haemost 1991;65:117–121.

335. Samlaska CP, James WD, Simel DL. Superficial migratory thrombophlebitis and factor XII deficiency. J Am Acad Dermatol 1990;22:939–943.

336. Hellstern P, Kohler M, Schmengler K et al. Arterial and venous thrombosis and normal response to streptokinase treatment in a young individual with severe Hageman factor deficiency. Acta Haematol 1983;69:123–126.

337. Dyerberg J, Stoffersen E. Recurrent thrombosis in a individual with factor XII deficiency. Acta Haematol 1980;63:278–282.

338. McPherson RA. Thromboembolism in Hageman trait. Am J Clin Pathol 1977;68:420–423.

339. Penny WJ, Colvin BT, Brooks N. Myocardial infarction with normal coronary arteries and factor XII deficiency. Br Heart J 1985;53:230–234.

340. Lodi S, Isa L, Pollini E et al. Defective intrinsic fibrinolytic activity in a individual with severe factor XII deficiency and myocardial infarction. Scand J Haematol 1984;33:80–82.

341. Glueck HI, Roehill W. Myocardial infarction in a individual with a Hageman (factor XII) defect. Ann Intern Med 1966;64:390–396.

342. Hoak JC, Swanson LW, Warner ED et al. Myocardial infarction associated with severe factor XII deficiency. Lancet 1966;ii:884–886.

343. Kluft C, Svendsen L, Los P. Direct assay of factor XIIa in plasma with synthetic chromogen substrates. Adv Exp Med Biol 1983;156:201–204.

344. Gordon EM, Donaldson VH, Saito H et al. Reduced titers of Hageman factor (factor XII) in Orientals. Ann Intern Med 1981;95:697–700.

345. Criel A, Collen D, Masson PL. A case of IgM antibodies which inhibit the contact activation of blood coagulation. Thromb Res 1978;12:883–892.

346. Zucker S, Zarrabi MH, Romano GS et al. IgM inhibitors of the contact activation phase of coagulation in chlorpromazine-treated individuals. Br J Haematol 1978;40:447–457.

347. Canoso RT, Hutton RA, Deykin D. A chlorpromazine-induced inhibitor of blood coagulation. Am J Hematol 1977;2:183–191.

348. Clyne LP, Farber LR, Chopyk RL. Procainamide-induced circulating anticoagulants in a congenitally-deficient factor XI individual. Folia Haematol Int Mag Klin Morphol Blutforsch 1989;116:239–244.

349. Buchanan GR, Green DM, Handin RI. Combined von Willebrand's disease and Hageman factor deficiency. J Pediatr 1977;90:779–781.

350. Mant MJ. Combined factor IX and XII deficiencies in both male and female members of a single family. Thromb Haemost 1979;42:816–818.

351. Beard J, Dudley JM, Holland LJ et al. Combined von Willebrand's disease and factor XII deficiency in a carrier of haemophilia B. Clin Lab Haematol 1989;11:139–141.

352. Mannhalter CH. Biochemical and functional properties of factor XI and prekallikrein. Semin Thromb Hemost 1987;13:25–35.

353. Hathaway WE, Belhasen LP, Hathaway HS. Evidence for a new plasma thromboplastin factor. I. Case report, coagulation studies, and physiochemical properties. Blood 1965;26:521–532.

354. Wuepper KD. Prekallikrein deficiency in man. J Exp Med 1973;138: 1345–1355.

355. De Stefano V, Leone G, Teofili L et al. Association of Graves disease and prekallikrein congenital deficiency in a individual belonging to the first CRM+ prekallikrein-deficient Italian family. Thromb Res 1990;60:397–404.

356. Saito H, Goodnough LT, Soria J et al. Heterogeneity of human prekallikrein deficiency (Fletcher trait): evidence that 5 of 18 cases are positive for cross reacting material. N Engl J Med 1981;305:910–914.

357. Harris MG, Exner T, Rickard KA et al. Multiple cerebral thromboses in Fletcher factor (prekallikrein) deficiency: a case report. Am J Hematol 1985; 19:387–393.

358. Goodnough LT, Saito H, Ratnoff OD. Thrombosis or myocardial infarction in congenital clotting factor abnormalities and chronic thrombocytopenias: a report of 21 individuals and a Review of 50 previously reported cases. Medicine 1983;62:248–255.

359. Currimbhoy Z, Vinciguerra V, Palakavongs P et al. Fletcher factor deficiency and myocardial infarction. Am J Clin Pathol 1976;65:970–974.

360. Vennerod AM, Laake K. Prekallikrein and plasminogen proactivator: absence of plasminogen proactivator in Fletcher factor deficient plasma. Thromb Res 1976;8:519–522.

a probable second genotype inherited as an autosomal dominant characteristic. Blood 1972;40:412–415.

361. Hathaway WE, Wuepper KD, Weston WL et al. Clinical and physiologic studies of two siblings with prekallikrein (Fletcher factor) deficiency. Am J Med 1976;60:654–664.

362. Weiss AS, Gallin JI, Kaplan AP. Fletcher factor deficiency, a diminished rate of Hageman factor activation caused by absence of prekallikrein with abnormalities of coagulation, fibrinolysis, chemotactic activity and kinin generation. J Clin Invest 1974;53:622–633.

363. Hathaway WE, Alsever J. The relation of "Fletcher Factor" to factors XI and XII. Br J Haematol 1970;18:161–169.

364. Wong PY, Talamo RC, Williams GH. Kallikrein-kinin and renin-angiotensin systems in functional renal failure of cirrhosis of the liver. Gastroenterology 1977;73:1114–1118.

365. Edelman R, Nimmannitya S, Colman RW et al. Evaluation of the plasma kinin system in dengue hemorrhagic fever. J Lab Clin Med 1975;86:410–421.

366. Saito H, Ratnoff OD, Waldmann R et al. Fitzgerald trait: deficiency of a hitherto unrecognized agent, Fitzgerald factor, participating in surface mediated reactions of clotting, fibrinolysis, generation of kinins, and the property of diluted plasma enhancing vascular permeability (PF/DIL). J Clin Invest 1975;55:1082–1089.

367. Lacombe MJ, Varet B, Levy JP. A hitherto undescribed plasma factor acting at the contact phase of blood coagulation (Flaujeac factor): case report and coagulation studies. Blood 1975;46:761–768.

368. Wuepper KD, Miller DR, Lacombe MJ. Flaujeac trait. Deficiency of human plasma kininogen. J Clin Invest 1975;56:1663–1672.

369. Colman RW, Bagdasarian A, Talamo RC et al. Williams trait. Human kininogen deficiency with diminished levels of plasminogen proactivator and prekallikrein associated with abnormalities of the Hageman factor-dependent pathways. J Clin Invest 1975;56:1650–1662.

370. Robbins KC. A study on the conversion of fibrinogen to fibrin. Am J Physiol 1944;142:581–588.

371. Duckert F, Jung E, Shmerling DH. A hitherto undescribed congenital haemorrhagic diathesis probably due to fibrin stabilizing factor deficiency. Thromb Diath Haemorrh 1960;5:179–186.

372. Girolami A, Sartori MT, Simioni P. An updated classification of factor XIII defect. Br J Haematol 1991;77:565–566.

373. Girolami A, Cappellato MG, Lazzaro AR et al. Type I and type II disease in congenital factor XIII deficiency. A further demonstration of the correctness of the classification. Blut 1986;53:411–413.

374. Barbui T, Rodeghiero F, Dini E et al. Subunits A and S inheritance in four families with congenital factor XIII deficiency. Br J Haematol 1978;38:267–271.

375. Israels ED, Paraskevas F, Israels LG. Immunologic studies of coagulation factor XIII. J Clin Invest 1973;52:2398–2403.

376. Mikkola H, Muzbek L, Laiho E et al. Molecular mechanism of a mild phenotype in coagulation factor XIII (FXIII) deficiency: a splicing mutation permitting partial correct splicing of FXIII A-subunit mRNA. Blood 1997;89:1279–1287.

377. Izumi T, Hashiguchi T, Castaman G et al. Type I factor XIII deficiency is caused by a genetic defect of its b-subunit: insertion of triplet AAC in exon III leads to premature termination in the second sushi domain. Blood 1996;87:2769–2774.

378. Mikkola H, Yee VC, Syrjala M et al. Four novel mutations in deficiency of coagulation factor XIII: consequences to expression and structure of the A-subunit. Blood 1996;87:141–151.

379. Coggan M, Baker R, Miloszewski K et al. Mutations causing coagulation factor XIII subunit A deficiency: characterization of the mutant proteins after expression in yeast. Blood 1995;85:2455–2460.

380. Fear JD, Miloszewski KJ, Losowsky MS. Factor XIII levels in five families of individuals with inherited factor XIII deficiency: support for an autosomal recessive inheritance. Thromb Haemost 1983;50:588–590.

381. Kitchens CS, Newcomb TF. Factor XIII. Medicine 1979;58:413–429.

382. Lorand L, Urayama T, Atencio AC et al. Inheritance of deficiency of fibrin-stabilizing factor (factor 13). Am J Hum Genet 1970;22:89–95.

383. Board PG, Reid M, Serjeantson S. The gene for coagulation factor XIII A subunit (F13A) is distal to HLA on chromosome 6. Hum Genet 1984;67:406–408.

384. Lai TS, Greenberg CS. Factor XIII. In: High KA, Roberts HR eds. Molecular basis of thrombosis and hemostasis. New York: Marcel Dekker, 1995:287–308.

385. Duckert F, Beck EA. Clinical disorders due to the deficiency of factor XIII (fibrin stabilizing factor, fibrinase). Semin Hematol 1968;5:83–90.

386. Britten AF. Congenital deficiency of factor 13 (fibrin-stabilizing factor): report of a case and review of the literature. Am J Med 1967;43:751–761.

387. Thakker S, McGehee W, Quismorio FP Jr. Arthropathy associated with factor XIII deficiency. Arthritis Rheum 1986;29:808–811.

388. Greenberg LH, Schiffman S, Wong YS. Factor XIII deficiency. Treatment with monthly plasma infusions. JAMA 1969;209:264–265.

389. Barry A, Delage JM. Congenital deficiency of fibrin-stabilizing factor. N Engl J Med 1965;272:943–946.

390. Duckert F. The fibrin stabilizing factor. Ser Haematol 1965;5:58–69.

391. Duckert F. Documentation of the plasma factor XIII deficiency in man. Ann N Y Acad Sci 1972;202:190–199.

392. Fisher S, Rikover M, Nador S. Factor 13 deficiency with severe hemorrhagic diathesis. Blood 1966;28:34–39.

393. Ikkala E, Myllyla G, Nevanlinna HR. Transfusion therapy in factor XIII (FSF) deficiency. Scand J Haematol 1964;1:308–312.

394. Francis JL. The detection and measurement of factor XIII activity: a review. Med Lab Sci 1980;37:137–147.

395. Henriksson P, Stenberg P, Nilsson IM et al. A specific, fluorescent activity staining procedure applied to plasma and red blood cells in congenital factor XIII deficiency. Br J Haematol 1980;44:141–147.

396. Lorand L, Urayama T, De Kiewiet JW et al. Diagnostic and genetic studies on fibrin-stabilizing factor with a new assay based on amine incorporation. J Clin Invest 1969;48:1054–1064.

397. Schmer G. A solid-phase radioassay for factor XIII activity (fibrin stabilizing factor) in human plasma. Br J Haematol 1973;24:735–742.

398. Godal HC, Gravem K, Brosstad F et al. Quantitation of factor XIII by SDS polyacrylamide gel electrophoresis. Thromb Res 1984;35:577–582.

399. Krumdieck R, Shaw DR, Huang ST et al. Hemorrhagic disorder due to an isoniazid-associated acquired factor XIII inhibitor in a individual with Waldenstrom's macroglobulinemia. Am J Med 1991;90:639–645.

400. Otis PT, Feinstein DI, Rapaport SI et al. An acquired inhibitor of fibrin stabilization associated with isoniazid therapy: clinical and biochemical observations. Blood 1974;44:771–781.

401. Graham JE, Yount WJ, Roberts HR. Immunochemical characteristics of a human antibody to factor XIII. Blood 1973;41:661–669.

402. Godal HC, Ly B. An inhibitor of activated factor XIII inhibiting fibrin crosslinking but not incorporation of amine into casein. Scand J Haematol 1977;19:443–448.

403. Lewis JH. Hemorrhagic disease associated with inhibitors of fibrin cross-linkage. Ann N Y Acad Sci 1972;202:213–219.

404. Lopaciuk S, Bykowska K, McDonagh JM et al. Differences between type I autoimmune inhibitors of fibrin stabilization in two individuals with severe hemorrhagic disorders. J Clin Invest 1978;61:1196–1203.

405. Lorand L, Velasco PT, Rinne JR et al. Autoimmune antibody (IgG Kansas) against the fibrin stabilizing factor (factor XIII) system. Proc Natl Acad Sci U S A 1988;85:232–236.

406. Kamitsuji H, Tani K, Yasui M et al. Activity of blood coagulation factor XIII as a prognostic indicator in individuals with Henoch-Schönlein purpura. Efficacy of factor XIII substitution. Eur J Pediatr 1987;146:519–523.

407. Wisen O, Garlund B. Hemostasis in Crohn's disease: low factor XIII levels in active disease. Scand J Gastroenterol 1988;23:961–966.

408. Rasche H. Blutgerinnungsfaktor XIII und fibrinstabilisierung. Klin Wochenschr 1975;53:1137–1145.

409. Grand B, Blanco A, Riveros D et al. Congenital factor XIII deficiency associated with von Willebrand disease. Am J Hematol 1990;35:208–209.

410. Fear JD, Miloszewski KJ, Losowsky MS. The half life of factor XIII in the management of inherited deficiency. Thromb Haemost 1983;49:102–105.

411. Ikkala E. Transfusion therapy in congenital deficiencies of plasma factor XIII. Ann N Y Acad Sci 1972;202:200–203.

412. Stenbjerg S. Prophylaxis in factor XIII deficiency [Letter]. Lancet 1980;ii:257.

413. Amris CJ, Hilden M. Treatment of factor XIII deficiency with cryoprecipitate. Thromb Diath Haemorrh 1968;20:528–533.

414. Daly HM, Haddon ME. Clinical experience with a pasteurized human plasma concentrate in factor XIII deficiency. Thromb Haemost 1988;59:171–174.

415. Winkelman L, Sims GE, Haddon ME et al. A pasteurized concentrate of human plasma factor XIII for therapeutic use. Thromb Haemost 1986;55:402–405.

416. Lorand L, Losowsky MS, Miloszewski KJ. Human factor XIII: fibrin stabilizing factor. Prog Hemost Thromb 1980;5:245–290.

417. Kobayashi T, Terao T, Kojima T et al. Congenital factor XIII deficiency with treatment of factor XIII concentrate and normal vaginal delivery. Gynecol Obstet Invest 1990;29:235–238.

418. Rodeghiero F, Castaman GC, Di Bona E et al. Successful pregnancy in a woman with congenital factor XIII deficiency treated with substitutive therapy. Report of a second case. Blut 1987;55:45–48.

419. Godal HC. An inhibitor to fibrin-stabilizing factor (FSF, factor XIII). Scand J Haematol 1970;7:43–48.

420. Soff GA, Levin J, Bell WR. Familial multiple coagulation factor deficiencies. II. Combined factor VIII, IX, and XI deficiency and combined factor IX, and XI deficiency: two previously uncharacterized familial multiple factor deficiency syndromes. Semin Thromb Hemost 1981;7:149–169.

421. Brown JM, Selik NJ, Voelpel MJ et al. Combined factor V/VIII deficiency: a case report including levels of factor V and VIII coagulant and antigen as well as protein C inhibitor. Am J Hematol 1985;20:401–407.

422. Canfield WM, Kisiel W. Evidence of normal functional levels of activated protein C inhibitor in combined Factor V/VIII deficiency disease. J Clin Invest 1982;70:1260–1272.

423. Marwaha N, Sarode R, Marwaha RK et al. Combined factors V and VIII deficiency. Indian Pediatr 1990;27:630–632.

424. McMillan CW, Roberts HR. Congenital combined deficiency of coagulation factors II, VII, IX and X. N Engl J Med 1966;274:1313–1315.

425. Vicente V, Maia R, Alberca I et al. Congenital deficiency of vitamin K-dependent coagulation factors and protein C. Thromb Haemost 1984;51:343–346.

426. Goldsmith GH Jr, Pence RE, Ratnoff OD et al. Studies on a family with combined functional deficiencies of vitamin K-dependent coagulation factors. J Clin Invest 1982;69:1253–1260.

427. Johnson CA, Chung KS, McGrath KM et al. Characterization of a variant prothrombin in an individual congenitally deficient in factor II, VII, IX and X. Br J Haematol 1980;44:461–469.

428. Chung KS, Bezeaud A, Goldsmith JC et al. Congenital deficiency of blood clotting factors II, VIII, IX and X. Blood 1979;53:776–787.

429. Brenner B, Tavori S, Zivelin A et al. Hereditary deficiency of all vitamn K-dependent procoagulants and anticoagulants. Br J Haematol 1990;75:537–542.

430. Soff GA, Levin J, Bell WR. Combined factor IX and factor XI deficiency; familial multiple factor deficiency VI (FMFD VI). Semin Thromb Hemost 1981;7:149–169.

431. Oeri J, Matter M, Isenchmed H et al. An geborener Mangel an faktor V (parahemophilie) verbunden mitechter hemophilie A bei zwei brudern. Mod Probl Pediatr 1954;1:575–588.

432. Nichols WC, Seligsohn U, Zivelin A et al. Linkage of combined factor V and VIII deficiency to chromosome 18q by homozygosity mapping. J Clin Invest 1997;99:596–601.

433. Sane DC, Pizzo SV, Greenberg CS. Elevated urokinase-type plasminogen activator level and bleeding in amyloidosis: case report and literature Review. Am J Hematol 1989;31:53–57.

434. Meyer K, Williams EC. Fibrinolysis and acquired alpha-2-plasmin inhibitor deficiency in amyloidosis. Am J Med 1985;79:394–396.

435. Liebman H, Chinowsky M, Valdin J et al. Increased fibrinolysis and amyloidosis. Arch Intern Med 1983;143:678–682.

436. Takahashi H, Koike T, Yoshida N et al. Excessive fibrinolysis in suspected amyloidosis: demonstration of plasmin-α2-plasmin inhibitor complex and von Willebrand factor fragment in plasma. Am J Hematol 1986;23:153–166.

437. Mazurier C, Parquet-Gernez A, Descamps J et al. Acquired von Willebrand's syndrome in the course of Waldenström's disease. Thromb Haemost 1980;44:115–118.

438. Henstell HH, Kligerman M. A new theory of interference with the clotting mechanism: the complexing of euglobulin with factor V, factor VII, and prothrombin. Ann Intern Med 1958;49:371–387.

439. Gruber A, Blasko G, Sas G. Functional deficiency of protein C and skin necrosis in multiple myeloma. Thromb Res 1986;42:579–581.

440. Sanchez-Avalos J, Soong BC, Miller SP. Coagulation disorders in cancer. II. Multiple myeloma. Cancer 1969;23:1388–1398.

441. Coleman M, Vigliano EM, Weksler ME et al. Inhibition of fibrin monomer polymerization by lambda myeloma globulins. Blood 1972;39:210–223.

442. Wisloff F, Michaelsen TE, Godal HC. Inhibition or acceleration of fibrin polymerization by monoclonal immunoglobulins and immunoglobulin fragments. Thromb Res 1984;35:81–90.

443. Gabriel DA, Smith LA, Folds JD et al. The influence of immunoglobulin (IgG) on the assembly of fibrin gels. J Lab Clin Med 1983;101:545–552.

444. Lackner H, Hunt V, Zucker MB et al. Abnormal fibrin ultrastructure, polymerization and clot retraction in multiple myeloma. Br J Haematol 1970;18:625–636.

445. Frick PG. Inhibition of conversion of fibrinogen to fibrin by abnormal proteins in multiple myeloma. Am J Clin Pathol 1955;25:1263–1273.

446. Glueck HI, Coots MC, Benson M et al. A monoclonal immunoglobulin A(kappa) factor VIII: C inhibitor associated with primary amyloidosis: identification and characterization. J Lab Clin Med 1989;113:269–277.

447. Mohri H, Noguchi T, Kodama F et al. Acquired von Willebrand disease due to inhibitor of human myeloma protein specific for von Willebrand factor. Am J Clin Pathol 1987;87:663–668.

448. Bovill EG, Ershler WB, Golden EA et al. A human myeloma-produced monoclonal protein directed agianst the active subpopulation of von Willebrand factor. Am J Clin Pathol 1986;85:115–123.

449. Kelsey PR, Leyland MJ. Acquired inhibitor to factor VIII associated with paraproteinemia and subsequent development of chronic lymphatic leukaemia. Br Med J 1982;285:174–175.

450. Castaldi PA, Penny R. A macroglobulin with inhibitory activity against coagulation factor VIII. Blood 1970;35:370–376.

451. Elezovic I, Djukanovic R, Rolovic Z. Successful treatment of hemorrhagic syndrome due to an acquired, combined deficiency of factors VII and X in a individual with multiple myeloma and amyloidosis [Letter]. Eur J Haematol 1989;42:105–106.

452. Gastineau DA, Gertz MA, Daniels TM et al. Inhibitor of the thrombin time in systemic amyloidosis: a common coagulation abnormality. Blood 1991;77:2637–2640.

453. Greipp PR, Kyle RA, Bowie EJ. Factor X deficiency in amyloidosis: a critical Review. Am J Hematol 1981;11:443–450.

454. Galbraith PA, Sharma N, Parker WL et al. Acquired factor X deficiency. Altered plasma antithrombin activity and associations with amyloidosis. JAMA 1974;230:1658–1660.

455. Bernhart B, Valletta M, Brook J et al. Amyloidosis with factor X deficiency. Am J Med Sci 1972;264:411–414.

456. Barth WF, Willerson JT, Waldmann TA et al. Primary amyloidosis. Clinical, immunochemical and immunoglobulin metabolism. Studies in fifteen individuals. Am J Med 1969;47:259–273.

457. Pechet L, Kastrul JJ. Amyloidosis associated with factor X (Stuart) deficiency. Ann Intern Med 1964;61:315–318.

458. Howell M. Acquired factor X deficiency associated with systematized amyloidosis—a report of a case. Blood 1963;21:739–744.

459. Korsan-Bengtsen K, Hjort F, Ygge J. Acquired factor X deficiency in a individual with amyloidosis. Thromb Diath Haemorrh 1962;7:558–566.

460. Lucas FV, Fishleder AJ, Becker RC et al. Acquired factor X deficiency in systemic amyloidosis. Cleve Clin J Med 1987;54:399–406.

461. Fair DS, Edgington TS. Heterogeneity of hereditary and acquired factor X deficiencies by combined immunochemical and functional analyses. Br J Haematol 1985;59:235–248.

462. Triplett DA, Bang NU, Harms CS et al. Mechanism of acquired factor X deficiency in primary amyloidosis [Abstract]. Blood 1977;50(Suppl):285.

463. Spero JA, Lewis JH, Hasiba U et al. Treatment of amyloidosis associated factor X deficiency. Thromb Haemost 1976;35:377–381.

464. Rosenstein ED, Itzkowitz SH, Penziner AS et al. Resolution of factor X deficiency in primary amyloidosis following splenectomy. Arch Intern Med 1983;143:597–599.

465. Camoriano JK, Greipp PR, Bayer GK et al. Resolution of acquired factor X deficiency and amyloidosis with melphalan and prednisone therapy. N Engl J Med 1987;316:1133–1135.

466. Beardell FV, Varma M, Martinez J. Normalization of plasma factor X levels in amyloidosis after plasma exchange. Am J Hematol 1997;54:68–71.

467. Moroi M, Aoki N. Isolation and characterization of α2-plasmin inhibitor from human plasma. A novel proteinase inhibitor which inhibits activation induced clot lysis. J Biol Chem 1976;251:5956–5965.

468. Aoki N. α2-Plasmin inhibitor. In: High KA, Roberts HR, eds. Molecular basis of thrombosis and hemostasis. New York: Marcel Dekker, 1995:545–560.

469. Kluft C, Nieukienhuis HK, Rijken DC et al. Alpha2A-antiplasmin Enschede: dysfunctional α2-antiplasmin molecule associated with an autosomal recessive hemorrhagic disorder. J Clin Invest 1987;80:1391–1400.

470. Collen D, Lijnen HR. Molecular basis of fibrinolysis, as relevant for thrombolytic therapy. Thromb Haemost 1995;74:167–171.

471. Kato A, Hirosawa S, Toyota S et al. Localization of the human α2-plasmin inhibitor gene (PLI) to 17p13. Cytogenet Cell Genet 1993;62:190–191.

472. Toyota S, Hirosawa S, Aoki N. Secretion of α2-plasmin inhibitor is impaired by amino acid deletion in a small region of the molecule. J Biochem 1994;115:293–297.

473. Koie E, Kamiya T, Ogata K et al. α2-Plasmin-inhibitor deficiency (Miyasato disease). Lancet 1978;ii:1334–1336.

474. Aoki N, Saito H, Kamiya T et al. Congenital deficiency of α2-plasmin inhibitor associated with severe hemorrhagic tendency. J Clin Invest 1979;63:877–884.

475. Kluft C, Vellenga E, Brommer EJ. Homozygous α2-antiplasmin deficiency [Letter]. Lancet 1979;ii:206.

476. Saito H. Alpha2-plasmin inhibitor and its deficiency states. J Lab Clin Med 1988;112:671–678.

477. Kordich L, Feldman L, Porterie P et al. Severe hemorrhagic tendency in heterozygous α2-antiplasmin deficiency. Thromb Res 1985;40:645–651.

478. Lijnen HR, Collen D. Congenital and acquired deficiencies of components of the fibrinolytic system and their relation to bleeding or thrombosis. Fibrinolysis 1989;3:67–76.

479. Collen D, Bounameaux H, De Cock F et al. Analysis of coagulation and fibrinolysis during intravenous infusion of recombinant human tissue-type plasminogen activator in individuals with acute myocardial infarction. Circulation 1986;73:511–517.

480. Wiman B, Lijnen HR, Collen D. On the specific interaction between the lysine-binding sites in plasmin and complementary sites in α2-antiplasmin and in fibrinogen. Biochem Biophys Acta 1979;579:142–154.

481. Owen MC, Brennan SO, Lewis JH et al. Mutation of antitrypsin to antithrombin: α1-antitrypsin Pittsburgh (358 Met leads to Arg), a fatal bleeding disorder. N Engl J Med 1983;309:694–698.

482. Vidaud D, Emmerich J, Alhenc-Gelas M et al. Met 358 to Arg mutation of alpha1-antitrypsin associated with protein C deficiency in a individual with mild bleeding tendency. J Clin Invest 1992;89:1537–1543.

483. Lewis JH, Iammarino RM, Spero JA et al. Antithrombin Pittsburgh: an α1-antitrypsin variant causing hemorrhagic disease. Blood 1978;51:129–137.

484. Emmerich J, Alhenc-Gelas M, Gandrille S et al. Mechanism of protein C deficiency in a individual with arginine 358 α1-antitrypsin (Pittsburgh mutation): role in the maintenance of hemostatic balance. J Lab Clin Med 1995;125:531–539.

485. Scott CF, Schapira M, James HL et al. Inactivation of factor XIa by plasma protease inhibitors: predominant role of α1-protease inhibitor and protective effect of high molecular weight kininogen. J Clin Invest 1982;69:844–852.

486. Heeb MJ, Bischoff R, Courtney M et al. Inhibition of activated protein C by recombinant α1-antitrypsin variants with substitution of arginine or leucine for methionine-358. J Biol Chem 1990;265:2365–2369.

487. Scott CF, Carrell RW, Glaser CB et al. Alpha-1-antitrypsin-Pittsburgh. A potent inhibitor of human plasma factor XIa, kallikrein, and factor XIIf. J Clin Invest 1986;77:631–634.

488. Schapira M, Ramus MA, Jallat S et al. Recombinant α1-antitrypsin Pittsburgh (Met-358 → Arg) is a potent inhibitor of plasma kallikrein and activated factor XII fragment. J Clin Invest 1986;77:635–637.

# CHAPTER 37

# FACTOR VIII AND OTHER COAGULATION FACTOR INHIBITORS

David Green

Although infrequently encountered, coagulation inhibitors (i.e., circulating anticoagulants) cause considerable morbidity and mortality. They may be paraproteins secreted by myeloma cells, heparinlike proteoglycans liberated during hemodialysis, or, most often, antibodies directed against specific clotting factors.

There are three types of antibodies: alloantibodies, autoantibodies, and xenoantibodies. Alloantibodies that arise in patients with congenital factor deficiencies who are treated with native or recombinant proteins are most common. They are distinct from the autoantibodies that appear spontaneously in persons without inherited coagulopathies. Xenoantibodies develop in patients exposed to clotting factors of animal origin, such as porcine factor (F) VIII or the bovine F V and thrombin used in preparing fibrin glue.

Autoantibodies are the main focus of this chapter. They are suspected when there is unexplained bleeding or abnormal coagulation tests, and there may be a history of an autoimmune disease such as systemic lupus erythematosus (SLE). There also may be a history of malignancy (usually lymphoma or myeloma) or exposure to drugs such as penicillin (F VIII and F XIII inhibitors), streptomycin or gentamicin (F V inhibitor), and isoniazid (F XIII inhibitor). Some antibodies are noted immediately postpartum (F VIII and F IX inhibitors). Most, however, occur in elderly persons of either sex, and most are idiopathic. Laboratory tests demonstrate depressed levels of one or more clotting factors depending on the assay used. Diluting the patient's plasma results in higher rather than lower clotting factor levels, thus suggesting an inhibitor is being weakened by dilution. The diagnosis is confirmed when the addition of patient plasma, serum, or immunoglobulin prolongs the clotting time of normal plasma.

Autoantibodies complicating SLE, malignancy, or drugs have remitted with effective management of the associated disorder. Some that are idiopathic in origin may disappear spontaneously, whereas others may persist for years and lead to the patient's demise. Because the risk of bleeding is unpredictable, efforts to eliminate the antibody are usually warranted. In some patients, drugs such as prednisone, cyclophosphamide, and cyclosporine have been effective. In others, neutralizing the antibody with clotting factor concentrate, binding it to anti-idiotypic antibodies, or removing it with plasmapheresis or immunoadsorption may tide the patient over a major hemorrhage or provide adequate surgical hemostasis.

Of all clotting inhibitors, those that inactivate F VIII are most common (Fig. 37.1). Therefore, most of this chapter discusses F VIII inhibitors. For the other inhibitors, brief descriptions of clinical presentation, diagnostic approaches, and therapeutic considerations are provided. Inhibitors in patients with lupus anticoagulant are discussed in Chapter 38.

## FACTOR VIII INHIBITORS IN PATIENTS WITHOUT HEMOPHILIA

### INCIDENCE

In those without hemophilia, F VIII inhibitors are detected infrequently; the incidence is approximately one in a million (1). Both sexes are affected equally, usually

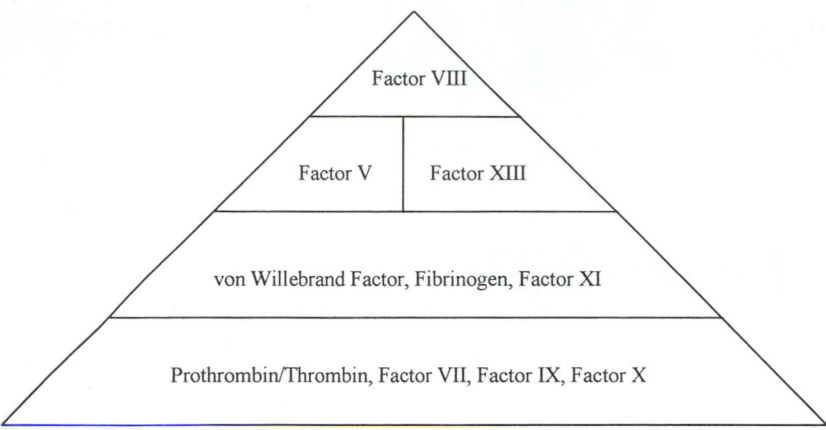

**FIGURE 37.1.** Hierarchy of clotting factor inhibitors based on prevalence.

after the fifth decade of life (2, 3), but there is an association with pregnancy (4). Possibly related disorders in other patients are SLE, rheumatoid arthritis, asthma, allergic reactions to medications, and solid tumors. Some associations may be coincidental, however, because many of these conditions are common in the elderly population.

## IMMUNOLOGY

The F VIII inhibitors are autoantibodies and almost always immunoglobulin G (IgG) molecules. Most are $IgG_1$ and $IgG_4$ (5), of kappa or mixed light chain specificity, and they do not bind complement. They are usually directed against the $A_2$ domain (on the heavy chain), $C_2$ domain (on the light chain), or both, of the F VIII molecule. Those reacting with the $C_2$ domain may interfere with binding of F VIII to phosphatidylserine (6), von Willebrand factor (7), or both. Scandella et al (8) showed that inhibitors binding to amino acids 2303 through 2332 of the $C_2$ domain inhibit binding of F VIII to synthetic phospholipid membranes. They suggest that the anticoagulant activity of these inhibitors results from their interference with the membrane binding of activated F VIII, which is required for its integration into the developing tenase complex (see Chapter 1). Inhibitors binding to the $A_2$ domain may prevent activation of F X by the tenase complex.

More detailed epitope localization studies have also been reported by Scandella et al (9). They compared 28 alloantibody and autoantibody inhibitors using immunoblotting and immunoprecipitation assays, and they examined the ability of the $A_2$ and $C_2$ domains to neutralize the functional activity of inhibitors in the Bethesda assay. Immunoblotting studies of 15 autoantibodies revealed binding to the $A_2$ domain by six, the $C_2$ domain by eight, and both domains by one. When examined using immunoprecipitation methods, two bound to the $A_2$ domain, four to the $C_2$ domain, and nine to both. Thus, with the more sensitive immunopre-

cipitation assay, 60% of patients had multiple F VIII antibodies. Neutralization studies, however, showed that only one fragment was usually required to neutralize inhibitor activity. Thus, many antibodies are directed toward nonfunctional regions of the F VIII molecule. Furthermore, levels of antibody varied widely among inhibitor plasmas, with a 10,000-fold range of anti-light chain antibody concentration detected using a quantitative immunoprecipitation assay. Similar results were obtained for alloantibodies. Both Scandella et al (9) and Fulcher et al (10) noted that the epitope specificities of any given inhibitor plasma can change over time and probably relates to patient exposure to various clotting factor concentrates.

## CLINICAL MANIFESTATIONS

The most common presenting complaint is bleeding into the skin or muscles (Table 37.1). During the course of the illness, however, bleeding may occur at any site. Many patients have mucous membrane bleeding, and there may be recurrent, recalcitrant epistaxis or persistent bleeding after dental procedures. Others have melena or hematochezia and become weak from blood-loss anemia. Because F VIII inhibitors develop in mostly elderly persons, many of whom have a history of cardiac disease, this anemia may provoke angina or signs of heart failure. In addition, some patients have persistent hematuria, especially if they also have bladder infections or prostate disease.

Enlarging muscle hematomas of the arm or leg occur after trivial trauma. These hematomas may produce a compartment syndrome, with nerve compression or compromise of the blood supply to the hand or foot. Hemarthroses are less common in patients with acquired inhibitors than in patients with hemophilia, but they do occur. The affected joints are warm, swollen, tender, and have a restricted range of motion because of pain.

Persistent vaginal bleeding may be a major problem

**TABLE 37.1.**   Presenting Sites of Bleeding in 46 Patients with F VIII Autoantibodies[a]

| Site | Patients (n [%]) |
|---|---|
| Muscle | 20 (44) |
| Skin | 6 (13) |
| Genitourinary tract | 4 (9) |
| Gastrointestinal tract | 4 (9) |
| Joint | 3 (6) |
| Surgical wound | 3 (6) |
| Oropharynx and hypopharynx | 2 (4) |
| Other | 4 (9) |
|    Subconjunctival | |
|    Nose | |
|    Periodontal | |
|    Pleural | |
| Total | 46 (100) |

*Reprinted with permission from Green D. Inhibitors of factor VIII in non-hemophiliacs. In: Green D, ed. Anticoagulants, physiologic, pathologic, and pharmacologic. Boca Raton: CRC Press, 1994: 97–112.*
[a] *Data from Nilsson et al (42) and Uehlinger et al (43).*

in postpartum patients. In others, persistent bleeding from trauma or surgical wounds may defy attempts at local hemostasis. Retroperitoneal hemorrhages may be massive and may result in death from blood loss. Intracranial bleeding is infrequent but devastating. Overall, major bleeding occurs in more than 80% of patients, and approximately 20% die, either directly or indirectly from the autoantibody and its effects (2).

Because the presence of an F VIII inhibitor is rare and the diagnosis often unsuspected, iatrogenic bleeding is common. Major bleeding may be encountered after minor procedures, such as placement of a venous catheter or pacemaker. In patients with compartment syndromes, difficulty in controlling oozing from the fasciotomy wound may complicate surgery to relieve neurovascular compression. Needle aspiration of hemarthroses may be associated with persistent bleeding from the puncture wound, and joint infection may supervene. In summary, an F VIII inhibitor should be strongly considered in elderly patients with spontaneous hemorrhages or bleeding after relatively minor trauma, and invasive procedures should be withheld until basic laboratory tests of hemostasis (discussed later) have been performed.

## DIAGNOSIS

Table 37.2 presents an algorithm for diagnosis. The hallmark of antibodies directed against F VIII is a prolonged partial thromboplastin time (PTT), with no effect on the

**TABLE 37.2.**   Algorithm for Diagnosis of F VIII Inhibitors

1. *Obtain activated PTT and prothrombin time*
   PTT is prolonged; prothrombin time is normal.
2. *Exclude heparin as cause for prolonged PTT*
   Treat plasma with enzyme or resin to remove heparin and repeat PTT; should still be prolonged.
3. *Demonstrate presence of anticoagulant*
   Mix equal volumes of patient plasma with normal plasma; include citrate–saline control; test immediately and after 60 minutes of incubation at 37°C. PTT of the mixture should be >4 seconds longer than the PTT of the control—if not initially, then always at 60 min.
4. *Differentiate from lupus anticoagulant*
   Add freeze-thawed platelets or diluted thromboplastin to the mixture, and repeat the PTT. (Note: patient plasma must be platelet-free, either filtered or double-spun.) Minimal correction of the PTT of the mixture is observed.
5. *Document low F VIII level*
   Perform F VIII assay. Both one-stage and two-stage assays will give low values; if lupus anticoagulant is present, two-stage assay will be normal.
6. *Quantitate strength of inhibitor*
   Perform Bethesda assay using the Nijmegen modification. With appropriate dilutions, the inhibitor titer can be reasonably approximated.

prothrombin time. This pattern also typifies patients with hemophilia, von Willebrand disease, or deficiencies of contact activation factors. However, these disorders may be distinguished from F VIII inhibitors by mixing tests (see Chapter 26). In patients with deficiencies, addition of normal plasma corrects the PTT, but when normal plasma is mixed with plasma containing an inhibitor, the PTT is prolonged. Testing should be performed immediately after mixing and also after incubation at 37°C for 1 hour. This allows weak inhibitors that require time for F VIII inactivation to be recognized. Contamination of the sample with heparin may prolong the PTT and affect mixing tests; if so, it can be removed from the sample with enzyme or resin absorption and the plasma retested.

The mixing test provides suggestive evidence for an F VIII inhibitor, but the Bethesda assay (see Chapter 26) establishes the diagnosis and provides important quantitative information (11). Dilutions of patient plasma are incubated with normal pooled plasma for 2 hours at 37°C, then the residual F VIII in the pooled plasma is measured. One Bethesda Unit (B.U.) is defined as the reciprocal of the patient plasma dilution yielding 50% residual F VIII activity in the test system.

The Bethesda method presumes a linear relationship between the plasma dilution and residual F VIII activity; in other words, the greater the dilution, the more residual F VIII activity. This is true for F VIII inhibitors in patients with hemophilia, but the relationship is nonlinear with most autoantibodies from patients without hemophilia. Their plasma must be considerably diluted before residual F VIII climbs above baseline levels (12). Thus, the Bethesda assay tends to underestimate the ability of nonhemophilic antibodies to inactivate F VIII. The clinical consequences are that substantially more F VIII must be infused to obtain hemostatic levels of the clotting factor.

The interested reader is referred to Kessler (13), White (14), and Chapter 26 for further discussion of the Bethesda assay and other quantitative methods for studying F VIII autoantibodies. A recent innovation has been use of buffered rather than unbuffered normal plasma for incubation with patient plasma and replacing buffer with immunodepleted F VIII plasma in the control mixture (i.e., Nijmegen modification) (15).

## TREATMENT

### Acute Bleeding

Table 37.3 presents an algorithm for treatment of bleeding in patients with F VIII inhibitors. Typically, the clinician is confronted by persistent bleeding in an elderly patient. The PTT is prolonged, the prothrombin time is normal, and mixing studies are consistent with presence of a clotting inhibitor. It may be possible to obtain an F VIII assay in some centers, but a Bethesda assay probably will not be available. Therefore, treatment decisions usually are influenced by the severity of bleeding. If hemorrhage is mild to moderate, desmopressin (DDAVP), 0.3 µg/kg body weight in 50 mL of saline, is given intravenously over 20 minutes. Peak F VIII levels are anticipated 45 to 90 minutes after the dose, which may be repeated every 24 hours. Anecdotal evidence suggests DDAVP raises F VIII levels in patients with low-titer inhibitors and controls bleeding (16, 17). Adverse reactions are infrequent, especially if dosing is limited to once every 24 hours (18, 19).

For more serious bleeding, porcine F VIII (Hyate-CR) should be administered. Most inhibitors cross-react with porcine F VIII in much lower titer (10–20% lower) than with human F VIII (20). Viral-transmissible diseases have not been reported with the porcine product, and large clinical trials have shown it to be safe and effective (3, 21, 22). The dose is 50–100 U/kg repeated every 8-12 hrs or 4 U/kg/hr given by continuous infusion (23). Morrison et al (24) examined use of porcine F VIII for 74 bleeding episodes in 65 patients with acquired inhibitors. They found that initial inhibitor titers to human F VIII ranged from 1.2 to 1024.0 B.U., but titers

**TABLE 37.3.** Algorithm for Treatment of Bleeding in Patients with F VIII Inhibitors

1. If bleeding is not life- or limb-threatening, give DDAVP, 0.3 µg/kg IV. Measure PTT or F VIII after 60 minutes. Clinical response or F VIII increased >25%; may repeat DDAVP every 24 hrs as necessary.

2. If no response, give human F VIII if bleeding is not life- or limb-threatening; otherwise, give porcine F VIII. Begin with bolus of 50–100 U/kg and follow with a continuous infusion (human, 10 U/kg/hr; porcine, 4 U/kg/hr). Monitor with clinical response, PTT, or F VIII level. (Note: always have porcine F VIII in reserve should patient become refractory to human F VIII.)

3. If no response, increase dose of porcine F VIII (bolus, 100–200 U/kg; continuous infusion, 10 U/kg/hr). Adverse reactions more likely with higher dose; check for platelet clumping on peripheral blood films.

4. If no response, give prothrombin complex concentrate, 50–75 U/kg every 8–12 hours. Avoid use in postoperative or septic patients potentially at risk for thrombosis.

5. In patients continuing to bleed despite these measures, attempt to obtain:
   a. rFVIIa. Give in doses of 90 µg/kg every 2–3 hours until clinical improvement.
   b. Plasmapheresis or extracorporeal immunoadsorbtion, accompanied by infusions of porcine or human F VIII. (Requires placement of large bore catheter, with potential for bleeding and infection.)

6. All patients should be given prednisone, 1 mg/kg, for at least 3 weeks. Monitor F VIII and inhibitor levels.

7. Also recommended is at least one course of IVIg, 1 g/kg daily for 2 days. Monitor F VIII and inhibitor levels.

*Adapted with permission from Suggestions for the Management of Hemophiliacs and Non-Hemophiliacs with Factor VIII Inhibitors. Prepared by the Subcommittee on Coagulation Factor Inhibitor Development for the Association of Hemophilia Centre Directors of Canada, July 1995.*

of only 0 to 15 B.U. were recorded to porcine F VIII. The mean initial dose was 84 U/kg, and good or excellent objective clinical responses were observed in 78%. Adverse reactions were infrequent but included one episode of anaphylaxis, which was nonfatal. Other adverse effects, such as rigors and back pain, are more common. A recent survey reported the incidence rate of these reactions as 10 per 1000 infusions in patients receiving less than 100 U/kg and 82 per 1000 infusions in those receiving higher doses (25). Another side effect noted with porcine F VIII is thrombocytopenia (21, 26), which appears to be a pseudothrombocytopenia resulting from platelet aggregation *ex vivo* (27).

Refractoriness to porcine F VIII also may occur and be detected by a modified Bethesda assay using Hyate-CR diluted to 1 U/mL activity when compared with a human plasma F VIII standard (28). In the study of Morrison et al (24), poor or no response was observed in 22% of patients. This lack of response could not be predicted by the pretreatment inhibitor titer to porcine F VIII. Following administration of either human or porcine F VIII, inhibitor titers may rise over several days, and complete refractoriness to these concentrates is evident. Following exposure to porcine F VIII, Hay et al (25) noted anamnestic (i.e., recall) inhibitor responses in 60% of patients; interestingly, 38% had no such responses despite receiving multiple courses of therapy.

When there is time to wait for Bethesda assay results, therapy is based on the inhibitor titer. If the titer is less than 5 B.U., human F VIII should be administered, beginning with a bolus of 100 U/kg and followed by a continuous infusion of 10 U/kg/hr until bleeding is controlled or it is clear the treatment is ineffective. Continuous infusion appears to be more efficient for maintaining hemostatic blood levels of F VIII (29). Blood samples should be obtained 4 to 6 hours after initiating therapy to ascertain that plasma concentrations of greater than 0.25 U/ml are being achieved. Persistence of bleeding, poor recovery of F VIII, or both suggests either the potency of the inhibitor has been underestimated by the Bethesda assay (discussed earlier) or the F VIII in the concentrate is unduly susceptible to inactivation by the inhibitor. F VIII in concentrates with high levels of von Willebrand factor (i.e., intermediate purity concentrates) may be protected from inactivation by certain inhibitors (30), which appear to be those that bind specifically to the $C_2$ domain of F VIII (31). Therefore, treatment should be switched to such human F VIII concentrates or porcine F VIII.

If bleeding is not controlled by F VIII concentrates, there are two alternatives: recombinant F VIIa (rFVIIa), and prothrombin complex concentrate. The first, rFVIIa, offers several potential advantages (32). It is mainly effective at initiating clot formation when complexed with tissue factor (33), whereas prothrombin complex concentrate is exposed at the site of injury (i.e., bleeding). Thus, it acts locally and should have minimal systemic thrombogenicity. Its hemostatic effectiveness also is independent of F VIII and, therefore, should not be affected by F VIII inhibitors. It is not prepared from blood, so the risk of transmitting infectious agents is low. Clinical experience with rFVIIa has been summarized by Glazer et al (34) and included 1270 bleeding episodes in 240 patients, 18 of which were patients without hemo-

philia and with inhibitors. Effective responses were reported in 74 to 100% of patients, depending on type of bleed; for critical bleeds, the effective response rate was 91%. Adverse effects were infrequent, with hypertension, skin reactions, fever, headache, and epistaxis reported. Only two transient cardiovascular events occurred, however, and the frequency of serious events was only 0.8% overall (35). The recommended dose of rFVIIa is an intravenous bolus injection of 90 µg/kg. Because the half-life of rFVIIa is only 2.9 hrs, injections must be given at 2 to 3 hour intervals for 1 to 2 days or until clinical improvement is apparent. At this writing, rFVIIa is still under evaluation by the U.S. Food and Drug Administration (FDA), but it is available from Novo Nordisk (Princeton, NJ) for compassionate use if other, currently approved measures have failed.

Prothrombin complex concentrates are approved by the FDA for use in patients with F VIII inhibitors. Two activated products are available: Autoplex, at 50 U/kg; or FEIBA, at 50–75 U/kg. Doses are repeated every 8 to 12 hours. Bleeding is controlled in many patients with these doses, but others require more intensive therapy (36). Escalated doses, however, carry a major risk of thrombosis (37). Events such as myocardial infarction and disseminated intravascular coagulation are more frequent in patients given repeated, high doses. These should be avoided in patients prone to thrombosis because of major surgery, crush injuries, or large muscle hemorrhages. Furthermore, antifibrinolytic agents should not be given while patients are receiving prothrombin complex concentrates. These products are prepared from human blood and, therefore, have the potential to transmit infectious agents. The viral inactivation processes used, however, have effectively prevented infection with human immunodeficiency and hepatitis B and C viruses. Other adverse reactions, such as hives, pruritus, and fever, are uncommon.

Efforts to remove inhibitors should also be considered. Given intravenously, immune globulin (IVIg) has induced dramatically decreased inhibitor titers in some patients (38, 39). In a multicenter trial, two of 19 patients had a rapid decline in inhibitor titers, and four others had more gradual responses over several months (40). Adverse reactions were infrequent (11%) and mild, including headache, aching, dizziness, itching, and wheezing. Doses given were either 1 g/kg daily for 2 days or 0.4 g/kg daily for 5 days. The mechanism of effect has been studied and attributed to anti-idiotypic antibodies in the pools of normal immunoglobulin used to prepare the IVIg (41). These anti-idiotypic antibodies are directed against the patient's autoantibody. Targeted anti-idiotypic antibodies are not yet clinically available, and outcomes with current preparations of IVIg are largely unpredictable.

Other options include plasmapheresis or immunoadsorption. Simple plasma exchange usually is ineffective because of large extravascular antibody reservoirs. Immunoadsorption entails use of extracorporeal columns containing Sepharose coupled to immunoglobulin-adsorbing proteins. Protein A–Sepharose has been used in the past (42, 43), but polyclonal sheep antibodies to human immunoglobulin coupled to Sepharose have been investigated more recently (44). In three patients with antibody titers of 29, 132, and 313 B.U., the average titer reduction was 76% during a 4 hour session. After four sessions, antibody titers were less than 1 B.U. in all three subjects. No adverse effects were noted. Thus, a few strategically located centers equipped with this technology could offer this potentially life-saving treatment to all bleeding patients with high titer inhibitors.

A general principle in the treatment of patients with F VIII inhibitors is to avoid trauma, particularly invasive procedures such as catheter insertion, intramuscular injections, and vigorous physical therapy. Occasionally, however, surgery cannot be deferred. Prevention of bleeding under these circumstances requires knowledge of the patient's inhibitor titer and previous response to therapeutic concentrates. Perioperative bleeding may be controlled by plasma exchange and bolus doses of concentrates, but delayed bleeding from wounds is common, persistent, and usually serious. Such bleeding generally becomes apparent 7 to 14 days after surgery, when inhibitor titers to human or porcine F VIII have increased substantially. As indicated, giving a prothrombin complex concentrate in this setting may lead to intravascular coagulation and organ infarction. A better choice is rFVIIa, which has been effective in 81% of major surgical procedures and had few adverse effects (32).

## Long-term Treatment

The factors responsible for the development of autoantibodies are unknown, and in approximately one-third of cases, the antibodies will spontaneously disappear (45). Loss of the antibody may take months or years, however, during which the patient is at risk for serious hemorrhage and may be denied important procedures such as cataract extraction and transurethral resection for prostatic hypertrophy. Therefore, measures to eliminate the autoantibody should be initiated as early as possible.

When the diagnosis of an inhibitor is confirmed, prednisone, 1 mg/kg orally, should be administered. A satisfactory response is a decline in inhibitor titer in 3 weeks to less than 50% of the initial value. If this occurs, prednisone should be continued until the inhibitor disappears and normal levels of F VIII reappear. This result was observed in one-third of patients in a prospective, randomized, multi-institutional clinical trial (46). Patients who responded to treatment had significantly lower inhibitor titers than patients who did not respond (3 B.U. versus 50 B.U., respectively) and higher baseline

levels of F VIII (9% versus 1%). In the two-thirds with persistence of the inhibitor, there are several choices:

1. Stop prednisone and give cyclophosphamide, 2 mg/kg orally, for 3 to 6 weeks;
2. Continue prednisone and add cyclophosphamide;
3. Give bolus doses of F VIII concurrently with intravenous cyclophosphamide (47, 48); or
4. Use combination chemotherapy with prednisone, intravenous cyclophosphamide, and intravenous vincristine (49).

These regimens each have their champions. The last is more toxic, however, and is reserved for patients with more recalcitrant antibodies.

Should antibodies persist, another option is cyclosporine. Patients refractory to other regimens have responded to this agent given in doses up to 5 mg/kg/day to achieve plasma levels ranging from 150 to 350 ng/ml (50). Careful monitoring of creatinine clearance is essential when using this drug.

Inhibitors that appear postpartum are an important subset of the F VIII autoantibody problem. These inhibitors may arise because of differences in the F VIII of the patient, father, and newborn, but polymorphisms of the F VIII gene have not been reported in this setting (51). A recent review of 51 published cases indicated these inhibitors are most commonly associated with first pregnancies, provoke vaginal or other bleeding immediately postpartum, and tend not to recur with subsequent pregnancies (52). Almost all cases resolve within 30 months. While steroid treatment was found to be unhelpful, other immunosuppressive drugs such as cyclophosphamide were noted to shorten the time to complete remission.

# FACTOR VIII INHIBITORS IN PATIENTS WITH HEMOPHILIA

## INCIDENCE

Much has been learned about the incidence of F VIII antibodies in patients with hemophilia and the factors predisposing to inhibitor development in them. This is largely because of randomized, controlled clinical trials of clotting factor preparations, often given to previously untreated patients. Approximately 25% of patients exposed to exogenous F VIII develop antibodies, usually after a median of 9 exposure-days (53, 54). These studies have been performed using recombinant F VIII, but similar results have been shown with F VIII derived from plasma (55). Briet et al (56) performed a meta-analysis of eight trials involving crude or intermediate-purity F VIII given to 451 patients. The cumulative incidence of high titer inhibitors was 20% by 18 years of age; however, these figures probably underestimate the true incidence of antibody formation for two reasons. First, the inhibitors in some patients may be transient. Second, the antibodies may be directed toward nonfunctional determinants of the F VIII molecule, so they are clinically inapparent (57, 58).

Development of an antibody in a particular patient is governed by several factors, including type of mutation responsible for the hemophilia, characteristics of the exogenous F VIII used for treatment, number of exposure-days, and perhaps other, as yet unrecognized factors. Regarding genetic factors, one analysis of 364 mutations showed stop mutations, large deletions, and intrachromosomal recombinations in over 90% of patients with inhibitors, whereas missense mutations and small deletions were found in less than 10% (59). Thus, inhibitors more often occur in families with more extensive alterations in the F VIII gene.

The frequency of inhibitor development is similar for most concentrates, including those produced by recombinant technology, but a few preparations have a clearly associated, increased inhibitor risk. One specific concentrate (Factor VIII-P or CPS-P), which is pasteurized in the fluid phase, has induced an approximately fivefold increase in patients expected to develop inhibitors (60, 61). Another (Bisinact), which was subject to solvent-detergent and pasteurization at 63°C for 10 hours, resulted in development of inhibitor in eight of 140 previously responsive, multitransfused patients (62). Reasons for the antigenicity of these preparations are unclear. Barrowcliffe et al (63), however, found a small amount of activated F VIII in CPS-P, which might indicate some of the factor had undergone limited proteolysis.

## CLINICAL MANIFESTATIONS

Development of F VIII inhibitors in patients with severe hemophilia is insidious. There may be no increase in the frequency or severity of bleeding, but specific inquiry may elicit the information that larger or more frequent doses of clotting factor are required to manage the patient's usual bleeding episodes. Often, however, the antibody is first recognized during an invasive procedure, when the patient bleeds excessively despite previously adequate clotting factor therapy. The relatively rare development of an inhibitor in patients with previously mild to moderate hemophilia may result in more frequent bleeds or in hemorrhages into joints formerly free of disease.

## DIAGNOSIS

Because formation of F VIII antibodies is often insidious, most hemophilia centers recommend annual testing for the presence of inhibitors. In addition, it is prudent to check for an inhibitor before invasive procedures such as joint aspiration or surgery. The Bethesda assay (11, 15), as previously described, is the method used most often for detecting and quantifying inhibitors.

## TREATMENT

Treatment of hemorrhage is influenced by the titer of F VIII inhibitor. Patients with less than 5 B.U. usually respond well to bolus doses of 50 to 100 U/kg of human or porcine F VIII concentrate, whereas those with higher titers may be completely refractory to such concentrates. After exposure to F VIII, most patients experience an anamnestic rise in their antibody titer to more than 10 B.U. and, within a week, become totally resistant to F VIII. These patients are designated as "high responders." Those designated as "low responders" demonstrate little rise in their inhibitor titers and remain responsive to F VIII (64). The decision to expose high responder patients to F VIII must be carefully considered, because once titers become elevated, they may remain high for many months. During this period, treatment of bleeding episodes is often unsatisfactory.

To retain responsiveness to F VIII, methods for inducing immune tolerance have been developed (65, 66). These are best applied as soon as inhibitors are detected and while titers are still low (67). Various regimens have been used, but daily F VIII doses of 100 U/kg are most effective. Doses of less than 50 U/kg/day, however, have been successful in some series as well (68). In patients with high titer inhibitors, reduction of the titer is attempted using combinations of serial plasmapheresis, immune adsorption, cyclophosphamide, and IVIg along with bolus or continuous infusions of F VIII (69). Following the development of immune tolerance, many patients continue receiving F VIII on an every-other-day schedule.

Restoring responsiveness to F VIII in patients with inhibitors is a worthy objective, but inducing immune tolerance requires long-term, intravenous access and considerable amounts of F VIII concentrate. Immune tolerance is best reserved for those who meet the following criteria:

1. High responder,
2. Recently detected inhibitor,
3. Adequate venous access,
4. Cooperative family, and
5. Sufficient supply of F VIII concentrate.

This profile best fits young children who develop an inhibitor after one of their first exposures to F VIII. Algorithms for inhibitor management and tolerance induction are presented in detail in a manual prepared by the Subcommittee on Coagulation Factor Inhibitor Development for the Association of Hemophilia Centre

Directors of Canada (available from Dr Georges Rivard, Hopital Ste-Justine, 3175 Cote Ste Catherine, Montreal, Quebec H3T 1C5, Canada).

For patients refractory to human and porcine F VIII, hemorrhagic events may be treated with prothrombin complex concentrates (70). Clinical trials have found response rates of up to 60% for hemarthroses, and other types of bleeding also may be amenable to this therapy. Doses range from 50 to 75 U/kg and are given at 8- to 12-hour intervals, depending on the severity of bleeding (71). These concentrates are not generally used for patients undergoing elective surgery because their effectiveness is unpredictable. As noted, frequent dosing may be associated with myocardial infarction and other evidence of thrombogenicity.

As described, rFVIIa offers a safe and effective therapy for patients with inhibitors. Clinical trials and anecdotal experience have documented control of hemarthroses and bleeding after trauma (34), and adverse effects have been infrequent (35). Available in Canada, rFVIIa has not yet received FDA approval at this writing.

Prednisone and antifibrinolytic agents are useful adjuncts in treatment of patients with inhibitors. A short, intensive course of corticosteroids, along with an effective dose of clotting factor concentrate, may shorten the duration of pain and swelling accompanying hemarthrosis. Antifibrinolytic agents, again in association with clotting factor concentrate, may decrease bleeding from the mouth or gastrointestinal tract. Chapter 53 discusses these drugs in more detail.

Immunosuppressive agents such as cyclophosphamide or azathioprine are almost always ineffective in decreasing titers of inhibitors in patients with hemophilia, except when used as part of immune tolerance regimens. This is contrary to experience in patients without hemophilia.

# VON WILLEBRAND FACTOR INHIBITORS

Deficiencies of von Willebrand factor may be congenital or acquired (see Chapter 34). Some acquired deficiencies result from autoantibodies, and others are associated with disorders such as hypothyroidism, myeloproliferative disease, congenital heart disease, Wilm's tumor, and glycogen storage disease (72). The autoantibodies may be idiopathic or complicate diseases such as SLE (73) or malignancy (74). In one patient with a lymphoproliferative disorder, the autoantibody bound to the $A_3$ and glycoprotein Ib binding domains of the von Willebrand protein, thus inhibiting adherence to collagen (75).

The diagnosis is made on the basis of a prolonged bleeding time, impaired ristocetin-induced platelet aggregation, and decreased high-molecular-weight mul-

timers of von Willebrand factor. It has been very difficult to develop a functional method to measure autoantibody activity, but an enzyme-linked immunosorbent assay has recently been described (51). Treatment with steroids diminishes or eliminates the autoantibody in some persons; however, in a patient with chronic lymphocytic leukemia, extracorporeal immunoadsorption was required (76).

# FACTOR V INHIBITORS

Rarely, inhibitors to F V develop in persons without congenital F V deficiency. Possible predisposing factors include exposure to aminoglycoside antibiotics (e.g., streptomycin, gentamicin), systemic infections, surgery and transfusions (77, 78), and even celiac disease (79). Similar to F VIII autoantibodies, F V inhibitors are usually polyclonal IgG antibodies, but other types have been reported in the older literature. They may cause bleeding by interfering with critical functions of F V. For example, Ortel et al (80) described an inhibitor that prevented prothrombinase formation by interfering with binding of the $C_2$ domain of F V to procoagulant phospholipids. These investigators subsequently examined 11 other F V inhibitors (six autoantibodies and five in patients exposed to bovine F V) (81). All 11 bound to the light chain of F V, and seven of eight inhibitors that were associated with clinical bleeding bound specifically to the amino terminal third of the $C_2$ domain of F V.

The diagnosis is suspected on the basis of a prolonged PTT and prothrombin time that does not correct with the addition of normal plasma. Low levels of F V may be observed with lupus anticoagulants and with specific F V inhibitors. The levels of other clotting factors will be normal in the latter, however, and the platelet neutralization test will be negative. Bleeding in patients with F V autoantibodies ranges from trivial to life-threatening. If treatment is required (e.g., preoperatively), platelet transfusions may be effective because platelet F V is sheltered from circulating F V antibodies (82, 83).

Fibrin glue is a mixture of cryoprecipitated autologous or homologous plasma, calcium, and a bovine thrombin preparation used to enhance local hemostasis during cardiothoracic operations, neurosurgery, or extensive orthopedic procedures (84). The topical thrombin usually employed (Thrombostat; Parke-Davis, Morris Plains, NJ) contains bovine F V as well as thrombin (85). Weeks to months after surgery, patients may have prolonged thrombin times and decreased levels of F V, because antibodies form against the bovine proteins and cross-react with the corresponding human proteins (86, 87). Usually, these antibodies are discovered when preoperative coagulation tests are abnormal, but those directed against F V may be associated with severe bleeding (62). A history of fibrin glue used during recent surgery is the major clue to the diagnosis. Most of these antibodies gradually subside, but plasmapheresis may rapidly reduce antibody titers and restore hemostasis in bleeding patients (62).

# FACTOR VII INHIBITORS

Inhibitors of F VII are extremely rare. A man with this disorder was reported by Campbell et al (88) in 1980. The patient had metastatic carcinoma and positive tests for SLE, and he bruised with venipuncture but had no other bleeding. The PTT was normal and the prothrombin time prolonged; the prolongation increased with incubation. Normal plasma did not correct the prothrombin time when added *in vitro* or after infusion *in vivo*. The level of F VII was 30% of normal. The levels of factors V, IX, and X were normal. Inhibitor neutralization studies indicated that the inhibition of the prothrombin time resulted from an IgG-class antibody.

A second report described a severely affected, 62-year-old man with no associated disorder (89). This patient's F VII level declined to less than 0.01 U/mL, and he experienced an intracranial hemorrhage. Bleeding was eventually controlled with plasma exchange and F VII concentrate. The IgG antibody disappeared coincident with treatment using prednisone and cyclophosphamide.

# FACTOR IX INHIBITORS

Factor IX inhibitors are almost exclusively observed in F IX hemophilia. Of the few reports involving patients without hemophilia, most have had associated autoimmune disease (90) or SLE (91). Similar to cases of F VIII inhibitors, some have occurred postpartum (92, 93). Most that have been studied are polyclonal IgG immunoglobulins, and they may be identified and quantitated using a modified Bethesda assay (94).

In the differential diagnosis of F IX deficiency, one should first consider inherited F IX deficiency or carriership of F IX hemophilia. Acquired causes of low F IX levels are liver disease, vitamin K deficiency, and warfarin therapy; rarely, F IX may be lost through urine in patients with nephrotic syndrome (95, 96). F IX also may be adsorbed to amyloid deposits in patients with myeloma, but most reported cases involve F X (discussed later). Finally, low levels of F IX have been recorded in patients with Gaucher disease, and it has been suggested that cerebroside in the plasma samples alters F IX activity when measured *in vitro* (97). Lack of bleeding in these patients lends support to this theory.

Treatment of patients with autoimmune F IX inhibitors is similar to that for patients with F VIII autoanti-

bodies. It includes use of F IX concentrates to neutralize the antibody, activated prothrombin complex concentrates if the antibody cannot be neutralized, and plasmapheresis or immunoadsorption in particularly refractory cases (98). IVIg and immunosuppressive medications may provide long-term control.

# FACTOR X INHIBITORS

Autoantibodies directed against F X are rare. Lankiewicz and Bell (99) described an 84-year-old woman with extensive skin and gastrointestinal bleeding and a prolonged PTT, prothrombin time, and Russell viper venom time. A modified Bethesda assay showed 5.4 inhibitor units. The anti-F X activity was localized to the patient's IgG fraction, and it was neutralized with antihuman IgG. Bleeding subsided with $\epsilon$-aminocaproic acid therapy. After a few months, the inhibitor spontaneously disappeared.

Another anti-F X IgG inhibitor bound to the light chain of F X, thus preventing F X activation by the VIIa/tissue factor complex, IXa/VIIIa/phospholipid complex, and Russell viper venom (100). Other functions of F Xa were also impaired, such as prothrombin activation, activation of F VII in tissue factor/VII complex, and ability of the tissue factor pathway inhibitor/Xa complex to inhibit the VIIa/tissue factor complex. Bleeding in this patient gradually subsided, and the inhibitor disappeared during a 5-week course of prednisone therapy.

More often, F X deficiency occurs during amyloid disease of the AL variety (101), with lambda VI light chains (102). Bleeding is usually mucosal and responds poorly to infused F X, either in plasma or prothrombin complex concentrates, because F X adsorbs to the amyloid fibrils and quickly disappears from the circulation (103). The PT and PTT are prolonged but may correct with *in vitro* addition of normal plasma. Splenectomy (104), melphalan and prednisone (105), and vincristine-loaded platelets (106) have produced remissions in this disorder.

# FACTOR XI INHIBITORS

A prolonged PTT, low F XI level, and no correction after mixing with normal plasma should raise suspicion of an F XI inhibitor. However, on further investigation platelet neutralization test and dilute Russell Viper Venom test (i.e., the diagnosis of "lupus anticoagulant" usually becomes apparent) (see Chapter 38). As was reported years ago, these "anticoagulants" are associated with thrombosis rather than with bleeding (107). Some patients have had bleeding, however, and may have had true autoantibodies to F XI (108).

Patients with congenital deficiencies of factor XI

who develop antibodies because of transfusion usually experience significant bleeding in association with surgery or trauma (109).

# PROTHROMBIN AND THROMBIN INHIBITORS

Antiprothrombin antibodies can be found in most patients with lupus anticoagulants (110). Those that complex with prothrombin may accelerate clearance of prothrombin (111), but bleeding is unusual and occurs only if the hypoprothrombinemia is severe. On the other hand, inhibitors of thrombin are associated with bleeding. An elderly patient with no evidence of lupus anticoagulant or other underlying illness had a prolonged thrombin time and massive hemorrhage (112), and an IgG antibody that bound to thrombin but not prothrombin was discovered, thus suggesting the antibody was directed to an active site of the thrombin molecule. Binding of the autoantibody to thrombin is reminiscent of the attachment of hirudin to the exosite and catalytic domains of thrombin (113).

Other reported thrombin inhibitors have been heparinlike and discovered in patients with multiple myeloma (114, 115), transitional cell carcinoma of the genitourinary tract (116, 117), during suramin therapy (118), and in patients undergoing hemodialysis (119). Most are negatively charged glycosaminoglycans that prolong the thrombin time but not the reptilase time (120). Mixtures of heparan sulfate, chondroitin sulfate, and dermatan sulfate, as well as abnormal proteoglycans, appear in increased concentrations in the patient plasma. Bleeding is usually mucocutaneous and from venipuncture wounds and other surgical sites. Bleeding may be controlled by infusion of protamine sulfate, which transiently neutralizes the negatively charged anticoagulant molecules.

# INHIBITORS OF FIBRINOGEN–FIBRIN

The conversion of fibrinogen to fibrin is a multistep process involving cleavage of fibrinopeptides, fibrin monomer aggregation and polymerization, and cross linking of the polymer (see Chapter 6). Inhibitors that interfere with this process may act at any point, but most interfere with fibrin monomer aggregation. Such inhibitors are usually macroglobulins arising in patients with multiple myeloma or macroglobulinemia (121–123). Patients tend to have oozing from various sites. The disorder is suspected when *in vitro* clots are bulky and gelatinous, with poor clot retraction, and turbidity measurements reveal these clots are composed of fibers significantly thinner than normal (124). Plasmapheresis is often effec-

tive in lowering immunoglobulin concentration and controlling bleeding until a response to chemotherapy is achieved.

Other reports have described patients with antibodies that delay the release of fibrinopeptide A from the α-chain of fibrinogen (125) or inhibit the association of fibrin monomers (126). All clotting tests are typically prolonged in the presence of these antibodies, and the patient serum or plasma alters the clotting time of normal fibrinogen. When the patient plasma is diluted, the thrombin clotting time shortens, thus showing the dependence of inhibition on the anticoagulant concentration.

# FACTOR XIII INHIBITORS

After activation by thrombin and calcium, F XIII then cross links the γ- and α-chains of fibrin (see Chapter 6). Antibodies may interfere with F XIII activation or fibrin cross linking. Bleeding occurs because the clot is fragile and readily undergoes lysis, and the diagnosis should be suspected in patients with clinical evidence of bleeding but normal clotting times. It should be confirmed by the observation that clots formed by recalcifying patient plasma are soluble in 5 M urea or 1% monochloroacetic acid.

Lorand (127) recently reviewed the literature and summarized 22 cases. Most patients were elderly, and men and women were affected equally. The inhibitors were IgG antibodies, and in seven cases, they appeared in conjunction with isoniazid therapy. Isoniazid reacts with a variety of proteins and can modify the transaminase, thus rendering it immunogenic (128). In many of the patients reported by Lorand (128), bleeding was severe; six (27%) experienced fatal hemorrhage.

Green et al (129) recently described a 67-year-old man who presented with spontaneous large ecchymoses. An IgG inhibitor was discovered that mainly prevented cross linking of the α-chains of fibrinogen. The patient had unstable angina and required coronary revascularization. He was prepared for surgery with a F XIII concentrate (Fibrogammin®), which was given immediately preoperatively. This neutralized the antibody and normalized the clot solubility. No untoward bleeding occurred, and the patient made an uneventful recovery from the operation. The inhibitor has persisted in low titer, however.

# REFERENCES

1. Green D. Inhibitors of factor VIII in non-hemophiliacs. In: Green D, ed. Anticoagulants: physiologic, pathologic, and pharmacologic. Boca Raton: CRC Press, 1994:97–112.
2. Green D, Lechner K. A survey of 215 non-hemophilic individuals with inhibitors to factor VIII. Thromb Haemost 1981;45:200–203.
3. Kessler CM, Ludlam CA. The treatment of acquired factor VIII inhibitors: worldwide experience with porcine factor VIII concentrate. Semin Hematol 1993;30(Suppl 1):22–27.

4. Hauser I, Schneider B, Lechner K. Post-partum factor VIII inhibitors. Thromb Haemost 1995;73:1–5.

5. Fulcher CA, Mahoney S, Zimmerman TS. FVIII inhibitor IgG subclass and FVIII polypeptide specificity determined by immunoblotting. Blood 1987;69:1475–1480.

6. Arai M, Scandella D, Hoyer LW. The molecular basis of factor VIII inhibition by human antibodies: antibodies that bind to the factor VIII light chain prevent the interaction of factor VIII with phospholipid. J Clin Invest 1989;83:1978–1984.

7. Shima M, Scandella D, Yoshioka A et al. A factor VIII neutralizing monoclonal antibody and a human inhibitor alloantibody recognizing epitopes in the C₂ domain inhibit factor VIII binding to von Willebrand factor and to phosphatidylserine. Thromb Haemost 1993;69:240–246.

8. Scandella D, Gilbert GE, Shima M et al. Some factor VIII inhibitor antibodies recognize a common epitope corresponding to C₂ domain amino acids 2248 through 2312, which overlap a phospholipid-binding site. Blood 1995;86:1811–1819.

9. Scandella D, Kessler C, Esmon P et al. Epitope specificity and functional characterization of factor VIII inhibitors. In: Aledort LM, Hoyer LW, Lusher JM et al, eds. Inhibitors to coagulation factors. New York: Plenum Press, 1995:47–63.

10. Fulcher CA, Lechner K, deGraff Mahoney SG. Immunoblot analysis shows changes in factor VIII inhibitor chain specificity in factor VIII inhibitor individuals over time. Blood 1988;72:1348–1356.

11. Kasper CK, Aledort LM, Counts RB et al. A more uniform measurement of factor VIII inhibitors. Thromb Diath Haemorrh 1975;34:869–872.

12. Green D. Spontaneous inhibitors of factor VIII. Br J Haematol 1968;15:57–75.

13. Kessler CM. An introduction to factor VIII inhibitors: the detection and quantitation. Am J Med 1991;91(Suppl 5A):1S–5S.

14. White GC II. Factor VIII inhibitor assay: quantitative and qualitative assay limitations and development needs. Semin Hematol 1994;31(Suppl 4):6–10.

15. Verbruggen B, Novakova I, Wessels H, Boezeman J, van den Berg M, Mauser-Bunschoten E. The Nijmegen modification of the Bethesda assay for factor VIII:C inhibitors: improved specificity and reliability. Thromb Haemost 1995;73:247–251.

16. de la Fuente B, Panek S, Hoyer LW. The effect of 1-deamino-8-D-arginine vasopressin (DDAVP) in a non-hemophilic individual with an acquired type II factor VIII inhibitor. Br J Haematol 1985;59:127–131.

17. Naorose-Abidi SM, Bond LR, Chitolie A, Bevan DH. Desmopressin therapy in individuals with acquired factor VIII inhibitors [Letter]. Lancet 1988;i:366.

18. Mannucci PM. Desmopressin: a nontransfusional form of treatment for congenital and acquired bleeding disorders. Blood 1988;72:1449–1455.

19. Mannucci PM, Carlsson S, Harris AS. Desmopressin, surgery and thrombosis [Letter]. Thromb Haemost 1994;71:154–155.

20. Kasper CK. Cross-reactivity of human factor VIII allo- and auto-antibodies to porcine F VIII is similar [Abstract]. Haemophilia 1996;2(Suppl 1):105.

21. Hay C, Lozier JN. Porcine factor VIII therapy in individuals with factor VIII inhibitors. In: Aledort LM, Hoyer LW, Lusher JM et al., eds. Inhibitors to coagulation factors. New York: Plenum Press, 1995:143–151.

22. Kessler CM. The treatment of acquired hemophilia with porcine factor VIII concentrate. In: Green D, ed. Anticoagulants: physiologic, pathologic, and pharmacologic. Boca Raton: CRC Press, 1994:113–124.

23. Bona RD, Ribeno M, Klatsky AV, Panck S, Magnifico M, Rickles FR. Continuous infusion of porcine factor VIII for the treatment of individuals with factor VIII inhibitors. Semin Hematol 1993;30(Suppl 1):32–35.

24. Morrison AE, Ludlam CA, Kessler C. Use of porcine factor VIII in the treatment of individuals with acquired hemophilia. Blood 1993;81:1513–1520.

25. Hay CRM, Lozier JN, Lee CA et al. Safety profile of porcine factor VIII and its use as hospital and home-therapy for individuals with haemophilia-A and inhibitors: the results of an international survey. Thromb Haemost 1996;75:25–29.

26. Gringeri A, Santagostine E, Tradati F, Giangrande PLF, Mannucci PM. Adverse effects of treatment with porcine F VIII. Thromb Haemost 1991;65:245–247.

27. Green D, Tuite DF Jr. Declining platelet counts and platelet aggregation during porcine VIII:C infusions. Am J Med 1989;86:222–224.

28. Kasper CK. Treatment of factor VIII inhibitors. In: Coller BM, ed. Progress in hemostasis and thrombosis. Philadelphia: WB Saunders, 1989:57–86.

29. Bona RD, Weinstein RA, Weisman SJ, Bartolomeo A, Rickles FR. The use of continuous infusion of factor concentrates in the treatment of hemophilia. Am J Hematol 1989;32:8–13.

30. Berntorp E, Ekman M, Gunnarsson M, Nilsson IM. Variation in factor VIII inhibitor reactivity with different commercial factor VIII preparations. Haemophilia 1996;2:95–99.

31. Suzuki T, Arai M, Amano K, Kagawa K, Fukutake K. Factor VIII inhibitor antibodies with C₂ domain specificity are less inhibitory to factor VIII complexed with von Willebrand factor. Thromb Haemost 1996;76:749–754.

32. Glazer S, Hedner U, Falch JF. Pathologic inhibitors: management with factor VIIa. In: Green D, ed. Anticoagulants: physiologic, pathologic, and pharmacologic. Boca Raton: CRC Press, 1994:131–141.

33. Nemerson Y. The function of factor VIIa in hemophilia A: an hypothesis. In: Aledort LM, Hoyer LW, Lusher JM et al., eds. Inhibitors to coagulation factors. New York: Plenum Press, 1995:157–161.

34. Glazer S, Hedner U, Falch JF. Clinical update on the use of recombinant factor VII. In: Aledort LM, Hoyer LW, Lusher JM et al, eds. Inhibitors to coagulation factors. New York: Plenum Press, 1995:163–174.

35. Roberts H. Clinical experience with recombinant factor VIIa (NovoSeven): summary of efficacy and safety [Abstract]. Haemophilia 1996;2(Suppl 1):63.

36. Penner JA. Overview of factor VIII inhibitors. In: Green D, ed. Anticoagulants: physiologic, pathologic, and pharmacologic. Boca Raton: CRC Press, 1994:69–80.

37. Lusher JM. Prediction and management of adverse events associated with the use of factor IX complex concentrates. Semin Hematol 1993;30(Suppl 1):36–40.

38. Sultan Y, Maisonneuve P, Kazatchkine MD, Nydegger UE. Anti-idiotypic suppression of autoantibodies to factor VIII by high-dose intravenous gammaglobulin. Lancet 1984;ii:765–768.

39. Green D, Kwaan HC. An acquired factor VIII inhibitor responsive to high dose gammaglobulin. Thromb Haemost 1987;58:1005–1007.

40. Schwartz RS, Gabriel DA, Aledort LM, Green D, Kessler CM. A prospective study of treatment of acquired (autoimmune) factor VIII inhibitors with high-dose intravenous gammaglobulin. Blood 1995;86:797–804.

41. Dietrich G, Algiman M, Sultan Y, Nydegger UE, Kazatchkine MD. Origin of anti-idiotypic activity against anti-factor VIII autoantibodies in pools of normal human immunoglobulin G (IVIg). Blood 1992;79:2946–2951.

42. Nilsson I, Sundquist S, Freiburghaus C. Extracorporeal protein A-sepharose and specific affinity chromatography for removal of antibodies. Prog Clin Biol Res 1984;150:225–241.

43. Uehlinger J, Button GR, McCarthy J, Forster A, Watt R, Aledort LM. Immunoadsorption for coagulation factor inhibitors. Transfusion 1991;31:265–269.

44. Knobl P, Derfler K, Korninger L et al. Elimination of acquired factor VIII antibodies by extracorporeal antibody-based immunoadsorption (Ig-Therasorb). Thromb Haemost 1995;74:1035–1038.

45. Lottenberg R, Kentro TB, Kitchens CS. Acquired hemophilia: a natural history study of 16 individuals with factor VIII inhibitors receiving little or no therapy. Arch Intern Med 1987;147:1077–1081.

46. Green D, Rademaker AW, Briet E. A prospective, randomized trial of prednisone and cyclophosphamide in the treatment of individuals with factor VIII autoantibodies. Thromb Haemost 1993;70:753–757.

47. Green D. Suppression of an antibody to factor VIII by a combination of factor VIII and cyclophosphamide. Blood 1971;37:381–387.

48. Herbst KD, Rapaport SI, Kenoyer DG et al. Syndrome of an acquired inhibitor of factor VIII responsive to cyclophosphamide and prednisone. Ann Intern Med 1981;95:575–578.

49. Lian EC-Y, Larcada AF, Chiu AY-Z. Combination immunosuppressive therapy after factor VIII infusion for acquired factor VIII inhibitor. Ann Intern Med 1989;110:774–778.

50. Schulman S, Langevitz P, Livneh A, Martinowitz U, Seligsohn U, Varon D. Cyclosporine therapy for acquired factor VIII inhibitor in a individual with systemic lupus erythematosus. Thromb Haemost 1996;76:344–346.

51. Coller BS, Hultin MB, Hoyer LW et al. Normal pregnancy in a individual with a prior postpartum factor VIII inhibitor: with observations on pathogenesis and prognosis. Blood 1981;58:619–624.

52. Hauser I, Schneider B, Lechner K. Post-partum factor VIII inhibitors. Thromb Haemost 1995;73:1–5.

53. Lusher JM, Arkin S, Abildgaard CF, Schwartz RS. Recombinant factor VIII for the treatment of previously untreated individuals with hemophilia A. Safety, efficacy, and development of inhibitors. Kogenate Previously Untreated Individual Study Group. N Engl J Med 1993;328:453–459.

54. Bray GL, Gomperts ED, Courter S et al. A multicenter study of recombinant factor VIII (recombinate): safety, efficacy, and inhibitor risk in previously untreated individuals with hemophilia A. Blood 1994;83:2428–2435.

55. de Biasi R, Rocino A, Papa ML, Salerno E, Mastrullo L, De Blasi D. Incidence of factor VIII inhibitor development in hemophilia A individuals treated with less pure plasma derived concentrates. Thromb Haemost 1994;71:544–547.

56. Briet E, Rosendaal FR, Kreuz W et al. High titer inhibitors in severe haemophilia A: a meta-analysis based on eight long-term follow-up studies concerning inhibitors associated with crude or intermediate purity factor VIII products. Thromb Haemost 1994;72:162–164.

57. Nilsson IM, Berntop E, Zettervall O, Dahlback B. Noncoagulation inhibitory factor VIII antibodies after induction of tolerance to factor VIII in hemophilia A individuals. Blood 1990;75:378–383.

58. Gilles JGG, Arnout J, Vermylen J, Saint-Remy J-MR. Anti-factor VIII antibodies of hemophiliac individuals are frequently directed towards nonfunctional determinants and do not exhibit isotypic restriction. Blood 1993;82:2452–2461.

59. Schwaab R, Brackmann HH, Meyer C et al. Haemophilia A: mutation

type determines risk of inhibitor formation. Thromb Haemost 1995;74: 1402–1406.

60. Rosendaal FR, Nieuwenhuis HK, van den Berg HM et al. A sudden increase in factor VIII inhibitor development in multitransfused hemophilia A individuals in the Netherlands. Blood 1993;81:2180–2186.

61. Peerlinck K, Arnout J, Gilles JG, Saint-Remy J-M, Vermylen J. A higher than expected incidence of factor VIII inhibitors in multitransfused haemophilia A individuals treated with an intermediate purity pasteurized factor VIII concentrate. Thromb Haemost 1993;69:115–118.

62. Peerlinck K, Arnout J, Di Giambattista M et al. Factor VIII inhibitors in previously treated haemophilia A individuals with a double virus-inactivated plasma derived factor VIII concentrate. Thromb Haemost 1997;77: 80–86.

63. Barrowcliffe TW, Kemball-Cook G, Tubbs JE. Inhibitor development and activated factor VIII in concentrates. Thromb Haemost 1993;70:1065–1066.

64. Allain JP, Frommel D. Antibodies to factor VIII. V. Patterns of immune response to factor VIII in hemophilia A. Blood 1976;47:973–982.

65. Brackmann HH. Induced immunotolerance in factor VIII inhibitor individuals. Prog Clin Biol Res 1986;150:181–195.

66. Nilsson IM, Berntorp E, Zettervall O. Induction of immune tolerance in individuals with hemophilia and antibodies to FVIII by combined treatment with intravenous IgG, cyclophosphamide and FVIII. N Engl J Med 1988;328:947–950.

67. Mariani G, Scheibel E, Nogao T et al. Immunetolerance as treatment of alloantibodies to factor VIII in hemophilia. Semin Hematol 1994;31(Suppl 4):62–64.

68. Gill JC, Leissinger C, Kasper CK, Sexauer C, Inwood M, Cohen A, and other HRS Inhibitor Registry Investigators. Hemophilia inhibitors in the 80's and 90's: a first look at the Hemophilia Research Society (HRS) inhibitor registry. Blood 1996;86(Suppl 1):330A.

69. Kucharski W, Scharf R, Nowak T. Immune tolerance induction in haemophiliacs with inhibitor to FVIII: high- or low-dose programme. Haemophilia 1996;2:224–228.

70. Lusher JM. Use of prothrombin complex concentrates in management of bleeding in hemophiliacs with inhibitors—benefits and limitations. Semin Hematol 1994;31(Suppl 4):49–52.

71. Penner JA. Treatment of inhibitor individuals with activated prothrombin complex concentrates. In: Hoyer LW, ed. Factor VIII inhibitors. New York: Alan R Liss, 1984:291–308.

72. Soff GA. Acquired von Willebrand's disease. In: Green D, ed. Anticoagulants: physiologic, pathologic, and pharmacologic. Boca Raton: CRC Press, 1994:157–168.

73. Soff GA, Green D. Autoantibody to von Willebrand factor in systemic lupus erythematosus. J Lab Clin Med 1993;121:424–430.

74. Jakway JL. Acquired von Willebrand's disease in malignancy. Semin Thromb Hemost 1992;18:434–439.

75. van Genderen PJJ, Vink T, Michiels JJ, van't Veer MB, Sixma JJ, van Vliet HDM. Acquired von Willebrand disease caused by an autoantibody selectively inhibiting the binding of von Willebrand factor to collagen. Blood 1994;84:3378–3384.

76. Uehlinger J, Rose E, Aledort LM, Lerner R. Successful treatment of an acquired von Willebrand factor antibody by extracorporeal immunoadsorption. N Engl J Med 1989;320:254–255.

77. Green D. Acquired inhibitors of blood coagulation. In: Bloom AL, Thomas DP, eds. Thromb Haemost and thrombosis. New York: Churchill Livingstone, 1987:547–548.

78. Ewenstein BM. Factor VIII and other coagulation factor inhibitors. In: Loscalzo J, Schafer AI, eds. Thrombosis and hemorrhage. Boston: Blackwell Scientific Publications, 1994:740–741.

79. Taillan B, Fuzibet J-G, Vinti H et al. Factor V inhibitor in celiac disease. Am J Med 1989;87:360.

80. Ortel TL, Quinn-Allen MA, Charles LA, Devore-Carter D, Kane WH. Characterization of an acquired inhibitor to coagulation factor V. J Clin Invest 1992;90:2340–2347.

81. Ortel TL, Moore KD, Quinn-Allen MA, Kane WH. Factor V inhibitors associated with hemorrhagic symptoms bind to a limited region of the factor Va light chain [Abstract]. J Invest Med 1996;44:233A.

82. Chediak J, Ashenhurst JB, Garlick I, Desser RK. Successful management of bleeding in a individual with factor V inhibitor by platelet transfusions. Blood 1980;56:835–841.

83. Nesheim ME, Nichols WL, Cole TL et al. Isolation and study of an acquired inhibitor of human coagulation factor V. J Clin Invest 1986;77:405–415.

84. Green D, Wong CA, Twardowski P. Efficacy of hemostatic agents in improving surgical hemostasis. Transfusion Med Rev 1996;10:171–182.

85. Zehnder JL, Leung LLK. Development of antibodies to thrombin and factor V with recurrent bleeding in a individual exposed to topical bovine thrombin. Blood 1990;76:2011–2016.

86. Stricker BV, Lane PK, Leffert JD, Rodgers GM, Shuman MA, Corash L. Development of antithrombin antibodies following surgery in individuals with prosthetic cardiac valves. Blood 1988;72:1375–1380.

87. Banninger H, Hardegger T, Tobler A et al. Fibrin glue in surgery: frequent development of inhibitors of bovine thrombin and human factor V. Br J Haematol 1993;85:528–532.

88. Campbell E, Sanal S, Mattson J et al. Factor VII inhibitor. Am J Med 1980; 68:962–964.

89. Delmer A, Horellou M-H, Andreu G et al. Life-threatening intracranial bleeding associated with the presence of an antifactor VII autoantibody. Blood 1989;74:229–232.

90. Largo R, Sigg P, von Felten A, Straub PW. Acquired factor IX inhibitor in a non-haemophilic individual with autoimmune disease. Br J Haematol 1974;26:129–140.

91. Castro O, Farber LR, Clyne LP. Circulating anticoagulants against factors IX and XI in systemic lupus erythematosus. Ann Intern Med 1972;77: 543–548.

92. Ozsoylu S, Ozer FL. Acquired factor IX deficiency. Acta Haematologica 1973;50:305–314.

93. Shapiro SS, Hultin M. Acquired inhibitors to the blood coagulation factors. Semin Thromb Hemost 1975;1:336–385.

94. Kasper CK. Blood—its derivatives and its problems: factor IX. Ann N Y Acad Sci 1975;240:172–180.

95. Natelson EA, Lynch EC, Hettig RA, Alfrey CP. Acquired factor IX deficiency in the nephrotic syndrome. Ann Intern Med 1970;73:373–378.

96. Green D, Arruda J, Honig G, Muehrcke RC. Urinary loss of clotting factors due to hereditary membranous glomerulopathy. Am J Clin Pathol 1976; 65:376–383.

97. Boklan BF, Sawitsky A. Factor IX deficiency in Gaucher disease. Arch Intern Med 1976;136:489–492.

98. Nilsson IM, Jonsson S, Sundqvist S-B, Ahlberg A, Bergentz S-E. A procedure for removing high titer antibodies by extracorporeal protein-A-Sepharose adsorption in hemophilia: substitution therapy and surgery in a individual with hemophilia B and antibodies. Blood 1981;58:38–44.

99. Lankiewicz MW, Bell WR. A unique circulating inhibitor with specificity for coagulation factor X. Am J Med 1992;93:343–346.

100. Rao LVM, Zivelin A, Iturbe I, Rapaport SI. Antibody-induced acute factor X deficiency: clinical manifestations and properties of the antibody. Thromb Haemost 1994;72:363–371.

101. Glenner GG. Factor X deficiency and systemic amyloidosis. N Engl J Med 1977;297:108–109.

102. Cohen D, Pras M, Franklin EC, Frangione B. Characterization of amyloid deposits and P component from a individual with factor X deficiency reveals protein derived from a lambda VI light chain. Am J Med 1983;74: 513–518.

103. Furie B, Voo L, McAdam KPWJ, Furie BC. Mechanism of factor X deficiency in systemic amyloidosis. N Engl J Med 1981;304:827–830.

104. Greipp PR, Kyle RA, Bowie EJW. Factor X deficiency in primary amyloidosis: resolution after splenectomy. N Engl J Med 1979;301:1050–1051.

105. Camoriano JK, Greipp PR, Bayer GK, Bowie EJW. Resolution of acquired factor X deficiency and amyloidosis with melphalan and prednisone therapy. N Engl J Med 1987;316:1133–1135.

106. Bletry O, Andreu G, Horellou MH, N'Guyen L, Cherin P, Godeau P. Amyloidosis and acquired factor X deficiency: treatment with vinca-loaded platelets. Eur J Int Med 1990;1:307–309.

107. Aberg H, Nilsson IM. Recurrent thrombosis in a young woman with a circulating anticoagulant directed against factor XI and XII. Acta Med Scand 1972;192:419–425.

108. Rolovic Z, Elezovic I, Obrenovic B, Rizza CR. Life-threatening bleeding due to an acquired inhibitor to factor XII-XI successfully treated with activated prothrombin complex concentrate (FEIBA) [Letter]. Br J Haematol 1982;51:659.

109. Schnall SF, Duff TP, Clyne LP. Acquired factor XI inhibitors in congenitally deficient individuals. Am J Hematol 1987;26:323–328.

110. Fleck RA, Rapaport SI, Rao VM. Anti-prothrombin antibodies and the lupus anticoagulant. Blood 1988;72:512–519.

111. Bajaj SP, Rapaport SI, Fierer DS, Herbst KD, Schwartz DB. A mechanism for the hypoprothrombinemia of the acquired hypoprothrombinemia-lupus anticoagulant syndrome. Blood 1983;61:684–692.

112. La Spada AR, Skalhegg BS, Henderson R, Schmer G, Pierce R, Chandler W. Brief report: fatal hemorrhage in a individual with an acquired inhibitor of human thrombin. N Engl J Med 1995;33:494–497.

113. Rydel TJ, Ravichandran KG, Tulinski A et al. The structure of a complex of recombinant hirudin and human a-thrombin. Science 1990;249:277–280.

114. Khoory MS, Nesheim ME, Bowie EJW, Mann KG. Circulating heparin sulfate proteoglycan anticoagulant from a individual with a plasma cell disorder. J Clin Invest 1980;65:666–674.

115. Palmer RN, Rick ME, Rick PD, Zeller JA, Gralnick HR. Circulating heparan sulfate anticoagulant in a individual with a fatal bleeding disorder. N Engl J Med 1984;310:1696–1699.

116. Tefferi A, Owen BA, Nichols WL, Witzig TE, Owen WG. Isolation of a heparin-like anticoagulant from the plasma of a individual with metastatic bladder carcinoma. Blood 1989;74:252–254.

117. Horne MK III, Chao ES, Wilson OJ, Scialla SJ, Lynch MA, Kragel PJ. A heparin-like anticoagulant as part of global abnormalities of plasma glycosaminoglycans in a individual with transitional cell carcinoma. J Lab Clin Med 1991;118:250–260.

118. Horne MK III, Stein CA, LaRocca RV, Myers CE. Circulating glycosaminoglycan anticoagulants associated with suramin treatment. Blood 1988; 71:273–279.
119. Delorme MA, Saeed N, Sevcik A et al. Plasma dermatan sulfate proteoglycan in a individual on chronic hemodialysis. Blood 1993;82:3380–3385.
120. Tefferi A, Nichols WL, Bowie EJW. Circulating heparin-like anticoagulants: report of five consecutive cases and a review. Am J Med 1990;88: 184–188.
121. Cohen I, Amir J, Ben-Shaul Y, Pick A, de Vries A. Plasma cell myeloma associated with an unusual myeloma protein causing impairment of fibrin aggregation and platelet function in a individual with multiple malignancy. Am J Med 1970;48:766–776.
122. Coleman M, Vigliano EN, Weksler ME, Nachman RL. Inhibition of fibrin monomer polymerization by lambda myeloma globulins. Blood 1972;39: 210–223.
123. Lackner H. Hemostatic abnormalities associated with dysproteinemias. Semin Hematol 1973;10:125–133.

124. Carr ME Jr, Dent RM, Carr SL. Abnormal fibrin structure and inhibition of fibrinolysis in individuals with multiple myeloma. J Lab Clin Med 1996; 128:83–88.
125. Marciniak E, Greenwood MF. Acquired coagulation inhibitor delaying fibrinopeptide release. Blood 1979;53:81–92.
126. Hoots WK, Carrell NA, Wagner RH, Cooper HA, McDonagh J. A naturally occurring antibody that inhibits fibrin polymerization. N Engl J Med 1981; 304:857–861.
127. Lorand L. Acquired inhibitors of fibrin stabilization: a class of hemorrhagic disorders of diverse origins. In: Green D, ed. Anticoagulants: physiologic, pathologic, and pharmacologic. Boca Raton: CRC Press, 1994:169–191.
128. Lorand L, Campbell LK, Robertson BJ. Enzymatic coupling of isoniazid to proteins. Biochemistry 1972;11:434–438.
129. Green D, Sanders J, Wong C, Velasco PT, Lorand L. Coronary revascularization in the presence of an inhibitory antibody to factor XIII. Bull Intens Crit Care 1996;3:14–16.

# CHAPTER 38

# ANTIPHOSPHOLIPID SYNDROME, LUPUS ANTICOAGULANTS, AND ANTICARDIOLIPIN ANTIBODIES

## Barbara M. Alving

Antiphospholipid antibodies (APA), which are now recognized to be antiphospholipid–protein antibodies, were initially discovered more than 40 years ago because of their interference in routine phospholipid-dependent clotting assays (1–4). Because plasma from some individuals with systemic lupus erythematosus (SLE) demonstrated anticoagulant activity resulting from APA, the term *lupus anticoagulant* (LA) was coined to describe the antibody activity. However, plasma with LA activity usually came from individuals without underlying SLE (5–9). In 1963, Bowie et al (9) reported the association of the antibodies with thrombosis in four individuals with SLE; this association was soon confirmed in additional individuals with no other apparent illness (8, 10, 11).

In 1983, Harris et al (12) developed a radioimmunoassay, later converted to an enzyme-linked immunosorbent assay (ELISA), to measure the LA quantitatively and to determine their isotype. The negatively charged phospholipid cardiolipin was chosen as the antigen, because individuals with LA had a biologic false-positive test with the Venereal Disease Research Laboratory (VDRL) reagent, which contains cardiolipin. The immunoassay was 200–400-fold more sensitive than the VDRL precipitation test in detecting the antibodies (12).

In 1990, three groups reported that antibodies against phospholipids were really directed against a complex of phospholipid with a protein such as $\beta_2$-glycoprotein I ($\beta_2$-GP I) (13–15). Galli et al (14) also suggested that some antibodies could be directed against $\beta_2$-GP I alone. Thus, the ELISA was really detecting antibodies against the complex of cardiolipin and $\beta_2$-GP I, which was in the diluted individual sera or protein solutions used in the assay.

Development of tests for APA resulted in several different terms to define their activities (Table 38.1). APA can be detected by an ELISA that contains cardiolipin and a standardized concentration of $\beta_2$-GP I or by assays for LA. Individuals may have immunoglobulin (Ig) G, IgM, or even IgA APA, but measurements for the latter isotype have not been well standardized (16). Approximately 90% of individuals testing positive for LA also have anticardiolipin antibody (ACA) activity (17). However, there is no direct correlation between potency of the LA activity and concentration of the ACA, which may reflect the heterogeneity of the APA (16–18). Despite the difficulties of comparing studies in which only a test for LA or an ELISA has been used, associations between well-defined clinical problems and APA have emerged. This chapter reviews the clinical features and treatment of individuals with APA, recent developments in the pathophysiology and immunology of APA, and the coagulation assays and ELISAs commonly used for their detection.

## CLINICAL MANIFESTATIONS OF ANTIPHOSPHOLIPID SYNDROME

Initial studies with quantitative immunoassays for APA found that individuals with SLE and arterial or venous

**TABLE 38.1.**    Common Terms for Anti-phospholipid Antibodies

*Antiphospholipid–protein antibodies* (APA) or, formerly, *antiphospholipid antibodies*

> IgG, IgM, or IgA antibodies now recognized as being antibodies against proteins such as prothrombin or $\beta_2$-GPI that bind to phospholipids. (Proposed new terms are *anti–phospholipid-protein antibodies* or *auto-antibodies to phospholipid-binding plasma proteins.*) APA are often described as lupus anticoagulants or anticardiolipin antibodies according to the assay procedure used for their detection.

*Antiphospholipid syndrome*

> Characterized by venous or arterial thrombosis, thrombocytopenia, and recurrent fetal loss in association with APA.

*Lupus anticoagulant*

> Antibody against a phospholipid-binding protein such as prothrombin or $\beta_2$-GPI that prolongs clotting in a phospholipid-dependent assay.

*Anticardiolipin antibodies* (ACA)

> Antibodies against $\beta_2$-GPI detected in an ELISA containing cardiolipin as the phospholipid that binds $\beta_2$-GPI in patient sera or blocking fluids. Some ACA (in sera from patients with syphilis) recognize and bind to cardiolipin without $\beta_2$-GPI. The two types of ACA cannot be differentiated in commercially available ELISAs.

thrombosis, recurrent spontaneous abortion, or thrombocytopenia frequently tested positive for moderate to high titers of ACA (12). This constellation of clinical symptoms with LA or ACA is known as the *antiphospholipid syndrome* (Table 38.2) (16, 18–26). The syndrome manifests by at least one of the following clinical conditions: venous thrombosis, arterial thrombosis (e.g., stroke, myocardial infarction, gangrene), recurrent pregnancy loss, or thrombocytopenia. In addition, the individual must also test positive for LA or for moderate to high levels of ACA (IgG or IgM) on two occasions more than 12 weeks apart (19–22). The requirement for sustained APA positivity is indicated as well, because in many instances, tests may be transiently positive and unrelated to clinical symptoms. In a study of normal subjects followed for 1 year (27), the prevalence was 6.5% and 9.4% for IgG ACA and IgM ACA, respectively; at the end of the year, 7% of those who tested positive initially remained positive for ACA.

When antiphospholipid syndrome occurs without SLE or other autoimmune connective tissue disorders, it is known as *primary antiphospholipid syndrome.* Many individuals with primary antiphospholipid syndrome do not develop SLE with time. Other features of the

syndrome, including migraine headaches, livedo reticularis, Coombs' test–positive hemolytic anemia, and cardiac abnormalities (23, 24), have yet to be fully accepted as major criteria, because they can occur in association with underlying autoimmune connective tissue disorders. Vianna et al (28) compared the clinical manifestations of primary and secondary antiphospholipid syndrome in 114 individuals during a 2-year period. The clinical manifestations were similar in both groups, but valvular cardiac disease, hemolytic anemia, neutropenia, and decreased levels of C4 were more common in individuals with secondary antiphospholipid syndrome.

Approximately 34 to 54% of individuals with primary antiphospholipid syndrome also have deep venous thrombosis, which may be multiple or bilateral (19, 25); 25 to 44% can have arterial occlusions, including strokes, transient ischemic events, and multi-infarct dementia, and 34% of female individuals may have recurrent fetal losses (19, 25). Approximately 50% of individuals with this syndrome also have vasculitic rashes and arthralgias. Other complications have been reported as well, including necrosis of digits, pulmonary hypertension, and cutaneous skin necrosis (26).

Thrombocytopenia occurs in 30 to 50% of individuals with primary antiphospholipid syndrome, and 50% have elevated levels of antinuclear antibodies (ANA). The IgG antiphospholipid antibody, which is usually measured as ACA, has a high titer in 60% and is detectable at lower levels in others. Some individuals have only a positive LA, which is usually measured with a phospholipid dilution assay (19, 25). For individuals with

**TABLE 38.2.**    Major Features of Antiphospholipid Syndrome

*Clinical*
Venous thromboembolism
> Deep venous thrombosis
> Pulmonary embolism

Arterial thromboses
> Stroke
> Transient ischemic attack
> Myocardial infarction

Recurrent fetal loss

*Laboratory*
Thrombocytopenia
Moderate- to high-positive ACA IgG or IgM or positive LA on two occasions (12 weeks apart)

*Other serology*
ANA may be present in low titer (1:40 to 1:160)
Antibodies to single-stranded DNA are frequent
Occasional Coombs' positivity and hemolytic anemia
Antibodies to double-stranded DNA and extractable nuclear antigen are negative

primary antiphospholipid syndrome, the female:male ratio is 2:1. The female:male ratio for individuals with SLE and the antiphospholipid syndrome is 9:1, which is the same as that for individuals with SLE alone.

# PRIMARY ANTIPHOSPHOLIPID SYNDROME AND THROMBOSIS

In a natural history study, Finazzi et al (29) followed 360 consecutive, unselected individuals originally evaluated for clinical manifestations of APA or for LA discovered incidentally. In these individuals, the risk factors for thrombosis were a previous thrombotic event (relative risk, 4.9) and a moderately or highly positive IgG ACA titer (relative risk, 3.7). In a prospective nested case-control study drawn from the Physicians' Health Study (30), which included men between the ages of 40 and 84 years, those with ACA IgG antibody titers above the 95th percentile had a relative risk of 5.3 for developing venous thrombosis; LA was not measured in this study.

In another study of individuals without SLE (31), the odds ratio for the association between LA and venous thrombosis was 9.4. No association was found for ACA and thrombosis (odds ratio, 0.7) because of the high frequency of positive ACA assays in individuals without venous thromboembolism. Of the individuals who presented with venous thromboembolism, 14% tested positive for LA. In this study, LA was defined as positive if the results of one or more of the following tests were positive: dilute Russell viper venom time (RVVT), dilute prothrombin time (PT), or prolongation of the activated partial thromboplastin time (aPTT), with both screening and confirmatory tests abnormal.

In an additional study of individuals without SLE but with deep venous thrombosis (32), 8.5% had LA. In contrast, LA was not present in any individual with a normal venogram. The odds ratio for an acute venous thrombosis in individuals with LA was 10.7. Individuals with other clotting disorders were excluded from this study.

Recently, six individuals without SLE but with recurrent arterial or venous thromboembolism were found to have antibodies against human or bovine $\beta_2$-GP I alone (33). However, these individuals did not have positive ELISAs with cardiolipin as the coating antigen, thus suggesting that the antibodies did not recognize $\beta_2$-GP I when bound to cardiolipin (33). Additional studies are needed to determine if this laboratory observation truly identifies an immunologically unique group of individuals.

# ANTIPHOSPHOLIPID SYNDROME WITH SLE

An initial study of individuals with SLE indicated that 61% had elevated levels of at least one ACA antibody isotype and that 49% had detectable levels of LA (12). The overlap between LA and ACA was quite significant, because ACA levels were increased in 91% of individuals testing positive for LA. Subsequent prospective (34–36) and retrospective (37) analyses have confirmed that LA and ACA antibodies are detectable in approximately 50% of individuals with SLE. However, at least one report has stated that LA and ACA positivity may be as low as 7 and 25%, respectively (38).

There is a high incidence of APA among relatives of individuals with SLE, thus indicating the predisposition to antibody formation may be genetically determined in some situations (39). There is also an increased frequency of HLA-DQw7 in individuals with SLE and LA, thereby suggesting the existence of distinct subgroups of individuals with SLE and APA (40).

Several studies of individuals with SLE have documented a significant correlation between positive tests for APA (measured as LA or ACA) and thromboembolic events, including cerebral thrombosis (12, 34, 35, 37, 38, 41, 42). In one report on individuals with SLE, 55% of those with central nervous system (CNS) disease (transient ischemic attacks, strokes, epilepsy, psychiatric disorders) were positive for APA, compared with 20% of control subjects ($P < .001$) (43). Control subjects were individuals with SLE but no evidence of CNS disorders. Furthermore, 50% of the individuals with CNS manifestations had no other evidence of lupus activity; however, other studies have not found this association (36, 44). One explanation for this discrepancy is that even without antibodies to phospholipid, 40% of individuals with SLE will have thromboembolic events during their illness (35). Individuals with SLE and persistently elevated ACA levels, defined as testing positive on two separate occasions at least 3 months apart, have a significantly increased odds ratio (5.4) for a peripheral thromboembolic event compared with those who test positive for APA on only one occasion (35, 42).

Occlusive ocular vascular disease has been found in 8% of individuals with SLE and high titers of predominantly IgG ACA (45). Most of these individuals also have other features of the antiphospholipid syndrome, such as transient ischemic attacks, thrombocytopenia, and deep venous thrombosis.

The value of IgG ACA in identifying individuals with thrombosis was also assessed in a retrospective analysis of individuals with SLE (46). The posttest probability of thrombosis increased from 0.2 for individuals with moderately positive IgG ACA values to 0.75 for individuals with highly positive values. The authors concluded that IgG ACA identifies well the potential for thrombosis in individuals with SLE, but that IgM and IgA ACA have poor diagnostic accuracy.

In a retrospective study of individuals with SLE and thrombosis, Horbach et al (47) found that LA was the strongest risk factor for venous and arterial thromboses (odds ratio, 6.6 and 9.8, respectively). ACA levels also were associated with thrombosis; mean titers of IgG and IgM ACA were significantly higher in thrombotic than in asymptomatic individuals. In addition, antibody activity was assessed by ELISAs that contained only $\beta_2$-GP I or prothrombin as the antigen. These tests, however, provided no additional information or association regarding thrombotic risk.

One study evaluated the interaction between thrombotic risk associated with resistance to activated protein C (factor V Leiden) (see Chapter 40) and LA in individuals with SLE (48). In this population, factor V Leiden was a risk factor for venous thrombosis (odds ratio, 4.9), and LA was a risk factor for both venous thrombosis (odds ratio, 6.4) and arterial thrombosis (odds ratio, 7.1). LA and factor V Leiden were independent risk factors for venous thrombosis. For arterial thrombosis, a significant risk factor was high-titer IgM ACA (odds ratio, 6.5) and moderate- to high-titer IgG ACA (odds ratio, 2.9).

A significant correlation between IgG ACA and thrombocytopenia has been reported as well. In one study of individuals with thrombocytopenia and SLE or related autoimmune disorders, IgG ACA and IgM ACA levels were increased in 72% and 44% of individuals, respectively (49). For those individuals without thrombocytopenia, these values were 38% and 20%, respectively. The association between either isotype and thrombocytopenia was statistically significant. In contrast, elevated levels of IgG and IgM ACA were present in 15% and 28% of individuals with idiopathic immune thrombocytopenia (ITP) (see Chapter 30) (50). There was no correlation between levels of either isotype and of platelet-associated immunoglobulin. Others have found positive APA tests in as many as 46% of individuals with ITP (51). APA does not appear to affect outcome, but in most individuals with ITP and APA who experience resolution of thrombocytopenia after prednisone therapy, APA titers have remained elevated.

# NEUROLOGIC MANIFESTATIONS OF ANTIPHOSPHOLIPID SYNDROME

Neurologic manifestations of antiphospholipid syndrome include single or recurrent cerebral infarcts, severe vascular headaches, transient ischemic attacks, and visual disturbances (Table 38.3) (52). These may include amaurosis fugax, retinal arterial or venous occlusion, and migrainelike symptomatology. Sneddon's syndrome, which is defined as stroke (without systemic disease) and livedo reticularis in individuals with APA, can result in vascular dementia (53). Recurrent strokes are more likely

**TABLE 38.3.** Neurologic Manifestations of Antiphospholipid Syndrome

Relatively young age (usually <55 years)
One or more episodes of the following:
    Vascular dementia
    Cerebral infarction
    Transient ischemic attack
    Amaurosis fugax
    Retinal infarction
    Myelopathy
    Acute ischemic encephalopathy
Sneddon's syndrome (progressive dementia and livedo reticularis)

in individuals with antiphospholipid syndrome and hypertension or other risk factors for cerebrovascular disease, such as cigarette smoking and hyperlipidemia (52). As many as 80% of individuals with primary antiphospholipid syndrome have at least one of these additional risk factors. Cerebral angiography performed on such individuals shows large-vessel occlusion or stenosis without evidence of vasculitis (52). These individuals also may have mild thrombocytopenia and elevated ANA levels (52). Approximately 80% will have only IgG ACA, 10% will have only IgM ACA, and 10% will have both isotypes.

Several prospective studies have determined the frequency of antiphospholipid syndrome in individuals hospitalized with cerebral ischemia or transient ischemic attacks (54–59). The frequency of antibodies varies from 6% overall in this individual population (56) to 46% (54) in individuals younger than 50 years. In one study, ACA-positive individuals with cerebrovascular ischemia could be classified into two groups (59). The first, comprised of individuals older than 60 years, had risk factors for thrombosis such as hypertension and cigarette smoking as well as low-positive titers of ACA without underlying autoimmune disorder. These individuals had no short-term risk for recurrence. The second group, comprised of individuals 60 years or younger, had medium- to high-positive titers of IgG ACA and a history of other symptoms of antiphospholipid syndrome, such as livedo reticularis and malar rash. These individuals had a greater risk for recurrence of cerebrovascular events. This conclusion is supported by Nencini et al (60), who in a prospective study found that 18% of young adults (age range, 15–44 years) with sustained ischemic stroke or transient ischemic attacks tested positive for ACA. The individuals with ACA had a higher probability of recurrent events than those who did not have the antibody.

The decreased association of ACA with stroke in older individuals is also supported by a nested, case-controlled study of men with stroke who were enrolled in the Physicians' Health Study, which was comprised of men from 40 to 84 years of age. IgG ACA levels in 61 participants with ischemic stroke were not significantly different from those in control subjects ($P > .2$), and there was no evidence of increased risk for stroke in those with higher APA levels (30). This is still a controversial area, however, because others have found no evidence in prospective studies that ACA is an independent risk for stroke in young persons but rather that it increases nonspecifically in older individuals and those with atherosclerosis or cardiovascular disease (61). Despite the conflicting data, testing for ACA and LA is warranted in individuals with transient ischemic attacks at a young age and in those for whom these events are associated with other features of antiphospholipid syndrome. Indiscriminate testing of a general individual population with cerebrovascular events, however, is not recommended.

## APA AND CARDIAC VALVE DYSFUNCTION

Individuals with SLE and APA as well as those with primary antiphospholipid syndrome have an increased incidence of cardiac valvular lesions and myocardial dysfunction (62–66). The valvular abnormalities include bland, verrucous endocardial lesions comprised of leukocytes, plasma cells, fibrous tissue, fibrin, and platelets. The lesions appear as small clusters on the edge of cardiac valves, and they frequently affect the mitral valves (Fig. 38.1). The lesions may produce no symptoms or cause valvular insufficiency or stenosis (62–69).

In three prospective studies that used two-dimensional echocardiography to determine the prevalence of cardiac valvular lesions in individuals with SLE, a significant association was found between elevated APA levels and valvular lesions, which primarily involved thickened mitral valves. The incidence of valvular disease was 40% in individuals with SLE and elevated APA levels, compared with 12 to 14% in individuals with SLE but no detectable antibodies (63, 64). At least 50% of the individuals with cardiac lesions had other features of the antiphospholipid syndrome as well (62). Serial studies in these individuals indicated that hemodynamically significant cardiac valvular disease can develop with time (64), and that these individuals may have an increased risk for cerebroembolic events (70, 71). Intramural cardiac thrombosis occurs rarely (72). Studies also suggest that all individuals with SLE or the antiphospholipid syndrome should undergo echocardiography (66). Individuals with asymptomatic vegetations should receive antibiotic prophylaxis before dental or surgical work; however, anticoagulation does not appear to be routinely indicated (66).

APA has also been associated with myocardial vasculopathy sufficiently severe to induce myocardial in-

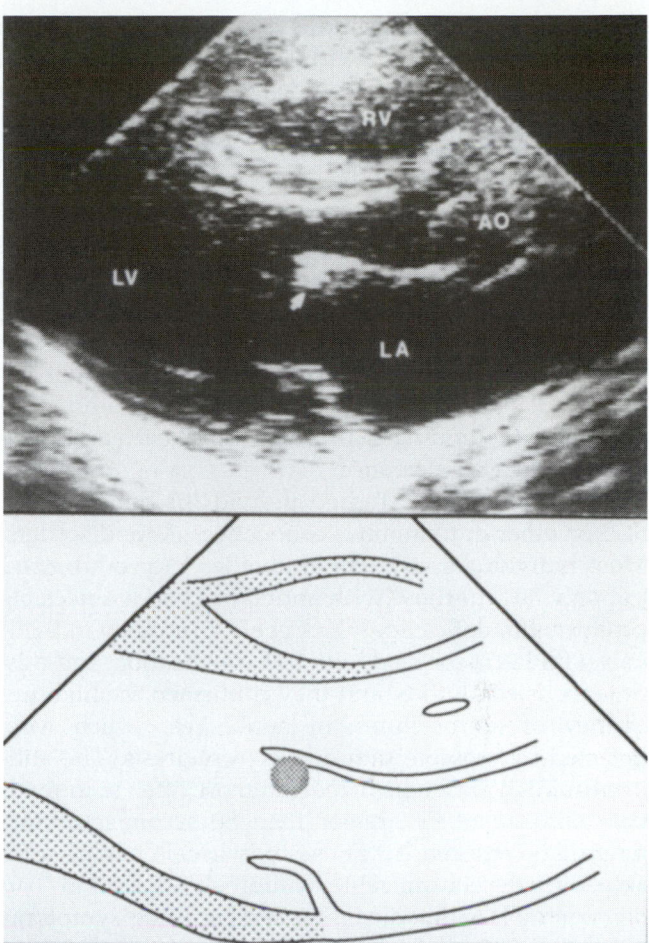

**FIGURE 38.1.**  Cardiac valvular lesion in a patient with SLE and elevated antiphospholipid antibodies. The two-dimensional echocardiogram (parasternal long-axis view) shows verrucous thickening of anterior leaflet of the mitral valve (arrow). *AO,* aorta; *LA,* left atrium; *LV,* left ventricle; *RV,* right ventricle. (Reprinted with permission from Leung WH, Wong KL, Lau CP, et al Association between antiphospholipid antibodies and cardiac abnormalities in patients with systemic lupus erythematosus. Am J Med 1990;89:411–419.)

farction, even with normal coronary arteries (68). However, in a cohort study of myocardial infarction survivors divided into those younger and those older than 51 years, ACA (measured as both IgG and IgM isotypes) was not an independent risk factor for overall mortality, reinfarction, or thrombotic stroke (70). The multivariate analysis in this study was adjusted for age and high-density lipoprotein cholesterol.

## ASSOCIATION OF LA WITH PROTHROMBIN DEFICIENCY

The mechanism for prothrombin deficiency in individuals with LA, although recognized at least 30 years ago, was not fully described until 1983, when Bajaj et al (73) studied two individuals with LA and prothrombin levels of 6% and less than 1%, respectively. Plasma from both individuals contained IgG antibodies that selectively bound prothrombin *in vitro* without neutralizing its activity. The antibodies, which could be detected by immunodiffusion, had relatively high affinities for prothrombin (Kd $10^{-10}$ M and $10^{-9}$ M). The antibodies did not bind to the aminoterminal end of prothrombin, where the sites for phospholipid and factor Va binding are located, and they did not interfere with either the proteolytic cleavage of prothrombin or the activity of thrombin. They appeared to induce true prothrombin deficiency by binding to prothrombin *in vivo* and causing its increased clearance.

Edson et al (74) studied individuals with LA and SLE or other autoimmune connective tissue disorders. Most individuals had IgG antibodies to prothrombin, but only 30% of those with antibodies had a detectable prothrombin deficiency. Fleck et al (75) studied individuals with LA associated with SLE, medication, and miscellaneous conditions, and they confirmed the high frequency of antiprothrombin antibodies, which were detected by crossed immunoelectrophoresis. The antiprothrombin antibodies occurred more often in individuals with an aPTT greater than 50 seconds (normal range, 22–30 seconds). Those individuals having a PT exceeding the control value by more than 2 seconds had demonstrable antibodies (75), and bleeding symptoms correlated with the level of functional prothrombin and occurred in individuals with a prothrombin activity of 10% or less.

Antibody production can be easily suppressed by administration of corticosteroids and azathioprine, as demonstrated in one individual with a normal PT 7 days after the initiation of treatment (73). In another study, corticosteroids alone increased the prothrombin level even while the prothrombin-antibody complexes were still detectable (76). Presumably, this increase resulted from the blocking of mononuclear phagocytic activity. For an actively bleeding patient, the prothrombin deficiency requires treatment with fresh frozen plasma or factor concentrates containing prothrombin.

Antibodies to prothrombin can also be detected in individuals with infections and LA. In one series of seven such individuals, approximately 20% had antibodies to prothrombin detected by ELISA, but none had hypoprothrombinemia (77). At least eight cases of LA and clinically significant hypoprothrombinemia have occurred in children younger than 17 years in association with a viral illness (78). In these individuals, the diagnosis is made on the basis of clinical symptomatology, and individuals improve as the antibody spontaneously disappears. In one patient, a 3-year-old girl with a history of a nonspecific viral illness, severe hypoprothrombinemia that resulted in epistaxis and gastrointestinal hemorrhage was treated successfully with intravenous methylprednisolone, 30 mg/kg/day for 3 days, followed by oral prednisone (79).

## LA AS A LABORATORY ABNORMALITY

Other conditions associated with LA include carcinoma, autoimmune disorders such as rheumatoid arthritis (80) and Sjögren's syndrome, infection (6–8), and medications (81–85). Drugs such as procainamide, hydralazine, chlorpromazine, quinidine, isoniazid, and methyldopa have been associated with the development of SLE (86). The most common cause of drug-induced SLE in the United States is procainamide. Onset of symptomatology relates to the rate at which the drug can be acetylated in a given patient. Individuals who rapidly acetylate the drug develop symptoms or serologic changes much later than those who are slow acetylators (86, 87).

The first report of LA in a individual with procainamide-induced SLE was in 1977 (84). Thromboembolic events have been described in several individuals who developed LA in association with procainamide (88–90). Most are asymptomatic, however, and the true incidence of thromboembolic events is not known (84, 85, 91). LA activity, which can be associated with the IgG or IgM isotype (85), may be detected for months after procainamide has been discontinued (91).

Detected as LA or in ELISAs, APA develops in approximately 40% of individuals receiving chlorpromazine (81, 83), and it may occur as early as 3 months after the initiation of treatment (83). One group reported that phenothiazines other than chlorpromazine did not induce LA; however, LA in individuals receiving chlorpromazine persisted when those individuals were switched to other phenothiazines (83). Other investigators have found APA in 27% of individuals receiving phenothiazines other than chlorpromazine (81).

Individuals may have APA detected as LA only or as ACA, which is usually of the IgM isotype (81, 82). Additional frequent immunologic abnormalities include positive tests for ANA (83, 92) and antibodies to native DNA (92). LA positivity is probably not a risk factor for thrombosis in these individuals. Of 110 individuals receiving phenothiazines with either LA or ACA, only 3% had a history of thrombosis (81–83).

LA frequently is associated with bacterial infections (7). Elevated ACA levels have also been measured in individuals infected with human immunodeficiency virus (93), Lyme disease (94), ornithosis, adenovirus, rubella, chickenpox, and in those who have undergone vaccination against smallpox (95) or have syphilis. LA does not increase the risk for thrombosis in these individuals. In another study (96), sera from 114 individuals with infections (syphilis, tuberculosis, *Klebsiella* sp.)

were tested for IgG antibodies against $\beta_2$-GP I and ACA. All individuals tested negative for antibodies to $\beta_2$-GP I, and the incidence of antibodies to cardiolipin in individuals was: syphilis, 64%; tuberculosis, 6%; and *Klebsiella* sp., 5%.

# PATHOGENESIS OF THROMBOSIS IN PATIENTS WITH APA

Arnout (97) postulated that the pathogenesis of antiphospholipid syndrome is similar to that of heparin-induced thrombocytopenia, because in both settings, antibodies are directed against a protein complexed with a polysaccharide or a phospholipid localized on a cell surface. The Fc portion of the antibody can then activate platelets through the FcII receptors. In addition, in both syndromes, initial vascular damage is an integral part of the thrombotic process, resulting in venous thrombosis, arterial thrombosis, or both. A double hit, such as vascular injury and immune complex formation, is needed in both as well. Greaves et al (98) have suggested that because antiendothelial cell antibodies are a common aspect of antiphospholipid syndrome, they may result in endothelial injury, thereby inducing tissue factor production and membrane damage with exposure of phospholipid. Then, circulating $\beta_2$-GP I could bind to the exposed phospholipid and, in turn, the APA could bind to the complex, thus inducing further damage. Other investigators have shown that APA can also recognize heparin or heparin bound to $\beta_2$-GP I, thus inhibiting the interaction of heparin with antithrombin III (99–101). None of these theories has gained universal acceptance, however. It is possible that APA is a marker for other antibodies or processes that promote thrombosis.

Results of several *in vitro* studies suggest that APA promote thrombosis by inhibiting the activation or function of protein C, which is an essential regulator of hemostasis (Fig. 38.2). In conjunction with free protein S, activated protein C prevents thrombosis by inhibiting factors Va and VIIIa. Protein C is converted to its active form by thrombin that is bound to the receptor thrombomodulin on endothelial cells (102). Activation of protein C is enhanced by binding to phospholipids, which increases the proximity of thrombin to protein C (103). IgG or IgM immunoglobulins with LA activity can inhibit protein C activation *in vitro* (103–105), and plasma or purified immunoglobulins from individuals with LA can inhibit activated protein C in the presence or absence of protein S (106–108).

Inactivation of factors Va and VIIIa occurs on a phospholipid surface, and the extent of interference by APA in this process depends in part on the type and concentration of phospholipid in the system (106–108). The phospholipid composition of the membrane can

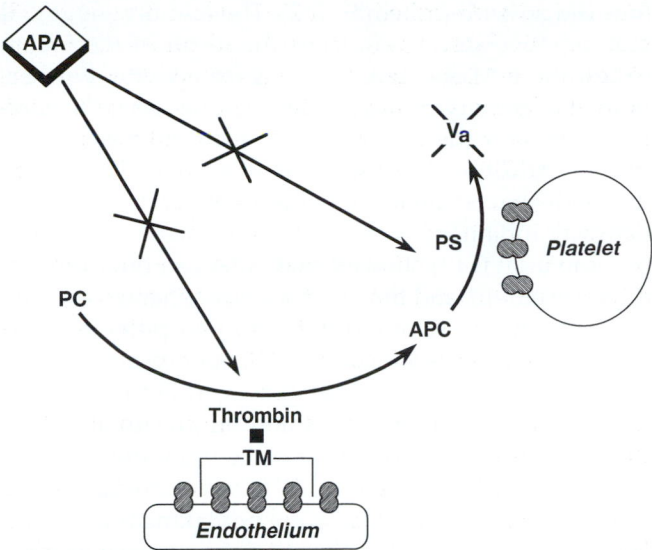

**FIGURE 38.2.** Possible mechanism of action of antibodies against phospholipid-binding proteins (APA). When thrombin binds to thrombomodulin (TM), it converts protein C to an activated form (APC) that in turn inhibits factors Va and VIIIa with protein S (PS) on a phospholipid (PL) surface, such as a platelet. *In vitro* studies have shown that APA can reduce the ability of APC to inactivate factors Va on a phospholipid surface. APA can also inhibit the activation of protein C (PC).

determine the relative activity of a particular enzymic reaction in the protein C system. Incorporation of phosphatidylethanolamine into vesicles containing phosphatidylserine potentiates the ability of activated protein C to inhibit factor Va by tenfold (109). In contrast, phosphatidylethanolamine has little influence on the activation of prothrombin (109). Additional studies have identified several individuals with LA whose plasma inhibited the anticoagulant activity of activated protein C in membranes containing phosphatidylethanolamine. This inhibition did not result from LA binding to protein C or protein S. The inhibitory activity could be removed by adsorption with liposomes containing phosphatidylethanolamine, and the ability to inhibit activated protein C did not correlate with LA activity. Thus, the composition of the membrane component is essential for optimal expression of activated protein C activity, but it is also the target for the immune complex that decreases the expression of activated protein C (110).

The importance of activated protein C is evident in individuals with an increased risk for venous thrombosis because of resistance to activated protein C (also known as factor V Leiden). Factor V Leiden is an Arg506Gln mutation in factor V that renders factor Va relatively resistant to inhibition by activated protein C (111). In a study of 30 IgG fractions from individuals with APA and thrombosis, three purified IgG fractions inhibited activated protein C activity, and an additional four did so with protein S (112). The authors suggested that negative studies could be the result of the failure to test the IgM and IgA fractions for activity. Furthermore, the activity may have declined between the clinical event and the sera for IgG purification being obtained. Additionally, the antibodies may have been directed against other proteins, such as tissue factor pathway inhibitor.

Rao et al (113) showed that APA can bind directly to prothrombin, and that the complex enhances the subsequent binding of prothrombin to phosphatidylserine or phosphatidylethanolamine. The significance of this enhanced binding is unclear, however, because it may not increase thrombin generation. In one small, retrospective, clinical study, seven of 11 individuals with a history of fetal wastage and APA had decreased levels of free protein S when they were not taking oral contraceptives or were pregnant (114). This decrease was not familial, and the individuals did not have antibodies to protein S as assessed by Western blotting. The authors suggested that protein S deficiency could be an additional factor in the increased risk for thrombosis in individuals with APA.

Sera from individuals with SLE contain IgG antiendothelial cell antibodies as well as IgG complexes that can bind to endothelial cells (115, 116). These might initiate vascular injury (115). However, no correlation between these antibodies and clinical features attributed to antiphospholipid syndrome has been found (117).

Immunoglobulins from individuals with APA may increase procoagulant activity by enhancing tissue factor expression on monocytes through their interaction with membrane phospholipids (118). The resulting thrombin generation could then activate platelets. APA may directly induce tissue factor expression in unprimed monocytes (119), or may increase the expression of tissue factor in monocytes primed with endotoxin (120). *In vitro* studies have shown that APA from individuals with SLE potentiate the procoagulant activity of endothelial cells with tumor necrosis factor.

Annexin V is a phospholipid-binding protein with antithrombotic activity that is synthesized by placental trophoblasts (121). Placentas from women with antiphospholipid syndrome and pregnancy losses have reduced annexin V immunostaining on the placental villous surfaces, thus suggesting that APA may block the transport of annexin V to the cell surfaces (121). More recent *in vitro* studies with endothelial cells as well as cultured primary trophoblasts have demonstrated that both cell lines have reduced levels of annexin V and reduced anticoagulant activity with APA (122). Kaburaki et al (123) found that in individuals with SLE and anti–annexin V antibodies, the incidence of venous and arterial thrombosis as well as fetal loss is increased above that for individuals with SLE who do not test positive for the antibodies (123).

Initial reports suggested that APA inhibits endothelial-derived prostaglandin $I_2$ (prostacyclin), a potent antagonist of platelet aggregation. In several *in vitro* studies, sera containing high-titer ACA or purified ACA alone inhibited the production of prostacyclin by thrombin-stimulated endothelial cells (124) or by fresh rings of rat aorta (125). Depending on the stimulus used, however, endothelial prostacyclin production can be decreased (126) or increased (104, 126) with APA.

At least two groups have reported that APA can bind directly to circulating platelets without necessarily inducing platelet activation or aggregation (127, 128). Others have shown that APA can bind to activated platelets, but this binding does not affect the release reaction or aggregation (129). Most human hybridoma LA do not bind to resting platelets *in vitro* (130). Galli et al (131) reported that 40% of individuals with antiphospholipid syndrome and thrombocytopenia had antibodies against glycoprotein GP IIb-IIIa, GP Ib-IX, or both, and that APA did not bind to resting platelets. APA is detected in sera from as many as 46% of individuals with ITP, but it does not appear to have a physiologic role in this disorder (51).

Direct evidence of a role for APA in inducing thrombosis comes from two reports in which the infusion of monoclonal or polyclonal APA into mice increased fetal resorption (132, 133) and decreased the fertility rate (133). Fetal loss resulted from a necrotizing, decidual vasculopathy and decidual necrosis that occurred on the maternal side of the circulation (132). Olee et al (134) have produced two human monoclonal IgG antibodies with ACA positivity from a individual with antiphospholipid syndrome. They demonstrated that one of the antibodies is thrombogenic in an anesthetized mouse model, in which a standardized injury is developed by pinching an exposed femoral vein.

# IMMUNOLOGY OF APA

As early as 1959, Loeliger (135) postulated that the antigen for antibodies against phospholipid also involved prothrombin. The idea that proteins and phospholipids (or proteins alone) were the targets for "antiphospholipid" antibodies, however, did not gain wide acceptance until 1990, after simultaneous reports that the antibodies may actually be directed against $\beta_2$-GP I (13–15). Thus, terminology of the antibodies as well as recognition of the antigens against which they are directed have been redefined and are still evolving.

APA is now recognized as being directed against $\beta_2$-GP I and prothrombin, but protein S and protein C may be antigens as well. The test systems and clinical associations are listed in Table 38.4. Cardiolipin alone is an antigen, but only in individuals with syphilis or other infections and no clinical sequelae.

In 1990, McNeil et al (13) and Galli et al (14) reported

**TABLE 38.4.** Detection of Antigens for APA

| Antigen | LA | ELISA$_a$ | Disease | Clinical Association |
|---|---|---|---|---|
| Prothrombin | Yes | No | Infections, antiphospholipid syndrome | Potential decrease in prothrombin with bleeding; thrombosis |
| $\beta_2$-GPI | | | | |
|   Type A | Yes | Yes | Antiphospholipid syndrome | Thrombosis |
|   Type B | No | Yes | Antiphospholipid syndrome | Thrombosis |
| Protein C | No | No | | Thrombosis |
| Protein S | No | No | | Thrombosis |
| Phospholipid, cardiolipin | No | Yes | Syphilis, other infections | None |

$^a$ *Cardiolipin.*

that purified antibodies with anticardiolipin activity bound to columns of phosphatidylserine or cardiolipin or to liposomes containing these phospholipids only with a plasma cofactor, which was identified as $\beta_2$-GP I. To bind with cardiolipin, antibodies from individuals with SLE required a cofactor, but antibodies from individuals with syphilis did not require the cofactor (15). The cofactor suppressed antibody binding in the latter case, thus suggesting it was competing with the antibody for binding sites on cardiolipin. McNeil et al (13) provided evidence that the APA may be directed to a complex of $\beta_2$-GP I and an anionic phospholipid or to a new epitope exposed by this protein binding to phospholipids, thereby enhancing the antigen–antibody interaction. $\beta_2$-GP I is a 50 kDa, proline-rich glycoprotein that can bind to negatively charged domains on lipoproteins, heparin, and platelets. At concentrations as low as 1 $\mu$g/ml, $\beta_2$-GP I displays cofactor activity in an ELISA (13, 14); normal plasma values are 200 $\mu$g/ml. Therefore, the cofactor is uniformly present at sufficient concentration in diluted individual plasma or serum to complex with cardiolipin in ELISAs, and it enhances APA binding. Immunization of mice and rabbits with human $\beta_2$-GP I induced antibodies that reacted as human autoantibodies in an ELISA with cardiolipin as antigen (and a source of $\beta_2$-GP I in the diluted sera) (136).

Hunt et al (137) identified the C-terminal region as important for lipid binding and cofactor activity. $\beta_2$-GP I contains five repeat motifs of approximately 60 amino acids; lipid binding depends on an intact region including Lys-317 and Thr-318. Furthermore, Hunt and Krilis (138) showed that the peptide Cys281–Cys288 was critical for binding to phospholipid. By expressing mutants of $\beta_2$-GP I in a baculovirus system, Igarashi et al (139) confirmed that the binding site for $\beta_2$-GP I to negatively charged phospholipid was in domain V (comprised of 82 amino acids), and that the epitope for the antibodies is cryptic and may require domain IV for exposure.

Matsuura et al (140) found that APA could recognize $\beta_2$-GP I without phospholipid if the protein was coated onto an oxygen-modified polystyrene surface. Oxygen atoms were introduced onto the polystyrene surface by irradiation with electron or gamma radiation, thus producing C-O and C=O groups on the oxidized surfaces. Roubey et al (141) additionally confirmed that IgG APA are low-affinity antibodies to $\beta_2$-GP I. The ability of antibodies to bind to $\beta_2$-GP I alone on a solid phase without cardiolipin depends on the density of the immobilized antigen, which must be sufficiently high to allow bivalent binding of the antibodies. Irradiation of solid-phase plates provides 1.5-fold more binding of $\beta_2$-GP I than untreated plates. Thus, antibodies do not bind to $\beta_2$-GP I in the fluid phase, but they will bind to an antigen of sufficient density to permit interaction with both antigen-binding sites of the IgG molecule. This is achieved by immobilization on cardiolipin-treated plates, cardiolipin-containing liposomes, or irradiated plates. Confirmation of antibody binding to $\beta_2$-GP I alone has been achieved with polyvinylchloride plates and processed polystyrene or COOH–surface polystyrene plates (142).

*In vitro*, $\beta_2$-GP I can inhibit contact activation (143) and the ability of platelets and phosphatidylserine/phosphatidylcholine liposomes to generate prothrombinase activity. This inhibition probably occurs when the protein binds to the negatively charged phospholipid, which results in rearrangement of the liposome, thereby reducing its prothrombinase activity; however, this rearrangement has not been demonstrated with platelets (144).

Although APA does not bind to neutral phospholipids such as phosphatidylethanolamine, they will bind to this particular phospholipid when it is presented in the hexagonal (II) phase (145). In this phase, phosphatidylethanolamine is comprised of lipid cylinders, with aqueous channels formed by the polar head groups (146). The LA activity of human hybridomas (146) or of immunoglobulins in individual plasma can be neutralized by phosphatidylethanolamine in a hexagonal, but not a bilayer, phase. Furthermore, mice immunized with phosphatidylethanolamine in the hexagonal phase develop APA that react with phosphatidylethanolamine and cardiolipin. Immunization with bilayer-phase phosphatidylethanolamine does not induce similar antibody formation (147).

The APA that develop in individuals with syphilis have several characteristics that differ from those of APA in individuals with SLE (148, 149). APA induced by syphilis do not demonstrate LA activity (150), and they appear to have a lower avidity for cardiolipin than those induced by SLE (151, 152). The syphilis-induced APA demonstrate greater reactivity with cardiolipin when it is formulated as a VDRL reagent, which is a mixture of phosphatidylcholine, cholesterol, and cardiolipin in an approximate mole ratio of 1.00 : 8.70 : 0.07. Using nuclear magnetic resonance (NMR) techniques, the physical nature of the VDRL antigen has been found to differ from that of cardiolipin in liposomal form (153). In one study, $IgG_1$ and $IgG_3$ with kappa chain predominated in individuals with syphilis, and $IgG_2$ and $IgG_4$ with lambda light chain were more prominent in individuals with SLE (152). This was confirmed by Arvieux et al (154), who reported that anti-$\beta_2$-GP I antibodies are primarily of the $IgG_2$ subclass in individuals with autoimmune disorders, whereas the ACA in individuals with infections is of the $IgG_3$ subclass.

Galli et al (155, 156) have described APA as antibodies that recognize the human prothrombin/phospholipid complex and, thus, have LA activity only or as ACA directed against $\beta_2$-GP I on anionic surfaces. They further postulated that some ACA (type A) inhibit coagulation reactions by increasing the binding of $\beta_2$-GP I to phospholipid, and that ACA type B have no anticoagulant activity (Table 38.4). In addition, they found that individuals with LA activity had a lower incidence of thromboembolic complications compared to those with ACA type A antibodies (21% versus 73%, respectively). The LA-type APA were more sensitive to the kaolin clotting time (KCT), whereas the ACA type A were more sensitive to dilute RVVT. The authors suggested that characterizing the properties of APA (as LA or as ACA type A) could help to identify individuals at risk for thromboembolic events.

Further proof of an antibody against $\beta_2$-GP I having LA activity was provided by Matsuda et al (157), who raised heterologous antibodies to human $\beta_2$-GP I and showed that the antibodies prolonged the dilute RVVT and KCT in human plasma containing $\beta_2$-GP I. These findings were confirmed by Roubey et al (158), who showed that anticardiolipin reactivity was $\beta_2$-GPI-dependent in individuals with autoimmune disease and also acted as an anticoagulant in plasmas containing $\beta_2$-GP I. In contrast, APA from one individual with syphilis had only anticardiolipin reactivity and did not act as an anticoagulant. This was also confirmed using rabbit

antihuman $\beta_2$-GP I and mouse monoclonal antibodies against $\beta_2$-GP I (159). In another study, the dilute phospholipid aPTT demonstrated higher sensitivity and the dilute RVVT greater specificity for detecting APA (160). These data depend on the reagents used in the assays, however, and therefore can vary.

## ELISA FOR APA (CARDIOLIPIN ASSAY) (SEE CHAPTER 26)

The cardiolipin assay is designed to measure the level of APA in individual sera quantitatively, using microtiter plates coated with cardiolipin or another negatively charged phospholipid (12, 23, 161, 162). Cardiolipin has been used primarily as the phospholipid, but other negatively-charged phospholipids such as phosphatidylserine provide similar reactivity (163, 164). The plates are blocked with bovine serum albumin or other appropriate reagents, and then individual sera diluted in fetal calf serum or adult bovine serum are added (23). The diluent for the individual sera should contain $\beta_2$-GP I to maximize binding of the antibody to the phospholipid antigen. Most test procedures now contain a known concentration of $\beta_2$-GP I. After an incubation period, the plates are washed and the APA detected by labeled antihuman IgG or IgM antibodies (23).

Test results are expressed in units of mpl or GPL. One mpl is equal to 1 μg of IgM APA, and 1 GPL is equal to 1 μg of IgG APA. The current recommendation is that assay results be described as "high positive" (>80 GPL or >60 mpl U/mL), "moderately positive" (20–80 GPL or 20–60 mpl U/mL), or "low positive" (<20 GPL or mpl U/mL). Samples with less than 10 GPL or mpl U/mL are considered to be negative (165–167). Concordance among laboratories for high-positive and negative IgG and IgM ACA is 90%; for medium-positive and low-positive results, agreement is greater than 75% (164).

Recurrent fetal loss and other thrombotic tendencies are most often associated with IgG in the moderately positive range (≥40 GPL U/mL). Ninety-percent of individuals with clinical symptoms have IgG ACA either alone or in association with IgM; 10% of such individuals have IgM alone (164). Although elevated levels of IgA ACA have been reported in association with thrombosis, the quantitation is undergoing standardization and the clinical significance is not yet defined.

## TESTING FOR LA (SEE CHAPTER 26)

Negatively-charged phospholipids greatly accelerate the rate of *in vitro* clotting by providing binding surfaces for factors II, VII, IX, and X (i.e., the vitamin K-dependent factors), and for factors Va and VIIIa (168, 169). The major source of phospholipids *in vivo* is platelets. *In vitro* assays such as the aPTT use bovine or rabbit brain phospholipids, which are called *partial thromboplastins*, because they do not contain tissue factor. The active phospholipid in these preparations is phosphatidylserine, but it comprises only a small fraction of the total phospholipid content. Crude sources of partial thromboplastins can be replaced by liposomes comprised of phosphatidylserine/phosphatidylcholine (170–172), freeze-thawed platelets, or even the neutral phospholipid phosphatidylethanolamine in the negatively charged (173) or the hexagonal phase (146, 174, 175). The PT assay uses rabbit brain thromboplastin, which contains tissue factor and phospholipids.

LA are APA that prolongs the clotting time of phospholipid-dependent coagulation assays by blocking the binding of coagulation factors to the acidic phospholipid surfaces or by enhancing the binding of $\beta_2$-GP I to the procoagulant phospholipid surface (156, 176). Initially, LA was identified by a prolonged aPTT that was not corrected by mixing individual and normal plasma. However, not all aPTT reagents are equally sensitive to the anticoagulant effect of APA (177). Therefore, LA is now described as an IgG or IgM antibody with inhibitory activity in a phospholipid-dependent assay (178). In individuals with a prolonged aPTT, addition of a

phospholipid such as platelets (179) or rabbit brain partial thromboplastin (180) to the test system shortens the aPTT if LA is present. The aPTT will remain prolonged, however, if a factor deficiency or an inhibitor other than LA is the cause of the abnormality (179, 180).

The criteria for LA were recently reviewed by a subcommittee of the Scientific and Standardisation Committee of the International Society on Thrombosis and Thromb Haemost (181). Recognizing that new LA assays are now available and that no single assay detects all APA, the committee suggested that more than one study be performed, followed by alteration of phospholipid (either increase or decrease) as a confirmatory test. In one study, detection of LA increased from 73% with one test to 90% with two tests (182). Assays based on a single concentration of phospholipid are screening tests, but in some situations, a screening and a confirmatory test cannot be separated. Knowledge of the patient's medical history is essential. Phospholipid dilution assays are currently used to detect LA, especially in individuals with a normal or only minimally prolonged aPTT (178, 183). The major tests for LA, which are described in more detail in Chapter 26, are listed in Table 38.5; their characteristics are listed in Table 38.6.

Perhaps the most sensitive test for LA is the kaolin clotting time (KCT). This assay, which does not require addition of phospholipid, measures the clotting time of plasma with the contact activator kaolin and calcium

**TABLE 38.5.  Assays to Detect and Verify LA**

| Test | | | | | Effect of LA |
|---|---|---|---|---|---|
| aPTT | Patient plasma | + Contact activator | + PL | → CaCl$_2$ | Normal or ↑ |
| KCT | Plasma | + Kaolin | + No PL | → CaCl$_2$ | ↑↑↑ |
| Dilute PL:aPTT | Plasma | + Silica | + Dilute PL | → CaCl$_2$ | ↑↑ |
| PNP | Plasma | + Activator | + Increased PL | → CaCl$_2$ | Normal |
| Dilute RVVT | Plasma | + RVV | + Dilute PL | → CaCl$_2$ | ↑↑ |
| TTI | Plasma | + Dilute thromboplastin | | → CaCl$_2$ | ↑↑ |

*Dilute PL:aPPT, dilute phospholipid aPTT; PNP, platelet neutralization procedure; TTI, tissue thromboplastin inhibition test; KCT, kaolin clotting time; RVVT, Russell viper venom time.*

**TABLE 38.6.  Characteristics of Assays for LA**

| | PNP | dRVVT | dPL-aPTT | KCT | TTI |
|---|---|---|---|---|---|
| Phospholipid | Added | Diluted | Diluted | None | Diluted |
| False positive with heparin | Yes | Yes | Yes | Yes | No |
| False positive with factor deficiency | No | No[a] | No[a] | No[a] | No[a] |
| False positive with factor inhibitors | No | Yes | Yes | Yes | Yes |
| Detects LA in plasmas with normal aPTT | No | Yes | Yes | Yes | Perhaps |

*dPL-aPTT, dilute phospholipid aPTT; dRVVT, dilute RVVT; PNP, platelet neutralization procedure; KCT, kaolin clotting time; TTI, tissue thromboplastin inhibition test.*
[a] *Test must be performed with a mixture of normal and patient plasma.*

(184, 185). The assay is influenced by residual platelets in plasma, especially if plasma has been exposed to a freeze–thaw cycle (186).

Assays using dilute phospholipid include the dilute RVVT (187–189) and the dilute phospholipid aPTT (17, 160, 170), both of which involve only a single dilution of phospholipid, such as phosphatidylserine/phosphatidylcholine liposomes (160). The dilute RVVT is a phospholipid dilution assay in which Russell viper venom, which activates factor X, is used to initiate coagulation with dilute phospholipid and calcium (187). One laboratory reported a sensitivity of 97% and a specificity of 100% in detecting LA when two tests were used (the dilute RVVT and the dilute aPTT-LA [American Bioproducts, Parsippany, New Jersey] (189).

The dilute phospholipid aPTT is essentially a modified aPTT, in which a dilute phospholipid is used to enhance sensitivity. The dilute phospholipid aPTT is sensitive to heparin, but it can also be used for individuals receiving warfarin if the individual plasma is first mixed with normal plasma to restore sufficient levels of coagulation factors (160).

The thromboplastin inhibition assay is a PT performed with a dilution of the thromboplastin reagent (7). It has been modified to provide increased sensitivity (190), but this modification has resulted in false-positive tests with heparin. The dilute PT has achieved increased sensitivity when a recombinant tissue thromboplastin has been used (Innovin; Baxter Diagnostics, Miami, FL) (191).

A newer assay based on a ratio of the clotting times of individual plasma obtained with the venom textarin to that of the venom ecarin has recently been developed as well (192). Textarin activates prothrombin in a phospholipid-dependent fashion, whereas ecarin does not require phospholipid. Thus, the ratio of the clotting times is increased in the plasma of individuals with APA having anticoagulant activity. The test can be falsely positive, however, if individual plasma contains heparin or antibodies against factor V.

There is no standard for LA, so the sensitivity and specificity of a given assay can be compared against arbitrary standards only, especially if the aPTT is normal or only minimally prolonged (187). Estimates for the percentage of plasma samples testing positive for LA that are also positive in ACA assays range from 60% (193) to 90% (17). Many plasma samples that test positive for LA will have low levels of ACA (17). Thus, the poor correlation between the LA and ACA assays in detecting plasma that is positive for APA may result from the boundaries established for abnormal values in the ACA assay among individual laboratories.

In the general population, prolonged aPTT most frequently results from LA (194). Correction studies frequently are not helpful in determining the presence of

LA since they can be normal even in the presence of LA (195, 196). LA usually does not increase prolongation of the aPTT with time, because the antibody is directed against the phospholipid added to the assay. In some cases, however, inhibition is time dependent (197), which could suggest an antibody to a specific factor, such as factor VIII (198).

Even although LA may appear to be the cause of a prolonged aPTT, factor levels are measured to exclude a true factor deficiency or another inhibitor. If individual plasma has a prolonged aPTT and a normal PT, then levels of factors VIII, IX, XI, and XII are measured. Frequently, LA are sufficiently potent to induce an apparent decrease in these coagulation factors; in this case, factor activity should increase toward the true value when measured in serial dilutions of the individual plasma. The dilution of the plasma also dilutes the inhibitory activity of the LA and allows for more accurate determination of the factor activity. If the individual has a true factor deficiency, such as of factor VIII, that results from an antibody directed against the factor, then determination of the factor level will not be influenced by the dilution at which the plasma is tested.

If the PT is also prolonged, then factors II, V, VII, and X should be measured. In plasma with LA, the PT occasionally can be slightly prolonged without a true factor deficiency (195, 196). The most common true factor deficiency that is associated with the LA is prothrombin deficiency, as described earlier.

# TREATMENT OF ANTIPHOSPHOLIPID SYNDROME OR LABORATORY MANIFESTATIONS OF APA

A major goal in treatment of antiphospholipid syndrome is to reduce other risk factors for thrombosis, such as uncontrolled hypertension, smoking, and use of oral contraceptives (199). Treatment of asymptomatic individuals with LA or with moderate or high titers of ACA is controversial. Some physicians prescribe low-dose aspirin (75 mg/day), then use anticoagulation with warfarin or heparin at times of increased risk for thrombosis (199). The role of corticosteroids or plasmapheresis has not been documented for individuals with the antiphospholipid syndrome, however, and they are reserved for "catastrophic antiphospholipid syndrome," which is defined as acute, multiorgan failure in individuals with APA (200). In this rare syndrome, the mortality rate is 60% (200). Plasmapheresis may be beneficial in individuals who do not respond to heparin, corticosteroids, or immunosuppressive agents.

A randomized study (Warfarin Aspirin Recurrent

**TABLE 38.7.** Antithrombotic Treatments for Patients with APA and Thrombosis

| Treatment | Patient-years | Events per Year of Follow-up | References |
|---|---|---|---|
| None | 161 | 0.19 | 202 |
| | 281 | 0.29 | 203 |
| Aspirin[a] | 28 | 0.36 | 202 |
| | 240 | 0.18 | 203 |
| Warfarin (INR) | | | |
| ≤1.9 | 11 | 0.57 | 202 |
| <3.0 | 141 | 0.23 | 203 |
| 2.0–2.9 | 41 | 0.07 | 202 |
| ≥3.0 | 110[b] | 0.000 | 202 |
| | 197[c] | 0.015 | 203 |
| Nonfatal | | 0.031 | 202 |
| bleeding[d] | | 0.071 | 203 |

[a] Aspirin doses were 80–325 mg and daily in Rosove and Brewer (202) and 75 mg daily in Khamashka et al (203).
[b] Some patients also received aspirin.
[c] Patients received no aspirin.
[d] Associated with INR above 3 in patients receiving warfarin.

Stroke Study) to estimate the rate of recurrent thrombosis in individuals with neurologic events resulting from antiphospholipid syndrome, and to determine the relative efficacies of aspirin and warfarin, is currently underway (201). At present, however, there is no consensus regarding the best means of anticoagulation. Some individuals with brief, focal neurologic manifestations such as migraine auras have been successfully treated with phenytoin or carbamazepine in addition to their anticoagulation (201).

Individuals with antiphospholipid syndrome and arterial or venous thromboembolism are at high risk for recurrence if anticoagulation is discontinued after the first episode of thrombosis (Table 38.7) (202, 203). In one retrospective study, the recurrence rate was highest (1.30 per patient-year) in the first 6 months after discontinuation (203). In contrast, continuation of warfarin (INR ≥ 3.0) and low-dose aspirin (75 mg daily) resulted in 100% freedom from thrombosis during 40 patient years of follow-up. In a prospective study comparing the clinical manifestations of individuals with primary and secondary antiphospholipid syndrome during a 2-year period, seven of eight individuals who developed recurrent thrombosis while on warfarin had INR values of less than 3 (28). The value of anticoagulation is high with an INR of 3.0; however, the degree of anticoagulation must be judged according to the risk for bleeding.

A prospective study of the clinical relevance of APA in individuals with venous thromboembolism but without SLE showed no recurrence in individuals receiving warfarin at INR intensities of between 2.0 and 2.9 and no difference in the recurrence rate in individuals with and individuals without APA (31). However, these authors evaluated a individual population different from that described in Table 38.7. Thus, their conclusions may not be valid for individuals with underlying primary or secondary antiphospholipid syndrome (31).

Controlled, prospective studies are underway, but in the meantime, an INR of 3 is recommended for individuals with antiphospholipid syndrome and thrombosis if there are no contraindications. Low-dose aspirin may or may not be added, depending on whether thrombotic manifestations such as superficial thrombophlebitis persist. Individuals with LA or ACA associated with underlying infections or using medications are not at risk for thrombosis and do not require anticoagulation (82, 83, 89).

## SUMMARY

The most exciting advances in APA have been identification of the antigens for antibody recognition and new approaches to its management. APA is actually directed against epitopes of phospholipid-binding proteins such as $\beta_2$-GP I and prothrombin. Additional proteins may be recognized in future studies. The ways that the complexes promote thrombosis are still not well defined, however, and additional immune or nonimmune mechanisms may be involved.

Standardized tests for LA are being developed. However, because of the heterogeneity of the antibodies, one test will not detect all APA or even all antibodies with potential LA activity. At present, laboratory assessment of LA includes measuring the APA by ELISA whenever there is a question regarding an underlying thrombotic disorder or antiphospholipid syndrome. Correlation between potency of the LA and titer of the ACA is poor. Assays using prothrombin or $\beta_2$-GP I alone may not offer additional benefits over those using cardiolipin combined with a known concentration of $\beta_2$-GP I. For individuals presenting with LA as an incidental finding in association with a history of an infection or medication known to induce LA, quantitative measurement of ACA is not necessary.

Retrospective studies have shown that recurrent thrombosis in individuals with antiphospholipid syndrome can be successfully prevented by maintaining anticoagulation with warfarin at an INR of 3. Aspirin can be used as well if additional symptoms such as superficial phlebitis are noted. Slowly, questions concerning the antiphospholipid syndrome are being answered through laboratory investigations and empiric observations of individual response to treatment. Eventually, investigations at these different levels may clearly establish the pathophysiology of the antiphospholipid syndrome.

# REFERENCES

1. Conley CL, Rathbun HK, Morse WI II et al. Circulating anticoagulant as a cause of hemorrhagic diathesis in man. Bull Johns Hopkins Hosp 1948; 83:288–296.
2. Conley CL, Hartmann RC. A hemorrhagic disorder caused by circulating anticoagulant in patients with disseminated lupus erythematosus [Abstract]. J Clin Invest 1952;31:621–622.
3. Mueller JF, Ratnoff O, Heinle RW. Observations on the characteristics of an unusual circulating anticoagulant. J Lab Clin Med 1951;38:254–261.
4. Margolius A Jr, Jackson DP, Ratnoff OD. Circulating anticoagulants: a study of 40 cases and a review of the literature. Medicine 1961;40:145–202.
5. Feinstein DI, Rapaport SI. Acquired inhibitors of blood coagulation. Prog Hemost Thromb 1972;1:75–95.
6. Boxer M, Ellman L, Carvalho A. The lupus anticoagulant. Arthritis Rheum 1976;19:1244–1248.
7. Schleider MA, Nachman RL, Jaffe EA et al. A clinical study of the lupus anticoagulant. Blood 1976;48:499–509.
8. Elias M, Eldor A. Thromboembolism in patients with the 'lupus'-type circulating anticoagulant. Arch Intern Med 1984;144:510–515.
9. Bowie EJW, Thompson JH Jr, Pascuzzi CA et al. Thrombosis in systemic lupus erythematosus despite circulating anticoagulants. J Lab Clin Med 1963;62:416–430.
10. Mueh JR, Herbst KD, Rapaport SI. Thrombosis in patients with the lupus anticoagulant. Ann Intern Med 1980;92:156–159.
11. Gastineau DA, Kazmier FJ, Nichols WL et al. Lupus anticoagulant: an analysis of the clinical and laboratory features of 219 cases. Am J Hematol 1985;19:265–275.
12. Harris EN, Gharavi EA, Boey ML et al. Anticardiolipin antibodies: detection by radioimmunoassay and association with thrombosis in systemic lupus erythematosus. Lancet 1983;ii:1211–1214.
13. McNeil HP, Simpson RJ, Chesterman CN et al. Anti-phospholipid antibodies are directed against a complex antigen that includes a lipid-binding inhibitor of coagulation: beta 2-glycoprotein I (apolipoprotein H). Proc Natl Acad Sci U S A 1990;87:4120–4124.
14. Galli M, Comfurius P, Maassen C et al. Anticardiolipin antibodies (ACA) directed not to cardiolipin but to a plasma protein cofactor. Lancet 1990; 335:1544–1547.
15. Matsuura E, Igarashi Y, Fujimoto M et al. Anticardiolipin cofactor(s) and differential diagnosis of autoimmune disease. Lancet 1990;336:177–178.
16. Sammaritano LR, Gharavi AE, Lockshin MD. Antiphospholipid antibody syndrome: immunologic and clinical aspects. Semin Arthritis Rheum 1990; 20:81–96.
17. Alving BM, Barr CF, Tang DB. Correlation between lupus anticoagulants
and anticardiolipin antibodies in patients with prolonged activated partial thromboplastin times. Am J Med 1990;88:112–116.
18. McNeil HP, Chesterman CN, Krilis SA. Immunology and clinical importance of antiphospholipid antibodies. Adv Immunol 1991;49:193–280.
19. Asherson RA, Khamashta MA, Ordi-Ros J et al. The "primary" antiphospholipid syndrome: major clinical and serological features. Medicine 1989; 68:366–374.
20. Harris EN. The anti-phospholipid syndrome—an introduction. In: Harris EN, Exner T, Hughes GR, Asherson RA, eds. Phospholipid-binding antibodies. Boston: CRC Press, 1991:373–376.
21. Asherson RA. A "primary" antiphospholipid syndrome? J Rheumatol 1988;15:1742–1745.
22. Asherson RA. "Primary" anti-phospholipid syndrome. In: Harris EN, Exner T, Hughes GRV, Asherson RA, eds. Phospholipid-binding antibodies. Boston: CRC Press, 1991:378–386.
23. Harris EN. Antiphospholipid antibodies. Br J Haematol 1990;74:1–9.
24. Hughes GRV, Harris EN, Gharavi AE. The anticardiolipin syndrome. J Rheumatol 1986;13:486–489.
25. Mackworth-Young CG, Loizou S, Walport MJ. Primary antiphospholipid syndrome: features of patients with raised anticardiolipin antibodies and no other disorder. Ann Rheum Dis 1989;48:362–367.
26. Asherson RA. Anti-phospholipid antibodies. Clinical complications reported in medical literature. In: Harris EN, Exner T, Hughes GRV, Asherson RA, eds. Phospholipid-binding antibodies. Boston: CRC Press, 1991: 388–402.
27. Vila P, Hernández MC, López-Hernández MF et al. Prevalence, follow-up and clinical significance of the anticardiolipin antibodies in normal subjects. Thromb Haemost 1994;72:209–213.
28. Vianna JL, Khamashta MA, Ordi-Ros J et al. Comparison of the primary and secondary antiphospholipid syndrome: a European multicenter study of 114 patients. Am J Med 1994;96:3–9.
29. Finazzi G, Brancaccio V, Moia M et al. Natural history and risk factors for thrombosis in 360 patients with antiphospholipid antibodies: a four-year prospective study from the Italian registry. Am J Med 1996;100: 530–536.
30. Ginsburg KS, Liang MH, Newcomer L et al. Anticardiolipin antibodies and the risk for ischemic stroke and venous thrombosis. Ann Intern Med 1992;117:997–1002.
31. Ginsberg JS, Wells PS, Brill-Edwards P et al. Antiphospholipid antibodies and venous thromboembolism. Blood 1995;86:3685–3691.
32. Simioni P, Prandoni P, Zanon E et al. Deep venous thrombosis and lupus anticoagulant. A case-control study. Thromb Haemost 1996;76:187–189.
33. Cabral AR, Amigo MC, Cabiedes J et al. The antiphospholipid / cofactor syndromes: a primary variant with antibodies to $\beta_2$-glycoprotein I but no antibodies detectable in standard antiphospholipid assays. Am J Med 1996;101:472–481.
34. Boey ML, Colaco CB, Gharavi AE et al. Thrombosis in systemic lupus erythematosus: striking association with the presence of circulating lupus anticoagulant. Br Med J (Clin Res) 1983;287:1021–1023.
35. Long AA, Ginsberg JS, Brill-Edwards P et al. The relationship of antiphospholipid antibodies to thromboembolic disease in systemic lupus erythematosus: a cross-sectional study. Thromb Haemost 1991;66:520–524.
36. Cronin ME, Biswas RM, Van der Straeton C et al. IgG and IgM anticardiolipin antibodies in patients with lupus with anticardiolipin antibody associated clinical syndromes. J Rheumatol 1988;15:795–798.
37. Love PE, Santoro SA. Antiphospholipid antibodies: anticardiolipin and the lupus anticoagulant in systemic lupus erythematosus (SLE) and in non-SLE disorders. Ann Intern Med 1990;112:682–698.
38. Petri M, Rheinschmidt M, Whiting-O'Keefe Q et al. The frequency of lupus anticoagulant in systemic lupus erythematosus: a study of sixty consecutive patients by activated partial thromboplastin time, Russell viper venom time, and anticardiolipin antibody level. Ann Intern Med 1987;106: 524–531.
39. Mackworth-Young C, Chan J, Harris N et al. High incidence of anticardiolipin antibodies in relatives of patients with systemic lupus erythematosus. J Rheumatol 1987;14:723–726.
40. Arnett FC, Olsen ML, Anderson KL et al. Molecular analysis of major histocompatibility complex alleles associated with the lupus anticoagulant. J Clin Invest 1991;87:1490–1495.
41. Harris EN, Chan JKH, Asherson RA et al. Thrombosis, recurrent fetal loss and thrombocytopenia. Arch Intern Med 1986;146:2153–2156.
42. Ishii Y, Nagasawa K, Mayumi T et al. Clinical importance of persistence of anticardiolipin antibodies in systemic lupus erythematosus. Ann Rheum Dis 1990;49:387–390.
43. Toubi E, Khamashta MA, Panarra A et al. Association of antiphospholipid antibodies with central nervous system disease in systemic lupus erythematosus. Am J Med 1995;99:397–401.
44. Alarcon-Segovia D, Deleze M, Oria CV et al. Antiphospholipid antibodies and the antiphospholipid syndrome in systemic lupus erythematosus. A prospective analysis of 500 consecutive patients. Medicine 1989;68: 353–365.
45. Asherson RA, Merry P, Acheson JF et al. Antiphospholipid antibodies: a risk factor for occlusive ocular vascular disease in systemic lupus erythe-

matosus and the 'primary' antiphospholipid syndrome. Ann Rheum Dis 1989;48:358–361.

46. Escalante A, Brey RL, Mitchell BD et al. Accuracy of anticardiolipin antibodies in identifying a history of thrombosis among patients with systemic lupus erythematosus. Am J Med 1995;98:559–565.

47. Horbach DA, van Oort E, Donders RC et al. Lupus anticoagulant is the strongest risk factor for both venous and arterial thrombosis in patients with systemic lupus erythematosus. Comparison between different assays for the detection of antiphospholipid antibodies. Thromb Haemost 1996; 76:916–924.

48. Fijnheer R, Horbach DA, Donders RC. Factor V Leiden, antiphospholipid antibodies and thrombosis in systemic lupus erythematosus. Thromb Haemost 1996;76:514–517.

49. Harris EN, Asherson RA, Gharavi AE et al. Thrombocytopenia in SLE and related autoimmune disorders: association with anticardiolipin antibody. Br J Haematol 1985;59:227–230.

50. Harris EN, Gharavi AE, Hegde U et al. Anticardiolipin antibodies in autoimmune thrombocytopenic purpura. Br J Haematol 1985;59:231–234.

51. Stasi R, Stipa E, Masi M et al. Prevalence and clinical significance of elevated antiphospholipid antibodies in patients with idiopathic thrombocytopenic purpura. Blood 1994;84:4203–4208.

52. Levine SR, Deegan MJ, Futrell N et al. Cerebrovascular and neurologic disease associated with antiphospholipid antibodies: 48 cases. Neurology 1990;40:1181–1189.

53. Coull BM, Levine SR, Brey RL. The role of antiphospholipid antibodies in stroke. Neurol Clin 1992;10:125–143.

54. Brey RL, Hart RG, Sherman DG et al. Antiphospholipid antibodies and cerebral ischemia in young people. Neurology 1990;40:1190–1196.

55. Olsen ML, O'Conner S, Arnett FC et al. Autoantibodies and rheumatic disorders in a neurology inpatient population: a prospective study. Am J Med 1991;90:479–488.

56. Trimble M, Bell DA, Brien W et al. The antiphospholipid syndrome: prevalence among patients with stroke and transient ischemic attacks. Am J Med 1990;88:593–597.

57. Kushner MJ. Prospective study of anticardiolipin antibodies in stroke. Stroke 1990;21:295–298.

58. Montalban J, Codina A, Ordi J et al. Antiphospholipid antibodies in cerebral ischemia. Stroke 1991;22:750–753.

59. Hess DC, Krauss J, Adams RJ et al. Anticardiolipin antibodies: a study of frequency in TIA and stroke. Neurology 1991;41:525–528.

60. Nencini P, Baruffi MC, Abbate R et al. Lupus anticoagulant and anticardiolipin antibodies in young adults with cerebral ischemia. Stroke 1992;23: 189–193.

61. Muir KW, Squire IB, Alwan W et al. Anticardiolipin antibodies in an unselected stroke population. Lancet 1994;344:452–456.

62. Leung WH, Wong KL, Lau CP et al. Association between antiphospholipid antibodies and cardiac abnormalities in patients with systemic lupus erythematosus. Am J Med 1990;89:411–419.

63. Nihoyannopoulos P, Gomez PM, Joshi J et al. Cardiac abnormalities in systemic lupus erythematosus. Association with raised anticardiolipin antibodies. Circulation 1990;82:369–375.

64. Khamashta MA, Cervera R, Asherson RA et al. Association of antibodies against phospholipids with heart valve disease in systemic lupus erythematosus. Lancet 1990;335:1541–1544.

65. Galve E, Ordi J, Barquinero J et al. Valvular heart disease in the primary antiphospholipid syndrome. Ann Intern Med 1992;116:293–298.

66. Gleason CB, Stoddard MF, Wagner SG et al. A comparison of cardiac valvular involvement in the primary antiphospholipid syndrome versus anticardiolipin-negative systemic lupus erythematosus. Am Heart J 1993; 125:1123–1129.

67. Ford PM, Ford SE, Lillicrap DP. Association of lupus anticoagulant with severe valvular heart disease in systemic lupus erythematosus. J Rheumatol 1988;15:597–600.

68. Kattwinkel N, Villanueva AG, Labib SB et al. Myocardial infarction caused by cardiac microvasculopathy in a patient with the primary antiphospholipid syndrome. Ann Intern Med 1992;116:974–976.

69. Chartash EK, Lans DM, Paget SA et al. Aortic insufficiency and mitral regurgitation in patients with systemic lupus erythematosus and the antiphospholipid syndrome. Am J Med 1989;86:407–412.

70. Sletnes KE, Smith P, Abdelnoor M et al. Antiphospholipid antibodies after myocardial infarction and their relation to mortality, reinfarction, and non-haemorrhagic stroke. Lancet 1992;339:451–453.

71. Pope JM, Canny CL, Bell DA. Cerebral ischemic events associated with endocarditis, retinal vascular disease, and lupus anticoagulant. Am J Med 1991;90:299–309

72. Leventhal LJ, Borofsky MA, Bergey PD et al. Antiphospholipid antibody syndrome with right atrial thrombosis mimicking an atrial myxoma. Am J Med 1989;87:111–113.

73. Bajaj SP, Rapaport SI, Fierer DS et al. A mechanism for the hypoprothrombinemia of the acquired hypoprothrombinemia-lupus anticoagulant syndrome. Blood 1983;61:684–692.

74. Edson JR, Vogt JM, Hasegawa DK. Abnormal prothrombin crossed-immu-

75. Fleck RA, Rapaport SI, Rao LV. Anti-prothrombin antibodies and the lupus anticoagulant. Blood 1988;72:512–519.

76. Bajaj SP, Rapaport SI, Barclay S et al. Acquired hypoprothrombinemia due to non-neutralizing antibodies to prothrombin: mechanism and management. Blood 1985;65:1538–1543.

77. Arvieux J, Darnige L, Caron C et al. Development of an ELISA for autoantibodies to prothrombin showing their prevalence in patients with lupus anticoagulants. Thromb Haemost 1995;74:1120–1125.

78. Lee MT, Nardi MA, Hu G et al. Transient hemorrhagic diathesis associated with an inhibitor of prothrombin with lupus anticoagulant in a 1½-year-old girl: report of a case and review of the literature. Am J Hematol 1996; 51:307–314.

79. Bernini JC, Buchanan GR, Ashcraft J. Hypoprothrombinemia and severe hemorrhage associated with a lupus anticoagulant. J Pediatr 1993;123: 937–939.

80. Keane A, Woods R, Dowding V et al. Anticardiolipin antibodies in rheumatoid arthritis. Br J Rheumatol 1987;26:346–350.

81. Lillicrap DP, Pinto M, Benford K et al. Heterogeneity of laboratory test results for antiphospholipid antibodies in patients treated with chlorpromazine and other phenothiazines. Am J Clin Pathol 1990;93:771–775.

82. Canoso RT, de Oliveira RM. Chlorpromazine-induced anticardiolipin antibodies and lupus anticoagulant: absence of thrombosis. Am J Hematol 1988;27:272–275.

83. Canoso RT, Sise HS. Chlorpromazine-induced lupus anticoagulant and associated immunologic abnormalities. Am J Hematol 1982;13:121–129.

84. Bell WR, Boss GR, Wolfson JS. Circulating anticoagulant in the procainamide-induced lupus syndrome. Arch Intern Med 1977;137:1471–1473.

85. Edwards RL, Rick ME, Wakem CJ. Studies on a circulating anticoagulant in procainamide-induced lupus erythematosus. Arch Intern Med 1981;141: 1688–1690.

86. Hess E. Drug-related lupus. N Engl J Med 1988;318:1460–1462.

87. Reidenberg MM. Aromatic amines and the pathogenesis of lupus erythematosus. Am J Med 1983;75:1037–1042.

88. Li GC, Greenberg CS, Currie MS. Procainamide-induced lupus anticoagulants and thrombosis. South Med J 1988;81:262–264.

89. List AF, Doll DC. Thrombosis associated with procainamide-induced lupus anticoagulant. Acta Haematol 1989;82:50–52.

90. Asherson RA, Zulman J, Hughes GR. Pulmonary thromboembolism associated with procainamide induced lupus syndrome and anticardiolipin antibodies. Ann Rheum Dis 1989;48:232–235.

91. Heyman MR, Flores RH, Edelman BB et al. Procainamide-induced lupus anticoagulant. South Med J 1988;81:934–936.

92. Zarrabi MH, Zucker S, Miller F et al. Immunologic and coagulation disorders in chlorpromazine-treated patients. Ann Intern Med 1979;91:194–199.

93. Cohen AJ, Philips TM, Kessler CM. Circulating coagulation inhibitors in the acquired immunodeficiency syndrome. Ann Intern Med 1986;104: 175–180.

94. Mackworth-Young CG, Harris EN, Steere AC et al. Anticardiolipin antibodies in Lyme disease. Arthritis Rheum 1988;31:1052–1056.

95. Vaarala O, Palosuo T, Kleemola M et al. Anticardiolipin response in acute infections. Clin Immunol Immunopathol 1986;41:8–15.

96. McNally T, Purdy G, Mackie IJ et al. The use of an anti-β₂-glycoprotein I assay for discrimination between anticardiolipin antibodies associated with infection and increased risk of thrombosis. Br J Haematol 1995;91: 471–473.

97. Arnout J. The pathogenesis of the antiphospholipid syndrome: a hypothesis based on parallelisms with heparin-induced thrombocytopenia. Thromb Haemost 1996;75:536–541.

98. Greaves M, Hill MB, Phipps J et al. The pathogenesis of the antiphospholipid syndrome. Thromb Haemost 1996;76:817–818.

99. Santoro SA. Antiphospholipid antibodies and thrombotic predisposition: underlying pathogenetic mechanisms. Blood 1994;83:2389–2391.

100. Pengo V, Biasiolo A, Fior MG. Binding of autoimmune cardiolipin-reactive antibodies to heparin: a mechanism of thrombosis? Thromb Res 1995;78: 371–378.

101. Shibata S, Harpel PC, Gharavi A et al. Autoantibodies to heparin from patients with antiphospholipid antibody syndrome inhibit formation of antithrombin III-thrombin complexes. Blood 1993;83:2532–2540.

102. Esmon CT. The regulation of natural anticoagulant pathways. Science 1987;235:1348–1352.

103. Freyssinet M, Wiesel ML, Gauchy J et al. An IgM lupus anticoagulant that neutralizes the enhancing effect of phospholipid on purified endothelial thrombomodulin activity—a mechanism for thrombosis. Thromb Haemost 1986;55:309–313.

104. Cariou R, Tobelem G, Bellucci S et al. Effect of lupus anticoagulant on antithrombogenic properties of endothelial cells—inhibition of thrombomodulin-dependent protein C activation. Thromb Haemost 1988;60:54–58.

105. Tsakiris DA, Settas L, Makris PE et al. Lupus anticoagulant-antiphospholipid antibodies and thrombophilia. Relation to protein C-protein S-thrombomodulin. J Rheumatol 1990;17:785–789.

106. Marciniak E, Romond EH. Impaired catalytic function of activated protein

C: a new *in vitro* manifestation of lupus anticoagulant. Blood 1989;74:2426–2432.

107. Malia RG, Kitchen S, Greaves M et al. Inhibition of activated protein C and its cofactor protein S by antiphospholipid antibodies. Br J Haematol 1990;76:101–107.

108. Lo SC, Salem HH, Howard MA et al. Studies of natural anticoagulant proteins and anticardiolipin antibodies in patients with the lupus anticoagulant. Br J Haematol 1990;76:380–386.

109. Smirnov MD, Esmon CT. Phosphatidylethanolamine incorporation into vesicles selectively enhances factor Va inactivation by activated protein C. J Biol Chem 1994;269:816–819.

110. Smirnov MD, Triplett DT, Comp PC et al. On the role of phosphatidylethanolamine in the inhibition of activated protein C activity by antiphospholipid antibodies. J Clin Invest 1995;95:309–316.

111. Bertina RM, Koeleman BP, Koster T et al. Mutation in blood coagulation factor V associated with resistance to activated protein C. Nature 1994;369:64–67.

112. Oosting JD, Derksen RH, Bobbink IWG, Hackeng TM, Bouma BN, de Groot PG. Antiphospholipid antibodies directed against a combination of phospholipids with prothrombin, protein C, or protein S: an explanation for their pathogenic mechanism? Blood 1993;81:2618–2625.

113. Rao LVM, Hoang AD, Rapaport SI. Mechanism and effects of the binding of lupus anticoagulant IgG and prothrombin to surface phospholipid. Blood 1996;88:4173–4182.

114. Parke AL, Weinstein RE, Bona RD et al. The thrombotic diathesis associated with the presence of phospholipid antibodies may be due to low levels of free protein S. Am J Med 1992;93:49–56.

115. Cines DB, Lyss AP, Reeber M et al. Presence of complement-fixing anti-endothelial cell antibodies in systemic lupus erythematosus. J Clin Invest 1984;73:611–625.

116. Hashemi S, Smith CD, Izaguirre CA. Anti-endothelial cell antibodies: detection and characterization using a cellular enzyme-linked immunosorbent assay. J Lab Clin Med 1987;109:434–440.

117. Vismara A, Meroni PL, Tincani A et al. Relationship between anti-cardiolipin and anti-endothelial cell antibodies in systemic lupus erythematosus. Clin Exp Immunol 1988;74:247–253.

118. Reverter JC, Tassies D, Font J et al. Hypercoagulable state in patients with antiphospholipid syndrome is related to high induced tissue factor expression on monocytes and to low free protein S. Arteriosclerosis Thromb Vasc Biol 1996;6:1319–1326.

119. Kornberg A, Blank M, Kaufman S et al. Induction of tissue factor-like activity in monocytes by anti-cardiolipin antibodies. J Immunol 1994;153:1328–1332.

120. Schved JF, Gris JC, Ollivier V et al. Procoagulant activity of endotoxin or tumor necrosis factor activated monocytes is enhanced by IgG from patients with lupus anticoagulant. Am J Hematol 1992;41:92–96.

121. Rand JH, Wu XX, Guller S et al. Reduction of annexin-V (placental anticoagulant protein-I) on placental villi of women with antiphospholipid antibodies and recurrent spontaneous abortion. Am J Obstet Gynecol 1994;171:1566–1572.

122. Rand JH, Wu XX, Andree HAM et al. Pregnancy loss in the antiphospholipid-antibody syndrome–a possible thrombogenic mechanism. N Engl J Med 1997;337:154–160.

123. Kaburaki J, Kuwana M, Yamamoto M et al. Clinical significance of anti-annexin V antibodies in patients with systemic lupus erythematosus. Am J Hematol 1997;54:209–213.

124. Watson KV, Schorer AE. Lupus anticoagulant inhibition of *in vitro* prostacyclin release is associated with a thrombosis-prone subset of patients. Am J Med 1991;90:47–53.

125. Carreras LO, Vermylen JG. "Lupus" anticoagulant and thrombosis-possible role of inhibition of prostacyclin formation. Thromb Haemost 1982;48:38–40.

126. Hasselaar P, Derksen RH, Blokzijl L et al. Thrombosis associated with antiphospholipid antibodies cannot be explained by effects on endothelial and platelet prostanoid synthesis. Thromb Haemost 1988;59:80–85.

127. Out HJ, de Groot PG, van Vliet M et al. Antibodies to platelets in patients with anti-phospholipid antibodies. Blood 1991;77:2655–2659.

128. Lin YL, Wang CT. Activation of human platelets by the rabbit, anticardiolipin antibodies. Blood 1992;80:3135–3143.

129. Shi W, Chong BH, Chesterman CN. β$_2$-Glycoprotein I is a requirement for anticardiolipin antibodies binding to activated platelets: differences with lupus anticoagulant. Blood 1993;81:1255–1262.

130. Rauch J, Meng QH, Tannenbaum H. Lupus anticoagulant and antiplatelet properties of human hybridoma autoantibodies. J Immunol 1987;139:2598–2604.

131. Galli M, Daldossi M, Barbui T. Anti-glycoprotein 1b/1x and IIb/IIIa antibodies in patients with antiphospholipid antibodies. Thromb Haemost 1994;71:571–575.

132. Branch DW, Dudley DJ, Mitchell MD et al. Immunoglobulin G fractions from patients with antiphospholipid antibodies cause fetal death in BALB/c mice. A model for autoimmune fetal loss. Am J Obstet Gynecol 1990;163:210–216.

133. Blank M, Cohen J, Toder V et al. Induction of anti-phospholipid syndrome in naive mice with mouse lupus monoclonal and human polyclonal anti-cardiolipin antibodies. Proc Natl Acad Sci U S A 1991;88:3069–3073.

134. Olee T, Pierangeli SS, Handley HH et al. A monoclonal IgG anticardiolipin antibody from a patient with the antiphospholipid syndrome is thrombogenic in mice. Proc Natl Acad Sci U S A 1996;93:8606–8611.

135. Loeliger A. Prothrombin as co-factor of the circulating anticoagulant in systemic lupus erythematosus? Thromb Diath Haemorrh 1959;3:237–256.

136. Gharavi AE, Sammaritano LR, Wen J et al. Induction of antiphospholipid autoantibodies by immunization with β$_2$-glycoprotein I (apolipoprotein H). J Clin Invest 1992;90:1105–1109.

137. Hunt JE, Simpson RJ, Krilis SA. Identification of a region of β$_2$-glycoprotein I critical for lipid binding and anti-cardiolipin antibody cofactor activity. Proc Natl Acad Sci U S A 1993;90:2141–2145.

138. Hunt J, Krilis S. The fifth domain of B$_2$-glycoprotein I contains a phospholipid binding site (Cys 281-Cys 288) and a region recognized by anticardiolipin antibodies. J Immunol 1994;152:653–659.

139. Igarashi M, Matsura E, Igarashi Y et al. Human β$_2$-glycoprotein I as an anticardiolipin cofactor determined using mutants expressed by a baculovirus system. Blood 1996;87:3262–3270.

140. Matsuura E, Igarashi Y, Yasuda T et al. Anticardiolipin antibodies recognize β$_2$-glycoprotein I structure altered by interacting with an oxygen modified solid phase surface. J Exp Med 1994;179:457–462.

141. Roubey RA, Eisenberg RA, Harper MF et al. "Anticardiolipin" autoantibodies recognize β$_2$-glycoprotein I in the absence of phospholipid. J Immunol 1995;154:954–960.

142. Pengo V, Biasiolo A, Fior MG. Autoimmune antiphospholipid antibodies are directed against a cryptic epitope expressed when β$_2$-glycoprotein I is bound to a suitable surface. Thromb Haemost 1995;73:29–34.

143. Schousboe I. β$_2$-glycoprotein I: a plasma inhibitor of the contact activation of the intrinsic blood coagulation pathway. Blood 1985;66:1086–1091.

144. Nimpf J, Bevers EM, Bomans PH et al. Prothrombinase activity of human platelets is inhibited by β$_2$-glycoprotein-I. Biochim Biophys Acta 1986;884:142–149.

145. Rauch J, Janoff AS. Role of monoclonal antibodies in understanding the interactions between anti-phospholipid antibodies and phospholipids. In: Harris EN, Exner T, Hughes GRV, Asherson RA, eds. Phospholipid-binding antibodies. Boston: CRC Press, 1991:107–122.

146. Rauch J, Tannenbaum M, Tannenbaum H et al. Human hybridoma lupus anticoagulants distinguish between lamellar and hexagonal phase lipid systems. J Biol Chem 1986;261:9672–9677.

147. Rauch J, Janoff AS. Phospholipid in the hexagonal II phase is immunogenic: evidence for immunorecognition of nonbilayer lipid phases *in vivo*. Proc Natl Acad Sci U S A 1990;87:4112–4114.

148. Colaco CB, Male DK. Anti-phospholipid antibodies in syphilis and a thrombotic subset of SLE: distinct profiles of epitope specificity. Clin Exp Immunol 1985;59:449–456.

149. Harris EN, Gharavi AE, Wasley GD et al. Use of an enzyme-linked immunosorbent assay and of inhibition studies to distinguish between antibodies to cardiolipin from patients with syphilis or autoimmune disorders. J Infect Dis 1988;157:23–31.

150. Johansson EA, Lassus A. The occurrence of circulating anticoagulants in patients with syphilitic and biologically false positive antilipoidal antibodies. Ann Clin Res 1974;6:105–108.

151. Harris EN, Gharavi AE, Tincani A et al. Affinity purified anti-cardiolipin and anti-DNA antibodies. J Clin Lab Immunol 1985;17:155–162.

152. Levy RA, Gharavi AE, Sammaritano LR et al. Characteristics of IgG antiphospholipid antibodies in patients with systemic lupus erythematosus and syphilis. J Rheumatol 1990;17:1036–1041.

153. Janoff AS, Rauch J. The structural specificity of anti-phospholipid antibodies in autoimmune disease. Chem Phys Lipids 1986;40:315–332.

154. Arvieux J, Roussel B, Ponard D et al. IgG$_2$ subclass restriction of anti-β$_2$ glycoprotein I antibodies in autoimmune patients. Clin Exp Immunol 1994;95:310–315.

155. Galli M, Comfurius P, Barbui T et al. Anticoagulant activity of β$_2$-glycoprotein I is potentiated by a distinct subgroup of anticardiolipin antibodies. Thromb Haemost 1992;68:297–300.

156. Galli M, Finazzi G, Bevers EM et al. Kaolin clotting time and dilute Russell's viper venom time distinguish between prothrombin-dependent and β$_2$-glycoprotein I-dependent antiphospholipid antibodies. Blood 1995;86:617–623.

157. Matsuda J, Gohchi K, Tsukamoto M et al. Anticoagulant activity of an anti-β$_2$-glycoprotein I antibody is dependent on the presence of β$_2$-glycoprotein I. Am J Hematol 1993;44:187–191.

158. Roubey RA, Pratt CW, Buyon JP et al. Lupus anticoagulant activity of autoimmune antiphospholipid antibodies is dependent upon β$_2$-glycoprotein I. J Clin Invest 1992;90:1100–1104.

159. Brandt JT. Antibodies to β$_2$-glycoprotein I inhibit phospholipid-dependent coagulation reactions. Thromb Haemost 1993;70:598–602.

160. Alving BM, Barr CF, Johansen LE et al. Comparison between a one-point dilute phospholipid APTT and the dilute Russell viper venom time for verification of lupus anticoagulants. Thromb Haemost 1992;67:672–678.

161. Loizou S, McCrea JD, Rudge AC et al. Measurement of anti-cardiolipin

antibodies by an enzyme-linked immunosorbent assay (ELISA): standardization and quantitation of results. Clin Exp Immunol 1985;62:738–745.

162. Smolarsky M. A simple radioimmunoassay to determine binding of antibodies to lipid antigens. J Immunol Methods 1980;38:85–93.

163. Falcon CR, Hoffer AM, Forastiero RR et al. Clinical significance of various ELISA assays for detecting antiphospholipid antibodies. Thromb Haemost 1990;64:21–25.

164. Gharavi AE, Harris EN, Asherson RA et al. Anticardiolipin antibodies: isotype distribution and phospholipid specificity. Ann Rheum Dis 1987; 46:1–6.

165. Harris EN. The second international anti-cardiolipin standardization workshop/the Kingston Anti-Phospholipid Antibody Study (KAPS) Group. Am J Clin Pathol 1990;94:476–484.

166. Lockshin MD. Antiphospholipid antibody and antiphospholipid antibody syndrome. Curr Opin Rheumatol 1991;3:797–802.

167. Stewart MW, Etches WS, Russell AS et al. Detection of antiphospholipid antibodies by flow cytometry: rapid detection of antibody isotype and phospholipid specificity. Thromb Haemost 1993;70:603–607.

168. Zwaal RFA. Membrane and lipid involvement in blood coagulation. Biochim Biophys Acta 1978;515:163–205.

169. Zwaal RFA, Bevers EM, Rosing J. Phospholipids and the clotting process. In: Harris EN, Exner T, Hughes GRV, Asherson RA, eds. Phospholipid-binding antibodies. Boston: CRC Press, 1991:32–56.

170. Alving BM, Baldwin PE, Richards RL et al. The dilute phospholipid APTT: a sensitive assay for verification of lupus anticoagulants. Thromb Haemost 1985;54:709–712.

171. Kelsey PR, Stevenson KJ, Poller L. The diagnosis of lupus anticoagulants by the activated partial thromboplastin time—the central role of phosphatidyl serine. Thromb Haemost 1984;52:172–175.

172. Ueno M, Kimura M, Nozima Y et al. Effect of phospholipid vesicles in the blood coagulation process in vitro. Chem Pharm Bull 1982;30:4570–4572.

173. Bangham AD. A correlation between surface charge and coagulant action of phospholipids. Nature 1961;192:1197–1198.

174. Exner T, Triplett DA, Taberner DA et al. Comparison of test methods for the lupus anticoagulant: international survey on lupus anticoagulants-I (ISLA-1). Thromb Haemost 1990;64:478–484.

175. Rauch J, Tannenbaum M, Janoff AS. Distinguishing plasma lupus anticoagulants from anti-factor antibodies using hexagonal (II) phase phospholipids. Thromb Haemost 1989;62:892–896.

176. Pengo V, Thiagarajan P, Shapiro SS et al. Immunological specificity and mechanism of action of IgG lupus anticoagulants. Blood 1987;70:69–76.

177. Brandt JT, Triplett DA, Musgrave K et al. The sensitivity of different coagulation reagents to the presence of lupus anticoagulants. Arch Pathol Lab Med 1987;111:120–124.

178. Exner T, Triplett DA, Taberner D et al. Guidelines for testing and revised criteria for lupus anticoagulants. SSC Subcommittee for the standardization of lupus anticoagulants. Thromb Haemost 1991;65:320–322.

179. Triplett DA, Brandt JT, Kaczor D et al. Laboratory diagnosis of lupus inhibitors: a comparison of the tissue thromboplastin inhibition procedure with a new platelet neutralization procedure. Am J Clin Pathol 1983;79: 678–682.

180. Rosove MH, Ismail M, Koziol BJ et al. Lupus anticoagulants: improved diagnosis with a kaolin clotting time using rabbit brain phospholipid in standard and high concentrations. Blood 1986;68:472–478.

181. Brandt JT, Triplett DA, Alving B et al. Criteria for the diagnosis of lupus anticoagulants: an update on behalf of the subcommittee on lupus anticoagulant/antiphospholipid antibody of the scientific and standardisation committee of the ISTH. Thromb Haemost 1995;74:1185–1190.

182. Anonymous. Comparison of a standardized procedure with current laboratory practices for the detection of lupus anticoagulant in France. Working group on hemostasis of the Société Francaise de Biologie Clinique. Thromb Haemost 1993;70:781–786.

183. Lo SC, Oldmeadow MJ, Howard MA et al. Comparison of laboratory tests used for identification of the lupus anticoagulant. Am J Hematol 1989;30: 213–220.

184. Exner T, Rickard KA, Kronenberg H. A sensitive test demonstrating lupus anticoagulant and its behavioural patterns. Br J Haematol 1978;40:143–151.

185. Exner T. Comparison of two simple tests for the lupus anticoagulant. Am J Clin Pathol 1985;83:215–218.

186. Anonymous. Detection of lupus-like anticoagulant: current laboratory practice in the United Kingdom. The lupus anticoagulant working party. J Clin Pathol 1990;43:73–75.

187. Thiagarajan P, Pengo V, Shapiro SS. The use of the dilute Russell viper venom time for the diagnosis of lupus anticoagulants. Blood 1986;68: 869–874.

188. Exner T, Papadopoulos G, Koutts J. Use of a simplified dilute Russell's viper venom time (DRVVT) confirms heterogeneity among 'lupus and anticoagulants.' Blood Coagul Fibrinolysis 1990;1:259–266.

189. Schjetlein R, Wisloff F. An evaluation of two commercial test procedures for the detection of lupus anticoagulant. Am J Clin Pathol 1995;103: 108–111.

190. Liu HW, Wong KL, Lin CK et al. The reappraisal of dilute tissue thromboplastin inhibition test in the diagnosis of lupus anticoagulant. Br J Haematol 1989;72:229–234.

191. Forastiero RR, Cerrato GS, Carreras LO. Evaluation of recently described tests for detection of the lupus anticoagulant. Thromb Haemost 1994;72: 728–733.

192. Triplett DA, Stocker KF, Unger GA et al. The textarin/ecarin ratio: a confirmatory test for lupus anticoagulants. Thromb Haemost 1993;70:925–931.

193. Triplett DA, Brandt JT, Musgrave KA et al. The relationship between lupus anticoagulants and antibodies to phospholipid. JAMA 1988;259:550–554.

194. Kitchens CS. Prolonged activated partial thromboplastin time of unknown etiology: a prospective study of 100 consecutive cases referred for consultation. Am J Hematol 1988;27:38–45.

195. Lazarchick J, Kizer J. The laboratory diagnosis of lupus anticoagulants. Arch Pathol Lab Med 1989;113:177–180.

196. Triplett DA, Brandt JT, Maas RL. The laboratory heterogeneity of lupus anticoagulants. Arch Pathol Lab Med 1985;109:946–951.

197. Clyne LP, White PF. Time dependency of lupuslike anticoagulants. Arch Intern Med 1988;148:1060–1063.

198. Kasper CK, Aledort LM, Counts RB et al. A more uniform measurement of factor VIII inhibitors. Thromb Diath Haemorrh 1975;34:869–872.

199. Khamashta MA. Management of thrombosis in the antiphospholipid syndrome. Lupus 1996;5:463–466.

200. Asherson RA, Piette JC. The catastrophic antiphospholipid syndrome 1996: acute multi-organ failure associated with antiphospholipid antibodies: a review of 31 patients. Lupus 1996;5:414–417.

201. Brey RL, Levine SR. Treatment of neurologic complications of antiphospholipid antibody dyndrome. Lupus 1996;5:473–476.

202. Rosove MH, Brewer PMC. Antiphospholipid thrombosis: clinical course after the first thrombotic event in 70 patients. Ann Intern Med 1992;117: 303–308.

203. Khamashta MA, Cuadrado MJ, Mujic F et al. The management of thrombosis in the antiphospholipid-antibody syndrome. N Engl J Med 1995;332: 993–997.

# SECTION 9

# THROMBOTIC DISORDERS

# CHAPTER 39

# THE RELATIONSHIP BETWEEN THROMBOSIS AND ATHEROSCLEROSIS

David R. Dobroski, LeRoy E. Rabbani, and Joseph Loscalzo

## INTRODUCTION

Coronary artery disease and cerebral artery disease continue to be the leading causes of mortality and morbidity in the western world, accounting for up to 50% of all deaths in the United States, Europe, and Japan (1). The underlying pathogenesis of these clinical entities is atherosclerotic vascular disease, which is marked by the chronic evolution of atheromata during a clinically quiescent phase, followed by an acute thrombotic or thromboembolic event that renders the heretofore quiescent atherosclerotic plaque "active." Intermittent plaque rupture and thrombosis, with subsequent neointima formation, play a critical role in the temporal progression of atherosclerotic lesions. This process ultimately precipitates acute ischemic syndromes, such as unstable angina, and myocardial as well as cerebral infarction (1–3). Fig. 39.1 depicts the events contributing to the temporal progression of atherosclerotic lesion development. Although the relationship between atherosclerosis and thrombosis has long been recognized, it is only recently that major emphasis has been placed on the important role of thrombosis in both the prolonged evolutionary phase of the atherosclerotic plaque, as well as its acute, clinically active phase (2).

## HISTORICAL BACKGROUND

There have historically been two major classes of hypotheses to explain atherogenesis (4). In 1856, Virchow first proposed the imbibition theory of atherosclerosis, which suggested that blood lipids transudate into the arterial wall, where they interact with arterial wall components and affect cellular proliferation, resulting in atherosclerotic plaque formation (4–6). The second class of hypotheses was based on the so-called encrustation theory of atherosclerosis (4). Originally proposed by von Rokitansky in 1852 and modified by Duguid in 1946, this theory argued that thrombosis plays a major role in the atherosclerotic process, and that atherosclerotic plaque pathogenesis results from the abnormal deposition of fibrin and other blood components into the arterial intima (4, 7, 8).

The evolution of these initial attempts to explain atherogenesis has led to the currently prevailing theory of atherosclerosis, Ross' widely held revised response-to-injury model, which posits that the crucial initiating event in atherosclerosis is actually endothelial cell injury, occurring as a result of various factors such as hypertension and hypercholesterolemia (3, 9). As summarized in Fig. 39.2, endothelial cell injury initiates a cascade of cellular events, including growth factor secretion, monocyte attachment to the endothelium, monocyte growth factor secretion, subendothelial migration of monocytes, foam cell and fatty streak formation, and further release of mitogens, resulting in formation of the atheromatous plaque (1, 3). Indeed, the multifaceted nature of the response-to-injury hypothesis underscores the fact that the classic imbibition and encrustation theories of atherosclerosis may not have been mutually exclusive, and in fact demonstrated remarkable insight

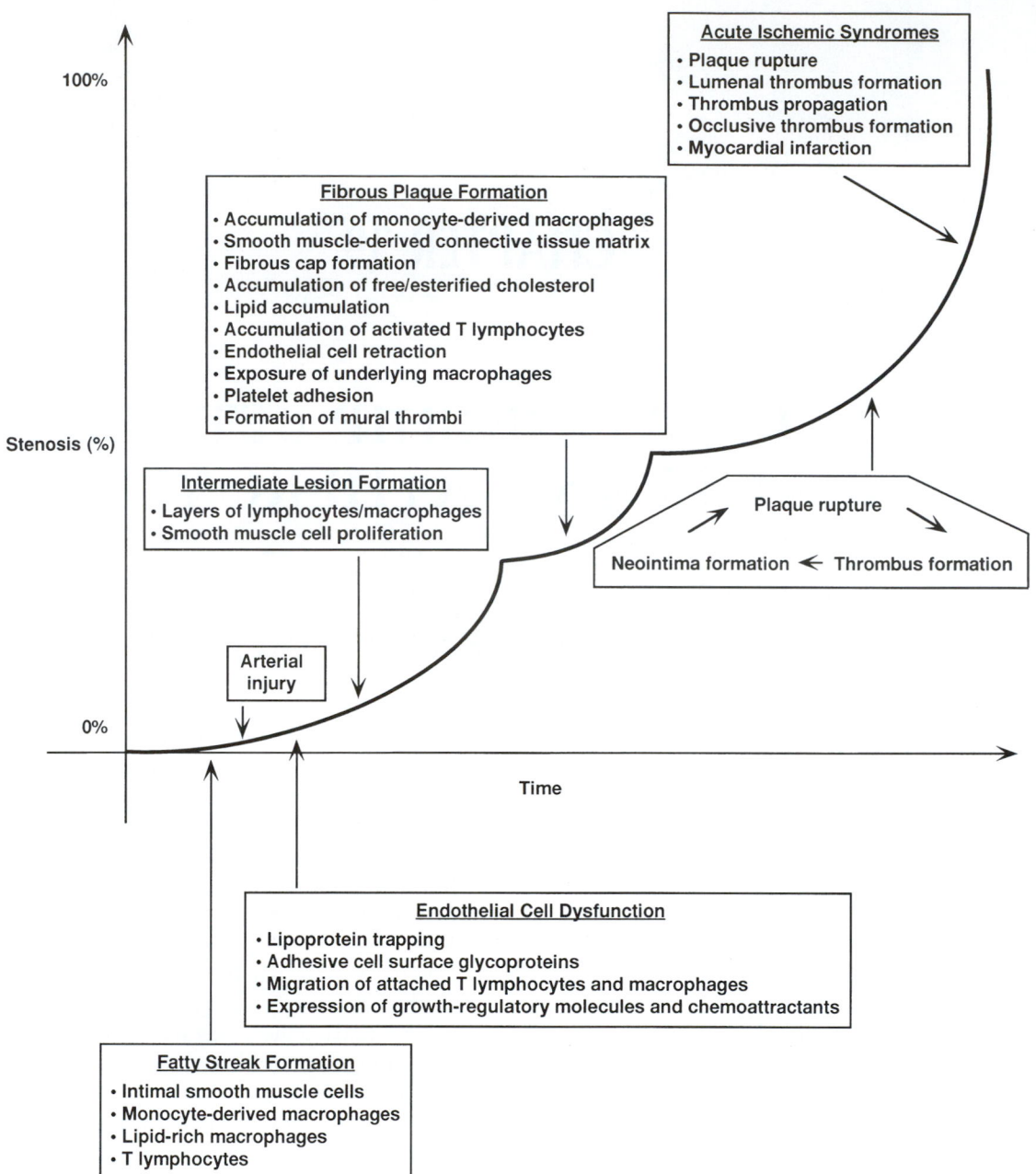

**FIGURE 39.1.** Development of the atherosclerotic lesion. Initial fatty streak formation subsequently leads to intermediate lesion formation after the accumulation of macrophages, T lymphocytes, and the proliferation of smooth muscle cells. Further accumulation of lipid, macrophages, and activated T lymphocytes, along with the formation of a smooth muscle cell-derived connective tissue matrix and fibrous cap, result in the formation of the fibrous plaque. Endothelial cell retraction and injury result in the formation of mural thrombi, which, if not occlusive, are subsequently covered by neointima formation. Continued proliferation of smooth muscle cells results in additional growth of the lesion. Acute ischemic syndromes result when plaque rupture leads to the formation of an occlusive thrombus, with the resultant Q-wave or non–Q-wave myocardial infarction.

into this complex disease process (4). More recently, both *in vitro* and *in vivo* studies have established that low-density lipoprotein (LDL) can undergo an oxidative modification that targets it for uptake by the macrophage through the acetyl LDL, or scavenger, receptor (5). Oxidized LDL, as well as other postsecretory modifi-cations of LDL, increases its atherogenicity, and un-doubtedly plays a significant role in enhancing athero-sclerosis (5). These more recent observations have led to further modification of the response-to-injury hy-pothesis, accounting for this important role of oxidized LDL in atherogenesis (9).

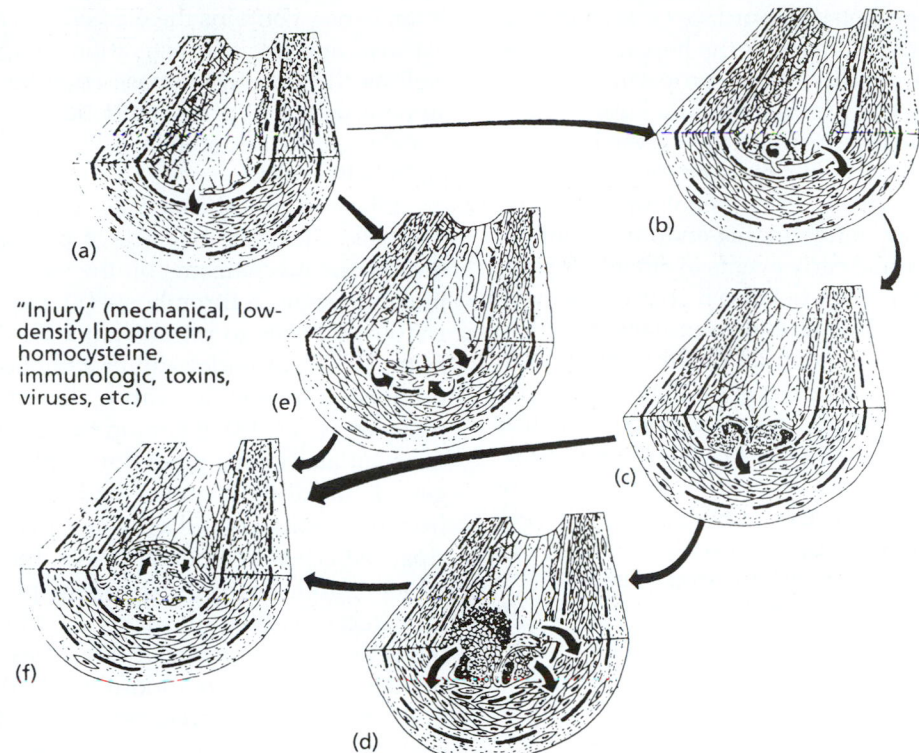

"Injury" (mechanical, low-density lipoprotein, homocysteine, immunologic, toxins, viruses, etc.)

**FIGURE 39.2.**   The response-to-injury hypothesis of atherosclerosis. Injury to the endothelium, from a variety of sources, leads to endothelial cell dysfunction. This results in the increased adherence of monocytes/macrophages and T lymphocytes to the endothelium, which subsequently migrate and localize subendothelially. Lipid accumulation by macrophages results in the formation of large foam cells, and these, along with T cells and smooth muscle cells, form a fatty streak. In this way, the initial fatty streak can progress to form an intermediate fibrofatty lesion, ultimately forming a fibrous lesion, then a fibrous plaque. As cells accumulate within the lesions, some of the lipid-laden macrophages can separate the endothelial cells and migrate back into the bloodstream. These sites then become a nidus for the formation of platelet mural thrombi, especially at locations such as vascular branch sites and bifurcations, where irregular blood flow can occur. Platelets within these thrombi then release potent growth-regulatory molecules, which join with those released by activated macrophages and, possibly, smooth muscle cells. This process results in the establishment of a cell network within the lesion, consisting of platelets, activated macrophages, smooth muscle cells, T lymphocytes, and endothelium, all releasing growth-regulatory molecules and cytokines, which contribute to the progression of these lesions of atherosclerosis to fibrous plaques or to advanced, complicated lesions. (Adapted with permission from Ross R. The pathogenesis of atherosclerosis—an update. N Engl J Med 1986;314:488–500.)

# THE FOUR MAJOR CELL TYPES OF ATHEROSCLEROSIS: THEIR INTERACTION WITH THE CO-AGULATION/FIBRINOLYTIC SYSTEMS

The revised response-to-injury hypothesis of atherosclerosis highlights the importance of four major cell types involved in the pathogenesis of atherosclerosis: endothelial cells, monocyte/macrophages, vascular smooth muscle cells, and platelets (1, 3, 9). Each of these four cell types is capable of secreting various mitogens that are crucial to the initiation and progression of the atherosclerotic plaque (1, 9). In addition, each participates in several important interactions with the blood components of both the coagulation and fibrinolytic systems.

## ENDOTHELIUM

One of the critical functions of the normal vascular endothelium (see Chapter 13) is the maintenance of thromboresistance (1, 10). In this regard, normal endothelium is capable of releasing prostacyclin (PGI$_2$), endothelium-derived relaxing factor (EDRF), or nitric oxide (NO), and plasminogen activators, and expressing ecto-ADPase activity. Endothelium also facilitates the vascular uptake and degradation of prothrombotic vasoactive amines, and binds, inactivates, and cleaves thrombin (1, 11). Moreover, thrombomodulin, a cofactor for the thrombin-catalyzed activation of the antithrombotic protein C, is expressed on the endothelial cell surface (1, 11). Furthermore, glycosaminoglycans such as the heparan sulfates, which also possess antithrombotic properties, are expressed on the surface of vascular endothelium (1, 12).

These thromboresistant properties of the endothelium, however, are markedly reduced by endothelial dysfunction or injury (1, 12). Endothelial injury leading to denudation, or even nondenuding endothelial injury, both believed to be initial early events in atherosclerosis, are capable of altering endothelial cell structure as well as function, thus rendering the endovascular surface less thromboresistant (1). An example of this alteration in endothelial function is the observation that the vascular production of prostacyclin is reduced in experimental atherosclerosis in the rabbit (13). Advanced atherosclerotic plaques have been shown to possess decreased endothelial-dependent production of PGI$_2$ and EDRF (14).

Under certain conditions, the vascular endothelium not only loses its thromboresistant properties, but also directly participates in prothrombotic processes (1). In this regard, endothelium is able to bind coagulation factors and promote activation of both factor X and prothrombin (1, 11). Moreover, von Willebrand factor (vWF), a polymeric protein necessary for platelet adhesion to the vessel wall, is secreted by endothelial cells in response to thrombin generation, most notably under conditions of high shear stress (15). Factor XIa and the factor VIIa-tissue factor pathway can activate factor IX bound to endothelium (1, 16). Endothelial cell-bound factor IXa can activate factor X in the presence of factor VIII and calcium (1, 16). Furthermore, cultured endothelial cells *in vitro* are able to secrete factor V, as well as serve as an exogenous phospholipid source, thereby catalyzing thrombin generation (1). The vascular endothe-

lium, hence, contains the elements to assemble both the extrinsic and intrinsic activation complex of factor X, as well as the prothrombinase complex (1, 11). Fig. 39.3 summarizes the prothrombotic changes in dysfunctional (injured) endothelial cells, compared with normal endothelial cells.

Injury of endothelial cells, as occurs early in atherosclerosis, alters the balance of procoagulant and antithrombotic mechanisms on the surface of the endothelium, in favor of thrombosis (1). Exposure of cultured endothelial cells to interleukin-1 (IL-1), tumor necrosis factor (TNF), or endotoxin *in vitro* induces tissue factor production thereby activating the extrinsic coagulation pathway (1, 17, 18). It should be noted that interleukin-1, an inflammatory mediator implicated in the pathogenesis of atherosclerosis, and TNF are both derived from macrophages and activated T cells, which are principal cell types in atherosclerosis. Interleukin-1 also inhibits endothelial cell-dependent protein C activation (17). Recently, IL-4, also a product of activated T cells, has been found to neutralize the downregulation of endothelial cell thrombomodulin activity caused by IL-1, TNF, and lipopolysaccharide, but not to affect the increase in endothelial cell tissue factor activity caused by those cytokines (19). Fig. 39.4 depicts the role of inflammatory cytokines in the endothelial cell response to injury.

## MACROPHAGES

Peripheral blood monocytes/macrophages participate in blood coagulation via numerous mechanisms (20). A major role in this process is played by tissue factor

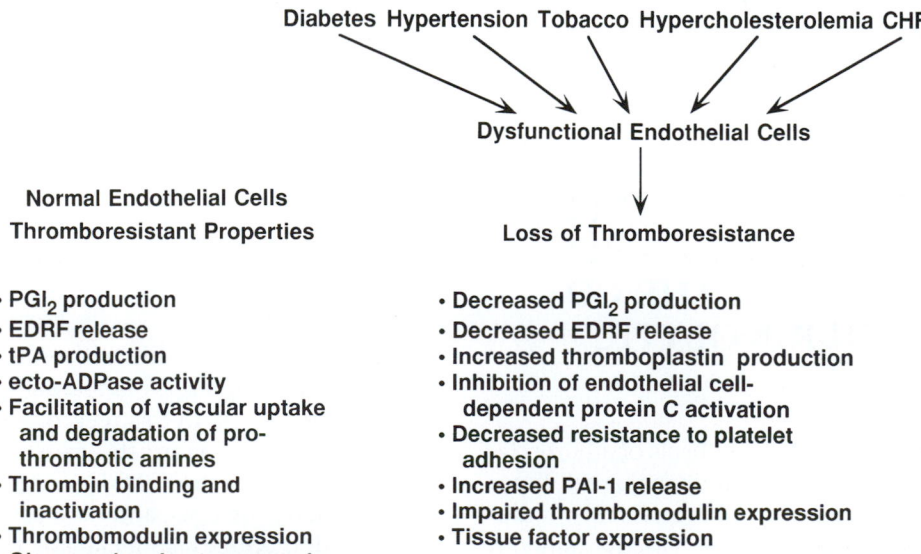

**FIGURE 39.3.** Thromboresistant properties of normal and dysfunctional endothelial cells. Endothelial cell injury from a variety of causes (hypertension, diabetes, hypercholesterolemia, tobacco, congestive heart failure) results in the loss of these thromboresistant properties.

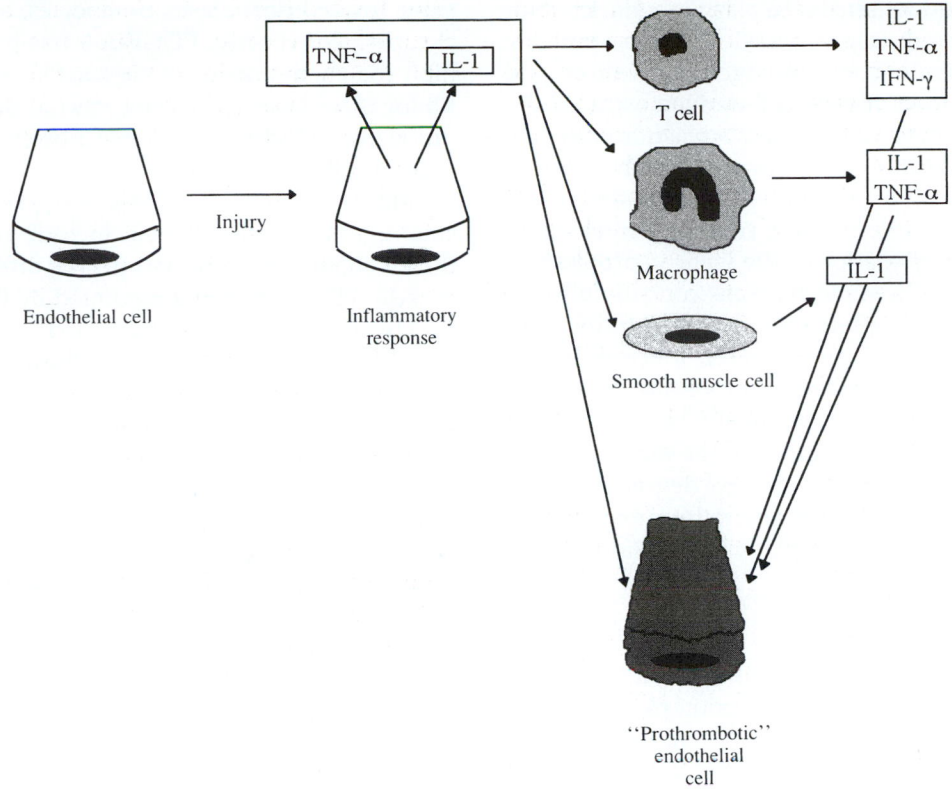

**FIGURE 39.4.**   The role of cytokines in the process of atherothrombosis. Endothelial cell injury leads to an inflammatory response by the endothelial cell, resulting in the production of the cytokine TNF-α and IL-1. These cytokines, in turn, stimulate T cells, macrophages, and smooth muscle cells to produce IL-1, TNF-α, and interferon-γ (IFN-γ). These then act on the endothelial cell to induce a ''prothrombotic'' state, characterized by activities that include the secretion of PDGF-AA and PDGF-BB, tissue factor expression (which causes activation of the extrinsic coagulation pathway), decreased endothelial cell-dependent protein C activation, and increased release of PAI-1.

(thromboplastin), a requisite cofactor in the factor VIIa-catalyzed activation of factors IX and X (see Chapter 4) (20). Monocyte tissue factor expression is low or absent normally, but may increase dramatically in response to various pathologic stimuli, such as endotoxin (20–22). Monocyte-initiated blood coagulation is composed of factor VII/VIIa binding to tissue factor on the cell surface, resulting in factor Xa formation (20, 23, 24). Monocytes can activate factor X, independently of tissue factor, via the Mac-1 (CDIIb/CD18) receptor (20, 25). Furthermore, monocyte cell surface expression of factor V/Va activity promotes the formation of the prothrombinase complex (Chapter 1), and thereby, fibrin (20, 26–28). In addition, macrophages isolated from carotid artery plaques of individuals undergoing carotid endarterectomy have enhanced factor V and factor VII-dependent procoagulant activity (29). Monocyte procoagulant activity can be neutralized by the lipoprotein-associated inhibitor of the tissue factor/factor VIIa complex, termed tissue factor pathway inhibitor (TFPI) (see Chapter 4) (20, 30). TFPI is linked to dense LDL, and minimal oxidation of the LDL-bound TFPI has been demonstrated to inactivate TFPI's

anticoagulant effect (31). The stable prostacyclin analog iloprost and prostaglandin $E_1$ inhibit monocyte procoagulant activity *in vitro*, suggesting that endothelium-derived prostacyclin may be a physiologic modulator of monocyte tissue factor expression (20).

Monocytes/macrophages are intimately involved with the fibrinolytic system. Exposure of monocytes to stimuli such as bacterial lipopolysaccharide (endotoxin) or phorbol esters results in augmented secretion of plasminogen activator inhibitor-type 2 (PAI-2) (32–34). There is differential regulation of tissue factor and PAI-2 by human mononuclear cells, as evidenced by divergent tissue factor and PAI-2 responses of monocytes exposed to alloantigen (35). Macrophages are also capable of manifesting profibrinolytic activity, as evidenced by their secretion of urokinase-type plasminogen activator (34). The activation of plasminogen by macrophages has been implicated in the activation of matrixins (tissue metalloproteinases) and the consequent degradation by macrophages of insoluble collagen, fibrin, elastin, and cell-derived extracellular matrices (36). In addition, it was recently shown that IL-4 can stimulate human monocytes to produce tissue-type plasminogen activator (t-PA) (37, 38). Interestingly, acetyl-LDL can stimulate macrophage-dependent plasminogen activation and degradation of smooth muscle cell-derived extracellular matrix (36). Monocytes also possess a plasmin-independent alternative fibrinolytic pathway through which fibrinogen is bound to the integrin receptor Mac-1 (CD11b/CD18) and internalized, resulting in its subsequent lysosomal degradation by the aspartyl protease cathepsin D (39, 40). These mechanisms contribute to the integral role that macrophage fibrinolytic activity plays in the atherothrombotic process (41). Macrophage fibrinolytic activity appears to be an important contributor to atherosclerotic lesion development from a number of standpoints: to facilitate the entry of the monocyte into the evolving plaque, to induce matrix degradation and consequent plaque weakening, and to promote the exodus of the macrophage during plaque regression (41, 42).

## SMOOTH MUSCLE CELLS

Smooth muscle cell proliferation within the intima is one of the cardinal features in the evolution of the chronic atheromatous plaque (1). The principal mitogen for smooth muscle cell migration is platelet-derived growth factor (PDGF) (1), which plays a role in smooth muscle cell proliferation as well (1). Platelet-derived growth factor is a highly cationic protein present in the α-granules of megakaryocytes and platelets, its secretion from platelets occurring within the milieu of platelet activation (1). There is extensive homology between PDGF and the c-sis gene product, the cellular homologue of the simian sarcoma virus v-sis oncogene (43–46). In addition, activated endothelial cells, monocytes, and smooth muscle cells themselves produce PDGF or PDGF-like mitogens (1). Along with its role in smooth muscle cell migration, PDGF stimulates smooth muscle cell proliferation via induction of insulin growth factor-1 (IGF-1) as well as thrombospondin expression (47–49).

The structure of PDGF has been extensively studied and characterized (50, 51). Two distinct PDGF chains have been identified, which are coded by different genes and termed "A" and "B," resulting in three different isoforms: the AA and BB homodimers, and an AB heterodimer (52). All three isoforms have been observed *in vivo* and possess biological activity *in vitro*, the AA homodimer appearing to possess the least cellular mitogenic activity (52). Each of these isoforms binds to a high-affinity cell surface receptor composed of two different subunits, each subunit possessing specificity for one or the other of the peptide chains of PDGF (53). The capacity of the different isoforms of PDGF to induce mitogenesis depends on the specific PDGF isoform and the relative number of receptor subunits present on the surface of the responding cell (53). In this respect, PDGF-AB and PDGF-BB are both chemotactic as well as mito-

genic toward fibroblasts, monocytes, and smooth muscle cells. Conversely, PDGF-AA has been shown to inhibit the chemotactic activity of PDGF-AB and PDGF-BB for fibroblasts and monocytes (50, 53). Moreover, the mitogenic activity of IL-1 for fibroblasts and smooth muscle cells appears to be indirect, being mediated by the induction of the PDGF A-chain gene (53). Additional smooth muscle cell mitogens include angiotensin II and thrombin, the proliferative effect of thrombin on smooth muscle cells likely being mediated by the production of IL-1 by activated macrophages (54).

Vascular smooth muscle cell growth can be inhibited by endothelial cell-derived heparan sulfate (43, 55), and heparan has been shown to inhibit thrombospondin binding to smooth muscle cells (47, 56). A human platelet heparitinase is responsible for cleaving endothelial cell surface heparan sulfates into fragments that inhibit smooth muscle cell growth (43, 57). Another platelet α-granule component, platelet factor 4, inhibits endothelial cell heparan sulfate activity by complexing with the glycosaminoglycan (34, 58).

Smooth muscle cell apoptosis has recently been shown to play an important role in the regulation of cell accumulation during the early, proliferative phase of atherosclerotic lesion development (59). Apoptosis itself is regulated by specific growth factors. In particular, IGF-1 and PDGF have been shown to suppress apoptosis in normal smooth muscle cells (60). Recent work has demonstrated involvement of interleukin-1 β-converting enzyme (ICE) in smooth muscle cell death in the fibrous regions of complex atheromata, and also in macrophage death in the lipid rich core of the lesion (59). Also, EDRF or NO has been shown to promote smooth muscle cell apoptosis (61). Observations such as these have led to the hypothesis that the apoptosis seen in plaque smooth muscle cells may ultimately contribute to plaque rupture and, hence, to the clinical sequelae of acute plaque activation (59, 60). Smooth muscle cells may play an early role in the genesis of the prelesional fatty streaks; immunohistochemistry with monoclonal antibodies for smooth muscle cells and macrophages has revealed that some of the foam cells in the fatty streak are smooth muscle cells, while the majority are macrophages (1, 62). In this regard, several experimental models have revealed that fibrin-rich thrombus on the vessel wall is, in fact, more effective than endothelial denudation in promoting smooth muscle cell growth, as well as lipid accumulation by macrophages and smooth muscle cells (63). Photographs of coronary arteries following injection with a silicone polymer have demonstrated the presence of an extensive network of vasa vasorum in the region of arterial wall surrounding atherosclerotic plaques (64). This abnormal proliferation of the adventitial vasa vasorum, a process that plays an integral role in atherosclerotic lesion development, is contributed to, in large part, by smooth muscle cells (65). Vascular endothelial growth factor (VEGF) and basic fibroblast growth factor (bFGF), both of which have been shown to be synthesized by smooth muscle cells, are important elements in this process, inducing angiogenesis by a direct effect on vascular endothelial cells (65, 66). Tissue hypoxia is a potent stimulus of VEGF expression, and it is thought that this growth factor may, therefore, be one of the principal mediators of hypoxia-induced angiogenesis (66). Moreover, several other growth factors have recently been shown to exert a synergistic up-regulation of this hypoxia-induced smooth muscle cell VEGF expression, namely bFGF and transforming growth factor-β (TGF-β), along with PDGF-BB (66–68).

## PLATELETS

The role of platelets in atherosclerotic lesion development was noted as early as the 1970s when Friedman and Stemerman demonstrated that intimal thickening was dramatically suppressed in balloon-injured aortae of rabbits with experimentally induced thrombocytopenia when compared with controls having normal platelet counts (69). The revised response-to-injury hypothesis of atherosclerosis suggests a role for platelets after endothelial injury. Following injury, platelets adhere to the exposed underlying subendothelium (3). Platelets subsequently release vasoactive substances, as well as PDGF, thereby inducing smooth muscle cell migration and proliferation (70). Platelets also contribute to the progression of the atherosclerotic plaque through other major mechanisms. They can directly enhance macrophage cholesterol esterification and cholesteryl ester accumulation (70, 71). Platelets are a potential source of cholesterol for esterification by macrophages because they contain high levels of free cholesterol and adhere to macrophages early during atherogenesis. Platelets also elicit cholesterol accumulation in cultured smooth muscle cells (72). Evidence exists to suggest that the ability of platelets to serve as cholesterol donors for macrophages increases in proportion to plasma cholesterol levels; however, platelets may affect foam cell formation even in the absence of severe hypercholesterolemia (73). This role of platelets may in part explain the observation that vascular injury can elicit foam cell formation even in the absence of hyperlipidemia (73). Indeed, Mendelsohn and Loscalzo found that activated platelets from normocholesterolemic human donors stimulated cholesteryl ester formation by U-937 cells (a human monocyte-derived cell line) (73). Interestingly, they observed that platelet cholesterol was equipotent with normal human LDL cholesterol in donating cholesterol to the U-937 cells for esterification (73). Furthermore, increasing plasma cholesterol levels in hypercholesterolemic donors direcly correlated with the ability of hypercholesterolemic platelets to support cholesteryl ester formation by U-937 cells (73).

The effects of hyperlipidemia on platelets have been extensively investigated. Hyperlipidemic conditions, specifically hypercholesterolemia, have been reported to enhance platelet activity (74). Augmented platelet adhesion, aggregation, and serotonin release have been identified in individuals with primary hypercholesterolemia, marked by reduced bleeding times and elevated levels of circulating platelet aggregates (74). Platelet hypersensitivity has also been demonstrated in experimental animals with diet-induced hypercholesterolemia, which is primarily due to elevations of β-very low-density lipoprotein (β-VLDL), but has not been demonstrated in platelets from Watanabe Heritable Hyperlipidemic rabbits, which have elevations of LDL only (75, 76). Platelets isolated from cholesterol-fed rabbits hypersensitively aggregate, owing to thromboxane $A_2$ ($TxA_2$), as well as thrombin (independent of $TxA_2$) (75). The latter mechanism may be the result of increased inositol triphosphate formation induced by thrombin (77). The major circulating lipoproteins, particularly VLDL, can mediate *in vitro* platelet adhesion through platelet integrin receptors (74). Although platelet adhesion is promoted *in vitro* by VLDL, LDL, and high-density lipoprotein (HDL), platelet adhesion is maximal when induced by VLDL (74). Ethylenediaminetetraacetic acid (EDTA), RGD-containing peptides, and monoclonal antibodies directed against platelet membrane glycoprotein IIb-IIIa are capable of inhibiting *in vitro* platelet adhesion (74). Moreover, individuals with Glanzmann's thrombasthenia, a disorder characterized by platelets that lack the glycoprotein IIb-IIIa receptor, have a 50% reduction in adhesion mediated by VLDL when compared to adhesion with VLDL in normal individuals, thereby implicating these platelet integrin receptors in VLDL-mediated platelet adhesion (74).

Platelet adhesion to the vessel wall in flowing blood is mediated by vWf (1). von Willebrand factor (see Chapter 16) circulates as an array of multimers and is derived from megakaryocytes and endothelial cells, which secrete it both luminally and abluminally into the subendothelium in response to thrombin (1, 78, 79). A role for vWf in the pathogenesis of occlusive arterial thrombosis and myocardial infarction has been inferred from several studies comparing normal and von Willebrand disease (vWD) pigs, which are severely deficient in vWf (80). von Willebrand disease pigs tend to develop less atherosclerosis of the abdominal aorta than normal pigs in response to a high fat and cholesterol diet (80–82); however, the relationship of vWf deficiency to coronary atherosclerosis remains controversial (83). von Willebrand factor does appear to be necessary for occlusive thrombosis, even in the presence of coronary atherosclerosis and hypercholesterolemia (80), but it is not essential for atherosclerotic lesion development in this model (83). Both the coronary and carotid arteries in pigs with vWd are protected from experimentally induced occlusive thrombosis (80). Moreover, the progression of nonocclusive platelet-fibrin microthrombi to occlusive thrombosis in this pig model appears to depend on vWf (80). A recent study examining plasma levels of vWf and serum lipid profiles in cynomolgus monkeys on an atherogenic diet failed to correlate changes in plasma vWf levels with atherogenesis (84). However, early during atherogenesis in this model, there appeared to be a temporal relationship among serum phospholipids, triglycerides, and levels of plasma factor XIII, which is noncovalently bound to circulating vWf (84). A recent clinical study does, however, support a relationship between plasma vWf and the risk of coronary heart disease, specifically in individuals with angina pectoris (85).

Platelets may also contribute to atherosclerosis by their ability to affect vasomotor tone (70). Aggregating platelets and their products, such as platelet activating factor and serotonin, can evoke endothelium-dependent relaxation (70). The vascular endothelium mediates relaxation of the underlying arterial smooth muscle, primarily by generating the potent vasodilator EDRF, which is thought to be either NO or a chemically related free radical species (see Chapter 19) (86, 87). In addition, EDRF also inhibits platelet aggregation as well as platelet adhesion to the endothelium or subendothelial matrix (88, 89). It has been observed that intracoronary infusion of acetylcholine results in endothelium-dependent dilation of normal human coronary arteries but paradoxical vasoconstriction of atherosclerotic coronary arteries, whereas intracoronary nitroglycerin dilates both atherosclerotic and normal coronary arteries (90). Concurrent with this are observations that coronary risk factors, such as hypercholesterolemia, are associated with an impairment of endothelium-dependent relaxation (see Chapter 41). The advent of paradoxical vasoconstriction is therefore likely to be an index of endothelial dysfunction that precedes atherosclerosis or an early marker of atherosclerosis not detectable by coronary angiography (91). This endothelial cell damage, which accompanies the development of atherosclerotic lesions, thus results in the decreased production of EDRF (70). In atherosclerotic vessels with areas of damaged endothelium lacking EDRF, platelet aggregation will therefore be augmented by uninhibited contact with subendothelial collagen (70, 92). In this setting, aggregating platelets will then release adenosine triphosphate (ATP), adenosine 5'-diphosphate (ADP), serotonin, thromboxane $A_2$, platelet activating factor, and vasopressin, and also provide an activated surface to promote the coagulation cascade, resulting in the production of thrombin, a substance which has been shown to promote vasoconstriction in atherosclerotic arteries (70, 92); all of these substances will therefore promote paradoxical vasoconstriction and proliferation of vascular smooth muscle (54, 70, 92).

Activation of the platelet glycoprotein IIb-IIIa receptor for fibrinogen and vWf is the final common pathway of all platelet agonists. Recently, an inherited genetic polymorphism of the platelet glycoprotein IIb-IIIa receptor has been identified as a potent risk factor for coronary thrombosis (93). The frequency of this $Pl^{A2}$ polymorphism of the glycoprotein IIIa gene in the general U.S. population is 19% (93). Yet, in individuals with unstable angina or acute myocardial infarction, the frequency is 39%, and in individuals with acute ischemic events before age 60, the prevalence of $Pl^{A2}$ is 50% (93).

# THE ROLE OF THROMBOSIS IN THE CHRONIC DEVELOPMENT OF THE ATHEROSCLEROTIC PLAQUE

## CLINICAL STUDIES

Although there are several independent risk factors for atherosclerosis, they have nonetheless failed to identify the majority of individuals who will ultimately suffer an acute thrombotic event (94). Indeed, the United Kingdom Heart Disease Prevention Project showed that individuals who were "high risk" for a future myocardial infarction because of hypertension, smoking, or hypercholesterolemia, represented only one-third of future infarctions (94, 95). In the early 1980s, the advent of seminal studies establishing the presence of thrombus in acute ischemic syndromes (96, 97) resulted in many investigations of hemostatic risk factors for atherosclerosis (94). Of these, the best studied have been the plasma fibrinogen level, coagulation factor VII activity, and the total white blood cell count.

In spite of its role as an acute-phase reactant, plasma fibrinogen level has been identified as an independent cardiovascular risk factor that also makes a major contribution to plasma viscosity (98, 99). This inference of fibrinogen as a cardiovascular risk factor is based on a number of clinical observations. Coronary artery disease individuals with angina pectoris have elevated fibrinogen levels (98, 100, 101). Moreover, as the number of involved coronary arteries increases, there is an increase in fibrinogen levels (100–103). Individuals with multivessel coronary artery disease have significantly higher fibrinogen levels than those with normal arteries or even single vessel disease (94, 103). Elevations in fibrinogen levels and plasma viscosity occur in myocardial infarction, with the extent of myocardial necrosis correlating with the degree of fibrinogen increase (98, 104, 105). However, the fact that fibrinogen is also an acute phase reactant has hampered interpretations of studies associating fibrinogen level elevations with myocardial infarction (94, 98). One case report has described an individual with unstable angina who had a gradual increase in fibrinogen levels prior to a myocardial infarction (98, 106). In a prospective trial investigating fibrinogen levels in individuals with myocardial infarction, reinfarction occurred only in individuals whose initial fibrinogen level was higher than 750 mg/dL (98, 107).

After cerebrovascular accidents, fibrinogen levels increase, although once again the interpretation of this phenomenon is limited by the fact that fibrinogen is an acute-phase reactant synthesized by the liver (98, 108–110). The contention that elevated fibrinogen levels may contribute to the etiology of stroke is buttressed by the finding that individuals with transient ischemic attacks have increased red blood cell aggregation and plasma viscosity owing to hyperfibrinogenemia (98, 111).

Patients with peripheral vascular disease also have elevated fibrinogen levels (98, 112, 113), and fibrinogen levels have proven to be effective as a screening test for the presence of peripheral vascular disease in middle aged men (114). The deleterious effects of fibrinogen on blood rheology are thought to adversely affect the peripheral vascular circulation in the same manner as the coronary artery and cerebral circulations (98, 115).

What factors determine an individual's fibrinogen level? There appears to be a genetic predilection for elevated fibrinogen levels (98, 116, 117). In addition, fibrinogen levels have been shown to increase with age (98, 118). Hyperlipidemia is strongly related to hyperfibrinogenemia (98, 119). Rats fed high cholesterol diets develop increased fibrinogen levels (98, 119). Hyperfibrinogenemia is manifest in individuals with hypercholesterolemia and hypertriglyceridemia (98, 120, 121). Even in studies of asymptomatic healthy males, there is a positive correlation between the levels of plasma cholesterol and fibrinogen (98, 122). Cigarette smoking causes a dose-dependent and reversible increase in fibrinogen levels in healthy subjects (98, 123–126). In an animal model using greyhound dogs, nicotine in cigarettes was found to increase the retention of fibrinogen by the arterial wall (127).

Several studies have confirmed that fibrinogen levels are higher in individuals with essential hypertension than in normotensive controls (98, 128). In addition, hypertensive individuals have elevated plasma viscosity levels (98, 129). Individuals with insulin-dependent diabetes mellitus or non insulin-dependent diabetes mellitus have hyperfibrinogenemia, particularly those who have evidence of microvascular involvement (98, 130, 131). Elevated fibrinogen levels and plasma viscosity are also found in obese individuals (98, 132). Oral contraceptives induce a dose-dependent increase in fibrinogen levels (98). After menopause, a sharp rise in plasma fibrinogen parallels the increase in cardiovascular risk

(98, 133). Finally, elevated fibrinogen levels have been associated with lower social class and increased stress (63, 132). A recent cross-sectional population study of men revealed that the strongest risk factors for an elevated fibrinogen level are smoking, social class, LDL cholesterol, and HDL cholesterol (134).

Plasma fibrinogen levels may be lowered in several ways. Many lifestyle interventions that reduce the risk of conventional atherosclerotic risk factors also lower fibrinogen levels and plasma viscosity. For example, vigorous exercise reduces fibrinogen levels (98, 135). A vegetarian diet also is associated with low plasma fibrinogen levels (98, 136). Moderate alcohol intake may have a beneficial effect as well (98). Unfortunately, the pharmacologic methods for treating hyperfibrinogenemia are fairly limited. Fish oil decreases plasma fibrinogen levels (63, 137). Bezafibrate, a lipid-lowering drug of the fibric acid class, also reduces plasma fibrinogen (63, 138).

In addition to the aforementioned observational clinical studies inferring fibrinogen as a cardiovascular risk factor, several prospective epidemiologic studies have firmly established the relationship between hyperfibrinogenemia and atherosclerotic disease. Of these, the most notable is the Northwick Park Heart Study, which involved 1500 white men and revealed that higher fibrinogen levels were predictive of individuals who subsequently suffered an ischemic event or cardiovascular death (Table 39.1) (94, 139, 140). It is important to note that the correlation between fibrinogen levels and ischemic events or cardiovascular mortality was independent of the other coronary risk factors examined (94). Moreover, fibrinogen levels could predict future ischemic events as well as blood cholesterol levels (94). In another prospective trial of about 300 men aged 40 to 69 years, fibrinogen emerged as the single strongest predictor of future ischemic events, followed by age, systolic blood pressure, cholesterol, obesity index, number of cigarettes per day, and VLDL level (98, 141). Two analyses of the Framingham Heart Study of 1315 men and women with a 14-year follow-up have further strengthened the notion that fibrinogen is an independent coronary artery disease risk factor in men and women and a risk factor for stroke in men alone (98, 142, 143). Finally, the Goteborg Study followed 792 Swedish men aged 54 years for 13.5 years, demonstrating that fibrinogen levels could predict subsequent myocardial infarction and stroke (98, 144). These findings notwithstanding, elevations in fibrinogen may in fact be a surrogate for elevated IL-6, a cytokine which plays a critical role in regulating fibrinogen production (145). Interleukin-6 also regulates the production of tumor necrosis factor-$\alpha$ (TNF-$\alpha$), an inflammatory cytokine known to activate endothelial cells (146). Furthermore, elevated levels of IL-6 have been found in individuals with unstable angina (147). These levels correlated with C-reactive protein levels and were linked to prog-

**TABLE 39.1.** Independent Associations with Ischemic Heart Disease (IHD) for Events Occurring within 5 Years and in Total Follow-up Period

| Event | Age | Factor VII | Fibrinogen | Cholesterol | Systolic BP |
|---|---|---|---|---|---|
| *IHD death* | | | | | |
| ≤5years | | | | | |
| SRE | 1.92 | 1.55 | 1.67 | 1.36 | 1.21 |
| *P* | 0.006 | 0.04 | 0.02 | NS | NS |
| Total | | | | | |
| SRE | 2.00 | 1.32 | 1.39 | 1.27 | 1.17 |
| *P* | <0.0001 | 0.03 | 0.02 | 0.07 | NS |
| *Non-fatal IHD* | | | | | |
| ≤5 years | | | | | |
| SRE | 1.18 | 1.28 | 1.68 | 1.16 | 1.14 |
| *P* | 0.04 | NS | 0.004 | NS | NS |
| Total | | | | | |
| SRE | 1.43 | 1.00 | 1.60 | 1.12 | 1.35 |
| *P* | 0.02 | NS | 0.002 | NS | 0.04 |
| *All IHD* | | | | | |
| ≤5 years | | | | | |
| SRE | 1.54 | 1.37 | 1.57 | 1.17 | 1.27 |
| *P* | 0.006 | 0.03 | 0.003 | NS | 0.09 |
| Total | | | | | |
| SRE | 1.65 | 1.14 | 1.41 | 1.18 | 1.32 |
| *P* | <0.0001 | NS | 0.0002 | NS | 0.008 |

*All five variables included in regression whether or not they were significantly associated with IHD in stepwise analyses.*

BP, *blood pressure;* NS, *not significant;* SRE, *standard regression effect. (Reproduced with permission from Mead TW, Mellows S, Brozovic M, et al. Haemostatic function and ischaemic heart disease: Principal results of The Northwick Park Heart Study. Lancet 1986;2:533–537.*

nosis (147). Taken together, these data suggest a possible direct role for IL-6 in plaque development and acute ischemic syndromes, mediated in part through its effects on fibrinogen synthesis.

Coagulation factor VII has also emerged as a prothrombotic marker which confers an independent risk for ischemic heart disease (94). The Northwick Park Heart Study revealed a 62% increased risk of ischemic heart disease within 5 years in individuals with elevated factor VII coagulant (factor VII:C) activity, which was distinct from the 47% increased risk associated with elevated serum cholesterol (Table 39.1) (140, 148). Interestingly, dietary lipids profoundly influence factor VII:C levels by mediating extrinsic coagulation pathway activation via VLDL and chylomicrons (148–154). Miller et al reported that plasma factor VII activity is enhanced acutely, but only transiently, by postprandial triglyceridemia, regardless of dietary fat composition (155, 156). These findings were further confirmed by another study, which indicated that the ratio of polyunsaturated to saturated fatty acids did not affect plasma VII:C levels (156, 157). Dietary influence on plasma triglyceride concentration directly influences levels of phospholipid-factor VII complexes in plasma (156, 158). One current hypoth-

esis to explain the mechanism by which triglyceride-rich lipoproteins such as VLDL activate factor VII is that the negatively charged surfaces of these large lipoproteins utilize activated factor $XII_a$ to activate the intrinsic coagulation pathway and, hence, factor VII (156).

As is the case with fibrinogen, there are several other determinants of factor VII:C levels besides dietary lipid intake (148). For example, higher factor VII:C levels are present in women who use oral contraceptives and at the advent of menopause (118, 122, 148). Additionally, both age and body mass index are related to elevated factor VII:C levels (118, 122, 148). In contrast to its marked influence on fibrinogen levels, cigarette smoking does not influence factor VII:C levels (126, 148). Moreover, unlike fibrinogen, factor VII:C is not an acute-phase reactant (148). Although there is substantial intra-individual variation in factor VII:C levels, almost half the total variance in factor VII:C levels reflects inter-individual variability (122, 148, 159). These variances have been linked to a common DNA polymorphism in the human factor VII gene on chromosome 13 (148).

As described in Chapter 4, TFPI is a Kunitz-type protease inhibitor, synthesized principally by the endothelium, that regulates the factor $VII_a$-tissue thromboplastin complex (160–165). Sandset et al studied individuals with heterozygous familial hypercholesterolemia treated with simvastatin, a hydroxymethylglutaryl CoA (HMGCoA) reductase inhibitor (165). Simvastatin treatment resulted in a significant decrease in TFPI activity, which was found to correlate with LDL cholesterol, total cholesterol, apoB, and apoA-1 (165). Multiple stepwise regression analysis demonstrated that the most important predictor of TFPI activity is LDL cholesterol, thereby suggesting that a majority of plasma TFPI activity is LDL-associated (165).

Two more recent clinical studies have further delineated the important role played by the hemostatic system in both atherosclerosis and acute coronary syndromes (85, 166). The Atherosclerosis Risk in Communities (ARIC) study demonstrated that individuals with early atherosclerosis, defined by increased carotid artery intima-media thickness by ultrasound, had higher circulating levels of t-PA, PAI-1, and fibrin D-dimer than a group of controls (166). The European Concerted Action on Thrombosis (ECAT) Study, a prospective study of more than 3000 individuals with angina, revealed that levels of fibrinogen, vWf, and t-PA antigen were independent predictors of subsequent acute coronary syndromes (85).

Yet another "hemostatic" marker for ischemic heart disease appears to be the leukocyte count (94). Although white blood cell counts are more elevated in cigarette smokers than nonsmokers, several studies have established that white blood cell count is an independent predictor of coronary heart disease and sudden death (94, 167–170). Indeed, the prospective combined Caerphilly and Speedwell Collaborative Heart Disease studies of 4860 middle-aged men during a period of 3 to 5 years revealed that, by multivariate analysis, white blood cell count is an independent risk factor for ischemic heart disease, as is either fibrinogen or viscosity, or perhaps both (Table 39.2) (171). Futhermore, a model to predict ischemic heart disease consisting of age, smoking, fibrin-

ogen, viscosity, and white blood cell count was as efficacious as a model consisting of total cholesterol, body mass index, and diastolic blood pressure (171).

Consonant with the role of the white blood cell count as a hemostatic marker for ischemic heart disease, there is a growing body of evidence supporting a relationship between the inflammatory response, thrombosis, and atherosclerotic lesion development. Monocyte-derived cytokines, such as IL-6, are in part responsible for the elevations of plasma fibrinogen that accompany inflammation (145, 172). In this regard, interleukin-1 has been shown to exert a negative modulating influence on IL-6 (172). Conversely, TGF-$\beta$ attenuates fibrinogen levels, primarily through its modulating effects on IL-6 (173). Cytokines also regulate the expression of adhesion molecules, including vascular cell adhesion molecule-1 (VCAM-1), essential for the recruitment of leukocytes to lesions (174). Interleukin-1 and TNF-$\alpha$ regulate the production of monocyte chemoattractant protein-1 (MCP-1), a potential signal for the migration of monocytes into the intima (174). In addition, TNF-$\alpha$ and IL-1 are also capable of inducing tissue factor-like procoagulant activity on the surface of endothelial cells (175).

## BASIC STUDIES

There is a plethora of histopathologic evidence confirming the importance of mural thrombi in the chronic evolution and progression of the often clinically quiescent chronic atheromatous plaque (176). Schwartz et al have enumerated the histologic features of atheromatous plaques that may be subsumed within the rubric of fibrous plaque-induced mural thrombus organization and subsequent endothelialization: smooth muscle cell intimal proliferation, fibrosis, endothelialization, plaque vascularization, deposition of hemosiderin, plaque fibrinoid layer formation, plaque lamination, and the presence of plaque platelet and fibrin antigens, transitional lesions, and monocytes, as well as foam cells (Table 39.3) (176).

**TABLE 39.2.**   Mean Levels of Fibrinogen, Viscosity, and White Blood Cell Count, and Incidence of Major Ischemic Heart Disease (IHD)

| | Incidence* | | Age- and Area-standardized Difference | |
| | No major IHD (*n* = 4408) | Major IHD (*n* = 233) | Mean | 95% CI |
|---|---|---|---|---|
| Fibrinogen (g/L) | 3.66 ± 0.82 | 4.09 ± 0.92 | 0.38 | 0.28 –0.49 |
| Viscosity (cp) | 1.688 ± 0.096 | 1.735 ± 0.099 | 0.045 | 0.032–0.057 |
| WBCs (10⁹/L) | 7.02 ± 2.01 | 7.86 ± 2.22 | 0.84 | 0.57 –1.10 |

CI, *confidence interval*; WBCs, *white blood count*.

* Values are area-standardized and given as mean ± SD.

(Adapted with permission from Yarnell JW, Barker IA, Sweetnam PM, et al. Fibrinogen, viscosity, and white blood cell count are major risk factors for ischemic heart disease. The Caerphilly and Speedwell collaborative heart disease studies. Circulation 1991;83:836–844.)

Mural thrombi are not limited solely to the atheromatous plaque but can become endothelialized, existing in the arterial intima as evidenced by a histologic study of plaque-free areas of the human aorta, which identified intimal fibrin in one-fourth of sites visualized (176, 177). Immunohistochemical and electron microscopic techniques have been used to establish definitively the presence of fibrinogen or fibrin, either within or on the surface of plaques, as well as fatty streaks (176, 178–183). Woolf and Carstairs utilized antiplatelet antibody staining to identify platelet antigens in approximately one-half of advanced fibrous atherosclerotic plaques (183). Studies using antifibrin antibody have noted diffuse antifibrin antibody fluorescence, reflecting the transendothelial passage of plasma fibrinogen to the intima (176, 183). Bini et al have shown that fibrin II (formed by thrombin cleavage of both fibrinogen bonds A$\alpha$16-17 and B$\beta$14-15 and release of both fibrinopeptides A and B), not fibrin I (formed by thrombin cleavage of the fibrinogen bond A$\alpha$16-17 and release of fibrinopeptide A only), is the major component in human atherosclerotic thrombotic areas (184, 185). Conversely, normal aortic samples contained only fibrinogen and fibrin I (184). With increasing severity of the atherosclerotic lesions, fibrin II concentration increased while fibrinogen concentration decreased (184).

Fig. 39.5 shows the relative amounts of fibrinogen, fibrin I, fibrin II, and fragment X, the first product of plasmin-induced fibrinogen digestion, in acute and organized thrombi (Fig. 39.5A) versus complicated, fibrous, fatty plaques, as well as normal aortae (Fig. 39.5B) (184). Using monoclonal antibodies, Bini et al were able to demonstrate that normal aortae contained little fibrinogen/fibrin I or fibrin II, and absolutely no fibrin(ogen) degradation products (185). However, fibrinogen/fibrin I and fibrin II were situated in long threads surrounding macrophages and smooth muscle cells in early lesions, as well as fibrous plaques, which were devoid of fibrin(ogen) degradation products (185). Fibrinogen/fibrin I, fibrin II, and fibrin(ogen) degradation products appeared diffusely in thrombus, surrounding cholesterol crystals, and in areas of loose connective tissue in fibrous and advanced atherosclerotic plaques (185). These intriguing results suggested that augmented fibrin formation, as well as degradation, occur during the evolution of the chronic atheromatous plaque, and that the cells in the lesion may actively contribute to the fibrinogen-to-fibrin transformation within the arterial vessel wall (185). Other studies have confirmed the continuous generation of crosslinked fibrin by plaques, as well as the presence of continuous fibrinolysis within plaques, generating fibrin(ogen) degradation products (186).

**TABLE 39.3.** Histologic Features of the Atherosclerotic (Fibrous) Plaques Compatible with a Thrombotic Component in Plaque Development

Smooth muscle cell proliferation in intima
Fibrosis
Endothelialization
Plaque vascularization
Hemosiderin deposition
Fibrinoid or fibrinous layers within the plaque
Plaque lamination
Presence of platelet and fibrin antigens within the plaque
Presence of transitional lesions
Presence of mononuclear phagocytes and foam cells

*(Adapted with permission from Schwartz CJ, Valente AJ, Kelley JL, et al. Thrombosis and the development of atherosclerosis: Rokitansky revisited. Semin Thromb Hemost 1988;14:189–195.)*

**FIGURE 39.5.** **(a)** Reveals the relative amounts of fibrinogen, fibrin I, fibrin II, and fragment X, expressed as a percentage of the NH$_2$-terminal disulfide knot of fibrinogen (NDSK), for acute and organized thrombi. **(b)** demonstrates the relative amounts of fibrinogen, fibrin I, fibrin II, and fragment X for complicated, fibrous and fatty plaques, and normal aortae. (Adapted with permission from Bini A, Fenoglio JJ Jr, Sobel J, et al. Immunochemical characterization of fibrinogen, fibrin I, and fibrin II in human thrombi and atherosclerotic lesions. Blood 1987; 69:1038–1045.)

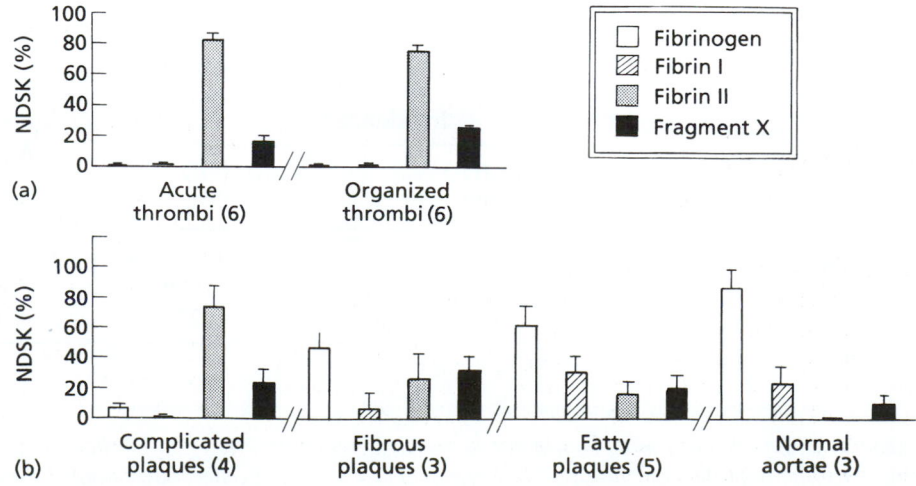

The presence of multiple fibrin(ogen) degradation products in the evolving plaque may actually be critical for the initiation and progression of the plaque (186). Fibrin has been shown to promote aortic smooth muscle cell proliferation (186–188). In addition, fibrinogen, as well as fibrin, are chemotactic for vascular smooth muscles *in vitro,* suggesting that they may perform a similar *in vivo* role, attracting smooth muscle cells from the media into the intima at the very early stages of atherogenesis (189). In this regard, fibrinopeptide B, as well as other fragments, are capable of being chemotactic for monocytes (186, 189). Fibrin and fibrin(ogen) degradation products can damage endothelium, thereby disrupting the monolayer (186, 187). The addition of fibrin(ogen) degradation products to endothelial cells and smooth muscle cells *in vitro* can also impair prostacyclin synthesis (187, 190). Fibrin may also be capable of binding to and causing localization of LDL within the plaque (95). Thus, fibrin and fibrinogen, as well as their degradation products, possess the ability to interact with each of the four major cell types involved in atherosclerosis at each stage in the progression of the plaque, including the earliest stages.

## THE RELATIONSHIP BETWEEN IMPAIRED FIBRINOLYSIS, HYPERLIPIDEMIA, AND OTHER RISK FACTORS IN THE EVOLUTION OF THE CHRONIC ATHEROMATOUS PLAQUE

The complexity of the fibrinolytic system is displayed in Fig. 39.6 (191) and is discussed in detail in Chapter 7. Several of the well-defined risk factors for ischemic heart disease and atherosclerosis have been associated with impaired fibrinolytic activity (192). Cigarette smoking has been linked to decreased fibrinolytic activity (192, 193). Impaired fibrinolytic function, secondary to elevations in the activity of plasma PAI-1, a rapidly acting specific inhibitor of t-PA, has been correlated with hypertriglyceridemia (156, 194–196). Several studies examining the effects of dietary intervention in reducing serum triglyceride levels have revealed a concomitant amelioration, if not normalization, of fibrinolytic function (120, 121, 156, 197, 198). Moreover, gemfibrozil-induced lowering of serum triglycerides in individuals with postmyocardial infarction was associated with restoration of fibrinolytic potential (156, 199). However, obesity has also been related to low vascular fibrinolytic activity (192, 200), and interpretation of the aforementioned studies of dietary-induced reduction in serum triglycerides, with concomitant improvement in fibrinolysis, must be tempered by the fact that weight loss occurred in all individuals who had reduced serum triglyceride levels (156). Indeed, Sundell et al demonstrated that modest weight loss, in the absence of a reduction in serum triglycerides, can effect a reduction of elevated PAI-1 levels (156, 201). As opposed to the case with triglycerides, although there are weak yet significant correlations between serum cholesterol and t-PA and PAI-1 (156, 202), cholesterol and LDL alterations do not appear to perturb the t-PA/PAI-1 balance (156).

To investigate further the association between hypertriglyceridemia and raised PAI-1 levels, Stitko-Rahm et al exposed cultured human umbilical vein endothelial cells (HUVEC) to purified lipoproteins isolated from normal and hypertriglyceridemic individuals (192). Very low density lipoprotein from both sets of individuals stimulated the secretion of PAI-1 from HUVEC, although hypertriglyceridemic VLDL proved to be a better stimulus than normotriglyceridemic VLDL (Fig. 39.7) (156, 192). In addition, the VLDL-induced secretion of PAI-1 depends on the binding of VLDL particles to apoB/E receptors of endothelial cells (192). Furthermore, LDL induces secretion of PAI-1 by endothelial cells as well as the hepatoma cell line Hep G2 cells (156, 203). These observations have now been extended to include acetylated LDL, which is a potent stimulus for endothelial cell secretion of PAI-1 (156, 204).

There appears to be strong clinical relevance for the hyperlipidemia-PAI-1 relationship and for the role of attenuated fibrinolysis in atherosclerotic risk (156). PAI-1 levels are elevated in individuals with coronary artery disease (4, 205), and Hamsten et al discovered that increased PAI-1 levels were present in young survivors of myocardial infarction and predisposed to reinfarction in a prospective study of 109 men with a first myocardial infarction before the age of 45 (4, 194, 206).

Ridker et al have demonstrated an association between elevated t-PA antigen levels and future risk of

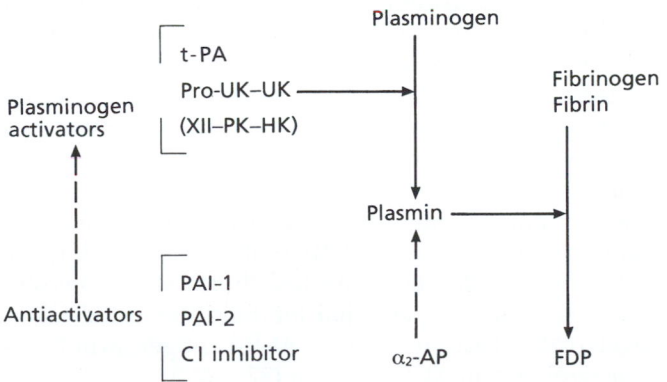

**FIGURE 39.6.**  The complexity of the fibrinolytic system. *UK,* urokinase; *XII,* factor XII; *PK,* prekallikrein; *HK,* high molecular weight kininogen; PAI-1, plasminogen activator inhibitor; *CI inh,* CI inhibitor; $\alpha_2$AP, $\alpha_2$-antiplasmin; *FDP,* fibrinogen degradation products. (Adapted with permission from Juhan-Vague I, Alessi MC, Vague PH. Increased plasminogen activator inhibitor 1 levels. A possible link between insulin resistance and atherothrombosis. Diabetologia 1991;34:457–462.)

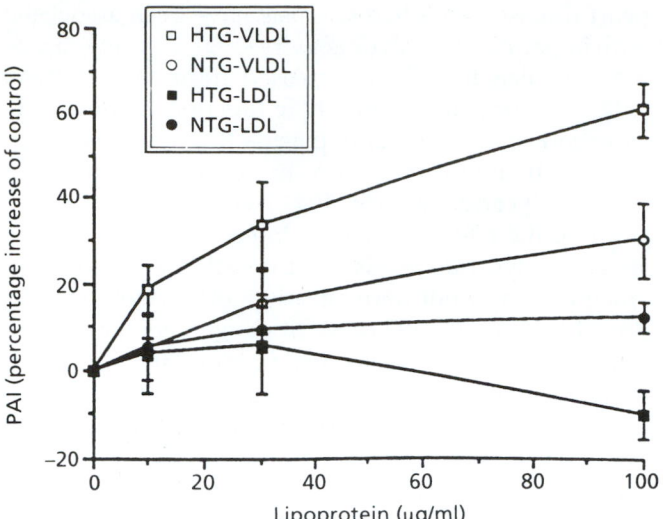

**FIGURE 39.7.** The effects of normotriglyceridemic (NTG) and hypertriglyceridemic (HTG), VLDL, and LDL on the PAI-1 release from endothelium. Confluent endothelial cells were exposed to HTG-VLDL, NTG-VLDL, HTG-LDL, or NTG-LDL for 48 hours. The amount of PAI-1 in the culture medium was then determined. The values indicate the mean ± SE of 18 determinations performed with lipoproteins from six different subjects for HTG-VLDL, nine determinations with lipoproteins from three different subjects for NTG-VLDL, and six determinations with lipoproteins from two different subjects for HTG-LDL and NTG-LDL. All values are shown as the percents of controls incubated without lipoproteins. (Adapted with permission from Stiko-Rahm A, Wiman B, Hamsten A, et al. Secretion of plasminogen activator inhibitor-1 from cultured human umbilical vein endothelial cells is induced by very low density lipoprotein. Arteriosclerosis 1990; 10:1067–1073.)

myocardial infarction, suggesting that elevated t-PA levels represent a potential marker for subsequent coronary events (207). Owing to earlier studies suggesting reduced fibrinolytic activity in survivors of an initial myocardial infarction (194), these data suggest that elevations in t-PA are accompanied and exceeded by concomitant elevations in its endothelial-derived inhibitor, PAI-1, with resultant elevation of circulating t-PA PAI-1 complexes (208). Indeed, the association between high t-PA antigen levels and both coronary artery disease and myocardial infarction is a reflection of high plasma PAI-1 activity, and reduced rather than augmented fibrinolytic activity (208). Moreover, increased PAI-1 gene expression has been demonstrated in the intima of atherosclerotic human arteries (209, 210).

Reaven's syndrome, or syndrome X, is the grouping of hypertriglyceridemia with central abdominal obesity, hypertension, and hypoalphalipoproteinemia and defines a subset of individuals at particularly high risk for coronary artery disease (156, 211). Hyperinsulinemia is a major index of the insulin resistance that defines syn-

drome X (191) and is a risk factor for myocardial infarction (191, 212, 213). Individuals with insulin resistance and syndrome X also have elevated PAI-1 levels (191, 195, 214–217). Moreover, fasting plasma insulin levels and PAI-1 levels have been correlated in the normal population, obese individuals, type II non-insulin-dependent diabetics, and individuals with angina pectoris (191). Measures aimed at lowering insulin resistance, including fasting, weight loss, dietary interventions, and the drug metformin, all result in a concomitant reduction of PAI-1 and plasma insulin levels (191).

It has been argued that plasma insulin may in fact be the chief physiologic regulator of plasma PAI-1 activity (156, 218). Alessi et al have demonstrated that insulin affects a dose-dependent elevation of hepatocellular Hep G2 cell secretion of PAI-1 *in vitro*, without a similar effect of insulin on endothelial cell secretion of PAI-1 (156, 218). The underlying mechanism for this phenomenon appears to be a specific increase in PAI-1 messenger RNA levels induced by insulin, as evidenced by *in vitro* studies with primary cultures of human hepatocytes (156, 219). Euglycemic clamp technique studies in individuals with abdominal obesity have established a significant inverse correlation between plasma PAI-1 activity and insulin sensitivity (156, 220). Alternatively, elevated PAI-1 levels may reflect insulin resistance "*per se*", independent of plasma insulin levels (156, 221).

Plasma PAI activity is influenced by variation of the PAI-1 gene on chromosome 7 (156). Dawson et al compared genotypes of young postmyocardial infarction individuals and population-based controls with respect to two PAI-1 locus polymorphisms (156, 222). Their results showed that the positive relationships of insulin and VLDL with PAI-1 appeared to be genotype-specific (156, 222). Plasminogen activator inhibitor-1 activity is also mediated by components of the renin-angiotensin system. Vaughan et al demonstrated increased PAI-1 mRNA and antigen levels after exposing cultured bovine endothelial cells to angiotensin II, an effect noted to be mediated via a pharmacologically distinct form of endothelial receptor (223). Subsequent work demonstrated this receptor to be specific for angiotensin IV (224). Moreover, Hamdan et al observed diminished PAI-1 expression in the neointima of balloon-injured rat aorta in the angiotensin converting enzyme (ACE) inhibitor, captopril (225). In this respect, placebo-controlled clinical studies involving survivors of myocardial infarction revealed lower levels of PAI-1 activity, as well as t-PA antigen, in individuals receiving an ACE inhibitor (226, 227).

## THE EFFECT OF LIPIDS ON PROSTACYCLIN IN THE PATHOGENESIS OF ATHEROSCLEROSIS

Endothelial cell prostacyclin is a potent vasodilator and inhibitor of platelet aggregation through its ability to raise intracellular cyclic adenosine monophosphate (cAMP), and thereby block the formation of platelet thromboxane $A_2$ (228, 229). Prostacyclin also inhibits platelet PDGF release, reduces foam cell cholesteryl esters, and enhances HDL-mediated reverse transport of cholesterol to the liver (230). Decreased production of prostacyclin has been found in advanced atherosclerotic plaques (13, 228, 230). Moreover, hyperlipidemic serum and lipid peroxides have been demonstrated to injure endothelial cells, thereby inactivating prostacyclin synthetase and causing decreased prostacyclin generation (228). Conversely, Yui et al have identified a serum prostacyclin stabilizing factor that is identical to apolipoprotein A-I (Apo A-I), a major component of the antiatherogenic molecule HDL (231). Not only does HDL promote endothelial cell release of prostacyclin (229, 232), it facilitates stabilization of circulating prostacyclin (which has a half-life of 3 minutes *in vitro*) (229, 233). In this regard, individuals with both unstable angina and acute myocardial infarction have a decreased prostacyclin half-life owing to reduced apo A-I levels (233). More recently, Morishita et al used arterial smooth muscle cells to demonstrate that HDL augments prostacyclin-mediated lysosomal and cytosolic hydrolysis of cholesteryl ester, as well as the reduction of cholesteryl ester cellular content, via high levels of intracellular cAMP (234).

## LIPOPROTEIN(a)

As shown in Fig. 39.8, lipoprotein(a) [Lp(a)] is a unique lipoprotein composed of the LDL apolipoprotein B-100 particle, linked to the glycoprotein apo(a), which bears significant homology to plasminogen (2, 235). Lipoprotein(a) has been shown to be qualitatively associated with coronary artery disease and quantitatively associated with both coronary artery and cerebrovascular disease, by retrospective as well as prospective studies (2). Dahlen et al prospectively demonstrated that Lp(a) is an independent risk factor for coronary artery disease, conferring a relative risk of 1.6 to 3.6 (2, 236). In particular, Lp(a) levels powerfully predicted the presence of angiographic coronary artery disease in women of all ages and in men younger than age 56 (2, 236). Elevated Lp(a) levels are also associated with an augmented risk for coronary artery bypass venous graft stenosis (2, 237). Yet it should also be noted that Ridker et al, using subjects from the Physician's Health Study, more recently demonstrated no association between elevated Lp(a) levels and future risk of myocardial infarction (238). This, however, represented a selected population for whom other classic coronary artery disease risk factors, such as family history and elevated cholesterol, also failed to impart an increased risk for myocardial infarction (238).

One potential atherogenic mechanism for Lp(a) resides in its role in cholesterol metabolism (2). Lipoprotein(a) binds to the classic LDL receptor in cultured fi-

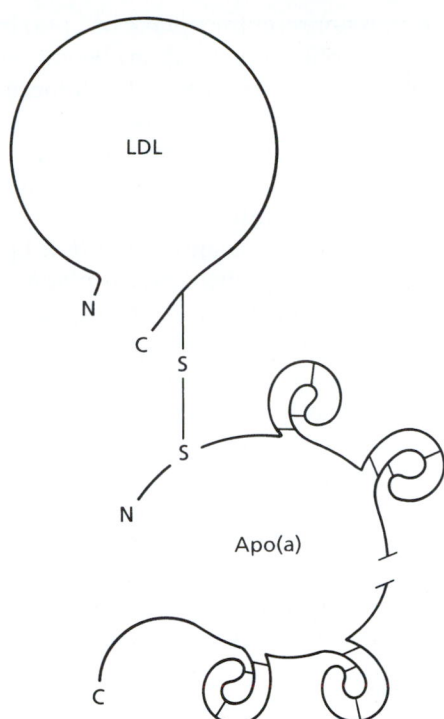

**FIGURE 39.8.** The structure of Lp(a). The apolipoprotein(a) moiety is shown in the lower portion of the diagram with four of its kringle (triple-loop) domains. A single disulfide bridge links Apo(a) to LDL. (Adapted with permission from Loscalzo J. Lipoprotein(a). A unique risk factor for atherothrombotic disease. Arteriosclerosis 1990;10:672–679.)

broblasts, albeit with a lower affinity than LDL itself (2, 239, 240). Once bound, Lp(a) inhibits HMGCoA reductase, indicating that Lp(a) enters cells and releases its component cholesterol, regulating *de novo* cholesterol synthesis in a manner similar to LDL (2). Moreover, lipoprotein(a) is removed from plasma by similar mechanisms as LDL, as evidenced by fractional catabolic rate studies of Lp(a) in normal individuals, and in individuals with familial hypercholesterolemia (2, 240). A more relevant *in vivo* role for Lp(a) in cholesterol metabolism involves its interaction with the macrophage scavenger pathway. Although macrophage cell culture studies have failed to demonstrate that unmodified Lp(a) is preferentially taken up by the scavenger pathway, malondialdehyde modification of Lp(a) enhances uptake and degradation by 60-fold over that of unmodified Lp(a) (2, 241). Therefore, modified Lp(a) may be atherogenic and may contribute to foam cell formation in a manner similar to that of modified LDL (2). Moreover, Lp(a) is much less efficiently cleared by the liver than is LDL in the presence of estrogen-induced apo B/E receptor up-regulation (2, 242), and familial hypercholesterolemia, as well as atherogenic apo(a) phenotypes, synergistically elevate plasma levels of Lp(a) (2, 243).

Another possible proatherogenic mechanism for

Lp(a) is through nonreceptor uptake of Lp(a) by the endothelium (2). Apolipoprotein(a) has been found in the neointima of venous grafts, where it is colocalized with apo B (2, 244). Moreover, in another study, Lp(a) was also extant extracellularly, and in a largely undegraded state, in the arterial wall of coronary bypass individuals (2, 245). Beisiegel et al studied fresh human arterial wall biopsies and autopsy tissue and found that Lp(a) accumulates in the intima, particularly in plaque areas, in an extracellular fashion (246). A strong colocalization was also observed for apo(a) and apo(B), and for apo(a) and fibrin (246). Studies of monkeys with diet-induced atherosclerosis revealed striking accumulations of Lp(a) in coronary artery atherosclerotic lesions (247). There is a significant correlation between aortic wall Lp(a) and serum Lp(a) levels, but serum cholesterol levels failed to correlate with either aortic Lp(a) or serum Lp(a) levels (247). Lipoprotein(a) also binds more avidly than LDL to glycosaminoglycans and proteoglycans present in the arterial wall (248). The apo(a) portion of Lp(a) binds to the carboxyterminal heparin-binding domain of fibronectin, and Lp(a) proteolytically cleaves fibronectin (249), although with kinetics that may not be of any relevance *in vivo*. Smith and Cochran have demonstrated preferential immobilization of Lp(a), as opposed to LDL, in fibrous lipid plaques, via fibrin binding (250). Moreover, a significant fraction of Lp(a) present in carotid endarterectomy specimens is associated with tissue macrophages (2). Therefore, after transport into the subendothelium, Lp(a) may interact with a variety of extracellular matrix components, undergo chemical modification, and consequently serve as a ligand for scavenger receptor uptake by macrophages during atherogenesis (2).

Another major atherogenic mechanism of Lp(a) is its deleterious effect on fibrinolysis (2). Lipoprotein(a) bears striking homology to plasminogen (2, 251–252), yet it does not generate plasmin-like activity when exposed to plasminogen activators because of a substitution of serine for arginine at the equivalent activation site (2). However, Loscalzo et al demonstrated that Lp(a) inhibits the fibrin-dependent enhancement of t-PA activity (253). Through its multiple kringle 4-like domains located on the apo(a) molecule, Lp(a) binds to fibrin(ogen) and thus attenuates the fibrin-mediated enhancement of t-PA activation of plasminogen (253). Lipoprotein(a) diminishes the fibrin-dependent enhancement of t-PA conversion of plasminogen to plasmin by acting as a noncompetitive inhibitor ($K_i = 15$ nM) (253, 254). Lipoprotein(a) binds to fibrin immobilized on an inert surface and in solution, and it competes with plasminogen and t-PA for fibrin binding (2, 253, 254). However, low density lipoprotein, which is devoid of apo(a), is unable to exhibit any of these effects (2). Amino acid substitutions, which result in variable numbers of plasminogen kringle 4-type repeats and polymorphisms in kringle structure, can impart varying affinities of Lp(a) for fibrinogen (255). In this regard, certain kringle mutations, by conferring a reduced affinity of Lp(a) for fibrinogen, may therefore impart a relatively reduced risk for atherosclerotic cardiovascular disease (255). In addition, Lp(a) attenuates clot lysis in plasma (254); individuals with high levels of Lp(a) have significantly reduced endogenous clot lysis in plasma *ex vivo* (2). Moreover, plasmin treatment of immobilized fibrin(ogen) augments the binding of Lp(a) to that ligand (2, 256, 257). In this regard, Wolf et al have shown that apo(a) colocalizes with fibrin(ogen) in human coronary atheromata (258).

Lipoprotein(a) also inhibits plasminogen binding to endothelial cells and, thus, the generation of plasmin, thereby impairing endothelial cell surface-mediated fibrinolysis (259, 260). Lipoprotein(a) increases levels of human endothelial cell PAI-1 antigen activity, and steady-state mRNA levels, without affecting t-PA activity or mRNA levels, or causing generalized endothelial cell activation (261). Therefore, Lp(a) appears to be capable of inducing an endothelial cell "prothrombotic phenotype" (262). Taken together, these numerous studies suggest that Lp(a) may promote atherosclerosis, not only by altering cholesterol metabolism, but also by interfering with fibrinolysis through multiple mechanisms (2). A hypothetical model for the role of Lp(a) in the pathogenesis of atherothrombotic disease is shown in Fig. 39.9 (2).

# THROMBOSIS AND THE ACUTE ISCHEMIC SYNDROMES

The acute ischemic syndromes of unstable angina, both non-Q-wave and Q-wave acute myocardial infarction, and sudden ischemic death, all share the common etiologic basis of atherosclerotic plaque rupture, resulting in thrombus formation (262–269). Atherosclerotic plaque morphology can be either concentric, resulting in a fixed degree of obstruction, or eccentric, involving an arc of the vessel wall (270). A lipid-rich plaque causing eccentric stenosis is shown in Fig. 39.10 (270). In addition, although plaques may be solid or fibrous, they may also possess extracellular cholesterol (270). Individuals with coronary artery disease frequently have a mixture of all of the aforementioned plaque types (270). Endothelium overlying plaques is both dysfunctional and often manifests localized denudation injury, with a platelet monolayer adhering to the denuded site (270). Davies has noted that larger thrombi result from superficial intimal injury, or from deep intimal injury caused by plaque rupture (fissuring) (270). As a result of both superficial and deep intimal injury, underlying collagen and vWf are exposed to platelets, thus creating a nidus for throm-

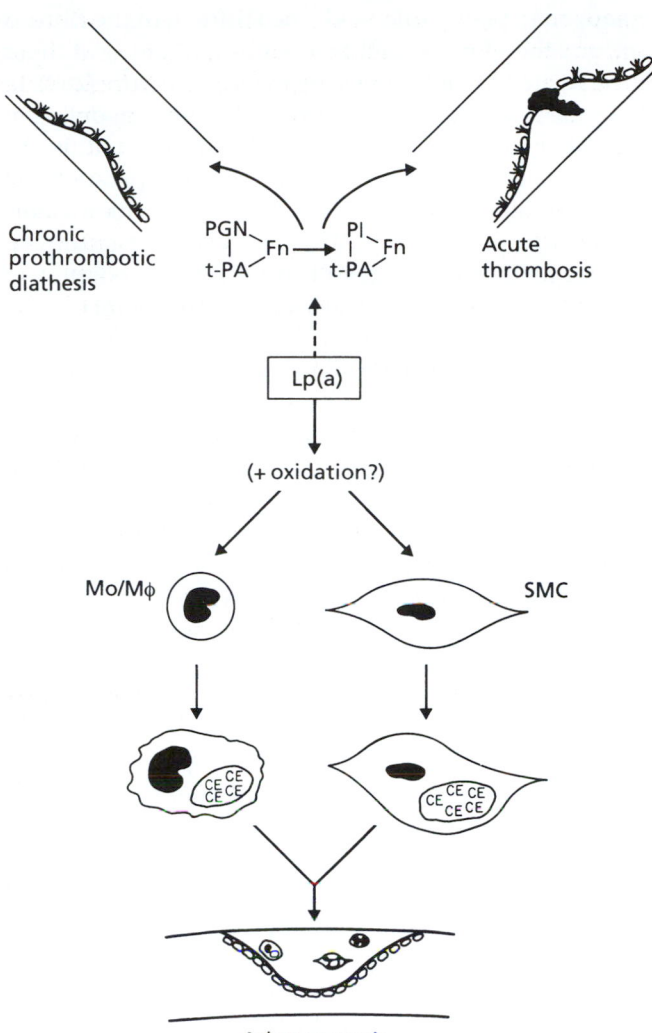

**FIGURE 39.9.**   Proposed role for Lp(a) in the etiology of atherothrombotic disease. The effect of Lp(a) on both thrombotic processes (**upper part of figure**) and atherogenic processes (**lower part of figure**) is depicted. Lipoprotein(a) may contribute to both the chronic prothrombotic diathesis of the atheromatous lesion and the acute thrombotic event occurring after plaque rupture by inhibiting (*dashed arrow*) t-PA-mediated activation of plasminogen. As a cholesterol-laden particle containing apolipoprotein B, Lp(a)'s influence on foam cell formation is also shown. *CE*, cholesterol ester; *Fn*, fibronectin; *PGN*, plasminogen; *Pl*, plasmin; *MO/Mϕ*, monocyte/macrophage; *SMC*, smooth muscle cell. (Adapted with permission from Loscalzo J. Lipoprotein(a). A unique risk factor for atherothrombotic disease. Arteriosclerosis 1990;10:672–679.)

presence of luminal thrombus, which can be either mural or occlusive (270). Indeed, during the course of an acute ischemic syndrome, individuals may have frequent transformations between mural and occlusive thrombi, owing to the activity of endogenous fibrinolytic mechanisms (270).

It should be noted, however, that as many as two-thirds of individuals who develop unstable angina or myocardial infarction have angiographic coronary lesions, which are only mild to moderate in severity (262, 271–273). Thus, small plaques, which may not necessarily cause a significant reduction in overall lumen diameter, may nonetheless play a critical role in the genesis of acute ischemic syndromes upon their rupture (262). This contention is further supported by the fact that although more severe angiographic coronary artery lesions are more likely to progress to total occlusion of the vessel than less severe lesions, they are not more likely to result in acute myocardial infarction, most likely owing to the presence of collateral blood flow (262). Fig. 39.11 shows a histologic cross-section of major plaque rupture (Fig. 39.11A), and a corresponding diagram (Fig. 39.11B).

Pathologic studies have revealed that atherosclerotic plaques, which are most prone to rupture, are the so-called "soft" plaques, which have a high cholesterol content (262, 263). Moreover, eccentrically located extracellular intimal lipid is often present at the site of plaque rupture, which tends to develop at the junction of the thin fibrous cap with the normal vessel wall (262, 274, 275). Davies and Thomas have also observed that plaque rupture is preceded by thinning of the fibrous cap that covers the lipid core (262, 263). Macrophages may play an important role in plaque rupture, owing to their ability to generate toxic free radicals and lipid peroxides, as well as to secrete elastase and collagenase (matrix metalloproteinases, or matrixins) (262, 274, 276). Macrophages also stimulate the secretion of matrixins by vascular smooth muscle cells through an IL-1-dependent mechanism (277). In particular, dysfunctional vascular

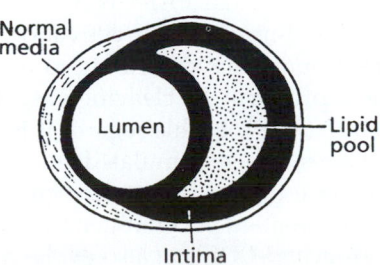

**FIGURE 39.10.**   Transverse section of a lipid-rich plaque causing eccentric stenosis. (Adapted with permission from Davies MJ. A macro and micro view of coronary vascular insult in ischemic heart disease [review]. Circulation 1990; 82(Suppl):II-38–II-46.)

bus formation (270). As a result of deep intimal injury, the tears often stretch into a lipid pool deep within the intima, the subsequent thrombus expanding the volume of the plaque and distorting its morphology (270). Although many fissures will reseal, the result nonetheless is a larger plaque (270). Moreover, Davies has noted that a percentage of plaque ruptures are complicated by the

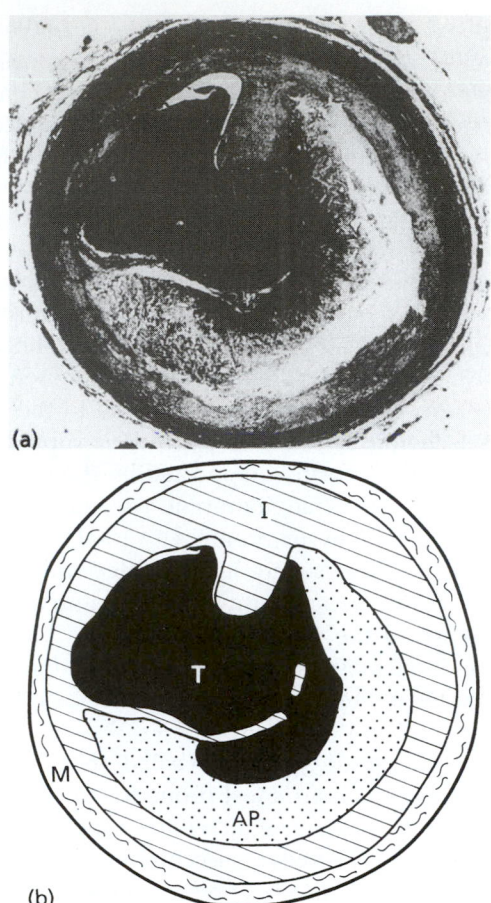

**FIGURE 39.11.** Histologic cross-section of a major plaque rupture (**a**) and accompanying diagram (**b**) are depicted. The plaque (AP) has a major defect in the fibrous cap, through which a thrombus mass has formed, part being within the plaque, and part occluding the lumen. *I*, neo(intima); *M*, media; *T*, thrombus. (Adapted with permission from Davies MJ, Thomas AC. Plaque fissuring–the cause of acute myocardial infarction, sudden ischaemic death, and crescendo angina [review]. Br Heart J 1985;53:363–373.)

endothelium results in elevations in t-PA, which can, in turn, lead to increased local conversion of plasminogen to plasmin (provided that PAI-1 is not in excess). Matrixins require plasmin for their activation (278). Once activated, these matrixins contribute to overall plaque destabilization, primarily by cleaving vascular wall matrix proteins (276, 279). In this regard, it is noteworthy that macrophages, when stimulated with IL-4, secrete not only urokinase-type plasminogen activator, but also t-PA with its consequent plasmin-generating effects (37, 38). Moreover, acetyl-LDL can also evoke macrophage-dependent plasminogen activation, resulting in extracellular matrix degradation (36).

These insights into subsequent events notwithstanding, the exact mechanism(s) underlying plaque rupture remains largely unknown (262). External stress on the plaque may play a role, with the stiffness of the fibrous cap, and therefore, its ability to withstand physical stress being related to the plaque's histologic structure (280). In this regard, Richardson et al used computer modeling to show that at systole, eccentric pools of lipid within the plaque concentrated stress on the plaque cap, especially near the edge at the junction of the plaque with the normal vessel wall (262, 275). This suggests that accumulations of foam cells can result in focal weak points and tears in the cap that are not necessarily at the point of maximum mechanical stress (275). Moreno et al used antihuman macrophage monoclonal antibody to demonstrate a high macrophage content in lesions from individuals with unstable angina and non–Q-wave myocardial infarction, suggesting that macrophage-rich sclerotic tissue may represent a nidus for plaque rupture (281). Furthermore, tissue factor content is increased in plaques from individuals with unstable angina as compared to stable angina, with tissue factor levels correlating to areas of smooth muscle cells and, particularly, macrophages in the atheromatous gruel (282).

Aside from the cellular properties of plaques, their mechanical behavior and response to external stress are also likely to play a role in determining a plaque's susceptibility to rupture. Lee et al showed that fibrous cap stiffness increases in proportion to heart rate frequency in its physiologic range, a finding that may in part explain the protective effect of β-adrenergic receptor blockers (280). The distribution of circumferential tensile stress within the diseased vessel is likely to be of critical importance, although plaque rupture is not always observed to occur at the regions of highest tensile stress, again supporting the notion that the local histologic composition of the plaque plays an essential part in defining its susceptibility to rupture (283, 284). It is likely that structural subintimal plaque features such as fibrous cap thickness are in fact more important in the distribution of stress than actual stenosis severity. This view is supported by the finding that reducing fibrous cap thickness dramatically increases peak circumferential stress, whereas an increase in stenosis severity actually decreases peak stress within the plaque (285). Severe, eccentric stenoses may lead to plaque rupture by lowering local transmural pressure so as to cause arterial collapse, resulting in highly concentrated compressive and tensile stress (286).

A relationship has been described between circadian variation, physical or mental stress, and the onset of myocardial infarction or sudden cardiac death (287). These findings lend support to the notion that mental or physical stress can lead to plaque rupture which, along with increases in coagulability and vasoconstriction triggered by daily activities, results in occlusive coronary thrombosis (287). Increasing levels of habitual physical activity have been associated with progressively lower relative risks of myocardial infarction during periods of heavy physical exertion (288). However, the fact that exercise stress testing in individuals with advanced coronary disease rarely triggers an acute coronary syndrome or myocardial infarction suggests that plaque vulnerability ultimately plays a more important role in plaque rupture than triggers or physiologic stress (289). Hence, the exact moment and location of atherosclerotic plaque rupture is likely a result of the dynamic interplay of plaque histologic composition, external mechanical stress, and the triggering effect of circadian variation and daily activities.

In spite of the relative paucity of insight surrounding the mechanisms of plaque rupture, Fuster et al have delineated the pathophysiology of acute ischemic syndromes (262). Unstable angina appears to be due to atherosclerotic plaque rupture, with a decrease in coronary flow owing to the subsequent thrombus formation that occurs at the rupture site (262). Angina that occurs at rest may result from transient episodes of thrombotic vessel occlusion at the site of plaque rupture, but spontaneous lysis of this labile thrombus, occurring as a result of endogenous thrombolytic mechanisms, thereby staves off progression to an acute myocardial infarction (262, 267). Furthermore, platelet aggregation and localization at the site of injury induces vasospasm, which serves to reduce coronary blood flow (262, 290). Fig. 39.12 depicts a ruptured plaque with subsequent thrombus formation and propagation, leading to vessel occlusion.

Plaque rupture also precedes non-Q-wave acute myocardial infarction (262, 266). Angiographic studies have confirmed that as many as one-fourth of individuals with this entity have a totally occluded infarct-related vessel that is well supplied distally by an extensive collateral network (262, 291). The remaining individuals also most likely undergo a total occlusion of the infarct vessel by thrombus (262). However, in these individuals the thrombus is endogenously lysed early (within the first 2 hours) after occlusion, thus aborting full-thickness damage to the myocardium (262). Early resolution of vasospasm may also contribute to the denouement of this entity (262, 292, 293).

Acute Q-wave myocardial infarction is marked by plaque rupture with concomitant deep arterial injury or ulceration, leading to the formation of a fixed thrombus (262). Although spontaneous or therapeutic lysis of the thrombus may ultimately intervene, the residual mural thrombus is often highly thrombogenic, thereby predisposing to recurrent thrombotic occlusion of the infarct-related vessel (262, 294, 295). Finally, ischemic sudden death also usually entails plaque rupture, with subsequent thrombosis resulting in decreased coronary perfusion, and resultant lethal ventricular arrhythmias (97, 262, 269). Platelet microemboli or the absence of adequate distal collateral flow may also be involved in the pathogenesis of ischemic sudden death (262, 269).

## CONCLUSION

Since the initial attempts of Virchow and von Rokitansky to delineate the basic pathophysiologic mechanisms underlying atherosclerotic lesion development, tremendous progress has been achieved in understanding the interface between atherosclerosis with thrombosis, not only in the acute ischemic syndromes, but also in the chronic evolution of the clinically quiescent atherothrombotic plaque. In particular, it appears that each of the four major cell types involved in the development of the atherothrombotic plaque (monocytes/macrophages, smooth muscle cells, endothelium, and platelets) are closely associated with the procoagulant and fibrinolytic systems at a fundamental level. Work at the basic level has highlighted the important role played by mural thrombus in chronic plaque development, and several clinical and epidemiologic studies have emphasized the importance of independent thrombotic risk factors, such as fibrinogen, factor VII:C, and the white blood count, in predicting atherosclerotic disease of clinical consequence. Recent histopathologic studies have underscored the crucial role played by fibrin(ogen) and its degradation products in almost every facet of the development of the atherosclerotic plaque, extending to even the earliest stages of fatty streak formation, or even prelesional endothelial dysfunction.

Several studies have provided insights into the impaired fibrinolytic system extent in atherosclerosis. In-

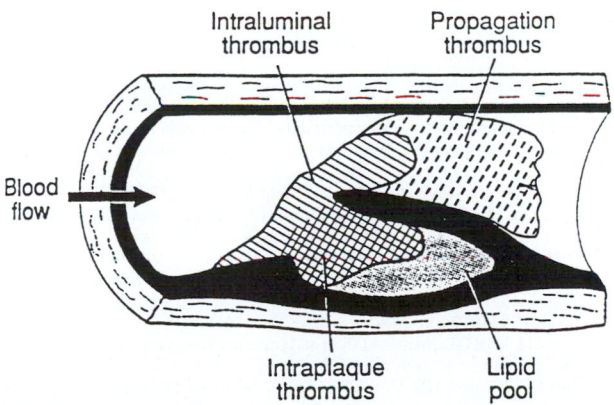

**FIGURE 39.12.** Diagrammatic representation of a longitudinal section of artery reconstructed from step histologic sections, containing an occluding thrombus that failed to respond to thrombolytic therapy. The dark area represents plaque fibrous cap, with intercurrent rupture at the shoulder region. The shaded area represents lipid pool, whereas the stippled areas represent the progressive states of thrombus formation. (Adapted with permission from Davies MJ. A macro and micro view of coronary vascular insult in ischemic heart disease [review]. Circulation 1990;82(Suppl):II-38–II-46.)

deed, the complicated relationships among hyperlipidemia, insulin resistance, and the fibrinolytic system have been elucidated by revelations that VLDL, LDL, and insulin affect *in vitro* secretion of PAI-1. Conversely, HDL, an antiatherogenic lipoprotein, promotes the release of prostacyclin and facilitates stabilization of this endogenous vasodilator and antiplatelet agent.

Lastly, Lp(a) is a molecule that has generated enormous interest in that it integrates thrombosis with atherosclerosis on several different levels. Among its many potential atherogenic mechanisms are its involvement in cholesterol metabolism, its interaction with extracellular matrix components, and its ability to undergo modification, thereby promoting scavenger receptor uptake by macrophages. Moreover, it has several deleterious effects on the fibrinolytic system, including its attenuation of fibrin-mediated enhancement of t-PA activation of plasminogen and thereby diminution of clot lysis, its impairment of endothelial cell surface-mediated fibrinolysis, and its ability to induce an endothelial cell "prothrombotic phenotype" by regulating endothelial cell expression of PAI-1. Discoveries such as these have brought Lp(a) to the fore as an independent risk factor for coronary artery disease. These and future insights into the link between atherosclerosis and thrombosis will provide not only a better understanding of the pathogenesis of this intricate disease process, but will also lead to improved therapeutic approaches at multiple levels, from the prevention of atherothrombotic lesion development to enhanced therapies for acute ischemic syndromes.

# REFERENCES

1. Scharf RE, Harker LA. Thrombosis and atherosclerosis: Regulatory role of interactions among blood components and endothelium. Blut 1987;55:131–144.
2. Loscalzo J. Lipoprotein(a). A unique risk factor for atherothrombotic disease. Arteriosclerosis 1990;10:672–679.
3. Ross R. The pathogenesis of atherosclerosis–an update. N Engl J Med 1986;314:488–500.
4. Collen D, Juhan-Vague I. Fibrinolysis and atherosclerosis. Semin Thromb Hemost 1988;14:180–183.
5. Steinberg D, Parthasarathy S, Carew TE et al. Beyond cholesterol. Modifications of low-density lipoprotein that increase its atherogenicity. N Engl J Med 1989;320:915–924.
6. Virchow RLK. Cellular pathology as based upon physiological and pathological histology. New York: Dover Publications, 1971;230.
7. Rokitansky K. A manual of pathological anatomy. London: Sydenham Society, 1852;4:271–273.
8. Duguid JB. Thrombosis as a factor in the pathogenesis of aortic atherosclerosis. J Pathol Bacteriol 1946;58:207–212.
9. Ross, R. The pathogenesis of atherosclerosis: A perspective for the 1990's. Nature 1993;362:801–809.
10. Harker LA, Schwartz SM, Ross R. Endothelium and arteriosclerosis. Clin Haematol 1981;10:283–296.
11. Nawroth P, Kisiel W, Stern D. The role of endothelium in the homeostatic balance of haemostasis. Clin Haematol 1985;14:531–546.
12. Rosenberg RD. Role of heparin and heparinlike molecules in thrombosis and atherosclerosis. Fed Proc 1985;44:404–409.
13. Dembinska-Kiec A, Gryglewska T, Zmuda A et al. The generation of prostacyclin by arteries and by the coronary vascular bed is reduced in experimental atherosclerosis in rabbits. Prostaglandins 1977;14(6):1025–1034.
14. Loscalzo, J. Endothelial injury, vasoconstriction, and its prevention. Tex Heart Inst J 1995;22:180–184.
15. Levine JD, Harlan HM, Harker LA et al. Thrombin-mediated release of factor VIII antigen from human umbilical vein endothelial cells in culture. Blood 1982;60:531–534.
16. Stern DM, Drillings M, Kisiel W et al. Activation of factor IX bound to cultured bovine aortic endothelial cells. Proc Natl Acad Sci U S A 1984;81:913–917.
17. Nawroth PP, Handley DA, Esmon CT et al. Interleukin 1 induces endothelial cell procoagulant while suppressing cell-surface anticoagulant activity. Proc Natl Acad Sci U S A 1986;83:3460–3464.
18. Nawroth PP, Stern DM. Modulation of endothelial cell hemostatic properties by tumor necrosis factor. J Exp Med 1986;163:740–745.
19. Kapiotis S, Besemer J, Bevec D et al. Interleukin-4 counteracts pyrogen-induced down-regulation of thrombomodulin in cultured human vascular endothelial cells. Blood 1991;78:410–415.
20. Crutchley DJ, Hirsh MJ. The stable prostacyclin analog, iloprost, and prostaglandin E$_1$ inhibit monocyte procoagulant activity *in vitro*. Blood 1991;78:382–386.
21. Edwards RL, Rickles FR. Macrophage procoagulants. Prog Hemost Thromb 1984;7:183–209.
22. Gregory SA, Morrissey JH, Edgington TS. Regulation of tissue factor gene expression in the monocyte procoagulant response to endotoxin. Mol Cell Biol 1989;9:2752–2755.
23. Broze GJ Jr. Binding of human factor VII and VIIa to monocytes. J Clin Invest 1982;70:526–535.
24. Drake TA, Ruf W, Morrissey JH et al. Functional tissue factor is entirely cell surface expressed on lipopolysaccharide-stimulated human blood monocytes and a constitutively tissue factor-producing neoplastic cell line. J Cell Biol 1989;109:389–395.
25. Altieri DC, Morrissey JH, Edgington TS. Adhesive receptor Mac-1 coordinates the activation of factor X on stimulated cells of monocytic and myeloid differentiation: An alternative initiation of the coagulation protease cascade. Proc Natl Acad Sci U S A 1988;85:7462–7466.
26. Tracy PB, Rohrbach MS, Mann KG. Functional prothrombinase complex assembly on isolated monocytes and lymphocytes. J Biol Chem 1983;258:7264–7267.
27. Altieri DC, Edgington TS. Sequential receptor cascade for coagulation proteins on monocytes. Constitutive biosynthesis and functional prothrombinase activity of a membrane form of factor V/Va. J Biol Chem 1989;264:2969–2972.
28. Hogg N. Human monocytes are associated with the formation of fibrin. J Exp Med 1983;157:473–485.
29. Tipping PG, Malliaros J, Holdsworth SR. Procoagulant activity expression by macrophages from atheromatous vascular plaques. Atherosclerosis 1989;79:237–243.
30. Rana SV, Reimers HJ, Pathikonda MS et al. Expression of tissue factor and factor VIIa/tissue factor inhibitor activity in endotoxin or phorbol ester stimulated U937 monocyte-like cells. Blood 1988;71:259–262.
31. Lesnik P, Dentan C, Vonica A et al. Tissue factor pathway inhibitor activity associated with LDL is inactivated by cell-and copper-mediated oxidation. Arterioscler Thromb Vasc Biol 1995;15:1121–1130.
32. Saksela O, Hovi T, Vaheri A. Urokinase-type plasminogen activator and its inhibitor secreted by cultured human monocyte-macrophages. J Cell Physiol 1985;122:125–132.
33. Schwartz BS, Monroe MC, Levin EG. Increased release of plasminogen activator inhibitor type 2 accompanies the human mononuclear cell tissue factor response to lipopolysaccharide. Blood 1988;71:734–741.
34. Vassalli JD, Dayer JM, Wohlwend A et al. Concomitant secretion of pro-urokinase and of a plasminogen activator-specific inhibitor by cultured human monocytes-macrophages. J Exp Med 1984;159:1653–1668.
35. Schwartz BS, Bradshaw JD. Differential regulation of tissue factor and plasminogen activator inhibitor by human mononuclear cells. Blood 1989;74:1644–1650.
36. Falcone DJ, Ferenc MJ. Acetyl-LDL stimulates macrophage-dependent plasminogen activation and degradation of extracellular matrix. J Cell Physiol 1988;135:387–396.
37. Hart PH, Vitti GF, Burgess DR et al. Human monocytes can produce tissue-type plasminogen activator. J Exp Med 1989;169:1509–1514.
38. Hart PH, Burgess DR, Vitti GF et al. Interleukin-4 stimulates human monocytes to produce tissue-type plasminogen activator. Blood 1989;74:1222–1225.
39. Simon DI, Ezratty AM, Francis SA et al. Fibrin(ogen) is internalized and degraded by activated human monocytoid cells via Mac-1 (CD11b/CD18): A nonplasmin fibrinolytic pathway. Blood 1993;82:2414–2422.
40. Simon DI, Ezratty AM, Loscalzo J. The fibrin(ogen)olytic properties of cathepsin D. Biochemistry 1994;33:6555–6563.
41. Rabbani LE, Loscalzo J. Recent observations on the role of hemostatic determinants in the development of the atherosclerotic plaque. Atherosclerosis 1994;105:1–7.
42. Schaub RG, Bree MP, Hayes LL et al. Recombinant human macrophage colony-stimulating factor reduces plasma cholesterol and carrageenan granuloma foam cell formation in Watanabe heritable hyperlipidemic rabbits. Arterioscler Thromb 1994;14:70–76.
43. Weksler BB. Platelet interactions with the blood vessel wall. In: Colman

RW, Hirsh J, Marder VJ, Salzman EW, eds. Hemostasis and thrombosis. Philadelphia: JB Lippincott Co, 1987;804–815.

44. Waterfield MD, Scrace GT, Whittle N et al. Platelet-derived growth factor is structurally related to the putative transforming protein p$^{28}$sis of simian sarcoma virus. Nature 1983;304:35–39.

45. Doolittle RF, Hunkapiller MW, Hood LE et al. Simian sarcoma virus onc gene, v-sis, is derived from the gene (or genes) encoding a platelet-derived growth factor. Science 1983;221:275–277.

46. Robbins KC, Antoniades HN, Devare SG et al. Structural and immunological similarities between simian sarcoma virus gene product(s) and human platelet-derived growth factor. Nature 1983;305:605–608.

47. Cercek B, Sharifi B, Barath P et al. Growth factors in the pathogenesis of coronary arterial restenosis. Am J Cardiol 1991;68:24c–33c.

48. Giannella-Neto D, Kamyar A, Sharifi B et al. Platelet-derived growth factor isoforms decrease insulin-like growth factor I gene expression in rat vascular smooth muscle cells and selectively stimulate the biosynthesis of insulin-like growth factor. Circ Res 1992;71:646–656.

49. Majack RA, Mildbrandt J, Dixit VM. Induction of thrombospondin messenger RNA levels occurs as an immediate primary response to platelet-derived growth factor. J Biol Chem 1987;262:8821–8825.

50. Siegbahn A, Hammacher A, Westermark B et al. Differential effects of the various isoforms of platelet-derived growth factor on the chemotaxis of fibroblasts, monocytes and granulocytes. J Clin Invest 1990;85:916–920.

51. Hosang M, Rouge M, Wipf B et al. Both homodimeric isoforms of PDGF (AA and BB) have mitogenic and chemotactic activity and stimulate phosphoinositol turnover. J Cell Physiol 1989;140:558–564.

52. Meyer-Ingold W, Eichner W. Platelet-derived growth factor. Cell Biol Int 1995;19:389–398.

53. Raines EW, Dower SK, Ross R. Interleukin-1 mitogenic activity for fibroblasts and smooth muscle cells is due to PDGF-AA. Science 1989;243: 393–396.

54. Loscalzo J. The relation between atherosclerosis and thrombosis. Circulation 1992;86(suppl III):III95–III99.

55. Castellot JJ Jr, Favreau LV, Karnovsky MJ et al. Inhibition of vascular smooth muscle cell growth by endothelial cell-derived heparin. Possible role of a platelet endoglycosidase. J Biol Chem 1982;257:11256–11260.

56. Majack RA, Cook SC, Bornstein P. Platelet-derived growth factor and heparin-like glycosaminoglycans regulate thrombospondin synthesis and deposition in the matrix by smooth muscle cells. J Cell Biol 1985;101: 1059–1070.

57. Yahalom J, Eldor A, Fuks Z et al. Degradation of sulfated proteoglycans in the subendothelial extracellular matrix by human platelet heparitinase. J Clin Invest 1984;74:1842–1849.

58. Goldberg ID, Stemerman MB, Handin RI. Vascular permeation of platelet factor 4 after endothelial injury. Science 1980;209:611–612.

59. Geng YJ, Libby P. Evidence for apoptosis in advanced human atheroma. Colocalization with interleukin-1 beta-converting enzyme. Am J Pathol 1995;147:251–266.

60. Bennett MR, Evan GI, Schwartz SM. Apoptosis of human vascular smooth muscle cells derived from normal vessels and coronary atherosclerotic plaques. J Clin Invest 1995;95:2266–2274.

61. Welch G, Zhao Z, Loscalzo J et al. Oxidative stress induces apoptosis in vascular smooth muscle cells that is attenuated by glutathione. J Invest Med 1996;44:263A.

62. Gown AM, Tsukada T, Ross R. Human atherosclerosis. II. Immunocytochemical analysis of the cellular composition of human atherosclerotic lesions. Am J Pathol 1986;125:191–207.

63. Thompson WD, Smith EB. Atherosclerosis and the coagulation system. J Pathol 1989;159:97–106.

64. Barger AC, Beeuwkes R 3d, Lainey LL et al. Hypothesis: Vasa vasorum and neovascularization of human coronary arteries. A possible role in the pathophysiology of atherosclerosis. N Engl J Med 1984;310:175–177.

65. Ferrara N, Winer J, Burton T. Aortic smooth muscle cells express and secrete vascular endothelial growth factor. Growth Factors 1991;5:141–148.

66. Stavri GT, Zachary IC, Baskerville PA et al. Basic fibroblast growth factor upregulates the expression of vascular endothelial growth factor in vascular smooth muscle cells. Synergistic interaction with hypoxia. Circulation 1995;92:11–14.

67. Stavri GT, Hong Y, Zachary IC et al. Hypoxia and platelet-derived growth factor-BB synergistically upregulate the expression of vascular endothelial growth factor in vascular smooth muscle cells. FEBS Lett 1995;358:311–315.

68. Brogi E, Wu T, Namiki A et al. Indirect angiogenic cytokines upregulate VEGF and bFGF gene expression in vascular smooth muscle cells, whereas hypoxia upregulates VEGF expression only. Circulation 1994;90:649–652.

69. Friedman RJ, Stemerman MB, Wenz B et al. The effect of thrombocytopenia on experimental atherosclerotic lesion formation in rabbits. Smooth muscle cell proliferation and re-endothelialization. J Clin Invest 1977;60: 1191–1201.

70. Hoak JC. Platelets and atherosclerosis. Semin Thromb Hemost 1988;14: 202–205.

71. Curtiss LK, Black AS, Takagi Y et al. New mechanism for foam cell generation in atherosclerotic lesions. J Clin Invest 1987;80:367–373.

72. Kruth HS. Platelet-mediated cholesterol accumulation in cultured aortic smooth muscle cells. Science 1985;227:1243–1245.

73. Mendelsohn ME, Loscalzo J. Role of platelets in cholesteryl ester formation by U-937 cells. J Clin Invest 1988;81:62–68.

74. Kowalska MA, Tuszynski GP, Capuzzi DM. Plasma lipoproteins mediate platelet adhesion. Biochem Biophys Res Commun 1990;172:113–118.

75. Gross PL, Rand ML, Barrow DV et al. Platelet hypersensitivity in cholesterol-fed rabbits: Enhancement of thromboxane A$_2$-dependent and thrombin-induced, thromboxane A$_2$-independent platelet responses. Atherosclerosis 1991;88:77–86.

76. Gross PL, Rand ML, Barrow DV et al. Platelet function in Watanabe heritable hyperlipidemic rabbits. Decreased sensitivity to thromboxane A$_2$. Arterioscler Thromb 1991;11:610–616.

77. Winocour PD, Vickers JD, Kinlough-Rathbone RL et al. Thrombin-induced inositol phosphate production by platelets from rats with diet-induced or genetically determined hypercholesterolemia. J Lab Clin Med 1990;115: 241–248.

78. Levine JD, Harlan JM, Harker LA et al. Thrombin-mediated release of factor VIII antigen from human umbilical vein endothelial cells in culture. Blood 1982;60:531–534.

79. Nichols TC, Bellinger DA, Reddick RL et al. Role of von Willebrand factor in arterial thrombosis: Studies in normal and von Willebrand disease pigs. Circulation 1991;83(Suppl):IV56–IV64.

80. Nichols TC, Bellinger DA, Tate DA et al. von Willebrand factor and occlusive arterial thrombosis. A study in normal and von Willebrand's disease pigs with diet-induced hypercholesterolemia and atherosclerosis. Arteriosclerosis 1990;10:449–461.

81. Fuster W, Bowie EJ, Lewis JC et al. Resistance to arteriosclerosis in pigs with von Willebrand's disease. Spontaneous and high cholesterol diet-induced arteriosclerosis. J Clin Invest 1978;61:722–730.

82. Fuster V, Lie JT, Badimon L et al. Spontaneous and diet-induced coronary atherosclerosis in normal swine and swine with von Willebrand disease. Arteriosclerosis 1985;5:67–73.

83. Griggs TR, Reddick RL, Sultzer D et al. Susceptibility to atherosclerosis in aortas and coronary arteries of swine with von Willebrand's disease. Am J Pathol 1981;102:137–145.

84. Baron BW, Lyon RT, Zarins CK et al. Changes in plasma factor VIII complex and serum lipid profile during atherogenesis in cynomolgus monkeys. Arteriosclerosis 1990;10:1074–1081.

85. Thompson SG, Kienast J, Pyke SD et al. Hemostatic factors and the risk of myocardial infarction or sudden death in individuals with angina pectoris. European Concerted Action on Thrombosis and Disabilities Angina Pectoris Study Group. N Engl J Med 1995;332:635–641.

86. Furchgott RF, Zawadzki JV. The obligatory role of endothelial cells in the relaxation of arterial smooth muscle by acetylcholine. Nature 1980;288: 373–376.

87. Palmer RM, Ferrige AG, Moncada S. Nitric oxide release accounts for the biological activity of endothelium-derived relaxing factor. Nature 1987; 327:524–526.

88. Ware A, Heistad DD. Platelet-endothelium interactions. Seminars in medicine of the Beth Israel Hospital, Boston. N Engl J Med 1993;328:628–635.

89. Radomski MW, Palmer RM, Moncada S. Endogenous nitric oxide inhibits human platelet adhesion to vascular endothelium. Lancet 1987;2: 1057–1058.

90. Ludmer PL, Selwyn AP, Shook TL et al. Paradoxical vasoconstriction induced by acetylcholine in atherosclerotic coronary arteries. N Engl J Med 1986;315:1046–1051.

91. Vita JA, Treasure CB, Nabel EG et al. Coronary vasomotor response to acetylcholine relates to risk factors for coronary artery disease. Circulation 1990;81:491–497.

92. Vanhoutte PM. Could the absence or malfunction of vascular endothelium precipitate the occurrence of vasospasm? J Mol Cell Cardiol 1986;18: 679–689.

93. Weiss EJ, Bray PF, Tayback M et al. A polymorphism of a platelet glycoprotein receptor as an inherited risk factor for coronary thrombosis. N Engl J Med 1996;334:1090–1094.

94. Ridker PM, Hennekens CH. Hemostatic risk factors for coronary heart disease. Circulation 1991;83:1098–1100.

95. Heller RF, Chinn S, Pedoe HD et al. How well can we predict coronary heart disease? Findings in the United Kingdom Heart Disease Prevention Project. Br Med J 1984;288:1409–1411.

96. DeWood MA, Spores J, Notske R et al. Prevalence of total coronary artery occlusion during the early hours of transmural myocardial infarction. N Engl J Med 1980;303:897–902.

97. Davies MJ, Thomas A. Thrombosis and acute coronary-artery lesions in sudden cardiac ischemic death. N Engl J Med 1984;310:1137–1140.

98. Ernst E. Plasma fibrinogen—An independent cardiovascular risk factor. J Int Med 1990;277:365–372.

99. Barras JP. Blood rheology—A general review. Bibl Haematol 1969;33: 277–297.

100. Rainer C, Kawanishi DT, Chandraratna AN et al. Changes in blood rheology in individuals with stable angina pectoris as a result of coronary artery disease. Circulation 1987;76:15–20.

101. O'Connor NTJ, Cederholm-Williams S, Copper S et al. Hypercoagulability and coronary artery disease. Br Heart J 1984;52:614–616.

102. Nicolaides AN, Horbourne T, Bowers R et al. Blood viscosity, red cell flexibility, haematocrit and plasma-fibrinogen in individuals with angina. Lancet 1977;2:943–945.

103. Lowe GDO, Drummond MM, Lorimer AR. Relation between extent of coronary artery disease and blood viscosity. Br Med J 1980;280:673–674.

104. Dormandy J, Ernst E, Matrai A, Flute P. Hemorrhagic changes following acute myocardial infarction. Am Heart J 1982;104:1364–1367.

105. Hamsten A, Blomback M, Wiman B et al. Haemostatic function in myocardial infarction. Br Heart J 1986;55:58–66.

106. Volger E. Bedeutung der Flieszeigenschaften des Blutes bei drohendem myokardinfarkt. Haemostaseologie 1986;6:118–123.

107. Fulton RM, Duckett K. Plasma-fibrinogen and thromboemboli after myocardial infarction. Lancet 1976;2:1161–1164.

108. Eisenberg S. Blood viscosity and fibrinogen concentration following cerebral infarction. Circulation 1966 (Suppl 2):33:10–14.

109. Todd M, McDevitt E, McDowell F. Stroke and blood coagulation. Stroke 1973;4:400–405.

110. Pilgeram LO, Chee AN, Von dem Bussche G. Evidence for abnormalities in clotting and thrombolysis as a risk factor for stroke. Stroke 1973;4(4): 643–657.

111. Ernst E, Matrai A, Marshall M. Blood rheology in individuals with transient ischemic attacks. Stroke 1988;19:634–636.

112. Dormandy JA, Hoare E, Colley J et al. Clinical, haemodynamic, rheological, and biochemical findings in 126 individuals with intermittent claudication. Br Med J 1973;4:576–581.

113. Ernst E, Matrai A. Intermittent claudication, exercise, and blood rheology. Circulation 1987;76:1110–1114.

114. Baxter K, Wiseman S, Powell J et al. Pilot study of a screening test for peripheral arterial disease in middle aged men: Fibrinogen as a possible risk factor. Cardiovasc Res 1988;22:300–302.

115. Dormandy J. Cardiovascular diseases. In: Chien S, Dormandy J, Ernst E, Matrai A, eds. Clinical Hemorheology. Dordrecht: M. Nijhoff, 1987; 165–194.

116. Humphries SE, Cook M, Dubowitz M et al. Role of genetic variation at the fibrinogen locus in determination of plasma fibrinogen concentrations. Lancet 1987;1:1452–1455.

117. Hamsten A, Iselius L, deFaire U, Blomback M. Genetic and cultural inheritance of plasma fibrinogen concentration. Lancet 1987;2:988–991.

118. Balleisen L, Bailey J, Epping PH et al. Epidemiological study on factor VII, factor VIII and fibrinogen in an industrial population. I. Baseline data on the relation to age, gender, body weight, smoking, alcohol, pill-using and menopause. Thromb Haemost 1985;54:475–479.

119. Merskey C, Wohl H. Changes in blood coagulation and fibrinolysis in rats fed atherogenic diets. Thromb Diath Haemorrh 1964;10:295.

120. Elkeles RS, Chakrabarti R, Vickers M et al. Effect of treatment of hyperlipidaemia on haemostatic variables. Br Med J 1980;281:973–974.

121. Simpson HC, Mann JI, Meade TW et al. Hypertriglyceridaemia and hypercoagulability. Lancet 1983;1:786–790.

122. Meade TW, North WR, Chakrabarti R et al. Population-based distributions of haemostatic variables. Br Med Bull 1977;33:283–288.

123. Ernst E, Matrai A, Schmolzl C et al. Dose-effect relationship between smoking and blood rheology. Br J Haematol 1987;65:485–487.

124. Wilkes HC, Kelleher C, Meade TW. Smoking and plasma fibrinogen [Letter]. Lancet 1988;1:307–308.

125. Ernst E, Matrai A. Abstention from chronic cigarette smoking normalizes blood rheology. Atherosclerosis 1987;64:75–77.

126. Meade TW, Imeson J, Stirling Y. Effects of changes in smoking and other characteristics on clotting factors and the risk of ischaemic heart disease. Lancet 1987;2:986–988.

127. Allen DR, Browse NL, Rutt DL. Effects of cigarette smoke, carbon monoxide and nicotine on the uptake of fibrinogen by the canine arterial wall. Atherosclerosis 1989;77:83–88.

128. Letcher RL, Chien S, Pickering TG et al. Direct relationship between blood pressure and blood viscosity in normal and hypertensive subjects. Role of fibrinogen and concentration. Am J Med 1981;70:1195–1202.

129. Koenig W, Sund M, Ernst E et al. Is increased plasma viscosity a risk factor for high blood pressure? Angiology 1989;40:153–163.

130. Barnes AJ, Locke P, Scudder PR et al. Is hyperviscosity a treatable component of diabetic microcirculatory disease? Lancet 1977;2:789–791.

131. Hill MA, Court JM, Mitchell GM. Blood rheology and microalbuminuria in type I diabetes mellitus [Letter]. Lancet 1982;2:985.

132. Ernst E, Weihmayr T, Schmid M et al. Cardiovascular risk factors and hemorheology. Physical fitness, stress and obesity. Atherosclerosis 1986; 59:263–269.

133. Kannel WB, Hjortland MC, McNamara PM et al. Menopause and the risk of cardiovascular disease: the Framingham Study. Ann Intern Med 1976; 85:447–452.

134. Moller L, Kristensen TS. Plasma fibrinogen and ischemic heart disease risk factors. Arterioscler Thromb 1991;11:344–350.

135. Ernst E. Influence of regular physical activity on blood rheology. Eur Heart J 1987;8(Suppl):59–62.

136. Ernst E, Pietsch L, Eisenberg J et al. Blood rheology in vegetarians. Br J Nutr 1986;56:555–560.

137. Hostmark AT, Bjerkedal T, Kierulf P et al. Fish oil and plasma fibrinogen. Br Med J 1988;297:180–181.

138. Niort G, Bulgarelli A, Cassader M et al. Effect of short-term treatment with bezafibrate on plasma fibrinogen, fibrinopeptide A, platelet activation and blood filterability in atherosclerotic hyperfibrinogenemic individuals. Atherosclerosis 1988;71:113–119.

139. Meade TW, North WR, Chakrabarti R et al. Haemostatic function and cardiovascular death: Early results of a prospective study. Lancet 1980;1: 1050–1054.

140. Meade TW, Mellows S, Brozovic M et al. Haemostatic function and ischaemic heart disease: Principal results of the Northwick Park Heart Study. Lancet 1986;2:533–537.

141. Stone MC, Thorp JM. Plasma fibrinogen—A major coronary risk factor. J R Coll Gen Pract 1985;35:565–569.

142. Kannel WB, D'Agostino RB, Belanger AJ. Fibrinogen, cigarette smoking, and risk of cardiovascular disease: Insights from the Framingham Study. Am Heart J 1987;113:1006–1010.

143. Kannel WB, Wolf PA, Castelli WP et al. Fibrinogen and risk of cardiovascular disease. The Framingham Study. JAMA 1987;258:1183–1186.

144. Wilhelmsen L, Svardsudd K, Korsan-Bengtsen K et al. Fibrinogen as a risk factor for stroke and myocardial infarction. N Engl J Med 1984;311: 501–505.

145. Andus T, Geiger T, Hirano T et al. Action of recombinant human interleukin 6, interleukin 1β and tumor necrosis factor α on the mRNA induction of acute-phase proteins. Eur J Immunol 1988;18:739–746.

146. Remick DG, Kunkel RG, Larrick JW et al. Acute *in vivo* effects of human recombinant tumor necrosis factor. Lab Invest 1987;56:583–590.

147. Biasucci LM, Vitelli A, Luizzo G et al. Elevated levels of interleukin-6 in unstable angina. Circulation 1996;94:874–877.

148. Green F, Kelleher C, Wilkes H et al. A common genetic polymorphism associated with lower coagulation factor VII levels in healthy individuals. Arterioscler Thromb 1991;11:540–546.

149. Mitropoulos KA, Esnouf MP, Meade TW. Increased factor VII coagulant activity in the rabbit following diet-induced hypercholesterolaemia. Evidence for increased conversion of VII to -VII and higher flux within the coagulation pathway. Atherosclerosis 1987;63:43–52.

150. Mitropoulos KA, Esnouf MP. Turnover of factor X and of prothrombin in rabbits fed on a standard or cholesterol-supplemented diet. Biochem J 1987;244:263–269.

151. Miller GJ, Walter SJ, Stirling Y et al. Assay of factor VII activity by two techniques: Evidence for increased conversion of VII to α-VIIa in hyperlipidaemia, with possible implications for ischaemic heart disease. Br J Haematol 1985;59:249–258.

152. Miller GJ, Martin JC, Webster J et al. Association between dietary fat intake and plasma factor VII coagulant activity—A predictor of cardiovascular mortality. Atherosclerosis 1986;60:269–277.

153. Mitropoulos KA, Miller GJ, Reeves BE et al. Factor VII coagulant activity is strongly associated with the plasma concentration of large lipoprotein particles in middle-aged men. Atherosclerosis 1989;76:203–208.

154. Miller GJ, Cruickshank JK, Ellis LJ et al. Fat consumption and factor VII coagulant activity in middle-aged men. An association between a dietary and thrombogenic coronary risk factor. Atherosclerosis 1989;78:19–24.

155. Miller GJ, Martin JC, Mitropoulos KA et al. Plasma factor VII is activated by postprandial triglyceridaemia, irrespective of dietary fat composition. Atherosclerosis 1991;86:163–171.

156. Hamsten A. Coagulation factors and hyperlipidaemia. Curr Opin Lipidol 1991;2:266–271.

157. Marckmann P, Sandstrom B, Jespersen J. Effects of total fat content and fatty acid composition in diet on factor VII coagulant activity and blood lipids. Atherosclerosis 1990;80:227–233.

158. Skartlien AH, Lyberg-Beckmann S, Holme I et al. Effect of alteration in triglyceride levels on factor VII-phospholipid complexes in plasma. Arteriosclerosis 1989;9:798–801.

159. Thompson SG, Martin JC, Meade TW. Sources of variability in coagulation factor assays. Thromb Haemost 1987;58:1073–1077.

160. Rao LV, Rapaport SI. Studies of a mechanism inhibiting the initiation of the extrinsic pathway of coagulation. Blood 1987;69:645–651.

161. Sandset PM, Abildgaard U, Pettersen M. A sensitive assay of extrinsic coagulation pathway inhibitor (EPI) in plasma and plasma fractions. Thromb Res 1987;47:389–400.

162. Broze GJ Jr, Warren LA, Novotny WF et al. The lipoprotein-associated coagulation inhibitor that inhibits the factor VII-tissue factor complex also inhibits factor Xa: Insight into its possible mechanism of action. Blood 1988;71:335–343.

163. Wun TC, Kretzmer KK, Girard TJ et al. Cloning and characterization of a cDNA coding for the lipoprotein-associated coagulation inhibitor shows that it consists of three tandem Kunitz-type inhibitory domains. J Biol Chem 1988;263:6001–6004.

164. Bajaj MS, Kuppuswamy MN, Saito H et al. Cultured normal human hepatocytes do not synthesize lipoprotein-associated coagulation inhibitor: Evi-

dence that endothelium is the principal site of its synthesis. Proc Natl Acad Sci U S A 1990;87:8869–8873.

165. Sandset PM, Lund H, Norseth J et al. Treatment with hydroxymethylglutaryl coenzyme A reductase inhibitors in hypercholesterolemia induces changes in the components of the extrinsic coagulation system. Arterioscler Thromb 1991;11:138–145.

166. Salomaa V, Stinson V, Kark JD et al. Association of fibrinolytic parameters with early atherosclerosis. The ARIC Study. Atherosclerosis Risk in Communities Study. Circulation 1995;91:281–290.

167. Friedman GD, Klatsky AL, Siegelaub AB. The leukocyte count as a predictor of myocardial infarction. N Engl J Med 1974;290:1275–1278.

168. Friedman GD, Klatsky AL, Siegelaub AB. Predictors of sudden cardiac death. Circulation 1975;52:(Suppl):III164–III169.

169. Grimm RH Jr, Neaton JD. Prognostic importance of the white blood cell count for coronary, cancer, and all-cause mortality. JAMA 1985;254:1932–1937.

170. Prentice RL, Szatrowski TP, Fujikura T et al. Leukocyte counts and coronary heart disease in a Japanese cohort. Am J Epidemiol 1982;116:496–509.

171. Yarnell JW, Barker IA, Sweetnam PM et al. Fibrinogen, viscosity, and white blood cell count are major risk factors for ischemic heart disease. The Caerphilly and Speedwell collaborative heart disease studies. Circulation 1991;83:836–844.

172. Conti P, Bartle L, Barbacane RC et al. The down-regulation of IL-6-stimulated fibrinogen steady state mRNA and protein levels by human recombinant IL-1 is not PGE2-dependent: Effects of IL-1 receptor antagonist (IL-1RA). Mol Cell Biochem 1995;142:171–178.

173. Mackiewicz A, Ganapathi MK, Schultz D et al. Transforming growth factor beta 1 regulates production of acute phase proteins. Proc Natl Acad Sci U S A 1990;87:1491–1495.

174. Libby P, Sukhova G, Lee RT et al. Cytokines regulate vascular functions related to stability of the atherosclerotic plaque. J Cardiovasc Pharmacol 1995;25(Suppl):S9–S12.

175. Bevilacqua MP, Pober JS, Majeau GR et al. Recombinant tumor necrosis factor induces procoagulant activity in cultured human vascular endothelium: Characterization and comparison with the actions of interleukin-1. Proc Natl Acad Sci U S A 1986;83:4533–4537.

176. Schwartz CJ, Valente AJ, Kelley JL et al. Thrombosis and the development of atherosclerosis: Rokitansky revisited. Semin Thromb Hemost 1988;14:189–195.

177. Crawford T, Levene CI. The incorporation of fibrin in the aortic intima. J Pathol Bacteriol 1952;64:523–528.

178. Woolf N, Crawford T. Fatty streaks in the aortic intima studied by an immuno-histochemical technique. J Pathol Bacteriol 1960;80:405–408.

179. Woolf N. The distribution of fibrin within the aortic intima. An immunohistochemical study. Am J Pathol 1961;39:521–532.

180. Wyllie JC, More RH, Haust MD. Demonstration of fibrin in the white plaque by the fluorescent antibody technique. Am J Pathol 1964;44:255–267.

181. Haust MD, Wyllie JC, More RH. Electron microscopy of fibrin in human atherosclerotic lesions. Immunohistochemical and morphologic identification. Exp Mol Pathol 1965;4:205–216.

182. Walton KW, Williamson N. Histological and immunofluorescent studies on the evolution of the human atheromatous plaque. J Atheroscler Res 1968;8:599–624.

183. Woolf N, Carstairs KC. Infiltration and thrombosis in atherogenesis. A study using immunofluorescent techniques. Am J Pathol 1967;51:373–386.

184. Bini A, Fenoglio JJ Jr, Sobel J et al. Immunochemical characterization of fibrinogen, fibrin I, and fibrin II in human thrombi and atherosclerotic lesions. Blood 1987;69:1038–1045.

185. Bini A, Fenoglio JJ Jr, Mesa-Tejada R et al. Identification and distribution of fibrinogen, fibrin, and fibrin(ogen) degradation products in atherosclerosis. Use of monoclonal antibodies. Arteriosclerosis 1989;9:109–121.

186. Smith EB, Keen GA, Grant A et al. Fate of fibrinogen in human arterial intima. Arteriosclerosis 1990;10:263–275.

187. Shekhonin BV, Tararak EM, Samokhin GP et al. Visualization of apo B, fibrinogen/fibrin, and fibronectin in the intima of normal human aorta and large arteries and during atherosclerosis. Atherosclerosis 1990;82:213–226.

188. Ishida T, Tanaka K. Effects of fibrin and fibrinogen-degradation products on the growth of rabbit aortic smooth muscle cells in culture. Atherosclerosis 1982;44:161–174.

189. Naito M, Hayashi T, Kuzuya M et al. Effects of fibrinogen and fibrin on the migration of vascular smooth muscle cells in vitro. Atherosclerosis 1990;83:9–14.

190. Watanabe K, Ishida T, Yoshitomi F et al. Fibrinogen degradation products influence PGI2 synthesis by cultured porcine aortic endothelial and smooth muscle cells. Atherosclerosis 1984;51:151–161.

191. Juhan-Vague I, Alessi MC, Vague PH. Increased plasminogen activator inhibitor 1 levels. A possible link between insulin resistance and atherothrombosis. Diabetologia 1991;34:457–462.

192. Stiko-Rahm A, Wiman B, Hamsten A et al. Secretion of plasminogen activator inhibitor-1 from cultured human umbilical vein endothelial cells is induced by very low density lipoprotein. Arteriosclerosis 1990;10:1067–1073.

193. Meade TW, Chakrabarti R, Haines AP et al. Characteristics affecting fibrinolytic activity and plasma fibrinogen concentrations. Br Med J 1979;1:153–156.

194. Hamsten A, Wiman B, de Faire U, Blomback M. Increased plasma levels of rapid inhibitor of tissue plasminogen activator in young survivors of myocardial infarction. N Engl J Med 1985;313:1557–1563.

195. Juhan-Vague I, Vague P, Alessi MC et al. Relationships between plasma insulin triglyceride, body mass index, and plasminogen activator inhibitor 1. Diabetes Metab 1987;13:331–336.

196. Mehta J, Mehta P, Lawson D et al. Plasma tissue plasminogen activator inhibitor levels in coronary artery disease: Correlation with age and serum triglyceride concentrations. J Am Coll Cardiol 1987;9:263–268.

197. Andersen P, Nilsen DW, Lyberg Beckmann S et al. Increased fibrinolytic potential after diet intervention in healthy coronary high-risk individuals. Acta Med Scand 1988;223:449–506.

198. Mehrabian M, Peter JB, Barnard RJ et al. Dietary regulation of fibrinolytic factors. Atherosclerosis 1990;84:25–32.

199. Andersen P, Smith P, Seljeflot I et al. Effects of gemfibrozil on lipids and haemostasis after myocardial infarction. Thromb Haemost 1990;63:174–177.

200. Almer LO, Janzon L. Low vascular fibrinolytic activity in obesity. Thromb Res 1975;6:175–175.

201. Sundell IB, Dahlgren S, Ranby M et al. Reduction of elevated plasminogen activator inhibitor levels during modest weight loss. Fibrinolysis 1989;3:51–53.

202. Crutchley DJ, McPhee GV, Terris MF et al. Levels of three hemostatic factors in relation to serum lipids. Monocyte procoagulant activity, tissue plasminogen activator, and type-1 plasminogen activator inhibitor. Arteriosclerosis 1989;9:934–939.

203. Latron Y, Alessi MC, Anfosso F et al. Effect of low density lipoproteins on secretion of plasminogen activator inhibitor-1 (PAI-1) by human endothelial cells and hepatoma cells. Fibrinolysis 1990;4(Suppl 2):82–83.

204. Mussoni L, Maderna P, Carrera M et al. Atherogenic lipoproteins and release of plasminogen activator inhibitor-1 (PAI-1) by endothelial cells. Fibrinolysis 1990;4(Suppl 2):79–81.

205. Paramo JA, Colucci M, Collen D et al. Plasminogen activator inhibitor in the blood of individuals with coronary artery disease. BMJ 1985;291:573–574.

206. Hamsten A, de Faire U, Walldius G et al. Plasminogen activator inhibitor in plasma: Risk factor for recurrent myocardial infarction. Lancet 1987;2:3–9.

207. Ridker PM, Vaughan DE, Stampfer MJ et al. Endogenous tissue-type plasminogen activator and risk of myocardial infarction. Lancet 1993;341:1165–1168.

208. Hamsten A. Hemostatic function and coronary artery disease. N Engl J Med 1995;332:677–678.

209. Schneiderman J, Sawdey MS, Keeton MR et al. Increased type 1 plasminogen activator inhibitor gene expression in atherosclerotic human arteries. Proc Natl Acad Sci U S A 1992;89:6998–7002.

210. Raghunath PN, Tomaszewski JE, Brady ST et al. Plasminogen activator system in human coronary atherosclerosis. Arterioscler Thromb Vasc Biol 1995;15:1432–1443.

211. Reaven GM. Banting Lecture 1988. Role of insulin resistance in human disease. Diabetes 1988;37:1595–1607.

212. Stout RW, Vallance-Owen J. Insulin and atheroma. Lancet 1969;1:1078–1080.

213. Ducimetiere P, Eschwege E, Papoz L et al. Relationship of plasma insulin levels to the incidence of myocardial infarction and coronary heart disease mortality in a middle-aged population. Diabetologia 1980;19:205–210.

214. Juhan-Vague I, Alessi MC, Joly P et al. Plasma plasminogen activator inhibitor in angina pectoris. Influence of plasma insulin and acute-phase response. Arteriosclerosis 1989;9:362–367.

215. Vague P, Juhan-Vague I, Aillaud MF et al. Correlation between blood fibrinolytic activity, plasminogen activator inhibitor-1 level, plasma insulin level and relative body weight in normal and obese subjects. Metabolism 1986;35:250–253.

216. Vague P, Juhan-Vague I, Chabert V et al. Fat distribution and plasminogen activator inhibitor activity in nondiabetic obese women. Metabolism 1989;38:913–915.

217. Juhan-Vague I, Roul C, Alessi MC et al. Increased plasminogen activator inhibitor activity in noninsulin dependent diabetic individuals—Relationship with plasma insulin. Thromb Haemost 1989;61:370–373.

218. Alessi MC, Juhan-Vague I, Kooistra T et al. Insulin stimulates the synthesis of plasminogen activator inhibitor 1 by the human hepatocellular cell line Hep G2. Thromb Haemost 1988;60:491–494.

219. Kooistra T, Bosma PJ, Tons HA et al. Plasminogen activator inhibitor 1: Biosynthesis and mRNA levels are increased by insulin in cultured human hepatocytes. Thromb Haemost 1989;62:723–728.

220. Landin K, Stigendal L, Eriksson E et al. Abdominal obesity is associated with an impaired fibrinolytic activity and elevated plasminogen activator inhibitor-1. Metabolism 1990;39:1044–1048.

221. Grant PJ, Kruithof EK, Felley CP et al. Short-term infusions of insulin, triacylglycerol and glucose do not cause acute increases in plasminogen activator inhibitor-1 concentrations in man. Clin Sci 1990;79:513–516.

222. Dawson S, Hamsten A, Wiman B et al. Genetic variation at the plasminogen activator inhibitor-1 locus is associated with altered levels of plasma plasminogen activator inhibitor-1 activity. Arterioscler Thromb 1991;11: 183–190.

223. Vaughan DE, Lazos SA, Tong K. Angiotensin II regulates the expression of plasminogen activator inhibitor-1 in cultured endothelial cells. A potential link between the renin-angiotensin system and thrombosis. J Clin Invest 1995;95:995–1001.

224. Kerins DM, Hao W, Vaughan DE. Angiotensin induction of PAI-1 expression in endothelial cells is mediated by the hexapeptide angiotensin IV. J Clin Invest 1995;96:2515–2520.

225. Hamdan AD, Quist WC, Gagne JB et al. Angiotensin-converting enzyme inhibition suppresses plasminogen activator inhibitor-1 expression in the neointima of balloon-injured rat aorta. Circulation 1996;93:1073–1078.

226. Wright RA, Flapan AD, Alberti KG et al. Effects of captopril therapy on endogenous fibrinolysis in men with recent, uncomplicated myocardial infarction. J Am Coll Cardiol 1994;24:67–73.

227. Jansson JH, Boman K, Nilsson TK. Enalapril-related changes in the fibrinolytic system in survivors of myocardial infarction. Eur J Clin Pharmacol 1993;44:485–488.

228. Wang JA, Zhen EZ, Guo ZZ et al. Effect of hyperlipidemic serum on lipid peroxidation, synthesis of prostacyclin and thromboxane by cultured endothelial cells: Protective effect of antioxidants. Free Radic Biol Med 1989; 7:243–249.

229. Lefer AM. Prostacyclin, high density lipoproteins, and myocardial ischemia. Circulation 1990;81:2013–2015.

230. Gryglewski RJ, Dembinska-Kiec A, Zmuda A et al. Prostacyclin and thromboxane A$_2$ biosynthesis capacities of heart, arteries, and platelets at various stages of experimental atherosclerosis in rabbits. Atherosclerosis 1978;31:385–394.

231. Yui Y, Aoyama T, Morishita H et al. Serum prostacyclin stabilizing factor is identical to apolipoprotein A-I (Apo A-I). A novel function of Apo A-I. J Clin Invest 1988;82:803–807.

232. Eldor A, Falcone DJ, Hajjar DP et al. Diet-induced hypercholesterolemia inhibits the recovery of prostacyclin production by injured rabbit aorta. Am J Pathol 1982;107:186–190.

233. Aoyama T, Yui Y, Morishita H et al. Prostaglandin I$_2$ half-life regulated by high density lipoprotein is decreased in acute myocardial infarction and unstable angina pectoris. Circulation 1990;81:1784–1791.

234. Morishita H, Yui Y, Hattori R et al. Increased hydrolysis of cholesteryl ester with prostacyclin is potentiated by high density lipoprotein through the prostacyclin stabilization. J Clin Invest 1990;86:1885–1891.

235. Scanu AM, Lawn RM, Berg K. Lipoprotein(a) and atherosclerosis. Ann Intern Med 1991;115:209–218.

236. Dahlen GH, Guyton JR, Attar M et al. Association of levels of lipoprotein Lp(a), plasma lipids, and other lipoproteins with coronary artery disease documented by angiography. Circulation 1986;74:758–765.

237. Hoff HF, Beck GJ, Skibinski CI et al. Serum Lp(a) level as a predictor of vein graft stenosis after coronary artery bypass surgery in individuals. Circulation 1988;77:1238–1244.

238. Ridker PM, Hennekens CH, Stampfer MJ. A prospective study of lipoprotein(a) and the risk of myocardial infarction. JAMA 1993;270:2195–2199.

239. Floren CH, Albers JJ, Bierman EL. Uptake of Lp(a) lipoprotein by cultured fibroblasts. Biochem Biophys Res Commun 1981;102:636–639.

240. Krempler F, Kostner GM, Roscher A et al. Studies on the role of specific cell surface receptors in the removal of lipoprotein(a) in man. J Clin Invest 1983;71:1431–1441.

241. Haberland ME, Fless G, Scanu AM et al. Modification of Lp(a) by malondialdehyde leads to avid uptake by human monocyte-macrophages [Abstract]. Circulation 1989;80(Suppl II):II-163.

242. Harkes L, Jurgens G, Holasek A et al. *In vivo* studies on the binding sites for lipoprotein(a) in parenchymal and non-parenchymal rat liver cells. FEBS Lett 1988;227:27–31.

243. Utermann G, Hoppichler F, Dieplinger H et al. Defects in the low density lipoprotein receptor gene affect lipoprotein(a) levels: Multiplicative interaction of two gene loci associated with premature atherosclerosis. Proc Natl Acad Sci U S A 1989;86:4171–4174.

244. Cushing GL, Gaubatz JW, Nava ML et al. Quantitation and localization of apolipoprotein[a] and B in coronary artery bypass vein grafts resected at re-operation. Arteriosclerosis 1989;9:593–603.

245. Rath M, Niendorf A, Reblin T et al. Detection and quantification of lipoprotein(a) on the arterial wall of 107 coronary bypass individuals. Arteriosclerosis 1989;9:579–592.

246. Beisiegel U, Niendorf A, Wolf K et al. Lipoprotein(a) in the arterial wall. Eur Heart J 1990;11(Suppl):174–183.

247. Nachman RL, Gavish D, Azrolan N et al. Lipoprotein(a) in diet-induced atherosclerosis in nonhuman primates. Arterioscler Thromb 1991;11: 32–38.

248. Kostner GM, Bihari-Varga M. Is the atherogenicity of Lp(a) caused by its reactivity with proteoglycans? Eur Heart J 1990;11(Suppl):184–189.

249. Ehnholm C, Jauhiainen M, Metso J. Interaction of lipoprotein(a) with fibronectin and its potential role in atherogenesis. Eur Heart J 1990;11(Suppl): 190–195.

250. Smith EB, Cochran S. Factors influencing the accumulation in fibrous plaques of lipid derived from low density lipoprotein II. Preferential immobilization of lipoprotein(a) (Lp[a]). Atherosclerosis 1990;84:173–181.

251. Eaton DL, Fless GM, Kohr WJ et al. Partial amino acid sequence of apolipoprotein(a) shows that it is homologous to plasminogen. Proc Natl Acad Sci U S A 1987;84:3224–3228.

252. McLean JW, Tomlinson JE, Kuang WJ et al. cDNA sequence of human apolipoprotein(a) is homologous to plasminogen. Nature 1987;330: 132–137.

253. Loscalzo J, Fless GM, Scanu AM. Lipoprotein(a) inhibits fibrin dependent enhancement of tissue plasminogen activator activity [Abstract]. Blood 1988;72:374a.

254. Loscalzo J, Weinfeld M, Fless GM et al. Lipoprotein(a), fibrin binding, and plasminogen activation. Arteriosclerosis 1990;10:240–245.

255. Scanu AM. Identification of mutations in human apolipoprotein(a) kringle 4-37 from the study of DNA of peripheral blood lymphocytes: Relevance to the role of lipoprotein(a) in atherothrombosis. Am J Cardiol 1995;75: 58B–61B.

256. Brandstrom A, Dahlen GH, Ranby M. Lipoprotein(a): *In vitro* effects on t-PA mediated fibrinolysis [Abstract]. Fibrinolysis 1988;1(Suppl):140.

257. Harpel PC, Gordon BR, Parker TS. Plasmin catalyzes binding of lipoprotein(a) to immobilized fibrinogen and fibrin. Proc Natl Acad Sci U S A 1989;86:3847–3851.

258. Wolf K, Rath M, Niendorf A et al. Morphological colocalization of apoprotein(a) and fibrin(ogen) in human coronary atheromas. Circulation 1989; 80(Suppl II):II-522.

259. Hajjar KA, Gavish D, Breslow JL et al. Lipoprotein(a) modulation of endothelial cell surface fibrinolysis and its potential role in atherosclerosis. Nature 1989;339:303–305.

260. Miles LA, Fless GM, Levin EG et al. A potential basis for the thrombotic risks associated with lipoprotein(a). Nature 1989;339:301–303.

261. Fuster V, Stein B, Ambrose JA et al. Atherosclerotic plaque rupture and thrombosis. Evolving concepts [Review]. Circulation 1990;82(Suppl):II-47–II-59.

262. Etingin OR, Hajjar DP, Hajjar KA et al. Lipoprotein(a) regulates plasminogen activator inhibitor-1 expression in endothelial cells. A potential mechanism in thrombogenesis. J Biol Chem 1991;266:2459–2465.

263. Davies MJ, Thomas AC. Plaque fissuring–the cause of acute myocardial infarction, sudden ischaemic death, and crescendo angina [Review]. Br Heart J 1985;53:363–373.

264. Falk E. Plaque rupture with severe pre-existing stenosis precipitating coronary thrombosis. Characteristics of coronary atherosclerotic plaques underlying fatal occlusive thrombi. Br Heart J 1983;50:127–134.

265. Ambrose JA, Winters SL, Stern A et al. Angiographic morphology and the pathogenesis of unstable angina pectoris. J Am Coll Cardiol 1985;5: 609–616.

266. Ambrose JA, Hjemdahl-Monsen CE, Borrico S et al. Angiographic demonstration of a common link between unstable angina pectoris and non-Q-wave acute myocardial infarction. Am J Cardiol 1988;61:244–247.

267. Sherman CT, Litvack F, Grundfest W et al. Coronary angioscopy in individuals with unstable angina pectoris. N Engl J Med 1986;315:913–919.

268. Levin DC, Fallon JT. Significance of the angiographic morphology of localized coronary stenoses: histopathologic correlations. Circulation 1982;66: 316–320.

269. Falk E. Unstable angina with fatal outcome: Dynamic coronary thrombosis leading to infarction and/or sudden death. Autopsy evidence of recurrent mural thrombosis with peripheral embolization culminating in total vascular occlusion. Circulation 1985;71:699–708.

270. Davies MJ. A macro and micro view of coronary vascular insult in ischemic heart disease [Review]. Circulation 1990;82(Suppl):II-38–II-46.

271. Ambrose JA, Winters SL, Arora RR et al. Angiographic evolution of coronary artery morphology in unstable angina. J Am Coll Cardiol 1986;7: 472–478.

272. Ambrose JA, Tannenbaum MA, Alexopoulos D et al. Angiographic progression of coronary artery disease and the development of myocardial infarction. J Am Coll Cardiol 1988;12:56–62.

273. Little WC, Constantinescu M, Applegate RJ et al. Can coronary angiography predict the site of a subsequent myocardial infarction in individuals with mild-to-moderate coronary artery disease? Circulation 1988;78: 1157–1166.

274. Davies MJ. Thrombosis and coronary atherosclerosis. In: Julian DG, Kubler W, Norris RM, Swan HJ, Collen D, Verstraete M, eds. Thrombolysis in cardiovascular disease. New York: Marcel Dekker, 1989:25–43.

275. Richardson PD, Davies MJ, Born GV. Influence of plaque configuration and stress distribution on fissuring of coronary atherosclerotic plaques. Lancet 1989;2:941–944.

276. Shah PK, Falk E, Badimon JJ et al. Human monocyte-derived macrophages induce collagen breakdown in fibrous caps of atherosclerotic plaques. Potential role of matrix-degrading metalloproteinases and implications for plaque rupture. Circulation 1995;92:1565–1569.

277. Lee E, Grodzinsky AJ, Libby P et al. Human vascular smooth muscle cell-monocyte interactions and metalloproteinase secretion in culture. Arterioscler Thromb Vasc Biol 1995;15:2284–2289.

278. Jean-Claude J, Newman KM, Li H et al. Possible key role for plasmin in the pathogenesis of abdominal aortic aneurysms. Surgery 1994;116:472–478.

279. Galis ZS, Zukhova GK, Lark MW et al. Increased expression of matrix metalloproteinases and matrix degrading activity in vulnerable regions of human atherosclerotic plaques. J Clin Invest 1994;94:2493–2503.

280. Lee RT, Grodzinsky AJ, Frank EH et al. Structure-dependent dynamic mechanical behavior of fibrous caps from human atherosclerotic plaques. Circulation 1991;83:1764–1770.

281. Moreno PR, Falk E, Palacios IF et al. Macrophage infiltration in acute coronary syndromes. Implications for plaque rupture. Circulation 1994;90:775–778.

282. Moreno PR, Bernardi VH, Lopez-Cuellar J et al. Macrophages, smooth muscle cells, and tissue factor in unstable angina. Implications for cell-mediated thrombogenicity in acute coronary syndromes. Circulation 1996;94:3090–3097.

283. Cheng GC, Loree HM, Kamm RD et al. Distribution of circumferential stress in ruptured and stable atherosclerotic lesions. A structural analysis with histopathological correlation. Circulation 1993;87:1179–1187.

284. Lee RT, Loree HM, Fishbein MC. High stress regions in saphenous vein bypass graft atherosclerotic lesions. J Am Coll Cardiol 1994;24:1639–1644.

285. Loree HM, Kamm RD, Stringfellow RG et al. Effects of fibrous cap thickness on peak circumferential stress in model atherosclerotic vessels. Circulation 1992;71:850–858.

286. Aoki T, Ku DN. Collapse of diseased arteries with eccentric cross section. J Biomech 1993;26:133–142.

287. Muller JE, Tofler GH. Triggering and hourly variation of onset of arterial thrombosis. Ann Epidemiol 1992;2:393–405.

288. Mittleman MA, Maclure M, Tofler GH et al. Triggering of acute myocardial infarction by heavy physical exertion. Protection against triggering by regular exertion. Determinants of Myocardial Infarction Onset Study Investigators. N Engl J Med 1993;329:1677–1683.

289. Falk E. Why do plaques rupture [review]? Circulation 1992;86:III30–III42.

290. Willerson JT, Golino P, Eidt J et al. Specific platelet mediators and unstable coronary artery lesions. Experimental evidence and potential clinical implications [Review]. Circulation 1989;80:198–205.

291. DeWood MA, Stifter WF, Simpson CS et al. Coronary arteriographic findings soon after non-Q wave myocardial infarction. N Engl J Med 1986;315:417–423.

292. Gibson RS, Beller GA, Gheorghiade M et al. The prevalence and clinical significance of residual myocardial ischemia 2 weeks after uncomplicated non-Q wave infarction: A prospective natural history study. Circulation 1986;73:1186–1198.

293. Timmis AD, Griffin B, Crick JC et al. The effects of early coronary patency on the evolution of myocardial infarction: A prospective arteriographic study. Br Heart J 1987;58:345–351.

294. Harrison DG, Ferguson DW, Collins SM et al. Rethrombosis after reperfusion with streptokinase: Importance of geometry of residual lesions. Circulation 1984;69:991–999.

295. Gash AK, Spann JF, Sherry S et al. Factors influencing reocclusion after coronary thrombolysis for acute myocardial infarction. Am J Cardiol 1986;57:175–177.

# CHAPTER 40

# INHERITED AND ACQUIRED HYPERCOAGULABLE STATES

Kenneth A. Bauer

Chapter 24 presented a clinical approach to identifying risk factors in individuals with thrombosis along with general guidelines for managing such individuals. Individuals with a tendency to thrombosis are defined as having thrombophilia, and the term inherited thrombophilia is applied to individuals with genetic defects that predispose them towards thromboembolism (1, 2). Due to the episodic nature of thrombosis, the manifestation of symptoms may require the presence of other prothrombotic mutations or conditions (see Fig. 24.2, Chapter 24). This chapter will provide a detailed description of the hereditary thrombotic disorders or primary hypercoagulable states (Table 24.1, Chapter 24) as well as the major acquired or secondary hypercoagulable states (malignancy, paroxysmal nocturnal hemoglobinuria, hyperviscosity syndromes, drug-induced hypercoagulable states, lupus anticoagulants, and antiphospholipid antibody syndrome) (Table 24.2, Chapter 24). Several of these topics and other hypercoagulable states are discussed in other chapters in this text, including thrombotic microangiopathies in Chapter 27, heparin-associated thrombocytopenia with thrombosis in Chapter 29, myeloproliferative disorders in Chapter 31, lupus anticoagulants and antiphospholipid syndrome in Chapter 38, disseminated intravascular coagulation in Chapter 44, pregnancy/oral contraceptives in Chapter 46, and veno-occlusive disease in Chapter 49. In addition, thrombosis in pediatric individuals is specifically discussed in Chapter 47. Although this chapter includes information regarding management of these disorders, more thorough coverage of antithrombotic therapy is provided in Chapters 24 and 54–57.

Prior to 1993, the diagnosis of a hereditary disorder could be established in only about 15% of individuals under age 50 presenting with venous thromboembolism. The major disorders known at that time were deficiencies of antithrombin III, protein C, or protein S. With the discovery that many individuals with unexplained venous thrombosis have activated protein C resistance due to the factor V Leiden mutation and more recently a prothrombin gene mutation, it is currently possible to define genetic risk factors in a much larger percentage of individuals in all age groups presenting with unexplained venous thrombosis. It has also been recognized that hyperhomocysteinemia, which is determined by genetic as well as dietary factors, is a common risk factor for venous and arterial thrombosis.

## INHERITED THROMBOTIC DISORDERS

### ANTITHROMBIN III DEFICIENCY

In 1965, Egeberg (3) described a Norwegian family in which certain individuals who had a history of thrombosis had plasma concentrations of antithrombin III (see Chapter 3) that were 40 to 50% of normal. Subsequently, other investigators described additional families with a similar constellation of clinical and laboratory abnormalities (4–12).

Antithrombin III deficiency is usually inherited in an autosomal dominant fashion, and thus, affects both sexes equally. Two major types of inherited antithrom-

**TABLE 40.1.**   Assay Measurements in Heterozygous Antithrombin III (ATIII) Deficiency

| Types | Antigen | Activity | |
|---|---|---|---|
| | | **Heparin Cofactor** | **Progressive ATIII** |
| I ("Classic") | Low | Low | Low |
| II | | | |
|   Active site defect | Normal | Low | Low |
|   Heparin-binding site defect | Normal | Low | Normal |

bin III deficiency have been delineated (Table 40.1). The classic deficiency state (type I) is a result of reduced synthesis of biologically normal protease inhibitor molecules (13). In these cases, the antigenic and functional activity of antithrombin III in the blood are reduced in parallel. The molecular basis of this disorder is either a deletion of a major segment of the antithrombin III gene or, more commonly, the occurrence of small deletions/insertions (less than 22 base pairs), or single-base substitutions (14–28). These mutations will introduce a frameshift (plus premature termination codon), a direct termination codon, a change in mRNA processing, or unstable translation products. The most recent update of the antithrombin III mutation database includes 80 distinct mutations in individuals with a type I deficiency (29). The second type of antithrombin III deficiency is produced by a discrete molecular defect within the protease inhibitor (type II). The plasma levels of antithrombin III are greatly reduced as judged by functional activity, whereas antithrombin III immunologic activity is essentially normal. Among nine unrelated antithrombin III-deficient individuals of a cohort of 210 individuals presenting with a history of venous thromboembolism before the age of 40 years or recurrent venous thrombosis, five had a type I deficiency and four had a type II deficiency (30).

Using only an immunoassay for measuring antithrombin III levels in the blood, initial estimates of the deficiency state in the general population were one in 2,000 to 5,000 (31, 32). However, recent studies employing functional assays that measure antithrombin III-heparin cofactor activity have found that the prevalence of antithrombin III deficiency in the general population is one in 250 to 500 (33, 34). Interestingly, the majority of the antithrombin III-deficient individuals identified in these studies did not have a personal or familial history of thrombosis and had a type II defect with mutations at the heparin-binding site (Table 40.2) (35). On rare occasions, some of these molecular defects came to clinical attention when homozygous children of consangui-

neous parents who were asymptomatic carriers of such a defect developed severe venous or arterial thrombosis in association with plasma antithrombin III-heparin cofactor levels of less than 10% (36, 37).

Reviews of published cases of familial antithrombin III deficiency indicate that approximately 55% of affected individuals experience venous thrombotic episodes (38, 39). The initial clinical manifestations occur apparently spontaneously in about 42% of subjects, but are related to pregnancy, parturition, oral contraceptive ingestion, surgery, or trauma in the remaining 58% of individuals (38). The most common sites of disease are the deep veins of the leg and the mesenteric veins. Approximately 60% of individuals develop recurrent thrombotic episodes, and clinical signs of pulmonary embolism are evident in 40% (38). Although cases have been reported in which antithrombin III-deficient infants sustain cerebral venous thrombosis (12, 40, 41), affected children rarely develop thrombotic episodes before puberty. At this time, thrombotic events start to occur with some frequency and the risk of thrombosis increases substantially with advancing age (38).

The first family with a functional deficiency of antithrombin III due to the presence of an abnormal protein (type II) was reported by Sas in 1974 (42). Many families with this type of deficiency state have now been reported and they have been further subcategorized on the basis of two different functional assays of antithrombin III activity. The first is the antithrombin III-heparin cofactor assay which measures the ability of heparin to bind to lysyl residues on the inhibitor and catalyze the neutralization of coagulation enzymes such as thrombin and factor Xa. The second test is the progressive antithrombin III activity assay, which quantifies the capacity of this inhibitor to neutralize the enzymatic activity of thrombin in the absence of heparin.

Heparin cofactor II is another protein in human plasma that exhibits heparin cofactor activity (43–45). In contrast to antithrombin III, this inhibitor does not inhibit factor Xa or other serine proteases and requires concentrations of heparin of at least 1 U/mL in the reaction mixture in order to function as an efficient inhibitor of thrombin; it therefore probably plays a minimal role when heparin is used clinically as an anticoagulant (44). As many functional antithrombin III assays use heparin concentrations greater than 1 U/mL, an assay based on factor Xa inhibition is likely to be more specific than one based on thrombin inhibition to identify individuals with a congenital deficiency of antithrombin III (46). Heparin cofactor II can also interact with another glycosaminoglycan, dermatan sulfate, and this binding dramatically accelerates the neutralization of thrombin by this inhibitor. Several individuals have been described with inherited deficiencies of heparin cofactor II and thrombotic phenomena (47, 48), but the causal relationship remains uncertain (49).

**TABLE 40.2.**   Point Mutations in Antithrombin III Deficiency (Type III)

| City or Region of Propositus | Substitution | Effect of Mutation |
|---|---|---|
| Rouen 3 (64) | Ile 7—Asn | Defective heparin binding, new carbohydrate attachment site |
| Rouen 4 (62) | Arg 24—Cys | Defective heparin binding |
| Basel (59), Clichy (52), Dublin II (60), Franconville (61) | Pro 41—Leu | Defective heparin binding |
| Toyama (50), Tours (51), Alger (36), Paris 1 (52), Paris 2 (52), Barcelona 2 (53), Kumamoto (37), Padua 2 (63), Amiens (65) | Arg 47—Cys | Defective heparin binding |
| Rouen 1 (54), Padua 1 (55), Bligny (56) | Arg 47—His | Defective heparin binding |
| Rouen 2 (57) | Arg 47–Ser | Defective heparin binding |
| Budapest 3 (66) | Leu 99—Phe | Defective heparin binding |
| Southport (68) | Leu 99—Val | Defective heparin binding |
| Nagasaki (67) | Ser 116—Pro | Defective heparin binding |
| Vienna (68) | Gln 118—Pro | Defective heparin binding |
| Geneva (58) | Arg 129—Gln | Defective heparin binding |
| Rouen VI (90) | Asn 187—Asp | Defective serine protease inhibition |
| Glasgow III (91) | Asn 187—Lys | Defective serine protease inhibition |
| Truro (29) | Glu 237—Lys | Defective heparin binding |
| Unnamed (92) | Met 251—Ile | Defective serine protease inhibition |
| Haslar (29) | Ile 284—Asn | Defective serine protease inhibition |
| Unnamed (29) | Glu 302—Lys | Defective serine protease inhibition |
| Hamilton (72), Glasgow-II (74) | Ala 382—Thr | Defective serine protease inhibition |
| Charleville (52), Cambridge 1 (75), Vicenza (81), Sudbury (80) | Ala 384—Pro | Defective serine protease inhibition |
| Cambridge 2 (82) | Ala 384—Ser | Defective serine protease inhibition |
| Stockholm (83) | Gly 392—Asp | Defective serine protease inhibition |
| Glasgow (78, 84), Sheffield (86), Chicago (87), Waikato (88), Avranches (52) | Arg 393—His | Defective serine protease inhibition |
| Northwick Park (78), Milano 1 (77), Frankfurt 1 (79) | Arg 393—Cys | Defective serine protease inhibition |
| Pescara (89) | Arg 393—Pro | Defective serine protease inhibition |
| Denver (70), Milano 2 (71) | Ser 394—Leu | Defective serine protease inhibition |
| Rosny (98) | Phe 402—Cys | These mutations result in the presence of trace amounts of the abnormal antithrombin III in individual's plasma. |
| Torino (98) | Phe 402—Ser | |
| Maisons, Lafitte (100, 101) | Phe 402—Leu | |
| Oslo (97) | Ala 404—Thr | |
| La Rochelle (100) | Asn 405—Lys | |
| Kyoto (99) | Arg 406—Met | |
| Unnamed (29) | Arg 406—Gly | |
| Utah (95) | Pro 407—Leu | |
| Budapest 5 (100) | Pro 407—Thr | |
| Unnamed (29) | Arg 425—Thr | Abnormal heparin binding and reduced thrombin inhibitory activity. |
| Budapest (103) | Pro 429—Leu | |

The antithrombin III-heparin cofactor and progressive antithrombin III activity assays have identified antithrombin III-deficient individuals with reductions in heparin cofactor activity with or without concordant decrements in progressive antithrombin III activity. Several abnormal antithrombin III molecules have been identi-fied with isolated reductions in heparin cofactor activity that have defects at a heparin binding site (Table 40.2). These variants generally have mutations at the aminoter-minal end of the molecule (36, 37, 50–68). In one of these variants, the substitution of asparagine for isoleucine at residue 7 produces a new glycosylation site and the resultant protein has a reduced affinity for heparin (64). Variants with decreased activity in both antithrombin III functional assays generally have mutations near the thrombin binding site at the carboxyterminal end of the molecule (Table 40.2) (29, 52, 69–92). All antithrombin III variants can not be neatly characterized by this schema, as single amino acid substitutions can affect both functional domains of the molecule. This is perhaps best illustrated by a mutation in which arginine is replaced by histidine at residue 393 (52, 77, 78, 84–88). This mutation markedly decreases the ability of the protein to inhibit thrombin, but also leads to increased heparin affinity.

Another type of mutation has been described at the carboxyterminal end of the antithrombin III molecule between amino acids 402 and 429 (Table 40.2). These type II variants are called pleiotropic as they exhibit multiple functional defects (29). In a large Utah family, trace amounts of an electrophoretically and functionally abnormal inhibitor molecule have been identified (93). Leucine is substituted for proline at position 407 in the antithrombin III molecules of the affected members of this kindred (94, 95). Small amounts of an electrophoretically abnormal inhibitor species have also been observed in the plasma of antithrombin III-deficient members of the Oslo kindred first reported by Egeberg (3, 96). In this case, threonine replaces alanine at position 404 in the abnormal protein (97). Mutations at positions 402, 405, 406, and 407 apparently also lead to a similar type of defect (29, 98–101). The antithrombin III deficient subjects in the Utah and Oslo pedigrees appear, however, to have a type I deficiency state as determined by routine laboratory testing. The similar characteristics of these mutations suggest that the region of residues 402 to 407 is important for the maintenance of normal plasma levels of antithrombin III antigen (95). The mutant inhibitor molecules synthesized by the liver of these deficient individuals may be susceptible to increased intracellular degradation, decreased extracellular export, or increased clearance upon entry into the circulation. Finally, the mutation in the first reported antithrombin III variant, Budapest (42), is replacement of a proline by leucine at residue 429, leading to a molecular defect that affects both the heparin and thrombin binding sites (102, 103).

The prevalence of thrombosis appears to be different in heterozygous individuals with type II defects at the heparin binding site as compared to the thrombin binding site (104). As noted earlier, individuals with plasma antithrombin III-heparin cofactor activity measurements of approximately 50% and normal progressive antithrombin III activity (heparin binding site defects) have infrequent thrombotic episodes (54, 57). In contrast to these observations, heterozygous type II individuals with both diminished progressive antithrombin III activity and antithrombin III-heparin cofactor activity (thrombin binding site defects) sustain venous thromboembolism as often as type I individuals.

The mean concentration of antithrombin III in normal pooled plasma is approximately 140 μg/mL. In plasmas from normal individuals, the range of antithrombin III concentrations as determined by immunologic or functional tests is reasonably narrow. Most laboratories report a normal range between 80 and 120% for antithrombin III-heparin cofactor determinations (105) and a somewhat wider range for immunoassay results (106). The antithrombin III-heparin cofactor assay will detect all the different subtypes of the familial deficiency state currently recognized and is, therefore, the best single laboratory screening test for the disorder.

Healthy newborns have about half the normal adult concentration of antithrombin III (107, 108) and gradually reach the adult level by 6 months of age (109). The levels may be considerably lower in infants born after 30 to 36 weeks of gestation (109) and are even further reduced in infants with respiratory distress, necrotizing enterocolitis, sepsis, or disseminated intravascular coagulation (DIC) (110). Thromboembolic events are rare in children with hereditary antithrombin III deficiency. In the absence of heparin, antithrombin III contributes approximately 80% of the thrombin-neutralizing capacity of normal adult plasma (111, 112). The levels of a second thrombin inhibitor, $\alpha_2$-macroglobulin, are higher during the first two decades of life than in adults, and this may lessen the risk of thromboembolic complications in antithrombin III-deficient individuals during childhood (113).

A variety of pathophysiologic conditions can reduce the concentration of antithrombin III in the blood. Acute thrombosis infrequently lowers antithrombin III levels substantially (114), but DIC usually reduces the level of this inhibitor (115). Lowered antithrombin III concentrations occur in individuals with liver disease (mainly cirrhosis) due to decreased protein synthesis (116). Decreased antithrombin III levels are also observed in individuals with the nephrotic syndrome as a consequence of urinary excretion (117). Furthermore, modest reductions in plasma antithrombin III concentration are found in users of oral contraceptives (118, 119), as well as in individuals receiving estrogen for other purposes (38, 120). The levels of antithrombin III do not change substantially during normal pregnancies (118, 119), but may decrease significantly in women with pregnancy-induced hypertension, pre-eclampsia, or eclampsia (121). Infusions of L-asparaginase, a chemotherapeutic agent used in the treatment of acute lymphocytic leukemia, can substantially lower the plasma concentration of this inhibitor (122). In addition, the administration of heparin decreases plasma antithrombin III levels (123), presumably on the basis of accelerated *in vivo* clearance. Evaluation of plasma samples from individuals during a period of heparinization can therefore potentially lead to an erroneous diagnosis of antithrombin III deficiency.

Due to the number of clinical disorders that can be associated with reductions in the plasma concentration of antithrombin III, definitive diagnosis of the hereditary deficiency state is often difficult. Whereas an antithrombin III level in the normal range is usually sufficient to exclude the disorder, low levels should be confirmed by obtaining another sample at a subsequent time. This determination is ideally performed when the individual is no longer receiving oral anticoagulants, as these medications have occasionally been reported to raise plasma antithrombin III concentrations into the normal range in individuals with the hereditary deficiency state (5). In such situations, clinical assessment of the individual's risk of recurrent thrombosis will determine whether this approach is feasible. In most antithrombin III-deficient subjects, however, this effect of oral anticoagulants is not of sufficient magnitude to obscure the diagnosis (124). Confirmation of the hereditary nature of the disorder requires the investigation of other family members. Diagnosis of other affected family members also allows for appropriate counseling regarding the need for prophylaxis against venous thrombosis.

The indications for thrombolytic therapy in individuals with heterozygous antithrombin III deficiency are similar to those in other individuals with acute venous thromboembolic episodes. These individuals can usually be treated successfully with intravenous heparin (125), although in some situations unusually high doses of the drug are required to achieve adequate anticoagulation. Indeed, the diagnosis of antithrombin III deficiency is usually considered in the differential diagnosis of "heparin resistance."

In antithrombin III-deficient individuals receiving heparin for the treatment of acute thrombosis, the adjunctive role of antithrombin III concentrate purified from human plasma is not clearly defined, as controlled trials have not been performed (125, 126). This product (see Chapter 52) should probably be administered when difficulty is encountered in achieving adequate heparinization, or recurrent thrombosis is observed despite adequate anticoagulation. It is also reasonable to treat antithrombin III-deficient subjects with concentrate before major surgeries or in obstetrical situations where the risks of bleeding from anticoagulation are unacceptable. The manufacturing processes used to prepare antithrombin III concentrate result in a product that is more than 95% pure; hepatitis B virus and human immunodeficiency virus-I are also inactivated (127, 128). Hence, it is preferable to administer antithrombin III concentrate rather than fresh frozen plasma.

The biological half-life of antithrombin III is approximately 48 hours (13). The infusion of 50 U of antithrombin III concentrate per kilogram of body weight (1 U is defined as the amount of antithrombin III in 1 mL of pooled normal human plasma) will usually raise the plasma antithrombin III level to approximately 120% in a congenitally deficient individual with a baseline level of 50% (128, 129). Plasma levels should be monitored to ensure that they remain above 80%; the administration of 60% of the initial dose at 24-hour intervals is recommended to maintain inhibitor levels in the normal range (129).

Oral anticoagulants are highly effective in the management of individuals with antithrombin III deficiency. Warfarin should be continued indefinitely in individuals with recurrent venous thrombosis. Asymptomatic antithrombin III individuals from thrombophilic kindreds are not generally anticoagulated prophylactically unless they are exposed to situations that predispose them to developing thrombosis (e.g., prolonged immobilization, surgery, pregnancy, etc.) (39).

The management of pregnancies in women with congenital antithrombin III deficiency poses special problems (130). The incidence of thrombotic complications during pregnancy and the postpartum period appears to be greater in women with antithrombin III deficiency than in those with deficiencies of protein C or protein S (131). During pregnancy, adjusted-dose heparin administered by the subcutaneous route is the antithrombotic regimen of choice because its efficacy and safety are established (132). Antithrombin III-deficient individuals with a history of previous thrombotic episodes should definitely receive treatment throughout pregnancy, whereas affected women who have not yet experienced such events should probably receive treatment.

In women who are planning pregnancy during long-term oral anticoagulant therapy, several approaches can be taken to minimize the risk of both thrombotic complications and warfarin embryopathy. One is to stop warfarin and commence subcutaneous heparin therapy; this potentially exposes the individual to many months of heparin therapy while she is trying to conceive. Another approach is to use replacement therapy with antithrombin III concentrates until conception. This product, however, is costly and needs to be administered intravenously at frequent intervals. Finally, warfarin therapy could be continued with the performance of pregnancy tests on a frequent basis. As soon as pregnancy is diagnosed and before the sixth week of gestation, oral anticoagulants must be discontinued and heparin therapy initiated. Although the risk of warfarin embryopathy appears to be quite small during the first 6 weeks of pregnancy (133), even the small risk of this complication makes this the least preferable of the three approaches.

Anabolic steroids such as stanozolol and danazol raise plasma antithrombin III levels in individuals with normal (134) as well as with reduced levels of this inhibitor (135). In spite of this effect, these drugs have not been shown to prevent thrombosis in individuals with hereditary antithrombin III deficiency (135). Stanozolol and danazol also have the potential for raising the levels of vitamin K-dependent procoagulant factors, which could lead to a lack of therapeutic benefit.

## PROTEIN C DEFICIENCY

In 1981, Griffin et al described the first kindred in which several individuals had plasma levels of protein C antigen of approximately 50% of normal and a history of recurrent thrombotic events (136). Subsequently, other investigators (137–141) have reported numerous other families with heterozygous protein C deficiency.

Heterozygous protein C deficiency is inherited in an autosomal dominant fashion, whereas a more severe form of protein C deficiency is an autosomal recessive disorder. The phenotype of individuals with heterozygous protein C deficiency is similar to hereditary antithrombin III deficiency. In severely affected families, about 75% of protein C-deficient individuals experienced one or more thrombotic events. The initial episode occurs apparently spontaneously in approximately 70%. The remaining 30% have the usual associated risk factors at the time they develop acute thrombotic events (for example, pregnancy, parturition, contraceptive pill use, surgery, or trauma). However, individuals are infrequently symptomatic until their early twenties, with increasing numbers of individuals experiencing thrombotic events as they reach the age of 50. The most common sites of disease are the deep veins of the legs, the iliofemoral veins, and the mesenteric veins. Approximately 63% of affected individuals develop recurrent venous thrombosis and about 40% exhibit signs of pulmonary embolism (142). Investigators from the Netherlands noted a high frequency of superficial thrombophlebitis of the leg veins (138), as well as several cases of cerebral venous thrombosis in their protein C-deficient individuals (143). There have also been reports of nonhemorrhagic arterial stroke in young adults with hereditary protein C deficiency (144–146), but additional studies will be required to determine a causal relationship.

Miletich et al (147) determined that the frequency of heterozygous protein C deficiency is one per 200 to 300 in healthy adult blood donors while Tait et al reported a prevalence of one per 500 in a healthy general population (148). None of the affected individuals in this population had histories of thrombosis before being tested. Although the inclusion criteria used for these studies do not permit estimation of the relative thrombotic risk conferred by protein C deficiency, they demonstrated that protein C deficiency can have markedly different clinical phenotypes depending on how individuals are selected. The data also suggested that other factors modulate the phenotypic expression of heterozygous protein C deficiency (149), which has become clear with the identification of other frequent prothrombotic mutations such as factor V Leiden. Data from the Leiden Thrombophilia Study (see below) indicate that individuals from the general population with heterozygous protein C deficiency have about a sevenfold increased risk of an initial episode of deep vein thrombosis as compared to normal subjects (150).

Warfarin-induced skin necrosis (see Chapter 43) has been associated with the presence of heterozygous protein C deficiency (151–153). This syndrome typically occurs during the first several days of warfarin therapy, often in association with the administration of large loading doses of the medication. The skin lesions occur on the extremities, breasts, and trunk, as well as the penis and marginate over a period of hours from an initial central erythematous macule. If a product containing protein C is not rapidly administered, the affected cutaneous areas become edematous, develop central purpuric zones, and ultimately become necrotic. Biopsies demonstrate fibrin thrombi within cutaneous vessels with interstitial hemorrhage. The dermal manifestations of warfarin-induced skin necrosis are clinically and pathologically similar to those seen in infants with purpura fulminans due to severe protein C deficiency (see below).

The pathogenesis of warfarin-induced skin necrosis is attributable to the emergence of a transient hypercoagulable state. The initiation of the drug at standard doses leads to a decrease in protein C anticoagulant activity levels to approximately 50% of normal within one day (154). Although factor VII activity measurements follow a pattern similar to that of protein C, the levels of the other vitamin K-dependent factors decline at slower rates, consistent with their longer half-lives (Fig. 40.1). Increased thrombin generation has been documented in individuals during this early phase of warfarin therapy using a sensitive immunochemical assay for fragment $F_{1+2}$, an index of the *in vivo* activation of prothrombin mediated by factor Xa (155). During this period, the drug's suppressive effect on protein C seems to have a greater influence on the hemostatic mechanism than its reduction in factor VII. These effects are likely to be augmented when greater than 10 mg of warfarin daily is administered to initiate oral anticoagulation or the individual has an underlying hereditary deficiency of protein C. Only approximately one-third of individuals with warfarin-induced skin necrosis, however, have an underlying inherited deficiency of protein C (156), and this complication is only infrequently reported in individuals with the heterozygous deficiency state. A case report has also described this syndrome in association with an acquired functional deficiency of protein C (157).

Two major subtypes of heterozygous protein C deficiency have been delineated using immunologic and functional assays (Table 40.3). The classic, or type I, deficiency state is the most common form and is characterized by a reduction in both the immunologic and bio-

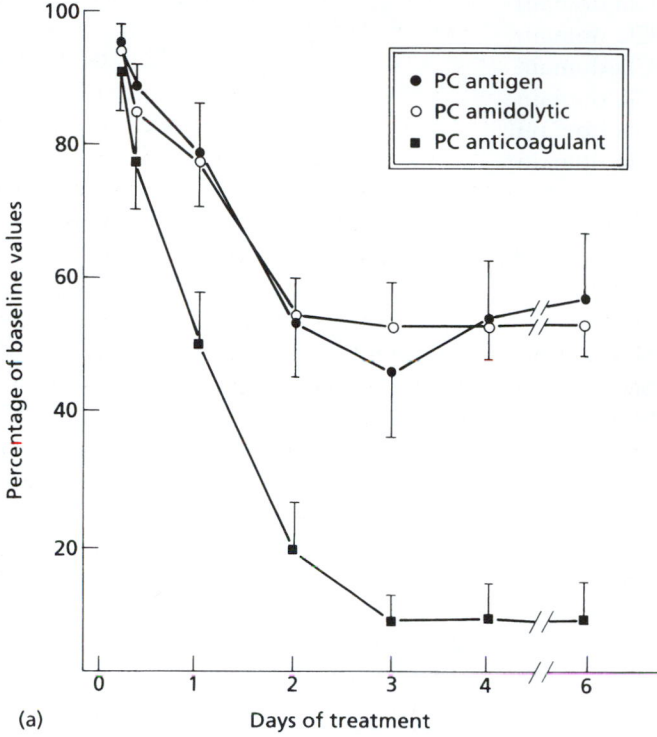

(a)

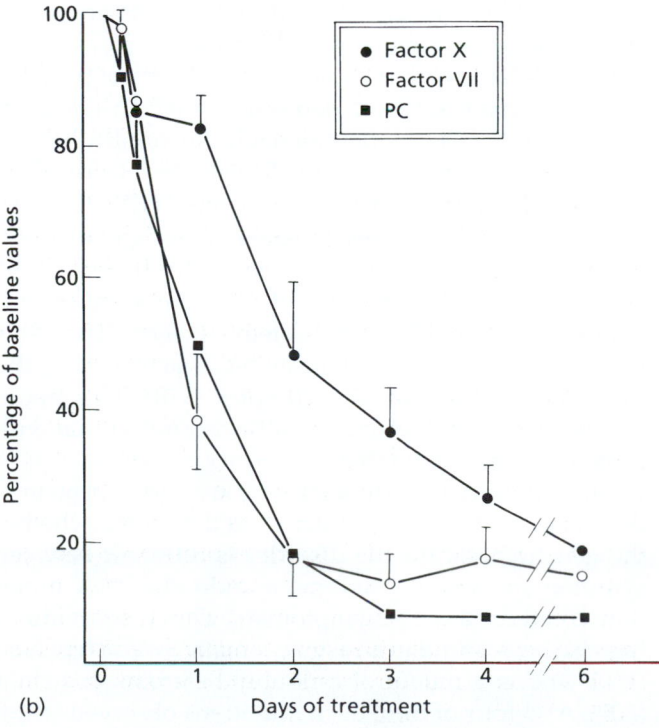

(b)

**TABLE 40.3.** Assay Measurements in Heterozygous Protein C Deficiency

| Types | Antigen | Activity | |
| | | Amidolytic | Coagulant |
|---|---|---|---|
| I ("Classic") | Low | Low | Low |
| II | Normal | Low | Low |
| | Normal | Normal | Low |

logic activity of plasma protein C to approximately 50% of normal (142). Studies of the genetic defects in individuals with protein C deficiency have led to the identification of more than 160 different mutations (158). In individuals with a type I deficiency, missense and nonsense mutations are most common (158–160). In several Dutch families, the linkage between a rare polymorphism and a particular mutation with the deficiency state has indicated the presence of a founder effect (that is, the families are related) (161). Other types of mutations resulting in type I protein C deficiency include promoter mutations, splice site abnormalities, in-frame deletions, frameshift deletions, in-frame insertions, and frameshift insertions (158, 162–166). In families with a type II deficiency state, affected individuals have normal protein C levels on immunologic examination, yet possess lowered functional levels of the zymogen (154, 167–169). The point mutations that have been identified in individuals with type II protein C deficiency are shown in Table 40.4 (164, 165, 170–180).

A clinical disorder has been reported in which newborns develop a syndrome that has been described as purpura fulminans (although the long-established syndrome of purpura fulminans complicates meningococcal infection in children) and laboratory evidence of disseminated intravascular coagulation in association with protein C antigen levels less than 1% of normal (see

**FIGURE 40.1.** Mean levels of protein C (PC) anticoagulant activity, factor VII activity, factor X activity, protein C amidolytic activity, and protein C antigen after the initiation of warfarin therapy in individuals with deep venous thrombosis. Individuals were maintained on heparin infusions, and 10 mg of warfarin was administered for the first 3 days. Dosages were subsequently adjusted based on the prothrombin time. Measurements are expressed as percentages of prewarfarin levels. (Adapted with permission from the publisher from D'Angelo SV, Comp PC, Esmon CT et al. Relationship between protein C antigen and anticoagulant activity during oral anticoagulation and in selected disease states. J Clin Invest 1986; 77:416–425.)

**TABLE 40.4.** Point Mutations in Protein C Deficiency (Type II)

| City or Country of Propositus | Substituion | Domain of Mutation |
|---|---|---|
| Paris (176) | Arg-5—Try | |
| Malakoff (176) | Arg-1—His | Propeptide cleavage site |
| Paris (176) | Arg-1—Cys | Complexation with other plasma proteins through free SH group |
| Spain (171) | Arg 9—Cys | Gla domain |
| Netherlands (158); Paris (172) | Arg 15—Try | Gla domain |
| Yonago (174) | Arg 15—Gly | Gla domain |
| Vermont I (175) | Gln 20—Ala | Gla domain |
| Mie (178) | Glu 26—Lys | Gla domain |
| Vermont I (175) | Val 34—Met | Gla domain |
| La Jolla I (173) | His 66—Asn | |
| La Jolla III (158) | Arg 147—Trp | |
| Japan (170); London 1 (199) | Arg 169—Try | Thrombin-thrombomodulin cleavage site |
| Austria (158) | Arg 169—Gln | |
| Spain (171) | Arg 178—Gln | |
| Austria (158) | His 211—Gln | Serine protease domain |
| Spain (171) | Arg 229—Try | Serine protease domain |
| Marseille (176) | Arg 229—Gln | Serine protease domain |
| Paris (176) | Ser 252—Asn | Serine protease domain |
| Austria (158) | Met 343—Ileu | Serine protease domain |
| Osaka 9 (179) | Gly 350—Arg | Serine protease domain |
| Netherlands (158) | Arg 352—Try | Serine protease domain |
| Netherlands (158); La Jolla II | Asp 359—Asn | Serine protease domain |
| Italy (158) | Gly 381—Ser | Serine protease domain |
| Cadiz (177, 208) | Gly 383—Cys | Serine protease domain |
| Osaka 3 (180) | Gly 385—Arg | Serine protease domain |
| Purmerend (158) | Gly 391—Ser | Serine protease domain |

Chapter 47) (181–190). In some instances, there was a history of consanguinity in the family, making it highly likely that many of the affected infants were homozygous for the deficiency state (182, 185, 188). These newborns can also be double heterozygotes, as was demonstrated in a Chinese individual (186), who had a 5 nucleotide deletion in one protein C allele and a missense mutation in the other (191). The heterozygous parents of these infants only infrequently had thromboses, in contrast to individuals with thrombotic histories and a hereditary partial deficiency of protein C. However, a number of case reports have documented older individuals with homozygous or doubly heterozygous protein C deficiency in whom the lesions resembling purpura fulminans were not present. These individuals generally had protein C levels under 20% of normal in the absence of oral anticoagulant therapy, and their clinical presentation was oftentimes similar to that of severely affected subjects from thrombophilic kindreds with the heterozygous deficiency state (192, 193). Genotyping of such homozygous individuals has led to the identification of missense mutations in the protein C gene (194–197); the variant protein C molecules produced by these individuals are either synthesized at a decreased rate or rapidly cleared from the circulation. The parents of these subjects and infants with the so-called syndrome of purpura fulminans have a type I deficiency state. In addition, individuals have been identified who are doubly heterozygous for both type I and type II alleles that were inherited separately from each of the parents (170, 171, 197, 198). In one of these cases, Japanese investigators determined that a type II defect was coded for by one of the alleles resulting in replacement of arginine by tryptophan at position 12 of the protein's heavy chain. This residue is the site at which protein C is activated by the thrombin-thrombomodulin complex (170). This mutation has also been detected in a British individual with protein C deficiency (199).

In individuals with heterozygous type I protein C deficiency, it has been of interest to determine whether the genetic basis for the disorder is different between symptomatic and asymptomatic individuals. A mutation common among symptomatic Dutch individuals has also been found in an asymptomatic Swedish person (160) who is a parent of a doubly heterozygous child (200). Also four of the eleven mutations observed in homozygotes, whose parents are frequently asymptomatic, have been found in symptomatic heterozygotes (197). Whereas unique mutations have been reported in asymptomatic kindreds with heterozygous protein C deficiency (147, 201), the nature of the defects in the protein C gene alone will not explain the marked phenotypic variability among type I individuals.

A variety of immunologic and functional techniques have been developed to measure protein C levels in plasma samples (see Chapter 26). The most common procedures for antigen determination are electroimmunoassay (136, 137), enzyme-linked immunosorbent assay (ELISA) (202), and radioimmunoassay (203, 204). Functional assays have used either thrombin (167, 205) or the thrombin-thrombomodulin complex (168, 206) to activate protein C. Other methods have used the thrombin-thrombomodulin complex to first activate protein C in plasma, followed by immunoadsorption of the enzyme with goat antihuman protein C IgG-agarose (168). Alternatively, the protein C is first adsorbed with a calcium-dependent monoclonal antibody and subsequently activated by the thrombin-thrombomodulin complex (154). The activity of the enzyme is then assessed using either a chromogenic substrate (167, 168, 206) or by measuring its anticoagulant activity in a factor Xa one-stage clotting assay (154). The development of simpler functional assays has been facilitated by the observation that the venom of the Southern copperhead snake, *Agkistrodon contortrix,* is able to activate protein C in plasma (207). After activation of protein C by this venom, the enzyme's amidolytic activity can be measured using a suitable chromogenic substrate, or its anticoagulant activity can be measured in a clotting assay.

Functional assays utilizing amidolytic and clotting endpoints may give useful information regarding the nature of the molecular defect in individuals with type II protein C deficiency. Several individuals have been described with normal protein C antigen measurements who have substantial reductions in protein C anticoagulant activity, but normal or near-normal amidolytic activity (154). These defects may potentially reflect a reduced ability of activated protein C to interact with platelet membranes, or its substrates such as factor V and factor VIII. The molecular abnormality in one of these families (175) has been determined and is characterized by two $\gamma$-carboxyglutamic acid (Gla) domain mutations (Glu$_{20}$ to Ala and Val$_{34}$ to Met). On the other hand, abnormal protein C molecules that are normally activated by the thrombin-thrombomodulin complex, but fail to exhibit proteolytic activity as measured by amidolytic or anticoagulant assays, have been reported (169, 208). This suggests that the mutations reside near the active site of the protein.

Protein C circulates in human plasma at an average concentration of 4 $\mu$g/mL. The logarithms of the values for protein C antigen in healthy adults are normally distributed with 95% of the values ranging from 70 to 140% (147). There is no significant gender dependence, but mean protein C concentrations increase by approximately 4% per decade. The relatively wide normal range of protein C measurements in the general population occasionally makes it difficult to identify a given individual as having heterozygous protein C deficiency (209). If medical and pharmacologic causes of low levels are excluded (see below), individuals with a protein C value of less than 55% are very likely to have the genetic abnormality, whereas levels from 55 to 65% are consistent with either a deficiency state or the lower end of the normal distribution (147). To document the presence of protein C deficiency with confidence, it is useful to obtain repeat laboratory determinations as well as to perform family studies to identify an autosomal dominant inheritance pattern.

Protein C levels in newborns are 20 to 40% of normal adult levels (210, 211). Preterm infants have even lower levels (212), and babies with significant perinatal thrombosis can have levels suggestive of the homozygous deficiency state (213). Acquired protein C deficiency occurs in liver disease (154, 210, 214, 215); severe infection and septic shock (216); DIC (154, 210, 214, 217, 218); adult respiratory distress syndrome (210, 219); the postoperative state (210); breast cancer individuals receiving cyclophosphamide, methotrexate, and 5-fluorouracil (220, 221); and in association with L-asparaginase therapy (222). A particularly severe form of acquired protein C deficiency has been reported in association with purpura fulminans and DIC in individuals with acute viral or bacterial infections (223–225). In contrast to antithrombin III, the antigenic concentrations of vitamin K-dependent plasma proteins, including protein C, are often elevated in individuals with the nephrotic syndrome (226, 227). Most individuals with uremia have low levels of protein C anticoagulant activity but normal levels of protein C amidolytic activity and antigen (228, 229). This is attributable to a dialyzable moiety in uremic plasma that interferes with most clotting assays for protein C activity (229).

Warfarin therapy reduces functional (154, 167, 206) and, to a lesser extent, immunologic measurements of protein C (136, 137), making it difficult to diagnose individuals with heterozygous protein C deficiency in this setting. Several research laboratories have used a reduced ratio of protein C antigen to prothrombin or factor X antigen to identify individuals with a type I deficiency state (136, 137). This approach, however, can only be used in subjects in a stable phase of oral anticoagulation, and the diagnostic criteria for the disorder vary with the intensity of warfarin therapy (137). Other groups have successfully used protein C activity assays in conjunction with functional measurements of factor VII, a vitamin K-dependent zymogen with a similar plasma half-life (230, 231). In practice, it is preferable to investigate individuals suspected of having the deficiency state after oral anticoagulation has been discontinued for at least 1 week and to perform family studies. If it is not possible to discontinue warfarin due to the severity of the thrombotic diathesis, such individuals can be studied while receiving heparin therapy, which does not alter plasma protein C levels.

An acquired inhibitor of protein C has been documented in an Australian individual (232). This individual had a bleeding diathesis for several years and developed purpura fulminans before his death. An autopsy showed arterial and venous thrombi in many organs. Laboratory evaluation demonstrated the presence of chronic DIC. The IgG fraction of the subject's plasma completely inhibited the functional anticoagulant activity of activated protein C.

The acute management of thromboembolic events in heterozygous protein C-deficient individuals is similar to that of subjects without this disorder. It is advisable to keep the subject fully anticoagulated with heparin during the initiation of oral anticoagulation, and large loading doses of warfarin should clearly be avoided as has been recommended in other individual populations. Oral anticoagulants are effective in managing individuals with protein C deficiency, and the recommendations for its use in such individuals, who have either sustained recurrent venous thrombosis or are asymptomatic, are similar to those in individuals with congenital antithrombin III deficiency. Many of the general guidelines for the management of pregnancies in women with this latter disorder are also relevant to this situation in protein C-deficient women. A case report described the successful treatment of a protein C-deficient woman with purified protein C concentrate (233).

Stanozolol and danazol raise protein C levels substantially in heterozygous individuals with type I protein C deficiency (234–236) and in women without protein C deficiency (237). In a individual doubly heterozygous for both type I and II deficiency states, danazol treatment resulted in an increase in protein C antigen concentration from 66 to 98%, but no change in anticoagulant activity (198). However, these drugs do not prevent thrombosis in individuals with this disorder (236), and an increase in fragment $F_{1+2}$ levels, a measure of the *in vivo* activity of factor Xa upon prothrombin, has been observed in conjunction with the rise in protein C levels in two protein C-deficient individuals who received stanozolol for 4 weeks (235).

The infrequent occurrence of warfarin-induced skin necrosis, the relatively high frequency of asymptomatic hereditary protein C deficiency, and the diagnostic difficulty in making a rapid and definitive laboratory diagnosis of the deficiency state are arguments against the routine measurement of plasma protein C levels in all individuals with thrombosis before the initiation of oral anticoagulants. If, however, one is starting oral anticoagulants in a individual who is already known or likely to be protein C deficient, it would seem prudent to start the drug under the cover of full heparinization and also to increase the dose of warfarin gradually, starting from a relatively low level (for example, 2 mg for the first 3 days and then increasing the daily dose by 2 to 3 mg daily until therapeutic anticoagulation is achieved). A case report has reported the successful oral anticoagulation of a individual with heterozygous protein C deficiency and an earlier history of warfarin-induced skin necrosis (152). Therapeutic doses of heparin, and protein C replacement in the form of fresh frozen plasma were used to prevent the development of this complication. Infusions of purified protein C concentrate have also been given to initiate warfarin therapy successfully at full doses in a individual with severe protein C deficiency (238).

## PROTEIN S DEFICIENCY

In 1984, members from several kindreds who exhibited reduced levels of protein S were described who had a striking history of recurrent venous thrombotic disease (239, 240). Subsequently, many additional families with this disorder have been reported (241–248).

Heterozygous protein S deficiency is inherited in an autosomal dominant fashion, whereas a more severe form of protein S deficiency is an autosomal recessive disorder. The clinical presentation of individuals with heterozygous protein S deficiency is similar to that outlined for antithrombin III or protein C deficiency. Among 71 protein S-deficient members from 12 Dutch pedigrees (245), 74%, 72%, and 38% of the individuals have sustained deep venous thrombosis, superficial thrombophlebitis, or pulmonary emboli, respectively. The mean age of the first thrombotic event was 28 years with a range between 15 and 68; 56% of the episodes were apparently spontaneous and the remainder were precipitated by an identifiable factor. Thrombosis has also been reported in the axillary, mesenteric, and cerebral veins. Warfarin-induced skin necrosis has been described in a individual with heterozygous protein S deficiency (249).

Several case reports have described young individuals with arterial thrombosis and hereditary protein S deficiency (250–253). In a cohort of 37 consecutive young adults (younger than 45 years of age) presenting with arterial occlusive disease, three had hereditary protein S deficiency (254). However, the occurrence of arterial thromboembolic events was not increased in protein S deficient relatives of these people as compared to their biochemically unaffected family members. Further studies will therefore be required to determine whether protein S deficiency is a risk factor for the development of arterial thrombosis.

Under normal conditions, approximately 60% of the total protein S antigen in plasma is complexed to a complement component, C4b-binding protein (see Chapter 3). Only the free 40% is functionally active as a cofactor in mediating the anticoagulant effects of activated protein C (241). This observation has led to the development of methods for measuring total (240, 255, 256) and free protein S antigen (244) (see Chapter 26). The most reliable measurements of total protein S antigen are by radioimmunoassay (255–257) and ELISA techniques, which involve dilution of plasma samples, thereby favoring dissociation of the protein S-C4b-binding protein complexes. After removing protein S-C4b-binding protein complexes from plasma by polyethylene glycol precipitation (244, 258), free protein S may be quantified by immunoassay of the supernatant fractions. It is also now possible to measure free protein S specifically using a monoclonal antibody-based immunoenzymatic assay that uses antibodies specific for the free form (259). Functional assay methods require protein S-deficient plasma, immobilized monoclonal antibodies to protein S (239, 260–263), or both. They are based on the ability of protein S to serve as a cofactor for the anticoagulant effect of activated protein C. Some of these assays, however, are not specific for protein S and are sensitive to the defect characterized by resistance to activated protein C (see below), and their use can lead to an erroneous diagnosis of functional protein S deficiency (264).

The classic deficiency state is associated with approximately 50% of the normal total S antigen level (240, 242), and greater reductions in free protein S antigen and protein S functional activity (244) (Table 40.5). The molecular genetic analysis of mutations in individuals with protein S deficiency was initially complicated by the presence of a protein S pseudogene (265–268), but mutations can now be identified in about 70% of thrombophilic families with protein S deficiency using mutation screening strategies (269). Molecular analysis has identified only three cases of large deletions of the protein S gene (270–272). Among 69 candidate causal mutations identified in individuals with the "classic" type of protein S gene deficiency, 51% are missense mutations, 25% are microinsertions or deletions of base pairs, 14%

are premature stop codons, and 9% affect a splice site (273–284). Mutations in the protein S promoter have yet to be identified.

Another type of hereditary deficiency state has been described in which total protein S antigen measurements are in the normal range, but levels of free protein S and protein S functional activity are disproportionately reduced to less than about 40% of normal (Table 40.5). Whereas the mutations in the "classic" type of protein S deficiency are distributed throughout the coding sequence, it has only been possible to identify protein S gene mutations in 44% of individuals with this phenotype, raising the possibility that some cases represent acquired abnormalities (269). Among French individuals with the low free protein S phenotype in which mutations could be identified, 82% had a single mutation, Ser 460 to Pro, in the sex-hormone-binding globulin domain of protein S (275). The low free plasma protein S may result from increased binding of this abnormal protein S molecule to C4b-binding protein (244, 285). It is not, however, clear that the Ser 460 to Pro mutation (also termed protein S Heerlen) is associated with an increase in thrombotic risk as it has been identified with similar frequency in Dutch individuals with thrombosis (0.7%) and the general population (0.5%) (286). The situation is further complicated by a report of 14 Swedish thrombophilic families in whom laboratory evaluation demonstrated the coexistence of the "classic" deficiency state along with the low free protein S phenotype; these data led the authors to propose that the two types of protein S deficiency are phenotypic variants of the same genotype (287). In summary, the above data suggest that the low free protein S phenotype may not confer the same degree of thrombotic risk as the "classic" type of protein S deficiency, and this possibility should be taken into account in the management of such individuals.

A third type of protein S deficiency is characterized by normal total and free protein S levels, but diminished protein S functional activity (Table 40.5). This phenotype has been identified infrequently, which suggests that current functional assays may not screen for all such defects. Interestingly, all five mutations found in such individuals are located in the aminoterminal end of the protein S molecule, which includes the domains that interact with activated protein C (288). Two of the mutations are located in the propeptide at positions $-2$ (Arg to Leu) and $-1$ (Arg to His) (274). A substitution of Lys 9 by Glu has been identified, which may alter the conformation of protein S or interfere with carboxylation of the molecule's $\gamma$-carboxyglutamic acid domain (276). The other two mutations result in substitution of Thr 103 by Asn and Lys 155 by Glu in the first and second epidermal growth factor domains of protein S, respectively (274, 289, 290).

Recurrent venous thromboembolic disease can occur

**TABLE 40.5.**   Assay Measurements in Heterozygous Protein S Deficiency

| | Protein S Antigen Total | Free | Protein S Activity |
|---|---|---|---|
| "Classic" | Low | Low | Low |
| | Normal | Low | Low |
| | Normal | Normal | Low |

in association with doubly heterozygous or homozygous protein S deficiency (241). The parents of the individuals were asymptomatic and had laboratory studies consistent with the classic protein S deficient state. Neonatal purpura fulminans has been described in association with homozygous protein S deficiency (291, 292).

The average concentration of total protein S antigen in normal adults is 23 µg/mL (255). The levels increase with advancing age and are significantly lower and more variable in females than males (293, 294). These factors have confounded the reliable estimation of the prevalence of heterozygous protein S deficiency in the normal population. Thus, it is difficult to make the diagnosis of heterozygous protein S deficiency by performing only a single assay. Repeat sampling, as well as family studies, are usually required to establish the diagnosis firmly.

Acquired protein S deficiency occurs during pregnancy (257, 258) and in association with the use of oral contraceptives (293, 295). Reduced protein S levels have also been noted in individuals with DIC (261, 296, 297) and acute thromboembolic disease (261). C4b-binding protein is an acute phase protein and the declines in protein S activity in the latter two conditions, as well as in other inflammatory disorders, is attributable to a shift of the protein to the complexed, inactive form (261). The levels of total and especially free protein S are significantly reduced in men with HIV infection (298) (see Chapter 48). Total protein S antigen measurements are generally increased in individuals with the nephrotic syndrome (226, 227, 299), although functional assays give reduced values. This is, in part, due to the loss of free protein S in the urine and elevations in C4b-binding protein levels. Total and free protein S antigen concentrations are moderately decreased in liver disease (256, 261) and in association with L-asparaginase chemotherapy (222). An acquired severe deficiency of protein S has also been reported in association with cutaneous necrosis (300). In a individual with thromboembolic disease recovering from chickenpox, a transient isolated deficiency of protein S has been reported due to the presence of an autoantibody (301).

Interpretation of protein S measurements in individuals on oral anticoagulants is complicated inasmuch as the antigenic and functional levels of the protein drop substantially. A few groups have used reductions in the ratio of protein S antigen to prothrombin antigen to infer a diagnosis of the classic type of protein S deficient state; this is accomplished by using a strategy similar to that described for protein C-deficient subjects (240, 242).

Total protein S antigen values in healthy newborns at term are 15 to 30% of normal, whereas C4b-binding protein is reduced to less than 20%. Thus, the free form of the protein predominates in this setting and functional levels are only slightly reduced as compared to those in normal adults (302–304).

The recommendations for the treatment of protein S-deficient individuals with anticoagulants and thrombolytic agents are similar to those in individuals without this disorder. Heparin therapy is generally effective for the acute treatment of thrombotic episodes and standard warfarin schedules appear to be effective in preventing recurrent venous thromboembolism. Protein S concentrates have not yet been developed for clinical use. Anabolic steroids such as danazol or stanozolol have not been shown to have a role in the treatment of protein S-deficient individuals.

## ACTIVATED PROTEIN C RESISTANCE

In 1993, Dahlbäck (305) identified a novel mechanism for familial thrombophilia. He identified individuals with unexplained personal and familial histories of venous thromboembolism whose plasmas exhibited a poor response to activated protein C (APC) in an activated partial thromboplastin time (aPTT) assay. Recognized mechanisms for APC resistance were excluded, such as functional protein S deficiency or inhibitors to APC. Other clinically affected relatives of the probands demonstrated APC resistance in the aPTT test, suggesting that the abnormality was hereditary. Poor anticoagulant responses to APC were also demonstrable in the probands in factor IXa- and factor Xa-based assays. Based on these observations, Dahlbäck hypothesized that these individuals were deficient in an unrecognized plasma cofactor that functions in concert with protein S to support the anticoagulant activity of APC.

The observations of Dahlbäck facilitated the development of an aPTT-based assay to screen for APC resistance. Svensson and Dahlbäck (306) screened 104 consecutive Swedish individuals referred for evaluation of venous thrombosis and found that the plasmas of 33% of the subjects showed APC resistance (defined as an anticoagulant response in the aPTT-based assay below the fifth percentile of controls). Precipitating factors for thrombosis, such as pregnancy and the use of oral contraceptives, were identified in 60% of their individuals. Family studies revealed that relatives with APC resistance had a significantly higher frequency of thrombosis than relatives without the defect. In a U.S. referral population of individuals younger than age 50 with unexplained venous thromboembolic disease, Griffin et al (307) found that approximately 50% had APC resistance. Other groups in Italy and Austria confirmed that APC resistance was a frequent laboratory abnormality in individuals with unexplained venous thrombosis (264, 308).

A major contribution to our understanding of the molecular basis and clinical relevance of APC resistance was made by Dutch investigators from Leiden. In 1987, they initiated the Leiden Thrombophilia Study, a large case-control study to investigate risk factors for first episodes of venous thrombosis in the general population of the Netherlands (309). This effort grew from an attempt to define the true risk of venous thrombosis asso-

**TABLE 40.6.** The Leiden Thrombophilia Study Data: Relative and Absolute Risks of an Initial Episode of Deep Venous Thrombosis in the General Population due to Common Risk Factors

|  | Risk | Incidence/100 person years | Reference |
|---|---|---|---|
| Normal | — | 0.008 | |
| Hyperhomocysteinemia | 2.5× ↑ | 0.02 | 437 |
| Prothrombin gene mutation | 2.8× ↑ | 0.022 | 346 |
| Oral contraceptives | 4× ↑ | 0.03 | 460 |
| Factor V Leiden heterozygotes | 7× ↑ | 0.057 | 310 |
| Oral contraceptives + factor V Leiden | 35× ↑ | 0.285 | 460 |
| Factor V Leiden homozygotes | 80× ↑ | 0.5–1 | 319 |

ciated with protein C deficiency. As noted above, there was a seeming paradox in that referred individuals from families with protein C deficiency had a high frequency of venous thrombosis, but the deficiency state is present in 1 in 200 to 500 healthy blood donors. The criteria for accruing subjects into these studies was felt to be a major factor underlying this difference.

After the initial observations of Dahlbäck, the group in Leiden screened 301 unselected consecutive individuals for APC resistance who had been entered into the Leiden Thrombophilia Study after the completion of anticoagulant therapy (310). Entry criteria were a first episode of deep venous thrombosis in outpatients under age 70 with the diagnosis having been confirmed by objective testing. Individuals with malignancy were excluded. Each individual with thrombosis was matched with a healthy age-matched and sex-matched control. Activated protein C (APC) resistance was found in 21% of thrombosis individuals and 5% of controls. Individuals with APC resistance were calculated to have a sevenfold increased risk of venous thrombosis as compared to controls (Table 40.6). The lower frequency of resistance to APC in this study as compared to other studies of referral populations cited earlier is primarily attributable to different selection criteria for the thrombosis cohorts.

It was subsequently shown that a defect in factor V involving the mutation of arginine-506 to glutamine-506 (Arg506Gln or factor V Leiden) is most often the cause of APC resistance (311–314). This is the site at which APC cleaves factor Va, and this sequence alteration makes the mutant factor Va molecule biochemically resistant to inactivation by the enzyme (311, 315, 316). The Arg506Gln substitution was found to be the cause of APC resistance in about 90% of Dutch individuals with APC resistance in the aPTT assay (311), and the mutation was found in 2 to 4% of healthy Dutch controls. Most individuals with APC resistance are heterozygous for the factor V Leiden mutation, but a number of homozygous individuals with heightened APC resistance in

aPTT assays have been identified (311, 317, 318). Homozygotes are at higher thrombotic risk than heterozygotes (Table 40.4) (318, 319), as are individuals with heterozygous resistance to APC combined with mutations in the genes for protein C, antithrombin III, and probably protein S (320–324). The genes for factor V and antithrombin III are both located on the long arm of chromosome 1, allowing for coinheritance of the factor V Leiden mutation and an antithrombin III mutation within all affected members of a family. This situation is expected to lead to an even more severe thrombotic diathesis (322).

Although the factor V Leiden mutation is the dominant mechanism underlying APC resistance, data exist to support the original hypothesis of Dahlbäck that a second plasma cofactor supports the anticoagulant activity of APC (305, 325). Interestingly, factor V itself, but not purified factor Va, is able to enhance the inactivation of factor VIIIa by APC (326, 327). Factor V Leiden is significantly less effective than normal factor V in mediating this effect (328).

The U.S. Physician's Health Study has also provided valuable data regarding factor V Leiden as a risk factor for venous as well as arterial thrombosis. In a retrospective case-control study of 14,916 healthy men older than age 40 with a mean follow-up of 8.6 years, heterozygosity for the factor V Leiden mutation was identified in 12% of subjects (14 of 121) with a first episode of deep venous thrombosis or pulmonary embolism and 6% of controls (329). The relative risk of venous thromboembolism was increased 3.5-fold in those individuals with no concomitant risk factors, but surprisingly was reduced to 1.7-fold in those with pre-existent cancer or recent surgery. This study also showed that elderly individuals with venous thrombosis frequently have the mutation (329, 330). Among men over age 60 with initial episodes of venous thrombosis and no identifiable triggering factors, 26% (8 of 31) were heterozygotes for factor V Leiden (329).

There has been considerable interest in determining whether a prevalent prothrombotic risk factor such as factor V Leiden might lead to an increased risk for arterial events. As mentioned previously, there are no convincing data that other thrombophilic states such as deficiencies of antithrombin III, protein C, and protein S confer an increased risk of arterial thrombosis, but evaluation of this association is complicated by the relative infrequency of these defects. In a cohort of men over age 40 in which there was a low prevalence of smoking, the Physician's Health Study did not find an association between the factor V Leiden mutation and myocardial infarction or stroke. In a younger cohort of Italian individuals with myocardial infarction prior to age 45, an increased incidence of the factor V Leiden mutation also was not found vis a vis controls (331). Furthermore, a report of 36 French homozygous individuals with the mutation did not identify a tendency for the development of arterial thrombosis (332).

However, recent data from a case-control study suggest that heterozygosity for factor V Leiden is a risk factor for myocardial infarction in young women (18 to 44 years old) but only in the presence of other cardiac risk factors (333). The presence of the factor V Leiden mutation was associated with a 2.4-fold increased risk of myocardial infarction after adjustment for age (8 of 79 or 9.5% of individuals with myocardial infarction as compared to 4.1% in controls). The risk of myocardial infarction associated with factor V Leiden however was observed only among current cigarette smokers in whom the mutation conferred a threefold increased risk. In comparison to women who did not smoke and did not carry factor V Leiden, women who smoked and carried the mutation had a 30-fold increased risk of myocardial infarction. Interestingly, while other cardiac risk factors such as older age, obesity, hypercholesterolemia, hypertension, diabetes, family history of ischemic heart disease, and post-menopausal status (surgically induced) were associated with cardiac events, the use of low-dose oral contraceptives was not. Data from this cohort indicate that the prothrombin gene mutation (see below) is also a risk factor for myocardial infarction, but again only in current cigarette smokers (334).

The prevalence of heterozygosity for the factor V Leiden mutation in Caucasians, including European, Jewish, Israeli, Arab, and Indian populations, ranges between 1 to 8.5%. The mutation is apparently not present in African Blacks, Chinese, Japanese, or Native American populations (335). Using dimorphic sites in the factor V gene to do haplotype analysis, Zivelin et al (336) provided data for the existence of a founder effect as the basis for the mutation in Caucasians of differing ethnic backgrounds. It was also estimated that the mutation originated approximately 30,000 years ago, which came after the evolutionary divergence of Caucasian, African, and Oriental populations (336). Thus far, no genetic abnormalities in the factor V gene other than the Leiden mutation or in the factor VIII gene have been identified to cause APC resistance.

There have been reports of individuals in which there is cosegregation of heterozygous APC resistance due to the factor V Leiden mutation and type I factor V deficiency (337–340). The plasma of these individuals manifests severe APC resistance in aPTT assays similar to homozygous factor V Leiden individuals (that is, they are pseudohomozygous). These individuals were seemingly more thrombosis prone than heterozygous relatives with factor V Leiden alone, suggesting that their clinical phenotype is similar to homozygous factor V Leiden individuals.

Several polymorphisms are present in the factor V gene (341, 342). Two amino acid substitutions, Leu1257-Ile and His1299Arg, and a codon dimorphism for Ser1240 are present in exon 13, which codes for the protein's B domain and is removed upon activation (341). In an Italian population, the frequency of the allele encoding Arg1299 (R2) was 30% in individuals with partial factor V deficiency and 7.5% in control subjects (341). Interestingly, an extended factor V gene haplotype (HR2) containing the R2 polymorphism, distinct from that encoding Arg506Gln, contributes to a mild APC resistant phenotype (342); it also contains nucleotide transversions resulting in the amino acid substitutions, Arg830Lys and Arg837His. Despite its association with mild APC resistance and its increased frequency in factor V Leiden-positive individuals with the lowest APC resistance ratios, the HR2 haplotype has not yet been shown to confer an increased risk of venous thrombosis.

The initial observations of Dahlbäck (305) facilitated the development of an aPTT-based assay that serves as a screening test for APC resistance (see also Chapter 26). The aPTT is run in the presence or absence of a standardized amount of APC, and the two clotting times are converted to an APC ratio. Results can be interpreted by comparing the ratio to the normal range, or by normalizing it to the APC resistance ratio obtained using normal pooled plasma. Whereas this "first generation" APC resistance assay was conceptually quite simple and easy to perform in a coagulation laboratory, it required careful standardization and determination of the normal range in at least 50 controls. The level of activated protein C, the aPTT reagent, and the instrumentation used for clot detection affected the performance characteristics of the assay. Some assays using this format therefore had inadequate sensitivity and specificity for the factor V Leiden mutation. Also, individuals receiving anticoagulants or with an abnormal aPTT due to other coagulation defects could not be investigated with this assay, and the test was not validated in individuals with acute thrombotic events or in pregnant women.

The discovery that factor V Leiden apparently underlies all cases of APC resistance facilitated "second generation" coagulation tests, which with proper standardization, can give nearly 100% sensitivity and 100%

specificity for the mutation. This was achieved by diluting individual plasma in a sufficient volume of factor V-deficient plasma and then performing either an aPTT-based assay or a tissue factor-dependent factor V assay (343). This modification also permits the evaluation of plasmas of individuals receiving anticoagulants or demonstrating abnormal aPTT results due to coagulation factor deficiencies other than factor V.

The fact that the only presently known mutation underlying APC resistance is factor V Leiden also makes it attractive to diagnose this defect by analyzing genomic DNA in peripheral blood mononuclear cells. This can be readily accomplished by amplifying a DNA fragment containing the factor V mutation site by polymerase chain reaction (PCR) and analyzing the cleavage products on ethidium bromide-stained agarose gels after restriction enzyme digestion with MnlI (311). The substitution of an A for a G at nucleotide 1691 in the factor V cDNA (CGA to CAA) results in the Arg506Gln mutation and the loss of a MnlI cleavage site. Other diagnostic approaches include hybridization with allele-specific oligonucleotide probes.

At present, the most cost-effective approach to diagnosing individuals with factor V Leiden is to test for APC resistance using a "second generation" coagulation assay. Individuals with low APC resistance ratios should then be genotyped for the mutation, although it can be argued that such confirmatory testing is unnecessary in labs that have perfect concordance between the results of their APC resistance assays and factor V Leiden genotype.

Using the "first generation" aPTT-based assay for APC resistance, some individuals with APC resistance without the factor V Leiden mutation could be identified. The clinical implications of this type of APC resistance are uncertain. The use of such assays to identify such individuals is therefore best restricted to thrombosis research centers. Two groups have reported individuals with cerebrovascular disease in association with APC resistance that is not due to the factor V Leiden mutation (344, 345). In one of the studies, the investigators divided individuals into five categories of responsiveness to APC as opposed to the usual practice of using a cut-off value for optimal separation of carriers and non-carriers of the mutation (345). Statistical analysis showed that a low response to APC was associated with an increased risk of cerebrovascular disease independent of the factor V Leiden mutation.

The acute management of thrombosis in individuals with APC resistance is no different than other individuals. Due to the prevalence of this disorder, data have emerged regarding the recurrence risk following an initial venous thrombotic episode in association with the factor V Leiden mutation. This information is presented, along with its implications with respect to long-term anticoagulation in such individuals, in Chapter 24.

## PROTHROMBIN GENE MUTATION

In 1996, investigators from Leiden reported that a G to A substitution at nucleotide 20210 in the 3'-untranslated region of the prothrombin gene is associated with elevated plasma prothrombin levels and an increased risk of venous thrombosis (346). This mutation, which was discovered by directly sequencing the prothrombin gene of selected individuals with venous thrombosis, is located at the last position of the 3'-untranslated region at or near the cleavage site for polyadenylation of prothrombin mRNA. There is not yet experimental evidence whether this mutation results in increased prothrombin biosynthesis by the liver or whether it is linked to another sequence variation in the prothrombin gene that was not detected by sequence analysis. In any case, it is likely that the increased thrombotic risk is attributable to the elevated plasma prothrombin concentration.

Investigation of a referral population with a personal and family history of venous thrombosis demonstrated that 18% had the mutation in the 3'-untranslated region of the prothrombin gene while it was present in only 1 of 100 healthy controls (346). Among these thrombosis individuals, 40% also carried the factor V Leiden mutation, again emphasizing the current view of venous thrombosis as a multigene disorder (see Chapter 24).

In the Leiden Thrombophilia Study, 6.2% of venous thrombosis individuals and 2.3% of healthy matched controls had the prothrombin gene mutation (346). This mutation independently confers a 2.8-fold increased risk of venous thrombosis (see Table 40.6) and the effect is operative in both sexes and all age groups. Among heterozygotes with the prothrombin gene mutation, 87% of thrombosis individuals and controls in the study had prothrombin activity levels that were greater than 1.15 U/mL, whereas only 23% of those with a normal prothrombin genotype were elevated to this degree. Investigators in Sweden, England, and Italy have recently confirmed that the prothrombin 20210 mutation is a common risk factor for venous thrombosis in unselected outpatients as well as individuals with other inherited thrombotic disorders (347–349). The allele frequency of 1.2% for the prothrombin gene mutation in the Dutch population is approximately half that of factor V Leiden, making it the second most common genetic risk factor for venous thrombosis.

## DYSFIBRINOGENEMIAS

Qualitative abnormalities of fibrinogen are usually inherited in an autosomal dominant manner. The dysfibrinogenemias are a heterogeneous group of disorders that may present with either no clinical symptoms, a bleeding diathesis, or a history of recurrent venous or arterial thromboembolism (350). Fewer than twenty cases of variant fibrinogens have been reported to be associated with thrombotic complications. These defects can be detected with thrombin and reptilase times, which are often prolonged. In one instance, the thrombin time has been substantially shortened (351, 352). Functional fibrinogen measurements are usually substantially lower than antigenic measurements in the plasmas of these individuals. An occasional individual with a dysfibrinogenemia may have a prolonged prothrombin time or aPTT, and the inability of some abnormal fibrinogens to clot completely *in vitro* can result in false-positive results in fibrin(ogen) degradation product tests.

The functional and biochemical defects of a number of abnormal fibrinogens associated with thromboembolic disease have been characterized (350). The conversion of fibrinogen to fibrin by thrombin results in the proteolytic cleavage of fibrinopeptides A and B from the molecule. Defects in the release of these two peptides (353–357) or abnormalities in fibrin polymerization (358–360) have been reported. Such functional defects do not, however, offer a ready explanation for the thrombotic diathesis seen in these subjects. Abnormalities in the binding of thrombin to fibrin have also been found in some dysfibrinogenemias (361–363). In one of these kindreds, three homozygous siblings with a Bβ chain substitution of Ala by Thr at position 68 had a severe clinical phenotype sustaining both arterial and venous thrombosis at a young age (363, 364). It has been suggested that decreased binding of thrombin by this mutant fibrinogen may lead to the presence of excessive thrombin in the circulation and the occurrence of thrombosis (364). Other fibrinogen mutants have been shown to cause abnormal fibrin polymerization (358–360, 362). Some of the abnormal fibrinogens have been evaluated for their ability to resist or promote fibrinolysis upon incorporation into a fibrin clot. The fibrin formed from fibrinogen "Chapel Hill III" has been demonstrated to be abnormally resistant to lysis by plasmin (358). Plasminogen activation is decreased in the presence of the fibrin formed from fibrinogen "Dusart," despite normal tissue-type plasminogen activator binding to the substrate (365–368). These abnormalities clearly have the potential for decreasing fibrinolytic activity *in vivo*, which results in a familial thrombotic diathesis in biochemically affected persons.

## INHERITED ABNORMALITIES OF FIBRINOLYSIS

Whereas investigators have identified a few individuals with inherited abnormalities of the fibrinolytic mechanism and recurrent venous thromboembolism, the clinical association is considerably less striking than that in many kindreds with deficiencies of antithrombin III, protein C, or protein S, or with APC resistance due to the factor V Leiden mutation and the prothrombin gene

mutation. Dysplasminogenemia or hypoplasminogenemia has been reported in approximately 20 individuals with thromboembolic disease (369–382). The first case of an abnormal plasminogen was identified in Japan by Aoki et al (369). The propositus had a history of recurrent thrombosis, and family studies demonstrated that the biochemical abnormality followed an autosomal dominant inheritance pattern. Despite the hereditary nature of the defect, none of the other biochemically affected members of the kindred had thrombotic events. Other Japanese pedigrees without thrombosis have since been described with the same biochemical defect (371, 372, 383) and the gene frequency of this abnormality in Japan is 0.018 (384). Population studies in the United States have not uncovered any cases of this dysplasminogenemia. A study of two unrelated Japanese families with reduced functional and antigenic levels of plasminogen was unable to demonstrate a significant correlation between the deficiency state and thrombosis (385). The non-Japanese cases of dysplasminogenemias and hypoplasminogenemias have also been remarkable for the lack of thrombotic episodes in biochemically affected family members other than the propositi.

A few reports have documented the existence of thrombophilic families with inherited abnormalities of fibrinolysis (386–388). Individuals from these kindreds were initially observed to have reduced fibrinolytic potential after venous occlusion (386) and subsequently they were noted to have high levels of plasminogen activator inhibitor (389, 390). Re-evaluation of two of these families (386–388) has recently demonstrated the presence of hereditary protein S deficiency and no association between PAI-1 activity and a history of thrombosis (248, 391). These data provide further evidence that the association between defective fibrinolysis and familial thrombosis has not been established (392, 393).

Immunochemical methods for the measurement of tissue-type plasminogen activator and functional assays for its inhibitors have been applied to the study of individuals with documented venous thromboembolism. These studies have suggested that defective synthesis or release of tissue-type plasminogen activator, as well as increased levels of plasminogen activator inhibitor-1, may be important pathogenetic factors in as many as one-third of these individuals (394–399). Reduced fibrinolytic activity due to increased plasma levels of a rapid inhibitor of tissue-type plasminogen activator has been found in young survivors of myocardial infarction (400, 401). The measurements of this inhibitor correlated strongly with serum concentrations of triglycerides.

## FACTOR XII DEFICIENCY (see Chapter 36).

Factor XII is the zymogen of a serine protease that initiates the contact activation reactions and intrinsic blood coagulation *in vitro* (see Chapter 5). The first individual with a deficiency of factor XII, or Hageman factor, was reported by Ratnoff and Colopy (402) in 1955. Subjects with severe factor XII deficiency (factor XII activity less than 1% of normal) have markedly prolonged aPTTs, but do not exhibit a bleeding diathesis (403). The absence of a hemostatic defect in individuals with a severe deficiency of factor XII, prekallikrein, or high-molecular-weight kininogen indicates that these factors are not required for *in vivo* hemostasis. However, there have been a number of cases of venous thromboembolism or myocardial infarction in factor XII-deficient individuals (404), including the initial individual described with the abnormality (405). This thrombophilic tendency has been attributed to reduced plasma fibrinolytic activity (406). A literature review of 121 individuals with factor XII deficiency found an 8% incidence of thromboembolism, including several myocardial infarctions in relatively young individuals (404). Interpretation of such data is difficult, as such complications are likely to be reported in the literature as compared to the asymptomatic individual with factor XII deficiency. This has led some groups to perform cross-sectional analyses of thromboembolic events in larger numbers of unselected families with factor XII deficiency (407, 408). In Swiss families with factor XII deficiency, two of 18 homozygous or doubly heterozygous individuals had sustained deep venous thrombosis, although each occurred at a time that other predisposing thrombotic risk factors were present (407). Among heterozygotes with factor XII deficiency, only one of 45 heterozygotes had a possible history of venous thrombosis. These investigators concluded that heterozygous factor XII deficiency does not constitute a major thrombotic risk factor, whereas a severe deficiency may predispose some affected persons to venous thrombosis. Other groups have found a 10 to 20% incidence of thrombotic episodes in heterozygotes (408, 409). Thus, it remains uncertain as to whether an increased thrombotic risk is associated with factor XII deficiency.

## OTHER DEFECTS

The thrombomodulin gene is a potential candidate for prothrombotic mutations. A individual with a single episode of pulmonary embolism and his asymptomatic son were found to have a point mutation in the thrombomodulin gene resulting in Asp468Tyr (410). Additional studies are required to evaluate whether this mutation alters the structure of thrombomodulin in such a way as to either reduce its cell surface expression or functional activity as well as to determine whether thrombomodulin mutations increase the risk of thrombosis.

Two brothers with thrombotic strokes during childhood were found to have deficient amounts of the extracellular isoform of glutathione peroxidase in their plasma, thereby resulting in a functional deficiency of

nitric oxide (411). Both individuals had impaired platelet inhibition in response to nitric oxide secondary to impaired metabolism of reactive oxygen species.

## HYPERHOMOCYSTEINEMIA

While premature atherosclerosis and arterial thrombosis was associated with severe hyperhomocysteinemia almost 30 years ago (412), it has only been in the last several years that mild or moderate hyperhomocysteinemia has been established as an independent risk factor for atherosclerosis as well as thrombosis (413, 414) (see Chapter 39).

Homocysteine is a sulfur-containing amino acid that is formed from methionine (Fig. 40.2). It is converted back to methionine by one of two remethylation pathways or undergoes transulfuration to cysteine. In remethylation catalyzed by the enzyme methionine synthase, homocysteine acquires a methyl group from 5-methyltetrahydrofolate and vitamin $B_{12}$ (cobalamin) acts as a cofactor. In a secondary pathway, betaine is the methyl donor in a reaction catalyzed by betaine-homocysteine methyltransferase. In transulfuration, homocysteine condenses with serine to form cystathionine in a reaction catalyzed by cystathionine-β-synthase followed by hydrolysis by the enzyme γ-cystathionase to cysteine and α-ketobutyrate. Vitamin $B_6$ (pyridoxine) is a cofactor in both of these reactions.

The normal plasma homocysteine concentration is 5 to 16 μmol/L. As a result of impaired intracellular metabolism of homocysteine, increased amounts of the amino acid accumulate in the blood, leading to hyperhomocysteinemia. Homocystinuria refers to a group of rare inborn errors of metabolism resulting in severe hyperhomocysteinemia (>100 μmol/L) and the excretion of high levels of homocysteine in the urine. The most frequent cause is homozygous cystathionine-β-synthase deficiency, which has a frequency in the general population of approximately 1 in 250,000 (415). Affected individuals exhibit premature atherosclerosis and venous thromboembolism along with mental retardation, ectopic lenses, and skeletal abnormalities. A small number of cases are due to homozygous defects encoding methylenetetrahydrofolate reductase (MTHFR), and these individuals are similarly afflicted with premature vascular disease and thrombosis along with neurologic problems.

Mild (16 to 24 μmol/L) or moderate (25 to 100 μmol/L) hyperhomocysteinemia results from genetic and acquired abnormalities. Whereas heterozygous cystathionine-β-synthase deficiency is found in only approximately 0.3% of the general population, a MTHFR variant with an alanine to valine substitution at amino acid 677 is more common (416) and can be present in 1.4 to 15% of the population depending on their origin (414). This mutation causes thermolability of MTHFR and a 50% reduction in its specific activity. The most

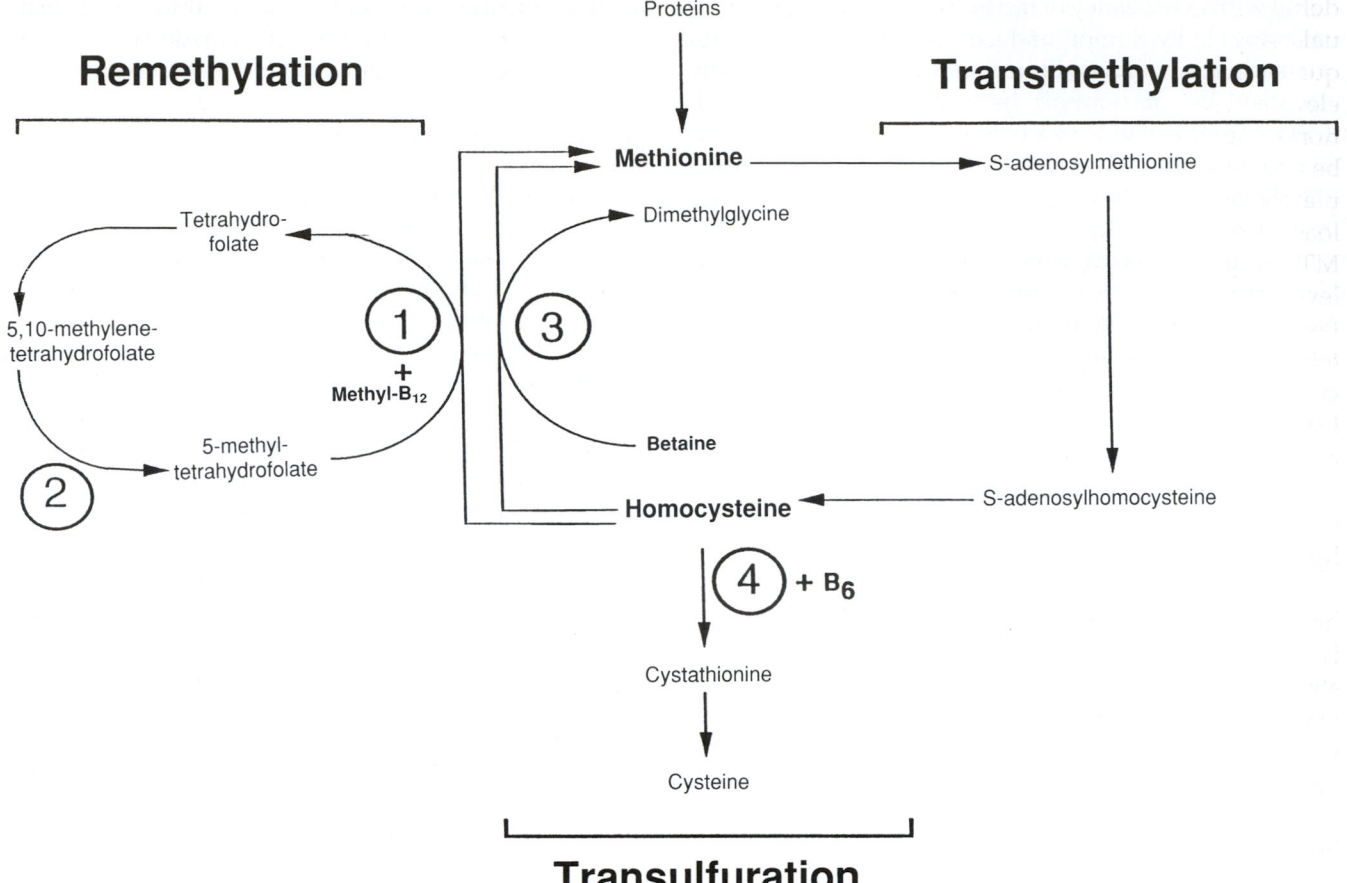

**FIGURE 40.2.** Intracellular metabolism of homocysteine occurs through remethylation to methionine or transulfuration to cysteine. Numbered circles indicate the enzymes involved: 1 = methionine synthase, 2 = methylenetetrahydrofolate reductase (MTHFR), 3 = betaine-homocysteine methyltransferase, 4 = cystathionine beta-synthase. (Adapted with permission from De Stefano V, Finazzi G, Mannucci PM. Inherited thrombophilia: Pathogenesis, clinical syndromes, and management. Blood 1996; 87:3531–3544.)

common causes of acquired hyperhomocysteinemia are deficiencies of vitamin $B_{12}$, folate, or vitamin $B_6$ which are cofactors in homocysteine metabolism. There is a strong inverse correlation between hyperhomocysteinemia and folate levels and to a lesser extent with vitamin $B_{12}$ and $B_6$ concentrations (417). Elderly individuals frequently have elevated plasma homocysteine concentrations even in the absence of vitamin deficiencies, as do individuals with renal failure. Cigarette smoking is also associated with acquired hyperhomocysteinemia.

The mechanisms by which hyperhomocysteinemia acts as an atherogenic and thrombogenic risk factor have only been partially elucidated, but the major effect is on the vessel wall. *In vitro*, homocysteine is able to promote vascular smooth muscle cell proliferation (418) and inhibit endothelial cell growth (419). In primates, it was shown that the infusion of homocysteine causes endothelial cell desquamation, smooth muscle cell proliferation, and intimal thickening (420). Recent data indicate that moderate hyperhomocysteinemia induced by dietary

manipulation leads to vascular dysfunction with impaired vasomotor responses as well as decreased thrombomodulin activity in the aorta (421). The thrombogenic effects of hyperhomocysteinemia that have been demonstrated *in vitro* include induction of tissue factor expression (422), inhibition of heparan sulfate expression (423), inhibition of nitric oxide and prostacyclin release (424, 425), inhibition of tissue-type plasminogen activator binding (426), and inhibition of thrombomodulin-dependent protein C activation (427, 428). However, most of these studies were carried out at homocysteine concentrations that were considerably higher than are encountered in individuals with severe hyperhomocysteinemia, thereby raising questions about their relevance to the prothrombotic diathesis associated with this defect.

Hyperhomocysteinemia is usually diagnosed by measuring plasma levels of homocysteine by high-pressure liquid chromatography with electrochemical or fluorescent detection. Whereas individuals with homozygous homocystinuria due to cystathionine-β-synthase deficiency have levels greater than 100 μmol/L, individuals with heterozygous defects in this gene or inadequate vitamin $B_6$ levels may have normal or only slightly elevated levels of fasting homocysteine. The discrimination of such individuals from normal individuals can be improved by demonstrating an abnormal increase in plasma homocysteine 4 hours after an oral methionine load. Defects in the remethylation pathway due to MTHFR gene defects or inadequate folate or vitamin $B_{12}$ levels tend to cause elevated homocysteine levels under fasting conditions. The prevalence of hyperhomocysteinemia is almost twice as high when based on homocysteine measurements performed after methionine loading as when based on fasting levels. It is also possible to test for the common Ala677Val mutation in MTHFR genetically, but this is not recommended in the initial evaluation of individuals suspected of having hyperhomocysteinemia.

Mild or moderate hyperhomocysteinemia due to inherited enzyme defects or acquired vitamin deficiencies is an independent risk factor for myocardial infarction, stroke, and carotid arterial disease (429–431). Case-control studies have found that up to 40% of individuals with atherosclerotic coronary or cerebrovascular disease have mild to moderate elevations in plasma homocysteine. Prospective data have shown that elevated plasma homocysteine concentrations predict for coronary events and especially mortality among individuals with established coronary artery disease (432). An association between fasting plasma homocysteine levels and arterial thrombotic events has also been shown prospectively in individuals with systemic lupus erythematosus (433).

A relationship between hyperhomocysteinemia and venous thrombosis is also now appreciated. Studies of individuals with an initial episode of venous thrombosis before age 45 demonstrate that 13 to 18% have moderate hyperhomocysteinemia based on homocysteine measurements done fasting and following an oral methionine load (434, 435). Many of these individuals had a history of familial thrombosis in association with hyperhomocysteinemia. A Dutch study showed that 25% of individuals with recurrent venous thrombosis had homocysteine levels above the 90th percentile of the control distribution, and the presence of this abnormality conferred a twofold increased risk of recurrence (see Table 40.6) (436).

Case-control studies have provided strong evidence that hyperhomocysteinemia is also an independent risk factor for initial episodes of venous thrombosis in the general population. These studies did not perform homocysteine levels after methionine loading and in some instances did not even obtain homocysteine levels in the fasting state, thereby underestimating the disorder's prevalence. In the Leiden Thrombophilia Study, an elevated homocysteine level exceeding the 95th percentile

of the control group was found in 10% of individuals and conferred a twofold increased risk of thrombosis (see Table 40.6) (437). However, only women older than age 50 showed a statistically significant association, although a trend was present in both sexes and all age groups. In an older male population, the Physician's Health Study demonstrated a weak association between total plasma homocysteine level and venous thromboembolism, but this was confined to those with so-called "idiopathic" events (that is, no acquired risk factors) (438). The risk of thrombosis was increased 20-fold in individuals with "idiopathic thrombosis" who were both hyperhomocysteinemic and had the factor V Leiden mutation. This markedly increased thrombotic risk is consistent with a report of individuals with hereditary homocystinuria in whom only those who carried factor V Leiden had sustained venous thrombosis (439).

The fact that lower plasma levels of folate, and to a lesser extent, vitamin $B_6$ or vitamin $B_{12}$, are associated with hyperhomocysteinemia makes it attractive to prescribe vitamin supplements to slow atherogenesis, as well as to reduce the risk of arterial and venous thrombosis (417). Indeed appropriate vitamin supplements can normalize plasma homocysteine levels, but the clinical efficacy of this approach has not yet been demonstrated in controlled clinical trials. However, because vitamins are inexpensive and have almost no side effects, it is at present reasonable to treat symptomatic hyperhomocysteinemic individuals with appropriate doses of folate, vitamin $B_6$, or vitamin $B_{12}$ to lower their levels of homocysteine.

# ACQUIRED THROMBOTIC DISORDERS (SEE TABLE 24.1, CHAPTER 24)

## PREGNANCY AND ORAL CONTRACEPTIVES (SEE ALSO CHAPTER 46)

Pregnancy is associated with about a sixfold increased risk of venous thromboembolism (440). Whereas the incidence of deep vein thrombosis and pulmonary embolism has been estimated to be as high as 1%, the true incidence is unknown due to difficulties in performing screening radiologic studies in pregnant women. Although relatively rare, pulmonary embolism causes 12 deaths per million pregnancies in the state of Massachusetts and is estimated to account for 12% of fatalities during pregnancy (441).

The puerperium, defined as the 6-week period following delivery, is associated with a higher rate of thrombosis than pregnancy itself. Risk factors for thrombosis in pregnancy include increasing age, Caesarian delivery, prolonged immobilization, obesity, and prior thromboembolism (440). Coexistent thrombophilia represents a major risk factor, particularly during pregnancy itself (442). In Sweden, 46 to 59% of women with venous thromboembolism had APC resistance and 65 to 75% of the thrombotic events occurred during pregnancy (443, 444). Among a referral population of Italian women with APC resistance managed without anticoagulant prophylaxis, 28% sustained venous thrombosis and 62% of the events occurred postpartum (445).

Thrombosis during pregnancy and the puerperium is attributable to pregnancy-induced alterations in hemostasis as well as venous stasis in the lower extremities caused by the gravid uterus. Trauma to the pelvic veins during vaginal delivery or tissue injury during Caesarian section also contribute to the hypercoagulable state. Compression of the left iliac vein by the crossing right iliac artery is a local, mechanical factor that is believed to underlie the threefold higher incidence of deep vein thrombosis in the left leg as compared to the right (446).

There are important changes in the coagulation mechanism during pregnancy (447). Increased levels of markers of coagulation system activation can be detected in the systemic circulation by the end of the first trimester. The elevations in thrombin generation likely arise from the uteroplacental circulation, as the placenta is rich in tissue factor. The vasculature of the placenta is unique from other tissues in that it is lined by chorionic villi which are covered by trophoblast tissue, rather than endothelium, which is in direct contact with maternal blood. The levels of most procoagulant factors increase during pregnancy with fibrinogen rising from a nonpregnant normal level of 250 to 400 mg/dL to 600 mg/dL by late pregnancy. Among the natural anticoagulant proteins, there is a significant decline in the level of free and total protein S in the second trimester (257, 258). At the same time, fibrinolytic system activity declines progressively during pregnancy, in large part due to the generation of plasminogen activator-2 (PAI-2) by the placenta (448). In addition, platelet activation and increased platelet turnover also probably occur during pregnancy; mild thrombocytopenia, possibly due to increased consumption, occurs in 8.3% of healthy women at term (449). The net effect of these hemostatic changes is to promote blood coagulation to provide adequate hemostasis at the time of placental separation. The altered levels of hemostatic proteins return to normal within 4 weeks after delivery, whereas fibrinolytic activity rapidly returns to nonpregnant levels within hours after placental separation (450).

Since the early 1960s, it has been known that oral contraceptive use is associated with an increased risk of venous and arterial thrombosis. It subsequently became apparent that the risk of venous thrombosis was related to the estrogen dose (451), and most oral contraceptives prescribed in the U.S. contain less than 50 μg of ethinylestradiol in combination with a progestational agent (combined oral contraceptives). The use of low-dose estrogen preparations containing older progestational agents (levonorgestrel, lynestrenol, and norethisterone), however, still confers about a fourfold increased risk of venous thromboembolism as compared to nonusers (see Table 40.6) (452). The risk of myocardial infarction and stroke is less (453–455), which is in part related to estrogen's effect in lowering low-density lipoprotein cholesterol and raising high-density lipoprotein cholesterol levels. Unexpectedly, the introduction of newer progestogens (desogestrel, gestodene, and norgestimate) with more beneficial effects on lipid profiles carries a higher risk of venous thromboembolism than the previous generation of combined oral contraceptives (456–459). This risk is particularly high among carriers of the factor V Leiden mutation (460, 461) and women with a family history of thrombosis. It is not yet known whether oral contraceptives containing the newer progestogens are associated with any increase in risk of myocardial infarction, which is an extremely rare event in young women (453).

The mechanisms by which oral contraceptives induce a prothrombotic state are incompletely understood. Oral contraceptive use is associated with changes in many coagulation factors, which are qualitatively similar to those found during pregnancy (462). It has recently been suggested that oral contraceptives induce a state of "acquired" APC resistance (463).

## THE POSTOPERATIVE STATE AND TRAUMA

Deep vein thrombosis and pulmonary embolism occur with increased frequency in postoperative individuals; the thrombotic risk, however, depends on the type of surgery performed. Deep vein thrombosis in this population is usually asymptomatic, requiring the use of reliable noninvasive tests or lower limb venography to establish the diagnosis. Based on individual characteristics and the type of surgery, the postoperative thrombotic risk can be estimated and an assessment made of the need for prophylactic anticoagulation (464). Risk factors associated with higher rates of thrombosis include older age, previous venous thromboembolism, the coexistence of malignancy or medical illness (for example, cardiac disease), thrombophilia, and longer surgical and immobilization times. In individuals older than age 40, the incidence of deep vein thrombosis after general or gynecologic surgical procedures is approximately 20 to 25% and clinically significant pulmonary embolism occurs in 1 to 2%. For urologic surgery, the incidence of deep vein thrombosis ranges from 10% for transurethral procedures and up to 40% for radical prostatectomies. Orthopedic procedures on the hip and lower extremities are among the most thrombogenic surgical procedures. In the absence of prophylaxis, the risk of deep vein thrombosis after total knee replacement ranges from 45 to 70%, and fatal pulmonary embolism has been reported to occur in 1 to 3% of individuals undergoing hip surgery. The increased thrombotic risk is not confined to the immediate postoperative period and continues for several weeks (465).

Deep vein thrombosis and pulmonary embolism are also commonly encountered after major trauma. A study of individuals admitted to a Canadian regional trauma unit demonstrated that 58% of individuals had lower extremity deep vein thrombosis, which was usually asymptomatic (466). Risk factors for thrombosis in this setting were older age, the need for surgery or blood transfusions, and the presence of lower extremity fractures or spinal cord injury. Pulmonary embolism occurs in 2 to 22% of trauma individuals, and is the third most common cause of death in those who survive the first 24 hours (467).

The mechanism of activation of the coagulation system following surgery or trauma has not been elucidated, but the exposure of tissue factor from injured tissue or activated monocytes is the most likely pathway for increased thrombin generation in these settings. In postoperative individuals, the occurrence of thrombosis is determined by the balance between coagulation and fibrinolytic system function (468). In a study of neurosurgical individuals undergoing craniotomy, Owen and associates (469) found that individuals developing venous thrombosis exhibit increased levels of fibrinopeptide A, a marker of thrombin-mediated fibrinogen proteolysis, relative to levels of Bβ 1-42, a marker of plasmin action on non-crosslinked fibrin, for several days before thrombus visualization as compared to controls. Minor alterations in a number of hemostatic parameters have been reported in postoperative individuals, including elevated levels of fibrinogen and von Willebrand factor and decreased levels of antithrombin III and protein C. Decreased venous blood flow in the lower extremities also contributes to postoperative hypercoagulability (470). In hip replacement surgery, the femoral vein in the operated leg may kink, thereby stimulating proximal venous thrombosis in the absence of pre-existent calf vein thrombosis (471).

## OBESITY

Although obesity is an independent risk factor for atherosclerosis and cardiovascular disease, the evidence regarding its role in venous thrombosis is equivocal. An early study by Kakkar et al (472) suggested that overweight individuals had an increased incidence of venous thrombosis. More recent studies have shown that this association disappears when account is taken of other risk factors such as age, history of venous thrombosis, and the type of surgery (473). Obesity may, however, be a risk factor for chronic venous insufficiency (474).

## MALIGNANCY

The incidence of clinical thromboembolic disease in the cancer population has been estimated to be as high as 11% (475). Autopsy series have described even higher rates of thrombosis for certain tumor types. One autopsy study found a 30% incidence of thrombosis in individuals who died of pancreatic cancer and over 50% with tumors in the body or tail of the pancreas (476). Other tumor types commonly associated with thromboembolic complications are carcinomas of the gastrointestinal tract, ovary, prostate, and lung. By virtue of its prevalence, lung cancer accounts for the largest number of thromboembolic events (477).

Patients with malignancy also have a higher rate of postoperative venous thrombotic complications than the general population, with an incidence of approximately 40% (472). Careful attention should therefore be paid to prophylaxis of deep vein thrombosis in such individuals undergoing major abdominal or pelvic surgical procedures.

In some instances, thrombosis manifests itself prior to the diagnosis of an underlying malignancy, and may predate the diagnosis by several years (see Chapter 24). In Trousseau's syndrome, which is classically characterized by migratory superficial phlebitis involving the upper or lower extremities (phlegmasia alba dolens) (478), it is not unusual for a premortem diagnostic evaluation for an underlying malignancy to be unsuccessful. For years it was debated whether the presence of a venous thrombotic event identifies individuals at significantly increased risk of developing cancer. Several studies demonstrated an excess risk of cancer in individuals who present with pulmonary embolism or deep vein thrombosis (479, 480), but other investigators were unable to document an increased risk of developing cancer after an idiopathic thrombotic episode. These observations, however, were obtained from small or retrospective clinical trials.

A significant and clinically important association between idiopathic venous thrombosis and the subsequent development of clinical cancer was established in 1992. Prandoni et al (481) investigated 250 consecutive individuals with symptomatic deep vein thrombosis that was objectively documented by venogram. Cancer was identified at the time of diagnosis of the thrombotic event in 3.3% (5 of 153) of individuals with idiopathic venous thrombosis (no other known risk factors), but no cases were found in individuals with secondary venous thrombosis (presence of other risk factors such as prolonged immobilization, leg trauma, hereditary thrombotic disorder, etc.). During a 2-year follow-up period, cancer was diagnosed in 7.6% (11 of 145) of the individuals with idiopathic venous thrombosis and in 1.9% (2 of 105) of individuals with secondary venous thrombosis. The incidence of cancer was considerably higher in individuals with recurrent idiopathic venous thrombosis. The probability of detecting an occult neoplasm in individuals with a documented thrombotic event was also evaluated by Monreal et al (482, 483), who found a malignant lesion in 7 of 31 (22.6%) individuals with idiopathic deep vein thrombosis in contrast to 5 of 82 (6.1%) individuals with secondary thrombosis and in 9 of 78 (11.5%) individuals with pulmonary embolism. The higher incidence of cancer reported by this group is most likely due to a more aggressive diagnostic approach, which included chest radiography, upper gastrointestinal endoscopy, abdominal ultrasound, and computed tomography scan.

For individuals who present with idiopathic venous thromboembolism, recommendations have varied as to the extent of evaluation for malignancy that is appropriate (484). Decisions regarding diagnostic testing should be based upon the status of the individual individual; however, a complete physical examination including digital rectal examination and testing for fecal occult blood, pelvic examination in women, and routine laboratory testing (CBC, chemistry panel including electrolytes, renal function tests, liver function tests and calcium, urinalysis, chest radiograph) should be performed in all individuals presenting with thrombosis. Prospective studies are required to assess if an aggressive diagnostic approach will result in improved survival.

Nonbacterial thrombotic endocarditis (NBTE), sterile vegetations composed of platelets and fibrin on heart valves, is highly associated with malignant disorders. In autopsy series, cancer was found in as many as 75% of cases of NBTE (485). The majority of cases of NBTE are in individuals with adenocarcinomas, and its incidence among lung cancer individuals may run as high as 7% (486). Laboratory evidence for DIC is often present. The aortic and mitral valves are most commonly affected. The diagnosis of NBTE can be difficult to make antemortem, because less than 50% of individuals have audible cardiac murmurs, and small lesions may not be identified by echocardiography. The major clinical manifestations are due to systemic emboli from the vegetations on the heart valve(s) rather than from valvular dysfunction itself. Common sites of embolization include the spleen, kidney, and extremities, with the most significant morbidity arising from emboli to the central nervous system and coronary arteries. Nonbacterial thrombotic endocarditis is not an uncommon disorder and should be considered in all individuals with cancer who develop an acute stroke syndrome, as well as in others who have cerebral embolism with an unknown etiology (487).

Disseminated intravascular coagulation is the cardinal coagulopathy associated with malignancy and results from generalized activation of the coagulation system (see Chapter 44). Malignancy is the third most common cause of DIC after infection and trauma, and

accounts for 7% of cases. Disseminated intravascular coagulation is a common coagulopathic complication in cancer individuals, and has been reported in as many as 15% of individuals with malignancy. Disseminated intravascular coagulation occurs in virtually all individuals with acute promyelocytic leukemia. The leukemic promyelocytes contain procoagulants that can trigger DIC, as well as fibrinolytic activators. The cell lysis that results from conventional chemotherapy releases these enzymes and can exacerbate the coagulopathy. Other disease entities, particularly sepsis, that may *per se* be responsible or may contribute to the development of DIC in cancer individuals, should be ruled out.

Various patterns of DIC are seen in association with malignancy. Acute forms of DIC are rare and usually present with minor bleeding from mucosal or cutaneous surfaces, and/or extensive life-threatening hemorrhage involving visceral sites. As described in Chapters 26 and 44, laboratory evaluation demonstrates prolongation of the prothrombin time (PT), aPTT, thrombin time, and reptilase time, decreased fibrinogen concentration, thrombocytopenia, and elevated levels of fibrin degradation products (FDPs). More common in cancer individuals are chronic forms of DIC. Many such individuals are asymptomatic, and laboratory data often show modest reductions in fibrinogen and platelet count, elevated FDPs, and minimal changes in the PT or aPTT. Others may have more obvious evidence of platelet, fibrinogen, and coagulation factor consumption. These individuals often are hypercoagulable, and can manifest deep vein thrombosis, Trousseau's syndrome, or NBTE.

Thrombotic microangiopathy (TM) is the descriptive term of a syndrome that is characterized by hemolytic anemia, thrombocytopenia, pathognomonic microvascular thrombotic lesions, and the involvement of various specific organs. Depending on the differences in organ involvement, TM is commonly described as thrombotic thrombocytopenic purpura (TTP) or as hemolytic uremic syndrome (HUS). The syndrome is described in detail in Chapter 27. Severe TM, in association with thrombocytopenia, may occur in as many as 5.7% of individuals with metastatic carcinomas, most frequently with gastric, breast, or lung primary sites. Despite the classical manifestations of a Coombs'-negative hemolytic anemia and severe thrombocytopenia, individuals usually present with neurologic abnormalities, including headache, confusion, or paresis, and occasionally signs of DIC. Renal failure is an uncommon feature of carcinoma-associated TM. The mainstay in the treatment of malignancy-related TM is to decrease the tumor burden, because other treatment modalities, such as corticosteroids, plasma exchange, or plasma infusion, only result in a moderate and transient improvement of the clinical symptoms.

The association of neoplasia and thrombotic disorders has led to the isolation of substances from animal and human tumors that are directly active with respect to components of the hemostatic mechanism and, once released from the tumor, may trigger intravascular activation of the coagulation system. In 1958, it was shown that a variety of human cancers contain a lipid-protein complex that could initiate fibrin formation in and around the tumor nidus. During the past 20 years, considerable attention has been focused on the identification of procoagulants in animals and humans that are able to convert factor X to factor Xa. In 1975, a substance from human and animal neoplasms was identified that did not require the presence of factor VII and tissue factor to directly activate factor X (488). This cancer procoagulant was subsequently characterized as a cysteine protease (489) and purified from rabbit V2 carcinoma extracts (490). There is also evidence that this procoagulant is present in extracts of cells obtained from tumors of individuals with malignant melanoma and acute myelocytic leukemia (AML) (491, 492). To date, only a small amount of sequence has been obtained for this cancer procoagulant, and its cDNA has not been cloned.

Another major group of factor X activators includes the tissue factor-like procoagulants, which enhance factor VII activity in clotting assays. These procoagulants have been studied in greatest detail in the leukocytes of individuals with AML. High amounts of a tissue factor-like procoagulant have been found in the leukocytes of individuals with acute promyelocytic leukemia (APML) (493) and other AML subtypes (494, 495). It should be noted that myeloid precursor cells from normal bone marrow do not possess procoagulant activity (496). Tissue factor-like activity has also been described in cells derived from a variety of human and animal tumors (477).

In addition to the above direct mechanisms by which tumor procoagulants may activate the coagulation cascade, the expression of tissue factor could be detected on various malignant cell tissues by localizing the tissue factor antigen with a monospecific rabbit anti-human tissue factor IgG (497). Intense immunohistochemical reactivity was found in the tissues of lung carcinomas, gastrointestinal malignancies, squamous cell carcinomas of the neck and head, and bladder carcinomas, all of which are known to be frequently associated with Trousseau's syndrome. It has also been reported that unstimulated peripheral blood mononuclear cells from individuals with lung cancer express increased tissue factor activity *in vitro* as compared to cells from normal controls, and that this activity could be correlated with *in vivo* generation of thrombin as measured by fibrinopeptide A (498). It has been suggested that this procoagulant is generated by the host's immune system in response to the tumor, but several other factors appear to be involved in the modulation of this activity, including the presence of T lymphocytes (499), cytokines

(500, 501), and lipoproteins (502). Furthermore, there may be non-tissue factor-dependent molecular species associated with monocytes that are able to mediate the activation of factor Xa (503).

Data indicating the importance of tissue factor expressed on tumor cells as a procoagulant must still be interpreted with some caution, because the expression of tissue factor antigen and activity depends heavily on the source of the malignant tissue (504). For example, tissue factor expression is frequently studied in cell culture, and this milieu may not be representative of that found *in vivo* (505).

Substances have also been obtained from various animal and human tumors that can directly aggregate platelets (506–508). However, efforts to recover and purify the active species from detergent-solubilized tumor cell membranes have thus far been unsuccessful. It is postulated that platelet proaggregatory moieties may lead to clot formation on the vascular subendothelium, thereby stimulating hemostatic activation in cancer individuals.

It has been reported that increased levels of tumor necrosis factor (TNF) can occur in as many as 50% of cancer individuals with active disease (509). However, several other groups have only infrequently observed elevated TNF levels in this population (510, 511). Tumor necrosis factor is able to dramatically enhance the procoagulant and suppress the anticoagulant properties of cultured vascular endothelial cells (512, 513). These effects are mediated by an increase in tissue factor activity, a decrease in thrombomodulin expression leading to diminished protein C activation, and suppression of endothelial fibrinolytic activity. It has also been shown that TNF causes a rise in biochemical markers of coagulability (514) and is potentially an important mediator in the hypercoagulability of individuals with cancer.

Likely contributing to the thrombotic tendency in cancer individuals are clinical factors such as vascular stasis due to obstruction of blood flow by the tumor or individual immobility, hepatic involvement and dysfunction, sepsis, advanced age, other comorbid conditions, and certain antineoplastic agents (see below). Thus, the exact details of the mechanisms underlying coagulation activation in malignancy remain uncertain and may be a complex interaction of several of the above mechanisms as well as others yet to be identified.

## NEPHROTIC SYNDROME

The nephrotic syndrome results from a variety of pathologic processes that cause excessive kidney glomerular leakage of plasma proteins into the urine. It is clinically characterized by edema, proteinuria, hypoalbuminemia, and hyperlipidemia. Thrombosis is a major cause of morbidity in individuals with the nephrotic syndrome, with the renal veins being the most commonly affected site. Renal vein thrombosis occurs in approximately 35% of cases (515) but varies considerably based on the underlying renal pathology and the severity and duration of the proteinuria. The incidence of thrombosis in other sites is approximately 20% (515, 516); in adults, deep vein thrombosis and pulmonary embolism are the most common thrombotic complications. Arterial thrombosis is seemingly more common in children with nephrotic syndrome, resulting in stroke, mesenteric infarction, or limb ischemia.

Alterations in many blood coagulation parameters have been reported in individuals with the nephrotic syndrome, although some abnormalities are inconsistently reported, of relatively minor magnitude, and poorly correlated with thrombotic events. The variability in findings is attributable to the complex nature of the nephrotic syndrome itself and the resultant stimulation of hepatic protein biosynthesis.

Among the natural anticoagulant proteins, plasma antithrombin III levels are often decreased due, at least in part, to urinary excretion (117, 517). As noted previously, the antigenic levels of protein C and protein S are generally increased (226, 227, 299). Plasma levels of several components of the coagulation cascade, factors XII, XI, and X, are reported to be decreased due to urinary excretion, whereas factors XIII, X, VIII, VII, and V are characteristically elevated in these individuals. There are data that platelet hyperreactivity (518) or increased whole blood viscosity (519) may contribute to the thrombotic diathesis in the nephrotic syndrome.

## PAROXYSMAL NOCTURNAL HEMOGLOBINURIA

Paroxysmal nocturnal hemoglobinuria (PNH) is a rare acquired clonal disorder of bone marrow stem cells. Individuals generally manifest chronic intravascular hemolysis with episodes of gross hemoglobinuria accompanied by leukopenia and thrombocytopenia. Many have a prior history of aplastic anemia. Despite the presence of thrombocytopenia, thrombosis is more commonly encountered than bleeding. Indeed, thrombosis can be a presenting feature of PNH, as well as an important cause of morbidity and mortality in this disorder. A diagnosis of PNH should be suspected in individuals with a negative family history of thrombosis with evidence of pancytopenia, an elevated reticulocyte count, or iron studies consistent with iron deficiency.

A unique feature of PNH is the predilection for thrombosis to occur in the intra-abdominal venous network (mesenteric, hepatic, portal, splenic, and renal veins) and cerebral vessels as opposed to deep vein thrombosis or pulmonary embolism. Arterial events such as myocardial infarction and stroke have been reported rarely. Acute thrombotic episodes should be treated with heparin or low-molecular-weight heparin.

Fibrinolytic agents have been used successfully to treat acute intra-abdominal venous thrombosis. Long-term oral anticoagulation should be considered in individuals with thrombosis in association with PNH.

The abnormality of PNH erythrocytes that leads to hemolysis is their increased sensitivity to complement-mediated lysis. Deficiencies of a number of membrane proteins have been observed in PNH, including acetylcholinesterase, leukocyte alkaline phosphatase, "decay accelerating factor," CD59 (membrane inhibitor of reactive lysis) antigen, homologous restriction factor, CD58, 5'-ectonucleotidase, CD16, urokinase-type plasminogen activator, and CD14 antigen. These proteins are all attached to the cells via a glycosylphosphatidylinositol (GP I) anchor, and PNH appears to be the consequence of somatic mutations in the X-linked PIG-A (phosphatidylinositol glycan class A) gene, which participates in an early step in GP I anchor synthesis (520). Several of the membrane abnormalities involve proteins that modulate complement function, and the absence of CD59 antigen on erythrocytes appears to be the most critical defect (521). Granulocytes and platelets, like red cells, show increased sensitivity to complement-mediated lysis. Although it has been suggested that the membrane abnormalities in PNH may lead to increased platelet activation by complement, there is no adequate explanation for the thrombotic tendency in this disease. Indeed, there is no apparent association between hemolytic and thrombotic episodes, nor does the onset of thrombosis correlate with the duration or degree of hemolysis.

## HYPERVISCOSITY

Thrombosis can be a manifestation of diseases associated with hyperviscosity. Hyperviscosity of the blood may be due to increased plasma viscosity, an increased number of red or white blood cells, or decreased deformability of cells.

Increased plasma viscosity can result from hypergammaglobulinemia or hyperfibrinogenemia. Hypergammaglobulinemia associated with the hyperviscosity syndrome is most commonly encountered in individuals with Waldenström's macroglobulinemia or multiple myeloma. Presenting symptoms of the hyperviscosity syndrome include bleeding due to platelet dysfunction, visual disturbances, and neurologic defects. Thrombosis in hypergammaglobulinemic states is attributable to abnormal rheology.

Hyperviscosity plays an important role in the pathogenesis of thrombosis in polycythemia vera, which is a major complication of this disorder. Individuals with elevated hematocrits have increased whole blood viscosity, and these have been inversely correlated with cerebral blood flow. Acquired qualitative platelet defects have also been implicated in the pathogenesis of the hemostatic defects in polycythemia vera. Common thrombotic complications in this disorder include cerebrovascular accidents, myocardial infarction, peripheral arterial occlusion, deep venous thrombosis, pulmonary embolism, and portal and hepatic vein thrombosis (Budd-Chiari syndrome).

In the myeloid and monocytic leukemias, the presence of very elevated white blood counts (generally greater than 100,000/mm$^3$) can increase the viscosity in the microcirculation, which can play a role in the pathogenesis of thrombosis. Small-vessels in the lungs, brain, and less commonly in other organs may be obstructed by high levels of immature leukocytes.

In sickle cell disease, the increase in blood viscosity secondary to sickled erythrocytes may contribute to the occlusion of small blood vessels. Enhanced adhesion of sickle erythrocytes to vascular endothelium, along with increased coagulation and platelet activation, promote vascular occlusion (522).

## DRUG-INDUCED THROMBOSIS

The contribution of cancer chemotherapy to the development of thrombotic events is difficult to evaluate as the neoplasm itself and other risk factors described above predispose cancer individuals to thromboembolic complications.

Thrombotic events have been reported with induction chemotherapy regimens for acute lymphoblastic leukemia (ALL) that include L-asparaginase. Intracranial thrombosis with hemorrhage is observed most frequently, but deep venous thrombosis and pulmonary embolism can also occur (523–525). In one large series of children receiving L-asparaginase as part of induction chemotherapy for ALL, the incidence of thrombotic complications was 1.2%. Generalized bleeding episodes have only rarely been observed.

The inhibition of protein synthesis by L-asparaginase causes deficiencies of numerous plasma proteins, including albumin, thyroxine-binding globulin, and various coagulation proteins. Decreased levels of prothrombin, factors V, VII, VIII, IX, X, XI, fibrinogen, antithrombin III, protein C, protein S, and plasminogen have all been described secondary to L-asparaginase chemotherapy (122, 526). This results in prolongation of the prothrombin time, aPTT, and thrombin time, as well as hypofibrinogenemia with levels often less than 100 mg/dL. These coagulation abnormalities resolve within 1 to 2 weeks after cessation of the drug.

It is difficult to assess the role of the substantial reductions in the levels of natural anticoagulant proteins such as antithrombin III, protein C, and protein S in the pathogenesis of the thrombotic events. Both procoagulant and anticoagulant protein synthesis in the liver are decreased by L-asparaginase, leading to uncertainty as to whether there is an alteration in the balance of the opposing forces of the hemostatic mechanism. In one study of children with ALL receiving L-asparaginase, prednisone, and vincristine, no correlation was found between protein C, protein S, or antithrombin III levels and the presence or absence of thrombosis (222). Other clinical factors may contribute to the pathogenesis of thrombotic complications that are observed in these individuals including immobility or the concurrent presence of sepsis.

There are data now that women with breast cancer receiving certain chemotherapy regimens are at increased risk for developing thrombosis. The availability of large numbers of individuals receiving standard adjuvant chemotherapy programs as well as appropriate matched, untreated control populations has facilitated studies of this association. A 1981 study found a 5% incidence of symptomatic venous thrombosis among individuals with stage II breast cancer treated with chemotherapy regimens that included cyclophosphamide, methotrexate, and 5-fluorouracil (CMF) (527). All of the thrombotic events occurred while the individuals were receiving chemotherapy. In the posttreatment follow-up period, no clinically evident thromboses were observed. Goodnough et al (528) reported a 17.6% incidence of thrombosis in a series of individuals with metastatic breast cancer receiving chemotherapy, the majority of the events being pulmonary embolism or deep vein thrombosis. Levine et al (529) randomized 205 individuals receiving adjuvant chemotherapy for stage II breast cancer to either a 12-week or 36-week course of chemotherapy after primary surgical treatment. During the first 12 weeks of chemotherapy, there were similar numbers of thrombotic events; however, during the next 24 weeks, there were five additional thrombotic events in the 36-week treatment group, whereas no further thromboses were seen in the 12-week treatment group that had already completed therapy. Thus, 6.8% of the individuals had a thromboembolic event while on chemotherapy, but no further thrombotic events were detected during the more than 2400 individual-months of follow-up after chemotherapy. No relationships were found in this study between the development of thrombosis and estrogen or progesterone receptor status, age, number of involved lymph nodes, or subsequent tumor recurrence.

The association of arterial thrombosis and cancer therapy was shown in studies by Wall et al (530) and Saphner et al (531). The Cancer and Acute Leukemia Group B (CALGB) study (530) found a 1.3% incidence of arterial thrombosis, either peripheral arterial or cerebrovascular, in 1014 individuals during treatment for stage II or III breast cancer on two separate chemotherapy protocols. All except one of the thrombotic events occurred while individuals were receiving chemotherapy. In the study by Saphner et al (531) including 2352 individuals, a significant increase in arterial thrombosis was found in premenopausal women who received combined chemohormonal therapy, whereas no higher risk for arterial thrombosis was seen in postmenopausal women either receiving tamoxifen alone or in combination with chemotherapy. In both studies, arterial thrombotic events tended to occur early in the course of treatment.

The pathophysiologic basis for the thrombogenicity of chemotherapy in breast cancer individuals is not well understood. In a prospective study of individuals receiving adjuvant chemotherapy for breast cancer, no alterations in antithrombin III levels were detected. Rogers et al (220) found a statistically significant decrease in protein C and protein S levels during CMF chemotherapy. Some of these individuals had decrements in protein C and S levels that fell below the range of values seen in hereditary thrombotic disorders. Decreases in factor VII and fibrinogen levels were also reported. None of the individuals in this small study, however, had clinically evident thrombosis. Other investigators have observed significant declines in protein C concentration during CMF chemotherapy, which returned to baseline values after the completion of therapy (221). Possible explanations for these chemotherapy-induced abnormalities include impairment of vitamin K metabolism, inhibition of DNA/RNA synthesis leading to a decrease in protein synthesis by the liver, and initiation of intravascular coagulation.

Hormonal therapies, such as estrogen therapy for prostate carcinoma, have clearly been linked to an increased incidence of thromboembolic disease. In the Veterans Administration Cooperative Urologic Research Group's studies of estrogen therapy in individuals with prostate cancer, higher death rates from cardiovascular events were reported in those receiving 5 mg of diethylstilbestrol daily as compared to those receiving a 1-mg daily dose (532). The antitumor effect of these two dosages was similar.

## LUPUS ANTICOAGULANTS AND THE ANTIPHOSPHOLIPID SYNDROME (SEE CHAPTER 38)

Lupus anticoagulants are antibodies (usually IgG, IgM, or both) that prolong phospholipid-dependent clotting assays *in vitro*. These immunoglobulins do not directly inhibit the activity of specific plasma coagulation factors.

The term "lupus anticoagulant" is a misnomer, as this laboratory abnormality frequently occurs in individuals without systemic lupus erythematosus. It has been observed in other autoimmune diseases, after exposure to drugs or various infectious agents, in malignancy, and in some individuals without any apparent underlying disease (533, 534). Furthermore, individuals with lupus anticoagulants do not suffer from a bleeding diathesis unless other hemostatic defects, such as thrombocytopenia or prothrombin deficiency, are present. Paradoxically, the presence of lupus anticoagulants increases the apparent risk of both arterial and venous thromboembolism (535, 536), and there is conflicting evidence whether recurrent events occur in the same distribution (arterial or venous) as the initial episode (537, 538). Compilation of published reports suggests that about one-third of individuals with such inhibitors will have thrombotic events (534). This is likely to be an overestimate, because thrombophilic individuals with this abnormality are more likely to be studied than asymptomatic subjects. Prospective clinical studies have not yet been carried out to determine the risk of thrombosis in asymptomatic individuals with lupus anticoagulants. Reports have also appeared describing cutaneous lesions in association with lupus anticoagulants. These include livedo reticularis (539) and skin necrosis (540), which likely represent manifestations of thrombosis in underlying vessels. Livedo reticularis with cerebral thrombosis is known as Sneddon's syndrome.

In coagulation tests, lupus anticoagulants are generally detected by finding a prolonged aPTT. Other coagulation assays that have been used to screen individuals for the presence of lupus anticoagulants are the dilute Russell viper venom time (541), the kaolin clotting time (542), and the tissue thromboplastin inhibition test (543). It is currently popular to confirm abnormal screening tests using a hexagonal phospholipid assay. If a lupus anticoagulant is present, the antibody will be neutralized by the addition of hexagonal-phase phospholipid and the clotting time will normalize. Further details of these laboratory tests are provided in Chapters 26 and 38.

The presence of lupus anticoagulants has also been associated with the presence of biological false-positive tests for syphilis, as the VDRL assay depends on the presence of cardiolipin (544). Some of these antibodies react with anionic phospholipids (545, 546), but it has recently been found that the binding of most antiphospholipid antibodies to cardiolipin requires the presence of a plasma cofactor, $\beta_2$-glycoprotein I (apolipoprotein H) (547–549). Sensitive radioimmunoassays (550) or ELISAs (551) have been developed for the detection of antiphospholipid antibodies that are considerably more sensitive than the VDRL test. The relationship between the presence of lupus anticoagulants, antiphospholipid antibodies, and a thrombotic predisposition are complex, and there are conflicting data as to which test result is associated with increased thrombotic risk. A study by Triplett et al (552) demonstrated that antiphospholipid antibodies are not present in all individuals with lupus anticoagulants, and the presence of such immunoglobulins does not necessarily confer an increased thrombotic risk on these individuals. However, in individuals with systemic lupus erythematosus, persistently elevated levels of IgG anticardiolipin antibodies appear to correlate more strongly with thrombosis and fetal loss than do abnormalities in clotting assays for lupus anticoagulants (553–555). The opposite was shown in another study with respect to venous or arterial thrombosis (556). There are conflicting data with respect to the risk of arterial and venous thrombosis in such individuals. Additional evidence that the presence of IgG anticardiolipin antibodies constitutes a thrombotic risk factor comes from a case-control study of healthy adult men participating in the U.S. Physicians Health Study (557). An antibody titer above the 95th percentile was a significant risk factor for venous thromboembolism, but not for ischemic stroke. This study, however, did not test for the presence of lupus anticoagulants. A prospective Canadian study showed that the presence of a lupus anticoagulant conferred a 9.4-fold increased risk of venous thrombosis, but the anticardiolipin antibody titer was not a significant risk factor (558).

From both the clinical and laboratory standpoint, individuals with lupus anticoagulants constitute a very heterogeneous population. It is not surprising that many different mechanisms have been implicated in the pathogenesis of thrombosis in these subjects. It was shown that IgG from the plasma of a individual with arterial thrombosis and a lupus anticoagulant inhibited prostacyclin production by endothelial cells (559). Other investigators have reported that immunoglobulins from such individuals either increase prostacyclin production (560, 561), or have no effect (562). One study of individuals with the lupus anticoagulant provided evidence that excessive platelet activation can occur without a compensatory increment in the vascular biosynthesis of prostacyclin (563). Immunoglobulins from some individuals with lupus anticoagulants inhibit protein C activation mediated by the thrombin-thrombomodulin complex on endothelial cell surfaces (560, 564) and interfere with the inactivation of factor Va by APC in plasma (565) or on phospholipid surfaces (566). There are also data that antiphospholipid antibodies interfere with APC function on phosphatidylethanolamine-containing surfaces (567). Abnormalities of the heparan sulfate-antithrombin III (568) or fibrinolytic mechanisms (569) have also been suggested as explanations for the thrombotic tendency associated with lupus anticoagulants. Recently, antiphospholipid antibodies were found to reduce the levels of annexin V, a phospholipid-binding protein with potent anticoagulant activity, thereby accelerating the coagulation of plasma on cultured trophoblasts and endothelial cells (570).

The management of acute venous thromboembolism in individuals with lupus anticoagulants is similar to that of other individuals without this laboratory abnormality. However, the initial treatment of such subjects is complicated by the fact that the aPTT cannot be used reliably to monitor unfractionated heparin dosage unless proper *in vitro* calibration studies are done by adding known amounts of heparin into plasma samples and measuring the response of the aPTT. Thus, it is preferable to monitor anticoagulant therapy in these individuals by performing an activated whole blood clotting time (which usually is not affected by the lupus anticoagulant) or plasma heparin measurements, using either factor Xa or thrombin and a suitable chromogenic substrate of these enzymes. These problems are obviated by the use of low-molecular-weight heparin, which does not require monitoring. The presence of lupus anticoagulants can also interfere with heparin monitoring during cardiac surgery (571). Warfarin is effective in preventing recurrent thrombosis but requires that a relatively high international normalized ratio (INR) be maintained (537, 538).

The clinical heterogeneity of the individual populations that develop lupus anticoagulants makes it difficult to generalize regarding the long-term antithrombotic management of such individuals. Although the relationship between thrombosis and the lupus anticoagulant appears to be strong in individuals with systemic lupus erythematosus (554), the significance of the association in individuals without this disorder is more ambiguous (572). Indeed, individuals who develop transient lupus anticoagulants in association with infections do not usually sustain thromboembolic episodes, and it is unclear whether drug-associated lupus anticoagulants are associated with thrombosis. Thus, the presence of a persistent lupus anticoagulant, a high-titer antiphospholipid antibody, or both in an asymptomatic subject with no prior thrombotic history is not currently an indication for anticoagulant or antiplatelet medications. However, inasmuch as it is not currently possible to determine reliably the risk of thrombosis in an asymptomatic individual with these laboratory abnormalities, all such individuals should receive appropriate prophylaxis in conjunction with major surgical procedures (573) or prolonged immobilization, unless there is a strong contraindication to such treatment. Corticosteroids can normalize clotting assay times or reduce antiphospholipid antibody titers in individuals with lupus anticoagulants. However, these and other immunosuppressive medications may not prevent recurrent thrombosis.

As discussed in Chapter 46, the presence of lupus anticoagulants, anticardiolipin antibodies, or both has also been reported in women with obstetric complications such as habitual abortions, intrauterine death, and fetal growth retardation (559, 574–577). In some cases, pathological examination of the placenta demonstrates infarction due to decidual vessel thrombosis (575). In a cross-sectional study of unselected women with systemic lupus erythematosus, Ginsberg et al (555) could establish a significant association between persistently positive tests for lupus anticoagulants and anticardiolipin antibodies and pregnancy loss. However, in women without systemic lupus erythematosus, a prospective study did not demonstrate a relationship between the presence of a lupus anticoagulant and anticardiolipin antibodies and an initial episode of spontaneous abortion or fetal death (578).

Data from small studies indicated that corticosteroid administration (40 to 60 mg per day of prednisone) might be helpful in preventing recurrent fetal death in asymptomatic pregnant women with high antiphospholipid antibody titers and prior fetal deaths (577). However, studies with larger numbers of individuals demonstrated that this treatment was not efficacious and might even be detrimental (579). A recent prospective study randomized 202 pregnant women with a history of fetal loss and antiphospholipid antibodies to receive either prednisone (0.5 to 0.8 mg/kg body weight daily) and aspirin (100 mg daily) or placebo for the duration of the pregnancy. Treatment with prednisone and aspirin was found to be ineffective in promoting live births, and actually increased the risk of prematurity (580). Aspirin alone or full-dose heparin have also been suggested as beneficial therapeutic modalities to improve the outcome of pregnancies in women with lupus anticoagulants and poor obstetric histories (581). A case report has appeared in which a woman with a lupus anticoagulant and recurrent fetal loss was successfully treated with intravenous gammaglobulin (582).

# REFERENCES

1. Lane DA, Mannucci PM, Bauer KA et al. Inherited thrombophilia: Part 1 [Review]. Thromb Haemost 1996;76:651–662.
2. Lane DA, Mannucci PM, Bauer KA et al. Inherited thrombophilia: Part 2 [Review]. Thromb Haemost 1996;76:824–834.
3. Egeberg O. Inherited antithrombin deficiency causing thrombophilia. Thromb Diath Haemorrh 1965;13:516–530.
4. Van der Meer J, Stoepman-van Dalen EA, Jansen JM. Antithrombin-III deficiency in a Dutch family. J Clin Pathol 1973;26:532–538.
5. Marciniak E, Farley CH, DeSimone PA. Familial thrombosis due to antithrombin III deficiency. Blood 1974;43:219–231.
6. Gruenberg JC, Smallridge RC, Rosenberg RD. Inherited antithrombin-III deficiency causing mesenteric venous infarction: a new clinical entity. Ann Surg 1975;181:791–794.
7. Carvalho A, Ellman L. Hereditary antithrombin III deficiency. Effect of antithrombin III deficiency on platelet function. Am J Med 1976;61:179–183.
8. Stathakis NE, Papayannis AG, Antonopoulos M et al. Familial thrombosis due to antithrombin III deficiency in a Greek family. Acta Haematol 1977;57:47–54.
9. Mackie M, Bennett B, Ogston D et al. Familial thrombosis: inherited deficiency of antithrombin III. Br Med J 1978;1:136–138.
10. Gyde OHB, Middleton MD, Vaughan GR et al. Antithrombin III deficiency, hypertriglyceridaemia and venous thrombosis. Br Med J 1978;1:621–622.
11. Pitney WR, Manoharan A, Dean S. Antithrombin III deficiency in an Australian family. Br J Haematol 1980;46:147–149.
12. Ambruso DR, Jacobson LJ, Hathaway WE. Inherited antithrombin III deficiency and cerebral thrombosis in a child. Pediatrics 1980;65:125–131.
13. Ambruso DR, Leonard BD, Bies RD et al. Antithrombin III deficiency: decreased synthesis of a biochemically normal molecule. Blood 1982;60:78–83.
14. Prochownik EV, Antonarakis S, Bauer KA et al. Molecular heterogeneity of inherited antithrombin III deficiency. N Engl J Med 1983;308:1549–1552.
15. Bock SC, Prochownik EV. Molecular genetic survey of 16 kindreds with hereditary antithrombin III deficiency. Blood 1987;70:1273–1278.
16. Olds RJ, Lane DA, Finazzi G et al. A frameshift mutation leading to type I antithrombin deficiency and thrombosis. Blood 1990;76:2182–2186.
17. Olds RJ, Lane DA, Ireland H et al. Novel point mutations leading to type 1 antithrombin deficiency and thrombosis. Br J Haematol 1991;78:408–413.
18. Gandrille S, Vidaud D, Emmerich J et al. Molecular basis for hereditary antithrombin III quantitative deficiencies: a stop codon in exon IIIa and a frameshift in exon VI. Br J Haematol 1991;78:414–420.
19. Grundy CB, Thomas F, Millar DS et al. Recurrent deletion in the human antithrombin III gene. Blood 1991;78:1027–1032.
20. Vidaud D, Emmerich J, Sirieix ME et al. Molecular basis for antithrombin III type I deficiency: three novel mutations located in exon IV. Blood 1991;78:2305–2309.
21. Lane DA, Ireland H, Olds RJ et al. Antithrombin III: a database of mutations. Thromb Haemost 1991;66:657–661.
22. Daly M, Perry DJ, Harper PL et al. Insertions/deletions in the antithrombin gene: 3 mutations associated with non-expression. Thromb Haemost 1992;67:521–525.
23. Tomonari A, Iwahana H, Yoshimoto K et al. Two new nonsense mutations in type Ia antithrombin III deficiency at Leu 140 and Arg197. Thromb Haemost 1992;68:378–485.
24. Olds RJ, Lane DA, Chowdhury V et al. Complete nucleotide sequence of the antithrombin gene: evidence for homologous recombination causing thrombophilia. Biochemistry 1993;32:4216–4224.
25. Chowdhury V, Olds RJ, Lane DA et al. Identification of nine novel mutations in type I antithrombin deficiency by heteroduplex screening. Br J Haematol 1993;84:656–661.
26. van Boven HH, Olds RJ, Thein SL et al. Hereditary antithrombin deficiency: heterogeneity of the molecular basis and mortality in Dutch families. Blood 1994;84:4209–4213.
27. Jochmans K, Lissens W, Vervoort R et al. Antithrombin-Gly 424 Arg: a novel point mutation responsible for type I antithrombin deficiency and neonatal thrombosis. Blood 1994;83:146–151.
28. Jochmans K, Lissens W, Yin T et al. Molecular basis for type I antithrombin deficiency: identification of two novel mutations and evidence for a de novo splice site mutation. Blood 1994;84:3742–3748.
29. Lane DA, Bayston T, Olds RJ et al. Antithrombin mutation database: 2nd (1997) update. For the Plasma Coagulation Inhibitors Subcommittee of the Scientific and Standardization Committee of the International Society on Thrombosis and Haemostasis [Review]. Thromb Haemost 1997;77:197–211.
30. Harper PL, Luddington RJ, Daly M et al. The incidence of dysfunctional antithrombin variants: four cases in 210 individuals with thromboembolic disease. Br J Haematol 1991;77:360–364.
31. Rosenberg RD. Actions and interactions of antithrombin and heparin [Review]. N Engl J Med 1975;292:146–151.
32. Odegard OR, Abildgaard U. Antithrombin III: critical review of assay methods. Significance of variations in health and disease [Review]. Haemostasis 1978;7:127–134.
33. Meade TW, Dyer S, Howarth DJ et al. Antithrombin III and procoagulant activity: Sex differences and effects of the menopause. Br J Haematol 1990;74:77–81.
34. Tait RC, Walker ID, Davidson JF et al. Antithrombin III activity in healthy blood donors: age and sex related changes and the prevalence of asymptomatic deficiency [Letter]. Br J Haematol 1990;75:141–142.
35. Tait RC, Walker ID, Perry DJ et al. Prevalence of antithrombin III deficiency subtypes in 4000 healthy blood donors [Abstract]. Thromb Haemost 1992;65:839.
36. Brunel F, Duchange N, Fischer AM et al. Antithrombin III Alger: a new case of Arg47-Cys mutation. Am J Hematol 1987;25:223–224.
37. Ueyama H, Murakami T, Nishiguchi S et al. Antithrombin III Kumamoto: identification of a point mutation and genotype analysis of the family [Review]. Thromb Haemost 1990;63:231–234.
38. Thaler E, Lechner K. Antithrombin III deficiency and thromboembolism. In: Prentice CRM, ed. Clinics in haematology. London: Saunders, 1981;10:369–380.
39. Demers C, Ginsberg JS, Hirsh J et al. Thrombosis in antithrombin-III-deficient persons. Report of a large kindred and literature review [Review]. Ann Intern Med 1992;116:754–761.
40. Winter JH, Fenech A, Ridley W et al. Familial antithrombin III deficiency. Q J Med 1982;51:373–395.
41. Brenner B, Fishman A, Goldsher D et al. Cerebral thrombosis in a newborn with a congenital deficiency of antithrombin III. Am J Hematol 1988;27:209–211.
42. Sas G, Blasko G, Banhegyi D et al. Abnormal antithrombin III (antithrombin III "Budapest") as a cause of familial thrombophilia. Thromb Diath Haemorrh 1974;32:105–115.
43. Tollefsen DM, Blank MK. Detection of a new heparin-dependent inhibitor of thrombin in human plasma. J Clin Invest 1981;68:589–596.
44. Tollefsen DM, Majerus DW, Blank MK. Heparin cofactor II. Purification and properties of a heparin-dependent inhibitor of thrombin in human plasma. J Biol Chem 1982;257:2162–2169.
45. Wunderwald P, Schrenk WJ, Port H. Antithrombin BM from human plasma: an antithrombin binding moderately to heparin. Thromb Res 1982;25:177–191.
46. Demers C, Henderson P, Blajchman MA et al. An antithrombin III assay based on factor Xa inhibition provides a more reliable test to identify

congenital antithrombin III deficiency than an assay based on thrombin inhibition. Thromb Haemost 1993;69:231–235.

47. Sie P, Dupouy D, Pichon J et al. Constitutional heparin cofactor II deficiency associated with recurrent thrombosis. Lancet 1985;2:414–416.

48. Tran TH, Marbet GA, Duckert F. Association of hereditary heparin cofactor II deficiency with thrombosis. Lancet 1985;2:413–414.

49. Bertina RM, van der Linden IK, Engesser L et al. Hereditary heparin cofactor II deficiency and the risk of development of thrombosis. Thromb Haemost 1987;57:196–200.

50. Koide T, Odani S, Takahashi K et al. Antithrombin III Toyama: replacement of arginine-47 by cysteine in hereditary abnormal antithrombin III that lacks heparin-binding ability. Proc Natl Acad Sci U S A 1984;81:289–293.

51. Duchange N, Chasse J, Cohen GN et al. Molecular characterization of the antithrombin III Tours deficiency. Thromb Res 1987;45:115–121.

52. Molho-Sabatier P, Aiach M, Gaillard I et al. Molecular characterization of antithrombin III (ATIII) variants using polymerase chain reaction. Identification of the ATIII Charleville as an Ala 384 Pro mutation. J Clin Invest 1989;84:1236–1242.

53. Owen MC, Shaw GJ, Grau E et al. Molecular characterization of antithrombin Barcelona-2: 47 arginine to cysteine. Thromb Res 1989;55:451–457.

54. Owen MC, Borg JY, Soria C et al. Heparin binding defect in a new antithrombin III variant: Rouen, 47 Arg to His. Blood 1987;69:1275–1279.

55. Caso R, Lane DA, Thompson E et al. Antithrombin Padua I: impaired heparin binding caused by an Arg47 to His (CGT to CAT) substitution. Thromb Res 1990;58:185–190.

56. Wolf M, Boyer-Neumann C, Molho-Sabatier P et al. Familial variant of antithrombin III (AT III Bligny, 47Arg to His) associated with protein C deficiency. Thromb Haemost 1990;63:215–219.

57. Borg JY, Owen MC, Soria C et al. Proposed heparin binding site in antithrombin based on arginine 47. A new variant Rouen-II, 47 Arg to Ser. J Clin Invest 1988;81:1292–1296.

58. Gandrille S, Aiach M, Lane DA et al. Important role of Arg 129 in heparin binding site of antithrombin III: identification of a novel mutation Arg 129 to glutamine. J Biol Chem 1990;265:18997–19001.

59. Chang JY, Tran TH. Antithrombin III Basel. Identification of a Pro-Leu substitution in a hereditary abnormal antithrombin with impaired heparin cofactor activity. J Biol Chem 1986;261:1174–1176.

60. Daly M, Ball R, O'Meara A et al. Identification and characterisation of an antithrombin III mutant (AT Dublin 2) with marginally decreased heparin activity. Thromb Res 1989;56:503–513.

61. de Roux N, Chadeuf G, Molho-Sabatier P et al. Clinical and biochemical characterization of antithrombin III Franconville, a variant with Pro 41 Leu mutation. Br J Haematol 1990;75:222–227.

62. Borg JY, Brennan SO, Carrell RW. Antithrombin Rouen-IV 24Arg-Cys. The aminoterminal contribution to heparin binding. FEBS Lett 1990;266:163–166.

63. Olds RJ, Lane DA, Caso R et al. Antithrombin III Padua 2: a single base substitution in exon 2 detected with PCR and direct genomic sequencing. Nucleic Acids Res 1990;18:1926.

64. Brennan SO, Borg JY, George PM et al. New carbohydrate site in mutant antithrombin (7 Ile—-Asn) with decreased heparin affinity. FEBS Lett 1988;237:118–122.

65. Roussel B, Dieval J, Delobel J et al. Antithrombin III-Amiens: a new family with an Arg47-Cys inherited variant of antithrombin III with impaired heparin cofactor activity. Am J Hematol 1991;36:25–29.

66. Olds RJ, Lane DA, Boisclair M et al. Antithrombin Budapest 3: an antithrombin variant with reduced heparin affinity resulting from the substitution L99F. FEBS Lett 1992;300:241–246.

67. Okajima K, Abe H, Maeda S et al. Antithrombin III Nagasaki (Ser116-Pro): a heterozygous variant with defective heparin binding associated with thrombosis. Blood 1993;81:1300–1305.

68. Chowdhury V, Mille B, Olds RJ et al. Antithrombins Southport (Leu99 to Val) and Vienna (Gln118 to Pro): two novel antithrombin variants with abnormal heparin binding. Br J Haematol 1995;89:602–609.

69. Sambrano JE, Jacobson LJ, Reeve EB et al. Abnormal antithrombin III with defective serine protease binding (antithrombin III "Denver"). J Clin Invest 1986;77:877–893.

70. Stephens AW, Thalley BS, Hirs CHW. Antithrombin-III Denver, a reactive site variant. J Biol Chem 1987;262:1044–1048.

71. Olds RJ, Lane D, Caso R et al. Antithrombin III Milano 2: a single base substitution in the thrombin binding domain detected with PCR and direct genomic sequencing. Nucleic Acids Res 1989;17:10511.

72. Devraj-Kizuk R, Chu DH, Prochownik EV et al. Antithrombin-III-Hamilton: a gene with a point mutation (guanine to adenine) in codon 382 causing impaired serine protease reactivity. Blood 1988;72:1518–1523.

73. Austin RC, Rachubinski RA, Ofosu FA et al. Antithrombin-III-Hamilton, Ala 382 to Thr: an antithrombin-III variant that acts as a substrate but not an inhibitor of alpha-thrombin and factor Xa. Blood 1991;77:2185–2189.

74. Ireland H, Lane DA, Thompson E et al. Antithrombin III Glasgow II: alanine 382 to threonine mutation in the serpin P12 position, resulting in a substrate reaction with thrombin. Br J Haematol 1991;79:70–74.

75. Perry DJ, Harper PL, Fairham S et al. Antithrombin Cambridge, 384 Ala to Pro: a new variant identified using the polymerase chain reaction. FEBS Lett 1989;254:174–176.

76. Erdjument H, Lane DA, Ireland H et al. Formation of a covalent disulfide-linked antithrombin-albumin complex by an antithrombin variant, antithrombin "Northwick Park." J Biol Chem 1987;262:13381–13384.

77. Erdjument H, Lane DA, Ireland H et al. Antithrombin Milano, single amino acid substitution at the reactive site, Arg 393 to Cys. Thromb Haemost 1988;60:471–475.

78. Erdjument H, Lane DA, Panico M et al. Single amino acid substitutions in the reactive site of antithrombin leading to thrombosis. Congenital substitution of arginine 393 to cysteine in antithrombin Northwick Park and to histidine in antithrombin Glasgow. J Biol Chem 1988;263:5589–5593.

79. Ireland H, Lane DA, Thompson EA et al. Antithrombin Frankfurt I: arginine to cysteine substitution at the reactive site and formation of a variant antithrombin-albumin covalent complex [Abstract]. Thromb Haemost 1991;65:913.

80. Pewarchuk WJ, Fernandez-Rachubinski F, Rachubinski RA et al. Antithrombin III Sudbury: an Ala 384-Pro mutation with abnormal thrombin-binding activity and thrombotic diathesis. Thromb Res 1990;59:793–797.

81. Caso R, Lane DA, Thompson EA et al. Antithrombin Vicenza, Ala 384 to Pro (GCA to CGA) mutation, transforming the inhibitor into a substrate. Br J Haematol 1991;77:87–92.

82. Perry DJ, Daly M, Harper PL et al. Antithrombin Cambridge II, 384 Ala to Ser. Further evidence of the role of the reactive centre loop in the inhibitory function of the serpins. FEBS Lett 1991;285:248–250.

83. Blajchman MA, Fernandez-Rachubinski F, Sheffield WP et al. Antithrombin-III-Stockholm: a codon 392 (Gly-Asp) mutation with normal heparin binding and impaired serine protease reactivity. Blood 1992;79:1428–1434.

84. Owen MC, Beresford CH, Carrell RW. Antithrombin Glasgow, 393 Arg to His: a P1 reactive site variant with increased heparin affinity but no thrombin inhibitory activity. FEBS Lett 1988;231:317–320.

85. Thein SL, Lane DA. Use of synthetic oligonucleotides in the characterization of antithrombin III Northwick Park (393 CGT—TGT) and antithrombin III Glasgow (393 CGT—CAT). Blood 1988;72:1817–1821.

86. Lane DA, Erdjument H, Flynn A et al. Antithrombin Sheffield: amino acid substitution at the reactive site (Arg 393 to His) causing thrombosis. Br J Haematol 1989;71:91–96.

87. Erdjument H, Lane DA, Panico M et al. Antithrombin Chicago, amino acid substitution of arginine 393 to histidine. Thromb Res 1989;54:613–619.

88. Owen MC, Beresford CH, Carrell RW. Antithrombin Glasgow, 393 Arg to His: a P1 reactive site variant with increased heparin affinity but no thrombin inhibitory activity. FEBS Lett 1988;231:317–320.

89. Lane DA, Erdjument H, Thompson E et al. A novel amino acid substitution in the reactive site of a congenital variant antithrombin. Antithrombin Pescara Arg393 to Pro, caused by a CGT to CCT mutation. J Biol Chem 1989;264:10200–10204.

90. Bruce D, Perry DJ, Borg JY et al. Thromboembolic disease due to thermolabile conformational changes of antithrombin Rouen-VI (187 Asn ? Asp). J Clin Invest 1994;94:2265–2274.

91. Perry DJ, Marshall C, Borg JY et al. Two novel antithrombin variants, Asn187Asp and Asn187Lys, indicate a functional role for asparagine 187. Blood Coagul Fibrinolysis 1995;6:51–54.

92. Millar DS, Wacey AI, Ribando J et al. Three novel missense mutations in the antithrombin III (AT3) gene causing recurrent venous thrombosis. Hum Genet 1994;94:509–512.

93. Cosgriff TM, Bishop DT, Hershgold EJ et al. Familial antithrombin III deficiency: its natural history, genetics, diagnosis and treatment. Medicine 1983;62:209–220.

94. Bock SC, Harris JF, Schwartz CE et al. Hereditary thrombosis in a Utah kindred is caused by a dysfunctional antithrombin III gene. Am J Hum Genet 1985;37:32–41.

95. Bock SC, Marrinan JA, Radziejewska E. Antithrombin III Utah: proline-407 to leucine mutation in a highly conserved region near the inhibitor reactive site. Biochemistry 1988;27:6171–6178.

96. Hultin MB, McKay J, Abildgaard U. Antithrombin Oslo: type Ib classification of the first reported antithrombin-deficient family, with a review of hereditary antithrombin variants [Review]. Thromb Haemost 1988;59:468–473.

97. Bock SC, Silberman JA, Wikoff W et al. Identification of a threonine for alanine substitution at residue 404 of antithrombin III Oslo suggests integrity of the 404-407 region is important for maintaining normal plasma inhibitor levels [Abstract]. Thromb Haemost 1989;62:494.

98. Olds RJ, Thein SL, Ireland H et al. Identification of 402 phenylalanine as a functionally important residue in antithrombin [Abstract]. Thromb Haemost 1991;65:670.

99. Nakagawa M, Tanaka S, Tsuji H et al. Congenital antithrombin-III deficiency (ATIII Kyoto): identification of a point mutation altering arginine-406 to methionine behind the reactive site. Thromb Res 1991;64:101–108.

100. Lane DA, Old RJ, Conard J et al. Pleiotropic effects of antithrombin strand 1C substitution mutations. J Clin Invest 1992;90:2422–2433.

101. Emmerich J, Chadeuf G, Coetzee MJ et al. A phenylalanine 402 to leucine mutation is responsible for a stable inactive conformation of antithrombin. Thromb Res 1994;76:307–315.

102. Sas G, Pepper DS, Cash JD. Further investigations on antithrombin III in the plasmas of individuals with the abnormality of "antithrombin III Budapest." Thromb Diath Haemorrh 1975;33:564–572.

103. Olds RJ, Lane DA, Caso R et al. Antithrombin III Budapest: a single amino acid substitution (429Pro to Leu) in a region highly conserved in the serpin family. Blood 1992;79:1206–1212.

104. Finazzi G, Caccia R, Barbui T. Different prevalence of thromboembolism in the subtypes of congenital antithrombin deficiency: review of 404 cases [Letter]. Thromb Haemost 1987;58:1094.

105. Odegard OR, Lie M, Abildgaard U. Heparin cofactor activity measured with an amidolytic method. Thromb Res 1975;6:287–294.

106. Fagerhol MK, Abildgaard U. Immunological studies on human antithrombin III. Influence of age, sex and use of oral contraceptives on serum concentration. Scand J Haematol 1970;7:10–17.

107. McDonald MM, Hathaway WE, Reeve EB et al. Biochemical and functional study of antithrombin III in newborn infants. Thromb Haemost 1982;47:56–58.

108. Andrew M, Paes B, Milner R et al. Development of the human coagulation system in the full-term infant. Blood 1987;70:165–172.

109. Andrew M, Paes B, Milner R et al. Development of the human coagulation system in the healthy premature infant. Blood 1988;72:1651–1657.

110. Manco-Johnson MJ. Neonatal antithrombin III deficiency [Review]. Am J Med 1989;87 (Suppl 3B):49S–52S.

111. Rosenberg RD, Damus PS. The purification and mechanism of action of human antithrombin-heparin cofactor. J Biol Chem 1973;248:6490–6505.

112. Downing MR, Bloom JW, Mann KG. Comparison of the inhibition of thrombin by three plasma protease inhibitors. Biochemistry 1978;17:2649–2653.

113. Mitchell L, Piovella F, Ofosu F et al. a-2-macroglobulin may provide protection from thromboembolic events in antithrombin III-deficient children. Blood 1991;78:2299–2304.

114. de Boer AC, van Riel LA, den Ottolander GJ. Measurement of antithrombin III, a2-macroglobulin and a1-antitrypsin in individuals with deep venous thrombosis and pulmonary embolism. Thromb Res 1979;15:17–25.

115. Damus PS, Wallace GA. Immunologic measurement of antithrombin III-heparin cofactor and a2-macroglobulin in disseminated intravascular coagulation and hepatic failure coagulopathy. Thromb Res 1975;6:27–38.

116. von Kaulla E, von Kaulla KN. Antithrombin III and diseases. Am J Clin Pathol 1967;48:69–80.

117. Kauffman RH, Vetlkamp JJ, Van Tilburg NH et al. Acquired antithrombin III deficiency and thrombosis in the nephrotic syndrome. Am J Med 1978;65:607–613.

118. Panicucci F, Sagripanti A, Conte B et al. Antithrombin III, heparin cofactor and antifactor Xa in relation to age, sex and pathological condition. Haemostasis 1980;9:297–302.

119. Weenink GH, Kahle LH, Lamping RJ et al. Antithrombin III in oral contraceptive users and during normotensive pregnancy. Acta Obstet Gynecol Scand 1984;63:57–61.

120. Caine YG, Bauer KA, Barzegar S et al. Coagulation activation following estrogen administration to postmenopausal women. Thromb Haemost 1992;68:392–395.

121. Weenink GH, Treffers PE, Vijn P et al. Antithrombin III levels in preeclampsia correlate with maternal and fetal morbidity. Am J Obstet Gynecol 1984;148:1092–1097.

122. Buchanan GR, Holtkamp CA. Reduced antithrombin III levels during L-asparaginase therapy. Med Ped Oncol 1980;8:7–14.

123. Marciniak E, Gockerman JP. Heparin-induced decrease in circulating antithrombin-III. Lancet 1977;2:581–584.

124. Kitchens CS. Case report: amelioration of antithrombin III deficiency by coumarin administration. Am J Med Sci 1987;293:403–406.

125. Schulman S, Tengborn L. Treatment of venous thromboembolism in individuals with congenital deficiency of antithrombin III. Thromb Haemost 1992;68:628–783.

126. Lechner K, Kyrle PA. Antithrombin III concentrates—are they clinically useful? [Review] Thromb Haemost 1995;73:340–348.

127. Hoffman DL. Purification and large-scale preparation of antithrombin III. Am J Med 1989;87(Suppl 3B):23S–26S.

128. Menache D, O'Malley JP, Schorr JB et al. Evaluation of the safety, recovery, half-life, and clinical efficacy of antithrombin III (human) in individuals with hereditary antithrombin III deficiency. Cooperative Study Group. Blood 1990;75:33–39.

129. Schwartz RS, Bauer KA, Rosenberg RD et al. Clinical experience with antithrombin III concentrate in treatment to congenital and acquired deficiency of antithrombin. The Antithrombin III Study Group [Review]. Am J Med 1989;87(Suppl 3B):53S–60S.

130. Hirsh J, Piovella F, Pini M. Congenital antithrombin III deficiency. Incidence and clinical features [Review]. Am J Med 1989;87(Suppl 3B):34S–38S.

131. Conard J, Horellou MH, Van Dreden P et al. Thrombosis and pregnancy in congenital deficiencies in ATIII, protein C or protein S: study of 78 women [Letter]. Thromb Haemost 1990;63:319–320.

132. Ginsberg JS, Hirsh J. Anticoagulants during pregnancy. Annu Rev Med 1989;40:79–86.

133. Iturbe-Alessio I, Fonseca MC, Mutchinik O et al. Risks of anticoagulant therapy in pregnant women with artificial heart valves. N Engl J Med 1986;315:1390–1393.

134. Walker ID, Davidson JF, Young P et al. Effect of anabolic steroids on plasma antithrombin III a2macroglobulin and a1antitrypsin levels. Thromb Diath Haemorrh 1975;34:106–114.

135. Winter JH, Fenech A, Bennett B et al. Prophylactic antithrombotic therapy with stanazolol in individuals with familial antithrombin III deficiency. Br J Haematol 1984;57:527–537.

136. Griffin JH, Evatt B, Zimmerman TS et al. Deficiency of protein C in congenital thrombotic disease. J Clin Invest 1981;68:1370–1373.

137. Bertina RM, Broekmans AW, van der Linden IK et al. Protein C deficiency in a Dutch family with thrombotic disease. Thromb Haemost 1982;48:1–5.

138. Broekmans AW, Veltkamp JJ, Bertina RM. Congenital protein C deficiency and venous thromboembolism. A study of three Dutch families. N Engl J Med 1983;309:340–344.

139. Horellou MH, Conard J, Bertina RM et al. Congenital protein C deficiency and thrombotic disease in nine French families. Br Med J (Clin Res Ed) 1984;289:1285–1287.

140. Pabinger-Fasching I, Bertina RM, Lechner K et al. Protein C deficiency in two Austrian families. Thromb Haemost 1983;50:810–813.

141. Bovill EG, Bauer KA, Dickerman JD et al. The clinical spectrum of heterozygous protein C deficiency in a large New England kindred. Blood 1989;73:712–717.

142. Broekmans AW, Bertina RM. Protein C. In: Poller L, ed. Recent advances in blood coagulation. New York: Churchill Livingstone, 1985;4:117–137.

143. Wintzen AR, Broekmans AW, Bertina RM et al. Cerebral hemorrhagic infarction in young individuals with hereditary protein C deficiency: evidence for "spontaneous" cerebral venous thrombosis. Br Med J (Clin Res Ed) 1985;290:350–352.

144. Kohler J, Kasper J, Witt I et al. Ischemic stroke due to protein C deficiency. Stroke 1990;21:1077–1080.

145. Grewal RP, Goldberg MA. Stroke in protein C deficiency [Letter]. Am J Med 1990;89:538–539.

146. Camerlingo M, Finazzi G, Casto L et al. Inherited protein C deficiency and nonhemorrhagic arterial stroke in young adults. Neurology 1991;41:1371–1373.

147. Miletich J, Sherman L, Broze G Jr. Absence of thrombosis in subjects with heterozygous protein C deficiency. N Engl J Med 1987;317:991–996.

148. Tait RC, Walker ID, Reitsma PH et al. Prevalence of protein C deficiency in the healthy population. Thromb Haemost 1995;73:87–93.

149. Miletich JP, Prescott SM, White R et al. Inherited predisposition to thrombosis [Review]. Cell 1993;72:477–480.

150. Koster T, Rosendaal FR, Briët E et al. Protein C deficiency in a controlled series of unselected outpatients: an infrequent but clear risk factor for venous thrombosis (Leiden Thrombophilia Study). Blood 1995;85:2756–2761.

151. McGehee WG, Klotz TA, Epstein DJ et al. Coumarin necrosis associated with hereditary protein C deficiency. Ann Intern Med 1984;101:59–60.

152. Zauber NP, Stark MW. Successful warfarin anticoagulation despite protein C deficiency and a history of warfarin necrosis. Ann Intern Med 1986;104:659–660.

153. Bauer KA. Coumarin-induced skin necrosis [Editorial]. Arch Dermatol 1993;129:766–768.

154. D'Angelo SV, Comp PC, Esmon CT et al. Relationship between protein C antigen and anticoagulant activity during oral anticoagulation and in selected disease states. J Clin Invest 1986;77:416–425.

155. Conway EM, Bauer KA, Barzegar S et al. Suppression of hemostatic system activation by oral anticoagulants in the blood of individuals with thrombotic diatheses. J Clin Invest 1987;80:1535–1544.

156. Broekmans AW, Teepe RG, van der Meer FJM et al. Protein C (PC) and coumarin-induced skin necrosis [Abstract]. Thromb Res 1986;6:137.

157. Teepe RG, Broekmans AW, Vermeer BJ et al. Recurrent coumarin-induced skin necrosis in a individual with an acquired functional protein C deficiency. Arch Dermatol 1986;122:1408–1412.

158. Reitsma PH, Bernardi F, Doig RG et al. Protein C deficiency: a database of mutations, 1995 update. On behalf of the Subcommittee on Plasma Coagulation Inhibitors of the Scientific and Standardization Committee of the ISTH [Review]. Thromb Haemost 1995;73:876–879.

159. Romeo G, Hassan HJ, Staempfli S et al. Hereditary thrombophilia: identification of nonsense and missense mutations in the protein C gene. Proc Natl Acad Sci U S A 1987;84:2829–2832.

160. Reitsma PH, Poort SR, Allaart CF et al. The spectrum of genetic defects in a panel of 40 Dutch families with symptomatic protein C deficiency type I: heterogeneity and founder effects. Blood 1991;78:890–894.

161. Reitsma PH, te Lintel Hekkert W, Koenhen E et al. Application of two neutral MspI DNA polymorphisms in the analysis of hereditary protein C deficiency. Thromb Haemost 1990;64:239–244.

162. Grundy C, Plendl H, Grote W et al. A single base-pair deletion in the protein C gene causing recurrent thromboembolism. Thromb Res 1991;61:335–340.

163. Bernardi F, Patracchini P, Gemmati D et al. Rapid detection of a protein C mutation present in the asymptomatic and not in the thrombosis-prone lineage. Br J Haematol 1992;81:277–282.

164. Reitsma PH, Poort SR, Bernardi F et al. Protein C deficiency: a database of mutations. For the Protein C & S Subcommittee of the Scientific and Standardization Committee of the International Society on Thrombosis and Hemostasis. Thromb Haemost 1993;69:77–84.

165. Poort SR, Pabinger-Fasching I, Mannhalter C et al. Twelve novel and two recurrent mutations in 14 Austrian families with hereditary protein C deficiency. Blood Coagul Fibrinolysis 1993;4:273–280.

166. Lind B, van Solinge WW, Schwartz M et al. Splice site mutation in the human protein C gene associated with venous thrombosis: demonstration of exon skipping by ectopic transcript analysis. Blood 1993;82:2423–2432.

167. Bertina RM, Broekmans AW, Krommenhoek-van Es C et al. The use of a functional and immunologic assay for plasma protein C in the study of the heterogeneity of congenital protein C deficiency. Thromb Haemost 1984;51:1–5.

168. Comp PC, Nixon RR, Esmon CT. Determination of functional levels of protein C, an antithrombotic protein, using thrombin-thrombomodulin complex. Blood 1984;63:15–21.

169. Faioni EM, Esmon CT, Esmon NL et al. Isolation of an abnormal protein C molecule from the plasma of a individual with thrombotic diathesis. Blood 1988;71:940–946.

170. Matsuda M, Sugo T, Sakata Y et al. A thrombotic state due to an abnormal protein C. N Engl J Med 1988;319:1265–1268.

171. Sala N, Poort SR, Bertina RM. Identification of two deletions and four point mutations in the protein C gene of 6 unrelated Spanish individuals with protein C deficiency [Abstract]. Thromb Haemost 1991;65:1197.

172. Gandrille S, Vidaud M, Aiach M et al. Six previously undescribed mutations in 9 families with protein C quantitative deficiency [Abstract]. Thromb Haemost 1991;65:646.

173. Tsay W, Greengard JS, Montgomery RR et al. Genetic mutations in 10 unrelated American individuals with symptomatic type I protein C deficiency. Blood Coagul Fibrinolysis 1993;4:791–796.

174. Iijima K, Fukuda C, Nakamura K et al. A new hereditary abnormal protein C (protein C Yonago) with a dysfunctional Gla-domain. Thromb Res 1991;63:249–257.

175. Bovill EG, Tomczak JA, Grant B et al. Protein CVermont: symptomatic type II protein C deficiency associated with two GLA domain mutations. Blood 1992;79:1456–1465.

176. Gandrille S, Alhenc-Gelas M, Gaussem P et al. Five novel mutations located in exons III and IX of the protein C gene in individuals presenting with defective protein C anticoagulant activity. Blood 1993;82:159–168.

177. Marchetti G, Patracchini P, Gemmati D et al. Symptomatic type II protein C deficiency caused by a missense mutation (Gly 381 ? Ser) in the substrate-binding pocket. Br J Haematol 1993;84:285–289.

178. Ido M, Ohiwa M, Hayashi T et al. A compound heterozygous protein C deficiency with a single nucleotide G deletion encoding Gly-381 and an amino acid substitution of Lys for Gla-26. Thromb Haemost 1993;70:636–641.

179. Zheng YZ, Sakata T, Matsusue T et al. Six missense mutations associated with type I and type II protein C deficiency and implications obtained from molecular modelling. Blood Coagul Fibrinolysis 1994;5:687–696.

180. Miyata T, Zheng YZ, Sakata T et al. Three missense mutations in the protein C heavy chain causing type I and type II protein C deficiency. Thromb Haemost 1994;71:32–37.

181. Branson HE, Katz J, Marble R et al. Inherited protein C deficiency and coumarin-responsive chronic relapsing purpura fulminans in a newborn infant. Lancet 1983;2:1165–1168.

182. Seligsohn U, Berger A, Abend M et al. Homozygous protein C deficiency manifested by massive venous thrombosis in the newborn. N Engl J Med 1984;310:559–562.

183. Sills RH, Marlar RA, Montgomery RR et al. Severe homozygous protein C deficiency. J Pediatr 1984;105:409–413.

184. Estelles A, Garcia-Plaza I, Dasi A et al. Severe inherited "homozygous" protein C deficiency in a newborn infant. Thromb Haemost 1984 52:53–56.

185. Marciniak E, Wilson HD, Marlar RA. Neonatal purpura fulminans: a genetic disorder related to the absence of protein C in blood. Blood 1985;65:15–20.

186. Yuen P, Cheung A, Lin HJ et al. Purpura fulminans in a Chinese boy with congenital protein C deficiency. Pediatrics 1986;77:670–676.

187. Rappaport ES, Speights VO, Helbert B et al. Protein C deficiency. South Med J 1987;80:240–242.

188. Peters C, Casella JF, Marlar RA et al. Homozygous protein C deficiency: observations on the nature of the molecular abnormality and the effectiveness of warfarin therapy. Pediatrics 1988;81:272–276.

189. Tarras S, Gadia C, Meister L et al. Homozygous protein C deficiency in a newborn. Clinicopathologic correlation. Arch Neurol 1988;45:214–216.

190. Pegelow CH, Curless R, Bradford B. Severe protein C deficiency in a newborn. Am J Pediatr Hematol Oncol 1988;10:326–329.

191. Sugahara Y, Miura O, Yuen P et al. Protein C deficiency Hong Kong 1 and 2: hereditary protein C deficiency caused by two mutant alleles, a 5-nucleotide deletion and a missense mutation. Blood 1992;80:126–133.

192. Bauer KA, Broekmans AW, Bertina RM et al. Hemostatic enzyme generation in the blood of individuals with hereditary protein C deficiency. Blood 1988;71:1418–1426.

193. Melissari E, Kakkar VV. Congenital severe protein C deficiency in adults. Br J Haematol 1989;72:222–228.

194. Grundy CB, Melissari E, Lindo V et al. Late-onset homozygous protein C deficiency [Letter]. Lancet 1991;338:575–576.

195. Conard J, Horellou MH, van Dreden, P et al. Homozygous protein C deficiency with late onset and recurrent coumarin-induced skin necrosis [letter]. Lancet 1992;339:743–744.

196. Yamamoto K, Matsushita T, Sugiura I et al. Homozygous protein C deficiency: identification of a novel missense mutation that causes impaired secretion of the mutant protein C. J Lab Clin Med 1992;119:682–689.

197. Aiach M, Gandrille S, Emmerich J. A Review of mutations causing deficiencies of antithrombin protein C and protein S [Review]. Thromb Haemost 1995;74:81–89.

198. Gruppo RA, Leimer P, Francis RB et al. Protein C deficiency resulting from possible double heterozygosity and its response to danazol. Blood 1988;71:370–374.

199. Grundy C, Chitolie A, Talbot S et al. Protein C London 1: recurrent mutation at Arg 169 (CGG-TGG) in the protein C gene causing thrombosis. Nucleic Acids Res 1989;17:10513.

200. Petrini P, Segnestam K, Ekelund H et al. Homozygous protein C deficiency in two siblings [Review]. Pediatr Hematol Oncol 1990;7:165–175.

201. Tsuda S, Reitsma P, Miletich J. Molecular defects causing heterozygous protein C deficiency in three asymptomatic kindreds [Abstract]. Thromb Haemost 1991;65:647.

202. Boyer C, Rothschild C, Wolf M et al. A new method for the estimation of protein C by ELISA. Thromb Res 1984;36:579–589.

203. Epstein DJ, Begum PW, Bajaj SP et al. Radioimmunoassays for protein C and factor X. Plasma antigen levels in abnormal hemostatic states. Am J Clin Pathol 1984;82:573–581.

204. Bauer KA, Kass BL, Beeler DL et al. Detection of protein C activation in humans. J Clin Invest 1984;74:2033–2041.

205. Francis RB Jr, Patch MJ. A functional assay for protein C in human plasma. Thromb Res 1983;32:605–613.

206. Sala N, Owen WG, Collen D. A functional assay for protein C in human plasma. Blood 1984;63:671–675.

207. Francis RB Jr, Seyfert U. Rapid amidolytic assay of protein C in whole plasma using an activator from the venom of Agkistrodon contortrix. Am J Clin Pathol 1987;87:619–625.

208. Sala N, Borrell M, Bauer KA et al. Dysfunctional activated protein C (PC Cadiz) in a individual with thrombotic disease. Thromb Haemost 1987;57:183–186.

209. Pabinger I, Allaart CF, Hermans J et al. Hereditary protein C-deficiency: laboratory values in transmitters and guidelines for the diagnostic procedure. Report on a study of the SSC subcommittee on protein C and protein S. Thromb Haemost 1992;68:470–474.

210. Mannucci PM, Vigano S. Deficiencies of protein C, an inhibitor of blood coagulation. Lancet 1982;2:463–467.

211. Polack B, Pouzol P, Amiral J et al. Protein C level at birth. Thromb Haemost 1984;52:188–191.

212. Karpatkin M, Mannucci PM, Bhogal M et al. Low protein C in the neonatal period. Br J Haematol 1986;62:137–142.

213. Manco-Johnson MJ, Marlar RA, Jacobson LJ et al. Severe protein C deficiency in newborn infants. J Pediatr 1988;113:359–363.

214. Griffin JH, Mosher DF, Zimmerman TS et al. Protein C, an antithrombotic protein, is reduced in hospitalized individuals with intravascular coagulation. Blood 1982;60:261–264.

215. Rodeghiero F, Mannucci PM, Vigano S et al. Liver dysfunction rather than intravascular coagulation as the main cause of low protein C and antithrombin III in acute leukemia. Blood 1984;63:965–969.

216. Hesselvik JF, Malm J, Dahlback B et al. Protein C, protein S and C4b-binding protein in severe infection and septic shock. Thromb Haemost 1991;65:126–129.

217. Marlar RA, Endres-Brooks J, Miller C. Serial studies of protein C and its plasma inhibitor in individuals with disseminated intravascular coagulation. Blood 1985;66:59–63.

218. Mimuro J, Sakata Y, Wakabayashi K et al. Level of protein C determined by combined assays during disseminated intravascular coagulation and oral anticoagulation. Blood 1987;69:1704–1711.

219. Sheth SB, Carvalho AC. Protein S and C alterations in acutely ill individuals. Am J Hematol 1991;36:14–19.

220. Rogers JS, II, Murgo AJ, Fontana JA et al. Chemotherapy for breast cancer decreases plasma protein C and protein S. J Clin Oncol 1988;6:276–281.

221. Feffer SE, Carmosino LS, Fox RL. Acquired protein C deficiency in individuals with breast cancer receiving cyclophosphamide, methotrexate, and 5-fluorouracil. Cancer 1989;63:1303–1307.

222. Pui CH, Chesney CM, Bergum PW et al. Lack of pathogenic role of protein C and S in thrombosis associated with asparaginase-prednisone-vincristine therapy for leukemia. Br J Haematol 1986;64:283–290.

223. Auletta MJ, Headington JT. Purpura fulminans. A cutaneous manifestation of severe protein C deficiency. Arch Dermatol 1988;124:1387–1391.

224. Ozsoylu S, Cengiz B, Karabent A. Purpura fulminans in a case of protein C deficiency. Eur J Pediatr 1988;147:209–210.

225. Gerson WT, Dickerman JD, Bovill EG et al. Severe acquired protein C

deficiency in purpura fulminans associated with disseminated intravascular coagulation: treatment with protein C concentrate. Pediatrics 1993;91:418–422.

226. Vigano-D'Angelo S, D'Angelo A, Kaufman CE Jr et al. Protein S deficiency occurs in the nephrotic syndrome. Ann Intern Med 1987;107:42–47.

227. Cosio FG, Harker C, Batard MA et al. Plasma concentrations of the natural anticoagulants protein C and protein S in individuals with proteinuria. J Lab Clin Med 1985;106:218–222.

228. Sorensen PJ, Knudsen F, Nielsen AH et al. Protein C activity in renal disease. Thromb Res 1985;38:243-249.

229. Faioni EM, Franchi F, Krachmalnicoff A et al. Low levels of the anticoagulant activity of protein C in individuals with chronic renal insufficiency: an inhibitor of protein C is present in uremic plasma. Thromb Haemost 1991;66:420–425.

230. Pabinger I, Kyrle PA, Speiser W et al. Diagnosis of protein C deficiency in individuals on oral anticoagulant treatment: comparison of three different functional protein C assays. Thromb Haemost 1990;63:407–412.

231. Jones DW, Mackie IJ, Winter M et al. Detection of protein C deficiency during oral anticoagulant therapy-use of the protein C:factor VII ratio. Blood Coagul Fibrinolysis 1991;2:407–411.

232. Mitchell CA, Rowell JA, Hau L et al. A fatal thrombotic disorder associated with an acquired inhibitor of protein C. N Engl J Med 1987;317:1638–1642.

233. Manco-Johnson M, Nuss R. Protein C concentrate prevents peripartum thrombosis. Am J Hematol 1992;40:69–70.

234. Gonzalez R, Alberca I, Sala N et al. Protein C deficiency-response to danazol and DDAVP. Thromb Haemost 1985;53:320–322.

235. Broekmans AW, Conard J, van Weyenberg RG et al. Treatment of hereditary protein C deficiency with stanozolol. Thromb Haemost 1987;57:20–24.

236. De Stefano V, Leone G, Teofili L et al. Transient ischemic attack in a individual with congenital protein-C deficiency during treatment with stanozolol. Am J Hematol 1988;29:120–121.

237. Thorisdottir H, Evans JA, Schwartz HJ et al. Some clotting factors in plasma during danazol therapy: free and total protein S, but not C4b-binding protein, are elevated by danazol therapy. J Lab Clin Med 1992;119:698–701.

238. De Stefano V, Mastrangelo S, Schwarz HP et al. Replacement therapy with a purified protein C concentrate during initiation of oral anticoagulation in severe protein C congenital deficiency. Thromb Haemost 1993;70:247–249.

239. Comp PC, Esmon CT. Recurrent venous thromboembolism in individuals with a partial deficiency of protein S. N Engl J Med 1984;311:1525–1528.

240. Schwarz HP, Fischer M, Hopmeier P et al. Plasma protein S deficiency in familial thrombotic disease. Blood 1984;64:1297–1300.

241. Comp PC, Nixon RR, Cooper MR et al. Familial protein S deficiency is associated with recurrent thrombosis. J Clin Invest 1984;74:2082–2088.

242. Broekmans AW, Bertina RM, Reinalda-Poot J et al. Hereditary protein S deficiency and venous thrombo-embolism. A study in three Dutch families. Thromb Haemost 1985;53:273–277.

243. Kamiya T, Sugihara T, Ogata K et al. Inherited deficiency of protein S in Japanese family with recurrent venous thrombosis: a study of three generations. Blood 1986;67:406–410.

244. Comp PC, Doray D, Patton D et al. An abnormal plasma distribution of protein S occurs in functional protein S deficiency. Blood 1986;67:504–508.

245. Engesser L, Broekmans AW, Bri't E et al. Hereditary protein S deficiency: clinical manifestations. Ann Intern Med 1987;106:677–682.

246. Broekmans AW, van Rooyen W, Westerveld BD et al. Mesenteric vein thrombosis as presenting manifestation of hereditary protein S deficiency. Gastroenterology 1987;92:240–242.

247. Cros D, Comp PC, Beltran G et al. Superior sagittal sinus thrombosis in a individual with protein S deficiency. Stroke 1990;21:633–636.

248. Bolan CD, Krishnamurti C, Tang DB et al. Association of protein S deficiency with thrombosis in a kindred with elevated levels of plasminogen activator-1. Ann Intern Med 1993;119:779–785.

249. Friedman KD, Marlar RA, Houson JG et al. Warfarin-induced skin necrosis in a individual with protein S deficiency [Abstract]. Blood 1986;68(suppl 1):333a.

250. Coller BS, Owen J, Jesty J et al. Deficiency of plasma protein S, protein C or antithrombin III and arterial thrombosis. Arteriosclerosis 1987;7:456–462.

251. Israels SJ, Seshia SS. Childhood stroke associated with protein C or protein S deficiency. J Pediatr 1987;111:562–564.

252. Girolami A, Simioni P, Lazzaro AR et al. Severe arterial cerebral thrombosis in a individual with protein S deficiency (moderately reduced total and markedly reduced free protein S): a family study. Thromb Haemost 1989;61:144–147.

253. Green D, Otoya J, Oriba H et al. Protein S deficiency in middle-aged women with stroke. Neurology 1992;42:1029–1033.

254. Allaart CF, Aronson DC, Ruys T et al. Hereditary protein S deficiency in young adults with arterial occlusive disease. Thromb Haemost 1990;64:206–210.

255. Fair D, Revak DJ. Quantitation of human protein S in the plasma of normal and warfarin-treated individuals by radioimmunoassay. Thromb Res 1984;36:527–535.

256. Bertina RM, van Wijngaarden A, Reinalda-Poot J et al. Determination of plasma protein S-the protein factor of activated protein C. Thromb Haemost 1985;53:268–272.

257. Comp PC, Thurnau GR, Welsh J et al. Functional and immunologic protein S levels are decreased during pregnancy. Blood 1986;68:881–885.

258. Malm J, Laurell M, Dahlback B. Changes in the plasma levels of vitamin K-dependent proteins C and S and of C4B-binding protein during pregnancy and oral contraception. Br J Haematol 1988;68:437–443.

259. Amiral J, Grosley B, Boyer-Neumann C et al. New direct assay of free protein S antigen using two distinct monoclonal antibodies specific for the free form. Blood Coagul Fibrinolysis 1994;5:179–186.

260. Van de Waart P, Preissner KT, Bechtold JR et al. A functional test for protein S activity in plasma. Thromb Res 1987;48:427–437.

261. D'Angelo A, Vigano-D'Angelo S, Esmon CT et al. Acquired deficiencies of protein S. Protein S activity during oral anticoagulation, in liver disease, and in disseminated intravascular coagulation. J Clin Invest 1988;81:1445–1454.

262. Wolf M, Boyer-Neumann C, Martinoli JL et al. A new functional assay for human protein S activity using activated factor V as substrate [Letter]. Thromb Haemost 1989;62:1144–1145.

263. Preda L, Tripodi A, Valsecchi C et al. A prothrombin time-based functional assay of protein S. Thromb Res 1990;60:19–32.

264. Faioni EM, Franchi F, Asti D et al. Resistance to activated protein C in nine thrombophilic families: interference in a protein S functional assay. Thromb Haemost 1993;70:1067–1071.

265. Ploos van Amstel HK, van der Zanden AL, Bakker E et al. Two genes homologous with protein S cDNA are located on chromosome 3. Thromb Haemost 1987;58:982–987.

266. Schmidel DK, Tataro AV, Phelps LG et al. Organization of the human protein S genes. Biochemistry 1990;29:7845–7852.

267. Ploos van Amstel HK, Reitsma PH, van der Logt CPE et al. Intron-exon organization of the active protein S gene PS alpha and its pseudogene PSb: duplication and silencing during primate evolution. Biochemistry 1990;29:7853–7861.

268. Edenbrandt CM, Lundwall A, Wydro R et al. Molecular analysis of the gene for vitamin K-dependent protein S and its pseudogene. Cloning and partial gene organization. Biochemistry 1990;29:7861–7868.

269. Borgel D, Gandrille S, Aiach M. Protein S deficiency. Thromb Haemost 1997;78:351–356.

270. Ploos van Amstel HK, Huisman MV, Reitsma PH et al. Partial protein S gene deletion in a family with hereditary thrombophilia. Blood 1989;73:479–483.

271. Schmidel DK, Nelson RM, Broxson EH Jr et al. A 5.3-kb deletion including exon XIII of the protein S a gene occurs in two protein S-deficient families. Blood 1991;77:551–559.

272. Holmes ZR, Bertina RM, Reitsma PH. Characterization of a large chromosomal deletion in the PROS1 gene of a individual with protein S deficiency type I using long PCR. Br J Haematol 1996;92:986–991.

273. Gomez E, Ledford MR, Pegelow CH et al. Homozygous protein S deficiency due to a one base pair deletion that leads to a stop codon in exon III of the protein S gene. Thromb Haemost 1994;71:723–726.

274. Gandrille S, Borgel D, Eschwege-Gufflet V et al. Identification of 15 different candidate causal point mutations and three polymorphisms in 19 individuals with protein S deficiency using a scanning method for the analysis of the protein S active gene. Blood 1995;85:130–138.

275. Borgel D, Duchemin J, Alhenc-Gelas M et al. Molecular basis for protein S hereditary deficiency: genetic defects observed in 118 individuals with type I and type IIa deficiencies. The French Network on Molecular Abnormalities Responsible for Protein C and Protein S Deficiencies. J Lab Clin Med 1996;128:218–227.

276. Simmonds RE, Ireland H, Kunz G et al. Identification of 19 protein S gene mutations in individuals with phenotypic protein S deficiency and thrombosis. Blood 1996;88:4195–4204.

277. Reitsma PH, Ploos van Amstel HK, Bertina RM. Three novel mutations in five unrelated subjects with hereditary protein S deficiency type I. J Clin Invest 1994;93:486–492.

278. Gomez E, Poort SR, Bertina RM et al. Identification of eight point mutations in protein S deficiency type I: Analysis of 15 pedigrees. Thromb Haemost 1995;73:750–755.

279. Mustafa S, Pabinger I, Mannhalter C. Protein S deficiency type I: identification of point mutations in 9 of 10 families. Blood 1995;86:3444–3451.

280. Duchemin J, Borg JY, Borgel D et al. Five novel mutations of the protein S active gene (PROS1) in 8 Norman families. Thromb Haemost 1996;75:437–444.

281. Beauchamp NJ, Daly ME, Cooper PC et al. Molecular basis of protein S deficiency in three families also showing independent inheritance of factor V leiden. Blood 1996;88:1700–1707.

282. Andersen BD, Lind B, Philips M et al. Two mutations in exon XII of the protein S alpha gene in four thrombophilic families resulting in premature stop codons and depressed levels of mutated mRNA. Thromb Haemost 1996;76:143–150.

283. Okamoto Y, Yamazaki T, Katsumi A et al. A novel nonsense mutation associated with an exon skipping in a individual with hereditary protein S deficiency type I. Thromb Haemost 1996;75:877–882.

284. Yamazaki T, Katsumi A, Kagami K et al. Molecular basis of a hereditary type I protein S deficiency caused by a substitution of Cys for Arg474. Blood 1996;87:4643–4650.

285. Duchemin J, Gandrille S, Borgel D et al. The Ser 460 to Pro substitution of the protein S alpha (PROS1) gene is a frequent mutation associated with free protein S (type IIa) deficiency. Blood 1995;86:3436–3443.

286. Bertina RM, Ploos van Amstel HK, van Wijngaarden A et al. Heerlen polymorphism of protein S, an immunologic polymorphism due to dimorphism of residue 460. Blood 1990;76:538–548.

287. Zöller B, Garcia de Frutos P, Dahlbäck B. Evaluation of the relationship between protein S and C4b-binding protein isoforms in hereditary protein S deficiency demonstrating type I and type III deficiencies to be phenotypic variants of the same genetic disease. Blood 1995;85:3524–3531.

288. Dahlbäck B. Protein S and C4b-binding protein: components involved in the regulation of the protein C anticoagulant system [Review]. Thromb Haemost 1991;66:49–61.

289. Shigekiyo T, Uno Y, Kawauchi S et al. Protein S Tokushima: an abnormal protein S found in a Japanese family with thrombosis. Thromb Haemost 1993;70:244–246.

290. Hayashi T, Nishioka J, Shigekiyo T et al. Protein S Tokushima: abnormal molecule with a substitution of Glu for Lys-155 in the second epidermal growth factor-like domain of protein S. Blood 1994;83:683–690.

291. Mahasandana C, Suvatte V, Chuansumrit A et al. Homozygous protein S deficiency in an infant with purpura fulminans. J Pediatr 1990;117:750–753.

292. Pegelow CH, Ledford M, Young JN et al. Severe protein S deficiency in a newborn. Pediatrics 1992;89:674–676.

293. Boerger LM, Morris PC, Thurnau GR et al. Oral contraceptives and gender affect protein S status. Blood 1987;69:692–694.

294. Miletich JP, Broze GJ Jr. Age and gender dependence of total protein S antigen in the normal adult population [Abstract]. Blood 1988;72:371a.

295. Gilabert J, Fernandez JA, Espana F et al. Physiological coagulation inhibitors (protein S, protein C and antithrombin III) in severe preeclamptic states and in users of oral contraceptives. Thromb Res 1988;49:319–329.

296. Heeb MJ, Mosher D, Griffin JH. Activation and complexation of protein C and cleavage and decrease of protein S in plasma of individuals with intravascular coagulation. Blood 1989;73:455–461.

297. Madden RM, Gill JC, Marlar RA. Protein C and protein S levels in two individuals with acquired purpura fulminans. Br J Haematol 1990;75:112–117.

298. Stahl CP, Wideman CS, Spira TJ et al. Protein S deficiency in men with long-term human immunodeficiency virus infection. Blood 1993;81:1801–1807.

299. Gouault-Heilmann M, Gadelha-Parente T, Levent M et al. Total and free protein S in nephrotic syndrome. Thromb Res 1988;49:37–42.

300. Alessi MC, Aillaud MF, Boyer-Neumann C et al. Cutaneous necrosis associated with acquired severe protein S deficiency [Letter]. Thromb Haemost 1993;69:524–526.

301. D'Angelo A, Della Valle P, Crippa L et al. Brief report: autoimmune protein S deficiency in a boy with severe thromboembolic disease. N Engl J Med 1993;328:1753–1757.

302. Schwarz HP, Muntean W, Watzke H et al. Low total proteins antigen but high protein S activity due to decreased C4b-binding protein in neonates. Blood 1988;71:562–565.

303. Malm J, Bennhagen R, Holmberg L et al. Plasma concentrations of C4b-binding protein and vitamin K-dependent protein S in term and preterm infants: low levels of protein S-C4b-binding protein complexes. Br J Haematol 1988;68:445–449.

304. Melissari E, Nicolaides KH, Scully MF et al. Protein S and C4b-binding protein in fetal and neonatal blood. Br J Haematol 1988;70:199–203.

305. Dahlbäck B, Carlsson M, Svensson PJ. Familial thrombophilia due to a previously unrecognized mechanism characterized by poor anticoagulant response to activated protein C. Proc Natl Acad Sci U S A 1993;90:1004–1008.

306. Svensson PJ, Dahlback B. Resistance to activated protein C as a basis for venous thrombosis. N Engl J Med 1994;330:517–522.

307. Griffin JH, Evatt B, Wideman C et al. Anticoagulant protein C pathway defective in majority of thrombophilic individuals. Blood 1993;82:1989–1993.

308. Halbmayer WM, Haushofer A, Schon R et al. The prevalence of poor anticoagulant response to activated protein C (APC resistance) among individuals suffering from stroke or venous thrombosis and among healthy subjects. Blood Coagul Fibrinolysis 1994;5:51–57.

309. van der Meer FJM, Koster T, Vandenbroucke JP et al. The Leiden Thrombophilia Study (LETS). Thromb Haemost 1997;78:631–635.

310. Koster T, Rosendaal FR, de Ronde H et al. Venous thrombosis due to poor anticoagulant response to activated protein C: Leiden Thrombophilia Study. Lancet 1993;342:1503–1506.

311. Bertina RM, Koeleman BPC, Koster T et al. Mutation in blood coagulation factor V associated with resistance to activated protein C. Nature 1994;369:64–67.

312. Greengard JS, Sun X, Xu X et al. Activated protein C resistance caused by Arg506Gln mutation in factor Va. Lancet 1994;343:1361–1362.

313. Voorberg J, Roelse J, Koopman R et al. Association of idiopathic venous thromboembolism with single point-mutation at Arg506 of factor V. Lancet 1994;343:1535–1536.

314. Zöller B, Dahlbäck B. Linkage between inherited resistance to activated protein C and factor V gene mutation in venous thrombosis. Lancet 1994;343:1536–1538.

315. Sun X, Evatt B, Griffin JH. Blood coagulation factor Va abnormality associated with resistance to activated protein C in venous thrombophilia. Blood 1994;83:3120–3125.

316. Kalafatis M, Bertina RM, Rand MD et al. Characterization of the molecular defect in Factor VR506Q. J Biol Chem 1995;270:4053–4057.

317. Greengard JS, Eichinger S, Griffin JH et al. Brief report: variability of thrombosis among homozygous siblings with resistance to activated protein C due to an Arg→Gln mutation in the gene for factor V. N Engl J Med 1994;331:1559–1561.

318. Zöller B, Svensson PJ, He X et al. Identification of the same factor V gene mutation in 47 out of 50 thrombosis-prone families with inherited resistance to activated protein C. J Clin Invest 1994;94:2521–2524.

319. Rosendaal FR, Koster T, Vandenbroucke JP et al. High risk of thrombosis in individuals homozygous for factor V Leiden (activated protein C resistance). Blood 1995;85:1504–1508.

320. Koeleman BP, Reitsma PH, Allaart CF et al. Activated protein C resistance as an additional risk factor for thrombosis in protein C-deficient families. Blood 1994;84:1031–1035.

321. Gandrille S, Greengard JS, Alhenc-Gelas M et al. Incidence of activated protein C resistance caused by ARG 506 GLN mutation in factor V in 113 unrelated symptomatic protein C-deficient patients. The French Network on the behalf of INSERM. Blood 1995;86:219–224.

322. van Boven HH, Reitsma PH, Rosendaal FR et al. Factor V Leiden (FV R506Q) in families with inherited antithrombin deficiency. Thromb Haemost 1996;75:417–421.

323. Zöller B, Berntsdotter A, Garcia de Frutos P et al. Resistance to activated protein C as an additional genetic risk factor in hereditary deficiency of protein S. Blood 1995;85:3518–3523.

324. Koeleman BPC, van Rumpt D, Hamulyak K et al. Factor V Leiden: an additional risk factor for thrombosis in protein S deficient families? Thromb Haemost 1995;74:580–583.

325. Dahlbäck B, Hildebrand B. Inherited resistance to activated protein C is corrected by anticoagulant cofactor activity found to be a property of factor V. Proc Natl Acad Sci U S A 1994;91:1396–1400.

326. Shen L, Dahlbäck B. Factor V and protein S as synergistic cofactors to activated protein C in degradation of factor VIIIa. J Biol Chem 1994;269:18735–18738.

327. Lu D, Kalafatis M, Mann KG et al. Comparison of activated protein C/protein S-mediated inactivation of human factor VIII and factor V. Blood 1996;87:4708–4817.

328. Varadi K, Rosing J, Tans G et al. Factor V enhances the cofactor function of protein S in the APC-mediated inactivation of factor VIII: influence of the factor VR506Q mutation. Thromb Haemost 1996;76:208–214.

329. Ridker PM, Hennekens CH, Lindpaintner K et al. Mutation in the gene coding for coagulation factor V and the risk of myocardial infarction, stroke, and venous thrombosis in apparently healthy men. N Engl J Med 1995;332:912–917.

330. Ridker PM, Glynn RJ, Miletich JP et al. Age-specific incidence rates of venous thromboembolism among heterozygous carriers of factor V Leiden mutation. Ann Intern Med 1997;126:528–531.

331. Ardissino D, Peyvandi F, Merlini PA et al. Factor V (Arg506TGln) mutation in young survivors of myocardial infarction. Thromb Haemost 1996;75:701–702.

332. Emmerich J, Alhenc-Gelas M, Aillaud MF et al. Clinical features in 36 individuals homozygous for the ARG 506TGLN factor V mutation. Thromb Haemost 1997;77:620–623.

333. Rosendaal FR, Siscovick DS, Schwartz SM et al. Factor V Leiden (resistance to activated protein C) increases the risk of myocardial infarction in young women. Blood 1997;89:2817–2821.

334. Rosendaal FR, Siscovick DS, Schwartz SM et al. A common prothrombin variant (20210 G >A) increases the risk of myocardial infarction in young women [Abstract]. Blood 1997;90:1747–1750.

335. Rees DC, Cox M, Clegg JB. World distribution of factor V Leiden. Lancet 1995;346:1133–1134.

336. Zivelin A, Griffin JH, Xu X et al. A single genetic origin for a common Caucasian risk factor for venous thrombosis. Blood 1997;89:397–402.

337. Greengard JS, Alhenc-Gelas M, Gandrille S et al. Pseudo-homozygous activated protein C resistance due to coinheritance of heterozygous factor V-506Q and type I factor V deficiency associated with thrombosis [Abstract]. Thromb Haemost 1995;73:1361.

338. Simione P, Scoudeller A, Radossi P et al. "Pseudo homozygous" activated protein C resistance due to double heterozygous factor V defects (factor V Leiden mutation and type I quantitative factor V defect) associated with thrombosis: report of two cases belonging to two unrelated kindreds. Thromb Haemost 1996;75:422–426.

339. Zehnder JL, Jain M. Recurrent thrombosis due to compound heterozygos-

ity for the factor V Leiden and factor V deficiency. Blood Coagul Fibrinolysis 1996;7:361–362.

340. Guasch JF, Lensen RP, Bertina RM. Molecular characterization of a type I quantitative factor V deficiency in a thrombosis individual that is "pseudo homozygous" for activated protein C resistance. Thromb Haemost 1996; 77:252–257.

341. Lunghi B, Iacoviello L, Gemmati D et al. Detection of new polymorphic markers in the factor V gene: association with factor V levels in plasma. Thromb Haemost 1996;75:45–48.

342. Bernardi F, Faioni EM, Castoldi E et al. A factor V genetic component differing from factor V R506Q contributes to the activated protein C resistance phenotype. Blood 1997;90:1552–1557.

343. Le DT, Griffin JH, Greengard JS et al. Use of a generally applicable tissue factor-dependent factor V assay to detect activated protein C-resistant factor Va in individuals receiving warfarin and in individuals with a lupus anticoagulant. Blood 1995;3:1704–1711.

344. Fisher M, Fernández JA, Ameriso SF et al. Activated protein C resistance in ischemic stroke not due to factor V arginine$^{506}$→glutamine mutation. Stroke 1996;27:1163–1166.

345. van der Bom JG, Bots ML, Haverkate F et al. Reduced response to activated protein C is associated with increased risk for cerebrovascular disease. Ann Intern Med 1996;125:265–269.

346. Poort SR, Rosendaal FR, Reitsma PH et al. A common genetic variation in the 3'-untranslated region of the prothrombin gene is associated with elevated prothrombin levels and an increase in venous thrombosis. Blood 1996;88:3698–3703.

347. Hillarp A, Svensson P, Dahlbäck B. Prothrombin gene mutation and venous thrombosis in unselected outpatients [Abstract]. Thromb Haemost 1997(suppl):378–379.

348. Cooper PC, Beauchamp NJ, Daly ME et al. The prothrombin 20210 GTA variant is associated with increased levels of prothrombin and increased incidence of venous thrombosis [Abstract]. Thromb Haemost 1997(suppl): 379.

349. Ferraresi P, Legnani C, Quaglio S et al. Study of a G/A variation in the 3'-untranslated region of prothrombin mRNA in Italian individuals with venous thrombosis [Abstract]. Thromb Haemost 1997;(suppl):379.

350. McDonagh J, Carrell N, Lee MH. Dysfibrinogenemia and other disorders of fibrinogen structure and function. In: Colman RW, Hirsh J, Marder VJ, Salzman EW, eds. Hemostasis and thrombosis: basic principles and clinical practice. 3rd ed. Philadelphia: JB Lippincott, 1994;314–334.

351. Egeberg O. Inherited fibrinogen abnormality causing thrombophilia. Thromb Diath Haemorrh 1967;17:175–187.

352. Thorsen LI, Brosstad F, Solum NO et al. Increased binding to ADP-stimulated platelets and aggregation effect of the dysfibrinogen Oslo I as compared with normal fibrinogen. Scand J Haematol 1986;36:203–210.

353. Beck EA, Charache P, Jackson DP. A new inherited coagulation disorder caused by an abnormal fibrinogen "(fibrinogen Baltimore)." Nature 1965; 208:143–145.

354. Beck EA, Shainoff JR, Vogel A et al. Functional evaluation of an inherited abnormal fibrinogen: fibrinogen "Baltimore." J Clin Invest 1971;50: 1874–1884.

355. Hansen MS, Clemmensen I, Winther D. Fibrinogen Copenhagen: An abnormal fibrinogen with defective polymerization and release of fibrinopeptide A, but normal absorption of plasminogen. Scand J Clin Lab Invest 1980;40:221–226.

356. Henschen A, Kehl M, Southan C et al. Genetically abnormal fibrinogens—Some current characterization strategies. In: Haverkate F, Henschen A, Nieuwenhuizen W, Straub PW, eds. Fibrinogen-structure, functional aspects, metabolism: Proceedings, Workshop on Fibrinogen, May 1982, Leiden, The Netherlands. Berlin: Walter de Gruyter, 1983;2: 125–144.

357. Andes WA. Fibrinogen New Orleans II: a new dysfibrinogenemia with venous thrombosis [Abstract]. Thromb Haemost 1983;50:337.

358. Carrell N, Gabriel DA, Blatt PM et al. Hereditary dysfibrinogenemia in a individual with thrombotic disease. Blood 1983;62:439–447.

359. Carrell N, McDonagh J. Functional defects in abnormal fibrinogens. In: Henschen A, Hessel B, McDonagh J, Saldeen T, eds. Fibrinogen, structural variants and interactions: Proceedings, Workshop on Fibrinogen, May 1994, Stockholm, Sweden. Berlin: Walter de Gruyter, 1985;3:155–164.

360. Soria J, Soria C, Samama M et al. Fibrinogen Haifa: fibrinogen variant with absence of protective effect of calcium on plasmin degradation of gamma chains. Thromb Haemost 1987;57:310–313.

361. Al-Mondhiry H, Bilezikian SB, Nossel HL. Fibrinogen "New York"—An abnormal fibrinogen associated with thromboembolism: functional evaluation. Blood 1975;45:607–619.

362. Soria J, Soria C, Samama M et al. Study of 10 cases of congenital dysfibrinogenemia. Clinical and molecular biological aspects. In: Henschen A, Hessel B, McDonagh J, Saldeen T, eds. Fibrinogen: structural variants and interactions. Berlin: Walter de Gruyter, 1985;3:165–183.

363. Haverkate F, Koopman J, Kluft C et al. Fibrinogen Milano II: a congenital dysfibrinogenemia associated with juvenile arterial and venous thrombosis. Thromb Haemost 1986;55:131–135.

364. Koopman J, Haverkate F, Lord ST et al. The molecular basis of fibrinogen

Naples associated with defective a-thrombin binding and congenital thrombophilia: homozygous substitution of Bb 68 Ala-Thr [Abstract]. Thromb Haemost 1991;65:809.

365. Soria J, Soria C, Caen JP. A new type of congenital dysfibrinogenemia with defective fibrin lysis-Dusard syndrome: possible relation to thrombosis. Br J Haematol 1983;53:575–586.

366. Lijnen HR, Soria J, Soria C et al. Dysfibrinogenemia (fibrinogen Dusard) associated with impaired fibrin-enhanced plasminogen activation. Thromb Haemost 1984;51:108–109.

367. Koopman J, Haverkate F, Grimbergen J et al. Molecular basis for fibrinogen Dusart (Aa 554 Arg-Cys) and its association with abnormal fibrin polymerization and thrombophilia. J Clin Invest 1993;91:1637–1643.

368. Collet JP, Soria J, Mirshahi M et al. Dusart syndrome: a new concept of the relationship between fibrin clot architecture and fibrin clot degradability: Hypofibrinolysis related to an abnormal clot structure. Blood 1993;82: 2462–2469.

369. Aoki N, Moroi M, Sakata Y et al. Abnormal plasminogen. A hereditary abnormality found in a individual with recurrent thrombosis. J Clin Invest 1978;61:1186–1195.

370. Sakata Y, Aoki N. Molecular abnormality of plasminogen. J Biol Chem 1980;255:5442–5447.

371. Miyata T, Iwanaga S, Sakata Y et al. Plasminogen Tochigi: inactive plasmin resulting from replacement of alanine-600 by threonine in the active site. Proc Natl Acad Sci U S A 1982;79:6132–6136.

372. Miyata T, Iwanaga S, Sakata Y et al. Plasminogens Tochigi II and Nagoya: two additional molecular defects with Ala-600—Thr replacement found in plasmin light chain variants. J Biochem 1984;96:277–287.

373. Wohl RC, Summaria L, Robbins KC. Physiological activation of the human fibrinolytic system. Isolation and characterization of human plasminogen variants, Chicago I and Chicago II. J Biol Chem 1979;254:9063–9069.

374. Kazama M, Tahara C, Suzuki Z et al. Abnormal plasminogen, a case of recurrent thrombosis. Thromb Res 1981;21:517–522.

375. Wohl RC, Summaria L, Chediak J et al. Human plasminogen variant Chicago III. Thromb Haemost 1982;48:146–152.

376. Soria J, Soria C, Bertrand O et al. Plasminogen Paris I: congenital abnormal plasminogen and its incidence in thrombosis. Thromb Res 1983;32: 229–238.

377. Lottenberg R, Dolly FR, Kitchens CS. Recurring thromboembolic disease and pulmonary hypertension associated with severe hypoplasminogenemia. Am J Hematol 1985;19:181–193.

378. Mannucci PM, Kluft C, Traas DW et al. Congenital plasminogen deficiency associated with venous thromboembolism: therapeutic trial with stanozolol. Br J Haematol 1986;63:753–759.

379. Scharrer IM, Wohl RC, Hach V et al. Investigation of a congenital abnormal plasminogen, Frankfurt I, and its relationship to thrombosis. Thromb Haemost 1986;55:396–401.

380. Liu Y, Lyons RM, McDonagh J. Plasminogen San Antonio: an abnormal plasminogen with a more cathodic migration, decreased activation and associated thrombosis. Thromb Haemost 1988;59:49–53.

381. Dolan G, Greaves M, Cooper P et al. Thrombovascular disease and familial plasminogen deficiency: a report of three kindreds. Br J Haematol 1988; 70:417–421.

382. Azuma H, Uno Y, Shigekiyo T et al. Congenital plasminogen deficiency caused by a Ser$^{572}$ to Pro mutation. Blood 1993;82:475–480.

383. Barbui T, Rodeghiero F. Hereditary dysfunctional antithrombin III (AT-III variant) [Letter]. Thromb Haemost 1981;45:97.

384. Aoki N, Tateno K, Sakata Y. Differences of frequency distributions of plasminogen phenotypes between Japanese and American populations: new methods for the detection of plasminogen variants. Biochem Genet 1984; 22:871–881.

385. Shigekiyo T, Uno Y, Tomonari A et al. Type I congenital plasminogen deficiency is not a risk factor for thrombosis. Thromb Haemost 1992;67: 189–192.

386. Johansson L, Hedner U, Nilsson IM. A family with thromboembolic disease associated with deficient fibrinolytic activity in vessel wall. Acta Med Scand 1978;203:477–480.

387. Jorgensen M, Mortensen JZ, Madsen AG et al. A family with reduced plasminogen activator activity in blood associated with recurrent venous thrombosis. Scand J Haematol 1982;29:217–223.

388. Stead NW, Bauer KA, Kinney TR et al. Venous thrombosis in a family with defective release of vascular plasminogen activator and elevated plasma factor VIII/von Willebrand's factor. Am J Med 1983;74:33–39.

389. Nilsson IM, Tengborn L. Impaired fibrinolysis. New evidence in relation to thrombosis. In: Jespersen J, Kluft C, Korsgaard O, eds. Clinical aspects of fibrinolysis. South Jutland University Press, 1983;273–291.

390. Jorgensen M, Bonnevie-Nielsen V. Increased concentration of the fast-acting plasminogen activator inhibitor in plasma associated with familial thrombosis. Br J Haematol 1987;65:175–180.

391. Zöller B, Dahlbäck B. Protein S deficiency in a large family with thrombophilia previously characterized as having an inherited fibrinolytic defect [Abstract]. Thromb Haemost 1993;69:1256.

392. Malm J, Laurell M, Nilsson IM et al. Thromboembolic disease-critical evaluation of laboratory investigation. Thromb Haemost 1992;68:7–13.

393. Prins MH, Hirsh J. A critical Review of the evidence supporting a relationship between impaired fibrinolytic activity and venous thromboembolism. Arch Intern Med 1991;151:1721–1731.
394. Nilsson IM, Ljungner H, Tengborn L. Two different mechanisms in individuals with venous thrombosis and defective fibrinolysis: low concentration of plasminogen activator or increased concentration of plasminogen activator inhibitor. Br Med J 1985;290:1453–1456.
395. Wiman B, Ljungberg B, Chmielewska J et al. The role of the fibrinolytic system in deep venous thrombosis. J Lab Clin Med 1985;105:265–270.
396. Juhan-Vague I, Valadier J, Alessi MC et al. Deficient t-PA release and elevated PA inhibitor levels in individuals with spontaneous or recurrent deep venous thrombosis. Thromb Haemost 1987;57:67–72.
397. Nguyen G, Horellou MH, Kruithof EKO et al. Residual plasminogen activator activity after venous stasis as a criterion for hypofibrinolysis: a study in 83 individuals with confirmed deep venous thrombosis. Blood 1988;72:601–605.
398. Engesser L, Brommer EJP, Kluft C et al. Elevated plasminogen activator inhibitor (PAI), a cause of thrombophilia?—A study in 203 individuals with familial or sporadic venous thrombophilia. Thromb Haemost 1989;62:673–680.
399. Grimaudo V, Bachmann F, Hauert J et al. Hypofibrinolysis in individuals with a history of idiopathic deep venous thrombosis and/or pulmonary embolism. Thromb Haemost 1992;67:397–401.
400. Hamsten A, Wiman B, de Faire U et al. Increased plasma levels of a rapid inhibitor of tissue plasminogen activator in young survivors of myocardial infarction. N Engl J Med 1985;313:1557–1563.
401. Hamsten A, Walldius G, Szamosi A et al. Plasminogen activator inhibitor in plasma: risk factor for recurrent myocardial infarction. Lancet 1987;2:3–9.
402. Ratnoff OD, Colopy JE. Familial hemorrhagic trait associated with deficiency of clot-promoting fraction of plasma. J Clin Invest 1955;34:602–613.
403. Saito H. Contact factors in health and disease. Semin Thromb Haemost 1987;13:36–49.
404. Goodnough LT, Saito H, Ratnoff OD. Thrombosis or myocardial infarction in congenital clotting factor abnormalities and chronic thrombocytopenias: a report of 21 individuals and a review of 50 previously reported cases [Review]. Medicine 1983;62:248–255.
405. Ratnoff OD, Busse RJ Jr, Sheon RP. The demise of John Hageman. N Engl J Med 1968;279:760–761.
406. Lodi S, Isa L, Pollini E et al. Defective intrinsic fibrinolytic activity in a individual with severe factor XII deficiency and myocardial infarction. Scand J Haematol 1984;33:80–82.
407. Lämmle B, Wuillemin WA, Huber I et al. Thromboembolism and bleeding tendency in congenital factor XII deficiency—A study on 74 subjects from 14 Swiss families. Thromb Haemost 1991;65:117–121.
408. Rodeghiero F, Castaman G, Ruggeri M et al. Thrombosis in subjects with homozygous and heterozygous factor XII deficiency [Letter]. Thromb Haemost 1992;67:590.
409. Mannhalter C, Fischer M, Hopmeier P et al. Factor XII activity and antigen concentrations in individuals suffering from recurrent thrombosis. Fibrinolysis 1987;1:259–263.
410. Öhlin AK, Marlar RA. The first mutation identified in the thrombomodulin gene in a 45-year-old man presenting with thromboembolic disease. Blood 1995;85:330–336.
411. Freedman JE, Loscalzo J, Benoit SE et al. Decreased platelet inhibition by nitric oxide in two brothers with a history of arterial thrombosis. J Clin Invest 1996;97:979–987.
412. McCully KS. Vascular pathology of homocysteinemia: implications for the pathogenesis of arteriosclerosis. Am J Pathol 1969;56:111–128.
413. De Stefano V, Finazzi G, Mannucci PM. Inherited thrombophilia: pathogenesis, clinical syndromes, and management. Blood 1996;87:3531–3544.
414. D'Angelo A, Selhub J. Homocysteine and thrombotic disease [Review]. Blood 1997;90:1–11.
415. Mudd SH, Levy HL, Skovby F. Disorders of transsulfuration. In: Scriver CR, Beaudet AL, Sly WS, Valle D, eds. The metabolic and molecular bases of inherited disease. 7th ed. New York: McGraw-Hill, 1995;1:1279–1327.
416. Frosst P, Blom HJ, Milos R et al. A candidate genetic risk factor for vascular disease: a common mutation in methylenetetrahydrofolate reductase. Nat Genet 1995;10:111–113.
417. Selhub J, Jacques PF, Wilson PWF et al. Vitamin status and intake as primary determinants of homocysteinemia in an elderly population. JAMA 1993;270:2693–2698.
418. Tsai JC, Perrella MA, Yoshizumi M et al. Promotion of vascular smooth muscle cell growth by homocyst(e)ine: a link to atherosclerosis. Proc Natl Acad Sci U S A 1996;91:6369–6373.
419. Starkebaum G, Harlan JM. Endothelial cell injury due to copper-catalyzed hydrogen peroxide generation from homocysteine. J Clin Invest 1986;77:1370–1376.
420. Harker LA, Ross R, Slichter SJ et al. Homocystine-induced arteriosclerosis: the role of endothelial cell injury and platelet response in its genesis. J Clin Invest 1976;58:731–741.
421. Lentz SR, Sobey CG, Piegors DJ et al. Vascular dysfunction in monkeys with diet-induced hyperhomocyst(e)inemia. J Clin Invest 1996;98:24–29.
422. Fryer RH, Wilson BD, Gubler DB et al. Homocysteine, a risk factor for premature vascular disease and thrombosis, induces tissue factor activity in endothelial cells. Arterioscler Thromb 1993;13:1327–1333.
423. Nishinaga M, Ozawa T, Shimada K. Homocysteine, a thrombogenic agent, suppresses anticoagulant heparan sulfate expression in cultured porcine aortic endothelial cells. J Clin Invest 1993;92:1381–1386.
424. Stamler JS, Osborne JA, Jaraki O et al. Adverse vascular effects of homocysteine are modulated by endothelium-derived relaxing factor and related oxides of nitrogen. J Clin Invest 1993;91:308–318.
425. Wang J, Dudman NP, Wilken DE. Effects of homocysteine and related compounds on prostacyclin production by cultured human vascular endothelial cells. Thromb Haemost 1993;70:1047–1052.
426. Hajjar KA. Homocysteine-induced modulation of tissue plasminogen activator binding to its endothelial cell membrane receptor. J Clin Invest 1993;91:2873–2879.
427. Rodgers GM, Conn MT. Homocysteine, an atherogenic stimulus, reduces protein C activation by arterial and venous endothelial cells. Blood 1990;75:895–901.
428. Lentz SR, Sadler JE. Inhibition of thrombomodulin surface expression and protein C activation by the thrombogenic agent homocysteine. J Clin Invest 1991;88:1906–1914.
429. Stampfer MJ, Malinow MR, Willett WC et al. A prospective study of plasma homocyst(e)ine and risk of myocardial infarction in US physicians. JAMA 1992;268:877–881.
430. Perry IJ, Refsum H, Morris RW et al. Prospective study of serum total homocysteine concentration and risk of stroke in middle-aged British men. Lancet 1995;346:1395–1398.
431. Selhub J, Jacques PF, Bostom AG et al. Association between plasma homocysteine concentrations and extracranial carotid-artery stenosis. N Engl J Med 1995;332:286–291.
432. Nygård O, Nordrehaug JE, Refsum H et al. Plasma homocysteine levels and mortality in individuals with coronary artery disease. N Engl J Med 1997;337:230–236.
433. Petri M, Roubenoff R, Dallal GE et al. Plasma homocysteine as a risk factor for atherothrombotic events in systemic lupus erythematosus. Lancet 1996;348:1120–1124.
434. Falcon CR, Cattaneo M, Panzeri D et al. High prevalence of hyperhomocyst(e)inemia in individuals with juvenile venous thrombosis. Arterioscler Thromb 1994;14:1080–1083.
435. Fermo I, D'Angelo SV, Paroni R et al. Prevalence of moderate hyperhomocysteinemia in individuals with early-onset venous and arterial occlusive disease. Ann Intern Med 1995;123:747–753.
436. Den Heijer M, Blom HJ, Gerrits WBJ et al. Is hyperhomocysteinaemia a risk factor for recurrent venous thrombosis. Lancet 1995;345:882–885.
437. Den Heijer M, Koster T, Blom HJ et al. Hyperhomocysteinemia as a risk factor for deep-vein thrombosis. N Engl J Med 1996;334:759–762.
438. Ridker PM, Hennekens CH, Selhub J et al. Interrelation of hyperhomocyst(e)inemia, factor V Leiden, and risk of future venous thromboembolism. Circulation 1997;95:1777–1782.
439. Mandel H, Brenner B, Berant M et al. Coexistence of hereditary homocystinuria and factor V Leiden-effect on thrombosis. N Engl J Med 1996;334:763–768.
440. Letsky EA, de Swiet M. Maternal hemostasis: coagulation problems of pregnancy. In: Loscalzo J, Schafer AI, eds. Thrombosis and hemorrhage. 1st ed. Boston: Blackwell Scientific Publications, 1994:965–998.
441. Sachs BP, Brown DA, Driscoll SG et al. Maternal mortality in Massachusetts. Trends and prevention. N Engl J Med 1987;316:667–672.
442. de Boer K, Boller HR, ten Cate JW et al. Deep vein thrombosis in obstetric patients: diagnosis and risk factors. Thromb Haemost 1992;67:4–7.
443. Hellgren M, Svensson PJ, Dahlbäck B. Resistance to activated protein C as a basis for venous thromboembolism associated with pregnancy and oral contraceptives. Am J Obstet Gynecol 1995;173:210–213.
444. Bokarewa MI, Bremme K, Blombäck M. Arg$^{506}$-Gln mutation in factor V and risk of thrombosis during pregnancy. Br J Haematol 1996;92:473–478.
445. De Stefano V, Mastrangelo S, Paciaroni K et al. Thrombotic risk during pregnancy and puerperium in women with APC-resistance-effective subcutaneous heparin prophylaxis in a pregnant individual [Letter]. Thromb Haemost 1995;74:793–794.
446. Hull RD, Raskob GE, Carter CJ. Serial impedance plethysmography in pregnant individuals with clinically suspected deep-vein thrombosis. Clinical validity of negative findings. Ann Intern Med 1990;112:663–667.
447. Delorme MA, Burrow RF, Ofosu FA et al. Thrombin regulation in mother and fetus during pregnancy [Review]. Sem Thromb Hemost 1992;18:81–90.
448. Booth NA, Reith A, Bennett B. A plasminogen activator inhibitor (PAI-2) circulates in two molecular forms during pregnancy. Thromb Haemost 1988;59:77–79.
449. Burrows RF, Kelton JG. Incidentally detected thrombocytopenia in healthy mothers and their infants. N Engl J Med 1988;319:142–145.
450. Hellgren M, Blomback M. Blood coagulation and fibrinolysis in pregnancy, during delivery and in the puerperium. I. Normal condition. Gynecol Obstet Invest 1981;12:141–154.
451. Gerstmann BB, Piper JM, Tomita DK et al. Oral contraceptive estrogen

dose and the risk of deep venous thromboembolic disease. Am J Epidemiol 1991;133:32–37.

452. Helmerhorst FM, Bloemenkamp KWM, Rosendaal FR et al. Oral contraceptives and thrombotic disease: risk of venous thromboembolism. Thromb Haemost 1997;78:327–333.

453. Thorogood M. Oral contraceptives and myocardial infarction: new evidence leaves unanswered questions. Thromb Haemost 1997;78:334–338.

454. Lidegaard O. Oral contraception and risk of a cerebral thromboembolic attack: results of a case-control study. Br Med J 1996;306:956–963.

455. Petitti DB, Sidney S, Bernstein A et al. Stroke in users of low-dose oral contraceptives. N Engl J Med 1996;335:8–15.

456. Anonymous. Venous thromboembolic disease and combined oral contraceptives: results of international multicentre case-control study. World Health Organization Collaborative Study of Cardiovascular Disease and Steroid Hormone Contraception. Lancet 1995;346:1575–1582.

457. Anonymous. Effect of different progestagens in low oestrogen oral contraceptives on venous thromboembolic disease. World Health Organization Collaborative Study of Cardiovascular Disease and Steroid Hormone Contraception. Lancet 1996;346:1582–1588.

458. Jick H, Jick SS, Gurewich V et al. Risk of idiopathic cardiovascular death and nonfatal venous thromboembolism in women using oral contraceptives with differing progestagen components. Lancet 1995;346:1589–1593.

459. Spitzer WO, Lewis MA, Heinemann LA et al. Third generation oral contraceptives and risk of venous thromboembolic disorders: an international case-control study. Transnational Research Group on Oral Contraceptives and the Health of Young Women. Br Med J 1996;312:83–88.

460. Vandenbroucke JP, Koster T, Bri't E et al. Increased risk of venous thrombosis in oral-contraceptive users who are carriers of factor V Leiden mutation. Lancet 1994;344:1453–1457.

461. Bloemenkamp KWM, Rosendaal FR, Helmerhorst FM et al. Enhancement by factor V Leiden mutation of risk of deep-vein thrombosis associated with oral contraceptives containing a third-generation progestagen. Lancet 1995;346:1593–1596.

462. Kluft C, Lansink M. Effect of oral contraceptives on haemostasis variables. Thromb Haemost 1997;78:315–326.

463. Olivieri O, Friso S, Manzato F et al. Resistance to activated protein C in healthy women taking oral contraceptives. Br J Haematol 1995;91:465–470.

464. Anonymous. Prevention of venous thrombosis and pulmonary embolism. NIH Consensus Conference. JAMA 1986;256:744–749.

465. Bergqvist D, Benoni G, Bjorgell O et al. Low-molecular-weight heparin (enoxaparin) as prophylaxis against venous thromboembolism after total hip replacement. N Engl J Med 1996;335:696–700.

466. Geerts WH, Code KI, Jay RM et al. A prospective study of venous thromboembolism after major trauma. N Engl J Med 1994;331:1601–1606.

467. Geerts WH, Jay RM, Code KI et al. A comparison of low-dose heparin with low-molecular-weight heparin as prophylaxis against venous thromboembolism after major trauma. N Engl J Med 1996;335:701–707.

468. Nossel HL. Relative proteolysis of the fibrinogen B beta chain by thrombin and plasmin as a determinant of thrombosis. Nature 1981;291:165–167.

469. Owen J, Kvam D, Nossel HL et al. Thrombin and plasmin activity and platelet activation in the development of venous thrombosis. Blood 1983;61:476–482.

470. McNally MA, Molan RA. Total hip replacement, lower limb blood flow and venous thrombogenesis. J Bone Joint Surg Br 1993;75:640–644.

471. Planes A, Vochelle N, Fagola M. Total hip replacement and deep vein thrombosis: a venographic and necropsy study. J Bone Joint Surg Br 1990;72:9–13.

472. Kakkar VV, Howe CT, Nicolaides AN et al. Deep vein thrombosis of the leg. Is there a "high risk" group? Am J Surg 1970;120:527–530.

473. Salzman EW, Hirsh J. The epidemiology, pathogenesis, and natural history of venous thrombosis. In: Colman RW, Hirsh J, Marder VJ, Salzman EW, eds. Hemostasis and thrombosis: basic principles and clinical practice. 3rd ed. Philadelphia: JB Lippincott, 1994;1275–1296.

474. Scott TE, LaMorte WW, Gorin DR et al. Risk factors for chronic venous insufficiency: a dual case-control study. J Vasc Surg 1995;22:622–628.

475. Sack GH Jr, Levin J, Bell WR. Trousseau's syndrome and other manifestations of chronic disseminated coagulopathy in individuals with neoplasms: clinical, pathophysiologic, and therapeutic features. Medicine 1977;56:1–37.

476. Sproul EE. Carcinoma and venous thrombosis: the frequency of association of carcinoma in the body or tail of the pancreas with multiple venous thrombosis. Am J Cancer 1938;34:566–585.

477. Rickles FR, Edwards RL. Activation of blood coagulation in cancer: Trousseau's syndrome revisited. Blood 1983;62:14–31.

478. Bell WR, Starksen NF, Tong S et al. Trousseau's syndrome: devastating coagulopathy in the absence of heparin. Am J Med 1985;79:423–430.

479. Goldberg RJ, Seneff M, Gore JM et al. Occult malignant neoplasm in individuals with deep venous thrombosis. Arch Intern Med 1987;147:251–253.

480. Gore JM, Appelbaum JS, Greene HL et al. Occult cancer in individuals with acute pulmonary embolism. Ann Intern Med 1982;96:556–560.

481. Prandoni P, Lensing AW, Buller HR et al. Deep-vein thrombosis and the incidence of subsequent symptomatic cancer. N Engl J Med 1992;327:1128–1133.

482. Monreal M, Lafoz E, Casals A et al. Occult cancer in individuals with deep venous thrombosis. A systematic approach. Cancer 1991;67:541–545.

483. Monreal M, Casals A, Inaraja L et al. Occult cancer in individuals with acute pulmonary embolism. A prospective study. Chest 1993;103:816–819.

484. Prins MH, Lensing AWA, Hirsh J. Idiopathic deep venous thrombosis. Arch Intern Med 1994;154:1310–1312.

485. Deppisch LM, Fayemi AO. Nonbacterial thrombotic endocarditis. Am Heart J 1976;92:723–729.

486. Rosen P, Armstrong D. Nonbacterial thrombotic endocarditis in individuals with malignant neoplastic diseases. Am J Med 1973;54:23–29.

487. Graus F, Rogers LR, Posner JB. Cerebrovascular complications in individuals with cancer. Medicine 1985;64:16–35.

488. Gordon SG, Franks JJ, Lewis B. Cancer procoagulant A: a factor X activating procoagulant from malignant tissue. Thromb Res 1975;6:127–137.

489. Gordon SG, Cross BA. A factor X-activating cysteine protease from malignant tissue. J Clin Invest 1981;67:1665–1671.

490. Falanga A, Gordon SG. Isolation and characterization of cancer procoagulant: a cysteine proteinase from malignant tissue. Biochemistry 1985;24:5558–5567.

491. Donati MB, Gambacorti-Passerini C, Casali B et al. Cancer procoagulant in human tumor cells: evidence from melanoma individuals. Cancer Res 1986;46:6471–6474.

492. Falanga A, Alessio MG, Donati MB et al. A new procoagulant in acute leukemia. Blood 1988;71:870–875.

493. Koyama T, Hirosawa S, Kawamata N et al. All-trans retinoic acid upregulates thrombomodulin and downregulates tissue-factor expression in acute promyelocytic leukemia cells: distinct expression of thrombomodulin and tissue factor in human leukemia cells. Blood 1994;84:3001–3009.

494. Guarini A, Gugliotta L, Timoncini C et al. Procoagulant cellular activity and disseminated intravascular coagulation in acute non-lymphoid leukemia. Scand J Haematol 1985;34:152–156.

495. Wada H, Nagano T, Tomeoku M et al. Coagulant and fibrinolytic activates in the leukemic cell lysates. Thromb Res 1985;30:315–322.

496. Guarini A, Gugliotta L, Valvassori L et al. Human myeloid precursor cells do not possess or produce procoagulant activity (PCA). Exp Hematol 1986;14:72–74.

497. Callander NS, Varki N, Rao LVM. Immunohistochemical identification of tissue factor in solid tumors. Cancer 1992;70:1194–1201.

498. Edwards RL, Rickles FR, Cronlund M. Abnormalities of blood coagulation in individuals with cancer: mononuclear cell tissue factor generation. J Lab Clin Med 1981;98:917–928.

499. Edwards RL, Edwards FR, Bobrove AM. Mononuclear cell tissue factor: cell of origin and requirements for activation. Blood 1979;54:359–370.

500. Conkling PR, Greenberg CS, Weinberg JB. Tumor necrosis factor induces tissue factor-like activity in human leukemia cell line U937 and peripheral blood monocytes. Blood 1988;72:128–133.

501. Gregory SA, Kornbluth RS, Helin H et al. Monocyte procoagulant inducing factor: a lymphokine involved in the T cell-instructed monocyte procoagulant response to antigen. J Immunol 1986;137:3231–3239.

502. Levy GA, Schwartz BS, Curtiss LK et al. Plasma lipoprotein induction and suppression of the generation of cellular procoagulant activity in vitro. Requirements for cellular collaboration. J Clin Invest 1981;67:1614–1622.

503. Altieri DC, Edgington TS. The saturable high affinity association of factor X to ADP-stimulated monocytes defines a novel function of the Mac-1 receptor. J Biol Chem 1988;263:7007–7015.

504. Zucchella M, Pacchiarini L, Tacconi F et al. Different expression of procoagulant activity in human cancer cells cultured "in vitro" or in cells isolated from human tumor tissues. Thromb Haemost 1993;69:335–338.

505. Curatola L, Alessio MG, Casali B et al. Procoagulant activity of mouse transformed cells: different expression in freshly isolated or cultured cells. In Vitro Cell Dev Biol 1988;24:1154–1158.

506. Gasic GJ, Gasic TB, Galanti N et al. Platelet-tumor cell interactions in mice. The role of platelets in the spread of malignant disease. Int J Cancer 1973;11:704–718.

507. Hara Y, Steiner M, Baldini MG. Characterization of the platelet-aggregating activity of tumor cells. Cancer Res 1980;40:1217–1222.

508. Pearlstein E, Salk PL, Yogeeswaran G et al. Correlation between spontaneous metastatic potential, platelet-aggregating activity of cell surface extracts, and cell surface sialylation in 10 metastatic-variant derivates of a rat renal sarcoma line. Proc Natl Acad Sci U S A 1980;77:4336–4339.

509. Balkwill F, Burke F, Talbot FD et al. Evidence for tumor necrosis factor/cachectin production in cancer. Lancet 1987;2:1229–1232.

510. Scuderi P, Lam KS, Ryan KJ et al. Raised serum levels of tumor necrosis factor in parasitic infections. Lancet 1986;2:1364–1365.

511. Waage A, Espevik T, Lamvik J. Detection of tumor necrosis factor-like cytotoxicity in serum from individuals with septicaemia but not from untreated cancer individuals. Scand J Immunol 1986;24:739–743.

512. Bevilacqua MP, Pober JS, Majeau GR et al. Recombinant tumor necrosis factor induces procoagulant activity in cultured human vascular endothelium: characterization and comparison with the actions of interleukin 1. Proc Natl Acad Sci U S A 1986;83:4533–4537.

513. Nawroth PP, Stern DM. Modulation of endothelial cell hemostatic properties by tumor necrosis factor. J Exp Med 1986;163:740–745.

514. Bauer KA, ten Cate H, Barzegar S et al. Tumor necrosis factor infusions have a procoagulant effect on the hemostatic mechanism of humans. Blood 1989;74:165–172.

515. Llach F. Hypercoagulability, renal vein thrombosis, and other thrombotic complications of the nephrotic syndrome [Review]. Kidney Int 1985;28:429–439.

516. Harris RC, Ismail N. Extrarenal complications of the nephrotic syndrome [Review]. Am J Kidney Dis 1994;23:477–497.

517. Varizi N, Paule P, Toohey J. Acquired deficiency and urinary excretion of antithrombin III in nephrotic syndrome. Arch Intern Med 1984;144:1802–1803.

518. Adler AJ, Lundin AP, Feinroth MV. Beta-thromboglobulin levels in the nephrotic syndrome. Am J Med 1980;69:551–554.

519. Ozanne P, Francis RB, Meiselman HJ. Red blood cell aggregation in nephrotic syndrome. Kidney Int 1983;23:519–525.

520. Rosse WF, Ware RE. The molecular basis of paroxysmal nocturnal hemoglobinuria. Blood 1995;86:3277–3286.

521. Wilcox LA, Ezzell JL, Bernshaw NJ et al. Molecular basis of the enhanced susceptibility of the erythrocytes of paroxysmal nocturnal hemoglobinuria to hemolysis in acidified serum. Blood 1991;78:820–829.

522. Hebbel RP, Boogaerts MAB, Eaton JW et al. Erythrocyte adherence to endothelium in sickle cell anemia. A possible determinant of disease severity. N Engl J Med 1980;302:992–995.

523. Priest JR, Ramsay NK, Latchaw RE et al. Thrombotic and hemorrhagic strokes complicating early therapy for childhood acute lymphoblastic leukemia. Cancer 1980;46:1548–1554.

524. Priest JR, Ramsay NK, Steinherz PG et al. A syndrome of thrombosis and hemorrhage complicating L-asparaginase therapy for childhood acute lymphoblastic leukemia. J Pediatr 1982;100:984–989.

525. Steinherz PG, Miller LP, Ghavimi F et al. Dural sinus thrombosis in children with acute lymphoblastic leukemia. JAMA 1981;246:2837–2839.

526. Conard J, Horellou MH, Van Dreden P et al. Decrease in protein C in L-asparaginase-treated individuals. Br J Haematol 1985;59:725–727.

527. Weiss RB, Tormey DC, Holland JF et al. Venous thrombosis during multimodal treatment of primary breast carcinoma. Cancer Treat Rep 1981;65:677–679.

528. Goodnough LT, Saito H, Manni A et al. Increased incidence of thromboembolism in stage IV breast cancer treated with a five-drug chemotherapy regimen. A study of 159 individuals. Cancer 1984;54:1264–1268.

529. Levine MN, Gent M, Hirsh J et al. The thrombogenic effect of anticancer drug therapy in women with stage II breast cancer. N Engl J Med 1988;318:404–407.

530. Wall JG, Weiss RB, Norton L et al. Arterial thrombosis associated with adjuvant chemotherapy for breast carcinoma: a Cancer and Leukemia Group B study. Am J Med 1989;87:501–504.

531. Saphner T, Tormey DC, Gray R. Venous and arterial thrombosis in individuals who received adjuvant therapy for breast cancer. J Clin Oncol 1991;9:286–294.

532. Byar DP. Proceedings: The Veterans Administration Cooperative Urologic Research Group's studies of cancer of the prostate. Cancer 1973;32:1126–1130.

533. Triplett DA, Brandt JT. Lupus anticoagulants: misnomer, paradox, riddle, epiphenomenon. Hematol Pathol 1988;2:121–143.

534. Lechner K. Lupus anticoagulants and thrombosis. In: Verstraete J, Vermylen J, Lijnen R, Arnout J, eds. Thrombosis and haemostasis. Leuven: Leuven University Press, 1987:525–547.

535. Mueh JR, Herbst KD, Rapaport SI. Thrombosis in individuals with the lupus anticoagulant. Ann Intern Med 1980;92:156–159.

536. Gastineau DA, Kazmier FJ, Nichols WL et al. Lupus anticoagulants: an analysis of the clinical and laboratory feature of 219 cases. Am J Hematol 1985;19:265–275.

537. Rosove MH, Brewer PM. Antiphospholipid thrombosis: clinical course after the first thrombotic event in 70 individuals. Ann Intern Med 1992;117:303–308.

538. Khamashta MA, Cuadrado MJ, Mujic F et al. The management of thrombosis in the antiphospholipid-antibody syndrome. N Engl J Med 1995;332:993–997.

539. Weinstein C, Miller MH, Axtens R et al. Livedo reticularis associated with increased titers of anticardiolipin antibodies in systemic lupus erythematosus. Arch Dermatol 1987;123:596–600.

540. Dodd HJ, Sarkany I, O'Shaughnessy D. Widespread cutaneous necrosis associated with lupus anticoagulant. Clin Exp Dermatol 1985;10:581–586.

541. Thiagarajan P, Pengo V, Shapiro SS. The use of the dilute Russell viper venom time for the diagnosis of lupus anticoagulants. Blood 1986;68:869–874.

542. Exner T, Rickard KA, Kronenberg H. A sensitive test demonstrating lupus anticoagulant and its behavioral patterns. Br J Haematol 1978;40:143–151.

543. Schleider MA, Nachman RL, Jaffe EA et al. A clinical study of the lupus anticoagulant. Blood 1976;48:499–509.

544. Johansson EA, Lassus A. The occurrence of circulating anticoagulants in individuals with syphilitic and biologically false positive antilipoidal antibodies. Ann Clin Res 1974;6:105–108.

545. Pengo V, Thiagarajan P, Shapiro SS et al. Immunological specificity and mechanism of action of IgG lupus anticoagulants. Blood 1987;70:69–76.

546. Thiagarajan P, Shapiro SS, DeMarco L. Monoclonal immunoglobulin M-lambda coagulation inhibitor with phospholipid specificity. Mechanism of a lupus anticoagulant. J Clin Invest 1980;66:397–405.

547. McNeil HP, Simpson RJ, Chesterman CN et al. Anti-phospholipid antibodies are directed against a complex antigen that includes a lipid-binding inhibitor of coagulation: beta 2-glycoprotein I (apolipoprotein H). Proc Natl Acad Sci U S A 1990;87:4120–4124.

548. Galli M, Comfurius P, Maassen C et al. Anticardiolipin antibodies (ACA) directed not to cardiolipin but to a plasma protein cofactor. Lancet 1990;335:1544–1547.

549. Roubey RA, Pratt CW, Buyon JP et al. Lupus anticoagulant activity of autoimmune antiphospholipid antibodies is dependent upon beta 2-glycoprotein I. J Clin Invest 1992;90:1100–1104.

550. Harris EN, Gharavi AE, Boey ML et al. Anticardiolipin antibodies: detection by radioimmunoassay and association with thrombosis in systemic lupus erythematosus. Lancet 1983;2:1211–1214.

551. Loizou S, McCrea JD, Rudge AC et al. Measurement of anti-cardiolipin antibodies by an enzyme-linked immunosorbent assay (ELISA): standardization and quantitation of results. Clin Exp Immunol 1985;62:738–745.

552. Triplett DA, Brandt JT, Musgrave KA et al. The relationship between lupus anticoagulants and antibodies to phospholipid. JAMA 1988;259:550–554.

553. Lam LH, Silbert JE, Rosenberg RD. The separation of active and inactive forms of heparin. Biochem Biophys Res Commun 1976;69:570–577.

554. Long AA, Ginsberg JS, Brill-Edwards P et al. The relationship of antiphospholipid antibodies to thromboembolic disease in systemic lupus erythematosus: a cross-sectional study. Thromb Haemost 1991;66:520–524.

555. Ginsberg JS, Brill-Edwards P, Johnston M et al. Relationship of antiphospholipid antibodies to pregnancy loss in individuals with systemic lupus erythematosus: a cross-sectional study. Blood 1992;80:975–980.

556. Abu-Shakra M, Gladman DD, Urowitz MB. Anticardiolipin antibodies in systemic lupus erythematosus: clinical and laboratory correlations. Am J Med 1995;99:624–628.

557. Ginsburg KS, Liang MH, Newcomer L et al. Anticardiolipin antibodies and the risk for ischemic stroke and venous thrombosis. Ann Intern Med 1992;117:997–1002.

558. Ginsberg JS, Wells PS, Brill-Edwards P et al. Antiphospholipid antibodies and venous thromboembolism. Blood 1995;86:3685–3691.

559. Carreras LO, Defreyn G, Machin SJ et al. Arterial thrombosis, intrauterine death and "lupus" anticoagulant: detection of immunoglobulin interfering with prostacyclin formation. Lancet 1981;1:244–246.

560. Cariou R, Tobelem G, Bellucci S et al. Effect of lupus anticoagulant on antithrombogenic properties of endothelial cells-inhibition of thrombomodulin-dependent protein C activation. Thromb Haemost 1988;60:54–58.

561. Petraiuolo W, Bovill E, Hoak J. The lupus anticoagulant stimulates the release of prostacyclin from human endothelial cells. Thromb Res 1988;50:847–855.

562. Rustin MH, Bull HA, Machin SJ et al. Effects of the lupus anticoagulant in individuals with systemic lupus erythematosus on endothelial cell prostacyclin release and procoagulant activity. J Invest Dermatol 1988;90:744–748.

563. Lellouche F, Martinuzzo M, Said P et al. Imbalance of thromboxane/prostacyclin biosynthesis in individuals with lupus anticoagulant. Blood 1991;78:2894–2899.

564. Freyssinet JM, Wiesel ML, Gauchy J et al. An IgM lupus anticoagulant that neutralizes the enhancing effect of phospholipid on purified endothelial thrombomodulin activity-a mechanism for thrombosis. Thromb Haemost 1986;55:309–313.

565. Marciniak E, Romond EH. Impaired catalytic function of activated protein C: a new in vitro manifestation of lupus anticoagulant. Blood 1989;74:2426–2432.

566. Oosting JD, Derksen RHWM, Bobbick IWG et al. Antiphospholipid antibodies directed against a combination of phospholipids with prothrombin, protein C, or protein S. An explanation for their pathogenic mechanism. Blood 1993;81:2618–2625.

567. Smirnov MD, Triplett DT, Comp PC et al. On the role of phosphatidylethanolamine in the inhibition of activated protein C activity by antiphospholipid antibodies. J Clin Invest 1995;95:309–316.

568. Faaber P, Rijke TP, Van de Putte LB et al. Cross reactivity of human and murine anti-DNA antibodies with heparan sulfate. The major glycosaminoglycan in glomerular basement membranes. J Clin Invest 1986;77:1824–1830.

569. Angles-Cano E, Sultan Y, Clauvel JP. Predisposing factors to thrombosis in systemic lupus erythematosus: possible relation to endothelial cell damage. J Lab Clin Med 1979;94:312–323.

570. Rand JH, Wu XX, Andree HA et al. Pregnancy loss in the antiphospholipid-antibody syndrome—A possible thrombogenic mechanism. N Engl J Med 1997;337:154–160.

571. Wanger GP, Roberts W, Brandt JT. Misleading heparin monitoring leading to protamine sulphate overdose in a individual with a lupus anticoagulant [Letter]. Lancet 1981;2:1112.

572. Love PE, Santoro SA. Antiphospholipid antibodies: anticardiolipin and the lupus anticoagulant in systemic lupus erythematosus (SLE) and in non-SLE disorders. Prevalence and clinical significance [Review]. Ann Intern Med 1990;112:682–698.

573. Ahn SS, Kalunian K, Rosove M et al. Postoperative thrombotic complications in individuals with the lupus anticoagulant: increased risk after vascular procedures. J Vasc Surg 1988;7:749–756.

574. Nilsson IM, Astedt B, Hedner U et al. Intrauterine death and circulating anticoagulant, ("antithromboplastin"). Acta Med Scand 1975;197:153–159.

575. de Wolf F, Carreras LO, Moerman P et al. Decidual vasculopathy and extensive placental infarction in a individual with repeated thromboembolic accidents, recurrent fetal loss, and a lupus anticoagulant. Am J Obstet Gynecol 1982;142:829–834.

576. Lockshin MD, Druzin ML, Goei S et al. Antibody to cardiolipin as a predictor of fetal distress or death in pregnant individuals with systemic lupus erythematosus. N Engl J Med 1985;313:152–156.

577. Branch DW, Scott JR, Kochenour NK et al. Obstetric complications associated with the lupus anticoagulant. N Engl J Med 1985;313:1322–1326.

578. Infante-Rivard C, David M, Gauthier R et al. Lupus anticoagulants, anticardiolipin antibodies, and fetal loss. A case-control study. N Engl J Med 1991;325:1063–1066.

579. Lockshin MD, Druzin ML, Qamar T. Prednisone does not prevent recurrent fetal death in women with antiphospholipid antibody. Am J Obstet Gynecol 1989;160:439–443.

580. Laskin CA, Bombardier C, Hannah ME et al. Prednisone and aspirin in women with autoantibodies and unexplained recurrent fetal loss. N Engl J Med 1997;337:148–153.

581. Rosove MH, Tabsh K, Wasserstrum N et al. Heparin therapy for pregnant women with lupus anticoagulant or anticardiolipin antibodies. Obstet Gynecol 1987;75:630–663.

582. Carreras LO, Perez GN, Vega HR et al. Lupus anticoagulant and recurrent fetal loss: successful treatment with gammaglobulin [Letter]. Lancet 1988;2:393–394.

# CHAPTER 41

# ENDOTHELIOPATHIES: CLINICAL MANIFESTATIONS OF ENDOTHELIAL DYSFUNCTION

Noyan Gokce, John F. Keaney, Jr., and Joseph A. Vita

The vascular system is more than just a passive conduit for the flow of blood. Cellular components of the vessel wall actively participate in the maintenance of normal blood flow and fluidity. At the interface between blood and the vessel wall, the endothelium acts through a complex interplay of tightly regulated paracrine and autocrine interactions to control vascular tone and growth, the balance between thrombosis and fibrinolysis, and entry of inflammatory cells into the vessel wall. The term *endotheliopathy*, which was coined by Mendelsohn and Loscalzo (1), refers to disease states in which these regulatory functions are perturbed, thus promoting vasospasm, thrombosis, intimal growth, plaque rupture, and leading to tissue ischemia and infarction. A partial list of such disease states is provided in Table 41.1

This chapter briefly summarizes the normal homeostatic functions of the vascular endothelium (Table 41.2). Using atherosclerosis as a paradigm, it reviews how endothelial dysfunction contributes to the clinical expression of vascular disease, then discusses the mechanisms and clinical expression of endothelial dysfunction in other disease states, including hypertension, diabetes, congestive heart failure (CHF), and arterial injury. Finally, therapeutic interventions that ameliorate endothelial dysfunction and the mechanisms underlying their effects are reviewed. Considering the crucial regulatory functions of the endothelium, therapy designed to restore endothelial function has great promise in individuals with vascular disease.

## NORMAL ENDOTHELIAL FUNCTIONS (see Chapter 13)

### CONTROL OF VASOMOTOR TONE

In 1980, Furchgott and Zawadzki (2) reported that acetylcholine-mediated relaxation of isolated rabbit aorta segments is lost after "unintentional rubbing of its intimal surface against foreign surfaces during its preparation." This seminal observation led them to postulate that acetylcholine and other factors stimulate release of a vasodilator from intact endothelium, which they termed *endothelium-derived relaxing factor*. Subsequent studies have identified endothelium-derived relaxing factor as nitric oxide (NO) (3, 4) or a closely related S-nitrosothiol compound (5) and emphasized the primary importance of the endothelium in regulating blood vessel tone.

Endothelial production of NO and NO actions are outlined in Fig. 41.1. In endothelial cells, a constitutive, membrane-associated NO synthase (eNOS), which derives from the NO synthase type 3 gene (*Nos3*), catalyzes conversion of the amino acid L-arginine to NO and L-citrulline (6). Endothelial production of NO by eNOS is tightly controlled and depends on cytosolic ionized calcium concentration. Several agonists, including acetylcholine, catecholamines, bradykinin, substance P, and products of aggregating platelets such as adenosine diphosphate (ADP) and serotonin, act on specific endothelial cell membrane receptors, thereby leading to in-

**TABLE 41.1.** Partial List of Disease States Associated with Endothelial Dysfunction

Atherosclerosis and associated risk factors
    Cigarette smoking
    Diabetes mellitus
    Hypercholesterolemia
    Hypertension
Congestive heart failure
Hyperhomocysteinemia
Infectious diseases
    Endotoxemia
    Rickettsial infection
Ischemia/reperfusion
Posttransplantation vasculopathy
Pulmonary hypertension
Vascular injury/regenerated endothelium

**TABLE 41.2.** Major Endothelial Products and Regulatory Functions

*Vasomotor Tone*
**Vasodilators**
    Nitric oxide
    Prostacyclin
    Endothelial-derived hyperpolarizing factor
**Vasoconstrictors**
    Endothelin
    Prostaglandin $H_2$
    Endothelium-derived constricting factor
    Angiotensin II
    Platelet-derived growth factor
    Thromboxane $A_2$
*Fibrinolysis*
**Profibrinolytic factors**
    Tissue plasminogen activator (t-PA)
    Urokinase-type plasminogen activator
**Antifibrinolytic factors**
    Plasminogen activator inhibitor-1
*Thrombosis*
**Anticoagulants**
    Thrombomodulin
    Heparan sulfate
    Dermatan sulfate
**Platelet inhibitors**
    Nitric oxide
    Prostacyclin
    Ecto-ADPase
**Procoagulants**
    Tissue factor
    von Willebrand factor
**Platelet activators**
    von Willebrand factor
    Platelet-activating factor
*Cell growth*
**Growth inhibition**
    Nitric oxide
    Heparan sulfate
    Prostacyclin
**Growth promotion**
    Angiotensin II
    Platelet-derived growth factor
    Endothelin
*Inflammation*
**Anti-inflammatory factors**
    Nitric oxide
**Proinflammatory factors**
    E-selectin
    Intercellular adhesion molecule-1 (ICAM-1)
    Vascular cell adhesion molecule-1 (UCAM-1)
    Monocyte chemotactic protein-1 (MCP-1)
    Interleukin-8

*ADP = adenosine diphosphate*

creased cytosolic ionized calcium concentration, activation of eNOS, and increased NO production (6). Increased shear stress at the endothelial surface resulting from increased blood flow (see Chapter 20) also is an important and clinically relevant stimulus for NO production (7, 8). This close regulation in endothelial cells differs from the control of NO production in other cell types. For example, in leukocytes, fibroblasts, and vascular smooth muscle cells, inducible NOS (iNOS), which derives from the *Nos2* gene, may catalyze NO production in a manner not dependent on cytosolic ionized calcium concentration, and the large amounts of NO produced under these circumstances may have pathologic effects (6, 9).

Like exogenous nitrovasodilators, endothelium-derived NO (EDNO) primarily induces vasodilation by activating soluble guanylyl cyclase in vascular smooth muscle cells and increasing intracellular cyclic 3, 5′-guanosine monophosphate (cGMP) as a second messenger (10). NO-dependent inhibition of platelet adhesion and aggregation also is mediated by a guanylyl cyclase-dependent mechanism (11). In addition, EDNO may directly activate calcium-dependent potassium channels in vascular smooth muscle, thus hyperpolarizing the cell and inducing relaxation (12). When the endothelium is rubbed off or rendered dysfunctional in pathologic conditions, certain agonists, such as acetylcholine or serotonin, may act directly on vascular smooth muscle to induce vasoconstriction, which no longer is opposed by EDNO (13).

Endothelium-derived NO is an important regulator of arterial tone in humans. Infusion of acetylcholine induces vasodilation in normal human coronary arteries (14) and peripheral arteries (15). As discussed later, normal vasodilation to acetylcholine may be replaced by

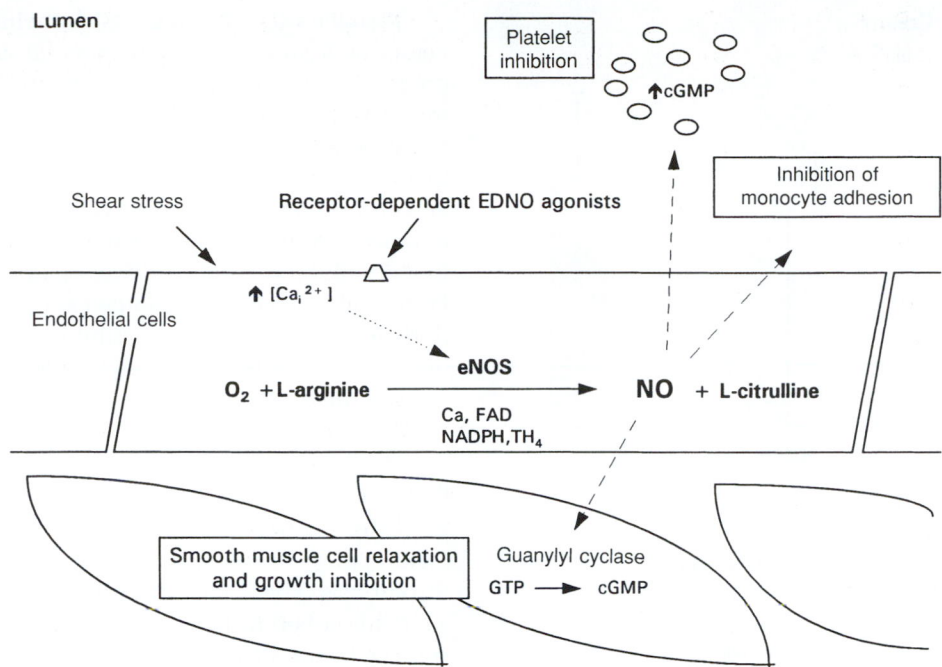

**FIGURE 41.1.** Schematic representation of endothelium-derived nitric oxide (EDNO) production and action. *cGMP,* guanosine 3,5'-cyclic monophosphate; *eNOS,* endothelial nitric oxide synthase; *FAD,* flavin adenine dinucleotide; *GTP,* guanosine 5'-triphosphate; *NADPH,* nicotinamide adenine dinucleotide phosphate; *TH₄,* tetrahydrobiopterin.

vasoconstriction in hypercholesterolemia and other endotheliopathies (14, 16), reflecting in part the impairment of EDNO action. Normal acetylcholine-induced arterial dilation (17) or flow-mediated dilation (18, 19) can be inhibited by concurrent infusion of $N^G$-monomethyl-L-arginine (L-NMMA), which inhibits NO synthase (Fig. 41.2). Infusion of L-NMMA alone induces dose-dependent vasoconstriction and hypertension, reflecting the inhibition of basal EDNO release (17).

Other endothelium-derived vasodilator substances, such as prostacyclin (PGI₂) (20) and endothelium-derived hyperpolarizing factor (EDHF) (21), may act independently or in conjunction with NO to produce vasodilation. First discovered in 1976 (22), PGI₂ activates adenylyl cyclase and increases levels of cyclic adenosine monophosphate (cAMP) in smooth muscle cells and platelets, thereby leading to vasodilation and inhibiting platelet aggregation, respectively (23). The relative importance of these other endothelium-derived vasodilators in comparison with NO remains uncertain in humans. Results of one recent study (19) suggest that NO, not PGI₂, is mainly responsible for flow-mediated vasodilation, because it is inhibited by L-NMMA but not aspirin, an inhibitor of PGI₂ synthesis (19). In addition, EDHF-dependent dilation may compensate for loss of EDNO in pathologic conditions (21).

Under certain conditions, endothelial cells also may synthesize and release vasoconstrictor substances, including endothelin (24), angiotensin II (25), platelet-derived growth factor (PDGF) (26, 27), thromboxane A₂ (28), and cyclo oxygenase derived endothelium-derived constricting factors (29). Endothelin also may stimulate EDNO production as well, which in a counter-regulatory manner opposes endothelin-induced vasoconstriction. Thus, physiologic regulation of vessel tone is determined by the delicate interplay of endothelium-derived vasodilator and vasoconstrictor substances. In pathologic states, imbalance of these mechanisms may favor vasospasm.

## ENDOTHELIAL REGULATION OF FIBRINOLYSIS AND THROMBOSIS

Another function of normal endothelium is to regulate fibrinolysis and thrombosis via precise production of fibrinolytic mediators, inhibitors, and anticoagulant factors. Endothelial cells produce at least two immunologically distinct plasminogen activators: tissue-type plasminogen activator (t-PA), and urokinase-type plasminogen activator, which convert inactive plasminogen to plasmin and promote degradation of fibrin (30) (see Chapter 7). Release of t-PA from endothelial cells is augmented by physiologic stimuli, including shear stress (31) and receptor-dependent agonists such as histamine and thrombin (32). Endothelial cells also express t-PA and urokinase receptors, which localize the fibrinolytic effects of plasminogen activators to the endothelial surface (33).

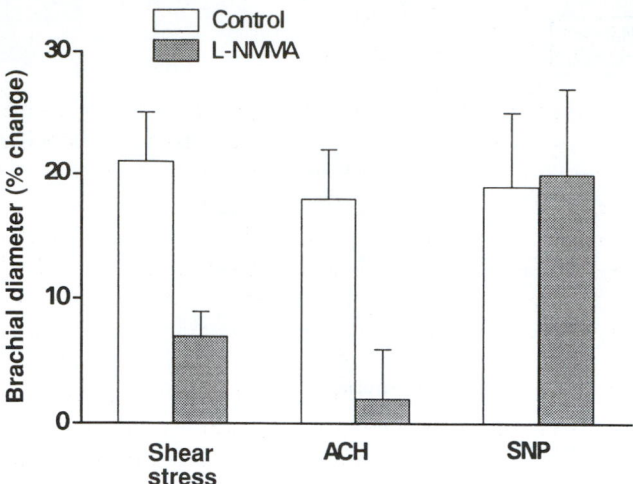

**FIGURE 41.2.** Brachial artery flow-mediated dilation depends on NO synthesis. Using high-resolution brachial ultrasonography, change in brachial diameter was measured in response to increased shear stress (produced by increased blood flow associated with reactive hyperemia), infusion of acetylcholine (ACH), and infusion of sodium nitroprusside (SNP). Extent of dilation is expressed as the percentage change from baseline (± SEM). Infusion of L-NMMA, which inhibits eNOS, inhibited shear stress-mediated dilation and acetylcholine-mediated dilation, thus confirming their dependence on NO synthesis. L-NMMA had no effect on nitroprusside-mediated dilation. (Adapted with permission from Lieberman EH, Gerhard MD, Uehata A, et al Flow-induced vasodilation of the human brachial artery is impaired in individuals <40 years of age with coronary artery disease. Am J Cardiol 1996;78:1210–1214.)

In addition to producing plasminogen activators, endothelial cells express antifibrinolytic factors, including the primary inhibitor of t-PA in plasma, plasminogen activator inhibitor-1 (PAI-1) (30, 34). PAI-1 expression is modulated by various factors, including lipoproteins, inflammatory cytokines, angiotensin II, and thrombin (30, 32, 35–38). The plasma balance of t-PA and PAI-1 is critical in determining response to thrombus formation in the vascular milieu. Normally, this balance favors fibrinolysis. As discussed later, however, in pathologic conditions, including atherosclerosis, relative production of PAI-1 may be increased, thus limiting fibrinolysis and promoting thrombosis.

The endothelium has several other antithrombotic functions (see Chapter 3), including production of thrombomodulin, which is a cell surface protein that promotes thrombin-mediated activation of protein C (a vitamin K-dependent anticoagulant) and inhibits thrombin-mediated platelet aggregation (39, 40). Inhibition of thrombomodulin activity may contribute to the prothrombotic state associated with hyperhomocystinemia (41). Production of heparan and dermatan sulfate at the endothelial surface further contributes to an antithrombotic milieu (42).

Platelet adhesion to subendothelial elements in the vessel wall and subsequent platelet activation and aggregation are among the initial events leading to arterial thrombosis. Endothelial cells play an important role in this process. Intact endothelium blocks platelet exposure to subendothelial sites, including collagen, fibronectin, and von Willebrand factor (vWf) (43), and thus prevents platelet adhesion to the normal vessel wall. In addition, EDNO inhibits platelet adhesion, and both EDNO and $PGI_2$ inhibit subsequent platelet aggregation (11, 44). Endothelial cells may further inhibit platelet reactivity by inactivating ADP, a platelet product that promotes platelet aggregation, through the action of an ecto-ADPase (45).

In addition to its antithrombotic functions, the endothelium also produces several prothrombotic factors. In pathologic conditions, synthesis of these prothrombotic factors may be induced, thus increasing the risk of thrombosis. These factors include vWf, which serves as a site for subendothelial platelet adhesion and as a carrier for factor VIII in plasma (see Chapter 16). Several disease states are associated with increased or altered vWf production, including rickettsial infection (46) and atherosclerosis (47). Tissue factor (see Chapter 4), which activates the extrinsic coagulation pathway, also may be produced by endothelial cells following exposure to oxidized low-density lipoprotein (LDL) (48), homocysteine (49), and cytokines (50).

In summary, healthy endothelial cells inhibit platelet reactivity and activation of the coagulation cascade, and they promote fibrinolysis. Pathologic states alter these endothelial functions, thereby promoting thrombosis and inhibiting fibrinolysis.

## ENDOTHELIAL REGULATION OF INFLAMMATION AND INTIMAL GROWTH

The endothelium is important to the inflammatory response (see Chapter 15). Normally, an intact endothelial layer limits entry of leukocytes into the subendothelial space by providing a physical barrier and through the effects of endothelial products, including EDNO (51). Exposure to cytokines such as tumor necrosis factor–α or interleukin-1β(IL-1β) however, may "activate" endothelial cells, thus resulting in new gene expression and fundamental alteration in phenotype. Endothelial cell activation is characterized by increased expression of endothelial–leukocyte adhesion molecules, such as intercellular adhesion molecule-1 (ICAM-1), vascular cell adhesion molecule-1 (VCAM-1), and E-selectin, as well as leukocyte chemoattractants, such as interleukin-8 and monocyte chemotactic protein-1 (MCP-1) (52). These products control leukocyte adhesion to the endothelial surface and their eventual retention in the subendothelial space. Cytokine-stimulated expression of VCAM-1 occurs via activation of the redox-sensitive transcription factor nuclear factor-κB (NFκB) in endothelial cells (53), and NO may inhibit leukocyte adhesion, in part by inhibiting activation of NFκB (54).

Endothelial cell activation may be an adaptive component of the normal immune response, but the resulting inflammatory events may contribute to the pathogenesis of disease. For example, activation of endothelial cells leads to expression of adhesion molecules (55), accumulation of monocytes in the subendothelial space, and formation of foam cells, which are the initial events in formation of the fatty streak (52). Other consequences include increased production of tissue factor (56, 57), PAI-1 (58), and endothelin (59), as well as changes in endothelial cell morphology that lead to increased permeability (56). These mechanisms also may contribute to the pathogenesis of atherosclerosis.

Finally, an intact, normally functioning endothelium limits the growth of underlying vascular smooth muscle; endothelial denudation stimulates intimal growth (60). Antiproliferative products of the endothelium include NO (61–63) and heparan sulfate (64). Furthermore, by inhibiting platelet activation, EDNO indirectly prevents release of platelet-derived chemotactic and mitogenic cytokines that stimulate the vascular smooth muscle cells, including transforming growth factor-β (TGF-β), basic fibroblastic growth factor, and PDGF (65). When activated, endothelial cells also produce growth factors, including PDGF (66). Other endothelial products, including the vasoconstrictors endothelin and angiotensin II, may stimulate growth of smooth muscle cells as well (67). Thus, in pathologic conditions, the growth-inhibitory properties of the endothelium are replaced by a growth-promoting phenotype, which may relate to atherogenesis and the vascular response to injury.

# ENDOTHELIAL DYSFUNCTION IN VASCULAR DISEASE

As discussed, the endothelium is important to the regulation of vasomotor tone, thrombosis, platelet activity, inflammation, and intimal growth. In this discussion, the term *endothelial dysfunction* denotes the general abnormality of many, or all, of these functions in certain disease states, which contributes to their pathogenesis and clinical expression. Specific abnormalities of endothelial function in five inter-related vascular disease states are reviewed. These include: atherosclerosis/hypercholesterolemia, diabetes mellitus, hypertension, CHF, and arterial injury. Available information about the mechanisms of endothelial dysfunction and clinical importance of these abnormalities are discussed, and potential interventions to reverse endothelial dysfunction are reviewed.

## ATHEROSCLEROSIS/HYPERCHOLESTEROLEMIA

Atherosclerosis is a disease of large and medium arteries that begins with development of fatty streaks in specific, lesion-prone areas of the arterial tree. The fatty streak consists of local intimal collections of lipid-laden macrophages (i.e., foam cells). According to the "oxidative modification hypothesis of atherosclerosis" (68), LDL undergoes oxidative modification in the intimal space, then is taken up in an unregulated manner by macrophages, thus leading to foam cell formation (69). Oxidized LDL (ox-LDL) further contributes to atherosclerosis, because it is chemotactic and chemostatic for monocytes (70) and stimulates monocyte binding to the endothelium, thereby leading to intimal macrophage accumulation (71). In a slowly evolving process, these initial lesions progress to fibrous plaques containing foam cells covered by connective tissue. Subsequently, following migration and proliferation of smooth muscle cells and development of a necrotic lipid-laden core, advanced lesions form. Ox-LDL is cytotoxic to vascular cells, and by promoting the release of lipids and lysosomal enzymes into the intimal space, it further increases progression of atherosclerosis and necrotic core formation (72, 73).

In the coronary circulation, atherosclerotic lesions may remain clinically silent for decades before undergoing plaque rupture, mural hemorrhage, formation of an occlusive or near-occlusive thrombus, and vasoconstriction, which eventually precipitate clinical events such as acute myocardial infarction or unstable angina (74). Abnormalities of endothelial function are present in the earliest stages of atherosclerosis, and they contribute to the initial phases of the atherogenic process and to the clinical activity of advanced coronary artery disease (CAD).

### Impaired NO Bioactivity

In 1986, Ludmer et al (14) reported that the normal vasodilator response to intracoronary acetylcholine infusion is replaced by a paradoxic constriction in individuals with early or advanced coronary atherosclerosis. The vasodilator response to nitroglycerin, a non-endothelium-dependent NO donor, remains intact. These findings suggest that atherosclerosis is associated with a loss of effective EDNO release, not impaired function of the vascular smooth muscle. EDNO-dependent dilation is similarly impaired in isolated coronary arterial tissue collected from individuals with CAD and in arterial tissue from cholesterol-fed animals (75).

Results of numerous studies in humans have confirmed and extended these initial observations. Impaired endothelium-dependent coronary dilation is lost in hypercholesterolemia before development of atherosclerosis, as assessed by angiography (16) or intravascular ultrasonography (76). Impaired flow-mediated dilation has been demonstrated in the brachial and femoral arteries of children (age range, 7–17 years) with familial hypercholesterolemia (77). Acetylcholine-mediated increases in blood flow also are impaired in humans with hypercholesterolemia, a finding that reflects impaired EDNO-dependent dilation of microvessels in the coronary and peripheral circulations (15, 17). Vasodilator responses to other stimuli for EDNO release, including serotonin (78), substance P (79), and shear stress (Fig. 41.3) (80), also are impaired in CAD. Loss of receptor-dependent EDNO release occurs early in atherosclerosis, whereas loss of flow-mediated dilation occurs later in the disease (81).

Coronary risk factors, including cigarette smoking (82), exposure to secondhand cigarette smoke (83), age (16), gender (16), diabetes mellitus (84), and hypertension (85), are associated with impaired EDNO-dependent dilation as well. Recently, noninvasive ultrasound-based methods have been developed to examine EDNO-dependent dilation in the brachial and femoral arteries

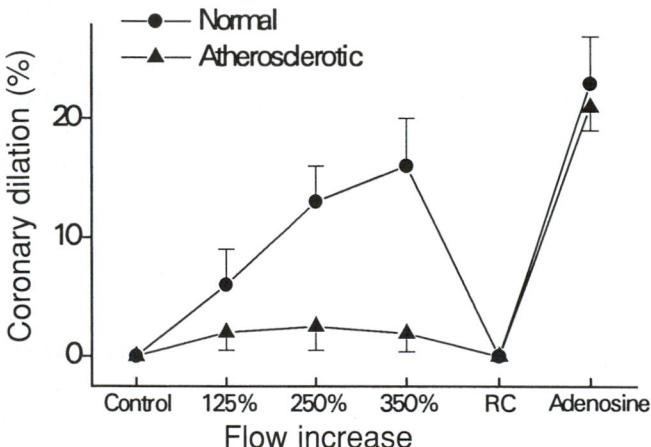

**FIGURE 41.3.** Atherosclerosis impairs NO-dependent flow-mediated dilation in the epicardial coronary arteries. In individuals undergoing cardiac catheterization, adenosine was infused (final concentration, $10^{-6}$ to $10^{-4}$ M) into the distal coronary artery, thus producing the indicated increases in coronary blood flow. Diameter measurements were made of a segment proximal to the point of infusion (exposed to increased flow but not to adenosine) using quantitative angiography. Angiographically normal segments demonstrated flow-mediated dilation, which depended on the degree of flow increase. Subjects with early atherosclerosis (i.e., luminal irregularities but no stenosis > 30%) demonstrated a loss of flow-mediated dilation. Coronary diameter returned to baseline during a 5-minute recontrol infusion (RC). Atherosclerosis had no effect on non-endothelium-dependent dilation to adenosine. (Adapted with permission from Cox DA, Vita JA, Treasure CB, et al Atherosclerosis impairs flow-mediated dilation of coronary arteries in humans. Circulation 1989;80:458–465.)

(86). Anderson et al (87) reported a close correlation between ultrasound-determined, flow-mediated dilation in the brachial artery and the vasomotor response to acetylcholine in the coronary arteries of individuals who had endothelial function studied in both the brachial artery and the coronary artery (87). These concordant responses in separate vascular beds suggest that vasomotor function in a peripheral artery may reflect the coronary physiology. These findings are not surprising, because the brachial artery is similar in size to the proximal coronary arteries (i.e., 2–4 mm). Also, like the coronary artery, it can develop nonobstructive atherosclerosis (88). Development of this noninvasive technique has permitted examination of endothelial vasomotor function in large groups of individuals and lower-risk populations. It also is ideally suited for repeated studies in the same individual and, thus, has great potential for studying interventions to improve endothelial function.

Studies in animal models have provided insight into the mechanisms of impaired EDNO vasodilation in hypercholesterolemia and atherosclerosis. In rabbits, arterial relaxation in response to acetylcholine and other receptor-dependent agonists is impaired as early as 2 weeks after cholesterol feeding is initiated (89). Relaxation in response to receptor-independent agonists for EDNO release, such as the calcium ionophore A23187, however, is spared (75). In swine, NO release by agonists dependent on receptors coupled to a pertussis toxin-sensitive $G_{i-2}$ protein (e.g., serotonin, thrombin, and $\alpha_2$-adrenergic receptors) is impaired early in cholesterol feeding, but the response to agonists dependent on other signal transduction mechanisms (e.g., bradykinin, ADP) may be spared (90). Following more prolonged hypercholesterolemia, loss of EDNO action may be more generalized.

Loss of EDNO in hypercholesterolemia may contribute to the atherosclerotic process itself. Inhibition of NO synthesis promotes monocyte adhesion to the endothelial surface (91) and worsens lesion formation in cholesterol-fed rabbits (92). Administration of the NOS substrate L-arginine inhibits monocyte adhesion to the endothelium and limits lesion formation in cholesterol-fed rabbits (91) and in LDL receptor knockout mice (93). These effects relate to NO-mediated inhibition of monocyte adhesion to the endothelial surface, in part through inhibition of adhesion molecule expression (54). In addition, NO also may inhibit oxidative modification of LDL (94).

Abnormalities of endothelial function in atherosclerosis and hypercholesterolemia are not restricted to impaired EDNO activity. Individuals with atherosclerosis demonstrate increased levels of plasma endothelin (95), which may contribute to acetylcholine-mediated coronary vasoconstriction (96). Fibrinolytic activity also is reduced in individuals with hypercholesterolemia (97).

Both t-PA and PAI-1 antigen levels are elevated in individuals with atherosclerosis (98), but studies consistently demonstrate that t-PA activity is reduced and PAI-1 activity increased in individuals with CAD (99, 100). Thus, atherosclerosis is associated with alterations in the vasomotor and antithrombotic functions of the endothelium that have the potential to contribute to the pathogenesis of CAD.

## Oxidative Stress and Endothelial Dysfunction

Recent studies indicate that increased vascular oxidative stress, which is defined as an imbalance between endogenous oxidants and antioxidants in favor of the former, is a unifying mechanism of endothelial dysfunction in hypercholesterolemia and atherosclerosis (101). These observations further support the concept that increased oxidative stress is central to the atherogenic process.

The first form of increased oxidative stress to consider is increased production of reactive oxygen species, including superoxide anion. Superoxide anion is produced by vascular cells as a consequence of normal oxidative metabolism (102–104), and it rapidly reacts with NO and eliminates its biologic activity (105). Inhibiting endogenous copper-zinc superoxide dismutase (SOD) in normal vascular tissue decreases NO bioactivity (106).

Hypercholesterolemia is associated with increased vascular production of superoxide anion. Arterial tissue isolated from rabbits fed a hypercholesterolemic diet release increased amounts of superoxide anion, and this increase is associated with impaired EDNO-dependent dilation (107, 108). In humans, an infusion of recombinant human SOD improved acetylcholine-mediated coronary dilation further supporting the importance of increased superoxide anion production as a mechanism of endothelial dysfunction (109).

The enzymatic source of increased superoxide production in hypercholesterolemia and atherosclerosis remains controversial, but xanthine oxidase (107, 110), NADPH (nicotinamide-adenine dinucleotide phosphate, reduced) oxidase (111), and eNOS (112) have been implicated. There also is evidence that lysophosphatidylcholine stimulates superoxide production in vascular tissue (113).

Another aspect of increased oxidative stress relevant to endothelial vasomotor dysfunction is formation of ox-LDL, which impairs EDNO action and other endothelial functions by several mechanisms. Ox-LDL is cytotoxic to endothelial cells (114) and may induce endothelial cell apoptosis via activation of CPP32-like proteases (115). Ox-LDL inhibits receptor-dependent stimulation of EDNO production coupled to the $G_{i-2}$ protein (116), which is attributable to the formation of lysophosphatidylcholine (117). In addition, ox-LDL may decrease transcription of the *Nos3* gene and destabilize the *Nos3* message (118). Finally, ox-LDL may inactivate NO directly (119).

That therapy directed toward inhibiting LDL oxidation, including the lipid-soluble antioxidants α-tocopherol (120) and probucol (108), prevents the development of endothelial dysfunction further supports for the importance of increased oxidative stress as a mechanism of endothelial vasomotor dysfunction. These agents may preserve EDNO action via alternative mechanisms, however, including prevention of superoxide anion production, prevention of cytotoxicity, and inhibition of cell-mediated LDL oxidation (121).

Additionally, ox-LDL may alter other functions of the endothelium. Exposure of endothelial cells to lysophosphatidylcholine, which is a product of LDL oxidation, activates endothelial cells and promotes expression of ICAM-1 (55) and growth factor (66). Ox-LDL also decreases t-PA production, and increases PAI-1 (36) and tissue factor (122) production.

Thus, during increased oxidative stress, endothelial cells lose their protective phenotype and express procoagulant, proinflammatory, and vasoconstrictor factors instead. Loss of EDNO bioavailability and expression of cytokines and endothelial surface adhesion molecules promote leukocyte accumulation in the vessel wall. In turn, intimal leukocytes may contribute to increased production of reactive oxygen species and further LDL oxidation. In addition, products of inflammatory cells may promote the migration and proliferation of smooth muscle cells and, thus, accelerate the atherosclerotic process.

## Endothelial Dysfunction and Clinical Expression of Coronary Artery Disease

In addition to promoting atherogenesis, impaired endothelial function may contribute to the clinical manifestations of advanced atherosclerosis, including chronic and acute coronary syndromes. The presence or anatomic severity of coronary artery stenoses does not fully predict the risk for clinical ischemia or coronary events (74, 123). The level of physical effort required to provoke ischemia may vary from day to day in individuals with chronic stable angina and does not relate to angiographic severity of the atherosclerotic lesions (124). Acute myocardial infarction and unstable angina occur following activation of atherosclerotic lesions, which leads to plaque rupture, mural hemorrhage, vasospasm, and formation of an obstructive thrombus (74, 123). These events typically involve mildly stenosed coronary arteries (125). The mechanisms of lesion activation remain incompletely understood, but they probably represent a fundamental lapse in vessel homeostasis. Endothelial dysfunction may be an important contributor to these processes.

In individuals with stable angina and obstructive atherosclerotic lesions, impaired endothelial vasomotor function may contribute to the pathophysiology of myocardial ischemia by aggravating the supply-demand mismatch that occurs during exercise or other clinical stimuli for angina. Atherosclerotic coronary arteries with impaired release of EDNO develop coronary artery constriction during exercise (126), exposure to cold (127), or mental stress (128). These complex clinical stimuli for ischemia also are associated with increased circulating catecholamines levels and coronary blood flow (128, 129). In individuals with coronary atherosclerosis, loss of EDNO action produces increased sensitivity to the constrictor effects of catecholamines (130) and impaired flow-mediated dilation (80). In stenosed vessels, these effects generally worsen the severity of the stenosis and further limit coronary blood flow during stimuli that also increase myocardial oxygen demand. Thus, an intervention that improves EDNO-dependent vasodilation has the potential to lessen the severity of ischemia.

Along with contributing to the pathophysiology of stable coronary syndromes, impaired endothelial vasomotor function also may be involved in unstable angina and acute myocardial function. Loss of flow-mediated dilation and increased coronary vasoconstriction in response to catecholamines may lead to elevated shear stress at an atherosclerotic lesion, thus increasing the likelihood of plaque rupture (131, 132). Following plaque rupture, activation of platelets and the clotting cascade leads to local generation of serotonin, thrombin, and other potential vasoconstrictors. Because these vasoconstrictors also stimulate release of EDNO, endothelial function may determine the vasomotor response to intra-arterial thrombus formation. In isolated coronary arteries of atherosclerotic swine, loss of EDNO action is associated with loss of normal vasodilation following exposure to aggregating platelets or thrombin (133). In individuals with CAD, the normal coronary vasodilator response to intracoronary infusion of serotonin infusion is lost, and it is replaced by coronary constriction (78). Thus, loss of EDNO-dependent dilation may lead to a more severe constrictor response and contribute to the development of myocardial ischemia. That acetylcholine-induced vasoconstriction is greater for infarct-related coronary arteries compared with similarly stenosed, non–infarct-related lesions in humans supports this hypothesis (134). Similarly, individuals with unstable angina demonstrate more severe vasoconstriction during exercise and the cold-pressor test as compared to individuals with stable angina (135).

Other aspects of endothelial dysfunction in atherosclerosis may also contribute to plaque activation, rupture, and arterial thrombosis. Adhesion molecule expression promotes monocyte accumulation in plaques. Metalloproteinases expressed by inflammatory cells may degrade collagen and other structural elements of the plaque, thus increasing the risk for rupture

(136). The degree of endothelial dysfunction may vary within groups of individuals with coronary atherosclerosis (137), within different portions of the coronary tree in the same individual (138, 139), and within individual individuals over time, particularly following interventions such as lipid-lowering therapy (140). At the local level, endothelial dysfunction may contribute to the activation of an individual atherosclerotic plaque, but the mechanisms for activation of one lesion and not another remain unknown. Furthermore, the prothrombotic and vasospastic phenotype associated with endothelial activation (i.e., increased release of tissue factor, PAI-1, and endothelin), together with loss of the vasodilator and antiplatelet effects of EDNO, may contribute to the extent of coronary thrombosis and vasospasm following plaque rupture (123). Thus, endothelial dysfunction has the potential to increase both the risk and the severity of acute coronary events, and it is a potentially important target for therapy.

## DIABETES MELLITUS

Vascular diseases, specifically macrovascular atherosclerosis and microvascular retinopathy and nephropathy, are the major causes of morbidity and mortality in individuals with diabetes mellitus (141). Moreover, atherosclerosis occurs prematurely, and it generally is more severe and diffuse in individuals with diabetes compared to non-diabetic individuals (142, 143). Intensive control of hyperglycemia reduces the risk of microvascular disease, but whether such therapy reduces atherosclerosis risk is unclear (144). The mechanisms for increased risk of atherosclerosis in diabetes are incompletely understood and likely multifactorial. Dyslipidemia, hypertension, and obesity are more prevalent in individuals with diabetes, but they only account for approximately 25% of the excess coronary risk (145).

Endothelial dysfunction is a feature of human diabetes mellitus. Subjects with both type 1 and type 2 diabetes display impaired EDNO-dependent dilation in response to acetylcholine in the coronary arteries before development of angiographically apparent atherosclerosis (84). In the forearms of individuals with type 1 diabetes and poor glucose control (hemoglobin $A_{1C}$, $11.9 \pm 0.6\%$), EDNO-dependent flow response to methacholine infusion is impaired (146), but individuals with better glucose control (hemoglobin $A_{1C}$, 6.7–9.2%) have preserved responses to infusion of a muscarinic agonist (147–149). Several groups also have reported impaired flow responses during infusion of sodium nitroprusside, indicating that NO may be inactivated or the ability of vascular smooth muscle to respond to NO in diabetes may be impaired (146, 148, 150). Hyperreactivity to nitrovasodilators, possibly resulting from autonomic dysfunction or hypersensitivity of vascular smooth muscle cells, has been reported as well (151, 152). Preserved flow responses to muscarinic agonists with impaired responses to an NO donor is consistent with compensatory release of other endothelium-dependent vasodilators in response to methacholine, such as EDHF, but evidence for such a mechanism is lacking in humans (21). Forearm blood flow responses are impaired in subjects with type 2 diabetes mellitus (153, 154), and endothelial vasomotor dysfunction correlates with both the duration (155) and severity of diabetes (156) as well as with the LDL level (155). Finally, insulin itself is a stimulus for EDNO in humans (157), and insulin deficiency or resistance could lead to loss of the beneficial EDNO effects.

In animal models of diabetes mellitus, endothelial vasomotor function also is impaired. Short-term exposure of isolated arterial segments to glucose (44 mM) impairs acetylcholine-induced relaxation compared with that in normoglycemic vessels (5.5 mM), but it has no effect on the responses to calcium ionophore A23187 or sodium nitroprusside (28). Similar findings have been reported in chronic hyperglycemia associated with experimental diabetes induced by streptozotocin or alloxan (158, 159).

The prostaglandin system may contribute to endothelial dysfunction in animal models of diabetes. Increased production of vasoconstrictor prostaglandins may impair arterial relaxation in hyperglycemia and in diabetic animals (28). Inhibitors of prostaglandin synthesis or a prostaglandin $H_2$-thromboxane $A_2$ antagonist restore endothelium-dependent relaxation (158). Prostaglandin H synthase is a source of superoxide anion production (160), and its activity may contribute to NO inactivation in experimental diabetes. In hyperglycemic vessels, EDNO-dependent dilation may be restored by SOD, catalase, or the hydroxyl radical scavenger deferoxamine, which also implicates NO inactivation by reactive oxygen species as a pathogenic mechanism (161). EDNO action in diabetes mellitus is improved by allopurinol (161), which inhibits xanthine oxidase and may be a source of superoxide production in hypercholesterolemia (107). Relaxation in response to authentic NO gas also is impaired in diabetic vessels and may be restored by SOD, thus further supporting the idea that superoxide anion-mediated inactivation of NO is a pathogenic mechanism (162). Probucol, which may reduce superoxide production and inhibit LDL oxidation in hypercholesterolemia (108), also prevents development of endothelial vasomotor dysfunction in diabetic rabbits (161). In individuals with type 2 diabetes, a high concentration of ascorbic acid, which may scavenge superoxide anion, improves the vasodilator response to methacholine infusion (154).

Diabetic vascular disease is associated with several other forms of increased oxidative stress, all of which may interfere with EDNO and promote atherogenesis. Individuals with diabetes have higher plasma levels of thiobarbituric acid-reactive substances, which may indicate increased lipid peroxidation *in vivo* (163). LDL exposed to hyperglycemic conditions *in vitro* (164) and LDL isolated from diabetic individuals (165) are more susceptible to oxidation. These observations are consistent with the finding that LDL may undergo nonenzymatic glycosylation, leading to the formation of advanced glycosylation end products that may facilitate lipid peroxidation (166). The dyslipidemia associated with type 2 diabetes mellitus (i.e., hypertriglyceridemia and low high-density lipoprotein [HDL] cholesterol) also may reflect an alteration in LDL metabolism rendering it more susceptible to oxidation (167). As discussed, ox-LDL may interfere with EDNO action through several mechanisms and contribute to atherogenesis by activating endothelial cells and increasing adhesion molecule expression. Advanced glycosylation end products may have other effects on endothelial cell function, leading to increased vascular permeability, inflammatory cell recruitment, and directly inactivating NO (168, 169). Finally, hyperglycemia increases vascular oxidative stress through the aldose reductase pathway, which catalyzes the conversion of glucose to sorbitol (170). This pathway leads to an increased ratio of reduced to oxidized nicotinamide-adenine dinucleotide ($NADH$:-$NAD^+$), which has a number of metabolic consequences, including increased production of superoxide anion via mitochondrial NADH oxido-reductases and prostaglandin synthase, and activation of protein kinase C (170). Recent evidence implicates vascular endothelial growth factor in mediating vascular dysfunction induced by hyperglycemia and increased sorbitol pathway activity (171). Long-term treatment of diabetic rabbits with an aldose reductase inhibitor normalizes EDNO action (172).

Diabetes mellitus is associated with other abnormalities of endothelial function that may contribute to atherogenesis and thrombosis. These abnormalities include increased production of VCAM-1 (173), PAI-1 (174), and vWf (175). Thus, the risk for premature, diffuse atherosclerosis and its ischemic complications in diabetes mellitus may result, at least in part, from impaired vasodilator, antithrombotic, and anti-inflammatory properties of the vascular endothelium.

## HYPERTENSION

Atherosclerotic vascular disease and its associated ischemic complications in the coronary, cerebral, and renal circulations are important features of hypertension. Endothelial dysfunction is a prominent finding in these individuals and in animal models, and it may contribute to the pathogenesis of these complications. Individuals with essential hypertension display impaired epicardial and coronary resistance vessel dilation in response to EDNO agonists, including acetylcholine, but

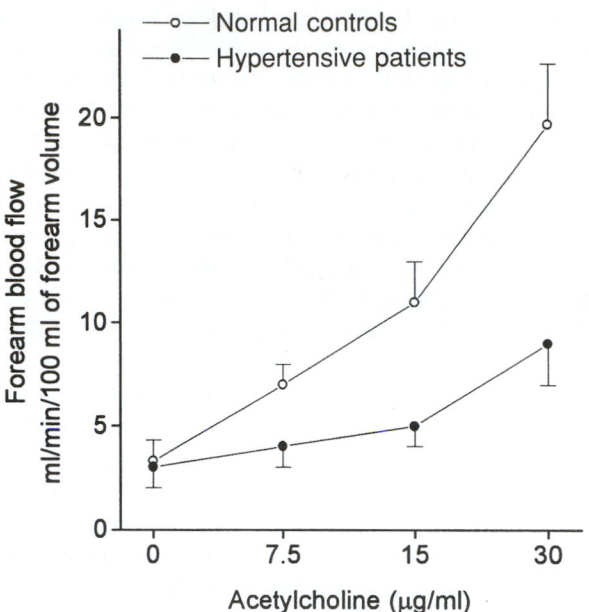

**FIGURE 41.4.** Impaired endothelial function in the forearm microvasculature of individuals with essential hypertension. Forearm blood flow was determined at baseline and during intrabrachial artery acetylcholine infusion in 18 normal control subjects (○) and 18 individuals with hypertension (●) using venous occlusion plethysmography. Flow response was lower in individuals with hypertension ($P < .0001$). Data are mean ± SEM. (Adapted with permission from Panza JA, Quyyumi AA, Brush JE Jr, et al Abnormal endothelium-dependent vascular relaxation in individuals with essential hypertension. N Engl J Med 1990;323:22–27.)

their vasodilator response to exogenous NO donors is preserved (85, 176, 177). Microvascular EDNO-dependent dilation has been reported to be impaired in the forearm circulation of some (Fig. 41.4) (178, 179), but not all (180), individual populations. Infusion of L-NMMA produces less reduction of resting flow in individuals with hypertension than in individuals who are normotensive, thus suggesting that basal EDNO action also is impaired in hypertension (181, 182). In the forearm of individuals with hypertension, impaired endothelium-dependent vasodilation is not improved by L-arginine, which suggests there is no absolute or relative deficiency of NOS substrate (183). In addition, individuals with essential hypertension experience a generalized reduction of the vasodilator responses to acetylcholine, substance P, and bradykinin (184), which suggests that impaired release of EDNO is not restricted to a single signal transduction pathway, as has been suggested for hypercholesterolemia (117).

Studies in hypertensive animals have provided further information about impaired EDNO action in hypertension, but the findings depend on the experimental model being used (185, 186). In Dahl salt-sensitive rats,

a high-salt diet induces hypertension and impairs the aortic relaxation responses to acetylcholine; blood pressure and vasodilator responses are normal when these animals consume a low-salt diet (187). In this model, L-arginine prevents hypertension, and this effect can be overcome by an inhibitor of iNOS (188). Salt and water excretion depends on renal vascular production of NO, and inhibition of NO synthesis with C-NMMA produces a salt-sensitive phenotype in normal rats (189). Endothelial vasomotor dysfunction in isolated aortic rings from salt-fed animals, however, can be prevented with antihypertensive therapy (i.e., reserpine, hydralazine, hydrochlorothiazide), thus suggesting that endothelial vasomotor dysfunction in extrarenal vessels of Dahl rats results from—and does not cause—hypertension (187). Forearm blood flow responses to isoproterenol, which depend in part on EDNO release, are impaired in normotensive blacks who display an increased incidence of salt-sensitive hypertension (190). Even so, a direct relationship between impaired renal vascular NO synthesis and salt-sensitive hypertension has not been demonstrated in humans.

Spontaneously hypertensive rats also develop endothelial vasomotor dysfunction, but the operative mechanisms in these animals are different. L-Arginine does not prevent hypertension (186), and even although acetylcholine-induced relaxation of aortic tissue is impaired, relaxation from other EDNO agonists, including thrombin and histamine, is intact or enhanced (29). In this model, acetylcholine stimulates endothelium-dependent vessel contraction that can be blocked by indomethacin (29), and results of subsequent studies suggest this effect is attributable to prostaglandin $H_2$ synthesis (191). Furthermore, administration of copper-zinc-SOD fusion protein targeted to endothelial cells reduces blood pressure in spontaneously hypertensive rats, thus suggesting that acetylcholine-induced production of superoxide anion and inactivation of NO may contribute to hypertension in this model (192).

Impaired arterial relaxation from acetylcholine and increased production of superoxide anion also are features of angiotensin II-induced, but not of catecholamine-induced, hypertension (193). Administration of angiotensin II in rats elevates blood pressure and increases vascular superoxide production. This effect depends on activation of membrane-associated NADH/NADPH oxidase (194). In this model, relaxation from nitroglycerin is impaired as well, which is consistent with superoxide anion-mediated inactivation of both EDNO and exogenous NO. The increased superoxide production and impaired vessel relaxation during infusion of angiotensin II could be prevented with concurrent administration of losartan, thereby suggesting that activation of NADH/NADPH oxidase occurs through an angiotensin II receptor-dependent mechanism (194). In individuals with essential hypertension, infusion of recombinant SOD fails to restore EDNO-dependent dilation, but this discrepancy could result from inability of the enzyme to access the intracellular sources of superoxide anion production during short-term infusion (195). That short-term treatment (7–8 weeks) with angiotensin-converting enzyme (ACE) inhibitors in individuals with hypertension fails to improve EDNO-dependent dilation (196), whereas long-term treatment (2 years) has a beneficial effect (197), further complicates this issue. Thus, the importance of angiotensin II-induced superoxide production for impaired action of EDNO in human hypertension remains unclear.

Finally, evidence supports the idea that loss of EDNO action is more than just a consequence of elevated blood pressure and, instead, is involved in pathogenesis of the disease. In rats, blockade of NO synthesis by long-term administration of L-NMMA produces severe hypertension (198) with a high mortality rate (186). In addition, mice deficient in the *Nos3* gene are hypertensive (199, 200). As mentioned, antihypertensive treatment may restore normal EDNO action in some animal models (187), thus suggesting this abnormality is a secondary phenomenon. Attempts to show a similar effect in humans, however, have yielded mixed results (196, 197, 201). Normotensive offspring of individuals with essential hypertension have impaired vasodilator responses to acetylcholine that can be improved by administration of L-arginine (202), thereby implying a primary abnormality and genetic basis for a defect in the NO pathway in human hypertension. This interpretation remains speculative, however, and longitudinal studies will determine whether this early functional abnormality is a marker for individuals who will develop clinical hypertension.

Much is known about the importance of EDNO in hypertension, but less is known about other abnormalities of endothelial function in this disease. Endothelin levels are not consistently elevated, although there is evidence for increased susceptibility to its vasoconstrictor effects (185). Other vascular vasodilator products may contribute to blood pressure regulation in hypertension as well. For example, heme oxygenase-mediated production of carbon monoxide has been implicated in the control of blood pressure and is altered in hypertensive animals (203).

Endothelial control of fibrinolysis also may be disturbed in this disease. Several investigators have described decreased t-PA activity and increased PAI-1 activity in individuals with essential hypertension (204, 205). That angiotensin II stimulates PAI-1 production in humans provides a possible mechanism for this observation (206). Thus, human hypertension is associated with impaired EDNO action as well as other abnormalities of endothelial cell function that may contribute to ischemic complications and, possibly, be involved in pathogenesis of the disease.

## CONGESTIVE HEART FAILURE

Deterioration of left ventricular function is associated with reflex activation of neuroendocrine pathways, such as the renin–angiotensin and the sympathetic nervous systems. These compensatory mechanisms maintain blood pressure and tissue perfusion during reduced cardiac output (207). Endothelial dysfunction in CHF may produce loss of counterregulatory responses to vasoconstrictor stimuli, thus resulting in altered tissue perfusion (208). In addition, EDNO may have paracrine effects on myocardial function.

Results of several studies have shown impaired EDNO-dependent dilation in the peripheral and coronary circulation of individuals with CHF. The coronary blood flow response to acetylcholine is impaired in those with dilated cardiomyopathy, thus reflecting a loss of EDNO action in the coronary resistance vessels (209). Similarly, blood flow responses to EDNO agonists are blunted in the upper and lower extremities of such individuals (210–213). The underlying etiology of CHF does not predict impaired EDNO action because impaired vasodilator responses are observed in individuals with either idiopathic cardiomyopathy or ischemic heart disease (210). Inherent abnormalities of oxygen use in the skeletal muscle have been described, but blunted endothelium-dependent dilation of peripheral vessels may be responsible for impaired perfusion of skeletal muscle and peripheral tissues and, thus, may contribute to reduced exercise tolerance in individuals with CHF (214). Even although stimulated EDNO action is impaired in CHF, infusion of L-NMMA decreases blood flow in an exaggerated fashion in this setting, thereby suggesting that basal release of EDNO is maintained or even enhanced (215). Plasma endothelin levels are threefold higher in individuals with CHF compared with normal controls (216), thus suggesting a more generalized abnormality of endothelial function. The direct relationship between elevated levels of this vasoconstrictor and loss of EDNO-dependent dilation, however, remains uncertain. Investigators have hypothesized that increased EDNO production in CHF may be a counterregulatory mechanism that limits the vasoconstrictor effects of increased angiotensin II and endothelin levels (208, 217, 218).

The mechanisms of impaired EDNO action in CHF remain uncertain. In these individuals, oral L-arginine supplementation has no effect on impaired acetylcholine responses in the forearm circulation (219). Indomethacin improves EDNO-dependent dilation in CHF, thus suggesting that increased production of vasoconstrictor prostanoids may play a role (213). As in atherosclerosis, diabetes mellitus, and hypertension, increased oxidative stress may contribute to endothelial dysfunction in CHF. Increased prostaglandin synthesis is associated with increased production of reactive oxygen species (160). This effect may lead to inactivation of NO as discussed earlier for diabetes mellitus (161). CHF is associated with decreased plasma levels of antioxidant thiols and increased levels of malondialdehyde, which provides further indirect evidence that CHF is associated with increased oxidative stress (220). ACE inhibitors improve acetylcholine-mediated vasodilation in CHF (221), and angiotensin II-stimulated superoxide production and NO inactivation may be involved in pathogenesis of the endothelial vasomotor dysfunction in CHF, as discussed earlier for hypertension (194). In addition to catalyzing the conversion of angiotensin I to angiotensin II, ACE also degrades bradykinin and, thus, decreases bradykinin-stimulated EDNO production (222). Increased ACE activity in CHF may decrease bradykinin availability, and ACE inhibitors may oppose this process.

The novel β/α-blocker carvedilol reduces morbidity and mortality rates in CHF (223–225). Interestingly, in addition to its antisympathetic and vasodilator actions, carvedilol inhibits lipid peroxidation, scavenges oxygen radicals, protects endogenous antioxidant reserves, and inhibits LDL oxidation (226, 227). The relevance of these antioxidant properties to the beneficial effects of carvedilol is unclear. The effect of carvedilol on endothelial function in humans has not been examined, but the ability of carvedilol to scavenge superoxide anion correlates with improved EDNO action in isolated rat aortas (227).

Finally, evidence is increasing that EDNO directly regulates myocardial function. Synthesized in microvessels as a result of local bradykinin action, EDNO inhibits oxygen consumption by myocardial and skeletal muscle cells (228, 229). Furthermore, ACE inhibitors may reduce oxygen consumption by inhibiting ACE-mediated bradykinin metabolism (230). Investigators have proposed that in individuals with CHF, increased oxygen consumption in the setting of decreased tissue perfusion, resulting from circulating vasoconstrictor substances, may lead to a mismatch between myocardial oxygen supply and demand. This effect may contribute to the pathogenesis of myocardial dysfunction (229, 230). Inhibition of NO synthesis augments myocardial contractile responses to β-adrenergic stimulation (231). This observation further supports the concept of a regulatory role for NO in myocardial function. Overexpression of NO because of iNOS activity is believed to contribute to left ventricular dysfunction associated with septic shock (6). Inhibition of NO synthesis increases myocardial fibrosis during stimulation by angiotensin II (232), thus indicating that EDNO also regulates myocardial tissue composition. Thus, in addition to regulation of myocardial perfusion, close regulation of normal EDNO production is critical for normal myocardial function and growth. Therefore, loss of normal EDNO in CHF may contribute to myocardial dysfunction through several mechanisms.

## VASCULAR INJURY AND RESTENOSIS

Restenosis following coronary angioplasty is a paradigm for endothelial dysfunction and intimal growth following vascular injury. Angioplasty results in endothelial denudation and exposure of the thrombogenic subendothelial surface to the circulation (233). During the acute period following angioplasty, mechanical loss of the endothelium may lead to platelet adhesion and thrombotic occlusion of the vessel, but adjunctive use of heparin and other antithrombin and antiplatelet therapy largely has curtailed this problem (234). Platelet activation also leads to the release of various growth factors that promote smooth muscle cell proliferation and migration, thereby resulting in obstruction of the arterial lumen at the site of balloon angioplasty. To some extent, luminal narrowing occurs in all individuals. In 30 to 40% of individuals, however, this process produces a diameter stenosis of 50% or more, thus meeting the definition of "restenosis" and often necessitates repeat angioplasty (60, 233, 234).

Ample evidence suggests that products of intact endothelium play an important role in inhibiting intimal growth. Mechanical removal of the endothelium is a standard experimental method to induce intimal proliferation (60). NO donors (62, 63, 235) and L-arginine (236) inhibit intimal proliferation through several mechanisms, including the inhibition of platelet adhesion to the denuded vessel (62, 235) and direct effects on smooth muscle cells to inhibit their proliferation and migration (63, 236). To date, human studies using NO donors have been disappointing (237); however, adequate delivery of NO to the injury site may be a problem. PGI$_2$ (238) and endothelium-derived heparan sulfate (64) inhibit smooth muscle proliferation as well. Thus, loss of endothelium following balloon injury makes an important contribution to the restenotic process.

The endothelium is regenerated within 2 to 4 weeks following denudation (60), but this regenerated endothelium is both morphologically and functionally abnormal. In the rabbit aorta, regenerated endothelium is irregularly shaped and lacks the typical alignment of cells (i.e., with the direction of blood flow) (61). Vessels containing regenerated endothelium demonstrate impaired relaxation in response to acetylcholine, whereas the response to sodium nitroprusside remains intact (61). In swine coronary arteries, regenerated endothelium displays impaired EDNO-dependent relaxation in response to G protein-dependent stimuli, as observed in animal models of hypercholesterolemia or atherosclerosis (239). These abnormalities are well documented in animal models, but whether dysfunction of regenerated endothelium in humans is clinically relevant for restenosis, graft patency after vascular surgery, or recurrent events following plaque rupture is not known.

# INTERVENTIONS TO IMPROVE ENDOTHELIAL FUNCTION

As previously discussed, endothelial dysfunction occurs in several important vascular diseases and contributes to their clinical expression. Understanding the importance of endothelial dysfunction in vascular syndromes provides insight into the mechanisms of action of several interventions already known to improve individual outcome. In addition, results of studies on the mechanisms of endothelial dysfunction have suggested new therapies with the potential to improve individual outcome through their effects on endothelial function, but these remain to be tested in well-controlled trials examining clinical endpoints. A list of these potential interventions is provided in Table 41.3.

## LIPID-LOWERING THERAPY

Results of several large, randomized, placebo-controlled primary and secondary prevention trials have convincingly demonstrated that treatment of hyperlipidemia with a 3-hydroxyl-3-methylglutaryl-coenzyme A (HMG-CoA) reductase inhibitor reduces both the number of cardiovascular events (240–242) and the overall mortality rate (240). These results fit well with those of many previous studies that used less potent lipid-lowering therapy and also demonstrated reduced cardiovascular events. When the results of the earlier studies were pooled by meta-analysis, they also were suggestive of important effects on cardiovascular and overall mortality in both primary and secondary prevention (243, 244).

Lipid-lowering therapy decreases the incidence of

**TABLE 41.3.** Potential Interventions to Improve Endothelial Function

Lipid-lowering therapy
Angiotensin-converting enzyme inhibitors
Estrogen replacement therapy
Exercise
α-Tocopherol
Probucol
Ascorbic acid
Glutathione repletion
Pyrrolidine dithiocarbamate
L-Arginine
Tetrahydrobiopterin
Smoking cessation
?Glucose control
?Blood pressure control
?Folate

cardiovascular events, but the mechanisms underlying these observed benefits remain unclear. Because hypercholesterolemia is an independent risk factor for CAD and is integral to lesion development, one might speculate that lipid-lowering therapy would result in atherosclerotic lesion regression or halt lesion progression. Indeed, nearly a dozen angiographic studies have been performed to demonstrate such an effect. In general, however, the effects of even the most potent lipid-lowering therapy have been minimal and unlikely explanations of the dramatic effects on clinical outcome (123). This lack of relationship fits well with our understanding of the importance of plaque activation rather than lesion severity in the pathogenesis of acute coronary events as discussed earlier.

Several investigators have proposed that the improvement of endothelial function with lipid-lowering therapy provides an alternative explanation for these beneficial effects (123, 245, 246). As outlined in Table 41.4, five human studies have examined the effect of lipid-lowering therapy on coronary endothelial vasomotor function. In general, more prolonged treatment of individuals with higher baseline cholesterol levels was associated with clear improvement in the coronary vasomotor response to acetylcholine. Several studies also demonstrated an improvement in brachial artery flow-mediated dilation with HMG-CoA reductase inhibitor therapy (247, 248). Improvement in EDNO action may occur as early as after 1 to 3 months of therapy (248, 249). Lipid-lowering therapy also may decrease the number of episodes of ambulatory ischemia (250) and reduce the severity of persantine-induced ischemia (251) in individuals with CAD over the same short period of time. These findings suggest that lipid lowering therapy improves vascular function.

In addition to NO, lipid-lowering therapy improves other aspects of endothelial function as well. Therapy with pravastatin lowers levels of circulating PAI-1 in individuals with hypercholesterolemia (252). Plasma levels of soluble cell adhesion molecules are elevated in hypercholesterolemia, and in one study (253), 42 weeks of pravastatin therapy reduced levels of soluble E-selectin but not of soluble VCAM-1 or soluble ICAM-1. Even so, questions remain about whether these soluble markers accurately reflect the expression of endothelial cell adhesion molecule.

Lipid-lowering therapy also may have other effects that could reduce the risk for plaque rupture, including reducing the lipid content of lesions (123, 254). The combination of increased plaque stability and improved endothelial function may explain the observed reduction in acute coronary events associated with lipid-lowering therapy (123). These agents reduce the need for revascularization by coronary angioplasty or coronary bypass surgery (240–242). Improved endothelial function may

**TABLE 41.4.** Studies of Lipid-lowering/Endothelial Function

| Study | Agent | Baseline Total Chol (mg/ml) | Duration | Benefit |
|-------|-------|------------------------------|----------|---------|
| Leung et al (339) | Cholestyramine | 278 | 6 months | + |
| Egashira et al (340) | Pravastatin | 272 | 6 months | + |
| Treasure et al (140) | Lovastatin | 230 | 6 months | + |
| Anderson et al (308) | Lovastatin | 210 | 1 year | ± |
| Yeung et al (341) | Simvastatin | 205 | 6 months | − |

also explain this reduction in more stable symptoms in individuals with CAD (123). It remains unknown whether examination of endothelial function will identify a subset of individuals who would benefit from lipid-lowering therapy.

## ANGIOTENSIN-CONVERTING ENZYME INHIBITION

Therapy with ACE inhibitors improves outcome in individuals with CHF (255). The reduced event rate in individuals with left ventricular dysfunction treated with ACE inhibitors is independent of the effect on left ventricular function, thus supporting the idea that such intervention has direct effects on the vasculature (256). Observational reports have linked high plasma renin concentrations, and presumably high angiotensin II concentrations, to an increased risk for myocardial infarction (257). It now is known that ACE inhibitors reduce the risk of myocardial infarction in individuals with CAD and previous infarction (258).

As noted, therapy with ACE inhibitors improves endothelium-dependent dilation in the forearm circulation of individuals with CHF (221). In individuals with hypertension, the vasodilator responses of microvessel specimens obtained by gluteal fat biopsy improve after 2 years of treatment with cilazapril, but not with atenolol, despite an equivalent reduction in blood pressure (197). In the coronary circulation, vasomotor response to acetylcholine in individuals with CAD improves following treatment with quinapril for 6 months (259), and short-term administration of the ACE inhibitor perindoprilat improves coronary vasodilation during the cold-pressor test, which likely reflects improved EDNO action (260). Thus, ACE inhibitors can improve endothelial vasomotor function in a variety of diseases.

The effects of ACE inhibitors on the vasculature are complex, and they may influence endothelial function at several levels. ACE catalyzes the formation of angiotensin II from angiotensin I and the conversion of bradykinin to inactive fragments. Reduction of angiotensin II formation by ACE inhibitors may have several effects. Angiotensin II stimulates expression of PAI-1 in cul-

tured endothelial cells (38), and it increases levels of circulating PAI-1 in humans (206) and, thus, could increase the risk for thrombotic events. Angiotensin II also stimulates expression of endothelin from cultured cells (261). As discussed earlier, angiotensin II may stimulate superoxide anion production via receptor-dependent stimulation of NADH/NADPH oxidase and, therefore, may lead to NO inactivation (194). Thus, by limiting angiotensin II formation, ACE inhibitors may improve the vasomotor and fibrinolytic functions of the endothelium. Because bradykinin stimulates production of NO, inhibition of ACE-mediated bradykinin metabolism also may favorably affect basal EDNO release. One recent study (262) suggested that ACE inhibitors may improve flow-mediated vasodilation via a bradykinin-dependent mechanism.

Angiotensin II has several other proatherosclerotic effects that may be unrelated to its effects on endothelial function. For example, angiotensin II stimulates the growth of vascular smooth muscle cells (263), and it may stimulate leukocyte infiltration into injured arterial tissue by inducing MCP-1 expression in monocytes and vascular smooth muscle cells (264). Thus, whether the beneficial effects of therapy with ACE inhibitors relate to improved endothelial cell function or other effects on the vascular wall remains speculative.

## ESTROGEN

The prevalence of coronary disease is low in premenopausal women, but it rises sharply after menopause (265). That estrogen is cardioprotective is supported by the observations from more than 30 epidemiologic studies linking use of estrogen to a reduced prevalence of coronary disease in women (266). In addition to its role in primary prevention, estrogen replacement therapy also improves individual outcome in women with established coronary disease, thus suggesting that estrogen does more than simply inhibit atherogenesis (267). Estrogen favorably alters the lipid profile, but the results of multivariate analyses suggest that only 25 to 50% of the reduction in coronary events can be explained by these effects (268).

Estrogen favorably influences endothelial function. Treatment with 17β-estradiol improves EDNO-dependent arterial relaxation in oophorectomized, normocholesterolemic rabbits (269) and in hypercholesterolemic monkeys (270) and swine (271). In postmenopausal (272) and oophorectomized (273) women, long-term estrogen replacement improves brachial artery flow-mediated dilation. Trials are underway to determine whether long-term hormone replacement therapy improves coronary artery endothelial function in postmenopausal women.

How estrogen affects endothelial vasomotor function remains incompletely understood. Estrogen may have direct vasodilator effects and inhibit endothelin-mediated vasoconstriction (274). One study (275) demonstrated increased eNOS expression in cultured endothelial cells exposed to 17β-estradiol, but another (276) demonstrated no such effect. There also is evidence that the antioxidant effects of estrogen are relevant to its protective effects. Estrogens directly inhibit LDL oxidation in superphysiologic concentrations (277), and exposure of LDL to physiologic concentrations of 17β-estradiol in a plasma milieu results in the incorporation of estradiol derivatives into LDL and protection against oxidation (278). Inhibition of LDL oxidation may prevent ox-LDL–mediated impairment of EDNO action, as discussed earlier. LDL isolated from oophorectomized swine (271) and postmenopausal women receiving (279) 17β-estradiol is more resistant to oxidation compared with that isolated from untreated controls, and this protection is associated with improved endothelium-dependent dilation (271). In cultured cells, 17β-estradiol reduces superoxide anion production and increases cGMP production without altering the total NO production, thus suggesting that estrogen can improve EDNO action by limiting superoxide-mediated inactivation of NO (276).

Estrogens may favorably influence other aspects of endothelial function as well. For example, PGI$_2$ production in vascular tissue may be enhanced (280). 17β-Estradiol also inhibits interleukin-1–mediated induction of VCAM-1 and E-selectin expression in cultured human endothelial cells by an estrogen receptor–dependent mechanism (281). In postmenopausal women, estrogen replacement therapy reduces PAI-1 activity (282). Similarly, postmenopausal women as well as men have higher plasma levels of PAI-1 and lower t-PA levels than premenopausal women and women receiving hormone replacement therapy (283). Thus, estrogens improve the vasomotor, anti-inflammatory, and fibrinolytic functions of the vascular endothelium, and these effects likely contribute to the cardioprotective effects of estrogen in women.

## EXERCISE

Results of epidemiologic studies suggest that regular exercise reduces the incidence of cardiovascular disease (284, 285). Exercise training has several potentially beneficial effects, including weight loss, decreased body fat, increased HDL cholesterol, decreased glucose intolerance, and decreased release of catecholamines, renin, aldosterone, and vasopressin (286). Collectively, these beneficial effects may reduce the risk of CAD.

In addition, recent data suggest that exercise training favorably influences arterial structure and function (286). Exercise is associated with chronic and repetitive increases in coronary and peripheral artery blood flow, and there is evidence this stimulus influences the endothelial control of vasomotion. Seven days of treadmill exercise has improved coronary vasodilator responses to acetylcholine in dogs, and the response was eliminated by L-NMMA, thus confirming that it depends on NO synthesis (287). Similar observations have been made in exercise-trained swine (288) and rats (289). Four weeks of handgrip training in individuals with heart failure improved radial artery flow-mediated dilation, and L-NMMA blocked this improvement (290). A preliminary study of 15 young military recruits found improvement of brachial artery flow-mediated dilation after 10 weeks of exercise (291). To date, however, no large study has examined the effects of exercise training on coronary artery endothelial vasomotor function in humans.

Long-term exercise training improves other aspects of endothelial function as well, such as increasing t-PA activity and decreasing PAI-1 activity (292). Repetitive increases in blood flow during exercise also may influence arterial growth. In animal models, a long-term increase or decrease in blood flow stimulates an increase or decrease in vessel size, respectively, and there is evidence these changes are endothelium dependent (293, 294). In individuals, observational studies demonstrate a larger epicardial vessel size in those who are physically active (286). Similarly, Masai tribesmen with a physically active lifestyle who died of noncardiovascular causes had similar degrees of atherosclerosis as U.S. men but greater arterial patency at autopsy because of larger coronary arteries (295). The mechanism of how endothelium transduces the signal of chronic changes in blood flow into an altered vessel size remains incompletely understood (286).

Regarding the effect of exercise on endothelial function, cultured endothelial cells exposed to laminar shear stress (see Chapter 20) respond with increased expression of eNOS (296, 297). Expression of the *eNOS* gene also is increased in the coronary arteries of dogs subjected to long-term exercise (298). There is a shear stress-responsive element within the promoter region of the *eNOS* gene; similarly, there are shear stress-responsive elements in the promoter regions of other endothelial cell genes, including those for t-PA, TGF-β, PDGF-β, and endothelin (286). Even so, laminar shear stress does not enhance expression of the endothelin gene in cultured cells (297). In animal models, shear stress also increases $PGI_2$ synthesis (299), but in humans, NO plays a more prominent role than $PGI_2$ as a mediator of flow-mediated dilation (19).

In general, the endothelium responds to both acute and chronic increases in shear stress by increased blood vessel size and, as a result, reduced shear stress at the endothelial surface (132). Acutely, this response is achieved by NO, $PGI_2$-induced vasodilation, or both. With chronically increased shear stress, arterial vessel growth and increased capacity for NO-mediated dilation may have a similar effect. Thus, the endothelium adapts to blood flow changes within local vascular beds through these shear stress-dependent changes in function. Because increased vessel size, development of new collaterals, and improvement in EDNO action may be beneficial in coronary atherosclerosis, improved endothelial function may contribute to the known reduction in cardiovascular risk associated with exercise.

## ANTIOXIDANTS

### Lipid-soluble Antioxidants

Considering the importance of increased oxidative stress as a mechanism of endothelial cell dysfunction in atherosclerosis, hypercholesterolemia, diabetes, and hypertension, it is logical to hypothesize that antioxidant therapy would be beneficial. Increased dietary intake of lipid-soluble antioxidants, and particularly of vitamin E, reduces the risk of CAD in both men and women (300, 301). In a randomized, double-blind, placebo-controlled trial, vitamin E, 50 mg/day (75 IU/day), modestly decreased the risk of angina pectoris in previously asymptomatic men (302). There was no effect on overall mortality, however. In the recently published Cambridge Heart Antioxidant Study (CHAOS), vitamin E, 400 to 800 IU/day, reduced the combined endpoint of nonfatal myocardial infarction and cardiovascular death by 47% compared with placebo (303).

As discussed regarding lipid-lowering therapy, it is difficult to attribute the beneficial effects of antioxidants solely to a reduced severity of atherosclerotic lesions. One study (304) demonstrated less progression of carotid artery intimal thickness, as assessed by vascular ultrasonography, in individuals consuming more than 45 mg/day of $\alpha$-tocopherol; however, this effect was modest. In the CHAOS study (303), the reduction in nonfatal myocardial infarction was observed after only 200 days of follow-up, which likely is too short for significant lesion regression.

Lipid-soluble antioxidant therapy prevents the endothelial vasomotor dysfunction in animal models. For example, in rabbits, addition of $\alpha$-tocopherol (120), $\beta$-carotene (120), or probucol (108, 121) to a hypercholes-

terolemic diet prevents endothelial vasomotor dysfunction. These effects may be attributed to the inhibition of LDL oxidation, because $\alpha$-tocopherol and probucol treatment is associated with increased resistance of LDL to *ex vivo* oxidation (108, 120). $\beta$-Carotene, however, does not provide antioxidant protection for LDL (120). Furthermore, although low-dose $\alpha$-tocopherol (110 IU/day) preserves endothelial function and protects LDL against oxidation, a higher dose (1100 IU/day) actually worsens endothelial function despite enhanced antioxidant protection of LDL. Thus, alternative mechanisms for the beneficial effects of lipid-soluble antioxidants on endothelial function must be considered (121).

Lipid-soluble antioxidants accumulate in vascular tissue, and tissue-specific actions likely contribute to their beneficial effects. Probucol prevents the increased production of vascular superoxide anion associated with hypercholesterolemia (108). $\alpha$-Tocopherol prevents impaired release of EDNO following exposure of vessels to ox-LDL, in part by preventing ox-LDL-mediated stimulation of protein kinase C (305). $\alpha$-Tocopherol, $\beta$-carotene, and probucol reduce the ability of cells to oxidize LDL and stimulate MCP-1 production in cell coculture systems (306). Lipid-soluble antioxidants may influence other aspects of endothelial cell function. For example, $\alpha$-tocopherol and probucol inhibits E-selectin mRNA levels, cell surface E-selectin protein expression, and monocyte adhesion following activation of cultured endothelial cells (307). Thus, lipid-soluble antioxidants may improve endothelial cell function by preventing LDL oxidation and by direct effects on endothelial cells.

Lipid-soluble antioxidants also may improve endothelial function in humans, but data are conflicting. Treatment of individuals with CAD using a combination of probucol and lovastatin significantly improved the coronary artery vasomotor response to acetylcholine infusion (308). One small study (309) suggested that vitamin E, 400 IU/day for 3 months, improved forearm blood flow response to acetylcholine in individuals with previous myocardial infarction; however, 1 month of vitamin E, $\beta$-carotene, and vitamin C had no effect on forearm blood flow response to acetylcholine in individuals with hypercholesterolemia (310). Which individuals and which lipid-soluble antioxidant regimens, if any, will convincingly improve endothelial vasodilator function remain to be determined. Vitamin E has other potentially important effects as well, including inhibition of platelet aggregation (311) and of smooth muscle cell proliferation (312). These effects may provide alternative explanations for the observed, beneficial effects against CAD events.

### Water-soluble Antioxidants

Ascorbic acid improves endothelial function in several diseases (154, 313–316). These observations support the

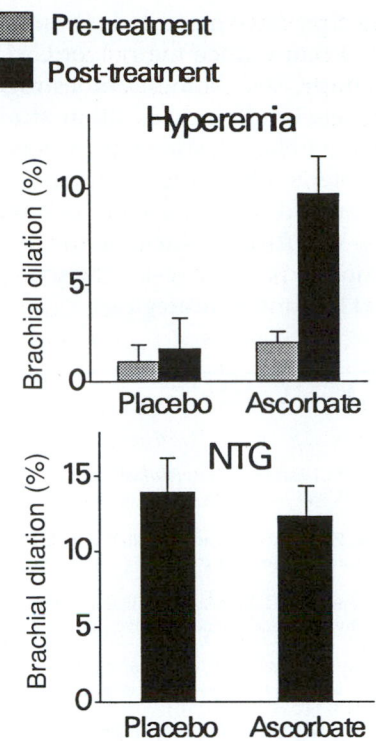

**FIGURE 41.5.** Ascorbic acid improves brachial artery flow-mediated dilation in individuals with CAD. Brachial artery dilation in response to increased flow (upper panel) and nitroglycerin (lower panel) was measured using high-resolution ultrasonography in individuals with CAD and impaired baseline response (less than 5% increase in arterial diameter). Mean ($\pm$ SEM) flow-mediated dilation was the same before (gray bars) and 2 hours after (black bars) placebo administration, whereas flow-mediated dilation markedly improved 2 hours after oral administration of 2 g of ascorbic acid ($P = .003$) compared with placebo. Ascorbic acid had no effect on nitroglycerin-mediated dilation. (Adapted with permission from Levine GN, Frei B, Koulouris SN, et al Ascorbic acid reverses endothelial vasomotor dysfunction in individuals with coronary artery disease. Circulation 1996;96:1107–1113.)

idea that increased oxidative stress is a pathophysiologic mechanism of endothelial dysfunction. A single oral dose of ascorbic acid that increases the plasma ascorbic acid levels within the physiologic range (50–150 µM) improves brachial artery flow-mediated dilation in individuals with angiographically proved CAD (Fig. 41.5) (313). In individuals with type 2 diabetes mellitus (154) and in chronic cigarette smokers (314), improvements in forearm blood flow response to methacholine are produced by intra-arterial infusion of ascorbic acid designed to raise the final plasma concentration to between 5 and 10 mM. In experimental models, supplementation with ascorbic acid within the physiologic range also inhibits binding of monocytes to the endothelial surface,

thus suggesting that other endothelial cell functions may be influenced by ascorbic acid as well (315, 316).

Altered availability of other intracellular antioxidant species also may influence EDNO action. Along with ascorbic acid, the principal water-soluble antioxidant in cells is glutathione (GSH). Intracellular GSH status is closely coupled with intracellular ascorbic acid status, and each water-soluble antioxidant can substitute for the other *in vivo* (317). In cultured human endothelial cells, GSH depletion reduces EDNO production in a dose-dependent manner, whereas bolstering cellular GSH enhances EDNO production (318). Augmentation of intracellular GSH with L-2-oxo-4-thiazolidine carboxylate improves brachial artery flow-mediated dilation in individuals with CAD (319).

The mechanisms by which GSH and ascorbic acid improve EDNO-dependent dilation remain unclear. GSH protects endothelial cells against the cytotoxic effects of ox-LDL (320). Furthermore, GSH may enhance NOS activity through direct effects on the enzyme (321, 322), thus preventing enzyme inactivation by reactive oxygen species (321), sparing essential NOS cofactors (322), and maintaining substrate availability (323). Furthermore, GSH may facilitate stabilization and bioavailability of NO through formation of S-nitrosothiol compounds (5). Ascorbic acid could improve EDNO action in atherosclerosis by sparing intracellular GSH (317) or preserving the NOS cofactor terahydrobiopterin (321). In high concentrations, ascorbic acid may scavenge superoxide anion (324) and prevent NO inactivation. Thus, loss of intracellular antioxidant species in atherosclerosis may lead to impaired EDNO action.

Other water-soluble antioxidants have the potential to improve endothelial function as well. Thiols in plasma may act as antioxidants, and one study (325) demonstrated a relationship between reduced total plasma thiol concentration and unstable angina. The thiol antioxidant compounds pyrrolidine dithiocarbamate and $N$-acetylcysteine prevent activation of nuclear factor B and induction of VCAM-1 expression in cultured endothelial cells (53). The relevance of these findings to human disease, however, remains unknown. A short-term infusion of $N$-acetylcysteine had no effect on the forearm blood flow response to methacholine (326); however, increasing intracellular thiol status may play a more important role (319).

## OTHER INTERVENTIONS

Several other interventions also may improve endothelial function in individuals with various vascular diseases. Cigarette smoking and exposure to secondhand cigarette smoke are associated with impaired EDNO-dependent dilation (83, 327), and smoking cessation may improve endothelial function (327). Because hyperglycemia is associated with impaired EDNO action in animal models, long-term reduction of blood glucose levels could improve endothelial function in individuals with diabetes. To date, however, no study has examined this issue. Similarly, blood pressure control may improve endothelial function, but as discussed, studies examining the effect of blood pressure control on endothelial function have provided conflicting information.

L-Arginine, the precursor for NO synthesis, is a potential therapy to improve endothelial function and benefit individuals with vascular disease. Under normal circumstances, L-arginine is not a rate-limiting substrate for NOS because of its high intracellular concentration compared with the $K_m$ of eNOS. In individuals with hypercholesterolemia, however, elevated levels of endogenous competitive NOS inhibitors such as asymmetric dimethyl-L-arginine (ADMA) may reduce NO synthesis and impair endothelial function (328). This effect of ADMA might be overcome through bolstering the intracellular substrate L-arginine concentrations via exogenous supplementation. In animal models, L-arginine reduces atherogenesis (329) and xanthoma development (93). Short-term L-arginine administration improves coronary and forearm EDNO-dependent dilation (330, 331), and long-term oral L-arginine therapy improves brachial artery flow-mediated dilation in young adults with hypercholesterolemia (332). Furthermore, L-arginine reduces platelet reactivity in individuals with hypercholesterolemia (333) and inhibits monocyte adhesion to vascular endothelium (334, 335). To date, however, no study has shown a beneficial effect of L-arginine therapy on clinical ischemia in subjects with atherosclerosis.

In addition, there is evidence that hyperhomocystinemia (see Chapter 40) is associated with impaired endothelial vasomotor function (336, 337). Folate treatment, which reduces plasma homocysteine levels in individuals with this disease, also may improve endothelial function, and studies examining this issue are currently in progress. Finally, tetrahydrobiopterin, which is a cofactor for NOS, restores endothelial function in individuals with hypercholesterolemia (338), but the long-term effects remain unknown.

## CONCLUSIONS

Endothelial dysfunction is a feature of vascular diseases, including hypercholesterolemia, atherosclerosis, diabetes mellitus, hypertension, CHF, and arterial injury. There is strong evidence that impaired vasodilator, antithrombotic, fibrinolytic, and anti-inflammatory properties of the endothelium contribute to pathogenesis of these diseases. There also is growing information about the mechanisms of endothelial dysfunction in these diseases. These mechanistic studies have provided data on potential interventions to improve endothelial function.

Furthermore, they have increased our understanding of how therapies that reduce the risk of CAD (e.g., lipid-lowering therapy, ACE inhibitors, estrogen, exercise) exert their beneficial effect. In addition, studies on mechanisms of endothelial dysfunction in vascular disease have led to potential therapies that may improve endothelial function and be beneficial in individuals. Future studies likely will further elucidate the role of endothelial dysfunction in pathogenesis of vascular disease and lead to novel treatment strategies.

## REFERENCES

1. Mendelsohn ME, Loscalzo J. The endotheliopathies. In: Loscalzo J, Creager MA, Dzau VJ, eds. Vascular medicine. Boston: Little, Brown, 1992: 279–306.
2. Furchgott RF, Zawadzki JV. The obligatory role of endothelial cells in the relaxation of arterial smooth muscle by acetylcholine. Nature 1980;288: 373–376.
3. Palmer RM, Ferrige AG, Moncada S. Nitric oxide release accounts for the biological activity of endothelium-derived relaxing factor. Nature 1987; 327:524–526.
4. Ignarro LJ, Buga GM, Wood KS et al. Endothelium-derived relaxing factor produced and released from artery and vein is nitric oxide. Proc Natl Acad Sci U S A 1987;84:9265–9269.
5. Stamler JS, Singel DJ, Loscalzo J. Biochemistry of nitric oxide and its redox-activated forms. Science 1992;258:1898–1902.
6. Moncada S, Higgs A. The L-arginine nitric oxide pathway. N Engl J Med 1993;329:2002–2012.
7. Cooke JP, Rossitch E Jr, Andon NA et al. Flow activates an endothelial potassium channel to release an endogenous nitrovasodilator. J Clin Invest 1991;88:1663–1671.
8. Olesen SP, Clapham DE, Davies PF. Haemodynamic shear stress activates a K+ current in vascular endothelial cells. Nature 1988;331:168–170.
9. Nathan C. Nitric oxide as a secretory product of mammalian cells. FASEB J 1992;6:3051–3064.
10. Ignarro LJ. Endothelium-derived nitric oxide: actions and properties. FASEB J 1989;3:31–36.
11. Radomski MW, Palmer RM, Moncada S. The role of nitric oxide and cGMP in platelet adhesion to vascular endothelium. Biochem Biophys Res Commun 1987;148:1482–1489.
12. Bolotina VM, Najibi S, Palacino JJ et al. Nitric oxide directly activates calcium-dependent potassium channels in vascular smooth muscle. Nature 1994;368:850–853.
13. Furchgott RF. Role of endothelium in responses of vascular smooth muscle. Circ Res 1983;53:557–573.
14. Ludmer PL, Selwyn AP, Shook TL et al. Paradoxical vasoconstriction induced by acetylcholine in atherosclerotic coronary arteries. N Engl J Med 1986;315:1046–1051.
15. Creager MA, Cooke JP, Mendelsohn ME et al. Impaired vasodilation of forearm resistance vessels in hypercholesterolemic humans. J Clin Invest 1990;86:228–234.
16. Vita JA, Treasure CB, Nabel EG et al. Coronary vasomotor response to acetylcholine relates to risk factors for coronary artery disease. Circulation 1990;81:491–497.
17. Quyyumi AA, Dakak N, Andrews NP et al. Nitric oxide activity in the human coronary circulation. Impact of risk factors for coronary atherosclerosis. J Clin Invest 1995;95:1747–1755.
18. Lieberman EH, Gerhard MD, Uehata A et al. Flow-induced vasodilation of the human brachial artery is impaired in individuals <40 years of age with coronary artery disease. Am J Cardiol 1996;78:1210–1214.
19. Joannides R, Haefeli WE, Linder L et al. Nitric oxide is responsible for flow-dependent dilatation of human peripheral conduit arteries in vivo. Circulation 1995;91:1314–1319.
20. Moncada S, Vane JR. Pharmacology and endogenous roles or prostaglandin endoperoxides, thromboxane A₂, and prostacyclin. Pharmacol Rev 1978;30:293–331.
21. Cohen RA, Vanhoutte PM. Endothelium-dependent hyperpolarization. Beyond nitric oxide and cyclic GMP. Circulation 1995;92:3337–3349.
22. Moncada S, Gryglewski R, Bunting S et al. An enzyme isolated from arteries transforms prostaglandin endoperoxides to an unstable substance that inhibits platelet aggregation. Nature 1976;263:663–665.
23. Vane JR, Anggard EE, Botting RM. Regulatory functions of the vascular endothelium. N Engl J Med 1990;323:27–36.
24. Yanagisawa M, Kurihara H, Kimura S et al. A novel potent vasoconstrictor

peptide produced by vascular endothelial cells. Nature 1988;332: 411–415.

25. Dzau VJ. Circulating versus local renin-angiotensin system in cardiovascular homeostasis. Circulation 1988;77:I4–I13.

26. Fox PL, DiCorleto PE. Regulation of production of a platelet-derived growth factor-like protein by cultured bovine aortic endothelial cells. J Cell Physiol 1984;121:298–308.

27. Berk BC, Alexander RW, Brock TA et al. Vasoconstriction: a new activity for platelet-derived growth factor. Science 1986;232:87–90.

28. Tesfamariam B, Brown ML, Deykin D et al. Elevated glucose promotes generation of endothelium-derived vasoconstrictor prostanoids in rabbit aorta. J Clin Invest 1990;85:929–932.

29. Luscher TF, Vanhoutte PM. Endothelium-dependent contractions to acetylcholine in the aorta of the spontaneously hypertensive rat. Hypertension 1986;8:344–348.

30. Hekman CM, Loskutoff DJ. Fibrinolytic pathways and the endothelium. Semin Thromb Hemost 1987;13:514–527.

31. Wiman B, Mellbring G, Ranby M. Plasminogen activator release during venous stasis and exercise as determined by a new specific assay. Clin Chim Acta 1983;127:279–288.

32. Hanss M, Collen D. Secretion of tissue-type plasminogen activator and plasminogen activator inhibitor by cultured human endothelial cells: modulation by thrombin, endotoxin, and histamine. J Lab Clin Med 1987;109: 97–104.

33. Hajjar KA, Hamel NM. Identification and characterization of human endothelial cell membrane binding sites for tissue plasminogen activator and urokinase. J Biol Chem 1990;265:2908–2916.

34. Loskutoff DJ, Edgington TE. Synthesis of a fibrinolytic activator and inhibitor by endothelial cells. Proc Natl Acad Sci U S A 1977;74:3903–3907.

35. Stiko-Rahm A, Wiman B, Hamsten A et al. Secretion of plasminogen activator inhibitor-1 from cultured human umbilical vein endothelial cells is induced by very low density lipoprotein. Arteriosclerosis 1990;10:1067–1073.

36. Kugiyama K, Sakamoto T, Misumi I et al. Transferable lipids in oxidized low-density lipoprotein stimulate plasminogen activator inhibitor-1 and inhibit tissue-type plasminogen activator release from endothelial cells. Circ Res 1993;73:335–343.

37. Collen D, Juhan-Vague I. Fibrinolysis and atherosclerosis. Semin Thromb Hemost 1988;14:180–183.

38. Vaughan DE, Shen C, Lazo S. Angiotensin II induces plasminogen activator inhibitor synthesis *in vitro*. Circulation 1992;83:645–651.

39. Esmon NL, Owen WG, Esmon CT. Isolation of a membrane-bound cofactor for thrombin-catalyzed activation of protein C. J Biol Chem 1982;257: 859–864.

40. Esmon NL, Carroll RC, Esmon CT. Thrombomodulin blocks the ability of thrombin to activate platelets. J Biol Chem 1983;258:12238–12242.

41. Lentz SR, Sadler JE. Inhibition of thrombomodulin surface expression and protein C activation by the thrombogenic agent homocysteine. J Clin Invest 1991;88:1906–1914.

42. Marcum JA, Rosenberg RD. Heparin like molecules with anticoagulant activity are synthesized by cultured endothelial cells. Biochem Biophys Res Commun 1985;126:365–372.

43. Coller BS. Platelets and thrombolytic therapy. N Engl J Med 1990;322: 33–42.

44. Higgs EA, Moncada S, Vane JR et al. Effect of prostacyclin (PGI2) on platelet adhesion to rabbit arterial subendothelium. Prostaglandins 1978; 16:17–22.

45. Marcus AJ, Broekman MJ, Drosopoulos JHF et al. The endothelial cell ecto-ADPase responsible for inhibition of platelet function is CD39. J Clin Invest 1997;99:1351–1360.

46. Rao AK, Schapira M, Clements ML et al. A prospective study of platelets and plasma proteolytic systems during the early stages of Rocky Mountain spotted fever. N Engl J Med 1988;318:1021–1028.

47. Blann AD, Dobrotova M, Kubisz P et al. von Willebrand factor, soluble P-selectin, tissue plasminogen activator and plasminogen activator inhibitor in atherosclerosis. Thromb Haemost 1995;74:626–630.

48. Weis JR, Pitas RE, Wilson BD et al. Oxidized low-density lipoprotein increases cultured human endothelial cell tissue factor activity and reduces protein C activation. FASEB J 1991;5:2459–2465.

49. Fryer RH, Wilson BD, Gubler DB et al. Homocysteine, a risk factor for premature vascular disease and thrombosis, induces tissue factor activity in endothelial cells. Arteriosclerosis Thromb 1993;13:1327–1333.

50. Bierhaus A, Zhang Y, Deng Y et al. Mechanism of the tumor necrosis factor alpha-mediated induction of endothelial tissue factor. J Biol Chem 1995;270:26419–26432.

51. Kubes P, Suzuki M, Granger DN. Nitric oxide: an endogenous modulator of leukocyte adhesion. Proc Natl Acad Sci U S A 1991;88:4651–4655.

52. Collins T. Endothelial nuclear factor-kB and the initiation of the atherosclerotic lesion. Lab Invest 1993;68:499–508.

53. Marui N, Offermann MK, Swerlick R et al. Vascular cell adhesion molecule-1 (VCAM-1) gene transcription and expression are regulated through an antioxidant-sensitive mechanism in human vascular endothelial cells. J Clin Invest 1993;92:1866–1874.

54. De Caterina R, Libby P, Peng HB et al. Nitric oxide decreases cytokine-induced endothelial activation. Nitric oxide selectively reduces endothelial expression of adhesion molecules and proinflammatory cytokines. J Clin Invest 1995;96:60–68.

55. Kume N, Cybulsky MI, Gimbrone MA Jr. Lysophosphatidylcholine, a component of atherogenic lipoproteins, induces mononuclear leukocyte adhesion molecules in cultured human and rabbit arterial endothelial cells. J Clin Invest 1992;90:1138–1144.

56. Horvath CJ, Ferro TJ, Jesmok G et al. Recombinant tumor necrosis factor increases pulmonary vascular permeability independent of neutrophils. Proc Natl Acad Sci U S A 1988;85:9219–9223.

57. Stern DM, Kaiser E, Nawroth PP. Regulation of the coagulation system by vascular endothelial cells. Haemostasis 1988;18:202–214.

58. Martin NB, Jamieson A, Tuffin DP. The effect of interleukin-4 on tumor necrosis factor-alpha induced expression of tissue factor and plasminogen activator inhibitor-1 in human umbilical vein endothelial cells. Thromb Haemost 1993;70:1037–1042.

59. Klemm P, Warner TD, Hohlfeld T et al. Endothelin 1 mediates *ex vivo* coronary vasoconstriction caused by exogenous and endogenous cytokines. Proc Natl Acad Sci U S A 1995;92:2691–2695.

60. Clowes AW, Reidy MA, Clowes MM. Kinetics of cellular proliferation after arterial injury. I. Smooth muscle growth in the absence of endothelium. Lab Invest 1983;49:327–333.

61. Weidinger FF, McLenachan JM, Cybulsky MI et al. Persistent dysfunction of regenerated endothelium after balloon angioplasty of rabbit iliac artery. Circulation 1990;81:1667–1679.

62. Marks DS, Vita JA, Folts JD et al. Inhibition of neointimal proliferation in rabbits after vascular injury by a single treatment with a protein adduct of nitric oxide. J Clin Invest 1995;96:2630–2638.

63. Garg UC, Hassid A. Nitric oxide-generating vasodilators and 8-bromo-cyclic guanosine monophosphate inhibit mitogenesis and proliferation of cultured rat vascular smooth muscle cells. J Clin Invest 1989;83: y1774–1777.

64. Castellot JJ Jr, Addonizio ML, Rosenberg R et al. Cultured endothelial cells produce a heparin like inhibitor of smooth muscle cell growth. J Cell Biol 1981;90:372–379.

65. Schwartz SM, Gajdusek CM, Selden SC III. Vascular wall growth control: the role of the endothelium. Arteriosclerosis 1981;1:107–126.

66. Kume N, Gimbrone MA Jr. Lysophosphatidylcholine transcriptionally induces growth factor gene expression in cultured human endothelial cells. J Clin Invest 1994;93:907–911.

67. Berk BC, Alexander RW. Vasoactive effects of growth factors [Review]. Biochem Pharmacol 1989;38:219–225.

68. Witztum JL, Steinberg D. Role of oxidized low density lipoprotein in atherogenesis. J Clin Invest 1991;88:1785–1792.

69. Steinberg D, Parthasarathy S, Carew TE et al. Beyond cholesterol. Modifications of low-density lipoprotein that increase its atherogenicity. N Engl J Med 1989;320:915–924.

70. Quinn MT, Parthasarathy S, Fong LG et al. Oxidatively modified low density lipoproteins: a potential role in recruitment and retention of monocyte/macrophages during atherogenesis. Proc Natl Acad Sci U S A 1987;84:2995–2998.

71. Frostegard J, Haegerstrand A, Gidlund M et al. Biologically modified LDL increases the adhesive properties of endothelial cells. Atherosclerosis 1991; 90:119–126.

72. Cathcart MK, Morel DW, Chisolm GM III. Monocytes and neutrophils oxidize low density lipoprotein making it cytotoxic. J Leukocyte Biol 1985; 38:341–350.

73. Schwartz CJ, Valente AJ, Sprague EA et al. The pathogenesis of atherosclerosis: an overview. Clin Cardiol 1991;14:I1–I16.

74. Fuster V, Badimon L, Badimon JJ et al. The pathogenesis of coronary artery disease and the acute coronary syndromes (Part 1). N Engl J Med 1992; 326:242–250.

75. Bossaller C, Habib GB, Yamamoto H et al. Impaired muscarinic endothelium-dependent relaxation and cyclic guanosine 5′-monophosphate formation in atherosclerotic human coronary artery and rabbit aorta. J Clin Invest 1987;79:170–174.

76. Reddy KG, Nair RN, Sheehan HM et al. Evidence that selective endothelial dysfunction may occur in the absence of angiographic or ultrasound atherosclerosis in individuals with risk factors for atherosclerosis. J Am Coll Cardiol 1994;23:833–843.

77. Sorensen KE, Celermajer DS, Georgakopoulos D et al. Impairment of endothelium-dependent dilation is an early event in children with familial hypercholesterolemia and is related to the lipoprotein (a) level. J Clin Invest 1994;93:50–55.

78. Golino P, Piscione F, Willerson JT et al. Divergent effects of serotonin on coronary artery dimensions and blood flow in individuals with coronary atherosclerosis and control individuals. N Engl J Med 1991; 324:641–648.

79. Crossman DC, Larkin SW, Dashwood MR et al. Responses of atherosclerotic human coronary arteries *in vivo* to the endothelium-dependent vasodilator substance P. Circulation 1991;84:2001–2010.

80. Cox DA, Vita JA, Treasure CB et al. Atherosclerosis impairs flow-mediated dilation of coronary arteries in humans. Circulation 1989;80:458–465.

81. Zeiher AM, Drexler H, Wollschlager H et al. Modulation of coronary vaso-motor tone in humans. Progressive endothelial dysfunction with different early stages of coronary atherosclerosis. Circulation 1991;83:391–401.

82. Kugiyama K, Yasue H, Ohgushi M et al. Deficiency in nitric oxide bioactiv-ity in epicardial coronary arteries of cigarette smokers. J Am Coll Cardiol 1996;28:1161–1167.

83. Celermajer DS, Adams MR, Clarkson P et al. Passive smoking and im-paired endothelium-dependent arterial dilatation in healthy young adults. N Engl J Med 1996;334:150–154.

84. Nitenberg A, Valensi P, Sachs R et al. Impairment of coronary vascular reserve and ACh-induced coronary vasodilation in diabetic individuals with angiographically normal coronary arteries and normal left ventricu-lar systolic function. Diabetes 1993;42:1017–1025.

85. Treasure CB, Manoukian SV, Klein JL et al. Epicardial coronary artery responses to acetylcholine are impaired in hypertensive individuals. Circ Res 1992;71:776–781.

86. Vita JA, Keaney JF Jr. Ultrasound assessment of endothelial vasomotor function. In: Lanzer P, Lipton M, eds. Diagnostics of vascular diseases: principals and technology. Berlin: Springer, 1996:49–259.

87. Anderson TJ, Uehata A, Gerhard MD et al. Close relation of endothelial function in the human coronary and peripheral circulations. J Am Coll Cardiol 1995;26:1235–1241.

88. Sorensen KE, Kristensen IB, Celermajer DS. Atherosclerosis in the human brachial artery. J Am Coll Cardiol 1997;29:318–322.

89. Osborne JA, Lento PH, Siegfried MR et al. Cardiovascular effects of acute hypercholesterolemia in rabbits. Reversal with lovastatin treatment. J Clin Invest 1989;83:465–473.

90. Flavahan NA, Vanhoutte PM. Endothelial cell signaling and endothelial dysfunction. Am J Hypertens 1995;8:28S–41S.

91. Tsao PS, McEvoy LM, Drexler H et al. Enhanced endothelial adhesiveness in hypercholesterolemia is attenuated by L-arginine. Circulation 1994;89:2176–2182.

92. Cayette AJ, Palacino JJ, Horten K et al. Chronic inhibition of nitric oxide production accelerates neointima formation and impairs endothelial func-tion in hypercholesterolemic rabbits. Arteriosclerosis Thromb 1994;14:753–759.

93. Aji W, Ravalli S, Szabolcs M et al. L-arginine prevents xanthoma develop-ment and inhibits atherosclerosis in LDL receptor knockout mice. Circula-tion 1997;95:430–437.

94. Jessup W, Mohr D, Gieseg SP et al. The participation of nitric oxide in cell free- and its restriction of macrophage-mediated oxidation of low-density lipoprotein. Biochim Biophys Acta 1992;1180:73–82.

95. Lerman A, Edwards BS, Hallett JW et al. Circulating and tissue endothelin immunoreactivity in advanced atherosclerosis. N Engl J Med 1991;325:997–1001.

96. Lerman A, Holmes DR Jr, Bell MR et al. Endothelin in coronary endothelial dysfunction and early atherosclerosis in humans. Circulation 1995;92:2426–2431.

97. Andersen P, Arnesen H, Hjermann I. Hyperlipoproteinaemia and reduced fibrinolytic activity in healthy coronary high-risk men. Acta Med Scand 1981;209:199–202.

98. Ridker PM, Vaughan DE, Stampfer MJ et al. Endogenous tissue-type plas-minogen activator and risk of myocardial infarction. Lancet 1993;341:1165–1168.

99. Hamsten A, Wiman B, de Faire U et al. Increased plasma levels of a rapid inhibitor of tissue plasminogen activator in young survivors of myocardial infarction. N Engl J Med 1985;313:1557–1563.

100. Aznar J, Estelles A, Tormo G et al. Plasminogen activator inhibitor activity and other fibrinolytic variables in individuals with coronary artery dis-ease. Br Heart J 1988;59:535–541.

101. Keaney JF Jr, Vita JA. Atherosclerosis, oxidative stress and antioxidant protection in endothelium-derived relaxing factor action. Prog Cardiovasc Dis 1995;38:129–154.

102. Rosen GM, Freeman BA. Detection of superoxide generated by endothelial cells. Proc Natl Acad Sci U S A 1984;81:7269–7273.

103. Heinecke JW, Baker L, Rosen H et al. Superoxide-mediated modification of low density lipoprotein by arterial smooth muscle cells. J Clin Invest 1986;77:757–761.

104. Hiramatsu K, Rosen H, Heinecke JW et al. Superoxide initiates oxidation of low density lipoprotein by human monocytes. Arteriosclerosis 1987;7:55–60.

105. Gryglewski RJ, Palmer RM, Moncada S. Superoxide anion is involved in the breakdown of endothelium-derived vascular relaxing factor. Nature 1986;320:454–456.

106. Mugge A, Elwell JH, Peterson TE et al. Release of intact endothelium-derived relaxing factor depends on endothelial superoxide dismutase ac-tivity. Am J Physiol 1991;260:C219–C225.

107. Ohara Y, Peterson TE, Harrison DG. Hypercholesterolemia increases en-dothelial superoxide anion production. J Clin Invest 1993;91:2546–2551.

108. Keaney JF Jr, Xu A, Cunningham D et al. Dietary probucol preserves endo-thelial function in cholesterol-fed rabbits by limiting vascular oxidative stress and superoxide generation. J Clin Invest 1995;95:2520–2529.

109. Meredith IT, Anderson TJ, Yeung AC et al. Superoxide dismutase restores endothelial vasodilator function in human coronary arteries in vivo. Circu-lation 1993;88:I467.

110. White CR, Darley-Usmar V, Berrington WR et al. Circulating plasma xan-thine oxidase contributes to vascular dysfunction in hypercholesterolemic rabbits. Proc Natl Acad Sci U S A 1996;93:8745–8749.

111. Pagano PJ, Ito Y, Tornheim K et al. An NADPH oxidase superoxide-gener-ating system in the rabbit aorta. Am J Physiol 1995;268:H2274–2280.

112. Pritchard KA Jr, Groszek L, Smalley DM et al. Native low-density lipopro-tein increases endothelial cell nitric oxide synthase generation of superox-ide anion. Circ Res 1995;77:510–518.

113. Ohara Y, Peterson TE, Zheng B et al. Lysophosphatidylcholine increases vascular superoxide anion production via protein kinase C activation. Ar-teriosclerosis Thromb 1994;14:1007–1013.

114. Nègre-Salvayre A, Pieraggi MT, Mabile L et al. Protective effect of 17-beta-estradiol against the cytotoxicity of minimally oxidized LDL to cultured bovine aortic endothelial cells. Atherosclerosis 1993;99:207–217.

115. Dimmeler S, Haendeler J, Galle J et al. Oxidized low-density lipoprotein induces apoptosis of human endothelial cells by activation of CPP32-like proteases: a mechanistic clue to the 'response to injury' hypothesis. Circu-lation 1997;95:1760–1763.

116. Liao JK, Clark SL. Regulation of G protein alpha i2 subunit expression by oxidized low-density lipoprotein. J Clin Invest 1995;95:1457–1463.

117. Kugiyama K, Kerns SA, Morrisett JD et al. Impairment of endothelium-dependent arterial relaxation by lysolecithin in modified low-density lipo-proteins. Nature 1990;344:160–162.

118. Liao JK, Shin WS, Lee WY et al. Oxidized low-density lipoprotein de-creases the expression of endothelial nitric oxide synthase. J Biol Chem 1995;270:319–324.

119. Chin JH, Azhar S, Hoffman BB. Inactivation of endothelium-derived relax-ing factor by oxidized lipoproteins. J Clin Invest 1992;89:10–18.

120. Keaney JF Jr, Gaziano JM, Xu A et al. Dietary antioxidants preserve endo-thelium-dependent vessel relaxation in cholesterol-fed rabbits. Proc Natl Acad Sci U S A 1993;90:11880–11884.

121. Diaz MN, Frei B, Vita JA et al. Antioxidants and atherosclerotic heart disease. N Engl J Med 1997;337:408–416.

122. Drake TA, Hannani K, Fei HH et al. Minimally oxidized low-density lipo-protein induces tissue factor expression in cultured human endothelial cells. Am J Pathol 1991;138:601–607.

123. Levine GN, Keaney JF Jr, Vita JA. Cholesterol reduction in cardiovascular disease: clinical benefits and possible mechanisms. N Engl J Med 1995;332:512–521.

124. Folland ED, Vogel RA, Hartigan P et al. Relation between coronary artery stenosis assessed by visual, caliper, and computer methods and exercise capacity in individuals with single-vessel coronary artery disease. Circula-tion 1994;89:2005–2014.

125. Ambrose JA, Winters SL, Arora RR et al. Coronary angiographic morphol-ogy in myocardial infarction: a link between the pathogenesis of unstable angina and myocardial infarction. J Am Coll Cardiol 1985;6:1233–1238.

126. Gordon JB, Ganz P, Nabel EG et al. Atherosclerosis influences the vasomo-tor response of epicardial coronary arteries to exercise. J Clin Invest 1989;83:1946–1952.

127. Nabel EG, Ganz P, Gordon JB et al. Dilation of normal and constriction of atherosclerotic coronary arteries caused by the cold pressor test. Circula-tion 1988;77:43–52.

128. Yeung AC, Vekshtein VI, Krantz DS et al. The effect of atherosclerosis on the vasomotor response of coronary arteries to mental stress. N Engl J Med 1991;325:1551–1556.

129. Dimsdale JE, Moss J. Plasma catecholamines in stress and exercise. JAMA 1980;243:340–342.

130. Vita JA, Treasure CB, Yeung AC et al. Individuals with evidence of coro-nary endothelial dysfunction as assessed by acetylcholine infusion demon-strate marked increase in sensitivity to constrictor effects of catechola-mines. Circulation 1992;85:1390–1397.

131. Loree HM, Kamm RD, Stringfellow RG et al. Effects of fibrous cap thick-ness on peak circumferential stress in model atherosclerotic vessels. Circ Res 1992;71:850–858.

132. Vita JA, Treasure CB, Ganz P et al. Control of shear stress in the epicardial coronary arteries of humans: impairment by atherosclerosis. J Am Coll Cardiol 1989;14:1193–1199.

133. Shimokawa H, Vanhoutte PM. Impaired endothelium-dependent relaxa-tion to aggregating platelets and related vasoactive substances in porcine coronary arteries in hypercholesterolemia and atherosclerosis. Circ Res 1989;64:900–914.

134. Okumura K, Yasue H, Matsuyama K et al. Effect of acetylcholine on the highly stenotic coronary artery: difference between the constrictor re-sponse of the infarct-related coronary artery and that of the noninfarct-related artery. J Am Coll Cardiol 1992;19:752–758.

135. Bogaty P, Hackett D, Davies G et al. Vasoreactivity of the culprit lesion in unstable angina. Circulation 1994;90:5–11.

136. Libby P. Molecular basis of the acute coronary syndromes. Circulation 1995;91:2844–2850.

137. Werns SW, Walton JA, Hsia HH et al. Evidence of endothelial dysfunction in angiographically normal coronary arteries of individuals with coronary artery disease. Circulation 1989;79:287–291.

138. el-Tamimi H, Mansour M, Wargovich TJ et al. Constrictor and dilator responses to intracoronary acetylcholine in adjacent segments of the same coronary artery in individuals with coronary artery disease. Endothelial function revisited. Circulation 1994;89:45–51.

139. McLenachan JM, Vita J, Fish DR et al. Early evidence of endothelial vasodilator dysfunction at coronary branch points. Circulation 1990;82:1169–1173.

140. Treasure CB, Klein JL, Weintraub WS et al. Beneficial effects of cholesterol-lowering therapy on the coronary endothelium in individuals with coronary artery disease. N Engl J Med 1995;332:481–487.

141. Ruderman NB, Gupta S, Sussman I. Hyperglycemia, diabetes and vascular disease: an overview. In: Ruderman NB, Williamson J, Brownless M, eds. Hyperglycemia, diabetes and vascular disease. New York: Oxford Press, 1992:3–20.

142. Nathan DM. Long-term complications of diabetes mellitus. N Engl J Med 1993;328:1676–1685.

143. Krolewski AS, Warram JH, Valsania P et al. Evolving natural history of coronary artery disease in diabetes mellitus. Am J Med 1991;90:56S–61S.

144. Anonymous. The effect of intensive treatment of diabetes on the development and progression of long-term complications in insulin-dependent diabetes mellitus. The Diabetes Control and Complications Trial Research Group. N Engl J Med 1993;329:977–986.

145. Bierman EL. George Lyman Duff Memorial Lecture. Atherogenesis in diabetes [Review]. Arteriosclerosis Thromb 1992;12:647–656.

146. Johnstone MT, Creager SJ, Scales KM et al. Impaired endothelium-dependent vasodilation in individuals with insulin-dependent diabetes mellitus. Circulation 1993;88:2510–2516.

147. Smits P, Kapma JA, Jacobs MC et al. Endothelium-dependent vascular relaxation in individuals with type I diabetes. Diabetes 1993;42:148–153.

148. Calver A, Collier J, Vallance P. Inhibition and stimulation of nitric oxide synthesis in the human forearm arterial bed of individuals with insulin-dependent diabetes. J Clin Invest 1992;90:2548–2554.

149. Halkin A, Benjamin N, Doktor HS et al. Vascular responsiveness and cation exchange in insulin-dependent diabetes. Clin Sci 1991;81:223–232.

150. Khan F, Cohen RA, Ruderman NB et al. Vasodilator responses in the forearm of individuals with diabetes mellitus. Vasc Med 1996;1:187–193.

151. Makimattila S, Mantysaari M, Groop H et al. Hyperactivity to nitrovasodilators in forearm vasculature is related to autonomic dysfunction in insulin-dependent diabetes mellitus. Circulation 1997;95:618–625.

152. Steinberg HO, Baron AD. Insulin-dependent diabetes mellitus and nitrovasodilation: important and complex interactions. Circulation 1997;95:560–561.

153. McVeigh GE, Brennan GM, Johnston GD et al. Impaired endothelium-dependent and independent vasodilation in individuals with type 2 (non-insulin-dependent) diabetes mellitus. Diabetologia 1992;35:771–776.

154. Ting HH, Timimi FK, Boles KS et al. Vitamin C improves endothelium-dependent vasodilation in individuals with non-insulin-dependent diabetes mellitus. J Clin Invest 1996;97:22–28.

155. Clarkson P, Celermajer DS, Donald AE et al. Impaired vascular reactivity in insulin-dependent diabetes mellitus is related to disease duration and low density lipoprotein cholesterol levels. J Am Coll Cardiol 1996;28:573–579.

156. Elliott TG, Cockcroft JR, Groop PH et al. Inhibition of nitric oxide synthesis in forearm vasculature of insulin-dependent diabetic individuals: blunted vasoconstriction in individuals with microalbuminuria. Clin Sci 1993;85:687–693.

157. Scherrer U, Randin D, Vollenweider P et al. Nitric oxide release accounts for insulin's vascular effects in humans. J Clin Invest 1994;94:2511–2515.

158. Tesfamariam B, Jakubowski JA, Cohen RA. Contraction of diabetic rabbit aorta caused by endothelium-derived PGH2/TXA2. Am J Physiol 1989;257:H1327–H1333.

159. Oyama Y, Kawasaki H, Hattori Y et al. Attenuation of endothelium-dependent relaxation in aorta from diabetic rats. Eur J Pharmacol 1986;132:75–78.

160. Kukreja RC, Kontos HA, Hess ML et al. PGH synthase and lipoxygenase generate superoxide in the presence of NADH or NADPH. Circ Res 1986;59:612–619.

161. Tesfamariam B, Cohen RA. Free radicals mediate endothelial cell dysfunction caused by elevated glucose. Am J Physiol 1992;263:H321–H326.

162. Hattori Y, Kawasaki H, Abe K et al. Superoxide dismutase recovers altered endothelium-dependent relaxation in diabetic rat aorta. Am J Physiol 1991;261:H1086–H1094.

163. Nishigaki I, Hagihara M, Tsunekawa H et al. Lipid peroxide levels of serum lipoprotein fractions of diabetic individuals. Biochem Med 1981;25:373–378.

164. Kawamura M, Heinecke JW, Chait A. Pathophysiological concentrations of glucose promote oxidative modification of low density lipoprotein by a superoxide-dependent pathway. J Clin Invest 1994;94:771–778.

165. Tsai EC, Hirsch IB, Brunzell JD et al. Reduced plasma peroxyl radical trapping capacity and increased susceptibility of LDL to oxidation in poorly controlled IDDM. Diabetes 1994;43:1010–1014.

166. Bucala R, Makita Z, Koschinsky T et al. Lipid advanced glycosylation: pathway for lipid oxidation *in vivo*. Proc Natl Acad Sci U S A 1993;90:6434–6438.

167. Selby JV, Austin MA, Newman B et al. LDL subclass phenotypes and the insulin resistance syndrome in women. Circulation 1993;88:381–387.

168. Vlassara H, Bucala R, Striker L. Pathogenic effects of advanced glycosylation: biochemical, biologic, and clinical implications for diabetes and aging. Lab Invest 1994;70:138–151.

169. Bucala R, Tracey KJ, Cerami A. Advanced glycosylation products quench nitric oxide and mediate defective endothelium-dependent vasodilatation in experimental diabetes. J Clin Invest 1991;87:432–438.

170. Williamson JR, Chang K, Frangos M et al. Hyperglycemic pseudohypoxia and diabetic complications. Diabetes 1993;42:801–813.

171. Tilton RG, Kawamura T, Chang KC et al. Vascular dysfunction induced by elevated glucose levels in rats is mediated by vascular endothelial growth factor. J Clin Invest 1997;9:2192–2202.

172. Tesfamariam B, Palacino JJ, Weisbrod RM et al. Aldose reductase inhibition restores endothelial cell function in diabetic rabbit aorta. J Cardiovasc Pharmacol 1993;21:205–211.

173. Richardson M, Hadcock SJ, DeReske M et al. Increased expression *in vivo* of VCAM-1 and E-selectin by the aortic endothelium of normolipemic and hyperlipemic diabetic rabbits. Arteriosclerosis Thromb 1994;14:760–769.

174. Auwerx J, Bouillon R, Collen D et al. Tissue-type plasminogen activator antigen and plasminogen activator inhibitor in diabetes mellitus. Arteriosclerosis 1988;8:68–72.

175. Colwell JA, Winocour PD, Lopes-Virella M et al. New concepts about the pathogenesis of atherosclerosis in diabetes mellitus. Am J Med 1983;75:67–80.

176. Treasure CB, Klein JL, Vita JA et al. Hypertension and left ventricular hypertrophy are associated with impaired endothelium-mediated relaxation in human coronary resistance vessels. Circulation 1993;87:86–93.

177. Brush JE Jr, Faxon DP, Salmon S et al. Abnormal endothelium-dependent coronary vasomotion in hypertensive individuals. J Am Coll Cardiol 1992;19:809–815.

178. Panza JA, Quyyumi AA, Brush JE Jr et al. Abnormal endothelium-dependent vascular relaxation in individuals with essential hypertension. N Engl J Med 1990;323:22–27.

179. Linder L, Kiowski W, Buhler FR et al. Indirect evidence for release of endothelium-derived relaxing factor in human forearm circulation *in vivo*. Circulation 1990;81:1762–1767.

180. Cockcroft JR, Chowienczyk PJ, Benjamin N et al. Preserved endothelium-dependent vasodilation in individuals with essential hypertension. N Engl J Med 1994;330:1036–1040.

181. Calver A, Collier J, Moncada S et al. Effect of local intra-arterial NG-mono-methyl-L-arginine in individuals with hypertension: the nitric oxide dilator mechanism appears normal. J Hypertens 1992;10:1025–1031.

182. Panza JA, Casino PR, Kilcoyne CM et al. Role of endothelium-derived nitric oxide in the abnormal endothelium-dependent vascular relaxation of individuals with essential hypertension. Circulation 1993;87:1468–1474.

183. Panza JA, Casino PR, Badar DM et al. Effect of increased availability of endothelium-derived nitric oxide precursor on endothelium-dependent vascular relaxation in normal subjects and in individuals with essential hypertension. Circulation 1993;87:1475–1481.

184. Panza JA, Garcia CE, Kilcoyne CM et al. Impaired endothelium-dependent vasodilation in individuals with essential hypertension. Evidence that nitric oxide abnormality is not localized to a single signal transduction pathway. Circulation 1995;91:1732–1738.

185. Luscher TF. Heterogeneity of endothelial dysfunction in hypertension. Eur Heart J 1992;13:D50–D55.

186. Arnal JF, Michel JB, Harrison DG. Nitric oxide in the pathogenesis of hypertension. Curr Opin Nephrol Hypertens 1995;4:182–188.

187. Luscher TF, Vanhoutte PM, Raij L. Antihypertensive treatment normalizes decreased endothelium-dependent relaxations in rats with salt-induced hypertension. Hypertension 1987;9:III193–III197.

188. Chen PY, Sanders PW. L-arginine abrogates salt-sensitive hypertension in Dahl/Rapp Rats. J Clin Invest 1991;88:1559–1567.

189. Shultz PJ, Tolins JP. Adaptation to increased dietary salt intake in the rate: role of endogenous nitric oxide. J Clin Invest 1993;91:642–650.

190. Lang CC, Stein CM, Brown RM et al. Attenuation of isoproterenol-mediated vasodilation in blacks. N Engl J Med 1995;333:155–160.

191. Luscher TF, Boulanger CM, Dohi Y et al. Endothelium-derived contracting factors. Hypertension 1992;19:117–130.

192. Nakazono K, Watanabe N, Matsuno K et al. Does superoxide underlie the pathogenesis of hypertension? Proc Natl Acad Sci U S A 1991;88:10045–10048.

193. Laursen JB, Rajagopalan S, Galis Z et al. Role of superoxide in angiotensin II-induced but not catecholamine-induced hypertension. Circulation 1997;95:588–593.

194. Rajagopalan S, Kurz S, Munzel T et al. Angiotensin II-mediated hypertension in the rat increases vascular superoxide production via membrane NADH/NADPH oxidase activation. J Clin Invest 1996;97:1916–1923.

195. Garcia CE, Kilcoyne CM, Cardillo C et al. Effect of copper-zinc superoxide dismutase on endothelium-dependent vasodilation in individuals with essential hypertension. Hypertension 1995;26:863–868.

196. Creager MA, Roddy MA. Effect of captopril and enalapril on endothelial function in hypertensive individuals. Hypertension 1994;24:499–505.

197. Schiffrin EL, Deng LY. Comparison of effects of angiotensin I-converting enzyme inhibition and beta blockade for 2 years on function of small arteries from hypertensive individuals. Hypertension 1995;25:699–703.

198. Arnal JF, Warin L, Michel JB. Determinants of aortic cyclic guanosine monophosphate in hypertension induced by chronic inhibition of nitric oxide synthase. J Clin Invest 1992;90:647–652.

199. Shesely EG, Maeda N, Kim HS et al. Elevated blood pressure in mice lacking endothelial nitric oxide synthase. Proc Natl Acad Sci U S A 1996; 93:13176–13181.

200. Huang PL, Huang Z, Mashimo H et al. Hypertension in mice lacking the gene for endothelial nitric oxide synthase. Nature 1995;377:239–242.

201. Panza JA, Quyyumi AA, Callahan TS et al. Effect of antihypertensive treatment on endothelium-dependent vascular relaxation in individuals with essential hypertension. J Am Coll Cardiol 1993;21:1145–1151.

202. Taddei S, Virdis A, Mattei P et al. Defective L-arginine-nitric oxide pathway in offspring of essential hypertensive individuals. Circulation 1996; 94:1298–1303.

203. Johnson RA, Lavesa M, DeSeyn K et al. Heme oxygenase substrates acutely lower blood pressure in hypertensive rats. Am J Physiol 1996;271: H1132–H1138.

204. Palermo A, Bertalero P, Pizza N et al. Decreased fibrinolytic response to adrenergic stimulation in hypertensive individuals. J Hypertens 1989; 7(Suppl):S162–S163.

205. Gleerup G, Vind J, Winther K. Platelet function and fibrinolytic activity during rest and exercise in borderline hypertensive individuals. Eur J Clin Invest 1995;25:266–270.

206. Ridker PM, Gaboury CL, Seely EW et al. Stimulation of plasminogen activator inhibitor in vivo by infusion of angiotensin II. Evidence of a potential interaction between the renin-angiotensin system and fibrinolytic function. Circulation 1993;87:1969–1973.

207. Cohn JN. The management of chronic heart failure. N Engl J Med 1996; 335:490–498.

208. Treasure CB, Alexander RW. The dysfunctional endothelium in heart failure. J Am Coll Cardiol 1993;22(Suppl A):129A–134A.

209. Treasure CB, Vita JA, Cox DA et al. Endothelium-dependent dilation of the coronary microvasculature is impaired in dilated cardiomyopathy. Circulation 1990;81:772–779.

210. Kubo SH, Rector TS, Bank AJ et al. Endothelium-dependent vasodilation is attenuated in individuals with heart failure. Circulation 1991;84: 1589–1596.

211. Katz SD, Biasucci L, Sabba C et al. Impaired endothelium-mediated vasodilation in the peripheral vasculature of individuals with congestive heart failure. J Am Coll Cardiol 1992;19:918–925.

212. Lindsay DC, Holdright DR, Clarke D et al. Endothelial control of lower limb blood flow in chronic heart failure. Heart 1996;75:469–476.

213. Katz SD, Schwarz M, Yuen J et al. Impaired acetylcholine-mediated vasodilation in individuals with congestive heart failure. Role of endothelium-derived vasodilating and vasoconstricting factors. Circulation 1993;88: 55–61.

214. Drexler H. Changes in the peripheral circulation in heart failure. Curr Opin Cardiol 1995;10:268–273.

215. Drexler H, Hayoz D, Munzel T et al. Endothelial function in chronic congestive heart failure. Am J Cardiol 1992;69:1596–1601.

216. Cody RJ, Haas GJ, Binkley PF et al. Plasma endothelin correlates with the extent of pulmonary hypertension in individuals with chronic congestive heart failure. Circulation 1992;85:504–509.

217. Drexler H, Hornig B. Importance of endothelial function in chronic heart failure. J Cardiovasc Pharmacol 1996;27(Suppl 2):S9–S12.

218. Kiowski W, Sutsch G, Hunziker P et al. Evidence of endothelin-1-mediated vasoconstriction in severe chronic heart failure. Lancet 1995;346:732–736.

219. Chin-Dusting JP, Kaye DM, Lefkovits J et al. Dietary supplementation with L-arginine fails to restore endothelial function in forearm resistance arteries of individuals with severe heart failure. J Am Coll Cardiol 1996; 27:1207–1213.

220. Belch JJ, Bridges AB, Scott N et al. Oxygen free radicals and congestive heart failure. Br Heart J 1991;65:245–248.

221. Drexler H, Kurz S, Jeserich M et al. Effect of chronic angiotensin-converting enzyme inhibition on endothelial function in individuals with chronic heart failure [Review]. Am J Cardiol 1995;76:13E–18E.

222. Ng KK, Vane JR. Some properties of angiotensin converting enzyme in the lung in vivo. Nature 1970;225:1142–1144.

223. Packer M, Colucci WS, Sackner-Bernstein JD et al. Double-blind, placebo-controlled study of the effects of carvedilol in individuals with moderate to severe heart failure. The PRECISE Trial. Prospective Randomized Evaluation of Carvedilol on Symptoms and Exercise. Circulation 1996;94: 2793–2799.

224. Packer M, Bristow MR, Cohn JN et al. The effect of carvedilol on morbidity and mortality in individuals with chronic heart failure. US Carvedilol Heart Failure Study Group. N Engl J Med 1996;334:1349–1355.

225. Olsen SL, Gilbert EM, Renlund DG et al. Carvedilol improves left ventricular function and symptoms in chronic heart failure: a double-blind randomized study. J Am Coll Cardiol 1995;25:1225–1231.

226. Feuerstein GZ, Ruffolo RR Jr. Carvedilol, a novel vasodilating beta-blocker with the potential for cardiovascular organ protection [Review]. Eur Heart J 1996;17(Suppl B):24–29.

227. Lopez BL, Christopher TA, Yue TL et al. Carvedilol, a new beta-adrenoreceptor blocker antihypertensive drug, protects against free-radical-induced endothelial dysfunction. Pharmacology 1995;51:165–173.

228. Shen W, Hintze TH, Wolin MS. Nitric oxide. An important signaling mechanism between vascular endothelium and parenchymal cells in the regulation of oxygen consumption. Circulation 1995;92:3505–3512.

229. Xie YW, Shen W, Zhao G et al. Role of endothelium-derived nitric oxide in the modulation of canine myocardial mitochondrial respiration in vitro. Implications for the development of heart failure. Circ Res 1996;79: 381–387.

230. Laursen JB, Harrison DG. Modulation of myocardial oxygen consumption through ACE inhibitors: no effect? Circulation 1997;95:14–16.

231. Keaney JF Jr, Hare JM, Balligand JL et al. Inhibition of nitric oxide synthase augments myocardial contractile responses to beta-adrenergic stimulation. Am J Physiol 1996;271:H2646–H2652.

232. Hou J, Kato H, Cohen RA et al. Angiotensin II-induced cardiac fibrosis in the rat is increased by chronic inhibition of nitric oxide synthase. J Clin Invest 1995;96:2469–2477.

233. Landau C, Lange RA, Hillis LD. Percutaneous transluminal coronary angioplasty. N Engl J Med 1994;330:981–993.

234. Gokce N, Loscalzo J. Are newer antithrombotic drugs better than aspirin after angioplasty? Cardiol Rev 1996;4:5:271–277.

235. Groves PH, Lewis MJ, Cheadle HA et al. SIN-1 reduces platelet adhesion and platelet thrombus formation in a porcine model of balloon angioplasty. Circulation 1993;87:590–597.

236. McNamara DB, Bedi B, Aurora H et al. L-arginine inhibits balloon catheter-induced intimal hyperplasia. Biochem Biophys Res Commun 1993;193: 291–296.

237. Lablanche JM, Grollier G, Lusson JR et al. Effect of the direct nitric oxide donors linsidomine and molsidomine on angiographic restenosis after coronary balloon angioplasty. The ACCORD Study. Circulation 1997;95: 83–89.

238. Koh E, Morimoto S, Jiang B et al. Effects of beraprost sodium, a stable analogue of prostacyclin, on hyperplasia, hypertrophy and glycosaminoglycan synthesis of rat aortic smooth muscle cells. Artery 1993;20:242–252.

239. Shimokawa H, Flavahan NA, Vanhoutte PM. Loss of endothelial pertussis toxin-sensitive G protein function in atherosclerotic porcine coronary arteries. Circulation 1991;83:652–660.

240. Anonymous. Randomized trial of cholesterol lowering in 4444 individuals with coronary heart disease. The Scandinavian Simvastatin Survival Study (4S). Lancet 1994;344:1383–1389.

241. Shepherd J, Cobbe SM, Ford I et al. Prevention of coronary heart disease with pravastatin in men with hypercholesterolemia. West of Scotland Coronary Prevention Study Group. N Engl J Med 1995;333:1301–1307.

242. Sacks FM, Pfeffer MA, Moye LA et al. The effect of pravastatin on coronary events after myocardial infarction in individuals with average cholesterol levels. Cholesterol and Recurrent Events Trial Investigators. N Engl J Med 1996;335:1001–1009.

243. Yusuf S, Wittes J, Friedman L. Overview of results of randomized clinical trials in heart disease. II. Unstable angina, heart failure, primary prevention with aspirin, and risk factor modification. JAMA 1988;260:2259–2263.

244. Law MR, Wald NJ, Thompson SG. By how much and how quickly does reduction in serum cholesterol concentration lower risk of ischaemic heart disease? Br Med J 1994;308:367–372.

245. Brown G, Albers JJ, Fisher LD et al. Regression of coronary artery disease as a result of intensive lipid-lowering therapy in men with high levels of apolipoprotein B. N Engl J Med 1990;323:1289–1298.

246. Loscalzo J. Regression of coronary atherosclerosis. N Engl J Med 1990;323: 1337–1339.

247. Drury J, Cohen JD, Veerendrababu B et al. Brachial artery endothelium-dependent vasodilation in individuals enrolled in the Cholesterol and Recurrent Events (CARE) Study [Abstract]. Circulation 1996;94:I402.

248. Vogel RA, Corretti MC, Plotnick GD. Changes in flow-mediated brachial artery vasoactivity with lowering of desirable cholesterol levels in healthy, middle-aged men. Am J Cardiol 1996;77:37–40.

249. O'Driscoll G, Green D, Taylor RR. Simvastatin, an HMG-coenzyme A reductase inhibitor, improves endothelial function within 1 month. Circulation 1997;95:1126–1131.

250. Andrews TC, Raby K, Barry J et al. Effect of cholesterol reduction on myocardial ischemia in individuals with coronary disease. Circulation 1997;95:324–328.

251. Gould KL, Martucci JP, Goldberg DI et al. Short-term cholesterol lowering decreases size and severity of perfusion abnormalities by positron emission tomography after dipyridamole in individuals with coronary artery

disease. A potential noninvasive marker of healing coronary endothelium. Circulation 1994;89:1530–1538.

252. Wada H, Mori Y, Kaneko T et al. Elevated plasma levels of vascular endothelial cell markers in individuals with hypercholesterolemia. Am J Hematol 1993;44:112–116.

253. Hackman A, Abe Y, Insull W Jr et al. Levels of soluble cell adhesion molecules in individuals with dyslipidemia. Circulation 1996;93: 1334–1338.

254. Badimon JJ, Badimon L, Fuster V. Regression of atherosclerotic lesions by high density lipoprotein fraction in the cholesterol-fed rabbit. J Clin Invest 1990;85:1234–1241.

255. Anonymous. Effects of enalapril on mortality in severe congestive heart failure. Results of the Cooperative North Scandinavian Enalapril Survival Study (CONSENSUS). The CONSENSUS Trial Study Group. N Engl J Med 1987;316:1429–1435.

256. Yusuf S, Pepine CJ, Garces C et al. Effect of enalapril on myocardial infarction and unstable angina in individuals with low ejection fractions. Lancet 1992;340:1173–1178.

257. Alderman MH, Madhavan S, Ooi WL et al. Association of the renin-sodium profile with the risk of myocardial infarction in individuals with hypertension. N Engl J Med 1991;324:1098–1104.

258. Pfeffer MA, Braunwald E, Moye LA et al. Effect of captopril on mortality and morbidity in individuals with left ventricular dysfunction after myocardial infarction. Results of the survival and ventricular enlargement trial. The SAVE Investigators. N Engl J Med 1992;327:669–677.

259. Mancini GBJ, Henry GC, Macaya C et al. Angiotensin-converting enzyme inhibition with quinapril improves endothelial vasomotor dysfunction in individuals with coronary artery disease. Circulation 1996;94:258–265.

260. Antony I, Lerebours G, Nitenberg A. Angiotensin-converting enzyme inhibition restores flow-dependent and cold pressor test-induced dilations in coronary arteries of hypertensive individuals. Circulation 1996; 94:3115–3122.

261. Paul M, Zintz M, Bocker W et al. Characterization and functional analysis of the rat endothelin-1 promoter. Hypertension 1995;25:683–693.

262. Hornig B, Kohler C, Drexler H. Role of bradykinin in mediating vascular effects of angiotensin-converting enzyme inhibitors in humans. Circulation 1997;95:1115–1118.

263. Rosendorff C. The renin-angiotensin system and vascular hypertrophy. J Am Coll Cardiol 1996;28:803–812.

264. Hernandez-Presa M, Bustos C, Ortego M et al. Angiotensin-converting enzyme inhibition prevents arterial nuclear factor-kappa B activation, monocyte chemoattractant protein-1 expression, and macrophage infiltration in a rabbit model of early accelerated atherosclerosis. Circulation 1997; 95:1532–1541.

265. Barrett-Connor E, Bush TL. Estrogen and coronary heart disease in women. JAMA 1991;265:1861–1867.

266. Grodstein F, Stampfer M. The epidemiology of coronary heart disease and estrogen replacement in postmenopausal women. Prog Cardiovasc Dis 1995;38:199–210.

267. Sullivan JM, Vander Zwaag R, Hughes JP et al. Estrogen replacement and coronary artery disease. Effect on survival in post-menopausal women. Arch Intern Med 1990;150:2557–2562.

268. Bush TL, Barrett-Connor E, Cowan LD et al. Cardiovascular mortality and noncontraceptive use of estrogen in women: results from the Lipid Research Clinics Program Follow-up Study. Circulation 1987;75: 1102–1109.

269. Gisclard V, Miller VM, Vanhoutte PM. Effect of 17 beta-estradiol on endothelium-dependent responses in the rabbit. J Pharmacol Exp Ther 1988; 244:19–22.

270. Williams JK, Adams MR, Klopfenstein HS. Estrogen modulates responses of atherosclerotic coronary arteries. Circulation 1990;81:1680–1687.

271. Keaney JF Jr, Shwaery GT, Xu A et al. 17 beta-estradiol preserves endothelial vasodilator function and limits low-density lipoprotein oxidation in hypercholesterolemic swine. Circulation 1994;89:2251–2259.

272. Lieberman EH, Gerhard MD, Uehata A et al. Estrogen improves endothelium-dependent, flow mediated vasodilation in post menopausal women. Ann Intern Med 1994;121:936–941.

273. Pinto S, Virdis A, Ghiadoni L et al. Endogenous estrogen and acetylcholine-induced vasodilation in normotensive women. Hypertension 1997;29: 268–273.

274. Jiang C, Sarrel PM, Poole-Wilson PA et al. Acute effect of 17-beta estradiol on rabbit coronary artery contractile responses to endothelin-1. Am J Physiol 1992;263:H271–H275.

275. Hishikawa K, Nakaki T, Marumo T et al. Up-regulation of nitric oxide synthase by estradiol in human aortic endothelial cells. FEBS Lett 1995; 360:291–293.

276. Arnal JF, Clamens S, Pechet C et al. Ethinylestradiol does not enhance the expression of nitric oxide synthase in bovine endothelial cells but increases the release of bioactive nitric oxide by inhibiting superoxide anion production. Proc Natl Acad Sci U S A 1996;93:4108–4113.

277. Mazière C, Auclair M, Ronveaux MF et al. Estrogens inhibit copper and cell-mediated modification of low density lipoprotein. Atherosclerosis 1991;89:175–182.

278. Shwaery GT, Vita JA, Keaney JF Jr. Antioxidant protection of LDL by physiological concentrations of 17-beta estradiol. Circulation 1997;95: 1378–1385.

279. Sack MN, Rader DJ, Cannon RO 3rd. Oestrogen and inhibition of oxidation of low-density lipoproteins in postmenopausal women. Lancet 1994;343: 269–270.

280. Wakasugi M, Noguchi T, Kazama YI et al. The effects of sex hormones on the synthesis of prostacyclin (PGI2) by vascular tissues. Prostaglandins 1989;37:401–410.

281. Caulin-Glaser T, Watson CA, Pardi R et al. Effects of 17beta-estradiol on cytokine-induced endothelial cell adhesion molecule expression. J Clin Invest 1996;98:36–42.

282. Koh KK, Mincemoyer R, Bui MN et al. Effects of hormone replacement therapy on fibrinolysis in postmenopausal women. N Engl J Med 1997; 336:683–690.

283. Gebara OC, Mittleman MA, Sutherland P et al. Association between increased estrogen status and increased fibrinolytic potential in the Framingham Offspring Study. Circulation 1995;91:1952–1958.

284. Paffenbarger RS Jr, Hyde RT, Wing AL et al. The association of changes in physical-activity level and other lifestyle characteristics with mortality among men. N Engl J Med 1993;328:538–545.

285. Blair SN, Kohl HW III, Barlow CE et al. Changes in physical fitness and all-cause mortality. A prospective study of healthy and unhealthy men. JAMA 1995;273:1093–1098.

286. Niebauer J, Cooke JP. Cardiovascular effects of exercise: role of endothelial shear stress. J Am Coll Cardiol 1996;28:1652–1660.

287. Wang J, Wolin MS, Hintze TH. Chronic exercise enhances endothelium-mediated dilation of epicardial coronary artery in conscious dogs. Circ Res 1993;73:829–838.

288. Muller JM, Myers PR, Laughlin MH. Vasodilator responses of coronary resistance arteries of exercise-trained pigs. Circulation 1994;89:2308–2314.

289. Sun D, Huang A, Koller A et al. Short-term daily exercise activity enhances endothelial NO synthesis in skeletal muscle arterioles of rats. J Appl Physiol 1994;76:2241–2247.

290. Hornig B, Maier V, Drexler H. Physical training improves endothelial function in individuals with chronic heart failure. Circulation 1996;93:210–214.

291. Clarkson P, Montgomery H, Donald A et al. Exercise training enhances endothelial function in young men [Abstract]. J Am Coll Cardiol 1996; 288A.

292. Stratton JR, Chandler WL, Schwartz RS et al. Effects of physical conditioning on fibrinolytic variables and fibrinogen in young and old healthy adults. Circulation 1991;83:1692–1697.

293. Kamiya A, Togawa T. Adaptive regulation of wall shear stress to flow change in the canine carotid artery. Am J Physiol 1980;239:H14–H21.

294. Langille BL, O'Donnell F. Reduction in arterial diameter produced by chronic decreases in blood flow are endothelium-dependent. Science 1986; 231:405–407.

295. Mann GV, Spoerry A, Gray M et al. Atherosclerosis in the Masai. Am J Epidemiol 1972;95:26–37.

296. Sessa WC, Harrison JK, Barber CM et al. Molecular cloning and expression of a cDNA encoding endothelial cell nitric oxide synthase. J Biol Chem 1992;267:15274–15276.

297. Noris M, Morigi M, Donadelli R et al. Nitric oxide synthesis by cultured endothelial cells is modulated by flow conditions. Circ Res 1995;76: 536–543.

298. Sessa WC, Pritchard K, Seyedi N et al. Chronic exercise in dogs increases coronary vascular nitric oxide production and endothelial cell nitric oxide synthase gene expression. Circ Res 1994;74:349–353.

299. Koller A, Huang A, Sun D et al. Exercise training augments flow-dependent dilation in rat skeletal muscle arterioles: role of endothelial nitric oxide and prostaglandins. Circ Res 1995;76:544–550.

300. Stampfer MJ, Hennekens CH, Manson JE et al. Vitamin E consumption and the risk of coronary disease in women. N Engl J Med 1993;328:1444–1449.

301. Rimm EB, Stampfer MJ, Ascherio A et al. Vitamin E consumption and the risk of coronary heart disease in men. N Engl J Med 1993;328:1450–1456.

302. Rapola JM, Virtamo J, Haukka JK et al. Effect of vitamin E and beta carotene on the incidence of angina pectoris. A randomized, double-blind, controlled trial. JAMA 1996;275:693–698.

303. Stephens NG, Parsons A, Schofield PM et al. Randomised controlled trial of vitamin E in individuals with coronary disease: Cambridge Heart Antioxidant Study (CHAOS). Lancet 1996;347:781–786.

304. Kritchevsky SB, Shimakawa T, Tell GS et al. Dietary antioxidants and carotid artery wall thickness: the ARIC study. Circulation 1995;92: 2142–2150.

305. Keaney JF Jr, Guo Y, Cunningham D et al. Vascular incorporation of alpha-tocopherol prevents endothelial dysfunction due to oxidized LDL by inhibiting protein kinase C stimulation. J Clin Invest 1996;98: 386–394.

306. Navab M, Imes SS, Hama SY et al. Monocyte transmigration induced by modification of low density lipoprotein in cocultures of human aortic wall cells is due to induction of monocyte chemotactic protein 1 synthesis and is abolished by high density lipoprotein. J Clin Invest 1991;88: 2039–2046.

307. Faruqi R, De La Motte C, Dicorleto PE. Alpha-tocopherol inhibits agonist-induced monocytic cell adhesion to cultured human endothelial cells. J Clin Invest 1994;94:592–600.

308. Anderson TJ, Meredith IT, Yeung AC et al. The effect of cholesterol lowering and antioxidant therapy on endothelium-dependent coronary vasomotion. N Engl J Med 1995;332:488–493.

309. Elliott TG, Barth JD, Mancini GB. Effects of vitamin E on endothelial function in men after myocardial infarction. Am J Cardiol 1995;76:1188–1190.

310. Gilligan DM, Sack MN, Guetta V et al. Effect of antioxidant vitamins on low density lipoprotein oxidation and impaired endothelium-dependent vasodilation in individuals with hypercholesterolemia. J Am Coll Cardiol 1994;24:1611–1617.

311. Freedman JE, Farhat JH, Loscalzo J et al. Alpha-tocopherol inhibits aggregation of human platelets by a protein kinase C-dependent mechanism. Circulation 1996;94:2434–2440.

312. Boscoboinik D, Szewczyk A, Azzi A. Alpha-tocopherol (vitamin E) regulates vascular smooth muscle cell proliferation and protein kinase C activity. Arch Biochem Biophys 1991;286:264–269.

313. Levine GN, Frei B, Koulouris SN et al. Ascorbic acid reverses endothelial vasomotor dysfunction in individuals with coronary artery disease. Circulation 1996;96:1107–1113.

314. Heitzer T, Just H, Munzel T. Antioxidant vitamin C improves endothelial dysfunction on chronic smokers. Circulation 1996;94:6–9.

315. Weber C, Erl W, Weber K et al. Increased adhesiveness of isolated monocytes to endothelium is prevented by vitamin C intake in smokers. Circulation 1996;93:1488–1492.

316. Lehr HA, Frei B, Arfors KE. Vitamin C prevents cigarette smoke-induced leukocyte aggregation and adhesion to endothelium *in vivo*. Proc Natl Acad Sci U S A 1994;91:7688–7692.

317. Meister A. Glutathione-ascorbic acid antioxidant system in animals. J Biol Chem 1994;269:9397–9400.

318. Ghigo D, Alessio P, Foco A et al. Nitric oxide synthesis is impaired in glutathione-depleted human umbilical vein endothelial cells. Am J Physiol 1993;265:C728–C732.

319. Vita JA, Frei B, Holbrook M et al. Endothelial function in coronary artery disease is sensitive to intracellular Redox state [Abstract]. Circulation 1997;95:I–286.

320. Kuzuya M, Naito M, Funaki C et al. Protective role of intracellular glutathione against oxidized low density lipoprotein in cultured cells. Biochem Biophys Res Commun 1989;163:1466–1472.

321. Hofmann H, Schmidt HH. Thiol dependence of nitric oxide synthase. Biochemistry 1995;34:13443–13452.

322. Komori Y, Hyun J, Chiang K et al. The role of thiols in the apparent activation of rat brain nitric oxide synthase (NOS). J Biochem 1995;117:923–927.

323. Patel JM, Abeles AJ, Block ER. Nitric oxide exposure and sulfhydryl modulation alter L-arginine transport in cultured pulmonary artery endothelial cells. Free Radic Biol Med 1996;20:629–637.

324. Briviba K, Sies H. Nonenzymatic antioxidant defense systems. In: Frei B, ed. Natural antioxidants in human health and disease. San Diego: Academic Press, 1994:107–128.

325. McMurray J, Chopra M, Abdullah I et al. Evidence for oxidative stress in unstable angina. Br Heart J 1992;68:454–457.

326. Creager MA, Roddy MA, Boles K et al. N-acetylcysteine does not influence the activity of endothelium derived relaxing factor *in vivo*. Hypertension 1997;29:668–672.

327. Celermajer DS, Sorensen KE, Georgakopoulos D et al. Cigarette smoking is associated with dose-related and potentially reversible impairment of endothelium-dependent dilation in healthy young adults. Circulation 1993;88:2149–2155.

328. Cooke JP, Tsao PS. Arginine: a new therapy for atherosclerosis. Circulation 1997;95:311–312.

329. Cooke JP, Singer AH, Tsao P et al. Antiatherogenic effects of L-arginine in the hypercholesterolemic rabbit. J Clin Invest 1992;90:1168–1172.

330. Drexler H, Zeiher AM, Meinzer K et al. Correction of endothelial dysfunction in coronary microcirculation of hypercholesterolemic individuals by L-arginine. Lancet 1991;338:1546–1550.

331. Creager MA, Gallagher SJ, Girerd XJ et al. L-arginine improves endothelium-dependent vasodilation in hypercholesterolemic humans. J Clin Invest 1992;90:1248–1253.

332. Clarkson P, Adams MR, Powe AJ. Oral L-arginine improves endothelium-dependent dilation in hypercholesterolemic young adults. J Clin Invest 1994;67:1989–1994.

333. Wolf A, Zalpour C, Theilmeier G et al. Dietary L-arginine supplementation normalizes platelet aggregation in hypercholesterolemic humans. J Am Coll Cardiol 1997;29:479–485.

334. Adams MR, Jessup W, Hailstones D et al. L-arginine reduces human monocyte adhesion to vascular endothelium and endothelial expression of cell adhesion molecules. Circulation 1997;95:662–668.

335. Lefer AM. Nitric oxide: nature's naturally occurring leukocyte inhibitor. Circulation 1997;95:553–554.

336. Celermajer DS, Sorensen K, Ryalls M et al. Impaired endothelial function occurs in the systemic arteries of children with homozygous homocystinuria but not in their heterozygous parents. J Am Coll Cardiol 1993;22:854–858.

337. Tawakol A, Omland T, Gerhard M et al. Hyperhomocyst (e) inemia is associated with impaired endothelium-dependent vasodilation in humans. Circulation 1997;95:1119–1121.

338. Stroes E, Kastelein J, Cosentino F et al. Tetrahydrobiopterin restores endothelial function in hypercholesterolemia. J Clin Invest 1997;99:41–46.

339. Leung WH, Lau CP, Wong CK. Beneficial effect of cholesterol-lowering therapy on coronary endothelium-dependent relaxation in hypercholesterolemic individuals. Lancet 1993;341:1496–1500.

340. Egashira K, Hirooka Y, Kai H et al. Reduction in serum cholesterol with pravastatin improves endothelium-dependent coronary vasomotion in individuals with hypercholesterolemia. Circulation 1994;89:2519–2524.

341. Yeung A, Hodgson JM, Winniford M et al. Assessment of coronary vascular reactivity after cholesterol lowering [Abstract]. Circulation 1996;94:I402.

# CHAPTER 42

# INTERACTION OF BLOOD AND ARTIFICIAL SURFACES

## Brian Richard Smith and Kenneth A. Ault

## INTRODUCTION

During normal resting physiology, the circulating coagulation and immune systems must maintain a state of readiness but at the same time fail to respond to minor alterations in the intravascular and extravascular environment of the host. This requires a delicately balanced homeostasis that involves the interaction of the endothelium with both soluble and cellular components of the blood. Modern medical practice routinely violates that balance under several circumstances that force blood components to make contact with nonendothelialized surfaces. These include procedures in which artificial organs are implanted, simple or complex catheters are inserted transiently or permanently into the individual, and in processes such as hemodialysis and extracorporeal circulation, which require the blood to leave the vasculature for extended periods but to return ultimately to the individual in a (hopefully) minimally altered state. Even procedures such as implantation of orthopedic appliances result in a gradual exposure of blood elements to a nonendothelial, "nonself" surface. A "biocompatible" material would perfectly substitute for the endothelium so that soluble and cellular blood components would remain entirely naive of its foreign presence. The first biomaterial used in clinical practice was a stainless steel hip nail used before World War II, and the first implantable cardiovascular device was a methylmethacrylate ball valve used to treat aortic regurgitation by Charles Hufnagel in 1953 (1). Although biomaterial science has advanced sufficiently in the past 45

years to allow all the aforementioned modern techniques to occur on a routine basis, true biocompatibility of artificial surfaces remains a relatively distant and elusive goal (2). The clinical consequences of a failure to achieve biocompatability include excessive thrombogenicity and proinflammatory diathesis of these artificial surfaces. These, in turn, result in neurologic, vascular, and other complications from local and distant thrombus as well as local and distant embolization; pulmonary and other inflammatory complications from the vascular egress and activation of phagocytes (with "reperfusion injury" and multiorgan failure syndrome); and local and distant bleeding related to the induction of platelet dysfunction or activated fibrinolysis. In complex clinical settings, such as cardiopulmonary bypass, these interactions at the blood-biomaterial interface have been described as generating a "whole body inflammatory response" (3). In addition to these directly generated pathophysiologies, imperfect biomaterials are also a constant stimulatory nidus for infection (4, 5). Contact with currently used artificial surfaces results in direct activation of both soluble protein and cellular homeostatic systems, including a) the complement system (predominantly via the alternative pathway but often also involving the classical system); b) the soluble protein contact system (kallikrein and related molecules); c) the intrinsic and extrinsic coagulation cascades; d) platelets; e) leukocytes (including granulocytes, monocytes, and lymphocytes); and, indirectly, f) nearby endothelial cells. Some of these interactions are illustrated schematically in Fig. 42.1. In most clinical settings involving arti-

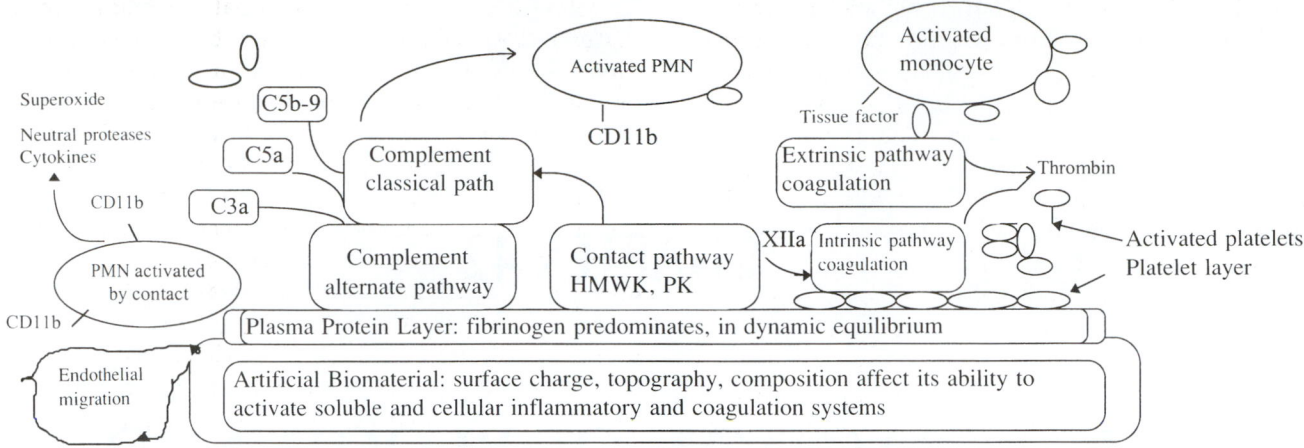

**FIGURE 42.1.** Schematic of the interactions of blood with artificial surfaces. The interactions of blood with artificial membranes are complex and include deposition of a plasma protein layer composed predominantly of conformationally altered fibrinogen with overlayering of adherent platelets. Complement is activated via the alternative pathway and indirectly through the classic pathway generating anaphylotoxins and the membrane attack complex. The contact system is similarly activated and helps drive the intrinsic pathway of coagulation. Platelet, neutrophil, and monocyte activation occur both through direct interactions with the artificial membrane and via soluble intermediates. Activated monocytes help drive the extrinsic (tissue factor) coagulation pathway, and both monocytes and granulocytes themselves release a variety of cytokines and reactive intermediates. Over time, endothelialization of the biomaterial occurs if left in place. *PMN,* polymorphonuclear leukocyte; *HMWK,* high-molecular-weight kininogen; *PK,* prekallikrein.

ficial surface pathophysiology, there are a myriad of ongoing related processes that also activate these soluble and cellular systems. For example, in cardiopulmonary bypass and extracorporeal membrane oxygenation, heparinization, and subsequent protamine administration, administration of ventilatory gases and anesthesia, tissue hypoxia, and blood transfusion all contribute to the end result observed in the individual. In hemodialysis, uremia and concomitant medication may directly alter components of the soluble and cellular systems. The effects of transient exposure to an artificial surface may last for days to weeks after this exposure. Finally, it has become clearer in recent years that none of the immune and coagulation systems are separate; rather, they constantly interact at both a soluble and cellular level (6). This chapter will focus on the best understood subsets of these alterations in normal circulatory physiology induced by artificial surfaces and will attempt to emphasize the most clinically relevant features of these phenomena.

# BIOMATERIAL COMPOSITION, ALTERATION OVER TIME, AND BIOCOMPATIBILITY

Understanding the pathobiology of the blood-biomaterial interface would be far simpler if different artificial surfaces were interchangeable with respect to their pathophysiologic effects, were inert and did not alter

with time in the individual, and generated their interactions with blood components through direct contact of blood with the nonblood surface. Unfortunately, none of these assumptions is correct. Biomaterials that contact the blood vary widely in their innate composition. For example, dialysis membranes may be composed of regenerated cellulose and variants, such as cuprophan, or of a host of other materials including polysulfone, polyacrylonitrile (PAN), and polymethylmethacrylate (PMMA). Similarly, transient and permanent intravascular and extravascular tubing may consist of knitted dacron (polyethylene terephthalate), woven dacron, polycarbonate, polyvinylchloride, polyurethane, expanded polytetrafluorethylene (teflon, PTFE), silicone rubber (polydimethyl sioloxane, PDMS), or high density polyethylene, to name just a few. Even materials that are placed in an extravascular location will be significantly influenced by blood-biomaterial interactions. For example, orthopedic devices made of titanium or PMMA, although not designed to have significant interaction with vascular components, in fact appear to do so over time. This occurs in part via particulate biomaterial phagocytosis by infiltrating monocyte-macrophages, which subsequently release important mediators such as interleukin (IL)-1β, IL-6, and prostaglandin E2(PGE2), all of which may then go on to participate in subsequent osteolysis (7).

All these biomaterials are far from being completely "biostable" and inert. They may degrade significantly over time and, through that erosive process, establish new blood-biomaterial interactions. This degradation process itself is often related to prolonged interaction with blood components. For example, the polyetherurethanes used as insulation on cardiac pacemaker wires undergo "environmental stress cracking," which may be caused by interacting phagocytes secreting chlorine and nitric oxide based oxidants (8). Some biomaterials are designed to be biodegradable for use in devices such as intravascular stents; the poly(organo)-phosphazenes are a good example of this class of materials (9, 10). In these cases, the routinely expected degradation products also often have their own unique aspects of interacting with soluble and cellular elements of the blood (8). Plasticizers, such as di-2-ethyl-hexyl-phthalate, that are used in the production of many polymers, may leach from the material over time and affect platelets and other cells (11). Finally, the relative prothrombotic and proinflammatory properties of different materials, when used in humans, may be difficult to predict from animal models. For example, although metal (tantalum) stents in small-vessels are associated with a significant restenosis rate, covering these stents with polyethylacrylate/PMMA has actually led to an increased thrombotic tendency in some studies (12), emphasizing the difficulty in creating biocompatible materials. Although it is convenient to consider all of these biomaterials as representing a single class of stable compounds that interact similarly in the individual, this is clearly not an accurate picture.

The interactions of blood components with a foreign biomaterial are also sometimes implicitly considered to involve direct, unadulterated contact with the foreign surface. This is seldom, if ever, the case. Plasma proteins are adsorbed onto the surface of foreign biomaterials very rapidly (within seconds) and form a protein layer that is approximately 200 Å thick (13–15). This adsorption, the detailed molecular basis for which is not yet well worked out, is selective. Fibrinogen is generally adsorbed in the highest concentration; once adsorbed its conformational structure appears to be altered (16, 17). Adsorption differs between biomaterials with hydrophobic surfaces adsorbing more fibrinogen than hydrophilic surfaces. The location and the conformation of deposited fibrinogen may also relate to shear forces imparted to the blood as it circulates over the artificial surface (18). In addition to fibrinogen, albumin, gamma globulin, fibronectin, lipoproteins, thrombospondin, factor XII, high molecular weight kininogen, prekallikrein, plasminogen, and von Willebrand factor/factor VIII complex are all also adsorbed onto artificial surfaces. These proteins are in a dynamic equilibrium with those in the plasma (19). For example, over time, fibrinogen is partially replaced with high molecular weight kininogen, a process referred to as the "Vroman effect" (13, 20).

The presence of these adsorbed blood proteins has a profound effect on the biocompatibility of a specific material and its interaction with blood components. Thus, polyether-polyurethane is more effective at spontaneously inducing superoxide production by neutrophils compared to expanded PTFE when in direct contact with the granulocyte, but the reactions on both materials are markedly diminished when the biopolymer is first allowed to incubate with normal plasma proteins. By contrast, woven dacron shows no or minimal direct activation of neutrophils (measured by superoxide production) by itself, yet will vigorously activate the granulocytes after preincubation with plasma proteins (19). As a rule, gamma globulin and fibrinogen promote platelet and leukocyte adhesion and possibly activation, whereas albumin tends to neutralize these effects (21). Thus the relative capacity of an artificial surface to affect blood components may change significantly based on the adsorbed protein composition of its blood-exposed surfaces.

Topographic aspects of the biomaterial and the particular clinical application for the foreign substance also greatly influence the observed pathophysiology. For example, in cardiac bypass, bubble oxygenators result in the generation of more reactive intermediates, such as C3a and C5a, than do membrane oxygenators (22). Hemodialysis membranes may differ with respect to generation of reactive intermediates based on the particular material from which they are constructed and on their pore size (23). Many artificial surfaces not only result in generation of soluble reactive intermediates. They may adsorb these same intermediates onto their surface and neutralize their activity (23–25). The final clinical result will reflect the net sum of this addition and subtraction kinetic process.

Finally, there is no single definition of overall "biocompatibility" of an artificial surface. As will be discussed further, artificial surfaces produce several effects on soluble and cellular blood components, and different materials may be more or less interactive with any one of those systems. An attempt will be made to define some of the key physiochemical determinants to interactions at the biomaterial-blood interface for each of the affected homeostatic systems as those separate systems are discussed.

# COMPLEMENT ACTIVATION BY ARTIFICIAL SURFACES

## MECHANISMS OF COMPLEMENT ACTIVATION AND COMPLEMENT-MEDIATED CELL DAMAGE

One of the major homeostatic systems affected by artificial surfaces is the complement cascade (Fig. 42.2). The

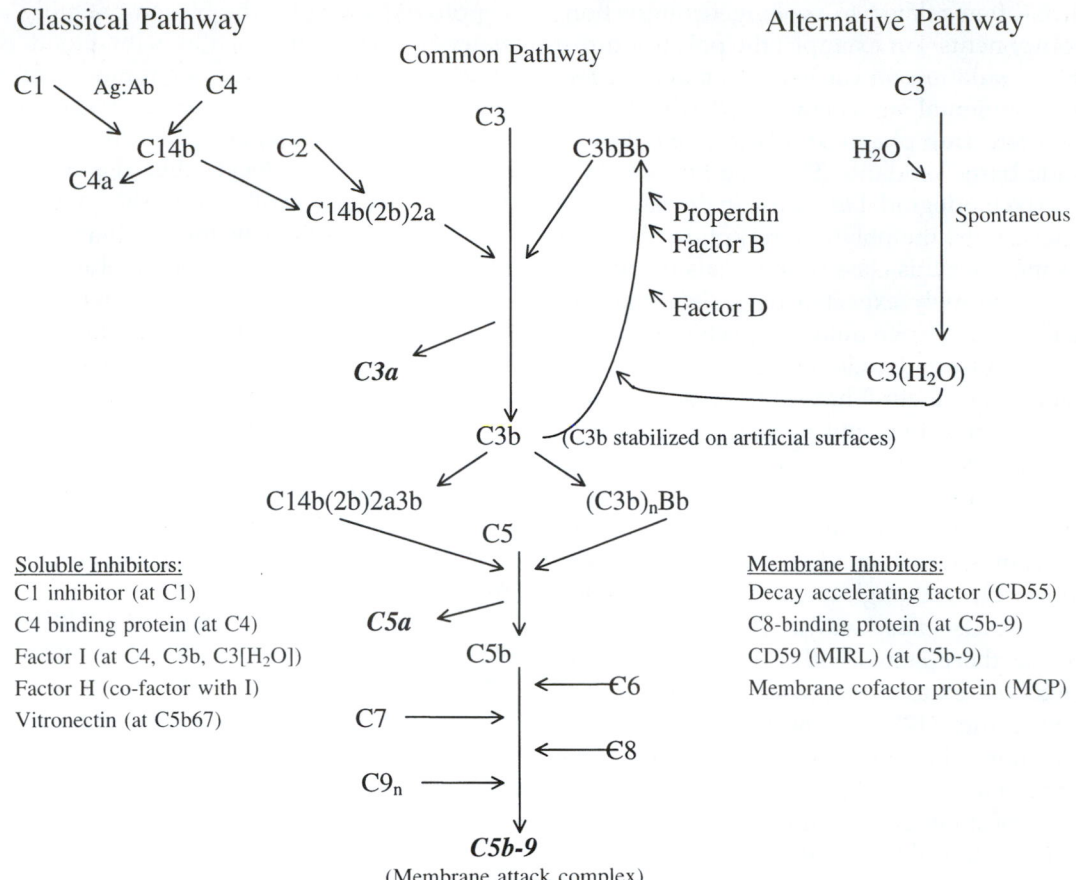

**FIGURE 42.2.** Schematic of the complement system. Complement activation occurs either via the classic pathway, initiated by antigen:antibody (Ag:Ab) complexes and by some other molecular complexes such as heparin:protamine and involving the generation of C3 convertase activity by interaction of C1, C4 and C2, or via the alternate pathway. C3 undergoes continuous low grade hydrolysis in plasma and, with C3b affixed to a cell or artificial membrane surface, will interact with properdin, factor B, and factor D to form a potent C3 convertase. C3 convertase leads to generation of the anaphylatoxin C3a and well as C3b; the latter undergoes further interactions to generate C5 convertase activity with production of anaphylatoxin C5a as well as C5b. Further complement component interactions in the common pathway generate the membrane attack complex, C5b-9. Inhibitors of the complement cascade include both soluble and cell membrane species. MIRL, membrane inhibitor of reactive lysis.

major mechanism by which complement is directly activated in the presence of an artificial surface is believed to involve the alternative complement pathway. This is not to say that under specific clinical circumstances (such as cardiopulmonary bypass), the classic pathway may not also be involved or perhaps even predominate as the initiator of complement-mediated injury. Although it is not within the scope of this chapter to review the complement system in detail, a brief explanation of the likely pathways involved is nonetheless appropriate here (26, 27).

The central actor in the complement cascade is component C3; this molecule is the prime target and central propagator of both the alternative and the classic pathways. Activation of C3, which involves its proteolysis into C3a and C3b components, takes place through a relatively straightforward cascade mechanism in the case of the classic pathway, with the initiating antibody-

antigen complexes providing nonself specificity and resulting in activation of C1, C2, and C4 and their association to form a C3 convertase. The alternative pathway of C3 activation is a more complex system that depends heavily on a balance of inhibitory and activating components and on solid versus fluid phase reactivity. The alternative pathway uses a much less rigorous means of distinguishing self from nonself. The following is a simplification of our current knowledge of a complex and still imperfectly understood alternative pathway.

Complement component C3 likely undergoes continuous low-level hydrolysis in the blood, resulting in generation of a fluid phase C3 convertase that can cleave C3 molecules into C3a and C3b components. For this reaction to be significantly self-perpetuating requires C3b to be stabilized, preferably on a nucleophilic membrane or other biological or artificial surface. Thereafter, C3b is able to participate in further elements of the reaction sequence. C3a, by contrast, is more stable and can exist for prolonged periods in the fluid phase. Also in the fluid phase, factor D converts factor B into Ba and Bb fragments. Bb fragments can combine with C3b to form C3bBb, a relatively potent C3 convertase. Further clustering of these moieties (C3b(n)Bb) also results in formation of C5 convertase activity, perpetuating the reaction sequence. Properdin (factor P) stabilizes the solid phase components of the C3 and C5 convertases generated by these pathways. Counteracting these activities is factor H, an alternative pathway inhibitor that acts in either the fluid or cell-bound phase and that, when attached to C3b, prevents further interaction of factor B with C3b. Another participant in the inhibitory arm, factor I, can cleave C3b after C3b has associated with factor H, generating iC3b, which is impotent with regard to participation in C3 convertase activity. Additional fluid-phase regulators include C1 inhibitor, which removes C1r and C1s from the C1 complex; C4b binding protein, which accelerates decay of C4b2a and is a factor I cofactor; anaphylatoxin inactivator, which inactivates C3a, C4a and C5a; and S-protein (vitronectin), which binds C5b-7, preventing it from attaching to cell membranes (see below). The ultimate activity of complement both directly on the involved solid phase and in terms of activated, long-lived components that are released into the fluid phase depends on the balance between these activating and inhibitory pathways. Some of these components are summarized in Table 42.1.

It should be clear on the basis of these mechanistic considerations that the alternative pathway is suboptimal in distinguishing self from nonself and may indiscriminately deposit C3 components on cell membranes. Mammalian cells use many mechanisms to control the C3 convertase activity that may be generated on their surface. These include expression of the gylocophosphatidyl (gpi)-linked proteins decay accelerating factor (DAF or CD55), which accelerates decay of C4b2a and C3bBb complexes, and membrane inhibitor of reactive lysis (MIRL or CD59), which binds C8 and C9, preventing formation of the membrane attack complex (MAC). Also included in the cell membrane's intrinsic protective repertoire is the iC3b receptor CD11b/CD18, homologous restriction factor or C8 binding protein, complement receptor 1 (CR1), and membrane cofactor protein (MCP, CD46). Some of these proteins' roles in regulation is summarized in Table 42.2. The importance of these membrane-bound regulatory molecules is illustrated by the acquired, clonal disorder, paroxysmal nocturnal hemoglobinuria (PNH). Patients with PNH cannot express DAF and MIRL on the surface of their clonally abnormal hematopoietic cells because of a universal defect in one or more enzymes crucial to the production of the gpi link. Hence these individuals develop severe consequences of unopposed comple-

**TABLE 42.1.** Active Mediator Components of the Complement System

**Initiation of the Classical Pathway**

| | | |
|---|---|---|
| C1 | C1q | Binds to antigen-antibody complex, activates C1r |
| | C1r | Cleaves C1s to an active protease form |
| | C1s | Cleaves both C4 and C2 |

**Propagation of the Classical Pathway**

| | | |
|---|---|---|
| C4 | C4a | Weak anaphylatoxin |
| | C4b | Binds C2 to promote cleavage by C1s; Opsonin—covalently binds to pathogens |
| C2 | C2a | Unknown function |
| | C2b | Active enzyme for the classical pathway C3/C5 convertase |

**Initiation and Propagation of the Alternate Pathway**

| | | |
|---|---|---|
| C3 | C3b | Binds to cell surfaces, binds B for cleavage by D |
| | C3Bb | Active alternate pathway C3/C5 convertase |
| B | Ba | Unknown function |
| | Bb | The active enzyme of the C3Bb convertase |
| D | D | Serine protease, cleaves B bound to C3b to Ba and Bb |

**Common Pathway**

| | | |
|---|---|---|
| C3 | C3a | Anaphylatoxin, persists as both soluble and cell-bound |
| | C3b | Binds to cell surfaces, opsonizes, initiates alternate pathway amplification, binds C5 for cleavage by C2b |

**Terminal Components**

| | | |
|---|---|---|
| C5 | C5a | Anaphylotoxin, rapidly degraded if not surface-bound |
| | C5b | Initiates assembly of membrane attack complex (MAC) |
| C6 | C6 | Binds C5b, acceptor for C7 |
| C7 | C7 | Binds C5bC6, amphiphilic complex inserts into membrane |
| C8 | C8 | Binds C5b67, initiates polymerization of C9 |
| C9 | C9 | Polymerizes with other MAC components to form the membrane spanning, lytic channel (MAC) |

ment activation on the cell surface, including red cell hemolysis and platelet activation resulting in hypercoagulability.

Once C3 and C5 convertase activity has been established in the fluid phase or on the cell surface, the major effector complement molecules are produced (Table 42.1

## TABLE 42.2. Regulatory Components of the Complement System

**Soluble Regulatory Proteins**

| | |
|---|---|
| C1 Inhibitor | Binds to activated C1rC1s, removing it from C1q |
| C4-binding protein | Binds C4b replacing C2b; cofactor for C4b cleavage by I |
| H | Binds C3b displacing Bb; cofactor for I |
| I | Serine protease that cleaves C3b aided by H, MCP, or CR1 |
| CR1 | Binds C4b, displacing C2b; cofactor for C4b cleavage by I |

**Cell Surface Regulatory Proteins**

| | |
|---|---|
| DAF (CD55) | Displaces Bb from C3b and C2b from C4b |
| MCP | Promotes C3b and C4b inactivation by I |
| MIRL (CD59) | Prevents formation of MAC on homologous cells |

**Cell Surface Complement Receptors**

| | |
|---|---|
| CR1 | Binds C3b and C4b promoting decay, stimulates phagocytosis |
| CR2 | Binds C3d, C3dg, iC3b; binds Epstein-Barr Virus |
| CR3 (CD11b/CD18) | Binds iC3b, stimulates phagocytosis, multiple functions |
| CR4 (CD11c/CD18) | Binds iC3b, stimulates phagocytosis |
| C1q Receptor | Binds immune complexes to phagocytes |

and Fig. 42.2). In terms of the principal participants in the clinical consequences of artificial membrane-induced pathophysiology, there are two major categories: the anaphylotoxins C3a and C5a and the MAC proteins C5b through C9 (C5b-9). C4a is also an anaphylatoxin, albeit of far less potency than C3a or C5a. The anaphylotoxins have promiscuous proinflammatory biological activity. They cause increased vascular permeability, enhanced smooth muscle contraction, and enhanced histamine release. They demonstrate potent chemotactic activity, the ability to promote release of oxidative products from phagocytes, and have important opsonization properties. The membrane attack complex is formed from the combination of C5b in loose association with the C3b of the convertase along with C6 and C7. The resultant C5b-7 complex dissociates from the con-

vertase and can transiently bind to cell membranes; a hydrophilic to amphiphilic transition occurs that permits attack complex insertion into the membrane. The addition of C8 results in the triggering for polymerization of up to eighteen C9 molecules that then form the ring-like C5b-9 membrane attack complex. Once formed, the MAC provides a channel for indiscriminate entry of electrolytes into the cell, causing cell lysis.

## INITIATION OF COMPLEMENT ACTIVATION BY BIOMATERIALS

Artificial membranes obviously do not have the protective proteins that normally control complement activation on the surface of human cells. Hence, they are likely to allow C3 convertase and C5 convertase activity to occur in a relatively unopposed fashion once appropriate complement components have been deposited on their surfaces. With respect to such deposition of the continually formed fluid-phase complement components, artificial membranes appear to mimic natural stimuli for alternative pathway activation, such as bacterial cell walls and other eukaryotic and prokaryotic "foreign" membranes. In particular, the physical and ionic charge configuration of the artificial luminal wall of polymer biomaterials provides a very stable solid-phase surface for the binding of C3b and for the conformational change that reduces the affinity of C3b for factor H. Once this occurs, the lack of regulatory molecules on the solid phase allows for relatively unopposed participation of C3b and the other alternative pathway components in enhanced activation of the complement cascade. Thus, many biomaterials provide an unfortunately ideal substrate for complement activation via the alternative pathway.

The precise physiochemical properties of naturally occurring membranes that favor C3 and C5 convertase activity are not fully known. In the case of artificial membranes, exposed amino- and hydroxyl-groups contribute toward increased complement generation, whereas negatively charged species such as $SO_3$-favor association of factor H with C3b and are anticomplementary (28–30). The relationship of structure to complement activation is clearly a complex one. It is known, for example, that two membranes that generate similar amounts of C3a may not generate the same quantities of C5a, implying that C5 convertase activity on artificial surfaces may be separable from C3 convertase activity (30). The net effect of an artificial membrane on the individual will relate to the capacity of that membrane to support complement activation and to the ability of the surface to adsorb activated complement components and remove them from the individual's circulation after they have been generated. For example, some dialysis membranes, such as those composed of acrylonitrile and sodium methylsulfonate copolymers, activate complement but produce relatively low levels of fluid phase-activated components because of their ability to adsorb C3 and C3a efficiently (23–25).

## COMPLEMENT ACTIVATION IN CLINICAL CIRCUMSTANCES INVOLVING ARTIFICIAL SURFACES

Complement is significantly activated during extracorporeal circulation (31) and is also significantly activated during hemodialysis. It is activated to a greater extent when dialysis is undertaken with cellulose-based membranes such as cuprophan when compared with the activation associated with polysulfone membranes (32–36). Although the primary pathway for this activation by artificial surfaces is believed to be the alternative complement sequence, it should be noted that the artificial surfaces involved in cardiopulmonary bypass (and in hemodialysis) also activate the soluble protein contact system, which may in turn activate complement via the classic pathway (see below). In cardiac bypass, as well as in other clinical scenarios where heparin is used as a transient anticoagulant to prevent thrombosis during artificial surface exposure, another stimulant of the complement system must be considered. At the end of bypass, protamine is administered to neutralize heparin; heparin-protamine complexes activate the complement cascade via the classic pathway (37). Based on these considerations, classic pathway complement activation has been considered by some as the primary means of activating complement during cardiac bypass extracorporeal circulation (31, 38).

Complement activation, in turn, results in activation of leukocytes, of platelets, and likely of endothelial cells. In the case of hemodialysis, complement-mediated activation of leukocytes, which is accompanied by up-regulation of CD11b/CD18 through mobilization of intracellular granules, explains the neutropenia that is frequently observed in this setting (35, 36, 39–41). The incidence and degree of leukopenia observed correlates with the ability of a given dialysis membrane to activate complement—in particular, the alternate complement pathway. Reused cuprophane membranes that are treated with formaldehyde stabilize C3b-like molecules on their surface, prevent new C3b deposition, and attenuate complement activation and its resultant leukopenia (42). The $\beta_2$ integrins and the selectins are the two classes of molecules whose role in neutrophil and other phagocyte adhesion has been well established. Complement is believed to mediate the adhesive and perhaps aggregatory effects of hemodialysis by initially stimulating functional and quantitative up-regulation of CD11b/CD18 (43–48) on neutrophils, resulting in increased adhesion and margination. This is then followed by down-regulation of L-selectin and CD43 (44, 46) with consequent rebound leukocytosis.

Complement activation in the clinical setting affects more than just vascular tone and granulocyte adhesion and activation. The complement anaphylatoxins including C5a can also directly affect monocytes, leading to IL-1 production and priming for tumor necrosis factor (TNF)-$\alpha$ production (49, 50). Complement activation that extends all the way to generation of the MAC is likewise a potent platelet activator. C5b-9 results in calcium mobilization, activation of protein kinases, granule secretion, vesiculation, and generation of platelet microparticles (51–54). This platelet activation may contribute to both local prothrombotic events as well as transient bleeding resulting from the circulation of previously activated ("spent") platelets. Complement, in particular C5a and C5b-9, is also a potent endothelial cell stimulant (55–57) that results in cytokine and reactive intermediate production as well as alteration in expression of important adhesive moieties such as P-selectin.

Defining which complement components cause the most problems in the clinical arena is important in devising appropriate therapeutic strategies and for understanding the basic biology of these processes. Several studies suggest that it is the terminal complement components (C5 and beyond) that are the most crucial, at least in the cardiopulmonary bypass (CPB) setting (58, 59). In simulated CPB, blockade of complement activation at C5 ameliorates CD11b/CD18 up-regulation on phagocytes, prevents platelet $\alpha$-granule release, and results in preservation of granulocyte and platelet counts (59). Thus it is possible that therapeutic intervention targeted at late complement components would preserve some of the beneficial aspects of the early complement components in staving off infection while ameliorating some of the clinical problems associated with the CPB "whole body inflammatory response" (13). This latter entity includes pulmonary and coronary dysfunction associated with CPB that bears a pathophysiologic relationship to "reperfusion injury" and to adult respiratory distress syndrome, neurologic dysfunction that may also relate to changes in vascular tone, and the full spectrum of abnormal coagulation. The details of CPB induced inflammatory and coagulation pathobiology are included in Chapter 50.

In the case of hemodialysis, complement activation by the artificial membrane plays an important role clinically in "first use" granulocytopenic syndrome (60) via the mechanisms outlined earlier. In addition, the generation of homotypic leukocyte aggregation has been associated with reversible embolic phenomena (61). Leukocyte adherence to pulmonary endothelium may result in clinically measurable hypoxemia during dialysis (62), which again occurs more frequently when complement-activating dialysis membranes are used. Some data also suggest that chronic neutrophil activation may result in relatively "spent" neutrophils with a higher threshold for zymosan activation, and this might result in an increased incidence of infectious complications (63). Lymphocyte subsets and function are also altered during both cardiopulmonary bypass and dialysis, although the role that complement may play here and the clinical significance of such alterations is unknown (59, 64–66). Finally, the chronic hemodialysis syndrome of renal osteodystrophy and $\beta_2$-microglobulin amyloid deposition has been attributed partly to chronic leukocyte activation by the dialysis membrane. This syndrome usually develops after 5 to 15 years of hemodialysis and is associated with carpal tunnel syndrome, arthropathy, and lytic bone lesions, some resulting in pathologic fractures (67). The combination of increased $\beta_2$-microglobulin production and decreased excretion may contribute to its pathogenesis (68, 69).

# CONTACT SYSTEM ACTIVATION BY ARTIFICIAL SURFACES

Similar to activation of complement via the alternate pathway, the soluble contact system is directly activated by foreign biomaterials, especially negatively charged surfaces, which to some extent mimic naturally occurring materials such as extracellular matrix and bacterial lipopolysaccharides (70). Again, the precise physiochemical requirements for this activation are incompletely understood (37, 71–72), although protein coating of the foreign surface probably helps to induce a conformational change in surface-bound factor XII that accelerates the conversion of factor XII into factor XIIa and other fragments (often collectively designated factor XIIf). This conversion occurs in the presence of prekallikrein and high-molecular-weight kininogen (13). Factor XIIa, a serine protease, cleaves prekallikrein to form kallikrein and high-molecular-weight kininogen to form bradykinin. Again reminiscent of the alternative complement system, a feedback loop is created as kallikrein accelerates conversion of factor XII, and the amplification cascade is initiated. Also similar to the complement system, plasma inhibitors are normally available to dampen these reactions. Those protease inhibitors include C1 inhibitor, $\alpha$2-macroglobulin, and even antithrombin III. Factor XIIa can directly stimulate the complement cascade via the classical pathway; kallikrein directly stimulates neutrophils; bradykinin is a potent vasoactive peptide; and factor XIIa can also initiate the intrinsic pathway of coagulation (71, 73, 74). More detailed discussion of the contact system may be found in Chapter 5.

Evidence for participation of activated contact system components in the initiation of biomaterial pathophysiology has been reported most clearly in cardiopulmonary bypass (13, 75). Here, in simulated systems and during *in vivo* bypass, circulating levels of kallikrein-C1-inhibitor and C1-C1-inhibitor complex rise significantly (75). Aprotinin effectively inhibits much of this contact system activation (37). The contact activation pathway has also been implicated in anaphylactoid reactions that occur during hemodialysis, especially in individuals taking angiotensin-converting enzyme (ACE) inhibitors (76). Thus generation of a self-sustaining contact pathway cascade on the surface of a biomembrane generates its own set of vasoactive compounds that may result in pathophysiology that contributes to a diffuse inflammatory response. It also acts to initiate and maintain the complement and coagulation cascades.

# COAGULATION SYSTEM ACTIVATION BY ARTIFICIAL SURFACES

One of the first effects of introducing a foreign biomaterial into a individual without accompanying systemic anticoagulation is the development of local thrombus. In addition, even under conditions of high-dose heparinization such as is used in CPB, systemic thrombin activation still occurs at a remarkable rate (77, 78). The major stimulus for thrombin generation, both locally and systemically, is considered to be a predominant effect on the intrinsic pathway of coagulation by the artificial surface (79). As noted above, activation of the contact pathway by an artificial surface initiates factor XII conversion to factor XIIa, with the subsequent initiation of the coagulation cascade. Contact activation also participates in conversion of plasminogen to plasmin (75). Thus, the physiochemical parameters that result in biomaterial activation of the contact system are similar to those initiating the soluble clotting system, and fibrinolysis is also initiated to some extent at the same time. Thrombin itself may be efficiently adsorbed onto the protein-coated surface of a biomaterial, which further propagates a clot (80). Nevertheless, thrombus formation on an artificial surface as a whole is far more complex. From the macroscopic point of view, thrombus formation on biomaterials usually involves both platelet and soluble coagulation pathway participation [although for some biomaterials minimal platelet participation in red thrombus formation has been described (81)]. This participation of platelets, with aggregation and release of granule contents, is crucial to the cascade, as will be outlined further below. Recall especially that although heparin can effectively blunt a variety of factors in the coagulation cascade in the presence of adequate quantities of antithrombin III, platelet adherence is not blunted by this agent and platelets may even be aggregated by heparin and enhanced in terms of their ability to release platelet factor 4 (82). High-dose heparin has now also been demonstrated to decrease nitric oxide production by endothelial cells, potentially resulting in a further increase in local platelet aggregability (83). Thus heparin has platelet procoagulatory effects that are important in the pathobiology of extracorporeal circulation.

Recent evidence suggests an important role for the extrinsic (tissue factor) coagulation pathway in the thrombogenesis that occurs in at least some biomaterial-associated pathophysiology. Direct measurement of factor VIIa during cardiopulmonary bypass, for example, is consistent with extrinsic pathway activation (84) as is the fact that changes in F1.2 (prothrombin activation products) correlate poorly with factor XIIa generation (85). Careful analysis of a individual with severe factor XII deficiency undergoing bypass has demonstrated thrombin generation equivalent to that seen in factor XII-sufficient individuals (86). A number of studies also provide grounds for understanding in part how the extrinsic pathway may be initiated in these clinical circumstances. Analysis of tissue factor expression by nonendothelial cells has demonstrated that: a) monocytes adherent to the CPB circuit may upregulate surface expression of tissue factor and associated procoagulant activity several hours into simulated extracorporeal circulation (87); and b) in clinical bypass, pericardial blood monocytes upregulate tissue factor, and this is associated with high factor VIIa/factor VII ratios in pericardial fluid (84). Monocyte-macrophages with upregulated tissue factor can be found in the heart-lung machine circuit itself (84). It is possible for monocytes to provide the procoagulant stimulus to the extrinsic pathway. There are also many potential sources for extrinsic pathway activation in these clinical circumstances, including activation by processes occurring in the surgical wound itself (84), possibly promoted further by stimulation of the extrinsic pathway by myocytes that constituitively express tissue factor (88). The up-regulation of tissue factor on monocytes is particularly intriguing, because this could occur due to a direct interaction with the protein-coated foreign biomaterial resulting in tissue factor up-regulation, as a consequence of cytokine production during bypass, or, possibly, through indirect stimulation of the monocyte by circulating activated platelets. These potential etiologies will be discussed below.

In some clinical scenarios that prominently involve artificial surface thrombotic pathobiology such as CPB there is concomitant activation of the fibrinolytic system (89). This could occur both via effects of the contact system on plasminogen or via endothelial cell interaction with thrombin resulting in tissue-type plasminogen activator generation (89). The fact that simulated cardiopulmonary bypass (where the circuit essentially is formed into a "closed loop" without the presence of the individual or the endothelium) is not accompanied by significant plasmin generation strongly suggests that it is the endothelium that is the predominent source of fibrinolytic activity in the individual (75). There is minimal change in plasminogen activator inhibitor (90) during clinical cardiac bypass.

# CELLULAR ACTIVATION BY ARTIFICIAL SURFACES

## PLATELET ADHESION TO AND ACTIVATION BY ARTIFICIAL SURFACES

Platelets may adhere to biomaterials and may be directly activated by this contact. Possible mechanisms include shear stress-induced activation during the relatively turbulent flow around a foreign surface, mechanical disturbance associated with direct foreign material contact, or interaction of platelet fibrinogen receptors (predominantly GP IIb-IIIa) with the fibrinogen coating of the foreign biomaterial (91–93). All three processes contribute *in vivo*, although a coherent generalizable explanation of the specific physiochemical properties associated with platelet attachment and activation on an artificial membrane remains elusive. This is one area in which extraneous variables such as temperature, type of anticoagulation used either *in vivo* or in the experimental setting, and exact topography of the *in vivo* or *in vitro* membrane (and not just its chemical composition) all have such a profound influence on the quality and quantity of the platelet activation observed that it may be nearly impossible to predict clinical results based on any specific *in vitro* experiment.

Platelets usually attach to the biomaterial itself and spread during the initial 15-minute to 90-minute period of blood-biomaterial contact (94, 95). During this time, activated platelets generally appear in the circulating blood, presumably reflecting both platelets activated by surface contact that did not achieve attachment as well those in the circulation that are secondarily activated by soluble products of the attached platelets. Platelet attachment may be accompanied by extensive spreading and degranulation in some cases. In other circumstances, attachment may occur with relatively modest effects on shape and granule content. After the platelet attachment phase, most biomaterials become resistant to further platelet attachment (96, 97), a phenomenon sometimes referred to as "passivation." However, some materials (for example, hydrogel poly [vinyl alcohol]) result in continuous activation of platelets that fail to adhere to the surface of the biomaterial; under those circumstances "passivation" fails (98) and the material may be less suitable for intravascular use. Other materials have been described that show very little platelet activation at all (98), at least under specific temperature and flow conditions. Some evidence suggests that the degree and quality of platelet adhesion to artificial surfaces relate directly to the conformation of fibrinogen adsorbed to the surface (99) and to the presence or absence of other plasma protein constituents (100). It is reasonable to speculate that relative composition of the protein layer in terms of other extracellular matrix molecules and coagulation factors will affect platelet attachment and activation. In some clinical circumstances, fragmentation of platelets may also occur. For example, the generation of platelet microparticles has been observed in cardiac bypass (101, 102), where it is likely that shear forces and complement activation play a significant role in the generation of these potentially procoagulant entities. Nonetheless, morphologic evidence suggests that some nonpassivating biomaterials may permit transient attachment of platelets followed by partial release of the platelet after this contact and the consequent generation of microparticles, both on the biomaterial surface and in the blood (98).

Indirect mechanisms may play an equal or even greater role in the activation of platelets by artificial membranes, especially for the production of circulating activated platelets. As noted earlier, C5b-9 activates platelets and may lead to the production of prothrombotic platelet microparticles (101, 103). In the setting of simulated extracorporeal circulation, blockade of C5b-9 production results in marked abrogation of the increase normally seen in circulating activated platelets (59). Plasmin formation has also been suggested as a means of stimulating platelets to activate and lose GP Ib, and activation of the contact system results in platelet alteration that may be prevented by aprotonin (38, 52, 75, 104, 105). The participation of secondary processes in platelet activation may also help to explain why some clinical scenarios, such as CPB, produce significant platelet activation whereas others, such as hemodialysis, produce lower levels.

Coating of artificial membranes by platelets participates in the capacity of the membrane to continually activate the intrinsic coagulation system by supplying an appropriate surface for the solid phase reactions. Platelet activation may also have a variety of additional effects. The presence of activated "spent" platelets and increased platelet clearance may lead to inadequate hemostasis in some settings (suggested, for example, for cardiac bypass and for some complications of prosthetic valves) (93, 106, 107). Platelet microparticles may add to the prothrombotic diathesis associated with artificial membrane use. Activated platelets and their products may also stimulate the endothelium at a distance from the site of the biomaterial. Finally, activated platelets may further interact with other hematopoietic-derived cells in a proinflammatory and procoagulant manner, as discussed below.

## LEUKOCYTE ACTIVATION BY ARTIFICIAL SURFACES

Contact of leukocytes with foreign biomaterials results in activation, as measured by several parameters. Neutrophils generate a number of regulatory cytokines, including IL-1 and TNF-$\alpha$ (108–112), after biomaterial contact. In addition, neutral proteases, including elastase, cathepsin G, and lactoferrin are released during hemodialysis and cardiac bypass (13, 113). Granulocytes and monocytes (but not lymphocytes) extensively upregulate important adhesion receptors, especially CD11b/CD18, during clinical conditions involving biomembrane use, including CPB (104), implantation of vascular prostheses (114), and hemodialysis (45, 46). Production of reactive oxygen intermediates routinely occurs in these settings (40, 115), with consequent lipid peroxidation and other adverse consequences (116, 118). Although all of these events occur under clinical conditions in which multiple pathophysiologies are active, data from *in vitro* experiments strongly suggest that direct contact with the foreign membrane is sufficient, although not necessary, for most of these processes to occur (46, 59, 111, 119–121). Other contributing factors include complement (especially the anaphylatoxins), contact system components, and possibly endothelium-derived products. Even in settings where significant vascular flow is not present, such as the use of orthopedic and dental devices, various prosthetic coatings such as hydroxyapatite result in activation of monocytes with secretion of multiple cytokines (TNF-$\alpha$, IL-1$\beta$, IL-6) as well as prostaglandins (e.g., PGE$_2$) (122).

The precise biochemical mechanism by which this direct activation occurs and the important signaling pathways are not clear. The pathways may even differ depending on the biomaterial being investigated. For example, some data suggest that rises in intracellular calcium concentration must occur to generate neutrophil degranulation by cuprophane, PMMA, and hemophane dialysis membranes, but degranulation in response to polyamide or polysulfone membranes may not involve calcium or inositol intermediates; other studies are not so clear (58).

The clinical consequences of these inflammatory reactions have been outlined previously. However, in recent years it has become clearer that leukocytes participate in inflammatory reactions and in the coagulation system (6). Neutrophils regulate surface expression of the $\beta_2$ integrin CD11b/CD18, which is a receptor for factor X, high-molecular-weight kininogen and fibrinogen (123–125). Monocyte CD11b/CD18 has been proposed as an important alternate fibrin(ogen)olytic pathway: fibrinogen bound to CD11b is internalized and degraded (126). The proteolytic products of activated granulocytes, especially elastase, may also affect the extrinsic coagulation pathway by cleaving tissue factor pathway inhibitor (TFPI) (127). Activated monocytes play a crucial role in initiation of the extrinsic pathway of coagulation by expressing tissue factor and allowing factor VII assembly (128), binding factor Va (129), synthesizing factor XIII (130), and expressing CD11b/CD18 which, as noted above, is a cell-cell adhesion and complement receptor. CD116 also binds fibrinogen and factor X (125, 131) and enhances tissue factor expression (132). As noted earlier, expression of tissue factor by monocytes could be an important mechanism contributing to graft occlusion after cardiac bypass and in other settings where a biomaterial-blood interface is established.

Thus the activation of leukocytes by artificial surfaces, directly and via soluble intermediates such as complement and contact pathway components, contributes to an overall proinflammatory state and contributes to the coagulation disturbances associated with the biomaterial-blood interface.

## PLATELET-LEUKOCYTE INTERACTIONS ASSOCIATED WITH ARTIFICIAL SURFACES

Artificial membranes stimulate a host of homeostatic protective systems that then interact through a host of common intermediates. One aspect of these interactions that has received increasing recognition over the recent past is the role that platelet-leukocyte adhesion can play in propagating the inflammatory and coagulation systems. Platelets and leukocytes adhere to endothelium (131–133, 134) and to one another (59). Although this adhesion can occur between resting platelets and resting leukocytes (6, 135–138), the reaction of direct relevance to artificial membrane pathobiology is the interaction of activated platelets with leukocytes. When platelets are activated, the neoantigen P-selectin (CD62P, GMP-140) is expressed on the external membrane of the platelet after α-granule fusion with the surface membrane (139–142). P-selectin mediates binding of the activated platelet to neutrophils, monocytes, and some subsets of lymphocytes, predominantly using P-selectin glycoprotein ligand-1 (PSGL-1) as a counterligand (143, 144). This adhesion appears to be a dynamic process, and simultaneous activation of neutrophils alters the interaction by redistributing PSGL-1 and lowering the affinity of activated granulocytes for activated platelets. However, activation of monocytes does not appear to adversely affect the adhesion (145–147).

The functional significance of platelet-leukocyte adhesion likely includes targeting the conjugates of both cell types to areas of inflammation and hemostatic injury (59, 148), providing a mechanism to support transcellular metabolism and functional alteration of the involved cells (6). P-selectin-expressing platelets are capable of modulating superoxide anion release by monocytes and neutrophils (149, 150). After P-selectin-mediated adhesion, neutrophils and monocytes may upregulate functional expression of CD11b/CD18 and possibly CD11c/

CD18 (148–150). Monocytes secrete IL-8 and monocyte chemotactic peptide-1 after P-selectin-mediated platelet adhesion in a process that depends on secretion of the chemokine RANTES by the platelet (154). Moreover, P-selectin is also an important stimulus for the up-regulation of tissue factor expression on monocytes (155, 156). The up-regulation of surface tissue factor by monocytes after activated platelet adhesion to these cells provides an ideal substrate for extrinsic coagulation pathway activation.

There is increasing evidence to suggest that these platelet-leukocyte heterotypic interactions promote the pathobiology associated with the blood-biomaterial interface. For example, in clinical CPB, platelet-leukocyte conjugates can be demonstrated to form in the circulation as platelets are activated (102). This is illustrated in Fig. 42.3. Blockade of complement component C5 blocks the formation of these conjugates in a simulated cardiac bypass model (58). Similarly, angioplasty is associated with the generation of circulating platelet-leukocyte conjugates (157) and the increase in platelet-leukocyte conjugates observed in acute myocardial infarction may directly relate to the generation of ischemic injury, partly mediated by further induction of local cytokine production (IL-1β, IL-8, monocyte chemotactic peptide-1) (158). One hypothetical scenario envisions the activation of platelets by artificial biomaterials as a prime mover in activation of both the extrinsic (tissue factor) pathway of coagulation and of transmigration, reactive oxygen species production, and cytokine generation by leukocytes (see Fig 42.1).

## ENDOTHELIAL ALTERATIONS INDUCED BY ARTIFICIAL SURFACES

Although most of the consideration given to the effect of biomaterials on the soluble and cellular circulatory systems revolves around the direct interaction of these elements with the foreign surface, this physiology can be altered due to the indirect effects of the biomaterial on the underlying endothelium with which it may come in contact. This is of most concern in those circumstances in which foreign material contact extends for more than just a brief period, that is, in the use of stents, vascular repair, or artificial organs more than in extracorporeal circulation. Neointimal proliferation occurs in all these circumstances. In the case of some materials a dramatic, acute, histiolymphocytic and fibromuscular reaction may be observed. In most others, endothelialization occurs in a much more ordered manner with little infiltration by inflammatory cells, usually with endothelial migration occurring over 1 to 8 weeks depending on the surface area to be covered and whether the arterial or venous side of the circulation is disturbed (9, 81, 159–162). In the case of endovascular grafts, fibrointimal hyperplasia and atherosclerosis may occur and become

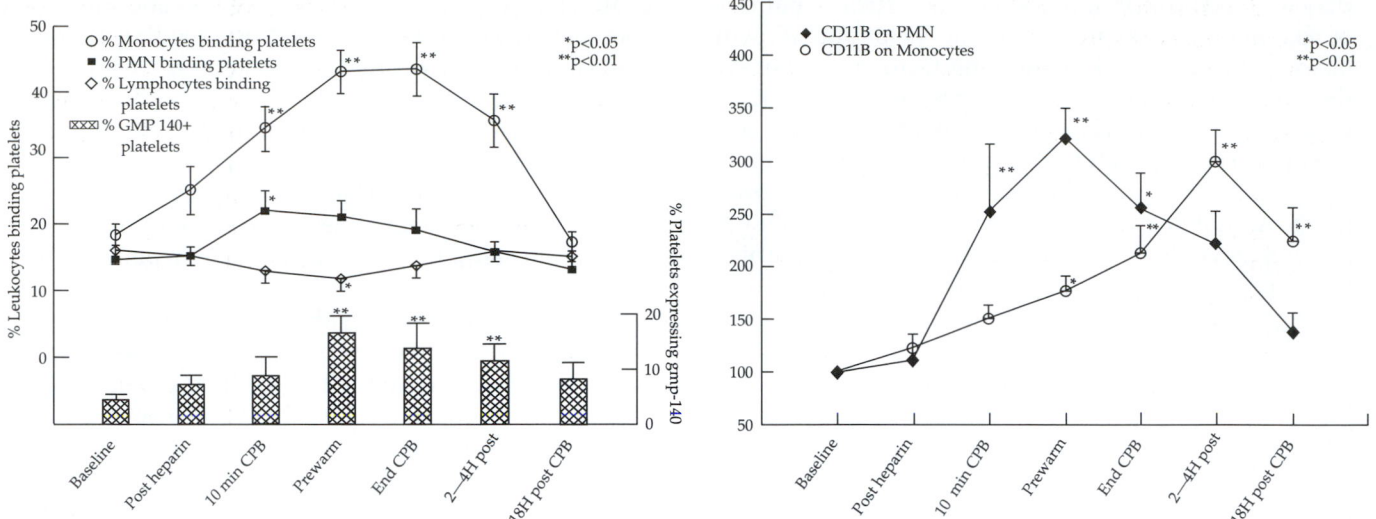

**FIGURE 42.3.** Cellular activation by cardiopulmonary bypass (CPB). **A,** Platelet activation measured by expression of CD62P (GMP-140) increases over time on bypass. Simultaneously, platelet-monocyte and platelet-neutrophil conjugates (heterophilic aggregates) form. Platelet-neutrophil conjugates are lost relatively rapidly, presumably due either to margination and egress or to loss of the platelet ligand on the neutrophil as the neutrophil undergoes activation. Platelet-monocyte conjugates persist into the post-bypass period. **B,** CD11b/CD18 is upregulated on both neutrophils (PMN) and monocytes during bypass but with very different time courses. Up-regulation of this receptor on leukocytes, platelet activation, and platelet-leukocyte conjugate formation are all inhibited by complement component C5 blockade. *H,* hour; *Min,* minute (Reprinted from Rinder CS, Bonan JL, Rinder HM, Mathew J, Hines R, Smith BR. Cardiopulmonary bypass induces leukocyte-platelet adhesion. Blood 1992;79:1201-1205.)

clinically detectable 1 to 2 years after graft placement (163, 164, 166).

Endothelial cells appear to be activated during those processes that involve transient exposure of the circulation to a foreign material, such as CPB and hemodialysis. This is to be expected, based on the ability of many of the activated soluble and cellular compounds discussed earlier to perturb the endothelium. Prostacyclin (PGI$_2$), endothelin-1, soluble P-selectin, and PAF all increase in concentration in the circulation during CPB (165–168).

The major contributing factors to these changes in the endothelium, whether in the case of transient biomaterial introduction or more permanent insertions remain uncertain. All of the previously described soluble and cellular activations could play a role.

# IMPROVING BIOCOMPATABILITY OF ARTIFICIAL MEMBRANES

## METHODS THAT ALTER THE BIOMATERIAL

There are a number of approaches that have been used to increase the "biocompatability" of artificial membranes. Biocompatability is a complex phenomenon. Although diminished complement activation has been touted as a potential surrogate for measuring enhanced

biocompatability (169), it is not at all clear that reducing the ability of an artificial membrane to activate complement will always reduce its thrombogenicity or its pro-inflammatory potential at the same time. Indeed, in actual industrial practice, multiple *in vitro* measurements of biocompatibility may be made, including morphologic examination after blood contact, radiolabeling of cells and proteins, and measurement of several released products of activated platelets and leukocytes, as well as measurement of hemolysis as an index of erythrocyte damage (20, 170). Nonetheless, modifications of artificial surfaces have tended to affect all these parameters in a similar direction.

Chemical modification of artificial surfaces can result in significant reduction in their potential to activate complement. Some investigators have modified cuprophane membranes by covalently coupling protamine to the -OH groups on the membrane that appear to be most important for complement activation (2, 171). Alteration of other terminal chemical groups on prosthetic grafts and artificial organs and development of new modified polymer surfaces have produced modest improvement in biocompatability (2, 172). Net surface charge of a particular polymer is one important determinant of its ability to activate soluble and cellular inflammatory pathways (173). For example, in one study, altering net charge of a poly(ether)urethane base material through sulfonation resulted in alteration in TNF-α producing monocyte-macrophage infiltration (174).

Another approach to improving biocompatability is to coat prosthetic surfaces with various, naturally occurring extracellular matrix and proteins, including serum albumin, fibronectin, and fibrinogen. Such approaches partially mimic what happens to successful grafts over time; the long-term place of such manipulations remains uncertain. Much effort has also gone into the coating of these surfaces with natural and other anticoagulants, such as heparin, hirudin, urokinase, thrombomodulin, and prostaglandin derivatives (2, 175). The idea is to provide a less thrombogenic material, one less able to activate the other soluble and cellular systems induced by artificial membranes. Perhaps one of the best studied systems is the use of heparin-coated circuits in cardiopulmonary bypass. Many studies have been carried out with such materials either *in vitro*, *in vivo*, or both (176–182). Although decreased soluble and cellular activation accompanies this manipulation, overall efficacy in terms of reduction of complement activation, platelet preservation, reduction in dose of systemic heparinization required *in vivo*, and reduction in platelet and leukocyte activation have varied significantly among studies and remain somewhat controversial. This suggests that although there is a salutary effect of this manipulation, it may be relatively modest, and its overall utility in clinical management remains somewhat uncertain (180–184). Conflicting results between studies of this type illustrate that the complexity of the clinical problem may require "combination therapy" to result in improvement in biocompatability.

Low-molecular-weight heparin has also been considered for the coating of foreign biomaterial surfaces. This compound appears to result in less fibrin deposition, at least on hemodialysis membranes (185). Interestingly, when introduced into the blood during simulated extracorporeal circulation, it is an excellent inhibitor of the complement system (186); whether these observations will have long-term clinical application is unknown.

The above approaches are well suited to clinical situations involving transient exposure of blood to artificial membranes, in which acute protein coating may occur but for which the issues of neovascularization and long-term foreign body reactivity are minimal. For long term implantable devices, however, one approach to devising a "completely natural" nonthrombogenic surface is to "seed" endothelial cells onto the foreign material (187, 188). This is perhaps being most vigorously studied as a solution to the problem of creating artificial small-diameter vascular prosthetic grafts. A recent variation on this concept has been to use genetically modified endothelial cells designed to express the tissue-type plasminogen activator gene or other antithrombotic proteins (189–193). Significant technical problems remain, however, and the long-term applicability of the concept in clinical practice is currently unknown. Another alternative or adjunct to actual seeding is to make the biomaterial itself more conducive to endothelial cell migration. Removal of gas nuclei (which normally represent nearly 70% of volume of some biomaterials), treatment with cationic surfactants, and attachment of fibronectin or short RGD containing peptides all hold promise in this area (194).

## METHODS FOR TRANSIENT INTERVENTION TO ABROGATE BIOMATERIAL-BLOOD INTERACTIONS

For circumstances in which exposure of the circulation to foreign materials is time limited, such as in CPB, hemodialysis, or, in a slightly more extended fashion, extracorporeal membrane oxygenation, it may be possible to intervene beneficially to prevent complications inherent in the pathophysiology of biomaterial-blood interactions by systemic administration of salutory agents. This includes the routine administration of relatively high-dose heparin during these procedures; unfortunately, standard heparin administration only blocks thrombin generation partially and does not beneficially affect complement, leukocyte, platelet, and contact system activation. Some interesting recent work suggests that low-molecular-weight heparins may be potent complement pathway inhibitors (186). The role of these compounds in cardiopulmonary bypass must still be determined, because unlike heparin, which is easily reversed by protamine, low-molecular-weight heparin cannot be rapidly counteracted.

As noted earlier, one mechanism of platelet activation and circuit adhesion involves interaction of GP IIb-IIIa with coated fibrinogen on the foreign surface (195). It is reasonable to postulate that interference with this process might help preserve platelet counts and reduce abnormal platelet function. Disintegrins are low-molecular-weight peptides isolated from snake venoms that contain the arg-gly-asp (RGD) sequence responsible for this adhesive interaction. Early studies suggest that such compounds may find a clinical role in extracorporeal circulation (196–198). Therapy using a disintegrin plus Iloprost may be an attractive combination in cardiac bypass (199).

Prostanoids, although theoretically attractive, have so far not met with great success in this setting because of their associated vascular reactivity effects (159, 160). Aprotinin has moved into clinical practice. Although it was initially given during cardiopulmonary bypass primarily for its antifibrinolytic effect in reducing overall operative blood loss, it is also an inhibitor of the contact system and of leukocyte and platelet activation (38, 96).

The possibility of using specific inhibitors of complement to prevent many of the coagulation and inflammatory complications of hemodialysis and cardiopulmonary bypass remains attractive. Soluble complement receptor 1 has shown some promise in this regard (200), as has an anti-C5 monoclonal antibody (59). Again, as with all these experimental manipulations, long-term utility will only be established after extensive clinical trials.

# REFERENCES

1. Edmunds LH Jr. Hastings lecture. Breaking the blood-biomaterial barrier. ASAIO J 1995;41:824–830.
2. Didisheim P. Current concepts of thrombosis and infection in artificial organs. ASAIO J 1994;40:230–237.
3. Kirklin JK, Westaby S, Blackstone EH et al. Complement and damaging effects of cardiopulmonary bypass. J Thorac Cardiovasc Surg 1983;86:845–857.
4. Edwards WH Jr, Martin RS 3d, Jenkins JM et al. Primary graft infections. J Vasc Surg 1987;6:235–239.
5. Sapatnekar S, Kieswetter KM, Merritt K et al. Blood-biomaterial interactions in a flow system in the presence of bacteria: Effect of protein adsorption. J Biomed Mater Res 1995;29:247–256.
6. Smith BR, Rinder HM. Interactions of platelets and endothelial cells with erythrocytes and leukocytes in thrombotic thrombocytopenic purpura. Semin Hematol 1997;34:90–97.
7. Shanbhag AS, Jacobs JJ, Black J et al. Human monocyte response to particulate biomaterials generated *in vivo* and *in vitro*. J Orthop Res 1995;13:792–801.
8. Sutherland K, Mahoney JR 2d, Coury AJ et al. Degradation of biomaterials by phagocyte-derived oxidants. J Clin Invest 1993;92:2360–2367.
9. De Scheerder IK, Wilczek KL, Verbeken EV et al. Biocompatibility of biodegradable and nonbiodegradable polymer-coated stents implanted in porcine peripheral arteries. Cardiovasc Intervent Radiol 1995;18:227–232.
10. Crommen JH, Schacht EH, Mense EH. Biodegradable polymers. II. Degradation characteristics of hydrolysis-sensitive poly(organo)phosphazenes. Biomaterials 1992;13:601–611.
11. Courtney JM, Irvine L, Jones C et al. Biomaterials in medicine—A bioengineering perspective. Int J Artif Organs 1993;16:164–171.
12. Tepe G, Duda SH, Hanke H et al. Covered stents for prevention of restenosis. Experimental and clinical results with different stent designs. Invest Radiol 1996;31:223–229.
13. Edmunds LH Jr. Why cardiopulmonary bypass makes individuals sick: Strategies to control the blood-synthetic surface interface. Adv Card Surg 1995;6:131–167.
14. Baier RE, Dutton RC. Initial events in interactions of blood with a foreign surface. J Biomed Mater Res 1969;3:191–206.
15. George JN. Direct assessment of platelet adhesion to glass: A study of the forces of interaction and the effects of plasma and serum factors, platelet function, and modification of the glass surface. Blood 1972;40:862–874.
16. Uniyal S, Brash JL. Patterns of adsorption of proteins from human plasma onto foreign surfaces. Thromb Haemost 1982;47:285–290.
17. Brash JL, Scott CF, ten Hove P et al. Mechanism of transient adsorption of fibrinogen from plasma to solid surfaces: role of the contact and fibrinolytic systems. Blood 1988;71:932–939.
18. Ryu GH, Kim J, Ruggeri ZM et al. Effect of shear stress on fibrinogen adsorption and its conformational change. ASAIO J 1995;41:M384–M388.
19. Kaplan SS, Basford RE, Jeong MH et al. Mechanisms of biomaterial-induced superoxide release by neutrophils. J Biomed Mater Res 1994;28:377–386.
20. Courtney JM, Forbes CD. Thrombosis on foreign surfaces. Br Med Bull 1994;50:966–981.
21. Engbers GH, Feijen J. Current techniques to improve the blood compatibility of biomaterial surfaces. Int J Artif Organs 1991;14:199–215.
22. Cavarocchi NC, Pluth JR, Schaff HV et al. Complement activation during cardiopulmonary bypass. Comparison of bubble and membrane oxygenators. J Thorac Cardiovasc Surg 1986;91:252–258.
23. Momoi T, Ono M, Takagi T et al. The effects of hemodialysis (HD) membranes on interleukin 1-beta (IL-1 beta) production from peripheral blood mononuclear cells (PBMC). Clin Nephrol 1995;44(Suppl 1):S24–S28.
24. Cheung AK. Biocompatibility of hemodialysis membranes. J Am Soc Nephrol 1990;26:150–161.
25. Cheung AK, Chenoweth DE, Otsuka D et al. Compartmental distribution of complement activation products in artificial kidneys. Kidney Int 1986;30:74–80.
26. Homeister JW, Lucchesi BR. Complement activation and inhibition in myocardial ischemia and reperfusion injury. Annu Rev Pharmacol Toxicol 1994;34:17–40.
27. Janeway CA, Travers P. The complement system in humoral immunity. In: Janeway CA, Travers P, eds. Immunobiology. New York: Garland Publishing, Inc. 1994;8:35–56.
28. Chenoweth DE. Complement activation in extracorporeal circuits. Ann N Y Acad Sci 1987;516:306–313.
29. Chenoweth DE. The properties of human C5a anaphylatoxin. The significance of C5a formation during hemodialysis. Contrib Nephrol 1987;59:51–71.
30. Chenoweth DE. Complement activation produced by biomaterials. Artif Organs 1988;12:508–510.
31. Chenoweth DE, Cooper SW, Hugli TE et al. Complement activation during cardiopulmonary bypass: Evidence for generation of C3a and C5a anaphylatoxins. N Engl J Med 1981;304:497–503.
32. Arnaout MA, Hakim RM, Todd RF et al. Increased expression of an adhesion-promoting surface glycoprotein in the granulocytoprotenia of hemodialysis. N Engl J Med 1985;312:457–462.
33. Aljama P, Bird PA, Ward MK et al. Hemodialysis-induced leukopenia and activation of complement: effects of different membranes. Proc Eur Dial Transplant Assoc 1978;15:144–153.
34. Carney DF, Lang TJ, Shin ML. Multiple signal messengers generated by terminal complement complexes and their role in terminal complement complex elimination. J Immunol 1990;145:623–629.
35. Craddock PR, Fehr J, Dalmasso AP et al. Hemodialysis leukopenia. Pulmonary vascular leukostasis resulting from complement activation by dialyzer cellophane membranes. J Clin Invest 1977;59:879–888.
36. Hakim RM, Breillatt J, Lazarus JM et al. Complement activation and hypersensibility reactions to dialysis membranes. N Engl J Med 1984;311:878–882.
37. Wachtogel YT, Kucich U, Hack CE et al. Aprotinin inhibits the contact, neutrophil, and platelet activation systems during simulated extracorporeal perfusion. J Thorac Cardiovasc Surg 1993;106:1–9.
38. Kirklin JK, Chenoweth DE, Naftel DC et al. Effects of protamine administration after cardiopulmonary bypass on complement, blood elements, and the hemodynamic state. Ann Thorac Surg 1986;41:193–199.
39. Combe C, Pourtein M, de Precigout V et al. Granulocyte activation and adhesion molecules during hemodialysis with cuprophan and a high-flux biocompatible membrane. Am J Kidney Dis 1994;24:437–442.
40. Himmelfarb J, Lazarus JM, Hakim R. Reactive oxygen species production by monocytes and polymorphonuclear leukocytes during dialysis. Am J Kidney Dis 1991;17:271–276.
41. Hakim RM. Clinical implications of hemodialysis membrane biocompatibility. Kidney Int 1993;44:484–494.
42. Chenoweth DE, Cheung AK, Ward DM et al. Anaphylatoxin formation during hemodialysis: Comparison of new and re-used dialyzers. Kidney Int 1983;24:770–774.
43. Arnaout MA. Structure and function of the leukocyte adhesion molecules CD11/CD18. Blood 1990;75:1037–1050.
44. Alvarez V, Pulido R, Campanero MR et al. Differentially regulated cell surface expression of leukocyte adhesion receptors on neutrophils. Kidney Int 1991;40:899–905.
45. Arnaout MA, Hakim RM, Todd RF 3d et al. Increased expression of an adhesion-promoting surface glycoprotein in the granulocytopenia of hemodialysis. N Engl J Med 1985;312:457–462.
46. Himmelfarb J, Zaoui P, Hakim RM et al. Modulation of granulocyte LAM-1 and MAC-1 during dialysis—A prospective, randomized controlled trial. Kidney Int 1992;41:388–395.
47. Tonnesen MG, Anderson DC, Springer TA et al. Adherence of neutrophils to cultured human microvascular endothelial cells. Stimulation by chemotactic peptides and lipid mediators and dependence upon the Mac-1, LFA-1, p150,95 glycoprotein family. J Clin Invest 1989;83:637–646.
48. Fletcher MP, Stahl GL, Longhurst JC. C5a-induced myocardial ischemia: Role for CD18-dependent PMN localization and PMN-platelet interactions. Am J Physiol 1993;265 (Heart Circ Physiol 34):H1750–H1761.
49. Schindler R, Linnenweber S, Schulze M et al. Gene expression of interleukin-1b during hemodialysis. Kidney Int 1993;43:712–721.
50. Chollet-Martin S, Stamatakis G, Bailly S et al. Induction of tumor necrosis factor-α during hemodialysis. Influence of the membrane type. Clin Exp Immunol 1991;83:329–333.
51. Wiedmer T, Esmon CT, Sims PJ. On the mechanisms by which complement proteins C5b-9 increase platelet prothrombinase activity. J Biol Chem 1986;261:14587–14592.
52. Rinder CS, Bohnert J, Rinder HM et al. Platelet activation and aggregation during cardiopulmonary bypass. Anesthesiology 1991;75:388–393.
53. Wiedmer T, Sims PJ. Participation of protein kinases in complement C5b-9-induced shedding of platelet plasma membrane vesicles. Blood 1991;78:2880–2886.
54. Sims PJ, Wiedmer T, Esmon CT et al. Assembly of the platelet prothrombinase complex linked to vesiculation of the platelet plasma membrane. Studies in Scott Syndrome: An isolated defect in platelet procoagulant activity. J Biol Chem 1989;264:17049–17057.

55. Foreman KE, Vaporciyan AA, Bonish BK et al. C5a-induced expression of P-selectin in endothelial cells J Clin Invest 1994;94:1147–1155.

56. Hattori R, Hamilton KK, McEver RP et al. Complement proteins C5b-9 induce secretion of high molecular with multimers of endothelial von Willebrand factor and translocation of granule membrane protein GMP-140 to the cell surface. J Biol Chem 1989;264:9053–9060.

57. Hamilton KK, Hattori R Esmon CT et al. Complement proteins C5b-9 induce vesiculation of the endothelial plasma membrane and expose catalytic surface for assembly of the prothrombinase complex. J Biol Chem 1990;265:3809–3814.

58. Haag-Weber M, Mai B, Deppisch R et al. Studies of biocompatibility of different dialyzer membranes: Role of complement system, intracellular calcium and inositol-triphosphate. Clin Nephrol 1994;41:245–251.

59. Rinder CS, Rinder HM, Smith BR et al. Blockade of C5a and C5b-9 generation inhibits leukocyte and platelet activation during extracorporeal circulation. J Clin Invest 1995;96:1564–1572.

60. Himmelfarb J, Gerard NP, Hakim RM. Intradialytic modulation of granulocyte C5a receptors. J Am Soc Nephrol 1991;2:920–926.

61. Arora N, Lambrou FH Jr, Steward MW et al. Sudden blindness associated with central nervous symptoms in a hemodialysis individual. Nephron 1991;59:490–492.

62. Davenport A, Williams AJ. The effect of dialyzer reuse on peak expiratory flow rate. Respir Med 1990;84:17–21.

63. Vanholder R, Ringoir S, Dhondt A et al. Phagocytosis in uremic and hemodialysis individuals: a prospective and cross sectional study. Kidney Int 1991;39:320–327.

64. Zaoui P, Hakim RM. Natural killer-cell function in hemodialysis individuals: Effect of the dialysis membrane. Kidney Int 1993;43:1298–1305.

65. Zaoui P, Green W, Hakim RM. Hemodialysis with cuprophane membrane modulates interleukin-2 receptor expression. Kidney Int 1991;39:1020–1026.

66. Rinder CS, Mathew JP, Rinder HM et al. Lymphocyte and monocyte subset changes during cardiopulmonary bypass: Effects of aging and gender. J Lab Clin Med 1997; 129: 592–602.

67. Stone WJ, Hakim RM. Beta-2-microglobulin amyloidosis in long-term dialysis individuals. Am J Nephrol 1989;9:177–183.

68. Van Ypersele de Strihou C, Jadoul M, Malghem J et al. Effect of dialysis membrane and individual's age on signs of dialysis-related amyloidosis. Kidney Int 1991;5:1012–1019.

69. Zaoui PM, Stone WJ, Hakim RM. Effects of dialysis of membranes on beta 2-microglobulin production and cellular expression. Kidney Int 1990;38:962–968.

70. Williams DF. Blood physiology and biochemistry: Hemostasis and thrombosis. In: Williams DF, ed. Blood compatibility. Boca Raton: CRC Press, 1987;1:5–36.

71. Colman RW. Surface-mediated defense reactions. The plasma contact activation system. J Clin Invest 1984;73:1249–1253.

72. Irvine L, Sundaram S, Courtney JM et al. Monitoring of factors XII activity and granulocyte elastase release during cardiopulmonary bypass. ASAIO Trans 1991;37:566–571.

73. Wachtfogel YT, Kucich U, James HL. Human plasma kallikrein releases neutrophil elastase during blood coagulation. J Clin Invest 1983;72:1672–1677.

74. Laurel MT, Ratnoff OD, Everson B. Inhibition of the activation of Hageman factor (factor XII) by aprotinin (Trasylol). J Lab Clin Med 1992;119:580–585.

75. Wachtfogel YT, Harpel PC, Edmunds LH Jr et al. Formation of C1s-C1-inhibitor, kallikrein-C1-inhibitor and plasmin-alpha 2-plasmin-inhibitor complexes during cardiopulmonary bypass. Blood 1989;73:468–471.

76. Schulman G, Hakim R, Aries R, et al. Bradykinin generation by dialysis membranes: Possible role in anaphylactic reactions. J Am Soc Nephrol 1993;3:1563–1569.

77. Brister SJ, Ofosu FA, Buchanan MR. Thrombin generation during cardiac surgery: Is heparin the ideal anticoagulant? Thromb Haemost 1993;70:259–262.

78. Boisclair MD, Lane DA, Philippou H et al. Thrombin production, inactivation and expression during open heart surgery measured by assays for activation fragments including a new ELISA for prothrombin fragment F1 + 2. Thromb Haemost 1993;70:253–258.

79. Cenni E, Ciapetti G, Cervellati M et al. Activation of the plasma coagulation system induced by some biomaterials. J Biomed Mater Res 1996;31:145–148.

80. Chuang HY, Mohammad SF, Sharma NC et al. Interaction of human thrombin with artificial surfaces and reactivity of adsorbed thrombin. J Biomed Mater Res 1980;14:467–476.

81. Kambayashi J, Watase M, Itoh T et al. Blood compatibility of venous prosthesis made of textile or non-textile material. Thromb Res 1992;66:365–372.

82. Mohammad SF, Anderson WH, Smith JB et al. Effects of heparin on platelet aggregation and release reaction and thromboxane A2 production. Am J Pathol 1981;104:132–141.

83. Upchurch GR Jr, Welch GN, Freedman JE et al. High-dose heparin decreases nitric oxide production by cultured bovine endothelial cells. Circulation 1997;95:2115-2121.

84. Chung JH, Gikakis N, Rao AK et al. Pericardial blood activates the extrinsic coagulation pathway during clinical cardiopulmonary bypass. Circulation 1996;93:2014–2018.

85. Boisclair MD, Philippou H, Lane DA. Thrombogenic mechanisms in the human: fresh insights obtained by immunodiagnostic studies of coagulation markers. Blood Coagul Fibrinolysis 1993;4:1007–1021.

86. Burman JF, Chung HI, Lane DA et al. Role of factor XII in thrombin generation and fibrinolysis during cardiopulmonary bypass. Lancet 1994;344:1192–1193.

87. Kappelmayer J, Bernabei A, Edmunds LH Jr et al. Tissue factor is expressed on monocytes during simulated extracorporeal circulation. Circ Res 1993;72:1075–1081.

88. Drake TA, Morrissey JH, Edgington TS. Selective cellular expression of tissue factor in human tissues. Am J Pathol 1989;134:1087–1097.

89. Gram J, Janetzko T, Jespersen J et al. Enhanced effective fibrinolysis following the neutralization of heparin in open heart surgery increases the risk of post-surgical bleeding. Thromb Haemost 1990;63:241–245.

90. Niewiarowski S, Senyi AF, Gillies P. Plasmin-induced platelet aggregation and platelet release reaction. Effects on hemostasis. J Clin Invest 1973;52:1647–1659.

91. Gluszko P, Rucinski B, Musial J et al. Fibrinogen receptors in platelet adhesion to surfaces of extracorporeal circuit. Am J Physiol 1987;252:H615–H621.

92. Moroz LA, Gilmore NJ. A rapid and sensitive $^{125}$I-fibrin solid-phase fibrinolytic assay for plasmin. Blood 1975;46:543–553.

93. Wenger RK, Lukasiewicz H, Mikuta BS et al. Loss of platelet fibrinogen receptors during clinical cardiopulmonary bypass. J Thorac Cardiovasc Surg 1989;97:235–239.

94. Merhi Y, Bernier J, Marois Y et al. Acute thrombogenicity of arterial prostheses exposed to reduced blood flow in dogs: Effects of heparin, aspirin, and prostacyclin. J Cardiovasc Pharmacol 1995;26:1–5.

95. Schoephoerster RT, Oynes F, Nunez G et al. Effects of local geometry and fluid dynamics on regional platelet deposition on artificial surfaces. Arterioscler Thromb 1993;13:1806–1813.

96. Edmunds LH Jr. Blood-surface interactions during cardiopulmonary bypass. J Card Surg 1993;8:404–410.

97. Zucker MB, Vroman L. Platelet adhesion induced by fibrinogen adsorbed onto glass. Proc Soc Exp Biol Med 1969;131:318–320.

98. Haycox CL, Ratner BD. In vitro platelet interactions in whole human blood exposed to biomaterial surfaces: insights on blood compatibility. J Biomed Mater Res 1993;27:1181–1193.

99. Shiba E, Lindon JN, Kushner L et al. Antibody-detachable changes in fibrinogen adsorption affecting platelet activation on polymer surfaces. Am J Physiol 1991;260:C965–C974.

100. Sheppard JI, McClung WG, Feuerstein IA. Adherent platelet morphology on adsorbed fibrinogen: Effects of protein incubation time and albumin addition. J Biomed Mater Res 1994;28:1175–1186.

101. George JN, Pickett EB, Saucerman S et al. Platelet surface glycoprotein. Studies on resting and activated platelets and platelet membrane microparticles in normal subjects, and observations in individuals during adult respiratory distress syndrome and cardiac surgery. J Clin Invest 1986;78:340–348.

102. Musial J, Niewiarowski S, Hershock D et al. Loss of fibrinogen receptors from the platelet surface during simulated extracorporeal circulation. J Lab Clin Med 1985;105:514–522.

103. Abrams CS, Ellison N, Budzynski AZ et al. Direct detection of activated platelets and platelet-derived microparticles in humans. Blood 1990;75:128–138.

104. Rinder CS, Bonan JL, Rinder HM et al. Cardiopulmonary bypass induces leukocyte-platelet adhesion. Blood 1992;79:1201–1205.

105. Adelman B, Michelson AD, Loscalzo J et al. Plasmin effect on platelet glycoprotein Ib-von Willebrand factor interactions. Blood 1985;65:32–40.

106. Harker LA, Malpass TW, Branson HE et al. Mechanism of abnormal bleeding in individuals undergoing cardiopulmonary bypass: Acquired transient platelet dysfunction associated with selective alpha-granule release. Blood 1980;56:824–834.

107. Pumphrey CW, Dawes J. Platelet alpha granule depletion: findings in individuals with prosthetic heart valves and following cardiopulmonary bypass surgery. Thromb Res 1983;130:257–264.

108. Haeffner-Cavaillon N, Roussellier N, Ponzio O et al. Induction of interleukin-1 production in individuals undergoing cardiopulmonary bypass. J Thorac Cardiovasc Surg 1989;98:1100–1106.

109. Steinberg JB, Kapelanski DP, Olson JD et al. Cytokine and complement levels in individuals undergoing cardiopulmonary bypass. J Thorac Cardiovasc Surg 1993;106:1008–1016.

110. Hebelin A, Nguyen AT, Zingraff J et al. Influence of uremia and hemodialysis on circulating interleukin-1 and tumor necrosis factor a. Kidney Int 1990;37:116–125.

111. Schindler R, Lonnemann G, Shaldon S et al. Transcription, not synthesis, of interleukin-1 and tumor necrosis factor by complement. Kidney Int 1990;37:85–93.

112. Betz M, Haensch GM, Rauterberg EW et al. Cupramonium membranes stimulate interleukin 1 release and arachidonic acid metabolism in monocytes in the absence of complement. Kidney Int 1988;34:67–73.

113. Schaefer RM, Herfs N, Ormanns W et al. Change of elastase and cathepsin G content in polymorphonuclear leukocytes during hemodialysis. Clin Nephrol 1988;29:307–311.

114. Jakubiec B, Roy R, Isles MB et al. Measurement of CD11/CD18 integrin expression on the polymorphonuclear cell surface after incubation with synthetic vascular prostheses. ASAIO J 1994;40:M616–M618.

115. Himmelfarb J, Ault KA, Holbrook D et al. Intradialytic granulocyte reactive oxygen species production: a prospective, crossover trial. J Am Soc Nephrol 1993;4:178–186.

116. Davies SW, Duffy JP, Wickens DG et al. Time-course of free radical activity during coronary artery operations with cardiopulmonary bypass. J Thorac Cardiovasc Surg 1993;105:979–987.

117. Toivonen HJ, Ahotupa M. Free radical reaction products and antioxidant capacity in arterial plasma during coronary artery bypass grafting. J Thorac Cardiovasc Surg 1994;108:140–147.

118. Pyles LA, Fortney JE, Kudlak JJ et al. Plasma antioxidant depletion after cardiopulmonary bypass in operations for congenital heart disease. J Thorac Cardiovasc Surg 1995;110:165–171.

119. Rosenkranz AR, Templ E, Traindl O et al. Reactive oxygen product formation by human neutrophils as an early marker for biocompatibility of dialysis membranes. Clin Exp Immunol 1994;98:300–305.

120. Kaplan SS, Basford RE, Mora E et al. Biomaterial-induced alterations of neutrophil superoxide production. J Biomed Mater Res 1992;26:1039–1051.

121. DeFife KM, Yun JK, Azeez A et al. Adhesion and cytokine production by monocytes on poly (2-methacryloyloxyethyl phosphorylcholine-co-alkyl methacrylate)-coated polymers. J Biomed Mater Res 1995;29:431–439.

122. Harada Y, Wang JT, Doppalapudi VA et al. Differential effects of different forms of hydroxyapatite and hydroxyapatite/tricalcium phosphate particulates on human monocyte macrophages *in vitro*. J Biomed Mater Res 1996;31:19–26.

123. Altieri DC, Bader R, Mannucci PM et al. Oligospecificity of the cellular adhesion receptor MAC-1 encompasses an inducible recognition specificity for fibrinogen. J Cell Biol 1988;107:1893–1900.

124. Wright SD, Weitz JI, Huang AJ et al. Complement receptor type three (CD11b/CD18) of human polymorphonuclear leukocytes recognizes fibrinogen. Proc Natl Acad Sci U S A 1988;85:7734–7738.

125. Altieri DC, Morrissey JH Edgington TS. Adhesive receptor Mac-1 coordinates the activation of factor X on stimulated cells of monocytic and myeloid differentiation: An alternative initiation of the coagulation cascade. Proc Natl Acad Sci U S A 1988;85:7462–7466.

126. Simon DI, Ezratty AM, Francis SA et al. Fibrin(ogen) is internalized and degraded by activated human monocytoid cells via Mac-1: A nonplasmin fibrinolytic pathway. Blood 1993; 82:2414–2422.

127. Petersen LC, Bjorn SE, Nordfang O. Effect of leukocyte proteinases on tissue factor pathway inhibitor. Thromb Haemost 1992;67:537–541.

128. Broze GJ Jr. Binding of human factor VII and VIIa to monocytes. J Clin Invest 1982;70:527–535.

129. Tracy PB, Eide LL, Mann KG. Human prothrombinase complex assembly and function on isolated peripheral blood cell populations. J Biol Chem 1985;260:2119–2124.

130. Weisberg LJ, Shiu DT, Conkling PR et al. Identification of normal human peripheral monocytes and liver as sites of synthesis of coagulation factor XII Ia-chain. Blood 1987;70:579–582.

131. Bitzan M, Richardson S, Huang C et al. Evidence that verotoxins (shiga-like toxins) from E coli bind to P blood group antigens of human erythrocytes *in vitro*. Infect Immun 1994;62:3337–3347.

132. Fan ST, Edgington TS. Coupling of the adhesive receptor CD11b/CD18 to functional enhancement of effector macrophage tissue factor response. J Clin Invest 1991;87:50–57.

133. Carlos TM, Harlan JM. Leukocyte-endothelial adhesion molecules. Blood 1994;84:2068–2078.

134. McEver RP, Moore KL, Cummings RD. Leukocyte trafficking mediated by selectin-carbohydrate interactions. J Biol Chem 1995;270:11025–11028.

135. Rinder HM, Bonan JL, Rinder CS et al. Activated and unactivated platelet adhesion to monocytes and neutrophils. Blood 1991;78:1760–1769.

136. Rinder HM, Bonan JL, Rinder CS et al. Dynamics of leukocyte-platelet adhesion in whole blood. Blood 1991;78:1730–1737.

137. Diacovo TG, deFougerolles AR, Bainton DF et al. functional integrin ligand on the surface of platelets: Intercellular adhesion molecule-2. J Clin Invest 1994;94:1243–1251.

138. Silverstein RL, Asch AS, Nachman RL. Glycoprotein IV mediates thrombospondin-dependent platelet-monocyte adhesion and platelet-U937 adhesion. J Clin Invest 1989;84:546–549.

139. Hamburger SA, McEver RP. GMP-140 mediates adhesion of stimulated platelets to neutrophils. Blood 1990;75:550–554.

140. Larsen E, Celi A, Gilbert GE et al. PADGEM protein: A receptor that mediates the interaction of activated platelets with neutrophils and monocytes. Cell 1989;59:305–312.

141. Rinder HM, Ault KA, Jatlow P et al. Platelet alpha-granule release in cocaine users. Circulation 1994;90:1162–1167.

142. Rinder CS, Student LA, Bonan JL et al. Aspirin does not inhibit adenosine diphosphate-induced platelet a-granule release. Blood 1993;82:505–512.

143. Moore KL, Stults NL, Diaz S et al. Identification of a specific glycoprotein ligand for P-selectin on myeloid cells. J Cell Biol 1992;118:445–456.

144. Furie B, Furie BC. The molecular basis of platelet and endothelial cell interaction with neutrophils and monocytes: Role of P-selectin and P-selectin ligand, PSGL-1. Thromb Haemost 1995;74:224–227.

145. Dore M, Burns AR, Hughes BJ et al. Chemoattractant-induced changes in surface expression and redistribution of a functional ligand for P-selectin on neutrophils. Blood 1996;87:2029–2037.

146. Lorant DE, McEver RP, McIntyre TM et al. Activation of polymorphonuclear leukocytes reduces their adhesion to P-selectin and causes redistribution of ligands for P-selectin on their surfaces. J Clin Invest 1995;96: 171–182.

147. Rinder HM, Tracey JL, Rinder CS et al. Neutrophil but not monocyte activation inhibits P-selectin mediated platelet adhesion. Thromb Haemost 1994;72:750–756.

148. Kirchhofer D, Riederer MA, Baumgartner HR. Specific accumulation of circulating monocytes and polymorphonuclear leukocytes in platelet thrombi in a vascular injury model. Blood 1997;89:1270–1278.

149. Nagata K, Tsuji T, Todoroki N et al. Activated platelets induce superoxide anion release by monocytes and neutrophils through P-selectin (062). J Immunol 1993;151:3267–3273.

150. Wong CS, Gamble JR, Skinner MP et al. Adhesion protein GMP140 inhibits superoxide release by human neutrophils. Proc Natl Acad Sci U S A 1991; 88:2397–2401.

151. Furie B, Furie BC. The molecular basis of platelet and endothelial cell interaction with neutrophils and monocytes: Role of P-selectin and the P-selectin ligand, PSGL-1. Thromb Haemost 1995; 74: 224–227.

152. Evangelista V, Manarini S, Rotondo S et al. Platelet/polymorphonuclear leukocyte interaction in dynamic conditions: Evidence of adhesion cascade and cross talk between P-selectin and the $\beta_2$ integrin CD11b/CD18. Blood 1996;88:4183–414.

153. Sheikh S, Nash GB. Continuous activation and deactivation of integrin CD11b/CD18 during *de novo* expression enables rolling neutrophils to immobilize on platelets. Blood 1996;87:5040–5050.

154. Weyrich AS, Elstad ER, McEver RP et al. Activated platelets signal chemokine synthesis by human monocytes. J Clin Invest 1996;97:1525–1534.

155. Celi A, Pellegrini G, Lorenzet R et al. P-selectin induces the expression of tissue factor on monocytes. Proc Natl Acad Sci U S A 1994;91:8767–8771.

156. Palabrica T, Lobb R, Furie BC et al. Leukocyte accumulation promoting fibrin deposition is mediated *in vivo* by P-selectin on adherent platelets. Nature 1992;359:848–851.

157. Mickelson JK, Lakkis NM, Villarreal-Levy G et al. Leukocyte activation with platelet adhesion after coronary angioplasty: A mechanism for recurrent disease? J Am Coll Cardiol 1996;28:345–353.

158. Neumann FJ, Marx N, Gawaz M et al. Induction of cytokine expression in leukocytes by binding of thrombin stimulated platelets. Circulation 1997;95:2387–2394.

159. Addonizio VP Jr, Strauss JF, Macarak EJ et al. Preservation of platelet number and function with prostaglandin E1 during total cardiopulmonary bypass in rhesus monkey. Surgery 1978;83:619–625.

160. Kappa JR, Fisher CA, Todd B et al. Intraoperative management of individuals with heparin-induced thrombocytopenia. Ann Thorac Surg 1990;49: 714–723.

161. Mackenzie DC, Loewenthal J. Endothelial growth in nylon vascular grafts. Brit J Surg 1961;48:212–217.

162. Halpert B, O'Neal RM, Jordan GL Jr et al. Vasa vasorum of Dacron prosthesis in canine aorta. Arch Pathol 1966;81:412–417.

163. Manfredi RA, Allison EJ Jr. Vascular prostheses. Emerg Med Clin North Am 1994;12:657–677.

164. Souttuirai VS, Yao JS, Flinn WR et al. Intimal hyperplasia and neointima: An ultrastructural analysis of thrombosed grafts in humans. Surgery 1983; 93:809–817.

165. Downing SW, Edmunds LH Jr. Release of vasoactive substances during cardiopulmonary bypass. Ann Thorac Surg 1992;54:1236–1243.

166. Hashimoto K, Miyamoto H, Suzuki K et al. Evidence of organ damage after cardiopulmonary bypass. The role of elastase and vasoactive mediators. J Thorac Cardiovasc Surg 1992;104:666–673.

167. Faymonville ME, Deby-Dupont G, Larbuisson R et al. Prostaglandin E$_2$, prostacyclin, and thromboxane changes during nonpulsatile cardiopulmonary bypass in humans. J Thorac Cardiovasc Surg 1986;91:858–866.

168. Hoshikawa-Fujimura AY, Auler JO Jr, Da Rocha TR et al. PAF-acether, superoxide anion and beta-glucuronidase as parameters of polymorphonuclear cell activation associated with cardiac surgery and cardiopulmonary bypass. Braz J Med Biol Res 1989;22:1077–1082.

169. Deppisch R, Schmitt V, Sommer J et al. Fluid phase generation of terminal complement complex as a novel index of bioincompatibility. Kidney Int 1990;37:696–706.

170. Courtney JM, Sundaram S, Forbes CD. Extracorporeal circulation: Biocompatibility of biomaterials. In: Forbes CE, Cushieri A, eds. Management of bleeding disorders in surgical practice. Oxford: Blackwell Scientific, 1993; 236–276.

171. Fu YY, Yang VC. A means to improve the biocompatibility of celluosic dialyzer membranes [Abstract]. ASAIO 1993;22:84a.

172. Tomizawa Y, Moon MR, DeAnda A et al. Coronary bypass grafting with biological grafts in a canine model. Circulation 1994;90:II160–166.

173. Grasel TG, Cooper SL. Properties and biological interactions of polyurethane aninonmers: Effect of sulfonate incorporation. J Biomed Mater Res 1989;23:311–338.

174. Hunt JA, Flanagan BF, McLaughlin PJ et al. Effect of biomaterial surface charge on the inflammatory response: evaluation of cellular infiltration and TNF alpha production. J Biomed Mater Res 1996;31:139–144.

175. Kishida A, Akatsuka Y, Yanagi M et al. *In vivo* and *ex vivo* evaluation of the antithrombogenicity of human thrombomodulin immobilized biomaterials. ASAIO J 1995;41:M369–M374.

176. Jansen PG, te Velthuis H, Huybregts RA et al. Reduced complement activation and improved postoperative performance after cardiopulmonary bypass with heparin-coated circuits. J Thorac Cardiovasc Surg 1995;110:829–834.

177. Ovrum E, Mollnes TE, Fosse E et al. Complement and granulocyte activation in two different types of heparinized extracorporeal circuits. J Thorac Cardiovasc Surg 1995;110:1623–1632.

178. Redmond JM, Gillinov AM, Stuart RS et al. Heparin-coated bypass circuits reduce pulmonary injury. Ann Thorac Surg 1993;56:474–478.

179. Steinberg BM, Grossi EA, Schwartz DS et al. Heparin bonding of bypass circuits reduces cytokine release during cardiopulmonary bypass. Ann Thorac Surg 1995;60:525–529.

180. Edmunds LH Jr. Surface-bound heparin—Panacea or peril? Ann Thorac Surg 1994;58:285–286.

181. Gorman RC, Ziats N, Rao AK et al. Surface-bound heparin fails to reduce thrombin formation during clinical cardiopulmonary bypass. J Thorac Cardiovasc Surg 1996;111:1–11.

182. Aldea GS, Doursounian M, O'Gara P et al. Heparin-bonded circuits with a reduced anticoagulation protocol in primary CABG: A prospective, randomized study. Ann Thorac Surg 1996;62:410–417.

183. Kuitunen AH, Heikkila LJ, Salmenpera MT. Cardiopulmonary bypass with heparin-coated circuits and reduced systemic anticoagulation. Ann Thorac Surg 1997;63:438–444.

184. Moen O, Hogasen K, Fosse E et al. Attenuation of changes in leukocyte surface markers and complement activation with heparin-coated cardiopulmonary bypass. Ann Thorac Surg 1997;63:105–111.

185. Bambauer R, Rucker S, Weber U et al. Comparison of low-molecular-weight heparin and standard heparin in hemodialysis. ASAIO Trans 1990;36:M646–M649.

186. Gikakis N, Khan MM, Hiramatsu Y et al. Effect of factor Xa inhibitors on thrombin formation and complement and neutrophil activation during *in vitro* extracorporeal circulation. Circulation 1996;94(9 Suppl):II341–II346.

187. Herring M, Gardner A, Glover J. A single-staged technique for seeding vascular grafts with autogenous endothelium. Surgery 1978:84:498–504.

188. Carabasi RA, Williams SK, Jarrell BE. Cultured and immediately procured endothelial cells: Current and future clinical applications. Ann Vasc Surg 1991;5:477–484.

189. Wilson JM, Birinyi LK, Salomon RN et al. Implantation of vascular grafts lined with genetically modified endothelial cells. Science 1989;244:1344–1346.

190. Podrazik RM, Whitehill TA, Ekhterae D et al. High-level expression of recombinant human t-PA in cultivated canine endothelial cells under varying conditions of retroviral gene transfer. Ann Surg 1992;216:446–452.

191. Sackman JE, Freeman MB, Petersen MG et al. Synthetic vascular grafts seeded with genetically modified endothelium in the dog: Evaluation of the effect of seeding technique and retroviral vector on cell persistence *in vivo*. Cell Transplant 1995;4:219–235.

192. Dichek DA, Neville RF, Zwiebel J et al. Seeding of intravascular stents with genetically engineered endothelial cells. Circulation 1989;80:1347–1353.

193. Dunn PF, Newman KD, Jones M et al. Seeding of vascular grafts with genetically modified endothelial cells. Secretion of recombinant TPA results in decreased seeded cell retention *in vitro* and *in vivo*. Circulation 1996;93:1439–1446.

194. Wigod MD, Klitzman B. Quantification of *in vitro* endothelial cell adhesion to vascular graft material. J Biomed Mater Res 1993;27:1057–1062.

195. Gluszko P, Rucinski B, Musial J et al. Fibrinogen receptors in platelet adhesion to surfaces of extracorporeal circuit. Am J Physiol 1987;252:H615–H621.

196. Shigeta O, Gluszko P, Downing SW, et al. Protection of platelets during long-term extracorporeal membrane oxygenation in sheep with a single dose of a disintegrin. Circulation 1992;86:II398–II404.

197. Musial J, Niewiarowski S, Rucinski B et al. Inhibition of platelet adhesion to surfaces of extracorporeal circuits by disintegrins. RGD-containing peptides from viper venoms. Circulation 1990;82:261–273.

198. Dennis MS, Henzel WJ, Pitti RM et al. Platelet glycoprotein IIb-IIIa protein antagonists from snake venoms: Evidence for a family of platelet aggregation inhibitors. Proc Natl Acad Sci U S A 1990;87:2471–2475.

199. Bernabei A, Gikakis N, Kowalska MA, et al. Iloprost and echistatin protect platelets during simulated extracorporeal circulation. Ann Thorac Surg 1995;59:149–153.

200. Cheung AK, Parker CJ, Hohnholt M. Soluble complement receptor type 1 inhibits complement activation induced by hemodialysis membranes *in vitro*. Kidney Int 1994;46:1680–1687.

# SECTION 10

# OTHER DISORDERS OF HEMOSTASIS

# CHAPTER 43

# VASCULAR PURPURA AND DISEASES OF BLOOD VESSELS

Martin D. Phillips and Moise L. Levy

Purpura results from the incompetence of platelets and dermal capillaries or small blood vessels to retain erythrocytes within the vascular space. Vascular (i.e., nonthrombocytopenic) purpura results from abnormalities of the vasculature and integument. They must be distinguished from lesions caused by abnormal platelet number or function, defects in the humoral coagulation pathways, or abnormal vascular structures. The appearance of erythrocytes in the dermis or mucous membranes, other than the pink color of normal capillaries, may be a source of concern for individuals or a sign of disease to physicians. The differential diagnosis is simplified by a logical approach, including appropriate individual history, physical examination, and laboratory testing (Table 43.1).

When lesions are present, the physician should determine whether the blood is intravascular or extravascular. This can be ascertained by whether the lesions blanch on pressure. Numerous methods have been proposed for this test, but the easiest is stretching the skin around the lesions between the thumb and index finger. Alternatively, the lesion can be pressed gently under a glass microscope slide. The disappearance of a colored lesion is termed *blanching*, and blanching indicates that the erythrocytes are contained within competent vessels. Release of pressure permits vascular refilling and reappearance of such colored lesions. Conversely, lesions that do not blanch contain extravasated erythrocytes.

Extravasated blood can appear as red or purplish-green patches ranging from millimeters to centimeters in size. These lesions are classified mostly by size, but the pathophysiology is always a failure of endothelial cells and platelets to maintain vascular integrity. If subsequent lesions are smaller than 3 mm in diameter, they are termed *petechiae* (Fig. 43.1; see color plate Fig. 43.1); larger leaks or coalescence of petechiae are termed *purpura* (Fig. 43.2; see color plate 43.2). Larger lesions, which usually result from incisions or ruptured arterioles, venules, or larger vessels, are termed *ecchymoses* (i.e., bruises) and rapidly attain a purplish to greenish hue as they age and heme is metabolized (Fig. 43.3; see color plate 43.3).

Integrity of the vascular barrier depends on a sufficient number of normally functioning platelets and on the integrity of endothelial cells and their subendothelial connective tissue matrix (Fig. 43.4). Inflammatory mediators produced by leukocytes or a humoral immune response may render the endothelial barrier permeable to fluid and protein, causing local edema. When combined with the extravasation of erythrocytes, the palpable purpura of vasculitis ensue. Increased transmural pressure, which is observed in dependent regions of the body during Valsalva maneuvers, coughing, or at high altitude, can exacerbate extravasation.

Locally dilated blood vessels may appear as red lesions of the skin and mucous membranes. If vascular integrity to erythrocytes is maintained, these lesions will blanch on pressure. They may result from the physiologic response to inflammation (i.e., the "wheal and flare" reaction) or abnormal vascular malformations that are either congenital, the result of trauma, or related to systemic illness such as liver disease.

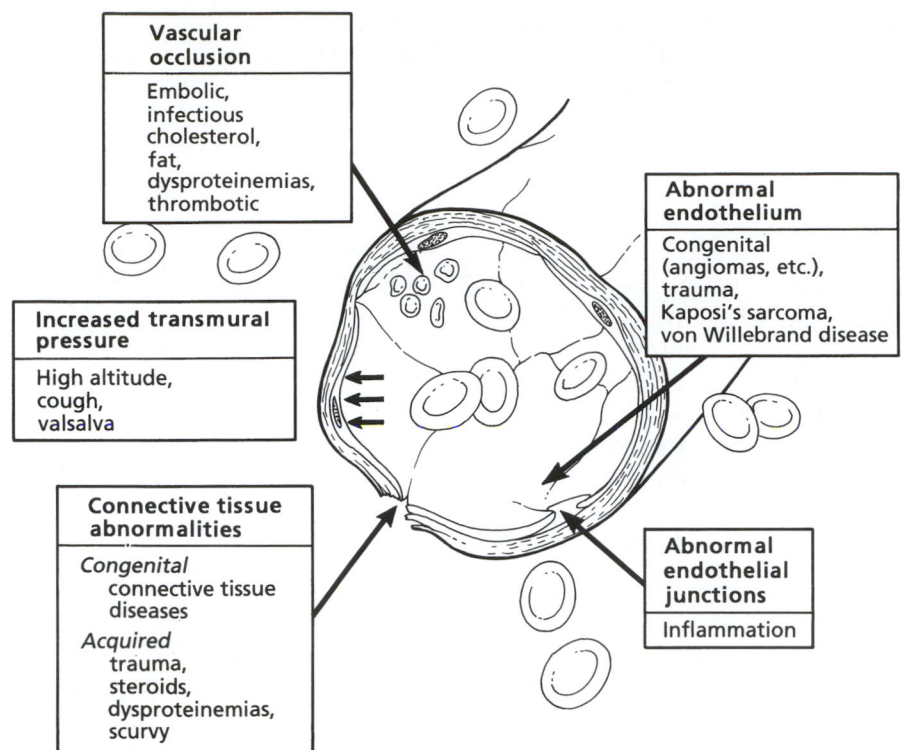

**FIGURE 43.4.** Pathophysiology of vascular purpura. (Platelet dysfunction and thrombocytopenic purpura are discussed in other chapters.)

**TABLE 43.1.** Causes of Vascular Purpura

| | |
|---|---|
| Nonpalpable | Connective tissue disorders |
|   Mechanical | Dysproteinemia |
|   Senile | Purpura fulminans |
|   Metabolic | Palpable |
|   Pigmented |   Vasculitis |
| Infections | Psychogenic |
|   Viral | Telangiectasia |
|   Bacterial | Kaposi's sarcoma |
|   Fungal | |
|   Protozoal | |

# PATIENT EVALUATION

## HISTORY

As for most individuals with hemostatic and vascular diseases, the medical history is paramount. Onset of the lesions will help to distinguish congenital from acquired causation. Temporal and visual evaluation of the lesions includes size, color, affected areas, exacerbations, remissions, previous episodes, and their relationship to trauma as well as animal or insect bites, all of which aid in further classification. Associated fever may relate to infection or vasculitis, and other manifestations of hem-

orrhage, including epistaxis, gingival, gastrointestinal, or postsurgical bleeding that suggest a systemic coagulopathy, should be sought. Remote or recent transfusion of blood products may be relevant as well.

A history of concurrent medical conditions such as uremia, infection, endocrinopathy, or inflammatory disease should be sought, and all medications being used, especially corticosteroids, aspirin, and nonsteroidal anti-inflammatory drugs (NSAIDs), should be suspected. Topical corticosteroids may cause local dermal changes. Potent, long-acting congeners, when used topically in large amounts, may be absorbed and have systemic effects. Many nonprescription and prescription formulations contain aspirin, and individuals may not consider a trade-name aspirin product to be aspirin. NSAIDs temporarily induce the same platelet defect as aspirin.

Any history of allergy, especially to medications, is essential, and a family history is important to determine if relatives are affected. A social history, with special attention to vocational or avocational exposure to chemicals or trauma, use of alcohol or nonmedicinal drugs, and sexual habits placing the individual at risk for acquired immunodeficiency syndrome (AIDS), should be obtained as well. Travel to high altitudes or areas where certain infectious diseases are endemic may be relevant, and a dietary and nutritional history may reveal vitamin deficiency. Finally, the review of systems may remind individuals of a seemingly irrelevant yet pathophysiologically related condition, such as systemic lupus erythematosus, malabsorption, and liver disease or malignancy.

## PHYSICAL EXAMINATION

A complete physical examination should be performed to evaluate for any coexisting abnormalities. A thorough dermatologic examination should include inspection of the scalp, oral mucous membranes, conjunctivae, nailbeds (e.g., for "splinter hemorrhages"), and all other areas of the body, especially those inaccessible to individual self-examination. The nature and extent of all skin lesions should be noted.

## LABORATORY EVALUATION

Laboratory tests should be used to confirm any possible diagnoses suggested by the individual history and physical examination. At minimum, the laboratory evaluation should include a complete blood count, leukocyte count with differential, platelet count, and peripheral blood smear. A prothrombin time (PT) and activated partial thromboplastin time (aPTT) should be performed to evaluate the integrity of the humoral coagulation system.

Abnormal results for any of these tests may explain the lesions. A modestly decreased platelet count in individuals with palpable purpura suggests vasculitis or autoimmune disease. Fragmented erythrocytes with thrombocytopenia indicate microangiopathy accompanying thrombotic thrombocytopenic purpura, hemolytic-uremic syndrome, disseminated intravascular coagulation (DIC), renovascular disease of scleroderma, or malignant hypertension. A prolonged aPTT or PT indicates primary humoral coagulopathy and, when accompanied by thrombocytopenia, suggests advanced liver disease or consumption coagulopathy. von Willebrand disease may manifest as easy bruising. (These conditions are discussed fully in other chapters.)

Other specialized laboratory tests also may be indicated. Platelet dysfunction with adequate platelet number or abnormal morphology should evaluated using platelet aggregation studies. These studies examine the ability of platelets to agglutinate or aggregate in response to various stimuli, and they can define congenital or acquired platelet abnormalities. Examples of such conditions, which may include hemorrhagic skin lesions, are Bernard-Soulier syndrome (deficiency of platelet glycoprotein Ib); Glanzmann thrombasthenia (deficiency of glycoprotein IIb-IIIa); platelet "storage pool" or granule-release defects, including the aspirin-induced defect (1); and other platelet defects resulting

in large, dysfunctional platelets with or without mild thrombocytopenia, including the May-Hegglin anomaly or Montreal platelet syndromes. Platelet function studies require technical expertise, however, and should be performed by a specialized laboratory (see Chapters 23 and 26).

Delayed postoperative or posttraumatic ecchymosis may result from factor XIII deficiency, which produces poorly crosslinked, friable fibrin clots. This deficiency is not evident on screening tests of coagulation, however, and its assay must be specifically requested (see Chapters 6 and 26). Other uncommon causes of delayed ecchymoses are deficiencies or abnormalities of fibrinogen or the fibrinolytic system.

The forearm bleeding time deserves special mention, because its usefulness is quite limited. The test is designed to measure combined platelet–vascular function, and its methods and interpretation are discussed in detail in Chapter 23. Because thrombocytopenia prolongs the bleeding time, this test of platelet or vessel wall functional integrity is difficult to interpret with platelet counts less than 100,000 cells/µl. There are reports of abnormal fibrinogen function affecting the results (2, 3), and the limited usefulness of the bleeding time as a screening test or predictor of hemorrhage has been previously reviewed (4). Frequently, it does not add any useful information to the more specific tests detailed earlier. Use of this test may be justified, however, in selected individuals as a general measure of platelet–vascular hemostatic function (5).

# EASY BRUISING

The syndrome of "easy bruising" may be particularly difficult to evaluate (6). Much of this difficulty arises from the subjective nature of its symptoms and signs. There is a considerable degree of biologic variation between individuals in their response to trauma, and there are no methods to quantify the severity of an injury. A history of easy bruising is said to be more indicative of psychiatry than of medicine: one who bruises on minimal provocation is delicate, whereas one who withstands trauma with no visible effect is robust. This statement is an oversimplification, but a individual's self-image does affect the reporting of symptoms. Similarly, a individual's personal experience also affect the perception of bruising. For example, individuals with congenital coagulopathy may be accustomed to large ecchymoses developing spontaneously or after minimal provocation.

On a somber note, physicians should be aware that easy bruising may be a presenting complaint or an explanation offered for physical abuse of mates or children. Physicians should be sensitive to this possibility, and they should structure their interview to allow consideration of this diagnosis.

## PATIENT HISTORY AND PHYSICAL EXAMINATION

The individual history should seek the frequency of bruising, the severity of insult necessary to produce bruising, and the size of the bruise that ensues. Comparing the size of a bruise to a coin or asking individuals to demonstrate the extent of bruises on their bodies may be helpful. A complete history, as outlined earlier, should be taken, with emphasis on the time course and progression of symptoms, use of medications, and other hemorrhagic phenomena.

A lifelong history of bruising may indicate a congenital coagulopathy or vasculopathy (i.e., connective tissue disorders). Mild von Willebrand disease is common and particularly likely to present as bruising. Coexistence of muscular or joint hemorrhage may suggest systemic coagulopathy, and dermal or skeletal abnormalities may suggest a congenital connective tissue abnormality. Whether any relatives are affected should be determined as well; a defect in maternally related males may indicate an X-linked abnormality such as factor VIII or IX deficiency. As many as one-third of classic hemophilias arise as spontaneous mutations (7, 8), so a negative family history does not rule out congenital coagulopathy.

Alternatively, recent onset of easy bruising after apparently normal responses to past trauma increases the likelihood of acquired coagulopathy. It may be the presenting sign of immune thrombocytopenic purpura or Cushing syndrome, especially in younger individuals, or of an acquired coagulation inhibitor in older individuals.

Again, medication use is important. Systemic or topical steroids, as used in Cushing syndrome, may result in bruising. Consumption of aspirin or NSAIDs is a leading cause of acquired coagulopathy associated with easy bruising. These drugs are universally available without prescription, and their use should be documented. An exacerbation of easy bruising associated with use of aspirin may indicate a mild, previously subclinical, underlying coagulopathy (e.g., von Willebrand disease). In some individuals, concomitant use of ethanol and aspirin or NSAIDs markedly prolongs the bleeding time (9, 10). It also has been implicated in some hemorrhagic events. Modest ethanol intake alone does not measurably affect hemostasis.

Age and sex of the individual are significant. The cumulative effects of aging and exposure to ultraviolet irradiation can lead to a syndrome of impaired vascular integrity, which is termed *senile purpura* (discussed later). There is a poorly understood phenomenon of easy bruising associated with the menstrual cycle of some young women, but bruising is not associated with any particular phase of that cycle. The laboratory evaluation is uniformly normal in these individuals as well. There is scant research on this problem, but the explanations suggested so far do not offer a biochemical basis for the observation beyond ''hormonal changes.'' As with any excessive bruising, the complaint should be considered seriously and evaluated appropriately.

The syndromes of psychogenic purpura, which usually occur in individuals with abnormal psychologic development (discussed later), also may present as easy bruising. These syndromes have many unexplained features, and they result in painful, frequently raised, and slowly healing ecchymoses. An unusual or inappropriate affect, slowly healing bruises at locations the individual may predict and sense, or the suggestion of self-infliction should raise this diagnostic possibility. Psychogenic purpura is a serious psychiatric problem that manifests most visibly as bruising in otherwise normal individuals. Responsible evaluation and treatment entail counseling and support.

## LABORATORY EVALUATION

Laboratory evaluation of easy bruising should be dictated by the individual history and physical examination. If evidence suggests a true coagulopathy, then a complete blood count, platelet count, peripheral blood smear with emphasis on platelet morphology, PT, aPTT, and ristocetin cofactor assay for von Willebrand factor (vWf) activity are necessary. Platelet function (aggregation) studies should be considered as well. Chemical or serologic tests (e.g., for steroid excess or systemic lupus erythematosus) or imaging procedures to evaluate for connective tissue disorders should be obtained as appropriate.

Several hemostatic abnormalities should be considered in individuals with excessive bleeding after injury but normal screening tests of hemostasis (see Chapter 23). In individuals with bleeding symptoms truly out of proportion to injury and normal results for commonly available tests, consideration should be given to plasminogen activator inhibitor deficiency, especially PAI-1 (11–13); abnormal fibrinogen unusually sensitive to plasmin degradation; or plasmin inhibitor deficiencies (e.g., $\alpha_2$-antiplasmin) (14). If individuals have had hemostatic challenges without excessive bleeding, other than easy bruising, and their physical examination and laboratory evaluation are unremarkable, the physician should reassure that the likelihood of a serious problem is small. Therefore, it is permissible for them to lead a normal lifestyle and even undergo surgery as needed.

# NONPALPABLE PURPURA
## MECHANICAL PURPURA

Mechanical purpura is induced by local trauma or barotrauma and appear as classic, nonblanching lesions. By definition, it is localized to the area directly involved in the trauma. In the unusual syndrome of high-altitude purpura, however, it may be more generalized. Before this purpura can be ascribed to strictly mechanical phenomena, it must be ascertained that the platelet number and function are normal. A common early manifestation of autoimmune or other thrombocytopenias is petechiae in dependent areas or at the line of tightly fitting clothing, such as belts, socks, or brassieres.

Mechanical purpura results from disrupted capillary integrity, with subsequent leakage of erythrocytes into the dermis. This phenomenon is the basis of the "capillary fragility" or Rumple-Leeds test, which is variously positive in many vascular or thrombocytopenic purpuric conditions and no longer is used. The mechanical insult may be a hydrostatic pressure differential, such as with high altitude (15, 16), cardiopulmonary resuscitation (17), suction or pressure applied to skin during aggressive and prolonged kissing or other intimate contacts (18), or suction-cup purpura (19, 20). Paroxysms of coughing in whooping cough (i.e., *Bordetella pertussis* bronchitis) may cause mechanical purpura on the head and torso. Alternatively, petechiae and purpura may occur in or around any area that has been mechanically or chemically traumatized (21), such as from exposure to sunlight (22), Scottish dancing (23), debris from a grass trimmer (24), vigorous handshaking (25), exposure to more than 5g in the cockpit of fighter aircraft (26), and "target lesions" in individuals shot with paint-pellet guns during recreational war simulations (27). A special case is snakebite with envenomation, which may bear the hallmark of a pair of puncture wounds with surrounding petechiae, resulting from the platelet-fibrinogen receptor–blocking agents in venom, in addition to a local inflammatory response. Vigorous exercise also has been reported to cause petechiae over the torso without apparent hematopathology (28).

## SENILE PURPURA/PURPURA SIMPLEX

Localized areas of purpura, which usually are seen over the exposed skin of the arms and legs, may occur in elderly individuals or after exposure to solar radiation or corticosteroid therapy (29, 30). Senile purpura/purpura simplex is considered to result from lack of support of the capillaries because of alterations in the connective tissue. The collagen in such individuals shows elastosis and atrophy, with the vessels generally appearing unaffected. Acceleration of cutaneous aging, including senile purpura, is associated with hemodialysis, possibly secondary to hypoproteinemia (31). Lesions may appear spontaneously after minor trauma, and the amount of pressure required declines with age, from 300 to 400 mm Hg in young adults to 150 mm Hg in elderly individuals (20). The differential diagnoses of easy bruising should be considered. There is no specific treatment for this symptom.

## METABOLIC PURPURA

Metabolic purpura is a systemic condition that causes impaired capillary integrity and erythrocyte extravasation. Examples are vitamin C deficiency (i.e., scurvy) and steroid excess. Uremia and use of aspirin or other drugs may affect platelet function and result in purpura fitting the broad definition of "metabolic purpura," but these entities primarily affect platelet function and are discussed in detail in other chapters. Historically, diabetes, pernicious anemia, and liver disease have been considered causes of metabolic purpura, but there is no evidence these diseases result in purpura by mechanisms other than those described here.

### Scurvy

Scurvy, a disease of defective collagen synthesis resulting from vitamin C deficiency, is rare in developed countries. Vitamin C is a cofactor in hydroxylation of lysine and proline residues, which account for one-quarter of the amino acids in collagen. There is a generalized blood vessel and connective tissue defect, and painful subperiosteal bleeding may be present. Typically, the petechial hemorrhage is perifollicular. The collagen defect also affects hair growth, so "corkscrew" hairs are a common finding (Fig. 43.5; see color plate 43.5).

### Steroid Excess

Corticosteroids impair synthesis of collagen and connective tissue, possibly because nuclear steroid hormone–receptor complexes inhibit collagen mRNA production (32). This effect has several clinical consequences, including poor wound healing, abdominal striae, and purpura. Thin skin and purpura are seen in autonomous adrenal hypersecretion and exogenous administration of corticosteroids (Cushing syndrome), as is endogenous overproduction of steroids resulting from adrenocorticotropic hormone hypersecretion by the pituitary gland (Cushing disease). Purpura and ecchymosis occasionally are presenting signs of these disorders (Fig. 43.6; see color plate 43.6).

### Cholesterol Emboli

Cholesterol embolization from atherosclerotic plaques may occur spontaneously or after vascular instrumentation (33). Some cases have occurred after initiation of oral warfarin therapy. The emboli may occlude any arterial vessel, with resultant ischemia. Cholesterol crystals may be apparent in the retinal arteries on fundoscopic examination and are associated with an increased risk of cerebral infarction (34). Characteristically, the dermatologic appearance of cholesterol emboli is petechiae, especially on the lower half of the body. Livedo reticularis and large areas of purplish discoloration have been observed as well (Fig. 43.7; see color plate 43.7) (35). These findings may suggest vasculitis and the need for biopsy (36). Biopsy specimens may reveal characteristic crystals occluding small arterial vessels (37, 38) and cholesterol clefts in the lumina of larger arteries at the junction of the dermis and subcutaneous fat (35).

### Fat Emboli

Petechiae from fat emboli result from occlusion of the microvasculature, as occurs with cholesterol emboli. The characteristic clinical triad is petechiae, diffuse central nervous system dysfunction, and hypoxia following long-bone fracture. The emboli are caused by fat globules released from the bone marrow (39–42); more recently, the syndrome has been observed after liposuction (43). For unknown reasons, petechiae characteristically are noted in the axillae and subconjunctivae, but they are also sometimes observed in many nondependent areas (44). The petechiae may occur without thrombocytopenia and DIC, or they may coexist, especially after traumatic fracture. Fat globules in the plasma or urine are helpful in suggesting the diagnosis, and bronchoalveolar lavage demonstrates fat droplets in two-thirds of individuals (45). Treatment should be supportive. Ethanol, heparin, and dextrans have been used, but their efficacy is not established (43, 44, 46). The fat globules eventually will be cleared by lipases and macrophages as well as via the urine.

### Ethylmalonic Aciduria

A syndrome of defective fatty acid oxidation resulting in encephalopathy, relapsing petechiae, orthostatic acrocyanosis, and ethylmalonic aciduria has been described (47). Cytochrome $c$ oxidase in muscle also is deficient (48, 49), but the relationship of the biochemical defects and dermatologic findings in this syndrome is not known.

## PIGMENTED PURPURA

Pigmented purpura is a group of benign disorders usually seen clinically as red-brown papules or plaques over the lower extremities. These lesions also have been called purpura simplex, but this nonspecific term should be reserved for the syndrome of senile purpura (discussed earlier). Histopathologically, pigmented purpura reveals dilatation of the superficial dermal capillaries with swelling of the endothelium and extravasation of erythrocytes. In older lesions, hemosiderin may replace the erythrocytes seen previously (Fig. 43.8; see color plate 43.8) (50).

Attempts have been made to separate these disorders into distinct clinical entities, such as Schamberg disease, Majocchi disease, pigmented purpuric lichenoid dermatitis of Gougerot and Blum, and the eczematoid-like purpura of Doucas and Kapetanakis (50, 51). Each of these entities may begin with punctate areas of erythema and telangiectasia, which evolve into red-brown patches or plaques, most often on the lower extremities. More diffuse cutaneous presentations may be seen. There also exist localized variants, known as lichen aureus, and unilateral linear capillaritis (52).

Hematologic indices are normal in the entire spectrum of disease. The cause of these disorders is unknown, but cell-mediated hypersensitivity phenomena and immune complex deposition have been considered. Several drugs have been implicated as well (53), including aminoglutethimide (54) and streptokinase (55). PUVA and oral griseofulvin have shown some therapeutic success (56, 57). Treatment is difficult, however, and no specific therapy is available.

## PURPURA RESULTING FROM INFECTION

Many infectious diseases cause purpuric lesions. There are several potential mechanisms: direct invasion of the vasculature by organisms, septic emboli with local inflammation and infarction, immune complex vasculitis, DIC with thrombocytopenia, and other poorly defined possibilities. It is not apparent, however, how often petechiae result from bacterial infection without DIC and thrombocytopenia.

Virtually any infection may cause purpuric lesions, but several agents are classically associated with purpura (Table 43.2). In candidemia, clumps of nondeformable organisms produce local occlusion of small blood vessels. The "spots" of Rocky Mountain spotted fever, a rickettsial infection transmitted by tick bites, are petechiae. The organisms proliferate within the capillary endothelium and activate complement (58, 59), and a prospective study of *Rickettsia rickettsii* infection (60) demonstrated subclinical activation of the plasma procoagulant and fibrinolytic systems. The mean nadir platelet count was 170,000 cells/$\mu$l, and the lowest nadir was 130,000 cells/$\mu$l, thus indicating that endothelial cell perturbation, not thrombocytopenia, is the cause of petechiae in this disease.

Severe *Neisseria meningitidis* infection is classically associated with petechiae and purpura (Fig. 43.2; see color plate 43.2), but this sign is neither sensitive nor specific diagnostically. In a prospective study of children with fever and petechiae (61), infections with *Neisseria* sp., with or without meningitis, accounted for only 7% of individuals with these presenting signs. *Haemophilus influenza* type B, *Streptococcus pneumoniae*, and *Capnocytophaga* sp. (formerly DF-2) also are causes of petechiae with bacteremia. "Brazilian purpuric fever" is caused by *H. influenza aegyptius* (62), and *S. pyogenes* pharyngitis

**TABLE 43.2.** Infectious Causes of Purpura

Bacteria
    *Niesseria* sp. (61)
    *Haemophilus* sp. (61, 62)
    *Streptococcus* sp. (61)
    *Capnocytophaga* sp. (58)
    *Bordetella* sp.
    Rickettsia (60)
Viruses (65, 89)
    Enterovirus
    ECHO virus
    Coxsackievirus
    Respiratory syncytial virus
    Rubella
    Measles
    Hepatitis A (76)
    Hepatitis B (77, 78)
    Parvovirus B19 (79, 80)
    Cytomegalovirus (85)
    Varicella (87)
Vaccines
    Killed measles (66)
    Influenza (74)
    Diphtheria-pertussis-tetanus (75)
Fungi
    *Candida* sp.
    *Trichosporon* sp. (241)
Protozoa
    *Strongyloides* sp. (82, 83)
    Malaria (86)

may cause petechiae without bacteremia (61, 63). Numerous viruses can cause a petechial rash, but the most common are enterovirus, ECHO viruses, coxsackievirus, respiratory syncytial virus, rubella, and measles. Petechiae are part of the "TORCH" syndrome as well (64). The cause usually is immune complex vasculitis, but this frequently is difficult to prove (65). "Atypical" measles occurring after administration of killed measles vaccine also has been reported to cause a hemorrhagic rash (66).

Several infections may be part of the "papular-purpuric gloves and socks syndrome" (67). These include infections with parvovirus B19 (68, 69), measles (70), hepatitis B (71), or unknown agents (72, 73). There may be associated minor hematologic abnormalities or mucous membrane ulceration. This syndrome is similar to Gianotti-Crosti syndrome (papular acrodermatitis of childhood) and is self-limited.

Many cases of more rare infectious agents associated with petechiae have been reported. Vasculitis and normal platelet counts have occurred in individuals after influenza (74) or diphtheria-tetanus-pertussis (75) vacci-

nation; viral infections, including relapsing hepatitis A (76), hepatitis B (77, 78), or parvovirus B19 (79, 80); or brucellosis (81). *Strongyloides stercoralis* (82–84) is presumed to occlude small-vessels, with local inflammation, and primary cytomegalovirus infection (85) and malaria (86) have caused petechiae. No mechanisms have been proposed for the latter infections, however. Varicella causes petechiae by diverse mechanisms (87), some of which indicate serious underlying coagulopathy (88). Numerous other viruses not mentioned here are associated with immune thrombocytopenia as well (89).

# CONNECTIVE TISSUE DISORDERS

## EHLERS-DANLOS SYNDROME

Coagulation defects have occurred in the Ehlers-Danlos syndrome (EDS) (90), which is a group of inherited diseases of varying molecular pathogenesis. Ten subtypes have been reported to date (91, 92). All are characterized by soft, lax, velvety skin as well as joint hypermobility, scarring, and bleeding tendency. The bleeding tendency is worst in type IV, or the ecchymotic variety of EDS, which can be fatal in the third to fifth decades of life. In this variety, collagen type III synthesis is defective, resulting from a variety of mutations (93); accurate diagnosis can be made from a skin biopsy specimen (93). Bruising also may occur in types I, II, V, VIIc, VIII, and X. Some abnormalities in humoral coagulation factors and platelet function have been associated with EDS (90), but these defects are almost certainly coincidental. EDS may be misdiagnosed as "variant hemophilia."

## OTHER CONNECTIVE TISSUE SYNDROMES

Two additional heritable disorders of type I collagen synthesis—osteogenesis imperfecta (especially type I or dominant inheritance with blue sclerae) and Marfan syndrome—may be complicated by bruising. This is a minor clinical feature compared with the skeletal defects, however. Pseudoxanthoma elasticum, another connective tissue disorder of unknown pathophysiology (94), causes prolonged bleeding times and may be associated with gastrointestinal hemorrhage (95). Yellow papular skin lesions and ocular angioid streaks are characteristic.

# DYSPROTEINEMIAS

Several dysproteinemic diseases cause petechiae and purpura (96). These include Waldenstrom's macroglobulinemia, which is the malignant lymphoid disease accompanied by a monoclonal immunoglobulin (Ig) M paraprotein; the benign (polyclonal) hypergammaglobulinemic purpura of Waldenstrom's (97); cold insoluble protein syndromes; and amyloidosis, especially of the AL (acquired light chain) type but rarely of the AA (reactive) type may result in purpura. The infamous finding for this syndrome is "postproctoscopic periorbital purpura," which was first recognized during the era when rectal biopsies to diagnose amyloidosis were performed by rigid sigmoidoscopy, with the individual in a head-down position. The increased hydraulic pressure of the Valsalva maneuver in this position frequently caused fragile vessels around the ocular orbits to rupture. A specific mechanism is lacking, but the abnormal, AL-type protein that accumulates around dermal capillaries as amorphous, uniformly staining globules disrupts the normal capillary integrity (98). There also is a report of purpura and vasculopathy resulting from deposition of λ light-chain crystals within small-vessels (99). Skin biopsy specimens from individuals with AA amyloid may demonstrate protein deposition deeper in the dermis, thus accounting for the rarity of visible skin lesions in this population (96). In systemic amyloidosis, involvement of other organ systems may be evident, and common findings are orthostatic hypotension, excessive fatigue, congestive heart failure, hepatosplenomegaly, and nephrotic syndrome or renal insufficiency. On physical examination, the skin may appear yellow or waxy and hairless because of amyloid deposits damaging the hair follicles.

Two syndromes of cold-insoluble plasma proteins result in purpura. The first, cryoglobulinemia, results from cold-precipitable immunoglobulins, frequently IgM with anti-IgG specificity (cryorheumatoid factor). Cryoglobulins are classified as type I (monoclonal protein only), type II (monoclonal and polyclonal), or type III (polyclonal proteins only) (100). The second, cryofibrinogenemia, results from a mixture of cold-insoluble fibrinogen, fibrin and fibrin degradation products, vWf, and factor XIII (101). Either syndrome may occur secondary to chronic inflammation or malignancy, especially lymphoid malignancy, as well as idiopathically. Type I cryoglobulinemia often is associated with lymphoid malignancy, and many cases of type II cryoglobulinemia are associated with hepatitis C infection (102, 103). The purpuric lesions result from occlusion of small arterioles by the cryoprecipitate.

These syndromes should not be confused with cold agglutinin disease, however, which is caused by IgM antibodies of anti-Ii blood group specificity that agglutinate erythrocytes. Cold agglutinins are either idiopathic or secondary to infection with *Mycoplasma pneumoniae*, Epstein-Barr virus, or to lymphoproliferative disease. Cold agglutinins do not cause petechial hemorrhage, but they may occur in conjunction with cryoglobulins.

Normally, several large plasma proteins, including fibrinogen, vWf (with associated factor VIII), IgM, fibronectin, and factor XIII, may be precipitated from plasma through freezing followed by thawing at 4°C. In contrast, abnormal cryoglobulins and cryofibrinogens that cause disease precipitate on incubation of plasma at 4°C for 24 to 72 hours. The biochemical reason for the abnormal cold precipitation of these proteins is not known. Some polyclonal cryoglobulins have an amino acid homology in the variable region, which may relate to a cold-induced, antigen-binding structural domain. A temperature-dependent conformational change has been postulated in monoclonal cryoglobulins (104).

Typically, lesions are purpurae or ecchymoses on the distal digits, earlobes, lower extremities, and genitalia, possibly because lower temperature of these distal regions causes cryoprecipitation (105). Reticulate purpura (i.e., livedo reticularis) also may be seen (106). Symptoms are worse among individuals in cold climates.

Another cause of urticaria and livedo reticularis on exposure to cold is familial cold urticaria. The cause of this rare disorder is unknown, but transmission is autosomal dominant (107). Rarely, Waldenstrom's macroglobulinemia may present with cold-induced purpura (108).

Laboratory evaluation may reveal anemia, typically from chronic disease; abnormal serum protein electrophoresis with monoclonal or polyclonal gammopathy; and damage to other organ systems. Levels of antibodies to hepatitis C and hepatitis C viral RNA should be measured and an assay for cryoglobulin and cryofibrinogen performed. These can be quantitated loosely by chilling plasma to 4°C for 24 to 72 hours, followed by centrifugation at 4°C in a capillary tube. The volume of white precipitate is the "cryocrit." In severe disease, the cryocrit may be more than 10%, but there is only a moderate correlation between cryocrit and disease activity. It sometimes may be helpful to perform immunofixation electrophoresis on the cryoprecipitated protein to accentuate a small monoclonal band. In amyloidosis, the PT or aPTT may be prolonged because of amyloid adsorption of factor X or other vitamin K-dependent factors (see Chapter 36). Skin biopsy of an affected area is diagnostic, with the specimen demonstrating either amorphous, globular protein deposition or green birefringence of a Congo Red–stained section in amyloidosis. As described in Chapter 33, paraproteins may also affect platelet function directly (109–113).

Treatment of paraproteinemia requires elucidation of the underlying disorder, and appropriately directed therapy. Use of stanozolol has been effective in idiopathic cryofibrinogenemia (114, 115).

# PURPURA FULMINANS

Purpura fulminans refers to the massive ecchymoses that may occur in acute or congenital deficiencies of protein C or protein S (see Chapter 40). Such deficiency may occur during DIC or severe infections, early in the administration of warfarin (i.e., warfarin skin necrosis) (Fig. 43.9; see color plate 43.9) (see Chapter 55), or at birth because of a congenital homozygous deficiency state (116, 117). Purpura fulminans has been reported in a individual with chronic alcohol abuse and acetaminophen ingestion (118). This combination probably diminished glutathione production in the liver, resulting in decreased protein C and S levels as well as purpura. Skin necrosis also has been reported with hypersensitivity to heparin (119–122) and with antiphospholipid antibodies (123–125). The skin necrosis observed with heparin is another manifestation of the heparin-dependent platelet autoantibody syndrome, which is caused by antibodies against heparin complexed with platelet factor 4 (124, 126, 127). Cholestasis with deficient vitamin K absorption has been implicated as well (128).

The early clinical appearance is transient flushing followed by petechiae, with or without edema. At presentation, the appearance usually is of massive bruising. The lesion periphery may be hyperemic, and the center may be replaced by hemorrhagic bullae and necrosis of the skin, with sparing of the subjacent muscle (129). Dependent areas typically are involved, but the predilection for areas such as the breast, fatty tissue, and penis is not understood. Areas of pressure also may be involved.

The histopathology is thrombosis of the dermal capillaries and venules, with hemorrhagic infarction. The arteries and arterioles are spared. The thrombi are composed of fibrin, platelets, or a mixture of the two (129).

Several pathogenetic theories were advanced before the 1970s. More recently, however, there has been general agreement that purpura fulminans results from an imbalance of procoagulants and the natural vitamin K-dependent anticoagulant proteins C and S. Neonatal purpura fulminans is associated with a severe, congenital deficiency of either protein. In DIC, these proteins may be consumed. Additionally, numerous cases have occurred after warfarin administration, especially when a loading dose has been employed. The incidence is highest during the first 3 days of drug administration, because both proteins C and S have short half-lives (6–9 hours) compared with the procoagulant factors IX, X, and II. Twenty-four hours after the rate of vitamin K-dependent posttranslational protein modification is decreased, levels of functional proteins C and S may be less than 10% of normal, whereas levels of functional procoagulant vitamin K-dependent factors (other than factor VII) are still greater than 50% of normal. The problem is accentuated in individuals heterozygous for protein C deficiency, who may account for as much as 2% of the general population (130). Local coagulation and fibrinolysis can lead to endothelial release of interleukin-1 and tumor necrosis factor, both of which propagate the cellular injury by recruiting inflammatory cells (117). In individuals with normal protein C and S levels, antiphospholipid antibodies may simulate a deficiency state by interfering with the activation of protein C by thrombomodulin (123, 124).

If a deficiency of protein C or S is suspected, it is common practice, and theoretically sound, to begin warfarin therapy while the individual is heparinized. Anecdotal evidence of skin necrosis even in this setting, however, has been reported. The most important method of prevention is use of low initial doses of warfarin. A loading dose has no physiologic advantage and is not justified (see Chapter 55).

# PALPABLE PURPURA

The hallmark finding of small-vessel vasculitis is palpable purpura. Many diseases with differing pathogenesis produce this finding (131), including Henoch-Schöenlein purpura, leukocytoclastic angiitis, allergic purpura, anaphylactoid purpura, and serum sickness. Allergic reactions to drugs typically manifest as diffuse palpable purpura, and contact dermatitis may cause local purpura (Fig. 43.10; see color plate 43.10).

Palpable purpura results from local release of cytokines and vasoactive substances, which cause capillary leakage of proteinaceous fluid and erythrocytes. The specific factors causing edema formation are not known, but experimental evidence suggests that platelet-activating factor and tumor necrosis factor are pathogenetically involved (132). The need for biopsy to confirm the diagnosis of vasculitis is dictated by the clinical situation. Granulomata, emboli, tissue immunoglobulin, or organisms may be helpful findings in selected cases (133). Panniculitis has been demonstrated rarely (134).

Of particular hematologic concern is vasculitis associated with hairy-cell leukemia. Individuals with this disease also commonly have cutaneous vasculitis (135), but isolated cerebral (136) and testicular (137) vasculitis have been reported as well. The pathogenesis of vasculitis associated with hairy-cell leukemia is not known. There is a strong association with an underlying infection, however, which may be bacterial, mycobacterial, or fungal (135). The vasculitis usually responds to treatment of the leukemia. Any infection, if documented, also should be treated.

Sweet's syndrome (i.e., acute febrile neutrophilic dermatosis) is associated with hematologic and nonhematologic malignancies as well as some medicines, including granulocyte colony-stimulating factor (138). The clinical and histopathologic features of Sweet's syndrome easily distinguish it from purpura during individual evaluation. Generally, the syndrome presents with discrete, erythematous papules and plaques, which may appear to be vesiculated (139). Fever, arthralgias, and myalgias may be present. Skin biopsy of representative lesions fails to reveal true leukocytoclastic vasculitis with vascular necrosis, but such specimens do show vascular edema, some extravasation of erythrocytes, and prominent neutrophilic infiltrates (139, 140).

# PSYCHOGENIC AND FACTITIOUS PURPURA

The skin lesions of psychogenic and factitious purpura are the outward manifestation of maladaptive psychiatric disorders. Psychogenic purpura has been cogently reviewed by Ratnoff (141, 142), and the reader is referred to these articles for a thorough historical, medical, and psychiatric perspective on these disorders. Various explanations have been proposed to explain the neuroendocrine mechanisms of causation (143). Four of these disorders are grouped together:

1. Factitious or directly self-induced lesions,
2. Religious stigmatization,
3. Autoerythrocyte sensitization, and
4. Autosensitization to DNA.

## FACTITIOUS PURPURA

Factitious purpura, which also is called dermatitis artefacta, results from self-abuse and concealment of the cause from physicians and other health care providers. This may be for secondary gain or the satisfaction of deceiving one's physician (i.e., a form of Münchausen syndrome). Individuals may be wiley in their deception. Clues may be found, however, in the individual's affect toward the disorder, the location of purpura and bruises (i.e., restricted to locations accessible to the individual), lesions that take the shape of the object used to inflict them, the lack of any excessive bleeding after trauma or surgery, and entirely normal results of laboratory studies. Occasionally, the individual may be caught inflicting a lesion or in a logical inconsistency, but this disorder is difficult to diagnose accurately.

In a similar disorder, individuals have surreptitiously ingested warfarin analogues (144) or quinidine (145), with consequent deficiencies of vitamin K-dependent clotting factors or platelets. These individuals exhibit abnormalities of hemostasis and abnormal laboratory results.

## RELIGIOUS STIGMATA

Religious stigmata are bruises or hemorrhages from the skin associated with a belief they are divinely induced. They have been reported to occur on days of special religious significance or in the distribution of wounds inflicted by the crucifixion of Christ. In some of these rare cases, individuals can indicate the religious association of their lesions.

## AUTOERYTHROCYTE AND DNA AUTOSENSITIZATION

In 1955, Gardner and Diamond (146) reported a syndrome of painful bruises in women with no definable coagulopathy and who had not sustained trauma. Their report related these bruises to a hypersensitivity to autologous erythrocytes. Paradoxically, some individuals were protected from bruising by the intramuscular injection of erythrocytes.

Subsequently, numerous investigators have attempted to elicit bruises in similar individuals by injecting erythrocytes, erythrocyte stroma, phosphatidyl serine (i.e., a phospholipid in erythrocyte membranes), serum, human and bovine DNA, histamine and chemicals promoting histamine release, and saline (142, 147–151). In aggregate, the results have been equivocal (152–154). The pathogenesis of these lesions is not known; therefore, it has been proposed that the syndrome be named "painful bruising syndrome" (151).

There is evidence for psychosomatic causation in some individuals, and virtually all have a history of psychiatric dysfunction, often related to severe emotional trauma (152). In one case, there was a clear correlation of widespread, typical skin lesions with use of a copper-containing intrauterine device, but not with use of a nonmetallic device (142). A local lesion has even been induced with a copper penny taped to the skin (155).

### Clinical Characteristics

Most individuals are female, most commonly adolescents or young adults. They are afflicted with painful, warm, raised, red to purple lesions. Frequently, there are associated, vague somatic or nervous complaints, and there may or may not be acknowledged antecedent trauma to the area. Characteristically, there is a prodrome of local pain, and the individual can sense development of a hematoma. Other hemorrhage, especially gastrointestinal, has been reported as well. Exacerbations and remissions are unpredictable and may be associated with emotional stress.

### Diagnosis and Therapy

Results of laboratory tests are uniformly normal. When large hematomas have been surgically drained, histologic examination has demonstrated extravasated erythrocytes and modest or absent angiitis. There also may be a mononuclear cell infiltrate late in the course of disease. Rarely, objects such as splinters or needles have been found, but surgical exploration of lesions should be undertaken only to prevent compromise of vital structures or to remove documented foreign objects. Delayed wound healing and scarring are frequent (156).

Attempts have been made to inject individuals with erythrocytes, erythrocyte fractions, DNA, tuberculin purified protein derivative, histamine, and various chemicals as a definitive challenge to provoke lesion formation (142, 147–151). In some individuals, the saline control injections also produced painful bruises. In a series of 59 individuals (142), 35 developed typical lesions at the injection sites, and the author has discontinued use of the diagnostic challenge in favor of clinical criteria. Others have advocated use of a diagnostic intradermal challenge in the emergency department (157). The usefulness of this test is limited, however. Development of painful bruises after an intradermal challenge indicates the syndrome of autoerythrocyte sensitization, but a negative challenge does not rule it out. Finally, some authors have made a distinction between DNA and autoerythrocyte sensitization (158).

There is no specific therapy for psychogenic and factitious purpura (142). If it is appropriate and the individual amenable, psychotherapy should be undertaken. These lesions are painful, and the individual may be accustomed to receiving narcotics. Therefore, limits for narcotic use should be decided early in the course of disease, and the physician should be aware the individual may be obtaining prescriptions from more than one source.

# TELANGIECTASIA/ ANGIOMATA

Telangiectasia/angiomata are best considered to represent proliferative vascular lesions, as distinguished from true vascular malformations. The latter generally are present at birth and grow in a fashion commensurate with the individual (159); an example is the port-wine stain birthmark. Vascular malformations may be purely capillary, venous, lymphatic, or arterial in origin, or they may occur in mixed forms. Hemangiomas are distinguished histologically by their prominent endothelium (during the proliferative phase) and occur during infancy or later in life. As the lesions progress, numerous dilated capillaries may be seen, and occasionally, they enlarge dramatically and cause erythrocyte fragmentation, DIC, and compromise of adjacent structures (i.e., Kasabach-Merritt syndrome) (see Chapter 44). Tissue from such lesions may be propagated *in vitro*, and the lesion growth can be modified by use of a variety of cytokines and growth factors (160).

## HEREDITARY HEMORRHAGIC TELANGIECTASIA

Hereditary hemorrhagic telangiectasia (HHT), also known as Rendu-Osler-Weber syndrome, is a familial disease of proliferative telangiectasia in the skin, mucosal surfaces, and solid organs (Fig. 43.11; see color plate 43.11) (161–163). The cosmetic problem of small telangiectasias is mild, but larger lesions may cause chronic blood loss, systemic emboli, hypoxemia, hepatic dysfunction, or high-output cardiac failure. HHT has been reported in all races, and the transmission is autosomal dominant. An association with the haplotype HLA-A2Bw17 has been noted in one family (164).

## Pathogenesis

The pathogenesis of these lesions is not known. Careful ultrastructural studies using computerized reconstructions of micrographs (165), however, have demonstrated that the earliest stage is a dilation of postcapillary venules in dermal zones 1 and 2 (i.e., those closest to the epidermis). Subsequently, direct arteriovenous connections form without any resistance vessels separating arterioles and dilated venules. This may relate to the profuse hemorrhage that is observed. A prominent histologic feature is perivascular infiltration of lymphocytes, with normal-appearing endothelium and endothelial junctions (165). This raises the possibility of an abnormal angiogenic factor resulting from the lymphocytic infiltrate contributing to development of the lesions (166–168).

Three genetic mutations are associated with HHT. All are in proteins associated with the signal transduction of transforming growth factor–β (TGF-β). TGF-β is a potent angiogenic factor and mediator of vascular remodeling (169), and abnormal TGF-β metabolism might contribute to the development of vascular abnormalities. HHT1 (or ORW1) is a mutation of endoglin, a TGF-β–binding protein. The gene resides on chromosome 9 (9q3.3-3.4) (169, 170). ORW2 has been mapped to an interval on chromosome 12q that contains the activin receptor–like kinase 1 gene (ALK-1). ALK-1 is a receptor for the TGF-β superfamily. Several ALK-1 mutations are linked to HHT in affected kindreds (171, 172), and a third locus, 3p2.2, also is linked to HHT. The TGF-βII receptor gene is located in this region (173).

Clinically and histologically similar telangiectatic lesions occur in the CREST variant of scleroderma, although with a lesser degree of lymphocytic infiltrate (174). Bleeding is not a feature of telangiectasia in CREST.

The lesions of HHT usually first appear during the second and third decades of life (175), but presentations in individuals ranging from infants to octogenarians have been reported. Penetrance depends on age and is nearly complete (97%) by age 40. Typically, the lesions are blanching, punctate, red "spots" from 0.5 to 3.0 mm in size. They usually occur on the face and lips, in the nares, and on the tongue and oral mucosa. The clinical presentation frequently is recurrent epistaxis, which is the most common complication of the syndrome and occurs in 90% of affected individuals (176). There is painless upper or lower gastrointestinal bleeding in half of these individuals and hematuria in one-sixth. Skin lesions are the hallmark of HHT, but the disease may present as gastrointestinal bleeding, iron deficiency anemia, hemoptysis, opacities in chest radiographs because of vascular ectasias, or other organ hemorrhage.

Virtually every organ may be affected, either directly or indirectly, by telangiectasias. Pulmonary arteriovenous fistulae (PAVF) occur in 15% of individuals and may lead to hypoxemia, clubbing, right-to-left shunting (without cardiomegaly), and thrombotic or septic cerebral emboli. Worsening of PAVF during pregnancy has been observed (177, 178), and individuals with the ORW1 mutation are at the highest risk for PAVF (179–181). Recommendations for screening tests vary (162, 182).

Hepatic involvement may lead to high-output congestive heart failure, cirrhosis (183), or pseudocirrhosis (184). A single case of hepatocellular carcinoma has been reported (185), and the hepatic manifestations of HHT have been reviewed by Martini (186).

Ocular involvement includes conjunctival telangiectasia (35%), which is benign but for causing bloody tears. More significant is retinal telangiectasia, which occurs in 10% of individuals and may cause retinal hemorrhage (187). Neurologic involvement, reviewed by Press and Ramsey (188), consists of thromboemboli, hyperviscosity resulting from polycythemia, air emboli, vascular spasm, rupture of intracerebral arteriovenous fistulae, altered mental status because of hypoxemia, portosystemic encephalopathy, and septic embolization. The most common organisms are anaerobic and microaerophilic streptococci (188).

## Differential Diagnosis

The most difficult differential diagnosis is distinguishing HHT from the CREST (or REST) variant of scleroderma. Telangiectasia in these variants may precede other symptoms of scleroderma by more than 10 years. Some features that help to differentiate these entities and suggest the diagnosis of HHT include a strong family history of typical HHT; absence of other features of scleroderma; a history of bleeding from telangiectasias, which is common in HHT but not in CREST (189); and a negative serologic test for anticentromere antibodies (190), which likely will be positive in the scleroderma variants.

Unilateral nevoid telangiectasia may occur over the trunk or upper extremities also with thin-walled vessels without inflammation being seen in the upper dermis on biopsy. Telangiectasia macularis eruptiva perstans is a rare mastocytosis that sometimes is marked by prominent telangiectasia and hyperpigmentation (191). The lesions commonly occur on the trunk, and they may be extensive. Urticaria that develop on pressure (i.e., Darier sign), as seen in other forms of cutaneous mastocytosis, is unusual. Another diagnostic consideration is essential telangiectasia, which is a vascular process marked by grouped, macular telangiectatic mats that usually involve the legs and buttocks.

Once the diagnosis of HHT is made, screening of family members is encouraged. One large study found that one-third of relatives tested had HHT (192); pulmonary and cerebral lesions were found in 44% of the affected individuals.

## Therapy

Treatment of HHT largely is supportive. Because of the universal involvement of endothelial beds and pervasive course of the syndrome, cure or eradication of the lesions is not feasible. Only symptomatic lesions should be treated. Control of hemorrhage, both short-term and long-term, can be technically taxing, and long-range planning is essential. Individuals with mucosal blood loss (nasopharyngeal, gastrointestinal, or urothelial) should receive iron and folic acid supplementation. It may not be possible for endogenous erythrocyte production to keep up with a brisk, gastrointestinal bleed. Transfusions are frequently required; therefore, individuals should receive recombinant hepatitis B vaccine. In addition, they should undergo complete blood group typing (i.e., major and minor antigens) to facilitate later management of multiple transfusions. Desmopressin (see Chapter 53) may supplant transfusion therapy in some cases (193), and danazol has been used with anecdotal success (194). ε-Aminocaproic acid, which inhibits fibrinolysis, has been used for alimentary tract lesions (195, 196); however, the effectiveness of this therapy is unpredictable.

Some specific interventions are worth consideration. Nasal septal dermoplasty and laser ablative therapy are beneficial in individuals with severe epistaxis (197), and carefully selected individuals may experience significant symptomatic improvement for several years. Because the pathophysiologic factors affect all areas of the skin, lesions eventually can recur in autologous tissue grafts. Therefore, long observation periods are necessary before a "cure" can be assumed (197).

McCue et al (198) suggested that PAVF be treated aggressively with early catheter embolization because of the high frequency of central nervous system complications from the pulmonary lesions. In addition, symptoms of hypoxemia resulting from right-to-left shunting, including fatigue, polycythemia, and clubbing, may be reversed if the shunt fraction is significantly reduced. In one individual, embolization of PAVF has been used to complete a pregnancy successfully (177). This modality should be considered, especially for large or symptomatic lesions.

The role of estrogen and progesterone therapy is controversial (199). Much of the supporting evidence is anecdotal, and a placebo-controlled, double-blind, randomized study (200) demonstrated no clinical or histologic improvement in oronasal lesions after 3 months of estrogen therapy. In some studies (165, 200), histologic endothelial abnormalities were not observed in the pretreatment phase, but another (201) showed estrogen therapy to reverse signs of endothelial activation. Another histologic study (202) found that estrogens induced squamous metaplasia, leading to keratinization of the squamous epithelium. This has not been universally observed, however.

There may be a physiologic basis for a response to estrogens. Receptors for both estrogen and progesterone were demonstrated on involved skin biopsy specimens from two female individuals (203), but for progesterone only in two male individuals. Appropriate controls did not have sex-steroid receptors present. In addition, patients with positive biopsies for progesterone or estrogen/progesterone had decreased mucosal bleeding during estrogen or progesterone therapy. The cellular response to occupancy of these receptors, however, is not known.

Side effects of estrogen and progesterone therapy are substantial, including increased risk of venous thrombosis. In women, endometrial bleeding occurs, and there is a risk of endometrial cancer. In men, symptoms of feminization, including testicular atrophy, gynecomastia, and decreased libido, may be intolerable. Overall, estrogens may be beneficial in a few individuals, especially to decrease gastrointestinal bleeding, but the side effects and lack of uniform efficacy preclude their general use.

## Associated Abnormalities

There has been much speculation about the relationship of HHT to coagulation abnormalities. The simultaneous occurrence of HHT and coagulopathy is a formidable problem. The association of vWf abnormalities and HHT has been reported (204–207), and a genetic linkage or common defect has been postulated. For each case in which families were studied, however, there was not complete concordance of both diseases. In 1991, Iannuzzi et al (208) analyzed restriction fragment length polymorphisms (RFLPs) and performed allele-specific polymerase chain reaction on a family with type IIa von Willebrand disease. This pedigree had no association between the von Willebrand disease mutation (Ile 865 → Thr) and the RFLPs that assorted with HHT. In this family, it can be inferred that the vWf and HHT loci are completely distinct (208), which is consistent with the three known loci associated with HHT. The gene for vWf is on the short arm of chromosome 12.

Other reported coagulopathies are a moderate deficiency of factor VIII (209) (although vWf activity was not mentioned) and an acquired inhibitor of factor VIII

that responded to immunosuppression (210). A local increase of fibrinolysis has been postulated to enhance the hemorrhagic diathesis of HHT (211), but other investigators have not demonstrated this phenomenon (212). Consumptive coagulopathy may be observed in other diseases associated with arteriovenous malformations but is not a feature of HHT. One series (213) demonstrated laboratory evidence of DIC in HHT.

## KAPOSI'S SARCOMA

Kaposi's sarcoma (KS) occurs in four distinct clinical settings (214):

1. The "classic" variety;
2. The endemic form seen among children in Africa;
3. The epidemic form seen with HIV infection; and
4. The form that develops in iatrogenically immunosuppressed individuals.

There is evidence of immunologic aberration in each of these groups.

Classic KS was initially described in 1872 (214). The disease generally occurs in those older than 50 years and in males. Most often, the process is localized and presents as a blue-purple tumor over the lower extremities (215). Dark-brown patches and lymphedema also may be seen (Fig. 43.12; see color plate 43.12) (216). This is a slowly progressive disease, with only rare involvement of viscera or death. There is an increased frequency of HLA-DR5 in individuals with this disease (217, 218) as well as a decreased frequency of HLA-B8 and HLA-DR3 and an increased frequency of homozygosity of the Gm haplotype 3; 5, 13 (217). Other studies, however, refute any association of HLA-antigen with classic KS (219).

When related to AIDS (see Chapter 48), KS has a younger age of onset (average, 34 years). This disease often is widespread in a given individual and can be quite aggressive. The lower extremities, as distinguished from classic KS, are less commonly involved than other skin or mucous membranes, gastrointestinal tract, and lymph nodes (215).

Widespread lesions of KS have been observed in individuals who are immunosuppressed for renal transplantation (220, 221), after cyclosporine therapy (222), with rheumatoid arthritis (223), and in one individual receiving intra-articular and epidural corticosteroid injections (224). This form regresses after immunosuppression is reduced.

The clinical forms of KS do not differ hisopathologically. Vascular proliferation with prominent endothelium and spindle-cell formation is seen in well-defined lesions; early lesions may appear somewhat granulomatous (216).

Human herpesvirus-8 or KS-associated herpesvirus (KSHV) DNA is in KS lesions of all varieties (225–228), thus suggesting a possible etiologic role. However, these findings are not specific to KS. The virus has been found in AIDS-associated lymphomas (229), Castleman disease (230), basal cell carcinomas, squamous cell carcinomas, actinic and seborrheic keratoses, and warts (231). In one study (232), KSHV was in the peripheral blood monocytes in 52% of individuals with KS and in none of 160 controls. Antibodies to KSHV nuclear antigen develop before KS lesions (233). KSHV can be cultured from active KS lesions (234), and KSHV detection is correlated with low CD4 counts.

Response of KS to treatment depends on the clinical setting. Classic KS frequently does not require therapy or, alternatively, responds well to single-agent vinblastine (235). KS arising during immunosuppression responds best to withdrawal of the immunosuppressive agent. In AIDS-related KS, individual lesions have been treated successfully with cryotherapy, radiotherapy, and intralesional injections of chemotherapeutic agents. For disseminated disease, recombinant interferon-α and systemic chemotherapy have been used.

Interferon-$\alpha_{2A}$ induces a complete response in 30 to 35% of individuals with AIDS-related KS. The response is better in individuals without other opportunistic infections and with CD4 counts greater than 300 cells/μl (236, 237). As single agents, vinblastine, vincristine, anthracyclines, or podophyllotoxin derivatives have poor response rates in AIDS-related KS (238, 239). A regimen of low-dose doxorubicin, bleomycin, and vincristine has a combined complete and partial remission rate of 88% (240).

# REFERENCES

1. Rao AK. Congenital disorders of platelet function. Hematol Oncol Clin North Am 1990;4:65–86.
2. Lacombe M, Soria J, Soria C et al. Fibrinogen Montreal. A new case of congenital dysfibrinogenemia with defective aggregation of monomers. Thromb Diath Haemorrh 1973;29:536–546.
3. Weiss HJ, Rogers J. Fibrinogen and platelets in the primary arrest of bleeding. Studies in two individuals with congenital afibrinogenemia. N Engl J Med 1971;285:369–374.
4. Rodgers RP, Levin J. A critical reappraisal of the bleeding time. Semin Thromb Hemost 1990;16:1–20.
5. Lind SE. Prolonged bleeding time. Am J Med 1984;77:305–312.
6. Sham RL, Francis CW. Evaluation of mild bleeding disorders and easy bruising [Review]. Blood Rev 1994;8:98–104.
7. Hartmann JR, Diamond LK. Natural history of seventy-three individuals with hemophilia and related hemorrhagic diseases. Am J Dis Child 1955;90:594–595.
8. Youssoufian H, Kazazian HH Jr, Phillips DG et al. Recurrent mutations in haemophilia A give evidence for CpG mutation hotspots. Nature 1986;324:380–382.
9. Deykin D, Janson P, McMahon L. Ethanol potentiation of aspirin-induced prolongation of the bleeding time. N Engl J Med 1982;306:852–854.
10. Fiore LD, Brophy MT, Lopez A et al. The bleeding time response to aspirin. Identifying the hyperresponder. Am J Clin Pathol 1990;94:292–296.
11. Lee MH, Vosburgh E, Anderson K et al. Deficiency of plasma plasminogen activator inhibitor 1 results in hyperfibrinolytic bleeding. Blood 1993;81:2357–2362.
12. Fay WP, Shapiro AD, Shih JL et al. Brief report: complete deficiency of plasminogen-activator inhibitor type 1 due to a frame-shift mutation. N Engl J Med 1992;327:1729–1733.
13. Dieval J, Nguyen G, Gross S et al. A lifelong bleeding disorder associated with a deficiency of plasminogen activator inhibitor type 1. Blood 1991;77:528–532.
14. Aoki N, Saito H, Kamiya T et al. Congenital deficiency of α2-plasmin inhibitor associated with severe hemorrhagic tendency. J Clin Invest 1979;63:877–884.
15. Hunter DJ, Smart JR, Whitton L. Increased capillary fragility at high altitude. Br Med J (Clin Res) 1986;292:98.
16. Forster PJ. Microvascular fragility at high altitude [Letter]. Br Med J (Clin Res) 1988;296:1004–1005.
17. Hood I, Ryan D, Spitz WU. Resuscitation and petechiae. Am J Forensic Med Pathol 1988;9:35–37.
18. Gewirtzman GB. Sweetheart's syndrome: purpura of a pleasant nature. Cutis 1985;35:359.
19. Metzker A, Merlob P. Suction purpura. Arch Dermatol 1992;128:822–824.
20. Gough GR. Capillary resistance to suction in hypertension. Blood 1962;28:19–33.
21. Yates VM. Factitious purpura. Clin Exp Dermatol 1992;17:238–239.
22. Leung AK. Purpura associated with exposure to sunlight. J R Soc Med 1986;79:423–424.
23. Finlay AY, Finlay IG, Paton EL et al. Antecubital fossa petechiae in Scottish country dancers [Letter]. Lancet 1985;ii:1191.
24. Hendricks WM. Grass-trimmer's purpura [Letter]. N Engl J Med 1986;315:199–200.
25. Litt JZ. "Pastoral" purpura. J Am Acad Dermatol 1989;20:851–852.
26. Whinnery JE. Comparative distribution of petechial haemorrhages as a function of aircraft cockpit geometry. J Biomed Eng 1987;9:201–205.
27. Siegel DM, Goldberg LH, Altman AR et al. Paint pellet purpura: a peril for pistol-packing paramilitary personnel [Letter]. JAMA 1986;255:3367.
28. Leung AK, Grant RM, Truscott R. Exercise-induced purpura. J Sports Med Phys Fitness 1990;30:329–330.
29. Champion RH. Purpura. In: Rook A, Wilkinson DS, Ebling FBJ, eds. Textbook of dermatology. 5th ed. Oxford: Blackwell Scientific Publications, 1992:1881–1892.
30. Menditto V, Borrelli L. Bateman's disease. Pathologica 1994;86:645–648.
31. Tercedor J, Lopez-Hernandez B, Rodenas JM et al. Multivariate analysis of cutaneous markers of aging in chronic hemodialyzed individuals. Int J Dermatol 1995;34:546–550.
32. Oikarinen AI, Vuorio EI, Zaragoza EJ et al. Modulation of collagen metabolism by glucocorticoids. Receptor-mediated effects of dexamethasone on collagen biosynthesis in chick embryo fibroblasts and chondrocytes. Biochem Pharmacol 1988;37:1451–1462.
33. Nasser TK, Mohler ER III, Wilensky RL et al. Peripheral vascular complications following coronary interventional procedures [Review]. Clin Cardiol 1995;18:609–614.
34. Bruno A, Jones WL, Austin JK et al. Vascular outcome in men with asymptomatic retinal cholesterol emboli. A cohort study. Ann Intern Med 1995;122:249–253.
35. Kalter DC, Rudolph A, McGavran M. Livedo reticularis due to multiple cholesterol emboli. J Am Acad Dermatol 1985;13:235–242.
36. Peat DS, Mathieson PW. Cholesterol emboli may mimic systemic vasculitis. Br Med J 1996;313:546–547.
37. Richards AM, Eliot RS, Kanjuh VI et al. Cholesterol embolism: a multisystem disease masquerading as polyarteritis nodosa. Am J Cardiol 1965;15:696–707.
38. Pierce JR, Wren MV, Cousar JB Jr. Cholesterol embolism: diagnosis antemortem by bone marrow biopsy. Ann Intern Med 1978;89:937–938.
39. Fabian TC, Hoots AV, Stanford DS et al. Fat embolism syndrome: prospective evaluation in 92 fracture individuals. Crit Care Med 1990;18:42–46.
40. Miller JD. Fat embolism: a clinical diagnosis. Am Fam Physician 1987;35:129–134.
41. Pell AC, Hughes D, Keating J et al. Brief report: fulminating fat embolism syndrome caused by paradoxical embolism through a patent foramen ovale. N Engl J Med 1993;329:926–929.
42. Fabian TC. Unraveling the fat embolism syndrome. N Engl J Med 1993;329:961–963.
43. Laub DR Jr, Laub DR. Fat embolism syndrome after liposuction: a case report and Review of the literature. Ann Plast Surg 1990;25:48–52.
44. Levy D. The fat embolism syndrome [Review]. Clin Orthop 1990;261:281–286.
45. Chastre J, Fagon JY, Soler P et al. Bronchoalveolar lavage for rapid diagnosis of the fat embolism syndrome in trauma individuals. Ann Intern Med 1990;113:583–588.
46. Ganong RB. Fat emboli syndrome in isolated fractures of the tibia and femur. Clin Orthop 1993;291:208–214.
47. Burlina AB, Dionisi-Vici C, Bennett MJ et al. A new syndrome with ethylmalonic aciduria and normal fatty acid oxidation in fibroblasts. J Pediatr 1994;124:79–86.
48. Garcia-Silva MT, Campos Y, Ribes A et al. Encephalopathy, petechiae, and acrocyanosis with ethylmalonic aciduria associated with muscle cytochrome c oxidase deficiency [Letter]. J Pediatr 1994;125:843–844.
49. Burlina AB. Encephalopathy, petechiae, and acrocyanosis with ethylmalonic aciduria associated with muscle cytochrome c oxidase deficiency [Reply]. J Pediatr 1994;843.

50. Lever WF, Schaumberg-Lever G. Vascular diseases. In: Histopathology of the skin. 7th ed. Philadelphia: JB Lippincott, 1990:185–209.

51. Newton RC, Raimer SS. Pigmented purpuric eruptions. Dermatol Clin 1985;3:165–169.

52. Riordan CA, Darley C, Markey AC et al. Unilateral linear capillaritis. Clin Exp Dermatol 1992;17:182–185.

53. Pang BK, Su D, Ratnam KV. Drug-induced purpura simplex: clinical and histological characteristics. Ann Acad Med Singapore 1993;22:870–872.

54. Stratakis CA, Chrousos GP. Capillaritis (purpura simplex) associated with use of aminoglutethimide in Cushing's syndrome. Am J Hosp Pharm 1994; 51:2589–2591.

55. Smithson JE, Kennedy CT, Hughes S. A new skin lesion associated with intravenous streptokinase. Br Med J 1993;306:973.

56. Krizsa J, Hunyadi J, Dobozy A. PUVA treatment of pigmented purpuric lichenoid dermatitis (Gougerot-Blum). J Am Acad Dermatol 1992;27: 778–780.

57. Tamaki K, Yasaka N, Osada A et al. Successful treatment of pigmented purpuric dermatosis with griseofulvin [Letter]. Br J Dermatol 1995;132: 159–160.

58. Musher DM. Cutaneous manifestations of bacterial sepsis. Hosp Pract (Off Ed) 1989;71–75, 80–82, 92.

59. Silverman DJ, Bond SB. Infection of human vascular endothelial cells by Rickettsia rickettsii. J Infect Dis 1984;149:201–206.

60. Rao AK, Schapira M, Clements ML et al. A prospective study of platelets and plasma proteolytic systems during the early stages of Rocky Mountain spotted fever. N Engl J Med 1988;318:1021–1028.

61. Baker RC, Seguin JH, Leslie N et al. Fever and petechiae in children. Pediatrics 1989;84:1051–1055.

62. Musser JM, Selander RK. Brazilian purpuric fever: evolutionary genetic relationships of the case clone of Haemophilus influenzae biogroup aegyptius to encapsulated strains of Haemophilus influenzae. J Infect Dis 1990; 161:130–133.

63. Goldenhersh MA. Petechiae caused by streptococcal pharyngitis. J Am Acad Dermatol 1992;27:456–457.

64. Epps RE, Pittelkow MR, Su WP. TORCH syndrome. Semin Dermatol 1995; 14:179–186.

65. Sams WM Jr. Hypersensitivity angiitis. J Invest Dermatol 1989;93(Suppl 2):78–81.

66. Kallick CA. A febrile child with a peripheral hemorrhagic rash. Infect Med 1991;15–16.

67. Feldmann R, Harms M, Saurat JH. Papular-purpuric "gloves and socks" syndrome. J Am Acad Dermatol 1990;23:850–854.

68. Evans LM, Grossman ME, Gregory N. Koplik spots and a purpuric eruption associated with parvovirus B19 infection. J Am Acad Dermatol 1992; 27:466–467.

69. Halasz CL, Cormier D, Den M. Petechial glove and sock syndrome caused by parvovirus B19. J Am Acad Dermatol 1992;27:835–838.

70. Perez-Ferriols A, Martinez-Aparicio A, Aliaga-Boniche A. Papular-purpuric "gloves and socks" syndrome caused by measles virus [Letter]. J Am Acad Dermatol 1994;30:291–292.

71. Guibal F, Buffet P, Mouly F et al. Papular-purpuric gloves and socks syndrome with hepatitis B infection [Letter]. Lancet 1996;347:473.

72. Feldmann R, Harms M, Saurat JH. Papular-purpuric 'gloves and socks' syndrome: not only parvovirus B19. Dermatology 1994;188:85–87.

73. Person DA. Gloves and socks syndrome [Letter]. Lancet 1996;347: 1125–1126.

74. Molina M, Ortega G, Galvez J et al. Leukocytoclastic vasculitis secondary to flue vaccination [Letter]. Med Clin 1990;95:78.

75. Lewis K, Jordan SC, Cherry JD et al. Petechiae and urticaria after DTP vaccination: detection of circulating immune complexes containing vaccine-specific antigens. J Pediatr 1986;109:1009–1012.

76. Glikson M, Galun E, Oren R et al. Relapsing hepatitis A. Review of 14 cases and literature survey [Review]. Medicine 1992;71:14–23.

77. Zurn A, Schmied E, Saurat JH. Cutaneous manifestations of infection due to hepatitis B virus. Schweiz Rundsch Med Prax 1990;79:1254–1257.

78. Gocke DJ, Hsu K, Morgan C et al. Vasculitis in association with Australia antigen. J Exp Med 1971;134(Suppl):330S–336S.

79. Anonymous. Human parvovirus and purpura [Letter]. Lancet 1985;ii: 730–731.

80. Li-Loong TC, Coyle PV, Anderson MJ et al. Human serum parvovirus associated vasculitis. Postgrad Med J 1986;62:493–494.

81. Yrivarren JL, Lopez LR. Cryoglobulinemia and cutaneous vasculitis in human brucellosis. J Clin Immunol 1987;7:471–474.

82. Berenson CS, Dobuler KJ, Bia FJ. Fever, petechiae, and pulmonary infiltrates in an immunocompromised Peruvian man. Yale J Biol Med 1987; 60:437–445.

83. Kalb RE, Grossman ME. Periumbilical purpura in disseminated strongyloidiasis. JAMA 1986;256:1170–1171.

84. Purvis RS, Beightler EL, Diven DG et al. Strongyloides hyperinfection presenting with petechiae and purpura. Int J Dermatol 1992;31:169–171.

85. Merrien D, Raffi F, Barbier JH. Febrile purpura disclosing primary cytomegalovirus infection [Letter]. Presse Med 1990;19:1681–1682.

86. Agarwal N, Arora RC, Sood P et al. Malaria presenting as purpura [Letter]. J Assoc Physicians India 1987;35:804.

87. Maness DL, Rogers DY. Hemorrhagic complications of varicella. Am Fam Physician 1987;35:151–155.

88. Miller HC, Stephan M. Hemorrhagic varicella: a case report and Review of the complications of varicella in children [Review]. Am J Emerg Med 1993;11:633–638.

89. Cosgriff TM. Viruses and hemostasis. Rev Infect Dis 1989;11(Suppl 4): S672–S688.

90. Anstey A, Mayne K, Winter M et al. Platelet and coagulation studies in Ehlers-Danlos syndrome. Br J Dermatol 1991;125:155–163.

91. Byers PH. Ehlers-Danlos syndrome type IV: a genetic disorder in many guises [Editorial]. J Invest Dermatol 1995;105:311–313.

92. Byers PH. Ehlers-Danlos syndrome: recent advances and current understanding of the clinical and genetic heterogeneity. J Invest Dermatol 1994; 103(Suppl):47–52.

93. Byers PH. Disorders of collagen biosynthesis and structure. In: Scriver CR, Beaudet AL, Sly WS, Valle D, eds. Metabolic and molecular bases of inherited disease. 7th ed. New York: McGraw-Hill, 1995;4029–4078.

94. Lebwohl M, Neldner K, Pope FM et al. Classification of pseudoxanthoma elasticum: report of a consensus conference. J Am Acad Dermatol 1994; 30:103–107.

95. Spinzi G, Strocchi E, Imperiali G et al. Pseudoxanthoma elasticum: a rare cause of gastrointestinal bleeding. Am J Gastroenterol 1996;91: 1631–1634.

96. Piette WW. Myeloma, paraproteinemias, and the skin [Review]. Med Clin North Am 1986;70:155–176.

97. Kyle RA, Gleich GJ, Bayrid ED et al. Benign hypergammaglobulinemic purpura of Waldenstrom. Medicine 1971;50:113–123.

98. Brownstein MH, Helwig EB. The cutaneous amyloidoses. II. Systemic forms. Arch Dermatol 1970;102:20–28.

99. Stone GC, Wall BA, Oppliger IR. A vasculopathy with deposition of lambda light chain crystals. Ann Intern Med 1989;110:275–278.

100. Davis MD, Su WP. Cryoglobulinemia: recent findings in cutaneous and extracutaneous manifestations. Int J Dermatol 1996;35:240–248.

101. Jantunen E, Soppi E, Neittaanmaki H et al. Essential cryofibrinogenaemia, leukocytoclastic vasculitis and chronic purpura. J Intern Med 1993;234: 331–333.

102. Gumber SC, Chopra S. Hepatitis C: a multifaceted disease. Review of extrahepatic manifestations. Ann Intern Med 1995;123:615–620.

103. Miescher PA, Huang YP, Izui S. Type II cryoglobulinemia [Review]. Semin Hematol 1995;32:80–85.

104. Wang AC. Molecular basis for cryoprecipitation. Springer Semin Immunopathol 1988;10:21–34.

105. Ireland TA, Werner DA, Rietschel RL et al. Cutaneous lesions in cryofibrinogenemia. J Pediatr 1984;105:67–69.

106. Speight EL, Lawrence CM. Reticulate purpura, cryoglobulinaemia and livedo reticularis. Br J Dermatol 1993;129:319–323.

107. Zip CM, Ross JB, Greaves MW et al. Familial cold urticaria. Clin Exp Dermatol 1993;18:338–341.

108. Torok L, Borka I, Szabo G. Waldenstrom's macroglobulinaemia presenting with cold urticaria and cold purpura. Clin Exp Dermatol 1993;18:277–279.

109. Pachter MR, Basinski DH, Johnson SA. The effect of macroglobulins and their dissociation units on release of platelet factor 3. Thromb Diath Haemorrh 1959;3:501–509.

110. Cohen I, Amir J, Ben-Shaul Y et al. Plasma cell myeloma associated with an unusual myeloma protein causing impairment of fibrin aggregation and platelet function in a individual with multiple malignancy. Am J Med 1970;48:766–776.

111. Perkins HA, MacKenzie MR, Fudenberg HH. Hemostatic defects in dysproteinemias. Blood 1970;35:695–707.

112. Penny R, Castaldi PA, Whitsed HM. Inflammation and haemostasis in paraproteinaemias. Br J Haematol 1971;20:35–44.

113. DiMinno G, Coraggio F, Cerbone AM et al. A myeloma paraprotein with specificity for platelet glycoprotein IIIa in a individual with a fatal bleeding disorder. J Clin Invest 1986;77:157–164.

114. Kirsner RS, Eaglstein WH, Katz MH et al. Stanozolol causes rapid pain relief and healing of cutaneous ulcers caused by cryofibrinogenemia. J Am Acad Dermatol 1993;28:71–74.

115. Helfman T, Falanga V. Stanozolol as a novel therapeutic agent in dermatology [Review]. J Am Acad Dermatol 1995;32:254–258.

116. Francis RB Jr. Acquired purpura fulminans. Semin Thromb Hemost 1990; 16:310–325.

117. Adcock DM, Brozna J, Marlar RA. Proposed classification and pathologic mechanisms of purpura fulminans and skin necrosis. Semin Thromb Hemost 1990;16:333–340.

118. Guccione JL, Zemtsov A, Cobos E et al. Acquired purpura fulminans induced by alcohol and acetaminophen. Arch Dermatol 1993;129:1267–1269.

119. Stricker H, Lammle B, Furlan M et al. Heparin-dependent in vitro aggregation of normal platelets by plasma of a individual with heparin-induced skin necrosis: specific diagnostic test for a rare side effect. Am J Med 1988; 85:721–724.

120. Hartman AR, Hood RM, Anagnostopoulos CE. Phenomenon of heparin-

induced thrombocytopenia associated with skin necrosis. J Vasc Surg 1988; 7:781–784.

121. O'Toole RD. Heparin toxicity: adverse reaction. Ann Intern Med 1973;79: 759.

122. White PW, Sadd JR, Nensel RE. Thrombotic complications of heparin therapy. Ann Surg 1979;190:595–608.

123. Freyssinet JM, Cazenave JP. Lupus-like anticoagulants, modulation of the protein C pathway and thrombosis. Thromb Haemost 1987;58:679–681.

124. Cariou R, Tobelem G, Bellucci S et al. Effect of lupus anticoagulant on antithrombogenic properties of endothelial cells—inhibition of thrombomodulin-dependent protein C activation. Thromb Haemost 1988;60:54–58.

125. Grob JJ, Bonerandi JJ. Cutaneous manifestations associated with the presence of the lupus anticoagulant. A report of two cases and a Review of the literature. J Am Acad Dermatol 1986;15:211–219.

126. Chong BH. Heparin-induced thrombocytopenia. Br J Haematol 1995;89: 431–439.

127. Visentin GP, Ford SE, Scott JP et al. Antibodies from individuals with heparin-induced thrombocytopenia/thrombosis are specific for platelet factor 4 complexed with heparin or bound to endothelial cells. J Clin Invest 1994;93:81–88.

128. Michiels JJ, Bertina RM. Thrombo-hemorrhagic skin necrosis due to rapid development of severe vitamin K deficiency associated with cholestasis [Abstract]. Thromb Haemost 1987;58:1512.

129. Adcock DM, Hicks MJ. Dermatopathology of skin necrosis associated with purpura fulminans. Semin Thromb Hemost 1990;16:283–292.

130. Miletich J, Sherman L, Broze G. Absence of thrombosis in subjects with heterozygous protein C deficiency. N Engl J Med 1987;317:991–996.

131. Hunder G. Vasculitis: diagnosis and therapy [Review]. Am J Med 1996; 100(Suppl 2A):37S–45S.

132. Braquet P, Hosford D, Braquet M et al. Role of cytokines and platelet-activating factor in microvascular immune injury. Int Arch Allergy Appl Immunol 1989;88:88–100.

133. Gibson LE. Cutaneous vasculitis: approach to diagnosis and systemic associations. Mayo Clin Proc 1990;65:221–229.

134. Murray JC, Mahoney DH Jr, Dominey AM. Panniculitis in the differential diagnosis of recurrent purpura and hematomata in children [Letter]. Am J Hematol 1993;43:327–328.

135. Farcet JP, Weschsler J, Wirquin V et al. Vasculitis in hairy-cell leukemia. Arch Intern Med 1987;147:660–664.

136. Lowe J, Russell NH. Cerebral vasculitis associated with hairy-cell leukemia. Cancer 1987;60:3025–3028.

137. Lie JT. Isolated polyarteritis of the testis in hairy cell leukemia. Arch Pathol Lab Med 1988;112:646–647.

138. Jain KK. Sweet's syndrome associated with granulocyte colony-stimulating factor [Review]. Cutis 1996;57:107–110.

139. Moragas JM, Pujol RM. Neutrophilic dermatoses. Curr Opin Dermatol 1997;4:13–20.

140. Barnhill RL, Busam KJ. Vascular Diseases. In: Elder D, Elenitsas R, Jaworski C, Johnson B Jr, eds. Lever's histopathology of the skin. 8th ed. Philadelphia: Lippincott-Raven, 1997:204–206.

141. Ratnoff OD. The psychogenic purpuras: a Review of autoerythrocyte sensitization, autosensitization to DNA, "hysterical" and factitial bleeding, and the religious stigmata. Semin Hematol 1980;17:192–213.

142. Ratnoff OD. Psychogenic purpura (autoerythrocyte sensitization): an unsolved dilemma. Am J Med 1989;87(Suppl 3N):16–21.

143. Panconesi E, Hautmann G. Stress, stigmatization and psychosomatic purpuras. Int Angiol 1995;14:130–137.

144. Weitzel JN, Sadowski JA, Furie BC. Surreptitious ingestion of a long-acting vitamin K antagonist/rodenticide, brondifacoum: clinical and metabolic studies of three cases. Blood 1990;76:2555–2559.

145. Reid DM, Shulman NR. Drug purpura due to surreptitious quinidine intake. Ann Intern Med 1988;108:206–208.

146. Gardner FH, Diamond LK. Autoerythrocyte sensitization: a form of purpura producing painful bruising following autosensitization to red blood cells in certain women. Blood 1955;10:675–690.

147. Groch GS, Finch SC, Rogoway W et al. Studies in the pathogenesis of autoerythrocyte sensitization syndrome. Blood 1966;28:19–33.

148. Kremer WB, Mengel CE, Nowlin JB et al. Recurrent ecchymoses and cutaneous hyperreactivity to hemoglobin: a form of autoerythrocyte sensitization. Blood 1967;30:62–73.

149. Shulman NR, Feigon JH, Bithell TC. The role of histamine in the pathogenesis of a disease characterized by ecchymoses and systemic symptoms. Clin Res 1959;7:216.

150. Starink TM. Painful bruising syndrome. Dermatology 1974;149:191–192.

151. Hersle K, Mobacken H. Autoerythrocyte sensitization syndrome (painful bruising syndrome). Report of two cases and review of literature. Br J Dermatol 1969;81:574–587.

152. McDuffie FC, McGuire FL. Clinical and psychological patterns in autoerythrocyte sensitivity. Ann Intern Med 1965;63:255–265.

153. Stocker WW, McIntyre R, Clendenning WE. Psychogenic purpura. Arch Dermatol 1977;113:606–609.

154. Meister MM, Bodner AC. Autoerythrocyte sensitization—a psychogenic purpura? Cutis 1977;19:221–224.

155. Grossman RA. Autoerythrocyte sensitization worsened by a copper-containing IUD. Obstet Gynecol 1987;70:526–528.

156. Koblenzer PJ, Koblenzer CS. Psychogenic purpura: a most distressing case. Cutis 1990;45:60–61.

157. Tomec RJ, Walsh M, Garcia JC et al. Diagnosis of autoerythrocyte sensitization syndrome in the emergency department. Ann Emerg Med 1989;18: 780–782.

158. Berman DA, Roenigk HH, Green D. Autoerythrocyte sensitization syndrome (psychogenic purpura). J Am Acad Dermatol 1992;27:829–832.

159. Mulliken JB. Classification of vascular birthmarks. In: Mulliken JB, Young A, eds. Vascular birthmarks. Philadelphia: WB Saunders, 1988:24–37.

160. Folkman J, Klagsburn M. Angiogenic factors. Science 1987;235:442–447.

161. Peery WH. Clinical spectrum of hereditary hemorrhagic telangiectasia (Osler-Weber-Rendu Disease). Am J Med 1987;82:989–997.

162. Guttmacher AE, Marchuk DA, White RI Jr. Hereditary hemorrhagic telangiectasia. N Engl J Med 1995;333:918–924.

163. Haitjema T, Westermann CJ, Overtoom TT et al. Hereditary hemorrhagic telangiectasia (Osler-Weber-Rendu disease): new insights in pathogenesis, complications, and treatment [Review]. Arch Intern Med 1996;156: 714–719.

164. Kissel P, Raffoux C, Faure G et al. HLA antigens and hereditary hemorrhagic telangiectasia. Int Arch Allergy Appl Immunol 1977;54:281–284.

165. Braverman IM, Keh A, Jacobson BS. Ultrastructure and three-dimensional organization of the telangiectases of hereditary hemorrhagic telangiectasia. J Invest Dermatol 1990;95:422–427.

166. Auerbach R, Sidky YA. Nature of the stimulus leading to lymphocyte-induced angiogenesis. J Immunol 1979;123:751–754.

167. Leibovich SJ, Polverini PJ, Shephard HM et al. Macrophage-induced angiogenesis is mediated by tumor necrosis factor-alpha. Nature 1987;329: 630–632.

168. Malhotra R, Stenn KS, Fernandez LA et al. Angiogenic properties of normal and psoriatic skin associate with epidermis, not dermis. Lab Invest 1989;61:162–165.

169. McAllister KA, Grogg KM, Johnson DW et al. Endoglin, a TGF-beta binding protein of endothelial cells, is the gene for hereditary haemorrhagic telangiectasia type 1. Nat Genet 1994;8:345–351.

170. Heutink P, Haitjema T, Breedveld GJ et al. Linkage of hereditary haemorrhagic telangiectasia to chromosome 9q34 and evidence for locus heterogeneity. J Med Genet 1994;31:933–936.

171. Johnson DW, Berg JN, Baldwin MA et al. Mutations in the activin receptor-like kinase 1 gene in hereditary haemorrhagic telangiectasia type 2. Nat Genet 1996;13:189–195.

172. Johnson DW, Berg JN, Gallione CJ et al. A second locus for hereditary hemorrhagic telangiectasia maps to chromosome 12. Genome Res 1995;5: 21–28.

173. Vincent P, Plauchu H, Hazan J et al. A third locus for hereditary haemorrhagic telangiectasia maps to chromosome 12q. Hum Mol Genet 1995;4: 945–949.

174. Braverman IM, Ken-Yen A. Ultrastructure and three-dimensional reconstruction of several macular and papular telangiectases. J Invest Dermatol 1983;81:489–497.

175. Olsen T. Peripheral vascular diseases, necrotizing vasculitis, and vascular related diseases. In: Moschella SL, Hurley HS, eds. Dermatology. 2nd ed. Philadelphia: WB Saunders, 1985:1050–1051.

176. AAssar OS, Friedman CM, White RI Jr. The natural history of epistaxis in hereditary hemorrhagic telangiectasia. Laryngoscope 1991;101:977–980.

177. Gammon RB, Miksa AK, Keller FS. Osler-Weber-Rendu disease and pulmonary arteriovenous fistulas. Deterioration and embolotherapy during pregnancy. Chest 1990;98:1522–1524.

178. Swinburne AJ, Fedullo AJ, Gangemi R et al. Hereditary telangiectasia and multiple pulmonary arteriovenous fistulas. Clinical deterioration during pregnancy. Chest 1986;89:459–460.

179. Berg JN, Guttmacher AE, Marchuk DA et al. Clinical heterogeneity in hereditary haemorrhagic telangiectasia: are pulmonary arteriovenous malformations more common in families linked to endoglin? J Med Genet 1996;33:256–257.

180. Porteous ME, Curtis A, Williams O et al. Genetic heterogeneity in hereditary haemorrhagic telangiectasia. J Med Genet 1994;31:925–926.

181. McAllister KA, Lennon F, Bowles-Biesecker B et al. Genetic heterogeneity in hereditary haemorrhagic telangiectasia: possible correlation with clinical phenotype. J Med Genet 1994;31:927–932.

182. Shovlin CL, Hughes JM. Hereditary hemorrhagic telangiectasia [Letter]. N Engl J Med 1996;334:330–331.

183. Deviere J, Brohee D, Hiden M et al. Hepatic telangiectasia and cirrhosis. J Clin Gastroenterol 1988;10:111–114.

184. Cooney T, Sweeney EC, Coll R et al. 'Pseudocirrhosis' in hereditary haemorrhagic telangiectasia. J Clin Pathol 1977;30:1134–1141.

185. Jameson CF. Primary hepatocellular carcinoma in hereditary haemorrhagic telangiectasia: a case report and literature review. Histopathology 1989;15:550–552.

186. Martini GA. The liver in hereditary haemorrhagic telangiectasia: an inborn error of vascular structure with multiple manifestations: a reappraisal. Gut 1978;19:531–537.

187. Brant AM, Schachat AP, White RI. Ocular manifestations in hereditary hemorrhagic telangiectasia (Rendu-Osler-Weber disease). Am J Ophthalmol 1989;107:642–646.

188. Press OW, Ramsey PG. Central nervous system infections associated with hereditary hemorrhagic telangiectasia. Am J Med 1984;77:86–92.

189. Allende HD, Ona FV, Noronha AI. Bleeding gastric telangiectasia. Complications of Raynaud's phenomenon, esophageal motor dysfunction, sclerodactyly and telangiectasia (REST) syndrome. Am J Gastroenterol 1981;75:354–356.

190. Fritzler MJ, Arlette JP, Behm AR et al. Hereditary hemorrhagic telangiectasia versus CREST syndrome: can serology aid diagnosis? J Am Acad Dermatol 1984;10:192–196.

191. Denis DJ. Mast cell disease. In: Denis DJ, ed. Clinical dermatology. Philadelphia: JB Lippincott, 1990:1–27.

192. Haitjema T, Disch F, Overtoom TT et al. Screening family members of individuals with hereditary hemorrhagic telangiectasia. Am J Med 1995;99:519–524.

193. Quitt M, Froom P, Veisler A et al. The effect of desmopressin on massive gastrointestinal bleeding in hereditary telangiectasia unresponsive to treatment with cryoprecipitate. Arch Intern Med 1990;150:1744–1746.

194. Haq AU, Glass J, Netchvolodoff CV et al. Hereditary hemorrhagic telangiectasia and danazol [Letter]. Ann Intern Med 1988;109:171.

195. Saba HI, Morelli GA, Logrono LA. Brief report: treatment of bleeding in hereditary hemorrhagic telangiectasia with aminocaproic acid. N Engl J Med 1994;330:1789–1790.

196. Korzenik JR, Topazian MD, White R. Treatment of bleeding in hereditary hemorrhagic telangiectasia with aminocaproic acid [Letter]. N Engl J Med 1994;331:1236.

197. Siegel MB, Keane WM, Atkins JF Jr et al. Control of epistaxis in individuals with hereditary hemorrhagic telangiectasia. Otolaryngol Head Neck Surg 1991;105:675–679.

198. McCue CM, Hartenberg M, Nance WE. Pulmonary arteriovenous malformations related to Rendu-Osler-Weber syndrome. Am J Med Genet 1984;19:19–27.

199. Lewis BS, Kornbluth A. Hormonal therapy for bleeding from angiodysplasia: chronic renal failure. Am J Gastroenterol 1990;85:1649–1651.

200. Vase P, Lorentzen M. Histological findings following oestrogen treatment of hereditary haemorrhagic telangiectasia. A controlled double-blind investigation. J Laryngol Otol 1983;97:427–429.

201. Menefee MG, Flessa HC, Glueck HI et al. Hereditary hemorrhagic telangiectasia (Osler-Weber-Rendu disease). An electron microscopic study of the vascular lesions before and after therapy with hormones. Arch Otolaryngol 1975;101:246–251.

202. Harrison DF. Use of estrogen in treatment of familial hemorrhagic telangiectasia. Laryngoscope 1982;92:314–320.

203. Richtsmeier W, Weaver G, Streck W et al. Estrogen and progesterone receptors in hereditary hemorrhagic telangiectasia. Otolaryngol Head Neck Surg 1984;92:564–570.

204. Quick AJ. Telangiectasia: its relationship to the Minot-von Willebrand syndrome. Am J Med Sci 1967;254:585–601.

205. Ahr DJ, Rickles FR, Hoyer LW et al. von Willebrand's disease and hemorrhagic telangiectasia: association of two complex disorders of hemostasis resulting in life-threatening hemorrhage. Am J Med 1977;62:452–458.

206. Conlon CL, Weinger RS, Cimo PL et al. Telangiectasia and von Willebrand's disease in two families. Ann Intern Med 1978;89:921–924.

207. Hanna W, McCarroll D, Lin D et al. A study of a Caucasian family with variant von Willebrand's disease in association with vascular telangiectasia and haemoglobinopathy. Thromb Haemost 1984;51:275–278.

208. Iannuzzi MC, Hidaka N, Boehnke M et al. Analysis of the relationship of von Willebrand disease (vWd) and hereditary hemorrhagic telangiectasia and identification of a potential type IIA vWd mutation (IIe865 to Thr). Am J Hum Genet 1991;48:757–763.

209. Esham RH, Skilling FC Jr, Dodson WH et al. Hereditary hemorrhagic telangiectasia and factor VIII deficiency. Arch Intern Med 1974;134:327–329.

210. Sudarshan A, Natelson EA, Gordon C. Hereditary hemorrhagic telangiectasia and factor VIII inhibitor. South Med J 1985;78:623–624.

211. Kwaan HC, Silverman S. Fibrinolytic activity in lesions of hereditary hemorrhagic telangiectasia. Arch Dermatol 1973;107:571–573.

212. Sureda A, Cesar J, Garcia-Frade LJ et al. Hereditary hemorrhagic telangiectasia: analysis of platelet aggregation and fibrinolytic system in seven individuals. Acta Haematol 1991;85:119–123.

213. Bick RL. Hereditary hemorrhagic telangiectasia and disseminated intravascular coagulation: a new clinical syndrome. Ann N Y Acad Sci 1981;370:851–854.

214. Ziegler JL, Dorfman RF. Overview of Kaposi's sarcoma: history, epidemiology, and biomedical features. In: Ziegler JL, Dorfman RF, eds. Kaposi's sarcoma: pathophysiology and clinical management. New York: Marcel Dekker, 1988:1–22.

215. Schwartz JJ, Dias BM, Safai B. HIV-related malignancies. Dermatol Clin 1991;9:503–515.

216. Lever WF, Schaumberg-Lever G. Tumors of vascular tissue. In: Anonymous. Histopathology of the skin. 7th ed. Philadelphia: JB Lippincott, 1990:689–721.

217. Pollack MS, Safai B, Myskowski PL et al. Frequencies of HLA and Gm immunogenetic markers in Kaposi's sarcoma. Tissue Antigens 1983;21:1–8.

218. Contu L, Cerimele D, Bonu G et al. Kaposi's sarcoma and HLA in Sardinia. In: Cerimele D, ed. Kaposi's sarcoma. New York: Medical & Scientific Books, 1985:29–38.

219. Tzfoni EE, Scherman L, Battat S et al. No HLA antigen is significant in classic Kaposi's sarcoma. J Am Acad Dermatol 1993;28:118–119.

220. Shmueli D, Shapira Z, Yussim A et al. The incidence of Kaposi sarcoma in renal transplant individuals and its relation to immunosuppression. Transplant Proc 1989;21:3209–3210.

221. Smith JL, Wilkinson AH, Hunsicker LG et al. Increased frequency of post-transplant lymphomas in individuals treated with cyclosporin, azathioprine, and prednisone. Transplant Proc 1989;21:3199–3200.

222. Penn I. Cancers after cyclosporin therapy. Transplant Proc 1988;20(Suppl 1):276–279.

223. Schottstaedt MW, Hurd ER, Stone MJ. Kaposi's sarcoma in rheumatoid arthritis. Am J Med 1987;82:1021–1026.

224. Trattner A, Hodak E, David M et al. Kaposi's sarcoma with visceral involvement after intraarticular and epidural injections of corticosteroids. J Am Acad Dermatol 1993;29:890–894.

225. Chang Y, Cesarman E, Pessin MS et al. Identification of herpes virus-like DNA sequences in AIDS-associated Kaposi's sarcoma. Science 1994;266:1865–1869.

226. Dupin N, Grandadam M, Calvez V et al. Herpesvirus-like DNA sequences in individuals with Mediterranean Kaposi's sarcoma. Lancet 1995;345:761–762.

227. Huang YQ, Li JJ, Kaplan MH et al. Human herpesvirus-like nucleic acid in various forms of Kaposi's sarcoma. Lancet 1995;345:759–761.

228. Moore PS, Chang Y. Detection of herpesvirus-like DNA sequences in Kaposi's sarcoma in individuals with and without HIV infection. N Engl J Med 1995;332:1181–1185.

229. Cesarman E, Chang Y, Moore PS et al. Kaposi's sarcoma-associated herpesvirus-like DNA sequences in AIDS-related body-cavity-based lymphomas. N Engl J Med 1995;332:1186–1191.

230. Soulier J, Grollet L, Oksenhendler E et al. Kaposi's sarcoma-associated herpesvirus-like DNA sequences in multicentric Castleman's disease. Blood 1995;86:1276–1280.

231. Rady PL, Yen A, Rollefson JL et al. Herpesvirus-like DNA sequences in non-Kaposi's sarcoma skin lesions of transplant individuals. Lancet 1995;345:1339–1340.

232. Whitby D, Howard MR, Tenant-Flowers M et al. Detection of Kaposi sarcoma associated herpesvirus in peripheral blood of HIV-infected individuals and progression to Kaposi's sarcoma. Lancet 1995;346:799–802.

233. Gao SJ, Kingsley L, Hoover DR et al. Seroconversion to antibodies against Kaposi's sarcoma-associated herpesvirus-related latent nuclear antigens before the development of Kaposi's sarcoma. N Engl J Med 1996;335:233–241.

234. Foreman KE, Friborg J Jr, Kong WP et al. Propagation of a human herpesvirus from AIDS-associated Kaposi's sarcoma. N Engl J Med 1997;336:163–171.

235. Volberding PA. Chemotherapy. In: Anonymous. Kaposi's sarcoma: pathophysiology and clinical management. New York: Marcel Dekker, 1988:249–260.

236. Rozenbaum W, Gharakhanian S, Navarette MS et al. Long-term follow-up of 120 individuals with AIDS-related Kaposi's sarcoma treated with interferon alpha-2a. J Invest Dermatol 1990;95(Suppl 6):161S–165S.

237. Safai B, Bason M, Friedman-Birnbaum R et al. Interferon in the treatment of AIDS-associated Kaposi's sarcoma: the American experience. J Invest Derm 1990;95(Suppl 6):166S–169S.

238. Schwartsmann G, Sprinz E, Kronfeld M et al. Phase II study of teniposide in individuals with AIDS-related Kaposi's sarcoma. Eur J Cancer 1991;27:1637–1639.

239. Northfelt DW, Kahn JO, Volberding PA. Treatment of AIDS-related Kaposi's sarcoma. Hematol Oncol Clin North Am 1991;5:297–310.

240. Gill PS, Rarick M, McCutchan JA et al. Systemic treatment of AIDS-related Kaposi's sarcoma: results of a randomized trial. Am J Med 1991;90:427–433.

241. Nahass GT, Rosenberg SP, Leonardi CL et al. Disseminated infection with trichosporon beigelii: report of a case and Review of the cutaneous and histologic manifestations [Review]. Arch Dermatol 1993;129:1020–1023.

# CHAPTER 44

# DISSEMINATED INTRAVASCULAR COAGULATION

## Eliot Williams

## INTRODUCTION

Disseminated intravascular coagulation (DIC), also called defibrination syndrome and consumptive coagulopathy, can be defined as formation of soluble fibrin and accelerated degradation of fibrin and fibrinogen resulting from uncontrolled protease activity in the blood. The causes of DIC are many (Table 44.1) and its clinical consequences variable, ranging from none at all to life-threatening bleeding or thrombosis. This chapter considers the pathophysiology, clinical consequences, diagnosis, and treatment of DIC.

## PATHOPHYSIOLOGY

DIC is not simply a disseminated extension of physiological clotting. Physiological clot formation and lysis are the consequence of a series of tightly-regulated and exquisitely balanced interactions among platelets, plasma proteases, protease inhibitors, enzyme cofactors, and various cells that results in the controlled formation and breakdown of a localized, platelet-associated fibrin gel. In most cases this process is confined to the extravascular space. DIC occurs when the processes that regulate coagulation break down (Fig. 44.1). This usually happens as a consequence of the generation of thrombin, plasmin, and plasma proteases in quantities sufficient to overwhelm normal regulatory mechanisms. Fibrin formation and platelet activation become dissociated: fibrin forms soluble oligomers that circulate in the blood

(Fig. 44.2) (1), and platelets are activated in the circulation instead of on the subendothelium of an injured vessel, so that an adherent platelet plug does not form. Plasminogen activators are released into the blood, bind to soluble fibrin, and catalyze widespread plasmin formation. Depending on the absolute and relative rates of fibrin formation and fibrinolysis, DIC may be asymptomatic or it may cause severe bleeding, large- or small-vessel thrombosis, or simultaneous bleeding and thrombosis.

## INITIATION OF DIC

In most cases DIC begins when circulating blood is exposed to tissue factor. Tissue factor (see Chapter 4) is an apolipoprotein most abundant in vascular adventitia, mucosal epithelium, epidermis, brain, and placenta (2, 3). Although small amounts of tissue factor can be detected in the plasma of healthy people (4–6), most of it is normally confined to the extravascular space, where it is responsible for triggering thrombin formation when blood enters this space. Many, but not all, individuals with DIC have higher than normal levels of tissue factor in their plasma; the level is about two to four times normal on average (4–6). Tissue factor may enter the circulation as a result of disruption of endothelium or it may be exposed to blood on the surface of circulating cells. Breakdown of the endothelial barrier may result directly from tissue injury, or when endothelial permeability in the microcirculation is altered by inflammatory cytokines (Fig. 44.3) (7). Circulating monocytes express tis-

## TABLE 44.1. Some Causes of DIC

**Infection**
Gram-negative bacteria
   *Neisseria meningitidis*
   *Enterobacteriaceae* sp.
   *Salmonella* sp.
   *Haemophilus* sp.
   *Pseudomonas* sp.
Gram-positive bacteria
   Pneumococcus
   Staphylococci
   Hemolytic streptococci
Anaerobes
   *Clostridium* sp.
*Mycobacterium tuberculosis*
Ehrlichiosis
Bacterial meningitis
Septic shock
Postsplenectomy sepsis
Toxic shock syndrome
Fungi
   *Aspergillus* sp.
   *Histoplasma* sp.
   *Candida* sp.
Rocky Mountain spotted fever
Viruses
Protozoa
   Malaria
   Visceral leishmaniasis (kala-azar)
   Babesiosis
**Neoplasia**
Solid tumors
   Adenocarcinoma
   Lymphoma
Leukemia
   Promyelocytic
   Acute myelogenous
   Chronic myelogenous
   Acute lymphoblastic
**Vascular disease**
Aortic aneurysm
Giant hemangioma (Kasabach-Merritt syndrome)
Vascular tumors
Multiple telangiectasias
Acute myocardial infarction
Intracardiac tumors and thrombi
Aortic balloon pump
Cholesterol embolism
Vasculitis
**Liver disease**
Fulminant hepatic failure
Cirrhosis
Reye's syndrome
Biliary obstruction
**Obstetric complications**
Amniotic fluid embolism
Abruptio placentae
Mid-trimester abortion

Septic abortion
Uterine rupture
Retained dead fetus
Toxemia of pregnancy
Hydatidiform mole
**Transfusion reactions**
Acute hemolytic transfusion reaction
Massive transfusion
**Surgery**
Vascular surgery
Cardiac bypass surgery
Liver transplantation
Peritoneovenous shunt
**Envenomation**
Rattlesnakes, other vipers
Keel-back snake (*Rhabdophis subminiatus*)
Insects (caterpillars of *Lonomia achelous*)
**Trauma and tissue injury**
Brain injury
Crush injury
Burns
Hyperthermia
Hypothermia
Asphyxia/hypoxia
Ischemia/infarction
Rhabdomyolysis
Fat embolism
**Shock**
**Respiratory distress syndromes**
**Inherited disorders**
Antithrombin III deficiency
Homozygous protein C deficiency
Homozygous protein S deficiency
Hyperlipoproteinemia types II and IV
**Drugs/therapeutic agents**
Fibrinolytic agents
Heparin-associated thrombocytopenia
Ancrod
Warfarin (in Trousseau syndrome, protein C deficiency)
Intravenous lipid emulsion
Clotting factor concentrates
   Factor IX
   Activated factor IX
   Factor XI
Immune drug reaction
OKT3 monoclonal antibody
Interleukin-2
**Miscellaneous**
Amyloidosis
Inflammatory bowel disease
Acute intravascular hemolysis
Histiocytic disorders
Anaphylaxis
Kawasaki disease
Pancreatitis
Graft-versus-host disease

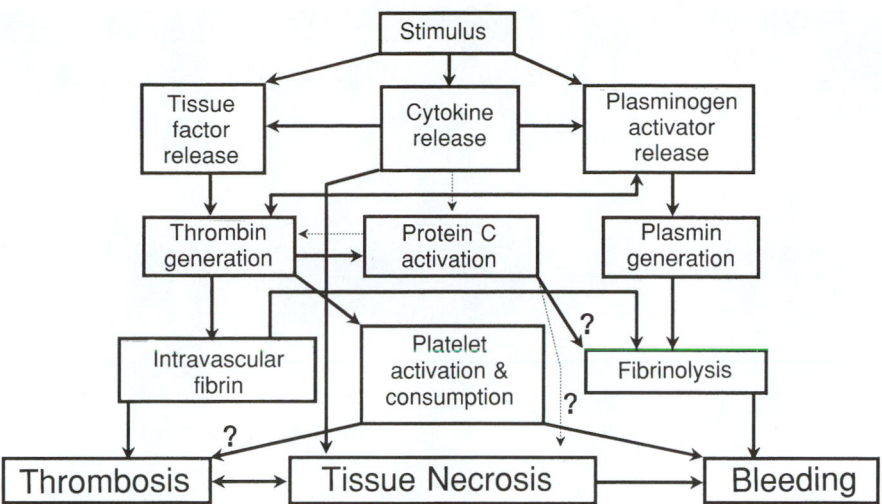

**FIGURE 44.1.**  Pathophysiology of disseminated intravascular coagulation. Solid arrows indicate positive or stimulatory influences and dashed arrows indicate negative or inhibitory influences. The initial events may include release of tissue factor, plasminogen activators and plasminogen activator inhibitors (PAI) (not shown) and inflammatory cytokines into the blood by monocytes, endothelial cells, and other cells. These substances promote formation of plasma proteases including thrombin and plasmin, which in turn cause consumption of protease inhibitors (not shown). Cytokines inhibit protein C activation, and protein C is consumed as a consequence of thrombin formation; decreased availability of activated protein C increases thrombin formation. Thrombin generates soluble intravascular fibrin, causes platelet activation and consumption, and amplifies the fibrinolytic response. Note the reciprocal relationship between thrombin formation and fibrinolysis; either pathway can activate the other. Fibrinolysis and thrombocytopenia promote bleeding, while intravascular fibrin promotes both fibrinolysis and thrombosis. Intravascular thrombosis, cytokines, protein C deficiency, and tissue hypoperfusion (shock) all promote tissue necrosis, which may in turn exacerbate local bleeding or thrombosis.

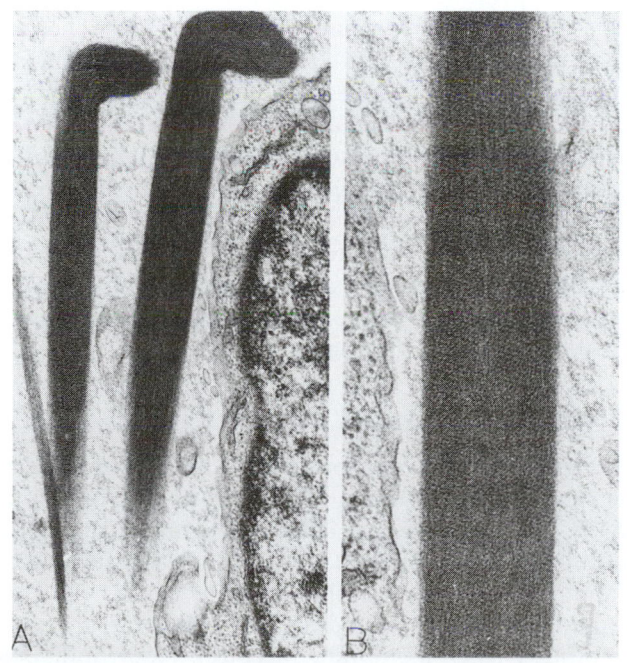

**FIGURE 44.2.**  Soluble fibrin in the peripheral blood of a individual with acute myelogenous leukemia. Note the periodicity of the fibrin, and the absence of platelets, at higher magnification **(B)**. From Dvorak AM. Fibrin in the peripheral blood of a patient with acute myelocytic leukemia. Blood 1996;87;2648.

sue factor when stimulated by bacterial endotoxin or cytokines (2), and circulating malignant cells often express tissue factor constitutively (8). If sufficient tissue factor enters the blood, rapid and widespread generation of thrombin occurs. Thrombin, in turn, causes formation of soluble fibrin, activation of circulating platelets, and secondary fibrinolysis, i.e., DIC (Fig. 44.1).

The role of procoagulants other than tissue factor in the initiation of DIC is not clear. The intrinsic coagulation pathway is activated in sepsis, producing kinins that contribute to the hemodynamic abnormalities of septic shock (9), and which could in theory generate thrombin and cause DIC. However, data from humans (10, 11) and baboons (12) suggest that the intrinsic (contact activation) system is not a major contributor to thrombin generation in DIC. Endothelial cells express a protease capable of activating prothrombin when exposed to endotoxin or inflammatory cytokines (13); its role in DIC is unknown. Several substances with procoagulant activity have been described in cancer cells (14). A cysteine protease that directly activates factor X is expressed in amniotic tissue and by some malignant cells (15, 16), and therefore might contribute to DIC associated with cancer and amniotic fluid embolism. Extracts of mucus also contain factor X-activating activity that could contribute to DIC in individuals with mucin-producing adenocarcinomas (17).

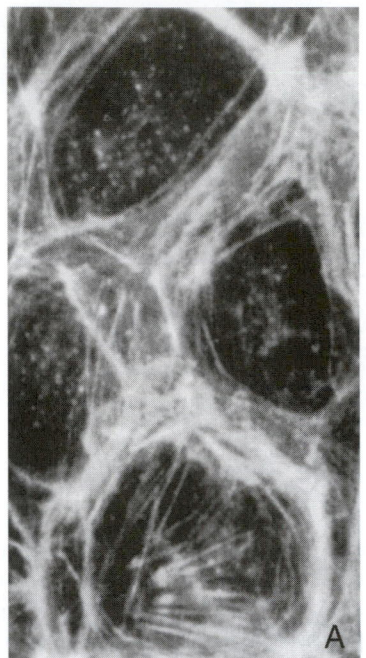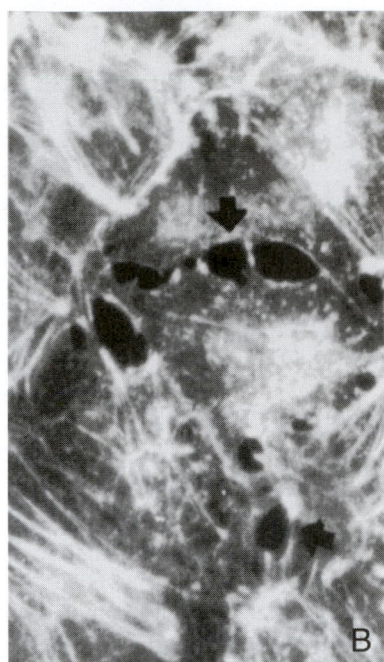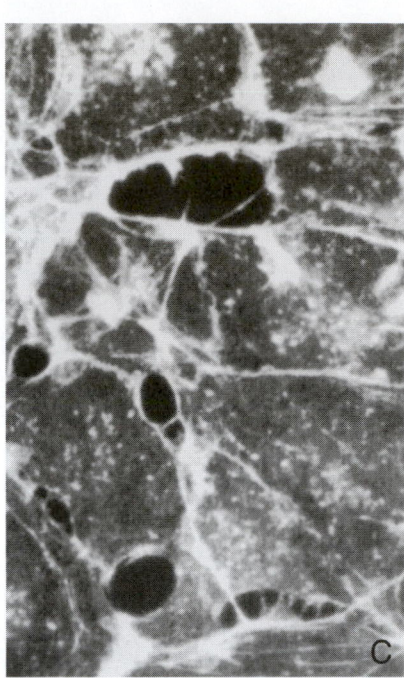

**FIGURE 44.3.** Effects of incubation with tumor necrosis factor (TNF) on cultured endothelial cells. **A,** Control monolayer; **B,** culture exposed to TNF (5 nM) for 90 min. Note retraction of cell margins and gap formation (arrows); **C,** culture exposed to TNF for 24 hours. Brett J, Gerlach H, Nawroth P et al. Tumor necrosis factor/cachectin increases permeability of endothelial cell monolayers by a mechanism involving regulatory G proteins. J Exp Med 1989;169:1977–1991.

## FIBRINOLYSIS IN DIC

Increased fibrinolytic activity is a *sine qua non* of DIC, since it is an inevitable consequence of intravascular thrombin formation (see Fig. 44.1); its contribution to the coagulopathy is, however, quite variable. Endothelial cells exposed to thrombin release tissue-type plasminogen activator (t-PA) (18, 19), and so blood levels of t-PA are high in DIC (20, 21). Fibrinolysis may also be initiated by thrombin-independent mechanisms. Endotoxin (18), tumor necrosis factor-α (TNF-α) (22), or other mediators cause release of t-PA from endothelial cells and urokinase-type plasminogen activator (u-PA) from monocytes (23). Enzymes of the intrinsic coagulation system can act as plasminogen activators and promote fibrinolysis (24). Leukemic blasts and other malignant cells also express u-PA (25).

Soluble fibrin in DIC plasma enhances activation of plasminogen by t-PA. Soluble fibrin and fibrin degradation products are excellent catalysts for plasmin formation (26), particularly in the absence of platelets, which normally retard clot lysis by releasing plasminogen activator inhibitor-1 (PAI-1) (27) and thrombospondin (28). Actin filaments released from injured tissue also enhance plasminogen activation (29). The liberation of large amounts of plasminogen activator into a milieu that strongly favors plasmin formation may generate enough plasmin to overwhelm its major inhibitor, α$_2$-antiplasmin, the plasma concentration of which is only about half that of plasminogen. When this occurs, systemic fibrinolysis and fibrinogenolysis may occur at rates disproportionate to that of fibrin formation (30–32). The term "primary fibrinolysis" has been applied to this state (33, 34). However, it is very difficult to exclude thrombin formation as a contributing factor to fibrinolysis, except perhaps in the case of thrombolytic drug administration. Furthermore, because plasminogen activators themselves promote thrombin formation (35, 36), it is unlikely that systemic fibrinolysis ever occurs in the absence of at least some intravascular coagulation. Therefore, for the purpose of this discussion, coagulopathy that is predominantly fibrinolytic is considered part of the spectrum of DIC.

## OTHER PROTEASES

Endogenous and exogenous proteases not normally associated with coagulation or fibrinolysis may contribute to DIC. Elastase released from leukocytes during endotoxemia (37), or from leukemic blasts (38), can degrade fibrinogen (38, 39) or other clotting factors (40) and either enhance (41) or reduce (42) platelet aggregation by proteolysis of membrane receptors. Neutrophil elastase also enhances the effects of thrombin and plasmin by complexing with or degrading inhibitors of coagulation and fibrinolysis (43, 44). In acute pancreatitis, trypsin may degrade fibrinogen or other clotting factors (40, 45, 46).

Exogenous proteins with procoagulant, profibrino-lytic, or fibrinogenolytic activity may cause DIC-like syndromes. Examples include defibrination due to pit viper envenomation and thrombolytic therapy with streptokinase. Small amounts of such "foreign" enzymes can sometimes cause considerable damage, perhaps because the blood lacks specific inhibitors for them.

## LEUKOCYTES AND INFLAMMATORY CYTOKINES

Blood leukocytes (neutrophils and monocytes) are important participants in DIC, particularly in the setting of inflammation (47). In experimental animals, induction of leukopenia prevents endotoxin-induced DIC (48). There is some evidence that leukopenia protects humans with sepsis from DIC (49). Activated neutrophils produce elastase and other enzymes that may have a variety of effects on coagulation as noted above. Activated monocytes promote coagulation in several ways. They provide a surface for assembly of the prothrombinase complex (50), and they secrete inflammatory mediators including TNF-$\alpha$, interleukin-1 (IL-1), interleukin-6 (IL-6), and platelet activating factor that exert profound effects on the coagulation system. TNF-$\alpha$ and IL-1 increase expression of tissue factor, plasminogen activators, and plasminogen activator inhibitor-1 (PAI-1) by a variety of cells and reduce protein C activation by reducing endothelial cell expression of thrombomodulin (47, 51, 52). TNF-$\alpha$, IL-1, and platelet activating factor all increase endothelial permeability and may thereby expose blood to subendothelial tissue factor (7, 53, 54) (Fig. 44.3). The mechanism by which IL-6 promotes DIC is unknown, but may in part involve the induction of fibrinogen synthesis by the hepatocyte; administration of antibodies to IL-6 greatly reduces thrombin formation in experimental endotoxin-induced DIC (55). The net effect of inflammatory cytokines in DIC is to promote fibrin formation and diminish fibrinolysis (37, 47, 56–58).

## LIVER, ENDOTHELIUM AND BONE MARROW

The severity and clinical course of DIC are strongly influenced by the functional status of the liver, since it produces both clotting factors and their inhibitors, and clears protease-inhibitor complexes and fibrin degradation products from the circulation (see Chapter 45). In the face of DIC a diseased liver is less able to replace clotting factors as they are consumed (59). More importantly, rates of inhibition of activated clotting factors and plasmin, and clearance of these enzymes from the blood, are also reduced (60, 61). This causes more rapid fibrinogen consumption and fibrinolysis, increasing the risk

of hemorrhage (31, 62, 63). Altered hepatic synthesis of clotting factors and protease inhibitors in response to inflammation also affects the course of DIC. For example, both fibrinogen and $\alpha_2$-antiplasmin are acute-phase reactants (64). When their blood levels increase in conditions such as infection and cancer, fibrin formation is promoted while fibrinolysis is retarded. If DIC occurs in this setting the likelihood of thrombosis is enhanced.

Alterations of the normally antithrombotic, profibrinolytic properties of the endothelium also have a profound effect on the severity and outcome of DIC. As noted above, inflammatory cytokines increase endothelial expression of tissue factor and PAI-1 and decrease expression of thrombomodulin; bacterial endotoxin has similar effects, which are likely mediated at least in part by cytokines (18, 47, 57, 65). An IL-1- and endotoxin-inducible prothrombin activator in human endothelial cells that is distinct from tissue factor has recently been described (13). Hypoxemia (66) and the complement membrane attack complex (67) also have prothrombotic effects on vascular endothelium.

If bone marrow function is impaired, the rate at which platelets are replenished in DIC is reduced and thrombocytopenia may become severe. Leukopenia due to impaired marrow production may attenuate DIC in individuals with sepsis (49).

## CHRONIC DIC

The spectrum of DIC includes acute and chronic syndromes. Chronic (compensated) DIC refers to a state in which the rates of consumption of clotting factors and platelets do not exceed the rates of their production. Clotting times are usually normal (or shorter than normal), and fibrin degradation product levels are increased with a normal or elevated fibrinogen level. Chronic DIC may simply reflect the presence of a low-grade stimulus, in which case it is likely to produce few clinical manifestations. However, chronic DIC can occur despite significant thrombin formation if production of fibrinogen and other coagulation factors is increased and the fibrinolytic response is blunted by enhanced endothelial PAI-1 release or accelerated $\alpha_2$-antiplasmin synthesis, as may occur during inflammation. In this setting fibrin formation is rapid and its clearance is slow, creating an imbalance that increases the likelihood of thrombosis.

## THE SHWARTZMAN REACTION AND ENDOTOXIN-INDUCED DIC

It has long been recognized that bacterial lipopolysaccharide (endotoxin) promotes coagulation and can cause DIC (53). Shwartzman injected a cell-free bacterial extract into rabbit skin and noted infiltration of neutrophils and monocytes at the injection site. When a second, intravenous, injection was given 24 hours later, multiple fibrin thrombi in small dermal vessels developed within

15 minutes at the site of the preparatory injection, followed by hemorrhagic necrosis of the skin (68). Subsequently, other investigators found that two intravenous injections of endotoxin given 24 hours apart caused shock, DIC associated with widespread formation of fibrin microthrombi, renal cortical necrosis, and death (the generalized Shwartzman reaction) (69, 70).

Fibrin formation in the local and generalized Shwartzman reactions is a consequence of tissue factor expression by monocytes and of leukocyte-mediated damage to endothelial cells (71–73). Leukocytes are essential to the reaction, since the phenomenon does not occur during leukopenia (48, 70) or if leukocyte adhesion to endothelium is inhibited (72). The priming injection (which can be endotoxin or one of a variety of other immunostimulatory agents) releases cytokines that stimulate tissue factor synthesis by monocytes and causes expression of adhesion molecules on the surface of neutrophils and endothelium. The second endotoxin injection exposes the newly synthesized tissue factor to the blood and induces adhesion of activated neutrophils to endothelium, resulting in vascular damage and intravascular coagulation.

The effects of endotoxin administration to healthy human subjects have been studied in detail. A single dose of endotoxin causes rapid increases in blood levels of TNF-$\alpha$ and IL-6, accompanied by flu-like symptoms, fever, and tachycardia (10). Subsequently there is a brief increase in fibrinolytic activity manifested by increased t-PA and plasmin-antiplasmin complex levels, which is quickly counteracted by an increase in PAI-1 concentration (10, 37). Activation of coagulation, as measured by plasma prothrombin activation peptide and thrombin-antithrombin complex levels, occurs more slowly but is more long-lasting (10). Plasma von Willebrand factor and neutrophil elastase levels also rise (10, 37). These studies show that endotoxin has a net procoagulant effect in humans, and suggest that this effect is mediated by cytokines.

Studies in which *Escherichia coli* are injected into baboons indicate that endotoxin-induced tissue damage may occur independently of DIC. Inhibition of thrombin formation by infusion of active site-inhibited factor Xa completely blocks DIC in this experimental model, but does not prevent hemorrhagic necrosis of tissue or renal cortical necrosis (74). Protein C apparently provides protection from this endotoxin-induced tissue damage: infusion of activated protein C prevents both DIC and organ damage, while inhibition of protein C by infusion of antiprotein C antibody, or neutralization of protein S by infusion of C4b-binding protein, have an opposite effect (75, 76).

# COMPLICATIONS OF DIC

Mortality in severe DIC is high; death rates as high as 85% have been reported (77). Although death and mor-

bidity are usually due to the underlying disease, three serious clinical complications may result from DIC *per se:* bleeding, thrombosis, and purpura fulminans.

## BLEEDING

Bleeding is the most feared complication of DIC and the most common, with a reported incidence of 75–85% in some series (77, 78). Bleeding may be limited to sites of injury (e.g., surgical incisions, gastric ulcers, etc.). In more severe cases complete breakdown of hemostasis occurs, with diffuse oozing of blood from mucosal surfaces and venipuncture sites, hematuria, pulmonary hemorrhage (79), and sometimes intracranial hemorrhage.

Bleeding in DIC is caused by a combination of hyperfibrinolysis, depletion of clotting factors, thrombocytopenia, and inhibition of fibrin polymerization by fibrin degradation products (FDP) (80, 81). Several lines of evidence indicate that hyperfibrinolysis is the most important of these factors. For example, induction of hyperfibrinolysis without hypofibrinogenemia with streptokinase or t-PA (82) causes much more bleeding than does induction of profound hypofibrinogenemia without hyperfibrinolysis with the snake venom enzyme ancrod (83). A high rate of fatal bleeding (over 50%) occurs in transgenic mice that transiently secrete high levels of u-PA (84). Patients with DIC who have very low plasma $\alpha_2$-antiplasmin activity (an indicator of hyperfibrinolysis) have a markedly higher incidence of severe bleeding than do individuals without this finding (31).

## THROMBOSIS

Large-vessel thrombosis is unusual in DIC, despite extensive fibrin formation (77, 79). This is not surprising, since fibrin polymers in DIC tend to be small, soluble, and short-lived. Fibrin "microthrombi" and platelet aggregates become trapped in small-vessels, particularly in the lungs and kidneys (79, 85, 86). Clinically apparent organ dysfunction as a result of this phenomenon is unusual (79), although renal cortical necrosis is a rare complication (87). Large-vessel thrombosis may occur when endothelial damage or an intravascular catheter offer a site where adherent platelets can provide the foundation for a stable clot (79). Antifibrinolytic drug therapy has also been implicated as a cause of thrombosis in DIC (79, 88–90). Chronic DIC caused by some kinds of cancer (see Chapter 40) is associated with a high incidence of thromboembolism (Trousseau syndrome) (91).

## PURPURA FULMINANS

DIC is occasionally complicated by gangrene of digits or entire extremities and hemorrhagic infarction of the

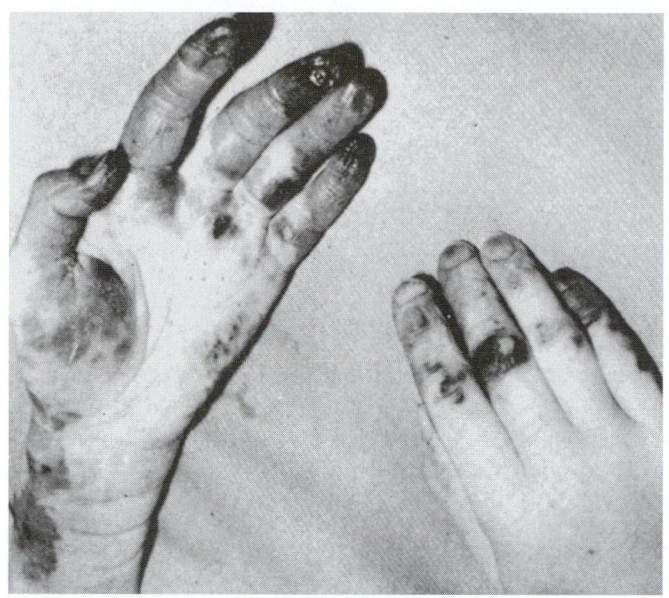

**FIGURE 44.4.** Symmetric gangrene of the fingers (purpura fulminans) in a individual with disseminated intravascular coagulation due to *Staphylococcus aureus* septicemia. Adapted with permission from Robboy SJ, Mihm MC, Colman RW et al. The skin in disseminated intravascular coagulation. Prospective analysis of thirty-six cases. Br J Dermatol 1973;88:221–229.

skin due to extensive formation of fibrin thrombi (Fig. 44.4) (92–94). Hemorrhagic necrosis of the adrenal glands (Waterhouse-Friderichsen syndrome) (95) and renal cortical necrosis (87) may also occur, although such lesions are probably not due entirely to DIC (74). Purpura fulminans may complicate high-grade bacteremia, particularly that caused by *Neisseria meningitidis* or *Streptococcus pneumoniae* (96, 97). In children and (rarely) in adults, it may occur during or shortly after viral upper respiratory infection, varicella, or streptococcal infection (for example, scarlet fever) (93, 98). It is also a rare complication of noninfectious hyper-immune reactions (99).

A mounting body of evidence suggests that acquired defects in the protein C anticoagulant pathway play an important role in the pathogenesis of purpura fulminans. Protein C protects experimental animals from endotoxin-induced hemorrhagic tissue necrosis (75, 76). Congenital absence of either protein C or protein S (see Chapter 40) causes spontaneous purpura fulminans in neonates (100–102), and low levels of proteins C and S are often found in individuals with purpura fulminans associated with bacterial sepsis (103–105). Deficiency of protein S caused by autoantibodies has been demonstrated in children with post-infectious purpura fulminans (106, 107) and an acquired inhibitor of protein C has been found in an adult with this syndrome (108).

Purpura fulminans associated with sepsis is similar

to the generalized Shwartzman reaction caused by endotoxin in rabbits (see above) (109). As with the Shwartzman reaction, it seems to be a manifestation of the prothrombotic effects of cytokines produced in response to bacterial toxins (10, 47, 94, 110). Consumption of protein C (111), diminished protein C activation as a consequence of reduced endothelial cell thrombomodulin expression (65), and reduced protein S activity (112) may contribute to tissue necrosis. Tissue hypoperfusion due to shock and iatrogenic peripheral vasoconstriction caused by pressor administration (113) are probably important contributing factors as well. Post-infectious purpura fulminans, on the other hand, may be caused by autoimmune destruction of protein C or protein S and therefore analogous to the coagulopathy associated with congenital severe deficiency of either protein.

# DIAGNOSIS OF DIC

Diagnosing DIC is not usually difficult. If there is evidence of accelerated fibrinolysis accompanied by low or declining levels of coagulation factors and platelets in a individual with a disease known to cause DIC, the syndrome is probably present. Scoring systems for diagnosing and grading DIC have been proposed (114, 115), but in most instances the diagnosis is made by combining clinical judgment with several simple, well-standardized laboratory tests (see Chapter 26). Prenatal diagnosis of DIC has been described (116).

## SCREENING FOR DIC

Clinically significant DIC is unlikely if there is no biochemical evidence of accelerated fibrinolysis. Such evidence may be provided by either a latex agglutination test for FDP or a D dimer assay, which measures only crosslinked fibrin degradation products (see Chapter 26). Of these two tests the D dimer test is the more specific (117); depending on the assay used, it may also be more sensitive. The D dimer test measures fibrin, but not fibrinogen, degradation products. This probably does not make much difference, since fibrinogen degradation products make only a minor contribution to total FDP (118). The D dimer test has the advantage of being applicable to both plasma and serum, and is not susceptible to artifacts due to incomplete clotting of the test sample, which may cause a false positive FDP result.

In addition to an FDP or D dimer test, screening tests for DIC should include a prothrombin time (PT), a functional fibrinogen assay, and a platelet count. Levels of most clotting factors decrease in acute DIC; activities of the components of the extrinsic (tissue factor) pathway (factors VII X, V, and prothrombin) are most likely to be low (78), so that the PT is often prolonged. Prolongation of the PT has prognostic as well as diagnostic significance in DIC (119). In contrast, the plasma factor VIII activity is often higher than normal in DIC (78), probably due to the presence of circulating activated factor and because von Willebrand factor released from damaged endothelial cells complexes and stabilizes factor VIII (120). This shortens the activated partial thromboplastin time (aPTT), which is therefore less useful than the PT in screening for or monitoring DIC (121, 122). The thrombin clotting time (thrombin time) is often prolonged in DIC, due to a combination of hypofibrinogenemia and impairment of fibrin polymerization by circulating FDP (81). However, the thrombin time is not well standardized, and it does not give any information about the severity of DIC in addition to that provided by measurement of fibrinogen and FDP/D-dimer levels. It is useful as a screen for heparin contamination of blood samples, which may cause prolonged clotting times.

Although the platelet count usually is low in acute DIC, and is often the earliest detectable abnormality in DIC associated with sepsis, it is not a particularly sensitive or specific screening test. The platelet count may drop for reasons unrelated to DIC (e.g., antibody-mediated destruction in sepsis) (123–126), and it may remain stable despite a high FDP titer and low fibrinogen level in predominantly fibrinolytic states. The presence of schistocytes on the peripheral blood smear suggests intravascular fibrin deposition (127), but this finding is neither sensitive nor specific for DIC (128, 129). If marked red cell fragmentation is found, the possibility of a microangiopathic disorder such as thrombotic thrombocytopenic purpura should be entertained (see Chapter 27).

In individuals with chronic or compensated DIC the FDP/D-dimer titer is elevated. However, clotting factor and platelet levels may be normal or even elevated. Tests for circulating fibrin or prothrombin activation peptide (see below) may help to establish the diagnosis.

## OTHER TESTS (SEE CHAPTER 26)

Plasma antithrombin and plasminogen activities are often low in DIC, and are useful in estimating the severity of the coagulopathy (130, 131). Low $\alpha_2$-antiplasmin activity almost always accompanies extreme hyperfibrinolysis, and may be associated with a high bleeding risk (31). Assays for soluble fibrin or "fibrin monomer" should in theory have high specificity for DIC. Older methods for detecting soluble fibrin such as the ethanol gelation (132), protamine paracoagulation (133), and cryofibrinogen (134) tests were poorly standardized and had limited sensitivity. Newer methods, including various immunoassays and a hemagglutination assay using fibrin-coated red cells, show less variability, with good sensitivity and specificity for DIC in clinical testing (135, 136). Measurement of plasma fibrinopeptide A, which

is generated during conversion of fibrinogen to fibrin, is a very sensitive, but nonspecific, test for DIC that has been used (primarily in research) to follow the course of the coagulopathy (137). Measurement of plasma prothrombin activation peptide ($F_{1.2}$) allows estimation of the rate of thrombin generation. While not a specific indicator of DIC (36), the plasma $F_{1.2}$ level appears to be a sensitive measure of DIC severity (138–140). The plasma thrombin-antithrombin complex level is also proportional to the rate of thrombin formation, while measurement of plasmin-antiplasmin complexes provides information about the rate of plasmin formation (141–143). Assays for the B$\beta$1-42 peptide of fibrinogen and the B$\beta$1-42 peptide of fibrin (56, 144) reflect rates of fibrinogenolysis and fibrinolysis, respectively; these are used primarily for research purposes at present.

# DIFFERENTIAL DIAGNOSIS

Several disorders that may cause, or be associated with, serious illness produce laboratory findings similar to those found in DIC (Table 44.2).

## LOCALIZED INTRAVASCULAR COAGULATION

Local thrombosis may result in high FDP titers and platelet and clotting factor consumption. These changes are qualitatively similar to those in DIC; they tend to be smaller in magnitude, but in massive thrombosis the picture may be indistinguishable from DIC (33). Localized thrombosis and DIC can usually be differentiated by the clinical findings.

## LIVER DISEASE (SEE CHAPTER 45)

Severe liver disease causes decreased synthesis of coagulation factors and inhibitors (59, 145), increased FDP or D dimer titers (146), and thrombocytopenia due to splenic platelet sequestration (59). DIC is often difficult to diagnose or rule out in the presence of liver disease (147). As is the case in DIC, plasma factor VIII activity is often normal or elevated in liver disease; measurement of individual clotting factor levels (e.g., factors V and VIII) cannot reliably distinguish liver disease from DIC. Tests for soluble fibrin and those that detect activation of clotting enzymes (e.g., plasma $F_{1.2}$ peptide and thrombin-antithrombin complex) may be useful in this setting. Serial measurements should be done to show the progressive changes in clotting factors, inhibitors, and FDP or D dimer levels characteristic of DIC.

## OTHER CAUSES OF CLOTTING FACTOR DEFICIENCY OR THROMBOCYTOPENIA

Patients with bacterial sepsis may become thrombocytopenic in the absence of DIC (123–126). Vitamin K defi-

**TABLE 44.2.** Differential Diagnosis of DIC

| Condition | Elevated FDP or D-dimer Level | Prolonged PT | Decreased Platelet Count | Decreased Fibrinogen Level | Decreased Antithrombin or Antiplasmin Level | Elevated $F_{1.2}$ or TAT Level | Soluble Fibrin |
|---|---|---|---|---|---|---|---|
| DIC | Yes | Variable | Common | Variable | Variable | Yes | Common |
| Vitamin K deficiency | No | Yes | No | No | No | No | No |
| Thrombocytopenia of sepsis | No | No | Yes | No | No | No | No |
| Liver disease | Variable | Yes | Yes | Yes | Yes | Variable | No |
| Localized coagulation | Yes | Rare | Rare | Rare | Rare | Yes | Rare |
| Microangiopathy | Variable | No | Yes | No | No | Variable | No |
| Lupus anticoagulant | No | Variable | Variable | No | No | Variable | No |
| Hemodilution | No | Yes | Yes | Yes | Yes | No | No |

*FDP*, fibrin degradation products; *PT*, prothrombin time; $F_{1.2}$, prothrombin activation peptide $F_{1.2}$; *TAT*, thrombin–antithrombin complex.

ciency (see Chapter 45) may cause prolonged clotting times in individuals with a variety of acute illnesses (148, 149). After massive blood transfusions or cardiopulmonary bypass surgery, low levels of clotting factors and inhibitors are usually caused by hemodilution rather than by DIC (150, 151).

## MICROANGIOPATHIC DISORDERS (SEE CHAPTER 27)

Thrombotic thrombocytopenic purpura, hemolytic uremic syndrome, and other forms of microangiopathy are characterized by acute, multisystem illness and thrombocytopenia. However, they typically do not cause much clotting factor consumption, and fibrinolytic activity as measured by FDP titer is usually only mildly increased (152, 153). Increased FDP and D dimer titers are found in individuals with sickle cell crisis (154), but other laboratory manifestations of DIC are usually absent.

## OTHER CAUSES OF INCREASED FDP TITER

Since FDP are cleared in part by the kidneys, renal failure causes increased FDP titers in the absence of DIC (155). Products of intraperitoneal fibrinolysis enter the blood during peritoneal dialysis and thereby increase the FDP titer (156). False-positive latex agglutination tests for FDP and D dimer occur in serum containing rheumatoid factor (157) or cryoglobulin (158). Incomplete removal of fibrinogen from a blood sample due to the presence of heparin (159) (if thrombin is used to defibrinate the sample) or dysfibrinogenemia (42) may also cause a false-positive FDP result.

## LUPUS ANTICOAGULANTS (SEE CHAPTER 38)

These antiphospholipid antibodies interfere with phospholipid-dependent thrombin generation *in vitro*, and thereby prolong the aPTT and sometimes the PT. They are occasionally associated with hypoprothrombinemia (160), immune thrombocytopenia, hemolytic anemia, arterial and venous thrombosis, and vasculitis (161). The effects of a lupus anticoagulant can usually be distinguished from those of DIC by performing appropriate mixing studies and clotting factor assays (see Chapters 26 and 38).

# CLINICAL SYNDROMES

## INFECTION

Infection is the most common cause of DIC. DIC occurs in a variety of bacterial, fungal, or viral infections (see Table 44.1). It is most common in Gram-negative sepsis; 10–20% of individuals with Gram-negative bacteremia have laboratory evidence of DIC (162, 163). DIC may also complicate pneumococcal sepsis, particularly if clearance of the responsible organism from the blood is delayed, as is the case in asplenic individuals (164). DIC is an early manifestation of Rocky Mountain spotted fever (165), although it rarely becomes severe. It is probably due to infection of endothelial cells by *Rickettsia rickettsii*. Systemic fungal infection, particularly by an angioinvasive pathogen such as *Aspergillus*, may cause DIC associated with small and large-vessel thrombosis (79). DIC may occur as a result of endothelial cell damage in viral hemorrhagic fevers (166) and hantavirus infection (167). Infection is the most common cause of purpura fulminans in adults (see above). Hyperfibrinolysis and bleeding are relatively uncommon in infection associated DIC (31, 78, 162, 168), possibly because levels of $\alpha_2$-antiplasmin and PAI-1 are usually high in septic individuals (169).

## CARCINOMA (SEE CHAPTER 40)

Accelerated fibrin formation and fibrinolysis are frequently found in individuals with carcinoma (8). Most individuals with carcinoma have elevated blood fibrino-peptide A levels at the time of diagnosis, and these levels tend to increase in parallel with the growth of the malignancy (170). Levels of tissue factor and $F_{1.2}$ peptide are also elevated in the blood of carcinoma individuals (11). Not all of the coagulation changes associated with cancer are caused by events in the blood. Fibrin formation around neoplastic cells in the extravascular compartment (171, 172), rather than DIC, probably accounts for most of the increase in fibrinogen turnover accompanying metastatic cancer (173). In some cases FDP and fibrinopeptide A in the blood of individuals with cancer may represent "spillover" from the extravascular compartment. Clearly, however, many individuals with cancer have DIC (174). Up to 50% of cancer individuals referred for coagulation testing have evidence of soluble fibrin in the blood (132, 175). Many of these individuals have normal or elevated levels of platelets and fibrinogen, i.e., chronic (compensated) DIC (see above) (175).

DIC caused by carcinoma may lead to bleeding (particularly in prostate carcinoma) (176, 177) or to thrombosis. Thrombotic syndromes associated with chronic DIC in carcinoma include recurrent thrombophlebitis (Trousseau syndrome) (91) and arterial embolism secondary to nonthrombotic bacterial endocarditis, which is characterized by fibrin formation on cardiac valves (178). Microangiopathic hemolytic anemia may occur as a consequence of intravascular fibrin deposition and/or endothelial damage by circulating neoplastic cells (179).

Carcinoma cells express several substances that might cause or contribute to DIC if secreted into the bloodstream (14, 180, 181). These include molecules with tissue factor-like activity (182), a cysteine protease ("cancer procoagulant") that directly activates factor X (183), u-PA and t-PA, and plasminogen activator inhibitors (182). They secrete molecules that induce tissue factor expression by monocytes and endothelial cells and that increase microvascular permeability, thereby exposing subendothelial tissue factor to the blood (184, 185). Other factors that may play a role in the coagulopathy include the presence of liver metastases (186) and damage to endothelial cells caused by circulating cancer cells (179). Plasmin-antiplasmin complex levels in individuals with cancer and DIC are low compared to thrombin-antithrombin complex levels (142). This suggests that in cancer individuals the fibrinolytic response to thrombin generation is diminished, creating a predisposition toward thrombosis.

Carcinoma-associated DIC often responds favorably to the administration of low doses of intravenous heparin (91, 187). Improvement with heparin may occur even when laboratory findings suggest that fibrinolysis is the dominant process (91, 177). An unusual and unexplained aspect of the coagulopathy associated with carcinoma is paradoxical deterioration that sometimes accompanies warfarin therapy. Administration of warfarin can cause a significant increase in FDP levels in individuals with carcinoma who do not have overt DIC or clinically evident thrombosis (188). Some individuals with Trousseau syndrome treated with warfarin develop recurrent superficial or deep venous thrombosis, skin necrosis (189), and, in extreme cases, severe defibrination and widespread arterial and venous thrombosis resembling purpura fulminans (190).

## ACUTE LEUKEMIA

Biochemical evidence for DIC is present in most individuals with acute leukemia (191, 192). Various substances expressed by leukemic cells or released as a consequence of cell lysis may contribute to DIC. These include tissue factor (193, 194), the cysteine protease "cancer procoagulant" (15, 195), u-PA and t-PA (196, 197), leukocyte elastase (37), and cytokines capable of modulating endothelial cell coagulant function (198). Leukemic blasts may damage endothelial cells or infiltrate other tissues and cause tissue factor release into the circulation. Impaired marrow function often causes severe thrombocytopenia, and liver dysfunction may exacerbate hypofibrinogenemia and deficiencies of other coagulation factors or inhibitors (199). The risk of bleeding is high in leukemia-associated DIC (undoubtedly due in part to associated thrombocytopenia and the effects of leukostasis) (200), but thrombosis may also occur (201–203).

The incidence and severity of DIC are particularly high in the promyelocytic (M3) variant of the acute non-lymphoblastic leukemias (acute promyelocytic leukemia or APML) (204, 205). Promyelocytes have more profibrinolytic activity than other leukemic cells (206, 207), and DIC in APML usually manifests itself as hyperfibrinolysis, with hypofibrinogenemia and depletion of $\alpha_2$-antiplasmin (30, 208, 209) and PAI-1 (210). However, the rate of thrombin generation (as reflected by the blood level of prothrombin activation peptide $F_{1.2}$) is also elevated (138), indicating that a "pure" fibrinolytic state is not present. The coagulopathy may become worse during induction chemotherapy due to the release of proteases during leukemic cell lysis (210). A number of deaths from intracranial bleeding have been reported (204, 211, 212). Successful management of DIC in APML by aggressive transfusion of platelets, fresh frozen plasma, and cryoprecipitate has been reported (213). Treatment of DIC in APML with heparin has been advocated; this recommendation, which is based on anecdotal reports (214, 215) and retrospective studies (211), has been disputed (213). Patients who bleed despite intensive blood component therapy may benefit from the administration of an antifibrinolytic drug, either with or without heparin (208, 216). Treatment of APML with all-trans retinoic acid (ATRA), which induces differentiation of leukemic promyelocytes without massive cell lysis, reverses hyperfibrinolysis more rapidly than does treatment with cytotoxic drugs (217) and may reduce the risk of bleeding. However, there are several reports describing persistent thrombin generation and thrombosis in individuals with APML treated with ATRA (218, 219).

## VASCULAR DISEASE

Large aortic aneurysms can cause chronic DIC (220, 221). Subclinical DIC is common after aneurysm resection (222), and some individuals develop severe coagulopathy (223). Activation of coagulation is probably a consequence of ulceration of an atherosclerotic plaques and exposure of blood to adventitial tissue factor. DIC also occurs with other extensive endothelial lesions (e.g., intracardiac thrombi) (224). Low-dose heparin therapy can reverse chronic DIC caused by an aneurysm (221). In individuals with ruptured abdominal aortic aneurysm, the presence of DIC predicts a substantially higher mortality rate (225).

Giant hemangiomas and other vascular malformations may cause activation of coagulation, hyperfibrinolysis and platelet consumption (Kasabach-Merritt syndrome) (226) (see color plate 44.5). Although this syndrome seems to be due to localized rather than disseminated intravascular coagulation, it is indistinguishable from DIC in most respects. Kasabach-Merritt syndrome usually occurs in infants and young children (227), but is occasionally seen in adults (228, 229). In many cases the coagulopathy begins after a hemangioma that has been present for some time enlarges suddenly (227). Eradication of the lesion by surgical removal, embolization, or radiotherapy is curative. The coagulopathy may improve with administration of heparin (228) or an antifibrinolytic drug (227, 229, 230). In addition, antifibrinolytic therapy may help eliminate the vascular lesion by promoting local thrombosis (229, 231). Hemangiomas may also shrink after glucocorticoid (227) or interferon (232) treatment, or without any treatment. Chronic and acute DIC responsive to low-dose heparin treatment have been described in individuals with hereditary hemorrhagic telangiectasia (233). A recent report describes the prenatal diagnosis of congenital DIC caused by a large vascular tumor of the umbilical cord (116).

## LIVER DISEASE (SEE CHAPTER 45)

As described above, hepatic failure has many effects on the coagulation system that predispose to DIC, and that make the diagnosis of DIC difficult. There is controversy as to whether or not severe liver disease itself causes DIC (147). While it is clear that decreased synthesis of coagulation proteins is the main reason for coagulation

abnormalities in most individuals with cirrhosis (59), activation of the coagulation and fibrinolytic pathways is also enhanced (61, 63, 234–236). Intravascular coagulation in cirrhosis may occur in the portal circulation, since the splenic cords often contain fibrin deposits and levels of coagulation proteins and platelets in cirrhosis increase after splenectomy (237). Administration of oral nonabsorbable antibiotics attenuates DIC in cirrhosis, suggesting that endotoxemia due to impaired hepatic clearance of endotoxin may help trigger the coagulopathy (236). In acute hepatic failure, release of tissue factor from injured hepatocytes may trigger DIC (238, 239). DIC associated with biliary tract obstruction is probably a consequence of endotoxemia (240, 241). Low-dose heparin (242) or antithrombin III infusion (60) may partially correct coagulation defects in cirrhotic individuals. Heparin treatment has been recommended for individuals with acute hepatic failure and DIC (238). However, heparin administration did not significantly affect outcome in a controlled trial involving individuals with acetaminophen-induced acute hepatic necrosis (243).

## OBSTETRIC COMPLICATIONS (SEE CHAPTER 46)

Pregnancy causes changes in plasma proteins and endothelial function that favor thrombin generation (244, 245), and may in fact cause low level intravascular coagulation (246). These changes set the stage for DIC if there is a strong procoagulant stimulus. The placenta and uterine contents are rich in procoagulants, and acute DIC is a frequent complication of abruptio placentae and amniotic fluid embolism (247, 248). DIC can also occur after second-trimester saline abortion (137, 249), septic abortion, or intrauterine infection (250).

Retained dead fetus can cause chronic or subacute DIC. Coagulopathy usually follows fetal death by at least 5 weeks, and gradually worsens with time (251). Delivery of a fetus that has been dead for over 5 weeks may precipitate acute DIC with hemorrhage (251, 252). Amelioration of DIC by administration of heparin prior to delivery has been reported (253).

Toxemia of pregnancy and its variants may cause microangiopathic hemolytic anemia, thrombocytopenia, and DIC. Syndromes in this category include preeclampsia/eclampsia (254, 255), acute fatty liver of pregnancy (256, 257), the so-called HELLP syndrome (*h*emolysis, *e*levated *l*iver enzymes, and *l*ow *p*latelets) (258), and postpartum renal failure (259). As is the case in other microangiopathic disorders (see below), endothelial dysfunction seems to be the primary process in these pregnancy-related syndromes (260). DIC occurs in about 20% of cases (261), but seems to be a secondary phenomenon (262); it is more likely to become severe if there is associated hepatic failure (257, 263). The treatment of choice is to empty the uterus; there is no evidence that administration of heparin is beneficial.

## MICROANGIOPATHIC DISORDERS (SEE CHAPTER 27)

In thrombotic thrombocytopenic purpura (TTP), hemolytic-uremic syndrome, vasculitis associated with systemic lupus erythematosus and scleroderma, toxemia of pregnancy (see above), and heparin-induced thrombotic thrombocytopenia, deposits of fibrin and platelets in small blood vessels cause organ dysfunction and intravascular hemolysis (264). Patients with microangiopathy often have elevated plasma levels of thrombin-antithrombin and plasmin-antiplasmin complexes consistent with the presence of low-grade DIC (153). However, in most cases clotting factor consumption is minimal, soluble fibrin is not found in the blood, and levels of FDP are only slightly elevated (152). As discussed in Chapter 27, the evidence suggests that the primary process is an endothelial cell abnormality possibly leading to von Willebrand factor mediated platelet agglutination (265), rather than release of tissue factor and thrombin-mediated formation of intravascular fibrin.

## TRANSFUSION REACTION

Acute hemolytic transfusion reaction is often complicated by severe DIC (266–268). Endothelial damage caused by cytokines (268), leukocyte proteases (269), activated complement (67), and products of hemolysis (e.g., heme iron [270]) is probably the responsible mechanism. Low levels of clotting factors and platelets after massive transfusion are usually due to hemodilution (151). However, a few massively transfused individuals develop a bleeding diathesis and biochemical signs of DIC (271); it is not clear whether this is due to transfusion *per se* or to the underlying disease.

## SURGERY

Compensated DIC is common after major surgery; over 80% of individuals have elevated FDP titers, and 30–50% have positive tests for circulating fibrin (272). Acute DIC in the perioperative period may occur as a consequence of major trauma, shock, or sepsis (273). The possibility of DIC secondary to an acute hemolytic transfusion reaction should be considered when generalized bleeding occurs in an anesthetized individual (274). Intraoperative blood salvage and autotransfusion has been proposed as a cause of DIC due to activation of leukocytes and platelets in the cell saver centrifuge bowl (275), but high grade DIC resulting from blood salvage seems to be quite rare in practice (276).

Patients undergoing cardiopulmonary bypass (Chapter 50) exhibit increased blood fibrinolytic activity (277) and thrombin generation (278), and some individuals who require prolonged bypass develop frank DIC with bleeding (279). However, most of the coagulation changes accompanying cardiopulmonary bypass are the result of hemodilution and platelet "exhaustion" rather than DIC (150, 280), and most bleeding complications are due to a surgically correctable lesion (i.e., a severed blood vessel) (281). The antifibrinolytic drugs ε-aminocaproic acid and aprotinin (Chapter 53) have been shown in controlled studies to reduce blood loss during cardiopulmonary bypass (282, 283).

Liver transplantation (Chapter 45) causes significant hemostatic derangement (284). Most individuals have preexisting coagulation defects due to underlying liver disease. During the anhepatic phase of transplantation, plasma fibrinolytic activity is increased. This is probably due to high t-PA activity (285), the effects of which are amplified by absent hepatic clearance of t-PA and depletion of the limited plasma $\alpha_2$-antiplasmin reserves. The coagulopathy intensifies after hepatic reperfusion, as ischemic tissue in the transplanted organ releases tissue factor and/or plasminogen activator (286). Increased plasma endotoxin levels and leukocyte activation products released from the graft liver may also contribute to DIC at this stage (287, 288). Complications that may ensue include intracranial bleeding (289) and respiratory failure caused by platelet aggregates in pulmonary vessels (290). Orthotopic liver transplantation, in which the host liver is removed, is more likely to cause DIC than is heterotopic liver transplantation, in which the host liver is left in place and the anhepatic phase of the procedure thereby avoided (291).

DIC may complicate placement of a peritoneovenous shunt for cirrhotic (292, 293) or malignant (294, 295) ascites. Substances found in ascitic fluid that might cause DIC include tissue factor (296), endotoxin (293), plasminogen activator (297), and collagen derivatives that activate platelets (298). Hemodilution, FDP and fibrin monomer in ascitic fluid, and the underlying liver disease also contribute to postshunt coagulation changes (295, 299). Discarding the ascitic fluid present at the time of surgery, rather than reinfusing it, has been recommended as a method for preventing DIC (296). Administration of ε-aminocaproic acid is reportedly of benefit in the treatment of postshunt coagulopathy (297), while treatment with antithrombin III concentrate is not (300).

## ENVENOMATION

Bites from crotalid snakes (rattlesnakes) and other vipers cause a coagulopathy with many of the characteristics of DIC. The most dangerous snakes in the United States in this regard are the eastern and western diamondback rattlesnakes, because of their large size and the quantity of venom they can inject. Coagulation changes observed following snake bites include thrombocytopenia, and profound and prolonged hypofibrinogenemia; the blood is rendered incoagulable in some cases (301, 302). Although bleeding may occur, its severity is often less than would be expected on the basis of the laboratory findings (301, 302). Snake venoms contain a wide variety of substances that can affect coagulation (303, 304). These include: phospholipases that release arachidonic acid from cell membranes (305); peptides that inhibit (306) or promote (307) platelet aggregation; enzymes that activate prothrombin and many other clotting proteins (308, 309); proteases with thrombin-like activity (310); and enzymes that degrade fibrinogen (311). The absence of specific inhibitors in human plasma enhances the potency of venom proteases. Venom also contains toxins that increase endothelial permeability and cause tissue necrosis (312), leading to release of endogenous tissue factor and plasminogen activators (302, 313). Management of snakebite coagulopathy is primarily supportive; administration of polyvalent antivenin may speed recovery from the coagulation abnormalities (314–316). Heparin is of little benefit, since it does not block the effects of venom proteases (317, 318).

## TRAUMA AND TISSUE INJURY

The likelihood of DIC following injury is a function of the extent of injury and the tissue factor content of the injured tissue. Brain is rich in tissue factor (2), and so individuals with traumatic brain injury are especially prone to develop DIC (319, 320). DIC may also accompany generalized tissue injury due to hypoxia (321), rhabdomyolysis (322), heat stroke (323, 324), or hypothermia (325). Fat embolism may cause DIC after a major fracture (326).

## SHOCK

Experimentally induced hypovolemic shock in animals causes coagulation abnormalities that resemble DIC (327). Decreased levels of clotting factors and platelets also occur in association with shock from a variety of causes in humans (328). These changes are due in part to internal fluid shifts and fluid administration, which lead to hemodilution (151, 329), but activation of coagulation and fibrinolysis may also contribute (330). Endotoxemia, which occurs in hemorrhagic as well as septic shock (331), and the adverse effects of hypotension on the endothelium and liver are all potential causes of DIC associated with shock.

## RESPIRATORY DISTRESS SYNDROMES

Many conditions that cause DIC can also cause adult respiratory distress syndrome (ARDS), so that there is significant overlap between the two syndromes. ARDS occurs in about 20% of individuals with DIC (332), and laboratory evidence of DIC is found in up to 20% of individuals with ARDS (333). A similar relationship exists between DIC and infant respiratory distress syndrome (334, 335). Patients with ARDS and DIC have a worse prognosis than those with ARDS alone (333, 336).

DIC may result from the illness that causes ARDS, or it may be a result of acute lung injury itself. Damage to pulmonary vascular endothelium and altered vascular permeability are common in respiratory distress syndromes (337); this is likely to expose blood to tissue factor and thereby cause DIC. DIC has also been proposed as a cause of lung injury in acute respiratory failure (338). In experimental animals, acute lung injury can be induced by administering intravenous thrombin along with an inhibitor of fibrinolysis (339, 340), and endotoxin-induced acute lung injury can be prevented by administering a thrombin inhibitor (341). However, there is no evidence that administration of anticoagulants prevents ARDS, and clinical data do not support the idea that DIC causes ARDS (342).

## INHERITED DISORDERS

Homozygous protein C deficiency causes a potentially lethal form of purpura fulminans, which usually begins shortly after birth (101, 343) (Chapter 40). In individuals with antithrombin III deficiency, DIC has been described in association with acute thrombotic episodes (344, 345). Inherited deficiency of $\alpha_2$-antiplasmin results in a tendency towards hyperfibrinolysis and bleeding; however, afflicted individuals do not have elevated FDP levels or other biochemical evidence of DIC (346). Chronic, low-grade intravascular coagulation occurs in inherited hyperlipoproteinemia types II and IV; its clinical significance is unclear (347).

## DRUG-INDUCED DIC

Several drugs and therapeutic agents can cause DIC or a DIC-like state. Thrombolytic drugs such as streptokinase and recombinant t-PA induce systemic hyperfibrinolysis. They generate large amounts of plasmin, which may in turn consume enough $\alpha_2$-antiplasmin to allow free plasmin to appear in the blood. A hirudin-inhibitable increase in fibrinopeptide A level occurs after t-PA administration; this has been attributed to local exposure of clot-bound thrombin during clot lysis, rather than DIC (348). However, there is also evidence that plasminogen activators directly promote thrombin formation (35, 36). Bleeding is the most important complication of thrombolytic treatment (349, 350). Ancrod is an enzyme which is derived from snake venom and used as an anticoagulant. It cleaves the fibrinopeptides A from fibrinogen, creating friable, fibrin-like particles which cannot be clotted by thrombin, and causing a small or moderate increase in fibrinolytic activity. In therapeutic doses Ancrod causes hypofibrinogenemia, but little bleeding (83). Pharmacologic preparations of procoagulant precursors such as prothrombin complex concentrate (which contains factors II, VII, X, and IX and is used to treat hemophilia B) and factor XI concentrate contain a proportion of activated clotting factors. These products can cause thrombosis and, on occasion, DIC (351–353). Many hemophiliacs have coexisting liver disease, which promotes the coagulopathy. High-purity factor IX is less likely to cause DIC than prothrombin complex concentrate (354). Heparin can cause a syndrome of thrombotic thrombocytopenia with secondary DIC (355, 356). Drug induced immune damage to endothelial cells may be responsible (357). Warfarin treatment may precipitate DIC or a purpura fulminans-like syndrome in individuals with protein C deficiency or cancer (190, 358, 359). Hyperfibrinolysis and bleeding have been reported as a complication of intravenous lipid emulsion administration, the cause for which is unknown (360). Agents such as glycine or dextran solution that are used to distend the uterus during hysteroscopy can cause DIC if they enter the bloodstream (361, 362). Hypersensitivity reactions to a variety of other drugs have been reported to cause DIC.

## "PRIMARY" FIBRINOLYSIS

This term has been applied to cases of DIC in which the laboratory and clinical manifestations are dominated by the effects of fibrinolysis (25, 33). These cases are characterized by marked hypofibrinogenemia, very high FDP levels (which may reflect plasminolysis of fibrinogen as well as fibrin) (118), absence of detectable $\alpha_2$-antiplasmin activity in plasma, and, in many instances, life-threatening bleeding (31). Some individuals with these findings have nearly normal platelet counts and antithrombin III levels, indicating that thrombin activity in their blood is not increased in proportion to plasmin activity. Except for cases of coagulopathy induced by the administration of streptokinase, t-PA, or u-PA (34, 349), however, it is difficult to be certain that fibrinolysis is really the "primary" event. In many instances there is laboratory or clinical evidence indicating that fibrinolysis is associated with or dependent upon thrombin formation. For example, in the hyperfibrinolytic state associated with promyelocytic leukemia the blood level of the prothrombin activation peptide ($F_{1.2}$) increases significantly (138). Hyperfibrinolysis associated with prostate cancer can sometimes be extinguished by heparin administration, indicating that plasmin formation in such cases is largely secondary to thrombin and fibrin

formation (177). Many cases of "primary" fibrinolysis would therefore be more accurately described as "predominant" fibrinolysis.

## DIC OF UNCERTAIN CAUSE

The cause of DIC can usually be deduced by considering the clinical setting in which it occurs, although assigning a specific etiology may be difficult in a individual with several serious medical problems. Occasionally, bleeding or thrombosis associated with DIC is the initial sign of an illness. In most instances the underlying cause (e.g., sepsis) becomes apparent quickly. Occult cancer sometimes presents with compensated DIC and thrombosis (91) or with hyperfibrinolysis and bleeding (particularly in prostatic carcinoma [363]). A syndrome of unknown etiology characterized by the sudden onset of hyperthermia, shock, cerebral edema, and defibrination has been described in infants and young children (364, 365). Other causes of DIC that may elude quick diagnosis include toxic shock syndrome (366), Kawasaki syndrome (367), postinfectious purpura fulminans (368), any of the viral hemorrhagic fevers (166, 369), and amyloidosis (370). DIC for which no cause can be determined after extensive investigation has been described (33), however it is quite rare.

# TREATMENT OF DIC

Morbidity and mortality in individuals with DIC are usually due to the effects of the underlying disease rather than to DIC itself (77). Eliminating the cause should therefore be the primary concern when DIC is encountered. Measures to counteract circulatory and respiratory failure, if these are present, must also take priority. Many individuals with DIC require no specific therapy for the coagulopathy, either because it is self-limited or because it is not severe enough to present a major risk of bleeding or thrombosis. At the other end of the clinical spectrum, however, there are individuals with profound hyperfibrinolysis or hypercoagulability for whom treatment of DIC can be lifesaving. Two types of treatment are available for them: blood products that replace those factors missing from their blood, and drugs that block the enzyme pathways responsible for coagulation and fibrinolysis.

## REPLACEMENT THERAPY

Blood component therapy in DIC helps restore hemostatic balance by repletion of clotting factors, inhibitors of coagulation and fibrinolysis, and platelets. Fears that such therapy might "feed the fire" and contribute to organ damage by increasing intravascular fibrin formation have not been borne out in clinical practice.

Several products derived from plasma are available for replacement of coagulation proteins (see Chapter 52). Fresh frozen plasma (FFP) provides virtually all coagulation factors and inhibitors (371). Transfusion of one unit of FFP to an adult (in the absence of DIC) raises blood levels of most coagulation proteins by about 3% of normal. Cryoprecipitate is a plasma fraction enriched in fibrinogen, von Willebrand factor, and fibronectin. It usually contains between 200 and 300 mg of fibrinogen per bag (372). Concentrates of factors VIII and IX used to treat hemophilia are not useful in DIC. In the case of factor VIII, this is because levels of the factor are not usually low in DIC (78, 120). Factor IX concentrate (prothrombin complex concentrate) is potentially thrombogenic and may itself cause DIC because it contains activated clotting factors (351). Antithrombin III concentrate has a 50-fold higher concentration of this protease inhibitor than plasma (373). It ameliorates experimentally induced DIC in dogs (374), but to date there is no convincing evidence that it is of benefit in human DIC (375, 376). Protein C concentrate, which contains about 100-fold more protein C than plasma, has recently become available (377). There is anecdotal evidence suggesting that it may be of benefit in infectious purpura fulminans (378, 379).

The need for blood component replacement therapy in DIC is determined by the extent of depletion of the factors in question and the risk of bleeding. The prothrombin time (expressed as the international normalized ratio or INR) is the best overall indicator of the severity of clotting factor depletion. If the INR is greater than 2.0, administration of FFP is reasonable, particularly if the individual is bleeding or at high risk for bleeding (e.g., after surgery). The amount of FFP needed is a function of the degree of prolongation of the prothrombin time and the rates of clotting factor consumption and synthesis, which must be determined empirically. If there is hyperfibrinolysis with a low plasma fibrinogen level ($< 100$ mg/dl), cryoprecipitate may be given along with FFP. Ten units of cryoprecipitate per 2–3 units of FFP is usually sufficient. Patients with marked thrombocytopenia (platelets $< 10,000$–$20,000/$ $\mu l$), or with moderate thrombocytopenia (platelets $<50,000/\mu l$) and active bleeding or a high risk of bleeding, should be given platelet transfusions (1–2 U/10 kg per day). The risks of volume overload and transmission of infectious agents must always be borne in mind when giving large quantities of blood products. Clotting factor depletion due to vitamin K deficiency (148, 149) and thrombocytopenia due to folic acid deficiency (380) may arise in the clinical setting of DIC, and so empiric treatment with these vitamins is advisable.

Plasma or whole blood exchange has been advocated as a treatment for individuals with overwhelming sepsis and DIC (381), and there is anecdotal evidence that it may be beneficial in this setting (382–384). Plasma exchange allows administration of larger volumes of plasma and should be considered as an option in individuals with profound coagulation defects resistant to simple plasma replacement. Whether it provides any additional benefit by removing toxins or activated clotting factors remains an open question.

## DRUG THERAPY

The role of pharmacologic inhibitors of coagulation and fibrinolysis in the treatment of DIC is controversial. Heparin (Chapter 55) is the drug most often used to treat DIC (385, 386). Among its many biologic effects is the ability to catalyze inhibition of thrombin and other procoagulant enzymes by antithrombin III (387). In theory this might prevent large- and small-vessel thrombosis, and prevent bleeding by reducing the rates of both clotting factor consumption and secondary fibrinolysis. However, heparin might also increase the risk of bleeding by virtue of its anticoagulant effect.

Treatment of purpura fulminans with heparin has been advocated (93, 99, 385). This recommendation is based on the assumption that such treatment will help prevent tissue damage due to thrombosis; the supporting data are anecdotal (93, 94, 99). The clinical benefit of heparin in purpura fulminans is generally not dramatic (96, 99, 388). It should be kept in mind that factors other than thrombosis may be responsible for much of the tissue damage that accompanies severe DIC (74), which casts doubt on the rationale for giving heparin to prevent such damage.

Heparin therapy clearly benefits some individuals with DIC caused by cancer (91, 177, 190). This is particularly true if the individual has chronic, compensated DIC and recurrent thrombosis (91, 191), but there are reports of improvement after heparin treatment in individuals with hyperfibrinolysis and bleeding as well (178). Chronic DIC from other causes, such as large aneurysms (221), Kasabach-Merritt syndrome (228), and retained dead fetus (99, 253), may also improve with heparin treatment. Patients with Trousseau syndrome who have deep venous thrombosis and DIC should be treated initially with anticoagulant doses of heparin (sufficient to prolong the aPTT to at least 1½ times normal). In other individuals with chronic DIC, however, low doses (5–10 U/kg per hour) of heparin may be sufficient to reverse the coagulopathy (131, 389).

There is presently no convincing evidence that giving heparin reduces morbidity or mortality in acute DIC. Because individuals with DIC are heterogeneous in terms of associated diseases and disease severity and tend to be subjected to many different types of treatment, controlled prospective trials comparing different treatments in DIC are practically nonexistent. For the same reasons, conclusions about treatment efficacy that are derived from retrospective data analysis must be regarded with caution. Such analyses have produced conflicting opinions as to the efficacy of heparin in DIC. Colman et al., based upon a review of the literature, concluded that administration of heparin to individuals with acute DIC was associated with less bleeding and increased chance of survival (122). In contrast, Corrigan reviewed the literature and concluded that administration of heparin was of no benefit in children with acute DIC due to sepsis (390). Mant and King reviewed 47 cases of acute, severe DIC treated at a single institution and concluded that administration of heparin was of no benefit, and might even have worsened bleeding (77). Several retrospective studies involving small numbers of individuals have concluded that heparin helps to control DIC associated with APML (211, 214, 215, 391). However, two larger retrospective studies found no evidence of improved outcome with heparin treatment in APML (212, 227). There are anecdotal reports that present convincing evidence that heparin treatment was beneficial to individual individuals with acute DIC (187). All that can be concluded about the role of heparin in treating acute DIC is that while some individuals may benefit from such treatment, it should be used with caution, and usually at a low dose.

The role of other anticoagulants such as low-molecular-weight heparin derivatives and hirudin in treating DIC is unclear. A single controlled trial comparing dalteparin (a low-molecular-weight heparin) to low-dose unfractionated heparin showed a trend toward improved survival in the individuals receiving dalteparin, although the difference was not statistically significant (392). In an uncontrolled trial, improvement in laboratory indicators of DIC after treatment with hirudin has been described (393).

Antifibrinolytic drugs such as ε-aminocaproic acid (EACA) and tranexamic acid are lysine analogs that inhibit binding of plasmin, plasminogen, and t-PA to fibrin and fibrinogen, and can diminish bleeding caused by hyperfibrinolysis (Chapter 53). However, their use in DIC is considered contraindicated by many authors because of the potential for thrombosis due to unopposed fibrin formation (394). Indeed, administration of EACA can cause increased tissue injury due to thrombosis in experimental DIC (339, 340, 395), and there are clinical reports of thrombosis in DIC following EACA therapy (79, 89). In addition, it is possible that treatment with lysine analogs could enhance some of the pathological effects of hyperfibrinolysis, since at low concentrations they increase activation of plasminogen by u-PA and t-PA (396, 397). On the other hand, in experimental DIC induced by thrombin infusion, infusion of EACA together with heparin is more effective than treatment with heparin alone in controlling the coagulopathy

(398), and tranexamic acid prevents neutrophil sequestration and increased vascular permeability in the lungs (399, 400).

The benefits of antifibrinolytic drug therapy may outweigh the risks when there is profound hyperfibrinolysis with bleeding, particularly if there does not seem to be very much thrombin or fibrin formation (33, 350, 401). This is often the situation in APML, and several reports suggest that the administration of EACA or tranexamic acid to individuals with APML can reduce bleeding without creating a high risk of thrombosis (208, 216, 402). EACA has been used with favorable results in individuals with DIC caused by prostate cancer (403) or after peritoneovenous shunt placement (297), and to prevent bleeding after cardiac bypass surgery (282). It has also been used successfully in treating DIC secondary to vascular malformations (Kasabach-Merritt syndrome). This represents a special case, since thrombosis of the abnormal vessels is a desired consequence of such treatment (229, 231). In other individuals with DIC, antifibrinolytic therapy should be considered as a last resort in individuals who have profound hyperfibrinolysis and who bleed despite aggressive blood component therapy (31). Concomitant administration of low-dose intravenous heparin may decrease the chance of thrombosis. Doses of 10–15 mg/kg per hour of EACA and 8–10 U/kg per hour of heparin are appropriate (208). Heparin and EACA can be mixed together and administered through the same intravenous line, if necessary.

Aprotinin is a naturally occurring inhibitor of trypsin, plasmin, and kallikrein (404, 405) that has been shown to reduce blood loss after cardiac surgery, a benefit presumably related to the drug's antifibrinolytic activity (283) (see Chapters 50 and 53). However, there are also reports of generalized microvascular thrombosis following aprotinin administration (406, 407), suggesting that it should be used with caution in coagulopathic individuals. Gabexate is a synthetic inhibitor of thrombin, factor Xa, plasmin, and kallikrein (408); it is not available in the U.S., but has been used with some success in Japan to treat DIC (409).

# REFERENCES

1. Dvorak AM. Fibrin in the peripheral blood of a patient with acute myelocytic leukemia. Blood 1996;87:2648.
2. Drake TA, Morrissey JH, Edgington TS. Selective cellular expression of tissue factor in human tissues. Implications for disorders of hemostasis and thrombosis. Am J Pathol 1989;134:1087–1097.
3. Faulk WP, Labarrere CA, Carson SD. Tissue factor: identification and characterization of cell types in human placentae. Blood 1990;76:86–96.
4. Koyama T, Nishida K, Ohdama S et al. Determination of plasma tissue factor antigen and its clinical significance. Br J Haematol 1994;87:343–347.
5. Takahashi H, Satoh N, Wada K et al. Tissue factor in plasma of patients with disseminated intravascular coagulation. Am J Hematol 1994;46:333–337.
6. Wada H, Nakase T, Nakaya R et al. Elevated plasma tissue factor antigen level in patients with disseminated intravascular coagulation. Am J Hematol 1994;45:232–236.

7. Brett J, Gerlach H, Nawroth P et al. Tumor necrosis factor/cachectin increases permeability of endothelial cell monolayers by a mechanism involving regulatory G proteins. J Exp Med 1989;169:1977–1991.

8. Rickles FR, Edwards RL. Activation of blood coagulation in cancer: trousseau's syndrome revisited. Blood 1983;62:14–31.

9. Colman RW. Formation of human plasma kinin. N Engl J Med 1974;291: 509–515.

10. van Deventer SJ, Buller HR, ten Cate TW et al. A. Experimental endotoxemia in humans: analysis of cytokine release and coagulation, fibrinolytic, and complement pathways. Blood 1990;76:2520–2526.

11. Kakkar AK, DeRuvo N, Chinswangwatanakul V et al. Extrinsic-pathway activation in cancer with high factor VIIa and tissue factor. Lancet 1995; 346:1004–1005.

12. Pixley RA, De La Cadena R, Page JD et al. The contact system contributes to hypotension but not disseminated intravascular coagulation in lethal bacteremia. In vivo use of a monoclonal anti-factor XII antibody to block contact activation in baboons. J Clin Invest 1993;91:61–68.

13. Lui L, Rodgers G. Characterization of an inducible endothelial cell prothrombin activator. Blood 1997;88:2989–2994.

14. Edwards RL, Silver J, Rickles FR. Human tumor procoagulants: registry of the Subcommittee on Haemostasis and Malignancy of the Scientific and Standardization Committee, International Society on thrombosis and hemostasis. Thromb Haemost 1993;69:205–213.

15. Falanga A, Alessio MG, Donati MB et al. A new procoagulant in acute leukemia. Blood 1988;71:870–875.

16. Gordon SG. Cancer cell procoagulants and their implications. Hematol Oncol Clin North Am 1992;6:1359–1374.

17. Pineo GF, Regoeczi E, Hatton MW et al. The activation of coagulation by extracts of mucus: a possible pathway of intravascular coagulation accompanying adenocarcinomas. J Lab Clin Med 1973;82:255–266.

18. Hanss M, Collen D. Secretion of tissue-type plasminogen activator and plasminogen activator inhibitor by cultured human endothelial cells: modulation by thrombin, endotoxin, and histamine. J Lab Clin Med 1987;109: 97–104.

19. Levin EG, Marzec U, Anderson J et al. Thrombin stimulates tissue plasminogen activator release from cultured human endothelial cells. J Clin Invest 1984;74:1988–1995.

20. Bennett B, Croll A, Ferguson K et al. Complexing of tissue plasminogen activator with PAI-1, alpha 2-macroglobulin, and C1-inhibitor: studies in patients with defibrination and a fibrinolytic state after electroshock or complicated labor. Blood 1990;75:671–676.

21. Giles AR, Nesheim ME, Herring SW et al. The fibrinolytic potential of the normal primate following the generation of thrombin in vivo. Thromb Haemost 1990;63:476–481.

22. van Hinsbergh VW, Bauer KA, Kooistra T et al. Progress of fibrinolysis during tumor necrosis factor infusions in humans. Concomitant increase in tissue-type plasminogen activator, plasminogen activator inhibitor type-1, and fibrin(ogen) degradation products. Blood 1990;76:2284–2289.

23. Philippe J, Offner F, Declerck PJ et al. Fibrinolysis and coagulation in patients with infectious disease and sepsis. Thromb Haemost 1991;65: 291–295.

24. Jansen PM, Pixley RA, Brouwer M et al. Inhibition of factor XII in septic baboons attenuates the activation of complement and fibrinolytic systems and reduces the release of interleukin-6 and neutrophil elastase. Blood 1996;87:2337–2344.

25. Bennett B, Booth NA, Croll A et al. The bleeding disorder in acute promyelocytic leukaemia: fibrinolysis due to u-PA rather than defibrination. Br J Haematol 1989;71:511–517.

26. Weitz JI, Leslie B, Ginsberg J. Soluble fibrin degradation products potentiate tissue plasminogen activator-induced fibrinogen proteolysis. J Clin Invest 1991;87:1082–1090.

27. Keijer J, Linders M, van Zonneveld AJ et al. The interaction of plasminogen activator inhibitor 1 with plasminogen activators (tissue-type and urokinase-type) and fibrin: localization of interaction sites and physiologic relevance. Blood 1991;78:401–409.

28. Hogg PJ, Stenflo J, Mosher DF. Thrombospondin is a slow tight-binding inhibitor of plasmin. Biochemistry 1992;31:265–269.

29. Lind SE, Smith CJ. Actin accelerates plasmin generation by tissue plasminogen activator. J Biol Chem 1991;266:17673–17678.

30. Booth NA, Bennett B. Plasmin-alpha 2-antiplasmin complexes in bleeding disorders characterized by primary or secondary fibrinolysis. Br J Haematol 1984;56:545–556.

31. Williams EC. Plasma alpha 2-antiplasmin activity. Role in the evaluation and management of fibrinolytic states and other bleeding disorders. Arch Intern Med 1989;149:1769–1772.

32. Okajima K, Kohno I, Soe G et al. Direct evidence for systemic fibrinogenolysis in patients with acquired alpha 2-plasmin inhibitor deficiency. Am J Hematol 1994;45:16–24.

33. Merskey C, Johnson AJ, Kleiner GJ et al. The defibrination syndrome: clinical features and laboratory diagnosis. Br J Haematol 1967;13:528–549.

34. Harker LA, Slichter SJ. Platelet and fibrinogen consumption in man. N Engl J Med 1972;287:999–1005.

35. Brommer EJ, Meijer P. Thrombin generation induced by the intrinsic or

extrinsic coagulation pathway is accelerated by streptokinase, independently of plasminogen. Thromb Haemost 1993;70:995–997.

36. Bruhn HD, Conard J, Mannucci M et al. Multicentric evaluation of a new assay for prothrombin fragment F1 + 2 determination. Thromb Haemost 1992;68:413–417.

37. Suffredini AF, Harpel PC, Parrillo JE. Promotion and subsequent inhibition of plasminogen activation after administration of intravenous endotoxin to normal subjects. N Engl J Med 1989;320:1165–1172.

38. Eckhardt T, Koch M. Fibrinogen–proteolysis in acute myelogenous leukemia (AML). Blut 1986;53:39–48.

39. Brower MS, Harpel PC. Alpha-1-antitrypsin-human leukocyte elastase complexes in blood: quantification by an enzyme-linked differential antibody immunosorbent assay and comparison with alpha-2-plasmin inhibitor-plasmin complexes. Blood 1983;61:842–849.

40. Schmidt W, Egbring R, Havemann K. Effect of elastase-like and chymotrypsin-like neutral proteases from human granulocytes on isolated clotting factors. Thromb Res 1975;6:315–329.

41. Kornecki E, Ehrlich YH, De Mars DD et al. Exposure of fibrinogen receptors in human platelets by surface proteolysis with elastase. J Clin Invest 1986;77:750–756.

42. Brower MS, Levin RI, Garry K. Human neutrophil elastase modulates platelet function by limited proteolysis of membrane glycoproteins. J Clin Invest 1985;75:657–666.

43. Higuchi DA, Wun TC, Likert KM et al. The effect of leukocyte elastase on tissue factor pathway inhibitor. Blood 1992;79:1712–1719.

44. Wu K, Urano T, Ihara H et al. The cleavage and inactivation of plasminogen activator inhibitor type 1 by neutrophil elastase: the evaluation of its physiologic relevance in fibrinolysis. Blood 1995;86:1056–1061.

45. Wilde JT, Thomas WE, Lane DA et al. Acquired dysfibrinogenaemia masquerading as disseminated intravascular coagulation in acute pancreatitis. J Clin Pathol 1988;41:615–618.

46. Kwaan HC, Anderson MC, Gramatica L. A study of pancreatic enzymes as a factor in the pathogenesis of disseminated intravascular coagulation during acute pancreatitis. Surgery 1971;69:663–672.

47. Schwager I, Jungi TW. Effect of human recombinant cytokines on the induction of macrophage procoagulant activity. Blood 1994;83:152–160.

48. Horn RG, Collins RD. Studies on the pathogenesis of the generalized Schwartzman reaction. The role of granulocytes. Lab Invest 1968;18: 101–107.

49. Okajima K, Yang WP, Okabe H et al. Role of leukocytes in the activation of intravascular coagulation in patients with septicemia. Am J Hematol 1991;36:265–271.

50. Robinson RA, Worfolk L, Tracy PB. Endotoxin enhances the expression of monocyte prothrombinase activity. Blood 1992;79:406–416.

51. Bevilacqua MP, Pober JS, Majeau GR et al. Recombinant tumor necrosis factor induces procoagulant activity in cultured human vascular endothelium: characterization and comparison with the actions of interleukin 1. Proc Natl Acad Sci U S A 1986;83:4533–4537.

52. Nawroth PP, Stern DM. Modulation of endothelial cell hemostatic properties by tumor necrosis factor. J Exp Med 1986;163:740–745.

53. Morrison DC, Ryan JL. Endotoxins and disease mechanisms. Annu Rev Med 1987;38:417–432.

54. Ryan J, Brett J, Tijburg P et al. Tumor necrosis factor-induced endothelial tissue factor is associated with subendothelial matrix vesicles but is not expressed on the apical surface. Blood 1992;80:966–974.

55. van der Poll T, Levi M, Hack CE et al. Elimination of interleukin 6 attenuates coagulation activation in experimental endotoxemia in chimpanzees. J Exp Med 1994;179:1253–1259.

56. Nossel HL. Fibrinogen proteolysis by thrombin, plasmin and platelet release in relation to disseminated intravascular coagulation. Bibl Haematol 1983;49:151–162.

57. Heyderman RS. Sepsis and intravascular thrombosis. Arch Dis Child 1993; 68:621–623.

58. Bauer KA, ten Cate H, Barzegar S et al. Tumor necrosis factor infusions have a procoagulant effect on the hemostatic mechanism of humans. Blood 1989;74:165–172.

59. Stein SF, Harker LA. Kinetic and functional studies of platelets, fibrinogen, and plasminogen in patients with hepatic cirrhosis. J Lab Clin Med 1982; 99:217–230.

60. Schipper HG, ten Cate JW. Antithrombin III transfusion in patients with hepatic cirrhosis. Br J Haematol 1982;52:25–33.

61. Takahashi H, Tatewaki W, Wada K et al. Thrombin and plasmin generation in patients with liver disease. Am J Hematol 1989;32:30–35.

62. Fletcher A, Biederman O, Moore D et al. Abnormal plasminogen-plasmin system activity (fibrinolysis) in patients with hepatic cirrhosis: its cause and consequences. J Clin Invest 1964;43:681–695.

63. Hersch SL, Kunelis T, Francis RB, Jr. The pathogenesis of accelerated fibrinolysis in liver cirrhosis: a critical role for tissue plasminogen activator inhibitor. Blood 1987;69:1315–1319.

64. Matsuda M, Wakabayashi K, Aoki N et al. Alpha 2-Plasmin inhibitor is among acute phase reactants. Thromb Res 1980;17:527–532.

65. Moore KL, Andreoli SP, Esmon NL et al. Endotoxin enhances tissue factor

and suppresses thrombomodulin expression of human vascular endothelium in vitro. J Clin Invest 1987;79:124–130.

66. Ogawa S, Gerlach H, Esposito C et al. Hypoxia modulates the barrier and coagulant function of cultured bovine endothelium. Increased monolayer permeability and induction of procoagulant properties. J Clin Invest 1990; 85:1090–1098.

67. Hamilton KK, Hattori R, Esmon CT et al. Complement proteins C5b-9 induce vesiculation of the endothelial plasma membrane and expose catalytic surface for assembly of the prothrombinase enzyme complex. J Biol Chem 1990;265:3809–3814.

68. Shwartzman G. Phenomenon of local tissue reactivity and its immunological, pathological and clinical significance. London, Oxford University Press; 1937.

69. Apitz K. A study of the generalized Shwartzman phenomenon. J Immunol 1935;29:255–266.

70. Thomas L, Good R. Studies on the generalized Shwartzman reaction. I. General observations concerning the phenomenon. J Exp Med 1952;96: 605–623.

71. Rothberger H, Dove FB, Lee TK et al. Procoagulant activity of lymphocyte-macrophage populations in rabbits: selective increases in marrow, blood, and spleen cells during Shwartzman reactions. Blood 1983;61:712–717.

72. Argenbright LW, Barton RW. Interactions of leukocyte integrins with intercellular adhesion molecule 1 in the production of inflammatory vascular injury in vivo. The Shwartzman reaction revisited. J Clin Invest 1992;89: 259–272.

73. Zivelin A, Rao VM, Rapaport SI. Evidence for an essential role of tissue factor dependent blood coagulation in the pathogenesis of the local Shwartzman reaction. Blood Cells Mol Dis 1995;21:9–19.

74. Taylor FB, Jr., Chang AC, Peer GT et al. DEGR-factor Xa blocks disseminated intravascular coagulation initiated by Escherichia coli without preventing shock or organ damage. Blood 1991;78:364–368.

75. Taylor FB, Jr., Chang A, Esmon CT et al. Protein C prevents the coagulopathic and lethal effects of Escherichia coli infusion in the baboon. J Clin Invest 1987;79:918–925.

76. Taylor F, Chang A, Ferrell G et al. C4b-binding protein exacerbates the host response to Escherichia coli. Blood 1991;78:357–363.

77. Mant MJ, King EG. Severe, acute disseminated intravascular coagulation. A reappraisal of its pathophysiology, clinical significance and therapy based on 47 patients. Am J Med 1979;67:557–563.

78. Spero JA, Lewis JH, Hasiba U. Disseminated intravascular coagulation. Findings in 346 patients. Thromb Haemost 1980;43:28–33.

79. Robboy SJ, Major MC, Colman RW et al. Pathology of disseminated intravascular coagulation (DIC). Analysis of 26 cases. Hum Pathol 1972;3: 327–343.

80. Fletcher A, Alkjaersig N, Sherry S. Pathogenesis of the coagulation defect developing during pathological plasma proteolytic ("fibrinolytic") states. I. The significance of fibrinogen proteolysis and circulating fibrin breakdown products. J Clin Invest 1962;41:896–916.

81. Alkjaersig N, Fletcher A, Sherry S. Pathogenesis of the coagulation defect developing during pathological plasma proteolytic ("fibrinolytic") states. II. The significance, mechanism and consequences of defective fibrin polymerization. J Clin Invest 1962;41:917–934.

82. Rao AK, Pratt C, Berke A et al. Thrombolysis in Myocardial Infarction (TIMI) Trial–phase I: hemorrhagic manifestations and changes in plasma fibrinogen and the fibrinolytic system in patients treated with recombinant tissue plasminogen activator and streptokinase. J Am Coll Cardiol 1988; 11:1–11.

83. Latallo ZS. Retrospective study on complications and adverse effects of treatment with thrombin-like enzymes–a multicenter trial. Thromb Haemost 1983;50:604–609.

84. Heckel JL, Sandgren EP, Degen JL et al. Neonatal bleeding in transgenic mice expressing urokinase-type plasminogen activator. Cell 1990;62: 447–456.

85. Bleyl U. Morphologic diagnosis of disseminated intravascular coagulation: histologic, histochemical and electron microscopic studies. Semin Thromb Hemost 1977;3:247–267.

86. Taylor FB. Role of tissue factor and factor VIIa in the coagulant and inflammatory response to LD100 Escherichia coli in the baboon. Haemostasis 1996;26 (suppl):83–91.

87. Matlin RA, Gary NE. Acute cortical necrosis. Case report and review of the literature. Am J Med 1974;56:110–118.

88. McKay DG, Muller-Berghaus G. Therapeutic implications of disseminated intravascular coagulation. Am J Cardiol 1967;20:392–410.

89. Charytan C, Purtilo D. Glomerular capillary thrombosis and acute renal failure after epsilon-amino caproic acid therapy. N Engl J Med 1969;280: 1102–1104.

90. Naeye R. Thrombotic state after a hemorrhagic diathesis, a possible complication of therapy with epsilon-aminocaproic acid. Blood 1962;19: 694–701.

91. Sack GH, Jr., Levin J, Bell WR. Trousseau's syndrome and other manifestations of chronic disseminated coagulopathy in patients with neoplasms: clinical, pathophysiologic, and therapeutic features. Medicine 1977;56: 1–37.

92. Robboy SJ, Mihm MC, Colman RW et al. The skin in disseminated intravascular coagulation. Prospective analysis of thirty-six cases. Br J Dermatol 1973;88:221–229.

93. Spicer TE, Rau JM. Purpura fulminans. Am J Med 1976;61:566–571.

94. Francis RB, Jr. Acquired purpura fulminans. Semin Thromb Hemost 1990; 16:310–325.

95. Margaretten W, Nakai H, Landing B. Septicemic adrenal hemorrhage. Am of Child 1963;105:64–69.

96. Giraud T, Dhainaut JF, Schremmer B et al. Adult overwhelming meningococcal purpura. A study of 35 cases, 1977-1989. Arch Intern Med 1991;151: 310–316.

97. Hautekeete ML, Berneman ZN, Bieger R et al. Purpura fulminans in pneumococcal sepsis. Arch Intern Med 1986;146:497–499.

98. Antley RM, McMillan CW. Sequential coagulation studies in purpura fulminans. N Engl J Med 1967;276:1287–1290.

99. Molos MA, Hall JC. Symmetrical peripheral gangrene and disseminated intravascular coagulation. Arch Dermatol 1985;121:1057–1061.

100. Marciniak E, Wilson HD, Marlar RA. Neonatal purpura fulminans: a genetic disorder related to the absence of protein C in blood. Blood 1985;65: 15–20.

101. Seligsohn U, Berger A, Abend M et al. Homozygous protein C deficiency manifested by massive venous thrombosis in the newborn. N Engl J Med 1984;310:559–562.

102. Mahasandana C, Suvatte V, Marlar RA et al. Neonatal purpura fulminans associated with homozygous protein S deficiency. Lancet 1990;335:61–62.

103. Powars DR, Rogers ZR, Patch MJ et al. Purpura fulminans in meningococemia: association with acquired deficiencies of proteins C and S. N Engl J Med 1987;317:571–572.

104. Madden RM, Gill JC, Marlar RA. Protein C and protein S levels in two patients with acquired purpura fulminans. Br J Haematol 1990;75:112–117.

105. Fijnvandraat K, Peters M, Derkx B et al. Endotoxin induced coagulation activation and protein C reduction in meningococcal septic shock. Prog Clin Biol Res 1994;388:247–254.

106. Levin M, Eley BS, Louis J et al. Postinfectious purpura fulminans caused by an autoantibody directed against protein S. J Pediatr 1995;127:355–363.

107. Manco-Johnson M, Nuss R, Key N et al. Lupus anticoagulant and protein S deficiency in children with postvaricella purpura fulminans or thrombosis. J Pediatr 1997;128:319–323.

108. Mitchell CA, Rowell JA, Hau L et al. A fatal thrombotic disorder associated with an acquired inhibitor of protein C. N Engl J Med 1987;317:1638–1642.

109. Margaretten W, McAdams A. An appraisal of fulminant meningococcemia with reference to the Shwartzman phenomenon. Am J Med 1958;25: 868–876.

110. Girardin E, Grau GE, Dayer JM et al. Tumor necrosis factor and interleukin-1 in the serum of children with severe infectious purpura. N Engl J Med 1988;319:397–400.

111. Marlar RA, Endres-Brooks J, Miller C. Serial studies of protein C and its plasma inhibitor in patients with disseminated intravascular coagulation. Blood 1985;66:59–63.

112. D'Angelo A, Vigano-D'Angelo S, Esmon CT et al. Acquired deficiencies of protein S. Protein S activity during oral anticoagulation, in liver disease, and in disseminated intravascular coagulation. J Clin Invest 1988;81: 1445–1454.

113. Hayes MA, Yau EH, Hinds CJ et al. Symmetrical peripheral gangrene: association with noradrenaline administration. Intensive Care Med 1992; 18:433–436.

114. Kobayashi N, Maekawa T, Takada M et al. Criteria for diagnosis of DIC based on the analysis of clinical and laboratory findings in 345 DIC patients collected by the Research Committee on DIC in Japan. Bibl Haematol 1983; 49:265–275.

115. Bick RL. Disseminated intravascular coagulation. Objective laboratory diagnostic criteria and guidelines for management. Clin Lab Med 1994; 14.729–768.

116. Richards DS, Lutfi E, Mullins D et al. Prenatal diagnosis of fetal disseminated intravascular coagulation associated with umbilical cord arteriovenous malformation. Obstet Gynecol 1995;85(Pt 2):860–862.

117. Carr JM, McKinney M, McDonagh J. Diagnosis of disseminated intravascular coagulation. Role of D-dimer. Am J Clin Path 1989;91:280–287.

118. Koppert PW, Kuipers W, Hoegee-de Nobel B et al. A quantitative enzyme immunoassay for primary fibrinogenolysis products in plasma. Thromb Haemost 1987;57:25–28.

119. Pati HP, Saraya AK, Charan VD et al. Prognostic role of screening tests of haemostasis and underlying diseases in acute disseminated intra-vascular coagulation in adults. Clin Lab Haematol 1994;16:9–13.

120. Lombardi R, Mannucci PM, Seghatchian MJ et al. Alterations of factor VIII von Willebrand factor in clinical conditions associated with an increase in its plasma concentration. Br J Haematol 1981;49:61–68.

121. Colman RW, Robboy SJ, Minna JD. Disseminated intravascular coagulation (DIC): an approach. Am J Med 1972;52:679–689.

122. Colman RW, Robboy SJ, Minna JD. Disseminated intravascular coagulation: a reappraisal. Annu Rev Med 1979;30:359–374.

123. Neame PB, Kelton JG, Walker IR et al. Thrombocytopenia in septicemia: the role of disseminated intravascular coagulation. Blood 1980;56:88–92.

124. Kelton JG, Neame PB, Gauldie J et al. Elevated platelet-associated IgG in the thrombocytopenia of septicemia. N Engl J Med 1979;300:760–764.
125. Iberti TJ, Rand JH, Benjamin E et al. Thrombocytopenia following peritonitis in surgical patients. A prospective study. Ann Surg 1986;204:341–345.
126. Riedler GF, Straub PW, Frick PG. Thrombocytopenia in septicemia. A clinical study for the evaluation of its incidence and diagnostic value. Helv Med Acta 1971;36:23–38.
127. Bull BS, Kuhn IN. The production of schistocytes by fibrin strands (a scanning electron microscope study). Blood 1970;35:104–111.
128. Visudhiphan S, Piankijagum A, Sathayapraseart P et al. Erythrocyte fragmentation in disseminated intravascular coagulation and other diseases [Letter]. N Engl J Med 1983;309:113.
129. Bessman JD. Red blood cell fragmentation. Improved detection and identification of causes. Am J Clin Pathol 1988;90:268–273.
130. Cembrowski GS, Griffin JH, Mosher DF. Diagnostic efficacy of six plasma proteins in evaluating consumptive coagulopathies. Use of receiver operating characteristic curves to compare antithrombin III, plasminogen, alpha 2-plasmin inhibitor, fibronectin, prothrombin, and protein C. Arch Intern Med 1986;146:1997–2002.
131. Bick RL, Bick MD, Fekete LF. Antithrombin III patterns in disseminated intravascular coagulation. Am J Clin Pathol 1980;73:577–583.
132. Haselager EM, Vreeken J. Clinical significance of "circulating fibrin monomers." J Clin Pathol 1981;34:468–472.
133. Niewiarowski S, Gurewich V. Laboratory identification of intravascular coagulation. The serial dilution protamine sulfate test for the detection of fibrin monomer and fibrin degradation products. J Lab Clin Med 1971;77:665–676.
134. Mosesson MW, Colman RW, Sherry S. Chronic intravascular coagulation syndrome. N Engl J Med 1968;278:815–821.
135. Wada H, Wakita Y, Nakase T et al. Increased plasma-soluble fibrin monomer levels in patients with disseminated intravascular coagulation. Am J Hematol 1996;51:255–260.
136. Wieding JU, Hosius C. Determination of soluble fibrin: a comparison of four different methods. Thromb Res 1992;65:745–756.
137. Nossel HL, Wasser J, Kaplan KL et al. Sequence of fibrinogen proteolysis and platelet release after intrauterine infusion of hypertonic saline. J Clin Invest 1979;64:1371–1378.
138. Bauer KA, Rosenberg RD. Thrombin generation in acute promyelocytic leukemia. Blood 1984;64:791–796.
139. van der Poll T, Buller HR, ten Cate H et al. Activation of coagulation after administration of tumor necrosis factor to normal subjects. N Engl J Med 1990;322:1622–1627.
140. Asakura H, Shiratori Y, Jokaji H et al. Changes in plasma levels of prothrombin fragment F 1 + 2 in cases of disseminated intravascular coagulation. Acta Haematol 1993;89:22–25.
141. Harpel PC. Alpha2-plasmin inhibitor and alpha2-macroglobulin-plasmin complexes in plasma. Quantitation by an enzyme-linked differential antibody immunosorbent assay. J Clin Invest 1981;68:46–55.
142. Takahashi H, Tatewaki W, Wada K et al. Thrombin vs. plasmin generation in disseminated intravascular coagulation associated with various underlying disorders. Am J Hematol 1990;33:90–95.
143. Hoek JA, Sturk A, ten Cate JW et al. Laboratory and clinical evaluation of an assay of thrombin-antithrombin III complexes in plasma. Clin Chem 1988;34:2058–2062.
144. Weitz JI, Koehn JA, Canfield RE et al. Development of a radioimmunoassay for the fibrinogen-derived peptide B beta 1-42. Blood 1986;67:1014–1022.
145. Aoki N, Yamanaka T. The alpha2-plasmin inhibitor levels in liver diseases. Clin Chim Acta 1978;84:99–105.
146. vanDeWater L, Carr JM, Aronson D et al. Analysis of elevated fibrin(ogen) degradation product levels in patients with liver disease. Blood 1986;67:1468–1473.
147. Carr JM. Disseminated intravascular coagulation in cirrhosis. Hepatology 1989;10:103–110.
148. Alperin JB. Coagulopathy caused by vitamin K deficiency in critically ill, hospitalized patients. JAMA 1987;258:1916–1919.
149. Mant MJ, Hirsh J, Pineo GF et al. Prolonged prothrombin time and partial thromboplastin time in disseminated intravascular coagulation not due to deficiency of factors V and VIII. Br J Haematol 1973;24:725–734.
150. Mammen EF, Koets MH, Washington BC et al. Hemostasis changes during cardiopulmonary bypass surgery. Semin Thromb Hemost 1985;11:281–292.
151. Hewson JR, Neame PB, Kumar N et al. Coagulopathy related to dilution and hypotension during massive transfusion. Crit Care Med 1985;13:387–391.
152. Jaffe EA, Nachman RL, Merskey C. Thrombotic thrombocytopenic purpura–coagulation parameters in twelve patients. Blood 1973;42:499–507.
153. Takahashi H, Tatewaki W, Wada K et al. Thrombin generation in patients with thrombotic thrombocytopenic purpura. Am J Hematol 1989;32:255–257.
154. Devine DV, Kinney TR, Thomas PF et al. Fragment D-dimer levels: an objective marker of vaso-occlusive crisis and other complications of sickle cell disease. Blood 1986;68:317–319.

155. Lane DA, Ireland H, Knight I et al. The significance of fibrinogen derivatives in plasma in human renal failure. Br J Haematol 1984;56:251–260.
156. Gries E, Kopp J, Thomae U et al. Relation of intraperitoneal and intravascular coagulation and fibrinolysis related antigens in peritoneal dialysis. Thromb Haemost 1990;63:356–360.
157. Rutstein JE, Holahan JR, Lyons RM et al. Rheumatoid factor interference with the latex agglutination test for fibrin degradation products. J Lab Clin Med 1978;92:529–535.
158. Hammouda W, Moroz LA. False-positive reaction for fibrin degradation products due to a monoclonal (IgM lambda) cryoglobulin with warm-reactive antibody activity for rabbit IgG. Am J Med 1987;82:1263–1268.
159. Connaghan DG, Francis CW, Ryan DH et al. Prevalence and clinical implications of heparin-associated false positive tests for serum fibrin(ogen) degradation products. Am J Clin Pathol 1986;86:304–310.
160. Bajaj SP, Rapaport SI, Barclay S et al. Acquired hypoprothrombinemia due to non-neutralizing antibodies to prothrombin: mechanism and management. Blood 1985;65:1538–1543.
161. Alarcon-Segovia D. Pathogenetic potential of antiphospholipid antibodies. J Rheumatol 1988;15:890–893.
162. Kreger BE, Craven DE, McCabe WR. Gram-negative bacteremia. IV. Reevaluation of clinical features and treatment in 612 patients. Am J Med 1980;68:344–355.
163. Bone RC. Modulators of coagulation. A critical appraisal of their role in sepsis. Arch Intern Med 1992;152:1381–1389.
164. Zarrabi MH, Rosner F. Serious infections in adults following splenectomy for trauma. Arch Intern Med 1984;144:1421–1424.
165. Rao AK, Schapira M, Clements ML et al. A prospective study of platelets and plasma proteolytic systems during the early stages of Rocky Mountain spotted fever. N Engl J Med 1988;318:1021–1028.
166. Cosgriff TM. Viruses and hemostasis. Rev Infect Dis 1989;11:Suppl 4:S672–S688.
167. Zaki SR, Greer PW, Coffield LM et al. Hantavirus pulmonary syndrome. Pathogenesis of an emerging infectious disease. Am J Pathol 1995;146:552–579.
168. Laursen B, Faber V, Brock A et al. Disseminated intravascular coagulation, antithrombin III, and complement in meningococcal infections. Acta Med Scand 1981;209:221–227.
169. Pralong G, Calandra T, Glauser MP et al. Plasminogen activator inhibitor 1: a new prognostic marker in septic shock. Thromb Haemost 1989;61:459–462.
170. Rickles FR, Edwards RL, Barb C et al. Abnormalities of blood coagulation in patients with cancer. Fibrinopeptide A generation and tumor growth. Cancer 1983;51:301–307.
171. Brown LF, Van de Water L, Harvey VS et al. Fibrinogen influx and accumulation of crosslinked fibrin in healing wounds and in tumor stroma. Am J Pathol 1988;130:455–465.
172. Brown LF, Dvorak AM, Dvorak HF. Leaky vessels, fibrin deposition, and fibrosis: a sequence of events common to solid tumors and to many other types of disease. Am Rev Respir Dis 1989;140:1104–1107.
173. Mombelli G, Roux A, Haeberli A et al. Comparison of 125I-fibrinogen kinetics and fibrinopeptide A in patients with disseminated neoplasias. Blood 1982;60:381–388.
174. Colman RW, Rubin RN. Disseminated intravascular coagulation due to malignancy. Semin Oncol 1990;17:172–186.
175. Sun NC, Bowie EJ, Kazmier FJ et al. Jr. Blood coagulation studies in patients with cancer. Mayo Clin Proc 1974;49:636–641.
176. Mertens BF, Greene LF, Bowie EJ et al. Fibrinolytic split products (FSP) and ethanol gelation test in preoperative evaluation of patients with prostatic disease. Mayo Clin Proc 1974;49:642–646.
177. Straub PW, Riedler G, Frick PG. Hypofibrinogenaemia in metastatic carcinoma of the prostate: suppression of systemic fibrinolysis by heparin. J Clin Pathol 1967;20:152–157.
178. Schwartzman RJ, Hill JB. Neurologic complications of disseminated intravascular coagulation. Neurology 1982;32:791–797.
179. Antman KH, Skarin AT, Mayer RJ et al. Microangiopathic hemolytic anemia and cancer: a review. Medicine 1979;58:377–384.
180. Costantini V, Zacharski LR. Fibrin and cancer. Thromb Haemost 1993;69:406–414.
181. Dvorak HF, Quay SC, Orenstein NS et al. Tumor shedding and coagulation. Science 1981;212:923–924.
182. Cajot JF, Kruithof EK, Schleuning WD et al. Plasminogen activators, plasminogen activator inhibitors and procoagulant analyzed in twenty human tumor cell lines. Int J Cancer 1986;38:719–727.
183. Gordon SG, Cross BA. A factor X-activating cysteine protease from malignant tissue. J Clin Invest 1981;67:1665–1671.
184. Clauss M, Murray JC, Vianna M et al. A polypeptide factor produced by fibrosarcoma cells that induces endothelial tissue factor and enhances the procoagulant response to tumor necrosis factor/cachectin. J Biol Chem 1990;265:7078–7083.
185. Clauss M, Gerlach M, Gerlach H et al. Vascular permeability factor: a tumor-derived polypeptide that induces endothelial cell and monocyte procoagulant activity, and promotes monocyte migration. J Exp Med 1990;172:1535–1545.

186. Nand S, Fisher SG, Salgia R et al. Hemostatic abnormalities in untreated cancer: incidence and correlation with thrombotic and hemorrhagic complications. J Clin Oncol 1987;5:1998–2003.

187. Gurewich V, Lipinski B. Case report: low-dose intravenous heparin in the treatment of disseminated intravascular coagulation. Am J Med Sci 1977; 274:83–86.

188. Edwards RL, Rickles FR, Moritz TE et al. Abnormalities of blood coagulation tests in patients with cancer. Am J Clin Pathol 1987;88:596–602.

189. Stone MS, Rosen T. Acral purpura: an unusual sign of coumarin necrosis. J Am Acad Dermatol 1986;14:(Pt 1):797–802.

190. Bell WR, Starksen NF, Tong S et al. Trousseau's syndrome. Devastating coagulopathy in the absence of heparin. Am J Med 1985;79:423–430.

191. Myers TJ, Rickles FR, Barb C et al. Fibrinopeptide A in acute leukemia: relationship of activation of blood coagulation to disease activity. Blood 1981;57:518–525.

192. Sarris AH, Kempin S, Berman E et al. High incidence of disseminated intravascular coagulation during remission induction of adult patients with acute lymphoblastic leukemia. Blood 1992;79:1305–1310.

193. Andoh K, Kubota T, Takada M et al. Tissue factor activity in leukemia cells. Special reference to disseminated intravascular coagulation. Cancer 1987;59:748–754.

194. Hair GA, Padula S, Zeff R et al. Tissue factor expression in human leukemic cells. Leuk Res 1996;20:1–11.

195. Donati MB, Falanga A, Consonni R et al. Cancer procoagulant in acute non lymphoid leukemia: relationship of enzyme detection to disease activity. Thromb Haemost 1990;64:11–16.

196. Tapiovaara H, Alitalo R, Stephens R et al. Abundant urokinase activity on the surface of mononuclear cells from blood and bone marrow of acute leukemia patients. Blood 1993;82:914–919.

197. Wilson EL, Jacobs P, Dowdle EB. Secretion of plasminogen activators by human myeloid leukemic cells: modulation and therapeutic correlations. Hamatol Bluttransfus 1983;28:78–80.

198. Cozzolino F, Torcia M, Miliani A et al. Potential role of interleukin-1 as the trigger for diffuse intravascular coagulation in acute nonlymphoblastic leukemia. Am J Med 1988;84:240–250.

199. Rodeghiero F, Mannucci PM, Vigano S et al. Liver dysfunction rather than intravascular coagulation as the main cause of low protein C and antithrombin III in acute leukemia. Blood 1984;63:965–969.

200. Rossle A, Ostermann H. What's new in the causes of hemorrhage in acute myelogenous leukemia? Pathol Res Prac 1990;186:415–420.

201. Needleman SW, Stein MN, Hoak JC. Pulmonary embolism in patients with acute leukemia and severe thrombocytopenia. West J Med 1981;135: 9–13.

202. Riccio JA, Colley AT, Cera PJ. Hepatic vein thrombosis (Budd-Chiari syndrome) in the microgranular variant of acute promyelocytic leukemia. Am J Clin Path 1989;92:366–371.

203. Sarris A, Cortes J, Kantarjian H et al. Disseminated intravascular coagulation in adult acute lymphoblastic leukemia: frequent complications with fibrinogen levels less than 100 mg/dl. Leuk Lymphoma 1996;21:85–92.

204. Sultan C, Heilmann-Gouault M, Tulliez M. Relationship between blast-cell morphology and occurrence of a syndrome of disseminated intravascular coagulation. Br J Haematol 1973;24:255–259.

205. Tallman MS, Kwaan HC. Reassessing the hemostatic disorder associated with acute promyelocytic leukemia. Blood 1992;79:543–553.

206. Gralnick HR, Abrell E. Studies of the procoagulant and fibrinolytic activity of promyelocytes in acute promyelocytic leukaemia. Br J Haematol 1973; 24:89–99.

207. Wijermans PW, Rebel VI, Ossenkoppele GJ et al. Combined procoagulant activity and proteolytic activity of acute promyelocytic leukemic cells: reversal of the bleeding disorder by cell differentiation. Blood 1989;73: 800–805.

208. Schwartz BS, Williams EC, Conlan MG et al. Epsilon-aminocaproic acid in the treatment of patients with acute promyelocytic leukemia and acquired alpha-2-plasmin inhibitor deficiency. Ann Intern Med 1986;105:873–877.

209. Sakata Y, Murakami T, Noro A, Mori K et al. The specific activity of plasminogen activator inhibitor-1 in disseminated intravascular coagulation with acute promyelocytic leukemia. Blood 1991;77:1949–1957.

210. Fibach E, Treves A, Korenberg A et al. In vitro generation of procoagulant activity by leukemic promyelocytes in response to cytotoxic drugs. Am J Hematol 1985;20:257–265.

211. Kantarjian HM, Keating MJ, Walters RS et al. Acute promyelocytic leukemia. M.D. Anderson Hospital experience. Am J Med 1986;80:789–797.

212. Rodeghiero F, Avvisati G, Castaman G et al. Early deaths and anti-hemorrhagic treatments in acute promyelocytic leukemia. A GIMEMA retrospective study in 268 consecutive patients. Blood 1990;75:2112–2117.

213. Goldberg MA, Ginsburg D, Mayer RJ et al. Is heparin administration necessary during induction chemotherapy for patients with acute promyelocytic leukemia? Blood 1987;69:187–191.

214. Gralnick HR, Bagley J, Abrell E. Heparin treatment for the hemorrhagic diathesis of acute promyelocytic leukemia. Am J Med 1972;52:167–174.

215. Collins AJ, Bloomfield CD, Peterson BA et al. Acute promyelocytic leukemia. Management of the coagulopathy during daunorubicin-prednisone remission induction. Arch Intern Med 1978;138:1677–1680.

216. Avvisati G, ten Cate JW, Buller HR et al. Tranexamic acid for control of haemorrhage in acute promyelocytic leukaemia. Lancet 1989;2:122–124.

217. Falanga A, Iacoviello L, Evangelista V et al. Loss of blast cell procoagulant activity and improvement of hemostatic variables in patients with acute promyelocytic leukemia administered all-trans-retinoic acid. Blood 1995; 86:1072–1081.

218. Dombret H, Scrobohaci ML, Daniel MT et al. In vivo thrombin and plasmin activities in patients with acute promyelocytic leukemia (APL): effect of all-trans retinoic acid (ATRA) therapy. Leukemia 1995;9:19–24.

219. Escudier S, Kanrarjian H, Estey E. Thrombosis in patients with acute promyelocytic leukemia treated with and without all-trans retinoic acid. Leuk Lymphoma 1996;20:435–439.

220. Gibney EJ, Bouchier-Hayes D. Coagulopathy and abdominal aortic aneurysm. Eur J Vasc Surg 1990;4:557–562.

221. Diskin CJ, Weitberg AB. Minidose heparin therapy. Treatment of chronic intravascular coagulation syndrome. Arch Intern Med 1980;140:263–266.

222. Mulcare RJ, Royster TS, Phillips LL. Intravascular coagulation in surgical procedures on the abdominal aorta. Surg Gynecol Obstet 1976;143: 730–734.

223. Mulcare RJ, Royster TS, Weiss HJ et al. Disseminated intravascular coagulation as a complication of abdominal aortic aneurysm repair. Ann Surg 1974;180:343–349.

224. McIlraith DM, Mant MJ, Brien WF. Chronic consumptive coagulopathy due to intracardiac thrombus. Am J Med 1987;82:135–136.

225. Davies MJ, Murphy WG, Murie JA et al. Preoperative coagulopathy in ruptured abdominal aortic aneurysm predicts poor outcome. Br J Surg 1993;80:974–976.

226. Kasabach H, Merritt K. Capillary hemangioma with extensive purpura: report of a case. Am J Dis Child 1940;59:1063–1070.

227. Larsen EC, Zinkham WH, Eggleston JC et al. Kasabach-Merritt syndrome: therapeutic considerations. Pediatrics 1987;79:971–980.

228. Mewes T, Moldenhauer H, Pfeifer J et al. The Kasabach-Merritt syndrome: severe bleeding disorder caused by celiac arteriography—reversal by heparin treatment. Am J Gastroenterol 1989;84:965–971.

229. Warrell RP Jr. Kempin SJ. Treatment of severe coagulopathy in the Kasabach-Merritt syndrome with aminocaproic acid and cryoprecipitate. N Engl J Med 1985;313:309–312.

230. Bell AJ, Chisholm M, Hickton M. Reversal of coagulopathy in Kasabach-Merritt syndrome with tranexamic acid. Scand J Haematol 1986;37: 248–252.

231. Poon MC, Kloiber R, Birdsell DC. Epsilon-aminocaproic acid in the reversal of consumptive coagulopathy with platelet sequestration in a vascular malformation of Klippel-Trenaunay syndrome. Am J Med 1989;87: 211–213.

232. Ezekowitz RA, Mulliken JB, Folkman J. Interferon alfa-2a therapy for life-threatening hemangiomas of infancy. N Engl J Med 1992;326:1456–1463.

233. Bick RL. Hereditary hemorrhagic telangiectasia and disseminated intravascular coagulation: a new clinical syndrome. Ann N Y Acad Sci 1981; 370:851–854.

234. Coccheri S, Mannucci PM, Palareti G et al. Significance of plasma fibrinopeptide A and high molecular weight fibrinogen in patients with liver cirrhosis. Br J Haematol 1982;52:503–509.

235. Leebeek FW, Kluft C, Knot EA et al. A shift in balance between profibrinolytic and antifibrinolytic factors causes enhanced fibrinolysis in cirrhosis. Gastroenterology 1991;101:1382–1390.

236. Violi F, Ferro D, Basili S et al. Association between low-grade disseminated intravascular coagulation and endotoxemia in patients with liver cirrhosis. Gastroenterology 1995;109:531–539.

237. Kamisasa I, Hidai K, Sugiura M et al. Effects of splenectomy on blood coagulation and fibrinolysis in patients with liver cirrhosis: possible role of the spleen in haemostasis. Thromb Haemost 1980;42:1529–1535.

238. Rake MO, Flute PT, Shilkin KB et al. Early and intensive therapy of intravascular coagulation in acute liver failure. Lancet 1971;2:1215–1218.

239. Hillenbrand P, Parbhoo SP, Jedrychowski A et al. Significance of intravascular coagulation and fibrinolysis in acute hepatic failure. Scand J Gastroenterol Suppl 1973;19:133–134.

240. Takeda S, Takaki A, Ohsato K. Occurrence of disseminated intravascular coagulation (DIC) in obstructive jaundice and its relation to biliary tract infection. Surg Today 1977;7:82–89.

241. Semeraro N, Montemurro P, Chetta G et al. Increased procoagulant activity of peripheral blood monocytes in human and experimental obstructive jaundice. Gastroenterology 1989;96:892–898.

242. Cordova C, Musca A, Violi F et al. Improvement of some blood coagulation factors in cirrhotic patients treated with low doses of heparin. Scand J Haematol 1982;29:235–240.

243. Gazzard BG, Clark R, Borirakchanyavat V et al. A controlled trial of heparin therapy in the coagulation defect of paracetamol-induced hepatic necrosis. Gut 1974;15:89–93.

244. Stirling Y, Woolf L, North WR et al. Haemostasis in normal pregnancy. Thromb Haemost 1984;52:176–182.

245. Gerbasi FR, Bottoms S, Farag A et al. Increased intravascular coagulation associated with pregnancy. Obstet Gynecol 1990;75:385–389.

246. Bremme K, Ostlund E, Almqvist I et al. Enhanced thrombin generation

and fibrinolytic activity in normal pregnancy and the puerperium. Obstet Gynecol 1992;80:132–137.

247. Pritchard JA, Brekken AL. Clinical and laboratory studies on severe abruptio placentae. Am J Obstet Gynecol 1967;97:681–700.

248. Weiner CP. Disseminated intravascular coagulopathy associated with pregnancy. In: Clark SL, Cotton DB, Hankins GDV, Phelan JP, eds: Critical care obstetrics. Boston, Blackwell Scientific Publications; 1991:180–198.

249. White PF, Coe V, Dworsky WA et al. Disseminated intravascular coagulation following midtrimester abortions. Anesthesiology 1983;58:99–101.

250. Swingler GR, Bigrigg MA, Hewitt BG et al. Disseminated intravascular coagulation associated with group A streptococcal infection in pregnancy. Lancet 1988;1:1456–1457.

251. Pritchard J. Fetal death in utero. Obstet Gynecol 1959;14:573–580.

252. Hatch RL, Barke JI, Barke MW. Coagulopathy associated with dilatation and evacuation for intrauterine fetal death. Obstet Gynecol 1985;66:463–467.

253. Romero R, Duffy TP, Berkowitz RL et al. Prolongation of a preterm pregnancy complicated by death of a single twin in utero and disseminated intravascular coagulation. Effects of treatment with heparin. N Engl J Med 1984;310:772–774.

254. Lopez-Llera M, de la Luz Espinosa M, Diaz de Leon M et al. Abnormal coagulation and fibrinolysis in eclampsia. A clinical and laboratory correlation study. Am J Obstet Gynecol 1976;124:681–687.

255. Borok Z, Weitz J, Owen J et al. Fibrinogen proteolysis and platelet alpha-granule release in preeclampsia/eclampsia. Blood 1984;63:525–531.

256. Kaplan MM. Acute fatty liver of pregnancy. N Engl J Med 1985;313:367–370.

257. Liebman HA, McGehee WG, Patch MJ et al. Severe depression of antithrombin III associated with disseminated intravascular coagulation in women with fatty liver of pregnancy. Ann Intern Med 1983;98:330–333.

258. Weinstein L. Syndrome of hemolysis, elevated liver enzymes, and low platelet count: a severe consequence of hypertension in pregnancy. Am J Obstet Gynecol 1982;142:159–167.

259. Hayslett JP. Current concepts. Postpartum renal failure. N Engl J Med 1985;312:1556–1559.

260. Roberts JM, Taylor RN, Musci TJ et al. Preeclampsia: an endothelial cell disorder. Am J Obstet Gynecol 1989;161:1200–1204.

261. Sibai BM, Ramadan MK, Usta I et al. Maternal morbidity and mortality in 442 pregnancies with hemolysis, elevated liver enzymes, and low platelets (HELLP syndrome). Am J Obstet Gynecol 1993;169:1000–1006.

262. Pritchard JA, Cunningham FG, Mason RA. Coagulation changes in eclampsia: their frequency and pathogenesis. Am J Obstet Gynecol 1976;124:855–864.

263. Castro MA, Goodwin TM, Shaw KJ et al. Disseminated intravascular coagulation and antithrombin III depression in acute fatty liver of pregnancy. Am J Obstet Gynecol 1996;174:(Pt 1):211–216.

264. Brain M, Dacie J, Hourihane D. Microangiopathic haemolytic anaemia: the possible role of vascular lesions in pathogenesis. Br J Haematol 1962;8:358–374.

265. Kelton JG, Moore J, Santos A et al. The detection of a platelet-agglutinating factor in thrombotic thrombocytopenic purpura. Ann Intern Med 1984;101:589–593.

266. McKay D, Hardaway R, Wahle G et al. Alterations in blood coagulation mechanism after incompatible blood transfusion. Clinical and experimental observations. Am J Surg 1955;89:583–592.

267. Goldfinger D. Acute hemolytic transfusion reactions–a fresh look at pathogenesis and considerations regarding therapy. Transfusion 1977;17:85–98.

268. Capon SM, Goldfinger D. Acute hemolytic transfusion reaction, a paradigm of the systemic inflammatory response: new insights into pathophysiology and treatment [Review]. Transfusion 1995;35:513–520.

269. Butler J, Parker D, Pillai R et al. Systemic release of neutrophil elastase and tumour necrosis factor alpha following ABO incompatible blood transfusion. Br J Haematol 1991;79:525–526.

270. Balla G, Vercellotti GM, Muller-Eberhard U et al. Exposure of endothelial cells to free heme potentiates damage mediated by granulocytes and toxic oxygen species. Lab Invest 1991;64:648–655.

271. Ciavarella D, Reed RL, Counts RB et al. Clotting factor levels and the risk of diffuse microvascular bleeding in the massively transfused patient. Br J Haematol 1987;67:365–368.

272. Egan EL, Bowie EJ, Kazmier FJ et al. Effect of surgical operations on certain tests used to diagnose intravascular coagulation and fibrinolysis. Mayo Clin Proc 1974;49:658–664.

273. Dyke C, Sobel M. The management of coagulation problems in the surgical patient. Adv Surg 1991;24:229–257.

274. Friesen SR, Nelson RM. The occurrence of massive generalized wound bleeding during operation. With reference to the possible role of blood transfusions in its etiology. Am Surg 1951;17:609–622.

275. Bull BS, Bull MH. The salvaged blood syndrome: a sequel to mechano-chemical activation of platelets and leukocytes? Blood Cells 1990;16:5–20.

276. Tawes RL, Jr., Duvall TB. Is the "salvaged-cell syndrome" myth or reality? Am J Surg 1996;172:172–174.

277. Kucuk O, Kwaan HC, Frederickson J et al. Increased fibrinolytic activity

278. Boisclair MD, Lane DA, Philippou H et al. Mechanisms of thrombin generation during surgery and cardiopulmonary bypass. Blood 1993;82:3350–3357.

279. Al-Mondhiry H, Pierce WS, Richenbacher W et al. Hemostatic abnormalities associated with prolonged ventricular assist pumping: analysis of 24 patients. Am J Cardiol 1984;53:1344–1348.

280. Woodman RC, Harker LA. Bleeding complications associated with cardiopulmonary bypass. Blood 1990;76:1680–1697.

281. Bachmann F, McKenna R, Cole ER et al. The hemostatic mechanism after open-heart surgery. I. Studies on plasma coagulation factors and fibrinolysis in 512 patients after extracorporeal circulation. J Thorac Cardiovasc Surg 1975;70:76–85.

282. DelRossi AJ, Cernaianu AC, Botros S Prophylactic treatment of postperfusion bleeding using EACA. Chest 1989;96:27–30.

283. Rocha E, Hidalgo F, Llorens R et al. Randomized study of aprotinin and DDAVP to reduce postoperative bleeding after cardiopulmonary bypass surgery. Circulation 1994;90:921–927.

284. Porte RJ, Knot EA, Bontempo FA. Hemostasis in liver transplantation. Gastroenterology 1989;97:488–501.

285. Dzik WH, Arkin CF, Jenkins RL et al. Fibrinolysis during liver transplantation in humans: role of tissue-type plasminogen activator. Blood 1988;71:1090–1095.

286. Dinbar A, Rangel DM, Fonkalsrud EW. Effects of hepatic ischemia in coagulation in primates. Application to liver transplantation. Surgery 1970;68:269–275.

287. Miyata T, Yokoyama I, Todo S et al. Endotoxaemia, pulmonary complications, and thrombocytopenia in liver transplantation. Lancet 1989;2:189–191.

288. Himmelreich G, Jochum M, Bechstein WO et al. Mediators of leukocyte activation play a role in disseminated intravascular coagulation during orthotopic liver transplantation. Transplantation 1994;57:354–358.

289. Estol CJ, Pessin MS, Martinez AJ. Cerebrovascular complications after orthotopic liver transplantation: a clinicopathologic study. Neurology 1991;41:815–819.

290. Gosseye S, van Obbergh L, Weynand B et al. Platelet aggregates in small lung vessels and death during liver transplantation. Lancet 1991;338:532–534.

291. Bakker CM, Metselaar HJ, Gomes MJ et al. Intravascular coagulation in liver transplantation—is it present or not? A comparison between orthotopic and heterotopic liver transplantation. Thromb Haemost 1993;69:25–28.

292. Harmon DC, Demirjian Z, Ellman L et al. Disseminated intravascular coagulation with the peritoneovenous shunt. Ann Intern Med 1979;90:774–776.

293. Ragni MV, Lewis JH, Spero JA. Ascites-induced LeVeen shunt coagulopathy. Ann Surg 1983;198:91–95.

294. Tempero MA, Davis RB, Reed E et al. Thrombocytopenia and laboratory evidence of disseminated intravascular coagulation after shunts for ascites in malignant disease. Cancer 1985;55:2718–2721.

295. Gleysteen JJ, Hussey CV, Heckman MG. The cause of coagulopathy after peritoneovenous shunt for malignant ascites. Arch Surg 1990;125:474–477.

296. Addonizio VP, Jr., Fisher CA, Strauss JF 3d et al. Preliminary characterization of the procoagulant material in human ascites. Surgery 1987;101:753–762.

297. LeVeen HH, Ip M, Ahmed N et al. Coagulopathy post peritoneovenous shunt. Ann Surg 1987;205:305–311.

298. Salem HH, Koutts J, Handley C et al. The aggregation of human platelets by ascitic fluid: a possible mechanism for disseminated intravascular coagulation complicating LeVeen shunts. Am J Hematol 1981;11:153–157.

299. Hoefs J, Barnes T, Halle P. Intraperitoneal coagulation in chronic liver disease ascites. Dig Dis Sci 1981;26:518–522.

300. Buller HR, ten Cate JW. Antithrombin III infusion in patients undergoing peritoneovenous shunt operation: failure in the prevention of disseminated intravascular coagulation. Thromb Haemost 1983;49:128–131.

301. Weiss HJ, Allan S, Davidson E et al. Afibrinogenemia in man following the bite of a rattlesnake (Crotalus adamanteus). Am J Med 1969;47:625–634.

302. Budzynski AZ, Pandya BV, Rubin RN et al. Fibrinogenolytic afibrinogenemia after envenomation by western diamondback rattlesnake (Crotalus atrox). Blood 1984;63:1–14.

303. Hawgood BJ. Physiological and pharmacological effects of rattlesnake venoms. In: Tu AT ed. Rattlesnake venoms: their actions and treatment. New York: Marcel Dekker, 1982:121–162.

304. Marsh N. Inventory of haemorrhagic factors from snake venoms. Registry of Exogenous Hemostatic Factors. Scientific and Standardization Committee of the International Society on thrombosis and hemostasis. Thromb Haemost 1994;71:793–797.

305. Teng CM, Chen YH, Ouyang CH. Effect of Russell's viper venom phospholipase A on blood coagulation and platelet aggregation. Semin Thromb Hemost 1985;11:367–372.

306. Teng CM, Huang TF. Inventory of exogenous inhibitors of platelet aggregation. For the Subcommittee on Nomenclature of Exogenous Hemostatic Factors of the Scientific and Standardization Committee of the Interna-

tional Society on thrombosis and hemostasis. Thromb Haemost 1991;65: 624–626.

307. Smith SV, Brinkhous KM. Inventory of exogenous platelet-aggregating agent derived from venoms. Thromb Haemost 1991;66:259–263.

308. Rosing J, Tans G. Inventory of exogenous prothrombin activators. For the Subcommittee on Nomenclature of Exogenous Hemostatic Factors of the Scientific and Standardization Committee of the International Society on thrombosis and hemostasis. Thromb Haemost 1991;65:627–630.

309. Stocker K. Inventory of exogenous hemostatic factors affecting the prothrombin activating pathways. For the Registry of Exogenous Hemostatic Factors of the Scientific and Standardization Committee of the International Society on thrombosis and hemostasis. Thromb Haemost 1994;71: 257–260.

310. Pirkle H, Stocker K. Thrombin-like enzymes from snake venoms: an inventory. For the Subcommittee on Nomenclature of Exogenous Hemostatic Factors of the Scientific and Standardization Committee of the International Society on thrombosis and hemostasis. Thromb Haemost 1991;65: 444–450.

311. Markland FS, Jr. Inventory of alpha- and beta-fibrinogenases from snake venoms. For the Subcommittee on Nomenclature of Exogenous Hemostatic Factors of the Scientific and Standardization Committee of the International Society on thrombosis and hemostasis. Thromb Haemost 1991; 65:438–443.

312. Ohsaka A. Hemorrhagic, necrotizing and edema-forming effects of snake venoms. In: Lee C, ed. Snake venoms. New York: Springer-Verlag, 1979: 480–546.

313. Simon TL, Grace TG. Envenomation coagulopathy in wounds from pit vipers. N Engl J Med 1981;305:443–447.

314. Kitchens CS, Van Mierop LH. Mechanism of defibrination in humans after envenomation by the Eastern diamondback rattlesnake. Am J Hematol 1983;14:345–353.

315. Glass TG. Management of the western diamondback rattlesnake bite. In Tu At, ed. Rattlesnake venoms: their actions and treatment. New York, Marcel Dekker; 1982:339–360.

316. White RR, 4th, Weber RA. Poisonous snakebite in central Texas. Possible indicators for antivenin treatment. Ann Surg 1991;213:466–471.

317. Schaeffer RC, Jr., Briston C, Chilton SM et al Disseminated intravascular coagulation following Echis carinatus venom in dogs: effects of a synthetic thrombin inhibitor. J Lab Clin Med 1986;107:488–497.

318. Tin Na Swe, Myint Lwin, Khin Ei Han et al. Heparin therapy in Russell's viper bite victims with disseminated intravascular coagulation: a controlled trial. Southeast Asian J Trop Med Public Health 1992;23:282–287.

319. Goodnight SH, Kenoyer G, Rapaport SI et al. Defibrination after brain-tissue destruction: A serious complication of head injury. N Engl J Med 1974;290:1043–1047.

320. Olson JD, Kaufman HH, Moake J et al. The incidence and significance of hemostatic abnormalities in patients with head injuries. Neurosurgery 1989;24:825–832.

321. Bartsch P, Haeberli A, Hauser K et al. Fibrinogenolysis in the absence of fibrin formation in severe hypobaric hypoxia. Aviat Space Environ Med 1988;59:428–432.

322. Better OS, Stein JH. Early management of shock and prophylaxis of acute renal failure in traumatic rhabdomyolysis. N Engl J Med 1990;322:825–829.

323. Beard ME, Hickton CM. Haemostasis in heat stroke. Br J Haematol 1982; 52:269–274.

324. el-Kassimi FA, Al-Mashhadani S, Abdullah AK et al. Adult respiratory distress syndrome and disseminated intravascular coagulation complicating heat stroke. Chest 1986;90:571–574.

325. Mahajan SL, Myers TJ, Baldini MG. Disseminated intravascular coagulation during rewarming following hypothermia. JAMA 1981;245: 2517–2518.

326. Fabian TC, Hoots AV, Stanford DS et al. Fat embolism syndrome: prospective evaluation in 92 fracture patients. Crit Care Med 1990;18:42–46.

327. Turpini R, Stefanini M. The nature and mechanism of the hemostatic breakdown in the course of experimental hemorrhagic shock. J Clin Invest 1959;38:53–65.

328. Attar S, Hanashiro P, Mansberger A et al. Intravascular coagulation–reality or myth? Surgery 1970;68:27–33.

329. Hewson JR, Prodger D, Roberts RS et al. Prolonged hemorrhagic shock does not impair regeneration of plasma coagulant masses in the rabbit. Crit Care Med 1991;19:253–259.

330. Garcia-Barreno P, Balibrea JL, Aparicio P. Blood coagulation changes in shock. Surg Gynecol Obstet 1978;147:6–12.

331. Rush BF, Jr., Sori AJ, Murphy TF et al. Endotoxemia and bacteremia during hemorrhagic shock. The link between trauma and sepsis? Ann Surg 1988; 207:549–554.

332. Fowler AA, Hamman RF, Good JT et al. Adult respiratory distress syndrome: risk with common predispositions. Ann Intern Med 1983;98:(Pt 1): 593–597.

333. Bone RC, Francis PB, Pierce AK. Intravascular coagulation associated with the adult respiratory distress syndrome. Am J Med 1976;61:585–589.

334. Groniowski J. Thrombotic arteriolar lesions in lungs of newborn. Arch Pathol 1963;75:144–155.

335. Schmidt B, Vegh P, Weitz J et al. Thrombin/antithrombin III complex formation in the neonatal respiratory distress syndrome. Am Rev Respir Dis 1992;145:Pt 1):767–770.

336. Bell RC, Coalson JJ, Smith JD Johanson WG, Jr. Multiple organ system failure and infection in adult respiratory distress syndrome. Ann Intern Med 1983;99:293–298.

337. Rinaldo JE, Rogers RM. Adult respiratory-distress syndrome: changing concepts of lung injury and repair. N Engl J Med 1982;306:900–909.

338. Hasegawa N, Husari AW, Hart WT Role of the coagulation system in ARDS. Chest 1994;105:268–277.

339. Saldeen T. Trends in microvascular research. The microembolism syndrome. Microvasc Res 1976;11:227–259.

340. Malik AB, van der Zee H. Thrombin induced pulmonary insufficiency. Thromb Res 1977;11:497–506.

341. Hoffmann H, Siebeck M Spannagl M et al. Effect of recombinant hirudin, a specific inhibitor of thrombin, on endotoxin-induced intravascular coagulation and acute lung injury in pigs. Am Rev Respir Dis 1990;142:782–788.

342. Garber BG, Hebert PC, Yelle JD, Hodder RV McGowan J. Adult respiratory distress syndrome: a systematic overview of incidence and risk factors. Crit Care Med 1996;24:687–695.

343. Branson HE, Katz J, Marble R Griffin JH. Inherited protein C deficiency and coumarin-responsive chronic relapsing purpura fulminans in a newborn infant. Lancet 1983;2:1165–1168.

344. Cosgriff TM, Bishop DT, Hershgold EJ et al. Familial antithrombin III deficiency: its natural history, genetics, diagnosis and treatment. Medicine 1983;62:209–220.

345. Okajima K, Ueyama H, Hashimoto Y et al. Homozygous variant of antithrombin III that lacks affinity for heparin, AT III Kumamoto. Thromb Haemost 1989;61:20–24.

346. Saito H. Alpha 2-plasmin inhibitor and its deficiency states. J Lab Clin Med 1988;112:671–678.

347. Carvalho AC, Lees RS, Vaillancourt RA et al. Intravascular coagulation in hyperlipidemia. Thromb Res 1976;8:843–857.

348. Owen J, Friedman KD, Grossman BA et al. Thrombolytic therapy with tissue plasminogen activator or streptokinase induces transient thrombin activity. Blood 1988;72:616–620.

349. Collen D, Verstraete M. alpha 2-Antiplasmin consumption and fibrinogen breakdown during thrombolytic therapy. Thromb Res 1979;14:631–639.

350. Sane DC, Califf RM, Topol EJ et al. Bleeding during thrombolytic therapy for acute myocardial infarction: mechanisms and management. Ann Intern Med 1989;111:1010–1022.

351. Conlan MG, Hoots WK. Disseminated intravascular coagulation and hemorrhage in hemophilia B following elective surgery. Am J Hematol 1990; 35:203–207.

352. Hadley T, Djulbegovic B. Disseminated intravascular coagulation after factor IX complex resolved using purified factor IX concentrate. Ann Intern Med 1991;115:621–622.

353. Bolton-Maggs PH, Colvin BT, Satchi BT et al. Thrombogenic potential of factor XI concentrate. Lancet 1994;344:748–749.

354. Santagostino E, Mannucci PM, Gringeri A et al. Markers of hypercoagulability in patients with hemophilia B given repeated, large doses of factor IX concentrates during and after surgery. Thromb Haemost 1994;71:737–740.

355. Bell WR, Royall RM. Heparin-associated thrombocytopenia: a comparison of three heparin preparations. N Engl J Med 1980;303:902–907.

356. Zalcberg JR, McGrath K, Dauer R et al. Heparin-induced thrombocytopenia with associated disseminated intravascular coagulation. Br J Haematol 1983;54:655–657.

357. Cines DB, Tomaski A, Tannenbaum S. Immune endothelial-cell injury in heparin-associated thrombocytopenia. N Engl J Med 1987;316:581–589.

358. Francis RB, Jr., McGehee WG. Defibrination during warfarin therapy in a man with protein C deficiency. Thromb Haemost 1985;53:249–251.

359. Comp PC, Elrod JP, Karzenski S. Warfarin-induced skin necrosis. Semin Thromb Hemost 1990;16:293–298.

360. Haber LM, Hawkins EP, Seilheimer DK et al. Fat overload syndrome. An autopsy study with evaluation of the coagulopathy. Am J Clin Pathol 1988; 90:223–227.

361. Goldenberg M, Zolti M, Seidman DS et al. Transient blood oxygen desaturation, hypercapnia, and coagulopathy after operative hysteroscopy with glycine used as the distending medium. Am J Obstet Gynecol 1994;170: (Pt 1)25–29.

362. Brandt RR, Dunn WF, Ory SJ. Dextran 70 embolization. Another cause of pulmonary hemorrhage, coagulopathy, and rhabdomyolysis. Chest 1993; 104:631–633.

363. Lowe FC, Somers WJ. The use of ketoconazole in the emergency management of disseminated intravascular coagulation due to metastatic prostatic cancer. Microvasc Res 1987;137:1000–1002.

364. Levin M, Hjelm M, Kay JD et al. Haemorrhagic shock and encephalopathy: a new syndrome with a high mortality in young children. Lancet 1983;2: 64–67.

365. Weibley RE, Pimentel B, Ackerman NB. Hemorrhagic shock and encephalopathy syndrome of infants and children. Crit Care Med 1989;17:335–338.

366. Fisher RF, Goodpasture HC, Peterie JD et al. Toxic shock syndrome in menstruating women. Ann Intern Med 1981;94:156–163.

367. Burns JC, Glode MP, Clarke SH et al. Coagulopathy and platelet activation in Kawasaki syndrome: identification of patients at high risk for development of coronary artery aneurysms. J Pediatr 1984;105:206–211.

368. Glass RD. Purpura gangrenosa: report of a case, with a discussion of the Shwartzman phenomenon. Med J Austr 1962;2:300–302.

369. Lee M, Kim BK, Kim S et al. Coagulopathy in hemorrhagic fever with renal syndrome (Korean hemorrhagic fever). Rev Infect Dis 1989;11(Suppl 4):S877–S883.

370. Meyer K, Williams EC. Fibrinolysis and acquired alpha-2 plasmin inhibitor deficiency in amyloidosis. Am J Med 1985;79:394–396.

371. NIH consensus conference. Fresh-frozen plasma. Indications and risks. JAMA 1985;253:551–553.

372. Hoffman M, Jenner P. Variability in the fibrinogen and von Willebrand factor content of cryoprecipitate. Implications for reducing donor exposure. Am J Clin Pathol 1990;93:694–697.

373. Nunez H, Drohan WN. Purification of antithrombin III (human). Semin Hematol 1991;28:24–30.

374. Mammen EF, Miyakawa T, Phillips TF et al. Human antithrombin concentrates and experimental disseminated intravascular coagulation. Semin Thromb Hemost 1985;11:373–383.

375. Lechner K, Kyrle PA. Antithrombin III concentrates–are they clinically useful? Thromb Haemost 1995;73:340–348.

376. Menache D, Grossman BJ, Jackson CM. Antithrombin III: physiology, deficiency, and replacement therapy. Transfusion 1992;32:580–588.

377. Conard J, Bauer KA, Gruber A et al. Normalization of markers of coagulation activation with a purified protein C concentrate in adults with homozygous protein C deficiency. Blood 1993;82:1159–1164.

378. Gerson WT, Dickerman JD, Bovill EG et al. Severe acquired protein C deficiency in purpura fulminans associated with disseminated intravascular coagulation: treatment with protein C concentrate. Pediatrics 1993;91:418–422.

379. Rivard GE, David M, Farrell C et al. Treatment of purpura fulminans in meningococcemia with protein C concentrate. J Pediatr 1995;126:646–652.

380. Mant MJ, Connolly T, Gordon PA et al. Severe thrombocytopenia probably due to acute folic acid deficiency. Crit Care Med 1979;7:297–300.

381. Scharfman WB, Tillotson JR, Taft EG et al. Plasmapheresis for meningococcemia with disseminated intravascular coagulation. N Engl J Med 1979;300:1277–1278.

382. Churchwell KB, McManus ML, Kent P et al. Intensive blood and plasma exchange for treatment of coagulopathy in meningococcemia. J Clin Apheresis 1995;10:171–177.

383. Stegmayr BG. Plasma exchange in patients with septic shock including acute renal failure. Blood Purif 1996;14:102–108.

384. van Deuren M, Santman FW, van Dalen R et al. Plasma and whole blood exchange in meningococcal sepsis. Clin Infect Dis 1992;15:424–430.

385. Feinstein DI. Diagnosis and management of disseminated intravascular coagulation: the role of heparin therapy. Blood 1982;60:284–287.

386. Rubin RN, Colman RW. Disseminated intravascular coagulation. Approach to treatment. Drugs 1992;44:963–971.

387. Hirsh J. Heparin. N Engl J Med 1991;324:1565–1574.

388. Lo SS, Hitzig WH, Frick PG. Clinical experience with anticoagulant therapy in the management of disseminated intravascular coagulation in children. Acta Haematol 1971;45:1–16.

389. Feinstein DI. Treatment of disseminated intravascular coagulation. Semin Thromb Hemost 1988;14:351–362.

390. Corrigan JJ, Jr. Heparin therapy in bacterial septicemia. J Pediatr 1977;91:695–700.

391. Hoyle CF, Swirsky DM, Freedman L et al. Beneficial effect of heparin in the management of patients with APL. Br J Haematol 1988;68:283–289.

392. Sakuragawa N, Hasegawa H, Maki M et al. Clinical evaluation of low-molecular-weight heparin (FR-860) on disseminated intravascular coagulation (DIC)—a multicenter co-operative double-blind trial in comparison with heparin. Thromb Res 1993;72:475–500.

393. Saito M, Asakura H, Jokaji H et al. Recombinant hirudin for the treatment of disseminated intravascular coagulation in patients with haematological malignancy. Blood Coagul Fibrinolysis 1995;6:60–64.

394. Ratnoff OD. Epsilon aminocaproic acid—dangerous weapon. N Engl J Med 1969;280:1124–1125.

395. Yamamoto K, Loskutoff DJ. Fibrin deposition in tissues from endotoxin-treated mice correlates with decreases in the expression of urokinase-type but not tissue-type plasminogen activator. J Clin Invest 1996;97:2440–2451.

396. Peltz SW, Hardt TA, Mangel WF. Positive regulation of activation of plasminogen by urokinase: differences in Km for (glutamic acid)-plasminogen and lysine-plasminogen and effect of certain alpha, omega-amino acids. Biochemistry 1982;21:2798–2804.

397. Urano T, Sator de Serrano V, Gaffney PJ et al. Effectors of the activation of human [Glu1]plasminogen by human tissue plasminogen activator. Biochemistry 1988;27:6522–6528.

398. Minn SK, Mandel EE. Experimental disseminated intravascular coagulation effect of heparin and epsilon-aminocaproic acid on tests of hemostatic function. Thromb Res 1975;6:235–246.

399. Lo SK, Ryan TJ, Gilboa N et al. Role of catalytic and lysine-binding sites in plasmin-induced neutrophil adherence to endothelium. J Clin Invest 1989;84:793–801.

400. Malik AB, Horgan MJ. Mechanisms of thrombin-induced lung vascular injury and edema. Am Rev Respir Dis 1987;136:467–470.

401. Boulton FE, Letsky E. Obstetric haemorrhage: causes and management. Clinics in Haematology 1985;14:683–728.

402. Keane TJ, Gorman AM, O'Connell LG et al. epsilon-Amino-caproic acid in the management of acute promyelocytic leukaemia. Acta Haematol 1976;56:202–204.

403. Cooper DL, Sandler AB, Wilson LD et al. Disseminated intravascular coagulation and excessive fibrinolysis in a patient with metastatic prostate cancer. Response to epsilon-aminocaproic acid. Cancer 1992;70:656–658.

404. Verstraete M. Clinical application of inhibitors of fibrinolysis. Drugs 1985;29:236–261.

405. Neuhaus P, Bechstein WO, Lefebre B et al. Effect of aprotinin on intraoperative bleeding and fibrinolysis in liver transplantation. Lancet 1989;2:924–925.

406. Milne AA, Drummond GB, Paterson DA et al. Disseminated intravascular coagulation after aortic aneurysm repair, intraoperative salvage autotransfusion, and aprotinin. Lancet 1994;344:470–471.

407. Saffitz JE, Stahl DJ, Sundt TM et al. Disseminated intravascular coagulation after administration of aprotinin in combination with deep hypothermic circulatory arrest. Am J Cardiol 1993;72:1080–1082.

408. Umeki S, Adachi M, Watanabe M et al. Gabexate as a therapy for disseminated intravascular coagulation. Arch Intern Med 1988;148:1409–1412.

409. Wada H, Wakita Y, Nakase T et al. Outcome of disseminated intravascular coagulation in relation to the score when treatment was begun. Mie DIC Study Group. Thromb Haemost 1995;74:848–852.

# CHAPTER 45

# COAGULOPATHY OF LIVER FAILURE AND VITAMIN K DEFICIENCY

## Jose Martinez and Carl Barsigian

Laboratory tests of individuals with liver disease frequently show abnormalities of the hemostatic system, and in some, these biochemical alterations manifest clinically as a hemorrhagic tendency (1–5). The pathophysiologic mechanisms underlying the coagulopathy of liver failure and vitamin K deficiency are multifactorial. The hemostatic alterations can be attributed to the liver being the principal organ responsible for the biosynthesis of most proteins in the coagulation and fibrinolytic systems as well as of several blood coagulation and fibrinolysis inhibitors. Moreover, hemostatic abnormalities resulting from impaired liver synthesis of coagulation factors can be compounded by increased consumption of specific blood coagulation proteins. These mechanisms can produce greater changes in certain factors, thus leading to gross imbalances in the coagulation and fibrinolytic systems. Such imbalances can have profound clinical significance.

In addition to qualitative and quantitative abnormalities of the protein blood coagulation factors synthesized by the liver, individuals with liver disease may have diminished platelet counts and defects in platelet function. Such platelet abnormalities frequently contribute to the associated coagulopathy, and they usually can be attributed to pooling in the spleen or to intrinsic defects, respectively. The combination of clotting factor deficiencies and platelet abnormalities is important in bleeding episodes, which may be either spontaneous or associated with various diagnostic and surgical procedures.

## LIVER FAILURE

### ANATOMIC CAUSES OF BLEEDING

Anatomic causes of bleeding include esophageal varices and portal hypertensive gastropathy as well as congestive splenomegaly.

### Esophageal Varices and Portal Hypertensive Gastropathy

In individuals with liver disease, bleeding episodes, which may be severe enough to cause serious complications and even death, frequently are precipitated by anatomic and hemodynamic factors. Bleeding from the upper gastrointestinal tract occurs in 26% of individuals with portal hypertension and esophageal varices (6). Variceal bleeding usually is associated with the size of the varices, but other factors, such as liver dysfunction, mucosal color changes indicating submucosal hemorrhage, plasma volume expansion, and development of ascites, also can be predictive of which individuals are prone to hemorrhage (6–8).

Some investigators have found a correlation between variceal bleeding and a hypercoagulable state or intravascular coagulation (9, 10), but others have failed to confirm these observations (11). Because the biosynthetic capacity of the liver often is preserved in portal hypertension, individuals with esophageal varices occasionally do not exhibit a significantly altered coagulation system (except as noted later, under "Congestive Splenomegaly.")

Dilation of the hemorrhoidal veins is a common manifestation of portal hypertension, but severe hemorrhage from this site is rare. When it does occur, however, it is difficult to control. In contrast to hemorrhage from esophageal varices or the gastric mucosa, which can occur without pronounced alterations in the coagulation factors (12–15), hemorrhagic manifestations involving the skin or mucosa, such as ecchymosis, hematomas, or epistaxis, and bleeding through puncture sites are associated with severe alterations in blood coagulation and fibrinolysis (11).

Primary liver disease is the most frequent cause of portal hypertension and variceal bleeding. Occasionally, however, portal hypertension results from a myeloproliferative syndrome that can cause hepatic vein thrombosis (i.e., Budd-Chiari syndrome) or portal vein or splenic vein thrombosis, or both, which may result from activation of the coagulation system (16–19). That the hypercatabolism of prothrombin and fibrinogen seen in these individuals returns to normal following therapeutic reduction of platelet counts supports this concept (20).

Other disorders of bone marrow stem cells, such as paroxysmal nocturnal hemoglobinuria, also are associated with hepatic, portal, splenic, or portal and splenic vein thrombosis (21, 22). Identification of these disorders is important, because therapy should aim to correct the pathogenic mechanisms involved in the primary disorder (16). Thrombosis of the hepatic or portal veins also occurs with the use of oral contraceptives (23, 24) and can be associated with other disorders, such as inflammatory bowel disease.

## Congestive Splenomegaly

Splenomegaly resulting from liver cirrhosis and portal hypertension often is accompanied by thrombocytopenia, which can be mild or moderate, with platelet counts as low as 40,000 cells/mm$^3$ (25–27). Normally, the spleen contains approximately 30% of the extramedullary pool of platelets (26, 28), and it can release large numbers of platelets into the circulation when stimulated by epinephrine (28). The most important parameter relating to the degree of thrombocytopenia is the size of the spleen. In individuals with marked splenomegaly, approximately 90% of the platelets can be stored in the spleen (26, 29), but even in these individuals, platelet counts of approximately 30,000 to 40,000 cells/mm$^3$ do not necessarily cause spontaneous bleeding (30).

Increased pooling of platelets in the spleen is the major cause of thrombocytopenia in individuals with congestive splenomegaly, but sometimes the mechanism is more complex. In bone marrow, the number of megakaryocytes usually is either increased or normal (30), but platelet production occasionally is impaired (25). Furthermore, serum thrombopoietin levels are normal in individuals with thrombocytopenia secondary to liver cirrhosis with splenomegaly, thus suggesting that in this group, platelet production is not increased as the total platelet mass, although present mainly in the enlarged spleen, is normal (31). Platelet survival usually is normal (see Chapter 9), but in one-third of individuals with chronic liver disease, both platelet and fibrinogen survival times are shortened. Whereas administration of heparin corrects the half-life of fibrinogen, survival of the platelets is not affected, thereby indicating factors other than activation of the coagulation system (27). In some individuals, the short survival time of platelets can relate to platelet-bound immunoglobulins (33), but the precise cause of this shortened platelet survival is unknown.

## PATHOPHYSIOLOGY OF COAGULOPATHY

Pathophysiology of the coagulopathy of liver failure can be broadly divided into two categories: abnormalities in the protein coagulation factors, and alterations in the formed elements (i.e., platelets) of coagulation.

## Coagulation Factor Abnormalities

Alterations of the coagulation system relate to the hepatocyte being the cell that synthesizes all coagulation factors—with the exceptions of von Willebrand factor, which is produced by endothelial cells (34), and of factor VIII, which also is synthesized by the spleen (3, 35). In addition, the liver dampens the coagulation system by producing specific coagulation inhibitors, such as antithrombin III (AT III), protein C, and protein S, and by removing activated clotting factors from the circulation. The liver also synthesizes several components of the fibrinolytic system, particularly plasminogen and $\alpha_2$-antiplasmin. Therefore, individuals with liver disease may have altered fibrinolysis superimposed on the primary coagulation defects. In some instances, such as during disseminated intravascular coagulation (DIC), increased use of these factors also may play a role in decreasing their plasma concentration. Finally, the low plasma concentration of some factors may be accompanied by qualitative abnormalities of these proteins.

Posttranslational modification of the vitamin K-dependent factors, which is crucial for expression of their biologic activity, is catalyzed by a vitamin K-dependent γ-carboxylase present in the hepatocyte. Therefore, alterations of the vitamin K-dependent factors can have a dual origin, consisting of defects in polypeptide precursor synthesis and abnormal vitamin K-dependent γ-carboxylation resulting from an intrinsic enzymatic defect of the hepatocyte or a deficiency of vitamin K (36).

Factors II, VII, IX, and X are vitamin K-dependent procoagulants, and protein C and protein S are vitamin K-dependent inhibitors of blood coagulation. In acute or chronic parenchymal liver disease, low levels of factors II, VII, and X commonly are seen and reflected by a prolonged prothrombin time (PT), whereas concentrations of factor IX usually are normal or slightly decreased (1, 37–39). Factor VII is the most sensitive vitamin K-dependent factor; showing the greatest reduction in plasma levels during both acute and chronic liver disease (37–39). Furthermore, because of its short plasma half-life of approximately 5 hours, factor VII deficiency is one of the earliest markers of coagulation abnormalities in liver disease. Also, because the plasma concentration is not affected by inflammation or DIC, the factor VII assay reflects the synthetic capacity of the hepatocyte and can be used as a prognostic indicator in liver disease (40). This assay does not offer any advantage over the PT, however, especially if the thromboplastin used is sufficiently sensitive to detect mildly depressed levels of factor VII (41).

Most individuals with acute or chronic liver disease have impaired γ-carboxylation of the vitamin K-dependent factors, which is reflected by depressed levels of des-γ-carboxyprothrombin compared with that of the native molecule (42). Moreover, administration of vitamin K to these individuals does not eliminate the abnormal molecule from the plasma (36–42). The des-γ-carboxyprothrombin molecule also is present in more than 90% of individuals with primary hepatocarcinoma (i.e., hepatoma), and the plasma concentration of this molecule is even higher than that in individuals with other liver diseases. Furthermore, levels of the abnormal prothrombin drop following surgical removal of the tumor or chemotherapy (43). The plasma concentration of abnormal prothrombin in these individuals is too low to play a clinical role in the coagulopathy of liver disease, but high levels of des-γ-carboxyprothrombin may be a marker for hepatoma (43).

Factors V and VIII share common functional properties as cofactors in the assembly of the prothrombinase complex and the tenase complex, respectively, but their behaviors in liver disease are distinct. Low plasma levels of factor V commonly are seen in acute and chronic parenchymal liver disease and in hepatoma (1, 39, 44), mainly resulting from impaired synthesis. Sometimes, however, increased use and degradation because of DIC and hyperfibrinolysis also play a role in the low levels of these factors (37). In severe parenchymal liver disease, the level of factor V can be markedly decreased, thus contributing to a poor prognosis (45). Biliary disorders are associated with normal or even high concentrations of factor V, however, as in biliary cirrhosis (1, 39, 44, 46).

Unlike factor V, plasma levels of functional factor VIII usually are normal or increased in a variety of liver diseases, including acute and chronic hepatocellular disease, hepatoma, and obstructive jaundice (11, 47, 48).

The very high levels of factor VIII coagulant activity, which occur in individuals with fulminant hepatitis (48), may reflect enhanced synthesis by cells other than hepatocytes, such as cells in the spleen (3, 35). Similarly, levels of von Willebrand factor are increased in individuals with liver disease (47), and a disproportionate increase in von Willebrand factor or factor VIII antigen as compared with the functional activities of these proteins sometimes is observed (3, 35).

Of the contact activation factors studied, levels of factor XI and factor XII are slightly decreased in advanced liver disease and hepatitis (37), but they are normal or increased in obstructive jaundice (37). These subtle changes do not play a role in the bleeding episodes of advanced liver dysfunction.

The A-chain of factor XIII is synthesized mainly by hepatocytes (49), and plasma factor XIIIa activity therefore is reduced in approximately 30% of individuals with acute hepatitis, liver cirrhosis (1, 37, 50), or hepatoma (1). In obstructive jaundice, levels of factor XIII are normal, and the clinical significance of the low factor XIII levels in liver disease is questionable (4), especially as equally low values in other conditions do not involve alterations in the hemostatic mechanism.

## Dysfibrinogenemia

The fibrinogen abnormalities in liver disease may be both quantitative and qualitative. The liver has a large synthetic capacity for fibrinogen and can maintain a normal plasma concentration of fibrinogen until the very advanced stages of liver disease. Fibrinogen concentrations less than 100 mg/dL usually occur in fulminant hepatitis or severe decompensated liver cirrhosis (1, 37, 51). In addition to the impaired compensatory capacity of the liver regarding fibrinogen synthesis, low fibrinogen concentrations also may result from accelerated fibrinogen metabolism caused by intravascular coagulation and hyperfibrinolysis. Fibrinogen is an acute phase reactant; therefore, its plasma concentration can be elevated in inflammatory disorders such as acute or chronic hepatocellular disorders (1, 37), obstructive jaundice, biliary cirrhosis, and hepatoma as well as metastatic tumors (46, 52).

In addition to quantitative abnormalities of fibrinogen, the synthesized molecule can exhibit abnormal functional properties. The dysfibrinogenemia of individuals with hepatoma (53–55) also occurs in hepatitis, alcoholic liver cirrhosis, postnecrotic cirrhosis, and toxic hepatitis (56–60). The reported incidence varies between 50% in liver cirrhosis and nearly 100% in individuals with acute liver failure (57, 59). Accurate estimates are difficult, however, because the incidence depends on individual selection and the methods used to detect the abnormal fibrinogen molecule.

Formation of a stabilized fibrin clot entails three principal events, as discussed in Chapter 6:

1. Thrombin-mediated proteolytic cleavage of fibrinopeptides from fibrinogen to form fibrin monomers,
2. Polymerization of fibrin monomers to form fibrin fibrils and fibers, and
3. Factor XIIIa–mediated covalent stabilization of the fibrin matrix.

Thus, functional defects of fibrinogen may affect any of these steps. Prolonged thrombin and reptilase times, with normal fibrinogen concentrations and levels of fibrinogen degradation products, typically occur in liver disease. A prolonged thrombin time (Fig. 45.1) results from defective fibrin monomer aggregation (Fig. 45.2), and thrombin cleavage of fibrinopeptides is entirely normal (60). The contribution of the fibrin polymerization defect to the abnormal bleeding manifestations in these individuals is difficult to evaluate, because the abnormal molecule also is detected in individuals with other hemostatic system defects. Most individuals with congenital dysfibrinogenemias involving fibrin polymerization defects, especially those with moderate defects, do not bleed excessively (61, 62), however, so the dysfibrinogenemia of liver disease alone probably will not lead to clinically apparent bleeding disorders. Finally, this type of dysfibrinogenemia is characteristic of disorders affecting the hepatocyte, and individuals with obstructive jaundice manifest completely normal fibrin polymerization (58).

Structurally, the dysfibrinogenemia of liver disease is characterized by an increased sialic acid content (61), which correlates with and is responsible for the functional defect (60, 61) as portrayed in Fig. 45.1. Increased branching of oligosaccharides rather than additional carbohydrate linkages to the protein backbone occurs in dysfibrinogenemia of liver disease (63), including hepatoma (55). The precise biochemical lesion responsible for the hyperglycosylation of fibrinogen has not been elucidated, but tissue levels of sialyltransferase, galactosyltransferase, and N-acetylglucosaminyltransferase are elevated in hepatocellular disorders (64). Moreover, fetal fibrinogen exhibits functional and structural properties similar to those of the abnormal fibrinogen in liver disease (65). Hyperglycosylation or hypoglycosylation of other plasma proteins also is present in individuals with liver disease (64).

## Inhibitors of Blood Coagulation

Antithrombin III (AT III) is an endogenous inhibitor of thrombin, factor Xa, and factor IXa. Heparin and certain heparan sulfate proteoglycans of the vessel wall markedly enhance its inhibitory action (see Chapter 3). Because AT III is synthesized by hepatocytes, its levels often are low in individuals with liver parenchymal disorders such as hepatitis, cirrhosis, or the fatty liver of pregnancy (66–69). The low AT III level primarily results from impaired synthesis (70), but the increased catabolism associated with DIC also may contribute to de-

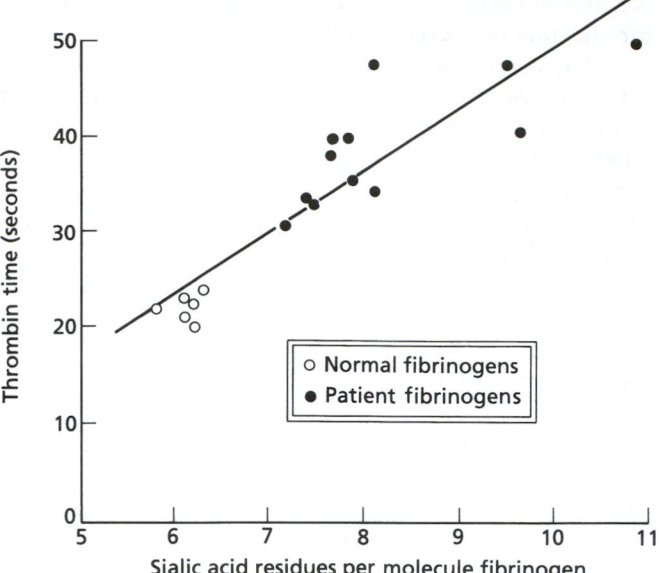

**FIGURE 45.1.** Comparison of sialic acid content versus thrombin time of purified normal (○) and individual (●) fibrinogens. Linear regression analysis of the data revealed a correlation coefficient of +0.91. The equation of the thrombin time versus sialic acid content is $Y = 6.51 \times -15.32$. (Reprinted with permission from Martinez J, Palascak JE, Kwasniak D. Abnormal sialic acid content of the dysfibrinogenemia associated with liver disease. J Clin Invest 1978;61:535–538.)

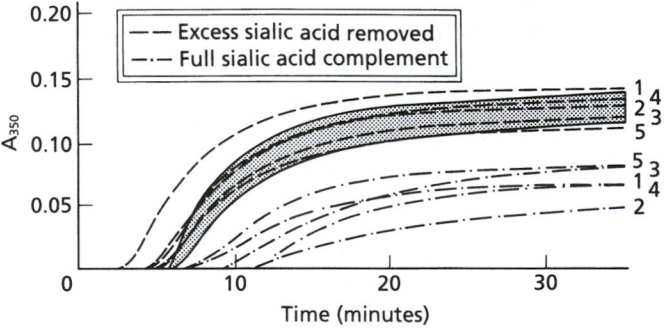

**FIGURE 45.2.** Aggregation of fibrin monomers of purified normal and individual fibrinogens. Shaded areas represent the range of aggregation of five normal controls. Dashed lines represent the fibrin monomer aggregation of five individual fibrinogens with their full sialic acid complement and after removal of their excess sialic acid. (Reprinted with permission from Martinez J, MacDonald KA, Palascak JE. The role of sialic acid in the dysfibrinogenemia associated with liver disease: distribution of sialic acid on the constituent chains. Blood 1983;61:1196–1202.)

pressed levels (71). In addition, increased extravascular distribution may cause secondary decreases in the plasma level of AT III (71). In nonparenchymal liver disorders such as biliary cirrhosis and obstruction of the common bile duct, plasma AT III concentrations usually are normal or increased (37, 46).

The clinical significance of low plasma AT III levels in liver disease is unclear; however, the concentration may be insufficient to inhibit adequately the excessively active coagulation system in some of these individuals. That the increased catabolism of fibrinogen in some individuals with liver disease returns to normal after the infusion of AT III supports this concept (70).

Protein C and protein S are vitamin K-dependent proteins that also function as endogenous inhibitors of the coagulation pathway. Activated protein C possesses proteolytic activity, and in conjunction with its cofactor protein S, it cleaves factor Va and factor VIIIa (see Chapter 3). Levels of protein C are decreased by as much as 80% in individuals with acute viral hepatitis and liver cirrhosis (72, 73), but normal levels are present in early biliary cirrhosis and chronic hepatitis (73). An abnormal protein C molecule manifesting defective γ-carboxylation is seen in individuals with hepatoma, and the alteration is not corrected by administration of vitamin K (74). In contrast to individuals with genetic deficiencies of protein C, individuals with liver disease rarely experience thrombotic events despite having very low levels of the protein.

Protein S circulates through the plasma in two forms. One is bound to a component of the complement system, C4b, and one is a free form serving as a cofactor for protein C (see Chapter 3). Although levels of the free fraction of protein S antigen are moderately reduced in liver disease, this abnormality is modest compared with those of other vitamin K-dependent factors (75, 76). The decreased functional activity of protein S may result from abnormal γ-carboxylation in the liver or synthesis of noncarboxylated forms from extrahepatic sites such as endothelial cells (75).

Tissue factor pathway inhibitor (TFPI) (see Chapter 4), a coagulation inhibitor, was initially referred to as LACI, for lipoprotein-associated coagulation inhibitor, or EPI, for extrinsic pathway inhibitor. TFPI binds to factor Xa and to the complex formed by tissue factor and VIIa, and it interferes with the activation of coagulation. At least *in vitro*, the TFPI molecule is synthesized by endothelial cells and hepatoma cell lines. In individuals with severe liver disease, plasma concentrations of TFPI are normal (77, 78); however, in one study in which TFPI levels were normal to markedly reduced, there was no correlation between the TFPI level and the PT (79). Therefore, plasma levels of TFPI may not reflect the synthetic capacity of hepatocytes because of compensation through synthesis by endothelial cells (79).

## Disseminated Intravascular Coagulation and Fibrinolysis

Coagulation abnormalities in individuals with liver disease can resemble those in DIC, and some individuals with liver disease manifest clinical and laboratory findings nearly indistinguishable from those in DIC (see Chapter 44). Furthermore, abnormalities of the fibrinolytic system are common in advanced liver disease, but hemorrhagic manifestations secondary to hyperfibrinolysis are rare. Even so, bleeding manifestations may develop when hyperfibrinolysis occurs in conjunction with profoundly decreased levels of circulating procoagulants secondary to impaired synthesis by the diseased liver (11). Occasionally, these complexities make the approach to individuals with coagulopathy of liver disease difficult.

Identification of the underlying disorder responsible for the liver disease or DIC, along with careful analysis of appropriate laboratory tests, can be useful in differentiating the coagulopathy of liver disease without DIC from overt DIC with another cause. Table 45.1 lists some of the important laboratory parameters that can distinguish the coagulopathy of liver disease from overt DIC. In liver disease, the standard liver indices of albumin and transaminases are changed more markedly than those in DIC, with albumin decreased and transaminases increased. Of the standard coagulation tests, PT is most useful, because it is more prolonged in liver disease than in DIC, probably because of the dramatic decreases in factor V and factor VII. In overt DIC, levels of fibrin(ogen) degradation products, D-dimer, and fibrinopeptide A, are increased more than in liver disease.

**TABLE 45.1.** Laboratory Values in Individuals with Liver Failure Without Overt DIC Compared with Values in Individuals with DIC of Other Cause

| | Type of Disease | |
| Laboratory Parameters | Severe Liver Disease | DIC |
| --- | --- | --- |
| Albumin | ⇃⇃ | N/↓ |
| Transaminases | ↑/↑↑ | N/↑ |
| Platelets[a] | N/↓ | ↓ |
| PT | ↑↑ | ↑ |
| aPTT | ↑ | ↑ |
| Thrombin time | ↑ | ↑ |
| Fibrinogen | N/↓ | N/↓ |
| FDP | ↑ | ↑↑ |
| D-Dimer | N/↑ | ↑↑ |
| Fibrinopeptide A | N/↑ | ↑↑ |
| Factor VII | ↓↓ | ↓ |
| Factor VIII | ↑/↑↑ | N/↓ |
| Factor V | ↓/↓↓ | ↓ |

*FDP*, fibrin/fibrinogen degradation product; *N*, normal; ↑, increased; ↑↑, marked increase; ↓, decrease; ↓↓, marked decrease.

[a] Decrease may result from hypersplenism.

The decreases in fibrinogen levels, however, are not as dramatic and therefore are of more limited usefulness.

Assessment of the laboratory parameters in Table 45.1 provides a useful framework to analyze the contribution of liver disease itself to the coagulopathy in individuals with severe liver disease. These tests should be carefully scrutinized, and sound clinical judgment should be applied considering the inherent complexities in their interpretation. For example, the relationship between low fibrinogen levels and DIC in individuals with liver disease is unclear. Some attribute the diminution in plasma fibrinogen concentration to impaired synthesis by the diseased liver and to altered distribution of fibrinogen between the intravascular and extravascular pools (80). Others favor increased consumption as the major cause (51, 81, 82). Individuals with a variety of hepatocellular diseases often manifest a shortened plasma fibrinogen half-life with an increased catabolic rate (27, 51, 81–83), thus indicating that fibrinogen is consumed. That heparin prolongs the plasma half-life of fibrinogen and increases its concentration (27, 51, 81–83) supports this concept. Administration of heparin, however, does not result in normalization of platelet survival (27), because this process possibly results from increased platelet adhesion to the damaged vascular bed of the diseased liver rather than to DIC. Furthermore, infusion of AT III into these individuals increases fibrinogen survival, thus suggesting that increased catabolism of fibrinogen results from activation of the coagulation system (71, 84). AT III concentrates, however, have failed to improve the clinical picture or alter laboratory parameters of individuals with coagulopathy of liver failure, and there currently is no basis to recommend AT III replacement therapy in individuals with acquired deficiency of AT III (85, 86). Finally, inhibition of fibrinolysis is unable to correct fibrinogen hypercatabolism, thereby indicating that hyperfibrinolysis plays a minor role in hypofibrinogenemia among these individuals (81).

Analysis of other clotting factors and the relationship of changes in multiple factors can aid the evaluation of coagulopathy in liver disease. For example, low levels of factor VIII favor the diagnosis of overt DIC, especially when in conjunction with high levels of fibrin(ogen) degradation products, particularly D-dimer (87). High levels of fibrinopeptide A, which can be normalized by heparin therapy, occur in DIC and reflect the *in vivo* formation of thrombin (88). Elevated levels of fibrinopeptide A also occur in individuals with liver cirrhosis (88), but these increases are not substantial and the role of DIC in the coagulopathy of liver cirrhosis has been questioned (89). The discrepancies in levels of fibrinopeptide A, fibrin(ogen) derivatives, and fibrin monomers in plasma may result from impaired removal of these peptides by the diseased liver (88). Another hallmark of DIC is visceral microthrombi, and micro-

thrombi also are found in biopsy specimens of the liver and other organs in individuals with acute hepatic failure (90).

Apart from secondary activation of the fibrinolytic system in response to DIC, primary activation of fibrinolytic mechanisms may also occur in liver disease. For example, increased fibrinolytic activity occurs in individuals with acute hepatitis and liver cirrhosis (11, 91–93), which may be associated with mucosal bleeding (11), hemorrhage into soft tissues, and rarely, bleeding into the central nervous system (94). In contrast, fibrinolytic activity is diminished in individuals with obstructive jaundice (95). The enhanced fibrinolytic activity that occurs in liver cirrhosis may result from elevated plasma levels of tissue plasminogen activator, which in turn result from impaired clearance by the diseased liver (96–98) or from decreased levels of a tissue plasminogen–activator inhibitor (96). Decreased levels of plasminogen (4, 37) and $\alpha_2$-antiplasmin (99) also occur in individuals with hepatitis or advanced liver cirrhosis, probably secondary to impaired hepatic synthesis of plasminogen (4, 37) and $\alpha_2$-antiplasmin (100). Increased consumption of plasminogen also may be involved in certain individuals secondary to increased activity of the coagulation system, as suggested by the reversal of plasminogen use with administration of heparin (101).

The causes of intravascular coagulation in viral or toxic hepatitis (51), postnecrotic liver cirrhosis (83), or alcoholic liver cirrhosis (81) are unclear. Implicated mechanisms include the release of thromboplastic material from necrotic hepatic cells (51), systemic endotoxemia resulting from impaired removal of endotoxins originating from the bowel (102), and the slow removal of activated coagulation factors by the liver.

Disseminated intravascular coagulation also can arise following placement of the LeVeen shunt to relieve intractable ascites (27) (see Chapter 44). Severe bleeding can develop, and laboratory evidence of DIC is present while the shunt is patent (103–105), with return to normal laboratory results when the flow of ascitic fluid ceases (103). Thus, the DIC may arise from failure of the diseased liver to rapidly clear the procoagulant-rich ascitic fluid introduced into the systemic circulation by the shunt (103). Whether heparin prevents bleeding or improves shunt function, however, is unclear, and most authors recommend shunt ligation when DIC is evident (103).

## Thrombocytopenia and Platelet Dysfunction

Congestive splenomegaly is the most common cause of thrombocytopenia in liver disease, but other pathogenic mechanisms also may be involved. Heavy consumption of alcohol, for example, can cause thrombocytopenia, which can become severe (106, 107). The mechanism relates to the ability of alcohol to suppress production of platelets by bone marrow (106–108). This suppression is reversible, however, and platelet counts return to normal a few days after discontinuation of alcohol consumption (106, 107). Individuals with alcoholism also frequently have folic acid deficiency. Therefore, thrombocytopenia in this population can be multifactorial, involving splenomegaly in conjunction with bone marrow depression and folic acid deficiency (106–109).

In contrast to the frequent thrombocytopenia in alcoholic liver disease, aplastic anemia with severe thrombocytopenia is a rare complication of viral hepatitis. There is no correlation between severity of liver involvement and onset of bone marrow failure, but the occurrence of aplasia carries a very poor prognosis (110–112). Mild thrombocytopenia commonly is seen with toxic or viral hepatitis, and this thrombocytopenia usually resolves as the liver function recovers (45).

In addition to thrombocytopenia, qualitative platelet abnormalities occur in some individuals with liver dysfunction (see Chapter 33). Abnormal platelet aggregation in response to adenosine diphosphate has occurred in individuals with liver cirrhosis, and platelet-poor plasma from these individuals has decreased the adenosine diphosphate–induced aggregation of normal platelets (113). The factor or factors responsible for the abnormal platelet aggregation remain unidentified; however, defective signal transduction in thrombin- or collagen-stimulated platelets has been reported (114). Both structural and functional platelet abnormalities occur in severe hepatitis and cirrhosis, and both improve with recovery of the liver (115).

## LIVER TRANSPLANTATION

Liver transplantation is commonly performed for the treatment of end-stage liver disease (116, 117), and severe bleeding both during and immediately following this surgery is a significant cause of mortality (118, 119). Moreover, the type of liver disease correlates with the severity of bleeding during transplantation and influences clinical outcome. Individuals with coagulopathies secondary to liver cirrhosis bleed more and, therefore, need more intraoperative blood transfusions than individuals with biliary cirrhosis (120).

Hemostatic abnormalities during liver transplantation have been analyzed in relation to the three stages of the procedure (121). Stage I begins at the start of anesthesia and continues to the occlusion of hepatic blood flow. Stage II, the anhepatic phase, continues from this point until the donor liver is reperfused by the individual's blood. Stage III begins with the circulation of individual blood through the transplanted liver and continues until the end of the procedure. Platelet counts, PTs, activated partial thromboplastin times (aPTTs), assays of coagulation factors (e.g., factors VII, V, and VIII), fibrinogen levels, and euglobulin clot lysis times are good preoperative predictors of bleeding (120–122). Thromboelastography also has been used during the procedure to rapidly assess coagulation parameters and aid in selecting replacement therapy (123).

During stage I, the coagulation profile usually is similar to that of the preoperative period. Some individuals with cirrhosis, however, exhibit enhanced fibrinolysis, as evidenced by a shortened euglobulin clot lysis time (120, 122). In addition, the plasma concentration of fibrinogen decreases during stage I and continues to fall during stage II.

During stage II, the PT and aPTT are prolonged, because the absence of a liver results in decreased plasma concentrations of factor V and the vitamin K–dependent coagulation factors. The factor VIII level, which usually is elevated preoperatively secondary to increased synthesis by splenic endothelial cells, decreases to a normal value in this period (121, 122). Absence of a liver also results in decreased clearance of activated clotting factors, thereby favoring thrombosis. Overt DIC, however, does not contribute to the coagulation pattern during stage II (122), and because it can induce bleeding, heparin is not used in stage II.

The hemostatic alterations that occur during stage III depend on the degree of ischemic changes in the grafted liver (122). Early in stage III, levels of the vitamin K–dependent factors as well as of factor V, fibrinogen, and platelets continue to decline (121, 122), but there is no evidence of DIC or platelet microthrombi in biopsy specimens from the newly transplanted liver (124). Release of tissue plasminogen activator from the grafted liver may account for the increased fibrinolytic activity seen in some individuals (125). In individuals being transplanted for liver failure secondary to biliary cirrhosis, the perioperative coagulopathy is less severe than in those with cirrhosis from another cause, and during the anhepatic phase, these individuals generate more thrombin with attenuated enhancement of fibrinolytic activity (126). The altered hemostatic parameters usually return to normal by the third day after transplantation, provided that the new liver functions properly (127). Thrombosis of the hepatic artery can occur and is more frequent in children (128), and sudden death because of platelet aggregation in the pulmonary vasculature also can occur in children during transplantation (128). Administration of AT III concentrates does not improve laboratory values, transfusion requirements, or clinical manifestations of coagulopathy during stages II or III in orthotopic liver transplantations (129). Finally, transplantation can confer to the recipient any inherited disorders of the donor's coagulation system, as recently described for the transmission of thrombotic tendencies following liver transplantation from a donor with protein C deficiency (130).

## CLINICAL MANIFESTATIONS AND DIFFERENTIAL DIAGNOSIS

Hemorrhagic manifestations in individuals with liver disease frequently can be severe, and bleeding often is a cause of death. In some instances, hemorrhagic manifestations may not be obvious, however. A thorough individual history is necessary, in which splenomegaly and stigmata of liver disease provide clinically useful markers of individuals with liver disease and associated underlying disorders of coagulation. Gastrointestinal bleeding, which is expressed clinically by hematemesis, melena, or both, most often results from esophageal varices or portal hypertensive gastropathy. Hemorrhage from other mucosal sites, as manifested by ecchymoses, epistaxis, gingival bleeding, menorrhagia, or blood in the stool, should alert physicians to the possibility of a coagulopathy involving aberrations in both the coagulation and the fibrinolytic systems (1–5, 11). Hemorrhage into the central nervous system (94) or retroperitoneal space (90) has occurred, and bleeding has been found to account for 20% of the deaths associated with hepatic failure (90). In one study of acute viral hepatitis (45), bleeding occurred in approximately 58% of individuals with liver failure and was associated with both a poor prognosis and a mortality rate of 73%. In another study of individuals with hepatic cirrhosis (5), 19 of 59 individuals had bleeding, and all 19 individuals had a prolonged PT (5).

Liver disease-induced alterations in the plasma levels of specific coagulation factors depend mainly on the type and severity of disease. These alterations are tabulated in Table 45.2 and discussed in greater detail under "Laboratory Testing." In general, however, the changes seen in hepatitis may differ from those in cirrhosis or obstructive jaundice, and within each category, differences also may arise relative to the severity of the disease, the liver failure, or both. On the other hand, the degree of thrombocytopenia will relate principally to portal hypertension causing splenomegaly.

Because vitamin K deficiency may be associated with parenchymal liver disease, the PT and levels of specific vitamin K-dependent coagulation factors should be determined after the parenteral administration of vitamin K. Improvement of the PT has occurred in individuals with parenchymal liver disease after vitamin K therapy, thus indicating these individuals also had some degree of vitamin K deficiency (5). Moreover, biliary tract diseases, such as stones, tumors, and inflammation, may lead to severe coagulopathy that can be reversed by parenteral administration of vitamin K. In biliary diseases, levels of vitamin K-dependent factors are depressed, whereas levels of factor V, fibrinogen, and AT III remain normal or elevated (1, 39, 44–46). Hereditary deficiency of factor VII has been associated with congenital hyperbilirubinemias, such as Dubin-Johnson syndrome and Gilbert syndrome (130, 131); in these individuals, plasma levels of factor VII do not rise following parenteral administration of vitamin K (131).

## LABORATORY TESTING

Coagulopathy associated with liver disease can be detected by routine coagulation assays, such as the platelet count, PT, aPTT, and thrombin time (TT) (1–5). When analyzing the results of these assays, however, it is important to know the sensitivity of the test systems and any other limitations or distinguishing features. For example, mild reductions of factor VII levels will be detected by the PT if the thromboplastin being used is sufficiently sensitive (41). Use of Normotest, which measures factors VII, X, and prothrombin and is sensitive to mild reductions of factor VII, may be more predictable than the PT (69). To account for the different activities of thromboplastin reagents commercially available for use in the PT, it now is common to report the International Normalized Ratio (INR). This method has been useful for standardizing the PT in individuals treated with oral anticoagulants. In individuals with liver failure, however, the INR has been reported to give variable results and to not adequately reflect the severity of liver failure, especially in individuals with very prolonged PTs (132). On the other hand, Robert and Chazouilleres (133) found that PT expressed as a percentage was more accurate in differentiating mild from severe alterations of liver failure, and it is possible that hepatic synthesis of vitamin K independent as well as vitamin K-dependent coagulation factors impaired by the diseased liver may be responsible for these discrepancies.

**TABLE 45.2.** Abnormalities of Coagulation Parameters in Liver Disease

| Coagulation Parameter | Type of Liver Disease | | | |
| --- | --- | --- | --- | --- |
| | Hepatitis | | Cirrhosis | |
| | Acute[a] | Chronic | Hepatic[b] | Biliary[b] |
| PT | ↑ | ↑ | N/↑ | N/↑ |
| aPTT | ↑ | ↑ | N/↑ | N/↑ |
| Thrombin time | ↑ | ↑ | N/↑ | N |
| Clot lysis | ↓ | N/↓ | ↓ | ↓/N |
| Fibrinogen | ↓ | ↓ | N/↓ | ↑/N |
| Factor V | ↓ | ↓ | ↓ | N/↓ |
| Factor VII | ↓ | ↓ | ↓ | N/↓ |
| Factor VIII | ↑ | N/↑ | N/↑ | N/↑ |
| AT III | ↓ | ↓ | ↓ | N/↑ |

N, normal; ↑, increased; ↓, decreased.

[a] With liver failure; values are normal without failure.

[b] Advanced; values are normal in early stages of cirrhosis.

Measuring the plasma levels of specific vitamin K-dependent factors provides more information than the PT alone. For example, because the half-life of factor VII is only a few hours, diminution of factor VII levels can be detected very early in acute hepatocellular damage. Levels of vitamin K-dependent factors should be assayed before and after administration of vitamin K to assess the potential contribution of vitamin K deficiency to the coagulopathy of liver disease, as discussed under "Abnormalities of the Coagulation Factors."

The aPTT is less sensitive to alterations in the tissue factor (i.e., extrinsic) pathway than the PT, and it does not measure factor VII. An aPTT that is disproportionately prolonged when compared with the PT in individuals without genetic deficiencies of coagulation factors suggests coagulation inhibitors, such as antiphospholipid antibodies or inhibitors to factors VIII, IX, and XI. The thrombin time can be helpful, because it can detect low levels of fibrinogen and dysfibrinogenemias and elevated levels of fibrin(ogen) degradation products, as described under "Disseminated Intravascular Coagulation and Fibrinolysis."

Liver disease-induced changes in coagulation assays and in the plasma levels of specific coagulation factors are listed in Table 45.2. Coagulation abnormalities in viral or drug-induced acute hepatitis vary and depend on the degree of liver damage. The PT is prolonged in approximately half of individuals with hepatitis without liver failure and in all with hepatitis accompanied by liver failure (45).

In chronic active or persistent hepatitis, individuals frequently have an abnormal PT with low levels of AT III, both of which correlate with the clinical evolution of the disorder (134). Moreover, the PT is elevated in proportion to the deficiencies of vitamin K-dependent factors in general and of factor VII in particular (41).

In individuals with liver cirrhosis, the state of the coagulation system depends on the extent of parenchymal damage; there is no correlation with the cause. There may be alterations in the levels of specific coagulation proteins, but these result in an abnormal PT only in approximately 70% of these individuals (5). The PT also is elevated in 75 to 85% of individuals with cirrhosis secondary to right-sided heart failure (135). Compensated liver cirrhosis presents a normal coagulation profile, with minimally prolonged PT and aPTT (5). In individuals with advanced (i.e., decompensated) cirrhosis (Table 45.2), changes in the coagulation system are more pronounced, and the PT and aPTT frequently are prolonged to a greater degree than in compensated cirrhosis (5). Individuals with advanced cirrhosis and liver failure also have decreased levels of AT III, protein C, and protein S (68, 69, 72, 75, 76), along with enhanced activity of the fibrinolytic system with low levels of $\alpha_2$-antiplasmin (102). DIC can be detected by measuring the plasma lev-

els of fibrin(ogen) degradation products, especially fibrin D-dimer and also fibrinopeptide A. The depressed biosynthesis of procoagulants and enhanced fibrinolytic activity correlate with bleeding into the skin and mucosa (11). Coagulation abnormalities in individuals with hepatoma may reflect changes caused by cirrhosis, which frequently is present in this population.

In primary biliary cirrhosis (early stages) or obstructive jaundice, levels of all coagulation factors and inhibitors usually are normal or slightly increased (Table 45.2), provided there is no concurrent vitamin K deficiency (37, 46). This is an interesting observation, because there also is a simultaneous decrease in the circulating levels of other proteins, such as albumin and cholinesterase, which are synthesized by the liver (136). The underlying mechanism possibly involves stimulation of procoagulant synthesis by the hyperlipemic condition, which frequently results from obstructive jaundice (95). Even although levels of procoagulants are increased, there is no resulting increase in the incidence of thrombotic complications following surgery (37, 46).

In addition to quantitative abnormalities in the levels of circulating coagulation factors during liver disease, qualitative abnormalities of coagulation proteins occur as well. These changes occur with the vitamin K-dependent factors, most notably prothrombin and protein C, and they result from an impaired $\gamma$-carboxylation process (42, 43). Qualitative abnormalities of fibrinogen also are present and are characterized by an excess sialic acid content, which can be detected by a prolonged thrombin time, as shown in Fig. 45.1 (56, 62). In addition, similar qualitative abnormalities of prothrombin, protein C, and fibrinogen are seen in individuals with hepatoma (43, 52–55, 74).

Laboratory testing also is a valuable prognostic indicator in individuals with liver disease. In acute hepatitis, the PT offers a better index than measurements of serum transaminases or serum albumin, with a PT of less than 30% associated with poor prognosis (136). As discussed, some authors have reported that a factor VII level was more informative than the PT regarding prognosis (40), but this finding has not been verified (41). The PT has been valuable in acute hepatitis resulting from acetaminophen poisoning, in which individuals with a PT ratio of greater than 2.2 lapsed into coma (137, 138). Measurements of coagulation inhibitors are useful as well (139, 140). Low AT III concentrations are common in acute hepatitis, and values of less than 60% have been associated with poor prognosis (139). Furthermore, 84% of individuals with liver cirrhosis have low AT III levels (66), and the degree of depression in the plasma AT III concentration correlates with severity of the liver disease (66, 140).

Regarding liver cirrhosis, a prolonged PT is a useful predictor of fatal outcome (141, 142). The death rate for individuals with a PT of less than 58% of normal is markedly increased compared to that for individuals with a PT above 58% of normal (142), and the predictive value is enhanced when PT is combined with analysis of serum albumin levels (142). Dysfibrinogenemia also is a negative prognostic indicator in individuals with compensated liver cirrhosis (143).

## ASSESSMENT OF BLEEDING RISK DURING INVASIVE PROCEDURES

Individuals with advanced liver disease and coagulopathy often require liver biopsy and invasive diagnostic or therapeutic procedures. These procedures can trigger severe bleeding, which may be unresponsive to replacement therapy with platelets or coagulation factors. Therefore, a thorough evaluation of the hemostatic system is required.

Clinical reports on the risk for hemorrhagic complications of percutaneous liver biopsy in individuals with liver disease are conflicting. For example, the incidence of bleeding associated with biopsy has been reported to increase in individuals with a 3-second (144) to 4-second (145) prolongation of the PT and platelet counts of 50,000 (145) to 80,000 cells/mm$^3$ (144). In contrast, no increase in bleeding for individuals with liver disease and a 4-second prolongation of the PT or a 9-second prolongation of the aPTT above the midrange of normal has also been reported (146). Similarly, other studies have reported that platelet counts of greater than 50,000/mm$^3$ (147) or of 60,000 to 90,000 cells/mm$^3$ (147) are not associated with an increased incidence of bleeding. The incidence of hemorrhagic complications is increased, however, in individuals with a platelet count of 30,000 to 60,000 cells/mm$^3$ (147). In light of these findings, it is recommended that individuals with a PT prolonged by 3 seconds and a platelet count of less than 70,000 cells/mm$^3$ receive prophylactic therapy with fresh frozen plasma and platelet concentrates (144, 145). Platelet transfusions in individuals with counts of greater than 50,000 cells/mm$^3$ are not in accordance with the guidelines of a consensus conference for platelet transfusion therapy (148), but individuals with thrombocytopenia and coagulopathy of liver disease frequently have multiple qualitative and quantitative abnormalities involving platelets and coagulation factors, which justify transfusion therapy because of their high risk for bleeding.

Technical difficulties of the biopsy, number of passes, underlying liver pathology, and ascites play more significant roles than coagulation abnormalities in the safety of biopsy, and they may account for half of the bleeding episodes (146). Accordingly, alternatives to standard percutaneous biopsy have been recommended. For example, both a transvenous approach via the jugular vein and percutaneous biopsy followed by insertion of a hemostatic sponge plug appear to be adequate and safe in individuals with coagulopathy (149). More recently, laparoscopic liver biopsy has been shown to be effective and safe in individuals with mild to moderate coagulopathies (150, 151) and PT ratios of less than 2.1 and platelet counts of greater than 55,000 cells/mm$^3$ (150) or with PTs prolonged up to 2.5 seconds and platelet counts of less than 50,000 cells/mm$^3$ (151). Moreover, bleeding following laparoscopic liver biopsy is not related to the PT or platelet count (150), and portal hypertension and ascites do not adversely affect outcome following laparoscopic liver biopsy in individuals with coagulopathy (151).

Individuals with liver disease frequently require invasive diagnostic and therapeutic procedures, including placement of invasive vascular lines, thoracentesis, and pleural biopsy. Commonly, blood components have been given prophylactically to individuals with coagulopathies before the placement of invasive lines. A recent retrospective chart review of intensive care individuals receiving arterial, pulmonary artery, and central venous lines, however, revealed that rates of hemorrhage are low even without correction of coagulation abnormalities before the procedure, and that rates of hemorrhage closely relate to the experience of the physician placing the lines (152). This suggests that blood component replacement therapy in these individuals is not necessary before placement of invasive lines.

Both thoracentesis and pleural biopsy have a low incidence of complications, but specific guidelines for assessing the influence of platelet counts or coagulation tests on the potential for hemorrhage have not been established (153). The American College of Physicians views a platelet count of less than 50,000 cells/mm$^3$ or significant coagulopathy as contraindications for thoracentesis (154). Information regarding the safety of paracentesis in this group, however, is sparse (154). One study of thoracentesis and paracentesis (156) demonstrated that significant blood loss or decreases in hemoglobin of more than 2 g/dL did not occur in individuals with platelet counts of greater than 50,000 cells/mm$^3$ or with a PT or aPTT of between 1.5 to 2.0 seconds greater than the midrange of normal (i.e., PT corresponding to an INR of from 2.2 to 3.8). An increased incidence of bleeding was observed, however, in individuals with uremia (156).

Liver dysfunction severe enough to be marked by hemostatic abnormalities causes increased morbidity and mortality with a variety of surgical procedures (157). Surgical risk in individuals with liver disease is difficult to estimate, because the available data derive from retrospective analysis of a limited number of case studies (157). Furthermore, in many cases, clinical descriptions of the degree of liver impairment are insufficient to evaluate the associated hemostatic abnormalities properly. Nevertheless, a clear evaluation of these studies is helpful in appreciating the seriousness of the surgical risks in this group. Surgical procedures involving the biliary system carry high morbidity and mortality rates because of excessive bleeding (158). When performed in individuals with a PT prolonged by 2.5 seconds from that of controls, these procedures are associated with 83% mortality rate because of sepsis, hepatic encephalopathy, and bleeding from intraoperative sites despite use of platelets and plasma (159). However, when performed in individuals with a PT prolonged by less than 2.5 seconds, the mortality rate was 9% (159). Thus, this type of surgery should be performed only in life-threatening situations.

High rates of morbidity and mortality (30%) also are associated with a variety of abdominal surgical procedures, such as peptic ulcer surgery, colectomy, or biliary tract exploration, and multivariate analysis of these individuals, excluding Child's classification, shows that a low albumin level, infection, or mildly prolonged PT (1.5 seconds) are independent predictors of complications associated with these procedures (160). A PT prolonged by greater than 1.5 seconds was associated with an increase in morbidity and mortality of from 30 to 63% (160). In other procedures, such as portocaval shunt surgery, increased fibrinolytic activity was a good predictor of oozing during surgery, and ε-aminocaproic acid was useful in controlling the hemorrhage (98). The studies cited here indicate a high mortality rate in these individuals, but more recent reports have stated the incidence of mortality to be somewhat lower (161, 162). It is important to note, however, that even in those individuals in whom the hemostatic abnormalities are corrected by plasma and platelet transfusions, the severe alteration of liver function causes high morbidity and mortality, mainly because of infections, hepatic encephalopathy, and kidney failure (157–162). Thus, a thorough evaluation of hemostatic parameters is important in preoperative evaluation, and correction of any underlying hemostatic alterations may result in a more favorable surgical outcome.

## TREATMENT

The need to correct the coagulopathy of liver disease may arise under two different clinical settings. These are: (a) for treatment of overt hemorrhagic manifestations, and (b) for improvement of coagulation parameters before invasive procedures, such as liver or pleural biopsy or lumbar puncture, which can be associated with serious hemorrhagic complications.

Fresh frozen plasma (see Chapter 52) is the mainstay of therapy for coagulopathy of liver disease. Such treatment has the advantage of containing all coagulation factors, with the exception of platelets, as well as all coagulation inhibitors. Therefore, it can be used to reestablish hemostatic balance. Even so, use of fresh frozen plasma is associated with two major disadvantages: (a) the large volumes required for adequate correction of severe coagulopathy, and (b) the brief duration of action after infusion. For example, one study showed that administration of fresh frozen plasma at a dose of 12 mL/kg body weight corrected the PT to an acceptable range in individuals manifesting mild coagulopathy (163). This was true even when the coagulation studies were done within 15 minutes of the infusion (163). Similarly, 600 mL of fresh frozen plasma administered before liver biopsy corrected the PT to within 3 seconds of the control value in three of 15 individuals (164), and levels of factor VII fell 20 hours after the infusion (164). In addition, some individuals require large volumes (15–20 mL/kg) of fresh frozen plasma to decrease their PT to an acceptable range (165), and even this volume will not correct the PT and aPTT in everyone. Furthermore, some coagulation factors have a short half-life, so transfusing one-third of the initial volume of fresh frozen plasma administered every 8 to 12 hours may be necessary (165). These large volumes and frequent administration may cause fluid overload, especially in individuals with renal disease. Therefore, the total volume of plasma to be infused to maintain adequate levels of coagulation factors must be reduced.

Therapeutic plasmapheresis has been recommended as an adjunct to administration of fresh frozen plasma to circumvent fluid overload. Indeed, one study of 19 individuals with liver failure (166) demonstrated marked improvement in several coagulation parameters, such as reduction of the PT from a mean of 28 seconds to a mean of 17 seconds, after a plasma exchange of 36 mL/kg. Therapeutic plasmapheresis also has been successful prophylactically before percutaneous liver biopsy (166). Hemostatic improvements in individuals with acute liver failure have been achieved through extensive plasma exchange (45, 166), but additional clinical studies are necessary to fully evaluate the clinical efficacy of this therapy.

In the past, prothrombin complex concentrates have been used to treat coagulopathy of liver disease. These preparations contain all the vitamin K-dependent factors, but because they do not contain factor V, correction of the coagulopathy is only partial (164, 167). In another study (163), combination therapy with prothrombin complex concentrates and fresh frozen plasma provided greater correction of the PT. More recent studies, however, indicate that infusion of these concentrates is associated with a high incidence of thromboembolic events (168–170) and DIC (171, 172). The thrombogenic effect may relate to trace amounts of activated vitamin K-dependent factors in these preparations (173). Moreover, the activated factors may have increased plasma half-lives because of impaired clearance by the diseased liver (91). In addition, the decreased plasma concentration of

AT III may contribute to the induction of DIC or thromboembolism. Administration of AT III concentrates to individuals with liver failure and DIC, however, has not improved disease manifestations or clinical outcomes (86). Similar results have been obtained in individuals with DIC secondary to placement of a LeVeen shunt (86).

Another problem with use of prothrombin complex concentrates is the potential for transmission of viral hepatitis. The incidence of this infection is decreasing, however, because of better donor screening, availability of tests to detect viruses in donor plasma or concentrates, and newer methods of preparing the concentrates (see Chapter 52). Because of the risks of viral infection and induction of thromboembolic episodes, DIC, or both, vitamin K-dependent factor concentrates are no longer recommended for treatment of the coagulopathy associated with liver disease.

Heparin administration has been another means of reversing some coagulation abnormalities in individuals with liver disease, especially the increased consumption of clotting factors resulting from excessive activation of the coagulation system (81–84). Heparin increases both the half-life and the plasma levels of fibrinogen as well as of other procoagulants (81–83), but its use remains controversial. Evidence for clinical improvement in individuals is sparse. For example, in one study of acetaminophen-induced acute hepatitis (174), individuals treated with heparin demonstrated no improvement in their recovery or final outcome compared with individuals who were not anticoagulated. Aside from its questionable therapeutic efficacy, use of heparin in individuals with multiple coagulation abnormalities and local predisposing factors, such as esophageal varices or gastritis, adds a significant risk of bleeding. For these reasons, most authorities do not recommend heparin in these individuals, even with evidence of DIC (80).

Antifibrinolytic agents, such as $\epsilon$-aminocaproic acid (see Chapter 53), can inhibit the hyperfibrinolysis associated with liver disease, and it improves the diffuse bleeding present in some individuals during porta-systemic shunts (98). Because these individuals also may exhibit excessive activation of the coagulation system, however, use of antifibrinolytic drugs may cause thrombotic complications (2, 81).

Vitamin K administration is recommended by some authorities for treatment of individuals with hepatocellular diseases, because these individuals may have deficiencies of this vitamin (5). To identify individuals with this deficiency, parenteral doses of 10 mg of vitamin $K_1$ should be given to determine the therapeutic response (discussed under "Vitamin K Deficiency"). A shortening of the PT and an increase in the level of vitamin K-dependent factors after administration is helpful in verifying vitamin K deficiency and in distinguishing obstructive biliary diseases of the liver from hepatocellular disorders (136).

Platelet transfusions (see Chapter 51) are indicated for individuals with bleeding manifestations and platelet counts of less than 50,000 cells/mm$^3$. Because of platelet pooling in the spleen and shortened platelet half-life, however, transfusions with platelet concentrates seldom increase counts to the levels expected for a given number of units, and it is difficult to achieve the therapeutic goal of maintaining the platelet count at greater than 70,000 cells/mm$^3$. Prophylactic platelet transfusions before invasive procedures are indicated as well. Guidelines for platelet transfusions have been discussed, but there is no consensus regarding therapy when the platelet count is from 70,000 to 80,000 cells/mm$^3$. Even so, platelets should be administered immediately before the procedure when the platelet count is less than 50,000 cells/mm$^3$ (144–148).

Neither splenectomy nor shunting procedures generally are advocated as a means of increasing platelet counts in individuals with thrombocytopenia from splenomegaly secondary to liver disease (175), even although such procedures increase platelet counts in one-third of these individuals (176). Desmopressin (see Chapter 53) shortens the bleeding time in individuals with cirrhosis (177, 178), and this therapy may have a beneficial effect similar to that described in individuals with alterations of the factor VIII complex. However, because the shortening of the bleeding time does not predict bleeding during surgery (179, 180), the clinical usefulness of this agent in liver disease remains to be demonstrated. Clinical trials are necessary to assess whether treatment with desmopressin reduces the risk of bleeding during invasive procedures in this group (177).

# VITAMIN K DEFICIENCY
## METABOLISM AND FUNCTION

As discussed, several blood coagulation factors are referred to as vitamin K-dependent factors. These include factors II, VII, IX and X, which function as procoagulants, and protein C and protein S, which function as inhibitors of the coagulation cascade. These factors are synthesized by hepatocytes and undergo post-translational modification involving the addition of carboxyl groups to specific glutamic acid residues located in the N-terminal regions of the molecules. Vitamin K is required for hepatocytes to perform the enzymatic addition of these carboxyl groups to the proteins (see Chapter 55).

The term *vitamin K* refers to a group of fat-soluble vitamins required for normal functioning of the hemostatic mechanism (181, 182). Dietary vitamin K occurs naturally in two major forms (Fig. 45.3). These are the vitamin $K_1$ family (i.e., phylloquinone), which is found exclusively in plants, and vitamin $K_2$ family (i.e., menaquinone), which is a series of chemical congeners syn-

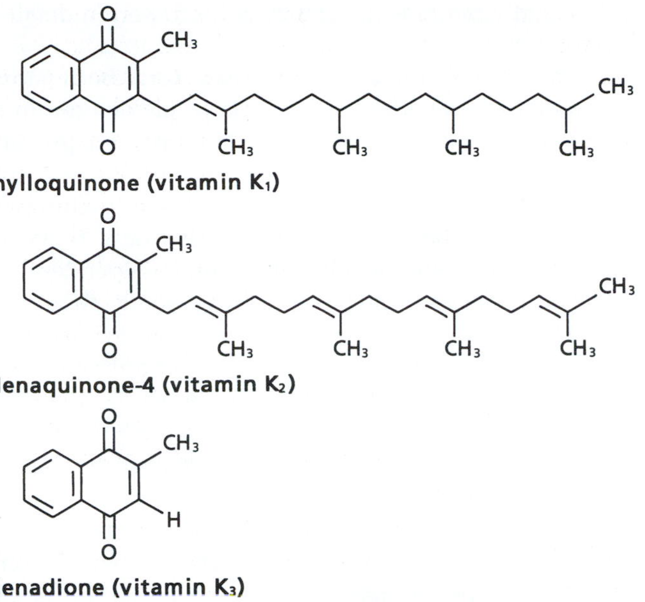

**FIGURE 45.3.**   Structure of the various forms of vitamin K.

thesized by Gram-positive bacteria in the human gastrointestinal tract and also found at high concentrations in putrefied fish meal. These congeners differ from one another in the length of the isoprenyl units that are substituted at the quinone ring. The natural vitamin $K_2$ found in fish meal has seven isoprenyl units and is known as menaquinone-7. Menadione (i.e., vitamin $K_3$, or menaquinone-0) lacks an isoprenyl substituent at this position (Fig. 45.3) and, therefore, is a provitamin, which is converted to an active vitamin K (i.e., menaquinone-4) in the microsomes of the liver.

The vitamin K content of selected foods is listed in Table 45.3 (182, 183). In general, green leafy vegetables are high in vitamin $K_1$ (183), meat and dairy products are intermediate, and cereals and fruits are low. Vitamin K is absorbed in the small bowel and colon, with phytonadione absorbed primarily in the proximal small bowel and the menaquinones and menadione in the distal small bowel and colon. Phytonadione and the menaquinones predominantly enter the lymphatics, and they require bile salts and pancreatic juice for maximal absorption, which ranges from 40 to 80% depending on the source (184). Menadione, which is water soluble and enters the blood, is well absorbed even without bile salts. When oral doses of vitamin $K_1$ are given, the peak plasma concentration occurs in approximately 2 hours, with a decrease to the fasting level of 1 to 3 ng/mL occurring over 2 to 3 days (185, 186). Approximately 30 to 50% of the administered dose is recovered in the feces over a 5-day period, with smaller amounts of between 8 and 30% appearing in the urine as polar metabolites. Because it is fat soluble, the absorption of vitamin K is significantly retarded by coadministration of nonabsorbable lipids, such as mineral oil.

When administered parenterally, approximately 50% of the phylloquinone dose appears in the liver within 1 hour (187). Within the hepatocyte, the largest concentration of vitamin $K_1$ appears in the microsomal fraction, with the second largest in the cytosol (187). Other major uptake sites of this vitamin include the skin and muscle, and concentrations in these tissues reach a maximum approximately 24 hours after parenteral administration (187).

The body pool of vitamin K is not large, and its turnover is rapid (188, 189). Distribution in the body involves two phases. The initial disappearance from the plasma occurs with a half-life of approximately 25 minutes, and the longer, second phase with a half-life of approximately 160 minutes (188). The fractional turnover rate is 0.4 per hour, thus indicating that the body pool turns over approximately once every 2.5 hours (189).

## CLINICAL SETTINGS

Dietary sources of vitamin K are absorbed primarily in the small bowel, and bile salts and pancreatic juice are necessary for absorption. The minimal daily requirement has been estimated as between 0.03 and 1.50 $\mu$g/kg/day, with a portion being contributed through biosynthesis of menaquinone forms of vitamin K by the intestinal flora (190). Because body stores of vitamin K are small, partial depletion without clinical consequences can occur after 1 week of dietary insufficiency. As mentioned, however, vitamin K is synthesized by the bacterial flora of the intestine, and the amounts from

**TABLE 45.3.**   Vitamin K Content of Selected Foods

| Food | Vitamin K Content ($\mu$g/100 g) |
|---|---|
| Bacon | 46 |
| Beef liver | 93 |
| Broccoli | 175 |
| Butter | 30 |
| Cabbage | 125 |
| Cheese | 35 |
| Chicken liver | 7 |
| Coffee | 38 |
| Eggs | 11 |
| Lettuce | 129 |
| Milk | 1 |
| Pork liver | 25 |
| Soybean oil | 193 |
| Spinach | 415 |
| Tea, green | 712 |

**TABLE 45.4.** Clinical Conditions Associated with Vitamin K Deficiency

Hemorrhagic disease of newborns
Dietary insufficiency combined with administration of broad-spectrum antibiotics
Total parenteral nutrition
Malabsorption of lipid-soluble vitamins because of obstructive jaundice (intrahepatic or extrahepatic)
Malabsorption because of intrinsic diseases of the bowel:
    Celiac disease
    Sprue
    Inflammatory bowel disease
    Short-bowel syndrome

this source are adequate to prevent hemorrhagic manifestations. Indeed, for a deficiency to become clinically apparent, low dietary intake and reduced synthesis by decreased or abnormal intestinal flora must occur concurrently (190). In addition, malabsorption resulting from intrinsic diseases of the bowel or to lack of bile salts may lead to decreased vitamin K availability.

Clinical conditions associated with vitamin K deficiency are listed in Table 45.4. Hemorrhagic disease of newborns results from vitamin K deficiency, which in turn results from the low vitamin K content of mother's milk coupled with insufficient synthesis by the sparse bacterial flora in the newborn's colon. The vitamin K content of mother's milk is very low (1–2 µg/l), whereas the requirements of infants for this vitamin are approximately 1 µg/kg/day (191). Thus, there is a higher incidence of vitamin K deficiency among breast-fed than among formula-fed babies or babies who receive supplementation (191–193).

During the first 2 or 3 days after birth, plasma prothrombin levels of infants are approximately 30% of normal, but they gradually increase thereafter with adequate dietary vitamin K. Because breast-fed infants do not receive adequate levels of vitamin K, hemorrhagic episodes usually appear during the first weeks of life, and most frequently when levels of prothrombin and other vitamin K-dependent factors are less than 10% of normal (194). Mucosal bleeding and bleeding following circumcision are common, but intracranial and retroperitoneal bleeding also may occur (195). Premature infants and babies born to mothers receiving anticonvulsant therapy with hydantoins are more prone to develop vitamin K deficiency (196), and affected newborns have a prolonged PT because of defective γ-carboxylation of the vitamin K-dependent factors. Prophylactic use of vitamin K at doses of 0.1 to 1 mg immediately after birth has prevented the appearance of this disorder (197, 198).

(Neonatal vitamin K deficiency is discussed in detail in Chapter 47.)

Low dietary intake can decrease total body stores of vitamin K, but adequate plasma levels of vitamin K-dependent clotting factors are still maintained, presumably through the vitamin K synthesized by gut flora (199). If low dietary intake occurs during a course of therapy with bowel-sterilizing antibiotics, however, markedly depressed levels of vitamin K-dependent coagulation factors ensue (190). Even so, it should be stressed that dietary vitamin K deficiency can affect nonhepatic tissues, such as bone, before any noticeable effect on γ-carboxylation of the vitamin K-dependent clotting factors, which are synthesized by hepatocytes, occurs. This is because the liver preferentially absorbs vitamin K from the circulation, thus depriving bone tissue when the plasma level may be within normal limits (181). That circulating osteocalcin is undercarboxylated in some healthy postmenopausal women, while the levels and functional activity of prothrombin are normal, supports this concept (200). In addition, administration of phylloquinone corrects the carboxylation abnormality of osteocalcin. More extensive studies are required, however, to assess the optimum concentration of vitamin K for the normal carboxylation of bone proteins.

It is difficult for clinically significant vitamin K deficiency to occur, because there usually must be concurrent antibiotic therapy and dietary insufficiency before levels of the vitamin K-dependent clotting factors fall low enough to elicit bleeding. Hemorrhagic manifestations caused by vitamin K deficiency, however, can occur in specific situations, such as individuals in the intensive care setting (201) with renal failure, and recovering from abdominal surgery who receive a diet low in vitamin K because of the omission of green leafy vegetables (202, 203). These individuals can experience bleeding disorders that manifest clinically as epistaxis, hematuria, retroperitoneal bleeding, and postsurgical wound bleeding. Uremia also can increase the hemorrhagic tendency of these individuals (202, 203). A special case of vitamin K deficiency is represented by individuals receiving parenteral nutrition for long periods of time (204, 205). Accordingly, these individuals require supplementation of their parenteral diet with approximately 150 µg of parenteral vitamin K per day.

Deficient absorption of vitamin K is associated with malabsorption of lipids and other fat-soluble vitamins, a process that usually occurs secondary to obstructive jaundice, lack of bile salts in the bowel, or intrinsic bowel diseases. Individuals with obstructive jaundice can manifest excessive bleeding from mucosa or during surgery (206). This hemorrhagic tendency can be easily reversed by parenteral administration of vitamin K. During severe bleeding, these individuals may need fresh frozen plasma, because correction of the coagulation abnormality in response to vitamin K administration may be delayed for 12 to 24 hours.

Some individuals with hepatocellular diseases, biliary cirrhosis, or cholestatic hepatitis also may have a component of intrahepatic biliary obstruction that causes vitamin K deficiency (207). For this reason, it is advisable to give daily vitamin K doses of 5 mg for 3 days and to measure the effect of this therapy on the PT. Bowel diseases, such as celiac disease, ulcerative colitis, and regional ileitis, also can lead to vitamin K malabsorption requiring replacement therapy (208). Indeed, occult malabsorption of vitamin K secondary to subclinical celiac disease can manifest as ecchymoses or as a warfarin requirement of less than 1.3 mg daily when indicated for cardiac valve replacement (209). Moreover, certain surgical procedures of the bowel, such as ileojejunostomy, which occasionally is performed as a treatment for severe obesity, can induce malabsorption of fat-soluble vitamins; therefore, vitamin K replacement therapy should be used to avoid complications.

## TREATMENT

Treatment of vitamin K deficiency largely depends on the clinical condition responsible for the deficiency. When an inadequate diet is accompanied by an antibiotic-induced decrease in biosynthesis through the intestinal flora, oral supplementation with vitamin $K_1$ is sufficient. With malabsorption syndromes, however, the vitamin K should be administered parenterally (10 mg/day subcutaneously for 3 to 4 days) and the clinical response assessed by following the PT. Individuals with severe alterations of the hemostatic system should be treated with intravenous vitamin K preparations; absorption from subcutaneous tissue may be incomplete in those who are hypotensive because of hemorrhage. Commonly, 5 mg of phytonadione, (AquaMephyton, Merck & Co, West Point, PA) are given by slow intravenous administration to avoid potential adverse effects such as hypotension, burning sensations, and dizziness (210). The intramuscular route should be avoided, because it can lead to hematomas. Finally, individuals with overt gastrointestinal bleeding and gross hematuria, or those with bleeding into cavities resulting in the compromise of organ function (e.g., central nervous system, pleural cavity, and so on), should be treated with fresh frozen plasma, as outlined under "Treatment of the Coagulopathy of Liver Disease.")

## REFERENCES

1. Deutsch E. Blood coagulation changes in liver diseases. In: Popper H, Schaffner F, eds. Progress in liver diseases. New York: Grune & Stratton, 1965;2:69–83.
2. Flute PT. Clotting abnormalities in liver disease. Prog Liver Dis 1979;6:301–312.
3. Kelly DA, Tuddenham EG. Haemostatic problems in liver disease. Gut 1986;27:339–349.
4. Walls WD, Losowsky MS. The hemostatic defect of liver disease. Gastroenterology 1971;60:108–119.
5. Spector I, Corn M. Laboratory tests of hemostasis: the relation to hemorrhage in liver disease. Arch Intern Med 1967;119:577–582.
6. Anonymous. Prediction of the first variceal hemorrhage in individuals with cirrhosis of the liver and esophageal varices. A prospective multicenter study. The North Italian Endoscopic Club for the Study and Treatment of Esophageal Varices. N Engl J Med 1988;319:983–989.
7. Rector WG Jr. Portal hypertension: a permissive factor only in the development of ascites and variceal bleeding. Liver 1986;6:221–226.
8. Snady H, Feinman L. Prediction of variceal hemorrhage: a prospective study. Am J Gastroenterol 1988;83:519–525.
9. Hiller E, Hegemann F, Possinger K. Hypercoagulability in acute esophageal variceal bleeding. Thromb Res 1981;22:243–251.
10. Bertaglia E, Belmont P, Vertolli U et al. Bleeding in cirrhotic individuals: a precipitating factor due to intravascular coagulation or to hepatic failure? Haemostasis 1983;13:328–334.
11. Boks AL, Brommer EJ, Schalm SW et al. Hemostasis and fibrinolysis in severe liver failure and their relation to hemorrhage. Hepatology 1986;6:79–86.
12. Vigneri S, Termini R, Piraino A et al. The stomach in liver cirrhosis: endoscopic, morphological, and clinical correlations. Gastroenterology 1991;101:472–478.
13. Hosking SW. Congestive gastropathy in portal hypertension: variations in prevalence. Hepatology 1989;10:257–258.
14. Poynard T, Cales P, Pasta L et al. Beta-adrenergic-antagonist drugs in the prevention of gastrointestinal bleeding in individuals with cirrhosis and esophageal varices. N Engl J Med 1991;324:1532–1538.
15. Perez-Ayuso RM, Pique JM, Bosch J et al. Propranolol in prevention of recurrent bleeding from severe portal hypertensive gastropathy in cirrhosis. Lancet 1991;337:1431–1434.
16. Schafer AI. Bleeding and thrombosis in the myeloproliferative disorders. Blood 1984;64:1–12.
17. Valla D, Casadevall N, Lacombe C et al. Primary myeloproliferative disorder and hepatic vein thrombosis. Ann Intern Med 1985;103:329–334.
18. Mitchell MC, Biotnott KJ, Kaufman S et al. Budd-Chiari syndrome: etiology, diagnosis and management. Medicine (Baltimore) 1982;61:199–218.
19. Knox TA, Kaplan MM. Myeloproliferative disorders in portal vein thrombosis in adults. Hepatology 1989;10:392–393.
20. Martinez J, Shapiro SS, Holburn RR. Metabolism of human prothrombin and fibrinogen in individuals with thrombocytosis secondary to myeloproliferative states. Blood 1973;42:35–46.
21. Peytremann R, Rhodes RS, Hartmann RC. Thrombosis in paroxysmal nocturnal hemoglobinuria (PNH) with particular reference to progressive, diffuse hepatic venous thrombosis. Ser Haematol 1972;5:115–136.
22. Hartmann RC, Luther AB, Jenkins DE Jr et al. Fulminant hepatic venous thrombosis (Budd-Chiari syndrome) in paroxysmal nocturnal hemoglobinuria: definition of a medical emergency. Johns Hopkins Med J 1980;146:247–254.
23. Schafer AI. The hypercoagulable states. Ann Intern Med 1985;102:814–828.
24. Lewis JH, Tice HL, Zimmerman HJ. Budd-Chiari syndrome associated with oral contraceptives steroids: review of treatment of 47 cases. Dig Dis Sci 1983;28:673–683.
25. Cohen P, Gardner FH, Barnett GO. Reclassification of the thrombocytopenias by the Cr-51 labeling method for measuring platelet life span. N Engl J Med 1961;264:1294–1299.
26. Toghill PJ, Green S, Ferguson F. Platelet dynamics in chronic liver disease with special reference to the role of the spleen. Clin Pathol 1977;30:367–371.
27. Stein SF, Harker LA. Kinetic and functional studies of platelets, fibrinogen, and plasminogen in individuals with hepatic cirrhosis. J Lab Clin Med 1982;99:217–230.
28. Aster RH. Pooling of platelets in the spleen: role in the pathogenesis of "hypersplenic" thrombocytopenia. J Clin Invest 1966;45:645–657.
29. Wadenvik H, Jacobsson S, Kutti J et al. In vitro and in vivo behavior of $^{111}$In-labelled platelets: an experimental study of healthy male volunteers. Eur J Haematol 1987;38:415–425.
30. Desforges JF, Bigelow FS, Chalmers TC. The effects of massive gastrointestinal hemorrhage on hemostasis. J Lab Clin Med 1954;43:501–510.
31. Shimodaira S, Ishida F, Ichikawa N et al. Serum thrombopoietin (c-Mpl ligand) levels in individuals with liver cirrhosis. Thromb Haemost 1996;76:545–548.
32. Lozner EL. Seminars on blood coagulation. Differential diagnosis, pathogenesis and treatment of the thrombocytopenic purpuras. Am J Med 1953;14:449–468.
33. Barrison IG, Knight ID, Viola L et al. Platelet associated immunoglobulins on chronic liver disease. Br J Haematol 1981;48:347–350.
34. Jaffe EA, Hoyer LW, Nachman RL. Synthesis of antihemophilic factor antigen by cultured human endothelial cells. J Clin Invest 1973;52:2757–2764.
35. Kelly DA, Summerfield JA, Tuddenham EGD. Localization of factor VIIIC:

antigen in guinea-pig tissues and isolated liver cell fractions. Br J Haematol 1984;56:535–543.

36. Furie B, Furie BC. Molecular basis of vitamin K-dependent g-carboxylation. Blood 1990;75:1753–1762.
37. Lechner K, Niessner H, Thaler E. Coagulation abnormalities in liver disease. Semin Thromb Hemost 1977;4:40–56.
38. Kuppfer HG, Gee W, Ewald AT et al. Statistical correlation of liver function tests with coagulation factor deficiencies in Laennec's cirrhosis. Thromb Diath Haemorrh 1964;10:317–331.
39. Rapaport SI, Ames SB, Mikkelsen AS et al. Plasma clotting factors in chronic hepatocellular disease. N Engl J Med 1960;263:278–282.
40. Dymock IW, Tucker JS, Woolf IL et al. Coagulation studies as a prognostic index in acute liver failure. Br J Haematol 1975;29:385–395.
41. Green G, Poller L, Thomson JM et al. Factor VII as a marker of hepatocellular synthetic function in liver disease. J Clin Pathol 1976;29:971–975.
42. Blanchard RA, Furie BC, Jorgensen M. Acquired vitamin K-dependent carboxylation deficiency on liver disease. N Engl J Med 1981;305:242–248.
43. Liebman HA, Furie BC, Tong MJ et al. Des-g-carboxy (abnormal) prothrombin as a serum marker of primary hepatocellular carcinoma. N Engl J Med 1984;310:1427–1431.
44. Owren PA. The diagnostic and prognostic significance of plasma prothrombin and factor V levels in parenchymatous hepatitis and obstructive jaundice. Scand J Lab Clin Invest 1949;1:131–140.
45. Izumi S, Langley PG, Wendon J et al. Coagulation factor V levels as a prognostic indicator in fulminant hepatic failure. Hepatology 1996;23:1507–1511.
46. Cederblad G. Observations of increased levels of blood coagulation factors and other plasma proteins in cholestatic liver disease. Scand J Gastroenterol 1976;11:391–396.
47. Green AJ, Ratnoff OD. Elevated antihemophilic factor (AHF, factor VIII) procoagulant activity and AHF-like antigen in alcoholic cirrhosis of the liver. J Lab Clin Med 1974;83:189–197.
48. Meili EO, Straub PW. Elevation of factor VIII in acute fatal liver necrosis. Thromb Diath Haemorrh 1970;24:161–174.
49. Nussbaum M, Morse BS. Plasma fibrin stabilizing factor activity in various diseases. Blood 1964;23:669–678.
50. Biland L, Duckert F, Prisender S et al. Quantitative estimation of coagulation factors in liver disease: the diagnostic and prognostic value of factor XIII, factor V, and plasminogen. Thromb Haemost 1978;39:646–656.
51. Rake MO, Pannell G, Flute PT. Intravascular coagulation in acute hepatic necrosis. Lancet 1970;i:533–537.
52. van der Walt JA, Gomperts ED, Kew MC. Hemostatic factors in primary hepatocellular cancer. Cancer 1977;40:1593–1603.
53. von Felten A, Straub PW, Frick PG. Dysfibrinogenemia in a individual with primary hepatoma. First observation of an acquired abnormality of fibrin monomer aggregation. N Engl J Med 1969;280:405–409.
54. Verhaeghe R, Van Damme B, Molla A et al. Dysfibrinogenaemia associated with primary hepatoma. Scand J Haematol 1972;9:451–458.
55. Gralnick HR, Givelber H, Abrams E. Dysfibrinogenemia associated with hepatoma: increased carbohydrate content of the fibrinogen molecule. N Engl J Med 1978;299:221–226.
56. Soria J, Soria C, Samama M et al. Dysfibrinogénémies acquises dans les atteintes hépatiques sévères. Coagulation 1970;3:37–44.
57. Green G, Thomson JM, Dymock IW et al. Abnormal fibrin polymerization in liver disease. Br J Haematol 1976;34:427–439.
58. Lane DA, Scully MF, Thomas DP et al. Acquired dysfibrinogenaemia in acute and chronic liver disease. Br J Haematol 1977;35:301–308.
59. Francis JL, Armstrong DJ. Acquired dysfibrinogenaemia in liver disease. J Clin Pathol 1982;35:667–672.
60. Palascak JE, Martinez J. Dysfibrinogenemia associated with liver disease. J Clin Invest 1977;60:89–95.
61. Martinez J, Palascak JE, Kwasniak D. Abnormal sialic acid content of the dysfibrinogenemia associated with liver disease. J Clin Invest 1978;61:535–538.
62. Martinez J, MacDonald KA, Palascak JE. The role of sialic acid in the dysfibrinogenemia associated with liver disease: distribution of sialic acid on the constituent chains. Blood 1983;61:1196–1202.
63. Martinez J, Keane PM, Gilman PB et al. The abnormal carbohydrate composition of the dysfibrinogenemia associated with liver disease. Ann N Y Acad Sci 1983;408:388–396.
64. Martinez J, Barsigian C. Carbohydrate abnormalities of N-linked plasma glycoproteins in liver disease. Lab Invest 1987;57:240–257.
65. Galanakis DK, Martinez J, McDevitt C et al. The role of sialic acid on human fetal fibrinogen function. Symposium on fibrinogen. Ann N Y Acad Sci 1983;408:640–643.
66. Duckert F. Behaviour of antithrombin III in liver disease. Scand J Gastroenterol Suppl 1973;19:109–112.
67. Rodzynek JJ, Preux C, Leautaud P et al. Diagnostic value of anti-thrombin III and aminopyrine breath test in liver disease. Arch Intern Med 1986;146:677–680.
68. Mosvold J, Abildgaard U, Jenssen H et al. Low antithrombin III in acute hepatic failure at term. Scand J Haematol 1982;29:48–50.
69. Mannucci L, Dioguardi N, Del Ninno E et al. Value of normotest and

antithrombin III in the assessment of liver function. Scand J Gastroenterol Suppl 1973;19:103–107.
70. Chan V, Lai CL, Chan TK. Metabolism of antithrombin III in cirrhosis and carcinoma of the liver. Clin Sci 1981;60:681–688.
71. Schipper HG, tenCate JW. Antithrombin III transfusion in individuals with hepatic cirrhosis. Br J Haematol 1982;52:25–33.
72. Mannucci PM, Vigano S. Deficiencies of protein C, an inhibitor of blood coagulation. Lancet 1982;ii:463–467.
73. Vigano S, Mannucci PM, D'Angelo A et al. The significance of protein C antigen in acute and chronic liver biliary disease. Am J Clin Pathol 1985;84:454–458.
74. Yoshikawa Y, Sakata Y, Toda G et al. The acquired vitamin K-dependent g-carboxylation deficiency in hepatocellular carcinoma involves not only prothrombin, but also protein C. Hepatology 1988;8:524–530.
75. D'Angelo A, Vigano-D'Angelo S et al. Comp PC. Acquired deficiencies of protein S. Protein S activity during oral anticoagulation, in liver disease, and in disseminated intravascular coagulation. Clin Invest 1988;81:1445–1454.
76. Wolf M, Boyer-Neumann C, Leroy-Matheron C et al. Functional assay of protein S in 70 individuals with congenital and acquired disorders. Blood Coagulation Fibrinolysis 1991;2:705–712.
77. Bajaj MS, Rana SV, Wysolmerski RB et al. Inhibitor of the factor VIIa-tissue factor complex is reduced in individuals with disseminated intravascular coagulation but not in individuals with severe hepatocellular disease. J Clin Invest 1987;79:1874–1878.
78. Novotny WF, Brown SG, Miletich JP et al. Plasma antigen levels of the lipoprotein-associated coagulation inhibitor in patient samples. Blood 1991;78:387–393.
79. Warr TA, Rapaport SI. Human plasma extrinsic tathway inhibitor activity: II. Plasma levels in disseminated intravascular coagulation and hepatocellular disease. Blood 1989;74:994–998.
80. Straub PW. Diffuse intravascular coagulation in liver disease? Semin Thromb Hemost 1977;4:29–39.
81. Tytgat GN, Collen D, Verstraete M. Metabolism of fibrinogen in cirrhosis of the liver. J Clin Invest 1971;50:169–701.
82. Clark RD, Gazzard BG, Lewis ML et al. Fibrinogen metabolism in acute hepatitis and active chronic hepatitis. Br J Haematol 1975;30:95–102.
83. Coleman M, Bettigole RE, Pasmantier N. Fibrinogen survival in cirrhosis: improvement by 'low dose' heparin. Ann Intern Med 1975;83:79–81.
84. Laursen B, Mortensen JZ, Frost L et al. Disseminated intravascular coagulation in hepatic failure treated with antithrombin III. Thromb Res 1981;22:701–704.
85. Langley PG, Hughes RD, Forbes A et al. Controlled trial of antithrombin III supplementation in fulminant hepatic failure. J Hepatol 1993;17:326–331.
86. Lechner K, Kyrle PA. Antithrombin III concentrates—are they clinically useful? Thromb Haemost 1995;73:340–348.
87. Paramo JA, Rifon J, Fernandez J et al. Thrombin activation and increased fibrinolysis in individuals with chronic liver disease. Blood Coagulation Fibrinolysis 1991;2:227–230.
88. Coccheri S, Mannucci PM, Palareti G et al. Significance of plasma fibrinopeptide A and high molecular weight fibrinogen in individuals with liver cirrhosis. Br J Haematol 1982;52:503–509.
89. Mombelli G, Fiori G, Monotti R et al. Fibrinopeptide A in liver cirrhosis: evidence against a major contribution of disseminated intravascular coagulation to coagulopathy of chronic liver disease. J Lab Clin Med 1993;121:83–90.
90. Gazzard BG, Portmann B, Murray-Lyon IM et al. Causes of death in fulminant hepatic failure and relationship to quantitative histological assessment of parenchymal damage. Q J Med 1975;44:615–626.
91. Goodpasture EW. Fibrinolysis in chronic hepatic insufficiency. Johns Hopkins Hosp Bull 1914;25:330–336.
92. Ratnoff OD. Studies on a proteolytic enzyme in human plasma. IV. The rate of lysis of plasma clots in normal and diseased individuals, with particular reference to hepatic disease. Bull Johns Hopkins Hosp 1949;84:29–42.
93. Tytgat G, Collen D, De Vreker R et al. Investigations on the fibrinolytic system in liver cirrhosis. Acta Haematol 1968;40:265–274.
94. Francis RB Jr, Feinstein DI. Clinical significance of accelerated fibrinolysis in liver disease. Haemostasis 1984;14:460–465.
95. Dioguardi N, Mari D, Del Ninno E et al. Fibrinolysis in cholestatic jaundice. Br Med J 1973;2:778–779.
96. Violi F, Ferro D, Basili S et al. Hyperfibrinolysis resulting from clotting activation in patients with different degrees of cirrhosis. Hepatology 1993;17:78–83.
97. Hersch SL, Kunelis T, Francis RB Jr. The pathogenesis of accelerated fibrinolysis in liver cirrhosis: a critical role for tissue plasminogen activator inhibitor. Blood 1987;69:1315–1319.
98. Grossi CE, Rousselot LM, Panke WF. Coagulation defects in individuals with cirrhosis of the liver undergoing porta-systemic shunts. Am J Surg 1962;104:512–526.
99. Aoki N, Yamanka T. The a2-plasmin inhibitor levels in liver diseases. Clin Chim Acta 1978;84:99–105.

100. Knot EA, Drijfhout HR, ten Cate JW et al. a2-Plasmin inhibitor metabolism in individuals with liver cirrhosis. J Lab Clin Med 1985;105:353–358.
101. Collen D, Rouvier J, Chamone DA et al. Turnover of radiolabelled plasminogen and prothrombin in cirrhosis of the liver. Eur J Clin Invest 1978;8:185–188.
102. Violi F, Ferro D, Basili S et al. Ongoing prothrombotic state in the portal circulation of cirrhotic patients. Thromb Haemost 1997;77;44–47.
103. Harmon DC, Demirjian Z, Ellman L et al. Disseminated intravascular coagulation with the peritoneovenous shunt. Ann Intern Med 1979;90:774–776.
104. Lerner RG, Nelson JC, Corines P et al. Disseminated intravascular coagulation. Complications of LeVeen peritoneovenous shunts. JAMA 1978;240–2066.
105. Gleysteen JJ, Hussey CV, Heckman MG. The cause of coagulopathy after peritoneovenous shunt for malignant ascites. Arch Surg 1990;125:474–477.
106. Cowan DH. Effect of alcoholism on hemostasis. Semin Hematol 1980;17:137–147.
107. Post RM, Desforges JF. Thrombocytopenia and alcoholism. Ann Intern Med 1968;68:1230–1236.
108. Sullivan LW, Herber V. Suppression of hematopoiesis by ethanol. J Clin Invest 1964;43:2048–2062.
109. Lindenbaum J. Folate and vitamin B12 deficiences in alcoholism. Semin Hematol 1980;17:119–129.
110. Levy RN, Sawitsky A, Florman A et al. Fatal aplastic anemia after hepatitis. Report of five cases. N Engl J Med 1965;273:1118–1123.
111. Rubin E, Gottlieb C, Vogel P. Syndrome of hepatitis and aplastic anemia. Am J Med 1968;45:88–97.
112. Camitta BM, Nathan DG, Forman EN et al. Posthepatic severe aplastic anemia—an indication for early bone marrow transplantation. Blood 1974;43:473–483.
113. Thomas DP, Ream VJ, Stuart RK. Platelet aggregation in individuals with Laennec's cirrhosis of the liver. N Engl J Med 1967;276:1344–1348.
114. Laffi G, Cominelli F, Ruggiero M et al. Molecular mechanism underlying impaired platelet responsiveness in liver cirrhosis. FEBS Lett 1987;220:217–219.
115. Rubin MH, Weston MJ, Bullock G et al. Abnormal platelet function and ultrastructure in fulminant hepatic failure. Q J Med 1977;46:339–352.
116. Starzl TE, Demetris AJ, Van Thiel DH. Liver transplantation. N Engl J Med 1989;10:1014–1099.
117. Maddrey WC, Van Thiel DH. Liver transplantation: an overview. Hepatology 1990;8:948–959.
118. Bontempo FA, Lewis JH, Van Thiel DH et al. The relation of preoperative coagulation findings to diagnosis, blood usage, and survival in adult liver transplantation. Transplantation 1985;39:532–536.
119. Van Thiel DH, Tarter R, Gavaler JS et al. Liver transplantation in adults. An analysis of costs and benefits at the University of Pittsburgh. Gastroenterology 1986;90:211–216.
120. Palareti G, Legnani C, Maccaferri M et al. Coagulation and fibrinolysis in orthotopic liver transplantation: role of the recipient's disease and use of antithrombin III concentrates. Orsola Working Group on Liver Transplantation. Haemostasis 1991;21:68–76.
121. Owen CA Jr, Rettke SR, Bowie EJ. Hemostatic evaluation of individuals undergoing liver transplantation. Mayo Clin Proc 1987;62:761–772.
122. Lewis JH, Bontempo FA, Awad SA et al. Liver transplantation: intraoperative changes in coagulation factors in 100 first transplants. Hepatology 1989;9:710–714.
123. Clayton DG, Miro AM, Kramer DJ et al. Quantification of thrombelastographic changes after blood component transfusion in individuals with liver disease in the intensive care unit. Anesth Analg 1995;81:272–278.
124. Hutchison DE, Genton E, Porter KA et al. Platelet changes following clinical and experimental hepatic homotransplantation. Arch Surg 1968;97:27–33.
125. Dzik WH, Arkin CF, Jenkins RL et al. Fibrinolysis during liver transplantation in humans: role of tissue-type plasminogen activator. Blood 1988;71:1090–1095.
126. Segal H, Cottam S, Potter D et al. Coagulation and fibrinolysis in primary biliary cirrhosis compared with other liver disease and during orthotopic liver transplantation. Hepatology 1997;25:683–688.
127. Stahl RL, Duncan A, Hooks MA et al. A hypercoagulable state follows orthotopic liver transplantation. Hepatology 1990;12:553–558.
128. Gosseye S, Van Obbergh L, Weynand B et al. Platelet aggregates in small lung vessels and death during liver transplantation. Lancet 1991;338:532–534.
129. Coccheri S, Palareti G. Antithrombin III replacement in orthotopic liver transplantation. Semin Thromb Hemost 1993;19:268–272.
130. Cransac M, Carles J, Bernard PH et al. Heterozygous protein C deficiency and dysfibrinogenemia acquired by liver transplantation. Transpl Int 1995;8:307–311.
131. Seligsohn U, Shani M, Ramot B. Gilbert syndrome and factor VII deficiency. Lancet 1970;i:1398.
132. Kovacs MJ, Wong A, MacKinnon K et al. Assessment of the validity of the INR system for individuals with liver impairment. Thromb Haemost 1994;71:727–730.
133. Robert A, Chazouilleres O. Prothrombin time in liver failure: time, ratio, activity percentage, or international normalized ratio? Hepatology 1996;24:1392–1394.
134. Coccheri S, Gasbarrini G. The relevance of blood clotting tests in chronic aggressive hepatitis. Scand J Gastroenterol Suppl 1973;19:97–101.
135. Fried MW. The liver in systemic illness. In: Zakim D, Boyer TD, eds. Hepatology: a textbook of liver disease. 3rd ed. Philadelphia: WB Saunders, 1996:1706–1726.
136. Koller F. Theory and experience behind the use of coagulation tests in diagnosis and prognosis of liver disease. Scand J Gastroenterol Suppl 1973;19:51–61.
137. Clark R, Rake MO, Flute PT et al. Coagulation abnormalities in acute liver failure: pathogenetic and therapeutic implications. Scand J Gastroenterol 1973;19:63–70.
138. Clark R, Borirakchanyavat V, Gazzard BG et al. Disordered hemostasis in liver damage from paracetamol overdose. Gastroenterology 1973;65:788–795.
139. Boyadjian H. Changes in antithrombin III activity in the various clinical forms of viral hepatitis. Folia Med 1981;23:11–17.
140. Sato S, Murakami A, Yoshida T et al. Usefulness of antithrombin III and a2-plasmin inhibitor in early differentiation of fulminant hepatitis and severe form of acute hepatitis. Gastroenterol Jpn 1983;18:128–136.
141. Christensen E, Schlichting P, Fauerholdt L et al. Changes of laboratory variables with time in cirrhosis: prognostic and therapeutic significance. Hepatology 1985;5:843–853.
142. Tygstrup N. The prognostic value of laboratory tests in liver disease. Scand J Gastroenterol Suppl 1973;19:47–50.
143. Lurie B, Creter D. Coagulation studies for severe liver disease detection in a gastroenterologic department. Digestion 1981;21:244–247.
144. Sherlock S. Needle biopsy of the liver. In: Sherlock S, ed. Diseases of the liver and biliary system. Oxford: Blackwell Scientific Publications, 1989;36–48.
145. Ishak KG, Schiff ER, Schiff L. Needle biopsy of the liver. In: Schiff L, Schiff ER, eds. Diseases of the liver. Philadelphia: JB Lippincott, 1987:399–441.
146. McVay PA, Toy PT. Lack of increased bleeding after liver biopsy in individuals with mild hemostatic abnormalities. Am J Clin Pathol 1990;94:747–753.
147. Sharma P, McDonald GB, Banaji M. The risk of bleeding after percutaneous liver biopsy: relation to platelet count. J Clin Gastroenterol 1982;4:451–453.
148. Consensus conference. Platelet transfusion therapy. JAMA 1987;257:1777–1780.
149. Sawyerr AM, McCormick PA, Tennyson GS et al. A comparison of transjugular and plugged-percutaneous liver biopsy in individuals with impaired coagulation. J Hepatol 1993;17:81–85.
150. Dillon JF, Simpson KJ, Hayes PC. Liver biopsy bleeding time: an unpredictable event. J Gastroenterol Hepatol 1994;9:269–271.
151. Inabnet WB, Deziel DJ. Laparoscopic liver biopsy in individuals with coagulopathy, portal hypertension, and ascites. Am Surg 1995;61:603–606.
152. DeLoughery TG, Liebler JM, Simonds V, Goodnight SH. Invasive line placement in critically ill individuals: do hemostatic defects matter? Transfusion 1996;36:827–831.
153. Sokolowski JW Jr, Burgher LW, Jones FL Jr et al. Guidelines for thoracentesis and needle biopsy of the pleura. Am Rev Respir Dis 1989;140:257–258.
154. Health and Public Policy Committee, American College of Physicians. Diagnostic thoracentesis and pleural biopsy in pleural effusions. Ann Intern Med 1985;103:799–802.
155. Runyon BA. Paracentesis of ascitic fluid. A safe procedure. Arch Intern Med 1986;146:2259–2261.
156. McVay PA, Toy PTCY. Lack of increased bleeding after paracentesis and thoracentesis in patients with mild coagulation abnormalities. Transfusion 1991;31:164–171.
157. Friedman LS, Maddrey WC. Surgery in the individual with liver disease. Med Clin North Am 1987;71:453–476.
158. Schwartz SI. Biliary tract surgery and cirrhosis: a critical combination. Surgery 1981;90:577–583.
159. Aranha GV, Sontag SJ, Greenlee HB. Cholecystectomy in cirrhotic individuals: a formidable operation. Am J Surg 1982;143:55–60.
160. Garrison RN, Cryer HM, Howard DA, Polk HC Jr. Clarification of risk factors for abdominal operations in individuals with hepatic cirrhosis. Ann Surg 1984;199:648–655.
161. Aranha GV, Greenlee HB. Intra-abdominal surgery in individuals with advanced cirrhosis. Arch Surg 1986;121:275–277.
162. Doberneck RC, Sterling WA Jr, Allison DC. Morbidity and mortality after operation in nonbleeding cirrhotic individuals. Am J Surg 1983;146:306–309.
163. Mannucci PM, Franchi F, Dioguardi N. Correction of abnormal coagulation in chronic liver disease by combined use of fresh frozen plasma and prothrombin complex concentrates. Lancet 1976;ii:542–545.
164. Gazzard BG, Henderson JM, Williams R. The use of fresh frozen plasma

or a concentrate of factor IX as replacement therapy before liver biopsy. Gut 1975;16:621–625.

165. Jagathambal K, Grunwald HW, Rosner F. Evaluation and management of the bleeding patient. Med Clin North Am 1981;65:133–146.

166. Munoz SJ, Ballas SK, Moritz MJ et al. Perioperative management of fulminant and subfulminant hepatic failure with therapeutic plasmapheresis. Transplant Proc 1989;21:3535–3536.

167. Sandler SG, Rath CE, Ruder A. Prothrombin complex concentrates in acquired hypoprothrombinemia. Ann Intern Med 1973;79:485–491.

168. Blatt PM, Lundblad RL, Kingdon HS et al. Thrombogenic materials in prothrombin complex concentrates. Ann Intern Med 1974;81:766–770.

169. Kasper CK. Thromboembolic complications. Thromb Diath Haemorrh 1975;33:640–644.

170. Marassi A, Manzullo V, di Carlo V et al. Thromboembolism following prothrombin complex concentrates and major surgery in severe liver disease. Thromb Haemost 1978;39:787–788.

171. Cederbaum AI, Blatt PM, Roberts HR. Intravascular coagulation with use of human prothrombin complex concentrates. Ann Intern Med 1976;84:683–687.

172. Davey RJ, Shashaty GG, Rath CE. Acute coagulopathy following infusion of prothrombin complex concentrate. Am J Med 1976;60:719–722.

173. Hultin MB. Activated clotting factors in factor IX concentrates. Blood 1979;54:1028–1038.

174. Gazzard BG, Clark R, Borirakchanyavat V et al. A controlled trial of heparin therapy in the coagulation defect of paracetamol-induced hepatic necrosis. Gut 1974;15:89–93.

175. el-Khishen MA, Henderson JM, Millikan WJ Jr et al. Splenectomy is contraindicated for thrombocytopenia secondary to portal hypertension. Surg Gynecol Obstet 1985;160:233–238.

176. Sullivan BH, Tumen HJ. The effect of portocaval shunt on thrombocytopenia associated with portal hypertension. Ann Intern Med 1961;55:598–603.

177. Mannucci PM, Vicente V, Vianello L et al. Controlled trial of desmopressin in liver cirrhosis and other conditions associated with a prolonged bleeding time. Blood 1986;67:1148–1153.

178. Burroughs AK, Matthews K, Qadiri M et al. Desmopressin and bleeding time in individuals with cirrhosis. Br Med J (Clin Res) 1985;291:1377–1381.

179. Lind SE. The bleeding time does not predict surgical bleeding. Blood 1991;77:2547–2552.

180. Rodgers RP, Levin J. A critical reappraisal of the bleeding time. Semin Thromb Hemost 1990;16:1–20.

181. Vermeer C, Hamulyak K. Pathophysiology of vitamin K-deficiency and oral anticoagulants. Semin Thromb Haemost 1991;66:153–159.

182. Bjornsson TD. Vitamin K and vitamin K antagonists. Drugs Nutrients 1984;12:429–473.

183. Seifert RM. Analysis of vitamin K1 in some green leafy vegetables by gas chromatography. J Agric Food Chem 1979;27:1301–1304.

184. Blomstrand R, Forsgren L. Vitamin K1-3H in man. Its intestinal absorption and transport in the thoracic duct lymph. Int Z Vitaminforsch 1968;38:45–64.

185. Wiss O, Gloor H. Absorption, distribution, storage and metabolites of vitamin K and related quinones. Vitam Horm 1966;24:575–586.

186. Shearer MJ, Barkhan P, Webster GR. Absorption and excretion of an oral dose of tritiated vitamin K1 in man. Br J Haematol 1970;18:297–308.

187. Bell RG, Matschiner JT. Intracellular distribution of vitamin K in the rat. Biochim Biophys Acta 1969;184:597–603.

188. Bjornsson TD, Meffin PJ, Swezey SE et al. Disposition and turnover of vitamin K1 in man. In: Suttie JW, ed. Vitamin K metabolism and vitamin K-dependent proteins. Baltimore: Baltimore Park Press, 1980;328–332.

189. Bjornsson TD, Meffin PJ, Swezey SE et al. Effects of clofibrate and warfarin alone and in combination on the disposition of vitamin K1. J Pharmacol Exp Ther 1979;210:322–326.

190. Frick PG, Riedler G, Brogli H. Dose response and minimal daily requirement for vitamin K in man. J Appl Physiol 1967;23:387–389.

191. Haroon Y, Shearer MJ, Rahim S et al. The content of phylloquinone (vitamin K1) in human milk, cows' milk, and infant formula foods determined by high-performance liquid chromatography. J Nutr 1982;112:1105–1117.

192. Dam H, Dyggve H, Larsen H et al. Relation of vitamin K deficiency to hemorrhagic disease of the newborn. Adv Pediatr 1952;5:129–153.

193. Keenan WJ, Jewett T, Glueck HI. Role of feeding and vitamin K in hypoprothrombinemia of the newborn. Am J Dis Child 1971;121:271–277.

194. Brinkhous KM, Smith HP, Warner ED. Plasma prothrombin level in normal infancy and in hemorrhagic disease of the newborn. Am J Med Sci 1937;193:475–480.

195. Sutherland JM, Glueck HI, Glesser G. Hemorrhagic disease of the newborn. Breast feeding as a necessary factor in the pathogenesis. Am J Dis Child 1967;113:524–533.

196. Evans AR, Forrester RM, Discombe C. Neonatal hemorrhage following maternal anticonvulsant therapy. Lancet 1970;i:517–518.

197. Committee on Nutrition, American Academy of Pediatrics. Vitamin K supplementation for infants receiving milk substitute infant formulas and for those with fat malabsorption. Pediatrics 1971;48:483–487.

198. Seeler RA. Vitamin K deficiency—revisited. IMJ 1975;147:59–61,82.

199. Olson, RE, Meyer RG, Chao J et al. The vitamin K requirement in man [Abstract]. Circulation 1984;70(II):97.

200. Knapen MH, Hamulyak K, Vermeer C. The effect of vitamin K supplementation on circulating osteocalcin (bone Gla-protein) and urinary calcium excretion. Ann Intern Med 1989;111:1001–1005.

201. Chakraverty R, Davidson S, Peggs K et al. The incidence and cause of coagulopathies in an intensive care population. Br J Haematol 1996;93:460–463.

202. Ansell JE, Kumar R, Deykin D. The spectrum of vitamin K deficiency. JAMA 1977;238:40–42.

203. Pineo GF, Gallus AS, Hirsh J. Unexpected vitamin K deficiency in hospitalized patients. Can Med Assoc J 1973;109:880–883.

204. Dudrick SJ, Wilmore DW, Vars HM et al. Long-term total parenteral nutrition with growth, development and positive nitrogen balance. Surgery 1968;64:134–142.

205. Ryan JA Jr. Complication of total parenteral nutrition. In: Fischer E, ed. Total parenteral nutrition. Boston: Little, Brown, 1976:55–100.

206. Boland EW. Pathologic data in cases of jaundice and fatal hemorrhage. Proc Staff Meet Mayo Clinic 1938;13:70–72.

207. Kaplan MM, Elta GH, Furie B et al. Fat soluble vitamin nutriture in primary biliary cirrhosis. Gastroenterology 1988;95:787–792.

208. Krasinski SD, Russell RM, Furie BC et al. The prevalence of vitamin K deficiency in chronic gastrointestinal disorders. Am J Clin Nutr 1985;41:639–643.

209. Avery RA, Duncan WE, Alving BM. Severe vitamin K deficiency induced by occult celiac disease BR96-026 [Letter]. Am J Hematol 1996;53:55.

210. Barash P, Kitahata LM, Mandel S. Acute cardiovascular collapse after intravenous phytonadione. Anesth Analg 1976;55:304–306.

# CHAPTER 46

# MATERNAL HEMOSTASIS: COAGULATION PROBLEMS OF PREGNANCY

Bryan T. Oshiro and D. Ware Branch

## INTRODUCTION

For the vast majority of women, the risk of thrombosis or hemorrhage is greater during pregnancy than at any other time in their lives. Pregnancy is recognized as a "thrombogenic state," and thromboembolic disease is a leading cause of obstetric morbidity and mortality in western countries. What most physicians would consider frank hemorrhage occurs routinely with vaginal birth. Bleeding from the placenta, uterus, or lower genital tract may complicate pregnancy before, during, or after delivery. The physiologic alterations in maternal hemostatic and cardiovascular systems are primarily responsible for the increased risk of thrombosis and hemorrhage, but inherited or acquired predispositions may also play a key role. Concerns about the fetus, especially with regard to medical treatment of disorders of hemostasis, influence maternal and physician decisions in management.

## HEMOSTASIS IN NORMAL PREGNANCY

Vascular and hematologic systems work together to maintain blood flow under physiologic circumstances and to halt the loss of blood rapidly when the integrity of the vascular system is breached. The importance of normal blood circulation for survival has led to a num-

ber of integrated and overlapping hemostatic mechanisms. These include the vasculature, cellular components of the blood, circulating procoagulants, anticoagulant, and fibrinolytic factors. The physiologic role of each in hemostasis is reviewed elsewhere in this text. Traditionally, pregnancy is considered a "hypercoagulable state" owing to an increase in the circulating concentrations of specific procoagulant factors, a decrease in the circulating concentrations of selected anticoagulant proteins, and a decrease in fibrinolysis.

One of the most important hemostatic elements of the vasculature is the endothelium. Under normal physiologic circumstances, this extremely active tissue serves a primarily anticoagulant role by separating circulating procoagulant factors and cells from underlying tissues with which they react. The endothelium favors vasodilation through the synthesis and secretion of prostacyclin ($PGI_2$) and nitric oxide (NO), inhibiting coagulation through synthesis and secretion of thrombomodulin and heparan sulfate, inhibiting platelet aggregation through $PGI_2$ and NO, and promoting fibrinolysis by synthesis and secretion of tissue-type plasminogen activator. Under certain circumstances, the endothelium may become activated or dysfunctional and take on a procoagulant role by synthesizing and secreting tissue factor, plasminogen activator inhibitor, and von Willebrand factor (vWf). In addition, certain stimuli cause a reduction in endothelial thrombomodulin content.

Pregnancy comprises a time of considerably increased cardiac output and increased blood volume. In conjunction with this, there is relative vasodilation in both the arterial and venous circulations. Increased concentrations of progesterone and other hormones likely play a role, and endothelial production of $PGI_2$ is increased twofold.

In the first phase of hemostasis, platelets, the primary cellular elements of clotting, adhere to exposed subendothelial tissues and secrete procoagulant substances that result in the formation of a platelet aggregate and thrombus (see Chapter 12). The platelet surface glycoprotein (GP) Ib complexed with GP IX binds to vWf, an interaction that is crucial for platelet aggregation to subendothelium under high shear rate conditions. Activated platelets secrete their contents in response to thrombin, adenosine diphosphate, collagen, thromboxane $A_2$, and epinephrine, all of which have surface receptors on platelets. The platelet granules contain serotonin, adenosine triphosphate and diphosphate, vWf, factor V, high-molecular-weight kininogen, fibronectin, and other substances with vasoactive and thrombogenic properties. Activation of platelets by a variety of substances induces secretion of these products. Platelet GP IIb complexed with GP IIIa then binds to fibrinogen, as well as vWf, fibronectin, and vitronectin leading to aggregation.

In pregnancy, there is a slight decline in the platelet count toward term, although the mean values fall within the normal range (1–3). Part of this decline in platelet count may be due to a low-grade, chronic consumption of platelets. Increased levels of the platelet secretory product β-thrombomodulin in the latter half of pregnancy (4, 5) or postpartum (6) support this assumption. Platelet activation and aggregation are slightly increased in pregnancy (7, 8). One group measured an increased production of platelet-derived thromboxane $A_2$ in the first half of pregnancy (9). An alternative explanation for the fall in the mean platelet count in pregnancy is that approximately 7 to 8% of seemingly normal pregnant women have an "incidental" thrombocytopenia of pregnancy (10), possibly due to an immune-mediated consumption of the platelets or to a "low-grade" intravascular coagulopathy in the uteroplacental circulation. The interaction of platelets with the vascular wall is intact in normal pregnancy as evidenced by normal or slightly subnormal bleeding times in pregnant women (11).

The second phase of hemostasis involves the formation of a stable fibrin clot. Circulating and locally produced coagulation factors are primary participants in blood coagulation *in vivo* and cooperate in a system characterized by conversion of zymogens to enzymes and by feedback potentiation and inhibition. The critical component for clotting after vascular injury is tissue factor (TF). TF is found in the subendothelial matrix and on vascular smooth muscle walls. When exposed on endothelial membrane surfaces after endothelial activation, TF serves as a cofactor for factor VIIa. In simplistic terms, as described in detail in Chapter 4, the TF-factor VIIa complex activates factor IX and factor X. The procoagulant activity of factor VII is enhanced by factor XIIa and factor IXa, with the former being activated by a complex of factor XIIa and high-molecular-weight kininogen. Factor IXa in concert with factor VIIIa also converts factor X to factor Xa. Factor Xa, operating in concert with its cofactor, factor Va, converts prothrombin to thrombin. Thrombin, in turn, hydrolyzes the peptide bonds of soluble fibrinogen, releasing fibrinopeptides A and B, allowing the fibrin monomers to polymerize. Thrombin also activates factor XIII, which then forms covalent bonds to crosslink the fibrin clot (see Chapter 6). At several steps in the process, phospholipid surfaces, probably derived from cell membranes, act as templates on which the coagulation proteins interact in a timely fashion (see Chapter 1). In addition, at several steps in the process, negative feedback by procoagulant proteins or inhibitory effects of anticoagulant proteins come into play.

In pregnancy, the circulating levels of factors VII, X, and fibrinogen increase substantially beginning in the first trimester. By term, the increases in factor VII levels and fibrinogen levels are particularly marked at 80 and 70%, respectively. Factor VIII, which exists in plasma mostly in a noncovalent complex with vWf, also increases beginning early in pregnancy. By term, the coagulant activity of factor VIII is twice that of the nonpregnant state. Levels of factors IX and XII are slightly increased, whereas, levels of factor XI decrease slightly. Factor XIII levels rise in the first half of pregnancy and tend to fall toward normal as pregnancy advances. Factor V levels are largely unchanged. Prekallikrein and high-molecular-weight kininogen levels increase in pregnancy.

Fibrinolysis, which is set into action concomitantly with fibrin formation, serves to regulate unbridled clot formation. As described in detail in Chapter 7, circulating plasminogen is activated by tissue-type plasminogen activator, primarily derived from endothelial cells, and other activators. The activated product, plasmin, cleaves crosslinked fibrin into soluble fragments. This process, in turn, is regulated by inhibitors such as $\alpha_2$-plasmin inhibitor and plasminogen activator inhibitors 1 and 2. In normal pregnancy, the fibrinolytic activity of plasma, even in response to physiologic stimulation (12), is diminished, probably due to a substantial increase in the levels of plasminogen activator inhibitors 1 and 2, the latter of which is made in abundance by the placenta (13). The net effect is a greater than 50% reduction in plasma fibrinolytic activity by term.

Two important systems that inhibit coagulation

have been identified, as described in detail in Chapter 3. These include the antithrombin III (ATIII) system and the thrombomodulin-protein C (PC) system. ATIII, which is produced by the liver, is a serine protease inhibitor that binds directly to thrombin and other activated coagulation factors. Thrombomodulin is an endothelial cell surface protein that binds thrombin and thereby limits its activity. The thrombin-thrombomodulin complex also binds to and activates PC, a vitamin K-dependent hepatic protein. Activated PC, in the presence of its cofactor, protein S (PS), inhibits factors V and VIII through a series of cleavages. Activated PC also enhances fibrinolysis. Neither circulating ATIII concentrations nor ATIII activity change substantially during pregnancy, although the production of ATIII is increased to keep up with the gestational plasma volume expansion. Circulating PC concentrations remain stable or increase slightly during pregnancy, and PC activity falls within the normal nonpregnant range. Total PS antigen may decrease somewhat during pregnancy or remain unchanged (14). However, free PS levels fall by nearly 50% by the mid-to-late second trimester, leading to a decrease in PS activity (15, 16).

There are dramatic changes in hemostasis that occur with delivery of the fetus, separation of the placenta, and the postpartum period (17–19). Immediately following delivery, markers of platelet aggregation increase. Shortened clotting tests suggest increased thrombin generation. Levels of factor XII, prekallikrein, and high-molecular-weight kininogen fall dramatically, while levels of fibrin split products and other measurable products of fibrin formation increase. Within hours, however, plasma fibrinolytic activity returns to that of the normal nonpregnant state, probably because of the rapid decline in plasminogen activator inhibitor 2 after delivery of the placenta. Factor VIII coagulant activity increases and then decreases. Within a few days, the platelet count normalizes, and the concentrations of factor VII, VIII, and fibrinogen return to those of the nonpregnant state.

# VENOUS THROMBOEMBOLISM (SEE CHAPTER 40)

## OCCURRENCE AND PREDISPOSITIONS

Venous thromboembolism is a leading cause of maternal morbidity and mortality during pregnancy and the puerperium (20–22). Death from pulmonary embolism (PE), which may be determined with precision, occurs in 0.03 per 10,000 vaginal births and in 0.5 per 10,000 Caesarian deliveries (23). The rate of deep vein thrombosis (DVT) and nonfatal thromboembolism is more difficult to determine with certainty because of variability in diagnostic criteria and methodology used. The overall

rate of PE during pregnancy (fatal and nonfatal) is estimated at 0.2 to 1 per 1000 pregnancies (24, 25). Estimates of the rate of DVT associated with pregnancy range widely. In various reports, the estimated rate of DVT in pregnancy or the puerperium is 0.013 to more than 1 per 100 gravidas (26–29). In a prospective study using venography in symptomatic individuals, investigators found the rate of antepartum thrombosis was 0.7 per 100 (30).

Medical reports and clinical experience indicate that DVT and PE are more common in the postpartum period than in the antepartum period. In the past, this may have been due to the common obstetric practices of the time, such as prolonged bed rest after delivery and the use of estrogen compounds to suppress lactation. A recent retrospective study (25) found that 75% of DVTs occurred before delivery, with half of the cases occurring in the first or early second trimester. Other investigators found that the rate of DVT is similar in each trimester of pregnancy (30–32). In contrast, two-thirds of the PEs occur postpartum (25).

The rate of DVT or thromboembolism during pregnancy and the puerperium is increased by numerous factors, including increased maternal age, increasing parity, obesity, a blood group other than O, bed rest or immobilization, dehydration, and other illnesses. For example, the rate of maternal death from PE is significantly increased with a fourth child or a subsequent child in any age group over 30 (23). The influence of pregnancy itself and the mode of delivery is impressive—pregnancy increases a woman's risk of thromboembolism fivefold to sixfold, and the ratio of deaths from PE after Caesarian section to those after vaginal delivery is in excess of 10:1 (33).

The increased venous stasis incurred by pregnancy, which begins in the first trimester, undoubtedly plays an important role in the increased rate of DVT and thromboembolism. The pregnant uterus impedes venous return from the lower extremities, especially in later pregnancy. This factor plays a relatively minor role, however, because one-third to one-half of the thrombotic events occur before week 15 of gestation (25, 30, 32). The left lower extremity is involved far more frequently than the right (30, 34).

Seven to 15% of women with a history of thrombosis or thromboembolism during a prior pregnancy will have a thrombotic event in a subsequent pregnancy (35, 36). The risk of thrombosis during subsequent pregnancy in women with a history of thrombosis related to oral contraceptives, surgery, major trauma or most other provoking factors is uncertain. A questionnaire study found that the risk of recurrent venous thrombosis in pregnancy was similar whether or not the prior event was related to oral contraceptive use or pregnancy (36).

Thrombophilic conditions pose a unique concern for

pregnancy, but there are no prospective studies of the risk of thrombosis in women with thrombophilias. In one retrospective analysis (37), women with protein C and S deficiency *without* prior thrombosis had a 5 and 9% rate of thrombosis during pregnancy, respectively. For women *with* prior thrombosis, the rate of thrombosis during pregnancy was 17 and 22%, respectively. Antithrombin III deficiency may represent an especially dangerous situation. Even without prior thrombosis, women with antithrombin III deficiency may have a thrombosis rate of 29% during pregnancy. The risk of thrombosis during pregnancy in women with activated protein C resistance is uncertain. In the two largest series of women with antiphospholipid syndrome, 5 and 12% of individuals suffered a venous or arterial thrombosis during pregnancy (38, 39).

## DIAGNOSIS (SEE CHAPTER 25)

### DVT

Our ability to diagnose DVT by history and physical examination is modest at best and is further hampered by the discomfort and edema that normally accompanies pregnancy. Concerns regarding radiation exposure to the fetus create a reluctance to make the diagnosis of DVT by venography. Finally, the pelvic veins, although to be a relatively common source of PE associated with pregnancy, are poorly accessed by noninvasive, nonradiation methods.

### Ultrasonographic Techniques

Most clinicians use sonographic techniques as the first line diagnostic studies in symptomatic individuals suspected of having a lower extremity DVT. Real-time sonography may allow visualization of the clot in the proximal deep veins of the leg; visualization of the clot has virtually 100% positive predictive value for proximal DVT. The failure of the vein to collapse under gentle transducer pressure ("compression ultrasonography") is an exceedingly sensitive technique (40) that also has a positive predictive value of 84% for proximal DVT in nonpregnant individuals (41). Importantly, the predictive accuracy of ultrasound critically depends on the expertise of the technician performing the study.

Real-time sonography is now commonly supplemented with sonographic Doppler flow imaging, a technique that identifies alterations in venous flow. The combination of real-time ultrasonographic imaging and Doppler flow studies is more than 90% sensitive and specific for the detection of proximal DVTs in nonpregnant, symptomatic individuals (42, 43). Care must be taken to displace the uterus from the vena cava when imaging the lower extremity venous system using Doppler ultrasound flow imaging.

Real-time and Doppler sonography are less satisfactory for the evaluation of the lower leg (calf), with each having a sensitivity of approximately 50% in nonpregnant individuals. Likewise, these sonographic techniques have limited utility in the diagnosis of thrombosis above the inguinal ligament, especially in pregnancy. One caveat, however, is that poor venous flow in the proximal deep venous system of the symptomatic leg can be a sign of thrombosis in the iliac vessels. Sonographic studies are less sensitive, although quite specific, for the diagnosis of proximal or distal DVT in asymptomatic individuals.

There are no large, well-designed studies of the use of combined real-time and Doppler ultrasound to diagnose DVT in pregnancy, but althoughtful analysis (44) and clinical experience strongly support the ultrasonographic evaluation of pregnant women with suspected proximal DVT. It is unlikely that ultrasonographic methods will ever be compared with venography in formal study of pregnant women with suspected DVT.

### Impedance Plethysmography (IPG)

In IPG, the electrical impedance between two electrodes around the calf is measured. Engorgement of the leg with blood due to venous obstruction proximal to the electrodes results in decreased electrical impedance and delays the normal increase in impedance when a thigh tourniquet is deflated. In pregnancy, it is important to position the individual in the lateral recumbent position to avoid occlusion of flow by the gravid uterus (45). The accuracy of the technique hinges on the degree of venous occlusion and the capacity of collateral venous drainage.

In experienced hands, the sensitivity and specificity of IPG for the diagnosis of proximal DVT in symptomatic individuals are in excess of 90%, although recent studies suggest a lower sensitivity (46, 47). One study has demonstrated the utility of IPG in symptomatic pregnant women (48). Of 152 individuals, 139 had repeatedly negative IPG studies (on days 3, 5, 7, 10, and 14 after the initial study) and received no anticoagulation treatment. None developed additional clinical features of DVT or clinically apparent PE. Like sonographic studies, IPG is a relatively insensitive tool for the diagnosis of distal extremity DVT and thrombosis above the inguinal ligament.

### Venography

Venography (phlebography) is widely considered the gold standard for the diagnosis of proximal and distal DVT. While it is technically cumbersome to perform, venography is cost effective in symptomatic nonpregnant individuals (49) because of the high sensitivity, specificity, and predictive values. Side effects include discomfort associated with contrast injection and peripheral vein contrast-induced thrombosis in 2 to 3% of individuals (50).

Most physicians consider venography relatively contraindicated in pregnancy because of the risk of ionizing radiation to the fetus. However, using judicious technique, the amount of radiation exposure to the fetus is less than 500 μGy (51). Thus, in suspected cases in which the results of sonographic or plethysmography studies are negative or equivocal, venography should be used to rule out thrombosis. In addition, venography is virtually the only practical method for the diagnosis of thrombosis in the iliac vessels or inferior vena cava during pregnancy.

## Pulmonary Embolism (PE)

Results from the Prospective Investigation of Pulmonary Embolism Diagnosis (PIOPED) study show that a normal or high probability ventilation-perfusion scan may be used with confidence for clinical decision making in individuals with suspected PEs (52). In pregnancy, the estimated fetal radiation exposure from ventilation-perfusion scanning is well within acceptable limits (less than 350 μGy) (43).

When the results of the ventilation-perfusion scanning are either low- or intermediate-probability, or the clinical situation is particularly suspicious, further studies are required. Some clinicians initially perform noninvasive tests of the legs; if the results are positive, treatment is initiated. If the results are negative, pulmonary angiography is indicated, especially in pregnancy wherein embolic thrombi may emanate from the pelvic veins. Other clinicians favor moving directly to pulmonary angiography when low- or intermediate-probability ventilation-perfusion scanning results are obtained. Concerns about radiation risk to the fetus during pulmonary angiography seem unwarranted because the estimated radiation exposure to the fetus is less than 500 μGy using a brachial approach (43).

## TREATMENT

## Acute Thrombosis or Thromboembolism

The treatment of acute thrombosis or thromboembolism is anticoagulation with heparin. Molecules of neither unfractionated nor low-molecular-weight heparin cross the placenta (53), and most authorities agree that heparin is safe for the fetus. The regimen of heparin in pregnancy does not differ from that used in the nonpregnant state. For uncomplicated DVT, a loading dose of 5000 IU of unfractionated heparin (UFH) is administered intravenously. This is followed by a continuous infusion of heparin (concentration of 40 IU per milliliter) at an hourly rate that achieves 31,000 to 32,000 IU per 24 hours (54–56). At 6 hours after the initial bolus of heparin, the activated partial thromboplastin time (aPTT) is measured, and the dose of heparin is adjusted to maintain an aPTT of 1.5 to 2.5 times the control mean.

In nonpregnant individuals, it is probably unnecessary to administer continuous infusion UFH for more than 4 to 5 days before switching over to oral anticoagulants (54, 57, 58). In pregnant individuals, however, authorities recommend running continuous infusion UFH for 5 to 10 days before beginning a regimen of intermittently injected subcutaneous UFH (59).

Following initial treatment of acute DVT in pregnancy with continuous infusion UFH, most authorities recommend subcutaneous UFH administered every 12 hours. In a given individual, the initial dose of subcutaneous UFH should be the same as that required for continuous infusion therapy per 24 hours. The dose of subcutaneous UFH should be adjusted to keep the aPTT 6 hours after the dose (i.e., at mid-interval) at 1.5 times the control mean.

These recommendations of authorities notwithstanding, it is important to recognize that studies of heparin pharmacokinetics and pharmacodynamics in pregnancy are remarkably few. In one study (60), pregnant women (24 to 30 weeks' gestation) and nonpregnant controls were administered UFH subcutaneously at a dose of 143 units/kg (about 8500 to 11,500 units). Compared to the nonpregnant controls, the pregnant women demonstrated a significantly longer time to peak heparin concentrations (113 ± 20 versus 222 ± 21 minutes), longer time to peak aPTT (137 ± 31 versus 230 ± 26 seconds), lower peak plasma heparin concentration (0.11 ± 0.017 versus 0.23 ± 0.036 units), and lower peak aPTT (30.3 ± 1.7 versus 50 ± 4.0 seconds). The investigators noted that the peak heparin effect in a pregnant woman should be determined about 2 hours after a subcutaneous dose and that the trough plasma concentration was reached 4.5 to 5 hours after the dose. In a differently designed study (59), another group studied heparin levels in women receiving a thromboprophylactic subcutaneous dose of UFH every 12 hours. Measuring mid-interval heparin levels, they found that only four of nine women were in the therapeutic range (0.05 to 0.25 units/mL) using 7500 unit doses in the second trimester. All other subjects required higher doses. In the third trimester, only four of 13 women achieve the desired heparin levels using 10,000 units twice a day; all others required higher doses (60).

The implications of these two studies for the use of UFH in pregnancy are important. First, subcutaneous UFH should be administered more frequently than the standard every 12 hour regimen often used if one is to achieve the desired effect throughout the day, and probably as often as every 6 to 8 hours. One reasonable strategy for following the anticoagulation status of pregnant women on subcutaneous heparin is to aim for a peak heparin aPTT effect at 2 to 3 hours after injection of 2 to 2.5 times the control mean and a trough heparin aPTT effect of 10 to 15 seconds above the control mean (59, 61).

Heparin may be administered by continuous subcutaneous infusion using a medication pump, an approach that would appear to have several advantages over intermittent injections. However, initial reports indicated an unacceptably high rate of bleeding complications (62–64). More favorable results were recently reported in a small, randomized, crossover trial (65). Intermittent injections of UFH are quite inexpensive compared to continuous subcutaneous infusion via a medication pump. At this time, heparin administration via a continuous infusion pump cannot be recommended over intermittent injections.

Recent studies have demonstrated the effectiveness and safety of low-molecular-weight heparin (LMWH) in the treatment of acute venous thrombosis (66, 67). LMWH does not cross the placenta, and there is every reason to consider it safe for use in pregnancy (68–70). Like UFH, formal, well-designed studies of the pharmacokinetics and pharmacodynamics of LMWH in pregnancy are lacking. Anecdotal experience suggests that enoxaparin may be dosed according to a per kilogram basis in pregnancy to achieve the desired anticoagulation effect. Twice-daily injections will be required to maintain anticoagulation. Given the lack of clinical experience with LMWH in pregnancy, it would be prudent to monitor peak (2 to 3 hours after injection) and trough (just prior to next dose) heparin (antifactor Xa) levels.

For acute venous thrombosis or thromboembolism in pregnancy, the American College of Chest Physicians recommends continuing full anticoagulation for the duration of pregnancy (71). However, this recommendation is controversial, and some authorities believe that heparin treatment may be adjusted to thromboprophylactic doses after 3 months of full anticoagulation (72). Following delivery, thromboprophylaxis with heparin or warfarin should be maintained for at least 6 weeks.

## Peripartum Anticoagulation

The peripartum management of anticoagulation therapy rarely poses a significant problem, although concerns abound. There are three acceptable approaches, and the choice will be influenced primarily by the degree of concern in a given individual, rather than scientific proof that one approach is superior to another. For most individuals, subcutaneous heparin treatment may be discontinued with the onset of uterine contractions or 6 to 12 hours prior to induction of labor or Caesarian section. A second approach is to continue subcutaneous heparin injections through labor at a dose of 5000 IU every 12 hours (73). A third approach is to continue intravenous heparin treatment at a dose adjusted to maintain the aPTT 1.3 to 1.5 times the control mean, turning the infusion off as delivery becomes imminent. Excessive bleeding with vaginal delivery is unusual, especially when heparin levels are less than 0.4 IU/mL (73, 74). Heparin treatment should be restarted 4 to 6 hours

following delivery when the individual is clinically stable.

## Thromboprophylaxis

Most clinicians believe that women with a history of prior venous thrombosis after no more than minor perturbation should be treated with thromboprophylactic doses of heparin (either UFH or LMWH) during pregnancy (71, 73, 75), although not all agree (76). The need for thromboprophylaxis in pregnancy for women with a history of thrombosis after major perturbation (e.g., major trauma) is controversial. For most clinicians, the degree of residual venous damage or insufficiency will be an important consideration. Finally, the need for thromboprophylaxis in asymptomatic women with an inherited thrombophilia is uncertain, although retrospective studies suggest an unacceptably high rate of thrombosis during pregnancy (see above). Based on series and case reports, the risk of thrombosis during pregnancy in women with antiphospholipid syndrome, ATIII deficiency, or paroxysmal nocturnal hemoglobinuria warrants thromboprophylaxis (see above).

The American College of Chest Surgeons recommends thromboprophylaxis during pregnancy using 5000 IU of UFH injected subcutaneously twice daily (71). The findings of two studies (see above) (59, 60) raise serious doubts about the adequacy of this approach. Firstly, dosing UFH every 12 hours in a pregnant woman likely leaves many hours of the day "uncovered" with regard to measurable heparin activity in plasma. Thrice daily injections probably provide better coverage. Secondly, the dose of UFH required to achieve measurable heparin effect in plasma is considerably higher in pregnancy. In one study, investigators found that a subcutaneous dose of UFH averaging 225 IU per kilogram of body weight per 24 hours was required to maintain an antifactor Xa activity level of 0.08 to 0.15 IU/mL (73); this totals just over 14,000 IU per day in a 65-kilogram pregnant woman. LMWH has a longer half-life than UFH, but no one has determined its optimal dose or dose interval for thromboprophylaxis in pregnancy. For enoxaparin (Lovenox), doses of at least 40 mg per day are required to achieve thromboprophylactic levels of heparin (68, 70). It is likely, although not proven, that twice daily dosing will be required for adequate thromboprophylaxis using enoxaparin.

## Complications of Heparin in Pregnancy

The three clinically important adverse effects of heparin use in pregnancy are hemorrhage, osteoporosis with risk of fracture, and heparin-induced thrombocytopenia (HIT). The issue of hemorrhage as a complication of heparin is discussed in Chapter 55. Osteoporosis with risk of fracture is a genuine concern in obstetric uses of heparin since individuals tend to be on long-term treatment regimens (76–78). A great majority of symptomatic fracture cases involve the use of UFH, but at least one individual treated with LMWH has been reported to suffer a symptomatic fracture (39). In one study of 70 women undergoing heparin treatment or prophylaxis, 12% had radiographic evidence of osteopenia and 2% had vertebral fractures (79). One fracture occurred in a woman on 15,000 units per day of UFH for 7 weeks! The overall risk of heparin-induced osteopenia with fracture is uncertain, but may be as high as 1 to 2% in pregnant women treated with heparin (79). Whether or not LMWH differs from UFH with regard to this risk is unknown.

Bone loss attributable to heparin treatment during pregnancy is probably reversible over time (79, 80). In an attempt to avoid severe osteoporosis, women treated with heparin should be encouraged to take supplemental calcium and vitamin D (e.g., prenatal vitamins) daily. It also seems prudent to encourage axial skeleton weight-bearing exercise (e.g., walking) daily. If a woman who needs heparin during pregnancy seeks preconceptional counseling, it seems prudent to advise that calcium and vitamin D supplementation and weight-bearing exercise be started immediately. It also seems prudent to maintain a program aimed at good bone health after pregnancy in women treated with heparin during gestation.

Heparin-induced thrombocytopenia (HIT), the most dreaded complication of heparin therapy, occurs in up to 5% of individuals (81). Fortunately, the most severe form of HIT, which includes life-threatening thromboembolism, is less frequent. The management of HIT is covered in Chapter 29. It has recently been shown that LMWH is less likely to be associated with HIT, a major relative safety feature compared to unfractionated sodium heparin (82). Some authorities believe that HIT is less common in pregnant individuals than in nonpregnant individuals, although there are a handful of case reports (83–85).

### Thrombolysis in Pregnancy

Experience with thrombolytic therapy during pregnancy is quite limited. Theoretically, the use of these agents, which usually result in systemic fibrinolysis and an anticoagulant effect, may cause bleeding from the placental implantation site. Thus the use of thrombolytic agents in pregnancy should be limited to life-threatening situations (86–90).

### Warfarin in Pregnancy (See Chapter 55)

Warfarin is teratogenic in humans and is therefore contraindicated in pregnancy. A first trimester embryopathy involving stippling of the epiphyses and nasal and limb hypoplasia occurs in about 10 to 25% of exposed embryos (90–92). The critical period of exposure is between 6 and 9 weeks' gestation (90). Warfarin use in the second or third trimesters has been associated with central nervous system abnormalities, including dorsal midline dysplasia (agenesis of the corpus callosum, Dandy-Walker malformation, midline cerebellar atrophy, optic atrophy, and encephalocele) or ventral midline dysplasia (optic atrophy). In the only prospective study of warfarin use in pregnancy (92), none of these central nervous system abnormalities were found. The American Academy of Pediatrics considers warfarin to be compatible with breast feeding in term infants because (1) warfarin does not enter breast milk (93), and (2) no adverse neonatal effects have been detected in breast-fed infants of women on warfarin.

## THROMBOPHILIA AND PREGNANCY (SEE CHAPTER 40)

### INHERITED THROMBOPHILIC DISORDERS

More than one-quarter of individuals with new onset DVT will be found to have an inherited predisposition. For uncertain reasons, the rate of thrombosis in individuals with an inherited thrombophilia is low until adolescence, when the rate begins to climb with advancing age (12). Some 50% of thrombotic episodes in individuals with inherited thrombophilia occur in identifiable thrombogenic circumstances, such as with the use of oral contraceptives or in association with pregnancy or surgery.

Activated protein C (APC) resistance is by far the most commonly recognized inherited thrombophilia. At least 80% of cases of APC resistance are due to a mutation in factor V (Arg506Gln), known as the Leiden mutation, which renders factor Va less susceptible to initial cleavage by APC (94–99). APC resistance occurs in 6 to 8% of northern Europeans and 4 to 5% of American Caucasians (100). In the general, predominantly Caucasian population, APC resistance is found in association with 20 to 50% of DVT cases (101–105). The risk of thrombosis during pregnancy in individuals with APC resistance is unknown. However, in one study of DVT in pregnancy, APC resistance was found in nearly 60% of cases (106). Individuals homozygous for the Leiden mutation have higher rates of thrombosis than heterozygotes (97).

Heterozygous deficiencies in ATIII, PC, and PS are found in less than 10% of individuals with DVT (107, 108). There are two major types of ATIII deficiency. Type I is characterized by reduced synthesis of the molecule and is accompanied by decreased circulating ATIII antigen and ATIII function. In type II ATIII deficiency, a discrete molecular abnormality in the ATIII molecule results in reduced function of ATIII, although circulating concentrations of ATIII antigen are normal. A large number of families with type II ATIII deficiency have been described, each with a different molecular mutation. Not surprisingly, the rate of thrombosis among affected individuals varies with the nature of the mutation. Individuals heterozygous for a mutation near the thrombin-binding site of ATIII, have rates of thrombosis similar to those with type I deficiency (109). Using functional assays to determine ATIII-heparin cofactor activity, investigators have found that about one in 250 to 500 individuals in the general population have measurable abnormalities in ATIII (109–111). Since most of these individuals do not have a history of thrombosis, the prevalence of clinically important ATIII deficiency would appear much less, probably no more than one in 1000 to 2000.

Like ATIII deficiency, PC deficiency is classified into two subtypes. The type I disorder involves proportionately decreased functional activity and antigenic concentrations of PC. Type II PC deficiency is characterized by decreased functional PC activity but normal concentrations of PC antigen. A number of type II PC deficiency molecular variants have been described, and the severity of the specific abnormality is likely related to how much it interferes with the protein's interaction with thrombin-thrombomodulin, factor Va, or factor VIIIa (112). Type I PC deficiency occurs in one in 200 to 300 apparently healthy individuals (109).

PS circulates in bound and free forms. Type I PS deficiency is characterized by reduced functional and antigenically determined total and free PS concentrations. In type II PS deficiency, individuals have normal total PS levels, but reduced free PS levels and functional PS activity. This may be due to a defect in either protein S or its binding protein, C4b-binding protein.

The overall contribution of ATIII, PC, or PS deficiency to thrombosis in pregnancy is uncertain, although these deficiencies likely account for less than 10% of DVTs in pregnancy. Retrospective analyses have attempted to determine the rates of thrombosis during pregnancy in women with known deficiencies. In one study, women with protein C and S deficiency without prior thrombosis had a 5 and 9% rate of thrombosis, respectively, in association with pregnancy. For women with a prior thrombosis, the rate of thrombosis in association with pregnancy was 17 and 22%, respectively. In another study, investigators found that 7% of women with PC deficiency had thrombosis during pregnancy and that 19% had thrombosis in the postpartum period (113).

Among women with ATIII deficiency, the rate of thrombosis in association with pregnancy appears higher than for other inherited thrombophilias, although the rate likely varies according to the type of ATIII deficiency and the molecular mutation involved. In retrospective studies, from 44 to 94% of untreated women with ATIII deficiency have a thrombotic episode during pregnancy (113–115).

The relatively high frequency of thrombosis during and after pregnancy in women with ATIII, PC, and PS deficiencies is generally considered an indication for thromboprophylaxis, even in women with no history of previous thrombosis. However, in women with APC resistance, the frequency of thrombosis in association with pregnancy is uncertain; thus the need for thromboprophylaxis in individuals with APC resistance but no history of prior thrombosis is debatable. Depending on the indication, due consideration should be given to continuing thromboprophylaxis for 4 to 8 weeks following delivery.

Two issues related to treatment in cases of inherited thrombophilia deserve special comment. First, by the very nature of the problem, some women with ATIII deficiency do not respond to heparin as readily as women with normal ATIII levels and function, and a small proportion do not respond at all. For this reason, some investigators have suggested using sufficient subcutaneously administered heparin to achieve full anticoagulation during pregnancy in individuals with ATIII deficiency (115). For some individuals, this approach may require doses of heparin in the range of 45,000 to 50,000 units per day. Others have used subcutaneously administered heparin in doses sufficient to prolong the mid-interval aPTT by 5 to 10 seconds (114). Individuals who fail to respond to heparin with an elevation in their aPTT should either be treated with warfarin or administered AT-III concentrate. The latter is so expensive that treatment throughout pregnancy may not be an option. In these cases, a reasonable alternative would be treatment with ATIII concentrate during the first 12 to 14 weeks of pregnancy to avoid the teratogenic effects of warfarin, switching to warfarin treatment in the second and third trimesters. Many investigators have proposed that the risk of thrombosis in the peripartum period be managed with ATIII concentrate (116, 117). Heparin is discontinued, and ATIII concentrate sufficient to increase the functional level of plasma ATIII to 120% of normal is given. This is repeated in 24 hours if restarting heparin is for some reason contraindicated.

A second point deserving emphasis is that women with PC deficiency are at risk for warfarin-induced skin necrosis. This infrequently occurring condition is due to further suppression of PC concentrations by warfarin before an adequate anticoagulant effect is achieved. It may be avoided by overlapping the slow initiation of warfarin (2 mg per day for 3 days and then increasing by 2 to 3 mg per day) with adequate heparinization.

An expanding body of evidence suggests that inherited thrombophilic disorders may be associated with preeclampsia, fetal growth impairment, and pregnancy loss, perhaps somewhat analogous to these clinical conditions being associated with antiphospholipid syndrome. Two groups have shown that the frequency of APC resistance is significantly elevated among women with preeclampsia (100, 118). One group found that APC resistance was associated with second trimester fetal death (119); they and others found no relationship between APC resistance and early (first trimester) spontaneous pregnancy loss (100, 119). Whether treatment with antiplatelet agents or anticoagulants has a beneficial effect on these clinical problems is unknown.

## ACQUIRED THROMBOPHILIAS

Antiphospholipid syndrome (APS) is associated with thrombosis, autoimmune thrombocytopenia, and fetal loss (see Chapter 38). The relationship between the latter clinical problem and antiphospholipid antibodies was first established by case reports and small case series (120). All these reports were retrospective and the individuals were highly selected. Most individuals had underlying conditions such as systemic lupus erythematosus, prior fetal death, or a history of thrombosis. Most recent studies have focused on unselected individuals with recurrent pregnancy loss, most of whom had recurrent preembryonic or embryonic losses. Data from these series indicate that up to 20% of women with recurrent pregnancy loss have either lupus anticoagulant or anticardiolipin antibodies, which are the two best characterized antiphospholipid antibodies, if low-positive anticardiolipin results are included (121–127). In the largest series of women presenting with recurrent pregnancy loss (128), 9.6% were persistently (tested twice) positive for lupus anticoagulant. Approximately 3 and 2% of individuals were persistently positive for IgG and IgM anticardiolipin antibodies, respectively.

Some investigators have emphasized that the type of pregnancy loss most specific to APS is fetal death (death of the conceptus after 10 weeks from the last menstrual period), rather than preembryonic or embryonic loss. In one review of case reports and small series, 20% of antiphospholipid-related pregnancy losses were found to be second- or early third-trimester fetal death (120). A retrospective analysis of women with well-characterized APS showed that 27 or 195 (41%) previous pregnancies were fetal deaths (38). More recently, Oshiro et al (129) analyzed the obstetric histories of 366 women with two ore more consecutive pregnancy losses who were tested for lupus anticoagulant and anticardiolipin antibodies. Seventy-six of the individuals in this highly selected referral population had clinically relevant levels of antiphospholipid antibodies (lupus anticoagulant present or medium-to-high positive IgG anticardiolipin antibodies). Fully 50% of the previous pregnancy losses in this group were fetal deaths; whereas only 10% of the losses in the 290 women without significant levels of antiphospholipid antibodies were fetal deaths. Moreover, over 80% of the women

with clinically significant levels of antiphospholipid antibodies had suffered at least one fetal death compared with 24% in women without antiphospholipid antibodies.

It should be noted that positive tests for antiphospholipid antibodies may be found, albeit infrequently, among otherwise normal pregnant women. Two studies each have included more than 1000 unselected obstetric individuals. In one, less than 2% of obstetric individuals had IgG anticardiolipin antibodies, while 4% had IgM (130). More than 80% of the positive results were in the low-positive range, with only 0.2% of IgG results and 0.7% of IgM results being in the medium- or high-positive range. In the other study, 3.5 and 0.94% of women had IgG and IgM anticardiolipin antibodies, respectively (131). Again, most women had low-positive results.

Some investigators believe that fetal loss in women with APS is due to placental thrombosis, although this is disputed (132). The immediate cause of fetal deaths in women with APS is due to spiral artery vasculopathy (133, 134), with subsequent inadequate blood flow to the intervillous space of the placenta.

The favored treatment used to avoid fetal loss is a combination of heparin, administered in thromboprophylactic doses, and low-dose aspirin (38). Two prospective studies indicate that this treatment is efficacious in preventing pregnancy loss (135, 136), although 15 to 30% of individuals so treated will miscarry or suffer fetal death (38, 135, 136).

APS is widely recognized as predisposing to thrombosis during pregnancy. In the two largest studies of women with well-characterized APS (38, 39), the rates of thrombosis associated with prospectively followed pregnancies were 5 and 12%, respectively. Some of the individuals with thrombosis were on doses of heparin considered thromboprophylactic. Importantly, APS poses a risk for arterial events, including stroke. Among the 142 prospectively followed pregnancies in women with APS, two women had strokes and one died. Treatment of APS during pregnancy requires adequate thromboprophylactic heparin, probably no less than 15,000 to 20,000 units per day in divided doses.

Paroxysmal nocturnal hemoglobinuria (PNH) is associated with a substantial risk of thrombosis in association with pregnancy. Hepatic venous thrombosis leading to Budd-Chiari syndrome is a particular concern in PNH; it accounts for 50% of all deaths in women with PNH. At a minimum, thromboprophylactic doses of heparin should be administered during pregnancy and in the postpartum state of women with PNH. However, DVT has been reported in pregnant PNH cases on low doses of heparin (137). Given the relatively high likelihood of thrombosis and the serious nature of Budd-Chiari syndrome, a case can be made for full anticoagulation with heparin in women with PNH.

# PLATELET DISORDERS IN PREGNANCY

## THROMBOCYTOPENIA IN PREGNANCY

In a pregnant woman presenting with thrombocytopenia, it is imperative to examine a peripheral smear to exclude a spuriously low platelet count from platelet clumping (see Chapter 23 for a discussion of pseudo-thrombocytopenia). Viral infections, especially HIV and CMV, should be considered—both may have serious fetal effects. If deemed necessary, bone marrow aspiration may be done in pregnancy without special concerns for maternal or fetal safety. Autoimmune diseases must be considered, especially antiphospholipid syndrome, which has important fetal consequences. All pregnant women beyond 18 to 20 weeks' gestation with thrombocytopenia should be meticulously evaluated for preeclampsia.

### Incidental Thrombocytopenia of Pregnancy

Based on automated platelet counts done on admission to labor and delivery, the overall incidence of maternal thrombocytopenia in pregnancy is 7 to 8% (137). Most of these individuals have what is now known as incidental thrombocytopenia of pregnancy—asymptomatic thrombocytopenia occurring in otherwise normal pregnant women with no history of bleeding or prior nongestational thrombocytopenia. Platelet counts in this condition usually range between $95 \times 10^9/L$ and $150 \times 10^9/L$, but some women may have counts in the range of $80 \times 10^9/L$ to $95 \times 10^9/L$. Although an occasional woman with incidental thrombocytopenia may have a platelet count of $40 \times 10^9/L$ to $80 \times 10^9/L$, such low platelet counts are suspicious for other diagnoses. In incidental thrombocytopenia, maternal platelet counts return to normal within a few days after delivery (138). The neonates born to women with incidental thrombocytopenia have mean cord platelet counts that do not differ from those of neonates born of normal, nonthrombocytopenic gravidas.

The importance of recognizing incidental thrombocytopenia of pregnancy lies in its benignity. In the largest study of the condition, only one infant born to 756 women with incidental thrombocytopenia of pregnancy had a cord blood platelet count of under $50 \times 10^9/L$, and no infants had hemorrhagic morbidity (139). In addition, the mothers themselves had normal outcomes. There is no medical rationale for Caesarian section, treatment with glucocorticoids or other medications, or platelet transfusions in these individuals. In an otherwise normal pregnant woman with no prior history of thrombocytopenia, the discovery of mild, asymptomatic thrombocytopenia during pregnancy requires no treatment or invasive diagnostic studies. At most, platelets can be monitored weekly or bi-weekly to ascertain that the thrombocytopenia is not worsening.

## Autoimmune Thrombocytopenia (ATP) (See Chapter 30)

This condition, also known as idiopathic thrombocytopenic purpura or immune thrombocytopenic purpura (ITP), occurs in one to two women per 10,000 pregnancies (140). As in the nonpregnant individual, the diagnosis of ATP in pregnancy is one of exclusion and requires careful clinical judgment. None of the diagnostic features of ATP are particularly specific. The mean platelet volume is increased in ATP, but it is also increased in incidental thrombocytopenia of pregnancy (138). About 90% of women with ATP have platelet associated IgG, but such antibodies may be found in otherwise normal pregnant women (141).

The maternal risks of ATP are those related to thrombocytopenia. Easy bruising and petechiae are the typical early signs of thrombocytopenia when platelet counts fall below $50 \times 10^9/L$. With platelet counts under 10 to $20 \times 10^9/L$, spontaneous epistaxis, gingival bleeding, and mucosal surface blood vesicles may appear. The most serious forms of bleeding are genitourinary, gastrointestinal, and intracranial.

Pregnancy-related increased blood flow to many maternal tissues, the risk of delivery-associated hemorrhage, and anxiety about the well-being of the fetus influence treatment decisions. Once the diagnosis of ATP is established, it is reasonable to initiate treatment in the pregnant individual when the platelet count falls below $50 \times 10^9/L$, regardless of whether or not she has hemorrhagic symptoms. The mainstay of treatment in gravidas with ATP is prednisone. While an increased frequency of cleft palate has been found in the offspring of glucocorticoid-treated laboratory animals, a wealth of human experience and several studies indicate that the risk for human teratogenesis is very low. The risk of neonatal adrenal suppression following maternal treatment with hydrocortisone or prednisolone is very low, having been only rarely reported. One reason for the relative safety of these glucocorticoids in the human is the abundance of 11-β dehydrogenase in the human placenta. This enzyme converts hydrocortisone or prednisolone into the relatively inactive 11-keto forms, leaving no more than 10% of the active drug to reach the fetus. Glucocorticoids with fluorine at the 9α position are considerably less well metabolized by the placenta and should not be administered chronically during pregnancy unless it is the intent to treat the fetus with glucocorticoids. Treatment is started at a dose of 1 to 1.5 mg per kg per day and continued until there is a clear response or for 3 to 4 weeks. Once a good response is noted, the dose is tapered as it would be in nonpregnant individuals to the smallest dose that will maintain the platelet count above

50 × 10$^9$/l. Usually, glucocorticoids are continued through the remaining course of pregnancy, and decisions about when to discontinue them are made after delivery. Individuals will require "stress" doses of steroids in labor or at the time of Caesarian section.

Pregnant women who do not respond to glucocorticoids within 3-4 weeks of starting therapy should be treated with high-dose intravenous immune globulin (IVIG). The dose is either 400 mg/kg/day for 5 consecutive days or 1 g/kg/day for 2 consecutive days; this is repeated every 3-4 weeks, and prednisone can be tapered. A response to IVIG should be noted within 4 to 6 days.

A small percentage of individuals will not respond to these therapies. If near or at term, these individuals should be delivered and treatment reassessed thereafter. If remote from term, splenectomy may be required. The procedure may be done in the second trimester with good surgical exposure. If splenectomy is to be done, pneumococcal vaccination is indicated and may be given in pregnancy. The physician should be prepared for surgical or postpartum hemorrhage in all women with ATP.

Since ATP is mediated by IgG autoantibodies, transplacental passage of the antibodies with resultant fetal-neonatal thrombocytopenia is a possibility. Overall, the rate of fetal or neonatal thrombocytopenia ranges from 10 to 50%, but the median rate of severe fetal thrombocytopenia (<50 × 10$^9$/l) is only 12% (142). Clinicians have devised several strategies to minimize or avoid fetal bleeding. Glucocorticoids (143–146) and IVIG (147) administered to the mother have been tried, but neither are consistently effective in preventing fetal-neonatal thrombocytopenia.

Some physicians suggested that labor and vaginal delivery posed the greatest risk for precipitating dangerous hemorrhage in fetuses with thrombocytopenia; therefore Caesarian section was indicated in women with ATP (147–149). However, less than half of infants born to women with ATP have thrombocytopenia, and fewer than 15% have severe thrombocytopenia (<50 × 10$^9$/l). The reliable and safe identification of fetuses at greatest risk for hemorrhage has been problematic. Maternal characteristics such as the degree of thrombocytopenia, the presence of platelet associated antibodies, and the severity of past disease correlate poorly with the risk for fetal-neonatal thrombocytopenia (142). Discordant platelet counts in twin pregnancy complicated by ATP have been reported (150, 151). More invasive procedures, including fetal cordocentesis prior to labor and fetal scalp blood sampling in labor to determine the fetal platelet count, have been proposed and used (152–155). Properly done, these are reliable for determining the fetal platelet count. However, cordocentesis is associated with a fetal loss rate of 1 to 2% (156–157), and fetuses with thrombocytopenia may be at greater risk.

Fetal scalp blood sampling poses little risk to mother or fetus, but falsely low platelet counts occur in up to 50% of cases (145, 158, 159).

Recent analyses have emphasized the low risk of fetal hemorrhagic complications. One group found that only 14 of 447 (3.1%) reported neonates born to women with ATP had a bleeding complication and only 4 (0.9%) had intracranial hemorrhage (142). The authors suggested that these figures probably overstated the risk of fetal hemorrhagic complications. Not only were some infants with neonatal, rather than cord-blood, thrombocytopenia included, older studies did not exclude possible neonatal alloimmune thrombocytopenia. In a recent, well-designed, population-based study of more than 15,000 pregnancies, no infant born to a woman with ATP suffered a bleeding complication (139). For these reasons, many authorities do not recommend fetal platelet count assessment prior to delivery in women with ATP and allow labor with vaginal delivery (142, 160).

## Neonatal Alloimmune Thrombocytopenia (NAIT) (See Chapter 28)

NAIT is a syndrome of fetal-neonatal thrombocytopenia due to maternal immunization to alloantigens present on the paternal platelets, with subsequent transplacental transfer of IgG antiplatelet alloantibodies. It is analogous to hemolytic (Rh) disease of the fetus and newborn, and is estimated to complicate one in 1000 to 5000 pregnancies (161, 162).

The most common platelet antigen involved in NAIT is the HPA-1a (PL$^{A1}$) antigen, being responsible for up to 75% of cases (maternal immunizations in Caucasians) (163–165). This antigen is present in 97% of the population, and 70% of individuals are homozygous. There are two allelic variants (HPA-1a and HPA-1b), but HPA-1a is the most immunogenic. Immune response genes influence alloantibody formation in women negative for HPA-1a antigen—women with HLA-DR3 alloantigen make up the majority of cases (166). Other platelet antigens that may cause NAIT include HPA-3a (Bak$^a$), HPA-4a (Pen$^a$), HPA-4b (Pen$^b$), HPA-5a (Br$^a$), and HPA-5b (Br$^b$).

NAIT presents with unexpected, moderate-to-severe neonatal thrombocytopenia; the maternal platelet count is normal. Other causes of neonatal thrombocytopenia must be excluded, and platelet typing and maternal antipaternal platelet antibody testing performed. Unlike Rh disease, NAIT often presents in a first pregnancy. Some 75% of subsequent pregnancies by the same mating are also affected (165, 167), and the degree of neonatal thrombocytopenia is as severe or more severe than in the prior pregnancy (168).

Without question, NAIT is the most common cause of serious fetal-neonatal thrombocytopenia. Serious bleeding has been reported in up to 25% of cases, and serious morbidity or mortality may occur in up to 15% of infants (165, 169). Intracranial hemorrhage is estimated to occur in 10 to 20% of cases due to HPA-1a alloimmunization (167) and may occur before the onset of labor, although rarely before the third trimester. With these risks in mind, the obstetric management goals are to (a) identify pregnancies at risk for NAIT; (b) to treat current, serious fetal thrombocytopenia that might result in intrauterine hemorrhage; (c) properly select a safe mode of delivery, depending on the fetal platelet count; and (d) assist in preparation for treatment of the neonate if serious thrombocytopenia is present at birth.

The occurrence of neonatal thrombocytopenia in an infant should raise suspicion of possible NAIT and must be properly investigated. If the diagnosis is uncertain, maternal and paternal blood samples should be sent to a laboratory well versed in evaluation for NAIT. A diagnosis of NAIT is confirmed if the mother is negative for a pertinent platelet antigen, the father is positive for the same antigen, and the mother's serum contains alloantibodies to paternal platelets and other platelets positive for the same antigen. In some suspected cases, maternal alloantibodies to paternal platelets will be found, but no specific antigenic difference between maternal and paternal platelets can be identified. The proper interpretation of such results requires the advice of expert pathologists.

Once a pregnancy at risk is identified, current antenatal management involves determining whether or not the fetus is at risk, either by demonstrating that the fetus has the pertinent antigen or by demonstrating that the fetus is thrombocytopenic. For cases in which the pertinent antigen is HPA-1a, the fetal antigen status can be determined by polymerase chain reaction using amniotic fluid cells (170, 171). This is unnecessary if the father is known to be homozygous for HPA-1a and paternity is certain. Initially, investigators recommended confirming that the fetus is thrombocytopenic by cordocentesis performed in the mid-trimester before starting therapy (167, 172). This approach is not without risk, and at least five thrombocytopenic neonates have died from complications of cordocentesis (173). To avoid this problem, most maternal-fetal medicine specialists now have washed maternal platelets available for intravascular umbilical vein infusion when performing a cordocentesis for suspected fetal thrombocytopenia. Not all experts initiate potentially dangerous diagnostic studies or expensive therapy in the mid-second trimester because antepartum hemorrhage is rare before 28 weeks' gestation.

Fetal-neonatal outcomes appear improved by treatment of the mother with IVIG. In the largest published series (172), investigators found that antenatal IVIG treatment (1 g/kg/wk) started in the mid-to-late second trimester was associated with nearly 85% of infants hav-

ing platelet counts in excess of $30 \times 10^9/l$ and no cases of intracranial hemorrhage. By comparison, 48% of siblings born previously had intracranial hemorrhage and 16 of 20 had platelet counts $<30 \times 10^9/l$ at birth.

Cordocentesis should be used in preparation for delivery. If the fetal platelet count is less than $50 \times 10^9/l$, Caesarian delivery or fetal platelet transfusion with immediate induction and attempted vaginal delivery is indicated. With or without antenatal treatment, it is imperative that the obstetrician aid in preparing for possible neonatal thrombocytopenia by arranging plateletpheresis of the mother immediately prior to delivery. These platelets, which do not bear the offending antigen, will raise the neonatal platelet count for several days.

# PREECLAMPSIA

Preeclampsia is a unique form of hypertensive disease that occurs only during pregnancy and is most common among young primigravidae, occurring in up to 7%. The triad of symptoms includes hypertension, proteinuria, and generalized edema. Individuals are considered to have mild disease until they have evidence of end organ damage (see Table 46.1). The etiology of preeclampsia is unknown; however, it is quite clear that vasospasm plays a primary role in the pathophysiology of the hypertension itself. Doppler flow studies indicate that abnormalities of the uteroplacental circulation are evident early in gestation, well before the onset of maternal hypertension. Histopathologic features include diminished or absent physiologic alterations of the terminal (myometrial and decidual) segments of the spiral arteries, which feed the intervillous spaces of the placenta. Normally, these unique vessels undergo a degeneration of the muscular layer in their terminal segments, leaving them unresponsive to circulating vasopressors. In preeclampsia, the muscular layer of many or most terminal spiral arteries remains intact and is presumably susceptible to vasopressors (174). Other abnormalities of the

| **TABLE 46.1.** Criteria for Severe Preeclampsia |
|---|

1. Blood pressure >160 mm Hg systolic or >110 mm Hg diastolic
2. Proteinuria >5 grams/24 hours
3. Oliguria <500 cc/24 hours
4. The development of pulmonary edema
5. Hemolysis
6. Elevated liver enzymes, epigastric pain, or right-upper-quadrant pain
7. Intrauterine growth retardation or oligohydramnios
8. Headache, visual disturbances
9. Seizures

terminal spiral arteries include fibrinoid necrosis, accumulation of lipid-laden macrophages suggestive of an atherosclerotic-like condition (175), and endothelial damage (176). The net effect is to cause a reduction in blood flow to the intervillous space with more severe cases resulting in fetal growth impairment or fetal death.

There also is an alteration in the balance between plasminogen activators and plasminogen activator inhibitors in pregnancies complicated by preeclampsia (177–179). In normal pregnancy, there is a progressive increase in both plasminogen activators and inhibitors. However, in pregnancies complicated by preeclampsia, there is a larger increase of plasminogen activator inhibitor than that of plasminogen activator leading to a depression of fibrinolysis. This may account for the formation of microthrombi in the terminal capillary system in the placental bed of preeclamptic pregnancies.

Angiotensin II levels increase during normal pregnancy. However, as pregnancy progresses, this increase in angiotensin II is accompanied by an increased refractoriness to the effects of angiotensin II (180). Gant et al found that women destined to develop preeclampsia lost this refractoriness to angiotensin II several weeks before the development of hypertension (181). Invasive monitoring studies have shown systemic vascular resistance to be significantly elevated in preeclampsia (182, 183). Several groups of investigators have found a shift toward an increase in thromboxane production relative to prostacyclin production in pregnancies complicated by preeclampsia (184, 185). Other imbalances involving potent mediators of vascular tone have also been reported. Endothelium-derived relaxing factor (nitric oxide), a potent vasodilator, has been found to be decreased in individuals with preeclampsia (186) while endothelin, a potent vasoconstrictor, was found to be elevated (187). Recently, Schobel et al have reported a substantial increase in sympathetic vasoconstrictor activity in preeclamptic women compared to normotensive pregnant and nonpregnant women and nonpregnant women with chronic hypertension (188).

In addition to vasospasm leading to an increase in peripheral vascular resistance, an increase in cardiac output also seems to contribute to elevated blood pressures in preeclamptic women. Progressive increases in the cardiac output were reported in preeclamptic women (189), as well as increases in left ventricular stroke work index (181). At the same time, the normal robust expansion of plasma volume normally seen in pregnancy is reduced in individuals with preeclampsia, with the net effect being one of reduced intravascular volume.

Endothelial damage or activation may play a primary role in the development of preeclampsia. Serum from preeclamptic women has been found to be cytotoxic to endothelial cells (190). Plasma levels of ED+

cellular fibronectin, which is mainly confined to the endothelium, were found to be increased in the first and second trimester of women who later developed preeclampsia (191). Thrombomodulin levels in preeclamptic women have been found to be increased indicating endothelial cell damage (192). Others found elevated levels of thrombomodulin, tissue plasminogen activator inhibitor type 1 and fibronectin in women with preeclampsia. These latter two are nonspecific as they are synthesized in cells other than the endothelium; nevertheless, their presence supports the evidence that endothelial cell damage or activation plays a role in the pathophysiology of preeclampsia.

## HEMATOLOGIC EFFECTS

Probably as a result of plasma volume contraction, the mean hematocrit is higher in women with preeclampsia than in normotensive pregnant individuals or nonpregnant women (40.5, 34.7, and 38.2%, respectively) (193). Thrombocytopenia is another common feature in preeclampsia and platelet counts of less than $100,000/\mu L$ may occur in up to 50% of women with severe disease (194, 195). Platelet life span is also reduced, suggesting that the thrombocytopenia is consumptive in nature. In addition, some investigators (196, 197) have detected platelet function abnormalities, although clinically important platelet dysfunction is exceedingly unusual in preeclampsia.

On average, thrombocytopenia takes 60 hours to resolve after delivery; virtually all individuals with preeclampsia and thrombocytopenia have platelet counts above $100,000/\mu L$ by 96 hours postpartum (198). The etiology of the thrombocytopenia is althought to be secondary to endothelial damage causing a low-grade coagulopathy. Some authors have proposed an immune mechanism for thrombocytopenia, and others have proposed activation of platelets (199). Samuel et al (200) found increased platelet antibodies during pregnancy in women with preeclampsia, with normalization of the test 6 weeks postpartum. Others found an increase in platelet aggregation and increase of beta-thromboglobulin and other platelet factors (199, 201, 202).

Fibrin degradation products, plasma fibrinopeptide A, factor VIII antigen/activity ratio, and thrombin-antithrombin complexes are increased in women with preeclampsia (203). Antithrombin III levels are reduced (204). The hemolysis is microangiopathic in nature, mimicking the hemolysis seen in hemolytic uremic syndrome and thrombotic thrombocytopenic purpura, however, in these two entities the antithrombin III levels are not decreased (205).

## HELLP SYNDROME

A subcategory of severe preeclampsia consisting of *he*molysis, *e*levated *liver* enzymes, and *low* *p*latelets has been termed the HELLP syndrome (see Chapter 46). The anemia of HELLP syndrome is rarely severe. Although most individuals with HELLP syndrome have obvious preeclampsia, clinicians should recognize that HELLP syndrome may occur in the absence of obvious or substantial hypertension (206). Distinguishing HELLP syndrome from other causes of thrombocytopenia or elevated hepatocellular enzymes is imperative, and a high index of suspicion for HELLP syndrome is warranted.

The incidence of HELLP syndrome in preeclampsia varies from 2 to 21% (207, 208). The risk of recurrence for HELLP syndrome has been estimated to be 20 to 25% (207). Laboratory evidence of disseminated intravascular coagulation is found in 20 to 35% of individuals with HELLP syndrome, but in only 5% of HELLP individuals without abruptio placentae, peripartum hemorrhage, or subcapsular hematomas (206).

## CLINICAL MANAGEMENT

Delivery is the definitive treatment for preeclampsia. In individuals with mild preeclampsia at term, delivery is indicated and intravenous magnesium sulfate should be given as seizure prophylaxis during the peripartum period. Close attention to urinary output is mandatory since magnesium overdose may occur with renal impairment. If mild preeclampsia occurs at a preterm gestation, the individual may be managed expectantly but with vigilant observation for signs or symptoms of severe preeclampsia.

Temporizing measures have been used by some experts in extremely premature pregnancies (<28 weeks' gestation) with severe preeclampsia. In such cases, high dose corticosteroids and/or antihypertensive medications have been used in an attempt to ameliorate concerning clinical features (209, 210). Laboratory parameters often improve in individuals with HELLP syndrome after corticosteroid administration. One group reported an average prolongation of 19.4 days in pregnancies between 24 to 27 weeks who were managed with bed rest, antihypertensive medications, and close maternal and fetal monitoring (211).

During labor, the goal of antihypertensive therapy is to keep the diastolic blood pressure below 110-mm Hg diastolic (212). Intravenous hydralazine, labetolol, and oral or sublingual calcium channel blocking agents have been used to control blood pressure in preeclampsia. If these agents fail to control blood pressure adequately, sodium nitroprusside or another potent antihypertensive should be used. Central hemodynamic monitoring is indicated for marked hypertension requiring continuous infusion of antihypertensive agents. Other indications for central monitoring include oliguria refractory to intravenous fluid administration and pulmonary edema (213). Because of the endothelial damage and extravasation of fluid into the extravascular compartment, care must be taken to avoid fluid overload with its potential adverse sequela of pulmonary edema.

## SEPTIC PELVIC THROMBOPHLEBITIS

Puerperal infection may spread through the pelvic venous system and result in septic pelvic thrombophlebitis (SPT). Although rare, the condition is often quite serious. The presumed etiology is infection of myometrial veins following delivery complicated by myometritis. The ovarian veins may become involved because they drain the upper uterus. SPT usually presents within the first week postpartum in a individual with hectic fever spikes despite antibiotic therapy following Caesarian delivery. Pain is usually present on the involved side, but is not easily distinguished from the pain of myometritis alone. Although a tender adnexal mass may be found in some cases, the pelvic examination is often nondiagnostic (214, 215). Computed tomographic or magnetic resonance imaging studies may demonstrate phlebitis. When SPT is suspected, the individual should be treated presumptively with heparin therapy. Most clinicians believe that fever generally subsides within 48 to 72 hours after anticoagulation is initiated (214). At present there is no consensus as to the duration of therapy required to treat the condition. Certainly antibiotic treatment and heparin should be continued until the individual is afebrile for 24 to 48 hours. The need for further anticoagulation therapy or future thromboprophylaxis is uncertain.

## ARTIFICIAL HEART VALVES IN PREGNANCY

Patients with artificial heart valves are at risk for systemic embolism and require lifelong anticoagulant therapy. Pregnancy represents a particularly high-risk time for thromboembolism, not only because of its thrombogenic nature, but also because of the difficulty in anticoagulant management imposed by pregnancy. There are no randomized, controlled trials evaluating the efficacy of various thromboprophylaxis regimens in pregnancy. However, Salazar et al (216) demonstrated that antiplatelet agents alone were inadequate as prophylactic agents. Cerebral embolic events were diagnosed in 17 of 68 individuals treated with antiplatelet agents alone, and three individuals died as a result of valvular thromboembolism.

In a nonrandomized study, Iturbe-Alesio et al (92) prospectively evaluated 72 pregnancies divided into three groups based on differing treatment regimens. All women were taking warfarin at the time of conception, and most women were treated with heparin after the 38th week of pregnancy. In the first group, individuals were administered 5000 U of subcutaneous unfractionated heparin twice daily from the 6th through the 12th week of gestation in place of warfarin. In the second group, individuals were converted over to heparin after the seventh week of gestation. In the third group, warfarin was given until the 37th week of gestation. Nearly 9% of women in the first group sustained massive valve thrombosis, suggesting the superiority of warfarin over low-dose heparin in the prevention of thromboembolism. However, as discussed previously, slightly more than 25% of infants exposed to warfarin between 6 and 12 weeks of gestation developed warfarin embryopathy.

Other studies also have shown that low-dose heparin is inadequate in preventing thrombotic events in pregnant individuals with prosthetic valves (217, 218). Some investigators have suggested that heparin administered in doses adequate to keep the activated partial thromboplastin time (aPPT) between 1.5 and 2.0 times control may be efficacious in preventing thromboembolism (219, 220). Others have indicated that a minimum aPPT ratio of 1.5 is too low and recommend that the aPTT should be kept between 2 and 3 times the control (221, 222).

Salazar et al (223) prospectively evaluated 40 pregnancies in 37 individuals with prosthetic heart valve who were converted from acenocoumarol to therapeutic doses of subcutaneous heparin during the period between 6 and 12 weeks of gestation and reported a higher failure rate while on heparin. The heparin dose was adjusted to keep the aPTT ratio between 1.5 and 2.5. Two individuals developed fatal massive thrombosis of their Björk-Shiley valves while on heparin anticoagulation. One individual on acenocoumarol therapy died from gastrointestinal bleeding and one neonatal death (2.5%) occurred due to intracranial hemorrhage. However, no individuals on oral anticoagulants developed thrombosis.

In one study of 49 pregnant individuals with mainly newer generation prosthetic heart valves, investigators found a low incidence in individuals despite inadequate anticoagulation (224). This is consistent with studies in nonpregnant individuals, which also indicated that the incidence of thromboembolism is lower with the use of newer generation mechanical prosthetic valves (225, 226).

Anticoagulation in pregnant individuals with mechanical prosthetic heart valves poses a risk not only for the mother, but also for the unborn child. The use of warfarin poses the risk of warfarin embryopathy, central nervous system abnormalities, and intracranial bleeding in the fetus. Heparin does not cross the placenta and therefore the fetus is protected from these risks, but recent information indicates that thromboembolic complications may be increased with heparin compared with warfarin therapy (223, 227).

However, the information obtained thus far has been compromised by either small numbers of individuals, retrospective nature of the studies, possible inadequate heparin therapy, or lack of consideration of newer developments, such as newer generation prosthetic valves, continuous subcutaneous heparin therapy via a programmable pump, and low-molecular-weight heparin. Therefore a definitive statement regarding optimal anticoagulation therapy cannot be made in individuals with mechanical prosthetic valves at this time.

The American College of Chest Physicians recommends subcutaneous heparin therapy until the 13th week of gestation, followed by warfarin anticoagulation until the middle of the third trimester, then converting back to heparin therapy until delivery. The European Society of Cardiology recommends either (a) anticoagulation with heparin until the end of the 13th week of pregnancy, followed by warfarin anticoagulation until the 37th week, converting back to heparin therapy until delivery; or (b) continuous treatment with warfarin until the 37th or 38th week of pregnancy, then switching to heparin until delivery (228).

# OBSTETRIC HEMORRHAGE

Since the 1950s, maternal mortality from hemorrhage has decreased by almost 50%, although it continues to be a leading cause of maternal death. Currently, postpartum hemorrhage accounts for approximately 10% of maternal deaths annually in the United States, and if ectopic pregnancy is included, hemorrhage is the leading cause of maternal death (229).

The increase in blood volume during pregnancy fortunately provides enough vascular reserve to accommodate a moderate-to-excessive amount of blood loss without threat of serious morbidity (230). With additional bleeding, however, compensatory mechanisms may be overwhelmed, and the individual may rapidly decompensate. When obstetric hemorrhage occurs, medical personnel must work swiftly and efficiently to prevent catastrophe. As in any case of hemorrhage, the first concern is to maintain sufficient intravascular volume while preparations are made to correct the source of bleeding. Whole blood replacement would be ideal in cases of severe obstetric hemorrhage, but is rarely available today. Therefore crystalloid should be administered to maintain adequate circulatory volume and tissue perfusion until packed red blood cells are available.

In massive obstetric hemorrhage unrelated to an underlying coagulopathy, platelet and coagulation factor replacement is generally not necessary unless more than 8 to 10 units of packed red cells are replaced. Volume replacement with crystalloid and packed red cells alone may result in a "dilutional" coagulopathy. In this situation blood for hematocrit, platelet count, aPTT, PT, fibrinogen, and fibrin degradation products should be obtained. In such a scenario, the most common deficiency is that of platelets (231) and these should be replaced along with the coagulation factors. In bleeding individuals with thrombocytopenia, platelets should be administered to keep the platelet count above $50 \times 10^9$/L. All the coagulation factors are found in fresh frozen plasma, and it should be used to correct coagulation factor depletion.

# DISSEMINATED INTRAVASCULAR COAGULATION IN OBSTETRICS

Disseminated intravascular coagulation (DIC) is discussed in Chapter 44. In brief, DIC results when the coagulation and fibrinolytic pathways are activated on a systemic rather than local level. Pregnancy and delivery pose an increased risk for the development of DIC, and several obstetric conditions are well known to be associated with DIC. These include abruptio placentae, amniotic fluid embolism, puerperal infection, and retained dead fetus (see Table 46.2). Rarely, preeclampsia is associated with clinically apparent DIC. The various etiologies of DIC in obstetrics are listed in Table 46.2.

Clinically, DIC may present with hemorrhagic complications such as ecchymoses, hematuria, hemorrhage, and hypovolemic shock, or with thrombotic complications involving the brain, kidneys, lungs, and intestines. The clinically most useful diagnostic tests in obstetric DIC are the platelet count, fibrinogen level, and a test to determine the presence of fibrin degradation products. It is worth noting that the fibrinogen level is considerably increased in pregnancy such that values under 300 mg/dL may represent DIC. Fibrin degradation products will be detectable in cases of low-grade DIC where other laboratory tests are still within normal ranges. Soluble fibrin-fibrinogen dimers are also increased with DIC. Prothrombin and activated partial thromboplastin times may not be abnormal until the fibrinogen levels decrease below 100-mg/dL (232).

The most important principle of treatment in obstetric-related DIC is to identify and eliminate the underlying cause. For example, in cases of abruptio placentae, delivery should be effected as soon as possible. In addition, depleted coagulation factors and platelets must be replaced to promote hemostasis. Heparin should not be used in obstetric DIC when hemorrhage is present as this may exacerbate the bleeding. One clinical situation in which heparin may be useful is when DIC occurs with an intact vascular system such as occurs with intrauterine fetal demise (233).

## INTRAUTERINE FETAL DEMISE

Intrauterine fetal demise is a rare cause of DIC, and it rarely if ever occurs in cases of fetal death before 20 to 22 weeks' gestation. In general, the dead fetus must be retained *in utero* for several weeks before DIC develops (234). It is believed that release of thromboplastic substances from the dead fetus produce a decline in fibrinogen by activation of the clotting cascade. Approximately one-third of individuals who retain a dead fetus for more than 4 weeks will develop DIC (235). In individuals who do develop DIC with an intact circulatory system, intravenous heparin therapy may be considered to interrupt the coagulation cascade while plans for delivery are made. Normalization of platelet count and levels of coagulation factors may take up to 48 hours with continuous heparin infusion (236). Once delivery is effected, the thromboplastic nidus is removed and the coagulopathy will be corrected. Romero et al reported a case of a single fetal demise in a twin pregnancy in which DIC developed. The individual was treated successfully with heparin therapy with subsequent reversal of the coagulopathy. A healthy infant was delivered 8 weeks later (233).

## AMNIOTIC FLUID EMBOLISM

Amniotic fluid embolism (AFE) is a rare, but highly lethal condition. The reported incidence of AFE ranges from one in 8000 to one in 80,000 pregnancies. AFE is one of the most common causes of immediate peripartum death, accounting for approximately 10% of all maternal deaths in the United States (240). Maternal mortality has been as high as 86% in some series (237). A national registry of AFE cases established by Clark reported a maternal mortality rate of 61% with only 15% of survivors neurologically intact (239). Neonatal outcome was nearly as dismal with only a 39% neurologically intact survival rate reported (239).

### Risk Factors

Recent evaluations of AFE have shown that maternal age, race, parity, obstetric history, weight gain, blood

---

**TABLE 46.2.** Obstetrical Causes of Disseminated Intravascular Coagulation

Induced abortion
Septic abortion
Abruptio placentae
Intrauterine fetal demise
Hemorrhage
Preeclampsia/HELLP syndrome
Amniotic fluid embolism
Acute fatty liver of pregnancy

pressure, labor characteristics, and oxytocin use are no different in individuals with AFE compared with the uncomplicated individuals (237, 239, 241). Data from the national registry found that AFE occurred during labor in 70% and during Caesarian section in 19% of cases. In addition, 39% of individuals were nulliparous. Interestingly, 41% of individuals reported a history of drug allergy or atopy, and there was a significant association with male fetuses (67%) (239).

## Pathophysiology

The etiology and the early pathophysiology of AFE remain uncertain. Because of the rarity of the condition and the rapidity of its onset and evolution, there are few hemodynamic data available in humans to evaluate the early changes of AFE. The scant hemodynamic, hematologic, and respiratory data available suggest that AFE may be similar to anaphylactic or septic shock, with maternal exposure to fetal antigen(s) hypothesized as the inciting event. Animal models of AFE have also shown a temporal sequence of events similar to what is seen with anaphylactic shock and suggests a common pathophysiologic mechanism. Recently, Hankins et al have developed an animal model using pregnant goats by injecting them with aliquots of autologous amniotic fluid (242). His group demonstrated that amniotic fluid injected into the pulmonary artery caused a rapid rise in the pulmonary arterial pressure and pulmonary vascular resistance. These effects were increased with administration of meconium containing amniotic fluid. In addition, there was a significant drop in maternal cardiac output and PaO$_2$, an increase in the pulmonary capillary wedge pressure, and acute left ventricular failure. The data are consistent with the hypothesis that amniotic fluid or meconium contains vasoactive pressor agents or myocardial depressants or both.

Rat hearts perfused with human amniotic fluid have shown a decrease in coronary artery flow with marked fluctuations of left ventricular function. Richards et al speculated that the ventricular failure seen in individuals with AFE may be due to coronary artery vasospasm with resultant ischemia (243). Based on the accumulated clinical and experimental evidence, it appears that AFE is not strictly an embolic event. Some authorities have suggested that the term AFE be discarded in favor of *Anaphylactoid Syndrome of Pregnancy* to emphasize that this syndrome is most likely caused by endogenous mediators similar to those found in anaphylaxis or sepsis.

## Diagnosis

Patients generally present with acute cardiopulmonary collapse, peripartum hypoxia, and coagulopathy (see

**TABLE 46.3.**  Signs and Symptoms in Individuals with Amniotic Fluid Embolism

| Sign or Symptom | Number of Individuals | Percent |
|---|---|---|
| Hypotension | 43 | 100 |
| Fetal distress[a] | 30 | 100 |
| Pulmonary edema or ARDS[b] | 28 | 93 |
| Cardiopulmonary arrest | 40 | 87 |
| Cyanosis | 38 | 83 |
| Coagulopathy[c] | 38 | 83 |
| Dyspnea[d] | 22 | 49 |
| Seizure | 22 | 48 |
| Atony | 11 | 23 |
| Brochospasm[e] | 7 | 15 |
| Transient hypertension | 5 | 11 |
| Cough | 3 | 7 |
| Headache | 3 | 7 |
| Chest pain | 1 | 2 |

*Reproduced with permission from Clark SL, Hankins GD, Dudley DA et al Amniotic fluid embolism: analysis of the national registry. Am J Obstet Gynecol 1995;172:1158–1167.*

[a] *n = 30. Includes all live fetuses in utero at time of event.*

[b] *n = 30. Eighteen individuals did not survive long enough for these diagnoses to be confirmed.*

[c] *n = 38. Eight individuals did not survive long enough for this diagnosis to be confirmed.*

[d] *n = 45. One individual was intubated at the time of the event and could not be assessed.*

[e] *Difficult ventilation was noted during cardiac arrest in six individuals, and wheezes were auscultated in one individual.*

Table 46.3) (223). Classically the diagnosis has been made at autopsy with the finding of fetal squamous cells in the pulmonary vascular bed. However, only 73% of individuals dying from AFE have fetal squamous cells in the pulmonary circulation. Furthermore, these cells can also be found in the pulmonary vasculature of laboring pregnant women without evidence of AFE (239, 244, 245). Therefore the diagnosis is based on clinical and laboratory findings with the absence of other potential explanations for the observed findings. The stringent criteria developed by the national registry for the diagnosis of AFE are listed in Table 46.4 (239).

## Treatment

Immediate respiratory support is essential. Following respiratory stabilization, shock should be treated with intravascular volume and inotropic support (246). If the individual survives the initial insult, DIC will ensue and must be treated.

**TABLE 46.4.** Amniotic Fluid Embolism Registry Entry Criteria

1. Acute hypotension or cardiac arrest
2. Acute hypoxia, deafined as dyspnea, cyanosis, or respiratory arrest
3. Coagulopathy, defined as laboratory evidence of intravascular consumption or fibrinolysis or severe clinical hemorrhage in the absence of other explanations[a]
4. Onset of the above during labor, caesarian section, or dilation and evacuation, or within 30 minutes postpartum
5. Absence of any other significant confounding condition or potential explanation for the signs and symptoms observed
6. Occurrence within 5 years of registry opening

*Reproduced with permission from Clark SL, Hankins GD, Dudley DA et al Amniotic fluid embolism: analysis of the national registry. Am J Obstet Gynecol 1995;172:1158–1167.*

[a] *Patients meeting all other criteria, including abrupt cardiorespiratory arrest, who died before coagulopathy could be assessed were included in the primary analysis.*

## ABORTION

DIC has been reported in individuals undergoing therapeutic abortion performed using urea and hypertonic saline. The cause of DIC in these cases is the release of thromboplastic materials into the maternal circulation from the damaged placenta. DIC has been reported with other forms of termination including first trimester suction dilatation and curettage, as well as third trimester abortions (246, 247). Volume replacement and replacement of blood and coagulation factors should be instituted promptly.

## ACUTE FATTY LIVER OF PREGNANCY

Acute fatty liver of pregnancy (AFLP) is a rare but potentially fatal condition first categorized as a distinct clinical entity by Sheehan in 1940 (248). It generally occurs in the third trimester with an incidence of between one in 9000 and one in 13,000 pregnancies (249, 250). Earlier reports indicated a high maternal and fetal mortality rate of more than 80% (251, 252), but recent studies have shown a maternal survival rate of more than 90% and a perinatal survival rate of more than 85% (253, 254).

Patients with AFLP commonly present with signs of a viral-like illness. The most frequently reported symptoms include nausea, vomiting, malaise, dyspnea, or myalgias (254). Individuals may also present with jaundice, asterixis, abdominal pain, fever, headache, pruritus, polydipsia, edema, proteinuria, hypertension, and mental confusion (250, 251, 253).

Laboratory abnormalities include thrombocytopenia, leukocytosis, profound hypoglycemia, hyperbilirubinemia, elevated serum ammonia, increased blood urea nitrogen and serum creatinine, and abnormal coagulation tests (254, 255). Ames, Castro et al found evidence of DIC in all 28 individuals with AFLP in their series. Unlike other obstetric conditions associated with DIC, abnormal coagulation tests persisted up to 2 weeks postpartum in individuals with AFLP (255). These investigators postulated that the persistence of the coagulopathy may have been due to the profound decrease in antithrombin III levels.

The differential diagnosis of AFLP includes preeclampsia, HELLP syndrome, viral- or drug-induced hepatitis, cholestasis of pregnancy, gall bladder disease, and Reyes syndrome. However, the unique constellation of symptoms and laboratory findings, particularly severely depressed antithrombin III activity (11% of normal), should lead to an accurate diagnosis in most cases. Pregnancy does not generally affect antithrombin III activity (89% ± 13%), and antithrombin III activity is decreased only mildly in preeclampsia and HELLP syndrome. Clinically confusing cases may require liver biopsy to make the diagnosis of AFLP. Magnetic resonance imaging, ultrasonography, or computed tomography examination of the liver have been proposed to detect fatty changes. However, the utility of these diagnostic modalities is disputed (254, 256, 257).

Full recovery can be expected once the individual is delivered. After the diagnosis of AFLP is made, the individual's neurologic, cardiovascular, hematologic, renal, and hepatic function should be monitored closely while delivery is undertaken. Glucose solutions should be infused to correct hypoglycemia, and fresh frozen plasma or cryoprecipitate may be used to correct clotting-factor deficiencies. Antithrombin III replacement has been suggested to decrease the morbidity and mortality and to hasten the resolution of DIC; however, Ames Castro et al did not find empiric antithrombin III transfusion to be of benefit in improving the clinical course of the disease (255). In individuals with severe bleeding complications, antithrombin III replacement may be beneficial.

# REFERENCES

1. Fay RA, Hughes AO, Farron NT. Platelets in pregnancy: hyperdestruction in pregnancy. Obstet Gynaecol 1983;61:238–240.
2. Sill PR, Lind T, Walker W. Platelet values during normal pregnancy. Br J Obstet Gynaecol 1985;92:480–483.
3. Tygart SG, McRoyan DK, Spinnato JA et al. Longitudinal study of platelet indices during normal pregnancy. Am J Obstet Gynecol 1986;154:883–887.
4. Douglas JT, Shah M, Lowe GD et al. Plasma fibrinopeptide A and beta-thrombomodulin in pre-eclampsia and pregnancy hypertension. Thromb Haemost 1982;47:54–55.
5. Suarez CR, Gonzalez J, Menendez C et al. Neonatal and maternal platelets: activation at time of birth. Am J Hematol 1988;29:18–21.
6. Leuschen MP, Davis RB, Boyd D et al. Comparative evaluation of antepartum and post-partum platelet function in smokers and nonsmokers. Am J Obstet Gynecol 1986;155:1276–1280.

7. Burgess-Wilson ME, Morrison R, Heptinstall S. Spontaneous platelet aggregation in heparinised blood during pregnancy. Thromb Res 1986;41:385–393.

8. Louden KA, Broughton-Pipkin F, Heptinstall S et al. Platelet reactivity and serum thromboxane $B_2$ production in whole blood in gestational hypertension and pre-eclampsia. Br J Obstet Gynaecol 1991;98:1239–1244.

9. Fitzgerald DJ, Mayo G, Catella F et al. Increased thromboxane biosynthesis in normal pregnancy is mainly derived from platelets. Am J Obstet Gynecol 1987;157:325–330.

10. Burrows RF, Kelton JG. Incidentally detected thrombocytopenia in healthy mothers and their infants. N Engl J Med 1988;319:142–145.

11. Beller FK, Ebert C. The coagulation and fibrinolytic enzyme system in pregnancy and in the puerperium. Eur J Obstet Gynecol Reprod Biol 1982;13:177–197.

12. Ballegeer V, Mombaerts P, Declerk PJ et al. Fibrinolytic response to venous occlusion and fibrin fragment D-dimer levels in normal and complicated pregnancy. Thromb Haemost 1987;58:1030–1032.

13. Booth NA, Reith A, Bennett B et al. A plasminogen activator inhibitor (PAI-2) circulates in two molecular forms during pregnancy. Thromb Haemost 1988;59:77–79.

14. Faught W, Garner P, Jones G et al. Changes in protein C and protein S levels in normal pregnancy. Am J Obstet Gynecol 1995;172:(1 Pt 1)147–150.

15. Warwick R, Hutton RA, Goff L et al. Changes in protein C and free protein S during pregnancy and following hysterectomy. J R Soc Med 1989;82:591–594.

16. Comp PC, Thurnau GR, Welsh J et al. Functional and immunologic protein S levels are decreased during pregnancy. Blood 1986;68:881–885.

17. Suzuki S, Sakamoto W. The kinetics of blood coagulability: fibrinolytic and kallikrein-kinin system at the onset of and during labor. Eur J Obstet Gynecol Reprod Biol 1984;17:209–218.

18. Hellgren M, Blomback M. Studies on blood coagulation and fibrinolysis in pregnancy, during delivery and in the puerperium. I. Normal condition. Gynecol Obstet Invest 1981;12:141–154.

19. Suarez CR, Menendez CE, Walenga JM et al. Neonatal and maternal hemostasis: value of molecular markers in the assessment of hemostatic status. Semin Thromb Hemost 1984;10:280–284.

20. Rochat RW, Koonin LM, Atrash HK et al. Maternal mortality in the United States: report from the Maternal Mortality Collaborative. Obstet Gynecol 1988;72:91–97.

21. Franks AL, Atrash HK, Lawson HW et al. Obstetrical pulmonary embolism mortality, United States, 1970–85. Am J Public Health 1990;80:720–722.

22. Sachs BP, Brown DA, Driscoll SG et al. Maternal mortality in Massachusetts. Trends and prevention. N Engl J Med 1987;316:667–672.

23. Department of Health and Social Security. Report on confidential enquiries in maternal deaths in England and Wales, 1979–81. London: Her Majesty's Stationery Office, 1986.

24. de Swiet M, Fidler J, Howell R et al. Thromboembolism in pregnancy. In: Jewell D, ed. Advanced medicine. London: Pitman Medical, 1981; pp. 309–317.

25. Rutherford S, Montoro M, McGehee W et al. Thromboembolic disease associated with pregnancy: an 11-year Review [Abstract]. Am J Obstet Gynecol 1991;164(Suppl):286a.

26. Hellgren M, Nygards EB. Long-term therapy with subcutaneous heparin during pregnancy. Gynecol Obstet Invest 1982;13:76–89.

27. Kierkegaard A. Incidence and diagnosis of deep vein thrombosis associated with pregnancy. Acta Obstet Gynecol Scand 1983;62:239–243.

28. Toglia MR, Weg JG. Venous thromboembolism during pregnancy. N Engl J Med 1996;335:108–114.

29. Barbour LA, Pickard J. Controversies in thromboembolic disease during pregnancy: a critical review. Obstet Gynecol 1995;86(4 Pt 1):621–633.

30. Bergqvist A, Bergqvist D, Hallbook T. Deep vein thrombosis during pregnancy. A prospective study. Acta Obstet Gynecol Scand 1983;62:443–448.

31. Bergqvist D, Hedner U. Pregnancy and venous thrombo-embolism. Acta Obstet Gynecol Scand 1983;62:449–453.

32. Ginsberg JS, Brill-Edwards P, Burrows RF et al. Venous thrombosis during pregnancy: leg and trimester of presentation. Thromb Haemost 1992;67:519–520.

33. Hathaway WE, Bonnar J. Thrombotic disorders in pregnancy and the newborn infant. In: Hathaway WE, Bonnar J, ed. Hemostatic disorders of the pregnant woman and newborn infant. New York: Elsevier, 1987; pp. 151–184.

34. Hull RD, Raskob GE, Carter CJ. Serial impedance plethysmography in pregnant individuals with clinically suspected deep-vein thrombosis. Clinical validity of negative findings. Ann Intern Med 1990;112:663–667.

35. Tengborn L, Bergqvist D, Matzsch T et al. Recurrent thromboembolism in pregnancy and puerperium: is there a need for thromboprophylaxis? Am J Obstet Gynecol 1989;160:90–94.

36. Badaracco MA, Vessey MP. Recurrence of venous thromboembolic disease and use of oral contraceptives. Br Med J 1974;1:215–217.

37. Vicente V, Rodriguez C, Soto I et al. Risk of thrombosis during pregnancy and post-partum in hereditary thrombophilia. Am J Hematol 1994;46:151–152.

38. Branch DW, Silver RM, Blackwell JL et al. Outcome of treated pregnancies in women with antiphospholipid syndrome: an update of the Utah experience. Obstet Gynecol 1992;80:614–620.

39. Lima F, Khamashta MA, Buchanan NM et al. A study of sixty pregnancies in patients with the antiphospholipid syndrome. Clin Exp Rheumatol 1996;14:131–136.

40. Cogo A, Lensing AW, Prandoni P et al. Distribution of thrombosis in individuals with symptomatic deep vein thrombosis. Implications for simplifying the diagnostic process with compression ultrasound. Arch Intern Med 1993;153:2777–2780.

41. Heijboer H, Buller HR, Lensing AWA et al. A comparison of real-time compression ultrasonography with impedance plethysmography for the diagnosis of deep-vein thrombosis in symptomatic outpatients. N Engl J Med 1993;329:1365–1369.

42. Killewich LA, Bedford GR, Beach KW et al. Diagnosis of deep venous thrombosis. A prospective study comparing duplex scanning to contrast venography. Circulation 1989;79:810–814.

43. White RH, McGahan JP, Daschbach MM et al. Diagnosis of deep-vein thrombosis using duplex ultrasound. Ann Intern Med 1989;111:297–304.

44. Greer IA, Barry J, Mackon N et al. Diagnosis of deep venous thrombosis in pregnancy: a new role for diagnostic ultrasound. Br J Obstet Gynaecol 1990;97:53–57.

45. Nicholas GG, Lorenz RP, Botti JJ et al. The frequent occurrence of false-positive results in phleborheography during pregnancy. Surg Gynecol Obstet 1985;161:133–135.

46. Anderson DR, Lensing AW, Wells PS et al. Limitations of impedance plethysmography in the diagnosis of clinically suspected deep-vein thrombosis. Ann Intern Med 1993;118:25–30.

47. Heijboer H, Buller HR, Lensing AW et al. A comparison of real-time compression ultrasonography with impedance plethysmography for the diagnosis of deep-vein thrombosis in symptomatic outpatients. N Engl J Med 1993;329:1365–1369.

48. Hull RD, Hirsh J, Carter CJ et al. Diagnostic efficacy of impedance plethysmography for clinically suspected deep-vein thrombosis. A randomized trial. Ann Intern Med 1985;102:21–28.

49. Hull R, Hirsh J, Sackett DL et al. Cost effectiveness of clinical diagnosis, venography, and noninvasive testing in individuals with symptomatic deep-vein thrombosis. N Engl J Med 1981;304:1561–1567.

50. Bonnar J. Venous thromboembolism and pregnancy. Clin Obstet Gynecol 1981;8:455–473.

51. Ginsberg JS, Hirsh J, Rainbow AJ et al. Risks to the fetus of radiologic procedures used in the diagnosis of maternal venous thromboembolic disease. Thomb Haemost 1989;61:189–196.

52. Verstraete M. The diagnosis and treatment of deep-vein thrombosis. N Engl J Med 1993;329:1418–1420.

53. Forestier F, Sole Y, Aiach M et al. Absence of transplacental passage of fragmin (Kabi) during the second and third trimesters of pregnancy [Letter]. Thromb Haemost 1992;67:180–181.

54. Hirsh J. Heparin. N Engl J Med 1991;324:1565–1574.

55. Cruickshank MK, Levine MN, Hirsh J et al. A standard heparin nomogram for the management of heparin therapy. Arch Intern Med 1991;151:333–337.

56. Hull RD, Raskob GE, Rosenbloom D et al. Optimal therapeutic level of heparin therapy in individuals with venous thrombosis. Arch Intern Med 1992;152:1589–1595.

57. Gallus A, Jackaman J, Tillett J et al. Safety and efficacy of warfarin started early after submassive venous thrombosis of pulmonary embolism. Lancet 1986;2:1293–1296.

58. Hull RD, Raskob GE, Rosenbloom D et al. Heparin for 5 days as compared with 10 days in the initial treatment of proximal venous thrombosis. N Engl J Med 1990;322:1260–1264.

59. Barbour LA, Smith JM, Marlar RA. Heparin levels to guide thromboembolism prophylaxis during pregnancy. Am J Obstet Gynecol 1995;173:1869–1873.

60. Brancazio LR, Roperti KA, Stierer R et al. Pharmacokinetics and pharmacodynamics of subcutaneous heparin during the early third trimester of pregnancy. Am J Obstet Gynecol 1995;173:1240–1245.

61. Sipes SL, Weiner CP. Venous thromboembolic disease in pregnancy. Semin Perinatol 1990;14:103–118.

62. Barss VA, Schwartz PA, Greene MF et al. Use of the subcutaneous heparin pump during pregnancy. J Reprod Med 1985;30:899–901.

63. Hahn CL. Pulsatile heparin administration in pregnancy: a new approach. Am J Obstet Gynecol 1986;155:283–287.

64. Floyd RC, Gookin KS, Hess LW et al. Administration of heparin by subcutaneous infusion with a programmable pump. Am J Obstet Gynecol 1991;165:931–933.

65. Anderson DR, Ginsberg JS, Brill-Edwards P et al. The use of an indwelling Teflon catheter for subcutaneous heparin administration during pregnancy. A randomized crossover study. Arch Intern Med 1993;153:841–844.

66. Prandoni P, Lensing AW, Buller HR et al. Comparison of subcutaneous low-molecular-weight heparin with intravenous standard heparin in proximal deep-vein thrombosis. Lancet 1992;339:441–445.

67. Hull RD, Raskob GE, Pineo GF et al. Subcutaneous low-molecular-weight heparin compared with continuous intravenous heparin in the treatment of proximal-vein thrombosis. N Engl J Med 1992;326:975–982.

68. Dulitzki M, Pauzner R, Langevitz P et al. Low-molecular-weight heparin during pregnancy and delivery: preliminary experience with 41 pregnancies. Obstet Gynecol 1996;87:380–383.

69. Fejgin MD, Lourwood DL. Low-molecular-weight heparins and their use in obstetrics and gynecology. Obstet Gynecol Surv 1994;49:424–431.

70. Sturridge F, de Swiet M, Letsky E. The use of low-molecular-weight heparin for thromboprophylaxis in pregnancy. Br J Obstet Gynaecol 1994;101:69–71.

71. Ginsberg JS, Hirsh J. Use of antithrobotic agents during pregnancy. Chest 1995;108(4 Suppl): 305S–311S.

72. Barbour LA, Pickard J. Controversies in thromboembolic disease during pregnancy: a critical review. Obstet Gynecol 1995;86(4 Pt 1):621–633.

73. Dahlman TC, Hellgren MS, Blomback M. Thrombosis prophylaxis in pregnancy with use of subcutaneous heparin adjusted by monitoring heparin concentration in plasma. Am J Obstet Gynecol 1989;161:420–425.

74. Weinmann EE, Salzman EW. Deep-vein thrombosis. N Engl J Med 1994;331:1630–1641.

75. Colvin BT, Barrowcliff TW. The British Society for Haematology Guidelines on the use and monitoring of heparin 1992: second revision. J Clin Pathol 1993;46:97–103.

76. Howell R, Fidler J, Letsky E et al. The risks of antenatal subcutaneous heparin prophylaxis: a controlled trial. Br J Obstet Gynaecol 1983;90:1124–1128.

77. Wise PH, Hall AJ. Heparin-induced osteopenia in pregnancy. Br Med J 1980;281:110–111.

78. Griffiths HT, Liu DT. Severe heparin osteoporosis in pregnancy. Postgrad Med J 1984;60:424–425.

79. Dahlman TC. Osteoporotic fractures and the recurrence of thromboembolism during pregnancy and the puerperium in 184 women undergoing thromboprophylaxis with heparin. Am J Obstet Gynecol 1993;168:1265–1270.

80. Dahlman T, Lindavall N, Hellgren M. Osteopenia in pregnancy during long-term heparin treatment: a radiological study post partum. Br J Obstet Gynaecol 1990;97:221–228.

81. Kelton JG, Levine MN. Heparin-induced thrombocytopenia. Semin Thromb Hemost 1986;12:59–62.

82. Warkentin TE, Levine MN, Hirsh J et al. Heparin-induced thrombocytopenia in individuals treated with low-molecular-weight heparin or unfractionated heparin. N Engl J Med 1995;332:1330–1335.

83. Hatjis CG. Heparin-induced thrombocytopenia in pregnancy. A case report. J Reprod Med 1984;29:337–338.

84. Copplestone A, Oscier DG. Heparin-induced thrombocytopenia in pregnancy. Br J Haematol 1987;65:248.

85. van Besien K, Hoffman R, Golichowski A. Pregnancy associated with lupus anticoagulant and heparin induced thrombocytopenia: management with a low-molecular-weight heparinoid. Thromb Res 1991;62:23–29.

86. Delclos GL, Davila F. Thrombotic therapy for pulmonary embolism in pregnancy: a case report. Am J Obstet Gynecol 1986;155:375–376.

87. Baudo F. Emergency treatment with recombinant tissue plasminogen activator of pulmonary embolism in a pregnant woman with antithrombin-III deficiency. Am J Obstet Gynecol 1990;163(4 Pt 1):1274–1275.

88. Flossdorf T. Successful treatment of massive pulmonary embolism with recombinant tissue plasminogen activator in a pregnant woman with intact gravidity and preterm labor. Int Care Med 1990;16:454–456.

89. Kramer WB. Successful urokinase treatment of massive pulmonary embolism in pregnancy. Obstet Gynecol 1995;86:660–665.

90. Hall JG, Pauli RM, Wilson KM. Maternal and fetal sequelae of anticoagulation during pregnancy. Am J Med 1980;68:122–140.

91. Ginsberg JS, Hirsh J, Turner DC et al. Risks to the fetus of anticoagulant therapy during pregnancy [Review]. Thromb Haemost 1989;61:197–203.

92. Iturbe-Alessio I, Fonseca MC, Mutchinik O et al. Risks of anticoagulant therapy in pregnant women with artificial heart valves. N Engl J Med 1986;315:1390–1393.

93. Orme ML, Lewis PJ, de Swiet M et al. May mothers given warfarin breast-feed their infants? Br Med J 1977;1:1564–1565.

94. Bertina RM, Koeleman BPC, Koster T et al. Mutation in blood coagulation factor V associated with resistance to activated protein C. Nature 1994;369:64–67.

95. Greengard JS, Sun X, Xu X et al. Activated protein C resistance caused by Arg506Gln mutation in factor Va [Letter]. Lancet 1994;343:1361–1362.

96. Voorberg J, Roelse J, Koopman R et al. Association of idiopathic venous thromboembolism with single point–mutation at Arg506 of factor V. Lancet 1994;343:1535–1536.

97. Zoller B, Svensson PJ, He X et al. Identification of the same factor V gene mutation in 47 out of 50 thrombosis-prone families with inherited resistance to activated protein C. J Clin Invest 1994;94:2521–2524.

98. Zoller B, Dahlback B. Linkage between inherited resistance to activated protein C and factor V gene mutation in venous thrombosis. Lancet 1994;343:1536–1538.

99. Sun X, Evatt B, Griffin JH. Blood coagulation factor Va abnormality associated with resistance to activated protein C in venous thrombophilia. Blood 1994;83:3120–3125.

100. Dizon-Townson DS, Nelson LM, Easton K et al. The factor V leiden mutation may predispose women to severe preeclampsia. Am J Obstet Gynecol 1996;175:902–905.

101. Griffin JH, Evatt B, Wideman C et al. Anticoagulant protein C pathway defective in majority of thrombophilic patients. Blood 1993;82:1989–1993.

102. Koster T, Rosendaal FR, de Ronde H et al. Venous thrombosis due to poor anticoagulant response to activated protein C: Leidin Thrombophilia Study. Lancet 1993;342:1503–1506.

103. Faioni EM, Franchi F, Asti D et al. Resistance to activated protein C in nine thrombophilic families: interference in a protein S functional assay. Thromb Haemost 1993;70:1067–1071.

104. Svensson PJ, Dahlback B. Resistance to activated protein C as a basis for venous thrombosis. N Engl J Med 1994;330:517–522.

105. Halbmayer WM, Haushofer A, Schon R et al. The prevalence of poor anticoagulant response to activated protein C (APC resistance) among individuals suffering from stroke or venous thrombosis and among healthy subjects. Blood Coagul Fibrinolys 1994;5:51–57.

106. Hellgren M, Svensson PJ, Dahlback B. Resistance to activated protein C as a basis for venous thromboembolism associated with pregnancy and oral contraceptives. Am J Obstet Gynecol 1995;173:210–213.

107. Heijboer H, Brandjes DP, Buller HR et al. Deficiencies of coagulation-inhibiting and fibrinolytic proteins in outpatients with deep vein thrombosis. N Engl J Med 1990;323:1512–1516.

108. Finazzi G, Caccia R, Barbui T. Different prevalence of thromboembolism in subtypes of congenital antithrombin deficiency: Review of 404 cases [Letter][Review]. Thromb Haemost 1987;58:1094.

109. Meade TW, Dyer S, Howarth DJ et al. Antithrombin III and procoagulant activity: sex differences and effects of the menopause. Br J Haematol 1990;74:77–81.

110. Tait RC, Walker ID, Davidson JF et al. Antithrombin III activity in healthy blood donors: age and sex related changes and the prevalence of asymptomatic deficiency [Letter]. Br J Haematol 1990;75:141–142.

111. Wells PS, Blajchaman MA, Henderson P et al. Prevalence of antithrombin deficiency in healthy blood donors: a cross-sectional study. Am J Hematol 1994;45:321–324.

112. Miletich J, Sherman L, Broze GJ Jr. Absence of thrombosis in subjects with heterozygous protein C deficiency. N Engl J Med 1987;317:991–996.

113. Conard J, Horellou MH, van Dreden P et al. Thrombosis and pregnancy in congenital deficiencies in AT III, protein C or protein S: study of 78 women. Thromb Haemost 1990;63:319–320.

114. Hellgren M, Hagnevik K, Robbe H et al. Severe acquired antithrombin III deficiency in relation to hepatic and renal insufficiency and intrauterine fetal death in late pregnancy. Gynecol Obstet Invest 1983;16:107–118.

115. Winter JH, Fenech A, Ridley W et al. Familial antithrombin III deficiency. Q J Med 1982;51:373–395.

116. Brandt P, Stenbjerg S. Subcutaneous heparin for thrombosis in pregnant women with hereditary antithrombin deficiency [Letter]. Lancet 1979;1:100–101.

117. Samson D, Stirling Y, Woolf L et al. Management of planned pregnancy in a individual with congenital antithrombin III deficiency. Br J Haematol 1984;56:243–249.

118. Dekker GA, de Vries JIP, Doelitzsch PM et al. Underlying disorders associated with severe early-onset preeclampsia. Am J Obstet Gynecol 1995;173:1042–1048.

119. Rai R, Regan L, Hadley E et al. Second-trimester pregnancy loss is associated with activated C resistance. Br J Haematol 1996;92:489–490.

120. Branch DW. Althoughts on the mechanism of pregnancy loss associated with the antiphospholipid syndrome [Review]. Lupus 1994;3:275–280.

121. Petri M, Golbus M, Anderson R et al. Antinuclear antibody, lupus anticoagulant, and anticardiolipin antibody in women with idiopathic habitual abortion. A controlled prospective study of forty-four women. Arthritis Rheum 1987;30:601–606.

122. Out HJ, Bruinse HW, Christiaens GC et al. Prevalence of antiphospholipid antibodies in individuals with fetal loss. Ann Rheum Dis 1991;50:553–557.

123. Parazzini F, Acaia B, Facen D et al. Antiphospholipid antibodies and recurrent abortion. Obstet Gynecol 1991;77:854–858.

124. Parke AL, Wilson D, Maier D. The prevalence of antiphospholipid antibodies in women with recurrent spontaneous abortion, women with successful pregnancies, and women who have never been pregnant. Arthritis Rheum 1991;34:1231–1235.

125. Plouffe L Jr, White EW, Tho SP et al. Etiologic factors of recurrent abortion and subsequent reproductive performance of couples: have we made any progress in the past 10 years? Am J Obstet Gynecol 1992;167:313–320.

126. Yetman DL, Kutteh WH. Antiphospholipid antibody panels and recurrent pregnancy loss: prevalent of anticardiolipin antibodies compared with other antiphospholipid antibodies. Fertil Steril 1996;66:540–546.

127. Branch DW, Silver R, Pierangeli S et al. Antiphospholipid antibodies other than lupus anticoagulant and anticardiolipin antibodies in women with recurrent pregnancy loss, fertile controls, and antiphospholipid syndrome. Obstet Gynecol 1997;98:549–555.

128. Rai RS, Regan L, Clifford K et al. Antiphospholipid antibodies and beta 2-glycoprotein-1 in 500 women with recurrent miscarriage: results of a comprehensive screening approach. Hum Reprod 1995;10:2001–2005.

129. Oshiro BT, Silver RM, Scott JR et al. Antiphospholipid antibodies and fetal death. Obstet Gyecol 1996;87:489–493.

130. Harris EN, Spinnato JA. Should anticardiolipin tests be performed in

otherwise healthy pregnancy women? Am J Obstet Gynecol 1991;165:1272–1277.

131. Robinson RD, Polzin WJ, Kozakowski MH et al. The incidence of antiphospholipid antibodies in the obstetric population [Abstract]. Proceedings of the Annual Clinical Meeting of the American College of Obstetricians and Gynecologists, Las Vegas, 1992.

132. Branch DW. Althoughts on the mechanism of pregnancy loss associated with the antiphospholipid syndrome [Review]. Lupus 1994;3:275–280.

133. De Wolf F, Carreras LO, Moerman P et al. Decidual vasculopathy and extensive placental infarction in a individual with repeated thromboembolic accidents, recurrent fetal loss, and a lupus anticoagulant. Am J Obstet Gynecol 1982;142:829–834.

134. Erlendsson K, Steinsson K, Johannsson JH et al. Relation of antiphospholipid antibody and placental bed inflammatory vascular changes to the outcome of pregnancy in successive pregnancies of 2 women with systemic lupus erythematosus. J Rheumatol 1993;20:1779–1785.

135. Kutteh WH. Antiphospholipid antibody-associated recurrent pregnancy loss: treatment with heparin and low-dose aspirin is superior to low-dose aspirin alone. Am J Obstet Gynecol 1996;174:1584–1589.

136. Rai R, Cohen H, Dave M et al. Randomised controlled trial of aspirin and aspirin plus heparin in pregnant women with recurrent miscarriage associated with phospholipid antibodies (or antiphospholipid antibodies). BMJ 1997;314:253–257.

137. Spencer JA. Paroxysmal nocturnal haemoglobinuria in pregnancy. Br J Obstet Gynaecol 1980;87:246–248.

138. Burrows RF, Kelton JG. Thrombocytopenia at delivery: a prospective survey of 6715 deliveries. Am J Obstet Gynecol 1990;162:731–734.

139. Burrows RF, Kelton JG. Fetal thrombocytopenia and its relation to maternal thrombocytopenia. N Engl J Med 1993;329:1463–1466.

140. Kessler I, Lancet M, Borenstein R et al. The obstetrical management of individuals with immunologic thrombocytopenic purpura. Int J Gynaecol Obstet 1982;20:23–28.

141. Hart D, Dunetz C, Nardi M et al. An epidemic of maternal thrombocytopenia associated with elevated antiplatelet antibody. Platelet count and antiplatelet antibody in 116 consecutive pregnancies: relationship to neonatal platelet count. Am J Obstet Gynecol 1986;154:878–883.

142. Silver RM, Branch DW, Scott JR. Maternal thrombocytopenia in pregnancy: time for a reassessment. Am J Obstet Gynecol 1995;173:479–482.

143. Yin CS, Scott JR. Unsuccessful treatment of fetal immunologic thrombocytopenia with dexamethasone. Am J Obstet Gynecol 1985;152:316–317.

144. Kaplan C, Daffos F, Forestier F et al. Fetal platelet counts in thrombocytopenic pregnancy. Lancet 1990;336:979–982.

145. Cook RL, Miller RC, Katz VL et al. Immune thrombocytopenic purpura in pregnancy: a reappraisal of management [Review]. Obstet Gynecol 1991;78:578–583.

146. Christiaens GC, Nieuwenhuis HK, Von Dem Borne AE. Idiopathic thrombocytopenic purpura in pregnancy: a randomized trial on the effect of antenatal low dose corticosteroids on neonatal platelet count. Br J Obstet Gynaecol 1990;97:893–898.

147. Carloss HW, McMillan R, Crosby WH. Management of pregnancy in women with immune thrombocytopenic purpura. JAMA 1980;224:2756–2758.

148. Murray JM, Harris RE. The management of the pregnant individual with idiopathic thrombocytopenic purpura. Am J Obstet Gynecol 1976;126:449–451.

149. Territo M, Finklestein J, Oh W et al. Management of autoimmune thrombocytopenia in pregnancy and the neonate. Obstet Gynecol 1973;41:579–584.

150. Scott JR, Rote NS, Cruikshank DP. Antiplatelet antibodies and platelet counts in pregnancies complicated by autoimmune thrombocytopenic purpura. Am J Obstet Gynecol 1983;145:932–939.

151. Moise KJ Jr, Cotton DB. Discordant fetal platelet counts in a twin gestation complicated by idiopathic thrombocytopenic purpura. Am J Obstet Gynecol 1987;156:1141–1142.

152. Scott JR, Cruikshank DP, Kochenour NK et al. Fetal platelet counts in the obstetric management of immunologic thrombocytopenic purpura. Am J Obstet Gynecol 1980;136:495–499.

153. Moise KJ Jr, Carpenter RJ Jr, Cotton DB et al. Percutaneous umbilical cord blood sampling in the evaluation of fetal platelet counts in pregnant individuals with autoimmune thrombocytopenic purpura. Obstet Gynecol 1988;72:346–350.

154. Scioscia AL, Grannum PA, Copel JA et al. The use of percutaneous umbilical blood sampling in immune thrombocytopenic purpura. Am J Obstet Gynecol 1988;159:1066–1068.

155. De Carolis S, Noia G, DeSantis M et al. Immune thrombocytopenic purpura and percutaneous umbilical blood sampling: an open question. Fetal Diagn Ther 1993;87:154–160.

156. Weiner CP, Wenstrom KD, Sipes SL et al. Risk factors for cordocentesis and fetal intravascular transfusion. Am J Obstet Gynecol 1991;165:1020–1025.

157. Ghidini A, Sepulveda W, Lockwood CJ et al. Complications of fetal blood sampling [Review]. Am J Obstet Gynecol 1993;168:1339–1344.

158. Hunter S, Merrill D, Weiner C. Fetal scalp platelet sampling in the obstetrical management of idiopathic thrombocytopenic purpura (ITP) pregnancies [Abstract]. Am J Obstet Gynecol 1993;168:412.

159. Adams DM, Bussel JB, Druzin ML. Accurate intrapartum estimation of fetal platelet count by fetal scalp sample smear. Am J Perinatol 1994;11:42–45.

160. Weiner CP. Why the fuss over diagnosing fetal thrombocytopenia secondary to ITP? Contrib Gynecol Obstet 1995;40(8):45–50.

161. Blanchette VS, Chen L, de Friedberg ZS et al. Alloimmunization to the PlA1 platelet antigen: results of a prospective study. Br J Haematol 1990;74:209–215.

162. Pillai M. Platelets and pregnancy. Br J Obstet Gynaecol 1993;100:201–204.

163. Pearson HA, Shulman NR, Marder VJ et al. Isoimmune neonatal thrombocytopenic purpura. Clinical and therapeutic considerations. Blood 1964;23:154–177.

164. Katz J, Hodder FS, Aster RS et al. Neonatal isoimmune thrombocytopenia. The natural course and management and the detection of maternal antibody. Clin Pediatr 1984;23:159–162.

165. Mueller-Eckhardt G, Kiefel V, Grubert A et al. 348 cases of suspected neonatal alloimmune thrombocytopenia. Lancet 1989;1:363–366.

166. De Waal LP, Van Dalen CM, Engelfriet CP et al. Alloimmunization against the platelet-specific Zwᵃ antigen, resulting in neonatal thrombocytopenia or posttransfusion purpura, is associated with the supertypic DRw52 antigen including DR3 and DRw6. Hum Immunol 1986;17:45–53.

167. Bussel JB, Berkowitz RL, McFarland JG et al. Antenatal treatment of neonatal alloimmune thrombocytopenia. N Engl J Med 1988;319:1374–1378.

168. Reznikoff-Etievant MF. Management of alloimmune neonatal and antenatal thrombocytopenia [Review]. Vox Sang 1988;55:193–201.

169. Blanchette VS. Neonatal alloimmune thrombocytopenia: a clinical perspective [Review]. Curr Stud Hematol Blood Transfus 1988;54:112–126.

170. Kuijpers RW, Faber NM, Kanhai HH et al. Typing of fetal platelet alloantigens when platelets are not available [Letter]. Lancet 1990;336:1319.

171. McFarland JG, Aster RH, Bussel JB et al. Prenatal diagnosis of neonatal alloimmune thrombocytopenia using allele-specific oligonucleotide probes. Blood 1991;78:2276–2282.

172. Lynch L, Bussel JB, McFarland JG et al. Antenatal treatment of alloimmune thrombocytopenia. Obstet Gynecol 1992;80:67–71.

173. Paidas MJ, Berkowitz RL, Lynch L et al. Alloimmune thrombocytopenia: fetal and neonatal losses related to cordocentesis. Am J Obstet Gynecol 1995;172:475–479.

174. Khong TY, De Wolf F, Robertson WB et al. Inadequate maternal vascular response to placentation in pregnancies complicated by pre-eclampsia and by small-for-gestational-age infants. Br J Obstet Gynaecol 1986;93:1049–1059.

175. Frusca T, Morassi L, Pecorelli S et al. Histological features of uteroplacental vessels in normal and hypertensive patients in relation to birthweight. Br J Obstet Gynaecol 1989;96:835–839.

176. Shanklin DR, Sibai BM. Ultrastructural aspects of preeclampsia. I. Placental bed and uterine boundary vessels. Am J Obstet Gynecol 1989;161:735–741.

177. Kolben M, Lopens A, Blaser J et al. Proteases and their inhibitors are indicative in gestational disease. Eur J Obstet Gynecol Reprod Biol 1996;65:59–65.

178. Gao M, Nakabayashi M, Sakura M et al. The imbalance of plasminogen activators and inhibitor in preeclampsia. J Obstet Gynaecol Res 1996;22:9–16.

179. Abdul-Karim R, Assali NS. Pressor response to angiotonin in pregnant and nonpregnant women. Am J Obstet Gynecol 1961;82:246–251.

180. Gant NF, Jimenez JM, Whalley PJ et al. A prospective study of angiotensin II pressor responsiveness in pregnancies complicated by chronic essential hypertension. Am J Obstet Gynecol 1977;127:369–375.

181. Mabie WC, Ratts TE, Sibai BM. The central hemodynamics of severe preeclampsia. Am J Obstet Gynecol 1989;161:1443–1448.

182. Cotton DB, Lee W, Huhta JC et al. Hemodynamic profile of severe pregnancy-induced hypertension. Am J Obstet Gynecol 1988;158:523–529.

183. Walsh SW, Parisi VM. The role of arachidonic acid metabolites in preeclampsia. Semin Perinatol 1986;10:335–355.

184. Walsh SW. Preeclampsia: an imbalance in placenta prostacyclin and thromboxane production. Am J Obstet Gynecol 1985;152:335–340.

185. Moodley J, Norman RJ, Reddi K. Central venous concentrations of immunoreactive prostaglandins E, F, and 6-keto-PGF1α in eclampsia. Br Med J (Clin Res Ed) 1984;288:1487–1489.

186. Pinto A, Sorrentino R, Sorrentino P et al. Endothelial-derived relaxing factor released by endothelial cells of human umbilical vessels and its impairment in pregnancy-induced hypertension. Am J Obstet Gynecol 1991;164:507–513.

187. Clark BA, Halvorson L, Sachs B et al. Plasma endothelin levels in preeclampsia: elevation and correlation with uric acid levels and renal impairment. Am J Obstet Gynecol 1992;166:962–968.

188. Schobel HP, Fischer T, Heuszer K et al. Preeclampsia—a state of sympathetic overactivity. N Engl J Med 1996;335:1480–1485.

189. Easterling TR, Benedetti TJ, Schmucker BC et al. Maternal hemodynamics in normal and preeclamptic pregnancies: a longitudinal study. Obstet Gynecol 1990;76:1061–1069.

190. Rodgers GM, Taylor RN, Roberts JM. Preeclampsia is associated with a serum factor cytotoxic to human endothelial cells. Am J Obstet Gynecol 1988;159:908–914.

191. Lockwood CJ, Peters JH. Increased plasma levels of ED1 + cellular fibronectin precede the clinical signs of preeclampsia. Am J Obstet Gynecol 1990;162:358–362.

192. Hsu CD, Copel JA, Hong SF et al. Thrombomodulin levels in preeclampsia, gestational hypertension, and chronic hypertension. Obstet Gynecol 1995; 86:897–899.

193. Pritchard JA, Cunningham FG, Mason RA. Coagulation changes in eclampsia: their frequency and pathogenesis. Am J Obstet Gynecol 1976; 124:855–864.

194. Sibai BM, Watson DL, Hill GA et al. Maternal-fetal correlations in individuals with severe preeclampsia/eclampsia. Obstet Gynecol 1983;62: 745–750.

195. Leduc L, Wheeler JM, Kirshon B et al. Coagulation profile in severe preeclampsia. Obstet Gynecol 1992;79:14–18.

196. Rakoczi I, Tallian F, Bagdany S et al. Platelet lifespan in normal pregnancy and pre-eclampsia as determined by non-radioisotope technique. Thromb Res 1979;15:553–556.

197. Socol ML, Weiner CP, Louis G et al. Platelet activation in preeclampsia. Am J Obstet Gynecol 1985;151:494–497.

198. Neiger R, Contag SA, Coustan DR. The resolution of preeclampsia-related thrombocytopenia. Obstet Gynecol 1991;77:692–695.

199. Inglis TCM, Stuart J, George AJ et al. Haemostatic and rheological changes in normal pregnancy and pre-eclampsia. Br J Haematol 1982;50:461–465.

200. Samuels P, Bussel JB, Braitman LE et al. Estimation of the risk of thrombocytopenia in the offspring of pregnant women with presumed immune thrombocytopenic purpura. N Engl J Med 1990;323:229–235.

201. Borok Z, Weitz J, Owen J et al. Fibrinogen proteolysis and platelet α-granule release in pre-eclampsia/eclampsia. Blood 1984;63:525–531.

202. Pekonen F, Rasi V, Ammala M et al. Platelet function and coagulation in normal and pre-eclamptic pregnancy. Thromb Res 1986;43:553–560.

203. Perry KG Jr, Martin JN Jr. Abnormal hemostasis and coagulopathy in preeclampsia and eclampsia [Review]. Clin Obstet Gynecol 1992;35: 338–350.

204. Weiner CP, Kwaan HC, Xu C et al. Antithrombin III activity in women with hypertension during pregnancy. Obstet Gynecol 1985;65:301–306.

205. Weinstein L. Syndrome of hemolysis, elevated liver enzymes, and low platelet count: a severe consequence of hypertension in pregnancy. Am J Obstet Gynecol 1982;142:159–167.

206. Sibai BM, Ramadan MK, Usta I et al. Maternal morbidity and mortality in 442 pregnancies with hemolysis, elevated liver enzymes, and low platelets (HELLP syndrome). Am J Obstet Gynecol 1993;169:1000–1006.

207. Audibert F, Friedman SA, Frangieh AY et al. Clinical utility of strict diagnostic criteria for the HELLP (hemolysis, elevated liver enzymes, and low platelets) syndrome. Am J Obstet Gynecol 1996;175:460–464.

208. Sibai BM, Akl S, Fairlie F et al. A protocol for managing severe preeclampsia in the second trimester. Am J Obstet Gynecol 1990;163:733–738.

209. Clark SL, Phelan JR, Allen SH et al. Antepartum reversal of hematologic abnormalities with the HELLP syndrome. A report of three cases. J Reprod Med 1986;31:70–72.

210. Magann EF, Bass D, Chauhan SP et al. Antepartum corticosteroids: disease stabilization in individuals with the syndrome of hemolysis, elevated liver enzymes, and low platelets (HELLP). Am J Obstet Gynecol 1994;171: 1148–1153.

211. Sibai BM, Akl S, Fairlie F et al. A protocol for managing severe preeclampsia in the second trimester. Am J Obstet Gynecol 1990;163:773–778.

212. Sibai BM. Treatment of hypertension in pregnant women [Review]. N Engl J Med 1996;335:257–265.

213. Fox DB, Troiano NH, Graves CR. Use of the pulmonary artery catheter in severe preeclampsia: a Review [Review]. Obstet Gynecol Surv 1996;51: 684–695.

214. Duff P, Gibbs RS. Pelvic vein thrombophlebitis: diagnostic dilemma and therapeutic challenge [Review]. Obstet Gynecol Surv 1983;38:365–373.

215. Cohen MB, Pernoll ML, Gevirtz CM et al. Septic pelvic thrombophlebitis: an update. Obstet Gynecol 1983;62:83–89.

216. Salazar E, Zajarias A, Gutierrez N et al. The problem of cardiac valve prostheses, anticoagulants and pregnancy. Circulation 1984;70(Suppl I): 169–177.

217. Ben Ismail MB, Abid F, Trabelsi S et al. Cardiac valve prostheses, anticoagulation, and pregnancy. Br Heart J 1986;55:101–105.

218. Wang RY, Lee PK, Chow JS et al. Efficacy of low dose, subcutaneously administered heparin in treatment of pregnant women with artificial heart valves. Med J Aust 1983;2:126–128.

219. Levine HJ, Pauker SG, Salzman EW. Antithrombotic therapy in valvular heart disease [Review]. Chest 1986;89(Suppl 2):36S–45S.

220. Cheseboro JH, Adams PC, Fuster V. Antithrombotic therapy in individuals with valvular heart disease and prosthetic heart valves [Review]. J Am Coll Cardiol 1986;8(6 Suppl B):41B–56B.

221. Brill-Edwards P, Ginsberg JS, Johnston M et al. Establishing a therapeutic range for heparin therapy. Ann Intern Med 1993;119:104–109.

222. Ginsberg JS, Barron WM. Pregnancy and prosthetic heart valves. Lancet 1994;334:1170–1172.

223. Salazar E, Izagurine R, Verdejo J et al. Failure of adjusted doses of subcutaneous heparin to prevent thromboembolic phenomena in pregnant individuals with mechanical cardiac valve prostheses. J Am Col Cardiol 1996; 27:1698–1713.

224. Sareli P, England MJ, Berk MR et al. Maternal and fetal sequelae of anticoagulation during pregnancy in individuals with mechanical heart valve prosthesis. Am J Cardiol 1989;63:1462–1465.

225. Butchart EG, Lewis PA, Gunkemeier GL et al. Low risk of thrombosis and serious emobic events despite low-intensity anticoagulation. Experience with 1,004 Medtronic Hall valves. Circulation 1988;88(Suppl I):I-66–I-77.

226. Kopf GS, Hammond GL, Geha AS et al. Long-term performance of the St. Jude Medical Valve: low incidence of thromboembolism and hemorrhagic complications with modest doses of warfarin. Circulation 1987;79(Suppl III):III-132–III-136.

227. Sbarouni E, Oakley CM. Outcome of pregnancy in women with valve prostheses. Br Heart J 1997;71:196–201.

228. Ad Hoc Committee of the Working Group on Valvular Heart Disease. European Society of Cardiology. Guidelines for prevention of thromboembolic events in valvular heart disease. J Heart Valve Dis 1993;2:398–410.

229. Turner LM. Vaginal bleeding during pregnancy [Review]. Emerg Med Clin North Am 1994;12:45–54.

230. Combs CA, Murphy EL, Laros RK Jr. Factors associated with postpartum hemorrhage with vaginal birth. Obstet Gynecol 1991;77:69–76.

231. Wilson RF, Mammen E, Walt AJ. Eight years of experience with massive blood transfusions. J Trauma 1971;11:275–285.

232. Richey ME, Giltrap LC III, Ramin SM. Management of disseminated intravascular coagulopathy [Review]. Clin Obstet Gynecol 1995;38:514–520.

233. Romero R, Duffy TP, Berkowitz RL et al. Prolongation of a preterm pregnancy complicated by death of a single twin in utero and disseminated intravascular coagulation. Effects of treatment with heparin. N Engl J Med 1984;310:772–774.

234. Hodgkinson CR, Thompson RJ, Hodari AA. Dead fetus syndrome. Clin Obstet Gynecol 1964;7:349–358.

235. Pritchard JA. Fetal death in utero. Obstet Gynecol 1959;14:573–580.

236. Bonnar J. Hemorrhagic disorders during pregnancy. In: Hathaway WE, Bonnar J, eds. Hemostatic disorders of the pregnant woman and newborn infant. Chichester: John Wiley, 1987; pp. 76–103.

237. Morgan M. Amniotic fluid embolism [Review]. Anaesthesia 1979;34: 20–32.

238. Martin RW. Amniotic fluid embolism [Review]. Clin Obstet Gynecol 1996; 39:101–106.

239. Clark SL, Hankins GD, Dudley DA et al. Amniotic fluid embolism: analysis of the national registry. Am J Obstet Gynecol 1995;172:1158–1167.

240. Atrash HK, Koonin LM, Lawson HW et al. Maternal mortality in the United States 1979–1986. Obstet Gynecol 1990;76:1055–1060.

241. Burrows A, Khoo SK. The amniotic fluid embolism syndrome: 10 years' experience at a major teaching hospital. Aust N Z J Obstet Gynaecol 1994; 35:245–250.

242. Hankins GD, Snyder RR, Clark SL et al. Acute hemodynamic and respiratory effects of amniotic fluid embolism in the pregnant goat model. Am J Obstet Gynecol 1993;168:1113–1129.

243. Richards DS, Carter LS, Corke B et al. The effect of human amniotic fluid on the isolated perfused rat heart. Am J Obstet Gynecol 1988;158:210–214.

244. Clark SL, Pavlova Z, Greenspoon J et al. Squamous cells in the maternal pulmonary circulation. Am J Obstet Gynecol 1986;154:104–106.

245. Clark SL, Montz FJ, Phelan JP. Hemodynamic alterations associated with amniotic fluid embolism: a reappraisal. Am J Obstet Gynecol 1985;151: 617–621.

246. Goss AS Jr. Disseminated intravascular coagulation syndrome after vacuum curettement for first trimester abortion. South Med J 1978;71:967–968.

247. Kafrissen ME, Barke MW, Workman P et al. Coagulopathy and induced abortion methods: rates and relative risks. Am J Obstet Gynecol 1983;147: 344–345.

248. Sheehan HL. The pathology of acute yellow atrophy and delayed chloroform poisoning. J Obstet Gynaecol Br Empire 1940;47:49–61.

249. Pockros PJ, Peters RL, Reynolds TB. Idiopathic fatty liver of pregnancy: findings in ten cases. Medicine 1984;63:1–11.

250. Purdie JM, Walters BN. Acute fatty liver of pregnancy: clinical features and diagnosis. Aust N Z Obstet Gynecol 1988;28:62–67.

251. Kaplan MM. Acute fatty liver of pregnancy [Review]. N Engl J Med 1985; 313:367–70.

252. Moise KJ Jr, Shah DM. Acute fatty liver of pregnancy: etiology of fetal distress and fetal wastage. Obstet Gynecol 1987;69:482–485.

253. Watson WJ, Seeds JW. Acute fatty liver of pregnancy [Review]. Obstet Gynecol Surv 1990;45:585–591.

254. Usta IM, Barton JR, Amon EA et al. Acute fatty liver of pregnancy: an experience in the diagnosis and management of fourteen cases. Am J Obstet Gynecol 1994;171:1342–1347.

255. Castro MA, Goodwin TM, Shaw KJ et al. Disseminated intravascular coagulation and antithrombin III depression in acute fatty liver of pregnancy [Review]. Am J Obstet Gynecol 1996;174:211–216.

256. Campillo B, Bernuau J, Witz MO et al. Ultrasonography in acute fatty liver of pregnancy. Ann Intern Med 1986;105:383–384.

257. McKee CM, Weir PE, Foster JH et al. Acute fatty liver of pregnancy and diagnosis by computed tomography. Br Med J (Clin Res Ed) 1986;292: 291–292.

# CHAPTER 47

# HEMORRHAGE, THROMBOSIS, AND ANTITHROMBOTIC THERAPY IN CHILDREN

## Michael J. Rohrer, Maureen Andrew, and Alan D. Michelson

## INTRODUCTION

Both thrombotic and hemorrhagic problems are relatively common in the newborn period. Although thrombotic and hemorrhagic events are less common in older pediatric age groups, they are, nonetheless, important clinical problems that often have limb threatening and life threatening potential. The focus of this chapter is to describe a clinical approach to deal with hemorrhage and thrombosis in neonatal and pediatric individuals, as well as to provide guidelines for the use of anticoagulants and thrombolytic agents in these individuals. Before discussing specific clinical problems, it is essential to gain an understanding of the maturation of the hemostatic system with regard to molecular and cellular mechanisms, as well as to review laboratory methods relevant to understanding the uniqueness of neonatal and pediatric hemorrhagic and thrombotic problems.

## THE MATURATION OF THE HEMOSTATIC SYSTEM

### COAGULATION PROTEINS

The hemostatic system of neonates and infants differs in a number of important ways from that of older children and adults. In a study of 118 healthy full-term babies from birth 6 months of age, Andrew et al (1) demonstrated that coagulation test results varied with the postnatal age of the infant and that different coagulation factors show different postnatal patterns of maturation. Adult values are achieved in most components by 6 months of age. These reference values for normal full-term babies are shown in Tables 47.1 and 47.2. The importance of knowing the laboratory methodology used to determine the test results is illustrated by the fact that previous studies utilizing kaolin as a reagent resulted in marked prolongation of the activated partial thromboplastin time (aPTT) in term babies (2, 3). The near-adult values for the aPTT shown in Table 47.1 were obtained using ellagic acid rather than kaolin as the activating agent.

A separate study of 137 healthy preterm neonates, also by Andrew et al (4), resulted in identification of normal reference ranges for hemostatic proteins in these individuals (Tables 47.3 and 47.4). The overall pattern of the coagulation system was similar in premature and full-term babies. The differences between premature and full-term babies, although frequent, were minor compared with the large differences between neonates and adults. In general, the postnatal maturation of the coagulation system is accelerated in preterm infants as compared with full-term infants. Thus, by 6 months of age, full-term and preterm infants show equivalent levels for all but four of the measured components of the coagulation system, with mean values well within the normal adult range.

Normal reference ranges for the coagulation param-

**TABLE 47.1.** Reference Values for Coagulation Tests in Healthy Full-Term Infants During the First 6 Months of Life, Compared with Values for Adults

| Coagulation Tests | Day 1 Mean (boundary) | Day 5 Mean (boundary) | Day 30 Mean (boundary) | Day 90 Mean (boundary) | Day 180 Mean (boundary) | Adults Mean (boundary) |
|---|---|---|---|---|---|---|
| PT(s) | 13.0 (10.1–15.9)* | 12.4 (10.0–15.3)* | 11.8 (10.0–14.3)* | 11.9 (10.0–14.2)* | 12.3 (10.7–13.9)* | 12.4 (10.8–13.9) |
| aPTT(s) | 42.9 (31.3–54.5) | 42.6 (25.4–59.8) | 40.4 (32.0–55.2) | 37.1 (29.0–50.1)* | 35.5 (28.1–42.9)* | 33.5 (26.6–40.3) |
| TCT(s) | 23.5 (19.0–28.3)* | 23.1 (18.0–29.2) | 24.3 (19.4–29.2)* | 25.1 (20.5–29.7)* | 25.5 (19.8–31.2)* | 25.0 (19.7–30.3) |
| Fibrinogen (g/l) | 2.83 (1.67–3.99)* | 3.12 (1.62–4.62)* | 2.70 (1.62–3.78)* | 2.43 (1.50–3.79)* | 2.51 (1.50–3.87)* | 2.78 (1.56–4.00) |
| II (U/ml) | 0.48 (0.26–0.70) | 0.63 (0.33–0.93) | 0.68 (0.34–1.02) | 0.75 (0.45–1.05) | 0.88 (0.60–1.16) | 1.08 (0.70–1.46) |
| V (U/ml) | 0.72 (0.34–1.08) | 0.95 (0.45–1.45) | 0.98 (0.62–1.34) | 0.90 (0.48–1.32) | 0.91 (0.55–1.27) | 1.06 (0.62–1.50) |
| VII (U/ml) | 0.66 (0.28–1.04) | 0.89 (0.35–1.43) | 0.90 (0.42–1.38) | 0.91 (0.39–1.43) | 0.87 (0.47–1.27) | 1.05 (0.67–1.43) |
| VIII (U/ml) | 1.00 (0.50–1.78)* | 0.88 (0.50–1.54)* | 0.91 (0.50–1.57)* | 0.79 (0.50–1.25)* | 0.73 (0.50–1.09) | 0.99 (0.50–1.49) |
| vWF (U/ml) | 1.53 (0.50–2.87) | 1.40 (0.50–2.54) | 1.28 (0.50–2.46) | 1.18 (0.50–2.06) | 1.07 (0.50–1.97) | 0.92 (0.50–1.58) |
| IX (U/ml) | 0.53 (0.15–0.91) | 0.53 (0.15–0.91) | 0.51 (0.21–0.81) | 0.67 (0.21–1.13) | 0.86 (0.36–1.36) | 1.09 (0.55–1.63) |
| X (U/ml) | 0.40 (0.12–0.68) | 0.49 (0.19–0.79) | 0.59 (0.31–0.87) | 0.71 (0.35–1.07) | 0.78 (0.38–1.18) | 1.06 (0.70–1.52) |
| XI (U/ml) | 0.38 (0.10–0.66) | 0.55 (0.23–0.87) | 0.53 (0.27–0.79) | 0.69 (0.41–0.97) | 0.86 (0.49–1.34) | 0.97 (0.67–1.27) |
| XII (U/ml) | 0.53 (0.13–0.93) | 0.47 (0.11–0.83) | 0.49 (0.17–0.81) | 0.67 (0.25–1.09) | 0.77 (0.39–1.15) | 1.08 (0.52–1.64) |
| PK (U/ml) | 0.37 (0.18–0.69) | 0.48 (0.20–0.76) | 0.57 (0.23–0.91) | 0.73 (0.41–1.05) | 0.86 (0.56–1.16) | 1.12 (0.62–1.62) |
| HK (U/ml) | 0.54 (0.06–1.02) | 0.74 (0.16–1.32) | 0.77 (0.33–1.21) | 0.82 (0.30–1.46)* | 0.82 (0.36–1.28)* | 0.92 (0.50–1.36) |
| XIII$_a$ (U/ml) | 0.79 (0.27–1.31) | 0.94 (0.44–1.44)* | 0.93 (0.39–1.47)* | 1.04 (1.36–1.72)* | 1.04 (0.46–1.62)* | 1.05 (0.55–1.55) |
| XIII$_b$ (U/ml) | 0.76 (0.30–1.22) | 1.06 (0.32–1.80)* | 1.11 (0.39–1.73)* | 1.16 (0.48–1.84)* | 1.10 (0.50–1.70)* | 0.97 (0.57–1.37) |

*Adapted with permission from Andrew M, Paes B, Milner R et al. Development of the human coagulation system in the full-term infant. Blood 1987;70:165–172.*

*PT = prothrombin time; aPTT = activated partial thromboplastin time; TCT = thrombin clotting time; VIII = factor VIII procoagulant; vWf = von Willebrand factor; PK = prekallikrein; HK = high-molecular-weight kininogen.*

*All factors, except fibrinogen, are expressed as units per milliliter (U/ml), where pooled plasma contains 1.0 U/ml. All values are expressed as the mean, followed by the lower and upper boundary encompassing 95% of the population. Between 40 and 77 samples were assayed for each value for the newborn. Some measurements were skewed due to a disproportionate number of high values. The lower limit, which excludes the lower 2.5% of the population, has been given.*

*All babies received vitamin K at birth.*

*\* Values that are indistinguishable from those of the adult.*

**TABLE 47.2.** Reference Values for the Inhibitors of Coagulation in Healthy Full-Term Infants During the First 6 Months of Life, Compared with Values for Adults

| Coagulation Inhibitors | Day 1 Mean (boundary) | Day 5 Mean (boundary) | Day 30 Mean (boundary) | Day 90 Mean (boundary) | Day 180 Mean (boundary) | Adults Mean (boundary) |
|---|---|---|---|---|---|---|
| ATIII (U/ml) | 0.63 (0.39–0.87) | 0.67 (0.41–0.93) | 0.78 (0.48–1.08) | 0.97 (0.73–1.21)* | 1.04 (0.84–1.24)* | 1.05 (0.79–1.31) |
| $\alpha_2$M (U/ml) | 1.39 (0.95–1.83) | 1.48 (0.98–1.98) | 1.50 (1.06–1.94) | 1.76 (1.26–2.26) | 1.91 (1.49–2.33) | 0.86 (0.52–1.20) |
| C$_1$E-INH (U/ml) | 0.72 (0.36–1.08) | 0.90 (0.60–1.20)* | 0.89 (0.47–1.31) | 1.15 (0.71–1.59) | 1.41 (0.89–1.93) | 1.01 (0.71–1.31) |
| $\alpha_1$AT (U/ml) | 0.93 (0.49–1.37)* | 0.89 (0.49–1.29)* | 0.62 (0.36–0.88) | 0.72 (0.42–1.02) | 0.77 (0.47–1.07) | 0.93 (0.55–1.31) |
| HCII (U/ml) | 0.43 (0.10–0.93) | 0.48 (0.10–0.96) | 0.47 (0.10–0.87) | 0.72 (0.10–1.46) | 1.20 (0.50–1.90) | 0.96 (0.66–1.26) |
| Protein C (U/ml) | 0.43 (0.17–0.53) | 0.42 (0.20–0.64) | 0.43 (0.21–0.65) | 0.54 (0.28–0.80) | 0.59 (0.37–0.81) | 0.96 (0.64–1.28) |
| Protein S (U/ml) | 0.36 (0.12–0.60) | 0.50 (0.22–0.78) | 0.63 (0.33–0.93) | 0.86 (0.54–1.18)* | 0.87 (0.55–1.19)* | 0.92 (0.60–1.24) |

*Adapted with permission from Andrew M, Paes B, Milner R et al. Development of the human coagulation system in the full-term infant. Blood 1987;70:165–172.*

*ATIII = antithrombin III; $\alpha_2$M = $\alpha_2$-macroglobulin; C$_1$E-INH = C$_1$-esterase inhibitor; $\alpha_1$AT = $\alpha_1$-antitrypsin; HCII = heparin cofactor II.*

*All values are expressed in units per milliliter (U/ml), where pooled plasma contains 1.0 U/ml. All values are given as a mean, followed by the lower and upper boundary encompassing 95% of the population. Between 40 and 75 samples were assayed for each value for the newborn. Some measurements were skewed due to a disproportionate number of high values. The lower limits, which exclude the lower 2.5% of the population, have been given.*

*\* Values that are indistinguishable from those of the adult.*

eters of preterm infants of less than 30 weeks gestation are not available since the majority of these infants have postnatal complications and cannot be considered completely normal (5). However, Riverdian-Moalic et al (6) measured levels of the blood coagulation proteins and inhibitors by direct puncture of the umbilical cord using ultrasonographic guidance in 285 healthy fetuses be-

tween 19 and 38 weeks gestation (Tables 47.5 and 47.6). Low levels of the vitamin K-dependent factors (II, VII, IX, X), contact factors (XI, XII, prekallikrein and high-molecular-weight kininogen), factor V, factor VII, and fibrinogen all contribute to the prolonged PT and aPTT observed. Low levels of antithrombin III (ATIII), heparin cofactor II, protein C, protein S, and tissue factor path-

**TABLE 47.3.** Reference Values for Coagulation Tests in Healthy Premature Infants (30–36 Weeks Gestation) During the First 6 Months of Life, Compared with Those in Adults

| Coagulation Tests | Day 1 Mean (boundary) | Day 5 Mean (boundary) | Day 30 Mean (boundary) | Day 90 Mean (boundary) | Day 180 Mean (boundary) | Adults Mean (boundary) |
|---|---|---|---|---|---|---|
| PT (s) | 13.0 (10.6–16.2)* | 12.5 (10.0–15.3)* | 11.8 (10.0–13.6)* | 12.3 (10.0–14.6)* | 12.5 (10.0–15.0)* | 12.4 (10.8–13.9) |
| aPTT (s) | 53.6 (27.5–79.4)† | 50.5 (26.9–74.1)† | 44.7 (26.9–62.5) | 39.5 (28.3–50.7) | 37.5 (27.1–53.3)* | 33.5 (26.6–40.3) |
| TCT (s) | 24.8 (19.2–30.4)* | 24.1 (18.8–29.4)* | 24.4 (18.8–29.9)* | 25.1 (19.4–30.8)* | 25.2 (18.9–31.5)* | 25.0 (19.7–30.3) |
| Fibrinogen (g/l) | 2.43 (1.50–3.73)*,† | 2.80 (1.60–4.18)*,† | 2.54 (1.50–4.14)* | 2.46 (1.50–3.52)* | 2.28 (1.50–3.60) | 2.78 (1.56–4.00) |
| II (U/ml) | 0.45 (0.20–0.77) | 0.57 (0.29–0.85)† | 0.57 (0.36–0.95)† | 0.68 (0.30–1.06) | 0.87 (0.51–1.23) | 1.08 (0.70–1.46) |
| V (U/ml) | 0.88 (0.41–1.44)*,† | 1.00 (0.46–1.54)* | 1.02 (0.48–1.56)* | 0.99 (0.59–1.39)* | 1.02 (0.58–1.46)* | 1.06 (0.62–1.50) |
| VII (U/ml) | 0.67 (0.21–1.13) | 0.84 (0.30–1.38) | 0.83 (0.21–1.45) | 0.87 (0.31–1.43) | 0.99 (0.47–1.51)* | 1.05 (0.67–1.43) |
| VIII (U/ml) | 1.11 (0.50–2.13)* | 1.15 (0.53–2.05)*,† | 1.11 (0.50–1.99)*,† | 1.06 (0.58–1,88)*,† | 0.99 (0.50–1.87)*,† | 0.99 (0.50–1.49) |
| vWF (U/ml) | 1.36 (0.78–2.10) | 1.33 (0.72–2.19) | 1.36 (0.66–2.16) | 1.12 (0.75–1.84)* | 0.98 (0.54–1.58)* | 0.92 (0.50–1.58) |
| IX (U/ml) | 0.35 (0.19–0.65)† | 0.42 (0.14–0.74)† | 0.44 (0.13–0.80) | 0.59 (0.25–0.93) | 0.81 (0.50–1.20) | 1.09 (0.55–1.63) |
| X (U/ml) | 0.41 (0.11–0.71) | 0.51 (0.19–0.83) | 0.56 (0.20–0.92) | 0.67 (0.35–0.99) | 0.77 (0.35–1.19) | 1.06 (0.70–1.52) |
| XI (U/ml) | 0.30 (0.08–0.52)† | 0.41 (0.13–0.69)† | 0.43 (0.15–0.71)† | 0.59 (0.25–0.93)† | 0.78 (0.46–1.10) | 0.97 (0.67–1.27) |
| XII (U/ml) | 0.38 (0.10–0.66)† | 0.39 (0.09–0.69)† | 0.43 (0.11–0.75) | 0.61 (0.15–1.07) | 0.82 (0.22–1.42) | 1.08 (0.52–1.64) |
| PK (U/ml) | 0.33 (0.09–0.57) | 0.45 (0.25–0.75) | 0.59 (0.31–0.87) | 0.79 (0.37–1.21) | 0.78 (0.40–1.16) | 1.12 (0.62–1.62) |
| HK (U/ml) | 0.49 (0.09–0.89) | 0.62 (0.24–1.00)† | 0.64 (0.16–1.12)† | 0.78 (0.32–1.24) | 0.83 (0.41–1.25)* | 0.92 (0.50–1.36) |
| XIII$_a$ (U/ml) | 0.70 (0.32–1.08) | 1.01 (0.57–1.45)* | 0.99 (0.51–1.47)* | 1.13 (0.71–1.55)* | 1.13 (0.65–1.61)* | 1.05 (0.55–1.55) |
| XIII$_b$ (U/ml) | 0.81 (0.35–1.27) | 1.10 (0.68–1.58)* | 1.07 (0.57–1.57)* | 1.21 (0.75–1.67) | 1.15 (0.67–1.63) | 0.97 (0.57–1.37) |

Adapted with permission from Andrew M, Paes B, Milner R et al. Development of the human coagulation system in the healthy premature infant. Blood 1988;72:1651–1657.

PT = prothrombin time; aPTT = activated partial thromboplastin time; TCT = thrombin clotting time; VIII = factor VIII procoagulant; vWf = von Willebrand factor; HK = high-molecular-weight kininogen; PK = prekallikrein.

All factors, except fibrinogen, are expressed as units per milliliter (U/ml), where pooled plasma contains 1.0 U/ml. All values are given as a mean, followed by the lower and upper boundary encompassing 95% of the population (boundary). Between 40 and 96 samples were assayed for each value for the newborn. Some measurements were skewed due to a disproportionate number of high values. The lower limits, which exclude the lower 2.5% of the population, have been given.

* Values that are indistinguishable from the adult.

† Values different from those of full-term infants.

**TABLE 47.4.** Reference Values for the Inhibitors of Coagulation in Healthy Premature Infants (30–36 Weeks Gestation) During the First 6 Months of Life, Compared With Those in Adults

| Coagulation Inhibitors | Day 1 Mean (boundary) | Day 5 Mean (boundary) | Day 30 Mean (boundary) | Day 90 Mean (boundary) | Day 180 Mean (boundary) | Adults Mean (boundary) |
|---|---|---|---|---|---|---|
| ATIII (U/ml) | 0.38 (0.14–0.62)* | 0.56 (0.30–0.82) | 0.59 (0.37–0.81)* | 0.83 (0.45–1.21)* | 0.90 (0.52–1.28)* | 1.05 (0.79–1.31) |
| $\alpha_2$M (U/ml) | 1.10 (0.56–1.82)* | 1.25 (0.71–1.77) | 1.38 (0.72–2.04) | 1.80 (1.20–2.66) | 2.09 (1.10–3.21) | 0.86 (0.52–1.20) |
| C$_1$E-INH (I/ml) | 0.65 (0.31–0.99) | 0.83 (0.45–1.21) | 0.74 (0.40–1.24)* | 1.14 (0.60–1.68)† | 1.40 (0.96–2.04) | 1.01 (0.71–1.31) |
| $\alpha_1$AT (U/ml) | 0.90 (0.36–1.44)† | 0.94 (0.42–1.46)† | 0.76 (0.38–1.12)* | 0.81 (0.49–1.13)*,† | 0.82 (0.48–1.16)† | 0.93 (0.55–1.31) |
| HCII (U/ml) | 0.32 (0.10–0.60)* | 0.34 (0.10–0.69) | 0.43 (0.15–0.71) | 0.61 (0.20–1.11) | 0.89 (0.45–1.40)*,† | 0.96 (0.66–1.26) |
| Protein C (U/ml) | 0.28 (0.12–0.44)* | 0.31 (0.11–0.51) | 0.37 (0.15–0.59)* | 0.45 (0.23–0.67)† | 0.57 (0.31–0.83) | 0.96 (0.64–1.28) |
| Protein S (U/ml) | 0.26 (0.14–0.38)* | 0.37 (0.13–0.61) | 0.56 (0.22–0.90) | 0.76 (0.40–1.12)† | 0.82 (0.44–1.20) | 0.92 (0.60–1.24) |

Adapted with permission from Andrew M, Paes B, Milner R et al. Development of the human coagulation system in the healthy premature infant. Blood 1988;72:1651–1657.

ATIII = antithrombin III; $\alpha_2$M = $\alpha_2$-macroglobulin; C$_1$E-INH = C$_1$-esterase inhibitor; $\alpha_1$AT = $\alpha_1$-antitrypsin; HCII = heparin cofactor II.

* Values that are different from those of the full-term infant.

† Values that are indistinguishable from those of the adult.

way inhibitor were found, thus maintaining a balanced level of hemostasis throughout prenatal development. In addition to the above described quantitative changes, fibrinogen (7–9) and von Willebrand factor (10) have distinct fetal molecular forms.

Coagulation proteins do not cross the placenta from mother to fetus (5), so a knowledge of the above noted normal ranges is essential for the accurate diagnosis congenital and acquired hemostatic disorders. The data in Tables 47.1 and 47.2 demonstrate that the severe forms of hemophilia A (factor VIII deficiency) and hemophilia B (factor IX deficiency), as well as the moderate and mild

**TABLE 47.5.**   Values for Coagulation Screening Tests and Coagulation Factor Levels in Fetuses, Compared with Those of Adults

| Parameter | Fetuses (Weeks' Gestation) | | | Newborns (n = 60) | Adults (n = 40) |
|---|---|---|---|---|---|
| | 19–23 (n = 20) | 24–29 (n = 22) | 30–38 (n = 22) | | |
| PT (s) | 32.5 (19–45) | 32.2 (19–44)† | 22.6 (16–30)† | 16.7 (12.0–23.5)* | 13.5 (11.4–14.0) |
| PT (INR) | 6.4 (1.7–11.1) | 6.2 (2.1–10.6)† | 3.0 (1.5–5.0)* | 1.7 (0.9–2.7)* | 1.1 (0.8–1.2) |
| aPTT (s) | 168.8 (83–250) | 154.0 (87–210)† | 104.8 (76–128)† | 44.3 (35–52)* | 33.0 (25–39) |
| TCT (s) | 34.2 (24–44)* | 26.2 (24–28) | 21.4 (17.0–23.3) | 20.4 (15.2–25.0)† | 14.0 (12–16) |
| Factor | | | | | |
| I (g/L Von Clauss) | 0.85 (0.57–1.50) | 1.12 (0.65–1.65) | 1.35 (1.25–1.65) | 1.68 (0.95–2.45)† | 3.0 (1.78–4.50) |
| 1 Ag (g/L) | 1.08 (0.75–1.50) | 1.93 (1.56–2.40) | 1.94 (1.30–2.40) | 2.65 (1.68–3.60)† | 3.5 (2.50–5.20) |
| IIc (%) | 16.9 (10–24) | 19.9 (11–30)* | 27.9 (15–50)† | 43.5 (27–64)† | 98.7 (70–125) |
| VIIc (%) | 27.4 (17–37) | 33.8 (18–48)* | 45.9 (31–62) | 52.5 (28–78)† | 101.3 (68–130) |
| IXc (%) | 10.1 (6–14) | 9.9 (5–15) | 12.3 (5–24)† | 31.8 (15–50)† | 104.8 (70–142) |
| Xc (%) | 20.5 (14–29) | 24.9 (16–35) | 28.0 (16–36)† | 39.6 (21–65)† | 99.2 (75–125) |
| Vc (%) | 32.1 (21–44) | 36.8 (25–50) | 48.9 (23–70)† | 89.9 (50–140) | 99.8 (65–140) |
| VIIIc (%) | 34.5 (18–50) | 35.5 (20–52) | 50.1 (27–78)† | 94.3 (38–150) | 101.8 (55–170) |
| XIc (%) | 13.2 (8–19) | 12.1 (6–22) | 14.8 (6–26)† | 37.2 (13–62)† | 100.2 (70–135) |
| XIIc (%) | 14.9 (6–25) | 22.7 (6–40) | 25.8 (11–50)† | 69.8 (25–105)† | 101.4 (65–144) |
| PK (%) | 12.8 (8–19) | 15.4 (8–26) | 18.1 (8–28)† | 35.4 (21–53)† | 99.8 (65–135) |
| HK (%) | 15.4 (10–22) | 19.3 (10–26) | 23.6 (12–34)† | 38.9 (28–53)† | 98.8 (68–135) |

*Adapted with permission from Reverdiau-Moalic P, Delahousse B, Body G et al. Evolution of blood coagulation activators and inhibitors in the healthy human fetus. Blood 1996;88:900–906.*

*Values are the mean, followed in parentheses by the lower and upper boundaries including 95% of the population.*

*PT = prothrombin time; INR = international normalized ratio; aPTT = activated partial thromboplastin time; TCT = thrombin clotting time; Ag = antigenic value; c = coagulant activity; PK = prekallikrein; HK = high-molecular-weight kininogen.*

*\* P < .05.*

*† P < .01.*

**TABLE 47.6.**   Levels of Blood Coagulation Inhibitors in Fetuses, Compared with Adult Values

| Parameter | Fetuses (Weeks' Gestation) | | | Newborns (n = 60) | Adults (n = 40) |
|---|---|---|---|---|---|
| | 19–23 (n = 20) | 24–29 (n = 22) | 30–38 (n = 22) | | |
| ATIII (%) | 20.2 (12–31)* | 30.0 (20–39) | 37.1 (24–55)† | 59.4 (42–80)† | 99.8 (65–130) |
| HCII (%) | 10.3 (6–16) | 12.9 (5.5–20) | 21.1 (11–33)† | 52.1 (19–99)† | 101.4 (70–128) |
| TFPI (ng/mL)‡ | 21.0 (16.0–29.2) | 20.6 (13.4–33.2) | 20.7 (10.4–31.5)† | 38.1 (22.7–55.8)† | 73.0 (50.9–90.1) |
| PC Ag (%) | 9.5 (6–14) | 12.1 (8–16) | 15.9 (8–30)† | 32.5 (21–47)† | 100.8 (68–125) |
| PC Act (%) | 9.6 (7–13) | 10.4 (8–13) | 14.1 (8–18)* | 28.2 (14–42)† | 98.8 (68–129) |
| Total PS (%) | 15.1 (11–21) | 17.4 (14–25) | 21.0 (15–30)† | 38.5 (22–55)† | 99.6 (72–118) |
| Free PS (%) | 21.7 (13–32) | 27.9 (19–40) | 27.1 (18–40)† | 49.3 (33–67)† | 98.7 (72–128) |
| Ratio of free PS to total PS | 0.82 (0.75–0.92) | 0.83 (0.76–0.95) | 0.79 (0.70–0.89)† | 0.64 (0.59–0.98)† | 0.41 (0.38–0.43) |
| C4b-BP (%) | 1.8 (0–6) | 6.1 (0–12.5) | 9.3 (5–14) | 18.6 (3–40)† | 100.3 (70–124) |

*Adapted with permission from Reverdiau-Moalic P, Delahousse B, Body G et al. Evolution of blood coagulation activators and inhibitors in the healthy human fetus. Blood 1996;88:900–906.*

*Values are the mean, followed in parentheses by the lower and upper boundaries including 95% of the population.*

*ATIII = antithrombin III; HCII = heparin cofactor II; TFPI = tissue factor pathway inhibitor; PC = protein C; Ag = antigen; Act = activity; PS = protein S; C4b-BP = C4b-binding protein.*

*\* P < .05.*

*† P < .01.*

*‡ Twenty samples were assayed for each group, but only 10 for 19- to 23-week-old fetuses.*

**TABLE 47.7.** Fibrinolytic System of the Newborn Compared With Older Children and Adults

| Component | Blood Level |
| --- | --- |
| Plasminogen | Low |
| Plasminogen activators | Similar or high |
| Plasminogen activator inhibitor | Similar |
| $\alpha_2$-Antiplasmin | Similar |
| $\alpha_2$-Macroglobulin | High |
| Fibrin split products | Similar |

*Adapted with permission from Corrigan JJ Jr. Neonatal thrombosis and the thrombolytic system: pathology and therapy. Am J Pediatr Hematol Oncol 1988;10:83–91.*

forms of hemophilia A, can be reliably diagnosed in the immediate postnatal period. In contrast, the diagnosis of factor XI deficiency should be deferred because of the low levels of factor XI in normal neonates. The diagnosis of mild von Willebrand disease should also be deferred because of the high level of von Willebrand factor and the transient appearance of unusually large von Willebrand factor multimers in normal neonates (10, 11). Alternatively, the polymerase chain reaction can be used to diagnose von Willebrand disease in the neonatal period (12). Although the homozygous states for deficiencies of antithrombin, proteins C, and protein S can be diagnosed at birth, diagnosis of the heterozygous states cannot be reliably made by standard clinical tests in the early postnatal period.

## THE FIBRINOLYTIC SYSTEM

The plasma levels of components of the fibrinolytic system of newborns are compared with older children and adults in Table 47.7 (13). Neonatal fibrinolytic activity is far lower than that observed in adults. Phillips and Skrodelis (14) found that functional plasminogen levels in full-term and premature neonates are only 25 and 12% of maternal levels, respectively. Several other studies (1, 15–17) have also found that neonatal plasminogen levels were markedly reduced compared with adult levels. The decreased plasminogen levels and lower activity of neonatal plasminogen explain the prolonged thrombus lysis times seen in neonates in response to urokinase administration (18).

The amino acid sequences of neonatal and adult plasminogen are identical (19). Like adults, neonates have two glycoforms of plasminogen (types 1 and 2), but both have significantly more mannose and sialic acid than the adult forms. This difference in carbohydrate composition appears to be the basis of the decreased functional activity of neonatal plasminogen (19).

## PLATELETS

Platelet counts of healthy neonates are similar to normal adult values (20, 21) and bleeding times in neonates are the same or slightly shorter than in older children and adults (21, 22). However, neonatal platelets have been reported to be less reactive than adult platelets to adenosine diphosphate (ADP), epinephrine, collagen, thrombin, and arachidonic acid (23–26), but not to ristocetin (25, 27). Aspirin intake by the mother aggravates the defective aggregation in the neonate (28). It has been reported that neonatal platelets have decreased α-adrenergic receptors (24). The deficient collagen response in neonatal platelets may result from a relative defect in the transduction signal from the collagen receptor to phospholipases $A_2$ and C (29). Neonatal platelets also demonstrate an impaired dense granule release (30, 31). It has been reported that neonatal platelets are activated, based on assays of the plasma concentrations of β-thromboglobulin, platelet factor 4, and thromboxane $B_2$ (32), suggesting that this state of platelet activation may account for the lack of responsiveness of neonatal platelets to agonists. However, other investigators have found that neonatal platelets respond as well as adult platelets to ADP, collagen, and arachidonic acid (27, 33, 34). The contradictory results obtained in the above studies may be explained by the fact that they were all performed with platelet-rich plasma or washed platelets. Separation of platelets from whole blood may result in artifactual *in vitro* platelet activation (35) and this, in turn, may result in refractoriness of platelets to exogenous agonists (36). To circumvent these problems, platelet activation has been studied in normal newborns by whole blood flow cytometry with a panel of platelet activation-dependent monoclonal antibodies (37, 38), demonstrating that neonatal platelets do not circulate in an activated state and are hyporeactive to exogenous agonists in whole blood (39). Furthermore, the hyporeactivity of the platelets of very low birth weight neonates is more profound than the hyporeactivity of the platelets of term neonates (40). This decrease raises the possibility that the degree of platelet hyporeactivity may be a factor in the propensity of very low birth weight, preterm neonates, but not term neonates, to have intraventricular hemorrhage (41, 42).

# LABORATORY METHODS

Laboratory testing in older children is similar to that performed in adults (see Chapter 26). However, accurate testing in neonates and small babies is complicated by their small size, difficulty in obtaining appropriate samples of blood, and their limited blood volumes, which precludes using the relatively large volumes of blood that would be casually drawn in older children or adults. Micromethods are widely available for determination of plasma fibrinogen, aPTT, prothrombin time (PT), and thrombin time, but not all nurseries, especially those physically located within a general (adult) hospital, have such methods available. Whole blood methods to measure the aPTT (43) and the PT (44) of capillary blood samples have recently been introduced and should be applicable to neonates, although high hematocrits may complicate measurement of the coagulation tests. Recently developed whole blood flow cytometric techniques utilizing a panel of platelet activation-dependent monoclonal antibodies make possible precise assessment of platelet function in less than 5 μL of peripheral or capillary blood (39, 40, 45). In addition, DNA genomic analysis using PCR technology on small volumes of blood is used to diagnose many genetic conditions (46).

Blood samples from neonates are frequently obtained by heel stick because of the convenience of obtaining a capillary blood sample. Because of excessive pressure on tissues during specimen collection, blood for anticoagulation monitoring may be contaminated by the presence of tissue factor, which will alter coagulation testing results. Similarly, tissue factor may contaminate samples if there are repeated venipuncture attempts with the same needle or if there is slow flow through the catheter used to draw the venous blood.

Heparin may contaminate blood specimens when samples are obtained from arterial or venous catheters that have been flushed with heparin-containing fluids. As little as 0.05 units of heparin per mL of blood will result in prolongation of the aPTT and the thrombin time. Withdrawal of up to 4 mL of blood from the catheter prior to obtaining the test sample may reduce the heparin contamination. The reptilase time is useful in determining whether a prolonged thrombin time is due to heparin, because the reptilase time is not altered by heparin. Others have described using small measured amounts of protamine (4 μg per mL of blood drawn) to neutralize residual heparin associated with withdrawal of blood from arterial lines, even after initial withdrawal of 4 mL of blood. This protocol successfully eliminated the artifactual elevation of the aPTT after correction for the 9% increase in the aPTT and PT induced by the protamine (47).

Since newborns, especially term and small-for-gestational-age babies, are relatively polycythemic, the amount of anticoagulant in the test tube should be decreased in proportion to the increased hematocrit since less plasma is available for testing in the sample. Nomograms are available to make this correction (48).

Evaluation of platelet number and function in the neonate is complicated by several practical considerations. Before a diagnosis of thrombocytopenia is made, a stained peripheral blood smear should be examined for platelet clumping especially when blood is obtained from a capillary sample. Platelet clumping is a common *in vitro* artifact in blood obtained from heel stick capil-

lary blood collections, and is most frequently observed at the edges of the blood smear. Sphygmomanometer application for bleeding time determination is complicated by the neonate's small size and lower blood pressure. Consequently, rather than the 40 mm Hg used for adults and older children, the sphygmomanometer pressure used for the bleeding time is 20 mm Hg for babies weighing less than 1 kg, 25 mm Hg for babies weighing 1 to 2 kg, and 30 mm Hg for babies weighing greater than 2 kg (22, 49). Automated bleeding time devices that are specifically designed for the newborn have been described (22, 49).

# HEMORRHAGIC PROBLEMS IN CHILDREN

In the following sections, neonatal hemorrhage will be considered first from the perspective of common clinical presentations and then from the perspective of the clinical conditions that are associated with an increased risk of neonatal hemorrhage.

## CLINICAL PRESENTATIONS OF NEONATAL HEMORRHAGE

### Intraventricular Hemorrhage

Intraventricular hemorrhage (IVH) is more common in preterm neonates than in term neonates, with a historical incidence between 40 and 90% in neonates born at less than 34 weeks gestation (41, 42). IVH usually originates in the subependymal region from vessels in the germinal matrix overlying the caudate nucleus. Rupture of the subependymal hemorrhage through the walls of the lateral ventricles results in IVH. Four levels of increasing severity of IVH have been defined by ultrasound for low birth weight infants (50): grade I is bleeding confined to the subependymal matrix; grade II indicates intraventricular bleeding; grade III includes grade II plus intraventricular dilation; grade IV includes grade III plus intracerebral bleeding (Fig. 47.1).

IVH occurs at a median age of 38 hours postnatally (51). In more than half of affected neonates, IVH is clinically silent (52). In the remainder, there may be a sudden catastrophic deterioration manifested by alterations in consciousness, a full fontanel, abnormal eye movements, and/or respiratory irregularities (50). The standard method of diagnosis of neonatal IVH is ultrasonography, which can be performed at the bedside. Magnetic resonance imaging and computerized tomography cannot be performed at the bedside and are therefore less practical given the risks of transporting sick premature neonates. Furthermore, serial studies, which are easily performed using ultrasound, are often helpful.

The pathogenesis of IVH remains poorly understood but appears to be multifactorial. Factors that have

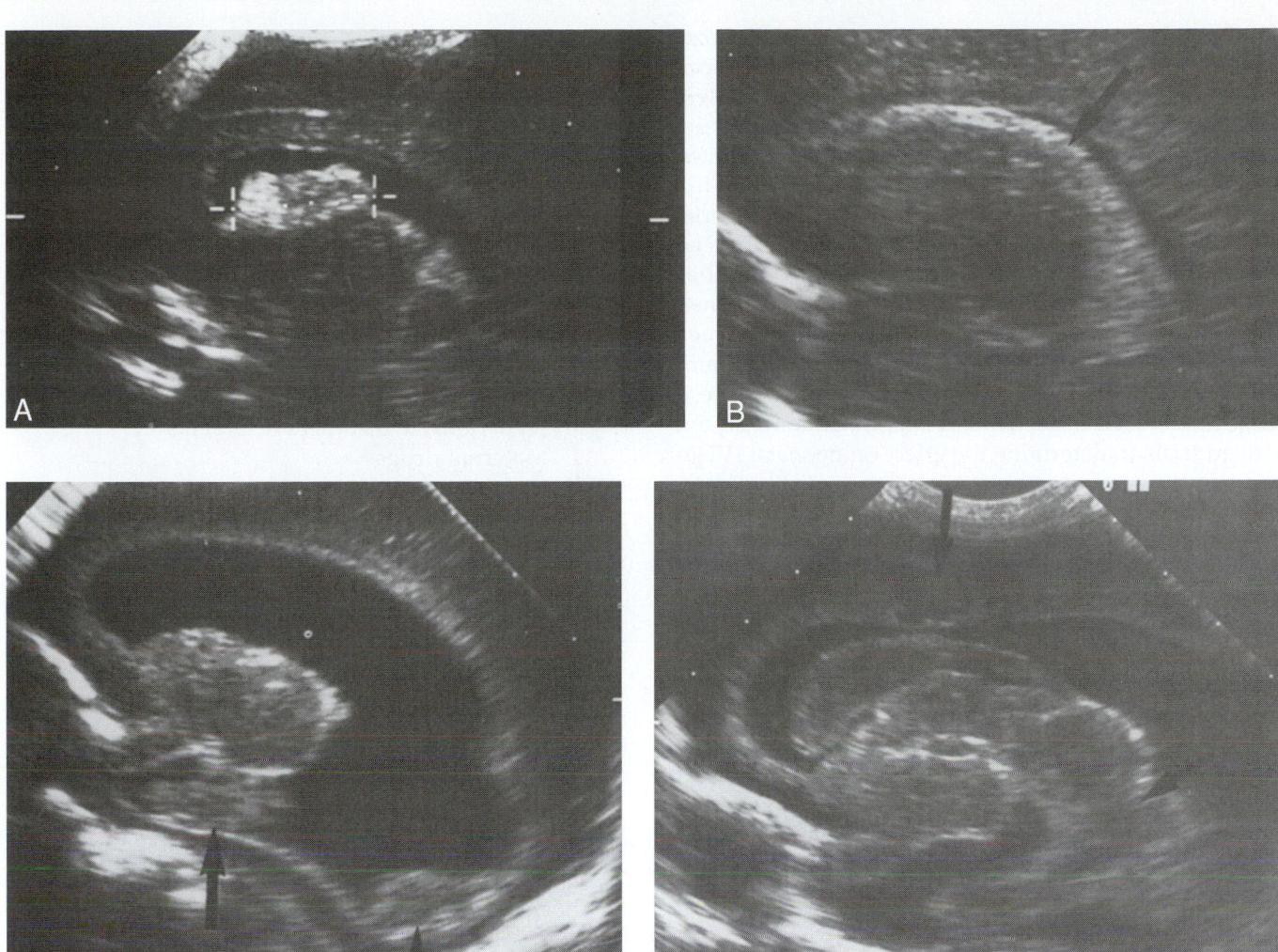

**FIGURE 47.1.**   Neonatal intraventricular hemorrhage as shown by ultrasonography. All panels show sagittal views of lateral ventricles (left = anterior; right = posterior). **A,** Grade I: bleeding is confined to the subependymal matrix (between the cursors), and there is no ventricular dilation. **B,** Grade II: the ventricle is filled with blood (arrow), but there is no ventricular dilation. **C,** Grade III: intraventricular clots (as indicated by arrows) with ventricular dilation. **D,** Grade IV: the ventricle is filled with blood; a huge retracting clot (lower arrow) within massively dilated ventricle; porencephalic cyst (upper arrow) developing as a result of intracerebral bleeding. (Ultrasounds courtesy of Jacqueline L. Wellman, M.D., Department of Radiology, Medical Center of Central Massachusetts, Worcester, MA.)

been associated with IVH include prematurity, hypoxia, fragility of the germinal matrix capillaries, abnormal regulation of cerebral blood flow with decreased perfusion of brain tissue, hypercapnia, hypernatremia, hyperosmolality, hypothermia, rapid colloid infusions, increased venous pressure, and alterations in hemostasis (50, 53–56). Whether the physiologic immaturity of the hemostatic system of the newborn contributes to the occurrence and extent of IVH is unknown. Premature infants with IVH have been reported to have a higher incidence of hemostatic abnormalities than premature infants without IVH, including low factor VIII levels, hypofibrinogenemia, low antithrombin levels, increased

fibrin/fibrinogen degradation products, prolonged whole blood clotting times, prolonged thrombin times, thrombocytopenia, impaired platelet aggregation, and prolonged bleeding times (57–61). However, no causal relationship has been established. In one study by Malloy and Cutter (62), there was an increased risk of IVH in neonates exposed to greater doses of heparin, which was typically administered as an adjunct to maintain umbilical artery catheter patency. Although the association between exposure to heparin and IVH was a strong one, it is possible that the observations were actually a reflection of the severity of illness in the infant rather than a causal relationship.

Treatment of neonatal IVH with fresh frozen plasma, cryoprecipitate, prothrombin complex concentrate, platelet transfusion, or exchange transfusion with fresh whole blood has often been successful at correcting hemostatic defects but has not resulted in a consistent beneficial effect on morbidity or mortality (63, 64). The capillary stabilizing drug ethamsylate has been reported to reduce the incidence of IVH (65–67). Some, but not all, randomized controlled trials to determine the effect of indomethacin on neonatal IVH have shown benefit (68–72). Results of several trials of prevention of neonatal IVH with antenatal administration of phenobarbital have been promising (73, 74). Trials of the use of vitamin E (75) have been inconsistent. Randomized controlled trials to determine the effect on neonatal IVH of the administration of vitamin K antenatally to the mother have produced conflicting results (76–78). The available data do not allow general recommendations with regard to any of the above therapies.

## Pulmonary Hemorrhage

Pulmonary hemorrhage is more common in preterm neonates than in term babies. The incidence of massive pulmonary hemorrhage has been reported to be 6% in neonates with a birth weight less than 2 kg (79). Although hemostatic defects may aggravate pulmonary hemorrhage, they are probably not the initiating cause because evidence for intravascular consumption, when documented, has usually followed the onset of the pulmonary hemorrhage (53).

## Gastrointestinal Hemorrhage

Approximately 30% of all episodes of apparent gastrointestinal bleeding in neonates are in fact due to swallowed maternal blood (80). As little as 3 mL of ingested maternal blood can produce one or more bloody stools in the neonate 7 to 17 hours after the ingestion. Maternal blood can be distinguished from fetal blood in vomitus, gastric aspirate, or stool by the Apt (alkali denaturation) test (81). In those cases in which there is true fetal blood loss, less than 25% of infants have detectable hemostatic abnormalities (82). Although underlying abnormalities of the gastrointestinal tract can be detected in some of these bleeding episodes, in many cases no cause for the hemorrhage can be found.

## CLINICAL CONDITIONS ASSOCIATED WITH AN INCREASED RISK OF NEONATAL HEMORRHAGE

The clinical conditions associated with an increased risk of neonatal hemorrhage are listed in Table 47.8. When bleeding is observed in a neonate who is otherwise well, the most likely possibilities are vitamin K deficiency,

**TABLE 47.8.** Clinical Conditions Associated with an Increased Risk of Neonatal Hemorrhage

Coagulation disorders
  Vitamin K deficiency
  Liver disease
  Congenital deficiencies of coagulation factors
Platelet disorders
  Thrombocytopenia
    Immune-mediated
      Neonatal alloimmune thrombocytopenia
      Maternal autoimmune thrombocytopenia
      Hypertensive disorders of pregnancy
      Maternal drugs
    Infections
      Bacterial
      Viral
    Congenital megakaryocytic hypoplasia
      Amegakaryocytic thrombocytopenia
      Thrombocytopenia with absent radii (TAR syndrome)
    Bone marrow disease
      Congenital leukemia
      Leukemoid reactions
      Neuroblastoma
    Miscellaneous
      Hypersplenism
      Extensive localized thrombosis
      Polycythemia
      Inherited metabolic disorders
      Wiskott-Aldrich syndrome
      Kasabach-Merritt syndrome
      Erythroblastosis fetalis
  Platelet function disorders
    Inherited
      Bernard-Soulier syndrome
      Glanzmann's thrombasthenia
    Acquired
      Maternal or neonatal drugs
  von Willebrand disease
Mixed disorders
  Disseminated intravascular coagulation
  Cyanotic congenital heart disease
  Cardiopulmonary bypass surgery
  Extracorporeal membrane oxygenation (ECMO)
Trauma

inherited disorders of coagulation, immune or drug-mediated thrombocytopenia, or trauma (83). In contrast, when bleeding is observed in a neonate who is "sick," the most likely possibilities are disseminated intravascular coagulation (DIC) or liver disease (83). Initial laboratory tests should include a platelet count, PT, and aPTT.

1 If gastrointestinal tract only, exclude swallowed maternal blood (Apt test).
2 Complete history (family, maternal, and birth).
3 Platelet count, prothrombin time (PT), activated partial thromboplastin time (aPTT)

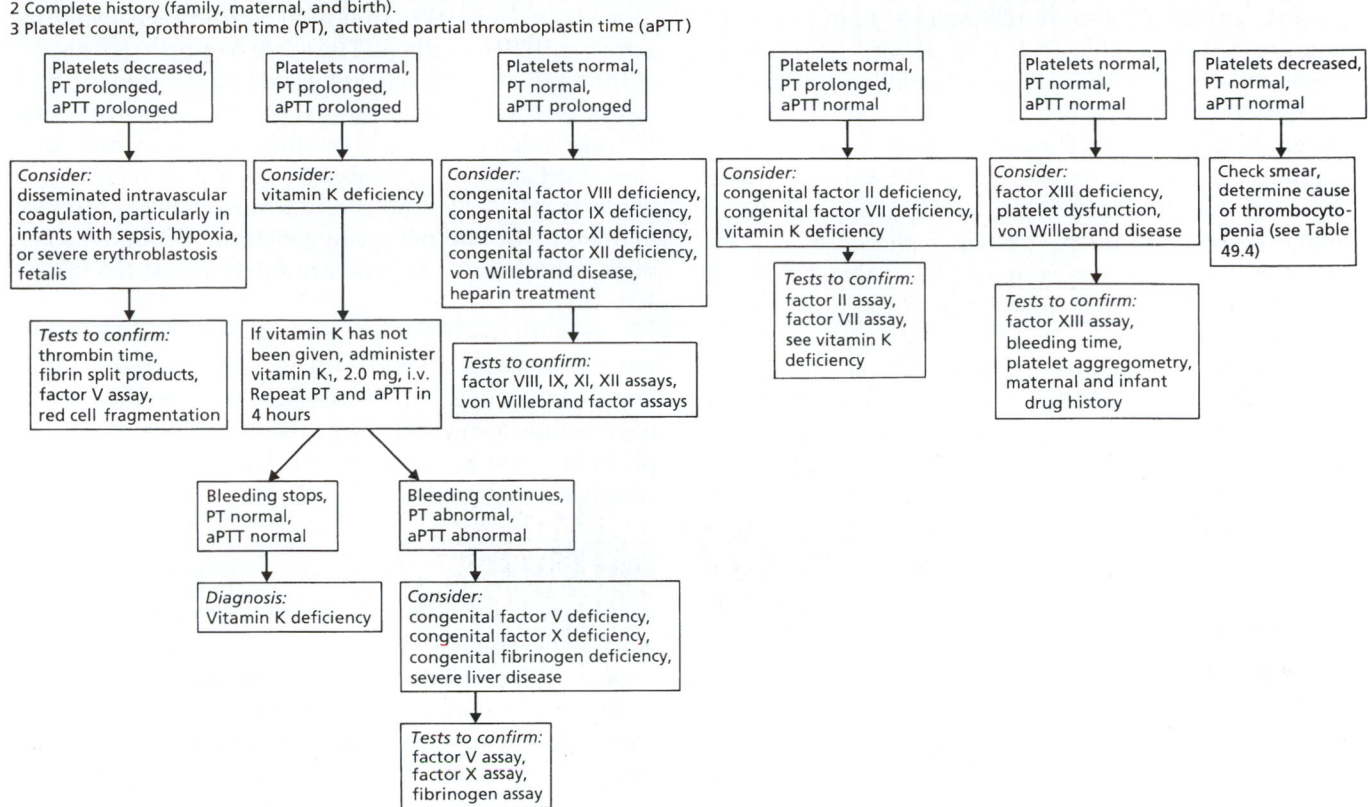

**FIGURE 47.2.**   A diagnostic approach to the bleeding newborn. Adapted with permission from Oski FA. Blood coagulation and its disorders in the newborn. Adapted with permission from Oski FA, Naiman JL, eds. Hematologic problems in the newborn. 3rd ed. Philadelphia: WB Saunders, 1982; pp. 137–174.

A diagnostic approach to bleeding in the newborn, based on the results of these screening tests, is presented in Fig. 47.2.

## Coagulation Disorders

### Vitamin K Deficiency

Vitamin K deficiency (see Chapter 45) in the neonatal period ("hemorrhagic disease of the newborn") typically presents in the first 5 days of life with evidence of bleeding from multiple sites such as diffuse ecchymoses, gastrointestinal hemorrhage, or cephalhematoma (Fig. 47.3) in an otherwise healthy infant. The vitamin K-dependent coagulation factors (II, VII, IX, and X) are known to be physiologically low in the neonatal period (Tables 47.1, 47.3, and 47.5) and a vitamin K deficiency further reduces the coagulant activity of these factors. The factors contributing to neonatal vitamin K deficiency include a low transplacental transfer of vitamin K (86, 87), a low intake of milk in the first few days of life, and breast-feeding because breast milk has a lower vitamin K content than cow's milk (88, 89) and other commercially available formulas (90). Furthermore, there is a lack of intestinal bacterial synthesis of vitamin

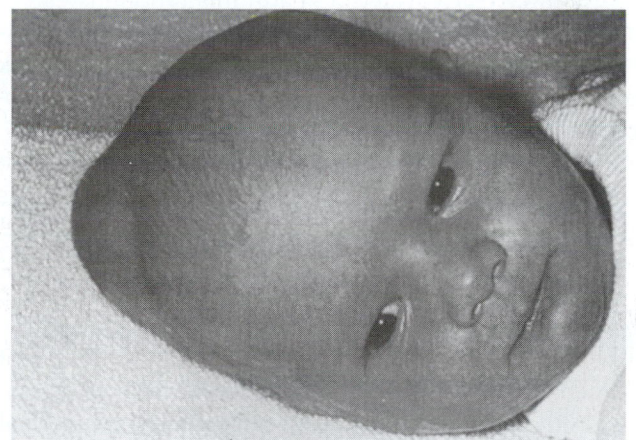

**FIGURE 47.3.**   Cephalohematoma. Adapted with permission from Simon C, Janner M. Color atlas of pediatric diseases. Toronto: BC Dekker, 1987.

K because the neonatal gut is not yet colonized. Vitamin K deficiency becomes more pronounced as the maternally derived stores of vitamin K are depleted during the first day of life.

The combination of a prolonged aPTT, prolonged PT, and normal platelet count suggests vitamin K deficiency. Bleeding infants with these laboratory findings should receive vitamin $K_1$ 1 mg subcutaneously or intravenously (91). The PT and aPTT should begin to normalize within 3 hours and clinical bleeding should stop. If bleeding does not stop and the aPTT and PT remain abnormal, other diagnoses such as liver disease and congenital coagulation factor deficiency should be considered. Since vitamin K is responsible for the carboxylation of the coagulation factors II, VII, IX, and X, a specific aid to the diagnosis of vitamin K deficiency is measurement of the decarboxylated forms of these vitamin K-dependent factors (PIVKA) (91). Alternatively, factor levels can be measured to detect a difference between coagulant activities (which will be reduced) and immunologic concentrations (which will be almost normal) (89). In the unusual event of a life-threatening hemorrhage secondary to vitamin K deficiency, fresh frozen plasma (15 cc/kg) or prothrombin complex should be infused in addition to administration of vitamin K.

Hemorrhagic disease of the newborn has almost disappeared as a clinical problem in the United States because of the routine administration of vitamin $K_1$ to all newborns, but may occur if vitamin K prophylaxis is not given at birth either because of accidental omission or due to parental refusal. At most centers, vitamin K is administered as an intramuscular injection (0.5 to 1.0 mg) (92, 93). Alternatively, some authors have noted no diagnoses of vitamin K deficiency related hemorrhage in healthy infants receiving an oral dose of vitamin K (94), and have advocated oral administration instead of intramuscular injection (95). Some centers will also routinely administer vitamin K one or two times each week to ill preterm babies and infants receiving broad spectrum antibiotics or total parenteral nutrition (82).

Vitamin K deficiency occasionally occurs in the first 24 hours of life in infants born to mothers taking drugs such as warfarin, anticonvulsants, rifampin, or isoniazid (96). Since warfarin crosses the placenta and interferes with neonatal vitamin K metabolism (95), infants born to mothers receiving warfarin may have a coagulopathy. Warfarin is not generally administered to pregnant women since maternal exposure to warfarin is associated with an embryopathy, especially during gestational weeks 6 to 12 (95). However, pregnant women who are receiving warfarin near term should be switched to heparin several days before anticipated delivery because heparin does not cross the placenta (97) and can be stopped during labor to promptly reverse the associated coagulopathy. Although the precise risk of developing vitamin K deficiency in an infant of an epileptic mother receiving anticonvulsant therapy is unknown, a reasonable approach may be to give the mother 20 mg of oral vitamin K daily for 2 weeks prior to delivery (98).

Vitamin K deficiency can also present beyond the immediate neonatal period with hemorrhage, including intracranial hemorrhage. This "late hemorrhagic disease of the newborn" may be associated with antibiotic therapy or diseases causing fat malabsorption such as cystic fibrosis, biliary atresia, hepatitis, $\alpha_1$-antitrypsin deficiency, celiac disease, or abetalipoproteinemia (99). Late hemorrhagic disease of the newborn is more common in infants who did not receive vitamin K prophylaxis at birth, especially those who are solely breast-fed (88, 89, 100, 101).

Vitamin K administration to the newborn has been reported to be associated with an increased risk of childhood cancers (102), but subsequent extensive studies have yielded no evidence of a relationship between prophylactic use of vitamin K and the later occurrence of childhood malignancy (95, 102, 103).

## Liver Disease

Bleeding related to liver dysfunction can occur in association with neonatal liver disease of any cause such as hypoxia, hypotension, viral hepatitis, and inherited metabolic defects. As in adults with liver disease (see Chapter 45), the hemorrhagic diathesis can be multifactorial in origin and can be from failure of hepatic synthesis of coagulation factors, activation of the coagulation and fibrinolytic systems, delayed clearance of activated coagulation factors and activators of fibrinolysis, loss of hemostatic proteins into ascitic fluid, and thrombocytopenia secondary to hypersplenism or disseminated intravascular coagulation (DIC). DIC in association with liver disease is common in fulminant hepatitis and acute liver necrosis.

Laboratory abnormalities associated with liver disease include a prolonged aPTT, prolonged PT, thrombocytopenia, increased fibrinolysis, and evidence of DIC such as the presence of high levels of fibrinogen/fibrin split products that may be present because of decreased hepatic clearance, even in the absence of DIC. Laboratory abnormalities that may distinguish liver disease from DIC are the presence of normal levels of factor VIII, a normal platelet count (in the absence of hypersplenism), and the absence of microangiopathic changes on the peripheral blood smear. Differentiation between liver disease and DIC is obviously impossible if the two conditions coexist.

The management of the hemostatic defect of liver disease includes treatment of the underlying cause of the liver disease, administration of parenteral vitamin K if there is fat malabsorption, and, for active bleeding, fresh frozen plasma (e.g., 10 cc/kg every 12 hours). Factor concentrates containing factors II, VII, IX, and X are best avoided in neonates with liver disease because of the thrombogenic potential of these concentrates and the impaired ability of the neonate to clear activated clotting factors. Platelet concentrates should be transfused only if there is active bleeding in association with significant thrombocytopenia.

## Congenital Deficiencies of Coagulation Factors

Congenital deficiencies of coagulation factors may not be clinically apparent in the newborn period. As discussed previously, a knowledge of the normal neonatal plasma levels of coagulation factors is essential to the diagnosis of congenital deficiencies of coagulation factors since some factor levels are normally low in the neonatal period. These disorders are discussed in detail elsewhere in this book.

### Hemophilia (Chapters 35 and 36)

Factor VIII deficiency (hemophilia A) and factor IX deficiency (hemophilia B or Christmas disease) are X-linked inherited disorders and therefore essentially affect only males. Hemophilia may present in the neonatal period with cephalhematoma, gastrointestinal hemorrhage, bleeding from the umbilical stump, or bleeding following circumcision. Interestingly, severe bleeding such as intracranial hemorrhage as a result of hemophilia is unusual in the neonatal period (104, 105), and only 40% of infants with hemophilia bleed excessively following circumcision (106). After the neonatal period, clinical bleeding does not usually occur until intramuscular immunizations are given or until the child begins to crawl. The diagnosis of hemophilia is made by the presence of a prolonged aPTT and a specific deficiency in the plasma level of either factor VIII or factor IX. The limitations of these methods in the diagnosis of hemophilia in the neonatal period have been previously discussed. The management of hemophilia is discussed in detail in Chapters 35 and 36, but includes genetic counseling to the family, hepatitis B immunization, and factor replacement therapy. Immunizations should be given subcutaneously followed by a local ice pack.

### Factor XIII Deficiency (Chapter 36)

Factor XIII deficiency in the neonate is clinically typically characterized by delayed and persistent bleeding from the umbilical stump. Screening tests of hemostasis (aPTT, PT, platelet count, bleeding time) are all normal. The diagnosis is made by a urea clot solubility test (see Chapters 23 and 26). Infusion of fresh frozen plasma will replace factor XIII and correct the coagulopathy.

## Platelet Disorders

Bleeding as a result of platelet disorders is typically petechial and superficial (skin and mucosal), in contrast to the larger ecchymoses and deep tissue hemorrhages typical of coagulation disorders.

## Thrombocytopenia

Neonatal thrombocytopenia is the most common hemostatic disease of the newborn (107). The incidence may be as high as 1% in healthy term babies, and 20% in infants in the neonatal intensive care unit (108). In a prospective study of 807 consecutive infants admitted to a regional intensive care unit, Castle et al (109) found thrombocytopenia in 22%. In 58% of these thrombocytopenic infants the platelet count was less than 100,000/mm$^3$ and in 20% it was less than 50,000/mm$^3$. The thrombocytopenia typically began by day 2 of life, reached a nadir by day 4 of life, and recovered to normal values (greater than 150,000/mm$^3$) by approximately day ten. This high incidence of neonatal thrombocytopenia coupled with its association with the most severe grades of intraventricular hemorrhage (110, 111) make it one of the most important hematologic problems encountered in the newborn (112). Increased destruction is probably the predominant mechanism of neonatal thrombocytopenia (113). The specific causes of thrombocytopenia in the neonatal period are listed in Table 47.8. The most common causes of neonatal thrombocytopenia are immune-mediated, infectious, and DIC.

### Neonatal Alloimmune Thrombocytopenia (see Chapter 28)

Neonatal alloimmune thrombocytopenia is analogous to hemolytic disease of the newborn due to Rh or ABO incompatibility. Thus, *in utero*, fetal platelets enter the maternal circulation and stimulate antibody production against a fetal platelet antigen that the mother lacks. This antibody does not affect maternal platelets but it crosses the placenta and destroys fetal platelets. The mother therefore has neither thrombocytopenia nor a clinical bleeding problem (in contrast to neonatal thrombocytopenia secondary to maternal autoimmune thrombocytopenia [see below]). The antigen to which the maternal antibody is raised is usually HPA-1a (previously known as PL$^{A1}$ and Zw$^a$) (114), which is absent in 2% of the population. The second most common antigen implicated in neonatal alloimmune thrombocytopenia is HPA-5b (previously known as Br$^a$) (115). In contrast to hemolytic disease of the newborn, approximately half of all cases of neonatal alloimmune thrombocytopenia occur with first pregnancies (116).

The overall incidence of neonatal alloimmune thrombocytopenia is approximately one in 2500 live births (114). An affected baby is usually full term and otherwise well. Clinical evidence of bleeding may include petechiae, gastrointestinal bleeding, cephalhematoma, and hematuria. Intracranial hemorrhage occurs in approximately 10% of reported cases of neonatal alloimmune thrombocytopenia (117). The intracranial hemorrhage may occur *in utero* (118, 119) and result in severe neurologic sequelae including porencephalic cysts (118) and optic hypoplasia (120). The thrombocytopenia typically persists for approximately 3 weeks before resolving spontaneously.

Platelet antigen typing of the parents will reveal whether the mother's platelets lack an antigen that is present on the platelets of the baby and the father. Antibodies directed against this antigen can usually be identified in the mother's serum by indirect immunofluorescence assays (121, 122) or enzyme-linked immunoassays (123).

Platelet transfusions are indicated for severe neonatal alloimmune thrombocytopenia. The source of the transfused platelets should be maternal platelets washed free of antibody-containing plasma, or platelets obtained from other individuals known to lack the offending antigen (124, 125). If possible, the platelets should be gamma-irradiated prior to transfusion to prevent graft-versus-host disease caused by maternal lymphocytes (126). If compatible platelets are not available, random donor platelets may be temporarily effective and should be infused if the baby has a major hemorrhagic event (125). In less urgent circumstances, high dose intravenous gamma globulin therapy will usually result in an increased platelet count within 24 to 48 hours (127–131).

With regard to subsequent deliveries, a father who is homozygous for the implicated antigen will always pass the antigen on to the fetus. A heterozygous father will pass the antigen to the fetus in approximately 50% of cases. Unfortunately, the inability to detect a platelet-specific alloantibody in maternal serum does not preclude the diagnosis of neonatal alloimmune thrombocytopenia (132, 133). Percutaneous umbilical vein sampling can be performed as early as 20 weeks of gestation, thereby allowing the fetal platelet count to be directly measured or, if sufficient blood can be obtained, platelet antigen typing to be performed (132, 134). Newly available methodology utilizes approximately 1 mL of fetal blood or 5 mL of amniotic fluid to determine the fetal platelet alloantigen genotype by allele-specific oligonucleotide probes of polymerase chain reaction-amplified fetal genomic DNA (135, 136). If severe fetal thrombocytopenia is present, maternal intravenous gamma globulin therapy appears to improve the fetal platelet count and prevent fetal intracranial hemorrhage (134, 137, 138). The possible benefit of maternal corticosteroids remains to be determined (134, 137, 139). A more invasive approach is to infuse the severely thrombocytopenic fetus weekly with antigen-negative platelets (132). The transfused platelets should be gamma-irradiated and, if they are obtained from the mother, washed. Direct administration of intravenous immunoglobulin to the fetus does not appear to have a role in management (140). Ultrasound of the fetus at regular intervals can be used to monitor for intracranial hemorrhage. Caesarian

section is recommended for all affected neonates to plan the postnatal management and, possibly, to prevent birth trauma. Maternal platelets for transfusion can be obtained the day before a planned delivery of an affected neonate.

## Maternal Autoimmune Thrombocytopenia

As a result of the passive transfer of autoantibodies, infants of mothers with immune thrombocytopenic purpura (ITP) may have thrombocytopenia (see Chapter 30). A similar autoimmune thrombocytopenia occasionally occurs in association with maternal systemic lupus erythematosus, lymphoproliferative disorder, or hypothyroidism (141, 142). In contrast to the situation in neonatal alloimmune thrombocytopenia, the maternal antibodies are directed against antigens common to both maternal and neonatal platelets.

Maternal thrombocytopenia secondary to ITP must be distinguished from the frequent occurrence of thrombocytopenia in healthy pregnant women at term (143). The absence of a history of ITP before pregnancy or the presence of negative results on circulating platelet antibody testing in pregnant women indicates a minimal risk of severe neonatal thrombocytopenia in their offspring (143, 144).

Approximately half of the infants born to mothers with active ITP or a history of ITP have thrombocytopenia (145). Neonatal thrombocytopenia can occur in babies of women who have a normal platelet count after a splenectomy for ITP. There are no reliable predictors of severe thrombocytopenia in affected infants except the direct determination of the platelet count by cordocentesis, which, in view of the generally mild clinical course, is rarely if ever indicated (54). Fetal scalp monitoring has a high technical failure rate and falsely low platelet counts may result in unnecessary caesarian sections (146). Neither maternal platelet count nor maternal platelet associated IgG accurately predict neonatal thrombocytopenia (144, 145, 147). After birth, the diagnosis is established by neonatal thrombocytopenia associated with a maternal history of ITP and elevated levels of IgG on the surface of the neonatal platelets.

Affected infants are usually full-term and generally healthy. The clinical course of neonatal thrombocytopenia secondary to maternal ITP is usually milder than neonatal alloimmune thrombocytopenia (54). Bleeding is rarely severe and is usually confined to the first few days of life. In contrast to neonatal alloimmune thrombocytopenia (see above), antenatal intracranial hemorrhage is extremely uncommon (148). Spontaneous resolution of the neonatal thrombocytopenia occurs within approximately 3 weeks of birth.

On the basis of case reports of intracranial hemorrhage in infants affected by maternal ITP, recommendations for delivery by caesarian section and monitoring of the fetal platelet count prenatally have been made in the hope of lowering infant morbidity and mortality (149, 150). However, the study by Burrows and Kelton (146) casts doubt on these recommendations. This study suggested that neonatal platelet counts at birth are rarely below 50,000/mm$^3$, intracranial hemorrhage rarely occurs prenatally, and intracranial hemorrhage is not clearly related to birth trauma. Prenatal administration of corticosteroids or high dose intravenous gamma globulin have also been advocated to reduce the incidence and severity of neonatal thrombocytopenia, but the response to these treatments is uncertain and unpredictable (145, 151, 152).

Infants born to mothers with ITP should be monitored closely because the platelet count falls in the immediate postnatal period (151). If there is significant bleeding or a platelet count of less than 20,000/mm$^3$, intravenous gamma globulin should be infused. Intravenous gamma globulin 1 g/kg on 2 successive days results in a significant rise in the platelet count in approximately 80% of affected infants (153, 154). The response rate to gamma globulin is faster than to corticosteroids (54). However, if there is no response to gamma globulin, prednisone, 2 mg/kg daily, should be instituted (54). If the infant is bleeding, random donor platelet transfusions may be transiently helpful.

## Hypertensive Disorders of Pregnancy (see Chapter 46)

In a prospective study of cord blood from 520 infants of 607 consecutive hypertensive mothers, neonatal thrombocytopenia was present in 9.2%, as compared with 2.2% of infants of normotensive mothers (155). In the hypertensive group, preterm birth was the major risk factor for neonatal thrombocytopenia (155). In fact, term infants of hypertensive mothers were no more likely to be thrombocytopenic than control infants (155). The degree of thrombocytopenia was modest in most infants, and only two infants, both preterm, had cord blood platelet counts less than 50,000/mm$^3$ (155). Although obstetric interventions are not warranted, the rate of thrombocytopenia in preterm infants born to hypertensive women justifies neonatal scrutiny.

## Maternal Drugs

Drug-induced thrombocytopenia in the mother (see Chapter 29) may also affect the newborn, but significant bleeding is rare. It is difficult to document maternal drug ingestion as a cause of neonatal thrombocytopenia if maternal platelets are unaffected.

## Infections

Thrombocytopenia is frequently associated with bacterial sepsis (156). Other systemic infections that can be associated with thrombocytopenia include human immunodeficiency virus (157), cytomegalovirus, rubella, herpes, toxoplasmosis, syphilis, and echovirus type II. When associated with infection, thrombocytopenia is usually not the only abnormality, nor is it the major problem. Hepatosplenomegaly is a common clinical finding that is rarely found in association with the other causes of neonatal thrombocytopenia. The mechanism of the development of thrombocytopenia associated with infection is multifactorial. DIC, inhibition of megakaryocyte production of platelets, platelet sequestration as a result of reticuloendothelial hyperplasia, and a direct effect of the infective agent on platelets resulting in platelet removal from the circulation are all contributory (82). In the absence of DIC, the degree of thrombocytopenia is rarely severe enough to cause serious bleeding. However, platelet transfusions may occasionally be necessary.

## Congenital Megakaryocytic Hypoplasia

Congenital megakaryocytic hypoplasia is rare. Bone marrow examination reveals the megakaryocytic hypoplasia. If necessary, the resultant thrombocytopenia can be treated with platelet transfusions. Congenital amegakaryocytic thrombocytopenia sometimes occurs with absent radii, referred to as the TAR (thrombocytopenia with absent radii) syndrome. The only hemopoietic cell line affected is the megakaryocytic series and the onset of the thrombocytopenia is in the neonatal period. In contrast, Fanconi's anemia involves all hematopoietic cell lines, is associated with other congenital anomalies, and the pancytopenia, including the thrombocytopenia, does not usually have its onset until later childhood.

## Bone Marrow Disease

Bleeding due to thrombocytopenia may be the presenting sign of congenital leukemia. Typically, the infant looks clinically ill, has hepatosplenomegaly, and blasts are found in the peripheral blood and bone marrow. Leukemoid reactions, which usually occur secondary to infections or Down's syndrome, are associated with thrombocytopenia. Neuroblastoma metastatic to the bone marrow can also result in thrombocytopenia. If necessary, the thrombocytopenia can be treated with platelet transfusions.

## Miscellaneous Causes of Thrombocytopenia

Some neonates with thrombocytopenia have evidence of hypersplenism (113). In other cases thrombocytopenia can be associated with extensive localized thrombosis, for example, renal vein thrombosis, necrotizing enterocolitis, indwelling vascular catheters, and intracardiac thrombosis. Polycythemia is commonly associated with thrombocytopenia but the etiology is unclear (158). Thrombocytopenia has been associated with several inherited metabolic disorders: isovaleric acidemia, holocarboxylase synthetase deficiency, methylmalonic acidemia and ketotic glycinemia (158). Wiskott-Aldrich syndrome, an X-linked disorder characterized by thrombocytopenia, small platelets, eczema, and an increased susceptibility to infection, rarely presents in the neonatal period.

Occasionally, giant hemangiomas are associated with thrombocytopenia, referred to as the Kasabach-Merritt syndrome (159) (Fig. 47.4; see color plate 47.4) (see Chapter 44). The etiology of the thrombocytopenia is sequestration and destruction of platelets within the vascular tumor (160). In some cases, there is also laboratory evidence of chronic DIC. Most commonly, hemangiomas appear in the neonatal period, enlarge during the first few months of life, and then begin to decrease in size. Thrombocytopenia is therefore usually most pronounced at a time beyond the immediate neonatal period. Corticosteroids, chemotherapy, angiographic embolization, and surgical excision have all been used with short-term beneficial effects. Alpha interferon has also been used with success at controlling the potentially life-threatening thrombocytopenia (161).

Severe erythroblastosis fetalis may be associated with thrombocytopenia. The mechanism of the thrombocytopenia is not entirely clear but may be related to DIC (162). Thrombocytopenia may also occur following exchange transfusion, but this can be partly prevented by the use of fresh whole blood (158).

Heparin-induced thrombocytopenia is clinically associated with thrombosis and will be discussed in the subsequent section.

## Platelet Function Disorders

### Inherited Platelet Function Disorders (Also See Chapter 32)

Although hereditary platelet function defects are rare, they should be suspected in a child with characteristic historical and clinical findings (163). Unfortunately, the bleeding time test is not a reliable means to identify or exclude a platelet function defect, and therefore platelet aggregometry or flow cytometry should be performed to establish the diagnosis.

Bernard-Soulier syndrome, described in detail in Chapter 32, is a rare autosomal recessive deficiency of platelet membrane glycoproteins Ib, V, and IX (164). The clinical features include petechiae, giant platelets on blood smear, mild thrombocytopenia, marked prolongation of the bleeding time, and lack of ristocetin-induced platelet agglutination. Glanzmann's thrombasthenia, also described in detail in Chapter 32, is a rare autosomal recessive deficiency of platelet membrane glycoproteins IIb and IIIa (164). The clinical features include petechiae, normal platelet count and morphology, prolongation of the bleeding time, absent clot retraction, and absent platelet aggregation in response to all ago-

nists. These inherited disorders of platelet function sometimes present in the neonatal period (165).

von Willebrand factor (see Chapter 16) is central to the process of platelet adhesion. von Willebrand factor binds to a receptor on platelets (166) and to subendothelial components exposed by damage to the blood vessel wall, thereby forming an adhesive bridge (167). von Willebrand disease (see Chapter 34), an inherited defect in von Willebrand factor, therefore results in defective platelet adhesion to damaged vessel walls. However, individuals with von Willebrand disease rarely present with clinical hemorrhage in the neonatal period. The diagnosis of von Willebrand disease in the neonatal period is discussed above.

### Acquired Platelet Function Disorders (Also See Chapter 33)

Drug administration to the mother or the baby is the most common cause of acquired platelet dysfunction. Aspirin ingestion by the mother within 2 or 3 days of delivery produces neonatal platelet dysfunction that may be associated with bleeding, for example, cephalhematoma and melena (28, 168, 169). The clinical effect of the neonatal platelet dysfunction apparently induced by other maternal drugs, for example, promethazine or meperidine (28), remains unclear.

## Mixed Hemorrhagic Disorders

### Diffuse Intravascular Coagulation (DIC) (Also See Chapter 44)

DIC is an acquired pathophysiologic process characterized by intravascular consumption of platelets and plasma clotting factors. This widespread coagulation within the vasculature results in both the deposition of fibrin thrombi and, as a result of depletion of coagulation proteins, a hemorrhagic state. Fibrin accumulation in the microcirculation results in mechanical injury to erythrocytes, resulting in red cell fragmentation and a microangiopathic hemolytic anemia.

Conditions that predispose to DIC in the neonatal period include placental abruption, placenta previa, birth asphyxia, hypoxia, sepsis, acidosis, shock, and hypothermia (170–172). DIC is an extremely common problem in sick preterm neonates because of the frequency of the conditions that predispose to DIC in this population. The neonate's ability to respond to DIC is compromised by the limited capacity of the neonatal reticuloendothelial system to clear activated clotting factors from the circulation, and the relative lack of compensatory synthesis of clotted factors because of hepatic immaturity.

Unlike bleeding secondary to vitamin K deficiency or inherited coagulation factor deficiencies, DIC occurs in "sick" infants. Clinical features of DIC may include oozing from needle puncture sites, gastrointestinal blood loss, or bleeding from the umbilical stump. Other manifestations include petechiae, signs of pulmonary, cerebral, or intraventricular hemorrhage, and purpura fulminans.

The diagnosis of DIC is based on the presence of one or more of the known predisposing causes of DIC, together with the following laboratory abnormalities: a microangiopathic hemolytic anemia with fragmented red cells on peripheral blood smear; thrombocytopenia; a prolonged aPTT, PT, and thrombin time; elevated fibrin split products; and hypofibrinogenemia. Other laboratory abnormalities present in DIC include low plasma levels of clotting factors V and VIII, elevated circulating levels of fibrin monomer, thrombin-antithrombin complexes, and D-dimers; and low plasma levels of inhibitors of clotting (antithrombin, heparin cofactor II, protein C). A combination of tests should be utilized in the diagnosis of DIC because individual tests can be abnormal in the absence of DIC. For example, infants with large hematomas may have a positive D-dimer test secondary to fibrin degradation.

The most important approach to infants with DIC is treatment of the underlying cause such as administration of antibiotics for bacterial sepsis, and correction of hypoxia, acidosis, and hypotension. Although there are few studies to clearly support its use, replacement therapy with fresh frozen plasma and platelet transfusions is usually administered (173). In severe cases of DIC, exchange transfusion can be used to replace hemostatic factors, but the procedure has significant risks and the effect is transient. Heparin, with (174, 175) or without (176, 177) the concomitant infusion of antithrombin concentrates, has been used in the treatment of neonatal DIC, but its efficacy remains uncertain. Heparin has been advocated when the predominant clinical presentation of DIC is thrombotic, as is the case in purpura fulminans (53, 82). In these circumstances, in order not to provide substrate for further thrombus formation, it is theoretically preferable to give the heparin prior to plasma and platelet replacement therapy (82).

## Cyanotic Congenital Heart Disease

Infants with cyanotic congenital heart disease may have underlying hemostatic defects (178). The reported abnormalities include: thrombocytopenia (179–181); a prolonged bleeding time (even in the face of a normal platelet count) (179); diminished platelet aggregation in response to ADP, epinephrine, and collagen (182, 183); platelet release abnormalities (184); and coagulation defects that may be secondary to low-grade, chronic, intravascular coagulation (179, 181).

Some children with noncyanotic congenital heart disease have an acquired loss of the largest von Willebrand factor multimers from plasma (185) that is likely a result of increased von Willebrand factor release from the endothelium caused by the elevated shear stress levels of high cardiac output states. This abnormality normalizes after surgical correction of the cardiac defect (185).

## Cardiac Surgery Requiring Cardiopulmonary Bypass (CPB)

Operations are frequently performed on newborn babies with congenital heart disease. There is a hemorrhagic diathesis associated with the use of CPB, as discussed in detail in Chapter 50. Defective hemostasis during and after CPB is related to multiple factors including mechanical sources of bleeding, thrombocytopenia, a platelet function defect, a fibrinolytic state, hypothermia, and the underlying hemostatic disorder associated with congenital heart disease (178, 186, 187).

Preoperative screening tests have not proved to be a reliable predictor of postoperative hemorrhage (188). Nevertheless, because of the hemostatic defects associated with congenital heart disease, and because an underlying hemostatic defect may not be clinically manifest in nonambulatory children, some pediatric cardiac surgery centers perform a preoperative laboratory evaluation of hemostasis that includes a platelet count, bleeding time, PT, aPTT, and a factor XIII screen (urea clot lysis).

The management of bleeding associated with CPB is discussed in detail in Chapter 50. However, there are a number of specific issues with regard to the management of bleeding after cardiac surgery on neonates and children utilizing cardiopulmonary bypass.

### Surgical Blood Loss

A localized defect in surgical hemostasis is a common cause of bleeding following CPB. Surgical bleeding is more common in the presence of adhesions from previous operations and cyanotic heart disease, which results in the development of multiple collateral vessels that are often fragile.

### Hypothermia

Neonates are particularly prone to hypothermia because of their large surface area to body mass ratio. Adequate rewarming and maintenance of normothermia is an important first measure in the prevention and treatment of excessive blood loss (189–191). Rewarming a hypothermic bleeding individual may reduce the need for the less safe alternative of transfusion of platelets and other blood components (191).

### Transfusion of Blood Components

Red blood cell transfusions should be administered for specific clinical indications, including the presence of significant bleeding. Although conventional practice in adults is to transfuse red blood cells to maintain hematocrits greater than 30% (192), children with cyanotic congenital heart disease whose intraoperative hemoglobin values were lowered to less than 10 g/dL by hemodilution had more normal coagulation tests, experienced 45% less bleeding, and required 54% fewer blood components than children whose intraoperative hemoglobin remained above 10 g/dL (193). This finding is consistent with the fact that in children with cyanotic congenital heart disease the degree of polycythemia is directly proportional to the underlying hemostatic defect (179, 181) and to postoperative bleeding after repair of the defect (194–196).

Transfusion of fresh whole blood (less than 48 hours old) is associated with less postoperative blood loss than the separate transfusion of packed red blood cells, fresh frozen plasma (FFP), and platelets in children (especially those less than 2 years of age) who undergo CPB surgery (197, 198). This difference may be due to better functioning platelets (197). Because the circulating blood volume of approximately 250 mL in the neonate is greatly exceeded by the 750 mL volume of the priming solution in the extracorporeal perfusion system, fresh whole blood is often included in the priming solution to lessen the hemodilution in neonates (199).

Platelet transfusions are indicated for individuals with excessive bleeding following CPB in the presence of thrombocytopenia and/or prolongation of the bleeding time. In these circumstances, transfusion of 1 unit of random donor platelets per 10 kilograms body weight has been recommended (200). However, in infants less than 10 kilograms in whom there is massive hemodilution, 2 units of platelets may be preferable (199). Because of the dilutional effect of standard platelet concentrates in small infants, specially prepared concentrates with a higher platelet concentration are advantageous in this population.

In general, there is no evidence to support the prophylactic transfusion of either fresh frozen plasma (FFP) or cryoprecipitate during or after CPB (201), although in neonates several of the factor levels are low enough to cause bleeding that may be helped by the administration of FFP (202). FFP administration is not indicated for factor replacement in individuals receiving massive transfusions, because none of the coagulation factors usually decrease to levels sufficiently low to cause abnormal bleeding (192). FFP administration is also not indicated for volume expansion, nutritional support, or wound healing (201). Administration of FFP should generally be reserved for individuals with acquired deficiencies of vitamin K-dependent coagulation factors such as in individuals receiving warfarin (192). Although there are no controlled studies to support its use, cryoprecipitate, with its smaller volume relative to coagulation factors, has been considered to be useful in neonates with a hemostatic defect in association with massive hemodilution after CPB (199).

## Pharmacologic Agents

The infusion during CPB of aprotinin (Trasylol), an inhibitor of plasmin, kallikrein, and urokinase (see Chapter 53), results in markedly decreased blood loss in adult individuals (203, 204). However, the effectiveness of aprotinin in children undergoing cardiac operations requiring CPB is controversial. Several studies have demonstrated a decrease in the amount of bleeding and the need for postoperative transfusion associated with the use of aprotinin (205, 206). Others have concluded that the use of aprotinin does not reduce blood loss or offer any other clinical benefit (207–209). In one study, individuals receiving aprotinin were noted to have an increased number of thrombotic complications such as superior vena cava thrombosis and lower extremity deep venous thrombosis (205). Profound hypotension has been reported in association with the use of aprotinin in a child undergoing CPB surgery (210).

Desmopressin acetate (1-deamino-8-D-arginine vasopressin; DDAVP) (see Chapter 53) has been reported to decrease blood loss after cardiac surgery in adults by some (211, 212), but this conclusion has been challenged by others (213–216). A prospective, randomized, double-blind trial of intraoperative desmopressin infusion during CPB in 60 children failed to demonstrate a reduction in blood loss (217). Furthermore, in individuals with cyanotic congenital heart disease, the decrease in peripheral vascular resistance induced by desmopressin may be life-threatening (218).

The antifibrinolytic agent epsilon aminocaproic acid (EACA, Amicar) (see Chapter 53) resulted in no overall benefit in a prospective, randomized, double-blind study of children undergoing CPB for correction of congenital heart defects (219). However, in this study there was a significant reduction of postoperative blood loss in children with cyanotic congenital heart disease and in those with pump times greater than 60 minutes, with the greatest difference in blood loss occurring between the discontinuation of CPB and the completion of surgery.

## Extracorporeal Membrane Oxygenation (ECMO)

ECMO has become the treatment of choice for critically ill newborns with reversible pulmonary disease that is unresponsive to conventional ventilatory support. Heparin anticoagulation is required for ECMO and is partly responsible for the high frequency of hemorrhagic complications during ECMO in neonates (220, 221). However, the incidence of hemorrhagic complications during ECMO does not correlate with the activated clotting time or the amount of heparin used (220). Thus, as with cardiac surgical procedures utilizing cardiopulmonary bypass, the etiology of the hemorrhagic diathesis during ECMO is multifactorial and includes thrombocytopenia, a platelet function defect, and, especially in the first 24 hours after initiation of ECMO, a consumptive coagulopathy (222). The types of hemorrhage that occur during ECMO include intracranial (220, 223–226), endobronchial (220), and incisional (220). The particularly high incidence of intracranial hemorrhage during ECMO may be the result of increased cerebral blood flow velocity and vasodilation of cerebral vessels at high flow rates (227). Infants under 2 kg and 34 weeks gestation have a higher incidence of intracerebral hemorrhage (223). Platelet transfusions are usually given to maintain the platelet count above 50,000/mm$^3$ during ECMO (228).

# NEONATAL AND PEDIATRIC THROMBOSIS

Thrombosis in newborn infants is probably more common than at any other period of life (229). Guidelines for the prevention, diagnosis, and treatment of thrombotic disease in adult individuals cannot necessarily be extrapolated to the neonatal period, because there are marked differences in the causes, natural history, and localization of thrombi, as well as in the normal hemostatic system and response to antithrombotic and thrombolytic agents (230–232). Infants with suspected or proven thrombotic disease should be managed in a neonatal intensive care unit where supportive care and anticoagulant, thrombolytic, or surgical therapy can be administered and monitored (233).

Organ or limb dysfunction as a result of thrombosis is the most important indication for anticoagulant, thrombolytic, or surgical intervention. The lack of strong evidence for the benefits of antithrombotic therapy and the propensity of neonatal thrombi to resolve spontaneously do not usually justify anticoagulant, thrombolytic, or surgical therapy for asymptomatic thrombosis (233). Before anticoagulant and/or thrombolytic therapy is prescribed, intracranial hemorrhage or hemorrhagic infarction should be excluded by cranial ultrasound or computerized tomography.

## THE LABORATORY EVALUATION OF HYPERCOAGULABILITY

In the absence of indwelling catheters, thrombotic complications in neonates and children are unusual. When they do occur, a search for an inherited or acquired hypercoagulable state should be undertaken. The panel of laboratory tests ordered should include a complete blood count and platelet count, the PT and aPTT, protein

**TABLE 47.9.** Laboratory Testing for the Evaluation of a Potential Hypercoagulable State

General studies
   CBC and platelet count
   Activated partial thromboplastin time (aPTT)
   Prothrombin time (PT)
Tests for inherited hypercoagulable states
   Protein C activity
   Protein S total and free
   Antithrombin III activity
   Factor V Leiden assay (activated protein C resistance)
   Urine for homocystine
Tests for acquired hypercoagulable states
   Lupus anticoagulant
   Anticardiolipin antibodies

**TABLE 47.10.** Common Clinical Presentations of Neonatal Thrombosis

Aortic thrombosis
Renal artery thrombosis
Renal vein thrombosis
Disseminated intravascular coagulation/purpura fulminans

C activity, protein S (total and free), antithrombin activity, a Factor V Leiden assay (hereditary resistance to activated protein C), assays for the presence of a lupus anticoagulant and anticardiolipin antibodies, and urine for homocystine (Table 47.9). It is important to consider the presence of a hypercoagulable state before initiating therapy so that appropriate laboratory studies can be drawn, since the administration of heparin will change measured antithrombin III levels and the use of warfarin will not only decrease the levels of the vitamin K-dependent factors II, VII, IX, and X, but will also decrease circulating levels of protein C and protein S.

## CLINICAL PRESENTATIONS OF NEONATAL THROMBOSIS (TABLE 47.10)

### Aortic Thrombosis

Thrombosis of the aorta is a potentially lethal condition, the incidence of which has increased in critically ill neonates in parallel with the widespread use of umbilical artery catheters, the tip of which is usually in the thoracic aorta (234). A prospective sonographic study of 81 consecutive neonates who had an umbilical artery catheter found detectable aortic thrombosis in 26%, of which two-thirds were symptomatic (235).

Clinical signs of aortic thrombosis include blanching and cyanosis of the lower extremities, decreased femoral artery pulses, hematuria, oliguria or anuria, hypertension, congestive heart failure, and multiorgan failure (234–237). Hepatic infarction is common in association with major aortic thrombosis (236). Underlying clinical conditions that have been reported in association with aortic thrombosis include umbilical artery catheters (234, 238–243), calcium in the umbilical artery catheter infusate (235), perinatal asphyxia (236), and congenital antithrombin deficiency (244).

Contrast angiography, usually via the umbilical artery catheter, was the "gold standard" for diagnosis of aortic thrombosis (230), but it is not without risk in critically ill infants. Ultrasonography has become the most popular diagnostic method for aortic thrombosis (234) (Fig. 47.5), but has been reported to have a false negative rate of 20% (236). Radionuclide renography-scintigraphy demonstrates abnormal renal perfusion in virtually all cases (236). Aortic thrombosis is first diagnosed at postmortem in approximately 24% of cases (230).

Although the successful use of heparin (234, 236), thrombolytic therapy (urokinase, streptokinase, or tissue plasminogen activator) (236, 238, 245–247), and surgical thrombectomy (234, 236, 237, 248) have been reported in case studies, there are insufficient data in the literature to allow general recommendations for the treatment of aortic thrombosis (230, 236). Thus the treatment must be individualized. Thrombolytic agents are contraindicated in the presence of active bleeding or intracranial hemorrhage.

Although most individuals with minor or moderate degrees of aortic thrombosis recover, the mortality rate is high in the presence of complete aortic occlusion (236, 249). Long term follow-up of survivors is necessary to detect hypertension, decreased renal function, and leg growth abnormalities (237, 249, 250).

## Renal Artery Thrombosis

Until the advent of routine umbilical artery catheterization in critically ill newborns, thrombosis of the renal artery was uncommon, with an incidence that was much less than renal vein thrombosis (251). Approximately 15% of critically ill newborns with umbilical artery catheters develop renal artery thrombosis (251). The incidence of renal artery thrombosis is related to the duration of catheterization (243), the presence or absence of heparin anticoagulation (252–254), the type of catheter used (243, 255), and the type of fluid infused.

Renal artery thrombosis is often clinically silent, but may be associated with hypertension, renal failure, or congestive heart failure. In sick newborns with umbilical artery catheters, renal artery thrombosis is often associated with thrombosis in the aorta, renal, mesenteric, and other arteries. In addition to umbilical artery catheterization, extracorporeal membrane oxygenation (ECMO) is a predisposing cause of renal artery thrombosis (256–258).

As with aortic thrombosis, heparin, thrombolytic therapy, and surgical thrombectomy have been reported to be successful therapies, but these modalities have not been compared in controlled clinical trials (251). In survivors, hypertension often persists for weeks or months but usually resolves by 2 years of age (259). Some survivors have renal atrophy and decreased renal function (259), however case reports document restoration of normal renal growth and function after 5 days of warm ischemia time reversed with thrombolysis (260).

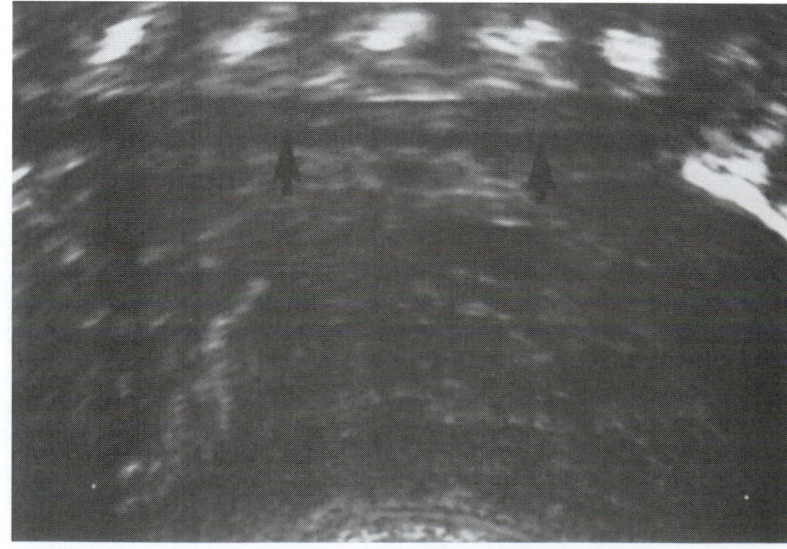

**FIGURE 47.5.** Diagnosis of neonatal aortic thrombosis by ultrasonography. Coronal view. The arrows point to a thrombus that extends from the diaphragm to the aortic bifurcation. (Ultrasound courtesy of Jacqueline L. Wellman, M.D., Department of Radiology, Medical Center of Central Massachusetts, Worcester, MA.)

## Renal Vein Thrombosis

Renal vein thrombosis occurs predominantly in the newborn period, and males are affected twice as often as females (261). Typical clinical signs of renal vein thrombosis are a palpably enlarged, hard kidney (60% of infants); metabolic acidosis (50%); hematuria (49%); oliguria or anuria (30%); and shock (251, 261). Elevated blood urea nitrogen, thrombocytopenia, microangiopathic hemolytic anemia, elevated fibrin split products, and lowered plasminogen level may occur (251, 261, 262). Associated renal calcification has been observed as early as the first day of life, indicating that renal vein thrombosis can occur prenatally (263). Underlying clinical conditions that have been reported in association with renal vein thrombosis include maternal diabetes (263–265), birth asphyxia (262), hypovolemia due to dehydration (266), hyperosmolality (261, 262), and neonatal nephrotic syndrome (267–269).

No single method has been generally accepted as the "gold standard" for the diagnosis of renal vein thrombosis (230). The radiologic modalities that have been used include contrast venography, renal scintigraphy, excretory urography, ultrasonography with or without Doppler, computerized tomography, and magnetic resonance imaging.

Although the use of heparin, thrombolytic therapy, surgical thrombectomy, and nephrectomy have been reported in case studies, there are insufficient data in the literature to allow specific recommendations for the treatment of renal vein thrombosis (230), although Nuss et al (270) suggest that renal dysfunction is not prevented in the majority of individuals treated with heparin alone. The mortality rate of renal vein thrombosis is approximately 12% (230). In survivors, long term complications can include renal fibrosis with renal insufficiency (271), calyceal clubbing (272), renal atrophy (272), renal calcification (272), hypertension (251), and renal tubular dysfunction (273). In addition to the renal veins, neonatal venous thrombosis can occur in the vena cava (Fig. 47.6) and the adrenal veins.

## Portal Vein Thrombosis

Thrombosis of the portal and hepatic veins can occur secondary to umbilical venous catheterization. When untreated, this can result in the development of portal hypertension with the subsequent formation of esophageal varices that can be a source of upper gastrointestinal bleeding, ascites, and hypersplenism (274). Case reports have described successful use of thrombolytic therapy using streptokinase administered through the umbilical vein catheter (275).

## Deep Vein Thrombosis of the Lower Extremities and Pulmonary Embolism

Deep venous thrombosis (DVT), a very common problem in the hospitalized adult population, is unusual in

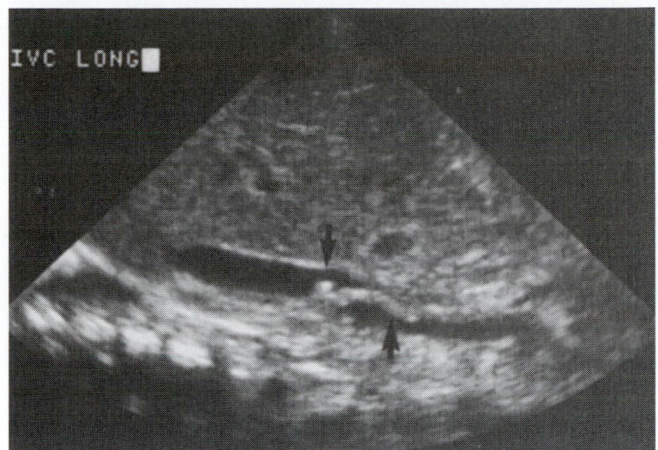

**FIGURE 47.6.** Thrombosis of the inferior vena cava in a neonate, as demonstrated by ultrasonography. Right parasagittal view. The arrows point to the thrombus. (Ultrasound courtesy of Paul K. Kleinman, M.D., Department of Radiology, University of Massachusetts Medical Center, Worcester, MA.)

individuals in the pediatric age group in the absence of lower extremity central venous catheterization. A retrospective study by Radecki et al (276) of disabled pediatric individuals at a rehabilitation hospital documented a risk of developing DVT of only 2.2%. The highest risk group were older children between the ages of 15 to 18 who were hospitalized following spinal cord injury and had a risk of developing DVT of 10%. Children with spinal cord injuries, who were less than 15 years old, had a risk of developing DVT of only 5%. Andrew et al (277) have reported the results of an analysis of the Canadian registry of DVT and pulmonary embolism (PE) in children. Of the cases of DVT identified, 50 episodes of upper extremity DVT were noted and 79 cases involved the lower extremities. Associated risk factors for the development of DVT were identified in 96% of the individuals, including central venous lines in one-third of the cases. In fact, 90% of the identified cases of DVT had two or more risk factors for the development of DVT. The mortality rate attributed to the presence of thromboembolic disease was 2.2%. In a prospective trial by Rohrer et al (278) of 59 pediatric inpatients with two or more risk factors for the development of DVT, only one episode of lower extremity DVT was identified in a 17 year old with a spinal cord injury and other risk factors. Based on the low observed incidence of deep venous thrombosis, DVT prophylaxis and surveillance were not recommended for hospitalized children who had two or fewer risk factors for the development of DVT. However, older children at very high risk may benefit from the use of measures to prevent the formation of DVT.

As in adults, DVT can be diagnosed by venography,

but venous duplex scanning is more readily available, less invasive, and has no risk of contrast induced nephrotoxicity (see Chapter 25).

Pulmonary embolism has been reported in 3 to 5% of children with hematologic malignancies (279, 280). The incidence is higher in children with acute myeloid leukemia. Potential sources of emboli include not only the lower extremities, but also thrombosis of the upper extremity great veins precipitated by the inevitable presence of the long-term indwelling central venous catheter.

## Stroke

Strokes, although more common in adults than children, are an important cause of neurologic morbidity. In contrast to adults in whom the etiology of the stroke can almost always be identified, an underlying problem can be identified in only approximately two-thirds of children who present with a stroke (281). The pathophysiology of strokes can be broadly classified as embolic, thrombotic, or hemorrhagic. Embolic strokes in children are usually associated with an underlying cardiac anatomic abnormality as a source of thrombus formation that may embolize to the cerebral circulation. The thrombotic complications of a hypercoagulable state can lead to cerebral infarction, as can intracranial hemorrhage as the result of a hemorrhagic diathesis (281, 282). Freedman et al have recently identified a hypercoagulable state in two brothers who suffered strokes related to a platelet insensitivity to nitric oxide that is a consequence of a deficiency of plasma glutathione peroxidase (283).

## Purpura Fulminans

Purpura fulminans (Fig. 47.7; see color plate 47.7) is a life-threatening disorder characterized histologically by microvascular thrombosis in the dermis followed by perivascular hemorrhage (284, 285). Clinically, rapidly progressive purpuric skin lesions and diffuse oozing from skin puncture sites are observed, often within hours of birth. The skin lesions often begin at heel or venous blood sampling sites. These lesions are initially red and flat, quickly become indurated and necrotic, form an eschar, and may result in gangrene (286). The known underlying causes of neonatal purpura fulminans are DIC, for example, in response to group B β-hemolytic streptococcal disease (287), homozygous protein C deficiency (288–293), homozygous protein S deficiency (294–296), and homozygous factor V Leiden (297, 298).

## CLINICAL CONDITIONS ASSOCIATED WITH AN INCREASED RISK OF NEONATAL AND PEDIATRIC THROMBOSIS (TABLE 47.11)

## Umbilical Arterial and Venous Catheters in Neonates

Arterial and venous catheters are the commonest predisposing cause of thrombosis in neonates (234, 299). In a

**TABLE 47.11.**   Clinical Conditions Associated with an Increased Risk of Neonatal and Pediatric Thrombosis

Umbilical artery and vein catheters in neonates
Central venous catheters
Deficiency of protein C or protein S
Factor V Leiden (activated protein C resistance)
Antithrombin III deficiency
Homocystinuria
Congenital nephrotic syndrome
Antiphospholipid antibodies
Heparin induced thrombocytopenia
Infants of diabetic mothers
Respiratory distress syndrome
Necrotizing enterocolitis
Extracorporeal membrane oxygenation (ECMO)
Polycythemia
Birth asphyxia
Dehydration
Idiopathic

retrospective study of 4000 babies who underwent umbilical artery catheterization, severe symptomatic vessel obstruction was observed in 1% of cases (239). The incidence of clinically silent thrombosis in association with umbilical artery catheterization is greater; between 3 and 59% of cases have postmortem evidence of catheter-related thrombosis (229). In six prospective angiographic studies, the incidence of thrombosis varied from 10 to 95% (240–242, 300–302).

Umbilical arterial and venous catheters have been shown to damage the vascular endothelium mechanically (303, 304) (Fig. 47.8). The interaction of flowing blood with the exposed subendothelium and the synthetic catheter results in thrombus formation. Regardless of the vessel and type of catheter used, the insertion of an intravascular catheter in a newborn infant carries a risk of thrombosis (230). However, silicone rubber catheters have been reported to have a lesser tendency toward thrombus formation than catheters made from polyethylene, polyurethane, or Teflon (257, 305).

Thrombotic complications in association with arterial catheters occur most commonly in the aorta and renal artery (discussed above), but also occur in femoral, mesenteric, pulmonary, temporal, and radial arteries. The acute complications of thrombosis associated with umbilical artery catheterization include renal hypertension, intestinal necrosis, and peripheral gangrene (54).

The appropriate level of umbilical artery catheter tip placement ("high" or "low") is controversial. In a randomized, prospective study, Mokrohisky et al (301) reported increased thrombotic complications with cath-

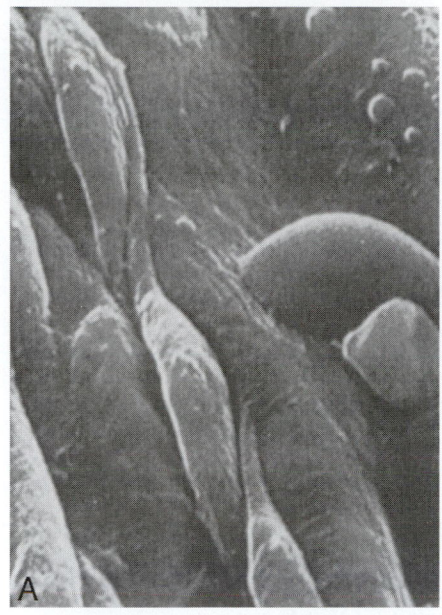
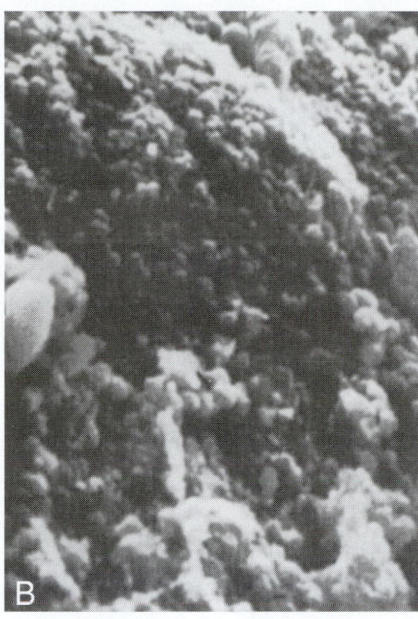

**FIGURE 47.8.** Catheter-induced damage to aortic vascular endothelium, as shown by scanning electron microscopy. **A,** Normal rabbit endothelium. **B,** Rabbit endothelium 24 hours after removal of umbilical artery catheter; note the accumulation of platelets and red cells intermixed with fibrin. Original magnification x2000. Adapted with permission from Chidi CC, King DR, Boles ET Jr. An ultrastructural study of the intimal injury induced by an indwelling umbilical artery catheter. J Pediatr Surg 1983;18:109–115.

eter tips placed at the level of the third or fourth lumbar segment. Fletcher et al (306), in a multicenter trial, defined a significant relationship between positioning a catheter tip in the abdominal aorta and removal due to complications of the presence of the catheter. Adelman et al (259), however, reported an increased incidence of renal artery thrombosis with catheters placed above the level of the renal arteries.

Umbilical venous catheters, like umbilical artery catheters, are associated with a high risk of thrombosis. A unique feature of umbilical venous catheterization is the predisposition to hepatic necrosis when hyperosmolar solutions are injected directly into the portal or hepatic systems. Portal vein thrombosis, as a result of umbilical venous catheterization, can subsequently lead to portal hypertension in association with splenomegaly and gastric and esophageal varices (54). Vena cava thrombosis can also occur.

Administration of low doses of heparin is widely used in newborn infants with intravascular catheters (307). One double-blind, randomized, controlled trial (254) and three nonblinded trials (252, 253, 308) have shown that low-dose heparin prolongs the patency of umbilical artery catheters. However, none of these trials demonstrated a reduction in the rate of catheter-associated thrombosis (252–254, 308). The effect of low-dose heparin on the incidence of intraventricular hemorrhage (IVH) in preterm babies remains unknown.

## Central Venous Catheters

Indwelling central venous catheters are used commonly in pediatric individuals to facilitate administration of medications and to serve as a source of venous access for blood drawing. These catheters are associated with a substantial risk of inducing thrombosis of the great veins. One study of 38 Hickman central venous catheters in individuals with malignancy revealed an incidence of thrombosis of 74% (309). A venographic study of 12 children with indwelling central lines for long term parenteral nutrition revealed chronic thrombosis in two-thirds of the individuals (310). Right atrial thrombi were diagnosed by echocardiography in 8.8% of 156 children with central venous lines and cancer, several of which required surgical atriotomy and thrombectomy because of venous obstruction and a compromise of tricuspid valve inflow (311). Atrial thrombi were observed to be more likely to form on catheters that had their tips located in the atrium than on catheters with their tips in the superior vena cava (311). Heparin bonding has been demonstrated to result in fewer catheter related thrombotic complications in individuals with short term central venous lines placed from a femoral venous approach (312). Interestingly, positive blood cultures related to line sepsis have been noted to be far more common in individuals with line related thrombosis compared with those who were thrombus free (309), with an incidence more than 10 times higher in one study (312). Whether or not thrombolytic therapy would decrease the incidence of line sepsis is presently unknown.

## Deficiency of Protein C or Protein S

As discussed in detail in Chapters 3 and 40, protein C and protein S are naturally occurring vitamin K-dependent anticoagulants. Thrombin, acting together with endothelial-bound thrombomodulin, cleaves protein C, thereby activating it (313). Activated protein C forms a complex with protein S, which binds to activated factors

V and VIII, causing these factors to be inactivated and thereby diminishing plasma procoagulant activity (313). Activated protein C bound to protein S also impairs the action of plasminogen activator inhibitor, type 1 (314).

Protein C and protein S deficiency states are inherited as autosomal recessive traits (see Chapter 40). Infants who are homozygous for protein C or protein S deficiency may present during the newborn period or during the first few days of life with a potentially fatal syndrome of purpura fulminans (285, 289–296) or, less commonly, massive venous thrombosis (285, 288, 292). Intrauterine, intraocular, and intracerebral thrombosis may occur (292, 293, 295). Screening coagulation tests are typical of DIC. Immunologic and functional assays of protein C or protein S reveal undetectable levels in the propositus and heterozygous levels in the parents.

Purpura fulminans and the associated DIC typically resolve rapidly with the administration of heparin and fresh frozen plasma, 8 to 12 ml/kg every 12 hours, which contains proteins C and S (292, 315). Although infusions of a highly purified protein C concentrate have been used successfully for the treatment of neonatal purpura fulminans and for long term replacement therapy in an infant with homozygous protein C deficiency (316), and infusions of cryoprecipitate have been infused for a child with homozygous protein S deficiency (294, 295), these children can be successfully maintained on warfarin without the need for long term plasma infusions (292, 293). The recommended dose of warfarin is that which maintains the international normalized ratio (INR) at 2.5 to 4.4 (292). Liver transplantation in a 20 month old child with homozygous protein C deficiency has resulted in complete reconstitution of protein C activity and resolution of the thrombotic condition (317).

In contrast to the fulminant thrombotic process seen in homozygotes for protein C or protein S deficiency, heterozygotes rarely present with thrombotic complications before their teenage years (318) and typically present with venous thromboembolic events. Since the risk of recurrent thrombotic events is higher than 60%, lifelong warfarin anticoagulation following initial anticoagulation with heparin is recommended (318).

An acquired form of protein S deficiency has been observed to occur due to the development of autoantibodies directed against protein S, typically after varicella infections in otherwise healthy children (319, 320). This form of protein S deficiency fails to respond to administration of exogenous protein S in the form of fresh frozen plasma since the circulating antibody binds to the newly administered protein S as well.

Severe deficiencies of protein C have been reported in neonates as an apparently transient phenomenon both in the presence (321, 322) and absence (321) of thrombosis. Family studies failed to document parental carrier status (321). Thus, assay of protein C beyond the neonatal period and parental studies are necessary before a final diagnosis of homozygous protein C deficiency can be made.

In a prospective study, protein C levels were assayed in cord blood collected at 193 deliveries (321). Protein C levels of less than 0.1 units/mL were found most frequently in preterm infants with respiratory distress, infants of diabetic mothers, and infants of twin gestations (321). Independent of other variables, protein C levels less than 0.1 units/mL correlated significantly with the subsequent development of thrombosis (321).

## Factor V Leiden (Hereditary Resistance to Activated Protein C)

As discussed in detail in Chapter 40, resistance to the thrombosis modulating feedback of activated protein C (APC) has recently been described, is the most common inherited hypercoagulable state, and is present in 20 to 30% of all adult individuals with deep venous thrombosis (323, 324). A mutation resulting in the substitution of glutamine for arginine 506 (R506Q mutation) on the factor V molecule (Factor V Leiden) is the most prevalent form of APC resistance in both adults and children (325) and prevents the normal inactivation of activated factor V by activated protein C (324).

Deep venous thrombosis is the most common presentation in individuals with APC resistance. However, APC resistance can present as neonatal purpura fulminans (298). The diagnosis can be made by polymerase chain reaction (PCR) assay to detect the presence of the R506Q mutation, or alternatively using an activated protein C resistance functional assay.

## Antithrombin III Deficiency

Congenital antithrombin III (ATIII) deficiency has been reported in association with aortic thrombosis (244). An inherited heterozygous ATIII deficiency is well recognized as a predisposing factor to thrombosis in adults (see Chapter 40), but thrombosis is althought to be rare in childhood (326). This lower risk of thromboembolic complications in children with congenital ATIII deficiency may result in part from the protective effect of elevated levels of plasma $\alpha_2$-macroglobulin throughout childhood (326), although the incidence of ATIII deficiency as a factor contributing to neonatal and pediatric thrombotic episodes is probably underestimated (327).

The low functional and immunologic levels of neonatal ATIII are further diminished in sick preterm infants (328), including those with respiratory distress syndrome and necrotizing enterocolitis (328, 329). Although it is not possible to isolate the effect of ATIII levels from other coexistent clinical factors, infants with the lowest levels of ATIII have a higher mortality rate and a higher incidence of both thrombotic and hemorrhagic complications (329). Treatment includes transfusion of fresh frozen plasma or ATIII concentrates to provide a substrate for the subsequent administration of heparin (327).

## Homocystinuria

Homocystinuria is an inherited disorder that predisposes to arterial thromboembolism, typically in the third decade of life (see Chapter 40). Thromboembolism in the neonatal period is very rare in this disorder and uncommon in young children (330).

## Congenital Nephrotic Syndrome

The presence of congenital nephrotic syndrome may lead to the development of renal vein thrombosis (267–269). Other thrombotic problems encountered include venous thrombosis, pulmonary embolization, and arterial thrombotic events (331). Sepsis may be an important etiologic factor in the genesis of renal vein thrombosis in this clinical setting (269).

## Antiphospholipid Antibodies

The antiphospholipid antibody syndrome has been described in children and may present as arterial thromboses with digital ischemia, stroke, and adrenal insufficiency, as well as venous thrombotic events with deep venous thrombosis and pulmonary embolization (332, 333). Systemic lupus erythematosus is present in 25 to 50% of children with the presence of antiphospholipid antibodies, and can be the presenting symptom of the disease (332, 333). Interestingly, antibody titers do not correlate well with the severity of the clinical disease (332). Anticoagulation with warfarin to achieve an INR of greater than 2.0 is effective at preventing further thrombotic episodes (333). The lupus anticoagulant and antiphospholipid antibody syndromes of adults are discussed in Chapter 38.

Maternal lupus anticoagulant has been associated with thrombotic events in the neonate (334, 335).

## Heparin-Induced Thrombocytopenia (HIT)

The use of heparin in hospitalized individuals of all ages is ubiquitous. Although therapeutic anticoagulation is not required for the majority of individuals, heparin in small quantities is used as an adjunct to maintain the patency of arterial and venous lines (336, 337). Heparin binds to platelets, and between 3 and 11% of adult individuals will develop antibodies to this heparin-platelet combination (338–340). The binding of this antibody to platelets can result in platelet activation and aggregation causing the measured platelet count to fall. The profound platelet activation can lead to thrombotic complications that are typically arterial in location (341). Exposure to even the minute amounts of heparin in an arterial or venous line flush can precipitate the development of antibodies, and the syndrome has been reported to be triggered even by the trace amounts of heparin present on heparin bonded central line catheters (342). Although primarily a disease seen in adults, heparin induced thrombocytopenia (HIT) has been reported in the newborn (343) and older children (344, 345).

Management of HIT includes the immediate cessation of heparin and the use of alternative forms of anticoagulation if needed. In some cases, low-molecular-weight heparin can be used without furthering the thrombotic process, but in some cases the formed antibodies can cross react with the lower-molecular-weight heparin fractions (346). Ancrod, a defibrinogenating drug, or Orgaran, a glycosaminoglycuronan, may be able to be used to achieve anticoagulation in individuals with HIT. Orgaran has only a 12 % cross reactivity with the HIT serum antibody (347).

All individuals receiving heparin in any form should undergo periodic platelet counts to identify the potential development of this process. A fall in the platelet count to less than 100,000 $mm^3$ or a precipitous drop in the platelet count should lead to platelet aggregation or other studies to identify the presence of a heparin induced antiplatelet antibody. This topic is reviewed in detail in Chapter 29.

## Infants of Diabetic Mothers

Maternal diabetes is associated with thrombosis in the prenatal and neonatal periods (263–265, 348). In a series of 4,000 neonatal autopsies, venous thrombosis was present in 1.1% of all infants, compared with 15.8% of infants of diabetic mothers (349). Although maternal diabetes is particularly associated with neonatal renal vein thrombosis (263–265), arterial thrombosis (348) and embolization (264) can also occur. Infants of diabetic mothers are also at increased risk for thrombotic complications from umbilical vessel catheterization (348). Lower levels of protein C (321), decreased prostacyclin production (350), and increased levels of antiplasmin (351) in infants of diabetic mothers may contribute to their propensity to thrombosis.

## Respiratory Distress Syndrome

Histologically, the respiratory distress syndrome is characterized by intraalveolar and intravascular fibrin deposition (352). The hypoxia associated with respiratory distress syndrome may result in DIC (329). Furthermore, lower levels of protein C are found in preterm infants with respiratory distress syndrome and, independent of other variables, a protein C level of less than 0.1 units/mL correlates significantly with the subsequent onset of thrombosis (321). The low functional and immunologic levels of neonatal antithrombin III are further diminished in infants with respiratory distress syndrome (328, 329). Although it is not possible to isolate the effect of antithrombin III levels from other coexistent clinical factors, infants with the lowest levels of antithrombin III have a higher mortality rate and a higher incidence of both thrombotic and hemorrhagic complications (329). Thrombin-antithrombin complexes, specific markers of increased thrombin generation, were found to be increased in severe neonatal respiratory distress syndrome (353).

The above-described biochemical and pathologic abnormalities associated with the respiratory distress syndrome provide a rationale for clinical trials of thrombolytic therapy or heparin in an attempt to decrease fibrin deposition. Although clinical trials have reported a beneficial effect of infusion of urokinase-activated plasmin (354) and plasminogen (355), these trials were performed prior to the institution of modern intensive care management. Clinical trials with heparin have not resulted in a clear improvement in outcome (177, 356). A clinical trial of infusion of an antithrombin III concentrate did not result in benefit for infants with the respiratory distress syndrome (357).

### Necrotizing Enterocolitis

The low functional and immunologic levels of neonatal antithrombin are further diminished in infants with necrotizing enterocolitis (329). Necrotizing enterocolitis may also be associated with DIC (329).

### Extracorporeal Membrane Oxygenation (ECMO)

ECMO is increasingly used in the management of neonatal respiratory failure. Although hemorrhage related to anticoagulation with heparin is the major complication of ECMO (220, 224), thromboembolic phenomena are also common in this setting (256–258) (Fig. 47.9). The most common site of origin of thrombus formation is the membrane oxygenator bypass circuit (257). An autopsy study of nonsurvivors of ECMO revealed evidence of pulmonary, renal, and cerebral infarcts, thromboembolism of external and internal carotid arteries, and thrombi in the lungs, kidneys, brain, and coronary arteries (257). In another study, fibrin thrombi or thromboemboli were found at autopsy in 22 of 23 infants with respiratory failure who had been treated with ECMO (256). In addition, 12 of these infants had distinctive, aluminum-containing emboli that were considered to be the result of aluminum fragments formed after the wearing away of the silicone coating of the heat exchanger (256).

### Other Conditions Associated with an Increased Risk of Neonatal Thrombosis

Intrauterine growth retardation and polycythemia are risk factors for neonatal thrombosis (231). Perinatal as-

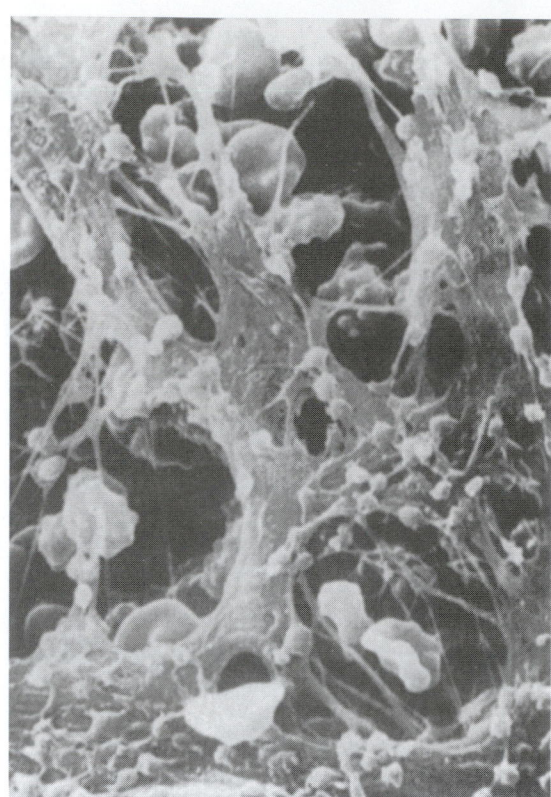

**FIGURE 47.9.** Thrombus formation during ECMO (extracorporeal membrane oxygenation) as shown by scanning electron microscopy. A segment of the bypass tubing shows platelets and red cells within a fibrin meshwork. Adapted with permission from Fink SM, Bockman DE, Howell CG et al. Bypass circuits as the source of thromboemboli during extracorporeal membrane oxygenation. J Pediatr 1989;115:621–624.

phyxia predisposes to both aortic thrombosis (236) and renal vein thrombosis (262). Renal vein thrombosis has been reported in association with dehydration (266). Finally, thromboses can present in otherwise well infants without any known underlying cause (13, 231).

Thrombocytosis in childhood is uncommon and usually secondary to other processes such as infection or the response to trauma or operation, especially splenectomy. If the only risk factor for thrombosis is a high platelet count, thrombotic complications are rare and antithrombotic prophylaxis is not necessary (358).

## ANTITHROMBOTIC THERAPY IN CHILDREN

The treatment and prophylaxis of thrombotic problems in children have historically been based on loosely extrapolated recommendations for anticoagulant therapy for adults, which will be discussed in detail in the last section of this textbook. However, optimal treatment of children with thromboembolic problems differs from that of adults because of features of the neonatal and pediatric hemostatic system that affect both the pathophysiology of the thrombotic process and the response to antithrombotic agents (232, 359).

## HEPARIN ANTICOAGULATION

As discussed in Chapter 55, the anticoagulant properties of heparin are derived from its ability to bind to antithrombin III and induce a conformational change in the ATIII molecule that greatly increases its ability to inactivate thrombin (360). As previously noted, plasma concentrations of ATIII are physiologically low at birth and increase to adult levels by 3 months of age (1, 4, 5). ATIII levels are even lower in sick neonates (4). These variable levels of the substrate for the action of heparin may complicate the administration of appropriate doses of heparin.

### Dosage and Monitoring

Optimal therapeutic heparin levels in adults are typically considered to be between 0.2 and 0.4 U/mL (360). Since a direct assay of heparin concentrations is not readily available in most hospitals, this is not a practical means of monitoring ongoing anticoagulation therapy. Therefore the aPTT is generally relied on to guide titration of heparin therapy. Elevations of the aPTT to 2.0 to 2.5 times the control level generally provide therapeutic heparin levels (360). In pediatric individuals, a therapeutic aPTT value correctly predicts appropriate heparin concentrations 70% of the time (361).

Heparin bolus and maintenance requirements for children are generally higher (on a U/kg basis) than those required for therapeutic anticoagulation in adults. This is due to the low levels of ATIII seen in neonates, infants and young children (1, 4, 5), as well as the fact that clearance of plasma heparin has been shown to be faster in neonates (362, 363). An initial bolus of 75 to 100 U/kg results in therapeutic aPTT values in 90% of children (232). Average maintenance heparin doses are age dependent and are outlined in Tables 47.12 and 47.13. The rate of the continuous heparin infusion should be titrated to maintain the aPTT between 60 and 85 seconds. A nomogram has been developed to standardize and simplify the management of heparin administration for children (Table 47.14).

The use of low-molecular-weight heparin to achieve anticoagulation in children is an attractive possibility. Its more predictable bioavailability from subcutaneous injections makes establishment of intravenous access and frequent blood drawing for monitoring and dose adjustment unnecessary (365). Its use does require subcutaneous injections, however. Massicotte et al (365) established recommendations for the dosing of low-mo-

**TABLE 47.12.**   Suggested Heparin Dosage Schedule for Neonatal Thrombosis

|  | Bolus (U/kg) | Maintenance (U/kg/hour) |
|---|---|---|
| Preterm less than 28 weeks | 25 | 15 |
| Preterm between 28 and 36 weeks | 50 | 20 |
| Full term | 100 | 25 |

*Adapted with permission from Manco-Johnson MJ. Diagnosis and management of thromboses in the perinatal period [Review]. Semin Perinatol 1990;14:393–409.*

**TABLE 47.13.**   Initiation of Heparin Anticoagulation in Children

|  | Initial Bolus of Heparin | Maintenance Dose of Heparin |
|---|---|---|
| Infants (less than 1 yr) | 75 U/kg i.v. over 10 min | 28 U/kg/hr |
| Young children | 75 U/kg i.v. over 10 min | 20 U/kg/hr |
| Older children | 75 U/kg i.v. over 10 min | 18 U/kg/hr |
| Adults (364) | 75 U/kg i.v. over 10 min | 18 U/kg/hr |

*Adapted with permission from Michelson AD, Bovill E, Andrew M. Antithrombotic therapy in children [Review]. Chest 1995;108: 506S–522S.*

lecular-weight heparin in children based on the measurement of anti-factor Xa activity. They found that newborn infants required 1.6 mg/kg of the low-molecular-weight heparin Enoxaparin twice daily, while older children required a dose of 1.0 mg/kg twice daily, the same dose used in adults. The frequency of needle punctures in these children was minimized by placing a subcutaneous catheter for a duration of 1 week at a time, which facilitated the twice daily administration of the low-molecular-weight heparin.

### Complications

The most common complication of heparin anticoagulation is bleeding (366). However, in experienced hands the incidence of bleeding complications has been reported to be as low as 2% (367). Depending on the source of the hemorrhage, bleeding will usually cease when the heparin infusion is stopped. If more rapid reversal of the effect of heparin is required, then protamine sulfate may be administered to neutralize the heparin. The dose

**TABLE 47.14.** Nomogram for Adjustment of Heparin Anticoagulation in Children

| APTT Value (Seconds) | Heparin Bolus (U/kg) | Hold Drip (Minutes) | Percent Heparin Rate Change | Repeat aPTT |
|---|---|---|---|---|
| <50 | 50 | 0 | +10 | 4 hr |
| 50–59 | 0 | 0 | +10 | 4 hr |
| 60–85 | 0 | 0 | 0 | Next day |
| 86–95 | 0 | 0 | −10 | 4 hr |
| 96–120 | 0 | 30 | −10 | 4 hr |
| >120 | 0 | 60 | −15 | 4 hr |

*Adapted with permission from Michelson AD, Bovill E, Andrew M. Antithrombotic therapy in children [Review]. Chest 1995;108:506S–522S.*

**TABLE 47.15.** Calculation of Protamine Dose Required to Reverse Heparin

| Time Since Last Heparin Dose (min) | Protamine Dose (mg per 100 U of Heparin Received) |
|---|---|
| <30 | 1.0 |
| 30–60 | 0.50–0.75 |
| 60–120 | 0.375–0.50 |
| >120 | 0.25–0.375 |

*Adapted with permission from Michelson AD, Bovill E, Andrew M. Antithrombotic therapy in children [Review]. Chest 1995;108: 506S–522S.*

of protamine required is based on the amount of heparin administered and the time since the most recent dose (Table 47.15). Protamine can be administered at a concentration of 10 mg/mL at a rate not to exceed 5 mg/min (232) because of the high frequency of associated hypotensive reactions. Hypersensitivity reactions are more likely to occur in individuals with an allergy to fish, or those who receive NPH insulin or have been exposed to protamine in the past (232).

An important adverse effect of heparin relates to the formation of heparin associated antiplatelet antibodies, the hallmark of which is the development of thrombocytopenia (see Chapter 29). Paradoxically, this condition can be associated with pathologic thrombosis secondary to platelet activation despite what is often a profound thrombocytopenia. In the absence of an alternative explanation for the thrombocytopenia, pediatric individuals should be evaluated for the presence of heparin associated antiplatelet antibodies and treated with alternative forms of anticoagulation as outlined for adult individuals (368).

Long-term administration of heparin in adults has been shown to cause osteoporosis in adults, and it therefore seems prudent to avoid long-term use of heparin in children (232).

## WARFARIN ANTICOAGULATION

Warfarin is the nearly universally used oral anticoagulant that functions by reducing the plasma concentrations of the active forms of the vitamin K-dependent factors II, VII, IX, and X (see Chapter 55). Use of warfarin in neonates and young children is complicated by the fact that at the time of birth levels of the vitamin K-dependent coagulant factors, as well as the naturally occurring coagulation inhibitors protein C and protein S, are approximately 50% of normal adult values (1, 4, 5, 369). The presence of a vitamin K deficiency, which can be seen in neonates, increases the sensitivity of the child to the effect of warfarin and therefore increases the risk of hemorrhage relating to the use of oral anticoagulants. Breast fed infants, in particular, are potentially very sensitive to oral anticoagulants because of the low concentrations of vitamin K in breast milk. In contrast, some children may be remarkably resistant to oral anticoagulation because of problems with impaired intestinal absorption of the drug from the gastrointestinal tract or the presence of vitamin K in commercially available formulas. Furthermore, infants and children who are maintained on total parenteral nutrition frequently have vitamin K supplements added to the formulation, which can result in a relative resistance to the effect of warfarin.

### Dosage and Monitoring

The most commonly used test to monitor the intensity of warfarin anticoagulation therapy is the prothrombin time (PT), now reported as an international normalized ratio (INR) to correct for the variable sensitivity of the reagents used in different laboratories and to allow the results of different clinical laboratories to be directly compared. Current therapeutic INR recommendations are directly extrapolated from recommendations for

**TABLE 47.16.** Average Warfarin Requirements by Age Group

| Age Group | Average Maintenance Warfarin Dose (mg/kg) |
| --- | --- |
| Infants | 0.32 |
| Children | 0.20 |
| Teenagers | 0.09 |
| Adults | 0.04–0.08 |

*Adapted with permission from Michelson AD, Bovill E, Andrew M. Antithrombotic therapy in children [Review]. Chest 1995;108: 506S–522S.*

**TABLE 47.17.** Protocol for Oral Anticoagulation Therapy to Maintain an INR between 2 and 3 for Pediatric Patients

I. Day 1: If the baseline INR is 1.0 to 1.3, dose = 0.2 mg/kg orally

II. Loading days 2–4:

| INR | Action |
| --- | --- |
| 1.1–1.3 | Repeat loading dose |
| 1.4–1.9 | 50% of loading dose |
| 2.0–3.0 | 50% of loading dose |
| 3.1–3.5 | 25% of loading dose |
| >3.5 | Hold until INR < 3.5, then restart at 50% less than previous dose |

III. Maintenance oral anticoagulation dose guidelines:

| INR | Action |
| --- | --- |
| 1.1–1.4 | Increase by 20% of dose |
| 1.5–1.9 | Increase by 10% of dose |
| 2.0–3.0 | No change |
| 3.1–3.5 | Decrease by 10% of dose |
| >3.5 | Hold dose, check INR daily until INR < 3.5, then restart at 20% less than previous dose |

*Adapted with permission from Michelson AD, Bovill E, Andrew M. Antithrombotic therapy in children [Review]. Chest 1995;108: 506S–522S.*

adult individuals because there are no clinical trials in children to assess clinical outcomes based on different intensities of anticoagulation. In general, the recommended therapeutic range of anticoagulation for the treatment of venous thromboembolic disease is an INR of 2 to 3 and for children with prosthetic cardiac valves, an INR of 2.5 to 3.5 (232).

Maintenance doses of warfarin to maintain therapeutic INR levels are age dependent, with infants having the highest and teenagers having the lowest warfarin requirements on a mg/kg basis (Table 47.16). Algorithms have been established to help guide the initiation and maintenance of warfarin anticoagulation based on the results of the INR determinations. Of importance is the fact that the impact of a particular dose of warfarin is reflected in the INR result approximately 36 hours after the dose has been administered. It is therefore important to maintain a working flow sheet of the doses of warfarin administered and the resulting INR to help tailor the dose of warfarin for each individual individual. One practical implication of the delayed onset of the effect of the warfarin is that the medication can be conveniently administered at the same time each evening, and INR values can be checked each morning. This is advantageous administratively because it provides the flexibility of having all day to check the results of the INR before having to calculate the dose of warfarin to be administered that evening. Nomograms and protocols provide a useful starting point for the administration of warfarin (Table 47.17), but variation amongst individuals is great because of their nutritional state and interaction with diet and concurrent medical problems This requires a significant degree of dosage adjustment based on experience learned from the daily INR results. Warfarin regulation is further complicated by its frequent interaction with other medications, which can either inhibit or potentiate the effect of the oral anticoagulant. For this reason, INR values should be checked frequently when medications are either initiated or stopped in anticoagulated individuals.

Longitudinal studies have shown that safe outpatient oral anticoagulation is feasible in children whose warfarin requirements are moderately predictable and whose control is no more erratic than that of adults (370). Home management of warfarin anticoagulation has been facilitated by the recent availability of capillary whole blood PT monitoring, which allows an assessment of the INR with a fingerstick sample of blood (371).

## Complications

Bleeding is the most important complication of anticoagulation with warfarin (372). Minor bleeding that does not result in any significant morbidity, such as bruising and minor nosebleeds, occurs in approximately 20% of children requiring oral anticoagulants (370). More serious bleeding in individuals anticoagulated at an intensity appropriate for the presence of a mechanical heart valve have bleeding complications at a rate of 3.2 per 100 individual-years (232).

Vitamin K can be administered to reverse bleeding associated with the administration of warfarin, although the INR returns toward normal only as new coagulation factors are synthesized. More rapid reversal of the bleeding diathesis can be accomplished by the administration of normal coagulation factors as fresh frozen plasma or prothrombin complex concentrates. This approach may also be practical if reinstitution of the warfarin is antici-

| **TABLE 47.18.** | Reversal of Oral Anticoagulation Therapy |
|---|---|

I. No bleeding
   A. Rapid reversal of oral anticoagulation is necessary and the individual **will** require oral anticoagulants again in the near future: give vitamin $K_1$, 0.5 to 2.0 mg subcutaneously or i.v. (not intramuscularly), depending on the individual's size.
   B. Rapid reversal of oral anticoagulation is necessary and the individual **will not** require oral anticoagulants again: vitamin $K_1$, 2 to 5 mg subcutaneously or i.v. (not intramuscularly).
II. Significant bleeding
   A. Significant bleeding that is not life threatening and will not cause morbidity: treat with vitamin $K_1$ as in 1A, plus FFP 20 mL/kg i.v.
   B. Significant bleeding that is life threatening and will cause morbidity: treat with vitamin $K_1$ i.v. (5 mg) by slow infusion over 10 to 20 min because of the risk of anaphylactic shock. Give vitamin $K_1$ replacement therapy. Consider giving prothrombin concentrate (containing factors II, VII, IX, X) 50 U/kg i.v. rather than FFP (20 mL/kg i.v.).

*Adapted with permission from Michelson AD, Bovill E, Andrew M. Antithrombotic therapy in children [Review]. Chest 1995;108: 506S–522S.*

| **TABLE 47.19.** | Contraindications to Thrombolytic Therapy |
|---|---|

Absolute contraindications
• Active internal bleeding
• Recent (within 2 months) cerebrovascular accident or other active intracranial process
Relative major contraindications
• Recent (<10 days) major surgery, obstetric delivery, organ biopsy, previous puncture of noncompressible vessels
• Recent serious gastrointestinal bleeding
• Recent serious trauma
• Severe arterial hypertension
Relative minor contraindications
• Recent minor trauma, including cardiopulmonary resuscitation
• High likelihood of left heart thrombus
• Bacterial endocarditis
• Hemostatic defects, including those associated with severe hepatic or renal disease
• Pregnancy
• Age over 75 years
• Diabetic hemorrhagic retinopathy

*Adapted with permission from Anonymous. Thrombolytic therapy in thrombosis: a National Institutes of Health consensus development conference. Ann Intern Med 1980;93;141–144*

pated since the administration of large doses of vitamin K may complicate reanticoagulation with warfarin in the near future. Guidelines for the reversal of anticoagulation therapy are outlined in Table 47.18.

Nonhemorrhagic complications of oral anticoagulation such as tracheal calcification (373) or hair loss (232) have been described on rare occasions in children. Warfarin should not be administered to sexually active women of childbearing age without adequate birth control measures in place because of the teratogenic effects of warfarin (102, 372).

## THROMBOLYTIC AGENTS

In contrast to the anticoagulants heparin and warfarin, which function to prevent fibrin clot formation, the thrombolytic agents act to dissolve established thrombus by converting endogenous plasminogen to plasmin, which can lyse existing thrombus (see Chapter 56). Plasminogen levels in neonates are only approximately 50% of adult levels, and consequently the efficacy of thrombolytic agents is decreased in these individuals (18, 361).

The three most commonly used thrombolytic agents are streptokinase (SK), urokinase (UK), and tissue plasminogen activator (tPA). The latter two agents act directly to cleave plasminogen to plasmin. SK binds to a plasminogen molecule to create an active complex that can then act to cleave unbound plasminogen to plasmin (374).

There are numerous contraindications to thrombolytic therapy including ongoing hemorrhage or recent operation or stroke (375). Other important contraindications include recent invasive procedures, especially involving areas of the body that cannot be readily observed for signs of bleeding, such as liver biopsies. A National Institutes of Health consensus conference has developed a list of contraindications to the use of thrombolytic agents that have been classified by the degree of risk (Table 47.19) (376). Although it is the least expensive of the thrombolytic agents, the use of SK is limited by the associated risk of significant anaphylactic reactions (374, 377). Furthermore, efficacy of the drug can be limited by the present of antistreptococcal antibodies derived from previous SK use or streptococcal infection (374, 377).

## Dosage and Monitoring

In contrast to the anticoagulant agents, there is no fixed therapeutic range for the administration of thrombolytic agents and a wide range of dosing regimens have been reported (378). Instead, the agents are administered and titrated to the thrombolytic effect observed. The most commonly used dosage regimens for the use of thrombolytic agents in children are outlined in Table 47.20. Fre-

**TABLE 47.20.**   Thrombolytic Therapy for Pediatric Patients

| | Low Dose for Blocked Catheters | |
| | Regimen | Monitoring |
| --- | --- | --- |
| Instillation | UK (5000 U/mL) 1.5–3.0 mL/lumen for 2–4 hr | None |
| Infusion | UK (150 U/kg/h) per lumen for 12–48 h | Fibrinogen, TCT PT, aPTT |

| | Systemic Thrombolytic Therapy[a] | | |
| Agent | Load (U/kg) | Maintenance | Monitoring |
| --- | --- | --- | --- |
| UK | 4000 | 4000 U/kg/hr for 6 hr | Fibrinogen, TCT PT, aPTT |
| SK | 4000 (maximum 250,000 units) | 2000 U/kg/hr for 6 hr | Same |
| tPA | None | 0.5 mg/kg/hr for 6 hr | Same |

*Adapted with permission from Michelson AD, Bovill E, Andrew M. Antithrombotic therapy in children [Review]. Chest 1995;108:506S–522S.*

*TCT = thrombin clotting time; UK = urokinase; SK = streptokinase; t-PA = tissue plasminogen activator.*

[a] *Start heparin therapy either during or immediately on completion of thrombolytic therapy. A loading dose of heparin may be omitted. The length of time for optimal maintenance is uncertain. Values provided are starting suggestions: some individuals may respond to longer or shorter courses of therapy.*

quent measurements of the fibrinogen level is valuable since the risk of bleeding complications rises substantially when fibrinogen levels fall below 100 mg/dL (232).

## Complications

As with anticoagulants, the most common complication associated with the use of thrombolytic agents is hemorrhage (377). The incidence of bleeding requiring transfusion associated with the use of thrombolytic agents in children is approximately 20% (232). Although the risk of life threatening central nervous system bleeding is difficult to ascertain from the literature, its reported incidence is less than 3% (232).

Treatment of minor bleeding associated with the use of thrombolytic agents, such as oozing from catheter puncture sites, can be treated with the application of pressure and supportive care. Significant bleeding should be treated by cessation of the thrombolytic agent, as well as other antithrombotic agents. Cryoprecipitate can be used to restore levels of fibrinogen.

## INDICATIONS FOR THE USE OF ANTITHROMBOTIC THERAPY IN CHILDREN

The following recommendations for antithrombotic therapy in the infant and child are derived from data generated for the Fourth Consensus Conference on Antithrombotic Therapy of the American College of Chest Physicians (Tucson, Arizona, USA, March 31 to April 1, 1995) (232). MEDLINE searches of the literature were

conducted for the period 1966–1995 using combinations of key words (children, newborns, heparin, warfarin, aspirin, antiplatelet agents, thrombolysis, thrombosis, embolism, mechanical and biologic prosthetic heart valves) and supplemented by additional references located through the bibliographies of listed articles. Because of the current paucity of pediatric studies with high levels of evidence, modified adult guidelines remain a primary source of pediatric recommendations. The consensus conference recommendations are as follows (232):

Treatment of Venous Thromboembolism in Children

1. Children (older than 2 months of age) with deep vein thrombosis or pulmonary embolism should be treated with intravenous heparin sufficient to prolong the activated partial thromboplastin time (aPTT) to a range that corresponds to an anti-factor Xa level of 0.3 to 0.7 U/mL.

2. It is recommended that treatment with heparin should be continued for 5 to 10 days and that treatment with oral anticoagulation should be overlapped with heparin for 4 to 5 days. For many individuals, heparin and warfarin therapy can be started together and heparin therapy discontinued on day 6 if the prothrombin time (PT) (international normalized ratio [INR]) is therapeutic. For massive pulmonary embolism or extensive deep vein thrombosis, a longer period of heparin therapy should be considered.

3. Long-term anticoagulant therapy should be continued for at least 3 months using oral

anticoagulants to prolong the PT to an INR of 2.0 to 3.0.

4. Indefinite oral anticoagulant therapy with an INR of 2.0 to 3.0, low-dose anticoagulant therapy (INR <2.0), or close monitoring should be considered for children with a first recurrence of venous thrombosis or an initial venous thrombosis and a continuing risk factor, such as a central venous line, hereditary resistance to activated protein C, protein C deficiency, protein S deficiency, antithrombin III deficiency, or lupus anticoagulant.

5. Indefinite oral anticoagulant therapy with an INR of 2.0 to 3.0 should be considered for children with a second recurrence of venous thrombosis or a first recurrence of a venous thrombosis and a continuing risk factor, such as a central venous line, hereditary resistance to activated protein C, protein C deficiency, protein S deficiency, antithrombin III deficiency, or lupus anticoagulant.

6. The use of thrombolytic agents in the treatment of venous thromboembolism continues to be highly individualized. Further clinical investigation is needed before definitive recommendations can be made.

7. Children with congenital prothrombotic disorders should receive short-term prophylactic anticoagulation in high-risk situations such as immobility, significant surgery, or trauma.

Treatment of Venous/Arterial Thromboembolism in Newborns

1. The use of anticoagulation therapy in the treatment of newborns with deep vein thrombosis, pulmonary embolism, or arterial thrombosis continues to be individualized. Further clinical investigation is needed before definitive recommendations can be made.

2. If short-term anticoagulation therapy is not used, the thrombus should be closely monitored with objective tests and, if extending, anticoagulation therapy instituted.

3. If anticoagulation is used, a short course (10 to 14 days) of intravenous heparin should be sufficient to prolong the aPTT to the therapeutic range that corresponds to an anti-factor Xa level of 0.3 to 0.7 U/mL. The thrombus should be closely monitored with objective tests for evidence of extension or recurrent disease. This grade C recommendation is based on unpublished data. If the thrombus extends following discontinuation of heparin therapy, oral anticoagulation therapy should be considered.

4. The use of thrombolytic agents in the treatment of venous thromboembolism continues to be

individualized. Further clinical investigation is needed before more definitive recommendations can be made. Supplementation with plasminogen (fresh frozen plasma) may be helpful.

## Prophylaxis for Cardiac Catheterization in Children and Newborns

Newborns and children requiring cardiac catheterization via an artery should undergo prophylaxis with bolus intravenous heparin 100 to 150 U/kg.

Mechanical Prosthetic Heart Valves in Children
1. It is strongly recommended that children with mechanical prosthetic heart valves receive oral anticoagulation therapy.
2. Levels of oral anticoagulation therapy that prolong the INR to 2.5 to 3.5 are recommended based on recommendations in adults.
3. Children with mechanical prosthetic heart valves who suffer systemic embolism despite adequate therapy with oral anticoagulation therapy may benefit from the addition of aspirin 6 to 20 mg/kg per day (adult level I study). Dipyridamole 2 to 5 mg/kg per day, in addition to oral anti-coagulation therapy, is an alternative option.
4. When full-dose oral anticoagulation therapy is contraindicated, long-term therapy with oral anticoagulation therapy sufficient to increase the INR 2.0 to 3.0 in combination with aspirin 6 to 20 mg/kg per day and dipyridamole 2 to 5 mg/kg per day may be used.

## Biologic Prosthetic Heart Valves in Children

Children rarely have biologic prosthetic heart valves. Further clinical investigation is needed before definitive recommendations can be made. One option is to treat children with biologic prosthetic valves according to adult recommendations (379).

## Kawasaki Disease

In addition to intravenous gamma globulin (2 g/kg as a single dose), children with Kawasaki disease should receive aspirin 80 to 100 mg/kg per day during the acute phase (up to 14 days) as an anti-inflammatory agent, then aspirin 3 to 5 mg/kg per day for 7 weeks or longer to prevent the formation of coronary aneurysm thrombosis.

## Fontan Operations

Further clinical investigation is needed before definitive recommendations can be made. One option is to initially administer therapeutic amounts of heparin followed by oral anticoagulation therapy to achieve an INR of 2.0 to

3.0 for 3 months. Patients with fenestrations may benefit from treatment until closure.

## Blalock-Taussig Shunts

Further clinical investigation is needed before definitive recommendations can be made. One option is to initially administer therapeutic amounts of heparin, followed by aspirin 3 to 5 mg/kg per day indefinitely.

## Patients With Homozygous Deficiency of Protein C or Protein S

1. It is recommended that newborns with purpura fulminans due to homozygous deficiency of protein C or S should be treated initially with replacement therapy (either fresh frozen plasma or protein C concentrate) for approximately 6 to 8 weeks until the skin lesions have healed.

2. Following resolution of the skin lesions, and under cover of replacement therapy, oral anticoagulation therapy can be introduced with target INR values of approximately 3.0 to 4.5. Treatment duration with oral anticoagulants is indefinite. Recurrent skin lesions should be treated with replacement therapy of protein C or S.

3. For individuals with homozygous protein C or S deficiency, but with measurable plasma concentrations, low-molecular-weight heparin is a therapeutic option.

# REFERENCES

1. Andrew M, Paes B, Milner R et al. Development of the human coagulation system in the full-term infant. Blood 1987;70:165–172.
2. Hathaway WE. The bleeding newborn. Semin Hematol 1975;12:175–188.
3. Andrew M, Karpatkin M. A simple screening test for evaluating prolonged partial thromboplastin times in newborn infants. J Pediatr 1982;101: 610–612.
4. Andrew M, Paes B, Milner R et al. Development of the human coagulation system in the healthy premature infant. Blood 1988;72:1651–1657.
5. Andrew M, Paes B, Johnston M. Development of the hemostatic system in the neonate and young infant. Am J Pediatr Hematol Oncol 1990;12: 95–104.
6. Reverdiau-Moalic P, Delahousse B, Body G et al. Evolution of blood coagulation activators and inhibitors in the healthy human fetus. Blood 1996; 88:900–906.
7. Galanakis DK, Mosesson MW. Evaluation of the role of in vivo proteolysis (fibrinogenolysis) in prolonging the thrombin time of human umbilical cord fibrinogen. Blood 1976;48:109–118.
8. Hasegawa N, Sasaki S. A deficiency in A alpha chain's N-terminal alanine residue as a major cause of the slow coagulation of fetal fibrinogen. Thromb Res 1989;54:595–602.
9. Seydewitz HH, Witt I. The fraction of high molecular weight (HMW) fibrinogen and phosphorylated fibrinopeptide A in fetal fibrinogen. Thromb Res 1989;55:785–790.
10. Katz JA, Moake JL, McPherson PD et al. Relationship between human development and disappearance of unusually large von Willebrand factor multimers from plasma. Blood 1989;73:1851–1858.
11. Weinstein MJ, Blanchard R, Moake JL et al. Fetal and neonatal von Willebrand factor (vWf) is unusually large and similar to the vWf in individuals with thrombotic thrombocytopenic purpura. Br J Haematol 1989;72:68–72.
12. Mannhalter C, Kyrle PA, Brenner B et al. Rapid neonatal diagnosis of type IIB von Willebrand disease using the polymerase chain reaction. Blood 1991;77:2539–2540.
13. Corrigan JJ Jr. Neonatal thrombosis and the thrombolytic system: pathophysiology and therapy. Am J Pediatr Hematol Oncol 1988;10:83–91.
14. Phillips LL, Skrodelis V. A comparison of the fibrinolytic system enzyme system in maternal and umbilical blood. Pediatrics 1958;22:715–726.
15. Suarez CR, Walenga J, Mangogna LC et al. Neonatal and maternal fibrinolysis: activation at time of birth. Am J Hematol 1985;19:365–372.
16. Ekelund H, Hedner U, Nilsson IM. Fibrinolysis in newborns. Acta Paediatr Scand 1970;59:33–43.
17. Caccamo ML, Rossi E, Salmoiraghi MG et al. The fibrinolytic system in the newborn: role of histidine-rich glycoprotein. Biol Neonate 1992;61: 281–284.
18. Ries M, Zenker M, Klinge J et al. Age-related differences in a clot lysis assay after adding different plasminogen activators in a plasma milieu in vitro. J Pediatr Hematol Oncol 1995;17:260–264.
19. Edelberg JM, Enghild JJ, Pizzo SV et al. Neonatal plasminogen displays altered cell surface binding and activation kinetics. Correlation with increased glycosylation of the protein. J Clin Invest 1990;86:107–112.
20. Corrigan JJ. Neonatal coagulation disorders. In: Alter BP, ed. Perinatal hematology. New York: Churchill Livingstone, 1989:165–193.
21. Hathaway WE. Haemostatic disorders in the newborn. In: Bloom AL, Thomas DP, eds. Haemostasis and thrombosis. 2nd ed. Edinburgh: Churchill Livingstone, 1987:554–569.
22. Feusner JH. Normal and abnormal bleeding times in neonates and young children utilizing a fully standardized template technic. Am J Clin Pathol 1980;74:73–77.
23. Mull MM, Hathaway WE. Altered platelet function in newborns. Pediatr Res 1970;4:229–237.
24. Corby DG, O'Barr TP. Decreased alpha-adrenergic receptors in newborn platelets: cause of abnormal response to epinephrine. Dev Pharmacol Ther 1981;2:215–225.
25. Ts'ao CH, Green D, Schultz K. Function and ultrastructure of platelets of neonates: enhanced ristocetin aggregation of neonatal platelets. Br J Haematol 1976;32:225–233.
26. Andrews NP, Broughton Pipkin F, Heptinstall S. Blood platelet behaviour in mothers and neonates. Thromb Haemost 1985;53:428–432.
27. Gader AM, Bahakim H, Jabbar FA et al. Dose-response aggregometry in maternal/neonatal platelets. Thromb Haemost 1988;60:314–318.
28. Corby DG, Schulman I. The effects of antenatal drug administration on aggregation of platelets of newborn infants. J Pediatr 1971;79:307–313.
29. Israels SJ, Daniels M, McMillan EM. Deficient collagen-induced activation in the newborn platelet. Pediatr Res 1990;27:337–343.
30. Whaun JM. The platelet of the newborn infant. 5-Hydroxytryptamine uptake and release. Thromb Diath Haemorrh 1973;30:327–333.
31. Corby DG, Zuck TF. Newborn platelet dysfunction: a storage pool and release defect. Thromb Haemost 1976;36:200–207.
32. Suarez CR, Gonzalez J, Menendez C et al. Neonatal and maternal platelets: activation at time of birth. Am J Hematol 1988;29:18–21.
33. Ahlsten G, Ewald U, Tuvemo T. Arachidonic acid-induced aggregation of platelets from human cord blood compared with platelets from adults. Biol Neonate 1985;47:199–204.
34. Jones CR, McCabe R, Hamilton CA et al. Maternal and fetal platelet responses and adrenoceptor binding characteristics. Thromb Haemost 1985; 53:95–98.
35. Levine SP. Secreted platelet proteins as markers for pathological disorders. In: Phillips DR, Shuman MA, eds. Biochemistry of platelets. Orlando: Academic Press, 1986:378–415.
36. Kinlough-Rathbone RL, Packham MA, Mustard JF. Platelet aggregation. In: Harker LA, Zimmerman TS, eds. Measurements of platelet function. New York: Churchill Livingstone, 1983:64–91.
37. Michelson AD, Ellis PA, Barnard MR et al. Downregulation of the platelet surface glycoprotein Ib-IX complex in whole blood stimulated by thrombin, adenosine diphosphate or an in vivo wound. Blood 1991;77:770–779.
38. Kestin AS, Ellis PA, Barnard MR et al. Effect of strenuous exercise on platelet activation state and reactivity. Circulation 1993;88:1502–1511.
39. Rajasekhar D, Kestin AS, Bednarek FJ et al. Neonatal platelets are less reactive than adult platelets to physiological agonists in whole blood. Thromb Haemost 1994;72:957–963.
40. Rajasekhar D, Barnard MR, Bednarek FJ et al. Platelet hyporeactivity in very low birthweight neonates. Thromb Haemost 1997;77:1002–1007.
41. Ahmann PA, Lazzara A, Dykes FD et al. Intraventricular hemorrhage in the high-risk preterm infant: incidence and outcome. Ann Neurol 1980;7: 118–124.
42. Bejar R, Curbelo V, Coen RW et al. Diagnosis and follow-up of intraventricular and intracerebral hemorrhages by ultrasound studies of infant's brain through the fontanelles and sutures. Pediatrics 1980;66:661–673.
43. Ansell J, Tiarks C, Hirsh J et al. Measurement of the activated partial thromboplastin time from a capillary (fingerstick) sample of whole blood. A new method for monitoring heparin therapy. Am J Clin Pathol 1991; 95:222–227.
44. Lucas FV, Duncan A, Jay R et al. A novel whole blood capillary technic for measuring the prothrombin time. Am J Clin Pathol 1987;88:442–446.
45. Michelson AD. Flow cytometry: a clinical test of platelet function. Blood 1996;87:4925–4936.

46. Marshall LR, Jones C, Munro TE. Prediction of neonatal alloimmune thrombocytopenia using PCR. Pathology 1994;26:46–47.

47. Ellis MR 3rd. Coagulopathy screening in children with heparinized central venous catheters. Pediatrics 1993;91:1147–1150.

48. Hellum AJ. The adhesiveness of human platelets *in vitro*. Scand J Clin Lab Invest 1960;51(Suppl):1–117.

49. Andrew M, Paes B, Bowker J et al. Evaluation of an automated bleeding time device in the newborn. Am J Hematol 1990;35:275–277.

50. Menkes JH. Intracranial hemorrhage: pathogenesis and pathology. In: Taeusch HW, Ballard RA, Avery ME, eds. Diseases of the newborn. 6th ed. Philadelphia: WB Saunders, 1991:422–425.

51. Tsiantos A, Victorin L, Relier JP et al. Intracranial hemorrhage in the prematurely born infant. Timing of clots and evaluation of clinical signs and symptoms. J Pediatr 1974;85:854–859.

52. Dubowitz LM, Levene MI, Morante A et al. Neurologic signs in neonatal intraventricular hemorrhage: a correlation with real-time ultrasound. J Pediatr 1981;99:127–133.

53. Stuart MJ. Bleeding in the newborn and pediatric individual. In: Colman RW, Hirsh J, Marder VJ, eds. Hemostasis and thrombosis. Basic principles and clinical practice. 2nd ed. Philadelphia: Lippincott, 1987:942–959.

54. Andrew M. An approach to the management of infants with impaired haemostasis. Baillières Clin Haematol 1991;4:251–289.

55. Levene MI, Fawer CL, Lamont RF. Risk factors in the development of intraventricular haemorrhage in the preterm neonate. Arch Dis Child 1982; 57:410–417.

56. Van de Bor M, Van Bel F, Lineman R et al. Perinatal factors and periventricular-intraventricular hemorrhage in preterm infants. Am J Dis Child 1986; 140:1125–1130.

57. Gray OP, Ackerman A, Fraser AJ. Intracranial haemorrhage and clotting defects in low-birth-weight infants. Lancet 1968;1:545–548.

58. Chessells JM, Wigglesworth JS. Coagulation studies in preterm infants with respiratory distress and intracranial haemorrhage. Arch Dis Child 1972;47:564–570.

59. Setzer ES, Webb IB, Wassenaar JW et al. Platelet dysfunction and coagulopathy in intraventricular hemorrhage in the premature infant. J Pediatr 1982;100:599–605.

60. McDonald MM, Johnson ML, Rumack CM et al. Role of coagulopathy in newborn intracranial hemorrhage. Pediatrics 1984;74:26–31.

61. Beverley DW, Chance GW, Inwood MJ et al. Intraventricular haemorrhage and haemostasis defects. Arch Dis Child 1984;59:444–448.

62. Malloy MH, Cutter GR. The association of heparin exposure with intraventricular hemorrhage among very low birth weight infants. J Perinatol 1995; 15:185–191.

63. Volpe JJ. Neurology of the newborn. 2nd ed. Philadelphia: WB Saunders, 1987.

64. Anonymous. A randomized trial comparing the effect of prophylactic intravenous fresh frozen plasma, gelatin or glucose on early mortality and morbidity in preterm babies. The Northern Neonatal Nursing Initiative [NNNI]. Eur J Pediatr 1996;155:580–588.

65. Morgan ME, Benson JW, Cooke RW. Ethamsylate reduces the incidence of periventricular haemorrhage in very low birth-weight babies. Lancet 1981;2:830–831.

66. Benson JW, Drayton MR, Hayward C et al. Multicentre trial of ethamsylate for prevention of periventricular haemorrhage in very low birthweight infants. Lancet 1986;2:1297–1300.

67. Rennie JM, Doyle J, Cooke RW. Ethamsylate reduces immunoreactive prostacyclin metabolite in low birthweight infants with respiratory distress syndrome. Early Hum Dev 1986;14:239–244.

68. Ment LR, Duncan CC, Ehrenkranz RA et al. Randomized indomethacin trial for prevention of intraventricular hemorrhage in very low birth weight infants. J Pediatr 1985;107:937–943.

69. Rennie JM, Doyle J, Cooke RW. Early administration of indomethacin to preterm infants. Arch Dis Child 1986;61:233–238.

70. Hanigan WC, Kennedy G, Roemisch F et al. Administration of indomethacin for the prevention of periventricular-intraventricular hemorrhage in high-risk neonates. J Pediatr 1988;112:941–947.

71. Bandstra ES, Montalvo BM, Goldberg RN et al. Prophylactic indomethacin for prevention of intraventricular hemorrhage in premature infants. Pediatrics 1988;82:533–542.

72. Bada HS, Green RS, Pourcyrous M et al. Indomethacin reduces the risks of severe intraventricular hemorrhage. J Pediatr 1989;115:631–637.

73. Morales WJ. Antenatal therapy to minimize neonatal intraventricular hemorrhage. Clin Obstet Gynecol 1991;34:328–335.

74. Abdel-Rahman AM, Rosenberg AA. Prevention of intraventricular hemorrhage in the premature infant. Clin Perinatol 1994;21:505–521.

75. Volpe JJ. Intraventricular hemorrhage in the premature infant—current concepts. II. Ann Neurol 1989;25:109–116.

76. Pomerance JJ, Teal JG, Gogolok JF et al. Maternally administered antenatal vitamin K1: effect on neonatal prothrombin activity, partial thromboplastin time, and intraventricular hemorrhage. Obstet Gynecol 1987;70:235–241.

77. Morales WJ, Angel JL, O'Brien WF et al. The use of antenatal vitamin K in the prevention of early neonatal intraventricular hemorrhage. Am J Obstet Gynecol 1988;159:774–779.

78. Kazzi NJ, Ilagan NB, Liang KC et al. Maternal administration of vitamin K does not improve the coagulation profile of preterm infants. Pediatrics 1989;84:1045–1050.

79. DeSa DJ, MacLean BS. An analysis of massive pulmonary haemorrhage in the newborn infant in Oxford, 1948-68. J Obstet Gynaecol Br Commonw 1970;77:158–163.

80. Sherman NJ, Clatworthy HW Jr. Gastrointestinal bleeding in neonates: a study of 94 cases. Surgery 1967;62:614–619.

81. Apt L, Downey WS Jr. "Melena" neonatorum: swallowed blood syndrome; simple test for the differentiation of adult and fetal hemoglobin in bloody stools. J Pediatr 1955;47:6–10.

82. Glader BE, Amylon MD. Hemostatic disorders in the newborn. In: Taeusch HW, Ballard RA, Avery ME, eds. Diseases of the newborn. 6th ed. Philadelphia: WB Saunders, 1991:777–790.

83. Glader BE, Buchanan GR. Care of the critically ill child: the bleeding neonate. Pediatrics 1976;58:548–555.

84. Oski FA. Blood coagulation and its disorders in the newborn. In: Oski FA, Naiman JL, eds. Hematologic problems in the newborn. 3rd ed. Philadelphia: WB Saunders, 1982:137–174.

85. Simon C, Janner M. Color atlas of pediatric diseases. Toronto: Marcel Dekker, 1987.

86. Hiraike H, Kimura M, Itokawa Y. Determination of K vitamins (phylloquinone and menaquinones) in umbilical cord plasma by a platinum-reduction column. J Chromatogr 1988;430:143–148.

87. Mandelbrot L, Guillaumont M, Leclercq M et al. Placental transfer of vitamin K1 and its implications in fetal hemostasis. Thromb Haemost 1988; 60:39–43.

88. von Kries R, Shearer MJ, Gobel U. Vitamin K in infancy. Eur J Pediatr 1988;147:106–112.

89. Widdershoven J, Lambert W, Motohara K et al. Plasma concentrations of vitamin K1 and PIVKA-II in bottle-fed and breast-fed infants with and without vitamin K prophylaxis at birth. Eur J Pediatr 1988;148:139–142.

90. Greer FR. Vitamin K deficiency and hemorrhage in infancy. Clin Perinatol 1995;22:759–777.

91. Hathaway WE. Vitamin K deficiency. Southeast Asian J Trop Med Public Health 1993;24(Suppl 1):5–9.

92. Vietti TJ, Murphy TP, James JA et al. Observations on the prophylactic use of vitamin K in the newborn. J Pediatr 1960;56:343–346.

93. Sutherland JM, Glueck HI, Gleser G. Hemorrhagic disease of the newborn. Breast feeding as a necessary factor in the pathogenesis. Am J Dis Child 1967;113:524–533.

94. Clark FI, James EJ. Twenty-seven years of experience with oral vitamin K1 therapy in neonates. J Pediatr 1995;127:301–304.

95. Brousson MA, Klein MC. Controversies surrounding the administration of vitamin K to newborns: a review. Can Med Assoc J 1996;154:307–315.

96. Mountain KR, Hirsh J, Gallus AS. Neonatal coagulation defect due to anticonvulsant drug treatment in pregnancy. Lancet 1970;1:265–268.

97. Hirsh J, Cade JF, O'Sullivan EF. Clinical experience with anticoagulant therapy during pregnancy. Br Med J 1970;1:270–273.

98. Deblay MF, Vert P, Andre M et al. Transplacental vitamin K prevents haemorrhagic disease of infant of epileptic mother [Letter]. Lancet 1982; 1:1247.

99. Lane PA, Hathaway WE. Vitamin K in infancy. J Pediatr 1985;106:351–359.

100. Motohara K, Endo F, Matsuda I. Screening for late neonatal vitamin K deficiency by acarboxyprothrombin in dried blood spots. Arch Dis Child 1987;62:370–375.

101. Lulseged S. Haemorrhagic disease of the newborn: a review of 127 cases. Ann Trop Paediatr 1993;13:331–338.

102. Astedt B. Antenatal drugs affecting vitamin K status of the fetus and newborn. Semin Thromb Hemost 1995;21:364–370.

103. von Kries R, Gobel U, Hachmeister A et al. Vitamin K and childhood cancer: a population based case-control study in Lower Saxony, Germany. Br Med J 1993;13:199–203.

104. Bray GL, Luban NL. Hemophilia presenting with intracranial hemorrhage. An approach to the infant with intracranial bleeding and coagulopathy. Am J Dis Child 1987;141:1215–1217.

105. Yoffe G, Buchanan GR. Intracranial hemorrhage in newborn and young infants with hemophilia. J Pediatr 1988;113:333–336.

106. Baehner RL, Strauss HS. Hemophilia in the first year of life. N Engl J Med 1966;275:524–528.

107. Menell JS, Bussel JB. Antenatal management of the thrombocytopenias. Clin Perinatol 1994;21:591–614.

108. George D, Bussel JB. Neonatal thrombocytopenia. Semin Thromb Hemost 1995;21:276–293.

109. Castle V, Andrew M, Kelton J et al. Frequency and mechanism of neonatal thrombocytopenia. J Pediatr 1986;108:749–755.

110. Van de Bor M, Bri't E, Van Bel F et al. Hemostasis and periventricular-intraventricular hemorrhage in the newborn. Am J Dis Child 1986;140:1131–1134.

111. Andrew M, Castle V, Saigal S et al. Clinical impact of neonatal thrombocytopenia. J Pediatr 1987;110:457–464.

112. Murray NA, Roberts IA. Circulating megakaryocytes and their progenitors in early thrombocytopenia in preterm neonates. Pediatr Res 1996;40:112–119.

113. Castle V, Coates G, Kelton JG et al. 111In-oxine platelet survivals in thrombocytopenic infants. Blood 1987;70:652–656.

114. Blanchette VS, Peters MA, Pegg-Feige K. Alloimmune thrombocytopenia. Review from a neonatal intensive care unit. Curr Stud Hematol Blood Transfus 1986;52:87–96.

115. Kaplan C, Morel-Kopp MC, Kroll H et al. HPA-5b (Br[a]) neonatal alloimmune thrombocytopenia: clinical and immunological analysis of 39 cases. Br J Haematol 1991;78:425–429.

116. Pearson HA, Shulman NR, Marder VJ et al. Isoimmune neonatal thrombocytopenic purpura: Clinical and therapeutic considerations. Blood 1964;23:154–177.

117. Mueller-Eckhardt C, Kiefel V, Grubert A et al. 348 cases of suspected neonatal alloimmune thrombocytopenia. Lancet 1989;1:363–366.

118. Herman JH, Jumbelic MI, Ancona RJ et al. In utero cerebral hemorrhage in alloimmune thrombocytopenia. Am J Pediatr Hematol Oncol 1986;8:312–317.

119. Udom-Rice I, Bussel JB. Fetal and neonatal thrombocytopenia. Blood Rev 1995;9:57–64.

120. Davidson JE, McWilliam RC, Evans TJ et al. Porencephaly and optic hypoplasia in neonatal isoimmune thrombocytopenia. Arch Dis Child 1989;64:858–860.

121. von dem Borne AE, van Leeuwen EF, von Riesz LE et al. Neonatal alloimmune thrombocytopenia: detection and characterization of the responsible antibodies by the platelet immunofluorescence test. Blood 1981;57:649–656.

122. Mueller-Eckhardt C, Kayser W, Forster C et al. Improved assay for detection of platelet-specific PlA1 antibodies in neonatal alloimmune thrombocytopenia. Vox Sang 1982;43:76–81.

123. Kiefel V, Santoso S, Katzmann B et al. A new platelet-specific alloantigen Bra. Report of 4 cases with neonatal alloimmune thrombocytopenia. Vox Sang 1988;54:101–106.

124. Adner MM, Fisch GR, Starobin SG et al. Use of "compatible" platelet transfusions in treatment of congenital isoimmune thrombocytopenic purpura. N Engl J Med 1969;280:244–247.

125. Katz J, Hodder FS, Aster RS et al. Neonatal isoimmune thrombocytopenia. The natural course and management and the detection of maternal antibody. Clin Pediatr (Phila) 1984;23:159–162.

126. Sanders MR, Graeber JE. Posttransfusion graft-versus-host disease in infancy. J Pediatr 1990;117:159–163.

127. Sidiropoulos D, Straume B. The treatment of neonatal isoimmune thrombocytopenia with intravenous immunoglobin (IgG i.v.). Blut 1984;48:383–386.

128. Derycke M, Dreyfus M, Ropert JC et al. Intravenous immunoglobulin for neonatal isoimmune thrombocytopenia. Arch Dis Child 1985;60:667–669.

129. Suarez CR, Anderson C. High-dose intravenous gammaglobulin (IVG) in neonatal immune thrombocytopenia. Am J Hematol 1987;26:247–253.

130. Massey GV, McWilliams NB, Mueller DG et al. Intravenous immunoglobulin in treatment of neonatal isoimmune thrombocytopenia. J Pediatr 1987;111:133–135.

131. Bussel JB, Berkowitz RL, Lynch L et al. Antenatal management of alloimmune thrombocytopenia with intravenous gamma globulin: a randomized trial of the addition of low-dose steroid to intravenous gamma globulin. Am J Obstet Gynecol 1996;174:1414–1423.

132. Kaplan C, Daffos F, Forestier F et al. Management of alloimmune thrombocytopenia: antenatal diagnosis and in utero transfusion of maternal platelets. Blood 1988;72:340–343.

133. McFarland JG, Frenzke M, Aster RH. Testing of maternal sera in pregnancies at risk for neonatal alloimmune thrombocytopenia. Transfusion 1989;29:128–133.

134. Bussel JB, Berkowitz RL, McFarland JG et al. Antenatal treatment of neonatal alloimmune thrombocytopenia. N Engl J Med 1988;319:1374–1378.

135. McFarland JG, Aster RH, Bussel JB et al. Prenatal diagnosis of neonatal alloimmune thrombocytopenia using allele-specific oligonucleotide probes. Blood 1991;78:2276–2282.

136. Kuijpers RW, Faber NM, Kanhai HH et al. Typing of fetal platelet alloantigens when platelets are not available. Lancet 1990;336:1319.

137. Lynch L, Bussel JB, McFarland JG et al. Antenatal treatment of alloimmune thrombocytopenia. Obstet Gynecol 1992;80:67–71.

138. Kornfeld I, Wilson RD, Ballem P et al. Antenatal invasive and noninvasive management of alloimmune thrombocytopenia. Fetal Diagn Ther 1996;11:210–217.

139. Bussel JB, McFarland JG, Lynch L et al. Antenatal treatment of alloimmune thrombocytopenia [Abstract]. Blood 1991;78:1540a.

140. Weiner E, Zosmer N, Bajoria R et al. Direct fetal administration of immunoglobulins: another disappointing therapy in alloimmune thrombocytopenia. Fetal Diagn Ther 1994;9:159–164.

141. Karpatkin S, Strick N, Karpatkin MB et al. Cumulative experience in the detection of antiplatelet antibody in 234 individuals with idiopathic thrombocytopenic purpura, systemic lupus erythematosus and other clinical disorders. Am J Med 1972;52:776–785.

142. de Swiet M. Maternal autoimmune disease and the fetus. Arch Dis Child 1985;60:794–797.

143. Burrows RF, Kelton JG. Incidentally detected thrombocytopenia in healthy mothers and their infants. N Engl J Med 1988;319:142–145.

144. Samuels P, Bussel JB, Braitman LE et al. Estimation of the risk of thrombocytopenia in the offspring of pregnant women with presumed immune thrombocytopenic purpura. N Engl J Med 1990;323:229–235.

145. Aster RH. "Gestational" thrombocytopenia: a plea for conservative management. N Engl J Med 1990;323:264–266.

146. Burrows RF, Kelton JG. Low fetal risks in pregnancies associated with idiopathic thrombocytopenic purpura. Am J Obstet Gynecol 1990;163:1147–1150.

147. Blanchette VS, Sacher RA, Ballem PJ et al. Commentary on the management of autoimmune thrombocytopenia during pregnancy and in the neonatal period. Blut 1989;59:121–123.

148. Bussel JB. Management of infants of mothers with immune thrombocytopenic purpura. J Pediatr 1988;113:497–499.

149. Territo M, Finklestein J, Oh W et al. Management of autoimmune thrombocytopenia in pregnancy and in the neonate. Obstet Gynecol 1973;41:579–584.

150. Daffos F, Forestier F, Kaplan C et al. Prenatal diagnosis and management of bleeding disorders with fetal blood sampling. Am J Obstet Gynecol 1988;158:939–946.

151. Karpatkin M, Porges RF, Karpatkin S. Platelet counts in infants of women with autoimmune thrombocytopenia: effects of steroid administration to the mother. N Engl J Med 1981;305:936–939.

152. Christiaens GC, Nieuwenhuis HK, von dem Borne AE et al. Idiopathic thrombocytopenic purpura in pregnancy: a randomized trial on the effect of antenatal low dose corticosteroids on neonatal platelet count. Br J Obstet Gynecol 1990;97:893–898.

153. Ballin A, Andrew M, Ling E et al. High-dose intravenous gamma globulin therapy for neonatal autoimmune thrombocytopenia. J Pediatr 1988;112:789–792.

154. Blanchette V, Andrew M, Perlman M et al. Neonatal autoimmune thrombocytopenia: role of high-dose intravenous immunoglobulin G therapy. Blut 1989;59:139–144.

155. Burrows RF, Andrew M. Neonatal thrombocytopenia in the hypertensive disorders of pregnancy. Obstet Gynecol 1990;76:234–238.

156. Oren H, Irken G, Oren B et al. Assessment of clinical impact and predisposing factors for neonatal thrombocytopenia. Indian J Pediatr 1994;61:551–558.

157. Rigaud M, Leibovitz E, Quee CS et al. Thrombocytopenia in children infected with human immunodeficiency virus: long-term follow-up and therapeutic considerations. J Acquir Immune Defic Syndr 1992;5:450–455.

158. Naiman JL. Disorders of the platelets. In: Oski FA, Naiman JL, eds. Hematologic problems of the newborn. 3rd ed. Philadelphia: WB Saunders, 1982:175–222.

159. Kasabach HH, Merritt KK. Capillary hemangioma with extensive purpura. Am J Dis Child 1940;59:1063–1070.

160. Kontras SB, Green OC, King L et al. Giant hemangioma with thrombocytopenia: case report with survival and sequestration studies of platelet labeled with chromium 51. Am J Dis Child 1963;105:188–192.

161. Hatley RM, Sabio H, Howell CG et al. Successful management of an infant with a giant hemangioma of the retroperitoneum and Kasabach-Merritt syndrome with alpha-interferon. J Pediatr Surg 1997;28:1356–1357.

162. Chessells JM, Wigglesworth JS. Haemostatic failure in babies with rhesus isoimmunization. Arch Dis Child 1971;46:38–45.

163. Bick RL. Laboratory evaluation of platelet dysfunction. Clin Lab Med 1995;15:1–38.

164. George JN, Nurden AT, Phillips DR. Molecular defects in interactions of platelets with the vessel wall. N Engl J Med 1984;311:1084–1098.

165. George JN, Caen JP, Nurden AT. Glanzmann's thrombasthenia: the spectrum of clinical disease. Blood 1990;75:1383–1395.

166. Michelson AD, Loscalzo J, Melnick B et al. Partial characterization of a binding site for von Willebrand factor on glycocalicin. Blood 1986;67:19–26.

167. Roth GJ. Developing relationships: arterial platelet adhesion, glycoprotein Ib, and leucine-rich glycoproteins. Blood 1991;77:5–19.

168. Bleyer WA, Breckenridge RT. Studies on the detection of adverse drug reactions in the newborn. II. The effects of prenatal aspirin on newborn hemostasis. JAMA 1970;213:2049–2053.

169. Haslam RR, Ekert H, Gillam GL. Hemorrhage in a neonate possibly due to maternal ingestion of salicylate. J Pediatr 1974;84:556–557.

170. Edson JR, Blaese RM, White JG et al. Defibrination syndrome in an infant born after abruptio placentae. J Pediatr 1968;72:342–346.

171. Chessells JM, Wigglesworth JS. Coagulation studies in severe birth asphyxia. Arch Dis Child 1971;46:253–256.

172. Corrigan JJ Jr, Ray WL, May N. Changes in the blood coagulation system associated with septicemia. N Engl J Med 1968;279:851–856.

173. Gross SJ, Filston HC, Anderson JC. Controlled study of treatment for disseminated intravascular coagulation in the neonate. J Pediatr 1982;100:445–448.

174. Hanada T, Abe T, Takita H. Antithrombin III concentrates for treatment of

disseminated intravascular coagulation in children. Am J Pediatr Hematol Oncol 1985;7:3–8.

175. von Kries R, Stannigel H, Gobel U. Anticoagulant therapy by continuous heparin-antithrombin III infusion in newborns with disseminated intravascular coagulation. Eur J Pediatr 1985;144:191–194.

176. Corrigan JJ Jr, Jordan CM. Heparin therapy in septicemia with disseminated intravascular coagulation. N Engl J Med 1970;283:778–782.

177. Gobel U, von Voss H, Jurgens H et al. Efficiency of heparin in the treatment of newborn infants with respiratory distress syndrome and disseminated intravascular coagulation. Eur J Pediatr 1980;133:47–49.

178. Michelson AD. Bleeding associated with cardiopulmonary bypass in children. Int J Pediatr Hematol Oncol 1994;1:147–158.

179. Ekert H, Gilchrist GS, Stanton R et al. Hemostasis in cyanotic congenital heart disease. J Pediatr 1970;76:221–230.

180. Gross S, Keefer V, Liebman J. The platelets in cyanotic congenital heart disease. Pediatrics 1968;42:651–655.

181. Komp DM, Sparrow AW. Polycythemia in cyanotic congenital heart disease–a study of altered coagulation. J Pediatr 1970;76:231–236.

182. Maurer HM, McCue CM, Caul J et al. Impairment in platelet aggregation in congenital heart disease. Blood 1972;40:207–211.

183. Ware JA, Reaves WH, Horak JK et al. Defective platelet aggregation in individuals undergoing surgical repair of cyanotic congenital heart disease. Ann Thorac Surg 1983;36:289–294.

184. Ekert H, Dowling SV. Platelet release abnormality and reduced prothrombin levels in children with cyanotic congenital heart disease. Aust Paediatr J 1977;13:17–21.

185. Gill JC, Wilson AD, Endres-Brooks J et al. Loss of the largest von Willebrand factor multimers from the plasma of individuals with congenital cardiac defects. Blood 1986;67:758–761.

186. Michelson AD. Pathomechanism of defective hemostasis during and after extracorporeal circulation: The role of platelets. In: Friedel N, Hetzer R, Royston D, eds. Blood use in cardiac surgery. Darmstadt: Steinkopff Verlag, 1991:16–26.

187. Saatvedt K, Lindberg H, Michelsen S et al. Activation of the fibrinolytic, coagulation and plasma kallikrein-kinin systems during and after open heart surgery in children. Scand J Clin Lab Invest 1995;55:359–367.

188. Marengo-Rowe AJ, Lambert CJ, Leveson JE et al. The evaluation of hemorrhage in cardiac individuals who have undergone extracorporeal circulation. Transfusion 1979;19:426–433.

189. Khuri SF, Wolfe JA, Josa M et al. Hematologic changes during and after cardiopulmonary bypass and their relationship to the bleeding time and nonsurgical blood loss. J Thorac Cardiovasc Surg 1992;104:94–107.

190. Valeri CR, Khabbaz K, Khuri SF et al. Effect of skin temperature on platelet function in individuals undergoing extracorporeal bypass. J Thorac Cardiovasc Surg 1992;104:108–116.

191. Michelson AD, MacGregor H, Barnard MR et al. Reversible inhibition of human platelet activation by hypothermia *in vivo* and *in vitro*. Thromb Haemost 1994;71:633–640.

192. Woodman RC, Harker LA. Bleeding complications associated with cardiopulmonary bypass [Review]. Blood 1990;76:1680–1697.

193. Milam JD, Austin SF, Nihill MR et al. Use of sufficient hemodilution to prevent coagulopathies following surgical correction of cyanotic heart disease. J Thorac Cardiovasc Surg 1985;89:623–629.

194. Bahnson HT, Ziegler RF. A consideration of the cause of death following operation for congenital heart disease of the cyanotic type. Surg Gynecol Obstet 1950;90:60–66.

195. Ekert H, Sheers M. Preoperative and postoperative platelet function in cyanotic heart disease. J Thorac Cardiovasc Surg 1974;67:184–190.

196. Maurer HM, McCue CM, Robertson JW et al. Correction of platelet dysfunction and bleeding in cyanotic congenital heart disease by simple red cell volume reduction. Am J Cardiol 1975;35:831–835.

197. Manno CS, Hedberg KW, Kim HC et al. Comparison of the hemostatic effects of fresh whole blood, stored whole blood, and components after open heart surgery in children. Blood 1991;77:930–936.

198. Guay J, Rivard GE. Mediastinal bleeding after cardiopulmonary bypass in pediatric individuals [Review]. Ann Thorac Surg 1996;62:1955–1960.

199. Kern FH, Morana NJ, Sears JJ et al. Coagulation defects in neonates during cardiopulmonary bypass. Ann Thorac Surg 1992;54:541–546.

200. Anonymous. Consensus conference: Platelet transfusion therapy. Office of Medical Applications of Research. National Institutes of Health. JAMA 1987;257:1777–1780.

201. Anonymous. Consensus conference: Fresh frozen plasma. Indications and risks. Office of Medical Applications of Research. National Institutes of Health. JAMA 1985;253:551–553.

202. Chan AK, Leaker M, Burrows FA et al. Coagulation and fibrinolytic profile of paediatric individuals undergoing cardiopulmonary bypass. Thromb Haemost 1997;77:270–277.

203. Royston D, Bidstrup BP, Taylor KM et al. Effect of aprotinin on need for blood transfusion after repeat open-heart surgery [Letter]. Lancet 1987;2:1289–1291.

204. Bidstrup BP, Royston D, Sapsford RN et al. Reduction in blood loss and blood use after cardiopulmonary bypass with high dose aprotinin (Trasylol). J Thorac Cardiovasc Surg 1989;97:364–372.

205. Penkoske PA, Entwistle LM, Marchak BE et al. Aprotinin in children undergoing repair of congenital heart defects. Ann Thorac Surg 1995;60(Suppl):S529–S532.

206. D'Errico CC, Shayevitz JR, Martindale SJ et al. The efficacy and cost of aprotinin in children undergoing reoperative open heart surgery. Anesth Analg 1996;83:1193–1199.

207. Boldt J, Knothe C, Zickmann B et al. Comparison of two aprotinin dosage regimens in pediatric individuals having cardiac operations. Influence on platelet function and blood loss. J Thorac Cardiovasc Surg 1993;105:705–711.

208. Davies MJ, Allen A, Kort H et al. Prospective, randomized, double-blind study of high-dose aprotinin in pediatric cardiac operations. Ann Thorac Surg 1997;63:497–503.

209. Boldt J, Knothe C, Zickmann B et al. Aprotinin in pediatric cardiac operations: platelet function, blood loss, and use of homologous blood. Ann Thorac Surg 1993;55:1460–1466.

210. Bohrer H, Bach A, Fleischer F et al. Adverse haemodynamic effects of high-dose aprotinin in a paediatric cardiac surgical individual. Anaesthesia 1990;45:853–854.

211. Salzman EW, Weinstein MJ, Weintraub RM et al. Treatment with desmopressin acetate to reduce blood loss after cardiac surgery. A double-blind randomized trial. N Engl J Med 1986;314:1402–1406.

212. Czer LS, Bateman TM, Gray RJ et al. Treatment of severe platelet dysfunction and hemorrhage after cardiopulmonary bypass: reduction in blood product usage with desmopressin. J Am Coll Cardiol 1987;9:1139–1147.

213. Rocha E, Llorens R, Paramo JA et al. Does desmopressin acetate reduce blood loss after surgery in individuals on cardiopulmonary bypass? Circulation 1988;77:1319–1323.

214. Hackmann T, Gascoyne RD, Naiman SC et al. A trial of desmopressin (1-desamino-8-D-arginine vasopressin) to reduce blood loss in uncomplicated cardiac surgery. N Engl J Med 1989;321:1437–1443.

215. Horaow JC, Van Riper DF, Strong MD et al. Hemostatic effects of tranexamic acid and desmopressin during cardiac surgery. Circulation 1991;84:2063–2070.

216. Reynolds LM, Nicolson SC, Jobes DR et al. Desmopressin does not decrease bleeding after cardiac operation in young children. J Thorac Cardiovasc Surg 1993;106:954–958.

217. Seear MD, Wadsworth LD, Rogers PC et al. The effect of desmopressin acetate (DDAVP) on postoperative blood loss after cardiac operations in children. J Thorac Cardiovasc Surg 1989;98:217–219.

218. Israels SJ, Kobrinsky NL. Serious reaction to desmopressin in a child with cyanotic heart disease. N Engl J Med 1989;320:1563–1564.

219. McClure PD, Izsak J. The use of epsilon-aminocaproic acid to reduce bleeding during cardiac bypass in children with congenital heart disease. Anesthesiology 1974;40:604–608.

220. Sell LL, Cullen ML, Whittlesey GC et al. Hemorrhagic complications during extracorporeal membrane oxygenation: prevention and treatment. J Pediatr Surg 1986;21:1087–1091.

221. Zwischenberger JB, Cox CS Jr. ECMO in the management of cardiac failure. ASAIO J 1992;38:751–753.

222. Urlesberger B, Zobel G, Zenz W et al. Activation of the clotting system during extracorporeal membrane oxygenation in term newborn infants. J Pediatr 1996;129:264–268.

223. Cilley RE, Zwischenberger JB, Andrews AF et al. Intracranial hemorrhage during extracorporeal membrane oxygenation in neonates. Pediatrics 1986;78:699–704.

224. Taylor GA, Fitz CR, Miller MK et al. Intracranial abnormalities in infants treated with extracorporeal membrane oxygenation: imaging with US and CT. Radiology 1987;165:675–678.

225. Bui KC, LaClair P, Vanderkerhove J et al. ECMO in premature infants. Review of factors associated with mortality. ASAIO Trans 1991;37:54–59.

226. Bulas DI, Taylor GA, Fitz CR et al. Posterior fossa intracranial hemorrhage in infants treated with extracorporeal membrane oxygenation: sonographic findings. AJR Am J Roentgenol 1991;156:571–575.

227. Van de Bor M, Walther FJ, Gangitano ES et al. Extracorporeal membrane oxygenation and cerebral blood flow velocity in newborn infants. Crit Care Med 1990;18:10–13.

228. Hansen T, Corbet A. Principles of respiratory monitoring and therapy. In: Taeusch HW, Ballard RA, Avery ME, eds. Diseases of the newborn. 6th ed. Philadelphia: WB Saunders, 1991:488–497.

229. Schmidt B, Zipursky A. Thrombotic disease in newborn infants [Review]. Clin Perinatol 1984;11:461–488.

230. Schmidt B, Andrew M. Neonatal thrombotic disease: prevention, diagnosis, and treatment [Review]. J Pediatr 1988;113:407–410.

231. Manco-Johnson MJ. Diagnosis and management of thromboses in the perinatal period [Review]. Semin Perinatol 1990;14:393–409.

232. Michelson AD, Bovill E, Andrew M. Antithrombotic therapy in children [Review]. Chest 1995;108:506S–522S.

233. Schmidt B, Andrew M. Report of scientific and standardization subcommittee on neonatal hemostasis. Diagnosis and treatment of neonatal thrombosis. Thromb Haemost 1992;67:381–382.

234. Colburn MD, Gelabert HA, Quinones-Baldrich W. Neonatal aortic thrombosis [Review]. Surgery 1992;111:21–28.

235. Seibert JJ, Taylor BJ, Williamson SL et al. Sonographic detection of neonatal umbilical-artery thrombosis: clinical correlation. AJR Am J Roentgenol 1987;148:965–968.

236. Vailas GN, Brouillette RT, Scott JP et al. Neonatal aortic thrombosis: recent experience. J Pediatr 1986;109:101–108.

237. Payne RM, Martin TC, Bower RJ et al. Management and follow-up of arterial thrombosis in the neonatal period. J Pediatr 1989;114:853–858.

238. Smith PK, Miller DA, Lail S et al. Urokinase treatment of neonatal aortoiliac thrombosis caused by umbilical artery catheterization: a case report [Review]. J Vasc Surg 1991;14:684–687.

239. O'Neill JA Jr, Neblett WW 3d, Born ML. Management of major thromboembolic complications of umbilical artery catheters. J Pediatr Surg 1981;16:972–978.

240. Goetzman BW, Stadalnik RC, Bogren HG et al. Thrombotic complications of umbilical artery catheters: A clinical and radiographic study. Pediatrics 1975;56:374–379.

241. Olinsky A, Aitken FG, Isdale JM. Thrombus formation after umbilical arterial catheterisation. An angiographic study. S Afr Med J 1975;49:1467–1470.

242. Wesstrom G, Finnstrom O, Stenport G. Umbilical artery catheterization in newborns. I. Thrombosis in relation to catheter type and position. Acta Paediatr Scand 1979;68:575–581.

243. Jackson JC, Truog WE, Watchko JF et al. Efficacy of thromboresistant umbilical artery catheters in reducing aortic thrombosis and related complications. J Pediatr 1987;110:102–105.

244. Bjarke B, Herin P, Blomback M. Neonatal aortic thrombosis. A possible clinical manifestation of congenital antithrombin 3 deficiency. Acta Paediatr Scand 1974;63:297–301.

245. Hustead VA, Wicklund BM. Treatment of neonatal aortic thrombosis with urokinase. Am J Pediatr Hematol Oncol 1990;12:336–339.

246. Kennedy LA, Drummond WH, Knight ME et al. Successful treatment of neonatal aortic thrombosis with tissue plasminogen activator. J Pediatr 1990;116:798–801.

247. Goldberg RE, Cohen AM, Bryan PJ et al. Neonatal aortic thrombosis treated with intra-arterial urokinase therapy. Can Assoc Radiol J 1989;40:55–56.

248. Martin JE Jr, Moran JF, Cook LS et al. Neonatal aortic thrombosis complicating umbilical artery catheterization: successful treatment with retroperitoneal aortic thrombectomy [Review]. Surgery 1989;105:793–796.

249. Caplan MS, Cohn RA, Langman CB et al. Favorable outcome of neonatal aortic thrombosis and renovascular hypertension. J Pediatr 1989;115:291–295.

250. Seibert JJ, Northington FJ, Miers JF et al. Aortic thrombosis after umbilical artery catheterization in neonates: prevalence of complications on long-term follow-up. AJR Am J Roentgenol 1991;156:567–569.

251. Anand SK, Aaberg RA, Koyle MA. Renal vascular thrombosis and renal cortical and medullary necrosis. In: Taeusch HW, Ballard RA, Avery ME, eds. Diseases of the newborn. 6th ed. Philadelphia: WB Saunders, 1991;898–904.

252. Bosque E, Weaver L. Continuous versus intermittent heparin infusion of umbilical artery catheters in the newborn infant. J Pediatr 1986;108:141–143.

253. Horgan MJ, Bartoletti A, Polansky S et al. Effect of heparin infusates in umbilihemostatic effects of fresh wholncy of thrombotic complications. J Pediatr 1987;111:774–778.

254. Rajani K, Goetzman BW, Wennberg RP et al. Effect of heparinization of fluids infused through an umbilical artery catheter on catheter patency and frequency of complications. Pediatrics 1979;63:552–556.

255. Caeton AJ, Goetzman BW. Risky business. Umbilical arterial catheterization [Editorial]. Am J Dis Child 1985;139:120–121.

256. Vogler C, Sotelo-Avila C, Lagunoff D et al. Aluminum-containing emboli in infants treated with extracorporeal membrane oxygenation. N Engl J Med 1988;319:75–79.

257. Fink SM, Bockman DE, Howell CG et al. Bypass circuits as the source of thromboemboli during extracorporeal membrane oxygenation. J Pediatr 1989;115:621–624.

258. Anonymous. Complications of neonatal extracorporeal membrane oxygenation. [Letter] J Pediatr 1990;116:1005–1007.

259. Adelman RD, Merten D, Vogel J et al. Nonsurgical management of renovascular hypertension in the neonate. Pediatrics 1978;62:71–76.

260. Molteni KH, George J, Messersmith R et al. Intrathrombic urokinase reverses neonatal renal artery thrombosis. Pediatr Nephrol 1993;7:413–415.

261. Arneil GC. Renal venous thrombosis. Contrib Nephrol 1979;15:21–29.

262. Mocan H, Beattie TJ, Murphy AV. Renal venous thrombosis in infancy: long-term follow-up. Pediatr Nephrol 1991;5:45–49.

263. Sanders LD, Jequier S. Ultrasound demonstration of prenatal renal vein thrombosis. Pediatr Radiol 1989;19:133–135.

264. Duncan ND, Adzick NS, Longaker MT et al. *In utero* arterial embolism from renal vein thrombosis with successful postnatal thrombolytic therapy. J Pediatr Surg 1991;26:741–743.

265. Katzman GH. Thrombosis and thromboembolism in an infant of a diabetic mother. J Perinatol 1989;9:137–140.

266. Clatworthy HW Jr, Dickens DR, McClave CR. Renal thrombosis complicating epidemic diarrhea in the newborn: Nephrectomy with recovery. N Engl J Med 1953;248:628–632.

267. Kaplan BS, Chesney RW, Drummond KN. The nephrotic syndrome and renal vein thrombosis. Am J Dis Child 1978;132:367–370.

268. Elliott GB, Grant-Tyrell J, Ringer G. Congenital lipoid nephrosis with left renal vein thrombosis and Chiari's syndrome. J Can Assoc Radiol 1979;30:175–176.

269. Tinaztepe K, Buyan N, Tinaztepe B et al. The association of nephrotic syndrome and renal vein thrombosis: a clinicopathological analysis of eight pediatric individuals. Turk J Pediatr 1989;31:1–18.

270. Nuss R, Hays T, Manco-Johnson M. Efficacy and safety of heparin anticoagulation for neonatal renal vein thrombosis. Am J Pediatr Hematol Oncol 1994;16:127–131.

271. Keating MA, Althausen AF. The clinical spectrum of renal vein thrombosis. J Urol 1985;133:938–945.

272. Sutton TJ, Leblanc A, Gauthier N et al. Radiological manifestations of neonatal renal vein thrombosis on follow-up examinations. Radiology 1977;122:435–438.

273. Stark H, Geiger R. Renal tubular dysfunction following vascular accidents of the kidneys in the newborn period. J Pediatr 1973;83:933–940.

274. Karrer FM. Portal hypertension. Semin Pediatr Surg 1992;1:134–144.

275. Rehan VK, Cronin CM, Bowman JM. Neonatal portal vein thrombosis successfully treated by regional streptokinase infusion. Eur J Pediatr 1994;153:456–459.

276. Radecki RT, Gaebler-Spira D. Deep vein thrombosis in the disabled pediatric population. Arch Phys Med Rehabil 1994;75:248–250.

277. Andrew M, David M, Adams M et al. Venous thromboembolic complications (VTE) in children: first analysis of the Canadian Registry of VTE. Blood 1994;83:1251–1257.

278. Rohrer MJ, Cutler BS, MacDougall E et al. A prospective study of the incidence of deep venous thrombosis in hospitalized children. J Vasc Surg 1996;24:46–49.

279. Uderzo C, Faccini P, Rovelli A et al. Pulmonary embolism in childhood leukemia: 8-years' experience in a pediatric hematology center. J Clin Oncol 1995;13:2805–2812.

280. Uderzo C, Marraro G, Riva A et al. Pulmonary thromboembolism in leukaemic children undergoing bone marrow transplantation. Bone Marrow Transplant 1993;11:201–203.

281. Riela AR, Roach ES. Etiology of stroke in children. J Child Neurol 1993;8:201–220.

282. Nicolaides P, Appleton RE. Stroke in children. Dev Med Child Neurol 1996;38:172–180.

283. Freedman JE, Loscalzo J, Benoit SE et al. Decreased platelet inhibition by nitric oxide in two brothers with a history of arterial thrombosis. J Clin Invest 1996;97:979–987.

284. Weinberg S, Prose NS. Color atlas of dermatology. 2nd ed. New York: McGraw-Hill, 1990.

285. Marlar RA, Neumann A. Neonatal purpura fulminans due to homozygous protein C or protein S deficiencies. Semin Thromb Hemost 1990;16:299–309.

286. Hathaway WE, Manco-Johnson M. Disorders of coagulation and platelets in the newborn. In: Hoffman R, Benz EJ, Shattil SJ et al eds. Hematology. Basic principles and practice. New York: Churchill Livingstone, 1409–1415.

287. Lynn NJ, Pauly TH, Desai NS. Purpura fulminans in three cases of early-onset neonatal group B streptococcal meningitis. J Perinatol 1991;11:144–146.

288. Seligsohn U, Berger A, Abend M et al. Homozygous protein C deficiency manifested by massive venous thrombosis in the newborn. N Engl J Med 1984;310:559–562.

289. Branson HE, Katz J, Marble R et al. Inherited protein C deficiency and coumarin-responsive chronic relapsing purpura fulminans in a newborn infant. Lancet 1983;2:1165–1168.

290. Marciniak E, Wilson HD, Marlar RA. Neonatal purpura fulminans: a genetic disorder related to the absence of protein C in blood. Blood 1985;65:15–20.

291. Sills RH, Marlar RA, Montgomery RR et al. Severe homozygous protein C deficiency. J Pediatr 1984;105:409–413.

292. Marlar RA, Montgomery RR, Broekmans AW. Diagnosis and treatment of homozygous protein C deficiency. Report of the Working Party on Homozygous Protein C Deficiency of the Subcommittee on Protein C and Protein S, International Committee on Thrombosis and Haemostasis. J Pediatr 1989;114:528–534.

293. Hartman KR, Manco-Johnson M, Rawlings JS et al. Homozygous protein C deficiency: early treatment with warfarin. Am J Pediatr Hematol Oncol 1989;11:395–401.

294. Mahasandana C, Suvatte V, Marlar RA et al. Neonatal purpura fulminans associated with homozygous protein S deficiency. Lancet 1990;335:61–62.

295. Mahasandana C, Suvatte V, Chuansumrit A et al. Homozygous protein S deficiency in an infant with purpura fulminans. J Pediatr 1990;117:750–753.

296. Pegelow CH, Ledford M, Young JN et al. Severe protein S deficiency in a newborn. Pediatrics 1992;89:674–676.

297. Brenner B, Zivelin A, Lanir N et al. Venous thromboembolism associated with double heterozygosity for R506Q mutation of factor V and for T298M mutation of protein C in a large family of a previously described homozygous protein C-deficient newborn with massive thrombosis. Blood 1996; 88:877–880.

298. Pipe SW, Schmaier AH, Nichols WC et al. Neonatal purpura fulminans in association with factor V R506Q mutation. J Pediatr 1996;128:706–709.

299. Schmidt B, Andrew M. Neonatal thrombosis: report of a prospective Canadian and international registry. Pediatrics 1995;96:939–943.

300. Neal WA, Reynolds JW, Jarvis CW et al. Umbilical artery catheterization: demonstration of arterial thrombosis by aortography. Pediatrics 1972;50: 6–13.

301. Mokrohisky ST, Levine RL, Blumhagen JD et al. Low positioning of umbilical-artery catheters increases associated complications in newborn infants. N Engl J Med 1978;299:561–564.

302. Saia OS, Rubaltelli FF, D'Elia RD et al. Clinical and aortographic assessment of the complications of arterial catheterization. Eur J Pediatr 1978; 128:169–179.

303. Chidi CC, King DR, Boles ET Jr. An ultrastructural study of the intimal injury induced by an indwelling umbilical artery catheter. J Pediatr Surg 1983;18:109–115.

304. Cilley RE. Arterial access in infants and children [Review]. Semin Pediatr Surg 1992;1:174–180.

305. Boros SJ, Thompson TR, Reynolds JW et al. Reduced thrombus formation with silicone elastomere (silastic) umbilical artery catheters. Pediatrics 1975;56:981–986.

306. Fletcher MA, Brown DR, Landers S et al. Umbilical arterial catheter use: report of an audit conducted by the Study Group for Complications of Perinatal Care. Am J Perinatol 1994;11:94–99.

307. Gilhooly JT, Lindenberg JA, Reynolds JW. Survey of umbilical artery catheter practices [Abstract]. Clin Res 1986;34:142A.

308. David RJ, Merten DF, Anderson JC et al. Prevention of umbilical artery catheter clots with heparinized infusates. Dev Pharmacol Ther 1981;2: 117–126.

309. Barzaghi A, Dell'Orto M, Rovelli A et al. Central venous catheter clots: incidence, clinical significance and catheter care in individuals with hematologic malignancies. Pediatr Hematol Oncol 1995;12:243–250.

310. Andrew M, Marzinotto V, Pencharz P et al. A cross-sectional study of catheter-related thrombosis in children receiving total parenteral nutrition at home. J Pediatr 1995;126:358–363.

311. Korones DN, Buzzard CJ, Asselin BL et al. Right atrial thrombi in children with cancer and indwelling catheters. J Pediatr 1996;128:841–846.

312. Krafte-Jacobs B, Sivit CJ, Mejia R et al. Catheter-related thrombosis in critically ill children: comparison of catheters with and without heparin bonding. J Pediatr 1995;126:50–54.

313. Clouse LH, Comp PC. The regulation of hemostasis: the protein C system [Review]. N Engl J Med 1986;314:1298–1304.

314. D'Angelo A, Lockhart MS, D'Angelo SV et al. Protein S is a cofactor for activated protein C neutralization of an inhibitor of plasminogen activation released from platelets. Blood 1987;69:231–237.

315. Marlar RA, Montgomery RR, Broekmans AW. Report on the diagnosis and treatment of homozygous protein C deficiency. Report of the Working Party on Homozygous Protein C Deficiency of the ICTH-Subcommittee on Protein C and Protein S. Thromb Haemost 1989;61:529–531.

316. Dreyfus M, Magny JF, Bridey F et al. Treatment of homozygous protein C deficiency and neonatal purpura fulminans with a purified protein C concentrate. N Engl J Med 1991;325:1565–1568.

317. Casella JF, Lewis JH, Bontempo FA et al. Successful treatment of homozygous protein C deficiency by hepatic transplantation. Lancet 1988;1: 435–438.

318. Pabinger I, Schneider B. Thrombotic risk in hereditary antithrombin III, protein C, or protein S deficiency–A cooperative retrospective study. Arterioscler Thromb Vasc Biol 1996;16:742–748.

319. Manco-Johnson MJ, Nuss R, Key N et al. Lupus anticoagulant and protein S deficiency in children with postvaricella purpura fulminans or thrombosis. J Pediatr 1996;128:319–323.

320. Levin M, Eley BS, Louis J et al. Postinfectious purpura fulminans caused by an autoantibody directed against protein S [Review]. J Pediatr 1995; 127:355–363.

321. Manco-Johnson MJ, Abshire TC, Jacobson LJ et al. Severe neonatal protein C deficiency: prevalence and thrombotic risk. J Pediatr 1991;119:793–798.

322. Minutillo C, Pemberton PJ, Willoughby ML et al. Neonatal purpura fulminans and transient protein C deficiency [Letter]. Arch Dis Child 1990;65: 561–562.

323. Zuber M, Toulon P, Marnet L et al. Factor V Leiden mutation in cerebral venous thrombosis. Stroke 1996;27:1721–1723.

324. Emmerich J, Alhenc-Gelas M, Aiach M et al. Resistance to activated protein C: role in venous and arterial thrombosis [Review]. Biomed Pharmacother 1996;50:254–260.

325. Nowak-Gottl U, Auberger K, Gobel U et al. Inherited defects of the protein C anticoagulant system in childhood thrombo-embolism [Review]. Eur J Pediatr 1996;155:921–927.

326. Mitchell L, Piovella F, Ofosu F et al. Alpha-2-macroglobulin may provide protection from thromboembolic events in antithrombin III-deficient children. Blood 1991;78:2299–2304.

327. Seguin J, Weatherstone K, Nankervis C. Inherited antithrombin III deficiency in the neonate. Arch Pediatr Adolesc Med 1994;148:389–393.

328. Andrew M, Massicotte-Nolan P, Mitchell L et al. Dysfunctional antithrombin III in sick premature infants. Pediatr Res 1985;19:237–239.

329. Manco-Johnson MJ. Neonatal antithrombin III deficiency [Review]. Am J Med 1989;87(Suppl):49S–52S.

330. Mudd SH, Skovby F, Levy HL et al. The natural history of homocystinuria due to cystathionine beta-synthase deficiency. Am J Hum Genet 1985;37: 1–31.

331. Andrew M, Brooker LA. Hemostatic complications in renal disorders of the young [Review]. Pediatr Nephrol 1996;10:88–99.

332. Von Scheven E, Athreya BH, Rose CD et al. Clinical characteristics of antiphospholipid antibody syndrome in children. J Pediatr 1996;129: 339–345.

333. Manco-Johnson MJ, Nuss R. Lupus anticoagulant in children with thrombosis. Am J Hematol 1995;48:240–243.

334. Finazzi G, Cortelazzo S, Viero P et al. Maternal lupus anticoagulant and fatal neonatal thrombosis [Letter]. Thromb Haemost 1987;57:238.

335. Sheridan-Pereira M, Porreco RP, Hays T et al. Neonatal aortic thrombosis associated with the lupus anticoagulant. Obstet Gynecol 1988;71: 1016–1018.

336. Moclair A, Bates I. The efficacy of heparin in maintaining peripheral infusions in neonates. Eur J Pediatr 1995;154:567–570.

337. Wright A, Hecker J, McDonald G. Effects of low-dose heparin on failure of intravenous infusions in children. Heart Lung 1997;24:79–82.

338. Shorten GD, Comunale ME. Heparin-induced thrombocytopenia [Review]. J Cardiothorac Vasc Anesth 1996;10:521–530.

339. Kibbe MR, Rhee RY. Heparin-induced thrombocytopenia: pathophysiology [Review]. Semin Vasc Surg 1996;9:284–291.

340. Dryjski M, Bentley DP. Heparin induced thrombocytopenia [Review]. Eur J Vasc Endovasc Surg 1996;11:260–269.

341. King DJ, Kelton JG. Heparin-associated thrombocytopenia. Ann Intern Med 1984;100:535–540.

342. Laster J, Silver D. Heparin-coated catheters and heparin-induced thrombocytopenia. J Vasc Surg 1988;7:667–672.

343. Spadone D, Clark F, James E et al. Heparin-induced thrombocytopenia in the newborn. J Vasc Surg 1992;15:306–311.

344. Murdoch IA, Beattie RM, Silver DM. Heparin-induced thrombocytopenia in children. Acta Paediatrica 1993;82:495–497.

345. Potter C, Gill JC, Scott JP et al. Heparin-induced thrombocytopenia in a child. J Pediatr 1992;121:135–138.

346. Gouault-Heilmann M, Huet Y, Adnot S et al. Low-molecular-weight heparin fractions as an alternative therapy in heparin-induced thrombocytopenia. Haemostasis 1987;17:134–140.

347. Chong BH, Magnani HN. Orgaran in heparin-induced thrombocytopenia. Haemostasis 1992;22:85–91.

348. Van Allen MI, Jackson JC, Knopp RH et al. *In utero* thrombosis and neonatal gangrene in an infant of a diabetic mother. Am J Med Genet 1989; 33:323–327.

349. Oppenheimer EH, Esterly JR. Thrombosis in the newborn: comparison between infants of diabetic and non-diabetic mothers. J Pediatr 1965;67: 549–556.

350. Stuart MJ, Sunderji SG, Allen JB. Decreased prostacyclin production in the infant of the diabetic mother. J Lab Clin Med 1981;98:412–416.

351. Ambrus CM, Ambrus JL, Courey N et al. Inhibitors of fibrinolysis in diabetic children, mothers, and their newborn. Am J Hematol 1979;7:245–254.

352. Gajl-Peczalska K. Plasma protein composition of hyaline membrane in the newborn as studied by immunofluorescence. Arch Dis Child 1964;39: 226–231.

353. Schmidt B, Shah J, Andrew M et al. Thrombin formation is increased in severe neonatal respiratory distress syndrome (RDS) [Abstract]. Pediatr Res 1990;27:224A.

354. Ambrus CM, Weintraub DH, Ambrus JL. Studies on hyaline membrane disease.3. Therapeutic trial of urokinase-activated human plasmin. Pediatrics 1966;38:231–243.

355. Ambrus CM, Choi TS, Cunnanan E et al. Prevention of hyaline membrane disease with plasminogen. A cooperative study. JAMA 1977;237: 1837–1841.

356. Markarian M, Lubchenco LO, Rosenblut E et al. Hypercoagulability in premature infants with special reference to the respiratory distress syndrome and hemorrhage. II. The effect of heparin. Biol Neonate 1971;17: 98–111.

357. Muntean W, Rosegger H. Antithrombin III concentrate in preterm infants with IRDS: An open, controlled randomized clinical trial [Abstract]. Thromb Haemost 1989;62:288.

358. Sutor AH. Thrombocytosis in childhood [Review]. Semin Thromb Hemost 1995;212:330–339.

359. Andrew M. Developmental hemostasis: relevance to hemostatic problems during childhood [Review]. Semin Thromb Hemost 1995;21:341–356.

360. Hirsh J. Heparin [Review]. N Engl J Med 1991;324:1565–1574.

361. Andrew M, Brooker L, Leaker M et al. Fibrin clot lysis by thrombolytic agents is impaired in newborns due to a low plasminogen concentration. Thromb Haemost 1992;68:325–330.

362. McDonald MM, Jacobson LJ, Hay WW Jr et al. Heparin clearance in the newborn. Pediatr Res 1981;15:1015–1018.
363. McDonald MM, Hathaway WE. Anticoagulant therapy by continuous heparinization in newborn and older infants. J Pediatr 1982;101:451–457.
364. Raschke RA, Reilly BM, Guidry JR et al. The weight-based heparin dosing nomogram compared with a "standard care" nomogram. A randomized controlled trial. Ann Intern Med 1993;119:874–881.
365. Massicotte P, Adams M, Marzinotto V et al. Low-molecular-weight heparin in pediatric individuals with thrombotic disease: a dose finding study. J Pediatr 1996;128:313–318.
366. Kelton JG, Hirsh J. Bleeding associated with antithrombotic therapy. Semin Hematol 1980;17:259–291.
367. Andrew M, Marzinotto V, Massicotte P et al. Heparin therapy in pediatric individuals: a prospective cohort study. Pediatr Res 1994;35:78–83.
368. Warkentin TE, Kelton JG. Heparin and platelets [Review]. Hematol Oncol Clin North Am 1990;4:243–264.
369. Hathaway W, Corrigan J. Report of Scientific and Standardization Subcommittee on Neonatal Hemostasis. Normal coagulation data for fetuses and newborn infants. Thromb Haemost 1991;65:323–325.
370. Andrew M, Marzinotto V, Brooker LA et al. Oral anticoagulation therapy in pediatric individuals: a prospective study. Thromb Haemost 1994;71:265–269.
371. Massicotte P, Marzinotto V, Vegh P et al. Home monitoring of warfarin therapy in children with a whole blood prothrombin time monitor. J Pediatr 1995;127:389–394.
372. Hirsh J. Oral anticoagulant drugs [Review]. N Engl J Med 1991;324:1865–1875.
373. Taybi H, Capitanio MA. Tracheobronchial calcification: an observation in three children after mitral valve replacement and warfarin sodium therapy. Radiology 1990;176:728–730.
374. Verstraete M, Collen D. Thrombolytic therapy in the eighties [Review]. Blood 1986;67:1529–1541.
375. Bovill EG, Becker R, Tracy RP. Monitoring thrombolytic therapy [Review]. Prog Cardiovasc Dis 1992;34:279–294.
376. Anonymous. Thrombolytic therapy in thrombosis: a National Institutes of Health consensus development conference. Ann Intern Med 1980;93:141–144.
377. Nazari J, Davison R, Kaplan K et al. Adverse reactions to thrombolytic agents. Implications for coronary reperfusion following myocardial infarction [Review]. Med Toxicol Adverse Drug Exp 1987;2:274–286.
378. Giacoia GP. High-dose urokinase therapy in newborn infants with major vessel thrombosis [Review]. Clin Pediatr (Phila) 1993;32:231–237.
379. Stein PD, Alpert JS, Copeland J et al. Antithrombotic therapy in individuals with mechanical and biological prosthetic heart valves [Review]. Chest 1995;108:371S–379S.

# CHAPTER 48

# HEMOSTATIC COMPLICATIONS OF HIV INFECTION

## James D. Levine and Jerome E. Groopman

The introduction of combination therapy including protease inhibitors for the treatment of HIV-1 infection has significantly improved morbidity and mortality. However, opportunistic infections and neoplasms continue to constitute the major source of complications, and these newer strategies have not yet been shown to impact significantly on the abnormalities of hemostasis that are commonly seen in individuals with HIV-1 infection.

The acquired abnormalities of hemostasis that occur in HIV-1-infected individuals are not unique to these individuals and are often seen in noninfected individuals. They do, however, add to the morbidity and complicate the management of individuals with HIV-1 disease.

The most common hemostatic abnormalities observed in individuals with HIV-1 infection are thrombocytopenia and acquired circulating anticoagulants such as anticardiolipin antibodies (ACA), lupus-like inhibitors, or lupus anticoagulants (LA). Other, less common abnormalities include thrombotic thrombocytopenic purpura (TTP) and the hemolytic-uremic syndrome (HUS).

## THROMBOCYTOPENIA

Thrombocytopenia was one of the first manifestations of the HIV-1 infection to be described. In 1982, 1983, and 1985 a series of now classic papers describing the association of thrombocytopenia with what we now know as acquired immunodeficiency syndrome (AIDS) or HIV-1 infection were published by Morris et al (1), Rattnoff, et al (2), and Savona, et al (3). These descriptions of thrombocytopenia were in homosexual males, classic hemophiliacs, and intravenous drug addicts, respectively.

The pathophysiology of classic thrombocytopenia results from either decreased platelet production or increased platelet destruction (shortened platelet half-life). Evidence for both mechanisms of thrombocytopenia exists in individuals infected with HIV-1.

## THROMBOCYTOPENIA SECONDARY TO DECREASED PRODUCTION

Infection with HIV-1 often is associated with significant defects in hematopoiesis (4–6). The resulting cytopenias include leukopenia, anemia, and thrombocytopenia. The precise mechanism of this bone marrow suppression has yet to be explained. There are however, much experimental data that give insight into possible mechanisms.

HIV-1 is able to infect normal cells by first binding to the CD4 receptor on the surface of the cell (7). In theory, therefore, any cell that expresses the CD4 receptor on its surface membrane is capable of becoming infected. T lymphocytes, monocytes, and macrophages are the most commonly infected cells and may act as a reservoir for the virus, transmitting it to other cell types. Bone marrow stromal cells (8), bone marrow progenitor cells (9), and myeloid progenitor cells (10) have been reported to be capable of being infected with HIV-1 by undefined mechanisms. This infection is speculated to be associated with bone marrow suppression and the resulting cytopenias, either by a direct effect of the virus or indirectly through perturbation of the bone marrow microenvironment.

There is evidence that HIV-1 can infect bone marrow megakaryocytes and may, thereby, adversely affect thrombopoiesis. The CD4 structure has been found on the surface of megakaryocytes (11). In addition, using *in situ* hybridization techniques, Zucker-Franklin and Cao (12) have found HIV sequences in bone marrow megakaryocytes from individuals infected with the virus. In other studies, this same laboratory has demonstrated the transfer of virus from HIV-1-infected H9 T cells to normal human megakaryocytes in culture. Viral particles were visualized within both megakaryocytes and platelets using electron microscopic techniques (Fig. 48.1) (13).

More recently, infection of megakaryocytes with two separate strains of HIV-1 has been demonstrated using the CMK cell line derived from a individual with megakaryoblastic leukemia (14). In addition, others have shown that some strains of the virus may be cytopathic without either viral replication or CD4 binding (15). In a comparison of HIV-1 infected thrombocytopenic individuals and noninfected individuals with immune thrombocytopenic purpura (ITP) or normals, Zauli et al (16) have shown that there was significantly increased apoptosis in the GP IIb/IIIa positive megakaryocytic bone marrow cells of HIV-1 infected individuals. This may explain in part the decrease in platelet production in these individuals. Further indirect data suggesting that the thrombocytopenia of HIV-1 infection is at least par-

tially caused by suppression of megakaryocytes can be demonstrated by measuring mean platelet volume-platelet number relationships (17). In a retrospective study of individuals infected with HIV, 92% of thrombocytopenic individuals had an inappropriately low mean platelet volume for their platelet count (17), a finding others have reported to correlate with bone marrow suppression. Thus, a direct suppressive effect on the megakaryocyte by the virus or a reaction to infection may be a more likely explanation than direct viral infection.

Other investigators have addressed the issue of HIV-1 infection of blood progenitor cells. In experiments using the polymerase chain reaction (PCR) to assay for HIV-DNA in single myeloid and erythroid (but not megakaryocyte) colonies, none could be found in colonies derived from the bone marrows of HIV-1-infected individuals (18). In addition, these researchers could not demonstrate HIV-DNA in the normal bone marrow progenitors exposed to high inocula of various strains of HIV *in vitro*. von Laer et al (19) have made similar observations using PER on populations of cells separated by fluorescence-activated cell sorting (FACS). These investigators found only one of 14 individuals with HIV-1 infection to be positive for retroviral DNA in CD34' progenitor cells. In other experiments performed to compare the early progenitor cells from the marrows of HIV-1 infected individuals with normals, Marandin et al (20) found that the pool of more primitive progenitor fractions (CD34 + /CD38− and CD34+ /Thy-1+) were significantly decreased when compared to uninfected controls. In addition, in a long-term culture initiating cell assay (LTC-IC) to assess production of more committed clonogenic progenitors (BFU-E, CFU-GK) the output from HIV-1 infected individuals' bone marrow was four to twelve times lower than controls. These same investigators then failed to demonstrate evidence of viral infection of these progenitor cells by PCR using both *gag* and *env* primers. Thus early progenitors may not be infected with the virus although they may be decreased in number, and this decrease, along with possible infection of more mature progenitors, probably accounts for decreases in platelet production.

Infection of stem cells or inhibition of early precursors may not be the only reason for cytopenias in HIV-1-infected individuals. Other possible causes of marrow suppression by the virus include defective modulation of progenitor cells by T-helper and suppressor cells or an imbalance of hemopoietic growth or suppressor factors. When T cells were depleted from the bone marrow of infected individuals prior to culture, an increase in growth of all lineages, including colony-forming unit megakaryocyte (CFU-Meg), was observed compared with colony growth before T cell depletion (21).

There may be additional circulating factors that contribute to the impaired production of blood cells. For

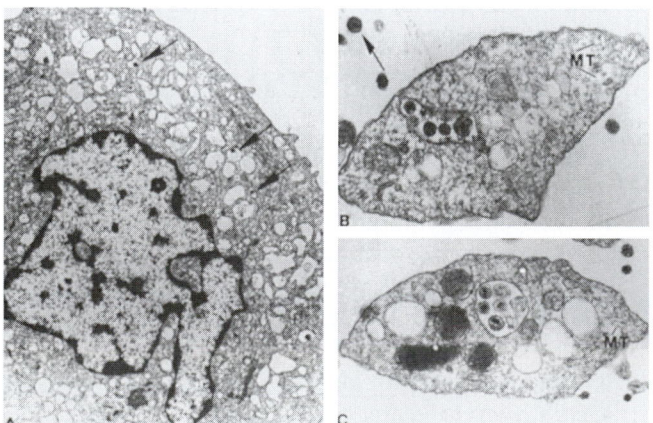

**FIGURE 48.1.** Electron micrographs of megakaryocytes and platelets after incubation with HIV-1-infected H9 monocytes. From Zucker-Franklin et al [13]. **A**, Human megakaryocyte showing HIV (arrows) within the channels of the demarcation membrane system. **B**, HIV particles (arrow) in extracellular medium and within platelet canalicular system. © Platelet with HIV within vacuole: G, α-granule; MT, microtubules.

instance, serum from AIDS individuals has been demonstrated to inhibit myeloid and erythroid progenitor growth in bone marrow from HIV-1-infected individuals (22). Antibodies in the IgG fraction appeared to be the active serum component, possibly antibody against the GP 120 antigen of the virus (a component of the viral envelope). Possible mediators of this impaired production are cytokines such as transforming growth factor or others, as proposed by Zauli et al (23, 24).

The issues regarding mechanisms of bone marrow inhibition are not clear; however, there appear to be multiple factors involved, and decreased platelet production probably results from a combination of infection of more committed progenitors, megakaryocytes, stroma, and from the effects of abnormal cytokine production and other plasma factors that affect hematopoiesis. In addition to direct and indirect effects of HIV-1, many of the drugs used in the care of infected individuals are known to be associated with bone marrow suppression. For example, one of the most common toxicities of zidovudine (AZT) is impaired hemopoiesis (25). This toxicity usually results in leukopenia and anemia more often than thrombocytopenia, and can be a confusing issue as zidovudine is often used to treat immune thrombocytopenia (ITP) in HIV-1 infection, as discussed below. In addition, drugs such as ganciclovir, trimethoprim-sulfa, pyrimethamine, interferon, and various chemotherapeutic agents are commonly used drugs in HIV-1-infected individuals that are also potential marrow suppressants.

Other causes of bone marrow suppression in these individuals include other coinfecting viruses, opportunistic infection that results in a marrow infiltrative process, such as tuberculosis, *Mycobacterium avium intracellulare* infection, or the involvement of marrow with tumor, usually non-Hodgkin's lymphoma. These factors are often difficult to sort out from each other, and require careful evaluation with appropriate microbiologic cultures and stains. Multifactorial mechanisms are frequently operative in HIV-infected individuals.

## THROMBOCYTOPENIA DUE TO INCREASED PERIPHERAL DESTRUCTION

Thrombocytopenia was one of the first manifestations of HIV-1 infection to be reported (1–3). These original reports described thrombocytopenia due to increased peripheral destruction. The thrombocytopenia was felt to be immune-mediated in each of these reports, i.e., there were adequate bone marrow megakaryocytes and no splenomegaly or evidence for other immune disorders such as systemic lupus erythematosus. What was unusual, however, was that the individuals were males and classic immune thrombocytopenia in adults is more commonly a disease of females (see Chapter 30).

Early in the descriptions of this disorder many individuals in the risk group for AIDS had thrombocytopenia alone without a concomitant AIDS-defining illness (26). In a multi-center study of homosexual and bisexual men with no AIDS-defining illnesses, thrombocytopenia was four times more likely to occur in seropositive than in seronegative men (27). The major correlating factor found among the seropositive men was the absolute CD4 (or T4) lymphocyte count. Thrombocytopenia was more likely in the cohort of individuals with CD4-lymphocyte counts of less than $250/\mu L$ (10.8%) than in the cohort with more than $750/\mu L$ CD4-lymphocytes (2.8%). These data are similar to those found in an Italian study of 657 HIV-1-positive individuals (28). These investigators noted that thrombocytopenia was the most frequently reported hematologic abnormality, occurring in 72 of 657 individuals (approx. 11%). They also noted that among the 72 individuals with thrombocytopenia, 58 (81%) exhibited thrombocytopenia alone while in 14 of 72 (19%) thrombocytopenia occurred in association with other cytopenias such as anemia or leukopenia. Neither this study nor any other (29–31) has demonstrated an increased rate of progression to AIDS in HIV-1-positive individuals with thrombocytopenia.

As discussed in Chapters 29 and 30, classic immune thrombocytopenia is thought to be mediated by two basic processes. Immune destruction results from the removal of platelets from the circulation by the reticuloendothelial system because they have antibody binding to a specific platelet antigen or, as in the case of some drug-induced immune thrombocytopenias, a platelet-hapten complex, or because antibody-antigen complexes are associated nonspecifically with the platelet surface. Classic autoimmune thrombocytopenia (Chapter 30) is an example of the first mechanism, and sera from these individuals contain platelet membrane-binding antibody to platelet antigens. Immune thrombocytopenia secondary to some drugs (Chapter 29) occurs because of hapten-antigen induced antibody. Most other forms of immune thrombocytopenia result from the binding of antibody-antigen complex to the platelet membrane, which results in the removal of these coated cells from the circulation at a rapid rate. Evidence for both autoimmune and antibody-antigen complex mechanisms has been reported in the immune thrombocytopenia of HIV-1 infection.

All of the risk groups for HIV-1 infection with thrombocytopenia studied to date have, depending on methods used, demonstrated increased levels of platelet-associated antibody, which is usually immunoglobulin G (IgG) and circulating immune complexes. In general, intravenous drug addicts had the highest detected levels of circulating complexes (32), although there was no association between titer and level of thrombocytopenia (33). This observation may reflect the likelihood of heavy intravenous antigen stimulation.

In one study comparing 33 homosexual men with thrombocytopenia who were assumed to be HIV-1 positive with eight men and 15 women with non-HIV-1 associated thrombocytopenia, a 3.8-fold higher level of platelet-associated IgG and a 4.2-fold higher level of platelet-associated complement was seen in the individuals presumed to be HIV-1 positive (33).

Stricker et al (34) have reported a specific antibody to a 25 Kda platelet antigen in the serum of homosexual individuals with thrombocytopenia. This finding has since been retracted (35) and the 25 Kda band has also been seen in the serum of individuals without AIDS or AIDS-related conditions. In addition, other investigators have failed to identify antibodies against the above mentioned 25 Kda platelet antigen in HIV-1-positive individuals with thrombocytopenia (36–38).

Others have found anti-HIV-1 antibody complex in the polyethylene glycol-precipitable immune complexes and platelet eluates from individuals with HIV-associated thrombocytopenia (39). These complexes bound to normal platelets, although the anti-HIV-1 alone did not. These same investigators have also discovered circulating anti-HIV-1 GP 120 antiidiotype-like complexes that were capable of binding to platelets (40). Others have shown that the platelet count correlated inversely with the amount of antiplatelet antibody present.

Several groups of investigators have found crossreactivity between antibody to HIV-1 and anti-platelet antibodies. Gonzalez-Conejero (41) and others have found autoantibodies against platelet membrane glycoproteins GP Ib/IX and GP IIb-IIIa in HIV-1 positive intravenous drug users. In this group of individuals with thrombocytopenia 50% of the anti-HIV-1 antibodies also bound to normal platelets. Bettaieb (42) and associates demonstrated that the IgG with anti-GP IIb/IIIa activity from HIV-1 infected thrombocytopenic individuals also crossreacted with HIV-gp120. Further work by these investigators showed that there was crossreactive antibody between HIV-1 gp120 and platelet GP IIIa in many of these individuals, though the specific epitope could not be identified. These studies support the hypothesis that the crossreactive antibody recognizes the conformational structure of HIV-1 gp120. Thus, perhaps the development of antibody to the virus leads to immune complex formation which, in turn, binds nonspecifically to the platelet membranes, resulting in platelet destruction and thrombocytopenia in individuals who, for other reasons related to viral infection, cannot increase platelet production to compensate for the now-shortened platelet half-life.

The site of peripheral destruction has been investigated by Dominguez et al (43) who found, in studies using [111]In-labeled platelets, that platelet uptake was most prominent in the spleen, followed by liver and rarely the bone marrow. These authors suggest that the most influential factors governing sequestration were the presence of antiplatelet antibodies in the case of splenic uptake and the presence of circulating immune complexes in the case of liver and marrow uptake.

The exact pathophysiology of HIV-1-related thrombocytopenia requires further definition, although it is likely that thrombocytopenia in HIV-1-infected individuals is multifactorial and involves both immune-mediated destruction by various mechanisms as well as alterations in bone marrow production of platelets.

## THROMBOTIC THROMBOCYTOPENIC PURPURA

TTP and HUS are discussed in greater detail in Chapter 27. They are both uncommon and poorly understood disorders characterized by the pentad of waxing and waning neurologic symptoms, renal insufficiency, thrombocytopenia, microangiopathic hemolytic anemia, and fever (in the former) and the triad of thrombocytopenia, acute renal failure, and microangiopathic hemolytic anemia (in the latter). Diagnosis of both disorders is based on clinical information and no single confirmatory test is available. Both have been associated with bacterial and viral infections. In addition, they are described in individuals with neoplastic disorders, with certain forms of chemotherapy, and in a small number of AIDS or HIV-1 infected individuals (44–47). The incidence appears to be increased in individuals with HIV-1 infection and AIDS, although the contribution of concurrent bacterial and fungal infections or neoplastic disease is as yet unclear. The mortality from TTP in individuals with HIV-1 infection may be as high as 33% (48, 49), which is higher than seen in the non-infected population (50). It is not clear yet if earlier diagnosis and treatment of TTP in HIV-1 infected individuals will bring this number closer to the non-infected mortality rate.

The etiologic agent in TTP and HUS is unclear, as is the pathophysiology; however, biotoxins such as verocytotoxin produced by certain strains of *Escherichia coli* 0157: H7 have been isolated in a individual stricken with HUS who had AIDS (51) and another individual is reported to have developed TTP during the course of rectosigmoiditis secondary to *Shigella flexneri* (52). In light of the increased infection rate in HIV individuals these agents may be found in more significant numbers if looked for. It is possible that the HIV-1 virus is alone responsible for causing TTP. Del Arco et al (53) reported finding HIV-1 p24 antigen in the endothelial cells of a woman infected with the virus who developed TTP, raising the possibility that the virus itself has a more direct role. This is of interest because it has been postulated that at least in some cases endothelial cell infection by viruses has an etiologic role in the development of TTP.

There have been no studies to define the best therapy in HIV-1 infected individuals with TTP/HUS, but from the above literature it would appear that standard therapy (see Chapter 27), including plasma exchange, is the mainstay, as is the case in classic TTP/HUS. Other modalities, such as corticosteroids, cytotoxic agents, and antiplatelet agents have also been used in these individuals, although recent reports (54, 55) would suggest that they are not of significant utility, and plasma exchange remains the treatment of choice. As in the case of ITP, Zidovudine (AZT) has also been used successfully to achieve a sustained remission in one individual with relapsing TTP while receiving standard therapy (56).

# TREATMENT OF HIV-1-ASSOCIATED THROMBOCYTOPENIA

The treatment of HIV-1-associated thrombocytopenia, and immune thrombocytopenia in particular, is not significantly different from treatment in noninfected individuals. There are, however, circumstances due to the viral infection that must be taken into account when deciding on a course of action in a particular individual.

A bone marrow examination can help determine whether the thrombocytopenia is secondary to decreased production, an infiltrative process, or decreased

platelet survival. If drug toxicity is suspected, the offending drug should be discontinued, if possible. This is not always necessary for individuals with mild thrombocytopenia and no bleeding history, and in the case of a drug used to treat life-threatening illness. Drugs commonly implicated are the penicillins, trimethoprim-sulfamethoxazole, pentamidine, and gancyclovir.

Treatment modalities commonly used in HIV-1 associated thrombocytopenia include corticosteroids, splenectomy, danazol, intravenous immunoglobulin, intravenous anti-D antibody (anti-Rh-D, rhogam), AZT, vincristine, *Staphylococcus aureus* protein-A column, dapsone, interferons, and expectant follow-up (Table 48.1). Most physicians involved in the treatment of HIV-1-infected individuals individualize treatment according to individual circumstances; however, certain general policies can be recommended.

The effectiveness of glucocorticoids in classic ITP (see Chapter 30) is well documented, with response rates in the range of 60–80%. The durability of these responses in adults, however, is disappointing, and many adults require further therapy upon failing steroids or because of toxicity. Similar response rates are seen in individuals with HIV-1-associated thrombocytopenia, although in some reported studies the response rate was less than would have been expected in classic ITP (57). Short

**TABLE 48.1.** Commonly Used Regimens in the Treatment of HIV-associated Thrombocytopenia

| Treatment | Dose or Regimen | Response Rate (%) | Comments |
|---|---|---|---|
| Zidovudine | 500–1200 mg/day in divided doses | 30–50 | Optimal agent for individual with CD4 < 500 cells/μL |
| Intravenous Ig | 400 mg/kg to 3 g/kg for 1–4 days | 80–90 | Response usually rapid, although short-lived |
| Splenectomy | | 60–80 | For individuals with good performance status and higher CD4 level |
| Danazol | 200–1200 mg/day in divided doses | 40–60, depending on concurrent steroid usage | May be used with steroids to decrease steroid dose; hepatic toxicity |
| Interferon-α | 3 million U subcutaneously | 70–80 | Response may be as early as 3 weeks; may be delayed; appears effective in thrombocytopenic individuals who fail zidovudine |
| Dapsone | 50–125 mg/day | Insufficient data | Also effective for PCP prophylaxis |
| Vincristine | 2 mg/w intravenously | 50 | Neurologic toxicity |
| Intravenous anti-Rh Ig | 20–75 μg × 1–6 days intravenously | 70–90 | Mild RBC hemolysis is common; response may be delayed a few weeks; use reduced dose if individual already anemic |
| Prednisone | 1–2 mg/kg/day; taper after maximum response | ≤80% | Relapse common after discontinuation; immunosuppressive |

PCP, *Pneumocystic carinii pneumonia*; RBC, *red blood cell.*

courses of steroids may be given without significant detriment. However, since short courses rarely, if ever, result in long-term remission, steroids are not usually the initial therapy in HIV-infected individuals, particularly because of concern about further immunologic suppression. Although there are no randomized studies demonstrating a negative clinical effect (58), some evidence exists implicating long-term corticosteroid use in increasing oral candidiasis and mucocutaneous herpes infection (59). In addition, individuals with concomitant Kaposi's sarcoma and thrombocytopenia have been reported to have progression of the Kaposi's sarcoma (60) if treated with steroids.

Splenectomy is the usual step taken in classical ITP individuals who have failed or are intolerant to steroids. This modality is also effective in individuals with HIV-associated ITP. Response rates of 60–100% and durable responses of between 40% and 82% have been reported, depending on the individual population in question (61–64). In 15 HIV-1-infected individuals treated with splenectomy, 14 responded initially with platelet counts of greater than 150,000/μL (48). Over a mean follow-up period of 12.4 months, nine of these individuals (60%) had a durable remission and, with the addition of adjunctive therapy, an additional two individuals achieved a durable remissions for a total of 11 (73%) individuals. In another group of individuals, only 1 of 8 had a complete response and 5 had a partial response (62). The average preoperative and postoperative platelet counts in a group of 11 individuals undergoing splenectomy for HIV-1-related thrombocytopenia were 19,700/μL and 498,000/μL , respectively (63). All had normal platelet counts at follow-up of an average of 12.4 months (range 1–37 months). More recently, 30 HIV-infected individuals with thrombocytopenia were followed prospectively for a mean period of 42 months following splenectomy: 21 individuals had a persistent complete response, six had a partial response and remained asymptomatic, and only three showed no response. There were no perioperative deaths and morbidity was minimal (65). In a group of 11 severe hemophiliacs with HIV-related thrombocytopenia who underwent splenectomy there was a sustained remission rate (platelet count > 100,000/μL) in 82% over a mean follow-up time of 54 months (64).

There is concern by some that splenectomy might result in progression of HIV disease or a decrease in survival (66). None of the above-cited studies reported a detrimental effect of splenectomy with regard to AIDS progression, and others have also reported on the safety of the procedure with respect to both progression of AIDS (67) and susceptibility to infection with encapsulated organisms (62). Interestingly, there is at least one case report (68) of an increase in the CD4 lymphocyte counts in adult HIV infected individuals after splenectomy for HIV-1 associated thrombocytopenia. The one caveat with regard to splenectomy is that it does not appear to be of benefit to individuals infected with *Mycobacterium avium-intracellulare* or active cytomegalovirus infection (69), and the authors of the reported failures considered these infections to be a contraindication to splenectomy. In addition to the expected increase in platelet count after splenectomy in HIV-associated thrombocytopenia, Ravikumar et al reported long-term remission from both thrombocytopenia and pancytopenia in 14 of 15 individuals who underwent splenectomy (70).

One of the most rapidly effective treatments of immune thrombocytopenias is intravenous immunoglobulin (see Chapter 30). This therapy has been used to raise the platelet count before invasive procedures such as splenectomy, or to correct bleeding problems in individuals with HIV-1-associated thrombocytopenia. High doses of between 1.0 and 3.0 g/kg given over the course of 1–4 days are reported to be effective in raising the platelet count from ranges of less than 20,000/μL to greater than 150,000/μL. Pollak et al reported a successful response in three individuals. Their review of the literature as of 1988 revealed a response rate of about 88% (71) among a total of 60 reported individuals. Reports from a larger group from a single institution revealed a response rate of 86%, with 19 of 22 individuals achieving a platelet count of greater than 50,000/μL and 77% obtaining a platelet count of greater than 100,000/μL (72). These individuals received a total dose of intravenous immunoglobulin of 2.0 g/kg over a period of 2–5 days followed by maintenance infusions of 0.5–1.0 g/kg as a single dose if the platelet count fell below 20,000–30,000/μL. These investigators found that the majority of individuals (19 of 22) could be maintained with a platelet count of greater than 50,000/μL with single infusions not more often than every 2 weeks. Jahnke et al (73) found similar results in a placebo controlled crossover study of 12 individuals, although they note that no individual responded to placebo and the incremental platelet count improvement ranged from 15,000/μL to 358,000/μL (mean 180,000/μL). Essentially no toxicity was noted, and no individual developed an opportunistic infection. Unfortunately, as has been seen in classic ITP treated with intravenous immunoglobulin, very few individuals demonstrated complete remissions that allowed discontinuation of the therapy.

A more specific immunoglobulin, anti-Rh immunoglobulin (anti-D), has also been used in the treatment of classic ITP and has demonstrated efficacy in HIV-1-associated thrombocytopenia (74). A few caveats can be gleaned from the literature: (i) the preparation does not appear to be effective in individuals who are Rh-negative or who have had a splenectomy; (ii) it causes some mild hemolysis but not to the degree that might be expected; (iii) both the intramuscular and intravenous preparations appear to be effective, although recent studies reported are of the intravenous preparation (Win Rho lca); (iv) the rise in platelet count usually occurs within a few days of administration but can be delayed by as long as 3 weeks; (v) higher doses appear to be more effective than low doses (reported dose ranges from 10 to 60 mg/kg); and (vi) as with intravenous immunoglobulin, some individuals treated with anti-D demonstrate a prolonged response or can be maintained in remission if repeated doses were administered (74, 75). The best results have been seen in individuals who are Rh-positive, unless Rh-negative individuals were first given plasma containing anti-c antibodies (76), and in individuals who have not undergone splenectomy (75). Response rates as high as 90% have been reported using doses between 20 to 75 μg/kg. In individuals with a low hemoglobin it is recommended that a reduced dose of 25 to 40 μg/kg be used to minimize the risk of worsening the anemia. The mechanism of action of all immunoglobulin preparations has been thought to be Fc-receptor blockade; however, investigations using anti-D have suggested that this is not the only mechanism, and that possibly an antiidiotype antibody may be active.

Mintzer et al (77) reported the results of 23 individuals treated with vincristine for AIDS-associated Kaposi's sarcoma. They noted that all three individuals with concurrent thrombocytopenia responded with a significant increase in platelet count. The efficacy of vincristine in classic ITP is well documented (Chapter 30). The disadvantage of using this regimen in HIV-1-infected individuals is the potential for further immunosuppression or induction of peripheral neuropathy, a well described complication of vincristine. However, this regimen is reasonable in individuals requiring concurrent therapy for Kaposi's sarcoma.

One observation during the initial trials of zidovudine (AZT) was that individuals with HIV-1-associated thrombocytopenia responded with increased platelet counts (78–80). Since these initial observations, a non-randomized study of AZT in thrombocytopenic HIV-1-infected individuals who had not previously been treated with an antiretroviral agent has been published. Patients were given AZT at either 1.0 or 1.5 g/day, and response rates of 30% and 50% were seen in the low-dose group and high-dose group, respectively (81). In another uncontrolled report, 3 of 3 individuals receiving 1.2 g of AZT per day had a significant rise in platelet counts with a subsequent fall when AZT was discontinued (82). A Swiss group performed a randomized study (83) and reported a response rate of about 50%. In addition, they reported that in some individuals the increase in platelet count was sustained despite discontinuation of AZT. It is clear that zidovudine is an effective agent in the treatment of HIV-1-associated thrombocytopenia. The studies reported have used higher doses of zido-

vudine than are now recommended (1,000–1,200 mg vs. 500–600 mg), and it remains to be seen whether these lower doses will have the same platelet raising effect. One study reported in abstract form (84) suggests that doses of 600 mg/day are effective, although others indicate that a dose response exists (78). A more recently reported open, randomized multicenter study of 84 individuals with severe HIV-related thrombocytopenia indicated that a higher dose (1000 mg/day) of AZT was more effective and more rapid in raising the platelet count than a lower dose (500 mg/day) (85). There are, however, no known predictive factors for a response, and some individuals become more pancytopenic on the drug (86), especially when AZT is used at higher doses. Understanding the mechanism of action of AZT in this situation may lead to a more complete elucidation of the role of viral infection in this complex disorder. There is some experimental evidence that AZT's effect is to enhance platelet production or release without affecting platelet survival, perhaps by decreasing the suppressive effects of the viral infection (87) on megakaryocytes. The clear benefit of AZT is that it treats both the thrombocytopenia and the retroviral infection.

Durand et al (88) reported the successful use of dapsone in a small group of previously treated thrombocytopenic HIV infected individuals (88) without AIDS-defining illness. Of 11 individuals treated, six improved to a persistent platelet count above 50,000/μL. Thrombocytopenia recurred upon cessation of the drug, but a second remission could be induced by reinstitution of the therapy. The regimen was well tolerated and has been used as prophylaxis for *Pneumocystis carinii* pneumonia in certain individuals. The authors speculate that the mechanism of action may be by an effect on phagocyte-mediated cytotoxicity.

Danazol has been effective for the treatment of classic ITP, and is also effective in individuals with HIV-1-related thrombocytopenia, although only 2 of 18 individuals responded in Oksenhendler's study group (57). In addition, the associated drug toxicity, especially hepatic, makes it less than optimal therapy in many of these individuals.

Ellis et al (89) reported that administration of recombinant α-2a interferon has been used successfully in HIV-1-infected individuals with thrombocytopenia. The interferon was administered for several months, although others have demonstrated that a shorter course might be as effective (90). In 13 severe immune thrombocytopenic individuals, none of whom had HIV-1 infection (90), 3 million units of α-2a interferon for 12 doses resulted in improved platelet counts in 11 individuals following the course of therapy. One individual developed improved platelet counts during therapy. In the majority of individuals this short course of interferon is well tolerated. In a prospective placebo controlled trial

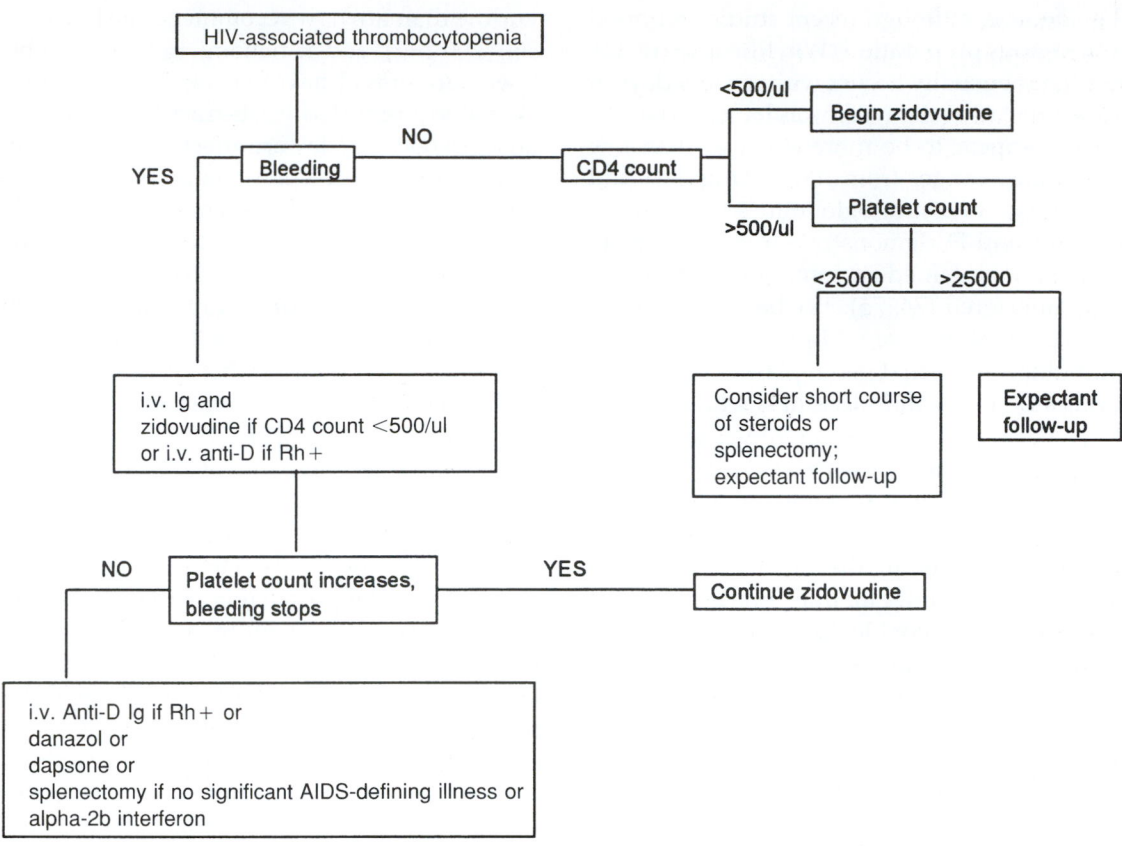

**FIGURE 48.2.** Treatment considerations in HIV-associated thrombocytopenia. i.v.lg, intravenous immunoglobulin.

of three million units of interferon-α in individuals with HIV-1 associated thrombocytopenia who were refractory to zidovudine, Marroni et al (91) found a significant increase in platelet counts by four weeks of therapy. Simi-lar results were reported in another trial using the same 3 million unit dose of interferon-α, given to HIV-1 infected individuals who had failed other ITP therapies, over 16 weeks (92). This form of biologic response modifier therapy is attractive for HIV-1-infected individuals with thrombocytopenia because α-2a interferon has been shown to be effective in decreasing viral replication and is also of benefit in treating AIDS individuals with Kaposi's sarcoma. Soubrane et al (93) recently reported successful treatment of a individual with refractory HIV-related ITP with anti-CD16 (anti-low affinity Fc-γ receptor) monoclonal antibody; this response was associated with simulation of natural killer (NK) function and elevation of CD4 lymphocytes.

The use of *Staphylococcus aureus* protein-A immunoadsorption columns for the treatment of immune mediated thrombocytopenia is a somewhat labor-intensive yet effective method of treating thrombocytopenia, and has been used in treating both classical and HIV-associated thrombocytopenia (94).

The most important rule in the treatment of individuals with HIV-1-associated thrombocytopenia is to treat the individual rather than the platelet count. In many instances expectant follow-up is adequate as most of these individuals, with the exception of hemophiliacs, do not have significant bleeding problems. Fig. 48.2 is an example of an approach to the individual used in our institution. We cannot, however, overemphasize the importance of individualized treatment, as the clinical situation can vary so greatly in this complex group of individuals.

## LUPUS ANTICOAGULANTS AND ANTICARDIOLIPIN ANTIBODIES

The presence of both lupus anticoagulant (LA) and anticardiolipin antibodies (ACA) has been described in individuals infected with HIV-1. For the purposes of this discussion, LA or lupus inhibitors are those phenomena discovered because of a prolonged activated partial thromboplastin time (aPTT) that does not correct with mixing studies, and on further evaluation is not caused by a specific coagulation factor inhibitor. Other common assays used to identify or confirm LA are the tissue thromboplastin inhibition time (TTI) (95) or the dilute Russell's viper venom time (DRVVT) (96). These tests are discussed in detail in Chapters 26 and 38. ACA are antibodies to the phospholipid components of the various reagents used in intrinsic pathway coagulation screening tests. They are usually present in individuals found to have lupus inhibitors (LAs) but may be present in individuals with a normal aPTT or any of the other assays used to define LAs. These antibodies are considered to be the result of abnormal immune responses and are often seen in, but not limited to, individuals with other immunologic disorders such as systemic lupus erythematosus; they commonly occur in HIV-1-infected individuals.

Reports of the incidence and prevalence of these phenomena depend upon the screening test and sensitivity of the aPTT reagents employed to identify affected individuals. In much of the available literature the presence of LAs or ACA has been based on first finding a prolonged aPTT that does not correct with a 1:1 mix with normal plasma. LAs, as defined by an abnormal aPTT, positive TTI, or abnormal kaolin clotting times (KCT), are much less common than ACA. Detailed discussion of these problems can be found in Chapter 38.

If a prolonged APTT that does not correct after incubation with an equal volume of normal plasma (1:1 mix) is used to define the presence of circulating anticoagulants, then as many as 43% of HIV-1-positive individuals will demonstrate the presence of a circulating anticoagulant (97). Using this same criterion, 24 of 34 consecutively tested HIV-1 antibody-positive individuals (70%) reported by Bloom et al had LA (98). In this series all individuals also had a prolonged RVVT. In a series from Belgium (99), there were no prolonged aPTT results from among 142 nonhospitalized HIV-positive individuals and 10% had ACA. If individuals were hospitalized, ACA was much more commonly found (30%) and the presence of a prolonged aPTT was found in about 17%; however, in none of these individuals could a lupus inhibitor be demonstrated by the TTI or KCT.

The most common finding is the presence of ACA, which may be present in as many as 94% of HIV-1-infected individuals (100). ACA are found commonly in individuals infected with the HIV-1 virus and in individuals at risk for infection. In a study of 73 homosexual men, high levels of IgG-ACA were found in 23 of 28 individuals with AIDS and in 12 of 14 individuals with AIDS-related complex, but in none of the 13 men who tested negative for the virus (101). In this group of men, 5 of 10 who were clinically well but HIV-1 antibody positive also had high titers of IgG-ACA. None of the individuals in this group had a history of thrombosis. In a study of hemophiliacs, all HIV-1-infected individuals were found to have increased ACA levels. However, ACA were also found in 13 of 21 HIV-1-negative hemophiliacs (102). Four years later, the ACA levels in the HIV-1-positive group decreased or disappeared in 9 of the original 34. Another study of hemophiliacs failed to

demonstrate ACA in any HIV-1-negative subjects, and only 10 of 43 HIV-1 antibody-positive individuals were positive for ACA (103). In addition, this group did not show a correlation between progression to AIDS and the presence of ACA in the infected group. When the DRVVT is used to identify the presence of LA in hemophiliacs, 58% of 22 individuals studied with mild to severe hemophilia was found to be LA-positive (104). Nine of these (75%) were positive for ACA of either IgG or IgM or both subtypes. In this group the presence of ACA was associated with a diagnosis of *Pneumocystis carinii* pneumonia; however, others have not found a similar correlation (105).

The presence of both LA and ACA in HIV-1-infected individuals appears to be a common occurrence. As opposed to the situation in individuals with systemic lupus erythematosus where the presence of ACA and LA is associated with an increased incidence of thrombosis, HIV-1-infected individuals with ACA and LA do not appear to be thrombosis-prone. However, there are case reports of antiphospholipid syndrome-like events such as transient ischemic attacks, stroke, and deep venous thrombosis in HIV-1-infected individuals with ACA or LA. Keeling et al reported transient ischemic attacks and a thrombotic stroke in an HIV-1-infected individual who had ACA but no LA (106). However, given the high incidence of LA and ACA in HIV disease, one would expect that if a correlation with stroke or other thromboembolic or thrombotic events was present it would have been recognized by now. Nevertheless, in a report from Germany (107) ACA were found to be associated with cerebral perfusion abnormalities in HIV-1 infected individuals, though the clinical significance of this finding remains to be determined.

Other causes of thrombotic events have been suggested in HIV-1-infected individuals, such as the possible association with acquired protein S deficiency (108, 109). Both free protein S and bound protein S are frequently decreased in some individuals infected with the virus and there may be a correlation between elevated IgG ACA and decreased free protein S levels, although no correlation with disease progression has been noted (108).

# SUMMARY

Thrombocytopenia and LA or ACA are commonly seen in individuals infected with HIV-1. Thrombocytopenia may be the result of either the suppressive effects of viral infection on hemopoiesis or the immunologically mediated shortening of platelet half-life. TTP and HUS also occur with increased frequency, although the contribution of associated viral and bacterial infections is not understood. The LA and ACA commonly found may also result from the disordered immune response induced by HIV-1 infection. There does not appear to be an increased incidence of thrombotic events in HIV-1-infected individuals with LA and ACA. The response to treatment of thrombocytopenia in HIV-infected individuals is very similar to that of individuals with classical ITP, with the exception of the response to zidovudine. Treatment of HIV-1-infected individuals differs only with respect to the concern for added immune suppressive effects of therapy and comorbid illness. By virtue of these factors, therapy to address hemostatic abnormalities in HIV-1 infection must be carefully tailored to individual individual circumstances.

# REFERENCES

1. Morris L, Distenfeld A, Amorosi E et al. Autoimmune thrombocytopenic purpura in homosexual men. Ann Intern Med 1982;96:714–717.
2. Ratnoff OD, Menitove JE, Aster RH et al. Coincident classic hemophilia and "idiopathic" thrombocytopenic purpura in individuals under treatment with concentrates of antihemophilic factor (factor VIII). N Engl J Med 1983;308:439–442.
3. Savona S, Nardi MA, Lennette ET et al. Thrombocytopenic purpura in narcotics addicts. Ann Intern Med 1985;102:737–741.
4. Scadden DT, Zon LI, Groopman JE. Pathophysiology and management of HIV-associated hematologic disorders. Blood 1989;74:1455–1463.
5. Spivak JL, Bender BS, Quinn TC. Acquired immune deficiency syndrome and pancytopenia. JAMA 1983;250:3084–3087.
6. Treacy M, Lai L, Costello C et al. Peripheral blood and bone marrow abnormalities in individuals with HIV-related disease. Br J Haematol 1987;65:289–294.
7. Klatzmann D, Champagne E, Chamaret S et al. T-lymphocyte T4 molecule behaves as the receptor for human retrovirus LAV. Nature 1984;312:767–768.
8. Scadden DT, Zeira M, Woon A et al. HIV infection of human bone marrow stromal fibroblasts. Blood 1990;76:317–322.
9. Steinberg HN, Crumpacker CS, Chatis PA. In vitro suppression of normal human bone marrow progenitor cells by human immunodeficiency virus. J Virol 1991;65:1765–1769.
10. Folks TM, Kessler SW, Orenstein JM et al. Infection and replication of HIV-1 in purified progenitor cells of normal human bone marrow. Science 1988;242:919–922.
11. Kouri YH, Borkowsky W, Nardi M et al. Human megakaryocytes have a CD4 molecule capable of binding human immunodeficiency virus-1. Blood 1993;81:2664–2670.
12. Zucker-Franklin D, Cao Y. Megakaryocytes of human immunodeficiency virus infected individuals express viral RNA. Proc Natl Acad Sci U S A 1989;86:5595–5599.
13. Zucker-Franklin D, Seremetis S, Zheng ZY. Internalization of human immunodeficiency virus type I and other retroviruses by megakaryocytes and platelets. Blood 1990;75:1920–1923.
14. Sakaguchi M, Sato T, Groopman JE. Human immunodeficiency virus infection of megakaryocytic cells. Blood 1991;77:481–485.
15. Kunzi MS, Groopman JE. Identification of a novel human immunodeficiency virus strain cytopathic to megakaryocytic cells. Blood 1993;81:3336–3342.
16. Zauli G, Catani L, Gibellini D et al. Impaired survival of bone marrow GP IIb-IIIa+ megakaryocytic cells as an additional pathogenetic mechanism of HIV-1 related thrombocytopenia. Br J Haematol 1996;92:711–717.
17. Koenig C, Sidhu GS, Schoentag RA. The platelet volume–number relationship in individuals infected with the human immunodeficiency virus. Am J Clin Pathol 1991;96:500–503.
18. Molina JM, Scadden DT, Sakaguchi M et al. Lack of evidence for infection of or effect on growth of hematopoietic progenitor cells after in vivo or in vitro exposure to human immunodeficiency virus. Blood 1990;76:2476–2482.
19. von Laer D, Hufert FT, Fenner TE et al. CD34+ hematopoietic progenitor cells are not a major reservoir of the human immunodeficiency virus. Blood 1990;76:1281–1286.
20. Marandin A, Katz A, Oksenhendler E et al. Loss of primitive hematopoietic progenitors in individuals with human immunodeficiency virus infection. Blood 1996;88:4568–4578.
21. Stella CC, Ganser A, Hoelzer D. Defective in vitro growth of the hemopoietic progenitor cells in the acquired immunodeficiency syndrome. J Clin Invest 1987;80:286–293.
22. Donahue RE, Johnson MM, Zon LI et al. In vitro suppression of hematopoiesis after human immunodeficiency virus infection. Nature 1987;326:200–203.
23. Zauli G, Vitale M, Gibellini D Capitani S. Inhibition of purified CD34+ hematopoietic progenitor cells by human immunodeficiency virus 1 or gp120 mediated by endogenous transforming growth factor beta1. J Exp Med 1996;183:99–108.
24. Zauli G, Vitale M, Re MC et al. In-Vitro exposure to HIV-1 induces apoptotic cell death of the factor-dependent TF-1 hematopoietic cell line. Blood 1994;83:167–175.
25. Richman DD, Fischl MA, Grieco MH et al. The toxicity of azidothymidine (AZT) in the treatment of individuals with AIDS and AIDS-related complex. A double-blind, placebo-controlled trial. N Engl J Med 1987;317:192–197.
26. Walsh C, Krigel R, Lennette E et al. Thrombocytopenia in homosexual individuals. Ann Intern Med 1985;103:542–545.
27. Kaslow RA, Phair JP, Friedman HB et al. Infection with the human immunodeficiency virus: clinical manifestations and their relationship to immune deficiency. A report of the multicenter AIDS Cohort Study. Ann Intern Med 1987;107:474–480.
28. Rossi G, Gorla R, Stellini R et al. Prevalence, clinical, and laboratory features of thrombocytopenia among HIV-infected individuals. AIDS Res Hum Retroviruses 1990;2:261–269.
29. Holtzman RS, Walsh CM, Karpatkin S. Risk for the acquired immunodeficiency syndrome among thrombocytopenic and non thrombocytopenic homosexual men seropositive for the human immunodeficiency virus. Ann Intern Med 1987;106:383–386.
30. Eyster ME, Rabkin CS, Hilgartner MW et al. Human immunodeficiency virus-related conditions in children and adults with hemophilia: rates, relationship to CD4 counts, and predictive value. Blood 1993;81:828–834.
31. Galli M, Musicco M, Gervasoni C et al. No evidence of a higher risk of progression to AIDS in individuals with HIV-1 related severe thrombocytopenia. J Acquir Immune Defic Syndr Hum Retrovirol 1996;12:268–275.
32. Savona S, Nardi MA, Lennette ET et al. Thrombocytopenic purpura in narcotic addicts. Ann Intern Med 1985;102:737–741.
33. Walsh CM, Nardi MA, Karpatkin S. On the mechanism of thrombocytopenic purpura in sexually active homosexual men. N Engl J Med 1984;311:635–639.
34. Stricker RB, Abrams DI, Corash L et al. Target platelet antigen in homosexual men with immune thrombocytopenia. N Engl J Med 1985;313:1375–1380.
35. Shuman MA, Corash L, Abrams DI et al. Retraction. Target platelet antigen in homosexual men with immune thrombocytopenia. N Engl J Med 1991;325:1487.
36. Bettaieb A, Oksenhendler E, Fromont P et al. Immunochemical analysis of platelet autoantibodies in HIV-related thrombocytopenic purpura: a study of 68 individuals. Br J Haematol 1989;73:241–247.
37. Klaassen RJ, van der Lelie J, Vlekke AB et al. The serology and immunochemistry of HIV-induced platelet bound immunoglobulin. Blut 1989;59:75–81.
38. Magnac C, de Saint Martin J, Pidard D et al. Platelet antibodies in serum of individuals with human immunodeficiency virus (HIV) infection. AIDS Res Hum Retroviruses 1990;6:1443–1449.
39. Karpatkin S, Nardi M, Lennette ET et al. Anti-human immunodeficiency virus type 1 antibody complexes on platelets of seropositive thrombocytopenic homosexuals and narcotic addicts. Proc Natl Acad Sci U S A 1988;85:9763–9767.
40. Karpatkin S, Nardi M. Autoimmune anti-HIV-1gp120 antibody with anti-idiotype-like activity in sera and immune complexes of HIV-1-related immunologic thrombocytopenia. J Clin Invest 1992;89:356–364.
41. Gonzalez-Conejero A, Rivera J, Rosillo MC et al. Association of autoantibodies against platelet glycoproteins Ib/IX and IIb/IIIa, and platelet-reactive anti-HIV antibodies in thrombocytopenic narcotic addicts. Br J Haematol 1996;93:464–471.
42. Bettaieb A, Oksenhendler E, Duedari N et al. Crossreactive antibodies between HIV-gp120 and platelet gpIIIa (CD61) in HIV-related immune thrombocytopenic purpura. Clin Exp Immunol 1996;103:19–23.
43. Dominguez A, Gamallo G, Garcia R et al. Pathophysiology of HIV related thrombocytopenia: an analysis of 41 individuals. J Clin Pathol 1994;47:999–1003.
44. Boccia RV, Gelmann EP, Baker CC et al. A hemolytic-uremic syndrome with the acquired immunodeficiency syndrome [Letter]. Ann Intern Med 1984;101:716–717.
45. Leaf AN, Laubenstein LJ, Raphael B et al. Thrombotic thrombocytopenic purpura associated with human immunodeficiency virus type 1 (HIV-1) infection. Ann Intern Med 1988;109:194–197.
46. Nair JMG, Bellevue R, Bertoni M et al. Thrombotic thrombocytopenic purpura in individuals with the acquired immunodeficiency syndrome (AIDS)-related complex. A report of two cases. Ann Intern Med 1988;109:209–212.
47. Botti AC, Hyde P, DiPillo F. Thrombotic thrombocytopenic purpura in a individual who subsequently developed the acquired immunodeficiency syndrome (AIDS). Ann Intern Med 1988;109:242–243.
48. Rarick MU, Espina B, Mocharnuk R et al. Thrombotic thrombocytopenic purpura in individuals with human immunodeficiency virus infection: a

report of three cases and Review of the literature. Am J Hematol 1992;40:103–109.

49. Chu QD, Medeiros LJ, Fisher AE et al. Thrombotic thrombocytopenic purpura and HIV infection. South Med J 1995;88:82–86.

50. Torok TJ, Holman RC, Chorba TL. Increasing mortality from thrombotic thrombocytopenic purpura in the United States—analysis of national mortality data, 1968-1991. Am J Hematol 1995;50:84–90.

51. Farina C, Gavazzeni G, Caprioli A et al. Hemolytic uremic syndrome associated with verocytotoxin-producing Escherichia coli infection in acquired immunodeficiency syndrome [Letter]. Blood 1990;75:2465.

52. Beris P, Dunand V, Isoz C et al. Association of thrombotic thrombocytopenic purpura and human immunodeficiency virus infection. Nouv Rev Fr Hematol 1990;32:277–280.

53. del Arco A, Martinez MA, Pena JM et al. Thrombotic thrombocytopenic purpura associated with human immunodeficiency virus infection: demonstration of p24 antigen in endothelial cells. Clin Infect Dis 1993;17:360–363.

54. Bell WR, Braine HG, Ness PM et al. Improved survival in thrombotic thrombocytopenic purpura-hemolytic uremic syndrome. Clinical experience in 108 individuals. N Engl J Med 1991;325:398–403.

55. Henon P. Treatment of thrombotic thrombocytopenic purpura. Results of a multicenter randomized clinical study. Presse Med 1991;20:1761–1767.

56. Salem G, Terebelo H, Raman S. Human immunodeficiency virus associated with thrombotic thrombocytopenic purpura: successful treatment with zidovudine. South Med J 1991;84:493–495.

57. Oksenhendler E, Bierling P, Farcet JP et al. Response to therapy in 37 individuals with HIV-related thrombocytopenic purpura. Br J Haematol 1987;66:491–495.

58. Shafer RW, Offit K, Macris NT et al. Possible risk of steroid administration in individuals at risk for AIDS [Letter]. Lancet 1985;1:934–935.

59. Abrams DI, Kiprov DD, Goedert JJ et al. Antibodies to human T-lymphotropic virus type III and development of the acquired immunodeficiency syndrome in homosexual men presenting with immune thrombocytopenia. Ann Intern Med 1986;104:47–50.

60. Gill PS, Loureiro C, Bemstein-Singer M et al. Clinical effect of glucocorticoids on Kaposi's sarcoma related to acquired immunodeficiency syndrome (AIDS). Ann Intern Med 1989;87:57–61.

61. Schneider PA, Abrams DI, Rayner AA et al. Immunodeficiency-associated thrombocytopenic purpura (IDTP). Response to splenectomy. Arch Surg 1987;122:1175–1178.

62. Tyler DS, Shaunak S, Bartlett JA et al. HIV-1-associated thrombocytopenia. The role of splenectomy. Ann Surg 1990;211:211–217.

63. Ferguson CM. Splenectomy for immune thrombocytopenia related to human immunodeficiency virus. Surg Gynecol Obstet 1988;167:300–302.

64. Brown SA, Majumdar G, Harrington C et al. Effect of splenectomy on HIV-related thrombocytopenia and progression of HIV infection in individuals with severe haemophilia. Blood Coagul Fibrinolysis 1994;5:393–397.

65. Alonso M, Gossot D, Bourstyn E et al. Splenectomy in human immunodeficiency virus-related thrombocytopenia. Br J Surg 1993;80:330–333.

66. Barbui T, Cortelazzo S, Minetti B et al. Does splenectomy enhance risk of AIDS in HIV-positive individuals with chronic thrombocytopenia? Lancet 1987;2:342–343.

67. Landonio G, Galli M, Nosari A et al. HIV-related severe thrombocytopenia in intravenous drug users: prevalence, response to therapy in a medium term follow-up, and pathologic evaluation. AIDS 1990;4:29–34.

68. Tunkel AR, Kelsall B, Rein MF et al. Case report: increase in CD4 lymphocyte counts after splenectomy in HIV-infected individuals. Am J Med Sci 1993;306:105–110.

69. Mathew A, Raviglione MC, Niranjan U et al. Splenectomy in individuals with AIDS. Am J Hematol 1989;32:184–189.

70. Ravikumar TS, Allen JD, Bothe A Jr et al. Splenectomy, the treatment of choice for human immunodeficiency virus-related immune thrombocytopenia? Arch Surg 1989;124:625–628.

71. Pollak AN, Janinis J, Green D. Successful intravenous immune globulin therapy for human immunodeficiency virus-associated thrombocytopenia. Arch Intern Med 1988;148:695–697.

72. Bussel JB, Haimi JS. Isolated thrombocytopenia in individuals infected with HIV: treatment with intravenous gammaglobulin. Am J Hematol 1988;28:79–84.

73. Jahnke L, Applebaum S, Sherman LA et al. An evaluation of intravenous immunoglobulin in the treatment of human immunodeficiency virus-associated thrombocytopenia. Transfusion 1994;34:759–764.

74. Salama A, Mueller-Eckhardt C. Use of Rh antibodies in the treatment of autoimmune thrombocytopenia. Transfus Med Rev 1992;7:17–25.

75. Bussel JB, Graziano JN, Kimberly RP et al. Intravenous anti-D treatment of immune thrombocytopenic purpura: analysis of efficacy, toxicity and mechanism of effect. Blood 1991;77:1884–1893.

76. Oksenhendler E, Bierling P, Brossard Y et al. Anti-RH immunoglobulin therapy for human immunodeficiency virus-related immune thrombocytopenic purpura. Blood 1988;71:1499–1502.

77. Mintzer DM, Real FX, Jovino L et al. Treatment of Kaposi's sarcoma and thrombocytopenia with vincristine in individuals with the acquired immunodeficiency syndrome. Ann Intern Med 1985;102:200–202.

78. Gottlieb MS, Wolfe PR, Chafey S. Case report: response of AIDS-related thrombocytopenia to intravenous and oral azidothymidine (3' azido-3'-deoxythymidine). AIDS Res Human Retroviruses 1987;3:109–114.

79. Hymes KB, Greene JB, Karpatkin S. The effect of azidothymidine on HIV-related thrombocytopenia [Letter]. N Engl J Med 1988;318:516–517.

80. Pomeroy C. Zidovudine therapy of HIV-associated thrombocytopenia: from MAIDS to AIDS [Editorial]. J Lab Clin Med 1993;121:536–538.

81. Oksenhendler E, Bierling P, Ferchal F et al. Zidovudine for thrombocytopenic purpura related to human immunodeficiency virus (HIV) infection. Ann Intern Med 1989;110:365–368.

82. Pottage JC Jr, Benson CA, Spear JB et al. Treatment of human immunodeficiency virus-related thrombocytopenia with zidovudine. JAMA 1988;260:3045–3048.

83. Anonymous. Zidovudine for the treatment of thrombocytopenia associated with human immunodeficiency virus (HIV). Swiss Group for Clinical Studies on the Acquired Immunodeficiency Syndrome (AIDS). Ann Intern Med 1988;109:718–721.

84. Montaner J, Le T, Gelman K et al. The effect of zidovudine on platelet count in HIV associated thrombocytopenia. V International Conference on AIDS, Montreal, Canada [Abstract]. June 1989;204.

85. Landonio G, Cinque P, Nosari A et al. Comparison of two dose regimens of zidovudine in an open, randomized, multicentre study for severe HIV-related thrombocytopenia. AIDS 1993;7:209–212.

86. Richman DD, Fischl MA, Grieco MH et al. The toxicity of azidothymidine (AZT) in the treatment of individuals with AIDS and AIDS-related complex. A double-blind, placebo-controlled trial. N Engl J Med 1987;317:192–197.

87. Ballem PJ, Belzberg A, Devine D et al. Pathophysiology of thrombocytopenia associated with HIV infection in homosexual men. A preliminary report. Blut 1989;59:111–114.

88. Durand JM, Lefevre P, Hovette P et al. Dapsone for thrombocytopenic purpura related to human immunodeficiency virus infection. Am J Med 1991;90:675–677.

89. Ellis ME, Neal KR, Leen CL et al. Alpha-2a recombinant interferon in HIV associated thrombocytopenia. BMJ Clin Res 1987;295:1519–1522.

90. Proctor SJ, Jackson G, Carey P et al. Improvement of platelet counts in steroid-unresponsive idiopathic immune thrombocytopenic purpura after short-course therapy with recombinant alpha-2b interferon. Blood 1989;74:1894–1897.

91. Marroni M, Gresele P, Landonio G et al. Interferon-alpha is effective in the treatment of HIV-1-related, severe, zidovudine-resistant thrombocytopenia. A prospective, placebo-controlled, double-blind trial. Ann Intern Med 1994;121:423–429.

92. Northfelt DW, Charlebois ED, Mirda MI et al. Continuous low-dose interferon-alpha for HIV-related immune thrombocytopenic purpura. J Acquir Immune Defic Syndr Hum Retrovirol 1995;8:45–50.

93. Soubrane C, Tourani JM, Andrieu JM et al. Biologic response to anti-CD16 monoclonal antibody therapy in a human immuno-deficiency virus-related immune thrombocytopenic purpura individual. Blood 1993;81:15–19.

94. Mittelman A, Bertram J, Henry DH et al. Treatment of individuals with HIV thrombocytopenia and hemolytic uremic syndrome with protein A (Prosorba Column) immunoadsorption. Semin Hematol 1989;26(Suppl):15–18.

95. Schleider MA, Nachman RL, Jaffe EA et al. A clinical study of the lupus anticoagulant. Blood 1976;48:499–509.

96. Thiagarajan P, Pengo V, Shapiro SS. The use of the dilute Russell viper venom time for diagnosis of lupus anticoagulants. Blood 1986;68:869–874.

97. Lefrere JJ, Gozin D, Lerable J. Circulating anticoagulant in asymptomatic persons seropositive for human immunodeficiency virus (HIV) [Letter]. Ann Intern Med 1988;108:771.

98. Bloom EJ, Abrams DI, Rodgers G. Lupus anticoagulant in the acquired immunodeficiency syndrome. JAMA 1986;256:491–493.

99. Capel P, Janssens A, Clumeck N et al. Anticardiolipin antibodies (ACA) are most often not associated with lupus-like anticoagulant (LLAC) in human immunodeficiency virus (HIV) infection. Am J Hematol 1991;37:234–238.

100. Stimmler MM, Quismorio FP Jr., McGehee WG et al. Anticardiolipin antibodies in acquired immunodeficiency syndrome. Arch Intern Med 1989;149:1833–1835.

101. Canoso RT, Zon LI, Groopman JE. Anticardiolipin antibodies associated with HTLV-1 infection. Br J Haematol 1987;65:495–498.

102. Panzer S, Stain C, Harti H et al. Anticardiolipin antibodies are elevated in HIV-1 infected haemophiliacs but do not predict for disease progression. Thromb Haemost 1989;61:81–85.

103. Naimi N, Plancherel C, Bosser C et al. Anticardiolipin antibodies in HIV-negative and HIV-positive haemophiliacs. Blood Coag Fibrinolysis 1990;1:5–8.

104. Cohen H, Mackie IJ, Anagnostopoulos N et al. Lupus anticoagulant, anticardiolipin antibodies, and human immunodeficiency virus in haemophilia. J Clin Pathol 1989;42:629–633.

105. Zon LI, Groopman JE. Hematologic manifestations of the human immune deficiency virus (HIV). Semin Hematol 1988;25:208–218.
106. Keeling DM, Birley H, Machin SJ. Multiple transient ischaemic attacks and a mild thrombotic stroke in a HIV-positive individual with anticardiolipin antibodies. Blood Coag Fibrinolysis 1990;1:333–335.
107. Rubbert A, Bock E, Schwab J et al. Anticardiolipin antibodies in HIV infection: association with cerebral perfusion defects as detected by 99mTc-HMPAO SPECT. Clin Exp Immunol 1994; 98:361–368.
108. Stahl CP, Wideman CS, Spira TJ et al. Protein S deficiency in men with long-term human immunodeficiency virus infection. Blood 1993;81: 1801–1807.
109. Laing RB, Brettle RP, Leen CL. Venous thrombosis in HIV infection [Editorial]. Int J STD AIDS 1996;7:82–85.

# CHAPTER 49

# HEMOSTATIC COMPLICATIONS OF BLOOD AND BONE MARROW TRANSPLANTATION

Philip L. McCarthy, Jr., and Michael H. Kroll

Allogeneic and autologous blood or bone marrow transplantation (BMT) are used for treatment of various hematologic, immunologic, and malignant disorders (1–3). Hemostatic complications commonly occur after high-dose chemotherapy and radiation therapy given to prepare individuals for BMT. This chapter reviews some of the common as well as unusual hemorrhagic and thrombotic complications of BMT.

## CATHETER COMPLICATIONS

Long-term intravenous catheters have facilitated treatment of individuals undergoing intensive chemotherapy and radiation therapy followed by bone marrow rescue (4–6). Generally, these catheters are tunneled subcutaneously through the upper infraclavicular chest wall into the subclavian vein, terminating in the right atrium (Fig. 49.1A). For BMT, a multi-lumen, external-port catheter, such as the Hickman or Groshong catheter, typically is required. These catheters are comparable except for their termini: the Groshong catheter has a pressure-sensitive, two-way valve that prevents backflow of blood when the line is dormant (Fig. 49.1B). Another type has its port placed subcutaneously (e.g,. the Portacath® or Mediport®). Usually, however, this type is not recommended for these individuals, because puncture of the catheter port through the skin increases the risk of local bleeding and infection during neutro-

penic and thrombocytopenic periods (Fig. 49.1C). Even so, these catheters may be left in place during the transplant period.

The type of anticoagulant used to maintain a long-term intravenous catheter depends on the type of catheter and the clinical situation. Catheters with external lumens require daily or twice-daily flushes with heparin (10–100 U/mL) or saline. Subcutaneously implanted catheters require no more than monthly heparin flushes. Groshong catheters may be flushed with saline because of the valve system in the catheter. Because of the small risk of heparin-induced thrombocytopenia, saline flushes may be an advantage (7); no data demonstrate conclusively that anticoagulant flushes are superior to saline flushes (8). There does not appear to be an increased number of catheter thromboses associated with saline flushes if the lines are in continuous use, but small clots may develop when the line is capped or used infrequently. An alternate strategy could be the addition of low-dose warfarin, which prevented catheter-related thromboses in a group of non-BMT individuals (9). Low-molecular-weight heparin may be a useful alternative to low-dose warfarin and has been used successfully for veno-occlusive disease (VOD) prophylaxis without increased bleeding complications (10).

Serious infections, thromboses, or both complicate clinical use of indwelling catheters in fewer than 5% of individuals (11, 12). Most thromboses require simple aspiration of the line to clear the obstruction. Failing this,

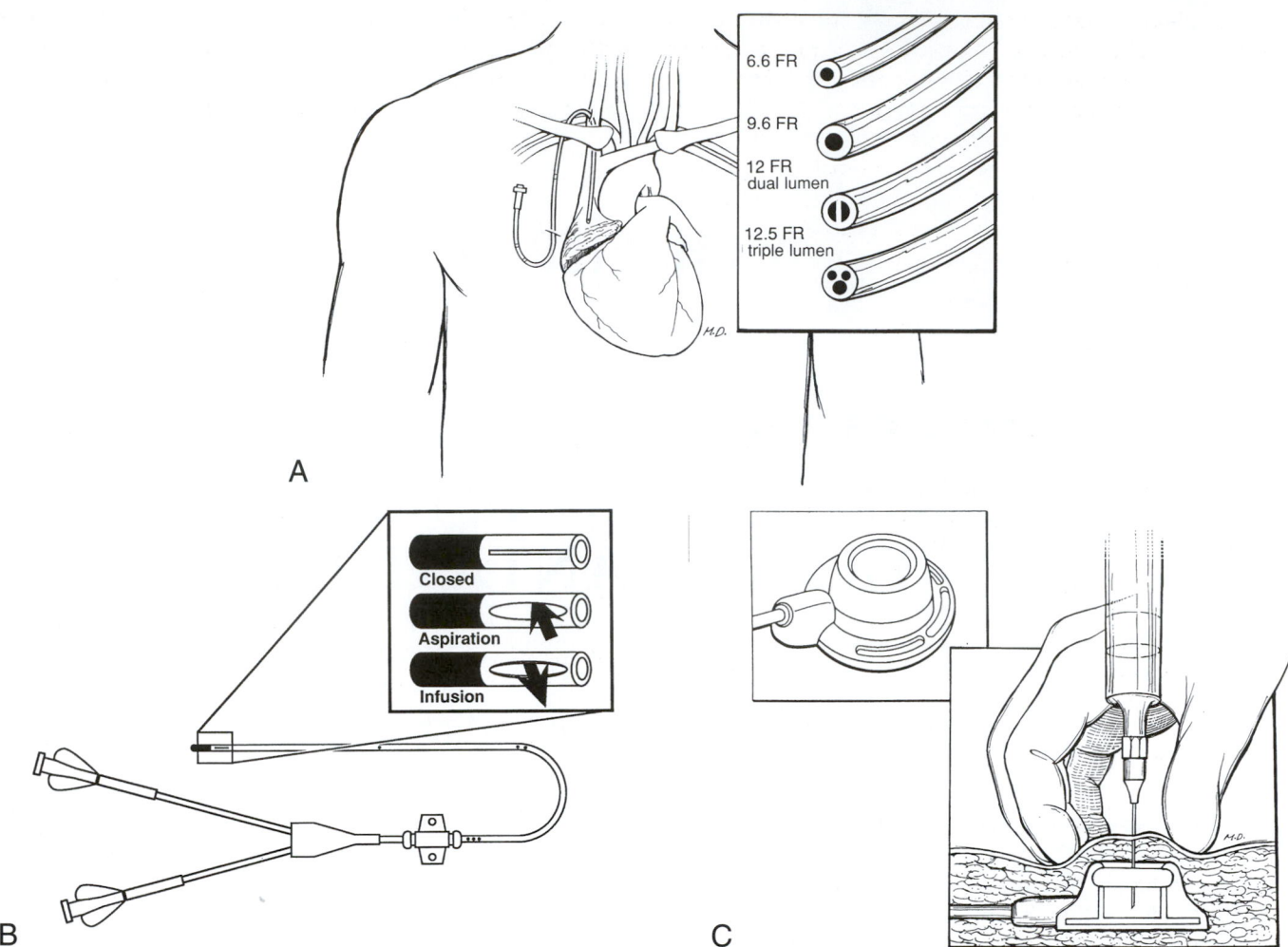

**FIGURE 49.1.** **A,** The preferred catheter type for long-term use in individuals receiving BMT. The catheter generally is inserted surgically into the subclavian vein, with its terminus in the right atrium and its ports (of varying number and diameter) external to the chest wall. These catheters require careful maintenance, including flushing, to minimize the risks of thrombosis and infection. FR, French. **B,** Backflow and stasis leading to catheter thrombosis may be decreased in the Groshong catheter, which has a terminal-segment valve that functions as shown. **C,** The subcutaneously implanted catheter is not recommended for individuals receiving BMT. It has easier maintenance, which still includes monthly flushes, but it provides fewer access ports and is more susceptible to hemorrhagic complications. FR, French.

instillation of 1 to 2 mL of urokinase (5000 IU/mL) usually will lyse the thrombus; irreversibly thrombosed catheters are predisposed to infection and must be removed. Thrombolytic therapy after catheter removal seldom is required unless there is persistent arm edema or a potentially dangerous thrombosis (e.g., superior vena cava syndrome). Clinically significant catheter thrombosis rarely is associated with distal embolization. These more serious catheter-related thromboembolic events usually are associated with placement of two or more ipsilateral catheters or a catheter inserted into an extremity with poor vascular drainage because of multiple previous catheter placements or previous surgical axillary dissection. Persistent or recurrent thrombosis or thromboembolism also should raise the possibility of a deficiency in the natural anticoagulants protein C, pro-

tein S, and antithrombin III or of abnormalities in factor V (see Chapter 40). Use of a narrow catheter with a single lumen decreases the incidence of thrombotic complications, but the advantage of a double-lumen or triple-lumen catheter capable of providing venous access for multiple infusions and blood drawing usually outweighs that of a single-lumen catheter. Very-narrow-lumen catheters, such as the Broviac, often present additional problems because of difficulty with aspiration, blood sampling, or large-volume infusions.

Treatment with granulocyte-monocyte colony-stimulating factor or granulocyte colony-stimulating factor is associated with thrombosis in individuals undergoing apheresis for hematopoietic stem-cell harvest (13). This complication probably relates to the elevated level of circulating leukocytes that develops in response to hematopoietic progenitor stimulation. These thromboses often are subclinical or confined solely to the catheter, and individuals seldom require anticoagulant therapy. Although associated with an increased risk of infection, temporary placement of a femoral catheter is not associated with an increased risk of thrombosis. There also is no increased incidence of thrombosis associated with use of short-term catheters placed directly into a central vein compared with long-term catheters tunneled subcutaneously.

# HEPATIC VOD

A distinct histopathologic syndrome, VOD is characterized by certain clinical features and is associated with several physical and chemical insults. Hepatic VOD frequently occurs following BMT as a complication of the preparative regimen. Its pathogenesis largely is unknown, but the histopathologic features suggest the endothelium may be the site of the primary lesion. Hepatic pathology typical of VOD was first reported in 1905 by Alfred Hess (14). This individual presented with jaundice, hepatomegaly, and ascites resulting from an obliterative endophlebitis of the liver. This was considered to be a variant of "Chiari syndrome" (i.e., thrombosis of the portal vein, hepatic vein, or both), and its cause was never discovered. The pathogenetic basis for hepatic VOD did not emerge until 1951, with the publication of "Senecio poisoning exhibiting as Chiari's syndrome," by Selzer and Parker (15). These authors reported six deaths in South Africa following ingestion of the fungus "ragwort," which manifested clinically by nausea, vomiting, painful hepatomegaly, and ascites. The pathology of each individual's liver was remarkably similar, with necrosis of the lining endothelial cells in the central and sublobular veins associated with a fibrocytic infiltrate of the lumina without significant thrombosis. Absence of thrombosis was a hallmark of this disease, and this suggested a nosologic entity distinct from "Chiari syndrome."

"Veno-occlusive disease" of the liver was first reported in 1954 among Jamaicans drinking "bush tea" and who developed hepatomegaly and ascites associated with progressive obliteration of hepatic-vein radicals (16). Six years later, hepatic VOD was first reported as a complication of therapy for hematologic malignancies in two individuals receiving 6-mercaptopurine for acute myelogenous leukemia (17). Since then, it has been established that hepatic VOD is an important potential side effect of therapy for many malignant disorders, including allogeneic and autologous BMT (18–35).

In addition to hepatic VOD, other vasculopathies can develop after BMT, including pulmonary VOD, ischemic lesions of the ocular fundus, and microangiopathic syndromes that resemble thrombotic thrombocytopenic purpura (TTP) and hemolytic-uremic syndrome (HUS) (36–40). Occurrence of these diverse and clinically important vascular processes suggests that pathologic factors related to BMT may be affecting the endothelium. Vascular endothelium in the liver is particularly vulnerable to this toxicity of BMT.

## HISTOPATHOLOGY

The histology of hepatic VOD is unique and distinguishable from those of other liver diseases that develop after BMT, such as graft-versus-host disease (GVHD) and infectious hepatitis. Hepatic VOD mainly involves the centrilobular region of the liver acinus (i.e., Rappaport zone 3) (41), and it often occurs in a patchy distribution throughout the liver. Fig. 49.2 shows typical features representing the progression of hepatic VOD. In its early stages, hepatic VOD is characterized by concentric subintimal thickening, representing subendothelial edema, with the endothelium separating from the basement membrane. This is associated with extensive centrilobular congestion, hepatocellular necrosis, and a mild inflammatory cell infiltrate comprised predominantly of hemosiderin-laden macrophages and loose connective tissue that begins to fill the lumen of the centrilobular and sublobular veins (Fig. 49.2A). The fibrosis progresses centripetally and the hepatocellular necrosis centrifugally, thereby resulting in concentric deposition of loose connective tissue along the intimal margin of the blood vessel (Fig. 49.2B). The hepatic-vein radicals eventually may become replaced with dense, fibrous tissue, thus creating an obliterative endophlebitis associated with necrosis of hepatocytes and loss of normal hepatic architecture in the vicinity of the affected hepatic veins (Fig. 49.2C).

In late or chronic VOD, fibrosis may bridge the centrilobular and sublobular regions, thereby resulting in the appearance of radial fibrosis on cut sections. This pathology usually is confined to the pericentral region, with the remainder of the liver spared except during advanced chronic VOD, in which portal fibrosis and micronodular cirrhosis develop. Following recovery from clinically significant VOD, the central vein becomes recanalized and lined with a monolayer of regenerated endothelial cells. Inflammatory debris is cleared, and new hepatocytes form the structural elements of the regenerating lobule (Fig. 49.3).

The histopathology of hepatic VOD differs from those of Budd-Chiari syndrome, viral infections, and GVHD. Compared with Budd-Chiari syndrome, VOD demonstrates no thrombi in the central and sublobular veins and no involvement of the large hepatic veins or the intrahepatic branches of the inferior vena cava. Compared with viral hepatitis, VOD is associated with minimal inflammation and absence of cytomegaly, intranuclear inclusions, and bile duct abnormalities (42). Acute GVHD of the liver, which may coexist with hepatic VOD in approximately 10% of individuals after allogeneic

BMT (27), almost always involves the bile ducts, with epithelial cell dropout, necrosis, and cholestasis (43). Hepatic venous and arterial endothelial cells are affected in acute hepatic GVHD, and the early inflammatory infiltrate of acute hepatic GVHD is predominantly luminal (i.e., leukocytes attaching to the vascular intima) rather than abluminal (i.e., subendothelial), as in VOD. Shulman et al (44) examined the liver histology in 76 autopsy specimens from individuals who underwent allogeneic BMT, finding severe VOD in 32. Clinically severe VOD was correlated with several centrilobular (zone 3 acinar) changes, including occluded hepatic venules, frequency of occluded hepatic venules and degree of occlusion, eccentric luminal narrowing or phlebosclerosis, sinusoidal fibrosis, and hepatocyte necrosis. As these authors noted, there is a constellation of histologic findings that should be correlated with the clinical course of the individual, and there is no single histologic feature of VOD that is diagnostic.

The histopathology of pulmonary VOD, which rarely occurs following allogeneic BMT, is similar to that of hepatic VOD. The pulmonary veins and venules demonstrate minimal inflammation without thrombus formation. The most striking histopathologic features, however, are endothelial cell proliferation with partial to complete occlusion of the vessel lumen by loose fibrous tissue (36). The histopathology of optic ischemic microvasculopathy following allogeneic BMT has been examined only at its end stage, when the retinal capillary network is atrophic and acellular, thus suggesting this advanced lesion begins with vaso-occlusion that results in ischemia of the optic disc (37).

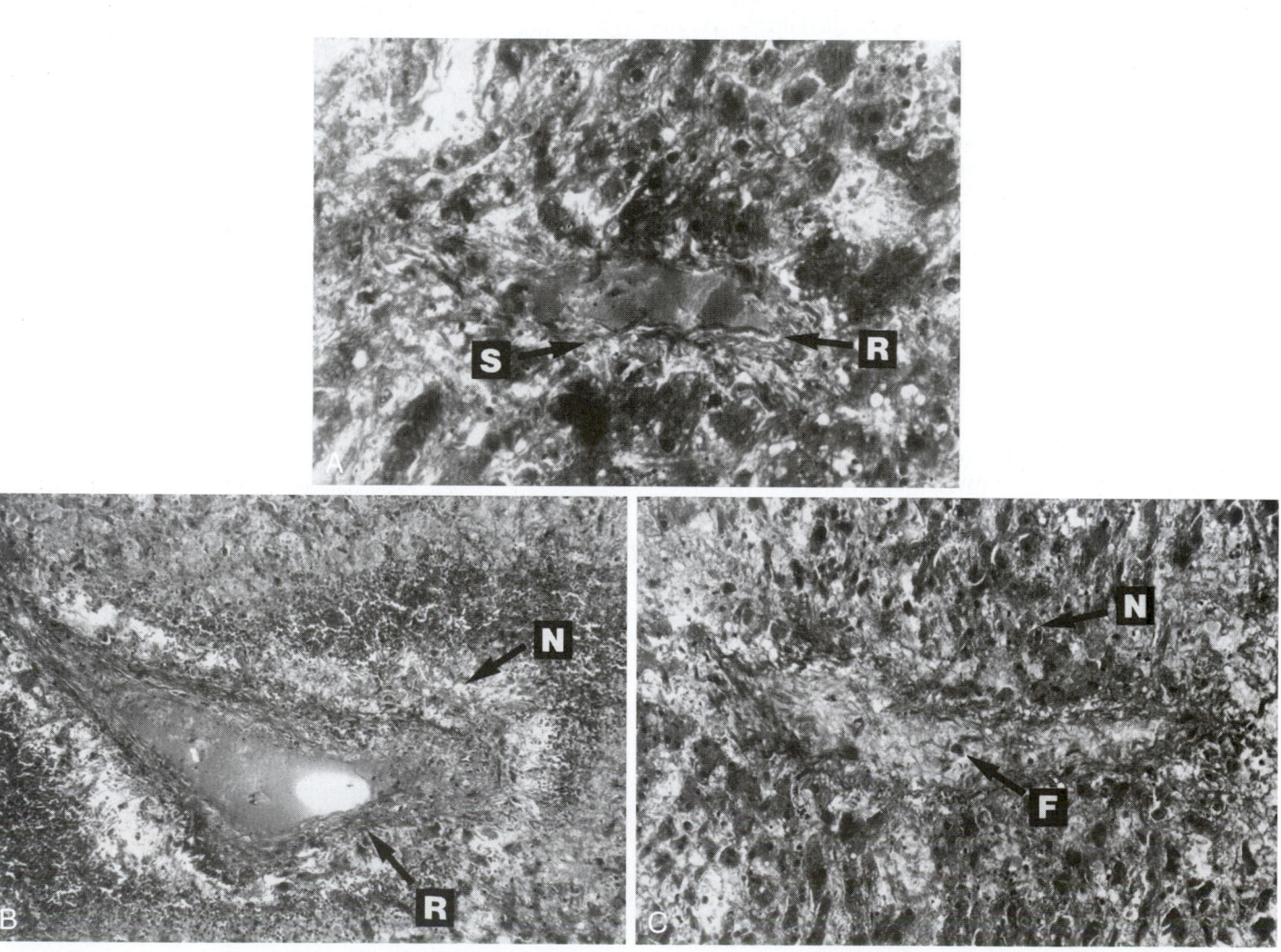

**FIGURE 49.2.** The histopathology of hepatic VOD as demonstrated, through the evolution of structural changes at the region of the central vein in individuals with clinical VOD after BMT. **A,** Shows early VOD with mild reticulin deposition in the vascular space (R) accompanied by perivenular swelling (S). (Original magnification 300x of Masson Trichrome–stained specimen.) **B,** Centripetal fibrosis by reticulin deposition (R) and centrifugal necrosis (N) of adjacent hepatocytes. (Original magnification 200x of Masson Trichrome–stained specimen.) **C,** Full-blown VOD with an obliterative endophlebitis resulting from complete occlusion of the central vein by fibrosis (F) accompanied by extensive hepatocellular necrosis (N). (Original magnification 300x of Masson Trichrome–stained specimen.)

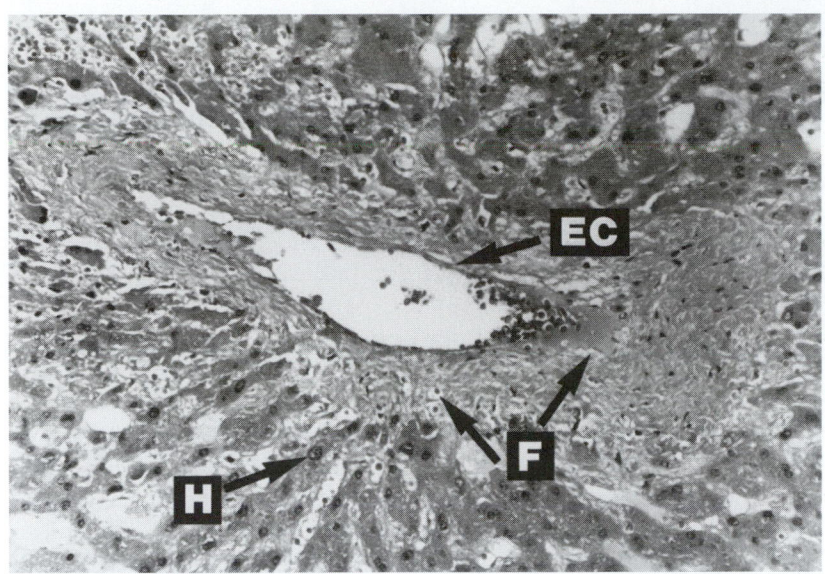

**FIGURE 49.3.** The histopathology of healed hepatic VOD. There is dense fibrosis (F) around a patent central vein accompanied by endothelial cell (EC) and hepatocyte (H) regeneration. (Original magnification 200x of specimen stained with hematoxylin and eosin.)

## CLINICAL FEATURES

Hepatic VOD typically develops within the first 21 days after BMT. Pre-BMT risk factors include elevated serum transaminase levels, ongoing therapy for bacterial or viral infection at the time of BMT, liver metastases, previous liver radiation therapy, previous BMT, and intensity and type of the conditioning regimen (30–35, 44). Other factors that may be associated with an increased risk of VOD include use of methotrexate for GVHD prophylaxis (34) and allogeneic versus autologous BMT (35).

Clinical signs of weight gain, hepatomegaly, or liver tenderness may occur during the conditioning regimen and before the infusion of hematopoietic stem cells. An elevation of the serum bilirubin level along with a mild elevation of serum aminotransferase levels usually occur 1 week after BMT. Occasionally, the alkaline phosphatase level will be elevated, but the serum bilirubin level is disproportionately elevated relative to other liver function tests. Laboratory abnormalities are followed by evidence of further hepatic dysfunction, including fluid retention, hepatomegaly, ascites, and multiorgan failure.

If the initial signs of weight gain, hepatomegaly, and elevated bilirubin level subside, the illness usually is self-limited. Approximately one-third of individuals die, with death often being heralded by encephalopathy and accompanying multiorgan failure. Approximately 10% of surviving individuals have chronic liver dysfunction.

Based on retrospective analyses of the clinical course and pathologic material derived primarily from autopsy studies, the overall incidence of hepatic VOD following BMT ranges from 1 to 54%. Data from three series with a total of 548 individuals reveal the incidence following allogeneic BMT to be approximately 20% (28–30). Other analyses of hepatic VOD following autologous BMT in 402 individuals among four series reveals a similar average incidence, although one of these studies found a very low incidence of 4% (29–31). A large, multivariate analysis found a 54% incidence of VOD in individuals with autologous or allogeneic BMT (33). These variations in the incidence of VOD may result from differing clinical definitions of VOD. The prevalence of subclinical hepatic VOD following BMT cannot be determined precisely because of the infrequency of liver biopsy during the early posttransplant period, but studies suggest it is less than 5%.

Many clinical features are designated as being risk factors for hepatic VOD and provide insight into possible pathogenic mechanisms. Preexisting liver disease of any cause is the most important risk factor. Among individuals beginning BMT, VOD developed in almost 50% of those with elevated aminotransferase levels, compared with fewer than 15% of those with normal aminotransferase levels (30–33). Viral hepatitis or hepatic metastases at transplant further increase the risk of hepatic VOD (30, 31). Some investigators consider active viral hepatitis to be a contraindication to BMT (30, 31), but this view has been challenged (45). Serologic evidence of previous hepatitis B or C infection are not major risk factors for the subsequent development of VOD following BMT (45–47).

Another risk factor is intensity of the conditioning regimen, particularly use of multiple alkylating agents (33, 34). The European Group for Blood and Marrow Transplantation reports increased risk for VOD in individuals receiving busulfan/cyclophosphamide conditioning compared with individuals receiving cyclophosphamide/total-body irradiation (48). Variability in the dose and absorption of busulfan may account for discor-

**TABLE 49.1.** Diagnostic Criteria for VOD

| Seattle Criteria | Baltimore Criteria |
|---|---|
| *Two of the following:* | *Bilirubin > 2.0 mg/dL and 2 of the following:* |
| 1. Bilirubin > 1.5 mg/dL | 1. Hepatomegaly |
| 2. Hepatomegaly and right-upper-quadrant pain | 2. Ascites |
| 3. Ascites, unexplained weight gain > 5% from baseline, or both | 3. Unexplained weight gain > 5% from baseline |

dant findings when comparing busulfan/cyclophosphamide versus cyclophosphamide/total-body irradiation regimens. Busulfan dose schedules directed at lowering steady-state serum concentrations without decreasing the total dose may mitigate the risk of VOD from busulfan-containing preparative regimens (32). The hepatotoxicity of total-body irradiation, in contrast, decreases with a total dose of less than 12 Gy (33). Used as part of combination cytotoxic chemotherapy, unfractionated BCNU (carmustine) and busulfan are associated with increased risk of subsequent VOD compared with chemotherapy given in divided doses (31, 49). Avoiding simultaneous therapies probably diminishes the risk associated with preparative regimens containing multiple alkylating agents; however, this has not been demonstrated conclusively.

Other factors that have been associated with increased risk for VOD include age, female sex, amount of pretreatment before transplantation, pretransplant diagnosis, unrelated or mismatched donor, second transplants, cytomegalovirus seropositivity, and GVHD therapy, particularly cyclosporine (50, 51). The vascular toxicity of cyclosporine is well known, and in a retrospective analysis (52), individuals with aplastic anemia receiving cyclophosphamide without cyclosporine had a lower incidence of VOD than those receiving cyclosporine for GVHD prophylaxis. Patients receiving T-cell depletion therapy of the donor bone marrow also had a lower incidence of VOD, perhaps because of less intensive GVHD prophylaxis and treatment (53). Multivariate analyses, however, have not demonstrated an increased risk for allogeneic versus syngeneic or autologous transplantation (54).

## DIAGNOSIS

The diagnosis of hepatic VOD usually is made on the basis of clinical findings. Two sets of criteria have been developed for the clinical diagnosis of VOD (Table 49.1). McDonald et al (29) have applied a triad of clinical criteria, including:

1. Jaundice (bilirubin level, >1.5 mg/dL [27 mmole/l]),
2. Hepatomegaly and right-upper-quadrant pain, and

3. Ascites, and/or unexplained weight gain of more than 5% from baseline.

The presence of two of these criteria within 30 days of transplant, without other identifiable causes of liver dysfunction, establishes the diagnosis. Alternative criteria offered by Jones et al (3), however, may provide a more accurate method. The Jones criteria are a bilirubin level greater than 2 mg/dL (34 mmole/l) plus any two of the following:

1. Hepatomegaly,
2. Ascites, and
3. Weight gain of more than 5% from baseline.

Hyperbilirubinemia, although often associated with poor outcome, is not invariably associated with VOD (55); therefore, establishing the cause of an elevated bilirubin level is critical. A logistic regression analysis has been developed to predict the severity of VOD, but the model does not capture all individuals who develop severe VOD (56).

The diagnosis of hepatic VOD is not facilitated by any specific radiologic or radionuclide study. It also rarely is made on the basis of liver histology, because percutaneous liver biopsy at onset of the clinical syndrome usually is considered too risky. In addition, percutaneous needle biopsy of the liver may provide a specimen that is insufficient to establish the diagnosis of hepatic VOD; in one small series (30), the liver biopsy specimen was "inadequate to make a specific diagnosis" in 50% of individuals. Hepatic venous pressure measurements and transvenous liver biopsy, however, may be useful for establishing the diagnosis (57). The pathology of the liver is extremely specific, with biopsy specimens from individuals with clinical evidence of VOD almost always demonstrating concentric subendothelial thickening and fibrous luminal narrowing involving the sublobular and terminal hepatic veins.

Most individuals develop VOD within the first 30 days after BMT, and VOD is the most common cause of liver dysfunction that develops in this period. In one early series of 53 individuals (58), the mean intervals to the development of weight gain (49 individuals), hyperbilirubinemia (52 individuals), and ascites (27 individuals) were 6, 7, and 12 days, respectively. In another detailed analysis of 190 individuals (33), the mean time to onset of weight gain (>2%) and for hepatomegaly to occur was before the end of the first day after BMT. The differential diagnosis of hepatic VOD during the immediate post-BMT period is important for determining therapeutic options, and it includes drug injury, acute GVHD, fungal or viral infection, right-sided heart failure, total parenteral nutrition–associated fatty infiltration of the liver, acalculous cholecystitis, peritonitis, and pericardial effusion.

In the intermediate post-BMT period (i.e., 30–100 days), VOD is a less common cause of liver dysfunction. During this period, additional diagnostic considerations include acute GVHD, nodular regenerative hyperplasia, and viral or fungal infections (59). Liver dysfunction that develops in the late stage of BMT (i.e., >100 days) most often results from chronic GVHD. Other causes include viral diseases, chronic VOD, and drug-induced hepatitis. Any of these conditions may lead to chronic cholestasis (60). Chronic hepatic GVHD involves additional organ systems in at least 90% of individuals and usually can be identified. Liver biopsies can be performed safely during this phase, and they are particularly important for assessment of pathogenetic factors associated with poorer prognoses, such as chronic active hepatitis or cirrhosis. Late hepatic VOD is rare.

## PULMONARY VOD

Pulmonary VOD following BMT was first reported in 1984 (61). A child who received allogeneic BMT for acute lymphoblastic leukemia died 44 days later from respiratory failure. Pathologic examination showed eccentric intimal fibrosis of the pulmonary and interlobular veins, without intraluminal thrombosis. Another report described two pediatric individuals with pulmonary VOD following BMT that manifested by symptomatic pulmonary hypertension (36). In one, the pulmonary VOD was fatal; in the other, it responded to high-dose corticosteroid therapy.

Pulmonary VOD has been associated with administration of combination chemotherapy, single-agent nitrosourea therapy, combined chemotherapy and radiation therapy, autoimmune disorders, viral infections, and described as a familial syndrome (61–69). The pathogenesis of pulmonary VOD may relate to direct pulmonary venous endothelial cell toxicity from chemical, physical, or infectious agents. Pulmonary VOD is very rare following BMT, but it should be considered in individuals with clinical evidence of pulmonary hypertension, normal left atrial pressures, and no identifiable infectious cause of deteriorating lung function associated with radiographic abnormalities resembling those of adult respiratory distress syndrome. Diagnosis is made on the basis of an open-lung biopsy specimen.

## PATHOGENESIS

A large body of clinical and experimental data support the hypothesis that hepatic VOD results from direct hepatic venular endothelial cytotoxicity. The histopathologic localization of VOD within the liver results from an intrinsic property of central and pericentral venular regions of the liver, which renders them susceptible to pleiotropic chemical and physical agents. This susceptibility reflects the functional heterogeneity of the normal liver lobule. The pericentral region of the liver lobule is the primary site of microsomal biotransformation by the cytochrome P-450 system (70). Active metabolites of many drugs, including cyclophosphamide, epidophyllotoxins, nitrosoureas, and dacarbazine, concentrate in this zone; cyclophosphamide is perhaps the best studied. It is transformed by the microsomal cytochrome P-450 system of the liver to the active metabolite aldophosphamide, which then is oxidized to inactive compounds by other liver enzymes. Liver cell injury in the pericentral region of the lobule may selectively affect activity of the aldophosphamide-metabolizing enzymes, thus causing a buildup of toxic substrate. Histologic studies of animals receiving related compounds confirm this region is most vulnerable to drug injury (71, 72). Fatal human poisonings with pyrrolizidine alkaloids are accompanied by hepatic VOD, and liver microsomal biotransformation may result in generation of toxic pyrroles that interfere with RNA synthesis of the surrounding hepatocytes (73–75). The toxic effect of many compounds metabolized by the liver cytochrome P-450 system increases when generation of reduced thiols such as glutathione decreases, thereby demonstrating that toxicity involves generation of reactive oxygen species (76). Because hepatic veins are lined by a fenestrated endothelium without a basement membrane, they may be more susceptible to damage by toxins that reach their vicinity by diffusion as they move down the normal hepatic blood flow gradient.

The antimetabolites azathioprine, 6-mercaptopurine, and 6-thioguanine are metabolized primarily by liver xanthine oxidase. This metalloenzyme is localized to the centrilobular region of the liver, and its activity results in generation of superoxide anions. Anthracyclines potentiate the hepatotoxicity of the purine antimetabolites, presumably by enhancing lipid peroxidation. High-dose busulfan causes hepatic VOD associated with irregularly birefringent busulfan crystals in the centrilobular sinusoids of the diseased liver, thus suggesting a direct toxic effect of concentrated busulfan; as stated, monitoring busulfan blood levels and adjusting the dose may decrease hepatotoxicity and the incidence of VOD (77, 78). Cytosine arabinoside and methotrexate are indiscriminate hepatotoxins that predispose to VOD, particularly when given in high doses. Methotrexate-containing GVHD prophylaxis regimens and, in a similar manner, cyclosporine-containing GVHD prophylaxis regimens may increase the risk of hepatic VOD. Cyclosporine is metabolized by the cytochrome P-450 system of the liver to metabolites that are directly toxic to the vascular endothelium (79). Radiation therapy can lead to hepatic VOD, and the small hepatic vein radicles are vulnerable to irradiation derived from either x-rays or gamma rays. Hepatic venous injury occurs predictably in more than 50% of individuals within 30 days after delivery of a single dose of 1000 cGy or fractionated doses totaling approximately 3500 cGy (18).

The hypothesis that venous endothelial cell injury mediates VOD is supported by clinical studies demonstrating markers of endothelial injury after BMT. Plasma levels of von Willebrand factor and tissue-type plasminogen activator (t-PA) increase during the first 2 weeks after BMT, thereby suggesting the vascular endothelium actively secretes or leaks these proteins following BMT (80–82). In addition, von Willebrand factor (and fibrinogen) have been localized to the pores through which hepatic sinusoids empty into the terminal venules (83).

Several abnormalities in the coagulation cascade occur in individuals with VOD (84–90). Changes in the levels of protein S, protein C, antithrombin III, serum procollagen type III, plasminogen-activator inhibitor–1, and factor VII have been noted in individuals undergoing BMT. Changes such as decreased levels of the anticoagulant proteins antithrombin III and protein C suggest the possibility of a coagulation imbalance favoring thrombosis. Alternatively, low levels of these natural anticoagulant proteins simply may reflect decreased hepatic synthesis. Other investigators have found no correlation between coagulation protein levels and the incidence of VOD (91, 92). Gordon et al (93) found that as many as 25% of individuals have decreased levels of functional protein C after BMT because of incomplete gamma carboxylation, thus implying that thrombotic complications of BMT (including VOD) might result from disordered as well as decreased synthesis of liver-derived anticoagulant proteins.

There is indirect evidence that altered host immunity contributes to hepatic VOD, and that this may contribute to its development following BMT. Hepatic VOD has been associated with systemic lupus erythematosus and a familial deficiency of immunoglobulin A, thus suggesting that endothelial cell injury sometimes may involve regulatory T-cell dysfunction (94, 95). There also is indirect evidence that inflammatory cytokines participate in hepatic VOD after BMT (discussed later in this section), but the degree to which they are involved in the initiation of the lesion is not known. The striking fibrosis that develops within the lumen of the veins suggests that mitogens or fibrosis-inducing cytokines (e.g., platelet-derived growth factor, fibroblast growth factor, transforming growth factor β) participate in the pathologic response to the initial toxic insult. Elevated levels of transforming growth factor β early in autologous BMT have been associated with VOD and pulmonary toxicity (96).

## THERAPY

Standard therapy for VOD includes limiting excess volume and sodium intake, paracentesis of symptomatic ascites, and diuresis. Diuretics are used cautiously to avoid intravascular volume depletion, and red-blood-cell transfusions often are used to maintain intravascular volume, even in cases of mild anemia. Once significant liver failure develops in association with renal failure, however, the prognosis is poor, even with intensive clinical interventions such as hemofiltration. Liver transplantation has been attempted but is a limited therapeutic option (97–101). In addition, for allogeneic BMT individuals, the risk of graft rejection and relapse of the primary disease are concerns in individuals receiving allogeneic liver transplants. Both allogeneic and autologous BMT individuals have a risk for transplant-associated GVHD after allogeneic liver transplantation (101). Shunting procedures have been used for the treatment of VOD; transjugular intrahepatic shunting is less invasive and may have greater benefit than hepatorenal shunting (102, 103).

Several prophylaxis regimens against VOD have demonstrated variable success. Because of the possible role of excessive procoagulant activity in the pathogenesis of VOD, anticoagulants have been used to prevent development of VOD after BMT. Heparin infused at both standard and low doses showed no effect in one study (104). A second study (105), however, employing regular low-dose heparin (100 U/kg body weight per 24 hours) showed it to be quite useful, and hepatic VOD after allogeneic BMT was completely prevented by this treatment (none of 39 treated individuals versus seven of 38 untreated individuals). In a recent, small randomized study (10), low-molecular-weight heparin was effective in preventing VOD. The vasodilatory and platelet inhibitory agent prostaglandin $E_1$ ($PGE_1$) has been studied as a prophylactic agent (106–108). In one study (106), continuous-infusion $PGE_1$ was given pretransplant and continued until day 30 after allogeneic BMT, and VOD incidence was compared with that of historical controls. The actuarial incidence of VOD was 12.2% in the $PGE_1$ group and 25.5% in the control group, suggesting a benefit. $PGE_1$ toxicity (i.e., hypotension) is quite severe and in general limits its use (107). A recent preliminary study using both low-dose heparin and lower doses of $PGE_1$ demonstrated the efficacy of this combination (108).

Another early intervention for VOD is a thrombolytic agent such as recombinant t-PA, which has demonstrated efficacy in a small number of individuals with established VOD (109), prompting further clinical trials. Published results, however, have varied (110–116). Early therapy for suspected VOD with t-PA may be beneficial in preventing severe progressive disease, but the timing and dosages are not clearly defined—whereas the risk of bleeding in these individuals is established. Therapy with t-PA cannot be recommended at present outside the setting of a clinical trial. Recently, combined antithrombin III and t-PA treatment has been used successfully for VOD (117), and another novel treatment has been plasma exchange combined with t-PA (118). Defibrotide, which is a nucleotide derivative that modulates fibrinolysis, also is a potential therapeutic agent for established VOD (119).

Another approach to prevention and treatment of VOD is inhibition of oxidant-induced hepatic and endothelial cell damage caused by chemotherapeutic agents. Glutathione monoethyl ester, which readily diffuses into cells and raises intracellular glutathione levels, protected the livers of mice receiving high-dose chemotherapy (120). There was no pathologic evidence of VOD in control animals that died of liver disease, however, emphasizing the difficulty of analyzing a disease with no consistent animal model analogous to human VOD. One *in vitro* model demonstrates that hepatic endothelial cells are more sensitive than hepatocytes to the lethal effects of dacarbazine, and that this sensitivity is reversed by agents that increase intracellular glutathione levels (76). This suggests that agents which modulate the redox state of susceptible tissues may be beneficial.

Immune mechanisms also may be involved in pathogenesis of VOD (94–96). Consistent with this are reports describing successful use of azathioprine or prednisone in pulmonary VOD (121). Immune cytokines may be involved in pathogenesis of hepatic VOD. Inflammatory molecules such as tumor necrosis factor–$\alpha$, interleukin (IL)-1$\beta$, and soluble IL-2 receptor are elevated during inflammatory disorders associated with BMT, including VOD (122–125). To date, however, anti-inflammatory agents have not proved useful for prophylaxis (126–128).

Another novel approach to prevention of VOD has been use of ursodiol, which is a hydrophilic bile salt used to treat cholesterol gallstones, primary biliary cirrhosis, and chronic active hepatitis. A pilot study (129) has demonstrated that ursodiol prevents VOD following BMT. The mechanism of action for this is not known, but it may relate to its oxygen-scavenging properties or its effects on cholesterol metabolism.

# MICROANGIOPATHIC SYNDROMES (SEE CHAPTER 27)

Microangiopathic syndromes during BMT occur nearly exclusively in allogeneic BMT individuals, but a single case of a individual undergoing autologous BMT has been reported (130). Risk factors for microangiopathy include cyclosporine, total-body irradiation, and OKT3 antibody for the treatment of GVHD (131, 132). Endothelial damage from use of cyclosporine may result in the release of procoagulant factors and a resultant prothrombotic state, and use of cyclosporine is associated with two overlapping syndromes that develop after BMT.

The first is a fulminant illness similar to TTP and often associated with GVHD. This usually is present with renal failure associated with hemolysis and thrombocytopenia and, despite its clinical similarity to TTP, responds poorly to all therapeutic maneuvers, including plasma exchange (133). A rising lactate dehydrogenase level and schistocytes on the peripheral blood smear herald the onset of this syndrome. No specific therapeutic interventions, are predictably effective. Tacrolimus (FK506) may be substituted for cyclosporine with resolution of clinical hemolysis, thrombocytopenia, and renal insufficiency (134). This alternate regimen is not always successful, however, because FK506 also may cause microangiopathy. Experimental treatment approaches should be considered for this serious complication of BMT.

The second type of BMT-related microangiopathy is similar to HUS. It occurs late after BMT (i.e., 4–12 months) and is associated with total-body irradiation and cyclosporine (39). It usually is self-limited and manifested by hemolysis, renal insufficiency, and occasionally, thrombocytopenia. Patients often benefit from discontinuation of cyclosporine. Thrombocytopenia and hemolysis usually resolve completely, but some degree of chronic renal insufficiency may remain. The renal pathology of individuals who develop cyclosporine nephropathy consists of glomerular collapse, tubular atrophy, interstitial fibrosis, and thrombotic depositions in the glomeruli and arterioles, thereby demonstrating the endothelial toxicity associated with this agent (135). An animal model for HUS/TTP has been developed and may be useful for testing therapeutic maneuvers to prevent and treat these complications of allogeneic BMT (136). Several investigators have proposed classification and grading systems for HUS/TTP after BMT (137, 138) to standardize and measure the effectiveness of clinical interventions.

# BLEEDING AND THROMBOCYTOPENIA

Hemorrhage is a common complication of BMT because of the prolonged aplasia related to the preparative regimen. Prolonged thrombocytopenia is a significant problem, and there currently is no U.S. Food and Drug Administration–approved growth factor or cytokine that enhances platelet recovery (see Chapter 8). In individuals with petechiae or signs of mild bleeding such as oral mucosal hemorrhage, platelet transfusions maintain the platelet count at greater than 20,000 cells/$\mu$l. Single-donor platelet products are preferable to decrease the incidence of alloimmunization. In individuals with severe hemorrhage, an attempt should be made to maintain the platelet count at greater than 50,000 cells/μl. In individuals without evidence of spontaneous hemorrhage, platelet transfusions can be used judiciously to maintain the platelet count at a lower level, which usually is physician or institution defined and often in the range of 10,000 to 20,000 cells/μl (139). HLA-matched platelets may be used in individuals who do not respond to single-donor platelet transfusions. As with all blood products, platelet transfusions must be irradiated to prevent transfusion-associated GVHD in allogeneic BMT recipients.

Intensive chemotherapy also may cause acquired platelet functional defects that occur before development of thrombocytopenia (140). It is uncertain, however, whether these defects are clinically significant.

Mucosal hemorrhage should be evaluated carefully, because mucositis can be severe after BMT conditioning. Mucositis after BMT usually is self-limited with supportive care, and severe bleeding because of mucositis is unusual unless the individual has profound thrombocytopenia unresponsive to platelet transfusions. Most episodes of gastrointestinal bleeding relate to an anatomic lesion, such as a gastric ulcer or an intestinal polyp, this is unmasked by thrombocytopenia. In allogeneic BMT recipients, cytomegalovirus enterocolitis and intestinal GVHD can cause life-threatening hemorrhage requiring surgical intervention. Epistaxis often occurs during the immediate posttransplant period, even when the platelet count is greater than 20,000 cells/μl. This may result in part from the lack of atmospheric humidity in a laminar flow or high-exchange, filtered-air environment. Local care prevents this type of bleeding, which can be severe enough to require nasal packing and topical vasoconstriction along with platelet transfusions. Antifibrinolytic agents such as ε-aminocaproic acid or tranexamic acid have been used occasionally in individuals with severe refractory thrombocytopenia and bleeding, but they should be avoided in individuals with hematuria. In individuals with severe alloimmunization, high-dose intravenous immunoglobulin G therapy may enhance the survival of transfused platelets.

Platelet recovery usually occurs 10 to 28 days after stem-cell or marrow infusion. Autologous recovery can be delayed for months in heavily pretreated individuals, however, or after *in vitro* chemotherapeutic purging of autologous bone marrow with agents such as 4-hydroperoxycyclophosphamide. Chronic thrombocytopenia associated with chronic GVHD is considered to be an indicator of an unfavorable prognosis (141).

# COAGULOPATHY

Coagulation abnormalities manifested by an elevated prothrombin time (PT), activated partial thromboplastin time (aPTT), and thrombin time are seen in individuals with severe VOD or GVHD. This type of coagulopathy often is a premorbid event related to liver failure complicating multiorgan failure. Plasma infusions have a temporary benefit. Deficiencies of factors VII, X, XII, and of protein C have been reported in a series of autologous BMT individuals (142) and may be secondary to endothelial cell damage and coagulation factor consumption, liver dysfunction, or both. An isolated elevated PT may represent vitamin K deficiency secondary to bowel "rest" and broad-spectrum antibacterial antibiotics (see Chapter 45), and parenteral vitamin K should be administered routinely in this setting. If a coagulation profile is obtained from the catheter, an elevated aPTT may result from residual heparin in the line.

# HEMORRHAGIC CYSTITIS

Hemorrhagic cystitis is a complication of high-dose cyclophosphamide or ifosfamide therapy (143–146). It usually occurs within the first 2 months after transplantation, and it manifests by hematuria, bladder pain, and dysuria. Severe hemorrhagic cystitis may result in intractable bleeding, clot formation, urinary obstruction, and renal failure. Other risk factors include busulfan as part of the conditioning regimen, younger age, allogeneic BMT, and viruria (145–154). Viruria, in particular the polyoma virus JK or adenoviruses, predisposes to hemorrhagic cystitis despite preventive measures such as forced diuresis or uroprotection with the drug mesna (154). Therapeutic approaches consist of prophylaxis against hemorrhagic cystitis and treatment of established disease.

Standard prophylaxis consists of continuous bladder irrigation (CBI), forced diuresis, mesna administration, or some combination during cyclophosphamide treatment (151–161). For adults, forced diuresis generally consists of vigorous intravenous hydration of 6 to 8 l/day in conjunction with diuretic administration to maintain urine output. CBI involves placement of a three-way bladder catheter and CBI. There is some controversy regarding the efficacy of CBI alone as prophylaxis (160, 161). In addition, individual acceptance of bladder catheterization and irrigation is low; most prefer forced diuresis or mesna. For prophylaxis against hemorrhagic cystitis, treatment with mesna is equivalent to forced diuresis and to CBI in two large studies (157, 158).

Despite these maneuvers, as many as 25% of individuals receiving high-dose cyclophosphamide will develop hemorrhagic cystitis, and between 1 and 5% will have hemorrhagic cystitis complicated by severe dysuria, clot formation, and urinary blockage (145, 154). Diagnostic procedures include urine viral culture and urinalysis. Ultrasonography of the bladder is useful for indirect assessment of bladder pathology (162), and cystoscopy may be necessary for fulguration of localized lesions to control bleeding. Initial treatment consists of hyperhydration and diuresis along with blood-product administration. CBI may be necessary in individuals with large clot formation and danger of obstruction. Instillation of alum or formalin may be required in individuals with uncontrollable hemorrhagic cystitis (143, 144). Life-threatening disease may be controlled by cystectomy or suprapubic cystotomy (163). Prostaglandins have been used for treatment and may allow control of bleeding without surgical intervention (164), and there are case reports of hemorrhagic cystitis associated with adenovirus and polyoma virus responding to ribavirin therapy (167, 168).

# PULMONARY HEMORRHAGE

Interstitial pneumonitis is a complication of autologous and allogeneic BMT. Interstitial pneumonitis resulting from an infectious cause, such as a viral, fungal, and bacterial pathogen, often was the case during the formative years of BMT, before the newer antiviral and antifungal agents became available. The diagnosis often was made on the basis of bronchoalveolar lavage (BAL) or lung biopsy (169–172). Some of these individuals had a hemorrhagic BAL that was although to be secondary to thrombocytopenia or some other unknown cause.

The syndrome of diffuse alveolar hemorrhage (DAH) was defined as a distinct interstitial pneumonitis by Robbins et al (173). DAH is an inflammatory complication of the lung that develops 7 to 28 days after BMT and is characterized by a hemorrhagic and inflammatory BAL (174). It manifests as an asymptomatic decrease in oxygen saturation, followed by an increase in the respiratory rate, progressive dyspnea, and cough. Diffuse infiltrates and consolidation are observed on chest radiographs. Risk factors include fever, older age, BMT for solid tumor, and neutrophil recovery (173), and the latter risk factor suggests that a "cytokine-release syndrome" may be associated with the DAH. One recent report (175) noted an association between microangiopathy and DAH, suggesting that endothelial cell damage may be a common pathogenetic factor. Herpes-virus or cytomegalovirus may predispose to development of this syndrome (176, 177).

The incidence of DAH approaches 7% following either allogeneic or autologous BMT, and it is associated with a high mortality rate (~50%). High-dose corticosteroid therapy may be effective in some of these individuals, and DDAVP (desmopressin) as well as antifibrinolytic agents given with high-dose corticosteroids may be beneficial if started early in the disorder (178, 179).

# CONCLUSION

A variety of hemorrhagic and thrombotic complications occur following BMT, and recent discoveries place us on the verge of effective control for many of them. With development of growth factors to enhance the platelet recovery, the time period of hemorrhagic complications resulting from thrombocytopenia may be shortened. Cytokines or drugs that decrease or modulate the toxic effects of chemotherapy and radiation therapy may be beneficial in preventing or treating many of these disorders as well. Less well understood, however, is the role of endothelial cells and the plasma coagulation system in the pathogenesis of BMT-related coagulation disturbances. Further work is required to establish whether endothelial cell damage, coagulation abnormalities, or both are pathophysiologically significant disorders or clinically irrelevant epiphenomena. Distinguishing their importance should elucidate the pathogenic mechanisms of BMT-related hemorrhage and thrombosis and, perhaps, lead to new therapeutic approaches.

# REFERENCES

1. Forman SJ, Blume KG, Thomas ED, eds. Bone marrow transplantation. 1st ed. Boston: Blackwell Scientific Publications, 1994.
2. Atkinson K, ed. Clinical bone marrow transplantation. 1st ed. Cambridge: Cambridge University Press, 1995:1–9.
3. Armitage JO, Antman KH, eds. High-dose cancer therapy: pharmacology, hematopoietins, stem cells. 2nd ed. Baltimore: Williams & Wilkins, 1995.
4. Broviac J, Cole JJ, Schribner BH. A silicone rubber atrial catheter for prolonged parenteral alimentation. Surg Gynecol Obstet 1973;136:602–606.
5. Hickman RO, Buckner CD, Clift RA et al. A modified right atrial catheter for access to the venous system in marrow transplant recipients. Surg Gynecol Obstet 1979;148:871–875.
6. Haire WD. Hickman line management. In: Armitage JO, Antman KH, eds. High-dose cancer therapy: pharmacology, hematopoietins, stem cells. 2nd ed. Baltimore: Williams & Wilkins, 1995:461–480.
7. Rama BN, Haake RE, Bander SJ et al. Heparin-flush associated thrombocytopenia-induced hemorrhage: a case report. Nebr Med J 1991;76:392–394.
8. Garrelts JC, LaRocca J, Ast D et al. Comparison of heparin and 0.9% sodium chloride injection in the maintenance of indwelling intermittent i.v. devices. Clinical Pharmacology 1989;8:34–39.
9. Bern MM, Lokich JJ, Wallach SR et al. Very low doses of warfarin can prevent thrombosis in central venous catheters. A randomized prospective trial. Ann Intern Med 1990;112:423–428.
10. Or R, Nagler A, Shpilberg O et al. Low-molecular-weight heparin for the prevention of veno-occlusive disease of the liver in bone marrow transplantation individuals. Transplantation 1996;61:1067–1071.
11. Press OW, Ramsey PG, Larson EB et al. Hickman catheter infections in individuals with malignancies. Medicine 1984;63:189–200.
12. Raaf JH. Vascular access prostheses in the management of cancer individuals. Clin Bull (MSK Cancer Center) 1980;10:91–101.
13. Stephens LC, Haire WD, Schmidt-Pokorny K et al. Granulocyte macrophage colony-stimulating factor: high incidence of apheresis catheter thrombosis during peripheral stem cell collection. Bone Marrow Transplant 1993;11:51–54.
14. Hess AF. Fatal obliterative endophlebitis of the hepatic veins. Am J Med Sci 1905;130:986–1001.
15. Selzer G, Parker RGF. Senecio poisoning exhibiting as Chiari's syndrome. Am J Pathol 1951;27:885–907.
16. Bras G, Jelliffe DB, Stuart KL. Veno-occlusive disease of the liver with non-portal type of cirrhosis, occurring in Jamaica. Arch Pathol 1954;57: 285–300.
17. Clark PA, Hsia YE, Huntsman RG. Toxic complications of treatment with 6-mercaptopurine: 2 cases with hepatic necrosis and interstitial ulceration. Br Med J 1960;1:393–395.
18. Reed GB Jr, Cox AJ Jr. The human liver after radiation injury. A form of veno-occlusive disease. Am J Pathol 1966;48:597–611.

19. Fajardo LF, Colby TV. Pathogenesis of veno-occlusive liver disease after radiation. Arch Pathol Lab Med 1980;104:584–588.
20. Marubbio AT, Danielson B. Hepatic venocclusive disease in a renal transplant individual receiving azathioprine. Gastroenterology 1975;69:739–743.
21. Griner PF, Elbadawi A, Packman CH. Veno-occlusive disease of the liver after chemotherapy of acute leukemia. A report of two cases. Ann Intern Med 1976;85:578–582.
22. Erichsen C, Jonsson PE. Veno-occlusive liver disease after dacarbazine therapy for melanoma. J Surg Oncol 1984;27:268–270.
23. Penta JS, VonHoff DD, Muggia FM. Hepatotoxicity of combination chemotherapy for acute myelocytic leukemia. Ann Intern Med 1977;87:247–248.
24. Jacobs P, Miller JL, Uys CJ et al. Fatal veno-occlusive of the liver after chemotherapy, whole body irradiation, and bone marrow transplantation for refractory acute leukemia. S Afr Med J 1979;55:5–10.
25. Berk PD, Popper H, Krueger GR et al. Veno-occlusive disease of the liver after bone marrow transplantation: a possible association with graft-versus-host disease. Ann Intern Med 1979;90:158–164.
26. Woods WG, Dehner LP, Nesbit ME et al. Fatal veno-occlusive disease of the liver following high dose chemotherapy, irradiation and bone marrow transplantation. Am J Med 1980;68:285–290.
27. Shulman HM, McDonald GB, Matthews D et al. An analysis of hepatic venocclusive disease and centrilobular hepatic degeneration following bone marrow transplantation. Gastroenterology 1980;79:1178–1191.
28. D'Cruz CA, Wimmer RS, Harcke HT et al. Veno-occlusive disease of the liver in children following chemotherapy for acute myelocytic leukemia. Cancer 1983;52:1803–1807.
29. McDonald GB, Sharma P, Matthews DE et al. Venocclusive disease of the liver after bone marrow transplantation: diagnosis, incidence, and predisposing factors. Hepatology 1984;4:116–122.
30. Jones RJ, Lee KSK, Beschorner WE et al. Venoocclusive disease of the liver following bone marrow transplantation. Transplantation 1987;44:778–783.
31. Ayash LJ, Hunt M, Antman K et al. Hepatic venoocclusive disease in autologous bone marrow transplantation of solid tumors and lymphomas. J Clin Oncol 1990;8:1699–1706.
32. Shulman HM, Hinterberger W. Hepatic veno-occlusive disease—liver toxicity syndrome after bone marrow transplantation. Bone Marrow Transplant 1992;10:197–214.
33. McDonald GB, Hinds MS, Fisher LD et al. Veno-occlusive disease of the liver and multiorgan failure after bone marrow transplantation: a cohort study of 355 individuals. Ann Intern Med 1993;118:255–267.
34. Bearman SI. The syndrome of hepatic veno-occlusive disease after marrow transplantation. Blood 1995;85:3005–3020.
35. Gluckman E. Veno-occlusive disease. In: Atkinson K, ed. Clinical bone marrow transplantation. 1st ed. Cambridge: Cambridge University Press, 1995:356–359.
36. Hackman RC, Madtes DK, Petersen FB et al. Pulmonary venoocclusive disease following bone marrow transplantation. Transplantation 1989;47:989–992.
37. Bernauer W, Gratwohl A, Keller A et al. Microvasculopathy in the ocular fundus after bone marrow transplantation. Ann Intern Med 1991;115:925–930.
38. Holler E, Kolb HJ, Hiller E et al. Microangiopathy in individuals on cyclosporine prohylaxis who developed acute graft-versus-host disease after HLA-identical bone marrow transplantation. Blood 1989;73:2018–2024.
39. Chappell ME, Keeling DM, Prentice HG et al. Haemolytic uremic syndrome after bone marrow transplantation: an adverse effect of total body irradiation? Bone Marrow Transplant 1988;3:339–347.
40. Schriber JR, Herzig GP. Transplantation-associated thrombotic thrombocytopenic purpura and hemolytic uremic syndrome. Semin Hematol 1997;34:1–6.
41. Rappaport AM, Knoblauch M, Zelin S et al. Experimental hepatic veno-occlusive disease. *In vivo* microcirculatory study. Adv Microcirc 1969;2:69–79.
42. Beschorner WE, Pino J, Boitnott JK et al. Pathology of the liver with bone marrow transplantation. Am J Pathol 1980;99:369–385.
43. Snover DC, Weisdorf SA, Ramsay NK et al. Hepatic graft versus host disease: a study of the predictive value of liver biopsy in diagnosis. Hepatology 1984;4:123–130.
44. Shulman HM, Fisher LB, Schoch HG et al. Veno-occlusive disease of the liver after marrow transplantation: histological correlates of clinical signs and symptoms. Hepatology 1994;19:1171–1181.
45. Locasciulli A, Bacigalupo A, Alberti A et al. Predictability before transplant of hepatic complications following allogeneic bone marrow transplantation. Transplantation 1989;48:68–72.
46. Locasciulli A, Bacigalupo A, VanLint MT et al. Hepatitis B virus infection and liver disease after allogeneic bone marrow transplantation: a report of 30 cases. Bone Marrow Transplant 1990;6:25–29.
47. Locasciulli A, Bacigalupo A, VanLint MT et al. Hepatitis C virus infection in individuals undergoing allogeneic bone marrow transplantation. Transplantation 1991;52:315–318.
48. Ringden O, Labopin M, Tura S et al. A comparison of busulphan versus total body irradiation combined with cyclophosphamide as conditioning for autograft or allograft bone marrow transplantation in individuals with acute leukaemia. Acute Leukemia Working Party of the European Group for Blood and Marrow Transplantation. Br J Haematol 1996;93:637–645.
49. Meresse V, Hartmann O, Vassal G et al. Risk factors for hepatic veno-occlusive disease after high-dose busulfan-containing regimens followed by autologous bone marrow transplantation: a study in 136 children. Bone Marrow Transplant 1992;10:135–141.
50. Shuhart MC, McDonald GB. Gastrointestinal and hepatic complications. In: Forman SJ, Blume KG, Thomas ED, eds. Bone marrow transplantation. 1st ed. Boston: Blackwell Scientific Publications, 1994:454–481.
51. Ayash LJ. Hepatic complications of bone marrow transplantation. In: Armitage JO, Antman KH, eds. High-dose cancer therapy: pharmacology, hematopoietics, stem cells. 2nd ed. Baltimore: Williams & Wilkins, 1995:543–562.
52. Deeg HJ, Shulman HM, Schmidt E et al. Marrow graft rejection and veno-occlusive disease of the liver in individuals with aplastic anemia conditioned with cyclophosphamide and cyclosporine. Transplantation 1986;42:497–501.
53. Soiffer RJ, Dear K, Rabinowe SN et al. Hepatic dysfunction following T-cell-depleted allogeneic bone marrow transplantation. Transplantation 1991;52:1014–1019.
54. Rozman C, Carreras E, Qian C et al. Risk factors for hepatic veno-occlusive disease following HLA-identical sibling bone marrow transplants for leukemia. Bone Marrow Transplant 1996;17:75–80.
55. Cunningham I, Marmaduke D, Copelan E et al. Hyperbilirubinemia as a predictor of post-BMT mortality [Abstract]. Blood 1991;78:949A.
56. Bearman SI, Anderson GL, Mori M et al. Venocclusive disease of the liver: development of a model for predicting fatal outcome after marrow transplantation. J Clin Oncol 1993;9:1729–1736.
57. Shulman HM, Gooley T, Dudley MD et al. Utility of transvenous liver biopsies and wedged hepatic venous pressure measurements in sixty marrow transplant recipients. Transplantation 1995;59:1015–1022.
58. McDonald GB, Sharma P, Matthews DE et al. The clinical course of 53 individuals with venocclusive disease of the liver after marrow transplantation. Transplantation 1985;39:603–608.
59. Snover DC, Weisdorf S, Bloomer J et al. Nodular regenerative hyperplasia of the liver following bone marrow transplantation. Hepatology 1989;9:443–448.
60. Bertheau P, Hadengue A, Cazals-Hatem D et al. Chronic cholestasis in individuals after allogeneic bone marrow transplantation: several diseases are often associated. Bone Marrow Transplant 1995;16:261–265.
61. Troussard X, Bernaudin JF, Cordonnier C et al. Pulmonary veno-occlusive disease after bone marrow transplantation. Thorax 1984;39:956–957.
62. Williams LM, Fussell S, Veith RW et al. Pulmonary veno-occlusive disease in an adult following bone marrow transplantation. Case report and Review of the literature. Chest 1996;109:1388–1391.
63. Joselson R, Warnock M. Pulmonary veno-occlusive disease after chemotherapy. Hum Pathol 1983;14:88–91.
64. Knight BK, Rose AG. Pulmonary veno-occlusive disease after chemotherapy. Thorax 1985;40:874–875.
65. Lombard CM, Churg A, Winokur S. Pulmonary veno-occlusive disease following therapy for malignant neoplasms. Chest 1987;92:871–876.
66. Liang MH, Stern S, Fortin PR et al. Fatal pulmonary veno-occlusive disease secondary to a generalized venulopathy: a new syndrome presenting with facial swelling and pericardial tamponade. Arthritis Rheum 1991;34:228–233.
67. Heath D, Scott O, Lynch J. Pulmonary veno-occlusive disease. Thorax 1971;26:663–674.
68. Voordes CG, Kuipers JRG, Elema JD. Familial pulmonary veno-occlusive disease: a case report. Thorax 1977;32:763–766.
69. Wagenvoort CA. Pulmonary veno-occlusive disease. Entity or syndrome? Chest 1976;69:82–86.
70. Willson RA, Hart JR. In vivo drug metabolism and liver lobule heterogeneity in the rat. Gastroenterology 1981;81:563–569.
71. Ungar H. Venoocclusive disease of the liver and phlebectatic peliosis in the golden hamster exposed to dimethylnitrosamine. Pathol Res Pract 1986;181:180–187.
72. Shulman HM, Luk K, Deeg HJ et al. Induction of hepatic veno-occlusive disease in dogs. Am J Pathol 1987;126:114–125.
73. Feigen M. Fatal veno-occlusive disease of the liver associated with herbal tea consumption and radiation. Aust N Z J Med 1984;14:61–62.
74. Ridker PM, Ohkuma S, McDermott WV et al. Hepatic venooclusive disease associated with the consumption of pyrrolizidine-containing dietary supplements. Gastroenterology 1985;88:1050–1054.
75. Mattocks AR. Toxicity of pyrrolizidine alkaloids. Nature 1968;217:723–728.
76. De Leve LD, Wang X, Kuhlenkamp JF et al. Toxicity of azathioprine and monocrotaline in murine sinusoidal endothelial cells and hepatocytes: the role of glutathione and relevance to hepatic venoocclusive disease. Hepatology 1996;23:589–599.
77. Grochow LB, Jones RJ, Brundett RB et al. Pharmacokinetics of busulfan: correlation with veno-occlusive disease in individuals undergoing bone marrow transplantation. Cancer Chemother Pharmacol 1989;25:55–61.

78. Grochow LB. Busulfan disposition: the role of therapeutic monitoring in bone marrow transplantation induction regimens. Semin Oncol 1993; 20(Suppl 4):18–25.

79. Kahan BD. Cyclosporine. N Engl J Med 1989;321:1725–1738.

80. Gordon B, Haire W, Kessinger A et al. High frequency of antithrombin III and protein C deficiency following autologous bone marrow transplantation for lymphoma. Bone Marrow Transplant 1991;8:497–502.

81. Scrobohaci ML, Drouet L, Baudin B. Hemostasis tests as markers of hepatic and endothelial toxicity in chemotherapy. Nouv Rev Franc D Hematol 1988;30:109–114.

82. Tsakiris DA, Huser B, Gratwohl A et al. Tendency to thrombosis following bone marrow transplantation? J Suisse Med 1991;121:341–343.

83. Shulman HM, Gown AM, Nugent DJ. Hepatic veno-occlusive disease after bone marrow transplantation. Immunohistochemical identification of the material within occluded central venules. Am J Pathol 1987;127:549–558.

84. Harper PL, Jarvis J, Jennings I et al. Changes in the natural anticoagulants following bone marrow transplantation. Bone Marrow Transplant 1990;5: 39–42.

85. Gordon B, Haire W, Dessinger A et al. High frequency of antithrombin 3 and protein C deficiency following autologous bone marrow transplantation for lymphoma. Bone Marrow Transplant 1991;8:497–502.

86. Scrobohaci ML, Drouet L, Monem-Mansi A et al. Liver veno-occlusive disease after bone marrow transplantation changes in coagulation parameters and endothelial markers. Thromb Res 1991;63:509–519.

87. Heikinheimo M, Halila R, Fasth A. Serum procollagen type III is an early and sensitive marker for veno-occlusive disease of the liver in children undergoing bone marrow transplantation. Blood 1994;83:3036–3040.

88. Eltumi M, Trivedi P, Hobbs JR et al. Monitoring of veno-occlusive disease after bone marrow transplantation by serum aminopropeptide of type III procollagen. Lancet 1993;342:518–521.

89. Salat C, Holler E. Reinhardt B et al. Parameters of the fibrinolytic system in individuals undergoing BMT: elevation of PAI-1 in veno-occlusive disease. Bone Marrow Transplant 1994;14:747–750.

90. Faioni EM, Krachmalnicoff A, Bearman SI et al. Naturally occurring anticoagulants and bone marrow transplantation: plasma protein C predicts the development of venocclusive disease of the liver. Blood 1993;81: 3458–3462.

91. Collins P, Roderick A, O'Brien D et al. Factor VIIa and other haemostatic variables following bone marrow transplantation. Thromb Haemost 1994; 72:28–32.

92. Catani L, Gugliotta L, Mattioli Belmonte M et al. Hypercoagulability in individuals undergoing autologous or allogeneic BMT for hematological malignancies. Bone Marrow Transplant 1993;12:253–259.

93. Gordon B, Haire W, Ruby E et al. Prolonged deficiency of protein C following hematopoietic stem cell transplantation. Bone Marrow Transplant 1996; 17:415–419.

94. Pappas SC, Malone DG, Rabin L et al. Hepatic venoocclusive disease in a individual with systemic lupus erythematosis. Arthritis Rheum 1984;27: 104–108.

95. Mellis C, Bale P. Familial hepatic venoocclusive disease with probable immune deficiency. J Pediatr 1976;88:236–242.

96. Murase T, Anscher MS, Petros WP et al. Changes in plasma transforming growth factor beta in response to high-dose chemotherapy for stage II breast cancer: possible implications for the prevention of hepatic venoocclusive disease and pulmonary drug toxicity. Bone Marrow Transplant 1995;15:173–178.

97. Nimer SD, Milewicz AL, Champlin RE et al. Successful treatment of hepatic venoocclusive disease in a bone marrow transplant individual with orthotopic liver transplantation. Transplantation 1990;49:819–821.

98. Rapoport AP, Doyle HR, Starzl T et al. Orthotopic liver transplantation for life-threatening veno-occlusive disease of the liver after allogeneic bone marrow transplant. Bone Marrow Transplant 1991;8:421–424.

99. Bunin N, Leahey A, Dunn S. Related donor liver transplant for veno-occlusive disease following T-depleted unrelated donor bone marrow transplantation. Transplantation 1996;27:664–666.

100. Hagglund H, Ringden O, Ericzon BG et al. Treatment of hepatic venoocclusive disease with recombinant human tissue plasminogen activator or orthotopic liver transplantation after allogeneic bone marrow transplantation. Transplantation 1996;62:1076–1080.

101. Schlitt HJ, Tischler HJ, Ringe B et al. Allogeneic liver transplantation for hepatic veno-occlusive disease after bone marrow transplantation-clinical and immunological considerations. Bone Marrow Transplant 1995;16: 473–478.

102. Michielsen PP, Pelckmans PA, d'Archambeau OC et al. Transjugular intrahepatic portosystemic shunt improves liver function in veno-occlusive disease. J Hepatol 1994;21:685–686.

103. Fried MW, Connaghan DG, Sharma S et al. Transjugular intrahepatic portosystemic shunt for the management of severe venoocclusive disease following bone marrow transplantation. Hepatology 1996;24:588–591.

104. Bearman SI, Hinds MS, Wolford JL et al. A pilot study of continuous infusion heparin for the prevention of hepatic veno-occlusive disease after bone marrow transplantation. Bone Marrow Transplant 1990;5:407–411.

105. Attal M, Huguet F, Rubie H et al. Prevention of hepatic veno-occlusive disease after bone marrow transplantation by continuous infusion of low-dose heparin: a prospective, randomized trial. Blood 1992;79:2834–2840.

106. Gluckman E, Jolivet I, Scrobohaci ML et al. Use of prostaglandin E1 for prevention of liver veno-occlusive disease in leukaemic individuals treated by allogeneic bone marrow transplantation. Br J Haematol 1990; 74:277–281.

107. Bearman SI, Shen DD, Hinds MS et al. A phase I/II study of prostaglandin E1 for the prevention of hepatic venocclusive disease after bone marrow transplantation. Br J Haematol 1993;84:724–730.

108. Schriber JR, Milk BJ, Baer MR et al. A randomized phase II trial comparing heparin (Hep) ± prostaglandin E1 (PG) to prevent hepatotoxicity following bone marrow transplantation: preliminary results [Abstract]. Blood 1996;88:413A.

109. Baglin TP, Harper P, Marcus RE. Veno-occlusive disease of the liver complicating ABMT successfully treated with recombinant tissue plasminogen activator (rt-PA). Bone Marrow Transplant 1990;5:439–441.

110. Bearman SI, Shuhart MC, Hinds MS et al. Recombinant human tissue plasminogen activator for the treatment of established severe venocclusive disease of the liver after bone marrow transplantation. Blood 1992;80: 2458–2462.

111. Laporte JP, Lesage S, Tilleul P et al. Alteplase for hepatic veno-occlusive disease complicating bone marrow transplantation. Lancet 1992;339:1057.

112. Rosti G, Bandini G, Belardinelli A et al. Alteplase for hepatic veno-occlusive disease after bone marrow transplantation. Lancet 1992;339: 1481–1482.

113. Ringden O, Wennberg L, Ericzon BG et al. Alteplase for hepatic veno-occlusive disease after bone marrow transplantation. Lancet 1992;340: 546–547.

114. Yu LC, Malkani I, Regueira O et al. Recombinant tissue plasminogen activator (rt-PA) for veno-occlusive liver disease in pediatric autologous bone marrow transplant individuals. Am J Hematol 1994;46:194–198.

115. Hagglund H, Ringden O, Ljungman P et al. No beneficial effects, but severe side effects caused by recombinant human tissue plasminogen activator for treatment of hepatitic veno-occlusive disease after allogeneic bone marrow transplantation. Transplant Proc 1995;27:3535.

116. Bearman SI, Jung LL, Baron AE et al. Treatment of hepatic venocclusive disease with recombinant human tisue plasminogen activator and heparin in 42 marrow transplant individuals. Blood 1997;89:1501–1506.

117. Patton DF, Harper JL, Wooldridge TN et al. Treatment of veno-occlusive disease of the liver with bolus tissue plasminogen activator and continuous infusion antithrombin III concentrate. Bone Marrow Transplant 1996; 17:443–447.

118. Espigado I, Rodriguez JM, Parody R et al. Reversal of severe hepatic veno-occlusive disease by combined plasma exchange and rt-PA treatment. Bone Marrow Transplant 1995;16:313–316.

119. Richardson P, Krishnan A, Wheeler C et al. The use of defibrotide in BMT-associated veno-occlusive disease. Blood 1995;86:221A.

120. Teicher BA, Crawford JM, Holden SA et al. Glutathione monoethyl ester can selectively protect liver from high dose BCNU or cyclophosphamide. Cancer 1988;62:1275–1281.

121. Sanderson JE, Spiro SG, Hendry AT et al. A case of pulmonary veno-occlusive disease responding to treatment with azathioprine. Thorax 1977; 32:140–148.

122. Holler E, Kolb HJ, Moller A et al. Increased serum levels of tumor necrosis factor alpha precede major complications of bone marrow transplantation. Blood 1990;75:1011–1016.

123. Tanaka J, Imamura M, Kasai M et al. Cytokine gene expression in peripheral blood mononuclear cells during graft-versus-host disease after allogeneic bone marrow transplantation. Br J Haematol 1993;85:558–565.

124. Castenskiold EC, Kelsey SM, Collins PW et al. Functional hyperactivity of monocytes after bone marrow transplantation: possible relevance for the development of post-transplant complications or relapse. Bone Marrow Transplant 1995;15:879–884.

125. Remberger M, Ringden O. Increased levels of soluble interleukin-2 receptor in veno-occlusive disease of the liver after allogenic bone marrow transplantation. Transplantation 1995;60:1293–1299.

126. Attal M, Huguet F, Rubie H et al. Prevention of regimen-related toxicities after bone marrow transplantation by pentoxifylline: a prospective, randomized trial. Blood 1993;82:732–736.

127. Clift RA, Bianco JA, Appelbaum FR et al. A randomized controlled trial of pentoxifylline for the prevention of regimen-related toxicities in individuals undergoing allogeneic marrow transplantation. Blood 1993;82: 2025–2030.

128. Clarke E, Rice GC, Weeks RS et al. Lisofylline inhibits transforming growth facor beta release and enhances trilineage hematopoietic recovery after 5-fluorouracil treatment in mice. Cancer Res 1996;56:105–112.

129. Essell JH, Thompson JM, Harman GS et al. Pilot trial of prophylactic ursodiol to decrease the incidence of veno-occlusive disease of the liver in allogeneic bone marrow transplant individuals. Bone Marrow Transplant 1992; 10:367–372.

130. Wassmann B, Martin H, Elsner S et al. Microangiopathic hemolytic anemia and renal impairment following autologous bone marrow transplantation:

a case of hemolytic uremic syndrome? Bone Marrow Transplant 1994;14:849–851.

131. Kalhs P, Brugger S, Schwarzinger I et al. Microangiopathy following allogeneic marrow transplantation. Association with cyclosporine and methylprednisolone for graft-versus-host disease prophylaxis. Transplantation 1995;60:949–957.

132. Gleixner B, Kolb HJ, Holler E et al. Treatment of aGVHD with OKT3: clinical outcome and side-effects associated with release of TNF alpha. Bone Marrow Transplant 1991;8:93–98.

133. Sarode R, McFarland JG, Flomenberg N et al. Therapeutic plasma exchange does not appear to be effective in the management of thrombotic thrombocytopenic purpura hemolytic uremic syndrome following bone marrow transplantation. Bone Marrow Transplant 1995;16:271–275.

134. McCauley J, Bronsther O, Fung J et al. Treatment of cyclosporin-induced haemolytic uraemic syndrome with FK506. Lancet 1989;ii:1516.

135. Nizze H, Mihatsch MJ, Zollinger HU et al. Cyclosporine-associated nephropathy in individuals with heart and bone marrow transplants. Clin Nephrol 1988;30:248–260.

136. Hillyer CD, Duncan A, Ledford M et al. Chemotherapy-induced hemolytic uremic syndrome—description of a potential animal model. J Med Primatol 1995;24:68–73.

137. Zeigler ZR, Shadduck RK, Nemunaitis J et al. Bone marrow transplant-associated thrombotic microangiopathy: a case series. Bone Marrow Transplant 1995;15:247–253.

138. Pettitt AR, Clark RE. Thrombotic microangiopathy following bone marrow transplantation. Bone Marrow Transplant 1994;14:495–504.

139. Beutler E. Platelet transfusions: the 20,000/1 trigger. Blood 1993;81:1411–1413.

140. Panella TJ, Peters W, White JG et al. Platelets acquire a secretion defect after high-dose chemotherapy. Cancer 1990;65:1711–1716.

141. First LR, Smith BR, Lipton J et al. Isolated thrombocytopenia after allogeneic bone marrow transplantation: existence of transient and chronic thrombocytopenic syndromes. Blood 1985;65:368–374.

142. Kaufman PA, Jones RB, Greenberg CS et al. Autologous bone marrow transplantation and factor XII, factor VII, and protein C deficiencies. Report of a new association and its possible relationship to endothelial cell injury. Cancer 1990;66:515–521.

143. Stillwell TJ, Benson RC Jr. Cyclophosphamide-induced hemorrhagic cystitis. Cancer 1988;61:451–457.

144. Efros MD, Ahmed T, Coombe N et al. Urologic complications of high-dose chemotherapy and bone marrow transplantation. Urology 1994;43:355–360.

145. Sencer SF, Haake RJ, Weisdorf DJ. Hemorrhagic cystitis after bone marrow transplantation. Risk factors and complications. Transplantation 1993;56:875–879.

146. Yang CC, Hurd DD, Case LD et al. Hemorrhagic cystitis in bone marrow transplantation. Urology 1994;44:322–328.

147. Ost L, Lonnqvist B, Eriksson L et al. Hemorrhagic cystitis—a manifestation of graft versus host disease? Bone Marrow Transplant 1987;2:19–25.

148. Thomas AE, Patterson J, Prentice HG et al. Haemorrhagic cystitis in bone marrow transplantation individuals: possible increased risk associated with prior busulphan therapy. Bone Marrow Transplant 1987;1:347–355.

149. Ringden O, Ruutu T, Remberger M et al. A randomized trial comparing busulfan with total body irradiation as conditioning in allogeneic marrow transplant recipients with leukemia: a report from the Nordic Bone Marrow Transplant Group. Blood 1994;83:2723–2730.

150. Arthur RR, Shah KV, Baust SJ et al. Association of BK viruria with hemorrhagic cystitis in recipients of bone marrow transplants. N Engl J Med 1986;315:230–234.

151. Ambinder RF, Burns W, Forman M et al. Hemorrhagic cystitis associated with adenovirus infection in bone marrow transplantation. Arch Intern Med 1986;146:1400–1401.

152. Apperley JF, Rice SJ, Bishop JA et al. Late-onset hemorrhagic cystitis associated with urinary excretion of polyomaviruses after bone marrow transplantation. Transplantation 1987;43:108–112.

153. Spach DH, Bauwens JE, Myerson D et al. Cytomegalovirus-induced hemorrhagic cystitis following bone marrow transplantation. Clin Infect Dis 1993;16:142–144.

154. Bedi A, Miller CB, Hanson JL et al. Association of BK virus with failure of prophylaxis against hemorrhagic cystitis following bone marrow transplantation. J Clin Oncol 1995;13:1103–1109.

155. Ehrlich RM, Freedman A, Goldsobel AB et al. The use of sodium 2-mercaptoethane sulfonate to prevent cyclophosphamide cystitis. J Urol 1984;131:960–962.

156. Hows JM, Mehta A, Ward L et al. Comparison of mesna with forced diuresis to prevent cyclophosphamide induced haemorrhagic cystitis in marrow transplantation: a prospective randomised study. Br J Cancer 1984;50:753–756.

157. Shepherd JD, Pringle LE, Barnett MJ et al. Mesna versus hyperhydration for the prevention of cyclophosphamide-induced hemorrhagic cystitis in bone marrow transplantation. J Clin Oncol 1991;9:2016–2020.

158. Vose JM, Reed EC, Pippert GC et al. Mesna compared with continuous bladder irrigation as uroprotection during high-dose chemotherapy and transplantation: a randomized trial. J Clin Oncol 1993;11:1306–1310.

159. Meisenberg B, Lassiter M, Hussein A et al. Prevention of hemorrhagic cystitis after high-dose alkylating agent chemotherapy and autologous bone marrow support. Bone Marrow Transplant 1994;14:287–291.

160. Turkeri LN, Lum LG, Uberti JP et al. Prevention of hemorrhagic cystitis following allogeneic bone marrow transplant preparative regimens with cyclophosphamide and busulfan: role of continuous bladder irrigation. J Urol 1995;153:637–640.

161. Atkinson K, Biggs JC, Golovsky D et al. Bladder irrigation does not prevent haemorrhagic cystitis in bone marrow transplant recipients. Bone Marrow Transplant 1991;7:351–354.

162. Cartoni C, Arcese W, Avvisati G et al. Role of ultrasonography in the diagnosis and follow-up of hemorrhagic cystitis after bone marrow transplantation. Bone Marrow Transplant 1993;12:463–467.

163. Baronciani D, Montesi M, Angelucci E et al. Suprapubic cystotomy as treatment for severe hemorrhagic cystitis after bone marrow transplantation. Bone Marrow Transplant 1995;16:267–270.

164. Miller LJ, Chandler SW, Ippoliti CM. Treatment of cyclophosphamide-induced hemorrhagic cystitis with prostaglandins. Ann Pharmacother 1994;28:590–594.

165. Chapman C, Flower AJ, Durrant ST. The use of vidarabine in the treatment of human polyomavirus associated acute haemorrhagic cystitis. Bone Marrow Transplant 1991;7:481–483.

166. Liles WC, Cushing H, Holt S et al. Severe adenoviral nephritis following bone marrow transplantation: successful treatment with intravenous ribavirin. Bone Marrow Transplant 1993;12:409–412.

167. Murphy GF, Wood DP Jr, McRoberts JW et al. Adenovirus-associated hemorrhagic cystitis treated with intravenous ribavirin. J Urol 1993;149:565–566.

168. Kitabayashi A, Hirokawa M, Kuroki J et al. Successful vidarabine therapy for adenovirus type 11-associated acute hemorrhagic cystitis after allogeneic bone marrow transplantation. Bone Marrow Transplant 1994;14:853–854.

169. Stover DE, Zaman MB, Hajdu SI et al. Bronchoalveolar lavage in the diagnosis of diffuse pulmonary infiltrates in the immuno suppressed host. Ann Intern Med 1984;101:1–7.

170. Springmeyer SC, Hackman RC, Holle R et al. Use of bronchoalveolar lavage to diagnose acute diffuse pneumonia in the immunocompromised host. J Infect Dis 1986;154:604–610.

171. Cordonnier C, Bernaudin JF, Bierling P et al. Pulmonary complications occurring after allogeneic bone marrow transplantation. A study of 130 consecutive transplanted individuals. Cancer 1986;58:1047–1054.

172. Cordonnier C, Bernaudin JF, Fleury J et al. Diagnostic yield of bronchoalveolar lavage in pneumonitis occurring after allogeneic bone marrow transplantation. Am Rev Respir Dis 1985;132:1118–1123.

173. Robbins RA, Linder J, Stahl MG et al. Diffuse alveolar hemorrhage in autologous bone marrow transplant recipients. Am J Med 1989;87:511–518.

174. Sisson JH, Thompson AB, Anderson JR et al. Airway inflammation predicts diffuse alveolar hemorrhage during bone marrow transplantation in individuals with Hodgkin disease. Am Rev Respir Dis 1992;146:439–444.

175. Srivastava A, Gottlieb D, Bradstock KF. Diffuse alveolar haemorrhage associated with microangiopathy after allogeneic bone marrow transplantation. Bone Marrow Transplant 1995;15:863–867.

176. Vercellotti GM, Kotasek D, Jacob HS. Excessive vulnerability of herpes-infected endothelium to lymphokine-activated lymphocytes: a possible role in lethal viral pneumonitis following bone marrow transplantation. Trans Assoc Am Phys 1988;101:310–313.

177. Mandanas RA, Saez RA, Selby GB et al. Cytomegalovirus surveillance and prevention in allogeneic bone marrow transplantation—examination of a preemptive plan of ganciclovir therapy. Am J Hematol 1996;51:104–111.

178. Chao NJ, Duncan SR, Long GD et al. Corticosteroid therapy for diffuse alveolar hemorrhage in autologous bone marrow transplant recipients. Ann Intern Med 1991;114:145–146.

179. Metcalf JP, Rennard SI, Reed EC et al. Corticosteroids as adjunctive therapy for diffuse alveolar hemorrhage associated with bone marrow transplantation. University of Nebraska Medical Center Bone Marrow Transplant Group. Am J Med 1994;96:327–334.

# CHAPTER 50

# EFFECTS OF CARDIOPULMONARY BYPASS ON HEMOSTASIS

Shukri F. Khuri, Alan D. Michelson, and C. Robert Valeri

Most cardiac surgeries are performed with use of cardiopulmonary bypass (CPB). Blood contact with the extracorporeal circuit used during CPB elicits a wide spectrum of pathophysiologic changes that affect a variety of organ systems. The hematologic changes brought about by CPB probably are the most important of these, because they result in the most pronounced clinical abnormality (i.e., increased postoperative bleeding) and affect several of the abnormal clinical manifestations of other organ systems (e.g., increased capillary permeability leading to respiratory abnormalities). CPB results in abnormal hemostasis, which leads to increased postoperative bleeding. The exact nature of this hemostatic abnormality, however, remains the subject of intense investigation, although abnormalities of platelet function and hyperfibrinolysis contribute to it significantly. This chapter describes our current knowledge of the hematologic changes observed during CPB, reviews our understanding of the nature of the hemostatic defect elicited by contact with the extracorporeal circuit, and addresses clinical issues related to postoperative blood loss.

## EFFECTS ON BLOOD ELEMENTS

### PLATELETS AND THE VESSEL WALL

#### Normal Platelet Physiology

Platelets are essential for normal hemostasis. The main functions of platelets are adhesion to damaged vessel walls, aggregation to form a platelet plug, and promotion of fibrin clot formation (Fig. 50.1). The mechanisms of platelet activation are detailed in other chapters; the following summary provides necessary background for understanding the clinical abnormalities of CPB.

The adhesive molecule von Willebrand factor (vWf), which binds both to a specific receptor on the platelet surface, glycoprotein (GP) Ib-IX complex, and to exposed subendothelial components, primarily mediates platelet adhesion (1, 2). Fibrinogen binding to its receptor on the platelet surface GP IIb-IIIa complex primarily mediates platelet-to-platelet association (i.e., aggregation) (3). Normal circulating platelets are in a resting state, and they do not bind to plasma vWf or plasma fibrinogen. *In vitro*, the cationic antibiotic ristocetin induces binding of vWf to its receptor on GP Ib (1), but the *in vivo* analogue of ristocetin remains uncertain. Shear stress, fibrin (i.e., monomer) interacting with vWf, or both may be the physiologic stimulus to initiate GP Ib–vWf interaction. Thrombin and other physiologic platelet agonists (e.g., adenosine 5′-diphosphate [ADP], epinephrine) induce exposure of the fibrinogen receptor on the platelet surface GP IIb-IIIa complex (3). These agonists also stimulate platelets to change shape, secrete the contents of their granules (e.g., β-thromboglobulin [β-TG], platelet factor 4, thrombospondin), and aggregate. Secreted thrombospondin binds to a receptor on the platelet surface membrane and to fibrinogen, thereby stabilizing platelet aggregates (4). P-selectin (5), which also is known as CD62P and previously known as granule membrane protein–140 (6) as well as platelet activator–dependent granule to external membrane

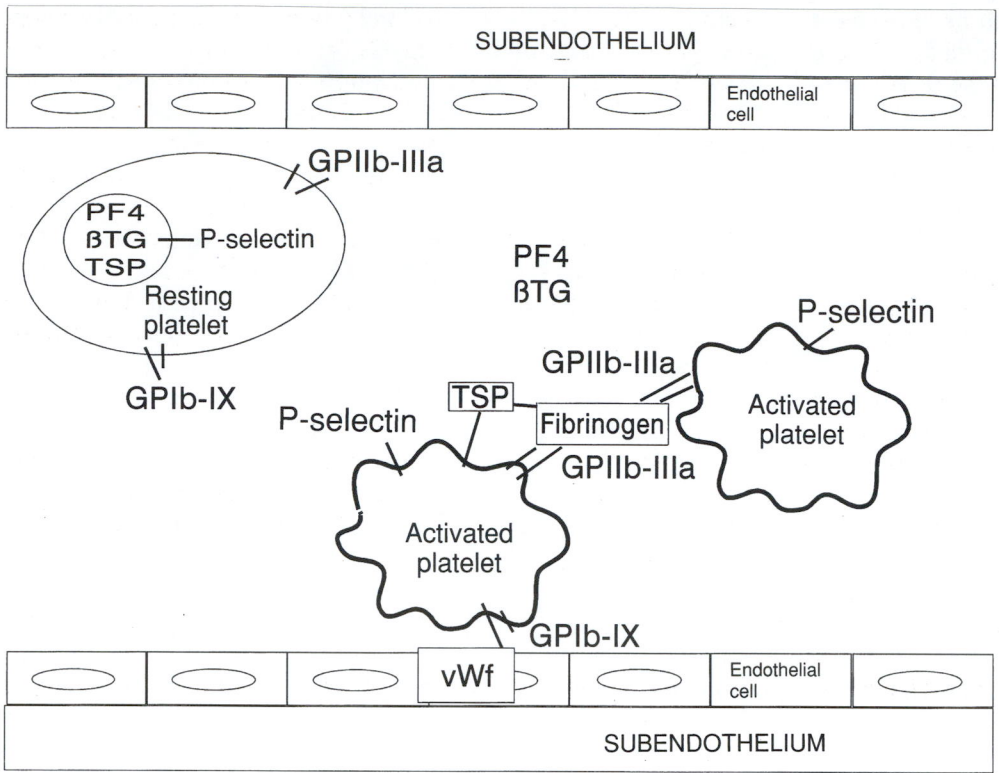

**FIGURE 50.1.** Normal platelet physiology. β-TG, β-thromboglobulin; *GP*, glycoprotein; *PF4*, platelet factor 4; *P-selectin*, granule membrane protein–140; *TSP*, thrombospondin; *vWf*, von Willebrand factor.

protein (7), is a component of the α-granule membrane of resting platelets, and it is expressed on the platelet plasma membrane after platelet activation and secretion (8). Therefore, platelet surface expression of P-selectin is a marker of platelet degranulation. Platelet surface P-selectin mediates the adherence of degranulated platelets to leukocytes in thrombi (9–11) and induces expression of tissue factor on monocytes (12). In contrast to its effect on P-selectin and the fibrinogen receptor on the GP IIb-IIIa complex, thrombin decreases the platelet surface expression of the vWf receptor on the GP Ib-IX complex (13–16).

## Time Course of Changes in Platelet Parameters

### Bleeding Time

Bleeding time is markedly prolonged during hypothermic CPB (17–19), but it normalizes within 24 hours postoperatively (17). The operator dependence and temperature dependence (20) of this measurement have contributed to a lack of consistency in the data reported. As shown by uniform measurements in 87 individuals undergoing uncomplicated myocardial revascularization procedures, systemic anticoagulation with 3 mg of heparin per kilogram of body weight before institution of CPB elicits a modestly but significantly prolonged

bleeding time (Fig. 50.2). Bleeding time is markedly prolonged during CPB and remains so for 2 hours after bypass. Although it essentially returns to normal between 2 and 24 hours after CPB, it may not normalize until 72 hours postoperatively (Fig. 50.2). The markedly prolonged bleeding time in CPB and its subsequent reversal suggest that platelet dysfunction is the primary culprit in the hemostatic defect induced by CPB.

### Platelet Count

Decreased platelet count is consistently observed both during and after CPB (17, 18, 21–23) (Table 50.1). It occurs as early as 5 minutes after institution of CPB (23), and reaches its nadir by 25 minutes (18). The platelet count remains depressed throughout the postoperative period (Table 50.1) and may continue to be depressed for several days after the procedure (17, 23).

Hemodilution and platelet adhesion to synthetic surfaces are the two primary contributors to thrombocytopenia observed during CPB. During extracorporeal circulation for cardiac surgery, blood dilution results from priming the extracorporeal perfusion system with either crystalloid or colloid solutions. This hemodilution generally is considered to be the major cause of thrombocytopenia during CPB (21, 22), but the thrombocytopenia observed both during and after CPB is more severe than might be expected from hemodilution alone (18, 24). During CPB, a loss of platelets occurs that is proportional to the flow rate and the surface area of the extracorporeal circuit (25). Platelets have been shown on scanning electron micrographs to adhere to extracorporeal synthetic surfaces (26), and fibrinogen is the most important cofactor in platelet adhesion to synthetic surfaces (27), just as it is for platelet aggregation (3). Plasma fibrinogen is preferentially adsorbed onto synthetic surfaces (28, 29). Platelet reactivity with these surfaces is directly proportional to the adsorbed fibrinogen concentration (30), but this supposition has been disputed (31). The mechanism by which platelets are initially activated within extracorporeal perfusion systems is not completely clear, but possible causes include direct surface contact, thrombin formation, and ADP release. Thrombin, which is generated in small amounts despite the presence of heparin during CPB surgery (32), is adsorbed onto synthetic surfaces (33) and probably binds to the adsorbed fibrinogen on the extracorporeal surface. ADP is stored in platelet-dense granules and released by platelet lysis and platelet activation; hemolysis of red cells also releases ADP.

Platelet activation exposes fibrinogen binding sites on the GP IIb-IIIa complex (34) and permits binding to fibrinogen molecules previously adsorbed onto the surface (35). Gluszko et al (31) showed that exposure of fibrinogen receptors associated with the GP IIb-IIIa complex contributes to platelet consumption during CPB. They also demonstrated that individuals with Glanzmann thrombasthenia, an inherited deficiency of the GP IIb-IIIa complex, had reduced the severity of CPB-induced thrombocytopenia. Individuals with the Bernard-Soulier syndrome, an inherited deficiency of the GP Ib-IX-V complex, did not.

Along with adhering to the synthetic surfaces of CPB tubing, activated platelets are more likely to adhere to injured vascular surfaces and to deposit in the heart after cardioplegic arrest than circulating unactivated platelets (36). That platelet activation and adherence are important in the etiology of thrombocytopenia during CPB is supported by findings that infusion of prostaglandin E$_1$ (PGE$_1$), prostacyclin (PGI$_2$), iloprost, or dipyridamole (i.e., drugs that inhibit platelet activation) during CPB can result in markedly reduced platelet adherence to the synthetic surfaces, maintenance of platelet counts at near-normal levels, and reduced postoperative blood loss (31, 37–44). An adsorbed protein layer that reduces the affinity of synthetic surfaces for platelets eventually may form (45, 46). The exact physiologic basis for this process, which is termed *passivation* (21), remains unclear, but the results of studies with PGI$_2$ support this concept. When PGI$_2$ was used to inhibit platelets during 2 hours of recirculation in a membrane oxygenator system, platelet activation was inhibited during the first hour (37, 38). PGI$_2$ is unstable in plasma, and after 1 hour, recirculated platelets regain their ability to aggregate with ADP and epinephrine yet do not react with the synthetic surface (37, 38).

Oxygenators, and to a lesser extent filters, contain the largest surface areas in contact with blood; therefore, they are the most prominent sites of platelet deposition (21). The degree of thrombocytopenia observed during CPB relates more to the turbulence, flow rate, and amount of suction in the circuit (25, 47, 48) than to the type of oxygenator employed (18, 49).

Three less common causes of thrombocytopenia during CPB are disseminated intravascular coagulation (DIC), heparin-induced thrombocytopenia, and cyanotic congenital heart disease. Although probably uncommon compared with primary fibrinolysis (50), DIC is a cause of thrombocytopenia and, possibly, of increased bleeding after CPB (51, 52). DIC rarely is encountered during CPB but is more likely to occur later, in association with sepsis or low cardiac output (21). Heparin-induced thrombocytopenia is discussed later in this chapter and in Chapter 29. The mechanism of the association between cyanotic congenital heart disease and thrombocytopenia is unclear (53, 54).

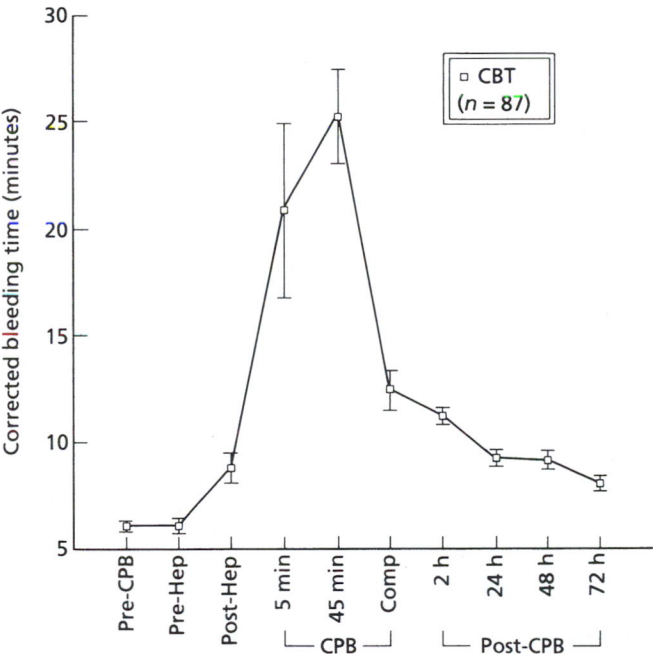

**FIGURE 50.2.** Means ± SEM of bleeding times (corrected for skin temperature) in 87 individuals undergoing isolated coronary artery revascularization at the Brockton/West Roxbury VA Medical Center. Blood samples were obtained in a subgroup of 24 individuals. *CBT,* corrected bleeding time; *CPB,* cardiopulmonary bypass; *Pre-CPB,* before cardiopulmonary bypass; *Pre-Hep,* before administration of heparin; *Post-Hep,* 5 minutes after administration of heparin and before institution of CPB; *min,* minutes after institution of CPB; *Comp,* at completion of CPB; *Post-CPB,* hours after completion of CPB.

**TABLE 50.1.**    Hematologic Changes Before, During, and After Cardiopulmonary Bypass in Individuals Undergoing Cardiac Surgery[a]

| Variable | n | Before CPB | During CPB | After CPB 2 Hours | After CPB 24 Hours | After CPB 48 Hours |
|---|---|---|---|---|---|---|
| Platelet count ($\times 10^3/mm^3$) | 54 | 206 ± 7 | 104 ± 5 | 128 ± 6 | 123 ± 6 | 109 ± 6 |
| Mean platelet volume ($\mu m^3$) | 54 | 8.3 ± 0.2 | 7.7 ± 0.2 | 7.2 ± 0.3 | 8.0 ± 0.3 | 8.5 ± 0.3 |
| Plasma β-TG (ng/mL) | 54 | 59 ± 5 | 285 ± 29 | 291 ± 39 | 58 ± 5 | 59 ± 18 |
| Plasma $TxB_2$ (pg/0.1 mL) | 54 | 88 ± 9 | 91 ± 5 | 75 ± 7 | 59 ± 4 | 59 ± 4 |
| Shed blood $TxB_2$ (pg/0.1 mL) | 54 | 571 ± 43 | — | 245 ± 30 | 405 ± 46 | 457 ± 37 |
| Shed blood 6-keto (pg/0.1 mL) | 54 | 15.6 ± 2.0 | — | 30.7 ± 3.2 | 17.9 ± 3.6 | 13.4 ± 1.9 |
| Hematocrit (vol %) | 40 | 37.7 ± 0.5 | 21 ± 0.5 | 33.9 ± 0.8 | 30.8 ± 0.7 | 29.8 ± 0.5 |
| Albumin (g/dL) | 40 | 3.5 ± 0.1 | 1.8 ± 0.9 | 2.8 ± 0.9 | 3.0 ± 0.1 | 2.9 ± 0.1 |
| Complement (mg/dL) | 40 | 148 ± 6 | 61 ± 2 | 90 ± 4 | 80 ± 4 | 94 ± 4 |
| Fibronectin (μ/mL) | 40 | 450 ± 41 | 219 ± 11 | 318 ± 17 | 258 ± 12 | 273 ± 17 |
| Immunoglobulin M (mg/mL) | 40 | 136 ± 13 | 50 ± 5 | 81 ± 9 | 67 ± 7 | 66 ± 7 |
| Immunoglobulin G (mg/mL) | 40 | 977 ± 41 | 437 ± 21 | 681 ± 37 | 605 ± 32 | 579 ± 34 |
| Fibrinogen (mg/dL) | 40 | 357 ± 15 | 208 ± 10.6 | 266 ± 18 | 356 ± 17 | 511 ± 24 |
| FVII:C (%N) | 40 | 109 ± 11 | — | 102 ± 9 | 121 ± 10 | 158 ± 12 |
| FVIII-vWf (μ/mL) | 40 | 1.62 ± 0.1 | 0.77 ± 0.1 | 1.77 ± 0.2 | 1.94 ± 0.2 | 2.65 ± 0.2 |
| Plasminogen (%) | 40 | 105 ± 3 | 56 ± 2 | 78 ± 2 | 67 ± 2 | 68 ± 2 |
| Antithrombin III (%) | 40 | 105 ± 2 | 60 ± 3 | 78 ± 2 | 74 ± 3 | 76 ± 2 |
| D-dimer (μg/mL) | 22 | 0.6 ± 0.1 | 0.9 ± 0.17 | 3.0 ± 0.37 | 1.6 ± 0.18 | 1.1 ± 0.16 |

*Reprinted with permission from Khuri SF, Wolfe JA, Josa M, et al Hematologic changes during and after cardiopulmonary bypass and their relationship to the bleeding time and nonsurgical blood loss. J Thorac Cardiovasc Surg 1992;104:94–107.*

[a] *Changes within each row were statistically significant by repeated measures of analysis of variance (MANOVA).*

[b] *Denotes a statistically significant difference from the preoperative value by paired student's t test ($P < .05$).*

*β-TG, β–thromboglobulin; $TxB_2$, thromboxane $B_2$; FVIII:C, factor VIII clotting protein; FVIII-vWf, factor VIII-related antigen/von Willebrand factor.*

## MEAN PLATELET VOLUME AND PLATELET MASS

Mean platelet volume (MPV) decreases significantly after institution of CPB and reaches its nadir approximately 2 hours after discontinuation of bypass (Table 50.1). MPV increases progressively and significantly between 2 and 72 hours postoperatively and is accompanied by a significant rise in platelet mass (18), thus suggesting that larger platelets are selectively removed during extracorporeal circulation (18, 55). This is important because platelet size directly relates to platelet function, with larger platelets being more hemostatically competent than smaller platelets (56). An increased MPV between 2 and 72 hours postoperatively, accompanied by a relatively stable platelet count, suggests that a postoperative release of large platelets into the peripheral circulation is responsible, at least in part, for the improvement in bleeding time during this period.

### α-Granule Release

When platelets adhere to synthetic surfaces, they are activated and the contents of their α-granules released into the circulation. Plasma levels of β-TG and platelet factor 4, both of which are contained within α-granules, are markedly increased both during and immediately after CPB (17, 57–61), but they return to normal within the 24-hour postoperative period (Table 50.1) (17, 18). These changes in the plasma levels of platelet-specific proteins may reflect an initial, irreversible activation and lysis of a small number of platelets, which are removed from the circulation within the first 24 hours after CPB (62).

### Thromboxane $B_2$ and 6-Keto Prostaglandin $F_{1\alpha}$

Studies of baboons and humans in which thromboxane $B_2$, which is the stable derivation product of thromboxane $A_2$, and 6-keto prostaglandin $F_{1\alpha}$ ($GF_{1\alpha}$), which is the stable derivation product of prostacyclin, were measured in blood shed from the skin at the site of the bleeding-time test have yielded valuable information on platelet function (63–65). In individuals undergoing CPB, a markedly reduced level of thromboxane $B_2$ in the shed blood occurs soon after institution of CPB and is indicative of platelet dysfunction (Table 50.1) (18, 20). Within 2 to 24 hours after discontinuation of CPB, the level of thromboxane $B_2$ in shed blood is significantly increased, whereas the systemic plasma level of thromboxane $B_2$ is decreased (Table 50.1) (18, 19). The increased postoperative level of thromboxane $B_2$ in shed blood does not reflect changes in the plasma concentration of this product. Rather, it reflects the progressive improvement in platelet function postoperatively, which is paralleled by improved bleeding time and increased MPV. Changes in the shed blood level of 6-keto $PGF_{1\alpha}$, both during and after CPB (Table 50.1), generally are opposite to those observed in the shed blood level of thromboxane $B_2$, and they probably reflect systemic changes in plasma 6-keto $PGF_{1\alpha}$ (18).

## Platelet Aggregation

Blood samples obtained from individuals during CPB show markedly reduced platelet aggregation in response to *in vitro* stimulation with various agonists (22, 49, 66–70). However, the *in vitro* nature of this test, the wide variability in reported responses to the various agonists, and the wide variability in data reported by various investigators underscore the unreliability of this measurement in quantifying the degree of platelet dysfunction elicited by CPB.

## Role of Platelets in the Hemostatic Defect Induced by CPB

The bleeding time is markedly prolonged during CPB (17–19). Three possible causes are:

1. Reduced vWf level,
2. Thrombocytopenia, and
3. A platelet function defect.

During CPB, the plasma level of vWf is either normal (71) or increased (72, 73), and the modest degree of thrombocytopenia that occurs (19) is insufficient to account for the prolonged bleeding time (74). Therefore, the prolonged bleeding time during CPB mainly results from a platelet function defect.

The cause of the platelet function defect during CPB is not entirely clear. Decreased platelet aggregation in response to ADP, epinephrine, and collagen as well as abnormalities in platelet release have been observed preoperatively in individuals with cyanotic congenital heart disease (75, 76). Possible causes of the platelet function defect are listed in Table 50.2. Circulating fibrin(ogen) degradation products (FDPs) are present in most individuals undergoing CPB (50) and may interfere with platelet function (77). A direct correlation between plasma levels of D-dimer and magnitude of platelet dysfunction has been reported in individuals undergoing cardiac surgery (18). Improved platelet aggregation has correlated with lower levels of D-dimer after CPB (78), and bleeding time at 2 hours after CPB has correlated with the corresponding level of plasma D-dimer. A cor-

**TABLE 50.2** Possible Causes of the Platelet Function Defect during Cardiopulmonary Bypass

| Cause | Reference |
|---|---|
| Contact with synthetic surfaces and shear force | 21, 26 |
| Hypothermia | 20 |
| Lack of availability of platelet agonists (e.g., thrombin and adenosine 5'-diphosphate) | 16, 34, 92 |
| Heparin | 177 |
| Hyperfibrinolysis (plasmin and fibrinogen degradation products) | 51 |
| Denatured plasma proteins | 21 |
| Protamine | 335 |
| Aspirin | 322 |
| Nitrovasodilators | 336 |
| Cyanotic congenital heart disease and the state of oxygenation | 51, 82 |

relation also has been observed between high concentrations of denatured plasma proteins and reduced platelet function during CPB (79), particularly with bubble oxygenator perfusion systems (80, 81) in which plasma proteins are denatured.

The variability in reported defects of platelet function both during and after bypass results in part from differences in equipment and techniques. Methodologic problems also may be involved. When separating platelets from whole blood for functional assays, platelets are susceptible to membrane alterations (82) and *ex vivo* activation. Use of the popular plasma assays of the secretion products of platelet $\alpha$-granules (platelet factor 4 and $\beta$-TG) to study the platelet defect in CPB is questionable, because 1% platelet secretion as a result of *in vitro* handling may cause as much as a 30-fold increase in the plasma platelet factor 4 level (83). Moreover, plasma assays of platelet factor 4 and $\beta$-TG reflect the number of circulating activated platelets, lysed platelets, and noncirculating activated platelets adherent to synthetic surfaces on the vessel wall.

To circumvent these problems, whole blood flow cytometric assays that do not involve separation or manipulation of platelets have been developed (84). As determined by these assays (19), CPB results in:

1. Markedly deficient platelet reactivity in response to an *in vivo* wound (Fig. 50.3),
2. Normal platelet reactivity *in vitro* (Fig. 50.4),
3. No loss of platelet surface GP Ib-IX or GP IIb-IIIa complexes (Fig. 50.5), and
4. A minimal number of circulating activated platelets (Fig. 50.4).

These data (19) suggest that the "platelet function defect" of CPB is not intrinsic to the platelet but rather an extrinsic, such as an *in vivo* lack of available platelet agonists. The near-universal use of heparin during CPB probably contributes substantially to this defect via inhi-

bition of thrombin, which is the preeminent platelet activator (85–87).

Heparin has two distinct effects on platelet function during CPB (19, 88, 89). First, it augments platelet activation in whole blood exposed to an exogenous platelet agonist *in vitro* (Fig. 50.4). Second, it suppresses platelet activation *in vivo*, as demonstrated by abrogation of the activation-induced increase in platelet surface P-selectin (Fig. 50.3), a prolonged bleeding time (19, 88), and a reduced level of shed blood thromboxane B$_2$ (19, 88). Presumably, these effects are mediated via inhibition of endogenous thrombin (19). Thus, even although heparin augments their activatibility, platelets cannot be activated *in vivo* during CPB, because thrombin, the preeminent agonist (85–87), is not available. Other extrinsic factors, such as hypothermia (18, 20, 90) and fibrinolytic activity (18, 75), also contribute to the platelet function defect associated with CPB (discussed below).

Earlier studies using washed platelets suggested a reduction in platelet surface GP Ib-IX (91) or GP IIb-IIIa complexes (92, 93) during CPB. The differences in the results of these studies and those of whole blood studies (19, 94), however, probably arise from artifactual *in vitro* changes in platelet membrane receptors caused by the separation procedures required to isolate platelets. Some whole blood studies have demonstrated modest reductions of platelet surface GP Ib-IX (13, 95) or GP IIb-IIa complexes (95), but these changes cannot explain the prolonged bleeding time during CPB. This is because individuals who are heterozygous for Bernard-Soulier syndrome and Glanzmann thrombasthenia (who lack 50% of platelet surface GP Ib-IX and GP IIb-IIIa complexes, respectively) do not have a bleeding diathesis and have a normal bleeding time.

Considering the modest increase in platelet surface P-selectin during CPB (19, 95, 96), the more profound increase in the plasma concentrations of soluble P-selectin, β-TG, and platelet factor 4 (17, 22, 97) during CPB may reflect one or more of the following:

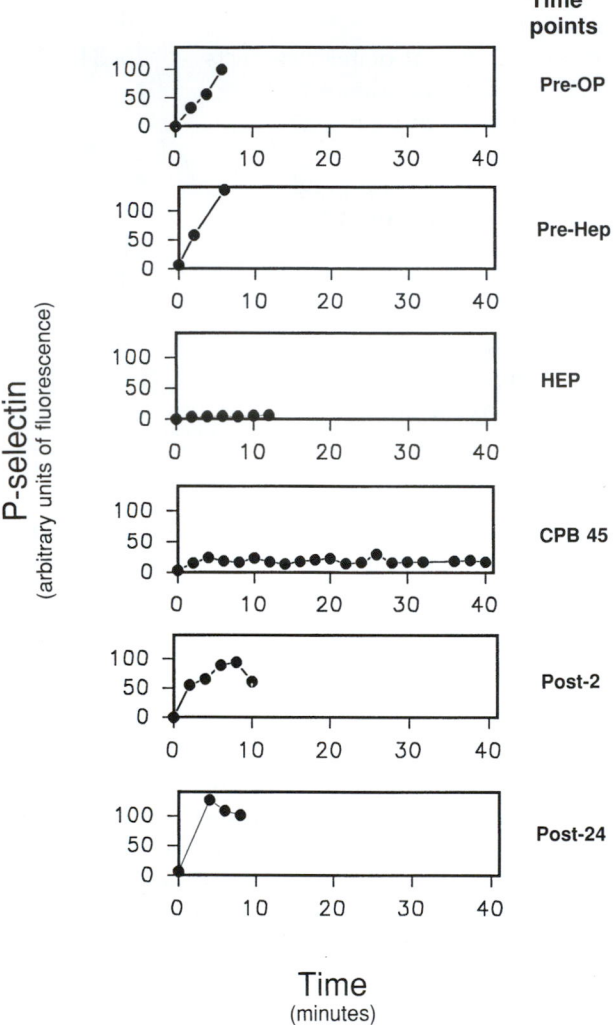

**FIGURE 50.3.** The effect of cardiopulmonary bypass (CPB) on activation-induced up-regulation of the platelet surface expression of P-selectin in whole blood *in vivo*. A standardized bleeding time was performed, and without touching the wound, shed blood was collected with a micropipet directly from the wound site at 2-minute intervals (as shown on the horizontal axis) until bleeding ceased. The sample was immediately anticoagulated, fixed, and analyzed by whole blood flow cytometry with P-selectin–specific monoclonal antibody S12. This experiment is representative of 14 separate experiments. *CPB 45,* 45 minutes on CPB; *HEP,* 5 minutes after heparin administration; *post 2,* 2 hours post CPB; *post 24,* 24 hours post CPB; *Pre-Hep,* before heparin administration: *Pre-OP,* before cardiopulmonary bypass. (Reprinted with permission from Kestin AS, Valeri CR, Khuri SF, et al. The platelet function defect of cardiopulmonary bypass. Blood 1993;82: 107–117.)

1. Platelet surface expression of P-selectin that results in formation of circulating monocyte–platelet aggregates or neutrophil–platelet aggregates, thus in turn resulting in loss of circulating single platelets expressing surface P-selectin (96);
2. Circulating degranulated platelets that rapidly lose surface P-selectin to the plasma pool but continue to circulate and function (98);
3. Noncirculating degranulated platelets that adhere to synthetic surfaces or the vessel wall;
4. Platelet lysis *in vivo* or *in vitro* (62); and
5. Artifactual *in vitro* degranulation and secretion as a result of separation of plasma from platelets before the performance of the assays (99).

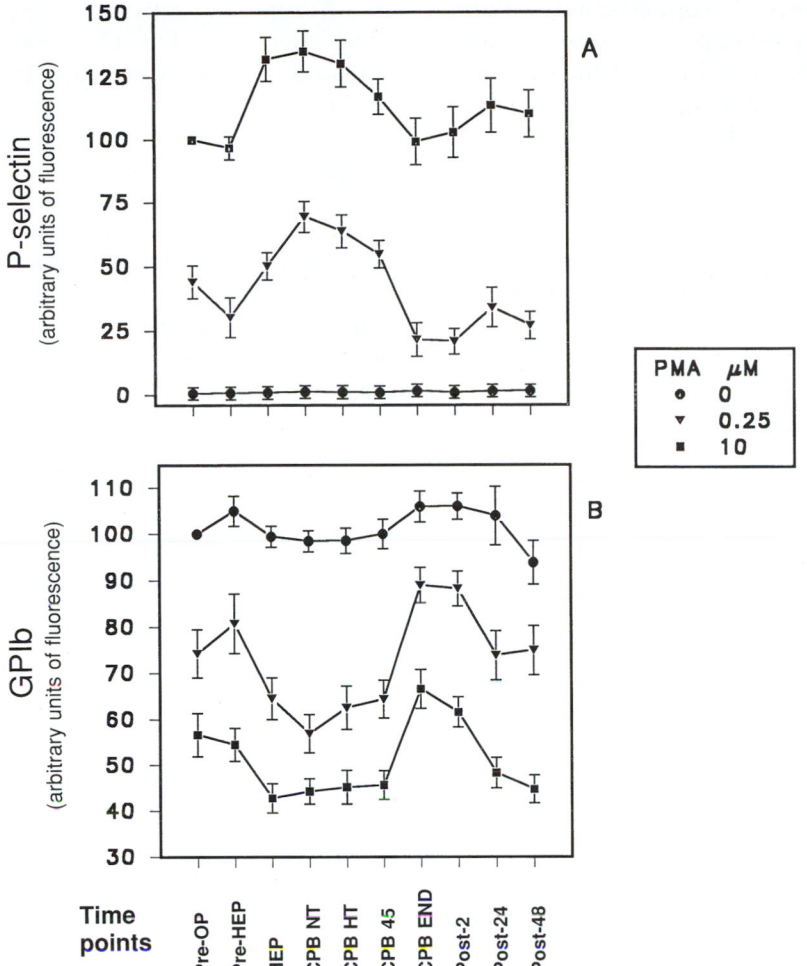

**FIGURE 50.4.**   Effect of cardiopulmonary bypass (CPB) on platelet reactivity to phorbol myristate acetate (PMA) as determined by whole blood flow cytometry. Peripheral blood samples were incubated with PMA 0 (circles), 0.25 (triangles), or 10 μM (squares). Data are mean ± SEM, $n = 16$. **A.** Platelet surface expression of P-selectin as determined by monoclonal antibody S12. **B.** Platelet surface glycoprotein (GP) Ib as determined by monoclonal antibody 6D1. *CPB END*, completion of CPB, immediately following protamine administration; *CPB HT*, beginning of maximal hypothermia on CPB; *CPB NT*, after the start of CPB (normothermic conditions); *HEP*, 5 minutes after heparin administration; *Post-2*, 2 hours after completion of CPB; *Post-24*, 24 hours after completion of CPB; *Post-48*, 48 hours after completion of CPB; *Pre-HEP*, before heparin administration; *Pre-OP*, before cardiopulmonary bypass. (Reprinted with permission from Kestin AS, Valeri CR, Khuri SF, et al. The platelet function defect of cardiopulmonary bypass. Blood 1993;82:107–117.)

CPB also is associated with a modest increase in the plasma concentration of platelet-derived microparticles (13, 100). This apparently results from turbulence and shear stress.

## FLUID PHASE: COAGULATION AND FIBRINOLYSIS

### Time Course of Changes in Plasma Proteins

Most plasma proteins are adsorbed to the CPB circuit in small and inconsequential amounts. Fibrinogen, however, is preferentially adsorbed to synthetic surfaces and is the dominant protein on them (28, 29). CPB elicits a nearly 50% decrease in the concentration of plasma proteins, mainly through hemodilution. Because of the

complexity of cardiac surgery and its demand for frequent administration of various fluids and blood components, the exact contribution of hemodilution to the observed concentration of the various plasma proteins both during and after CPB is difficult to ascertain. As reflected by changes in the hematocrit (Table 50.1), hemodilution is most pronounced within minutes after institution of CPB; it is sustained to a lesser degree for several days postoperatively. Protein concentrations, which fall during CPB and remain low throughout the initial postoperative period, may reflect hemodilution and not sustained intraoperative consumption.

Plasma protein changes both during and after CPB should be interpreted in light of the dilutional state. It is not appropriate, however, to correct for hemodilution simply by relating the plasma protein concentration to the corresponding hematocrit, because the proportion of plasma to whole blood differs from that of red cells to whole blood. Correcting for hemodilution without due consideration of this fact is another source of difficulty when interpreting published data on plasma protein concentration. The following equation is a more appropriate formula to calculate a plasma protein concentration independent of the dilutional effect of CPB:

$$DCP = BP \ (BL \ HCT/(BP \ HCT—BL \ HCT)/(1—BL \ HCT))$$

in which *DCP* is the dilution-corrected protein concentration during CPB, *BP* the actual protein concentration during CPB, *BL* the baseline (i.e., prebypass) value, and *HCT* the hematocrit.

## Oncotic and Opsonic Proteins

Total protein concentrations reflect the dilutional state observed during and after CPB (18). Albumin is minimally adsorbed to the extracorporeal circuit, and between 2 and 72 hours postoperatively, albumin remains depressed, paralleling the decline in hematocrit (Table 50.1). Levels of the opsonic proteins (i.e., immunoglobulin [Ig] G, IgM, C3, fibronectin) also decrease significantly and remain depressed for at least 3 days postoperatively (Table 50.1). The C3 level increases significantly during the 24- to 72-hour post-CPB period, but it does not return to its baseline value (Table 50.1). The decrease in opsonic protein levels is dilutional but also has been attributed to generalized opsonic consumption during prolonged CPB (101, 102), fibronectin-mediated removal of macrocellular aggregates by the reticuloendothelial system (103), protein degradation by proteolytic enzymes (104), and cold-induced precipitation of fibronectin with fibrinogen (105).

## Coagulation and Fibrinolytic Proteins

Plasma fibrinogen levels are elevated above normal in individuals with heart disease (106–108). Likewise, they are elevated preoperatively in individuals undergoing cardiac surgery (18, 57). Two hours after CPB, fibrinogen levels are decreased, but between 2 and 72 hours postoperatively, there is a progressive increase in the plasma fibrinogen level, thereby resulting in levels significantly higher than baseline (Table 50.1). Likewise, concentrations of factor VIII and vWf progressively increase between 2 and 72 hours after CPB, thereby resulting in levels significantly higher than baseline (Table 50.1). Thus, unlike opsonic protein levels, which remain depressed for several days postoperatively, coagulation protein levels increase well above baseline during this period (18, 109–112).

Fibrinolytic activity increases significantly during and after CPB (113–124), and this contributes to increased postoperative blood loss (50, 79, 113, 116, 119, 125). Fibrinolytic activity actually is observed shortly after systemic heparinization before institution of CPB. Heparin induces a significant rise in plasma plasmin activity (88, 121), which is sustained (although at a lower level, probably reflecting hemodilution) throughout the duration of CPB. Plasmin activity returns to normal at the completion of CPB. $\alpha_2$-antiplasmin, which is a specific inhibitor of plasmin, also is affected by systemic heparinization before institution of CPB. Both systemic heparinization and CPB produce a progressive decrease in antiplasmin activity, which is sustained throughout the first 24 hours postoperatively. The antiplasmin activity during bypass is significantly lower than that expected on the basis of hemodilution alone (121). Plasmin activity returns to normal immediately after discontinuation of CPB, but antiplasmin levels do not return to normal before 48 to 72 hours postoperatively.

The concentration of tissue-type plasminogen activator (t-PA) increases during CPB and returns to normal rapidly thereafter (114, 117, 119). It is not affected by systemic heparinization. This suggests that CPB is a major stimulus for release of t-PA from the vascular endothelium in addition to the other known stimuli, such as exercise, hypotensive shock, pharmacologic agents, and protein C (126). Levels of plasma plasminogen and antithrombin III decrease significantly during CPB and remain depressed from their baseline levels throughout the first 72 hours postoperatively (Table 50.1). They also parallel the changes in hematocrit and probably reflect the dilutional state (122).

Levels of FDPs and D-dimer increase during and after CPB (115, 116, 120, 123). At completion of CPB, the FDP level is markedly reduced, and no FDPs are detected beyond 2 hours post-CPB. The level of D-dimer, which is produced by degradation of crosslinked fibrin, increases after administration of protamine and reaches its peak 2 hours after discontinuation of CPB (Table 50.1).

## Role of Fibrinolytic and Coagulation Factors in the Hemostatic Defect

Several pathways could lead to increased fibrinolysis during surgery with CPB (127, 128). The contact of blood with a large artificial surface leads to activation of the contact phase of coagulation and generation of kallikrein (Chapter 5). Kallikrein, both directly and indirectly (via bradykinin), stimulates release of t-PA from endothelial cells (127, 128). Kallikrein also can convert the inactive zymogen prourokinase into urokinase. Release of t-PA from endothelial cells during CPB may be stimulated by the elevated levels of thrombin, epinephrine, angiotensin II, leukotrienes, and hypoxia (127). Heparin also can induce a significant rise in plasma plasmin ac-

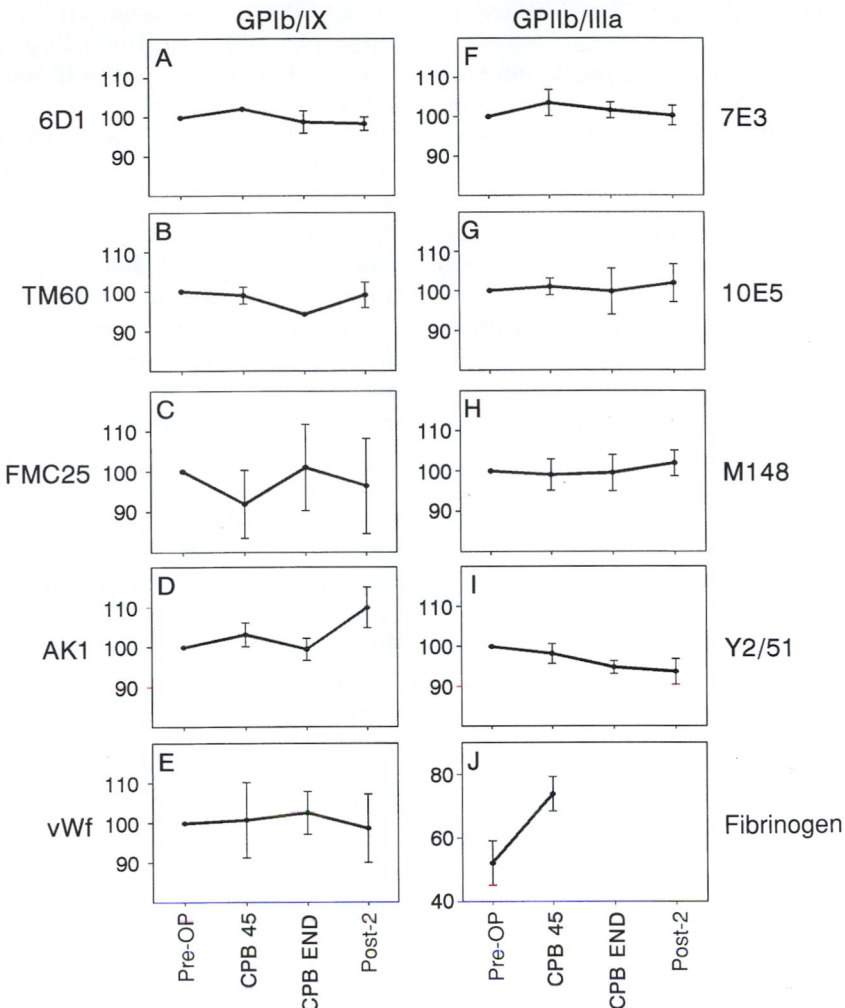

**FIGURE 50.5.** Effect of cardiopulmonary bypass (CPB) on platelet surface expression of the glycoprotein (GP) Ib-IX and GP IIb-IIIa complexes. Data are mean ± SEM, $n = 4$. **A through D.** Platelet binding of a panel of GP Ib-IX–specific monoclonal antibodies as determined by whole blood flow cytometry. Antibodies are directed against the von Willebrand factor (vWf)–binding site on GP Ib (6D1), the thrombin binding site on GP Ib (TM60), GP IX (FMC25), and the GP Ib-IX complex (AK1). **E.** Ristocetin-induced binding of exogenous vWf to washed platelets as determined by flow cytometry with a polyclonal anti-vWf antibody. **F through I.** Platelet binding of a panel of GP IIb-IIIa–specific monoclonal antibodies as determined by whole blood flow cytometry. Antibodies 7E3, 10E5, and M148 are directed against different epitopes near the fibrinogen site on the GP IIb-IIIa complex. Y2/51 is directed against the GP IIIa subunit. **J.** Binding site of exogenous radioiodinated fibrinogen to adenosine 5′-diphosphate (ADP)–stimulated, washed platelets. Fibrinogen binding is expressed as molecules $\times 10^3$ per platelet. *CPB 45,* 45 minutes after the start of CPB (hypothermic conditions); *CPB END,* completion of CPB, immediately follwing administration of protamine; *Post-2,* 2 hours after completion of CPB; *Pre-OP,* preoperative. (Reprinted with permission from Kestin AS, Valeri CR, Khuri SF, et al The platelet function defect of cardiopulmonary bypass. Blood 1993;82:107–117.)

tivity and FDPs before institution of CPB (88, 89, 121). In addition to the fibrinolytic state *per se,* circulating FDPs can interfere with thrombin activity, fibrin polymerization, and platelet function (50). Blood in the pericardial cavity activates the extrinsic coagulation pathway (129) and the fibrinolytic system (130). Hyperfibrinolysis resulting from stasis of blood and clots in the pericardial cavity (130) can produce a vicious cycle, leading to increased blood loss in the immediately postoperative period and prompting the individual's re-

turn to the operating room for control of bleeding. Often, no discrete bleeders are found in these individuals on reexploration, but evacuation of blood clots from the pericardial cavity will lead to cessation of excessive postoperative bleeding. That increased fibrinolysis is important in the genesis of the CPB-induced hemostatic defect is confirmed by studies relating blood levels of fibrinolysis products to the magnitude of post-CPB blood loss (18, 78) and by numerous placebo-controlled studies demonstrating the remarkable efficacy of antifibrinolytic agents at reducing post-CPB blood loss (discussed later).

Reductions in the plasma levels of coagulation factors during surgery with CPB primarily result from hemodilution (17, 131). Only factor V levels decrease to less than than that predicted by dilution alone (17, 22). For all coagulation factors, including factor V, levels observed during surgery with CPB rarely fall into a range in which hemostasis would be compromised (18, 22, 50, 51, 122).

There are conflicting results regarding concentration of vWf during and after CPB (18, 71–73, 132). The level of vWf decreases during CPB, but not to less than that considered to be adequate for hemostasis (18, 132). Preoperatively, high-molecular-weight multimers of vWf may be selectively deficient in individuals with valvular heart disease and noncyanotic congenital heart disease (132, 133).

## THE IMMUNE-INFLAMMATORY RESPONSE

Activation of platelets and the fibrinolytic and coagulation systems during CPB are part of a "whole body inflammatory response" (134, 135) attributed to CPB. This response also includes activation of complement and white blood cells and generation of inflammatory mediators such as tumor necrosis factor–$\alpha$, interleukin-6, and interleukin-8 (136–141). During cardiac surgery, complement is activated via both the classical and the alternative pathways. Blood contact with the artificial surfaces initiates complement activation through the alternative pathway, and administration of protamine to reverse the heparin effect after discontinuation of CPB results in formation of immune complexes that trigger complement activation through the classical pathway. Complement activation results in complex adverse sequelae, including activation and aggregation of granulocytes. For example, blockade of C5a and C5b-9 generation inhibits leukocyte and platelet activation during extracorporeal circulation (136). A detailed description of the effect of artificial surfaces, including CPB, on complement activation, leukocyte function, and inflammatory mediators is provided in Chapter 42.

# HYPOTHERMIA: ITS ROLE IN HEMOSTASIS

Surgeons have recognized intuitively that hypothermia tends to increase bleeding in surgical individuals and that rewarming individuals improves hemostasis. Until recently, however, individual studies elucidating the effect of hypothermia on hemostasis have been scarce. Canine studies have demonstrated that hypothermia at a temperature of 20°C causes thrombocytopenia, sequestration of platelets in the hepatic sinusoids, and a

marked decrease in collagen-induced platelet aggregability (142, 143). In addition, hypothermia in dogs causes a marked activation of the fibrinolytic system (143). In baboons, local hypothermia significantly increases the bleeding time and decreases the concentration of thromboxane $B_2$ in blood shed from the bleeding time measurement site (63). These changes are completely reversed with rewarming (63). Rewarming beyond 37°C, however, does not elicit any further changes in bleeding time or shed blood thromboxane $B_2$.

These observations in hypothermic baboons were confirmed in a clinical study of 25 individuals undergoing CPB with systemic hypothermia (25°C) (20). In these individuals, one arm was kept warm with a water-jacketed cuff throughout the intraoperative and postoperative periods; the temperature in the other arm reflected the systemic changes. As Fig. 50.6 shows, the bleeding time was significantly prolonged in the cold arm compared with the warm arm. Likewise, the concentration of shed blood (from the bleeding time measurement site) thromboxane $B_2$ was significantly lower in the cold arm than in the warm arm. These reversible changes in platelet function provided the first definitive demonstration in humans, the effect of hypothermia on hemostatic parameters during CPB. Along with recent data demonstrating relationships between temperature and postoperative blood loss (discussed later), this underscores the importance of adequate rewarming after CPB to prevent platelet dysfunction and to reduce blood loss after the surgical procedures.

The effect of moderate and profound hypothermia on hemostatic mechanism in humans cannot be investigated safely without CPB. Hence, it is difficult to differentiate clinically between the effects of hypothermia and the effects of CPB *per se* on the hemostatic mechanism. Hypothermia, however, reversibly inhibits human platelet activation in normal volunteers both *in vitro* and *in vivo* (90). These results suggest that rewarming a hypothermic, bleeding individual can reduce the need for transfusion of platelets and other blood components. Systemic hypothermia, hemodilution, and administration of heparin during CPB protect the individual somewhat from the adverse effects of complement activation by reducing both generation of C3a/C5a and the subsequent cellular response of neutrophil activation (144).

# CLINICAL CONSIDERATIONS

## ANTICOAGULATION

### Systemic Anticoagulation with Heparin

Anticoagulation with heparin is central to CPB. As described in Chapter 55, heparin elicits its anticoagulant effect by catalyzing the action of antithrombin, with re-

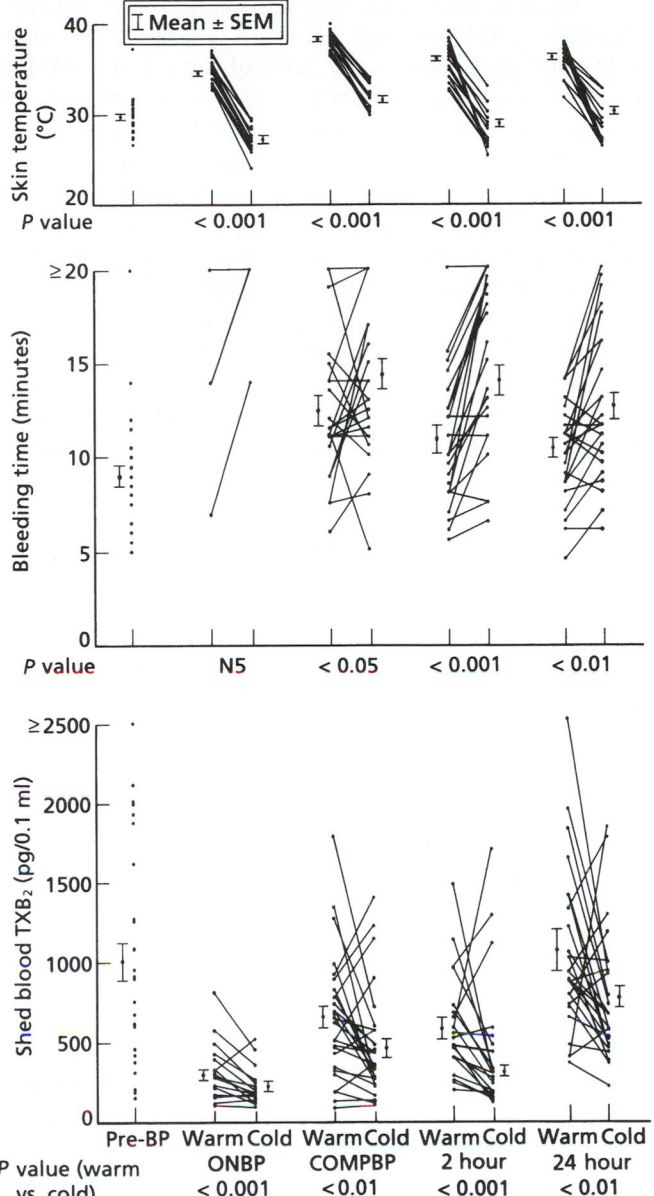

**FIGURE 50.6.** Shed blood thromboxane $B_2$ (TXB$_2$) level, skin temperature, and bleeding time measured simultaneously from the warm and cold arms during and after hypothermic cardiopulmonary bypass (CPB) in 37 individuals undergoing CPB surgery. One arm (Warm) was kept warm with a water-filled blanket set at 40°C; the other arm (Cold) was allowed to follow the systemic temperature. Hypothermia resulted in a significantly prolonged bleeding time and significantly reduced the TXB$_2$ level in blood shed from the bleeding time site. *Pre-BP*, pre bypass; *ONBP*, 20 minutes after institution of CPB; *COMPBP*, at completion of CPB. (Reprinted with permission from Valeri CR, Khabbaz K, Khuri SF, et al. Effect of skin temperature on platelet function in individuals undergoing extracorporeal bypass. J Thorac Cardiovasc Surg 1992;104: 108–116.)

sultant inhibition of thrombin and factor IXa, Xa, and XIa activity. The anticoagulant response to heparin is influenced by platelets, fibrin, vascular surfaces, and plasma proteins (145); it also is influenced by hypothermia and hemodilution. The response among individuals varies and depends disproportionately on the dose and duration of treatment (145). Individuals receiving intravenous infusions of heparin before cardiac surgery require larger-than-usual doses to achieve adequate anticoagulation during CPB. The plasma biologic half-life of an intravenous heparin injection is dose-dependent and not uniform (146, 147). For a dose of 100 U/kg (i.e., 1 mg/kg), the half-life is 56 minutes; for a dose of 400 U/kg (i.e., 4 mg/kg), the half-life is 152 minutes (147). Intravenous nitroglycerin may induce heparin resistance (148, 149), but this is still uncertain.

Heparin is administered before institution of CPB at an initial intravenous dose of 250 to 300 U/kg. The activated clotting time (ACT) is the most widely used measure of anticoagulation with heparin during extracorporeal circulation. Routine use of the ACT to gauge required doses of heparin during CPB offers distinct advantages over unmonitored, protocol-directed administration (150). Baseline ACT levels, to which post-heparin-reversal levels are compared, must be established after induction of anesthesia and opening of the chest, because anesthesia and surgery reduce the ACT (151, 152).The optimal ACT level during CPB has been debated, but after the initial dose of heparin, the ACT is maintained at greater than 480 seconds in most centers by periodic heparin administration.

The anticoagulant effect of heparin is reversed at the termination of CPB by protamine sulfate, which is given in incremental doses until the ACT returns to its preheparinization level. Protamine must be administered slowly because of its frequent adverse hemodynamic effects, including hypotension (153). Contrary to previous beliefs, rapid administration of protamine into the aorta is not safer than administration into the central venous system, and it does not prevent or reduce adverse hemodynamic effects (154, 155).

Administration of protamine may elicit a severe hemodynamic derangement characterized by marked pulmonary vasoconstriction, acute pulmonary hypertension, and peripheral vascular collapse. Such an event is uncommon but can be treated effectively with intravenous administration of PGE$_1$ (156). Protamine sulfate has been shown to elicit complement activation by the classic pathway, and the severity of complement activation correlates with subsequent hemodynamic derangements (157–160). High levels of antiprotamine IgE antibody have been identified in sera of a sensitized individual with protamine-induced fatal anaphylaxis and of individuals with diabetes who received insulin-containing protamine, thus indicating that routine administration of protamine in such susceptible individuals is not advisable (161).

Administration of heparin and protamine are guided by the ACT in most individuals undergoing CPB, but it remains uncertain whether monitoring the ACT alone ensures optimal heparin and protamine doses both during and after the procedure. The correlation between the ACT and plasma heparin levels, particularly during CPB, is debatable. In some studies, ACT levels correlated well with actual heparin levels (162) and provided for adequate treatment during long-term anticoagulation for extracorporeal respiratory assistance (163, 164). More recent studies, however, have shown a poor correlation between ACT levels and heparin concentrations during CPB (165, 166). This poor correlation results in part from the effect of hypothermia and hemodilution, both of which prolong the ACT during CPB (165–167).

To ensure more optimal dosing of heparin and protamine during cardiac surgery, a new heparin management system (HMS) has been proposed. The Hepcon/HMS device (Medtronic Blood Management, Parker, CO), which measures both the ACT and the whole-blood heparin concentration (168), uses heparin/protamine titration (126) to determine quantitatively the targeted heparin concentration for each individual. During the operation, heparin is administered to maintain the targeted levels of both the heparin concentration and the ACT (169, 170). This more precise institution, monitoring, and reversal of anticoagulation improves hemostasis and reduces blood loss as well as the need for transfusions (169, 171). The reliability of the Hepcon system in accurately reflecting the plasma heparin concentration, however, has been questioned (170). Wang et al (166) have proposed a new test, the high-dose thrombin time (HiTT), for monitoring the adequacy of anticoagulation, and showed a direct correlation between HiTT and heparin concentration throughout the period of CPB. HiTT also was unaffected by hypothermia and hemodilution.

## Limitations of Systemic Anticoagulation with Heparin

Heparin is universally employed for anticoagulation during CPB, but several adverse effects limit its ability to achieve optimal and safe anticoagulation. As noted, heparin administered before institution of CPB causes significant platelet dysfunction and elicits a fibrinolytic process that, in turn, augments the platelet dysfunction (88, 89). Because administration of protamine is unlikely to completely reverse these adverse effects, the hemostatic dysfunction attributed to CPB may result in part from heparin. In addition, post-CPB mediastinal drainage correlates strongly with increased heparin concentration during CPB (152).

Heparin also does not completely prevent prothrombin activation and thrombin activity during CPB (32, 152, 172, 173). Despite heparin concentrations adequate to maintain the ACT at greater than 400 seconds, levels of prothrombin fragment 1.2 (a byproduct of the cleavage of prothrombin to thrombin), fibrinopeptide A (the first thrombin cleavage product of fibrinogen), thrombin–antithrombin III complex, and fibrin monomer all increase significantly during CPB (Fig. 50.7). Of note is the twofold increase in prothrombin fragment 1.2, which occurs several hours after termination of CPB and administration of protamine (Fig. 50.7). This increase, which may still be observed 24 hours postoperatively, reflects a marked increase in thrombin generation compared with the pre-CPB baseline. As such, it may indicate a post-CPB hypercoagulable state, which hypothetically may contribute to postoperative thrombotic events such as acute myocardial infarction and cerebrovascular accidents (173).

Increased bleeding after CPB may occur secondary to "heparin rebound," which may result from:

1. Increased circulating levels of heparin,
2. Increased levels of antithrombin, or
3. Heparin–protamine complexes formed as a result of excess protamine (174).

One probable frequent cause of heparin rebound is the transfer of cold, heparin-containing extracellular fluid from the periphery into the central circulation, which results from postoperative rewarming and vasodilation. Inadequate systemic rewarming before termination of CPB predisposes individuals to this phenomenon. Still another possible cause is transfusion of fresh frozen plasma, which may provide an increase in antithrombin levels. Heparin also may remain complexed with excess protamine but is subsequently liberated as the protamine is metabolized, thereby resulting in increased antithrombin activity. By itself, an increased protamine level does not have an anticoagulant effect, although when protamine is complexed with heparin, heparin rebound with increased postoperative bleeding may occur (174). Teoh et al (175) investigated the mechanism of heparin rebound by using chemically modified heparin that lacked anticoagulant activity but could displace protein-bound heparin with anticoagulant activity. Their data suggest that after administration to individuals undergoing cardiac surgery, heparin binds to plasma proteins and is incompletely removed by protamine. After protamine is cleared, the protein-bound heparin slowly dissociates and produces an anticoagulant effect by increasing antithrombin activity (175). When chemical rather than biologic measurements of post-CPB heparin levels were made in samples from 27 individuals undergoing routine coronary revascularization, there was no evidence of persistent heparin in 99.6%, thus raising doubts as to the actual concept of heparin rebound (176). It is increasingly

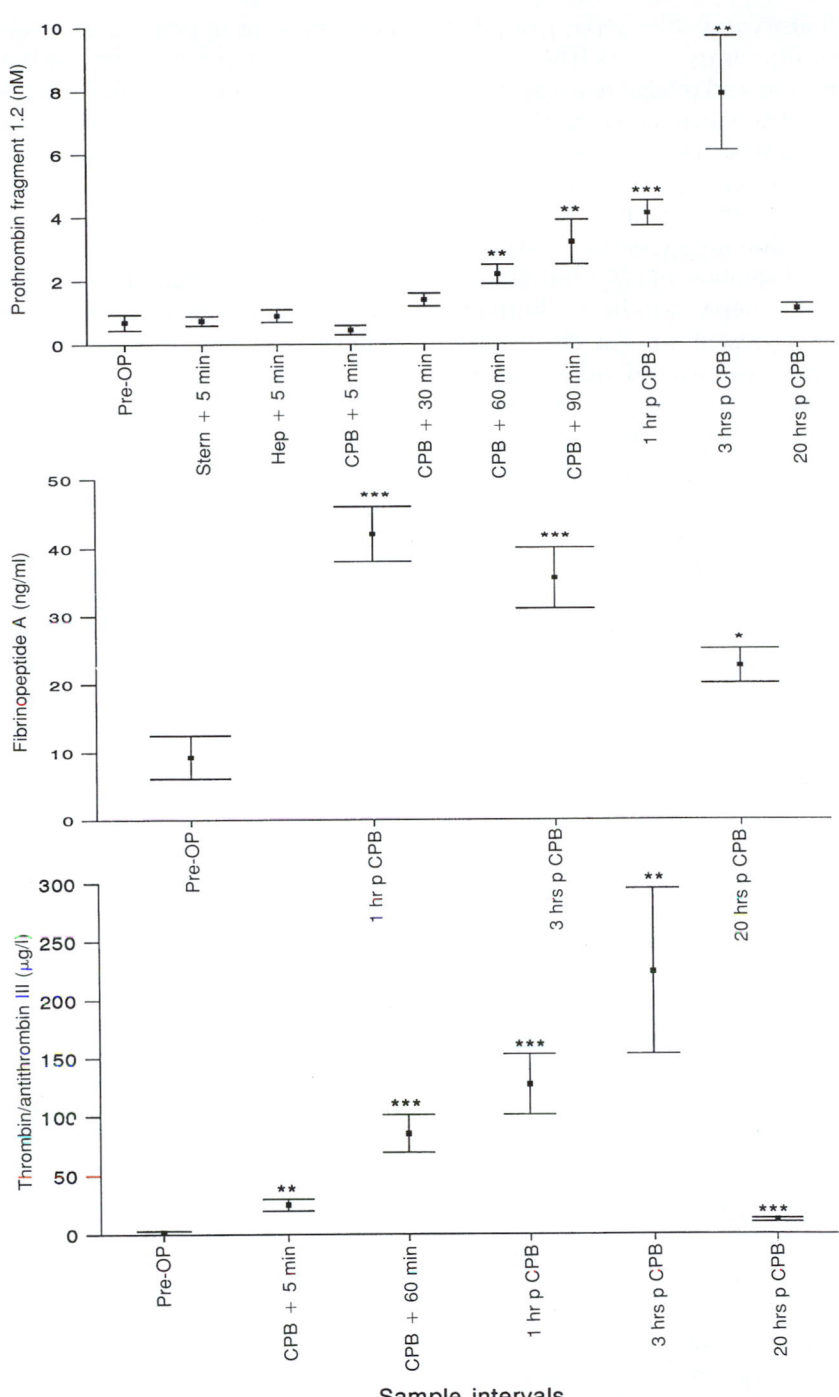

**FIGURE 50.7.** Perioperative plasma concentration of **(A)** prothrombin fragment 1.2, **(B)** thrombin–antithrombin III complex, and **(C)** fibrinopeptide A. P, post. **CPB**, cardiopulmonary bypass; **P**, post. Statistically significant changes from the preoperative value: *P < 005; **P = .01; ***P = .001. *Hep*, administration of heparin; *p CPB*, post cardiopulmonary bypass; *Pre-OP*, preoperative; *Stern*, sternal opening. (Modified with permission from Slaughter TF, LeBleu TH, Douglas JM Jr, et al. Characterization of prothrombin activation during cardiac surgery by hemostatic molecular markers. Anesthesiology 1994;80:520–526.)

evident that heparin rebound is unlikely to occur among individuals in whom systemic normothermia is maintained during CPB and in whom dosing of heparin and protamine is determined more precisely by titration and monitoring with an HMS.

The most serious limitation of heparin in cardiac surgery is heparin-induced thrombocytopenia and its sequela of intravascular thrombosis. There are two types of heparin-induced thrombocytopenia (see Chapter 29) (177). One is a transient thrombocytopenia of immediate onset and mild degree that accompanies heparin therapy in approximately 5% of individuals (177). The mechanism probably is nonimmune and related to a direct proaggregatory effect of heparin on platelets (178). The other type occurs much less frequently in individuals receiving heparin and is a delayed, severe, and probably an immune-mediated thrombocytopenia that may occur in association with platelet activation, aggregation, and on occasion, massive arterial thrombosis (177). Individuals known to be predisposed to heparin-induced thrombocytopenia and thrombosis present a major challenge if CPB is needed. Management of such individuals has included pretreatment with aspirin and dipyridamole (179), pretreatment with iloprost (41), and anticoagulation with low-molecular-weight heparins and heparinoids (180–184), but these heparin congeners still may induce the syndrome. Of particular promise is use of ancrod (185, 186) or hirudin (187–189) instead of heparin for anticoagulation during CPB.

## Heparin-Coated Extracorporeal Circuits

Both *in vitro* and animal studies have documented the biocompatibility of oxygenators and tubings coated with endpoint–attached heparin (190–199). These experimental studies also have demonstrated that compared with noncoated circuits, heparin-coated surfaces result in reduced complement and platelet activation, increased hematocrit and platelet count, decreased plasma hemoglobin level, improved intraoperative hemodynamics, decreased pulmonary injury, and reduced postoperative blood loss and transfusion requirements. Most clinical studies comparing heparin-coated surfaces to conventional circuits in individuals undergoing cardiac surgery (172, 200–211) have demonstrated advantages of heparin-coated over conventional surfaces. These studies fall into one of two categories:

1. Studies employing standard heparin doses in both the heparin-coated and the conventional surface groups, targeting an ACT of >400/480 seconds (172, 200–205); and
2. Studies employing low-dose heparin in the heparin-coated group, targeting an ACT of >250 seconds in that group (141, 206–211).

Two important studies in the first category failed to demonstrate any major advantage of heparin-coated circuits. Gorman et al (172), in a randomized study of 20 individuals undergoing myocardial revascularization, found significantly improved platelet function among individuals in whom heparin-coated surfaces were employed. Their data showed no significant differences, however, between groups in fibrinopeptide A, prothrombin fragment 1.2, and thrombin–antithrombin complex concentrations. In addition, no significant differences were observed between groups in markers of

fibrinolysis or in postoperative clinical outcome parameters, including postoperative blood loss.

Muchrcke et al (205), in a randomized study of 50 individuals undergoing reoperative coronary artery surgery, also found no significant differences in hematologic parameters and clinical outcome variables. The authors of these two studies concluded that heparin-coated CPB circuits did not improve biochemical or clinical markers of biocompatibility in their respective individual populations. Several other clinical studies that used standard heparin doses, however, have provided contrasting data, which demonstrate, although not consistently, improved biocompatibility and outcomes in individuals subjected to heparin-coated surfaces (200–203).

The main advantage of heparin-coated circuits is among individuals in whom heparin coating is combined with administration of low-dose heparin and, hence, low-dose protamine. All studies that include such individuals (141, 206–211) have concluded that low-dose heparinization combined with heparin coating is safe and advantageous. Reduced systemic heparinization (ACT, >250 seconds) in individuals undergoing extracorporeal circulation with heparin-coated circuits decreases complement activation (207) and reduces postoperative morbidity (210), including postoperative blood loss (141, 207, 209, 210). It also does not increase thrombogenicity (208). Confirmatory studies are needed, however, to ensure that excessive thrombin is not generated with low-dose heparin combined with heparin-coated circuits.

## Alternatives to Systemic Anticoagulation with Heparin

Decreasing the average molecular weight of heparin decreases its antithrombin activity and retains its anti–factor Xa activity (180, 212). Hence, a variety of low-molecular-weight heparins, heparin fractions, and heparinoids are under investigation as alternatives to unfractionated heparin for anticoagulation during CPB. The ability of these compounds to anticoagulate blood is measured by their anti–factor Xa activity in U/kg. Experimental studies in animals, including dogs placed on CPB, demonstrated that these compounds are associated with a lower incidence of hemorrhage than occurs with standard heparin at an equivalent anti–factor Xa activity (213–215). However, low-molecular-weight heparins may produce complications when emergency neutralization procedures are required (216). When used as anticoagulants for CPB, severe postoperative hemorrhage has been encountered (181, 217). To date, use of fractionated low-molecular-weight heparins and heparinoids for anticoagulation during CPB has been restricted to situations in which a standard heparin regimen cannot be used, such as in individuals with severe heparin-induced thrombocytopenia and thrombosis

(183, 184). Low-molecular-weight heparin, however, reduces the risk of heparin-induced thrombocytopenia and thrombosis but does not totally eliminate it. Both *in vitro* (218) and *in vivo* studies in dogs (219, 220) and pigs (221) provide evidence that low-molecular-weight heparin compounds are safe and effective enough to be considered as alternatives to heparin in the future.

Other compounds also are being investigated as potential replacements for heparin during cardiac surgery. Hirudin and ancrod are two pharmacologic agents that have been used clinically, mostly in individuals with heparin-induced thrombocytopenia. Hirudin is an antithrombin-independent thrombin inhibitor that, unlike heparin, can inactivate thrombin bound to fibrin (222–224). Recombinant hirudin has been effective as an anticoagulant during CPB in experimental animals and in humans (187, 189, 219). Recent experimental studies in rats (225), however, have raised concerns about an increased hemorrhagic effect of hirudin compared with those other new anticoagulants. In addition, a recent clinical study (226) demonstrated persistent thrombin generation in humans, which was indicated by increased levels of prothrombin fragment 1.2, during specific thrombin inhibition with hirudin (226). Hence, even although the specificity of hirudin and hirudin congeners (e.g., bivalirudin or Hirulog™) for thrombin and their ability to penetrate formed clots make them promising heparin substitutes, more studies are needed before routine use can be advocated.

Ancrod is a defibrinogenating enzyme that has been demonstrated to be safe and effective as a heparin substitute during CPB in initial animal and human studies (227, 228). The ACT, however, is not reliable in monitoring the adequacy of anticoagulation with ancrod; therefore, measurement of fibrinogen concentration before, during, and after CPB may be the only useful method to determine the anticoagulant adequacy of ancrod (186). During CPB, ancrod is administered as a continuous infusion and is titrated to achieve plasma fibrinogen concentrations of between 0.2 and 0.7 g/l. To achieve adequate reduction in clotable fibrinogen, however, 12 to 24 hours of therapy are required, thus limiting its use in elective procedures. As with hirudin, clinical use of ancrod should be limited to individuals in whom anticoagulation with heparin is contraindicated.

Experimental studies in canine and porcine models have explored the potential of newer agents as possible alternatives to heparin anticoagulation during CPB. Some of the agents found to be promising in these studies include dermatan sulfate (229), a short-acting, oligonucleotide-based thrombin inhibitor (i.e., thrombin aptamer) (230); DuP 714, a synthetic peptide thrombin inhibitor (231); and CGP 39393, a specific peptide inhibitor of thrombin (232). Experimental studies also have demonstrated the feasibility of interposing in the bypass circuit an immobilized heparinized reactor filter (233) and an immobilized protamine bioreactor filter (234, 235), which would eliminate heparin from blood returned to the individual, reduce heparin anticoagulant activity, and reduce the need for systemic protamine (with its potential adverse reactions). This technology has yet to be applied clinically, however.

A promising adjunct to systemic heparinization is use of GP IIb-IIIa receptor inhibitors. Hiramatsu et al (236) found impressive preservation of platelet function and complete prevention of platelet loss in pigs subjected to CPB and treated with high-dose tirofiban, which is a nonpeptide inhibitor of platelet GP IIb-IIIa receptors. This novel approach to reduction of CPB-induced hemostatic dysfunction, however, awaits clinical confirmation.

Preliminary studies in baboons and humans have identified recombinant platelet factor 4 as a possible substitute for protamine in the reversal of heparin-induced anticoagulation (237–239). Data from these studies support future clinical trial of this endogenous antiheparin protein.

## NONSURGICAL BLOOD LOSS

### Types and Measurement of Postbypass Blood Loss

Clinically, the most important adverse effect of hemostatic dysfunction in individuals undergoing cardiac surgery is increased intraoperative and postoperative blood loss. Increased blood loss after institution of CPB may be defined loosely as either "surgical" or "nonsurgical" in nature. Blood loss from a specific anatomic site resulting from surgical procedure itself is "surgical," whereas diffuse blood loss not associated with a specific is anatomic site and that cannot be corrected surgically is "nonsurgical." The magnitude of postoperative nonsurgical blood loss can reflect the magnitude of hemostatic derangement in individuals undergoing open-heart surgery. It also can be used as an endpoint when evaluating the efficacy of interventions to reduce the CPB-induced hemostatic defect. For postoperative blood loss to reflect the magnitude of hemostatic dysfunction accurately, however, it must be quantified properly by observing the following guidelines:

1. Individuals in whom postoperative bleeding is surgical in nature should be excluded from the analysis (e.g., a individual returned to the operating room for repair of an obvious leak in the aortotomy suture line); and

2. Measurement of post-CPB blood loss should include the postoperative chest tube drainage in the intensive care unit and blood loss encountered in the operating room after administration of protamine and normalization of the ACT (i.e.,

**FIGURE 50.8.** Median blood loss following discontinuation of cardiopulmonary bypass (CPB) and heparin reversal in 170 individuals undergoing coronary artery bypass grafting (CABG; *n* = 144) and valve replacement with or without CABG (*n* = 26). Average age (± SD) of the individuals was 64.2 ± 9.5 years; duration of CPB was 124.7 ± 46.5 minutes. The two bar graphs represent the two main components of post-CPB blood loss: *OR,* the component incurred intraoperatively after the normalization of the ACT; and *SICU,* the component incurred through chest drainage in the surgical intensive care unit.

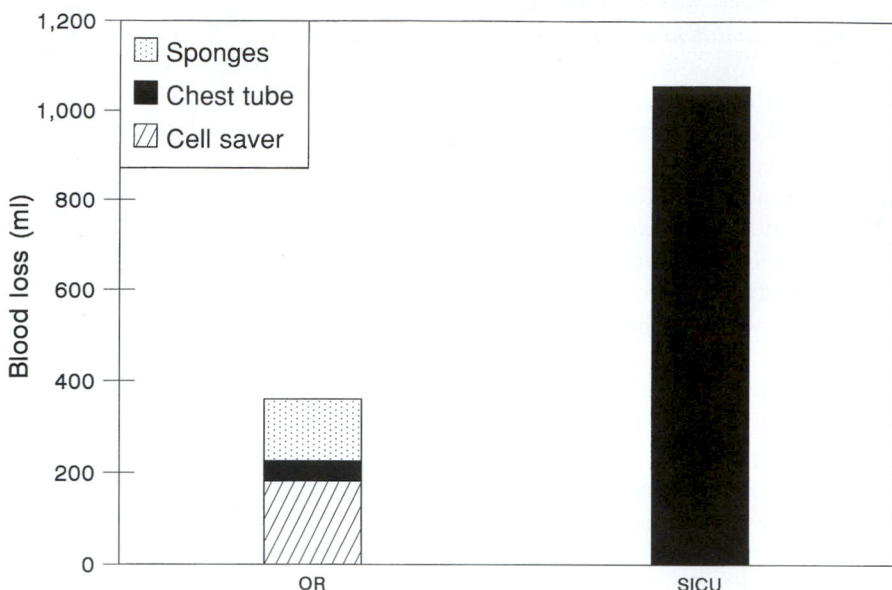

before the chest is closed and the individual transferred to intensive care).

Quantification of the intraoperative portion of post-CPB blood loss should include measurement of the blood volume aspirated into the wall suction or the Cell Saver during this period and that into mediastinal and chest tubes after their insertion. In addition, all sponges and laparotomy pads used during this period should be collected separately, weighed, and their blood contents recorded and added to the total blood loss. The weight differential of sponges and laparotomy pads can be transformed to milliliters of blood loss using the following formula:

$$\text{Blood loss (ml)} = \text{Weight (g)/Blood density}$$

where

$$\text{Blood density (g)} = 0.0692 \times \text{Hematocrit} + 1.0239$$

$$0.0692 = \text{Density of cells} - \text{Density of plasma}$$

$$1.0239 = \text{Density of plasma}$$

Fig. 50.8 shows the components of post-CPB blood loss as measured prospectively by a dedicated research assistant in 170 individuals undergoing CPB. In this individual population, the intraoperative component averaged 24.4% of the total blood loss (range, 2.4–69.9%). Ignoring this intraoperative component and restricting measurement to the chest tube drainage in the intensive care unit can jeopardize the validity of blood loss measurements. The intraoperative component is important in assessing the magnitude of the CPB-induced hemostatic dysfunction, because surgeons normally do not

close the chest and transfer the individual to intensive care until maximal control of the bleeding has been achieved in the operative field. Thus, blood loss during this period might provide more useful information about a individual's tendency to bleed than blood loss in the intensive care unit.

## Determinants of Postbypass Blood Loss

Surgical bleeding both during and after CPB primarily depends on expertise of the surgical team and adequacy of the surgical techniques employed. A consensus about the determinants of nonsurgical bleeding is difficult to achieve from the current literature because of the wide disparity in definitions, methods of measuring nonsurgical blood loss, and laboratory techniques. In a prospective study of 100 individuals that excluded surgical bleeders and was designed specifically to identify determinants of post-CPB blood loss in the first 4 hours (starting with the neutralization of protamine) (18), the following variables were noted to be significant in the univariate analyses (Fig. 50.9):

1. Duration of CPB,
2. Lowest esophageal temperature,
3. Platelet mass during CPB,
4. Wound temperature,
5. Hematocrit,
6. Platelet count, and
7. Bleeding time 2 hours post-CPB.

In the multivariate analysis, the two independent variables predictive of blood loss were duration of CPB and hematocrit 2 hours post-CPB. Many other studies have confirmed that duration of CPB (240, 241), hypothermia

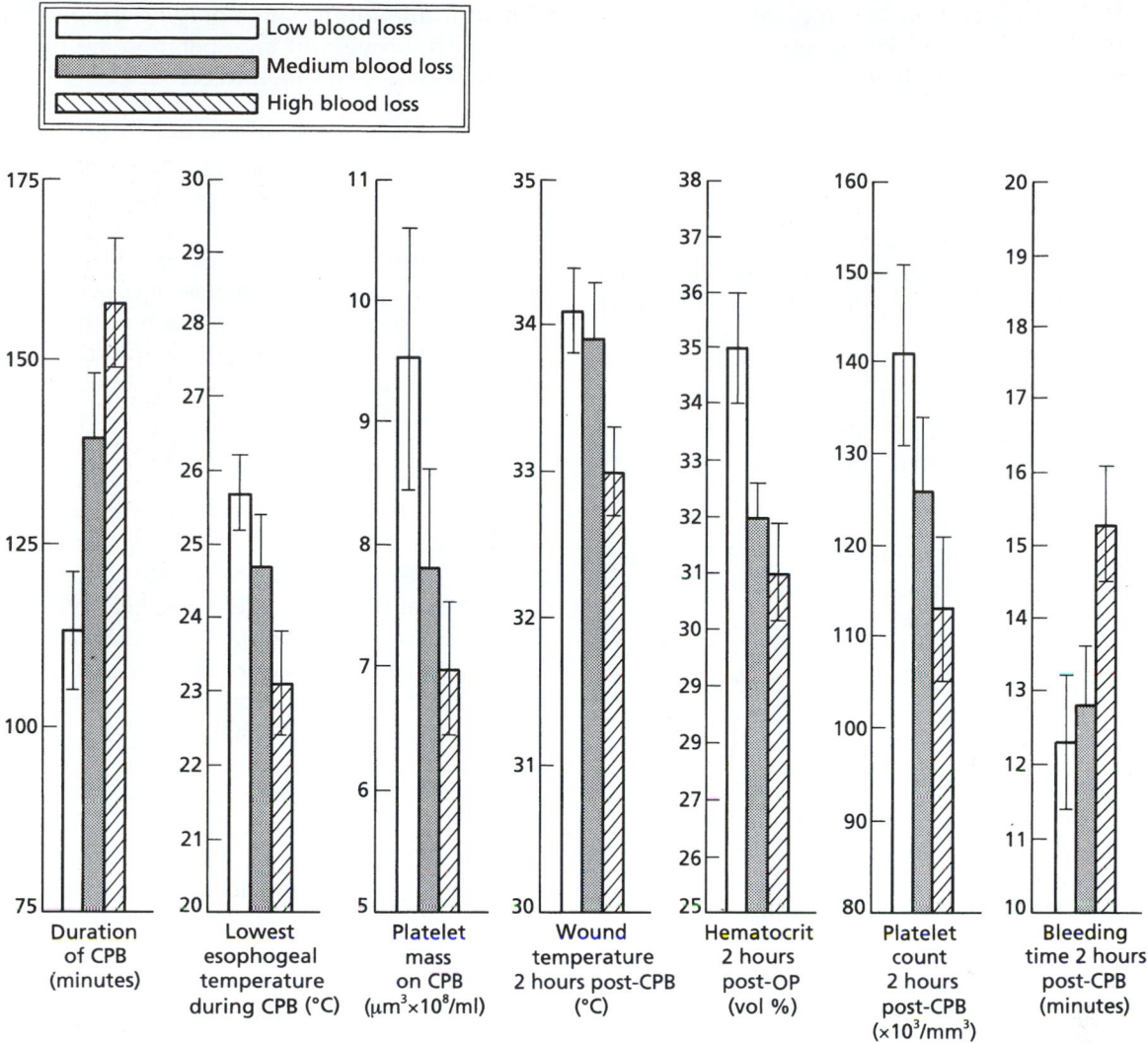

**FIGURE 50.9.** Preoperative, intraoperative, and postoperative variables in terciles of blood loss during the initial 4 hours after cardiopulmonary bypass (post-CPB) in 78 individuals undergoing valvular and coronary artery surgery. The designated tercile levels were: low, 215–790 mL, *n* = 26; medium, 805–1140 mL, *n* = 26; and high, 1235–2515 mL, *n* = 26. (Reprinted with permission from Khuri SF, Wolfe JA, Josa M, et al. Hematologic changes during and after cardiopulmonary bypass and their relationship to the bleeding time and nonsurgical blood loss. J Thorac Cardiovasc Surg 1992;104:94–107.)

(241, 242), and heparin concentration during CPB (207, 209) are important predictors of post-CPB blood loss. That hemodilution is a significant independent predictor of blood loss is an important finding, and it underscores the potential of red blood cell transfusion to reduce post-CPB blood loss.

Derangements in various laboratory measurements of blood coagulation and platelet function occur both during and after CPB (243, 244), but the role of these measurements in predicting post-CPB blood loss and the need for blood product transfusions is controversial. In particular, the role of bleeding time in predicting post-CPB blood loss is not fully defined (see Chapter 23). Under normal circumstances, the preoperative bleeding time does not predict the amount of postoperative blood

loss (18, 50, 72, 245–252); however, marked extensions in the preoperative bleeding time tend to result in increased postoperative blood loss (245). It is not established whether prolonged preoperative bleeding times in individuals receiving preoperative aspirin predict excessive bleeding after CPB. Data suggest that preoperative aspirin ingestion prolongs the preoperative bleeding time but does not influence the post-CPB bleeding time (253). Conversely, a blinded, randomized, placebo-controlled Veterans Administration Cooperative Study (254) demonstrated significantly increased post-CPB blood loss in individuals receiving preoperative aspirin. Unfortunately, no bleeding time measurements were obtained in that study, and the validity of published observations on this is further limited by:

1. Recent demonstration of the temperature dependence of bleeding time measurements and the need to correct bleeding times for temperature (20, 90, 255), and

2. Failure in most published studies to properly and prospectively differentiate and quantify nonsurgical blood loss.

In studies that carefully measured bleeding times and post-CPB blood loss, the postoperative bleeding time correlated with the magnitude of postoperative blood loss, thus providing a rationale for platelet transfusions in individuals with excessive postoperative bleeding and a significantly prolonged bleeding time (18, 256, 257).

Some investigators have identified a role for preoperative (240) and postoperative (241, 258) measurements of prothrombin time (PT) and activated partial thromboplastin time (aPTT) in the prediction and treatment of post-CPB blood loss (see Chapter 23). Most recent studies, however, have failed to associate pre-CPB and post-CPB measurements of PT and aPTT with magnitude of the post-CPB blood loss (18, 243, 244, 259). As stated by Brandt (257), the consensus of investigators addressing the merits of laboratory tests for coagulation, fibrinolysis, and platelet function in individuals undergoing CPB conveys two important messages:

1. Laboratory tests cannot be used to identify which individuals are likely to bleed, and

2. There is little indication for routinely performing an extensive battery of coagulation tests after CPB (257).

## Prevention and Treatment of Postbypass Blood Loss

### Preoperative Workup and Surgical Technique

An adequate preoperative workup of cardiac surgical individuals is important to prevent and treat post-CPB blood loss. The preoperative workup should include a thorough individual history to assess bleeding tendency and related family history. Preoperative ingestion of aspirin might increase post-CPB bleeding (253), but this need not deter the cardiac operation. Preoperatively, it is reasonable to obtain a partial thromboplastin time, PT, platelet count, and a template bleeding time (260). Considering the limitations of these tests in predicting postoperative blood loss, an alternative approach is to perform them only in individuals with increased risk of bleeding; protocols have been recently developed to identify such individuals preoperatively (261). In individuals with preoperative anemia, administration of recombinant human erythropoietin is useful in reducing postoperative blood loss (262–266).

Probably the single most important factor in preventing excessive post-CPB blood loss is meticulous attention to surgical technique. Performing an effective operation expeditiously, thereby reducing the period of CPB to a minimum, and applying proper hemostatic techniques throughout the operation are imperative to minimize post-CPB blood loss.

### Extracorporeal Perfusion Techniques

The conduct and conditions of extracorporeal perfusion influence the genesis and treatment of post-CPB blood loss. Adequate systemic rewarming and maintenance of systemic normothermia are important factors in the prevention and treatment of excessive postoperative blood loss. The rationale for this approach was elucidated earlier and is based on the observed relationships between temperature and post-CPB platelet function and blood loss. Because hematocrit is an important predictor of post-CPB blood loss, minimizing hemodilution during cardiac surgery likely will improve postoperative hemostatic function. The hematocrit can be raised during CPB through a combination of retrograde autologous priming (i.e., replacing the crystalloid prime with blood drained from the right side of the heart via the venous cannula immediately before institution of CPB [267]), interposition of a hemoconcentrator in the bypass circuit, and red blood cell transfusion.

Reducing the blood–gas interface by using a closed perfusion circuit and minimizing negative-pressure aspiration of blood from the surgical field into the extracorporeal circuit also can reduce hemostatic dysfunction and post-CPB blood loss (268). In addition, blood that is accumulated in the pericardial cavity and aspirated into the extracorporeal circuit causes increased thrombin generation (129) and increased fibrinolysis (130). Hence, during CPB, aspiration of blood accumulating in the pericardial cavity into the Cell Saver, instead of into the extracorporeal circuit, should reduce hemostatic dysfunction and decrease postoperative blood loss. Cell Saver blood is washed before it is retransfused at the end of CPB, thus ridding it of prothrombotic and profibrinolytic substances.

As discussed, reducing the ACT from 480 to 250 seconds by use of heparin-coated circuits is safe. It also is likely to reduce the heparin-induced hemostatic dysfunction and, therefore, post-CPB blood loss.

### Autologous and Homologous Blood Product Transfusions

Miscellaneous blood products should be transfused after significant blood loss. Autologous blood, collected over a period of 3 to 4 weeks preoperatively, is the optimal replacement, but it may not be feasible logistically in some individuals (269–271). Phlebotomy of whole blood immediately before institution of CPB and its subsequent postoperative reinfusion are not consistently beneficial (272–276), and routine use of homologous platelet transfusions in cardiac surgery is unnecessary (277). Newer methods and techniques have made possible sequestration of platelet-rich plasma, with retransfusion of the red cells, immediately before institution of CPB and reinfusion of this plasma postoperatively after discontinuation of bypass. This technique partially spares the platelets from being affected by the extracorporeal circuit. Preservation of platelet number, decreased postoperative blood loss, and decreased requirement for homologous blood transfusions have been reported with this technique (278–281). Cell Savers are used routinely during open-heart surgery, and washed red cells are autotransfused after completion of CPB. Blood shed from the pleura and mediastinum through the chest tubes during the first 24 hours is reinfused to reduce the need for postoperative homologous blood transfusion (272–285). Transfusing as much as 1 L of unwashed, shed mediastinal blood is safe, and except for its possible effect on the hematocrit, it does not affect any of the hematologic or related parameters in the recipient (286). The safety of larger transfusions of unwashed, shed mediastinal blood, however, has yet to be determined.

Treatment of excessive postoperative nonsurgical bleeding usually entails transfusion of platelets (see Chapter 51), cryoprecipitate, and fresh frozen plasma (see Chapter 52). These products should not be transfused before:

1. Heparin is adequately reversed,
2. Full systemic normothermia is achieved, and
3. The hematocrit is restored to a value exceeding 30% with red blood cell transfusions.

Observing these three conditions should reduce the need for postoperative fresh frozen plasma and platelet transfusions. Current storage techniques allow platelets to be transfused up to 5 days after pheresis, but platelet function progressively deteriorates during liquid storage. Actively bleeding individuals who lack adequate numbers of functional platelets should receive platelets that have been stored at room temperature for no more than 24 hours (287). Preliminary clinical data indicate that infusion of thawed, cryopreserved platelets (i.e., stored at −80°C) improves the function of platelets stored for an average of 289 days (median, 250 days; range, 30–720 days) compared with infusion of liquid-stored platelets and significantly reduces both postoperative blood loss and need for blood product transfusions (288).

## Pharmacologic Interventions

Various pharmacologic agents have been used to reduce bleeding after CPB. $PGE_1$ and $PGI_2$ reduce platelet loss during *in vitro* simulations of extracorporeal circulation (37, 38, 289). Randomized, double-blind, controlled trials of prophylactic $PGI_2$ administration in individuals undergoing CPB, however, have not shown a clear benefit (41, 42, 67, 68, 289–292). Furthermore, $PGI_2$ and its analogue iloprost cause severe vasodilation and hypotension (41, 42, 67, 68, 289). Studies in both dogs (43)

and humans (44) also have shown that preoperative administration of dipyridamole preserves the platelet count and reduces blood loss after cardiac surgery. Routine clinical use of these pharmacologic agents, however, has not been established (68).

It is established that antifibrinolytic agents (see Chapter 53) play a major role in reducing CPB-induced hemostatic dysfunction and post-CPB blood loss. The salutary role of these agents confirms the important role of hyperfibrinolysis in the genesis of hemostatic dysfunction during cardiac surgery. ε-aminocaproic acid (Amicar Elkins-Sinn, Inc, Cherry Hill, NJ) originally was used in selected individuals and proved to be effective in controlling excessive blood loss after CPB (119, 125, 293). The prophylactic intravenous administration of ε-aminocaproic acid (10 g before skin incision, 10 g after heparin administration, and 10 g at discontinuation of CPB; or 10 g at induction of anesthesia, followed by 2 g/hour infused for 5 hours) is safe and significantly reduces fibrinolysis and blood loss after cardiac surgery (94, 294). Prophylactic administration in a single dose of 5 g before institution of CPB also reduces blood loss when combined with postoperative administration of desmopressin (295). Tranexamic acid, which is an isomer of ε-aminocaproic acid, has seven to 10 times the inhibitory activity (296) and is effective in reducing blood loss when administered prophylactically to individuals undergoing cardiac surgery (297–301). Tranexamic acid may be less effective than ε-aminocaproic acid at preventing post-CPB blood loss (294), and its prophylactic administration to children is effective only in individuals with cyanotic heart disease (302).

Aprotinin, a protease inhibitor has consistently reduced postoperative blood loss in numerous clinical studies. Reductions of 40 to 60% were observed when this agent was administered in high doses before and during CPB (116, 303–308). Low-dose aprotinin (50–80% of the high dose), when administered before and during CPB, also effectively reduces the hemostatic dysfunction and postoperative blood loss in individuals undergoing cardiac surgery (308–313). It is increasingly evident that aprotinin, particularly when administered in a low dose, exerts its salutary effect mainly by inhibiting hyperfibrinolysis (116, 307, 311–315). Whether aprotinin has a protective effect on platelets during CPB remains controversial, but aprotinin has been reported to improve platelet function (91, 308, 316) and ultrastructure (309). Even so, a well-conducted, double-blind study provided convincing data indicating that aprotinin did not influence the change in platelet count, suppress β-TG release from platelets, prevent CPB-induced inhibition of platelet function, or influence plasma concentration of glycocalicin during and after CPB (314), and these results have been confirmed (317). A double-blind, randomized study of 106 individuals undergoing CPB (318) also found that the mechanism by which high-dose aprotinin reduced bleeding was independent of any effect on platelet function. This study did, however, demonstrate that aprotinin produced a greater reduction in bleeding among individuals whose condition was hemostatically compromised by preoperative platelet dysfunction.

Administration of aprotinin with heparin causes a prolonged ACT and aPTT. The prolonged ACT occurs when celite-activated tubes are used in obtaining this measurement; it is not observed when kaolin-activated tubes are used (319). This has prompted the use of kaolin instead of celite as the activating agent for measuring the ACT in individuals receiving aprotinin. Another study (306) has ascribed the prolonged celite-based ACT to an anticoagulant effect of aprotinin, and these authors have advocated use of celite rather than kaolin in these individuals. It is increasingly evident that both methods are equally reliable after anticoagulation in individuals receiving aprotinin, particularly in conjunction with the Hepcon/HMS (320, 321). Thrombin-based tests, such as the HITT, have been used to monitor the adequacy of anticoagulation in these individuals as well (322). The prolonged celite-based ACT and aPTT that occur with administration of aprotinin have led some investigators to hypothesize a synergistic relationship between aprotinin and heparin and to advocate reducing the usual heparin dose in individuals receiving aprotinin during CPB (323).

Concern had been expressed about the possibility of aprotinin causing a postoperative hypercoagulable state, thereby producing an increased incidence of postoperative aortocoronary graft occlusion. These concerns have been partially alleviated by the demonstration of decreased postoperative thrombin generation in adults and children receiving high-dose aprotinin (306, 307, 315). In addition, a placebo-controlled, double-blind study of 90 individuals showed that early (7–12 days) vein-graft patency was not adversely affected by high-dose aprotinin (324). Another recent study examined the *in vitro* vascular reactivity of coronary bypass grafts to a range of vasoconstrictor agents with and without aprotinin. In this study, use of aprotinin preserved endothelium-dependent responses to acetylcholine and decreased the vasoconstrictive response to the thromboxane analogue U46619. Hence, the investigators postulated that the decrease in vasoconstriction after administration of aprotinin could counteract potential prothrombotic adverse effects on graft patency (325). Renal dysfunction and intravascular coagulation also have been reported after administration of aprotinin in elderly individuals undergoing operations on the thoracic and thoracoabdominal aorta using CPB and hypothermic circulatory arrest (326).

Because it is an allogenic protein, aprotinin possesses antigenic properties. Dietrich et al (327) reported the incidence of adverse reactions to reexposure to be

2.8% (327). The severity of reactions to aprotinin in this series varied over a wide spectrum but did not result in any fatality. The authors recommend the following procedure for reexposure with high-dose aprotinin:

1. Delay of the first bolus injection of aprotinin until the surgeon is ready to begin CPB,
2. Administer a test dose of 10,000 Kallikrein inactivator units (KIU) aprotinin in all individuals with aprotinin treatment,
3. Initiated $H_1/H_2$ blockade in known or possible reexposures, and
4. Avoid of reexposure within the first 6 months after the last exposure to aprotinin (327).

Recent comparative studies have found aprotinin to be as effective as ε-aminocaproic acid (294), but more effective than tranexamic acid (294, 328), in reducing blood loss.

Intravenous DDAVP (desmopressin) (see Chapter 53) has been used to reduce post-CPB blood loss because of its potential to raise plasma levels of vWf and its multimers. Results, however, have been inconsistent and contradictory for postoperative use of this drug (73, 329–334). Salzman et al (329) reported DDAVP to be beneficial in increasing the vWf level and reducing postoperative blood loss in individuals undergoing complex valvular heart surgery. Subsequent studies in individuals undergoing routine coronary artery revascularization (73) and in children undergoing cardiac operations (332) found that the administration of DDAVP did not increase vWf levels more than the rise ordinarily observed postoperatively in the cardiac individuals, and it did not reduce postoperative blood loss. These latter results, along with the finding that the vWf level in a large group of individuals undergoing coronary and valvular operations did not correlate with post-CPB blood loss (18), indicate DDAVP should not be used as a routine adjunct in cardiac surgery. It might be useful in individuals known to have platelet dysfunction preoperatively (333, 334), however, or in combination with ε-aminocaproic acid (295).

# CONCLUSIONS

Institution of CPB elicits hemostatic abnormalities that result in increased postoperative blood loss. The two major CPB-induced hemostatic abnormalities are platelet dysfunction and hyperfibrinolysis.

Prolonged bleeding times during and after CPB and their reversal within 24 to 48 hours postoperatively indicate CPB-induced, reversible platelet dysfunction. Thrombocytopenia, which is observed both during and after CPB, results from hemodilution and loss of platelets, which are activated and degranulated through contact with and adhesion to synthetic surfaces. The thrombocytopenia observed during CPB is not severe enough to account for the prolonged bleeding time and the observed platelet dysfunction. Recent studies employing whole blood flow cytometry have shown that CPB results in:

1. Markedly deficient platelet reactivity in response to an *in vivo* wound,
2. Normal platelet reactivity *in vitro*,
3. No loss of platelet surface GP Ib-IX or GP IIb-IIIa complexes, and
4. Minimal circulating activated platelets.

Results of these studies also suggest that the "platelet function defect" of CPB is not intrinsic to the platelet; rather, it mostly results from a variety of extrinsic factors, some of which are still unidentified. Systemic hypothermia, fibrinolysis, and heparin are extrinsic factors that contribute to the platelet dysfunction during and after CPB.

Administration of heparin, institution of CPB, and blood stasis in the pericardial cavity result in increased fibrinolysis, which hinders post-CPB hemostasis. Prophylactic use of antifibrinolytic agents, in particular aprotinin and ε-aminocaproic acid, effectively reduces blood loss after CPB.

When measured properly, nonsurgical blood loss can reflect the magnitude of the hemostatic abnormality after institution of CPB. Quantification of this blood loss should begin intraoperatively, immediately after neutralization of heparin and normalization of the ACT. Nonsurgical blood loss after CPB is determined primarily by the duration of CPB and several other factors, including level of hemodilution, systemic and skin temperatures, heparin concentration (and adequacy of its reversal), and platelet mass both during and after CPB. Routine tests of coagulation do not consistently predict post-CPB blood loss. The preoperative bleeding time also does not predict postoperative blood loss, but the bleeding time during the initial postoperative period does predict blood loss during that period.

Clinical measures with a potential for limiting the hemostatic defect and reducing post-CPB blood loss include maintenance of systemic normothermia, complete reversal of systemic hypothermia, minimization of hemodilution, use of a closed perfusion circuit, avoidance of excessive aspiration of blood into the pump, avoidance of blood stasis in the pericardial cavity, and accurate monitoring of anticoagulation by use of an HMS. Heparin remains the universal anticoagulant for CPB. Heparin also has numerous adverse effects, however, and its use is limited in individuals with heparin-induced thrombocytopenia and thrombosis.

At its current clinical dose, heparin does not completely prevent thrombin generation during and, more importantly, after institution of CPB. Alternatives to heparin have been employed, but their use continues to be sporadic and limited to individuals who cannot receive heparin. Use of heparin-coated surfaces may enable the dose of heparin to be reduced during CPB. The safety and efficacy of low-dose heparin with heparin-coated surfaces is under investigation.

# REFERENCES

1. Roth GJ. Developing relationships: arterial platelet adhesion, glycoprotein Ib, and leucine-rich glycoproteins. Blood 1991;77:5–19.
2. Michelson AD, Loscalzo J, Melnick B et al. Partial characterization of a binding site for von Willebrand factor on glycocalicin. Blood 1986;67:19–26.
3. Phillips DR, Charo IF, Parise LV et al. The platelet membrane glycoprotein IIb-IIIa complex. Blood 1988;71:831–843.
4. Leung LL. Role of thrombospondin in platelet aggregation. J Clin Invest 1984;74:1764–1772.
5. Bevilacqua M, Butcher E, Furie B et al. Selectins: a family of adhesion receptors [Letter]. Cell 1991;67:233.
6. McEver RP. Properties of GMP-140, an inducible granule membrane protein of platelets and endothelium. Blood Cells 1990;16:73–80.
7. Hsu-Lin S, Berman CL, Furie BC et al. A platelet membrane protein expressed during platelet activation and secretion. Studies using a monoclonal antibody specific for thrombin-activated platelets. J Biol Chem 1984;259:9121–9126.
8. Stenberg PE, McEver RP, Shuman MA et al. A platelet alpha-granule membrane protein (GMP-140) is expressed on the plasma membrane after activation. J Cell Biol 1985;101:880–886.
9. Larsen E, Celi A, Gilbert GE et al. PADGEM protein: a receptor that mediates the interaction of activated platelets with neutrophils and monocytes. Cell 1989;59:305–312.
10. Hamburger SA, McEver RP. GMP-140 mediates adhesion of stimulated platelets to neutrophils. Blood 1990;75:550–554.
11. Palabrica T, Lobb R, Furie BC et al. Leukocyte accumulation promoting fibrin deposition is mediated *in vivo* by P-selectin on adherent platelets. Nature 1992;359:848–851.
12. Celi A, Pellegrini G, Lorenzet R et al. P-selectin induces the expression of tissue factor on monocytes. Proc Natl Acad Sci U S A 1994;91:8767–8771.
13. George JN, Pickett EB, Saucerman S et al. Platelet surface glycoproteins. Studies on resting and activated platelets and platelet membrane microparticles in normal subjects, and observations in individuals during adult respiratory distress syndrome and cardiac surgery. J Clin Invest 1986;78:340–348.
14. Michelson AD, Barnard MR. Thrombin-induced changes in platelet membrane glycoproteins Ib, IX, and IIb-IIIa complex. Blood 1987;70:1673–1678.
15. George JN, Torres MM. Thrombin decreases von Willebrand factor binding to platelet glycoprotein Ib. Blood 1988;71:1253–1259.
16. Michelson AD, Ellis PA, Barnard MR et al. Down-regulation of the platelet surface glycoprotein Ib-IX complex in whole blood stimulated by thrombin, adenosine diphosphate, or an *in vivo* wound. Blood 1991;77:770–779.
17. Harker LA, Malpass TW, Branson HE et al. Mechanism of abnormal bleeding in individuals undergoing cardiopulmonary bypass: acquired transient platelet dysfunction associated with selective α-granule release. Blood 1980;56:824–834.
18. Khuri SF, Wolfe JA, Josa M et al. Hematologic changes during and after cardiopulmonary bypass and their relationship to the bleeding time and nonsurgical blood loss. J Thorac Cardiovasc Surg 1992;104:94–107.
19. Kestin AS, Valeri CR, Khuri SF et al. The platelet function defect of cardiopulmonary bypass. Blood 1993;82:107–117.
20. Valeri CR, Khabbaz K, Khuri SF et al. Effect of skin temperature on platelet function in individuals undergoing extracorporeal bypass. J Thorac Cardiovasc Surg 1992;104:108–116.
21. Edmunds LH, Addonizio VP. Extracorporeal circulation. In: Colman RW, Hirsh J, Marder VJ, Salzman EW, eds. Hemostasis and thrombosis. Basic principles and clinical practice. Philadelphia: JB Lippincott, 1987:901–912.
22. Mammen EF, Koets MH, Washington BC et al. Hemostasis changes during cardiopulmonary bypass surgery. Semin Thromb Hemost 1985;11:281–292.
23. Colman RW. Platelet and neutrophil activation in cardiopulmonary bypass. Ann Thorac Surg 1990;49:32–34.
24. Martin JF, Daniel TD, Trowbridge EA. Acute and chronic changes in platelet volume and count after cardiopulmonary bypass induced thrombocytopenia in man. Thromb Haemost 1987;57:55–58.
25. Addonizio VP Jr, Colman RW, Edmunds LH Jr. The effect of blood flow rate and circuit surface area on platelet loss during extracorporeal circulation. Trans Am Soc Artif Intern Organs 1978;24:650–655.
26. Salzman EW, Lindon J, Brier D et al. Surface-induced platelet adhesion, aggregation and release. Ann N Y Acad Sci 1977;283:114–127.
27. George JN. Direct assessment of platelet adhesion to glass: a study of the forces of interaction and the effects of plasma and serum factors, platelet function and modification of the glass surface. Blood 1972;40:862–874.

28. Uniyal S, Brash JL. Patterns of adsorption of proteins from human plasma onto foreign surfaces. Thromb Haemost 1982;47:285–290.

29. Lindon JN, McManama G, Kushner L et al. Does the conformation of adsorbed fibrinogen dictate platelet interactions with artificial surfaces? Blood 1986;68:355–362.

30. Lindon JN, McManama G, Pekala R et al. Fibrinogen-platelet interactions on hydrophilic and hydrophobic surfaces [Abstract]. Circulation 1984;70: II-358.

31. Gluszko P, Rucinski B, Musial J et al. Fibrinogen receptors in platelet adhesion to surfaces of extracorporeal circuit. Am J Physiol 1987;252: H615–H621.

32. Slaughter TF, LeBleu TH, Douglas JM Jr et al. Characterization of pro-thrombin activation during cardiac surgery by hemostatic molecular markers. Anesthesiology 1994;80:520–526.

33. Chuang HY. In situ immunoradiometric assay of fibrinogen adsorbed to artificial surfaces. J Biomed Mater Res 1984;18:547–559.

34. Shattil SJ, Hoxie JA, Cunningham M et al. Changes in the platelet mem-brane glycoprotein IIb-IIIa complex during platelet activation. J Biol Chem 1985;260:11107–11114.

35. Musial J, Niewiarowski S, Hershock D et al. Loss of fibrinogen receptors from the platelet surface during simulated extracorporeal circulation. J Lab Clin Med 1985;105:514–522.

36. Teoh KH, Christakis GT, Weisel RD et al. Prevention of myocardial platelet deposition and thromboxane release with dipyridamole. Circulation 1986; 74:III-145–III-152.

37. Addonizio VP Jr, Macarak J, Nicolaou KC et al. Effects of prostacyclin and albumin on platelet loss during in vitro simulation of extracorporeal circulation. Blood 1979;53:1033–1042.

38. Addonizio VP Jr, Macarak EJ, Niewiarowski S et al. Preservation of human platelets with prostaglandin E₁ during in vitro simulation of cardiopulmo-nary bypass. Circ Res 1979,44:350–357.

39. Addonizio VP Jr, Fisher CA, Jenkin BK et al. Iloprost (ZK36374), a stable analogue of prostacyclin, preserves platelets during simulated extracorpo-real circulation. J Thorac Cardiovasc Surg 1985;89:926–933.

40. Addonizio VP Jr, Fisher CA, Kappa JR et al. Prevention of heparin-induced thrombocytopenia during open heart surgery with iloprost (ZK36374). Surgery 1987;102:796–807.

41. Walker ID, Davidson JF, Faichney A et al. A double blind study of prosta-cyclin in cardiopulmonary bypass surgery. Br J Haematol 1981;49:415–423.

42. Aren C, Feddersen K, Radegran K. Effects of prostacyclin infusion on platelet activation and postoperative blood loss in coronary bypass. Ann Thorac Surg 1983;36:49–54.

43. Teoh KH, Christakis GT, Weisel RD et al. Dipyridamole reduced myocar-dial platelet and leukocyte deposition following ischemia and cardi-oplegia. J Surg Res 1987;42:642–652.

44. Teoh KH, Christakis GT, Weisel RD et al. Dipyridamole preserved plate-lets and reduced blood loss after cardiopulmonary bypass. J Thorac Car-diovasc Surg 1988;96:332–341.

45. Packham MA, Evans G, Glynn MF et al. The effect of plasma proteins on the interaction of platelets with glass surfaces. J Lab Clin Med 1969;73: 686–697.

46. Salzman EW, Merrill EW, Binder A et al. Protein-platelet interaction on heparinized surfaces. J Biomed Mater Res 1969;3:69–81.

47. Edmunds LH Jr, Saxena NC, Hillyer P et al. Relationship between platelet count and cardiotomy suction return. Ann Thorac Surg 1978;25:306–310.

48. Boonstra PW, van Imhoff GW, Eysman L et al. Reduced platelet activation and improved hemostasis after controlled cardiotomy suction during clini-cal membrane oxygenator perfusions. J Thorac Cardiovasc Surg 1985;89: 900–906.

49. Edmunds LH Jr, Ellison N, Colman RW et al. Platelet function during cardiac operation: comparison of membrane and bubble oxygenators. J Thorac Cardiovasc Surg 1982;83:805–812.

50. Bick RL. Hemostasis defects associated with cardiac surgery, prosthetic devices, and other extracorporeal circuits. Semin Thromb Hemost 1985; 11:249–280.

51. Bachmann F, McKenna R, Cole ER et al. The haemostatic mechanism after open-heart surgery. I. Studies on plasma coagulation factors and fibrinoly-sis in 512 individuals after extracorporeal circulation. J Thorac Cardiovasc Surg 1975;70:76–85.

52. Young JA. Coagulation abnormalities with cardiopulmonary bypass. In: Utley JR, ed. Pathophysiology and techniques of cardiopulmonary bypass. Baltimore: Williams & Wilkins, 1982:88–105.

53. Ekert H, Gilchrist GS, Stanton R et al. Hemostasis in cyanotic congenital heart disease. J Pediatr 1970;76:221–230.

54. Gross S, Keefer V, Liebman J. The platelets in cyanotic congenital heart disease. Pediatrics 1968;42:651–658.

55. Laufer N, Merin G, Grover NB et al. The influence of cardiopulmonary bypass on the size of human platelets. J Thorac Cardiovasc Surg 1975;70: 727–731.

56. Thompson CB, Jakubowski JA, Quinn PG et al. Platelet size as a determi-nant of platelet function. J Lab Clin Med 1983;101:205–213.

57. Davey FR, Parker FB. Delayed hemostatic changes following cardiopulmo-nary bypass. Am J Med Sci 1976;271:171–178.

58. Cella G, Vittadello O, Gallucci V et al. The release of β-thromboglobulin and platelet factor 4 during extracorporeal circulation for open heart sur-gery. Eur J Clin Invest 1981;11:165–169.

59. Addonizio VP Jr, Smith JB, Strauss JF III et al. Thromboxane synthesis and platelet secretion during cardiopulmonary bypass with bubble oxy-genator. J Thorac Cardiovasc Surg 1980;79:91–96.

60. Mezzano D, Aranda E, Urzua J et al. Changes in platelet beta-thromboglo-bulin, fibrinogen, albumin, 5-hydroxytryptamine, ATP and ADP during and after surgery with extracorporeal circulation in man. Am J Hematol 1986;22:133–142.

61. Pumphrey CW, Dawes J. Platelet alpha granule depletion: findings in indi-viduals with prosthetic heart valves and following cardiopulmonary by-pass surgery. Thromb Res 1983;30:257–264.

62. Zilla P, Fasol R, Groscurth P et al. Blood platelets in cardiopulmonary bypass operations. Recovery occurs after initial stimulation, rather than continual activation. J Thorac Cardiovasc Surg 1989;97:379–388.

63. Valeri CR, Feingold H, Cassidy G et al. Hypothermia-induced reversible platelet dysfunction. Ann Surg 1987;205:175–181.

64. Thorngren M, Shafi S, Born GV. Thromboxane A2 in skin-bleeding-time blood and in clotted venous blood before and after administration of ace-tylsalicylic acid. Lancet 1983;i:1075–1078.

65. Gerrard JM, Taback S, Singhroy S et al. In vivo measurement of thrombox-ane B2 and 6-keto-prostaglandin F1a in humans in response to a standard-ized vascular injury and the influence of aspirin. Circulation 1989;79: 29–38.

66. Hennessy VL Jr, Hicks RE, Niewiarowski S et al. Function of human plate-lets during extracorporeal circulation. Am J Physiol 1977;232:H622–H628.

67. Longmore DB, Hoyle PM, Gregory A et al. Prostacyclin administration during cardiopulmonary bypass in man. Lancet 1981;i:800–804.

68. van den Dungen JJ, Karliczek GF, Brenken U et al. The effect of prostaglan-din E1 in individuals undergoing clinical cardiopulmonary bypass. Ann Thorac Surg 1983;35:406–414.

69. McKenna R, Bachmann F, Whittaker B et al. The hemostatic mechanism after open-heart surgery. II. Frequency of abnormal platelet functions dur-ing and after extracorporeal circulation. J Thorac Cardiovasc Surg 1975; 70:298–308.

70. Coppe D, Sobel M, Seamans L et al. Preservation of platelet function and number by prostacyclin during cardiopulmonary bypass. J Thorac Car-diovasc Surg 1981;81:274–278.

71. Mohr R, Golan M, Martinowitz U et al. Effect of cardiac operation on platelets. J Thorac Cardiovasc Surg 1986;92:434–441.

72. Jones DK, Luddington R, Higenbottam TW et al. Changes in factor VIII proteins after cardiopulmonary bypass in man suggest endothelial dam-age. Thromb Haemost 1988;60:199–204.

73. Hackmann T, Gascoyne RD, Naiman SC et al. A trial of desmopressin (1-desamino-8-D-arginine vasopressin) to reduce blood loss in uncompli-cated cardiac surgery. N Engl J Med 1989;321:1437–1443.

74. Harker LA, Slichter SJ. The bleeding time as a screening test for evaluation of platelet function. N Engl J Med 1972;287:155–159.

75. Ekert H, Dowling SV. Platelet release abnormality and reduced prothrom-bin levels in children with cyanotic congenital heart disease. Aust Paediatr J 1977;13:17–21.

76. Mauer HM, McCue CM, Caul J et al. Impairment in platelet aggregation in congenital heart disease. Blood 1972;40:207–216.

77. Kowalski E, Kopec M, Wegrzynowicz Z. Influence of fibrinogen degrada-tion products (FDP) on platelet aggregation, adhesiveness, and viscous metamorphosis. Thromb Diath Haemorrh 1963;10:406–423.

78. Ray MJ, Marsh NA, Hawson GA. Relationship of fibrinolysis and platelet function to bleeding after cardiopulmonary bypass. Blood Coagul Fibri-nolysis 1994;5:679–685.

79. Wallace HW, Liquiori EM, Stein TP et al. Denatured of plasma platelet function. Trans Am Soc Artif Intern Organs 1975;21:450–455.

80. Lee WH, Krumhaar D, Fonkalsrud E et al. Denaturation of plasma proteins as a cause of morbidity and death after intracardiac operations. Surgery 1961;50:29–39.

81. Pruitt KM, Stroud RM, Scott JW. Blood damage in the heart-lung machine. Proc Soc Exp Biol Med 1971;137:714–718.

82. George JN, Thoi LL, Morgan RK. Quantitative analysis of platelet mem-brane glycoproteins: effect of platelet washing procedures and isolation of platelet density subpopulations. Thromb Res 1981;23:69–77.

83. Levine SP, Krentz LS. Development of a radioimmunoassay for human platelet factor 4. Thromb Res 1977;11:673–686.

84. Michelson AD. Flow cytometry: a clinical test of platelet function [Review]. Blood 1996;87:4925–4936.

85. Hanson SR, Harker LA. Interruption of acute platelet-dependent thrombo-sis by the synthetic antithrombin PPACK. Proc Natl Acad Sci U S A 1988; 85:3184–3188.

86. Eidt JF, Allison P, Noble S et al. Thrombin is an important mediator of platelet aggregation in stenosed canine coronary arteries with endothelial injury. J Clin Invest 1989;84:18–27.

87. Kelly AB, Marzec UM, Krupski W et al. Hirudin interruption of heparin-resistant arterial thrombus formation in baboons. Blood 1991;77: 1006–1012.

88. Khuri SF, Valeri CR, Loscalzo J et al. Heparin causes platelet dysfunction and induces fibrinolysis before cardiopulmonary bypass. Ann Thorac Surg 1995;60:1008–1014.

89. Upchurch GR, Valeri CR, Khuri SF et al. Effect of heparin on fibrinolytic activity and platelet function *in vivo*. Am J Physiol 1996;271:H528–534.

90. Michelson AD, MacGregor H, Barnard MR et al. Reversible inhibition of human platelet activation by hypothermia *in vivo* and *in vitro*. Thromb Haemost 1994;71:633–640.

91. Van Oeveren W, Harder MP, Roozendaal KJ et al. Aprotinin protects platelets against the initial effect of cardiopulmonary bypass. J Thorac Cardiovasc Surg 1990;99:788–796.

92. Wenger RK, Lukasiewicz H, Mikuta BS et al. Loss of platelet fibrinogen receptors during clinical cardiopulmonary bypass. J Thorac Cardiovasc Surg 1989;97:235–239.

93. Dechavanne M, Ffrench M, Pages J et al. Significant reduction in the binding of a monoclonal antibody (LYP 18) directed against the IIb-IIIa glycoprotein complex to platelets of individuals having undergone extracorporeal circulation. Thromb Haemost 1987;57:106–109.

94. Vander Salm TJ, Kaur S, Lancey RA et al. Reduction of bleeding after heart operations through the prophylactic use of epsilon-amino caproic acid. J Thorac Cardiovasc Surg 1996;112:1098–1107.

95. Rinder CS, Mathew JP, Rinder HM et al. Modulation of platelet surface adhesion receptors during cardiopulmonary bypass. Anesthesiology 1991;75:563–570.

96. Rinder CS, Bonan JL, Rinder HM et al. Cardiopulmonary bypass induces leukocyte-platelet adhesion. Blood 1992;79:1201–1205.

97. Komai H, Haworth SG. Effect of cardiopulmonary bypass on the circulating level of soluble GMP-140. Ann Thorac Surg 1994;58:478–482.

98. Michelson AD, Barnard MR, Hechtman HB et al. *In vivo* tracking of platelets: circulating degranulated platelets rapidly lose surface P-selectin but continue to circulate and function. Proc Natl Acad Sci U S A 1996;93:11877–11882.

99. Levine SP. Secreted platelet proteins as markers for pathological disorders. In: Phillips DR, Shuman MA, eds. Biochemistry of platelets. Orlando: Academic Press, 1986:378–415.

100. Abrams CS, Ellison N, Budzynski AZ et al. Direct detection of activated platelets and platelet-derived micro particles in humans. Blood 1990;75:128–138.

101. Chenoweth DE, Cooper SW, Hugli TE et al. Complement activation during cardiopulmonary bypass: evidence for generation of C3a and C5a anaphylatoxins. N Engl J Med 1981;304:497–503.

102. Gotta AW, Carsons S, Abrams L et al. Fibronectin levels during cardiopulmonary bypass. N Y State J Med 1987;87:493–496.

103. Saba TM, Jaffe E. Plasma fibronectin (opsonic glycoprotein): its synthesis by vascular endothelial cells and role in cardiopulmonary integrity after trauma as related to reticuloendothelial function. Am J Med 1980;68:577–594.

104. Pourrat E, Sie PM, Desrez X et al. Changes in plasma fibronectin levels after cardiac and pulmonary surgery: role of cardiopulmonary bypass. Scand J Thorac Cardiovasc Surg 1985;19:63–67.

105. Deno DC, McCafferty MH, Saba TM et al. Mechanism of acute depletion of plasma fibronectin following thermal injury in rats. Appearance of a gelatin like ligand in plasma. J Clin Invest 1984;73:20–34.

106. Meade TW, North WR, Chakrabarti R et al. Haemostatic function and cardiovascular death: early results of a prospective study. Lancet 1980;i:1050–1054.

107. Lowe GD, Drummond MM, Lorimer AR et al. Relation between extent of coronary artery disease and blood viscosity. Br Med J 1980;8:673–674.

108. Di Minno G, Mancini M. Measuring plasma fibrinogen to predict stroke and myocardial infarction (review). Arteriosclerosis 1990;10:1–7.

109. Woods JE, Kirklin JW, Owen CA Jr et al. Effect of bypass surgery on coagulation-sensitive clotting factors. Mayo Clin Proc 1967;42:724–735.

110. Douglas AS, McNicol GP, Bain WH et al. The hemostatic defect following extracorporeal circulation [Review]. Br J Surg 1966;53:455–467.

111. Gralnick HR, Fischer RD. The hemostatic response to open-heart operations. J Thorac Cardiovasc Surg 1971;61:909–915.

112. Mustard JF, Hoeksema TD, Mustard WT et al. Activity of the clotting mechanism during the extracorporeal shunting of blood. Bibl Haematol 1962;13:84–89.

113. Holloway DS, Summaria L, Sandesara J et al. Decreased platelet number and function and increased fibrinolysis contribute to postoperative bleeding in cardiopulmonary bypass individuals. Thromb Haemost 1988;59:62–67.

114. Stibbe J, Kluft C, Brommer EJ et al. Enhanced fibrinolytic activity during cardiopulmonary bypass in open-heart surgery in man is caused by extrinsic (tissue-type) plasminogen activator. Eur J Clin Invest 1984;14:375–382.

115. Mori F, Nakahara Y, Kurata S et al. Late changes in hemostatic parameters following open-heart surgery. J Cardiovasc Surg (Torino) 1982;23:458–462.

116. Blauhut B, Gross C, Necek S et al. Effects of high-dose aprotinin on blood loss, platelet function, fibrinolysis, complement, and renal function after cardiopulmonary bypass. J Thorac Cardiovasc Surg 1991;101:958–967.

117. Tanaka K, Wada K, Morimoto T et al. The role of the protein C-thrombomodulin system in physiologic anticoagulation during cardiopulmonary bypass. ASAIO Trans 1989;35:373–375.

118. Kucuk O, Kwaan HC, Frederickson J et al. Increased fibrinolytic activity in individuals undergoing cardiopulmonary bypass operation. Am J Hematol 1986;23:223–229.

119. Sukhanov VA, Bauman NN, Levit AL. Hyperfibrinolysis: its express diagnosis and role in the development of haemorrhagic syndrome after cardiopulmonary bypass. Cor Vasa 1988;30:442–446.

120. Gando S, Tedo I, Goda Y et al. Increased fibrinolytic activity during surgery with cardiopulmonary bypass (in Japanese). Masui 1990;39:751–756.

121. Kongsgaard UE, Smith-Erichsen N, Geiran O et al. Changes in the coagulation and fibrinolytic systems during and after cardiopulmonary bypass surgery. Thorac Cardiovasc Surg 1989;37:158–162.

122. Kongsgaard UE, Smith-Erichsen N, Geiran O et al. Changes in the plasma protease systems during open-heart surgery with dextran vs. Ringer acetate as priming solution. Scand J Thorac Cardiovasc Surg 1989;23:253–258.

123. Giuliani R, Szwarcer E, Martinez Aquino E et al. Fibrin-dependent fibrinolytic activity during extracorporeal circulation. Thromb Res 1991;61:369–373.

124. Valen G, Eriksson E, Risberg B et al. Fibrinolysis during cardiac surgery. Release of tissue plasminogen activator in arterial and coronary sinus blood. Eur J Cardiothorac Surg 1994;8:324–330.

125. Lambert CJ, Marengo-Rowe AJ, Leveson JE et al. The treatment of postperfusion bleeding using epsilon-amino caproic acid, cryoprecipitate, fresh frozen plasma, and protamine sulfate. Ann Thorac Surg 1979;28:440–444.

126. Stead SW. Comparison of two methods for heparin monitoring: a semi-automated heparin monitoring device and activated clotting time during extracorporeal circulation. Int J Clin Monit Comput 1989;6:247–254.

127. Bachmann F, Parisi P. Fibrinolysis. In: Friedel N, Hetzer R, Royston D, eds. Blood use in cardiac surgery. Darmstadt: Steinkopff-Verlag, 1991:3–9.

128. Kluft C. Pathomechanisms of defective hemostasis during and after extracorporeal circulation: contact phase activation. In: Friedel N, Hetzer R, Royston D, eds. Blood use in cardiac surgery. Darmstadt: Steinkopff-Verlag, 1991:10–15.

129. Chung JH, Gikakis N, Rao AK et al. Pericardial blood activates the extrinsic coagulation pathway during clinical cardiopulmonary bypass. Circulation 1996;93:2014–2018.

130. Tabuchi N, de Haan J, Boonstra PW et al. Activation of fibrinolysis in the pericardial cavity during cardiopulmonary bypass. J Thorac Cardiovasc Surg 1993;106:828–833.

131. Brody JI, Pickering NJ, Fink GB. Concentrations of factor VIII-related antigen and factor XIII during open heart surgery. Transfusion 1986;26:478–480.

132. Weinstein M, Ware JA, Troll J et al. Changes in von Willebrand factor during cardiac surgery: effect of desmopressin acetate. Blood 1988;71:1648–1655.

133. Gill JG, Wilson AD, Endres-Brooks J et al. Loss of the largest von Willebrand factor multimers from the plasma of individuals with congenital cardiac defects. Blood 1986;67:758–761.

134. Butler J, Rocker GM, Westaby S. Inflammatory response to cardiopulmonary bypass. Ann Thorac Surg 1993;55:552–559.

135. Edmunds JH Jr. Why cardiopulmonary bypass makes individuals sick: strategies to control the blood-synthetic surface interface. In: Advances in cardiac surgery. St. Louis: Mosby–Year Book, 1995:6:131–167.

136. Rinder CS, Rinder HM, Smith BR et al. Blockade of C5a and C5b-9 generation inhibits leukocyte and platelet activation during extracorporeal circulation. J Clin Invest 1995;96:1564–1572.

137. Hennein HA, Ebba H, Rodriguez JL et al. Relationship of the proinflammatory cytokines to myocardial ischemia and dysfunction after uncomplicated coronary revascularization. J Thorac Cardiovasc Surg 1994;108:626–635.

138. Steinberg JB, Kapelanski DP, Olson JD et al. Cytokine and complement levels in individuals undergoing cardiopulmonary bypass. J Thorac Cardiovasc Surg 1993;106:1008–1016.

139. Kawamura T, Wakusawa R, Okada K et al. Elevation of cytokines during open heart surgery with cardiopulmonary bypass: participation of interleukin 8 and 6 in reperfusion injury. Can J Anaesth 1993;40:1016–1021.

140. Seghaye MC, Duchateau J, Grabitz RG et al. Effect of sodium nitroprusside on complement activation induced by cardiopulmonary bypass: a clinical and experimental study. J Thorac Cardiovasc Surg 1996;111:882–892.

141. Ovrum E, Mollnes TE, Fosse E et al. High and low heparin dose with heparin-coated cardiopulmonary bypass: activation of complement and granulocytes. Ann Thorac Surg 1995;60:1755–1761.

142. Pina-Cabral JM, Ribeiro-da-Silva A, Almeida-Dias A. Platelet sequestration during hypothermia in dogs treated with sulphinpyrazone and ticlopidine-reversibility accelerated after intra-abdominal rewarming. Thromb Haemost 1985;54:838–841.

143. Yoshihara H, Yamamoto T, Mihara H. Changes in coagulation and fibrinolysis occurring in dogs during hypothermia. Thromb Res 1985;37:503–512.

144. Moore FD Jr, Warner KG, Assousa S et al. The effects of complement activation during cardiopulmonary bypass. Attenuation by hypothermia, heparin and hemodilution. Ann Surg 1988;208:95–103.

145. Hirsh J. Heparin. N Engl J Med 1991;324:1565–1574.
146. Olsson P, Lagergren H, Ek S. The elimination from plasma of intravenous heparin: an experimental study on dogs and humans. Acta Med Scand 1963;173:619–630.
147. Bjornsson TD, Wolfram KM, Kitchell BB. Heparin kinetics determined by three assay methods. Clin Pharmacol Ther 1982;31:104–113.
148. Habbab MA, Haft JI. Heparin resistance induced by intravenous nitroglycerin [Abstract]. Circulation 1986;74(Suppl II):II-321.
149. Pizzulli L, Nitsch J, Luderitz B. Hemmung der Heparinwirkung durch glyceroltrinitrat. Dtsch Med Wochenschr 1988;133:1837–1840.
150. Lefemine AA, Lewis M. Activated clotting time for control of anticoagulation during surgery. Am Surg 1985;51:274–278.
151. Tuman KJ, Spiess BD, McCarthy RJ et al. Comparison of viscoelastic measures of coagulation after cardiopulmonary bypass. Anesth Analg 1989;69:69–75.
152. Gravlee GP, Whitaker CL, Mark LJ et al. Baseline activated coagulation time should be measured after surgical incision. Anesth Analg 1990;71:549–553.
153. Ovrum E, Lindberg H, Holen EA et al. Systemic and pulmonary circulatory effects of protamine following cardiopulmonary bypass in man. Scand J Thorac Cardiovasc Surg 1991;25:19–24.
154. Procaccini B, Clementi G, Bersanetti L et al. Cardiorespiratory effects of protamine sulphate in man: intra-aortic vs intra-right atrial rapid administration after cardiopulmonary bypass. J Thorac Surg (Torino) 1987;28:112–119.
155. Katz NM, Kim YD, Siegelman R et al. Hemodynamics of protamine administration. Comparison of right atrial, left atrial, and aortic injections. J Thorac Cardiovasc Surg 1987;94:881–886.
156. Whitman GJ, Martel D, Weiss M et al. Reversal of protamine-induced catastrophic pulmonary vasoconstriction by prostaglandin E1. Ann Thorac Surg 1990;50:303–305.
157. Kirklin JK, Chenoweth DE, Naftel DC et al. Effects of protamine administration after cardiopulmonary bypass on complement, blood elements, and the hemodynamic state. Ann Thorac Surg 1986;41:193–199.
158. Westaby S, Turner MW, Stark J. Complement activation and anaphylactoid response to protamine in a child after cardiopulmonary bypass. Br Heart J 1985;53:574–576.
159. Weiler JM, Gellhaus MA, Carter JG et al. A prospective study of the risk of an immediate adverse reaction to protamine sulfate during cardiopulmonary bypass surgery. J Allergy Clin Immunol 1990;85:713–719.
160. Cavarocchi NC, Schaff HV, Orszulak TA et al. Evidence for complement activation by protamine-heparin interaction after cardiopulmonary bypass. Surgery 1985;98:525–531.
161. Sharath MD, Metzer WJ, Richerson HB et al. Protamine-induced fatal anaphylaxis. Prevalence of antiprotamine immunoglobulin E antibody. J Thorac Cardiovasc Surg 1985;90:86–90.
162. Wolk LA, Wilson RF, Burdick M et al. Changes in antithrombin, antiplasmin, and plasminogen during and after cardiopulmonary bypass. Am Surg 1985;51:309–313.
163. Uziel L, Cugno M, Cacciabue E et al. Evaluation of tests for heparin control during long-term extracorporeal circulation. Int J Artif Organs 1986;9:111–116.
164. Uziel L, Cugno M, Fabrizi I et al. Physiopathology and management of coagulation during long-term extracorporeal respiratory assistance. Int J Artif Organs 1990;13:280–287.
165. Despotis GJ, Summerfield AL, Joist JH et al. Comparison of activated coagulation time and whole blood heparin measurements with laboratory plasma anti-Xa heparin concentration in individuals having cardiac operations. J Thorac Cardiovasc Surg 1994;108:1076–1082.
166. Wang JS, Lin CY, Karp RB. Comparison of high-dose thrombin time with activated clotting time for monitoring of anticoagulant effects of heparin in cardiac surgical individuals. Anesth Analg 1994;79:9–13.
167. Rohrer MJ, Natale AM. Effect of hypothermia on the coagulation cascade. Crit Care Med 1992;20:1402–1405.
168. Despotis GJ, Santoro SA, Spitznagel E et al. Prospective evaluation and clinical utility of on-site monitoring of coagulation in individuals undergoing cardiac operation. J Thorac Cardiovasc Surg 1994;107:271–279.
169. Despotis GJ, Joist JH, Hogue CW Jr et al. The impact of heparin concentration and activated clotting time monitoring on blood conservation. A prospective, randomized evaluation in individuals undergoing cardiac operation. J Thorac Cardiovasc Surg 1995;110:46–54.
170. Hardy JF, Belisle S, Robitaille D et al. Measurement of heparin concentration in whole blood with the Hepcon/HMS device does not agree with laboratory determination of plasma heparin concentration using a chromogenic substrate for activated factor X. J Thorac Cardiovasc Surg 1996;112:154–161.
171. Jobes DR, Aitken GL, Shaffer GW. Increased accuracy and precision of heparin and protamine dosing reduces blood loss and transfusion in individuals undergoing primary cardiac operations. J Thorac Cardiovasc Surg 1995;110:36–45.
172. Gorman RC, Ziats N, Rao AK et al. Surface-bound heparin fails to reduce thrombin formation during clinical cardiopulmonary bypass. J Thorac Cardiovasc Surg 1996;111:1–11.
173. Brister SJ, Ofosu FA, Buchanan MR. Thrombin generation during cardiac surgery: is heparin the ideal anticoagulant? Thromb Haemost 1993;70:259–262.
174. Shanberge JN, Murato M, Quattrociocchi-Longe T et al. Heparin-protamine complexes in the production of heparin rebound and other complications of extracorporeal bypass procedures. Am J Clin Pathol 1987;87:210–217.
175. Teoh KH, Young E, Bradley CA et al. Heparin binding proteins. Contributions to heparin rebound after cardiopulmonary bypass. Circulation 1993;88(5 Pt 2):II-420–II-425.
176. Gundry SR, Drongowski RA, Klein MD et al. Postoperative bleeding in cardiovascular surgery. Does heparin rebound really exist? Am Surg 1989;55:162–165.
177. Berndt MC, Chong BH, Andrews RK. Biochemistry of drug-dependent platelet autoantigens. In: Kunicki TJ, George JN, eds. Platelet immunobiology. Molecular and clinical aspects. Philadelphia: JB Lippincott, 1989:132–147.
178. Salzman EW, Rosenberg RD, Smith MH et al. Effect of heparin and heparin fractions on platelet aggregation. J Clin Invest 1980;65:64–73.
179. Makhoul RG, McCann RL, Austin EH et al. Management of individuals with heparin-associated thrombocytopenia and thrombosis requiring cardiac surgery. Ann Thorac Surg 1987;43:617–621.
180. Messmore HL. Clinical efficacy of heparin fractions: issues and answers. Crit Rev Clin Lab Sci 1986;23:77–94.
181. Dreyfus G, Massonnet-Castel S, Pelissier E et al. Etude d'une heparine de bas poids moleculaire au cours des circulations extracorporelles. Premieres applications cliniques. Arch Mal Coeur Vaiss 1986;79:1851–1857.
182. Rowlings PA, Mansberg R, Rozenberg MC et al. The use of a low-molecular-weight heparinoid (Org 10172) for extracorporeal procedures in individuals with heparin dependent thrombocytopenia and thrombosis. Aust N Z J Med 1991;21:52–54.
183. Altes A, Martino R, Gari M et al. Heparin-induced thrombocytopenia and heart operation: management with tedelparin. Ann Thorac Surg 1995;59:508–509.
184. Wilhelm MJ, Schmid C, Kececioglu D et al. Cardiopulmonary bypass in individuals with heparin-induced thrombocytopenia using Org 10172. Ann Thorac Surg 1996;61:920–924.
185. Teasdale SJ, Zulys VJ, Mycyk T et al. Ancrod anticoagulation for cardiopulmonary bypass in heparin-induced thrombocytopenia and thrombosis. Ann Thorac Surg 1989;48:712–713.
186. Spiekermann BF, Lake CL, Rich GF et al. Normal activated clotting time despite adequate anticoagulation with ancrod in a individual with heparin-associated thrombocytopenia and thrombosis undergoing cardiopulmonary bypass. Anesthesiology 1994;80:686–688.
187. Walenga JM, Bakhos M, Messmore HL et al. Potential use of recombinant hirudin as an anticoagulant in a cardiopulmonary bypass model. Ann Thorac Surg 1991;51:271–277.
188. Koza MJ, Walenga JM, Fareed J et al. A new approach in monitoring recombinant hirudin during cardiopulmonary bypass. Semin Thromb Hemost 1993;19(Suppl 1):90–96.
189. Schiele F, Vuillemenot A, Mouhat T et al. Traitement anti-thrombique par hirudine recombinante chez des individuals ayant une thrombopenie induite par l'heparine. Presse Med 1996;25:757–760.
190. Mollnes TE, Videm V, Gotze O et al. Formation of C5a during cardiopulmonary bypass: inhibition by precoating with heparin. Ann Thorac Surg 1991;52:92–97.
191. von Segesser LK, Turina M. Cardiopulmonary bypass without systemic heparinization. Performance of heparin-coated oxygenators in comparison with classic membrane and bubble oxygenators. J Thorac Cardiovasc Surg 1989;98:386–396.
192. Tong SD, Rolfs MR, Hsu LC. Evaluation of Duraflo II heparin immobilized cardiopulmonary bypass circuits. ASAIO Trans 1990;36:M654–M656.
193. Videm V, Nilsson L, Venge P et al. Reduced granulocyte activation with a heparin-coated device in an in vitro model of cardiopulmonary bypass. Artif Organs 1991;15:90–95.
194. Nilsson L, Storm KE, Thelin S et al. Heparin-coated equipment reduces complement activation during cardiopulmonary bypass in the pig. Artif Organs 1990;14:46–48.
195. von Segesser K, Weiss BM, Garcia E et al. Reduced blood loss and transfusion requirements with low systemic heparinization: preliminary clinical results in coronary artery revascularization. Eur J Cardiothorac Surg 1990;4:639–643.
196. von Segesser K, Turina M. Long term cardiopulmonary bypass without systemic heparinization. Int J Artif Organs 1990;13:687–691.
197. von Segesser LK, Weiss BM, Pasic M et al. Experimental evaluation of heparin-coated cardiopulmonary bypass equipment with low systemic heparinization and high-dose aprotinin. Thorac Cardiovasc Surg 1991;39:251–256.
198. Redmond JM, Gillinov AM, Stuart RS et al. Heparin-coated bypass circuits reduce pulmonary injury. Ann Thorac Surg 1993;56:474–478.
199. Wendel HP, Heller W, Gallimore MJ et al. Heparin-coated oxygenators significantly reduce contact system activation in an in vitro cardiopulmonary bypass model. Blood Coagul Fibrinolysis 1994;5:673–678.

200. van der Kamp KW, van Oeveren W. Contact, coagulation and platelet interaction with heparin treated equipment during heart surgery. Int J Artif Organs 1993;16:836–842.

201. te Velthuis H, Jansen PG, Hack CE et al. Specific complement inhibition with heparin-coated extracorporeal circuits. Ann Thorac Surg 1996;61:1153–1157.

202. Boonstra PW, Gu YJ, Akkerman C et al. Heparin coating of an extracorporeal circuit partly improves hemostasis after cardiopulmonary bypass. J Thorac Cardiovasc Surg 1994;107:289–292.

203. Shigemitsu O, Hadama T, Takasaki H et al. Biocompatibility of a heparin-bonded membrane oxygenator (Carmeda MAXIMA) during the first 90 minutes of cardiopulmonary bypass: clinical comparison with the conventional system. Artif Organs 1994;18:936–941.

204. Wagner WR, Johnson PC, Thompson KA et al. Heparin-coated cardiopulmonary bypass circuits: hemostatic alterations and postoperative blood loss. Ann Thorac Surg 1994;58:734–740.

205. Muehrcke DD, McCarthy PM, Kottke-Marchant K et al. Biocompatibility of heparin-coated extracorporeal bypass circuits: a randomized, masked clinical trial. J Thorac Cardiovasc Surg 1996;112:472–483.

206. Sellevold OF, Berg TM, Rein KA et al. Heparin-coated circuit during cardiopulmonary bypass. A clinical study using closed circuit, centrifugal pump and reduced heparinization. Acta Anaesthesiol Scand 1994;38:372–379.

207. Jones DR, Hill RC, Vasilakis A et al. Safe use of heparin-coated bypass circuits incorporating a pump-oxygenator. Ann Thorac Surg 1994;57:815–818.

208. Ovrum E, Brosstad F, Am Holen E et al. Effects on coagulation and fibrinolysis with reduced versus full systemic heparinization and heparin-coated cardiopulmonary bypass. Circulation 1995;92:2579–2584.

209. Ovrum E, Holen EA, Tangen G et al. Completely heparinized cardiopulmonary bypass and reduced systemic heparin: clinical and hemostatic effects. Ann Thorac Surg 1995;60:365–371.

210. Aldea GS, Doursounian M, O'Gara P et al. Heparin-bonded circuits with a reduced anticoagulation protocol in primary CABG: a prospective, randomized study. Ann Thorac Surg 1996;62:410–417.

211. von Segesser LK, Weiss BM, Pasic M et al. Risk and benefit of low systemic heparinization during open heart operations. Ann Thorac Surg 1994;58:391–397.

212. Messmore HL Jr. Clinical potential of low-molecular-weight heparins. Semin Thromb Hemost 1989;15:405–408.

213. Blajchman MA, Young E, Ofosu FA. Effects of unfractionated heparin, dermatan sulfate and low-molecular-weight heparin on vessel wall permeability in rabbits. Ann N Y Acad Sci 1989;556:245–254.

214. Hirsh J. From unfractionated heparins to low-molecular-weight heparins. Acta Chir Scand Suppl 1990;556:42–50.

215. Henny CP, ten Cate H, ten Cate JW et al. A randomized blind study comparing standard heparin and a new low-molecular-weight heparinoid in cardiopulmonary bypass surgery in dogs. J Lab Clin Med 1985;106:187–196.

216. Reber G, Schweizer A, de Moerloose P et al. Comparison between a low-molecular-weight and standard heparin for anticoagulation during extracorporeal CO$_2$ removal in the dog. Thromb Res 1988;49:157–168.

217. Doherty DC, Ortel TL, de Bruijn N et al. "Heparin-free" cardiopulmonary bypass: first reported use of heparinoid (Org 10172) to provide anticoagulation for cardiopulmonary bypass. Anesthesiology 1990;73:562–565.

218. Bagge L, Holmer E, Wahlberg T et al. Fragmin (LMWH) vs heparin for anticoagulation during in vitro recycling of human blood in cardiopulmonary bypass circuits: dose-dependence and mechanisms of clotting. Blood Coagul Fibrinolysis 1994;5:273–280.

219. Koza MJ, Messmore HL, Wallock ME et al. Evaluation of a low-molecular-weight heparin as an anticoagulant in a model of cardiopulmonary bypass surgery. Thromb Res 1993;70:67–76.

220. Walenga JM, Koza MJ, Park SJ et al. Evaluation of CGP 39393 as the anticoagulant in cardiopulmonary bypass operation in a dog model. Ann Thorac Surg 1994;58:1685–1689.

221. Bagge L, Wahlberg T, Holmer E et al. Low-molecular-weight heparin (Fragmin) versus heparin for anticoagulation during cardiopulmonary bypass in open heart surgery, using a pig model. Blood Coagul Fibrinolysis 1994;5:265–272.

222. Weitz JI, Hudoba M, Massel D et al. Clot-bound thrombin is protected from inhibition by heparin-antithrombin III but is susceptible to inactivation by antithrombin III-independent inhibitors. J Clin Invest 1990;86:385–391.

223. Heras M, Chesebro JH, Penny WJ et al. Effects of thrombin inhibition on the development of acute platelet-thrombus deposition during angioplasty in pigs. Heparin versus recombinant hirudin, a specific thrombin inhibitor. Circulation 1989;79:657–665.

224. Agnelli G, Pascucci C, Cosmi B et al. The comparative effects of recombinant hirudin (CGP 39393) and standard heparin on thrombus growth in rabbits. Thromb Haemost 1990;63:204–207.

225. Matthiasson SE, Lindblad B, Stjernquist U et al. The haemorrhagic effect of low-molecular-weight heparins, dermatan sulphate and hirudin. Haemostasis 1995;25:203–211.

226. Zoldhelyi P, Bichler J, Owen WG et al. Persistent thrombin generation in humans during specific thrombin inhibition with hirudin. Circulation 1994;90:2671–2678.

227. Zulys VJ, Teasdale SJ, Michel ER et al. Ancrod (Arvin) as an alternative to heparin anticoagulation for cardiopulmonary bypass. Anesthesiology 1989;71:870–877.

228. Smith RE, Townsend GE, Berry BR et al. Enoxaparin for unstable angina and ancrod for cardiac surgery following heparin allergy. Ann Pharmacother 1996;30:476–480.

229. Brister SJ, Ofosu FA, Heigenhauser GJ et al. Is heparin the ideal anticoagulant for cardiopulmonary bypass? Dermatan sulphate may be an alternate choice. Thromb Haemost 1994;71:468–473.

230. DeAnda A Jr, Coutre SE, Moon MR et al. Pilot study of the efficacy of a thrombin inhibitor for use during cardiopulmonary bypass. Ann Thorac Surg 1994;58:344–350.

231. Chomiak PN, Walenga JM, Koza MJ et al. Investigation of a thrombin inhibitor peptide as an alternative to heparin in cardiopulmonary bypass surgery. Circulation 1993;88(5 Pt 2):II-407–II-412.

232. Terrell MR, Walenga JM, Koza MJ et al. Efficacy of aprotinin with various anticoagulant agents in cardiopulmonary bypass. Ann Thorac Surg 1996;62:506–511.

233. Linhardt RJ, Langer R. New approaches for anticoagulation in extracorporeal therapy. Biomater Artif Cells Artif Organs 1987;15:91–100.

234. Yang VC, Teng CL, Kim JS. A filter device for the prevention of both heparin- and protamine-induced complications associated with extracorporeal therapy. Biomed Instrum Technol 1990;24:433–439.

235. Yang VC, Port FK, Kim JS et al. The use of immobilized protamine in removing heparin and preventing protamine-induced complications during extracorporeal blood circulation. Anesthesiology 1991;75:288–297.

236. Hiramatsu Y, Gikakis N, Anderson HL et al. Tirofiban provides "platelet anesthesia" during cardiopulmonary bypass in baboons. J Thorac Cardiovasc Surg 1997;113:182–193.

237. Williams RD, D'Ambra MN, Maione TE et al. Recombinant platelet factor 4 reversal of heparin in human cardiopulmonary bypass blood. J Thorac Cardiovasc Surg 1994;108:975–983.

238. Bernabei A, Gikakis N, Maione TE et al. Reversal of heparin anticoagulation by recombinant platelet factor 4 and protamine sulfate in baboons during cardiopulmonary bypass. J Thorac Cardiovasc Surg 1995;109:765–771.

239. Levy JH, Cormack JG, Morales A. Heparin neutralization by recombinant platelet factor 4 and protamine. Anesth Analg 1995;81:35–37.

240. Evans DA, Holder RL, Brawn WJ et al. Post-operative blood loss following cardiopulmonary bypass in children. Eur J Cardiothorac Surg 1994;8:25–29.

241. Despotis GJ, Filos KS, Zoys TN et al. Factors associated with excessive postoperative blood loss and hemostatic transfusion requirements: a multivariate analysis in cardiac surgical individuals. Anesth Analg 1996;82:13–21.

242. Tonz M, Mihaljevic T, von Segesser LK et al. Normothermia versus hypothermia during cardiopulmonary bypass: a randomized, controlled trial. Ann Thorac Surg 1995;59:137–143.

243. Gelb AB, Roth RI, Levin J et al. Changes in blood coagulation during and following cardiopulmonary bypass: lack of correlation with clinical bleeding. Am J Clin Pathol 1996;106:87–99.

244. Gravlee GP, Arora S, Lavender SW et al. Predictive value of blood clotting tests in cardiac surgery individuals. Ann Thorac Surg 1994;58:216–221.

245. Burns ER, Billett HH, Frater RW et al. The preoperative bleeding time as a predictor of postoperative hemorrhage after cardiopulmonary bypass. J Thorac Cardiovasc Surg 1986;92:310–312.

246. Marengo-Rowe AJ, Lambert CJ, Leveson JE et al. The evaluation of hemorrhage in cardiac individuals who have undergone extracorporeal circulation. Transfusion 1979;19:426–433.

247. Lind SE. The bleeding time does not predict surgical bleeding [Review]. Blood 1991;77:2547–2552.

248. Pillgram-Larsen J, Wisloff F, Jorgensen JJ et al. Effect of high dose ampicillin and cloxacillin on bleeding time and bleeding in open-heart surgery. Scand J Thorac Cardiovasc Surg 1985;19:45–48.

249. Ramsey G, Arvan DA, Stewart S et al. Do preoperative laboratory tests predict blood transfusion needs in cardiac operations? J Thorac Cardiovasc Surg 1983;85:564–569.

250. Ratnatunga CP, Rees GM, Kovacs IB. Preoperative hemostatic activity and excessive bleeding after cardiopulmonary bypass. Ann Thorac Surg 1991;52:250–257.

251. Ferraris VA, Berry W, Lough F. Routine template bleeding time determinations before cardiac procedures [Letter]. J Thorac Cardiovasc Surg 1987;93:474–476.

252. Ferraris VA, Gildengorin V. Predictors of excessive blood use after coronary artery bypass grafting. A multivariate analysis. J Thorac Cardiovasc Surg 1989;98:492–497.

253. Weksler BB, Pett SB, Alonso D et al. Differential inhibition by aspirin of vascular and platelet prostaglandin synthesis in atherosclerotic individuals. N Engl J Med 1983;308:800–805.

254. Goldman S, Copeland J, Moritz T et al. Improvement in early saphenous vein graft patency after coronary artery bypass surgery with antiplatelet therapy: results of a Veterans Administration Cooperative Study. Circulation 1988;77:1324–1332.

255. Valeri CR, MacGregor H, Pompei F et al. Acquired abnormalities of platelet function [Letter]. N Engl J Med 1991;324:1670.

256. Woodman RC, Harker LA. Bleeding complications associated with cardiopulmonary bypass [Review]. Blood 1990;76:1680–1697.

257. Brandt JT. The role of hemostasis laboratory in cardiopulmonary bypass surgery [Editorial]. Am J Clin Pathol 1996;106:3–5.

258. Nuttall GA, Oliver WC, Beynen FM et al. Determination of normal versus abnormal activated partial thromboplastin time and prothrombin time after cardiopulmonary bypass. J Cardiothorac Vasc Anesth 1995;9:355–361.

259. Nuttall GA, Oliver WC Jr, Beynen FM et al. Intraoperative measurement of activated partial thromboplastin time and prothrombin time by a portable laser photometer in individuals following cardiopulmonary bypass. J Cardiothorac Vasc Anesth 1993;7:402–409.

260. Rapaport SI. Preoperative hemostatic evaluation: which tests, if any? Blood 1983;61:229–231.

261. Magovern JA, Sakert T, Benckart DH et al. A model for predicting transfusion after coronary artery bypass grafting. Ann Thorac Surg 1996;61:27–32.

262. Schmoeckel M, Nollert G, Mempel M et al. Effects of recombinant human erythropoietin on autologous blood donation before open heart surgery. Thorac Cardiovasc Surg 1992;41:364–368.

263. Watanabe Y, Fuse K, Naruse Y et al. Subcutaneous use of erythropoietin in heart surgery. Ann Thorac Surg 1992;54:479–483.

264. Kulier AH, Gombotz H, Fuchs G et al. Subcutaneous recombinant human erythropoietin and autologous blood donation before coronary artery bypass surgery. Anesth Analg 1993;76:102–106.

265. Konishi T, Ohbayashi T, Kaneko T et al. Preoperative use of erythropoietin for cardiovascular operations in anemia. Ann Thorac Surg 1993;56:101–103.

266. Hayashi J, Kumon K, Takanashi S et al. Subcutaneous administration of recombinant human erythropoietin before cardiac surgery: a double blind, multicenter trial in Japan. Transfusion 1994;34:142–146.

267. Rosengart TK, DeBois W, Helm R et al. Retrograde autologous priming (RAP) for cardiopulmonary bypass: a safe and effective means of decreasing hemodilution and transfusion requirements [Abstract]. Circulation 1995;92(Suppl):I-763.

268. Schonberger JP, Everts PA, Hoffmann JJ. Systemic blood activation with open and closed venous reservoirs. Ann Thorac Surg 1995;59:1549–1555.

269. Love TR, Hendren WG, O'Keefe DD et al. Transfusion of predonated autologous blood in elective cardiac surgery. Ann Thorac Surg 1987;43:508–512.

270. Gluck D, Kubanek B, Ahnefeld FW. Eigenblut-transfusion. Ziele und nutzen, grenzen und risiken, dargestellt an einem praktikablen konzept. Anaesthesist 1988;37:565–571.

271. Anderson BV, Tomasulo PA. Current autologous transfusion practices. Implications for the future. Transfusion 1988;28:394–396.

272. Cohn LH, Fosberg AM, Anderson WP et al. The effects of phlebotomy, hemodilution and autologous transfusion on systemic oxygenation and whole blood utilization in open heart surgery. Chest 1975;68:283–287.

273. Kaplan JA, Cannarella C, Jones EL et al. Autologous blood transfusion during cardiac surgery. A re-evaluation of three methods. J Thorac Cardiovasc Surg 1977;74:4–10.

274. Moran JM, Babka R, Silberman S et al. Immediate centrifugation of oxygenator contents after cardiopulmonary bypass. Role in maximum blood conservation. J Thorac Cardiovasc Surg 1978;76:510–517.

275. Pliam MB, McGoon DC, Tarhan S. Failure of transfusions of autologous whole blood to reduce banked-blood requirements in open-heart surgical individuals. J Thorac Cardiovasc Surg 1975;70:338–343.

276. Aris A, Padro JM, Bonnin JO et al. Prediction of hematocrit changes in open heart surgery without blood transfusion. J Cardiovasc Surg (Torino) 1984;25:545–548.

277. Anonymous. Platelet transfusion therapy [Review]. National Institutes of Health Consensus Development Conference Statement. 1986;6:1–6.

278. Giordano GF, Rivers SL, Chung GK et al. Autologous platelet-rich plasma in cardiac surgery: effect on intraoperative and postoperative transfusion requirements. Ann Thorac Surg 1988;46:416–419.

279. Del Rossi AJ, Cernaianu AC, Vertrees RA et al. Platelet-rich plasma reduces postoperative blood loss after cardiopulmonary bypass. J Thorac Cardiovasc Surg 1990;100:281–286.

280. Jones JW, McCoy TA, Rawitscher RE et al. Effects of intraoperative plasmapheresis on blood loss in cardiac surgery. Ann Thorac Surg 1990;49:585–590.

281. Boldt J, von Bormann B, Kling D et al. Preoperative plasmapheresis in individuals undergoing cardiac surgery procedures. Anesthesiology 1990;72:282–288.

282. Schaff HV, Hauer JM, Bell WR et al. Autotransfusion of shed mediastinal blood after cardiac surgery: a prospective study. J Thorac Cardiovasc Surg 1978;75:632–641.

283. Johnson RG, Rosenkrantz KR, Preston RA et al. The efficacy of postoperative autotransfusion in individuals undergoing cardiac operations. Ann Thorac Surg 1983;36:173–179.

284. Griffith LD, Billman GF, Daily PO et al. Apparent coagulopathy caused by infusion of shed mediastinal blood and its prevention by washing of the infusate. Ann Thorac Surg 1989;47:400–406.

285. Thurer RL, Lytle BW, Cosgrove DM et al. Autotransfusion following cardiac operations: a randomized, prospective study. Ann Thorac Surg 1979;27:500–507.

286. Axford TC, Dearani JA, Ragno G et al. Safety and therapeutic effectiveness of reinfused shed blood after open heart surgery. Ann Thorac Surg 1993;57:615–622.

287. Valeri CR. Physiology of blood transfusion. In: Shires GT, Barie PS, eds. Surgical intensive care. Boston: Little, Brown, 1993:681–721.

288. Healey N, Khuri SF, Valeri CR et al. Platelets stored at -80°C for 1.3 years: a new option for post cardiopulmonary bypass transfusion therapy [Abstract]. Circulation 1995;92(Suppl):I-764.

289. Fish KJ, Sarnquist FH, van Steennis C et al. A prospective, randomized study of the effects of prostacyclin on platelets and blood loss during coronary bypass operations. J Thorac Cardiovasc Surg 1986;91:436–442.

290. Malpass TW, Amory DW, Harker LA et al. The effect of prostacyclin infusion on platelet hemostatic function in individuals undergoing cardiopulmonary bypass. J Thorac Cardiovasc Surg 1984;87:550–555.

291. Radegran K, Egberg N, Papaconstantinou C. Effects of prostacyclin during cardiopulmonary bypass in man. Scand J Thorac Surg 1981;15:263–268.

292. DiSesa VJ, Huval W, Lelcuk S et al. Disadvantages of prostacyclin infusion during cardiopulmonary bypass: a double-blind study of 50 individuals having coronary revascularization. Ann Thorac Surg 1984;38:514–519.

293. DelRossi AJ, Cernaiano AC, Botros S et al. Prophylactic treatment of post perfusion bleeding using EACA. Chest 1989;96:27–30.

294. Penta de Peppo A, Pierri MD, Scafuri A et al. Intraoperative antifibrinolysis and blood saving techniques in cardiac surgery. Prospective trial of 3 antifibrinolytic drugs. Tex Heart Inst J 1995;22:231–236.

295. Arom KV, Emery RW. Decreased postoperative drainage with addition of epsilon-amino-caproic acid before cardiopulmonary bypass. Ann Thorac Surg 1994;57:1108–1112.

296. Okamoto S, Sato S, Takeda Y et al. An active stereo-isomer (trans-form) of AMCHA and its antifibrinolytic (antiplasminic) action in vitro and in vivo. Keio J Med 1964;13:177–185.

297. Horrow JC, Hlavacek J, Strong MD et al. Prophylactic tranexamic acid decreases bleeding after cardiac operations. J Thorac Cardiovasc Surg 1990;99:70–74.

298. Shore-Lesserson L, Reich DL, Vela-Cantos F et al. Tranexamic acid reduces transfusions and mediastinal drainage in repeat cardiac surgery. Anesth Analg 1996;83:18–26.

299. Karski JM, Teasdale SJ, Norman P et al. Prevention of bleeding after cardiopulmonary bypass with high-dose tranexamic acid. Double-blind, randomized clinical trial. J Thorac Cardiovasc Surg 1995;110:835–842.

300. Nakashima A, Matsuzaki K, Fukumura F et al. Tranexamic acid reduces blood loss after cardiopulmonary bypass. ASAIO J 1993;39:M185–189.

301. Rousou JA, Engelman RM, Flack JE III et al. Tranexamic acid significantly reduces blood loss associated with coronary revascularization. Ann Thorac Surg 1995;59:671–675.

302. Zonis Z, Seear M, Reichert C et al. The effect of preoperative tranexamic acid on blood loss after cardiac operations in children. J Thorac Cardiovasc Surg 1996;111:982–987.

303. Royston D, Bidstrup BP, Taylor KM et al. Effect of aprotinin on need for blood transfusion after repeat open-heart surgery. Lancet 1987;ii:1289–1291.

304. Bidstrup BP, Royston D, Sapsford RN et al. Reduction in blood loss and blood use after cardiopulmonary bypass with high dose aprotinin (Trasylol). J Thorac Cardiovasc Surg 1989;97:364–372.

305. Lu H, Soria C, Commin PL et al. Haemostasis in individuals undergoing extracorporeal circulation: the effect of aprotinin (Trasylol). Thromb Haemost 1991;66:633–637.

306. Dietrich W, Dilthey G, Spannagl M et al. Influence of high-dose aprotinin on anticoagulation, heparin requirement and celite- and kaolin-activated clotting time in heparin-pretreated individuals undergoing open-heart surgery. A double-blind, placebo-controlled study. Anesthesiology 1995;83:679–689.

307. Dietrich W, Mossinger H, Spannagl M et al. Hemostatic activation during cardiopulmonary bypass with different aprotinin dosages in pediatric individuals having cardiac operations. J Thorac Cardiovasc Surg 1993;105:712–720.

308. Speekenbrink RG, Wildevuur CR, Sturk A et al. Low-dose and high-dose aprotinin improve hemostasis in coronary operations. J Thorac Cardiovasc Surg 1996;112:523–530.

309. Lavee J, Raviv Z, Smolinsky A et al. Platelet protection by low-dose aprotinin in cardiopulmonary bypass: electron microscopic study. Ann Thorac Surg 1993;55:114–119.

310. Bailey CR, Wielogorski AK. Randomized placebo controlled double blind

study of two dose aprotinin regimens in cardiac surgery. Br Heart J 1994; 71:349–353.

311. Liu B, Tengborn L, Larson G et al. Half-dose aprotinin preserves hemostatic function in individuals undergoing bypass operations. Ann Thorac Surg 1995;59:1534–1540.

312. Mastroroberto P, Chello M, Zofrea S et al. Suppressed fibrinolysis after administration of low-dose aprotinin: reduced level of plasmin-alpha2-plasmin inhibitor complexes and postoperative blood loss. Eur J Cardiothorac Surg 1995;9:143–145.

313. Kawasuji M, Ueyama K, Sakakibara N et al. Effect of low-dose aprotinin on coagulation and fibrinolysis in cardiopulmonary bypass. Ann Thorac Surg 1993;55:1205–1209.

314. Orchard MA, Goodchild CS, Prentice CR et al. Aprotinin reduces cardiopulmonary bypass-induced blood loss and inhibits fibrinolysis without influencing platelets. Br J Haematol 1993;85:533–541.

315. Lu H, Du Buit C, Soria J et al. Postoperative hemostasis and fibrinolysis in individuals undergoing cardiopulmonary bypass with or without aprotinin therapy. Thromb Haemost 1994;72:438–443.

316. Tabuchi N, Huet RC, Sturk A et al. Aprotinin preserves hemostasis in aspirin-treated individuals undergoing cardiopulmonary bypass. Ann Thorac Surg 1994;58:1036–1039.

317. Wahba A, Black G, Koksch M et al. Aprotinin has no effect on platelet activation and adhesion during cardiopulmonary bypass. Thromb Haemost 1996;75:844–848.

318. Ray MJ, Marsh NA, Just SJE et al. Preoperative platelet dysfunction increases the benefit of aprotinin in cardiopulmonary bypass. Ann Thorac Surg 1997;63:57–63.

319. Wang JS, Lin CY, Hung WT et al. *In vitro* effects of aprotinin on activated clotting time measured with different activators. J Thorac Cardiovasc Surg 1992;104:1135–1140.

320. Farooqi N, De Hert S, Vlaeminck R et al. Effects of low doses of aprotinin on clotting times activated with celite and kaolin. Acta Anaesthesiol Belg 1993;44:87–92.

321. Despotis GJ, Joist JH, Joiner-Maier D et al. Effect of aprotinin on activated clotting time, whole blood and plasma heparin measurements. Ann Thorac Surg 1995;59:106–111.

322. Huyzen RJ, Harder MP, Huet RC et al. Alternative perioperative anticoagulation monitoring during cardiopulmonary bypass in aprotinin-treated individuals. J Cardiothorac Vasc Anesth 1994;8: 153–156.

323. de Smet AA, Joen MC, van Oeveren W et al. Increased anticoagulation during cardiopulmonary bypass by aprotinin. J Thorac Cardiovasc Surg 1990;100:520–527.

324. Bidstrup BP. Effect of aprotinin (Trasylol) on aorto-coronary bypass graft patency. J Thorac Cardiovasc Surg 1993;105:147–152.

325. Allen S, Anastasiou N, Royston D et al. Effect of aprotinin on vascular reactivity of coronary bypass grafts. J Thorac Cardiovasc Surg 1997;113: 319–326.

326. Sundt TM III, Kouchoukas NT, Saffitz JE et al. Renal dysfunction and intravascular coagulation with aprotinin and hypothermic circulatory arrest. Ann Thorac Surg 1993;55:1418–1424.

327. Dietrich W, Spath P, Ebell A et al. Prevalence of anaphylactic reactions to aprotinin: analysis of two hundred forty-eight reexposures to aprotinin in heart operations. J Thorac Cardiovasc Surg 1997;113:194–201.

328. Blauhut B, Harringer W, Bettelheim P et al. Comparison of the effects of aprotinin and tranexamic acid on blood loss and related variables after cardiopulmonary bypass. J Thorac Cardiovasc Surg 1994;108:1083–1091.

329. Salzman EW, Weinstein MJ, Weintraub RM et al. Treatment with desmopressin acetate to reduce blood loss after cardiac surgery. A double-blind randomized study. N Engl J Med 1986;314:1402–1406.

330. Czer LSC, Bateman TM, Gray RJ et al. Treatment of severe platelet dysfunction and hemorrhage after cardiopulmonary bypass: reduction in blood product usage with desmopressin. J Am Coll Cardiol 1987;9: 1139–1147.

331. Tyers GF. Desmopressin: do we now know its role? Can J Surg 1990;33: 5–6.

332. Seear MD, Wadsworth LD, Rogers PC et al. The effect of desmopressin acetate (DDAVP) on postoperative blood loss after cardiac operations in children. J Thorac Cardiovasc Surg 1989;98:217–219.

333. Salzman EW, Weinstein MJ, Reilly D et al. Adventures in hemostasis. Desmopressin in cardiac surgery. Arch Surg 1993;128:212–217.

334. Sloand EM, Alyono D, Klein HG et al. 1-Deamino-8-D-arginine vasopressin (DDAVP) increases platelet membrane expression of glycoprotein Ib in individuals with disorders of platelet function and after cardiopulmonary bypass. Am J Hematol 1994;46:199–207.

335. Velders AJ, Wildevuur CRH. Platelet damage by protamine and the protective effects of prostacyclin: an experimental study in dogs. Ann Thorac Surg 1986;42:168–171.

336. Salzman EW. Hemostatic problems in surgical individuals. In: Colman RW, Hirsh J, Marder VJ, Salzman EW, eds. Hemostasis and thrombosis. Basic principles and clinical practice. Philadelphia: JB Lippincott, 1992.

# SECTION 11

# MANAGEMENT OF BLEEDING

# CHAPTER 51

# PLATELET TRANSFUSION THERAPY

Scott Murphy

## HISTORICAL PERSPECTIVE

Between 1980 and 1990 the use of platelet transfusions in the United States increased progressively, doubling between 1982 and 1989 (1, 2). In 1989 more than 6,000,000 units were infused. This liberal use and easy availability permitted and correlated with increasingly aggressive cytotoxic therapy of individuals with malignancy. There is evidence that the use of platelets has plateaued in the 1990s, perhaps due to a more rigorous evaluation of the indications for transfusion.

The first platelet transfusions were accomplished by direct transfer of whole blood without an anticoagulant from donors with thrombocytosis to recipients with thrombocytopenia (3). Clinical improvement of the recipient's bleeding tendency correlated with a sustained, measurable increase of the platelet concentration in the recipient's blood. The current work directed toward development of "platelet substitutes" will be discussed in a subsequent section. However, at this time intact platelets capable of circulating normally *in vivo* remain the product of choice to achieve hemostasis in the thrombocytopenic individual.

In the 1960s the development of appropriate plastic containers and centrifugation techniques allowed the sterile separation of platelets from the other blood cells in whole blood donations. Henceforth, these preparations will be referred to as whole blood derived platelet concentrates (PCs). In the second half of the 1970s apheresis procedures were developed for preparation of a therapeutic dose of platelets from a single donor at a single sitting (4). These preparations will be referred to as apheresis PCs. The progressively widespread use of

platelets in the early 1980s coincided with the development of methods for storage of PCs for 5 days. This storage capability allowed the cells to be widely and continuously available.

## TECHNIQUES FOR PLATELET COLLECTION
### WHOLE BLOOD DERIVED PCS
### Platelet-Rich-Plasma (PRP) Method

Traditionally, these products have been called random-donor PCs. When apheresis PCs were first developed, they were used primarily for refractory individuals who required products from specific donors generally selected on the basis of Human Leukocyte Antigen (HLA) typing. On the other hand, whole blood derived PCs were given "randomly." However, at this time, apheresis PCs are commonly given "randomly" to unselected individuals because of perceived advantages for all individuals.

PC prepared by the PRP method are obtained from routine donations of 450 to 500 mL (a unit) of whole blood anticoagulated with a citrate-based anticoagulant (Fig. 51.1, Pathway 1). The blood is held for up to 8 hours, and 200 to 250 mL of PRP are separated from the red cells and the buffy coat by low-speed centrifugation. The PRP is then centrifuged at high speed to produce a platelet pellet and all but approximately 50 mL of plasma is separated from the pellet, which is then resuspended in that plasma. The separated red cells are used for transfusion, while the plasma is used for transfusion or fractionation.

**FIGURE 51.1.** Three ways to prepare a pool of platelet concentrates (PCs) from units of whole blood. Pathway 1 is the platelet-rich plasma (PRP) method described in detail in the text. At this time, it is the only method used in the United States. Pathways 2 and 3 outline two methods for preparing PCs by the buffy-coat (BC) method, either as individual PCs (Pathway 2) or as a filtered pool (Pathway 3). The latter two methods, which are widely used in Europe, are also described in the text. RBC, red blood cells; PPP, platelet poor plasma. (Redrawn from Murphy S, Heaton WA, Rebulla P. Platelet production in the Old World—and the New. Transfusion 1996;36:751–754.)

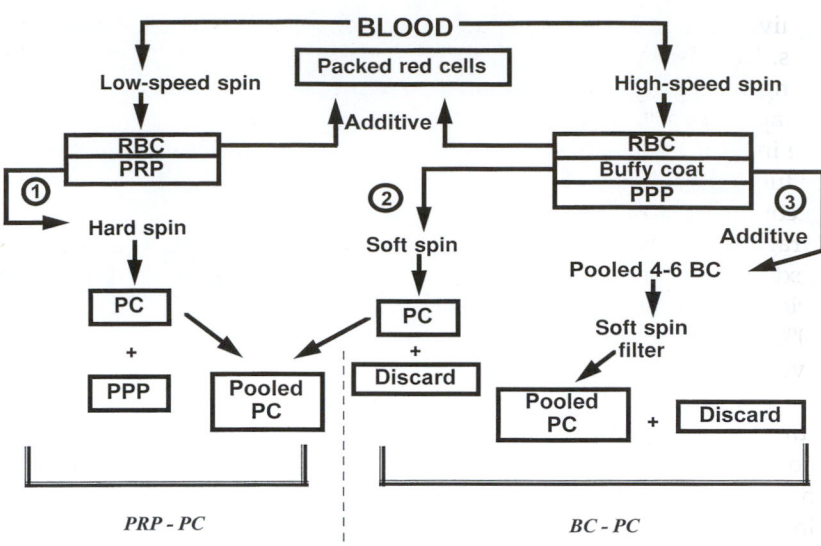

Whole blood and PRP are kept at ambient temperature until the platelets have been separated. The platelet pellet is allowed to "rest" for 1 to 2 hours before resuspension. If platelets are exposed to cold temperatures during processing or if the "rest" period is omitted, the platelets tend to clump irreversibly upon resuspension (5). These are empirical observations, and the nature of the events occurring during these first crucial hours has not been defined.

Over the past 20 years a variety of technical improvements have resulted in an increase in the number of platelets per unit from 5 to $6 \times 10^{10}$ in 1975 to possibly 9 to $10 \times 10^{10}$ in 1997 (6); 8 to $9 \times 10^{10}$ platelets represents 60 to 75% of the platelets in the original donation. Approximately 1 to $5 \times 10^8$ leukocytes, predominantly lymphocytes, will also be present. These leukocytes produce delayed hemolytic transfusion reactions, induce alloimmunization to HLA antigens, and transmit cytomegalovirus (CMV) infection, three of the major complications of platelet transfusion. One unit of platelets is adequate only for the transfusion of a small child less than 30 pounds in weight. To transfuse larger individuals, a sufficient number of these PCs are pooled to provide a therapeutic dose (4 to 8 units for adults).

## Buffy-Coat (BC) Method

PC prepared by the PRP method have been the standard platelet component in the United States for the last 20 to 25 years. For a variety of reasons many investigators, particularly in Europe, have been dissatisfied with the PRP method of separating blood components (7) and have developed the buffy-coat (BC) method. The whole-blood collection is given a high-speed spin so that the leukocytes and platelets are concentrated in the BC between the supernatant plasma and infranatant red cells. The platelets at the top of the bag fall to the BC, and the

platelets at the bottom of the bag rise to the BC; thus the majority of the platelets are in the BC.

One can suspend the BC in plasma and prepare individual PCs (8) by a soft spin of that suspension to remove contaminating red cells and leukocytes (Fig. 51.1, Pathway 2). These PCs can then be pooled as are PRP PCs. Alternatively, one can pool four to six BCs, add two to four volumes of an additive solution, centrifuge the pool at low speed to remove red cells and leukocytes, and push the supernatant through a leukoreduction filter to produce a therapeutic dose of platelets for an adult (9–11) (Fig. 51.1, Pathway 3).

The BC and PRP methods each have their advantages (7). The major drawback of the BC method is that approximately 20 to 25 mL of red cells (approximately 10% of those donated) are present in the BC and are lost with the discard portion. This is a disadvantage for the anemic individual who will be transfused with these red cells. On the other hand, the initial hard spin allows 70 to 80 extra mL of plasma to be collected with the BC method. This is an advantage for the individuals to be transfused with this plasma. In terms of platelet recovery, processing of individual PCs by the BC method (Fig. 51.1, Pathway 2) is less efficient than the PRP method. However, if pools of BC are processed according to Pathway 3 in Fig. 51.1, platelet recovery is identical to that of the PRP method. Furthermore, the final product has the advantage of being leukoreduced by filtration (see below).

## APHERESIS PCS

One can obtain 2.5 to $10 \times 10^{11}$ platelets (equivalent to 3 to >10 units of whole blood–derived PCs) by apheresis of donors over 1 to 2 hours using a variety of devices (12). The goal is to obtain a therapeutic dose for an adult equivalent to a 4- to 6-unit pool of whole blood derived PCs. This is an area in which technical advances are being made rapidly. There are two major advantages for apheresis PCs. First, the number of donors to which the individual is exposed is substantially reduced. This reduces the likelihood of transmission of viral diseases. Second, the apheresis technology lends itself to prestorage leukoreduction, which will be discussed in the next section. On the other hand, in the United States the price of apheresis PCs is generally set at approximately 50% more than an equivalent pool of whole blood derived PCs.

The number of platelets obtained during the procedure varies according to the platelet concentration in the blood of the donor, the duration of the donation, and the efficiency of the device. Since the platelet concentration in the blood of normal individuals varies in the range of 130,000 to 500,000 per $mm^3$, this is the major factor. The efficiency of the newest devices is such that one should expect to obtain at least 50% of the platelets that pass through them.

The wide range of potential platelet yields in the product creates a dilemma for the blood center. Products at the low end may provide an insufficient dose for some individuals (e.g., large adults), but administration of high-yield products to other individuals (e.g., small adults and children) may be wasteful. Many centers avoid such wastage by "splitting" high yield products so that two individuals may be treated with the platelets obtained from one donation.

In the long run it will be an improvement in the quality of the product if it contains a standard platelet content, and therefore potency, with minimal variation. In this way the clinician will be able to make sound judgments about individual response. If one standard product is to be produced, $4 \times 10^{11}$ (i.e., 5 whole blood derived units assuming $8 \times 10^{10}$ platelets per unit) with a range of 3 to $5 \times 10^{11}$ would seem to be a reasonable compromise. On the other hand, consideration could be given to the preparation of products containing two or more levels of platelet content, perhaps with means of $3.6 \times 10^{11}$ and $7.2 \times 10^{11}$ (i.e., approximately 4.5 and 9 whole blood derived units, respectively). The use of the products could be tailored to the needs of individual individuals. These issues will be discussed further in the section on platelet dose.

## LEUKOREDUCTION OF PLATELET PRODUCTS

As far as is known, there are no clinically significant differences among the platelets prepared by the procedures described above. However, there are major differences in leukocyte content. As will be described in greater detail in the section on complications of platelet transfusion, many of the unwanted side effects are mediated by contaminating leukocytes. A major goal at this

time in the United States is to reduce the level of leukocyte contamination to less than $5 \times 10^6$ leukocytes per transfusion dose for both red cells and platelets (13); the standard of $1 \times 10^6$ leukocytes is commonly used in Europe. These levels have been chosen somewhat arbitrarily as adequate to prevent alloimmunization and CMV transmission. Progressive improvement in the separation technology of the various apheresis devices has allowed those most recently available (14, 15) to produce products that are below $1 \times 10^6$ leukocytes essentially 100% of the time. Fig. 51.2 shows the experience of one blood center in this regard.

Apheresis products prepared with older separation technology and higher leukocyte contents must be filtered either in the blood center or at the bedside to achieve the benefits of leukoreduction. Prestorage leukoreduction at the blood center offers two advantages. First, it is carried out under standardized conditions, following current good manufacturing practices (cGMP)

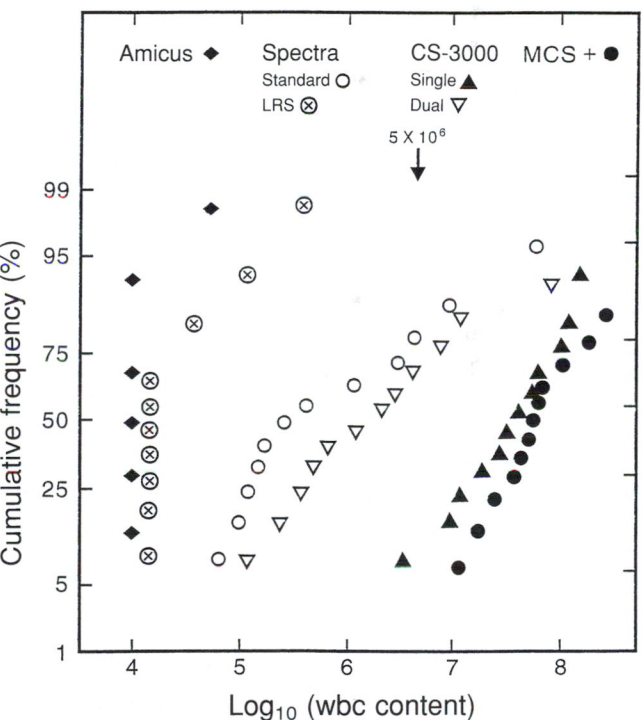

**FIGURE 51.2.** Cumulative frequency of leukocyte contents of apheresis PCs produced with six different apheresis methodologies: Fenwal Amicus, COBE Spectra (standard and leukocyte reduction system [LRS] versions), Fenwal CS-3000 (single and dual needle access), and Haemonetics MCS+. The newest procedures, the Amicus and Spectra LRS, produce >99% products with leukocyte content less than $5 \times 10^6$, the current standard in the United States. The older procedures have a 25% (standard Spectra, dual needle CS-3000) or 95% (single needle CS-3000, MCS+) failure rate. wbc, white blood cells. (Data from the American Red Cross Blood Services, Penn-Jersey Region.)

and performing appropriate quality control procedures. Such standardization is not possible at the bedside (16). Second, prestorage leukoreduction prevents the production of cytokines by leukocytes during storage (17–18). These cytokines are capable of producing febrile reactions in recipients. This will be discussed further in the section on complications of platelet transfusion.

Similarly, as mentioned above, pools of whole blood derived PCs prepared by the PRP method are heavily contaminated with leukocytes. If filtration is to be carried out at the bedside, it must be done with careful attention to technique to be certain that the required reduction of leukocyte content by three logs is achieved. There are reports in which bedside filtration has failed to achieve the expected beneficial results (19). Furthermore, there are reports of hypotensive reactions due to bradykinin generation during such filtration (20).

As mentioned above, the BC method of PC production offers the opportunity to achieve prestorage leukoreduction of whole blood derived PCs. There is also a system for the PRP method that inserts a leukocyte-reduction filter between the primary blood bag and the bag that accepts the PRP (21). Thus the PRP is leukoreduced at the time of its preparation. This approach is cumbersome for a busy manufacturing laboratory, and the expense of a filter is required for every PC produced. Thus, to date, this approach has not been widely used.

## PLATELET STORAGE

### LIQUID STORAGE OF PCS IN PLASMA AT 20 TO 24°C

Both whole blood derived and apheresis PCs may be stored for 5 days using the same principles: (a) the temperature must be 20 to 24°C; (b) the storage container must be constructed of a plastic material that allows adequate diffusion of oxygen to meet the cells' metabolic needs; and (c) the platelets must be agitated during storage.

### Assessment of Platelet Quality

In developing methods for the storage of platelets, maintenance of platelet viability has always been stressed, that is, the capacity of the cells to circulate *in vivo* without being removed by the recipient's phagocytic system because of cell damage. Although the ultimate test has always been the measurement of increments in platelet concentration in the blood of thrombocytopenic recipients, reliance has also been placed on autologous, radiolabeled reinfusion studies in normal volunteers using chromium-51 or indium-111 (22) (Fig. 51.3). In such a study platelets are stored by the method under investigation, radiolabeled after storage, and reinfused into the original donor. The data are generally presented as the percent recovery during the first few hours after infu-

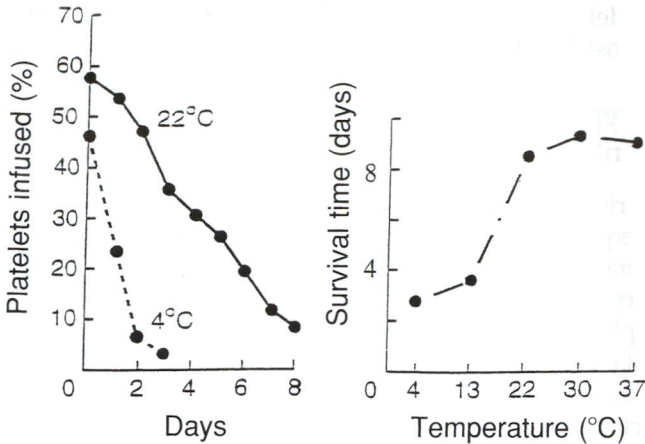

**FIGURE 51.3.** Autologous platelet survival after overnight storage of platelets at various temperatures. After storage at 22°C, the survival pattern is essentially identical to that of fresh platelets. The 50 to 60% recovery immediately after infusion is a result of physiologic pooling in the spleen (see Chapter 9) and not cell damage. On the other hand, survival time is substantially reduced when the storage has been at colder temperatures. (Adapted with permission from Murphy S. Platelet function, kinetics, and metabolism—impact on quality assessment, storage, and clinical use. In: McLeod B, Price TH, Drew MJ, eds. Apheresis: principles and practice. Bethesda: AABB Press, 1997.)

sion and the mean cell life (survival time) during the subsequent week.

### Temperature of Storage

In the 1960s platelets were stored at cold temperatures (1 to 6°C). It was recognized that they survived for only a few hours after infusion into individuals even after only one day of storage. Subsequently, using radiolabeling, it was found that survival was normal, even after several days of storage, if storage was carried out at room temperature (20 to 24°C) (23) (Fig. 51.3). Similar to observations during storage at 1 to 6°C, survival was also shortened after storage at 13°C for 18 hours and even at 18°C for 3 days (24). The superiority of storage at 20 to 24°C as opposed to 1 to 6°C has been confirmed in studies of thrombocytopenic individuals in whom both increments in platelet count and shortening of prolonged bleeding times have been measured (25, 26).

Many of these studies noted a correlation between decreased *in vivo* survival and loss of the normal discoid shape of the cell. Cells damaged by cold temperature assume a spherical shape that cannot be reversed by rewarming. In fact, the loss of discoid shape correlates with both degree and time of cooling. In one study (28) there was significant loss of discoid shape when the platelets were exposed to 16°C for >16 hours, to 12°C for >10 hours, and to 4°C for >6 hours. These data provide guidelines that can be used if the PCs are temporarily exposed to a low temperature inadvertently.

## Oxygen Requirements and the Storage Container

During storage in plasma at 20 to 24°C when there is adequate oxygen supply, platelets employ two major metabolic pathways that can generate energy and reconvert adenosine-5'-diphosphate (ADP) to adenosine-5'-triphosphate (ATP) (Fig. 51.4). In glycolysis, which does not require oxygen, one molecule of glucose is converted to two protons and two molecules of lactate such that lactate concentration rises by approximately 2.5 mM/day (29). Despite the availability of oxygen, little of the intermediate, pyruvate, enters the tricarboxylic acid (TCA) cycle. In the second pathway, plasma free fatty acids enter the mitochondria where beta-oxidation converts them to acetyl CoA, which is subsequently oxidized through the TCA cycle (30).

The rates of production of lactate and consumption of oxygen are approximately the same, 1.0 to 1.5 mmoles/day/$10^{12}$ platelets. Since the production of one lactate molecule fuels the regeneration of one ATP molecule and the consumption of one oxygen molecule fuels the regeneration of six ATP molecules, the cell derives 15% of its ATP regeneration through glycolysis and 85% through oxygen consumption. If the demand for oxygen is not met, the cell will compensate by increasing the rate of production of lactate molecules and protons.

The end product of oxidative metabolism is a gas, $CO_2$, which can leave the platelet suspension through the walls of the plastic container. The protons that accompany the production of lactate molecules cannot do so, and they must be buffered by bicarbonate, the only significant buffer in plasma. As each proton is buffered, bicarbonate is converted to water and $CO_2$. The latter leaves the PC through the walls of the container. There is only enough bicarbonate in plasma to accommodate the protons that accompany a rise in lactate concentration to 20 mM. Beyond that concentration, pH will fall, leading to progressive platelet swelling, disc-to-sphere transformation, agglutination and lysis (31). When labeled and reinfused, these platelets demonstrate marked decrease in recovery and survival (32).

As already mentioned, pooled PCs prepared by the BC method are commonly stored in an additive solution in Europe. Definition of the optimal solution is still in progress, but it appears that it can be relatively simple relying on the presence of acetate which can enter the TCA cycle for oxidation replacing the requirement for fatty acid (Fig. 51.4) (33–34). The oxidation of an organic anion such as acetate uses a proton from the medium, thus providing an alkalinizing effect. In fact, the vigorous oxidation of acetate (and consequent consumption of protons) eliminates any need to add bicarbonate to the medium.

Clearly, storage conditions must be such that there is adequate oxygen supply. Otherwise, the rates of proton production and bicarbonate consumption will increase so that pH will fall, even within the first 1 to 2 days of storage, thus jeopardizing the quality of the product. Plastics vary in the ease with which oxygen penetrates. During the first decade of platelet storage at 20 to 24°C, the plastic containers had inadequate oxygen permeability and pH fall was a major problem. However, since the mid 1980s adequate containers for whole blood derived PCs prepared by the PRP method have been available from many manufacturers (35–37). It is still not widely appreciated that some older storage containers for apheresis PCs and pooled BC PCs may have inadequate oxygen permeability. Fortunately, there are now newer containers available that are quite adequate (27, 38).

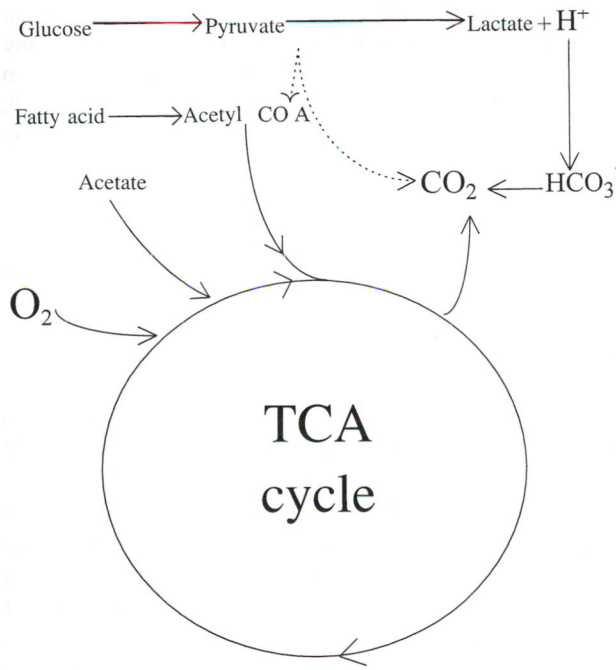

**FIGURE 51.4.**   Metabolic pathways utilized by platelets during storage at 20 to 24°C. Almost all glucose used passes through pyruvate to form lactate and a proton. Little, if any, pyruvate is decarboxylated to acetyl CoA. Thus that pathway is indicated by dashed lines. Rather, fatty acid provides the acetyl CoA, which enters the tricarboxylic acid (TCA) cycle for oxidation. When incorporated into a synthetic medium, acetate can also be oxidized through the TCA cycle. Protons produced from the metabolism of glucose are buffered by bicarbonate. $CO_2$ from this source and the TCA cycle leaves the PCs by passing through the walls of the container. (Redrawn from Murphy S. Platelet function, kinetics, and metabolism—impact on transfusion dose, quality assessment, and storage. In: McLeod B, Price TH, Drew MJ, eds. Principles of apheresis. Bethesda, MD: AABB Press, 1997.)

## Agitation During Storage

If PCs are not agitated during storage there is accelerated production of lactate and protons and a fall in pH (39). Even when pH does not fall, *in vivo* studies show that absence of agitation reduces *in vivo* recovery (40). Certain forms of agitation are superior to others. To summarize many studies (41–43), platform and "face-over-face" agitation have produced satisfactory results, while "elliptical" and "Ferris-wheel" forms have not. The scanty data available suggest that agitation may be discontinued for up to 24 hours without ill effects (44, 45).

## The Platelet Storage Lesion

Platelet viability is as satisfactory after 7 days of storage as it is after 5 days (46). However, storage is currently limited to 5 days because of concerns about bacterial overgrowth that will be discussed in the section on complications of platelet transfusion. During the 5 day storage interval many changes occur. Some authors have been unable to find any practical difference between fresh and stored platelets (47, 48), but most find a reduction in *in vivo* recovery and survival of approximately 25%. Furthermore, some authors have reported an even greater defect in the *in vivo* effectiveness of stored platelets relative to fresh platelets in sick individuals with fever, sepsis, splenomegaly, and disseminated intravascular coagulation (49, 50).

Many investigators have likened the platelet storage lesion to a form of activation (51). On activation with many agonists, platelets undergo disc-to-sphere transformation, secrete the contents of their granules, express P-selectin on the external face of the surface membrane, and release microparticles. All of these events occur to some extent during platelet storage at 22°C (52–55). After recovery from activation, platelets are less responsive to stimulation with agonists. Similarly, stored platelets have decreased reactivity to single aggregating agents such as thrombin (56), ADP, epinephrine, and collagen (57). However, these findings do not correlate with the function of stored platelets after infusion *in vivo*. The response of stored platelets to pairs of agonists is much less impaired (57), and response *in vivo* undoubtedly occurs in response to several stimuli at once. Furthermore, the responsiveness to single agents improves in the circulation after infusion (58).

Thus *in vitro* tests of stored platelets do not predict whether those platelets will have normal function *in vivo*. On the other hand, there are *in vitro* measurements that correlate with *in vivo* viability, that is, the capacity to circulate normally. A recent review of the literature (59) concluded that three assays correlate with *in vivo* recovery and survival: (a) the osmotic reversal reaction; (b) the extent of shape change; and (c) the morphology score by oil phase microscopy. Detailed methods for performing the first two assays have been published (60). Normal morphology score and extent of shape change reflect maintenance of the cell's disc shape. With few exceptions, platelets with normal discoid morphology will circulate normally after transfusion. Normal discoid shape is reflected by the "swirling" or "shimmering" appearance of well preserved PC during gross, visual inspection. A recent study indicated that this assessment could be performed in a reproducible manner and serve as a quick, cheap, quality control measure (61).

## OTHER APPROACHES TO PLATELET STORAGE AND REPLACEMENT

### Frozen Storage

The most widely used method for frozen storage employs controlled-rate freezing (1°C per minute) and 5% dimethyl sulfoxide (DMSO) as a cryoprotective agent. Viability after rapid thawing is approximately 40 to 50% relative to fresh platelets (62). Thus, this technology is both more expensive and less effective than liquid storage at 20 to 24°C (63). However, these preparations can be effective clinically (64) and may be particularly useful when used for autologous transfusion of individuals who are heavily alloimmunized and have no response to allogeneic transfusion. Autologous platelets may be obtained by apheresis, either before myelosuppressive therapy or during remission, and then frozen and used during subsequent periods of thrombocytopenia (65).

### Storage at 4°C

There has been a reawakening of interest in storing platelets at refrigerated temperatures to prolong storage beyond 5 days and to deal with the problem of bacterial contamination that will be described in the section concerning complications of platelet transfusion. A variety of second-messenger effectors (66) and stabilizers of platelet shape (67) are being evaluated in an attempt to overcome the damage to untreated platelets during storage in the cold. Studies demonstrating improved *in vivo* survival will be required for these approaches to be accepted. Concerns about toxicity of the additives after infusion in individuals will also have to be addressed.

### Fresh Whole Blood

There is very little evidence suggesting that the process of preparing PCs impairs platelet function in any clinically significant way. The only exception has been in the transfusion of children under the age of two who are undergoing complex cardiac bypass surgery. In one study (68) fresh whole blood provided a better hemostatic response than reconstituted blood components using PCs prepared and stored as described above.

However, this conclusion has not been confirmed in a second trial.

## Lyophilized Platelets and Membrane Microvesicles

Current methods of platelet storage are cumbersome and the storage duration of only 5 days creates shortages particularly after long holiday weekends. It would be ideal to have a dried preparation with a long shelf life that one could simply remove from the shelf, rehydrate, and infuse. Two approaches are being explored: whole platelets treated with paraformaldehyde and lyophilized (69) and lyophilized platelet membrane microvesicles (70). Both shorten the bleeding times of thrombocytopenic animals in some experimental situations. Such preparations also have the advantage that they can be sterilized to eliminate the possibility of transmission of viral disease. Appropriate clinical trials will be needed to compare these preparations with standard platelets preserved at 20 to 24°C. These will be difficult since the new preparations cannot be evaluated by increases in the platelet concentrations in the blood of recipients. Rather, there will have to be measurements of changes in rates of pathologic bleeding.

# CLINICAL RESPONSE TO PLATELET TRANSFUSION

## THEORETICAL OPTIMAL CLINICAL RESPONSE

As described in Chapter 9, approximately one-third of the total body platelet mass is pooled reversibly in a spleen of normal size. Therefore, the volume of distribution for transfused platelets is 50% greater than the recipient's blood volume. If one assumes that the average blood volume is 2.5 liters per m$^2$, the volume of distribution will be 3.75 liters per m$^2$. If one further assumes that the average unit of whole blood derived PCs contains 8 × 10$^{10}$ platelets, then the infusion of one unit should raise the platelet concentration in the blood by 21,000 per mm$^3$ in a individual with a surface area of 1 m$^2$.

Calculations of this type form the basis for a widely used method for assessing the response to platelet transfusion, the corrected count increment (CCI):

$$\frac{\text{Actual increase in platelet concentration} \times \text{BSA (m}^2)}{\text{Number of units infused (or number of platelets, } \times 10^{11})}$$

Under optimal circumstances, the response should be 21,000 per mm$^3$ per m$^2$ per unit infused or 26,000 per mm$^3$ per m$^2$ per 10$^{11}$ platelets infused.

## ACTUAL CLINICAL RESPONSE

In practice the average increment after transfusion is approximately one-half of that expected, 10,000 per mm$^3$ per unit infused per m$^2$ (71). Many studies have attempted to identify the factors responsible for this consistently less than optimal response (50, 71–76). Alloimmunization is clearly important and will be discussed as a complication of platelet transfusion. A variety of nonimmune factors have been incriminated including platelet storage, bacterial sepsis, concomitant use of antibacterial antibiotics and Amphotericin B, graft-versus-host disease, splenomegaly, disseminated intravascular coagulation, and simply having had a recent allogeneic bone marrow transplantation. It is of interest that no one factor predominates in the majority of studies, suggesting that the crucial factors vary with the populations of individuals being studied.

On average the 20-hour increment has been two-thirds of the 1-hour increment with adverse clinical factors affecting this measurement as well (77). Platelet survival is reduced in all individuals with thrombocytopenia, regardless of the cause, with progressive reduction as the platelet count falls (78). Thus, the duration of response and the time to next transfusion increase with the height of the platelet concentration achieved by the transfusion and, therefore, the dose of platelets administered (79, 80).

## PLATELET DOSE

If, as described above, the average individual has an increase in platelet concentration of 10,000 per mm$^3$ per unit of platelets infused per m$^2$ surface area, one can calculate an appropriate dose required for an individual individual after identifying the platelet concentration to be achieved. In a very common situation, the prophylactic transfusion of a myelosuppressed individual with a platelet count of 10,000 per mm$^3$, a reasonable goal would be to raise the platelet concentration to 40,000 per mm$^3$. This would require 6 units in a large adult (>2 m$^2$) and 4 units in a small adult. These doses are in the range that has commonly been used on an empiric basis.

To the author, it makes no sense to think of a standard dose that fits all individuals, regardless of size and the indication for transfusion. For example, in preparing this same individual for neurosurgery, one might want to double or even triple the dose to achieve a platelet concentration in the range of 50,000 to 100,000 per mm$^3$. In addition, if the individual has a very large spleen, one can predict that a larger dose will be required to achieve a given target because of the increased size of the exchangeable platelet pool in the spleen. It is appropriate to increase the dose in this situation. Finally, during outpatient transfusion, one might want to increase the dose to lengthen the interval between transfusions. In calculating the dose of apheresis PCs, one can go through the same thought processes with knowledge of the average platelet content of apheresis PCs being provided by the blood bank or regional blood center.

However, one has to remember that individuals vary dramatically in their responses. Therefore, the measurement of increments 1 and 24 hours after transfusion is a cost-effective way to modify the dose and frequency of transfusion based on the pathophysiology of the individual individual. In practice it has been shown that increments at 10 and 60 minutes after transfusion are not different (81). Measurements at 10 minutes are particularly convenient in the outpatient setting.

# INDICATIONS FOR PLATELET TRANSFUSION

## FAILURE OF PLATELET PRODUCTION

Aggressive cytoreductive therapy for individuals with malignancy results in hypoplasia of the bone marrow, thrombocytopenia, and the need for platelet transfusion. Clearly, a thrombocytopenic individual who is actively bleeding requires platelet transfusion. It is more difficult to judge the need for transfusion if the platelet count is simply very low without significant clinical sequelae. Clinical experience suggests that, if the platelet count is low enough for long enough, "spontaneous" hemorrhage, particularly into the central nervous system, may occur. Unfortunately, in an individual individual we do not know how low and how long. The fear of such disastrous, "spontaneous" hemorrhage is responsible for the use of most platelet transfusions worldwide.

Studies of children with acute leukemia carried out more than 30 years ago (prior to the availability of platelet transfusions) described the relationship between platelet concentration in the blood and clinical hemorrhage (82). Minor and major hemorrhage began when the platelet concentration fell to below 50,000 per $mm^3$ and 20,000 per $mm^3$, respectively. Major hemorrhage was observed in the range of 5000 to 20,000 per $mm^3$ but on only 3% of individual days. There was a rapid increase in the rate of major bleeding when the platelet concentration fell below 5000 per $mm^3$, reaching a frequency of one in every three individual days as the platelet concentration approached 0 per $mm^3$. Subsequently, the same group described the effect of prophylactic transfusion administered whenever the platelet concentration fell below 20,000 per $mm^3$ (83). There was a striking reduction in major hemorrhage when the platelet concentration (measured pretransfusion) was below 5000 per $mm^3$ but no substantial change in the range of 5000 to 20,000 per $mm^3$. It should be mentioned that many of these individuals were commonly treated with aspirin so these bleeding rates may be overestimates.

For many years this experience was used to justify prophylactic transfusions whenever the platelet concentration fell below 20,000 per $mm^3$, even although the therapy had not had a substantial effect in the range of 5000 to 20,000 per $mm^3$. More recently, clinical studies have strongly supported lowering the transfusion trigger to 10,000 per $mm^3$ (84, 85) or even 5000 per $mm^3$ (86). However, it is likely that it is as unjustified to choose a rigid transfusion trigger as it is to choose a rigid transfusion dose. It is commonly assumed (86, 87), probably correctly, that clinical factors increase the risk for hemorrhage at any given platelet concentration. These include fever and sepsis, administration of drugs that interfere with platelet function, coexistent abnormalities of plasma coagulation factors, anatomic lesions such as gastrointestinal ulceration due to therapy or disease, and high leukocyte concentrations in the blood. It is appropriate to raise the transfusion trigger in complicated, clinically ill individuals of this type.

## ANTICIPATION OF AN INVASIVE PROCEDURE

Data are scanty, but several studies (88, 89) indicate that it is safe to carry out an invasive procedure if the platelet concentration is >50,000 per $mm^3$. It may be that an even higher level is appropriate if the procedure is "blind" with no opportunity for the operator to achieve hemostasis mechanically, as in needle biopsy of the liver; if the surgery is in an area where even a small hemorrhage would be disastrous, as in neurosurgery; or if the surgical field is highly vascular, as in a site with extensive inflammation or portal hypertension. On the other hand, uncomplicated surgery can be carried out without platelet transfusion at levels <50,000 per $mm^3$ if the surgical field is not highly vascular and the surgeon can achieve hemostasis mechanically.

## OTHER FORMS OF THROMBOCYTOPENIA

### Massive Transfusion

Dilutional thrombocytopenia occurs when massive blood loss is replaced with stored red cells that lack viable platelets (see Chapter 23). Following replacement of one blood volume, the platelet concentration is reduced to one-third to one-half of the original concentration. Even when one to two blood volumes have been replaced, abnormal bleeding usually does not develop, and routine transfusion, simply because the platelet count is low, is not indicated (90). Platelets should be given to individuals who demonstrate bleeding that is out of proportion to the degree of thrombocytopenia.

### Cardiopulmonary Bypass (See Chapter 50)

For several days after cardiac surgery, the platelet concentration commonly falls to subnormal levels, occasionally as low as 50,000 per $mm^3$. There is an associated defect in platelet function. Prospective studies have shown no benefit from the prophylactic administration of platelet transfusions to such individuals (91). Similar to the situation with massive transfusion, they should be reserved for the individual who demonstrates bleeding out of proportion to the degree of thrombocytopenia.

## Splenomegaly

As mentioned above, individuals with massive splenomegaly have thrombocytopenia related predominantly to excessive sequestration in an expanded splenic platelet pool. The platelet concentration rarely falls below 30,000 per mm$^3$ due to this mechanism alone, so that platelet transfusion is rarely considered except in anticipation of invasive procedures such as surgery and needle biopsy of the liver.

## Idiopathic Thrombocytopenic Purpura (ITP)

In ITP, platelet transfusion is generally not used because the response to medical therapy is usually satisfactory and rapid (see Chapter 30). Furthermore, the survival of transfused platelets is relatively brief, similar to that of the individual's own platelets. Nonetheless, when there is critical bleeding or need for urgent surgery, 3 to 6 units of whole blood derived PCs per m$^2$ body surface area will often raise the platelet count for 12 to 48 hours (92). The same general principles apply to other diseases in which there is accelerated destruction of platelets such as thrombocytopenia associated with disseminated intravascular coagulation.

## Neonatal Alloimmune Thrombocytopenia

In this syndrome, the mother produces an alloantibody against fetal platelets that have crossed the placenta (see Chapter 28). The antibody in turn crosses the placenta, causing severe fetal and neonatal thrombocytopenia that may persist for weeks after delivery. Since the mother's platelets lack the antigen to which the antibody has been produced, platelets obtained from the mother by apheresis are an ideal product for transfusion of the newborn (93).

Unfortunately, it is often difficult to arrange for apheresis of the mother. The delivery may have been at a small hospital at a great distance from an appropriate facility and complicated by, for example, caesarian section. Surprisingly, a randomly selected unit of platelets may raise the neonate's platelet concentration substantially (94). If it does not, prompt serologic evaluation can identify the antigen to which the antibody has been formed, usually HPA-1a. Donors lacking HPA-1a (i.e., homozygous HPA-1b) can then be sought to support the infant (95).

## Hereditary Thrombocytopenia

These syndromes are generally not associated with severe bleeding (96). Since the survival of allogeneic platelets is normal irrespective of the kinetics of the individual's own platelets, platelet transfusion is quite effective and may be used for critical bleeding and surgery.

## Qualitative Platelet Disorders

In spite of normal platelet counts, individuals with qualitative platelet disorders have a clinical bleeding tendency associated with abnormal *in vitro* tests of platelet function and a prolonged bleeding time. The basis may be hereditary (see Chapter 32) or acquired (see Chapter 33). Platelet transfusion is generally not indicated when the cause is extrinsic to the platelet, as in uremia, von Willebrand disease, and hyperglobulinemia, since the transfused platelets will function no better than the individual's own platelets. There are exceptions in certain types of von Willebrand disease in which normal platelets can be used to deliver von Willebrand factor to a bleeding site (see Chapter 34). Most inherited intrinsic disorders are mild and do not require platelet transfusions even for surgery if the procedure is carried out under direct vision so that hemostasis may be achieved mechanically. If the bleeding tendency is more severe, as in thrombasthenia, platelet transfusions may be necessary for more severe bleeding and surgery. The acquired defects, as in the myeloproliferative and myelodysplastic syndromes, generally do not require platelet transfusion unless there is coexistent thrombocytopenia.

## POSSIBLE CONTRAINDICATIONS TO PLATELET TRANSFUSION

There is controversy in this area because there are no adequate data. Concern has been voiced that platelet transfusions should not be administered to individuals with forms of thrombocytopenia associated with thrombosis, such as thrombotic thrombocytopenic purpura (TTP) (see Chapter 27) and heparin-induced thrombocytopenia (see Chapter 29), since provision of platelets might worsen the thrombotic tendency (97, 98). Unfortunately, particularly in TTP, platelet transfusion is often requested prior to invasive procedures such as the insertion of intravenous catheters for therapy with apheresis. The author's experience has been that platelet transfusions are safe in this setting. However, it seems prudent not to administer *prophylactic* platelet transfusions for the thrombocytopenias of these diseases.

## COMPLICATIONS OF PLATELET TRANSFUSION

### ALLOIMMUNIZATION

## Lymphocytotoxic HLA Antibodies

Alloimmunization secondary to repeated exposure to allogeneic blood cells is a major cause of poor response to platelet transfusion. In most cases of alloimmunization to platelets, the alloantibodies responsible are directed against HLA antigens on the platelet surface. Alloimmunization should be suspected clinically if two or three consecutive transfusions produce a corrected count increment <3000 per mm$^3$ per m$^2$ (99). It can be confirmed in the laboratory by performing a lymphocytotoxicity (LCT) assay for HLA antibody in the individual's serum. The presence of such antibody has been a good predictor of poor response to platelets from randomly selected donors (100) and improved response when platelets are HLA-selected (101).

When individuals present for therapy of diseases requiring repeated platelet transfusions, 10% will already have LCT antibodies from prior transfusions or pregnancies (102). Another 30% become alloimmunized during therapy, and 60% never become immunized (102). There is no known difference between the individuals who do and do not become immunized. There is no dose-response relationship. Among individuals who are to become immunized, some do so after only two to four transfusions, whereas others require dozens of transfusions (103). Surprisingly, approximately 30% of immunized individuals will lose their antibodies over time in spite of continuing transfusions (104). Thus it is beneficial to monitor antibody levels during therapy since such individuals often regain responsiveness to

randomly selected platelets after long periods of refractoriness.

The pattern and intensity of immunization varies greatly from individual to individual. LCT antibody is assayed using a panel of cells from 50 to 100 donors. Thus each assay can be characterized by the percentage of the panel cells against which the individual's sera reacts, that is, the percent reactive antibody (PRA). Individuals may have PRAs at any level between 5 and 100% (Fig. 51.5). The LCT assay can also be used to identify the specific HLA antigens to which the individual has antibody, as well as the PRA. Except for the individuals who gradually lose antibody, the majority of alloimmunized individuals establish a level and specificity of immunization and tend to maintain that status in spite of repeated transfusions.

Cross-reactive groups (CREGs) of HLA antigens have been defined by serologic testing. Cross reactivity is based on the sharing of public epitopes by the antigens within each CREG (105). It is common for a individual with a moderate degree of immunization (40 to 60% PRA) to develop antibodies to only one or two public epitopes, that is, one or two CREGs (106). On the other hand, some moderately immunized individuals and most highly immunized individuals (90 to 100% PRA) often demonstrate intra-CREG antibodies, that is, anti-

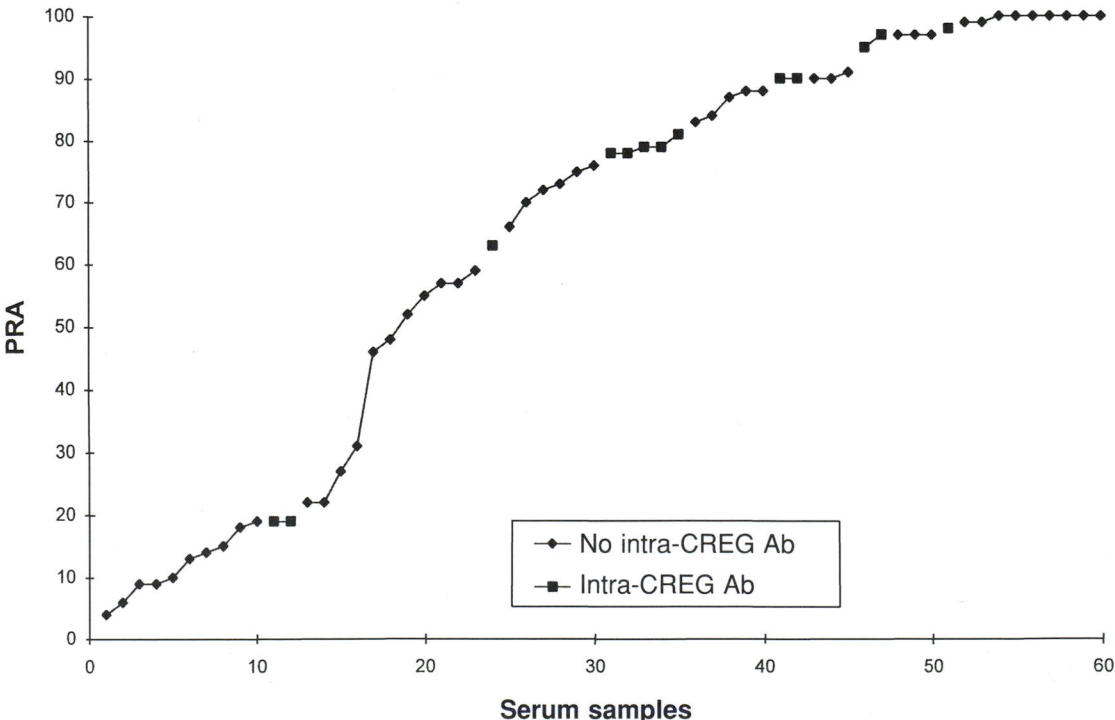

**FIGURE 51.5.** Cumulative frequency of percent reactive antibody (PRA) by lymphocytotoxicity (LCT) assay in serum samples from 108 thrombocytopenic individuals referred to a regional blood center for matched platelet support during a 6-month period. Fifty showed no reactivity, while 58 showed PRAs that varied from 4 to 100%. The squares indicate individuals who had demonstrable antibody against antigens within their own cross reactive groups (i.e., intra-CREG antibody). (Data provided by Dr. Susan Hsu, American Red Cross Blood Services, Penn-Jersey Region.)

bodies to antigens in the same CREGs as the individual's own antigens (107). These facts have a major impact on management.

## Antibody Detection Using the Platelet as Target

It is often a source of confusion that the LCT assay uses the T-lymphocyte as the target cell when the aim is to determine if a individual is responding poorly to platelet transfusion because of antibody to the transfused platelets. During the late 1980s and early 1990s, there were descriptions of many tests that used the platelet as the target cell (108–111). It was shown that HLA antibodies could be demonstrated by these techniques (108) and that there were correlations between positive and negative cross matches and poor and good corrected count increments. However, most of these studies were retrospective, and the tests were often expensive and not rapid enough to supply a useful product on an urgent basis. This situation changed in the early 1990s with the introduction of the solid phase red cell adherence (SPRCA) method for screening of donor sera (112) and for compatibility testing (113). This method was commercialized (Capture-P from Immucor Inc, Norcross, GA) and is now widely used in hospitals and blood centers (72). Other methods, particularly using flow cytometry (114), are also being reported.

## Antibody to Blood Group Determinants

ABO determinants are carried by both glycoproteins and glycolipids of platelets, as they are in red cells (115). Platelet cross matching methods, including the SPRCA assay, detect ABO IgG alloantibodies (116) if the titer is high enough. The relevance of these antibodies to ABO determinants needs better definition. Group O individuals commonly have excellent responses to platelets from group A donors, but in a subset of individuals the response is often poor (117) or very poor (118). It is not yet known whether one can distinguish the good from the poor responders among group O individuals by cross matching using the SPRCA method. For the present it seems wise to observe ABO compatibility when possible.

## Role of Platelet-Specific Antibody

It would seem reasonable that some cases of refractoriness to platelet transfusion on an immune basis might be related to the presence of platelet-specific alloantibody, that is, alloantibody to antigens on the platelet surface other than HLA antigens. There have been case reports (119–121), but on the whole most authors have found this to be a quite uncommon event (122–126). This area deserves further study. It has been technically difficult to identify platelet-specific antibodies when there is intense HLA alloimmunization as well. Techniques for

identifying platelet-specific antibodies in this setting are improving (127).

## Management of the Alloimmunized Individual

Strategies for selecting apheresis PCs for alloimmunized individuals may be antigen based, antibody based, or a combination of the two approaches. The initial approaches were antigen based. In 1969 it was shown that refractory individuals would respond to platelets from siblings who were identical for all four class I HLA antigens (128). Through the 1970s it was further shown that individuals could be supported by platelets from unrelated donors who were HLA-identical or closely matched (129). However, because of the great heterogeneity of the HLA antigens, many individuals had few identical matches even from within a pool of thousands of donors (130). Therefore, it became popular to choose donors who were selectively "mismatched" according to CREG classification (131). Table 51.1 demonstrates this approach based on choosing products from within the individual's CREGs.

Clearly, responses were better with such "matching" than they were to platelets selected randomly. However, it was striking that many BX matches failed while many C and D matches succeeded. Potential explanations for these findings may be derived from the patterns of alloimmunization that we have described in

**TABLE 51.1.** Classification of Donor/Recipient Pairs on the Basis of HLA Class I Matching

| | |
|---|---|
| A | All four antigens in donor identical to those of recipient. |
| B1U | Only three antigens detected in donor; all present in recipient. |
| B1X | Three donor antigens identical to recipient; fourth antigen cross reactive[a] with recipient. |
| B2U | Only two antigens detected in donor; both present in recipient. |
| B2UX | Only three antigens detected in donor; two identical with recipient, third cross reactive. |
| B2X | Two donor antigens identical to recipient; third and fourth antigens cross reactive with recipient. |
| C | One antigen of donor not present in recipient and non-cross-reactive with recipient. |
| D | Two antigens of donor not present in recipient and non-cross-reactive with recipient. |

*From Duquesnoy RJ, Filip DJ, Rodey GE et al. Successful transfusion of platelets "mismatched" for HLA antigens to alloimmunized thrombocytopenic individuals. Am J Hematol 1977;2:219–226.*

[a] *Antigen in a cross reactive group (CREG) that contains one of the individual's antigens.*

such individuals (Fig. 51.5). Some individuals develop antibody to a limited number of antigens, only one or two CREGs, so success with some C and D matches would be expected if the match happened to contain no CREG to which the individual had antibody. In addition, some HLA antigens are poorly expressed on platelets (132). On the other hand, some individuals develop intra-CREG antibody (Fig. 51.5). In these individuals failure of some BX matches would be expected. Finally, at the practical level, this antigen-based method generally required a great deal of time before a suitable product could be found. It was very uncommon to find an excellent match in inventory to respond to an urgent request. It often required days to recruit and pherese one or more well-matched donors from an HLA-typed donor file.

Because of these issues and the emerging availability of methods for cross-matching, antibody-based methods became popular in the late 1980s and early 1990s (133). Many centers found that they could simply cross-match individual's serum with products from approximately ten randomly selected donors to find a donor whose product would be successful *in vivo* (72, 134). They found this approach to be more cost-effective (135) than ordering platelets as "HLA matched" (72) from a regional blood center. Furthermore, a cross-match–compatible product could often be made available in a matter of hours rather than days. However, it has to be recognized that one may have to cross-match dozens of donors before finding a compatible product if the individual is highly immunized (i.e., PRA 90 to 100%).

One study directly compared a variety of cross-matching methods with HLA antigen matching (136). Provision of A and BU matches was the most successful strategy. Products that were less than an A or BU match and cross match-compatible products were comparable but not as effective as A and BU matches. The widely available and rapid SPRCA method was at least as successful as any other cross match method (137).

One other antibody-based method has emerged. If the PRA of the LCT assay is less than 100%, one should be able to identify the antigens to which the individual has not formed antibody using selected lymphocyte panels. Two groups (138, 139) have reported results equivalent to A and BU matches by supporting individuals with "antigen-negative" products, that is, platelets that lack the antigens to which the individual has antibody as determined by the LCT assay. If the results of the LCT assay are known, one can often provide a product from inventory on an urgent basis using this approach.

It is clear that the "art" of supporting alloimmunized individuals is evolving. If the PRA is <60%, successful support can usually be provided on an urgent

basis from an inventory of 30 to 50 products with cross matching alone (134) or by providing HLA matched products taking into account the specificities of the antibodies identified on the LCT assay. When the PRA is high (>80%), intra-CREG antibodies are frequently present and the blind provision of anything less than an A or BU match frequently fails. For such highly immunized individuals, a combination of methods is probably required. One can select for cross matching the best available, "antigen-negative" HLA matches (140). Surprisingly, cross matching sometimes identifies an effective donor who would not have been chosen by classical HLA criteria (141). Some individuals are best served by selective recruitment of A and BU matches from a large HLA-typed donor file. This requires advanced planning, a transfusion schedule, and constant communication between the blood center and the clinician. Some individuals with common HLA types (e.g., 1,2/7,8) will have dozens of A and BU matches available. Unfortunately, some individuals have rare HLA types, and they will have no A or BU match to recruit.

## Prevention of Alloimmunization

Blood cells vary dramatically in their capacity to induce alloimmunization to HLA. Although they express HLA class I antigens, platelets are very poor immunogens. Rather, a small population of leukocytes (monocytes, B lymphocytes, and dendritic cells) that express both class I and class II HLA antigens, as well as other costimulatory molecules, contains the major culprits (142). There is now abundant evidence that the incidence of alloimmunization can be reduced by the consistent use of leukocyte-reduced blood products (13). Red cell transfusions must also be leukocyte-reduced since leukocytes contained in them are quite capable of inducing alloimmunization (143).

However, there is still uncertainty as to the extent to which leukocyte reduction will influence the incidence and severity of HLA alloimmunization. One group (144) suggested that leukocyte reduction had almost no effect on the development of alloimmunization in individuals who had been previously exposed to leukocytes by pregnancy or previous transfusions that had not been leukoreduced. However, another trial (145) demonstrated some efficacy in such individuals. Ultimately, it may prove to be true that, in some highly sensitive individuals, platelets or very small numbers of leukocytes (i.e., less than $5 \times 10^6$) can stimulate secondary, if not primary (146), alloimmunization.

Another approach to the prevention of alloimmunization is irradiation of PCs with ultraviolet light (147). Such treatment apparently prevents the specific leukocytes involved from directly stimulating the recipient's immune system. While still investigational, efficacy has been clearly demonstrated in several studies (145).

## COMPLICATIONS UNIQUE TO PLATELET TRANSFUSION

### Bacterial Contamination

Storage of platelets at 20 to 24°C allows proliferation of bacteria that contaminate occasional units of blood or apheresis PCs at the time of collection (148). There have been many reports of clinical sepsis after transfusion of stored platelets (149–153). Although contamination may occur because of asymptomatic bacteremia in the donor, most episodes probably have their origin at the time of venipuncture because of inadequate decontamination of the skin or because of venipuncture through scarred or "dimpled" areas of the skin that may be colonized with surface and deep bacteria (153). Bacterial contamination that might not be clinically significant after 2 to 3 days of storage may become so after 5 to 7 days (151, 152). As previously mentioned, platelet storage is currently limited to 5 days because of these concerns.

The magnitude of this problem is commonly underestimated. Bacterial contamination of platelet products is probably the leading microbial cause of transfusion-related mortality in the United States (154). Estimates suggest that there is contamination of 5 to 10 per 10,000 whole blood derived PCs. There may be as many as 150 clinical episodes associated with severe morbidity or death in the United States per year (155). This is 50- to 250-fold higher than the risk for mortality from human immunodeficiency virus (HIV) or hepatitis B or C infection.

There are several potential approaches to reducing this risk. Because apheresis involves only one venipuncture, there may be less risk for apheresis PCs relative to pooled, whole blood derived PCs, although this has not been demonstrated conclusively. Under investigation are methods of viral inactivation (which also inactivate bacteria) (156), and methods for screening platelet products for bacteria before infusion (157).

### Cytokine Production

Prior to the availability of methods for leukoreduction, approximately 20% of individuals receiving platelet transfusions experienced febrile, nonhemolytic, transfusion reactions (158). Leukocyte reduction by filtration at the time of infusion has practically eliminated these reactions for red cells, but such bedside filtration has been much less effective for platelet transfusion (158, 159). It is now known that contaminating leukocytes produce a variety of cytokines, such as interleukin-1$\beta$, interleukin-6, interleukin-8, and tumor necrosis factor $\alpha$, during the 5-day storage of PCs at 20 to 24°C, a relatively high temperature at which leukocytes remain metabolically active (17, 18). Many reactions have been linked to these bioreactive substances in the plasma supernatant from which they are not removed by bedside filtration. These observations provide a strong argument for the routine "prestorage" removal of leukocytes from platelet products during or soon after preparation. Some febrile reactions to platelet transfusion, particularly those associated with allergic phenomena such as urticaria, are reactions to proteins present in the plasma at the time of donation (160). There are techniques for washing platelets free of plasma that can be used to alleviate these reactions (160).

## COMPLICATIONS COMMON TO ALL TRANSFUSIONS

Immunosuppressed individuals may develop graft-versus-host disease (GVHD) from T lymphocytes present in any transfusion. Thus, it is standard practice to irradiate PCs to inhibit proliferation of contaminating T lymphocytes when the recipient has been heavily immunosuppressed, as in bone marrow transplantation (161). Exposure to 5000 rad has no deleterious effect on platelets. It is important to emphasize that current methods of leukoreduction do not remove enough T cells to prevent GVHD.

During transfusion to girls or young women who are Rh-negative, one needs to be concerned about sensitization by Rh-positive red cells contaminating infused platelets. In practice, sensitization is rather uncommon in immunosuppressed individuals (162). However, one can administer Rh immunoglobulin (RhoGAM), about 20 $\mu$g intramuscularly per unit of platelets, so that the infused red cells will be cleared prior to sensitization of the recipient.

Platelet transfusion can transmit viruses such as hepatitis B and C and HIV. Recently improved methods of donor screening and testing have reduced but not eliminated this risk. As mentioned, methods for viral inactivation of platelet concentrates are being sought (156). Cytomegalovirus (CMV) represents a special situation. It is particularly dangerous for severely immunocompromised individuals such as those who have had allogeneic bone marrow transplantation. In asymptomatic carriers the virus resides in the nuclei of subsets of leukocytes, and there is little, if any, free in plasma. Studies indicate that provision of leukoreduced platelets and red cells is essentially equivalent to provision of blood products from CMV-negative donors in terms of CMV safety (163).

# ACKNOWLEDGMENT

The author thanks Dr. Charles Schiffer for many thoughtful suggestions concerning this manuscript.

# REFERENCES

1. Surgenor DM, Wallace EL, Hao SH et al. Collection and transfusion of blood in the United States, 1982–1988. N Engl J Med 1990;322:1646–1651.
2. Wallace EL, Surgenor DM, Hao HS et al. Collection and transfusion of blood and blood components in the United States. 1989. Transfusion 1993; 33:139–144.

3. Hirsch EO, Gardner FH. The transfusion of human blood platelets. With a note on the transfusion of granulocytes. J Lab Clin Med 1952;39:556–569.

4. Kurtz SR, McMican A, Carciero R et al. Plateletpheresis experience with the Haemonetics blood processor 30, the IBM Blood Processor 2997, and the Fenwal CS-3000 Blood Processor. Vox Sang 1981;41:212–218.

5. Mourad N. A simple method for obtaining platelet concentrates free of aggregates. Transfusion 1968;8:48.

6. Kelley DL, Fegan RL, Ng AT et al. High-yield platelet concentrates attainable by continuous quality improvement reduce platelet transfusion cost and donor exposure. Transfusion 1997;37:482–486.

7. Murphy S, Heaton WA, Rebulla P. Platelet production in the Old World—and the New. Transfusion 1996;36:751–754.

8. Pietersz RN, Loos JA, Reesink HW. Platelet concentrates stored in plasma for 72 hours at 22 degrees C prepared from buffycoats of citrate-phosphate-dextrose blood collected in a quadruple-bag saline-adenine-glucose-mannitol system. Vox Sang 1985;49:81–85.

9. Hogman CF, Eriksson L, Kristensen J. Leukocyte-depleted platelets prepared from pooled buffy coat. Post-transfusion increment and "in vitro bleeding time" using the Thrombostat 4000/2. Transfus Sci 1993;14:35–39.

10. Bertolini F, Rebulla P, Riccardi D. Evaluation of platelet concentrates prepared from buffy coats and stored in a glucose-free crystalloid medium. Transfusion 1989;29:605–609.

11. Bertolini F, Rebulla P, Marangoni F et al. Platelet concentrates stored in synthetic medium after filtration. Vox Sang 1992;62:82–86.

12. Simon TL. The collection of platelets by apheresis procedures [Review]. Transfus Med Rev 1994;8:132–145.

13. Meryman HT. Transfusion-induced alloimmunization and immunosuppression and the effects of leukocyte depletion [Review]. Transfus Med Rev 1989;3:180.

14. Fournel JJ, Zingsem J, Riggert J et al. A multicenter evaluation of the routine use of a new white cell-reduction apheresis system for collection of platelets. Transfusion 1997;37:487–492.

15. Yockey C, Murphy S, Eggers L et al. Evaluation of the Amicus separator for collection of apheresed platelets (AP) [Abstract #12]. Presented at the American Society for Apheresis, Washington, DC, 1997.

16. Popovsky MA. Quality of blood components filtered before storage and at the bedside: implications for transfusion practice. Transfusion 1996;36:470–474.

17. Heddle NM, Klama L, Singer J et al. The role of the plasma from platelet concentrates in transfusion reactions. N Engl J Med 1994;331:625–628.

18. Muylle L, Wouters E, Peetermans ME. Febrile reactions to platelet transfusion: the effect of increased interleukin 6 levels in concentrates prepared by the platelet-rich plasma method. Transfusion 1996;36:886–890.

19. Williamson LM, Wimperis JZ, Williamson P et al. Bedside filtration of blood products in the prevention of HLA alloimmunization—a prospective randomized study. Blood 1994;83:3028–3035.

20. Shiba M, Tadokoro K, Sawanobori M et al. Activation of the contact system by filtration of platelet concentrates with a negatively charged white cell-removal filter and measurement of venous blood bradykinin level in individuals who received filtered platelets. Transfusion 1997;37:457–462.

21. Sweeney JD, Holme S, Heaton WA et al. White cell-reduced platelet concentrates prepared by in-line filtration of platelet-rich plasma. Transfusion 1995;35:131–136.

22. Snyder EL, Moroff G, Simon T. Recommended methods for conducting radiolabeled survival studies. Transfusion 1986;26:37–42.

23. Murphy S, Gardner FH. Platelet preservation. Effect of storage temperature on maintenance of platelet viability–deleterious effect of refrigerated storage. N Engl J Med 1969;280:1094–1098.

24. Gottschall JL, Rzad L, Aster RH. Studies of the minimum temperature at which human platelets can be stored with full maintenance of viability. Transfusion 1986;26:460–462.

25. Slichter SJ, Harker LA. Preparation and storage of platelet concentrates. II. Storage variables influencing platelet viability and function. Br J Haematol 1976;34:403–419.

26. Filip DJ, Aster RH. Relative hemostatic effectiveness of human platelets stored at 4 degrees and 22 degrees C. J Lab Clin Med 1978;91:618–624.

27. Murphy S. Platelet function, kinetics, and metabolism—impact on quality assessment, storage, and clinical use. In: McLeod B, Price TH, Drew MJ, eds. Apheresis: principles and practice. Bethesda: AABB Press, 1997:123–139.

28. Holme S, Sawyer S, Heaton A et al. Studies on platelets exposed to or stored at temperatures below 20 degrees C or above 24 degrees C. Transfusion 1997;37:5–11.

29. Kilkson H, Holme S, Murphy S. Platelet metabolism during storage of platelet concentrates at 22 degrees C. Blood 1984;64:406–414.

30. Cesar J, DiMinno G, Alam I et al. Plasma free fatty acid metabolism during storage of platelet concentrates for transfusion. Transfusion 1987;27:434–437.

31. Holme S, Murphy S. Quantitative measurements of platelet shape by light transmission studies; application to storage of platelets for transfusion. J Lab Clin Med 1978;92:53–64.

32. Murphy S. Platelet storage for transfusion. Semin Hematol 1985;22:165–177.

33. Murphy S. The oxidation of exogenously added organic anions by platelets facilitates maintenance of pH during their storage for transfusion at 22 degrees C. Blood 1995;85:1929–1935.

34. Murphy S, Shimizu T, Miripol J. Platelet storage for transfusion in synthetic media: further optimization of ingredients and definition of their roles. Blood 1995;86:3951–3960.

35. Murphy S, Kahn RA, Holme S et al. Improved storage of platelets for transfusion in a new container. Blood 1982;60:194–200.

36. Simon TL, Nelson EJ, Carmen RL et al. Extension of platelet concentrate storage. Transfusion 1983;23:207–212.

37. Holme S, Heaton A, Momoda G. Evaluation of a new, oxygen-permeable, polyvinylchloride container. Transfusion 1989;29:159–164.

38. de Wildt-Eggen J, Schrijver JG, Bouter-Valk HJ et al. Improvement of platelet storage conditions by using new polyolefin containers. Transfusion 1997;37:476–481.

39. Murphy S, Gardner FH. Platelet storage at 22 degrees C: role of gas transport across plastic containers in maintenance of viability. Blood 1975;46:209–218.

40. Murphy S, Sayar SN, Gardner FH. Storage of platelet concentrates at 22 degrees C. Blood 1970;35:549–557.

41. Holme S, Vaidja K, Murphy S. Platelet storage at 22 degrees C: effect of type of agitation on morphology, viability, and function in vitro. Blood 1978;52:425–435.

42. Murphy S, Kahn RA, Holme S et al. Improved storage of platelets for transfusion in a new container. Blood 1982;60:194–200.

43. Snyder EL, Pope C, Ferri PM et al. The effect of mode of agitation and type of plastic bag on storage characteristics and in vivo kinetics of platelet concentrates. Transfusion 1986;26:125–130.

44. Mitchell SG, Hawker RJ, Turner VS. Effect of agitation on the quality of platelet concentrates. Vox Sang 1994;67:160–165.

45. Moroff G, George VM. The maintenance of platelet properties on limited discontinuation of agitation during storage. Transfusion 1990;30:427–430.

46. Hogge DE, Thompson BW, Schiffer CA. Platelet storage for 7 days in second-generation blood bags. Transfusion 1986;26:131–135.

47. Shanwell A, Larsson S, Aschan J et al. A randomized trial comparing the use of fresh and stored platelets in the treatment of bone marrow transplant recipients. Eur J Haematol 1992;49:77–81.

48. Leach MF, AuBuchon JP. Effect of storage time on clinical efficacy of single-donor platelet units. Transfusion 1993;33:661–664.

49. Peter-Salonen K, Bucher U, Nydegger UE. Comparison of post-transfusion recoveries achieved with either fresh or stored platelet concentrates. Blut 1987;54:207–212.

50. Norol F, Kuentz M, Cordonnier C et al. Influence of clinical status on the efficiency of stored platelet transfusion. Br J Haematol 1994;86:125–129.

51. Bode AP. Platelet activation may explain the storage lesion in platelet concentrates [Review]. Blood Cells 1990;16:109–125.

52. Holme S, Murphy S. Quantitative measurements of platelet shape by light transmission studies; application to storage of platelets for transfusion. J Lab Clin Med 1978;92:53–64.

53. Snyder EL, Pope C, Ferri PM et al. The effect of mode of agitation and type of plastic bag on storage characteristics and in vivo kinetics of platelet concentrates. Transfusion 1986;26:125–130.

54. Holme S, Sweeney JD, Sawyer S et al. The expression of p-selectin during collection, processing, and storage of platelet concentrates: relationship to loss of in vivo viability. Transfusion 1997;37:12–17.

55. Bode AP, Orton SM, Frye MJ et al. Vesiculation of platelets during in vitro aging. Blood 1991;77:887–895.

56. Lozano ML, Rivera J, Gonzalez-Conejero R et al. Loss of high-affinity thrombin receptors during platelet concentrate storage impairs the reactivity of platelets to thrombin. Transfusion 1997;37:368–375.

57. DiMinno G, Silver MJ, Murphy S. Stored human platelets retain full aggregation potential in response to pairs of aggregating agents. Blood 1982;59:563–568.

58. Owens M, Holme S, Heaton A et al. Post-transfusion recovery of function of 5-day stored platelet concentrates. Br J Haematol 1992;80:539–544.

59. Murphy S, Rebulla P, Bertolini F et al. In vitro assessment of the quality of stored platelet concentrates [Review]. Transfus Med Rev 1994;8:29–36.

60. Holme S, Moroff G, Murphy S. A multi-laboratory evaluation of platelet in vitro assays: the extent of shape change and response to hypotonic stress assays. Transfusion. In Press, 1997.

61. Bertolini F, Murphy S. A multicenter evaluation of reproducibility of swirling in platelet concentrates. Transfusion 1994;34:796–801.

62. Murphy S, Sayar SN, Abdou NL et al. Platelet preservation by freezing. Use of dimethylsulfoxide as cryoprotective agent. Transfusion 1974;14:139–144.

63. Towell BL, Levine SP, Knight WA 3d et al. A comparison of frozen and fresh platelet concentrates in the support of thrombocytopenic individuals. Transfusion 1986;26:525–530.

64. Lazarus HM, Kaniecki-Green EA, Warm SE et al. Therapeutic effectiveness of frozen platelet concentrates for transfusion. Blood 1981;57:243–249.

65. Schiffer CA, Aisner J, Wiernik PH. Frozen autologous platelet transfusion for individuals with leukemia. N Engl J Med 1978;299:7–12.

66. Connor J, Currie LM, Allan H et al. Recovery of in vitro functional activity

of platelet concentrates stored at 4 degrees C and treated with second-messenger effectors. Transfusion 1996;36:691–698.

67. Winokur R, Hartwig JH. Mechanism of shape change in chilled human platelets. Blood 1995;85:1796–1804.

68. Manno CS, Hedberg KW, Kim HC et al. Comparison of the hemostatic effects of fresh whole blood, stored whole blood, and components after open heart surgery in children. Blood 1991;77:930–936.

69. Read MS, Reddick RL, Bode AP et al. Preservation of hemostatic and structural properties of rehydrated lyophilized platelets: potential for long-term storage of dried platelets for transfusion. Proc Natl Acad Sci U S A 1995;92:397–401.

70. Chao FC, Kim BK, Houranieh AM et al. Infusible platelet membrane microvesicles: a potential transfusion substitute for platelets. Transfusion 1996;36:536–542.

71. Bishop JF, McGrath K, Wolf MM et al. Clinical factors influencing the efficacy of pooled platelet transfusions. Blood 1988;71:383–387.

72. Friedberg RC, Donnelly SF, Boyd JC et al. Clinical and blood bank factors in the management of platelet refractoriness and alloimmunization. Blood 1993;81:3428–3434.

73. Klumpp TR, Herman JH, Innis S et al. Factors associated with response to platelet transfusion following hematopoietic stem cell transplantation. Bone Marrow Transplant 1996;17:1035–1041.

74. Doughty HA, Murphy MF, Metcalfe P et al. Relative importance of immune and non-immune causes of platelet refractoriness. Vox Sang 1994;66:200–205.

75. Alcorta I, Pereira A, Ordinas A. Clinical and laboratory factors associated with platelet transfusion refractoriness: a case-control study. Br J Haematol 1996;93:220–224.

76. Bock M, Muggenthaler KH, Schmidt U et al. Influence of antibiotics on posttransfusion platelet increment. Transfusion 1996;36:952–954.

77. Bishop JF, Matthews JP, McGrath K et al. Factors influencing 20-hour increments after platelet transfusion. Transfusion 1991;31:392–396.

78. Hanson SR, Slichter SJ. Platelet kinetics in individuals with bone marrow hypoplasia: evidence for a fixed platelet requirement. Blood 1985;66:1105–1109.

79. Herman JH, Klumpp TR, Christman RA et al. The effect of platelet dose on the outcome of prophylactic platelet transfusion [Abstract]. Transfusion 1995;35:S181.

80. Norol F, Duedari N. Comparison of different doses of platelet transfusion [Abstract]. Blood 1995;86:353a.

81. O'Connell B, Lee EJ, Schiffer CA. The value of 10-minute posttransfusion platelet counts. Transfusion 1988;28:66–67.

82. Gaydos LA, Freireich EJ, Mantel N. The quantitative relation between platelet count and hemorrhage in individuals with acute leukemia. N Engl J Med 1962;266:905–909.

83. Freireich EJ, Kliman A, Lawrence AG et al. Response to repeated platelet transfusion from the same donor. Ann Intern Med 1963;59:277–287.

84. Wandt H, Frank M, Schneider C et al. The 10,000/L trigger compared to 20,000/L for prophylactic platelet transfusion in AML: a prospective comparative multicenter study [Abstract]. Blood 1996;88:443a.

85. GIMEMA Group. A prospective controlled study on bleeding risk in acute myeloblastic leukemia (AML) individuals randomized to be transfused at ≤10 versus ≤20 × 10⁹/l platelets. Interim report from the platelet transfusion trigger trial (PITT) [Abstract]. GIMEMA Group Blood 1996;88:443a.

86. Gmur J, Burger J, Schanz U et al. Safety of stringent prophylactic platelet transfusion policy for individuals with acute leukemia. Lancet 1991;338:1223–1226.

87. Creutzig U, Ritter J, Budde M et al. Early deaths due to hemorrhage and leukostasis in childhood acute myelogenous leukemia. Associations with hyperleukocytosis and acute monocytic leukemia. Cancer 1987;60:3071–3079.

88. McVay PA, Toy PT. Lack of increased bleeding after liver biopsy in individuals with mild hemostatic abnormalities. Am J Clin Pathol 1990;94:747–753.

89. McVay PA, Toy PT. Lack of increased bleeding after paracentesis and thoracentesis in individuals with mild coagulation abnormalities. Transfusion 1991;31:164–171.

90. Reed RL 2d, Ciavarella D, Heimbach DM et al. Prophylactic platelet administration during massive transfusion. A prospective, randomized, double-blind clinical study. Ann Surg 1986;203:40–48.

91. Simon TL, Akl Bechara F, Murphy W. Controlled trial of routine administration of platelet concentrates in cardiopulmonary bypass surgery. Ann Thorac Surg 1984;37:359–364.

92. Carr JM, Kruskall MS, Kaye JA et al. Efficacy of platelet transfusions in immune thrombocytopenia. Am J Med 1986;80:1051–1054.

93. McIntosh S, O'Brien RT, Schwartz AD et al. Neonatal isoimmune purpura: response to platelet infusions. J Pediatr 1973;82:1020–1027.

94. Win N. Provision of random-donor platelets (HPA-1a positive) in neonatal alloimmune thrombocytopenia due to anti HPA-1a alloantibodies. Vox Sang 1996;71:130–131.

95. Munizza M, Nance S, Keashen-Schnell MA et al. Provision of HPA-1a (PLᴬ¹) negative platelets for neonatal alloimmune thrombocytopenia

96. Murphy S. Hereditary thrombocytopenia. Clin Haematol 1972;1:359–368.

97. Bell WR, Braine HG, Ness PM et al. Improved survival in thrombotic thrombocytopenic purpura-hemolytic uremic syndrome. N Engl J Med 1991;325:398–403.

98. Warkentin TE, Kelton JG. Heparin and platelets [Review]. Hematol Oncol Clin North Am 1990;4:243–264.

99. Bishop JF, Matthews JP, Yuen K et al. The definition of refractoriness to platelet transfusions. Transfus Med 1992;2:35–41.

100. Hogge DE, Dutcher JP, Aisner J et al. Lymphocytotoxic antibody is a predictor of response to random donor platelet transfusion. Am J Hematol 1983;14:363–369.

101. McFarland JG, Anderson AJ, Slichter SJ. Factors influencing the transfusion response to HLA-selected apheresis donor platelets in individuals refractory to random donor platelet concentrates. Br J Haematol 1989;73:380–386.

102. Dutcher JP, Schiffer CA, Aisner J et al. Long-term follow-up of individuals with leukemia receiving platelet transfusions: identification of a large group of individuals who do not become alloimmunized. Blood 1981;58:1007–1011.

103. Dutcher JP, Schiffer CA, Aisner J et al. Alloimmunization following platelet transfusion: the absence of a dose-response relationship. Blood 1981;57:395–398.

104. Lee EJ, Schiffer CA. Serial measurement of lymphocytotoxic antibody and response to nonmatched platelet transfusion in alloimmunized individuals. Blood 1987;70:1727–1729.

105. Rodey GE, Neylan JF, Whelchel JD et al. Epitope specificity of HLA Class I alloantibodies. I. Frequency analysis of antibodies to private versus public specificities in potential transplant recipients. Hum Immunol 1994;39:272–280.

106. MacPherson BR, Hammond PB, Maniscalco CA. Alloimmunization to public HLA antigens in multi-transfused platelet recipients. Ann Clin Lab Sci 1986;16:38–44.

107. MacPherson BR. HLA antibody formation within the HLA-A1 crossreactive group in multitransfused platelet recipients. Am J Hematol 1989;30:228–232.

108. McGrath K, Holdsworth R, Veale M et al. Detection of HLA antibodies by platelet crossmatching techniques. Transfusion 1988;28:214–216.

109. Kickler TS, Ness PM, Braine HG. Platelet crossmatching. A direct approach to the selection of platelet transfusions for the alloimmunized thrombocytopenic individual. Am J Clin Pathol 1988;90:69–72.

110. McFarland JG, Aster RH. Evaluation of four methods for platelet compatibility testing. Blood 1987;69:1425–1430.

111. Freedman J, Garvey MB, Salomon de Friedberg ZS et al. Random donor platelet crossmatching: comparison of four platelet antibody detection methods. Am J Hematol 1988;28:1–7.

112. Lown JAG, Ivey JG. Evaluation of a solid phase red cell adherence technique for platelet antibody screening. Transfusion Med 1991;1:163–167.

113. Rachel JM, Summers TC, Sinor LT et al. Use of a solid phase red blood cell adherence method for pretransfusion platelet compatibility testing. Am J Clin Pathol 1988;90:63–68.

114. Kohler M, Dittmann J, Legler TJ et al. Flow cytometric detection of platelet-reactive antibodies and application in platelet crossmatching. Transfusion 1996;36:250–255.

115. Santoso S, Kiefel V, Mueller-Eckhardt C. Blood group A and B determinants are expressed on platelet glycoproteins IIa, IIIa, and Ib. Thromb Haemost 1991;65:196–201.

116. Ellinger PJ, Morgan LK, Malecek AC et al. Effect of ABO mismatching on a radioimmunoassay for platelet compatibility. Successful absorption of ABO alloantibodies with synthetic A and B substance. Transfusion 1989;29:134–138.

117. Lee EJ, Schiffer CA. ABO compatibility can influence the results of platelet transfusion. Results of a randomized trial. Transfusion 1989;29:384–389.

118. Brand A, Sintnicolaas K, Claas FH et al. ABH antibodies causing platelet transfusion refractoriness. Transfusion 1986;26:463–466.

119. Langenscheidt F, Kiefel V, Santoso S et al. Platelet transfusion refractoriness associated with two rare platelet-specific alloantibodies (anti-Bakᵃ and anti-P1ᴬ²) and multiple HLA antibodies. Transfusion 1988;28:597–600.

120. Ikeda H, Mitani T, Ohnuma M et al. A new platelet-specific antigen, Nakᵃ, involved in the refractoriness of HLA-matched platelet transfusion. Vox Sang 1989;57:213–217.

121. Saji H, Maruya E, Fujii H et al. New platelet antigen, Siba, involved in platelet transfusion refractoriness in a Japanese man. Vox Sang 1989;56:283–287.

122. Godeau B, Fromont P, Seror T et al. Platelet alloimmunization after multiple transfusions: a prospective study of 50 individuals. Br J Haematol 1992;81:395–400.

123. Kickler T, Kennedy SD, Braine HG. Alloimmunization to platelet-specific antigens on glycoproteins IIb-IIIa and Ib/IX in multiply transfused thrombocytopenic individuals. Transfusion 1990;30:622–625.

124. McGrath K, Wolf M, Bishop J et al. Transient platelet and HLA antibody formation in multitransfused individuals with malignancy. Br J Haematol 1988;68:345–350.

125. Uhrynowska M, Zupanska B. Platelet-specific antibodies in transfused individuals. Eur J Haematol 1996;56:248–251.

126. Kurz M, Greinix H, Hocker P et al. Specificities of anti-platelet antibodies in multitransfused individuals with haemato-oncological disorders. Br J Haematol 1996;95:564–569.

127. Kiefel V, Santoso S, Weisheit M et al. Monoclonal antibody–specific immobilization of platelet antigens (MAIPA): a new tool for the identification of platelet-reactive antibodies. Blood 1987;70:1722–1726.

128. Yankee RA, Grumet FC, Rogentine GN. Platelet transfusion. The selection of compatible platelet donors for refractory individuals by lymphocyte HL-A typing. N Engl J Med 1969;281:1208–1212.

129. Yankee RA, Graff KS, Dowling R et al. Selection of unrelated compatible platelet donors by lymphocyte HL-A matching. N Engl J Med 1973;288:760–764.

130. Schiffer CA, Keller C, Dutcher JP et al. Potential HLA-matched platelet donor availability for alloimmunized individuals. Transfusion 1983;23:286–289.

131. Duquesnoy RJ, Filip DJ, Rodey GE et al. Successful transfusion of platelets "mismatched" for HLA antigens to alloimmunized thrombocytopenic individuals. Am J Hematol 1977;2:219–226.

132. Schiffer CA, O'Connell B, Lee EJ. Platelet transfusion therapy for alloimmunized individuals: selective mismatching for HLA B12, an antigen with variable expression on platelets. Blood 1989;74:1172–1176.

133. von dem Borne AE, Ouwehand WH, Kuijpers RW. Theoretic and practical aspects of platelet crossmatching [Review]. Trans Med Rev 1990;4:265–278.

134. Gelb AB, Leavitt AD. Crossmatch-compatible platelets improve corrected count increments in individuals who are refractory to randomly selected platelets. Transfusion 1997;37:624–630.

135. Freedman J, Gafni A, Garvey MB et al. A cost-effectiveness evaluation of platelet crossmatching and HLA matching in the management of alloimmunized thrombocytopenic individuals. Transfusion 1989;29:201–207.

136. Moroff G, Garratty G, Heal JM et al. Selection of platelets for refractory individuals by HLA matching and prospective crossmatching. Transfusion 1992;32:633–640.

137. Moroff G, Garratty G, Heal JM et al. Evaluation of platelet crossmatching procedures [Abstract]. Transfusion 1989;29:45S.

138. Bryant PC, Vayntrub TA, Schrandt HA et al. HLA antibody enhancement by double addition of serum: use in platelet donor selection. Transfusion 1992;32:839–844.

139. Petz LD, Garratty G, Clark BD et al. The effectiveness of an antibody specificity prediction (ASP) method for selecting platelets for transfusion to alloimmunized individuals [Abstract]. Blood 1995;86:546a.

140. Edwards RL, Ells W, Stack G. Crossmatching HLA-selected platelet donors improves transfusion results in alloimmunized individuals [Abstract]. Transfusion 1993;33:15S.

141. O'Connell BA, Lee EJ, Rothko K et al. Selection of histocompatible apheresis platelet donors by cross-matching random donor platelet concentrates. Blood 1992;79:527–531.

142. Dzik WH. Leukoreduced blood components: laboratory and clinical aspects. In: Rossi EC, Simon TL, Moss GS et al, eds. Principles of transfusion medicine. Baltimore: Williams & Wilkins, 1996; pp. 353–373.

143. Friedman DF, Lukas MB, Jawad A et al. Alloimmunization to platelets in heavily transfused individuals with sickle cell disease. Blood 1996;88:3216–3222.

144. Sintnicolaas K, van Marwijk Kooij M, Van Prooijen HC et al. Leukocyte depletion of random single-donor platelet transfusions does not prevent secondary human leukocyte antigen-alloimmunization and refractoriness: a randomized prospective study. Blood 1995;85:824–828.

145. Trap Trail Study Group. Leukocyte-reduction and UV-B irradiation of platelets to prevent alloimmunization and refractoriness to platelet transfusions. Trial to reduce alloimmunization to platelets (TRAP) trial study group. N Engl J Med In press, 1998.

146. Novotny VM, van Doorn R, Witvliet MD et al. Occurrence of allogeneic HLA and non-HLA antibodies after transfusion of prestorage filtered platelets and red blood cells: a prospective study. Blood 1995;85:1736–1741.

147. Pamphilon DH, Blundell EL. Ultraviolet-B irradiation of platelet concentrates: a strategy to reduce transfusion recipient allosensitization [Review]. Semin Hematol 1992;29:113–121.

148. Klein HG, Dodd RY, Ness PM et al. Current status of microbial contamination of blood components: summary of a conference. Transfusion 1997;37:95–101.

149. Morrow JF, Braine HG, Kickler TS et al. Septic reactions to platelet transfusions. A persistent problem. JAMA 1991;266:555–558.

150. Arnow PM, Weiss LM, Weil D et al. Escherichia coli sepsis from contaminated platelet transfusion. Arch Intern Med 1986;146:321–324.

151. Yomtovian R, Lazarus HM, Goodnough LT et al. A prospective microbiologic surveillance program to detect and prevent the transfusion of bacterially contaminated platelets. Transfusion 1993;33:902–909.

152. Heal JM, Singal S, Sardisco E et al. Bacterial proliferation in platelet concentrates. Transfusion 1986;26:388–390.

153. Anderson KC, Lew MA, Gorgone BC et al. Transfusion-related sepsis after prolonged platelet storage. Am J Med 1986;81:405–411.

154. Dodd RY. Adverse consequences of blood transfusion: quantitative risk estimates. In: Nance ST, ed. Blood supply: risks, perceptions and prospects for the future. Bethesda, MD: AABB Press, 1994; pp. 1–24.

155. Svoboda R, Lipton KS. Bacterial contamination of blood components. AABB Assoc Bull 1996;96(6):2–4.

156. Lin L, Cook DN, Wiesehahn GP et al. Photochemical inactivation of viruses and bacteria in platelet concentrates by use of a novel psoralen and long-wavelength ultraviolet light. Transfusion 1997;37:423–435.

157. Burstain JM, Brecher ME, Workman K et al. Rapid identification of bacterially contaminated platelets using reagent strips: glucose and pH analysis as markers of bacterial metabolism. Transfusion 1997;37:255–258.

158. Mangano MM, Chambers LA, Kruskall MS. Limited efficacy of leukopoor platelets for prevention of febrile transfusion reactions. Am J Clin Pathol 1991;95:733–738.

159. Goodnough LT, Riddell J 4th, Lazarus H et al. Prevalence of platelet transfusion reactions before and after implementation of leukocyte-depleted platelet concentrates by filtration. Vox Sang 1993;65:103–107.

160. Buck SA, Kickler TS, McGuire M et al. The utility of platelet washing using an automated procedure for severe platelet allergic reactions. Transfusion 1987;27:391–393.

161. Leitman SF, Holland PV. Irradiation of blood products. Indications and guidelines [Review]. Transfusion 1985;25:293–303.

162. Goldfinger D, McGinniss MH. Rh-incompatible platelet transfusion–risks and consequences of sensitizing immunosuppressed individuals. N Engl J Med 1971;284:942–944.

163. Bowden RA, Slichter SJ, Sayers M et al. A comparison of filtered leukocyte-reduced and cytomegalovirus (CMV) seronegative blood products for the prevention of transfusion-associated CMV infection after marrow transplant. Blood 1995;86:3598–3603.

# CHAPTER 52

# PLASMA AND COMPONENT THERAPY

## Carlo Brugnara and W. Hallowell Churchill

Before World War II, the only plasma component available for therapy was convalescent sera. In 1930, E. J. Cohn's laboratory developed methods to fractionate animal plasma, and shortly before the onset of World War II, bovine plasma prepared with Cohn's methodology was used in humans. The severity of allergic reactions to bovine albumin, however, resulted in a shift to use of human plasma. Initial field trials of human serum albumin were performed with U.S. casualties at Pearl Harbor. The results were so impressive the Armed Services contracted with several pharmaceutical companies to produce human serum albumin, using Cohn's methods, for volume resuscitation of military casualties (1).

From these beginnings, the plasma industry has developed into a multibillion-dollar enterprise, which in 1986 used 12 million liters for both diagnostic and therapeutic products. Unlike all other sectors of the blood industry, however, more than half the plasma came from commercial sources that used paid donors. The remainder came from plasma recovered through volunteer donors.

After World War II, the standards for these plasma fractions initiated by E. J. Cohn, required as a condition of licensure that samples from all lots be sent to Cohn's laboratory at Harvard for quality control. This approach was later adopted by the U.S. Food and Drug Administration (FDA), and it forms the current basis for regulating this industry. On at least one occasion, this tight product control and central access to all lots has permitted a rapid solution to unexpected side effects from plasma protein fraction (2).

This chapter presents current products in the therapeutic armamentarium, along with their indications, composition (to the extent that it is known), and both infectious and noninfectious adverse effects. Other chapters include more detailed discussions of the hemostatic and thrombotic disorders for which these blood products are used.

## RISKS OF PLASMA AND COMPONENT THERAPY

### INFECTIOUS RISKS

Proof that human immunodeficiency virus (HIV) is transmitted through blood led to a remarkable reduction in the risk of infection by blood products during the past decade (3, 4). Table 52.1 provides estimates of the changes in risk per donor exposure between 1981 and 1997 for three of the most important blood-borne diseases: hepatitis C virus (HCV), hepatitis B virus (HBV), and HIV.

This reduction of risk was achieved by progress in donor selection, in tests to identify potentially infectious blood products, and in postcollection sterilization of products. Each has contributed to the safety of blood products. Donor selection has reduced the prevalence of infection in the donor pool and minimized the likelihood of an infected donor presenting while still seronegative. Postdonation testing for antibodies to disease vectors has provided an additional important laboratory screen (5). Postdonation viral inactivation of products has increased safety as well, especially for those products prepared from the pooled plasma of many donors. All of these methods contribute to increased safety, but the latter is most important for plasma derivatives.

**TABLE 52.1.** Estimate of Change in Risk of Viral Infections for the Period 1981–1992 and Current Risk from Blood Products[a]

| | Chance of Infection/Unit Transfused | | | | |
|---|---|---|---|---|---|
| Virus | 1981 | 1992 | Reduction | 1996[b] Risk (and Range) of Receiving an Infectious Donation | 1997[c] Estimated Risk by Reducing Window Period |
| HCV | 7–12% (10) | 0.03% (12) | 99.6% | 9.7 (3.5–36.1)/million | 2.7/million |
| HBV | 2.6% (5) | 0.002% (5) | 99.92% | 15.8 (6.8–32)/million | 9.1/million |
| HIV | 1.1% (6) | 0.00065% (3) | 99.93% | 2.0 (0.4–5.0)/million | 1.5/million |
| HTLV | — | — | — | 1.6 (0.5–3.9)/million | — |

[a] Data are estimates of seronegative donors who may be in the infectious window period at the time of donation, before becoming positive for the screened markers.

[b] 1996 data are from Schreiber et al. (4).

[c] 1997 data are estimates based on the efficiency of some of the proposed tests in reducing the window period for the donation of infective, seronegative units.

In 1982, the risk of infection with HIV in San Francisco was estimated to be 1.1% per unit (6). Donor education and voluntary exclusion of high-risk donors reduced this to 0.2% per unit before laboratory testing for HIV was introduced in March 1985. Testing and additional donor exclusion by predonation screening further reduced this risk to that of encountering a seronegative infectious donation (i.e., window period), which has been estimated at approximately 2.0 per million units (3, 4). Addition of testing for HIV antigen (p24) was projected to detect an additional seven "window period cases," which would produce a further 27% reduction in risk. Because of the possibility of further risk reduction, despite two large studies suggesting no benefit would derive from screening for p24 HIV antigen (7, 8), HIV-antigen testing was introduced in May 1996. Whether this additional risk reduction will be achieved, however, and if so, whether it justifies the costs incurred by HIV-antigen screening, is not known. In the first year of p24 HIV antigen testing in the U.S., only one donor was found to be p24 antigen-positive and anti-HIV-1 Ab negative. Thus the cost-effectiveness of this screening test may be much poorer than predicted (8a).

One study (9) examined the relationship between replacement therapy with factor concentrates and HIV positivity between 1979 and 1985, before the introduction of anti-HIV screening. Treatment with cryoprecipitate alone was associated with a 14% incidence of HIV infection, but with the use of even a single lot of coagulation concentrates, this rose to 48%. When individuals were treated exclusively with factor VIII or IX concentrates, 88 and 60% of individuals, respectively, became HIV positive. After introduction of HIV screening in March 1985, none of 55 individuals treated with cryoprecipitate ob-

tained from 71,173 screened donors was HIV positive. Subsequently, factor VIII and IX concentrates purified by immunoaffinity, heat, solvent/detergent, or heat and solvent/detergent have been shown to be free of HIV risk.

Risk for hepatitis C has been similarly reduced through donor selection and HCV-antibody testing. The combined effects of donor selection and surrogate markers reduced the risk from greater than 7 to 12% per unit to approximately 3% per unit. Testing for antibodies to HCV, which began in May 1990, further reduced this risk, which now, with a new and improved second-generation assay for hepatitis C, is approximately 1 in 103,000 (95% CI, 28,000–288,000) (4, 10–12). The number of false positive donations can be reduced by using a combination of two different anti-HCV screening assays (13). Studies based on identification of hepatitis C viral RNA with polymerase chain reaction (14) have revealed the presence of the virus in half the pre-1989 coagulation factor concentrates tested and the absence of viral material in concentrates with post-1989 expiration dates. Studies of the natural history of posttransfusion HCV (15) reveal an average interval of two decades from the infecting transfusion to the diagnosis of liver disease. Thereafter, the disease is progressive and severe, leading to liver failure or hepatocellular carcinoma in many individuals.

Sensitive tests for hepatitis B antigen have lowered the risk of hepatitis B to 1 in 63,000 (4). Testing of blood donors for antibodies to human T-cell lymphoma virus (HTLV) I/II leave the residual risk from screened units at approximately 1 per 641,000 units (4). Approximately half of the positive results of the HTLV I/II screening test are due to infection with HTLV II.

The current residual risk of blood-borne infection after screening is enormously reduced compared with that in 1980 (Table 52.1). Further risk reduction through screened blood depends on postdonation testing and improved detection of recent behavioral risks during the donor selection process. A recent study of risk factors undisclosed at the time of donation (16) found that 1.9% of donors retrospectively disclosed risks that would have excluded them had the information been available at the time of donation, and that for 21% of these donors, the risk-behavior occurred within 3 months of the donation. Detecting these donors will require continued efforts to improve the donor qualification process.

Neither predonation selection nor postdonation testing can protect against unrecognized new infections, which may have unknown clinical consequences. For example, hepatitis G RNA is detected in approximately 1% of normal blood donors and is transmitted by transfusion, but as yet, there is no recognizable chronic disease (17, 18). Even more problematic is Creutzfeld-Jakob disease and the theoretic yet unproved transmission by blood products or derivatives (e.g., factor concentrates, albumin) of the prion thought to cause this disease (19, 19a). Since 1994, lots containing thousands of units of albumin, factor VIII, and other derivatives have been recalled because a donor was identified who subsequently died of Creutzfeld-Jakob disease. Although not founded on experimental or epidemiologic evidence, such recalls have created product shortages and ethical dilemmas because of the lack of appropriate diagnostic tests and treatment. These risks will always be associated with transfusion of blood products and plasma derivatives, and they are one of many reasons why these products must be used on the basis of carefully identified, valid clinical indications. These considerations are particularly important for products that are prepared from plasma pooled from many donors (e.g., factor concentrates, albumin, pooled gamma globulin).

Because of limitations in donor selection and postdonation testing, several sterilization methods have been developed to further decrease the risk of transfusion-transmitted disease. Current methods are based on inactivation by heat, solvent/detergent extraction, or some combination of both (20–25).

Dry heat alone has been used at temperatures between 60 and 80°C for periods varying from 30 to 144 hours. Temperatures of 60°C inactivate HIV. When the temperature is raised to 80°C, the risk of HCV transmission is eliminated, but transmission of parvovirus remains possible. Temperatures of 80 and 90°C inactivate hepatitis A viruses (25, 26). Because of these varying effects, few products use this method exclusively to achieve sterilization.

Steam or vapor heating is not associated with HCV transmission, in contrast to unheated or dry-heated fac-

tor concentrates, which have an 84% incidence of seropositivity for HCV in children (27). To our knowledge, there are no reports of HIV or HBV transmission with vapor-heated products. Inactivation of hepatitis A virus ($8.7$–$10.4$ $\log_{10}$ reduction) by vapor heating has been demonstrated for several plasma-derived products manufactured by Immuno AG (Vienna, Austria) (28).

Pasteurization involves heating for 10 hours at 60°C in a solution containing sucrose and glycine. Long-term studies have found no transmission of HBV and HCV and no seroconversion for HIV-1 and HIV-2 in individuals using Humate P (Centeon, Kind of Prussia, PA), a pasteurized product (29).

Heating of heptane suspensions also has been used to prepare factor concentrates. HBV and HIV transmission have not been reported, but there have been reports of transmission of HCV with factor VIII concentrate undergoing this method of viral inactivation (21).

Solvent/detergent extraction is effective against viruses with lipid-containing envelopes (30). Methods of solvent/detergent extraction are based on use of either tri($n$-butyl)phosphate (TNBP) and sodium cholate, TNBP and Tween 80, or TNBP and Triton X-100. Transmission of HBV, HCV, and HIV-1 has not been reported with solvent/detergent-treated products. This technique can also be used with plasma (31), but not with cryoprecipitate because of the loss of von Willebrand factor (vWF) activity and antigen (32).

Some viruses, such as hepatitis A or parvovirus B19, are resistant to solvents and detergents because of the lack of lipids in their membranes. Transmission of human parvovirus B19, hepatitis A virus, or both have been reported with solvent/detergent-treated products (33–37). Double inactivation using solvent/detergent treatment followed by heating at 100°C for 30 minutes prevents transmission of the hepatitis A virus but not of parvovirus B19 (38).

Ultrafiltration is used in the manufacturing of Mononine (monoclonally purified factor IX; Centeon®). This product is rendered virus free through an ultrafiltration technique coupled with exposure to sodium thiocyanate as eluting agent. HIV is exquisitely sensitive to thiocyanate.

Recent studies have focused on photodecontamination of blood products with short wavelength ultraviolet light (UVC, 254 nm), which inactivates both enveloped and nonenveloped viruses (39). Adding quenchers of photoreactants (e.g., the flavonoid rutin) prevents UVC-induced protein degradation (40, 41). Photochemical treatment with psoralen S-59 and ultraviolet light also is effective in fresh frozen plasma (FFP) (42).

Preparations of recombinant factor VII, VIII, and IX are now available (see Chapters 35 and 36), and other recombinant factors will reach the market before the end of this decade. These products should be virtually free of any risk for transmission of blood-borne infections. Since human serum albumin is used as a stabilizing agent, however, the risk of blood-borne infections cannot be assumed to be zero. Therefore, the advantages of recombinant products must be weighed against their substantially increased cost and the excellent safety record of currently available factor concentrates. Beginning in 1987, the Seroconversion Surveillance Project (43) has monitored the risk of HIV transmission through clotting factor concentrates. Of 9496 individuals surveyed, 46% were seropositive. Only nine individuals, however, met the Centers for Disease Control (CDC) criteria for seroconversion, and no seroconversions were observed after use of products treated to inactivate viruses and made from HIV-tested plasma.

Certain blood-borne infections, such as cytomegalovirus (CMV), HTLV I/II, and Epstein-Barr virus, are only transmitted with blood cells. Consequently, they do not pose a risk when plasma or plasma derivatives are used.

## NONINFECTIOUS RISKS

Noninfectious risks include acute hemolytic transfusion reactions, alloimmunization, allergic reactions, and passive immunization. Rarely, anaphylaxis or transfusion-induced lung disease may also occur. Allergic reactions, anaphylaxis, transfusion-induced lung disease, and active or passive alloimmunization may be induced by plasma and some plasma derivatives.

The most common side effect, urticaria (4 per 100 transfusions), usually results from allergic reactions to plasma proteins. Anaphylactic reactions are rare (1 in 20, 000 to 1 in 47, 000) and usually occur in the presence of immunoglobulin (Ig) A deficiency in the recipient (44). IgA class-specific antibodies commonly are found in individuals who suffer anaphylaxis. The gene frequency for IgA deficiency is approximately 1 in 500 to 1 in 800, so many individuals with unrecognized IgA deficiency individuals presumably are transfused without difficulty. When an IgA-deficient individual is recognized, there is no definitive test for susceptibility to anaphylaxis (45). Consequently, some have recommended using plasma free components or administering transfusions in a setting that is equipped to handle anaphylactic reactions. In individuals known to be susceptible, IgA-deficient plasma can be obtained from rare donors through the American Red Cross.

Transfusion-induced lung disease usually results from passively transferred antibodies against recipient white cells, and it is characterized by clinical and laboratory findings of normal-pressure pulmonary edema (46). Passive immunization by transfer of antibodies against red cell antigens in pooled intravenous immune globulin (IVIG) may cause serologic difficulties in the Blood Bank. Rarely, passively transferred, incompatible ABO isoagglutinins may cause hemolysis (47).

Alloimmunization against Rh antigens has occurred when Rh-positive plasma was infused into Rh-negative recipients (48). Presumably, this results from residual red cell stroma and, thus, may be important to avoid in women of childbearing years.

Other risks of large volume plasma therapy, such as citrate toxicity, hypothermia, and metabolic alkalosis, are discussed in the section on plasma exchange and massive transfusion.

# PLASMA EXCHANGE

Plasma exchange has its origins in the mystical practice of "blood-letting," which was thought to provide therapy for a long list of ills. Writing about the practice of blood-letting, one contemporary observer said, "In letting of blood, the main cautions to be considered are who, how much, and when" (49).

Since automated exchange became widely available in 1968, a vast literature has attempted to answer these same questions. For a few diseases, plasma exchange provides effective treatment, and there is confidence about the replacement fluids. For more diseases, however, evidence for the therapeutic efficacy of plasma exchange is far less certain, because it is based on incompletely controlled trials or case reports. Assessing the efficacy of plasma exchange is hampered by the tendency of physicians to overestimate its therapeutic benefits (50). In such cases, the decision to use plasma exchange is influenced heavily by the potential risks, because the benefits are less well documented. Therefore, the technology and complications are reviewed here to provide a basis for risk assessment. Indications will then be described and classified in terms of the strength of the supporting studies of therapeutic efficacy.

## PLASMA EXCHANGE METHODOLOGY

Plasma exchange methodology is best classified according to whether the separation technique is centrifugal or membrane-based. Centrifugal techniques use centripetal forces to separate cells from plasma, after which the plasma fraction is removed and the replacement colloid is mixed with red cells, white cells, and platelets before being returned to the individual. Most often, this process is continuous, with the volume being removed linked to the volume being returned, so the volume out is maintained at an acceptably small amount. The availability of large, double-lumen catheters has made possible use of continuous-flow technology and, thereby, minimized fluid shifts during plasma exchange.

Plasma exchange with membrane technology is always continuous flow. It requires higher flow rates than those for centrifugal separation, but platelet and red cell losses are greater with centrifugal techniques than with membrane-based technology. With both techniques however, the extracorporeal volume can be maintained easily between 200 and 300 mL.

## COMPLICATIONS

Complications are best classified according to the replacement fluid and the method of anticoagulation used. Because of the large amounts of plasma removed, colloid replacement with 5% albumin or FFP is essential. Replacement with 5% albumin has no risk of blood-borne disease, minimal risk of allergic reactions, and a lower incidence of adverse effects compared with FFP (51). Use of 5% albumin causes dilution of all normal plasma constituents. In treating antibody-mediated diseases by plasma exchange, dilution of host immunoglobulin may be desirable. Dilution of normal coagulation components, however, regularly produces a

transient coagulopathy, which persists for 24 to 36 hours after exchange (52, 53). The effect of diluting coagulation components can be minimized by using an every-other-day schedule for plasma exchange. This schedule also allows the extravascular and intravascular pools of immunoglobulin to reequilibrate. If coagulation defects persist, FFP may be required to correct the coagulation abnormalities. Citrate toxicity is less likely with 5% albumin than with FFP, because at least half the citrate used for anticoagulation is removed with the discarded plasma and no additional citrate is returned. Citrate toxicity includes perioral tingling, abdominal cramps and, rarely, arrhythmias. If there is significant renal impairment, the increased blood citrate level may cause severe metabolic alkalosis (54).

The Canadian Apheresis Group (55) reported all complications observed during plasma exchanges for an entire calendar year (Table 52.2). A total of 5235 procedures were performed in 627 individuals. Reactions occurred during 12% of the procedures and were serious or life-threatening in 0.53%. This distribution is representative of complications reported in other studies as well. However, some of these complications, such as respiratory arrest, convulsions, chest pain, probably result from the illness being treated rather than from the plasma exchange.

## INDICATIONS FOR PLASMA EXCHANGE

In selecting individuals for plasma exchange, one needs to consider whether there is evidence that removal of a pathogenic factor(s) or replacement of a missing factor(s) is likely to influence the evolution of the disease process. When such a correlation can be made, there usually is good supporting evidence for the therapeutic effectiveness of plasma exchange.

Table 52.3 lists diseases with the clearest evidence justifying the use of plasma exchange. These diseases are classified according to whether the evidence comes from controlled clinical trials or from case reports. Neurologic and hematologic diseases are the most common

**TABLE 52.2. Complications of 5235 Plasma Exchange Procedures in 627 Individuals**

| Complication | Moderate or Severe (%) |
|---|---|
| Fever, chills, urticaria | 3.7 |
| Muscle cramps, paresthesias | 2.5 |
| Hypertension | 2.3 |
| Nausea and vomiting, abdominal pain | 1.6 |
| Headache | 1.2 |
| Chest pain | .23 |
| Cardiac arrhythmia | .11 |
| Dyspnea, bronchospasm | .11 |
| Convulsions | .04 |
| Respiratory arrest | .04 |
| Other | .76 |

*Adapted with from Sutton DM, Nair RC, Rock G. Complications of plasma exchange. Transfusion 1989;29:124–127.*

**TABLE 52.3. Indications for Plasma Exchange**

| Indications Based on Randomized Trials | Indications Based on Consensus and Case Reports | Possible Indications |
|---|---|---|
| Guillain-Barré syndrome | Myasthenia gravis | Pemphigus vulgaris |
| Chronic inflammatory polyneuropathy | Hyperviscosity | Goodpasture syndrome |
| Peripheral neuropathy associated with MGUS | Hemolytic-uremic syndrome | Autoimmune hemolytic anemia |
| Thrombotic thrombocytopenic purpura | Persistent HELLP syndrome | Antibody to coagulation factors |
| | Posttransfusion purpura | Idiopathic thrombocytopenic purpura |
| | Lupus nephritis | Cold agglutinin disease |
| | Cryoglobulinemia | |
| | Vasculitis | |
| | Familial hypercholesterolemia | |

HELLP, *hemolysis, elevated liver enzymes, low platelet count;* MGUS, *monoclonal gammopathy of unknown significance.*

indications. For example, in one study (55), the diagnostic categories were 38% neurologic, 31% hematologic, 14% connective tissue diseases, 10% renal diseases, 1.6% skin diseases, and 5.6% miscellaneous other diagnoses.

## Neurologic Diseases

In most neurologic diseases treated by plasma exchange, the antibody contributing to the pathogenesis of that disease has been identified. In myasthenia gravis, for example, the antibody is an IgG directed at the postsynaptic nicotinic acetylcholine receptor, and removal of that antibody by plasma exchange invariably leads to rapid clinical improvement. To sustain the clinical response, however, immunosuppression usually is required subsequent to plasma exchange. Normally, plasma exchange is performed on an every-other-day basis to allow equilibration with the extravascular IgG and to avoid depletion of coagulation factors. The replacement fluid is albumin. No controlled trials have been performed, but this therapy has been accepted on the basis of numerous case studies and the findings of a National Institutes of Health (NIH) consensus report (56–58).

Acute inflammatory polyradiculoneuropathy (i.e., Guillain-Barré syndrome) involves an anti-IgM directed against peripheral nerve myelin. Clinical improvement in this disease is associated with a fall in this antibody titer (59). A randomized prospective controlled trial provided clear evidence of clinical benefit from plasma exchange in Guillain-Barré syndrome (60). Individuals with disease of recent onset, sufficient severity to require respiratory support, or both are particularly likely to show therapeutic responses and may benefit from the more rapid depletion that daily plasma exchange provides (61). Similar therapeutic effects have been demonstrated in children, and IVIG also has been shown to be as efficacious as plasma exchange in this setting (62).

In chronic inflammatory polyneuropathy, the contribution of humoral and cellular immune processes is suspected. Treatment with corticosteroids, cyclophosphamide, or azathioprine has been attempted with variable success. Controlled trials have shown that plasma exchange is effective in this setting (63, 64). Plasma exchange also may lower the requirement for other forms of immunosuppression. Individuals with sensory-motor polyneuropathy and high titers of antimyelin-associated glycoprotein antibodies improve with plasma exchange (65); however, individuals with polyneuropathy associated with monoclonal gammopathy of unknown significance (MGUS) also demonstrate clinical improvement after plasma exchange, possibly because these monoclonal proteins contribute to neuromyelin injury. Some of these monoclonal proteins have antimyelin antibody specificity. A randomized, sham-controlled trial showed a short term benefit in individuals with IgA and IgG MGUS, but not in individuals with peripheral neuropathy and anti-IgM MGUS (66). This observation further

supports the use of plasma exchange in these individuals, but these trials need to be extended to a larger individual group.

The role of plasma exchange in multiple sclerosis remains controversial. In a multicenter trial involving individuals with acute intermittent relapsing multiple sclerosis (67), median time to recover preattack status was shorter in individuals receiving plasma exchange and immunosuppression (4 weeks) than in individuals receiving immunosuppression and sham-plasma exchange (13 weeks). Several controlled, prospective trials have involved individuals with chronic progressive multiple sclerosis, and the results of two such trials (68, 69) have suggested a therapeutic benefit. Another (70) showed a small improvement, and still another (71) showed no major benefit from plasma exchange.

## Hematologic Diseases

Hematologic diseases that may require plasma exchange are those associated with hyperviscosity, antibody-mediated diseases leading to destruction of the formed elements of blood, and the thrombotic microangiopathies.

The probability of hyperviscosity in individuals with monoclonal gammopathies depends on the concentration and class of the paraprotein. The larger size and intravascular distribution of IgM makes it the immunoglobulin most likely to cause hyperviscosity. IgA aggregates more readily than IgG and, thus, is also likely to produce hyperviscosity. Among the IgG subclasses, $IgG_3$ is most likely to cause symptoms because of its greater tendency toward aggregation. Measurements of *in vitro* serum viscosity only provide a rough guide because of *in vivo* flow differences between large and small-vessels. As a general rule, however, most individuals are symptomatic when serum viscosity is more than 4 to 6 times that of water. Because of the exponential relationship between protein concentration and symptoms, plasma exchange should rapidly reverse clinical hyperviscosity and should be reserved for this purpose, because chemotherapy for the gammopathy often can accomplish the same objectives both more slowly and for more sustained periods.

Renal failure associated with multiple myeloma can be reversed by plasma exchange if it is of recent onset (72). More studies are needed, however, before this can be considered as an established indication for plasma exchange.

Despite the central role of autoantibodies and alloantibodies in the pathogenesis of autoimmune and alloimmune anemia, thrombocytopenia, and neutropenia, no well-controlled studies have documented the therapeutic effectiveness of plasma exchange in these cytopenias. Case reports have appeared, however, documenting therapeutic efficacy in hemolytic anemia, chronic thrombocytopenia, and with acquired inhibitors of co-agulation. In some diseases, such as posttransfusion purpura (see Chapter 28), that are so rare as to make controlled trials impossible, clinical experience suggests plasma exchange using albumin as a replacement fluid significantly shortens the period of thrombocytopenia.

Treatment of thrombotic microangiopathies is discussed in detail in Chapter 27, in which the rationale for removing plasma as well as returning FFP is summarized. Such treatment has clearly improved individual survival (73). In the case of thrombotic thrombocytopenia purpura (TTP), a prospective controlled trial (74) compared plasma infusion with plasma exchange. Results of this trial indicate that plasma exchange is more effective than plasma infusion. However, this study does not completely settle the question, because the groups being treated with plasma infusion received a smaller dose of plasma than those being treated with plasma exchange. In a group of individuals with TTP and impaired renal function, 83% had a successful outcome following plasma exchange (75). Solvent/detergent-treated plasma also has been employed with success in pediatric and adult individuals with of TTP (76, 77). Such therapeutic success in individuals with TTP led to trials involving the thrombotic microangiopathy associated with pregnancy. No controlled trials have been performed as yet, but individuals with severe pre-eclampsia/eclampsia and HELLP syndrome who fail to improve after delivery may respond to plasma exchange (78).

## Antibody-mediated Renal, Muscular, and Cutaneous Diseases

In individuals with pemphigus vulgaris, a prospective comparison of those receiving prednisone and those receiving prednisone plus plasma exchange did not confirm the clinical effectiveness of plasma exchange (79). Similarly, in individuals with Goodpasture's syndrome, a prospective comparison of immunosuppression with or without plasma exchange (80) did not provide evidence favoring use of plasma exchange. Response to plasma exchange and immunosuppression has been reported, however, in individuals with idiopathic and rapidly progressive glomerulonephritis (81). A study of 39 individuals with polymyositis or dermatomyositis (82) showed that leukapheresis and plasma exchange were not more effective than sham apheresis.

## Diseases Associated with Immune Complexes

In 1982, a study of lymphoplasmapheresis demonstrated only minimal clinical benefit in individuals with rheumatoid arthritis, despite significant improvement in laboratory parameters (83). Subsequently, a con-trolled trial (84) showed that removal of plasma with replacement by 5% albumin produced no clinical benefit, despite marked changes in laboratory parameters. On the basis of these findings, plasma exchange in rheumatoid disease is limited to individuals with vasculitis that does not respond to other therapies.

In individuals with systemic lupus erythematosus, one controlled trial failed to show clinical benefit from plasma exchange; however, recent case reports suggest that plasma exchange combined with synchronous cyclophosphamide therapy in individuals with lupus nephritis is clinically useful (85, 86). Whether a similar approach might be effective in lupus vasculitis is not known. In these studies, the confounding factors of concurrent immunosuppression, either with cyclophosphamide or corticosteroids, make it difficult to interpret the effect of plasma exchange. A large randomized trial comparing a standard-therapy regimen consisting of prednisone and cyclophosphamide with the same regimen plus plasmapheresis (87) showed no benefit from the addition of plasmapheresis.

Cryoglobulins may circulate as single monoclonal proteins or as immune complexes. Clinically, their importance depends on the temperature at which these proteins precipitate. Although difficult technically, removal of the cryoglobulin by plasma exchange often modifies the clinical symptomatology.

## Metabolic Diseases

Plasma exchange and low-density lipoprotein (LDL)–apheresis are considered to be very effective treatments for reduction of LDL in individuals with familial hypercholesterolemia. LDL-apheresis comprises all procedures that allow a selective removal of plasma LDL cholesterol, such as filtration, immunoabsorption, heparin precipitation, and dextran sulfate cellulose absorption (88). LDL-apheresis can deplete the total cholesterol pool by 40 to 80% and stop the progression of coronary atherosclerosis; however, plasma exchange induces a much larger reduction than LDL-apheresis in high-density lipoprotein cholesterol (89). LDL-apheresis also effectively reduces LDL cholesterol in individuals with coronary artery disease and LDL-cholesterol of >200 mg/dl despite diet and drug therapy (90).

# USE OF PLASMA DERIVATIVES IN MASSIVE TRANSFUSION

Plasma exchange is the controlled removal of large volumes of plasma. Uncontrolled plasma exchange occurs in individuals undergoing transfusions of more than one total blood volume. The coagulopathy that develops during massive blood transfusions usually involves a dilutional component as well as disseminated intravascular coagulation (DIC) with secondary fibrinolysis and thrombocytopenia. Dilution of coagulation factors is best monitored by estimating the amount of blood loss. Thus, a one volume blood loss corresponds to an approximately 60% immediate loss of the coagulation factors. Clinically significant coagulation defects during massive transfusions usually relate to dilutional thrombocytopenia more than to dilution of coagulation factors (91, 92). Moreover, the prothrombin time (PT) and activated partial thromboplastin time (aPTT) have limited value as indicators of the extent of hemodilution or of bleeding propensity (93). During massive transfusions, diffuse microvascular bleeding generally is not associated with moderate deficiencies of clotting factors but rather with severe depletion of fibrinogen (<50 mg/dl) or clotting factor levels of less than 20% of normal (94). Therefore, mild or moderately prolonged PTs and aPTTs are not useful predictors of microvascular bleeding. The most accurate predictors in massively transfused individuals are a platelet count of less than 50,000 cells/μl, fibrinogen level of less than 50 mg/dl, and PT or aPTT ratios (patient/control) of greater than 1.8 (which correspond to a decrease to below 30% of normal of the factors involved) (94).

Potential side effects of rapid replacement with FFP are difficulties with temperature control, citrate toxicity, and occasionally, hyperkalemia. Problems with temperature control are best treated using blood warmers. Citrate toxicity can be easily treated by slowing the infusion rate or by infusing calcium. Hyperkalemia usually is only a transient problem, because the serum potassium level in most individuals falls either after or during massive transfusion.

# PLASMA AND ITS DERIVATIVES

## FRESH-FROZEN PLASMA

Plasma separated from red cells by centrifugation and frozen to $-18°C$ within 6 hours of collection is defined as "fresh frozen plasma." FFP can be stored in the frozen state for as long as 1 year after collection (95). In a 450-ml unit of blood with an hematocrit of 45%, the amount of plasma present is approximately 290 to 300 mL. This amount is diluted with 65 mL of anticoagulant, usually citrate-phosphate-dextrose. Therefore, in FFP the plasma actually is diluted by 20%. FFP can be thawed by immersion in a 37°C water bath or in a microwave oven (96, 97). Thawing time varies between 20 and 30 minutes with a waterbath and 7 minutes with a microwave oven. The temperature of the FFP after thawing usually is $15.4 \pm 3.3°C$ with a waterbath and $20.4 \pm 2.5°C$ with a microwave (97). After thawing, FFP can be maintained at 1 to 6°C for as long as 24 hours.

The number of units of FFP transfused each year in the United States has increased from 1.538 million in 1980 to 1.953 million in 1982 and has remained relatively constant thereafter, with a maximum of 2.257 million transfused in 1984 (98). Use of FFP increased by 4.9% between 1987 and 1989, from 2.056 to 2.157 million units (99).

Solvent/detergent-treated frozen plasma (SD-FP), which is a virally inactivated FFP (100), is a potential alternative to FFP. SD-FP is prepared by pooling several plasma units, which may increase the risk of transmitting nonenveloped viruses. Its coagulation factor content mirrors that of FFP, and clinical studies indicate efficacy in the treatment of individuals with congenital or acquired deficiencies of coagulation factors and those with TTP (76, 77). There is only a very small additional benefit from SD-FP, however, and it does not justify the higher cost compared with FFP (101).

## Indications

Indications for use of FFP were summarized by an NIH consensus conference in 1987 (102), by the British Society of Haematology in 1992 (103), and by a task force of the College of American Pathologists in 1994 (104). The availability of various factor concentrates with a high concentration of highly purified coagulation factors, has effectively narrowed these indications. The current indications are summarized here.

### Replacement of Isolated Coagulation Factor Deficiencies (see Chapter 36)

When therapy with a specific coagulation factor is not available or FFP is safer than existing concentrates, FFP can be used to treat isolated factor deficiencies. Possible indications are deficiencies of factors II, V, VII, X, XI, and XIII. Factor concentrates, however, are available (or will be in the near future) for most of these factors. Dosages and administration schedules are designed to account for the half-life of these factors and the plasma levels needed to achieve effective hemostasis.

### *Factor II (Prothrombin) Deficiency*

The half-life of transfused factor II is 2 to 3 days, and minimum plasma levels of between 10 and 40% of normal are required for hemostasis. FFP can be infused at 10 to 20 mL per kg of body weight daily.

### *Factor V Deficiency*

The half life of transfused factor V is 12 hours, and the plasma concentration required for hemostasis is at least 10 to 15% of normal. With acute bleeding, 10 to 20 mL of FFP per kg should be administered daily to maintain factor levels of between 25 and 30% of normal. Maintenance levels can be 50% lower, and FFP infusion can be repeated every 12 hours.

## Factor VII Deficiency

The half-life of transfused factor VII is from 2 to 6 hours, and minimum plasma levels between 5 and 10% of normal are required for hemostasis. The initial doses of from 10 to 20 mL of FFP per kg can be reduced for maintenance to 5 mL/kg every 4 to 6 hours.

## Factor X Deficiency

The half-life of transfused factor X is 2 days, and minimum plasma levels of between 10 and 15% of normal are needed for hemostasis. A loading dose of 10 to 20 mL of FFP per kg can be followed by 5 mL/kg every 12 hours.

## Factor XI Deficiency

The half-life of transfused factor XI is 3 days, and the required hemostatic level is 30% of normal. A loading dose of from 10 to 20 mL of FFP per kg can be followed by 5 to 10 mL/kg daily.

## Factor XIII Deficiency

Transfused factor XII has the longest half-life (6–10 days) and the lowest minimum plasma level (1–5% of normal) needed to achieve hemostasis. Very small amounts of FFP (2–3 mL/kg) are needed to correct this defect. Prophylactic administration can be repeated every 20 to 30 days.

## Reversal of the Warfarin Effect (see Chapter 55)

Anticoagulation with warfarin is characterized by depletion of coagulation factors that depend on vitamin K for their metabolism—specifically, factors II, VII, IX, and X as well as proteins C and S. Studies in individuals treated with oral anticoagulants for deep venous thrombosis have shown that the risk of bleeding increases when the PT ratio is greater than 1.5 (105). When therapy with warfarin is interrupted, the effect of the drug on coagulation factors disappears within 2 to 3 days. Vitamin K also reverses warfarin-induced anticoagulation, and its effect will begin at 6 to 12 hours and will be maximal in 36 hours. If the PT ratio is less than 1.5, intervention with FFP or vitamin K is not indicated; if the PT ratio is higher than 1.5 and surgery cannot be postponed until the PT returns to an acceptable value, FFP can be used to reverse the warfarin-induced coagulation. The goal of treatment in such cases is to raise levels of coagulation factors to between 30 and 50% of normal. To achieve this, a substantial volume of FFP (4–6 U) might be required, thereby leading to possible problems of volume overload. In addition, FFP may not satisfactorily correct an excessive increase in the international normalized ratio (INR). Use of factor concentrates such as prothrombin complex concentrate (PCC) has been shown to induce the desired correction in INR values (106); however, use of PCC should be weighed against the increased risk of inducing thrombosis and DIC.

## Massive Blood Transfusion (>1 blood volume within several hours)

Use of FFP in massive blood transfusions (>1 blood volume) was discussed previously under "Use of Plasma Derivatives in Massive Transfusion."

## Colloid Replacement

A 20- to 30-year long debate on the advantages and disadvantages of crystalloids and colloids has not yet reached a definitive conclusion (107). Because of the risks of blood-borne diseases, colloid replacement with FFP can be justified only when both coagulation factors and volume must be replaced. For colloid replacement alone, 5% albumin is as effective as FFP and does not carry any significant risk of infection. Several studies have shown it is possible to decrease the use of FFP, thus suggesting this product is overused. Education of the medical and surgical staff, coupled with administrative intervention, has the potential of greatly reducing use of FFP (108). Use of request forms that outline transfusion criteria also has been associated with a reduction in inappropriate transfusions of FFP (109).

## Treatment of TTP

The rationale for use of FFP in treatment of TTP is described in Chapter 27 and previously under "Indications for Plasma Exchange."

## Antithrombin Deficiency

Human antithrombin concentrates are safer than FFP. This is because of viral inactivation, which occurs during preparation of the concentrate.

## Congenital or Acquired Coagulopathy with Active Bleeding or before Invasive Procedures

Congenital or acquired coagulopathies should be treated with FFP if they are accompanied by an increase in PT to greater than 1.5 times the midpoint of the normal range, an increase in aPTT to greater than 1.5 times the upper limit of normal, or less than 25% factor activity with fibrinogen levels of greater than 100 mg/dl (104).

## Dosage

In adult individuals, two bags of FFP should be used. Some individuals may require doses of from 10 to 15 mL/kg. This should be repeated if the PT and aPTT remain greater than the limits detailed in the preceding section. If platelet concentrates are used in the same individual, it should be remembered that five to six units of pooled platelets or one unit of pheresis platelets have a plasma volume equivalent to that of one unit of FFP.

## Complications

Complications associated with use of FFP are similar to those described earlier for plasma and plasma derivatives. Aside from the infectious risks, side effects of FFP include allergic reactions (from urticaria to anaphylactoid reactions), occasional alloimmunization from contaminant red cells, and infrequently, transfusion-induced lung disease (i.e., noncardiogenic pulmonary edema).

## ALBUMIN

Albumin is a polypeptide of 584 amino acids with a molecular weight of 69,000 daltons. The total content of albumin of the human body is approximately 300 g, and 60% of this is in the interstitial space (110). Albumin accounts for approximately 50% of the circulating protein and provides up to 75% of the plasma oncotic pressure. The half-life of albumin is approximately 20 days, and in a 70-kg individual, 15 g are synthesized daily by the liver. Serum albumin levels can be used to estimate nutritional status, and mortality rates for inpatients increase when this level is below 2.0 g/dl (111). In individuals who are critically ill, the serum albumin level can decrease by 1 to 1.5 g/dl in 3 to 7 days (112). At normal plasma pH, albumin has a net negative charge of 19 and accounts for almost half of the normal anion gap. When the plasma concentration decreases by 1 g/dl, the anion gap decreases by 3 mEq/l, and plasma bicarbonate increases by 3.5 mEq/l (113).

Albumin is prepared by methods designed on the basis of the plasma fractionation procedure originally developed by Cohn (1). It is available in either a 5% or a 25% solution in saline (145 ± 15 mmol of NaCl per liter). A similar product, plasma protein fractions, contains a lower percentage of albumin and a higher amount of globulins (approximately 12% of alpha and beta globulins). Product safety is achieved by heat inactivation for 10 hours at 60°C. These products have not been associated with transmission of viral diseases (114); however, there has been a worldwide recall of Albuminar® and Plasma Plex® (Centeon™) because of a possible link with episodes of septicemia caused by *Enterobacter cloacae*.

## Indications

### Replacement for Colloid Osmotic Pressure

Albumin plays an essential role in determining colloid osmotic pressure and, thus, in regulating fluid exchange at the capillary level. This role is particularly critical for proper pulmonary function; however, in normal subjects, colloid osmotic pressure can be reduced greatly without affecting pulmonary function. Studies on the benefits of intravenous albumin in critically ill individuals and its effect on pulmonary function have produced conflicting results. Provided that an adequate volume of crystalloids is given, there is little difference if albumin is used rather than isotonic saline. Because a large portion of albumin is contained in the extravascular space, intravenous infusion of albumin will rapidly redistribute the infused product into the extravascular compartment, with reduced effect on the plasma colloid osmotic pressure. Despite the lack of well-conducted and definitive studies on the effect of intravenous albumin infusion, and probably because of the freedom from infectious risks, both 5% albumin and plasma protein fraction are products of choice for volume expansion by colloid. Therefore, 5% albumin and plasma protein fraction are used to maintain hemodynamic stability in individuals with increased vascular permeability such as septic shock, anaphylaxis, and adult respiratory distress syndrome.

### Refractory Ascites

Ascites can be treated with dietary restriction of sodium intake and proper use of diuretics in most individuals with hepatic failure. In individuals with cirrhosis and refractory ascites, use of paracentesis in conjunction with albumin infusion has been studied (115, 116), and comparison of large-volume paracentesis plus intravenous albumin with LeVeen peritoneovenous shunting showed that both treatments are effective in reducing ascites and had a similar incidence of complications and similar short-term survival rates (117). In that study, however, long-term control of ascites was more effective with shunting than with paracentesis and intravenous albumin replacement. Both survival rates and causes of death were not different in the two groups. Compared with paracentesis and intravenous albumin infusion, ascites recirculation (Rhodiascit apparatus) is associated with fewer complications and shortens hospital stay (118).

### Severe Burns

Severe burns are associated with massive edema leading to hypovolemia. Large volumes of isotonic crystalloid solutions usually are administered to maintain hemodynamic stability. One alternative approach is to use hypertonic solutions, which reduce tissue edema (119). After hemodynamic stabilization has been achieved, it is important to provide a high calorie, high protein diet to compensate for the increased metabolic rate. The serum albumin level decreases in individuals with severe burns, mostly because of increased capillary permeability but also because of increased catabolism and decreased synthesis. Administration of intravenous albumin is useful for maintaining adequate colloidosmotic pressure and hemodynamic stability. Because of the increased vascular permeability, however, a large fraction of the infused albumin will be distributed to the extravascular space. Severe burns can be managed without use of albumin and blood products if the appropriate diet is used, including iron supplementation, and the amount of blood drawn for laboratory testing is reduced (120). Thus, randomized studies are needed to determine if albumin has a useful role in the treatment of severe burns or if these individuals can be managed primarily with crystalloids.

## Intravenous Infusion of Drugs and Hormones

Use of a complex between cisplatin and albumin has been studied as a way to reduce the nephrotoxicity associated with cisplatin administration. In a group of individuals with end-stage squamous cell carcinoma of the head and neck (121), intravenous infusion of cisplatin-albumin complex was associated with fewer toxic events, but the median survival time was reduced compared to that with conventional cisplatin therapy. Addition of albumin during the intravenous infusion of interleukin-2 is associated with increased efficacy (122).

## Plasma Exchange

Use of albumin in plasma exchange was discussed previously under "Plasma Exchange."

## CRYOPRECIPITATE

Cryoprecipitate is obtained by thawing FFP at 4°C, which leads to formation of a small volume (10–20 mL) of precipitated plasma proteins. The precipitate contains fibrinogen, factor VIII, vWf, factor XIII, and fibronectin. The precipitate then is frozen at −18°C or lower and has a shelf-life of 1 year (95). The yield of this procedure varies, and its physicochemical bases are not understood.

Each bag of cryoprecipitate contains at least 80 U of factor VIII (i.e., procoagulant activity), 250 mg of fibrinogen, and 20 to 30% of the factor XIII as well as 40 to 70% of the vWf originally present. Cryoprecipitate is the only FDA-approved source of fibrinogen that provides a tenfold to twentyfold higher concentration than that in FFP. After thawing, cryoprecipitate can be stored for no more than 6 hours between 1 and 6°C; however, the fibrinogen in this preparation is stable for days (123).

## Indications

### Replacement of Depleted Plasma Fibrinogen

Rapid depletion of fibrinogen to levels of less than 100 mg/dl usually occurs because of an acute prothrombotic stimulus, such as amniotic fluid embolism, placenta accreta, or abruptio placentae. Less commonly, acute depletion of fibrinogen occurs during overwhelming sepsis, massive tissue injury, and incompatible blood transfusion. A low plasma fibrinogen level also may result from DIC or primary fibrinolysis (see Chapter 44).

Cryoprecipitate is the most concentrated source of fibrinogen available for replacement. One pool of cryoprecipitate from 10 donors contains approximately the same amount of fibrinogen as four units of FFP in roughly 20 to 25% of the volume. Concomitant with replacement, however, the primary goal of therapy is still removal of the underlying cause of DIC/fibrinolysis. Standard therapy for DIC has been replacement of consumed coagulation factors, but use of antithrombin concentrates may be considered, especially in individuals with the more acute forms of DIC (124). For conditions indicating cryoprecipitate, the dose must be estimated from the increment achieved by infusion of the first pool of cryoprecipitate.

In conditions associated with chronic DIC, such as in acute promyelocytic leukemia, Kasabach-Merrit syndrome, and cancer, plasma fibrinogen is typically greater than 100 mg/dl. Use of FFP, which provides all coagulation components, may be preferable in these cases. How rapidly to replete fibrinogen is a clinical decision, made on the basis of the measured levels of fibrinogen, severity of bleeding, and ability of the individual to tolerate volume replacement.

## Congenital Afibrinogenemia or Hypofibrinogenemia

If replacement therapy is needed because of bleeding, cryoprecipitate should be used at a dose of approximately four bags per 10 kg. Dosing must be evaluated, however, by postinfusion levels of fibrinogen (125).

## Fibrin Glue

*In situ* delivery of cryoprecipitate, calcium, and bovine thrombin produces a fibrin gel that facilitates local hemostasis. This technique has been used in a variety of surgical applications, mostly in cardiothoracic and general vascular surgery. The rate of clot formation can be controlled by adjusting the amount of thrombin, and it can vary from less than 5 seconds with 500 NIH units to several minutes with 4 NIH units. The amount of fibrinogen added affects the tensile strength of the "glue." In some settings, plasmin inhibitors such as aprotinin are added to retard local fibrinolysis. The major disadvantages of this technique are potential exposure to blood-borne infectious agents and the varying amount of fibrinogen in the cryoprecipitate preparations. Fibrin sealant preparations should be used if available (discussed earlier).

## Factor XIII Deficiency

Unless purified factor XIII is available (discussed earlier), replacement therapy with cryoprecipitate or FFP is adequate in individuals with factor XIII deficiency and significant bleeding.

## Fibronectin Replacement

Cryoprecipitate is the only concentrated source of fibronectin currently available. Evidence that increasing the fibronectin level modifies wound bleeding remains controversial, however, and use of cryoprecipitate to increase low plasma levels has not been shown to modify the underlying illness (126).

## von Willebrand Disease

Because of the risk of infection from cryoprecipitate, a safer alternative is to use factor VIII concentrates, which also contain vWf (Humate®-P: Centeon, in King of Prussia, PA; Koate-HP: Bayer Pharmaceutical, in West Haven, CT; Alphanate: Alpha Therapeutics Ca, in Los Angeles, CA). If the use of these preparations is not possible, factor VIII cryoprecipitate in a dose of 15 to 30 U/kg (approximately 20 bags in a 70-kg individual) usually is effective.

Recently, efforts have been made to obtain cryoprecipitate from single donors with plasma exchange after the infusion of desmopressin (DDAVP). This process has the advantage of reducing the number of donor exposures, and the concentration of factor VIII obtained through this procedure ranges from 20 to 30 IU/ml (127), which is higher than that of cryoprecipitate. In addition, the cost of this product per unit is substantially lower than that of commercial products.

## Complications

Aside from infection, the major risk of cryoprecipitate is passive transfer of isoagglutinins of the ABO system. During preparation of cryoprecipitate, plasma immunoglobulins remain at approximately the same concentration as that in FFP. Thus, if a large volume of cryoprecipitate is required, it may be necessary to use ABO-compatible cryoprecipitate. The risk of viral infections is proportional to the donor exposure; each pool of cryoprecipitate exposes a individual to 10 donors.

## CRYOPOOR PLASMA

Cryopoor plasma is the fraction remaining after cryoprecipitate is removed from FFP. In addition to being deficient in all factors found in cryoprecipitate, cryopoor plasma also may retain the ability to degrade ultralarge vWf multimers (128). Indications for this product are still evolving. Some individuals with TTP who are unresponsive to plasma exchange with FFP may respond when cryopoor plasma is used instead of FFP as the replacement colloid (see Chapter 27). A preliminary report (129) also suggests that cryopoor plasma might be useful in individuals with protein S deficiency. This benefit might result from the low fibrinogen content of cryopoor plasma, which in turn results in a lower risk of clotting during infusion.

# COAGULATION FACTOR CONCENTRATES

## FACTOR VIII CONCENTRATE

In the last two decades, the availability of factor VIII concentrates represented a major advance in therapy for hemophilia. The price paid for this advance, however, was that all individuals treated with these concentrates were exposed to viruses causing hepatitis and acquired immunodeficiency syndrome (AIDS). In one large study (130), 90% of the individuals treated with these concentrates had evidence of infection with HCV, and 50 to 90% were seropositive for HIV. In the past decade, however, progress in product purification and sterilization has reduced the risk of hepatitis and HIV infection to virtually zero (131).

## Indications

Factor VIII therapy in individuals with hemophilia (see Chapter 35) should be initiated for bleeding or to provide coverage for surgical procedures. Therapy is based on the half-life of factor VIII (8–12 hours) and on the volume of distribution of the infused products. In general, one unit of factor VIII per kilogram increases plasma factor VIII levels by 2%, or 0.02 U/ml in adults, although more may be required in children to achieve equivalent levels. The volume of distribution is 30% higher than the plasma volume, because the factor VIII infused does not distribute exclusively to the intravascular space (132). Postinfusion levels of factor VIII must be determined to adjust both the dose and schedule of administration (133). Recommended dosages are detailed in Chapter 35.

## Factor VIII Preparations Available (see Chapter 35)

Factor VIII preparations available in the United States can be divided into three general categories: partially purified, highly purified, and recombinant preparations. This classification is based on the concentration of clotting factor per mg of non-clotting protein.

### Partially Purified (Intermediate- and High-purity) Concentrates

Intermediate and high purity concentrates contain up to 50 and 150 mg of factor VIII per mg of non-clotting proteins, respectively. Humate-P® (Centeon) contains vWf multimers in an amount similar to that of normal plasma. Therefore, it can be used in treatment of von Willebrand disease. Humate®-P is heated in solution with high concentrations of sugar, which act as a stabilizing agent during pasteurization. Koate®-HP (Bayer Pharmaceutical in New Haven, CT) is treated with solvent/detergent. These factor concentrates have not been linked to infection with HIV, HBV, or HCV. A factor VIII concentrate preparation that is virally inactivated by exposure to hot vapor under high pressure is available outside the United States (Kryobulin; Immuno AG, Vienna, Austria). In a group of 35 previously untreated individuals, no recipient developed serologic markers of infection with HBV, HCV, or HIV with this product (134).

Alphanate™ (Alpha Therapeutic Co., Los Angeles, CA) is obtained from plasma through column purification that binds the heparin binding domain of the vWf-factor VIII complex and allows recovery of both factor VIII and native vWf. After column chromatography purification, the product is virally inactivated with solvent/detergent treatment (TNBP and polysorbate 80). The specific activity of this product is greater than 1000 IU per milligram of protein. Addition of a second viral inactivation step (dry heat at 80°C for 72 hours) induces adequate inactivation of nonlipid-enveloped viruses (135).

## Highly Purified (Very High or Ultra Purity) Concentrates

These concentrates contain more than 150 mg of factor VIII protein per mg of a non-clotting protein. Several very high (ultra) purity factor VIII concentrates are currently available. Some are obtained with immunoaffinity techniques, such as Monoclate-P® (Centeon™), Hemofil-M (Baxter), and Monarc-M (American Red Cross Blood Services, Washington, D.C.). Monarc-M is manufactured by Baxter Health Care Co. (Hyland Division) using plasma collected from American Red Cross volunteer donors. Stability in these products is achieved through addition of human albumin. The monoclonal antibody used for Monoclate-P is specific for vWf; the one used for Hemofil-M is specific for factor VIII. These products undergo a subsequent viral inactivation step (Monoclate-P, pasteurized for 10 hours at 60°C; Hemofil-M and Monarc-M with TNBP and Triton X-100). These two products contain much less vWf than partially purified factor VIII concentrates or Alphanate, and they are not indicated in von Willebrand disease (136). Individuals receiving monoclonally purified factor VIII may be exposed to contaminating mouse monoclonal antibody, which is used during the purification process. To date, however, induction of antibodies to mouse immunoglobulins in treated individuals has not been reported, although natural IgG against mouse IgG can be observed in some individuals (137).

MelAte (New York Blood Center) is a highly purified factor VIII concentrate that contains a total of 10 mg of protein per 1000 U. It has a specific activity of 50 to 200 U per milligram of protein.

## Recombinant Preparations (see Chapter 35)

Several recombinant factor VIII products are currently available. They contain more than 3000 mg of factor VIII protein per mg of non-clotting protein.

1. *Kogenate® (Bayer; also marketed as Helixate™ by Centeon®):* This factor is produced in R3 cells without need for addition of vWf, then is separated through immunoaffinity chromatography. A study using this recombinant factor VIII (138) showed this product can be used safely in both short- and long-term treatment of individuals with hemophilia. *In vivo* recovery, elimination half-lives, and projected annual consumption were similar to those for plasma-derived factor VIII concentrates. In another recent study (139), 16 of 81 individuals receiving recombinant factor VIII developed inhibitor antibodies, and in nine of these 16 individuals, inhibitor levels were or became low despite continued treatment with Kogenate. The inhibitors observed after Kogenate therapy have the same epitope specificity of those observed after infusion of factor VIII concentrates (140).

2. *Recombinate™ AHF (Baxter; also marketed as Bioclate™ by Centeon®):* Recombinate AHF is produced by Chinese hamster ovary cell lines transfected with the *vWF* gene. Both factors are produced, and the presence of vWf is required for stable production of factor VIII. vWf subsequently is removed; it not part of the final product. Studies using this preparation have shown its safety and efficacy, with development of inhibitors in 23.9% of individuals (141). This incidence of inhibitors is similar to that of other factor VIII concentrates, with three-fourths of the inhibitors having peak titers of 10 Bethesda Units (BU) or less and inhibitors disappearing in more than one-fourth of individuals after retesting. A more recent study (142) reported this recombinant factor exhibits similar pharmacokinetics and half-life to Hemofil-M, with no development of inhibitors in 65 individuals treated for as long as 30 months.

Some have argued that highly purified factor VIII concentrates should be used in individuals with HIV antibodies but no clinical symptoms of AIDS. This approach is based on the belief that these products are less likely to induce downregulation of the immune system, which may play a role in the subsequent development of full-blown AIDS (143). Several studies, however, have failed to show any significant difference among the various factor VIII concentrates in immune status and disease progression (144–146). There is no relationship between severity of hemophilia and progression to AIDS, but there is a negative association between mortality rates and progression to AIDS and the use of factor VIII concentrates, thus indicating a possible protective effect from the use of these preparations (147).

Infrequently, individuals needing therapy can be treated with a partially purified or high-purity factor VIII concentrate. For those needing more frequent therapy, with low titer inhibitors, or positive for HIV infection, highly purified or recombinant factors should be used. That the half-life of infused recombinant factor VIII depends on the presence of adequate plasma vWf levels also should be considered (148). The perceived, but not yet fully demonstrated advantage of higher purity preparations must be balanced against the increased cost of these products. The final choice may differ based on the availability of financial resources in different countries (149).

## Complications

### Development of Inhibitors

Development of inhibitors to coagulation factors (see Chapter 37) has been reported in 5 to 15% of individuals with hemophilia A treated with factor VIII concentrates (150). Inhibitors have also been reported in individuals receiving monoclonal antibody purified factor VIII (151) or recombinant factor VIII (152). In some individuals with inhibitors, factor VIII-reactive T lymphocytes have been demonstrated (153).

The risk of inhibitor development depends on the underlying genetic defect. Individuals with intron-22 inversions or complete absence of factor VIII because of large deletions or point mutations have a greater incidence of inhibitors (35%) than individuals with small deletions or missense mutations (7.4% and 4.3%, respectively) (154, 155). In individuals with the intron-22 inversion, HLA genotype has a small effect on inhibitor development (156, 157).

Inhibitors develop in approximately 5% for individuals receiving factor VIII concentrates, but this figure can reach 15% for some monoclonally derived factor VIII preparations and can be as high as 25% for some recombinant products (158). The clinical significance of this apparent increase of inhibitor development with more purified factor VIII concentrates, however, has not been established. Development of inhibitors depends on age; the incidence is highest in individuals younger than 5 or 6 years, in whom it can reach 33% (159). Data on the incidence of inhibitor development have not been collected systematically. Inhibitors often have been detected only by a reduced response to therapy. Thus, the incidence of transient, low titer inhibitors may be underestimated considerably. Reactivity with specific domains of the factor VII molecule has been demonstrated for inhibitors in individuals with hemophilia A, but these patterns of reactivity are complex and not specific for the factor VIII concentrate used (160). A sudden increase in the incidence of new inhibitors (from 4.4 to 20.1 per 1000 individual-years) was associated with introduction of a new factor VIII concentrate in the Netherlands (161), and Perlinck et al (162) reported another series of product-related inhibitor development. These inhibitors had complex inhibition kinetics, and their levels declined gradually when individuals were switched to other products. Whether these product-related inhibitors result from different viral inactivation techniques is not known. Some of the antibodies react specifically with the carboxylterminal end of the A2 heavy chain domains and the A3 and C2 domains of the factor VIII molecule, thus suggesting these regions could have been altered during preparation of the specific concentrate (163). A recombinant factor VIII molecule that lacks the B domain and does not require human albumin or other plasma-derived proteins is being developed by Pharmacia AB (Uppsala, Sweden).

### Downregulation of Immune Response

Patients treated with factor VIII concentrates have both *in vitro* and *in vivo* signs of downregulated immune systems not related to HIV infection. These include decreased interleukin-2 production, downregulation of Fc receptors on monocytes, and suppression of the mixed lymphocyte culture reaction (132–134). Other signs of a downmodulated immune system are reduced circulating T4+ cells, reduced cutaneous hypersensitivity, and reduced production of gamma interferon by monocytes (132–134). It is possible that these immunologic changes might lead to activation of latent HIV-1 in CD4+ lymphocytes. However the clinical significance of these laboratory findings is not clear. A randomized, prospective study comparing the immune status of asymptomatic, HIV-infected individuals with hemophilia treated with factor VIII concentrates of intermediate-purity (Kryobulin TIM 3; Immuno AG; specific activity, 1–2 U/mg) versus high-purity (Beriate P; Behring, Marburg, Germany; specific activity, 152–161 U/mg) found no differences in CD4 counts after 2 years (164).

### Transmission of Viral Diseases

Serologic testing and viral inactivation have reduced the transmission of viral disease to almost nil. A residual risk, however, remains for hepatitis A or parvovirus B19 infection because these viruses are insensitive to the solvent/detergent and heat inactivation methods. If infected with parvovirus B19, immunosuppressed individuals are susceptible to development of severe, persistent bone marrow failure (165). Seroconversion for parvovirus B19 has been reported for individuals treated with recombinant factor VIII, probably due to the use of human albumin in this product (165a).

### Other Complications

Infusion of high doses of recombinant factor VIII may result in depletion of vWf stores and laboratory signs similar to those of classic von Willebrand disease (166). Anaphylactic reactions to recombinant factor VIII also have been reported (167).

## VON WILLEBRAND FACTOR CONCENTRATE

Several factor VIII concentrates with a high vWf content can be used in therapy for von Willebrand disease. Dosages and indications are detailed in Chapter 34.

Humate®-P (Centeon) has a vWf multimer composition similar to that of normal plasma. The ratio of ristocetin cofactor to factor VIII activity is 3.80, whereas the ratio of ristocetin cofactor to vWf:Ag is 0.90.

In Koate®-HP (Bayer), the ratio of vWf to factor VIII varies between 0.8 to 1.7. The ratio of ristocetin cofactor to factor VIII is approximately 1.2.

Alphanate™ (Alpha Therapeutic Co.) is obtained from plasma through column purification, which binds the heparin-binding domain of the vWf-factor VIII complex and allows recovery of both factor VIII and native vWf. The vWf content of Alphanate is approximately half that of Humate-P.

These products have been used in the treatment of von Willebrand disease. They are not, however, officially licensed for this purpose (168).

A highly purified vWf preparation can be obtained through a three-step chromatographic procedure (169). The starting material is cryoprecipitate, and vWf is prepared as a byproduct in the purification of factor VIII. The procedure includes a solvent/detergent viral inactivation step, with 0.3% TNBP and 1% Tween 80. The final product has a multimer composition comparable to that of the original product, a vWf concentration 10,000-fold higher than that of plasma, and is active *in vitro,* as demonstrated by the ristocetin cofactor assay and collagen-binding activity. Preliminary reports on the safety and efficacy of this concentrate show that it reduces the prolonged bleeding time in individuals with von Willebrand disease and is associated with satisfactory hemostasis (170). Preparations with a high vWf content are available, or in the process of becoming available, in Europe, including two in France (FVIII-VHP-vWF and Facteur Willebrand; CRTS, Lille, France), one in Germany (Haemate P; Centeon), and one in Great Britain (8Y; Bio-Products Laboratory, Elstree, UK).

A study involving 10 individuals with severe von Willebrand disease (171) evaluated four of these high-vWF preparations. All were effective in correcting the deficiency of plasma factor VIII coagulant activity. The bleeding time was corrected by Humate-P in all individuals, but no individual showed a correction of bleeding time when the very high-purity vWf from Bio-Transfusion, Lille, France was used. A similar study (172) showed normalization of Duke bleeding time and multimeric patterns of plasma vWf after infusion of Haemate P.

No recombinant vWf preparations are yet available for clinical use. Recombinant vWf has been successfully produced in different cell types, however, using a vaccinia virus expression vector (173). Recombinant vWf is functionally active on the basis of binding to platelets in the presence of ristocetin and binding to collagen and factor VIII.

## FACTOR IX CONCENTRATE

The recent availability of purified factor IX concentrates has modified the therapeutic strategy for treatment of hemophilia B (see Chapter 36). These new preparations have substantially higher factor IX activity than PCC. They also have a reduced risk of inducing thrombotic complications, probably because they contain minimal amounts of activated factors II, VII, and X, which are thought to be involved in the thrombotic complications of PCC (174). A recombinant factor IX preparation is also available.

### Indications and Dosages

The volume of distribution of factor IX is larger than that of factor VIII. Thus, the recommended dosage of factor IX requires infusing an amount double that of factor VIII. Therefore, 1 U/kg will increase plasma factor IX levels by 1%. The expected increase in factor IX can also be calculated as follows:

$$\% \text{ expected increase} = \text{U administered} \times 1.0/\text{kg}$$

Animal studies have shown satisfactory plasma levels of factor IX following subcutaneous injection (175).

### Preparations Available (see Chapter 36)

Two purified factor IX products are currently available. One recombinant preparation is available as well.

AlphaNine SD (Alpha Therapeutic Co.) is a preparation of human factor IX that is solvent/detergent-treated (TNBP and polysorbate 80), virus filtered (15 nm), and purified through ion exchange chromatography and dual-affinity chromatography. The relative concentration of the other vitamin K-dependent factors compared with that of factor IX is reduced to less than 5% for factors II and X and to less than 4% for factor VII. Its efficacy has been demonstrated in 13 individuals with hemophilia B undergoing major orthopaedic, dental, or general surgery (176). It is nonthrombogenic in rabbit and porcine animal models (177), and preliminary results indicate therapeutic levels of factor IX can be achieved with extravascular administration of this concentrate (178).

Mononine™ (Centeon) is obtained through monoclonal antibody affinity immunopurification followed by aminohexyl-Sepharose chromatography incubation in sodium thiocyanate and ultrafiltration. In a study comparing Mononine with a PCC preparation (Konyne) in 10 individuals with hemophilia B (179), *in vivo* recovery of factor IX was similar for both. PCC, however, yielded increased plasma levels of factors II and X and elevated levels of prothrombin activation fragment ($F_{1+2}$), which remained all in the normal range with Mononine™. These results indicate this purified factor IX preparation does not activate intravascular coagulation as does PCC. The safety and efficacy of Mononine were demonstrated in a study of 32 previously untreated individuals with hemophilia B (180), in which only one individual (3%) developed a factor IX inhibitor.

BeneFix™ (Genetics Institute®, Cambridge, MA) is produced by Chinese hamster ovary cell lines and is purified through chromatography and ultrafiltration. Its specific activity is 200 or more IU per milligram of protein. BeneFix contains no preservatives or added animal or human components. Its efficacy has been demonstrated in both canine and human hemophilia B (181, 182).

## OTHER COAGULATION FACTOR CONCENTRATES

### Factor VII and X Concentrates

Factor VII and X concentrates have been produced as a byproduct of factor IX purification from PCC. Factor VII concentrates (Immuno AG, Vienna, Austria, Bio-Transfusion, Lille, France) and recombinant factor VIIa (NovoSeven; Novo Nordisk, Denmark) have been used in individuals with hemophilia and clinically significant inhibitors (183–185a) and congenital factor VII deficiencies (183–188). No antibodies against recombinant factor VIIa could be demonstrated in individuals with hemophilia or acquired inhibitors, but one seroconversion was observed in a child with factor VII deficiency (189, 190).

### Factor XI Concentrate

Factor XI concentrates have been produced from human plasma. One available preparation is obtained through modification of the heparin-Sepharose method used for antithrombin III purification (Blood Product Laboratories, Elstree, UK) (191). This concentrate is heat inactivated for 72 hours at 80°C and it has not been associated with transmission of viral infection (191). Infused factor XI has a mean recovery of 91% and a half-life of 52 hours (191). A dose of 1 U/kg will increase the plasma level of factor XI by 2%. Infusion of this product is associated with thrombotic complications (192) and increases the plasma levels of markers for coagulation activation (193), especially in individuals with preexisting vascular disease. Solvent/detergent treatment can be used for viral inactivation of factor XI concentrates (194).

### Factor XIII Concentrate

Factor XIII concentrate (Behringwerke AG, Germany) has been successful in the treatment of congenital factor XIII deficiency and in prophylaxis for intracranial hemorrhage in premature infants (195). Pasteurization is used for viral inactivation of this product, and placenta-derived factor XIII has been used instead of FFP or cryoprecipitate in the treatment of severe factor XIII deficiencies (196). Factor XIII concentrate in doses ranging from 1900 to 3200 U/kg have also been used successful in individuals with Henoch-Schonlein purpura (197).

### Protein C Concentrate

A protein C concentrate preparation is available from Immuno AG, Vienna, Austria. It is obtained through monoclonal antibody affinity chromatography of PCC. Viral inactivation is provided by vapor heating. This product has been used successfully in individuals with severe congenital protein C deficiencies (198–200) or acquired protein C deficiencies, such as the purpura fulminans of meningococcal sepsis (201) and warfarin-induced skin necrosis (202, 203). Indices of the *in vivo* activation of coagulation, such as D-dimer, $F_{1+2}$, and thrombin–antithrombin complexes, can be used to monitor therapy with this concentrate (204).

## PROTHROMBIN COMPLEX CONCENTRATE

PCC also is called "factor IX complex concentrate," because before the availability of purified factor IX concentrates (discussed earlier), it was used successfully in individuals with hemophilia B. Originally, this preparation was obtained through a fractionation method for vitamin K-dependent coagulation factors that was developed by Didisheim et al (205) in 1959. Today, anion exchange resins are used to prepare this product commercially. PCC mainly contains coagulation factors synthesized through a vitamin K-dependent process, including prothrombin, protein C, and factors VII, IX, and X. In addition, PCC contains a significant amount of activated factors and cell-derived phospholipids.

### Indications

In the past, these products have been used to treat individuals with hemophilia B and deficiencies of other vitamin K-dependent factors (i.e., factors VII and X). Given the current availability of purified factor IX preparations, however, indications for PCC now are limited to coagulation factor inhibitors and factor VII deficiency.

#### Coagulation Factor Inhibitors

Dosages are determined on the basis of the clinical condition; they cannot be calculated by laboratory tests.

Doses range from 50 to 125 U/kg, and the response should be monitored both clinically and by following the PT and aPTT. Considering the risk of thrombosis, however, excessive shortenings of the PT and aPTT should be avoided. Given the possible complications of PCC infusions, therapy with PCC should not exceed two or three standard doses during the first 36 to 48 hours; if there is no clinical response to this treatment, other therapeutic alternatives should be sought (see Chapter 37).

## Factor VII Deficiency

Treatment of factor deficiencies should be determined on the basis of the half-life of the factor involved and the plasma factor level required to achieve hemostasis. Factor VII has the shortest half-life (4–6 hours) of all coagulation factors, and in factor VII deficiency, infusions should be repeated every 4 to 6 hours with the dosages calculated as follows:

$$0.5 \text{ U/kg} \times \% \text{ desired increase in factor level}$$

In a 70 kg individual, 875 U will be needed to increase the factor VII level from 0 to 25% of normal. Plasma levels greater than 25% of normal are satisfactory to assure hemostasis, but some manufacturers suggest administering a dose calculated to attain a level 40 to 60% of normal.

## Preparations (see Chapter 36)

Products currently on the market use methods known to inactivate HIV and HBV. Four such products are discussed here.

Konyne 80® (Bayer) is heat treated at 80°C for 72 hours. It contains approximately 1000 U of factor IX dissolved in 40 mL, which is equivalent to the amount of factor IX in one liter of plasma.

Profilnine-SD® (Alpha Therapeutic Co.) is virally inactivated with a solvent/detergent step.

Proplex T (Baxter) is heat treated at 60°C for 144 hours, and it contains 1.5 U of heparin or less per milliliter as a stabilizing agent. This product is prepared using the cold-alcohol process (i.e., Cohn method) rather than through ion exchange chromatography.

Bebulin VH (Immuno AG) undergoes viral inactivation for 10 hours at 60°C and then for 1 hour at 80°C under pressure (i.e., vapor heating). It contains factors IX (2 IU per milligram of protein), II, and X, as well as low amounts of factor VII and small amounts of heparin (<0.15 IU per 1 IU of factor IX) (134).

## Complications

## Thrombosis

Use of PCC has been associated with an increased incidence of postoperative thrombosis (206), which may be as high as 30%. Thrombosis may result from activated factor IX or the marked and prolonged increase in plasma levels of factors II and X induced by the infusion (207). Administration of PCC also is associated with increased plasma levels of the prothrombin activation fragment ($F_{1+2}$). This phenomenon might result from the exogenous administration of these fragments, but it probably indicates that the coagulation cascade has been activated *in vivo* (184). Individuals with liver disease or surgical individuals are more likely to develop thrombotic complications (208). Individuals particularly at risk are those receiving large doses of PCC (100 U/kg) or those with factor VIII inhibitors. Addition of heparin to PCC or infusion of heparin with PCC has not been shown to reduce the risk of thrombosis (208).

## Hemorrhage and Disseminated Intravascular Coagulation

Hemorrhage and DIC are infrequent complications. Their incidence is higher in individuals with liver disease or when high doses are used. Monitoring individuals through measurement of functional levels of antithrombin III, fibrinopeptide A or B, and prothrombin fragment 1 + 2 has provided evidence in some, but not all, individuals that infusion of PCC is followed by intravascular activation of the coagulation cascade. These measurements have not been useful, however, in identifying individuals likely to develop complications after infusion. Fatal cases of acute myocardial infarction with transmural hemorrhage have been reported as well (208).

## Transmission of Viral Infection

Products inactivated with dry heat (72 hours at 80°C, or 144 hours at 60°C) have not been associated with transmission of HBV, HCV, or HIV.

## ACTIVATED PROTHROMBIN COMPLEX CONCENTRATE

### Indications

Indications for the use of activated PCC are limited to individuals with hemophilia A and B who have clinically significant inhibitors, and when use of PCC alone does not produce significant clinical improvement. The bypassing effect of activated PCC is mediated by the factors Xa and VII-VIIa contained in the product.

### Treatment of Factor VIII Inhibitors with Bleeding or before Surgery

In individuals with factor VIII inhibitor levels greater than 10 B.U. or with historical levels of greater than 10 B.U., the use of activated PCC rather than purified factor VIII is indicated. In individuals with actual or historical levels of factor VIII inhibitor between 2 and 10 B.U., activated PCC can be considered, but purified factor VIII and PCC also can be used.

## Treatment of Acquired Factor X Deficiency

Autoplex® T (Nabi, Boca Raton, FL), which is heat treated at 60°C for 144 hours, has been used successfully used in treatment of acquired factor X deficiency not responsive to PCC infusion (209).

## Preparations (see Chapter 36)

Two products are currently available. These are Autoplex® T and FEIBA VH.

Autoplex® T (Nabi, Boca Raton, FL) is administered as units of Hyland factor VIII correctional activity. The suggested dosage for inhibitor therapy is 25 to 100 Hyland factor VIII correctional units/kg. This infusion can be repeated after 6 hours if no response is noted.

FEIBA VH (Immuno AG) is an anti-inhibitor coagulant complex that contains factors II, IX, and X, mainly in the nonactivated form, and factor VII, mainly in the activated form. Viral inactivation is achieved through vapor heating at high pressure. Both the efficacy and safety of this product have been studied (210). Dosages of 50 U/kg every 12 hours were used for the treatment of bleeding episodes in individuals with inhibitor titers of at least 4 B.U., and doses of 70 U/kg were used for joint and muscle hemorrhages and for mucosal membrane bleeding. The frequency of administration was every 6 hours. These doses were associated with an 88% control rate of the various bleeding episodes. A recent study showed 81.3% success rate for FEIBA in the treatment of hemarthroses in individuals with high titer inhibitors (210a).

## ANTITHROMBIN

As discussed in Chapter 40, antithrombin deficiency can be acquired or inherited in an autosomal dominant fashion. Inherited deficiencies may result from decreased production or production of an abnormal antithrombin molecule. As described in Chapter 3, the inhibitory effects of this molecule on the coagulation cascade are greatest on thrombin and factor Xa, but other activated factors such as IXa, XIa, and XIIa are inhibited as well.

## Indications and Dosages

### Hereditary Deficiency

With the antithrombin concentrates currently available, 1 IU/kg will raise the circulating antithrombin level by 1 to 2%. Initial dosages can be calculated on the basis of the difference between the desired and the actual levels of antithrombin, multiplied by the individual's weight in kilograms. Therapeutic levels of antithrombin for hereditary deficiencies are 120% of normal for the initial loading dose and between 80 and 120% or normal for maintenance therapy. The half-life of the infused preparation varies from 43 to 77 hours, which is in the range of the biologic half-life of antithrombin (3 days), although shorter half-lives may be encountered during acute consumption or thrombotic episodes.

Clinical studies have demonstrated the efficacy of antithrombin concentrate in individuals with congenital antithrombin deficiency who present with acute thromboembolism (211). The efficacy of antithrombin concentrate for prophylaxis of thrombosis in antithrombin-deficient individuals also has been established (212). The range of dosages used for this purpose was 13 to 52 IU/kg for six surgical individuals (duration, 2–13 days; antithrombin range, 95–164% of normal) and 30 to 93 IU/kg for five pregnant individuals (during labor and for 5–6 days after delivery; maximum antithrombin levels, 137–208% of normal).

## Acquired Deficiency

Only small trials have attempted to evaluate the efficacy of antithrombin concentrate in the prevention of postoperative deep vein thrombosis. Antithrombin concentrate has been used for prophylaxis of venous thromboembolism in otherwise healthy individuals undergoing total hip or knee replacement (213). Preoperative dosages of 1500 U were followed by 1000 U/day for 5 days in association with low dose heparin. The incidence of venous thrombosis was reduced compared with reported data on low dose heparin prophylaxis alone. Until larger randomized studies are published, however, data on the efficacy of antithrombin concentrates for prevention of venous thrombosis in surgical individuals should be considered as inconclusive. Antithrombin concentrates also have been used in the hepatic veno-occlusive disease following bone marrow transplantation (214).

Reduced plasma antithrombin levels have been observed in individuals with preeclampsia. This reduction can be normalized by a constant infusion of antithrombin concentrate, which should be based on initial measurements of the half-life of the infused product (8.5 ± 1.2 hours) to maintain 100% activity during the 96 hours of infusion (mean infusion rate, 66.5 ± 9 U/hour) (215). The effectiveness of antithrombin concentrate compared with that of an injectable protease inhibitor was demonstrated in a study of 39 individuals with obstetric DIC (216), and no side effects were observed in the antithrombin concentrate group. Large, randomized studies are needed, however, to determine the effectiveness of antithrombin concentrates in obstetric individuals. Low levels of antithrombin also have been reported in sick preterm infants, and a low cord-blood level of antithrombin level is a predictor of poor outcome, higher mortality rate, and increased incidence of hemorrhagic

**TABLE 52.4.**   Antithrombin III Preparations

| Name | Manufacturer | Viral Inactivation | Composition |
|------|-------------|-------------------|-------------|
| ATnativ[a] | Kabi Pharmacia AB, Sweden | 10 hours at 60°C in solution | 500 IU in 10 mL |
| Thrombate-III | Bayer Pharmaceutical | 10 hours at 60°C | 500 IU in 10 mL |
| | | | 1000 IU in 20 mL |

[a] ATnativ is distributed by Hyland Division, Baxter Healthcare.

and thrombotic complications (217). No well-designed study on this potential use of antithrombin concentrates, however, has been conducted.

Low antithrombin levels have been reported in individuals with DIC as well. Antithrombin concentrates have been used to treat DIC (218), the rationale being that intravascular activation of coagulation leads to depletion of antithrombin. Experimental models of DIC have shown that thrombin formation and intravascular coagulation can be inhibited by administration of exogenous antithrombin and heparin (219). A randomized study showed that duration of symptoms was reduced by antithrombin in individuals with shock and DIC (220). These data are too preliminary, however, to indicate whether this might become a standard treatment for DIC (221).

## Preparations

A large-scale preparation method has been developed using material from Cohn fraction IV-1 to obtain antithrombin via heparin-affinity chromatography and subsequent heat inactivation (10 hours at 60°C). This process is followed by a second heparin-affinity chromatography run (222). Two products are currently available in the United States (Table 52.4).

ATnativ® is manufactured by Kabi Pharmacia AB (Sweden) and is distributed by Hyland (Baxter Healthcare Co.) and by the New York Blood Center. It is available in vials containing 500 IU of antithrombin suspended in 10 mL. The suggested intravenous infusion rate is 1 to 2 mL/min. The procedure used to prepare this product inactivates HIV (223).

Thrombate-III (Bayer) is a human antithrombin concentrate. It is virally inactivated through pasteurization (10 hours at 60°C).

## FIBRIN SEALANT

Fibrin sealant (i.e., fibrin glue) is a local hemostatic agent that contains all the components necessary to form a fibrin plug, namely fibrinogen, human thrombin, and sometimes, human factor XIII and bovine aprotinin

(224). Table 52.5 details the composition and characteristics of fibrin sealant preparations available in Europe and the United States (225). All preparations undergo viral inactivation, and many are applied from two connected syringes, one primarily containing highly concentrated fibrinogen, factor XIII, and aprotinin and the other containing thrombin. When combined, the two solutions quickly form a tightly crosslinked fibrin, which appears as a strong, rubberlike mass. The fibrinogen concentration of these preparations is substantially higher than that of cryoprecipitate; for example, the preparation from Immuno AG contains 70 to 100 mg/ml, compared with 2.6 to 25.0 mg/ml in cryoprecipitate. Fibrin glue also can be obtained through autologous plasmapheresis (226).

Formation of antibodies directed against bovine thrombin has been reported after use of fibrin glue (227, 228). These antithrombin antibodies can be associated with bleeding, thrombosis, or with no symptoms at all. In addition, exposure to bovine thrombin triggers formation of multiple autoantibodies against coagulation proteins (229).

## OTHER PLASMA CONCENTRATES

A virally inactivated concentrate of the inhibitor of the first component of complement is available for treatment of hereditary and acquired angioedema (230, 231). A concentrate preparation of $\alpha_1$-proteinase inhibitor (Prolastin; Bayer) obtained from human plasma is available for treatment of $\alpha_1$-antitrypsin deficiency (232).

# IMMUNOGLOBULINS

Immunoglobulin preparations are obtained with the cold-ethanol fractionation method. These products are not suitable for intravenous infusion, however, because of anticomplementary activity acquired during preparation. Treatment with pepsin at a pH of 4.0 has been used to make immunoglobulin (IG) suitable for intravenous use. This treatment also has enhanced viral inactivation (233). Several different viral inactivation procedures currently are used to eliminate the risk of viral transmission (see the section on infectious complications). Detailed

**TABLE 52.5.** Characteristics of Available Fibrin Sealant (Glue) Preparations

| Source | Human Fibrinogen (mg/ml) | Human Factor XIII (U/ml) | Human Thrombopoietin (U/ml) | Bovine Aprotinin (KIU/ml) | Virus-inactivated Fibrinogen | Virus-inactivated Thrombin |
|---|---|---|---|---|---|---|
| Immuno AG (Austria) | 70–115 | 10–50 (Europe) <1 (USA) | 4 and 500 (Europe) 500 (USA) | 3000 | Two-step vapor heat at 60 and 80°C | Two-step vapor heat at 60 and 80°C |
| Centeon Pharma GmbH (Germany) | 65–115 | 40–80 | 400–600 | 900–1100 | Wet heat, 10 hours at 60°C | Wet heat, 10 hours at 60°C |
| LFB-Lille (France) | 115 | 10–30 | 500 | 3000 | SD | SD |
| SNBTS (Scotland) | 40 | 10 | 200 | None | Dry heat, 72 hours at 80°C | SD |
| Haemacure Biotech (Canada) | 50–70 | 20–40 | 150–250 | None | SD, nanofilter, dry heat, 1 hour at 100°C | SD, nanofilter, dry heat, 1 hour at 100°C |
| Baxter/American Red Cross (USA) | 100 | 24 | 300 | None | SD | SD, nanofilter |
| Melville Biologics (USA) | 50–95 | 3–5 | 200 | None[a] | SD, UVC | SD, UVC |

*Adapted with permission from Alving BM, Weinstein MJ, Finlayson JS et al. Fibrin sealant: summary of a conference on characteristics and clinical uses. Transfusion 1995;35:783–790 (Updated in Transfusion 1996;36:845–846).*

SD, *Solvent-detergent treatment*; UVC, *ultraviolet C light*.

[a] *0.1 M ε-aminocaproic acid as excipient.*

characterization of the different IVIG preparations currently available in the United States has been published (234), and although differences exist among these preparations, all can be considered as therapeutically equivalent and interchangeable. Some of the differences do become relevant, however, when individuals cannot tolerate large osmotic glucose or acid loads.

## INDICATIONS FOR INTRAVENOUS IMMUNE GLOBULIN

Indications for IVIG were summarized by a NIH consensus conference (235) and by a University Hospital Consortium Expert Panel (236). Current indications are primary and secondary antibody immunodeficiency, immune thrombocytopenic purpura (ITP), and Kawasaki disease (236, 237). Many other possible indications have emerged, but these are still controversial because of the lack of properly controlled studies. IVIG is indicated in immunodeficiency states when the serum IgG is less than 2 g/l or with proven functional antibody

defects. Both the dose and frequency of IVIG should be tailored for each individual and monitored with serum IgG measurements to obtain a minimum IgG level of 5 g/l. The half-life of infused IgG is approximately 3 weeks, which is similar to that of the endogenous IgG (238). To attain therapeutic levels, 200 to 800 mg/kg every month often are necessary. This dosage should be adjusted for each individual, however, because the half-life of IVIG varies considerably among individuals.

## Primary and Secondary Immunodeficiency

### Primary Immunodeficiency

Patients with congenital agammaglobulinemia (239), common variable immunodeficiency, Wiskott-Aldrich syndrome, ataxia telangiectasia, X-linked immunodeficiency with hyperimmunoglobulinemia M, or severe combined immunodeficiency may benefit from IVIG therapy. Children with transient hypogammaglobulinemia should be evaluated for their ability to make specific antibodies to protein and polysaccharide antigens (240), and IVIG should be used when a significant defect in antibody formation is demonstrated. It should not be given, however, only to increase an abnormally low plasma IgG level.

## Chronic Lymphocytic Leukemia

In one study (241), prophylactic use of IVIG in individuals with chronic lymphocytic leukemia appeared to reduce infectious complications (241). When decision-analysis modeling was applied to these results, however, IVIG therapy did not result in improved quality or duration of life, and it was significantly more expensive than other, more cost-effective treatments (242).

## Bone Marrow Transplantation

In a study by Sullivan et al (243), use of IVIG in bone marrow transplantation has been associated with reduced incidence of graft-versus-host disease, reduced platelet usage, and reduced incidence of interstitial pneumonitis, Gram-negative sepsis, and local bacterial infections. The dosage used in this study was 500 mg/kg weekly to day 90, and then monthly to 1 year after transplantation. In individuals older than 20 years, IVIG was associated with a decreased number of deaths from transplant-related causes. Other studies have used doses as high as 1 g/kg weekly.

Another indication for IVIG is prevention of interstitial CMV pneumonia in recipients of bone marrow transplants (244). Availability of hyperimmune IVIG specific for CMV will add a new option to the prevention and treatment of this disease in such individuals (245). Use of hyperimmune intravenous CMV immunoglobulin already has been shown to be effective in prophylaxis of CMV infection in renal transplant recipients (246).

## Acquired Immunodeficiency Syndrome

A multicenter trial involving 327 children infected with HIV (mean age, 40 months) compared IVIG every 28 days (400 mg/kg) with placebo (247). IVIG resulted in longer infection-free times and reduced incidence of both serious and minor bacterial infections, with consequent reduction in the number of hospital admissions. These benefits were evident when the CD4+ cell count was greater than $0.2 \times 10^9$ cells/l (>200 cells/ml), and they were greatly reduced in individuals with CD4+ cell counts less than $0.2 \times 10^9$ cells/l or with a history of serious bacterial infections or AIDS-defining opportunistic infections. No difference in mortality rates between the two groups was found. In another study (248), IVIG-induced reduction of serious bacterial infections could be demonstrated only in children not receiving appropriate prophylaxis with trimethoprin-sulfamethoxazole. For adults, prophylaxis with IVIG has been shown to reduce the incidence of serious infections and hospitalization (249).

## Prevention of Sepsis in Premature Infants

Premature infants have low plasma levels of IgG. IVIG has been administered to low birth weight infants to increase circulating IgG levels; however, two large, randomized studies (250, 251) found no evidence for clinical effectiveness of IVIG in this setting. In one study involving 170 infants (252), administration of IVIG (750 mg/kg every 14 days) did not affect the hospital course, incidence of local or systemic infections, or the rate of necrotizing enterocolitis. IVIG does not modify either disease severity or infection rates by adenovirus and CMV (253). A multicenter, double-blind, randomized study of 588 neonates weighing 500 to 1750 g at birth (254) demonstrated that IVIG (500 mg/kg per day) is associated with reduced risk of first nosocomial infection and with length of hospitalization for infants in whom infection develops. Prophylactic use of IVIG, however, did not reduce either the morbidity or mortality rates.

## Prevention of Infection in the Surgical Intensive Care Unit

A major cause of death in individuals admitted to surgical intensive care units is infection. A double-blind study involving 320 individuals comparing IVIG (400 mg/kg weekly) with placebo (255) demonstrated that prophylactic IVIG was associated with a reduced incidence of infection (especially pneumonia from Gram-negative bacteria) and shorter intensive care unit and hospital stays. In this same study, a hyperimmunoglobulin directed against Gram-negative core lipopolysaccharide was not effective in preventing Gram-negative infections and their systemic complications.

## Prevention of Respiratory Syncytial Virus Infections

IVIG has been shown to reduce the incidence and the hospitalization rate for infections with respiratory syncytial virus in premature infants as well as infants with bronchopulmonary dysplasia (256, 257).

## Immunomodulation in Immune/Inflammatory Disorders

### Immune Thrombocytopenic Purpura (see Chapter 30)

Treatment with IVIG is indicated in pediatric (258) and adult individuals (259) with potentially life-threatening bleeding that results from ITP. Clinical practice guidelines for ITP published by the American Society of Hematology (260) have discussed the criteria for IVIG in both pediatric and adult ITP. Various regimens for IVIG administration can be used (see Chapter 30).

Antibodies against glycoprotein (GP) antigens of the platelet membrane are found in many individuals with

ITP (261). Possible mechanisms for the beneficial effects of IVIG in this setting are Fc-receptor blockade or anti-idiotypic interactions (262). One possible effect of the anti-idiotypic antibodies contained in IVIG was demonstrated toward idiotypes of autoantibodies against GP IIb-IIIa, but not toward alloantibodies against the same molecule (263). Use of IVIG before splenectomy may be appropriate in selected individuals, but it is not justified routinely. Individuals who respond well to IVIG are more likely to respond well to splenectomy (264). An intravenous preparation of anti-Rh(D) immunoglobulins (WinRho SD; Nabi, Boca Raton, FL) has been both safe and effective in the treatment of acute ITP (265).

### Kawasaki Syndrome

Administration of IVIG during the acute phase of Kawasaki syndrome decreases the incidence of coronary artery occlusions (266). The recommended therapeutic regimen for this disease includes aspirin and IVIG. The accepted standard regimens are 400 mg/kg daily for 4 days, or 1 or 2 g/kg in a single dose. A large study of 549 children (267) compared a single infusion of 2 g/kg of bodyweight over 10 hours with daily infusion of 400 mg/kg over 4 days. The results of this study indicate that administration of one large dose is associated with a reduced incidence of both clinical (fever) and laboratory (albumin, $\alpha_1$-antitrypsin and C-reactive protein levels) signs of inflammation. The prevalence of coronary occlusions also was reduced with the single dose, and the incidence of adverse effects was similar in the two groups. No significant differences in outcome are present with use of different types of IVIG (268).

### Other Inflammatory Disorders

IVIG has been used in chronic inflammatory demyelinating polyneuropathy (269), Guillain-Barré syndrome (62, 270), motor syndromes with anti-GM1 antibodies (271), polymyositis, refractory dermatomyositis (272), myasthenia gravis, steroid-dependent asthma, and posttransfusion purpura (236). A randomized study involving 147 individuals with Guillain-Barré syndrome compared IVIG with plasma exchange (273). Therapy with IVIG was associated with a reduced number of complications and reduced need for mechanical respiratory support. Improvement in symptomatology was better and more rapid in the IVIG group as well. There also have been reports of the successful use in pure red cell aplasia (274, 275).

### Acquired Circulating Coagulation Inhibitors

A response rate of between 25.0 and 37.5% has been reported for use of IVIG in 16 individuals with acquired factor VIII inhibitors (276).

## COMPLICATIONS

### Minor Side Effects

Minor side effects of IVIG include headache, back pain, chills, and fever in 2.5 to 15.0% of individuals. These symptoms often can be controlled by reducing the rate of infusion. There have been reports of severe respiratory difficulties and also of renal toxicity (277, 278), and increased viscosity has been reported following infusion (279).

### Aseptic Meningitis

Aseptic meningitis has been reported in 11% of individuals with autoimmune diseases receiving IVIG (280, 281). Aseptic meningitis is especially prevalent in individuals with a history of migraine.

### Anaphylactic Reactions

Anaphylactic reactions are very rare, but they occur more frequently in individuals with IgA deficiency. Screening individuals for IgA deficiency before use IVIG is advisable, especially in the setting of autoimmune diseases, in which production of anti-IgA autoantibodies can be induced. If IgA deficiency is confirmed, this may be an indication for IgA-depleted IVIG; the IVIG used in these circumstances should have an IgA concentration of less than 1.5 µg/ml.

### Neutropenia

Cases of transient neutropenia have been described with the use of IVIG (282). IVIG is obtained by pooling the plasma of many donors; the FDA Center for Biologics Evaluation and Research requires a minimum of 1000 donors in the pools used for manufacturing human immunoglobulin. This number usually is larger (typically 16,000 for Sandoglobulin, Novartis Pharmaceutical Co., East Hanover, NJ), and it therefore is possible that leukocyte antibodies might be present in the final preparation and lead to immune neutropenia.

### Immune Hemolysis

Immune hemolysis after IVIG administration has occurred. In one report (283), anti-A and anti-B antibodies of the IgG type were found in 12 of 20 IVIG lots tested. Most preparations induced hemagglutination at dilution titers of between 1:256 and 1:32. The individual with chronic ITP described in this report had a positive direct antiglobulin test, and anti-A was eluted from the individual's A cells, the serum showing the presence of anti-A. This was associated with the development of anemia.

### Positive Serologies

Use of IVIG may induce transiently positive serologic tests, which then revert to normal when the infused IgG is eliminated (284). This is a particular problem in transplant settings, in which passive transfer of antibodies against HCV and CMV leads to positive serologic tests aimed at detecting seroconversion and infection in seronegative individuals (285).

## Transmission of Viral Infections

Transmission of HCV has been demonstrated for IVIG manufactured with different methods by the Scottish National Blood Transfusion Service and for a Swedish column-fractionated preparation (286). In 1994, several cases of HCV infection were reported after the administration of IVIG (Gammagard and Polygam) manufactured by Baxter (287). Several different strains of HCV appear to have contaminated the Gammagard preparations (288–292), and these products as well as those from other manufacturers have been modified subsequently to include a solvent/detergent viral inactivation step.

# REFERENCES

1. Cohn EJ, Gurd FR, Surgenor DM et al. A system for the separation of the components of human blood. Qualitative procedures for the separation of the protein components of human plasma. J Am Chem Soc 1950;72:465–474.
2. Alving BM, Hojima Y, Pisano JJ et al. Hypotension associated with prekallikrein activator (Hageman-factor fragments) in plasma protein fraction. N Engl J Med 1978;299:66–70.
3. Lackritz EM, Satten GA, Aberle-Grasse J et al. Estimated risk of transmission of the human immunodeficiency virus by screened blood in the United States. N Engl J Med 1995;333:1721–1725.
4. Schreiber GB, Busch MP, Kleiman SH et al. The risk of transfusion-transmitted viral infections. N Engl J Med 1996;334:1685–1690.
5. Anonymous. Public Health Service inter-agency guidelines for screening donors of blood, plasma, organs, tissues, and semen for evidence of hepatitis B and hepatitis C. MMWR 1991;40(RR-4):1–17.
6. Busch MP, Young MJ, Samson SM et al. Risk of human immunodeficiency virus (HIV) transmission by blood transfusions before the implementation of HIV-l antibody screening. Transfusion 1991;31:4–11.
7. Alter HJ, Epstein JS, Swenson SG et al. Prevalence of human immunodeficiency virus type 1 p24 antigen in U.S. blood donors: an assessment of the efficacy of testing in donor screening. The HIV Antigen Study Group. N Engl J Med 1990;323:1312–1317.
8. Busch MP, Taylor PE, Lenes BA et al. Screening of selected male blood donors for p24 antigen of human immunodeficiency virus type 1. The Transfusion Safety Study Group. N Engl J Med 1990;323:1308–1312.
8a. Bush MP, Dodd AY, Lackritz EM et al. Value and cost-effectiveness of screening blood donors for antibody to hepatitis B core antigen as a way of detecting window-phase human immunodeficiency virus type 1 infections. Transfusion 1997;37:1003–1011.
9. Gjerset GF, Clements MJ, Counts RB et al. Treatment type and amount influenced human immunodeficiency virus seroprevalence of individuals with congenital bleeding disorders. Blood 1991;78:1623–1627.
10. Dienstag JL. Non-A, non-B hepatitis. I. Recognition, epidemiology, and clinical features. Gastroenterology 1983;85:439–462.
11. Alter HJ, Purcell RH, Shih JW et al. Detection of antibody to hepatitis C virus in prospectively followed transfusion recipients with acute and chronic non-A, non-B hepatitis. N Engl J Med 1989;321:1494–1500.
12. Donahue JG, Munoz A, Ness PM et al. The declining risk of post-transfusion hepatitis C virus infection. N Engl J Med 1992;327:369–373.
13. Allain JP, Kitchen A, Aloysius S et al. Safety and efficacy of hepatitis C virus antibody screening of blood donors with two sequential screening assays. Transfusion 1996;36:401–405.
14. Makris M, Garson JA, Ring CJ et al. Hepatitis C viral RNA in clotting factor concentrates and the development of hepatitis in recipients. Blood 1993;81:1898–1902.
15. Tong MJ, el-Farra NS, Reikes AR et al. Clinical outcomes after transfusion-associated hepatitis C. N Engl J Med 1995;332:1463–1466.
16. Williams AE, Thomson RA, Schreiber GB et al. Estimates of infectious disease risk factors in US blood donors. Retrovirus Epidemiology Donor Study. JAMA 1997;277:967–972.
17. Alter HJ, Nakatsuji Y, Melpolder J et al. The incidence of transfusion-associated hepatitis G virus infection and its relation to liver disease. N Engl J Med 1997;336:747–754.
18. Alter MJ, Gallagher M, Morris TT et al. Acute non-A-E hepatitis in the United States and the role of hepatitis G virus infection. Sentinel Counties Viral Hepatitis Study Team. N Engl J Med 1997; 336:741–746.
19. Collinge J, Sidle KC, Meads J et al. Molecular analysis of prion strain variation and the aetiology of "new variant" CJD. Nature 1996;383:685–690.
19a. Bush MP, Glynn SA, Schreiber GB. Potential increased risk of virus transmission due to exclusion of older donors because of concern over Creutzfeldt-Jacob disease. Transfusion 1997;37:996–1002.
20. Aronson DL. The development of the technology and capacity for the production of factor VIII for treatment of hemophilia A. Transfusion 1990;30:748–758.
21. Epstein JS, Fricke WA. Current safety of clotting factor concentrates. Arch Pathol Lab Med 1990;114:335–340.
22. Fricke WA, Lamb MA. Viral safety of clotting factor concentrates. Semin Thromb Hemost 1993;19:54–61.
23. Kasper CK, Lusher JM. Recent evolution of clotting factor concentrates for hemophilia A and B. Transfusion Practices Committee. Transfusion 1993;33:422–434.
24. Suomela H. Inactivation of viruses in blood and plasma products. Transfus Med Rev 1993;7:42–57.
25. Hart HF, Hart WG, Crossley J et al. Effect of terminal (dry) heat treatment on non-enveloped viruses in coagulation factor concentrates. Vox Sang 1994;67:345–350.
26. Lemon SM, Murphy PC, Smith A et al. Removal/neutralization of hepatitis A virus during manufacture of high purity, solvent/detergent factor VIII concentrate. J Med Virol 1994;43:44–49.
27. Blanchette VS, Vorstman E, Shore A et al. Hepatitis C infection in children with hemophilia A and B. Blood 1991;78:285–289.
28. Barrett PN, Meyer H, Wachtel I et al. Inactivation of hepatitis A virus in plasma products by vapor heating. Transfusion 1997;37:215–220.
29. Schimpf K, Brackmann HH, Kreuz W et al. Absence of anti-human immunodeficiency virus types 1 and 2 seroconversion after the treatment of hemophilia A or von Willebrand's disease with pasteurized factor VIII concentrate. N Engl J Med 1989;321:1148–1152.
30. Piet MP, Chin S, Prince AM et al. The use of tri(n-butyl)phosphate detergent mixtures to inactivate hepatitis viruses and human immunodeficiency virus in plasma and plasma's subsequent fractionation. Transfusion 1990;30:591–598.
31. Williamson LM, Allain JP. Virally inactivated fresh frozen plasma. Vox Sang 1995;69:159–165.
32. Keeling DM, Luddington R, Allain JP et al. Cryoprecipitate prepared from plasma virally inactivated by the solvent detergent method. Br J Haematol 1997;96:194–197.
33. Azzi A, Ciappi S, Zakvrzewska K et al. Human parvovirus B19 infection in hemophiliacs first infused with two high-purity, virally attenuated factor VIII concentrates. Am J Hematol 1992;39:228–230.
34. Mariani G, Di Paolantonio T, Baklaya R et al. Prospective study of the evaluation of hepatitis C virus infectivity in a high purity, solvent/detergent-treated factor VIII concentrate: parallel evaluation of the other markers for lipid-enveloped and non-lipid-enveloped viruses. Transfusion 1993;33:814–818.
35. Mannucci PM. Outbreak of hepatitis A among Italian patients with haemophilia [Letter]. Lancet 1992;339:819.
36. Peerlinck K, Vermylen J. Acute hepatitis A in patients with hemophilia A [Letter]. Lancet 1993;341:179.
37. Anonymous. Hepatitis A among persons with hemophilia who received clotting factor concentrate—United States, September—December 1995. MMWR 1996;45:29–32.
38. Santagostino E, Mannucci PM, Gringeri A et al. Transmission of parvovirus B10 by coagulation factor concentrates exposed to 100°C heat after lyophilization. Transfusion 1997;37:517–522.
39. Ben-Hur E, Moor AC, Margolis-Nunno H et al. The photodecontamination of cellular blood components: mechanisms and use of photosensitization in transfusion medicine. Transfus Med Rev 1996;10:15–22.
40. Marx G, Mou X, Freed R et al. Protecting fibrinogen with rutin during UVC irradiation for viral inactivation. Photochem Photobiol 1996;63:541–546.
41. Chin S, Williams B, Gottlieb P et al. Virucidal short wavelength ultraviolet light treatment of plasma and factor VIII concentrate: protection of proteins by antioxidants. Blood 1995;86:4331–4336.
42. Alfonso R, Lin C, Dupuis K et al. Inactivation of viruses with preservation of coagulation function in fresh frozen plasma. [Abstract]. Blood 1996;88:526A.
43. Fricke W, Augustyniak L, Lawrence D et al. Human immunodeficiency virus infection due to clotting factor concentrates: results of the Seroconversion Surveillance Project. Transfusion 1992;32:707–709.
44. Pineda AA, Taswell HF. Transfusion reactions associated with anti-IgA antibodies: report of four cases and review of the literature. Transfusion 1975;15:10–15.

45. Sandler SG, Mallory D, Malamut D et al. IgA anaphylactic transfusion reactions. Transfus Med Rev 1995;9:1–8.

46. Popovsky MA, Chaplin HC Jr, Moore SB. Transfusion-related acute lung injury: a neglected, serious complication of hemotherapy. Transfusion 1992;32:589–592.

47. Pierce RN, Reich LM, Mayer K. Hemolysis following platelet transfusion from ABO-incompatible donors. Transfusion 1985;25:60–62.

48. McBride JA, O'Hoski P, Blajchman MA et al. Rhesus alloimmunization following intensive plasmapheresis. Transfusion 1978;18:626A–627A.

49. Burton R. The anatomy of melancholy. New York: Oxford University Press 1989.

50. Noseworthy JH, Ebers GC, Vandervoort MK et al. The impact of blinding on the results of a randomized, placebo-controlled multiple sclerosis trial. Neurology 1994;44:16–20.

51. Bouget J, Chevret S, Chastang C et al. Plasma exchange morbidity in Guillan-Barre syndrome: results from the French prospective, randomized, multicenter study. The French Cooperative Group. Crit Care Med 1993; 21:651–658.

52. Wood L, Jacobs P. The effect of serial therapeutic plasmapheresis on platelet count, coagulation factors, plasma immunoglobulin and complement levels. J Clin Apheresis 1986;3:124–128.

53. Domen RE, Kennedy MS, Jones LL et al. Hemostatic imbalances produced by plasma exchange. Transfusion 1984;24:336–339.

54. Pearl RG, Rosenthal MH. Metabolic alkalosis due to plasmapheresis. Am J Med 1985;79:391–393.

55. Sutton DM, Nair RC, Rock G. Complications of plasma exchange. Transfusion 1989;29:124–127.

56. Nielsen VK, Paulson OB, Rosenkvist J et al. Rapid improvement of myasthenia gravis after plasma exchange. Ann Neurol 1982;11:160–169.

57. Kornfeld P, Ambinder EP, Papatestas AE et al. Plasmapheresis in myasthenia gravis: controlled study [Letter]. Lancet 1979;ii:629.

58. Anonymous. The utility of therapeutic plasmapheresis for neurologic disorders. NIH Consensus Development Conference Consensus Statement. JAMA 1986;256:1333–1337.

59. Koski CL, Gratz E, Sutherland J et al. Clinical correlation with anti-peripheral-nerve myelin antibodies in Guillain-Barre syndrome. Ann Neurol 1986;19:573–577.

60. Anonymous. Plasmapheresis and acute Guillain-Barre syndrome. Guillain-Barre Syndrome Study Group. Neurology 1985;35:1096–1104.

61. McKhann GM, Griffin JW, Cornblath DR et al. Plasmapheresis and Guillain-Barre syndrome: analysis of prognostic factors and the effect of plasmapheresis. Ann Neurol 1988;23:347–353.

62. Bril V, Ilse WK, Pearce R et al. Pilot trial of immunoglobulin versus plasma exchange in individuals with Guillain-Barré syndrome. Neurology 1996; 46:100–103.

63. Dyck PJ, Daube J, O'Brien P et al. Plasma exchange in chronic inflammatory demyelinating polyradiculoneuropathy. N Engl J Med 1986;314: 461–465.

64. Hahn AF, Bolton CF, Pillay N et al. Plasma exchange therapy in chronic inflammatory demyelinating polyneuropathy. A double-blind, sham-controlled, cross-over study. Brain 1996;119:1055–1066.

65. Blume G, Pestronk A, Goodnough LT. Anti-MAG antibody-associated polyneuropathies: improvement following immuntherapy with monthly plasma exchange and IV cyclophosphamide. Neurology 1995;45: 1577–1580.

66. Dyck PJ, Low PA, Windebank AJ et al. Plasma exchange in polyneuropathy associated with monoclonal gammopathy of undetermined significance. N Eng J Med 1991;325:1482–1486.

67. Weiner HL, Dau PC, Khatri BO et al. Double-blind study of true vs sham plasma exchange in individuals being treated with immunosuppression for acute attacks of multiple sclerosis. Neurology 1989;39:1143–1149.

68. Khatri BO, McQuillen MP, Harrington GJ et al. Chronic progressive multiple sclerosis: double-blind controlled study of plasmapheresis in individuals taking immunosuppressive drugs. Neurology 1985;35:312–319.

69. Gordon PA, Carroll DJ, Etches WS et al. A double-blind controlled pilot study of plasma exchange versus sham apheresis in chronic progressive multiple sclerosis. Can J Neurol Sci 1985;12:39–44.

70. Sorensen PS, Wanscher B, Szpirt W et al. Plasma exchange combined with azathioprine in multiple sclerosis using serial gadolinium-enhanced MRI to monitor disease activity: a randomized single-masked cross-over pilot study. Neurology 1996;46:1620–1625.

71. Anonymous. The Canadian cooperative trial of cyclophosphamide and plasma exchange in progressive multiple sclerosis. The Canadian Cooperative Multiple Sclerosis Study Group. Lancet 1991;337:441–446.

72. Zucchelli P, Pasquali S, Cagnoli L et al. Controlled plasma exchange trial in acute renal failure due to multiple myeloma. Kidney Int 1988;33: 1175–1180.

73. Bell WR, Braine HG, Ness PM et al. Improved survival in thrombotic thrombocytopenic purpura-hemolytic uremic syndrome. Clinical experience in 108 patients. N Engl J Med 1991;325:398–403.

74. Rock GA, Shumak KH, Buskard NA et al. Comparison of plasma exchange with plasma infusion in the treatment of thrombotic thrombocytopenic purpura. N Engl J Med 1991;325:393–397.

75. Rock G, Shumak K, Kelton J et al. Thrombotic thrombocytopenic purpura: outcome in 24 patients with renal impairment treated with plasma exchange. The Canadian Apheresis Study Group. Transfusion 1992;32: 710–714.

76. Moake J, Chintagumpala M, Turner N et al. Solvent/detergent treated plasma suppresses shear-induced platelet aggregation and prevents episodes of thrombotic thrombocytopenic purpura. Blood 1994;84:490–497.

77. Harrison CN, Lawrie AS, Iqbal A et al. Plasma exchange with solvent/detergent-treated plasma of resistant thrombotic thrombocytopenic purpura. Br J Haematol 1996;94:756–758.

78. Martin JN Jr, Files JC, Blake PG et al. Postpartum plasma exchange for atypical preeclampsia-eclampsia as HELLP syndrome. Am J Obstet Gynecol 1995;172:1107–1125.

79. Guillaume JC, Roujeau JC, Morel P et al. Controlled study of plasma exchange in pemphigus. Arch Dermatol 1988;124:1659–1663.

80. Johnson JP, Moore J Jr , Austin HA III et al. Therapy of anti-glomerular basement membranes antibody disease: analysis of prognostic significance of clinical, pathologic and treatment factors. Medicine 1985;64:219–227.

81. Gianviti A, Trompeter RS, Barratt TM et al. Retrospective study of plasma exchange in patients with idiopathic rapidly progressive glomerulonephritis and vasculitis. Arch Dis Child 1996;75:186–190.

82. Miller FW, Leitman SF, Cronin ME et al. Controlled trial of plasma exchange and leukapheresis in polymyositis and dermatomyositis. N Engl J Med 1992;326:1380–1384.

83. Wallace D, Goldfinger D, Lowe C et al. A double-blind, controlled study of lymphoplasmapheresis versus sham apheresis in rheumatoid arthritis. N Engl J Med 1982;306:1406–1410.

84. Dwosh IL, Giles AR, Ford PM et al. Plasmapheresis therapy in rheumatoid arthritis: a controlled, double-blind, crossover trial. N Engl J Med 1983; 308:1124–1129.

85. Schroeder JO, Euler HH, Loffler H. Synchronization of plasmapheresis and pulse cyclophosphamide in severe systemic lupus erythematosus. Ann Intern Med 1987;107:344–346.

86. Dau PC, Callahan J, Parker R et al. Immunologic effects of plasmapheresis synchronized with pulse cyclophosphamide in systemic lupus erythematosus. J Rheumatol 1991;18:270–276.

87. Lewis EJ, Hunsicker LG, Lan SP et al. A controlled trial of plasmapheresis therapy in severe lupus nephritis. N Engl J Med 1992;326:1373–1379.

88. Keller C. LDL-apheresis: results of long-term treatment and vascular outcome [Review]. Atherosclerosis 1991;86:1–8.

89. Berger GM, Firth JC, Jacobs P et al. Three different schedules of low-density lipoprotein apheresis compared with plasmapheresis in patients with homozygous familial hypercholesterolemia. Am J Med 1990;88: 94–100.

90. Seidel D, Armstrong VW, Schuff-Werner P. The HELP-LDL apheresis multicentre study, an angiographically assessed trial on the role of LDL-apheresis in the secondary prevention of coronary heart disease. I. Evaluation of safety and cholesterol-lowering effects during the first 12 months. HELP Study Group. Eur J Clin Invest 1991;21:375–383.

91. Miller RD, Robbins TO, Tong MJ et al. Coagulation defects associated with massive blood transfusions. Ann Surg 1971;174:794–801.

92. Counts RB, Haisch C, Simon TL et al. Hemostasis in massively transfused trauma patients. Ann Surg 1979;190:91–99.

93. Braunstein AH, Oberman HA. Transfusion of plasma components. Transfusion 1984;24:281–286.

94. Ciavarella D, Reed RL, Counts RB et al. Clotting factor levels and the risk of diffuse microvascular bleeding in the massively transfused patient. Br J Haematol 1987;67:365–368.

95. Klein HG. Standards for blood banks and transfusion services. 17th ed. Bethesda: American Association of Blood Banks, 1996.

96. Rock G, Tackaberry ES, Dunn JG et al. Rapid controlled thawing of fresh frozen plasma in a modified microwave oven. Transfusion 1984;24:60–65.

97. Churchill WH, Schmidt B, Lindsey J et al. Thawing fresh frozen plasma in a microwave oven. A comparison with thawing in a 37°C waterbath. Am J Clin Pathol 1992;97:227–232.

98. Surgenor DM, Wallace EL, Hao SH et al. Collection and transfusion of blood in the United States, 1982–1988. N Engl J Med 1990;322:1646–1651.

99. Wallace EL, Surgenor DM, Hao SH et al. Collection and transfusion of blood and blood components in the United States, 1989. Transfusion 1993; 33:139–144.

100. Horowitz B, Bonomo R, Prince AM et al. Solvent/detergent-treated plasma: a virus inactivated substitute for fresh frozen plasma. Blood 1992; 79:826–831.

101. Aubuchon JP, Birkmeyer JD. Safety and cost-effectiveness of solvent-detergent-treated plasma. In search of a zero-risk blood supply. JAMA 1994; 272:1210–1214.

102. Anonymous. Fresh frozen plasma: indications and risks. National Institutes of Health Consensus Conference. Transfus Med Rev 1987;1:201–204.

103. Contreras M, Ala FA, Greaves M et al. Guidelines for the use of fresh frozen plasma. British Committee for Standards in Haematology, Working Party of the Blood Transfusion Task Force. Transfus Med 1992;2:57–63.

104. Anonymous. Practice parameter for the use of fresh frozen plasma, cryoprecipitate, and platelets. Administration Practice Guidelines Develop-

ment Task Force of the College of American Pathologists. JAMA 1994;271: 777–781.

105. Hull R, Hirsh J, Jay R et al. Different intensities of oral anticoagulant therapy in the treatment of proximal-vein thrombosis. N Engl J Med 1982; 307:1676–1681.

106. Makris M, Greaves M, Phillips WS et al. Emergency oral anticoagulant reversal: the relative efficacy of infusion of fresh frozen plasma and clotting factor concentrate on correction of the coagulopathy. Thromb Haemost 1997;77:477–480.

107. Snyder AJ, Gottschall JL, Menitove JE. Why is fresh frozen plasma transfused? Transfusion 1986;26:107–112.

108. Solomon RR, Clifford JS, Gutman SI. The use of laboratory intervention to stem the flow of fresh frozen plasma. Am J Clin Pathol 1988;89:518–521.

109. Marshall BA, de Jongh TA, Moto TA. Improved use of fresh frozen plasma with a review of a pretransfusion worksheet [Abstract]. Transfusion 1991; 31:34S.

110. Doweiko JP, Nompleggi DJ. Role of albumin in human physiology and pathophysiology. JPEN J Parenter Enteral Nutr 1991;15:207–211.

111. Reinhardt GF, Myscofski JW, WIlkens DB et al. Incidence and mortality of hypoalbuminemic individuals in hospitalized veterans. JPEN J Parenter Enteral Nutr 1980;4:357–359.

112. Guthrie RD Jr, Hines C Jr. Use of intravenous albumin in the critically ill patient. Am J Gastroenterol 1991;86:255–263.

113. McAuliffe JJ, Lind LJ, Leith DE et al. Hypoproteineimic alkalosis. Am J Med 1986;81:86–90.

114. Lefrere JJ, Mariotti M, De la Croix I et al. Albumin batches and B19 parvovirus DNA. Transfusion 1995;35:389–391.

115. Smart HL, Triger DR. A randomised prospective trial comparing daily paracentesis and intravenous albumin with recirculation in diuretic refractory ascites. J Hepatol 1990;10:191–197.

116. Tito L, Gines P, Arroyo V et al. Total paracentesis associated with intravenous albumin management of individuals with cirrhosis and ascites. Gastroenterology 1990;98:146–151.

117. Gines P, Arroyo V, Vargas V et al. Paracentesis with intravenous infusion of albumin as compared with peritoneovenous shunting in cirrhosis with refractory ascites. N Engl J Med 1991;325:829–835.

118. Smart HL, Tiger DR. A randomised prospective trial comparing daily paracentesis and intravenous albumin with recirculation in diuretic refractory ascites. J Hepatol 1990;10:191–197.

119. Monafo WW. Initial management of burns. N Engl J Med 1996;335: 1581–1586.

120. Schlagintweit S, Snelling CF, Germann E et al. Major burns managed without blood or blood products. J Burn Care Rehabil 1990;11:214–220.

121. Holding JD, Lindup WE, Van Laer C et al. Phase I trial of a cisplatin-albumin complex for the treatment of cancer of the head and neck. Br J Clin Pharmacol 1992;33:75–81.

122. Cassidy J, Poole C, Sharkie E et al. The importance of added albumin during continuous intravenous infusion of interleukin-2 with alpha-interferon. Eur J Cancer 1991;27:1633–1634.

123. Howard PL, Bovill EG, Golden E. Post thaw stability of fibrinogen in cryoprecipitate stored between 1 and 6°C. Transfusion 1991;31:30–31.

124. Buller HR, ten Cate JW. Acquired antithrombin III deficiency: laboratory diagnosis, incidence, clinical implications, and treatment with antithrombin III concentrate. Am J Med 1989;87(SB):44S–48S.

125. Lusher JM. Diseases of coagulation: the fluid phase. In: Nathan D, Oski F, eds. Hematology of infancy and childhood. 3rd ed. Philadelphia: WB Saunders, 1987:1293–1342.

126. Powell FS, Doran JE. Current status of fibronectin in transfusion medicine: focus on clinical studies. Vox Sang 1991;60:193–202.

127. McLeod BC, Scott JP. Plasma exchange donation of cryoprecipitate after DDAVP stimulation: an alternative source of factor VIII. Prog Clin Biol Res 1990;324:189–198.

128. Byrnes JJ, Moake JL, Klug P et al. Effectiveness of the cryosupernatant fraction of plasma in the treatment of refractory thrombotic thrombobctopenic purpura. Am J Hematol 1990;34:169–174.

129. de Jongh RL. The regulation of hemostasis in a pediatric patient with inherited protein S deficiency using cryo-poor plasma [Abstract]. Transfusion 1991;31:S35.

130. Roberts HR. The treatment of hemophilia: past tragedy and future promise. N Engl J Med 1989;321:1188–1190.

131. Bloom AL. Progress in the clinical management of haemophilia. Thromb Haemost 1991;66:166–177.

132. Furie B, Limentani SA, Rosenfield CG. A practical guide to the evaluation and treatment of hemophilia. Blood 1994;84:3–9.

133. Gill JC. Therapy of Factor VIII deficiency. Semin Thromb Hemost 1993; 19:1–12.

134. Mannucci PM, Schimpf K, Abe T et al. Low risk of viral infection after administration of vapor-heated factor VIII concentrate. Transfusion 1992; 32:134–138.

135. Smith MP, Rice KM, Savidge GF. Successful clinical use of a plasma-derived, dual virus inactivated factor VIII concentrate incorporating solvent-detergent and dry heat treatment. Thromb Haemost 1997;77:406–407.

136. Morfini M, Mannucci PM, Tenconi PM et al. Pharmacokinetics of mono-

137. Davis HM, Brown SK, Nash DW et al. Lack of immune response to mouse IgG in hemophilia A individuals treated chronically with Monoclate, a monoclonal antibody affinity purified factor VIII preparation. Thromb Haemost 1990;63:386–391.

138. Schwartz RS, Abildgaard CF, Aledort LM et al. Human recombinant DNA-derived antohemophilic factor (factor VIII) in the treatment of hemophilia A. Recombinant Factor III Study Group. N Engl J Med 1990;323:1800–1805.

139. Lusher JM, Arkin S, Abildgaard CF et al. Recombinant factor VIII for the treatment of previously untreated patients with hemophilia A. Safety, efficacy, and development of inhibitors. Kogenate Previously Untreated Patient Study Group . N Engl J Med 1993;328:453–459.

140. Lusher J, Arkin S, Abildgaard CF et al. Kogenate treatment of previously untreated patients with hemophilia A: update on safety, efficacy, and inhibitor development after seven study years [Abstract]. Blood 1996;88: 442A.

141. Bray GL, Gomperts ED, Courter S et al. A multicenter study of recombinant factor VIII (Recombinate): safety, efficacy and inhibitor risk in previously untreated patients with hemophilia A. Blood 1994;83:2428–2435.

142. White GC, Courter S, Bray GL et al. A multicenter study of recombinant factor VIII (Recombinate) in previously treated patients with hemophilia A. Thromb Haemost 1997;77:660–667.

143. Mannucci PM. Effects of Factor VIII concentrates on the immune system of patients with hemophilia. Thromb Haemost 1995;74:437–439.

144. Mannucci PM, Brettler DB, Aledorf LM et al. Immune status of human immunodeficiency virus seropositive and seronegative hemophiliacs infused for 3.5 years with recombinant factor VIII. Blood 1994;83:1958–1962.

145. Gjerset GF, Pike MC, Mosley JW et al. Effect of low- and intermediate-purity clotting factor therapy on progression of human immunodeficiency virus infection in congenital clotting disorders. Blood 1994;84:1666–1671.

146. Varon D, Schulman S, Dardik R et al. High versus ultra-high purity factor VIII concentrate therapy: prospective evaluation of immunological and clinical parameters in HIV seronegative and seropositive hemophiliacs. Thromb Haemost 1994;72:359–362.

147. Montoro JB, Oliveras J, Lorenzo JI et al. An association between clotting factor concentrates use and mortality in human immunodeficiency virus–infected hemophilic patients. Blood 1995;86:2213–2219.

148. Fijnvandraat K, Peters M, Ten Cate JW. Inter-patient variation in half-life of infused recombinant factor VIII is related to pre-infusion von Willebrand factor antigen levels. Br J Haematol 1995;91:474–476.

149. Thomas DP. Clotting factor concentrated—whither purity? Thromb Haemost 1995;74:1604–1606.

150. Shapiro SS. Genetic predisposition to inhibitor formation. Prog Clin Biol Res 1984;150:44–55.

151. Lusher JM, Salzman PM, and the Monoclate® study group. Viral safety and inhibitor development associated with factors VIIIC ultra-purified from plasma in hemophiliacs previously unexposed to factor VIII concentrates. Semin Hematol 1990;27(Suppl 2):1–7.

152. Brettler DB. Comments on the development of inhibitor antibodies in patients using recombinant factor VIII concentrates. Semin Hematol 1991; 28:45–46.

153. Singer ST, Addiego JE Jr, Reason DC et al. T lymphocyte proliferative responses induced by recombinant factor VIII in hemophilia A patients with inhibitors. Thromb Haemost 1996;76:17–22.

154. Schwaab R, Brackmann HH, Meyer C et al. Haemophilia A: mutation type determines risk of inhibitor formation. Thromb Haemost 1995;74: 1402–1406.

155. Tizzano EF, Altisent C, Domenech M et al. Inhibitor development in haemophilia A patients with inversion of the intron 22 of the factor VIII gene. Thromb Haemost 1996;76:125–126.

156. Hay CRM, Ollier W, Pepper L et al. HLA class II profile: a weak determinant of factor VIII inhibitor development in severe haemophilia A. Thromb Haemost 1997;77:234–237.

157. Oldenburg J, Picard JK, Schwaab R et al. HLA genotype of patients with severe haemophilia A due to intron 22 inversion with and without inhibitors to Factor VIII. Thromb Haemost 1997;77:238–242.

158. Growe G, Poon MC, Scarth I. International symposium on recombinant factor VIII: report of the proceedings. Transfusion Med Rev 1992;6: 137–145.

159. Ehrenforth S, Kreuz W, Scharrer I et al. Incidence of development of factor VIII and factor IX inhibitors in haemophiliacs. Lancet 1992;339:594–598.

160. Prescott R, Nakai H, Saenko EL et al. The inhibitor antibody response is more complex in hemophilia A patients than in most nonhemophiliacs with factor VIII autoantiboodies. Blood 1997;89:3663–3671.

161. Rosendaal FR, Nieuwenhuis HK, van den Berg HM et al. A sudden increase in factor VIII inhibitor development in multitransfused hemophilia A patients in the Netherlands. Blood 1993;81:2180–2186.

162. Peerlinck K, Arnout J, Di Giambattista M et al. Factor VIII inhibitors in previously treated haemophilia A patients with a double virus-inactivated plasma derived factor VIII concentrate. Thromb Haemost 1997;77:80–86.

163. Gilles JG, Peerlinck K, Arnout J et al. Restricted epitope specificity of anti-

FVIII antibodies that appeared during a recent outbreak of inhibitors. Thromb Haemost 1997;77:938–943.

164. Mannucci PM, Gringeri A, deBiasi R et al. Immune status of asymptomatic HIV-infected hemophiliacs: randomized, prospective, two-year comparison of treatment with a high-purity or an intermediate-purity factor VIII concentrate. Thromb Haemost 1992;67:310–313.

165. Harris JW. Parvovirus B19 for the hematologist. Am J Hematol 1992;39:119–130.

165a. Pürsün-Aygören E, Scharrer E. A multicenter pharmaco surveillance study for the evaluation of the efficacy and safety of recombinant factor VIII in the treatment of patients with Hemophilia A. Thromb Haemost 1997;78:1352–1356.

166. Rock G, Adamkiewicz T, Blanchette V et al. Acquired von Willebrand factor deficiency during high-dose infusion of recombinant factor VIII. Br J Haematol 1996;93:684–687.

167. Shopnick RI, Kazemi M, Brettler DB et al. Anaphylaxis after treatment with recombinant factor VIII. Transfusion 1996;36:358–361.

168. Scott JP, Montgomery RR. Therapy of von Willebrand disease. Semin Thromb Hemost 1993;19:37–47.

169. Burnouf-Radosevich M, Burnouf T. Chromatographic preparation of a therapeutic highly purified von Willebrand factor concentrate from human cryoprecipitate. Vox Sang 1992;62:1–11.

170. Goudemand J, Mazurier C, Marey A et al. Clinical and biological evaluation in von Willebrand's disease of a von Willebrand factor concentrate with low factor VIII activity. Br J Haematol 1992;80:214–221.

171. Mannucci PM, Tenconi PM, Castaman G et al. Comparison of four virus-inactivated plasma concentrates for the treatment of severe von Willebrand disease: a cross-over randomized trial. Blood 1992;79:3130–3137.

172. Berntorp E. Plasma product treatment in various types of von Willebrand's disease. Haemostasis 1994;24:289–297.

173. Meulien P, Nishino M, Mazurier C et al. Processing and characterization of recombinant von Willebrand factor expressed in different cell types using a vaccinia virus vector. Thromb Haemost 1992;67:154–160.

174. Thompson AR. Factor IX concentrates for clinical use. Semin Thromb Hemost 1993;19:25–36

175. Gerrard AJ, Austen DEG, Brownlee GG. Subcutaneous injection of factor IX for the treatment of haemophilia B. Br J Haematol 1992;81:610–613.

176. Goldsmith JC, Kasper CK, Blatt PM et al. Coagulation factor IX: successful surgical experience with a purified factor IX concentrate. Am J Hematol 1992;40:210–215.

177. Herring SW, Abildgaard C, Shitanishi KT et al. Human coagulation factor IX: assessment of thrombogenicity in animal models and viral safety. J Lab Clin Med 1993;121:394–405.

178. Liles D, Landen CN, Monroe DM et al. Extravascular administration of factor IX: potential for replacement therapy of canine and human hemophilia B. Thromb Haemost 1997;77:944–948.

179. Kim HC, McMillan CW, White GC et al. Purified factor IX using monoclonal immunoaffinity technique: clinical trials in hemophilia B and comparison to prothrombin complex concentrates. Blood 1992;79:568–575.

180. Shapiro AD, Ragni MV, Lusher JM et al. Safety and efficacy of monoclonal antibody purified factor IX concentrate in previously untreated patients with hemophilia B. Thromb Haemost 1996;75:30–35.

181. Brinkhous KM, Sigman JL, Read MS et al. Recombinant human factor IX: replacment therapy, prophylaxis and pharmacokinetics in canine hemophilia B. Blood 1996;88:2603–2610.

182. White G, Lusher J, Shapiro A et al. Recombinant factor IX in the treatment of previously-treated patients with hemophilia B [Abstract]. Blood 1996;88:327A.

183. Hedner U, Glazer S, Falch J. Recombinant activated factor VII in the treatment of bleeding episodes in patients with inherited and acquired bleeding disorders. Transfus Med Rev 1993;7:78–83.

184. Warrier I, Lusher JM. Recombinant factor VIIa (NovoSeven) is the most appropriate treatment for children with hemophilia B complicated by inhibitor antibodies and anaphylaxis to F IX containing products [Abstract]. Blood 1996;88:442A.

185. Schulman S, Bech Jensen M, Varon D et al. Feasibility of using recombinant factor VIIa in continuous infusion. Thromb Haemost 1996;75:432–436.

185a. Hay CR, Negrier C, Ludlam CA. The treatment of bleeding in acquired haemophilia with recombinant factor VII: a multicentre study. Thromb Haemost 1997;78:1463–1467.

186. Stirling D, Ludlam CA. Therapeutic concentrates for the treatment of congenital deficiencies of factors VII, XI, and XIII. Semin Thromb Hemost 1993;19:48–53.

187. Cobos E, Keung YK, Akhter S et al. Use of recombinant factor VIIa for major elective surgery in a patient with factor VII deficiency, retroperitoneal fibrosis and hydronephrosis. Clin Appl Thromb/Hemost 1997;3:33–35.

188. Hedner U, Glazer S, Falch J. Recombinant activated factor VII in the treatment of bleeding episodes in individuals with inherited and acquired bleeding disorders. Transfus Med Rev 1993;7:78–83.

189. Nicolaisen EM. Long-term follow-up with regard to potential immunogenicity: clinical experience with NovoSeven (recombinant factor VIIa). Haemostasis 1996;26:98–101.

190. Nicolaisen EM, Hansen LL, Poulsen F et al. Immunological aspects of recombinant factor VIIa (rFVIIa) in clinical use. Thromb Haemost 1996;76:200–204.

191. Bolton-Maggs PH, Wensley RT, Kernoff PB et al. Production and therapeutic use of factor XI concentrate from plasma. Thromb Haemost 1992;67:314–319.

192. Bolton-Maggs PH, Colvin BT, Satchi BT et al. Thrombogenic potential of factor XI concentrate. Lancet 1994;344:748–749.

193. Richards EM, Makris MM, Cooper P et al. In vivo coagulation activation following infusion of highly purified factor XI concentrate. Br J Haematol 1997;96:293–297.

194. Burnouf-Radosevich M, Burnouf T. A therapeutic, highly purified factor XI concentrate from human plasma. Transfusion 1992;32:861–867.

195. Shirahata A, Nakamura T, Shimono M et al. Blood coagulation findings and the efficacy of factor XIII concentrate in premature infants with intracranial hemorrhages. Thromb Res 1990;57:755–763.

196. Stanton R, Kavulich L, Scialla S. Use of placenta derived factor XIII in the treatment of a prenatal patient. Transfusion 1991;31:S23.

197. Kamitsuji H, Tani K, Taniguchi A et al. Activity of blood coagulation factor XIII as a prognostic indicator in patients with Henoch-Schonlein purpura. Eur J Pediatr 1987;146:519–523.

198. Conard J, Bauer KA, Gruber A et al. Normalization of markers of coagulation activation with a purified protein C concentrate in adults with homozygous protein C deficiency. Blood 1993;82:1159–1164.

199. Minford AM, Parapia LA, Stainforth C et al. Treatment of homozygous protein C deficiency with subcutaneous protein C concentrate. Br J Haematol 1996;93:215–216.

200. Dreyfus M, Masterson M, David M et al. Replacement therapy with a monoclonal antibody purified protein C concentrate in newborns with severe congenital protein C deficiency. Semin Thromb Hemost 1995:21:371–381.

201. Rivard GE, David M, Farrell C et al. Treatment of purpura fulminans in meningococcemia with protein C concentrate. J Pediatr 1995;126:646–652.

202. Schramm W, Spannagl M, Bauer KA et al. Treatment of coumarin-induced skin necrosis with a monoclonal antibody purified protein C concentrate. Arch Dermatol 1993;129:753–756.

203. Lewandowski K, Zawilska K. Protein C concentrate in the treatment of warfarin-induced skin necrosis in the protein C deficiency [Letter]. Thromb Haemost 1994;71:395.

204. Muller FM, Ehrenthal W, Hafner G et al. Purpura fulminans in severe congenital protein C deficiency: monitoring of treatment with protein C concentrate. Eur J Pediatr 1996;155:20–25.

205. Didisheim P, Loeb J, Blatrix C et al. Preparation of a human plasma fraction rich in prothrombin, proconvertin, Stuart factor and PTC and a study of its activity and toxicity in rabbit and man. J Lab Clin Med 1959;53:322–330.

206. Lusher JM. Prediction and management of adverse events associated with the use of factor IX complex concentrates. Semin Hematol 1993;30:36–40.

207. Philippou H, Adami A, Lane DA et al. High purity factor IX and prothrombin complex concentrate (PCC): pharmacokinetics and evidence that factor IXa is the thrombogenic trigger in PCC. Thromb Haemost 1996;76:23–28.

208. Smith KJ. Factor IX concentrates: the new products and their properties. Transfus Med Rev 1992;6:124–136.

209. Henson K, Files JC, Morrison FS. Transient acquired factor X deficiency: report of the use of activated clotting concentrate to control a life-threatening hemorrhage. Am J Med 1989;87:583–585.

210. Hilgartner M, The FEIBA Study Group. Efficacy and safety of vapor-heated anti-inhibitor coagulant complex in hemophilia patients. Transfusion 1990;30:626–630.

210a. Negrier C, Goudemand J, Sultan Y et al. Multicenter retrospective study on the utilization of FEIBA in France in patients with factor VIII and factor IX inhibitors. Thromb Haemost 1997;77:1113–1119.

211. Schwartz RS, Bauer KA, Rosenberg RD et al. Clinical experience with antithrombin III concentrate in treatment of congenital and acquired deficiency of antithrombin. Am J Med 1989;87:3B-53S–60S.

212. Menache D, O'Malley JP, Schorr JB et al. Evaluation of the safety, recovery, half-life and clinical efficacy of antithrombin III (human) in patients with hereditary antithrombin III deficiency. Blood 1990;75:33–39.

213. Francis CW, Pellegrini VD Jr, Harris CM et al. Antithrombin III prophylaxis of venous thromboembolic disease after total hip or total knee replacement. Am J Med 1989;87:61S–66S.

214. Patton DF, Harper JL, Wooldridge TN et al. Treatment of veno-occlusive disease of the liver with bolus tissue plasminogen activator and continuous infusion antithrombin III concentrate. Bone Marrow Transplant 1996;17:443–447.

215. Weiner CP, Herrig JE, Pelzer GD et al. Elimination of antithrombin III concentrate in healthy pregnant and preeclamptic women with an acquired antithrombin III deficiency. Thromb Res 1990;58:395–401.

216. Maki M, Terao T, Ikenoue T et al. Clinical evaluation of antithrombin III concentrate (BI 6.013) for disseminated intravascular coagulation in obstetrics. Gynecol Obstet Invest 1987;23:230–240.

217. Manco-Johnson, MJ. Neonatal antithrombin III deficiency. Am J Med 1989;87:49S–52S.

218. Fuse S, Tomita H, Yoshida M et al. High dose of intravenous antithrombin

III without heparin in the treatment of disseminated intravascular coagulation and organ failure in four children. Am J Hematol 1996;53:18–21.

219. Spannagl M, Hoffmann H, Siebeck M et al. A purified antithrombin III-heparin complex as a potent inhibitor of thrombin in porcine endotoxin shock. Thromb Res 1991;61:1–10.

220. Blauhut B, Kramar H, Vinazzer H et al. Substitution of antithrombin III in shock and DIC: a randomized study. Thromb Res 1985;39:81–89.

221. Lechner K, Kyrle PA. Antithrombin III concentrates—are they clinically useful? Thromb Haemost 1995;73:340–348.

222. Hoffman DL. Purification and large-scale preparation of antithrombin III. Am J Med 1989;87:23S–26S.

223. Einarsson M, Perenius L, McDougal JS et al. Heat inactivation of human immunodeficiency virus in solutions of antithrombin III. Transfusion 1989; 29:148–152.

224. Gibble JW, Ness PM. Fibrin glue: the perfect operative sealant? Transfusion 1990;30:741–747.

225. Alving BM, Weinstein MJ, Finlayson JS et al. Fibrin sealant: summary of a conference on characteristics and clinical uses. Transfusion 1995;35: 783–790.

226. Casali B, Rodeghiero F, Tosetto A et al. Fibrin glue from single-donation autologous plasmapheresis. Transfusion 1992;32:641–643.

227. Flaherty MJ, Handerson R, Wener MH. Iatrogenic immunization with bovine thrombin: a mechanism of prolonged thrombin times after surgery. Ann Intern Med 1989;111:631–634.

228. La Spada AR, Skalhegg BS, Henderson R et al. Brief report: fatal hemorrhage in a patient with an acquired inhibitor of human thrombin. N Engl J Med 1995;333:494–497.

229. Chouhan VD, De La Cadena RA, Nagaswami C et al. Simultaneous occurrence of human antibodies directed against fibrinogen, thrombin, and factor V following exposure to bovine thrombin: effects on blood coagulation, protein C activation and platelet function. Thromb Haemost 1997;77: 343–349.

230. Cicardi M, Mannucci PM, Castelli R et al. Reduction in transmission of hepatitis C after the introduction of a heat-treatment step in the production of C1-inhibitor concentrate. Transfusion 1995;35:209–212.

231. Waytes TA, Rosen FS, Frank MM. Treatment of hereditary angioedema with a vapor-heated C1 inhibitor concentrate. N Engl J Med 1996;334: 1630–1634.

232. MacDonald JL, Johnson CE. Pathophysiology and treatment of alpha 1-antitrypsin deficiency. Am J Health Syst Pharm 1995;52:481–489.

233. Omar A, Kempf C, Immelmann A et al. Virus inactivation by pepsin treatment at pH 4.0 of IgG solutions: factors affecting the rate of virus inactivation. Transfusion 1996;36:866–872.

234. Siegel J. Intravenous immune globulins: therapeutic, pharmaceutical and cost considerations. Pharm Pract News 1997;24:33–35.

235. Anonymous. NIH consensus conference. Intravenous immunoglobulin. Prevention and treatment of disease [Review]. JAMA 1990;264:3189–3193.

236. Ratko TA, Burnett DA, Foulke GE et al. Recommendations for off-label use of intravenously administered immunoglobulin preparations. JAMA 1995;273:1865–1870.

237. Stiehm ER. New uses for intravenous immune globulin. N Engl J Med 1991;325:123–125.

238. Mankarious S, Lee M, Fisher S et al. The half-lives of IgG subclasses and specific antibodies in patients with primary immunodeficiency who are receiving intravenously administered immunoglobulin. J Lab Clin Med 1988;112:634–640.

239. Skull S, Kemp A. Treatment of hypogammaglobulinaemia with intravenous immunoglobulin, 1973–1993. Arch Dis Child 1996;74:527–530.

240. Buckley RH, Schiff RI. The use of intravenous immune globulin in immunodeficiency diseases. N Engl J Med 1991;325:110–117.

241. Anonymous. Intravenous immunoglobulin for the prevention of infection in chronic lymphocytic leukemia: a randomized, controlled clinical trial. Cooperative Group for the Study of Immunoglobulin in Chronic Lymphocytic Leukemia. N Engl J Med 1988;319:902–907.

242. Weeks JC, Tierney MR, Weinstein MC. Cost effectiveness of prophylactic intravenous immune globulin in chronic lymphocytic leukemia. N Engl J Med 1991;325:81–86.

243. Sullivan KM, Kopecky KJ, Jocom J et al. Immunomodulatory and antimicrobial efficacy of intravenous immunoglobulin in bone marrow transplantation. N Engl J Med 1990;323:705–712.

244. Filipovich AH, Peltier MH, Bechtel MK et al. Circulating cytomegalovirus (CMV) neutralizing activity in bone marrow transplant recipients: comparison of passive immunity in a randomized study of four intravenous IgG products administered to CMV-seronegative individuals. Blood 1992; 80:2656–2660.

245. Drobyski WR, Gottlieb M, Carrigan D et al. Phase I study of safety and pharmacokinetics of a human anticytomegalovirus monoclonal antibody in allogeneic bone marrow transplant recipients. Transplantation 1991;51: 1190–1196.

246. Snydman DR, Werner BG, Heinze-Lacey B et al. Use of cytomegalovirus immune globulin to prevent cytomegalovirus disease in renal-transplant recipients. N Engl J Med 1987;317:1049–1054.

247. Anonymous. Intravenous immune globulin for the prevention of bacterial

248. Spector SA, Gelber RD, McGrath N et al. A controlled trial of intravenous immune globulin for the prevention of serious bacterial infections in children receiving zidovudine for advance human immunodeficiency virus infection. N Engl J Med 1994;331:1181–1187.

249. Kiehl MG, Stoll R, Broder M et al. A controlled trial of intravenous immune globulin for the prevention of serious infections in adults with advanced human immunodeficiency virus infection. Arch Intern Med 1996;156: 2545–2550.

250. Baker CJ, Rench MA, Noya FJD et al. Role of intravenous immunoglobulins in prevention of late-onset infections in low-birth-weight neonates. Rev Infect Dis 1990;12:(Suppl 4):S463–S468.

251. Fanaroff AA, Korones SB, Wright LL et al. A controlled trial of intravenous immune globulin to reduce nosocomial infections in very-low-birth-weight infants. N Engl J Med 1994;330:1107–1113.

252. Kinney J, Mundorf L, Gleason C et al. Efficacy and pharmacokinetics of intravenous immune globulin administration to high-risk neonates. Am J Dis Child 1991;145:1233–1238.

253. Piedra PA, Kasel JA, Norton HJ et al. Evaluation of an intravenous immunoglobulin preparation for the prevention of viral infection among hospitalized low birth weight infants. Pediatr Infect Dis 1990;9:470–475.

254. Baker CJ, Melish ME, Hall RT et al. Intravenous immune globulin for the prevention of nosocomial infection in low-birth-weight neonates. N Engl J Med 1992;327:213–219.

255. Anonymous. Prophylactic intravenous administration of standard immune globulin as compared with core-lipopolysaccharide immune globulin in patients at high risk of postsurgical infection. The Intravenous Immunoglobulin-Collaborative Study Group. N Engl J Med 1992;327: 234–240.

256. Groothuis JR, Simoes EA, Levin MJ et al. Prophylactic administration of respiratory syncytial virus immune globulin to high-risk infants and young children. N Engl J Med 1993;329:1524–1530.

257. Anonymous. Reduction of respiratory syncytial virus hospitalization among premature infants and infants with bronchopulmonary dysplasia using respiratory syncytial virus immune globulin prophylaxis. The PREVENT study group. Pediatrics 1997;99:93–99.

258. Blanchette VS, Luke B, Andrew M et al. A prospective, randomized trial of high dose intravenous immune globulin G therapy, oral prednisone therapy, and no therapy in childhood acute immune thrombocytopenic purpura. J Pediatr 1993;123:989–995.

259. Godeau B, Lesage S, Divine M et al. Treatment of adult chronic autoimmune thrombocytopenic purpura with repeated high-dose intravenous immunoglobulin. Blood 1993;82:1415–1421.

260. George JN, Woolf SH, Raskob GE et al. Idiopathic thrombocytopenic purpura: a practice guideline developed by explicit methods for the American Society of Hematology. Blood 1996;88:3–40.

261. Berchtold P, Wenger M. Autoantibodies against platelet glycoproteins in autoimmune thrombocytopenic purpura: their clinical significance and response to treatment. Blood 1993;81:1246–1250.

262. Cardo LJ, Keenan JR, Bussel JB et al. Intravenous gammaglobulin contains anti-idiotypic antibodies to antiplatelet antibodies [Abstract]. Transfusion 1991;31:S30.

263. Berchtold P, Dale GL, Tani P et al. Inhibition of autoantibody binding to platelet glycoprotein IIb-IIIa by anti-idiotypic antibodies in intravenous gammaglobulin. Blood 1989;74:2414–2417.

264. Law C, Marcaccio M, Tam P et al. High-dose intravenous immune globulin and the response to splenectomy in patients with idiopathic thrombocytopenic purpura. N Engl J Med 1997;336:1494–1498.

265. Scaradavou A, Woo B, Woloski BM et al. Intravenous anti-D treatment of immune thombocytopenic purpura: experience in 272 patients. Blood 1997;89:2689–2700.

266. Furusho K, Kamiya T, Nakano H et al. High-dose intravenous gammaglobulin for Kawasaki disease. Lancet 1984;ii:1055–1058.

267. Newburger JW, Takahashi M, Beiser AS et al. A single intravenous infusion of gamma globulin as compared with four infusions in the treatment of acute Kawasaki syndrome. N Engl J Med 1991;324:1633–1639.

268. Rosenfeld EA, Shulman ST, Corydon KE et al. Comparative safety and efficacy of two immune globulin products in Kawasaki disease. J Pediatr 1995;126:1000–1003.

269. Hahn AF, Bolton CF, Zochodne D et al. Intravenous immunoglobulin treatment in chronic inflammatory demyelinating polyneuropathy. A double-blind, placebo-controled, cross-over study. Brain 1996;119:1067–1077.

270. Korinthenberg R, Monting JS. Natural history and treatment effects in Guillain-Barré syndrome: a multicentre study. Arch Dis Child 1996;74: 281–287.

271. Azulay JP, Blin O, Pouget J et al. Intravenous immunoglobulin treatment in patients with motor neuron syndromes associated with anti-GM1 antibodies: a double-blind, placebo-controlled study. Neurology 1994;44: 429–432.

272. Dalakas MC, Illa I, Dambrosia JM et al. A controlled trial of high dose

intravenous immune globulin infusions as treatment for dermatomyositis. N Engl J Med 1993;329:1993–2000.

273. Van der Meche FG, Schmitz PI. A randomized trial comparing intravenous immune globulin and plasma exchange in Guillain-Barré syndrome. Dutch Guillain-Barré study group. N Engl J Med 1992;326:1123–1129.

274. Kurtzman G, Frickhofen N, Kimball J et al. Pure red cell aplasia of 10 years' duration due to persistent parvovirus B19 infection and its cure with immunoglobulin therapy. N Engl J Med 1989;321:519–523.

275. Bodenstein H. Successful treatment of aplastic anemia with high-dose immunoglobulin. N Engl J Med 1991;324:1368–1369.

276. Schwartz RS, Gabriel DA, Aledort LM et al. A prospective study of treatment of acquired (autoimmune) factor VIII inhibitors with high-dose intravenous gammaglobulin. Blood 1995;86:797–804.

277. Rault R, Piraino B, Johnston JR et al. Pulmonary and renal toxicity of intravenous immunoglobulin. Clin Nephrol 1991;36:83–86.

278. Brannagan TH III, Nagle KJ, Lange DJ et al. Complications of intravenous immune globulin treatment in neurologic disease. Neurology 1996;47:674–677.

279. Dalakas MC. High-dose intravenous immunoglobulin and serum viscosity: risk of precipitating thromboembolic events. Neurology 1994;44:223–226.

280. Casteels-Van Daele M, Wijndaele L, Hunninck K et al. Intravenous immune globulin and acute aseptic meningitis. N Engl J Med 1990;323:614–615.

281. Sekul EA, Cupler EJ, Dalakas MC. Aseptic meningitis associated with high dose intravenous immunoglobulin therapy: frequency and risk factors. Ann Intern Med 1994;121:259–262.

282. Ben-Chetrit E, Putterman C. Transient neutropenia induced by intravenous immune globulin. N Engl J Med 1992;326:270–271.

283. Okubo S, Ishida T, Yasunaga K. Hemolysis after intravenous immune globulin therapy: relation to IgG subclasses of red cell antibody. Transfusion 1990;30:436–438.

284. Chambers LA, Pacinin DG, Malynn E et al. Antenatal intravenous immune globulin for neonatal alloimmune thrombocytopenia may jeopardize maternal donor suitability [Abstract]. Transfusion 1991;31:S32.

285. Horst HA, Schmitz N, Glinike C et al. Seroconversion for hepatitis C virus antibody in bone marrow recipients treated with immune globulin. N Engl J Med 1991;325:132–133.

286. Bussel J, Cunningham-Rundles C, Feldman C et al. Transmission of viral infection by preparations of intravenous immunoglobulin. Plasma Ther Transfusion Technol 1988;9:193–205.

287. Bjoro K, Froland SS, Yun Z et al. Hepatitis C infection in patients with primary hypogammaglobulinemia after treatment with contaminated immune globulin. N Engl J Med 1994;331:1607–1611.

288. Bresee JS, Mast EE, Coleman PJ et al. Hepatitis C virus infection associated with administration of intravenous immune globulin. A cohort study. JAMA 1996;276:1563–1567.

289. Jonas MM, Baron MJ, Bresee JS et al. Clinical and virologic features of hepatitis C virus infection associated with intravenous immunoglobulin. Pediatrics 1996;98:211–215.

290. Echevarria JM, Leon P, Domingo CJ et al. Laboratory diagnosis and molecular epidemiology of an outbreak of hepatitis C virus infection among recipients of human intravenous immunoglobulin in Spain. Transfusion 1996;36:725–730.

291. Healey CJ, Sabharwal NK, Daub J et al. Outbreak of acute hepatitis C following the use of anti-hepatitis C virus-screened intravenous immunoglobulin therapy. Gastroenterology 1996;110:1120–1126.

292. Widell A, Zhang YY, Andersson-Gäre et al. At least three hepatitis C virus strains implicated in Swedish and Danish patients with intravenous immunoglobulin-associated hepatitis C. Transfusion 1997;37:313–320.

# CHAPTER 53

# NONTRANSFUSIONAL MODALITIES

■

## Pier Mannuccio Mannucci

When excessive bleeding results from a recognizable defect of the hemostatic system, the treatment of choice is the specific correction of that defect. A typical example is replacement therapy for congenital coagulation disorders. Frequently, however, specific treatment cannot be given, either because there are multiple and complex hemostatic defects or because no cause can be recognized yet the individual bleeds excessively. In these situations, topical hemostatic agents can reduce or stop capillary bleeding when the bleeding site is identifiable and accessible, but such agents usually are not effective when bleeding occurs at high pressure from larger vessels. When bleeding is generalized or the bleeding site is not accessible, pharmacologic agents that facilitate hemostasis become important. Such "hemostatic agents" may be needed prophylactically when surgical operations are accompanied by large blood losses requiring multiple transfusions, which carry the risk of transmitting infectious agents (e.g., human immunodeficiency virus, hepatitis viruses). In addition, they may be needed to meet religious requests to avoid homologous transfusion (e.g., among Jehovah's Witnesses).

Several nontransfusional agents are reported to stop spontaneous bleeding and to prevent or reduce excessive blood loss, and a few have clinical value. This chapter discusses the therapeutic role of desmopressin, conjugated estrogens, erythropoietin, synthetic antifibrinolytic amino acids (i.e., ε-aminocaproic acid and tranexamic acid), and the protease-inhibitor aprotinin (Table 53.1). For each compound, the pharmacologic properties, mechanisms of action, clinical indications, dosages, and side effects are described. The therapeutic

applications of topical hemostatic agents also are mentioned briefly.

## DESMOPRESSIN
### BACKGROUND

Plasma factor VIII, the clotting factor that is either deficient or defective in hemophilia A, and von Willebrand factor, the adhesive protein that is deficient or defective in von Willebrand disease, can be increased for a short time by 1-deamino-8-D-arginine vasopressin (i.e., desmopressin [DDAVP]), which is an analogue of the antidiuretic hormone 8-L-arginine vasopressin (1). Unlike the parent hormone, DDAVP does not cause vasoconstriction, increase blood pressure, or contract the uterus or the gastrointestinal tract. DDAVP increases plasma levels of factor VIII and of von Willebrand factor in healthy individuals and in individuals with mild hemophilia and von Willebrand disease (1–3). These properties form the basis for its clinical use in these bleeding disorders (4–8). DDAVP also has been used successfully in disorders of hemostasis with no defect of factor VIII or von Willebrand factor; examples of these disorders include congenital defects of platelet function (7), uremia (9), liver cirrhosis (10), and hemostatic defects induced by anticoagulant and antiplatelet drugs (10–13). Finally, DDAVP also has been employed to reduce bleeding and transfusion requirements after surgical procedures characterized by large blood losses (14).

### PHARMACOLOGY

DDAVP can be given intravenously, subcutaneously, or intranasally. After intravenous and subcutaneous administration, the half-life and bioavalability are similar (15), which establishes that subcutaneous DDAVP is equivalent to intravenous DDAVP at the dose currently recommended for therapy (0.3 μg/kg body weight). The problem with subcutaneous DDAVP is that the most widely used formulation requires the injection of as much as 4 to 6 mL of fluid, which is impractical. More concentrated formulations (≤1 mL) are available in Europe. With intranasal administration, the bioavailability of DDAVP is 10%; accordingly, doses of approximately 10 times those given intravenously and subcutaneously (3 μg/kg) are needed to elicit the same biologic response (16). Such doses can be given through an intranasal spray using a concentrated formulation (17).

The effects of DDAVP on hemostasis are multiple (Table 53.2). The increase in the plasma levels of factor VIII and von Willebrand factor occurs in individuals with mild hemophilia and von Willebrand disease, in healthy individuals, and among individuals with already high levels of these factors (e.g., those with uremia or cirrhosis). Shortening of the activated partial thromboplastin time and the bleeding time probably results from the increased levels of factor VIII and von Willebrand factor, which have a rate-accelerating role in these global tests of intrinsic coagulation and primary hemostasis (Table 53.2). DDAVP has no effect on platelet count or aggregation. Release of large amounts of tissue-type plasminogen activator into plasma (1, 2) is another short-lived effect (Table 53.2). Plasminogen activation provokes generation of plasmin in vivo, but most of the plasmin generated is complexed to $\alpha_2$-antiplasmin and

---

**TABLE 53.1.** Nontransfusional Hemostatic Agents

Desmopressin (DDAVP)
Conjugated estrogens
Erythropoietin
Synthetic antifibrinolytic amino acids (ε-aminocaproic acid and tranexamic acid)
Aprotinin
Topical hemostatic agents

---

**TABLE 53.2.** Changes in Hemostatic Determinants following DDAVP

↑ Factor VIII
↑ von Willebrand factor
↑ Tissue-type plasminogen activator
↑ Urokinase-type plasminogen activator
↓ Activated partial thromboplastin time
↓ Bleeding time

---

does not produce fibrin(ogen)olysis in the circulating blood (18). Accordingly, administration of antifibrinolytic drugs with DDAVP usually is not necessary.

## MECHANISMS OF ACTION

DDAVP acts through its strong $V_2$ receptor–mediated agonist activity, because the hemostatic changes induced by DDAVP do not occur in individuals with nephrogenic diabetes insipidus who lack functioning $V_2$ receptors and, thus, are unresponsive to $V_2$ agonists (19). Anephric individuals respond normally to DDAVP (2), thus indicating that the $V_2$-like receptors involved in the hemostatic properties of DDAVP are not localized to the kidney.

The mechanisms governing increases in the plasma levels of factor VIII and von Willebrand factor after DDAVP administration are not completely understood. Because these increases are both rapid and transient, DDAVP probably triggers their release from storage sites, and because von Willebrand factor is both synthesized and stored in endothelial cells, the vascular endothelium probably is the source of von Willebrand factor. There is no release of von Willebrand factor after direct addition of DDAVP to cultured endothelial cells (20), but these cells may have lost specific $V_2$ receptors during culture and, therefore, may not be identical to native cells in the vessel wall. Release of von Willebrand factor from endothelial cells occurs after addition of DDAVP to peripheral mononuclear cells, which in turn produces an as-yet-unidentified, intermediate factor that acts on endothelial cells (21).

A puzzling and unresolved question is how DDAVP is effective in disorders other than hemophilia and von Willebrand disease that are characterized by normal or even high levels of von Willebrand factor. These favorable effects may be mediated by the supranormal levels of von Willebrand factor in the circulation and by hemostatically more effective, large multimers (22), which produced increased platelet adhesion to the vascular subendothelium and shortening of the bleeding time. On the other hand, the effect on the bleeding time is partially independent of von Willebrand factor (9, 10).

## CLINICAL INDICATIONS AND DOSAGES

### Congenital Bleeding Disorders

Since 1977, DDAVP has been used to prevent and treat bleeding in mild hemophilia and von Willebrand disease (4–7); individuals with severe deficiencies of factor VIII and von Willebrand factor do not respond to DDAVP. Intravenous or subcutaneous doses of 0.3 μg/kg, or an intranasal dose of 3 μg/kg, yield an optimal response. Lower doses are less effective, and higher doses are unnecessary. In individuals with mild factor VIII or von Willebrand factor deficiency (≥5 U/dl), levels of these factors increase on average to approximately three to five times basal levels, even although variability of responses among individuals is large (23). On the other hand, within-patient variability is small, so results of a test dose usually predict the overall response (23).

The peak response usually occurs 30 to 60 minutes after starting the intravenous infusion (which should last from 20 to 30 minutes), whereas it is delayed by 30 to 60 minutes after subcutaneous or intranasal DDAVP, probably because of slower absorption (23). The plasma half-lives of factor VIII and von Willebrand factor in individuals with hemophilia and von Willebrand disease vary between 5 and 8 hours for factor VIII and between 8 and 10 hours for von Willebrand factor (23). These data indicate that factors after DDAVP return to baseline more rapidly than after administration of plasma concentrates, but their persistence in the circulation is sufficient for therapeutic purposes.

In hemophilia (see Chapter 35), the hemostatic efficacy of DDAVP usually correlates with the postinfusion levels of plasma factor VIII. Accordingly, therapeutic indications are defined by the nature of the bleeding episode, baseline factor VIII levels, and the levels that must be attained and maintained for hemostasis in any given clinical situation. One limiting feature may be that factor VIII levels attained in some situations are not sufficient to control bleeding.

Most individuals with von Willebrand disease (see Chapter 34) respond to DDAVP with increased levels of factor VIII, similar to or greater than those seen in individuals with hemophilia (24), and with a shortened or normalized the bleeding time (4–8). The bleeding time in individuals with the homozygous, severe disease (3) or dysfunctional von Willebrand factor, however, usually is not shortened (22). Even so, there are individuals with type IIA and type IIB von Willebrand disease in whom DDAVP shortens the bleeding time. A test dose is the only way to differentiate responders from nonresponders. Table 53.3 summarizes the indications for DDAVP in individuals with von Willebrand disease.

DDAVP can be repeated at 24-hour intervals if necessary, but individuals with hemophilia who are treated repeatedly may become less responsive, or even unresponsive, perhaps because stores of factor VIII become exhausted (24). This phenomenon occurs to a lesser extent in individuals with von Willebrand disease (24). The clinical implication of this are that usefulness of DDAVP may be limited in some individuals with mild hemophilia, particularly when levels of factor VIII must be maintained above baseline for a prolonged period. In this situation, it is advisable to use plasma concentrates or to supplement them with DDAVP.

Because consistent responses are required before surgery and for treatment of severe hemorrhage, intravenous DDAVP is recommended, but subcutaneous

**TABLE 53.3. Indications for DDAVP in Different Types of von Willebrand Disease**

| | |
|---|---|
| Established[a] | Type I, "platelet normal" |
| | Type IIN |
| Possible[b] | Type I, "platelet low" and "platelet dysfunctional" |
| | Type IIA, IIB, IIC, IIM |
| Doubtful[c] | Type III (severe) |

[a] Those in which DDAVP normalizes the bleeding time and factor VIII levels and is clinically efficacious.

[b] Those in which the effect on the bleeding time is absent or inconsistent, with little data on clinical efficacy.

[c] Those in which DDAVP does not normalize factor VIII levels or the bleeding time and is not clinically efficacious.

DDAVP can be self-administered at home to prevent soft-tissue bleeding in individuals with hemophilia who participate in strenuous sports and in women with von Willebrand disease who bleed excessively during menstruation (25). Others prefer to use intranasal DDAVP in these situations, as well as for control of major spontaneous bleeding episodes and bleeding from surgical procedures (26).

DDAVP shortens or normalizes the bleeding time of individuals with congenital platelet dysfunctions (8, 10, 27) (see Chapter 32). Individuals with defects of the platelet-release reaction, cyclooxygenase deficiency, and isolated, unexplained prolongations of the bleeding time usually respond well. Most individuals with congenital storage-pool deficiency and the Bernard-Soulier syndrome also respond, but a few do not. Therefore, a test dose of DDAVP is recommended to identify those who will respond (10). Whether the effect on a laboratory measurement such as the bleeding time corresponds to a protective hemostatic effect is not well established. A few clinical studies, however, indicate that DDAVP can be used instead of blood products during or after surgery or delivery, thus ensuring satisfactory hemostasis (27). Individuals with Glanzmann's thrombasthenia usually do not respond to DDAVP (8, 10).

## Acquired Hemostatic Disorders

DDAVP has been used to treat acquired bleeding disorders in which levels of factor VIII and von Willebrand factor are normal or even high. After 0.3 μg/kg of DDAVP is infused intravenously, the prolonged bleeding time normalizes in approximately 75% of individuals with uremia (9), and it returns to pretreatment values after approximately 8 hours (9). In these individuals, DDAVP has prevented bleeding before invasive procedures (e.g., biopsy, major surgery) and stopped spontaneous bleeding (9). Closely spaced infusions, however, may progressively fail to shorten the bleeding time (29). Conjugated estrogens and recombinant erythropoietin are alternatives to DDAVP in individuals with uremia (discussed later).

Why the bleeding time is prolonged in some individuals with liver cirrhosis is not completely understood (see Chapter 45). There usually is mild or moderate thrombocytopenia, but platelet counts do not correlate (inversely) with bleeding times. Levels of factor VIII and von Willebrand factor in individuals with cirrhosis are in the high-normal range or higher, yet intravenous DDAVP shortens the bleeding time in these individuals (10, 30). Hence, DDAVP is a possible treatment for individuals with prolonged bleeding times who need invasive diagnostic procedures. DDAVP is not effective, however, in controlling acute variceal bleeding in individuals with cirrhosis (31).

DDAVP counteracts the antihemostatic effects of several antithrombotic drugs. It shortens the prolonged bleeding time in individuals taking the antiplatelet agents aspirin (8) and ticlopidine (10), the prolonged bleeding time and activated partial thromboplastin time in individuals receiving heparin (11), and the bleeding time in rabbits treated with aspirin and streptokinase or hirudin (12, 32). It also counteracts the antihemostatic effects of dextran without impairing the antithrombotic properties of this product (13). There is no clinical evidence that DDAVP can prevent or stop bleeding complications from developing in association with use of antithrombotic agents, but it may provide an opportunity to control drug-induced bleeding without discontinuing treatment and, perhaps, to avoid recurrence or progression of thrombosis.

## Reducing Surgical Blood Loss

Open-heart surgery with extracorporeal circulation (5) (see Chapter 50) is the epitome of operations associated with blood losses large enough to warrant blood saving techniques. In addition to techniques such as presurgical removal of autologous blood for postsurgical retransfusion, returning to the individual all oxygenator and tubing contents, and autotransfusion of mediastinal shed blood, hemostatic agents can be given prophylactically to further reduce the requirement for blood transfusion.

Since 1986, DDAVP has been evaluated extensively in clinical studies. In the first study (33), which involved individuals undergoing complex cardiac operations associated with large blood losses, DDAVP given at the time of chest closure (0.3 μg/kg) reduced both perioperative and early (12 hours) postoperative blood loss and transfusion requirements by approximately one-third (33). In contrast, two subsequent large studies of individuals undergoing less complex operations with lesser blood losses demonstrated no statistically significant differences in either total blood loss or transfusion requirements following DDAVP or placebo (34, 35). Results of these trials are summarized in Table 53.4. Other studies, mainly involving individuals undergoing coronary artery bypass grafting and uncomplicated valve replacement, have failed to establish any benefit of DDAVP in adults or in children (36, 37).

These conflicting outcomes in open-heart surgery might result from most trials having insufficient statistical power to detect true differences in blood loss. A meta-analysis of 17 randomized, double-blind, placebo-controlled trials, which included 1171 individuals undergoing open-heart surgery treated with DDAVP or placebo, has attempted to overcome this pitfall (38). Overall, these investigators found that DDAVP statistically significantly reduced postoperative blood loss by 9%, a value with little clinical impact. DDAVP had no blood saving effect when the mean blood loss in placebo-treated individuals were in the lower and middle thirds of distribution (687–1108 mL per 24 hours), but the compound reduced blood loss by 34% when blood losses were greater (38). Therefore, DDAVP appears to be beneficial only in cardiac operations associated with large blood losses. It is not easy to predict which individual will bleed more, but situations such as reoperation, presurgical use of antiplatelet agents, preexisting coagulation defects, and sepsis might help to identify such individuals for prophylaxis.

**TABLE 53.4.** Results of Major Clinical Trials of DDAVP to Reduce Blood Loss after Open-Heart Surgery

| Study | Mean Blood Loss (mL/24 hour) | | Patients (n) | Type of Operation |
|---|---|---|---|---|
| | DDAVP | Placebo | | |
| Salzman et al (33) | 1317[a] | 2210 | 70 | Valve replacement |
| Rocha et al (34) | 458 | 536 | 100 | Valve replacement |
| Hackman et al (35) | 865 | 738 | 150 | Valve replacement/coronary aortic bypass grafts |

[a] P < .01.

| **TABLE 53.5.** | Indications for DDAVP in the Treatment or Prevention of Bleeding |
|---|---|
| Established[a] | Mild and moderate hemophilia A von Willebrand disease (see Table 53.3) Congenital platelet dysfunctions Uremia |
| Possible[b] | Liver cirrhosis Drug-induced bleeding (e.g., heparin, hirudin, antiplatelet agents, dextran, streptokinase) Complicated cardiac surgery |
| Doubtful[c] | Uncomplicated cardiac surgery Thrombocytopenic bleeding |

[a] *Those in which the hemostatic efficacy of DDAVP has been demonstrated clinically.*

[b] *Those in which clinical data are too preliminary or inconclusive.*

[c] *Those in which DDAVP is not efficacious clinically.*

DDAVP is not the only blood saving agent used in open-heart surgery. Antifibrinolytic agents have been employed as well. One comparative study, for example, demonstrated that aprotinin is more efficacious than DDAVP in reducing blood loss (39). A more complete analysis is presented later.

The hemostatic effectiveness of DDAVP in operations other than cardiac surgery is not established, but there are some preliminary data. When given to hemostatically normal children before spinal fusion surgery for scoliosis, DDAVP reduced the average operative blood loss by approximately one-third (40). Reduced blood loss and red cell transfusion requirements also were found during surgery for lumbar fusion (41).

The main therapeutic indications for DDAVP are summarized in Table 53.5.

## SIDE EFFECTS

Frequent side effects of DDAVP include mild facial flushing, transient headache, a 10 to 20% increase in heart rate, and a slight decrease in systolic and diastolic blood pressure. Because of its potent antidiuretic effects and the large dose needed for hemostatic efficacy (approximately 15 times greater than that for diabetes insipidus), there is a risk of water retention, which could cause severe hyponatremia and seizures (42, 43). In individuals receiving more than one dose of DDAVP, monitoring plasma sodium levels, measuring body weight daily, and avoiding excessive fluid administration should be considered. Arterial thrombosis (sometimes fatal stroke and myocardial infarction) and venous

thromboembolism have occurred in some individuals treated with DDAVP, and in one healthy individual who injected himself with DDAVP for experimental purposes (44). A survey projecting the number of individuals with thrombosis compared to the number of individuals treated with DDAVP, however, indicates that thrombotic complications are rare (45). Most important, an analysis of DDAVP trials in individuals at high risk for thrombosis (e.g., those undergoing coronary artery bypass grafting) indicates no statistically significant increased thrombotic complications in individuals treated with DDAVP compared to untreated controls (46).

DDAVP has been given to pregnant women with diabetes insipidus with no evidence of teratogenicity. DDAVP also is used to increase factor VIII levels in hemophilia carriers before chorionic villus sampling with no complications observed (my unpublished observations).

## CONJUGATED ESTROGENS

### BACKGROUND

A preparation of conjugated estrogens was licensed as a hemostatic agent in the 1960s, but the lack of rigorous studies regarding its clinical efficacy led to a period of neglect for this preparation. In 1984, however, conjugated estrogens were revived by Liu et al (47), who showed that the compound often shortened or normalized the prolonged bleeding time in individuals with chronic renal insufficiency and also improved or arrested hemorrhage. These preliminary findings were confirmed in a double-blind, randomized trial (48).

### PHARMACOLOGY

The preparation is a mixture of estrone sulfate (50–60%) and equiline sulfate (20–30%), with smaller amounts of dihydroequiline sulfate, estroestriol sulfate, and 17β-estradiol, all of which are extracted from the urine of pregnant mares. 17β-Estradiol is the most active component (49). Conjugated estrogens are available for intravenous or intramuscular injection and for oral administration. In normal individuals and individuals with chronic renal insufficiency, conjugated estrogens have a plasma half-life of approximately 3 hours for estrone sulfate and equiline sulfate, and a dose-finding study established the regimen of conjugated estrogens that ensures an optimal effect on the bleeding time (50). After a single infusion of 0.6 mg/kg, which is repeated for 4 to 5 days, the bleeding time becomes shorter than the preinfusion values by approximately 50%, and the effect is sustained for at least 2 weeks (50). Given orally, conjugated estrogens at a daily dose of 50 mg shorten the prolonged bleeding time in individuals with uremia after an average of 7 days of treatment (51).

## MECHANISM OF ACTION

The mechanism whereby conjugated estrogens affect the bleeding time is not well established. Excessive production of prostacyclin, a potent platelet antiaggregatory and vasodilator agent, by uremic vessels is not reduced by the product (52). In individuals with uremia, conjugated estrogens activate blood platelets and improve defective release of the $\alpha$-granule substance, $\beta$-thromboglobulin, and production of the arachidonic acid metabolite thromboxane $B_2$ (53). The discrepancy between the short plasma half-life of conjugated estrogens and their long-lasting effects on the bleeding time suggests an estrogen receptor–mediated mechanism. The demonstration that two estrogen receptor antagonists, tamoxifen and clomiphene, block the shortening effect of conjugated estrogens on the bleeding time (49), and that zeranol, which has a structure resembling that of estrogens but weak hormonal activity, shortens the bleeding time as much as conjugated estrogens in uremic rats (54), supports this view.

## CLINICAL INDICATIONS AND DOSAGE

There are clinical cases indicating that conjugated estrogens (optimal daily dose, 0.6 mg/kg for 4–5 days) stops or prevents bleeding in individuals with uremia (47, 48), but no controlled trial has demonstrated hemostatic efficacy. Use of this compound rests on the well-demonstrated shortening of the prolonged bleeding time (47, 48) and on the relationship between the degree of prolongation in the bleeding time and the individual's tendency to bleed excessively (55). The chief advantage of the product over DDAVP is the longer duration of its effect on the bleeding time (10–15 days versus 6–8 hours). Hence, estrogens are the treatment of choice when long-lasting hemostatic competence is required, such as during surgical procedures or recurrent episodes of gastrointestinal bleeding or epistaxis. On the other hand, the time lag before conjugated estrogens are effective warrants use of DDAVP when an immediate effect on hemostasis is required (e.g., to stop acute bleeding or prevent bleeding during surgical procedures) (Table 53.6). These two products can be given concur-

rently, successfully exploiting the different timing of their maximal effects.

## SIDE EFFECTS

Conjugated estrogens are well tolerated, and side effects are negligible or absent. Because no more than five daily doses are recommended, side effects related to the hormonal activity of estrogens usually are avoided. Headache, nausea, and flushing have been recorded; therefore, slow infusion is recommended.

# ERYTHROPOIETIN

## BACKGROUND

In individuals with anemia and chronic renal insufficiency, recombinant erythroproietin causes a dose-dependent rise in the hematocrit and eliminates the need for blood transfusions (56, 57). On the basis of previous data indicating the rise in hematocrit induced by red cell transfusion shortens the prolonged bleeding time and stops bleeding symptoms in individuals with uremia (58), Moia et al (59) explored whether the efficacy of recombinant erythropoietin in correcting anemia was associated with improvement of the hemostatic defect. The progressive increases in hematocrit were paralleled by a pronounced shortening of bleeding times and improved platelet adhesion (59). These preliminary findings have been confirmed (60–62).

## PHARMACOLOGY

Chinese hamster ovary cells are used to produce the recombinant protein. This protein has a molecular weight of 30,400, the same amino acid composition as natural erythropoietin (i.e., 165 amino acid residues), and a similarly high content of carbohydrates (63).

The product can be given intravenously, subcutaneously, intramuscularly, or intraperitoneally. Intravenous erythropoietin is eliminated from plasma with a half-life of approximately 6 to 8 hours (64, 65). With subcutaneous injections, plasma levels are sustained for longer time, and the same rise in hematocrit is achieved with less fre-

**TABLE 53.6.** Nontransfusional Forms of Treatment for Uremic Bleeding

| Compound | Onset of Effect | Duration of Effect | Indications |
|---|---|---|---|
| DDAVP | Immediate | 6–8 hours | Acute hemorrhage<br>Before biopsy or minor surgery |
| Conjugated estrogens | Delayed | 10–15 days | Chronic, recurrent hemorrhage<br>Major surgery |
| Erythropoietin | Delayed | Sustained | Prevention of hemorrhage |

quent administration (i.e., twice weekly as opposed to thrice weekly) (64, 65).

## MECHANISM OF ACTION

In individuals with uremia, abnormalities of primary hemostasis are reflected by two main laboratory test results: prolonged bleeding time, and reduced platelet adhesion to the exposed subendothelium of human vessels (66). Both abnormalities progressively improve as the hematocrit rises in response to erythropoietin (59), perhaps because increasing the red cell concentration increases the rate of radial transport of centrally flowing platelets toward the vessel wall (67). In turn, greater margination facilitates platelet adhesion to the subendothelium, formation of the hemostatic plug, and shortening of the bleeding time (67, 68). Red cells also may metabolically enhance platelet reactivity via increased thromboxane production and adenosine diphosphate release (69, 70). In contrast, a direct effect of erythropoietin on platelet function cannot be excluded, because during treatment, changes such as a slight and transient increase in platelet count and volume, improvement of defective platelet aggregability, and heightened mobilization of intracellular free calcium (60, 71–73) also may account for improved hemostasis.

## CLINICAL INDICATIONS AND DOSAGE

Most individuals with chronic renal insufficiency are treated regularly with erythropoietin. This practice usually has led to sustained improvement of the hemostatic defect. Hence, little therapeutic role is left for short-acting agents such as DDAVP and conjugated estrogens, which remain indicated for individuals with acute or subacute renal failure who are not treated with or are unresponsive to erythropoietin (Table 53.7).

| **TABLE 53.7.** | Routes of Administration and Recommended Doses of Antifibrinolytic Amino Acids | |
|---|---|---|
| **Compound** | **Route of Administration** | **Recommended Daily Doses** |
| ε-Aminocaproic acid | Intravenous | 4.0 g every 4 hours |
| | Oral | 4.0 g every 4 hours |
| Tranexamic acid | Intravenous | 0.5–1.0 g every 8 hours |
| | Oral | 1.0–1.5 g every 8 hours |
| | Mouthwash | 1.0 g every 6 hours |

Erythropoietin should be started at low doses (e.g., 30–50 IU/kg three times weekly) and given as an intravenous bolus at the end of each routine dialysis treatment. Subcutaneous erythropoietin can be given twice weekly and is preferred in individuals with no ready venous access (e.g., those who have not yet begun hemodialysis, those treated with peritoneal dialysis). On average, these doses will produce a rise in hematocrit of approximately 1% per week. Larger doses induce greater and more rapid increases in hematocrit, but they usually are unnecessary and even may be dangerous. The target hematocrit values are from 27 to 32%, which ensure relief of the symptoms associated with anemia and, usually, a significant shortening of the bleeding time (59–62). To maintain the hematocrit at these levels, average doses of 25 U/kg twice weekly usually are sufficient. There are, however, individuals with prolonged bleeding times despite hematocrits of 30% or higher, thus indicating that low hematocrit is not the only cause of a prolonged bleeding time in individuals with uremia (58). In these individuals, it usually is futile to attempt to improve the bleeding time with larger doses of erythropoietin; DDAVP or conjugated estrogens are alternative therapeutic agents.

## SIDE EFFECTS

Aggravation of hypertension is the major adverse effect of raising the hematocrit in individuals with uremia. Hypertension generally can be minimized by increasing the hematocrit slowly and avoiding values greater than 30% (73, 74). Other side effects include decreased efficiency of dialysis, because the increase in hematocrit is accompanied by a decrease in plasma volume and, hence, in the amount of toxic substances that can be removed at each session. Partial or complete clotting in the dialysis lines and vascular access devices also may contribute to this decreased efficiency (73, 74). The risk of thrombus formation associated with erythropoietin is a cause for potential concern as well, but there is no evidence that correction of anemia is associated with an increased frequency of thrombosis in the coronary, cerebral, or peripheral blood vessels.

# SYNTHETIC ANTIFIBRINOLYTIC AMINO ACIDS

## BACKGROUND

Binding of plasminogen and plasmin to fibrin, which is a key reaction in fibrinolysis, is mediated by structures on the plasminogen molecule (i.e., lysine-binding sites) (see Chapter 7). Synthetic derivatives of lysine, such as 6-aminohexanoic acid (ε-aminocaproic acid [EACA]) and *trans-p*-aminomethyl-cyclohexane carboxylic acid (i.e., tranexamic acid), have strong antifibrinolytic activity at doses eliciting few side effects in humans (75, 76). Since the early 1960s, EACA and, subsequently, tranexamic acid have been used therapeutically in many clinical situations to control bleeding from local or systemic hyperfibrinolysis.

## PHARMACOLOGY

Both EACA and tranexamic acid can be given intravenously or orally, and they are eliminated through the kidney in chemically intact active forms (77, 78). They are highly concentrated in the urine (up to 100 times) and enter biologic fluids such as cerebrospinal fluid, semen, synovial fluid, and, through the placenta, umbilical cord blood (77, 78). Both amino acids enter the extravascular space and accumulate in tissues, in which they inhibit plasminogen activation. This probably forms the basis for their beneficial use in hemorrhagic conditions resulting from local hyperfibrinolysis.

The biological half-life of intravenous EACA is 60 to 90 minutes, with approximately 80% excreted within 3 to 4 hours (77). Oral EACA is absorbed rapidly from the gastrointestinal tract. Peak plasma levels are achieved within 1 to 2 hours after a therapeutic dose, with a half-life similar to that for intravenous administration (77). Because EACA is concentrated in the urine, its half-life becomes much greater when renal function is impaired, thus making necessary reduction in the dosage and frequency of administration.

On a molar basis, tranexamic acid is approximately 10 times more potent that EACA for inhibiting fibrinolysis. Accordingly, smaller doses can be given (Table 53.7), thus resulting in fewer gastrointestinal side effects (78). The half-life of tranexamic acid is similar to that of EACA, but the greater inhibitory potency makes possible administration at less frequent intervals (6–8 hours versus 3–4 hours) (78). Tranexamic acid, like EACA, can be given orally, but it is less readily absorbed (78). This explains why oral tranexamic acid must be given at approximately two to three times the intravenous dose to obtain the same antifibrinolytic effects (Table 53.7).

## MECHANISM OF ACTION

Both lysine analogues accelerate plasminogen activation through binding to the lysine-binding sites of the molecule (78–80). This interaction induces a conformational change that renders the zymogen more susceptible to the proteolytic action of activators, thus facilitating exposure of the enzymatic site. At the same time, however, occupancy of the lysine-binding site of plasminogen by the amino acids blocks binding of the zymogen to the substrate fibrin, which is necessary for full fibrinolytic

activity (79, 80). Hence, even although plasmin formation is not impeded by EACA or tranexamic acid, clot lysis is slowed or even blocked.

## CLINICAL INDICATIONS AND DOSAGES

Both EACA and tranexamic acid have been proposed as hemostatic agents in many clinical conditions characterized by excessive bleeding. Few studies have directly compared the two compounds, however, because the common mechanism of action indicates their therapeutic efficacy should be similar provided that the dosages are equivalent.

### Primary Menorrhagia

Excessive menstrual bleeding with no underlying uterine pathology is the most frequent cause of iron-deficiency anemia in women of fertile age. (Approximately 10% of women lose more than 80 mL of blood per menstrual period.) The most effective and practical treatment of menorrhagia is oral contraceptives, but tranexamic acid or EACA, given at the onset of menstruation, is effective in reducing blood loss. One randomized, controlled trial (81) demonstrated that tranexamic acid is superior to a hemostatic agent such as ethamsylate and a nonsteroidal anti-inflammatory drug such as mefenamic acid. Antifibrinolytic amino acids may act by inhibiting plasminogen activators present at high local concentrations in the endometrium during the secretory phase of the menstrual cycle.

Tranexamic acid and EACA should be considered only when organic lesions in the uterus are excluded and there are contraindications to oral contraceptives, which are easier to use and, probably, more efficacious. The recommended dose is 1 g of oral tranexamic acid every 8 hours or 4 g of oral EACA every 4 hours, beginning with the onset of menstruation, for 4 to 5 days (Table 53.8). These regimens also are useful for reducing excessive blood loss associated with use of intrauterine contraceptive devices.

### Epistaxis

Recurrent epistaxis in individuals with normal hemostasis rarely is dangerous, but it is unpleasant and can produce relevant morbidity. When recurrent epistaxis is severe and frequent enough to require hospital visits, tranexamic acid can stop or prevent bleeding; the same doses are recommended as those used for menorrhagia.

### Gastrointestinal Bleeding

The rationale leading to the evaluation of antifibrinolytic amino acids as treatment of bleeding in the gastrointestinal tract is that the local concentrations of plasminogen activators are abnormally high in individuals with gas-

**TABLE 53.8.** Clinical Indications for Anti-fibrinolytic Amino Acids

| | |
|---|---|
| Established | Primary menorrhagia |
| | Transurethral prostatectomy and other lower-urinary-tract operations |
| | Dental extraction in congenital bleeding disorders |
| | Open-heart surgery |
| Possible | Epistaxis |
| | Traumatic hyphema |
| | Mucosal bleeding in thrombocytopenia |
| | Promyelocytic leukemia |
| | Bleeding in association with thrombolytic agents |
| Doubtful | Gastrointestinal bleeding |
| | Subarachnoid bleeding |
| | Tonsillectomy and adenoidectomy |
| | Disseminated intravascular coagulation |

tric or duodenal ulcers, acute erosive gastritis, and ulcerative colitis. A double-blind study involving a large group of individuals evaluated endoscopically (82) demonstrated that even although tranexamic acid did not reduce rebleeding from benign lesions in the stomach and duodenum, significantly fewer blood transfusions were required (82). In individuals with rectal bleeding from ulcerative colitis, two double-blind trials (83, 84) produced contrasting results. Overall, however, there is no firm evidence that EACA or tranexamic acid is needed for treatment of bleeding in the upper and lower digestive tract, particularly as medical and endoscopic treatment has improved so dramatically in the last two decades.

## Urinary Tract Bleeding

Bleeding in the upper urinary tract responds well to EACA or tranexamic acid for at least two reasons. First, urine and the urinary tract mucosa are rich in plasminogen activators (i.e., urokinase-type and tissue-type plasminogen activators). Second, EACA and tranexamic acid are concentrated in urine. Clots formed during treatment, however, cannot be lysed and may obstruct the urinary tract, cause colicky pain, or both. The risk of irreversible renal insufficiency also should be kept in mind.

The most important indication for use of EACA or tranexamic acid is bleeding from the lower urinary tract, especially after transurethral prostatectomy. Following removal of the gland, urine comes into contact with hemostatic clots and tends to dissolve them, thus resulting in a long period of hematuria postoperatively. When elderly individuals undergo this operation, hematuria may lead to anemia, which in turn complicates the post-

operative course and slows individual recovery. Several controlled clinical trials have demonstrated consistently that EACA or tranexamic acid reduces the amount of blood loss and the duration of hematuria (85). The recommended dosage of tranexamic acid is 0.5 g every 8 hours intravenously, beginning immediately after surgery, for 3 days and switching to oral treatment thereafter (1.5 g every 8 hours). The corresponding doses of EACA are 4 g intravenously six times daily, followed by oral administration of the same dose at the same time intervals.

## Subarachnoid Bleeding

In contrast to the brain, the meninges and choroid plexus are rich in tissue-type plasminogen activator. Fibrinolytic activity, which is not present in normal cerebrospinal fluid, is high in the cerebrospinal fluid of individuals with subarachnoid bleeding from a ruptured arterial aneurysm, and it is a strong contributing cause of recurrent bleeding (86). Tranexamic acid accumulates in the cerebrospinal fluid, particularly when given intravenously in very large doses (15 mg/kg six times daily) (86, 87). The initial enthusiasm for antifibrinolytic agents was tempered by the results of clinical trials showing that despite a statistically significant lower prevalence of early rebleeding in individuals treated with EACA or tranexamic acid, overall mortality was not reduced because of a concurrent increase in late cerebral ischemia (88, 89). Hence, tranexamic acid should not be used in the early medical management of individuals with subarachnoid bleeding.

## Bleeding after Tonsillectomy and Adenoidectomy

Tonsillectomy and adnoidectomy are not associated with a high risk of hemorrhage, but a few individuals, particularly children, may rebleed 3 to 4 days after surgery, when the hemostatic clots clear. Along with the hypothesis that such bleeding may result from hyperfibrinolysis in the oral mucosa, this has led to use of antifibrinolytic amino acids both during and after surgery. A double-blind trial (90) demonstrated a reduction in blood loss and rebleeding, but the prophylactic regimen is not widely used.

## Traumatic Hyphema

Traumatic hyphema carries a high risk of rebleeding in the anterior chamber and the vitreous body. Such rebleeding occurs in approximately one-third of individuals, usually 5 to 7 days after the primary posttraumatic hemorrhage. A blind and painful eye is the consequence of secondary bleeding. On the assumption that rebleeding may result from local hyperfibrinolysis with premature removal of the hemostatic clot, antifibrinolytic agents have been used. Daily tranexamic acid (1 g every 8 hours) reduces the frequency of secondary hemorrhage after traumatic hyphema (91).

## Congenital Bleeding Disorders

There usually is no sign of systemic hyperfibrinolysis in individuals with hemophilia, but long-term inhibition of fibrinolysis might help hemostatic clots to become more stable, thereby reducing the frequency of spontaneous bleeding and the need for replacement therapy. Results of two double-blind trials with tranexamic acid, however, have provided contrasting results. One long-term study using a total dose of 2 g daily failed to show any benefit (92), whereas a trial using 3 g daily found a significant reduction in bleeding episodes (93). Prophylactic treatment with antifibrinolytic agents cannot be recommended.

The oral cavity is rich in plasminogen activators, present in the oral mucosa and saliva (94), which justifies use of antifibrinolytic agents as adjuvant therapy during dental extractions. Two double-blind trials found that both EACA and tranexamic acid substantially reduce rebleeding and the amount of blood products needed after dental extractions (95, 96). Usually, with these agents, one dose of factor concentrates must be given at the time of surgery, with no further therapy during the next few days. An oral dose of 4 g of EACA every 4 hours, or 1.5 g of tranexamic acid every 8 hours, is recommended for 8 to 10 days, until healing of the sockets is complete. When tranexamic acid is given topically as a mouthwash, it is not absorbed into blood; instead, it concentrates in the saliva, where it inhibits fibrinolytic activity for several hours (94). Mouthwashes of tranexamic acid (1 g) every 6 hours for 5 days, starting immediately after extraction, are recommended (97). Using this technique avoids inhibition of plasma fibrinolytic activity and the gastrointestinal effects related to systemic administration (94, 97). In addition, mouthwashes are essential for individuals with hemophilia B, because the concomitant systemic administration of prothrombin complex concentrates and antifibrinolytic amino acids may carry a high risk of thrombotic complications.

## Thrombocytopenic Bleeding

The rationale for using antifibrinolytic amino acids to prevent or treat bleeding in individuals with immune or nonimmune thrombocytopenia is that these agents may facilitate hemostasis by maintaining hemostatic clots. There are no double-blind, controlled studies examining this, but two studies do indicate that EACA successfully controls bleeding in individuals with thrombocytopenia, thus reducing the need for platelet transfusion (98, 99). Bleeding symptoms that respond more promptly to EACA are those in the mucosal tracts (i.e., epistaxis, vaginal, gastrointestinal) and those asso-

ciated with dental extractions. In the most recent of the two studies, EACA was effective at a lower dosage than that usually recommended (a loading dose of 5 g given orally or by intravenous infusion, followed by 1 g every 4 hours until the bleeding has stopped) (99).

## Disseminated Intravascular Coagulation

During disseminated intravascular coagulation, hyperfibrinolysis usually is secondary to thrombin formation and fibrin deposition. Hence, inhibition of fibrinolysis by EACA or tranexamic acid is unjustified and even may be dangerous, thus favoring fibrin deposition and organ failure.

Hyperfibrinolysis, however, may be important in the determination of bleeding in acute promyelocytic leukemia. A small, double-blind trial comparing individuals treated with a large daily dose of tranexamic acid (6 g/day by continuous intravenous infusion) with placebo (100) showed that the treated individuals had fewer hemorrhagic episodes, fewer transfusions of packed red cells, and less need for platelet concentrates. This study is small and does not address the most important issue—whether fatal episodes of bleeding are reduced by this treatment.

More recently, the efficacy of tranexamic acid in reducing bleeding and platelet transfusions during chemotherapy has been evaluated in individuals with acute myelogenous leukemia (101). During remission induction, there were no significant differences between treated and untreated individuals, but during consolidation chemotherapy, there was a significantly lower bleeding tendency in the individuals treated with tranexamic acid, thus resulting in a lower requirement for platelet transfusion (101). These results are promising but require confirmation before tranexamic acid can be recommended for all individuals with acute myelogenous leukemia.

## Bleeding after Thrombolytic Treatment

Extensive use of thrombolytic agents for treatment of individuals with myocardial infarction has reopened the problem of the best approach to bleeding complications from this treatment. Antifibrinolytic amino acids are effective for this purpose, and they should be given when bleeding is profuse and occurs in dangerous sites. In most individuals, however, there is no need for their use, because discontinuing infusion of the thrombolytic agent usually is sufficient to control bleeding.

## Reducing Surgical Blood Loss

In individuals undergoing open heart surgery (see Chapter 50), EACA or tranexamic acid reduces blood loss by 30 to 40% in the perioperative and the postoperative periods (102). The intravenous doses generally are large:

100–150 mg/kg for EACA, or 10–15 mg/kg of tranexamic acid, given in bolus before chest opening and usually repeated either as another bolus at chest closure or by continuous infusion throughout the operation. As mentioned, other drugs, such as DDAVP and aprotinin, can be used prophylactically to reduce bleeding.

Knee arthroplasty is another surgery associated with large losses of blood and transfusion requirements. Individuals treated with a single dose of tranexamic acid, 10 mg/kg, before releasing the tourniquet lost a smaller amount of blood than those treated with placebo (mean values, 730 ± 280 mL versus 1410 ± 480 mL) (103). This impressive reduction was accompanied by a statistically significant reduction in the units of blood transfused (103). Similar results were obtained in a smaller study (104). Whether this prophylactic treatment should be routine remains to be established by a cost–benefit analysis.

The main indications for antifibrinolytic amino acids are summarized in Table 53.8.

## SIDE EFFECTS

Side effects of EACA and tranexamic acid are dose-dependent and usually involve the gastrointestinal tract (e.g., nausea, abdominal pain, vomiting and diarrhea). Side effects related to the musculoskeletal and central nervous system are more rare and include myopathy, myoglobinuria, headache, diarrhea, and very rarely, delirium and seizures. Such side effects are less frequent with tranexamic acid, perhaps because its effective dosage is lower than that of EACA. Considering that established clinical indications for synthetic antifibrinolytic amino acids (Table 53.8) entail short periods of administration, side effects rarely are so intolerable that treatment must be interrupted.

There is concern that by inhibiting fibrinolysis, which is a naturally occurring defense mechanism against thrombus formation, EACA and tranexamic acid might carry a high risk of thrombotic complications. This risk has not been convincingly substantiated, however, even when the compounds were given in those situations accompanied by a high risk of thrombosis, such as prostatectomy, knee arthroplasty, and during pregnancy (103–106). Nevertheless, these compounds should be used with caution when elderly individuals undergoing prostatectomy have evidence of ischemic heart disease or cerebrovascular disease. With EACA or tranexamic acid, clots cannot be lysed by the fibrinolytic system. Hence, EACA and tranexamic acid are contraindicated in individuals with hematuria originating from the upper urinary tract. They also are contraindicated in association with infusion of prothrombin complex concentrates to individuals with hemophilia B, because the concomitant use of antifibrinolytic amino acids magnifies the risk of thrombotic complications. Animal studies have demonstrated that lysine analogues are teratogenic, so they should be avoided in women during the first months of pregnancy.

# APROTININ

## BACKGROUND

Aprotinin was first proposed as a hemostatic agent in the 1960s, then was neglected for two decades. Interest rekindled with new studies in the late 1980s. In earlier studies, the total daily doses ranged between 200,000 and 1 million U. Subsequently, Royston et al (107) gave a larger total dose (approximately 6–7 million U) to individuals undergoing repeat cardiac surgery. The results were dramatic. Average blood loss of individuals treated with aprotinin was 81% lower than that of controls, and mean blood transfusion requirements were reduced by 91%, with most individuals requiring no homologous blood transfusion. These results were confirmed in individuals undergoing coronary artery bypass grafting, the most frequent cardiac surgical procedure (108–111). Spectacular results in cardiac surgery led to use of high-dose aprotinin during liver transplantation (112, 113), in which there is great loss of blood, and peripheral vascular surgery (114).

## PHARMACOLOGY

Extracted from homogenates of bovine lungs or produced by recombinant technology, aprotinin is a basic polypeptide with a molecular weight of 6512 daltons and is composed of 58 amino acid residues (115). Its activity is expressed in kallikrein inhibitory units (KIU), with 1 KIU being the quantity of aprotinin that reduces the biologic activity of 2 U of kallikrein by 50%. One milligram of aprotinin is equivalent to 7143 KIU. Aprotinin is inactive when given orally. Elimination from plasma occurs with a half-life of 37 to 50 minutes (115). Therefore, the most effective method of administration, which produces stable plasma levels and makes possible reduction of the total dose, is continuous intravenous infusion preceded by bolus infusion.

## MECHANISM OF ACTION

A broad-spectrum inhibitor of serine proteases, aprotinin acts at several steps in the hemostatic system. The inhibitory effects on trypsin, chymotrypsin, plasmin, and kallikrein are well established (115, 116). By inhibiting kallikrein, aprotinin indirectly inhibits formation of factor XIIa and, hence, initiation of the coagulation cascade induced by contact of blood with foreign surfaces (117). Contact-phase activation via factor XIIa and kallikrein also activates the fibrinolytic system. Through the inhibition of kallikrein, aprotinin also reduces activation of the complement and angiotensin systems as well as the inflammatory responses initiated by kallikrein. Aprotinin inhibits another serine protease, activated protein C, that has anticoagulant and fibrinolytic properties (118).

High-dose aprotinin prevents the prolonged bleeding time that occurs after cardiac surgery (108). Aprotinin does not have a direct effect on platelet function. Glycoprotein Ib, which is the platelet receptor involved in the interaction of platelets with von Willebrand factor and in platelet adhesion to the damaged or dysfunctional endothelium of blood vessels, is destroyed during passage of blood through the cardiopulmonary bypass system (119). This destruction may be mediated by contact with the foreign surfaces of the oxygenator and by proteolytic enzymes, such as calpain and elastase, released from damaged platelets and leukocytes. Another possible mechanism for loss of glycoprotein Ib might relate to the transformation of plasminogen bound to platelet membranes and the action of plasmin formed *in situ* on this glycoprotein (120). Because these proteolytic enzymes are inhibited by aprotinin and glycoprotein Ib is preserved by the inhibitor during cardiopulmonary bypass (119), the mechanism of action for aprotinin in facilitating hemostasis may relate to its direct antiprotease effect and the resulting effects on platelets.

The mechanisms of action for aprotinin during liver transplantation (see Chapter 45) are not necessarily the same as those postulated for cardiac surgery. A brisk increase in plasminogen activator activity, particularly during the anhepatic phase and early reperfusion of the graft, probably is the main pathogenetic factor underlying the large blood losses occurring in these individuals. Aprotinin is not a direct inhibitor of tissue-type plasminogen activator, but it may reduce indirectly the increased production through inhibitory effects on kallikrein, which converts single-chain, tissue-type plasminogen activator into the two-chain form (121).

## CLINICAL INDICATIONS AND DOSAGES

In cardiac surgery, the highly effective dosage schedule first proposed by Royston et al (107), and subsequently validated in other studies, is recommended (Table 53.9).

**TABLE 53.9.** Dosage for Aprotinin in Cardiac Surgery

| | |
|---|---|
| Loading dose | 2 million KIU before surgery, infused slowly over 20 minutes |
| Maintenance dose | 500,000 KIU/hour during surgery, until the wound is closed |
| Oxygenator | 2 million KIU |

*Data from Royston D, Bidstrup B, Taylor KM, et al. Effect of aprotinin on need for blood transfusion after repeat open heart surgery. Lancet 1987;ii:1289–1219.*

Using this schedule, the total amount of aprotinin for a 5-hour operation in a 70-kg individual is 6.5 million KIU. The cost of this treatment is very high ($980). Lower-dose schedules are less expensive (2 million KIU only in the oxygenator prime volume, $300; or 30,000 KIU/kg in the oxygenator prime volume and 7500 KIU/kg/hr, $600) and may be equally effective (122, 123). Additional clinical studies, however, are needed to establish the effectiveness of these low-dose schedules. Cost-effectiveness should be assessed to see whether the high costs of aprotinin are recovered through the reduction of transfusion requirements and transfusion-related illness.

At this point, a few conclusive comments on the relative merits of different hemostatic agents in open-heart surgery are warranted. Interest in the pharmacologic reduction of bleeding after cardiac surgery increased in the 1980s following recognition that the acquired immunodeficiency syndrome could result from transfusion of blood products contaminated with the human immunodeficiency virus. Four drugs have been evaluated:

1. DDAVP,
2. EACA,
3. Tranexamic acid, and
4. Aprotinin.

A few direct comparisons and a meta-analysis have demonstrated that these agents reduce blood loss (102). The order of efficacy from greatest to least is aprotinin, tranexamic acid, EACA, and DDAVP; the order of costs also is the same. Cost-effectiveness analyses are necessary to help clinicians in making a choice. Limiting use of aprotinin to individuals at increased risk for massive blood loss may be reasonable, but there currently are few clinical and laboratory criteria to permit identification of such high-risk individuals. Such existing criteria include reoperation, preexisting hemostatic defects, use of antiplatelet agents, and sepsis.

In the original, small study by Neuhaus et al (112), aprotinin was given at a low dosage (2 million KIU) in orthotopic liver transplantation and led to a 35% reduction in blood loss and a 50% reduction in the number of units of homologous red cell and plasma transfused. In a more recent study, Grosse et al (124) studied a larger group of individuals (25 treated and 25 untreated) and gave a larger dose: 2 million KIU after induction of anesthesia, followed by infusion of 0.5 million KIU/hour during the entire operation. They found an average 50% reduction in the requirement for homologous red cell concentrates, a 59% reduction in the requirement for plasma, and a 54% reduction in the requirement for platelets. At this time, liver transplantation is not an established indication for use of aprotinin as an hemostatic agent.

## SIDE EFFECTS

Potential side effects of aprotinin relate to the heterologous source and, in theory, to the risk that such a powerful hemostatic agent could lead to thrombotic events (e.g., myocardial infarction, stroke, early graft occlusion). Overall, data on the frequencies of such events stemming from individual studies are inconclusive because of their limited statistical power. A meta-analysis demonstrated that aprotinin reduced perioperative death by 15 to 22% when compared with placebo (102). Because a clinically important excess of thrombotic events would produce and increased rate of operative mortality, the small, favorable effect on mortality of aprotinin is encouraging, but specific studies should be designed to resolve this issue.

Caution is recommended in the rare situations requiring the reuse of aprotinin, such as repeat cardiac surgery. The likelihood of hypersensitivity reactions should be explored through a test dose before anesthesia. Theoretically, inhibition of the coagulation cascade induced by aprotinin could potentiate the anticoagulant action of heparin during cardiopulmonary bypass. Some investigators suggest that anticoagulation by heparin can be enhanced and requirements for heparin reduced by use of aprotinin (125), but it usually is not necessary to change the scheme of heparinization in individuals and the extracorporeal circuit. Because the activated clotting time (ACT) of heparinized whole blood is prolonged *in vitro* by aprotinin in a dose-dependent manner (126), caution also should be exercised when interpreting the ACT during cardiopulmonary bypass, and heparin dosing should not depend on the ACT alone.

# TOPICAL HEMOSTATIC AGENTS

When bleeding occurs at low pressure and at well-identified sites, attempts to stop blood loss by suture or cautery may be successful. In the past, attempts to control localized bleeding have included use of substances that should facilitate hemostasis when applied directly in solution at the sites of bleeding or through carriers such as gelatin, methylcellulose, or oxidized cellulose (i.e., topical hemostatic agents). The most commonly used of these substances is bovine thrombin, which is licensed both in the United States and in Europe. Other substances include snake venoms with thrombin-like or factor Xa-like activity. The limitation of this approach is that on occasion, the hemostatic substances tend to be washed away by flowing blood before they achieve local concentrations sufficient to stop bleeding.

Recently, however, a major breakthrough in this field was achieved with the availability of fibrin sealants (127–129). The improvement relates to the availability of a highly concentrated solution containing human fibrinogen and aprotinin (i.e., sealer solution). Transformation of fibrinogen into fibrin is achieved by adding calcium chloride and thrombin to the sealer solution.

Varying the thrombin concentrations permits the rate of fibrin formation to be modulated. Optimally, these substances are mixed together and applied to the bleeding site with a special device made of two syringes mounted on a Y-connector, to which a disposable needle is attached. The solution is quickly transformed into a glue that adheres firmly to the surface of the wound and is resorbed completely during wound healing without a foreign-body reaction or extensive fibrosis. Fibrin sealants are commercially manufactured and licensed in Europe, but at the moment, there is no licensed preparation in the United States.

At present, fibrin sealants mainly are used in cardiovascular surgery (130). In a randomized, clinical trial in individuals undergoing reoperations (131), there was a 92% success rate for fibrin sealant in controlling localized bleeding, compared with a 12% success rate for conventional topical hemostatic agents (i.e., collagen, gelatin, and celluloses). There also was less postoperative blood loss, and the reoperation rate was lower. The fibrin sealant was particularly effective in control of diffuse bleeding from raw surfaces or damaged tissues, but it also was useful in control of oozing from puncture sites and suture lines. Fibrin sealant is valuable in middle-ear reconstructive surgery, nasal septum surgery, and to control posttonsillectomy hemorrhage in ear, nose, and throat surgery, to facilitate peripheral nerve reconstruction and repair dural defects in neurosurgery, to fix skin grafts without need for sutures in plastic surgery, to control bleeding from parenchymal organs abdominal surgery, and for repair of chondral and osteochondral injuries in orthopaedic surgery (127–129).

Fibrin sealants also are useful during minor surgical procedures in individuals with congenital bleeding disorders, typically dental extraction and circumcision. The topical application of these substances often permits reduction or avoidance of factor concentrate infusions, particularly if synthetic antifibrinolytic amino acids are given in combination, locally, or systemically (132). In addition, fibrin sealants are useful for minor surgery in individuals receiving oral anticoagulants (133); the advantage is that anticoagulants need not be discontinued and hospital admission can be avoided.

Fibrin sealants have few side effects. The risk of transmitting blood-borne viruses is minimized by accurate selection of donors and use of virucidal methods, such as pasteurization or steam heating, applied to the fibrinogen constituting the glue. To my knowledge, no case of blood-borne infection has been reported. As with all topical hemostatic preparations containing bovine thrombin, there is a small risk for development of antibodies that cross react with endogenous human coagulation proteins and that might prolong coagulation tests (134). The most consistent laboratory index for the occurrence of this abnormality is a prolonged bovine thrombin clotting time, which corrects, at least partially, when human thrombin is substituted for bovine thrombin. Some individuals exposed to fibrin sealants may develop factor V inhibitors that manifest as prolonged prothrombin and activated partial thromboplastin times (134). The clinical course of this complication varies from totally asymptomatic to life-threatening bleeding. Therapeutic intervention is largely empiric and depends on the clinical manifestations in the individual individual.

# REFERENCES

1. Cash JD, Gader AM, da Costa J. Proceedings: the release of plasminogen activator and factor VIII by LVP, AVP, DDAVP, AT III, and OT in man. Br J Haematol 1974;27:363–364.
2. Mannucci PM, Aberg M, Nilsson IM et al. Mechanism of plasminogen activator and factor VIII increase after vasoactive drugs. Br J Haematol 1975;30:81–93.
3. Mannucci PM, Pareti FI, Holmberg L et al. Studies on the prolonged bleeding time in von Willebrand disease. J Lab Clin Med 1976;88:662–671.
4. Mannucci PM, Ruggeri ZM, Pareti FI et al. 1-Deamino-8-D-arginine vasopressin: a new pharmacological approach to the management of haemophilia and von Willebrand's disease. Lancet 1977;i:869–872.
5. Warrier AI, Lusher JM. DDAVP: a useful alternative to blood components in moderate hemophilia A and von Willebrand disease. J Pediatr 1983; 102:228–233.
6. Mariana G, Ciavarella N, Mazzucconi MG et al. Evaluation of the effectiveness of DDAVP in surgery and bleeding episodes in hemophilia and von Willebrand's disease. A study of 43 patients. Clin Lab Hematol 1984;6: 229–238.
7. Kobrinsky NL, Israels ED, Gerrard JM et al. Shortening of bleeding time by 1-deamino-8-D-arginine vasopressin in various bleeding disorders. Lancet 1984;i:1145–1148.
8. de la Fuente B, Kasper CK, Rickles FR et al. Response of patients with mild and moderate hemophilia A and von Willebrand's disease to treatment with desmopressin. Ann Intern Med 1985;103:6–14.
9. Mannucci PM, Remuzzi G, Pusineri F et al. Deamino-8-D-arginine vasopressin shortens the bleeding time in uremia. N Engl J Med 1983;308:8–12.
10. Mannucci PM, Vicente V, Vianello L et al. Controlled trial of desmopressin (DDAVP) in liver cirrhosis and other conditions associated with a prolonged bleeding time. Blood 1986;67:148–1153.
11. Schulman S, Johnsson H. Heparin, DDAVP and the bleeding time. Thromb Haemost 1991;65:242–244.
12. Johnstone MT, Andrews T, Ware JA et al. Bleeding time prolongation with streptokinase and its reduction with 1-deamino-8-D-arginine vasopressin. Circulation 1990;82:2142–2151.
13. Flordal PA, Ljungstrom KG, Svensson J. Desmopressin reverses effects of dextran on von Willebrand factor. Thromb Haemost 1989;61:541.
14. Anonymous. Can drugs reduce surgical blood loss? Lancet 1988;i:155–156.
15. Mannucci PM, Vicente V, Alberca I et al. Intravenous and subcutaneous administration of desmopressin (DDAVP) to hemophiliacs: pharmacokinetics and factor VIII responses. Thromb Haemost 1987;58:1037–1039.
16. Lethagen S, Harris AS, Sjorin E et al. Intranasal and intravenous administration of desmopressin: effect on FVIII/vWf pharmacokinetics and reproducibility. Thromb Haemost 1987;58:1033–1036.
17. Lethagen S, Harris AS, Nilsson IM. Intranasal desmopressin (DDAVP) by spray in mild hemophilia A and von Willebrand's disease type I. Blut 1990;60:187–191.
18. Levi M, de Boer JP, Roem D et al. Plasminogen activation in vivo upon intravenous infusion of DDAVP. Quantitative assessment of plasmin-alpha 2-antiplasmin complex with a novel monoclonal antibody based radioimmunoassay. Thromb Haemost 1992;67:111–116.
19. Kobrinsky NL, Doyle JJ, Israels ED et al. Absent factor VIII response to synthetic vasopressin analogue (DDAVP) in nephrogenic diabetes insipidus. Lancet 1985;i:1293–1294.
20. Booyse FM, Osikowicz G, Feder S. Effects of various agents on ristocetin-Willebrand factor activity in long-term cultures of von Willebrand and normal human umbilical vein endothelial cells [Letter]. Thromb Haemost 1981;46:668.
21. Hashemi S, Tackaberry ES, Palmer DS et al. DDAVP-induced release of von Willebrand factor from endothelial cells in vitro: the effect of plasma and blood cells. Biochim Biophys Acta 1990;1052:63–70.
22. Ruggeri ZM, Mannucci PM, Lombardi R et al. Multimeric composition of factor VIII/von Willebrand factor following administration of DDAVP: implications for pathophysiology and therapy of von Willebrand's disease subtypes. Blood 1982;59:1272–1278.
23. Mannucci PM, Canciani MT, Rota L et al. Response of factor VIII/von Willebrand factor to DDAVP in healthy subjects and patients with haemophilia A and von Willebrand's disease. Br J Haematol 1981;47:283–293.
24. Mannucci PM, Bettega D, Cattaneo M. Patterns of development of tachyphylaxis in patients with haemophilia and von Willebrand disease after repeated doses of desmopressin (DDAVP). Br J Haematol 1992;82:87–93.
25. Rodeghiero F, Castaman G, Mannucci PM. Prospective multicenter study on subcutaneous concentrated desmopressin for home treatment of patients with von Willebrand disease and mild or moderate hemophilia A. Thromb Haemost 1996;76:692–696.
26. Rose EH, Aledort LM. Nasal spray desmopressin (DDAVP) for mild hemophilia A and von Willebrand disease. Ann Intern Med 1991;114:563–568.
27. DiMichele DM, Hathaway WE. Use of DDAVP in inherited and acquired platelet dysfunction. Am J Hematol 1990;33:39–45.
28. Gotti E, Mecca G, Valentino C et al. Renal biopsy in patients with acute renal failure and prolonged bleeding time. Lancet 1984;ii:978.
29. Canavese C, Salomone M, Paciti A et al. Reduced response of uraemic bleeding time to repeated doses of desmopressin. Lancet 1985;i:867.
30. Burroughs AK, Matthews K, Qadiri M et al. Desmopressin and bleeding time in patients with cirrhosis. Br Med J 1985;291:1377–1381.
31. de Franchis R, Arcidiacono PG, Carpinelli L et al. Randomized controlled trial of desmopressin plus terlipressin vs. terlipressin alone for the treatment of acute variceal hemorrhage in cirrhotic patients: a multicenter, double-blind study. Hepatology 1993;18:1102–1107.
32. Bove CM, Casey B, Marder VJ. DDAVP reduces bleeding during continued hirudin administration in the rabbit. Thromb Haemost 1996;75:471–475.
33. Salzman EW, Weinstein MJ, Weintraub RM et al. Treatment with desmopressin acetate to reduce blood loss after cardiac surgery. N Engl J Med 1986;314:1402–1406.
34. Rocha E, Llorens R, Paramo JA et al. Does desmopressin acetate reduce blood loss after surgery in patients on cardiopulmonary bypass? Circulation 1988;77:1319–1323.
35. Hackmann T, Gascoyne R, Naiman SC et al. A trial of desmopressin to reduce blood loss in uncomplicated cardiac surgery. N Engl J Med 1989; 321:1437–1443.
36. Andersson TL, Solem JO, Tengborn L et al. Effects of desmopressin acetate on platelet aggregation, von Willebrand factor and blood loss after cardiac surgery with extracorporeal circulation. Circulation 1990;81:872–878.
37. Seear MD, Wadsworth LD, Rogers PC et al. The effect of desmopressin acetate (DDAVP) on postoperative blood loss after cardiac operations in children. J Thorac Cardiovasc Surg 1989;98:217–219.
38. Cattaneo M, Harris AS, Stromberg U et al. The effect of desmopressin on reducing blood loss in cardiac surgery: a meta-analysis of double-blind, placebo-controlled trials. Thromb Haemost 1995;74:1064–1070.
39. Rocha E, Hidalgo F, Llorens R et al. Randomized study of aprotinin and DDAVP to reduce postoperative bleeding after cardiopulmonary surgery. Circulation 1994;90:921–927.
40. Kobrinsky NL, Letts RM, Patel LR et al. 1-Desamino-8-D-arginine vasopressin (desmopressin) decreases operative blood loss in patients having Harrington rod spinal fusion surgery. A randomized, double-blinded, controlled trial. Ann Intern Med 1987;107:446–450.
41. Johnson RG, Murphy JM. The role of desmopressin in reducing blood loss during lumbar fusion. Surg Gynecol Obstet 1990;171:223–226.
42. Shepherd LL, Hutchinson RJ, Worden EK et al. Hyponatremia and seizures after intravenous administration of desmopressin acetate for surgical hemostasis. J Pediatr 1989;114:470–472.
43. Smith TJ, Gill JC, Ambruso DR et al. Hyponatremia and seizures in young children given DDAVP. Am J Hematol 1989;31:99–202.
44. Anonymous. Desmopressin and arterial thrombosis [Editorial]. Lancet 1989;i:938–939.
45. Mannucci PM, Lusher JM. Desmopressin and thrombosis [Letter]. Lancet 1989;ii:675–676.
46. Mannucci PM, Carlsson S, Harris AS. Desmopressin, surgery and thrombosis. Thromb Haemost 1994;71:154–155.
47. Liu YK, Kosfeld RE, Marcum SG. Treatment of uremic bleeding with conjugated oestrogen. Lancet 1984;ii:887–890.
48. Livio M, Mannucci PM, Vigano G et al. Conjugated estrogens for the management of bleeding associated with renal failure. N Engl J Med 1986;315: 731–735.
49. Viganò G, Zoia C, Corna D et al. 17β-Estradiol is the most active component of the conjugated estrogen mixture active on uremic bleeding by a receptor mechanism. J Pharmacol Exp Ther 1990;252:344–348.
50. Viganò G, Gaspari F, Locatelli M et al. Dose-effect and pharmacokinetics of estrogens given to correct bleeding time in uremia. Kidney Int 1988;34: 853–858.
51. Shemin D, Elnour, Amarantes B et al. Oral estrogens decrease bleeding time and improve clinical bleeding in patients with renal failure. Am J Med 1990;89:436–440.
52. Zoja C, Viganò G, Bergamelli A et al. Prolonged bleeding time and increased vascular prostacyclin in rats with chronic renal failure: effects of conjugated estrogens. J Lab Clin Med 1988;112:380–386.

53. Heistinger M, Stockembuer F, Schneider B et al. Effect of conjugated estrogens on platelet function and prostacyclin generation in CRF. Kidney Int 1990;38:1181–1186.
54. Zoja C, Viganò G, Corna D et al. Oral zeranol shortens the prolonged bleeding time of uremic rats. Kidney Int 1990;38:96–100.
55. Steiner RW, Coggins C, Carvalho ACA. Bleeding time in uremia: a useful test to assess clinical bleeding. Am J Hematol 1979;7:107–117.
56. Winearls CG, Oliver DO, Pippard MJ et al. Effect of human erythropoietin derived from recombinant DNA on the anaemia of patients maintained by chronic haemodialysis. Lancet 1986;ii:1175–1178.
57. Eschbach JW, Egrie JC, Downing MR et al. Correction of the anemia of end-stage renal disease with recombinant human erythropoietin. N Engl J Med 1987;316:73–78.
58. Livio M, Gotti E, Marchesi D et al. Uraemic bleeding: role of anaemia and beneficial effect of red cell transfusions. Lancet 1982;ii:1013–1015.
59. Moia M, Mannucci PM, Vizzotto L et al. Improvement in the haemostatic defect of uraemia after treatment with recombinant human erythropoietin. Lancet 1987;ii:1227–1229.
60. van Geet C, Hauglustaine D, Verresen L et al. Haemostatic effects of recombinant human erythropoietin in chronic haemodialysis patients. Thromb Haemost 1989;61:117–121.
61. Zwaginga JJ, Ijsseldijk MJ, de Groot PG et al. Treatment of uremic anemia with recombinant erythropoietin also reduces the defects in platelet adhesion and aggregation caused by uremic plasma. Thromb Haemost 1991; 66:638–647.
62. Viganò G, Benigni A, Mendogni D et al. Recombinant human erythropoietin to correct uremic bleeding. Am J Kidney Dis 1991;18:44–49.
63. Krantz SB. Erythropoietin. Blood 1991;77:419–434.
64. Macdougall IC, Roberts DE, Neubert P et al. Pharmacokinetics of recombinant human erythropoietin in patients on continuous ambulatory peritoneal dialysis. Lancet 1989;i:425–427.
65. Bommer J, Ritz E, Weinrich T et al. Subcutaneous erythropoietin. Lancet 1988;ii:406.
66. Remuzzi G. Bleeding in renal failure. Lancet 1988;i:1205–1208.
67. Turitto VT, Baumgartner HR. Platelet interaction with subendothelium in a perfusion system: physical role of red blood cells. Microvasc Res 1975; 9:335–344.
68. Aarts PA, Bolhuis PA, Sakariassen KS et al. Red blood cell size is important for adherence of blood platelets to artery subendothelium. Blood 1983;62: 214–217.
69. Taylor JE, Henderson IS, Stewart WK et al. Erythropoietin and spontaneous platelet aggregation in haemodialysis patients. Lancet 1991;338: 1361–1362.
70. Valles J, Santos MT, Aznar J et al. Erythrocytes metabolically enhance collagen-induced platelet responsiveness via increased thromboxane production, adenosine diphosphate release and recruitment. Blood 1991;78: 154–162.
71. Van Geet C, Van Damme-Lombaerts R, Van Russelt M et al. Recombinant human erythropoietin increases blood pressure, platelet aggregability and platelet free calcium mobilisation in uraemic children: a possible link? Thromb Haemost 1990;64:7–10.
72. Gordge MP, Leaker B, Patel A et al. Recombinant human erythropoietin shortens the uraemic bleeding time without causing intravascular haemostatic activation. Thromb Res 1990;57:171–182.
73. Schaefer RM, Leschke M, Strauer BE et al. Blood rheology and hypertension in hemodialysis patients treated with erythropoietin. Am J Nephrol 1988;8:449–453.
74. Eschbach JW, Abdulhadi MH, Browne JK et al. Recombinant human erythropoietin in anemic patients with end-stage renal disease. Results of phase III multicenter clinical trials. Ann Intern Med 1989;111:992–1000.
75. Okamoto S, Hijikata A. Rational approach to proteinase inhibitors. Drug Design 1975;6:143–153.
76. Okamoto S, Nakajima T, Okamoto U et al. A suppressing effect of E-amino-n-caproic acid on the bleeding of dogs, produced with the activation of plasmin in the circulating blood. Keio J Med 1959;8:247–266.
77. McNicol GP, Fletcher AP, Alkjaersig N et al. The absorption, distribution and excretion of epsilon-aminocaproic acid following oral or intravenous administration to man. J Lab Clin Med 1962;59:15–21.
78. Andersson L, Nilsson IM, Nilhen JE et al. Experimental and clinical studies on AMCA, the antifibrinolytically active isomer of p-aminoethyl cyclohexane carboxylic acid. Scand J Hematol 1965;2:230–247.
79. Thorsen S. Differences in the binding to fibrin of native plasminogen and plasminogen modified by proteolytic degradation. Influence of omega-aminocarboxylic acids. Biochim Biophys Acta 1975;393:55–65.
80. Hoylaerts M, Lijnen HR, Collen D. Studies on the mechanism of antifibrinolytic action of tranexamic acid. Biochim Biophys Acta 1981;673:75–85.
81. Bonnar J, Sheppard BL. Treatment of menorrhagia during menstruation: randomized controlled trial of ethamsylate, mefenamic acid and tranexamic acid. Br Med J 1996;313:579–582.
82. Von Holstein CC, Eriksson SBS, Kallen R. Tranexamic acid as an aid to reducing blood transfusion requirements in gastric and duodenal bleeding. Br Med J 1987;294:7–10.
83. Mowatt NA, Douglas AS, Brunt PW et al. Epsilon-aminocaproic acid therapy in ulcerative colitis. Am J Dig Dis 1973;18:959–965.
84. Hollanders D, Thomson JM, Schofield PF. Tranexamic acid therapy in ulcerative colitis. Postgrad Med J 1983;58:87–91.
85. Miller RA, May MW, Hendry WF et al. The prevention of secondary haemorrhage after prostatectomy: the value of antifibrinolytic therapy. Br J Urol 1980;52:26–28.
86. Tovi D, Nilsson IM, Thulin CA. Fibrinolytic activity of the cerebrospinal fluid after subarachnoid haemorrhage. Acta Neurol Scand 1972;49:1–9.
87. Tovi D, Nilsson IM, Thulin CA. Fibrinolysis and subarachnoid hemorrhage. Inhibitory effect of tranexamic acid. A clinical study. Acta Neurol Scand 1972;48:393–402.
88. Vermeulen M, Lindsay KW, Murray GD et al. Antifibrinolytic treatment in subarachnoid hemorrhage. N Engl J Med 1984;311:432–437.
89. Adams HP Jr, Kassel NF, Torner JC et al. Predicting cerebral ischemia after aneurysmal subarachnoid hemorrhage: influences of clinical condition, CT results and antifibrinolytic therapy. A report of the Cooperative Aneurysm Study. Neurology 1987;37:586–1591.
90. Verstraete M, Tyberghein J, Degreef Y et al. Double-blind trials with ethamsylate, batroxobin or tranexamic acid on blood loss after adenotonsillectomy. Acta Clin Belg 1977;32:36–141.
91. Varnek L, Dalsgaard C, Hansen A et al. The effect of tranexamic acid on secondary haemorrhage after traumatic hyphaema. Acta Ophthalmol 1980;58:787–793.
92. Bennett AE, Ingram GI, Inglish PJ. Antifibrinolytic treatment in haemophilia: a controlled trial of prophylaxis with tranexamic acid. Br J Haematol 1973;24:83–88.
93. Rainsford SG, Jouhar AJ, Hall A. Tranexamic acid in the control of spontaneous bleeding in severe hemophilia. Thromb Diath Hemorrh 1973;30: 272–279.
94. Sindet-Pedersen S. Distribution of tranexamic acid to plasma and saliva after oral administration and mouth rinsing: a pharmacokinetic study. J Clin Pharmacol 1987;27:1005–1008.
95. Walsh PN, Rizza CR, Matthews JM et al. Epsilon-aminocaproic acid therapy for dental extraction in haemophilia and Christmas disease: a double-blind controlled trial. Br J Haematol 1971;20:463–475.
96. Forbes CD, Barr RD, Reid G et al. Tranexamic acid in control of haemorrhage after dental extraction in haemophilia and Christmas disease. Br Med J 1972;2:311–313.
97. Sindet-Pedersen S, Stenbjerg S. Effect of local antifibrinolytic treatment with tranexamic acid in hemophiliacs undergoing oral surgery. J Oral Maxillofac Surg 1986;44:703–707.
98. Gardner FH, Helmer RE. Aminocaproic acid. Use in control of hemorrhage in patients with amegakaryocytic thrombocytopenia. JAMA 1980;243: 35–37.
99. Bartholomew JR, Salgia R, Bell WR. Control of bleeding in patients with immune and nonimmune thrombocytopenia with aminocaproic acid. Arch Intern Med 1989;149:1959–1961.
100. Avvisati G, ten Cate JW, Buller HR et al. Tranexamic acid for control of haemorrhage in acute promyelocytic leukaemia. Lancet 1989;ii:122–124.
101. Shpilberg O, Blumenthal R, Sofer O et al. A controlled trial of tranexamic acid therapy for the reduction of bleeding during treatment of acute myeloid leukemia. Leuk Lymphoma 1995;19:141–144.
102. Fremes SE, Wong BI, Lee E et al. Metaanalysis of prophylactic drug treatment in the prevention of postoperative bleeding. Ann Thorac Surg 1994; 58:1580–1588.
103. Benoni G, Fredin H. Fibrinolytic inhibition with tranexamic acid reduces blood loss and blood transfusion after knee arthroplasty: a prospective, randomized, double blind study of 86 patients. J Bone Joint Surg Br 1996; 78:434–440.
104. Hiippala S, Strid L, Wennerstrand M et al. Tranexamic acid (Cyclokapron) reduces perioperative blood loss associated with total knee arthroplasty. Br J Anesth 1995;74:534–537.
105. Vinnicombe J, Shuttleworth KE. Aminocaproic acid in the control of haemorrhage after prostatectomy. A controlled trial. Lancet 1966;i:230–232.
106. Lindoff C, Rybo G, Astedt B. Treatment with tranexamic acid during pregnancy, and the risk of thrombo-embolic complications. Thromb Haemost 1993;70:238–240.
107. Royston D, Bidstrup B, Taylor KM et al. Effect of aprotinin on need for blood transfusion after repeat open heart surgery. Lancet 1987;ii: 1289–1291.
108. Bidstrup BP, Royston D, Sapsford RN, Taylor KM. Reduction in blood loss and blood use after cardiopulmonary bypass with high dose aprotinin. J Thorac Cardiovasc Surg 1989;97:364–372.
109. Fraedrich G, Weber C, Bernard C et al. Reduction of blood transfusion requirement in open heart surgery by administration of high doses of aprotinin-preliminary results. Thorac Cardiovasc Surg 1989;37:89–91.
110. Dietrich W, Spannagl M, Jochum M et al. Influence of high-dose aprotinin treatment on blood loss and coagulation patterns in patients undergoing myocardial revascularization. Anesthesiology 1990;73:1119–1126.
111. Harder MP, Eijsman L, Roozendaal KJ et al. Aprotinin reduces intraoperative and postoperative blood loss in membrane oxygenator cardiopulmonary bypass. Ann Thorac Surg 1991;51:936–941.

112. Neuhaus P, Bechstein WO, Lefebre B et al. Effect of aprotinin on intraoperative bleeding and fibrinolysis in liver transplantation. Lancet 1989;ii: 924–925.

113. Mallet SV, Cox D, Burroughs AK et al. Aprotinin and reduction of blood loss and transfusion requirements in orthotopic liver transplantation. Lancet 1990;336:886–887.

114. Thompson JF, Roath OS, Francis JL et al. Aprotinin in peripheral vascular surgery. Lancet 1990;335:911.

115. Fritz H, Wunderer G. Biochemistry and applications of aprotinin, the kallikrein inhibitor from bovine organs. Arzneimittelforschung 1983;33: 479–494.

116. Dubber AH, McNicol GP, Uttley D et al. *In vitro* and *in vivo* studies with trasylol, an anticoagulant and a fibrinolytic inhibitor. Br J Haematol 1968; 14:31–49.

117. Kluft C. Pathomechanisms of defective hemostasis during and after extracorporeal circulation: contact phase activation. In: Friedel N, Hetzer R, Royston D, eds. Blood use in cardiac surgery. New York: Steinkopff, Darmstadt, and Springer, 1991:10–15.

118. Espana F, Estelles A, Griffin JH et al. Aprotinin is a competitive inhibitor of activated protein C. Thromb Res 1989;56:751–756.

119. Van Oeveren W, Eijsman L, Roozendaal KJ et al. Platelet preservation by aprotinin during cardiopulmonary bypass. Lancet 1988;i:644.

120. Cramer EM, Lu H, Caen JP et al. Differential redistribution of platelet glycoproteins Ib and IIb-IIIa after plasmin stimulation. Blood 1991;77: 694–699.

121. Hunt BJ, Cottam S, Segal H et al. Inhibition by aprotinin of t-PA mediated fibrinolysis during orthotopic liver transplantation. Lancet 1990;336:381.

122. Lavee J, Raviv Z, Smolinsky A et al. Platelet protection by low-dose aprotinin in cardiopulmonary bypass: electron microscopic study. Ann Thorac Surg 1993;55:114–119.

123. Kawasuji M, Ueyama K, Sakakibora N et al. Effect of low-dose aprotinin on coagulation and fibrinolysis in cardiopulmonary bypass. Ann Thorac Surg 1993;55:1205–1209.

124. Grosse H, Lobles W, Frambach M et al. The use of high dose aprotinin in liver transplantation: the influence on fibrinolysis and blood loss. Thromb Res 1991;63:287–297.

125. de Smet AA, Joen MC, van Oeveren W et al. Increased anticoagulation during cardiopulmonary bypass by aprotinin. J Thorac Cardiovasc Surg 1990;100:520–527.

126. Hunt B, Segal H, Yacoub M. Monitoring heparin by the activated clotting time when aprotinin is used during cardiopulmonary bypass. Thromb Haemost 1991;65:1025.

127. Matras H. Fibrin seal: the state of the art. J Oral Maxillofac Surg 1985;43: 605–611.

128. Gibble JW, Ness PM. Fibrin glue: the perfect operative sealant? Transfusion 1990;30:741–747.

129. Brennan M. Fibrin glue. Blood Rev 1991;5:240–244.

130. Borst HG, Haverich A, Walterbusch G et al. Fibrin adhesive: an important hemostatic adjunct in cardiovascular operations. J Thorac Cardiovasc Surg 1982;84:548–553.

131. Rousou J, Levitsky S, Gonzales-Lavin L et al. Randomized clinical trial of fibrin sealant in patients undergoing resternotomy or reoperation after cardiac operations. A multicenter study. J Thorac Cardiovasc Surg 1989; 97:194–203.

132. Martinowitz U, Schulman S. Fibrin sealant in surgery of patients with a hemorrhagic diathesis. Thromb Haemost 1995;74:486–492.

133. Ginelli G, Bucciarelli P, Misani M et al. Fibrin glue plus tranexamic acid mouthwashing in patients on oral anticoagulants undergoing dental extractions [Abstract]. Thromb Haemost 1995;73:1464.

134. Ortel TL, Charles LA, Keller FG et al. Topical thrombin and acquired coagulation factor inhibitors: clinical spectrum and laboratory diagnosis. Am J Hematol 1994;45:128–135.

# SECTION 12

# MANAGEMENT OF THROMBOSIS

# CHAPTER 54

# PHARMACOLOGY OF ANTIPLATELET AGENTS

Carlo Patrono

## ASPIRIN

Acetylsalicylic acid, first synthesized by the German chemist Felix Hoffmann at Bayer AG in 1897, was introduced into medicine in 1899 under the name *aspirin*. The drug has a number of pharmacologic effects, which are characterized by markedly different dose–response relationships in man. Thus, an antiplatelet effect occurs with doses as low as 30 to 75 mg, analgesic and antipyretic effects require at least 300 mg, and an anti-inflammatory effect requires daily doses in excess of 2000 mg, and possibly even 4000 to 5000 mg (1). Moreover, these diverse pharmacologic effects have remarkably different durations, from a few hours to a few days. This is reflected in the drug being used once daily as an antiplatelet agent and four to six times daily as an analgesic or anti-inflammatory remedy. Such different dose and time relationships for the effects of aspirin are rather unusual, and they largely relate to its unique mechanism of action and short half-life in the human circulation.

## MECHANISM OF ACTION

Aspirin induces a long-lasting functional defect in platelets, which can be detectable clinically as a prolonged bleeding time. This appears to be primarily, if not exclusively, to permanent inactivation by aspirin of a key enzyme in platelet arachidonate metabolism. This enzyme, prostaglandin (PG) H-synthase, is responsible for the formation of $PGH_2$, the precursor of thromboxane (TX) $A_2$ (2). In human platelets, $TXA_2$ provides a mechanism

for amplifying the activation signal through its being synthesized and released in response to various platelet agonists (e.g., collagen, adenosine diphosphate [ADP], platelet-activating factor, thrombin) and, in turn, inducing irreversible aggregation (3) (see Chapter 12).

Aspirin selectively acetylates the hydroxyl group of a single serine residue at position 529 ($Ser^{529}$) within the polypeptide chain of platelet PGH-synthase (4, 5). This enzyme exhibits two distinct catalytic activities: a bisoxygenase (cyclo-oxygenase [COX]) involved in formation of $PGG_2$, and a hydroperoxidase allowing a net two-electron reduction in the 15-hydroperoxyl group of $PGG_2$, thus yielding $PGH_2$ (2). Through O-acetylation of $Ser^{529}$ by aspirin, the cyclooxygenase activity is lost permanently, whereas the hydroperoxidase activity is not affected (Fig. 54.1). Recently, an inducible form of PGH-synthase has been identified (6, 7) and termed *PGH-synthase 2* or *COX-2*. Aspirin inhibits the cyclooxygenase activity of PGH-synthase 2, but at higher concentrations than those required to inhibit PGH-synthase 1 or COX-1 (i.e., the constitutive enzyme). This may account, at least in part, for the different dose requirements of analgesic and anti-inflammatory versus antiplatelet effects of the drug.

Reduced formation of various eicosanoids (i.e., $TXA_2$, $PGE_2$, $PGI_2$) in different tissues probably accounts for the various pharmacologic effects of aspirin and forms the basis for both its therapeutic use and its toxicity (8). Because inactivation of PGH-synthase by aspirin is irreversible, *de novo* synthesis of the enzyme is required to restore normal eicosanoid formation. This oc-

**FIGURE 54.1.** Mechanism of the antiplatelet action of aspirin. Aspirin acetylates the hydroxyl group of a serine residue at position 529 (Ser$^{529}$) in the polypeptide chain of human platelet prostaglandin G/H synthase, resulting in the inactivation of its cyclooxygenase catalytic activity. Aspirin-induced blockade of prostaglandin $G_2$ synthesis results in decreased biosynthesis of prostaglandin $H_2$ and thromboxane $A_2$. (Adapted with permission from Patrono C. Aspirin as an antiplatelet drug. N Engl J Med 1994; 330:1287–1294.)

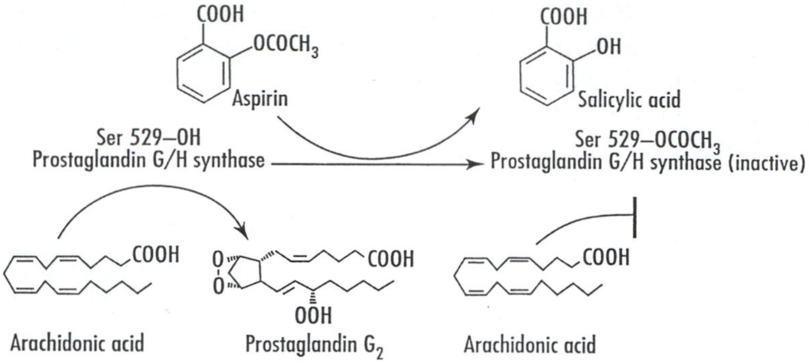

curs within hours in nucleated cells (e.g., endothelial cells), but cannot occur adequately in platelets that derive from fragmentation of the megakaryocyte cytoplasm and that have minimal protein synthesis. Thus, duration of the platelet and extraplatelet effects of a single dose varies considerably, ranging from several days to a few hours, respectively.

Alternative explanations have been proposed to explain the protective effect of aspirin against thrombosis (9–11). Thus, aspirin can acetylate other proteins, including the lysine residues of fibrinogen, although at higher concentrations and over longer periods of time than those required for acetylation of PGH-synthase. N-acetylated fibrinogen facilitates plasminogen activation and is less effective than unmodified fibrinogen at supporting platelet aggregation (11). Both the dose–response relationship and the clinical relevance of these additional effects, however, remain to be established. Similarly, high concentrations (>0.1 mM) of aspirin and sodium salicylate may have other effects *in vitro*, including inhibition of both DNA synthesis (12) and inducible nitric oxide synthase transcription (13) in fibroblasts, the relevance of which is largely unknown.

## PHARMACOKINETICS

Orally ingested aspirin is absorbed rapidly, partly from the stomach but mostly from the upper small intestine. This primarily occurs through passive diffusion of the nondissociated, lipid-soluble aspirin across the gastrointestinal membranes. Aspirin also is hydrolyzed by gastric and jejunal esterases and, therefore, is absorbed in part as salicylate. Such presystemic metabolism contributes to variable systemic bioavailability, which is a function of fluid and food ingestion. Systemic bioavailability of regular aspirin tablets is on the order of 40 to 50% in a range of doses from 20 to 1300 mg (14). Enteric-coated tablets and sustained-release microencapsulated preparations have a considerably lower bioavailability. Thus, different pharmaceutical formulations may deliver little, or even no, measurable aspirin to the systemic circulation. Because of acetylation of platelet PGH-synthase in

the presystemic circulation (14), however, the antiplatelet effect of aspirin is largely independent of systemic bioavailability. Both a controlled-release formulation (15) and a transdermal patch (16) of aspirin with very low systemic bioavailability have been developed to achieve selective inhibition of platelet $TXA_2$ production without suppressing systemic $PGI_2$ synthesis. The clinical relevance of the varying degrees of biochemical selectivity, however, remains to be established (discussed later).

The absorbed ester is rapidly hydrolyzed to salicylate in plasma, liver, lungs, and erythrocytes. The plasma half-life of aspirin is approximately 15 minutes. The plasma half-life for salicylate is dose-dependent and ranges from 2 to 12 hours.

Salicylate is further metabolized to salicyluric acid (i.e., the glycine conjugate), to the ether or phenolic glucuronide, and to the ester or acyl glucuronide. In addition, a small fraction is oxidized to 2,3-dihydroxybenzoic, 2,5-dihydroxybenzoic (i.e., gentisic acid), and 2,3,5-trihydroxybenzoic acids. With the possible exception of gentisic acid, no pharmacologic effects have been ascribed to these metabolites.

Salicylates are excreted mainly by the kidneys. The pharmacokinetics of aspirin have been approximated by an open, two-compartment model with first-order absorption, elimination, and metabolism from the central compartment.

## EFFECTS ON PLATELET BIOCHEMISTRY AND FUNCTION

The dose- and time-dependence of the antiplatelet effect of aspirin has been assessed using three distinct indices of platelet biochemistry and function: cyclooxygenase activity (17, 18), aggregation in response to various agonists (19), and forearm template bleeding time (20). Many studies assessing the pharmacodynamics of aspirin in humans have relied on measurements of serum $TXB_2$ as a reflection of thrombin-induced platelet $TXA_2$ production during whole blood clotting (17). This relatively simple method evaluates the capacity of platelets to synthesize $TXB_2$ in response to virtually maximal stimulation, and it by no means reflects the actual production rate of $TXB_2$ *in vivo*, which is several orders of magnitude lower (21).

When given orally to healthy subjects, aspirin inhibits $TXA_2$ production and $TXA_2$-dependent platelet function in a dose-dependent and time-dependent fashion (22, 23). A log-linear inhibition of platelet cyclooxygenase activity is found after single doses ranging from 10 to 100 mg. Moreover, such a dose–response relationship in healthy subjects is similar to that in individuals with atherosclerosis when assessed *ex vivo* by the same technique of determining $TXB_2$ production in whole blood. No consistent gender-related difference in the antiplatelet effect of aspirin has been described. The serum $TXB_2$ level is significantly reduced as early as 5 minutes after oral administration. Because no aspirin can be detected in peripheral venous blood at this time, acetylation of PGH-synthase during the first 5 minutes probably occurs by exposure of platelets to the drug in the presystemic circulation (14). Serum $TXB_2$ is maximally suppressed at between 30 and 60 minutes after oral aspirin, and it remains stable thereafter for as long as 24 hours, reflecting irreversible enzyme inactivation. There also is evidence that after a single dose of aspirin, the recovery of unacetylated platelet PGH-synthase (24) and enzyme activity (22) does not occur for approximately 48 hours. The 2-day lag in the return of functioning enzyme to the circulation indicates that aspirin acetylates PGH-synthase in the megakaryocyte.

Because of irreversible enzyme inactivation and lack of *de novo* enzyme synthesis in platelets, acetylation of platelet PGH-synthase and consequent inhibition of $TXA_2$ production by low-dose aspirin is cumulative with repeated dosing (22, 24). A log-linear relationship also exists between the oral dose of aspirin and inhibition of platelet $TXB_2$ production as measured at steady-state on repeated daily dosing (25). Comparing this dose–response relationship with that based on measurements performed after single dosing, an eightfold shift is apparent, with the $ID_{50}$ (dose required to inhibit enzyme activity by 50%) being approximately 3 and 26 mg, respectively (25). This finding suggests that the fractional dose necessary to achieve a given level of enzyme acetylation by virtue of cumulative effects, or for maintaining it after a full acetylating dose, approximately equals the fractional daily platelet turnover (i.e., 10–15% in healthy subjects) (25). Thus, for a given dose, both the rate at which cumulative acetylation occurs and its maximal extent essentially depend on the rate of platelet turnover and the dosing interval.

Given the greater variability of platelet aggregation measurements, relatively few investigators have correlated changes in platelet functional responses with variable degrees of $TXA_2$ inhibition as a function of aspirin

dosage. FitzGerald et al (23) studied five healthy subjects who received aspirin in daily doses of 20, 40, 80, 160, 325, 650, 1300, and 2600 mg. Each dose was given for 7 days, and ascending doses were administered in consecutive weeks. During this extended dose-ranging study, the aggregation response to ADP (maximal light transmittal [$T_{max}$] at 2.5, 5.0, and 10.0 μM) was measured as a marker of the platelet-inhibiting effect of aspirin. $T_{max}$ to ADP was reduced during the early weeks of the study, with the most pronounced changes in platelet response occurring at 20 to 80 mg/day. During the final 2 weeks (at 1300 and 2600 mg/day), however, the aggregation response returned to control values despite continuing inhibition of $TXA_2$ biosynthesis. This was not a controlled study, but the trend was evident at all ADP doses used and in all volunteers. These results suggest that acetylation of platelet membrane proteins other than PGH-synthase may render platelets more likely to aggregate during long-term, high-dose aspirin therapy.

De Caterina et al (26, 27) performed a randomized, double-blind, placebo-controlled study of 3-week aspiring therapy at 30, 50, or 324 mg/day in 20 individuals surviving an acute myocardial infarction. The secondary wave of ADP-induced aggregation, the epinephrine-induced, and the arachidonate-induced platelet aggregation were nearly maximally suppressed with respect to both basal and placebo measurements. No statistically significant differences were observed in platelet aggregation among the three groups, concomitant with 93 to 99% inhibition of serum $TXB_2$ levels.

Given the limitations of repeatedly measuring the bleeding time in the same subjects, the dose-dependence and time-dependence of aspirin effects on this parameter have not been examined with the same degree of accuracy. These studies were performed in relatively small groups of subjects ($n = 4–20$) and rarely had sufficient statistical power to detect small differences in bleeding time between different aspirin doses—if they even existed. Most of these studies did find a statistically significant increase in the bleeding time, however, ranging from 30% to approximately double the control measurements. These changes were obtained with single doses as low as 80 mg and with repeated daily dosing as low as 20 mg (23), coincident with greater than 90% suppression of serum $TXB_2$ levels. In the study by De Caterina et al (27), daily administration of 50 mg to individuals with coronary artery disease was associated with biochemical and functional changes indistinguishable from those achieved with 324 mg daily on reaching steady-state suppression of the platelet cyclooxygenase activity. Thus, the measurable *ex vivo* (i.e., inhibition of $TXA_2$-dependent platelet aggregation) and *in vivo* (i.e., prolongation of the bleeding time) effects from a standard dose of aspirin can be reproduced fully by a dose that reduces platelet cyclooxygenase activity by more than 95%. The only difference relates to the different rate at which such a maximal effect is achieved: over several days rather than instantaneously. Such a potential disadvantage of low-dose aspirin can be overcome by a loading dose (e.g., 120 mg) followed by a daily maintenance dose (e.g., 30–50 mg) (25, 26). Lesser degrees of inhibition would not be expected to prevent $TXA_2$-dependent platelet activation adequately, because substantial $TXA_2$ biosynthesis may occur *in vivo* with conventionally important (e.g., 80–90%), but incomplete, suppression of the platelet biosynthetic capacity.

Metabolically intact erythrocytes enhance platelet reactivity in an aspirin-sensitive fashion. Santos et al (28) recently suggested that an initial loading dose of 500 mg followed by 50 mg daily may neutralize the prothrombotic effect of erythrocytes. The loading dose should be repeated at 2-week intervals to prevent recovery of the erythrocyte capacity to promote platelet reactivity. The clinical relevance of these *ex vivo* measurements, however, remains to be demonstrated.

There are both theoretic and practical reasons to choose the lowest effective dose of aspirin (Table 54.1). The gastrointestinal side effects appear to be dose-dependent (29, 30), and for secondary prevention, treatment with aspirin is recommended for an indefinite period. There also are theoretic reasons to select a dose that inhibits $TXA_2$ synthesis without inhibiting the vascular synthesis of $PGI_2$. Thus, investigators have speculated that a low dose (e.g., 30 mg daily) might be more antithrombotic, because it inhibits $PGI_2$ biosynthesis to a lesser degree than a high dose. Attempts to identify a dosage (or dosing regimen) of aspirin that blocks $TXA_2$ production without inhibiting $PGI_2$ synthesis, however, have yielded conflicting results, largely depending on *ex vivo* versus *in vivo* assessment of $PGI_2$ production (30). The clinical relevance of the so-called "aspirin dilemma" probably has been overemphasized, but it seems likely that substantial $PGI_2$ production is maintained *in vivo* despite once-daily aspirin regimens. This would occur because of the 24-hour dosing interval, which would allow recovery of COX-1 activity in the vascular endothelial cells, and possibly because of endothelial

COX-2 induction in response to platelet activation (31). On the other hand, differences between the inhibiting effects of the aspirin doses studied (i.e., 30–1300 mg daily) are probably too small to test the hypothesis that inhibition of vascular $PGI_2$ synthesis is relevant clinically (30).

It has been claimed that the dose of aspirin needed to suppress platelet aggregation fully may be higher in individuals with cerebrovascular disease than in healthy subjects, and it may vary over time in the same individual. Terms such as *aspirin failure* or *aspirin resistance* have been used in these studies (32, 33) to designate less than complete inhibition of platelet aggregation. One important caveat when interpreting these measurements of platelet function is the uncontrolled nature of the studies, which does not recognize the contribution of:

1. Intrasubject variability of the aggregation measurements,
2. Lack of compliance with study medication, or
3. Drug interactions that potentially prevent acetylation of platelet PGH-synthase by aspirin.

A recent controlled study demonstrated the contribution of poor compliance in 10% of outpatients with ischemic cerebrovascular disease being treated with low-dose aspirin or ticlopidine (34). Certainly, questions about the effectiveness of aspirin therapy in blocking both platelet and nonplatelet prostanoid synthesis should continue to be raised. For example, enhanced $TXB_2$ metabolite excretion has been described in some individuals with unstable angina while receiving an intravenous low-dose aspirin regimen (35). This may reflect the contribution of extraplatelet $TXA_2$ biosynthesis, including the inducible expression of PGH-synthase 2 in monocytes and macrophages (36).

# OTHER CYCLO-OXYGENASE INHIBITORS

A variety of nonsteroidal anti-inflammatory drugs (NSAIDs) can inhibit $TXA_2$-dependent platelet function through competitive, reversible inhibition of PGH-synthase. When used at conventional anti-inflammatory dosage, these drugs generally inhibit platelet cyclooxygenase activity only by 70 to 85%. Such inhibition may be insufficient to block platelet aggregation adequately *in vivo*, however, because of the substantial biosynthetic capacity of human platelets to produce $TXA_2$ (21).

The only reversible cyclooxygenase inhibitors to be tested for antithrombotic efficacy in randomized, clinical trials are sulfinpyrazone, indobufen, and triflusal. Sulfinpyrazone is a uricosuric agent related structurally to the anti-inflammatory agent phenlybutazone. When used at the highest approved dosage (i.e., 200 mg four times a day), the drug inhibits platelet cyclooxygenase activity by approximately 60% after conversion from an

**TABLE 54.1.** Vascular Disorders for which Aspirin Is Effective

| Disorder | Minimum Effective Daily Dose (mg) |
|---|---|
| Stable angina | 75 |
| Unstable angina | 75 |
| Acute myocardial infarction | 160 |
| Transient cerebral ischemia and minor ischemic stroke | 50 |
| Acute ischemic stroke | 160 |

inactive sulfoxide to an active sulfide metabolite. The conflicting or negative results obtained in randomized, clinical trials of sulfinpyrazone in individuals with myocardial infarction or unstable angina, respectively, are not surprising considering the drug is a weak cyclooxygenase inhibitor with no other established antiplatelet mechanism of action.

Indobufen, in contrast, is a very effective inhibitor of platelet cyclooxygenase activity, and it has biochemical, functional, and clinical effects comparable to those of a standard dose of aspirin. Thus, at therapeutic plasma levels achieved after oral dosing of 200 mg two times a day, indobufen inhibits serum $TXB_2$ by more than 95% throughout the dosing interval (37). It also reduces urinary excretion of TX metabolite to an extent comparable to that of aspirin (38).

Triflusal, which is a derivative of salicylic acid, reversibly inhibits platelet cyclooxygenase activity after conversion to a long-lived metabolite, 2-hydroxy-4-trifluoromethyl-benzoic acid (39). The half-life of the parent compound is approximately 30 minutes, but that of the deacetylated metabolite is approximately 2 days. Triflusal is claimed to have negligible effects on vascular $PGI_2$ production; however, this probably reflects the experimental conditions used for assessment of $PGI_2$ production *ex vivo*.

None of these reversible cyclooxygenase inhibitors is approved as an antiplatelet drug in the United States.

# DIPYRIDAMOLE

Dipyridamole is a pyrimidopyrimidine derivative with both vasodilator and antiplatelet properties. Dipyridamole inhibits platelet aggregation in whole blood at lower concentrations than in plasma (40), but the mechanism of action for dipyridamole as an antiplatelet agent has been controversial (41). Both inhibition of cyclic nucleotide phosphodiesterase (i.e., the enzyme that degrades cyclic adenosine monophosphate (cAMP) to 5'-AMP), which results in intraplatelet accumulation of cAMP, and blockade of the uptake of adenosine, which acts at $A_2$ receptors for adenosine to stimulate platelet adenylyl cyclase, have been suggested. Moreover, direct stimulation of $PGI_2$ synthesis and protection against its degradation have been reported (41). The dipyridamole concentrations required to produce these effects, however, far exceed the low micromolar plasma levels that are achieved after oral administration of conventional doses (i.e., 100–400 mg daily). More recently, it has been suggested that dipyridamole potentiates platelet inhibition by nitric oxide through an action on the phosphodiesterase in platelets that breaks down cyclic guanosine 3,5'-monophosphate (cGMP) (42). Moreover, dipyridamole is a potent antioxidant (43) that can inhibit low-density lipoprotein oxidation at 1 to 10 μM (44).

Absorption of dipyridamole from conventional formulations varies, and it may result in low systemic bioavailability of the drug. A modified-release formulation of dipyridamole with improved bioavailability has been developed and used in association with a low dose of aspirin. Dipyridamole is eliminated primarily by biliary excretion as a glucuronide conjugate, and it is subject to enterohepatic recirculation. A terminal half-life of 10 hours has been reported, which is consistent with the most recent twice-daily regimen used in clinical studies (41).

The clinical efficacy of dipyridamole, whether used alone or in combination with aspirin, has been questioned on the basis of earlier randomized trials (41). The issue was reopened by the results of the recently published European Stroke Prevention Study 2 (45). Whether the favorable results obtained in that trial reflect the higher dose used (400 versus 225 mg daily) and the improved systemic bioavailability of the modified-release dipyridamole or the larger sample size and statistical power of the study itself remains to be established.

# THROMBOXANE-SYNTHASE INHIBITORS AND THROMBOXANE RECEPTOR ANTAGONISTS

TX-synthase is the enzyme that catalyzes synthesis of $TXA_2$ from its immediate precursor, $PGH_2$. Selective inhibitors of this enzyme have at least two theoretic advantages over cyclooxygenase inhibitors as potential antithrombotic agents (46). First, they do not prevent further metabolism of $PGH_2$ via other isomerases to form putatively beneficial eicosanoids, such as $PGI_2$ in the vasculature, gastric mucosa, and renal cortex and $PGE_2$ in the gastric mucosa and renal medulla. Second, $PGH_2$ that accumulates in platelets through the blockade of TX-synthase may be transferred to endothelial cells to serve as substrate for $PGI_2$-synthase at the site of platelet–vessel wall interaction, which is a process termed *endoperoxide steal* or *transcellular metabolism* (47). In fact, selective inhibition of $TXA_2$ biosynthesis coincident with enhanced $PGI_2$ formulation *in vivo* occurs after short-term administration of dazoxiben and CGS 13080 to healthy subjects (46).

Despite these attractive features and the efficacy of selective TX-synthase inhibitors in short-term animal models of thrombosis, the results of limited, phase II clinical studies have been largely disappointing. They also have led most pharmaceutical companies to discontinue clinical development of these compounds. Several factors may have contributed to such failure, including:

1. The clinical endpoints of the studies not necessarily being related to $TXA_2$-dependent phenomena,
2. Inadequate pharmacokinetic features of the compounds tested resulting in substantial recovery of $TXA_2$ synthesis during the dosing interval, and
3. Substitution for the biologic effects of $TXA_2$ by $PGH_2$ at the shared platelet and vascular receptors (46).

Given that selective inhibition of platelet $TXA_2$ formation can be achieved with novel aspirin formulations (discussed earlier), the value of TX-synthase inhibitors depends on enhancing vascular $PGI_2$ production, the clinical significance of which remains to be established.

The $TXA_2/PGH_2$ (TP) receptor is a G protein–coupled receptor, which on ligand stimulation results in activation of phospholipase C and subsequent increase in inositol 1,4,5-triphosphate, diacylglycerol, and intracellular $Ca^{2+}$ concentrations (see Chapters 11 and 12). The human TP complementary DNA originally was cloned from placenta and a plateletlike megakaryocyte cell line (48). A second form of the TP receptor recently was cloned from human umbilical vein endothelial cells (49). The endothelial receptor, which is known as TPβ, and the platelet/placental receptor, which is known as TPα, derive from an alternative splicing mechanism. They are identical for the first 328 amino acids but differ in their carboxylterminal cytoplasmic tails. Endothelial cells contain only TPβ; both TPα and TPβ are expressed in placental tissues and in platelets (49).

Potent ($K_d$ in the low nanomolar range) and long-lasting (half-life >20 hours) TP antagonists have been developed, including GR 32191, BMS-180291 (ifetroban), and BM 13.177 (sulotroban). Despite the antithrombotic activity demonstrated in various animal species and the interesting "cardioprotective" activity demonstrated in dogs and ferrets (50), these compounds have yielded disappointing results in phase II/III clinical trials (51–53). Before drawing definitive conclusions on the apparent failure of this approach, however, it should be mentioned that these studies suffer from severe limitations, including:

1. Unrealistic hypotheses of risk reduction being tested (e.g., a 50% reduction in the late clinical failure rate after successful coronary angioplasty);
2. Heterogeneous endpoints being pooled together, including "clinically important restenosis," for which no evidence of $TXA_2$-dependence was obtained during earlier aspirin trials; and
3. An anti-ischemic effect being tested in individuals with unstable coronary syndromes treated using standard therapy, including aspirin.

Clinical development of GR 32191 and sulotroban has been discontinued because of these disappoint-

ing—though largely predictable—results. It would be interesting to see at least one such compound developed through phase III clinical trials with adequate endpoints and realistic sample sizes. The potential advantages of potent TP antagonists compared with low-dose aspirin relate to the recent discovery of aspirin-insensitive agonists of the platelet receptor, such as $TXA_2$ derived from monocyte PGH-synthase 2 and the $F_2$-isoprostane, 8-epi-$PGF_2\alpha$, which is a product of free radical–catalyzed peroxidation of arachidonic acid (54). The latter can synergize with subthreshold concentrations of other platelet agonists to evoke a full aggregatory response, thus amplifying platelet activation in those clinical settings associated with enhanced lipid peroxidation (54).

Molecules that combine TX-synthase inhibition with TP antagonism have been developed as well after experimental evidence suggested a synergistic interaction between the two approaches (55). The only such molecule tested in clinical studies, ridogrel, lacks the desired balance of the two activities and, perhaps not surprisingly, has not lived up to expectations (56).

# TICLOPIDINE AND CLOPIDOGREL

Ticlopidine and clopidogrel are structurally related thienopyridines with platelet inhibitory properties (Fig. 54.2). Both drugs selectively inhibit ADP-induced platelet aggregation, with no direct effects on metabolism of arachidonic acid (57). Ticlopidine and clopidogrel also can inhibit platelet aggregation induced by collagen and thrombin, but these inhibitory effects are abolished by increasing the agonist concentration and, therefore, likely reflect blockade of ADP-mediated amplification of the response to other agonists.

Neither ticlopidine nor clopidogrel affect ADP-

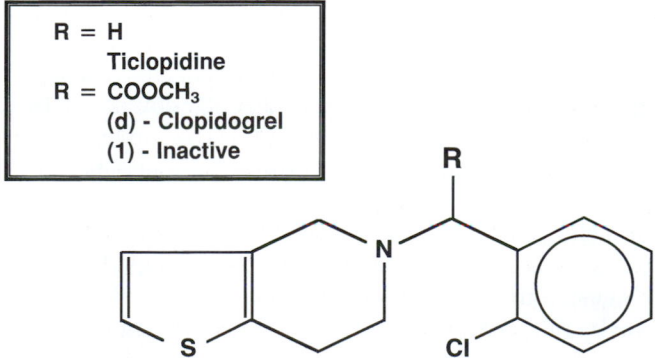

**FIGURE 54.2.** Chemical structure of ticlopidine and clopidogrel. (Adapted with permission from Dr. Jean-Marc Herbert, Sanofi Recherche, France.)

induced platelet aggregation when added *in vitro* up to 500 μM, thus suggesting that *in vivo* hepatic transformation to an active metabolite, or metabolites, is necessary for their antiplatelet effects. Molecular characterization of these metabolites, however, has remained elusive, nor has the molecular target of thienopyridine derivatives been elucidated. Evidence suggests that clopidogrel and, probably, ticlopidine induce irreversible alterations of the platelet ADP receptor mediating inhibition of stimulated adenylyl cyclase activity by ADP (58). Inhibition of platelet function by clopidogrel is associated with a selective reduction in ADP-binding sites, with no consistent change in the binding affinity (58). Permanent modification of an ADP receptor by thienopyridines is consistent with time-dependent, cumulative inhibition of ADP-induced platelet aggregation on repeated daily dosing and with slow recovery of platelet function on drug withdrawal (59).

As much as 90% of a single oral dose of ticlopidine is rapidly absorbed in humans (57). Peak plasma concentrations occur 1 to 3 hours after a single oral dose of 250 mg, and on repeated twice-daily dosing over 2 to 3 weeks, these concentrations increase by approximately threefold because of drug accumulation. More than 98% of ticlopidine is reversibly bound to plasma proteins, primarily albumin. Ticlopidine is metabolized rapidly and extensively, and 13 metabolites have been identified in humans. Of these, only the 2-keto derivative is a more potent inhibitor of ADP-induced aggregation than the parent compound (57).

The elimination half-life of ticlopidine is 24 to 36 hours after a single oral dose and as much as 96 hours after 14 days of repeated dosing (57). The recommended regimen is 250 mg twice per day, although how a twice-daily regimen relates to the pharmacokinetic and pharmacodynamic features noted earlier is not clear. In at least one clinical trial of ticlopidine, which involved individuals with unstable angina, a delayed antithrombotic effect was noted with no apparent protection during the first 2 weeks of drug administration (60).

A synergistic effect of ticlopidine and aspirin has been described in rats, both in terms of ADP-induced platelet aggregation *ex vivo* and in platelet-dependent thrombosis (61). Interestingly, the ticlopidine–aspirin combination produced only additive effects on the tail bleeding-time prolongation (61). The mechanism underlying these findings remains speculative, but the combination of these two agents is effective in preventing coronary stent thrombosis (62).

Major side effects of ticlopidine include bone marrow depression, rash, and diarrhea. In particular, ticlopidine may cause neutropenia (neutrophils $<1.2 \times 10^9/l$), for which the reported rate is approximately 2.4%, and severe neutropenia (neutrophils $<0.45 \times 10^9/l$), for which the reported rate is approximately 1%. In some countries, these serious side effects have restricted indications for ticlopidine to aspirin-intolerant individuals.

The pharmacokinetics of clopidogrel are somewhat different from those of ticlopidine. Thus, unchanged clopidogrel was not detectable in peripheral venous plasma after administration of single oral doses ($\leq$200 mg) or repeated doses ($\leq$100 mg daily) (59). Plasma concentrations of 1 to 2 ng/ml were measured in individuals receiving clopidogrel, 150 mg/day (twice the dose used in the Clopidogrel versus Aspirin in Individuals At Risk of Ischaemic Events [CAPRIE] study and likely to be approved) for 16 days. The main systemic metabolite of clopidogrel is the carboxylic acid derivative, SR 26334. From measurements of circulating levels of SR 26334, clopidogrel is inferred to be rapidly absorbed and extensively metabolized (59). The plasma elimination half-life of SR 26334 is approximately 8 hours, but as noted, clopidogrel, which is inactive *in vitro*, is metabolically transformed by the liver into a short-lived platelet inhibitor of unknown structure (58).

After single oral doses of clopidogrel, ADP-induced platelet aggregation was inhibited in a dose-dependent fashion in healthy volunteers, with an apparent ceiling effect (i.e., 40% inhibition) at 400 mg. Inhibited platelet aggregation was detectable 2 hours after oral dosing of 400 mg, and it remained relatively stable up to 48 hours (59). With repeated daily dosing of 50 to 100 mg in healthy volunteers, ADP-induced platelet aggregation was inhibited from the second day of treatment (25–30% inhibition) and reached a steady state (50–60% inhibition) after 4 to 7 days. Such maximal inhibition is comparable to that achieved with ticlopidine (500 mg daily). Ticlopidine, however, has shown a slower onset of antiplatelet effect compared with clopidogrel. No appreciable differences in the inhibitory effects of 50, 75, and 100 mg of clopidogrel were noted in this study, thus suggesting that 50 mg daily may be at, or close to, the top of the dose–response curve. It is interesting that 50 mg is only approximately 12% of the dose necessary to achieve maximal inhibition of ADP-induced platelet aggregation after single dosing. Given the short half-life of the putative active metabolite of clopidogrel, the active metabolite of clopidogrel is unlikely to accumulate to any substantial extent on repeated daily dosing of the parent compound.

The best available interpretation of these findings is that the active metabolite of clopidogrel has a pharmacodynamic pattern quite similar to that of aspirin in causing cumulative platelet inhibition on repeated daily low-dose administration. As with aspirin, platelet function returned to normal 7 days after the last dose. Both the cumulative nature of the inhibitory effects and the slow recovery rate of platelet function are consistent with the active moieties of aspirin (i.e., acetylsalicylic acid) and clopidogrel (i.e., metabolite X) causing a permanent defect in a platelet protein that cannot be repaired during the 24-hour dosing interval and can be replaced only through platelet turnover. This also justifies the once-

## Relative Risk-Reduction (%)

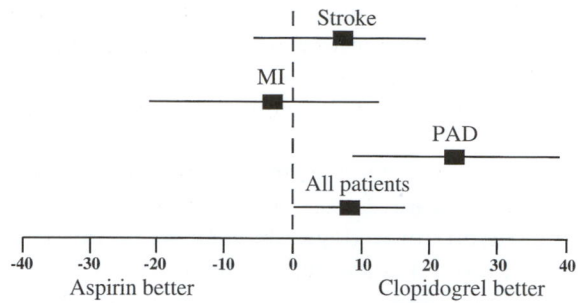

**FIGURE 54.3.** Relative risk reduction and 95% confidence interval by disease subgroup in the CAPRIE study. A test for heterogeneity of these three treatment effects was statistically significant ($P = .042$). *MI*, myocardial infarction; *PAD*, peripheral arterial disease. (Adapted with permission from CAPRIE Steering Committee. A randomized, blinded trial of clopidogrel versus aspirin in individuals at risk of ischaemic events (CAPRIE). Lancet 1996;348:1329–1339.)

daily regimen of both drugs despite their short half-life in the circulation. Bleeding times measured in the same multiple-dose study of clopidogrel described earlier (59) showed a comparable prolongation (by 1.5–2.0-fold over controls) at 50 to 100 mg daily or ticlopidine at 500 mg daily (59).

Clopidogrel has undergone an unusual clinical development, with limited phase II studies and a single large phase III trial (i.e., CAPRIE) to test its efficacy and safety at 75 mg daily compared with aspirin at 325 mg daily (63). The overall results indicate the two drugs are equally effective at preventing major vascular complications in individuals with a recent myocardial infarction or ischemic stroke (Fig. 54.3). Clopidogrel, however, was more effective than aspirin among individuals enrolled because of symptomatic peripheral arterial disease. This interesting and, perhaps, unexpected finding suggests the pathophysiologic importance of TXA$_2$ and ADP varies in that different clinical settings, and this may warrant further mechanistic studies exploring combined strategies based on the two best-characterized approaches to antiplatelet therapy. In the CAPRIE trial, the frequency of severe rash was higher with clopidogrel than with aspirin, as was the frequency of diarrhea, thus reproducing the characteristic side effects of ticlopidine. No excess neutropenia, however, was associated with clopidogrel, but the frequency of this serious complication was extremely low (0.05%) in this trial.

# GLYCOPROTEIN IIB/IIIA ANTAGONISTS

Given the redundancy of discrete pathways leading to platelet aggregation, the only partial clinical efficacy of

aspirin, ticlopidine, and clopidogrel is not surprising. While inhibiting TXA$_2$-mediated or ADP-mediated platelet aggregation, these drugs leave the activity of other platelet agonists such as thrombin largely unaffected. Following recognition that expression of functionally active glycoprotein (GP) IIb-IIIa ($\alpha_{IIb}\beta_3$) on the platelet surface is the final common pathway of platelet aggregation (Fig. 54.4) regardless of the initiating stimulus (see Chapter 11), this GP has become the target of novel antiplatelet drugs (64, 65). Inhibitors of GP IIb-IIIa include monoclonal antibodies against the receptor, naturally occurring RGD-containing peptides isolated from snake venoms, synthetic RGD-containing or KGD-containing peptides, and peptidomimetic as well as non-peptide RGD mimetics that compete with fibrinogen for occupancy of its platelet receptor. The mechanism of action for these compounds is illustrated in Fig. 54.5.

By developing murine monoclonal antibodies against platelet GP IIb-IIIa, Coller et al (66) demonstrated that fibrinogen-receptor blockade could induce a functional thrombasthenic phenotype. Approximately 40,000 antibody molecules bind to the surface of platelets, thus indicating there probably are 40,000 to 80,000 GP IIb-IIIa receptors per platelet (65). At antibody doses that decrease available receptors to less than 50% of normal, Coller (65) found that platelet aggregation was significantly inhibited. At approximately 80% receptor blockade, platelet aggregation was almost completely abolished, but the bleeding time was only mildly affected. Only with more than 90% receptor blockade will the bleeding time become extremely prolonged.

Because of concerns about immunogenicity of the original 7E3 antibody, a mouse/human chimeric 7E3 Fab was created for clinical development. After bolus

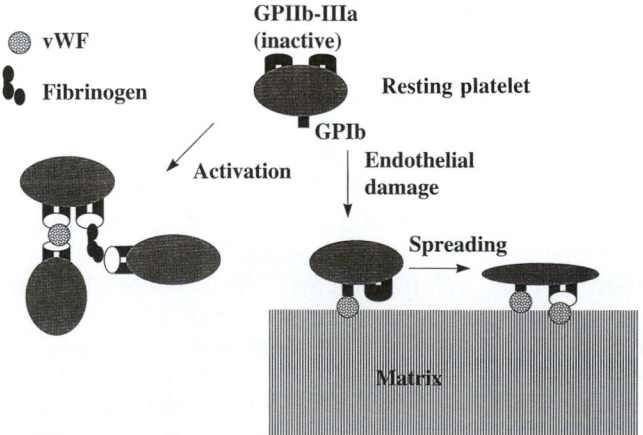

**FIGURE 54.4.** Expression and function of glycoprotein (GP) IIb-IIIa in mediating platelet–platelet and platelet–matrix adhesive interactions through von Willebrand factor (vWF) and fibrinogen. The resting and activated states of GP IIb-IIIa are indicated by the black and white representations, respectively.

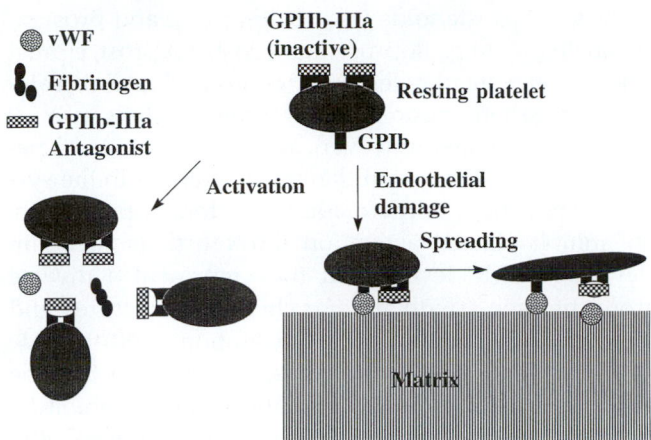

**FIGURE 54.5.** Occupancy of the platelet glycoprotein (GP) IIb-IIIa by antagonists of this receptor prevents platelet–platelet and platelet–matrix adhesive interactions. vWf, von Willebrand factor.

injection of c7E3 Fab, a dose-dependent inhibition of ADP-induced platelet aggregation was recorded in individuals at moderate to high risk of percutaneous transluminal coronary angioplasty (PTCA)–associated ischemic complications (67). A bolus dose of 0.25 mg/kg body weight resulted in more than 80% blockade of platelet receptors and reduced platelet aggregation in response to 20 µM ADP to less than 20% of baseline. A steep dose–response curve was apparent in this study, and peak effects on receptor blockade, platelet aggregation, and bleeding time were observed at the first sampling time of 2 hours after bolus administration of 0.25 mg/kg. Gradual recovery of platelet function then occurred over time, with the bleeding time returning to near-normal values by 12 hours. Administration of a 0.25 mg/kg bolus dose of c7E3 Fab, followed by a 12-hour infusion of 10 µg/min, demonstrated that receptor blockade, inhibition of platelet aggregation, and prolonged bleeding times could be maintained throughout the infusion (67).

This regimen was chosen for the pivotal phase III trial (EPIC), which demonstrated both short-term and long-term clinical efficacy of c7E3 Fab in reducing the incidence of ischemic events among individuals undergoing PTCA when added to conventional antithrombotic therapy. These results formed the basis for approval by the U.S. Food and Drug Administration of c7E3 Fab (abciximab, ReoPro) as adjunctive therapy for individuals undergoing high-risk PTCA and atherectomy.

The effect of c7E3 Fab in preventing vascular occlusion by suppressing platelet aggregation probably is the major mechanism of its beneficial effects, but the potent inhibition of thrombus formation by this antibody might result in decreased thrombin formation (68, 69). In fact,

c7E3 Fab produced dose-dependent inhibition of tissue factor–induced thrombin generation, reaching a plateau of 45 to 50% inhibition at concentrations of 15 µg/ml (68). Whether inhibition of thrombin generation by c7E3 Fab contributes to its immediate antithrombotic effect, its alleged effects on long-term vascular restenosis, or both (70), is not known.

Several RGD-containing, low-molecular-weight peptides that compete with fibrinogen for GP IIb-IIIa binding have been isolated from the venom of several species in the viper family. These peptides, known as "disintegrins," include trigramin, bitistatin, echistatin, kistrin, and applagin (71). The amino acid sequences for 25 different disintegrins are known (71).

These peptides provide insight regarding the structural requirements for GP IIb-IIIa antagonism, but their potential clinical application is hampered by their immunogenicity and propensity for causing transient thrombocytopenia. Moreover, RGD-containing disintegrins are not integrin specific, and they inhibit the adhesive functions of many other RGD-dependent integrins. The unique disintegrin peptide barbourin, which contains a conservative amino acid substitution of Lys (K) for Arg (R) in the RGD sequence, is highly specific for GP IIb-IIIa.

Integrin specificity can be mimicked by small, conformationally restrained peptides containing the KGD sequence (72). In addition to natural antagonists, a variety of RGD-containing and KGD-containing GP IIb-IIIa inhibitors have been synthesized. In a cyclic configuration, these synthetic peptides have markedly increased affinity for GP IIb-IIIa, comparable to that of the naturally occurring antagonists. Agents in this group include MK-852 and integrelin. The latter has undergone phase I and II testing and demonstrated rapid and profound suppression (>80%) of ADP-induced platelet aggregation in individuals undergoing PTCA and who were already receiving aspirin and heparin (73). Whether the higher specificity for GP IIb-IIIa receptors on platelets, shorter half-life, and lower immunogenicity of the synthetic antagonists compared with c7E3 Fab translates into improved efficacy or safety is not known (74). In fact, blockade of the $\alpha_v\beta_3$-vitronectin receptor in vascular cells by c7E3 Fab may contribute to an effect on "clinical restenosis" (70).

More recently, nonpeptide mimetics of the RGD sequence have been developed, including lamifiban, tirofiban, fradafiban, roxifiban, orbofiban, and xemilofiban. Both lamifiban and tirofiban have undergone extensive clinical testing in phase II, dose-ranging studies (75, 76). Similar to c7E3 Fab, these compounds inhibit ADP-induced platelet aggregation and prolong the bleeding time with a steep dose–response relationship, encompassing only a threefold to fivefold increase in dose and plasma concentrations.

These nonpeptide GP IIb-IIIa inhibitors are orally active and have the potential for long-term use, but several issues remain unsolved. These include:

1. Uncertainty regarding the optimal degree of GP IIb-IIIa receptor blockade that is compatible with superior efficacy compared with aspirin and acceptable bleeding risk during long-term administration,
2. The inadequacy of currently available surrogate markers for efficacy (i.e., ADP-induced platelet aggregation) and safety (i.e., skin bleeding time) on which dose-finding studies are based, and
3. The steep dose–response curve and consequent need for dose titration and monitoring.

In fact, there is a large discrepancy between state-of-the-art technology deployed in the design and clinical development of these novel antiplatelet drugs and the 1960s methodology used to assess their functional effects. Analytic measurement of mechanism-related biochemical endpoints has been crucial in defining the dose-dependence and time-dependence of the antiplatelet effects of aspirin, but no such development has occurred with the novel antiplatelet agents.

# OTHER DRUGS WITH ANTIPLATELET EFFECTS

A variety of other drugs possess antiplatelet effects *in vitro, ex vivo,* or both (Table 54.2). Although at some stage they were considered as potential candidates for new drug development by several pharmaceutical companies, none has reached a market with a specific labeling as an antiplatelet agent (with the possible exception of Japan), and the process of drug development has shifted toward other, more promising approaches.

Several prostanoids (e.g., $PGE_1$, $PGI_2$) and prostanoid analogues (e.g., iloprost, beraprost, cicaprost, ciprostene) can elevate platelet cAMP levels and inhibit platelet aggregation. Serious limitations to their use as antiplatelet agents, however, are the concomitant, peripheral vasodilation and their short half-life in the systemic circulation. Nitric oxide (NO) donors potentially can inhibit platelet activation through their effects in elevating cGMP levels, and they represent a diverse group of agents with unique chemical structures and biochemical requirements for generation of nitric oxide (77). Preliminary evidence for an *in vivo* effect of the nitric oxide donor S-nitrosoglutathione in inhibiting platelet activation has been reported in individuals with severe preeclampsia (78) and in those with acute coronary syndromes (79). This was associated, however, with detectable hemodynamic changes. Potent inhibitors of phosphodiesterase III also have been developed as potential antithrombotic agents, and a representative of this class, cilostazol, has been approved in Japan for the treatment of peripheral arterial disease. The spectrum of pharmacologic effects of this compound is quite wide, however, and includes bronchodilator and bronchoprotective effects *in vivo* (80) as well as suppressed mitogenesis of rat mesangial cells *in vitro* (81).

Ketanserin, which is a $5HT_2$ antagonist, has been developed as a potential antithrombotic agent through a large, phase III trial involving individuals with peripheral vascular disease, which produced largely negative results (82). Another $5HT_2$ antagonist, sarpogrelate, has been approved for the treatment of peripheral arterial disease in Japan. Other compounds are being developed for other indications such as migraine and anxiety.

Several potent and selective platelet-activating factor antagonists have been developed as well. Their primary indication is the treatment of asthma.

**TABLE 54.2.** Other Drugs with Antiplatelet Effects

| Products | Mechanism of Antiplatelet Action | Vascular Effects |
|---|---|---|
| Adenylyl cyclase activators (e.g., $PGI_2$ analogues) | ↑cAMP | Vasodilation |
| Guanylyl cyclase activators (e.g., nitric oxide donors) | ↑cGMP | Vasodilation |
| Phosphodiesterase III inhibitors (e.g., Cilostazol) | ↑cAMP | Vasodilation |
| $5HT_2$-antagonists (e.g., Ketanserin) | ↓Serotonin-induced aggregation | Vasodilation |
| PAF antagonists | ↓PAF-induced aggregation | Variable |
| Omega-3 fatty acids | ?Changes in membrane composition | Slight decrease in blood pressure |
| Vitamin E | ?PKC-dependent mechanism | Prevents endothelial dysfunction |

cAMP, *cyclic adenosine monophosphate;* cGMP, *cyclic guanosine monophosphate;* PAF, *platelet-activating factor;* PKC, *protein kinase C;* 5HT, *5-hydroxytryptamine.*

Omega-3 polyunsaturated fatty acids modulate a wide range of cellular responses, possibly including platelet function (83). There is no convincing evidence that they reduce platelet activation *in vivo*, however, and they may be exerting antiatherogenic effects by decreasing cytokine-induced expression of proatherogenic and proinflammatory proteins in endothelial cells (84).

Finally, platelet incorporation of α-tocopherol at levels attained with oral supplementation is associated with inhibited platelet aggregation through a protein kinase C–dependent mechanism (85). This may represent one potential mechanism for the beneficial effects of vitamin E supplementation in preventing myocardial infarction among individuals with ischemic heart disease (86). Pharmacologic doses of vitamin E can affect platelet as well as endothelial function through other mechanisms, however, possibly relating to its ability to inhibit low-density lipoprotein oxidation and to reduce nonenzymatic peroxidation of arachidonic acid to bioactive isoprostanes (87).

# REFERENCES

1. Patrono C. Aspirin and human platelets: from clinical trials to acetylation of cyclooxygenase and back. Trends Pharmacol Sci 1989;10:453–458.
2. Smith WL, Marnett LJ. Prostaglandin endoperoxide synthase: structure and catalysis. Biochim Biophys Acta 1991;1083:1–17.
3. FitzGerald GA. Mechanisms of platelet activation: thromboxane $A_2$ as an amplifying signal for other agonists. Am J Cardiol 1991;68:11B–15B.
4. Roth GJ, Stanford N, Majerus PW. Acetylation of prostaglandin synthetase by aspirin. Proc Natl Acad Sci U S A 1975;72:3073–3076.
5. DeWitt DL, Smith WL. Primary structure of prostaglandin G/H synthase from sheep vesicular gland determined from the complementary DNA sequence. Proc Natl Acad Sci U S A 1988;85:1412–1416.
6. Xie W, Chipman JG, Robertson DL et al. Expression of a mitogen-responsive gene encoding prostaglandin synthase is regulated by mRNA splicing. Proc Natl Acad Sci U S A 1991;88:2692–2696.
7. Kujubu DA, Fletcher BS, Varnum BC et al. TIS 10, a phorbol ester tumor promoter-inducible mRNA from Swiss 3T3 cells, encodes a novel prostaglandin synthase/cyclooxygenase homologue. J Biol Chem 1991;266:12866–12872.
8. Vane JR. Inhibition of prostaglandins as a mechanism of action for aspirin-like drugs. Nat New Biol 1971;231:232–235.
9. Bjornsson TD, Schneider DE, Berger H Jr. Aspirin acetylates fibrinogen and enhances fibrinolysis. Fibrinolytic effect is independent of changes in plasminogen activator levels. J Pharmacol Exp Ther 1989;250:154–161.
10. Ratnatunga CP, Edmondson SF, Rees GM et al. High-dose aspirin inhibits shear-induced platelet reaction involving thrombin generation. Circulation 1992;85:1077–1082.
11. Ezratty AM, Simon DI, Loscalzo J. Acetylated firbrinogen facilitates plasminogen activation and attenuates platelet aggregation [Abstract]. Clin Res 1992;40:201A.
12. Castaño E, Dalmau M, Martí M et al. Inhibition of DNA synthesis by aspirin in Swiss 3T3 fibroblasts. J Pharmacol Exp Ther 1997;280:366–372.
13. Farivar RS, Brecher P. Salicylate is a transcriptional inhibitor of the inducible nitric oxide synthase in cultured cardiac fibroblasts. J Biol Chem 1996;271:31585–31592.
14. Pedersen AK, FitzGerald GA. Dose-related kinetics of aspirin. Presystemic acetylation of platelet cyclooxygenase. N Engl J Med 1984;311:1206–1211.
15. Clarke RJ, Mayo G, Price P et al. Suppression of thromboxane $A_2$ but not systemic prostacyclin by controlled-release aspirin. N Engl J Med 1991;325:1137–1141.
16. McAdam B, Keimowitz RM, Maher M et al. Transdermal modification of platelet function: an aspirin patch system results in marked suppression of platelet cyclooxygenase. J Pharmacol Exp Ther 1996;277:559–564.
17. Patrono C, Ciabattoni G, Pinca E et al. Low dose aspirin and inhibition of thromboxane $B_2$ production in healthy subjects. Thromb Res 1980;17:317–327.
18. Thorngren M, Shafi S, Born GV. Thromboxane $A_2$ in skin bleeding-time blood and in clotted venous blood before and after administration of acetylsalicylic acid. Lancet 1983;i:1075–1078.
19. Born GV. Aggregation of blood platelets by adenosine diphosphate and its reversal. Nature 1962;194:927–929.
20. Harker LA, Slichter SJ. The bleeding time as a screening test for evaluation of platelet function. N Engl J Med 1972;287:155–159.
21. Patrono C, Ciabattoni G, Pugliese F et al. Estimated rate of thromboxane secretion into the circulation of normal humans. J Clin Invest 1986;77:590–594.
22. Patrignani P, Filabozzi P, Patrono C. Selective cumulative inhibition of platelet thromboxane production by low-dose aspirin in healthy subjects. J Clin Invest 1982;69:1366–1372.
23. FitzGerald GA, Oates JA, Hawiger J et al. Endogenous biosynthesis of prostacyclin and thromboxane and platelet function during chronic administration of aspirin in man. J Clin Invest 1983;71:676–688.
24. Burch JW, Stanford N, Majerus PW. Inhibition of platelet prostaglandin synthetase by oral aspirin. J Clin Invest 1978;61:314–319.
25. Patrono C, Ciabattoni G, Patrignani P et al. Clinical pharmacology of platelet cyclooxygeanse inhibition. Circulation 1985;72:1177–1184.
26. De Caterina R, Giannessi D, Bernini W et al. Low-dose aspirin in patients recovering from myocardial infarction. Evidence for a selective inhibition of thomboxane-related platelet function. Eur Heart J 1985;6:409–417.
27. De Caterina R, Giannessi D, Boem A et al. Equal antiplatelet effects of aspirin 50 or 324 mg/day in patients after acute myocardial infarction. Thromb Haemost 1985;54:528–532.
28. Santos MT, Valles J, Aznar J et al. Prothrombotic effects of erythrocytes on platelet reactivity. Reduction by aspirin. Circulation 1997;95:63–68.
29. Patrono C. Aspirin as an antiplatelet drug. N Engl J Med 1994;330:1287–1294.
30. Hirsh J, Dalen JE, Fuster V et al. Aspirin and other platelet-active drugs. The relationship among dose, effectiveness, and side effects. Chest 1995;108(Suppl 4):247S–257S.
31. Barry OP, Praticò D, Lawson JA et al. Transcellular activation of platelets and endothelial cells by bioactive lipids in platelet microparticles. J Clin Invest 1997;99:2118–2127.
32. Helgason CM, Hoff JA, Kondos GT et al. Platelet aggregation in patients with atrial fibrillation taking aspirin or warfarin. Stroke 1993;24:1458–1461.
33. Helgason CM, Bolin KM, Hoff JA et al. Development of aspirin resistance in persons with previous ischemic stroke. Stroke 1994;25:2331–2336.
34. Komiya T, Kudo M, Urabe T et al. Compliance with anti-platelet therapy in individuals with ischemic cerebrovascular disease. Stroke 1994;25:2337–2342.
35. Vejar M, Fragasso G, Hackett D et al. Dissociation of platelet activation and spontaneous myocardial ischemia in unstable angina. Thromb Haemost 1990;63:163–168.
36. Cipollone F, Patrignani P, Greco A et al. Differential suppression of thromboxane biosynthesis by indobufen and aspirin in patients with unstable angina. Circulation 1997;96:1109–1116.
37. Rebuzzi AG, Natale A, Bianchi C et al. Effects of indobufen on platelet thromboxane $B_2$ production in patients with myocardial infarction. Eur J Clin Pharmacol 1990;39:99–100.
38. Davi G, Patrono C, Catalano I et al. Inhibition of thromboxane biosynthesis and platelet function by indobufen in type II diabetes mellitus. Arterioscler Thromb 1993;13:1346–1349.
39. Ramis J, Torrent J, Mis R et al. Pharmacokinetics of triflusal after single and repeated doses in man. Int J Clin Pharmacol Ther Toxicol 1990;28:344–349.
40. Gresele P, Arnout J, Deckmyn H et al. Mechanism of the antiplatelet action of dipyridamole in whole blood: modulation of adenosine concentration and activity. Thromb Haemost 1986;55:12–18.
41. FitzGerald GA. Dipyridamole. N Engl J Med 1987;316:1247–1257.
42. Vane JR, Meade TW. Second European Stroke Prevention Study (ESPS 2): clinical and pharmacological implications. J Neurol Sci 1997;145(2):123–125.
43. Iuliano L, Pedersen JZ, Rotilio G et al. A potent chain-breaking antioxidant activity of the cardiovascular drug dipyridamole. Free Radic Biol Med 1995;18:239–247.
44. Iuliano L, Colavita AR, Camastra C et al. Protection of low density lipoprotein oxidation at chemical and cellular level by the antioxidant drug dipyridamole. Br J Pharmacol 1996;119:1438–1446.
45. Diener HC, Cunha L, Forbes C et al. European Stroke Prevention Study 2. Dipyridamole and acetylsalicylic acid in the secondary prevention of stroke. J Neurol Sci 1996;143:1–13.
46. FitzGerald GA, Reilly IA, Pedersen AK. The biochemical pharmacology of thromboxane synthase inhibition in man. Circulation 1985;72:1194–1201.
47. Marcus AJ, Weksler BB, Jaffe EA et al. Synthesis of prostacyclin from platelet derived endoperoxides by cultured human endothelial cells. J Clin Invest 1980;66:979–986.
48. Hirata M, Hayashi Y, Ushikubi F et al. Cloning and expression of the cDNA for a human thromboxane $A_2$ receptor. Nature 1991;349:617–620.
49. Raychowdhury MK, Yukawa M, Collins LJ et al. Alternative splicing produces a divergent cytoplasmic tail in the human endothelial thromboxane $A_2$ receptor. J Biol Chem 1994;269:19256–19261. (Published erratum appears in J Biol Chem 1995;270:7011.)

50. Gomoll AW, Grover GJ, Ogletree ML. Myocardial salvage efficacy of the thromboxane receptor antagonist ifetroban in ferrets and dogs. J Cardiovasc Pharmacol 1994;24:960–968.

51. Serruys PW, Rutsch W, Heyndrickx GR et al. Prevention of restenosis after percutaneous transluminal coronary angioplasty with thromboxane A$_2$-receptor blockade. A randomized, double-blind, placebo-controlled trial. Coronary Artery Restenosis Prevention on Repeated Thromboxane-Antagonism Study (CARPORT). Circulation 1991;84:1568–1580.

52. Savage MP, Goldberg S, Bove AA et al. Effect of thromboxane A$_2$ blockade on clinical outcome and restenosis after successful coronary angioplasty. Multi-Hospital Eastern Atlantic Restenosis Trial (M-HEART II). Circulation 1995;92:3194–3200.

53. Remme WJ. Prevention of ischaemic cardiac events in unstable angina and non-Q infarction. PRINCE, a placebo controlled trial with ifegatran-thromboxane A$_2$ receptor antagonist. Presented at the XVIIIth Congress of the European Society of Cardiology, Birmingham, UK, 1996.

54. Praticò D, Smyth EM, Violi F et al. Local amplification of platelet function by 8-epi prostaglandin F$_{2a}$ is not mediated by thromboxane receptor isoforms. J Biol Chem 1996;271:14916–14924.

55. Gresele P, Arnout J, Deckmyn H et al. Role of proaggregatory and antiaggregatory prostaglandins in hemostasis. Studies with combined thromboxane synthase inhibition and thromboxane receptor antagonism. J Clin Invest 1987;80:1435–1445.

56. Anonymous. Randomized trial of Ridogrel, a combined thromboxane A$_2$ synthase inhibitor and thromboxane A$_2$/prostaglandin endoperoxide receptor antagonist, versus aspirin as adjunct to thrombolysis in patients with acute myocardial infarction. The Ridogrel versus Aspirin Patency Trial (RAPT). Circulation 1994;89:588–595.

57. Ito MK, Smith AR, Lee ML. Ticlopidine: a new platelet aggregation inhibitor. Clin Pharm 1992;11:603–617.

58. Savi P, Heilmann E, Nurden P et al. Clopidogrel: an antithrombotic drug acting on the ADP-dependent activation pathway of human platelets. Clin Appl Thromb/Hemos 1996;2:35–42.

59. Herbert JM, Frehel D, Vallee E et al. Clopidogrel, a novel antiplatelet and antithrombotic agent. Cardiovasc Drug Rev 1993;11:180–198.

60. Balsano F, Rizzon P, Violi F et al. Antiplatelet treatment with ticlopidine in unstable angina: a controlled multicenter clinical trial. The Studio della Ticlopidina nell'Angina Instabile Group. Circulation 1990;82:17–26.

61. Herbert JM, Bernat A, Samama M et al. The antiaggregating and antithrombotic activity of ticlopidine is potentiated by aspirin in the rat. Thromb Haemost 1996;76:94–98.

62. More RS, Chauhan A. Antiplatelet rather than anticoagulant therapy with coronary stenting. Lancet 1997;349:146–147.

63. CAPRIE Steering Committee. A randomised, blinded, trial of clopidogrel versus aspirin in patients at risk of ischaemic events (CAPRIE). Lancet 1996;348:1329–1339.

64. Lefkovits J, Plow EF, Topol EJ. Platelet glycoprotein IIb-IIIa receptors in cardiovascular medicine. N Engl J Med 1995;332:1553–1559.

65. Coller BS. Platelet GP IIb-IIIa antagonists: the first anti-integrin receptor therapeutics. J Clin Invest 1997;99:1467–1471.

66. Coller BS, Peerschke EI, Scudder LE et al. A murine monoclonal antibody that completely blocks the binding of fibrinogen to platelets produces a thrombasthenic-like state in normal platelets and binds to glycoproteins IIb and/or IIIa. J Clin Invest 1983;72:325–338.

67. Tcheng JE, Ellis SG, George BS et al. Pharmacodynamics of chimeric glycoprotein IIb-IIIa integrin antiplatelet antibody Fab 7E3 in high-risk coronary angioplasty. Circulation 1994;90:1757–1764.

68. Reverter JC, Béguin S, Kessels H et al. Inhibition of platelet-mediated, tissue factor-induced thrombin generation by the mouse/human chimeric 7E3 antibody. Potential implications for effect of c7E3 Fab treatment on acute thrombosis and "clinical restenosis." J Clin Invest 1996;98:863–874.

69. Ammar T, Scudder LE, Coller BS. *In vitro* effects of the platelet glycoprotein IIb-IIIa receptor antagonist c7E3 Fab on the activated clotting time. Circulation 1997;95:614–617.

70. Topol EJ, Califf RM, Weisman HF et al. Randomised trial of coronary intervention with antibody against platelet IIb-IIIa integrin for reduction of clinical restenosis: results at six months. The EPIC Investigators. Lancet 1994;343:881–886.

71. Niewiarowski S, McLane MA, Kloczewiak M et al. Disintegrins and other naturally occurring antagonists of platelet fibrinogen receptors. Semin Hematol 1994;31:289–300.

72. Scarborough RM, Naughton MA, Teng W et al. Design of potent and specific integrin antagonists. Peptide antagonists with high-specificity for glycoprotein IIb-IIIa. J Biol Chem 1993;268:1066–1073.

73. Harrington RA, Kleiman NS, Kottke-Marchant K et al. Immediate and reversible platelet inhibition after intravenous administration of a peptide glycoprotein IIb-IIIa inhibitor during percutaneous coronary intervention. Am J Cardiol 1995;76:1222–1227.

74. Verheugt, FWA. In search of a superaspirin for the heart (commentary). Lancet 1997;349:1409–1410.

75. Théroux P, Kouz S, Roy L et al. Platelet membrane receptor glycoprotein IIb-IIIa antagonism in unstable angina. The Canadian Lamifiban Study. Circulation 1996;94:899–905.

76. Kereiakes DJ, Kleiman NS, Amborse J et al. Randomized, double-blind, placebo-controlled dose-ranging study of tirofiban (MK-383) platelet IIb-IIIa blockade in high risk patients undergoing coronary angioplasty. J Am Coll Cardiol 1996;27:536–542.

77. Hanson SR, Hutsell TC, Keefer LK et al. Nitric oxide donors: a continuing opportunity in drug design. Adv Pharmacol 1995;34:383–398.

78. Lees C, Langford E, Brown AS et al. The effects of S-nitrosoglutathione on platelet activation, hypertension, and uterine and fetal Doppler in severe preeclampsia. Obstet Gynecol 1996;88:14–19.

79. Langford EJ, Wainwright RJ, Martin JF. Platelet activation in acute myocardial infarction and unstable angina is inhibited by nitric oxide donors. Aterioscler Thromb Vasc Biol 1996;16:51–55.

80. Fujimura M, Kamio Y, Saito M et al. Bronchodilator and bronchoprotective effects of cilostazol in humans in vivo. Am J Respir Crit Care Med 1995;151:222–225.

81. Matousovic K, Grande JP, Chini CC et al. Inhibitors of cyclic nucleotide phosphodiesterase isozymes type-III and type-IV suppress mitogenesis of rat mesangial cells. J Clin Invest 1995;96:401-410.

82. Anonymous. Prevention of atherosclerotic complications: controlled trial of ketanserin. Prevention of Atherosclerotic Complications with Ketanserin (PACK) trial group. BMJ 1989;298:424–430.

83. Leaf A, Weber C. Cardiovascular effects of n-3 fatty acids. N Engl J Med 1988;318:549–557.

84. De Caterina R, Cybulsky MI, Clinton SK et al. The omega-3 fatty acid docosahexaenoate reduces cytokine-induced expression of proatherogenic and proinflammatory proteins in human endothelial cells. Aterioscler Thromb 1994;14:1829–1836.

85. Freedman JE, Farhat JH, Loscalzo J et al. Alpha-tocopherol inhibits aggregation of human platelets by a protein kinase C-dependent mechanism. Circulation 1996;94:2434–2440.

86. Stephens NG, Parsons A, Schofield PM et al. Randomised controlled trial of vitamin E in patients with coronary disease: Cambridge Heart Antioxidant Study (CHAOS). Lancet 1996;347:781–786.

87. Patrono C, FitzGerald GA. Isoprostanes: potential markers of oxidant stress in atherothrombotic disease. Arterioscler Thromb Vasc Biol 1997; in press.

# CHAPTER 55

# PHARMACOLOGY OF HEPARIN AND ORAL ANTICOAGULANTS

Walter Jeske, Harry L. Messmore, Jr., and Jawed Fareed

## INTRODUCTION

Despite major developments in anticoagulant and antithrombotic drugs, heparin and its derivatives and oral anticoagulant drugs have remained the therapy of choice for the management of thrombotic and cardiovascular disorders. It is, indeed, evident that unfractionated heparin exhibits certain unwanted side effects, such as heparin-induced thrombocytopenia and bleeding; however, in clinical settings it is difficult to find substitutes with a comparable therapeutic index at this time. Unfractionated heparin has also provided a surgical anticoagulant without which such procedures as open heart surgery and angioplasty would not be possible. The development of modified heparins such as the low-molecular-weight heparins has added a new spectrum to the prophylaxis and treatment of thrombotic and cardiovascular disorders. These agents have also provided a tool to understand the biology of heparin and the structure-activity relationships in this complex drug. Heparins exhibit several endogenous interactions and produce modulatory actions at cellular and plasmatic sites. Thus, the overall clinical effects of heparins represent a complex process involving several components.

Knowledge of the affinity of selected molecular components of heparin to antithrombin has led to the development of a chemically synthetic pentasaccharide. This drug is currently in clinical trials for the prophylaxis of deep venous thrombosis in individuals who have undergone hip surgery. In addition, since this agent has such a high affinity for antithrombin, at certain dosages, it is expected to saturate most cellular and plasmatic sites where antithrombin is present, providing an antithrombotic environment while minimizing heparin-induced thrombocytopenic or hemorrhagic manifestations. Additional features of heparin components such as the modulation of selectins and regulatory effects on the fibrinolytic system and TFPI may provide additional knowledge for the design of new drugs. While the clinical investigations with heparin, low-molecular-weight heparin, and pentasaccharide are expected to provide useful data on newer indications for these agents, basic pharmacologic information will continue to enhance our current knowledge of this drug.

Currently, warfarin is in clinical use because of its predictable pharmacodynamics and bioavailability characteristics. The introduction of the international normalized ratio (INR) for monitoring warfarin and the lowering of the therapeutic range to an INR of 2.0 to 3.0 represent significant advances in this area. Warfarin is effective in the prevention of venous thromboembolism, systemic thromboembolic disorders, and arterial thrombosis resulting in stroke or myocardial infarction. While bleeding is the main complication associated with warfarin therapy, the use of INR for monitoring and lowering of the dosage has resulted in a reduction in the incidence of bleeding. Despite major advances to develop additional oral anticoagulant drugs, there is not another drug that can parallel the effects of warfarin. Orally acting factor Xa and thrombin inhibitors are currently under development. Clinical trials are needed to validate their relative value in comparison to warfarin (1, 2).

## DISCOVERY OF HEPARIN

Heparin was discovered in 1916 by McLean during investigations into the procoagulant actions of phospholipids (3). Initially, heparin was although to be a phospholipid as it was isolated using procedures designed to separate phospholipids. Today it is known that heparin is a glycosaminoglycan structurally related to the dermatans and chondroitins. More specifically, heparin has been defined as " . . . a family of polysaccharide species, whose chains are made up of alternating 1-4 linked and variously sulfated residues of uronic acid and D-glucosamine" (4). The uronic acid residues are either L-iduronic acid or D-glucuronic acid. The glucosamine residues are either N-sulfated or N-acetylated. Typically, the iduronic acid moieties are 2-O sulfated whereas the glucosamine residues contain 6-O sulfate groups and a small proportion contain 3-O sulfates (5). The chemical structure of heparin is depicted in Fig. 55.1.

## CHEMISTRY OF HEPARIN

Heparin is synthesized by a number of tissues and mast cells as part of a high-molecular-weight proteoglycan (molecular mass ~ 750 to 1000 Kda). This proteoglycan consists of a peptide core that is composed of 20 to 25 residues each of glycine and serine (6). Attached to this peptide are 15 polysaccharide chains with molecular masses ranging from 60 to 100 Kda. The polysaccharide chains are attached to the peptide core via a galactosyl-galactosyl-xylosyl trisaccharide sequence (7).

The polysaccharide chains are formed by stepwise transfer of D-glucuronic acid and N-acetyl-D-glucosamine from their UDP sugar nucleotide forms to the non-reducing end of the polysaccharide chain (8–10). Presumably these sugar moieties are polymerized directly to the linkage region of the protein core. The alternating sequence of glucuronic acid and hexosamine is due to the substrate specificity of the glycosyl transferases (11). Following polysaccharide chain elongation, the polymer undergoes a series of modification reactions.

Heparin is structurally heterogeneous due to incomplete structural modifications. Four enzymatic modifications of the polysaccharide backbone occur following its synthesis. The majority of the N-acetyl groups on the glucosamine residues are removed (12) and the N-deacetylated glucosamines are subsequently sulfated. In the next step, D-glucuronic acid residues are epimerized to L-iduronic acid units by uronosyl C-5 epimerase (13, 14). During the epimerization process, most iduronic acids are 2-O sulfated. Finally, 3-O and 6-O sulfate groups are added onto the glucosamine units. N-sulfation allows more efficient O-sulfation to occur (11). More recent studies have indicated that chain elongation and modification may occur simultaneously during heparin synthesis (15, 16).

## BIOLOGIC EFFECTS OF HEPARIN—NONANTICOAGULANT

Heparin is a strongly anionic polyelectrolyte that at physiologic pH contains three acidic functional groups

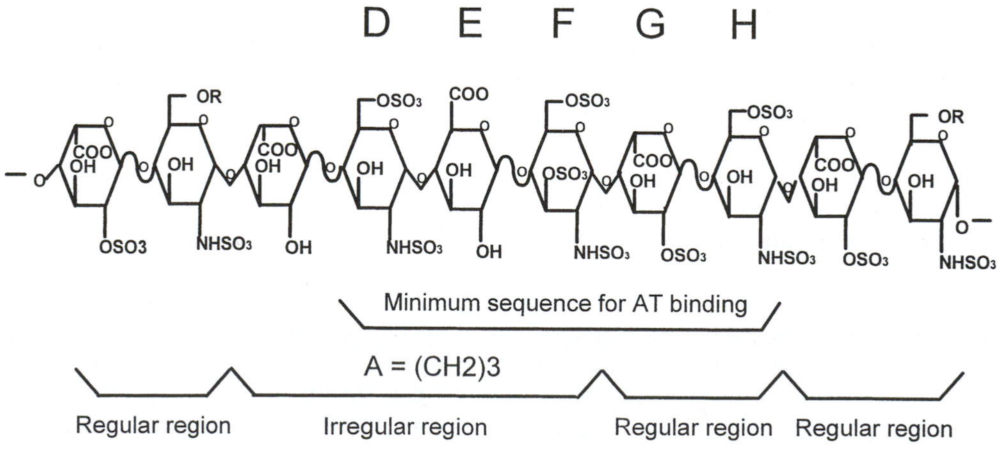

**FIGURE 55.1.**    Chemical structure of heparin. The regular regions of heparin are composed of repeating trisulfated disaccharide units made up of sulfated L-iduronic acid and sulfated glucosamine. Interspersed between the regular regions are heparin sequences composed of glucuronic acid, nonsulfated iduronic acid, and glucosamine. It is in these irregular regions that the 3-O sulfate group is required for high-affinity binding to antithrombin (AT) is present. The pentasaccharide sequence of heparin required for high-affinity binding to antithrombin is composed of saccharides from the regular (units G and H) and irregular units of heparin (units D, E, and F). (Adapted from Walenga JM. Doctoral thesis: Factor Xa inhibition in mediating antithrombotic actions: application of a synthetic heparin pentasaccharide. Universite Pierre et Marie Curie, 1987, with permission of J. Choay, Institut Choay, Paris, France.)

that are fully dissociated; $-OSO_3^-$, $-NHSO_3^-$, and $-COO^-$ (17). Owing to this fact, heparin exhibits a large number of sequence with nonspecific, charge dependent pharmacologic properties. Among these are its antilipemic and antihemolytic actions (18, 19). Heparin is also known to inhibit a variety of enzymes including myosin ATPase, RNA dependent DNA polymerase, elastase, and renin (20–22). Heparin inhibits tumor growth (23, 24). Additionally, heparin exhibits antibacterial and antiviral properties (25, 26).

## MECHANISMS OF ANTICOAGULANT ACTIONS OF HEPARIN

### Antithrombin

Heparin produces little anticoagulant or antithrombotic effect directly. Rather, its effects are mediated through several plasma proteins known as serpins (serine protease inhibitors). These serpins include antithrombin (or antithrombin III), heparin cofactor II, and the Kunitz-type inhibitor, tissue factor pathway inhibitor (TFPI).

In the beginning of this century, it was suspected that a natural inhibitor of thrombin was present in the plasma (27). The first hints of antithrombin's existence were detected shortly after the discovery of heparin when it was discovered that heparin required a cofactor to exhibit its anticoagulant activity (28, 29). At this point, the molecule was termed heparin cofactor (29). It was not until the late 1960s that Abildgaard demonstrated that the proteins antithrombin (or antithrombin III) and heparin cofactor were one and the same (30).

Antithrombin is a member of the serpin superfamily of proteins (MW = 58 Kda) (31), which includes the inhibitors $\alpha_2$-antiplasmin, $\alpha_1$-antichymotrypsin, and $\alpha_1$-proteinase inhibitor (32) (see Chapter 3). Antithrombin is considered to be the primary inhibitor of coagulation (33) and targets most coagulation proteases, as well as the enzymes trypsin, plasmin, and kallikrein (34, 35). Inhibition takes place when a stoichiometric complex between the active site serine of the protease and the Arg393-Ser294 bond of antithrombin forms (36–39).

The efficient inhibition of proteases by antithrombin requires heparin as a cofactor. Without heparin, the inhibition rate constants for thrombin and factor Xa have been estimated to be $1 \times 10^3$ and $3 \times 10^3$ L/mol sec$^{-1}$, respectively. In the presence of heparin, these rates of inhibition are accelerated to $3 \times 10^7$ and $4 \times 10^6$ L/mol sec$^{-1}$, respectively, for thrombin and factor Xa (40). The binding site for heparin is located on the N-terminal domain of the molecule.

Two mechanisms have been proposed to account for heparin's ability to catalyze the antiprotease actions of antithrombin. The first suggests that heparin binds to antithrombin and causes a conformational change at the active site, thereby making antithrombin more reactive (36). The second model, the ternary complex or template model, proposes that heparin acts catalytically by binding both antithrombin and the serine protease, thereby limiting their diffusion (34). Both models may be operative depending on the serine protease being inhibited. Conformational changes of antithrombin on heparin binding have been observed spectroscopically (36, 41, 42). Furthermore, the ability of a pentasaccharide region of heparin to promote the antithrombin-mediated inhibition of factor Xa supports this model, while the inhibition of thrombin is better explained by the template model. Conformational changes induced by heparin binding do not alter the reactivity of antithrombin toward thrombin (43). In addition, heparin pentasaccharides do not promote thrombin inhibition. Rather, chains of greater than 18 saccharide units are needed for this inhibition. Kinetic studies indicate that heparin must bind both thrombin and antithrombin to promote inhibition (44, 45), although it is not clear if the order of binding is important (46, 47). The inhibition of other coagulation factors by antithrombin such as factors IXa, VIIa, and XIa, is also promoted by heparin but to a lesser extent than factor Xa or thrombin.

### Heparin Cofactor II

Heparin cofactor II is a second plasma serpin (M.W. = 62 to 72 Kda) that has resemblance to antithrombin in that it is activatable by glycosaminoglycan binding. This protein has also been called antithrombin BM (48), dermatan sulfate cofactor (49), and human leuserpin 2 (50). The existence of this second inhibitor and heparin cofactor was first shown by Briginshaw in 1974 (51, 52). Whereas antithrombin is observed to have progressive antithrombin activity and to also inhibit factor Xa, the second cofactor exhibits only weak, progressive activity and does not inhibit factor Xa. Tollefsen observed two different thrombin inhibitor complexes, one of which could not be identified with antisera to known protease inhibitors (53). Several clinical studies observed a discrepancy between heparin cofactor activity levels and plasma antithrombin antigen levels (54, 55).

Like antithrombin, heparin cofactor II inhibits proteases by forming a 1:1 stoichiometric complex with the enzyme. The protease attacks the reactive site of heparin cofactor II located on the C-terminus, resulting in the formation of a covalent bond. Heparin cofactor II has a higher protease specificity than antithrombin, known only to inhibit thrombin due to the active site bond in the inhibitor (35).

As in the case of antithrombin, the inhibition of protease activity by heparin cofactor II is promoted by glycosaminoglycan binding. Whereas the activation of antithrombin depends on the presence of a specific sequence in the heparin chain, heparin cofactor II can be activated by a wide variety of agents. Heparins, heparans, and dermatan sulfate all promote thrombin inhibition via heparin cofactor II, whereas agents with relatively little sulfation such as chondroitin 4-O- or 6-O-sulfate, keratan sulfate, or hyaluronic acid do not activate heparin cofactor II. Heparan sulfate containing 0.97 sulfates per disaccharide has been shown to be a better activator of heparin cofactor II than heparan sulfate containing 0.67 sulfates per disaccharide (56). In addition, sulfated, synthetic agents are able to activate heparin cofactor II. Both pentosan polysulfate (57, 58) and dextran sulfate (59) have been shown to activate heparin cofactor II.

To study its heparin cofactor II binding characteristics, heparin has been fractionated by charge density and subsequently on an antithrombin-Sepharose column into high- and low-affinity fractions (60). It has been observed that for a given charge density, antithrombin affinity is unrelated to the ability of the fraction to activate heparin cofactor II. High- and low-affinity fractions equally activate heparin cofactor II if charge density is equal. To date, definitive data supporting the existence of a minimally required sequence to activate heparin cofactor II have not been reported.

## Tissue Factor Pathway Inhibitor

Tissue factor pathway inhibitor (TFPI) (see Chapter 4) is one of the coagulation protease inhibitors found endogenously within the vasculature and has alternatively been known as lipoprotein-associated coagulation inhibitor (LACI) or extrinsic pathway inhibitor (EPI). This 42 Kda inhibitor has been shown to contain three Kunitz domains tandemly linked between a negatively charged aminoterminus and a positively charged carboxyterminus (61). TFPI inhibits coagulation by simultaneously binding the factor VIIa-tissue factor complex and factor Xa via two of the Kunitz domains.

In normal tissues of the vasculature, TFPI is produced by megakaryocytes and the endothelium (62). Once produced, this TFPI is stored in three intravascular pools. These pools are located in the plasma, in platelets, and bound to the endothelium (63). The largest pool of TFPI is found bound to the endothelial surface (64–66); this pool can account for 50 to 90% of the total intravascular TFPI.

The TFPI pool bound to the endothelium has been shown to be heparin releasable in a number of studies (67–71). Venous occlusion (65) and agents such as DDAVP, which induce exocytosis of endothelial granular proteins (72), do not cause the release of TFPI. Repeated heparin administration is observed to release similar amounts of TFPI (67) with no tachyphylaxis. It is believed that the endothelial pool of TFPI is bound to glycosaminoglycans on the surface of the endothelium. Heparin injection is although to displace TFPI from the endogenous glycosaminoglycans. The amount of TFPI in the plasma following heparin administration is deter-

mined by the heparin concentration. TFPI levels twofold to tenfold above baseline have been reported following heparin and low-molecular-weight heparin administration. The chemical nature of the low-molecular-weight heparin also affects the degree of TFPI release. It has been shown that when different low-molecular-weight heparins are administered at the same anti-Xa unit dosage, plasma TFPI levels vary by as much as 30% (73). Neutralization of heparin by protamine sulfate or protamine chloride results in a dramatic decrease in plasma TFPI levels (74, 75).

TFPI acts *in vitro* as an anticoagulant when measured by a number of assays. Both the thromboplastin-induced clotting time and the activated partial thromboplastin time (aPTT) are prolonged by TFPI (76, 77). Factor Xa based assays such as the Heptest® and the amidolytic anti-Xa assay are also affected by recombinant TFPI (78). Higher amounts of TFPI are required in the prothrombin time (PT) and aPTT for prolongation of the clotting time than are needed in the Heptest®. The PT is a more sensitive assay for the anticoagulant effects of TFPI than is the aPTT, suggesting that the main *in vitro* inhibitory effect of TFPI is the inhibition of factor VIIa. Co-supplementation of heparin and rTFPI to plasma *in vitro* has differing effects depending on the assay used. Kristensen observed that heparin and rTFPI additively prolong the Heptest® clotting time. It has been shown that the prolongation of the aPTT and PT assays by heparin and TFPI is synergistic (79, 80). A study by Nordfang et al, however, suggests that the increased effect of TFPI in the presence of heparin is due to heparin-antithrombin complexes as addition of heparin exhibited no effect in antithrombin deficient plasma (81). The rate of Xa inhibition by rTFPI was observed to increase 2.5-fold on the addition of heparin (82), although not with full-length TFPI (83).

## PHARMACOKINETICS OF HEPARIN

Heparin is administered either by intravenous infusion or by subcutaneous injection. On entering the blood stream, heparin binds to a variety of plasma proteins, thereby lowering its bioavailability and producing a variable anticoagulant response (84). These proteins include histidine-rich glycoprotein, platelet factor 4, vitronectin, and von Willebrand factor (43, 85–90). Heparin exhibits complex pharmacokinetics and is cleared by two mechanisms. The rapid, saturable phase of elimination is although to be due to receptor mediated internalization of heparin by endothelial cells and macrophages (91–93). A slower, nonsaturable renal mechanism also clears heparin from the plasma (94–96). The anticoagulant effect of heparin is therefore not linearly related to dose when in the therapeutic range (97). The biologic half-life of heparin increases from 30 minutes following an intravenous bolus dose of 25 U/kg to 150 minutes following a dose of 400 U/kg (94–96). Bioavailability of heparin after subcutaneous administration is limited by the size of the molecule, with typical heparin preparations exhibiting a 20 to 30% subcutaneous bioavailability. Heparin does not exhibit significant bioavailability following oral administration. Administration by inhalation has been reported and results in a prolonged elimination half-life.

## CLINICAL USE OF HEPARIN

Heparin is used in the therapy of several cardiovascular disorders including prevention and treatment of venous thromboembolism, treatment of unstable angina, acute myocardial infarction, cardiac and vascular surgery, coronary angioplasty, stent implantation, and as an adjunctive agent during thrombolysis. Heparin is also the anticoagulant of choice during pregnancy.

Studies have demonstrated a reduction in mortality in individuals receiving heparin for the treatment of pulmonary embolism (98, 99). In addition, recurrent thrombosis was not common during the heparinization period, but increased significantly when heparin was stopped and no other anticoagulant therapy was utilized (100, 101). Heparin is effective in treating venous thrombosis. This effectiveness has been shown to depend on the anticoagulant effect achieved (102, 103). Heparin is also effective prophylactically, reducing the risk of venous thrombosis and pulmonary embolism by 60 to 70% (104, 105). Heparin is effective short-term in preventing acute myocardial infarction and recurrent refractory angina in individuals with unstable angina (106–108). This beneficial effect is lost on cessation of heparin therapy. In individuals with previous myocardial infarction, heparin administration has been shown to reduce reinfarction and death significantly when compared with untreated controls (109). Heparin has been tested as an adjunct in thrombolytic therapy where it appears to increase patency during the initial stages of recanalization by preventing rethrombosis (110, 111). Heparin is the anticoagulant of choice in pregnancy as it does not cross the placental barrier and is not known to cause teratogenic effects on the fetus (97, 112); however, its use in this setting does increase maternal bleeding risk.

The monitoring of the anticoagulant actions of heparin is necessary in order that drug concentrations remain in the therapeutic range and to minimize side effects. The therapeutic use of heparin is typically monitored using the aPTT assay, whereas the activated clotting time (ACT) is used in situations where high plasma concentrations of the drug are required. Because of variable responses of aPTT reagents to heparin, measurement of protamine titration heparin levels (therapeutic range of 0.2 to 0.4 U/ml) may be an alternative to measurement of aPTT ratios (therapeutic range of 1.5 to 2.5 times the control value) (113).

## EFFECT OF HEPARIN ON PLATELETS

The effect of heparin on platelet activation and aggregation is controversial. Studies by Ellison and Thomson have shown that heparin decreases the threshold for ADP- and epinephrine-induced aggregation and enhances the platelet release reactions by these agonists (114, 115). Treatment with heparin was also observed to increase platelet retention on cellophane membranes. Other studies have indicated the opposite effects on platelets. Besterman and Gillett showed that irreversible aggregation induced by collagen and epinephrine was reduced in individuals treated with 2500 to 5000 U of unfractionated heparin (116). In these same individuals, no effect to a slight increase in aggregation was observed with ADP (117). Heiden demonstrated a loss of [$^{14}$C]serotonin release in the platelet-rich plasmas of individuals treated with 100 U/kg heparin in response to collagen, epinephrine, and ADP (118). An indirect mechanism was suggested to account for this observation based on the finding that *in vitro* addition of heparin caused no effect on aggregation (119). Salzman et al have shown that concentrations of heparin as low as 10 µg/mL induce aggregation in platelet-rich plasma, but not in washed platelets (120).

## SIDE EFFECTS OF HEPARIN THERAPY

The most common side effect of heparin therapy is hemorrhage. The hemorrhagic effects associated with heparin therapy can range from minor to life-threatening and appear to be related to the total administered dose and the degree of prolongation of the aPTT rather than the route of administration. Heparin-induced thrombocytopenia (HIT) occurs in about 5% of individuals treated with heparin (see Chapter 29). Two types of HIT have been identified. Type I HIT occurs early in heparin treatment and causes a transient reduction in platelet count; this is believed to be due to a direct effect of heparin on the platelet and individuals usually remain asymptomatic. Type II HIT is a more severe thrombocytopenia and occurs with a delayed onset. This form of HIT often results in thrombosis and is associated with a high degree of morbidity and mortality (heparin-induced thrombocytopenia and thrombosis). While the mechanism of HIT has not been completely identified, it appears that an antibody is generated against the heparin/platelet factor 4 complex. Frequently these antibodies are IgG, although IgA and IgM antibodies have also been reported. The antibody-platelet factor 4-heparin complex binds to the FcRII receptor on the platelet surface, resulting in activation. Owing to the severity of the symptoms, heparin therapy must be discontinued.

Heparin therapy is associated with transient elevations in serum transaminase levels, which may or may not be of clinical importance. Long-term heparin therapy has also been shown to result in osteoporotic effects.

## CHEMICALLY MODIFIED HEPARINS

### Hypersulfated Heparins

Modification of the structure of heparin leads to differential pharmacologic effects. The anticoagulant and antithrombotic actions of heparins containing higher than normal degrees of sulfation have been examined in several studies. In a laser model of thrombosis, a supersulfated low-molecular-weight heparin was observed to require a tenfold lower dose than native heparin or low-molecular-weight heparin to achieve a comparable antithrombotic effect (121). In another study, oversulfation of low-molecular-weight heparin was observed to reduce the *ex vivo* anticoagulant activity relative to low-molecular-weight heparin that was not oversulfated. Addition of sulfate groups, however, did not affect the antithrombotic activity in a rat venous stasis-thrombosis model and did not significantly increase the bleeding time (122). The release of lipoprotein lipase by the supersulfated, low-molecular-weight heparin was twice that of heparin. In an *in vitro* system, the inhibition of thrombin via heparin cofactor II by supersulfated, low-molecular-weight heparin was approximately 100-fold greater than for low-molecular-weight heparin (123).

### Desulfated Heparins

*N*- and *O*-desulfated heparins have also been examined for a number of pharmacologic properties. In general, a

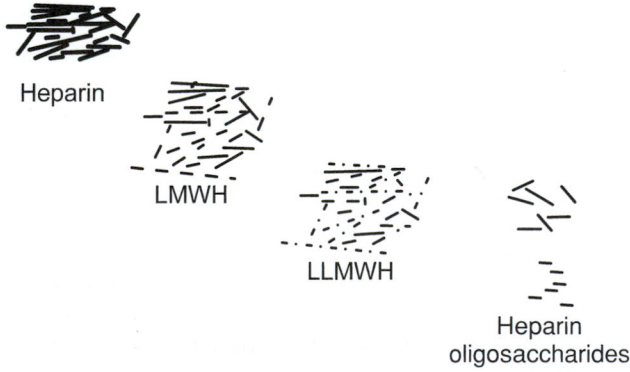

Heparin

LMWH

LLMWH

Heparin
oligosaccharides

**FIGURE 55.2.** Depicts a diagrammatic comparison of heparin, low-molecular-weight heparin (LMWH), lower low-molecular-weight heparin (LLMWH), and heparin oligosaccharides. Heparin is comprised of oligosaccharide chains ranging from 2 to 50 Kda with an apparent molecular weight of 13 Kda. The LMWHs vary in molecular weight, ranging from 4 to 8 Kda, with a mean mass of 5.2 Kda. The LLMWH exhibit a mean molecular weight of 3.4 Kda. The heparin oligosaccharides exhibit molecular weights from 1.5 to 5.2 Kda. The synthetic pentasaccharide mimicking the antithrombin binding sequence of heparin is 1.7 Kda.

reduction in the sulfation of heparin results in decreased biologic activity. *N*- and 6-*O*-desulfation significantly decreases the antiviral activity of heparin with respect to herpes simplex I binding (124). Heparin potentiates the binding of vascular endothelial growth factor (VEGF 165) to its cellular receptors, flk and flt. *O*- and *N*-desulfated heparins potentiate this binding to a lesser extent than unmodified heparin (125). Rajtar et al demonstrated that *N*-desulfated heparins were less effective at inhibiting platelet function than native heparin (126). Both fully desulfated heparin and *N*-desulfated heparin lack the ability to bind heparin binding growth factor (127).

The anticoagulant and antithrombotic effects of desulfated heparins have also been examined. A partially *N*-desulfated heparin has been shown to have no measurable anticoagulant or antiprotease activity, but to impair thrombogenesis dose-dependently *in vivo* (128). A completely *N*-desulfated heparin derivative lacked both *in vitro* and *in vivo* activity (129). Other investigators have shown that *N*-desulfated heparins have minimal anticoagulant activity (130, 131). *N*-desulfated heparin has been shown to be cleared approximately sixfold faster than native heparin (130). The weak anticoagulant activity is attributable to the lack of interaction with antithrombin (131).

## LOW-MOLECULAR-WEIGHT HEPARIN

The depolymerization of heparin either by nitrous acid degradation, benzylation-alkaline hydrolysis, peroxidative cleavage, heparinase, or physicochemically (gamma irradiation) results in the production of another clinically useful drug known as low-molecular-weight heparin (LMWH). This process, shown in Fig. 55.2, results in a material that is approximately one-third of the molecular weight of the parent unfractionated heparin. The largest heparin chains are not well absorbed following subcutaneous administration. Whereas the bioavailability of unfractionated heparin is only 20 to 30% (132), the bioavailability of LMWH is nearly 100% when measured using an amidolytic anti-Xa assay. The smaller molecular size of the LMWHs also has an effect on the biologic activity of these agents. The LMWHs have a lower anticoagulant potency than unfractionated heparin. This is a reflection of the lower antithrombin activity of these agents. Heparin exhibits a 1:1 ratio of antithrombin to anti-Xa activity whereas for LMWHs the ratio ranges from 1:2 to 1:4 depending on the molecular weight composition of the given LMWH (97).

LMWHs are depolymerized porcine mucosal heparin preparations with the exception of Fluxum (Opocrin Laboratories), which is obtained from beef mucosa. The first clinical batches of LMWHs were prepared by fractionation of heparin. However, due to cost and limited availability of sizable quantities of heparin for isolation of these agents, chemical and enzymatic depolymerization procedures were developed. Most LMWHs are cur-

**TABLE 55.1.** Currently Available Low-Molecular-Weight Heparins

| Agent | Manufacturer/Supplier | Method of Preparation |
|---|---|---|
| Fraxiparin (Seleparin) | Sanofi, Paris, France | Fractionation, optimized nitrous acid depolymerization |
| Enoxaparin (Clexane, Lovenox) | Rhone-Poulenc, Paris, France | Benzylation followed by alkaline hydrolysis |
| Dalteparin (Fragmin) | Pharmacia-Upjohn | Controlled nitrous acid depolymerization |
| Certoparin (Sandoparin) | Novartis, Basel, Switzerland | Isoamyl nitrite digestion |
| Tinzaparin (Logiparin, Innohep) | Novo-Nordisk/Leo, Copenhagen, Denmark | Heparinase digestion |
| Reviparin (Clivarin) | Knoll AG, Ludwigshafen, Germany | Nitrous acid digestion |
| Ardeparin (Normiflo) | Wyeth-Ayerst, Philadelphia, PA | Peroxidative cleavage |
| Parnaparin (Fluxum) | Opocrin, Corlo, Italy | Peroxidative cleavage |

**TABLE 55.2.** Structural Changes in Heparin Produced by Depolymerization

| Depolymerization Process | Chemical Change |
|---|---|
| Nitrous acid depolymerization | Deaminative cleavage resulting in the formation of 2,5-anhydro sugars at reducing end |
| Isoamyl nitrite depolymerization | Deaminative cleavage resulting in the formation of 2,5-anhydro sugars at reducing end |
| Benzylation + alkaline hydrolysis | Introduction of double bond at the reducing end |
| Peroxidative cleavage | Generation of labile glycosidic bonds |
| Heparinase digestion | Cleavage of $N$-sulfated glucosamine–L-iduronic acid linkages |

rently manufactured by chemical depolymerization with the exception of logiparin (Novo Nordisk, Copenhagen, Denmark), which is prepared by using the enzyme heparinase. More recently, physical methods such as gamma-irradiation have also been used to obtain LMWHs. A list of some of the commercially available products under development is given in Table 55.1.

Although each depolymerization process results in a lower molecular weight material (MW 4 to 8 Kda), these products exhibit differences in both their structural and functional properties. Table 55.2 lists chemical and structural modifications that occur as a result of the depolymerization procedures. As a rule, chemical depolymerization results in partial desulfation, a reduction in charge density, a reduction in the number of antithrombin binding sites, and other changes in the consensus sequences. Chemical and enzymatic degradation of heparin produces specific changes in heparin. End-residues of fragments are typical of the specific depolymerization method. The relative functional significance of these specific effects is unknown at this time. Heparinase usually cleaves glycosidic bonds between $N$-sulfated glucosamine and iduronic acid 2-sulfate, producing fragments terminating with 4,5-unsaturated iduronic acid 2-sulfate at the nonreducing end and $N$-sulfated glucosamine, (6-

sulfated) at the reducing end; this is exemplified in logiparin. Fragments terminating with unsaturated uronic acids are also produced by base-catalyzed depolymerization, such as that observed in enoxaparin.

Nitrous acid splits glycosidic bonds between $N$-sulfated glucosamine and any kind of uronic acid, resulting in fragments with 2,5 anhydromannose at the reducing end. For stabilization, these end-residues are frequently reduced to anhydromannitol. The depolymerized fraxiparin product represents these characteristics. Periodate oxidation splits the $C_2$-$C_3$ bonds of nonsulfated uronic acids, making the glycosidic bonds of modified residues labile to alkali, or (when reduced) to acid. Fluxum and ardeparin are prepared using these methods. Direct acid hydrolysis preferentially brings about $N$-desulfation. Fragments from $N$-desulfated heparin terminating with iduronic acid groups can be re-$N$-sulfated to restore the critical sulfamino functional groups. Fragments with these characteristics can be produced by ascorbic acid (or copper ion)—catalyzed depolymerization of heparin with hydrogen peroxide. Acid depolymerization and sulfation can be accomplished simultaneously with concentrated chlorosulphonic/sulfuric acid, producing "supersulfated" heparin fragments with one extra sulfate group per disaccharide unit.

The [$^{13}$C]-NMR spectra of fragments produced by different depolymerization procedures usually permit identification of end-residues and a checking of whether any "internal" structure has been modified by the fragmentation procedure. The spectra of fragments from depolymerization with heparinase clearly display signals from both end-residues, that is, the unsaturated uronic acid and the reducing glucosamine. Optimized methods are currently employed to prepare LMWHs that exhibit similar molecular profiles. However, owing to the significant differences in the chemical or enzymatic procedures, structural variations are found among these agents. These differences therefore exert significant influence on the biologic action of these products (133, 134). Well-designed clinical trials to compare the safety and efficacy of these agents are not available at this time. Initial attempts to standardize LMWHs on the basis of their biologic actions, such as anti-Xa potency, have failed; however, the European Pharmacopeial Commission has adopted this method for the potency evaluation of these agents. A potency designation on the basis of the anti-Xa actions only represents one of the several properties of these agents.

Recent biochemical and pharmacologic studies have shown that the materials obtained from each process exhibit chemical and pharmacologic differences as discussed. Chemical modification of the end groups and internal structures, charge density, and degree of desulfation during manufacturing, all add to the individuality displayed by the resulting products. Antithrombin binding sites can be modified during some depolymerization processes resulting in reduced activity. Heparin cofactor II, platelet factor 4 and protamine neutralization, and cellular interactions also vary from product to product. LMWHs also exhibit differences in their ability to release various mediators from the vascular lining.

Despite the clinical effectiveness of the LMWHs in the prophylaxis of postsurgical DVT, the mechanism of action of these agents is not completely understood. More recently, it has been suggested that endogenous release of a Kunitz-type inhibitor, TFPI, may be a contributing factor in the antithrombotic actions of these agents. It is interesting to note that most of the studies on LMWH have alluded to the relevance of the anti-Xa effect for the antithrombotic action of these agents. However, after subcutaneous administration of these agents, circulating anti-Xa activity is not detectable in samples collected 12 hours after the administration of prophylactic dosages. Despite this reduction in the anti-Xa activity, the individuals remain in an antithrombotic state. Thus additional mechanisms such as the release of TFPI may contribute to the overall action of these agents. LMWHs are also known to produce endothelial modulation and may release fibrinolytic activators, such as t-PA and antiplatelet substances, such as prostacyclin.

It has been suggested that repeated administration of LMWH results in the augmentation of its activity as an antithrombotic and antihemostatic drug. Thus this phenomenon needs to be investigated further to determine the implication of this finding for the therapeutic index of these agents.

## INDICATIONS FOR THE USE OF LMWHS

### Deep Vein Thrombosis (DVT) Prophylaxis

LeClerc et al have recently reported on the prevention of venous thrombosis after knee arthroplasty by LMWH (135). These authors concluded that a postoperative fixed dose of enoxaparin was more effective than adjusted dose warfarin in preventing venous thrombosis after knee surgery. No differences were seen in the incidence of proximal venous thrombosis or clinically overt hemorrhage.

In another study, Bergqvist et al reported on extended use of enoxaparin in the prevention of thrombotic events following hip surgery and concluded that extended duration of therapy may result in the decrease of postphlebitic syndrome (136). Levine et al have compared ardeparin administered twice daily after operation and found it safe and effective for the prevention of venous thrombosis in individuals who underwent major knee surgery. Heit et al compared ardeparin to warfarin and found that 50 anti–factor Xa U/kg administered subcutaneously twice daily resulted in significantly more blood loss than warfarin at an INR of 2.0 to 3.0 (137), whereas 35 anti–factor Xa U/kg subcutaneous twice daily may provide similar efficacy to the higher dose with reduced bleeding. Thus it is clear from the new trials, that LMWHs are effective in preventing venous thrombosis after orthopedic surgery (138).

There is a debate regarding the duration of postsurgical thrombotic risk and the appropriate duration of prophylaxis. Planes et al have endorsed a prolonged prophylactic treatment period with LMWHs of 35 days postsurgery (139). This approach was shown to reduce the postphlebitic syndrome considerably and has become the basis for a multicenter clinical trial (140). Dahl et al showed that dalteparin at 5000 IU once daily for 35 days (starting 7 days after surgery) significantly reduced the frequency of DVT compared with placebo in orthopedic individuals given the same thromboprophylaxis for the initial 7 postoperative days (141). The safety of high-dose (80 mg once daily for 3 months) certoparin has also been reported in the PARAT trial (J. Fareed, unpublished observation). No adverse effects, such as bleeding or heparin-induced thrombocytopenia, were observed in these individuals.

Low-dose subcutaneous heparin treatment for a 3-week period has been found to reduce the occurrence of nonfatal pulmonary embolism (PE) ($P <$ .0012) in nonsurgical individuals with infectious diseases (142). However, as mortality, the number of fatal PE, and the time from admission to death were not different between treatment and control groups, the overall findings of this study did not support the routine use of heparin prophylaxis in nonsurgical individuals. LMWHs have not been tested for this indication as yet.

## Cardiovascular Indications

Because of their favorable pharmacokinetic and pharmacodynamic properties, LMWHs are being developed for the initial treatment of thromboembolism (143), for the treatment of unstable angina, for the primary and secondary management of thrombotic and ischemic stroke, for the reduction of restenosis after interventional cardiac procedures, and for the maintenance of the late patency of peripheral arterial grafts. A recent study (FRISC) has been reported that tested the ability of dalteparin to prevent coronary events in individuals with unstable angina or non–Q wave myocardial infarction (144). At 120 IU/kg administered subcutaneously twice daily, dalteparin was shown to decrease death and myocardial infarction significantly in comparison with placebo. In comparison to unfractionated heparin (FRIC trial), dalteparin produced comparable beneficial effects and, thus, an advantage over heparin was not established (FRIC Investigators, unpublished).

Cohen recently reported on the use of enoxaparin for the management of unstable angina in the ESSENCE trial (145). In comparison to standard heparin, the LMWH was found to provide a better outcome in individuals treated with weight-adjusted dosages. This study has been favorably reviewed by the US FDA at a recent meeting. A second study of the use of enoxaparin for the treatment of unstable angina has also been reported (146).

LMWHs have also been used as adjunct anticoagulants in coronary stenting and other interventional cardiac procedures. The ENTICES trial demonstrated that enoxaparin, ticlopidine, and aspirin significantly reduced composite clinical endpoints (death, nonfatal myocardial infarction, coronary artery bypass surgery, repeat angioplasty) at 30 days compared with warfarin, heparin, dextran, dipyridamole, and aspirin after stent implantation (147). The synthetic heparin pentasaccharide has also been used successfully with percutaneous transluminal coronary angioplasty (PTCA) in one study (148).

## Outindividual Use

The efficacy of LMWH has been demonstrated in the treatment of preexisting thromboembolic conditions in five studies from 1992–1995 (149–153). Two studies have concluded that home therapeutic treatment (without laboratory monitoring) is feasible and as effective

and safe as continuous intravenous infusion of heparin in individuals with proximal deep vein thrombosis (154, 155). Hull et al have begun a multicenter, randomized clinical trial to study the effect of long-term, once-daily LMWH versus standard heparin treatment and warfarin on mortality in individuals with established proximal vein thrombosis (140).

Cancer can be associated with a prothrombotic state producing thromboembolic disorders in a significant number of individuals. Because cancer cells are capable of producing procoagulant substances, there are potentially a number of mechanisms involved in the production of cancer-associated thrombosis (see Chapter 40). Treatment of malignancy-associated thromboembolic disorders with LMWHs has become an issue in the design of clinical trials for these agents. The use of LMWHs as prophylactic or therapeutic agents in cancer has been reviewed by Godwin (156). Three studies in cancer individuals have shown that different LMWHs were either equal or superior to standard heparin in the prevention of DVT, with equivalent safety (157–159). In the treatment of cancer-associated thrombosis, Simonneau and Prandoni (153, 160) found that LMWH was equivalent to heparin, whereas Hull found equivalent efficacy but better safety with LMWH (149). In a meta-analysis the overall mortality has also been reportedly decreased in LMWH-treated cancer individuals. Thus LMWHs may be superior to standard heparin not only in decreasing thrombotic events but also in decreasing mortality in cancer individuals.

LMWHs have been used for the prevention of venous thrombosis in pregnant individuals (161). Since oral anticoagulants cross the placental barrier, these agents are contraindicated in pregnancy (162). Adjusted-dose subcutaneous heparin has been found to be ineffective for the prevention of thrombosis of mechanical valve prostheses during pregnancy (163). In one study, the use of heparin from the sixth to twelfth week of gestation did not show a decrease in the high incidence of fetal wastage associated with oral anticoagulant therapy (163). The use of LMWH, however, was found to be effective in two studies (164, 165). Postpartum osteoporotic fractures may develop in some individuals (164). Additional studies are needed to fully test the efficacy of all LMWHs in pregnancy.

## Additional Indications

The use of heparin in pediatric individuals has been reported to be problematic because of variations in responses and unpredictable efficacy. In a recent pilot study, LMWH was compared with standard heparin therapy in pediatric individuals with thrombotic disorders. Enoxaparin was shown to have several potential advantages over standard heparin in children (166). The superior efficacy of LMWH in children may be due to its pharmacokinetic characteristics. Studies in this population, however, are limited and require validation of safety and efficacy.

A high prevalence of thrombotic complications and vasoocclusive disorders has been reported in heart transplant individuals (167). The mechanism does not appear to be related only to platelet abnormalities, and thus the benefits of other antithrombotic therapies need to be considered. A clinical trial is currently in progress to investigate the usefulness of LMWHs for this indication. It is projected that preventive treatment started late in the first posttransplant year (to avoid bleeding complications) with LMWH, and potentially longer term treatment, may be useful in the prevention of thromboembolic events and transplant rejection.

For the management of bone marrow transplant associated venoocclusive (VOD) and microangiopathic disorders, enoxaparin has provided encouraging results in a pilot study (A. Eldor, personal communication). In 61 individuals randomized to LMWH or placebo prior to transplant and for 40 days thereafter, VOD parameters were significantly less frequent in the enoxaparin group and the time to platelet recovery was significantly shorter.

Heparin-induced thrombocytopenia (HIT) is a disease spectrum triggered by an immune response to heparin (see Chapter 29). The most dramatic clinical expression is arterial thrombosis leading to amputation or death. Owing to their smaller molecular size, it was postulated that LMWHs would be less immunogenic than heparin and could be used as an alternative anticoagulant in these individuals. *In vitro* and clinical experiences have shown that LMWHs produce platelet aggregation in about 85% of the cases positive to heparin (168–170). It appears from several trials with LMWHs published to date that HIT still occurs albeit with a lower incidence than with heparin (171).

It has been stated that from a clinical point of view, the difference in the safety and efficacy index of the LMWHs must be very small (173). It must be emphasized that most of the studies on the comparison between different drugs are primarily based on the clinical data obtained on the prophylaxis of thromboembolism in general surgery individuals at individually optimized low dosages (20 to 40 mg total dose). Thus this conclusion may only be pertinent to the prophylactic use of these agents. When LMWHs are used in therapeutic or cardiovascular indications at three- to ten-times-higher dosage in the intravenous and specialized delivery modes, product-based differences may become very evident. Thus any statement on the clinical equivalence amongst these LMWHs is not valid at this time. All LMWHs are, therefore, not the same and should be developed as distinct drugs in indication-specific clinical trials. Recognizing the clinical usefulness of LMWHs,

the American College of Chest Physicians 1995 Consensus Conference has endorsed the use of LMWHs for DVT phosphylaxis in high-risk major surgery, hip replacement, knee replacement, and high-risk multiple trauma (174). The consensus statement also includes favorable comments for LMWHs in contrast to the oral anticoagulant drugs for knee surgery. These recommendations are based on well-designed clinical trials and were objectively developed by a panel of experts. Such recommendations have taken into account product-specific clinical outcome.

There are several clinical trials in progress using different products in indication-specific protocols. Each of these trials was designed either empirically or by considering results of pilot trials of a given product. The dosages used are also product-specific. Some of these trials employ relatively high dosage for long periods of time. In these situations, each product will have its own clinical profile. The results of these trials should validate the notion that all LMWHs are not the same.

## LABORATORY MONITORING

Monitoring of heparin levels is important to minimize hemorrhagic side effects and maximize therapeutic efficacy. Heparin therapy is typically monitored using the activated partial thromboplastin time (aPTT) or amidolytic anti-Xa assays. When higher heparin levels are utilized, as in cardiac surgery or in interventional cardiologic procedures, the activated clotting time (ACT) is typically used to gauge the degree of anticoagulation. During heparin therapy, it is also important to determine platelet counts periodically to exclude the possibility of heparin-induced thrombocytopenia.

Because LMWHs produce weaker anticoagulant effects as measured by the aPTT or ACT, and the fact that these drugs have been proven to be safe at their effective prophylactic dosages, monitoring is generally not performed (175, 176). However, it is recommended that those individuals at higher risk of bleeding, or who are underweight or overweight, be monitored. In the case of therapeutic treatment or with interventional procedures where dosages are higher, monitoring can be performed by clot-based or chromogenic assays sensitive to factor Xa inhibition, such as the Heptest® or Hepaclot® (177). Even at the higher doses, LMWHs do not effectively prolong the aPTT or ACT assays. Platelet counts should be monitored periodically with long-term treatment.

## SYNTHETIC HEPARIN PENTASACCHARIDE

Early structural studies of heparin led to the knowledge that heparin binding to antithrombin produced inhibitory effects against thrombin and factor Xa (30, 178–180). In an effort to obtain defined anticoagulant agents, investigations into the structure-activity relationships in heparin continued. Natural heparin was separated into its components by various techniques based on molecular weight, charge density, solubility, or antithrombin affinity. Derivatives were subsequently obtained from heparin by chemical and enzymatic degradation coupled with the separation techniques. These derivatives were more homogeneous than heparin in structure and activity. A molecular weight dependence of heparin-antithrombin on the inhibition of several serine proteases of the coagulation system was determined (181–183). Subsequently, studies focused on a decasaccharide and an octasaccharide possessing high anti–factor Xa activity with no detectable inhibitory action against thrombin (factor IIa).

The essential role of the inhibition of factor Xa for eliciting an antithrombotic effect came to be questioned at that time since some of the heparin derivatives under investigation had been only partially effective at inhibiting thrombosis in experimental animal models (184–190). Thus it was suggested that the anti–factor IIa activity of heparin may have a more important role in producing the antithrombotic response than the anti–factor Xa activity.

The biochemical studies on heparin eventually led to the hypothesis that the minimal structure critical for binding to antithrombin that would elicit a high anti–factor Xa effect was represented by a hexasaccharide (191–193). Close inspection of the structure by [$^{13}$C]-NMR revealed a specific uronic acid leading to the hypothesis that the pentasaccharide located within the hexasaccharide was, therefore, the minimal heparin sequence that would bind antithrombin and elicit a high anti–factor Xa activity (194). A tetrasaccharide suggested by Rosenberg could not be conclusively proven to be responsible for anticoagulant activity (195).

The original pentasaccharide sequence was identified from natural heparin by fractionation procedures (191). A specific pentasaccharide (molecular weight 1714) of a predetermined sequence based on the above findings was subsequently synthesized by an innovative process of glycosaminoglycan synthesis (196, 197). The synthetic pentasaccharide structure was composed of a regular region (units G and H) and an irregular region of heparin (units D, E, and F) (Fig. 55.1—original pentasaccharide). [$^{13}$C]-NMR revealed the anticipated spectral characteristics and high-affinity antithrombin binding consistent within the derived pentasaccharide structure (198–199).

A certain degree of variability in the pentasaccharide structure was although to be compatible with antithrombin binding. However, four specific sulfate groups were shown to be critical for optimum binding: the 6-O sulfate on the D unit, the 3-O sulfate on the F unit, and two 2-N sulfates on the F and H units of the penta-

**Original pentasaccharide**

**SR 90107A/ORG 31540 - natural pentasaccharide**

**SanOrg 32701 - analogue of natural pentasaccharide**

**ORG 31550 - "super" pentasaccharide**

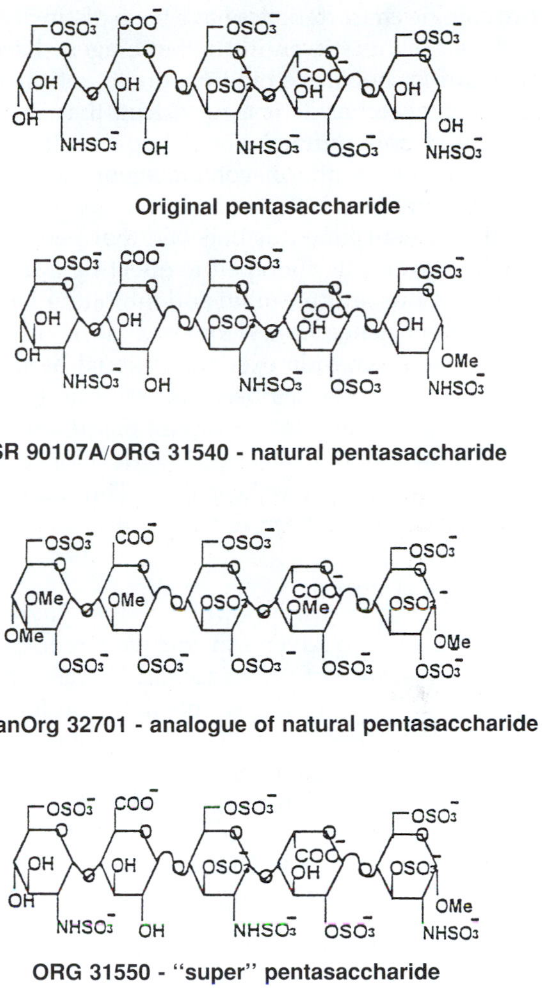

**FIGURE 55.3.** Chemical structures of the high anti-thrombin (AT) affinity binding pentasaccharide region of heparin and several of its synthetic derivatives. The original pentasaccharide binds to AT with high affinity due to the presence of a unique 3-O sulfate group. The alpha-methyl derivative (SR 90107A/ORG 31540) exhibits the same biologic effects as the original pentasaccharide and is currently under clinical investigation. Several highly sulfated derivatives (SanOrg 32701, ORG 31550) have also been synthesized.

saccharide (Fig. 55.3—original pentasaccharide) (191, 200, 201). In particular, in the irregular region of heparin important for binding to antithrombin, 25 to 30% of the glucosamine residues were found to contain a unique 3-O sulfate group. The relative positioning of the sulfated monosaccharides also proved to be of critical importance.

## POTENCY DESIGNATION, STANDARDIZATION, AND LABORATORY MONITORING

Pentasaccharide represents a homogeneous single targeted entity whose physicochemical, biochemical, and pharmacologic characteristics have been distinctly identified. It is a synthetic antithrombotic agent based on the structure of heparin's binding site to antithrombin. Because pentasaccharide is a new drug that is distinct from LMWH and unfractionated heparin, it must be treated as a unique pharmacologic agent with its own therapeutic profile.

At the present time it is believed that pentasaccharide mainly exerts its therapeutic effect by combining with endogenous antithrombin and inhibiting factor Xa and thrombin generation. However, it is not clear whether pentasaccharide exerts additional biologic effects. Pentasaccharide has been assessed and potency assignments in the amidolytic or clot-based anti–factor Xa assays, which have been originally developed for the assessment of LMWH, have been used. Thrombin generation assays have also been used.

## CLINICAL STUDIES

In phase I studies, no adverse events were reported and the general tolerance of pentasaccharide was excellent. The PT and aPTT were not significantly prolonged at even the highest doses studied. Only slight differences between healthy young and elderly subjects were noted in response to pentasaccharide. SR 90107A/Org 31540 can be safely administered subcutaneously by repeated twice daily injections up to 9 mg (6000 anti-Xa U) or by repeated single daily doses up to 12 mg (8000 anti-Xa U) (202).

# SYNOPSIS

Until now, unfractionated heparin has remained the anticoagulant-of-choice for most thrombotic and cardiovascular indications. Despite significant developments in the area of anticoagulants, it is expected that heparin will remain in use for various indications until a substitute drug becomes available. The development of LMWHs will continue and these agents will gradually replace the use of heparin for the prophylaxis of thromboembolic disorders, the treatment of DVT, and outindividual use in cardiovascular indications and thrombotic stroke. Because of their low anticoagulant activity, these agents may not be useful as surgical anticoagulants. LMWHs will likely be developed for several additional indications, some of which may be outside the area of thrombosis. Because of the heparin-induced thrombocytopenia potential of heparin and LMWH, the synthetic pentasaccharide may be developed for specific indications such as thromboprophylaxis and cardiovascular indications. It is unlikely that the pentasaccharide will be developed as an anticoagulant. Owing to its high affinity to antithrombin, pentasaccharide may turn out to be a highly effective antithrombotic agent with limited adverse effects compared with heparin and LMWH.

# ORAL ANTICOAGULANT DRUGS

The oral anticoagulants are one of the most important classes of drugs in clinical use today. They are highly effective but at the same time dangerous when not properly monitored. They are all derivatives of coumarin. The drug warfarin (Coumadin) is being used much more commonly than dicoumarol or indandione derivatives because of its more predictable dose response and favorable pharmacodynamics. The mechanism of action of these drugs and their metabolism is responsible for more drug interactions than any other commonly used drug, making it mandatory for the clinician to be aware of enhanced toxicity or diminished efficacy in the presence of other drugs.

## HISTORIC PERSPECTIVE

The development of coumarin derived oral anticoagulant drugs occurred as a result of four key discoveries between 1929 and 1941. The first of these was the linking of the hemorrhagic disease of cattle occurring in the Midwestern United States to the use of moldy sweet clover hay as cattle feed (203). The second event was the discovery by Henrik Dam that chicks developed a hemorrhagic disorder when fed a fat free diet. This led to his postulation of a vitamin, which he called vitamin K (koagulation) (204, 205). He was subsequently awarded the Nobel Prize for this work. The third important contribution occurring virtually simultaneously (1935) was the development of a coagulation test system by Armand Quick for the detection of low levels of "prothrombin" (206). This prothrombin time test has remained in clinical use in virtually the same form for the past 60 years. The fourth discovery was made by Link and associates in 1941. They isolated the substance in moldy sweet clover that caused the hemorrhagic disease in cattle (207). This was called dicoumarol, and was marketed as a rat poison by the Wisconsin Alumni Research Foundation. Subsequently, they developed the drug "warfarin," so named because it was marketed by the *Wisconsin Alumni Research Foundation.* It is now marketed by DuPont Chemical Company as Coumadin.

Since 1935, a number of research teams have studied the physiology of vitamin K, the role of bile in its absorption, and of the liver in its physiologic function (208). The similarities of the clotting defect produced by vitamin K deficiency, and the clotting defect induced by dicoumarol prompted the presumption that there was a relationship. Subsequently, it was shown that oral vitamin $K_1$ from plants (phytonadione) could correct the clotting defect induced by anticoagulant therapy (209).

It was learned that a chemical synthesized long before the discovery of vitamin K and dicumarol, menadi-

Vitamin K (quinone)

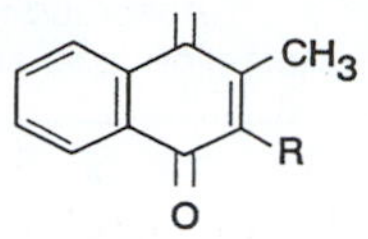

Warfarin sodium

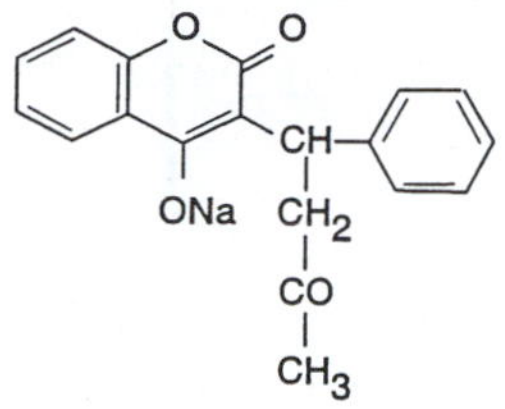

Dicumarol

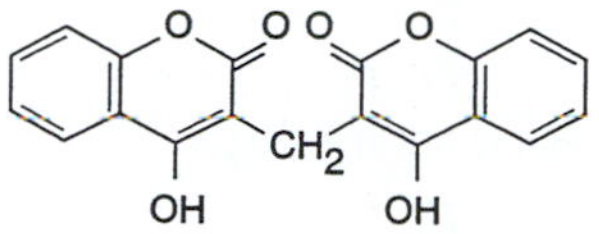

Phenprocoumon

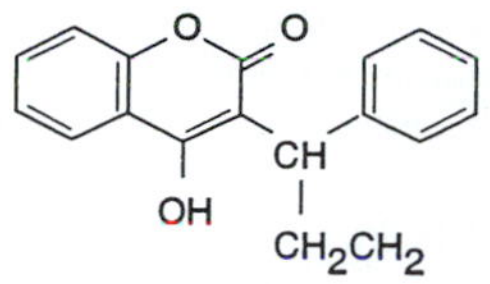

**FIGURE 55.4.** Chemical structure of vitamin K and various oral anticoagulant drugs.

one, could substitute for vitamin K in the diet. This was shown to be the ring structure of vitamin K (210, 211). Subsequently, the natural vitamin K (phytonadione) was extracted from plants and was found to have a phytate side chain at position 3. Vitamin $K_2$, which is synthesized by bacteria in the intestine, is capable of substituting for vitamin $K_1$. It has a farnesyl group in place of the phytyl group at position 3. In the animal, vitamin K is stored in various tissues, providing a dietary source for carnivores (212). The clarification of the mechanism of bleeding due to vitamin K deficiency in the review by Furie and Furie has made a strong contribution to our understanding of the physiology of vitamin K and the pharmacologic effects of oral anticoagulants (213).

## CHEMISTRY

The chemical structure of vitamin K (quinone) and the coumarin drugs that impair its regeneration in the liver are shown in Fig. 55.4. Warfarin is absorbed and metabolized differently from the other coumarins due to differences in the position 3 side chains. There are two meta-

bolically active stereoisomers, the R form and the S form. The R or S form determines the pathway of metabolism of the drug (214).

## PHARMACODYNAMICS

The mechanism by which oral anticoagulants interfere with the synthesis of vitamin K-dependent factors is shown in Fig. 55.5. The $\gamma$-carboxylation of glutamic acid occurs on the glutamic acid residues of the prozymogen near its aminoterminus. This makes possible the binding of calcium, which promotes the binding of the molecules to a lipid surface where the generation of active procoagulant enzymes occurs (215). The pharmacodynamics of warfarin are influenced by vitamin K levels, liver function, and the presence or absence of many other endogenous and exogenous (drug, chemical) factors (Tables 55.3 and 55.4).

Fig. 55.5 depicts the enzymatic recycling of vitamin K (quinone) to vitamin $KH_2$ (hydroquinone), which is the cofactor for the specific carboxylation of glutamic acid residues of the vitamin K-dependent clotting factors II, VII, IX, X protein C and protein S. Vitamin $KH_2$ is converted to vitamin K epoxide, which is subsequently reduced by vitamin K epoxide reductase to vitamin K. The affinity of the oral anticoagulants for the reductase enzymes in this pathway determines their efficacy as oral anticoagulants. The basic vitamin K ring structure, rather than the position 3 side chains, determines the affinity and specificity (213, 214).

**TABLE 55.3.** Endogenous Factors Enhancing the Effect of Warfarin on the Prothrombin Time

| | |
|---|---|
| Liver disease | Hyperthyroidism |
| Congestive heart failure | Poor nutrition |
| Fever | Vitamin K deficiency |

**TABLE 53.4.** Partial List of Drugs Enhancing the Effect of Warfarin on the Prothrombin Time

| | | |
|---|---|---|
| Acetaminophen | Cimetidine | Streptokinase |
| Alcohol | Clofibrate | Sulfonamides |
| Aspirin | Doxycycline | Tamoxifen |
| Allopurinol | Fenoprofen | Ticlopidine |
| Amiodarone | Fluconazole | Tolbutamide |
| Cefoxitin | Omeprazole | Urokinase |
| Ceftriaxone | Quinidine | Vitamin E |
| Chloral hydrate | Ranitidine | |

*From the Physicians Desk Reference, 1997.*

The rate of synthesis of the vitamin K-dependent clotting factors in the liver is modulated by factors affecting liver function, as well as the availability of vitamin K. The half-lives of these clotting factors are shown in Table 55.5. During oral anticoagulant therapy there may be wide discrepancies between individuals taking the same dose of oral anticoagulant drugs due to the many variables involved. Thus, it is mandatory to monitor therapy closely with the prothrombin time. The sensitivity of the thromboplastin reagent is a factor that is corrected for by the International Normalized Ratio (INR) (see Monitoring below).

## PHARMACOKINETICS

Warfarin transport and pharmacologic action and elimination involve the specific binding of warfarin to a chiral macromolecular complex. The position 3 side chains are important determinants of pharmacokinetics via this mechanism of binding to different macromolecules. Interaction of the warfarin molecule with the enzyme vitamin K epoxide reductase is less stereoselective than its interaction with cytochrome P 450 enzymes (214). This suggests that the lack of stereoselectivity in binding to vitamin $K_1$ epoxide reductase depends only on the 4-hydroxy coumarin ring of the drug (214). Thus the ring structure is important for enzyme inhibition, whereas the side chain determines the half-life of the drug. Plasma drug levels are determined using high-performance liquid chromatography, and is not clinically relevant except in toxicologic studies or research on pharmacokinetics.

The S-isomer of warfarin is two times more potent than the R-isomer in the inhibition of clotting factor synthesis. The plasma half-life of racemic warfarin is 36 to 42 hours. Maximal plasma levels are attained 90 minutes after ingestion. In plasma, warfarin is bound to albumin and is distributed in the albumin space. S warfarin is oxidized to 2-hydroxy S warfarin and is excreted in the bile, whereas the R form is reduced by conversion of the side chain to alcohols and excreted in the urine (214). The level of individual clotting factors will influence the

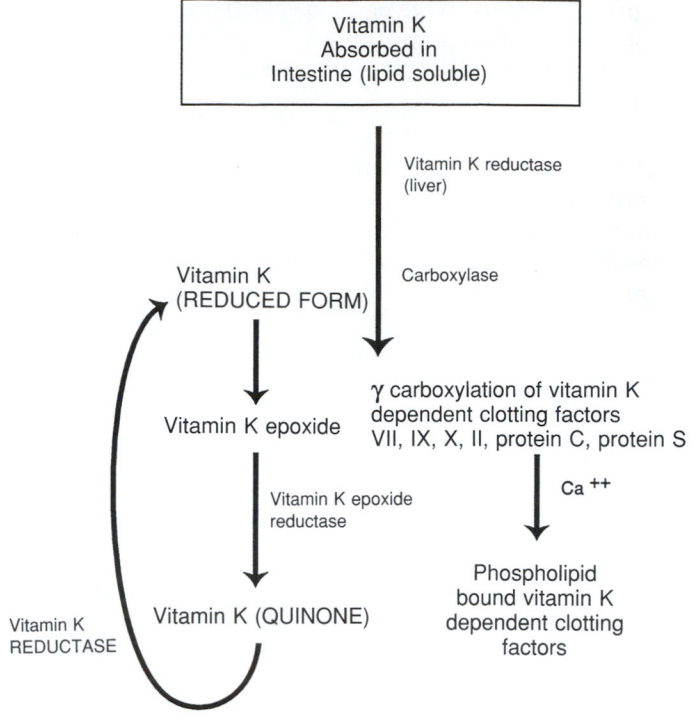

Vitamin K epoxide reductase and vitamin K reductase are blocked by warfarin and related drugs

**FIGURE 55.5.** Schematic of the mechanism by which oral anticoagulants interfere with the synthesis of vitamin K-dependent factors. Dietary vitamin K is a required cofactor for the carboxylation of coagulation factors VII, IX, X, II, protein C, and protein S. Warfarin and other oral anticoagulants prevent the synthesis of active coagulation factors by inhibiting the enzymes vitamin K epoxide reductase and vitamin K reductase.

time to onset of an abnormal prothrombin time, and thus is a variable in the study of the pharmacodynamics of the drug.

There are hereditary factors that result in familial resistance to warfarin. This may be due to a decreased affinity of the receptor in the liver to warfarin (214). Dietary intake of vitamin K, bile secretion, fat intake, and intestinal malabsorption syndromes all effect the pharmacokinetics by the oral route. Warfarin is available for intravenous use in the same dosage for those who cannot take it orally (214, 216). Drugs that influence the metabolism of warfarin are shown in Table 55.4. A more complete listing is available to physicians through their pharmacy or the Physicians Desk Reference (PDR). It is strongly advised that prescribed and over-the-counter drugs, habits (alcohol especially), diet and concomitant diseases (Table 55.3) be taken into account when warfarin is prescribed. It is of special interest that second and third generation cephalosporins can enhance the antico-

| TABLE 55.5. | Half-lives of Vitamin K-Dependent Clotting Factors |
| --- | --- |

| Factor | Half-life (hours) |
| --- | --- |
| Factor VII | 6 |
| Protein C | 8 |
| Factor IX | 24 |
| Protein S | 30 |
| Factor X | 36 |
| Prothrombin | 72 |

agulant effect of warfarin by blocking the cyclic inter-conversion of vitamin K (217).

Aspirin is particularly important because it acts on hemostasis by a separate mechanism. Aspirin increases the risk of gastrointestinal bleeding by production of gastric erosions. The combined effect of heparin and warfarin is to decrease the conversion of prothrombin to thrombin by prothrombinase, albeit by separate mechanisms. These two drugs are routinely used together during the first 4 to 5 days of heparin therapy for deep vein thrombosis. Bleeding risk may be enhanced by the combination, even although heparin in therapeutic doses has very little effect on the prothrombin time. It is important to consider whether there is an unusually low factor IX level if the activated partial thromboplastin time (aPTT) is inappropriately prolonged for the degree of prolongation of the prothrombin time (PT) of individuals taking warfarin.

## DOSING

Warfarin therapy is usually initiated at a dose of 5 to 10 mg in adults who have no risk factors for overanticoagulation (diet, nutrition, drugs, metabolic state). Doses as high as 20 mg/day have been employed to initiate therapy but studies have shown that it is no more effective than a 10 mg dose, and reversal of the drug effect is more difficult in case of bleeding (217). A study comparing 5 and 10 mg loading doses concluded that the 5 mg dose was less hazardous in terms of less rapid reduction of protein C, which should be reflected in fewer cases of warfarin-induced skin necrosis (218). The higher dose also brought about a more rapid change in the prothrombin time due entirely to factor VII depletion, but levels of factors X and prothrombin did not vary between the two groups (218).

## MONITORING

One of the most significant developments in the monitoring of oral anticoagulant therapy was the report by Hull and associates in 1982, which showed that the rabbit brain thromboplastin widely used in North America was much less sensitive to the reduction in vitamin K–dependent factors than was the thromboplastin commonly used in some European countries (219). Furthermore, the sources of rabbit thromboplastin also vary greatly. Thus research studies on efficacy and safety applied only to a given thromboplastin reagent. The result was that unnecessarily high doses of warfarin were needed on average to achieve the desired prothrombin time or prothrombin time ratio when the less sensitive thromboplastins were used.

This problem was resolved by adopting a system in which all commercial thromboplastin reagents were

compared by the manufacturer with an international standard reagent of a sensitive type that had an arbitrary sensitivity index of 1.0, and a sensitivity index was calculated. This is the International Sensitivity Index (ISI). Clinical laboratories could then report their results in terms of an International Normalized Ratio (INR) derived from the prothrombin time ratio (individual prothrombin time divided by the control for that hospital). When this ratio was raised to the power of the ISI, either by mathematical calculation or from a nomogram, an INR value could be reported for that individual. The World Health Organization has adopted this system and maintains international standard reagents (217). Since the sensitive human brain thromboplastin is considered neither safe nor practical, most thromboplastins in use today are rabbit brain or placental origin. Recombinant DNA methods have been used to produce human thromboplastins with an ISI near 1.0. When the ISI is 1.0, the PT ratio and the INR are the same. A table can be used in place of the calculation method utilizing the PT ratio for the individual and the ISI of the reagent (Table 55.6). In most laboratories using automated equipment the INR is automatically calculated. One problem with sensitive reagents is the rapid rise in the INR for a given dosage escalation. Thus there is a steeper dose response curve at or above the upper limit of the therapeutic range. The INR predicts efficacy for a given clinical disorder and gives an upper limit beyond which the risk of bleeding may be unacceptably high.

The current recommendations for INR ranges for various indications are shown in Table 55.7. The dosing and resultant INR are valid for individuals in a stable state of anticoagulation, usually 4 to 5 weeks after starting treatment, since plasmas used in the ISI determination were from such individuals. Until the prothrombin time is stable, frequent testing is advised, starting daily and then tapering to twice weekly, then weekly until stable. When INR values are stable, monthly monitoring is sufficient unless a new drug is introduced (antibiotic,

**TABLE 55.6.** Comparison of the INR at Two Therapeutic Ranges with the Prothrombin Time Ratio Using Thromboplastins with Increasing ISI

| INR | ISI 1.0 | ISI 1.4 | ISI 1.8 | ISI 2.3 | ISI 2.8 |
|---------|---------|---------|---------|---------|---------|
| 2.0–3.0 | 2.0–3.0 | 1.6–2.2 | 1.5–1.8 | 1.4–1.6 | 1.3–1.5 |
| 2.5–3.5 | 2.5–3.5 | 1.9–2.4 | 1.7–2.0 | 1.5–1.7 | 1.4–1.6 |

*Adapted from Hirsh J. Optimal intensity and monitoring of warfarin. Am J Cardiol 1995;75:39B–42B.*

*INR, International Normalized Ratio; ISI, International Sensitivity Index.*

**TABLE 55.7. Recommended Therapeutic Ranges of INR for Various Indications**

|  | INR |
| --- | --- |
| Deep vein thrombosis | 2–3 |
| Prophylaxis of DVT | 2–3 |
| Atrial fibrillation | 2–3 |
| Cardiac valve replacement |  |
|    Tissue valve | 2–3 |
|    Mechanical valve | 2.5–3.5 |
| Antiphospholipid antibody syndrome | 2.3–3.5 |
|    (recurrent DVT or arterial thrombosis) |  |
| Acute myocardial infarction (MI) | 2–3 |
|    (prevention of stroke, recurrent MI, |  |
|    and death) |  |

**TABLE 55.8. Risk of Bleeding with Oral Anticoagulants**

1. Duration of therapy: greater risk first few months
2. Level of the INR
3. Prior history of gastrointestinal bleeding
4. Comorbid disease
   Hypertension
   Cerebrovascular disease
   Atrial fibrillation
   Serious heart disease
   Renal insufficiency
   Liver disease
   Alcoholism
   Cancer
5. Drugs
   Aspirin in doses greater than 300 mg/day
   Nonaspirin platelet function inhibitors
   Heparin

etc.) or a new illness is present. Many large clinics and hospitals have established anticoagulation clinics, where monitoring and dosage adjustments are made. This has provided improved ability to achieve the desired therapeutic goal (219, 220) (Table 55.7).

## COMPLICATIONS OF THERAPY

Hemorrhage is by far the most frequent complication of warfarin, reflecting its very narrow efficacy-safety range. Many studies have been conducted to identify high-risk groups because of the concept that such individuals might be more safely managed with lower doses, lower INR ranges, or even treated with an alternate drug (221–227). Some of the identifiable risks are shown in Table 55.8. While there is a strong correlation

between the INR level and risk of bleeding, individual related factors are also of critical importance. Among these are age (controversial), history of gastrointestinal bleeding, hypertension, ischemic cerebrovascular disease, and cardioembolic disorders such as atrial fibrillation. In terms of age, it is accepted that lower doses of warfarin are usually adequate to achieve the desired INR in older individuals. Individuals at risk of falling may be at a higher risk taking the drug. Individual education is critical with these drugs, including written and verbal instructions regarding danger signs and when to seek medical attention are essential. Prescribing and dispensing errors and failure to act quickly when hemorrhage occurs may be fatal. There are guidelines regarding the management of individuals who are overanticoagulated but not bleeding, overanticoagulated and bleeding, or in the therapeutic range for the INR but are bleeding (Table 55.9).

Concomitant use of nonsteroidal antiinflammatory drugs is a concern because of their widespread usage. Aspirin is the most hazardous of these because it causes gastric erosions, particularly when the dose is 300 mg/

**TABLE 53.9. Management of Overanticoagulation with Warfarin and Bleeding**

1. *INR between upper limit and 6; individual not bleeding:*
   - Omit the drug until INR therapeutic
   - Resume therapy at a lower dose
2. *INR 6–10; individual not bleeding:*
   - Administer vitamin $K_1$, 1–2 mg subcutaneously
   - INR may be therapeutic within 12–24 hours
   - Alternatively, administer dilute vitamin $K_1$ intravenously over 10–20 minutes
   - Resume therapy at a lower dose if INR therapeutic; if not, vitamin $K_1$ 0.5 mg may be given
3. *INR greater than 10; individual not bleeding:*
   - Administer vitamin $K_1$, 3 mg parenterally
   - Repeat if no effect in 8 hours
4. *Overt bleeding or INR greater than 20:*
   - Administer vitamin $K_1$, 10 mg parenterally plus fresh frozen plasma or prothrombin-complex concentrates
   - Monitor INR and repeat vitamin $K_1$ if response not satisfactory at 12 hours
5. *Life-threatening bleeding or massive warfarin overdose with INR greater than 20:*
   - Administer prothrombin-complex concentrates and vitamin $K_1$, 10 mg parenterally
   - Repeat doses as necessary based on INR and/or continued bleeding, if INR has not normalized
6. *Reinstitute anticoagulation with heparin if urgently needed for thombotic disease or prosthetic valve*

day or more. Aspirin is not prohibitively hazardous when given in low doses with warfarin provided that very close control of the INR is maintained. Prior history of gastrointestinal bleeding is an added risk to be taken into account.

Management of massive hemorrhage requires the immediate restoration of intravascular volume with fluids and electrolytes, as well as the administration of fresh frozen plasma or prothrombin complex concentrates. Vitamin $K_1$ oxide should be given parenterally, but with the realization that it will not be of benefit for 6 to 24 hours, assuming normal liver function. Packed red cell transfusions are vital and should be given promptly as needed.

Warfarin-induced skin necrosis, is more frequent in females and in individuals with deficiency of protein C, activated protein C resistance (factor V Leiden) and protein S deficiency (228, 229). Family history of thrombosis suggesting a hereditary defect, prior thrombosis in the individual, or an unusual thrombotic presentation should prompt testing for these disorders. When it is suspected, initiation of therapy with heparin, followed by very low dose warfarin with gradual escalation of the dose may be safe (228). Routine testing for these defects in all individuals prior to initiation of oral anticoagulation is not advised at this time.

Blue toe syndrome is due to ischemia secondary to vascular or embolic disease. Some individuals on warfarin have experienced this syndrome and have been shown to have cholesterol crystals in the vessels of the toe. It is presumably due to release of cholesterol from plaques that have ulcerated in the aorta. Unless cholesterol crystals are demonstrated, it cannot be ascertained that the problem is related to warfarin therapy. Vasculitis, thrombocytopenia, myocardial infarction with embolism and diabetic vascular disease may be the cause (230).

Warfarin should be avoided in pregnancy because of its potential to cause embryopathy. Heparin has been shown to be a satisfactory alternative for most indications (prosthetic heart valves, deep vein thrombosis). The potential hazard of osteoporosis with prolonged heparin therapy should be considered in this setting (231).

## MANAGEMENT OF SURGICAL PATIENTS

Management of oral anticoagulant therapy in the individual undergoing an elective surgical procedure requires an understanding of the thrombotic and hemorrhagic risks involved in the perioperative period and the pharmacology of heparin and warfarin. There have been studies to evaluate various methods of management of these individuals, but recommendations have to be made based on pharmacology and the pathophysiology of hemorrhage and thrombosis. Reviews of clinical studies with recommendations for individual management have been recently published (232, 233). Some principles involved are the increased risk of thrombosis in individuals undergoing surgery and that the risk is greatest during the first 3 months after the thromboembolic event, whether it was venous or arterial. Likewise, the risk of bleeding may be higher in some individuals than in others, necessitating clinical judgment by knowledgeable clinicians.

If a individual on warfarin therapy for a thromboembolic event within the past month requires surgery on an elective basis, it is wise to postpone the surgery. If surgery cannot be postponed, then it is recommended that warfarin therapy be stopped 4 days prior to surgery and that heparin be given intravenously, beginning when the INR value reaches 1.5, which will be in 2 to 3 days. Heparin should be administered without an initial bolus and the aPTT maintained at therapeutic levels by frequent monitoring and dosage adjustment. The heparin should be stopped 6 hours before surgery. Following surgery, anticoagulation with warfarin and heparin without bolus should be resumed if there is no risk of bleeding. If reoperation within a day or so is a possibility, the warfarin should not be started until this risk is past. If heparin therapy is considered too dangerous, placement of a vena caval filter should be considered. Pneumatic intermittent pressure boots and elastic stockings should also be considered. If venous thromboembolism has occurred within 2 weeks of surgery, placement of a vena caval filter should be considered (232). If the venous thromboembolism has occurred 1 to 3 months prior, intravenous heparin before surgery is not advised, but warfarin should be stopped 4 days before surgery and the INR monitored to ensure that it is near normal at surgery. Following surgery, intravenous heparin and warfarin should be given in the same manner as for those whose thromboembolism was within the past month.

Individuals in whom venous thromboembolism occurred more than 3 months before surgery and were considered at high risk for recurrence do not require heparin before or after surgery, but standard heparin or low-molecular-weight heparin should be given postoperatively, subcutaneously at the dose recommended for prophylaxis of high-risk surgery.

Individuals with mechanical heart valves or arterial fibrillation should have warfarin stopped 4 days prior to surgery, with monitoring; small doses of vitamin K may be administered as necessary to ensure a near normal INR at surgery. Postoperatively, these individuals should be started on warfarin as soon as possible, and, if the bleeding risk is not too high, subcutaneous standard or low-molecular-weight heparin in the same dose as used for prophylaxis of deep vein thrombosis in high-risk surgical cases should be initiated (232, 233).

# REFERENCES

1. Hirsh J. Anticoagulants: the old and the new. Ham-Wasserman Lecture. Presented at the annual meeting of the American Society of Hematology, Orlando, 1996.
2. Breckenridge A, Orme M, Wesseling H et al. Pharmacokinetics and pharmacodynamics of the enantiomers of warfarin in man. Clin Pharmacol Ther 1974;15:424–430.
3. McLean J. The thromboplastic action of cephalin. Am J Physiol 1916;41: 250–257.
4. Casu B. Methods of structural analysis. In: Lane DA, Lindahl U, eds. Heparin: chemical and biological properties, clinical applications. London: Edward Arnold, 1989; pp. 25–50.
5. Lindahl U, Kjellen L. Heparin or heparan sulfate—what is the difference [Review]? Thromb Haemost 1991;66:44–48.
6. Robinson HC, Horner AA, Hook M et al. A proteoglycan form of heparin and its degradation to single-chain molecules. J Biol Chem 1978;253: 6687–6693.
7. Lindahl U, Rodén L. Carbohydrate-peptide linkages in proteoglycans of animal, plant and bacterial origin. In: Gottschalk A, ed. Glycoproteins. Their composition, structure, and function. Amsterdam: Elsevier, 1972; pp. 491–517.
8. Helting T, Lindahl U. Occurrence and biosynthesis of β-glucuronidic linkages in heparin. J Biol Chem 1971;246:5442–5447.
9. Helting T, Lindahl U. Biosynthesis of heparin. I. Transfer of N-acetylglucosamine and glucuronic acid to low-molecular-weight heparin fragments. Acta Chem Scand 1972;26:3515–3523.
10. Forsee WT, Roden L. Biosynthesis of heparin. Transfer of N-acetylglucosamine to heparan sulfate oligosaccharides. J Biol Chem 1981;256: 7240–7247.
11. Lindahl U. Biosynthesis of heparin and related polysaccharides. In: Lane DA, Lindahl U, eds. Heparin: chemical and biological properties, clinical applications. London: Edward Arnold, 1989; pp. 159–190.
12. Hook M, Lindahl U, Hallen A et al. Biosynthesis of heparin. Studies on the microsomal sulfation process. J Biol Chem 1975;250:6065–6071.
13. Lindahl U, Jacobsson I, Hook M et al. Biosynthesis of heparin. Loss of C-5 hydrogen during conversion of D-glucuronic to L-iduronic acid residues. Biochem Biophys Res Commun 1976;70:492–499.
14. Malmstrom A, Roden L, Feingold DS et al. Biosynthesis of heparin. Partial purification of the uronosyl C-5 epimerase. J Biol Chem 1980;255: 3878–3883.
15. Lidholt K, Kjellen L, Lindahl U. Biosynthesis of heparin. Relationship between the polymerization and sulphation processes. Biochem J 1989;261: 999–1007.
16. Lidholt K, Lindahl U. Biosynthesis of heparin. The D-glucuronyosy- and N-acetyl-D-glucosaminyltransferase reactions and their relation to polymer modification. Biochem J 1992;287:21–29.
17. Nieduszynski I. General physical properties of heparin. In: Lane DA, Lindahl U, eds. Heparin: chemical and biological properties, clinical applications. London: Edward Arnold, 1989; pp. 51–64.
18. Bradshaw RA, Wessler S, eds. Advances in experimental medicine and biology. Heparin: structure, function, and clinical implications. New York: Plenum Press, 1975.
19. Levy SW. Heparin and blood lipids. Rev Cand Biol 1958;17:1–61.
20. Cruz WO, Dietrich CP. Antihemostatic effect of heparin counteracted by adenosine triphosphate. Proc Soc Exp Biol Med 1967;126:420–426.
21. Neuhoff V, Schill WB, Sternbach H. Micro-analysis of pure deoxyribonucleic acid–dependent ribonucleic acid polymerase from Escherichia coli. Action of heparin and rifampicin on structure and function. Biochem J 1970;117:623–631.
22. Sealey JE, Gerten JN, Ledingham JG. Inhibition of renin by heparin. J Clin Endocrinol Metab 1967;27:699–705.
23. Folkman J. Tumor angiogenesis [Review]. Adv Cancer Res 1985;43: 175–203.
24. Lippman M. A proposed role for mucopolysaccharides in the initiation and control of cell division. Trans N Y Acad Sci 1965;27:343.
25. Corrigan JJ Jr. Heparin therapy in bacterial septicemia [Review]. J Pediatr 1977;91:695–700.
26. Vaheri A. Heparin and related polyanionic substances as virus inhibitors. Acta Pathol Microbiol Scand 1964;171:7.
27. Howell WH. The coagulation of blood. The Harvey Lectures 1918;12: 272–323.
28. Howell WH. The purification of heparin and its presence in blood. Am J Physiol 1925;71:553–562.
29. Brinkhous KM, Smith HP, Warmer ED et al. The inhibition of blood clotting: an unidentified substance which acts in conjunction with heparin to prevent the conversion of prothrombin into thrombin. Am J Physiol 1939; 125:683–687.
30. Abildgaard U. Highly purified antithrombin III with heparin cofactor activity prepared by disc electrophoresis. Scand J Clin Lab Invest 1968;21: 89–91.
31. Mourey L, Samama JP, Delarue M et al. Antithrombin III: structural and functional aspects [Review]. Biochemie 1990;72:599–608.
32. Pizzo SV. The physiologic role of antithrombin III as an anticoagulant. Semin Hematol 1994;31:4–7.
33. Pratt CW, Church FC. Antithrombin: structure and function. Semin Hematol 1991;28:3–9.
34. Björk I, Danielsson Å. Antithrombin and related inhibitors of coagulation proteinases. In: Barrett AJ, Salvesen G, eds. Proteinase inhibitors. Amsterdam: Elsevier, 1986:489–513.
35. Travis J, Salvesen GS. Human plasma proteinase inhibitors [Review]. Annu Rev Biochem 1983;52:655–709.
36. Rosenberg RD, Damus PS. The purification and mechanism of action of human antithrombin-heparin cofactor. J Biol Chem 1973;248:6490–6505.
37. Jornvall H, Fish WW, Bjork I. The thrombin cleavage site in bovine antithrombin. FEBS Lett 1979;106:358–362.
38. Damus PS, Hicks M, Rosenberg RD. Anticoagulant action of heparin. Nature 1973;246:355–357.
39. Owen WG. Evidence for the formation of an ester between thrombin and heparin cofactor. Biochim Biophys Acta 1975;405:380–387.
40. Jordan RE, Oosta GM, Gardner WT et al. The kinetics of hemostatic enzyme-antithrombin interactions in the presence of low-molecular-weight heparins. J Biol Chem 1980;255:10081–10090.
41. Shore JD, Olson ST, Craig PA et al. Kinetics of heparin action. Ann N Y Acad Sci 1989;556:75–80.
42. Villanueva G, Danishefsky I. Conformational changes accompanying the binding of antithrombin III to thrombin. Biochemistry 1979;18:810–817.
43. Peterson CB, Blackburn MN. Antithrombin conformation and the catalytic role of heparin. II. Is the heparin-induced conformational change in antithrombin required for rapid inactivation of thrombin? J Biol Chem 1987; 262:7559–7566.
44. Nesheim M, Blackburn MN, Lawler CM et al. Dependence of antithrombin III and thrombin binding stoichiometries and catalytic activity on the molecular weight of affinity purified heparin. J Biol Chem 1986;261: 3214–3221.
45. Hoylaerts M, Owen WG, Collen D. Involvement of heparin chain length in the heparin catalyzed inhibition of thrombin by antithrombin III. J Biol Chem 1984;259:5670–5677.
46. Griffith MJ. The heparin-enhanced antithrombin III/thrombin reaction is saturable with respect to both thrombin and antithrombin III. J Biol Chem 1982;257:13899–13902.
47. Pletcher CH, Nelsestuen GL. Two-substrate reaction model for the heparin-catalyzed bovine antithrombin protease reaction. J Biol Chem 1983; 258:1086–1091.
48. Wunderwald P, Schrenk WJ, Port H. Antithrombin BM from human plasma: an antithrombin binding moderately to heparin. Thromb Res 1982; 25:177–191.
49. Abildgaard U, Larsen ML. Assay of dermatan sulfate cofactor (heparin cofactor II) activity in human plasma. Thromb Res 1984;35:257–266.
50. Ragg H. A new member of the plasma protease inhibitor gene family. Nucleic Acids Res 1986;14:1073–1088.
51. Briginshaw GF, Shanberge JN. Identification of two distinct heparin cofactors in human plasma. II. Inhibition of thrombin and activated factor X. Thromb Res 1974;4:463–477.
52. Briginshaw GF, Shanberge JN. Identification of two distinct heparin cofactors in human plasma. Separation and partial purification. Arch Biochem Biophys 1974;161:683–690.
53. Tollefsen DM, Blank MK. Detection of a new heparin-dependent inhibitor of thrombin in human plasma. J Clin Invest 1981;68:589–596.
54. Friberger P, Egberg N, Holmer E et al. Antithrombin assay—the use of human or bovine thrombin and the observation of a "second" heparin cofactor. Thromb Res 1982;25:433–436.
55. Griffith MJ, Carraway T, White GC et al. Heparin cofactor activities in a family with hereditary antithrombin III deficiency: evidence for a second heparin cofactor in human plasma. Blood 1983;61:111–118.
56. Tollefsen DM. Heparin cofactor II. In: Lane DA, Lindahl U, eds. Heparin: chemical and biological properties, clinical applications. London: Edward Arnold, 1989; pp. 257–274.
57. Scully MF, Kakkar VV. Identification of heparin cofactor II as the principle plasma cofactor for the antithrombin activity of pentosan polysulfate (SP54). Thromb Res 1984;36:187–194.
58. Scully MF, Ellis V, Kakkar VV. Pentosan polysulfate: activation of heparin cofactor II or antithrombin III according to molecular weight fractionation. Thromb Res 1986;41:489–499.
59. Yamagishi R, Niwa M, Knodo S et al. Purification and biological property of heparin cofactor II: activation of heparin cofactor II and antithrombin III by dextran sulfate and various glycosaminoglycans. Thromb Res 1984; 36:633–642.
60. Hurst RE, Poon MC, Griffith MJ. Structure-activity relationships of heparin. Independence of heparin charge density and antithrombin-binding domains in thrombin inhibition by antithrombin and heparin cofactor II. J Clin Invest 1983;72:1042–1045.
61. Girard TJ, Warren LA, Novotny WF et al. Functional significance of the Kunitz-type inhibitory domains of lipoprotein-associated coagulation inhibitor. Nature 1989;338:518–520.
62. Werling RW, Zacharski LR, Kisiel W et al. Distribution of tissue factor pathway inhibitor in normal and malignant human tissues. Thromb Haemost 1993;69:366–369.

63. Lindahl AK, Sandset PM, Abildgaard U. The present status of tissue factor pathway inhibitor [Review]. Blood Coagul Fibrinolysis 1992;3:439–449.

64. Novotny WF, Palmier M, Wun TC et al. Purification and properties of heparin-releasable lipoprotein-associated coagulation inhibitor. Blood 1991;78:394–400.

65. Sandset PM, Abildgaard U, Larsen ML. Heparin induces release of extrinsic coagulation pathway inhibitor (EPI). Thromb Res 1988;50:803–813.

66. Lindahl AK, Abildgaard U, Stokke G. Release of extrinsic pathway inhibitor after heparin injection: increased response in cancer patients. Thromb Res 1990;59:651–656.

67. Ariens RA, Faioni EM, Mannucci PM. Repeated release of the tissue factor pathway inhibitor [Letter]. Thromb Haemost 1984;72:327–328.

68. Warn-Cramer BJ, Maki SL, Rapaport SI. Heparin-releasable and platelet pools of tissue factor pathway inhibitor in rabbits. Thromb Haemost 1993;69:221–226.

69. Bara L, Bloch MF, Zitoun D et al. Comparative effects of enoxaparin and unfractionated heparin in healthy volunteers on prothrombin consumption in whole blood during coagulation, and release of tissue factor pathway inhibitor. Thromb Res 1993;69:443–452.

70. Holst J, Lindblad B, Wedeberg E et al. Tissue factor pathway inhibitor (TFPI) and its response to heparin in patients with spontaneous deep vein thrombosis. Thromb Res 1993;72:467–470.

71. Novotny WF, Brown SG, Miletich JP et al. Plasma antigen levels of the lipoprotein-associated coagulation inhibitor in patient samples. Blood 1991;78:387–393.

72. Warr TA, Warn-Cramer BJ, Rao LV et al. Human plasma extrinsic pathway inhibitor activity: I. Standardization of assay and evaluation of physiological variables. Blood 1989;74:201–206.

73. Vogel GM, Meuleman DG, Bourgondien FG et al. Comparison of two experimental thrombosis models in rats—effects of four glycosaminoglycans. Thromb Res 1989;54:399–410.

74. Harenberg J, Siegele M, Dempfle CE et al. Protamine neutralization of the release of tissue factor pathway inhibitor activity by heparins. Thromb Haemost 1993;70:942–945.

75. Hoppensteadt DA, Fasanella A, Fareed J. Effect of protamine on heparin releasable TFPI antigen levels in normal volunteers. Thromb Res 1995;79:325–330.

76. Lindahl AK, Abildgaard U, Larsen ML et al. Extrinsic pathway inhibitor (EPI) released to the blood by heparin is a more powerful coagulation inhibitor than is recombinant EPI. Thromb Res 1991;62:607–614.

77. Lindahl AK, Abildgaard U, Staalesen R. The anticoagulant effect in heparinized blood and plasma resulting from interactions with extrinsic pathway inhibitor. Thromb Res 1991;64:155–168.

78. Kristensen HI, Ostergaard PB, Nordfang O et al. Effect of tissue factor pathway inhibitor (TFPI) in the HEPTEST assay and in an amidolytic anti factor Xa assay for LMW heparin. Thromb Haemost 1992;68:310–314.

79. Valentin S, Ostergaard P, Kristensen H et al. Simultaneous presence of tissue factor pathway inhibitor (TFPI) and low-molecular-weight heparin has a synergistic effect in different coagulation assays. Blood Coag Fibrinolysis 1991;2:629–635.

80. Wun TC. Lipoprotein-associated coagulation inhibitor (LACI) is a cofactor for heparin: synergistic anticoagulant action between LACI and sulfated polysaccharides. Blood 1992;79:430–438.

81. Nordfang O, Kristensen HI, Valentin S et al. The significance of TFPI in clotting assays—comparison and combination with other anticoagulants. Thromb Haemost 1993;70:448–453.

82. Broze GJ Jr, Warren LA, Novotny WF et al. The lipoprotein-associated coagulation inhibitor that inhibits the factor VII-tissue factor complex also inhibits factor Xa: insight into its possible mechanism of action. Blood 1988;71:335–343.

83. Wesselschmidt R, Likert K, Girard T et al. Tissue factor pathway inhibitor: the carboxyterminus is required for optimal inhibition of factor Xa. Blood 1992;79:2004–2010.

84. Hirsh J, van Aken WG, Gallus AS et al. Heparin kinetics in venous thrombosis and pulmonary embolism. Circulation 1976;53:691–695.

85. Lane DA, Pejler G, Flynn AM et al. Neutralization of heparin-related saccharides by histidine-rich glycoprotein and platelet factor 4. J Biol Chem 1986;261:3980–3986.

86. Lijnen HR, Hoylaerts M, Collen D. Heparin binding properties of human histidine-rich glycoprotein. Mechanism and role in the neutralization of heparin in plasma. J Biol Chem 1983;258:3803–3808.

87. Holt JC, Niewiarowski S. Biochemistry of alpha granule proteins [Review]. Semin Hematol 1985;22:151–163.

88. Preissner KT, Muller-Berghaus G. Neutralization and binding of heparin by S-protein/vitronectin in the inhibition of factor Xa by antithrombin III. Involvement of an inducible heparin-binding domain of S protein/vitronectin. J Biol Chem 1987;262:12247–12253.

89. Dawes J, Pavuk N. Sequestration of therapeutic glycosaminoglycans by plasma fibronectin [Abstract]. Thromb Haemost 1991;65:929.

90. Sobel M, McNeill PM, Carlson PL et al. Heparin inhibition of von Willebrand factor-dependent platelet function in vitro and in vivo. J Clin Invest 1991;87:1787–1793.

91. Glimelius B, Busch C, Hook M. Binding of heparin on the surface of cultured human endothelial cells. Thromb Res 1978;12:773–782.

92. Mahadoo J, Heibert L, Jacques LB. Vascular sequestration of heparin. Thromb Res 1978;12:79–90.

93. Friedman Y, Arsenis C. Studies on the heparin sulphamidase activity from rat spleen. Intracellular distribution and characterization of the enzyme. Biochem J 1979;139:699–708.

94. Bjornsson TD, Wolfram KM, Kitchell BB. Heparin kinetics determined by three assay methods. Clin Pharmacol Ther 1982;31:104–113.

95. de Swart CA, Nijmeyer B, Roelofs JM et al. Kinetics of intravenously administered heparin in normal humans. Blood 1982;60:1251–1258.

96. Olsson P, Lagergren H, Ek S. The elimination from plasma of intravenous heparin: an experimental study on dogs and humans. Acta Med Scand 1963;173:619–623.

97. Hirsh J, Fuster V. Guide to anticoagulant therapy. I. Heparin. Circulation 1994;89:1449–1468.

98. Barritt DW, Jordan SC. Anticoagulant drugs in the treatment of pulmonary embolism: a controlled trial. Lancet 1960;1:1309–1312.

99. Brandjes DP, Heijboer H, Butler HR et al. Acenocoumarol and heparin compared with acenocoumarol alone in the initial treatment of proximal-vein thrombosis. N Engl J Med 1992;327:1485–1489.

100. Hull R, Delmore T, Genton E et al. Warfarin sodium versus low-dose heparin in the long-term treatment of venous thrombosis. N Engl J Med 1979;301:855–858.

101. Lagerstedt CI, Olsson CG, Fagher BO et al. Need for long-term anticoagulant treatment in symptomatic calf-vein thrombosis. Lancet 1985;2:515–518.

102. Hull RD, Raskob GE, Hirsh J et al. Continuous intravenous heparin compared with intermittent subcutaneous heparin in the initial treatment of proximal-vein thrombosis. N Engl J Med 1986;315:1109–1114.

103. Turpie AG, Robinson JG, Doyle DJ et al. Comparison of high-dose with low-dose subcutaneous heparin to prevent left ventricular mural thrombosis in patients with acute transmural anterior myocardial infarction. N Engl J Med 1989;320:352–357.

104. Clagett GP, Reisch JS. Prevention of venous thromboembolism in general surgical patients. Results of meta-analysis [Review]. Ann Surg 1988;208:227–240.

105. Collins R, Scrimgeour A, Yusuf S et al. Reduction in fatal pulmonary embolism and venous thrombosis by perioperative administration of subcutaneous heparin. Overview of results of randomized trials in general, orthopedic, and urologic surgery [Review]. N Engl J Med 1988;318:1162–1173.

106. Theroux P, Ouimet H, McCans J. Aspirin, heparin, or both to treat acute unstable angina. N Engl J Med 1988;319:1105–1111.

107. Theroux P, Waters D, Lam J et al. Reactivation of unstable angina after the discontinuation of heparin. N Engl J Med 1992;327:141–145.

108. Neri Serneri GG, Gensini GF, Poggesi L. Effect of heparin, aspirin, or alteplase in reduction of myocardial ischaemia in refractory unstable angina. Lancet 1990;335:615–618.

109. Neri Serneri GG, Rovelli F, Gensini GF et al. Effectiveness of low-dose heparin in prevention of myocardial reinfarction. Lancet 1987;1:937–942.

110. Bleich SD, Nichols TC, Schumacher RR et al. Effect of heparin on coronary arterial patency after thrombolysis with tissue plasminogen activator in acute myocardial infarction. Am J Cardiol 1990;66:1412–1417.

111. de Bono DP, Simmons ML, Tijssen J et al. Effect of early intravenous heparin on coronary patency, infarct size, and bleeding complications after alteplase thrombolysis: results of a randomized double blind European Cooperative Study Group trial. Br Heart J 1992;67:122–128.

112. Hyers TM. Heparin therapy. Regimens and treatment considerations [Review]. Drugs 1992;44:738–749.

113. Brill-Edwards P, Ginsberg JS, Johnston M et al. Establishing a therapeutic range for heparin therapy. Ann Intern Med 1993;119:104–109.

114. Ellison N, Edmunds LH Jr, Colman RW. Platelet aggregation following heparin and protamine administration. Anesthesiology 1978;48:65–68.

115. Thomson C, Forbes CD, Prentice CR. The potentiation of platelet aggregation and adhesion by heparin in vitro and in vivo. Clin Sci Mol Med 1973;45:485–494.

116. Besterman EM, Gillett MP. Heparin effects on plasma lysolecithin formation and platelet aggregation. Atherosclerosis 1973;17:503–513.

117. Zucker MB. Heparin and platelet function [Review]. Fed Proc 1977;36:47–49.

118. Heiden D, Mielke CH Jr, Rodvien R. Impairment by heparin of primary haemostasis and platelet [$^{14}$C]5-hydroxytryptamine release. Br J Haematol 1977;36:427–436.

119. Eika C. On the mechanism of platelet aggregation induced by heparin, protamine and polybrene. Scand J Haemost 1972;9:248–257.

120. Salzman EW, Rosenberg RD, Smith MH et al. Effect of heparin and heparin fractions on platelet aggregation. J Clin Invest 1980;65:64–73.

121. Krupinski K, Breddin HK, Casu B. Anticoagulant and antithrombotic effects of chemically modified heparins and pentosanpolysulfate. Haemostasis 1990;20:81–92.

122. Naggi A, Torri G, Casu B et al. "Supersulfated" heparin fragments, a new type of low-molecular weight heparin. Physico-chemical and pharmacological properties. Biochem Pharmacol 1987;36:1895–1900.

123. Jeske W, Hoppensteadt D, Klauser R et al. Effect of repeated Aprosulate and Enoxaparin administration on tissue factor pathway inhibitor antigen levels. Blood Coagul Fibrinolysis 1995;6:119–124.

124. Herold BC, Gerber SI, Polonsky T et al. Identification of structural features of heparin required for inhibition of herpes simplex virus type 1 binding. Virology 1995;206:1108–1116.

125. Soker S, Goldstaub D, Svahn CM et al. Variations in the size and sulfation of heparin modulate the effect of heparin on the binding of VEGF165 to its receptors. Biochem Biophys Res Commun 1994;203:1339–1347.

126. Rajtar G, Marchim E, deGaetano G et al. Effects of glycosaminoglycans on platelet and leukocyte function: role of N-sulfation. Biochem Pharmacol 1993;46:958–960.

127. Belford DA, Hendry IA, Parish CR. Ability of different chemically modified heparins to potentiate the biological activity of heparin-binding growth factor 1: lack of correlation with growth factor binding. Biochemistry 1992;31:6498–6503.

128. Sache E, Maillard M, Malazzi P et al. Partially N-desulfated heparin as a non-anticoagulant heparin: some physico-chemical and biological properties. Thromb Res 1989;55:247–258.

129. Inoue Y, Nagasawa K. Selective N-desulfation of heparin with dimethyl sulfoxide containing water or methanol. Carbohydr Res 1976;46:87–95.

130. Bjornsson TD, Schneider DE, Hecht AR. Effects of N-deacetylation and N-desulfation of heparin on its anticoagulant activity and in vivo disposition. J Pharmacol Exp Ther 1988;245:804–808.

131. Danishefsky I, Ahrens M, Klein S. Effect of heparin modification on its activity in enhancing the inhibition of thrombin by antithrombin III. Biochim Biophys Acta 1977;498:215–222.

132. Fareed J. Basic and applied pharmacology of low-molecular-weight heparins. Pharm Ther 1995;(Suppl):16s–24s.

133. Fareed J, Walenga JM, Kumar A et al. A modified stasis thrombosis model to study the antithrombotic actions of heparin and its fractions. Semin Thromb Hemost 1985;11:155–175.

134. Fareed J, Walenga JM, Hoppensteadt D et al. Comparative study on the in vitro and in vivo activities of seven low-molecular-weight heparins [published erratum appears in Haemostasis 1988;18:389a]. Haemostasis 1988; 18(Suppl 3):3–15.

135. Leclerc JR, Geerts WH, Desjardins L et al. Prevention of venous thromboembolism after knee arthroplasty. A randomized, double-blind trial comparing enoxaparin with warfarin. Ann Intern Med 1996;124:619–626.

136. Bergqvist D, Benoni G, Bjorgell O et al. Low-molecular-weight heparin (enoxaparin) as prophylaxis against venous thromboembolism after total hip replacement. N Engl J Med 1996;335:696–700.

137. Heit JA, Berkowitz SD, Bona R et al. Efficacy and safety of low-molecular-weight heparin (ardeparin sodium) compared to warfarin for the prevention of venous thromboembolism after total knee replacement surgery: a double-blind, dose-ranging study. Ardeparin Arthroplasty Study Group. Thromb Haemost 1997;77:32–38.

138. Lassen MR, Borris LC. Low-molecular-weight heparin for the prevention of deep vein thrombosis following orthopedic surgery. Curr Opin Pulm Med 1996;2:300–304.

139. Planes A, Vochelle N, Darmon JY et al. Risk of deep-venous thrombosis after hospital discharge in individuals having undergone total hip replacement: double-blind randomised comparison of enoxaparin versus placebo. Lancet 1996;348:224–228.

140. Hull RD, Pineo GF, Brant RF. Effect of low-molecular-weight heparin versus warfarin sodium on mortality in long-term treatment of proximal vein thrombosis. Clin Appl Thromb/Hemost 1996;2(Suppl 1):S4–S11.

141. Dahl OE, Andreassen G, Aspelin T et al. Prolonged thromboprophylaxis following hip replacement surgery—results of a double-blind, prospective, randomised, placebo-controlled study with dalteparin (Fragmin®). Thromb Haemost 1997;77:26–31.

142. Gårdlund B. Randomised, controlled trial of low-dose heparin for prevention of fatal pulmonary embolism in individuals with infectious diseases. The Heparin Prophylaxis Study Group. Lancet 1996;347:1357–1361.

143. Anonymous. Low-molecular-weight heparin is an effective and safe treatment for deep-vein thrombosis and pulmonary embolism [Abstract]. The Columbus Investigators. Blood 1996;88(Suppl 1):626a.

144. Anonymous. Low-molecular-weight heparin during instability in coronary artery disease. Fragmin during Instability in Coronary Artery Disease (FRISC) study group. Lancet 1996;347:561–568.

145. Cohen M, Demers C, Gurfinkel E et al. Primary endpoint analysis from the ESSENCE trial: enoxaparin vs unfractionated heparin in unstable angina and non–Q wave infarction [Abstract]. Circulation 1996;94:I-554.

146. Antman EM, McCabe CH, Marble SJ et al. Dose-ranging trial of enoxaparin for unstable angina: results of TIMI 11A. The Thrombolysis in Myocardial Infarction (TIMI) 11A Trial Investigators. Circulation 1996;94:I-554.

147. Zidar J. New insights in the prevention of thrombosis in coronary stents—the ENTICES trial and the role of enoxaparin [Abstract]. Ann Hematol 1997;74(Suppl II):A152.

148. Schiele FJ, Vuillemenot AR, Meneveau NF et al. Initial experience of a sulphated pentasaccharide, a pure factor Xa inhibitor, in coronary angioplasty [Abstract]. Circulation 1996;94:I-742.

149. Hull RD, Raskob GE, Pineo GF et al. Subcutaneous low-molecular-weight heparin compared with continuous intravenous heparin in the treatment of proximal-vein thrombosis. N Engl J Med 1992;326:975–982.

150. Prandoni P, Lensing AW, Büller HR et al. Comparison of subcutaneous low-molecular-weight heparin with intravenous standard heparin in proximal deep-vein thrombosis. Lancet 1992;339:441–445.

151. Lopaciuk S, Meissner AJ, Filipecki S et al. Subcutaneous low-molecular-weight heparin versus subcutaneous unfractionated heparin in the treatment of deep vein thrombosis: a Polish multicenter trial. Thromb Haemost 1992;68:14–18.

152. Lindmarker P, Holmström M, Granqvist S et al. Comparison of once-daily subcutaneous Fragmin with continuous intravenous unfractionated heparin in the treatment of deep venous thrombosis. Thromb Haemost 1994; 72:186–190.

153. Simonneau G, Charbonnier B, Decousus H et al. Subcutaneous low-molecular-weight heparin compared with continuous intravenous unfractionated heparin in the treatment of proximal deep vein thrombosis. Arch Intern Med 1993;153:1541–1546.

154. Koopman MM, Prandoni P, Piovella F et al. Treatment of venous thrombosis with intravenous unfractionated heparin administered in the hospital as compared with subcutaneous low-molecular-weight heparin administered at home. The Tasman Study Group. N Engl J Med 1996;334:682–687.

155. Levine M, Gent M, Hirsh J et al. A comparison of low-molecular-weight heparin administered primarily at home with unfractionated heparin administered in the hospital for proximal deep-vein thrombosis. N Engl J Med 1996;334:677–681.

156. Godwin J. Use of low-molecular-weight heparins in malignancy-related thromboembolic disorders: a clinical review. Clin Appl Thrombosis/Hemostasis 1996;2(Suppl 1):S28–S34.

157. Fricker JP, Vergnes Y, Schach R et al. Low dose heparin versus low-molecular-weight heparin (Kabi 2165, Fragmin) in the prophylaxis of thromboembolic complications of abdominal oncological surgery. Eur J Clin Invest 1988;18:561–567.

158. Anonymous. Comparison of a low-molecular-weight heparin and unfractionated heparin for the prevention of deep vein thrombosis in patients undergoing abdominal surgery. The European Fraxiparin Study (EFS) Group. Br J Surg 1988;75:1058–1063.

159. Godwin JE, Comp P, Davidson B et al. Comparison of the efficacy and safety of subcutaneous RD heparin vs subcutaneous unfractionated heparin for the prevention of deep-vein thrombosis in patients undergoing abdominal or pelvic surgery for cancer [Abstract]. Thromb Haemost 1996; 69(Suppl):376.

160. Prandoni P, Lensing AW, Büller HR et al. Deep-vein thrombosis and the incidence of subsequent symptomatic cancer. N Engl J Med 1992;327: 1128–1133.

161. Monreal M, Lafoz E, Olive A et al. Comparison of subcutaneous unfractionated heparin with a low-molecular-weight heparin (Fragmin) in patients with venous thromboembolism and contraindications to coumarin. Thromb Haemost 1994;71:7–11.

162. Hirsh J, Hoak J. Management of deep vein thrombosis and pulmonary embolism. Circulation 1996;93:2212–2245.

163. Salazar E, Izaguirre R, Verdejo J et al. Failure of adjusted doses of subcutaneous heparin to prevent thromboembolic phenomena in pregnant patients with mechanical cardiac valve prostheses. J Am Coll Cardiol 1996; 27:1698–1703.

164. Hunt BJ, Doughty HA, Majumdar G et al. Thromboprophylaxis with low-molecular-weight heparin (Fragmin) in high risk pregnancies. Thromb Haemost 1997;77:39–43.

165. Boda Z, Laszlo P, Rejtō L et al. Low-molecular-weight heparin as thromboprophylaxis in familial thrombophilia during the whole period of pregnancy. Thromb Haemost 1996;76:128.

166. Massicotte P, Adams M, Marzinotto V et al. Low-molecular-weight heparin in pediatric patients with thrombotic disease: a dose finding study. J Pediatr 1996;128:313–318.

167. Forrat R, Ferrera R, Boissonnat P et al. High prevalence of thromboembolic complications in heart transplant recipients. Which preventive strategy? Transplantation 1996;61:757–762.

168. Walenga JM, Koza MJ, Lewis BE et al. Relative heparin-induced thrombocytopenic potential of low-molecular-weight heparins and new antithrombotic agents. Clin Appl Thrombosis/Hemostasis 1996;2(Suppl 1):S21–S27.

169. Greinacher A, Feigl M, Mueller-Eckhardt C. Crossreactivity studies between sera of patients with heparin associated thrombocytopenia and a new low-molecular-weight heparin, reviparin. Thromb Haemost 1994;72: 644–645.

170. Greinacher A, Alban S, Dummel V et al. Characterization of the structural requirements for a carbohydrate based anticoagulant with a reduced risk of inducing the immunological type of heparin-associated thrombocytopenia. Thromb Haemost 1995;74:886–892.

171. Warkentin TE, Levine MN, Hirsh J et al. Heparin-induced thrombocytopenia in patients treated with low-molecular-weight heparin or unfractionated heparin. N Engl J Med 1995;332:1330–1335.

172. Barrowcliffe TW. Annotation: low-molecular-weight heparins. Br J Hematol 1995;90:1.

173. Reference deleted.

174. Hirsh J, Raschke R, Warkentin TE et al. Heparin: mechanism of action, pharmacokinetics, dosing considerations, monitoring, efficacy, and safety [Review]. Chest 1995;108:258S–275S.

175. Boneu B. Low-molecular-weight heparin therapy: is monitoring needed? Thromb Haemost 1994;72:330–334.

176. Samama MM. Contemporary laboratory monitoring of low-molecular-weight heparins. Clin Lab Med 1995;15:119–123.

177. Hoppensteadt DA, Jeske W, Fareed J. Laboratory monitoring of new anticoagulant and antithrombotic drugs. In: Pifarré R, ed. New anticoagulants for the cardiovascular patient. Philadelphia: Hanley & Belfus, 1997; pp. 521–538.

178. Andersson LO, Barrowcliffe TW, Holmer E et al. Anticoagulant properties

of heparin fractionated by affinity chromatography on matrix-bound antithrombin III and by gel filtration. Thromb Res 1976;9:575–583.

179. Hook M, Bjork I, Hopwood J et al. Anticoagulant activity of heparin: separation of high-activity and low-activity heparin species by affinity chromatography on immobilized antithrombin. FEBS Lett 1976;66:90–93.

180. Lam LH, Silbert JE, Rosenberg RD. The separation of active and inactive forms of heparin. Biochem Biophys Res Commun 1976;69:570–577.

181. Holmer E, Kurachi K, Soderstrom G. The molecular-weight dependence of the rate-enhancing effect of heparin on the inhibition of thrombin, factor Xa, factor IXa, factor XIa, factor XIIa and kallikrein by antithrombin. Biochem J 1981;193:395–400.

182. Laurent TC, Tengblad A, Thunberg L et al. The molecular-weight-dependence of the anti-coagulant activity of heparin. Biochem J 1978;175:691–701.

183. Oosta GM, Gardner WT, Beeler DL et al. Multiple functional domains of the heparin molecule. Proc Natl Acad Sci U S A 1981;78:829–833.

184. Barrowcliffe TW, Johnson EA, Eggleton CA et al. Anticoagulant activities of high and low-molecular-weight heparin fractions. Br J Haematol 1979;41:573–583.

185. Choay J, Lormeau JC, Petitou M et al. Anti-Xa active heparin oligosaccharides. Thromb Res 1980;18:573–578.

186. Carter CJ, Kelton JG, Hirsh J et al. Relationship between the antithrombotic and anticoagulant effects of low-molecular-weight heparin. Thromb Res 1981;21:169–174.

187. Holmer E, Mattsson C, Nilsson S. Anticoagulant and antithrombotic effects of heparin and low-molecular-weight heparin fragments in rabbits. Thromb Res 1982;25:475–485.

188. Ockelford PA, Carter CJ, Mitchell L et al. Discordance between the anti-Xa activity and the antithrombotic activity in an ultra-low-molecular-weight heparin fraction. Thromb Res 1982;28:401–409.

189. Thomas DP, Merton RE, Lewis WE et al. Studies in man and experimental animals of a low-molecular-weight heparin fraction. Thromb Haemost 1981;45:214–218.

190. Thomas DP, Merton RE, Barrowcliffe TW et al. Effects of heparin oligosaccharides with high affinity for antithrombin III in experimental venous thrombosis. Thromb Haemost 1982;47:244–248.

191. Choay J, Lormeau JC, Petitou M et al. Structural studies on a biologically active hexasaccharide obtained from heparin. Ann NY Acad Sci 1981;370:644–649.

192. Thunberg L, Backstrom G, Lindahl U. Further characterization of the antithrombin-binding sequence in heparin. Carbohydr Res 1982;100:393–410.

193. Lindahl U, Backstrom G, Hook M et al. Structure of the antithrombin-binding site in heparin. Proc Natl Acad Sci U S A 1979;76:3198–3202.

194. Choay J, Petitou M, Lormeau JC et al. Structure-activity relationship in heparin: a synthetic pentasaccharide with high affinity for antithrombin III and eliciting high anti-factor Xa activity. Biochem Biophys Res Commun 1983;116:492–499.

195. Rosenberg RD, Lam L. Correlation between structure and function of heparin. Proc Natl Acad Sci U S A 1979;76:1218–1222.

196. Sinay P, Jaquinet JE, Petitou M et al. Total synthesis of a heparin pentasaccharide fragment having high affinity for antithrombin III. Carbohydr Res 1984;132:C5–C9.

197. Petitou M, Duchaussoy P, Lederman I et al. Synthesis of heparin fragments. A chemical synthesis of the pentasaccharide 0-(2-deoxy-2-sulfamido-6-O-sulfo-alpha-D-glucopyranosyl)-(1→4)-0-(beta-D-glucopyranosyluronic acid)-(1→4)-0-(2-deoxy-2-sulfamido-3, 6-di-0-sulfo-alpha-D-glucopyranosyl)-(1→4)-0-(2-O-sulfo-alpha-L-idopyranosyluronic acid)-(1→4)-2-deoxy-2-sulfamido-6-O-sulfo-D-glucopyranose decasodium salt, a heparin fragment having high affinity for antithrombin III. Carbohydr Res 1986;147:221–236.

198. Atha DH, Lormeau JC, Petitou M et al. Contribution of monosaccharide residues in heparin binding to antithrombin III. Biochemistry 1985;24:6723–6729.

199. Torri G, Casu B, Gatti G et al. Mono- and bidimensional 500 MHz ¹H-NMR spectra of a synthetic pentasaccharide corresponding to the binding sequence of heparin to antithrombin-III: evidence for conformational peculiarity of the sulfated iduronate residue. Biochem Biophys Res Comm 1985;128:134–140.

200. Lindahl U, Bäckström G, Thunberg L. The antithrombin-binding sequence in heparin. Identification of an essential 6-0 sulfate group. J Biol Chem 1983;258:9826–9830.

201. Riesenfeld J, Thunberg L, Hook M et al. The antithrombin-binding sequence of heparin. Location of essential N-sulfate groups. J Biol Chem 1981;256:2389–2394.

202. Boneu B, Necciari J, Cariou R et al. Pharmacokinetics and tolerance of the natural pentasaccharide (SR90107/ORG31540) with high affinity to antithrombin III in man. Thromb Haemost 1995;74:1468–1473.

203. Roderick LM. The pathology of sweet clover disease in cattle. J Am Vet Med Assoc 1929;74:314–315.

204. Dam H, Schonheyden F. The antihemorrhagic vitamin of the chick. Nature 1935;135:652–653.

205. Dam H, Schonheyden F, Tage-Hansen E. Studies on the mode of action of vitamin K. Biochem J 1936;30:1075–1079.

206. Quick AJ. The coagulation defect in sweet clover disease and in hemorrhagic chick disease of dietary origin. A consideration of the source of prothrombin. Am J Physiol 1937;118:260–266.

207. Campbell HA, Link KP. Studies on the hemorrhagic sweet clover disease. The isolation and crystallization of the hemorrhagic agent. J Biol Chem 1941;138:21–23.

208. Hawkins WB, Brinkhous KM. Prothrombin deficiency as the cause of bleeding in bile fistula dogs. J Exp Med 1936;63:795–801.

209. Cosgriff SW. The effectiveness of an oral vitamin K in controlling excessive hypoprothrombinemia during anticoagulant therapy. Ann Intern Med 1956;45:14–22.

210. Quick AJ, Stefanini M. Experimentally induced changes in the prothrombin level of the blood IV. The relation of vitamin K deficiency to the excess of vitamin A: with a simplified method for vitamin K assay. J Biol Chem 1948;175:945–950.

211. Quick AJ. The hemorrhagic diseases and the pathology of hemostasis. Springfield, IL: Charles C Thomas, 1974; p. 310.

212. Quick AJ. The hemorrhagic diseases and the pathology of hemostasis. Springfield, IL: Charles C Thomas, 1974; pp. 14–15.

213. Furie B, Furie BC. Molecular basis of vitamin K-dependent gamma-carboxylation. Blood 1990;75:1753–1762.

214. Park BK. Warfarin metabolism and mode of action. Biochem Pharmacol 1988;37:19–27.

215. Nelsestuen G. Role of gamma carboxy-glutamic acid. An unusual transition required for calcium-dependent binding of prothrombin to phospholipid. J Biol Chem 1976;251:5648–5665.

216. Physician's Desk Reference 1997; p. 944.

217. Hirsh J, Dalen J, Deykin D et al. Oral anticoagulants: mechanism of action, clinical effectiveness and optimal therapeutic range [Review]. Chest 1995;108(Suppl):231S–246S.

218. Harrison L, Johnston M, Massicotte P et al. Comparison of 5 mg and 10 mg loading doses in initiation of warfarin therapy. Ann Intern Med 1997;126:133–136.

219. Hull R, Hirsh J, Jay R et al. Different intensities of anticoagulant therapy in the long term treatment of proximal-vein thrombosis. N Engl J Med 1982;307:1676–1681.

220. Bern MM, Lokich JJ, Wallach SR et al. Very low doses of warfarin can prevent thrombosis in central venous catheters. A randomized prospective trial. Ann Intern Med 1990;112:423–428.

221. Clagett GP, Anderson FA Jr, Heit J et al. Prevention of venous thromboembolism [Review]. Chest 1995;108(Suppl):312S–331S.

222. Hirsh J. Optimal intensity and monitoring of warfarin. Am J Cardiol 1995;75:39B–42B.

223. Levine M, Raskob G, Landefeld S et al. Hemorrhagic complications of anticoagulant treatment [Review]. Chest 1995;108(Suppl):279S–290S.

224. Palareti G, Leali N, Coccheri S et al. Bleeding complications of oral anticoagulant treatment: an inception cohort, prospective collaborative study (ISCOAT) Italian Study on Complications of Oral Anticoagulant Therapy. Lancet 1996;348:423–428.

225. Van der Meer FJ, Rosendaal F, Van den Broucke et al. Bleeding complications in oral anticoagulant therapy: an analysis of risk factors. Arch Intern Med 1993;153:1557–1562.

226. Landefeld CS, Beyth RJ. Anticoagulant related bleeding: clinical epidemiology, prediction and prevention. Am J Med 1993;95:315–328.

227. Hirsh J, Fuster V. Guide to anticoagulant therapy. II. Oral anticoagulants. American Heart Association. Circulation 1994;89:1469–1480.

228. Jillella AP, Lutcher C. Reinstituting warfarin in individuals who develop warfarin skin necrosis. Am J Hematol 1996;52:117–119.

229. Makris M, Bardhan G, Preston FE. Warfarin-induced skin necrosis associated with activated protein C resistance. Thromb Haemost 1996;75:523–524.

230. Abdelmalek MF, Spittell PC. 79-year-old woman with blue toes. Mayo Clin Proc 1995;70:292–295.

231. Elkayam UR. Anticoagulation in pregnant women with prosthetic heart valves. A double jeopardy. J Am Coll Cardiol 1996;27:1704–1706.

232. Kearon C, Hirsh J. Management of anticoagulation before and after elective surgery. N Engl J Med 1997;336:1506–1511.

233. Brigdien ML. Oral anticoagulant therapy: practical aspects of management [Review]. Postgrad Med 1996;96:81–106.

# CHAPTER 56

# PHARMACOLOGY OF THROMBOLYTIC AGENTS

## Jane A. Leopold, John F. Keaney, Jr., and Joseph Loscalzo

The discovery and clinical development of novel thrombolytic agents has produced a wealth of knowledge about the pathophysiology and treatment of thrombotic vascular disease. Determining which mechanisms are involved in the action of thrombolytic agents has enhanced greatly our understanding of the fibrinolytic system and hemostatic regulation. This chapter discusses the pharmacology of thrombolytic agents, including a brief review of the relevant molecular mechanisms of fibrinolysis (see Chapter 7) and a more detailed description of the current clinical experience.

## STREPTOKINASE

Streptokinase (SK) is a single-chain protein product isolated from the broth of Lancefield group C β-hemolytic streptococci. SK was first isolated in 1933, and its *in vivo* fibrinolytic activity in humans was demonstrated in 1959 (1). The protein contains 414 amino acid residues and has a molecular size of 47.0 to 50.2 Kda. The 230 aminoterminal residues of SK share homology with trypsinlike serine proteases (2); however, SK has no active site serine residue and, therefore, lacks the properties commonly associated with serine proteases, including the ability to cleave peptide bonds and amidolytic activity against synthetic substrates (3). Use of differential scanning calorimetry has confirmed four independently folded domains within the SK protein (4). Specifically, there are three structurally autonomous regions and a less structured carboxyterminal tail (5) linked by

mobile segments of the protein chain (6). SK itself also may exist in several partially folded states (7).

The carboxyterminal and central domains of SK modulate plasminogen-binding and active site-generating functions; the aminoterminal domain predominantly serves in an activity-potentiating capacity (5). Analysis of truncated SK peptides has allowed functional properties to be localized to different regions of the SK protein. One of the two described plasminogen-binding sites is located in the region $Val_{143}$-$Lys_{293}$ (8). The second, high-affinity plasminogen-binding site is located in the aminoterminal region (i.e., residues 37–51) (9). The sequence $Ile_1$-$Lys_{59}$ is essential for conformational stability of the SK peptide, while the adjacent region, $Ser_{60}$-$Asn_{90}$, appears necessary for human plasminogen activation. The sequence $Val_{58}$-$Arg_{219}$ is required to induce conformational changes of human plasminogen to enzyme and, together with $Tyr_{252}$-$Ala_{316}$, results in the conversion of plasminogen to plasmin in the plasminogen-SK equimolar complex. Coordination of all regions is essential for enzyme formation as well as effective plasminogen activation (10).

### PLASMINOGEN ACTIVATION

Activation of plasminogen by SK is unusual among plasminogen activators in that SK itself possesses no enzymatic activity. The conversion of plasminogen to plasmin by SK is illustrated in Fig. 56.1. Initially, equimolar plasminogen and SK combine to form a complex that initiates a conformational change in the plasminogen moiety, thereby exposing an active site in plasminogen (i.e., reaction 1) (3). The active site formed in reaction 1 then catalyzes the conversion of plasminogen to plasmin (11) and of the SK-plasminogen complex to the SK-plasmin complex (i.e., reaction 2) through an intramolecular peptide bond cleavage (12). At this point, the SK and plasminogen moieties are subjected to progressive degradation into smaller fragments with resultant loss of plasminogen-activator activity (13–15).

## THE SK-PLASMINOGEN COMPLEX

The SK-plasminogen complex is formed rapidly on exposure of the two components in stoichiometric amounts, but it is short-lived in solution because of proteolytic cleavage (11). The plasminogen moiety undergoes rapid cleavage at two sites, the first located between $Arg_{560}$-$Val_{561}$ and the second located at the $Lys_{77}$-$Lys_{78}$ peptide bond (16, 17). The SK moiety of the SK-plasminogen com-

(1)  SK + PGN $\Rightarrow$ SK·PGN

(2)  SK·PGN + PGN $\Rightarrow$ SK·PGN + PI

(3)  SK·PGN $\Rightarrow$ SK·PI

(4)  SK·PI $\Rightarrow\Rightarrow\Rightarrow$ SKDPs

**FIGURE 56.1.** Streptokinase activation and degradation in plasma. *PGN,* plasminogen; *P1,* plasmin; *SK,* streptokinase; *SKDPs,* streptokinase degradation products. (Adapted with permission from Reddy KN. Mechanism of activation of human plasminogen by streptokinase. In: Kline DL, Reddy KNN, eds. Fibrinolysis. Boca Raton: CRC Press, 1980:71–94.)

plex also is cleaved proteolytically, thus giving rise to modified SK. Four different forms of modified SK have been identified, including $SK_A$ (40 Kda), $SK_B$ (36 Kda), $SK_C$ (31 Kda), and $SK_D$ (26 Kda) (13, 14, 18, 19). The type and stability of the modified SK molecules depend on both the duration of incubation and the species of plasminogen. For example, human plasminogen forms $SK_B$, but dog and rabbit plasminogen form $SK_D$ (13, 14, 18). Proteolytic modification of the SK moiety of the SK-plasminogen complex results in a threefold decrease in plasminogen activator activity (20, 21).

In contrast to SK alone, the SK-plasminogen complex possesses enzymatic activity toward synthetic substrates and plasminogen (11, 20, 22, 23). Formation of the SK-plasminogen complex from its constituent proteins follows first-order kinetics, with a $K_d$ of 0.05 nmol/l (15, 16). Similarly, activation of plasminogen by SK-plasminogen obeys Michaelis-Menten kinetics, with a $K_m$ of 1.4 μmol/l and a $k_{cat}$ of 21.8 per second, corresponding to a catalytic efficiency ($k_{cat}/K_m$) of 16 μmol/l per second (15, 16). Kinetic parameters for plasminogen activation by SK and its complexes are presented in Table 56.1.

Unlike plasmin, the SK-plasminogen complex has enzymatic activity specific for plasminogen as a substrate (11, 20). Furthermore, the SK-plasminogen complex activates Lys-plasminogen fourfold to sixfold more effectively than Glu-plasminogen on a molar basis (15). In addition, the particular plasminogen isoform that complexes with SK to form the SK-plasminogen complex influences the relative catalytic efficiency of plasminogen activation (Table 56.1) (15). In this regard, the SK-Lys-plasminogen complex activates plasminogen 50% more effectively than the SK-Glu-plasminogen complex (15, 24). Occupation of the lysine binding sites

**TABLE 56.1.** Kinetic Parameters of Streptokinase and Its Derivatives

| Plasminogen Activator | $K_m$ (μmol) | $k_{cat}$ (per second) | $k_{cat}/K_m$ (μmol/l per second) |
|---|---|---|---|
| *Glu-plasminogen activation* | | | |
| SK | 1.73 | 6.7 | 3.9 |
| B·SK | 2.75 | 19.0 | 6.9 |
| *Lys-plasminogen activation* | | | |
| SK | 1.27 | 26.7 | 21.0 |
| Glu-PGN·SK | 1.40 | 21.8 | 16.0 |
| Lys-PGN·SK | 1.03 | 22.6 | 22.0 |
| Lys-PI·SK | 1.12 | 16.6 | 15.0 |
| B·SK | 1.23 | 52.0 | 41.3 |

*Modified with permission from Wohl RC, Summaria L, Arzadon L, et al. Steady state kinetics of activation of human and bovine plasminogens by streptokinase and its equimolar complexes with various activated forms of human plasminogen. J Biol Chem 1978;253:1402–1407.*

B·SK, *Lys-plasminogen + SK B chain;* Glu-PGN, *Glu-plasminogen;* Lys-PGN, *Lys-plasminogen;* Lys-PI, *Lys-plasmin;* SK, *streptokinase.*

modulates the affinity of SK for plasminogen and changes in the environment of the catalytic site associated with SK-induced conformational activation (25).

## THE SK-PLASMIN COMPLEX

Proteolytic cleavage of the SK and plasminogen components of the SK-plasminogen complex results in formation of the SK-plasmin complex. Alternatively, the SK-plasmin complex forms on exposure of SK to plasmin in solution. This reaction proceeds with a rate constant of 3.0 to $4.7 \times 10^7$ mol/l per second and a $K_d$ of $5 \times 10^{-11}$ mol/l for the SK-plasmin complex (26, 27). The SK-plasmin complex retains the active site involving $His_{60}$, $Ser_{740}$, and $Asp_{645}$, and, therefore, bears enzymatic similarity to plasmin. In terms of catalytic efficiency, the SK-plasmin complex is twofold more effective than native plasmin in degrading fibrin (3).

Plasmin and SK-plasminogen have different enzymatic properties regarding their activity against plasminogen. Plasmin effectively hydrolyses the $Lys_{77}$-$Lys_{78}$ bond of (native) Glu-plasminogen to form Lys-plasminogen (28), but it is ineffective at converting plasminogen to plasmin. In contrast, the SK-plasmin complex activates plasminogen to plasmin both specifically and directly (27). Plasmin and the SK-plasmin complex are affected equally by the inhibitors diisopropyl fluorophosphate, pancreatic trypsin inhibitor, and tosyl-lysine-chloromethyl ketone (TLCK) (8). The *in vivo* plasmin inhibitors $\alpha_2$-antiplasmin and $\alpha_2$-macroglobulin are poor inhibitors of the SK-plasmin complex (26, 27, 29).

The conversion of plasminogen to plasmin by the SK-plasmin complex also follows Michaelis-Menten kinetics, with a $K_m$ of 1.12 $\mu$mol/l, a $k_{cat}$ of 16.6/second, and a catalytic efficiency ($k_{cat}/K_m$) of 15 $\mu$mol/l per second (15). Analogous to SK-plasminogen, the SK-plasmin complex is fourfold to sixfold more effective with (modified) as a substrate Lys-plasminogen then with Glu-plasminogen as a substrate (15). In terms of relative plasminogen activator activity, on a molar basis, SK-plasmin is one-third as potent as SK-plasminogen and equipotent to plasmin (20).

## MODULATION OF ACTIVITY

The activity of SK is enhanced by fibrinogen, fibrin, and the fibrin degradation products, fragments D and E (30–34). Fibrinogen both increases the formation rate of SK-plasminogen complex active sites (32) and stimulates the plasminogen activator activity of that complex (25, 33, 34). Specifically, fibrin enhances SK-plasminogen complex–mediated activation of Glu-plasminogen 6.5-fold, whereas fibrinogen provides only a twofold increase in activator activity (28). The overall descending order of plasminogen activator activity enhancement is: fibrin $\rightarrow$ fibrinogen $\rightarrow$ fragment D $\rightarrow$ fragment E (30). Stimulation of the SK-plasminogen complex by fibrin and fibrinogen also is reflected by increased amidolytic activity toward the synthetic substrate S-2251 (33). In contrast, micromolar concentrations of adenosine triphosphate and heparin oligosaccharides diminish both the amidolytic activity rate of the plasminogen-SK complex and its reciprocal plasminogen activating activity. This inhibition is readily reversed by calcium and magnesium. In addition, 6-aminohexanoic acid is a noncompetitive inhibitor of plasmin formation with a $K_i$ of 0.6 mmol/l (35).

## MECHANISM OF CLOT LYSIS

SK reacts with circulating plasminogen to form the SK-plasmin complex (Fig. 56.1). Fibrin binding of the SK-plasmin complex is accomplished by the five kringle regions in the plasmin moiety and affords localization of the complex to areas of fibrin deposition (11). Unlike the SK-plasminogen complex, the SK-plasmin complex is not subject to inhibition by $\alpha_2$-antiplasmin (27) and, therefore, can activate clot-bound plasminogen without impedance. Elaboration of plasmin serves two opposing functions. First, plasmin-mediated degradation of fibrin leads to stimulation of locally bound SK-plasmin and SK-plasminogen, thereby resulting in accelerated plasminogen activation and clot dissolution. Second, direct action of plasmin on the SK-plasmin complex leads to progressive degradation of both components, with subsequent reduction in plasminogen activator activity. Furthermore, circulating (free) SK-plasmin and SK-plasminogen act on circulating plasminogen to produce systemic plasminemia, consumption of fibrinogen, and activation of thrombin via the prothrombinase complex, either directly or indirectly through a calcium-dependent mechanism independent of plasminogen (36).

Onundarson et al (37) investigated SK-mediated clot lysability in individuals receiving SK for acute myocardial infarction. Five minutes after therapy was initiated, a lytic state was demonstrated. After 20 minutes, plasminogen levels decreased to 24% of baseline, $\alpha_2$-antiplasmin levels to 7% of baseline, and fibrinogen to 0.2 g/l. Lysis of radiolabeled clots decreased from 37% after 5 minutes to 21% at 10 minutes, and it was markedly diminished by 20 minutes. Clot lysability correlated positively with plasminogen concentration but not plasmin activity, thus suggesting clot lysability decreases in conjunction with development of a lytic state and the associated depletion of plasminogen.

SK further enhances clot lysis by indirectly creating a platelet aggregation defect. Gouin et al (38) performed *ex vivo* studies using human platelets incubated with SK at concentrations achievable during lytic therapy. Analysis of the platelet surface receptor glycoprotein (GP)

IIb-IIIa revealed that the aggregation defect relates to depleted levels of fibrinogen, coupled with accumulating amounts of fibrinogen degradation products which compete with fibrinogen, and not to degradation of the receptor itself.

## PHARMACOKINETICS

The pharmacokinetics of SK have been studied by several methods, including injection of radiolabeled protein (39) and assay of plasma amidolytic activity after SK administration (40). Early studies using radiolabeled SK demonstrated that SK clearance is biphasic, with an initial half-life of 11 to 17 minutes and a terminal half-life of 83 minutes (39). This suggests the initial clearance results from an antibody-mediated mechanism, with terminal clearance resulting from hepatic metabolism. Investigations with less contaminated preparations of SK revealed that plasma elimination is monophasic, with a half-life of 18 to 30 minutes (41–43).

In terms of biologic half-life, the plasminogen activator activity of SK is more enduring than the plasma half-life of the compound. Grierson et al (40) followed the plasma amidolytic activity of the activator complex in 13 individuals with acute myocardial infarction treated with SK. In these individuals, the biologic half-life of the compound was 82 minutes; however, other investigators (44) have demonstrated a half-life as long as 169 to 184 minutes in a similar individual population.

## THROMBOLYTIC THERAPY

Since its first therapeutic use in 1959 (1), SK has been used widely in the treatment of thrombotic disorders, including venous thrombosis (45–50), pulmonary embolism (51), peripheral arterial thrombosis (52), cerebral embolism (53), and acute myocardial infarction (54–64).

### Venous Thromboembolism (see Chapter 61)

Early clinical experience with SK focused on the treatment of venous thrombosis (45–50). Treatment with intravenous SK (10,000–100,000 IU/hour) was associated with complete, or near-complete, lysis of thrombus in 50 to 70% of individuals; standard heparin therapy resolved thrombus in less than 10% of individuals (45–50). Individuals with proximal, nonocclusive thrombi responded best to thrombolytic therapy with SK (48). Available evidence suggests that successful SK therapy diminishes the incidence of both postphlebitic syndrome and lower extremity ulcers, whereas heparin offers no benefit regarding these sequelae (47, 49, 65–69). SK therapy has demonstrated superior clinical efficacy compared with heparin, but individuals treated with SK have been more likely to experience adverse reactions, including fever and significant bleeding (45, 48–50). In

fact, the risk of significant hemorrhage with SK is three times that with heparin (50); rates as high as 25% have been reported. Decision analysis has revealed that individuals find this risk to be unacceptable despite the improved therapeutic profile of SK (70), and it supports heparin therapy alone for the treatment of venous thrombosis. Risk of pulmonary embolism in individuals with venous thrombosis treated with SK is similar to that in individuals treated with heparin (50).

SK also has been investigated as treatment for pulmonary embolism (71–74). Compared with heparin or warfarin, intravenous SK is associated with more rapid resolution of pulmonary emboli (53), pulmonary vascular reperfusion, and improved hemodynamic parameters (71, 72). After 1 year, individuals treated with SK manifest improved capillary blood volume and pulmonary gas exchange compared with heparin-treated individuals (75). In addition, these individuals demonstrate preserved normal pulmonary vascular response to exercise and less functional disability (76). Despite these obvious benefits, however, no clinical trial has confirmed improved individual survival with SK in the treatment of pulmonary embolism.

### Acute Myocardial Infarction (see Chapter 59)

Patients with acute myocardial infarction benefit from thrombolytic therapy. In the study by DeWood et al (77), coronary thrombus was present in most individuals with acute myocardial infarction who underwent coronary angiography early in their clinical course, thereby implicating coronary thrombosis as the cause of acute myocardial infarction. In light of this observation, several studies investigated the potential of intracoronary SK in acute myocardial infarction (54–60). Intracoronary SK (250,000–500,000 U over 1 hour) successfully resolved coronary thrombus and restored coronary flow in 49 to 79% of individuals; heparin or placebo resulted in arterial patency rates of only 0 to 15% (54–58). Subsequent comparison of intracoronary with intravenous SK (55–57) demonstrated that in sufficient doses (1.5 million U over 1–2 hours), intravenous SK produced infarct-related arterial patency rates near those of intracoronary SK (44–59% versus 49–79%, respectively) (55, 56) and could be delivered 1 to 2 hours earlier than intracoronary therapy. These two important findings set the stage for large scale trials of intravenous SK in the treatment of acute myocardial infarction.

The first such large scale, randomized trial of SK in acute myocardial infarction was the GISSI (Gruppo Italiano per lo studio della Streptochinasi nell'Infarto Miocardico) Study (61), in which 11,712 individuals presenting within the first 6 hours of suspected myocardial infarction were randomized to treatment with SK (1.5 million U over 1 hour) or placebo and followed clinically for 12 months. Therapy with SK was associated with a reduction in 1-year mortality from 19.0 to 17.2% ($P = .008$) and a 0.84% rate of cerebrovascular accident. Subsequent subgroup analysis revealed, however, that improved survival was restricted to those individuals with anterior myocardial infarction. The ISIS (International Study of Infarct Survival)-2 trial (62) later confirmed the GISSI findings, with the additional demonstration of improved survival among individuals treated with aspirin (160 mg/day), an effect which was additive to that seen with SK used alone. Results of several smaller studies of intravenous SK in myocardial infarction (56, 63, 64) have revealed improved preservation of left ventricular function among those individuals treated with SK compared to controls.

Thrombolytic therapy using SK also has been compared with primary percutaneous transluminal coronary angioplasty (PTCA) for acute myocardial infarction. Individuals randomized to treatment with SK suffered worse clinical outcomes, including higher rates of unstable angina and infarction (78). Furthermore, when stratified according to risk at presentation, those individuals determined to be low risk who received SK therapy had a higher composite incidence of death, nonfatal cerebrovascular events, and reinfarction at 6 months than individuals randomized to PTCA (79). Myocardial infarcts were 23% larger and left ventricular ejection fraction was consistently lower, and with worse regional wall motion in the infarct-related zones in the SK group (80). Individuals administered SK also sustained 60th higher in-hospital and long-term mortality rates (81) compared with individuals randomized to primary PTCA (11% vs. 5% at 9 months, respectively), and increased mortality from cardiac causes (28% vs. 7%, respectively) (82). Eighteen months after myocardial infarction, the relative risk of death from cardiac causes and nonfatal reinfarction in SK-treated individuals was 6.1 compared with PTCA-treated individuals (83). Therefore, SK therapy, when used as an adjunct to PTCA, did not enhance early preservation of left ventricular function, improve infarct related artery patency rates, or lower the rate of restenosis after primary PTCA for acute myocardial infarction (84).

## ADVERSE REACTIONS

In addition to bleeding complications, SK is associated with other side effects. Because of its bacterial origin, SK is immunogenic (85), and SK therapy is associated with development of both humoral and cellular immune responses. Anti-SK immunoglobulin (IgG) antibodies are well documented in the general population and have been implicated in reduced SK activity. As measured by fluorometric assay for plasmin and by a fibrin plate lysis assay, SK activity is decreased in the plasma of individuals with high levels of anti-SK IgG antibodies (86). Neutralizing antibody levels also have been monitored in individuals after SK therapy and have returned to near-baseline levels as early as 2 years after a single dose (87).

SK additionally activates the complement system, and the titer of anti-SK antibodies correlates to levels of $C_{3a}$ and $C_{5b-9}$ (88). In addition, T-cell clones recognize at least five different antigenic epitopes distributed along the SK polypeptide chain (89). Clinically, SK therapy in individuals with elevated anti-SK antibody titers are associated with a serum sickness-type syndrome (90, 91) as well as with hypotension (91), fever (56), rash (61), and bronchospasm (61).

## APSAC

The SK-plasmin complex demonstrates extreme catalytic efficiency in the conversion of fibrin-bound plasminogen to plasmin (30); however, this complex is inactivated rapidly in plasma, thereby limiting its therapeutic efficacy. To overcome this constraint (92), an SK derivative, in which SK is noncovalently associated with plasminogen and the active site is "protected" by the covalent addition of a $p$-anisoyl group, was chemically engineered. Known as *APSAC* (i.e., anisoylated plasminogen-SK activator complex), this compound retains fibrin-binding properties through the plasminogen moiety and possesses a prolonged chemical half-life of 94 minutes (92).

As shown in Fig. 56.2, APSAC is composed of two noncovalently bound species, SK and plasminogen, with a combined molecular weight of 131 Kda. The active center of the molecule, which is located in the plasminogen moiety, is protected by a $p$-anisoyl group covalently bound to $Ser_{740}$. Specific acylation of the active site is accomplished by use of $p$-amidinophenyl-$p'$-anisate-HCl (APAN), which is an inverse acylating agent. The reaction of APAN with the SK-plasminogen complex

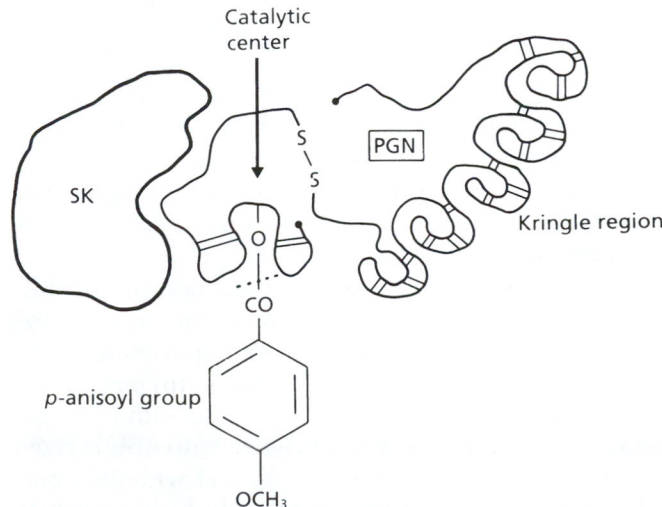

**FIGURE 56.2.** Structure of anisoylated plasminogen streptokinase activator complex (APSAC). *PGN*, plasminogen; *SK*, streptokinase.

**FIGURE 56.3.** Acylation of anisoylated plasminogen activator complex (APSAC) with the reverse acylating agent p-amidinophenyl-*p'*-anisate-HCl (APAN). (Adapted with permission from Anderson JL. Development and evaluation of anisoylated plasminogen streptokinase activator complex (APSAC) as a second generation thrombolytic agent (review). J Am Coll Cardiol 1987; 10:22B–27B.)

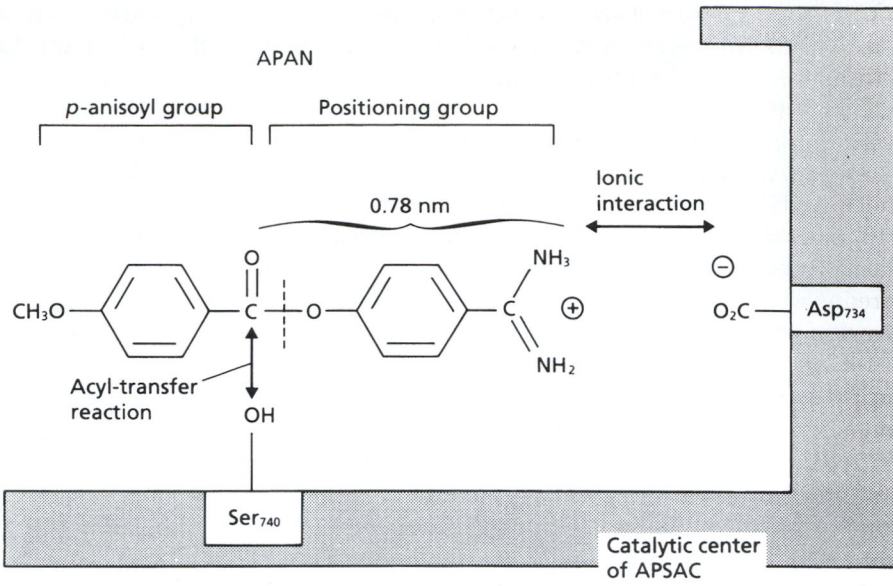

(93) is shown in Fig. 56.3. The cationic amidino group becomes positioned through an ionic interaction with $Asp_{734}$ in the catalytic center, thereby leaving the p-anisoyl group positioned near $Ser_{740}$. An acyl transfer reaction then accompanies the p-anisoylation of the catalytic center (92). The reaction of SK-plasmin with APAN results in a loss of enzymatic activity, which is regenerated by hydrolysis of the p-anisoyl group at the catalytic center. Studies using radiolabeled APAN have demonstrated that under basal conditions, the SK-plasmin complex does not undergo multiacylation (92).

Chemical modification of the active site occurs within the plasminogen moiety of the complex, which is distant from the kringle regions (92); as a result, the APSAC molecule retains fibrin binding properties similar to those of the SK-plasminogen complex (94). When injected intravenously, the enzymatically inert complex circulates to the site of fibrin deposition, where subsequent deacylation of the active site affords "fibrin-targeted" thrombolysis. This process is facilitated by APSAC resistance to inactivation by circulating $\alpha_2$-antiplasmin and $\alpha_2$-macroglobulin because of the inaccessible active center (95).

Alterations in the pharmacokinetics of the SK-plasmin complex conferred by p-anisoylation offer several advantages regarding clinical application of the molecule. The anisoylated SK-plasminogen complex can be administered rapidly as a single dose without hypotension (96), which often occurs when native SK is given as a bolus (97). Furthermore, compared with SK alone, APSAC demonstrates greater stability in plasma (92), has a longer circulation time in blood (98), possesses greater lytic potency (92), and retains similar fibrin-binding properties (97, 99).

## PHARMACOKINETICS

APSAC is administered as a rapid intravenous bolus, and once in the bloodstream, deacylation begins immediately, thus generating the active SK-plasminogen complex. The rate of deacylation follows first-order kinetics and depends on the solution milieu. Gemmill et al (100) compared the pharmacokinetic properties of APSAC (30 mg intravenous bolus) with those of SK (1.5 million U over 30 minutes) in individuals with acute myocardial infarction. SK was cleared more rapidly (36 versus 69 minutes) and demonstrated a shorter mean plasma residence time (46 versus 93 minutes). The precise mechanism for the prolonged half-life of APSAC remains unclear, but it may reflect slower hepatic clearance, less neutralization by plasma inhibitors, or both (95).

## FIBRIN SPECIFICITY

The fibrin binding capacity of APSAC, as measured through binding to forming clots, is similar to that of the SK-plasmin complex (97). This reflects the fact that fibrin binding is determined by the kringle regions on the plasminogen moiety of the complex. On deacylation, the SK-plasminogen complex derived from APSAC is thought to maintain properties similar to those of the native SK-plasminogen complex. In addition, at plasma concentrations producing 50 and 75% clot lysis, APSAC results in less marked fibrinogen depletion than SK-plasmin or urokinase, but more pronounced fibrinogen depletion than tissue-type plasminogen activator (t-PA) (97).

## THROMBOLYTIC PROPERTIES

Early clinical trials with APSAC demonstrated favorable results in terms of both thrombolytic efficacy and clinical safety. In these studies (101–109), therapy with intravenous APSAC (30 mg intravenous bolus) for suspected myocardial infarction produced infarct-related artery patency rates of 60 to 100%. A minimal dose of 30 mg was required to achieve acceptable patency rates but also was associated with marked fibrinogenolysis (101). The AIMS (APSAC Intervention Mortality Study) trial (110) randomized 1258 individuals with acute myocardial infarction to early treatment with APSAC. Compared with placebo, APSAC produced a 50.5% reduction in mortality at 30 days and a 43% reduction in mortality at 1 year. Compared with heparin alone, APSAC afforded improved preservation of left ventricular function and a 31% reduction in infarct size (111).

A clinical comparison of APSAC to SK demonstrated that APSAC was at least equivalent to SK and simpler to deliver (112). The Thrombolytic Trial of Eminase in Acute Myocardial Infarction (TEAM-2) study (113) compared APSAC (30 mg intravenous bolus) with SK (1.5 million U intravenously over 1 hour) and demonstrated no difference between therapies regarding rates of infarct-related artery patency (72 versus 77%, respectively), reocclusion (1%), bleeding complications (1%), and in-hospital mortality (5.9 versus 7.1%, respectively). This observation was confirmed in one arm of the ISIS-3 megatrial (114), which compared APSAC with SK in a subgroup of 41,299 individuals with suspected acute myocardial infarction. No difference in mortality rates between the groups occurred at either 30 days or 6 months, but APSAC-treated individuals suffered a higher rate of cerebrovascular accidents attributable to intracranial hemorrhage (0.24 vs. 0.55%, respectively).

Investigators comparing APSAC with t-PA have reported conflicting results regarding efficacy, morbidity, mortality, and hemorrhagic complications. Bassand et al (115) described equivalent coronary patency rates with APSAC and t-PA (72 versus 76%, respectively) 5 days after therapy in 183 individuals. These observations were supported by the TEAM-3 study (116), which evaluated left ventricular function, morbidity, and infarct-related artery patency 1 day after thrombolytic therapy. The ejection fraction was significantly higher after t-PA, but APSAC and t-PA were equivalent regarding other clinical endpoints. Similarly, the ISIS-3 trial (114) revealed no benefit regarding mortality from APSAC compared with t-PA (10.5 versus 10.3%, respectively) 35 days after therapy. In contrast, the TIMI (Thrombolysis in Myocardial Infarction) 4 trial (117), which compared APSAC with "front-loaded" t-PA, demonstrated significantly lower infarct-related artery patency rates at 60 minutes (59.5 versus 77.8%, respectively) and higher mortality rates at 6 weeks (8.8 versus 2.2%, respectively) in APSAC treated individuals. These findings were noted previously in

the rt-PA-APSAC Patency Study (TAPS) study (118), which was a randomized, multicenter trial of 421 individuals with acute myocardial infarction. Coronary angiography 90 minutes after initiation of APSAC or front-loaded t-PA revealed a patent infarct-related artery in 70.3 versus 84.4% of individuals, respectively. In addition, individuals treated with APSAC suffered more in-hospital deaths, presumably resulting from the increased number of hemorrhagic complications.

Additional review of these studies suggests the conflicting outcomes may be attributable to differences in t-PA dosing regimens and to the use of adjunctive antithrombin and antiplatelet therapies. The DUCCS (Duke University Clinical Cardiology Study)-II study (119) was designed to address these issues; however, the study was terminated prematurely when the results of the Global Use of Strategies to Open Occluded Coronary Arteries (GUSTO) trial, which demonstrated a mortality benefit of t-PA over SK, became available. The DUCCS-II study randomized 162 individuals to APSAC without heparin or front-loaded t-PA and weight-adjusted heparin. All individuals received aspirin in either a standard or a low dose. Despite early termination, data analysis revealed that individuals administered APSAC were not anticoagulated as well, yet suffered more hemorrhagic complications than those administered t-PA. In addition, a composite in-hospital morbidity profile favored treatment with t-PA over APSAC (25.4 versus 31.3%, respectively) (119).

## IMMUNOLOGIC COMPLICATIONS

Antibodies to SK (aSKa) have been implicated in the systemic inactivation of APSAC. In a study by Brugemann et al (120), approximately 14% of individuals with acute myocardial infarction treated using APSAC failed to achieve a systemic lytic state 1.5 hours after receiving thrombolytic therapy as measured by a decrease in the plasma fibrinogen level of less than 1 g/L. These individuals demonstrated elevated levels of aSKa before treatment, and they similarly manifested increased levels of fibrinogen, plasminogen, and $\alpha_2$-antiplasmin after APSAC administration. Measurements of aSKa at 1.5 and 48 hours after treatment revealed a dramatic decrease in antibody levels, thus suggesting the SK component of APSAC was binding aSKa and preventing successful thrombolysis.

IgG aSKa and neutralization titers have been demonstrated in individuals up to 54 months following thrombolytic therapy with APSAC. Anti-SK antibodies and neutralization titers were quantified in individuals within 5 days of therapy or 12 to 54 months following treatment. At 4 days, 19.4% of individuals demonstrated elevated antibody levels and neutralization titers, and by 12 to 54 months, 40% had antibody titers of 1:160 or greater, neutralization titers of more than 1.5 million U, or both, suggesting that readministration of APSAC should be avoided during this interval (121).

## ALLERGIC COMPLICATIONS

Because of its bacterial origin, APSAC is potentially allergenic, although the incidence of allergy related complications is low. The overall rate of allergic reactions in individuals receiving APSAC is 1.9%, which includes rash (0.8%), bronchospasm (0.5%), erythema (0.2%), and various other manifestations (0.2%) (122).

In summary, APSAC is a synthetic, noncovalent complex comprised of SK and plasminogen with a *p*-anisoyl group covalently bound to $Ser_{740}$ in its catalytic center. Anisoylation of the SK-plasminogen complex confers a prolonged serum half-life and, therefore, greater thrombolytic potency than the parent compound. APSAC demonstrated fibrin-binding properties similar to those of SK-plasminogen complex, with less tendency to produce fibrinogen depletion. Thus, chemical modification of the SK-plasminogen complex with a *p*-anisoyl group yields a specific and effective thrombolytic agent that is amenable to rapid administration as a single intravenous dose.

# UROKINASE

In mammalian systems, two main classes of plasminogen activators have been identified on the basis of their source (123). These activators have been derived mainly from tissue and vascular sources or from urine and kidney cells. By convention, plasminogen activators derived from tissues are denoted as tissue-type plasminogen activators (t-PA) and those derived from urine and kidney cells as urokinase-type plasminogen activators (u-PA).

## STRUCTURE

A serine protease similar to trypsin, urokinase is composed of two polypeptide chains, with molecular masses of 20 and 34 Kda, joined by a single disulfide bridge (124). Urokinase is synthesized in precursor form as a single-chain molecule, which is modified further to achieve enzymatic potency. The single-chain urokinase has been isolated from urine (125), plasma (126), and conditioned cell culture media (127).

Single-chain urokinase-type plasminogen activator (scu-PA) is a 411 amino acid GP with a molecular weight of 54 Kda (128) (Fig. 56.4). scu-PA is converted to the high-molecular-weight (HMW), two-chain u-PA derivative (tcu-PA) via limited hydrolysis of the $Lys_{158}$-$Ile_{159}$ peptide bond by plasmin and kallikrein (127). The aminoterminal (i.e., light) chain contains 158 amino acid residues, whereas the carboxyterminal (i.e., heavy)

chain contains 253 amino acids (129, 130) and includes the catalytic center, which is composed of $Asp_{255}$, $His_{204}$, and $Ser_{356}$ (131). Both chains are linked via the $Cys_{148}$-$Cys_{279}$ disulfide bond. scu-PA contains 12 additional disulfide bonds dispersed throughout the protein; disruption of these bonds in the catalytic region markedly perturbs fibrinolytic function only (132). A low-molecular-weight (LMW) scu-PA may be generated by hydrolysis of the $Glu_{143}$-$Leu_{144}$ peptide bond, thereby removing the aminoterminal 143 amino acids of scu-PA; however, LMW scu-PA is one to five times less active than scu-PA in a fibrin clot lysis assay and less sensitive to activation by plasmin (133). HMW tcu-PA also may be transformed to a LMW tcu-PA by an additional cleavage at $Lys_{135}$-$Lys_{136}$. This 33-kDa product manifests no enhancement in enzymatic activity with fibrin, and it is the urokinase commercially available in the United States.

Urokinase contains three distinct structural regions (134): an aminoterminal, receptor binding, epidermal growth factor–like domain; a central, kringle region; and a carboxyterminal, catalytic, serine protease domain (128, 131). Evaluating the secondary structure of these domains reveals that urokinase is arranged similarly to other plasminogen activators. The epidermal growth factor region resembles homologous peptides, and it is believed to contain particular structural differences that confer receptor binding properties on the molecule. This may explain, in part, why other growth factors show no appreciable affinity for the urokinase receptor (134). The kringle domain is similar to t-PA kringle 2, and structural analysis reveals two helices. The first, in the region $Ser_{40}$-$Gly_{46}$, is analogous to that described for t-PA kringle 2; the second, involving $Asn_{26}$-$Gln_{33}$, is unique to the urokinase kringle. In addition, three antiparallel β-sheets and three tight turns identical to that described for t-PA kringle 2 have been identified (135, 136). An extended binding site for anionic polysaccharides such as heparin has been localized to a flat facet of the molecule in this region (137), and resolution of the crystal structure of the serine protease domain has revealed the expected topology of a trypsinlike serine protease. The enzyme contains an S1 specificity pocket similar to trypsin; a restricted, less accessible, hydrophobic S2 pocket; and a solvent-accessible S3 pocket capable of accommodating a variety of residues. Notably, extra residues are inserted at six positions, one of which remains mobile despite being anchored by a disulfide bridge. This characteristic is shared by other serine proteases, namely t-PA, factor XII, and complement factor I (138).

## ENZYMATIC PROPERTIES

### HMW tcu-PA

Michaelis-Menten kinetics and the kinetic parameters listed in Table 56.2 describe the activation of plasmino-

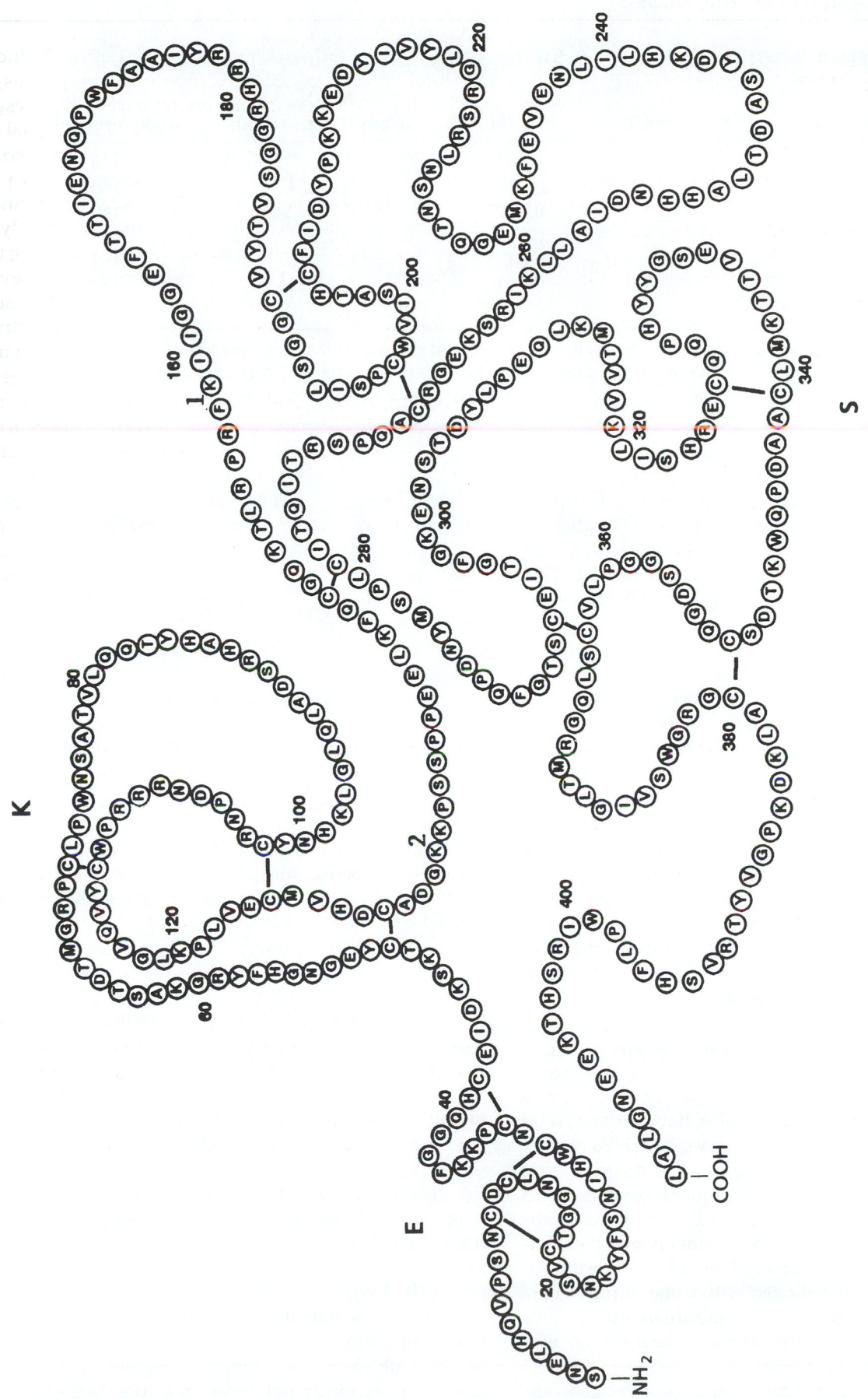

**FIGURE 56.4.** Structure of single-chain urokinase-type plasminogen activator (scu-PA). *E*, epidermal growth factor domain; *K*, kringle domain; *S*, serine protease domain; *1*, cleavage site for conversion of scu-PA to high-molecular-weight two-chain u-PA (HMW tcu-PA); *2*, cleavage site for conversion of HMW tcu-PA to LMW tcu-PA.

**TABLE 56.2.** Kinetic Constants for the Activation of Glu-plasminogen by u-PA

| Species | $K_m$ (μmol/l) | $k_{cat}$(S) | $k_{cat}/K_m$ (μmol/l per second) | Reference |
|---|---|---|---|---|
| HMW tcu-PA | 50 | 1.0 | 0.02 | 139 |
| nscu-PA | 70 | 0.0375 | 0.00054 | 150 |
| | 0.83 | 0.0009 | 0.00112 | 149 |
| rscu-PA-EC | 0.23 | 0.0170 | 0.07391 | 139 |
| rscu-PA-CHO | 1.0 | 0.0020 | 0.0020 | 152 |
| rscu-PA-$Glu_{158}$ | 87 | 0.010 | 0.00011 | 152 |
| rscu-PA-$Gly_{158}$ | 62 | 0.011 | 0.00018 | 152 |

nscu-PA, *native single-chain urokinase-type plasminogen activator;* rscu-PA-EC, *recombinant scu-PA derived from* Escherichia coli; rscu-PA-CHO, *recombinant scu-PA derived from Chinese hamster ovary cells;* rscu-PA-$Glu_{158}$, *and* rscu-PA-$Gly_{158}$, *recombinant scu-PA with glutamic acid and glycine substitutions at position 158, respectively, and* S = *seconds.*

gen by HMW tcu-PA. Regarding activation of Glu-plasminogen, recent studies have demonstrated the Michaelis constant ($K_m$) for HMW tcu-PA to be 50 μmol/l, with a catalytic rate constant ($k_{cat}$) of 1.0 per second. This provides a catalytic efficiency ($k_{cat}/K_m$) of 0.02 μmol/1 per second (139).

On a molar basis, HMW tcu-PA is threefold to 10-fold more effective than Gly-plasminogen in activating Lys-plasminogen (140). A similar increase in the rate of Glu-plasminogen activation by HMW tcu-PA occurs with fibrin (141, 142), fibrinogen (142), fibrinogen fragments D and E (143), and ω-aminocarboxylic acids (144) such as ϵ-aminocaproic acid and tranexamic acid (Table 56.2). This results from a conformational change in Glu-plasminogen induced through binding of these agents to lysine binding sites (145), which results in a modified Glu-plasminogen approximating the structure of Lys-plasminogen (144–146). Therefore, it is not unexpected that the activation rate of Lys-plasminogen by HMW tcu-PA is not significantly affected by fibrin, fibrinogen, FDPs, or ω-aminocarboxylic acids.

$$\text{I} \quad \text{scu-PA} + \text{PGN} \underset{}{\overset{K_m}{\rightleftharpoons}} \text{scu-PA} \cdot \text{PGN} \xrightarrow{k_2} \text{scu-PA} + \text{Pl}$$

$$\text{II} \quad \text{PGN} + \text{scu-PA} \overset{K'_m}{\rightleftharpoons} \text{Pl} \cdot \text{scu-PA} \xrightarrow{k'_2} \text{Pl} + \text{tcu-PA}$$

$$\text{III} \quad \text{tcu-PA} + \text{PGN} \overset{K''_m}{\rightleftharpoons} \text{tcu-PA} \cdot \text{PGN} \xrightarrow{k''_2} \text{tcu-PA} + \text{Pl}$$

**FIGURE 56.5.** Michaelis-Menten model depicting single-chain urokinase-type plasminogen activator (scu-PA)–mediated conversion of plasminogen (PGN) to plasmin (P1), with concomitant production of two-chain u-PA (tcu-PA). (Adapted with permission from Collen D, Zamarron C, Lijnen HR, et al. Activation of plasminogen by pro-urokinase II. Kinetics. J Biol Chem 1986;261:1259–1266.)

## Single-chain Urokinase-type Plasminogen Activator

The enzymatic properties of scu-PA have proved to be more difficult to elucidate than those of HMW tcu-PA because of extreme sensitivity of scu-PA to proteolytic activation by plasmin and subsequent conversion to HMW tcu-PA. In turn, HMW tcu-PA promotes additional plasmin generation, which enhances further scu-PA conversion to HMW tcu-PA. Under basal conditions, scu-PA is an inactive zymogen with some intrinsic amidolytic activity, estimated to be approximately 0.2 to 0.6% that of HMW tcu-PA, against plasminogen and LMW peptides (147).

The combination of scu-PA and plasminogen rapidly produces both plasmin and HMW tcu-PA. Plasmin inhibitors such as aprotinin block production of HMW tcu-PA but allow plasmin generation from plasminogen, thus suggesting that scu-PA may activate plasminogen directly (148). To describe better the conversion of plasminogen to plasmin by scu-PA, a three reaction model has been postulated (Fig. 56.5). Each reaction is described by Michaelis-Menten kinetics. In reaction I, scu-PA directly activates plasminogen, thereby producing plasmin that catalyzes the production of HMW tcu-PA from scu-PA in reaction II. The HMW tcu-PA thus formed initiates plasminogen activation directly via reaction III (139).

To examine the kinetic parameters of scu-PA formation of plasmin in isolation (139), the reaction was observed with excess plasmin chromogenic substrate (S-2251), which binds generated plasmin and competitively inhibits plasmin-mediated generation of HMW tcu-PA and Lys-plasminogen. Under these conditions scu-PA activated Glu-plasminogen with a $K_m$ of 0.83 $\mu$mol/l and a $k_{cat}$ of 0.0009 per second, thus yielding a catalytic efficiency ($k_{cat}/K_m$) of 0.0011 $\mu$mol/l per second (Table 56.2) (149). This catalytic efficiency is approximately 100-fold lower than that of HMW tcu-PA, thereby suggesting that low $K_m$ ($<1$ $\mu$mol/l) plays a role in determining the extent of direct activation of Glu-plasminogen by scu-PA. To evaluate further the activation of Glu-plasminogen by scu-PA, fluorescein-labeled aprotinin was used to block plasmin action (150), and under these conditions, the investigators demonstrated a $K_m$ of 70 $\mu$mol/l, a $k_{cat}$ of 0.0375 per second, and a catalytic efficiency ($k_{cat}/K_m$) of 0.00054 $\mu$mol/l per second. Activation of Lys-plasminogen by scu-PA is approximately 10-fold more efficient than that of Glu-plasminogen because of an increase in the catalytic rate constant ($k_{cat}$) (146, 151).

The catalytic efficiency of the 32-kDa form of scu-PA is similar to that of wild-type scu-PA (Table 56.2), thereby indicating that the aminoterminal 143 amino acid residues of scu-PA are not enzymatically important. Furthermore, the catalytic efficiency of scu-PA depends on the glycosylation state of the molecule. On a molar basis, recombinant nonglycosylated scu-PA derived from *Escherichia coli* is 15-fold to 20-fold more efficient than the glycosylated form derived from Chinese hamster ovary cells in activating plasminogen (152).

Plasmin-resistant mutants of scu-PA have been used to define the intrinsic plasminogen activator activity of scu-PA (152). Site-specific mutagenesis of $Lys_{158}$ to either $Gly_{158}$ or $Glu_{158}$ prevents the plasmin-mediated cleavage of scu-PA to HMW tcu-PA. The kinetic parameters for these recombinant proteins are listed in Table 56.2. Both mutant proteins have a catalytic efficiency ($k_{cat}/K_m$) of 0.00015 $\mu$mol/l per second, which corresponds to an intrinsic activity of 0.1 to 0.5% that of HMW tcu-PA. These values are consistent with the kinetic parameters of wild-type scu-PA obtained through inhibitors of secondary reactions (146). Thus, scu-PA, with its low intrinsic activity and resistance to HMW tcu-PA active site inhibitors, has properties consistent with those of a proenzyme.

## FIBRIN-SPECIFIC PLASMINOGEN ACTIVATION

In plasma, scu-PA is mostly inactive; however, with thrombus, scu-PA enriched human plasma is accompanied by plasminogen activation and clot lysis with production of HMW tcu-PA (153). Plasminogen activation in plasma by scu-PA requires fibrin (154, 155), despite the lack of direct fibrin binding to scu-PA (154).

The substitution of Lys-plasminogen for Glu-plasminogen in plasma leads to plasminogen activation without fibrin. Furthermore, exposure of Glu-plasminogen to $\omega$-aminocarboxylic acids or soluble fibrin results

in a conformational change approximating the structure of Lys-plasminogen, which is a phenomenon mediated by the lysine-binding sites of Glu-plasminogen (144–146, 156). Therefore, fibrin selectivity of scu-PA may, in part, result from a fibrin-induced conformational change in Glu-plasminogen.

On the basis of these observations, the mechanism by which fibrin mediates plasminogen activation by scu-PA probably involves limited plasmin digestion of fibrin, thus exposing "internal" carboxyterminal lysine binding sites of fibrin. Glu-plasminogen then binds to these carboxyterminal sites, which induces a conformational change that provides a favorable substrate for scu-PA. At this point, plasminogen activation by scu-PA proceeds, thereby leading to generation of HMW tcu-PA and additional carboxyterminal lysine residues and amplifying further the generation of plasmin and the activity of scu-PA (157, 158).

## RECEPTOR-MEDIATED PLASMIN FORMATION (SEE CHAPTERS 7 AND 18)

A urokinase-type plasminogen activator receptor (u-PAR) has been identified in several cell types, including endothelial cells (159, 160) and neutrophils (161). u-PAR is a single-chain, 55- to 60-kDa glycoprotein (162) anchored to the cell membrane by a glycophosphatidylinositol (GP I) moiety (163). The polypeptide contains 313 amino acids and 28 cysteine residues, the pattern of which defines three homologous repeats. The aminoterminal domain of u-PAR can be crosslinked covalently to the epidermal growth factor-like domain of urokinase after receptor-ligand interaction (164). Evidence suggests the receptor is localized to caveolae. Indirect immunofluorescence studies have demonstrated that u-PAR colocalizes with caveolin and that u-PAR, u-PA, and caveolin are found exclusively in the low-density detergent, insoluble fraction of cell lysates. The ultrastructural localization of u-PAR largely is restricted to small, non-clathrin-coated invaginations of the plasma membrane (165). u-PAR may modulate both u-PA proteolytic activity and internalization of u-PA-plasminogen activator-inhibitor complexes.

Once scu-PA is bound to its receptor, plasmin generation is enhanced by increasing the efficiency of plasminogen activation. Using the monocyte-like cell line U937 (166), investigators have demonstrated that nonsaturating concentrations of scu-PA accelerate Glu-plasminogen activation up to 16-fold. This can be abolished by addition of the lysine analog 6-aminohexanoic acid, which prevents plasminogen binding to U937 cells, thus indicating the observed increase in plasmin generation results from activation of cell bound plasminogen. Lys-plasminogen does not amplify plasmin production, which indicates the aminoterminal fragment of plasminogen plays a role in the interaction of this molecule with its cellular binding site. When the aminoterminal of tcu-PA was used as an antagonist of scu-PA binding, the increase in plasmin generation abated. These observations suggest both plasminogen and scu-PA binding to cells are required for the enhanced formation of plasmin (167).

Plasmin generation is additionally increased by improving the efficiency of reciprocal activation of scu-PA by cell localized plasmin. This was confirmed using U937 cells incubated with scu-PA, without aprotinin, to demonstrate a concentration dependent increase in the conversion of scu-PA to tcu-PA as measured using the chromogenic substrate pyro-Glu-Gly-Arg-$p$-nitroanilide for activation of cell bound plasmin (167). The catalytic efficiency of this reaction ($k_{cat}/K_m$) was 1700 $\mu$mol/l per minute with cells, compared to 35 $\mu$mol/l per minute without cells, thereby demonstrating a 50-fold cell-mediated enhancement in the conversion of scu-PA to tcu-PA.

scu-PA may undergo a reversible transformation between a latent and an active state. Binding of scu-PA to cellular and recombinant soluble u-PAR increases the $V_{max}$ of scu-PA fivefold, with little change in its $K_m$, and binding of scu-PA to soluble u-PAR stimulates its plasminogen activator activity approximately 50-fold by decreasing the $K_m$ for Glu-plasminogen from 1.15 $\mu$mol/l to 0.022 $\mu$mol/l and by increasing the $k_{cat}$ from 0.0015 to 0.022 to second (168). In contrast, an increase in the intrinsic activity of scu-PA after binding to soluble u-PAR has not been confirmed, and nonspecific proteolytic activation of scu-PA may be responsible for the soluble u-PAR–mediated induction of the activity observed (169).

tcu-PA generated from the conversion of scu-PA similarly binds to u-PAR, and it activates plasminogen with kinetic characteristics that differ from those of tcu-PA in the solution phase. Ellis et al (170) compared Glu-plasminogen activation by tcu-PA bound to U937 cells with activation by tcu-PA in solution. The catalytic efficiency of the reaction was sixfold higher with receptor-bound tcu-PA, mostly resulting from a 40-fold decrease in $K_m$ on receptor binding of tcu-PA. In addition, high-affinity Glu-plasminogen activation by receptor-bound tcu-PA was influenced strongly by plasminogen binding to the cell surface, as demonstrated by the diminished plasminogen activation with a plasminogen binding antagonist.

Ellis and Dano (171) used a murine IgG monoclonal antibody directed against urokinase to illustrate the role of surface localization of scu-PA and plasminogen in plasminogen activation. This antibody possesses a carboxyterminal lysine residue on the Ig $\gamma$ chain that represents a potential binding site for plasminogen. Plasminogen activation is enhanced by a novel mechanism in which the antibody serves as a specific template for the assembly of a ternary complex involving scu-PA/tcu-

PA and plasminogen, thus allowing them to act in a catalytically favorable manner. Addition of tcu-PA to the antibody produced a 50-fold increase in the overall reaction efficiency, primarily resulting from reduction in the $K_m$ from 20 to 0.1 $\mu$mol/l.

To demonstrate further the importance of cell surface localization, a modified urokinase molecule containing a sequence directing surface attachment via a GP I anchor was expressed in endothelial cells (172). This modified urokinase maintains both amidolytic and plasminogen activator activity, without receptor binding. The GP I-anchored scu-PA activated Glu-plasminogen threefold more efficiently than scu-PA released from the cell surface. When plasminogen was prevented from binding to the cell by 6-aminohexanoic acid, the rate of plasminogen activation diminished, thereby suggesting that augmented plasmin generation by GP I-anchored scu-PA depends on the simultaneous binding of plasminogen. GP I-anchored tcu-PA cleaved a peptide substrate at a rate equivalent to that of released tcu-PA. Using a kinetic model, the estimated $K_m$ for cell associated plasminogen activation by GP I-anchored tcu-PA was reduced to 0.15 $\mu$mol/l or less, compared with more than 10 $\mu$mol/l for activation of plasminogen in solution (i.e., an approximately 70-fold decrease) (172).

These observations suggest the cell surface is a template to assemble the components to stimulate urokinase-mediated plasmin generation. Once scu-PA/tcu-PA and plasminogen–plasmin are bound to their respective surface receptors, the reactants are colocalized in a catalytically favorable environment. Therefore, the physical approximation of scu-PA/tcu-PA to plasminogen/plasmin, not binding to the receptor that induces a change in the intrinsic activity of the scu-PA/tcu-PA, further enhances plasmin generation.

## MODULATION OF RECEPTOR MEDIATED PLASMIN FORMATION

Both circulating and receptor bound urokinase are susceptible to inhibition by the serine protease inhibitors, plasminogen activator inhibitor type-1 (PAI-1), plasminogen activator inhibitor type-2 (PAI-2), and protease nexin-1 (PN). Once these inhibitors bind, the complexes are readily internalized and degraded through a mechanism involving the multiligand receptor $\alpha_2$-macroglobulin/low density lipoprotein receptor-associated protein ($\alpha_2$-MR/LRP) (173, 174). This cell surface receptor consists of a 515-kDa heavy chain and an 85-kDa light chain, which derive proteolytically from a 600-kDa precursor. scu-PA and tcu-PA bind directly to LRP, which in turn mediates their internalization and degradation. This system is regulated by the action of the 39-kDa receptor-associated protein, which antagonizes ligand binding (175). Results of *in vitro* binding assays demonstrate that scu-PA and tcu-PA bind to LRP with a $K_d$ of 45 and 60 nmol/l, respectively, which is approximately 15-fold to 20-fold weaker than the affinity of the u-PA-PAI-1 complex for LRP ($K_d$, 3 nmol/l). Studies using $F_{ab}$ fragments with high relative affinity for the LRP receptor demonstrate the presence of an interaction site for scu-PA localized in the second cluster of cysteine-rich repeats (176). On u-PA-inhibitor internalization, u-PAR itself is endocytosed and recycled back to the cell surface.

scu-PA alone binds to $\alpha_2$-MR/LRP with low affinity ($EC_{50}$, 10 nmol/l). Efficient binding depends on contact with the A chain and the serine protease region. In contrast, when scu-PA is attached to u-PAR, it does not bind to $\alpha_2$-MR/LRP, and it is not internalized and degraded unless complexed to PAI-1 (177). Binding of PAI-1 to scu-PA/u-PAR complexes is reversible and can be overcome by increasing the concentration of plasminogen (178). Conversely, PAI-1 inhibits scu-PA enzymatic activity in a concentration-dependent manner with all detectable enzymatic activity being abolished by a 10-fold molar excess of PAI-1 (179).

Once the tcu-PA-PAI-1 complex is formed, it binds the $\alpha_2$-MR/LRP receptor with high affinity ($EC_{50}$ = 0.4 nmol/l) via contacts in both the PAI-1 moiety and the urokinase serine protease domain and A chain. The affinity of u-PAR-bound tcu-PA-PAI-1 complex for binding to $\alpha_2$-MR/LRP remains sufficient to allow rapid internalization and degradation (177).

Protease nexin I complexed to tcu-PA binds specifically to u-PAR, with a time course similar to that for u-PA-PAI-1. Using an anti-u-PAR monoclonal antibody and u-PAR antagonists, Conese et al (180) showed that internalization and degradation of tcu-PA requires initial binding to u-PAR to enhance subsequent binding to $\alpha_2$-MR/LRP.

## MODULATION OF ENZYMATIC ACTIVITY

Plasminogen activation by HMW tcu-PA is influenced by several endogenous compounds, including fibrin (141, 142), fibrinogen (142), FDPs (143, 147), long chain fatty acids such as oleic acid (178), and lysine analogues such as ω-aminocarboxylic acids (144). In each case, the catalytic efficiency of HMW tcu-PA is increased between twofold and 10-fold by a common mechanism involving a conformational change in Glu-plasminogen (144–146). scu-PA also is stimulated by fibrin as the exposure of carboxyterminal lysine residues allows more efficient plasminogen activation by scu-PA (153, 157).

Heparin influences the enzymatic activity of both forms of u-PA. Heparin stimulates a twofold increase in plasminogen activator activity, primarily by reducing the $K_m$ with no effect on the $k_{cat}$ (181). When chondroitin sulfate or hyaluronic acid is substituted for heparin, no effect is observed. Heparin also stimulates plasminogen activation by scu-PA to a much greater extent than that observed for tcu-PA (182). With heparin (1 U/ml), tcu-

PA leads to a fourfold increase in plasminogen activation, whereas scu-PA enhances activation by 100-fold. This may result from decreased inactivation by thrombin with heparin (183). Heparin and heparan sulfate also enhance the inhibitory activity of PAI-1 toward tcu-PA (184).

## PHARMACOKINETIC PROPERTIES

The pharmacokinetics of u-PA have been examined in several species, and the clearance characteristics are approximated by a two-compartment model consisting of intravascular and interstitial compartments (185, 186). In humans (187), scu-PA and HMW tcu-PA are cleared differently, with initial and terminal half-lives, respectively, of 12 and 60.8 minutes for HMW tcu-PA and of 69 and 26.5 minutes for scu-PA. The primary clearance site is the liver (188). The plasma half-life of u-PA is a property of the protein itself, not a consequence of inactivation by plasma inhibitors, as enzymatic activity, antigen, and [$^{125}$I]-labeled HMW tcu-PA are cleared in a similar manner (186). Both active site-blocked tcu-PA and scu-PA, which is unreactive toward inhibitors, demonstrate the same half-life as wild type HMW tcu-PA (188). Furthermore, the similar pharmacokinetics of scu-PA and its 32-kDa derivative indicate plasma clearance does not depend on the aminoterminal portion of the protein (186).

## THROMBOLYTIC THERAPY

Clinical application of u-PA in treating thrombotic vascular disease has been universal. This agent has successfully treated venous thrombosis (189, 190), pulmonary embolism (71, 72), peripheral arterial thrombosis (191–193), aortocoronary saphenous vein bypass graft occlusion (194), cerebrovascular thrombosis (195), unstable angina (196, 197), and acute myocardial infarction (198, 199). It also has been used to facilitate percutaneous transluminal coronary angioplasty (200–203).

### Venous Thrombosis

Early experience with tcu-PA in the treatment of venous thrombosis (1100–4400 IU/kg of body weight loading dose and 1100–50, 000 IU/kg/hour maintenance dose) produced partial to complete clot lysis in 26 to 92% of individuals (189). In one direct comparison with SK (192), LMW tcu-PA proved to be equally effective in resolving phlebographically documented venous thrombosis. Goldhaber et al (204) examined a novel bolus dosing regimen of urokinase (1 million IU over 10 minutes) administered three times during a 24-hour period with continuous infusion of heparin between bolus doses in individuals with deep venous thrombosis. This regimen produced clot lysis in 52% of individuals, without evidence of hemorrhagic complications. Bolus infusion, however, was associated with a high rate of rigors. To overcome this adverse reaction, Goldhaber et al. (205) evaluated recombinant u-Pa (ru-PA) with the same dosing schedule, but they failed to demonstrate any significant benefit compared with heparin therapy alone. Similarly, scu-PA has been investigated in the management of lower extremity deep venous thrombosis and found to be an effective thrombolytic agent in this setting (206).

Clinical use of u-PA in the treatment of pulmonary embolism has been evaluated in several trials. Therapy with LMW tcu-PA (4400 IU/kg loading dose followed by 10,000 IU/kg/hour maintenance dose) was associated with more rapid resolution of pulmonary emboli, improved hemodynamics, and restored pulmonary perfusion than therapy with heparin or warfarin alone (71, 72). One year after treatment, individuals treated with LMW tcu-PA demonstrated improved pulmonary gas exchange and capillary blood volume, but they showed no improvement in survival compared with individuals who received conventional therapy (207). Intrapulmonary infusion of a 500,000 IU bolus of u-PA followed by central administration of 1 million IU of u-PA resulted in significantly improved cardiac output, total pulmonary vascular resistance, and systolic, diastolic, and mean pulmonary vascular pressure (208).

## Peripheral Arterial Occlusive Disease

u-PA has been used extensively in the treatment of peripheral arterial thrombosis. In thrombosed native arteries, therapy with intra-arterial LMW tcu-PA (10,000–100,000 IU/hour) results in recanalization in 73 to 100% of individuals (191–193, 209) and reduces the incidence of both amputation and surgery (210). Urokinase is similarly effective in the treatment of acute (<14 days) peripheral graft occlusions, with successful thrombolysis leading to improved limb salvage and reduced magnitude of the planned surgery (211, 212). To evaluate further the role of (ru-PA) in treatment of peripheral arterial occlusion, the TOPAS (Thrombolysis or Peripheral Arterial Surgery) trial was conducted (213). This phase I trial assigned 213 individuals with acute lower extremity ischemia to treatment with catheter directed ru-PA at 2000, 4000, or 6000 IU/min for 4 hours and then 2000 IU/min up to 48 hours or to surgical intervention. Analysis revealed that 4000 IU/min delivered maximal thrombolytic efficacy (71% of individuals achieved complete lysis of thrombus) with fewer bleeding complications. At one-year follow-up, individuals treated with ru-PA fared no worse than surgical individuals regarding mortality and amputation-free survival rates.

u-PA also has been a successful adjunct to peripheral angioplasty in the treatment of thrombosed hemodialysis access grafts. u-PA infusion before mechanical intervention restored functional patency in 100 of 135 expanded polytetrafluoroethylene prosthetic grafts with few hemorrhagic complications (214). In individuals who failed previous surgical thrombectomy, pulse-spray pharmacomechanical thrombolysis with u-PA (250,000–1,000,000 IU) and heparin (2500 IU) for 17 to 33 minutes achieved graft recanalization without significant complications in approximately 75% of individuals (215). In addition, patency rates at 3 months compared favorably with those attained by surgical revascularization.

Saphenous vein aortocoronary bypass graft obstruction by thrombus has been relieved by local administration of u-PA. In one study (216), symptomatic individuals received low-dose u-PA (100,000 U/hour) infusion directly into the occluded graft. Once there was angiographic evidence of thrombus dissolution, balloon angioplasty was performed. Initial graft patency was achieved in 69% of individuals after a mean infusion duration of 25.4 hours; however, by 6 months, only 40% of grafts remained patent despite aggressive interim oral anticoagulant therapy. In another study (217), TIMI grade 2 or 3 flow after urokinase administration influenced successfully acute recanalization; however, the age of the graft, duration of occlusion up to 6 months, size of the distal native vessel, and site of stenosis did not predict outcome. Six-month graft patency was predicted by the presence of TIMI grade 3 flow and by the site of the lesion within the graft.

Thrombolytic therapy with u-PA also improves limb salvage and reduces limb ischemia in individuals with occluded lower extremity bypass grafts. Comerota et al (218) randomized individuals with both autogenous and prosthetic lower limb bypass grafts who presented with graft occlusion of up to 34 days of age to treatment with intra-arterial catheter directed thrombolysis or with surgical intervention. u-PA was administered as a 250,000 U bolus followed by an infusion of 4000 U/min for 4 hours and then 2000 U/min for up to 36 hours. Graft patency was restored by thrombolytic therapy alone in 84% of individuals and led to reduced magnitude of planned surgery in 42%; however, individuals assigned to surgical revascularization demonstrated a better composite clinical outcome at both 1 month and 1 year after treatment. This may result in part from limitations of catheter-based therapy. In the u-PA-treatment group, 39% of individuals failed catheter delivery and underwent subsequent surgical revascularization. Urokinase therapy did prove to be superior to surgical intervention in individuals who presented with an acute ischemic event. Individuals treated with a thrombolytic agent demonstrated a markedly reduced amputation rate compared with surgical individuals at both early and late follow-up.

## Acute Myocardial Infarction

Both tcu-PA and scu-PA have been evaluated for treatment of acute myocardial infarction. Therapy with intravenous LMW tcu-PA (960,000-3 million IU) produced infarct-related arterial patency in 41 to 66% of individuals with acute myocardial infarction (219–221), which is comparable to rates achieved with intracoronary LMW tcu-PA (221, 222). Similarly, intravenous administration of scu-PA (3-9 million IU) successfully restored infarct-related artery patency in 51 to 91% of individuals (223–227). In terms of preserved left ventricular function or mortality, neither scu-PA nor HMW tcu-PA treatment provides any distinct benefits compared with other thrombolytic agents (228). When administered to individuals with acute myocardial infarction, saruplase (Gruenthal Gmblt, Aachen, Germany), which is a recombinant, full-length, unglycosylated scu-PA, delivered higher angiographic patency rates at 60 minutes compared with SK (71.8 versus 48%, respectively) but failed to maintain this benefit at 90 minutes (229) or to improve significantly the left ventricular ejection fraction (230).

In contrast to other thrombolytic agents, therapy with scu-PA is greatly enhanced by pretreatment with small doses of other thrombolytic agents (228, 231–233). This phenomenon is attributable to accelerated plasminogen activation by scu-PA when plasminogen is bound to the carboxyterminal lysine residues of fibrin (158). The limited plasmin digestion of fibrin clots afforded by pretreatment with t-PA or tcu-PA exposes carboxyterminal lysine residues on fibrin (158, 234). The conformational change induced by plasminogen binding to carboxyterminal lysines of fibrin provides a more favorable substrate for scu-PA (156).

Clot lysis increased by 30% when a 41 mg dose of scu-PA was preceded by a 250,000 IU bolus of HMW tcu-PA (234). A similar result was obtained using t-PA as pretreatment (231, 235). Individuals who received a combination of low-dose tcu-PA (200,000 IU) and scu-PA (4.5 million IU) demonstrated fibrinolytic activity, as determined by fibrin plate assay at 24 hours, similar to individuals who received standard dose tcu-PA (2.5 million IU) (236). However, these individuals also had higher plasma fibrinogen and plasminogen levels, thus suggesting that combination therapy results in minor systemic fibrinolytic effects and, therefore, is clot specific.

Clinical trials to evaluate the efficacy of u-PA in individuals with acute myocardial infarction have yielded mixed results. Angiographic evaluation of early (90 min) coronary artery patency in 128 individuals who received either scu-PA (60 or 80 mg) or pretreatment with tcu-PA (250,000 IU) followed by infusion of scu-PA (60 mg) revealed no difference between regimens, with an average infarct-related artery patency rate of 73% (237). Similarly, early assessment of low dose recombinant t-PA (rt-PA) bolus (5–10 mg) followed by a 90-minute infusion of scu-PA (40 mg/hour) in 101 individuals demonstrated a 77% infarct-related artery patency at 90 minutes (238).

Follow-up angiography at 24 hours confirmed patency with TIMI grade 3 flow in 82% of individuals. Pilot studies using recombinant scu-PA (rscu-PA) in individuals primed with tcu-PA and those who were not revealed that this agent successfully achieved and maintained infarct-related artery patency (239). The SESAM (Study in Europe with Saruplase and Alteplase in Myocardial Infarction) study randomized 473 individuals with acute myocardial infarction to either saruplase (80 mg/hour) or rt-PA (100 mg every 3 hours) in addition to heparin and aspirin. Angiographic evaluation revealed similar infarct-related artery patency rates at 45, 60, and 90 minutes after therapy was initiated, with no significant difference between groups regarding reocclusion or complication rates (240).

In summary, u-PA is effective therapy for several thrombotic disorders; however, there is no evidence for any significant advantage compared with other available thrombolytic agents. The synergistic effect between scu-PA and other plasminogen activators is promising and may afford more efficient and rapid clot lysis at lower doses of thrombolytic agents.

# TISSUE-TYPE PLASMINOGEN ACTIVATOR

In 1979, plasminogen activator was purified from uterine tissue (234). Subsequently, an immunologic relationship was demonstrated among uterine, vascular, and blood plasminogen activators, with no discernible relationship to plasminogen activator from urine (235). Being derived from tissues, the plasminogen activator common to blood, uterine, and endothelial cells was designated tissue-type plasminogen activator (241). t-PA, which is now available commercially as a recombinant protein (242), is widely employed in the treatment of thrombotic disorders.

## PROTEIN STRUCTURE (SEE CHAPTER 7)

The amino acid sequence and proposed structure of t-PA is depicted in Fig. 52.6. t-PA is a single-chain serine protease composed of 527 amino acids with a molecular mass of 68 Kda (243). The molecule contains a free cysteine residue at position 83; the remaining cysteine residues comprise 17 disulfide bonds (244). The two-chain t-PA is generated by hydrolysis of the $Arg_{275}$-$Ile_{276}$ peptide bond, which is catalyzed by several endogenous proteases, including plasmin, kallikrein, and activated factor X (245, 246). The two chains of t-PA are denoted the *heavy* (A chain; residues 1–275) and *light* (B chain; residues 275–527) chain. The heavy chain includes the kringle regions, whereas the light chain contains the serine protease portion of the molecule.

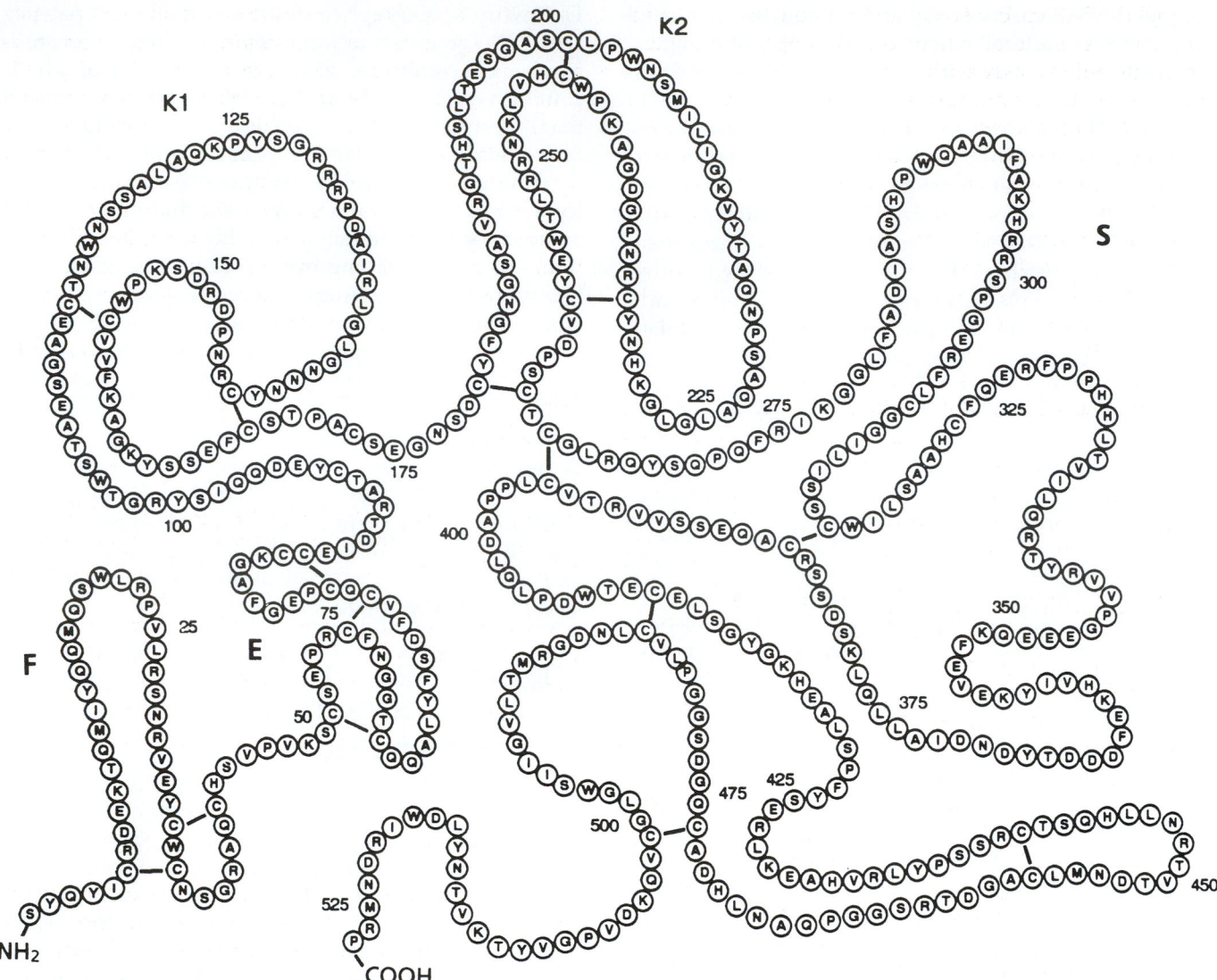

**FIGURE 56.6.** Structure of tissue-type plasminogen activator. *E*, epidermal growth factor-like region; *F*, finger domain; *K1* and *K2*, kringle regions 1 and 2; *S*, serine protease domain. (Adapted with permission from Pennica D, Holmes WE, Kohr WJ, et al. Cloning and expression of human tissue-type plasminogen activator cDNA in *E. coli*. Nature 1983;301:214–221.)

The structure of t-PA is divided into five domains on the basis of function and homology to other proteins. Residues 4-50 at the aminoterminal region are homologous to the (F) finger domain of fibronectin. Residues 50–87 are highly homologous to human epidermal growth factor (E). The K1 and K2 kringle domains, which consist of residues 87–176 and 176–262, respectively, share homology with and derive their name from the plasminogen kringle regions (246, 247). The serine protease domain includes residues 276–527 and is similar to other serine proteases. The catalytic center, which is located in the serine protease domain, is composed of His$_{322}$, Asp$_{371}$, and Ser$_{478}$ (243).

The solution structure of the F domain reveals that the amino acid sequence contains eight residues that are highly conserved in the type 1 finger domains of human fibronectin. The domain is folded similarly to the seventh type 1 repeat of human fibronectin, with side chains of conserved residues lying in similar conformations. The distinguishing characteristic of the t-PA F domain is that hydrophobic residues cover the exposed surface of the principal β-sheet (248). The F and E regions are linked by residues that form an extended β-strand, the carboxyterminal end of which contributes to the third strand of the major β-sheet of the E domain. These two regions maintain their orientation with respect to one another, and they combine with a fixed hydrophobic contact dominated by the side chain of Leu$_{22}$ (249). In this manner, they interact to bury the hydrophobic core (250).

($^1$H)-NMR spectroscopy and thermal stability studies demonstrate that when folded properly, kringle 1 interacts only weakly with $\omega$–amino acid effector molecules such as $\epsilon$-aminocaproic acid (251). In contrast, spectral comparisons reveal that kringle 2 binds both $\omega$–omega-amino acid molecules, peptides containing sequences found in the plasminogen aminoterminal, and the fibrinogen B$\beta$-chain. Furthermore, these ligands may share a common binding site within kringle 2. Two-dimensional spectra reveal that ligand binding is accomplished by the $Tyr_{36}$, $Trp_{62}$, $His_{64}$, $Trp_{72}$, and $Tyr_{74}$ aromatic rings and the aliphatic side chains of $Val_{35}$ and $Asp_{55}$ (252).

The structural arrangement of the kringle domain is functionally important. Mutant t-PA genes, in which the K2 region was placed in different positions such that K1 and K2 were reversed, were constructed and expressed in Chinese hamster ovary cells. The single-chain form of this protein demonstrated a 23 to 47% weaker interaction to lysyl-sepharose compared with rt-PA; however, deleting the F domain enhanced the interaction of K2 with lysyl-sepharose by 20 to 70% (253).

Recently, trigonal crystals of the catalytic domain of rt-PA have been analyzed, with the finding that the chain fold, active-site geometry, and $Ile_{276}$-$Asp_{477}$ bridge are similar to those observed for trypsin. The notable difference resulted from several surface-located insertion loops. Specifically, the disulfide bridge $Cys_{315}$-$Cys_{384}$, is incorporated without significant conformational changes, but the insertion loop preceding $Cys_{384}$ bulges on the molecular surface. The unique basic insertion loop $Lys_{296}$-$Arg_{304}$, which is important for PAI-1 binding and fibrin specificity, is partially disordered. Therefore, it can freely adapt to proteins docking at the active site. The S1 pocket of t-PA is almost identical to that of trypsin, whereas the S2 site is considerably reduced in size by the $Tyr_{368}$ side chain. The S3-S4 groove is hydrophobic. The structure of the proteinase domain of two-chain t-PA suggests that formation of a bridge between $Lys_{429}$ and $Asp_{477}$ may contribute to the unusually high catalytic activity of single-chain t-PA, thus stabilizing the catalytically active conformation without unmasking the $Ile_{276}$ aminoterminus. Modeling studies show that the covalently bound kringle 2 domain in full-length t-PA could interact with an extended hydrophobic groove in the catalytic domain; such a geometry would place the lysine binding site and the fibrin binding area of the catalytic domain in close proximity (254).

## ENZYMATIC PROPERTIES

Activation of plasminogen by t-PA proceeds directly and follows Michaelis-Menten kinetics. Hoylearts et al (255) have reported a Michaelis constant ($K_m$) of 65 $\mu$mol/l and a catalytic rate constant ($k_{cat}$) of 0.05 per second, thereby yielding a catalytic efficiency ($k_{cat}/K_m$) of 0.00076 $\mu$mol/l per second. Subsequent kinetic studies of t-PA catalyzed plasminogen activation have yielded $K_m$ values ranging from 1 mmol/l to 65 $\mu$mol/l, with $k_{cat}$ values of between 0.0005 and 0.05 per second, thus producing a wide range of values for catalytic efficiency (255–259). The range of Michaelis-Menten kinetic values noted here may reflect the relative content of single-chain t-PA in preparations used for kinetic studies. In the single-chain form, t-PA is less active than the two-chain form toward plasminogen in the absence of fibrin (256); however, with fibrin, the activities of single-chain and two-chain t-PA are comparable (260).

## MODIFICATION OF ENZYMATIC PROPERTIES

Initial reports that the $K_m$ for t-PA was approximately 65 $\mu$mol/l (255) proved to be perplexing, in that the endogenous concentration of plasminogen is 2 $\mu$mol/l. This suggests that, at least theoretically, endogenous plasminogen activation is unable to progress. Under normal conditions, t-PA mediated plasminogen activation does occur, mostly through enhanced catalytic efficiency of the reaction by a number of endogenous factors, thereby allowing for efficient plasminogen activation under both basal and therapeutic circumstances.

## FIBRIN BINDING

t-PA binds fibrin specifically with a stoichiometry of approximately 0.88 mol of t-PA per 1 mol of fibrin (261). Investigators have demonstrated that t-PA binds with high affinity to both the intact ($K_d$, 3.3 nmol/l) and the degraded ($K_d$, 1.2 nmol/l) surface of fibrin during ongoing thrombolysis. Binding of t-PA to the carboxyterminal lysine residues of degraded fibrin is efficiently competed for by physiologic concentrations of plasminogen (2 $\mu$mol/l), thereby indicating the affinity of t-PA for these residues is lower than that of plasminogen ($K_d$, 0.66 $\mu$mol/l) and does not relate to the high affinity of t-PA for specific binding sites on intact fibrin (262).

It is postulated that fibrin accelerates t-PA amidolytic activity through two different mechanisms. The first involves specific binding of fibrin, which results in increased catalytic efficiency for plasminogen activation by t-PA. In the presence of fibrin (257), the $K_m$ for t-PA activation of plasminogen decreases from 65 to 0.16 $\mu$mol/l with little change in $k_{cat}$, corresponding to a 1500-fold increase in catalytic efficiency ($k_{cat}/K_m$). The second mechanism, which is exclusive to single-chain t-PA, depends on formation of a ternary complex of fibrin, t-PA, and plasminogen, thus resulting in reduction of the $K_m$ of t-PA for plasminogen by a factor of 440 (258, 263). Similar results have been reported regarding the response to t-PA incubation with cyanide bromide (CNBr)-digested fibrinogen fragments (264). The resulting fibrin-induced enhancement of t-PA activity depends on the proper three-dimensional folding of fibrin. Additionally, without fibrin, t-PA continues to hydrolyze substrates modeled after the peptide sequence in plasminogen surrounding $Arg_{560}$-$Val_{561}$, with $(k_{cat}/K_m)$ values 28,000-fold to 210,000-fold lower than those obtained using trypsin. This suggests that despite homology to trypsin, the protease domain is inherently specific for recognition of one or more structural features displayed by native plasminogen (263).

Bauer et al (265) evaluated both fibrin structure and the stimulatory effect of fibrin on plasminogen activation during t-PA-mediated fibrinolysis using static and dynamic laser light scattering and cryotransmission electron microscopy. Three phases of fibrin formation and degradation were observed. The first was characterized by formation of protofibrils with an average length approximately 10 times that of fibrinogen. As local t-PA concentrations were increased, the duration of this phase was prolonged. During the second phase, sudden elongation and lateral aggregation of fibrin fibers occurred. This was most pronounced at low concentrations of t-PA and was associated with formation of fragment X. The third phase was dominated by disorganization of fibers and the formation of fibrin Y and D fragments. Plasmin internally degraded the fibers, thereby creating long, loose bundles that subsequently disintegrated into thin filaments. At high t-PA concentrations, plasmin generation occurred before onset of the rapid second phase of elongation and lateral aggregation of fibrin fibers; at low t-PA concentrations, this occurred later. The maximal rate of plasmin formation per mole of t-PA was equivalent at all concentrations of t-PA investigated, and it was achieved near the time of the peak generation of fragment X.

Lipid-induced modification of plasminogen activation by t-PA also has been demonstrated (266). Vesicles rich in negatively charged lipids lower the $K_m$ for plasminogen activation by sixfold to 20-fold, whereas neutral vesicles increase the $K_m$. These observations suggest that under the appropriate conditions, cell associated t-PA may be more effective than free t-PA at facilitating plasminogen activation, which is an observation that has been confirmed for platelets (267, 268), endothelial cells (269), and mononuclear cells (270). In addition, apo(a), which is homologous to plasminogen, may interfere with effective thrombolysis by binding to the lysine sites available for plasminogen on the surface of fibrin (271).

PAI-1 modulates fibrin-mediated acceleration of t-PA amidolytic activity. PAI-1, which accumulates within a forming clot, recognizes two binding sites on fibrin: a small number of high affinity sites ($K_d$, <1 nmol/l), and a large number of low affinity sites ($K_d$, 3.8

µmol/l). Studies using fibrin pretreated with activated PAI-1 demonstrated inhibition of t-PA-mediated plasmin degradation in a dose-responsive manner ($IC_{50}$ = 12.3 nmol/l), which was associated with partial occupancy of the low affinity PAI-1 binding site on fibrin (272). PAI-1 additionally binds to t-PA and inhibits the F and K2 domains from binding fibrin, possibly by creating steric interference (273).

## HEPARIN

Vascular endothelial cells also may participate in plasminogen activation through their synthesis of heparin-like proteoglycans. The heparan sulfate synthesized by endothelial cells is similar in both structure and anticoagulant activity to heparin (274), which binds to Glu-plasminogen ($K_d$, ≈120 µmol/l), Lys-plasminogen ($K_d$, ≈2.1 µmol/l) (275), and t-PA (276, 277). Plasminogen residues 422–790 and the B (light) chain of t-PA contain the binding sites for heparin (276). Heparin and fibrin do not share a common binding site, as revealed through studies using both monoclonal antibodies to t-PA fibrin-binding sites and 6-aminohexanoic (183). Furthermore, heparin enhances t-PA activity by approximately threefold, with attenuation of this effect with fibrin (1.7-fold increase in t-PA activity) (183). Heparin modulates t-PA-mediated plasminogen activation through a reduction in the Michaelis constant ($K_m$) (183, 277, 278). In contrast, other investigators (279) have attributed a 3.5-fold enhancement of t-PA on stimulation with heparin to an increase in the $k_{cat}$.

## PHARMACOKINETICS

The pharmacokinetic parameters of t-PA depend on both the t-PA (single-chain versus double-chain) and the glycosylation state of the molecule (279–281). Glycosylation depends on both protein folding and inhibition of disulfide bond formation (282). In animal models, unglycosylated t-PA demonstrates a longer half-life (5.6 versus 2.1 minutes, respectively) and a lower clearance rate (7.5 versus 22.2 mL/min per kg, respectively) than single-chain rt-PA (283). Once administered intravenously, t-PA circulates with a distribution volume of 3.5 to 5.4 L for the single-chain form and of 3.8 to 6.6 L for the two-chain form (280). Both the single-chain and the two-chain forms of t-PA are cleared from plasma in a manner best approximated by a two-compartment model (281, 283, 284). As a single species, t-PA has an initial half-life of 3.6 to 4.6 minutes and a terminal half-life of 39 to 53 minutes; the corresponding initial and terminal half-life values for the two-chain form are 4.1 to 6.3 and 41 to 50 minutes, respectively (285, 286). Bolus injection of single-chain t-PA achieves a mean steady-state plasma concentration during the initial 30 minutes of 3.2 µg/ml, which is 45% higher than that observed with standard infusion but does not alter the plasma half-life (287).

Mutant forms of t-PA have been engineered to increase the plasma residence time without compromising thrombolytic efficacy. For example, TNK–t-PA has substantially slower *in vivo* clearance (1.9 versus 16.1 mL/min per kg) compared with single-chain t-PA in an animal model, and it is eightfold more potent toward whole blood clots (288, 289). The plasma clearance of both single-chain and two-chain t-PA is mediated by the liver (286, 290, 291) and corresponds to 520-1000 and 450-640 mL/min, respectively (280). Two distinct pathways are involved. Liver endothelial cells and Kupffer cells clear rt-PA via the mannose receptor, and parenchymal cells clear rt-PA via the low-density lipoprotein receptor-related protein/$\alpha_2$-macroglobulin receptor (292, 293). Plasma clearance of t-PA also may depend on levels of PAI-1 as well as the formation of t-PA/PAI-1 complex. In individuals administered a 5 $\mu$g/kg bolus of t-PA, higher baseline levels of PAI-1 resulted in enhanced t-PA/PAI-1 complex formation, which was cleared more slowly than active t-PA (294).

## THROMBOLYTIC THERAPY

Clinical experience with t-PA is abundant and spans the entire spectrum of thrombotic disease, including venous thrombosis (295–297), pulmonary embolism (298–302), unstable angina (303), and acute myocardial infarction (304–309). In general, t-PA is at least equally effective as other thrombolytic agents, and it offers the marginal benefit of more rapid thrombolysis that occurs with other agents.

### Venous Thromboembolism

The role of t-PA in treatment of deep venous thrombosis is limited. Recombinant t-PA (rt-PA) (0.5 mg/kg for 4 hours) produces significant venous clot lysis in 60% of individuals (310). Lower doses (295, 296) are less effective at producing venous clot lysis as determined by both venography and phleborheography. Increasing the duration of the infusion (0.75 - 1.75 mg/kg per 24 hours) for 2 to 4 days is particularly effective in resolving deep venous thrombi. Compared with standard heparin infusion, the combination of rt-PA and heparin is superior in resolving lower extremity thrombosis (311).

In 36 individuals with angiographically documented pulmonary embolism, rt-PA (50 mg over 2 hours followed by 40 mg over 4 hours) resulted in successful thrombolysis in 34 (312). In addition, seven individuals who underwent serial echocardiography demonstrated resolution of pulmonary hypertension, decreased right ventricular diameter, improved left ventricular filling, and improved pulmonary perfusion as measured by radionuclide lung scanning (313).

Bolus administration of rt-PA in individuals with acute pulmonary embolism was evaluated in a prospective, open study in which 54 individuals received 1 mg/kg over 10 minutes (314). Improvements in perfusion defects were noted at both 48 hours and 10 days; however, major episodes of bleeding occurred in 15% of the individuals. To prevent hemorrhagic complications, a reduced bolus dose 0.6 mg/kg over 15 min was compared with standard dose rt-PA (100 mg over 2 hours) in 87 individuals (315). Between groups, there was no difference in mortality rates or episodes of major bleeding, and follow-up lung scans, angiograms, and echocardiograms were equivalent. In another, similar study (316), continuous monitoring of total pulmonary vascular resistance revealed improvement at 2 hours in individuals who received bolus rt-PA only, but by 12 hours, similar decreases were observed in both groups.

Compared with heparin alone, rt-PA restores both arterial oxygen tension and perfusion scans to near-baseline levels (317). In addition, right ventricular function is significantly improved (318). Combination therapy with rt-PA (10 mg bolus followed by 90 mg over 2 hours) followed by heparin also was compared to intravenous heparin at a continuous infusion rate of 1750 IU/hour alone (319). Vascular obstruction on pulmonary angiography and mean pulmonary artery pressures decreased in rt-PA treated individuals, with no significant difference in bleeding complications or mortality rates between groups.

Investigators have directly compared rt-PA (10 mg bolus followed by 90 mg over 2 hours) with urokinase (4400 U/kg bolus followed by 4400 U/kg per hour over 12 hours) (209). At 2 hours, rt-PA produced more complete resolution of pulmonary hypertension and pulmonary emboli than urokinase, although both agents were equivalent at 12 hours.

### Cerebrovascular Embolism

Thrombolytic therapy also has been used to treat individuals with acute embolic cerebrovascular accidents. Following neurologic evaluation and computed tomography of the brain, 74 individuals with confirmed acute ischemic stroke who presented within 90 minutes of the onset of symptoms received rt-PA (0.35 - 1.08 mg/kg) (320). Neurologic improvement was noted in 30% of individuals at 2 hours and in 46% by 24 hours, but this effect was not dose-dependent. In addition, individuals receiving doses of 0.85 mg/kg or greater suffered a higher incidence of intracranial hematoma (320, 321).

Hacke et al (322) compared rt-PA (1.1 mg/kg) to placebo in individuals who presented within 6 hours of the onset of symptoms. Evaluation of neurologic recovery using the Barthel Index and modified Rankin scale favored treatment with rt-PA, and recovery at 3 months was significantly improved in the rt-PA group. There was no difference in mortality rates between treatment groups; however, a large number of intracerebral hemorrhages occurred in the rt-PA individuals. These observations were confirmed in a randomized, double-blind, placebo-controlled trial (323) in which rt-PA was administered to individuals who presented within 3 hours of the onset of stroke. In this study, there was no discernible difference between groups at 24 hours, but neurologic improvement in rt-PA treated individuals was recognized by 3 months. These individuals were 30% more likely to have minimal disability at 3 months; however, rt-PA therapy also was associated with an increased incidence of symptomatic intracerebral hemorrhage.

## Myocardial Infarction

Early clinical trials of rt-PA in the treatment of acute myocardial infarction focused primarily on coronary artery patency in response to therapy. Table 56.3 details selected studies in which individuals received rt-PA, 50 to 100 mg/kg over 30 to 180 minutes. This dosing schedule produced infarct-related artery patency rates of 62 to 83%, as demonstrated by coronary angiography 90 minutes after initiation of therapy (298–302, 324, 325).

Patency of the infarct-related artery, however, is only one parameter by which to measure the success of thrombolytic agents. Residual left ventricular function remains an important predictor of survival after myocardial infarction (308). In early studies (309, 325, 326), therapy with rt-PA better preserved ejection fraction significantly more than placebo and resulted in lower end-systolic and end-diastolic left ventricular volumes (305).

Treatment with rt-PA also conferred mortality benefits on individuals with acute myocardial infarction in early studies (Table 56.4). In the ASSET (Anglo-Scandinavian Study of Early Thrombolysis) study (327), a 26% reduction in the mortality rate was associated with rt-PA therapy. These observations were confirmed by other investigators (305), who demonstrated a 51% decrease in the mortality rate among 355 individuals treated with rt-PA.

Subsequent trials have evaluated novel bolus dosing regimens and routes of administration. Using a front-loaded dosing schedule (100 mg over 90 minutes delivered as a 15 mg initial bolus followed by 50 mg infusion in the first 30 minutes and a 35 mg infusion over the next 60 minutes), infarct-related artery patency rates of 91% were achieved (118). This benefit extended to a decrease in predischarge mortality rates as well (328). Double bolus therapy consisting of two 50 mg infusions given 30 minutes apart resulted in infarct-related artery patency with TIMI grade 3 flow in 86% of individuals at 60 minutes and in 88% at 90 minutes (329). When administered via an intracoronary route, rt-PA achieved significant improvements in TIMI flow grade, with concomitant decreases in thrombus burden (330).

Traditionally, thrombolytic therapy has been restricted to individuals who presented within 6 hours of the onset of symptoms. The effects of thrombolysis provided between 6 and 24 hours from the beginning of symptoms were evaluated in the LATE (Late Assessment of Thrombolytic Efficacy) trial (331), which randomized 5711 individuals to rt-PA or placebo. Subgroup analysis revealed that treatment within 12 hours of symptoms provided a 25.6% relative reduction in the 35-day mortality rate in favor of rt-PA.

| **TABLE 56.3** | Early Trials Demonstrating Reduced Mortality with rt-PA | | |
|---|---|---|---|
| Trial (Reference) | Dose | Mortality Reduction (%) | Time of Analysis |
| ASSET (327) | 100 mg | 26 | 30 days |
| Van de Werf and Arnold (305) | 100 mg over 3 hours | 51<br>36 | 14 days<br>90 days |
| LATE (331) | 100 mg over 3 hours | 25.6 | 35 days |

| **TABLE 56.4.** | Infarct-related Artery Patency with rt-PA | | |
|---|---|---|---|
| Trial (Reference) | Dose | Patency Rate (%) | Time of Angiography |
| TIMI-I (232) | 50 mg over 90 minutes | 62 | 90 minutes after Rx |
| TIMI-II (234) | 100 mg over 90 minutes | 68 | 90 minutes after Rx |
| Smith et al. (250) | 50 mg intravenous bolus | 75 | 60 minutes after Rx |
| TAPS (118) | 15 mg intravenous bolus<br>50 mg over 30 minutes then 35 mg over 60 minutes | 91 | 90 minutes after Rx |
| Purvis (329) | 50 mg every 30 minutes | 86<br>88 | 60 minutes after Rx<br>90 minutes after Rx |

*Rx, treatment.*

Recombinant t-PA exists in several forms. On a milligram-for-milligram basis, Duteplase, a two-chain rt-PA, retains a specific activity regarding generation of plasmin in a kinetic, chromogenic substrate assay system similar to an equivalent amount of alteplase, which is a single-chain rt-PA (332).

Recently completed megatrials have compared rt-PA with other thrombolytic agents in terms of efficacy as well as infarct-related artery patency, left ventricular function, morbidity, and mortality. The GISSI-2 trial randomized 12,490 individuals with acute myocardial infarction to treatment with single-chain rt-PA or SK. At both 5 weeks and 6 months, rt-PA provided no survival advantage. Fewer individuals treated with rt-PA suffered reinfarction, but rt-PA was found to cause a significantly greater risk of hemorrhagic stroke (333).

The ISIS-3 study (114) compared two-chain rt-PA (0.6 mg/kg over 4 hours), SK (1.5 million IU over 1 hour), and APSAC (30 mg intravenous bolus). No differences between therapies were found regarding mortality rate or residual left ventricular function. An excess number of strokes, however, was noted in the rt-PA group.

The GUSTO trial (334) compared front-loaded, weight adjusted, single-chain rt-PA (≤100 mg over 90 minutes) with SK (1.5 million IU over 1 hour) and with combination therapy. All individuals received adjunctive therapy with heparin, either intravenous or subcutaneous. At 30 days, the rt-PA group demonstrated a significantly lower mortality rate compared with the SK regimens (6.3 versus 7.3%, pooled, respectively). Individuals who achieved TIMI grade 3 flow at 90 minutes had a significantly lower mortality rate compared with those who had TIMI grade 2 or 1 flow. The occurrence of all-cause mortality or nonfatal disabling stroke was significantly lower in the accelerated rt-PA group despite an increased incidence of total stroke in the rt-PA group. Infarct-related artery patency was higher in the rt-PA group at 90 minutes compared with the SK treated individuals. Measures of left ventricular function revealed that whereas the ejection fraction was similar between groups at 90 minutes and at 5 to 7 days, left ventricular end-systolic volume was lower in rt-PA treated individuals, and the proportion of individuals with normal wall motion was significantly higher.

Primary PTCA has been compared with rt-PA with variable results. A multicenter trial randomized 395 individuals who presented within 12 hours of the onset of myocardial infarction to primary PTCA or rt-PA followed by conservative care (335). In-hospital mortality rates were higher in the rt-PA than in the PTCA group (6.5 versus 2.6%, respectively), as were reinfarction rates. This observation persisted at 6 months. The GUSTO IIb trial (336) similarly randomized 1138 individuals presenting within 12 hours of acute myocardial infarction to primary PTCA or accelerated rt-PA and further supported these observations. Primary PTCA conferred an early therapeutic advantage on individuals with respect to a composite clinical outcome of death, nonfatal reinfarction, and nonfatal disabling cerebrovascular accident compared with thrombolytic therapy (9.6 versus 13.7%, respectively); however, by 6 months, there was no significant difference between groups. In contrast, other investigators have failed to demonstrate a difference between rt-PA and PTCA regarding myocardial salvage as assessed by technetium-99 sestamibi scan (337). In individuals with anterior myocardial infarction, rt-PA treated individuals had higher rates of in-hospital mortality, death or reinfarction, recurrent myocardial ischemia, and stroke (338). Individuals with infarcts in other areas demon trated similar in-hospital mortality profiles, but PTCA treated individuals had lower rates of recurrent ischemia (338).

# PRACTICAL ASPECTS OF THROMBOLYTIC ADMINISTRATION

Clinical application of thrombolytic therapy is easily accomplished. Maximum myocardial salvage is achieved when these agents are administered within 6 hours of the onset of symptoms; however, data suggest some individuals may benefit from therapy initiated up to 12 hours, and possibly up to 24 hours, following the onset of symptoms if their clinical course is characterized by unremitting or stuttering symptoms (331, 339). Candidates for reperfusion therapy should have symptoms suggestive of acute myocardial infarction and an electrocardiogram (ECG) demonstrating 1 mm or greater ST-segment elevation in at least two contiguous limb leads, or 2 mm or greater ST-segment elevation in two contiguous precordial leads that persist following administration of nitroglycerin to treat presumptive vasospasm. In this setting, individuals with left bundle branch block also should be considered as eligible for thrombolytic agents. Individuals without ST-segment changes, ST-segment depression (after posterior myocardial infarction has been excluded), or with only T-wave abnormalities, should be excluded from consideration for this treatment. Similarly, in an asymptomatic individual with an EKG suggestive of acute myocardial infarction, the diagnoses of pericarditis, previous infarction with aneurysm formation, or J-point elevation must be entertained (340, 341).

Before treatment is initiated, the individual must be rigidly screened for possible contraindications (Table 56.5) to thrombolytic therapy. Absolute contraindications include active internal bleeding, excluding menses, previous hemorrhagic stroke at any time or other cerebrovascular events within 1 year of presentation, intra-

**TABLE 56.5.** Contraindications to Thrombolytic Therapy

| Absolute | Relative |
| --- | --- |
| Active internal bleeding | Prolonged cardiopulmonary resuscitation |
| Hemorrhagic stroke | Severe hypertension |
| Nonhemorrhagic stroke within 1 year | Trauma (<2–4 weeks) |
| Intracranial neoplasm | Surgery (<3 weeks) |
| Suspected aortic dissection | Bleeding diathesis |
|  | Pregnancy |
|  | Active peptic ulcer disease |

cranial neoplasm, and suspected aortic dissection. Severe hypertension (either on presentation or historically), prolonged cardiopulmonary resuscitation, recent history of trauma (within 2–4 weeks) or surgery (within 3 weeks), bleeding diathesis, pregnancy, and active peptic ulcer disease are relative contraindications to treatment with thrombolytic agents (341). Using these accepted contraindications as guidelines, clinicians may judiciously screen individuals before selecting a thrombolytic agent as a reperfusion therapy.

Once a individual has been selected, the thrombolytic agent of choice may be administered. An agent can be selected on the basis of efficacy, morbidity and mortality rates, and side effect profiles (see the sections on SK and rt-PA) as well as on the local availability and cost. Current therapies include SK and rt-PA. SK is dosed as 1.5 million U infused over 60 minutes. Heparin is initially withheld in individuals receiving SK. Once the activated partial thromboplastin time (aPTT) falls below 2.0 times the control value, heparinization is initiated only in those individuals at high risk for systemic embolization, including those with an anterior or large myocardial infarction, atrial fibrillation, left ventricular thrombus, or history of embolic event. rt-PA is given in an accelerated or *front-loaded* dosing regimen consisting of a 15 mg intravenous bolus followed by a 50 mg or a 0.75 mg/kg intravenous infusion over 30 minutes and then a 35 mg or 0.5 mg/kg intravenous infusion over 60 minutes. Heparinization to maintain the aPTT at 1.5 to 2.0 times control is started simultaneously. In addition, all individuals should receive oral aspirin, and β-adrenoceptor blocker therapy should be considered (341).

During and immediately after thrombolytic administration, individuals should be observed closely for improvement of symptoms and signs of reperfusion. Repeat EKG monitoring may demonstrate resolution of ST-segment elevation, Q waves, or both. Return of the EKG to baseline has been considered a marker of reperfusion, and clinical studies have associated this finding with a lower mortality rate at 35 days (342). Q waves

on the EKG after thrombolytic therapy are predictive of regional left ventricular dysfunction, with a lower incidence of complete recovery of function (343). Reperfusion arrhythmias also have been considered to be markers of thrombolytic success. Attributed to the fluxes of potassium and calcium from ischemic cells, these arrhythmias may include idioventricular rhythms, ventricular tachycardia, or ventricular fibrillation (341).

Patients should be observed for adverse clinical events, including hemorrhagic complications associated with thrombolytic administration. The most common events relate to minor bleeding at puncture sites; however, major bleeding, including cerebrovascular hemorrhage, may occur and have serious sequelae. Treatment of these events depends on the degree of hemorrhage, but it may include cessation of the thrombolytic agent and heparin, reversal of the anticoagulant state with 6-aminohexanoic acid Amicar (Immunex Corp., Seattle, WA), protamine sulfate, and blood product transfusion. Interestingly, individuals who receive thrombolytic agents may develop a prothrombotic state and demonstrate clinical evidence of reocclusion, characterized by recurrent symptoms and ST-segment elevations on the EKG. If this occurs within 48 hours of the initial clinical event, these individuals are candidates for repeat therapy with half-dose rt-PA, which is administered as a 6 mg intravenous bolus followed by a 20 mg/hour intravenous infusion, for a total of 50 mg. If symptoms recur after 48 hours following initial therapy, full-dose rt-PA should be used. Because of the antigenic nature of SK, repeat SK infusion should be avoided. Anaphylactic reactions to SK are uncommon, but fever and rash are not and can be treated with intravenous corticosteroids and antihistamines. In addition, SK, but not rt-PA, is associated with hypotension during infusion, which usually responds to intravenous fluid or pressor support (341).

## IN SEARCH OF THE "PERFECT" THROMBOLYTIC AGENT

The perfect thrombolytic agent has not yet been found, although the desirable clinical and biochemical characteristics are reviewed in Table 56.6. When developing newer agents, it is important to consider these characteristics in design.

Insofar as formation of an occlusive thrombus is the triggering event in myocardial infarction (77), a thrombolytic agent should achieve rapid and specific clot lysis, preferably with a simple dosing scheme. In this regard, a model thrombolytic agent should possess high enzymatic efficiency for the activation of plasminogen, and it should bind specifically to the offending thrombus. Binding to the thrombus would produce a localized increase in concentration, thereby increasing enzymatic efficiency and preventing clearance via the liver and kidneys.

| TABLE 56.6. | Desirable Characteristics of a Thrombolytic Agent |
|---|---|
| **Feature** | **Benefit** |
| Enzymatic efficiency | Rapid and complete clot lysis |
| Fibrin binding | Enhanced local concentration |
| Prolonged half-life | Simple and rapid administration |
| Limited activation of thrombin | Limited reocclusion and enhanced activity |
| Substrate specificity fibrin ≫ fibrinogen thrombus ≫ plug | Intact hemostasis and reduced bleeding complications |
| Low antigenicity | Reduced allergic side effects |
| Low cost | Enhanced availability |

Adapted with permission from Ferres H. Preclinical pharmacological evaluation of anisoylated plasminogen streptokinase activator complex (review). Drugs 1987;33(Suppl):33–50.

An agent with a prolonged half-life would be desirable as well. A prolonged duration of action may help to prevent reocclusion (by maintaining a local "lytic state") and allow delivery by a single intravenous bolus. A simplified method of drug delivery would aid in rapid administration, possibly out-of-hospital, to reperfuse the affected organ as rapidly as possible. In addition, an agent with a prolonged storage life would be advantageous, in that delays when initiating treatment (i.e., preparing the agent) could be minimized, thus allowing more rapid reperfusion of the thrombosed vessel.

The "perfect" coronary thrombolytic agent also would possess a degree of specificity for an occlusive coronary thrombus, without significant effects on a protective hemostatic plug. This feature has proved to be particularly elusive, however, in that the intrinsic properties of an occlusive thrombus and a hemostatic plug are identical. Specific coronary clot lysis probably will require developments allowing localized delivery of thrombolytic agents to the coronary circulation.

Recently formed thrombi differ from "older" thrombi in at least two important respects. Recent thrombi contain fibrin polymers that are free of interstrand crosslinks, whereas more aged thrombi, through the action of activated factor XIII, are extensively crosslinked and, therefore, less susceptible to degradation by plasmin (344, 345). Furthermore, recent thrombi are rich in platelets and older thrombi less so. The "perfect" thrombolytic agent would bind preferentially to "newer" thrombi (by being selective for crosslinked fibrin and platelet membranes) and, thereby, offer some selectivity of clot lysis. This selectivity could be amplified further by the preferential stimulation of plasminogen activator activity through crosslinked fibrin and enhanced plasminogen activation with platelet membranes.

Thrombotic reocclusion within the first few hours after thrombolytic therapy limits the effectiveness of thrombolytic agents in individuals with acute myocardial infarction. The early reocclusion rate for individuals treated with t-PA is as high as 10 to 25% (346). Recent evidence suggests that early reocclusion may result from the enhanced thrombin activity seen with thrombolytic therapy (347). An agent that could achieve thrombolysis without extensive thrombin activation would certainly be desirable, but to date, no agent has this quality.

Unfortunately, the perfect thrombolytic agent has yet to be developed. The first effort at improving thrombolytic agents produced anisoylated plasminogen-streptokinase activator complex (APSAC), which is composed of the SK-plasminogen complex modified by the synthetic insertion of a p-anisoyl group in the active site, a feature which confers a prolonged serum half-life on the complex. Subsequent efforts at improving the performance of thrombolytic agents have been directed along two major lines. First, mutants or variants of existing plasminogen activators and chimeric proteins, which contain functional domains from different agents, have been designed to optimize thrombolytic potency (348–350). Second, adjunctive therapy with agents that inhibit clot formation (i.e., antiplatelet agents, antithrombin agents) have been used to promote thrombolysis and to prevent reocclusion (351, 352).

## MUTANTS AND VARIANTS OF scu-PA

Attempts have been made to design variants of scu-PA with improved pharmacokinetic and fibrinolytic profiles. To date, investigators have created mutants in which the plasmin cleavage site, the aminoterminal polypeptide chain, or the $Cys_{148}$-$Cys_{279}$ interchain disulfide bond are eliminated by site-specific mutagenesis. When evaluated in either a rabbit jugular vein thrombosis model or a human plasma milieu, however, these mutants failed to prove superior to native scu-PA regarding fibrinolytic potency (353, 354). Other mutants derive from the LMW scu-PA lacking the aminoterminal 143 residues, scu-PA-32k (353, 355), that was modified further by site-directed mutagenesis of clusters of charged amino acids with the highest solvent accessibility. Compared with scu-PA, these mutants possessed similar fibrinolytic activities, rates of plasminogen activation, clot lysis in a human plasma system, and plasma clearance (356).

## MUTANTS AND VARIANTS OF t-PA

Recombinant mutants of t-PA that contain amino acid substitutions in the both the finger and kringle 1 domains, resulting in a sixfold or 2.2-fold longer plasma half-life *in vivo,* respectively, have been constructed. When these mutant genes were combined and expressed as a single variant t-PA, the plasma half-life was markedly increased; however, this occurred at the expense of enzymatic potency (357).

Absence of the zymogen triad (i.e., $Asp_{194}$-$His_{40}$-$Ser_{32}$; chymotrypsin numbering) contributes to the enzymatic activity of single-chain t-PA. This was confirmed by construction of a zymogen triad containing an rt-PA mutant with reduced activity toward plasminogen. Further modification of the mutant t-PA was accomplished by creating a variant that contained the triad but was resistant to plasmin-mediated conversion into two-chain t-PA. Without fibrin, the zymogen region again depressed plasminogen activation; with fibrin, catalytic efficiency of the mutant t-PA toward plasminogen was increased by a factor of 130,000, thus suggesting that zymogenlike variants of t-PA may represent thrombolytic enzymes with enhanced "thrombus selectivity" (358).

A t-PA variant, t-PAΔFEK1, containing only the kringle-2 and serine protease domains has undergone clinical evaluation as r-PA or reteplase (Boehringer Mannehein Corp., Gaithersburg, MA) (359). This variant demonstrates fibrin binding, plasminogen activation, and *in vitro* thrombolysis. Using a canine coronary copper-coil model, t-PAΔFEK1 was compared with wild-type t-PA and found to produce more rapid reperfusion and less reocclusion. This was attributed to a prolonged serum half-life of 58 minutes, compared with 3 minutes for rt-PA (360).

Deletion mutants of rt-PA have a prolonged half-life: therefore, they may be administered as a single bolus. r-PA (reteplase) was compared with an accelerated, front-loaded infusion of rt-PA in 324 individuals to determine its efficacy regarding early coronary patency (361). Individuals received either 10-plus-10 megaunits double bolus of reteplase or front-loaded rt-PA in addition to standard aspirin and heparin therapy. TIMI grade 3 flow at both 60 and 90 minutes was significantly higher in individuals who received r-PA; however, this did not translate to a mortality benefit. These observations were confirmed in the larger-scale GUSTO III trial (362), which randomized more than 15,000 individuals to r-PA or rt-PA to evaluate mortality at 1 month after acute myocardial infarction. At 30 days, there was no significant difference between therapies regarding mortality or cerebrovascular events.

Clinical application of n-PA (lanoteplase) demonstrates comparable therapeutic efficacy with rt-PA. The InTIME (Intravenous nPA for Treating Infarcting Myocardium Early) trial (362) randomized individuals to four weight-adjusted doses of n-PA, and coronary angiography to evaluate TIMI flow revealed that higher doses achieved rates of TIMI grade 3 flow comparable to those with rt-PA at 30, 60, and 90 minutes. Combined TIMI grade 2 and grade 3 flow at 90 minutes, however, was significantly higher in individuals who received n-PA therapy.

The novel modified rt-PA E6010 is characterized by a Cys → Ser substitution at position 84. The compound possesses a half-life of 23 minutes or longer and is dosed similar to rt-PA as a single intravenous bolus. In a clinical comparison with native t-PA (tisokinase, 28.8 mg total, 2.88 mg over 1–2 minutes followed by the remainder infused over 60 minutes), E6010 (0.22 mg/kg over 1–2 minutes) demonstrated a shorter time to reperfusion and a higher angiographic patency rate at 15, 30, 45, and 60 minutes after initiation of therapy, without evidence of major hemorrhagic complications (363).

A t-PA mutant similar to wild-type t-PA, but with amino acid substitutions at three sites, has been designated TNK-TPA. This compound derives its name from the amino acid substitutions: a threonine (T) at position 103 is replaced by an asparagine, thereby adding a glycosylation site; an asparagine (N) at position 117 is replaced by glutamine, thereby removing a glycosylation site; and four amino acids, lysine (K), histidine, arginine, and arginine, are replaced by four alanines at positions 296–299. TNK-TPA is characterized by a prolonged half-life, improved fibrin specificity, and increased resistance to inhibition by PAI-1 (289). In a rabbit model that combined thrombogenic stimulation with increased PAI-1 activity (364), TNK-TPA prevented fibrin deposition.

The TIMI 10A trial was a phase 1, dose-ranging pilot trial designed to evaluate the efficacy of TNK-TPA in individuals with acute myocardial infarction in which 113 individuals presenting within 12 hours of the onset of symptoms received a single bolus of TNK-TPA (5–50 mg intravenously). The plasma half-life ranged from 11 to 20 minutes, compared with 3.5 minutes for wild-type t-PA. Systemic fibrinogen and plasminogen levels were decreased by 3% and 13%, respectively. Coronary angiography 90 minutes after infusion was initiated demonstrated TIMI grade 3 flow in 57 to 64% of individuals who received the highest doses of TNK-TPA. Hemorrhagic complications occurred in 6.2% of individuals, but these mostly were limited to the vascular access sites (365).

Recently, t-PA variants that demonstrate extreme resistance to PAI-1 have been identified. Single-chain t-PA with amino acid substitutions at positions 275, 298, 299, and 304 results in a mutant t-PA that PAI-1 inhibits 120,000 times less rapidly than it does native, single-chain t-PA. Similar substitutions in the two-chain t-PA also result in PAI-1 resistance, yet the magnitude of this response is diminished compared with the single-chain form. Further development of these mutant t-PAs may result in a thrombolytic agent with a significantly prolonged half-life and, therefore, a greater therapeutic efficacy (366).

# CHIMERIC THROMBOLYTIC AGENTS

The partial fibrin specificity and short plasma half-life of endogenous plasminogen activators has driven the search for thrombolytic agents with greater thrombolytic potency, fibrin specificity, or both. One approach to development of newer thrombolytic agents has included chimeric proteins, which contain functional domains arranged to maximize specific properties of endogenous plasminogen activators.

## PRODUCTION OF CHIMERIC PROTEINS

Chimeric proteins based on u-PA have been produced by disulfide crosslinkage of the plasmin $\alpha$ chain, which confers fibrin binding, to the u-PA $\beta$ chain (i.e., protease region) (367). Chimeric proteins of t-PA/u-PA have been produced through expression of complementary DNA (cDNA) fragments of t-PA spliced to scu-PA cDNA fragments (128, 243). Most of these recombinant proteins are enzymatically active, with some displaying fibrin affinity/specificity and some prolonged half-lives (348–350, 367–370).

Two t-PA based chimeric proteins comprised of the aminoterminal portion of t-PA (F, E, K1, K2 domains) and the serine protease (S) region of scu-PA (t-PA/scu-PA-e and t-PA/scu-PA-s) (369, 370) retained the catalytic efficiency and specific activity *in vitro* of u-PA while demonstrating partial fibrin affinity (371, 372). In terms of thrombolytic potency, these compounds produce similar dose-response curves compared with wild-type scu-PA in a rabbit jugular vein thrombosis model, thus suggesting fibrin affinity alone does not confer enhanced *in vivo* thrombolytic potency (373).

Nelles et al (374) examined the structure-function relationship between t-PA/u-PA chimeras using deletion/substitution mutations in the t-PA/scu-PA-e protein. The mutant t-PA $\Delta$FE–scu-PA-e, representing deletion of the F and E domains of the t-PA portion, possesses markedly reduced affinity for fibrin. Conversely, substitution of K1 by a second K2 (t-PA$\Delta$K1$\nabla$K2/scu-PA-e) results in enhanced fibrin and lysine-Sepharose binding. Despite differing degrees of fibrin binding, both deletion mutants were equipotent in an *in vitro* clot lysis system (374). *In vivo* studies using hamster, rabbit, and baboon thrombosis models further demonstrated that t-PA$\Delta$FE/scu-PA-e retained greater thrombolytic potency than wild-type scu-PA (374). The improved thrombolytic potency of t-PA$\Delta$FE/scu-PA-e results from diminished plasma clearance, not fibrin targeting (375).

Van den Werf et al (376) evaluated the *in vivo* efficiency of $K_1K_2P_u$, which is a t-PA/u-PA chimera comprised of kringles 1 and 2 of rt-PA and of the serine protease region of rscu-PA in individuals with acute myocardial infarction. Thrombolysis was achieved in two of four individuals administered 10 mg boluses with a 15 minute interval. This regimen did not induce a systemic lytic state, however, and $K_1K_2P_u$-related antigen was not detectable in plasma after 70 minutes, thereby indicating that the plasma clearance was 50 mL/min.

Modification of the t-PA A chain produces similar results. Deletion of the F and E domains of t-PA results in reduced fibrin affinity (377–380), reduced specific thrombolytic activity (381), and diminished plasma clearance (377, 378, 380–382). The sum total of these effects is marginally improved thrombolytic potency *in vivo* (381–383). Other recombinant chimeric plasminogen activators include FK$_2$tu-PA and K$_2$tu-PA, which are comprised of the t-PA finger and K$_2$ domain or the K$_2$ domain alone combined with the protease region of scu-PA. The K$_2$tu-PA chimera enhanced thrombolytic activity in a rabbit jugular vein thrombosis model compared with either t-PA or scu-PA (384).

The lack of correlation between specific thrombolytic activity (i.e., percentage of clot lysis per unit concentration of plasminogen activator in blood) and thrombolytic potency (i.e., percentage of lysis per unit dose per kilogram of body weight) further emphasizes the danger in extrapolating biochemical properties to potential clinical application. The domain-oriented structure of plasminogen activators exists in three dimensions, but our ability to modify protein structure in primary sequence has often unpredictable effects on global conformation and function. Therefore, the mere juxtaposition of functional domains does not ensure appropriate three-dimensional relationships. This shortcoming is supported by the experience with t-PA/scu-PA chimeric proteins.

A chimeric derivative comprised of the kringle and the protease domains of rscu-PA, coupled to an inhibitory sequence directed at the active site of thrombin and a fragment from the C-terminal region of hirudin, thereby conferring thrombus-specific properties on the molecule, has been constructed. Known as rscu-PA-40 Kda/Hir or M23, this molecular has an efficacy comparable to that of rscu-PA in canine femoral artery and saphenous vein thrombosis models. In contrast to rscu-PA, however, M23 is not associated with a significant decrease in plasma fibrinogen or $\alpha_2$-antiplasmin levels, or with an increase in the template bleeding time (385).

To promote more efficient thrombolysis, novel agents that target the offending thrombus have been synthesized. One such peptide, a rt-PA/P-selectin fusion protein, offers site directed thrombolysis along with inhibition of leukocyte binding native P-selectin on platelets and endothelial cells. *In vivo* efficacy studies of the construct protein have demonstrated significant reductions in cyclic flow variations compared with saline control in rat mesenteric arterial beds (386).

## CONJUGATES OF PLASMINOGEN ACTIVATORS AND ANTIFIBRIN MONOCLONAL ANTIBODIES

The increased fibrin specificity of a thrombolytic agent may be achieved by conjugating plasminogen activators with monoclonal antibodies that are fibrin specific and that do not cross react with fibrinogen (387). To accomplish this, monoclonal antibodies against the Bβ chain of fibrin (MA-59D8) or crosslinked human fibrin fragment D-dimer (MA-15C5) have been used (388).

A recombinant chimeric plasminogen activator composed of MA-15C5 and a 32 Kda scu-PA has a 12-fold higher fibrinolytic potency *in vitro* in a human plasma milieu (389). Compared with scu-PA *in vivo*, the conjugate MA-15C5/scu-PA demonstrated a 23-fold greater potency than scu-PA alone in a hamster pulmonary embolus model, an 11-fold greater potency in a rabbit jugular vein thrombosis model, and a fivefold greater potency in a baboon femoral vein system. In these animal models, clearance of MA-15C5/scu-PA was reduced, and therapy was not associated with depletion of fibrinogen or α$_2$-antiplasmin (390). With fibrin fragment-D dimer, clot lysis was diminished, thereby suggesting that increased fibrinolytic potency results antibody targeting (389).

Loop grafting, in which the amino acid sequence of a biologically active, flexible loop on one protein is used to replace a surface loop on another protein, was used to graft the complementarity-determining region of the monoclonal antibody, HCDR3 from Fab-9, an antibody selected to bind the β$_3$-integrins, to the epidermal growth factor region of t-PA (249). This mutant t-PA successfully bound α$_{IIb}$β$_3$ and retained full enzymatic activity.

## STAPHYLOKINASE

Isolated from *Staphylococcus* sp., staphylokinase is synthesized as an 18.5 Kda precursor peptide that is proteolytically modified to a 15.5 Kda protein before secretion (391). Analysis of the secondary structure reveals that the molecule consists of two folded domains of similar size, thus creating a flexible, dumbbell shape. Approximately 18% of the 163 amino acid residues are organized in helical structures, 30% are incorporated in β-sheets, and 20% form turns (392).

Staphylokinase forms a 1:1 stoichiometric complex with plasminogen, which after conversion to plasmin activates other plasminogen molecules to plasmin. The Met$_{26}$ residue is involved in staphylokinase-mediated plasminogen activation because substitutions at this site result in loss of fibrinolytic activity (393). In a plasma milieu, staphylokinase dissolves fibrin clots without associated fibrinogen degradation. In animal models, staphylokinase is equipotent to SK for dissolution of whole blood or plasma clots, but it is significantly more potent for dissolution of platelet-rich or retracted thrombi (394).

Without fibrin, α$_2$-antiplasmin inhibits staphylokinase-directed plasminogen activation by preventing generation of active plasmin-staphylokinase complex. Fibrin further stimulates plasminogen activation by staphylokinase via mechanisms involving the lysine-binding sites of plasminogen, thereby facilitating generation of the staphylokinase-plasmin complex and delaying its inhibition at the clot surface (395). Neutralization of the plasmin-staphylokinase complex by α$_2$-antiplasmin results in dissociation of functionally active staphylokinase from the complex and recycling of staphylokinase to other plasminogen molecules (396). Other protease inhibitors, including α$_2$-macroglobulin, C1-inhibitor, and α$_2$-antitrypsin, limit plasminogen activation by staphylokinase; however, the actions of these protease inhibitors are similarly diminished in the presence of fibrin (397, 398).

Staphylokinase-mediated plasminogen activation follows Michaelis-Menten kinetics, with a $K_m = 7.0$ μmol/l and a $k_{cat} = 1.5$ per second. In purified systems, α$_2$-antiplasmin inhibits the plasminogen-staphylokinase complex with a $K_i = 2.7 \times 10^6$ mol/l per second. Staphylokinase does not bind to fibrin, and fibrin stimulates the initial rate of plasminogen activation of staphylokinase by only 4-fold (399). When Lys-plasminogen is used as a substrate, the $k_{cat}/K_m$ is approximately 10 times higher than that obtained for Glu-plasminogen (400). In contrast, other investigators have demonstrated that the affinity of staphylokinase for Glu-plasminogen and Lys-plasminogen is comparable (401).

In a plasma system, platelet-rich plasma clots are lysed faster than platelet-poor plasma clots by staphylokinase. The plasminogen activation rate by staphylokinase is enhanced by the addition of washed platelets, and this effect is not attenuated by the addition of indomethacin, thus suggesting the platelet surface acts as a catalytic surface for assembly of the components of the plasminogen activator system (402). Shishido et al (403) used a rabbit jugular vein thrombosis model to evaluate the *in vivo* efficacy of staphylokinase. Approximately 50% thrombolysis, with no change in circulating fibrinogen levels, was observed 360 minutes after start of an intravenous infusion.

Compared with SK and t-PA in a plasma clot lysis system, staphylokinase produces high rates of clot lysis without significantly influencing fibrinogen, plasminogen, or α$_2$-antiplasmin levels in the plasma-containing clots. In contrast, SK at equimolar concentrations depletes these parameters in plasma despite low clot lysis rates. Low concentrations of t-PA successfully lyse clots, but at higher concentrations, plasminogen depletion diminishes this response (404).

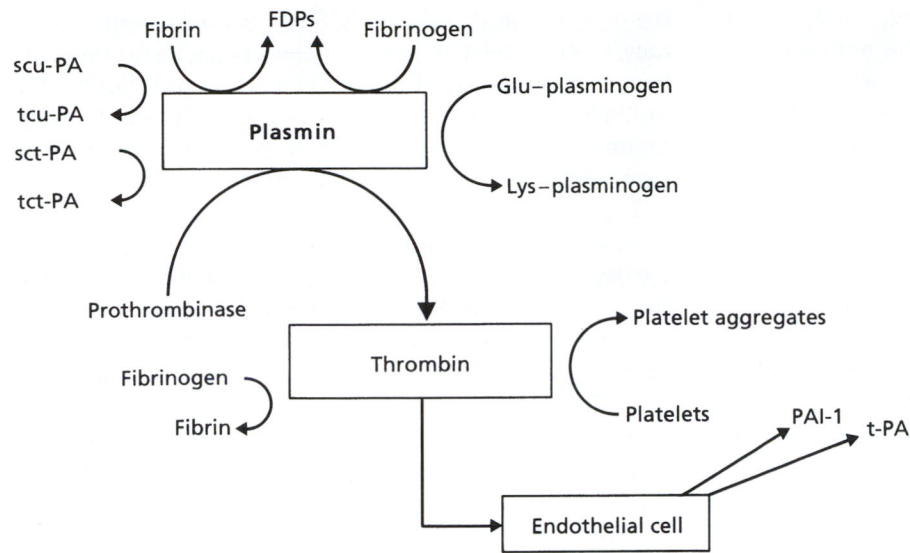

**FIGURE 56.7.** Effects of plasmin on hemostasis and fibrinolysis. *FDPs*, fibrinogen degradation products; *PAI-1*, plasminogen activator inhibitor 1; *sct-PA*, single-chain t-PA; *scu-PA*, single-chain urokinase-type plasminogen activator; *tct*, two-chain t-PA; *tcu-PA*, two-chain u-PA; *t-PA*, tissue-type plasminogen activator.

Recombinant staphylokinase (STAR) also has been evaluated in individuals with acute myocardial infarction. A multicenter trial to compare STAR with accelerated rt-PA (405) randomized 100 individuals to either STAR (10 or 20 mg intravenously over 30 minutes) or weight-adjusted rt-PA. Both groups received aspirin and heparin. At 90 minutes, TIMI grade 3 flow was achieved in 62% of the STAR group and in 58% of the rt-PA group. Fibrinogen levels were significantly reduced by rt-PA but were not affected by STAR. Treatment with STAR was not associated with an increased rate mortality or with hemorrhagic or allergic complications. In addition, STAR has been shown to restore vessel patency when administered intra-arterially to individuals with peripheral arterial occlusion (406).

Because staphylokinase is a bacterial plasminogen activator, it also is an antigenic thrombolytic agent in humans, with neutralizing antibodies still detectable 2 weeks after therapy (405). To attenuate the antigenicity of staphylokinase, two of its three immunodominant epitopes were altered by substituting clusters of two or three charged amino acids with alanine. This staphylokinase retains potency and fibrin specificity, but it is less antigenic than wild-type staphylokinase (407, 408) and, therefore, may be more amenable for clinical thrombolytic therapy.

## ADJUNCTIVE THERAPY FOR THROMBOLYSIS

The central event in thrombolysis is formation of plasmin from its zymogen precursor, plasminogen. Once formed, plasmin exerts a variety of effects that promote both fibrinolysis and hemostasis (Fig. 56.7). To enhance the thrombolytic potency and efficacy of therapeutic thrombolytic agents, adjunctive therapy has been

directed at specific components of the thrombolytic and hemostatic systems. Table 56.7 lists examples of potential adjunctive agents for thrombolytic therapy.

### Antiplatelet Agents (see Chapter 54)

#### 7E3

The antiplatelet agent 7E3 is a murine monoclonal antibody directed against the fibrinogen binding site of the

**TABLE 56.7. Adjunctive Agents for Thrombolytic Therapy**

| Agent | Class |
|---|---|
| *Antiplatelet agents* | |
| 7E3 | Glycoprotein IIb-IIIa antagonist |
| Integrelin | Glycoprotein IIb-IIIa antagonist |
| Bichistatin | RGD peptide |
| Eichistatin | RGD peptide |
| Kistrin | RGD peptide |
| Aspirin | Cyclooxygenase inhibitor |
| Sulatroban | Thromboxane $A_2$ receptor antagonist |
| Dazoxiban | Thromboxane synthase inhibitor |
| Ridogrel | Combined thromboxane $A_2$ receptor antagonist and thromboxane synthase inhibitor |
| Organic nitrates | Guanylyl cyclase stimulator |
| *Antithrombin agents* | |
| Heparin | Antithrombin III cofactor |
| Hirudin | Thrombin inhibitor |
| Hirulog | Synthetic thrombin inhibitor |
| Argatroban | Thrombin inhibitor |
| PPACK | Thrombin inhibitor |

platelet membrane (GP)-IIb-IIIa molecule (409). A chimeric form (i.e., human/murine) of the antibody has been developed (c7E3) and modified further by removing the Fc portion of the antibody molecule (c7E3 F[ab'2] or m7E3). This form is available commercially as abciximab (Eli Lilly & Co., Indianapolis, IN), and it has been investigated extensively as an adjunctive agent for thrombolytic therapy (410–415).

In a canine coronary thrombosis model (413), 7E3 (0.8 mg/kg) was effective in preventing reocclusion after successful t-PA-induced thrombolysis. Animals similarly treated with 7E3 and APSAC also demonstrated continued patency during a 2-hour observation period (416). The main effect of 7E3 is to inhibit reocclusion, without any effect on the rate of thrombolysis as determined in both arterial and venous thrombosis models. Notable side effects include thrombocytopenia and irreversible platelet inhibition (409).

The chimera c7E3 demonstrates markedly reduced immunogenicity compared with 7E3 and similar therapeutic profiles. Kohmura et al (417) studied the effects of a single intravenous bolus of c7E3 (0.45 mg/kg) on thrombolysis induced with rt-PA and reocclusion was studied in baboons with femoral arterial thrombosis and superimposed high-grade stenosis. This dose of c7E3-Fab blocked 96% of the platelet GP IIb-IIIa receptors, and it abolished adenosine diphosphate-induced aggregation. Reperfusion was obtained within 25 minutes and, compared with aspirin treated animals, was associated with delayed reocclusion.

The efficacy of 7E3 also was evaluated in a canine coronary model (418). Animals underwent electric current injury to the left circumflex artery to create an occlusive thrombus, which was aged for 30 minutes before t-PA was coadministered with a single dose of 7E3 (0.8 mg/kg intravenously) or placebo. *Ex vivo* platelet aggregation was inhibited for up to 48 hours after a single injection of 7E3, and vessel reocclusion and associated mortality were significantly reduced.

In the TAMI-8 study (419), 60 individuals treated with rt-PA, aspirin, and heparin for acute myocardial infarction also received 7E3 bolus injections in ascending doses at 3, 6, and 15 hours after initiation of thrombolytic therapy. Individuals treated with 7E3 Fab suffered less recurrent ischemia compared with controls (13 versus 20%, respectively) and sustained a higher rate of infarct-related artery patency (92 versus 56%, respectively).

## Other GP IIb-IIIa Receptor Antagonists

Platelet aggregation depends on fibrinogen binding to activated platelets via the membrane GP IIb-IIIa receptor. The receptor binding site recognizes the fibrinogen peptide sequence Arg-Gly-Asp (RGD) as well as a dodecapeptide sequence in the γ chain. A number of synthetic and naturally occurring peptides contain the RGD sequence; therefore, they are termed *RGD* peptides. By virtue of occupying the RGD binding site on the platelet surface, these platelets inhibit platelet aggregation and have been investigated as therapy to improve the efficacy and potency of existing thrombolytic agents. The receptor antagonist Ro-43-5054 was effective in a canine thrombolysis model in which a platelet rich coronary thrombus was induced by electrical stimulation (420). Animals were treated with t-PA and Ro-43-5054 (3 μg/kg per min). During a 120 minute observation period, Ro-43-5054 did not accelerate reperfusion compared with aspirin treated or heparin treated animals, although reocclusion was prevented after reinforcement of the thrombogenic stimulus. Thus, inhibition of platelet activation by the selective, nonpeptidic GP IIb-IIIa receptor antagonist Ro-43-5054 protected against early reocclusion after thrombolytic therapy better than aspirin.

Integrelin (COR Therapeutics, Inc., South San Francisco, CA), a platelet GP IIb-IIIa receptor antagonist, was evaluated in a canine coronary thrombosis model (421). Animals were treated with rt-PA in addition to either integrelin (5 μg/kg per min for 90 min) or saline. Integrelin-treated animals demonstrated enhanced lysis of the occlusive thrombus, thus causing full restoration of coronary blood flow for 29 minutes, compared with 5 minutes for saline control. In this setting, however, integrelin did not modify the reocclusion rate.

Integrelin also has been used with thrombolytic therapy in clinical trials. Ohman et al (422) reported on 132 individuals assigned to receive a bolus and a continuous infusion of one of six integrelin doses or placebo. Another 48 individuals received the highest integrelin dose in conjunction with accelerated rt-PA, aspirin, and intravenous heparin infusion. The highest integrelin dose delivered more complete reperfusion (TIMI grade 3, 66 versus 39% for placebo-treated individuals), with similar rates of in-hospital complications and severe bleeding.

FK 633, which is a novel GP IIb-IIIa receptor antagonist, has had similar results. FK 633 effectively inhibited *ex vivo* platelet aggregation with adenosine diphosphate (2.5 μmol/l) with an $IC_{50}$ of $5.4 \times 10^{-7}$ (423). In a hamster carotid artery injury model, FK 633 (0.3 or 1.0 mg/kg per hour), administered as an adjunct to rt-PA, improved late arterial patency compared with rt-PA alone. The high dose of FK 633, however, was associated with a prolonged bleeding time.

Bitistatin, which is isolated from the venom of the pit viper *Bitis arietans*, is an 83 amino acid polypeptide containing the RGD sequence at residues 64-66, and it possesses significant antiplatelet activity (424). In a canine coronary thrombolysis model, bitistatin (30 μg/kg bolus and 3 μg/kg per min infusion) accelerated t-PA induced thrombolysis 1.4-fold and reduced the reocclusion rate from 80 to 22% in combination with heparin (425, 426). Echistatin, a similar pit viper product, was investigated in a canine coronary thrombolysis model with electrically induced injury. Animals treated with echistatin (15 μg/kg per min) demonstrated improved t-PA-induced coronary thrombolysis compared with heparin alone (100 versus 60% lysis, respectively) and reduced rates of reocclusion (20 versus 100%, respectively). In addition, animals in the echistatin group retained less residual coronary thrombus than control animals (426). Kistrin, which is a 68 amino acid peptide isolated from the venom of the Malayan pit viper *Agkistrodon rhodostoma,* also contains the RGD sequence and effectively inhibits platelet GP IIb-IIIa. Kistrin (0.24 mg/kg) accelerated t-PA-induced thrombolysis sixfold and abolished reocclusion in a canine model of coronary thrombolysis (427). This therapy also was associated with a sevenfold increase in template bleeding time and inhibition of *ex vivo* adenosine disphosphate-induced and collagen-induced platelet aggregation.

SC-49992 is a mimetic of the tetrapeptide arginine-glycine-aspartic acid-phenylalanine, and it is a potent inhibitor of platelet aggregation. In a canine coronary artery lysis/reocclusion model designed to provide a platelet-rich, reoccluding thrombus (428), SC-49992 decreased the time to lysis in response to t-PA in a dose-dependent manner. The time to reocclusion was prolonged, and in those animals that demonstrated reocclusion, *ex vivo* platelet aggregation was inhibited 100% at reocclusion.

## Aspirin

Thrombolytic therapy is associated with thrombin generation and subsequent platelet activation. Aspirin exerts antiplatelet effects through irreversible acetylation of platelet cyclooxygenase, thereby preventing synthesis of thromboxane $A_2$. These platelet-inhibitory properties suggest aspirin would be a beneficial adjunct to thrombolytic therapy. Experimental results, however, are conflicting.

In an *in vitro* plasma clot lysis model, aspirin enhanced HMW tcu-PA-mediated clot lysis only if added before thrombus formation (429). Aspirin also significantly accelerated thrombolysis in a canine coronary thrombolysis model, although reocclusion occurred in 42% of animals within 90 minutes of the discontinuation of t-PA (430). In contrast, in a porcine carotid artery thrombolysis model, only two of six animals treated with t-PA and aspirin demonstrated evidence of reperfusion, and no animal was able to partially or completely eliminate residual thrombus (430a). This is supported by an *in vivo* study in rabbits that underwent shunt placement with a gore-tex graft containing $^{125}$I-fibrinogen-labeled thrombus (431), in which kinetic analysis revealed that aspirin offered no benefit over saline regarding the rate and extent of t-PA-mediated thrombolysis.

Aspirin also has been evaluated in clinical trials as an adjunct to thrombolytic therapy. The ISIS-2 trial (63) demonstrated improved survival in individuals with acute myocardial infarction treated with aspirin alone. Furthermore, the survival benefit associated with aspirin was additive to that observed with SK therapy alone. Meta-analysis of 419 individuals treated with aspirin revealed a lower rate of reocclusion and recurrent ischemic events, regardless of choice of thrombolytic agent (432). The APRICOT study further demonstrated that aspirin successfully reduced reinfarction and revascularization rates, improved event-free survival, and preserved left ventricular function compared with placebo in individuals with a patent infarct-related artery within 48 hours of thrombolytic therapy (432a).

## Thromboxane $A_2$ Receptor Antagonists

Elevated levels of urinary thromboxane $A_2$ metabolites have been detected after acute vessel reocclusion following thrombolytic therapy, thus suggesting these eicosanoids additionally enhance platelet activity (433–435). Thromboxane $A_2$, a potent platelet agonist secreted by activated platelets, may limit further the success of thrombolytic therapy by potentiating local thrombus formation. This suggests a role for thromboxane $A_2$ receptor antagonists as potential adjunctive agents in thrombolytic therapy.

Sulatroban, another thromboxane $A_2$ receptor antagonist, was administered with t-PA in a rabbit femoral artery thrombosis model (436). Sulatroban (1 mg/kg per hour intravenously) reduced the femoral artery clot lysis time from 65 to 29 minutes, with no effect on reocclusion. The thromboxane $A_2$ receptor antagonist vapiprost was evaluated in a guinea pig femoral artery model of photochemically induced thrombosis (437). Animals received a single bolus injection (0.3 mg/kg) coadministered with t-PA or 30 minutes after the thrombolytic infusion was completed. All animals received an additional oral dose (3 mg/kg) 120 minutes after the initial therapy. When vapiprost was given with t-PA, the clot lysis time was reduced from 28.4 to 9.1 minutes, and the frequency of reocclusion within 24 hours decreased from 70 to 37%. Delayed administration of vapiprost, however, conferred no additional benefit to t-PA.

Thromboxane receptor antagonism also reduces infarct size in cynomolgus monkeys. The thromboxane antagonist SQ 30,741 (2.1 mg/kg bolus and 0.5 mg/kg per hour infusion) was evaluated in a circumflex model of electrically induced thrombosis (438). Animals treated with the thromboxane antagonist demonstrated significantly reduced infarct size compared with saline control.

## Thromboxane Synthase Inhibitors

Thromboxane synthase inhibition has been evaluated as another adjunct to thrombolytic therapy. The effects of CGS 13080, which is a selective thromboxane synthase inhibitor, were studied in a rabbit femoral artery thrombosis model treated with rt-PA (439). Therapy with CGS

13080 (2 mg/kg infusion) was associated with accelerated thrombolysis, increased incidence of reperfusion, and enhanced blood flow after thrombolysis. These observations were confirmed in a canine copper-coil model of coronary thrombolysis (440), in which thromboxane synthase inhibition with dazoxiben (5 mg/kg bolus and 5 mg/kg per hour infusion) reduced the lysis time from 56 to 25 minutes without any effect on the incidence of reocclusion.

## Combined Thromboxane $A_2$ Receptor Antagonists and Thromboxane Synthase Inhibitors

To overcome the limitations of thromboxane $A_2$ receptor antagonist and thromboxane synthase inhibitor therapies, combination agents have been synthesized. Ridogrel (Janssen, Berse, Belgium), which is a potent inhibitor of thromboxane $A_2$ synthase at low concentrations and a competitive thromboxane $A_2$/prostaglandin endoperoxide receptor blocker at higher concentrations, has been evaluated in both animal models and clinical trials.

Ridogrel has superior efficacy in preventing arterial or coronary thrombosis compared with thromboxane $A_2$ synthase inhibition, thromboxane $A_2$/prostaglandin endoperoxide receptor blockade, or aspirin alone. When administered at higher doses in a canine platelet-rich coronary thrombosis model treated with rt-PA or SK, ridogrel reduced both time to reperfusion and incidence of reocclusion (441). Ridogrel also reduces infarct size independent of its effect on thrombolysis. A pilot study of 50 individuals with acute myocardial infarction who received ridogrel (300 mg) orally twice per day for 5 days in addition to rt-PA and heparin revealed patency rates of 86% at 90 minutes and of 94% between 6 and 24 hours (442). The RAPT (Ridogrel Versus Aspirin Patency) trial (443) compared ridogrel to aspirin in 907 individuals with acute myocardial infarction treated with SK. Coronary angiography performed 7 to 14 days after therapy demonstrated no difference in infarct-related vessel patency between groups.

## Organic Nitrates and Other Nitrosovasodilators

Organic nitrates and other nitrosovasodilators are potent inhibitors of platelet function and also influence vascular tone (444). In a canine carotid artery thrombolysis model (445), local infusion of nitroglycerin (1 μg/kg per min) reduced both formation of a primary thrombus after endothelial injury and incidence of rethrombosis after thrombolysis with APSAC. Nitroglycerin (10 μg/kg min), as an adjunct to rt-PA, heparin, and aspirin in a rabbit femoral arterial thrombosis model (446), did not accelerate reperfusion; however, animals treated with nitroglycerin revealed an increased magnitude of re-

stored flow and total patency duration after vessel recanalization. Pretreatment with the nitric oxide precursor L-arginine or the exogenous nitric oxide donor sodium nitroprusside delays thrombus formation, promotes thrombolysis with t-PA, and delays reocclusion (446).

Clinical studies have yielded differing results. Individuals with acute myocardial infarction receiving t-PA and nitroglycerin demonstrate less evidence of reperfusion, lower plasma levels of t-PA, and higher levels of PAI-1 than individuals receiving t-PA and saline control, suggesting that nitroglycerin impairs the thrombolytic efficacy of t-PA (447). Similarly, 63 individuals with an acute anterior myocardial infarction randomized to receive t-PA and nitroglycerin experienced delays in reperfusion, a greater incidence of reocclusion, and other in-hospital adverse events (448).

## Conclusions

A variety of antiplatelet agents have been evaluated as a means to enhance thrombolytic potency and efficacy. Currently available evidence suggests antiplatelet agents may enhance thrombolysis. All currently available thrombolytic agents that activate plasminogen also lead to activation of prothrombin (449, 450), and the thrombin produced in turn activates platelets. There is evidence supporting a role for thrombin activation in thrombotic reocclusion after thrombolytic therapy (449, 450). In this regard, antithrombin agents have become the subject of intense research as possible adjunctive agents for thrombolytic therapy, both to increase thrombolytic potency and to prevent thrombotic reocclusion.

## Antithrombin Agents (see Chapters 55 and 57)

Despite development of thrombolytic agents for the treatment of thrombotic disease, standard antithrombotic therapy is remarkably unchanged. Currently used antithrombotic agents include heparin and warfarin, which have been the standard of care for decades. Limitations in the efficacy, potency, and delivery of these drugs, however, have been the driving force behind the development of newer, more effective agents.

### Heparin

Historically, heparin has been the only parenteral antithrombotic agent with commercial preparations derived from either porcine intestine or bovine lung. Commercial preparations consist of a heterogeneous mixture of HMW and LMW glycosaminoglycan polymers (451, 452). The LMW fraction ($\leq$7 Kda) contains most of the anticoagulant activity with a high affinity for antithrombin III and factor Xa (453, 454). Heparin exerts its activity by catalyzing the formation of thrombin-antithrombin III complexes, which are inactive, thereby neutralizing the enzyme thrombin (454).

Use of heparin as an adjunct to thrombolytic therapy has been largely disappointing. Effects on *in vivo* t-PA-mediated thrombolysis were examined in a rabbit model (455), and heparin treatment (200 IU/kg) was associated with successful thrombolysis in five of seven animals, compared with one of seven animals treated with aspirin alone. In contrast, other investigators using rabbit (431, 456) and canine (430) models found heparin to be no more effective than saline as an adjunctive agent to t-PA.

Human studies on the efficacy of heparin as an adjunct to thrombolytic therapy have yielded differing results. One arm of the ISIS-2 pilot study (62) compared heparin with placebo in individuals receiving SK. Heparin therapy (1000 U/hour for 48 hours) was initiated 12 hours after completion of the SK infusion. Individuals treated with heparin demonstrated less reinfarction, with no change in the rates of bleeding complications or mortality. The DUCCS-I study (457) evaluated heparin in individuals who received APSAC. Individuals were randomized to receive heparin and aspirin or aspirin alone. There was no difference between groups regarding infarct-related artery patency rates or left ventricular function, but the overall bleeding rate was higher in the heparin group.

The LIMITS (Liquaemin in Myocardial Infarction During Thrombolysis with Saruplase) study (458) evaluated the effect of a prethrombolytic heparin bolus on the efficacy and safety of ru-PA in individuals with acute myocardial infarction. Individuals received heparin (5000 IU bolus) or saline within 6 hours of the onset of symptoms. Thirty minutes after the completion of thrombolysis, an intravenous heparin infusion was administered for 5 days. Individuals received an additional 5000 IU bolus before coronary angiography, which occurred within 6 to 12 hours after the start of lysis. At angiography, bolus individuals had a higher rate of patent infarct related arteries (78.6 versus 56.5%), with no appreciable increase in the risk of bleeding.

Heparin is effective at preventing reocclusion in t-PA treated individuals for acute myocardial infarction (459), but it has no effect on mortality (333). The European Cooperative Study Group treated individuals with t-PA, aspirin, and heparin (5000 U bolus followed by 1000 U/hour infusion) or placebo. Individuals received a continuous infusion until coronary angiography was performed at 48 to 120 hours. A small improvement in patency between groups was demonstrated, but this did not correlate with improved enzymatic infarct size or diminished incidence of recurrent ischemia. In contrast, subgroup analysis of the LATE trial (331) demonstrated that among individuals randomized to receive t-PA, those additionally receiving heparin benefited from a statistically significant reduction in the 35-day mortality rate.

The role of subcutaneous heparin as an adjunct to thrombolytic therapy was studied in large-scale studies such as the ISIS-3, GISSI-2, and the International Study Group trials, which randomized more than 62,000 individuals treated with thrombolytics to therapy with aspirin and delayed subcutaneous heparin (12,500 U twice daily) or aspirin alone. The heparin regimen was not associated with a clear reduction in either the 35-day mortality rate or the incidence of reinfarction or postinfarction angina. Importantly, there were significantly increased rates of bleeding in heparin-treated individuals. Compared with intravenous heparin in the GUSTO I trial, delayed subcutaneous heparin was not superior in individuals receiving SK, with no apparent difference in the 24-hour, 30-day, or 1-year mortality rates and with an increase in reinfarction noted among individuals given intravenous heparin (460).

LMW heparin also has been examined as adjunctive treatment to thrombolytic agents. In dogs with an electrically induced intracoronary thrombus, bolus administration of LMW heparin, 75 IU/kg, followed by intravenous t-PA resulted in significantly improved rates of coronary reocclusion, despite equivalent times to reperfusion compared with saline control (461).

LMW heparin has been compared with standard heparin therapy in animal models as well. In a canine coronary thrombosis model, intravenous rt-PA and aspirin were administered in combination with unfractionated heparin (200 IU/kg bolus followed by 100 IU/kg per hour) or three doses of the LMW heparin, nadroparin calcium (100 IU/kg bolus followed by 50 IU/kg per hour, 200 IU/kg bolus followed by 100 IU/kg per hour, or 300 IU/kg followed by 150 IU/kg hour). Coronary reperfusion was found in both the standard-heparin and the higher-dose LMW heparin groups. Measurements of thrombin-antithrombin III complex levels in plasma revealed that both heparins were effective in preventing new thrombin generation. At equivalent doses, nadroparin calcium was associated with a less prolonged aPTT and lower steady-state anti-Xa and anti-IIa activities (462). In a rabbit thrombosis model, animals were treated with t-PA alone or with standard intravenous heparin (200 IU bolus and 70 IU/hour) or subcutaneous LMW heparin fragmin (single dose of 500 IU/kg), before t-PA administration. Treatment with fragmin resulted in rates of recanalization similar to those seen with heparin; however, fragmin also resulted in improved persistent patency rates and prevented reocclusion (463).

To evaluate whether LMW heparin provides prophylaxis against recurrent myocardial infarction, 103 individuals were randomly assigned 5 days after acute myocardial infarction treated with SK to outpatient therapy with clexane (40 mg subcutaneously daily) for 25 days or no treatment (464). Reinfarction in the clexane group was significantly reduced over a 6-month period (4.6 versus 20%, respectively), as were episodes of angina. There was no difference between groups regarding major bleeding events.

## Hirudin

Hirudin is a 7 Kda polypeptide isolated from the salivary glands of the medicinal leech *Hirudo medicinalis* (465, 466). Analysis of the primary structure reveals a hydrophobic aminoterminal region, a hydrophilic carboxyterminus, and three disulfide bridges. At present, hirudin is available as a recombinant protein, which differs from the native protein only by the lack of sulfation at $Tyr_{63}$ (467). Use of hirudin as an adjunct to thrombolytic therapy has garnered considerable interest.

*In vitro* studies comparing the efficacy of hirudin to heparin have demonstrated hirudin to be more effective at inhibiting fibrin-bound thrombin (468). *In vivo* studies in a canine thrombolysis model have demonstrated that hirudin, at doses that prolong the aPTT from 1.5 to 2.0 times control, both accelerates clot lysis and prevents reocclusion (431). Furthermore, when used in conjunction with t-PA, hirudin was proved to be superior to heparin regarding both the rate of thrombolysis and the incidence of reocclusion (469).

Desulfatohirudin (REVASC) was compared with heparin as an adjunct to thrombolytic therapy with rt-PA in a canine model of coronary artery thrombosis (470). Animals were randomized to receive hirudin (2 mg/kg bolus followed by 2 mg/kg per hour) or intravenous heparin (120 IU/kg bolus followed by 80 IU/kg per hour infusion) 10 minutes before thrombolysis with rt-PA. Hirudin enhanced the time to reperfusion and completely prevented reocclusion. Coronary blood flow was improved by hirudin, as shown by a higher maximum blood flow after reperfusion, and a longer cumulative patency time was achieved.

Hirudin also has been evaluated extensively as an adjunct to thrombolytic therapy in individuals with acute myocardial infarction (471). A retrospective analysis of 183 individuals treated with t-PA and recombinant hirudin (bolus dose of 0.007, 0.1, 0.2, or 0.4 mg/kg followed by an infusion of 0.05, 0.06, 0.1, or 0.25 mg/kg per hour over 48 hours) demonstrated that optimal anticoagulation was achieved more frequently in the higher dose groups, and these individuals were more likely to have patency of the infarct related artery at 36 to 48 hours.

The TIMI 5 trial (472) was a randomized, dose-ranging pilot trial of hirudin versus heparin, administered with front-loaded t-PA and aspirin to 246 individuals with acute myocardial infarction. Individuals were assigned to one of four ascending dose regimens for 5 days. Coronary angiography was performed at 90 minutes and at 18 to 36 hours. TIMI grade 3 flow in the infarct related artery was achieved and preserved at

both 90 minutes and 18 to 36 hours in more individuals treated with hirudin than with heparin, with no difference between hirudin dosing regimens. Although not statistically significant, there was a trend toward less death and reinfarction in the hirudin group. The TIMI 6 trial (473) similarly compared hirudin with heparin in conjunction with SK and aspirin. Individuals received a 5-day infusion of heparin (5000 U bolus followed by infusion of 1000 U/hour) adjusted to a target aPTT or one of three doses of hirudin (0.15 mg/kg bolus plus 0.05 mg/kg per hour infusion; 0.3 mg/kg bolus plus 0.1 mg/kg per hour infusion; or 0.6 mg/kg bolus plus 0.2 mg/kg per hour infusion). Greater benefits regarding morbidity and mortality rates were seen with the two higher doses of hirudin.

The GUSTO IIa trial (474) planned to enroll 12,000 individuals to evaluate recombinant hirudin against standard heparin therapy. Individuals were randomized to receive heparin (5000 U bolus followed by infusion of 1000–1300 U/hour) adjusted to a target aPTT or hirudin (0.6 mg/kg bolus and 0.2 mg/kg per hour infusion) without adjustment. The trial was prematurely terminated after enrollment of 2,564 individuals because of an excess of intracerebral hemorrhagic events. The TIMI 9A study (475) similarly compared hirudin with heparin as an adjunct to thrombolytic therapy. Individuals received hirudin at a dose of 0.6 mg/kg bolus followed by a fixed-dose, 96-hour infusion of 0.2 mg/kg per hour or heparin at a weight-adjusted dose (5000 U bolus followed by infusion of 1000 U/hour for individuals less than 80 kg or 1300 U/hour those 80 kg or heavier). This trial also was stopped prematurely because of increased hemorrhage rates in both groups. Individuals who suffered a major bleeding complication were older and had higher aPTT values, particularly during the first 12 hours after thrombolysis.

The TIMI 9B trial (476) compared hirudin with heparin administered at lower doses than those associated with increased rates of bleeding. Individuals with acute myocardial infarction were treated with aspirin and either accelerated-dose t-PA or SK. Individuals were randomized within 12 hours of the onset of symptoms to receive either intravenous heparin (5000 U bolus followed by infusion of 1000 U/hour) or hirudin (0.1 mg/kg bolus followed by infusion of 0.1 mg/kg per hour). There was no difference between groups regarding death, recurrent nonfatal myocardial infarction, or development of congestive heart failure or cardiogenic shock at 30 days.

The GUSTO IIb trial (477) also compared hirudin with heparin administered at lower doses than those that caused increased bleeding rates in the GUSTO IIa trial. Individuals with acute myocardial infarction or unstable angina were randomized to either adjunctive heparin (5000 U bolus followed by infusion of 1000 U/hour) or hirudin (0.1 mg/kg bolus followed by infusion of 0.1 mg/kg per hour) therapy, both of which were administered for 72 hours. At 24 hours, the risk of death or myocardial infarction was significantly lower in the hirudin-treated individuals than in the heparin-treated individuals (1.3 versus 2.1%, respectively; $P$ = .001); however, this benefit diminished after 30 days (8.9 versus 9.8%; $P$ = .06).

Thus, the benefits of hirudin over heparin were marginal, at best, in these two large trials. There are several potential explanations for this lack of a more dramatic difference. First, activation of platelet by $\alpha$-thrombin cannot be inhibited as effectively by hirudin as the procoagulant activity of thrombin can (478). Second, heparin is more effective than hirudin in preventing thrombin activation after platelet activation in plasma (479). Third, hirudin is more effective than heparin at inactivating thrombin, but much more robust thrombin generation occurs when the thrombin inhibitory capacity of hirudin is exceeded than when that of heparin is exceeded (479).

Synthetic hirudin analogues are currently being investigated. Hirugen is a synthetic dodecapeptide fragment from the carboxyterminal region of hirudin, and this peptide binds to the anion binding exosite of thrombin and prevents thrombin-mediated cleavage of fibrinogen (480). Evidence suggests that hirugen enhances heparin-mediated inhibition of the thrombotic reocclusion, which often is seen with thrombolytic therapy (481). A second synthetic analogue, hirulog, which is a synthetic peptide containing hirugen linked by a polyglycine spacer to the serine protease inhibitor D-phenylalanyl-L-prolyl-L-arginyl chloromethyl ketone (PPACK), is similarly promising as an effective adjunctive antithrombin agent (482).

## Argatroban

Argatroban, or (2R,4R)-4-methyl-(N2-((3-methyl-1,2,3, 4-tetrahydro-8-quinolinyl)sulfonyl)-L-arginyl)-2-piperidinecarboxylic acid, is a potent thrombin inhibitor that binds to the catalytic site of thrombin (483). In humans, argatroban causes a dose-dependent increase in both the thrombin time and the aPTT with an anticoagulant half-life of approximately 25 minutes (484).

As an adjunct to thrombolytic therapy in a canine model of coronary thrombosis, argatroban (2.5 mg/kg per hour) significantly accelerates the rate of t-PA-induced thrombolysis and prevents reocclusion (485). In a guinea pig femoral artery model thrombotically occluded by photochemical reaction, animals receiving argatroban in conjunction with t-PA had a reduced time for vessel reopening and decreased frequency of reocclusion (437). In a similar model, argatroban (200 µg/kg per min) was compared with aspirin and 7E3 regarding t-PA-induced coronary thrombolysis (414), and argatroban

was associated with more complete reperfusion and less reocclusion than either of the other agents. Similar results were reported in a rabbit femoral artery model of thrombolysis (455), in which argatroban (100 µg/kg per min) significantly accelerated t-PA-induced thrombolysis and prevented thrombotic reocclusion compared with aspirin or heparin alone. Argatroban also was associated with less residual thrombus on pathologic examination. Furthermore, it provided protection against reocclusion even after its elimination from the circulation. More recently, enhanced thrombolysis and prevention of reocclusion with argatroban (1 mg/kg bolus and 3 mg/kg hour infusion) was demonstrated when used in conjunction with recombinant scu-PA (486).

Argatroban also has been evaluated as an adjunct to thrombolytic therapy in clinical trials. The AMI (Argatroban in Myocardial Infarction) trial was a phase II, double-blind, placebo-controlled study that randomized 910 individuals with acute myocardial infarction to low-dose or intermediate-dose argatroban or to placebo (362). The trial failed to demonstrate a significant difference between treatments when evaluating a composite 30 day endpoint consisting of death, reinfarction, cardiogenic shock, or congestive heart failure, but subgroup analysis revealed that individuals treated within 3 hours of the onset of symptoms with intermediate-dose argatroban received significant risk reduction compared with those randomized to placebo and low-dose therapy.

## PPACK

PPACK (D-phenylalanyl-L-prolyl-L-arginyl-chloromethyl ketone) is a synthetic antithrombin that inhibits thrombin through irreversible alkylation of the thrombin active-site histidine (487). PPACK is clinically useful as a thrombolytic agent, and it inhibits both free and clot-bound thrombin with equal potency (487, 488). *In vivo* experimentation thus far has been restricted to evaluating its usefulness for preventing platelet deposition on injured arterial segments and for preventing thrombosis (487–489).

In a rabbit deep vein thrombosis model, PPACK extended the thrombin clotting time 2.3-fold and prolonged both cuticle and ear bleeding times (490). In rat carotid arteries, occlusive thrombi were induced in 97% of PPACK-treated rats (491). PPACK (6 mg/kg intravenously) also decreased thrombus weight by 90% and was associated with improvements in either average blood flow or vessel patency.

## Other Thrombin Inhibitors

The thrombin inhibitor D-methyl-phenylalanyl-prolyl-arginyl (GYKI-14766) was compared with heparin in a canine arterial and venous rethrombosis model (492). Electrolytic injury was used to induce thrombus formation, and either heparin (300 U/kg), GYKI-14766 (0.5 mg/kg per hour) or saline was administered intravenously following APSAC. *Ex vivo* platelet aggregation and aPTT levels were similar between groups; however, GYKI-14766 did not increase bleeding time. GYKI-14766 did prevent cyclic flow variations and reocclusion in the artery and vein as well as reduce arterial thrombus weights. This suggests GYKI-14766 is effective at preventing occlusive rethrombosis in both the arterial and venous circulation after thrombolysis without prolonging the bleeding time.

Inogatran, which is a 439-kDa selective active site inhibitor of thrombin, was investigated in three rat thrombosis models (493). In the venous thrombosis model, inogatran inhibited thrombus formation in a dose-dependent fashion, with a greater than 80% antithrombotic effect at a plasma concentration of 0.45 μmol/l. In the arterial thrombosis model, inogatran similarly inhibited thrombus formation and preserved vessel patency and mean blood flow, again in a dose-dependent fashion. When t-PA was employed to initiate thrombolysis, the addition of inogatran improved the patency time and the cumulative blood flow compared with t-PA alone.

# CONCLUSIONS

The discovery and development of thrombolytic agents over the past two decades has provided exciting new information about the fibrinolytic system and contributed greatly to the treatment of vascular disease. The scope of these developments cannot be underestimated given the prevalence of atherosclerotic and thrombotic diseases in both developed and developing nations. Clinicians now have the tools to reverse vascular thrombosis rather than, as in the past, simply delay its progression. Furthermore, ongoing studies aimed at both improving thrombolytic agents and developing new adjunctive agents hold promise for further mitigating the mortality and morbidity rates associated with vascular disease.

# REFERENCES

1. Johnson AJ, McCarty WR. The lysis of artificially induced intravascular clots in man by intravenous infusion of streptokinase. J Clin Invest 1959; 38:1627–1643.
2. Jackson KW, Tang J. Complete amino acid sequence of streptokinase and its homology with serine proteases. Biochemistry 1982;21:6620–6625.
3. Reddy KN. Mechanism of activation of human plasminogen by streptokinase. In: Kline DL, Reddy KNN, eds. Fibrinolysis. Boca Raton: CRC Press, 1980:71–94.
4. Medved LV, Solovjov DA, Ingham KC. Domain structure, stability and interactions in streptokinase. Eur J Biochem 1996;239:333–339.
5. Parrado J, Conejero-Lara F, Smith RA et al. The domain organization of streptokinase: nuclear magnetic resonance, circular dichroism, and functional characterization of proteolytic fragments. Protein Sci 1996;5: 693–704.
6. Damaschun G, Damaschun H, Gast K et al. Streptokinase is a flexible multi-domain protein. Eur Biophys J 1992;20:355–361.
7. Malke H, Steiner K, Gase K et al. The streptokinase gene: allelic variation, genomic environment and expression control. Dev Biol Stand 1995;85: 183–193.
8. Rodriguez P, Fuentes P, Barro M et al. Structural domains of streptokinase involved in the interaction with plasminogen. Eur J Biochem 1995;229: 83–90.
9. Nihalani D, Sahni G. Streptokinase contains two independent plasminogen-binding sites. Biochem Biophys Res Commun 1995;217:1245–1254.
10. Young KC, Shi GY, Chang YF et al. Interaction of streptokinase and plasminogen. Studies with truncated streptokinase peptides. J Biol Chem 1995; 270:29601–29606.
11. Reddy KN, Markus G. Mechanism of activation of human plasminogen by streptokinase. Presence of an active center in streptokinase-plasminogen complex. J Biol Chem 1972;247:1683–1691.
12. Summaria L, Wohl RC, Boreisha IG et al. A virgin enzyme derived from human plasminogen. Specific cleavage of the arginyl-560-valyl peptide bond in the diisopropoxyphosphinyl virgin enzyme by plasminogen activators. Biochemistry 1982;21:2056–2059.
13. Markus G, Evers JL, Hobika GH. Activator activities of the transient forms of the human plasminogen streptokinase complex during its proteolytic conversion to the stable activator complex. J Biol Chem 1976;251: 6495–6504.
14. Siefring GE Jr, Castellino FJ. Interaction of streptokinase with plasminogen. Isolation and characterization of a streptokinase degradation product. J Biol Chem 1976;251:3913–3920.
15. Wohl RC, Summaria L, Arzadon L et al. Steady state kinetics of activation of human and bovine plasminogens by streptokinase and its equimolar complexes with various activated forms of human plasminogen. J Biol Chem 1978;253:1402–1407.
16. McClintock DK, Englert ME, Dziobkowski C et al. Two distinct pathways of the streptokinase-mediated activation of highly purified human plasminogen. Biochemistry 1974;13:5334–5344.
17. Bajaj AP, Castellino FJ. Activation of human plasminogen by equimolar levels of streptokinase. J Biol Chem 1977;252:492–498.
18. Reddy KN. Kinetics of active center formation in dog plasminogen by streptokinase and activity of a modified streptokinase. J Biol Chem 1979; 251:6624–6629.
19. Summaria L, Arzadon L, Bernabe P et al. The interaction of streptokinase with human, cat, dog, and rabbit plasminogens. The fragmentation of streptokinase in the equimolar plasminogen-streptokinase complexes. J Biol Chem 1974;249:4760–4769.
20. Reddy KN, Markus G. Esterase activities in the zymogen moiety of the streptokinase-plasminogen complex. J Biol Chem 1974;249:4851–4857.
21. Markus G, Evers JL, Hobika GH. Comparison of some properties of native (Glu) and modified (Lys) human plasminogen. J Biol Chem 1978;253: 733–739.
22. Sherry S, Alkjaersig N, Fletcher AP. Activity of plasmin and streptokinase-activator on substituted arginine and lysine esters. Thromb Diath Haemorrh 1966;16:18–31.
23. Claeson G, Aisell L, Karsson G et al. Substrate structure and activity relationships. In: Davidson R, Rowan R, Samama B, Desnoyers G, eds. Progress in Chemical Fibrinolysis and Thrombosis, Vol. 3. New York: Raven Press, 1978:299–304.
24. Fears R, Hibbs MJ, Smith RA. Kinetic studies on the interaction of streptokinase and other plasminogen activators with plasminogen and fibrin. Biochem J 1985;229:555–558.
25. Bock PE, Day DE, Verhamme IM et al. Analogs of human plasminogen that are labeled with fluorescence probes at the catalytic site of the zymogen. Preparation, characterization, and interaction with streptokinase. J Biol Chem 1996;271:1072–1080.
26. Cederholm-Williams SA, De Cock F, Lijnen HR et al. Kinetics of the reactions between streptokinase, plasmin, and α₂-antiplasmin. Eur J Biochem 1979;100:125–132.
27. Wiman B. On the reaction of plasmin or plasmin-streptokinase complex with aprotinin or α₂-antiplasmin. Thromb Res 1980;17:143–152.
28. Claeys H, Molla A, Verstraete M. Conversion of NH₂-terminal glutamic acid to NH₂-terminal lysine of human plasminogen by plasmin. Thromb Res 1973;3:515–523.
29. Rajagopalan S, Gonias SL, Pizzo SV. The temperature-dependent reaction between α₂-macroglobulin and streptokinase-plasmin(ogen) complex. J Biol Chem 1987;262:3660–3664.
30. Takada Y, Takada A. Kinetic analyses of potentiation of plasminogen activation by streptokinase in the presence of fibrin or its degradation products. Haemostasis 1987;16:1–7.
31. Chibber BA, Castellino FJ. Regulation of the streptokinase-mediated activation of human plasminogen by fibrinogen and chloride ions. J Biol Chem 1986;261:5289–5295.
32. Chibber BA, Morris JP, Castellino FJ. Effects of human fibrinogen and its cleavage products on activation of human plasminogen by streptokinase. Biochemistry 1985;24:3429–3434.
33. Takada A, Takada Y, Sugawara Y. The activation of Glu- and Lys-plasminogens by streptokinase: effects of fibrin, fibrinogen, and their degradation products. Thromb Res 1985;37:465–475.
34. Camiolo SM, Markus G, Evers JL et al. Augmentation of streptokinase activator activity by fibrinogen or fibrin. Thromb Res 1980;17:697–706.

35. Kosow DP. Kinetic mechanism of the activation of human plasminogen by streptokinase. Biochemistry 1975;14:4459–4465.
36. Brommer EJ, Meijer P. Thrombin generation induced by the intrinsic or extrinsic coagulation pathway is accelerated by streptokinase, independently of plasminogen. Thromb Haemost 1993;70:995–997.
37. Onundarson PT, Haraldsson HM, Bergmann L et al. Plasminogen depletion during streptokinase treatment or two-chain urokinase incubation correlates with decreased clot lysability *ex vivo* and *in vitro*. Thromb Haemost 1993;70:998–1004.
38. Gouin I, Lecompte T, Morel MC et al. *In vitro* effect of plasmin on human platelet function in plasma. Inhibition of aggregation caused by fibrinogenolysis. Circulation 1992;85:935–941.
39. Fletcher AP, Alkjaersig N, Sherry S. The clearance of heterologous protein from the circulation of normal and immunized man. J Clin Invest 1959;37:1306–1315.
40. Grierson DS, Bjornsson TD. Pharmacokinetics of streptokinase in individuals based on amidolytic activator complex activity. Clin Pharmacol Ther 1987;41:304–313.
41. Martin M. Streptokinase in chronic arterial disease. New York: CRC Press, 1982.
42. Mentzer RL, Budzynski AZ, Sherry S. High-dose, brief-duration intravenous infusion of streptokinase in acute myocardial infarction: description of effects in the circulation. Am J Cardiol 1986;57:1220–1226.
43. Robbins KC, Barlow GH, Nguyen G et al. Comparison of plasminogen activators [Review]. Semin Thromb Hemost 1987;13:131–138.
44. Col JJ, Col-De Beys CM, Renkin JP et al. Pharmacokinetics, thrombolytic efficacy and hemorrhagic risk of different streptokinase regimens in heparin-treated acute myocardial infarction. Am J Cardiol 1989;63:1185–1192.
45. Arnesen H, Heilo A, Jakobsen E et al. A prospective study of streptokinase and heparin in the treatment of deep vein thrombosis. Acta Med Scand 1978;203:457–463.
46. Porter JM, Seaman AJ, Common HH et al. Comparison of heparin and streptokinase in the treatment of venous thrombosis. Am Surg 1975;41:511–519.
47. Elliot MS, Immelman EJ, Jeffrey P et al. A comparative randomized trial of heparin versus streptokinase in the treatment of acute proximal venous thrombosis: an interim report of a prospective trial. Br J Surg 1979;66:838–843.
48. Thery C, Bauchart JJ, Lesenne M et al. Predictive factors of effectiveness of streptokinase in deep venous thrombosis. Am J Cardiol 1992;69:117–122.
49. Francis CW, Marder VJ. Fibrinolytic therapy for venous thrombosis [Review]. Prog Cardiovasc Dis 1991;34:193–204.
50. Goldhaber SZ, Buring JE, Lipnick RJ et al. Pooled analyses of randomized trials of streptokinase and heparin in phlebographically documented acute deep venous thrombosis. Am J Med 1984;76:393–397.
51. Ly B, Arnesen H, Eie H et al. A controlled clinical trial of streptokinase and heparin in the treatment of major pulmonary embolism. Acta Med Scand 1978;203:465–470.
52. Scott DJ, Wyatt MG, Wilson YG et al. Intra-arterial streptokinase infusion in acute lower limb ischaemia. Br J Surg 1991;78:732–734.
53. Frink RJ, Ostrach LH. Streptokinase in the treatment of an acute cerebral embolus—a case report. Angiology 1990;41:66–69.
54. Patel B, Kloner RA. Analysis of reported randomized trials of streptokinase therapy for acute myocardial infarction in the 1980s. Am J Cardiol 1987;59:501–504.
55. Valentine RP, Pitts DE, Brooks-Brunn JA et al. Intravenous versus intracoronary streptokinase in acute myocardial infarction. Am J Cardiol 1985;55:309–312.
56. Anderson JL, Marshall HW, Askins JC et al. A randomized trial of intravenous and intracoronary streptokinase in patients with acute myocardial infarction. Circulation 1984;70:606–618.
57. Rogers WJ, Mantle JA, Hood WP Jr et al. Prospective randomized trial of intravenous and intracoronary streptokinase in acute myocardial infarction. Circulation 1983;68:1051–1061.
58. Kennedy JW, Ritchie JL, Davis KB et al. Western Washington randomized trial of intracoronary streptokinase in acute myocardial infarction. N Engl J Med 1983;309:1477–1482.
59. Anderson JL, Marshall HW, Bray BE et al. A randomized trial of intracoronary streptokinase in the treatment of acute myocardial infarction. N Engl J Med 1983;308:1312–1318.
60. Khaja F, Walton JA Jr, Brymer JF et al. Intracoronary fibrinolytic therapy in acute myocardial infarction. Report of a prospective randomized trial. N Engl J Med 1983;308:1305–1311.
61. Anonymous. Long-term effects of intravenous thrombolysis in acute myocardial infarction: final report of the GISSI Study. Gruppo Italiano per lo Studio della Streptochi-nasi nell'Infarto Miocardico (GISSI). Lancet 1987;ii:871–874.
62. Anonymous. Randomised trial of intravenous streptokinase, oral aspirin, both, or neither among 17,187 cases of suspected acute myocardial infarction: ISIS-II (Second International Study of Infarct Survival) Collaborative Group. Lancet 1988;ii:349–360.
63. White HD, Norris RM, Brown MA et al. Effect of intravenous streptokinase on left ventricular function and early survival after acute myocardial infarction. N Engl J Med 1987;317:850–855.
64. Anonymous. A prospective trial of intravenous streptokinase in acute myocardial infarction (I.S.A.M.). Mortality, morbidity, and infarct size at 21 days. The I.S.A.M. Study Group. N Engl J Med 1986;314:1465–1571.
65. Common HH, Seaman AJ, Rosch J et al. Deep vein thrombosis treated with streptokinase or heparin. Follow-up of a randomized study. Angiology 1976;27:645–654.
66. Arnesen M, Hoiseth A, Ly B. Streptokinase of heparin in the treatment of deep vein thrombosis. Follow-up results of a prospective study. Acta Med Scand 1982;211:65–68.
67. Trubestein G. Can thrombolytics prevent post-phlebitic syndrome and thrombo-embolic disease? Haemostasis 1986;16(Suppl):38–50.
68. Widmer LK, Zemp E, Widmer MT et al. Late results in deep vein thrombosis of the lower extremity. Vasa 1985;14:264–268.
69. Eichlisberger R, Widmer MT, Widmer LK et al. Spatfolgen nach Becken-Bein-Venenthrombose—Basler Erfahrungen. Vasa Suppl 1987;20:95–103.
70. O'Meara JJ III, McNutt RA, Evans AT et al. A decision analysis of streptokinase plus heparin as compared with heparin alone for deep-vein thrombosis. New Engl J Med 1994;330:1864–1869.
71. Anonymous. Urokinase-streptokinase embolism trial. Phase 2 results. A cooperative study. JAMA 1974;229:1606–1613.
72. Anonymous. The urokinase pulmonary embolism trial. A national cooperative study. Circulation 1973;47(Suppl 2):1–108.
73. Anonymous. Etude multicentrique sur deux protocoles d'urokinase dans l'embolie pulmonarie grave. Groupe de recherche urokinase-embolie pulmonaire. Arch Mal Coeur Vaiss 1984;77:773–781.
74. Francois G, Charbonnier B, Raynaud P et al. Traitement de l'embolie pulmonaire aigue par urokinase comparee a l'association plasminogene-urokinase. A propos de 67 cas. Arch Mal Coeur Vaiss 1986;79:435–442.
75. Sharma GVRK, O'Connell DJ, Bleiko JS et al. Thrombolytic therapy in deep vein thrombosis. In: Paoletti R, Sherry S, eds. Thrombosis and urokinase. New York: Academic Press, 1977:181.
76. Sharma GVRK, Folland ED, McIntyre KM et al. Long-term hemodynamic benefit of thrombolytic therapy in pulmonary embolic disease [Abstract]. J Am Coll Cardiol 1990;15(Suppl A):65.
77. DeWood MA, Spores J, Notske R et al. Prevalence of total coronary occlusion during the early hours of transmural myocardial infarction. N Engl J Med 1980;303:897–902.
78. Zijlstra F, deBoer MJ, Hoorntje JC et al. A comparison of immediate coronary angioplasty with intravenous streptokinase in acute myocardial infarction. New Engl J Med 1993;328:680–684.
79. Zijlstra F, Beukema WP, van't Hof RW et al. Randomized comparison of primary coronary angioplasty with thrombolytic therapy in low risk patients with acute myocardial infarction. J Am Coll Cardiol 1997;29:908–912.
80. de Boer MJ, Suryapranata H, Hoorntje JC et al. Limitation of infarct size and preservation of left ventricular function after primary coronary angioplasty compared with intravenous streptokinase in acute myocardial infarction. Circulation 1994;90:753–761.
81. de Boer MJ, Hoorntje JC, Ottervanger JP et al. Immediate coronary angioplasty versus intravenous streptokinase in acute myocardial infarction: left ventricular ejection fraction, hospital mortality and reinfarction. J Am Coll Cardiol 1994;23:1004–1008.
82. Zijlstra F, de Boer MJ, Beukema WP et al. Mortality, reinfarction, left ventricular ejection fraction and costs following reperfusion therapies for acute myocardial infarction. Eur Heart J 1996;17:382–387.
83. Zijlstra F, de Boer MJ, Ottervanger JP et al. Primary coronary angioplasty versus intravenous streptokinase in acute myocardial infarction: differences in outcome during a mean follow-up of 18 months. Corornary Artery Dis 1994;5:707–712.
84. O'Neill WW, Weintraub R, Grines CL et al. A prospective, placebo-controlled, randomized trial of intravenous streptokinase and angioplasty versus lone angioplasty therapy of acute myocardial infarction. Circulation 1992;86:1710–1717.
85. Rosenschein U, Lenz R, Radnay J et al. Streptokinase immunogenicity in thrombolytic therapy for acute myocardial infarction. Isr J Med Sci 1991;27:541–545.
86. Lynch M, Pentecost BL, Littler WA et al. The significance of anti-streptokinase antibodies. Clin Exp Immunol 1994;96:427–431.
87. McGrath K, Hogan C, Hunt D et al. Neutralising antibodies after streptokinase treatment for myocardial infarction: a persisting puzzle. Br Heart J 1995;74:122–123.
88. Agostoni A, Gardinali M, Frangi D et al. Activation of complement and kinin systems after thrombolytic therapy in patients with acute myocardial infarction. A comparison between streptokinase and recombinant tissue-type plasminogen activator. Circulation 1994;90:2666–2670.
89. Bruserud O, Elsayed S, Pawelec G. At least five antigenic epitopes on the streptokinase molecule are recognized by human CD4+ TCR α-β+ T cells. Mol Immunol 1992;29:1097–1104.
90. Mosseri M, Hasin Y, Admon D et al. Thrombolytic therapy of a stenosed coronary vein bypass graft with continuous intragraft streptokinase drip. Cardiology 1990;77:318–321.

91. Lee HS, Yule S, McKenzie A et al. Hypersensitivity reactions to streptokinase in patients with high pre-treatment antistreptokinase antibody and neutralisation titres. Eur Heart J 1993;14:1640–1643.

92. Smith RA, Dupe RJ, English PD et al. Fibrinolysis with acyl-enzymes: a new approach to thrombolytic therapy. Nature 1981;290:505–508.

93. Anderson JL. Development and evaluation of anisoylated plasminogen streptokinase activator complex (APSAC) as a second generation thrombolytic agent [Review]. J Am Coll Cardiol 1987;10:22B–27B.

94. Smith RA, Dupe RJ, English PD et al. Acyl-enzymes as thrombolytic agents in a rabbit model of venous thrombosis. Thromb Haemost 1982;47:269–274.

95. Fears R, Ferres H, Standring R. The protective effect of acylation on the stability of anisoylated plasminogen streptokinase activator complex in human plasma. Drugs 1987;33(Suppl):57–63.

96. Green J, Dupe RJ, Smith RA et al. Comparison of the hypotensive effects of streptokinase-(human) plasmin activator complex and BRL 26921 (ρ-anisoylated streptokinase-plasminogen activator complex) in the dog after high dose, bolus administration. Thromb Res 1984;36:29–36.

97. Ferres H. Preclinical pharmacological evaluation of anisoylated plasminogen streptokinase activator complex [Review]. Drugs 1987;33(Suppl):33–50.

98. Ferres H, Hibbs M, Smith RA. Deacetylation studies in vitro on anisoylated plasminogen streptokinase activator complex. Drugs 1987;33(Suppl):80–82.

99. Fears R, Green JA, Smith RA et al. Induction of sustained fibrinolytic response by BRL 26921 in vitro. Thromb Res 1985;38:251–260.

100. Gemmill JD, Hogg KJ, Burns JM et al. A comparison of the pharmacokinetic properties of streptokinase and anistreplase in acute myocardial infarction. Br J Clin Pharmacol 1991;31:143–147.

101. Marder VJ, Rothbard RL, Fitzpatrick PG et al. Rapid lysis of coronary artery thrombi with anisoylated plasminogen: streptokinase activator complex. Treatment by bolus intravenous injection. Ann Intern Med 1986;104:304–310.

102. Hillis WS, Horning RS, Dunn FG. Coronary reperfusion following single dose intravenous BRL 26921 [Abstract]. Br Heart J 1985;53:78–79.

103. Horning RS, Walker D, Hogg KJ et al. Natural history of patients following intravenous thrombolytic therapy with acute myocardial infarction [Abstract]. Br Heart J 1985;53:662.

104. Been M, de Bono DP, Muir AL et al. Coronary thrombolysis with intravenous anisoylated plasminogen streptokinase complex BRL 26921. Br Heart J 1985;53:253–259.

105. Been M, Boulton FE, De Bono DP. Clinical and haematological effects of intravenous anisoylated plasminogen-streptokinase complex [Abstract]. Thromb Haemost 1985;54:212A.

106. Kasper W, Meinertz T, Just H. Fibrinolytic efficacy of a new acylated streptokinase-plasminogen activator complex (BRL 26921) in patients with acute myocardial infarction: comparison between intravenous and intracoronary administration [Abstract]. Thromb Haemost 1985;54:213 [Abstract.]

107. Hoffman JJ, Van Rey FJ, Bonnier JJ. Systemic effects of BRL 26921 during thrombolytic treatment of acute myocardial infarction. Thromb Res 1985;37:576–572.

108. Doenecke P, Hellstern P, Schwerdt H et al. Clinical efficacy of acylated streptokinase-plasminogen complex BRL 26921 in patients with acute myocardial infarction (AMI) [Abstract]. Thromb Haemost 1985;54:271.

109. Been M, de Bono DP, Muir AL et al. Clinical effects and kinetic properties of intravenous APSAC—anisoylated plasminogen streptokinase activator complex (BRL 26921) in acute myocardial infarction. Int J Cardiol 1986;11:53–61.

110. Anonymous. Long term effects of intravenous anistreplase in acute myocardial infarction: final report of the AIMS study. AIMS Trial Study Group. Lancet 1990;335:427–431.

111. Bassand JP, Machecourt J, Cassagnes J et al. Limitation of myocardial infarct size and preservation of left ventricular function by early administration of APSAC in myocardial infarction. Am J Cardiol 1989;64:18A–23A.

112. Anderson JL, Rothbard RL, Hackworthy RA et al. Multicenter reperfusion trial of intravenous anisoylated plasminogen streptokinase activator complex (APSAC) in acute myocardial infarction: controlled comparison with intracoronary streptokinase. J Am Coll Cardiol 1988;11:1153–1163.

113. Anderson JL, Sorensen SG, Moreno FL et al. Multicenter patency trial of intravenous anistreplase compared with streptokinase in acute myocardial infarction. The TEAM-2 Study Investigators. Circulation 1991;83:126–140.

114. Anonymous. ISIS-3: a randomised comparison of streptokinase vs tissue plasminogen activator vs anistreplase and of aspirin plus heparin vs aspirin alone among 41,299 cases of suspected acute myocardial infarction. ISIS-3 (Third International Study of Infarct Survival) Collaborative Group. Lancet 1992;339:753–770.

115. Bassand JP, Cassagnes J, Machecourt J et al. Comparative effects of APSAC and rt-PA on infarct size and left ventricular function in acute myocardial infarction. A multicenter randomized study. Circulation 1991;84:1107–1117.

116. Anderson JL, Becker LC, Sorenson SG et al. Anistreplase versus alteplase in acute myocardial infarction: comparative effects on left ventricular function, morbidity and 1-day coronary artery patency. The TEAM-3 Investigators. J Am Coll Cardiol 1992;20:753–766.

117. Cannon CP, McCabe CH, Diver DJ et al. Comparison of front-loaded recombinant tissue-type plasminogen activator, anistreplase and combination thrombolytic therapy for acute myocardial infarction: results of the Thrombolysis in Myocardial Infarction (TIMI) 4 trial. J Am Coll Cardiol 1994;24:1602–1610.

118. Neuhaus KL, von Essen R, Tebbe U et al. Improved thrombolysis in acute myocardial infarction with front-loaded administration of alteplase: results of the rt-PA-APSAC patency study (TAPS). J Am Coll Cardiol 1992;19:855–891.

119. O'Connor CM, Meese R, Carney R et al. A randomized trial of intravenous heparin in conjunction with anistreplase (anisoylated plasminogen streptokinase activator complex) in acute myocardial infarction: the Duke University Clinical Cardiology Study (DUCCS) 1. J Am Coll Cardiol 1994;23:11–18.

120. Brugemann J, van der Meer J, Bom VJ et al. Anti-streptokinase antibodies inhibit fibrinolytic effects of anistreplase in acute myocardial infarction. Am J Cardiol 1993;72:462–464.

121. Lee HS, Cross S, Davidson R et al. Raised levels of antistreptokinase antibody and neutralization titres from 4 days to 54 months after administration of streptokinase or anistreplase. Eur Heart J 1993;14:84–89.

122. Johnson ES, Cregeen RJ. An interim report of the efficacy and safety of anisoylated plasminogen streptokinase activator complex (APSAC). Drugs 1987;33(Suppl 3):298–311.

123. Collen D. Report of the Subcommittee on Fibrinolysis; San Diego, CA, July 13, 1985. Thromb Haemost 1985;54:893.

124. Robbins KC, Summaria L, Hseih B et al. The peptide chains of human plasmin: mechanism of activation of human plasminogen to plasmin. J Biol Chem 1967;242:2333–2342.

125. Husain S, Gurewich V, Lipinski B. Purification and partial characterization of a single-chain high-molecular-weight form of urokinase from human urine. Arch Biochem Biophys 1983;220:31–38.

126. Wun TC, Schleuning WD, Reich E. Isolation and characterization of urokinase from human plasma. J Biol Chem 1982;257:3276–3283.

127. Wun TC, Ossowski L, Reich E. A proenzyme form of human urokinase. J Biol Chem 1982;257:7262–7268.

128. Holmes WE, Pennica D, Blaber M et al. Cloning and expression of the gene for pro-urokinase in Escherichia coli. Biotechnology 1985;3:923–929.

129. Gunzler W, Steffens GJ, Otting F et al. The primary structure of high molecular mass urokinase from human urine. The complete amino acid sequence of the A chain. Hoppe Seylers Z Physiol Chem 1982;363:1155–1165.

130. Gunzler WA, Steffens GJ, Otting F et al. Structural relationship between human high and low molecular mass urokinase. Hoppe Seylers Z Physiol Chem 1982;363:133–141.

131. Riccio A, Grimaldi G, Verde P et al. The human urokinase-plasminogen activator gene and its promotor. Nucleic Acids Res 1985;13:2759–2771.

132. Hamelin J, Sarmientos P, Orsini G et al. Implication of cysteine residues in the activity of single chain urokinase-plasminogen activator. Biochem Biophys Res Commun 1993; 194:978–985.

133. de Munk GAW, Groeneveld E, Rijken DC. Comparison of the in vitro fibrinolytic activities of low and high molecular weight single-chain urokinase-type plasminogen activator. Thromb Haemost 1993;70:481–485.

134. Hansen AP, Petros AM, Meadows RP et al. Solution structure of the amino-terminal fragment of urokinase-type plasminogen activator. Biochemistry 1994;33:4847–4864.

135. Li X, Smith RA, Dobson CM. Sequential $^1$H NMR assignments and secondary structure of the kringle domain from urokinase. Biochemistry 1992;31:9562–9571.

136. Bokman AM, Jimenez-Barbero J, Llinas M. $^1$H NMR characterization of the urokinase kringle module. Structural, but not functional, relatedness to homologous domains. J Biol Chem 1993;268:13858–13868.

137. Li X, Bokman AM, Llinas M et al. Solution structure of the kringle domain from urokinase-type plasminogen activator. J Mol Biol 1994;235:1548–1559.

138. Spraggon G, Phillips C, Nowak UK et al. The crystal structure of the catalytic domain of human urokinase-type plasminogen activator. Structure 1995;3:681–691.

139. Collen D, Zamarron C, Lijnen HR et al. Activation of plasminogen by pro-urokinase II. Kinetics. J Biol Chem 1986;261:1259–1266.

140. Christensen U, Mullertz S. Kinetic studies of the urokinase catalysed conversion of $NH_2$-terminal lysine plasminogen to plasmin. Biochim Biophys Acta 1977;480:275–281.

141. Takada A, Takada Y, Sugawara Y. Effects of fibrinogen and fibrin on the activation of Glu- and Lys-plasminogen by urokinase. Thromb Res 1984;33:561–569.

142. Takada T, Watahiki Y, Takada Y. Release of the N-terminal peptides from Glu-plasminogen by plasmin in the presence of fibrin. Thromb Res 1986;41:819–827.

143. Lucas MA, Straight DL, Fretto LJ et al. The effects of fibrinogen and its

cleavage products on the kinetics of plasminogen activation by urokinase and subsequent plasmin activity. J Biol Chem 1983;258:12171–12177.

144. Markus G, Priore RL, Wissler FC. The binding of tranexamic acid to native (Glu) and modified (Lys) human plasminogen and its effect on conformation. J Biol Chem 1979;254:1211–1216.

145. Vali Z, Patthy L. The fibrin-binding site of human plasminogen. Arginines 32 and 34 are essential for fibrin affinity of the kringle 1 domain. J Biol Chem 1984;259:13690–13694.

146. Pannell R, Gurewich V. Activation of plasminogen by single-chain urokinase or by two-chain urokinase—a demonstration that single-chain urokinase has low catalytic activity (pro-urokinase). Blood 1987;69:22–26.

147. Liu JN, Gurewich V. Fragment E-2 from fibrin substantially enhances pro-urokinase-induced Glu-plasminogen activation. A kinetic study using the plasmin-resistant mutant pro-urokinase Ala-158-rpro-UK. Biochemistry 1992;31:6311–6317.

148. Lijnen HR, Zamarron C, Blaber M et al. Activation of plasminogen by pro-urokinase I. Mechanism. J Biol Chem 1986;261:1253–1258.

149. Stump DC, Lijnen HR, Collen D. Purification and characterization of single-chain urokinase-type plasminogen activator from human cell cultures. J Biol Chem 1986;261:1274–1278.

150. Ellis V, Scully MF, Kakkar VV. Plasminogen activation by single-chain urokinase in functional isolation—demonstration of a novel mechanism. Thromb Haemost 1987;58:108–112.

151. Lijnen HR, Zamarron C, Collen D. Characterization of the high affinity interaction between human plasminogen and pro-rokinase. Eur J Biochem 1985;150:141–144.

152. Nelles L, Lijnen HR, Collen D et al. Characterization of recombinant human single chain urokinase-ype plasminogen activator mutants produced by site-pecific mutagenesis of lysine 158. J Biol Chem 1987;262:5682–5689.

153. Pannell R, Gurewich V. Pro-urokinase: a study of its stability in plasma and of a mechanism for its selective fibrinolytic effect. Blood 1986;67:1215–1223.

154. Zamarron C, Lijnen HR, Van Hoef B et al. Biological and thrombolytic properties of proenzyme and active forms of urokinase-I. Fibrinolytic and fibrinogenolytic properties in human plasma in vitro of urokinases obtained from human urine or by recombinant DNA technology. Thromb Haemost 1984;52:19–23.

155. Gurewich V, Pannell R, Louie S et al. Effective and fibrin-specific clot lysis by a zymogen precursor form of urokinase (pro-urokinase). A study in vitro and in two animal species. J Clin Invest 1984;73:1731–1739.

156. Violand BN, Sodetz JM, Castellino FJ. The effect of ϵ-amino caproic acid on the gross conformation of plasminogen and plasmin. Arch Biochem Biophys 1975;170:300–305.

157. Pannell R, Black J, Gurewich V. Complementary modes of action of tissue-type plasminogen activator and pro-urokinase by which their synergistic effect on clot lysis may be explained. J Clin Invest 1988;81:853–859.

158. Gurewich V, Pannell R. Synergism of tissue-type plasminogen activator (t-PA) and single-chain urokinase-type plasminogen activator (scu-PA) on clot lysis in vitro and a mechanism for this effect [Letter]. Thromb Haemost 1987;57:372–373.

159. Miles LA, Levin EG, Plescia J et al. Plasminogen receptors, urokinase receptors, and their modulation on human endothelial cells. Blood 1988;72:628–635.

160. Pepper MS, Sappino AP, Stocklin R et al. Up-regulation of urokinase receptor expression on migrating endothelial cells. J Cell Biol 1993;122:673–684.

161. Plesner T, Ploug M, Ellis V et al. The receptor for urokinase-type plasminogen activator and urokinase is translocated from two distinct intracellular compartments to the plasma membrane on stimulation of human neutrophils. Blood 1994;83:808–815.

162. Nielsen LS, Kellerman GM, Behrendt N et al. A 55,000-60,000 Mr receptor protein for urokinase-type plasminogen activator. Identification in human tumor cell lines and partial purification. J Biol Chem 1988;236:2358–2363.

163. Ploug M, Ronne E, Behrendt N et al. Cellular receptor for urokinase plasminogen activator. Carboxylterminal processing and membrane anchoring by glycosyl-phosphatidylinositol. J Biol Chem 1991;266:1926–1933.

164. Ploug M, Kjalke M, Ronne E et al. Localization of the disulfide bonds in the NH₂-terminal domain of the cellular receptor for human urokinase-type plasminogen activator. A domain structure belonging to a novel superfamily of glycolipid-anchored membrane proteins. J Biol Chem 1993;268:17539–17546.

165. Stahl A, Mueller BM. The urokinase-type plasminogen activator receptor, a GP I-linked protein, is localized in caveolae. J Cell Biol 1995;129:335–344.

166. Plow EF, Freaney DE, Plescia J et al. The plasminogen system and cell surfaces: evidence for plasminogen and urokinase receptors on the same cell type. J Cell Biol 1986; 103:2411–2420.

167. Ellis V, Scully MF, Kakkar VV. Plasminogen activation initiated by single-chain urokinase-type plasminogen activator. Potentiation by U937 monocytes. J Biol Chem 1989;264:2185–2188.

168. Higazi AA, Cohen RL, Henkin J et al. Enhancement of the enzymatic activity of single-chain urokinase plasminogen activator by soluble urokinase receptor. J Biol Chem 1995;270:17375–17380.

169. Ellis V. Functional analysis of the cellular receptor for urokinase in plas-

170. Ellis V, Behrendt N, Dano K. Plasminogen activation by receptor-bound urokinase. A kinetic study with both cell-associated and isolated receptor. J Biol Chem 1991;266:12752–12758.

171. Ellis V, Dano K. Potentiation of plasminogen activation by an anti-urokinase monoclonal antibody due to ternary complex formation. A mechanistic model for receptor-mediated plasminogen activation. J Biol Chem 1993;268:4806–4813.

172. Lee SW, Ellis V, Dichek DA. Characterization of plasminogen activation by glycosylphosphatidylinositol-anchored urokinase. J Biol Chem 1994;269:2411–2418.

173. Heegaard CW, Simonsen AC, Oka K et al. Very low density lipoprotein receptor binds and mediates endocytosis of urokinase-type plasminogen activator-type-1 plasminogen activator inhibitor complex. J Biol Chem 1995;270:20855–20861.

174. Nykjaer A, Petersen CM, Moller B et al. Purified ₂-macroglobulin receptor / LDL receptor-related protein binds urokinase plasminogen activator inhibitor type-1 complex. Evidence that the ₂-macroglobulin receptor mediates cellular degradation of urokinase receptor-bound complexes. J Biol Chem 1992;267:14543–14546.

175. Stefansson S, Kounnas MZ, Henkin J et al. gp330 on type II pneumocytes mediates endocytosis leading to degradation of pro-urokinase, plasminogen activator inhibitor-1 and urokinase-plasminogen activator inhibitor-1 complex. J Cell Sci 1995;108:2361–2368.

176. Horn IR, Moestrup SK, van den Berg BM et al. Analysis of the binding of pro-urokinase and urokinase-plasminogen activator inhibitor-1 complex to the low density lipoprotein receptor-related protein using a F_ab fragment selected from a phage-displayed F_ab library. J Biol Chem 1995;270:11770–11775.

177. Nykjaer A, Kjoller L, Cohen RL et al. Regions involved in binding of urokinase-type-1 inhibitor complex and pro-urokinase to the endocytic α₂-macroglobulin receptor / low density lipoprotein receptor-related protein. Evidence that the urokinase receptor protects pro-urokinase against binding to the endocytic receptor. J Biol Chem 1994;269:25668–25676.

178. Higazi AA, Mazar A, Wang J et al. Single-chain urokinase-type plasminogen activator bound to its receptor is relatively resistant to plasminogen activator inhibitor type 1. Blood 1996;87:3545–3549.

179. Manchanda N, Schwartz BS. Interaction of single-chain urokinase and plasminogen activator inhibitor type 1. J Biol Chem 1995;270:20032–20035.

180. Conese M, Olson D, Blasi F. Protease nexin-1-urokinase complexes are internalized and degraded through a mechanism that requires both urokinase receptor and α₂-macroglobulin receptor. J Biol Chem 1994;269:17886–17892.

181. Fears R. Kinetic studies on the effect of heparin and fibrin on plasminogen activators. Biochem J 1988;249:77–81.

182. Lijnen HR, Collen D. Stimulation by heparin of the plasmin-mediated conversion of single-chain and two-chain urokinase-type plasminogen activator. Thromb Res 1986;43:687–690.

183. Dosne AM, Bendetowicz AV, Kher A et al. Marked potentiation of the plasminogenolytic activity of pro-urokinase by unfractionated heparin and a low-molecular-weight heparin. Thromb Res 1988;51:627–630.

184. Urano T, Serizawa K, Takada Y et al. Heparin and heparan sulfate enhancement of the inhibitory activity of plasminogen activator inhibitor type-1 toward urokinase type plasminogen activator. Biochim Biophys Acta 1994;1201:217–222.

185. Van de Werf F, Nobuhara M, Collen D. Coronary thrombolysis with human single-chain, urokinase-type plasminogen activator (pro-urokinase) in individuals with acute myocardial infarction. Ann Intern Med 1986;104:345–348.

186. Stump DC, Kieckens L, De Cock F et al. Pharmacokinetics of single-chain forms of urokinase-type plasminogen activator. J Pharmacol Exp Ther 1987;242:245–250.

187. Kohler M, Sen S, Miyashita C et al. Half-life of single-chain urokinase-type plasminogen activator (scu-PA) and two chain urokinase-type plasminogen activator (tcu-PA) in patients with acute myocardial infarction. Thromb Res 1991;62:75–81.

188. Collen D, De Cock F, Lijnen HR. Biological and thrombolytic properties of proenzyme and active forms of human urokinase-II. Turnover of natural and recombinant urokinase in rabbits and squirrel monkeys. Thromb Haemost 1984;52:24–26.

189. Mannucci PM. Thrombolytic therapy of acute deep vein thrombosis of the lower limbs: choices, indications and limits. [Review]. Ric Clin Lab 1984;14:593–599.

190. van de Loo JC, Kreissmann A, Trubestein G et al. Controlled multicenter pilot study of urokinase-heparin and streptokinase in deep venous thrombosis. Thromb Haemost 1983;50:660–663.

191. Valji K, Roberts AC, Davis GB et al. Pulsed-spray thrombolysis of arterial and bypass graft occlusions. Am J Roentgenol 1991;156:617–621.

192. Aburahma AF, Sadler D, Stuart P et al. Conventional versus thrombolytic therapy in spontaneous (effort) axillary-subclavian vein thrombosis. Am J Surg 1991;161:459–465.

minogen activation. Receptor binding has no influence on the zymogenic nature of the pro-urokinase. J Biol Chem 1996;271:14779–14784.

193. Eisenbud DE, Brener BJ, Shoenfeld R et al. Treatment of acute vascular occlusions with intra-arterial urokinase. Am J Surg 1990;160:160–164.

194. Hartmann JR, McKeever LS, O'Neill WW et al. Recanalization of chronically occluded aortocoronary saphenous vein bypass grafts with long-term, low dose direct infusion of urokinase (ROBUST): a serial trial. J Am Coll Cardiol 1996;27:60–66.

195. Jungreis CA, Wechsler LR, Horton JA. Intracranial thrombolysis via a catheter embedded in the clot. Stroke 1989;20:1578–1580.

196. Schoebel FC, Leschke M, Jax TW et al. Chronic-intermittent urokinase therapy in patients with end-stage coronary artery disease and refractory angina pectoris—a pilot study. Clin Cardiol 1996;19:115–120.

197. Schreiber TL, Macina G, McNulty A et al. Urokinase plus heparin versus aspirin in unstable angina and non-Q-wave myocardial infarction. Am J Cardiol 1989;64:840–844.

198. Rossi P, Bolognese L. Comparison of intravenous urokinase plus heparin versus heparin alone in acute myocardial infarction. Urochinasi per via Sistemica nell'Infarto Miocardico (USIM) Collaborative Group. Am J Cardiol 1991;68:585–592.

199. Wall TC, Phillips HR III, Stack RS et al. Results of high dose intravenous urokinase for acute myocardial infarction. Am J Cardiol 1990;65:124–131.

200. Goudreau E, DiSciascio G, Vetrovec GW et al. Intracoronary urokinase as an adjunct to percutaneous transluminal coronary angioplasty in patients with complex coronary narrowings or angioplasty-induced complications. Am J Cardiol 1992;69:57–62.

201. Morishita H, Hattori R, Aoyama T et al. The intracoronary administration of urokinase following direct PTCA for acute myocardial infarction reduces early restenosis. Am Heart J 1992;123:1153–1156.

202. Cecena FA. Urokinase infusion after unsuccessful angioplasty in patients with chronic total occlusion of native coronary arteries. Cathet Cardiovasc Diagn 1993;28:214–218.

203. Zidar FJ, Kaplan BM, O'Neill WW et al. Prospective, randomized trial of prolonged intracoronary urokinase infusion for chronic total occlusions in native coronary arteries. J Am Coll Cardiol 1996;27:1406–1412.

204. Goldhaber SZ, Polak JF, Feldstein ML et al. Efficacy and safety of repeated boluses of urokinase in the treatment of deep venous thrombosis. Am J Cardiol 1994;73:75–79.

205. Goldhaber SZ, Hirsch DR, MacDougall RC et al. Bolus recombinant urokinase versus heparin in deep venous thrombosis: a randomized controlled trial. Am Heart J 1996;132:314–318.

206. Moia M, Mannucci PM, Pini M et al. A pilot study of pro-urokinase in the treatment of deep vein thrombosis. Thromb Haemost 1994;72:430–433.

207. Meyer G, Sors H, Charbonnier B et al. Effects of intravenous urokinase versus alteplase on total pulmonary resistance in acute massive pulmonary embolism: a European multicenter double-blind trial. The European Cooperative Study Group for Pulmonary Embolism. J Am Coll Cardiol 1992;19:239–245.

208. Gonzalez-Juanatey JR, Valdes L, Amaro A et al. Treatment of massive pulmonary thromboembolism with low intrapulmonary dosages of urokinase. Short-term angiographic and hemodynamic evolution. Chest 1992;102:341–346.

209. Parent FN, Piotrowski JJ, Bernhard VM et al. Outcome of intraarterial urokinase for acute vascular occlusion. J Cardiovasc Surg 1991;32:680–689.

210. McNamara TO, Bomberger RA, Merchant RF. Intra-arterial urokinase as the initial therapy for acutely ischemic lower limbs. Circulation 1991;83(Suppl 2):I106–I119.

211. Comerota AJ, Weaver FA, Hosking JD et al. Results of a prospective, randomized trial of surgery versus thrombolysis for occluded lower extremity bypass grafts. Am J Surg 1996;172:105–112.

212. Ikeda Y, Rummel MC, Bhatnagar PK et al. Thrombolysis therapy in individuals with femoropopliteal synthetic graft occlusions. Am J Surg 1996;171:251–254.

213. Ouriel K, Veith FJ, Sasahara AA. Thrombolysis or peripheral arterial surgery: phase I results. TOPAS Investigators. J Vasc Surg 1996;23:64–73.

214. Cohen MA, Kumpe DA, Durham JD, Zwerdlinger SC. Improved treatment of thrombosed hemodialysis access sites with thrombolysis and angioplasty. Kidney Int 1994;46:1375–1380.

215. Berger MF, Aruny JE, Skibo LK. Recurrent thrombosis of polytetrafluoroethylene dialysis fistulas after recent surgical thrombectomy: salvage by means of thrombolysis and angioplasty. J Vasc Intervent Radiol 1994;5:725–730.

216. Hartmann JR, McKeever LS, O'Neill WW et al. Recanalization of chronically occluded aortocoronary saphenous vein bypass grafts with long-term, low dose direct infusion of urokinase (ROBUST): a serial trial. J Am Coll Cardiol 1996;27:60–66.

217. Hartmann JR. Urokinase recanalization of chronically occluded aortocoronary vein grafts. Coronary Artery Dis 1996;7:641–648.

218. Comerota AJ, Weaver FA, Hosking JD et al. Results of a prospective, randomized trial of surgery versus thrombolysis for occluded lower extremity bypass grafts. Am J Surg 1996; 172:105–112.

219. Neuhaus KL, Tebbe U, Gottwik M et al. Intravenous recombinant tissue plasminogen activator (rt-PA) and urokinase in acute myocardial infarction: results of the German Activator Urokinase Study (GAUS). J Am Coll Cardiol 1988;12:581–587.

220. Kanemoto N, Goto Y, Hirosawa K et al. Intravenous recombinant tissue-type plasminogen activator (rt-PA) and urokinase (UK) in patients with evolving myocardial infarction—a multicenter double-blind randomized trial in Japan. Jpn Circ J 1991;55:250–261.

221. Motomiya T, Tokuyasu Y, Watanabe K et al. Intracoronary urokinase in acute myocardial infarction: prevalence of total coronary occlusion during the early hours, effects on myocardial infarct size and left ventricular function, and outcome of residual coronary stenosis. Jpn Circ J 1988;52:702–708.

222. Kambara H, Kawai C, Kajiwara N et al. Randomized, double-blinded multicenter study. Comparison of intracoronary single-chain urokinase-type plasminogen activator, pro-urokinase (GE-0943), and intracoronary urokinase in patients with acute myocardial infarction. Circulation 1988;78:899–905.

223. Gulba DC, Fischer K, Reil GH et al. Potentiation of the thrombolytic efficacy of single-chain urokinase (pro-urokinase) by heparin. Thromb Haemost 1988;60:350–351.

224. Diefenbach C, Erbel R, Pop T et al. Recombinant single-chain urokinase-type plasminogen activator during acute myocardial infarction. Am J Cardiol 1988;61:966–970.

225. Kasper W, Hohnloser SH, Engler H et al. Coronary reperfusion studies with pro-urokinase in acute myocardial infarction: evidence for synergism of low dose urokinase. J Am Coll Cardiol 1990;16:733–738.

226. Anonymous. Randomised double-blind trial of recombinant pro-urokinase against streptokinase in acute myocardial infarction. PRIMI Trial Study Group. Lancet 1989;i:863–868.

227. Loscalzo J, Wharton TP, Kirshenbaum JM et al. Clot-selective coronary thrombolysis with pro-urokinase. Circulation 1989;79:776–782.

228. Bode C, Schoenermark S, Schuler G et al. Efficacy of intravenous prourokinase and a combination of prourokinase and urokinase in acute myocardial infarction. Am J Cardiol 1988;61:971–974.

229. Ostermann H, Schmitz-Huebner U, Windeler J et al. Rate of fibrinogen breakdown related to coronary patency and bleeding complications in patients with thrombolysis in acute myocardial infarction—results from the PRIMI trial. Eur Heart J 1992;13:1225–1232.

230. Schofer J, Lins M, Mathey DG et al. Time course of left ventricular function and coronary patency after saruplase vs streptokinase in acute myocardial infarction. The PRIMI Trial Study Group. Eur Heart J 1993;14:958–963.

231. Bode C, Schuler G, Nordt T et al. Intravenous thrombolytic therapy with a combination of single-chain urokinase-type plasminogen activator and recombinant tissue-type plasminogen activator in acute myocardial infarction. Circulation 1990;81:907–913.

232. Rijken DC, Wijngaards G, Zaal-De Jong M et al. Purification and partial characterization of plasminogen activator from human uterine tissue. Biochim Biophys Acta 1979;580:140–153.

233. Rijken DC, Wijngaards G, Welbergen J. Relationship between tissue plasminogen activator and the activators in blood and vascular wall. Thromb Res 1980;18:815–830.

234. Gurewich V, Black J. Pannell R. A mechanism for the potentiating effect of urokinase (UK) or tissue plasminogen activator (t-PA) on clot lysis by pro-urokinase (pro-UK). Thromb Haemost 1987;58:Abstract 1615.

235. Collen D, Van de Werf F. Coronary arterial thrombolysis with low-dose synergistic combinations of recombinant tissue-type plasminogen activator (rt-PA) and recombinant single-chain urokinase-type plasminogen activator (rscu-PA) for acute myocardial infarction. Am J Cardiol 1987;60:431–434.

236. Pindur G, Koehler M, Sen S et al. Fibrinolytic effects of pro-urokinase combined with low-dose urokinase compared to high-dose urokinase in individuals with acute myocardial infarction. Thromb Res 1992;67:191–200.

237. Weaver WD, Hartmann JR, Anderson JL et al. New recombinant glycosylated prourokinase for treatment of patients with acute myocardial infarction. Prourokinase Study Group. J Am Coll Cardiol 1994;24:1242–1248.

238. Zarich SW, Kowalchuk GJ, Weaver WD et al. Sequential combination thrombolytic therapy for acute myocardial infarction: results of the Pro-Urokinase and t-PA Enhancement of Thrombolysis (PATENT) Trial. J Am Coll Cardiol 1995;26:374–379.

239. Sasahara AA, Barker WM, Weaver WD et al. Clinical studies with the new glycosylated recombinant prourokinase. J Vasc Intervent Radiol 1995;6:84S–93S.

240. Bar FW, Meyer J, Vermeer F et al. Comparison of saruplase and alteplase in acute myocardial infarction. SESAM Study Group. The Study in Europe with Saruplase and Alteplase in Myocardial Infarction. Am J Cardiol 1997;79:727–732.

241. Levin EG, Loskutoff DJ. Cultured bovine endothelial cells produce both urokinase and tissue-type plasminogen activators. J Cell Biol 1982;94:631–636.

242. Collen D, Rijken DC, Van Damme J et al. Purification of human tissue-type plasminogen activator in centigram quantities from human melanoma cell culture fluid and its conditioning for use in vivo. Thromb Haemost 1982;48:294–296.

243. Pennica D, Holmes WE, Kohr WJ et al. Cloning and expression of human

tissue-type plasminogen activator cDNA in E. coli. Nature 1983;301: 214–221.

244. Lijnen HR, Collen D. Mechanisms of plasminogen activation by mammalian plasminogen activators. Enzyme 1988;40:90–96.

245. Pohl G, Einarsson M, Nilsson B et al. The size heterogeneity in melanoma tissue plasminogen activator is caused by carbohydrate differences. Thromb Res 1988;50:163–168.

246. Ichinose A, Kisiel W, Fujikawa K. Proteolytic activation of tissue plasminogen activator by plasma and tissue enzymes. FEBS Lett 1984;175:412–418.

247. Ny T, Elgh F, Lund B. The structure of the human tissue-type plasminogen activator gene: correlation of intron and exon structures to functional and structural domains. Proc Natl Acad Sci U S A 1984;81:5355–5359.

248. Downing AK, Driscoll PC, Harvey TS et al. Solution structure of the fibrin binding finger domain of tissue-type plasminogen activator determined by $^1$H nuclear magnetic resonance. J Mol Biol 1992;225:821–833.

249. Smith BO, Downing AK, Dudgeon TJ et al. Secondary structure of fibronectin type 1 and epidermal growth factor modules from tissue-type plasminogen activator by nuclear magnetic resonance. Biochemistry 1994;33: 2422–2429.

250. Smith BO, Downing AK, Driscoll PC et al. The solution structure and backbone dynamics of the fibronectin type I and epidermal growth factor-like pair of modules of tissue-type plasminogen activator. Structure 1995; 3:823–833.

251. De Serrano VS, Sehl LC, Castellino FJ. Direct identification of lysine-33 as the principal cationic center of the ω-amino acid binding site of the recombinant kringle 2 domain of tissue-type plasminogen activator. Arch Biochem Biophys 1992;292:206–212.

252. Byeon IJ, Kelley RF, Mulkerrin MG et al. Ligand binding to the tissue-type plasminogen activator kringle 2 domain: structural characterization by $^1$H-NMR. Biochemistry 1995;34:2739–2750.

253. Bakker AH, Rehberg EF, Marotti KR et al. The position of the structurally autonomous kringle 2 domain influences the functional features of tissue-type plasminogen activator. Protein Eng 1995;8:293–300.

254. Lamba D, Bauer M, Huber R et al. The 2.3 A crystal structure of the catalytic domain of recombinant two-chain human tissue-type plasminogen activator. J Mol Biol 1996;258:117–135.

255. Hoylaerts M, Rijken DC, Lijnen HR et al. Kinetics of the activation of plasminogen by human tissue plasminogen activator. Role of fibrin. J Biol Chem 1982;257:2912–2919.

256. Rijken DC, Hoylaerts M, Collen D. Fibrinolytic properties of one-chain and two-chain human extrinsic (tissue-type) plasminogen activator. J Biol Chem 1982;257:2920–2925.

257. Ranby M. Studies on the kinetics of plasminogen activation by tissue plasminogen activator. Biochim Biophys Acta 1982;704:461–469.

258. Nieuwenhuizen W, Voskuilen M, Vermond A et al. The influence of fibrin-(ogen) fragments on the kinetic parameters of the tissue-type plasminogen-activator-mediated activation of different forms of plasminogen. Eur J Biochem 1988;174:163–169.

259. Wallen P, Bergsdorf N, Ranby M. Purification and identification of two structural variants of porcine tissue plasminogen activator by affinity adsorption on fibrin. Biochim Biophys Acta 1982;719:318–328.

260. Loscalzo J. Structural and kinetic comparison of recombinant human single- and two-chain tissue plasminogen activator. J Clin Invest 1988;82: 1391–1397.

261. Rijken DC, Groeneveld E. Isolation and functional characterization of the heavy and light chains of human tissue-type plasminogen activator. J Biol Chem 1986;261:3098–3102.

262. Fleury V, Loyau S, Lijnen HR et al. Molecular assembly of plasminogen and tissue-type plasminogen activator on an evolving fibrin surface. Eur J Biochem 1993;216:549–556.

263. Madison EL, Coombs GS, Corey DR. Substrate specificity of tissue type plasminogen activator. Characterization of the fibrin independent specificity of t-PA for plasminogen. J Biol Chem 1995;270:7558–7562.

264. Zamarron C, Lijnen HR, Collen D. Kinetics of the activation of plasminogen by natural and recombinant tissue-type plasminogen activator. J Biol Chem 1984;259:2080–2083.

265. Bauer R, Hansen SL, Jones G et al. Fibrin structures during tissue-type plasminogen activator-mediated fibrinolysis studied by laser light scattering: relation to fibrin enhancement of plasminogen activation. Eur Biophys J 1994;23:239–252.

266. Soeda S, Kakiki M, Shimeno H et al. Some properties of tissue-type plasminogen activator reconstituted onto phospholipid and/or glycolipid vesicles. Biochem Biophys Res Commun 1987;146:94–100.

267. Stricker RB, Wong D, Shiu DT et al. Activation of plasminogen by tissue plasminogen activator on normal and thromboasthenic platelets: effects on surface proteins and platelet aggregation. Blood 1986;68:275–280.

268. Gao SW, Morser J, McLean K et al. Differential effect of platelets on plasminogen activation by tissue plasminogen activator, urokinase, and streptokinase. Thromb Res 1990;58:421–433.

269. Hajjar KA, Hamel NM, Harpel PC et al. Binding of tissue plasminogen activator to cultured human endothelial cells. J Clin Invest 1987;80: 1712–1719.

270. Felez J, Chanquia CJ, Levin EG et al. Binding of tissue plasminogen activator to human monocytes and monocytoid cells. Blood 1991;78:2318–2327.

271. Angles-Cano E. Hervio L, Rouy D et al. Effects of lipoprotein(a) on the binding of plasminogen to fibrin and its activation by fibrin-bound tissue-type plasminogen activator. Chem Phys Lipids 1994;67–68:369–380.

272. Reilly CF, Hutzelmann JE. Plasminogen activator inhibitor-1 binds to fibrin and inhibits tissue-type plasminogen activator-mediated fibrin dissolution. J Biol Chem 1992;267:17128–17135.

273. Kaneko M, Sakata Y, Matsuda M et al. Interactions between the finger and kringle-2 domains of tissue-type plasminogen activator and plasminogen activator inhibitor-1. J Biochem 1992;111:244–248.

274. Andrade-Gordon P, Strickland S. Interaction of heparin with plasminogen activators and plasminogen: effects on the activation of plasminogen. Biochemistry 1986;25:4033–4040.

275. Soeda S, Kakiki M, Shimeno H et al. Localization of the binding sites of porcine tissue-type plasminogen activator and plasminogen to heparin. Biochim Biophys Acta 1987;916:279–287.

276. Paques EP, Stohr HA, Heimburger N. Study on the mechanism of action of heparin and related substances on the fibrinolytic system: relationship between plasminogen activators and plasminogen. Thromb Res 1986;42: 797–807.

277. Soeda S, Sakaguchi S, Shimeno H et al. Tissue plasminogen activator catalyzed Lys-plasminogen activation on heparin-inserted phospholipid liposomes. Biochemistry 1990;29:5188–5194.

278. Edelberg JM, Pizzo SV. Kinetic analysis of the effects of heparin and lipoproteins on tissue plasminogen activator mediated plasminogen activation. Biochemistry 1990; 29:5906–5911.

279. Larsen GR, Metzger M, Henson K et al. Pharmacokinetic and distribution analysis of variant forms of tissue-type plasminogen activator with prolonged clearance in rat. Blood 1989; 73:1842–1850.

280. Garabedian HD, Gold HK, Leinbach RC et al. Comparative properties of two clinical preparations of recombinant human tissue-type plasminogen activator in patients with acute myocardial infarction. J Am Coll Cardiol 1987;9:599–607.

281. Collen D, Stassen JM, Marafino BJ Jr et al. Biological properties of human tissue-type plasminogen activator obtained by expression of recombinant DNA in mammalian cells. J Pharmacol Exp Ther 1984;231:146–152.

282. Allen S, Naim HY, Bulleid NJ. Intracellular folding of tissue-type plasminogen activator. Effects of disulfide bond formation on N-linked glycosylation and secretion. J Biol Chem 1995;270:4797–4804.

283. Martin U, Fischer S, Kohnert U et al. Pharmacokinetic and thrombolytic properties of unglycosylated recombinant tissue-type plasminogen activator (BM 06.021) produced in Escherichia coli. Naunyn-Schmiedebergs Arch Pharmakol 1992;346:108–113.

284. Kopia GA, Kopaciewicz LJ, Fong KL et al. Evaluation of the acute hemodynamic effects and pharmacokinetics of coronary thrombolysis produced by intravenous tissue-type plasminogen activator in the anesthetized dog. J Cardiovasc Pharmacol 1988;12:308–316.

285. Verstraete M, Su CA, Tanswell P et al. Pharmacokinetics and effects on fibrinolytic and coagulation parameters of two doses of recombinant tissue-type plasminogen activator in healthy volunteers. Thromb Haemost 1986;56;1–5.

286. Fuchs HE, Berger H Jr, Pizzo SV. Catabolism of human tissue plasminogen activator in mice. Blood 1985;65:539–544.

287. Tanswell P, Tebbe U, Neuhaus KL et al. Pharmacokinetics and fibrin specificity of alteplase during accelerated infusions in acute myocardial infarction. J Am Coll Cardiol 1992;19:1071–1075.

288. Paoni NF, Keyt BA, Refino CJ et al. A slow clearing, fibrin specific, PAI-1 resistant variant of t-PA (T103N, KHRR 296-299 AAAA). Thromb Haemost 1993;70:307–312.

289. Keyt BA, Paoni NF, Refino CJ et al. A faster-acting and more potent form of tissue plasminogen activator. Proc Natl Acad Sci U S A 1994;91:3670–3674.

290. Korninger C, Stassen JM, Collen D. Turnover of human extrinsic (tissue-type) plasminogen activator in rabbits. Thromb Haemost 1981;46:658–661.

291. Bounameaux H, Stassen JM, Seghers C et al. Influence of fibrin and liver blood flow on the turnover and the systemic fibrinogenolytic effects of recombinant human tissue-type plasminogen activator in rabbits. Blood 1986;67:1493–1497.

292. Camani C, Kruithof EK. Clearance receptors for tissue-type plasminogen activator [Review]. Int J Hematol 1994;60:97–109.

293. Orth K, Willnow T, Herz J et al. Low density lipoprotein receptor-related protein is necessary for the internalization of both tissue-type plasminogen activator-inhibitor complexes and free tissue-type plasminogen activator. J Biol Chem 1994;269:21117–21122.

294. Chandler WL, Alessi MC, Aillaud MF, Henderson P, Vague P, Juhan-Vague I. Clearance of tissue plasminogen activator (TPA) and TPA/plasminogen activator inhibitor type 1 (PAI-1) complex. Circulation 1997;96: 761–768.

295. Turpie AGG. Thrombolysis in deep vein thrombosis. In: Juhan D, Kubler W, Norms RM et al eds. Thrombolysis in cardiovascular disease. Basal/ New York: Marcel Dekker, 1989:397–416.

296. Turpie AGG. Thrombolysis in deep vein thrombosis. In: Julian D, Kubler

W, Norns RM et al., eds. Thrombolysis in cardiovascular disease. Basel/New York: Marcel Dekker, 1989:397.

297. Zimmerman R, Horn A, Harenberg J. Thrombolysetherapy der tiefen venosen thrombose mit rt-PA. Klin Wochenschr 1988;66(Suppl XII):137–142.

298. Collen D, Topol EJ, Tiefenbrunn AJ et al. Coronary thrombolysis with recombinant human tissue-type plasminogen activator: a prospective, randomized, placebo-controlled trial. Circulation 1984;70:1012–1017.

299. Anonymous. The thrombolysis in myocardial infarction (TIMI) trial. Phase I findings. N Engl J Med 1985;312:932–936.

300. Williams DO, Borer J, Braunwald E et al. Intravenous recombinant tissue-type plasminogen activator in patients with acute myocardial infarction: a report from the NHLBI thrombolysis in myocardial infarction trial. Circulation 1986;73:338–346.

301. Mueller HS, Rao AK, Forman SA. Thrombolysis in myocardial infarction (TIMI): Comparative studies of coronary reperfusion and systemic fibrinogenolysis with two forms of recombinant tissue-type plasminogen activator. J Am Coll Cardiol 1987;10:479–490.

302. Verstraete M, Arnold AE, Brower RW et al. Acute coronary thrombolysis with recombinant human tissue-type plasminogen activator: initial patency and influence of maintained infusion on reocclusion rate. Am J Cardiol 1987;60:231–237.

303. Gold HK, Johns JA, Leinbach RC et al. Thrombolytic therapy for unstable angina pectoris: rationale and results [Review]. J Am Coll Cardiol 1987; 10(Suppl B):91B–95B.

304. Marder VJ, Francis CW. Thrombolytic therapy for acute transmural myocardial infarction. Am J Med 1984;77:921–928.

305. Van de Werf F, Arnold AE. Intravenous tissue plasminogen activator and size of infarct, left ventricular function, and survival in acute myocardial infarction. Br Med J 1988;297:1374–1379.

306. Rentrop KP, Feit F, Blanke H. Effects of intracoronary streptokinase and intracoronary nitroglycerin infusion on coronary angiographic patterns and mortality in patients with acute myocardial infarction. N Engl J Med 1984;311:1457–1463.

307. Braunwald E. Myocardial reperfusion, limitation of infarct size, reduction of left ventricular dysfunction and improved survival. Should the paradigm be expanded? Circulation 1989;79:441–444.

308. Verdouw PD, Hagemeijer F, Dorp WG et al. Short-term survival after acute myocardial infarction predicted by hemodynamic parameters. Circulation 1975;52:413–419.

309. Guerci AD, Gerstenblith G, Brinker JA et al. A randomized trial of intravenous tissue plasminogen activator for acute myocardial infarction with subsequent randomization to elective coronary angioplasty. N Engl J Med 1987;317:1613–1618.

310. Turpie AG, Jay RM, Carter CJ et al. A randomized trial of recombinant tissue-type plasminogen activator for the treatment of proximal deep vein thrombosis. Circulation 1985;72:III-193.

311. Turpie AG, Levine MN, Hirsh J et al. Tissue plasminogen activator (rt-PA) vs heparin in deep vein thrombosis. Results of a randomized trial. Chest 1990;97(Suppl 4):172S–175S.

312. Goldhaber SZ, Vaughan DE, Markis JE et al. Acute pulmonary embolism treated with tissue plasminogen activator. Lancet 1986;ii:886–889.

313. Come PC, Kim D, Parker JA et al. Early reversal of right ventricular dysfunction in individuals with acute pulmonary embolism after treatment with intravenous tissue plasminogen activator. J Am Coll Cardiol 1987; 10:971–978.

314. Diehl JL, Meyer G, Igual J et al. Effectiveness and safety of bolus administration of alteplase in massive pulmonary embolism. Am J Cardiol 1992: 70:1477–1480.

315. Goldhaber SZ, Agnelli G, Levine MN. Reduced bolus alteplase vs conventional alteplase infusion for pulmonary embolism thrombolysis. An international multicenter randomized trial. The Bolus Alteplase Pulmonary Embolism Group. Chest 1994;106:718–724.

316. Sors H, Pacouret G, Azarian R et al. Hemodynamic effects of bolus versus 2-h infusion of alteplase in acute massive pulmonary embolism. A randomized controlled multicenter trial. Chest 1994;106:712–717.

317. Yamasawa F, Okada Y, Asano K et al. The role of recombinant human tissue-type plasminogen activator in the treatment of acute pulmonary thromboembolism. Intern Med 1992;31:885–888.

318. Goldhaber SZ, Haire WD, Feldstein ML et al. Alteplase versus heparin in acute pulmonary embolism: randomised trial assessing right-ventricular function and pulmonary perfusion. Lancet 1993;341:507–511.

319. Dalla-Volta S, Palla A, Santolicandro A et al. PAIMS 2: alteplase combined with heparin versus heparin in the treatment of acute pulmonary embolism. Plasminogen activator Italian multicenter study 2. J Am Coll Cardiol 1992;20:520–526.

320. Brott TG, Haley EC Jr, Levy DE et al. Urgent therapy for stroke. Part I. Pilot study of tissue plasminogen activator administered within 90 minutes. Stroke 1992;23:632–640.

321. Haley EC Jr, Levy DE, Brott TG et al. Urgent therapy for stroke. Part II. Pilot study of tissue plasminogen activator administered 91-180 minutes from onset. Stroke 1992;23:641–645.

322. Hacke W, Kaste M, Fieschi C et al. Intravenous thrombolysis with recombinant tissue plasminogen activator for acute hemispheric stroke. The Euro-

pean Cooperative Acute Stroke Study (ECASS). JAMA 1995;274: 1017–1025.

323. Anonymous. Tissue plasminogen activator for acute ischemic stroke. The National Institute of Neurological Disorders and Stroke rt-PA Stroke Study Group. New Engl J Med 1995;333:1581–1587.

324. Tebbe U, Tanswell P, Siefried E et al. Single-bolus injection of recombinant tissue-type plasminogen activator in acute myocardial infarction. Am J Cardiol 1989;64:448–453.

325. O'Rourke M, Baron D, Keogh A et al. Limitation of myocardial infarction by early infusion of recombinant tissue-type plasminogen activator. Circulation 1988;77:1311–1315.

326. Anonymous. Coronary thrombolysis and myocardial salvage by tissue plasminogen activator given up to 4 hours after onset of myocardial infarction. National Heart Foundation of Australia Coronary Thrombolysis Group. Lancet 1988;i:203–208.

327. Wilcox RG, von der Lippe G, Olsson CG et al. Trial of tissue plasminogen activator for mortality reduction in acute myocardial infarctions. Anglo-Scandinavian Study of Early Thrombolysis (ASSET). Lancet 1988;ii: 525–530.

328. Neuhaus KL, Feurer W, Jeep-Tebbe S et al. Improved thrombolysis with a modified dose regimen of recombinant tissue-type plasminogen activator. J Am Coll Cardiol 1989;14:1566–1569.

329. Purvis JA, McNeill AJ, Siddiqui RA et al. Efficacy of 100 mg of double-bolus alteplase in achieving complete perfusion in the treatment of acute myocardial infarction. J Am Coll Cardiol 1994;23:6–10.

330. Anonymous. Clinical experience with intracoronary tissue plasminogen activator: results of a multicenter registry. Intracoronary t-PA Registry Investigators. Cathet Cardiovasc Diagn 1995;34:196–201.

331. Anonymous. Late Assessment of Thrombolytic Efficacy (LATE) study with alteplase 6-24 hours after onset of acute myocardial infarction. Lancet 1993;342:759–766.

332. Berger H Jr, Pizzo SV. Preparation of polyethylene glycol-tissue plasminogen activator adducts that retain functional activity: characteristics and behavior in three animal species. Blood 1988;71:1641–1647.

333. Anonymous. GISSI-2: A factorial randomised trial of alteplase versus streptokinase and heparin versus no heparin among 12,490 individuals with acute myocardial infarction. Gruppo Italiano per lo Studio della Sopravvivenza nell'Infarto Miocardico. Lancet 1990;336:65–71.

334. Anonymous. An international randomized trial comparing four thrombolytic strategies for acute myocardial infarction. The GUSTO investigators. N Engl J Med 1993;329:673–682.

335. Grines CL, Browne KF, Marco J et al. A comparison of immediate angioplasty with thrombolytic therapy for acute myocardial infarction. The Primary Angioplasty in Myocardial Infarction Study Group. N Engl J Med 1993;328:673–679.

336. Anonymous. A clinical trial comparing primary coronary angioplasty with tissue plasminogen activator for acute myocardial infarction. The Global Use of Strategies to Open Occluded Coronary Arteries in Acute Coronary Syndromes (GUSTO IIb) Angioplasty Substudy Investigators. New Engl J Med 1997;336:1621–1628.

337. Gibbons RJ, Holmes DR, Reeder GS et al. Immediate angioplasty compared with the administration of a thrombolytic agent followed by conservative treatment for myocardial infarction. N Eng J Med 1993;328: 685–691.

338. Stone GW, Grines CL, Browne KF et al. Influence of acute myocardial infarction location on in-hospital and late outcome after primary percutaneous transluminal coronary angioplasty versus tissue plasminogen activator therapy. Am J Cardiol 1996;78:19–25.

339. Steinberg JS, Hochman JS, Morgan CD et al. Effects of thrombolytic therapy administered 6 to 24 hours after myocardial infarction on the signal-averaged ECG. Results of a multicenter randomized trial. LATE Ancillary Study Investigators. Late Assessment of Thrombolytic Efficacy. Circulation 1994;90:746–752.

340. Anderson HV, Willerson JT. Thrombolysis in acute myocardial infarction [Review]. N Engl J Med 1993;329:703–709.

341. Ryan TJ, Anderson JL, Antman EM et al. ACC/AHA guidelines for the management of patients with acute myocardial infarction. A report of the American College of Cardiology/American Heart Association Task Force on Practice Guidelines (Committee on Management of Acute Myocardial Infarction). Am Coll Cardiol 1996;28:1328–1428.

342. Schroder R, Wegscheider K, Schroder K et al. Extent of early ST segment elevation resolution: a strong predictor of outcome in patients with acute myocardial infarction and a sensitive measure to compare thrombolytic regimens. A substudy of the International Joint Efficacy Comparison of Thrombolytics (INJECT) trial. J Am Coll Cardiol 1996;26:1657–1664.

343. Isselbacher EM, Siu SC, Weyman AE et al. Absence of Q waves after thrombolysis predicts more rapid improvement in regional left ventricular dysfunction. Am Heart J 1996;131:649–654.

344. Shen LL, Hermans J, McDonagh J et al. Effects of calcium ion and covalent crosslinking on formation and elasticity of fibrin cells. Thromb Res 1975; 6:255–265.

345. Mosesson MW. The roles of fibrinogen and fibrin in hemostasis and thrombosis. Sem in Hematol 1992;29:177–188.

346. Anonymous. Comparison of invasive and conservative strategies after treatment with intravenous tissue-plasminogen activator in acute myocardial infarction (TIMI) phase II. The TIMI Study Group. N Engl J Med 1989; 320:618–627.

347. Eisenberg PR, Sherman LA, Jaffee AS. Paradoxic elevation of fibrinopeptide A after streptokinase: evidence for continued thrombosis despite intensive fibrinolysis. J Am Coll Cardiol 1987;10:527–529.

348. Krause J. Catabolism of tissue-type plasminogen activator (t-PA), its variants, mutants and hybrids. Fibrinolysis 1988;2:133–142.

349. Lijnen HR, Collen D. New strategies in the development of thrombolytic agents. Blut 1988;57:147–162.

350. Haber E, Quertermous T, Matsueda GR et al. Innovative approaches to plasminogen activator therapy [Review]. Science 1989;243:51–56.

351. Reed GL, Matsueda GR, Haber E. Inhibition of clot-bound $\alpha_2$-antiplasmin enhances in vivo thrombolysis. Circulation 1990;82:164–168.

352. Cercek B, Lew AS, Hod H et al. Ancrod enhances the thrombolytic effect of streptokinase and urokinase. Thromb Res 1987;47:416–426.

353. Stump DC, Lijnen HR, Collen D. Purification and characterization of a novel low-molecular-weight form of single-chain urokinase-type plasminogen activator. J Biol Chem 1986;261:17120–17126.

354. Lijnen HR, Li XK, Nelles L et al. Biochemical properties of recombinant single-chain urokinase-type plasminogen activator mutants with deletion of Asn$_2$ through Phe$_{157}$ and/or substitution of Cys$_{279}$ with Ala. Eur J Biochem 1992;205:701–709.

355. Collen D, Mao J, Stassen JM et al. Thrombolytic properties of Lys-158 mutants of recombinant single chain urokinase-type plasminogen activator (scu-PA) in rabbits with jugular vein thrombosis. J Vasc Med Biol 1989; 1:46–49.

356. Ueshima S, Holvoet P, Lijnen HR et al. Expression and characterization of clustered charge-to-alanine mutants of low Mr single-chain urokinase-type plasminogen activator. Thromb Haemost 1994;71:134–140.

357. Yahara H, Matsumoto K, Maruyama H et al. Recombinant variants of tissue-type plasminogen activator containing amino acid substitutions in the fibronectin finger-like domain and the kringle 1 domain. Thromb Haemost 1994;72:893–899.

358. Tachias K, Madison EL. Variants of tissue-type plasminogen activator which display substantially enhanced stimulation by fibrin. J Biol Chem 1995;270:18319–18322.

359. Burck PJ, Berg DH, Warrick MW et al. Characterization of a modified human tissue plasminogen activator comprising a kringle-2 and a protease domain. J Biol Chem 1990;265:5170–5177.

360. Jackson CV, Crowe VG, Craft TJ et al. Thrombolytic activity of a novel plasminogen activator, LY210825, compared with recombinant tissue-type plasminogen activator in a canine model of coronary artery thrombosis. Circulation 1990;82:930–940.

361. Bode C, Smalling RW, Berg G et al. Randomized comparison of coronary thrombolysis achieved with double-bolus reteplase (recombinant plasminogen activator) and front-loaded, accelerated alteplase (recombinant tissue plasminogen activator) in patients with acute myocardial infarction. The RAPID II Investigators. Circulation 1996;94:891–898.

362. Cody RJ. Results from late breaking clinical trials sessions ACC '97. J Am Coll Cardiol 1997;30:1–7.

363. Kawai C, Yui Y, Hosoda S et al. A prospective, randomized double-blind multicenter trial of a single bolus injection of the novel modified t-PA E6010 in the treatment of acute myocardial infarction: comparison with native t-PA. E6010 Study Group. J Am Coll Cardiol 1997;29:1447–1453.

364. Krishnamurti C, Keyt B, Maglasang P et al. PAI-1-resistant t-PA: low doses prevent fibrin deposition in rabbits with increased PAI-1 activity. Blood 1996;87:14–19.

365. Cannon CP, McCabe CH, Gibson M et al. TNK-tissue plasminogen activator in acute myocardial infarction. Results of the Thrombolysis in Myocardial Infarction (TIMI) 10A dose-ranging trial. Circulation 1997;95:351–356.

366. Tachias K, Madison EL. Variants of tissue-type plasminogen activator that display extraordinary resistance to inhibition by the serpin plasminogen activator inhibitor type-1. J Biol Chem 1997;272:14580–14585.

367. Robbins KC, Tanaka Y, Gulba DL et al. Covalent molecular weight ~92,000 hybrid plasminogen activator derived from human plasmin aminoterminal and urokinase carboxylterminal domains. Biochemistry 1986;25:3603–3611.

368. Pierard L, Garcia Quintana L, Reff ME et al. Production in eukaryotic cells and characterization of four hybrids of tissue-ype and urokinase-ype plasminogen activators. DNA 1989;8:321–328.

369. Pierard L, Jacobs P, Gheysen D et al. Mutant and chimeric recombinant plasminogen activators. Production in eukaryotic cells and preliminary characterization. J Biol Chem 1987;262:11771–11778.

370. Gheysen D, Lijnen HR, Pierard L et al. Characterization of a recombinant fusion protein of the finger domain of tissue-type plasminogen activator with a truncated single chain urokinase-type plasminogen activator. J Biol Chem 1987;262:11779–11784.

371. Nelles L, Lijnen HR, Collen D et al. Characterization of a fusion protein consisting of amino acids 1 to 263 of tissue-type plasminogen activator and amino acids 144 to 411 of urokinase-type plasminogen activator. J Biol Chem 1987;262:10855–10862.

372. Lijnen HR, Nelles L, Van Hoef B et al. Characterization of a chimeric plasminogen activator consisting of amino acids 1 to 274 of tissue-type plasminogen activator and amino acids 138 to 411 of single-chain urokinase-type plasminogen activator. J Biol Chem 1988;263:19083–19091.

373. Collen D, Stassen JM, Demarsin E et al. Pharmacokinetics and thrombolytic properties of chimeric plasminogen activators consisting of the NH$_2$-terminal region of human tissue-type plasminogen activator and the COOH-terminal region of human single-chain urokinase-type plasminogen activator. J Vasc Med Biol 1989;1:234–240.

374. Nelles L, Lijnen HR, Van Nuffelen A et al. Characterization of domain deletion and/or duplication mutants of a recombinant chimera of tissue-type plasminogen activator and urokinase-type plasminogen activator (rt-PA/u-PA). Thromb Haemost 1990;64:53–60.

375. Collen D, Lu HR, Lijnen HR et al. Thrombolytic and pharmacokinetic properties of chimeric tissue-type and urokinase-type plasminogen activators. Circulation 1991;84:1216–1234.

376. Van de Werf F, Lijnen HR, Collen D. Coronary thrombolysis with K$_1$K$_2$P$_u$, a chimeric tissue-type and urokinase-type plasminogen activator: a feasibility study in six patients with acute myocardial infarction. Coron Artery Dis 1993;4:929–933.

377. Kalyan NK, Lee SG, Wilhelm J et al. Structure-function analysis with tissue-type plasminogen activator. Effect of deletion of NH$_2$-terminal domains on its biochemical and biological properties. J Biol Chem 1988;263:3971–3978.

378. Larsen GR, Henson K, Blue Y. Variants of human tissue-type plasminogen activator. Fibrin binding, fibrinolytic, and fibrinogenolytic characterization of genetic variants lacking the fibronectin finger-like and/or the epidermal growth factor domains. J Biol Chem 1988;263:1023–1029.

379. Verheijen JH, Caspers MP, Chang GT et al. Involvement of finger domain and kringle-2 domain of tissue-type plasminogen activator in fibrin binding and stimulation of activity by fibrin. EMBO J 1986;5:3525–3530.

380. Browne MJ, Carey JE, Chapman CG et al. A tissue-type plasminogen activator mutant with prolonged clearance in vivo. Effect of removal of the growth factor domain. J Biol Chem 1988;263:1599–1602.

381. Collen D, Stassen JM, Larsen G. Pharmacokinetics and thrombolytic properties of deletion mutants of human tissue-type plasminogen activator in rabbits. Blood 1988;71:216–219.

382. Cambier P, Van de Werf F, Larsen GR et al. Pharmacokinetics and thrombolytic properties of a nonglycosylated mutant of human tissue-type plasminogen activator, lacking the finger and growth factor domains, in dogs with copper-coil induced coronary artery thrombosis. J Cardiovasc Pharmacol 1988;11:468–472.

383. Wu Z, Van de Werf F, Stassen T et al. Pharmacokinetics and coronary thrombolytic properties of two human tissue-type plasminogen activator variants lacking the finger-like, growth-factor-like, and first kringle domains (amino acids 6-173) in a canine model. J Cardiovasc Pharmacol 1990;16:197–203.

384. Agnelli G, Pascucci C, Colucci M et al. Thrombolytic activity of two chimeric recombinant plasminogen activators (FK2tu-PA and K2tu-PA) in rabbits. Thromb Haemost 1992;68:331–335.

385. Schneider J, Hauser R, Hennies HH et al. A novel chimaeric derivative of saruplase, rscu-PA-40 Kda/Hir, binds to thrombin and exerts thrombus-specific fibrinolysis in arterial and venous thrombosis in dogs. Thromb Haemost 1997;77:535–539.

386. Fujise K, Revelle BM, Stacy L et al. A tissue plasminogen activator/P-selectin fusion protein is an effective thrombolytic agent. Circulation 1997; 95:715–722.

387. Haber E, Quertermous T, Matsueda GR et al. Innovative approaches to plasminogen activator therapy [Review]. Science 1989;243:51–56.

388. Dewerchin M, Collen D. Enhancement of the thrombolytic potency of plasminogen activators by conjugation with clot-specific monoclonal antibodies. Bioconjug Chem 1991;2:293–300.

389. Vandamme AM, Dewerchin M, Lijnen HR et al. Characterization of a recombinant chimeric plasminogen activator composed of a fibrin fragment-D-dimer specific humanized monoclonal antibody and a truncated single-chain urokinase. Eur J Biochem 1992;205:139–146.

390. Dewerchin M, Vandamme AM, Holvoet P et al. Thrombolytic and pharmacokinetic properties of a recombinant chimeric plasminogen activator consisting of fibrin fragment D-dimer specific humanized monoclonal antibody and a truncated single-chain urokinase. Thromb Haemost 1992;68:170–179.

391. Sako T, Tsuchida N. Nucleotide sequence of the staphylokinase gene from Staphylococcus aureus. Nucleic Acids Res 1983;11:7679–7693.

392. Damaschun G, Damaschun H, Gast K et al. Physical and conformational properties of staphylokinase in solution. Biochim Biophys Acta 1993;1161:244–248.

393. Schlott B, Hartmann M, Guhrs KH et al. Functional properties of recombinant staphylokinase variants obtained by site-specific mutagenesis of methionine-26. Biochim Biophys Acta 1994;1204:235–242.

394. Collen D, Lijnen HR, Vanderschueren S. Staphylokinase: fibrinolytic properties and current experience in individuals with occlusive arterial thrombosis [Review]. Verh K Acad Geneeskd Belg 1995;57:183–196.

395. Silence K, Collen D, Lijnen HR. Regulation by $\alpha_2$-antiplasmin and fibrin of

the activation of plasminogen with recombinant staphylokinase in plasma. Blood 1993;82:1175–1183.

396. Silence K, Collen D, Lijnen HR. Interaction between staphylokinase, plasmin(ogen), and $\alpha_2$-antiplasmin. Recycling of staphylokinase after neutralization of the plasmin-staphylokinase complex by $\alpha_2$-antiplasmin. J Biol Chem 1993;268:9811–9816.

397. Shishido Y, Sakai M, Kaneda N et al. Involvement of protease inhibitors in staphylokinase-induced fibrin-specific fibrinolysis. Biol Pharm Bull 1994;17:1595–1598.

398. Lijnen HR, Van Hoef B, Matsuo O et al. On the molecular interactions between plasminogen-staphylokinase, $\alpha_2$-antiplasmin and fibrin. Biochim Biophys Acta 1992;1118:144–148.

399. Lijnen HR, Van Hoef B, De Cock F et al. On the mechanism of fibrin-specific plasminogen activation by staphylokinase. J Biol Chem 1991;266:11826–11832.

400. Shibata H, Nagaoka M, Sakai M et al. Kinetic studies on the plasminogen activation by the staphylokinase-plasmin complex. J Biochem (Tokyo) 1994;115:738–742.

401. Lijnen HR, De Cock F, Van Hoef B et al. Characterization of the interaction between plasminogen and staphylokinase. Eur J Biochem 1994;224:143–149.

402. Suehiro A, Tsujioka H, Yoshimoto H et al. Enhancing effect of platelets on staphylokinase-mediated clot lysis and plasminogen activation. Thromb Res 1995;80:135–142.

403. Shishido Y, Matsumoto T, Sakai M et al. Fibrin-specific fibrinolysis induced by recombinant staphylokinase. Biol Pharm Bull 1994;17:1060–1064.

404. Hauptmann J, Glusa E. Differential effects of staphylokinase, streptokinase and tissue-type plasminogen activator on the lysis of retracted human plasma clots and fibrinolytic plasma parameters in vitro. Blood Coagul Fibrinolysis 1995;6:579–583.

405. Vanderschueren S, Barrios L, Kerdsinchai P et al. A randomized trial of recombinant staphylokinase versus alteplase for coronary artery patency in acute myocardial infarction. The STAR Trial Group. Circulation 1995;92:2044–2049.

406. Vanderschueren S, Stockx L, Wilms G et al. Thrombolytic therapy of peripheral arterial occlusion with recombinant staphylokinase. Circulation 1995;92:2050–2057.

407. Vanderschueren S, Stassen JM, Collen D. Comparative antigenicity of recombinant wild-type staphylokinase (SakSTAR) and a selected mutant (SakSTAR.M38) in a baboon thrombolysis model. J Cardiovasc Pharmacol 1996;27:809–815.

408. Collen D, Bernaerts R, Declerck P et al. Recombinant staphylokinase variants with altered immunoreactivity. I: Construction and characterization. Circulation 1996;94:197–206.

409. Coller BS, Scudder LE, Beer J et al. Monoclonal antibodies to platelet glycoprotein IIb-IIIa as antithrombotic agents. Ann N Y Acad Sci 1991;614:193–213.

410. Mickelson JK, Simpson PJ, Cronin M et al. Antiplatelet antibody [7E3 F(b')2] prevents rethrombosis after recombinant tissue-type plasminogen activator-induced coronary artery thrombolysis in a canine model. Circulation 1990;81:617–627.

411. Gold HK, Coller BS, Yasuda T et al. Rapid and sustained coronary artery recanalization with combined bolus injection of recombinant tissue-type plasminogen activator and monoclonal antiplatelet GP IIb-IIIa antibody in a canine preparation. Circulation 1988;77:670–677.

412. Yasuda T, Gold HK, Leinbach RC et al. Lysis of plasminogen activator-resistant platelet-rich coronary artery thrombus with combined bolus injection of recombinant tissue-type plasminogen activator and antiplatelet GP IIb-IIIa antibody. J Am Coll Cardiol 1990;16:1728–1735.

413. Yasuda T, Gold HK, Yaoita H et al. Comparative effects of aspirin, a synthetic thrombin inhibitor and a monoclonal antiplatelet glycoprotein IIb-IIIa antibody on coronary artery reperfusion, reocclusion and bleeding with recombinant tissue-type plasminogen activator in a canine preparation. J Am Coll Cardiol 1990;16:714–722.

414. Yasuda T, Gold HK, Fallon JT et al. Monoclonal antibody against the platelet glycoprotein (GP) IIb-IIIa receptor prevents coronary artery reocclusion after reperfusion with recombinant tissue-type plasminogen activator in dogs. J Clin Invest 1988;81:1284–1291.

415. Spriggs D, Gold HK, Hashimoto Y et al. Absence of potentiation with murine antiplatelet GP IIb-IIIa antibody of thrombolysis with recombinant tissue-type plasminogen activator (rt-PA) in a canine venous thrombosis model. Thromb Haemost 1989;61:93–96.

416. Markland FS, Friedrichs GS, Pewitt SR et al. Thrombolytic effects of recombinant fibrolase or APSAC in a canine model of carotid artery thrombosis. Circulation 1994;90:2448–2456.

417. Kohmura C, Gold HK, Yasuda T et al. A chimeric murine/human antibody Fab fragment directed against the platelet GP IIb-IIIa receptor enhances and sustains arterial thrombolysis with recombinant tissue-type plasminogen activator in baboons. Arterioscler Thromb 1993;13:1837–1842.

418. Rote WE, Mu DX, Bates ER et al. Prevention of rethrombosis after coronary thrombolysis in a chronic canine model. I. Adjunctive therapy with monoclonal antibody 7E3 F(ab')2 fragment. J Cardiovasc Pharmacol 1994;23:194–202.

419. Kleiman NS, Ohman EM, Califf RM et al. Profound inhibition of platelet aggregation with monoclonal antibody 7E3 Fab after thrombolytic therapy. Results of the Thrombolysis and Angioplasty in Myocardial Infarction (TAMI) 8 Pilot Study. J Am Coll Cardiol 1993;22:381–389.

420. Roux SP, Tschopp TB, Kuhn H et al. Effects of heparin, aspirin and a synthetic platelet glycoprotein IIb-IIIa receptor antagonist (Ro 43-5054) on coronary artery reperfusion and reocclusion after thrombolysis with tissue-type plasminogen activator in the dog. J Pharmacol Exp Ther 1993;264:501–508.

421. Nicolini FA, Lee P, Rios G et al. Combination of platelet fibrinogen receptor antagonist and direct thrombin inhibitor at low doses markedly improves thrombolysis. Circulation 1994;89:1802–1809.

422. Ohman EM, Kleiman NS, Gacioch G et al. Combined accelerated tissue-plasminogen activator and platelet glycoprotein IIb-IIIa integrin receptor blockade with Integrilin in acute myocardial infarction. Results of a randomized, placebo-controlled, dose-ranging trial. IMPACT-AMI Investigators. Circulation 1997;95:846–854.

423. Kaida T, Matsuno H, Niwa M et al. Antiplatelet effect of FK633, a platelet glycoprotein IIb-IIIa antagonist, on thrombus formation and vascular patency after thrombolysis in the injured hamster carotid artery. Thromb Haemost 1997;77:562–567.

424. Shebuski RJ, Ramjit DR, Benson GH et al. Characterization and platelet inhibitory activity of bitistatin, a potent arginine-glycine-aspartic acid-containing peptide from the venom of the viper Bitis arietans. J Biol Chem 1989;264:21550–21556.

425. Shebuski RJ, Stabilito IJ, Sitko GR et al. Acceleration of recombinant tissue-type plasminogen activator-induced thrombolysis and prevention of reocclusion by the combination of heparin and the Arg-Gly-Asp-containing peptide bitistatin in a canine model of coronary thrombosis. Circulation 1990;82:169–177.

426. Holahan MA, Mellot MJ, Garsky VM et al. Prevention of reocclusion following tissue-type plasminogen activator-induced thrombolysis by the RGD-containing peptide, echistatin, in a canine model of coronary thrombosis. Pharmacology 1991;42:340–348.

427. Yasuda T, Gold HK, Leinbach RC et al. Kistrin, a polypeptide platelet GP IIb-IIIa receptor antagonist, enhances and sustains coronary arterial thrombolysis with recombinant tissue-type plasminogen activator in a canine preparation. Circulation 1991;83:1038–1047.

428. Feigen LP, Nicholson NS, King LW et al. SC-49992, a mimetic of the peptide arginine-glycine-aspartic acid-phenylalanine that blocks platelet aggregation, enhances recombinant tissue plasminogen activator-induced thrombolysis and prevents reocclusion in a canine model of coronary artery thrombosis. J Pharmacol Exp Ther 1993;267:1191–1197.

429. Terres W, Beythien C, Kupper W et al. Effects of aspirin and prostaglandin E1 on in vitro thrombolysis with urokinase. Evidence for a possible role of inhibiting platelet activity in thrombolysis. Circulation 1989;79:1309–1314.

430. Haskel EJ, Prager NA, Sobel BE et al. Relative efficacy of antithrombin compared with antiplatelet agents in accelerating coronary thrombolysis and preventing early reocclusion. Circulation 1991;83:1048–1056.

430a. Mruk JS, Zoldhelyi P, Webster MW et al. Does antithrombotic therapy influence residual thrombus after thrombolysis of platelet-rich thrombus? Effects of recombinant hirudin, heparin, or aspirin. Circulation 1996;93(4):792–799.

431. Rudd MA, George D, Johnstone MT et al. Effect of thrombin inhibition on the dynamics of thrombolysis and on platelet function during thrombolytic therapy. Circ Res 1992;70:829–834.

432. Roux S, Christeller S, Ludin E. Effects of aspirin on coronary reocclusion and recurrent ischemia after thrombolysis: a meta-analysis. J Am Coll Cardiol 1992;19:671–677.

432a. Meijer A, Verheught FW, Werter CJ et al. Aspirin versus coumadin in the prevention of reocclusion and recurrent ischemia after successful thrombolysis: a prospective placebo-controlled angiographic study. Results of the APRICOT study. Circulation 1993;87:1524–1530.

433. Rebuzzi AG, Natale A, Bianchi C et al. Importance of reperfusion on thromboxane A2 metabolite excretion after thrombolysis. Am Heart J 1992;123:560–566.

434. Fitzgerald DJ, Wright F, Fitzgerald GA. Increased thromboxane biosynthesis during coronary thrombolysis. Evidence that platelet activation and thromboxane $A_2$ modulate the response to tissue-type plasminogen activator in vivo. Circ Res 1989;65:83–94.

435. Kerins DM, Roy L, FitzGerald GA, Firtgerald DJ. Platelet and vascular function during coronary thrombolysis with tissue-type plasminogen activator. Circulation 1989;80:1718–1725.

436. Fujita T, Hasan S, Storer BL et al. Effect of selective endoperoxide/thromboxane $A_2$ receptor antagonism with sulotroban on t-PA-induced thrombolysis in a rabbit model of femoral arterial thrombosis. Fundam Clin Pharmacol 1989;3:643–653.

437. Nishiyama H, Umemura K, Saniabadi AR et al. Enhancement of thrombolytic efficacy of tissue-type plasminogen activator by adjuvants in the guinea pig thrombosis model. Eur J Pharmacol 1994;264:191–198.

438. Schumacher WA, Grover GJ. The thromboxane receptor antagonist SQ 30,741 reduces myocardial infarct size in monkeys when given during re-

perfusion at a threshold dose for improving reflow during thrombolysis. J Am Coll Cardiol 1990;15:883–889.

439. Shebuski RJ, Storer BL, Fujita T. Effect of thromboxane synthase inhibition on the thrombolytic action of tissue-type plasminogen activator in a rabbit model of peripheral arterial thrombosis. Thromb Res 1988;52:381–392.

440. Golino P, Rosolowsky M, Yao SK et al. Endogenous prostaglandin endoperoxides and prostacyclin modulate the thrombolytic activity of tissue plasminogen activator. Effects of simultaneous inhibition of thromboxane A$_2$ synthase and blockade of thromboxane A$_2$/prostaglandin H$_2$ receptors in a canine model of coronary thrombosis. J Clin Invest 1990;86:1095–1102.

441. Yao SK, Ober JC, Ferguson JJ et al. Combination of inhibition of thrombin and blockade of thromboxane A$_2$ synthetase and receptors enhances thrombolysis and delays reocclusion in canine coronary arteries. Circulation 1992;86:1993–1999.

442. Vandeplassche G, Hermans C, Somers Y et al. Combined thromboxane A$_2$ synthase inhibition and prostaglandin endoperoxide receptor antagonism limits myocardial infarct size after mechanical coronary occlusion and reperfusion at doses enhancing coronary thrombolysis by streptokinase. J Am Coll Cardiol 1993;21:1269–1279.

443. Anonymous. Randomized trial of ridogrel, a combined thromboxane A$_2$ synthase inhibitor and thromboxane A$_2$/prostaglandin endoperoxide receptor antagonist, versus aspirin as adjunct to thrombolysis in individuals with acute myocardial infarction. The Ridogrel Versus Aspirin Patency Trial (RAPT). Circulation 1994;89:588–595.

444. Werns SW, Rote WE, Davis JH et al. Nitroglycerin inhibits experimental thrombosis and reocclusion after thrombolysis. Am Heart J 1994;127: 727–737.

445. Kornowski R, Chernine A, Hasdai D et al. Beneficial effect of nitroglycerin on arterial rethrombosis after thrombolysis. Results from a rabbit thrombosis model. Eur Heart J 1995;16:177–183.

446. Yao SK, Akhtar S, Scott-Burden T et al. Endogenous and exogenous nitric oxide protect against intracoronary thrombosis and reocclusion after thrombolysis. Circulation 1995;92:1005–1010.

447. Nicolini FA, Ferrini D, Ottani F et al. Concurrent nitroglycerin therapy impairs tissue-type plasminogen activator-induced thrombolysis in patients with acute myocardial infarction. Am J Cardiol 1994;74:662–666.

448. Romeo F, Rosano GM, Martuscelli E et al. Concurrent nitroglycerin administration reduces the efficacy of recombinant tissue-type plasminogen activator in patients with acute anterior wall myocardial infarction. Am Heart J 1995;130:692–697.

449. Owen J, Friedman KD, Grossman BA et al. Thrombolytic therapy with tissue plasminogen activator or streptokinase induces transient thrombin activity. Blood 1988;72:616–620.

450. Eisenberg PR, Sherman LA, Jaffe AS. Paradoxic elevation of fibrinopeptide A after streptokinase: evidence for continued thrombosis despite intense fibrinolysis. J Am Coll Cardiol 1987;10:527–529.

451. Rosenberg RD. Biochemistry of heparin antithrombin interactions, and the physiologic role of this natural anticoagulant mechanism. Am J Med 1989; 87(Suppl 3B):2S–9S.

452. Rosenberg RD. Mechanism of antithrombin action and the structural basis of heparin's anticoagulant function. In: Bing DH, ed. The chemistry and physiology of the human plasma protein. New York: Pergamon Press, 1988:353–368.

453. Salzman EW, Rosenberg RD, Smith MH et al. Effect of heparin and heparin fractions on platelet aggregation. J Clin Invest 1980;65:64–73.

454. Choay J, Petitou M, Lormeau JC et al. Structure-activity relationship in heparin: a synthetic pentasaccharide with high affinity for antithrombin III and eliciting high anti-factor Xa activity. Biochem Biophys Res Commun 1983;116:492–499.

455. Jang IK, Gold HK, Leinbach RC et al. In vivo thrombin inhibition enhances and sustains arterial recanalization with recombinant tissue-type plasminogen activator. Circ Res 1990;67:1552–1561.

456. Agnelli G, Pascucci C, Cosmi B et al. Effects of therapeutic doses of heparin on thrombolysis with tissue-type plasminogen activator in rabbits. Blood 1990;76:2030–2036.

457. O'Connor CM, Meese R, Carney R et al. A randomized trial of intravenous heparin in conjunction with anistreplase (anisoylated plasminogen streptokinase activator complex) in acute myocardial infarction: the Duke University Clinical Cardiology Study (DUCCS) 1. J Am Coll Cardiol 1994;23: 11–18.

458. Tebbe U, Windeler J, Boesl I et al. Thrombolysis with recombinant unglycosylated single-chain urokinase-type plasminogen activator (saruplase) in acute myocardial infarction: influence of heparin on early patency rate (LIMITS study). Liquemin in Myocardial Infarction during Thrombolysis with Saruplase. J Am Coll Cardiol 1995;26:365–373.

459. de Bono DP, Simoons ML, Tijssen J et al. Effect of early intravenous heparin on coronary patency, infarct size, and bleeding complications after alteplase thrombolysis; results of a randomized double-blind study. European Cooperative Study Group. Br Heart J 1992;67:122–128.

460. Agnelli G. Thrombolytic and antithrombotic treatment in myocardial infarction. Main achievements and future perspectives. Int J Cardiol 1995; 49:S77–S87.

461. Nicolini FA, Nichols WW, Saldeen TG et al. Adjunctive therapy with low-

molecular-weight heparin with recombinant tissue-type plasminogen activator causes sustained reflow in canine coronary thrombosis. Am Heart J 1992;124:280–288.

462. Jun L, Arnout J, Vanhove P et al. Comparison of a low-molecular-weight heparin (nadroparin calcium) and unfractionated heparin as adjunct to coronary thrombolysis with alteplase and aspirin in dogs. Coronary Artery Dis 1995;6:257–263.

463. Kornowski R, Glikson M, Hasdai D et al. Low-molecular-weight heparin (Fragmin) prevents early reocclusion following femoral artery thrombolysis with rt-PA in rabbits. Eur Heart J 1994;15:541–546.

464. Glick A, Kornowski R, Michowich Y et al. Reduction of reinfarction and angina with use of low-molecular-weight heparin therapy after streptokinase (and heparin) in acute myocardial infarction. Am J Cardiol 1996;77: 1145–1148.

465. Markwardt F. Hirudin as an inhibitor of thrombin. Methods Enzymol 1991;45:669–676.

466. Harvey RP, Degryse E, Stefani L et al. Cloning and expression of a cDNA coding for the anticoagulant hirudin from the bloodsucking leech, Hirudo medicinalis. Proc Natl Acad Sci U S A 1986;83:1084–1088.

467. Dodt J, Schmitz T, Schafer T et al. Expression, secretion and processing of hirudin in E. coli using the alkaline phosphatase signal sequence. FEBS Lett 1986;202:373–377.

468. Mirshahi M, Soria J, Soria C et al. Evaluation of the inhibition of heparin and hirudin of coagulation activation during r-tPA-induced thrombolysis. Blood 1989;74:1025–1030.

469. Sitko GR, Ramjit DR, Stabilito II et al. Conjunctive enhancement of enzymatic thrombolysis and prevention of thrombotic reocclusion with the selective factor Xa inhibitor, tick anticoagulatnt peptide. Comparison to hirudin and heparin in a canine model of acute coronary artery thrombosis. Circulation 1992;85:805–815.

470. Martin U, Dorge L, Fischer S. Comparison of desulfatohirudin (REVASC) and heparin as adjuncts to thrombolytic therapy with reteplase in a canine model of coronary thrombosis. Br J Pharmacol 1996;118:271–276.

471. Zeymer U, von Essen R, Tebbe U et al. Frequency of "optimal anticoagulation" for acute myocardial infarction after thrombolysis with front-loaded recombinant tissue-type plasminogen activator and conjunctive therapy with recombinant hirudin (HBW 023). ALKK Study Group. Am J Cardiol 1995;76:997–1001.

472. Cannon CP, McCabe CH, Henry TD et al. A pilot trial of recombinant desulfatohirudin compared with heparin in conjunction with tissue-type plasminogen activator and aspirin for acute myocardial infarction: results of the Thrombolysis in Myocardial Infarction (TIMI) 5 trial. J Am Coll Cardiol 1994;23:993–1003.

473. Lee LV. Initial experience with hirudin and streptokinase in acute myocardial infarction: results of the Thrombolysis in Myocardial Infarction (TIMI) 6 trial. Am J Cardiol 1995;75:7–13.

474. Anonymous. Randomized trial of intravenous heparin versus recombinant hirudin for acute coronary syndromes. The Global Use of Strategies to Open Occluded Coronary Arteries (GUSTO) IIa Investigators. Circulation 1994;90:1631–1637.

475. Antman EM. Hirudin in acute myocardial infarction. Safety report from the Thrombolysis and Thrombin Inhibition in Myocardial Infarction (TIMI) 9A Trial. Circulation 1994;90:1624–1630.

476. Antman EM. Hirudin in acute myocardial infarction. Thrombolysis and Thrombin Inhibition in Myocardial Infarction (TIMI) 9B trial. Circulation 1996;94:911–921.

477. Anonymous. A comparison of recombinant hirudin with heparin for the treatment of acute coronary syndromes. The Global Use of Strategies to Open Occluded Coronary Arteries (GUSTO) IIb investigators. N Engl J Med 1996;335:775–782.

478. Liu L, Freedman J, Hornstein A et al. Thrombin binding to platelets and their activation in plasma. Br J Haematol 1994;88:592–600.

479. Gallistl S, Muntean W, Leis HJ. Effects of heparin and hirudin on thrombin generation and platelet aggregation after intrinsic activation of platelet-rich plasma. Thromb Haemost 1995;74:1163–1168.

480. Naski MC, Fenton JW II, Maraganore JM et al. The COOH-terminal domain of hirudin. An exosite-directed competitive inhibitor of the action of α-thrombin on fibrinogen. J Biol Chem 1990;265:13484–13489.

481. Yao SK, McNatt J, Anderson HV et al. Thrombin inhibition enhances tissue-type plasminogen activator-induced thrombolysis and delays reocclusion. Am J Physiol 1992;262(2 Pt 2):H374–H379.

482. Maraganore JM, Bourdon P, Jablonski J et al. Design and characterization of hirulogs: a novel class of bivalent peptide inhibitors of thrombin. Biochemistry 1990;29:7095–7101.

483. Kikumoto R, Tamao Y, Tezuka T et al. Selective inhibition of thrombin by (2R, 4R)-4-methyl-1-[N2-(3-methyl-1, 2, 3, 4-tetrahydro-8-quinolinyl + + I +)sulfonyl]-1-arginyl)-2-piperidine-carboxylic acid. Biochemistry 1984;23:85–90.

484. Clarke RJ, Mayo G, FitzGerald GA et al. Combined administration of aspirin and a specific thrombin inhibitor in man. Circulation 1991;83: 1510–1518.

485. Fitzgerald DJ, Fitzgerald GA. Role of thrombin and thromboxane A2 in

reocclusion following coronary thrombolysis with tissue-type plasminogen activator. Proc Natl Acad Sci U S A 1989;86:7585–7589.

486. Schneider J. Heparin and the thrombin inhibitor argatroban enhance fibrinolysis by infused or bolus-injected saruplase (r-scu-PA) in rabbit femoral artery thrombosis. Thromb Res 1991;64:677–689.

487. Hanson SR, Harker LA. Interruption of acute platelet-dependent thrombosis by the synthetic antithrombin D-phenylalanyl-L-prolyl-L-arginyl chloromethyl ketone. Proc Natl Acad Sci U S A 1988;85:3184–3188.

488. Schneider PA, Hanson SR, Harker LA. Permanent interruption of thrombus formation on carotid endarterectomy sites by short-term therapy with a synthetic antithrombin. Circulation 1988;78(Suppl II):II–311.

489. Kaplan AV, Leung LL, Leung WH et al. Roles of thrombin and platelet membrane glycoprotein IIb-IIIa in platelet-subendothelial deposition after angioplasty in an *ex vivo* whole artery model. Circulation 1991;84:1279–1288.

490. Hollenbach S, Sinha U, Lin PH et al. A comparative study of prothrombinase and thrombin inhibitors in a novel rabbit model of non-occlusive deep vein thrombosis. Thromb Haemost 1994;71:357–362.

491. Schumacher WA, Steinbacher TE, Heran CL et al. Effects of antithrombotic drugs in a rat model of aspirin-insensitive arterial thrombosis. Thromb Haemost 1993;69:509–514.

492. Sudo Y, Lucchesi BR. Antithrombotic effect of GYKI-14766 in a canine model of arterial and venous rethrombosis: a comparison with heparin. J Cardiovasc Pharmacol 1996;27:545–555.

493. Gustafsson D, Elg M, Lenfors S et al. Effects of inogatran, a new low-molecular-weight thrombin inhibitor, in rat models of venous and arterial thrombosis, thrombolysis and bleeding time. Blood Coagul Fibrinolysis 1996;7:69–79.

# CHAPTER 57

# NEW ANTITHROMBOTIC STRATEGIES

Jane E. Freedman, Jonathan S. Scharfstein, Herman K. Gold,
and Joseph Loscalzo

Clinicians recently have witnessed the advent of thrombolytic therapy for many clinical thrombotic disorders, including acute myocardial infarction and pulmonary embolism. Nevertheless, standard antithrombotic therapy has changed little. Heparin and warfarin (see Chapter 55) have been the mainstays of anticoagulant therapy for decades, and they remain the only widely available choices for clinicians treating a variety of cardiovascular and cerebrovascular diseases. The many limitations of these agents, however, have prompted an intense search for new drugs with improved efficacy and safety profiles.

New antithrombotic strategies have evolved in three general directions (Table 57.1, Fig. 57.1). The most investigated approach has been the development of direct inhibitors of specific coagulation factors. Direct inhibitors of thrombin (i.e., factor IIa) and factor Xa, which are two serine proteases with central roles in the coagulation cascade, have undergone clinical trials to define their role as adjuncts to thrombolysis and their use in preventing thrombosis after interventional cardiovascular procedures. Similarly, tissue factor pathway inhibitor (TFPI), which formerly was called lipoprotein-associated coagulation inhibitor or extrinsic pathway inhibitor and is a direct endogenous inhibitor of both factor Xa and the factor VIIa-tissue factor complex, has been produced in recombinant form and had limited clinical evaluation.

A second approach has been production of recombinant endogenous anticoagulants (see Chapter 3). These include recombinant forms of antithrombin III and heparin cofactor II, which are serine protease inhibitors that interact with the glycosaminoglycan cofactors, heparin, heparan sulfate, and dermatan sulfate to inhibit coagulation factors by complexation, and also activated protein C, which is a natural anticoagulant that inhibits factors Va and VIIIa through proteolytic degradation. In addition, recombinant TFPI has been developed as an endogenous anticoagulant.

A third strategy is manipulation or synthetic production of endogenous, natural anticoagulant cofactors. This includes modification of native glycosaminoglycans, such as heparan sulfate and dermatan sulfate, to enhance their anticoagulant activity.

Development of synthetic endogenous natural anticoagulants with enhanced potency and production of recombinant antithrombin cofactors for clinical use remain in the earliest stages of research. Some specific inhibitors of coagulation factors, however, already have completed clinical trials in humans. This chapter reviews these new approaches to antithrombotic therapy and summarizes the available clinical studies. More detailed analyses of some studies appear in other chapters devoted to the specific thrombotic disorders involved.

## COAGULATION CASCADE

hOne of the most promising new approaches to antithrombotic therapy targets different components of the coagulation cascade (Fig. 57.1). The complex network of reactions characterizing the coagulation cascade (see Chapter 1) classically has been considered as being composed of two pathways. The first, which originally was called the extrinsic pathway (see Chapter 4), begins with

**FIGURE 57.1.** New antithrombotic agents target various components of the coagulation cascade. Specific coagulation inhibitors include the antithrombins such as hirudin, hirugen, hirulog, D-Phe-Pro-Arg chloromethyl ketone (PPACK), argatroban, and single-stranded DNA (ssDNA) aptamers. New inhibitors of factor Xa include recombinant tick anti-coagulant peptide (rTAP), recombinant antistasin (rATS), mutant factor Xa (Asn$_{322}$–Ala$_{419}$), and tissue factor pathway inhibitor (TFPI). TFPI also inhibits the factor VIIa-tissue factor (TF) complex. The recombinant forms of the endogenous anticoagulants, antithrombin III and heparin cofactor II, also mediate inhibition of thrombin, but they require heparin, heparan sulfate, or dermatan sulfate as cofactors. Activated protein C is another native anticoagulant protein produced in recombinant form (rAPC), and this agent cleaves factors Va and VIIIa. The central role of thrombin in the coagulation process is highlighted. *PL,* phospholipid.

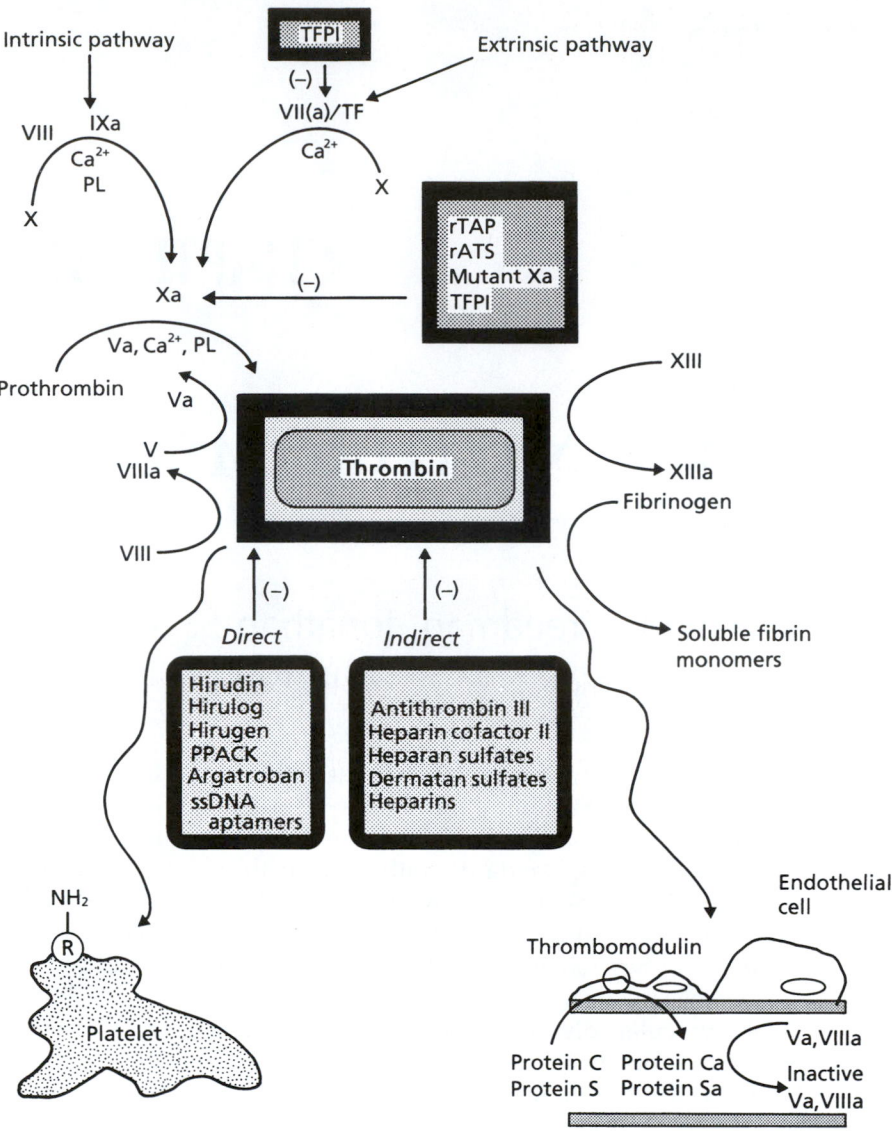

**TABLE 57.1.   New Antithrombotic Strategies**

*Specific coagulation factor inhibitors*
Thrombin inhibitors
Factor Xa inhibitors
Factor VIIa-tissue factor inhibitor

*Recombinant endogenous anticoagulants*
Antithrombin III
Heparin cofactor II
Activated protein C
Factor VIIa-tissue factor inhibitor

*Endogenous anticoagulant cofactors*
Glycosaminoglycan preparations

interaction of the proteolipid tissue factor with factor VIIa to form factor Xa. Factor Xa also can be generated by the second pathway, which originally was called the intrinsic pathway (see Chapter 5) and begins with activation of factor XII (Hageman factor) by surface contact (1). This simplistic view of the coagulation cascade recently was complicated by recognition of common amplification mechanisms and "cross-talk" between enzymatic and cofactor determinants of both pathways. Regardless of the mechanistic pathway involved, however, factor Xa is generated early during the coagulation process, and it occupies a central role in subsequent enzymatic reactions. Thrombin, which eventually is generated in the final steps of the coagulation cascade from prothrombin (factor II) by a complex of enzymes and cofactors assembled on a membrane surface (the prothrombinase complex), likewise has a pivotal role in the coagulation cascade.

**TABLE 57.2.** Specific Coagulation Factor Inhibitors

*Thrombin inhibitors*
Hirudin
Hirugen
Hirulogs
D-Phe-Pro-Arg-chloromethyl ketone
Argatroban
ssDNA aptamers

*Factor Xa inhibitors*
Tick anticoagulant peptide
Antistasin
Mutant factor Xa ($Asn_{322}$–$Ala_{419}$)
Tissue factor pathway inhibitor

*Factor VIIa-tissue factor inhibitors*
Tissue factor pathway inhibitor

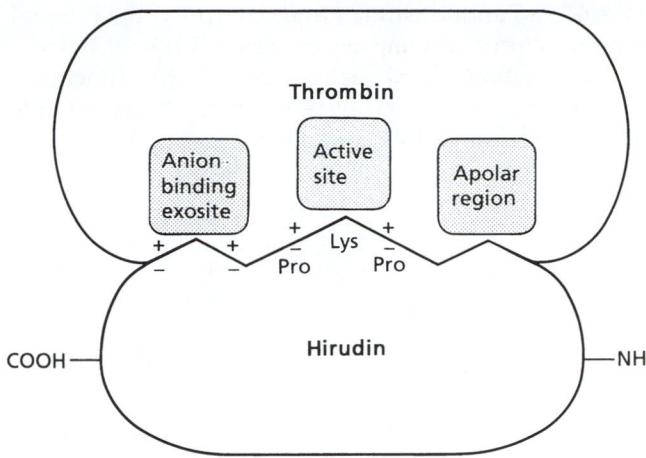

**FIGURE 57.2.** Model of the hirudin-thrombin interaction illustrating the trivalent binding of hirudin to thrombin. The aminoterminal region of hirudin binds to the apolar region of thrombin, the $Pro_{46}$-$Lys_{47}$-$Pro_{48}$ region of hirudin binds to the active site of thrombin, and the highly acidic carboxyterminal region of hirudin binds to the anion binding exosite of thrombin. (Adapted with permission from Scharfstein JS, Loscalzo J. Molecular approaches to antithrombotic therapy. Hosp Pract [Off Ed] 1992;27:77–86.)

# SPECIFIC COAGULATION FACTOR INHIBITORS

Both thrombin and factor Xa are ideally situated within the coagulation cascade to serve as targets of specific inhibitors designed to be potent antithrombotic agents (Table 57.2). A more detailed understanding of the molecular structure of both, however, is necessary to understand the mechanisms of their inhibition by novel anticoagulants. Full discussions of thrombin and factor Xa appear in Chapters 1 and 2; the following sections summarize these concepts as they relate to development of antithrombotic agents.

## THROMBIN

Thrombin is composed of 295 amino acids that comprise two polypeptide chains joined by a single disulfide bridge. α-Thrombin, which is the only human thrombin with potent clotting activity, has a molecular mass of 36 Kda. Its A chain is 36 amino acids in length, and its B chain, which possesses the serine protease domain, is 259 amino acids (2).

There are three distinct functional domains of the thrombin molecule (Fig. 57.3). The active or catalytic site, with its basic specificity pocket, binds arginine or lysine side chains of scissile peptide bonds (2). The anion binding exosite is composed of multiple basic amino acids, and it contains the fibrinogen recognition site (4). The third domain is the apolar binding site, which is located near the active site and also may be important to fibrin binding (4). Thrombin cleaves fibrinogen in two steps, thereby liberating fibrinopeptides A and B and forming fibrin monomers. Fibrin monomers polymerize end-to-

end and side-to-side to form fibrin thrombi (2, 5). The catalysis of fibrin formation is only one function of thrombin. Thrombin also activates a series of reactions that are important in hemostasis, including conversion of factor XIII to XIIIa, which irreversibly crosslinks fibrin polymers, and activation of factors V and VIII, which as potent nonenzymatic cofactors greatly amplify thrombin generation (1, 2, 3, 5).

Thrombin also is one of the most potent direct stimuli of platelet aggregation (see Chapter 12). The primary platelet thrombin receptor has been identified, cloned, and sequenced, and a unique mechanism characterizing its interaction with thrombin has been elucidated (6). The aminoterminal extracellular extension of this receptor possesses both a thrombin cleavage site and a secondary binding site resembling the carboxyterminal region of hirudin, which is a specific thrombin inhibitor. The basic specificity pocket of thrombin binds to the cleavage site of the receptor, and the anionbinding exosite binds to the hirudinlike sequence. Subsequent cleavage of the thrombin receptor leads to formation of a new aminoterminus, which functions as a receptor-attached (i.e., tethered) ligand for a unique receptor domain and leads to platelet activation (6).

Thrombin directly activates platelet membrane phospholipase C (7), and it initiates formation of thromboxane $A_2$, which is another potent stimulus for platelet aggregation. Thrombin also induces endothelial cells to release von Willebrand factor, plasminogen activator inhibitor-1 (8), endothelin (9), and to express the integral membrane procoagulant tissue factor (10).

In addition to these prothrombotic functions, thrombin also manifests antithrombotic effects. It binds to endothelial-bound thrombomodulin and, thereby, activates the natural anticoagulant protein C (11). Thrombin also stimulates endothelial cells to release tissue-type plasminogen activator (t-PA) (8), prostacyclin, and endothelium derived relaxing factor or nitric oxide.

## FACTOR Xa

Factor X is a glycoprotein with a molecular mass of 59 Kda. It is composed of two polypeptide chains of unequal size, which are connected by a disulfide bridge. The heavy chain contains the active site serine, which distinguishes the activated form of this coagulation factor as a member of the serine protease family (1).

Factor X is activated to factor Xa($\alpha$) by cleavage of an Arg-Leu peptide bond in the carboxyterminal region of the heavy chain. This reaction is catalyzed by the factor VIIa-tissue factor complex and by a complex of enzymes and cofactors composed of factor IXa, factor VIII, and calcium, all of which are arranged on a membrane surface. Factor Xa($\alpha$) can be modified further by autocatalytic cleavage of the carboxyterminus of its heavy chain to form factor Xa($\beta$), which is a serine protease with coagulant activity similar to that of its parent molecule (1).

Once formed, factor Xa participates in the coagulation process by serving as one component of the prothrombinase complex. This complex is a noncovalent assembly of enzymes and cofactors that cleaves prothrombin, thus generating thrombin. Also included in the prothrombinase complex are factor Va and calcium ions; these components are assembled on a phospholipid membrane surface (1).

# THROMBIN INHIBITORS

## HIRUDIN

Hirudin is a polypeptide found in the salivary glands of the leech *Hirudo medicinalis,* and it is the most potent natural thrombin inhibitor. Until cloning of its gene in 1986 (12–15), hirudin was isolated by extraction from homogenized leech heads and subsequent affinity chromatography using Sapharose (Pharmacia, Uppsala, Sweden) (16–18). With this technique, vast numbers of leeches (50,000 a year) were required to meet the demands of researchers for hirudin (18). The cumbersome extraction process and endangered species status of the medicinal leech (18), however, which limited the supply of hirudin, provided the impetus to develop the recombinant molecule.

Harvey et al (12) initiated production of recombinant desulfatohirudin (r-dsHIR) by constructing a complementary DNA (cDNA) library from homogenized leech-head regions. This library then was screened with oligonucleotide probes synthesized on the basis of the known amino acid sequence of hirudin. Using this technique, Harvey et al and others (13–15) identified a cDNA coding for hirudin. Initially, this cDNA was inserted into an *Escherichia coli* vector containing the bacteriophage PL promoter (12). Several investigators subsequently expressed r-dsHIR in the same vector with different promoters (4). Hirudin produced intracellularly with these systems spontaneously refolds into its appropriate tertiary structure after mechanical release from the host cell (4).

This expression system has been modified by Braun et al (19) by fusion of the hirudin gene to that coding for the signal peptide of the major outer membrane protein of *E. coli.* This modification leads to secretion of hirudin. Secretion of r-dsHIR also has been accomplished using a yeast vector in *Saccharomyces cerevisiae,* which expresses the folded, active gene product (20). The r-dsHIR produced in all these systems, however, lacks the sulfation of tyrosine 63, but it otherwise is identical to native hirudin (4).

At least three hirudin variants, which differ by a maximum of 13 amino acids, have been characterized and termed *HV-1, HV-2,* and *HV-3* (21, 22). Each is a polypeptide of 65 to 66 amino acids in length, with a molecular mass of approximately 7 Kda (21). Important features in the primary structure of hirudin include three disulfide bridges, an high overall content of glutamine and asparagine, and a sulfated tyrosine at position 63 (Fig. 57.4). Hirudin also possesses a hydrophobic aminoterminal region and a hydrophilic carboxyterminal region that is rich in acidic amino acids (21).

Stone and Hofsteenge (23) carefully studied the kinetics of thrombin inhibition by hirudin. They found that the hirudin-thrombin complex is formed rapidly and has a dissociation constant of approximately 20 fmol/l. Their kinetic analysis also showed that hirudin binds competitively to the active site of thrombin and to a second, lower affinity site.

Various biochemical and molecular biologic techniques have been used to study the specific nature of the hirudin-thrombin interaction and to guide the production of new and improved thrombin inhibitors. These include chemical modifications of thrombin (24), limited proteolytic digest experiments (24), use of specific antithrombin antibodies (25) and monoclonal antibodies to hirudin (26), and production of various recombinant hirudin mutants (27).

By chemically modifying thrombin, Stone et al (24) identified critical regions involved in binding to hirudin. The most important include the active-site $Ser_{205}$ and $His_{43}$ residues. The importance of the anion binding exosite domain of thrombin in mediating hirudin binding

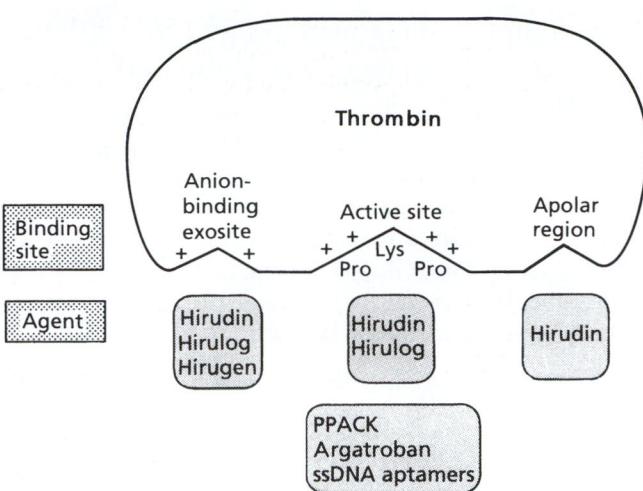

**FIGURE 57.3.** Thrombin inhibitors inactivate thrombin by interacting with one or more binding sites on the thrombin molecule. Hirudin binds to the anion binding exosite, the active site, and the apolar region. Hirulog exhibits bivalent binding properties, and hirugen binds to the anion binding exosite. D-Phe-Pro-Arg-chloromethyl ketone (PPACK), argatroban, and single-stranded DNA (ssDNA) aptamers all bind to the active site of thrombin.

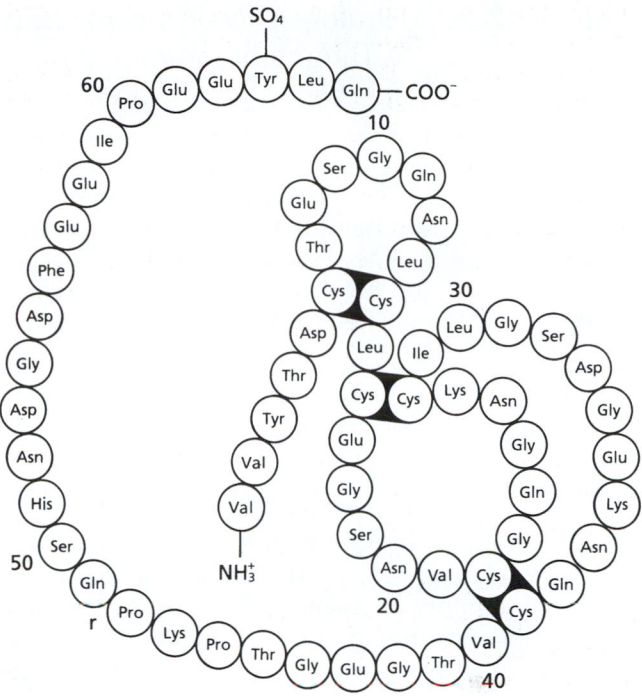

**FIGURE 57.4.** The primary structure of hirudin includes three disulfide bridges, a sulfated tyrosine at position 63, a hydrophobic aminoterminal region, and a hydrophilic carboxyterminal region. (Adapted with permission from Talbot M. Biology of recombinant hirudin (CGP 39393): a new prospect in the treatment of thrombosis (review). Semin Thromb Hemost 1989;15:293–301.)

is by removal of this region through limited proteolysis (24) or blockage of it with a site-specific antibody (25). Both cause large increases in the hirudin-thrombin dissociation constant.

Regions of hirudin important to its inhibition of thrombin have been identified with studies using r-dsHIR mutants and synthetic hirudin fragments. Marked increases in the dissociation constant produced by single point mutations in the aminoterminal region of hirudin demonstrated the importance of this region in thrombin inhibition (27). Similarly, r-dsHIR fragments entirely lacking the aminoterminal region showed a dramatic decrease in their affinity for thrombin (27).

Analogous studies using synthetic peptide fragments of the carboxyterminal region and r-dsHIR mutants of this region have confirmed that the carboxyterminus also is critical to inhibition of thrombin and interacts specifically with the fibrinogen recognition site of thrombin. By substituting the basic residues of hirudin with apolar or acidic amino acids, two groups (28, 29) were able to show that $Lys_{47}$ is the residue that interacts with the basic specificity pocket of thrombin.

These studies have led to a model that, at present, best characterizes the hirudin-thrombin complex (Figs. 57.2 and 57.4) (4, 21). The aminoterminal region of hirudin binds via hydrophobic interaction with the apolar binding site of thrombin. The carboxyterminal region appears to bind ionically to the anion binding exosite of thrombin, and the $Pro_{46}$-$Lys_{47}$-$Pro_{48}$ region of hirudin most likely occupies the basic specificity pocket of

thrombin. Direct interaction of hirudin with both the catalytic site and the anion binding exosite of thrombin probably accounts for its potent inhibition of all thrombin-mediated reactions. Furthermore, Weitz et al (29) have demonstrated this inhibition is equipotent toward free and fibrin-bound thrombin.

## HIRUGEN

Once the functional domains of hirudin were better understood, synthetic, hirudin-derived peptides that could inhibit thrombin were developed (30–33). Naski et al (31) first studied a dodecapeptide fragment of the carboxyterminal region of hirudin sulfated at tyrosine 63. Labeled as hirugen, this peptide binds to the anion binding exosite of thrombin and inhibits thrombin-mediated cleavage of fibrinogen. It is equally potent *in vitro* against fluid-phase and clot-bound thrombin (28). Because it lacks the second functional domain of hirudin, hirugen cannot inhibit the catalytic site of thrombin, and this may limit its effectiveness as an antithrombotic agent.

## HIRULOGS

Maraganore et al (32) also constructed an entire class of hirudin-derived thrombin inhibitors. Known as hiru-

**TABLE 57.3.** Hirulogs Contain a Thrombin Active-site Inhibitory Fragment, D-Phe-Pro-Arg-Pro, a Thrombin Anion-binding Exosite Recognition Sequence Analogue to Hirugen 53–64, and a Glycine Spacer of Variable Length

| | Sequence | $K_i$ (nmol/l) |
|---|---|---|
| Hirulog-1 | (D-Phe)-Pro-Arg-Pro-(Gly)$_4$-Asn-Gly-Asp-Phe-(Glu)$_2$-Ile-Pro-(Glu)$_2$-Tyr-Leu | 2.3 |
| Hirulog-2 | (D-Phe)-Pro-Arg-Pro-(Gly)$_2$-Asn-Gly-Asp-Phe-(Glu)$_2$-Ile-Pro-(Glu)$_2$-Tyr-Leu | 64.5 |
| Hirulog-3 | (D-Phe)-Pro-Arg-Pro-(Gly)$_6$-Asn-Gly-Asp-Phe-(Glu)$_2$-Ile-Pro-(Glu)$_2$-Tyr-Leu | 3.0 |
| Hirulog-4 | (D-Phe)-Pro-Arg-Pro-(Gly)$_8$-Asn-Gly-Asp-Phe-(Glu)$_2$-Ile-Pro-(Glu)$_2$-Tyr-Leu | 2.6 |
| Hirulog-5 | Phe-Pro-Arg-Pro-(Gly)$_4$-Asn-Gly-Asp-Phe-(Glu)$_2$-Ile-Pro-(Glu)$_2$-Tyr-Leu | 156.0 |

Reprinted with permission from Maraganore JM, Bourdon P, Jablonski J et al. Design and characterization of hirulogs: a novel class of bivalent peptide inhibitors of thrombin. Biochemistry 1990;29:7095–7101.

logs, they are synthetic peptides that contain the two distinct domains of hirudin with antithrombin activity (Table 57.3). Hirulog-1 (bivalirudin) contains a thrombin active-site inhibitory fragment, D-Phe-Pro-Arg-Pro, and a thrombin anion binding exosite recognition sequence that is analogous to hirugen (hirudin 53–64). These fragments are joined by a glycine spacer at least four residues in length. Although not quite as potent an inhibitor of thrombin as native hirudin, hirulog-l inhibits thrombin-mediated hydrolysis of a tripeptide (chromogenic) substrate with an inhibitory constant of 2.3 nmol/l (32). However, Kline et al (33) have found that subtle modifications of hirulogs can increase their affinity for thrombin to that of native hirudin.

## PPACK

PPACK (or D-Phe-Pro-Arg-chloromethyl ketone) specifically inhibits the catalytic site of thrombin by irreversibly alkylating the active-site histidine (34). Unlike hirugen, this monovalent thrombin inhibitor can inhibit thrombin-mediated platelet activation, and is useful clinically as an antithrombotic agent (34, 35). Like hirudin, PPACK inhibits both free and clot-bound thrombin with equal potency (Fig. 57.5) (29).

## ARGATROBAN

Another potent direct thrombin inhibitor is (2R,4R) 4-methyl-[N$^2$-(3-methyl-1,2,3,4-tetrahydro-8-quinolinyl) sulfonyl]-2-piperidinecarboxylic acid, or argatroban. This compound is a synthetic N$^2$-substituted arginine derivative that, like PPACK, binds to the catalytic site of thrombin with high affinity (36).

## SINGLE-STRANDED DNA APTAMERS

Bock et al (37) used a novel approach to develop specific segments of DNA that inhibit thrombin. Known as ap-

tamer, these segments are strands of single-stranded RNA, double-stranded DNA, or as these authors demonstrated for the first time, single-stranded DNA (ssDNA). They synthesized $10^{13}$ DNA oligonucleotides, each 96 nucleotides in length and containing a randomly generated, 60-nucleotide sequence. By amplifying these segments using the polymerase chain reaction, isolating ssDNA, and applying these strands repetitively to human thrombin that was coupled to concanavalin A-agarose, these investigators generated a bank of ssDNA aptamers that bound specifically to thrombin.

Sequence analysis of the thrombin-specific aptamers revealed in 31 of 32 clones a highly conserved hexamer sequence that appears to be responsible for thrombin binding. The thrombin aptamer binds to the anion binding exosite and inhibits the function of thrombin by competing with the exosite binding substrates fibrinogen and platelet thrombin receptor (38). Thrombin-aptamer binding was characterized by a dissociation constant of approximately 200 nmol/l (37).

The functional properties of these aptamers were assessed using an *in vitro* assay of thrombin-catalyzed conversion of fibrinogen to fibrin. Certain clones, or portions of clones, prolonged the time to fibrin formation by a factor of six when compared to unselected ssDNA sequence controls. The potency of the aptamers was diminished in plasma, but it could be restored by adding these agents in excess concentration. These findings suggest inactivation of aptamers in plasma by nucleases or other plasma proteins. The median effective dose [ED$_{50}$] for aptamer-induced inhibition of thrombin is approximately 25 nmol/l (37).

# FACTOR Xa INHIBITORS

Inhibitors of factor Xa are members of a novel class of antithrombotic agents. Their anticoagulant activity derives from direct inhibition of factor Xa and prevention of thrombin generation. These anticoagulants include tick anticoagulant peptide (TAP), leech-derived recom-

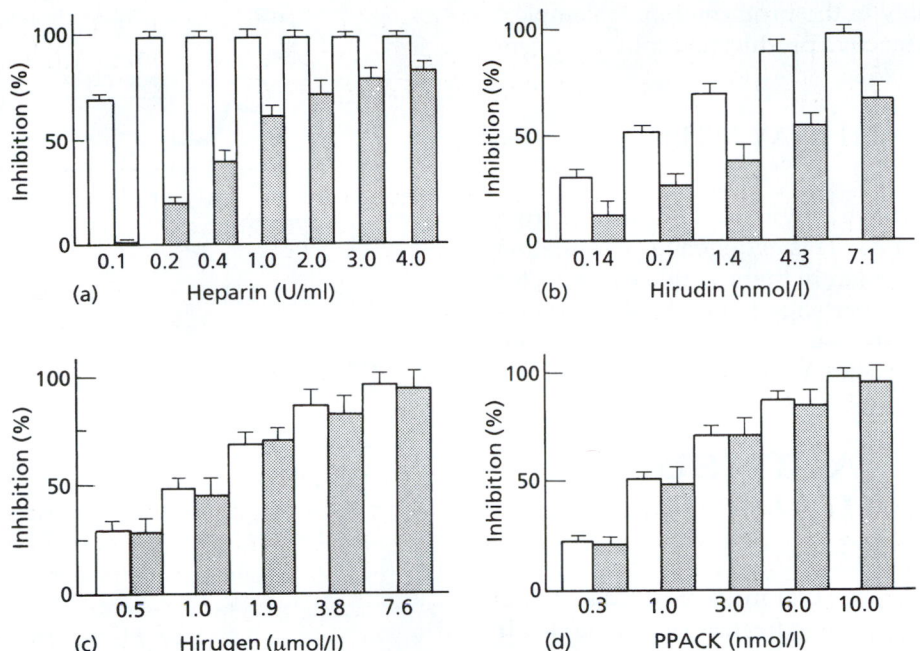

**FIGURE 57.5.**   Comparative *in vitro* effects of the direct thrombin inhibitors hirudin, hirugen, and PPACK and the indirect thrombin inhibitor heparin on clot-bound (filled bars) and fluid-phase (open bars) thrombin. **(a)**, Inhibition by heparin of clot-bound thrombin is markedly attenuated at low concentrations compared with inhibition by heparin of fluid-phase thrombin. The heparin concentration required to inhibit 70% of the activity of clot-bound thrombin (2.0 U/ml) is 20 times that necessary to similarly inhibit fluid-phase thrombin (0.1 U/ml). **(b)**, Hirudin is less effective against clot-bound thrombin than against fluid-phase thrombin, but this discrepancy is less marked than that for heparin. **(c)**, and **(d)**, Hirugen and PPACK (D-Phe-Pro-Arg-chloromethyl ketone) are equally effective at inhibiting clot-bound and fluid-phase thrombin. (Adapted with permission from Weitz JI, Hudoba M, Massel D et al. Clot-bound thrombin is protected from inhibition by heparin-antithrombin III but is susceptible to inactivation by antithrombin III-independent inhibitors. J Clin Invest 1990;86:385–391.)

binant antistasin (rATS), recombinant mutant factor Xa (Asn$_{322}$-Ala$_{419}$), and recombinant TFPI (rTFPI). TAP, rATS, and rTFPI inhibit the factor Xa molecule directly; recombinant mutant factor Xa (Asn$_{322}$-Ala$_{419}$) competes with factor Xa in assembly of the prothrombinase complex on a membrane surface. The crystal structure of factor Xa complexed to specific inhibitors of the bisamidino-aryl class (DX9065a) indicates the structural determinants of selective inhibition of the protease as being distinct from the inhibition of thrombin. These inhibitors exhibit an extended conformation along the active site, and this conformational requirement is distinctly different from the compact, folded structure observed with thrombin-specific inhibitors. Future development of specific factor Xa inhibitors should incorporate these structural features to ensure selectivity (39).

## TICK ANTICOAGULANT PEPTIDE

Initially, TAP was isolated from the tick *Ornithodoros moubata* by Waxman et al (40) in 1990. Later, a recombinant form (rTAP) was produced in *Saccharomyces cerevisiae* by Neeper et al (41). TAP is a single polypeptide composed of 60 amino acids and with a molecular mass

of 60 Kda. Its specific inhibition of factor Xa is dose-dependent, with an inhibition constant of 0.18 to 0.59 nmol/1 (40).

## ANTISTASIN

Antistasin was purified to homogeneity from the salivary glands of the Mexican leech *Haaementeria officinalis* by Nutt et al (42) in 1988. A polypeptide composed of 119 amino acids, it has a molecular mass of 15 Kda, is rich in cysteine residues, and contains several disulfide bridges (41). Dunwiddie et al (43) examined the kinetics of the antistasin-factor Xa interaction, and they showed that antistasin binds specifically and reversibly to factor Xa. The dissociation constant of the resulting complex is between 0.31 and 0.62 nmol/l. The active site of antistasin appears to be in the aminoterminal region. In addition, the cDNA for antistasin has been cloned, and rATS has been produced in baculovirus-infected Sf9 cells (44).

## MUTANT FACTOR XA (ASN$_{322}$-ALA$_{419}$)

Recombinant variants of proteolytically inactive factor Xa also have been developed as inhibitors of factor Xa. Mutant factor Xa (Asn$_{322}$-Ala$_{419}$) competes with native factor Xa for assembly in the prothrombinase complex, thereby forming an inactive product and inhibiting generation of thrombin (45).

## TISSUE FACTOR PATHWAY INHIBITOR (SEE CHAPTER 4)

Part of the anticoagulant activity of TFPI results from its inhibition of factor Xa. This endogenous coagulation inhibitor binds noncovalently to the active site of factor Xa, thus preventing its participation in the prothrombinase complex (46). The resulting TFPI–factor Xa complex also inhibits the factor VIIa–tissue factor complex (discussed later).

# FACTOR VIIA–TISSUE FACTOR INHIBITORS

## TISSUE FACTOR PATHWAY INHIBITOR

A polypeptide with a molecular mass of 38 Kda, TFPI is associated with the lipoprotein fraction of plasma (47). It can be prepared directly from plasma or from human HepG2 cells (i.e., a human hepatoma cell line) that secrete functional TFPI. The protein is purified from the media of these cells through affinity chromatography with factor Xa (47). Wun et al (48) cloned a cDNA for TFPI in 1988. Using rabbit polyclonal antibodies against TFPI, these investigators also screened the translation products of placental and fetal liver cDNA libraries, and they identified a 1.4-kb segment of DNA coding for TFPI. Detailed analysis of the cDNA nucleotide sequence has yielded important information about the primary structure of TFPI. The aminoterminus of this endogenous anticoagulant is rich in acidic amino acids, and the carboxyterminus contains many positively charged, basic amino acids. In addition, there are three Kunitz-type inhibitory domains in the central portion of the molecule.

As noted, TFPI directly inhibits factor Xa, and it serves as a cofactor for inhibition of the factor VIIa–tissue factor complex. As discussed in Chapter 4, Broze et al (47) proposed a model that unifies these two anticoagulant functions (Fig. 57.6), in which TFPI binds first to the active site of factor Xa, inhibiting this serine protease. This TFPI–factor Xa complex then binds to a preexisting factor VIIa–tissue factor-calcium complex assembled on a phospholipid membrane. The resulting inhibition of factor VIIa–tissue factor is an alternative mechanism to abrogate the coagulation cascade, thus adding yet another layer of complexity to the modulating factors of the coagulation process.

# CLINICAL STUDIES WITH COAGULATION FACTOR INHIBITORS

Numerous clinical trials have addressed the potential benefits of new antithrombotic strategies in individuals

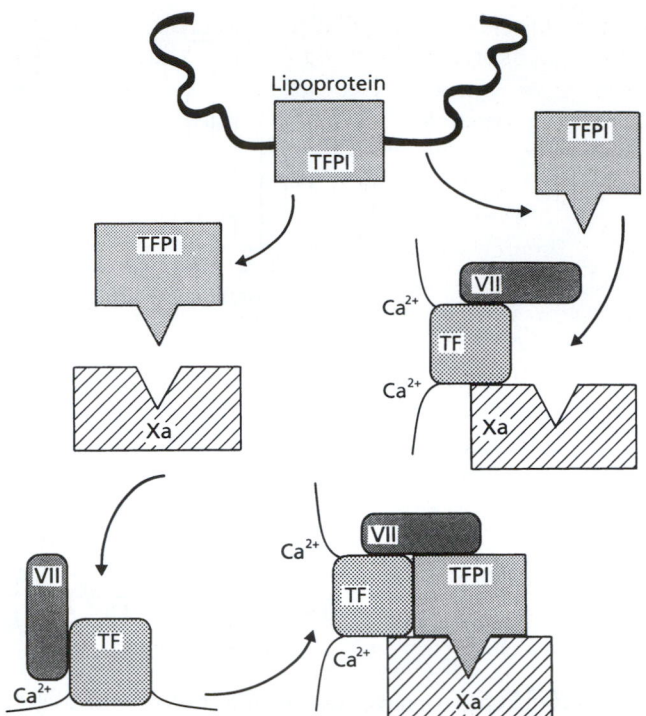

**FIGURE 57.6.** Tissue factor pathway inhibitor (TFPI) directly inhibits both factor Xa and the factor VIIa–tissue factor (TF) complex. TFPI first may bind to and inhibit factor Xa; this TFPI–factor Xa complex then may bind to the preformed factor VIIa–TF complex. Alternatively, TFPI may bind to a preassembled factor VIIa–TF-factor Xa complex. (Adapted with permission from Broze GJ Jr, Warren LA, Novotny WF, et al. The lipoprotein-associated coagulation inhibitor that inhibits the factor VII-tissue factor complex also inhibits factor Xa: insight into its possible mechanism of action. Blood 1988;71:335–343.)

with cardiovascular or cerebrovascular diseases. The interested reader is referred to Chapters 55, 56, 58, and 59 as well as to recent reviews of this topic published elsewhere (49–52). A summary of the most important of these trials is presented here.

## THROMBIN INHIBITORS

### Hirudin

Hirudin has been studied extensively *in vitro*, and its clinical use is under investigation. The most commonly used measures for the anticoagulant activity of hirudin are the thrombin time (TT) and the activated partial thromboplastin time (aPTT) (53). Hirudin does not have direct effects on platelet aggregation or secretion (54), and the bleeding time is not significantly prolonged by its use at antithrombotic doses (55, 56).

When administered intravenously to humans, hirudin follows first-order elimination kinetics and is excreted primarily by the kidney (57). Its plasma half-life is approximately 1 hour (57). Initial studies reported no side effects or significant bleeding with hirudin (55, 56), but in larger clinical trials (58, 59) high doses were associated with an increased rate of intracerebral hemorrhage (discussed later).

Hirudin also has been tested in several animal models of thrombosis. These include stasis-induced venous thrombosis (30, 60) and arterial thrombosis induced by vessel wall damage and deendothelialization (60–64). In each of these experimental systems, intravenous or subcutaneous administration of hirudin has effectively inhibited or completely eliminated thrombus formation.

In a baboon arterial thrombosis model using a thrombogenic arteriovenous shunt, Kelly et al (65) showed that hirudin infusions (5 and 20 nmol/kg per minute) significantly reduced both platelet and fibrin deposition compared with heparin (100 U/kg intravenous bolus followed by 10 U/kg per hour). Badimon et al (63) evaluated the antithrombotic efficacy of hirudin in an *ex vivo* system using vessel wall fragments perfused with flowing blood at different shear rates. In this limited study, hirudin (20 U/ml) significantly reduced thrombus formation (as measured by [$^{111}$In]-labeled platelet deposition) at high shear rates compared with heparin (dose-adjusted to prolong aPTT to 1.5 times control).

Recent efforts have focused on prevention of immediate thrombus formation after arterial angioplasty and subsequent restenosis. Heras et al (62) conducted a prospective study of 60 pigs subjected to carotid artery balloon angioplasty. These animals were treated with heparin (intravenous bolus followed by infusion) or r-dsHIR (1 mg/kg intravenous bolus followed by 1 mg/kg per hour), and thrombus formation was quantitatively measured by [$^{111}$In]-platelet and [$^{125}$I]-fibrin deposition at 1 hour. There was a significant inverse relationship of thrombus formation on deeply injured arterial segments with increasing heparin dosing regimens. Mean fibrin and platelet deposition in these segments, however was significantly lower in the hirudin group compared with the highest heparin dose group. Furthermore, mural thrombus was completely eliminated by hirudin.

Other investigators have studied the effect of hirudin on restenosis after angioplasty of focally stenosed rabbit femoral arteries (60, 64). Sarembock et al (64), for example, used rabbits treated with air desiccation injury to the femoral artery followed by a 2% cholesterol diet for 1 month. This protocol was followed by balloon angioplasty of the resulting stenosed arterial segment, immediately preceded by treatment with either heparin or r-dsHIR. As measured by quantitative angiography and quantitative histopathology at 4 weeks, restenosis was reduced in the r-dsHIR–treated group (1 mg/kg bolus followed by 1 mg/kg for 1 hour, then 0.5 mg/kg for 1 hour) compared with the group receiving a single bolus

of heparin (150 U/kg). This difference was statistically significant.

The results of these studies demonstrate the superiority of hirudin therapy compared with heparin for preventing thrombus formation after arterial injury in animal models. These results also suggest a role for generation of thrombin in the restenosis process. One factors that probably accounts for these findings is the ability of hirudin to inhibit clot-bound thrombin at therapeutic doses (Fig. 57.5). Weitz et al (29) showed *in vitro* that heparin cannot inhibit fibrin-bound thrombin unless the dose is increased 20-fold to 50-fold above standard doses (Fig. 57.5). One proposed mechanism that may account for diminished activity of heparin with preexisting thrombus is the steric hindrance and limitations on diffusion posed by the surrounding clot to formation of the heparin-antithrombin III complex. Because hirudin is a much smaller molecule that can directly inhibit thrombin independent of cofactors, it can interact more efficiently with clot-bound thrombin.

In addition to its potential for use with thrombotic disorders and as a possible inhibitor of restenosis after angioplasty, hirudin and other direct thrombin inhibitors are good candidates for adjunctive agents with thrombolytic therapy. Early reocclusion (within hours) limits the effectiveness of treatment with thrombolytic agents in individuals with acute myocardial infarction. The early reocclusion rate is reported to be as high as 10 to 25% for individuals treated with t-PA (66).

Substantial evidence indicates that early reocclusion may be secondary to the enhanced thrombin activity that occurs with this therapeutic approach. In a clinical study of individuals receiving intravenous streptokinase (750,000 U over 1 hour) for acute myocardial infarction, Eisenberg et al (67) found that 84% of individuals had a statistically significant increase in their levels of fibrinopeptide A (a sensitive and specific marker of thrombin activity) within 30 minutes (Fig. 57.7). This increase was still evident at 60 minutes and abruptly returned to baseline within 15 minutes of the administration of heparin.

Owen et al (68) followed fibrinopeptide A levels among individuals enrolled in the Thrombolysis in Myocardial Infarction (TIMI) trial, which was a randomized study of thrombolysis using t-PA or streptokinase in individuals presenting with acute myocardial infarction. In these individuals, plasma levels of fibrinopeptide A were significantly elevated 45 minutes after treatment with either agent despite receiving heparin before the initiation of thrombolytic therapy.

The source of this paradoxic rise in thrombin activity accompanying thrombolytic therapy is not clear. Thrombin may be liberated directly from the thrombus undergoing lysis. It also is likely that the underlying site of intimal injury continues to be a potent thrombogenic

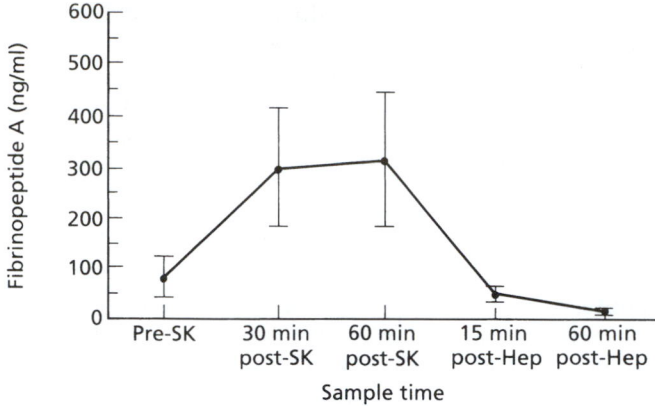

**FIGURE 57.7.** Paradoxically, thrombin activity increases with fibrinolytic therapy. Plasma levels of fibrinopeptide A increase within 30 minutes of intravenous streptokinase (SK) therapy for acute myocardial infarction, but this increase is abruptly abated with intravenous heparin (Hep) administration. (Adapted with permission from Eisenberg PR, Sherman LA, Jaffe AS. Paradoxic elevation of fibrinopeptide A after streptokinase: evidence for continued thrombosis despite intense fibrinolysis. J Am Coll Cardiol 1987;10:527–529.)

stimulus during thrombolysis. In addition, plasmin may lead directly to prothrombinase expression or indirectly to prothrombinase activity by activating platelets. Regardless of the mechanism, however, inhibition of this concomitant generation of thrombin could play a critical role in enhancing the speed of lysis and reducing the rate of early reocclusion after lysis, thus increasing the net patency achieved by activation or plasminogen. As a direct inhibitor of both free and clot-bound thrombin, hirudin is a good candidate for an adjunctive agent to accomplish this goal. Compared with heparin as adjunctive therapy to t-PA for treatment of acute myocardial infarction (69), hirudin produced a reduced rate of in-hospital death or reinfarction, as well as a trend toward fewer major hemorrhagic events. Similar results were obtained using hirudin as an adjunct to thrombolysis with streptokinase (70).

To study use of adjunctive hirudin and heparin in individuals with acute Q-wave myocardial infarction, two larger trials were conducted. Both the TIMI-9 and the Global Utilization of Strategies to Open Occluded Coronary Arteries (GUSTO) II trials compared a single dose of heparin with a single dose of hirudin. Importantly, both trials initially used high doses of hirudin (0.6 mg/kg bolus followed by 0.2 mg/kg per hour) and weight-adjusted heparin, and both trials were terminated prematurely because of an unacceptably high rate of intracerebral hemorrhage in both treatment arms (58, 59). These trials were continued as TIMI-9b and GUSTO IIb using lower doses of both hirudin (0.1 mg/kg bolus followed by 0.1 mg/kg per hour) and heparin (not weight-adjusted). Results from the TIMI-9b trial (71)

showed heparin and hirudin to be equally effective as adjunctive therapies for streptokinase or t-PA in individuals with acute Q-wave myocardial infarction, without a difference in bleeding events (71). Results of the GUSTO IIb trial (72) showed a marginally significant benefit of hirudin over heparin early after infarction in individuals with both Q wave and non-Q wave myocardial infarction; however, this effect lessened over time.

Hirudin also was studied clinically in individuals undergoing interventional coronary procedures. Compared with heparin in individuals undergoing coronary angioplasty, a continuous infusion of hirudin (20 mg bolus before angioplasty followed by continuous infusion of 0.16 mg/kg per hour for 24 hours) resulted in complete maintenance of perfusion and fewer acute cardiac or procedural complications than with heparin (73). The efficacy of hirudin in preventing restenosis also has been studied (74) in more than 1000 individuals undergoing angioplasty for unstable angina and given either heparin or hirudin. In this study, in-hospital clinical cardiac events were reduced in the hirudin group. After 7 months, however, angiographic restenosis and eventfree survival rates were not different, and the rate of bleeding complications was similar in both groups.

## Hirugen

Hirugen has undergone only limited clinical investigation. When administered to individuals, it causes a dose-dependent increase in aPTT, prothrombin time (PT), and TT, with the latter parameter being the most sensitive index of its effects (75, 76). Cadroy et al (77) observed that hirugen (0.5–75.0 mg/kg) caused a dose-dependent decrease in fibrin-rich (i.e., venous-type) thrombus formation in a baboon arteriovenous shunt model. Despite *in vitro* evidence that hirugen is a potent inhibitor of thrombin-induced platelet aggregation, this group did not observe a decrease in platelet-rich (i.e., arterial-type) thrombus formation in their model (30). This limited *in vivo* antithrombotic effect probably reflects the monovalent inhibition of thrombin by hirudin. It also demonstrates the importance of inhibiting the catalytic site, as well as the exosite, of thrombin in preventing arterial thrombus formation.

## Hirulog

Clinical studies with hirulog also have been limited in number. Because this synthetic peptide was constructed to include the critical antithrombin domains of hirudin, it probably will be as effective as r-dsHIR at inhibiting thrombin in clinical studies.

Hirulog (bivalirudin) was studied in a phase II clinical trial (78) involving individuals with presumed coronary artery disease undergoing cardiac catheterization. In this randomized study, intravenous hirulog-1 (0.05 mg/kg intravenous bolus followed by 0.2 mg/kg per hour infusion, or 0.15 mg/kg intravenous bolus followed by 0.6 mg/kg per hour infusion) or heparin (5000 U intravenous bolus) was administered during cardiac catheterization. Hirulog-1 caused a dose-dependent prolongation in the aPTT, PT, TT, and activated clotting time, which was similar to that found in the heparin group. The half-life for the anticoagulant effect of hirulog-1 was approximately 10 minutes. There were no side-effects reported with hirulog-1, and no clinical bleeding complications occurred in any treatment group.

A trial of hirulog in individuals under going coronary angioplasty confirmed its efficiency in preventing abrupt closure (3.9%) and its overall safety (79). In addition, among individuals undergoing percutaneous transluminal coronary angioplasty for unstable or post-infarction angina (80), hirulog was as effective as heparin but also was associated with a 61% reduction in hemorrhagic complications.

## PPACK

The ability of PPACK to inhibit thrombus formation has been studied in direct comparison to heparin in both rabbits and baboons. Using an *ex vivo* angioplasty model involving rabbit aortas mounted in a perfusion chamber, Kaplan et al (81) found that PPACK (10 μmol/l) was significantly more effective than heparin (2 U/ml) at inhibiting platelet deposition on injured arterial segments.

PPACK also has been tested in a primate model of arterial graft thrombosis. In this study (34), a continuous intravenous infusion (100 nmol/kg per minute) abolished [$^{111}$In]-platelet deposition on, and thrombosis of, freshly implanted vascular grafts. In this same model, treatment with heparin at conventional doses (100 U/kg) was not significantly more effective than control at inhibiting platelet deposition. Using a local delivery system in a swine model, Nunes et al (82) demonstrated that PPACK inhibited platelet-dependent thrombosis at doses less that those required for systemic administration.

## Argatroban

Studies with argatroban primarily have assessed its use as adjunctive therapy with thrombolytic agents in models of arterial thrombosis. In a dog coronary artery thrombosis model, Fitzgerald and FitzGerald (83) found that argatroban significantly accelerated the rate of recombinant t-PA (rt-PA)–induced thrombolysis at doses of 0.5 and 2.5 mg/kg per hour. In addition, at 2.5 mg/kg per hour, argatroban significantly delayed reocclusion, which was a universal endpoint in this model. Reocclusion could be completely abolished, however, in dogs treated with GR32191, which is a thromboxane A$_2$ antagonist, with a dose of 1 mg/kg over 10 minutes in addition to argatroban at 0.5 mg/kg per hour.

Yasuda et al (84) found similar results in their canine model of coronary artery thrombosis. Infusion of argatroban at a dose of 200 μg/kg per minute significantly accelerated the rate of rt-PA-induced thrombolysis. Compared with a 17 mg/kg intravenous bolus of aspirin in this model, argatroban also significantly improved the coronary artery patency rate at 2 hours. Similar results were obtained by Jang et al (85, 86) in a rabbit model of femoral artery thrombosis. Argatroban significantly reduces thrombosis of everted arterial segments compared with heparin (84) and is a superior adjunctive agent for thrombolytic therapy (86).

In a phase I clinical trial, Clarke et al (87) found that argatroban caused a dose-dependent increase in aPTT and TT. The half-life of the anticoagulant effect in humans is approximately 25 minutes when argatroban is used alone, and its administration is well tolerated and does not prolong the bleeding time (87). In a phase I dose-ranging trial involving individuals with unstable angina, argatroban (0.5–5.0 μg/kg per minute for 4 hours) was administered with no clinically significant bleeding (88). However, a rebound activation of angina, was precipitated by cessation of the argatroban infusion, and the clinical rebound phenomenon was accompanied by a 39-fold increase in thrombin-antithrombin III complex concentration within 2 hours after termination of the infusion. This rebound coagulation phenomenon may limit the effectiveness of argatroban as a clinical antithrombotic agent.

Suzuki et al (89) studied argatroban treatment in individuals after acute coronary occlusion following PTCA. All eight individuals studied had successful patency after redilation following argatroban infusion.

## Single-Stranded DNA Aptamers

A thrombin aptamer has been used as an anticoagulant during cardiopulmonary bypass in a canine model. In this study (90), a continuous infusion of 0.5 mg/kg per minute both before and during bypass led to a rise in the activated clotting time, which returned to normal levels within 5 minutes of discontinuing the infusion. In addition, minimal postoperative bleeding was associated with use of this agent.

## FACTOR Xa INHIBITORS

### Recombinant Tick Anticoagulant Peptide

rTAP has been studied *in vivo* in a rabbit model of venous thrombosis and in a dog coronary artery thrombosis model. Vlasuk et al (91) randomly administered rTAP (7–64 μg/kg per minute), rATS (0.625–5.000 μg/kg per minute), or heparin (30–100 U/kg per hour) to rabbits 60 minutes before inducing internal jugular vein thrombosis with rabbit brain thromboplastin. In this study, rTAP caused a dose-dependent decrease in clot formation (as measured by clot weight). These results were statistically significant compared with control rabbits at all but the lowest dose of rTAP. In addition, rTAP caused mild, dose-dependent prolongation of the aPTT and PT.

Sitko et al (92) studied rTAP as an adjunctive agent to thrombolysis with t-PA in a canine coronary artery thrombus model. In this study, rTAP and r-dsHIR (100 μg/kg per minute infusions) both statistically increased the incidence of reperfusion and accelerated its rate compared with saline control. Although not statistically significant, rTAP also reduced the incidence of reocclusion compared with control, r-dsHIR, and heparin. In another study comparing rTAP to r-dsHIR as adjunctive treatment with thrombolysis (93), rTAP was more effective than r-dsHIR at equimolar plasma concentrations in maintaining postthrombolysis vessel patency and reducing residual thrombus mass in a canine model of coronary thrombosis.

### Recombinant Antistasin

In the study by Vlasuk et al (91), rATS significantly reduced clot formation at infusions as low as 1.25 μg/kg per minute. rATS was approximately 10 times more potent than rTAP in this model. Compared with rTAP, rATS caused a more marked dose-dependent increase in the aPTT and PT. At the maximal infused dose of 5 μg/kg per minute, rATS caused a 3.7-fold rise in the aPTT and a 1.9-fold increase in the PT. In addition, plasma clearance of rATS was more prolonged compared with rTAP (91).

### Mutant Factor Xa ($Asn_{322}$-$Ala_{419}$)

No clinical investigations involving this agent have been published.

## FACTOR VIIa–TISSUE FACTOR INHIBITORS

### Recombinant Tissue Factor Pathway Inhibitor

Haskel et al (94) studied rTFPI in two canine models of femoral artery thrombosis. They demonstrated a statistically significant decrease in the incidence of reocclusion after t-PA-induced thrombolysis with adjunctive rTFPI in femoral arteries damaged by transluminal electrical injury. This model results in extensive transmural vascular injury, platelet-rich thrombi, and, presumably, exposure of tissue factor. In similar experiments involving femoral arteries damaged by the implantation of copper wires, which causes minimal damage to the vessel wall and produces fibrin-rich thrombi, rTFPI had no significant effect on the incidence of reocclusion (94). These studies suggest that extrinsic pathway activation also may be important in reocclusion after thrombolysis or

early restenosis, or both, after arterial angioplasty. Additional animal studies have demonstrated that high concentrations of rTFPI can prevent venous thrombosis in rabbits (95), and that a 24-hour infusion of rTFPI prevents restenosis in a hyperlipemic minipig model of angioplasty injury (96). It is not known, however, whether the efficacy of rTFPI in such models results from inhibition of factor Xa or factor VIIa–tissue factor activity. Results of a recently published canine study (97) suggest that rTFPI also can be used to maintain coronary patency following thrombolysis in a model of platelet-rich thrombi, and that it does so without marked perturbation of hemostatic determinants.

# ENDOGENOUS ANTICOAGULANTS

Heparan sulfate and dermatan sulfate are endogenous anticoagulant glycosaminoglycans that act as cofactors for serpins to efficiently inhibit thrombin, other coagulation factors, or both. These serpins are antithrombin III and heparin cofactor II, and glycosaminoglycans act as true chemical catalysts to facilitate interaction of these serpins with serine proteases. The endogenous anticoagulants are discussed in detail in Chapter 3.

## ANTITHROMBIN III

Antithrombin III has a molecular mass of 58.2 Kda and is 432 amino acids in length (98). The gene for this serpin is located on chromosome 1, and it has been characterized by Prochownik et al (99). It spans 19 kb, and it is composed of six exons and five introns. Despite significant amino acid homology between antithrombin III and other members of the serpin superfamily, introns within the antithrombin III gene do not show homology to other members of the superfamily.

Recombinant human antithrombin III has been expressed in Chinese hamster ovary cells by cotransfection of antithrombin III cDNA with an amplifiable mouse dihydrofolate reductase gene and subsequent exposure to methotrexate (100). The functional protein was purified through affinity chromatography with heparin-Sepharose and appears to be identical physiologically to native antithrombin III. Recombinant antithrombin III also has been expressed in mammalian cells derived from the green monkey kidney cell line (101). These initial systems were limited by low yields of functional antithrombin III, but Gillespie et al (102) overcame this problem by cotransfecting *Spodoptera frugiperda* (Sf9) insect cells with human antithrombin III cDNA inserted into a baculovirus vector and wild-type baculovirus. Successful transfection has resulted in cells that secrete 10 to 35 μg of recombinant antithrombin III per $10^6$ cells. This efficient system provides milligram quantities of recombinant protein that is functionally identical to native antithrombin III.

Antithrombin III is cofactor for the endogenous glycosaminoglycan heparan sulfate as well as for commercially prepared heparin. The resulting complex inhibits thrombin and thrombin-mediated activation of factors V and VIII as well as factors IXa, Xa, XIa, and XIIa (98, 102–104).

The anticoagulant mechanism of the heparin-antithrombin III complex has been studied in detail and is most clearly understood for its inhibition of thrombin. The active-site serine of thrombin interacts with an arginine residue in the carboxyterminal region of antithrombin III. This binding is greatly accelerated by heparin, which binds to lysyl residues of the aminoterminal region of antithrombin III (103, 104).

Two possible models characterizing this complex have been proposed (Fig. 57.8). One draws on the work of Danielsson et al (105), who used a panel of heparin-derived oligosaccharides of varying lengths to show that heparin binds simultaneously to thrombin and antithrombin III, thus forming a ternary complex. This intermediary complex brings the serine protease and its serpin in close proximity, thereby facilitating their interaction.

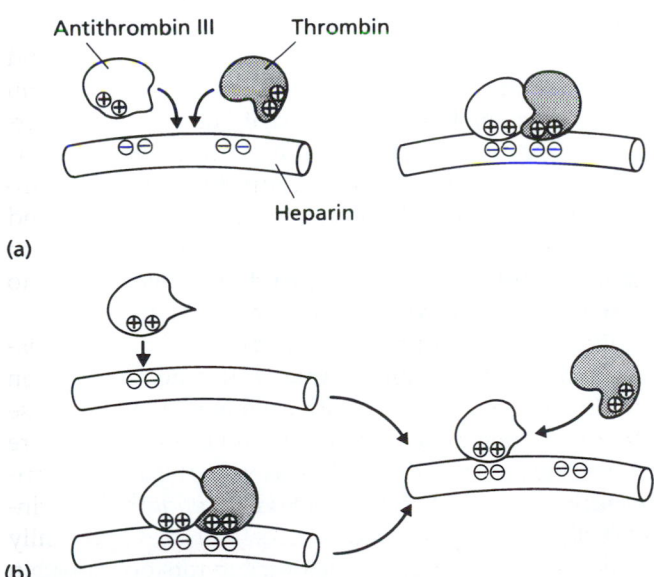

**(a)**

**(b)**

**FIGURE 57.8.** Two models characterizing the antithrombin III-mediated inhibition of thrombin have been proposed. **(a),** In the ternary complex model, antithrombin III and thrombin bind simultaneously to heparin. **(b),** In the conformational change model, heparin induces a conformational change in antithrombin III, thus exposing a critical arginine residue and facilitating interaction between antithrombin III and thrombin. (Adapted with permission from Scharfstein JS, Loscalzo J. Molecular approaches to antithrombotic therapy. Hosp Pract (Off Ed) 1992;27:77–86.)

Heparin may also induce a conformational change in antithrombin III, thus exposing the critical arginine residue and facilitating its binding to the active-site serine of thrombin (98, 103, 104). By itself, this conformational change may be sufficient to accelerate the inhibition of some serine proteases, such as factor Xa. However, the inhibition of thrombin also appears to require ternary complex formation (104). Regardless of the specific mechanism once antithrombin III is bound to thrombin (or other coagulation factors), it acts as a suicide substrate, with the subsequent covalent binding inactivating the coagulation factor. Heparin is then released from this complex and can catalyze additional thrombin-antithrombin III reactions (103, 104).

## HEPARIN COFACTOR II

Heparin cofactor II was initially purified through heparin Sepharose affinity chromatography. It is a glycoprotein and has a molecular mass of 65.6 Kda (106, 107). Herzog et al (108) cloned the gene for heparin cofactor II and localized it to chromosomal band 22q11.

There are several important biochemical differences between heparin cofactor II and antithrombin III. The active site residue cleaved by thrombin is a leucyl residue instead of arginine (107). In addition, the affinity of heparin cofactor II for thrombin is not as great as that of antithrombin III. Furthermore, unlike antithrombin III, heparin cofactor II does not mediate inhibition of any coagulation cascade serine protease other than thrombin (107). Therefore, heparin cofactor II is a specific cofactor for the inhibition of thrombin. This inhibition is mediated by heparin, heparan sulfate, and dermatan sulfate.

The physiologic importance and function of heparin cofactor II are not clear. Scattered cases of heparin cofactor II deficiency in individuals with venous thrombosis have been reported (see Chapter 40) (109, 110); However, in a study by Bertina et al (111) the incidence of heparin cofactor II deficiency (defined as a 90% probability of a heparin cofactor II level below the 95% tolerance limits of the normal distribution adjusted for age), in healthy volunteers was similar to the incidence in individuals with thrombosis. Thus, heparin cofactor II may represent an endogenous antithrombotic agent that inhibits thrombin in a specific vascular milieu rich in dermatan sulfate.

## ACTIVATED PROTEIN C

Activated protein C (APC) is a glycoprotein composed of two polypeptide chains, and its molecular mass is approximately 62 Kda (112). APC is formed by thrombin-mediated cleavage of the aminoterminal region of the protein C heavy chain. This proteolytic cleavage forms the new aminoterminus of the active protein, and releases an inactive dodecapeptide fragment (113). Endothelial-bound thrombomodulin is required as a cofactor for this enzymatic cleavage (112). As a serine protease, APC cleaves factors Va and VIIIa, thus inactivating these amplifiers of thrombin generation (1).

# CLINICAL STUDIES WITH ENDOGENOUS ANTICOAGULANTS

## ANTITHROMBIN III

Clinical studies of antithrombin III are few in number, and have been limited primarily to replacement therapy for individuals with acquired or congenital antithrombin III deficiency (see Chapters 40 and 52) (114, 115). There also are some data on the use of antithrombin III in normal individuals as prophylaxis for postoperative venous thromboembolism (116). Given with low-dose subcutaneous heparin (5000 U subcutaneously 2 hours before surgery followed by 5000 U every 12 hours for 5 days) to individuals undergoing total hip or knee replacements, intravenous administration of antithrombin III (1500 to 3000 U 2 hours preoperatively and 1000 to 2000 U daily for 5 postoperative days) was associated with a statistically significant decrease in venous thrombosis, as determined by venography, compared with dextran 40 (10 mL/kg over 12 hours starting 2 hours preoperatively followed by 7 mL/kg per 24 hours for 5.5 days) (116). This study did not compare antithrombin III treatment with a control group receiving heparin alone, but it did show intravenous administration of antithrombin III to be safe and free of side effects. A recent review of the available clinical trials involving treatment with antithrombin III concentrates (117) suggests these concentrates may be beneficial in specific clinical situations involving individuals with hereditary antithrombin III deficiency, such as delivery and postoperative thromboprophylaxis. Because of limited published data and the lack of randomized clinical trials, there are no proven indications for antithrombin III concentrates in acquired antithrombin III deficiency.

## HEPARIN COFACTOR II

Because the functional significance of heparin cofactor II is not clear and evidence that a deficiency in this glycoprotein causes a clinical thrombotic syndrome is lacking, there have been no clinical studies with this agent.

## ACTIVATED PROTEIN C

Both human APC and recombinant APC (rAPC) have been studied *in vivo* in a primate model of arterial thrombosis (118). Gruber et al (119) also studied rAPC in baboons with chronic femoral arteriovenous shunts containing inserts of thrombogenic graft material. rAPC (0.25 and 1 mg/kg per hour) significantly reduced the incidence of graft occlusion compared with controls. In addition, the higher dose of rAPC significantly decreased [$^{111}$In]-labeled platelet deposition in the grafts compared with controls. There was no significant prolongation of the bleeding time in this study, and there were no side effects from rAPC administration.

rAPC has also been studied in a canine model of coronary artery thrombosis as adjunctive therapy to thrombolytic treatment (120). After treatment with rTPA, a total rAPC dose of 0.6 mg/kg was given, thereby leading to prevention of coronary artery reocclusion. In a study by Arnljots and Dahlback (121), APC was given with protein S (0.5 mg/kg) in a rabbit model of microarterial thrombosis. Potentiation of the APC response was seen with protein S coadministration and without hemorrhagic side effects.

# ENDOGENOUS ANTICOAGULANT COFACTORS (SEE CHAPTER 3)

## HEPARAN SULFATE AND DERMATAN SULFATE

Extensive clinical experience with heparin as an anticoagulant cofactor has highlighted its many limitations. Heparin has a narrow therapeutic index, and it can cause immunologically mediated, heparin-induced thrombocytopenia (122). In addition, heparin is inactivated by platelet factor 4 (122) and has limited activity against clot-bound thrombin (29). These pitfalls have prompted the search for improved heparin preparations as well as modified preparations of the natural glycosaminoglycans heparan sulfate and dermatan sulfate.

Heparan sulfate, proteoglycans and dermatan sulfate are endogenous, heparinlike molecules with antithrombotic activity. These glycosaminoglycans are produced by many cell types, including endothelial cells (123), fibroblasts (124), and mast cells (125). Glycosaminoglycans are coagulation factor inhibitors operating at the cell surface or its surrounding milieu, and they probably play an important role in the balance of local thrombosis and fibrinolysis (122–126). Heparan sulfate inhibits serine proteases by catalyzing the formation of covalent complexes of a coagulation factor, such as thrombin, with either antithrombin III (98, 127) or heparin cofactor II (107, 127). Dermatan sulfate specifically catalyzes thrombin-heparin cofactor II complex formation (98, 99) and, unlike heparin, does not act through antithrombin III.

## TABLE 57.4. Endogenous Anticoagulant Cofactors; Glycosaminoglycan-derived Drugs

*Heparan sulfate preparations*
Lomoparan (ORG 10172)

*Dermatan sulfate preparations*
MF 701
OP 435
Desmin (OP 370)

*Pentosan polysulfate*

Development of these endogenous anticoagulant glycosaminoglycans as clinical antithrombotic agents is continuing (Table 57.4). These preparations usually are obtained as side products of the purification of heparin from mammalian tissues such as skin, intestine, pancreas, spleen, or kidney (128). As with commercial heparin, these glycosaminoglycans are heterogeneous in composition. One such preparation is ORG 10172 (lomoparan), which is a mixture of heparin, heparans, dermatans, and chondroitin sulfate (129). In addition, pentosan polysulfate (also known as PPS, SP54, PZ68, and hemoclar) is a semisynthetic glycosaminoglycan preparation derived from beechwood-tree shavings (130). Preparations composed mostly of dermatan sulfates include MF 701 (Mediolanum Laboratories, Milan, Italy), OP 435 (Opocrin Laboratories, Corlo, Italy) and OP 370 (desmin) (128). Several of these agents have been tested clinically and are currently in use as antithrombotic medications.

## LOMOPARAN

Lomoparan is extracted from porcine mucosa and has a molecular mass of 4 to 7 Kda (average, 4.9 Kda) (129). It is composed of a mixture of low-molecular-weight glycosaminoglycans, including heparan, dermatan, and chondroitin sulfates.

The anticoagulant actions of lomoparan are not well understood. *In vitro*, lomoparan causes a dose-dependent inhibition of factor Xa and thrombin; at equimolar concentrations of lomoparan, the inhibition of factor Xa is more pronounced (129). The ability of lomoparan to inhibit factor Xa depends on antithrombin III. In contrast, the inhibition of thrombin *in vitro* by lomoparan does not require antithrombin III as a cofactor (129). Lomoparan is a weak anticoagulant as measured by the PT, aPTT, and TT assays. The Heptest assay (Haemachem, St. Louis, MO) appears to be a more sensitive marker of its anticoagulant action; in this clot-based, anti-factor IIa/anti-factor Xa assay, lomoparan produces a dose-dependent prolongation of the clotting time. Lo-

moparan also exerts a weak effect on platelets as measured in the heparin-induced platelet activation and heparin-induced thrombocytopenia screening assays (129).

## PENTOSAN POLYSULFATE

Pentosan polysulfate (PPS) is a heterogeneous mixture of polysaccharides that is the only nonmammalian glycosaminoglycan currently under investigation. Derived from the beechwood tree, PPS has a molecular mass of 1.8 to 9.0 Kda (131). The antithrombotic mechanism of PPS is not well understood, but it prolongs the aPTT *in vitro* independent of heparin cofactor II or antithrombin III. PPS also inhibits generation of both thrombin and factor Xa in plasma (130). PPS may inhibit directly formation of the prothrombinase complex and thrombin-induced activation of factor VIII to factor VIIIa, which is a marker for one of the complexes responsible for activation of factor X.

## MF 701/DERMATAN SULFATE

MF 701 is a heterogeneous dermatan sulfate preparation that derives from porcine intestinal mucosa (131). It has a mean molecular mass of 36 Kda and, like endogenous dermatan sulfate, causes a heparin cofactor II–mediated inhibition of thrombin. Although often contaminated with traces of heparin and heparan sulfate, MF 701 is significantly less potent *in vitro* than unfractionated heparin as measured by its ability to prolong the aPTT (131).

## HEPARINS

Careful biochemical analyses of commercial heparin have revealed more details about its heterogeneous composition. Almost all heparin preparations extracted from porcine intestinal mucosa or bovine lung consist of both high-molecular-weight and low-molecular-weight fractions. The high-molecular-weight fraction (average molecular mass, 20 Kda) comprises 66% of a given preparation by mass, has a weak anticoagulant effect, and can activate platelets (132). The low-molecular-weight fraction (average molecular mass, 7 Kda) represents approximately 33% of a given preparation, possesses 85% of the total anticoagulant activity of the original sample (132), and causes little platelet activation (133).

The low-molecular-weight and high-molecular-weight fractions are each characterized by subspecies with low and high affinities for antithrombin III (132). The heparin species with high affinity for antithrombin III possesses a critical pentasaccharide sequence that mediates this interaction (134, 135). The low-molecular-weight heparin fraction with high affinity for antithrombin III represents that fraction with the most potent anticoagulant activity and the least platelet-stimulating activity (115). These detailed studies of heparin preparations led to development of low-molecular-weight heparins with enhanced potency for clinical use; a detailed discussion of these agents appears in Chapter 55.

# CLINICAL STUDIES WITH ENDOGENOUS ANTICOAGULANT COFACTORS

## LOMOPARAN

Lomoparan has been tested in animal models of thrombosis as well as in clinical trials. In a rabbit venous stasis model induced by activated prothrombin complex (129), lomoparan caused a dose-dependent antithrombotic affect when administered either intravenously ($ED_{50}$, ≈200 µg/kg) or subcutaneously ($ED_{50}$, ≈ 2.5 mg/kg). Significant bleeding was observed only at supratherapeutic intravenous doses of 5 and 10 mg/kg.

In humans, lomoparan has been tested as prophylaxis for postoperative deep venous thrombosis and as an anticoagulant during hemodialysis (129). In four randomized clinical trials comparing lomoparan with either placebo, subcutaneous heparin, dextran 70, or warfarin, lomoparan reduced the relative risk of postoperative deep venous thrombosis by at least 47%, and there were no significant side effects from treatment (129). During hemodialysis, lomoparan was an effective anticoagulant, but in at least one study, which involved individuals with chronic renal failure, it was associated with an unacceptable rate of late (24–36 hours) bleeding from puncture sites (129).

## PENTOSAN POLYSULFATE

In humans, PPS inhibits generation of factor Xa and thrombin *in vivo*. It mildly prolongs the PT and inhibits *ex vivo* platelet aggregation at high doses (130).

In animal models of venous thrombosis, PPS has been shown to be a weak antithrombotic agent (130). Its anticoagulant effect, however, can be enhanced dramatically by coadministration of heparin (130). At present, the molecular basis for this synergistic relationship is not clear.

## MF 701/DERMATAN SULFATE

There is limited clinical experience with dermatan sulfate as an antithrombotic agent, but it has been tested *in vivo* with animal models of venous thrombosis. In a limited study (131), MF 701 inhibited rabbit internal jugular vein thrombosis induced by thrombin and thromboplastin; it also limited extension of existing

thrombus. These results demonstrated that significant bleeding as a side effect of MF 701 is problematic only at supratherapeutic doses.

Limited human studies have been conducted with MF 701. When administered intravenously, the plasma half-life (≈1 hour) varies depending on the method used to assay this agent's effects. The drug is excreted by the kidney, with 90% clearance by 24 hours (131). MF 701 causes a dose-dependent increase in the aPTT and thrombin clotting time when given by this route. When given subcutaneously or intramuscularly, however, the plasma half-life is approximately 7 to 10 hours. In general, the drug is well tolerated.

Clinical trials with MF 701 have been initiated to assess its efficacy as prophylaxis for postoperative deep venous thrombosis in individuals undergoing elective orthopaedic surgery (136) and as an anticoagulant for hemodialysis. Studies have shown MF 701 to be an effective antithrombotic agent, with a trend toward less hemorrhagic potential than with heparin (131, 137). Dermatan sulfate also is being tested as an alternative to heparin during cardiopulmonary bypass, and in a pig model (138). Successful bypass could be achieved with dermatan sulfate at lower doses than heparin in a pig model.

# CONCLUSIONS

Development of recombinant DNA technology and improved protein chemistry techniques have opened new avenues for novel drugs and dramatically expanded the medical pharmacopeia. Virtually all classes of drugs have been affected by these advances. Although still in various stages of development, new antithrombotic agents are included in this pharmaceutical growth.

New antithrombotic drugs are particularly in demand given the extensive clinical need and the inadequacies of currently available anticoagulants. Each of the three strategies for developing antithrombotic agents outlined in this chapter have used, at least in part, molecular biologic techniques; as a result, promising new antithrombotic drugs have been produced. Of these, the specific coagulation factor inhibitors probably will find a niche in treatment of cardiovascular disorders. In that field, new drugs are needed as adjuncts to thrombolysis in acute myocardial infarction, as possible inhibitors of early reocclusion or late restenosis after arterial angioplasty, and as new therapeutic agents for unstable coronary syndromes. In addition, various glycosaminoglycan preparations are being used clinically for prophylaxis of postoperative deep venous thrombosis.

Importantly, the clinical studies discussed here reveal the potential limitations of direct thrombin inhibitors used in treatment of acute coronary syndromes. While inhibiting thrombin activity, these agents do not suppress ongoing thrombin generation. Development and further study of coagulation cascade enzyme inhibitors, therefore, may reveal a role as adjuncts to thrombolytic therapy. Despite potential limitations, heparin and warfarin probably soon will no longer represent the only clinically available choices for antithrombotic therapy.

# REFERENCES

1. Nemerson Y. Sequence of coagulation reactions. In: Williams WJ, Bentler E, Erstev AJ, Lichtman MA, eds. Hematology. 4th ed. New York: McGraw-Hill, 1990:1295–1304.
2. Fenton JW II, Landis BH, Walz DA et al. Human thrombin: preparative evaluation, structural properties, and enzymatic specificity. In: Bing DH, ed. The chemistry and physiology of the human plasma proteins. New York: Pergamon Press, 1979:151.
3. Scharfstein JS, Loscalzo J. Molecular approaches to antithrombotic therapy [Review]. Hosp Pract (Off Ed) 1992;27:77–86.
4. Johnson PH, Sze P, Winant R et al. Biochemistry and genetic engineering of hirudin [Review]. Semin Thromb Hemost 1989;15:302–315.
5. Bennett JS. Blood coagulation and coagulation tests [Review]. Med Clin North Am 1989;68:557–576.
6. Vu TK, Hung DT, Wheaton VI et al. Molecular cloning of a functional thrombin receptor reveals a novel proteolytic mechanism of receptor activation. Cell 1991;64:1057–1068.
7. Shukla SD, Franklin CC, Carter MG. Activation of phospholipase C in platelets by platelet activating factor and thrombin causes hydrolysis of a common pool of phosphatidylinositol 4,5-biphosphate. Biochim Biophys Acta 1987;929:134–141.
8. Van Hinsberg VW, Sprengers ED, Kooistra T. Effect of thrombin on the production of plasminogen activators and PA inhibitor-1 by human foreskin microvascular endothelial cells. Thromb Haemost 1987;57:148–153.
9. Kohno M, Yasunari K, Yokokawa K et al. Thrombin stimulates the production of immunoreactive endothelin-1 in cultured human umbilical vein endothelial cells. Metabolism 1990;39:1003–1005.
10. Galdal KS, Lyberg T, Evensen SA et al. Thrombin induces thromboplastin synthesis in cultured vascular endothelial cells. Thromb Haemost 1985;54:373–376.
11. Dittman WA, Majerus PW. Structure and function of thrombomodulin: a natural anticoagulant [Review]. Blood 1990;75:329–336.
12. Harvey RP, Degryse E, Stefani L et al. Cloning and expression of a cDNA coding for the anticoagulant hirudin from the bloodsucking leech, *Hirudo medicinalis*. Proc Natl Acad Sci U S A 1986;83:1084–1088.
13. Dodt J, Schmitz T, Schafer T et al. Expression, secretion and processing of hirudin in E. coli using the alkaline phosphatase signal sequence. FEBS Lett 1986;202:373–377.
14. Fortkamp E, Rieger M, Heisterberg-Moutses G et al. Cloning and expression in *Escherichia coli* of a synthetic DNA for hirudin, the blood coagulation inhibitor in the leech. DNA 1986;5:511–517.
15. Bergmann C, Dodt J, Kohler S et al. Chemical synthesis and expression of a gene coding for hirudin, the thrombin-specific inhibitor from the leech Hirudo medicinalis. Biol Chem Hoppe-Seyler 1986;367:731–740.
16. Markwardt F. The development of hirudin as an antithrombotic drug [Review]. Thromb Res 1994;74:1–23.
17. Bagdy D, Barabas E, Graf L et al. Hirudin. Methods Enzymol 1976;45:669–678.
18. Markwardt F. The comeback of hirudin as an antithrombotic agent [Review]. Semin Thromb Hemost 1991;17:79–82.
19. Braun PJ, Dennis S, Hofsteenge J et al. Use of site-directed mutagenesis to investigate the basis for the specificity of hirudin. Biochemistry 1988;27:6517–6522.
20. Riehl-Bellon N, Carvallo D, Acker M et al. Purification and biomedical characterization of recombinant hirudin produced by Saccharomyces cerevisiae. Biochemistry 1989;28:2941–2949.
21. Marki WE, Grossenbacher H, Grutter MG et al. Recombinant hirudin: genetic engineering and structure analysis [Review]. Semin Thromb Hemost 1991;17:88–93.
22. Walsmann P. Isolation and characterization of hirudin from Hirudo medicinalis [Review]. Semin Thromb Hemost 1991;17:83–87.
23. Stone SR, Hofsteenge J. Kinetics of the inhibition of thrombin by hirudin. Biochemistry 1986;25:4622–4628.
24. Stone SR, Braun PJ, Hofsteenge J. Identification of regions of α-thrombin involved in its interaction with hirudin. Biochemistry 1987;26:4617–4624.
25. Noe G, Hofsteenge J, Rovelli G et al. The use of sequence-specific antibodies to identify a secondary binding site in thrombin. J Biol Chem 1988;263:11729–11735.
26. Schlaeppi JM, Vekemans S, Rink H et al. Preparation of monoclonal antibodies to hirudin and hirudin peptides. A method for studying the hirudin–thrombin interaction. Eur J Biochem 1990;188:463–470.
27. Lazar JB, Winant RC, Johnson PH. Hirudin: aminoterminal residues play a major role in the interaction with thrombin. J Biol Chem 1991;266:685–688.
28. Dodt J, Kohler S, Baici A. Interaction of site specific hirudin variants with α-thrombin. FEBS Lett 1988;229:87–90.
29. Weitz JI, Hudoba M, Massel D et al. Clot-bound thrombin is protected from inhibition by heparin-antithrombin III but is susceptible to inactivation by antithrombin III-independent inhibitors. J Clin Invest 1990;86:385–391.
30. Kelly AB, Maraganore JM, Bourdon P et al. Antithrombotic effects of synthetic peptides targeting various functional domains of thrombin. Proc Natl Acad Sci U S A 1992;89:6040–6044.
31. Naski MC, Fenton JW II, Maraganore JM et al. The COOH-terminal domain of hirudin. An exosite-directed competitive inhibitor of the action of α-thrombin on fibrinogen. J Biol Chem 1990;265:13484–13489.
32. Maraganore JM, Bourdon P, Jablonski J et al. Design and characterization of hirulogs: a novel class of bivalent peptide inhibitors of thrombin. Biochemistry 1990;29:7095–7101.
33. Kline T, Hammond C, Bourdon P et al. Hirulog peptides with scissile bond replacements resistant to thrombin cleavage. Biochem Biophys Res Commun 1991;177:1049–1055.
34. Hanson SR, Harker LA. Interruption of acute platelet-dependent thrombosis by the synthetic antithrombin D-phenylalanyl-L-prolyl-L-arginyl chloromethyl ketone. Proc Natl Acad Sci U S A 1988;85:3184–3188.
35. Schneider PA, Hanson SR, Harker LA. Permanent interruption of thrombus formation on carotid endarterectomy sites by short term therapy with a synthetic antithrombin [Abstract]. Circulation 1988;78(Suppl II):311A.
36. Kikumoto R, Tamao Y, Tezuka T et al. Selective inhibition of thrombin by (2R, 4R)-4-methyl-1-[N2-(3-methyl-1, 2, 3, 4-tetrahydro-8-quinolinyl)-sulfonyl]-1-arginyl)]-2-piperidinecarboxylic acid. Biochemistry 1984;23:85–90.
37. Bock LC, Griffin LC, Latham JA et al. Selection of single-stranded DNA molecules that bind and inhibit human thrombin. Nature 1992;355:564–566.
38. Paborsky LR, McCurdy SN, Griffin LC et al. The single-stranded DNA aptamer-binding site of human thrombin. J Biol Chem 1993;268:20808–20811.
39. Stubbs MT, Huber R, Bode W. Crystal structures of factor Xa specific inhibitors in complex with trypsin: structural grounds for inhibition of factor Xa and selectivity against thrombin. FEBS Lett 1995;375:103–107.
40. Waxman L, Smith DE, Arcuri KE et al. Tick anticoagulant peptide (TAP) is a novel inhibitor of blood coagulation factor Xa Science 1990;248:593–596. (Published erratum appears in Science 1990;248:1473.)
41. Neeper MP, Waxman L, Smith DE et al. Characterization of recombinant tick anticoagulant peptide. A highly selective inhibitor of blood coagulation factor Xa. J Biol Chem 1990;265:17746–17752.
42. Nutt E, Gasic T, Rodkey J et al. The amino acid sequence of antistasin. A potent inhibitor of factor Xa reveals a repeated internal structure. J Biol Chem 1988;263:10162–10167.
43. Dunwiddie C, Thornberry NA, Bull HG et al. Antistasin, a leech-derived inhibitor of factor Xa. Kinetic analysis of enzyme inhibition and identification of the reactive site. J Biol Chem 1989;264:16694–16699.
44. Nutt EM, Jain D, Lenny AB et al. Purification and characterization of recombinant antistasin: a leech-derived inhibitor of coagulation factor Xa. Arch Biochem Biophys 1991;285:37–44.
45. Sinha U, Hancock TE, Lin P-H et al. Selective inhibition of the prothrombinase complex by the novel coagulation inhibitor, factor Xa (Asn$_{322}$-Ala$_{419}$) [Abstract]. Circulation 1991;84(Suppl II):580A.
46. Rapaport SI. Inhibition of factor VIIa/tissue factor-induced blood coagulation: with particular emphasis upon a factor Xa-dependent inhibitory mechanism [Review]. Blood 1989;73:359–365.
47. Broze GJ Jr, Warren LA, Novotny WF et al. The lipoprotein-associated coagulation inhibitor that inhibits the factor VII-tissue factor complex also inhibits factor Xa: insight into its possible mechanism of action. Blood 1988;71:335–343.
48. Wun TC, Kretzmer KK, Girard TJ et al. Cloning and characterization of a cDNA coding for the lipoprotein-associated coagulation inhibitor shows that it consists of three tandem Kunitz-type inhibitory domains. J Biol Chem 1988;263:6001–6004.
49. Philippides GJ, Loscalzo J. Potential advantages of direct-acting thrombin inhibitors [Review]. Coron Artery Dis 1996;7:497–507.
50. Bittl JA. Clinical trials of Hirulog in patients undergoing high-risk percutaneous transluminal coronary angioplasty [Review]. Coronary Artery Dis 1996;7:449–454.
51. Fitzgerald D, Murphy N. Argatroban: a synthetic thrombin inhibitor of low relative molecular mass [Review]. Coronary Artery Dis 1996;7:455–458.
52. Albers GW. Antithrombotic agents in cerebral ischemia [Review]. Am J Cardiol 1995;75:34B–38B.
53. Walenga JM, Hoppensteadt D, Koza M et al. Comparative studies on various assays for the laboratory evaluation of r-hirudin. Semin Thromb Hemost 1991;17:103–112.

54. Glusa E. Hirudin and platelets [Review]. Semin Thromb Hemost 1991;17:122–125.

55. Kaiser B. Anticoagulant and antithrombotic actions of recombinant hirudin [Review]. Semin Thromb Hemost 1991;17:130–136.

56. Zoldhesyi P, Chesebro JH, Webster MWI et al. Recombinant desulfato hirudin, a specific antithrombin, in individuals with chronic, stable coronary disease: effect on hemostatic parameters [Abstract]. J Am Coll Cardiol 1992;19:104A.

57. Nowak G. Pharmacokinetics of hirudin [Review]. Semin Thromb Hemost 1991;17:145–149.

58. Antman EM. Hirudin in acute myocardial infarction. Safety report from the Thrombolysis and Thrombin Inhibition in Myocardial Infarction (TIMI) 9A Trial. Circulation 1994;90:1624–1630.

59. Anonymous. Randomized trial of intravenous heparin versus recombinant hirudin for acute coronary syndromes. The Global Use of Strategies to Open Occluded Coronary Arteries (GUSTO) IIa Investigators. Circulation 1994;90:1631–1637.

60. Kaiser B, Simon A, Markwardt F. Antithrombotic effects of recombinant hirudin in experimental angioplasty and intravascular thrombolysis. Thromb Haemost 1990;63:44–47.

61. Lam JY, Chesebro JH, Steele PM et al. Antithrombotic therapy for deep arterial injury by angioplasty. Efficacy of common platelet inhibition compared with thrombin inhibition in pigs. Circulation 1991;84:814–820.

62. Heras M, Chesebro JH, Penny WJ et al. Effects of thrombin inhibition on the development of acute platelet-thrombus deposition during angioplasty in pigs. Heparin versus recombinant hirudin, a specific thrombin inhibitor. Circulation 1989;79:657–665.

63. Badimon L, Badimon J, Lassila R et al. Thrombin inhibition by hirudin decreases platelet thrombus growth on areas of severe vessel wall injury [Abstract]. J Am Coll Cardiol 1984;13:145A.

64. Sarembock IJ, Gertz SD, Gimple LW et al. Effectiveness of recombinant desulphatohirudin in reducing restenosis after balloon angioplasty of atherosclerotic femoral arteries in rabbits. Circulation 1991;84:232–243.

65. Kelly AB, Marzec UM, Krupski W et al. Hirudin interruption of heparin-resistant arterial thrombus formation in baboons. Blood 1991;77:1006–1012.

66. Roberts R. Heparin and aspirin in thrombolysis: biological and clinical issues. Clinical Challenges in Acute Myocardial Infarction 1992;1:1–7.

67. Eisenberg PR, Sherman LA, Jaffe AS. Paradoxic elevation of fibrinopeptide A after streptokinase: evidence for continued thrombosis despite intense fibrinolysis. J Am Coll Cardiol 1987;10:527–529.

68. Owen J, Friedman KD, Grossman BA et al. Thrombolytic therapy with tissue plasminogen activator or streptokinase induces transient thrombin activity. Blood 1988;72:616–620.

69. Cannon CP, McCabe CH, Henry TD et al. A pilot trial of recombinant desulfatohirudin compared with heparin in conjunction with tissue-type plasminogen activator and aspirin for acute myocardial infarction: results of the Thrombolysis in Myocardial Infarction (TIMI) 5 trial. J Am Coll Cardiol 1994;23:993–1003.

70. Lee LV. Initial experience with hirudin and streptokinase in acute myocardial infarction: results of the Thrombolysis in Myocardial Infarction (TIMI) 6 trial. Am J Cardiol 1995;75:7–13.

71. Antman EM. Hirudin in acute myocardial infarction. Thrombolysis and Thrombin Inhibition in Myocardial Infarction (TIMI) 9B trial. Circulation 1996;94:911–921.

72. Anonymous. A comparison of recombinant hirudin with heparin for the treatment of acute coronary syndromes. The Global Use of Strategies to Open Occluded Coronary Arteries (GUSTO) IIb investigators. N Engl J Med 1996;335:775–782.

73. van den Bos AA, Deckers JW, Heyndrickx GR et al. Safety and efficacy of recombinant hirudin (CGP 39 393) versus heparin in patients with stable angina undergoing coronary angioplasty. Circulation 1993;88:2058–2066.

74. Serruys PW, Herrman JP, Simon R et al. A comparison of hirudin with heparin in the prevention of restenosis after coronary angioplasty. Helvetica Investigators. N Engl J Med 1995;333:757–763.

75. Jakubowski JA, Maraganore JM. Inhibition of coagulation and thrombin-induced platelet activities by a synthetic dodecapeptide modeled on the carboxyterminus of hirudin. Blood 1990;75:399–406.

76. Maraganore JM, Chao B, Joseph ML et al. Anticoagulant activity of synthetic hirudin peptides. J Biol Chem 1989;264:8692–8698.

77. Cadroy Y, Maraganore JM, Hanson SR et al. Selective inhibition by a synthetic hirudin peptide of fibrin-dependent thrombosis in baboons. Proc Natl Acad Sci U S A 1991;88:1177–1181.

78. Cannon CP, Ganz P, Selwyn AP et al. Use of hirulog-1, a novel thrombin inhibitor, to anticoagulate patients during cardiac catheterization [Abstract]. J Am Coll Cardiol 1992;19:60A.

79. Topol EJ, Bonan R, Jewitt D et al. Use of a direct antithrombin, hirulog, in place of heparin during coronary angioplasty. Circulation 1993;87:1622–1629.

80. Bittl JA, Strony J, Brinker JA et al. Treatment with bivalirudin (Hirulog) as compared with heparin during coronary angioplasty for unstable or postinfarction angina. Hirulog Angioplasty Study Investigators. N Engl J Med 1995;333:764–769.

81. Kaplan AV, Leung LL, Leung W et al. Roles of thrombin and platelet membrane glycoprotein IIb-IIIa in platelet-subendothelial deposition after angioplasty in an *ex vivo* whole artery model. Circulation 1991;84:1279–1288.

82. Nunes GL, Hanson SR, King SB III et al. Local delivery of a synthetic antithrombin with a hydrogel-coated angioplasty balloon catheter inhibits platelet-dependent thrombosis. J Am Coll Cardiol 1994;23:1578–1583.

83. Fitzgerald DJ, FitzGerald GA. Role of thrombin and thromboxane A2 in reocclusion following coronary thrombolysis with tissue-type plasminogen activator. Proc Natl Acad Sci U S A 1989;86:7585–7589.

84. Yasuda T, Gold HK, Yaoita HK et al. Comparative effects of aspirin, a synthetic thrombin inhibitor and a monoclonal antiplatelet glycoprotein IIb-IIIa antibody on coronary artery reperfusion, reocclusion and bleeding with recombinant tissue-type plasminogen activator in a canine preparation. J Am Coll Cardiol 1990;16:714–722.

85. Jang IK, Gold HK, Ziskind AA et al. Prevention of platelet-rich arterial thrombosis by selective thrombin inhibition. Circulation 1990;81:219–225.

86. Jang IK, Gold HK, Leinbach RC et al. *In vivo* thrombin inhibition enhances and sustains arterial recanalization with recombinant tissue-type plasminogen activator. Circ Res 1990;67:1552–1561.

87. Clarke RJ, Mayo G, FitzGerald GA et al. Combined administration of aspirin and a specific thrombin inhibitor in man. Circulation 1991;83:1510–1518.

88. Gold HK, Torres FW, Garabedian HD et al. Evidence for a rebound coagulation phenomenon after cessation of a 4-hour infusion of a specific thrombin inhibitor in patients with unstable angina pectoris. J Am Coll Cardiol 1993;21:1039–1047.

89. Suzuki S, Sakamoto S, Adachi K et al. Effect of argatroban on thrombus formation during acute coronary occlusion after balloon angioplasty. Thromb Res 1995;77:369–373.

90. DeAnda A Jr, Coutre SE, Moon MR et al. Pilot study of the efficacy of a thrombin inhibitor for use during cardiopulmonary bypass. Ann Thorac Surg 1994;58:344–350.

91. Vlasuk GP, Ramjit D, Fujita T et al. Comparison of the *in vivo* anticoagulant properties of standard heparin and the highly selective factor Xa inhibitors antistasin and tick anticoagulant peptide (TAP) in a rabbit model of venous thrombosis. Thromb Haemost 1991;65:257–262.

92. Sitko GR, Ramjit DR, Stabilito II et al. Conjunctive enhancement of enzymatic thrombolysis and prevention of thrombotic reocclusion with the selective factor Xa inhibitor, tick anticoagulant peptide. Comparison to hirudin and heparin in a canine model of acute coronary artery thrombosis. Circulation 1992;85:805–815.

93. Lynch JJ Jr, Sitko GR, Mellott MJ et al. Maintenance of canine coronary artery patency following thrombolysis with front loaded plus low dose maintenance conjunctive therapy. A comparison of factor Xa versus thrombin inhibition. Cardiovasc Res 1994;28:78–85.

94. Haskel EJ, Torr SR, Day KC et al. Prevention of arterial reocclusion after thrombolysis with recombinant lipoprotein-associated coagulation inhibitor. Circulation 1991;84:821–827.

95. Holst J, Lindblad B, Bergqvist D et al. Antithrombotic effect of recombinant truncated tissue factor pathway inhibitor (TFPI1-161) in experimental venous thrombosis—a comparison with low-molecular-weight heparin. Thromb Haemost 1994;71:214–219.

96. Abendschein DR, Recchia D, Meng YY et al. Inhibition of thrombin attenuates stenosis after arterial injury in minipigs. J Am Coll Cardiol 1996;28:1849–1855.

97. Abendschein DR, Meng YY, Torr-Brown S et al. Maintenance of coronary patency after fibrinolysis with tissue factor pathway inhibitor. Circulation 1995;92:944–949.

98. Pratt CW, Church FC. Antithrombin: structure and function [Review]. Semin Hematol 1991;28:3–9.

99. Prochownik EV, Bock SC, Orkin SH. Intron structure of the human antithrombin III gene differs from that of other members of the serine protease inhibitor superfamily. J Biol Chem 1985;260:9608–9612.

100. Zettlmeissl G, Conradt HS, Nimtz M et al. Characterization of recombinant human antithrombin III synthesized in Chinese hamster ovary cells. J Biol Chem 1989;264:21153–21159.

101. Wasley LC, Atha DH, Bauer KA et al. Expression and characterization of human antithrombin III synthesized in mammalian cells. J Biol Chem 1987;262:14766–14772. (Published erratum appears in J Biol Chem 1988;263:6459.)

102. Gillespie LS, Hillesland KK, Knauer DJ. Expression of biologically active human antithrombin III by recombinant baculovirus in *Spodoptera frugiperda* cells. J Biol Chem 1991;266:3995–4001.

103. Rosenberg RD. Heparin, antithrombin, and abnormal clotting [Review]. Annu Rev Med 1978;29:367–378.

104. Rosenberg RD. Biochemistry of heparin antithrombin interactions, and the physiologic role of this natural anticoagulant mechanism [Review]. Am J Med 1989;87(Suppl 3B):2S–9S.

105. Danielsson A, Raub E, Lindahl U et al. Role of ternary complexes, in which heparin binds both antithrombin and proteinase, in the acceleration of the reactions between antithrombin and thrombin or factor Xa. J Biol Chem 1986;261:15467–15473.

106. Tollefsen DM, Sugimori T, Maimone MM. Effect of low-molecular-weight heparin preparations on the inhibition of thrombin by heparin cofactor II [Review]. Semin Thromb Hemost 1990;16(Suppl):66–70.

107. Pratt CW, Whinna HC, Meade JB et al. Physicochemical aspects of heparin cofactor II. Ann N Y Acad Sci 1989;556:104–115.

108. Herzog R, Lutz S, Blin N et al. Complete nucleotide sequence of the gene for human heparin cofactor II and mapping to chromosomal band 22qll. Biochemistry 1991;30:1350–1357.

109. Tran TH, Marbet GA, Duckert F. Association of hereditary heparin co-factor II deficiency with thrombosis. Lancet 1985;ii:413–414.

110. Sie P, Dupouy D, Pichon J et al. Constitutional heparin co-factor II deficiency associated with recurrent thrombosis. Lancet 1985;ii:414–416.

111. Bertina RM, Van der Linden IK, Engesser L et al. Hereditary heparin cofactor II deficiency and the risk of development of thrombosis. Thromb Haemost 1987;57:196–200.

112. Esmon CT, Owen WG. Identification of an endothelial cell cofactor for thrombin-catalyzed activation of protein C. Proc Natl Acad Sci U S A 1981; 78:2249–2252.

113. Kisiel W. Human plasma protein C: isolation, characterization, and mechanism of activation by alpha-thrombin. J Clin Invest 1979;64:761–769.

114. Schwartz RS, Bauer KA, Rosenberg RD et al. Clinical experience with antithrombin III concentrate in treatment of congenital and acquired deficiency of antithrombin. The Antithrombin III Study Group [Review]. Am J Med 1989;87(Suppl 3B):53S–60S.

115. Menache D. Replacement therapy in individuals with hereditary antithrombin III deficiency [Review]. Semin Hematol 1991;28:31–38.

116. Francis CW, Pellegrini VD Jr, Harris CM et al. Antithrombin III prophylaxis of venous thromboembolic disease after total hip or total knee replacement. Am J Med 1989;87(Suppl 3B):61S–66S.

117. Lechner K, Kyrle PA. Antithrombin III concentrates–are they clinically useful [Review]? Thromb Haemost 1995;73:340–348.

118. Gruber A, Griffin JH, Harker LA et al. Inhibition of platelet-dependent thrombus formation by human activated protein C in a primate model. Blood 1989;73:639–642.

119. Gruber A, Hanson SR, Kelly AB et al. Inhibition of thrombus formation by activated recombinant protein C in a primate model of arterial thrombosis. Circulation 1990;82:578–585.

120. Sakamoto T, Ogawa H, Yasue H et al. Prevention of arterial reocclusion after thrombolysis with activated protein C. Comparison with heparin in a canine model of coronary artery thrombosis. Circulation 1994;90:427–432.

121. Arnljots B, Dahlback B. Antithrombotic effects of activated protein C and protein S in a rabbit model of microarterial thrombosis. Arterioscler Thromb Vasc Biol 1995;15:937–941.

122. Hirsh J. Heparin [Review]. N Engl J Med 1991;324:1565–1574.

123. de Agostini AI, Watkins SC, Slayter HS et al. Localization of anticoagulantly active heparan sulfate proteoglycans in vascular endothelium: antithrombin binding on cultured endothelial cells and perfused rat aorta. J Cell Biol 1990;111:1293–1304.

124. Marcum JA, Conway EM, Youssoufian H et al. Anticoagulantly active heparin-like molecules from cultured fibroblasts. Exp Cell Res 1986;166: 253–258.

125. Marcum JA, Rosenberg RD. Anticoagulantly active heparin-like molecules from vascular tissue. Biochemistry 1984;23:1730–1737.

126. Marcum JA, McKenney JB, Rosenberg RD. Acceleration of thrombin-antithrombin complex formation in rat hindquarters via heparinlike molecules bound to the endothelium. J Clin Invest 1984;74:341–350.

127. Casu B. Structural features and binding properties of chondroitin sulfates, dermatan sulfate, and heparan sulfate [Review]. Semin Thromb Hemost 1991;17(Suppl 1):9–14.

128. Walenga JM, Hoppensteadt D, Fareed J. Non-heparin glycosaminoglycan-derived drugs: a biochemical and pharmacologic perspective [Review]. Semin Thromb Hemost 1991;17(Suppl 2):137–142.

129. Nurmohamed MT, Fareed J, Hoppensteadt D et al. Pharmacological and clinical studies with Lomoparan, a low-molecular-weight glycosaminoglycan [Review]. Semin Thromb Hemost 1991;17(Suppl 2):205–213.

130. Maffrand JP, Herbert JM, Bernat A et al. Experimental and clinical pharmacology of pentosan polysulfate [Review]. Semin Thromb Hemost 1991; 17(Suppl 2):186–198.

131. Gianese F, Lucchelli PE. A survey of the clinical experience with dermatan sulfate [Review]. Semin Thromb Hemost 1991;17(Suppl 2):199–204.

132. Rosenberg RD. Mechanism of antithrombin action and the structural basis of heparin's anticoagulant function. In: Bing DH, ed. The chemistry and physiology of the human plasma proteins. New York: Pergamon Press, 1979:353–368.

133. Salzman EW, Rosenberg RD, Smith MH et al. Effect of heparin and heparin fractions on platelet aggregation [Review]. J Clin Invest 1980;65:64–73.

134. Choay J, Lormeau JC, Petitou M et al. Structural studies on a biologically active hexasaccharide obtained from heparin. Ann N Y Acad Sci 1981;370: 644–649.

135. Choay J, Petitou M, Lormeau JC et al. Structure-activity relationship in heparin: a synthetic pentasaccharide with high affinity for antithrombin III and eliciting high anti-factor Xa activity. Biochem Biophys Res Commun 1983;116:492–499.

136. Agnelli G, Cosmi B, Di Filippo P et al. A randomised, double-blind, placebo-controlled trial of dermatan sulphate for prevention of deep vein thrombosis in hip fracture. Thromb Haemost 1992;67:203–208.

137. Ryan KE, Lane DA, Flynn A et al. Antithrombotic properties of dermatan sulphate (MF 701) in haemodialysis for chronic renal failure. Thromb Haemost 1992;68:563–569.

138. Brister SJ, Ofosu FA, Heigenhauser GJ et al. Is heparin the ideal anticoagulant for cardiopulmonary bypass? Dermatan sulphate may be an alternate choice. Thromb Haemost 1994;71:468–473.

# CHAPTER 58

# ANTITHROMBOTIC INTERVENTIONS IN CEREBROVASCULAR DISEASE

Gregory J. del Zoppo

Agents that inhibit thrombosis have played a central role in treatment of cerebrovascular disease. Cerebrovascular disease refers to fixed or transient neurologic deficits resulting from atherothrombotic events (40–57%), embolism (16–23%), transient ischemic attacks (TIAs) (10%), subarachnoid hemorrhage (10–19%), intracerebral hemorrhage (4–18%), lacunae (14%), and other potential causes (1–3). Atherothrombotic stroke refers to cerebrovascular occlusion secondary to *in situ* arterial thrombosis or to artery-to-artery emboli from intracranial arteries or the principal extracranial brain-supplying arteries.

In the latter case, platelet-fibrin thrombi on atheromata within the extracranial portion of the carotid artery (i.e., at the flow divider) or in the aortic arch can embolize downstream, predominantly into the middle and anterior cerebral arterial territories. A similar process can send emboli from atheromata at the subclavian-vertebral artery junctions into the basilar artery. Cardiac source emboli may originate from left ventricular mural thrombi formed during myocardial ischemia (MI), atrial thrombi formed in association with (nonvalvular) atrial fibrillation, valvular injury formed during rheumatic disease, or from prosthetic valves. Thrombosis of small, penetrating cerebral arteries leads to lipohyalinosis and formation of lacunae and is less common than atherothrombotic stroke (4).

Investigators have adopted one or more classification schemes, employing symptom-complex, temporal, and anatomic criteria (or some combination of these), for ischemia-related cerebrovascular disease. Symptom-complex definitions distinguish between carotid and vertebrobasilar territory ischemia, which may have significantly different prognoses. Temporal aspects of neurologic symptoms distinguish cerebrovascular ischemic events as being transient ischemic attacks (TIAs), reversible ischemic neurologic deficits (RINDs), or minor stroke, stroke-in-evolution, stroke-in-progression, and completed stroke (5). More recently, and particularly regarding acute intervention approaches, knowledge of the specific vascular anatomy and occlusion location has been valuable to understanding the fate of symptomatic occlusions and to defining clinical outcome. Studies employing angiography during the early hours of stroke have shown a high frequency of atherothrombotic or thromboembolic arterial occlusions in individuals who present within 6 hours of onset of symptoms (6–9). Anatomy-directed studies using computed tomographic (CT) scan, angiographic and Doppler ultrasonographic criteria have redefined the relative frequency of probable etiologies and the interpretation of neurologic outcome.

## CLASSIFICATION OF CEREBROVASCULAR DISEASE

This chapter uses the clinical temporal classification of cerebrovascular events in common usage, because most clinical trials have adopted these criteria. In many studies however, temporal criteria, which are useful for selecting the population under study, have limited the

| **TABLE 58.1.** Clinical Classification of Focal Cerebral Ischemia |
| --- |
| Transient ischemic attack (TIA) |
| Reversible ischemic neurologic deficit (RIND) |
| Minor stroke |
| Stroke-in-evolution |
| Stroke-in-progression |
| Completed stroke |
| Acute stroke |

treatment and, therefore, the outcomes of those studies. Vascular anatomy, thrombotic or embolic source, and timing of the signal event also are critical features of cerebrovascular ischemia not accounted for by these criteria. Here, TIAs refer to episodes of focal cerebral dysfunction of short duration, often lasting minutes but not more than 24 hours and leaving no detectable residual neurologic deficit. Minor strokes, RINDs, or TIAs with ischemic residua are episodes of focal cerebral dysfunction persisting longer than 24 hours and of intermediate severity, which resolve within 1 month. A completed stroke is a focal cerebral ischemic event with variable severity that is both fixed and persistent (Table 58.1). Improvement in function is not invariable, but recovery is gradual. The intermediate categories of stroke-in-progression, stroke-in-evolution, and partial stable stroke refer to neurologic deficits of ischemic origin that may increase in severity and to deficits of minor to moderate degree with stroke residua.

# NATURAL HISTORY OF CEREBRAL ATHEROTHROMBOTIC AND THROMBOEMBOLIC DISEASE

Prospective intervention trials have relied on epidemiologic studies to provide an overview for outcome expectations in individuals at risk for cerebral ischemia. In early trials, the anatomic basis for ischemic symptoms generally was not appreciated during assessments of natural history. Carotid territory TIAs often are accompanied by subsequent stroke or other cardiovascular disease, and completed stroke has been reported in 40 to 75% of individuals with one or more premonitory TIAs (10–12), with a prevalence of approximately 30% per year (13). Of individuals with a premonitory TIA, about 50% may have a stroke within the first year (13). Stroke-related death and cardiac death have been reported to occur in 28% and 37% of TIA individuals, respectively, indicating that cardiovascular mortality is significant (13). More recent evaluations, which have included data from placebo groups in large trials of anti-

thrombotic efficacy, suggest a lower mortality rate. For instance, the combined outcome events of stroke, myocardial infarction (MI), and death occurred in 14% of placebo-treated individuals over 2 years in the UK-TIA Study Group Trial (14). Approximately 64% of individuals with TIAs show evidence of infarction on their initial CT scan (15).

Patients with a primary stroke are at risk for recurrence, often within the same vascular territory. The 5 year cumulative incidence of secondary stroke was 42% among males in one prospective follow-up study (2). A separate study (16) noted a 32% 7 year cumulative incidence for recurrent stroke. Again, the highest recurrence rates for stroke are within the first year following the initial event.

Stroke-related mortality during the initial 7 days after ictus was examined prospectively by Silver et al (17). Cerebral edema from large, hemispheric ischemic lesions led to transtentorial herniation and death in 36 of 46 individuals (78%) who died in the first 7 days after the onset of stroke symptoms. This is consistent with the number of fatal events (82%) in one retrospective pathology study (18). Generally, however, mortality is not considered to be the primary outcome in current acute stroke intervention trials (discussed later) because of its low incidence and multifactorial basis.

Both neurologic presentation and outcome depend on the stroke subtype, and this has been well demonstrated by Wityk et al (19). Improvements in neurologic status among individuals surviving stroke without intervention are commonly observed. Furthermore, improvements in the mortality rate as recently documented among stroke populations result, at least in part, from risk-factor reduction. Both observations strongly indicate the need for concurrent controls in interventional stroke studies.

# HEMOSTASIS AND CEREBROVASCULAR ISCHEMIA

Thrombosis and thromboembolism play a central role in focal cerebral ischemia, as suggested by clinical, angiographic and laboratory observations. The findings of migrating retinal arterial thromboemboli and refractile bodies in individuals with focal cerebral ischemia (20–22) and of thrombi in cortical arteries at craniotomy (23) or during cerebral ischemia (24) and on affected carotid arteries at endarterectomy (25) support a pathogenic role for these thrombotic events.

Selective angiographic studies have documented cerebrovascular occlusions in individuals with acute focal ischemia. In three prospective studies (7–9), symptomatic occlusion of a brain-supplying artery within the carotid territory was documented in 81% of individuals undergoing angiography within 8 hours of symptom onset. Other angiographic studies have shown arterial occlusions in 59% at 24 hours (6) and in 41% at 1 week (26) after symptom onset in individuals with focal cerebral ischemia. Furthermore, results of angiographic studies support the view that focal ischemia after large-artery events in the carotid territory primarily are thrombotic or embolic in origin. Vertebrobasilar arterial ischemia more frequently results from *in situ* thrombosis on atheromata, similar to the finding of thrombotic coronary artery occlusion during the initial hours of acute MI (27).

Indirect evidence also emerged from studies of platelet, coagulation, and fibrinolytic system activation in individuals with thrombotic stroke and with transient cerebral ischemia (28–32). Spontaneous platelet aggregation and circulating platelet aggregates have been reported in individuals with atherothrombotic and thromboembolic cerebral ischemia. Several studies of acute ischemic cerebrovascular disease have reported accelerated activated partial thromboplastin times, decreased levels of plasminogen activator, increased levels of plasma fibrinogen and serum fragment E levels (FgE, E monomer), and increased levels of soluble fibrin monomer. Increased levels of fibrinopeptide A (FPA) and D-dimer levels also have been documented for up to 4 weeks after stroke, thus suggesting ongoing fibrin formation and fibrinolysis (32). β-thromboglobulin levels, which are a measure of platelet α-granule release, were not elevated in 24 individuals with "old CVA disease," but levels of fibrinopeptide A, fibrinogen B-β peptides, and D-dimer were normal in 13 "chronic stroke" individuals (31). While these findings may represent consequences rather than causes of cerebral infarction, reports of cerebral thromboembolic events in young individuals with hyperhomocystinemia and familial plasminogen activator deficiency also implicate altered hemostatic function as a predisposing factor in thrombus formation and dissolution in stroke, which supports a primary role for arterial thrombosis in the pathogenesis of ischemic stroke.

# HEMORRHAGIC TRANSFORMATION IN CEREBRAL ISCHEMIA

Hemorrhage accounts for approximately 10% of strokes (1, 33, 34), and hemorrhage in the neuraxis also may accompany use of antithrombotic agents. In otherwise normal individuals, neuropathologic changes probably underlie the very low, but significant, frequency of intracranial hemorrhage (e.g., 0.02% in individuals with acute MI [35]).

Hemorrhagic transformation of the ischemic lesion results naturally from thromboembolic stroke without antithrombotic therapy. Hemorrhagic transformation also may result from fragmentation and distal migration of thromboemboli that expose ischemic vessels to arterial pressure, thereby producing hemorrhage into the infarct (36). This concept was broadened by recent angiographic studies of thrombolytic agents in individuals with acute thrombotic stroke (8, 37–39), and the potential contribution of basal lamina degradation within the microvasculature to petechial hemorrhage has been emphasized (40). Furthermore, hemorrhagic transformation with persistent occlusion of the primary artery suggests that hemorrhage may occur from other vascular sources (e.g., collateral channels) (36, 41).

Hemorrhagic transformation can be classified as hemorrhagic infarction (HI), parenchymatous hematoma (PH), or both. HI refers to petechial or confluent petechial hemorrhage in the area of ischemic injury, typically involving cortical or basal ganglia gray matter. Postmortem studies (36, 41, 42) have described HI as a spectrum, from scattered petechiae to more confluent hemorrhage within a region of infarction, occurring in 50 to 70% of individuals. In CT studies (43, 44), HI has been noted in 10 to 43% of nonanticoagulated individuals with acute cerebral infarction, an incidence somewhat lower than that found at autopsy. HI usually appears within 2 to 4 days, but it rarely occurs during the first few hours after onset of stroke-related symptoms (45–47). Most commonly, HI occurs in association with cardioembolic stroke but not with *in situ* atherothrombotic vascular occlusions. In an angiographic study, Yamaguchi et al (48) described HIs in 45 of 120 cases (37.5%) with cardiogenic cerebral embolism, but in only two of 105 individuals (1.9%) with cerebral thrombosis in the carotid territory.

In contrast, parenchymatous hematoma (PH) is a homogeneous, discrete mass of blood that may displace brain tissue, thus shifting the midline structures, and that may extend to the ventricle. Radiographically, PH is a homogeneous, circumscribed mass of blood, often associated with shift of midline structures. Many reports of PH in individuals with cerebral embolism are associated with anticoagulant treatment (49–52). The mechanisms underlying the appearance of PH are not known, but they may include rupture of small penetrating arteries. The hemorrhagic potential of lacunae is not known.

Information about the mechanisms underlying formation of HI and PH in cerebrovascular ischemia as well as their relative risks is not complete. The cause of the ischemic event (e.g., thromboembolism, hypertension), its localization and extent, and other vascular features (e.g., collateral integrity) associated with ischemia all contribute to the risk of hemorrhagic transformation, and antithrombotic agents may augment this risk.

# ANTITHROMBOTIC AGENTS

Antiplatelets, anticoagulants, and fibrinolytics are the antithrombotic drugs used to treat cerebrovascular ischemia. Those agents either tested or currently used for the treatment of focal cerebral ischemia are considered here. The pharmacologic properties of these agents are detailed in Chapters 54, 55, and 56.

## ANTIPLATELET AGENTS (SEE CHAPTER 54)

Agents that inhibit any component essential for platelet activation and aggregation, that further interfere with platelet vascular reactivity, or both, may function as antiplatelet agents (53–55).

## ASPIRIN AND DIPYRIDAMOLE

Aspirin (ASA) interferes with platelet function by irreversible acetylation and inactivation of cyclooxygenase (56–58). In doing so, it inhibits production of thromboxane $A_2$. ASA inhibits collagen-stimulated adhesion at low shear stress, but it has little effect on adhesion or aggregation at high shear stress (59, 60).

Despite these observations, ASA has been employed in both primary and secondary prevention of thrombotic processes occurring at arterial flow rates. In most trials involving cerebral ischemia, ASA doses (300–1300 mg/day) exceed those at which the solitary antiplatelet effect occurs, thereby also contributing a potential vascular effect. In combination with other antiplatelet agents (e.g., dipyridamole), ASA may normalize the decreased platelet survival associated with various arterial thrombotic disorders (61). That dipyridamole may act synergistically with ASA to normalize platelet survival *in vivo* has led to use of combination ASA-dipyridamole therapy for carotid TIAs. The efficacy of this combination, however, has been challenged (62, 63). Dipyridamole also may act as an antioxidant at therapeutic doses, and its beneficial vascular effect may arise principally from this unique action.

## SULFINPYRAZONE

Sulfinpyrazone, a phenylbutazone derivative, has uricosuric properties *in vivo* and inhibits platelet aggregation *in vitro* by inhibiting cyclooxygenase and by other as yet poorly defined mechanisms (64). When used alone, sulfinpyrazone can normalize the decreased platelet survival times associated with TIAs, prosthetic heart valves and coronary artery disease (53).

## TICLOPIDINE

Ticlopidine is a potent antiplatelet agent not related to ASA, dipyridamole, or sulfinpyrazone (65, 66). Its proposed mechanisms of action are discussed in Chapter 54, and its pharmacology and potential uses in thrombotic disorders have been reviewed elsewhere (65). Leukope-

nia, which is consistently associated with use of ticlopidine in recent cerebral ischemia trials, demands careful monitoring in individuals receiving this agent (67, 68). Thrombocytopenia is a rare side effect that also warrants monitoring.

## CLOPIDOGREL

Clopidogrel is a thienopyridine derivative and a relative of ticlopidine. It irreversibly inhibits binding of adenosine diphosphate to its platelet receptor (69, 70). Studies of dose equivalence as measured on the basis of *ex vivo* platelet aggregation confirm the efficacy of single daily dosing. Leukopenia is rare.

## SULOCTIDIL

The antithrombotic effects of suloctidil result from inhibition of platelet aggregation induced by collagen and thrombin, serotonin leakage, and other mechanisms. Decreased fibrinogen level and whole blood viscosity as well as a hypocholesterolemic effect also occur. In addition, reduced thrombus extension in polyethylene catheters has been documented (71). Suloctidil functions as a peripheral vasodilator.

## PROSTACYCLIN

Prostacyclin ($PGI_2$), which is a product of endothelial cell metabolism of arachidonic acid, inhibits platelet aggregation both *in vitro* and *in vivo* by elevation of platelet cytoplasmic cyclic adenosine monophosphate (cAMP) levels. Small studies of individuals with completed stroke and other thrombotic disorders have failed to demonstrate a useful therapeutic role for prostacyclin. This also may result from symptom-dependent dosage restrictions. In addition, iloprost and other stable prostacyclin analogues have not found a lasting role in treatment of cerebrovascular disease.

## INHIBITORS OF PLATELET GLYCOPROTEIN IIb-IIIa

The potential use of glycoprotein IIb-IIIa (integrin $\alpha_{IIb}/\beta_3$) antagonists in individuals with acute stroke or other cerebrovascular disorders remains theoretical, and concerns regarding hemorrhagic risk are relevant (72). In one experimental study (M. Pierschbacher, personal communication), the peptide integrin $\alpha_{IIb}/\beta_3$ antagonist TP9201 produced a significant increase in microvascular patency compared with placebo during early reperfusion after middle cerebral artery occlusion. In clinical practice, use of monoclonal antibody integrin $\alpha_{IIb}/\beta_3$ antagonists is accompanied by a low but significant frequency of thrombocytopenia.

## ANTICOAGULANTS (SEE CHAPTER 55)

Use of anticoagulants limits thrombus formation and extension. Both heparin and warfarin have seen wide prophylactic use in individuals with cardiogenic embolism, and low-molecular-weight fractions of heparin are being tested for this indication. General clinical indications for the use of anticoagulants have been summarized elsewhere (73).

## HEPARIN

A collection of polydisperse glycosaminoglycans with antithrombotic properties, heparin requires the specific pentasaccharide sequence D-glucuronic-D-glucosamine (N-SO$_3$; 3-6-di-0-SO$_3$) for anticoagulant activity (74). When bound to large heparin oligosaccharides, antithrombin III maximally inhibits thrombin activity (75). The interaction with thrombin supersedes heparin-antithrombin III binding. A similar molecular weight-dependent inhibition of factor IXa and XIa by heparin has been observed, whereas inhibition of factor XIa probably does not involve an antithrombin III mechanism (76, 77). In addition to its antithrombin activity, lower-molecular-weight heparin fractions exhibit factor Xa neutralization.

## LOW-MOLECULAR-WEIGHT HEPARIN

Fractions containing low-molecular-weight oligosaccharides of heparin (4000–9000 ds) possess predominantly anti-factor Xa activity, with minimal antithrombin properties (78). Potential advantages to these preparations are their more reproducible anticoagulant activity, relative lack of thrombocytopenic effect, and reduced risk of associated hemorrhagic complications.

## LOW-MOLECULAR-WEIGHT HEPARINOIDS

Org 10172 (danaparoid) is a mixture of low-molecular-weight heparan, dermatan, and chondroitin sulfates that inhibits factor IX activation (more effectively than heparin) and factor X activation (equivalent to heparin) both *in vitro* and *in vivo*. This antithromberic also has a much greater anti-factor Xa:anti-factor IIa ratio than heparin (79, 80). In small animal thrombosis models and *in vivo*, Org 10172 has minimal effects on platelet plug formation (80). In clinical trials, Org 10172 is effective for treatment of deep venous thrombosis (DVT) (81, 82) and in prophylaxis for DVT in ischemic stroke individuals (83). Danaparoid has been used in a placebo-controlled trial of its efficacy in early (<24 hours) ischemic stroke (84–86).

## WARFARIN

As a vitamin K antagonist, warfarin inhibits the γ-carboxylation of terminal glutamic acid residues and, thereby, reduces plasma levels of functional factors II, VII, IX, and X as well as plasma levels of proteins C and S (87). Coumarin, warfarin, phenindione and other compounds with similar mechanisms of action also reduce the risk of thromboembolic stroke accompanying atrial fibrillation and cardiac valvular prostheses.

## PLASMINOGEN ACTIVATORS (SEE CHAPTER 56)

Thrombolytic agents currently in clinical use are obligate plasminogen activators. Their use in cerebrovascular disease is confined to the acute setting.

### Tissue-type Plasminogen Activator

A single-chain, 527 amino acid serine protease glycoprotein, tissue-type plasminogen activator (t-PA) is converted to the two-chain form by plasmin cleavage of the Arg$_{275}$-Isoleu$_{276}$ linkage (88, 89). The catalytic efficiency of single-chain and two-chain t-PA for *in vitro* conversion of plasminogen to plasmin is stimulated to similar activity by fibrin (90–92). These observations and the preferential cleavage of fibrin (in the presence of fibrin-bound plasminogen) over fibrinogen *in vivo* suggest that both species of t-PA have relative fibrin-selective properties (89, 93). In humans, infusion studies of both t-PA species have demonstrated a $t_{1/2}$ of 3 to 8 minutes, even although the biologic $t_{1/2}$ is believed to be somewhat longer. Recombinant t-PA (rt-PA) in single-chain (alteplase) or two-chain (duteplase) form has been used for the treatment of acute coronary artery thrombosis and the study of acute ischemic stroke, peripheral arterial thrombosis, acute pulmonary embolism, and DVT.

### Urokinase-type Plasminogen Activator

High-molecular-weight urokinase-type plasminogen activator (u-PA; 54,000 ds) is a fibrin-nonselective serine protease that directly converts plasminogen to plasmin by first order kinetics (94–97). u-PA exists as two separate species, both of which exhibit fibrin(ogen)olytic activity *in vitro* and *in vivo* (discussed later) (98). Infused u-PA has a plasma $t_{1/2}$ of 9 to 12 minutes.

### Single-chain Urokinase-type Plasminogen Activator

Single-chain u-PA (scu-PA or pro-UK) is a 54,000-d, endogenous, fibrin-selective proenzyme of u-PA that is unusual for generating plasmin at the thrombus surface (98–100). The relationship of scu-PA to u-PA is complex. Cleavage or removal of the Lys$_{158}$ of scu-PA produces the high-molecular-weight (54,000-d), two-chain u-PA, whereas further cleavages at Lys$_{135}$ and Arg$_{156}$ produce the low-molecular-weight (31,000-d) u-PA (89). Both high- and low-molecular-weight species are enzymatically active *in vivo*.

## Streptokinase

A 47,000-d glycoprotein product of *Streptococcus haemolyticus* (group G), streptokinase (SK) activates plasminogen to plasmin by complex kinetics. Active [SK/plasminogen] and [SK/plasmin] species are generated. Free circulating plasmin and complexed [SK/plasmin(ogen)] degrade both fibrinogen and fibrin, and they inactivate prothrombin, factor V, and factor VIII (101, 102), thereby producing a "systemic lytic state" similar to that for u-PA. Dose-rate adjustments with SK are difficult because of the nonstoichiometric generation of plasmin and, to a larger degree, the inactivation of an unknown quantity of infused SK by circulating antistreptococcal antibodies. Extreme hypoplasminogenemia may occur, thus limiting the activity of a SK infusion.

## Acylated Plasminogen Streptokinase Activator Complex

Acylated plasminogen streptokinase activator complex (APSAC) is an inactive complex of acylated human lys-plasminogen and streptokinase, with fibrin-binding properties from the lys-plasminogen kringles. Plasmin is generated by streptokinase within the complex by hydrolytic activation of the acyl-protected, plasminogen-active site (103). The biologic activity is believed to be longer than that of streptokinase (104, 105), and the hypofibrinogenemia and inactivation of factors V and VIII with APSAC are similar to those with streptokinase. APSAC has been used only in preliminary studies involving a small number of individuals with stroke.

The streptokinase-plasminogen complexes Fibrinolysin® and Thrombolysin® offer no advantages over streptokinase. They are of historical interest only.

## Novel Thrombolytic Agents

Several plasminogen activator constructs have been prepared to enhance thrombus lytic potency, shorten or extend $t_{1/2}$, alter clearance, and/or take advantage of known synergistic actions. These constructs include single-site t-PA mutants, t-PA–scu-PA and t-PA–u-PA chimeras (106), u-PA–antifibrin monoclonal antibody conjugates (107), and scu-PA deletion mutants (108). Mutants of t-PA, including TNK and r-PA, have altered clearance and, therefore, a longer $t_{1/2}$ than that of rt-PA. So far, none has been used clinically in individuals with cerebrovascular disease.

# ANTITHROMBOTIC INTERVENTIONS IN CEREBRAL ISCHEMIA

## GENERAL CONSIDERATIONS

The literature concerning use of antithrombotic agents in cerebrovascular disease is extensive, and the reader is referred to reviews examining various aspects of this problem (109–111). This section discusses use of antithrombotic agents in clinical trials following the example of Oczkowski and Turpie (109) and using the rules of evidence as summarized by Sackett (112).

## METHODOLOGIC ISSUES

In stroke intervention trials, statistical requirements demand large cohort sizes on which relatively secure treatment recommendations can be based (113). This is particularly cogent for treatment strategies carrying an associated presumed risk (e.g., hemorrhage with antithrombotic agents) and large expected individual withdrawal. One alternative view is that small cohort sizes may be required when known stroke pathophysiology is used as a selection criterion (9, 39). Still another suggests that a series of independently performed, similarly designed studies may be analyzed *in toto* by a meta-analysis to provide an overview of therapeutic trends and an indication of outcome significance (114). The five-rank classification of clinical trials on the basis of design features (i.e., "rules of evidence") may indicate the power of a given study (112). Randomized trials with a low chance of false-positive and false-negative errors (level I) have high power to evaluate the intervention of interest, whereas randomized trials with a high chance of such errors (level II) have low power. Nonrandomized trials may compare the outcomes of: cohorts that receive either active agent or placebo in parallel (level III); the active agent with a historical, untreated cohort (level IV); or a single treated cohort without control (level V).

Subgroup analysis, which may be instructive for future trial planning, demands larger cohort sizes. For instance, in the Canadian Cooperative Study Group trial, the predominant outcome of reduced events with ASA occurred among male individuals; however, male individuals accounted for 69.4% of those randomized, with females therefore having fewer events that could be evaluated (115, 116). In the subsequent UK-TIA Group Study (14), this led to a subgroup analysis on the basis of gender response in which no difference in outcome was observed, in part because of the small number of female individuals.

Attempts to evaluate several of the large comparative studies by a meta-analysis also have been made. The Antiplatelet Trialists' Collaboration (114) examined the effect of sustained antiplatelet treatment in 31 prospective trials for secondary prevention of vascular events in individuals with a history of TIAs, stroke, unstable angina, or MI. An odds ratio of 0.75 in favor of all antiplatelet regimens was devised for initial stroke, MI, or vascular death. For all cerebrovascular trials examined, a reduction in the odds ratio of 22% was computed in favor of the antiplatelet strategies for initial stroke, MI, or vascular death ($p < .0001$). This result was "driven" by the outcome of three prospective trials: the European Stroke Prevention Study Group Trial (117), the "AICLA" (118), and the UK-TIA Study (14). In this type of analysis, individual contributions from ASA, dipyridamole, suloctidil, and sulfinpyrazone were obscured, as were any anatomic considerations of the cerebrovascular events for the overall outcome.

A more limited examination of anticoagulant therapy in cerebral or retinal ischemia/infarction among controlled, nonsurgical studies up to 1987 also has been published (119). Among 10 studies enlisting individuals with stroke or TIAs, results from anticoagulant therapy were significantly worse than control in prevention of subsequent death or stroke. Only the Cerebral Embolism Study Group trial (120) indicated a benefit from immediate anticoagulation for cardiogenic embolism. This analysis (119) included level II and III studies, however, so an overall benefit of anticoagulation may have been underestimated.

Use of plasminogen activators in individuals with ischemic stroke has been the subject of a continuously updated meta-analysis (i.e., the Cochrane Collaboration) (121). On the basis of a small group of prospective studies using CT inclusion criteria, this analysis underscored the benefit of plasminogen activators in terms of mortality and disability, but also a risk of hemorrhage. The relative degree of benefit or risk cannot be estimated from this type of analysis, however. Furthermore, an implicit assumption in this analysis is that all studies have similar design features (i.e., level I or II) and employ agents of similar efficacy in similarly chosen individual populations.

## CEREBROVASCULAR DISEASE

Antiplatelet agents and anticoagulants have been used to limit the consequences of recent transient or fixed neurologic deficits. They also have been used as prophylaxis against second events (i.e., secondary prevention). In addition, anticoagulants have been used for treatment of sinus venous thrombosis and prevention of thromboembolic events originating in individuals with atrial fibrillation, acute MI, or cardiac valve injury. Fibrinolytic agents have been used successfully to treat acute symptomatic cerebral ischemia.

## TRANSIENT CEREBRAL ISCHEMIA (TRANSIENT ISCHEMIC ATTACKS)

### Antiplatelet Agents

A role for antiplatelet agents in individuals with transient ischemia was suggested by use of ASA reducing the frequency of transient monocular blindness (amaurosis fugax) in selected individuals (122, 123). ASA had a similar effect on the frequency of TIAs in 26 individuals with documented alterations (e.g., ulceration) at the carotid artery bifurcation (124).

The likelihood that ASA may affect sequelae of transient ischemia, including completed stroke, was addressed by two level II trials and three level III trials (Table 58.2). In the Aspirin in Transient Ischemic Attacks (AITIA) study (125), which involved 178 individuals with a 3-month history of TIAs not considered candidates for carotid endarterectomy by contemporary criteria, a reduced incidence of stroke and vascular death at 6 months among those randomized to ASA (1300 mg/day) was observed. There was a significant reduction in the combined outcome events of recurrent TIAs, cerebral/retinal infarction, and death among those receiving ASA ($n = 88$) over those receiving placebo ($n = 90$), but there was no reduction by life-table analysis at the 24 month follow-up. No difference in the incidence of stroke between the two groups occurred, and *post hoc* subgroup analyses revealed no meaningful relationships. A less substantial decrease in disabling stroke and death among those with TIA receiving ASA ($n = 101$; 1000 mg/day) over those receiving placebo (n = 102) was observed after a mean follow-up of 2.1 years in the subsequent Danish Cooperative Study (126). Both studies, however, suffered from limited power to distinguish principal outcome events between the treatment groups.

The Canadian Cooperative Study Group trial (115), which was a randomized, double-blind (level I), four-arm study comparing ASA (1300 mg/day), sulfinpyrazone (800 mg/day), and the combination of ASA and sulfinpyrazone with placebo, demonstrated a significantly reduced incidence of stroke and death among individuals with a history of TIAs who received ASA, with a mean follow-up of 2.2 years. No benefit was attributed to the sulfinpyrazone arm, and the risk reduction for stroke and death was most significant for male individuals receiving ASA. In this study, 66% of the ischemic episodes at entry were in the carotid territory alone, whereas 23% were isolated to the vertebrobasilar territory.

A reduced incidence of stroke, MI, and death was attributed to ASA in the three-arm, randomized, double-blind (level I) "AICLA" trial (118) of individuals presenting with a history of TIAs. In that study, individuals were randomized to ASA (990 mg/day, $n = 198$), the combination of ASA (990 mg/day) and dipyridamole (225 mg/day, $n = 202$), or placebo ($n = 204$).

The subsequent UK-TIA ASA aspirin trial randomized 2435 individuals with TIAs or minor ischemic stroke to ASA (1200 mg/day, $n = 815$), ASA (300 mg/day, $n = 806$, "low dose"), or placebo ($n = 814$) (14). With a mean follow-up of 4 years, a significant 18% reduction in nonfatal MI, nonfatal major stroke, and vascular or nonvascular death occurred in individuals receiving ASA (300–1200 mg/day, $n = 1621$). A central feature of the UK-TIA study was a comparison of two ASA dose regimens to address the issue of optimal antiplatelet effect.

**TABLE 58.2.    Transient Ischemic Attacks: Antiplatelet Agents**

| Study | Year | Agent | Dose (per day) | Patients (n) | Follow-up (years) | Stroke (n) | Mortality (n) Vascular[a] | Nonvascular | Total |
|---|---|---|---|---|---|---|---|---|---|
| AITIA Study (125) | 1977 | ASA | 1300 mg | 88 | 0.5 | 10 | 3 | — | 3 |
| | | Placebo | | 90 | | 12 | 6 | 1 | 7 |
| Danish Cooperative Study (126) | 1983 | ASA | 1000 mg | 101 | 2.1 | 18 | 6 | 1 | 7 |
| | | Placebo | | 102 | | 11 | 6 | 1 | 7 |
| Canadian Cooperative Trial Study Group (115) | 1978 | ASA/placebo 1 | 1300 mg/— | 144 | 2.2 | 22 | 4 | 0 | 4 |
| | | Sulfinpyrazone/placebo 2 | 800 mg/— | 156 | | 29 | 6 | 3 | 9 |
| | | ASA/sulfinpyrazone | 1300 mg/800 mg | 146 | | 14 | 4 | 2 | 6 |
| | | Placebo 1/placebo 2 | —/— | 139 | | 20 | 8 | 2 | 10 |
| AICLA (118) | 1983 | ASA/dipyridamole | 990 mg/225 mg | 202 | 3.0 | 18 | 5 | 3 | 8 |
| | | ASA | 990 mg | 198 | | 17 | 4 | 6 | 10 |
| | | Placebo | | 204 | | 31 | 4 | 3 | 7 |
| UK-TIA Study Group (14) | 1988 | ASA | 1200 mg | 815 | 4.0 | 66 | 84 | 27 | 111 |
| | | ASA | 300 mg | 806 | | 68 | 84 | 22 | 106 |
| | | Placebo | | 814 | | 88 | 86 | 36 | 122 |
| Dutch TIA Trial Study Group (127) | 1991 | ASA | 283 mg | 1576 | 2.6 | 109 | 107 | 44 | 151 |
| | | ASA | 30 mg | 1555 | | 90 | 105 | 55 | 160 |
| SALT (128) | 1991 | ASA | 75 mg | 676 | 2.7 | 93 | 48 | 13 | 61 |
| | | Placebo | | 684 | | 112 | 50 | 19 | 69 |
| Acheson et al. (131) | 1969 | Dipyridamole | 400–800 mg | 85/69[a] | 2.1 | 5/7[a] | — | — | 13 |
| | | Placebo | | 84/70[a] | | 7/4[a] | — | — | 9 |
| European Stroke Prevention Study Group (117) | 1987 | ASA/dipyridamole | 975 mg/225 mg | 1250 | 2.0 | 114[b] | 69 | 39 | 108 |
| | | Placebo | | 1250 | | 184[b] | 100 | 56 | 156 |
| American-Canadian Cooperative Study Group (132) | 1985 | ASA/dipyridamole | 1300 mg/300 mg | 448 | 1.5 | 53 | 29 | 17 | 46 |
| | | ASA | 1300 mg | 442 | | 60 | 29 | 9 | 38 |
| Matius-Guiu et al. (133) | 1987 | ASA/dipyridamole | 50 mg/300 mg | 115 | 1.75 | 3 | 1 | 1 | 2 |
| | | Dipyridamole | 400 mg | 71 | | 3 | 2 | 1 | 3 |
| Roden et al. (137) | 1981 | Sulfinpyrazone | 800 mg | 39[c] | 0.33 | 1 | 1 | — | 1 |
| | | Placebo | | 39[c] | | 3 | 1 | — | 1 |
| Candelise et al. (138) | 1982 | Sulfinpyrazone | 800 mg | 61 | 2.0 | 2 | 1 | — | — |
| | | ASA | 1000 mg | 63 | | 2 | 0 | — | — |
| Hass et al. (68) | 1991 | Ticlopidine | 500 mg | 1529 | 2.0–6.0 | 172 | 120 | 55 | 175 |
| | | ASA | 1300 mg | 1540 | | 212 | 116 | 80 | 196 |

ASA, aspirin.

[a] First evaluation/second evaluation.

[b] Intention-to-treat analysis.

[c] Cross-over format.

No dose-response from ASA for the outcome events was noted, but gastrointestinal side effects were more common with the high-dose regimen. Nine deaths were attributed to intracranial hemorrhage in the ASA-treated groups, whereas only one occurred in the placebo group.

An additional study of ASA dose on nonfatal stroke, nonfatal MI and vascular death (127) found no difference in outcome between individuals with TIAs or minor strokes treated with ASA at 30 mg/day ($n = 1555$) or 283 mg/day ($n = 1576$) at a mean follow-up of 2.6 years. Fewer major hemorrhagic events occurred with the lower dose, with six fatal cerebral hemorrhages in the low-dose group and nine in the high-dose group.

Confirming the benefit of low-dose ASA after signal TIAs, the Swedish Aspirin Low-Dose Trial (SALT) Collaborative Group (128) reported an 18% reduction in risk of stroke and death among 676 individuals with TIA who began ASA (75 mg/day) within 1 to 4 months of their initial symptoms as compared to 684 individuals who received placebo. A 16 to 20% reduction in risk of stroke, frequent TIAs and MI also was observed, thereby confirming that low-dose ASA can reduce the risk of stroke and death following TIA.

To summarize, results of four level I trials suggest a benefit from ASA on early stroke and vascular mortality in individuals with TIAs or minor ischemic events. The pathophysiologic basis for the relative benefit seen among ASA-treated individuals, however, is not evident.

Aspirin most often has been used in combination with dipyridamole because of synergism between the agents as in both preclinical and platelet survival studies of clinical vascular disease (54, 62, 63, 129, 130). Dipyridamole (400–800 mg/day) alone did not alter the incidence of stroke or related mortality compared with placebo in a single double-blind, randomized trial (level I) (131). Because of the limited power of that study, however, a clinical benefit from dipyridamole cannot be excluded.

In contrast, the combination of ASA and dipyridamole conferred a benefit over placebo in two randomized, double-blind controlled studies. The European Stroke Prevention Study (ESPS) Group (117) compared ASA (975 mg/day) and dipyridamole (225 mg/day) to placebo in equal patient groups ($n = 1250$). After a mean follow-up of 2 years, a 33% reduction in risk of stroke and death was apparent. A second comparison of ASA and dipyridamole ($n = 202$) and placebo ($n = 204$), which was derived from the three-arm "AICLA" study, also indicated benefit from the combination for individuals with TIA when the outcome events of stroke, MI, and mortality were combined. No difference in stroke or mortality was reported by the American-Canadian Cooperative Study Group (132) at 1.5 years follow-up when 448 individuals receiving ASA (1300 mg/day) and dipyridamole (300 mg/day) were compared with 442 individuals receiving ASA (1300 mg/day) alone. A similar relationship also was suggested by the "AICLA" study (118), which also tested ASA ($n = 198$) against ASA with dipyridamole ($n = 202$) for 3-year incidence of stroke, MI, and mortality. That study did not have sufficient power to exclude a type II error, however. Results of a small, open, non-randomized trial of 115 individuals receiving low-dose ASA (50 mg/day) and dipyridamole (300 mg/day) suggested no differential benefit from that of dipyridamole (400 mg/day) alone in 71 individuals with at least one atherothrombotic cerebral event for the outcome events of TIA, stroke and mortality (25 of 115 versus 15 of 71, respectively) at a mean follow-up of 1.75 years (133).

ESPS-2 (134), a recent product of the European Stroke Prevention Working Group, examined the relative efficacy of dipyridamole (400 mg/day), ASA (50 mg/day), and the combination of ASA and dipyridamole to limit stroke, death, or both in individuals presenting with TIAs or stroke in a 2 × 2 factorial design. In that randomized trial, ASA alone and dipyridamole alone (relative risk reductions for stroke, 15.8 and 17.7%, respectively) and the combination (relative risk reduction, 36.7%) were superior to placebo at 2 year follow-up (135). For individuals with a history of TIAs or recent stroke, the combination is superior to no treatment, but it is not substantially different from ASA alone for the outcomes of stroke, MI, and mortality.

The antiplatelet agents sulfinpyrazone and ticlopidine also have been studied in individuals with a history of TIAs or minor stroke in separate studies (Table 58.2). Following a report that sulfinpyrazone may significantly reduce episodes of amaurosis fugax and TIAs (136), the Canadian Cooperative Study Group compared ASA, sulfinpyrazone, and placebo. No significant difference in the incidence of stroke and mortality over 2.2 years of follow-up was observed between sulfinpyrazone (800 mg/day, $n = 156$) and placebo ($n = 139$) (115). Sulfinpyrazone (800 mg/day) and placebo also were tested in a double-blind, cross over trial (137), in which a nonsignificant reduction in transient cerebral ischemic episodes and in the outcome events of stroke and mortality at 4-month follow-up was recorded in individuals receiving sulfinpyrazone. Another level I study (138) comparing sulfinpyrazone (800 mg/day) to ASA (1000 mg/day) in individuals with TIAs concluded there was a higher incidence of stroke, MI, and vascular death in the sulfinpyrazone cohort at 11 month follow-up. Considering the small number of individuals involved in each study, however, a type II error cannot be excluded. These results also do not exclude the possibility that individual individuals may have benefited from sulfinpyrazone.

Ticlopidine has been tested in individuals with TIA/minor stroke (68) and in secondary stroke prevention (67). Individuals with transient ischemic symptoms were randomized to either ticlopidine (500 mg/day) or ASA (1300 mg/day). In the "intention-to-treat" analysis, ticlopidine was associated with a significant 12% reduction in risk of stroke and death from any cause ($P = .048$), and with a similar 21% reduction in the risk of secondary outcomes of stroke and stroke-related death ($P = .024$). Leukopenia, which was reversible, occurred in approximately 0.8% of individuals taking ticlopidine; gastrointestinal symptoms were more common in individuals receiving ASA. Intracerebral hemorrhage occurred equally among individuals in each group.

In summary, ASA reduces the risk of stroke, MI, and mortality in individuals with a history of TIAs or minor stroke. This risk reduction is not dose-dependent (14). The combination of ASA and dipyridamole also produces a substantial risk reduction (134, 135). Ticlopidine was somewhat more effective than ASA in preventing stroke and mortality after TIAs in one study (68). When used alone, dipyridamole and sulfinpyrazone have little benefit.

## Anticoagulation

Clinical studies of anticoagulation in individuals with TIA or minor stroke have been small and nonrandomized, thus providing low statistical power to support a positive outcome. Several such anticoagulation trials were undertaken between 1965 and 1975.

**TABLE 58.3.** Transient Ischemic Attacks: Anticoagulants

| Study | Year | Agent | Dose (per day) | Patients (n) | Follow-up (years) | Stroke (n) | Mortality (n) Vascular | Nonvascular | Total |
|---|---|---|---|---|---|---|---|---|---|
| Siekert et al. (144) | 1963 | Anticoagulation | — | 175 | >3.0 | 4 | 16 | 24 | 40 |
| | | Nil | | 160 | | 33 | 25 | 19 | 44 |
| MRC (149) | 1965 | Phenindione | 50 mg | 17 | | 1 | 0 | 0 | 0 |
| | | Phenindione | 1 mg | 20 | | 2 | 1 | 2 | 3 |
| Friedman et al. (145) | 1975 | Anticoagulation | — | 22 | 2.3 | 1 | — | — | — |
| | | Nil | | 22 | | 7 | — | — | — |
| Toole et al. (146) | 1975 | Warfarin | — | 21 | 0.1–4.0 | 6 | 5 | 0 | 5 |
| | | Nil | | 56 | | 7 | 10 | 1 | 11 |
| Baker et al. (147) | 1962 | Anticoagulation | — | 24 | 36.5[a] | 1 | 2[b] | — | 5 |
| | | Nil | | 20 | 34.2[a] | 4 | 1[b] | — | 2 |
| Baker et al. (148) | 1966 | Anticoagulation | — | 30 | 3.2 | 2 | 5 | 1 | 6 |
| | | Nil | | 30 | 3.4 | 4 | 4 | 1 | 5 |

[a] Per individual-year.

[b] Demise from cerebral infarction or cerebral hemorrhage.

Theoretically, generation of fibrin-rich thrombi in static or low flow (e.g., ventricular or atrial mural thrombi) should be appropriate for the action of anticoagulants. Unfortunately, no randomized, blinded, level I studies have evaluated the long-term outcome of anticoagulation in individuals with TIA or minor stroke, and lower level studies have provided mixed results. Several early, non-controlled reports suggested heparin may decrease the incidence of basilar artery TIAs (139, 140), and Fisher (141) observed a dramatic, transient reduction in the incidence of TIAs in 28 of 29 individuals treated with anticoagulants, with TIAs returning in 60% of those in whom anticoagulation was discontinued. Subsequent trials have provided disparate results.

In individuals with TIA receiving long-term anticoagulation, Fazekas et al (142) found no substantial decrease in the frequency of transient ischemic events consistent with vertebrobasilar insufficiency (142), whereas Olsson et al (143) found a decreased frequency of TIA frequency. In the latter, non-randomized study, 163 of 178 individuals with carotid (n = 105) or vertebrobasilar (n = 73) symptoms of transient ischemia, with or without residual deficits, received warfarin, then no anticoagulant in a longitudinal fashion. When trials assessing the outcome events of subsequent stroke, vascular events, and mortality are considered, a similar disparity in outcome is observed (Table 58.3). Long-term anticoagulation (agent unspecified) decreased the incidence of strokes and vascular death among 175 individuals with recent TIAs, compared with 160 individuals with TIAs receiving no therapy as reported by Siekert et al (144). A similar reduction in the incidence of stroke was reported among individuals with TIA receiving anticoagulation in a retirement community (145). In contrast, a third study (146), with a mean follow-up of 2.25 years, demonstrated a reduced frequency of TIAs among anticoagulated individuals that did not translate into a decreased

incidence of stroke or vascular death. Among 77 individuals with TIA who received either warfarin or no treatment, 42 (55%) had carotid artery abnormalities, and 13 (17%) had vertebrobasilar artery abnormalities.

Several small, randomized, level II trials with limited power have not clarified the role of anticoagulants in transient ischemia. In an open study, Baker et al (147) found a nonsignificant reduction in the incidence of stroke and death among individuals with TIA receiving anticoagulation (n = 24) over those not receiving anticoagulation (n = 20). No difference between anticoagulated and non-anticoagulated groups (n = 30 each) in the incidence of stroke and death was seen in a subsequent open, randomized trial with mean follow-up of 3 years (148). In a Medical Research Council (MRC) sponsored trial of phenindione (149), individuals with TIA receiving a fixed oral anticoagulant ("low dose," n = 20) had a somewhat lower incidence of vascular events, stroke, and death than those receiving an adjusted dose regimen ("high dose," n = 17). Both carotid and vertebrobasilar events were studied, and those results must be interpreted with caution, however, because of the small number of individuals involved.

Uncontrolled experience with anticoagulation for vertebrobasilar and carotid TIAs has been reviewed (150). Short-term use of heparin did not alter the frequency of TIAs in 12 of 74 individuals presenting with a history of TIAs (151); long-term outcome was not assessed. No difference in the incidence of cerebral infarction between individuals randomized to heparin or to ASA for recent TIAs was observed in a separate angiographic pilot study (152), in which vertebrobasilar TIAs were more likely to result in cerebral infarction.

Use of anticoagulants in transient ischemia carries a risk of intracerebral hemorrhage. Hemorrhage caused the demise of two anticoagulated individuals at the end of follow-up in one study (147), and an increase in fatal intracranial hemorrhage among anticoagulated individuals compared with untreated individuals (13 of 40 fatal events versus 7 of 44 fatal events) was noted by Siekert et al (144). The risk of symptomatic intracranial hemorrhage among individuals with TIAs receiving anticoagulants under the conditions of these studies is in accord with the increased incidence of fatal hemorrhagic complications noted among elderly individuals receiving anticoagulation (153).

In summary, excluding individuals with atrial fibrillation or cardiac valvular prostheses, results of the various small studies do not conclusively support a role for anticoagulation in individuals with TIA or minor stroke considering the risk of hemorrhage.

## Plasminogen Activators

There is no basis for the use of fibrinolytic agents in individuals with TIAs or cerebral ischemic episodes of limited extent. Use of fibrinolytic agents very early after the onset of symptoms of stroke, however, does not necessarily exclude treatment of individuals with TIA. This section considers use of these agents in cerebrovascular ischemia.

## STROKE-IN-PROGRESSION (EVOLUTION)

An attractive basis for anticoagulant intervention has been the possibility that symptom progression might result from anterograde extension of *in situ* thrombus to occlude critical arterial branches, or that it might result from recurrent embolism. Undoubtedly, this contributed to the early enthusiasm for the approach. The role of anticoagulation in individuals with stroke-in-progression remains unsettled, however, in part because of the absence of properly controlled, randomized trials with adequate power to test the concept, the difficulty in defining degree of progression at entry, and uncertainty regarding the pathogenesis of "evolving stroke."

In 1965, Millikan (154) reported that individuals with stroke and progressive symptoms who received anticoagulants were less likely to progress further or to succumb than their untreated counterparts (Table 58.4).

Use of historical controls was a significant weakness of this study. However, in support of this report was a previous, randomized comparison by Carter (155) of heparin-phenindione anticoagulation with no treatment in two groups ($n = 38$ each) of individuals with progressive neurologic deficits. The incidence of mortality and neurologic deterioration at 6 months were lower in individuals receiving anticoagulation. In contrast, the earlier randomized study of Marshall and Shaw (156) failed to show any difference in mortality between individuals who received heparin and then phenindione after angiography and individuals who received no treatment. That study was terminated, however, because of a twofold increase in deaths at 6 weeks among the anticoagulated group. Nearly 86% of those individuals had vascular abnormalities in the carotid territory. More recently, in a dose-rate comparison of two heparin regimens (adjusted dose, $n = 11$ versus fixed low dose, $n = 7$), a nonsignificant trend in favor of the fixed low-dose regimen was noted. The very small number of individuals in this study, however, has limited its impact.

With their potentially lower risk of hemorrhagic events, fractionated low-molecular-weight heparin or low-molecular-weight heparinoids have been used in individuals with cerebrovascular disease in, as yet, few studies. A report by ten Cate et al (158) indicated no exacerbation or extension of hemorrhage among five individuals with known intracerebral hemorrhage who received a heparinoid when plasma anti-factor Xa levels were maintained between 0.63 and 0.96 U/ml. In another study (159), symptomatic intracerebral hemorrhage occurred in two individuals (3.5%) who received the heparinoid, both with cardioembolic strokes presenting less than 24 hours from the onset of symptoms. Furthermore, several studies have demonstrated significant protection against development of DVT in several disorders including stroke (83). Results of a prospective level I comparison of the heparinoid Org 10172 with placebo in individuals with early stroke-in-progression have been presented as well (160). No advantage of Org 10172 over placebo regarding disability indices, neurologic status, or mortal-

## TABLE 58.4. Stroke-in-Progression: Anticoagulation

| Study | Year | Agent | aPTT (seconds) | Patients (n) | Follow-up (years) | Stroke (n) | Vascular | Nonvascular | Total |
|---|---|---|---|---|---|---|---|---|---|
| Marshall and Shaw (156) | 1960 | Heparin/Phenindione | — | 26 | 0.1 | — | — | — | 6 |
| | | No Treatment | | 25 | | — | — | — | 3 |
| Carter (155) | 1961 | Heparin/Phenindione | — | 38 | 0.5 | 9 | — | — | 3 |
| | | No Treatment | | 38 | | 12 | — | — | 7 |
| Millikan (154) | 1965 | Anticoagulation | — | 181 | 1.0 | 25 | 12 | — | 12 |
| | | No Treatment | | 60 | | 8 | 25 | — | 25 |
| Duke et al. (162) | 1986 | Heparin | 50–70 | 112 | 1.0 | 19 | — | — | 17 |
| | | Placebo | | 113 | | 22 | — | — | 8 |

aPTT, *activated partial thromboplastin time.*

**TABLE 58.5.** Completed Stroke: Antiplatelet Agents

| Study | Year | Agent | Dose (per day) | Patients (n) | Follow-up (years) | Stroke (n) | Mortality (n) | | |
|---|---|---|---|---|---|---|---|---|---|
| | | | | | | | Vascular | Nonvascular | Total |
| Swedish Cooperative Study (163) | 1987 | ASA | 1500 mg | 253 | 2.0 | 32 | 27 | 7 | 34 |
| | | Placebo | | 252 | | 32 | 25 | 12 | 37 |
| Gent et al. (164) | 1985 | Suloctidil | 600 mg | 218 | 1.7 | 29[a] | 4[a] | 9[a] | 13[a] |
| | | Placebo | | 220 | | 28[a] | 14[a] | 11[a] | 25[a] |
| Blakeley (166) | 1979 | Sulfinpyrazone | 800 mg | 145 | — | — | — | — | 25 |
| | | Placebo | | 145 | | — | — | — | 28 |
| Canadian-American Ticlopidine Study (67) | 1989 | Ticlopidine | 500 mg | 525 | 2.0 | 54 | 17[a] | 13[a] | 30[a] |
| | | Placebo | | 528 | | 89 | 29[a] | 8[a] | 38[a] |
| CAPRIE (167)[b] | 1996 | Clopidogrel | 75 mg | 3233 | 1.9 | 315 | 102 | — | — |
| | | ASA | 325 mg | 3198 | | 338 | 102 | — | — |
| IST (168) | 1997 | ASA[c] | 300 mg | 9720 | 0.5 | 362[d] | 855 | 17 | 872 |
| | | no ASA[c] | — | 9715 | | 452[d] | 896 | 13 | 909 |

ASA, aspirin.

[a] Eligible events only, excluding events >28 days after study drug was permanently discontinued.

[b] Stroke subgroup.

[c] Factorial design (include heparin ± ASA).

[d] 14-day outcomes.

ity was observed. A significant advantage for prevention of DVT, however, was detected.

In summary, the benefit of anticoagulation in individuals with progressive symptoms of focal cerebral ischemia rests on one level IV study. Until randomized trials including appropriate numbers of individuals with this rather elusive class of cerebral ischemic symptoms are undertaken, no definitive statement about the role of anticoagulation in this setting can be made.

## ACUTE PARTIAL STABLE STROKE

Acute partial stable stroke refers to focal cerebral ischemia with a persistent neurologic deficit of minor severity, which may be subject to symptomatic worsening (161). Following a limited comparison of subcutaneous heparin with placebo for this presentation (157), Duke et al (162) randomized 225 individuals in a placebo-controlled, double-blind format (level II) to intravenous, adjusted-dose heparin for 7 days (n = 112) or placebo (n = 113) (162). No significant difference between groups regarding progression of ischemic symptoms by 7 days or death was observed, although a trend favoring anticoagulation was suggested. The 1-year mortality rate, however, was significantly greater in the heparin group (P = .01). Symptomatic deterioration from intracerebral hemorrhage was not observed in either group. These findings are in accord with the equivocal reports regarding anticoagulants in the setting of stroke-in-evolution.

## COMPLETED STROKE
### Antiplatelet Agents

Antithrombotic intervention in completed stroke has been directed at preventing subsequent secondary focal cerebral ischemic events, MI, death, or vascular-related death. The approximate rate of the combined outcomes is 10 to 12% per year (67, 163, 164). A growing number of trials with acceptable power (levels I or II) have examined the effect of different antiplatelet agents in individuals presenting with fixed neurologic deficits. Benefit from ASA in individuals presenting with TIAs (and stroke) has been indicated in meta-analyses (165).

A level I study of ASA (163) found no difference in the outcomes of recurrent stroke or death between individuals treated early (≤3 weeks) after completed stroke who were assigned to receive ASA (1500 mg/day) or placebo. Mean follow-up in this study was 2 years (Table 58.5). HI was documented in one individual receiving ASA and in two receiving placebo.

Suloctidil (600 mg/day, n = 218) was compared with placebo (n = 220) for the outcomes of subsequent first stroke, MI, or vascular death in a randomized, double-blind format (164). At the 1.7 year follow-up, there was no significant difference between groups. Use of suloctidil in this setting, however, was accompanied by side effects, including reversible hepatitis, which resulted in individual withdrawal.

Sulfinpyrazone (800 mg/day) did not significantly reduce the mortality rate in individuals within 6 months of a presumed atherothrombotic or thromboembolic stroke (166). A trend favoring sulfinpyrazone was suggested, but the cohort sizes were insufficient to allow a clear difference to be seen.

The effect of ticlopidine (500 mg/day) on secondary stroke incidence in individuals with a signal thromboembolic stroke was tested by Gent et al (67). After a mean follow-up of 2 years, a significant decrease in the combined outcomes of stroke, MI, and vascular mortality was observed between individuals receiving ticlopidine ($n = 525$) over placebo ($n = 528$) in both efficacy and "intention-to-treat" analyses. Individuals were entered within 1 to 16 weeks of a signal completed stroke. Side effects related to ticlopidine occurred in 43 of 525 individuals (8%). These side effects consisted principally of reversible leukopenia, diarrhea, and rash.

The Clopidogrel versus Aspirin in Individuals at Risk of Ischaemic Events (CAPRIE) study (167), which was a prospective, randomized, blinded comparison of the thienopyridine derivative clopidogrel (75 mg/day, $n = 9577$) and ASA (325 mg/day, $n = 9566$) in individuals with signal thrombotic disease demonstrated an 8.7% reduction in relative risk in favor of clopidogrel ($P = .043$). Individuals with evidence of ischemic stroke (including lacunar disease), MI less than 35 days old, or symptomatic atherosclerotic peripheral arterial disease were randomized to treatment and followed for 1 year for the combined outcomes of ischemic stroke, MI, and vascular-related death. Adverse experiences were not significantly different between groups, with a near equivalent frequency of intracranial hemorrhage (clopidogrel, 0.33%; ASA, 0.47%). There was no difference in the incidence of clinically significant neutropenia.

To examine the effects of simple antithrombotic regimens in individuals with completed stroke, the International Stroke Trial (IST) randomized 19,436 individuals with presumed ischemic stroke within 48 hours of the onset of symptoms in a $3 \times 2$ factorial design to receive placebo, ASA (300 mg/day) alone, subcutaneous heparin (low dose, 10,000 IU/day; or medium dose, 25,000 IU/day), or both ASA and heparin for 14 days (168). ASA was associated with an overall significant reduction in total recurrent ischemic strokes within 14 days

($P < .001$), with no significant excess of intracranial hemorrhages over control. At 6 months, a modest decrease in the risk of death or dependency was seen. Heparin was associated with an increase in symptomatic intracranial hemorrhage. A study of similar intent, the Chinese Acute Stroke Trial (CAST), demonstrated similar outcomes (169). Together, the IST and CAST trials indicate that ASA is associated with a small reduction in the incidence of recurrent stroke and mortality in the first weeks after signal stroke.

In summary, on the basis of its salutary effects on stroke outcome in individuals with TIA, ASA is recommended for secondary prevention. Both ticlopidine and clopidogrel produce a significant further reduction in subsequent stroke, MI, or vascular related death over ASA in individuals with an initial completed stroke.

## Anticoagulants

Evidence of a salutary effect from heparin or long-term oral anticoagulation on the outcome of presumed atherothrombotic "completed" stroke is scant. Three randomized, controlled trials of oral anticoagulation have been reported (147, 170, 171) (Table 58.6). Baker et al (147) randomized 132 individuals with recently completed stroke to placebo ($n = 60$) or oral anticoagulation ($n = 72$). When normalized for individual follow-up, recurrent stroke occurred more often in those individuals receiving anticoagulation than in those receiving placebo. Three fatal intracerebral hemorrhages occurred in the anticoagulant group. A contemporaneous study (171) compared adjusted high-dose with fixed low-dose (1 mg) phenindione in individuals with hypertension and, in a separate subtrial, without hypertension. Follow-up in the two subtrials was a minimum of 1.75 and

### TABLE 58.6. Completed Stroke: Anticoagulation

| Study | Year | Agent | Dose (per day) | Patients (n) | Follow-up (years) | Stroke (n) | Mortality (n) Vascular | Nonvascular | Total |
|---|---|---|---|---|---|---|---|---|---|
| Baker et al. (170, 283) | 1962 | Anticoagulation | — | 72 | 65.2[a] | 12 | 8[b] | — | 18 |
| | | No treatment | | 60 | 81.5[a] | 6 | 5[b] | — | 15 |
| Hill et al. (171) | 1962 | Phenindione[c] | 50 mg | 71 | 1.75 | 9 | — | — | 8 |
| | | Phenindione[c] | 1 mg | 71 | | 4 | — | — | 1 |
| | | Phenindione[d] | 50 mg | 66 | 2.3 | 22 | — | — | 12 |
| | | Phenindione[d] | 1 mg | 65 | | 19 | — | — | 4 |
| FISS (177) | 1995 | Nadroparin[e] | 8200 aFXa/day | 100 | 0.5 | — | — | — | 45[e] |
| | | Nadroparin[e] | 4100 aFXa/day | 101 | | — | — | — | 53[e] |
| | | Placebo | — | 105 | | — | — | — | 68[e] |

aFXa, anti–factor Xa activity.

[a] Per individual-year.

[b] Demise from cerebral infarction or cerebral hemorrhage.

[c] Patients with hypertension included.

[d] Patients with mean diastolic pressure >110 mm Hg excluded.

[e] Death or dependency.

2.3 years, respectively. In both subtrials, secondary stroke and death occurred more frequently in the high-dose phenindione groups, and intracerebral hemorrhage was documented in six patients in each subtrial. Both studies suffered from low individual entry, however, and failure to exclude individuals with cardiogenic embolism (172). Results of other series have not improved on the overall impression that anticoagulant therapy does not prevent recurrent stroke in individuals with presumed atherothrombotic primary stroke (173–175). The frequency of symptomatic intracerebral hemorrhage has suggested caution regarding use of anticoagulant therapy in individuals with stroke. No study has attempted to define safety conditions for anticoagulant therapy in completed stroke, but several investigators have suggested clinical conditions for which anticoagulation might be beneficial (150, 176).

Very recently, a salutary report regarding the effect of subcutaneous low-molecular-weight heparin on 6 month mortality rates following stroke onset has appeared (177). Of 2750 individuals screened for the Fraxiparin in Stroke Study (FISS), 312 individuals were randomized to either "high-dose" nadroparin (8200 IU of anti-factor Xa per day), "low-dose" nadroparin (4100 IU/day), or placebo subcutaneously for 10 days beginning within 48 hours after the onset of stroke. A significant dose-dependent reduction in 6 month mortality and dependence was observed favoring low-molecular-weight heparin. Set against this first provocative report from FISS of a potential benefit from low-molecular-weight heparin on mortality in individuals with completed stroke are the results of the recently completed TOAST trial (160). The clinical significance of both reports, however, awaits corroboration by several ongoing, prospective trials of low-molecular-weight heparin.

## Plasminogen Activators

The association of thrombosis with cerebrovascular ischemia was the basis for early trials of plasminogen activators in individuals with completed stroke. In general, all level V studies failed to demonstrate efficacy when symptomatic improvement and death were considered as the primary outcomes. Eight clinical trials evaluating late intravenous infusion of thrombolytic agents in individuals with completed stroke have been reported (Table 58.7).

Clarke and Cliffton (178) as well as Herndon et al (179) treated seven and 13 individuals, respectively, with intravenous plasmin, and both found equivocal results. In a series of angiographically controlled studies comparing streptokinase (180) or Thrombolysin (51) with placebo, Meyer et al found no significant difference in the incidence of recanalization or in clinical outcome when individuals with stable symptoms were treated within 72 hours. A more recent angiographic study by Araki et al (181) demonstrated only an 8% incidence of

recanalization with systemic infusion of u-PA in individuals receiving treatment within 35 days of the onset of symptoms, and there was no improvement in clinical outcome for the u-PA-treated cohort. Fletcher et al (182) also observed no benefit in 31 individuals treated with u-PA treatment administered within 10 to 12 hours of symptom onset. Severe intracranial hemorrhage occurred in four individuals in this series, and five individuals died. On the basis of these results, a general contraindication to use of fibrinolytic agents in individuals with stroke has resulted (183). The long interval to treatment after stroke onset and the possibility that some neurologic deficits were caused by undiagnosed hemorrhage are common concerns with the early studies.

Two prospective, randomized, controlled studies of intravenous u-PA in individuals with stable focal neurologic deficits of less than 5 days duration demonstrated no difference in clinical outcome or incidence of symptomatic intracerebral hemorrhage (184, 185). Prospective, randomized (level II) comparisons of intravenous rt-PA with u-PA in individuals who received treatment within 3 days (186) or 5 days (187) suggested no difference in clinical outcome for these agents. More recent work indicates that plasminogen activators must be used within a much shorter interval from the onset of symptoms to limit hemorrhagic complications and enhance the possibility of favorable outcome.

## ACUTE STROKE

A significant change in the approach to stroke occurred in the early 1980s, when plasminogen activators were applied during the acute period (6–8 hours from symptom onset) (188). Acute intervention in individuals selected by strict CT and clinical criteria has shown evidence of benefit (189, 190).

## Plasminogen Activators

Experimental studies support the concept of a metastable, potentially reversible zone of neuronal injury in the ischemic vascular territory supplied by the occluded cerebral artery (Tables 58.8 and 58.9) (191, 192). The contributions of local vascular anatomy and collateral protection, as well as the predominantly thrombotic basis for focal cerebral ischemia, underlie attempts to achieve early recanalization with fibrinolytic agents (6). Acute, primary use of antiplatelet agents or anticoagulants within 6 hours of the onset of sypmtoms, however, has not been studied as yet.

## Intra-arterial Direct Infusion

Intra-arterial infusion studies are, perforce, angiographically controlled and have the advantage of defining both vascular anatomy and outcome. Zeumer et al

**TABLE 58.7.** Completed Stroke: Thrombolytic Agents

| Study | Year | Agent | Patients (n) | $\Delta$(T-O) (hours)[a] | Clinical Improvement (%)[b] | Hemorrhage (%)[b] |
|---|---|---|---|---|---|---|
| Clarke and Cliffton (178) | 1960 | F | 7 | 3–720 | 71.4 | — |
| Herndon et al. (179) | 1960 | F | 13 | <72 | 61.5 | — |
| Fletcher et al. (182) | 1976 | u-PA | 31 | <36 | 0.0 | 12.9 |
| Abe et al. (284) | 1981 | u-PA | 57 | <720 | 70.4 | 0.0 |
|  |  | C | 56 |  | 47.2 | 0.0 |
| Atarashi et al. (184) | 1985 | u-PA | 191 | <120 | 45.0 | 1.0 |
|  |  | C | 94 |  | 43.6 | 1.1 |
| Otomo et al. (185) | 1985 | u-PA | 176 | <120 | 51.8 | 1.1 |
|  |  | C | 188 |  | 41.0 | 0.5 |
| Otomo et al. (187) | 1988 | rt-PA | 171 | <120 | 59.3 | 1.1 |
|  |  | u-PA | 184 |  | 54.7 | 1.6 |
| Abe et al. (186) | 1990 | rt-PA | 145 | <72 | 66.2 | 2.0 |
|  |  | u-PA | 77 |  | 44.7 | 7.8 |

C, control; F, Fibrinolysin®; rt-PA, recombinant tissue-type plasminogen activator; u-PA, urokinase-type plasminogen activator.

[a] Time interval from symptom onset to treatment.

[b] % of individuals.

**TABLE 58.8.** Acute Stroke: Thrombolytic Agents

| Study[a] | Year | Agent | Patients (n) | $\Delta$(T-O) (hours)[b] | Recanalization (%) | Hemorrhage (%) |
|---|---|---|---|---|---|---|
| *Carotid territory: intra-arterial delivery* |  |  |  |  |  |  |
| del Zoppo et al. (38) | 1988 | SK/u-PA | 20 | 1–24 | 90.0 | 20.0 |
| Mori et al. (37) | 1988 | u-PA | 22 | 0.82–7.00 | 45.5 | 18.2 |
| Matsumoto et al. (199) | 1990 | u-PA | 40 | 1–24 | 60.0 | 32.5 |
| *Carotid territory: intravenous delivery* |  |  |  |  |  |  |
| Yamaguchi et al. (202) | 1990 | rt-PA | 52 | <6 | 38.5 | 28.6 |
| von Kummer et al. (201) | 1992 | rt-PA | 22 | <6 | 59.1 | 36.4 |
| del Zoppo et al. (210) | 1992 | rt-PA | 93 (104)[c] | <8 | 34.4[c] | 30.8 |
| Mori et al. (39) | 1992 | rt-PA | 19 | <6 | 47.4 | 52.6 |
|  |  | C | 12 |  | 16.7 | 41.7 |
| Yamaguchi (285) | 1993 | rt-PA | 47 (51) | <6 | 21.3 | 47.1 |
|  |  | C | 46 (47) |  | 4.4 | 46.8 |
| *Vertebrobasilar territory: intra-arterial delivery* |  |  |  |  |  |  |
| Hacke et al. (200) | 1988 | SK/u-PA | 43 | <24 | 44.2 | 9.3 |
| Zeumer et al. (193) | 1989 | u-PA | 7 | 4–48 | 100.0 | 14.3 |
| Matsumoto et al. (199) | 1990 | u-PA | 10 | 3–24 | 40.0 | 10.0 |
| Möbius et al. (286) | 1991 | SK/u-PA | 18 | 0.5–2.0 | 77.8 | 0.0 |
| *Vertebrobasilar territory: intravenous delivery* |  |  |  |  |  |  |
| Yamaguchi et al. (202) | 1990 | rt-PA | 5 | <6 | 80.0 | 0.0 |
| von Kummer et al. (201) | 1990 | rt-PA | 5 | <6 | 40.0 | 0.0 |

C, control; rt-PA, recombinant tissue-type plasminogen activator; SK, streptokinase; u-PA, urokinase-type plasminogen activator.

[a] Studies with angiographic control; angiography necessary for diagnosis.

[b] Time interval from symptom onset to treatment.

[c] Dose-rate finding study of recanalization (efficacy, 93 individuals; intention-to-treat, 104); recanalization % = cumulative overall dose rates.

**TABLE 58.9.**    Acute Stroke: Thrombolytic Agents

| Study[a] | Year | Agent | Patients (n) | $\Delta$(T-O) (hours)[b] | Clinical Improvement (%) | Hemorrhage | | | |
|---|---|---|---|---|---|---|---|---|---|
| | | | | | | nil | HI | PH | % |
| MAST-E (203) | 1995 | SK | 156 | <6.0 | 35.0 | 88 | 25 | 24 | 17.5 |
| | | C | 154 | | 18.1 | 116 | 13 | 4 | 0.3 |
| ASK (204) | 1995 | SK | 106 | <4.0 | 43.4 | — | — | — | — |
| | | C | 122 | | 22.1 | — | — | — | — |
| MAST-I (205) | 1995 | SK | 313 | <6.0 | 26.5 | 232 | 60 | 21 | 6.7 |
| | | C | 309 | | 11.7 | 280 | 27 | 2 | 0.7 |
| ECASS (190) | 1995 | rt-PA | 313 | <6.0 | 35.9 | 179 | 72 | 62 | 19.8 |
| | | C | 307 | | 29.3 | 184 | 93 | 30 | 6.5 |
| NINDS (Part 1) (287) | 1995 | rt-PA | 144 | ≤1.5, ≤3.0 | 1.2[c] | — | — | 13 | 5.6 |
| | | C | 147 | | | — | — | 3 | 0.0 |
| NINDS (Part 2) (287) | 1995 | rt-PA | 168 | ≤1.5, ≤3.0 | 50,[d] 31[e] | — | — | 21 | 7.1 |
| | | C | 165 | | 38,[d] 20[e] | — | — | 8 | 2.1 |

C, control; HI, hemorrhagic infarction; PH, parenchymatous hematoma; rt-PA, recombinant tissue-type plasminogen activator; SK, streptokinase.

[a] Randomized studies without vascular diagnosis.

[b] Time from symptom onset to treatment.

[c] Relative risk reduction.

[d] Barthel index.

[e] National Institutes of Health Stroke Scale (NIHSS).

and other investigators (193, 194) pioneered the use of flow-directed and guide wire-directed catheter techniques for delivery of thrombolytic agents in the cerebral circulation, which have led to several limited, level V case studies (178, 193, 195–198) (Table 58.8). Recanalization of symptomatic arterial occlusions in the carotid territory has been reported in 46 to 90% of individuals treated with intra-arterial infusion of streptokinase or u-PA within 8 hours (37, 38, 199). Among 82 individuals with carotid obstruction treated with u-PA or streptokinase, 55% underwent complete or partial recanalization following intra-arterial infusion, and hemorrhagic transformation in the carotid territory occurred in 18 to 33% of individuals treated (37, 38, 199). Regarding the vertebrobasilar territory, results of a single, retrospective comparison of clinical outcome in 43 individuals who received intra-arterial u-PA or streptokinase with that of 22 individuals who received conventional therapy (200) suggested a significant survival benefit in those individuals demonstrating recanalization who received the fibrinolytic agent. Hemorrhagic transformation occurred in four individuals treated with u-PA or streptokinase, of whom two deteriorated and died from the hemorrhage.

Only one prospective, randomized, controlled study of the intra-arterial delivery of a plasminogen activator in individuals with acute thrombotic stroke has been undertaken (9). This small, level I study compared recombinant scu-PA (rpro-UK) with placebo for recanalization and safety outcomes. A significant heparin-dependent increase in recanalization of M1 and M2 middle cerebral artery (MCA) occlusions by rpro-UK and an increase in hemorrhagic transformation were observed. The results of a clinical outcome study are awaited.

## Intravenous Systemic Infusion

Among intravenous infusion studies, partial or complete recanalization has been achieved in 34 to 59% of individuals with carotid occlusions treated within 6 to 8 hours of the onset of symptoms (8, 39, 201, 202) (Table 58.8). In three studies (8, 39, 202), recanalization of internal carotid artery occlusions was infrequent (0–25%) at the dose-rates employed. One prospective, open, multicenter dose-rate study (8) was unable to demonstrate an optimal intravenous dose-rate of rt-PA (duteplase) for recanalization, but early reperfusion of MCA division and branch occlusions occurred more frequently than internal carotid artery occlusions. In a placebo-controlled trial by Mori et al (39), individuals treated with 20 or 30 MIU of two-chain rt-PA (duteplase) demonstrated improved recanalization, a significantly better clinical improvement at 30 days than those treated with placebo (39). Individuals undergoing recanalization had a better neurologic outcome than non-recanalized individuals. In the series discussed (8, 39, 201, 202), hemorrhagic transformation occurred in 29 to 53% of treated individuals.

Three symptom-based, randomized, placebo-controlled trials of streptokinase in individuals with acute ischemic stroke (203–206) were terminated because of unacceptable symptomatic hemorrhage or early mortality (Table 58.9). The Multicenter Acute Stroke Trial-Europe (MAST-E) and the Australia Streptokinase (ASK) trials were terminated because of excessive early mortality and symptomatic intracranial hemorrhage in the streptokinase group (203, 204). The Multicentre Acute Stroke Trial-Italy (MAST-I) group also was terminated because of an excess 10 day case fatality rate associated with streptokinase with or without ASA ($P <$ .00001) (205, 206). Each study compared placebo with a single intravenous infusion of streptokinase (1.5 x $10^6$ IU). No dose-finding study that found a safe streptokinase dose preceded any of these trials (207, 208), and the excess of early mortality raises the issue of whether streptokinase–antibody complexes may enhance ischemic injury.

Results of two randomized safety and efficacy studies of rt-PA (alteplase) were more positive (Table 58.9). The European Cooperative Acute Stroke Study (ECASS), which was a prospective, level I study comparing intravenous infusion rt-PA (1.1 mg/kg to a maximum of 100 mg) with placebo within 6 hours, demonstrated no difference between groups regarding 90 day disability outcome (190). A *post hoc* analysis of the "target population" suggested an 11 to 12% absolute improvement in best modified-Rankin scale scores (0 and 1) in the rt-PA-treated group. A significantly higher proportion of individuals with intracerebral hemorrhage causing neurological deterioration or death (PH2), however, was observed with rt-PA (19 of 313 individuals) compared with placebo (seven of 307 individuals).

In contrast, a two-part, four-armed, placebo-controlled clinical outcome study of rt-PA (0.9 mg/kg) with entry at 90 minutes or sooner or at 91 to 180 minutes from the onset of symptoms was completed by the National Institutes of Neurological Disorders and Stroke rt-PA Stroke Study Group (NINDS) (198). In part 1, there was no difference at 24 hours in neurologic status between the rt-PA ($n = 144$) and placebo ($n = 147$) groups according to the National Institutes of Health Stroke Scale (NIHSS) score. In part 2, rt-PA ($n = 168$) recipients displayed a significant 11 to 13% absolute improvement in the Barthel index, modified Rankin scale score, Glasgow outcome scale score, and NIHSS, with minimal or no disability (i.e., deficit) at 3 months over that with placebo ($n = 165$). The frequency of symptomatic hemorrhage, however, was significantly greater among those individuals treated receiving rt-PA (6.4%, $P <$ .001) than among those who received placebo (0.6%) and contributed to demise.

Taken together, results of the ECASS and NINDS studies indicate the enormous importance of individual selection to reduce the hemorrhagic risk accompanying use of plasminogen activators in acute stroke (190, 198, 209). Today, rt-PA is available for treatment of ischemic stroke in appropriately selected individuals within 3 hours of the onset of symptoms.

Studies using intravenous infusions of rt-PA also have indicated significant contributors to hemorrhage risk. These include excessive time from the onset of symptoms to treatment (210), low body mass, diastolic hypertension (211), and older age (212).

In a separate setting, fibrinolytic agents have been used successfully in individuals with retinal artery and retinal vein occlusion (213). Partial visual recovery was observed when retinal vein occlusion was treated with intravenous streptokinase within 2 weeks of the onset of symptoms. Partial recovery of form vision was possible in some individuals with acute retinal artery occlusion (214, 215). Neither approach has been tested prospectively, however.

## Defibrinating Agents

One report (216) has supported the safety of the defibrinating agent ancrod in patinets with acute ischemic stroke when a reduction in fibrinogen of 100 mg/dl was maintained. A phase III study is currently in progress.

## SINUS VENOUS THROMBOSIS

Thrombosis of the sagittal sinus (SVT) and associated intracranial veins may produce transient or progressive focal symptoms, seizures, and profound, progressive alterations in consciousness. Until recently, therapy has been expectant. In a controlled study, Einhaupl et al (217) reported a significant improvement in clinical status at 72 hours and 3 months in those receiving continuous heparin infusion ($n = 10$) compared with those receiving no treatment ($n = 10$). Both the incidence and severity of hemorrhage associated with SVT, however, was not altered by heparin exposure. Two of three individuals with intracranial hemorrhage in the heparin group had complete clinical recovery. Despite its small size, results of this study, in juxtaposition to those of a single-site retrospective study, suggests a benefit to early use of heparin in individuals with SVT (217). Only very limited experience with thrombolytic agents in individuals with SVT has been reported (218).

## CAROTID ARTERY ATHEROTHROMBOTIC DISEASE

The carotid artery bifurcation is a predilection site for atheromatous change, which also may lead to cerebral ischemic symptoms. Endarterectomy of the extracranial portion of the carotid artery, with or without patch angioplasty, may resolve the local abnormality of the vascular flow, but cerebral ischemic symptoms may recur.

Results of both the North American Symptomatic Carotid Endarterectomy Trial (NASCET) and the MRC European Carotid Surgery Trial (ECST) have indicated significant survival benefit and symptomatic relief from endarterectomy over medical (i.e., antiplatelet agent) therapy for carotid stenosis of 70 to 99% (219, 220). Both trials were undertaken to resolve controversies arising from liberal use of this procedure in individuals with TIAs.

Trials of adjunctive antiplatelet treatment have sought to alter the incidence of stroke and death or to decrease the incidence of carotid restenosis after carotid endarterectomy. In one prospective double-blind trial among individuals who underwent carotid endarterectomy randomized to ASA (1300 mg/day, $n = 65$) or to placebo ($n = 60$) within 5 days of the procedure (221), the incidence of stroke or death at 6 months was greater in those receiving placebo than in those receiving ASA, but this difference did not reach statistical significance. In a separate trial (222), no significant difference at 2.1 year follow-up in the outcomes of stroke, MI, or vascular death was seen between individuals receiving ASA (50–100 mg/day, $n = 150$) or placebo ($n = 151$) within 1 to 12 weeks of carotid endarterectomy. Kretschmer et al (223) retrospectively examined 252 individuals undergoing carotid endarterectomy who had received either ASA (1500 mg/day) or no adjunctive treatment. The finding of significantly prolonged survival in the ASA group was the basis for a prospective comparison of pre-surgical ASA (1000 mg/day, $n = 32$) or no treatment ($n = 34$). Survival was prolonged in the ASA-treated group, although cerebral events occurred equally in both. The small number of individuals in all three trials, however, may have obscured any potential benefit to cerebrovascular outcome in the active arms.

At this time, there are no results of level I trials to support any recommendation for adjunctive antiplatelet therapy after endarterectomy. In the large ongoing endarterectomy trials, the practice has been to continue postendarterectomy individuals on ASA alone. A single trial of the effect from ASA and dipyridamole versus placebo on restenosis after endarterectomy was terminated when no significant difference was noted on the interim analysis (224). Finally, there is little information regarding a role for anticoagulants after endarterectomy, and fibrinolytic agents are contraindicated.

## CEREBRAL EMBOLISM FROM A CARDIAC SOURCE (SEE CHAPTERS 59 AND 60)

The principal cardiac embolic sources that lead to focal cerebral ischemia include mural thrombi associated with left ventricular dyskinesis in myocardial ischemia, valvular abnormalities including prosthetic valves and rheumatic vegetations, and thromboembolism in atrial fibrillation. Because of the thrombotic nature of most cardioembolic events, a role for anticoagulation has been suggested in both primary and secondary prevention.

## Cardioembolic Stroke in Acute Myocardial Infarction (see Chapter 59)

The incidence of systemic thromboembolism, including stroke, after MI without adjunctive therapy varies from 1 to 3% per year, but it may be as high as 3.7% during the first month after MI (i.e., the acute phase) (225–230). Anticoagulation during the acute in-hospital phase and in the chronic post-hospitalization phase significantly reduces the incidence of stroke. Evidence for this effect derives from a series of well conducted, randomized level I and II trials (Table 58.10).

Secondary prevention trials designed to determine the incidence of recurrent MI as the main outcome event also have examined the relative effect of long-term anticoagulation on the incidence of stroke. Four of 388 individuals randomized to long-term oral anticoagulation and nine of 359 individuals randomized to placebo had strokes within 1 to 5 years of their MI in the Veterans Administration Cooperative Study (226). This study entered individuals within 21 days of acute MI, and the trend favoring anticoagulation for stroke was mirrored by an overall reduction in the combined outcomes of stroke, second MI, and death. A similar trend was noted by Loeliger et al (227) in a double-blind, randomized trial of long-term oral anticoagulation (i.e., phenprocoumon) versus placebo when treatment was initiated at least 12 months after the acute MI. Two of 122 individuals receiving placebo and none of 128 individuals receiving anticoagulation suffered strokes during the 15 month follow-up period, but serious hemorrhage was more common in the active agent group.

More recently, the open German-Austrian Aspirin Trial (GAAT) (228), which also had a phenprocoumon arm, reported a decreased incidence of stroke in individuals receiving oral anticoagulation compared with placebo when treatment began within 42 days of MI. No significant difference in the outcome events of stroke, second MI, and death was apparent, however. The Sixty Plus Reinfarction Study (229) randomized individuals older than 60 years to oral anticoagulation or placebo in a double-blind fashion after recovery from a signal MI (229). Here, too, a trend toward lower incidence of stroke with anticoagulation was evident at 2 year follow-up. The incidence of second MI and death was similarly decreased.

All four of these level II studies (226–229) demonstrated an increased incidence of serious hemorrhagic complications, which contributed to morbidity or demise in the anticoagulated group. In the GAAT and the Sixty Plus Reinfarction studies, the number of serious hemorrhages, including intracerebral events, associated with anticoagulation was considered to be excessive.

Two level I trials, which assigned individuals surviving an acute MI to long-term oral anticoagulation or placebo, demonstrated a significantly reduced incidence in stroke in association with anticoagulation. Harvald

**TABLE 58.10.**   Acute Myocardial Infarction: Anticoagulation

| Study | Year | Agent | Dose (per day) | Patients (n) | Follow-up (years) | Stroke (n) | Mortality (n) Vascular | Mortality (n) Nonvascular | Total |
|-------|------|-------|----------------|--------------|-------------------|------------|-----------------------|--------------------------|-------|
| Harvald et al. (225) | 1962 | Dicoumarol | 10–25%[b] | 145 | 3.0 | 1 (9) | — | — | 34 |
|  |  | Placebo |  | 170 |  | 11 (17) | — | — | 45 |
| MRC (Long-term Anticoagulation) (231) | 1964 | Phenindione | | 195 | 2.1 | 3 | — | — | 29 |
|  |  | Phenindione | 1 mg | 180 |  | 1 | — | — | 40 |
| VA Cooperative Trial (226) | 1965 | Warfarin | — | 388 | 1.0–5.0 | 4 (10) | 82 | 5 | 87 |
|  |  | Placebo |  | 359 |  | 9 (17) | 90 | 7 | 97 |
| Loeliger et al. (227) | 1967 | Phenprocoumon | — | 128 | — | 0 | 8 | — | — |
|  |  | Placebo |  | 122 |  | 2 | 9 | — | — |
| MRC (Short-term Anticoagulation) (234) | 1969 | Heparin/Phenindione | 72 mg | 712 | — | 3 (34) | — | — | 115 |
|  |  | Phenindione | 1 mg | 715 |  | 7 (79) | — | — | 129 |
| Drapkin and Merskey (232) | 1972 | Heparin/Phenindione | — | 745 | 6.0 | 13 (75) | — | — | 111 |
|  |  | Placebo |  | 391 |  | 7 (44) | — | — | 83 |
| VA Cooperative Trial (233) | 1973 | Heparin/Warfarin | — | 500 | — | 4 (15) | 27 | 20 | 48 |
|  |  | Placebo |  | 499 |  | 19 (45) | 36 | 20 | 56 |
| Sixty-Plus Reinfarction Study (229) | 1980 | Phenprocoumon | INR, | 439 | 2.0 | 13 | 45 | 6 | 51 |
|  |  | Placebo | 2.7–4.5 | 439 |  | 21 | 63 | 6 | 69 |
| German-Austrian Aspirin Trial (228) | 1980 | Warfarin | — | 320 | 2.0 | 1 | 32 | 7 | 39 |
|  |  | ASA | 1500 mg | 317 |  | 0 | 18 | 9 | 27 |
|  |  | Placebo |  | 309 |  | 2 | 26 | 6 | 32 |
| WARIS (230) | 1990 | Warfarin | INR, | 607 | 3.1 | 20 | 82 | 12 | 94 |
|  |  | Placebo | 2.1–4.8 | 607 |  | 44 | 104 | 19 | 123 |

ASA, *aspirin;* INR, *international normalized ratio.*

[a] *Numbers in parentheses indicate systemic embolic events.*

[b] *Prothrombin–proconvertin activity.*

et al (225), in a trial based in Copenhagen, reported a significantly decreased incidence of stroke during a mean 3 year follow-up, from 11 events in 170 individuals receiving placebo to one event in 145 individuals receiving anticoagulation. The Warfarin Reinfarction Study (WARIS) (230) also reported a significant decrease (55% risk reduction, $P = .0015$) in the incidence of cerebrovascular accidents (secondary endpoint) at 3.1 year follow-up in individuals receiving warfarin over those receiving placebo. While the incidence of death and reinfarction (MI) was also reduced by warfarin in that study, no effect of anticoagulation on systemic embolism, second MI, death, or major hemorrhage was apparent in the earlier trial (225). Hemorrhage was more common in the active treatment group in both trials, and dramatically so in the former; importantly, ASA treatment was excluded in that trial.

Finally, a nonstatistically significant decrease in the number of systemic embolic events with (adjusted) high-dose phenindione at a mean follow-up of 2.1 years was reported from a randomized phenindione dose-comparison trial sponsored by the MRC (231). Serious hemorrhage also was more frequent in the high-dose phenindione group.

In summary, a reduced number of cerebrovascular events after recovery from MI accompanied the use of long-term anticoagulation, reaching statistical significance in two level I trials. In practice, however, concerns about the higher incidence of serious hemorrhagic events, including intracerebral hemorrhages, has prevented routine use of anticoagulants.

Similarly, a decreased incidence of stroke in the acute (i.e., in hospital) phase of myocardial ischemia was noted in three trials of anticoagulation. A trend favoring heparin/oral anticoagulation to decrease the number of embolic events was noted in individuals randomized to heparin ($n = 745$) or placebo ($n = 391$) within 24 hours of their MI. However, in this study there was no effect on the combined outcomes of stroke, second MI, and death (232). Subsequently, in a single-blind test in which male individuals were randomized to heparin/warfarin ($n = 500$) or placebo ($n = 499$) for 28 days after an acute MI, anticoagulation was associated with a significant decrease in strokes (233). Here, too, the combined outcomes of stroke, second MI, and death were not different between groups. To evaluate the effect of anticoagulant dose on MI recurrence or death, a separate level I trial sponsored by the MRC (234) randomized individuals within 14 days of acute MI to heparin/adjusted high-dose phenindione or heparin/fixed low-dose phenindione (1 mg) for 28 days, and although no difference in the incidence of principal outcome events was apparent, a significant decrease in the incidence of systemic embolism was seen in the high-dose group. Interestingly, both the incidence and severity of hemorrhagic complications accompanying anticoagulation during the acute phase of MI in those trials was quite low, with no deaths resulting from intracerebral hemorrhage reported overall. This experience has suggested a notable reduction in cerebrovascular ischemic events with use of anticoagulants during the acute phase of MI.

In only one dose-rate study (heparin/phenindione versus phenindione) was a correlation between frequency of hemorrhagic events and degree of anticoagulation reported (231). Despite a fourfold increase in extracranial hemorrhage, no difference in the number of cerebral hemorrhages between the low-dose and high-dose regimens (one each) was seen in this study. Unfortunately, the degree of anticoagulation at the time of an intracranial hemorrhagic event has not been reported in any other trial.

## Cardioembolic Stroke in Atrial Fibrillation (see Chapter 60)

Atrial fibrillation may be classified either as nonvalvular (i.e., nonrheumatic) atrial fibrillation or as atrial fibrillation associated with valvular dysfunction. The 2 year incidence of stroke in individuals with chronic nonvalvular atrial fibrillation is from 6.2 to 7.6% (235, 236). Atrial fibrillation is a significant risk factor for thromboembolic stroke, especially in elderly individuals (235),

and it may be first observed during stroke in up to 30% of individuals (237). Stroke recurrence also is associated with atrial fibrillation, especially early after the signal event (11, 237, 238).

## Primary Prevention

### All Classes of Atrial Fibrillation

Results of two prospective studies (239, 240) have suggested a decreased incidence of systemic emboli or death in individuals with valvular or nonvalvular atrial fibrillation receiving anticoagulation compared with those receiving no treatment. Both studies, however, suffer from the limitations of non-randomized trials, but they still support a protective role for anticoagulation in individuals with atrial fibrillation.

### Nonvalvular (Nonrheumatic) Atrial Fibrillation

The pathogenesis of stroke and the role of antithrombotic regimens in individuals with nonrheumatic atrial fibrillation have been reviewed (241). In a retrospective study, Sage et al (242) indicated that risk of cerebral infarction after an episode of nonvalvular atrial fibrillation may be 20% per year, with a mortality rate from the initial infarct of 38% (242). This is in accord with the experience of Hart et al (243), who reported a 34.8% incidence of symptomatic embolism (13% cerebral) in individuals not undergoing immediate anticoagulation. These, as well as other data, have suggested the need for prospective clinical trials (Table 58.11); the prospective

---

**TABLE 58.11.** Atrial Fibrillation (Nonvalvular): Antiplatelet Agents/Anticoagulants

| Study | Year | Agent | Dose or Range (per day) | Patients (n) | Follow-up (years) | Stroke (n)[a] | Mortality (n) Vascular | Mortality (n) Nonvascular | Mortality (n) Total |
|---|---|---|---|---|---|---|---|---|---|
| AFASAK (244) | 1989 | Warfarin | INR, 2.8–4.2 | 335 | 2.0 | 5 | 3 | — | — |
| | | ASA | 75 mg | 336 | | 17 (3) | 12 | — | — |
| | | Placebo | | 336 | | 19 (2) | 15 | — | — |
| SPAF (245) | 1990 | 1. Warfarin/ASA | INR, 2.0–3.5/325 mg | 393 | 1.13 | 7 | 6 | 2 | 14 |
| | | Placebo | | 195 | | 17 (1) | 5 | 1 | 8 |
| | | 2. ASA | 325 mg | 517 | 1.13 | 18 (1) | 15 | 10 | 31 |
| | | Placebo | | 528 | | 34 (4) | 15 | 14 | 39 |
| BAATAF (246) | 1990 | Warfarin | INR, 1.5–2.7 | 212 | 2.2 | 2 | 7 | 4 | 11 |
| | | Placebo | | 208 | | 13 | 13 | 13 | 26 |
| CAFA (87) | 1991 | Warfarin | INR, 2.0–3.0 | 187 | 1.26 | 4 (1) | 6 | 1 | 7 |
| | | Placebo | | 191 | | 9 (2) | 6 | 0 | 6 |
| SPAF-II (248) | 1994 | Warfarin[b] | INR, 2.0–4.5 | 358 | 2.3 | 13 (1) | 20 | 11 | 36 |
| | | ASA | 325 mg | 357 | | 19 (2) | 25 | 11 | 41 |
| | | Warfarin[c] | INR, 2.0–4.5 | 197 | — | 13 (1) | 16 | 7 | 26 |
| | | ASA | 325 mg | 188 | | 18 (0) | 14 | 7 | 24 |
| SPAF-III (249) | 1996 | Warfarin | INR, 2.0–3.0 | 523 | 1.1 | 11 (0) | 27 | 8 | 35 |
| | | Warfarin | INR, 1.2–1.5 | 521 | | 43 (1) | 27 | 12 | 42 |

ASA, aspirin; INR, international normalized ratio.

[a] Numbers in parentheses indicate systemic embolic events.

[b] Patients ≤ 75 years.

[c] Patients > 75 years.

clinical trials described here are discussed further in Chapter 60.

The AFASAK study (244), which was an open trial, randomized individuals with nonrheumatic, nonvalvular atrial fibrillation to warfarin ($n = 335$), ASA (75 mg/day, $n = 336$), or placebo ($n = 336$). A significant decrease in cerebral embolic events was apparent at 2 year follow-up in the warfarin group. Five of 335 warfarin-treated individuals versus 19 of 336 placebo-treated (and 17 of the ASA-treated) individuals had documented cerebral embolic events. Hemorrhagic complications were significantly more common in the warfarin group (21 of 335) than in the ASA or placebo groups.

That experience was supported by two additional trials of primary stroke prevention (245, 246). The Stroke Prevention in Atrial Fibrillation (SPAF) study (245) randomized 1244 individuals to warfarin, ASA, or placebo (group 1) if they were eligible for warfarin, or to ASA or placebo (group 2, double-blind) if they were not. This study was terminated at a mean follow-up of 1.13 years, however, when the warfarin and ASA arms of group 1 were shown to have a significant combined risk reduction (81%) for the outcomes of ischemic stroke and systemic embolism. The relative benefit of warfarin over ASA was not reported, but 10.9% of individuals randomly assigned to warfarin were withdrawn because of drug intolerance. The Boston Area Anticoagulation Trial for Atrial Fibrillation (BAATAF) trial (246) openly randomized individuals with nonrheumatic atrial fibrillation to long-term, low-dose warfarin ($n = 212$) or no therapy ($n = 208$). At a mean follow-up of 2.2 years, a significant risk reduction of 86% for stroke and death favored the warfarin group. The number of fatal hemorrhages in the warfarin and no therapy groups was identical.

Results of the AFASAK and SPAF studies led to premature termination of the Canadian Atrial Fibrillation Anticoagulation (CAFA) Study (247) in 1990. In that trial, a risk reduction of 44.8% for ischemic stroke and systemic thromboembolism was attributed to the warfarin group (six events) over the placebo group (11 events).

Concern regarding the risk of intracranial hemorrhage associated with warfarin fueled approaches using ASA (248) or incorporating low-dose oral anticoagulation (249). The SPAF-II trial (248) examined the relative efficacies of warfarin and ASA in individuals with nonvalvular atrial fibrillation. This study prospectively stratified individuals into two age cohorts: those 75 years old or older, and those younger than 75 years. A modest, but nonstatistically significant, reduction in ischemic stroke events was associated with warfarin over ASA. There was a significantly greater frequency of major hemorrhagic events, however, with warfarin in the older cohort than in the younger cohort ($P = .008$). One concern with this study is that the overall annual thromboembolic event rate was rather low.

Age greater than 80 years, intensity of anticoagulation, and prothrombin time prolonged from the therapeutic range all are contributors to increased bleeding risk (250). The SPAF-III trial (249) addressed this issue in individuals with nonvalvular atrial fibrillation. Individuals were randomized to either adjusted dose warfarin ($n = 523$) to maintain an INR of between 2.0 and 3.0 or to low-intensity warfarin with ASA (325 mg/day) to maintain an INR of between 1.2 and 1.5 ($n = 521$). This trial was terminated at a mean follow-up of 1.1 years, when the annual disabling stroke rate of the combination therapy exceeded that of adjusted-dose warfarin (5.6 versus 1.7%, respectively; $P = .0007$). When cumulative event rates were calculated, a nearly significant difference ($P = .07$) favoring warfarin seemed to support the results of previous studies (Table 58.11).

In summary, results of randomized, controlled trials of individuals with nonvalvular atrial fibrillation support use of warfarin at an INR of 2.0 to 3.0 for reduction in primary stroke incidence. The benefit of oral anticoagulation as a prophylactic measure must be weighed against the increased incidence of hemorrhagic complications with a higher INR and an unacceptable frequency of embolic events with inadequate anticoagulation.

## Secondary Prevention: All Classes of Atrial Fibrillation

Information from secondary prevention trials involving individuals with atrial fibrillation presenting with a signal stroke is scant. In an open trial of anticoagulation in individuals with stroke and nonvalvular atrial fibrillation, Lodder et al (251) found no difference in the incidence of second stroke or death at a mean follow-up of 2.25 years; death from serious hemorrhage occurred in six of the 70 anticoagulated individuals (18.6%). The Cerebral Embolism Study Group (120) performed a randomized, open trial of immediate versus delayed anticoagulation in individuals with atrial fibrillation individuals and a signal cardioembolic stroke for the principal outcome event of recurrent embolism. Anticoagulation was initiated immediately on signal stroke ($n = 24$) or 10 days after the first stroke ($n = 20$), and in this small series, two individuals in the delayed treatment group had second embolic events. From that experience, it is difficult to conclude a definite role for anticoagulants in secondary prevention of recurrent cerebral embolism in atrial fibrillation.

Three well-performed, prospective, level I trials indicate that anticoagulation in individuals with nonvalvular atrial fibrillation is associated with a decreased incidence of primary cerebral embolic events. Data regarding secondary prevention of stroke in populations with valvular or nonvalvular atrial fibrillation are equivocal, being compromised by the small and uncontrolled nature of the trials.

## VALVULAR CARDIOVASCULAR DISEASE

Cerebral embolism may occur with unattended rheumatic valvular disease, both mechanical and xenograft prosthetic cardiac valves, and calcified mitral annuli. Risk of cerebral embolism is greatly increased by concurrent atrial fibrillation (252–254). Coulshed et al (255) recorded a 3.7 and 1.9% yearly incidence of systemic embolism from untreated rheumatic mitral stenosis and mitral insufficiency, respectively. Recurrent embolism is frequent, most commonly occurring within 6 to 12 months after the signal embolism (252, 256). The incidence of systemic embolism from prosthetic cardiac valves is greater for mechanical devices than for xenograft prostheses, and modifications of device strut and annular design (257), use of fabric covering to reduce metal contact (258), and development of xenograft materials and valves (259) have been aimed at reducing the thrombogenicity and embolic risk. Use of antithrombotic strategies for protection against thromboembolic complications of valve prostheses has been reviewed elsewhere (253, 254).

### Mechanical Prosthetic Cardiac Valves

Antiplatelet and anticoagulant agents have been used as prophylaxis against embolic complications of mechanical valves (254). The more recent use of nonmechanical prostheses, however, has altered the approach to prophylaxis with anticoagulants.

In a retrospective review of 283 individuals having Starr-Edwards ball-valve prostheses with metal struts, Akbarian et al (260) reported a decreased frequency of systemic emboli at a mean follow-up 1.75 years in the anticoagulated group (Table 58.12). This decrease is greatest for individuals with aortic valve replacement; of 214 individuals with aortic valve prostheses (metal struts), there was an apparent reduction in the frequency of thromboembolic events at 2 years from 41 to 4% (261). Similarly, in a retrospective review, Barnhorst et al (258) confirmed that long-term anticoagulation with warfarin in 1684 individuals with Starr-Edwards prostheses in the aortic or mitral position was associated with a significant reduction in the rate of systemic embolism. Moggio et al (262) reported their experience with anticoagulation of individuals having cloth-covered aortic or metal Starr-Edwards valve prostheses. A reduction in the mean number of thromboembolic events from 4.0 to 2.1 per 100 patient years was observed with warfarin anticoagulation, but this advantage was lost when anticoagulants were discontinued after 1 year.

Beyond these level III studies, there has been some difficulty in interpretating reports of thromboembolic outcome, resulting at least in part from the absence of direct comparisons of anticoagulated and untreated individuals as well as from the level of anticoagulation undertaken (254). Generally, all individuals with mechanical prosthetic valves should be treated with long-term anticoagulation. A target INR of 3.5 (range, 3.0–4.5) has been recommended (263). A recent comparison of "high intensity" warfarin (INR, 9; $n = 125$) with "moderate intensity" warfarin (INR, 2.65; $n = 122$) indicated a significant increase in hemorrhagic episodes with the high-intensity regimen, without a further reduction in thromboembolic events (264). Loeliger (265) has suggested that a target INR of 4.0 for mechanical valves and 3.5 for tissue valves produces an acceptable reduction in hemorrhagic risk.

## TABLE 58.12. Cardiac Valvular Prostheses (Mechanical): Anticoagulation

| Study | Year | Agent | Dose | Valve Position | Patients (n) | Follow-up (years) | Thromboembolic Events (%) |
|---|---|---|---|---|---|---|---|
| Duvoisin et al. (261) | 1967 | Warfarin | — | Aortic | 177 | 2.0 | 4 |
| | | Nil | | | 37 | | 41 |
| Akbarian et al. (260) | 1968 | Warfarin | — | Aortic | 50 | 1.75 | 8 |
| | | Nil | | | 52 | | 56 |
| | | Warfarin | — | Mitral | 15 | — | 30 |
| | | Nil | | | 10 | | 27 |
| Moggio et al. (262) | 1978 | Coumadin | — | Aortic/Mitral | 48 | 2.0–3.8 | 1.2 |
| | | Nil | | | 58 | | 4.0 |
| Dale et al. (266) | 1977 | Warfarin/ASA | 1000 mg | Aortic | 75 | 2.0 | 1.8 |
| | | Warfarin | — | | 73 | | 9.3 |
| Altman et al. (267) | 1976 | Warfarin/ASA | —/500 mg | Aortic/mitral | 57 | 2.1 | 5 |
| | | Warfarin | — | | 65 | 1.9 | 20 |
| Sullivan et al. (268) | 1969 | Warfarin/Dipyridamole | —/400 mg | Aortic/mitral | 42 | 1.1 | 2 |
| | | Warfarin | — | | 50 | 1.2 | 14 |
| Chesebro et al. (270) | 1983 | Warfarin/Dipyridamole | —/400 mg | — | 181 | — | 2, 0.5[a] |
| | | Warfarin/ASA | —/500 mg | | 179 | | 4, 1.2[a] |

ASA, *aspirin.*

[a] *Number per 100 individual-years.*

Antiplatelet agents may augment the antithromboembolic protection afforded by anticoagulants alone. Two level I studies have demonstrated reduced thromboembolic risk in individuals receiving anticoagulation/ASA over anticoagulation alone. Dale et al (266) reported a decrease in thromboembolic events from 9.3 per 100 patient years in those receiving warfarin ($n = 73$) to 1.8 in those receiving warfarin and ASA (1000 mg/day, $n = 75$) in individuals with aortic prostheses at approximately 2 year followup. Most embolic events were cerebral (10 of 13 in the warfarin group, two of two in the warfarin/ASA group), of which three were fatal. Altman et al (267) noted a similar, 75% reduction in systemic thromboembolism and death in individuals with aortic or mitral Starr-Edwards valves randomized to warfarin and ASA (500 mg/day, $n = 57$) compared with those randomized to warfarin alone ($n = 65$) at a follow-up of 1.75 years. The incidence of gastrointestinal hemorrhage was not different in the groups, but the large number of hemorrhages in the earlier study led to discontinuation of ASA.

Considering the lower rate of gastrointestinal side effects of dipyridamole, studies using this agent are of interest. In two reports of a randomized, prospective, double-blind trial (268, 269), Sullivan et al indicated that addition of dipyridamole (400 mg/day) to warfarin produced a significant reduction in thromboembolism or death over warfarin and placebo. A similar finding was reported by Chesebro (270) in an open trial of individuals with mechanical prostheses randomized to warfarin and dipyridamole (400 mg/day, $n = 181$) or to warfarin and ASA (500 mg/day, $n = 170$). Addition of dipyridamole was favorable in individuals receiving ASA for reducing thromboembolic events in that study, and major hemorrhagic complications were significantly fewer with the addition of dipyridamole as well ($P = .001$). In general, use of dipyridamole with warfarin in level II and III studies and the combination of warfarin and ASA in level I studies (254) have been associated with a decreased incidence of cerebral thromboembolism in individuals with mechanical prosthetic cardiac valves; dipyridamole has been associated with fewer hemorrhagic events.

An additional challenge is provided by individuals who are pregnant and require valve replacement. Anticoagulation with warfarin, subcutaneous heparin, or standard intravenous heparin during pregnancy each have significant risks, which must be weighed against the thromboembolic risk of the valve itself (271, 272).

## Xenograft (Bio)Prosthetic Cardiac Valves

The incidence of systemic thromboembolic events associated with bioprostheses at 3 years is 4% in individuals with sinus rhythm (273) and 16% in individuals with atrial fibrillation (274). The incidence of embolic events associated with atrial fibrillation may be highest in those

individuals with a history of embolism or left atrial thrombus (274). Results of a few level V studies have suggested the greatest risk of thromboembolism occurs during the first 3 months after placement of the bioprosthesis (275, 276). A decreased incidence of major embolic events at 3 years was seen in individuals with porcine biosynthetic valves treated with dicumarol postoperatively for 6 to 12 weeks in one study (274), and in a level I study Turpie et al (259) demonstrated no significant difference in the incidence of systemic emboli in individuals with xenograft prostheses randomized to anticoagulant control at an INR of 2.00 to 2.25 or 2.5 to 4.0 (standard anticoagulation) for the initial 3 postoperative months. In that study, clinically significant hemorrhagic events were more numerous in the group receiving standard anticoagulation.

The lower incidence of thromboembolic events with xenograft valve prostheses as compared to that with mechanical prostheses implies that antiplatelet prophylaxis may have some benefit with lower hemorrhagic risk. Nuñez et al (277, 278) examined this scenario in two prospective, nonrandomized trials of warfarin versus ASA (1000 or 500 mg/day). In the first study (277), no embolic events were recorded among individuals in sinus rhythm who received warfarin ($n = 124$) or ASA ($n = 260$) at a mean follow-up of 1.9 years. In individuals with atrial fibrillation, the number of embolic events in the ASA group ($n = 135$) was somewhat lower than that in the warfarin group ($n = 151$). In a second, level III study of ASA prophylaxis following placement of mitral valve bioprostheses (278), individuals who received 500 mg every 2 days were less likely to have embolic events than those who received 1000 mg/day; this experience has remained unchallenged. Thus, with a mitral valve bioprosthesis, ASA may provide some protection against embolic events; however, this conclusion has not been rigorously tested. Generally accepted clinical practice requires anticoagulation of individuals with a bioprosthesis for the initial 3 postoperative months, when the thromboembolic risk is greatest.

## DEEP VENOUS THROMBOSIS IN STROKE

DVT is a common complication of stroke during the recuperation phase (279). Attempts to improve on the effects of prophylactic unfractionated heparin have entailed testing of heparinoids and low-molecular-weight heparins. Early experience with two low-molecular-weight heparin preparations as prophylaxis, however, was mixed (280–282). Twice daily subcutaneous treatment with one preparation was associated with significantly reduced frequency of DVT (282). Turpie et al (83) demonstrated an advantage to twice daily subcutaneous treatment with a low-molecular-weight heparinoid compared with low-dose subcutaneous heparin in decreasing DVT.

# CONCLUSIONS

Preservation or reconstitution of vascular patency and protection of neuronal function are two general approaches to minimizing permanent injury from cerebrovascular ischemia. The contribution of atherothrombosis and thromboembolism to acute cerebrovascular disease has supported the enthusiasm for using antithrombotic agents to preserve flow. Early explorations of such agents, however, were limited by small treatment cohorts, late intervention, and use of temporal clinical criteria for individual entry. Increased statistical power from larger cohorts and more specific definitions of study populations by anatomic and physiologic criteria (e.g., angiography in carotid endarterectomy trials) have characterized recent studies. Nevertheless, the difficulty of selecting individuals on clinical grounds alone remains a central limitation in many antithrombotic studies of cerebrovascular ischemia. Studies of antithrombotic prophylaxis against cardiovascular sources of thromboembolism have not suffered this restriction.

## ANTIPLATELET AGENTS

Antiplatelet agents may reduce risk in individuals with a history of recent TIAs for the combined outcomes of subsequent stroke, MI, and mortality. ASA is the most active antiplatelet agent in this setting. When TIAs are associated with carotid artery stenosis of 70 to 99%, carotid endarterectomy and ASA are superior to ASA alone in preventing subsequent stroke and stroke-related mortality. The combination of ASA and dipyridamole, however, is no better than ASA alone for TIAs. For secondary prevention of recurrent stroke in individuals presenting with a stable, recent focal cerebral deficit, ticlopidine and clopidogrel are beneficial, and ASA/dipyridamole also may be active.

## ANTICOAGULANTS

Anticoagulation has not been beneficial in individuals with TIAs, stroke-in-evolution, partial stable stroke, or completed stroke, even although one study showed subcutaneous heparin applied in early stroke to reduce the mortality rate at 6 months. Anticoagulation does decrease the incidence of both systemic and cerebral embolism in individuals with a signal MI, nonvalvular (i.e., nonrheumatic) atrial fibrillation, mechanical valve prosthesis, and xenograft (bio)prosthesis (for the initial 3 months after placement). Individuals with atrial fibrillation without a valvular abnormality may benefit from long-term anticoagulation, and early use of heparin in individuals with sinus venous thrombosis may produce clinical improvement.

## PLASMINOGEN ACTIVATORS

Plasminogen activators have a role in selected individuals with acute cerebral ischemia. Recanalization of symptomatic, documented carotid occlusions (except for the extracranial internal carotid artery) and vertebrobasilar arterial occlusions has been achieved by local intra-arterial and by intravenous delivery. A single study demonstrated clinical benefit at 3 month follow-up when rt-PA was given intravenously within 3 hours of the onset of symptoms and under stringent selection criteria. Other recent studies have underscored the need for careful individual selection, because fatal hemorrhage is a risk.

## FUTURE DIRECTIONS

Antithrombotic interventions have been used successfully in conditions with a known pathogenesis, natural history, and anatomy (e.g., cardiac valvular prostheses). Further evidence of beneficial roles for each class of antithrombotic agent in individuals with cerebrovascular disease will be aided by refinements in vascular diagnostic techniques and a better understanding of the relationship between vascular thrombosis and neuronal injury.

# REFERENCES

1. Mohr JP, Caplan LR, Melski JW et al. The Harvard Cooperative Stroke Registry: a prospective registry. Neurology 1978;28:754–762.
2. Sacco RL, Wolf PA, Kannel WB et al. Survival and recurrence following stroke. The Framingham study. Stroke 1982;13:290–295.
3. Mohr JP, Barnett HJM. Classification of ischemic strokes. In: Barnett HJM, Mohr JP, Stein BM, Yatsu FM, eds. Stroke: pathophysiology, diagnosis, and management. New York: Churchill Livingstone, 1986:281–291.
4. Fisher CM. The arterial lesions underlying lacunes. Acta Neuropathol (Berl) 1968;12:1–15.
5. Mohr JP, Pessin MS. Extracranial carotid artery disease. In: Barnett HJM, Mohr JP, Stein BM, Yatsu FM, eds. Stroke: pathophysiology, diagnosis, and management. New York: Churchill Livingstone, 1986:293–336.
6. Solis OJ, Roberson GR, Taveras JM et al. Cerebral angiography in acute cerebral infarction. Rev Interam Radiol 1977;2:19–25.
7. Fieschi C, Argentino C, Lenzi GL et al. Clinical and instrumental evaluation of patients with ischemic stroke within the first six hours. J Neurol Sci 1989;91:311–321.
8. Anonymous. An open safety/efficacy trial of rt-PA in acute thromboembolic stroke: final report [Abstract]. The rt-PA Acute Stroke Study Group. Stroke 1991;22:153.
9. del Zoppo GJ, Higashida RT, Furlan AJ et al. The Prolyse in Acute Cerebral Thromboembolism Trial (PROACT): results of 6 mg dose tier [Abstract]. Stroke 1996;27:164A.
10. Marshall J. The natural history of transient ischaemic cerebrovascular attacks. Q J Med 1964;33:309–324.
11. Wolf PA, Kannel WB, McGee DL et al. Duration of atrial fibrillation and imminence of stroke: the Framingham study. Stroke 1983;14:664–667.
12. Wolf PA, Kannel WB, McGee DL. Prevention of ischemic stroke: risk factors. In: Barnett HJM, Mohr JP, Stein BM, Yatsu FM, eds. Stroke: pathophysiology, diagnosis, and management. New York: Churchill Livingstone, 1986:967–988.
13. Whisnant JP, Matsumoto N, Elveback LR. Transient cerebral ischemic attacks in a community. Rochester, Minnesota, 1955 through 1969. Mayo Clin Proc 1973;48:194–198.
14. Anonymous. United Kingdom transient ischaemic attack (UK-TIA) aspirin trial: interim results. UK-TIA Study Group. Br Med J (Clin Res) 1988;296:316–320.
15. Caplan LR. Are terms such as completed stroke or RIND of continued usefulness? Stroke 1983;14:431–433.

16. Scmidt EV, Smirnov VE, Ryabova VS. Results of the seven-year prospective study of stroke patients. Stroke 1988;19:942–949.

17. Silver FL, Norris JW, Lewis AJ et al. Early mortality following stroke: a prospective review. Stroke 1984;15:492–496.

18. Shaw CM, Alvord EC Jr, Berry RG. Swelling of the brain following ischemic infarction with arterial occlusion. Arch Neurol 1959;1:161–177.

19. Wityk RJ, Pessin MS, Kaplan RF et al. Serial assessment of acute stroke using the NIH stroke scale. Stroke 1994;25:362–365.

20. Denny-Brown D. Recurrent cerebrovascular episodes. Arch Neurol 1960;2:194–210.

21. Russell RWR. Atheromatous retinal embolism. Lancet 1963;ii:1354–1356.

22. Hollenhorst RW. Vascular status of individuals who have cholesterol emboli in the retina. Am J Ophthalmol 1966;61:1159–1165.

23. Barnett HJ. The pathophysiology of transient cerebral ischemic attacks [Review]. Med Clin North Am 1979;63:649–679.

24. Marshall J. The management of cerebrovascular diseases. Oxford: Blackwell Scientific Publications, 1976:57–59.

25. Davis-Jones GAB, Preston FE, Temperly WR. Neurological complications in clinical hematology. Oxford: Blackwell Scientific Publications, 1980:176–177.

26. Irino T, Taneda M, Minami T. Angiographic manifestations in post-recanalized cerebral infarction. Neurology 1977;27:471–475.

27. DeWood MA, Spores J, Notske R et al. Prevalence of total coronary occlusion during the early hours of transmural myocardial infarction. N Engl J Med 1980;303:897–902.

28. Dougherty JH Jr, Levy DE, Weksler BB. Platelet activation in acute cerebral ischaemia. Serial measurements of platelet function in cerebrovascular disease. Lancet 1977;i:821–824.

29. Mettinger KL, Nyman D, Kjellin KG et al. Factor VIII related antigen, antithrombin III, spontaneous platelet aggregation and plasminogen activator in ischemic cerebrovascular disease: a study of stroke before 55. J Neurol Sci 1979;41:31–38.

30. de Boer AC, Turpie AG, Butt RW et al. Plasma beta thromboglobulin and serum fragment E in acute partial stroke. Br J Haematol 1982;50:327–334.

31. Cella G, Zahavi J, de Haas HA et al. β-Thromboglobulin, platelet production time, and platelet function in vascular disease. Br J Haematol 1979;43:127–136.

32. Feinberg WM, Bruck DC, Ring ME et al. Hemostatic markers in acute stroke. Stroke 1989;20:592–597.

33. Bogousslavsky J, Van Melle G, Regli F. The Lausanne Stroke Registry: analysis of 1,000 consecutive patients with first stroke. Stroke 1988;19:1083–1092.

34. Foulkes MA, Wolf PA, Price TR et al. The stroke data bank: design, methods, and baseline characteristics. Stroke 1988;19:547–554.

35. del Zoppo GJ, Mori E. Hematologic causes of intracerebral hemorrhage and their treatment [Review]. Neurosurg Clin North Am 1992;3:637–658.

36. Fisher M, Adams RD. Observations on brain embolism with special reference to the mechanism of hemorrhagic infarction. J Neuropathol Exp Neurol 1951;10:92–94.

37. Mori E, Tabuchi M, Yoshida T et al. Intracarotid urokinase with thromboembolic occlusion of the middle cerebral artery. Stroke 1988;19:802–812.

38. del Zoppo GJ, Ferbert A, Otis S et al. Local intra-arterial fibrinolytic therapy in acute carotid territory stroke. A pilot study. Stroke 1988;19:307–313.

39. Mori E, Yoneda Y, Tabuchi M et al. Intravenous recombinant tissue plasminogen activator in acute carotid artery territory stroke. Neurology 1992;42:976–982.

40. Hamann GF, Okada Y, Fitridge R et al. Microvascular basal lamina antigens disappear during cerebral ischemia and reperfusion. Stroke 1995;26:2120–2126.

41. Fisher CM, Adams RD. Observations on brain embolism with special reference to hemorrhage infarction. In: Furlan AJ, ed. The heart and stroke. Exploring mutual cerebrovascular and cardiovascular issues. New York: Springer-Verlag, 1987:17–36.

42. Jörgensen L, Torvik A. Ischaemic cerebrovascular diseases in an autopsy series. 2. Prevalence, location, pathogenesis, and clinical course of cerebral infarcts. J Neurol Sci 1969;9:285–320.

43. Okada Y, Yamaguchi T, Minematsu K et al. Hemorrhagic transformation in cerebral embolism. Stroke 1989;20:598–603.

44. Hornig CR, Dorndorf W, Agnoli AL. Hemorrhagic cerebral infarction—a prospective study. Stroke 1986;17:179–185.

45. Eisenberg HM, Suddith RL. Cerebral vessels have the capacity to transport sodium and potassium. Science 1979;206:1083–1085.

46. Hart RG. Cerebral embolism study group: timing of hemorrhagic transformation of cardioembolic stroke. In: Stober T, Schimrigk K, Ganten D, Sherman DG, eds. Central nervous system control of the heart. Boston: Martinus Nijhoff Publishing, 1986:229–232.

47. Lodder J, Krijne-Kubat B, Broekman J. Cerebral hemorrhagic infarction at autopsy: cardiac embolic cause and the relationship to the cause of death. Stroke 1986;17:626–629.

48. Yamaguchi T, Minematsu K, Choki J et al. Clinical and neuroradiological analysis of thrombotic and embolic cerebral infarction. Jpn Circ J 1984;48:50–58.

49. Anonymous. Immediate anticoagulation of embolic stroke: brain hemorrhage and management options. Cerebral Embolism Study Group. Stroke 1984;15:779–789.

50. Drake ME Jr, Shin C. Conversion of ischemic to hemorrhagic infarction by anticoagulant administration. Report of two cases with evidence from serial computed tomographic brain scans. Arch Neurol 1983;40:44–46.

51. Meyer JS, Gilroy J, Barnhart MI et al. Therapeutic thrombolysis in cerebral thromboembolism. Neurology 1963;13:927–93752.

52. Babikian VL, Kase CS, Pessin MS et al. Intracerebral hemorrhage in stroke individuals anticoagulated with heparin [Review]. Stroke 1989;20:1500–1503.

53. Kelton JG. Antiplatelet agents: rationale and results [Review]. Clin Haematol 1983;12:311–354.

54. Harker LA. Antiplatelet drugs in the management of patients with thrombotic disorders [Review]. Semin Thromb Hemost 1986;12:134–155.

55. Fuster V, Badimon L, Badimon J et al. Drugs interfering with platelet functions: mechanisms and clinical relevance. In: Verstraete M, Vermylen J, Lijnen R, Arnout J, eds. Thrombosis and haemostasis. Leuven, Belgium: Leuven University Press, 1987:349–418.

56. Roth GJ, Stanford N, Majerus PW. Acetylation of prostaglandin synthase by aspirin. Proc Natl Acad Sci U S A 1975;72:3073–3076.

57. Preston FE, Whipps S, Jackson CA et al. Inhibition of prostacyclin and platelet thromboxane $A_2$ after low-dose aspirin. N Engl J Med 1981;304:76–79.

58. Clarke RJ, Mayo G, Price P et al. Suppression of thromboxane $A_2$ but not of systemic prostacyclin by controlled-release aspirin. N Engl J Med 1991;325:1137–1141.

59. Baumgartner HR, Tschopp TB, Weiss HJ. Platelet interaction with collagen fibrils in flowing blood. II. Impaired adhesion-aggregation in bleeding disorders. A comparison with subendothelium. Thromb Haemost 1977;37:17–28.

60. Moake JL, Turner NA, Stathopoulos NA et al. Shear-induced platelet aggregation can be mediated by vWf released from platelets, as well as by exogenous large or unusually large vWf multimers, requires adenosine diphosphate and is resistant to aspirin. Blood 1988;71:1366–1374.

61. Harker LA, Slichter SJ. Studies of platelet and fibrinogen kinetics in patients with prosthetic heart valves. N Engl J Med 1970;283:1302–1305.

62. FitzGerald GA. Dipyridamole [Review]. N Engl J Med 1987;316:1247–1257.

63. Ranhosky A. Dipyridamole [Letter]. N Engl J Med 1987;317:1734.

64. Wiley JS, Chesterman CN, Morgan FJ et al. The effect of sulphinpyrazone on the aggregation and release reactions of human platelets. Thromb Res 1979;14:23–33.

65. McTavish D, Faulds D, Goa KL. Ticlopidine. An updated review of its pharmacology and therapeutic use in platelet-dependent disorders [Review]. Drugs 1990;40:238–259.

66. Panak E, Maffrand JP, Picard-Fraire C et al. Ticlopidine: a promise for the prevention and treatment of thrombosis and its complications. Haemostasis 1983;13(Suppl I):1–54.

67. Gent M, Blakely JA, Easton JD et al. The Canadian-American Ticlopidine Study (CATS) in thromboembolic stroke. Lancet 1989;i:1215–1220.

68. Hass WK, Easton JD, Adams HP Jr et al. A randomized trial comparing ticlopidine hydrochloride with aspirin for prevention of stroke in high-risk patients. Ticlopidine Aspirin Stroke Study Group. N Engl J Med 1989;321:501–507.

69. Herbert JM, Frehel D, Vallee E et al. Clopidogrel, a novel antiplatelet and antithrombotic agent. Cardiovasc Drug Rev 1993;11:180–198.

70. Savi P, Laplace MC, Maffrand JP et al. Binding of [$^3$H]-2-methylthio ADP to rat platelets: effect of clopidogrel and ticlopidine. J Pharmacol Exp Ther 1994;269:772–777.

71. Gurewich V, Lipinski B. Evaluation of antithrombotic properties of suloctidil in comparison with aspirin and dipyridamole. Thromb Res 1976;9:101–108.

72. Schror K. Antiplatelet drugs. A comparative review [Review]. Drugs 1995;50:7–28.

73. Hirsh J, Dalen JE, Poller L et al. Optimal Therapeutic Range for Oral Anticoagulants. Second ACCP Conference on Antithrombotic Therapy. Chest 19;95:5S–11S.

74. Björk I, Lindahl U. Mechanism of the anticoagulant action of heparin [Review]. Mol Cell Biochem 1982;48:161–182.

75. Nesheim ME. A simple rate law that describes the kinetics of the heparin-catalysed reaction between antithrombin III and thrombin. J Biol Chem 1983;258:14708–14717.

76. Holmer E, Kurachi K, Söderström G. The molecular weight dependence of the rate-enhancing effect of heparin on the inhibition of thrombin, factor Xa, factor IXa, factor XIa, factor XIIa and kallikrein by antithrombin. Biochem J 1981;193:395–400.

77. Damus PS, Hicks M, Rosenberg RD. Anticoagulant action of heparin. Nature 1973;246:355–357.

78. Johnson EA, Kirkwood TB, Stirling Y et al. Four heparin preparations: anti-Xa potentiating effect of heparin after subcutaneous injection. Thromb Haemost 1976;35:586–591.

79. Ofosu FA. Anticoagulant mechanisms of Orgaran (Org 10172) and its fraction with high affinity to antithrombin III (Org 10849). Haemostasis 1992;22:66–72.

80. Meuleman DG. Orgaran (Org 10172): its pharmacological profile in experimental models [Review]. Haemostasis 1992;22:58–65.
81. Boneu B. New antithrombotic agents for the prevention and treatment of deep vein thrombosis [Review]. Haemostasis 1996;26:368–378.
82. Gent M, Hirsh J, Ginsberg JS et al. Low-molecular-weight heparinoid orgaran is more effective than aspirin in the prevention of venous thromboembolism after surgery for hip fracture. Circulation 1996;93:80–84.
83. Turpie AG, Gent M, Cote R et al. A low-molecular-weight heparinoid compared with unfractionated heparin in the prevention of deep vein thrombosis in patients with acute ischemic stroke. A randomized, double-blind study. Ann Intern Med 1992;117:353–357.
84. Adams HP Jr, Woolson RF, Biller J et al. Studies of Org 10172 in patients with acute ischemic stroke. TOAST Study Group [Review]. Haemostasis 1992;22:99–103.
85. Madden KP, Karanjia PN, Adams HP Jr et al. Accuracy of initial stroke subtype diagnosis in the TOAST study. Trial of Org 10172 in Acute Stroke Treatment. Neurology 1995;45:1975–1979.
86. Davis PH, Clarke WR, Bendixen BH et al. Silent cerebral infarction in patients enrolled in the TOAST study. Neurology 1996;46:942–948.
87. Poller L. Oral anticoagulant therapy. In: Bloom AL, Thomas DP, eds. Haemostasis and thrombosis. Edinburgh: Churchill Livingstone, 1987:870–885.
88. Robbins KC, Summaria L, Hsieh B et al. The peptide chains of human plasmin. Mechanism of activation of human plasminogen to plasmin. J Biol Chem 1967;242:2333–2342.
89. Rijken DC. Structure/function relationships of t-PA. In: Kluft C, ed. Tissue type plasminogen activator (t-PA): physiological and clinical aspects. Vol 1. Boca Raton: CRC Press, 1988:101–122.
90. Ranby M, Bergsdorf N, Nilsson T. Enzymatic properties of the one- and two-chain form of tissue plasminogen activator. Thromb Res 1982;27:175–183.
91. Rijken DC, Hoylaerts M, Collen D. Fibrinolytic properties of one-chain and two-chain human extrinsic (tissue-type) plasminogen activator. J Biol Chem 1982;257:2920–2925.
92. Ranby M, Bergsdorf N, Norrman B et al. Tissue plasminogen activator kinetics. In: Davison JF, Bachmann F, Bouvier CA, Kruithof EKO, eds. Progress in fibrinolysis. New York: Churchill Livingstone, 1982:182.
93. Ehrlich HJ, Bang NW, Little SP et al. Biological properties of a kringleless tissue plasminogen activator (t-PA) mutant. Fibrinolysis 1987;1:75–81.
94. White WF, Barlow GH, Mozen MM. The isolation and characterization of plasminogen activators (urokinase) from human urine. Biochemistry 1966;5:2160–2169.
95. Bernik MB, Kwaan HC. Plasminogen activator activity in cultures from human tissues. An immunological and histochemical study. J Clin Invest 1969;48:1740–1753.
96. Fletcher AP, Alkjaersig N, Sherry S et al. The development of urokinase as a thrombolytic agent. Maintenance of a sustained thrombolytic state in man by its intravenous infusion. J Lab Clin Med 1965;65:713–731.
97. Stump DC, Mann KG. Mechanisms of thrombus formation and lysis. Ann Emerg Med 1988;17:1138–1147.
98. Gunzler WA, Steffens GJ, Otting F et al. Structural relationship between human high and low molecular mass urokinase. Hoppe Seylers Z Physiol Chem 1982;363:133–141.
99. Lijnen HR, Zamarron C, Blaber M et al. Activation of plasminogen by pro-urokinase. I. Mechanism. J Biol Chem 1986;261:1253–1258.
100. Bando H, Okada K, Matsuo O. Thrombolytic effect of prourokinase in vitro. J Fibrinolysis 1987;1:169–176.
101. Castellino FJ. A unique enzyme-protein substrate modifier reaction: plasmin/streptokinase interaction. Trends Biochem Sci 1979;4:1–5.
102. Brogden RN, Speight TM, Avery GS. Streptokinase: a review of its clinical pharmacology, mechanism of action, and therapeutic uses [Review]. Drugs 1973;5:357–445.
103. Smith RA, Dupe RJ, English PD et al. Fibrinolysis with acyl-enzymes: a new approach to thrombolytic therapy. Nature 1981;290:505–508.
104. Smith RA, Dupe FJ, English PD et al. Acyl-enzymes as thrombolytic agents in a rabbit model of venous thrombosis. Thromb Haemost 1982;47:269–274.
105. Matsuo O, Collen D, Verstraete M. On the fibrinolytic and thrombolytic properties of active-site p-anisoylated streptokinase-plasminogen complex (BRL 26921). Thromb Res 1981;24:347–358.
106. Pierard L, Jacobs P, Gheysen D et al. Mutant and chimeric recombinant plasminogen activators. Production in eukaryotic cells and preliminary characterization. J Biol Chem 1987;262:11771–11778.
107. Runge MS, Bode C, Matsueda GR et al. Antibody-enhanced thrombolysis: targeting of tissue plasminogen activator in vivo. Proc Natl Acad Sci U S A 1987;84:7659–7662.
108. Gheysen D, Lijnen HR, Pierard L et al. Characterization of a recombinant fusion protein of the finger domain of tissue-type plasminogen activator with a truncated single chain urokinase-type plasminogen activator. J Biol Chem 1987;262:11779–11784.
109. Oczkowski WJ, Turpie AG. Antithrombotic treatment of cerebrovascular disease [Review]. Baillieres Clin Haematol 1990;3:781–813.
110. Barnett HJM. Antithrombotic therapy in cerebral vascular disease; anti-spasmodics and fibrinolysis. In: Barnett HJM, Mohr JP, Stein BM, Yatsu EM, eds. Stroke: pathophysiology, diagnosis, and management. New York: Churchill Livingstone, 1986:989–1002.
111. Sherman DG, Dyken ML, Fisher M et al. Antithrombotic therapy for cerebrovascular disorders [Review]. Chest 1989;95(Suppl 2):140S–155S.
112. Sackett DL. Rules of evidence and clinical recommendations on the use of antithrombotic agents. Chest 1986;89(Suppl 2):2S–3S.
113. Barnett HJ. The contribution of multicenter trials to stroke prevention and treatment [Review]. Arch Neurol 1990;47:441–444.
114. Anonymous. Secondary prevention of vascular disease by prolonged antiplatelet treatment. Antiplatelet Trialists' Collaboration. Br Med J (Clin Res) 1988;296:320–331.
115. Anonymous. A randomized trial of aspirin and sulfinpyrazone in threatened stroke. The Canadian Cooperative Study Group. N Engl J Med 1978;299:53–59.
116. Gent M, Barnett HJ, Sackett DL et al. A randomized trial of aspirin and sulfinpyrazone in individuals with threatened stroke. Results and methodologic issues. Circulation 1980;62:V97–V105.
117. Anonymous. Principal endpoints. The ESPS Group. European Stroke Prevention Study (ESPS). Lancet 1987;ii:1351–1354.
118. Bousser MG, Eschwege E, Haguenau M et al. "AICLA" controlled trial of aspirin and dipyridamole in the secondary prevention of athero-thrombotic cerebral ischemia. Stroke 1983;14:5–14.
119. Jonas S. Anticoagulant therapy in cerebrovascular disease: review and meta-analysis [Review]. Stroke 1988;19:1043–1048.
120. Anonymous. Immediate anticoagulation of embolic stroke: a randomized trial. Cerebral Embolism Study Group. Stroke 1983;14:668–676.
121. Wardlaw JM, Yamaguchi T, del Zoppo GJ et al. The efficacy and safety of thrombolytic therapy in acute ischaemic stroke: a systematic review of the randomised trials comparing thrombolysis with control. In: Warlow C, Van Gijn J, Sandercock P, eds. Stroke module of the cochrane database of systematic reviews. London: BMJ Publishing Company, 1996.
122. Mundall J, Quintero P, von Kaulla KN et al. Transient monocular blindness and increased platelet aggregability treated with aspirin. A case report. Neurology 1972;22:280–285.
123. Harrison MJ, Marshall J, Meadows JC et al. Effect of aspirin in amaurosis fugax. Lancet 1971;ii:743–744.
124. Dyken ML, Kolar OJ, Jones FH. Differences in the occurrence of carotid transient ischemic attacks associated with antiplatelet aggregation therapy. Stroke 1973;4:732–736.
125. Fields WS, Lemak NA, Frankowski RF et al. Controlled trial of aspirin in cerebral ischemia. Stroke 1977;8:301–314.
126. Sorenson PS, Pedersen H, Marquardsen J et al. Acetylsalicylic acid in the prevention of stroke in patients with reversible cerebral ischemic attacks. A Danish Cooperative Study. Stroke 1983;14:15–22.
127. Anonymous. A comparison of two doses of aspirin (30 mg vs. 283 mg a day) in patients after a transient ischemic attack or minor ischemic stroke. The Dutch TIA Trial Study Group. N Engl J Med 1991;325:1261–1266.
128. Anonymous. Swedish Aspirin Low-Dose Trial (SALT) of 75 mg aspirin as secondary prophylaxis after cerebrovascular ischemic events. The SALT Collaborative Group. Lancet 1991;338:1345–1349.
129. Hirsch L. Anticoagulant and platelet antiaggregant agents. In: Barnett HJM, Mohr JP, Stein BM, Yatsu FM, eds. Stroke: pathophysiology, diagnosis and management. New York: Churchill Livingston, 1986;2:925–966.
130. Harker LA, Slichter SJ. Arterial and venous thromboembolism: kinetic characterization and evaluation of therapy. Thromb Diath Haemorrh 1974;31:188–203.
131. Acheson J, Danta G, Hutchinson EC. Controlled trial of dipyridamole in cerebral vascular disease. Br Med J 1969;1:614–615.
132. Anonymous. Persantine Aspirin Trial in cerebral ischemia. Part II: endpoint results. The American-Canadian Cooperative Study group. Stroke 1985;16:406–415.
133. Matias-Guiu J, Davalos A, Pico M et al. Low-dose acetylsalicylic acid (ASA) plus dipyridamole versus dipyridamole alone in the prevention of stroke in patients with reversible ischemic attacks. Acta Neurol Scand 1987;76:413–421.
134. Anonymous. Second European Stroke Prevention Study. ESPS-2 Working Group [Editorial]. J Neurol 1992;239:299–301.
135. Anonymous. Secondary stroke prevention: aspirin/dipyridamole combination is superior to either agent alone and to placebo The European Stroke Prevention Study (ESPS-2) Working Group. Stroke 1996;27:195.
136. Evans G. Effect of drugs that suppress platelet surface interaction on incidence of amaurosis fugax and transient cerebral ischemia. Surg Forum 1972;23:239–241.
137. Roden S, Low-Beer T, Carmalt M et al. Transient cerebral ischaemic attacks—management and prognosis. Postgrad Med J 1981;57:275–278.
138. Candelise L, Landi G, Perrone P et al. A randomized trial of aspirin and sulfinpyrazone in patients with TIA. Stroke 1982;13:175–179.
139. Campbell MH. Basilar artery syndrome. Can Med Assoc J 1953;69:314–315.
140. Millikan CH, Siekert RG, Shick RM. Studies in cerebrovascular disease. III. The use of anticoagulant drugs in the treatment of insufficiency or thrombosis within the basilar arterial system. Mayo Clin Proc 1955;30:116–126.

141. Fisher CM. The use of anticoagulants in cerebral thrombosis. Neurology 1958;8:311–332.

142. Fazekas JF, Alman RW, Sullivan JF. Vertebral-basilar insufficiency. Arch Neurol 1963;8:215–220.

143. Olsson JE, Müller R, Berneli S. Long-term anticoagulant therapy for TIAs and minor strokes with minimum residuum. Stroke 1976;7:444–451.

144. Siekert RG, Whisnant JP, Millikan CH. Surgical and anticoagulant therapy of occlusive cerebrovascular disease. Ann Intern Med 1963;58:637–641.

145. Friedman GD, Wilson WS, Mosier JM et al. Transient ischemic attacks in a community. JAMA 1969;210:1428–1434.

146. Toole JF, Janeway R, Choi K et al. Transient ischemic attacks due to atherosclerosis. A prospective study of 160 patients. Arch Neurol 1975;32:5–12.

147. Baker RN, Broward JA, Fang HC et al. Anticoagulant therapy in cerebral infarction. Neurology 1962;12:823–835.

148. Baker RN, Schwartz WS, Rose AS. Transient ischemic strokes. A report of a study of anticoagulant therapy. Neurology 1966;16:841–847.

149. Pearce JMS, Gubbay SS, Walton JN. Long-term anticoagulant therapy in transient cerebral ischemic attacks. Lancet 1965;i:6–9.

150. Estol CJ, Pessin MS. Anticoagulation: is there still a role in atherothrombotic stroke? [Review]. Stroke 1990;21:820–824.

151. Putnam SF, Adams HP Jr. Usefulness of heparin in initial management of patients with recent transient ischemic attacks. Arch Neurol 1985;42: 960–962.

152. Biller J, Bruno A, Adams HP Jr et al. A randomized trial of aspirin or heparin in hospitalized patients with recent transient ischemic attacks. A pilot study. Stroke 1989;20:441–447.

153. Walker AM, Jick H. Predictors of bleeding during heparin therapy. JAMA 1980;244:1209–1212.

154. Millikan CH. Anticoagulant therapy in cerebrovascular disease. In: Millikan CH, Siekert RG, Whisnant JP, eds. Cerebral vascular diseases. New York: Grune and Stratton, 1965:183.

155. Carter AB. Anticoagulant treatment in progressing stroke. Br Med J 1961; 2:70–73.

156. Marshall J, Shaw DA. Anticoagulant therapy in acute cerebrovascular accidents: a controlled trial. Lancet 1960;i:995–998.

157. Duke RJ, Turpie AG, Bloch RF et al. Clinical trial of low-dose subcutaneous heparin for the prevention of stroke progression: natural history of acute partial stable stroke. In: Reivich M, Hurtig HI, eds. Cerebrovascular disease. New York: Raven Press, 1983:399–405.

158. ten Cate H, Henny CP, Buller HR et al. Use of a heparinoid in patients with hemorrhagic stroke and thromboembolic disease. Ann Neurol 1984; 15:268–270.

159. Massey EW, Biller J, Davis JN et al. Large-dose infusions of heparinoid ORG 10172 in ischemic stroke. Stroke 1990;21:1289–1292.

160. Adams HP Jr. Trial of Org 10172 in Acute Stroke Treatment (TOAST). Presented at the 6th European Stroke Conference, Amsterdam, 1997.

161. Genton E, Barnett HJ, Felds WS et al. Cerebral ischemia: the role of thrombosis and of antithrombotic therapy. Study group on antithrombotic therapy. Stroke 1977;8:150–175.

162. Duke RJ, Bloch RF, Turpie AG et al. Intravenous heparin for the prevention of stroke progression in acute partial stable stroke. Ann Intern Med 1986; 105:825–828.

163. Anonymous. High-dose acetylsalicylic acid after cerebral infarction. A Swedish Cooperative Study. Stroke 1987;18:325–334.

164. Gent M, Blakely JA, Hachinski V et al. A secondary prevention, randomized trial of suloctidil in patients with a recent history of thromboembolic stroke. Stroke 1985;16:416–424.

165. Anonymous. Collaborative overview of randomised trials of antiplatelet therapy. I: Prevention of death, myocardial infarction, and stroke by prolonged antiplatelet therapy in various categories of individuals. Antiplatelet Trialists' Collaboration. Br Med J 1994;308:81–106.

166. Blakely JA. A prospective trial of sulfinpyrazone and survival after thrombotic stroke. Thromb Haemost 1979;42:382A.

167. Anonymous. A randomised, blinded, trial of clopidogrel versus aspirin in patients at risk of ischaemic events (CAPRIE). CAPRIE Steering Committee. Lancet 1996;348:1329–1339.

168. Anonymous. The International Stroke Trial (IST): a randomised trial of aspirin, subcutaneous heparin, both, or neither among 19,435 patients with acute ischaemic stroke. International Stroke Trial Collaborative Group. Lancet 1997;349:1569–1681.

169. Chen ZM, Xie JX, Peto R et al. CAST Collaborative Group. Chinese Acute Stroke Trial (CAST): Rationale, design and progress. Cerebrovasc Dis 1996; 6:23.

170. Fisher CM. Anticoagulant therapy in cerebral thrombosis and cerebral embolism. A national cooperative study, interim report. Neurology 1961; 11:119–131.

171. Hill AB, Marshall J, Shaw DA. Cerebrovascular disease: trial of long-term anticoagulant therapy. Br Med J 1962;2:1003–1006.

172. Brust JC. Transient ischemic attacks: natural history and anticoagulation [Review]. Neurology 1977;27:107–707.

173. McDowell F, McDevitt E. Treatment of the completed stroke with long-term anticoagulant. Six and one-half years' experience. In: Siekert RH,

174. Enger E, Boyesen S. Long-term anticoagulant therapy in patients with cerebral infarction. A controlled clinical study. Acta Med Scand 1965; 179(Suppl):1–61.

175. Baker RN. An evaluation of anticoagulant therapy in the treatment of cerebrovascular disease. Report of the Veterans Administration Cooperative Study of Atherosclerosis, Neurology Section. Neurology 1961;11: 132–138.

176. Miller VT. Transient ischemic attacks and ischemic stroke: indications for anticoagulation [Review]. Clin Cardiol 1990;13:VI-29–VI-30.

177. Kay R, Wong KA, Yu YL et al. Low-molecular-weight heparin for the treatment of acute ischemic stroke. N Engl J Med 1995;333:1588–1593.

178. Clarke RL, Cliffton EE. The treatment of cerebrovascular thrombosis and embolism with fibrinolytic agents. Am J Cardiol 1960;30:546–551.

179. Herndon RM, Meyer JS, Johnson JF et al. Treatment of cerebrovascular thrombosis with fibrinolysin. Preliminary report. Am J Cardiol 1960;30: 540–545.

180. Meyer JS, Gilroy J, Barnhart MI et al. Anticoagulants plus streptokinase therapy in progressive stroke. JAMA 1964;189:373.

181. Araki G, Minakami K, Mihara H. Therapeutic effect of urokinase on cerebral infarction. Rinsho To Kenkyu 1973;50:3317–3326.

182. Fletcher AP, Alkjaersig N, Lewis M et al. A pilot study of urokinase therapy in cerebral infarction. Stroke 1976;7:135–142.

183. Anonymous. Thrombolytic therapy in treatment: summary of an NIH Consensus Conference. Br Med J 1980;280:1585–1587.

184. Atarashi J, Otomo E, Araki G et al. Clinical utility of urokinase in the treatment of acute stage of cerebral thrombosis: multi-center double-blind study in comparison with placebo. Clin Eval 1985;13:659–709.

185. Otomo E, Araki G, Itoh E et al. Clinical efficacy of urokinase in the treatment of cerebral thrombosis. Clin Eval 1985;13:711–751.

186. Abe T, Terashi A, Tohgi H et al. Clinical efficacy of intravenous administration of SM-9527 (t-PA) in cerebral thrombosis. Clin Eval 1990;18:39–69.

187. Otomo E, Tohgi H, Hirai S et al. Clinical efficacy of AK-124 (tissue plasminogen activator) in the treatment of cerebral thrombosis: study by means of multi-center double blind comparison with urokinase. Yakuri To Chiryo 1988;16:3775–3821.

188. del Zoppo GJ, Zeumer H, Harker LA. Thrombolytic therapy in stroke: possibilities and hazards. Stroke 1986;17:595–607.

189. Anonymous. Tissue plasminogen activator for acute ischemic stroke. The National Institute of Neurological Disorders and Stroke rt-PA Stroke Study Group. N Engl J Med 1995;333:1581–1587.

190. Hacke W, Kaste M, Fieschi C et al. Intravenous thrombolysis with recombinant tissue plasminogen activator for acute hemispheric stroke. The European Cooperative Acute Stroke Study (ECASS). JAMA 1995;274: 1017–1025.

191. Astrup J, Siesjö BK, Symon L. Thresholds in cerebral ischemia—the ischemic penumbra. Stroke 1981;12:723–725.

192. Astrup J, Symon L, Branston NM et al. Cortical evoked potential and extracellular K+ and H+ at critical levels of brain ischemia. Stroke 1977; 8:51–57.

193. Zeumer H, Freitag HJ, Grzyska U et al. Local intra-arterial fibrinolysis in acute vertebrobasilar occlusion. Technical developments and recent results. Neuroradiology 1989;31:336–340.

194. Toni D, Fiorelli M, Gentile M et al. Progressing neurological deficit secondary to acute ischemic stroke. A study on predictability, pathogenesis, and prognosis. Arch Neurol 1995;52:670–675.

195. Atkin N, Nitzberg S, Dorsey J. Lysis of intracerebral thromboembolism with fibrinolysin. Report of a case. Angiology 1964;15:346–439.

196. Meyer JS, Herndon RM, Gotoh F et al. Therapeutic thrombolysis. In: Millikan CH, Siekert RG, Whisnant JP, eds. Cerebral vascular diseases, Third Princeton Conference. New York: Grune and Stratton, 1961:160–177.

197. Nenci GG, Gresele P, Taramelli M et al. Thrombolytic therapy for thromboembolism of vertebrobasilar artery. Angiology 1983;34:561–571.

198. Miyakawa T, Sakuragawa N. The cerebral vessels and thrombosis (in Japanese). Rinsho Ketsueki 1984;25:1018–1026.

199. Matsumoto K, Satoh K. Topical intraarterial urokinase infusion for acute stroke. In: Hacke W, del Zoppo GJ, Hirschberg M, eds. Thrombolytic therapy in acute ischemic stroke. Heidelberg: Springer-Verlag, 1991:207–212.

200. Hacke W, Zeumer H, Ferbert A et al. Intra-arterial thrombolytic therapy improves outcome in patients with acute vertebrobasilar occlusive disease. Stroke 1988;19:1216–1222.

201. von Kummer R, Forsting M, Sartor K et al. Intravenous recombinant tissue plasminogen activator in acute stroke. In: Hacke W, del Zoppo GJ, Hirschberg M, eds. Thrombolytic therapy in acute ischemic stroke. Heidelberg: Springer-Verlag, 1991:161–167.

202. Yamaguchi T. Intravenous rt-PA in acute embolic stroke. In: Hacke W, del Zoppo GJ, Hirschberg M, eds. Thrombolytic therapy in acute ischemic stroke. Heidelberg: Springer-Verlag, 1991:168–174.

Whisnant JR, eds. Cerebral vascular diseases, Fourth Princeton Conference. New York: Grune and Stratton, 1965:185–199.

203. Hommel M, Boissel JP, Cornu C et al. Termination of trial of streptokinase in severe acute ischemic stroke. MAST Study Group [Letter]. Lancet 1995; 345:578–579.

204. Donnan GA, Davis SM, Chambers BR et al. Trials of streptokinase in severe acute ischaemic stroke [Letter]. Lancet 1995;345:578–579.

205. Anonymous. Randomised controlled trial of streptokinase, aspirin, and combination of both in treatment of acute ischaemic stroke. Multicentre Acute Stroke Trial-Italy (MAST-I) Group. Lancet 1995;346:1509–1514.

206. Tognoni G, Roncaglioni MC. Dissent: an alternative interpretation of MAST-I Multicentre Acute Stroke Trial-Italy Group. Lancet 1995;346: 1504–1515.

207. Anonymous. Effectiveness of intravenous thrombolytic treatment in acute myocardial infarction. Gruppo Italiano per lo Studio della Streptochinasi nell'Infarto Miocardico (GISSI). Lancet 1986;i:397–401.

208. Anonymous. GISSI-2: A factorial randomized trial of alteplase versus streptokinase and heparin versus no heparin among 12,490 patients with acute myocardial infarction. Gruppo Italiano per lo Studio della Sopravvivenza nell'Infarto Miocardico (GISSI). Lancet 1990;336:65–71.

209. del Zoppo GJ. Acute stroke—on the threshold of a therapy? [Editorial]. N Engl J Med 1995;333:1632–1633.

210. del Zoppo GJ, Poeck K, Pessin MS et al. Recombinant tissue plasminogen activator in acute thrombotic and embolic stroke. Ann Neurol 1992;32: 78–86.

211. Levy DE, Brott TG, Haley EC Jr et al. Factors related to intracranial hematoma formation in patients receiving tissue-type plasminogen activator for acute ischemic stroke. Stroke 1994;25:291–297.

212. Larrue V, von Kummer R, del Zoppo GJ et al. Hemorrhagic transformation in acute ischemic stroke. Potential contributing factors in the European Cooperative Acute Stroke Study. Stroke 1997;28:957–960.

213. Kwaan HC. Thromboembolic disorders of the eye. In: Comerota AC, ed. Thrombolytic therapy. Orlando: Grune and Stratton, 1988:153–163.

214. Freitag HJ, Zeumer H, Knospe V. Acute central retinal artery occlusion and the role of thrombolysis. In: del Zoppo GJ, Mori E, Hacke W, eds. Thrombolytic therapy in acute ischemic stroke II. Heidelberg: Springer-Verlag, 1993:103–105.

215. Schmidt D, Schumacher M, Wakhloo AK. Microcatheter urokinase infusion in central retinal artery occlusion. Am J Ophthalmol 1992;113:429–434.

216. Anonymous. Ancrod for the treatment of acute ischemic brain infarction. The Ancrod Stroke Study Investigators. Stroke 1994;25:1755–1759.

217. Einhaupl KM, Villringer A, Meister W et al. Heparin treatment in sinus venous thrombosis. Lancet 1991;338:597–600.

218. Scott JA, Pascuzzi RM, Hall PV et al. Treatment of dural sinus thrombosis with local urokinase infusion. Case report. J Neurosurg 1988;68:284–287.

219. Anonymous. Beneficial effect of carotid endarterectomy in symptomatic patients with high-grade carotid stenosis. Northern American Symptomatic Carotid Endarterectomy Trial Collaborators. N Engl J Med 1991;325: 445–453.

220. Anonymous. MRC European Carotid Surgery Trial: interim results for symptomatic patients with severe (70-99%) or with mild (0-29%) carotid stenosis. European Carotid Surgery Trialists' Collaborative Group. Lancet 1991;337:1235–1243.

221. Fields WS, Lemak NA, Frankowski RF et al. Controlled trial of aspirin in cerebral ischemia. Part II. Surgical group. Stroke 1978;9:309–319.

222. Boysen G, Sorensen PS, Juhler M et al. Danish very-low-dose aspirin after carotid endarterectomy trial. Stroke 1988;19:1211–1215.

223. Kretschmer G, Pratschner T, Prager M et al. Antiplatelet treatment prolongs survival after carotid bifurcation endarterectomy. Analysis of the clinical series followed by a controlled trial. Ann Surg 1990;211:317–322.

224. Harker LA, Bernstein EF, Dilley RB et al. Failure of aspirin plus dipyridamole to prevent restenosis after carotid endarterectomy. Ann Intern Med 1992;116:731–736.

225. Harvald B, Hilden T, Lund E. Long-term anticoagulant therapy after myocardial infarction. Lancet 1962;ii:626–630.

226. Anonymous. Cooperative Study. Long-term anticoagulant therapy after myocardial infarction. JAMA 1965;193:929–934.

227. Loeliger EA, Hensen A, Kroes F et al. A double blind trial of long-term anticoagulant treatment after myocardial infarction. Acta Med Scand 1967; 182:549–566.

228. Breddin K, Loew D, Lechner K et al. The German-Austrian aspirin trial: a comparison of acetylsalicylic acid, placebo, and phenprocoumon in secondary prevention of myocardial infarction. On behalf of the German-Austrian Study Group. Circulation 1980;62(Suppl):V63–V72.

229. Anonymous. A double-blind trial to assess long-term anticoagulant therapy in elderly patients after myocardial infarction. Report of the Sixty-Plus Reinfarction Study Research Group. Lancet 1980;ii:989–994.

230. Smith P, Arnesen H, Holme I. The effect of warfarin on mortality and reinfarction after myocardial infarction. N Engl J Med 1990;323:147–152.

231. Anonymous. An assessment of long-term anticoagulant administration after cardiac infarction. Medical Research Council. Br Med J 1964;2: 837–843.

232. Drapkin A, Merskey C. Anticoagulant therapy after acute myocardial infarction. Relation of therapeutic benefit to patient's age, sex, and severity of infarction. JAMA 1972;222:541–548.

233. Anonymous. Anticoagulants in acute myocardial infarction. Results of a cooperative clinical trial. JAMA 1973;225:724–729.

234. Anonymous. Assessment of short-term anticoagulant administration after cardiac infarction. Report of the Working Party on Anticoagulant Therapy in Coronary Thrombosis to the Medical Research Council. Br Med J 1969; 1:335–342.

235. Wolf PA, Abbott RD, Kannel WB. Atrial fibrillation: a major contributor to stroke in the elderly. The Framingham study. Arch Intern Med 1987; 147:1561–1564.

236. Sherman DG, Goldman L, Whiting RB et al. Thromboembolism in patients with atrial fibrillation. Arch Neurol 1984;41:708–710.

237. Hinton RC, Kistler JP, Fallon JT et al. Influence of etiology of atrial fibrillation on incidence of systemic embolism. Am J Cardiol 1977;40:509–513.

238. Chesebro JH, Fuster V, Halperin JL. Atrial fibrillation-risk marker for stroke [Editorial]. N Engl J Med 1990;323:1556–1558.

239. Freeman I, Wexler J, Howard F. Anticoagulants for treatment of atrial fibrillation. JAMA 1963;184:1007–1010.

240. Roy D, Marchard E, Gagne P et al. Usefulness of anticoagulant therapy in the prevention of embolic complications of atrial fibrillation. Am Heart J 1987;112:1039–1043.

241. Cairns JA, Connolly SJ. Nonrheumatic atrial fibrillation. Risk of stroke and role of antithrombotic therapy [Review]. Circulation 1991;84:469–481.

242. Sage JI, Van Uitert RL. Risk of recurrent stroke in patients with atrial fibrillation and non-valvular heart disease. Stroke 1983;14:537–540.

243. Hart RG, Coull BM, Hart D. Early recurrent embolism associated with nonvalvular atrial fibrillation: a retrospective study. Stroke 1983;14: 688–693.

244. Petersen P, Boysen G, Godtfredsen J et al. Placebo-controlled randomised trial of warfarin and aspirin to prevention of thromboembolic complications in chronic atrial fibrillation. The Copenhagen AFASAK Study. Lancet 1989;i:175–179.

245. Anonymous. Preliminary report of the Stroke Prevention in Atrial Fibrillation Study. N Engl J Med 1990;322:863–868.

246. Anonymous. The effect of low-dose warfarin on the risk of stroke in patients with non-rheumatic atrial fibrillation. The Boston Area Anticoagulation Trial for Atrial Fibrillation Investigators. N Engl J Med 1990;323: 1505–1511.

247. Connolly SJ, Laupacis A, Gent M et al. Canadian Atrial Fibrillation Anticoagulation (CAFA) Study. J Am Coll Cardiol 1991;18:349–355.

248. Anonymous. Warfarin versus aspirin for prevention of thromboembolism in atrial fibrillation. Stroke Prevention in Atrial Fibrillation II Study. Lancet 1994;343:687–691.

249. Anonymous. Adjusted-dose warfarin versus low-intensity, fixed-dose warfarin plus aspirin for high-risk individuals with atrial fibrillation. Stroke Prevention in Atrial Fibrillation III randomised clinical trial. Lancet 1996;348:633–638.

250. Fihn SD, Callahan CM, Martin DC et al. The risk for and severity of bleeding complications in elderly patients treated with warfarin. The National Consortium of Anticoagulation Clinics. Ann Intern Med 1996;124:970–979.

251. Lodder J, Dennis MS, Van-Raak L et al. Cooperative study on the value of long-term anticoagulation in individuals with stroke and non-rheumatic atrial fibrillation. Br Med J (Clin Res) 1988;296:1435–1438.

252. Szekely P. Systemic embolism and anticoagulant prophylaxis in rheumatic heart disease. Br Med J 1964;1:1209–1212.

253. Levine HJ, Pauker SG, Salzman EW. Antithrombotic therapy in valvular heart disease [Review]. Chest 1989;95(Suppl):98S–106S.

254. Stein PD, Kantrowitz A. Antithrombotic therapy in mechanical and biological prosthetic heart valves and saphenous vein bypass grafts [Review]. Chest 1989;95(Suppl):107S–117S.

255. Coulshed N, Epstein EJ, McKendrick CS et al. Systemic embolism in mitral valve disease. Br Heart J 1970;32:26–34.

256. Daley R, Mattingly TW, Holt CI et al. Systemic arterial embolism in rheumatic heart disease. Am Heart J 1951;42:566–581.

257. Kopf GS, Hammond GL, Geha AS et al. Long-term performance of the St. Jude medical valve: low incidence of thromboembolism and hemorrhagic complications with modest doses of warfarin. Circulation 1987;76(Suppl): 132–136.

258. Barnhorst DA, Oxman HA, Connolly DC et al. Long-term follow-up of isolated replacement of the aortic or mitral valve with the Starr-Edwards prosthesis. Am J Cardiol 1975;35:228–233.

259. Turpie AG, Gunstensen J, Hirsh J et al. Randomised comparison of two intensities of oral anticoagulant therapy after tissue heart valve placement. Lancet 1988;i:1242–1245.

260. Akbarian M, Austen G, Yurchak PM et al. Thromboembolic complications of prosthetic cardiac valves. Circulation 1986;37:826–831.

261. Duvoisin GE, Brandenburg RO, McGoon DC. Factors affecting thromboembolism associated with prosthetic heart valves. Circulation 1967; 35(Suppl):I-70–I-76.

262. Moggio RA, Hammond GL, Stansel HC Jr et al. Incidence of emboli with cloth-covered Starr-Edwards valve without anticoagulation and with varying forms of anticoagulation. J Thorac Cardiovasc Surg 1978;75: 296–299.

263. Loeliger EA, Poller L, Samama M et al. Questions and answers on pro-

thrombin time standardization in oral anticoagulant control. Thromb Haemost 1985;54:515–517.

264. Saour JN, Sleek JO, Mamo LA et al. Trial of different intensities of anticoagulation in patients with prosthetic heart valves. N Engl J Med 1990;322:428–432.

265. Loeliger EA. Therapeutic target values in oral anticoagulation—justification of Dutch policy and a warning against the so-called moderate-intensity regimens. Ann Hematol 1992;64:60–65.

266. Dale J, Myhre E, Storstein O et al. Prevention of arterial thromboembolism with acetylsalicylic acid. A controlled clinical study in patients with aortic ball valves. Am Heart J 1977;94:101–111.

267. Altman R, Boullon F, Rouvier J et al. Aspirin and prophylaxis of thromboembolic complications in patients with substitute heart valves. J Thorac Cardiovasc Surg 1976;72:127–129.

268. Sullivan JM, Harken DE, Gorlin R. Effect of dipyridamole on the incidence of arterial emboli after cardiac valve replacement. Circulation 1969;39(Suppl):I-149–I-153.

269. Sullivan JM, Harken DE, Gorlin R. Pharmacologic control of thromboembolic complications of cardiac valve replacement. N Engl J Med 1971;284:1391–1394.

270. Chesebro JH, Fuster V, Elveback LR et al. Trial of combined warfarin plus dipyridamole or aspirin therapy in prosthetic heart valve replacement: danger of aspirin compared with dipyridamole. Am J Cardiol 1983;51:1537–1541.

271. Ferraris VA, Klingman RR, Dunn L et al. Home heparin therapy used in a pregnant patient with a mechanical heart valve prosthesis. Ann Thorac Surg 1994;58:1168–1170.

272. Thomas D, Boubrit K, Darbois Y et al. Grossesses chez les porteuses de protheses valvulaires cardiaques. Etude retrospective a propos de 40 grossesses. Ann Cardiol Angeiol 1994;43:313–321.

273. Cohn LH, Allred EN, DiSesa VJ et al. Early and late risk of aortic valve replacement. A 12-year concomitant comparison of the porcine bioprosthetic and tilting disc prosthetic aortic valves. J Thorac Cardiovasc Surg 1984;88:695–705.

274. Williams JB, Karp RB, Kirklin JW et al. Considerations in selection and management of patients undergoing valve replacement with gluteraldehyde-fixed porcine bioprostheses. Ann Thorac Surg 1980;30:247–258.

275. Oyer PE, Stinson EB, Griepp RB et al. Valve replacement with the Starr-Edwards and Hancock prostheses. Comparative analysis of late morbidity and mortality. Ann Surg 1977;186:301–309.

276. Ionescu MI, Smith DR, Hasan SS et al. Clinical durability of the pericardial xenograft valve: ten years experience with mitral replacement. Ann Thorac Surg 1982;34:265–277.

277. Nuñez L, Aguado MG, Celemin D et al. Aspirin or Coumadin as the drug of choice for valve replacement with porcine bioprosthesis. Ann Thorac Surg 1982;33:354–358.

278. Nuñez L, Gil Aguado M, Larrea JL et al. Prevention of thromboembolism using aspirin after mitral valve replacement with porcine bioprosthesis. Ann Thorac Surg 1984;37:84–87.

279. Oczkowski WJ, Ginsberg JS, Shin A et al. Venous thromboembolism in patients undergoing rehabilitation for stroke. Arch Phys Med Rehabil 1992;73:712–716.

280. Sandset PM, Dahl T, Stiris M et al. A double-blind and randomized placebo-controlled trial of low-molecular-weight heparin once daily to prevent deep-vein thrombosis in acute ischemic stroke. Semin Thromb Hemost 1990;16:25–33.

281. Elias A, Milandre L, Lagrange G et al. Prevention des thromboses veineuses profondes des membres inferieurs par une fraction d'heparine de tres bas poids moleculaire (CY 222) chez des individus porteurs d'une hemiplegie secondaire a un infarctus cerebral: etude pilote randomisee (30 patients). Rev Med Interne 1990;11:95–98.

282. Prins MH, Gelsema R, Sing AK et al. Prophylaxis of deep venous thrombosis with a low-molecular-weight heparin (Kabi 2165/Fragmin) in stroke patients. Haemostasis 1989;19:245–250.

283. Autieri MV, Feuerstein GZ, Yue TL et al. Use of differential display to identify differentially expressed mRNAs induced by rat carotid artery balloon angioplasty. Lab Invest 1995;72:656–661.

284. Abe T, Kazawa M, Naito I et al. Clinical effect of urokinase (60,000 units/day) on cerebral infarction. Comparative study by means of multiple center double blind test. Blood Vessel 1981;12:342–358.

285. Yamaguchi T. Intravenous tissue plasminogen activator in acute thromboembolic stroke: a placebo-controlled, double-blind trial. In: del Zoppo GJ, Mori E, Hacke W, eds. Thrombolytic therapy in acute ischemic stroke II. Heidelberg: Springer-Verlag, 1993:59–65.

286. Möbius E, Berg-Dammer E, Kühne D et al. Local thrombolytic therapy in acute basilar artery occlusion: experience with 18 patients. In: Hacke W, del Zoppo GJ, Hirschberg M, eds. Thrombolytic therapy in acute ischemic stroke. Heidelberg: Springer-Verlag, 1991:213–215.

287. Anonymous. Tissue plasminogen activator for acute ischemic stroke. The National Institutes of Neurological Disorders and Stroke rt-PA Stroke Study Group. N Engl J Med 1995;333:1581–1587.

# CHAPTER 59

# ANTITHROMBOTIC THERAPY IN CARDIOVASCULAR DISEASE

## Glenn N. Levine, Bernardo Stein, and M. Nadir Ali

The medicinal use of aspirin was first recognized by Hippocrates in 400 BC. Aspirin was first synthesized in 1853, and it was marketed for the treatment of various disorders in 1899. Only during the past several decades, however, have the potential roles of aspirin and other antithrombotic medications in cardiovascular disease been studied systematically. From the 1950s to early 1980s, research focused primarily on the effects of aspirin, warfarin, and heparin, and these studies established the widely beneficial effects of aspirin in all phases of ischemic heart disease. Studies of heparin supported the role of short-term use in many individuals with acute coronary syndromes. Longer-term anticoagulation with warfarin has some modest role in some cardiovascular disorders.

Over the last decade, research has begun defining the role of newer antiplatelet and antithrombotic agents. Ticlopidine is effective in individuals with unstable angina and now is standard therapy for individuals with intracoronary stents. Agents that block the platelet membrane receptor glycoprotein (GP) IIB/IIIa are beneficial in individuals with unstable angina and have multiple beneficial effects in individuals undergoing percutaneous revascularization. Initial research also suggests a role for these agents as adjunctive therapy in individuals with acute myocardial infarction treated using thrombolytic therapy. In contrast to the encouraging results with these GP IIb/IIIa receptor blockers, the initial promise of direct thrombin inhibitors has been challenged.

This chapter discusses studies of antithrombotic therapy in cardiovascular disorders. The role of these agents in treating the spectrum of ischemic heart disease, including primary prevention, unstable angina, acute myocardial infarction and prevention of left ventricular thrombus, coronary revascularization, and secondary prevention are assessed and recommendations presented.

## PRIMARY PREVENTION

Cardiovascular disease is the leading cause of death in both men and women, but the annual incidence of cardiovascular events in the asymptomatic population is modest. Thus, demonstration of a significant reduction in such events with a potential therapeutic intervention is daunting. Nevertheless, several trials have assessed the role of antithrombotic therapy in primary prevention of cardiovascular morbidity and mortality rates.

### PLATELET INHIBITORS

Two studies have evaluated the potential benefit of aspirin (see Chapter 54) as a primary preventive agent in men. The U.S. Physicians' Health Study (1, 2) was a two-by-two factorial design study of 22,071 male physicians in whom treatment with aspirin (325 mg every other day) was compared with placebo. The aspirin arm was terminated prematurely after approximately 5 years because of a significant beneficial effect from aspirin on myocardial infarction rates. Compared with placebo, aspirin reduced the incidence of myocardial infarction by 44%

**FIGURE 59.1.** Results of the Physicians' Health Study (US) (2), the British primary prevention trial (UK) (3), and combined data (US + UK) on the effects of aspirin for primary prevention. Aspirin significantly reduced nonfatal myocardial infarction (MI) by 32%. *NS*, not significant. *SD*, standard deviation. (Adapted with permission from Hennekens CH, Buring JE, Sandercock P, Collins R, Peto R. Aspirin and other antiplatelet agents in the secondary and primary prevention of cardiovascular disease. Circulation 1989; 80:749–756.)

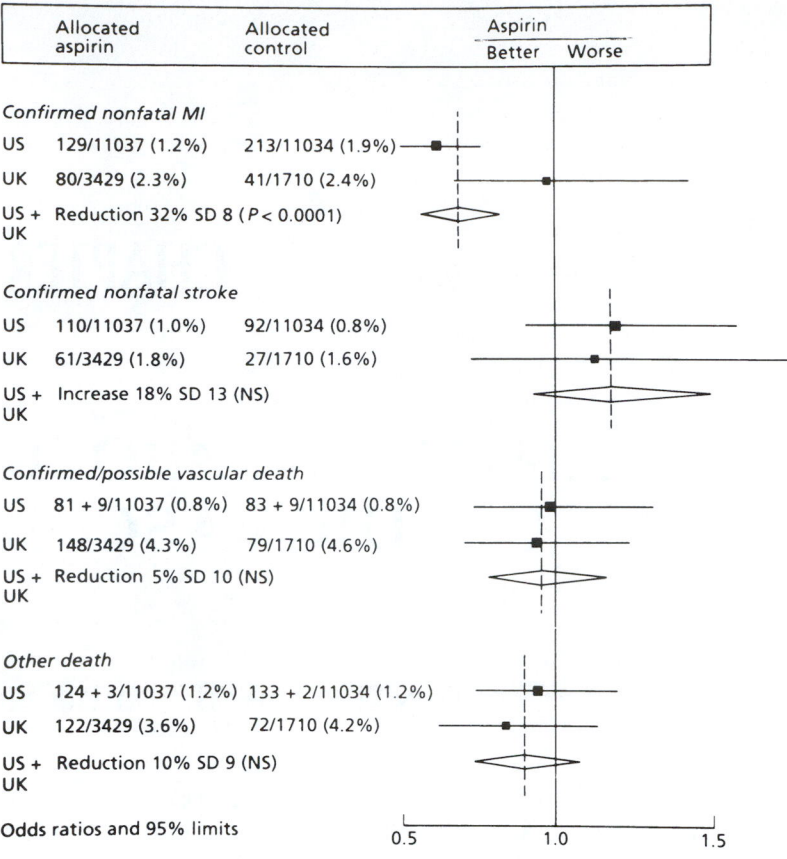

(from approximately 0.44 to 0.24% per year) and of death from myocardial infarction by 69%. The reduced risk of myocardial infarction was only apparent, however, in men at least 50 years of age. There was a slight increase in the number of hemorrhagic strokes among aspirin-treated subjects (23 vs. 12; P = .06). For the combined endpoint of all important vascular events (i.e., infarction, stroke, cardiovascular death), there was a statistically significant, 18% reduction among those individuals randomized to treatment with aspirin. No reduction in the total cardiovascular mortality rate, however, was demonstrated.

A British primary prevention trial of 5139 male physicians (3) randomly assigned two-thirds to aspirin (500 mg daily) and one-third to no-aspirin. No placebo was used. After 6 years, there were no differences in the rates of nonfatal or fatal myocardial infarction. Considering these two studies together, aspirin was associated with a significant 32% reduction in nonfatal myocardial infarction, a 13% decrease in any cardiovascular event, and no difference in total mortality. There also was a trend toward increased risk of stroke (Fig. 59.1) (4).

## ANTICOAGULANTS

On the basis of evidence that coronary events usually are thrombotic in origin and that increased levels of fibrinogen and factor VII coagulant activity are associated with a higher risk of myocardial ischemic events (5) (see Chapter 39), there has been widespread interest in testing the effects of anticoagulant therapy for individuals at high risk for coronary disease. A pilot study (6) demonstrated that warfarin (mean daily dose 4.6 mg; mean international normalized ratio [INR], 1.5) reduced factor VII coagulant activity from 115 to 75% without producing excessive bleeding. After these preliminary results, Meade et al (7) initiated a primary prevention study (the Thrombosis Prevention Trial) in high-risk individuals without overt coronary artery disease. Approximately 6000 middle-aged men are being treated for as long as 5 years with warfarin (aimed at achieving an INR of 1.5), low-dose aspirin (75 mg/day in a controlled-release preparation), both, or neither. An interim analysis of bleeding complications showed that the annual risk of serious bleeding (i.e., that requiring transfusion or surgery) with any treatment was approximately 1 in 500. There was no significant risk for bleeding complications of major or intermediate severity with combination therapy compared with either warfarin or aspirin alone (8). The results of this study should define what, if any, role anticoagulant therapy has in primary prevention.

## PRIMARY PREVENTION IN WOMEN

Past primary prevention studies excluded women, so as yet, no randomized data examining antithrombotic therapy in the primary prevention of cardiovascular disease in women are available. The results of three prospective observational studies (9–11) and one case-control study (12) of aspirin have yielded conflicting results. Two studies showed a reduced incidence of myocardial infarction (9, 12), one showed no effect on coronary heart disease (10), and another showed no effect on acute myocardial infarction but an increased risk of overall ischemic heart disease (11). To better assess the possible role of aspirin in primary prevention among women, the ongoing Women's Health Study has randomized approximately 40,000 apparently healthy women at least 45 years of age to aspirin (100 mg every other day) or placebo; the results of this study are eagerly anticipated.

## CURRENT RECOMMENDATIONS

Given the available data, aspirin cannot be universally recommended for primary prevention. On the basis of a risk–benefit analysis, aspirin (160–325 mg/day) is prudent for male individuals at least 50 years of age who have clear risk factors for coronary disease or evidence of atherosclerosis in other vascular territories (13, 14). For healthy individuals without risk factors, long-term aspirin therapy may be associated with a higher risk than benefit given the disconcerting increase in the incidence of stroke (14). The usefulness of warfarin by itself or in combination with low-dose aspirin is being investigated in men, and little data are currently available regarding antithrombotic therapy for primary prevention in women. Hopefully, the results of the Women's Health Study will correct this situation.

# UNSTABLE ANGINA

Results of both pathologic and clinical studies support the view that unstable angina is frequently, if not always, caused by fissuring or disruption of plaques within the epicardial circulation, thus leading to thrombus formation, change in configuration of the stenosis, or both. These processes often lead to acute reduction in myocardial perfusion. Usually, this reduction is only transient, but it may become sustained, thereby leading to myocardial infarction. Over the last several decades, research has focused on pharmacologic interventions to diminish the likelihood that individuals with unstable angina will develop acute myocardial infarction.

## PLATELET INHIBITORS

The acute effects of antiplatelet therapy in unstable angina were studied at the Montreal Heart Institute in a trial of 479 individuals comparing aspirin (325 mg twice daily), intravenous heparin, both, or neither in the treatment of unstable angina (15). Compared with placebo,

aspirin led to a significant 72% reduction in the in-hospital myocardial infarction rate (from 12 to 3%). In a larger study by the Research Group on Instability in Coronary Artery Disease (RISC), 796 men with unstable angina or non-Q-wave myocardial infarction were randomized to low-dose aspirin (75 mg/day), intermittent intravenous heparin for 5 days, both, or neither (16); after 5 days, aspirin was demonstrated to reduce the risk of myocardial infarction, death, or both by 57%.

The continued benefit of aspirin therapy in individuals with unstable angina was demonstrated by the RISC study and two other trials. Thirty-day follow-up in the RISC study demonstrated a continued, significant reduction in the risk of myocardial infarction, death, or both of 69% (Fig. 59.2) and at 3-month follow-up of 64%. In the Veterans Administration (VA) trial (17), 1266 men were randomly assigned to aspirin (324 mg/day) or placebo, and after 3 months, aspirin therapy had reduced the rate of mortality by 51% and of myocardial infarction by 55%. At 1-year follow-up, mortality remained significantly lower (by 43%) in aspirin-treated individuals. In the Canadian Multicenter Trial (18), 555 individuals were randomly assigned to aspirin (325 mg four times a day), sulfinpyrazone, both, or placebo; at a mean follow-up of 18 months, aspirin was found to reduce the cardiac mortality rate by 71% and cardiac death or nonfatal infarction by 50%.

In a study of the platelet inhibitor ticlopidine (see Chapter 54), Balsano et al (19) randomized 652 individuals with unstable angina to ticlopidine (250 mg twice daily) or placebo. At 6-month follow-up, ticlopidine was found to reduce the rate of myocardial infarction by

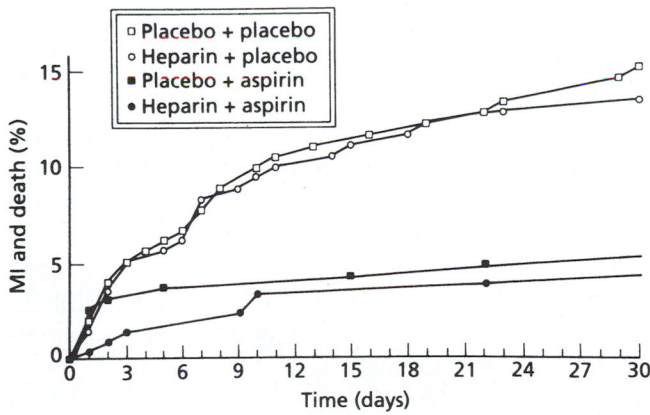

**FIGURE 59.2.** Efficacy of low-dose aspirin (75 mg/day) for prevention of myocardial infarction (MI) and death in individuals with unstable angina or non-Q-wave myocardial infarction. Aspirin exerted a highly beneficial effect compared with placebo or with placebo and intermittent heparin injections. (Adapted with permission from the RISC Group. Risk of myocardial infarction and death during treatment with low dose aspirin and intravenous heparin in men with unstable coronary artery disease. Lancet 1990;336:827–830.)

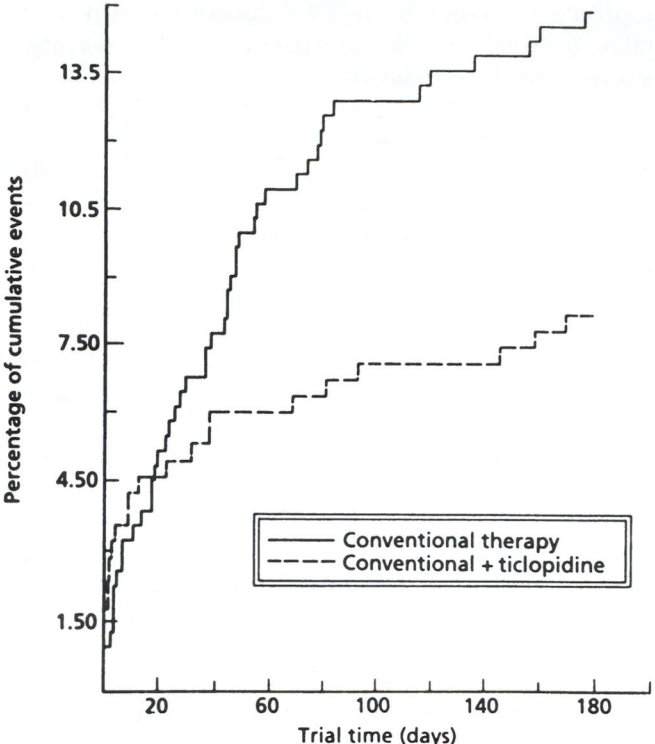

**FIGURE 59.3.**    Effects of ticlopidine in unstable angina. The graph shows the percentage of cumulative events (cardiovascular death and myocardial infarction) over time in individuals treated using conventional therapy compared with those treated using conventional therapy plus ticlopidine. Ticlopidine treatment was associated with a 46% reduction in the event rate. (Adapted with permission from Balsano F, Paolo P, Violi F, et al. Antiplatelet treatment with ticlopidine in unstable angina. Circulation 1990;82:17–26.)

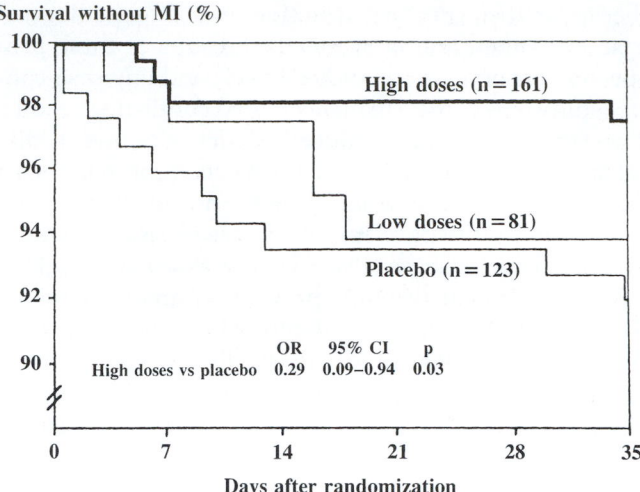

**FIGURE 59.4.**    Freedom from myocardial infarction and/or death in individuals treated with high-dose lamifiban (4 or 5 μg/min), low-dose lamifiban (1 or 2 μg/min), or placebo. The initial effect on adverse outcome achieved with all doses of lamifiban was sustained at 1 month in individuals treated with a high dose of lamifiban. *CI*, confidence intervals; *MI*, myocardial infarction; *OR*, odds ratio; *p*, p valve. (Adapted with permission from Theroux P, Kouz S, Roy L, et al. Platelet membrane receptor GP IIB/IIIa antagonism in unstable angina: the Canadian Lamifiban Study. Circulation 1996;94:899–905.)

53%, vascular mortality by 47%, and total cardiac events by almost 50% (Fig. 59.3).

As discussed in Chapter 54, new pharmacologic agents have been developed to block the platelet membrane fibrinogen receptor GP IIb/IIIa, which is the mediator in the final common pathway for platelet aggregation. In the Canadian Lamifiban Study (20), four different infusion concentrations (1, 2, 4, or 5 μg/min) of one such agent, the nonpeptide compound lamifiban, were compared among themselves and with placebo in 365 individuals with unstable angina. Individuals were treated with lamifiban or placebo infusion for 3 to 5 days. All individuals in the study received aspirin, and heparin was administered to 28%. Compared with placebo, lamifiban treatment at all four doses reduced the combined endpoint of death, nonfatal myocardial infarction, or need for urgent revascularization during the infusion period from 8.1 to 3.3% (*P* = 0.04). Bleeding complications were increased in those treated with lamifiban, but these occurred predominantly among individuals also treated with heparin and only in those treated

at one of the two higher doses. Furthermore, none of the bleeding complications was life-threatening. At 1-month follow-up, nonfatal myocardial infarction had occurred in 2.5% of individuals treated with one of the two high lamifiban doses, in 6.2% of individuals treated with one of the two low lamifiban doses, and in 8.1% of individuals treated with placebo (Fig. 59.4).

Three major phase III trials evaluating the role of GP IIb/IIIa inhibitors in individuals with unstable angina, non-Q-wave myocardial infarction, or both have completed individual enrollment, and preliminary results of two are available. The Platelet Receptor Inhibition for Ischemic Syndrome Management (PRISM) trial (21) randomized more than 3200 individuals presenting with chest pain and dynamic electrocardiographic changes to GP IIb/IIIa receptor blockade with Aggrastat (tirofiban [Merck Research Laboratories, Philadelphia, PA]) and a control heparin group. Individuals in the Aggrastat arm had a statistically significant, 36% reduction at 48 hours in the combined risk of death, reinfarction, and refractory ischemia. This in-hospital benefit was maintained at 30 days, at which time the Aggrastat arm significantly reduced death by 39% (3.6% in the heparin arm versus 2.3% in the Aggrastat arm). In the Platelet Receptor Inhibition for Ischemic Syndrome Management in Individuals Limited to very Unstable Signs and Symptoms (PRISM-PLUS) study (22), 773 individuals received Aggrastat plus heparin for up to 96 hours, and 797 individuals received heparin (22). Individuals in this study had documented electrocardiographic changes indicative of myocardial ischemia or elevated cardiac enzyme levels. Aggrastat produced a statistically significant, 34% reduction in the combined incidence of death, reinfarction, and refractory ischemia at 7 days when combined with heparin (17.9% event rate on heparin versus 12.9% with Aggrastat added). Analysis of the data at 30 days showed that the benefit of Aggrastat was sustained, with a statistically significant, 23% reduction in the combined risk of death, reinfarction, and refractory ischemia. These encouraging results are in accord with those reported in several preliminary studies of GP IIb/IIIa receptor–blocking agents (23–25) and in trials using these agents for individuals with unstable angina undergoing percutaneous revascularization (26–28) (discussed later).

## ANTICOAGULANTS

In the first randomized, double-blind, placebo-controlled trial of heparin therapy in individuals with unstable angina, Telford and Wilson (29) demonstrated that intravenous heparin reduced the rate of progression to myocardial infarction from 15 to 3% at 7 days, and that this benefit was maintained at 8-week follow-up. Because a large number of individuals were excluded from analysis, the validity of these findings remained unclear until results of the Montreal Heart Institute trial became available (15). As discussed, in the Montreal Heart Institute trial, individuals were treated with aspirin (650 mg immediately, then 325 mg twice daily), intravenous heparin (5000 U bolus, then 1000 U/hour), both, or neither. Compared with treatment using neither agent, treatment with heparin reduced the rate of progression to myocardial infarction from 12 to 0.8%.

The possibility of a "rebound" thrombotic process occurring in the first several days after discontinuation of intravenous heparin was first suggested by the RISC Study (16), which noted a small increase in the event rate on cessation of heparin treatment. Analysis of the Montreal Heart Institute study results (30) revealed that recurrent ischemic events, presumed to result from reactivation of the unstable coronary plaque, occurred significantly more frequently during the first three days after cessation of treatment in individuals given only heparin than in those individuals in the other three treatment groups. Analysis of the data from both these studies suggests that concomitant treatment with aspirin can diminish or prevent this phenomenon.

In a single-blinded study, Gurfinkel et al (31) evaluated the efficacy of the low-molecular-weight heparin nadroparin calcium in the treatment of unstable angina. A total of 219 individuals were randomized to treatment with either aspirin (200 mg/day), aspirin plus regular intravenous heparin (5000 U bolus, then intravenous infusion titrated to activated partial thromboplastin time [aPTT]), or aspirin plus low-molecular-weight heparin

(214 UIC/kg anti–Xa twice daily subcutaneously). The rate of recurrent angina was significantly lower in those treated with low-molecular-weight heparin, with recurrence rates in the three groups of 37, 44, and 21%, respectively. Both need for revascularization and incidence of progression to myocardial infarction were less frequent in the low-molecular-weight heparin group. Bleeding complications in all three groups were rare. To what extent the single-blinded nature of this study may have influenced the results is open to speculation.

Introduction of the direct thrombin inhibitors (see Chapter 57) hirudin, which is a polypeptide derived from leech saliva, and Hirulog (bivalirudin), which is a novel synthetic peptide, generated hope these agents would improve clinical outcomes in acute ischemic syndromes compared with those achieved using heparin. Pilot studies suggested that in individuals with unstable angina as well as those with other coronary syndromes, these agents were safe, led to therapeutic degrees of anticoagulation, and were associated with low rates of adverse outcomes (32–35). A study by Topol et al (36) of individuals with angiographic findings suggestive of coronary artery or saphenous vein-graft thrombus compared hirudin with heparin; treatment with hirudin led to greater improvement in coronary luminal cross-sectional area and lesser-percentage-diameter stenosis at the site of presumed thrombus.

The Global Use of Strategies to Open Occluded Coronary Arteries (GUSTO II) study (37) was designed as a large clinical trial to compare hirudin with heparin in the treatment of acute coronary syndromes. As such, it included individuals with unstable angina, non-Q-wave myocardial infarction, and transmural myocardial infarction, and it stratified individuals by the presence or absence of ST-segment elevation. After an excess of hemorrhagic strokes occurred in individuals with ST-segment elevation treated with thrombolytic therapy, doses of both hirudin and heparin were reduced with hirudin administered as a 0.1 mg/kg body weight bolus followed by a 0.1 mg/kg per hour infusion and heparin as a 5000 U bolus followed by a 1000 U/hour infusion. In the approximately 8000 individuals without ST-segment elevation (i.e., those with unstable angina or non-Q-wave myocardial infarction) treated with these modified regimens, the primary study endpoints of death or myocardial infarction at 30 days were not notably different between those treated with hirudin and those treated with heparin (8.3 versus 9.1%; $P = .22$). These investigators concluded that given these results the fact that heparin is both inexpensive and efficacious, heparin should continue to be the standard anticoagulant in individuals with acute coronary syndromes.

## ASPIRIN, HEPARIN, OR BOTH?

As discussed, aspirin and heparin are both efficacious in the treatment of unstable angina. Several studies, however, have evaluated whether individuals with unstable angina are best treated with only aspirin, only heparin, or with both. In the Montreal Heart Institute study (15), treatment with aspirin, heparin, or both decreased the rate of progression to myocardial infarction to 3, 0.8, and 1.6%, respectively; these results were not significantly different from one another. The incidence of bleeding was slightly higher in those treated with both agents, although bleeding complications were rare, usually not serious or life-threatening, and frequently related to cardiac catheterization procedures. In a follow-up to this study (38), an additional 245 individuals were randomized to either aspirin or heparin to facilitate statistically meaningful comparisons of these agents. Combining the results of these two studies, the rate of progression to acute myocardial infarction was 3.7% with aspirin and 0.8% with heparin ($P = .035$).

In the RISC study (16), progression to myocardial infarction or death was significantly reduced by aspirin but not by heparin. Individuals treated with both agents had the lowest rate of myocardial infarction. This trial has only modest use in comparing aspirin with heparin, however, in that heparin was administered using intermittent boluses and not a continuous infusion and aPTT levels were not monitored. Holdright et al (39) compared the effects of aspirin (150 mg daily) alone versus aspirin plus intravenous heparin (5000 U bolus, then a continuous infusion titrated to aPTT) on transient myocardial ischemia and development of myocardial infarction or death. No significant differences were detected between the two groups for these endpoints, but it has been argued that parameters of ischemic episodes were less in those treated with combination therapy and that statistically significant differences were not detected because of inadequate sample size (40). In the Antithrombotic Therapy in Acute Coronary Syndrome (ATACS) trial, aspirin (162.5 mg loading dose, then 162.5 mg daily) alone was compared with aspirin plus anticoagulation (initial intravenous heparin followed by warfarin) in the treatment of unstable angina or non-Q-wave myocardial infarction. After 14 days of treatment in those individuals classified as having unstable angina, ischemic events occurred in 29% of those treated with aspirin alone and in 21% of those treated with aspirin plus anticoagulation.

Oler et al (41) performed a meta-analysis of six randomized trials to compare risk for the combined endpoint of myocardial infarction or death in individuals treated with aspirin alone or with aspirin plus heparin. Compared with aspirin alone, combination therapy led to a 33% reduction in the occurrence of this combined endpoint.

## CURRENT RECOMMENDATIONS

Overall evaluation of trials examining the effects of aspirin, heparin, or combination therapy on progression to

myocardial infarction or death, as well as the observation that aspirin therapy may ameliorate rebound thrombosis after heparin discontinuation, suggest that most, if not all, individuals should be treated both with aspirin and intravenous heparin. Unless they have a true aspirin allergy or other strong contraindications, all individuals should be treated with aspirin (160–325 mg/day) (14, 42). In those individuals with true aspirin allergies, treatment with ticlopidine (250 mg twice daily) should be considered (14). Concomitant intravenous heparin therapy should be initiated unless there are strong contraindications (14, 42). Heparin should be administered in a weight-adjusted manner, with an initial bolus of approximately 80 mg/kg, followed by a continuous intravenous infusion at an initial dose of 18 mg/kg subsequently adjusted to maintain the aPTT at either 1.5 to 2.0 (14) or 1.5 to 2.5 (42) times control.

Early studies of GP IIb/IIIa receptor antagonists suggest these agents are highly effective, and their role in the treatment of unstable angina, including those individuals who are to undergo percutaneous revascularization, probably will expand over the next several years. Currently, however, there are insufficient data to recommend use of low-molecular-weight heparin over standard, unfractionated heparin. At this point, studies of direct thrombin inhibitors do not support routine use of such agents in the treatment of unstable angina.

# ACUTE MYOCARDIAL INFARCTION

Most myocardial infarctions result from disruption of an atherosclerotic plaque, thus leading to exposure of collagen, vessel media, and plaque elements to the circulating blood that in turn results in marked activation of platelets, the coagulation system, and thrombotic vascular occlusion. A substantial proportion of individuals with acute myocardial infarction also undergo either spontaneous or pharmacologically induced thrombolysis, which exposes a highly thrombogenic substrate to the circulation and may lead to rethrombosis, reinfarction, or death (43). The residual thrombus (after initial thrombolysis) contains active thrombin adsorbed to fibrin, and this thrombin, which is exposed during clot lysis, is a powerful activator of platelets and exerts a positive feedback on the coagulation cascade, thereby resulting in generation of more thrombin and fibrin. Rethrombosis and reinfarction after successful thrombolysis are associated with substantial morbidity. Therefore, the effects of antithrombotic agents in this setting have received great interest. This section discusses antithrombotic agents in individuals with acute myocardial infarction treated either conventionally or with thrombolytic therapy.

## ANTITHROMBOTIC TREATMENT WITHOUT THROMBOLYTIC THERAPY

### Platelet Inhibitors

The efficacy of aspirin therapy for evolving myocardial infarction was definitively demonstrated by the Second International Study of Infarct Survival (ISIS-2) (44). In this study, 17,187 individuals with suspected myocardial infarction were randomized in a placebo-controlled manner to either aspirin (325 mg chewed immediately, then 162 mg daily), streptokinase, both, or neither. At 5 weeks, aspirin reduced the rates of nonfatal reinfarction by 49%, of nonfatal stroke by 46%, and of vascular mortality by 23% (Fig. 59.5), without any increase in major bleeding episodes. The reduction in vascular deaths was similar whether aspirin was initiated 0 to 4 hours, 5 to 12 hours, or 13 to 24 hours after the onset of symptoms.

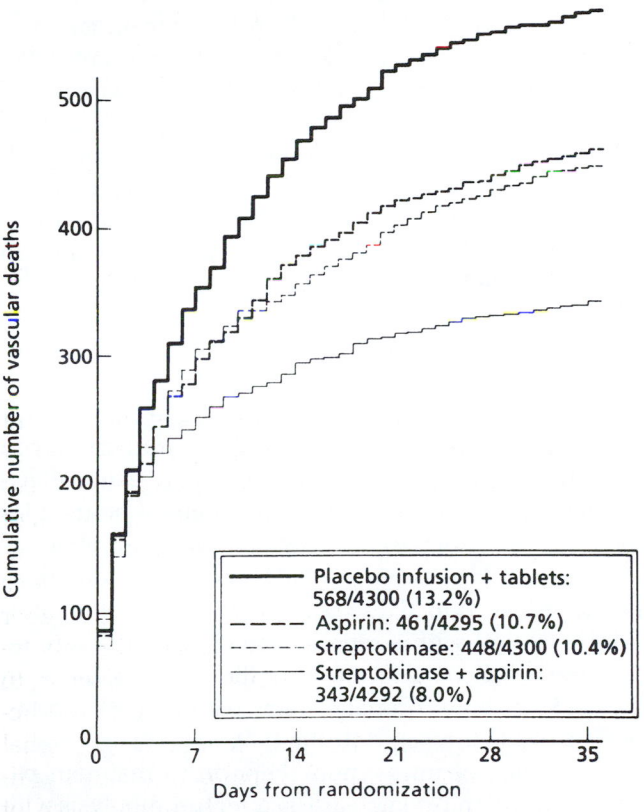

**FIGURE 59.5.**   Effects of platelet inhibition and thrombolysis on cardiovascular mortality within 5 weeks after acute myocardial infarction. The reductions in mortality were 23% with aspirin alone, 25% with streptokinase alone, and 42% for aspirin and streptokinase. Note that the benefit of aspirin was additive to that of streptokinase. (Adapted with permission from ISIS-2 [Second International Study of Infarct Survival] Collaborative Group. Randomized trial of intravenous streptokinase, oral aspirin, both, or neither among 17,187 cases of suspected acute myocardial infarction: ISIS-2. Lancet 1988;ii: 349–360.)

### Anticoagulants

The issue of benefit from short-term anticoagulation with heparin in individuals with acute myocardial infarction is still not completely settled. Of three large studies conducted in the late 1960s and early 1970s (45–47), only one (46) showed a statistically significant reduction in mortality. When the results of six randomized trials of anticoagulant therapy (with heparin, warfarin, and/or phenindione) were pooled, a significant 21% reduction in the mortality rate emerged (48). An overview restricted to heparin alone in acute myocardial infarction, which included approximately 5700 subjects, revealed a 22% reduction in nonfatal reinfarction, a 50% reduction in stroke, and a 17% reduction in mortality (49). Individuals included in these studies, however, were not treated routinely with other proven beneficial medications (including aspirin).

There are only limited data on what benefit heparin therapy might add in individuals with acute myocardial infarction treated with aspirin, and those data yield conflicting results. In the ISIS-2 study (44), there was no significant difference in mortality between those randomized to aspirin alone who were treated with intravenous heparin, subcutaneous heparin, or no heparin (10.9, 11.2, and 11.2%, respectively). In the Late Assessment of Thrombolytic Efficacy (LATE) trial (50), in which individuals with acute myocardial infarction presenting 6 to 24 hours after the onset of symptoms were randomized to aspirin alone or aspirin plus thrombolytic therapy, individuals in the aspirin-only arm who were also treated with heparin had a lower 35-day mortality rate than those who were not treated with heparin (8.7 versus 12.9%; $P < .001$). In neither trial, however, was heparin therapy randomized, and there probably were differences in baseline individual characteristics between those who were treated and those who were not treated with heparin (50).

## ADJUNCTIVE ANTITHROMBOTIC THERAPY WITH THROMBOLYTIC THERAPY

### Platelet Inhibitors

Results of the ISIS-2 trial (44) demonstrates the benefits of adjuvant treatment with aspirin in individuals receiving a thrombolytic agent. In this study, the effects of streptokinase and aspirin were additive, with the cardiovascular mortality rate reduced by 25% with streptokinase alone and by 42% with the combination of aspirin and streptokinase (Fig. 59.5). In addition, the excess in nonfatal reinfarction with streptokinase alone (compared with placebo) was eliminated by concomitant use of aspirin, probably because aspirin prevented thrombotic reocclusion.

Further support for aspirin in conjunction with thrombolytic therapy, particularly the supposition that aspirin prevents thrombotic reocclusion, comes from a meta-analysis of 32 trials (51). In this analysis, the angiographic reocclusion rate was 11% in individuals treated with aspirin, compared with 25% in untreated individuals. Recurrent ischemia occurred in 25% of the aspirin group and in 41% of those not receiving aspirin. Importantly, the beneficial effects of aspirin were similar regardless of the type of thrombolytic agent used.

Investigators now are exploring the adjunctive role of more potent antiplatelet agents in individuals treated with thrombolytic therapy (as well as with aspirin and heparin). The Thrombolysis and Angioplasty in Myocardial Infarction (TAMI) 8 pilot study (52) was a small, dose-ranging study to assess the safety of treatment with the monoclonal antibody GP IIb/IIIa inhibitor c7E3 Fab in conjunction with recombinant tissue-type plasminogen activator (t-PA) therapy in individuals with acute myocardial infarction. Rates of bleeding complications in this study were acceptable and comparable to those in control individuals. In individuals who underwent angiography for clinical indications, the infarct-related artery was patent (TIMI 2 or 3 flow) in 34 of 37 (92%) treated with c7E3 Fab and in five of nine (56%) treated with placebo. The incidence of recurrent ischemic events was lower in those treated with the two highest doses of c7E3 Fab than in those who received placebo (9.5 versus 20%, respectively).

The Evaluation of Integrelin in Individuals Receiving Thrombolytic Therapy for Acute Myocardial Infarction (IMPACT-AMI) phase I trial (53) was a dose-ranging study of the GP IIb/IIIa inhibitor integrelin in 85 individuals with acute myocardial infarction treated with recombinant t-PA. No severe bleeding complications occurred, and rates of overall bleeding rates were similar to those in placebo-treated individuals. Ninety-minute arterial patency, which was assessed as part of the study protocol, tended to be higher in those treated with integrelin (135 or 180 $\mu$g/kg bolus, then 0.75 $\mu$g/kg per minute) than in those treated with placebo. Clinical events were not significantly different between those treated with integrelin and those treated with placebo, but there was a general trend toward fewer events with integrelin. Ongoing studies should help to establish the role of these GP IIb/IIIa inhibitors in the treatment of acute myocardial infarction in individuals treated with thrombolytic therapy.

## Anticoagulants

The relative utility, if any, of additional heparin therapy in individuals treated with thrombolytic therapy and aspirin has been the subject of intense debate, even exceeding that concerning whether heparin can be administered subcutaneously or must be administered intravenously as a constant infusion. The International Study Group, in conjunction with the Gruppo Italiano per lo Studio della Sopravvivenze nell'Infarto Miocardico (GISSI-2), randomly assigned almost 21,000 individuals with suspected acute myocardial infarction to alteplase (t-PA) or streptokinase and to either subcutaneous heparin (12,500 U twice daily) or no heparin (54, 55). All individuals received aspirin. The in-hospital mortality rate was only 5% lower in the heparin arm, and reinfarction rates were similar. Bleeding, however, was twice as common in heparinized individuals. Heparin appeared to convey some modest benefit to those individuals treated with streptokinase but not those treated with alteplase. The results of this study are clouded somewhat, however, because heparin therapy (in those randomized to heparin) was initiated a full 12 hours after thrombolytic administration.

In the Third International Study of Infarct Survival (ISIS-3) trial (56), more than 41,000 individuals with suspected acute myocardial infarction were randomized to streptokinase, duteplase (t-PA), or anistreplase. In addition, half the individuals received subcutaneous heparin (12,500 U twice daily begun 4 hours after initiation of thrombolytic therapy) plus aspirin, and the rest received aspirin alone. Addition of heparin to aspirin was associated with a trend toward lower rates of in-hospital mortality and reinfarction but increased rates of major bleeding and definite or probable cerebral hemorrhage. Combining the results of the GISSI-2 and ISIS-3 two trials (Table 59.1), it appears that subcutaneous heparin slightly reduced the early mortality rate, but the benefit no longer was apparent at 30 days. In addition, heparin use was associated with a modest increased risk of bleeding complications.

The Global Utilization of Streptokinase and t-PA for Occluded Coronary Arteries (GUSTO I) study involved more than 41,000 individuals and compared subcutaneous heparin (12, 500 U twice daily begun 4 hours after initiation of thrombolytic therapy) with intravenous heparin (5000 U bolus, then 1000 U/hour infusion subsequently adjusted to aPTT) as adjunctive therapy in individuals treated with streptokinase (57). There were no significant differences between the two regimens in rates of 90-minute coronary artery patency (58), mortality (57), or hemorrhagic stroke (57).

The value of intravenous heparin to maintain patency of the infarct-related artery after thrombolysis with alteplase has been studied in several trials (Fig. 59.6). Heparin does not appear to improve early vessel patency when assessed angiographically 90 minutes after administration of alteplase (59). In contrast, in three trials (60–62), intravenous heparin appeared to be important in maintaining coronary patency as assessed 1 to 4 days after administration of alteplase. From this latter finding, many have concluded that heparin therapy is important in sustaining vessel patency (63). It should be noted, however, that in two of the latter three angiographic trials,

**TABLE 59.1.** Results of GISSI-2 and ISIS-3 Trials Comparing Heparin or No-heparin Therapy in Individuals with Acute Myocardial Infarction Treated using Thrombolytic Therapy and Aspirin

| Clinical Event | Aspirin Alone (%) | Aspirin + Heparin (%) | P |
|---|---|---|---|
| Death (in-hospital) | 7.3 | 6.8 | <.01 |
| Death (5 weeks) | 10.2 | 10.0 | NS |
| Reinfarction | 3.3 | 3.0 | NS |
| Stroke | 1.2 | 1.2 | NS |
| Cerebral hemorrhage | 0.4 | 0.5 | NS |
| Bleeding (requiring transfusion) | 0.7 | 1.0 | <.0001 |

*Adapted wth permission from ISIS-3 (Third International Study of Infarct Survival) Collaborative Group. ISIS-3: a randomized comparison of streptokinase vs tissue plasminogen activator vs anistreplase and of aspirin plus heparin vs aspirin alone among 41,299 cases of suspected acute myocardial infarction. Lancet 1992;339: 753–770.*

NS, *not significant.*

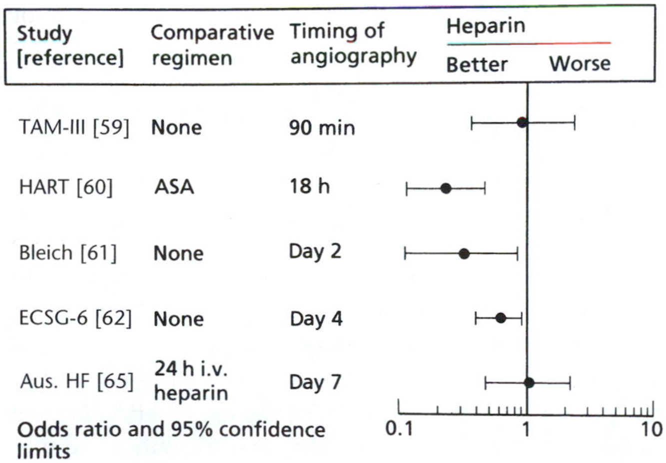

**FIGURE 59.6.** Influence of heparin on patency of the infarct-related artery in individuals with acute myocardial infarction treated with recombinant tissue-type plasminogen activator. Heparin did not enhance early vessel recanalization achieved with thrombolytics, but it show a benefit in maintaining patency after reperfusion. (Adapted with permission from Prins MH, Hirsh J. Heparin as an adjunctive treatment after thrombolytic therapy for acute myocardial infarction. Am J Cardiol 1991;67(Suppl A):3A–11A.)

individuals in the no-heparin group were treated with either no aspirin (61) or only 80 mg of aspirin (60), which is a dose althought to be inadequate for achieving a rapid clinical antithrombotic effect (64), which in turn is particularly relevant as angiography in this latter study was performed from 7 to 24 hours after treatment. Furthermore, in two studies in which individuals were treated with intravenous heparin for only 24 hours (65, 66), infarct-related artery patency at hospital discharge was similar to that among individuals treated with heparin for 3 to 5 days. Notably, in an overview of randomized trials involving intravenous heparin (67), no significant effect of intravenous heparin therapy on rates of recurrent ischemia or reinfarction or mortality in individuals treated with t-PA was observed, although these investigators noted this finding could have resulted from lack of statistical power, inappropriate levels of anticoagulation, or lack of benefit from heparin. Thus, at present, there are insufficient data to either support or refute use of intravenous heparin in individuals treated with t-PA.

Direct thrombin inhibitors, of which hirudin (see Chapter 57) is the prototype, were introduced as adjunctive agents to thrombolytic therapy with much enthusiasm. Early studies of hirudin and Hirulog™ (bivalirudin) in this role, which predominantly were conducted in small numbers of individuals, yielded results suggesting that direct thrombin inhibitors have acceptable safety profiles, potentiate thrombolysis, lead to high rates of infarct-related artery patency, and might lead to less adverse outcomes compared with heparin (68–73).

The Thrombin Inhibition in Myocardial Infarction (TIMI 9) (59) and GUSTO II (74) trials compared hirudin with intravenous heparin in individuals with acute myocardial infarction treated using thrombolytic therapy and aspirin (i.e., TIMI 9) or, as noted, in acute coronary syndromes, including unstable angina, myocardial infarction without ST-segment elevation, and myocardial infarction with ST-segment elevation (i.e., GUSTO II). In both trials, initial doses for heparin infusion and target aPTTs were set higher than those in previous trials, because standard heparin administration (beginning with a nonweight-adjusted infusion of 1000 U/hour) often did not lead to therapeutic aPTT levels in many individuals and weight adjustment of the heparin dose was required to maintain the aPTT in the desired range. Heparin therapy in these two studies consisted of a 5000 U bolus, then an initial infusion ranging from 1000 to 1300 U/hour, based on weight. Hirudin was administered as a 0.6 mg/kg bolus and a 0.2 mg/kg per hour infusion. Infusion rates for each agent subsequently were titrated to maintain an aPTT of from 60 to 90 seconds.

In each study, high rates of intracranial hemorrhage occurred in both treatment groups, and each study was halted and reconfigured at lower hirudin and heparin doses. Results at the higher doses were designated as

TIMI 9A and GUSTO IIa; results at the lower doses were designated as TIMI 9B and GUSTO IIb. In TIMI 9A, intracranial hemorrhage occurred in 1.9% of heparin-treated individuals and 1.7% of hirudin-treated individuals. In GUSTO IIa, among those treated with thrombolytic therapy, hemorrhagic stroke occurred in 1.5% of those treated with heparin and 2.2% of those treated with hirudin.

These initial results were echoed by those of the r-Hirudin for Improvement of Thrombolysis (HIT-III) study (75), which also compared hirudin (0.4 mg/kg bolus, then 0.15 mg/kg per hour) with heparin as adjunctive therapy in individuals treated using thrombolytic therapy. This study was terminated after enrollment of only several hundred individuals, however, because of a notable excess of fatal intracranial hemorrhages in those treated with hirudin (four of 148 individuals [2.7%]).

In the reconfigured TIMI 9B study (76), 3002 individuals were treated with hirudin, administered as a 0.1 mg/kg bolus followed by a 0.1 mg/kg infusion, or with heparin, administered as a 5000 U bolus followed by a 1000 U/hour infusion. In both treatment arms, infusion rates were titrated to target aPTTs of between 55 and 85 seconds. The primary endpoint (i.e., death, recurrent myocardial infarction, or severe congestive heart failure or cardiogenic shock) occurred in 12.9% of the hirudin group and 11.9% of the heparin group ($P$ = not significant [NS]). Intracranial hemorrhage occurred in 0.4% of the hirudin group and 0.9% of the heparin group.

The reconfigured GUSTO IIb study (37) used similar dosing regimens, the only difference being that infusions were titrated to aPTTs of between 60 to 85 seconds. In the 4131 individuals with ST-segment elevation, 74% of whom were treated with thrombolytic therapy, death or myocardial infarction at 30 days (the primary study endpoint) occurred in 9.9% of those treated with hirudin and 11.3% of those treated with heparin ($P$ = .058). Intracranial hemorrhages were rare with both therapies.

Taken together, these studies suggest only a very modest, if any, benefit from hirudin as an adjunct to thrombolytic and aspirin therapy, and they do not appear to support routine use of hirudin over heparin in individuals with acute myocardial infarction treated using thrombolytics and aspirin.

## CURRENT RECOMMENDATIONS

All individuals with acute myocardial infarction should be treated with an initial dose of 160 to 325 mg of aspirin (chewed to speed absorption) and then continued on a dose of 160 to 325 mg/day unless they have true aspirin allergy or strong contraindications to therapy (14, 77). Current data are insufficient to make specific recommendations regarding use of platelet membrane GP IIb/IIIa receptor–blocking agents in acute myocardial infarction. Preliminary data are encouraging, however,

and ongoing trials should help to define the role of these agents in acute myocardial infarction.

At present, it is recommended that in individuals not treated with thrombolytic therapy, subcutaneous heparin (7500 U twice daily) or intravenous heparin should be administered to those without contraindications to heparin therapy (14, 77). In those individuals at high risk of systemic emboli (i.e., those with large or anterior myocardial infarction, atrial fibrillation, previous embolus, or known left ventricular thrombus), intravenous heparin is recommended (14, 77). In individuals not at high risk of systemic emboli and treated with streptokinase, treatment with subcutaneous heparin (7500–12,500 U twice daily) should be considered (77). Individuals at high risk of systemic emboli should be treated with intravenous heparin (14, 77). In those individuals treated with t-PA, treatment for several days with intravenous heparin has been recommended, primarily on the basis of the angiographic studies discussed earlier (14, 77). Because of an increased risk of intracranial hemorrhage, high-dose, weight-adjusted heparin should not be used in conjunction with thrombolytic therapy. Heparin therapy should be titrated for target aPTT levels of 1.5 to 2.0 times control, and from the data currently available, direct thrombin inhibitors cannot be recommended in the routine care of individuals with acute myocardial infarction.

# SECONDARY PREVENTION IN PATIENTS WITH STABLE CORONARY ARTERY DISEASE

Disruption of atherosclerotic plaques within the coronary tree and subsequent thrombus formation are important in the development of unstable angina and acute myocardial infarction, and they also may contribute to progression of atherosclerosis in asymptomatic individuals and in those with stable angina. Results of autopsy studies suggest that organization of thrombi overlying ruptured plaques may play a role in progression of coronary disease (78). More recent studies have identified fibrinogen, fibrin, and their degradation products within advanced atherosclerotic plaques, thus raising the possibility that activation of the coagulation system is associated with development and growth of atheromas (79).

One plausible conclusion from these findings is that fissuring or rupture of small atherosclerotic plaques, with subsequent mural thrombosis and fibrotic organization of the thrombus, may contribute to progressive narrowing of coronary vessels without necessarily producing unstable angina or infarction. If so, this concept is of enormous clinical significance. No means are yet available to prevent plaque fissuring, but antithrombotic agents may inhibit the superimposed thrombotic process. In a 5-year study at the Mayo Clinic (80), 370 individuals with stable coronary disease received aspirin (975 mg/day) and dipyridamole (225 mg/day) or placebo. Individuals also underwent coronary angiographic assessment at the beginning and end of the trial. Treated individuals experienced fewer myocardial infarctions (5 versus 12%) and a lower incidence of new coronary lesions (23 versus 45%). No difference in progression of preexisting lesions, however, was observed.

The value of aspirin in individuals with stable angina has not been tested in large numbers of individuals. Of the 22,071 male physicians without a history of vascular disease enrolled in the Physicians' Health Study (81), 333 had a history of exertional angina. Over a 5-year follow-up, 21 of these men had confirmed myocardial infarction: seven of 178 (3.9%) who received aspirin, and 20 of 155 (12.9%) who received placebo (risk reduction, 70%; $P = .003$).

The Swedish Angina Pectoris Trial (SAPAT) group (82) enrolled 2035 individuals with stable angina. Individuals were randomly assigned to receive aspirin (75 mg daily) or placebo. Over a median follow-up of 15 months, there was a significant 34% reduction in the primary outcome of myocardial infarction and sudden death ($P = .003$) in the aspirin-treated group.

In conclusion, available data suggest that platelet inhibitor therapy with a daily dose of 160 to 325 mg of aspirin reduces the incidence of myocardial infarction in individuals with stable coronary disease. This benefit is at the cost, however, of an increase in the incidence of intracranial bleeding.

# SECONDARY PREVENTION AFTER MYOCARDIAL INFARCTION

Survivors of acute myocardial infarction already have demonstrated a substrate for acute coronary thrombosis. Thus, several trials in the last three decades have evaluated the role of antiplatelet and anticoagulant therapy in reducing the risk of death and reinfarction among this population. Proving a clear benefit from antithrombotic therapy in these individuals is difficult, however, because the risk of subsequent death in individuals after myocardial infarction relates to thrombotic episodes and is determined by the extent of left ventricular dysfunction and ventricular arrhythmias. In addition, none of these studies enrolled sufficient numbers of individuals (which is approximately 5000 individuals) to have an 80% chance of demonstrating a 20% relative risk reduction in mortality or reinfarction at a 0.05 level of significance.

## PLATELET INHIBITORS

Results of the seven major trials that prospectively assessed the efficacy of aspirin or of aspirin plus dipyrida-

mole in reduction of mortality and reinfarction rates (83–89) are summarized in Fig. 59.7. The dose of aspirin in these trials varied from 300 to 1500 mg/day, as did the interval from index infarction to enrollment, which ranged from 1 week to 5 years. The first six of these trials showed a nonsignificant survival benefit of aspirin therapy. Pooling data from these six trials showed a significant 21% reduction in reinfarction. Addition of dipyridamole to aspirin provided no additional benefit. The seventh and largest of these trials, the Aspirin Myocardial Infarction Study (AMIS) (89), had a 3-year mortality rate of 9.6% in the aspirin group, compared with 8.8% in the placebo group, and the failure of this large, randomized trial to demonstrate meaningful reductions in mortality and reinfarction rates has prompted experts to identify characteristics of the trial that may have led to these discordant results. Retrospective analysis of the earlier trials indicated a correlation between the interval between index infarction and entry into the trial with the subsequent survival benefit. Individuals enrolled within 6 weeks after infarction had a significantly lower mortality rate compared with those enrolled later. In the AMIS trial (89), only 12% of individuals were randomized within 6 months of their index infarction, and none were randomized within 6 weeks. In addition, despite random treatment allocation, high-risk individuals were randomized more frequently to receive aspirin than placebo. These differences in trials design and baseline characteristics could have contributed to the discrepant results of the AMIS trial.

A collaborative review of antiplatelet trials was reported by the Antiplatelet Trialists' Collaboration II in 1994 (90). This overview included 70,000 high-risk individuals with documented vascular disease enrolled in 145 randomized trials of antiplatelet therapy versus placebo. In approximately 20,000 survivors of myocardial infarction, a significant 25% risk reduction was reported with long-term aspirin treatment. The overview provided no evidence, however, that high-dose aspirin (900–1500 mg daily) is more beneficial than medium-dose (75–325 mg daily), although the latter was associated with less gastrointestinal toxicity. The protective effect of aspirin was most evident during the first 2 years of treatment, with insufficient data available to draw meaningful conclusions beyond 3 years (90).

The potential role of another antiplatelet agent, sulfinpyrazone, in the prevention of death and reinfarction among survivors of myocardial infarction was evaluated in two studies: the Anturane Reinfarction Trial (ART) (91), and the Anturane Reinfarction Italian Study (ARIS) (92). The ART study (91) showed a significant reduction in the mortality rate of treated individuals, mostly from a significant decrease in sudden deaths during the first 6 months. This study was criticized heavily, however, because of incomplete analysis of fatal cases.

**FIGURE 59.7.**   Long-term therapy with aspirin in survivors of myocardial infarction (MI). The odds ratios with 95% confidence intervals for mortality comparing coumadin versus placebo in the major randomized trials are shown. Pooling of data from all trials shows a significant but modest overall benefit from treatment. (*Enrollment time = months after myocardial infarction.) *F/U,* follow-up.

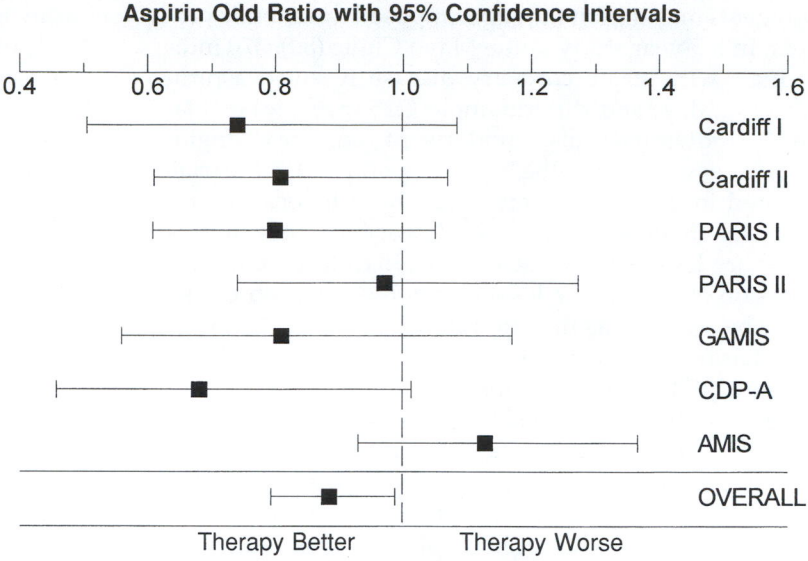

| Study [reference] | Year | Patients | Dose per Day | Months After MI* | Year(s) of F/U | Compliance (%) |
|---|---|---|---|---|---|---|
| Cardiff I [83] | 1971–72 | 1239 | 300 | 0–6 | 1 | 70 |
| Cardiff II [84] | 1974–77 | 1682 | 900 | 0–1 | 1 | 70 |
| PARIS I [87] | 1975–76 | 2026 | 972 | 2–60 | 3–4 | 70 |
| PARIS II [88] | 1980–83 | 3128 | 972 | 1–4 | 2 | 70 |
| GAMIS [86] | 1970–77 | 1340 | 1500 | 1–2 | 2 | 80 |
| CDP-A [85] | 1972–74 | 1529 | 972 | >60 | 2 | 80 |
| AMIS [89] | 1975–76 | 4524 | 1000 | 2–60 | 3 | 90 |

The ARIS trial (92) disclosed a significant decrease in the incidence of reinfarction with sulfinpyrazone, with no effect on the rates of cardiac mortality or sudden death. Some beneficial effect of sulfinpyrazone in the postinfarction period cannot be negated, but the conflicting findings of these trials, along with the potential side effects of the drug, have limited its value for secondary prophylaxis after myocardial infarction.

## ANTICOAGULANTS

Results of randomized clinical trials with warfarin in survivors of myocardial infarction are summarized in Fig. 59.8 (86, 93–96). In the early trials, the Medical Research Council (MRC) (93) and the VA Cooperative Study (94) showed a nonsignificant 5 to 30% reduction in total mortality. There was a significant relative risk reduction in reinfarction in the MRC study, with a favorable trend in the VA Cooperative Study. The German-Austrian Myocardial Infarction Study (GAMIS) (86) and Enquete de Prevention Secondaire de L'Infarctus du Myocarde (EPSIM) trial (97) compared the relative efficacy of aspirin versus warfarin in survivors of myocardial infarction, and mortality in the antiplatelet and anticoagulant

groups was identical in both studies. The Dutch Sixty Plus Reinfarction Study and the Warfarin Reinfarction Study (WARIS) were the first to show a significant 24% relative risk reduction for mortality in myocardial infarction survivors (95, 98); this was associated with significant reduction in the risk of reinfarction in both studies. The reason for the relative success of the Sixty Plus and WARIS trials is not certain, but the investigators suggest their success related to the higher degree of anticoagulation and maintenance of INR in the therapeutic range for a higher proportion of individuals. The high mortality rate of the placebo group in the WARIS study (20%), however, indicates that trial enrolled an excess of high-risk individuals, and it also may reflect the lack of aspirin use in these individuals. This does not negate the finding of the trial, but it does prevent generalization of its results to the average individual after myocardial infarction.

Before publication of the WARIS trial, the large-scale Anticoagulant in the Secondary Prevention of Events in Coronary Thrombosis (ASPECT) trial (96) was initiated. This trial randomized 3404 individuals (20% female) within the first 6 weeks after myocardial infarction to treatment with an oral anticoagulant regimen (target INR, 2.8–4.8) or placebo. At a mean follow-up of

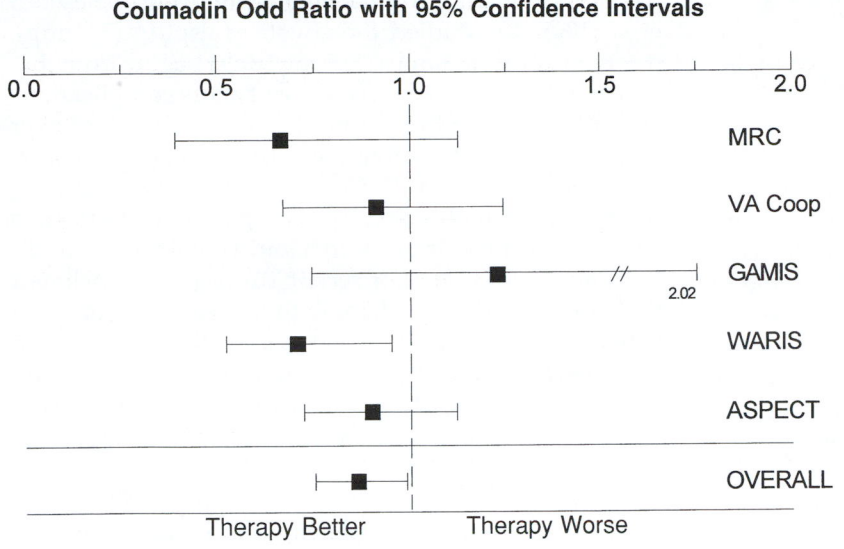

**Coumadin Odd Ratio with 95% Confidence Intervals**

**FIGURE 59.8.** Long-term therapy with warfarin in survivors of myocardial infarction (MI). The odds ratios with 95% confidence intervals for mortality comparing warfarin versus placebo in the major randomized trials spanning more than three decades are shown. Pooling of data from all trials shows a significant but modest overall benefit from treatment. (*Enrollment time = weeks after myocardial infarction.) *INR*, international normalized ratio.

| Study [reference] | Year | Patients | Target INR | Weeks after MI* | Year(s) of F/U | INR in Target Range (%) |
|---|---|---|---|---|---|---|
| MRC [93] | 1955–60 | 383 | 2.0–2.5 | 4–6 | 4 | 60 |
| VA Coop [94] | 1957–60 | 739 | 2.0–2.5 | 3 | 5 | 82 |
| GAMIS [86] | 1970–77 | 626 | 2.5–5.0 | 4–7 | 2 | 62–75 |
| WARIS [95] | 1983–86 | 1214 | 2.8–4.8 | 4 | 5 | 75 |
| ASPECT [96] | 1986–91 | 3404 | 2.8–4.8 | 2 | 3 | 74 |

37 months, a nonsignificant reduction in mortality of 10% was observed. This reduction was less, however, than that seen in the WARIS trial, and it possibly related to the lower mortality rate in the placebo group of the ASPECT trial.

The Italian Study Group on Prevention of Myocardial Infarction evaluated the potential efficacy of chronic, low-dose, subcutaneously administered calcium heparin (99), randomizing 728 individuals to 12,500 U daily of subcutaneous calcium heparin versus placebo for 23 months. Concurrent antiplatelet therapy was permitted. Heparin treatment reduced the cumulative death rate by 34% ($P$ = NS) and the occurrence of reinfarction by 61% ($P$ < .05). No increase in the rates of hemorrhage, osteoporosis, or thrombocytopenia were observed in the heparin group, and heparin treatment did not require laboratory monitoring of the aPTT. Despite its safety and a trend indicating its efficacy, however, this therapy generally is not implemented in clinical practice.

## CURRENT RECOMMENDATIONS

An overview of selected trials and meta-analyses supports the efficacy of both antiplatelet agents and anticoagulants for secondary prevention of cardiovascular morbidity and mortality in survivors of acute myocardial infarction. Aspirin in a single dose of 325 mg/day appears as effective as, and less toxic than, larger doses. Addition of dipyridamole to aspirin is unnecessary, and sulfinpyrazone may be reserved for individuals intolerant to aspirin. Ticlopidine is effective in unstable angina and stroke, but it has not been tested in individuals after myocardial infarction. Clear support for use of oral anticoagulants comes results of from the WARIS and Sixty Plus Study in addition to pooled data from several other trials.

Despite this large body of clinical data, controversy over the superiority and safety of aspirin versus oral anticoagulants in survivors of myocardial infarction continues. The magnitude of difference between these two agents probably is small. Thus, the answer to this question is not likely to be forthcoming in the near future, as it would require a clinical trial of enormous size. The benefit of aspirin probably is similar to that of oral anticoagulants but without the added costs, difficulty in administration, and associated risk of bleeding. The role of combined antiplatelet and anticoagulant therapy is currently being addressed in the Combination Hemotherapy and Mortality Prevention and Coumadin-Aspirin Reinfarction Study trials in the United States and by the WARIS II trial in Europe.

# PERCUTANEOUS CORONARY REVASCULARIZATION

## CORONARY ANGIOPLASTY

Major advances in coronary angioplasty have occurred with adjunctive antiplatelet therapy (i.e., GP IIb/IIIa inhibitors) and the devices (i.e., stents) used for interventions (100). These advances have expanded the role of percutaneous coronary interventions in the treatment of individuals with multivessel coronary artery disease and complex coronary anatomy. Dilatation of the stenosed coronary artery relieves luminal narrowing, but it also results in fracture of the atherosclerotic plaque and tears in the arterial media, which in turn expose highly thrombogenic surfaces. The resultant activation of the coagulation cascade with platelet–fibrin deposition at the site of dilatation has been implicated in acute ischemic complications (4–10% of cases) and in restenosis (30–45% of cases) (100).

## PREVENTION OF ACUTE ISCHEMIC COMPLICATIONS AFTER BALLOON ANGIOPLASTY

### Antiplatelet Agents

Clinical trials during the 1980s explored the use of conventional antiplatelet agents (i.e., aspirin, dipyridamole, ticlopidine) and antithrombins (i.e., unfractionated and low-molecular-weight heparin) for prevention of acute ischemic complications. Recent clinical trials have explored the role of potent, new antiplatelet agents (i.e., GP IIb/IIIa receptor antagonists) and direct antithrombins (i.e., hirudin, Hirulog™) to prevent periprocedural complications and restenosis.

Four published, prospective trials (101–104) evaluated the usefulness of antiplatelet therapy for the prevention of acute periprocedural complications (Table 59.2). Schwartz et al (101) randomized 376 individuals either to aspirin (990 mg) plus dipyridamole (225 mg) beginning 24 hours before angioplasty or to placebo. The main endpoint of this study was the effect of therapy on restenosis, but a retrospective review of periprocedural complications revealed the occurrence of postangioplasty Q-wave infarctions was significantly reduced by antiplatelet therapy (from approximately 7 to 2%). White et al (102) investigated the effects of aspirin (650 mg/day) plus dipyridamole (225 mg/day), ticlopidine (750 mg/day), or placebo beginning 4 to 5 days before percutaneous transluminal coronary angioplasty (PTCA) in 333 individuals. Abrupt occlusion, thrombosis, or major dissection usually necessitating urgent coronary artery bypass graft (CABG) surgery occurred in 14% of controls but in only 5% of the aspirin–dipyrida-

mole group and in 2% of the ticlopidine group. Chesebro et al (104) also studied the effects of aspirin (975 mg/day) plus dipyridamole (225 mg/day) begun 1 day before angioplasty on the incidence of acute complications and restenosis, and they found a trend toward a lower rate of acute complications (i.e., abrupt closure, myocardial infarction, repeat PTCA, or urgent CABG surgery) in treated individuals (11%) compared with controls (20%). These three trials used aspirin combined with dipyridamole, but another recent study (105) concluded that addition of dipyridamole to aspirin was not more beneficial than aspirin alone. In another prospective trial, Bertrand et al (103) found that ticlopidine (250 mg twice daily) markedly reduced the incidence of acute closure (from approximately 16 to 5%) in 266 individuals undergoing angioplasty.

To improve on these results from conventional antiplatelet agents, the role of chimeric monoclonal-antibody Fab fragment (c7E3 Fab) directed against the platelet GP IIb/IIIa receptor in individuals undergoing high-risk angioplasty was evaluated in the Evaluation of c7E3 Fab for Prevention of Ischemic Complication (EPIC) trial (26). In this prospective, randomized, double-blind trial, 2099 individuals received a bolus and an infusion of placebo, a bolus of c7E3 Fab and an infusion of placebo, or a bolus and an infusion of c7E3 Fab. The primary study endpoint was any of the following: death, nonfatal myocardial infarction, or urgent PTCA/CABG surgery within 30 days after the procedure. Results of this trial demonstrated that compared with placebo, c7E3 Fab bolus and infusion resulted in a 35% reduction in the rate of the primary endpoint (12.8 versus 8.3%; $P$ = .008). This efficacy in reduction of ischemic complications was associated with higher bleeding and transfusion rates in the group given c7E3 bolus and infusion. Considering this hemorrhagic risk, however, widespread use of c7E3 Fab during coronary angioplasty cannot be prescribed.

To reduce the risk of bleeding associated with c7E3 Fab administration during PTCA while still maintaining efficacy, a second trial (Evaluation of PTCA to Improve Longterm Outcomes by c7E3 Glycoprotein IIb-IIIa receptor blockade [EPILOG]) used lower doses of heparin (106). In this prospective, double-blind trial, 2792 individuals undergoing percutaneous coronary revascularization were randomized to one of three treatment groups: c7E3 Fab with standard-dose heparin (initial bolus, 100 U/kg), c7E3 Fab with low-dose heparin (bolus, 70 U/kg), or placebo with standard-dose heparin. The primary efficacy endpoint, which consisted of a composite of death, myocardial infarction, or urgent PTCA/CABG surgery within 30 days of randomization, was significantly reduced by 66 and 54%, respectively, in the two c7E3 Fab–treated groups compared with placebo. There were no significant differences between treatments regarding risk of major bleeding, and the rate of red-blood-cell transfusions among individuals receiv-

**TABLE 59.2.** Trials of Antiplatelet Agents for Prevention of Acute Complications during Coronary Angioplasty

| Study | Design | Patients (n) | Antiplatelet Agent | Rate of Acute Complications (%) | Results |
|---|---|---|---|---|---|
| Schwartz et al. (101) | Prospective, randomized | 376 | Aspirin + dipyridamole<br>Placebo | 1.6<br><br>6.9 | Reduction in acute MI (secondary endpoint, $P = .01$) |
| White et al. (102) | Prospective, randomized | 333 | Aspirin + dipyridamole<br>Ticlopidine<br>Placebo | 5.0<br><br>2.0<br>14.0 | Reduction in abrupt vessel closure, thrombosis or dissection ($P < .005$) |
| Chesebro et al. (104) | Prospective, randomized | 207 | Aspirin + dipyridamole<br>Placebo | 11.0<br><br>20.0 | Trend toward lower occlusion, infarction, repeat angioplasty or urgent CABG ($P = .07$) |
| Bertrand et al. (103) | Prospective, randomized | 266 | Ticlopidine<br>Placebo | 5.1<br>16.2 | Reduction in acute occlusion rate ($P < .01$) |
| EPIC (26) | Prospective, randomized | 2099 | c7E3 + aspirin<br>Aspirin alone | 8.3<br>12.8 | Reduction in composite endpoint of death, MI, and urgent revascularization or stent deployment for abrupt vessel closure at 30 days ($P < .008$) |
| EPILOG (106) | Prospective, randomized | 2792 | c7E3 + standard heparin<br>c7E3 + low-dose heparin<br>Placebo | 5.4<br><br>5.2<br><br>11.7 | Reduction in composite endpoint of death, MI, and urgent revascularization at 30 days ($P < .0001$) |
| IMPACT II (27) | Prospective, randomized | 4010 | Integrelin (high dose)<br>Integrelin (low dose)<br>Placebo | 10.0<br><br>9.1<br><br>11.6 | Trend toward reduction in 30-day composite endpoint of death, MI, and urgent revascularization or stent deployment for abrupt vessel closure ($P < .06$). Significant reduction early cardiac events,[b] 9.6 vs 6.6 & 6.9% in the two Integrelin groups ($P = .006$ and .01) |
| RESTORE (28) | Prospective, randomized | 2139 | Tirofiban<br>Placebo | 12.2<br>10.3 | Trend towards reduction in composite endpoint of death, MI, and urgent revascularization at 30 days ($P < .16$). Significant reduction in early cardiac events,[b] 8.7 vs 5.4% ($P = .005$) |

CABG, *coronary artery bypass graft surgery;* MI, *myocardial infarction*

[a] *Primary endpoint: effect of therapy on late restonosis.*

[b] *In-hospital death, myocardial infarction, or urgent revascularization.*

ing c7E3 Fab with low-dose heparin (1.9%) was significantly lower than with placebo (3.9%; $P = .013$).

The success of the EPIC trial and the potential drawbacks of c7E3 Fab (e.g., immunogenicity, rare cases of thrombocytopenia, extended duration of antiplatelet effect) created the impetus to evaluate other GP IIb/IIIa inhibitors (28) (see Chapter 54). Two phase III clinical trials using cyclic RGD peptides (integrelin) or nonpeptide RGD mimetics (tirofiban), both which compete with ligand binding to the GP IIb/IIIa receptor, have been reported (27, 28), and their results show a similar reduction in acute ischemic events during the first 24 to 48 hours after PTCA. Clinical efficacy with these shorter-acting agents, however, was not sustained at 30 days. In the Integrelin to Minimize Platelet Aggregation and Prevent Coronary Thrombosis (IMPACT) II trial, 4010 individuals were randomized to treatment with placebo or to high-dose or low-dose integrelin infusion for 24 hours. At 24 hours, there was a highly significant 30 to 35% reduction in the composite endpoint of death, nonfatal myocardial infarction, and urgent revascularization with both integrelin dosing strategies. At 30-day follow-up, however, reductions in the composite endpoint (13% for high-dose and 19% for low-dose integrelin infusion) were no longer statistically significant. Similar findings were observed in the Randomized Efficacy Study of Tirofiban for Outcomes and Restenosis (RESTORE) trial (28), a randomized trial that involved infusion of the nonpeptide disintegrin versus placebo for 36 hours after PTCA. Clinical efficacy at 48 hours was highly significant with a 38% reduction in ischemic events ($P = .005$); however, by 30 days, half the risk reduction was lost, with a final, nonsignificant relative reduction of 16% ($P = .16$).

Reasons for the differences in outcome with the three types of GP IIb/IIIa inhibitors are not uncertain. The c7E3 Fab acts like a cap over the entire GP IIb/IIIa integrin, whereas the mechanism of receptor inhibition by peptide disintegrins is via competitive binding to the RGD recognition site (see Chapter 54). The nonpeptide antagonists mimic the geometric, stereotactic, and charge characteristics of the RGD sequence and, thus, interfere with platelet aggregation. In addition, the chimeric monoclonal Fab fragment cross reacts with other integrin receptors (vitronectin and MAC-1 receptors), whereas the peptide and nonpeptide disintegrins are specific for the platelet GP IIb/IIIa receptor (107). These integrin receptors play a key role in modulation of the body's response to balloon injury.

## Anticoagulants

High doses of heparin have been used since the inception of angioplasty, and this practice has been reinforced by experimental evidence suggesting an inverse relationship between the dose of heparin and both platelet deposition and vascular mural thrombosis (108). Three retrospective clinical trials (109–111) showed that a lower intensity of anticoagulation during the procedure (activated coagulation time [ACT]) or an aPTT less than three times control during the first 24 hours after the procedure is associated with acute ischemic complications after PTCA. Ferguson et al (11) compared 103 consecutive individuals with an ischemic complication after PTCA to a control group of 400 individuals who underwent coronary intervention without complications, and they found that the postprocedure ACT was less than 250 seconds in 84% of individuals of ischemic complications, compared with 0% in the control. These retrospective trials do not address whether lower ACT and aPTT values in individuals with complications were the cause or the result of the adverse event. Ischemic complications after angioplasty increase the synthesis of heparin-binding proteins and potentiate local release of platelet factor 4 by platelets, which leads to heparin resistance and lower ACT and aPTT measurements. Therefore, the group with ischemic events possibly was less anticoagulated because of heparin resistance rather than because of suboptimal heparin dosing.

Inactivation of heparin by platelet-rich thrombi and heparin-binding proteins (112), as well as its inability to inhibit clot-associated thrombin (113), provided the impetus for testing direct thrombin inhibitors to prevent acute ischemic complications and restenosis after PTCA (Table 59.3). After encouraging results in preliminary studies, two prospective, randomized trials (114, 115) evaluated the direct thrombin inhibitors hirudin and Hirulog ™(bivalirudin) in individuals undergoing PTCA. The HELVETICA study (114) randomized 1141 individuals to treatment with standard heparin, hirudin bolus with infusion for 24 hours, or hirudin bolus followed by subcutaneous hirudin for 3 days. There was no difference between groups in the primary clinical endpoint of death, myocardial infarction, or repeat revascularization of the target lesion at 7 months, but there was a significant reduction in death, nonfatal myocardial infarction, and urgent revascularization at 96 hours, from 11% in the heparin arm to 7.9% and 5.6% in the two hirudin-treated groups. Similar results were obtained in the larger Hirulog Angioplasty Trial (115), which randomized 4010 individuals with unstable or postinfarction angina to either heparin or Hirulog™. After an initial bolus, an infusion of Hirulog was continued for 24 hours. The primary endpoint consisted of in-hospital death, nonfatal myocardial infarction, or urgent revascularization, but it was not different between the two groups. In the subgroup of individuals with postinfarction angina, however, there was a significant reduction in early in-hospital events, and there was a dramatic reduction in bleeding complications (~50%) in all individuals. In addition, a strategy of heparin versus hirudin in individuals with acute myocardial infarction undergoing primary angioplasty was reported

**TABLE 59.3.** Randomized Trials of Antithrombins for Prevention of Acute Complications during Coronary Angioplasty

| Study | Design | Patients (n) | Antithrombotic Agent | Rate of Acute Complications (%) | Results |
|---|---|---|---|---|---|
| HELVETICA (114) | Randomized | 1141 | Heparin<br>Hirudin (bolus + infusion)<br>Hirudin (bolus + SQ injections) | 11.0<br>7.9<br>5.6 | No difference in primary endpoint at 6 months but significant reduction in early (within 96 hours) cardiac events[a] in the combined hirudin groups.[b] |
| Hirulog Trial (115) | Randomized | 4010 | Heparin<br>Hirulog | 12.2<br>11.4 | No difference in early cardiac events[a] in the overall group. Significant reduction in early cardiac events in the subgroup with postinfarction angina.[c] |

SQ, subcutaneous.
[a] In-hospital death, myocardial infarction, or urgent revascularization.
[b] $P = .02$.
[c] $P = .04$ for event rate of 14.2% in heparin and 9.1% in Hirulog groups.

in the angiographic substudy of the GUSTO IIb trial (116), which enrolled 247 individuals in the hirudin arm and 256 individuals in the heparin arm. There was no significant difference in the combined endpoint of death, reinfarction, or disabling stroke at 30 days between the two antithrombins. The failure of these potent, direct thrombin inhibitors to show a significant advantage over heparin is multifactorial, but is partly attributed partly to continued generation of thrombin during treatment as well as a rebound increase in thrombin activity on cessation of infusion (117).

## ANTITHROMBOTIC THERAPY AFTER DEPLOYMENT OF INTRACORONARY STENTS

Significant advances also have occurred in the use of antithrombotic therapy after deployment of intracoronary stents, which are fenestrated, stainless-steel tubes. The stents provide an endovascular scaffold within the coronary artery that markedly improves luminal diameter and rheology. Initial studies of coronary stenting used high-intensity anticoagulation with warfarin (INR, 3.0–4.5) to prevent acute and subacute stent thrombosis, which occurred in 3 to 8% of individuals (118). Optimization of stent deployment using high-pressure balloon inflations, use of intravascular ultrasound guidance to embed the stent into the vessel wall, and use of combined antiplatelet therapy with aspirin and ticlopidine, however, have resulted in lowering the stent thrombosis rate to 0.6 to 1.5%. The relative contribution of refined techniques for stent deployment, which improves rheology, versus optimi-

zation of hemostasis with combination antiplatelet therapy toward reduction of stent thrombosis is not known. Results of recent clinical trials (119–121) show that combined antiplatelet therapy (aspirin plus ticlopidine) is significantly better than aspirin alone or standard anticoagulant therapy with warfarin and aspirin (Table 59.4). These findings recently were extended to individuals undergoing primary angioplasty along with intracoronary stenting for acute myocardial infarction but Schomig et al (123), who randomized 123 individuals after successful stenting for acute myocardial infarction to a strategy of aspirin plus ticlopidine or intense anticoagulation with aspirin plus warfarin (target INR, 3.5–4.5). Significant reduction in the clinical event rate (i.e., death, reinfarction, repeat intervention and hemorrhage) was observed with the combined antiplatelet regimen. The role of GP IIb/IIIa inhibitors in prevention of acute ischemic complications and restenosis after intracoronary stenting is currently being evaluated in the EPILOG stent trial.

The local delivery of heparin was explored in the BENESTENT II study (123), which was a nonrandomized trial evaluating the reduction in acute ischemic complications after deployment of a heparin-coated stent. The study, which enrolled 207 individuals, had a 0% incidence of stent thrombosis, along with a remarkably low 13% restenosis rate at 6 months. A randomized study evaluating a heparin-coated stent versus a conventional Palmaz-Schatz stent is currently underway to examine the need for local heparin delivery; there is some controversy that optimization of stent deployment techniques may obviate perfect control of hemostasis.

**TABLE 59.4.** Randomized Trials of Anticoagulant/Antiplatelet Agents for Prevention of Acute Complications after Intracoronary Stenting

| Study | Design | Patients (n) | Antithrombotic Agents | Rate of Acute Complications (%) | Results |
|---|---|---|---|---|---|
| Schomig et al. (120) | Randomized | 517 | Phenprocoumon + aspirin | 6.2 | Significant reduction in early cardiac events[a] ($P = .01$). |
| | | | Ticlopidine + aspirin | 1.6 | |
| Hall et al. (119) | Randomized | 226 | Aspirin alone | 3.9 | Trend toward a significant difference in early cardiac events [a] ($P = .1$). The relatively small sample size may have contributed to failure to detect a difference. |
| | | | Aspirin + ticlopidine | 0.8 | |
| STAR (121) | Randomized | 1652 | Aspirin alone | 3.6 | Significant reduction in early events[a] in the aspirin + ticlopidine arm |
| | | | Aspirin + ticlopidine | 0.6 | |
| | | | Warfarin + aspirin | 2.4 | |

[a] *In-hospital death, myocardial infarction, or urgent revascularization.*

## RESTENOSIS

Coronary restenosis involves the interaction of acute vessel recoil, mural thrombosis, neointimal smooth muscle cell proliferation, and vascular remodeling. An earlier hypothesis that the mural thrombus provides a scaffold for subsequent migration and proliferation of smooth muscle cells, thereby resulting in luminal narrowing or restenosis (124), has been challenged by the results of serial intravascular ultrasound studies (125, 126). Intravascular ultrasound allows transmural, tomographic imaging of coronary arteries in humans *in vivo* and has provided evidence that two-thirds of late-lumen loss results from arterial remodeling (i.e., vessel constriction), whereas the remaining one-third can be attributed to tissue proliferation in nonstented vessels after PTCA (125). Thus, it is not surprising that most trials using antiplatelet agents and antithrombins have yielded negative results (101–103, 127, 128).

The antiplatelet regimens tested clinically for prevention of restenosis have included aspirin (101), aspirin plus dipyridamole (102), and ticlopidine (103, 127). In these trials, rates of restenosis several months after angioplasty were essentially similar in the treated and the placebo groups. In the EPIC trial (129), which compared the GP IIb/IIIa inhibitor c7E3 Fab with placebo for high-risk angioplasty, there was a significant 26% reduction in the need for repeat revascularization of the target vessel, from 22.3 to 16.5%, at 6-month follow-up. In the EPILOG trial (106), in which the dose of heparin was lowered to reduce the incidence of bleeding complications (as was observed in the EPIC trial), there was a significant decrease in the composite clinical endpoint of death, nonfatal myocardial infarction, and repeat revascularization at 6-month follow-up between the c7E3 Fab group versus placebo. When repeat revascularization alone was analyzed, however, there was no significant difference in the c7E3 Fab versus the placebo groups. Similarly, the IMPACT II and RESTORE trials, which used peptide and nonpeptide disintegrins, found no significant difference in the composite clinical endpoint at 30 days after randomization (27, 28).

Potentiation of platelet antiaggregatory effect with ciprostene, which is a stable analogue of prostacyclin, was tested in 311 individuals undergoing PTCA (130). A beneficial trend toward reduced restenosis by ciprostene was observed, and the clinical endpoints of myocardial infarction, repeat PTCA, CABG, or death were significantly reduced (by 50%). Unfortunately, these preliminary findings were not confirmed by another trial, which tested the effects of short-term prostacyclin administration on restenosis (131). The encouraging results obtained with both heparin and direct antithrombins for prevention of restenosis in animal models prompted intensive clinical research with these agents (114, 115, 128, 132, 133, 134), and early trials used heparin as an infusion for 24 hours and low-molecular-weight heparin as subcutaneous injections for 6 months after PTCA (128, 134). Both failed to show any beneficial effect of the anticoagulants on prevention of restenosis. Similarly, the HELVETICA and Hirulog Angioplasty Trial, which used the potent, direct-acting antithrombins described here, failed to show any effect on the rate of coronary restenosis (114, 115).

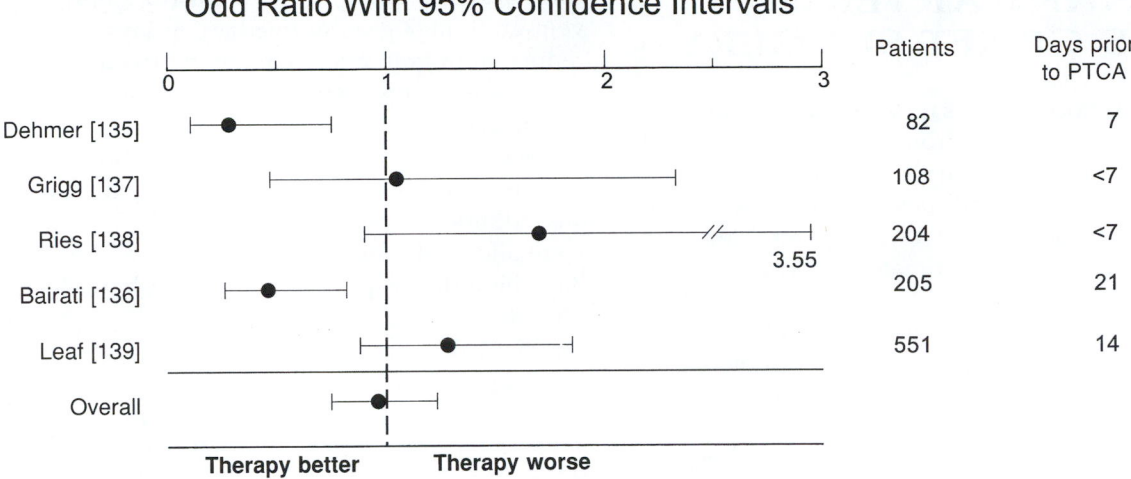

**FIGURE 59.9.** Overview of trials comparing omega-3 fatty acids with placebo for restenosis after percutaneous transluminal coronary angioplasty (PTCA). Results are shown as odd ratios with 95% confidence intervals. An odds ratio of less than 1 indicates of a lower restenosis rate among treated individuals and is statistically significant ($P < .05$) if the 95% confidence intervals do not cross the vertical hatched line (odds ratio, 1.0). An odds ratio of greater than 1 indicates a higher restenosis rate among treated individuals and is statistically significant ($P < .05$) if the 95% confidence intervals do not cross the vertical hatched line (odds ratio, 1.0). The number of individuals enrolled and days of therapy with omega-3 fatty acids before PTCA are shown on the right. (Data from Dehmer GJ, Popma JJ, van den Berg EK, et al. Reduction in the rate of early restenosis after coronary angioplasty by a diet supplemented with n-3 fatty acids. N Engl J Med 1988;319:733–740; Bairati I, Roy L, Meyer F. Double-blind, randomized, controlled trial of fish oil supplements in prevention of recurrence of stenosis after coronary angioplasty. Circulation 1992;85:950–956; Grigg LE, Kay TW, Valentine PA, et al. Determinants of restenosis and lack of effect of dietary supplementation with eicosapentaenoic acid on the incidence of coronary artery restenosis after angioplasty. J Am Coll Cardiol 1989;13:665–672; Reis GJ, Boucher TM, Sipperly ME, et al. Randomized trial of fish oil for prevention of restenosis after coronary angioplasty. Lancet 1989;ii:177–181; and Leaf A, Jorgensen MB, Jacobs AK, et al. Do fish oils prevent restenosis after coronary angioplasty? Circulation 1994;90:2248–2257.)

A different approach to restenosis consists of using fish oils (135–139), specifically omega-3 fatty acids (Fig. 59.9). These compounds affect the phospholipid composition of the membranes of platelets and leukocytes, thus resulting in platelet inhibitory and anti-inflammatory activity. In addition, they may improve endothelial-dependent relaxation and inhibit intimal hyperplasia after vessel injury. Initial studies yielded promising results (135, 136), but those of a subsequent large, prospective, randomized trial (139) using quantitative coronary angiography showed a restenosis rate of 52% in the fish-oil group versus 46% in the placebo group ($P = .37$). Thus, currently available data fail to support a role for omega-3 fatty acids in therapy for the prevention of coronary restenosis.

## CURRENT RECOMMENDATIONS

Conventional antiplatelet agents reduce the incidence of acute ischemic complications after coronary angioplasty. These regimens include aspirin, ticlopidine, and the combination of the two after intracoronary stenting. Soluble aspirin (325 mg daily) should be given both the day before and on the morning of the procedure.

As a higher ACT/aPTT is associated with a lower event rate, adequate heparinization (10,000–15,000 U bolus) is instrumental in reducing ischemic events. The optimal duration of heparin treatment after angioplasty largely is determined by the clinical status of the individual and the angiographic results. Optimization of luminal rheology with intracoronary stents reduces the need for prolonged in-hospital anticoagulation with heparin in most cases. The promising results obtained with direct thrombin inhibitors in animal models, however, have failed to translate into a clinical benefit in phase III trials. These agents have not been approved by the U.S. Food and Drug Administration for routine clinical use.

Recent clinical trials using GP IIb/IIIa inhibitors provide a new paradigm, suggesting that potent platelet inhibition is beneficial in reducing both acute and late complications after angioplasty without increasing bleeding rates. Whether the reduction in target-vessel revascularization observed with c7E3 Fab–mediated platelet inhibition is independent of the optimization of coronary luminal rheology, which now is feasible with use of intracoronary stents, is the subject of the ongoing EPILOG stent study.

# CORONARY ARTERY BYPASS GRAFT SURGERY

Occlusion of aortocoronary saphenous vein grafts is an important contributor to morbidity and mortality both early and late after CABG surgery. Vein-graft occlusion rates of 8 to 18% at 1-month postoperatively and 16 to 26% at 1-year postoperatively have been reported (140). At the end of 10 years, approximately 50% of vein grafts will be occluded.

Vein-graft disease can be divided into two general phases: an early, postoperative phase of thrombotic occlusion; and a late phase of accelerated intimal hyperplasia that eventually may lead to graft atherosclerosis not dissimilar to that affecting the native coronary arteries. Superimposed thrombus formation can occur at any time during the disease process. The results of antithrombotic therapy for prevention of early and late vein-graft disease are reviewed here.

## PREVENTION OF EARLY GRAFT OCCLUSION

Early vein-graft disease begins intraoperatively, as soon as the vein is removed from the leg, manipulated, sutured, and exposed abruptly to the high-pressure arterial system. Platelets, which are activated after passing through the extracorporeal pump and oxygenator, adhere to areas of damaged endothelium and release their thrombogenic factors. In addition, poor distal runoff or small-caliber vessels increase the potential for occlusion. Because early vein-graft disease is predominantly thrombotic in origin, under which circumstances platelets have a fundamental role, adequate perioperative antiplatelet therapy is essential.

Multiple studies (141–151) have demonstrated the importance of initiating platelet-inhibitor therapy during the perioperative period, preferably within 6 hours and no later than 48 hours after surgery (Table 59.5). Delaying institution of antiplatelet treatment results in an increased risk of graft closure. Indeed, when therapy was initiated more than 48 hours after surgery, no reduction in the vein-graft occlusion rate was seen (152–155).

Interest in the use of dipyridamole before surgery derived from both experimental and clinical evidence suggesting this agent decreased platelet activation by the extracorporeal pump, maintained platelet count during cardiopulmonary bypass, increased vein-graft blood flow, and unlike aspirin, did not increase intraoperative bleeding (156, 157). In a landmark placebo-controlled study (147), individuals received dipyridamole (400 mg/day) for 48 hours before surgery, followed by aspirin (325 mg) and dipyridamole (75 mg) three times daily started 7 hours after surgery and continued for 1 year. In this study, there was no increased incidence of bleeding

complications among the treatment group. At early vein-graft angiography (median, 8 days), a significant reduction in graft occlusion among treated individuals was evident, from 10 to 2% per graft and from 22 to 6% per individual.

Whether dipyridamole offers additional protection over aspirin alone has been questioned. In a large Veterans Affairs Cooperative Study (142), 772 individuals were allocated randomly to standard aspirin (325 mg/day), high-dose aspirin (975 mg/day), high-dose aspirin plus dipyridamole (225 mg/day), sulfinpyrazone (800 mg/day), or placebo. Treatment was started 2 days before surgery except for aspirin, which was given only 12 hours preoperatively. Early angiography at a median of 9 days after surgery revealed graft patency rates of from 92 to 94% in the aspirin groups, 90% in the sulfinpyrazone group, and 85% in the placebo group (Fig. 59.10). In a cluster analysis, the three aspirin-treatment groups had improved graft patency, but the group treated with sulfinpyrazone showed only a beneficial trend. No benefit resulted from use of high-dose over standard-dose aspirin or from addition of dipyridamole. Aspirin therapy, however, was associated with a significant increase in perioperative blood loss, need for transfusions, and reoperation rate (for bleeding complications). Sulfinpyrazone did not increase surgical bleeding, but its use was associated with transient renal insufficiency (5%).

Goldman et al (158) evaluated the need for preoperative aspirin to prevent graft occlusion. Grafts included saphenous vein grafts and mammary arteries. Individuals were randomized to aspirin (325 mg/day) starting either the night before or 6 hours after the operation. No significant differences in graft patency were seen for all individuals, but there was a trend toward higher patency in "Y" saphenous vein grafts and in internal mammary grafts in individuals who received aspirin before the operation. Preoperative aspirin resulted in increased bleeding complications and need for reoperation.

In the largest trial of platelet inhibitors in coronary surgery, Sanz et al (141) randomized 1112 individuals to aspirin (150 mg/day), aspirin (150 mg/day) plus dipyridamole (225 mg/day), or placebo. All individuals received dipyridamole (400 mg/day) for 48 hours before surgery, and assigned therapy was commenced 7 hours after operation. Angiography 10 days after surgery showed that graft occlusion rates were 18% in the placebo group, 14% in the aspirin group, and 13% in the aspirin-plus-dipyridamole group. Both hospital mortality and early reoperation rates were similar in all groups.

An even lower dose of aspirin (50 mg/day) was used by the Coronary Artery Bypass Graft Occlusion by Aspirin, Dipyridamole and Acenocoumarol Study (CABADAS) (150), in which 1-year angiographic vein-graft patency was evaluated in 948 individuals assigned to receive aspirin, aspirin plus dipyridamole (400 mg/

**TABLE 59.5.**   Trials of Platelet Inhibitors in Coronary Artery Surgery: Early Initiation of Therapy after Operation[a]

| Study | Patients (n) | Drug (mg/day) | Follow-up | Vein-graft Patency (%) | | P |
|---|---|---|---|---|---|---|
| | | | | Treatment | Control | |
| Chesebro et al. (147, 148) | 407 | Aspirin (975) + dipyridamole (225)[b] | 8 days | 97 | 90 | <.0001 |
| | | | 12 months | 89 | 75 | <.0001 |
| Baur et al. (149) | 255 | Sulfinpyrazone (800) | 1–2 months | 96 | 91 | <.03 |
| Rajah et al. (145) | 125 | Aspirin (990) + dipyridamole (225)[b] | 6 months | 92 | 75 | <.01 |
| Limet et al. (146) | 173 | Ticlopidine (500) | 10 days | 93 | 87 | <.05 |
| | | | 6 months | 85 | 76 | <.02 |
| | | | 12 months | 84 | 74 | <.01 |
| Goldman et al. (142) | 772 | Aspirin (325)[b] | 9 days | 94 | 85 | <.01 |
| | | Aspirin (975)[b] | | 92 | | <.05 |
| | | Aspirin (975) + dipyridamole (225)[b] | | 92 | | <.05 |
| | | Sulfinpyrazone (800)[b] | | 90 | | NS |
| Goldman et al. (143) | | Aspirin groups | 12 months | 84 | 77 | <.03 |
| | | Sulfinpyrazone | | 82 | | NS |
| Sanz et al. (141) | 1112 | Aspirin (150) | 10 days | 86 | 82 | .06 |
| | | Aspirin (150) + dipyridamole (225) | | 87 | | <.02[c] |
| Gavaghan et al. (144) | 237 | Aspirin (324) | 7 days | 98 | 94 | <.005 |
| | | | 12 months | 94 | 88 | .01 |
| CABADAS (150) | 948 | Aspirin (50) | 12 months | 85 | — | — |
| | | Aspirin (50) + dipyridamole (400)[b] | | 89 | | NS |
| | | | | 87 | | NS |
| | | Oral anticoagulant (INR, ~2.8–4.8) | | | | |
| CABADAS (151) Internal mammary | 494 | Aspirin (50) | 12 months | 95 | — | — |
| | | Aspirin (50) + dipyridamole (400)[b] | | 95 | | NS |
| Graft only | | Oral anticoagulant (INR, ~2.8–4.8) | | 93 | | NS |

INS, *international normalized ratio;* NS, *not significant.*

[a] *<48 hours.*

[b] *Preoperative initiation of therapy.*

[c] *Compared with control.*

day), or oral anticoagulants (INR, 2.8–4.8) in a prospective, randomized trial. Occlusion rates of distal anastomoses were 11% in the aspirin-plus-dipyridamole group, 15% in the aspirin group, and 13% in the oral anticoagulants group (*P* = NS). Thus, this large trial supports use of low-dose aspirin immediately after surgery for the prevention of early vein-graft occlusion. The addition of dipyridamole to aspirin, however, was only marginally beneficial, and compared with aspirin, oral anticoagulants provided no additional benefit.

The benefit of antiplatelet versus anticoagulant ther-

apy after internal mammary artery grafting was addressed by the CABADAS group as well (151). Angiographic internal mammary artery graft patency at 1 year was assessed in 494 individuals in whom this arterial conduit was used. Individuals were assigned to treatment with aspirin (50 mg/day), aspirin plus dipyridamole (400 mg/day), or oral anticoagulant agents (INR, 2.8–4.8). The occlusion rates of distal anastomoses were 5.3% in the aspirin group, 5.3% in the aspirin-plus-dipyridamole group, and 6.8% in the oral anticoagulant group (*P* = NS). Thus, internal mammary artery graft

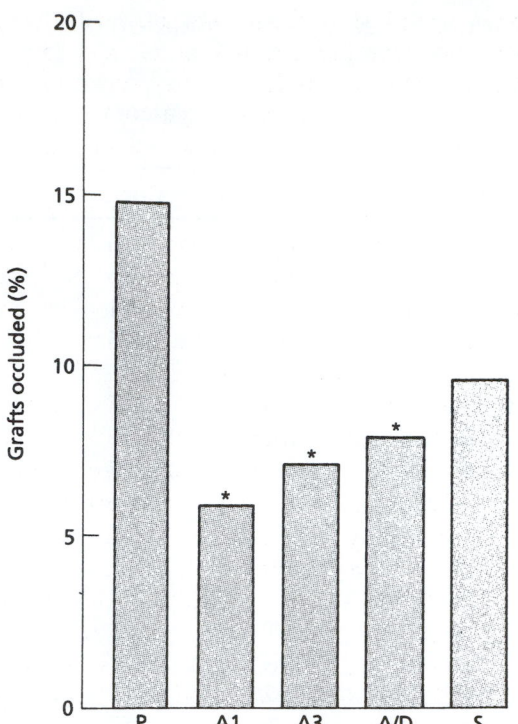

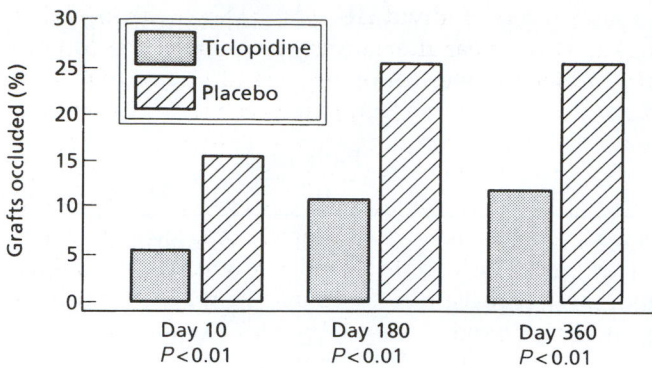

**FIGURE 59.11.** Effect of ticlopidine (250 mg twice a day) on early and late graft occlusion rates after coronary artery bypass surgery. Note that most of the beneficial effect from ticlopidine resulted from a reduction in early graft occlusion (at 10 days after operation). The initial benefit was maintained at 1-year follow-up. (Adapted with permission from Limet R, David JL, Magotteaux P, Larock MP, Rigo P. Prevention of aorta-coronary bypass graft occlusion. Beneficial effect of ticlopidine on early and late patency rates of venous coronary bypass grafts: a double-blind study. J Thorac Cardiovasc Surg 1987;94:773–783.)

**FIGURE 59.10.** Influence of platelet inhibitors for prevention of vein-graft occlusion after coronary bypass surgery. At early angiography, only the aspirin-containing regimens improved graft patency compared with placebo (P). A single dose of aspirin, 325 mg/day (A1), was as effective as aspirin three times a day (A3) or aspirin plus dipyridamole, each given three times a day (A/D). Only a beneficial trend was seen with sulfinpyrazone (S). *$P < .05$. (Adapted with permission from Goldman S, Copeland J, Moritz T, et al. Improvement in early saphenous vein graft patency after coronary artery bypass surgery with antiplatelet therapy: results of a Veterans Administration Cooperative Study. Circulation 1988;77:1324–1332.)

patency at 1 year is not improved by aspirin plus dipyridamole or oral anticoagulant agents over that obtained with low-dose aspirin alone.

One study (146) evaluated the effect of the antiplatelet agent ticlopidine (250 mg twice daily) on prevention of graft occlusion. In this study, the early graft occlusion rate was nearly twice as great in the placebo group as in the ticlopidine group (Fig. 59.11). Treatment with ticlopidine was fairly well tolerated. Neutropenia, which is a definite concern with ticlopidine, was observed in seven individuals on ticlopidine and in three on placebo; it was reversible in all cases.

## PREVENTION OF LATE VEIN-GRAFT DISEASE

The pathogenesis of late vein-graft disease, which occurs months to years after surgery, probably is multifactorial. Endothelial injury resulting from surgical manipulation and exposure to arterial shear forces favors platelet deposition and release of mitogenic factors from platelets and other cells. With time, this can lead to proliferation of smooth muscle cell, intimal hyperplasia, lipid accumulation, connective tissue synthesis by smooth muscle cells and fibroblasts, and development of fibrous or calcific plaques indistinguishable from native-vessel atherosclerosis. Mural or occlusive graft thrombosis commonly is seen at reoperation (159).

Currently available platelet inhibitors prevent neither platelet adherence to the injured endothelium nor release of mitogenic factors, which makes them ineffective for preventing intimal hyperplasia. Some studies, however, have shown that antithrombotic agents reduce late graft occlusion (144, 148, 160), which may be explained by their interference with superimposed thrombus formation rather than through direct inhibition of the occlusive proliferative process.

Whether antithrombotic agents are necessary beyond the early postoperative period is controversial (161). Results of some studies (143, 146) have suggested that the benefit is limited to the early phase of thrombotic occlusion. By contrast, in a randomized study that evaluated individuals assigned to antiplatelet or anticoagulant regimens for either 3 or 12 months after surgery (160), however, new graft occlusions at late angiographic follow-up were significantly reduced in the individuals who received long-term therapy, suggesting that antithrombotic agents may, indeed, prevent late graft occlusion.

Another recent study (162) evaluated the long-term (3 years) effectiveness of antiplatelet therapy after

CABG surgery. Individuals who received aspirin (325 mg/day) for 1 year after surgery and a 1-year postoperative cardiac catheterization were randomized to receive either aspirin (325 mg/day) or placebo for 2 additional years. At 3 years, coronary angiography was performed to determine saphenous vein-graft patency in 288 individuals and internal mammary graft patency in 167 individuals. For saphenous vein grafts that were patent at 1 year, the occlusion rate at 3 years was 4.8% in individuals treated with aspirin, compared with 4.2% in individuals who received placebo ($P$ = NS). For internal mammary artery grafts that were patent at 1 year, the occlusion rate at 3 years was 4.3% in individuals treated with aspirin, compared with 2.5% in individuals who received placebo ($P$ = NS). These data suggest aspirin does not improve vein or arterial conduit patency between 1 and 3 years after coronary bypass.

## CURRENT RECOMMENDATIONS

Platelet inhibitor therapy is mandatory for prevention of early vein-graft occlusion. Preoperative aspirin increases intraoperative bleeding (142) and is not more beneficial than aspirin started within a few hours after surgery (158). Therefore, for elective surgery and if the clinical situation permits, aspirin should be withheld until after the operation. Aspirin at a dose of 50 to 325 mg/day should be started immediately after surgery; treatment is ineffective if delayed for more than 48 hours after operation. Preoperative dipyridamole does not increase intraoperative bleeding, but its advantage over postoperative aspirin alone remains unproved.

The appropriate duration of therapy after surgery is still controversial. Studies suggest that antithrombotic therapy for at least 1 year reduces late graft occlusion. No benefit from antiplatelet therapy after the first year has been proved (162), but the beneficial effects of aspirin for secondary prevention of coronary disease argue that it be continued indefinitely in these individuals. Addition of dipyridamole to aspirin is unnecessary.

Ticlopidine also appears to be an effective antithrombotic agent. Its relative benefit compared with aspirin in individuals with coronary disease, however, needs to be assessed before definite recommendations can be made. The potential for serious side effects may limit its use to individuals who are intolerant of or allergic to aspirin.

# PREVENTION OF LEFT VENTRICULAR THROMBOEMBOLISM

## ACUTE MYOCARDIAL INFARCTION

The underlying substrate for ventricular mural thrombus formation after myocardial infarction is a large area of anterior or apical akinesis associated with failure of the coronary artery subtending that territory to recanalize. Consequently, mural thrombi frequently are associated with anterior wall infarctions (25–40%) and are rare in inferior infarctions (<5%) (163–165). Approximately 75% of mural thrombi develop within the first week after infarction. Early development of thrombi (within the first 2–3 days) portends a poor prognosis, probably because it reflects an underlying, large area of infarction and substantial impairment in ventricular function (166). In addition, thrombi constitute an important predisposing factor for arterial embolism.

Several published, randomized trials evaluated the effects of anticoagulant therapy on prevention of left ventricular thrombosis after anterior infarction (167–172) (Table 59.6). Results of the earlier, smaller studies were largely inconclusive (167–169); however, those of the recent, larger trials (171, 172) involving high-dose subcutaneous heparin (12,500 U every 12 hours) showed that this anticoagulant regimen reduces the incidence of mural thrombosis by 50 to 66%. Initiation of heparin therapy immediately after identification of an infarction is most effective at preventing formation of a ventricular thrombus, but it is less effective at enhancing its resolution (172), thus emphasizing the need for prophylactic therapy.

Thrombolytic therapy for acute myocardial infarction may reduce the incidence of ventricular thrombi, primarily because of the salutary effects of coronary recanalization on left ventricular function and remodeling, and it also may reduce the incidence of postinfarction ventricular dilatation (173). Studies evaluating the efficacy of thrombolytic therapy for prevention of mural thrombus formation (174) showed that early reperfusion of the coronary artery is associated with a low prevalence of thrombus formation (7%). Large anterior myocardial infarctions frequently are associated with ventricular thrombosis, but the highest prevalence of thrombus formation (75%) is seen when the left anterior descending coronary artery is occluded and no collateral blood vessels to the infarcted area are visualized on the coronary angiogram.

The incidence of systemic embolism can be as high as 20% in individuals with echocardiographic evidence of ventricular thrombus, especially if protrusion into the ventricular cavity or mobility are observed, compared with 2% in those individuals without a visualized thrombus (164). Oral anticoagulant therapy is effective in enhancing resolution of thrombi (163, 164, 175) and in protecting against systemic embolism (176). In contrast, the protective effects of antiplatelet agents in this situation are inconsistent; therefore, oral anticoagulants are advisable after infarction in individuals with left ventricular thrombi. Results from clinical trials of anticoagulant therapy after myocardial infarction, which have

**TABLE 59.6.** Randomized Trials of Anticoagulant Therapy in Acute Myocardial Infarction for Preventing Left Ventricular Thrombosis

| Study | Antithrombotic Regimen | Patients (n) | Left Ventricular Thrombi (%) | | P |
|---|---|---|---|---|---|
| | | | Treatment | Control | |
| Nordrehaug et al. (167) | Intravenous heparin followed by warfarin vs. placebo | 53 | 0 | 26 | <.01 |
| David and Ireland (168) | Intravenous heparin followed by warfarin vs. low-dose anticoagulants | 52 | 56 | 56 | NS |
| Gueret et al. (169) | Intravenous heparin followed by subcutaneous heparin vs. no anticoagulant | 46 | 38 | 52 | NS |
| Arvan and Boscha (170) | Intravenous heparin followed by warfarin vs. no anticoagulant | 30 | 31 | 35 | NS |
| Turpie et al. (171) | High-dose subcutaneous heparin (12,500 U) vs. low-dose (5000 U) every 12 hours | 183 | 11 | 32 | 0.0004 |
| SCATI (172) | High-dose subcutaneous heparin (12,500 U) every 12 hours vs. no anticoagulant | 200 | 18 | 36 | <.01[a] |

NS, *not significant.*

[a] *Some individuals admitted within 6 hours of infarction received streptokinase.*

shown that treatment reduces rates of thromboembolism and stroke by 50 to 75% provide support for this recommendation (93–95).

## DILATED CARDIOMYOPATHY

Postmortem studies (177) have found a high prevalence of right and left ventricular mural thrombi in individuals with idiopathic dilated cardiomyopathy. Blood stasis and low shear rates in a dilated, hypocontractile ventricle are thought to lead to activation of coagulation processes and thrombus formation, which in turn may result in systemic or cerebral embolism. One study of individuals with dilated cardiomyopathy who were not receiving anticoagulation (178) noted a high prevalence of ventricular thrombi (60%), particularly in individuals with severe ventricular contractile dysfunction. Left atrial thrombi also have been documented in a significant percentage of individuals with dilated cardiomyopathy by transesophageal echocardiography (179), and arterial embolism has been noted to be common in this group, occurring in 20% of these individuals. In a retrospective study (113), individuals treated with anticoagulants had no evidence of embolism, whereas those not anticoagulated had an embolic rate of 3.5% per year. Presence of atrial fibrillation increased the risk of embolism in this study (180).

## CHRONIC LEFT VENTRICULAR ANEURYSM

In contrast to the substantial risk of thromboembolism in individuals with acute anterior myocardial infarction or dilated cardiomyopathy, the incidence of embolism in individuals with chronic left ventricular aneurysm is low (0.35% per year) (181). This probably is because thrombi in acute infarction commonly are mobile and protrude into the ventricular cavity, whereas thrombi in ventricular aneurysms are laminated and more adherent to the endocardium. In addition, thrombi located within an aneurysmal sac, which is devoid of contractile fibers, are less prone to propulsion into the left ventricular outflow tract (182). Some investigators (183) have found a persistent risk of embolism in individuals with ventricular aneurysm after infarction, but it was the mobility and protrusion of the thrombus rather than the presence of an aneurysm that predicted embolic events.

## CURRENT RECOMMENDATIONS

In individuals with acute anterior myocardial infarction or large infarctions in other locations, immediate anticoagulation with intravenous heparin (aimed at prolonging the aPTT from 1.5–2.0 times control) or subcutaneous heparin (12,500 U twice daily) is indicated to prevent left ventricular mural thrombosis. Anticoagulation therapy with heparin should be initiated at the time of myocardial infarction, because waiting for echocardiographic confirmation of mural thrombi may result in missing the time period when preventive treatment is most effective. Heparin should be continued for several days after infarction, and a predischarge echocardiogram may help in risk stratification. Individuals at high risk, specifically those with left ventricular thrombi, severe left ventricular dysfunction, heart failure, or atrial fibrillation, probably will benefit from warfarin (target

INR, 2.0–3.0). The appropriate duration of anticoagulant treatment is not clear, but it should continue for at least 1 to 3 months, at which time the risk of embolism can be reassessed. In individuals at continuous risk, long-term anticoagulation therapy is indicated.

For individuals with dilated cardiomyopathy, chronic warfarin therapy should be individualized and cannot be routinely recommended. The benefits probably outweigh the risks, but no prospective data support its recommendation. The dose should be adjusted to an INR of 2.0 to 3.0. In cases of left ventricular aneurysm remote from acute infarction, the incidence of embolism is low, and chronic anticoagulant treatment probably is not necessary. It should be considered, however, for cases in whom mobile or protruding thrombi are evident on echocardiograms.

# CONCLUSIONS

The beneficial effects of acute and chronic antithrombotic therapy have been established in many cardiovascular disorders. Aspirin and heparin continue to be the mainstay, first-line agents in treatment of acute and chronic ischemic heart disease, but continued research should define the roles of newer antithrombotic agents in cardiovascular disease.

# REFERENCES

1. Steering Committee of the Physicians' Health Study Research Group. Final report on the aspirin component of the ongoing Physicians' Health Study. N Engl J Med 1989;321:129–135.
2. Steering Committee of the Physicians' Health Study Research Group. Preliminary report: findings from the aspirin component of the ongoing Physicians' Health Study. N Engl J Med 1988;318:262–264.
3. Peto R, Gray R, Collins R et al. Randomized trial of prophylactic daily aspirin in British male doctors. Br Med J 1988;296:313–316.
4. Hennekens CH, Buring JE, Sandercock P et al. Aspirin and other antiplatelet agents in the secondary and primary prevention of cardiovascular disease. Circulation 1989;80:749–756.
5. Meade TW, Mellows S, Brozovic M et al. Haemostatic function and ischaemic heart disease: principal results of the Northwick Park Heart Study. Lancet 1986;ii:533–537.
6. Meade TW, Wilkes HC, Stirling Y et al. Randomized controlled trial of low dose warfarin in the primary prevention of ischaemic heart disease in men at high risk: design and pilot study. Eur Heart J 1988;9:836–843.
7. Meade TW. Low-dose warfarin and low-dose aspirin in the primary prevention of ischemic heart disease. Am J Cardiol 1990;65(Suppl):7C–11C.
8. Meade TW, Miller GJ. Combined use of aspirin and warfarin in primary prevention of ischemic heart disease in men at high risk. Am J Cardiol 1995;75(Suppl):23B–26B.
9. Manson JE, Stampfer MJ, Colditz GA et al. A prospective study of aspirin use and primary prevention of cardiovascular disease in women. JAMA 1991;266:521–527.
10. Paganini-Hill A, Chao A, Ross RK et al. Aspirin use and chronic diseases: a cohort study of the elderly. Br Med J 1989;299:1247–1250.
11. Hammond EC, Garfinkel L. Aspirin and coronary heart disease: findings of a prospective study. Br Med J 1975;2:269–271.
12. Boston Collaborative Drug Surveillance Group. Regular aspirin intake and acute myocardial infarction. Br Med J 1974;1:440–443.
13. Fuster V, Cohen M, Halperin JL. Aspirin in the prevention of coronary disease. N Engl J Med 1989;321:183–185.
14. Cairns JA, Lewis D, Meade TW et al. Antithrombotic agents in coronary artery disease. Chest 1995;108(Suppl):380S–400S.
15. Theroux P, Ouimet H, McCans J et al. Aspirin, heparin, or both to treat acute unstable angina. N Engl J Med 1988;319:1105–1111.
16. The RISC Group. Risk of myocardial infarction and death during treatment with low dose aspirin and intravenous heparin in men with unstable coronary artery disease. Lancet 1990;336:827–830.
17. Lewis HD, Davis JW, Archibald DG et al. Protective effects of aspirin against acute myocardial infarction and death in men with unstable angina: results of a Veterans Administration Cooperative Study. N Engl J Med 1983;309:396–403.
18. Cairns JA, Gent M, Singer J et al. Aspirin, sulfinpyrazone, or both in unstable angina. N Engl J Med 1985;313:1369–1375.
19. Balsano F, Paolo P, Violi F et al. Antiplatelet treatment with ticlopidine in unstable angina. Circulation 1990;82:17–26.
20. Theroux P, Kouz S, Roy L et al. Platelet membrane receptor GP IIB/IIIa antagonism in unstable angina: the Canadian Lamifiban Study. Circulation 1996;94:899–905.
21. White HS. Late breaking clinical trials: platelet receptor inhibition for ischemic syndrome (PRISM). J Am Coll Cardiol 1997;30:2.
22. Teroux P. Late breaking clinical trials: GP IIb-IIIa antagonism with tirofoban in high-risk unstable angina Trial (PRISM-PLUS). J Am Coll Cardiol 1997;30:2.
23. Simoons M, de Boer MJ, van den Brand MJBM et al. Randomized trial of a GP IIb-IIIa platelet receptor blocker in refractory unstable angina. Circulation 1994;89:596–603.
24. Schulman SP, Goldschmidt-Clermont PJ, Navetta NC et al. Integrelin in unstable angina: a double-blind randomized trial [Abstract]. Circulation 1993;88(Suppl I):I-608.
25. Theroux P, Kleiman N, Shah PK et al. A double-blind, heparin-controlled study of MK-852 in unstable angina. Circulation 1993;88(Suppl I):I-201.
26. EPIC Investigators. Use of a monoclonal antibody directed against the platelet GP IIB/IIIa receptor in high-risk coronary angioplasty. N Engl J Med 1994;330.956–961.
27. Tcheng J, Lincoff A, Sigmon K et al. Platelet GP IIB/IIIa inhibition with integrelin during percutaneous coronary intervention: the IMPACT II trial [Abstract]. Circulation 1995;92(Suppl I):I-543.
28. Tcheng JE. Glycoprotein IIb-IIIa receptor inhibitors: putting the EPIC, IM-PACT II, RESTORE, and EPILOG trials into perspective. Am J Cardiol 1996;78:35–40.
29. Telford AM, Wilson C. Trial of heparin versus atenolol in prevention of myocardial infarction in intermediate coronary syndrome. Lancet 1981;i:1225–1228.
30. Theroux P, Waters D, Lam J et al. Reactivation of unstable angina after the discontinuation of heparin. N Engl J Med 1992;327:141–145.
31. Gurfinkel EP, Eustaquio EJ, Mejail RI et al. Low-molecular-weight heparin versus regular heparin or aspirin in the treatment of unstable angina and silent ischemia. J Am Coll Cardiol 1995;26:313–318.
32. Lidon RM, Theroux P, Juneau M et al. Initial experience with a direct antithrombin, Hirulog, in unstable angina: anticoagulant, antithrombotic, and clinical effects. Circulation 1993;99:1495–1501.
33. Fox KA. r-Hirudin in unstable angina pectoris: rationale and preliminary data from the APT pilot study. Eur Heart J 1995;16(Suppl D):28–32.
34. Sharma GV, Lapsley D, Vita JA et al. Usefulness and tolerability of Hirulog, a direct thrombin-inhibitor, in unstable angina pectoris. Am J Cardiol 1993;72:1357–1360.
35. Fuchs J, Cannon CP, and the TIMI 7 Investigators. Hirulog in the treatment of unstable angina: results of the Thrombin Inhibition in Myocardial Ischemia (TIMI) 7 Trial. Circulation 1995;92:727–733.
36. Topol EJ, Fuster V, Harrington RA et al. Recombinant hirudin for unstable angina pectoris: a multicenter, randomized angiographic trial. Circulation 1994;89:1557–1566.
37. Global Use of Strategies to Open Occluded Coronary Arteries (GUSTO) IIb Investigators. A comparison of recombinant hirudin with heparin for the treatment of acute coronary syndromes. N Engl J Med 1996;335:775–782.
38. Theroux P, Waters D, Qiu S et al. Aspirin versus heparin to prevent myocardial infarction during the acute phase of unstable angina. Circulation 1993;88:2045–2048.
39. Holdright D, Patel D, Cunningham D et al. Comparison of the effect of heparin and aspirin versus aspirin alone on transient myocardial ischemia and in-hospital prognosis in patients with unstable angina. J Am Coll Cardiol 1994;24:39–45.
40. Bodo I, Nemeth C, Littman L. Heparin and aspirin in unstable angina: insufficient sample size may lead to erroneous conclusions. J Am Coll Cardiol 1995;25:553–554.
40a. Cohen M, Adams PC, Parry G et al. Combination antithrombotic therapy in unstable rest angina and non-Q wave infarction in nonprior aspirin users. Circulation 1994;89:81–88.
41. Oler A, Whooley MA, Grady D. Adding heparin to aspirin reduces the incidence of myocardial infarction and death in patients with unstable angina: a meta-analysis. JAMA 1996;276:811–815.
42. Braunwald E, Jones RH, Mark DB et al. Diagnosing and managing unstable angina. Circulation 1994;90:613–622.
43. Fuster V, Badimon L, Cohen M et al. Insights into the pathogenesis of acute coronary syndromes. Circulation 1988;77:1213–1220.
44. ISIS-2 (Second International Study of Infarct Survival) Collaborative Group. Randomized trial of intravenous streptokinase, oral aspirin, both,

or neither among 17,187 cases of suspected acute myocardial infarction: ISIS-2. Lancet 1988;ii:349–360.

45. Report of the Working Party on Anticoagulation Therapy in Coronary Thrombosis to the Medical Research Council. Assessment of short-term anticoagulation administration after cardiac infarction. Br Med J 1969;1: 335–342.

46. Drapkin A, Merskey C. Anticoagulation therapy after acute myocardial infarction: relation of therapeutic benefit to patient's age, sex and severity of infarction. JAMA 1972;222:541–548.

47. Veterans Administration Hospital Investigators. Anticoagulants in acute myocardial infarction: results of a cooperative clinical trial. JAMA 1973; 225:724–729.

48. Chalmers TC, Matta RJ, Smith H et al. Evidence favoring the use of antico-agulants in the hospital phase of acute myocardial infarction. N Engl J Med 1977;297:1091–1096.

49. MacMahon S, Collins R, Knight C et al. Reduction in major morbidity and mortality by heparin in acute myocardial infarction. Circulation 1988; 78(Suppl 2):II-98.

50. O'Donnell CJ, Ridker PM, Hebert PR et al. Antithrombotic therapy for acute myocardial infarction. J Am Coll Cardiol 1995;25(Suppl 7):23S–29S.

51. Roux S, Christeller S, Ledin E. Effects of aspirin on coronary reocclusion and recurrent ischemia after thrombolysis: a meta-analysis. J Am Coll Cardiol 1992;19:671–677.

52. Kleiman N, Ohman M, Califf R et al. Profound inhibition of platelet aggre-gation with monoclonal antibody 7E3 Fab after thrombolytic therapy. Re-sults of the Thrombolysis and Angioplasty in Myocardial Infarction (TAMI)-8 pilot study. Circulation 1993;22:381–389.

53. Ohman E, Kleiman N, Talley J et al. Simultaneous platelet GP IIB/IIIa integrin blockade with accelerated tissue plasminogen activator in acute myocardial infarction [Abstract]. Circulation 1994;90(Suppl I):I-564.

54. Gruppo Italiano per lo Studio della Sopravvivenza nell'Infarto Miocardico. GISSI-2: a factorial randomized trial or alteplase versus streptokinase and heparin versus no heparin among 12,490 patients with acute myocardial infarction. Lancet 1990;336:65–71.

55. International Study Group. In-hospital mortality and clinical course of 20,891 patients with suspected acute myocardial infarction randomized between alteplase and streptokinase with or without heparin. Lancet 1990; 336:71–75.

56. ISIS-3 (Third International Study of Infarct Survival) Collaborative Group. ISIS-3: a randomized comparison of streptokinase vs tissue plasminogen activator vs anistreplase and of aspirin plus heparin vs aspirin alone among 41,299 cases of suspected acute myocardial infarction. Lancet 1992; 339:753–770.

57. The GUSTO Investigators. An international randomized trial comparing four thrombolytic strategies for acute myocardial infarction. N Engl J Med 1993;329:673–682.

58. The GUSTO Angiographic Investigators. The effects of tissue plasminogen activator, streptokinase, or both on coronary artery patency, ventricular function, and survival after acute myocardial infarction. N Engl J Med 1993;329:1615–1622.

59. Topol EJ, George BS, Kereiakes DJ et al. A randomized controlled trial of intravenous tissue plasminogen activator and early intravenous heparin in acute myocardial infarction. Circulation 1989;79:281–286.

60. Hsia J, Hamilton WP, Kleiman N et al. A comparison between heparin and low-dose aspirin as adjunctive therapy with tissue plasminogen acti-vator for acute myocardial infarction. N Engl J Med 1990;323:1433–1437.

61. Bleich SD, Nichols TC, Schumacher RR et al. Effect of heparin on coronary arterial patency after thrombolysis with tissue plasminogen activator in acute myocardial infarction. Am J Cardiol 1990;66:1412–1417.

62. de Bono DP, Simoons ML, Tijssen J et al. Effect of early intravenous hepa-rin on coronary patency, infarct size, and bleeding complications after alteplase thrombolysis: results of a randomized double blind European Cooperative Study Group trial. Br Heart J 1992;67:122–128.

63. Prins MH, Hirsh J. Heparin as an adjunctive treatment after thrombolytic therapy for acute myocardial infarction. Am J Cardiol 1991;67(Suppl A): 3A–11A.

64. Ridker PM, Hebert PR, Fuster V et al. Are both aspirin and heparin justi-fied as adjuncts to thrombolytic therapy for acute myocardial infarction? Lancet 1993;341:1574–1577.

65. Thompson PL, Aylward PE, Federman J et al. A randomized comparison of intravenous heparin with oral aspirin and dipyridamole 24 hours after recombinant tissue-type plasminogen activator for acute myocardial in-farction. Circulation 1991;83:1534–1542.

66. Kander NH, Holland KJ, Pitt B et al. A randomized pilot trial of brief versus prolonged heparin after successful reperfusion in acute myocardial infarction. Am J Cardiol 1990;65:139–142.

67. Mahaffey KW, Granger CB, Collins R et al. Overview of randomized trials of intravenous heparin in patients with acute myocardial infarction treated with thrombolytic therapy. Am J Cardiol 1996;77:551–556.

68. Haskel EJ, Prager NA, Sobel BE et al. Relative efficacy of antithrombin compared with antiplatelet agents in accelerating coronary thrombolytics and preventing early reocclusion. Circulation 1991;83:1048–1056.

69. Lidon RM, Theroux P, Lesperance J et al. A pilot, early angiographic pa-

tency study using a direct thrombin inhibitor as adjunctive therapy to streptokinase in acute myocardial infarction. Circulation 1994;89: 1567–1572.

70. Theroux P, Perez-Villa F, Waters D et al. Randomized double-blind com-parison of two doses of Hirulog with heparin as adjunctive therapy to streptokinase to promote early patency of the infarct-related artery in acute myocardial infarction. Circulation 1995;91:2132–2139.

71. Zeymer U, von Essen R, Tebbe U et al. Recombinant hirudin and front-loaded alteplase in acute myocardial infarction: final results of a pilot study. HIT-I (hirudin for the improvement of thrombolysis). Eur Heart J 1995;16(Suppl D):22–27.

72. Cannon CP, McCabe CH, Henry TD et al. A pilot trial of recombinant desulfatohirudin compared with heparin in conjunction with tissue-type plasminogen activator and aspirin for acute myocardial infarction: results of the Thrombolysis in Myocardial Infarction (TIMI) 5 trial. J Am Coll Cardiol 1994;23:993–1003.

73. Lee LV. Initial experience with hirudin and streptokinase in acute myocar-dial infarction: results of the Thrombolysis in Myocardial Infarction (TIMI) 6 trial. Am J Cardiol 1995;75:7–13.

74. Global Use of Strategies to Open Occluded Coronary Arteries (GUSTO) IIa Investigators. Randomized trial of intravenous heparin versus recombi-nant hirudin for acute coronary syndromes. Circulation 1994;90: 1631–1637.

75. Neuhaus KL, von Essen R, Tebbe U et al. Safety observations from the pilot phase of the randomized r-Hirudin for improvement of thrombolysis (HIT-III) study. Circulation 1994;90:1638–1642.

76. Antman EM, for the TIMI 9B Investigators. Hirudin in acute myocardial infarction: Thrombolysis and Thrombin Inhibition in Myocardial Infarc-tion (TIMI) 9B Trial. Circulation 1996;94:911–921.

77. Ryan TJ, Anderson JL, Antman EM et al. ACC/AHA guidelines for the management of patients with acute myocardial infarction. A report of the American College of Cardiology/American Heart Association Task Force on Practice Guidelines (Committee on Management of Acute Myocardial Infarction). J Am Coll Cardiol 1996;28:1328–1428.

78. Roberts WC, Buja LM. The frequency and significance of coronary arterial thrombi and other observations in fatal acute myocardial infarction: a study of 107 necropsy patients. Am J Med 1972;52:425–443.

79. Bini A, Fenoglio JJ Jr, Mesa-Tejada R et al. Identification and distribution of fibrinogen, fibrin, and fibrin(ogen) degradation products in atheroscle-rosis. Use of monoclonal antibodies. Arteriosclerosis 1989;9:109–121.

80. Chesebro J, Webster M, Smith H et al. Antiplatelet therapy in coronary disease progression: reduced infarction and new lesion formation [Ab-stract]. Circulation 1989;880(Suppl II):II-266.

81. Ridker PM, Manson JE, Gaziano JM et al. Low-dose aspirin therapy for chronic stable angina. A randomized, placebo-controlled clinical trial. Ann Intern Med 1991;114:835–839.

82. Juul-Moller S, Edvardsson N, Jahnmatz B et al. Double-blind trial of aspi-rin in primary prevention of myocardial infarction in patients with stable chronic angina pectoris. The Swedish Angina Pectoris Aspirin Trial (SAPAT) Group. Lancet 1992;340:1421–1425.

83. Elwood PC, Cochrane AL, Burr ML et al. A randomized controlled trial of acetyl salicylic acid in the secondary prevention of mortality from myo-cardial infarction. Br Med J 1974;1:436–440.

84. Elwood PC, Sweetnam PM. Aspirin and secondary mortality after myocar-dial infarction. Lancet 1979;ii:1313–1315.

85. The Coronary Drug Project Research Group. Aspirin in coronary heart disease. J Chronic Dis 1976;29:625–642.

86. Breddin K, Loew D, Lechner K et al. The German-Austrian aspirin trial: a comparison of acetylsalicylic acid, placebo and phenprocoumon in sec-ondary prevention of myocardial infarction. Circulation 1980;62:V63–V72.

87. The Persantine-Aspirin Reinfarction Study Research Group. Persantine and aspirin in coronary heart disease. Circulation 1980;62:449–461.

88. Klimt CR, Knatterud GL, Stamler J et al. Persantine-Aspirin Reinfarction Study. Part II. Secondary coronary prevention with persantine and aspirin. J Am Coll Cardiol 1986;7:251–269.

89. The Aspirin Myocardial Infarction Study Group. The aspirin myocardial infarction study: final results. Circulation 1980;62:V79–84.

90. Antiplatelet Trialists' Collaboration. Collaborative overview of random-ized trials of antiplatelet therapy—I: prevention of death, myocardial in-farction, and stroke by prolonged antiplatelet therapy in various categories of patients. Br Med J 1994;308:81–106.

91. The Anturane Reinfarction Trial Research Group. Sulfinpyrazone in the prevention of sudden death after myocardial infarction. N Engl J Med 1980;302:250–256.

92. Report from the Anturan Reinfarction Italian Study. Sulphinpyrazone in post-myocardial infarction. Lancet 1982;i:237–242.

93. Working Party on Anticoagulant Therapy in Coronary Thrombosis to the Medical Research Council. An assessment of long-term anticoagulant ad-ministration after cardiac infarction: second report. Br Med J 1964;2: 837–843.

94. Ebert RV. Long-term anticoagulant therapy after myocardial infarction. Final report of the Veterans Administration Cooperative Study. JAMA 1969;207:2263–2267.

95. Smith P, Arnesen H, Holme I. The effect of warfarin on mortality and reinfarction after myocardial infarction. N Engl J Med 1990;323:147–152.

96. Anticoagulants in the Secondary Prevention of Events in Coronary Thrombosis (ASPECT) Research Group. Effect of long-term oral anticoagulant treatment on mortality and cardiovascular morbidity after myocardial infarction. Lancet 1994;343:499–503.

97. The EPISM Research Group. A controlled comparison of aspirin and oral anticoagulants in prevention of death after myocardial infarction. N Engl J Med 1982;307:701–708.

98. Report of the Sixty Plus Reinfarction Study Research Group. A double-blind trial to assess long-term oral anticoagulant therapy in elderly patients after myocardial infarction. Lancet 1980;ii:989–994.

99. Neri Serneri GG, Rovelli F, Gensini GF et al. Effectiveness of low-dose heparin in prevention of myocardial reinfarction. Lancet 1987;i:937–942.

100. Bittl JA. Medical progress—advances in coronary angioplasty. N Engl J Med 1996;335:1290–1302.

101. Schwartz L, Bourassa MG, Lesperance J et al. Aspirin and dipyridamole in the prevention of restenosis after percutaneous transluminal coronary angioplasty. N Engl J Med 1988;318:1714–1719.

102. White C, Chaitman B, Lassar TA et al. Antiplatelet agents are effective in reducing the immediate complications of PTCA: Results from the ticlopidine multicenter trial [Abstract]. Circulation 1987;76(Suppl IV):IV-400.

103. Bertrand M, Allain H, Lablanche J. Results of a randomized trial of ticlopidine versus placebo for prevention of acute closure and restenosis after coronary angioplasty. The TACT study [Abstract]. Circulation 1990;82(Suppl III):III-90.

104. Chesebro J, Webster M, Lassar T et al. Coronary angioplasty: antiplatelet therapy reduces acute complications but not restenosis [Abstract]. Circulation 1989;82(Suppl II):II-64.

105. Lembo NJ, Black AJ, Roubin GS et al. Effect of pretreatment with aspirin versus aspirin plus dipyridamole on frequency and type of acute complications of percutaneous transluminal coronary angioplasty. Am J Cardiol 1990;65:422–426.

106. The EPILOG Investigators. Platelet glycoprotein IIb-IIIa receptor blockade and low-dose heparin during percutaneous coronary revascularization. N Engl J Med 1997;336:1689–1696.

107. Charo IF, Bekeart LS, Phillips DR. Platelet glycoprotein IIb-IIIa-like proteins mediate endothelial cell attachment to adhesive proteins and the extracellular matrix. J Biol Chem 1987;262:9935–9938.

108. Heras M, Chesebro JH, Penny WJ et al. Importance of adequate heparin dosage in arterial angioplasty in a porcine model. Circulation 1988;78:654–660.

109. McGarry TF Jr, Gottlieb RS, Morganroth J et al. The relationship of anticoagulation level and complications after successful percutaneous transluminal coronary angioplasty. Am Heart J 1992;123:1445–1451.

110. Ferguson JJ, Dougherty KG, Gaos CM et al. Relation between procedural activated coagulation time and outcome after percutaneous transluminal coronary angioplasty. J Am Coll Cardiol 1994;23:1061–1065.

111. Narins CR, Hillegass WB Jr, Nelson CL et al. Relation between activated clotting time during angioplasty and abrupt closure. Circulation 1996;93:667–671.

112. Eitzman DT, Chi L, Saggin L et al. Heparin neutralization by platelet-rich thrombi. Role of platelet factor 4. Circulation 1994;89:1523–1529.

113. Weitz JI, Hudoba M, Massel D et al. Clot-bound thrombin is protected from inhibition by heparin-antithrombin III but is susceptible to inactivation by antithrombin III-independent inhibitors. J Clin Inv 1990;86:385–391.

114. Serruys PW, Herrman JP, Simon R et al. A comparison of hirudin with heparin in the prevention of restenosis after coronary angioplasty. Helvetica Investigators. N Engl J Med 1995;333:757–763.

115. Bittl JA, Strony J, Brinker JA et al. Treatment with bivalirudin (Hirulog) as compared with heparin during coronary angioplasty for unstable or postinfarction angina. Hirulog Angioplasty Study Investigators. N Engl J Med 1995;333:764–769.

116. The GUSTO IIB Angiographic Substudy Investigators. A clinical trial comparing primary coronary angioplasty with tissue plasminogen activator for acute myocardial infarction. N Engl J Med 1997;336:1621–1628.

117. Ali MN, Villarreal-Levy G, Schafer AI. The role of thrombin and thrombin inhibitors in coronary angioplasty. Chest 1995;108:1409–1419.

118. Serruys PW, de Jaegere P, Kiemeneij F et al. A comparison of balloon-expandable-stent implantation with balloon angioplasty in patients with coronary artery disease. Benestent Study Group. N Engl J Med 1994;331:489–495.

119. Hall P, Nakamura S, Maiello L et al. A randomized comparison of combined ticlopidine and aspirin therapy versus aspirin therapy alone after successful intravascular ultrasound-guided stent implantation. Circulation 1996;93:215–222.

120. Schomig A, Neumann FJ, Kastrati A et al. A randomized comparison of antiplatelet and anticoagulant therapy after the placement of coronary-artery stents. N Engl J Med 1996;334:1084–1089.

121. Leon M, Baim D, Gordon P et al. Clinical and angiographic results from the Stent Anticoagulant Regimen Study (STARS) [Abstract]. Circulation 1996;96(Suppl I):I-685.

122. Schomig A, Neumann FJ, Walter H et al. Coronary stent placement in patients with acute myocardial infarction: comparison of clinical and angiographic outcome after randomization to antiplatelet or anticoagulant therapy. J Am Coll Cardiol 1997;29:28–34.

123. Serruys PW, Emanuelsson H, van der Giessen W et al. Heparin-coated Palmaz-Schatz stents in human coronary arteries. Early outcome of the Benestent-II Pilot Study. Circulation 1996;93:412–422.

124. Schwartz RS, Holmes DR Jr., Topol EJ. The restenosis paradigm revisited: an alternative proposal for cellular mechanisms. J Am Coll Cardiol 1992;20:1284–1293.

125. Mintz GS, Popma JJ, Hong MK et al. Intravascular ultrasound to discern device-specific effects and mechanisms of restenosis. Am J Cardiol 1996;78:18–22.

126. Mintz GS, Popma JJ, Pichard AD et al. Intravascular ultrasound predictors of restenosis after percutaneous transcatheter coronary revascularization. J Am Coll Cardiol 1996;27:1678–1687.

127. White C, Knudson M, Schmidt D et al. Neither ticlopidine nor aspirin-dipyridamole prevents restenosis post PTCA: results from a randomized placebo-controlled multicenter trial [Abstract]. Circulation 1987;76(Suppl IV):IV-213.

128. Ellis SG, Roubin GS, Wilentz J et al. Effect of 18- to 24-hour heparin administration for prevention of restenosis after uncomplicated coronary angioplasty. Am Heart J 1989;117:777–782.

129. Topol EJ, Califf RM, Weisman HF et al. Randomized trial of coronary intervention with antibody against platelet IIb-IIIa integrin for reduction of clinical restenosis: results at six months. The EPIC Investigators. Lancet 1994;343:881–886.

130. Raizner A, Hollman J, Abukhalil J et al. Ciprostene for restenosis revisited: Quantitative analysis of angiograms. J Am Coll Cardiol 1993;21(Suppl A):321A.

131. Knudtson ML, Flintoft VF, Roth DL et al. Effect of short-term prostacyclin administration on restenosis after percutaneous transluminal coronary angioplasty. J Am Coll Cardiol 1990;15:691–697.

132. Hanke H, Oberhoff M, Hanke S et al. Inhibition of cellular proliferation after experimental balloon angioplasty by low-molecular-weight heparin. Circulation 1992;85:1548–1556.

133. Sarembock IJ, Gertz SD, Gimple LW et al. Effectiveness of recombinant desulphatohirudin in reducing restenosis after balloon angioplasty of atherosclerotic femoral arteries in rabbits. Circulation 1991;84:232–243.

134. Faxon DP, Spiro TE, Minor S et al. Low-molecular-weight heparin in prevention of restenosis after angioplasty. Results of Enoxaparin Restenosis (ERA) Trial. Circulation 1994;90:908–914.

135. Dehmer GJ, Popma JJ, van den Berg EK et al. Reduction in the rate of early restenosis after coronary angioplasty by a diet supplemented with n-3 fatty acids. N Engl J Med 1988;319:733–740.

136. Bairati I, Roy L, Meyer F. Double-blind, randomized, controlled trial of fish oil supplements in prevention of recurrence of stenosis after coronary angioplasty. Circulation 1992;85:950–956.

137. Grigg LE, Kay TW, Valentine PA et al. Determinants of restenosis and lack of effect of dietary supplementation with eicosapentaenoic acid on the incidence of coronary artery restenosis after angioplasty. J Am Coll Cardiol 1989;13:665–672.

138. Reis GJ, Boucher TM, Sipperly ME et al. Randomized trial of fish oil for prevention of restenosis after coronary angioplasty. Lancet 1989;ii:177–181.

139. Leaf A, Jorgensen MB, Jacobs AK et al. Do fish oils prevent restenosis after coronary angioplasty? Circulation 1994;90:2248–2257.

140. Fuster V, Chesebro JH. Role of platelets and platelet inhibitors in aortocoronary artery vein-graft disease. Circulation 1986;73:227–232.

141. Sanz G, Pajaron A, Alegria E et al. Prevention of early aortocoronary bypass occlusion by low-dose aspirin and dipyridamole. Grupo Espanol para el Seguimiento del Injerto Coronario (GESIC). Circulation 1990;82:765–773.

142. Goldman S, Copeland J, Moritz T et al. Improvement in early saphenous vein graft patency after coronary artery bypass surgery with antiplatelet therapy: results of a Veterans Administration Cooperative Study. Circulation 1988;77:1324–1332.

143. Goldman S, Copeland J, Moritz T et al. Saphenous vein graft patency 1 year after coronary artery bypass surgery and effects of antiplatelet therapy. Results of a Veterans Administration Cooperative Study. Circulation 1989;80:1190–1197.

144. Gavaghan TP, Gebski V, Baron DW. Immediate postoperative aspirin improves vein graft patency early and late after coronary artery bypass graft surgery. A placebo-controlled, randomized study. Circulation 1991;83:1526–1533.

145. Rajah SM, Nair U, Rees M et al. Effects of antiplatelet therapy with indobufen or aspirin-dipyridamole on graft patency one year after coronary artery bypass grafting. J Thorac Cardiovasc Surg 1994;107:1146–1153.

146. Limet R, David JL, Magotteaux P et al. Prevention of aorta-coronary bypass graft occlusion. Beneficial effect of ticlopidine on early and late patency rates of venous coronary bypass grafts: a double-blind study. J Thorac Cardiovasc Surg 1987;94:773–783.

147. Chesebro JH, Clements IP, Fuster V et al. A platelet-inhibitor-drug trial

in coronary-artery bypass operations: benefit of perioperative dipyridamole and aspirin therapy on early postoperative vein-graft patency. N Engl J Med 1982;307:73–78.

148. Chesebro JH, Fuster V, Elveback LR et al. Effect of dipyridamole and aspirin on late vein-graft patency after coronary bypass operations. N Engl J Med 1984;310:209–214.

149. Baur HR, VanTassel RA, Pierach CA et al. Effects of sulfinpyrazone on early graft closure after myocardial revascularization. Am J Cardiol 1982; 49:420–424.

150. van der Meer J, Hillege HL, Kootstra GJ et al. Prevention of one-year vein-graft occlusion after aortocoronary-bypass surgery: a comparison of low-dose aspirin, low-dose aspirin plus dipyridamole, and oral anticoagulants. The CABADAS Research Group of the Interuniversity Cardiology Institute of the Netherlands. Lancet 1993;342:257–264.

151. van der Meer J, Brutel de la Riviere A et al. Effects of low dose aspirin (50 mg/day), low dose aspirin plus dipyridamole, and oral anticoagulant agents after internal mammary artery bypass grafting: patency and clinical outcome at 1 year. CABADAS Research Group of the Interuniversity Cardiology Institute of the Netherlands. Prevention of Coronary Artery Bypass Graft Occlusion by Aspirin, Dipyridamole and Acenocoumarol/Phenprocoumon Study. J Am Coll Cardiol 1994;24:1181–1188.

152. Brooks N, Wright J, Sturridge M et al. Randomized placebo controlled trial of aspirin and dipyridamole in the prevention of coronary vein graft occlusion. Br Heart J 1985;53:201–207.

153. Brown BG, Cukingnan RA, DeRouen T et al. Improved graft patency in patients treated with platelet-inhibiting therapy after coronary bypass surgery. Circulation 1985;72:138–146.

154. McEnany MT, Salzman EW, Mundth ED et al. The effect of antithrombotic therapy on patency rates of saphenous vein coronary artery bypass grafts. J Thorac Cardiovasc Surg 1982;83:81–89.

155. Pantely GA, Goodnight SH, Jr., Rahimtoola SH et al. Failure of antiplatelet and anticoagulant therapy to improve patency of grafts after coronary-artery bypass: a controlled, randomized study. N Engl J Med 1979;301: 962–966.

156. Josa M, Lie JT, Bianco RL, Kaye MP. Reduction of thrombosis in canine coronary bypass vein grafts with dipyridamole and aspirin. Am J Cardiol 1981;47:1248–1254.

157. Ekestrom SA, Gunnes S, Brodin UB. Effect of dipyridamole (Persantine) on blood flow and patency of aortocoronary vein bypass grafts. Scandinavian J Thor Cardiovasc Surg 1990;24:191–196.

158. Goldman S, Copeland J, Moritz T et al. Starting aspirin therapy after operation. Effects on early graft patency. Department of Veterans Affairs Cooperative Study Group. Circulation 1991;84:520–526.

159. Solymoss B, Nadeau P, Millette D et al. Late thrombosis of saphenous vein coronary bypass grafts related to risk factors. Circulation 1988; 78(Suppl I):I-140–I-143.

160. Pfisterer M, Burkart F, Jockers G et al. Trial of low-dose aspirin plus dipyridamole versus anticoagulants for prevention of aortocoronary vein graft occlusion. Lancet 1989;ii:1–7.

161. Pfisterer M, Burkart F, Jockers G et al. Prevention of aortocoronary vein bypass graft occlusion: which antithrombotic treatment and for how long? Thromb Res 1990;(Suppl 12):11–21.

162. Goldman S, Copeland J, Moritz T et al. Long-term graft patency (3 years) after coronary artery surgery. Effects of aspirin: results of a VA Cooperative study. Circulation 1994;89:1138–1143.

163. Keren A, Goldberg S, Gottlieb S et al. Natural history of left ventricular thrombi: their appearance and resolution in the posthospitalization period of acute myocardial infarction. J Am Coll Cardiol 1990;15:790–800.

164. Meltzer RS, Visser CA, Fuster V. Intracardiac thrombi and systemic embolization. Ann Intern Med 1986;104:689–698.

165. Nihoyannopoulos P, Smith GC, Maseri A et al. The natural history of left ventricular thrombus in myocardial infarction: a rationale in support of masterly inactivity. J Am Coll Cardiol 1989;14:903–911.

166. Kupper AJ, Verheugt FW, Peels CH et al. Left ventricular thrombus incidence and behavior studied by serial two-dimensional echocardiography in acute anterior myocardial infarction: left ventricular wall motion, systemic embolism and oral anticoagulation. J Am Coll Cardiol 1989;13: 1514–1520.

167. Nordrehaug JE, Johannessen KA, von der Lippe G. Usefulness of high-dose anticoagulants in preventing left ventricular thrombus in acute myocardial infarction. Am J Cardiol 1985;55:1491–1493.

168. Davis MJ, Ireland MA. Effect of early anticoagulation on the frequency of left ventricular thrombus after anterior wall acute myocardial infarction. Am J Cardiol 1986;57:1244–1247.

169. Gueret P, Dubourg O, Ferrier A et al. Effects of full-dose heparin anticoagulation on the development of left ventricular thrombosis in acute transmural myocardial infarction. J Am Coll Cardiol 1986;8:419–426.

170. Arvan S, Boscha K. Prophylactic anticoagulation for left ventricular thrombi after acute myocardial infarction: a prospective randomized trial. Am Heart J 1987;113:688–693.

171. Turpie AG, Robinson JG, Doyle DJ et al. Comparison of high-dose with low-dose subcutaneous heparin to prevent left ventricular mural thrombosis in patients with acute transmural anterior myocardial infarction. N Engl J Med 1989;320:352–357.

172. The SCATI (Studio sulla Calciparina nell'Angina e nella Trombosi Ventricolare nell'Infarto) Group. Randomized controlled trial of subcutaneous calcium-heparin in acute myocardial infarction. Lancet 1989;ii:182–186.

173. Marino P, Zanolla L, Zardini P. Effect of streptokinase on left ventricular modeling and function after myocardial infarction: the GISSI (Gruppo Italiano per lo Studio della Streptochinasi nell'Infarto Miocardico) Trial. J Am Coll Cardiol 1989;14:1149–1158.

174. Pizzetti G, Belotti G, Margonato A et al. Thrombolytic therapy reduces the incidence of left ventricular thrombus after anterior myocardial infarction. Relationship to vessel patency and infarct size. Eur Heart J 1996;17: 421–428.

175. Stratton JR, Nemanich JW, Johannessen KA et al. Fate of left ventricular thrombi in patients with remote myocardial infarction or idiopathic cardiomyopathy. Circulation 1988;78:1388–1393.

176. Kouvaras G, Chronopoulos G, Soufras G et al. The effects of long-term antithrombotic treatment on left ventricular thrombi in individuals after an acute myocardial infarction. Am Heart J 1990;119:73–78.

177. Roberts WC, Siegel RJ, McManus BM. Idiopathic dilated cardiomyopathy: analysis of 152 necropsy patients. Am J Cardiol 1987;60:1340–1355.

178. Falk RH, Foster E, Coats MH. Ventricular thrombi and thromboembolism in dilated cardiomyopathy: a prospective follow-up study. Am Heart J 1992;123:136–142.

179. Vigna C, Russo A, De Rito V et al. Frequency of left atrial thrombi by transesophageal echocardiography in idiopathic and in ischemic dilated cardiomyopathy. Am J Cardiol 1992;70:1500–1501.

180. Fuster V, Gersh BJ, Giuliani ER et al. The natural history of idiopathic dilated cardiomyopathy. Am J Cardiol 1981;47:525–531.

181. Lapeyre AC III, Steele PM, Kazmier FJ et al. Systemic embolism in chronic left ventricular aneurysm: incidence and the role of anticoagulation. J Am Coll Cardiol 1985;6:534–538.

182. Cabin HS, Roberts WC. Left ventricular aneurysm, intraaneurysmal thrombus and systemic embolus in coronary heart disease. Chest 1980;77: 586–590.

183. Stratton JR, Resnick AD. Increased embolic risk in patients with left ventricular thrombi. Circulation 1987;75:1004–1011.

# CHAPTER 60

# ANTICOAGULANTS IN ATRIAL FIBRILLATION

## Michael D. Ezekowitz, Ira S. Cohen, and Charles S. Gornick

Many controversies regarding use of anticoagulation in individuals with atrial fibrillation have been resolved by the results of seven randomized trials. These include five primary prevention trials (1–5), one secondary prevention trial (6), and the Stroke Prevention in Atrial Fibrillation Study (SPAF) III trial, which compared warfarin to warfarin combined with aspirin (7). A pooled analysis of the placebo-controlled, primary prevention trials defined subgroups of individuals at low and at high risk of stroke (8). This chapter discusses the approach to individuals with nonvalvular atrial fibrillation as well as to those with atrial fibrillation in association with rheumatic, congenital, and thyrotoxic heart disease.

## PREVALENCE AND SIGNIFICANCE AS A RISK FACTOR FOR EMBOLIC DISEASE

Atrial fibrillation occurs in only a fraction of a percent of the total population younger than 50 years (9) (Fig. 60.1). In Western countries, it usually occurs as an isolated phenomenon, without predisposing structural heart disease, hypertension, or diabetes. These individuals are termed *lone atrial fibrillators* and are at low risk for systemic embolism (10). Because nonrheumatic atrial fibrillation is a common condition in elderly individuals, however, care must be taken to exclude subclinical cardiac disease in this group. In the sixth decade of life, the prevalence of atrial fibrillation is approximately 3.8% for males and somewhat lower for females; in the seventh decade, the prevalence is estimated to be as high as 9% of the population (11). In a Minnesota community-based study, 16.1% of men and 12.2% of women older than 75 years had atrial fibrillation (12), which is a marker for both a higher incidence of stroke (more than five times that of comparable individuals in sinus rhythm) (13) and increased mortality (14). In addition to the associated embolic risk, the higher mortality probably relates to the underlying heart disease (15) and the potential proarrhythmic effect of some drugs used to maintain sinus rhythm (16).

The prevalence of atrial fibrillation should increase as the general population ages. Thus, the importance of atrial fibrillation as a source of systemic embolization and resultant cerebral infarction probably also will increase unless appropriate therapy is instituted. With better recognition and treatment of hypertension, which is the major risk factor for stroke, nonrheumatic atrial fibrillation eventually may become the most important etiologic factor for stroke in an aging population (17).

## ETIOLOGY

### ELECTROPHYSIOLOGIC CONSIDERATIONS

It has long been postulated that reentry is the underlying mechanism of atrial fibrillation (18). Generated by multiple wavelets of activation (19), reentry is affected by tissue mass, refractory periods, and conduction velocity. Other factors such as stretch (20), autonomic stimulation (21), and additional modulating influences also can affect the electrophysiologic properties of the atrium.

More recently, investigators using atrial-mapping studies have identified multiple intraatrial reentrant circuits, which form the pathophysiologic basis of the arrhythmia. Reentry is random, with individual wavelets lasting only a few hundred milliseconds (22).

In most cases, atrial fibrillation results from an initiating atrial premature beat (again supporting the role of reentry). Less commonly, retrograde conduction of a premature ventricular beat conducted into the atrium, or slowing of the rate of impulse generation within the sinus node, facilitates escape of ectopic atrial foci, which may precipitate the arrhythmia (18).

## ASSOCIATED CLINICAL CONDITIONS

An important minority of individuals has a predisposing cause for atrial fibrillation that is directly treatable. The most common of these are thyrotoxicosis, acute coronary ischemic syndromes, pulmonary embolism, acute hypoxia related to exacerbations of chronic pulmonary disease, acute cardiac decompensation, poorly controlled hypertension, and the use of drugs such as bronchodilators (Table 60.1). Individuals with mitral valve disease may revert to sinus rhythm after valve replacement or repair because of decreased left atrial size and hemodynamic improvement. The incidence of atrial fibrillation after cardiac surgery is high (30–60%), with a peak incidence from 2 to 4 days after operation (23). Fortunately, atrial fibrillation often is self-limiting in this setting, but it can prolong the length of hospital stay and morbidity. Age and discontinued β-blocker therapy after surgery are predisposing risk factors. Prophylactic treatment with β-blockers has been successfully used in this setting (24).

Hyperthyroidism should always be considered in individuals with atrial fibrillation without apparent underlying cardiac cause. This is especially true if the ventricular rate during the arrhythmia is rapid (25), difficult to control pharmacologically, or both.

Atrial fibrillation may occur as a chronic or a transient and recurring (i.e., paroxysmal) arrhythmia. In some individuals, paroxysmal atrial fibrillation is associated with the tachycardia-bradycardia (i.e., "sick sinus") syndrome (26). The transition from paroxysmal to chronic atrial fibrillation varies considerably, and it probably depends on the underlying cause of the atrial fibrillation itself. Takahashi et al (27) followed 94 individuals with paroxysmal atrial fibrillation. In 54.3% of these individuals, underlying hypertension, coronary artery disease, or both were present. Over a period of 1 year, 25% developed chronic atrial fibrillation.

Recently, three families from the same region in northern Spain were identified (28), in which 21 of 49 members have atrial fibrillation. Comparison of pooled DNA from those affected and those unaffected showed a molecular defect on chromosome 10q in the affected individuals. This is the first evidence of a potential genetic predisposition to atrial fibrillation.

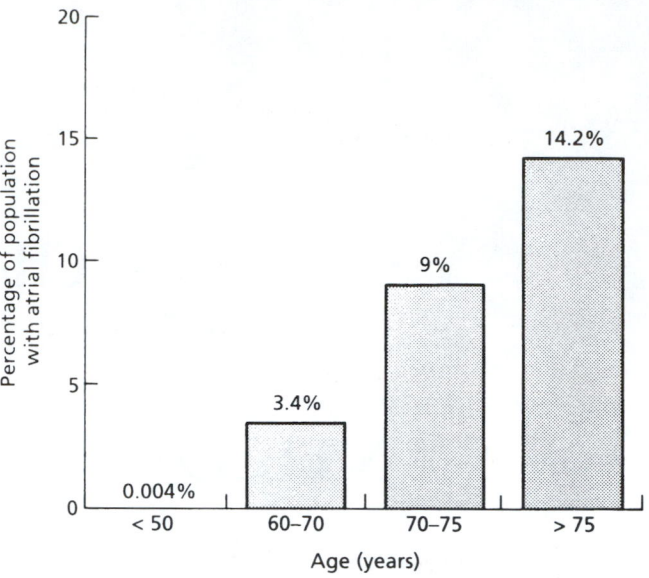

**FIGURE 60.1.**    Prevalence of atrial fibrillation by age.

**TABLE 60.1.    Conditions Associated with Atrial Fibrillation**

Age
Alcohol
Cardiac surgery
Cardiomyopathy
Cerebrovascular accident
Chronic pulmonary disease
Congenital heart disease
Electrocution
Electrolyte abnormalities
Emotional lability
Fever
Hypertension
Hypothermia
Hypovolemia
Ischemic heart disease (acute or chronic)
Lipomatous hypertrophy
Pericarditis
Preexcitation syndromes
Pregnancy
Swallowing
Tachycardia–bradycardia ("sick sinus") syndrome
Thyrotoxicosis
Trauma
Tumors
Valvular heart disease
Ventricular hypertrophy
Ventricular pacing

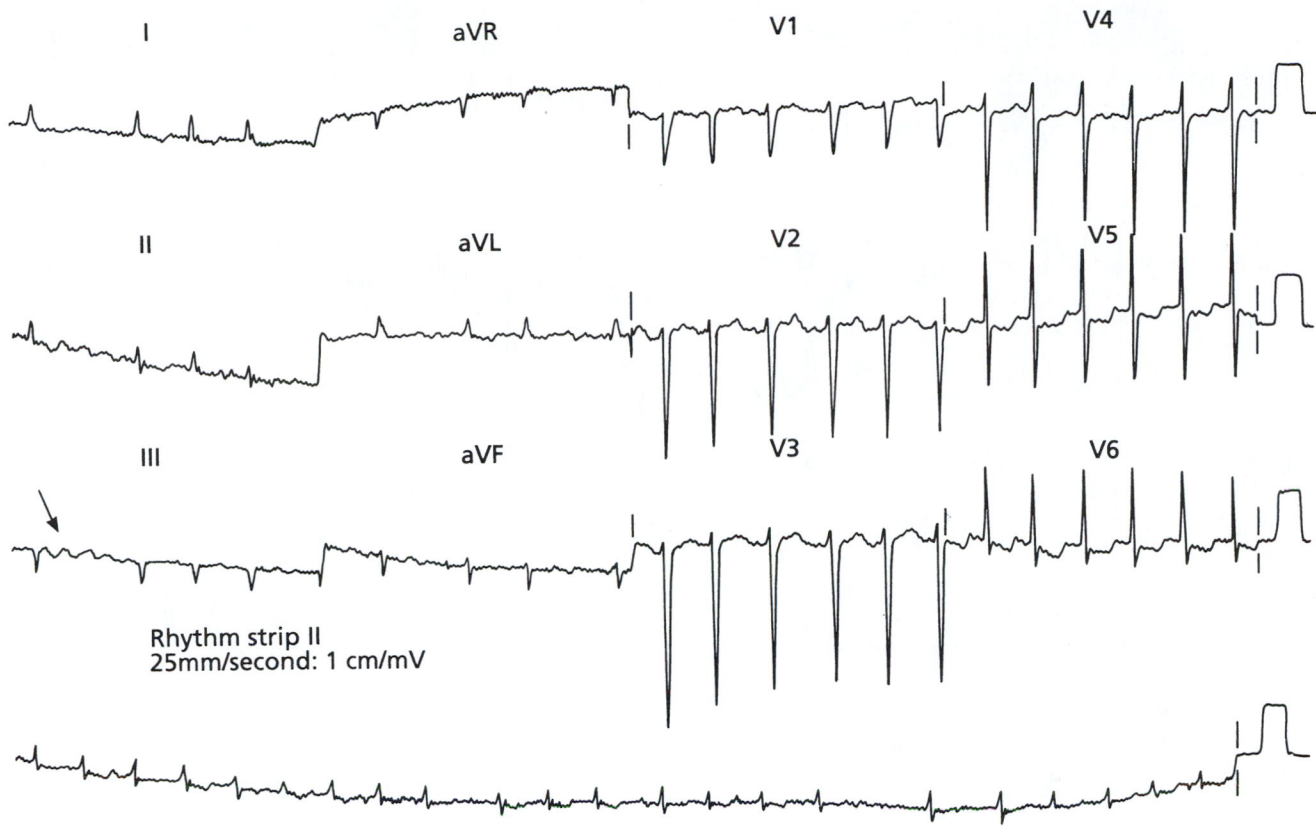

**FIGURE 60.2.**   Twelve-lead electrocardiogram demonstrating typical atrial fibrillation. The atria in individuals with atrial fibrillation are activated simultaneously in multiple areas, with impulses following a variety of routes. Consequently, the surface electrocardiogram demonstrates a markedly irregular and low-amplitude baseline. The arrow indicates a typical fibrillatory or "f" wave.

# DIAGNOSIS

The typical electrocardiogram (ECG) during atrial fibrillation shows the classic "irregularly irregular" ventricular rhythm superimposed on a baseline ranging from, essentially, a flat line to a "coarse," fibrillatory pattern as well as all the possible variants between these extremes (Fig. 60.2). The irregularity and rapidity of atrial stimuli reaching the atrioventricular (AV) node during atrial fibrillation results in variable penetrance of each and an irregularly irregular ventricular response. Most impulses do not reach the ventricles. Thus, the ventricular rate is slower than would be anticipated on the basis of the atrial rate (17).

During atrial fibrillation, intracardiac recordings are characterized by marked beat-to-beat variations in the atrial rate and impulse morphology. In some instances, the recordings can be discrete, with isoelectric baselines between deflections. In others, even including those in the same individual taken at different times, the intervening baseline can be chaotic, thus suggesting more rapid and disordered electrical activity. Differences in intracardiac recordings during atrial fibrillation may not be clinically significant, but they may be indicators of different factors affecting the substrate of the arrhythmia (16).

In individuals with preexcitation (e.g., Wolff-Parkinson-White syndrome), a pathway, or pathways, to the ventricles other than the AV node is present, with a shorter refractory period. In such individuals, rapid ventricular rates can occur. On the surface ECG, the QRS complexes can appear to be wide and bizarre because of the fusion of ventricular activation by antegrade conduction over one or more accessory connections and the AV node (Fig. 60.3). With this alternative pathway bypassing the "gating" function of the AV node, the "R-on-T" response can occur and, rarely, cause ventricular fibrillation and sudden cardiac death (22).

# CARDIOVERSION

## PREDICTORS OF SUCCESSFUL CARDIOVERSION

Echocardiographically determined left atrial size has been proposed as a predictor for successful long-term maintenance of sinus rhythm after cardioversion of

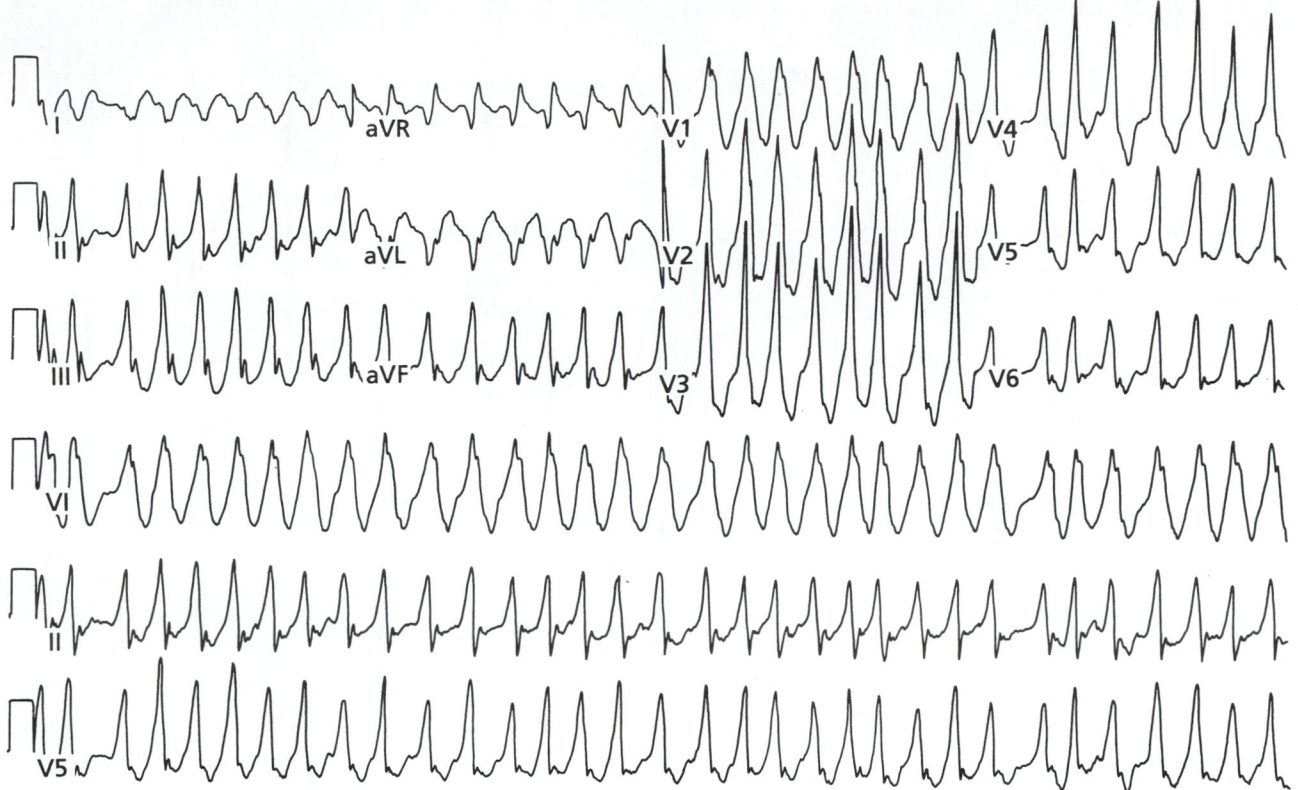

**FIGURE 60.3.**    Twelve-lead electrocardiogram demonstrating wide, bizarre QRS complexes during atrial fibrillation in a individual location with an accessory atrioventricular connection (in a left lateral location).

atrial fibrillation. Its reliability, however, has been controversial (29–32). Henry et al (29), using single-plane M-mode measurements of the left atrium in individuals with mitral, aortic, or hypertrophic disease, concluded that if left atrial size was greater than 4.5 cm, maintenance of sinus rhythm was unlikely at 6 months after cardioversion, with 75% of their individuals successfully cardioverted during atrial fibrillation. Other investigators (30) found that individuals with "lone atrial fibrillation" and a left atrial size greater than 4.5 cm were at increased risk for recurrence at 1 month after cardioversion, and Ewy et al (31) found that left atrial size predicted successful medical and electrical conversion.

A retrospective analysis by Dittrich et al (32) failed to show any predictive value for left atrial size on M-mode echocardiograms, for atrial dimensions on two-dimensional echocardiograms, or for either initial success or maintenance of sinus rhythm at 6 months. The best predictor for maintenance of sinus rhythm at 1 and 6 months, but not for successful cardioversion, was the prior duration of atrial fibrillation. Until the controversy is resolved, echocardiographically determined left atrial size should not be the sole criterion for attempted cardioversion. Cardioversion is unlikely to be successful if fibrillation has been present for 1 year or longer, and

this probably results from structural changes in the atria that have developed by that time.

## Methods of Cardioversion

Acute cardioversion can be achieved either pharmacologically (Fig. 60.2) or electrically. Electrical cardioversion is preferred if the individual is not stable (17). Intravenously administered ibutilide fumarate is a rapid (≤60 minutes of infusion) means of chemically cardioverting individuals with atrial fibrillation, with a conversion rate of approximately 50% (33).

A major consideration in treatment of atrial fibrillation is the proarrhythmic effects of certain pharmacologic agents used to maintain individuals in sinus rhythm. The clinical significance of these proarrhythmic properties is not known with certainty, but evidence suggests these drugs might pose a risk for death. A meta-analysis of studies using quinidine for control of atrial fibrillation demonstrated an increased mortality rate in the quinidine-treatment groups (16). Had there been one fewer death in the quinidine group, however, the mortality rate would not have been statistically different between groups. Results from several trials of antiarrhythmic drugs in individuals with atrial fibrillation suggest a proarrhythmic prevalence rate of between

**TABLE 60.2.** Dosage and Therapeutic Levels for Antiarrhythmic Drugs

| Drug | Oral Dose (mg) | Therapeutic Level (mg/ml) | Major Elimination Route | Primary Side Effects |
|------|----------------|---------------------------|-------------------------|----------------------|
| Amiodarone | 200–400 qd | 0.5–1.5 | Renal | Photosensitivity, liver/lung toxicity, thyroid abnormalities |
| Disopyramide | 200–400 q6–8 hours | 2–5 | Renal | Urinary retention, dry mouth, congestive failure |
| Ethmozine[a] | 200–300 q8 hours | — | Hepatic | CNS symptoms, GI upset, conduction disturbances |
| Flecainide | 100–200 q12 hours | 0.2–1.0 | Hepatic | Proarrhythmia, CNS symptoms |
| Procainamide | 750–1250 q6 hours | 4–10 | Renal | Lupus syndrome, GI upset |
| Propafenone | 150–300 q8–12 hours | 0.2–3.0 | Hepatic | Dysgensia, GI upset, conduction disturbances, CNS symptoms |
| Quinidine | 300–600 q6 hours | 3–6 | Hepatic | Diarrhea, GI upset, cinchonism, proarrhythmia |
| Sotalol | 80–160 q12 hours | — | Hepatic | CNS symptoms, conduction disturbances, proarrhythmia |
| Ibutilide | Only available intravenously | IV dose of 1 mg injected over 10 minutes followed by 1 mg (5–10 minute delay) | Hepatic | Proarrhythmic |

*Adapted with permission from Ezekowitz MD. Systemic cardiac embolism. New York: Marcel Dekker, 1993.*

CNS, *central nervous system;* GI, *gastrointestinal.*

[a] *Not available clinically.*

1 and 6% (34). In the SPAF I trial, which involved a population of individuals with atrial fibrillation, use of antiarrhythmics was associated with increased cardiac mortality (35, 36). In contrast to other antiarrhythmics, amiodarone decreases, or at least does not increase, mortality in individuals with heart failure and ventricular ectopy, including those who have sustained a myocardial infarction (37–39). This low risk of proarrhythmia and its apparent superior efficacy in maintaining sinus rhythm make amiodarone an attractive agent (40) despite the potential pulmonary, thyroid, hepatic, neurologic, and ocular side effects (41) (Table 60.2).

Rate control, both at rest and with exercise, usually can be achieved with use of digoxin, β-blockers, and those calcium channel blockers affecting the AV node (i.e., verapamil, diltiazem). When atrial fibrillation persists at an excessive ventricular rate despite optimal pharmacologic therapy and attempts at cardioversion, creation of a permanent AV block should be considered. Catheter ablation using direct current or, more recently, radiofrequency energy has been reported to be successful in 80 to 90% of individuals (42). In the remainder, although complete AV block is not achieved, modification of AV conduction results in better control of heart rate

without drugs or with use of previously ineffective drugs. Following a successful ablation, permanent cardiac pacing is required. Rate-responsive pacemakers are used to provide appropriate increases in heart rate with exercise (17). More recently, modification of AV conduction by lesions placed in the posteroinferior region of the tricuspid annulus have been used to better control ventricular rate during atrial fibrillation (43, 44). This procedure obviates permanent pacing. Long-term follow-up and comparison with individuals undergoing complete AV ablation will resolve the questions of efficacy.

Several other surgical procedures have been proposed as treatment of individuals with refractory atrial fibrillation. The so-called "corridor operation" creates an isolated strip of atrial tissue leading from the sinoatrial to the AV node (45). Unfortunately, this procedure does not provide for an atrial transport function, although it is useful in controlling heart rate. The atrial maze operation (46) and its modifications (47) provide similar success in heart rate control, and they are reported to preserve atrial transport function. Following the original atrial maze operation, 41% of individuals required insertion of rate-responsive, dual-chambered pacemakers (46). Subsequent modifications to the procedure have resulted in a 25% incidence of need for chronic pacing (47). To date, surgical procedures have been used in only a small group of selected individuals, with operative mortality rate of 2.4% (47).

Preliminary attempts to reproduce the maze procedure with catheter techniques using linear endocardial lesions produced by radiofrequency applications have been attempted (48, 49). Success has been achieved, but widespread use of this catheter-based approach awaits further technical refinement.

Catheter or surgical ablation of the AV node effectively controls heart rate, but it does not provide normal atrial contraction. Consequently, individuals treated with these methods remain at increased risk for thromboembolism and should undergo long-term anticoagulation therapy.

In individuals with sinus node dysfunction and bradycardia-induced atrial fibrillation, treatment with atrial pacing, coupled with ventricular pacing if required, can maintain a paced rate, which may prevent atrial fibrillation. When used to treat sinus node dysfunction (i.e., symptomatic bradycardia), ventricular pacing alone can result in a higher incidence of subsequent atrial fibrillation (50, 51).

Long term use of an implantable atrial defibrillator as a nonpharmacologic treatment of atrial fibrillation remains a challenge. Studies in humans have demonstrated its feasibility, but major issues still need to be addressed. These include individual discomfort related to the defibrillation shock, risk of inducing life-threatening ventricular arrhythmias, and cost-effectiveness (52).

## THROMBOEMBOLISM IN RELATIONSHIP TO CARDIOVERSION

Embolic risk is increased regardless of whether conversion is electrical or pharmacologic. The reported incidence is from 1 to 3% (53). Many studies have demonstrated a decreased incidence of embolization in individuals receiving anticoagulation therapy before cardioversion, but no randomized studies have documented its efficacy. Despite this lack of a definitive study, the catastrophic consequences of cerebral embolism demand serious consideration of anticoagulation in all individuals undergoing elective cardioversion, and the risk of major hemorrhage with anticoagulation must be weighed against the potential benefit. Anticoagulation usually is initiated 2 to 3 weeks before attempted cardioversion. This presumably prevents formation of new thrombi while allowing old thrombi to organize or lyse. Anticoagulation should be continued for at least 3 to 4 weeks after cardioversion because of late embolic events that may relate to a delayed return of normal atrial mechanical function (54) and atrial stunning after conversion. Evaluation of the left atrium using transesophageal echocardiography (TEE) for thrombi, spon-

taneous echocardiographic contrast, or both eventually may permit a more informed decision about the need for anticoagulation before cardioversion (55). The role of TEE has not been studied systematically in a large trial, however. Even so, echocardiographically detected left ventricular dysfunction was recently identified as an independent predictor of thromboembolic risk in individuals with chronic nonrheumatic atrial fibrillation (56).

## OVERALL TREATMENT STRATEGY

Cardioversion is attempted to improve hemodynamic status and prevent thromboembolic complications. Because long-term anticoagulation therapy can effectively reduce the risk of embolization, cardiac symptoms and medical contraindications to warfarin are the major indications for cardioversion to maintain sinus rhythm. In selected individuals with significant symptoms, an aggressive, staged approach to therapy can maintain sinus rhythm in more than 60% of individuals, at least in the short term (57). Individuals with noncompliant ventricles (e.g., chronic hypertensives with left ventricular hypertrophy) or with limited baseline cardiac reserve (e.g., cardiomyopathies) tend to benefit most from the resumption of normal atrial contraction (58). In these individuals, cardiac output may increase by 20 to 25%.

Controversy concerning the value of cardioversion continues. An ongoing National Institutes of Health-sponsored trial, the Atrial Fibrillation Follow-up Investigation of Rhythm Management (AFFIRM), has been initiated to study whether aggressive attempts at maintenance of sinus rhythm are preferable to rate control with anticoagulation in long-term treatment of individuals with atrial fibrillation. A similar study will begin soon as a Veterans Administration (VA) Cooperative Study. New surgical techniques also hold promise, but whether these will achieve the reported success rates in wider application is not known. Currently effective pharmacologic treatments that maintain sinus rhythm are associated with important morbidity, and they may increase the mortality rate because of their proarrhythmic effect. Hence, at present, aggressive attempts to convert individuals with atrial fibrillation and to maintain sinus rhythm should be reserved for individuals with significant symptoms and individuals in whom anticoagulation is contraindicated.

## PROPHYLAXIS AGAINST SYSTEMIC EMBOLIZATION (SEE CHAPTER 58)

Because reversible causes of atrial fibrillation are identified infrequently and many individuals with chronic or paroxysmal atrial fibrillation cannot be maintained in sinus rhythm, several independent clinical studies were designed to determine the most effective, safest pharmacologic approach to protecting individuals with atrial fibrillation from embolic risk. Each trial evaluated the efficacy of warfarin in low to intermediate doses (PT ratio, 1.7) (1) in preventing systemic embolization among individuals with atrial fibrillation. Two trials also formally evaluated aspirin as an alternative treatment (1, 2).

Three considerations prompted these clinical trials. First, atrial fibrillation is an important predisposing factor for systemic embolization and stroke. Second, atrial fibrillation increases with age and, thus, constitutes a constantly enlarging health-care problem. Finally, low-dose warfarin is as effective as conventional-dose warfarin, but is associated with substantially fewer bleeding complications, in treatment of individuals with deep-vein thrombosis (59).

The five primary prevention, placebo-controlled trials were the Atrial Fibrillation, Aspirin, Anticoagulation Study from Copenhagen, Denmark (AFASAK) (1); the SPAF II study from the United States (2); the Boston Area Anticoagulation Trial for Atrial Fibrillation (BAATAF) (3); the Canadian Atrial Fibrillation Anticoagulation Study (CAFA) (4); and the Stroke Prevention in Nonrheumatic Atrial Fibrillation Study (SPINAF) (5). The results of these trials have resolved many questions regarding antithrombotic and antiplatelet therapy in individuals with atrial fibrillation.

Each study had important similarities, but they also provided important and unique information. All were placebo-controlled, randomized trials and were terminated early. The studies comparing aspirin used different doses as well. The Danish study (1) used 75 mg/day, and the SPAF study (2) used 325 mg/day. The BAATAF study (3), which was not specifically designed to evaluate the role of aspirin, allowed individuals in the placebo group to undergo aspirin treatment at a dose of 325 mg/day. The Boston and Danish studies were not blinded (1, 3), and the SPAF study was blinded for aspirin but not for warfarin therapy (2). The remaining trials, the Canadian study (4) and the VA Cooperative Study (SPINAF) (5), specifically excluded use of aspirin or other nonsteroidal anti-inflammatory agents. These last two studies were unique in that they were double-blinded as well; to our knowledge, they were the first double-blinded studies of warfarin ever conducted in North America. Each study used stroke, or a variant thereof, as the primary endpoint (Table 60.3).

The characteristics of individuals in the nontreatment groups are shown in Fig. 60.4. In all the studies, hypertension, coronary artery disease, and heart failure were common. Individuals from the AFASAK study were older and more likely to have a history of heart failure. In the VA and AFASAK studies, intermittent atrial fibrillation was an exclusion. A major bleeding episode was, in general, classified in all the studies as that requiring a blood transfusion, hospitalization, interven-

**TABLE 60.3.**   End Points of Clinical Trials Comparing Prophylaxis against Embolism in Atrial Fibrillation

| | AFASAK (1) | SPAF (2) | BAATAF (3) | CAFA (4) | SPINAF (5) | EAFT (6) | SPAF III (7) |
|---|---|---|---|---|---|---|---|
| *Primary* | Systemic emboli, TIA, stroke | Ischemic stroke, systemic emboli | Ischemic stroke, intracranial hemorrhage | Ischemic stroke, systemic emboli | Cerebral infarction | Nonfatal stroke, nonfatal MI, nonfatal systemic embolism, vascular death | Cerebral infarction, systemic emboli |
| *Secondary* | Death | Death, myocardial infarction, TIA, unstable angina | Intracerebral bleed, major bleed | TIA, lacunar infarction, major bleeding, minor bleeding, death | Cerebral hemorrhage, death | Death (all causes), all strokes (fatal and nonfatal), major thromboembolic events | TIA, cerebral hemorrhage, major hemorrhage, death |
| *Intercurrent events* | | Minor hemorrhages | | | Noncerebral major hemorrhage, minor hemorrhage, TIA, myocardial infarction, venous thrombosis | TIA | None |

MI, *myocardial infarction;* TIA, *transient ischemic attack.*

**FIGURE 60.4.** Cumulative probability of cerebral infarction. The numbers below the figure are the numbers of individuals at risk for a cerebral infarction at each point. There was a significant reduction in risk in the warfarin group as compared with the placebo group (risk reduction, 0.79; $P = 0.001$). Adapted with permission from Ezekowitz MD, Bridgers SL, James KE, et al. Warfarin in the prevention of stroke associated nonrheumatic atrial fibrillation. Veterans Affairs Stroke Prevention in Nonrheumatic Atrial Fibrillation Investigators. N Engl J Med 1992;327:1406–1412.

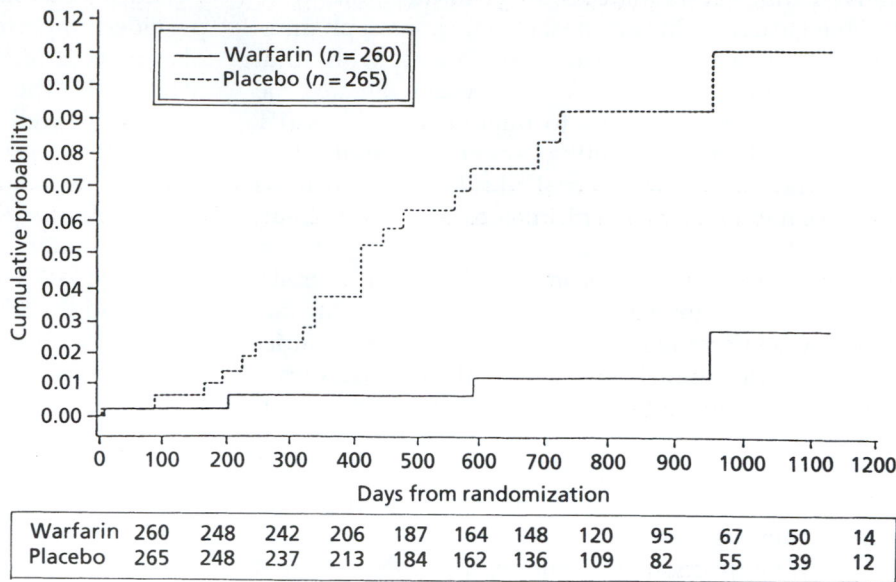

| | | | | | | | | | | | | |
|---|---|---|---|---|---|---|---|---|---|---|---|---|
| Warfarin | 260 | 248 | 242 | 206 | 187 | 164 | 148 | 120 | 95 | 67 | 50 | 14 |
| Placebo | 265 | 248 | 237 | 213 | 184 | 162 | 136 | 109 | 82 | 55 | 39 | 12 |

tion, or occurring in a critical location (e.g., intracranial). The primary analysis was the intention to treat for the SPAF, BAATAF, and SPINAF studies. For the AFASAK study, events were counted until individuals discontinued their study medication, and the CAFA study included all events occurring within 28 days of permanently discontinuing the study medication.

Each trial is reviewed here in the order in which the results were published. Tables are provided to facilitate comparison among their results.

## THE AFASAK STUDY

In the AFASAK study (1), 1007 individuals were randomized to receive warfarin, aspirin, or placebo. The characteristics of the individual population are provided in Fig. 60.4. The mean age was 74 years, which was several years older than mean ages in the other studies. An efficacy analysis found a highly statistically significant benefit afforded by warfarin compared with both placebo and aspirin (Tables 60.4 and 60.5). Bleeding complications were divided equally among the three groups. The results of this study are compelling; however, the unblinded nature of its design and that 38% of individuals assigned to the warfarin group withdrew from the trial, together with the analysis being an efficacy analysis, necessitate confirmation in other trials.

## THE SPAF STUDY

In the SPAF study (2), individuals determined to be randomizable to warfarin were assigned to a warfarin, aspirin, or placebo group. Individuals receiving aspirin or placebo were blinded; individuals receiving warfarin were not. Individuals otherwise eligible for the study

but who were determined not to be randomizable to warfarin were assigned, in a blinded manner, to either the aspirin or the placebo group. The study terminated prematurely because of a highly statistically significant benefit afforded by active treatment (either warfarin or aspirin) compared with placebo. These investigators planned a second phase of their study, involving direct comparison between warfarin and aspirin therapy, so the individual benefit of these two drugs was not revealed here. The investigators reported that individuals with lone atrial fibrillation ($n = 52$) had no cerebrovascular events during the short follow-up period, and that in individuals older than 75 years, aspirin had no benefit. It is noteworthy that the event rate in the placebo group (7.4% per year) was higher than event rates reported in the other studies.

## THE BAATAF STUDY

The BAATAF study (3) was an unblinded comparison of warfarin with placebo. Individuals receiving placebo were permitted to receive aspirin at a dose of 325 mg/day. The study demonstrated an 86% benefit in favor of warfarin therapy in preventing both systemic embolization and stroke and a 35% reduction in the mortality rate of individuals with chronic atrial fibrillation.

### The CAFA Study

The CAFA study (4) was a blinded comparison of warfarin with placebo. At the time the study was terminated prematurely, 378 individuals had been randomized. Analysis suggested a trend favoring warfarin in preventing systemic embolization, but this was not statistically significant. The investigators also found that bleed-

**TABLE 60.4.**   Event Rates (% Individuals per Year) Comparing Aspirin to Placebo

| | AFASAK (1) (n = 672) | | SPAF (2) (n = 1120) | |
|---|---|---|---|---|
| | Aspirin (n = 336) | Placebo (n = 336) | Aspirin (n = 552) | Placebo (n = 568) |
| Total individuals/year observation to death or end of study | 422 | 417 | 742 | 767 |
| Stroke | 3.9 | 4.8 | 3.2 | 5.7 |
| Systemic embolism | 0.2 | 0.5 | 0.4 | 0.7 |
| Intracerebral hemorrhage | 0 | 0 | 0.1 | 0 |
| Subdural hemorrhage | 0 | 0 | 0.1 | 0.3 |
| Subarachnoid hemorrhage | 0 | 0 | 0 | 0 |
| Transient ischemic attack | 0.5 | 0.7 | 1.4 | 2.3 |
| Death | 5.7 | 6.5 | 5.3 | 6.5 |
| Vascular | 4.0 | 4.1 | 3.2 | 3.6 |
| Nonvascular | 1.2 | 1.9 | 2.0 | 2.1 |
| Unknown | 0.5 | 0.5 | 0 | 0.8 |
| Myocardial infarction | NA | NA | 0.9 | 1.6 |
| Other bleeds | 0.3 | 0 | 1.1 | 1.2 |

NA, *not recorded.*

**TABLE 60.5.**   Event Rates (% Individuals per Year) Comparing Warfarin to Placebo

| | AFASAK (1) (n = 671) | | SPAF (2) (n = 421) | | BAATAF (3) (n = 420) | | CAFA (4) (n = 378) | | SPINAF (5) (n = 525) | |
|---|---|---|---|---|---|---|---|---|---|---|
| | Warfarin (n = 335) | Placebo (n = 336) | Warfarin (n = 210) | Placebo (n = 211) | Warfarin (n = 212) | Placebo (n = 208) | Warfarin (n = 187) | Placebo (n = 191) | Warfarin (n = 260) | Placebo (n = 265) |
| Total individuals/year observation to death or end of study | 423 | 417 | 271 | 259 | 487 | 435 | 239 | 251 | 456 | 440 |
| Stroke | 1.9 | 4.8 | 2.3 | 7.0 | 0.4 | 3.0 | 2.1 | 3.7 | 0.9 | 4.3 |
| Systemic embolism | 0 | 0.2 | 0 | 0.8 | 0 | 0 | 0.4 | 0.8 | 0.8 | 0.4 |
| Intracerebral hemorrhage | 0.2 | 0 | 0.4 | 0 | 0 | 0 | 0.4 | 0 | 0.2 | 0 |
| Subdural hemorrhage | 0 | 0 | 0.4 | 0.8 | 0.2 | 0 | 0 | 0 | 0 | 0 |
| Subarachnoid hemorrhage | 0 | 0 | 0 | 0 | 0 | 0 | 0 | 0 | 0 | 0 |
| Transient ischemic attack | 0.2 | 0.7 | 1.5 | 2.4 | 0.8 | 0.9 | 0.8 | 0.8 | 1.5 | 2.6 |
| Death | 4.7 | 6.5 | 2.2 | 3.1 | 2.3 | 6.0 | 4.2 | 3.2 | 3.3 | 5.0 |
| Vascular | 3.3 | 4.1 | 1.5 | 1.9 | 1.4 | 3.2 | 3.8 | 2.4 | | |
| Nonvascular | 1.4 | 1.9 | 0.4 | 0.8 | 0.8 | 2.8 | 0.4 | 0.8 | | |
| Unknown | 0 | 0.5 | 0.4 | 0.4 | 0 | 0 | 0 | 0 | | |
| Myocardial infarction | NA | NA | 0.7 | 0.8 | 0.8 | 0.7 | NA | NA | 0.4 | 1.5 |
| Major bleeds | 0.3 | 0 | 0.4 | 0.8 | 1.0 | 1.9 | 1.7 | 0.8 | 1.5 | 0.9 |

NA, *not recorded.*

ing complications were distributed fairly equally between the two groups, although two deaths related to hemorrhage in the warfarin group.

### The SPINAF Study

The SPINAF study (5), which was conducted under the auspices of the VA Cooperative Studies Program, was a double-blinded comparison of low-intensity anticoagulation therapy with a PT ratio of 1.2 to 1.5 with placebo. On the basis of a protocol-mandated interim analysis and results of other trials with similar goals (1–3), this study was terminated in March 1991. At that time, a total of 525 individuals with a mean age of 67 years had been randomized to either placebo or warfarin groups.

Nineteen individuals in the placebo group had a cerebral infarction, compared with four individuals in the warfarin group, for a risk benefit of 79% (Fig. 60.4). There were 10 major hemorrhages, all of which were gastrointestinal and one of which was fatal. Six of these were in the warfarin group; four were in the placebo group. Minor bleeding complications were more common in the warfarin group. In individuals older than 70 years, a similar benefit was seen.

## SUMMARY OF STUDY RESULTS

These studies have provided answers to important questions about the treatment of individuals with atrial fibrillation. All found warfarin to be effective at protecting individuals from systemic embolization. This was true for both chronic (1–5) and intermittent (2–4) atrial fibrillation. The general similarity of baseline characteristics and the comparable risk reduction among studies indicate these results have wide application. In the three unblinded warfarin studies, reduction in the risk of cerebral vascular events ranged from 67 to 86% (1–3). In the SPINAF study (5), there was a 79% reduction in the risk of cerebral infarction. The CAFA study (4), which was the only other double-blind, placebo-controlled trial, was terminated early on the basis of data from the other trials and without consideration of its own interim data. The study showed a nonstatistically significant trend, however, in favor of warfarin (4).

A major finding of these studies was that risk of major hemorrhage was similar for the warfarin and placebo groups (1, 4, 5). Minor hemorrhagic events were more common in the warfarin groups (5).

In contrast to the established efficacy of warfarin, the benefit of aspirin for prevention of stroke remains controversial. The AFASAK study (1) showed no benefit to aspirin compared with placebo. A preliminary report of the SPAF study (2) showed that individuals older than 75 years did not benefit from aspirin, whereas individuals younger than 75 did (incidence, 2.2% per year; risk reduction, 65%). In the overall SPAF population overall (60), the incidence of ischemic stroke and systemic embolism for aspirin-treated individuals was 3.6% per year, compared with 0.9% per year for cerebral infarction alone in the warfarin-treated individuals in the SPINAF study (5). Moreover, individuals in the placebo group of the BAATAF study (2) were permitted to use aspirin, and no benefit was found.

Thus, low-intensity anticoagulation therapy with warfarin is effective in preventing cerebral infarction among individuals with chronic atrial fibrillation, and it has an acceptable risk of major hemorrhage in individuals deemed to be suitable for anticoagulation. The benefit persists in individuals older than 75 years as well (5).

## EMBOLIC RISK STRATIFICATION

Identifying individuals at high risk for cerebral infarction is difficult. Each study found different variables predisposing to stroke. The SPINAF study (5), together with the BAATAF study (3), identified active angina as a possible risk factor. There was no unanimity, however, regarding mitral annular calcification (2, 3), recent history of heart failure (2), left atrial size (2), or reduced left ventricular function (3) as risk factors.

Lone atrial fibrillators (i.e., individuals without evidence for structural heart disease, hypertension, diabetes mellitus, or precipitating factors such as thyrotoxicosis) have a low incidence of systemic embolization. This group, when strictly defined, constitutes 2 to 4% of the population with chronic atrial fibrillation (1, 4, 32). The risk of embolization in this group is low, ranging from 1.3 to 1.4% per year (11, 35, 59), and not significantly different from that in the general population. The Framingham study demonstrated an increased risk of stroke, but this individual population was not strictly defined and included those older than 60 years as well as those with hypertension and diabetes (61). None of the 18 individuals in the SPINAF study (5) with lone atrial fibrillation had a cerebral infarction, which is consistent with the SPAF study (61), in which none of the 52 individuals with lone atrial fibrillation experience events. Thus, lone atrial fibrillators would not require anti coagulation therapy to reduce their risk of cerebral infarctions but probably would benefit from aspirin, although this has not been proved.

All five atrial fibrillation studies discussed here were terminated early by their respective Data Monitoring Boards (1–5), which precluded assessment of warfarin's long-term benefit. Each study demonstrated that cerebral infarction is a sporadic event in individuals with chronic atrial fibrillation (Fig. 60.4), and that the risk of an event persists even with long-standing atrial fibrillation. Thus, chronicity of atrial fibrillation does not attenuate the indication for anticoagulation, and individuals with long-standing atrial fibrillation would benefit from anticoagulation therapy.

## POOLED ANALYSIS

The principal investigators of the primary placebo-controlled trials pooled data from their control groups (8) and found that in aggregate, warfarin reduced the risk of stroke by 68% and aspirin by 36%. Most important, however, was the recognition that individuals with atrial fibrillation represented a heterogeneous group regarding development of a stroke. Thus, increasing age (and specifically age older than 65 years), history of high blood pressure, history of diabetes, and a previous transient ischemic attack or stroke were independent risk factors for the development of stroke in individuals with atrial fibrillation. In addition, from three studies in which transthoracic echocardiograms were available, very poor ventricular function was found to be an independent risk factor as well. Translating these findings into clinical practice, the risk of stroke is so low that anticoagulation therapy is not indicated in individuals younger than 65 years and without risk factors. In individuals younger than 65 years with risk factors or older than 65 years with or without risk factors, however, anticoagulation is indicated if the individual has no contraindications. Individuals who cannot tolerate anticoagulation should be treated with aspirin, and those at lower risk probably do well with aspirin therapy. Risk assessment of individuals with atrial fibrillation, however, is an ongoing process, because these individuals develop risk factors for stroke as they age and also develop comorbid processes that may increase their risk of bleeding.

Thus, on the basis of the SPINAF study, mortality related to atrial fibrillation is not related to thromboembolic phenomena but, primarily, to sudden, unexpected cardiac deaths that presumably are arrhythmic in etiology. This may result from the association of atrial fibrillation with other clinical entities that provide a substrate for dangerous ventricular arrhythmias (e.g., cardiomyopathy), or to the concomitant use of drugs such as quinidine that may have a proarrhythmic effect and predispose individuals to sudden death.

TEE is useful for identifying thrombi in the left atrium and the left atrial appendage. The effect of these findings on clinical decision making, however, is unclear. The presence of spontaneous echo contrast is an important marker for thrombus and embolic risk (62), but no studies have documented a clear embolic risk in individuals without these findings. A test at a particular point in time may not predict subsequent systemic embolization, because thrombi may form and resolve as part of a continuous process that would be difficult to monitor by repeated TEE. At present, it is premature to recommend TEE to stratify risk for systemic embolization with nonrheumatic atrial fibrillation; however, TEE may have a role in cardioversion (55).

Patients with intermittent atrial fibrillation were excluded by protocol from the AFASAK and the SPINAF studies (1, 5), but other investigators (2–4) have reported that risk of embolization is similar to that in individuals with chronic atrial fibrillation. Individuals with intermittent atrial fibrillation probably should be treated similar to those with chronic atrial fibrillation.

# SECONDARY PREVENTION OF EMBOLISM

The only published secondary prevention trial is the European Atrial Fibrillation Study (6). This was a large study involving 108 centers. The individual population consisted of 1007 individuals with nonrheumatic atrial fibrillation and a recent, transient ischemic attack or minor ischemic stroke. Individuals were randomized to open anticoagulation therapy or double-blind treatment with either aspirin, 300 mg/day, or placebo. Individuals with contraindications to anticoagulation were randomized to receive aspirin or placebo. The measure of outcome was death from vascular disease, any stroke, myocardial infarction, or systemic embolism.

There were 669 individuals eligible for anticoagulants; the remaining 338 were not. Individuals with chronic and poorly controlled hypertension, history of hemorrhagic cerebral infarction, retinopathy, chronic alcoholism, noncompliance, or refusal to use anticoagulants were not included in this study. During a mean follow-up of 2.3 years, the annual rate of outcome events was 8% in the anticoagulant group and 17% in the placebo group. The risk of stroke was reduced by warfarin from 12 to 4% per year (i.e., a 66% reduction). Among all individuals assigned to aspirin (in the placebo or anticoagulant group), the annual incidence of outcome events was 15%, compared with 19% among individuals on placebo. The on-treatment annual incidence of major bleeding complications was low in this study: 2.8% in the anticoagulant group, 0.9% in the aspirin group, and 0.7% in the placebo group. The absolute excess of major bleeds with anticoagulation, despite a mean individual age of 71 years, was 21 per 1000 treated individuals per year. No individual assigned to anticoagulation had an intracranial hemorrhage. Three fatal cerebral bleeds did occur, however, with one in the placebo group and two in the aspirin group.

These investigators concluded that in individuals with nonrheumatic atrial fibrillation and recent transient ischemic attack or minor stroke, anticoagulant treatment reduces the risk of recurrent stroke by two-thirds. In this study, the annual incidence of recurrent stroke was 12% in the placebo group—almost three times as much as that in the placebo groups of the primary prevention trials. This makes the value of anticoagulation for secondary prevention even more impressive in absolute terms: 90 vascular events were prevented per 1000 individuals treated for 1 year. In contrast, aspirin prevented 40 vascular events per 1000 individuals for 1 year.

Given the high efficacy of anticoagulation, treatment should begin as soon as possible. Several investigators, however, have recommended withholding anticoagulants during the first few days after a suspected stroke, especially if the infarct is large (64–66), to prevent hemorrhagic transformation (see Chapter 58).

# WARFARIN VERSUS ASPIRIN

## DIRECT COMPARISON

The SPAF II study (2) is the only direct comparison of warfarin with aspirin in individuals having atrial fibrillation. In this study, 1100 individuals were randomized to warfarin and aspirin therapy after being divided into two age groups: those younger than 75 years, and those 75 years or older. The SPAF II study was derived from the SPAF I study population. Those who had survived SPAF I without an event were rerandomized into SPAF II, and then additional individuals were recruited to complete the sample size. Using an intention-to-treat analysis, there was no statistically significant difference between warfarin and aspirin in both age groups. An on-treatment analysis, however, showed an approximately 50% benefit afforded by warfarin in both groups. The explanation for this is that individuals included in this study were at low risk, and because both treatment modalities are effective in preventing stroke, the study was underpowered to show a statistical difference under an intention-to-treat paradigm. Those 75 years or older had an increased risk of intracerebral bleeding estimated to be between 1.7 and 1.8% per year, as opposed to 0.3% per year in the other trials. This was directly attributable to the higher levels of anticoagulation used in this trial. Thus, in this regard, the trial proved to be valuable and highlighted that anticoagulation therapy in the elderly should be kept in a very narrow range, probably not exceeding an international normalized ratio (INR) of 3.0.

## WARFARIN AND ASPIRIN IN COMBINATION

The SPAF III study (7) evaluated 1044 individuals with atrial fibrillation who also had at least one risk factor for thromboembolic disease. Individuals were randomly assigned to a combination of low-intensity, fixed-dose warfarin, which was adjusted to an INR of 1.2 to 1.5 for initial dose adjustment, and aspirin, 325 mg/day, or to adjusted-dose warfarin for an INR of 2.0 to 3.0. In this unblinded study, the mean INR in the combination group was 1.3, compared with 2.4 for those taking adjusted-dose warfarin. The trial was terminated after a mean follow-up of 1.1 years, when the rate of ischemic stroke and systemic embolization in the combination-therapy group was 7.9% per year, as opposed to that of 1.9% per year in the dose-adjusted group. The difference between these groups was statistically significant ($P = .0001$). The rates of major bleeding were similar in both treatment groups. Thus, low-intensity, fixed-dose warfarin plus aspirin, following this regimen, was not sufficient to prevent stroke in individuals with nonvalvular atrial fibrillation considered to be at high risk for thromboembolic complications.

## IDEAL THERAPEUTIC RANGE FOR ANTICOAGULATION

From the results of several studies, anticoagulation therapy with warfarin should be monitored carefully, and an INR of between 2.0 and 3.5 is the optimum range for most indications. Among elderly individuals, however, an upper limit to the INR of approximately 3.0 is appropriate (67).

## ATRIAL FIBRILLATION IN SPECIFIC CARDIAC DISEASE STATES

### RHEUMATIC HEART DISEASE AND ATRIAL FIBRILLATION

The risk of stroke in individuals with rheumatic mitral valve disease and atrial fibrillation is three times greater than that in individuals with atrial fibrillation without mitral stenosis (13). No randomized, controlled studies have evaluated the efficacy of antithrombotic therapy in individuals with rheumatic heart disease in atrial fibrillation. Fukuda and Makamura (68) followed individuals with rheumatic valvular disease for a mean period of 22 months. They found that the incidence of thromboembolism without anticoagulation was 5.5% per year, and that this could be reduced to between 3 and 1% per year with warfarin therapy. Given this evidence as well as the efficacy of warfarin in nonrheumatic atrial fibrillation, long-term anticoagulation therapy with warfarin is recommended in individuals with rheumatic valvular disease and atrial fibrillation (68). Antiplatelet agents have not been adequately tested in this individual group (68).

### CONGENITAL HEART DISEASE

Patients with atrial and ventricular septal defects, corrected transposition of the great vessels, and Ebstein's anomaly are most likely to have atrial fibrillation. There are insufficient data to determine whether long-term anticoagulant therapy is indicated in individuals with congenital heart disease complicated by atrial fibrillation. Given the benefit of warfarin in individuals with nonrheumatic atrial fibrillation, however, it is reasonable to anticoagulate these individuals (68).

### THYROTOXIC HEART DISEASE AND ATRIAL FIBRILLATION

Atrial fibrillation occurs in approximately 10 to 30% of individuals with thyrotoxicosis (69–72). Of 1212 individuals with atrial fibrillation, Godtfredsen (73) found that 2.5% had thyrotoxicosis as the cause. A retrospective study of 163 individuals with a mean follow-up of 34 months (74) found that control of thyroid dysfunction alone resulted in spontaneous reversion to sinus rhythm in 101 individuals. If spontaneous reversion does not occur within 4 months, then cardioversion, either pharmacologic or electric, should be undertaken, because spontaneous reversion is unlikely (74). The frequency of systemic embolization in individuals with atrial fibrillation resulting from thyrotoxicosis is not known with accuracy, but it is at least as high as that in individuals who are euthyroid (75). Because the probability of embolization is sufficiently increased and warfarin is effective in individuals with nonrheumatic atrial fibrillation, anticoagulation is recommended in individuals with thyrotoxicosis and atrial fibrillation. It also is recommended that anticoagulation be continued for 4 weeks after conversion to normal sinus rhythm (76–78). The rationale for this recommendation is that the left atrium may not return to its normal contractile state immediately after reversion to sinus rhythm.

# CONCLUSIONS

It is strongly recommended that long-term warfarin therapy (INR, 2.0–3.5) be used in individuals with nonrheumatic atrial fibrillation who are eligible for anticoagulation. Exceptions are individuals with lone atrial fibrillation or with low risk for stroke (i.e., those younger than 65 years without a history of hypertension, diabetes, previous transient ischemic episode, or stroke). These individuals should not be anticoagulated; individuals with thyrotoxicosis, rheumatic heart disease, or congenital heart disease should be anticoagulated. Individuals with a contraindication to warfarin therapy should be treated with aspirin at a dose of 325 mg daily, because aspirin treatment is superior to placebo. This benefit remains controversial, however. Despite strong evidence favoring use of warfarin in atrial fibrillation, it continues to be underused (79). There also is a growing literature that silent cerebral infarction and dementia are associated with atrial fibrillation; however, whether warfarin modifies this incidence is not konwn (80, 81).

# REFERENCES

1. Petersen P, Boysen G, Godtfredsen J et al. Placebo-controlled, randomised trial of warfarin and aspirin for prevention of thromboembolic complications in chronic atrial fibrillation. The Copenhagen AFASAK Study. Lancet 1989;i:175–179.
2. Anonymous. Design of a multicenter randomized trial for the Stroke Prevention in Atrial Fibrillation Study. The Stroke Prevention in Atrial Fibrillation Investigators. Stroke 1990;21:538–545.
3. Anonymous. The effect of low-dose warfarin on the risk of stroke in nonrheumatic atrial fibrillation. The Boston Area Anticoagulation Trial for Atrial Fibrillation Investigators. N Engl J Med 1990;323:1505–1511.
4. Connolly SJ, Laupacis A, Gent M et al. Canadian Atrial Fibrillation Anticoagulation (CAFA) Study. J Am Coll Cardiol 1991;18:349–355.
5. Ezekowitz MD, Bridgers SL, James KE et al. Warfarin in the prevention of stroke associated with nonrheumatic atrial fibrillation. Veterans Affairs Stroke Prevention in Nonrheumatic Atrial Fibrillation Investigators. N Engl J Med 1992;327:1406–1412.
6. Anonymous. Secondary prevention in non-rheumatic atrial fibrillation after transient ischaemic attack or minor stroke. EAFT (European Atrial Fibrillation Trial) Study Group. Lancet 1993;342:1255–1262.
7. Anonymous. Adjusted-dose warfarin versus low intensity, fixed-dose warfarin plus aspirin for high-risk patients with atrial fibrillation: stroke
prevention in atrial fibrillation. III. Randomised clinical trial. Lancet 1996; 348:633–638.
8. Anonymous. Risk factors for stroke and efficacy of antithrombotic therapy in atrial fibrillation: analysis of pooled data from five randomized controlled trials. Atrial Fibrillation Investigators. Arch Intern Med 1994;154: 1449–1457.
9. Hiss RG, Lamb LE. Electrocardiographic findings in 122043 patients. Circulation 1962;25:947–961.
10. Kopecky SL, Gersh BJ, McGoon MD et al. The natural history of lone atrial fibrillation. A population-based study over three decades. N Engl J Med 1987;317:669–674.
11. Kannel WB, Abbott RD, Savage DD et al. Epidemiologic features of chronic atrial fibrillation. The Framingham study. N Engl J Med 1982;306: 1018–1022.
12. Phillips SJ, Whisnant JP, O'Fallon WM et al. Prevalence of cardiovascular disease and diabetes mellitus in residents of Rochester, Minnesota. Mayo Clin Proc 1990;65:344–359.
13. Wolf PA, Dawber TR, Thomas HE Jr et al. Epidemiologic assessment of chronic atrial fibrillation and risk of stroke: the Framingham study. Neurology 1978;28:973–977.
14. Kannel WB, Abbott RD, Savage DD et al. Epidemiologic features of chronic atrial fibrillation: the Framingham study. N Engl J Med 1982;306: 1018–1022.
15. Kaarisalo MM, Immonen-Raiha P, Marttila RJ et al. Atrial fibrillation and stroke. Mortality and causes of death after the first acute ischemic stroke [Review]. Stroke 1997;28:311–315.
16. Coplen SE, Antman EM, Berlin JA et al. Efficacy and safety of quinidine therapy for maintenance of sinus rhythm after cardioversion. A meta-analysis of randomized control trials. Circulation 1990;82:1106–1116.
17. Ezekowitz MD. Systemic cardiac embolism. New York: Marcel Dekker, 1993.
18. Moe G, Abidskov J. Atrial fibrillation as a self-sustaining arrhythmia independent of focal discharge. Am Heart J 1959;58:59–70.
19. Moe G. On the multiple wavelet hypothesis of atrial fibrillation. Arch Int Pharmacodyn Ther 1962;140:18:C3–188.
20. Kaseda S, Zipes D. Contraction-excitation feedback in the atria: a cause of changes in refractoriness. J Am Coll Cardiol 1988;11:1327–1336.
21. Corr PB, Yamada KA, Witkowski FX. Mechanisms controlling cardiac autonomic function and their relation to arrhythmogenesis. In: Fozzard H, ed. The heart and cardiovascular system. New York: Raven Press, 1986: 1343–1403.
22. Allessie M, Rensma P, Brigada J et al. Pathophysiology of atrial fibrillation. In: Zipes D, Jalife J, eds. Cardiac electrophysiology from cell to bedside. Philadelphia: WB Saunders, 1990:518–563.
23. Creswell LL, Schuessler RB, Rosenbloom M et al. Hazards of postoperative atrial arrhythmias. Ann Thorac Surg 1993;56:539–549.
24. Lauer MS, Eagle KA, Buckley MJ et al. Atrial fibrillation following coronary artery bypass surgery [Review]. Prog Cardiovasc Dis 1989;31: 367–378.
25. Forfar JC, Miller HC, Toft AD. Occult thyrotoxicosis: a correctable cause of "idiopathic" atrial fibrillation. Am J Cardiol 1979;44:9–12.
26. Kaplan BM, Langendorf R, Lev M et al. Tachycardia-bradycardia syndrome (so-called "sick sinus syndrome"). Pathology, mechanisms, and treatment. Am J Cardiol 1973;31:497–508.
27. Takahashi N, Seki A, Imataka K. Clinical features of paroxysmal atrial fibrillation. An observation of 94 patients. Jpn Heart J 1981;22:143–149.
28. Brugada R, Tapscott T, Czernuszewicz GZ et al. Identification of a genetic locus for familial atrial fibrillation. N Engl J Med 1997;336:905–911.
29. Henry WL, Morganroth J, Pearlman AS et al. Relation between echocardiographically determined left atrial size and atrial fibrillation. Circulation 1976;53:273–279.
30. Hoglund C, Rosenhamer G. Echocardiographic left atrial dimension as a predictor of maintaining sinus rhythm after conversion of atrial fibrillation. Acta Med Scand 1985;217:411–415.
31. Ewy GA, Ulfers L, Hager WD et al. Response of atrial fibrillation to therapy: role of etiology and left atrial diameter. J Electrocardiol 1980;13: 119–123.
32. Dittrich HC, Erickson JS, Schneiderman T et al. Echocardiographic and clinical predictors for outcome of elective cardioversion of atrial fibrillation. Am J Cardiol 1989;63:193–197.
33. Ellenbogen KA, Stambler BS, Wood MA et al. Efficacy of intravenous ibutilide for rapid termination of atrial fibrillation and atrial flutter: a dose-response study. J Am Coll Cardiol 1996;28:130–136.
34. Antman EM, Beamer AD, Cantillon C et al. Therapy of refractory symptomatic atrial fibrillation and atrial flutter: a staged care approach with new antiarrhythmic drugs. J Am Coll Cardiol 1990;15:698–707.
35. Anonymous. Stroke Prevention in Atrial Fibrillation Study: final results. The Stroke Prevention in Atrial Fibrillation Investigators. Circulation 1991; 84:527–539.
36. Flaker GC, Blackshear JL, McBride R et al. Antiarrhythmic drug therapy and cardiac mortality in atrial fibrillation. The Stroke Prevention in Atrial Fibrillation Investigators. J Am Coll Cardiol 1992;20:527–532.
37. Singh SN, Fletcher RD, Fisher SG et al. Amiodarone in patients with

congestive heart failure and asymptomatic ventricular arrhythmia. Survival Trial of Antiarrhythmic Therapy in Congestive Heart Failure. N Engl J Med 1995;333:77–82.

38. Doval HC, Nul DR, Grancelli HO et al. Randomised trial of low-dose amiodarone in severe congestive heart failure. Grupo de Estudio de la Sobrevida en la Insuficiencia Cardiaca en Argentina (GESICA). Lancet 1994;344:493–498.

39. Cairns JA, Connolly SJ, Gent M et al. Post-myocardial infarction mortality in individuals with ventricular premature depolarization. Canadian Amiodarone Myocardial Infarction Arrhythmia Trial Pilot Study. Circulation 1991;84:550–557.

40. Gosselink AT, Crijns HJ, Van Gelder IC et al. Low-dose amiodarone for maintenance of sinus rhythm after cardioversion of atrial fibrillation or flutter. JAMA 1992;267:3289–3293.

41. Hohnloser SH, Klingenheben T, Singh BN. Amiodarone-associated proarrhythmic effects. A review with special reference to torsade de pointes tachycardia. Ann Intern Med 1994;121:529–535.

42. Zipes D, Klein L, Miles W. Nonpharmacologic therapy: can it replace antiarrhythmic drug therapy? J Cardiovasc Electrophysiol 1991;2(Suppl): S225–S272.

43. Williamson BD, Man KC, Daoud E et al. Radiofrequency catheter modification of atrioventricular conduction to control the ventricular rate during atrial fibrillation. N Engl J Med 1994;331:910–917.

44. Feld GK, Fleck RP, Fujimura O et al. Control of rapid ventricular response by radiofrequency catheter modification of the atrioventricular node in patients with medically refractory atrial fibrillation. Circulation 1994;90: 2299–2307.

45. Defauw JJ, Guiraudon GM, van Hemel NM et al. Surgical therapy of paroxysmal atrial fibrillation with the "corridor" operation. Ann Thorac Surg 1992;53:564–570.

46. Guiraudon G, Klein G, Sharma A et al. Surgery for atrial flutter, atrial fibrillation, and atrial tachycardia. In: Zipes D, Jalife J, eds. Cardiac electrophysiology from cell to bedside. Philadelphia: WB Saunders, 1990: 915–920.

47. Cox JL, Boineau JP, Schuessler RB et al. Successful surgical treatment of atrial fibrillation. Review and clinical update. JAMA 1991;266:1976–1980.

48. Swartz JF, Pellersels G, Silvers J et al. A catheter-based curative approach to atrial fibrillation in humans [Abstract]. Circulation 1994;90:I-335.

49. Haissaguerre M, Gencel L, Fischer B et al. Successful catheter ablation of atrial fibrillation. J Cardiovasc Electrophysiol 1994;5:1045–1052.

50. Rosenqvist M, Brandt J, Schuller H. Atrial versus ventricular pacing in sinus node disease: a treatment comparison study. Am Heart J 1986;111: 292–297.

51. Sutton R, Kenny RA. The natural history of sick sinus syndrome [Review]. Pacing Clin Electrophysiol 1986;9:1110–1114.

52. Luderitz B, Pfeiffer D, Tebbenjohanns J et al. Nonpharmacologic strategies for treating atrial fibrillation [Review]. Am J Cardiol 1996;77:45A–52A.

53. Mancini GB, Goldberger AL. Cardioversion of atrial fibrillation: consideration of embolization, anticoagulation, prophylactic pacemaker, and long-term success. Am Heart J 1982;104:617–621.

54. Manning WJ, Leeman DE, Gotch PJ et al. Pulsed Doppler evaluation of atrial mechanical function after electrical cardioversion of atrial fibrillation. J Am Coll Cardiol 1989;13:617–623.

55. Manning WJ, Silverman Dl, Gordon SP et al. Cardioversion from atrial fibrillation without prolonged anticoagulation with use of transesophageal echocardiography to exclude the presence of atrial thrombi. N Engl J Med 1993;328:750–755.

56. Anonymous. Predictors of thromboembolism in atrial fibrillation: II. Echocardiographic features of patients at risk. The Stroke Prevention in Atrial Fibrillation Investigators. Ann Intern Med 1992;116:6–12.

57. Crijns HJ, Van Gelder IC, Van Gilst WH et al. Serial antiarrhythmic drug treatment to maintain sinus rhythm after electrical cardioversion for chronic atrial fibrillation or atrial flutter. Am J Cardiol 1991;68:335–341.

58. Lundstrom T, Ryden L. Chronic atrial fibrillation. Long-term results of direct current conversion. Acta Med Scand 1988;223:53–59.

59. Hull R, Hirsh J, Jay R et al. Different intensities of oral anticoagulant therapy in the treatment of proximal-vein thrombosis. N Engl J Med 1982; 307:1676–1681.

60. Sherman DG, Goldman L, Whiting RB et al. Thromboembolism in individuals with atrial fibrillation. Arch Neurol 1984;41:708–710.

61. Wolf PA, Kannel WB, McGee DL et al. Duration of atrial fibrillation and imminence of stroke: the Framingham study. Stroke 1983;14:664–667.

62. Daniel WG, Nellessen U, Schroder E et al. Left atrial spontaneous echo contrast in mitral valve disease: an indicator for an increased thromboembolic risk. J Am Coll Cardiol 1988;11:1204–1211.

63. Black IW, Hopkins AP, Lee LC et al. Left atrial spontaneous echo contrast: a clinical and echocardiographic analysis. J Am Coll Cardiol 1991;18: 398–404.

64. Kelley RE, Berger JR, Alter M et al. Cerebral ischemia and atrial fibrillation: prospective study. Neurology 1984;34:1285–1291.

65. Hart RG, Coull BM, Hart D. Early recurrent embolism associated with nonvalvular atrial fibrillation: a retrospective study. Stroke 1983;14: 688–693.

66. Anonymous. Cerebral embolism and anticoagulation [Letter]. Neurology 1983;33:1103–1106.

67. Hyleck EM, Skates SJ, Sheehan MA et al. An analysis of the lowest effective intensity of prophylactic anticoagulation for patients with nonrheumatic atrial fibrillation. N Engl J Med 1996;335:540–546.

68. Fukuda Y, Nakamura K. The incidence of thromboembolism and the hemocoagulative background in patients with rheumatic heart disease. Jpn Circ J 1984;48:59–66.

69. Laupacis A, Albers G, Dunn M et al. Antithrombotic therapy in atrial fibrillation [Review]. Chest 1992;102:426S–433S.

70. Barker PS, Bohning AL, Wilson FN. Auricular fibrillation in Grave's disease. Am Heart J 1932;8:121–127.

71. Yuen RW, Gutteridge DH, Thompson PL et al. Embolism in thyrotoxic atrial fibrillation. Med J Aust 1979;1:630–631.

72. Woeber KA. Thyrotoxicosis and the heart [Review]. N Engl J Med 1992; 327:94–98.

73. Godtfredsen J. Atrial fibrillation: etiology, course and prognosis: a follow-up study of 1212 cases [Thesis]. Copenhagen: University of Copenhagen, 1975.

74. Nakazawa HK, Sakurai K, Hamada N et al. Management of atrial fibrillation in the post-thyrotoxic state. Am J Med 1982;72:903–906.

75. Presti CF, Hart RG. Thyrotoxicosis, atrial fibrillation, and embolism revisited. Am Heart J 1989;117:976–977.

76. Navab A, La Due JS. Postconversion systemic arterial embolism. Am J Cardiol 1965;16:452–453.

77. Ikram H, Nixon PG, Arcan T. Left atrial function after electrical conversion to sinus rhythm. Br Heart J 1968;30:80–83.

78. DeSilva RA, Lown B. Cardioversion for atrial fibrillation—indications and complications. In: Kulbertus HE, Olsson SB, Schlepper M, eds. Atrial fibrillation. Molndal: AB Hassle, 1982:231–239.

79. Whittle J, Wickenheiser L, Venditti L. Is warfarin underused in the treatment of elderly persons with atrial fibrillation? Arch Intern Med 1997;157: 441–445.

80. Ott A, Breteler MM, de Bruyne MC et al. Atrial fibrillation and dementia in a population-based study. The Rotterdam Study. Stroke 1997;28:316–321.

81. Ezekowitz MD, James KE, Nazarian SM et al. Silent cerebral infarction in patients with nonrheumatic atrial fibrillation. The Veterans Affairs Stroke Prevention in Nonrheumatic Atrial Fibrillation Investigators. Circulation 1995;92:2178–2182.

# CHAPTER 61

# PREVENTION AND TREATMENT OF VENOUS THROMBOEMBOLIC DISEASE

## Charles W. Francis

Because of its high frequency as well as serious morbitidy and mortality, venous thromboembolic disease is a major health problem in the United States. Symptomatic disease results in approximately 260,000 hospital admissions per year (1), and asymptomatic calf-vein thrombosis occurs in as many as 20 to 30% of adult individuals following general surgery or during hospitalization with an acute medical illness (2). Anticoagulant treatment requires frequent laboratory tests, and it produces bleeding complications that also contribute to the high cost of care. Venous thrombosis often results in permanent vein damage. Chronic venous insufficiency develops in at least one-third of individuals (3). This manifests as leg swelling, pain, and ulceration, and it affects up to 500,000 individuals (4, 5). Deep vein thrombosis also is the precursor of pulmonary embolism, which causes 50,000 to 100,000 deaths per year and contributes to the deaths of many seriously ill and debilitated individuals (4–8).

## PREVENTION

Strategies for prevention include both primary and secondary prophylaxis as well as treatment of acute symptomatic episodes. Successful prophylaxis depends on consideration of disease incidence as well as the efficacy, safety, convenience, and cost of available treatment modalities. Thus, because of the high incidence of recurrence, secondary prophylaxis is needed after an initial episode of symptomatic deep vein thrombosis or pulmonary embolism. Strategies for pri-

mary prophylaxis have resulted from accurate epidemiologic information regarding incidence in at-risk groups and also from an understanding of the natural history of venous thrombosis.

The most widely used diagnostic technique in many studies of venous thrombosis has been the radioactive fibrinogen uptake test (RFUT). Although not routinely available clinically, this technique is noninvasive. The results also correlate well with venographic findings, thus making it suitable for screening large numbers of individuals. Results, however, correlate poorly with clinical symptoms of venous thrombosis, because most positive tests are caused by small, asymptomatic calf-vein thrombi. The clinical importance of such clots is controversial, and many resolve spontaneously. Therefore, many have been been skeptical regarding the value of prophylaxis based on studies using RFUT as the sole endpoint for efficacy. This is unjustified, however, when the findings are considered in relation to the good correlation with venography and the natural history of venous thrombosis, which has been studied carefully during the high-risk, postoperative period (9). Thrombi begin forming in calf-veins either during or soon after surgery. Most are asymptomatic at this stage, and many regress spontaneously. Without treatment, 20% extend to veins proximal to the knee, and this results in a significant risk of pulmonary embolism (9, 10), many of which are asymptomatic or may be misdiagnosed (11). The effectiveness of prophylaxis has been demonstrated in large studies with clinically relevant endpoints, the results of which have supported those of studies using RFUT.

The rapidly fatal outcome in many individuals with pulmonary embolism also supports the rationale for primary prevention. For example, reviewing the clinical records of 271 individuals shown at autopsy to have pulmonary embolism as the principal cause of death, Donaldson et al (12) revealed that 75% died during the first hour after the initial symptoms developed (Fig. 61.1). This study included only fatal cases, but it emphasizes that death from embolism may be too rapid for an accurate diagnosis and effective therapy in many individuals. Thus, many deaths could be prevented by prophylaxis.

## SURGICAL PATIENTS

### Postoperative Venous Thrombosis and Pulmonary Embolism

The simplest approach to postoperative venous thrombosis and pulmonary embolism would be treatment of clinically evident disease, but this is unacceptable in moderate-risk or high-risk groups. This is because postoperative deep vein thrombosis frequently is asymptomatic, and the initial presentation of pulmonary embolism may be sudden death. A second potential strategy would be routine monitoring with noninvasive tests, such as RFUT, ultrasonography, or plethysmography, followed by treatment of affected individuals only. This approach is both expensive and cumbersome, however, and it raises difficult problems in treatment of false-positive or false-negative results. The most effective approach, therefore, is primary prophylaxis in moderate-risk or high-risk individuals using either anticoagulants or methods to reduce venous stasis (Table 61.1).

Prophylaxis should be selected, at least in part, on the basis of the risks in specific surgical groups (13). Young individuals undergoing surgical procedures for less than 30 minutes with minimal immobility have the lowest risk. Individuals at moderate risk include those older than 40 years undergoing general abdominal or thoracic surgery for more than 30 minutes, with an incidence of total venous thrombosis of 20 to 30%, proximal vein thrombosis of 2 to 10%, and fatal pulmonary embolism of 0.1 to 0.7%. In certain high-risk orthopedic individual groups, the overall incidence of venous thrombosis is between 40 and 70%; of proximal vein thrombosis, 20%; of pulmonary embolism, 5 to 10%; and of fatal pulmonary embolism, 1 to 5% (13, 14).

**FIGURE 61.1.** Time of death in relation to the occurrence of initial symptoms in 271 individuals with pulmonary embolism identified at autopsy as the primary cause of death. (Adapted with permission from Donaldson GA, Williams C, Scannell JG, et al. A reappraisal of the application of the Trendelenburg Operation to massive pulmonary embolism. N Engl J Med 1963; 268:171–174.)

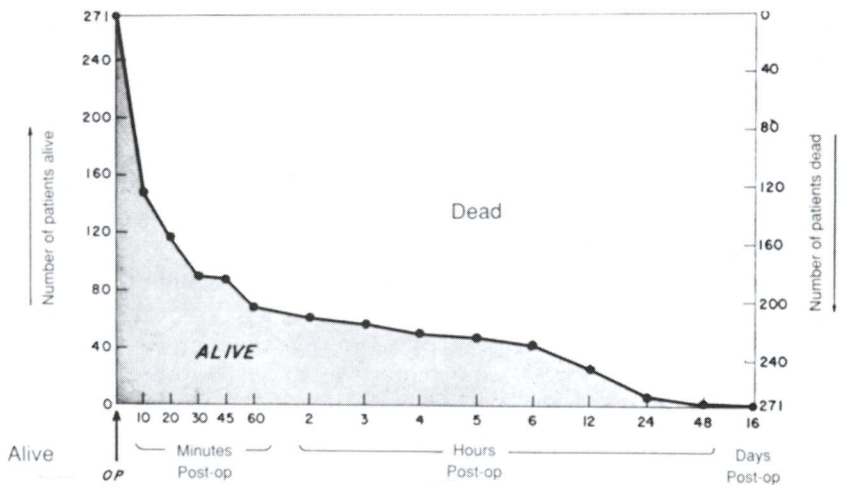

**TABLE 61.1.**    Rationale for Prevention of Venous Thrombosis

| Problem | Treatment | Action |
| --- | --- | --- |
| Venous stasis | Compression stockings | Decreases venous capacitance |
| | Early ambulation, leg exercises | Increases venous flow physiologically |
| | Pneumatic compression | Increases venous flow by external compression, stimulates local fibrinolysis |
| Hypercoagulability | Heparin | Accelerates antithrombin inhibition of factor Xa and thrombin |
| | Warfarin | Reduces vitamin K-dependent coagulation factors |
| | Dextran | Multiple |

**TABLE 61.2.** Results of the International Multicenter Trial of Prevention of Postoperative Venous Thromboembolic Disease with Low-dose Heparin (33)

|  | Control Group[a] | Heparin Group[b] | *P* |
|---|---|---|---|
| Fatal pulmonary emboli | 16/2076 (0.8%) | 2/2045 (0.1%) | <.005 |
| Clinically diagnosed pulmonary emboli | 24/2076 (1.2%) | 8/2075 (0.4%) | <.01 |
| Symptomatic DVT (confirmed by venography) | 32/2076 (1.5%) | 11/2075 (0.5%) | <.005 |
| Venous thrombosis by RFUT | 164/667 (25%) | 48/625 (8%) | <.005 |

*Data from Anonymous. Prevention of fatal postoperative pulmonary embolism by low doses of heparin. An international multicentre trial. Lancet 1975;ii:45–51.*

DVT, *deep vein thrombosis;* RFUT, *radioactive fibrinogen uptake test.*

[a] *No prophylaxis.*

[b] *Calcium heparin, 5000 U subcutaneously 2 hours before surgery and every 8 hours for 7 days.*

Anesthesia, operative pain, bed rest, and lack of muscle activity all reduce venous blood flow, thus predisposing individuals to thrombosis. Simple measures to counteract venous stasis that can be applied to nearly all individuals include leg and foot exercises while in bed as well as early ambulation. Elastic stockings may decrease venous capacitance, but their use has little documented benefit in preventing venous thrombosis. Graduated compression stockings that exert greater pressure at the ankles and lesser pressure proximally have value in low-risk or moderate-risk individuals (15–17), and external pneumatic compression employs active leg compression with inflatable boots or cuffs that rhythmically compress the calf or both the calf and thigh sequentially. This increases venous blood flow (18, 19) and raises blood fibrinolytic activity (20, 21), both of which may contribute to its efficacy. The absence of side effects makes it an attractive prophylactic modality, particularly in individuals with an increased risk of bleeding. External pneumatic compression is effective after general abdominal (22–24), urologic (25), neurologic (26), and gynecologic surgery (including that for malignancy [27]), and elective knee surgery (28). A mechanical system that rhythmically extends the foot, thereby causing plantar venous compression, also has also been effective in limited studies (29).

The largest experience with anticoagulant prophylaxis of postoperative venous thromboembolic disease has been with low doses of heparin, the rationale being that lower concentrations are needed to prevent than to treat venous thrombosis. Heparin in a dose of 5000 U subcutaneously results in a peak plasma level of 0.05 to 0.15 U/ml approximately 2 hours after injection (30, 31). This accelerates inhibition of factor Xa and thrombin by antithrombin, and it results in a slight but detectable increase in the activated partial thromboplastin time (aPTT) (32). Administering this dose every 8 to 12 hours, beginning 2 hours before general surgery, reduces the risk of venous thrombosis by 67% and of pulmonary embolism by 47% as determined by a meta-analysis of more than 70 controlled studies (14).

Clinical benefit also has been demonstrated by a single large trial involving individuals older than 40 years undergoing major surgery (33), which demonstrated a significant reduction in fatal pulmonary embolism (diagnosed at autopsy) in individuals who received low-dose heparin prophylaxis compared with control individuals (Table 61.2). This study also demonstrated a significant reduction in clinically diagnosed pulmonary emboli in symptomatic, venographically diagnosed deep vein thrombosis and in RFUT-diagnosed venous thrombosis. This study has been criticized and reinterpreted (34, 35), but its results are consistent with those of other studies and with the overall clinical experience. Side effects include bruising at injection sites, which can be minimized by proper technique, and a 2% increase in wound hematomas (14, 33). The generally accepted effectiveness and safety of this regimen have led to recommendations for its use in moderate-risk surgical individuals (13, 36). Surveys indicate, however, that only a minority of surgeons use low-dose heparin prophylaxis because of the perceived infrequency of clinically significant thromboembolic complications and the fear of perioperative bleeding (37–39). For example, a community-wide survey of 16 Central Massachusetts hospitals found that prophylaxis was provided for only 32% of high-risk individuals (40).

There have been several modifications of low-dose heparin prophylaxis to improve its effectiveness. Ergot, which is a venoconstricting agent, has been administered with heparin to decrease venous capacitance and stasis in leg veins and to improve efficacy (41, 42). This has not been widely accepted, however, because of occasional vasospastic side effects and limited evidence for superiority of the combination compared with low-dose heparin alone.

As described in Chapter 55, heparin preparations with a restricted, low-molecular-weight range (i.e., low-molecular-weight heparin) have a greater effect on the inhibition of factor Xa by antithrombin than on the inhibition of thrombin by antithrombin. Compared with unfractionated heparin, they have more complete and predictable absorption after subcutaneous administration and a longer plasma half-life (43). Several low-molecular-weight heparin preparations are effective in preventing venous thrombosis after general surgery, with only a small increase in bleeding complications (44–54). Data regarding their superiority over unfractionated heparin are conflicting, however, with both reviews and meta-analyses suggesting approximate equivalence to unfractionated heparin in prophylaxis for general surgery (13, 43, 55). These preparations do have the advantage of being more completely absorbed after subcutaneous administration (56), which permits once-daily injection rather than two or three times daily (as needed for unfractionated heparin).

Results of some studies suggest that adjusting the heparin dosage to slightly prolong the aPTT rather than administering a fixed dose may improve effectiveness, particularly in high-risk individuals (57, 58). The observation that antithrombin levels decline postoperatively led to consideration that heparin prophylaxis could be augmented with antithrombin. This was tested in two prospective, randomized studies following total hip (59) or knee (60) arthroplasty, which demonstrated the combination of antithrombin and heparin to be safe and also more effective than a standard regimen (i.e., dextran).

## High-risk Surgical Individuals

The protection afforded by low-dose heparin is insufficient in some surgical individuals with a particularly high risk of developing venous thrombosis, including those undergoing open prostatectomy, surgery for gynecologic malignancies, and especially, after certain orthopaedic procedures. For example, after hip fracture, total hip arthroplasty, or total-knee arthroplasty, risk of venous thrombosis without prophylaxis is between 40 and 70%, and fatal pulmonary embolism occurs in from 1 to 5% of individuals (13). Several prophylactic modalities have been tested in these high-risk individuals. Dextran is effective after total hip replacement or fracture (61–64), but it is not used widely because of the need for intravenous administration and occasional precipitation of congestive heart failure, especially in older individuals (who frequently require such procedures). In a limited number of studies, external pneumatic compression has been effective after elective knee surgery (28, 65, 66), prostatectomy (25), gynecologic surgery for malignancy (27), and neurosurgery (26). It is more effective than no prophylaxis after total hip replacement (67, 68), but it is less effective than warfarin in preventing proximal vein thrombosis (69). The usual low-dose heparin regimen has not been sufficiently effective in high-risk individu-

als, but it may be more effective when administered in a dose designed to increase aPTT to the upper-normal range (57, 58) or when given in combination with antithrombin (59, 60).

Oral anticoagulants have been consistently effective in preventing venous thrombosis in high-risk individuals. In a classic study, Sevitt and Gallagher (70) demonstrated reduced clinical and autopsy evidence of pulmonary embolism and deep vein thrombosis with coumarin prophylaxis as compared to a control group. The effectiveness of warfarin has been amply confirmed in subsequent studies, but concern over bleeding complications has limited its general acceptance for use in surgical individuals. Recent studies, however, have demonstrated that a lower intensity of anticoagulation is effective without increasing the risk of bleeding, even in surgical individuals. Francis et al (71) used a low dose of warfarin, which was begun 7 to 10 days before surgery, to increase the international normalized ratio (INR) to approximately 1.5 at the time of operation, then increased the dose postoperatively to achieve an INR of 2.5. In a prospective, randomized study after total hip replacement, this regimen was more effective than dextran in preventing venographically diagnosed thrombosis, and it was associated with a low risk of bleeding. A similar approach was effective in individuals after gynecologic surgery (72). Paiement et al (73) also have reported a low incidence of venous thrombosis and bleeding complications after hip replacement with warfarin begun the night before surgery and adjusted to keep the prothrombin time at less than 15 seconds. Warfarin also has been started postoperatively (74). A study comparing a warfarin regimen beginning 7 to 10 days preoperatively with one beginning the night before surgery found no difference in outcomes in individuals undergoing knee arthroplasty (75). Regarding use of warfarin in hip replacement, meta-analyses have identified deep vein thrombosis rates of 24% (76) and 19% (77), whereas large single studies have found rates of between 14% and 23% (69, 74, 78, 79). Warfarin has been less effective with knee replacement, with deep vein thrombosis rates of between 38 and 55% in recent studies (74, 75, 78). A single study also has shown that a "fixed mini-dose" warfarin regimen, administering 1 mg daily beginning 20 days preoperatively, was effective in preventing deep vein thrombosis after major gynecologic surgery (80).

Low-molecular-weight heparin is more effective than placebo in preventing deep vein thrombosis after hip replacement (81), and meta-analyses have identified deep vein thrombosis rates of between 12 and 17% (55, 76, 77). Large North American trials using low-molecular-weight heparin after total hip replacement found deep vein thrombosis as diagnosed with venography in between 14 and 50% of individuals (78, 81–84), and several studies have directly compared low-molecular-weight heparin with warfarin after hip replacement. In three (74, 78, 79), there was no significant difference in postoperative venous thrombosis rates, whereas one (85), showed a significantly lower rate with low-molecular-weight heparin (15%) than with warfarin (26%). Low-molecular-weight heparin also has been compared with unfractionated heparin in several trials following hip replacement (82–84), and meta-analyses of published trials indicate it is superior (55, 76, 77). Clinical trials have shown low-molecular-weight heparin to be superior to placebo (86), graduated compression stockings (87), and warfarin (74, 78, 79) after knee replacement. The optimum duration of prophylaxis after joint-replacement surgery is not certain, however, and the period of risk extends for several weeks postoperatively (88, 89). This raises particular problems, because many individuals currently are discharged after only a few days in the hospital. A recent double-blind study (90) demonstrated a significantly lower incidence of venous thrombosis 1 month after surgery when prophylaxis was extended postdischarge.

Hip fracture is associated with a high risk of postoperative venous thrombosis, similar to that with joint replacement. Low-intensity warfarin is effective in reducing risk (91–93), and low-molecular-weight heparin (94, 95) and dermatan sulfate (96) achieve comparable risk reduction. No studies directly comparing warfarin and low-molecular-weight heparin are available. Individuals suffering from multiple trauma are heterogeneous, but they also have a high risk of venous thrombosis. One recent prospective study (97) found an incidence of 58% in individuals admitted to a regional trauma unit. A prospective, randomized trial (98) demonstrated that low-molecular-weight heparin was more effective than unfractionated heparin for preventing deep vein thrombosis in individuals with multiple trauma.

## MEDICAL PATIENTS

Hospitalized medical individuals have a high incidence of asymptomatic venous thrombosis if they have risk factors such as bed rest, limb paralysis, congestive heart failure, obesity, malignancy, pregnancy, old age, or chronic inflammatory disease. Clinical studies in selected groups of medical individuals have demonstrated the effectiveness of low-dose heparin prophylaxis for venous thrombosis. Following acute myocardial infarction, there is a 10 to 40% incidence of deep vein thrombosis, which is significantly reduced by low-dose heparin (99–102). Individuals with stroke have a greater than 50% incidence of venous thrombosis, principally involving the paralyzed leg; prophylaxis with heparin (103), low-molecular-weight heparin (104–106), or a heparinoid (107) results in significant risk reduction. The very high incidence of venous thrombosis in paraplegic individuals (108, 109) also can be reduced by heparin prophylaxis, but adjusted-dose (58) or low-molecular-weight heparin (110) may be superior to fixed low-dose heparin. Results of a consecutive cohort study (111) suggest that prophylactic low-dose heparin also reduces the incidence of pulmonary embolism in individuals admitted to respiratory intensive care units. The effect of low-dose heparin prophylaxis on mortality rates among general medical individuals was studied in a prospective, randomized trial of individuals older than 40 years ad-

---

**TABLE 61.3.**  Recommendations for Prophylaxis of Deep Vein Thrombosis

| Risk | Patients | Recommendation |
|------|----------|----------------|
| Low | Surgical individuals under age 40, surgery lasting less than 30 minutes, no additional risk factors | Ambulation, leg exercises |
| | Hospitalized medical individuals without risk factors | Ambulation, leg exercises |
| Moderate | Surgical individuals over age 40 having abdominal or thoracic surgery lasting more than 30 minutes | Low-dose heparin[a] |
| | Hospitalized medical individuals with one or more risk factors (e.g., acute myocardial infarction, congestive heart failure, prolonged bed rest) | Low-dose heparin[a] |
| | Neurosurgery or other individuals with high bleeding risk | Pneumatic compression |
| High | Hip fracture | Warfarin[b] |
| | Hip replacement | LMWH, warfarin,[b] adjusted-dose heparin |
| | Knee replacement | LMWH, pneumatic compression |
| | Open prostatectomy | Pneumatic compression |
| | Gynecologic malignancy | Pneumatic compression, LWMH |

LMWH, low-molecular-weight heparin.

[a] 5000 U subcutaneously every 8 or 12 hours starting 2 hours preoperatively.

[b] Given in low-dose regimen.

mitted through the emergency room to a medical service (112); in 1358 consecutive individuals, the mortality rate among those who received low-dose heparin was 31% less than that in controls ($P = .025$). Congestive heart failure is associated with an increased risk of venous thrombosis, which is significantly reduced with low-dose heparin (113). Low-molecular-weight heparin also reduces deep vein thrombosis in elderly individuals hospitalized with various medical conditions (114).

## RECOMMENDATIONS

Recommendations for prophylaxis are listed in Table 61.3, in which individuals are classified into three risk groups. For individuals at low risk, early ambulation and leg exercises are recommended. If low-risk individuals have additional factors predisposing to thrombosis, such as a history of venous thromboembolic disease, congestive heart failure, severe obesity, or if they require prolonged bed rest, low-dose heparin is indicated. Individuals older than 40 years undergoing general abdominal or thoracic surgery lasting more than 30 minutes are at moderate risk, and low-dose heparin, 5000 U subcutaneously every 8 or 12 hours beginning 2 hours before surgery and continuing until the individual is fully ambulatory, is recommended. This regimen also is appropriate for high-risk medical inpatients, such as those with acute myocardial infarction, malignancy, or paralysis. After hip fracture or replacement, a low-dose warfarin regimen to minimize bleeding complications and low-molecular-weight heparin are effective. Low-molecular-weight heparin or pneumatic compression both are effective after knee replacement; warfarin is less effective. External pneumatic compression is recommended after surgery for gynecologic malignancy or open prostatectomy, or if there is a high risk of bleeding.

## TREATMENT

The goals in treating venous thromboembolic disease are to provide symptomatic relief, prevent disease extension or recurrence, and minimize structural damage to deep leg veins, thereby preventing long-term development of chronic venous insufficiency. This requires a choice to be made from several effective forms of anticoagulant, fibrinolytic, and surgical treatments to maximize individual benefit. When making such therapeutic choices, the risk–benefit ratio is of central importance, and it always involves difficult issues of clinical judgment focused on the individual individual, including considerations of disease extent, risk of bleeding, individual ability to comply with long-term therapy, and coexisting medical illnesses that contribute to thrombotic risk or influence drug response. Careful assessment of bleeding risk is particularly important, because

both anticoagulant and fibrinolytic therapies are associated with bleeding complications.

One critical element in providing appropriate therapy is an accurate diagnosis, and objective documentation is recommended in all individuals before therapy is initiated (see Chapter 25). The clinical presentation of both pulmonary embolism and venous thrombosis is nonspecific, and many individuals with suggestive clinical findings will not have thrombosis confirmed through objective diagnostic methods. Therefore, if a treatment is chosen on the basis of clinical suspicion alone and without objective confirmation, individuals without thrombotic disease will receive anticoagulant therapy, thus placing them at risk for bleeding and other complications and delaying therapy for the disorder actually causing symptoms. An additional benefit of objective diagnosis is that it helps to establish the extent and severity of disease, both of which are important considerations in designing the optimal therapeutic approach. For example, individuals with massive pulmonary embolism benefit more than individuals with smaller emboli from fibrinolytic therapy, and therapy for isolated calf-vein thrombosis differs from that for extensive proximal leg-vein thrombosis.

## ANTICOAGULANT THERAPY

### Short-term Anticoagulation

Pulmonary embolism and deep vein thrombosis most often are treated with short-term heparin, which is followed by a longer period of outpatient oral anticoagulation. Evidence for the efficacy of anticoagulant treatment derives from the overall clinical experience, descriptive studies (115–117), and results of single controlled trials in individuals with pulmonary embolism (118) or venous thrombosis (119). In a remarkable study (118), individuals with clinically diagnosed pulmonary embolism were allocated to groups receiving either anticoagulant or no anticoagulant treatment. The anticoagulant group was treated with heparin, given by an intravenous injection of 10,000 U every six hours for a total of six doses, without laboratory control. Coumarin was begun concurrently, and the dose was adjusted based on the prothrombin time. Without anticoagulation, fatal pulmonary embolism occurred in five of 19 individuals, an incidence that was significantly higher than that in the group receiving anticoagulation (0 of 54; $P = .0007$). The total incidence of fatal or nonfatal recurrent pulmonary embolism also was significantly less in the anticoagulated group (one of 54, compared with 10 of 19 in the control group; $P = 1.4 \times 10^{-6}$). This trial had major methodologic shortcomings, but its results are impressive. There have been no subsequent studies with an untreated control group.

In individuals with proximal deep vein thrombosis, a double-blind, prospective trial compared the use of intravenous heparin plus warfarin with warfarin alone for initial treatment (119). Symptomatic extension or recurrence occurred in 20% of individuals treated with warfarin alone but in only 7% of those who received heparin in addition ($P = .058$). Furthermore, asymptomatic extension as detected by repeat venography and lung scanning occurred in 40% of individuals not receiving heparin, compared with only 8% of those treated with heparin ($P < .001$).

The efficacy of heparin anticoagulation is further supported by clinical studies demonstrating a low incidence of pulmonary embolism or recurrent venous thrombosis in individuals adequately anticoagulated acutely with heparin, followed by either warfarin or adjusted-dose heparin (120–123). Recurrence rates are significantly higher if anticoagulation is inadequate during the acute (124, 125) or the outpatient (126) phase of treatment. The ability of heparin to prevent thrombus extension has been documented in two studies (127, 128) using pretreatment and posttreatment venography to quantitate thrombus size, which demonstrated no overall change in the mean extent of thrombosis after treatment with heparin. Of note, however, was extension of the thrombus in 33% of heparin-treated individuals in one study (127) and in 22% of the other (128), thereby indicating that extension can occur despite apparently adequate heparin anticoagulation.

An important determinant of the efficacy of initial anticoagulation is administration of sufficient heparin to prolong the aPTT to within the therapeutic range. Thus, Hull et al (125) correlated recurrence of venous thromboembolism with adequacy of anticoagulation in a randomized, prospective study comparing intravenous with subcutaneous heparin as initial treatment of proximal vein thrombosis. Recurrence was more frequent in those failing to achieve an aPTT of 1.5 times control or greater during the initial 24 hours of treatment. The association between an inadequately prolonged aPTT and recurrent venous thrombosis also was supported by Basu et al (124), who found that the mean aPTT in individuals with recurrent venous thrombosis was less than 1.5 times control and was significantly shorter than that in individuals who did not develop recurrence. The importance of prolonging the aPTT during initial treatment of venous thrombosis is especially relevant considering a survey of physician practices (129), which indicated that 60% of individuals treated for deep vein thrombosis or pulmonary embolism did not have a single aPTT greater than 1.5 times control within the first 24 hours of heparin therapy. In addition, not until the eighth day of treatment were 90% of aPTTs in the therapeutic range. The importance of adequate anticoagulation in preventing recurrence also is evident from studies evaluating chronic outpatient treatment

with subcutaneous heparin after an initial episode of symptomatic deep vein thrombosis. Administration of a fixed low dose of heparin was associated with a high incidence of recurrence (123), whereas a regimen adjusted to prolong the midinterval aPTT to 1.5 times control was as effective as warfarin (120). Use of a heparin-dosing nomogram with a weight-based (130) or fixed-dose (131) (Table 61.4) approach simplifies intravenous heparin administration and results in attaining a therapeutic level more rapidly.

## TABLE 61.4. Heparin Dosing Nomograms[a]

### Fixed-dose Nomogram

| aPTT (sec)[b] | Bolus Dose (units) | Stop Infusion (min) | Change Infusion Rate (ml/hr)[c] | Time to Repeat aPTT |
|---|---|---|---|---|
| <50 | 5000 | 0 | +3 | 6 hours |
| 50–59 | 0 | 0 | +3 | 6 hours |
| 60–85 | 0 | 0 | 0 | Next morning |
| 86–95 | 0 | 0 | −2 | Next morning |
| 96–120 | 0 | 30 | −2 | 6 hours |
| >120 | 0 | 60 | −4 | 6 hours |

[a] Modified with permission from Cruickshank MK, Levine MN, Hirsh J et al. A standard heparin nomogram for the management of heparin therapy. Arch Intern Med 1991;151:333–337.

[b] Normal range is 25–37 seconds. Therapeutic range is 60–85 seconds corresponding to a plasma heparin level of 0.2–0.4 U/ml by protamine sulfate neutralization.

[c] 1 ml/hr equals 40 U/hr.

### Weight-based Nomogram[a]

The initial dose is 80 U/kg as a bolus, then 18 U/kg per hour. The following dose adjustments are based on aPTT values obtained every 6 hours.

| aPTT (sec)[b] | Dose Adjustment Bolus Units/kg | Dose Adjustment Infusion Units/kg/hour |
|---|---|---|
| <35 | 80 | +4 |
| 35–45 | 40 | +2 |
| 46–70 | 0 | 0 |
| 71–90 | 0 | −2 |
| >90 | 0 | −3 (also hold 1 hour) |

[a] Adapted with permission from Raschke RA, Reilly BM, Guidry JR et al. The weight-based heparin dosing nomogram compared with a 'standard care' nomogram: a randomized control trial. Ann Intern Med 1993;119:874–881.

[b] Normal range 20–30 sec.

Two problems complicate laboratory monitoring of heparin therapy (see Chapter 55). First, multiple reagents with varying sensitivities to heparin are available for aPTT determination, and they are used with different coagulation systems. Consequently, the aPTT measured for a heparinized plasma sample may vary depending on the reagents and the system used in a particular laboratory; therefore, laboratories should standardize the therapeutic aPTT range for heparin to correspond with plasma heparin levels of 0.2 to 0.4 U/ml using protamine titration or 0.3 to 0.7 U/ml using an anti–factor Xa assay (132). After appropriate standardization, the aPTT can be used for monitoring therapy in most individuals. The second problem is the large interpatient variability in response to unfractionated heparin, resulting in part from effects of the acute-phase response that elevate levels of heparin-binding proteins and of factor VIII in ill individuals. These can decrease the aPTT during therapy and lead to "heparin resistance." Most individuals with subtherapeutic aPTTs despite high doses of heparin (>35,000 U per 24 hours) will have adequate plasma heparin levels if measured directly by protamine titration or anti–factor Xa. Such individuals can be treated adequately using plasma heparin assays to monitor therapy (133).

Bleeding is the most frequent complication of heparin. It occurs in approximately 10% of individuals, but the incidence varies greatly, with 1 to 33% rates of overall bleeding complications reported (134). This variability probably relates to differences in individual selection, dose, and adminstration methods. The risk of major bleeding complications in recent clinical studies of venous thromboembolism is less than 2% (134), and the incidence of bleeding with intermittent as compared to continuous heparin administration demonstrates a consistently lower risk from continuous administration (135–137). Weaker evidence suggests a higher risk of bleeding from higher daily doses of heparin and excessive aPTT prolongation. Overall, the most important predictors of bleeding are specific clinical features, including lower performance status, history of bleeding tendency, recent trauma or surgery, older age, hepatic dysfunction, and malignancy (138–141). Women may be at increased risk compared with men, as may heavy alcohol drinkers and individuals receiving aspirin (142).

Improvements in both convenience and cost-effectiveness have spurred studies examining the efficacy of subcutaneous heparin for initial treatment of acute venous thrombosis and of shorter durations for initial treatment. Results of several studies (143–146) and a meta-analysis (147) indicate that continuous intravenous as well as dose-adjusted subcutaneous heparin are equally effective in preventing recurrent venous thrombosis or pulmonary embolism when used as initial treatment of venous thrombosis. Attention to careful monitoring is necessary, however, because one study (125) found a high incidence of recurrence in association with inadequate early prolongation of the aPTT. Shortened hospital stay and attendant cost savings also can be realized by reducing the usual 10-day course of parenteral heparin therapy for initial treatment of venous thrombosis, and two studies have evaluated outcomes with a 4- or 5-day course of heparin with initiation of warfarin between the first and third days of treatment (123, 148). The frequency of objectively documented recurrence was not greater with shorter heparin therapy, which resulted in earlier hospital discharge and lower costs (149).

The superior pharmacologic properties of low-molecular-weight heparin (see Chapter 55) offer the possibility of treatment with subcutaneous administration without need for laboratory monitoring and dose adjustment. Meta-analyses (150–152) of many published trials indicate that subcutaneous low-molecular-weight heparin is more effective and produces fewer bleeding complications than therapy with intravenous heparin monitored using the aPTT. These findings are consistent with those of two large, randomized, prospective trials (153, 154). Both of these trials randomized individuals with acute proximal deep vein thrombosis to either twice-daily injections of low-molecular-weight heparin or heparin given intravenously with dose adjustment based on laboratory monitoring. Recurrent venous thromboembolism and bleeding complications were comparable in both groups in both studies, but the individuals assigned to low-molecular-weight heparin had markedly shorter hospital stays and improved quality-of-life measures. Use of low-molecular-weight heparin as primary therapy for deep vein thrombosis probably will result in simplified treatment and lower hospital use. Caution should be used, however, when generalizing the findings of these studies, which excluded many individuals and were conducted under carefully controlled conditions. Furthermore, some of the expected cost savings actually will be costs merely shifted to outpatient services (155).

## Long-term Anticoagulation

Patients with deep vein thrombosis or pulmonary embolism remain at risk for recurrence after initial heparin treatment, and they require continued anticoagulation. Oral anticoagulants effectively prevent recurrence and are convenient for outpatient treatment. Warfarin can be administered on the first day of therapy and heparin or low-molecular-weight heparin discontinued after 5 days, when a therapeutic level of oral anticoagulation has been achieved. Warfarin decreases all vitamin K-dependent proteins, including proteins C and S, which have anticoagulant properties, as well the procoagulant factors II, VII, IX, and X (see Chapter 55). During initiation of therapy, levels of factor VII and protein C decrease rapidly because of their short plasma half-lives, whereas the full anticoagulant effect depends on concomitant reduction of other procoagulants, including factor II. Therefore, prolonged PTs during the first 48 hours of therapy do not reflect adequate anticoagulation, and heparin should not be discontinued during this period despite prolongation of the PT. There is considerable individual variability in the response to warfarin, and the dose must be titrated carefully during initiation of therapy. Interaction with a number of foods and drugs also may alter the anticoagulant response (156).

The optimum intensity of oral anticoagulation to prevent recurrence while minimizing bleeding complications has been studied in clinical trials. These studies have demonstrated that a "less intense" regimen is equally effective as well as safer than higher-intensity regimens used previously. In a series of clinical studies, Hull et al (120, 121, 123, 126) determined the rates of recurrence and bleeding complications in individuals treated with several anticoagulant regimens after an acute episode of proximal deep vein thrombosis. They demonstrated that recurrent venous thromboembolism was prevented effectively at an intensity of anticoagulation corresponding to an INR of 3 or lower. More intense anticoagulation resulted in no therapeutic benefit but increased bleeding complicatons. Subcutaneous heparin also can be used for long-term outpatient treatment and is appropriate for individuals who are pregnant or cannot take warfarin. Given subcutaneously every 12 hours in a dose to prolong the midinterval aPTT to 1.5 times control, heparin is effective as warfarin in preventing recurrent thrombosis (120), but lower fixed-dose heparin is associated with an increased risk of recurrence (126). In addition, low-molecular-weight heparin has been a successful alternative to warfarin for outpatient treatment to prevent recurrence in small studies using doses of 5000 U doses of anti–factor Xa twice daily (157) or 4000 U of anti–factor Xa once daily (158).

Risk of recurrent venous thromboembolism declines with time after the acute event, as shown by Coon and Ellis (159), who observed the clinical course of 1539 individuals treated for acute venous thrombosis or pulmonary embolism. The recurrence rate was approximately 8% in the first week and 6% in the second, but it decreased progressively to less than 1% between the tenth and the sixteenth weeks. Recurrence was greatly reduced in individuals who received outpatient anticoagulant therapy. The optimal duration of anticoagulant therapy depends on the risk of recurrence after discontinuation and on both the complications and inconvenience of prolonged therapy. Several recent studies specifically addressed this issue (160–163), comparing shorter courses (4–6 weeks) with longer treatment (3–6 months). Overall, longer-duration therapy was associated with lower rates of recurrent venous thromboembolic disease. In addition, a multicenter trial (162) randomized 902 individuals with a first episode of venous thromboemoblism to 6 weeks or 6 months of oral anticoagulant therapy after initial treatment with heparin or low-molecular-weight heparin. After a 2-year follow-up, the recurrence rate was 18.1% in the 6-week group, compared with 9.5% in the 6-month group (*P* < .001). Recurrences in the shorter-treatment group were clustered shortly after discontinuation of treatment. In a similar study (160), the Research Committee of the British Thoracic Society randomly allocated individuals with deep vein thrombosis or pulmonary embolism to either 4 weeks or 3 months of oral anticoagulant treatment; in this study, recurrence rates were 4.0 versus 7.8%, respectively (*P* = .04). Duration of anticoagulation also was investigated in a prospective trial comparing 6-month with indefinite therapy using warfarin (164). In this study, those treated for 6 months experienced an eightfold increase in risk of recurrence and a decreased risk of major bleeding.

In these latter two studies, the rates of recurrence were lower in individuals with postoperative deep vein thrombosis or other transient, reversible risk factors, and they were higher in individuals for idiopathic venous thrombosis in individuals with a continuing predisposition. Prandoni et al (163) found a recurrence rate of 24% during 80 weeks of follow-up in individuals with idiopathic deep vein thrombosis, compared with 4.8% in other individuals. In addition, Levine et al (161) found a recurrence rate of 12.3% within 11 months in 212 individuals with continuing risk factors, compared with no recurrences in 89 individuals with transient risk factors (*P* = .0007) after initial therapy with warfarin.

Patients with venous thromboembolism associated with a transient risk (e.g., postoperative deep vein thrombosis) can be treated successfully with 4 to 6 weeks of oral anticoagulation. Individuals with venous thromboembolism without clear, predisposing factors have a greater risk and should be treated for 3 to 6 months. Longer treatment durations should be reserved for those with more extensive disease and shorter treatment durations for those with increased bleeding risk. Individuals with continuing risks (e.g., metastatic cancer) or inherited thrombophilia or recurrent episodes need prolonged treatment, as do individuals with recurrent venous thromboembolism.

## Calf-vein Thrombosis

Both the importance and treatment of isolated calf-vein thrombosis remain controversial. Symptomatic pulmonary emboli derive principally from proximal vein thrombosis (10). Calf-vein thrombosis may propagate to proximal veins, with resultant pulmonary emboli, and also may result in venous dysfunction and postphlebitic symptoms.

Kakkar et al (9) examined the natural history of postoperative asymptomatic venous thrombosis, and they observed that most calf thrombi resolved or remained confined to the calf. Approximately 20%, however, extended proximally, and of these, half caused pulmonary embolism. Lagerstedt et al (122) found a 29% incidence of recurrence in individuals with isolated calf-vein thrombosis treated using an initial course of heparin without subsequent oral anticoagulation, thus demonstrating the importance of adequate treatment. In addition, Pellegrini et al (165) found that four of 13 individuals with untreated, asymptomatic calf-vein thrombosis after total hip replacement subsequently developed symptomatic or fatal pulmonary embolism. These findings indicate that untreated, or inadequately treated, calf-vein thrombosis is associated with proximal extension, recurrence, and pulmonary embolism. Hemodynamic studies have demonstrated that valve incompetence in the perforating veins of the calf is the most common abnormality in individuals with postphlebitic syndrome (166, 167), and that calf-vein thrombosis may cause valve damage and incompetence. The high incidence of postphlebitic syndrome following calf-vein thrombosis, even after treatment, supports this possibility (168).

Thus, two strategies are appropriate for treatment of isolated calf-vein thrombosis. Because the greatest risk for significant pulmonary embolism is associated with proximal extension of thrombosis, individuals can be monitored with noninvasive tests and treatment withheld if there is no evidence of proximal extension. In two studies (169, 170), anticoagulant therapy was withheld in individuals having symptoms consistent with calf-vein thrombosis and who had negative serial impedance plethysmography (IPG) tests over a period of as long as 2 weeks. The incidence of pulmonary embolism was low, thereby indicating that anticoagulation can be withheld in individuals who are carefully monitored for proximal extension. Without careful serial monitoring, however, anticoagulant therapy is indicated.

## Recurrent Venous Thrombosis

Patients are at risk for recurrent venous thrombosis after an initial episode of venous thromboembolism, and both evaluation and treatment of suspected recurrence poses several problems. The diagnosis often is difficult to make, because the symptoms of acute recurrent venous thrombosis can be mimicked by the leg pain and swelling of postphlebitic syndrome. The symptoms and clinical findings are nonspecific; therefore, the diagnosis of recurrent venous thrombosis should be established with objective tests. Unfortunately, however, this is more difficult than the evaluation of an initial episode, because the structural and flow abnormalities resulting from previous thrombosis make interpretation of some tests less certain. Therefore, in individuals with recurrent symptoms, it is helpful to obtain a baseline venogram, ultrasound, or IPG during an asymptomatic interval for comparison when recurrent symptoms develop. Following proximal vein thrombosis, outflow obstruction as demonstrated by IPG returns to normal by 3 weeks in 30% of individuals and by 3 months in 70% (171).

Treatment depends on both the extent of thrombosis and whether the individual was receiving adequate anticoagulation at the time of recurrence. Full short-term heparinization is needed in individuals with recurrent pulmonary embolism or proximal venous thrombosis; it also is needed in some individuals with extensive calf-vein thrombosis. If recurrence develops when the individual is off treatment or receiving subtherapeutic anticoagulation, similar treatment can be given as for an initial episode, only the duration of oral anticoagulation should be longer. Indefinite anticoagulation may be needed in individuals with multiple recurrences. The most difficult to diagnose are individuals who have documented recurrence while on adequate anticoagulant therapy. Most can be treated successfully by altering or increasing the intensity of anticoagulation. Increasing the INR from between 2.0 and 3.0 to between 3.0 and 5.0 may prevent subsequent recurrence. Alternatively, a change in anticoagulation from warfarin to subcutaneous heparin may be successful, but this is difficult for extended periods because of inconvenience and the risk of osteoporosis (172). Placement of an inferior vena caval filter is needed in occasional individuals with recurrence despite optimal anticoagulation (discussed later).

## Recommendations

An accurate, objective diagnosis is the first consideration when choosing treatment for individuals with suspected venous thrombosis or pulmonary embolism. If an objective diagnosis is not immediately available, anticoagulant therapy can be started on the basis of clinical findings (unless there are contraindications) and discontinued later if the diagnosis is not confirmed. The choice between anticoagulant and fibrinolytic therapy should be considered carefully, however, and placement of an inferior vena caval filter sometimes will be needed in individuals with unacceptably high risk of bleeding or recurrence on optimal anticoagulant therapy.

If anticoagulant therapy is chosen, 5000 U of heparin can be administered intravenously, followed immediately by a constant infusion of 1200 U per hour (Table 61.5). The aPTT should be checked after 4 to 6 hours and the heparin infusion adjusted to prolong the aPTT to between 1.5 and 2.5 times control. The success of treatment depends on a prompt initial prolongation of the aPTT; therefore, repeated checks of the aPTT and dose adjustments should be made every 4 to 6 hours until the aPTT is adequately prolonged. Thereafter, the aPTT can be checked once daily. Because of the risk of thrombocytopenia, the platelet count should be monitored every other day while the individual is on heparin. Warfarin can be started during the first hospital day at a maintenance dose of 5 to 10 mg daily, depending on body weight. The prothrombin time should be checked daily and the

**TABLE 61.5.** Anticoagulant Therapy for Deep Vein Thrombosis and Pulmonary Embolism

*Initiate therapy with heparin*

Administer heparin, 5000 U intravenously, and start an infusion of 1200 U/hour.

Check aPTT after 4–6 hours, and adjust infusion to prolong the aPTT to 1.5–2.5 times control.

Alternatives:

Administer heparin subcutaneously every 12 hours beginning with an initial dose of 18,000 U. Check aPTT after 4 hours, and adjust subsequent doses to prolong aPTT to 1.5–2.5 times control.

Administer low-molecular-weight heparin, 100 anti–factor Xa units per kg subcutaneously every 12 hours.

*Maintenance anticoagulation*

Oral anticoagulants

Give warfarin, 5–10 mg, during first hospital day.

Check PT daily.

Adjust dose to prolong PT to an INR of 2–3.

Discontinue heparin after minimum of 5 days when INR reaches desired range.

Continue warfarin as an outpatient for 3–6 months.

Heparin

Heparin subcutaneous every 12 hours in a dose adjusted to prolong the midinterval aPTT to 1.5 times control.

---

aPTT, *activated partial thromboplastin time;* INR, *international normalized ratio;* PT, *prothrombin time.*

dose adjusted to prolong the INR to between 2.0 and 3.0. Heparin can be discontinued after a minimum of 5 days, when the INR is therapeutic. Warfarin should be continued for 6 weeks to 6 months, depending on the extent of thrombosis and individual predisposition to recurrence. For outpatients, the INR should be checked twice weekly until stable, and then weekly or biweekly as required. Adjustment of the warfarin dose often is needed after hospital discharge, because diets and medications differ compared with those in the hospital. Individuals should avoid medications containing aspirin and, because it may affect the warfarin dosage, report any change in medication to their physician.

Subcutaneous heparin is an alternative for both initial and long-term treatment of venous thrombosis. During initial treatment, higher subcutaneous doses of heparin are required compared with intravenous administration to achieve comparable prolongation of the aPTT. Heparin can be administered subcutaneously every 12 hours, with an initial dose of 18,000 U. The aPTT should be checked after 4 hours and subsequent doses adjusted as required to prolong the aPTT to between 1.5 and 2.5 times control. After this initial dose adjustment, the aPTT can be monitored once daily. The subcutaneous route has the advantages of not requiring an intravenous line and a constant-infusion device. It has the disadvantage that aPTT measurements must be timed in relation to the subcutaneous injections; with intravenous administration, aPTT measurements can be made whenever convenient. In addition, dose adjustment during initial treatment can be made more rapidly with intravenous therapy, and this can be especially important in individuals with pulmonary embolism or massive venous thrombosis, in whom adequate initial therapy must be assured. For outpatient anticoagulation, subcutaneous heparin every 12 hours also can be used. The dose should be adjusted initially to prolong the midinterval aPTT to 1.5 times control, and adjusted dose should be given every 12 hours for 3 to 6 months.

Low-molecular-weight heparin, administered in a weight-based dose every 12 or 24 hours, is at least as safe and effective as heparin for initial therapy, and it has the advantages of subcutaneous administration and lack of laboratory monitoring. The most frequently used dose has been approximately 100 U of anti–factor Xa per kg body weight twice daily.

## PREGNANCY (SEE CHAPTER 46)

The risk of venous thromboembolic disease increases during pregnancy, and particularly at parturition, and pulmonary embolism represents a leading cause of maternal death. Venous thrombosis and pulmonary embolism during pregnancy raises unique problems in both diagnosis and treatment (173). These include risks to the fetus from diagnostic tests and anticoagulant therapy as well as risks to the mother from hemorrhage, particularly at delivery. These risks, and the uncertainty of the clinical diagnosis, make an accurate, objective diagnosis especially important during pregnancy. Use of imaging modalities is limited, however, by concerns over potential adverse fetal effects from exposure to ionizing radiation with radiographic or scintigraphic procedures. In addition, noninvasive tests for venous thrombosis that rely on flow assessment, such as IPG and Doppler ultrasonography, may be abnormal during the third trimester because of extrinsic venous compression from the gravid uterus. Therefore, abnormal results of noninvasive tests during the third trimester are difficult to interpret, but normal test results are useful in excluding a diagnosis of venous thrombosis. Individuals with a positive noninvasive test can be treated either presumptively, thus accepting a possible false-positive risk, or the diagnosis may be confirmed with venography. Venography confined to the calf exposes the fetus to a very low dose of radiation. The exposure from a complete venogram of both the proximal and distal leg is greater, but this is estimated to be only 0.5 rad when adequate shielding is used (174). Fetal radiation exposure of less than 0.05 rads results from a ventilation-perfusion lung scan (174).

Anticoagulation during pregnancy is associated with significant risks to the mother and the fetus, because oral anticoagulants cross the placenta and enter the fetal circulation. Administration of warfarin during the first trimester, and particularly during the sixth to ninth weeks of gestation, can result in warfarin embryopathy, which is a syndrome characterized by nasal hypoplasia and stippling of epiphyses and is seen on radiographs primarily in the axial skeleton (175, 176). Central nervous system abnormalities may occur with exposure to warfarin at any time during pregnancy, resulting in developmental delay, dorsal midline dysplasia with agenesis of the corpus callosum, Dandy-Walker malformation, and midline cerebellar atrophy (sometimes associated with hydrocephalus). Ventral midline dysplasia with eye abnormalities, including optic atrophy, also may be seen (176). The fetal coagulation system is quite sensitive to the anticoagulant effect of warfarin, so appropriate levels of anticoagulation in the mother can result in fetal hemorrhage—and often in fetal loss (177). The frequency of these complications is difficult to determine. Most reports are retrospective, and large prospective studies are not available. However, a review of the published literature (176) found an incidence of warfarin embryopathy of 45 in 970 individuals (4.6%), and a prospective study of oral anticoagulants in 72 individuals with valvular heart disease found evidence of embryopathy in 14 of 49 individuals (29%) exposed between the seventh week and term (178). Because of these risks, warfarin should be avoided during pregnancy if possible.

Unlike warfarin, heparin does not cross the placenta and affect the fetus. One retrospective analysis (176) identified a high rate of fetal adverse effects associated with maternal heparin anticoagulation, but most could be attributed to maternal comorbid conditions leading to the anticoagulation or resulted in prematurity with a normal infant outcome. A reanalysis of published reports (177) suggested that the true frequency of adverse fetal outcomes was less than 4% in heparin-treated individuals, and that the prematurity rate was similar to that in the normal population. Other retrospective and prospective studies of heparin during pregnancy identified a rate of maternal bleeding complications similar to that in nonpregnant individuals and rates of prematurity, abortion, and stillbirths similar to those in the general population (177, 179, 180). Administration of heparin during the 24-hour period before delivery, however, may be associated with increased risk of maternal bleeding (181). An additional maternal risk from long-term heparin administration is symptomatic osteoporosis (172), which also may be accelerated by the high requirements for calcium during pregnancy. The incidence of clinical osteoporosis probably is low, but concerns remain regarding accelerated asymptomatic bone loss in heparinized, pregnant individuals.

Because of its effectiveness and greater safety, heparin is the anticoagulant of choice during pregnancy, and warfarin should be avoided. Like heparin, low-molecular-weight heparin does not cross the placenta, and a review of published obstetric experience (182) suggests it is a good alternative in pregnant individuals. Anticoagulation for acute venous thrombosis or pulmonary embolism can be provided using the guidelines for nonpregnant individuals, with the exception that subcutaneous heparin rather than warfarin should be used for long-term therapy. Heparin should be discontinued at the beginning of labor or 24 hours before elective delivery; it can be reinstituted between 24 and 48 hours postpartum. Warfarin can be used after delivery and is safe in nursing mothers, because it is not secreted in breast milk and results in no infant anticoagulation (183, 184). There is little experience with fibrinolytic therapy during pregnancy, but considering the potential for bleeding, its use should be restricted to life-threatening situations. Risks of venous thrombosis increase during pregnancy, and women with a previous documented episode of venous thrombosis are at significant risk of recurrence (185). Therefore, prophylaxis with low-dose subcutaneous heparin throughout pregnancy should be considered in women at high risk.

## SURGICAL THERAPY

Surgical approaches to venous thromboembolic disease are limited to specific situations in which anticoagulant or fibrinolytic therapy is ineffective or contraindicated. Surgical thrombectomy is a logical approach to reestablishing venous flow in a thrombosed vein, and it has the potential to rapidly relieve symptoms. There is a high rate of rethrombosis after thrombectomy, however, possibly resulting from a residual clot or injury to the vein wall, so postoperative anticoagulants are routinely required. Individual outcome may be as good with anticoagulant therapy alone as with surgery followed by anticoagulation, although no comparative studies are available. Thrombectomy is used in phlegmasia cerulea dolens, in which extensive venous thrombosis results in ischemia that threatens limb viability, and pulmonary embolectomy is a life-saving procedure in gravely ill individuals with massive embolism and severe cardiorespiratory compromise (186). There is, however, a high operative mortality, and the availability of an experienced operative team and surgical facilities for bypass are required, thereby further limiting its use. In individuals with massive embolism and shock, fibrinolytic therapy also can result in dramatic clinical improvement and is a better alternative. In addition, thromboembolectomy has been successful in treating individuals with chronic pulmonary hypertension caused by embolism (187, 188).

Surgical approaches have found wider application in the prevention of pulmonary embolism, and venous interruption proximal to a thrombus can prevent embolization in occasional individuals in whom anticoagulant or fibrinolytic therapy fails or is contraindicated. The first surgical approach to preventing embolization of a distal thrombus was femoral-vein ligation. This procedure rarely is used today, however, because it results in postoperative venous stasis and is associated with a high rate of recurrent pulmonary embolism (189), possibly from undetected thrombus proximal to the ligation site or in the other leg. Ligation of the inferior vena cava provides more complete protection from pulmonary embolism, but this procedure is associated with high surgical mortality and morbidity from distal venous obstruction. Recurrent pulmonary embolism also can occur after formation of collateral veins and from clots arising in the stagnant inferior vena caval cul-de-sac that results after ligation (190). Several techniques to compartmentalize the inferior vena cava use sutures or clips to avoid problems resulting from complete venous obstruction, but these still require general anesthesia and extensive surgery.

Such procedures largely have been replaced by devices that can be placed in the inferior vena cava through a vascular catheter. The catheter can be inserted into the jugular or femoral vein under local anesthesia and guided fluoroscopically to the proper location in the inferior vena cava, where the device then can be ejected from the catheter and fixed to the vein wall (191) (Fig. 61.2). The most frequently used device is the umbrella-shaped Greenfield filter, which consists of metal struts fixed to the vein wall by prongs. If embolization occurs, the filter traps the clot centrally and maintains flow near the vein periphery. In experienced hands, a long-term patency rate as high as 96% and a low rate of recurrent pulmonary emoblism can be achieved after placement of a Greenfield filter (192). The most frequent complications are sequelae of venous stasis, which occur in as many as 44% of individuals. Migration of the device rarely occurs.

Placement of an inferior vena cava umbrella should be considered in individuals with objectively documented proximal vein thrombosis and absolute contraindications to anticoagulant therapy, such as active gastrointestinal or high risk of central nervous system bleeding. Such umbrella devices also may be considered in individuals with relative contraindications, such as recent surgery, mild-to-moderate thrombocytopenia, recent history of gastrointestinal or genitourinary bleeding, and occult blood in the stool. Many of these latter individuals also can be treated successfully with carefully monitored, low-intensity anticoagulation therapy.

The second major indication for an inferior vena cava umbrella is recurrent proximal venous thrombosis or pulmonary embolism despite optimal anticoagulation. Before committing to the procedure, however, individual records should be reviewed carefully to document the adequacy of anticoagulant therapy, and the recurrence of venous thromboembolism should be documented objectively in comparison with previous studies. Few individuals require placement of vena caval umbrellas because of failed anticoagulation.

# FIBRINOLYTIC THERAPY

Bed rest with leg elevation and anticoagulation meet two goals of treatment for deep vein thrombosis and pulmonary embolism by providing relief of symptoms and preventing recurrence. They do not, however, accelerate the physiologic process of clot dissolution, which

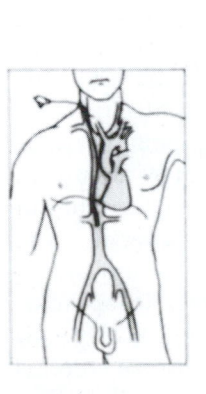
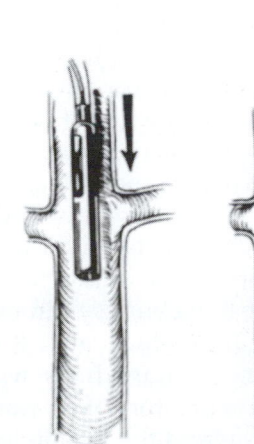
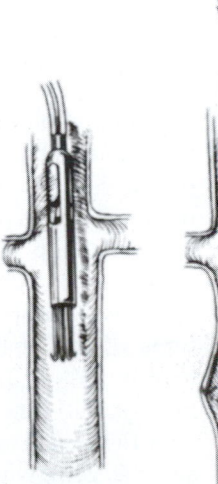
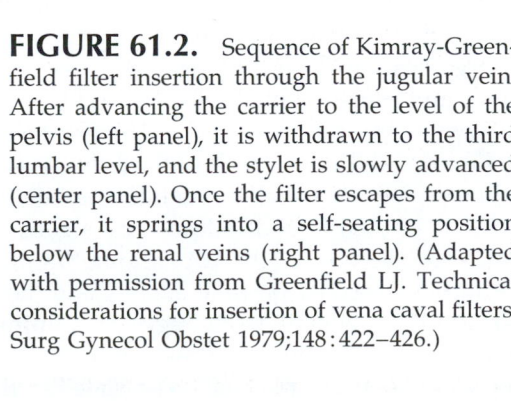

**FIGURE 61.2.** Sequence of Kimray-Greenfield filter insertion through the jugular vein. After advancing the carrier to the level of the pelvis (left panel), it is withdrawn to the third lumbar level, and the stylet is slowly advanced (center panel). Once the filter escapes from the carrier, it springs into a self-seating position below the renal veins (right panel). (Adapted with permission from Greenfield LJ. Technical considerations for insertion of vena caval filters. Surg Gynecol Obstet 1979;148:422–426.)

may be too slow to provide the rapid relief needed for individuals with pulmonary embolism and hemodynamic instability. Anticoagulant therapy also does little to prevent the valve damage and vein scarring that leads to abnormal venous hemodynamics and symptoms of the postphlebitic syndrome. In these individuals, fibrinolytic therapy is an attractive alternative, offering the potential for rapid clot dissolution to relieve vascular obstruction, improve hemodynamics, and prevent permanent vein damage.

Recent advances in fibrinolytic therapy (see Chapter 56) have improved our understanding of biochemical mechanisms and resulted in new fibrinolytic drugs and much wider application for arterial thrombosis, particularly in individuals with acute myocardial infarction. Despite these advances, however, the affect on treatment of venous thrombosis has been limited for several reasons. Fibrinolytic therapy for arterial thrombosis often results in dramatic clinical improvement. For example, in individuals with acute myocardial infarction, fibrinolytic therapy relieves symptoms, improves ventricular function, reduces mortality, and results in coronary reperfusion that can be observed angiographically. Such considerations do not apply to venous thrombosis, however, in which ischemia does not occur, the thrombus is much larger, and prevention of symptoms that may develop years later is an important goal. Frequently cited reasons for not using fibrinolytic therapy are increased risk of bleeding and lack of definitive evidence that mortality rates are improved in individuals with pulmonary embolism or that the postphlebitic syndrome can be prevented after acute venous thrombosis. Despite these appropriate concerns, there is a role for fibrinolytic therapy in the treatment of both acute pulmonary embolism and deep vein thrombosis.

## DEEP VEIN THROMBOSIS

Fibrinolytic therapy can be viewed as an initial phase of treatment, which is administered to rapidly dissolve a large amount of thrombus and to restore vessel patency and function. It then is followed by anticoagulant therapy to prevent recurrence. The greatest clinical experience with deep vein thrombosis has involved streptokinase, which usually is administered in a loading dose of 250,000 U and followed by a constant maintenance infusion of 100,000 U per hour. Streptokinase can be administered by peripheral vein, and there has been no apparent benefit from regional administration in treatment of leg vein thrombosis (193). Streptokinase results in a marked plasma "lytic state," with systemic plasminemia, depletion of plasminogen, and degradation of circulating fibrinogen. Kakkar et al (194, 195) have postulated that plasminogen depletion during fibrinolytic therapy may be important in limiting thrombolytic efficacy, and they have administered plasmino-

gen intermittently as an adjunct to therapy and achieved favorable results in small trials. Fewer studies have involved urokinase, which is given in a loading dose of 4400 U/kg and is followed by a maintenance infusion of 4400 U/kg per hour. Optimal duration of fibrinolytic therapy for venous thrombosis has not been established. Treatment for 3 days is often needed, but complete lysis of extensive venous thrombosis has been observed after only 12 hours (196).

Most controlled trials evaluating fibrinolytic therapy have compared the clinical or venographic outcome after treatment with anticoagulation alone to that with fibrinolytic therapy followed by anticoagulation. Short-term effectiveness has been evaluated by comparing pretreatment and posttreatment venograms from 11 prospective studies (127, 197–206). Critical evaluation is difficult, because these studies were small, randomization of treatment and interpretation of venograms varied, and treatment regimens as well as timing of outcome assessments differed. Despite these problems, however, the data suggest that clot lysis is greater in individuals who receive streptokinase. Ten randomized studies that used adequate pretreatment and posttreatment venography as the criteria for efficacy are summarized in Table 61.6. These included 400 individuals and documented substantial improvement in 47% of those who received streptokinase, compared with 4% of those who received heparin. No change or progression was noted in 74 and 5%, respectively, of those who received heparin, compared with 34 and 2%, respectively, of those who received streptokinase. Goldhaber et al (207) reported a similar analysis after pooling results from six randomized studies in which venography was used to confirm the diagnosis of venous thrombosis and to evaluate therapeutic efficacy. Their combined data indicated that thrombolysis was achieved 3.7 times more often among individuals treated with streptokinase than among those treated with heparin, with 95% confidence intervals of 2.5 to 5.7 ($P < .0001$).

Fibrinolytic therapy resulting in rapid clot dissolution may preserve venous valve function and prevent chronic venous insufficiency. An acute episode of symptomatic venous thrombosis can result in both venous functional abnormalities and the postphlebitic syndrome. Strandness et al (166) found symptoms of venous insufficiency in 67% of individuals within 39 months of an acute deep vein thrombosis, and Bauer (208) found symptoms in 91% of individuals 10 years after an acute episode. A more recent study, however, found symptoms of the postphlebitic syndrome only in approximately 25% of individuals after 8 years (3). Approximately half of all individuals with chronic venous insufficiency give a history of previous venous thrombosis (209, 210), whereas the remainder have their insufficiency either unexplained or attributed to subclinical

**TABLE 61.6.**   Comparison of Outcomes of Deep Vein Thrombosis Treated with Streptokinase Followed by Anticoagulation to Heparin Alone

### Short-term Venographic Evaluation[a]

| Therapy | Patients | Substantial Improvement | Partial Improvement | No Change | Progression |
|---|---|---|---|---|---|
| Streptokinase | 229 | 47% | 17% | 34% | 2% |
| Heparin | 171 | 4% | 17% | 74% | 5% |

### Long-term Venographic Evaluation[b]

| Therapy | Patients | Normal Venogram | Postthrombotic Changes |
|---|---|---|---|
| Streptokinase | 76 | 43 (57%) | 33 (43%) |
| Heparin | 65 | 5 (7%) | 60 (93%) |

### Clinical Evaluation[c]

| Therapy | Patients | Asymptomatic | Symptomatic |
|---|---|---|---|
| Streptokinase | 42 | 28 (67%) | 14 (33%) |
| Heparin | 46 | 14 (30%) | 32 (70%) |

[a] Repeat venography within 7 days (127, 197–206).

[b] Follow-up of 2–76 months (203, 205, 206, 214–216).

[c] Follow-up of 4–76 months (205, 214, 216).

thrombosis. Venous thrombosis also leads to objective evidence of valve dysfunction. For example, Ginsberg et al (211) found venous valve incompetence in 29 of 33 individuals (88%) with proximal vein thrombosis between 2 and 8 years after an acute episode, and Strandness et al (166) as well as Killewich et al (167) found a close association between symptoms of chronic venous insufficiency and valve damage and incompetence in the distal leg veins.

It has been difficult to demonstrate the benefit of fibrinolytic therapy in reducing subsequent symptomatic chronic venous insufficiency, both because of the necessary long-term follow-up and because additional episodes of venous thrombosis can occur during the follow-up period. In addition, venous insufficiency also occurs in individuals without a previous history of deep vein thrombosis (212, 213). Even so, long-term evaluation of individuals who received either fibrinolytic or anticoagulant therapy for deep vein thrombosis is available in several studies (203, 205, 206, 214–217) (Table 61.6). These results suggest a benefit from fibrinolytic therapy, even although the follow-up periods generally are too short to allow full development of postphlebitic syndrome. These studies also were small and suffered from methodologic shortcomings. Normal venograms were found in 57% of individuals treated with streptokinase, compared with only 7% of those treated with anti-

coagulants alone. Chronic postthrombotic changes, including residual fibrosis, collateral flow, or incompetent venous valves, were seen in 92% of anticoagulant-treated individuals, compared to 43% of streptokinase-treated individuals. The clinical evaluation supports the venographic findings, because there is a higher percentage of asymptomatic individuals among those treated with streptokinase followed by heparin (67%) as compared to those treated with heparin alone (30%).

This analysis disagrees with that of Kakkar and Lawrence (168) for 153 individuals treated with streptokinase or heparin and followed prospectively for 2 years. Severe hemodynamic impairment was seen in 20% of limbs with calf-vein thrombosis and 50% of those with proximal thrombi, and the proportion of affected individuals was the same in those treated with streptokinase and those treated with heparin. In addition, these investigators reported that complete clot dissolution during fibrinolytic therapy did not prevent subsequent hemodynamic deterioration.

To optimize the benefit of fibrinolytic therapy and minimize the risk, it is best to choose those individuals most likely to respond and avoid treating those with resistant thrombi or high risk of bleeding. The clearest predictor of outcome is the duration of symptoms before therapy, with the best success occurring with early treatment of newly formed thrombi. Recent evidence

(218–220) indicates that nonobstructing thrombi respond better, and Francis and Totterman (220) report that thrombi with magnetic resonance characteristics suggesting recent formation are more susceptible to fibrinolysis.

Several studies have evaluated therapy with recombinant tissue-type plasminogen activator (rt-PA) in individuals with venous thrombosis or pulmonary embolism; rt-PA is approved by the U.S. Food and Drug Administration for treatment of the latter condition. Prospective trials with pretreatment and posttreatment venography have used different dose regimens in deep vein thrombosis (219, 221–226), but an optimal regimen for rt-PA has not been established. The studies are small as well, with the largest including only 137 individuals treated using rt-PA (226). In general, the results show greater lysis of thrombus in individuals receiving rt-PA than in individuals receiving heparin alone, and they also suggest that a higher dose and longer duration of treatment result in greater response. Bleeding complications have been greater in individuals receiving rt-PA than in individuals receiving heparin. Additional studies are needed to define the optimum rt-PA regimen and the role of rt-PA in treatment of venous thrombosis.

Promising results have been reported in small trials involving catheter-directed thrombolysis of ileofemoral thrombosis using urokinase. The largest study (227) reported complete lysis in 18 of 25 and partial lysis in five of 25 treated limbs. In a second trial (228), lysis occurred in five of five individuals in whom the catheter could be positioned within the thrombus for drug infusion. This promising approach deserves further comparison with peripherally administered therapy.

## PULMONARY EMBOLISM

Fibrinolytic therapy can accelerate dissolution of pulmonary emboli and, thereby, rapidly improve arterial flow to occluded areas of lung. No placebo-controlled trials have demonstrated the effectiveness of thrombolytic therapy in pulmonary embolism, because of both the high mortality rate and the demonstrated effectiveness of heparin in preventing recurrence. Therefore, evidence for efficacy comes from clinical trials involving individuals treated with thrombolytic therapy or with heparin. This was the subject of two large, prospective, randomized trials sponsored by the National Institutes of Health. The Urokinase-Pulmonary Embolism Trial (UPET) (229) compared individual outcome after treatment with either heparin or fibrinolytic therapy given as urokinase for 12 hours. The subsequent Urokinase-Streptokinase Pulmonary Embolism Trial (USPET) (230) compared the efficacy of treatment with three fibrinolytic regimens: urokinase for 24 hours, urokinase for 12 hours, and streptokinase for 24 hours. Fibrinolytic ther-

apy in both these studies was followed by heparin and warfarin anticoagulation.

In these studies, dissolution of pulmonary emboli occurred more rapidly with fibrinolytic therapy than with anticoagulation. Treatment response was assessed by comparing pretreatment and immediate posttreatment pulmonary angiograms, which showed significantly greater clot lysis with urokinase than with heparin on the basis of quantitative scoring. Only 9% of heparin-treated individuals had moderate or greater improvement as shown on pulmonary angiograms at 24 hours, compared with 53% of urokinase-treated individuals. Accelerated lysis also was demonstrated by perfusion lung scans, which showed 22% greater perfusion on day one in individuals receiving urokinase, compared with 8% in individuals receiving heparin. This difference also was present on day two, but perfusion abnormalities were equal in the two groups after 5 days. Hemodynamic monitoring also confirmed the early benefits of fibrinolytic therapy, with a 28% decrease in total pulmonary resistance at 24 hours after urokinase, compared with no change after heparin.

Pulmonary embolism also has been treated with t-PA (231–234). In a prospective, randomized trial (233), 55 hemodynamically stable individuals with pulmonary embolism received heparin alone, and 46 received t-PA followed by heparin. Individuals treated with t-PA showed greater improvement in right ventricular wall motion and pulmonary perfusion on lung scans. A second, smaller study (231) confirmed greater short-term angiographic and hemodynamic improvement with tissue-type plasminogen activator (t-PA) than with heparin alone. Urokinase and t-PA have been compared in several trials as well (232, 234, 235). In two (234, 235), individuals were randomized to either 100 mg of t-PA given over 2 hours or urokinase given over 12 or 24 hours; short-term improvement in hemodynamics and pulmonary perfusion were better in the t-PA groups. A subsequent study (232), however, compared treatment using a 2-hour infusion of t-PA with a novel, accelerated-dose regimen of urokinase that also was given over 2 hours; the efficacy and safety of these two regimens were the same. These studies are important because of their focus on early, rapid fibrinolytic therapy, which may offer the greatest advantage for individuals with significant pulmonary artery obstruction and right ventricular dysfunction (236).

Fibrinolytic therapy accelerates dissolution of pulmonary emboli and improves perfusion and hemodynamics compared with anticoagulant therapy alone. Considering that the mortality rate is less than 10% among heparin-treated individuals, however, the available studies are too small to show a difference in the overall mortality. The mortality rate is higher in individuals with massive pulmonary embolism, especially with hemodynamic compromise, and in these tenuous individuals with extensive pulmonary arterial obstruction, the rapid clot lysis from thrombolytic therapy may be life-saving. Dramatic clinical improvement occurs in individuals with massive embolism and shock (237). Therefore, the best indication for fibrinolytic therapy in pulmonary embolism is severely affected individuals, and particularly those with hemodynamic compromise.

The clearest benefit from thrombolytic therapy is early acceleration of clot lysis, but Sharma et al (238) suggest an additional long-term effect on pulmonary function. In their prospective, randomized trial, individuals with pulmonary emboli were treated with heparin or fibrinolytic therapy, and the effects on pulmonary capillary blood volume and diffusing capacity were compared at 2 weeks and 1 year. The pulmonary capillary blood volume was abnormally low at both times in individuals receiving heparin, but it was normal in individuals receiving fibrinolytic therapy. Diffusing capacity at 1 year also was higher in individuals receiving thrombolytic therapy. The practical clinical significance of these findings is not clear, but they do reveal long-term adverse physiologic effects of pulmonary embolism that can be ameliorated by initial thrombolytic therapy.

## Bleeding Complications

Bleeding is more frequent with fibrinolytic than with anticoagulant therapy, and the risk–benefit ratio must be considered for individuals individually. Most episodes of bleeding during fibrinolytic therapy are minor and relate to previous invasive procedures. For example, in the UPET trial (230), the overall incidence of bleeding complications was 45% in the thrombolytic therapy group, compared with 27% in the heparin group. Both these rates were high, but careful analysis indicated that most bleeding episodes resulted from invasive procedures such as venipuncture, venous cutdowns, and arterial punctures for blood-gas determinations or catheterization. The same conclusion was reached in a recent analysis of bleeding with thrombolytic therapy for pulmonary embolism (239), with an estimated risk of bleeding with pulmonary angiography of 14% as compared to 4% with noninvasive diagnostic methods. Goldhaber et al (207) reviewed bleeding complications in three prospective, randomized studies of thrombolytic therapy for deep vein thrombosis, and they found the incidence varied from 8 to 38% in streptokinase-treated individuals and from zero to 12% in heparin-treated individuals. Analysis of pooled data indicated a relative risk of major bleeding 2.9 times greater in individuals who received streptokinase than in individuals who received heparin, with 95% confidence intervals of 1.8 to 8.1 ($P < .04$). The frequency of fatal bleeding or intracranial hemorrhage is sufficiently low

that available data from clinical trials of venous thrombosis are insufficient to provide a reliable estimate; however, extrapolating from the larger experience with acute myocardial infarction, an incidence of from 0.2 to 0.5% with streptokinase treatment is reasonable (240). The incidence may be higher with fibrinolytic therapy for venous thrombosis, because the duration of treatment is longer than that used for acute myocardial infarction.

## Monitoring

Monitoring implies that treatment can be modified on the basis of measuring a particular parameter to improve individual outcome. Ideally, the most important parameter to monitor during fibrinolytic therapy is thrombus size, because thrombus dissolution is the primary goal. This would allow dose adjustments on the basis of thrombus response, with treatment being discontinued either when dissolution occurred or no further lysis was seen. Repeat venography has been used in clinical trials but is impractical for routine use because of its invasiveness. Magnetic resonance imaging may be useful (220, 241), but its expense and limited availability are drawbacks. A preliminary study demonstrated that gadolinium-enhanced magnetic resonance angiography has promise in identifying pulmonary emboli (242), and ultrasonography also may have potential for following clot lysis. At present, however, no practical and inexpensive method of assessing clot response is readily available for routine use.

Routine monitoring of hemostasis has limited value in fibrinolytic therapy, which often results in systemic activation of the fibrinolytic system and, therefore, shortened euglobulin clot lysis times, decreased fibrinogen levels, increased fibrin(ogen) degradation products, prolonged thrombin clotting times, decreased plasminogen levels, and decreased $\alpha_2$-plasmin inhibitor levels, thus reflecting the "lytic state." The extent of these changes is greater with streptokinase than with more "fibrin-specific" agents, such as rt-PA. Generally, there has been little correlation between intensity of the lytic state and either treatment efficacy or the occurrence of complications. Thus, the UPET study (229) as well as that reported by Marder et al (127) showed no correlation between laboratory derangements of clotting test results and bleeding manifestations. Analysis of data from studies of thrombolytic therapy for acute myocardial infarction reinforces this interpretation. Overall, the risk of bleeding complications during therapy for acute myocardial infarction is the same with streptokinase as with rt-PA, although rt-PA induces a less intensive lytic state. A weak correlation has been reported in rt-PA–treated individuals between the occurrence of hemorrhagic complications and the drop in plasma fibrinogen level (243).

**TABLE 61.7.** Selection of Individuals for Thrombolytic Therapy

Treat those most likely to respond and benefit
  Deep vein thrombosis: Large, proximal thrombi with symptoms for less than 7 days.
  Pulmonary embolism: Massive or submassive embolism, especially with hemodynamic compromise.
Select individuals to avoid bleeding complications
  Major contraindications
    Risk of intracranial bleeding: Recent head trauma or central nervous sytem surgery, history of stroke or subarachnoid bleed, intracranial metastatic disease.
    Risk of major bleeding: Active gastrointestinal or genitourinary bleeding, major surgery or trauma within 7 days.
  Relative contraindications
    Remote history of gastrointestinal or genitourinary bleeding or of peptic ulcer or other lesion with potential for bleeding; recent minor surgery or trauma; severe, uncontrolled hypertension; coexisting hemostatic abnormalities.

In short, there is no substantial evidence that treatment outcome can be improved by routine monitoring of coagulation tests. The single exception is performance of coagulation tests early in fibrinolytic therapy to establish that the lytic state is present, particularly in individuals treated with streptokinase, because a small percentage of the general population will have high-titer antibodies that inactivate infused streptokinase. If there is no evidence of the lytic state, such as a prolonged thrombin clotting time or decreased fibrinogen level, then a repeat bolus of streptokinase can be administered or another agent used.

## RECOMMENDATIONS

Thrombolytic therapy should be reserved for those individuals most likely to respond and to benefit without bleeding complications (Table 61.7). Postphlebitic syndrome frequently develops in individuals with extensive proximal deep vein thrombosis, so thrombolytic therapy should be considered in this group. The clearest predictor of therapeutic outcome is clot age. Fresh, recent, nonobstructive thrombi respond best, and individuals with symptoms for more than 7 to 10 days are less likely to respond. The greatest benefit of thrombolytic therapy for pulmonary embolism is expected in individuals with large emboli and hemodynamic compromise, in whom the accelerated early clot lysis results in important clinical improvement.

Risk of bleeding also can be minimized through careful individual selection. Intracranial bleeding is the most serious complication, and individuals with recent head trauma, central nervous system surgery, or a history of stroke, subarachnoid bleed, or intracranial metastatic disease should not receive thrombolytic therapy. This therapy also should be avoided in individuals with a risk of major bleeding, such as those with active gastrointestinal or genitourinary bleeding or major surgery or trauma within 7 days. Less significant bleeding risks constitute relative contraindications, and thrombolytic therapy may be appropriate in selected individuals.

An objective diagnosis is important before administering thrombolytic therapy to establish the extent of disease and avoid unnecessary treatment. Treatment can involve streptokinase, urokinase, or rt-PA (Table 61.8). Unless serial noninvasive imaging is available, the progress of clot lysis can be monitored clinically, and treatment is continued for 12 to 24 hours in individuals with pulmonary embolism or longer in individuals with venous thrombosis, depending on response. Individuals should be observed carefully for signs of bleeding. Daily hematocrits should be obtained as well, because bleeding in the leg or retroperitoneum may initially be occult. To prevent recurrence, anticoagulation therapy should be instituted when fibrinolytic therapy is discontinued. A simple approach is to monitor the aPTT every 4 hours after stopping treatment and to begin heparin as a constant infusion without a loading dose when the aPTT is less than 2 times control.

## Upper Extremity Venous Thrombosis

Thrombosis of upper extremity veins is becoming more common among hospitalized individuals because of the increasing long-term use of central venous catheters in those needing parenteral nutrition, permanent transvenous cardiac pacemakers, antibiotics, or chemotherapy. Primary thrombosis of the axillary or subclavian veins also occurs in otherwise healthy individuals after trauma or associated with anatomic obstructions to venous flow. The clinical presentation is comparable to that of deep leg-vein thrombosis, with varying degrees of pain, swelling and venous engorgement of the arm, and symptoms occasionally involving the neck, head, or breasts if there is proximal extension of thrombosis. The diagnosis can be confirmed by venography, but compression ultrasonography and color-flow Doppler imaging also have good sensitivity and specificity (244). Treatment with anticoagulation, rest, and elevation may prevent extension and relieve acute symptoms, but individuals frequently suffer troublesome, chronic symptoms of arm pain, swelling, and weakness. The reported frequency of chronic symptoms varies from 35 to more than 90% with conservative therapy, including anticoagulation (245–250). Pulmonary embolism from arm-vein thrombosis occurs in 10 to 20% of individuals (249, 251,

**TABLE 61.8.** Systemic Thrombolytic Therapy for Venous Thrombosis and Pulmonary Embolism

*Streptokinase*
Dose
   250,000 U IV over 15–20 minutes, followed by a continuous infusion of 100,000 U/hour.
Duration
   12–24 hours for pulmonary embolism; 2–3 days or longer for deep vein thrombosis.
Advantages
   Largest experience; inexpensive.
Disadvantages
   Occasional allergic reactions; low percentage of population has high-titer neutralizing antibodies.

*Urokinase*
Dose
   4400 U/kg IV over 15–20 minutes, followed by a constant infusion of 4400 U/kg/hour.
Duration
   12–24 hours for pulmonary embolism; 2–3 days or longer for deep vein thrombosis.
Advantages
   Not antigenic.
Disadvantages
   More expensive than streptokinase.

*rt-PA[a]*
Dose
   100 mg IV as a constant infusion.
Duration
   2 hours.
Advantages
   Not antigenic; short treatment duration.
Disadvantages
   Least experience; more expensive; approved for pulmonary embolism only.

IV, *intravenously;* rt-PA, *recombinant tissue-type plasminogen activator.*

[a] *For pulmonary embolism only.*

252) and should be suspected in the appropriate clinical setting.

Most reports of fibrinolytic therapy for upper extremity thrombosis involve individual individuals or small series reviewed retrospectively. Systemic therapy with streptokinase administered by peripheral vein for 48 to 72 hours has been demonstrated as successful on the basis of venographic response and the absence of chronic symptoms (253–263). Therapy also be can delivered with a local infusion directly distal to, or especially into, the thrombus using streptokinase or urokinase at several possible doses. Additional therapy such as an-

gioplasty or rib resection may be required in some individuals (255, 260, 262, 263). The role of long-term anticoagulation therapy in preventing recurrence has not been established, but it may have value in individuals with a continuing predisposition, such as an indwelling catheter or vein stenosis.

Patients with catheter-related thrombosis differ from those with primary thrombosis, because the former often have chronic illnesses, including malignancies, and may be receiving chemotherapy. Thrombosis has been reported in as many as 45% of individuals (264–267) and is higher in those receiving chemotherapy, and thrombosis has been found in two-thirds of acutely ill individuals with pulmonary artery catheters placed for hemodynamic monitoring (268). Treatment including catheter removal, arm elevation, and anticoagulation usually results in symptomatic improvement. The optimal duration of oral anticoagulation has not been studied prospectively, but 4 to 6 weeks often are sufficient. Systemic or local fibrinolytic therapy also frequently is successful. In the largest reported study, Fraschini et al (269) administered urokinase locally and achieved complete lysis in 25 of 30 thrombi in which the catheter could be positioned for direct infusion into the thrombus. Therapy was less successful if the catheter could not be placed directly into the thrombus, or if there was active inflammation. Thrombosis did not recur in 10 of 16 individuals, even when the catheter was not removed.

Thrombotic catheter occlusion is a less serious but more frequent problem than venous thrombosis; however, it often precludes use of the catheter for infusion or blood sampling. In this setting, fibrinolytic agents are almost uniformly successful in restoring catheter patency using direct instillation of 5000 to 20,000 U of streptokinase or urokinase (270–272). Administration of very-low-dose of warfarin (1 mg daily) beginning 3 days before insertion of a central venous catheter significantly reduced the incidence of catheter-associated thrombosis without causing bleeding complications in a prospective, randomized trial (273).

## Abdominal Venous Thrombosis

### Renal Vein Thrombosis

Renal vein thrombosis occurs secondary to mechanical injury or tumor invasion, is associated with hypovolemia in infants, and also occurs in individuals with nephrotic syndrome. Early reports suggested a causal relation between renal vein obstruction and development of proteinuria, but prospective studies found that nephrotic syndrome usually predates the thrombosis. Renal vein thrombosis also can complicate renal transplantation, occurring in 4.1% of 558 individuals in one series (274). Llach et al (275) prospectively evaluated 151 individuals with nephrotic syndrome and found renal vein thrombosis in 22%; five individuals with nephrotic syndrome had documented normal renal veins and later developed renal vein thrombosis. In another cohort of 27 individuals with nephrotic syndrome resulting from membranous glomerulonephritis (276), there was a 50% incidence of renal vein thrombosis, and eight individuals had bilateral involvement.

The pathophysiology of renal vein thrombosis is not certain, but it has been related to hypercoagulability resulting from underlying inflammatory disease or from urinary loss of antithrombin. Kaufmann et al (277) found an association between the decrease in plasma antithrombin level and the incidence of renal vein thrombosis, with an 89% incidence in individuals who have antithrombin concentrations of less than 70%.

In a minority of individuals, renal vein thrombosis may present acutely with flank pain, costovertebral angle tenderness, and macroscopic hematuria. Most individuals have chronic thrombosis and no symptoms. Pulmonary embolism is common, with approximately 25% having an asymptomatic, positive ventilation-perfusion lung scan (275). The intravenous pyelogram can be of diagnostic value in acute renal vein thrombosis, showing unilateral enlargement and pelvicalyceal abnormalities, but no diagnostic findings are found in individuals with chronic renal vein thrombosis. The diagnosis requires a high index of suspicion, and it depends on identification of thrombus in the renal vein as shown on an inferior vena cavagram, renal venogram, ultrasound, or magnetic resonance image.

Anticoagulant therapy is used most commonly for, and is effective in, preventing embolic complications. Intravenous heparin followed by outpatient warfarin is indicated and, with a continuing proteinuria and thrombotic predisposition, may be required for a prolonged duration. Anticoagulation may result in some improvement of renal function in individuals with acute renal vein thrombosis, but the overall prognosis primarily is determined by progression of the renal parenchymal disease. The rate of decline in renal function is similar for individuals with or without renal vein thrombosis (275). Unless contraindicated, systemic fibrinolytic therapy should be considered in individuals with acute renal vein thrombosis; it has resulted in rapid and complete radiographic and clinical resolution (278–281). Fibrinolytic therapy also has successfully treated venous thrombosis in transplanted kidneys, which often results in graft loss (282, 283).

## Budd-Chiari Syndrome

Thrombotic obstruction of the major hepatic veins, often including the intrahepatic or infrahepatic vena cava, results in Budd-Chiari syndrome, which typically presents with rapidly developing ascites, abdominal pain, and a tender, enlarging liver (284, 285). The thrombosis may

relate to chronic myeloproliferative diseases, paroxysmal nocturnal hemoglobinuria or other hypercoagulable states, or involvement with tumor or anatomic obstruction of the vena cava by membranous webs or valves, with the latter being noted particularly in Asia (286). Diagnosis requires identifying the thrombus on contrast venograms of the hepatic veins or inferior vena cava, or on ultrasound or magnetic resonance images. Changes of venous congestion and dilatation of sinuses in liver biopsy specimens can suggest the diagnosis. Budd-Chiari syndrome must be distinguished, however, from hepatic venoocclusive disease, which involves smaller postsinusoidal vessels (see Chapter 25), and from venous obstruction resulting from right heart failure. Without effective therapy, the prognosis is poor, with progression to hepatic failure or symptomatic portal hypertension. Several surgical procedures, including angioplasty and placement of vascular stents and mesocaval, mesoatrial, and portosystemic shunts, have successfully relieved vascular obstruction (287, 288). Creation of a transjugular, intrahepatic portosystemic shunt also has been successful in some individuals (289). In several others, thrombolytic therapy has been successful (290–292), and it should be considered in individuals with acute thrombosis and no contraindications. Anticoagulants often are administered to limit thrombotic obstruction and prevent pulmonary embolism, but there is little evidence this favorably influences the course of the disease. Orthotopic liver transplantation is an alternative in individuals with refractory disease (293–295).

## Portal Vein Thrombosis

Acute portal vein thrombosis associated with trauma or intra-abdominal infection may present with acute development of ascites and pain resulting from venous inflammation or associated bowel ischemia. Both portal vein and splenic vein thrombosis can occur as a complication of splenectomy (296) and orthotopic liver transplantation (297). Thrombosis also may present subacutely in individuals with cirrhosis, pancreatitis, or involvement of the vein by tumor, infection, or trauma, or in individuals with hypercoagulable states, including paroxysmal nocturnal hemoglobinuria (298). The clinical presentation usually reflects sequelae of chronic portal hypertension with ascites, splenomegaly, and variceal bleeding.

Treatment involves therapy for ascites and recurrent variceal bleeding. Decompression of the portal system with portosystemic shunting controls variceal bleeding, with a better operative and long-term prognosis in individuals without cirrhosis (299, 300); however, this procedure requires identification of a suitable nonthrombosed vessel of adequate size to sustain the shunt without thrombosis. The value of anticoagulant therapy in individuals with chronic thrombosis is not certain, but it may prevent extension or thrombosis of shunts, particularly in individuals with a hypercoagulable state.

## Mesenteric Vein Thrombosis

Primarily a disease of elderly individuals, mesenteric vein thrombosis occurs with recent abdominal surgery or trauma, cirrhosis, abdominal infections, heart failure, or hypercoagulable states (301, 302). The thrombosis results in hemorrhagic bowel infarction and a nonspecific clinical presentation with intermittent, progressive abdominal pain, which may be out of proportion to findings on the physical examination. Abdominal distention, vomiting, melena, and fever occur with advanced disease. The diagnosis is difficult to establish, and it requires a high degree of suspicion. It is supported by radiographic evidence of an abnormal gas distribution or the finding of gas in the portal system or bowel wall. Paracentesis often shows serosanguinous peritoneal fluid, and peritoneoscopy with examination of the small bowel may establish the diagnosis. Treatment primarily is surgical, requiring resection of the infarcted bowel and administration of antibiotics. Anticoagulation therapy may prevent extension of thrombosis and development of recurrent infarction (303).

# REFERENCES

1. Anderson FA Jr, Wheeler HB, Goldberg RJ et al. A population-based perspective of the hospital incidence and case-fatality rates of deep vein thrombosis and pulmonary embolism. Arch Intern Med 1991;151:933–938.
2. Weinmann EE, Salzman EW. Deep-vein thrombosis. N Engl J Med 1994; 331:1630–1641.
3. Prandoni P, Lensing AW, Cogo A et al. The long-term clinical course of acute deep venous thrombosis. Ann Intern Med 1996;125:1–7.
4. Coon WW, Willis PW III, Keller JB. Thromboembolism and other venous disease in the Tecumseh Community Health Study. Circulation 1973;48: 839–846.
5. Coon WW. Epidemiology of venous thromboembolism. Ann Surg 1977; 186:149–164.
6. Lilienfeld DE, Chan E, Ehland J et al. Mortality from pulmonary embolism in the United States: 1962 to 1984. Chest 1990;98:1067–1072.
7. Soskolne CL, Wong AW, Lilienfeld DE. Trends in pulmonary embolism death rates for Canada and the United States, 1962–87. Can Med Assoc J 1990;142:321–324.
8. Alpert JS, Dalen JE. Epidemiology and natural history of venous thromboembolism. Prog Cardiovasc Dis 1994;36:417–422.
9. Kakkar VV, Howe CT, Flanc C et al. Natural history of postoperative deep vein thrombosis. Lancet 1969;ii:230–232.
10. Moser KM, LeMoine JR. Is embolic risk conditioned by location of deep venous thrombosis? Ann Intern Med 1981;94:439–444.
11. Moser KM, Fedullo PF, LitteJohn JK et al. Frequent asymptomatic pulmonary embolism in patients with deep venous thrombosis. JAMA 1994;271: 223–225.
12. Donaldson GA, Williams C, Scannell JG et al. A reappraisal of the application of the Trendelenburg Operation to massive pulmonary embolism. N Engl J Med 1963;268:171–174.
13. Clagett GP, Anderson FA Jr, Heit J et al. Prevention of venous thromboembolism. Chest 1995;108(Suppl):312–334.
14. Collins R, Scrimgeour A, Yusuf S et al. Reduction in fatal pulmonary embolism and venous thrombosis by perioperative administration of subcutaneous heparin. Overview of results of randomized trials in general, orthopedic and urologic surgery. N Engl J Med 1988;318:1162–1173.
15. Scurr JH, Ibrahim SZ, Faber RG et al. The efficacy of graduated compression stockings in the prevention of deep vein thrombosis. Br J Surg 1977; 64:371–373.
16. Fasting H, Andersen K, Nielsen HK et al. Prevention of postoperative deep venous thrombosis. Low-dose heparin versus graded pressure stockings. Acta Chir Scand 1985;151:245–248.
17. Wells PS, Lensing AW, Hirsh J. Graduated compression stockings in the prevention of postoperative venous thromboembolism. A meta-analysis. Arch Intern Med 1994;154:67–72.
18. Nicolaides AN, Fernandes e Fernandes J, Pollock AV. Intermittent sequential pneumatic compression of the legs in the prevention of venous stasis and postoperative deep venous thrombosis. Surgery 1980;87:69–76.
19. Muhe E. Intermittent sequential high-pressure compression of the leg: a new method of preventing deep vein thrombosis. Am J Surg 1984;147: 781–785.
20. Allenby F, Pflug JJ, Boardman L et al. Effects of external pneumatic intermittent compression on fibrinolysis in man. Lancet 1973;ii:1412–1414.
21. Knight MTN, Dawson R. Effect of intermittent compression of the arms on deep venous thrombosis in the legs. Lancet 1976;ii:1265–1268.
22. Sabri S, Roberts VC, Cotton LT. Prevention of early postoperative deep vein thrombosis by intermittent compression of the leg during surgery. Br Med J 1971;4:394–396.
23. Clark WB, MacGregor AB, Prescott RJ et al. Pneumatic compression of the calf and postoperative deep-vein thrombosis. Lancet 1974;ii:5–7.
24. Roberts VC, Cotton LT. Prevention of postoperative deep vein thrombosis in patients with malignant disease. Br Med J 1974;1:358–360.
25. Coe NP, Collins RE, Klein LA et al. Prevention of deep vein thrombosis in urological patients: a controlled, randomized trial of low-dose heparin and external pneumatic compression boots. Surgery 1978;83:230–234.
26. Skillman JJ, Collins RE, Coe NP et al. Prevention of deep vein thrombosis in neurosurgical patients: a controlled, randomized trial of external pneumatic compression boots. Surgery 1978;83:354–358.
27. Clarke-Pearson DL, Synan IS, Hinshaw WM et al. Prevention of postoperative venous thromboembolism by external pneumatic calf compression in patients with gynecologic malignancy. Obstet Gynecol 1984;63:92–98.
28. Hull R, Delmore TJ, Hirsh J et al. Effectiveness of intermittent pulsatile elastic stockings for the prevention of calf and thigh vein thrombosis in patients undergoing elective knee surgery. Thromb Res 1979;16:37–45.
29. Bradley JG, Krugener GH, Jager HJ. The effectiveness of intermittent plantar venous compression in prevention of deep venous thrombosis after total hip arthroplasty. J Arthroplasty 1993;8:57–61.
30. Kakkar VV, Spindler J, Flute PT et al. Efficacy of low doses of heparin in prevention of deep-vein thrombosis after major surgery. A double-blind randomised trial. Lancet 1972;ii:101–106.
31. Brozovic M, Stirling Y, Abbosh J. Plasma heparin levels after low dose subcutaneous heparin in patients undergoing hip replacement. Br J Haematol 1975;31:461–466.
32. Gallus AS, Hirsh J, Tuttle RJ et al. Small subcutaneous doses of heparin in prevention of venous thrombosis. N Engl J Med 1973;288:545–551.
33. Anonymous. Prevention of fatal postoperative pulmonary embolism by low doses of heparin. An international multicentre trial. Lancet 1975;ii: 45–51.
34. Gruber UF, Duckert F, Fridrich R et al. Prevention of postoperative thromboembolism by dextran 40, low doses of heparin, or xantinol nicotinate. Lancet 1977;i:207–210.
35. Kakkar VV, Corrigan TP, Fossard DP et al. Prevention of fatal post-operative pulmonary embolism by low doses of heparin: reappraisal of results of international multicentre trial. Lancet 1977;i:567–569.
36. Anonymous. Prevention of venous thrombosis and pulmonary embolism. Natl Inst Health Consens Dev Conf Consens Statement 1986;6:1–8.
37. Morris GK. Prevention of venous thromboembolism: a survey of methods used by orthopaedic and general surgeons. Lancet 1980;ii:572–574.
38. Conti S, Daschbach M. Venous thromboembolism prophylaxis: a survey of its use in the United States. Arch Surg 1982;117:1036–1040.
39. Paiement GD, Wessinger SJ, Harris WH. Survey of prophylaxis against venous thromboembolism in adults undergoing hip surgery. Clin Orthop 1987;223:188–193.
40. Anderson FA Jr, Wheeler HB, Goldberg RJ et al. Physician practices in the prevention of venous thromboembolism. Ann Intern Med 1991;115: 591–595.
41. Anonymous. Dihydroergotamine-heparin prophylaxis of post-operative deep vein thrombosis. A multicenter trial. Multicenter Trial Committee. JAMA 1984;251:2960–2966.
42. Gent M, Roberts RS. A meta-analysis of the studies of dihydroergotamine plus heparin in the prophylaxis of deep vein thrombosis. Chest 1986;89: 396S–400S.
43. Hirsh J, Levine MN. Low-molecular-weight heparin. Blood 1992;79:1–17.
44. Kakkar VV, Murray WJ. Efficacy and safety of low-molecular-weight heparin (CY216) in preventing postoperative venous thrombo-embolism: a cooperative study. Br J Surg 1985;72:786–791.
45. Bergqvist D, Burmark US, Frisell J et al. Low-molecular-weight heparin once daily compared with conventional low dose heparin twice daily. A prospective double-blind multicentre trial on prevention of postoperative thrombosis. Br J Surg 1986;73:204–208.
46. Caen JP. A randomized double-blind study between a low-molecular-weight heparin Kabi 2165 and standard heparin in the prevention of deep

vein thrombosis in general surgery. A French multicenter trial. Thromb Haemost 1988;59:216–220.

47. Anonymous. Comparison of a low-molecular-weight heparin and unfractionated heparin for the prevention of deep vein thrombosis in patients undergoing abdominal surgery. European Fraxiparin Study Group. Br J Surg 1988;75:1058–1063.

48. Bergqvist D, Matzsch T, Burmark VS et al. Low-molecular-weight heparin given the evening before surgery compared with conventional low dose heparin in prevention of thrombosis. Br J Surg 1988;75:888–891.

49. Samama M, Bernard P, Bonnardot JP et al. Low-molecular-weight heparin compared with unfractionated heparin in prevention of postoperative thrombosis. Br J Surg 1988;75:128–131.

50. Fricker JP, Vergnes Y, Schach R et al. Low dose heparin versus low-molecular-weight heparin (Kabi 2165, Fragmin®) in the prophylaxis of thromboembolic complications of abdominal oncological surgery. Eur J Clin Invest 1988;18:561–567.

51. Leizorovicz A, Picolet H, Peyrieux JC et al. Prevention of perioperative deep vein thrombosis in general surgery: a multicentre double-blind study comparing two doses of logiparin and standard heparin. HBPM Research Group. Br J Surg 1991;78:412–416.

52. Ockelford PA, Patterson J, Johns AS. A double-blind randomized placebo controlled trial of thromboprophylaxis in major elective general surgery using once daily injections of a low-molecular-weight heparin fragment (Fragmin). Thromb Haemost 1989;62:1046–1049.

53. Koppenhagen K, Adolf J, Matthes M et al. Low-molecular-weight heparin and prevention of postoperative thrombosis in abdominal surgery. Thromb Haemost 1992;67:627–630.

54. Kakkar VV, Cohen AT, Edmonson RA et al. Low-molecular-weight versus standard heparin for prevention of venous thromboembolism after major abdominal surgery. The Thromboprophylaxis Collaborative Group. Lancet 1993;341:259–265.

55. Nurmohamed MT, Rosendaal FR, Büller HR et al. Low-molecular-weight heparin versus standard heparin in general and orthopaedic surgery: a meta-analysis. Lancet 1992;340:152–156.

56. Bratt G, Törnebohm E, Lockner D et al. A human pharmacological study comparing conventional heparin and a low-molecular-weight heparin fragment. Thromb Haemost 1985;53:208–211.

57. Leyvraz PF, Richard J, Bachmann F et al. Adjusted versus fixed-dose subcutaneous heparin in the prevention of deep-vein thrombosis after total hip replacement. N Engl J Med 1983;309:954–958.

58. Green D, Lee MY, Ito VY et al. Fixed- vs adjusted-dose heparin in the prophylaxis of thromboembolism in spinal cord injury. JAMA 1988;260:1255–1258.

59. Francis CW, Pellegrini VD Jr, Marder VJ et al. Prevention of venous thrombosis after total hip arthroplasty. Antithrombin III and low dose heparin compared with dextran 40. J Bone Joint Surg [Am] 1989;71:327–335.

60. Francis CW, Pellegrini VD Jr, Stulberg BN et al. Prevention of venous thrombosis after total knee arthroplasty: comparison of antithrombin III plus low dose heparin to dextran. J Bone Joint Surg [Am] 1990;72:976–982.

61. Evarts CM, Feil EJ. Prevention of thromboembolic disease after elective surgery of the hip. J Bone Joint Surg [Am] 1971;53:1271–1280.

62. Bergquist E, Bergqvist D, Bronge A et al. An evaluation of early thrombosis prophylaxis following fracture of the femoral neck. A comparison between dextran and dicoumarol. Acta Chir Scand 1972;138:689–693.

63. Harris WH, Salzman EW, DeSanctis RW et al. Prevention of venous thromboembolism following total hip replacement. Warfarin vs dextran 40. JAMA 1972;220:1319–1322.

64. Harris WH, Salzman EW, Athanasoulis C et al. Comparison of warfarin, low-molecular-weight dextran, aspirin, and subcutaneous heparin in prevention of venous thromboembolism following total hip replacement. J Bone Joint Surg [Am] 1974;56:1552–1562.

65. Haas SB, Insall JN, Scuderi GR et al. Pneumatic sequential-compression boots compared with aspirin prophylaxis of deep-vein thrombosis after total knee arthroplasty. J Bone Joint Surg [Am] 1990;72:27–31.

66. Hodge WA. Prevention of deep vein thrombosis after total knee arthroplasty. Coumadin versus pneumatic calf compression. Clin Orthop 1991;271:101–105.

67. Gallus A, Raman K, Darby T. Venous thrombosis after elective hip replacement—the influence of preventive intermittent calf compression and of surgical technique. Br J Surg 1983;70:17–19.

68. Hull RD, Raskob GE, Gent M et al. Effectiveness of intermittent pneumatic leg compression for preventing deep vein thrombosis after total hip replacement. JAMA 1990;263:2313–2317.

69. Francis CW, Pellegrini VD Jr, Marder VJ et al. Comparison of warfarin and external pneumatic compression in prevention of venous thrombosis after total hip replacement. JAMA 1992;267:2911–2915.

70. Sevitt S, Gallagher NG. Prevention of venous thrombosis and pulmonary embolism in injured patients. Lancet 1959;ii:981–989.

71. Francis CW, Marder VJ, Evarts CM et al. Two-step warfarin therapy: prevention of postoperative venous thrombosis without excessive bleeding. JAMA 1983;249:374–378.

72. Taberner DA, Poller L, Burslem RW et al. Oral anticoagulants controlled

by the British comparative thromboplastin versus low-dose heparin in prophylaxis of deep vein thrombosis. Br Med J 1978;1:272–274.

73. Paiement G, Wessinger SJ, Waltman AC et al. Low-dose warfarin versus external pneumatic compression for prophylaxis against venous thromboembolism following total hip replacement. J Arthroplasty 1987;2:23–26.

74. Hull R, Raskob G, Pineo G et al. A comparison of subcutaneous low-molecular-weight heparin with warfarin sodium for prophylaxis against deep-vein thrombosis after hip or knee implantation. N Engl J Med 1993;329:1370–1376.

75. Francis CW, Pellegrini VD Jr, Leibert KM et al. Comparison of two warfarin regimens in the prevention of venous thrombosis following total knee replacement. Thromb Haemost 1996;75:706–711.

76. Imperiale TF, Speroff T. A meta-analysis of methods to prevent venous thromboembolism following total hip replacement. JAMA 1994;271:1780–1785.

77. Mohr DN, Silverstein MD, Murtaugh PA et al. Prophylactic agents for venous thrombosis in elective hip surgery. Meta-analysis of studies using venographic assessment. Arch Intern Med 1993;153:2221–2228.

78. Anonymous. RD heparin compared with warfarin for prevention of venous thromboembolic disease following total hip or knee arthroplasty. RD Heparin Arthroplasty Group. J Bone Joint Surg [Am] 1994;76:1174–1185.

79. Hamulyak K, Lensing AW, van der Meer J et al. Subcutaneous low-molecular-weight heparin or oral anticoagulants for the prevention of deep-vein thrombosis in elective hip and knee replacement? Fraxiparine Oral Anticoagulant Study Group. Thromb Haemost 1995;74:1428–1431.

80. Poller L, McKernan A, Thomson JM et al. Fixed minidose warfarin: a new approach to prophylaxis against venous thrombosis after major surgery. Br Med J 1987;295:1309–1312.

81. Turpie AG, Levine MN, Hirsh J et al. A randomized controlled trial of a low-molecular-weight heparin (enoxaparin) to prevent deep-vein thrombosis in patients undergoing elective hip surgery. N Engl J Med 1986;315:925–929.

82. Colwell CW Jr, Spiro TE, Trowbridge AA et al. Use of enoxaparin, a low-molecular-weight heparin, and unfractionated heparin for the prevention of deep venous thrombosis after elective hip replacement. A clinical trial comparing efficacy and safety. Enoxaparin Clinical Trial Group. J Bone Joint Surg [Am] 1994;76:3–14.

83. Levine MN, Hirsh J, Gent M et al. Prevention of deep vein thrombosis after elective hip surgery. A randomized trial comparing low-molecular-weight heparin with standard unfractionated heparin. Ann Intern Med 1991;114:545–551.

84. Spiro TE, Johnson GJ, Christie MJ et al. Efficacy and safety of enoxaparin to prevent deep venous thrombosis after hip replacement surgery. Enoxaparin Clinical Trial Group. Ann Intern Med 1994;121:81–89.

85. Francis CW, Pellegrini VD Jr, Marder VJ et al. Prevention of venous thrombosis after hip arthroplasty: comparison of warfarin and dalteparin. In press.

86. Leclerc JR, Geerts WH, Desjardins L et al. Prevention of deep vein thrombosis after major knee surgery—a randomized, double-blind trial comparing a low-molecular-weight heparin fragment (enoxaparin) to placebo. Thromb Haemost 1992;67:417–423.

87. Levine MN, Gent M, Hirsh J et al. Ardeparin (low-molecular-weight heparin) vs graduated compression stockings for the prevention of venous thrombosis. Arch Intern Med 1996;156:851–856.

88. Scurr JH. How long after surgery does the risk of thromboembolism persist? Acta Chir Scand 1990;556(Suppl):22–24.

89. Bergqvist D. Long-term prophylaxis following orthopaedic surgery. Haemostasis 1993;23(Suppl 1):27–31.

90. Bergqvist D, Benoni G, Björgell O et al. Low-molecular-weight heparin (enoxaparin) as prophylaxis against venous thromboembolism after total hip replacement. N Engl J Med 1996;335:696–700.

91. Bronge A, Dahlgren S, Lindquist B. Prophylaxis against thrombosis in femoral neck fractures: a comparison between dextran 70 and dicumarol. Acta Chir Scand 1971;137:29–35.

92. Bergquist E, Bergquist D, Bronge A et al. An evaluation of early thrombosis prophylaxis following fracture of the femoral neck. A comparison between dextran and dicoumarol. Acta Chir Scand 1972;138:689–693.

93. Powers PJ, Gent M, Jay RM et al. A randomized trial of less intense postoperative warfarin or aspirin therapy in the prevention of venous thromboembolism after surgery for fractured hip. Arch Intern Med 1989;149:771–774.

94. Monreal M, Lafoz E, Navarro A et al. A prospective double-blind trial of a low-molecular-weight heparin once daily compared with conventional low-dose heparin three times daily to prevent pulmonary embolism and venous thrombosis in patients with hip fracture. J Trauma 1989;29:873–875.

95. Bergqvist D, Kettunen K, Fredin H et al. Thromboprophylaxis in patients with hip fractures: a prospective, randomized, comparative study between ORG 10172 and dextran 70. Surgery 1991;109:617–622.

96. Agnelli G, Cosmi B, Di Fillipo P et al. A randomized double-blind, placebo-controlled trial of dermatan sulphate for prevention of deep vein thrombosis in hip fracture. Thromb Haemost 1992;67:203–208.

97. Geerts WH, Code KI, Jay RM et al. A prospective study of venous thrombo-embolism after major trauma. N Engl J Med 1994;331:1601–1606.

98. Geerts WH, Jay RM, Code KI et al. A comparison of low-dose heparin with low-molecular-weight heparin as prophylaxis again venous thrombo-embolism after major trauma. N Engl J Med 1996;335:701–707.

99. Warlow C, Terry G. Kenmure AC et al. A double-blind trial of low doses of subcutaneous heparin in the prevention of deep-vein thrombosis after myocardial infarction. Lancet 1973:934–936.

100. Emerson PA, Marks P. Preventing thromboembolism after myocardial infarction: effect of low-dose heparin or smoking. Br Med J 1971;1:18–20.

101. Nicolaides AN, Kakkar VV, Renney JT et al. Myocardial infarction and deep-vein thrombosis Br Med J 1971;1:432–434.

102. Handley AJ. Low dose heparin after myocardial infarction. Lancet 1972;ii:623–624.

103. McCarthy ST, Robertson D, Turner JJ et al. Low-dose heparin as a prophy-laxis against deep-vein thrombosis after acute stroke. Lancet 1977;ii:800–801.

104. Turpie AGG, Levine MN, Hirsh J et al. A double-blind randomized trial of ORG 10172 low-molecular-weight heparinoid in the prevention of deep vein thrombosis in thrombotic stroke. Lancet 1987;i:523–526.

105. Prins MH, den Ottolander GJ, Gelsema R et al. Deep vein thrombosis prophylaxis with a low-molecular-weight heparinoid in the prevention of deep vein thrombosis in thrombotic stroke. Lancet 1987;i:523.

106. Sandset PM, Dahl T, Stiris M et al. A double-blind and ransomized pla-cebo-controlled trial of low-molecular-weight heparin once daily to pre-vent deep vein thrombosis in acute ischemic stroke. Semin Thromb He-most 1990;16(Suppl):25–33.

107. Turpie AGG, Gent M, Cote R et al. A low-molecular-weight heparinoid compared with unfractionated heparin in the prevention of deep vein thrombosis in patients with acute ischemic stroke. Ann Intern Med 1992;117:353–357.

108. Todd JW, Frisbie JH, Rossier AB et al. Deep vein thrombosis in acute spinal cord injury: a comparison of $^{125}$I-fibrinogen leg scanning, imped-ance plethysmography, and venography. Paraplegia 1976;14:50–57.

109. Myllynen P, Kammonen M, Rokkanen P et al. Deep venous thrombosis and pulmonary embolism in patients with acute spinal cord injury: a com-parison with non-paralyzed patients immobilized due to spinal fractures. J Trauma 1985;25:541–543.

110. Green D, Lee MY, Lim AC et al. Prevention of thromboembolism after spinal cord injury using low-molecular-weight heparin. Ann Intern Med 1990;113:571–574.

111. Pingleton SK, Pingleton WW, Ruth WE et al. Prevention of pulmonary emboli in a respiratory intensive care unit. Efficacy of low-dose heparin. Chest 1981;79:647–650.

112. Halkin H, Goldberg J. Modan M et al. Reduction of mortality in general medical in-patients by low-dose heparin prophylaxis. Ann Intern Med 1982;96:561–565.

113. Belch JJ, Lowe GD, Ward AG et al. Prevention of deep-vein thrombosis in medical patients by low-dose heparin. Scott Med J 1981;26:115–117.

114. Dahan R, Houlbert D, Caulin C et al. Prevention of deep vein thrombosis in elderly in-patients by a low-molecular-weight heparin: a randomized double-blind trial. Haemostasis 1986;16:159–164.

115. Kernohan RJ, Todd C. Heparin therapy in thromboembolic disease. Lancet 1966;i:621–623.

116. Alpert JS, Smith R, Carlson J et al. Mortality in patients treated for pulmo-nary embolism. JAMA 1976;236:1477–1480.

117. Kanis JA. Heparin in the treatment of pulmonary thromboembolism. Thromb Diath Haemorrh 1974;32:519–527.

118. Barritt DW, Jordan SC. Anticoagulant drugs in the treatment of pulmonary embolism. A controlled trial. Lancet 1960;i:1309–1312.

119. Brandjes DPM, Heijboer H, Büller HR et al. Acenocoumarol and heparin compared with acenocoumarol alone in the initial treatment of proximal-vein thrombosis. N Engl J Med 1992;327:1485–1489.

120. Hull R, Delmore T, Carter C et al. Adjusted subcutaneous heparin versus warfarin sodium in the long-term treatment of venous thrombosis. N Engl J Med 1982;306:189–194.

121. Hull R, Hirsh J, Jay R et al. Different intensities of oral anticoagulant therapy in the treatment of proximal-vein thrombosis. N Engl J Med 1982;307:1676–1681.

122. Lagerstedt CI, Fagher BO, Olsson CG et al. Need for long-term anticoagu-lant treatment in symptomatic calf-vein thrombosis. Lancet 1985;ii:515–518.

123. Hull RD, Raskob GE, Rosenbloom D et al. Heparin for 5 days as compared with 10 days in the initial treatment of proximal venous thrombosis. N Engl J Med 1990;322:1260–1264.

124. Basu D, Gallus A, Hirsh J et al. A prospective study of the value of monitor-ing heparin treatment with the activated partial thromboplastin time. N Engl J Med 1972;287:324–327.

125. Hull RD, Raskob GE, Hirsh J et al. Continuous intravenous heparin com-pared with intermittent subcutaneous heparin in the initial treatment of proximal-vein thrombosis. N Engl J Med 1986;315:1109–1114.

126. Hull R, Delmore T, Genton E et al. Warfarin sodium versus low-dose heparin in the long-term treatment of venous thrombosis. N Engl J Med 1979;301:855–858.

127. Marder VJ, Soulen RL, Atichartakarn L et al. Quantitative venographic assessment of deep vein thrombosis in the evaluation of streptokinase and heparin therapy. J Lab Clin Med 1977;89:1018–1029.

128. Holm HA, Finnanger J, Hartmann A et al. Heparin treatment of deep venous thrombosis in 280 patients: symptoms related to dosage. Acta Med Scand 1984;215:47–53.

129. Wheeler AP, Jaquiss RD, Newman JH. Physician practices in the treatment of pulmonary embolism and deep venous thrombosis. Arch Intern Med 1988;148:1321–1325.

130. Raschke RA, Reilly BM, Guidry JR et al. The weight-based heparin dosing nomogram compared with a 'standard care' nomogram: a randomized controlled trial. Ann Intern Med 1993;119:874–881.

131. Cruickshank MK, Levine MN, Hirsh J et al. A standard heparin nomogram for the management of heparin therapy. Arch Intern Med 1991;151:333–337.

132. Hirsh J, Hoak J. Management of deep vein thrombosis and pulmonary embolism. A statement for healthcare professionals. Circulation 1996;93:2212–2245.

133. Levine MN, Hirsh J, Gent M et al. A randomized trial comparing activated thromboplastin time with heparin assay in patients with acute venous thromboembolism requiring large daily doses of heparin. Arch Intern Med 1994;154:49–56.

134. Levine MN, Raskob G, Landefeld S et al. Hemorrhagic complications of anticoagulant treatment. Chest 1995;108(Suppl):276–290.

135. Salzman EW, Deykin D, Shapiro RM et al. Management of heparin ther-apy, controlled prospective trial. N Engl J Med 1975;292:1046–1050.

136. Glazier RL, Crowell EB. Randomized prospective trial of continuous vs intermittent heparin therapy. JAMA 1976;236:1365–1367.

137. Wilson JR, Lampman J. Heparin therapy: a randomized prospective study. Am Heart J 1979;97:155–158.

138. Mant MJ, Thong KL, Birtwhistle RV et al. Haemorrhagic complications of heparin therpay. Lancet 1977;ii:1133–1135.

139. Landefeld CS, McGuire E III, Rosenblatt MW: A bleeding risk index for estimating the probability of major bleeding in hospitalized patients start-ing anticoagulant therapy. Am J Med 1990;89:569–578.

140. Nieuwenhuis HK, Albada J, Banga JD et al. Identification of risk factors for bleeding during treatment of acute venous thromboembolism with heparin or low-molecular-weight heparin. Blood 1991;78:2337–2343.

141. Wester JPJ, de Valk HW, Nieuwenhuis HK et al. Risk factors for bleeding during treatment of acute venous thromboembolism. Thromb Haemost 1996;76:682–688.

142. Walker AM, Jick H. Predictors of bleeding during heparin therapy. JAMA 1980;244:1209–1212.

143. Andersson G, Fagrell B, Holmgren K et al. Subcutaneous administration of heparin. A randomized comparison with intravenous administration of heparin to patients with deep-vein thrombosis. Thromb Res 1982;17:631–639.

144. Doyle DJ, Turpie AG, Hirsh J et al. Adjusted subcutaneous heparin or continuous intravenous heparin in patients with acute deep vein thrombo-sis. A randomized trial. Ann Intern Med 1987;107:441–445.

145. Walker MG, Shaw JW, Thomson GJ et al. Subcutaneous calcium heparin versus intravenous sodium heparin in treatment of established acute deep vein thrombosis of the legs: a multicentre prospective randomised trial. Br Med J 1987;294:1189–1192.

146. Pini M, Pattachini C, Quintavalla R et al. Subcutaneous vs intravenous heparin in the treatment of deep venous thrombosis—a randomized clini-cal trial. Thromb Haemost 1990;64:222–226.

147. Hommes DW, Bura A, Mazzolai L et al. Subcutaneous heparin compared with continuous intravenous heparin administration in the initial treat-ment of deep vein thrombosis. Ann Intern Med 1992;116:279–284.

148. Gallus A, Tillett J, Jackaman J et al. Safety and efficacy of warfarin started early after submassive venous thrombosis or pulmonary embolism. Lancet 1986;ii:1293–1296.

149. Rooke TW, Osmundson PJ. Heparin and the in-hospital management of deep venous thrombosis: cost considerations. Mayo Clin Proc 1986;61:198–204.

150. Leizorovicz A, Simonneau G, Decousus H et al. Comparison of efficacy and safety of low-molecular-weight heparins and unfractionated heparin in initial treatment of deep venous thrombosis: a meta-analysis. Br Med J 1994;309:299–304.

151. Lensing AW, Prins MH, Davidson BL et al. Treatment of deep venous thrombosis with low-molecular-weight heparins. Arch Intern Med 1995;155:601–607.

152. Siragusa S, Cosmi B, Piovella F et al. Low-molecular-weight heparins and unfractionated heparin in the treatment of patients with acute venous thromboembolism: results of a meta-analysis. Am J Med 1996;100:269–277.

153. Koopman MM, Prandoni P, Piovella F et al. Treatment of venous thrombo-sis with intravenous unfractionated heparin administered in the hospital as compared with subcutaneous low-molecular-weight heparin adminis-tered at home. N Engl J Med 1996;334:682–687.

154. Levine M, Gent M, Hirsh J et al. A comparison of low-molecular-weight

heparin administered primarily at home with unfractionated heparin administered in the hospital for proximal deep-vein thrombosis. N Engl J Med 1996;334:677–681.

155. Schafer AI. Low-molecular-weight heparin—an opportunity for home treatment of venous thrombosis. N Engl J Med 1996;334:724–725.

156. Wells PS, Holbrook AM, Crowther NR et al. Interactions of warfarin with drugs and food. Ann Intern Med 1994;121:676–683.

157. Monreal M, Lafoz E, Olive A et al. Comparison of subcutaneous unfractionated heparin with a low molecualr weight heparin (Fragmin®) in patients with venous thromboembolism and contraindications to coumarin. Thromb Haemost 1994;71:7–11.

158. Pini M, Aiello S, Manotti C et al. Low-molecular-weight heparin versus warfarin in the prevention of recurrences after deep vein thrombosis. Thromb Haemost 1994;72:191–197.

159. Coon WW, Willis PW III. Recurrence of venous thromboembolism. Surgery 1973;73:823–827.

160. Anonymous. Research Committee of the British Thoracic Society. Optimum duration of anticoagulation for deep-vein thrombosis and pulmonary embolism. Lancet 1992;340:873–876.

161. Levine MN, Hirsh J, Gent M et al. Optimal duration of oral anticoagulant therapy: a randomized trial comparing four weeks with three months of warfarin in patients with proximal deep vein thrombosis. Thromb Haemost 1995;74:606–611.

162. Schulman S, Rhedin AS, Lindmarker P et al. A comparison of six weeks with six months of oral anticoagulant therapy after a first epidose of venous thromboembolism. N Engl J Med 1995;332:1661–1665.

163. Prandoni P, Lensing AW, Büller HR et al. Deep-vein thrombosis and the incidence of subsequent symptomatic cancer. N Engl J Med 1992;327:1128–1133.

164. Schulman S, Granqvist S, Holmström M et al. The duration of oral anticoagulant therapy after a second episode of venous thromboembolism. N Engl J Med 1997;336:393–398.

165. Pellegrini VD Jr, Langhans MJ, Totterman S et al. Embolic complications of calf thrombosis following total hip arthroplasty. J Arthroplasty 1993;8:449–457.

166. Strandness DE Jr, Langlois Y, Cramer M et al. Long-term sequelae of acute venous thrombosis. JAMA 1983;250:1289–1292.

167. Killewich LA, Martin R, Cramer M et al. An objective assessment of the physiologic changes in the postthrombotic syndrome. Arch Surg 1985;120:424–426.

168. Kakkar VV, Lawrence D. Hemodynamic and clinical assessment after therapy for acute deep vein thrombosis. A prospective study. Am J Surg 1985;150:54–63.

169. Hull RD, Hirsh J, Carter CJ et al. Diagnostic efficacy of impedance plethysmography for clinically suspected deep-vein thrombosis. A randomized trial. Ann Intern Med 1985;102:21–28.

170. Huisman MV, Büller HR, ten Cate JW et al. Serial impedance plethysmography for suspected deep venous thrombosis in outpatients. The Amsterdam General Practitioner Study. N Engl J Med 1986;314:823–828.

171. Jay R, Hull R, Carter C et al. Outcome of abnormal impedance plethysmography results in patients with proximal-vein thrombosis: frequency of return to normal. Thromb Res 1984;36:259–263.

172. Ginsberg JS, Kowalchuk G, Hirsh J et al. Heparin effect on bone density. Thromb Haemost 1990;64:286–289.

173. Toglia MR, Weg JG. Venous thromboembolism during pregnancy. N Engl J Med 1996;335:108–114.

174. Ginsberg JS, Hirsh J, Rainbow AJ et al. Risks to the fetus of radiologic procedure used in the diagnosis of maternal venous thromboembolic disease. Thromb Haemost 1989;61:189–196.

175. Shaul WL, Hall JG. Multiple congenital anomalies associated with oral anticoagulants. Am J Obstet Gynecol 1977;127:191–198.

176. Hall, JG, Pauli RM, Wilson KM. Maternal and fetal sequelae of anticoagulation during pregnancy. Am J Med 1980;68:122–140.

177. Ginsberg JS, Hirsh J. Anticoagulants during pregnancy. Annu Rev Med 1989;40:79–86.

178. Iturbe-Alessio I, Fonseca MC, Mutchnik O et al. Risks of anticoagulant therapy in pregnant women with artificial heart valves. N Engl J Med 1986;315:1390–1393.

179. Hellgren M, Nygårds EB. Long-term therapy with subcutaneous heparin during prenancy. Gynecol Obstet Invest 1982;13:76–89.

180. Ginsberg JS, Kowalchuk G, Hirsh J et al. Heparin therapy during pregnancy. Risks to the fetus and mother. Arch Intern Med 1989;149:2233–2236.

181. Anderson DR, Ginsberg JS, Burrows R et al. Subcutaneous heparin therapy during pregnancy: a need for concern at the time of delivery. Thromb Haemost 1991;65:248–250.

182. Fejgin MD, Lourwood DL. Low-molecular-weight heparins and their use in obstetrics and gynecology. Obstet Gynecol Surv 1994;49:424–431.

183. Orme ML, Lewis PJ, DeSwiet M et al. May mothers given warfarin breastfeed their infants? Br Med J 1977;1:1564–1565.

184. McKenna R, Cole ER, Vasan U. Is warfarin sodium contraindicated in the lactating mother? J Pediatr 1983;103:325–327.

185. Badaracco MA, Vessey MP. Recurrence of venous thromboembolic disease and use of oral contraceptives. Br Med J 1974;1:215–217.

186. Turnier E, Hill JD, Kerth WJ et al. Massive pulmonary embolism. Am J Surg 1973;125:611–622.

187. Moser KM, Daily PO, Peterson K et al. Thromboendarterectomy for chronic, major-vessel thromboembolic pulmonary hypertension: immediate and long-term results in 42 patients. Ann Intern Med 1987;107:560–565.

188. Moser KM, Auger WR, Fedullo PF. Chronic major-vessel thromboembolic pulmonary hypertension. Circulation 1990;81:1735–1743.

189. Mozes M, Adar R, Bogokowsky H et al. Vein ligation in the treatment of pulmonary embolism. Surgery 1964;55:621–624.

190. Gurewich V, Thomas DP, Rabinov KR. Pulmonary embolism after ligation of the inferior vena cava. N Engl J Med 1966;274:1350–1354.

191. Greenfield LJ. Technical considerations for insertion of vena caval filters. Surg Gynecol Obstet 1979;148:422–426.

192. Greenfield LJ, Michna BA. Twelve-year clinical experience with Greenfield vena caval filter. Surgery 1988;104:706–712.

193. Schulman S, Lockner D. Local venous infusion of streptokinase in DVT. Thromb Res 1984;34:213–216.

194. Kakkar VV, Sagar S, Lewis M. Treatment of deep-vein thrombosis with intermittent streptokinase and plasminogen infusion. Lancet 1975;ii:674–676.

195. Kakkar VV, Scully MF. Intermittent plasminogen-streptokinase treatment of deep vein thrombosis. Haemostasis 1988;18:127–138.

196. Marder VJ, Bell WR. Fibrinolytic therapy. In: Colman RW, Hirsh J, Marder VJ, Salzman EW, eds. Hemostasis and thrombosis. Basic principles and clinical practice. Philadelphia: JB Lippincott, 1987:1393–1437.

197. Browse NL, Thomas ML, Pim HP. Streptokinase and deep vein thrombosis. Br Med J 1968;3:717–720.

198. Robertson BR, Nilsson IM, Nylander G. Thrombolytic effect of streptokinase as evaluated by phlebography of deep venous thrombi of the leg. Acta Chir Scand 1970;136:173–180.

199. Kakkar VV. Treatment of deep vein thrombosis: a comparative study of heparin, streptokinase and Arvin. Bull Schweiz Akad Med Wiss 1973;29:253–262.

200. Tsapogas MJ, Peabody RA, Wu KT et al. Controlled study of thrombolytic therapy in deep vein thrombosis. Surgery 1973;74:973–984.

201. Tibbutt DA, Williams EW, Walker MW et al. Controlled trial of ancrod and streptokinase in the treatment of deep vein thrombosis of lower limb. Br J Haematol 1974;27:407–414.

202. Duckert F, Müller G, Nyman D et al. Treatment of deep vein thrombosis with streptokinase. Br Med J 1975;1:479–481.

203. Rösch J, Dotter CT, Seaman AJ et al. Healing of deep venous thrombosis: venographic findings in a randomized study comparing streptokinase and heparin. Am J Roentgenol 1976;127:553–558.

204. Arnesen H, Heilo A, Jakobsen E et al. A prospective study of streptokinase and heparin in the treatment of deep vein thrombosis. Acta Med Scand 1978;203:457–463.

205. Elliot MS, Immelman EJ, Jeffrey P et al. A comparative randomized trial of heparin versus streptokinase in the treatment of acute proximal venous thrombosis: an interim report of a prospective trial. Br J Surg 1979;66:838–843.

206. Watz R, Savidge GF. Rapid thrombolysis and preservation of valvular venous function in high deep vein thrombosis. Acta Med Scand 1979;205:293–298.

207. Goldhaber SZ, Buring JE, Lipnick RJ et al. Pooled analyses of randomized trials of streptokinase and heparin in phlebographically documented acute deep venous thrombosis. Am J Med 1984;76:393–397.

208. Bauer GA. A roentgenological and clinical study of the sequelae of thrombosis. Acta Chir Scand 1942;74:1–86.

209. Birger I. Chronic (second) stage of thrombosis in lower extremities, its course into crural ulcer and its treatment. Acta Chir Scand 1947;95:13–110.

210. Negus D, Friedgood A. The effective management of venous ulceration. Br J Surg 1983;70:623–627.

211. Ginsberg JS, Shin A, Turpie AG et al. Detection of previous proximal venous thrombosis with Doppler ultrasonography and photoplethysmography. Arch Intern Med 1989;149:2255–2257.

212. Lindhagen A, Bergqvist D, Hallbook T et al. Venous function five to eight years after clinically suspected deep venous thrombosis. Acta Med Scand 1985;217:389–395.

213. Browse NL, Clemenson G, Thomas ML. Is the postphlebitic leg always postphlebitic? Relation between phlebographic appearances of deep-vein thrombosis and late sequelae. Br Med J 1980;281:1167–1170.

214. Bieger R, Boekhout-Mussert RJ, Hohmann F et al. Is streptokinase useful in the treatment of deep vein thrombosis? Acta Med Scand 1976;199:81–88.

215. Kakkar VV, Howe CT, Laws JW et al. Late results of treatment of deep vein thrombosis. Br Med J 1969;1:810–811.

216. Arnesen H, Hoiseth A, Ly B. Streptokinase or heparin in the treatment of deep vein thrombosis. Acta Med Scand 1982;211:65–68.

217. van de Loo JC, Kriessmann A, Trübestein G et al. Controlled multicenter pilot study of urokinase-heparin and streptokinase in deep vein thrombosis. Thromb Haemost 1983;50:660–663.

218. Thery C, Bauchart JJ, Lesenne M et al. Predictive factors of effectiveness of streptokinase in deep venous thrombosis. Am J Cardiol 1992;69:117–122.

219. Meyerovitz MF, Polak JF, Goldhaber SZ. Short-term response to thrombo-

lytic therapy in deep venous thrombosis: predictive value of venographic appearance. Radiology 1992;184:345–348.

220. Francis CW, Totterman S. Magnetic resonance imaging of deep vein thrombi correlates with response to thrombolytic therapy. Thromb Haemost 1995;73:386–391.

221. Verhaeghe R, Besse P, Bounameaux H et al. Multicenter pilot study of the efficacy and safety of systemic rt-PA administration in the treatment of deep vein thrombosis of the lower extremities and/or pelvis. Thromb Res 1989;55:5–11.

222. Goldhaber SZ, Meyerovitz MF, Green D et al. Randomized controlled trial of tissue plasminogen activator in proximal deep venous thrombosis. Am J Med 1990;88:235–240.

223. Turpie AG, Levine MN, Hirsh J et al. Tissue plasminogen activator (rt-PA) vs heparin in deep vein thrombosis. Results of a randomized trial. Chest 1990;97(Suppl):172–175.

224. Marder VJ, Brenner B, Totterman S et al. Comparison of dosage schedules of rt-PA in the treatment of proximal deep vein thrombosis. J Lab Clin Med 1992;119:485–495.

225. Bounameaux H, Banga JD, Bluhmki E et al. Double-blind, randomized comparison of systemic continuous infusion of 0.25 versus 0.50 mg/kg/24h of alteplase over 3 to 7 days for treatment of deep venous thrombosis in heparinized patients: results of the European Thrombolysis with rt-PA in Venous Thrombosis (ETTT) Trial. Thromb Haemost 1992;67:306–309.

226. Schwieder G, Grimm W, Siemens HJ et al. Intermittent regional therapy with rt-PA is not superior to systemic thrombolysis in deep vein thrombosis (DVT)—a German multicenter trial. Thromb Haemost 1995;74:1240–1243.

227. Semba CP, Dake MD. Iliofemoral deep venous thrombosis: aggressive therapy with catheter-directed thrombolysis. Radiology 1994;191:487–494.

228. Comerota AJ, Aldridge SC, Cohen G et al. A strategy of aggressive regional therapy for acute iliofemoral venous thrombosis with contemporary venous thrombectomy or catheter-directed thrombolysis. J Vasc Surg 1994;20:244–254.

229. Anonymous. The urokinase pulmonary embolism trial. A national cooperative study. Circulation 1973;47:1–108.

230. Anonymous. Urokinase-streptokinase embolism trial. Phase 2 results. JAMA 1974;229:1606–1613.

231. Dalla-Volta S, Palla A, Santolicandro A et al. PAIMS 2: alteplase combined with heparin versus heparin in the treatment of acute pulmonary embolism. Plasminogen activator Italian multicenter study 2. J Am Coll Cardiol 1992;20:520–526.

232. Goldhabert SZ, Kessler CM, Heit JA et al. Recombinant tissue-type plasminogen activator versus a novel dosing regimen of urokinase in acute pulmonary embolism: a randomized controlled multicenter trial. J Am Coll Cardiol 1992;20:24–30.

233. Goldhaber SZ, Haire WD, Feldstein ML et al. Alteplase versus heparin in acute pulmonary embolism: randomised trial assessing right-ventricular function and pulmonary perfusion. Lancet 1993;341:507–511.

234. Meyer G, Sors H, Charbonnier B et al. Effects of intravenous urokinase versus alteplase on total pulmonary resistance in acute massive pulmonary embolism: a European multicenter double-blind trial. J Am Coll Cardiol 1992;19:239–245.

235. Goldhaber SZ, Heit J, Sharma GV et al. Randomised controlled trial of recombinant tissue plasminogen activator versus urokinase in the treatment of acute pulmonary embolism. Lancet 1988;ii:293–298.

236. Lualdi JC, Goldhaber SZ. Right ventricular dysfunction after acute pulmonary embolism: pathophysiologic factors, detection, and therapeutic implications. Am Heart J 1995;130:1276–1282.

237. Gonzalez-Juanatey JR, Valdes L, Amaro A et al. Treatment of massive pulmonary thromboembolism with low intrapulmonary dosages of urokinase. Short-term angiographic and hemodynamic evolution. Chest 1992;102:341–346.

238. Sharma GV, Burleson VA, Sasahara AA. Effect of thrombolytic therapy on pulmonary-capillary blood volume in patients with pulmonary embolism. N Engl J Med 1980;303:842–845.

239. Stein PD, Hull RD, Raskob G. Risks for major bleeding from thrombolytic therapy in patients with acute pulmonary embolism. Ann Intern Med 1994;121:313–317.

240. Marder VJ, Sherry S. Thrombolytic therapy: current status. N Engl J Med 1988;318:1512–1520,1585–1595.

241. Francis CW, Foster TH, Totterman S et al. Monitoring of therapy for deep vein thrombosis using magnetic resonance imaging. Acta Radiol 1989;30:445–446.

242. Meaney JFM, Weg JG, Chenevert TL et al. Diagnosis of pulmonary embolism with magnetic resonance angiography. N Engl J Med 1997;336:1422–1427.

243. Rao AK, Pratt C, Berke A et al. Thrombolysis in myocardial infarction (TIMI) trial—phase I: hemorrhagic manifestations and changes in plasma fibrinogen and the fibrinolytic system in individuals treated with recombinant tissue plasminogen activator and streptokinase. J Am Coll Cardiol 1988;11:1–11.

244. Prandoni P, Polistena P, Bernardi E et al. Upper-extremity deep vein

245. Swinton NW Jr, Edgett JW Jr, Hall RJ. Primary subclavian-axillary vein thrombosis. Circulation 1968;38:737–745.

246. Adams JT, DeWeese JA. "Effort" thrombosis of the axillary and subclavian veins. J Trauma 1971;11:923–930.

247. Campbell CB, Chandler JG, Tegtmeyer CJ et al. Axillary, subclavian, and brachiocephalic vein obstruction. Surgery 1977;82:816–826.

248. Ameli FM, Minas T, Weiss M et al. Consequences of "conservative" conventional management of axillary vein thrombosis. Can J Surg 1987;30:167–169.

249. Donayre CE, White GH, Mehringer SM et al. Pathogenesis determines late morbidity of axillosubclavian vein thrombosis. Am J Surg 1986;152:179–184.

250. Tilney ML, Griffith HJ, Edwards EA. Natural history of major venous thrombosis of the upper extremity. Arch Surg 1970;101:792–796.

251. Monreal M, Lafoz E, Ruiz J et al. Upper-extremity deep venous thrombosis and pulmonary embolism: a prospective study. Chest 1991;99:280–283.

252. Horattas MC, Wright DJ, Fenton AH et al. Changing concepts of deep venous thrombosis of the upper extremity: report of a series and Review of the literature. Surgery 1988;104:561–567.

253. Rubenstein M, Creger WP. Successful streptokinase therapy for catheter-nduced subclavian vein thrombosis. Arch Intern Med 1980;140:1370–1371.

254. Bradof J, Sands MJ Jr, Lakin PC. Symptomatic venous thrombosis of the upper extremity complicating permanent transvenous pacing: reversal with streptokinase infusion. Am Heart J 1982;104:1112–1113.

255. Becker GJ, Holden RW, Rabe FE et al. Local thrombolytic therapy for subclavian and axillary vein thrombosis. Treatment of the thoracic inlet syndrome. Radiology 1983;149:419–423.

256. Appleby DH, Heller MS. Low-ose streptokinase therapy for subclavian vein thrombosis. South Med J 1984;77:536–537.

257. Collier PE, Diamond DL, Young JC. Axillary vein thrombosis. Vasc Surg 1984;18:174–178.

258. Painter TD, Karpf M. Deep venous thrombosis of the upper extremity five years experience at a university hospital. Angiology 1984;35:743–749.

259. Wilson JJ, Lesk D, Newman H. Subclavian-xillary vein thrombosis: successful treatment with streptokinase. Can Med Assoc J 1984;130:891–893.

260. Druy EM, Trout HH III, Giordano JM et al. Lytic therapy in the treatment of axillary and subclavian vein thrombosis. J Vasc Surg 1985;2:821–827.

261. Smith NL, Ravo B, Soroff HS et al. Successful fibrinolytic therapy for superior vena cava thrombosis secondary to long-erm total parenteral nutrition. JPEN J Parenter Enteral Nutr 1985;9:55–57.

262. Taylor LM Jr, McAllister WR, Dennis DL et al. Thrombolytic therapy followed by first rib resection for spontaneous ("effort") subclavian vein thrombosis. Am J Surg 1985;149:644–647.

263. Landercasper J, Gall W, Fischer M et al. Thrombolytic therapy of axillary-subclavian venous thrombosis. Arch Surg 1987;122:1072–1075.

264. Bozzetti F, Scarpa D, Terno G et al. Subclavian venous thrombosis due to indwelling catheters: a prospective study on 52 patients. JPEN J Parenter Enteral Nutr 1983;7:560–562.

265. Ross AH, Griffith CD, Anderson JR et al. Thromboembolic complications with silicone elastomer subclavian catheters. JPEN J Parenter Enteral Nutr 1982;6:61–63.

266. Blacklock HA, Pillai MV, Hill RS et al. Use of modified subcutaneous right-atrial catheter for venous access in leukaemic patients. Lancet 1980;i:993–994.

267. Haire WD, Lieberman RP, Edney J et al. Hickman catheter-induced thoracic vein thrombosis. Cancer 1990;66:900–908.

268. Chastre J, Cornud F, Bouchama A et al. Thrombosis as a complication of pulmonary-artery catheterization via the internal jugular vein. N Engl J Med 1982;306:278–281.

269. Fraschini G, Jadeja J, Lawson M et al. Local infusion of urokinase for the lysis of thrombosis associated with permanent central venous catheters in cancer patients. J Clin Oncol 1987;5:672–678.

270. Glynn MF, Jeejeebhoy KN, Langer B et al. Therapy for thrombotic occlusion of long-term intravenous alimentation catheters. JPEN J Parenter Enteral Nutr 1980;4:387–390.

271. Hurtubise MR, Bottino JC, Lawson M et al. Restoring patency of occluded central venous catheters. Arch Surg 1980;115:212–213.

272. Gale GB, O'Connor DM, Chu JY et al. Restoring patency of thrombosed catheters with cryopreserved urokinase. JPEN J Parenter Enteral Nutr 1984;8:298–299.

273. Bern MM, Lokich JJ, Wallach SR et al. Very low doses of warfarin can prevent thrombosis in central venous catheters. A randomized prospective trial. Ann Intern Med 1990;112:423–428.

274. Bakir N, Sluiter WJ, Ploeg RJ et al. Primary renal graft thrombosis. Nephrol Dial Transplant 1996;11:140–147.

275. Llach F, Papper S, Massry SG. The clinical spectrum of renal vein thrombosis: acute and chronic. Am J Med 1980;69:819–827.

276. Wagoner RD, Stanson AW, Holley KE et al. Renal vein thrombosis in idiopathic membranous glomerulopathy and nephrotic syndrome: incidence and significance. Kidney Int 1983;23:368–374.

277. Kauffmann RH, Veltkamp JJ, Van Tilburg NH et al. Acquired antithrombin

III deficiency and thrombosis in the nephrotic syndrome. Am J Med 1978; 65:607–613.

278. Burrow CR, Walker WG, Bell WR et al. Streptokinase salvage of renal function after renal vein thrombosis. Ann Intern Med 1984;100:237–238.

279. Rowe JM, Rasmussen RL, Mader SL et al. Successful thrombolytic therapy in two patients with renal vein thrombosis. Am J Med 1984;77:1111–1114.

280. Bromberg WD, Firlit CF. Fibrinolytic therapy for renal vein thrombosis in the child. J Urol 1990;143:86–88.

281. Markowitz GS, Brignol F, Burns ER et al. Renal vein thrombosis treated with thrombolytic therapy: case report and brief review. Am J Kidney Dis 1995;25:801–106.

282. Schwieger J, Reiss R, Cohen JL et al. Acute renal allograft dysfunction in the setting of deep venous thrombosis: a case of successful urokinase thrombolysis and a review of the literature. Am J Kidney Dis 1993;22:345–350.

283. Chiu AS, Landsberg DN. Successful treatment of acute transplant renal vein thrombosis with selective streptokinase infusion. Transplant Proc 1991;23:2297–2300.

284. Mitchell MC, Boitnott JK, Kaufman S et al. Budd-Chiari syndrome: etiology, diagnosis and management. Medicine 1982;61:199–218.

285. Mahmoud AE, Mendoza A, Meshikhes AN et al. Clinical spectrum, investigations and treatment of Budd-Chiari syndrome. QJM 1996;89:37–43.

286. Wang ZG, Zhu Y, Wang SH et al. Recognition and management of Budd-Chiari syndrome: report of one hundred cases. J Vasc Surg 1989;10:149–156.

287. Klein AS, Sitzmann JV, Coleman J et al. Current management of Budd-Chiari syndrome. Ann Surg 1990;212:144–149.

288. Lopez RR Jr, Benner KG, Hall L et al. Expandable venous stents for treatment of the Budd-Chiari syndrome. Gastroenterology 1991;100:1435–1441.

289. Tilanus HW. Budd-Chiari syndrome. Br J Surg 1995;82:1023–1030.

290. Greenwood LH, Yrizarry JM, Hallett JW Jr et al. Urokinase treatment of Budd-Chiari syndrome. Am J Roentgenol 1983;141:1057–1059.

291. Sholar PW, Bell WR. Thrombolytic therapy for inferior vena cava thrombosis in paroxysmal nocturnal hemoglobinuria. Ann Intern Med 1985;103:539–541.

292. McKee CM, Crothers JG, Mayne EE et al. Budd-Chiari syndrome treated with acylated streptokinase-plasminogen complex. J R Soc Med 1985;78:768–769.

293. Abdu RA, Zakhour BJ, Dallis DJ. Mesenteric venous thrombosis—1911 to 1984. Surgery 1987;101:383–388.

294. Gomez R, Moreno E, Colina F et al. Liver transplantation in patients with Budd-Chiari syndrome. Transplant Int 1995;8:312–316.

295. Hemming AW, Langer B, Greig P et al. Treatment of Budd-Chiari syndrome with portosystemic shunt or liver transplantation. Am J Surg 1996;171:176–180.

296. Rattner DW, Ellman L, Warshaw AL. Portal vein thrombosis after elective splenectomy. An underappreciated, potentially lethal syndrome. Arch Surg 1993;128:565–569.

297. Gayowski TJ, Marino IR, Doyle HR et al. A high incidence of native portal vein thrombosis in veterans undergoing liver transplantation. J Surg Res 1996;60:333–338.

298. Cohen J, Edelman RR, Chopra S. Portal vein thrombosis: a review. Am J Med 1992;173–182.

299. Grauer SE, Schwartz SI. Extrahepatic portal hypertension: a retrospective analysis. Ann Surg 1979;189:566–574.

300. Warren WD, Henderson JM, Millikan WJ et al. Management of variceal bleeding in patients with noncirrhotic portal vein thrombosis. Ann Surg 1988;207:623–634.

301. Abdu RA, Zakhour BJ, Dallis DJ. Mesenteric venous thrombosis—1911 to 1984. Surgery 1987;101:383–388.

302. Rhee RY, Gloviczki P, Mendonca CT et al. Mesenteric venous thrombosis: still a lethal disease in the 1990s. J Vasc Surg 1994;20:688–697.

303. Geelkerken RH, van Bockel JH. Mesenteric vascular disease: a review of diagnostic methods and therapies. Cardiovasc Surg 1995;3:247–260.

# CHAPTER 62

# GENE THERAPY OF THROMBOTIC AND HEMORRHAGIC DISORDERS

Elizabeth G. Nabel

Gene therapy derives from the remarkable progress in molecular biology during the latter half of this century. In the past 20 years, major scientific advances in viral genetics, eukaryotic gene expression, and cloning of human disease–related genes have laid the foundation for application of these methods to genetic therapies (1). Somatic gene therapy is defined as insertion of engineered genes into individual cells or tissues to correct an inherited or acquired disorder through *in vivo* synthesis of a missing or defective gene product. The genetic material used in gene transfer has included eukaryotic and prokaryotic genes, RNA molecules encoding intracellular and secreted polypeptides, synthetic oligonucleotides, and ribozymes. Progress in human gene therapy is attributable to the efforts of many investigators, who have made substantial advances in molecular biology and molecular genetics. Gene therapy remains in its infancy, however, dating back only to the mid-1980s, during which both viral and nonviral vectors have been developed. The principles of gene transfer have been established *in vitro* in numerous cell lines, and animal models have been created in which hypotheses concerning the pathophysiology of human diseases can be tested. Many of these hypotheses are now moving forward to testing in human gene therapy trials (2, 3).

At the National Institutes of Health, Anderson (4) and Blaese et al (5) initiated a first human gene therapy trial in 1990 to treat adenosine deaminase deficiency. In the 7 years since then, the field has expanded dramatically, with more than 125 trials of gene therapy now underway worldwide (6). These studies have enrolled more than 1600 individuals, and the results of early phase I trials have demonstrated the safety of current gene transfer technologies. Despite the favorable safety profile, there are only limited data supporting efficacy, however. This largely results from the need to expand phase I studies into multicenter phase II/III trials. The lack of rapid application to phase II/III trials reflects the current challenges in the field, which include definition of suitable disease targets for initial gene therapy trials, necessary improvements in vectors and delivery systems, and increased stability of gene expression in humans. Progress toward effective therapies may not be as rapid as initially anticipated, but early human gene transfer studies have produced a wealth of new information about the expression of recombinant genes in human tissues. The ability to express a recombinant gene directly in a cell type or tissue now permits direct testing of specific gene products in many human diseases. These advances in the basic science have been exciting.

This chapter summarizes our current understanding of gene therapy for thrombotic and hemorrhagic disorders. Current perspectives on viral and nonviral vectors are presented, and development of animal models to test hypotheses regarding the pathophysiology of thrombotic and hemorrhagic disorders is discussed. Finally, progress toward human gene therapies is presented. Throughout this discussion, hurdles to successful gene therapy that must still be overcome are highlighted.

# VECTORS

An ideal vector would have the following properties: efficient transduction; long-term, stable transgene expression in many cell types *in vivo*; little or no risk of persistent infection; lack of immunogenicity; no host-cell mutagenesis; and no individual-to-patient transmission. Many investigators had hoped such a vector could be constructed, but such an ideal vector is unlikely to exist (7–12). Instead, viral and nonviral vectors have been modified to fulfill certain niches. In other words, vectors with unique properties are being prepared that are suitable for the introduction of recombinant genes into specific cell types and expression of the recombinant gene for a sufficient period to treat the target diseases. When considering a vector, it is important to evaluate the following: the target disease, the candidate gene, the transduced cell type, the duration of gene expression, and the potential for toxicity in the cell type or tissue (12). Other factors include: efficiency of transduction of cell type both *in vitro* and *in vivo*, ability to target genetic material to specific cells, intracellular stability of the genetic material, ability to produce stable transcripts, and potential immunogenicity as well as cytotoxicity. The advantages and disadvantages of both viral and nonviral vectors are summarized in Table 62.1.

## VIRAL VECTORS

Two major viral vectors have been employed in human gene therapy studies: retroviral vectors, and adenoviral vectors. Recently, retroviral vectors have been modified as pseudotype retroviral vectors (13). Herpes simplex viruses also have been modified as vectors for use in the central nervous system, but these are not widely used for thrombotic and hemorrhagic disorders. Adeno-associated viral vectors have been developed more recently (10, 14).

### Retroviral Vectors

Retroviruses have been the most widely used vector in both animal and human gene therapy studies. Their initial use derived from the simplicity of their genome, their ability to infect many dividing mammalian cells, and their capacity to stably integrate their genome into the host chromosome, thereby providing long-term transgene expression (7, 9, 11, 15). The construction of retroviral vectors has been extensively reviewed elsewhere (16). Following infection of a mammalian cell with a retroviral vector, the RNA genome of the replication defective retroviral vector undergoes reverse transcription to yield a double-stranded DNA copy. This retroviral complementary DNA (cDNA) then randomly integrates into the host genome. Infection produces integration of from one to 10 copies of the viral genome per cell; following integration, the viral genome is transcribed either from the endogenous promoter in the 5′ untranslated region or from an internal promoter engineered into the vector. The integrated viral genome is replicated with the host chromosome and passed on to all progeny of the transduced cell.

The advantages of retroviral vectors include their ability to remove all viral genes and replace them with transgene sequences and transcriptional regulatory elements. The viral gene products necessary to generate an infectious particle are supplied *in trans* by the packaging cell line. A second advantage is the broad host range, which is determined by the envelope glycoprotein expressed in the packaging cell line.

Despite these advantages, retroviral vectors do have several limitations. First, retroviral vectors only infect dividing cells (17). Second, it is difficult to produce high viral titers (>$10^6$ particle-forming units [pfu]). Third, random integration of retroviral vectors poses a risk of insertional mutagenesis (18). Fourth, retroviral vectors are stably expressed in cultured cells *in vitro*, but transcription of these vectors is extinguished in primary cells *in vivo* after short periods of time. Initially, it was hoped that retroviral vectors could introduce and stably express recombinant genes in certain cell types to treat inherited disorders such as hemophilia A or B, but this hope has not been realized.

More recently, pseudotype retroviral particles containing the envelope glycoprotein from the vesicular stomatitis virus have been developed (19). These pseudotype viruses can be prepared at much higher titers than retroviral vectors (16). It also is possible to target retroviral vectors to specific cell types by modifying the envelope glycoprotein to contain recognition sites for lineage-specific cell surface receptors (20). Whether these pseudotype retroviral vectors will find common use in human gene therapy, however, remains to be determined. At present, retroviral vectors are unlikely to be used widely in gene therapy for thrombotic and hemorrhagic disorders.

### Adenoviral Vectors

During the past 8 years, replication-defective adenoviral vectors have been used widely for both animal and human gene therapy studies (8, 21–23). Adenoviruses are double-stranded, linear DNA viruses that cause a self-limited respiratory tract infection, and adenoviral vectors have several properties making them ideally suited for human gene therapy. Adenoviruses infect many replicating and nonreplicating mammalian cells both *in vitro* and *in vivo*. These vectors can be produced at titers as high as $10^{12}$ pfu/ml, thereby allowing efficient gene transfer *in vivo* with small volumes of virus. Adenoviral vectors do not integrate into the host genome, and they have not been associated with human

**TABLE 62.1.**   Advantages and Disadvantages of Viral and Nonviral Vectors

| Vector | Advantages | Disadvantages | Applications |
|---|---|---|---|
| *Viral* | | | |
| Retrovirus | Biology well understood<br>Stable integration into host cells<br>Efficient entry<br>No viral genes in vector | Low titer<br>Infection limited to dividing cells<br>Expression difficult to control and stabilize<br>Expensive and complex to prepare | Marker studies, *ex vivo* treatments, vaccines |
| Adenovirus | High titers<br>Efficient entry into most cell types<br>High level of expression<br>Infection of nondividing cells | Vectors contain viral genes<br>Immunogenic, stimulating T- and B-cell responses<br>Generation of replication-competent virus<br>Factors controlling tropism not well understood | Localized *in vivo* treatments: cystic fibrosis, short-term treatments such as cancer and cardiovascular disease |
| Adeno-associated virus | Integration at specific sites | Requires replicating adenovirus to grow<br>No helper cell line<br>Limited insert size | Similar to adenovirus |
| Herpesvirus | High titers<br>May be neurotropic | Complex construction<br>No packaging cell lines | Neurologic diseases |
| Pseudotype retrovirus | High titers<br>Higher efficiency of retrovirus infection<br>Broader host range | Similar to retrovirus | Not established; may be similar to retrovirus |
| *Nonviral* | | | |
| Naked DNA | Easy to prepare<br>No size constraints<br>High level of safety<br>No viral genes<br>Lack of integration | Inefficient entry and uptake<br>Limited persistence and lack of stability | Topical and/or mechanical applications, including skin and vasculature |
| DNA liposomes | Same as naked DNA<br>More efficient uptake of DNA | Limited persistence and lack of stability | Direct *in vivo* applications, cancer, cardiovascular disease, cystic fibrosis |
| Adenoviral polylysine DNA conjugates | Same as DNA liposomes<br>Targetable to specific cell types | Requires adenovirus<br>Complex to construct | Same as DNA liposomes |

*Adapted with permission from Nabel EG. Introduction to vectors. Current protocols in human genetics. New York: John Wiley & Sons, 1997.*

malignancies. Recombinant adenoviral vectors also accept large promoter and transgene cassettes (≤6 kb).

Current adenoviral vectors derive from adenovirus serotypes 2 and 5. Both serotypes are minimally pathogenic in humans (24). First-generation adenoviral vectors were constructed to be replication incompetent (8). The E1 region of the genome, which normally encodes two transcriptional regulatory proteins (E1A and E1B) required for expression of late viral genes and for induc-

tion of the lytic phase of the virus, are removed; this region is replaced by the desired transgene under transcriptional control of appropriate promoter and enhancer elements. Adenoviral vectors are propagated in permissive cell lines such as 293 cells, which stably express the E1 gene product *in trans* (25). Infectious particles are produced, but they are incapable of replication in host cells (26) (Fig. 62.1).

Adenoviral vectors have been widely used for cardi-

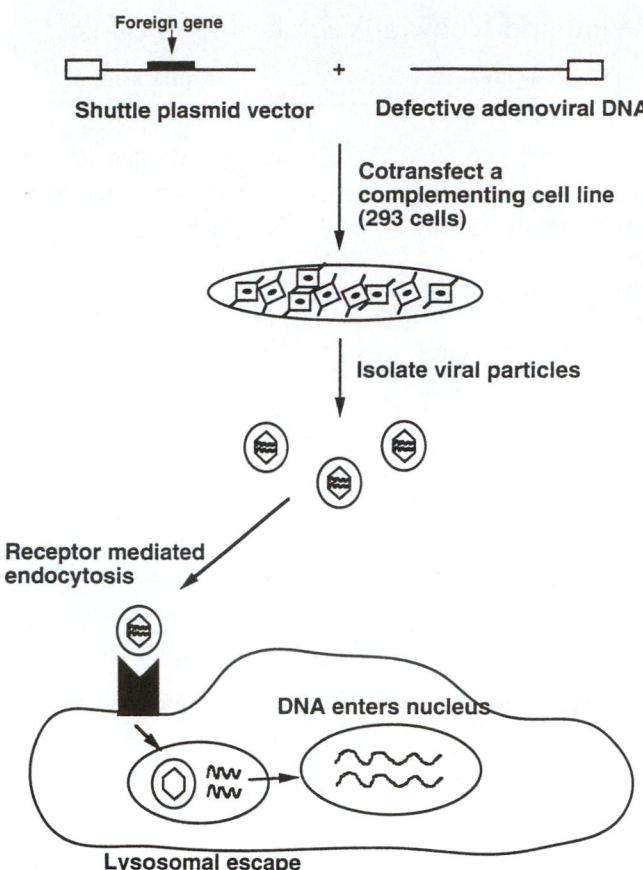

Foreign gene

Shuttle plasmid vector  +  Defective adenoviral DNA

Cotransfect a complementing cell line (293 cells)

Isolate viral particles

Receptor mediated endocytosis

DNA enters nucleus

Lysosomal escape

**FIGURE 62.1.** Principles of adenoviral gene transfer. Adenoviral plasmid is cotransfected with a defective adenoviral transcript into 293 cells, in which a replication-defective adenoviral particle is produced. Viral particles are used to infect cells and transfer the gene of interest to the host-cell nucleus. (Adapted with permission from Simari R, Nabel EG. Prevention of restenosis: genetic therapy. Semin Intervent Cardiol 1996;1:77–83.)

ovascular and hematologic applications, but first-generation adenoviral vectors have been limited by host inflammatory and immune responses that decrease transgene expression and preclude repeat vector administration (27, 28). Results from several laboratories have demonstrated that transient gene expression is complex because of immune responses involving non–antigen-specific inflammation caused by viral infection, cell death, and cellular and humoral immune responses directed against transgene proteins and viral proteins (29–34). Neutralizing antibodies produced against the viral capsid prevent readministration of the virus (34). Cytokine responses also may play a role in limiting the viral genome from host cells.

Several approaches have been used to modify first-generation adenoviral vectors. The first involves modifications in the viral genome (33). Second-generation and third-generation adenoviral vectors have been con-

structed to contain deletions in the *E2* and *E4* genes, which are required for late viral gene expression (35–37). Recently, a gutted viral vector has been produced in which all viral genes have been replaced with transgene sequences (38). A second approach involves transient immunosuppression of the host at the time of adenoviral administration. Immunosuppression with agents including α-CD4 and α-CD40 monoclonal antibodies, CTLA4-Ig, and cyclophosphamide plus cyclosporine have been used to prolong transgene expression in rodents (39). Long-term transgene expression may be required for inherited disorders in which gene expression is needed for the individual's entire lifetime; however, transient gene expression may be suitable for other diseases, such as vascular proliferative disorders and acute thrombosis.

In summary, adenoviral vectors have been used by many investigators to efficiently express recombinant genes in many cell types. Their current limitations preclude-long term transgene expression. Many groups are currently modifying adenoviral vectors, and improved versions of them likely will become readily available.

### Adeno-associated Viral Vectors

Adeno-associated virus (AAV) is a defective human parvovirus with attractive properties for gene transfer. This virus can be prepared at high titers, is not normally pathogenic in humans, and can infect many cell types *in vitro* (14). The AAV genome is a single-stranded, linear, 5 kb DNA molecule. The wild-type AAV integrates in a site-specific fashion into a single 7-kb region on human chromosome 19 (40). The AAV genome is flanked by 145 base pair–inverted terminal repeats containing the sequences required for packaging, DNA replication, and integration. The coating region contains two open reading frames, which can be deleted and replaced with one or more transgenes plus transcriptional regulatory units (41, 42). AAV vectors can accept transgene cassettes of only 4 to 5 kb; this limits the types of transgenes that can be used. Propagation of AAV vectors requires complex packaging, including AAV Rep and Cap proteins and five adenoviral proteins (i.e., E1A, E1B, E2A, E4, and VA). These complex packaging requirements have precluded construction of a helper cell line for AAV. Currently, vectors are constructed by cotransfection of cells with the AAV vector and a nonpackageable plasmid containing the AAV Rep and Cap proteins. This is followed by infection of the transfected cells with wild-type or mutant helper adenovirus. AAV then is separated from contaminating adenovirus by heat treatment and equilibrium density gradiation centrification. Protocols for constructing AAV vectors are described elsewhere (14).

AAV vectors infect a variety of cells *in vitro*, but their utility *in vivo* has not been established. Their ability to transduce vascular endothelial cells and smooth muscle cells remains unknown as well (43), and several problems are associated with their use. Lack of a packaging cell line and need for coinfection with adenovirus make it difficult to prepare large quantities of pure AAV vectors. Deletion of viral genes during vector construction limits the ability of these vectors to integrate in a site-specific manner, and it raises the possibility of insertional mutagenesis. AAV vectors are theoretically attractive, but considerable work is required before they can be implemented broadly (42).

## NONVIRAL VECTORS

### Plasmid DNA

Plasmid DNA has numerous advantages as a vector for gene therapy. Plasmids are easy to construct, and they can be produced both inexpensively and in large quantity (44). Use of a plasmid vector is safe and obviates an infectious viral vector. Injection of plasmid DNA into human tissues does not cause inflammation (45). Plasmid vectors encoding self-transgenes result in long-term transgene expression *in vivo*, and they have not been associated with immune responses to the transgene or DNA (46–49). This makes possible readministration of plasmid vectors to produce increased transgene expression.

Plasmid DNA is safe and easy to use, but its wide application has been limited by low efficiencies of transduction *in vitro*. In general, approximately 1 to 5% of cells surrounding the injection site have been shown to be transduced (46–50), and this low transduction efficiency reflects extensive cytoplasmic degradation and poor nuclear translocation following incorporation into the lysosome compartment. To date, modifications and expression vectors have been produced by optimizing the promoter and enhancer elements (51); however, the problem of lysosomal degradation has not been resolved.

The simplicity of plasmid DNA vectors continues to make them attractive vehicles for gene therapy. In the future, hybrid synthetic vectors that incorporate certain features of viral vectors likely will allow efficient *in vivo* gene delivery using plasmid DNA.

### Cationic Liposomes

One method to increase the efficiency of plasmid DNA is to incorporate it into a lipid moiety, which acts as a carrier to enhance uptake by fusion with a cell membrane or by receptor-mediated endocytosis (52–55). Significant degradation of DNA and lipid occurs in the lysosomal compartment with reduced nuclear translocation. Many groups also have modified the lipid moiety to improve cellular uptake and reduce lysosomal degradation (56, 57).

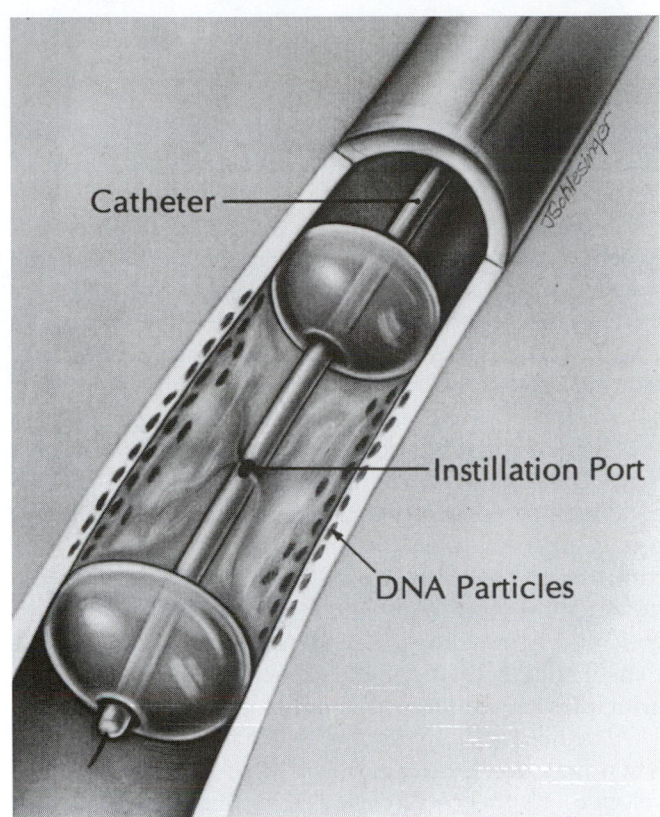

**FIGURE 62.2.** Catheter-mediated gene delivery. Catheters are modified to deliver recombinant genes and vectors to specific sites of vascular disease. (Adapted with permission from Nabel EG, Nabel GJ. Gene therapy for cardiovascular disease: potential applications. In: Braunwald E, ed. Heart disease: updates. New York: WB Saunders; 1994:1–13.)

Liposome-mediated gene transfer is attractive, because it does not require an infectious agent. Liposomes have been used to deliver a wide variety of DNA and RNA vectors to many cell types (2, 53). DNA liposome complexes can be targeted to cell lineages by incorporation of lineage-specific receptor binding proteins, but even although liposomes are attractive gene therapy vehicles, significant increases in transduction efficiency are required before they can be broadly applied to many human diseases. At present, their use is limited to local applications such as cancer therapy (44) and catheter-mediated vascular gene therapy (58–60) (Fig. 62.2).

## CELLULAR TARGETS

Many cell types have been employed as targets for cardiovascular gene therapy, including vascular endothelial and smooth muscle cells as well as cardiac myocytes and skeletal myocytes. This section discusses the issues involved in transducing each of these cell types both *in vitro* and *in vivo*. The three major cell types applicable to treatment of thrombotic and hemorrhagic disorders likely will be vascular endothelial and smooth muscle cells and skeletal myoblasts.

## EX VIVO VERSUS IN VIVO GENE TRANSFER

It is important to appreciate the practical differences between *ex vivo* and *in vivo* gene transfer. *Ex vivo* gene transfer involves removal of cells from a host and transduction of the cells in a culture medium *in vitro* (61). This is followed by transplantation of the genetically modified cells back into the host. Many initial gene therapy protocols used *ex vivo* gene transfer approaches, primarily because of the lack of efficient methods for direct *in vivo* gene transfer (62). *Ex vivo* gene transfer is a cumbersome process, however, requiring isolation and culture of primary cells from each individual. In the long run, this technique is unlikely to be practical for the treatment of large numbers of individuals with thrombotic and hemorrhagic disorders. Even so, *ex vivo* gene transfer has helped to be establish some of the initial principles of gene transduction (3).

The field of gene therapy took a major step forward when methods for direct *in vivo* gene transfer were developed. In the cardiovascular system, direct *in vivo* gene transfer involves development of novel vectors and catheters that allow investigators to deliver genes to the appropriate cardiovascular cells (58). Direct *in vivo* gene transfer is practical and, compared to *ex vivo* gene transfer, technically less complicated and likely to have greater utility in treating large numbers of individuals.

## ENDOTHELIAL CELLS

Endothelial cells are important regulators of vascular function *in vivo*. (See Chapter 13 for the role of these cells in maintaining vascular integrity and regulating hemostasis.) Results of initial gene transfer studies demonstrated it was possible both to transduce cultured endothelial cells *in vitro* using retroviruses or DNA liposome complexes and to reimplant these genetically modified cells onto denuded arteries or synthetic grafts *in vivo* (61, 63). Subsequent studies demonstrated efficient transduction of vascular endothelial cells *in vivo* using catheter mediated delivery of reporter genes with retroviral vectors, DNA liposomes, and adenoviral vectors (2, 64–66). The initial reports of direct *in vivo* gene transfer with retroviral vectors and DNA liposomes established the principles of gene transfection into vascular cells *in vivo*, but these studies were limited by low-level gene expression, in part resulting from limitations of the available vectors at the time (58).

Gene transfer into endothelial cells is an effective approach in gene therapy for thrombotic and hemorrhagic disorders. Gene expression in endothelial cells permits evaluation of the *in vivo* function of the hemostatic proteins. In addition, it was hoped that transduction of endothelial cells would permit efficient recombinant protein production and secretion into the systemic circulation, that might be used to treat systemic hemostatic disorders such as hemophilia (67). At present, however, high-level gene transduction in endothelial cells has not been achieved; hence, gene therapy for the hemophilias has focused more recently on use of skeletal myoblasts (68), as discussed later in this chapter. Nonetheless, local gene delivery into endothelial cells at sites of disease such as acute thrombosis still holds promise.

## SMOOTH MUSCLE CELLS

Vascular smooth muscle cells are important for regulating vascular tone. In addition, following vascular injury, these cells proliferate and contribute to the pathogenesis of vascular proliferative inflammatory disorders such as atherosclerosis and restenosis (Table 62.2). Therefore, expression of recombinant genes in smooth muscle cells permits study of the pathophysiology of vascular proliferative disorders; it also allows for a treatment strategy. Investigators recently have demonstrated that vascular smooth muscle cells can be transduced with highly level efficiencies *in vivo* by catheter-mediated gene delivery of adenoviral vectors and liposome DNA complexes (64, 65, 69–71). In addition, application of synthetic oligonucleotides in pluronic gels to the adventitia of blood vessels has yielded efficient vascular smooth muscle cell gene transduction *in vivo* (72). More recent efforts have focused on direct application of DNA onto hydrogel-coated balloons to directly transduce sites of vascular disease *in vivo* (73). Because the endothelium may constitute a barrier against intraluminal gene delivery to smooth muscle cells, the endothelial layer may need to be removed during gene delivery in certain applications. This does not appear to be a problem in gene therapy for atherosclerosis or restenosis, however, because endothelium already is either partially removed or dysfunctional (74). Even so, gene delivery to smooth muscle cells in normal vessels may require some manipulation

| **TABLE 62.2.** | Disease Targets for Intervention in Cardiovascular Diseases |
|---|---|

Thrombosis and hemostasis
Vascular cell proliferation
Plaque rupture
Endothelial cell dysfunction
Angiogenesis
Myocardial infarction
Cardiac arrhythmias

of the endothelium (75). Nonetheless, gene delivery to smooth muscle cells constitutes a major focus of current vascular gene therapy efforts.

## SKELETAL MYOCYTES

Skeletal myocytes are important new target cells for expression of recombinant proteins used to treat systemic disorders. Initial results demonstrated that genetically modified skeletal myocytes could stably deliver physiologic levels of recombinant proteins such as growth hormone to the systemic circulation of mice (76, 77). In these studies, skeletal myoblasts were transduced with retroviral vectors encoding growth hormone *in vitro*, and these genetically modified cells were injected intramuscularly into syngeneic mice. The injected myoblasts fused both with themselves and with endogenous myocytes to become stably incorporated into the muscle. Importantly, these transduced myoblasts secreted physiologic levels of growth hormone into the systemic circulation for at least 3 months. Additionally, Tripathy et al (33) have developed *in vivo* gene transfer approaches using skeletal muscle that may prove to be more useful for human gene therapies in contrast to injection of transduced myoblasts. These investigators showed that an intramuscular injection of adenoviral vectors encoding murine erythropoietin produced physiologically significant increases in erythropoietin levels that were stable for longer than 2 years. In terms of immunity, when mice were injected with recombinant adenoviral vectors encoding for murine proteins, immune responses did not eliminate transgene expression. More recently, this group has extended these studies to nonhuman primates and found similar results (unpublished data). These results suggest that intramuscular injection of adenoviral vectors can be used to treat systemic diseases, possibly including hemophilia and other serum protein deficiencies.

Intramuscular injection of plasmid DNA is a second approach to the treatment of serum protein disorders. One such injection of as little as 10 µg of plasmid DNA encoding erythropoietin resulted in physiologically significant levels of erythropoietin in the systemic circulation of mice (28). Erythropoietin expression is proportional to the dose of DNA and is stable for at least 90 days. Intramuscular injection of plasmid DNA has several advantages over intramuscular injection of adenoviral vectors. First, plasmid DNA is simpler to prepare (44). Second, immune responses are less of a problem with plasmid DNA compared with viral vectors (45, 78), including the possibility that repeat injections of plasmid DNA can be given to treat systemic thrombotic and hemorrhagic disorders. Third, injection of plasmid DNA does not present the risks of persistent or systemic injection or of individual-to-patient transmission. At present, however, intramuscular injection of plasmid

DNA is not as efficient as adenoviral injection, but with continued modifications of vectors, this may change in the next few years. Nonetheless, injection of recombinant genes using either plasmid DNA or adenoviral vectors into skeletal myocytes is emerging as a very important treatment of systemic protein deficiencies as well as of thrombotic and hemorrhagic disorders.

# DISEASE TARGETS

## HEMOPHILIAS

Gene therapy may become a favorable alternative to factor-replacement treatment in individuals with hemophilia. Such an approach would involve genetic modification of a limited number of individual cells to produce a continuous amount of the deficient protein, thereby preventing major bleeding episodes. Gene therapy for the hemophilias seems to be feasible, because even slight increases in plasma levels of factors VIII and IX can dramatically reduce disease severity (see Chapters 35 and 36).

The properties of factor VIII and IX proteins are reviewed extensively in Chapter 2. The factor VIII protein is synthesized as a single-chain polypeptide, which is converted by intracellular processing to generate a two-chain dimer consisting of an 80 Kda light chain and a 200-kDa heavy chain subunit. Proteolytic activation of the 80 Kda dimer is required to convert factor VIII to its active form. Once activated, factor VIII serves as an essential cofactor for the activation of factor X by factor IXa (79). In plasma, the persistence of factor VIII depends on complex formation with von Willebrand factor.

The factor IX protein is much smaller (55 Kda) and, on a weight basis, 30 times more abundant than factor VIII. Factor VIII has no intrinsic enzymatic activity, but factor IX can be activated to function as a serine protease that converts factor X to its activated form (factor Xa). Factor IX is secreted as a precursor protein and extensively modified. The first 12 glutamic acid residues of the Gla domain are γ-carboxylated posttranslationally; this modification is essential for calcium binding and critical to the function of factor IX.

At present, the best gene therapy for hemophilia probably is a gene addition strategy aimed at introducing an additional functional copy of the gene in some of the individual's cells. The new gene restores the cells' capacity to synthesize the factor VIII or factor IX protein. A small fraction of the normal activity should result in significant clinical improvement. For example, an increase in the factor VIII level to approximately 5% of normal would be sufficient to eliminate most clinical problems in individuals with severe hemophilia. Overexpression of factor VIII or factor IX should have no adverse effects.

Gene therapy of plasma protein deficiencies must

take into account that target tissue cells must have the cellular machinery required for proper posttranslational modification of the secreted protein. Modifications essential for the function of coagulation factors are glycosylation and sulphation of factor VIII, γ-carboxylation of glutamic residues of factor IX, and β-hydroxylation of aspartic residues in factor XIII. In addition, the secreted protein must have access to the circulation. Considering these limitations, endothelial cells and skeletal myocytes are the primary cell targets.

## Hemophilia A

Hemophilia A has received less attention from gene therapy researchers than hemophilia B, mainly because of the large size of the cDNA encoding the factor VIII protein and the problems of obtaining sufficiently high levels of expression (80). Initial studies have focused on developing efficient gene transfer methods, and several groups have used retroviral-mediated gene transfer of factor VIII cDNA into fibroblasts *in vitro* (81, 82). Retroviral vectors cannot be used to transfer full-length factor VIII cDNA, because this would yield a viral gene too large to be packaged efficiently into a virion. Therefore, cDNA clones have been used in which the region encoding the nonessential B-domain has been removed (80). Retrovirus-mediated transfer has been achieved in both human (81) and murine fibroblasts (80), endothelial cells (83), and progenitor bone marrow cells (84).

## Hemophilia B

Both *ex vivo* and *in vivo* strategies have been applied to gene therapy for factor IX deficiency. Initially, retroviral vectors were used in *ex vivo* approaches (85). Next, murine fibroblasts secreting human factor IX protein were embedded into collagen lattices and grafted under the epidermis of mice; human factor IX could be detected in recipient plasma for at least 10 to 12 days (86). The presence of human factor IX was transient, however, and the disappearance of expression could be not be explained by graft rejection. Circulating antibodies against human factor IX could be detected in some of the mice, thus providing a partial explanation (86). Palmer et al (87) also observed transient production of factor IX protein in both immune-incompetent and immune-deficient mice, showing that the vector was inactivated and could be overcome by use of the dihydrofolate reductase gene to drive transcription of the gene of interest (88). These results were initially promising, but plasma levels of factor IX in the mice were lower than would be expected on the basis of factor IX secretion in tissue culture.

After the demonstration that implantation of genetically modified fibroblasts could produce factor IX *in vivo*, other tissues were tested, including keratinocytes (89) and endothelial cells (67, 90). More recently, skeletal muscle has been an attractive target. Biopsies of skeletal muscle have been used to isolated myoblasts transduced with factor IX, and factor IX–producing myoblasts have been injected into skeletal muscle. The transduced myoblasts have fused with the existing myocytes and persist to produce factor IX. Initial results indicated that expression diminished several weeks after injection (68, 91). Use of retroviruses in which the transcription of factor IX cDNA is regulated by the enhancer of the murine muscle–specific creatine kinase gene, however, resulted in persistent expression of factor IX for at least 6 months (92). Thus, the feasibility of this approach should be confirmed through large animal models of hemophilia B.

*In vivo* strategies of gene therapy for hemophilia B have been developed as well. The natural target tissue of *in vivo* gene therapy for hemophilia is the liver. Both retroviral and adenoviral vectors have transduced hepatocytes in culture (93), and Kay et al (94) have used retroviral vectors containing the canine factor IX cDNA in factor IX–deficient dogs after partial hepatectomy. Low levels of canine factor IX could be detected in the recipients, but clotting and partial thromboplastin times were significantly reduced. Expression could be detected for at least 5 months. The major difficulty in this approach is the requirement for partial hepatectomy in order to render quiescent hepatocytes susceptible to retroviral infection. This approach is unlikely to be applied to individuals with hemophilia.

Adenoviral vectors have been applied to *in vivo* gene therapy for hemophilia B as well. Kay et al (95) generated an adenoviral vector expressing the canine factor IX cDNA. Intraportal infusion of replication-incompetent factor IX virus into factor IX–deficient hemophilic dogs resulted in normalization of bleeding tendency, coagulation, and hemostatic parameters. Levels of factor IX reached 300% of normal in dogs; however, as in other animal model systems, the *in vivo* synthesis of factor IX persisted but then declined below therapeutic levels 1 to 2 months after treatment. These data represent a step forward in gene therapy for hemophilia, because they demonstrate high-level recombinant protein expression in the serum for at least several months.

The *ex vivo* approach to gene therapy for hemophilia B is promising, but the plasma levels of factor IX obtained so far are too low to be therapeutic. The feasibility of an *ex vivo* approach still needs to be confirmed in studies of larger animal models. *In vivo* approaches have been more promising, although the current viral vectors require improvements to increase efficiency and longevity of gene expression. Long-term safety and efficacy also must be demonstrated in studies of large animal models before clinical implementation of gene therapy can be considered.

## LOCAL THROMBOSIS

The creation of transgenic and knockout mice has been a powerful new approach to investigating the role of fibrinolytic and thrombotic proteins in vascular diseases. Numerous murine models have been developed with effects on the fibrinolytic system, including mice deficient in fibrinogen (96), plasminogen (97), plasminogen-activator inhibitor type 1 (PAI-1) (98, 99), urokinase-type plasminogen activator and tissue-type plasminogen activator (100), factor V (101), tissue factor (96), a thrombin receptor (102), and thrombomodulin (103). These genetic models of hemorrhagic and thrombotic disorders are described in Chapter 22. Recent advances also have been made in applying gene transfer methods to these knockout mice. For example, recombinant gene transfer can be used to rescue a phenotype. These studies should be useful in further defining the role of specific gene products in the pathophysiology of thrombotic disorders.

Transgenic knockout mice also are being used to evaluate genetic contributions to complex traits such as atherosclerosis and to dissect the contribution of thrombosis to the pathophysiology of complex vascular diseases. One example is investigation of the role played by protease inhibitors in cell migration and proliferation. For example, mice deficient in PAI-1 demonstrate accelerated neointima formation after vascular injury compared with mice having normal PAI-1 levels (104). Mice deficient in urokinase-type plasminogen activator are protected and exhibit reduced intimal lesions after injury. Adenoviral-mediated gene transfer of PAI-1 to PAI-1 knockout mice results in rescue of the phenotype and reduction in neointima formation. Adenoviral gene transfer of a hirudin gene also reduces neointima hyperplasia in balloon-injured carotid arteries (105). It is important to recognize that gene transfer in the study and treatment of thrombotic disorders remains in its early phases. Gene transfer likely will be used in combination with transgenic and knockout mice to define further the pathophysiology of thrombotic disorders and to develop approaches to gene therapy for those disorders. Important unresolved issues include the efficiency of genetic versus protein therapies for local thrombotic disorders and the level of recombinant protein required locally to treat the thrombotic disease.

## CELL PROLIFERATION

A major focus of vascular gene therapies has been the proliferation of vascular cells, and primarily smooth muscle cells. Smooth muscle cell proliferation may not be implicated directly in pathogenesis of thrombotic and hemorrhagic disorders, but cell proliferation contributes to the pathophysiology of many vascular lesions. For example, resolution of organized thrombus results in secretion of growth factors and cytokines that stimulate smooth muscle cell migration, proliferation, and lesion formation (106).

Gene transfer also has been useful in probing regulatory pathways involved in the regulation of smooth muscle cell proliferation. After vascular injury, multiple growth factor and cytokine genes are induced to promote arterial repair. The expression of many growth factors leads to a single endpoint: intimal hyperplasia (107, 108). An inhibitor of a single growth factor or its receptor is unlikely to have significant effects on arterial repair by limiting intimal hyperplasia. This has led investigators to pursue regulators of the cell cycle as potential cell growth inhibitors.

In vascular smooth muscle cells, transit through the G1 phase of the cell cycle and entry into the S phase require the formation and activation of cyclin/cyclin-dependent kinase (CDK) complexes, predominately Cyclin E-Cdk2 and Cyclin D-Cdk4,6, which in turn phosphorylate the retinoblastoma product Rb (109, 110). cdk inhibitors (CKIs) are cellular proteins that inhibit cyclin-CDK activity and phosphorylation of Rb, thus resulting in G1 arrest (Fig. 62.3). CKIs directly implicated in mitogen-dependent cdk regulation are p21, p27, and p57.

Several approaches have been devised to inhibit proliferating cell nuclear antigen (PCNA) and cdk s using antisense oligonucleotides (72, 111–118). One al-

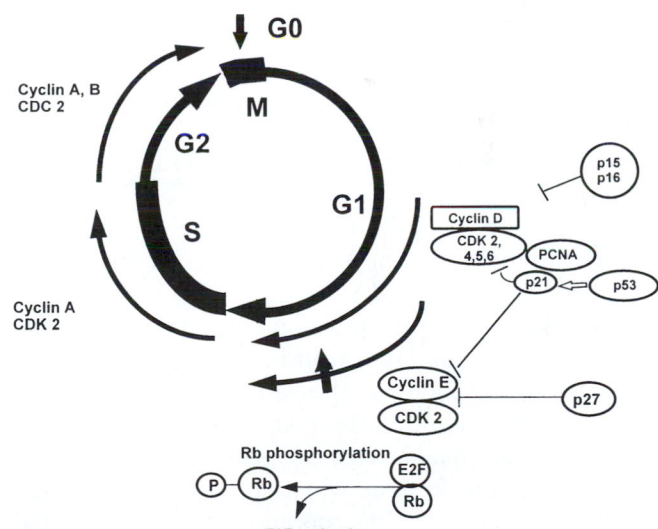

**FIGURE 62.3.**   Regulation of the cell cycle. Progression of the cell-cycle G1/S checkpoint is regulated by the assembly and activation of cyclins and cyclin-dependent kinases (CDKs) that phosphorylate and inactivate the retinoblastoma gene product (Rb). Cyclin-dependent kinase inhibitors (CKIs) complex with cyclin-CDKs to promote G1 arrest. (Adapted with permission from Tanner F, Yang Z, Simari RD et al. Gene transfer and vascular remodeling. In: Lafont A, Topol EJ, eds. Arterial remodeling: a critical factor in restenosis. Boston: Kluwer Academic Publishers, 1997:549–556.)

ternative is to overexpress natural inhibitors of cyclin-CDK complexes, the CKIs (e.g., p21, p27), by adenoviral-mediated gene transfer (119, 120). Chang et al (71) demonstrated that overexpression of a nonphosphorylatable, constitutively active Rb ($\Delta$Rb) inhibits growth factor–stimulated vascular smooth muscle cell proliferation *in vitro*. Local infection of injured rat and pig arteries with replication-defective adenoviral vectors encoding mutant Rb significantly reduced vascular cell proliferation and neointima formation in two animal models of restenosis (119, 120). More recent studies have examined the role of CKIs, including p21, p27, and p16, in regulating vascular cell growth. Adenovirus-mediated overexpression of human p21 in rat vascular smooth muscle cells inhibited growth factor stimulation of cell proliferation and arrested cells in the G1 phase of the cell cycle (119). Growth arrest of these smooth muscle cells was associated with inhibition of Rb phosphorylation and formation of p21-PCNA complexes. Growth arrest of pig vascular endothelial and smooth muscle cells *in vitro* also occurred after expression of p21 (120), and subsequent *in vivo* studies confirmed the importance of the CKIs p21 and p27 in regulating vascular smooth muscle cell proliferation after arterial injury. For example, in balloon-injured pig arteries, p21 and p27 are downregulated during mitogen-dependent stimulation of smooth muscle cell growth. During later phases of arterial injury, p21 and p27 are induced and probably mediated via collagen synthesis and integrin signaling to downregulate growth factor gene expression and to promote growth arrest (120). Thus, CKIs likely play major roles in growth regulation of vascular cells during arterial repair.

Other gene transfer approaches have been used to study growth regulation of vascular cells, and particularly smooth muscle cells and macrophages, within atherosclerotic plaques. The herpes simplex virus thymidine kinase gene (*HSV-tk*) and the nucleoside analogue ganciclovir have been examined in three models of restenosis: balloon-injured rat carotid arteries (121, 122), balloon-injured pig iliofemoral arteries (70), and balloon-injured atherosclerotic rabbit arteries (74). When expressed in mammalian cells, *HSV-tk* encodes for the enzyme thymidine kinase, which phosphorylates ganciclovir to a toxic form. Incorporation of phosphorylated ganciclovir into dividing cells leads to inhibition of DNA replication, resulting in cell death. Metabolites of the enzymatic reaction diffuse into adjacent cells and incorporate into dividing cells, thereby leading to disruption of DNA synthesis and cell death. This so-called "bystander effect" allows for cell death in dividing smooth muscle cells that do not express the thymidine kinase gene. The bystander effect also allows a greater number of cells to be eliminated than if the toxic metabolite remains intracellular; thus, gene transfer efficiency is less

critical. In balloon-injured rat and pig models, adenoviral gene transfer of *HSV-tk* and ganciclovir treatment are associated with significantly reduced smooth muscle cell proliferation and intimal hyperplasia (70, 121, 122). In addition, expression of *HSV-tk* and ganciclovir treatment are associated with significantly reduced intimal and medial cell proliferation in atherosclerotic rabbit arteries as well as with reduced intimal plaque size (74). Thus, the prodrug approach using *HSV-tk* gene transfer and ganciclovir treatment is an alternative in the treatment of vascular proliferative disorders. This approach likely produces its effect in the S-phase of the cell cycle by disrupting DNA synthesis.

Antisense oligonucleotides are another strategy used to suppress the function of specific gene products and vascular cells. Many initial studies examining the role of cell cycle regulatory proteins used antisense oligonucleotides to inhibit directly the cyclins, cdk s, or PCNA. For example, antisense oligonucleotides to *c-myb* were delivered to the adventitia of injured rat carotids with a pluronic gel and were associated with reduced mRNA and decreased neointima formation (72). Antisense *c-myc* also was delivered in a pluronic gel to the outer surface of injured arteries, where similar reductions in intimal hyperplasia were observed (113). A single intraluminal administration of antisense cdc2 kinase and PCNA with hemagglutinating virus of Japan (HVJ) liposomes resulted in a 6-week suppression of intimal thickening in balloon-injured rat carotid arteries (112). Other cellular targets that have been examined include cdk 2 kinase (116) and PCNA (115) in injured rat carotid arteries as well as *c-myc* in injured pig coronary arteries (114).

An important application of cell-cycle inhibitors has been in treatment of vein graft hyperplasia. When vein grafts are placed in the arterial position to bypass arterial stenoses, they become arterialized when subjected to hemodynamic pressures and shear stress from the arterial circulation. Normally, intimal hyperplasia develops in the vein, and these arterialized veins are subject to the same complications as arterial lesions (i.e., intimal hyperplasia and thrombosis). Treatment of rabbit veins with antisense oligonucleotides directed against cdc2 and PCNA before insertion in rabbit carotid arteries resulted in reduced intimal hyperplasia compared with veins treated using control oligonucleotides (123). On the basis of these preclinical results, a human trial to treat peripheral bypass vein grafts has been proposed (124). Individuals undergoing peripheral vascular surgery will be candidates, and veins will be harvested from their lower extremity and incubated with oligonucleotides, which function as transcription decoys to E2F for 10 minutes before placement in a bypass position. The primary endpoint of the study will be time from the initial bypass operation to the earliest adverse event, including occlusion of the index graft, invasive revision of the index graft, or restenosis in the index graft as measured by duplex ultrasonography. Theses studies will provide useful information about the introduction of oligonucleotides into human vascular cells, the efficacy of oligonucleotide therapies, and the utility of treatments to disrupt the G1 phase of the cell cycle and inhibit smooth muscle cell proliferation.

# CONCLUSIONS

The past 15 years have seen remarkable progress in somatic gene transfer and gene therapy. Development of multiple-vector systems and cloning of human disease–related genes have expanded the number of diseases that someday will be approached using gene transfer technologies. Both transgenic and gene targeting approaches have created important new animal models of human disease, which will be invaluable in developing novel gene therapies. These animal models are important for understanding disease pathogenesis and for establishing the principles of gene transfer.

Despite this extraordinary progress, however, important hurdles remain before these advances in vectors and gene delivery can be translated into successful human gene therapies. Safe vectors that efficiently program transgene expression into different cardiovascular cell types without evoking immune responses to either vector encoded or transgene proteins are required. In addition, as efficient vectors are developed, targeting these vectors to specific cardiovascular and hemostatic cells *in vitro* will be needed, including development of cell-specific promoters as well as regulated gene expression. Improved catheters for intravascular gene delivery are needed as well. Finally, a better understanding of the pathophysiology of hemostasis and thrombosis is required to design rational gene therapies for specific disorders. Significant hurdles remain, but genetics and gene therapy no doubt will play increasingly important roles in our understanding and treatment of hemorrhagic and thrombotic disorders, as well as of many other human diseases, in the 21st century.

# REFERENCES

1. Chien KR. Molecular cardiology in the postmolecular era: turning toward complexity. Trends Cardiovasc Med 1996;6:1–3.
2. Nabel EG. Gene therapy for cardiovascular disease [Review]. Circulation 1995;91:541–548.
3. Crystal RG. Transfer of genes to humans: early lessons and obstacles to success [Review]. Science 1995;270:404–410.
4. Anderson WF. Human gene therapy [Review]. Science 1992;256:808–813.
5. Blaese RM, Culver KW, Miller AD et al. T lymphocyte-directed gene therapy for ADA-SCID: initial trial results after 4 years. Science 1995;270:475–480.
6. Marcel T, Grausz JD. The TMC Worldwide Gene Therapy Enrollment Report (June 1996). Hum Gene Ther 1996;7:2025–2046.
7. Miller AD. Retroviral vectors [Review]. Curr Top Microbiol Immunol 1992;158:1–24.
8. Wilson JM. Adenoviruses as gene-delivery vehicles [Review]. N Engl J Med 1996;334:1185–1187.
9. Boris-Lawrie KL, Temin HM. Recent advances in retrovirus vector technology. Curr Opin Genet Dev 1993;3:102–109.
10. Muzyczka N. Use of adeno-associated virus as a general transduction vector for mammalian cells [Review]. Curr Top Microbiol Immunol 1992;158:97–129.
11. Kotani H, Newton PB III, Zhang S et al. Improved methods of retroviral vector transduction and production for gene therapy. Hum Gene Ther 1994;5:19–28.
12. Nabel EG. Vectors for gene therapy: introduction. In: Current protocols in human genetics. New York: John Wiley & Sons, 1996:12.0.1–12.0.3.
13. Yee J. Pseudotype-retroviral vectors. Current protocols in human genetics. New York: John Wiley & Sons, 1997:12.6.
14. Snyder RO, Xiao X. Production of recombinant adeno-associated viral vectors. In: Current protocols in human genetics. New York: John Wiley & Sons, 1996:12.1.1–12.1.20.
15. Friedman T. A brief history of gene therapy [Review]. Nat Genet 1992;2:93–98.
16. Miller AD. Production of retroviral vectors. In: Current protocols in human genetics. New York: John Wiley & Sons, 1996:12.5.1–12.5.19.
17. Miller AD. Retrovirus packaging cells [Review]. Hum Gene Ther 1994;5:567–575.
18. Otto E, Jones-Trower A, Vanin EF et al. Characterization of a replication-competent retrovirus resulting from recombination of packaging and vector sequences. Hum Gene Ther 1994;5:567–575.
19. Burns C, Friedmann T, Driever W et al. Vesicular stomatitis virus G glycoprotein pseudotyped retroviral vectors: concentration to very high titer and efficient gene transfer into mammalian and nonmammalian cells. Proc Natl Acad Sci U S A 1994;90:8033–8037.
20. Kasahara N, Dozy AM, Kan YW. Tissue-specific targeting of retroviral vectors through ligand-receptor interactions. Science 1994;266:1373–1376.
21. Berkner KL. Development of adenovirus vectors for the expression of heterologous genes [Review]. Biotechniques 1988;6:616–629.
22. Graham FL, Prevec L. Manipulation of adenovirus vectors. In: Murray EJ, ed. Gene transfer and expression protocols. Clifton, NJ: Humana, 1991:109–127.
23. Berkner KL. Expression of heterologous sequences in adenoviral vectors [Review]. Curr Top Microbiol Immunol 1992;58:39–66.
24. Horwitz MS. Virology. New York: Raven Press, 1990.
25. Graham FL, Smiley J, Russell WC et al. Characteristics of a human cell line transformed by DNA from human adenovirus type 5. J Gen Virol 1977;36:59–74.
26. Davis AR, Wilson JM. Adenoviral vectors. In: Boyle AL, ed. Current protocols in human genetics. New York: John Wiley & Sons, 1996:12.4.1–12.4.18.
27. Quantin B, Perricaudet LD, Tajbakhsh S et al. Adenovirus as an expression vector in muscle cells *in vivo*. Proc Natl Acad Sci U S A 1992;89:2581–2584.
28. Tripathy SK, Goldwasser E, Lu MM et al. Stable delivery of physiologic levels of recombinant erythropoietin to the systemic circulation by intramuscular injection of replication-defective adenovirus. Proc Natl Acad Sci U S A 1994;91:11557–11561.
29. Dai Y, Schwarz EM, Gu D et al. Cellular and humoral immune responses to adenoviral vectors containing factor IX gene: tolerization of factor IX and vector antigens allows for long-term expression. Proc Natl Acad Sci U S A 1995;92:1401–1405.
30. Smith TA, Mehaffey MG, Kayda DB. Adenovirus mediated expression of therapeutic plasma levels of human factor IX in mice. Nat Genet 1993;5:397–402.
31. Yang Y, Ertl HC, Wilson JM. MHC class 1–restricted cytotoxic lymphocytes to viral antigens destroy hepatocytes in mice infected with E1-deleted recombinant adenoviruses. Immunity 1994;1:433–442.
32. Yang Y, Nunes FA, Berencsi K. Cellular immunity to viral antigens limits E1-deleted adenoviruses for gene therapy. Proc Natl Acad Sci U S A 1994;91:4407–4411.
33. Tripathy SK, Black HB, Goldwasser E et al. Immune responses to transgene-encoded proteins limit the stability of gene expression after injection of replication-defective adenovirus vectors. Nat Med 1996;2:545–550.
34. Yang Y, Li Q, Ertl HC et al. Cellular and humoral immune response to viral antigens create barriers to lung-directed gene therapy with recombinant adenoviruses. J Virol 1995;69:2004–2015.
35. Yang Y, Nunes FA, Berencsi K et al. Inactivation of E2a in recombinant adenoviruses improves the prospect for gene therapy in cystic fibrosis. Nat Genet 1994;7:362–369.
36. Yeh P, Dedieu JF, Orsini C et al. Efficient dual transcomplementation of adenovirus E1 and E4 regions from a 293-derived cell line expressing a minimal E4 functional unit. J Virol 1996;70:559–565.
37. Wang Q, Finer MH. Second-generation adenovirus vectors [Review]. Nat Med 1996;2:714–716.
38. Kochanek S, Clemens PR, Mitani HH et al. A new adenoviral vector: replacement of all viral coding sequences with 28 kb of DNA independently expressing both full-length dystrophin and beta-galactosidase. Proc Natl Acad Sci U S A 1996;93:5731–5736.

39. Yang Y, Su Q, Grewal IS et al. Transient subversion of CD40 ligand function diminishes immune responses to adenovirus vectors in mouse liver and lung tissues. J Virol 1996;70:6370–6377.

40. Kotin RM, Linden RM, Berns KI. Characterization of a preferred site on human chromosome 19q for integration of adeno-associated virus DNA by nonhomologous recombination. EMBO J 1992;11:5071–5078.

41. Nahreini P, Larsen SH, Srivastava A. Cloning and integration of DNA fragments in human cells via the inverted terminal repeats of the adeno-associated virus 2 genome. Gene 1992;119:265–272.

42. Rolling F, Samulski RJ. AAV as a viral vector for human gene therapy. Generation of recombinant virus. Mol Biotechnol 1995;3:9–15.

43. Lynch CM, Hara PS, Leonard JC et al. Adeno-associated virus vectors for vascular gene delivery. Circ Res 1997;80:497–505.

44. Nabel GJ, Nabel EG, Yang ZY et al. Direct gene transfer with DNA liposome complexes in melanoma: expression, biologic activity and lack of toxicity in humans. Proc Natl Acad Sci U S A 1993;90:11307–11311.

45. Ulmer JB, Donnelly JJ, Parker SE et al. Heterologous protection against influenza by injection of DNA encoding a viral protein. Science 1993;259:1745–1749.

46. Wolff JA, Malone RW, Williams P et al. Direct gene transfer into mouse muscle in vivo. Science 1990;247:1465–1468.

47. Lin H, Parmacek MS, Morle G et al. Expression of recombinant genes in myocardium in vivo after direct injection of DNA. Circulation 1990;82:2217–2221.

48. Acsadi G, Jiao SS, Jani A. Direct gene transfer and expression into rat heart in vivo. New Biol 1991;3:71–81.

49. Kitsis RN, Buttrick PM, McNally EM et al. Hormonal modulation of a gene injected into rat heart in vivo. Proc Natl Acad Sci U S A 1991;88:4138–4142.

50. Gal D, Weir L, Leclerc G et al. Direct myocardial transfection in two animal models. Evaluation of parameters affecting gene expression and percutaneous gene delivery. Lab Invest 1993;68:18–25.

51. Simari RD, Yang X, Ling D et al. Splicing is required for enhanced transgene expression by untranslated sequences from the human cytomegalovirus immediate-early gene. Circulation 1996:I286.

52. Felgner PL, Gadek TR, Holm M et al. Lipofection: a highly efficient, lipid-mediated DNA-transfection procedure. Proc Natl Acad Sci U S A 1987;84:7413–7417.

53. Lasic DD, Papahadjopoulos D. Liposomes revisited [Review]. Science 1995;267:1275–1276.

54. Felgner PL, Holm M, Chan H. Cationic liposome mediated transfection. Proc West Pharmacol Soc 1989;32:115–121.

55. Felgner J, Bennett F, Felgner PL. Cationic lipid-mediated delivery of polynucleotides. Methods 1993;5:67–75.

56. Stephan DJ, Yang Z, San H et al. A new cationic liposome DNA complex enhances the efficiency of arterial gene transfer in vivo. Hum Gene Ther 1996;7:1803–1812.

57. Wheeler CJ, Felgner PL, Tsai YJ et al. A novel cationic lipid greatly enhances plasmid DNA delivery and expression in mouse lung. Proc Natl Acad Sci U S A 1996;93:11454–11459.

58. Nabel EG, Plautz G, Nabel GJ. Site-specific gene expression in vivo by direct gene transfer into the arterial wall. Science 1990;249:1285–1288.

59. Chapman GD, Lim CS, Gammon RS et al. Gene transfer into coronary arteries of intact animals with a percutaneous balloon catheter. Circ Res 1992;71:27–33.

60. Leclerc G, Gal D, Takeshita S et al. Percutaneous arterial gene transfer in a rabbit mode. Efficiency in normal and balloon-dilated atherosclerotic arteries. J Clin Invest 1992;90:936–944.

61. Nabel EG, Plautz G, Boyce FM et al. Recombinant gene expression in vivo within endothelial cells of the arterial wall. Science 1989;244:1342–1344.

62. Grossman M, Raper SE, Kozarsky K et al. Successful ex vivo gene therapy directed to liver in a patient with familial hypercholesterolaemia. Nat Genet 1994;6:335–341.

63. Wilson JM, Birinyi LK, Salomon RN. Implantation of vascular grafts lined with genetically modified endothelial cells. Science 1989;244:1344–1346.

64. Barr E, Carroll J, Kalynych AM et al. Efficient catheter-mediated gene transfer into the heart using replication-defective adenovirus. Gene Ther 1994;1:51–58.

65. Guzman RJ, Lemarchand P, Crystal RG et al. Efficient and selective adenovirus-mediated gene transfer into vascular neointima. Circulation 1993;88:2838–2848.

66. Lemarchand P, Jones M, Yamada I et al. In vivo gene transfer and expression in normal uninjured blood vessels using replication-deficient recombinant adenovirus vectors. Circ Res 1993;72:1132–1138.

67. Yao SN, Wilson JM, Nabel EG et al. Expression of human factor IX in rat capillary endothelial cells: toward somatic cell gene therapy for hemophilia B. Proc Natl Acad Sci U S A 1991;88:8101–8105.

68. Yao SN, Kurachi K. Expression of human factor IX in mice after injection of genetically modified myoblasts. Proc Natl Acad Sci U S A 1992;89:3357–3361.

69. Steg PG, Feldman LJ, Scoazec JY et al. Arterial gene transfer to rabbit endothelial and smooth muscle cells using percutaneous delivery of an adenoviral vector. Circulation 1994;90:1648–1656.

70. Ohno T, Gordon, San H et al. Gene therapy for vascular smooth muscle cell proliferation after arterial injury. Science 1994;265:781–784.

71. Chang MW, Barr E, Seltzer J et al. Cytostatic gene therapy for vascular proliferative disorders with a constitutively active form of the retinoblastoma gene product. Science 1995;267:518–522.

72. Simons M, Edelman ER, DeKeyser JL et al. Antisense c-myb oligonucleotides inhibit intimal arterial smooth muscle cell accumulation in vivo. Nature 1992;359:67–70.

73. Riessen R, Rhamizadeh H, Blessing E et al. Arterial gene transfer using pure DNA applied directly to a hydrogel-coated angioplasty balloon. Hum Gene Ther 1993;4:749–758.

74. Simari RD, San H, Rekhter M. Regulation of cellular proliferation and intimal formation following balloon injury in atherosclerotic rabbit arteries. J Clin Invest 1996;98:225–235.

75. Simari RD, San H, Nabel EG. Gene transfer to arteries. In: Boyle AL, ed. Current protocols in human genetics. New York: John Wiley & Sons, 1996: 13.1.1–13.1.10.

76. Barr E, Leiden JM. Systemic delivery of recombinant proteins by genetically modified myoblasts. Science 1991;254:1507–1509.

77. Dhawan J, Pan LC, Pavlath GK et al. Systemic delivery of human growth hormone by injection of genetically engineered myoblasts. Science 1991;254:1509–1512.

78. Shiver JW, Liu MA. DNA vaccination. In: Boyle AL, ed. Current protocols in human genetics. New York: John Wiley & Sons, 1996:13.2.1–13.2.6.

79. Van Dieijen G, van Rijn JL, Govers-Riemslag JW et al. Assembly of the intrinsic factor X activating complex-interactions between factor Ixa, factor VIIIa and phospholipid. Thromb Haemost 1985;53:396–400.

80. Israel DI, Kaufman RJ. Retroviral-mediated transfer and amplification of a functional human factor VIII gene. Blood 1990;75:1074–1080.

81. Hoeben RC, Van der Jagt RC, Schoute F et al. Expression of functional factor VIII in primary human skin fibroblasts after retrovirus-mediated gene transfer. J Biol Chem 1990;265:7318–7323.

82. Hoeben RC, van Tilburg N, Bri't E et al. Towards gene therapy in hemophilia A: expression factor VIII with a retroviral vector system [Abstract]. Thromb Haemost 1989;62:209.

83. Lynch CM, Israel DI, Miller AD. Towards somatic cell gene therapy using endothelial cells [Abstract]. J Cell Biochem 1990;14E:222.

84. Hoeben RC, Einerhand MP, Bri't E et al. Toward gene therapy in haemophilia A: retrovirus-mediated transfer of factor VIII gene into murine hematopoietic progenitor cells. Thromb Haemost 1992;67:341–345.

85. Anson DS, Hock RA, Austen D et al. Towards gene therapy for hemophilia B. Mol Biol Med 1987;411–420.

86. St Louis D, Verma IM. An alternative approach to somatic cell gene therapy. Proc Natl Acad Sci U S A 1988;85:3150–3154.

87. Palmer TD, Thompson AR, Miller AD. Production of human factor IX in animals by genetically modified skin fibroblasts: potential therapy for hemophilia B. Blood 1989;73:438–445.

88. Scharfmann R, Axelrod JH, Verma IM. Long-term in vivo expression of retrovirus-mediated gene transfer in mouse fibroblast implants. Proc Natl Acad Sci U S A 1991;88:4626–4630.

89. Gerrard AJ, Hudson DL, Brownlee GG et al. Towards gene therapy for haemophilia B using primary human keratinocytes. Nat Genet 1993;3:180–183.

90. Axelrod JH, Read MS, Brinkhous KM et al. Phenotypic correction of factor IX deficiency in skin fibroblasts of hemophilic dogs. Proc Natl Acad Sci U S A 1990;87:5173–5177.

91. Roman M, Axelrod JH, Dai Y et al. Circulating human or canine factor IX from retrovirally transduced primary myoblasts and established myoblast cell lines grafted into murine skeletal muscle. Somat Cell Mol Genet 1992;18:247–258.

92. Dai Y, Roman M, Naviaux RK. Gene therapy via primary myoblasts: long term expression of factor IX protein following transplantation in vivo. Proc Natl Acad Sci U S A 1992;89:10892–10895.

93. Armentano D, Thompson AR, Darlington G et al. Expression of human factor IX in rabbit hepatocytes by retrovirus-mediated gene transfer: potential for gene therapy of hemophilia. Proc Natl Acad Sci U S A 1990;87:6141–6145.

94. Kay MA, Rothenberg S, Landen CN et al. In vivo gene therapy of hemophilia B: sustained partial correction in factor IX-deficient dogs. Science 1993;262:117–119.

95. Kay MA, Landen CN, Rothenberg SR et al. In vivo hepatic gene therapy; complete albeit transient correction of factor IX deficiency in hemophilia B dogs. Proc Natl Acad Sci U S A 1994;91:2353–2357.

96. Suh TT, Holmback K, Jensen NJ et al. Resolution of spontaneous bleeding events but failure of pregnancy in fibrinogen-deficient mice. Genes Dev 1995;9:2020–2033.

97. Ploplis VA, Carmeliet P, Vazirzadeh S et al. Effects of disruption of the plasminogen gene on thrombosis, growth, and health in mice. Circulation 1995;92:2585–2593.

98. Carmeliet P, Kieckens L, Schoonjans L et al. Plasminogen activator inhibitor-1 gene-deficient mice. I. Generation by homologous recombination and characterization. J Clin Invest 1993;92:2746–2755.

99. Carmeliet P, Stassen JM, Schoonjans L et al. Plasminogen activator inhibi-

tor-1 gene-deficient mice. II. Effects on hemostasis, thrombosis, and thrombolysis. J Clin Invest 1993;92:2756–2760.

100. Carmeliet, Schoonjans L, Kieckens L et al. Physiological consequences of loss of plasminogen activator gene function in mice. Nature 1994;368:419–424.

101. Cui J, O'Shea KS, Purkayastha A et al. Fatal haemorrhage and incomplete block to embryogenesis in mice lacking coagulation factor V. Nature 1996;384:66–68.

102. Connolly AJ, Ishihara H, Kahn ML et al. Role of the thrombin receptor in development and evidence for a second receptor. Nature 1996;381:516–519.

103. Healy AM, Rayburn HB, Rosenberg RD et al. Absence of the blood-clotting regulator thrombomodulin causes embryonic lethality in mice before development of a functional cardiovascular system. Proc Natl Acad Sci U S A 1995;92:850–854.

104. Carmeliet P, Moons L, Ploplis V et al. Impaired arterial neointima formation in mice with disruption of the plasminogen gene. J Clin Invest 1997;99:200–208.

105. Rade JJ, Schulick AH, Virmani R et al. Local adenoviral-mediated expression of recombinant hirudin reduces neointima formation after arterial injury. Nat Med 1996;2:293–298.

106. Ross R. The pathogenesis of atherosclerosis: a perspective for the 1990's. Nature 1993;362:801–809.

107. Nabel EG, Yang Z, Liptay S et al. Recombinant platelet-derived growth factor B gene expression in porcine arteries induces intimal hyperplasia in vivo. J Clin Invest 1993;91:1822–1829.

108. Nabel EG, Yang ZY, Pautz G et al. Recombinant fibroblast growth factor-1 promotes intimal hyperplasia and angiogenesis in arteries in vivo. Nature 1993;362:844–846.

109. Sherr CJ. Mammalian G1 cyclins [Review]. Cell 1993;73:1059–1065.

110. Sherr CJ, Roberts JM. Inhibitors of mammalian G1 cyclin-dependent kinases [Review]. Genes Dev 1995;9:1149–1163.

111. Speir E, Epstein SE. Inhibition of smooth muscle cell proliferation by an antisense oligodeoxynucleotide targeting the messenger RNA encoding proliferating cell nuclear antigen. Circulation 1992;86:538–547.

112. Morishita R, Gibbons GH, Ellison KE et al. Single intraluminal delivery of antisense cdc2 and proliferating-cell nuclear antigen oligonucleotides results in chronic inhibition of neointimal hyperplasia. Proc Natl Acad Sci U S A 1993;90:8474–8478.

113. Bennett MR, Anglin S, McEwan Jr et al. Inhibition of vascular smooth muscle cell proliferation in vitro and in vivo by c-myc antisense oligodeoxynucleotides. J Clin Invest 1994;93:820–828.

114. Shi Y, Fard A, Galeo A et al. Transcatheter delivery of c-myc antisense oligomers reduces neointimal formation in a porcine model of coronary artery balloon injury. Circulation 1994;90:944–951.

115. Simons M, Edelman ER, Rosenberg RD. Antisense proliferating cell nuclear antigen oligonucleotides inhibit intimal hyperplasia in a rat carotid artery injury model. J Clin Invest 1994;93:2351–2356.

116. Morishita R, Gibbons GH, Ellison KE et al. Intimal hyperplasia after vascular injury is inhibited by antisense cdk 2 kinase oligonucleotides. J Clin Invest 1994;1458:1464.

117. Stein C, Cheng YC. Antisense oligonucleotides as therapeutic agents—is the bullet really magical [Review]? Science 1993;261:1004–1012.

118. Epstein SE, Speir E, Finkel T. Do antisense approaches to the problem of restenosis make sense [Editorial]? Circulation 1993;88:1351–1353.

119. Chang MW, Barr E, Lu MM et al. Adenovirus-mediated over-expression of the cyclin/cyclin-dependent kinase inhibitor, p21 inhibits vascular smooth muscle cell proliferation and neointima formation in the rat carotid artery model of balloon angioplasty. J Clin Invest 1995;96:2260–2268.

120. Yang ZY, Simari RD, Perkins ND et al. Role of the p21 cyclin-dependent kinase inhibitor in limiting intimal cell proliferation in response to arterial injury. Proc Natl Acad Sci U S A 1996;93:7905–7910.

121. Chang MW, Ohno T, Gordon D et al. Adenovirus-mediated transfer of the herpes simplex virus thymidine kinase gene inhibits vascular smooth muscle cell proliferation and neointima formation following balloon angioplasty of the rat carotid artery. Mol Med 1995;1:172–181.

122. Guzman RJ, Hirschowitz EA, Brody, SL et al. In vivo suppression of injury-induced vascular smooth muscle cell accumulation using adenovirus-mediated transfer of the herpes simplex thymidine kinase gene. Proc Natl Acad Sci U S A 1995;92:4502–4506.

123. Mann MJ, Gibbons GH, Kernoff RS et al. Genetic engineering of vein grafts resistant to atherosclerosis. Proc Natl Acad Sci U S A 1995;92:4502–4506.

124. Gibbons GH, Dzau VJ. Molecular therapies for vascular diseases [Review]. Science 1996;272:689–693.

# INDEX

References in *italics* denote figures; those followed by "t" denote tables

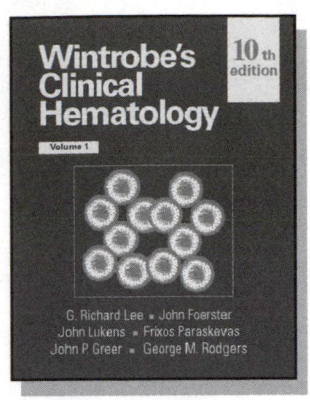
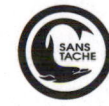